Canine Vaccination Guidelines

Modified from American Animal Hospital Association (AAHA) Canine Vaccination Task Force, et al: 2017 AAHA Canine Vaccination Guideli

Life Stage	Age	CDV	CAV2	lepto	CPiV	CPV	Rabies	Bb[2]	Lyme	CIV[6] H3N2	CIV[6] H3N8	C. atrox
Puppy	6-8 wks[1]	●	●		○	●		○[2]		○	○	
	9-11 wks[1]	●	●	○[4]	○	●		○[5]	○	○	○	
	14-16 wks[1]	●	●	○[4]	○	●	●		○			○[9]
First adult	1 yr, or 1st vaccination at > 16 wks	●[3]	●[3]	○[3]	○[3]	●[3]	●	○[3]	○[3]	○	○	○[9]
Adult booster	Annually when > 1 yr of age			○[3]	○[7]		●[8]	○[3]	○[3]	○	○	○[9]
	q 3 yr when > 1 yr of age	●	●		○[7]	●	●[8]					

LEGEND:

● Core vaccine: all dogs should receive core vaccines unless there is a specific reason to avoid vaccination.

○ Noncore vaccine: administered selectively based on assessment of risk-to-benefit ratio (e.g., environment, risk of exposure).

Bb, Bordetella bronchiseptica; C. atrox, Crotalus atrox (rattlesnake); *CAV2,* canine adenovirus 2 (infectious canine hepatitis); *CDV,* canine distemper virus; *lepto,* leptospirosis (4-serovar); *CIV,* canine influenza virus; *CPiV,* canine parainfluenza virus; *CPV,* canine parvovirus; MLV, modified live virus; wks, weeks; *yr,* year.

COMMENTS:

(1) Revaccinate q 3-4 weeks until 14-16 weeks of age. Dogs at high risk (e.g., exposure risk) may benefit from dose of CDV, CAV2, and CPV at 18-20 weeks of age.
(2) Options include SQ or mucosal routes (intranasal and oral). Two initial doses required for SQ vaccine, while a single initial dose of mucosal vaccine is adequate. Onset of efficacy more rapid with mucosal vaccine.
(3) When a dog receives the first vaccination of its life at >16 weeks of age, revaccination 3-4 weeks later is recommended.
(4) First vaccination should be given at 12 weeks, and again at 14-16 weeks.
(5) If first dose is between 6 and 8 weeks of age, second dose should be at 10-12 weeks of age.
(6) Monovalent or bivalent (H3N2 and H3N8) vaccines available.
(7) Intranasal vaccine, usually combined with Bb, may be given annually.
(8) Administration annually or triennially depends on product type and regional statutes.
(9) Dosing requirements and frequency vary among dogs depending on body weight and exposure risk.

Canine distemper: In the past, a single dose of measles vaccine IM was used in very young puppies to overcome maternal immunity, but newer recombinant CDV vaccines make this unnecessary. Recombinant and MLV vaccines perform similarly in the absence of maternal immunity.

Infectious canine hepatitis (adenovirus-2): Parenteral CAV2 vaccines protect from infectious canine hepatitis (adenovirus-1) and respiratory CAV2. Mucosal CAV2 does not protect from hepatitis.

Leptospirosis: For optimal response and lower risk of severe adverse effect, first dose should be given 12 weeks of age. Only vaccines that contain all 4 serovars (pomona, icterohaemorrhagiae, grippotyphosa, canicola) should be used.

Parainfluenza: Prevents clinical signs but has not been shown to prevent infection and viral shedding. Topical intranasal is safe at ≥ 3 weeks of age and is usually combined with Bb.

Parvovirus: MLV vaccine is recommended and should protect against any field variant, including CPV-2b and CPV-2c.

Rabies: Administration depends on product type and state, provincial, and local statutes. Read package insert and contact regional authorities for exact specifications.

Bordetella: Duration of immunity is 12-14 months after intranasal vaccination, while duration has not been published for SQ or oral routes. Mucosal vaccine for Bb may be administered as early as 3 weeks of age. **CAUTION:** Parenteral injection of mucosal vaccine preparation can cause acute liver injury.

Borreliosis/Lyme disease: Generally recommended only in dogs with a high risk of exposure.

Canine influenza: Monovalent or bivalent parenteral vaccines available. Initial vaccination should begin 4 weeks before potential exposure, with first booster 2 weeks before exposure.

Crotalus atrox: Only for use in dogs with high risk of exposure.

Feline Vaccination Guidelines

Recommendations for household pet cats, adapted from Scherk MA, et al: 2013 American Association of Feline Practitioners' Feline Vaccination Advisory Panel Report. J Feline Med Surg 15:785–808, 2013; and 2015 ABCD Recommendations for indoor/outdoor cats, rescue shelter cats and breeding catteries. J Feline Med Surg 17:583-587, 2015.

Life Stage	Age	FVRCP[1]	Rabies	FeLV	FIV	C. felis	Bb	FIP
Kitten	6-8 wks	●		○[6,7]			○	
	9-12 wks	●		○	○[6]	○	○	
	≥ 13 wks	●	◐[4,5]	○[8]	○[8]	○[8]	○	○[9]
First adult	1 yr of age, or first vaccination at >12 wks	●[3]	◐[4,5]	○[8]	○[8]	○[8]	○	○
Booster	Annually when >1 yr of age	●[3]	◐[5]	○	○	○[8]		○
	q 3 yr when > 1 yr of age[2]	●	◐[5]		○			

LEGEND:

● Core vaccine: highly recommended for all cats.

◐ Core in some locations.

○ Noncore vaccine: administered selectively based on assessment of risk-to-benefit ratio (e.g., environment, risk of exposure).

Bb, *Bordetella bronchiseptica; C. felis, Chlamydia felis;* FeLV, feline leukemia virus; FIP, feline infectious peritonitis; FIV, feline immunodeficiency virus; FVRCP, Feline herpesvirus-1 (feline viral rhinotracheitis)/calicivirus/panleukopenia; IN, intranasal vaccine (NOTE: *Never* administer a vaccine designed for parenteral injection via a mucosal route as it may cause disease); MLV, modified live virus; wks, weeks; yr, years.

COMMENTS:

(1) For pregnant queens, use inactivated rather than MLV; risks of MLV in retrovirus-positive cats are unknown.
(2) Presumes that adequate vaccination has occurred previously (e.g., 2 doses within 3-4 weeks of each other, beginning at ≥ 9 weeks of age). If not, or if uncertain, immediate vaccination is routinely warranted, followed by revaccination 3-4 weeks later, then 1 year later, and then every 3 years.
(3) Continue every 3-4 weeks until 16-20 weeks of age; if a cat first receives this vaccine at ≥ 12 weeks of age, then revaccination is warranted 3-4 weeks later, then 1 year later, then every 3 years; vaccination 7-10 days before boarding, stress, and/or group exposure if last vaccination was > 1 year earlier may be warranted.
(4) If a cat first receives this vaccine at age ≥ 12 weeks, a second vaccination is necessary 1 year later, then every 1 or 3 years according to product type and regional statutes.
(5) Consult regional statues for requirements as well as need for annual or triennial boosters (booster requirements also differ with vaccine products). Any cat with outdoor exposure in rabies endemic area should be vaccinated.
(6) Earliest age for vaccination = 8 weeks.
(7) FeLV vaccination, along with booster, are recommended for all kittens < 1 year of age. The need for subsequent vaccination is determined by individual risk.
(8) If a cat first receives this vaccine at ≥ 12 weeks of age, a second vaccination is necessary 3-4 weeks later, then annually if warranted by sustained risk of infection.
(9) FIP vaccine is administered intranasally at or after 16 weeks of age, by which time most cats reared in an endemic environment have already been exposed to feline coronavirus.

Feline viral rhinotracheitis (herpesvirus-1) and feline calicivirus: Kittens that are orphaned or at high risk of exposure may receive the first vaccination at age 4 weeks (parenteral) or at age 10-14 days (IN). If using IN vaccine and cat is ≥ 12 weeks of age, the second dose is not necessary until 1 year later (and then every 3 years). Multivalent calicivirus vaccines are appropriate in shelter settings where vaccinated cats are developing clinical signs of calicivirus infection (different strain).

Feline panleukopenia: Use killed vaccine if FeLV- or FIV-infected, < 4 weeks of age, or pregnant. Any cat should receive at least 1 panleukopenia vaccine parenterally.

Rabies: Considered core vaccine if rabies is endemic in area and/or vaccine is legally required.

Feline leukemia virus (FeLV): Serologic testing is recommended before vaccination; infected cats do not derive any benefit from vaccination. Vaccination is recommended for cats that are not restricted to a closed, indoor, FeLV-negative environment, especially if < 16 weeks of age.

Feline immunodeficiency virus (FIV): Vaccination for FIV is not routinely recommended but may be considered in high-risk cats (e.g., outdoor cats that fight, or FIV-negative cats in household contact with an FIV-positive cat). An FIV test is indicated before initial FIV vaccination.

Chlamydia felis: Vaccination is not recommended for routine use. Considered for use in cats in multiple-cat environments where *C. felis* infections are associated with clinical disease.

Bordetella bronchiseptica: Vaccination may be considered for use in cats in shelter environments where laboratory-proven *B. bronchiseptica* infections are associated with clinical disease. First dose of IN vaccine is given once at ≥ 4 weeks of age as single dose. **NOTE:** Dog vaccine should not be used in cats.

FIP: Vaccination is not recommended for routine use. Vaccine contains temperature-sensitive modified-live mutant coronavirus strain administered IN. There is controversy as to the efficacy of vaccination even in high-risk environments.

Vaccine site recommendations:

- FVRCP (with or without *Chlamydia felis*): right forelimb, distal to elbow.
- Rabies: right hindlimb, distal to stifle.
- FeLV: left hindlimb, distal to stifle.
- Injectable vaccine should be administered SQ or IM as labeled (if both are acceptable, then SQ is preferred).
- Injection sites of other medications should be recorded.

Antiparasitics in Small Animal Practice

Molecule(s)	Example Trade Name	Species	Heartworms	Roundworms	Hookworms	Whipworms	Tapeworms	Fleas (adults)	Fleas (immature)	Ticks	Ear mites	Scabies	Demodex
Afoxolaner	NexGard	D						●		●	●†	●†	●†
Amitraz	Mitoban	D										◐†	●
Epsiprantel	Cestex	D/C					●						
Fenbendazole	Panacur	D/C†		●	●	●	◐						
Fipronil	EasySpot	D/C						●		◐			
Fluralaner	Bravecto	D/C						●		●D ◐C	●†	●†	●†
Indoxacarb	Activyl	D/C						●					
Ivermectin*	Heartgard	D/C	●	●†	●†	◐†					●†	●†	●†
Lotilaner	Credelio	D						●		●			●
Lufenuron	Program	D/C							●				
Milbemycin	Interceptor	D/C	●	●	◐	●					●†	●†	◐†
Moxidectin	ProHeart6,‡ Coraxis	D	●	●‡	●‡	●‡						●†,‡	●†,‡
Nitenpyram	Capstar	D/C						●					
Praziquantel	Droncit	D/C					●						
Pyrantel	Strongid	D/C		●	●								
Sarolaner	Simparica	D/C						●		●	●	●	●
Selamectin	Revolution	D/C	●	●C	◐C			●	●	◐D	●	●D	●†
Spinetoram	Assurity	C						●					
Spinosad	Comfortis	D/C						●					
Dinotefuran and pyriproxyfen	Vectra	D/C						●	●				
Dinotefuran, pyriproxyfen, and permethrin	Vectra 3D	D						●	●	●	●†		
Dinotefuran, fipronil, and pyriproxyfen	Catego	C						●	●	●			
Fipronil and 5-methoprene	Frontline Plus	D/C						●	●	●		●D	
Fipronil and cyphenothrin	Parastar Plus	D						●		●		●†	
Fipronil, etofenprox, (s)-methoprene	Frontline Tritak	C						●	●	●			
Fipronil, (s)-methoprene, amitraz	Certifect	D						●	●	●		●	
Imidacloprid and flumethrin	Seresto	D/C						●	●	●		●	
Imidacloprid and permethrin	K9 Advantix	D						●	●	●			
Imidacloprid and pyriproxyfen	Advantage II	D/C						●	●				
Imidacloprid and Moxidectin	Advantage Multi	D/C	●	●	●	●D		●			●C	●D	●†D
Imidacloprid, pyriproxyfen, and permethrin	K9 Advantix II	D						●	●	●			
Indoxacarb and permethrin	Activyl Tick Plus	D						●		●			
Imidacloprid and moxidectin	Advantage multi	D	●	●	●	●		●				●	
Milbemycin and lufenuron	Sentinel	D	●	●	◐	●			●				
Milbemycin and spinosad	Trifexis	D	●	●	◐	●		●					
Milbemycin and praziquantel	Interceptor Plus	D	●	●	◐	●	●						
Pyrantel and praziquantel	Drontal	C		●	●		●						
Pyrantel, praziquantel, and febantel	Drontal Plus	D		●	●	●	●						
Selamectin and sarolaner	Revolution Plus	C	●	●	●			●	●	◐	●	●†	●†

*Dose-dependent effect.

D, Dog; *C*, cat; ● effective († no label claim); ◐ effective on some species or partial efficacy.

‡Low-dose injectable for prevention of heartworms lacks efficacy for other parasites.

Côté's

CLINICAL VETERINARY ADVISOR

DOGS AND CATS

FOURTH EDITION

Editors-in-Chief

Leah A. Cohn, DVM, PhD, DACVIM
(Small Animal Internal Medicine)
Professor of Veterinary Medicine and Surgery
Department of Veterinary Medicine and Surgery
University of Missouri College of Veterinary Medicine
Columbia, Missouri

Etienne Côté, DVM, DACVIM
(Cardiology, Small Animal Internal Medicine)
Professor, Department of Companion Animals
University of Prince Edward Island
Atlantic Veterinary College
Charlottetown, Prince Edward Island, Canada

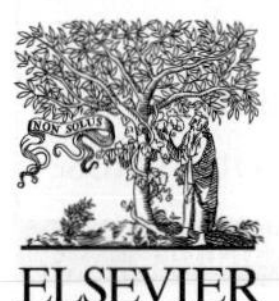

Elsevier
3251 Riverport Lane
St. Louis, Missouri 63043

CÔTÉ'S CLINICAL VETERINARY ADVISOR: DOGS AND CATS, FOURTH EDITION
ISBN: 978-0-323-55451-0

Notice

Practitioners and researchers must always rely on their own experience and knowledge in evaluating and using any information, methods, compounds or experiments described herein. Because of rapid advances in the medical sciences, in particular, independent verification of diagnoses and drug dosages should be made. To the fullest extent of the law, no responsibility is assumed by Elsevier, authors, editors or contributors for any injury and/or damage to persons or property as a matter of products liability, negligence or otherwise, or from any use or operation of any methods, products, instructions, or ideas contained in the material herein.

Previous editions copyrighted 2015, 2011, 2007.

International Standard Book Number: 978-0-323-55451-0

Director, Content Development: Rebecca Gruliow
Senior Content Strategist: Jennifer Catando
Senior Content Development Specialist: Jennifer Shreiner
Publishing Services Manager: Julie Eddy
Senior Project Manager: Jodi Willard
Design Direction: Paula Catalano

Printed in China

Last digit is the print number: 9 8 7 6 5

Section Editors

EDITORS-IN-CHIEF

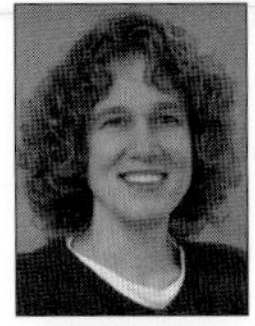

Leah A. Cohn, DVM, PhD, DACVIM (SAIM)
Professor of Veterinary Medicine and Surgery
Department of Veterinary Medicine and Surgery
University of Missouri College of Veterinary Medicine
Columbia, Missouri

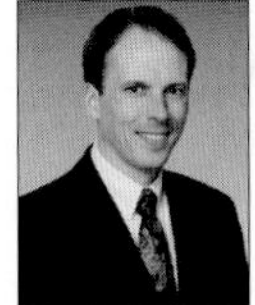

Etienne Côté, DVM, DACVIM (Cardiology, SAIM)
Professor, Department of Companion Animals
Atlantic Veterinary College
University of Prince Edward Island
Charlottetown, Prince Edward Island, Canada

EDITORS

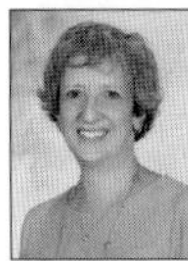

Ellen N. Behrend, VMD, PhD, DACVIM (SAIM)
Endocrinology
Joezy Griffin Endowed Professor and Alumni Professor
Department of Clinical Sciences
Auburn University College of Veterinary Medicine
Auburn, Alabama

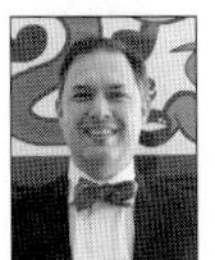

Benjamin M. Brainard, VMD, DACVAA, DACVECC
Emergency and Critical Care
Edward H. Gunst Professor of Small Animal Critical Care
Department of Small Animal Medicine and Surgery
University of Georgia College of Veterinary Medicine
Athens, Georgia

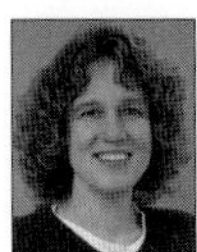

Leah A. Cohn, DVM, PhD, DACVIM (SAIM)
Chief Concerns
Nephrology / Urology
Other Topics
Professor of Veterinary Medicine and Surgery
Department of Veterinary Medicine and Surgery
University of Missouri College of Veterinary Medicine
Columbia, Missouri

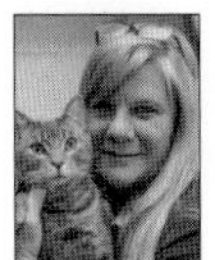

Gigi Davidson, BSPharm, DICVIP
Drug Compendium
Director of Pharmacy Services
Veterinary Teaching Hospital
North Carolina State University College of Veterinary Medicine
Raleigh, North Carolina

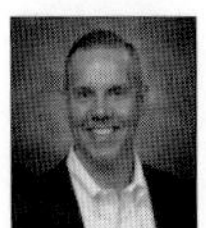

Jonathan E. Fogle, DVM, PhD, DACVIM (SAIM)
Hematologic / Immunologic Disease
Associate Professor of Immunology and Microbiology
Department of Population Health and Pathobiology
North Carolina State University College of Veterinary Medicine
Raleigh, North Carolina

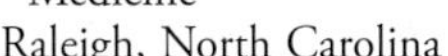

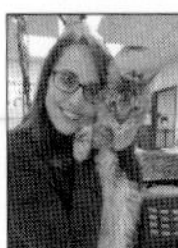

Megan Grobman, DVM, MS, DACVIM (SAIM)
Respiratory Disease
Clinical Instructor
Department of Veterinary Medicine and Surgery
University of Missouri College of Veterinary Medicine
Columbia, Missouri

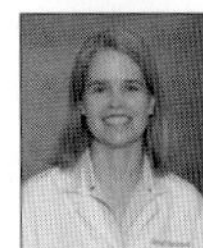

Diane V. H. Hendrix, DVM, DACVO
Ophthalmology
Professor of Ophthalmology
Department of Small Animal Clinical Sciences
University of Tennessee College of Veterinary Medicine
Knoxville, Tennessee

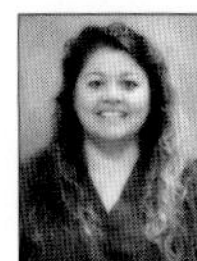

Michelle A. Kutzler, DVM, PhD, DACT
Theriogenology
Associate Professor
Department of Animal and Rangeland Sciences
Oregon State University
Corvallis, Oregon

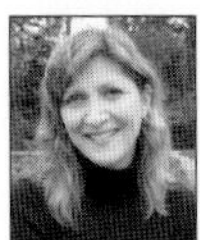

Jennifer A. Larsen, DVM, PhD, DACVN
Nutrition
Professor of Clinical Nutrition
Department of Veterinary Medicine: Molecular Biosciences
University of California-Davis School of Veterinary Medicine
Davis, California

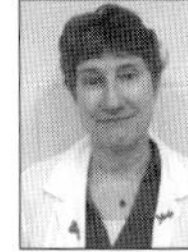

Kathleen Linn, DVM, MS, DACVS
Orthopedics
Associate Professor of Small Animal Surgery
Western College of Veterinary Medicine
University of Saskatchewan
Saskatoon, Saskatchewan, Canada

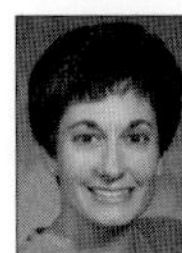

Karen R. Muñana, DVM, MS, DACVIM (Neurology)
Neurology
Professor of Neurology
Department of Clinical Sciences
North Carolina State University College of Veterinary Medicine
Raleigh, North Carolina

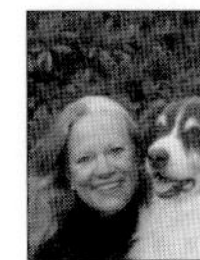

Karen L. Overall, VMD, MA, PhD, DACVB
Behavior
Senior Research Scientist
Department of Biology
University of Pennsylvania School of Veterinary Medicine
Philadelphia, Pennsylvania

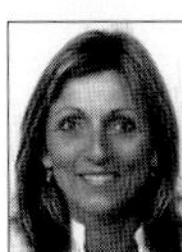

Manon Paradis, DMV, MVSc, DACVD
Dermatology
Professor of Dermatology
Department of Clinical Sciences
Faculté de Médecine Vétérinaire
University of Montreal
St-Hyacinthe, Québec, Canada

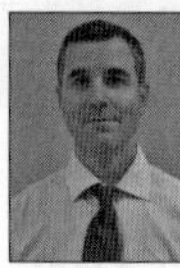

Kenneth Rassnick, DVM, DACVIM (Oncology)
Oncology
Director, Oncology Consultation Service
Veterinary Medical Center of Central New York
Syracuse, New York;
Director, Oncology Consultation Service
VCA Colonial Animal Hospital
Ithaca, New York

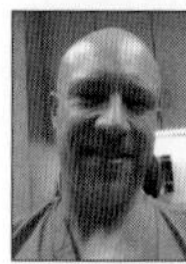

Alexander M. Reiter, DVM, Dr. med. vet., DAVDC, DEVDC
Dentistry / Oral Surgery
Professor of Dentistry and Oral Surgery
Department of Clinical Sciences and Advanced Medicine
University of Pennsylvania School of Veterinary Medicine
Philadelphia, Pennsylvania

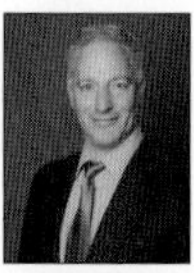

Keith Richter, DVM, MSEL, DACVIM (SAIM)
Hepatobiliary / Pancreatic Disease
Co-Founder/Board Member
Ethos Veterinary Health
San Diego, California

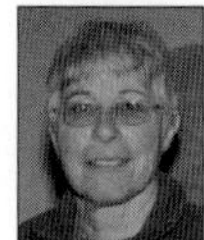

Lois Roth-Johnson, DVM, PhD, DACVP
Laboratory Tests
President
Dual Boarded, Inc
Needham Heights, Massachusetts

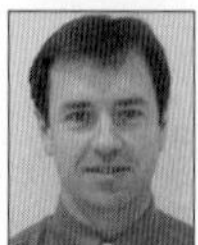

Rance K. Sellon, DVM, PhD, DACVIM (Oncology, SAIM)
Gastroenterology
Associate Professor
Department of Veterinary Clinical Sciences
Washington State University College of Veterinary Medicine
Pullman, Washington

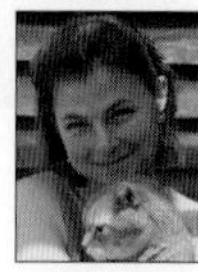

Meg M. Sleeper, VMD, DACVIM (Cardiology)
Cardiology
Clinical Professor of Cardiology
Department of Small Animal Clinical Sciences
University of Florida College of Veterinary Medicine
Gainesville, Florida

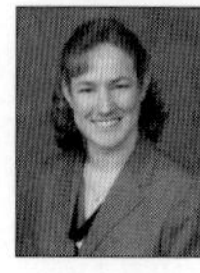

Elizabeth A. Swanson, DVM, MS, DACVS-SA
Soft-Tissue Surgery
Assistant Professor of Small Animal Surgery
Department of Clinical Sciences
Mississippi State University College of Veterinary Medicine
Mississippi State, Mississippi

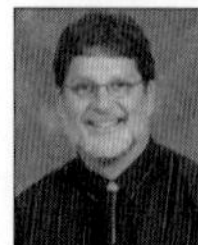

Joseph Taboada, DVM, DACVIM (SAIM)
Infectious Diseases
Professor, Small Animal Internal Medicine
Associate Dean, Academic Affairs
Louisiana State University School of Veterinary Medicine
Baton Rouge, Louisiana

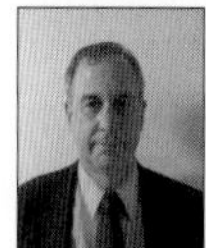

Mark S. Thompson, DVM, DABVP
Procedures and Techniques
Medical Director
Brevard Animal Hospital
Brevard, North Carolina

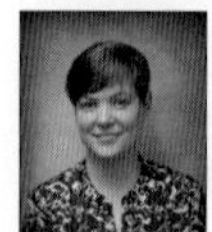

Tina Wismer, DVM, MS, DABVT, DABT
Toxicology
Medical Director
ASPCA Animal Poison Control Center
Urbana, Illinois

Contributors

Jonathan A. Abbott, DVM, DACVIM (Cardiology)
Associate Professor
Department of Small Animal Clinical Sciences
Virginia-Maryland College of Veterinary Medicine
Virginia Tech
Blacksburg, Virginia

Mark Acierno, MBA, DVM, DACVIM (SAIM)
Professor
Midwestern University College of Veterinary Medicine
Glendale, Arizona

Krista Adamovich-Rippe, DVM, DACVS-SA
Associate Surgeon
Department of Small Animal Surgery
Central Texas Veterinary Specialty & Emergency Hospital
Austin, Texas

Christopher Adin, DVM, DACVS
Professor and Department Chair
Department of Small Animal Clinical Sciences
University of Florida College of Veterinary Medicine
Gainesville, Florida

Darcy B. Adin, DVM, DACVIM (Cardiology)
Clinical Associate Professor, Cardiology
Department of Large Animal Clinical Sciences
University of Florida College of Veterinary Medicine
Gainesville, Florida

Arthur Rick Alleman Sr., DVM, PhD
CEO/Manager
Lighthouse Veterinary Consultants
Alachua, Florida

Marisa K. Ames, DVM, DACVIM (Cardiology)
Assistant Professor
Department of Clinical Sciences
Colorado State University
College of Veterinary Medicine and Biomedical Sciences
Fort Collins, Colorado

Erin L. Anderson, VMD, MSc, DACVIM (Cardiology)
Pittsburgh Veterinary Cardiology
Pittsburgh, Pennsylvania

Mary Aslanian, DVM, DACVECC
Department of Emergency and Critical Care
VCA Animal Diagnostic Clinic
Dallas, Texas

Harmeet Aulakh, BVSc & AH, MVSc, DACVIM (SAIM)
Visiting Assistant Professor
Department of Small Animal Internal Medicine
School of Veterinary Medicine
Louisiana State University
Baton Rouge, Louisiana

Lenore Bacek, DVM, MS, DACVECC
Clinical Associate Professor and Director, Emergency and Critical Care
Department of Clinical Sciences
Auburn University College of Veterinary Medicine
Auburn, Alabama

Jonathan F. Bach, DVM, DACVIM (SAIM), DACVECC
Clinical Associate Professor
Medical Sciences
University of Wisconsin School of Veterinary Medicine
Madison, Wisconsin

Dennis B. Bailey, DVM, DACVIM (Oncology)
Staff Oncologist
Department of Oncology
Oradell Animal Hospital
Paramus, New Jersey

Steven J. Bailey, DVM, DABVP (Feline)
Medical Director
ECats Veterinary Hospital
Waterford, Michigan;
Consultant, Feline Medicine
Veterinary Information Network
Davis, California;
Adjunct Professor
Department of Small Animal Clinical Sciences
Michigan State University College of Veterinary Medicine
East Lansing, Michigan

Raviv Balfour, DVM, DACVS
Staff Surgeon
Animal Specialty and Emergency Center
Los Angeles, California

Carsten Bandt, DVM, DACVECC
Canada West Veterinary Specialists
Vancouver, British Columbia, Canada

Gad Baneth, DVM, PhD, DECVCP
Professor of Veterinary Medicine
Director, Koret School of Veterinary Medicine
The Hebrew University of Jerusalem
Rehovot, Israel

Joseph W. Bartges, DVM, PhD, DACVIM (SAIM), DACVN
Professor of Medicine and Nutrition
Department of Small Animal Medicine and Surgery
Internist and Nutritionist
Veterinary Medical Center
The University of Georgia
Athens, Georgia

Ryan Baumwart, DVM, DACVIM (Cardiology)
Assistant Professor of Cardiology
Department of Veterinary Clinical Sciences
Oklahoma State University Center for Veterinary Health Sciences
Stillwater, Oklahoma

Jeff D. Bay, DVM, DACVIM (SAIM)
Staff Internist
Internal Medicine
Countryside Veterinary Medical Group
Queensbury, New York

Michaela J. Beasley, DVM, MS, DACVIM (Neurology)
Associate Clinical Professor
Neurology & Neurosurgery
Mississippi State University
Mississippi State, Mississippi

Sandra M. Bechtel, DVM, DACVIM (Oncology)
Associate Professor of Medical Oncology
Department of Small Animal Clinical Sciences
University of Florida College of Veterinary Medicine
Gainesville, Florida

Ellen N. Behrend, VMD, PhD, DACVIM (SAIM)
Joezy Griffin Professor
Department of Clinical Sciences
Auburn University College of Veterinary Medicine
Auburn, Alabama

Marie-Claude Belanger, DVM, MSc, DACVIM (SAIM)
Associate Dean, Clinical Programs
Professor of Small Animal Internal Medicine and Cardiology
Department of Clinical Sciences
Faculté de Médecine Vétérinaire
University of Montreal
St-Hyacinthe, Québec, Canada

Sara L. Bennett, DVM, MS, DACVB
Clinical Assistant Professor of Veterinary Behavior
North Carolina State University, College of Veterinary Medicine
Raleigh, North Carolina

Ellison Bentley, DVM, DACVO
Clinical Professor of Comparative Ophthalmology
Department of Surgical Sciences
University of Wisconsin-Madison School of Veterinary Medicine
Madison, Wisconsin

Allyson Berent, DVM, DACVIM (SAIM)
Director, Interventional Endoscopy Services
Internal Medicine
The Animal Medical Center
New York, New York

Frédéric Billen, DVM, MS, PhD, DECVIM-CA (Internal Medicine)
Senior Lecturer
Department of Veterinary Clinical Sciences of Companion Animals and Equine
University of Liège Faculty of Veterinary Medicine
Liège, Belgium

Adam J. Birkenheuer, DVM, PhD, DACVIM (SAIM)
Professor
Department of Clinical Sciences
North Carolina State University College of Veterinary Medicine
Raleigh, North Carolina

Marie-Claude Blais, DMV, DACVIM (SAIM)
Associate Professor in Small Animal Internal Medicine
Department of Clinical Sciences
Faculté de Médecine Vétérinaire
University of Montreal
St-Hyacinthe, Québec, Canada

Jason Bleedorn, DVM, MS, DACVS-SA
Clinical Associate Professor
Surgical Sciences, School of Veterinary Medicine
University of Wisconsin-Madison
Madison, Wisconsin

Shauna L. Blois, DVM, DVSc, DACVIM (SAIM)
Associate Professor
Department of Clinical Studies
Ontario Veterinary College
Guelph, Ontario, Canada

Manuel Boller, Dr. med. vet., MTR, DACVECC
Senior Lecturer, Emergency and Critical Care
Faculty of Veterinary and Agricultural Sciences
University of Melbourne
Melbourne, Victoria, Australia

John D. Bonagura, DVM, MS, DACVIM (Cardiology, SAIM)
Department of Clinical Sciences
College of Veterinary Medicine
North Carolina State University
Raleigh, North Carolina;
Professor Emeritus
College of Veterinary Medicine
The Ohio State University
Columbus, Ohio

Shannon D. Boveland, DVM, MS, DACVO
Associate Clinical Professor
Department of Clinical Sciences
Auburn University College of Veterinary Medicine
Auburn, Alabama

Søren Boysen, DVM, DACVECC
Professor
Department of Veterinary Clinical and Diagnostic Services
University of Calgary—Faculty of Veterinary Medicine
Calgary, Alberta, Canada

Benjamin M. Brainard, VMD, DACVAA, DACVECC
Edward H. Gunst Professor of Small Animal Critical Care
Department of Small Animal Medicine and Surgery
University of Georgia College of Veterinary Medicine
Athens, Georgia

Keith Branson, DVM, MS, DACVAA
Assistant Teaching Professor
Veterinary Medicine and Surgery
University of Missouri College of Veterinary Medicine
Columbia, Missouri

David Brewer, DVM, DACVIM (Neurology)
Neurologist
Hope Veterinary Specialists
Leesburg, Virginia

MAJ Desireé Broach, MS, DVM, DACVB
Veterinarian at US Army Veterinary Corps
Veterinary Medical Center Europe, Germany

Marjory B. Brooks, DVM, DACVIM (SAIM)
Section Director
Comparative Coagulation Laboratory
Cornell University
Ithaca, New York

Ginger Watts Brown, DVM
Senior Consulting Veterinarian in Clinical Toxicology
ASPCA Animal Poison Control Center
Urbana, Illinois

M. Raquel Brown, DVM, DACVIM (SAIM, Oncology)
Consultant in Oncology & Internal Medicine
IDEXX Laboratories
Westbrook, Maine

Stephanie R. Bruner, DVM, DACVD
Staff Dermatologist
Greater Cincinnati Veterinary Specialists and Emergency Services
Wilder, Kentucky

Jeffrey N. Bryan, DVM, MS, PhD, DACVIM (Oncology)
Professor of Oncology
Director, Comparative Oncology Radiobiology and Epigenetics Laboratory
Director, PET Imaging Center
Department of Veterinary Medicine and Surgery
University of Missouri College of Veterinary Medicine
Columbia, Missouri

James W. Buchanan, DVM, M Med Sci, DACVIM (Cardiology)
Emeritus Professor of Cardiology
Department of Clinical Studies
University of Pennsylvania School of Veterinary Medicine
Philadelphia, Pennsylvania

Gareth James Buckley, MA, VetMB, MRCVS, DACVECC
Clinical Assistant Professor, Emergency & Critical Care
Small Animal Clinical Sciences
University of Florida College of Veterinary Medicine
Gainesville, Florida

Melissa Bucknoff, DVM, DACVECC
Assistant Professor
Biomedical Sciences
Ross University School of Veterinary Medicine
Basseterre, Saint Kitts and Nevis

William J. Burkholder, DVM, PhD, DACVN
Veterinary Medical Officer
Division of Animal Feeds
Center for Veterinary Medicine
United States Food and Drug Administration
Rockville, Maryland

Erin N. Burton, DVM, MS, DACVP
Assistant Professor
Department of Veterinary and Biomedical Sciences
University of Minnesota College of Veterinary Medicine
St. Paul, Minnesota

Shelley Burton, DVM, MSc, DACVP
Professor of Clinical Pathology
Department of Pathology and Microbiology
Atlantic Veterinary College
University of Prince Edward Island
Charlottetown, Prince Edward Island, Canada

Christine D. Calder, DVM, DACVB
Assistant Clinical Professor
Veterinary Behavior and Community Veterinary Services
Mississippi State University College of Veterinary Medicine
Mississippi State, Mississippi

Lisa Carioto, DVM, DVSc, DACVIM (SAIM)
Internal Medicine Mobile Referral Service
Montreal, Quebec, Canada

Michelle Carlino, DVM
Consulting Veterinarian in Clinical Toxicology
ASPCA Animal Poison Control Center
Urbana, Illinois

Jodi Carlson, VMD, MS
Consulting Veterinarian in Clinical Toxicology
ASPCA Animal Poison Control Center
Urbana, Illinois

Khristen J. Carlson, DVM, MS
Guest Lecturer
Department of Clinical Sciences
Tuskegee University College of Veterinary Medicine
Tuskegee, Alabama

Ana Milena Carmona Gil, DVM, Spc., MVSc
Veterinary Dermatologist
DermaVet Center of Veterinary Dermatology;
Professor, Veterinary Immunology
Professor, Small Animal Endocrinology
Department of Small Animal Medicine
Universidad de Antioquia;
Member Colombian Association of Veterinary Dermatology ACDV
Medellín, Colombia

Sheila Carrera-Justiz, DVM, DACVIM (Neurology)
Clinical Assistant Professor
Small Animal Clinical Sciences
University of Florida College of Veterinary Medicine
Gainesville, Florida

Renee Carter, DVM, DACVO
Associate Professor, Ophthalmology
Veterinary Clinical Sciences
Louisiana State University School of Veterinary Medicine
Baton Rouge, Louisiana

Ana C. Castejon-Gonzalez, DVM, PhD, DAVDC, DEVDC
Lecturer, Dentistry and Oral Surgery Service
Department of Clinical Sciences and Advanced Medicine
University of Pennsylvania School of Veterinary Medicine
Philadelphia, Pennsylvania

Julie T. Cecere, DVM, MS, DACT
Clinical Assistant Professor, Theriogenology
Small Animal Clinical Sciences
Virginia-Maryland College of Veterinary Medicine
Blacksburg, Virginia

Serge Chalhoub, DVM, DACVIM (SAIM)
Senior Instructor
Department of Veterinary Clinical and Diagnostic Sciences
University of Calgary Faculty of Veterinary Medicine
Calgary, Alberta, Canada

Thomas Chen, DVM, MS, DACVO
Clinical Assistant Professor
Department of Small Animal Clinical Sciences
University of Tennessee College of Veterinary Medicine
Knoxville, Tennessee

Dennis J. Chew, DVM, DACVIM (SAIM)
Professor Emeritus
Veterinary Clinical Sciences
The Ohio State University College of Veterinary Medicine
Columbus, Ohio

Jane Cho, DVM, DACVO
Veterinary Ophthalmologist
Veterinary Eye Specialists, PLLC
Thornwood, New York

Ruthanne Chun, DVM, DACVIM (Oncology)
Associate Dean for Clinical Affairs
Director
UW Veterinary Care
Clinical Professor of Oncology
Department of Medical Sciences
University of Wisconsin School of Veterinary Medicine
Madison, Wisconsin

Cecile Clercx, DVM, PhD, DECVIM-CA
Professor of Companion Animal Internal Medicine
Department of Small Animal Clinical Sciences
University of Liège Faculté de Médecine Vétérinaire
Liège, Belgium

Joan R. Coates, DVM, MS, DACVIM (Neurology)
Professor
Department Veterinary Medicine and Surgery
University of Missouri College of Veterinary Medicine
Columbia, Missouri

Todd Cohen, DVM, DACVIM (SAIM)
Internal Medicine Specialist
VCA Animal Specialty and Emergency Center
Los Angeles, California

Leah A. Cohn, DVM, PhD, DACVIM (SAIM)
Professor of Veterinary Medicine and Surgery
Department of Veterinary Medicine and Surgery
University of Missouri College of Veterinary Medicine
Columbia, Missouri

Lynette K. Cole, DVM, MS, DACVD
Professor of Dermatology and Otology
Department of Veterinary Clinical Sciences
The Ohio State University College of Veterinary Medicine
Columbus, Ohio

Gary Conboy, DVM, PhD, DACVM
Professor of Parasitology
Department of Pathology and Microbiology
Atlantic Veterinary College
University of Prince Edward Island
Charlottetown, Prince Edward Island, Canada

Audrey K. Cook, BVM&S, MSc Vet Ed, MRCVS, DACVIM (SAIM), DECVIM-CA, DABVP (Feline)
Associate Professor
Department of Small Animal Clinical Sciences
Texas A&M College of Veterinary Medicine and Biomedical Sciences
College Station, Texas

Cynthia S. Cook, DVM, PhD, DACVO
Ophthalmologist
Veterinary Vision Animal Eye Specialists
San Carlos, California

Etienne Côté, DVM, DACVIM (Cardiology, SAIM)
Professor
Department of Companion Animals
Atlantic Veterinary College
University of Prince Edward Island
Charlottetown, Prince Edward Island, Canada

Susan M. Cotter, DVM, DACVIM (SAIM, Oncology)
Distinguished Professor Emerita
Department of Clinical Sciences
Cummings School of Veterinary Medicine at Tufts University
North Grafton, Massachusetts

Laura Ridge Cousins, DVM, MS, DACVIM (SAIM)
Internist
Upstate Veterinary Specialists
Greenville, South Carolina

Bronwyn Crane, DVM, MS, DACT
Assistant Professor
Health Management
Atlantic Veterinary College
University of Prince Edward Island
Charlottetown, Prince Edward Island, Canada

Kate E. Creevy, DVM, MS, DACVIM (SAIM)
Associate Professor
Department of Small Animal Medicine and Surgery
Texas A&M University College of Veterinary Medicine and Biomedical Sciences
College Station, Texas

Harry Cridge, MVB, MRCVS
Small Animal Internal Medicine, Resident
Department of Clinical Sciences
Mississippi State University College of Veterinary Medicine
Mississippi State, Mississippi

Elizabeth Cripe, DVM
Senior Consulting Veterinarian in Clinical Toxicology/Team Leader
ASPCA Animal Poison Control Center
Urbana, Illinois

Cheryl L. Cullen, DVM, MVetSc, DACVO
Owner/Operator
CullenWebb Animal Eye Specialists
Riverview, New Brunswick, Canada

Ronaldo Casimiro da Costa, DMV, MSc, PhD, DACVIM (Neurology)
Professor and Service Head of Neurology and Neurosurgery
Veterinary Clinical Sciences
The Ohio State University
Columbus, Ohio

Anne M. Dalby, DVM, DACVIM (SAIM)
Veterinary Internist
Internal Medicine
Animal Emergency and Specialty Center
Parker, Colorado

Sylvie Daminet, DMV, PhD, DACVIM (SAIM), DECVIM-CA
Professor
Companion Animal Clinic
Faculty of Veterinary Medicine—Ghent University
Ghent, Belgium

Autumn P. Davidson, DVM, MS, DACVIM (SAIM)
Clinical Professor
Veterinary Medical Teaching Hospital
University of California-Davis School of Veterinary Medicine
Davis, California

Gigi Davidson, BSPharm, DICVIP
Director of Pharmacy Services
Veterinary Teaching Hospital
North Carolina State University College of Veterinary Medicine
Raleigh, North Carolina

Deborah J. Davis, RT(T), RN
Department of Radiation Oncology
Southeast Veterinary Oncology & Internal Medicine
Orange Park, Florida;
Department of Progressive Care
Baptist Medical Center
Jacksonville, Florida

Deborah G. Davis, DVM, DACVP
Clinical Pathologist
IDEXX Laboratories
North Grafton, Massachusetts

Joao Felipe de Brito Galvao, MV, MS, DACVIM (SAIM)
Internal Medicine Specialist
Internal Medicine Department
VCA Arboretum View Animal Hospital,
Downers Grove, Illinois;
Adjunct Assistant Professor
Veterinary Clinical Sciences
The Ohio State University College of Veterinary Medicine
Columbus, Ohio

Camille DeClementi, VMD, DABT, DABVT
Vice President
ASPCA Animal Hospital
New York, New York

Amy E. DeClue, DVM, MS, DACVIM (SAIM)
Associate Professor, Small Animal Internal Medicine
Veterinary Medicine and Surgery
University of Missouri College of Veterinary Medicine
Columbia, Missouri

Andrea Dedeaux, DVM, DACVIM (SAIM)
Clinical Assistant Professor
Department of Small Animal Clinical Sciences
University of Tennessee College of Veterinary Medicine
Knoxville, Tennessee

Vincent E. Defalque, DVM, DACVD
Staff Dermatologist
North West Veterinary Dermatology Services
Vancouver, British Columbia, Canada

Alice M. Defarges, DVM, MSc, DACVIM (SAIM)
Associate Professor of Internal Medicine
Department of Clinical Studies
Ontario Veterinary College
University of Guelph
Guelph, Ontario, Canada

Teresa DeFrancesco, DVM, DACVIM (Cardiology), DACVECC
Professor of Cardiology and Critical Care
Department of Clinical Sciences
North Carolina State University College of Veterinary Medicine
Raleigh, North Carolina

Shannon D. Dehghanpir, DVM, MS, DACVP
Assistant Professor of Veterinary Clinical Pathology
Louisiana State University School of Veterinary Medicine
Baton Rouge, Louisiana

Caroline de Jaham, DMV, MScV, DACVD
CEO, DMV Veterinary Center
Montreal, Quebec, Canada

Alexander de Lahunta, DVM, PhD, DACVIM (Neurology), DACVP
James Law Professor of Anatomy, Emeritus
Department of Biomedical Sciences
Cornell University College of Veterinary Medicine
Ithaca, New York

Eric De Madron, DVM, DACVIM (Cardiology), DECVIM (Internal Medicine)
Head
Cardiology Service
Central Hospital for Veterinary Medicine
North Haven, Connecticut

Sage M. De Rosa, DVM
Resident
Department of Clinical Sciences and Advanced Medicine
University of Pennsylvania School of Veterinary Medicine
Philadelphia, Pennsylvania

Ravinder S. Dhaliwal, DVM, MS, DACVIM (Oncology), DABVP
Staff Oncologist
Oncology
Silicon Valley Veterinary Specialists
San Jose, California;
Consultant
Oncology
VCA Antech Diagnostics
Irvine, California

Sharon M. Dial, DVM, PhD, DACVP (Clinical and Anatomic Pathology)
Director, Arizona Veterinary Diagnostic Laboratory
Division of Agriculture, Life and Veterinary Sciences, and Cooperative Extension
University of Arizona
Tucson, Arizona

Ryan M. Dickinson, DVM, DACVP
Veterinary Clinical Pathologist
Adjunct Professor
Department of Veterinary Pathology
Western College of Veterinary Medicine
University of Saskatchewan
Saskatoon, Saskatchewan, Canada

Ursula M. Dietrich, Dr.med.vet., DACVO, DECVO, MRCVS
Senior Lecturer in Veterinary Ophthalmology
The Royal Veterinary College
Hatfield, United Kingdom

John R. Dodam, DVM, MS, PhD, DACVAA
Professor and Chair
Veterinary Medicine and Surgery
University of Missouri College of Veterinary Medicine
Columbia, Missouri

Kenneth J. Drobatz, DVM, MSCE, DACVIM (SAIM), DACVECC
Professor and Chief, Section of Critical Care
Department of Clinical Studies and Advanced Medicine
University of Pennsylvania School of Veterinary Medicine;
Director, Emergency Service
Matthew J. Ryan Veterinary Hospital of the University of Pennsylvania
Philadelphia, Pennsylvania

Felix Duerr, Dr. med. vet., MS, DACVS-SA, DECVS, DACVSMR
Associate Professor
Department of Clinical Sciences
Colorado State University
College of Veterinary Medicine and Biomedical Sciences
Fort Collins, Colorado

Yvan Dumais, DVM, DAVDC, FAVD
Clinical Instructor
Dentistry
Department of Clinical Sciences
Faculté de Médecine Vétérinaire
University of Montreal
St-Hyacinthe, Québec, Canada

Eric Dunayer, VMD, MS, DABT, DABVT
Associate Professor of Veterinary Clinical Sciences
St. Matthew's University School of Veterinary Medicine
Grand Cayman, Cayman Islands

Marilyn Dunn, DMV, MVSc, DACVIM (SAIM)
Professor
Department of Clinical Sciences
Faculté de Médecine Vétérinaire
University of Montreal
St-Hyacinthe, Québec, Canada

David Dycus, DVM, MS, CCRP, DACVS-SA
Orthopedic Staff Surgeon
Veterinary Orthopedic and Sports Medicine Group (VOSM)
Annapolis Junction, Maryland;
Co-Founder/Co-Director
Veterinary Sports Medicine and Rehabilitation Institute (VSMRI)
Severn, Maryland

Adam Eatroff, DVM, DACVIM (SAIM)
Staff Internist
Director of Hemodialysis Unit
ACCESS Specialty Animal Hospitals
Los Angeles, California

Bruce E. Eilts, DVM, MS, DACT
Professor Emeritus (Retired)
Louisiana State University School of Veterinary Medicine
Baton Rouge, Louisiana

Laura Eirmann, DVM, DACVN
Nutritionist
Oradell Animal Hospital
Paramus, New Jersey;
Veterinary Communications Manager
Nestle Purina Pet Care
St. Louis, Missouri

Amara H. Estrada, DVM, DACVIM (Cardiology)
Professor and Associate Chair
Department of Small Animal Clinical Sciences
University of Florida College of Veterinary Medicine
Gainesville, Florida

Michael Ethier, DVM, DVSc, DACVECC
Director of Emergency and Critical Care Medicine
Toronto Veterinary Emergency Hospital
Toronto, Ontario, Canada

Stephen J. Ettinger, DVM, DACVIM (SAIM, Cardiology)
Veterinary Consultant
VetCorp, Inc.
Los Angeles, California

Sue N. Ettinger, DVM, DACVIM (Oncology)
Medical Oncologist
Dr Sue Cancer Vet PLLC
Tarrytown, New York;
Medical Oncologist
Veterinary Referral and Emergency Center
Norwalk, Connecticut

James F. Evermann, MS, PhD
Professor, Infectious Diseases
Veterinary Clinical Sciences and Diagnostic Laboratory
Washington State University
Pullman, Washington

Patty J. Ewing, DVM, MS, DACVP
Director, Department of Pathology
Angell Animal Medical Center
Boston, Massachusetts

John Farrelly, DVM, MS, DACVIM (Oncology), DACVR
Oncologist/Radiation Oncologist
Blue Pearl Veterinary Partners
New York, New York

Wenche K. Farstad, DVM, Dr. Scient., PhD, DECAR
Department of Production Animal Clinical Sciences, Faculty of Veterinary Medicine
Norwegian University of Life Sciences
Oslo, Norway

Edward C. Feldman, DVM, DACVIM (SAIM)
Emeritus Professor of Medicine and Epidemiology
University of California-Davis School of Veterinary Medicine
Davis, California

Fidelia R. Fernandez, DVM, MS, DACVP
Veterinary Clinical Pathologist
Antech Diagnostics
Cary, North Carolina

Wendy D. Fife, DVM, MS, DACVR
Veterinary Radiologist
Bear Peak Veterinary Radiology;
Consultant, Eagle Eye Radiology
Boulder, Colorado

Linda S. Fineman, DVM, DACVIM (Oncology)
Vice President, Learning and Development
Ethos Veterinary Health
Woburn, Massachusetts;
Adjunct Professor of Veterinary Microbiology and Pathology
Washington State University College of Veterinary Medicine
Pullman, Washington

Courtney Fitzpatrick, DVM, DACVS
Small Animal Surgeon
Veterinary Specialties Referral Center
Pattersonville, New York

James A. Flanders, DVM, DACVS-SA
Associate Professor of Surgery
Department of Clinical Sciences
Cornell University
Ithaca, New York

Polly Arnold Fleckenstein, DVM, MS, CVA, cVSMT, CAC, CVPP
Pain Management and Emergency Services
Veterinary Medical Center of CNY
East Syracuse, New York;
Medical Officer, Disaster Response
National Veterinary Response Teams
U.S. Department of Health and Human Services
Washington, DC;
Medical Officer, Disaster Response
New York State Veterinary Medical Society
Albany, New York

Brian K. Flesner, DVM, MS, DACVIM (Oncology)
Assistant Professor
Department of Veterinary Medicine and Surgery
University of Missouri College of Veterinary Medicine
Columbia, Missouri

Daniel J. Fletcher, PhD, DVM, DACVECC
Associate Professor, Section of Emergency and Critical Care
Department of Clinical Sciences
Cornell University College of Veterinary Medicine
Ithaca, New York

Jon Fletcher, DVM, DACVIM (SAIM)
Associate Professor
Department of Veterinary Clinical Sciences
Louisiana State University School of Veterinary Medicine
Baton Rouge, Louisiana

Carrie L. Flint, DVM, DACVP
Clinical Pathologist
IDEXX Reference Laboratories
Delta, British Columbia, Canada

Andi B. Flory, DVM, DACVIM (Oncology)
Medical Oncologist
Veterinary Specialty Hospital
San Diego, California

Jonathan E. Fogle, DVM, PhD, DACVIM (SAIM)
Associate Professor of Immunology and Microbiology
Department of Population Health and Pathobiology
North Carolina State University College of Veterinary Medicine
Raleigh, North Carolina

Peter Foley, BSc, MSC, DVM, DACVIM (SAIM)
Associate Professor of Companion Animal Medicine
Companion Animals
Atlantic Veterinary College
University of Prince Edward Island
Charlottetown, Prince Edward Island, Canada

Marnin A. Forman, DVM, DACVIM (SAIM)
Head, Department of Internal Medicine
Cornell University Veterinary Specialists
Stamford, Connecticut

Lisa M. Freeman, DVM, PhD, DACVN
Professor
Department of Clinical Sciences
Cummings School of Veterinary Medicine at Tufts University
North Grafton, Massachusetts

Ryan C. Fries, DVM, DACVIM (Cardiology)
Assistant Professor
Department of Veterinary Clinical Medicine
University of Illinois College of Veterinary Medicine
Urbana, Illinois

Silvia Funes Sebastián, DVM, MS, DACVIM (SAIM)
Staff Internist
VCA Bay Area Veterinary Specialist
San Leandro, California

Sara Galac, DVM, PhD
Assistant Professor of Internal Medicine
Department of Clinical Sciences of Companion Animals
Utrecht University Faculty of Veterinary Medicine
Utrecht, The Netherlands

Laura D. Garrett, DVM, DACVIM (Oncology)
Clinical Professor of Oncology
Department of Veterinary Clinical Medicine
University of Illinois College of Veterinary Medicine
Urbana, Illinois

Frédéric Gaschen, Dr.med.vet., Dr.habil., DACVIM (SAIM), DECVIM-CA (IM)
Professor
Department of Veterinary Clinical Sciences
Louisiana State University School of Veterinary Medicine
Baton Rouge, Louisiana

Stephen D. Gaunt, DVM, PhD, DACVP
Professor of Veterinary Clinical Pathology
Section Chief, VTH Clinical Pathology Laboratory
Louisiana State University School of Veterinary Medicine
Baton Rouge, Louisiana

Joshua Gehrke, DVM, DACVIM (Neurology)
Assistant Professor and Service Chief
Department of Neurology & Neurosurgery
Michigan State University College of Veterinary Medicine
East Lansing, Michigan

Hans Gelens, DVM, MSc, DACVIM (SAIM)
University of Prince Edward Island
Companion Animals
Atlantic Veterinary College
University of Prince Edward Island
Charlottetown, Prince Edward Island, Canada

Anna R. M. Gelzer, Dr.med.vet., PhD, DACVIM (Cardiology), DECVIM-CA (Cardiology)
Associate Professor of Cardiology
Department of Clinical Sciences and Advanced Medicine
University of Pennsylvania School of Veterinary Medicine
Philadelphia, Pennsylvania

Anne J. Gemensky-Metzler, DVM, MS, DACVO
Professor—Clinical
Department of Veterinary Clinical Sciences
The Ohio State University College of Veterinary Medicine
Columbus, Ohio

Tracy Gieger, DVM, DACVIM (SAIM), DACVR
Clinical Associate Professor
Department of Clinical Sciences
North Carolina State University College of Veterinary Medicine
Raleigh, North Carolina

Peter Gilbert, BVSc (hons), MVetSc, MANZCVS, DACVS (SA)
Assistant Professor of Small Animal Orthopedics and Sports Medicine
Department of Veterinary Clinical Sciences
Washington State University College of Veterinary Medicine
Pullman, Washington

Mathieu Glassman, VMD, DACVS
Chief of Surgery
Friendship Hospital for Animals
Washington, DC

Tony M. Glaus, Dr. med. vet., Dr. habil., DACVIM (SAIM), DECVIM-CA (Internal Medicine, Cardiology)
Professor, Division of Cardiology
Clinic for Small Animal Internal Medicine
University of Zurich Vetsuisse Faculty
Zurich, Switzerland

Joseph C. Glennon, VMD, DACVS
Surgeon
Veterinary Specialties Referral Center
Pattersonville, New York;
Adjunct Associate Professor of Surgery
Albany Medical College
Albany, New York

Cristina Gobello, MV, DMV, DECAR
Laboratory of Reproductive Physiology
National University of La Plata
National Research Council,
La Plata, Argentina

Kristine L. Gonzales, DVM, DACT
Staff Veterinarian
Veterinary Clinic
Guide Dogs for the Blind
San Rafael, California

María Soledad González-Domínguez, MV, Esp, MSc
Associate Professor
Department of Veterinary Medicine and Zootechny;
Member, Colombian Association of Veterinary Dermatology;
INCA-CES Research Group
Veterinary Teaching Hospital
CES University
Medellín, Colombia

Lillian Good, DVM, DACVECC
Criticalist
Silicon Valley Veterinary Specialists
San Jose, California

Kinga Gortel, DVM, MS, DACVD
Staff Dermatologist
Westbank Animal Care Hospital
West Kelowna, British Columbia, Canada

Ruanna E. Gossett, DVM, PhD, DACVP
Clinical Pathologist
Grass Valley, California

Margherita Gracis, Med Vet, DAVDC, DEVC
Istituto Veterinario di Novara
Granozzo con Monticello (Novara), Italy;
Clinica Veterinaria San Siro
Milan, Italy

Carlos M. Gradil, DVM, MS, PhD, DACT
Professor and Equine Studies Program Coordinator
College of Veterinary and Animal Sciences
University of Massachusetts-Amherst
Amherst, Massachusetts

Britton J. Grasperge, BS, DVM, PhD, DACVP
Assistant Professor of Pathobiological Sciences
Louisiana State University School of Veterinary Medicine
Baton Rouge, Louisiana

Hillary Greatting, DVM, MS, DACVIM (Neurology), CCRT
Staff Neurologist
WestVet 24 Hour Emergency & Specialty Center
Boise, Idaho

Bradley A. Green, DVM, DACVIM (SAIM)
Chief, Department of Internal Medicine
Olympia Veterinary Specialists
Olympia, Washington;
Director
Washington Specialty VetMed
Poulsbo, Washington

Megan Grobman, DVM, MS, DACVIM (SAIM)
Clinical Instructor
Department of Veterinary Medicine and Surgery
University of Missouri College of Veterinary Medicine
Columbia, Missouri

Sophie A. Grundy, BVSc (Hons), MANZCVS, DACVIM (SAIM)
Internal Medicine Consultant
IDEXX Laboratories, Inc.
Westbrook, Maine

Julien Guevar, DVM, MVM, DECVN, MRCVS
Fellow, Neurology and Neurosurgery
Department of Clinical Sciences
North Carolina State University College of Veterinary Medicine
Raleigh, North Carolina

Sharon Gwaltney-Brant, DVM, PhD, DABVT, DABT
Consultant
Veterinary Information Network
Mahomet, Illinois;
Adjunct Assistant Professor
Department of Pathology, Immunology, and Laboratory Medicine
University of Florida College of Medicine
Gainesville, Florida

Devon Wallis Hague, DVM, DACVIM (Neurology)
Clinical Associate Professor
Department of Veterinary Clinical Medicine
University of Illinois College of Veterinary Medicine
Urbana, Illinois

Matt Haight, CVT
Internal Medicine Technician
University of Missouri College of Veterinary Medicine
Columbia, Missouri

Michael Hannigan, BVMS, CertSAD, MRCVS
Senior Manager, Veterinary Operations
Companion Animal Health
Zoetis, Inc., Kirkland
Kirkland, Quebec, Canada

Joseph Harari, DVM, MS, DACVS
Staff Surgeon
Small Animal Surgery
Veterinary Surgical Specialists
Spokane, Washington

Kenneth R. Harkin, DVM, DACVIM (SAIM)
Professor
Department of Clinical Sciences
College of Veterinary Medicine
Kansas State University
Manhattan, Kansas

Meghan Harmon, DVM, DACVECC
Staff Criticalist
BluePearl Veterinary Partners North Seattle
Seattle, Washington

Katrin Hartmann, Dr. med. vet., Dr. habil., DECVIM-CA (Internal Medicine)
Professor and Chair, Clinic of Small Animal Medicine
Medizinische Kleintierklinik
Centre of Clinical Veterinary Medicine
LMU
Munich, Germany

Cristine Hayes, DVM, DABT, DABVT
Senior Toxicologist
ASPCA Animal Poison Control Center
Urbana, Illinois

Timothy Hazzard, PhD, DVM
Instructor
Department of Animal and Rangeland Sciences
Oregon State University
Corvallis, Oregon

Geoff Heffner, DVM, DACVECC
Assistant Professor
Emergency and Critical Care Medicine
Colorado State University
College of Veterinary Medicine and Biomedical Sciences
Fort Collins, Colorado

Cailin R. Heinze, VMD, MS, DACVN
Associate Professor
Department of Clinical Sciences
Cummings School of Veterinary Medicine at Tufts University
North Grafton, Massachusetts

Alicia K. Henderson, DVM, DACVIM (SAIM)
Staff Internist
Internal Medicine
Garden State Veterinary Specialists
Tinton Falls, New Jersey

Charles M. Hendrix, DVM, PhD
Professor Emeritus of Parasitology
Department of Pathobiology
Auburn University College of Veterinary Medicine
Auburn, Alabama

Diane V. H. Hendrix, DVM, DACVO
Professor of Ophthalmology
Department of Small Animal Clinical Sciences
University of Tennessee College of Veterinary Medicine
Knoxville, Tennessee

Melanie Hezzell, MA, VetMB, PhD, DACVIM (Cardiology)
Senior Lecturer in Cardiology
Bristol Veterinary School
University of Bristol
Bristol, United Kingdom

Steve Hill, DVM, MS, DACVIM (SAIM)
Internist
Flagstaff Veterinary Internal Medicine Consulting (FLG VIM-C)
Flagstaff, Arizona

Mark E. Hitt, DVM, MS, DACVIM (SAIM)
Medical Director
Atlantic Veterinary Internal Medicine & Oncology
Annapolis, Maryland

Judy Holding, RN, BS, DVM
ASPCA Animal Poison Control Center
Urbana, Illinois

Steven R. Hollingsworth, DVM, DACVO
Professor of Clinical Ophthalmology
Department of Surgical and Radiological Sciences
University of California-Davis School of Veterinary Medicine
Davis, California

Fiona K. Hollinshead, BVSC (Hons), PhD, DACT
Associate Professor, Small Animal Theriogenology
Department of Clinical Sciences
College of Veterinary Medicine and Biomedical Sciences
Colorado State University
Fort Collins, Colorado

David Holt, BVSc, DACVS
Professor of Surgery
Department of Clinical Studies and Advanced Medicine
University of Pennsylvania School of Veterinary Medicine
Philadelphia, Pennsylvania

Katherine Albro Houpt, VMD, PhD, DACVB
Professor Emeritus
College of Veterinary Medicine
Cornell University
Ithaca, New York

Louis Huneault, DMV, MSc, DES, DACVS
Staff Surgeon
Centre Vétérinaire Rive-Sud
Brossard, Québec, Canada

K. David Hutcheson, DVM, DACVS-SA
Assistant Professor
Department of Small Animal Veterinary Medicine and Surgery
University of Missouri College of Veterinary Medicine
Columbia, Missouri

Jens Häggström, DVM, PhD, DECVIM-CA (Cardiology)
Professor of Internal Medicine
Department of Clinical Sciences
The Swedish University of Agricultural Sciences
Faculty of Veterinary Medicine
Uppsala, Sweden

Joanne L. Intile, DVM, MS, DACVIM (Oncology)
Clinical Assistant Professor of Medical Oncology
Department of Clinical Sciences
North Carolina State University College of Veterinary Medicine
Raleigh, North Carolina

Jared Jaffey, DVM, MS, DACVIM (SAIM)
Assistant Professor
Midwestern University
College of Veterinary Medicine
Phoenix, Arizona

Edward Jazic, DVM, DACVD
Veterinary Dermatologist
Department of Dermatology
Rochester Veterinary Specialists
Rochester, New York;
Department of Dermatology
Peak Veterinary Referral Center
Williston, Vermont

Albert E. Jergens, DVM, MS, PhD, DACVIM (SAIM)
Donn E. and Beth M. Bacon Professor of Small Animal Medicine and Surgery
Department of Veterinary Clinical Sciences
Iowa State University College of Veterinary Medicine
Ames, Iowa

Spencer A. Johnston, VMD, DACVS
James and Marjorie Waggoner Professor of Orthopedic Surgery
Department Head, Small Animal Medicine and Surgery
University of Georgia College of Veterinary Medicine
Athens, Georgia

Ashley E. Jones, DVM, DACVIM (Cardiology)
Staff Cardiologist
Veterinary Specialty Center
Buffalo Grove, Illinois

Soraya V. Juarbe-Diaz, DVM, DACVB
Veterinary Behaviorist
Affiliated Veterinary Specialists
Maitland, Florida

Aarti Kathrani, BVetMed (Hons), PhD, DACVIM (SAIM), DACVN
Senior Lecturer in Small Animal Internal Medicine
Royal Veterinary College
Hatfield, United Kingdom

Bruce W. Keene, DVM, MSc, DACVIM (Cardiology)
Jane Lewis Seaks Distinguished Professor of Companion Animal Medicine
Department of Small Animal Clinical Sciences
North Carolina State University College of Veterinary Medicine
Raleigh, North Carolina

Marc Kent, DVM, DACVIM (SAIM, Neurology)
Professor
Department of Small Animal Medicine and Surgery
University of Georgia College of Veterinary Medicine
Athens, Georgia

Marie E. Kerl, DVM, MPH, DACVIM (SAIM), DACVECC
Regional Medical Director, Central Group
VCA Inc.
Los Angeles, California

Safdar A. Khan, DVM, MS, PhD, DABVT
Associate Director
Global Regulatory Affairs
Zoetis Inc.
Kalamazoo, Michigan

Greg Kilburn, DVM, DACVIM (Neurology)
Staff Neurologist
Toronto Animal Health Partners Emergency and Specialty Hospital
Toronto, Ontario, Canada

Michael A. Kiselow, DVM, DACVIM (Oncology)
Associate Oncologist
Oncology
Sage Centers for Veterinary Specialty and Emergency Care
Campbell, California

Barbara E. Kitchell, DVM, PhD, DACVIM (SAIM, Oncology)
Director of Specialty Medicine
VCA Veterinary Care Animal Hospital and Referral Center
Albuquerque, New Mexico

Mandi Kleman, DVM, DACVIM (Cardiology)
Associate Cardiologist
IDEXX Laboratories
Atlanta, Georgia

Karen L. Kline, DVM, MS, DACVIM (Neurology)
Staff Neurologist
Veterinary Specialty Center of Seattle
Lynnwood, Washington

Tetsuya Kobayashi, DVM, MSpVM, DACVIM (Oncology, SAIM), DAiCVIM (Small Animal)
Director
Japan Small Animal Cancer Center
Tokorozawa, Japan

Kara A. Kolster, DVM, DACT
Staff Veterinarian
Springfield Veterinary Center
Glen Allen, Virginia

Lyndsay Kong, DVM
Resident in Cardiology
Department of Veterinary Medicine and Surgery
University of Missouri College of Veterinary Medicine
Columbia, Missouri

Hans S. Kooistra, DVM, PhD, DECVIM-CA
Professor of Internal Medicine
Department of Clinical Sciences of Companion Animals
Utrecht University Faculty of Veterinary Medicine
Utrecht, The Netherlands

Natali Krekeler, Dr. med. vet., PhD, DACT
Lecturer in Veterinary Reproduction
Department of Biomedical Sciences
The University of Melbourne
Melbourne, Victoria, Australia

Lyndsay Nichole Kubicek-Regev, DVM, DACVR
Staff Radiation Oncologist
Oncology
Angell Animal Medical Center
Boston, Massachusetts;
Adjunct Professor
Department of Radiation Oncology
University of Florida College of Veterinary Medicine
Gainesville, Florida

Sony Kuhn, DVM, DACVO
Veterinary Ophthalmologist
Animal Eye Clinic
Birmingham, Alabama

Lindsey M. Kurach, BSc, DVM, DACVS-SA
Veterinary Surgeon
Surgery Service
VCA Canada Guardian Veterinary Centre
Edmonton, Alberta, Canada

Michelle A. Kutzler, DVM, PhD, DACT
Associate Professor
Department of Animal and Rangeland Sciences
Oregon State University
Corvallis, Oregon

Tracy A. LaDue, DVM, DACVIM (Oncology), DACVR
Staff Oncologist
Southeast Veterinary Oncology and Internal Medicine
Orange Park, Florida

Elizabeth Laing, DVM, DVSc, DACVS
Consultant and Surgeon
Surgical Referral Service
Fort Atkinson, Wisconsin

Leigh A. Lamont, DVM, MS, DACVAA
Associate Dean of Academic and Student Affairs
Office of Academic and Student Affairs
Atlantic Veterinary College
University of Prince Edward Island
Charlottetown, Prince Edward Island, Canada

Selena Lane, DVM, DACVECC
Clinical Assistant Professor
Small Animal Medicine and Surgery
University of Georgia College of Veterinary Medicine
Athens, Georgia

Catherine E. Langston, DVM, DACVIM (SAIM)
Associate Professor of Small Animal Internal Medicine
Department of Veterinary Clinical Sciences
The Ohio State University College of Veterinary Medicine
Columbus, Ohio

Otto I. Lanz, DVM, DACVS
Professor
Department of Small Animal Clinical Sciences
Virginia-Maryland Regional College of Veterinary Medicine
Blacksburg, Virginia

Michael R. Lappin, DVM, PhD, DACVIM (SAIM)
The Kenneth W. Smith Professor
Department of Clinical Sciences
Colorado State University
College of Veterinary Medicine and Biomedical Sciences
Fort Collins, Colorado

Jennifer A. Larsen, DVM, PhD, DACVN
Professor of Clinical Nutrition
Department of Veterinary Medicine: Molecular Biosciences
University of California-Davis School of Veterinary Medicine
Davis, California

Nancy J. Laste, DVM, DACVIM (Cardiology)
Director of Medical Services
Departments of Cardiology, Dermatology, Diagnostic Imaging, and Internal Medicine
Angell Animal Medical Center
Boston, Massachusetts

Patty Lathan, VMD, MS, DACVIM (SAIM)
Associate Professor of Small Animal Internal Medicine
Department of Clinical Sciences
Mississippi State University College of Veterinary Medicine
Mississippi State, Mississippi

Susanne K. Lauer, Dr. med. vet., DACVS, DECVS, DACVSMR
Professor
Chirurgische u. Gynäkologische Kleintierklinik
Ludwig-Maximilians-Universität
Munich, Germany

James Lavely, DVM, DACVIM (Neurology)
Veterinary Neurologist
Department of Neurology and Neurosurgery
VCA Animal Care Center
Rohnert Park, California

Yuri A. Lawrence, DVM, PhD, MS, MA, DACVIM (SAIM)
Graduate Research Assistant
Department of Small Animal Clinical Sciences
Texas A&M University College of Veterinary Medicine and Biomedical Sciences
College Station, Texas

Elizabeth A. Layne, DVM, DACVD
Clinical Instructor
Division of Dermatology and Allergy
Department of Medical Sciences
University of Wisconsin–Madison School of Veterinary Medicine
Madison, Wisconsin

Mary Leissinger, DVM, MS, DACVP
Clinical Assistant Professor
University of Florida College of Veterinary Medicine
Gainesville, Florida

Jose A. Len, DVM, MS, PhD, DACT
Senior Lecturer in Theriogenology
School of Animal and Veterinary Sciences
The University of Adelaide
Roseworthy, South Australia, Australia

Britt Levy, VMD
Department of Clinical Sciences
North Carolina State University College of Veterinary Medicine
Raleigh, North Carolina

John R. Lewis, VMD, FAVD, DAVDC
Veterinary Dentistry Specialists
Silo Academy Education Center
Chadds Ford, Pennsylvania

Melissa J. Lewis, VMD, PhD, DACVIM (Neurology)
Assistant Professor of Neurology
Purdue University College of Veterinary Medicine
West Lafayette, Indiana

Christine C. Lim, DVM, DACVO
Eye Care for Animals Chicago
Chicago, Illinois

Kathleen Linn, DVM, MS, DACVS
Associate Professor of Small Animal Surgery
Western College of Veterinary Medicine
University of Saskatchewan
Saskatoon, Saskatchewan, Canada

Meryl P. Littman, VMD, DACVIM (SAIM)
Professor Emerita of Medicine
Clinician Educator, Department of Clinical Sciences & Advanced Medicine
University of Pennsylvania School of Veterinary Medicine
Philadelphia, Pennsylvania

Ingrid Ljungvall, DVM, PhD, DECVIM-CA (Cardiology)
Associate Professor of Internal Medicine
Department of Clinical Sciences
The Swedish University of Agricultural Sciences
Faculty of Veterinary Medicine
Uppsala, Sweden

Remo Lobetti, BVSc (Hons), MMedVet (Med), PhD, DECVIM-CA
Specialist Physician
Bryanston Veterinary Hospital
Bryanston, South Africa

Jennifer Locke, DVM, DACVIM (Oncology)
Medical Oncologist
Southeast Veterinary Oncology and Medicine
Orange Park, Florida

Dena L. Lodato, DVM, MS, DACVS-SA, CCRP
Department of Small Animal Surgery
South Paws Veterinary Surgical Specialists
Mandeville, Louisiana

Cheryl Lopate, MS, DVM, DACT
Co-Owner and Clinical Veterinarian
Reproductive Revolutions
Aurora, Oregon;
Co-Owner and Clinical Veterinarian
Wilsonville Veterinary Clinic
Wilsonville, Oregon

Andrew Lowe, DVM, MSc, DACVD
Staff Dermatologist
Alta Vista Animal Hospital
Ottawa, Ontario, Canada

Lori Ludwig, VMD, MS, DACVS
Department of Surgery
Veterinary Specialty Care
Mount Pleasant, South Carolina

Virginia Luis Fuentes, MA, VetMB, PhD, CertVR, DVC, DACVIM (Cardiology), DECVIM-CA
Professor of Veterinary Cardiology
Department of Clinical Science and Services
The Royal Veterinary College
Hatfield, Hertfordshire, United Kingdom

Jody P. Lulich, DVM, PhD, DACVIM (SAIM)
Professor
Department of Veterinary Clinical Sciences;
Co-Director
Minnesota Urolith Center
University of Minnesota College of Veterinary Medicine
St. Paul, Minnesota

Bertrand Lussier, DMV, MSc, DACVS
Professor of Surgery
Department of Clinical Sciences
Faculté de Médecine Vétérinaire
University of Montreal
St-Hyacinthe, Québec, Canada;
Associate Member
Research Group in Animal Pharmacology of Quebec-GREPAQ
Faculté de Médecine Vétérinaire
University of Montreal
St-Hyacinthe, Québec, Canada;
Associate Researcher
Osteoarthritis Research Unit,
University Hospital Research Centre (CRCHUM)
University of Montreal
Montreal, Québec, Canada

Jill K. Luther, DVM, MS, DACVS-SA
Assistant Teaching Professor of Small Animal Surgery
Department of Veterinary Medicine and Surgery
University of Missouri College of Veterinary Medicine
Columbia, Missouri

Alex Lynch, BVSc (Hons), DACVECC, MRCVS
Assistant Professor
Department of Clinical Sciences
North Carolina State University College of Veterinary Medicine
Raleigh, North Carolina

Janne G. Lyngby, DVM, DACVIM (SAIM)
Department of Veterinary Clinical Sciences
University of Copenhagen
Copenhagen, Denmark

Kristin A. MacDonald, DVM, PhD, DACVIM (Cardiology)
Veterinary Cardiologist
VCA Animal Care Center of Sonoma
Rohnert Park, California

Valerie Madden, DVM, DACVECC
Emergency and Critical Care
Western Veterinary Specialist and Emergency Center
Calgary, Alberta, Canada

David J. Maggs, BVSc (Hons), DACVO
Professor of Comparative Ophthalmology
Department of Surgical and Radiological Sciences
University of California-Davis School of Veterinary Medicine
Davis, California

Orla Mahony, MVB, DACVIM (SAIM), DECVIM
Department of Clinical Sciences
Cummings School of Veterinary Medicine at Tufts University
North Grafton, Massachusetts

Herbert W. Maisenbacher, III, VMD, DACVIM (Cardiology)
Veterinary Cardiologist
Veterinary Heart Care
Virginia Beach, Virginia

Rebecca L. Malakoff, DVM, DACVIM (Cardiology)
Staff Cardiologist
Cardiology Department
Angell Animal Medical Center West
Waltham, Massachusetts

Erin K. Malone, DVM, DACVIM (Oncology)
Staff Oncologist
Department of Medical Oncology
MedVet Medical and Cancer Centers for Pets
Worthington, Ohio

Steven Marks, BVSc, MS, MRCVS, DACVIM (SAIM)
Associate Dean and Director of Veterinary Medical Services
North Carolina State University College of Veterinary Medicine
Raleigh, North Carolina;
Clinical Professor
Department of Clinical Sciences
North Carolina State University College of Veterinary Medicine
Raleigh, North Carolina

Daniela A. Mauler, DVM, CCRP, DECVN
Veterinary Neurologist
Carolina Veterinary Specialists
Matthews, North Carolina

Katie D. Mauro, DVM
Resident
Department of Clinical Sciences & Advanced Medicine
University of Pennsylvania School of Veterinary Medicine
Philadelphia, Pennsylvania

Philipp D. Mayhew, BVM&S, DACVS
Professor of Small Animal Soft Tissue Surgery
Department of Surgical and Radiological Sciences
University of California-Davis School of Veterinary Medicine
Davis, California

Janet Kovak McClaran, DVM, DACVS, DECVS, MRCVS
Head of Surgery
Clinical Director
London Vet Specialists
London, United Kingdom

Brendan C. McKiernan, DVM, DACVIM (SAIM)
Professor Emeritus
Department of Veterinary Clinical Medicine
University of Illinois College of Veterinary Medicine
Urbana, Illinois

Nancy Johnstone McLean, DVM, DACVO
Veterinary Ophthalmologist
VCA Veterinary Care Animal Hospital and Referral Center
Albuquerque, New Mexico

Maureen A. McMichael, DVM, M.Ed., DACVECC
Professor of Veterinary Clinical Medicine
University of Illinois College of Veterinary Medicine
Urbana, Illinois

Irina D. Meadows, DVM, DABT
Toxicologist
ASPCA Animal Poison Control Center
Urbana, Illinois

Katrina L. Mealey, DVM, PhD, DACVCP, DACVIM (SAIM)
Professor
College of Veterinary Medicine
Washington State University
Pullman, Washington

Charlotte Means, DVM, MLIS, DABVT, DABT
Director of Toxicology
ASPCA Animal Poison Control Center
Urbana, Illinois

Valentina Merola DVM, MS, MPH, DABT, DABVT
Public Health Officer
United States Air Force
Robins AFB, Georgia

Kathryn E. Michel, DVM, MS, MSED, DACVN
Professor of Nutrition
Department of Clinical Sciences and Advanced Medicine
School of Veterinary Medicine, University of Pennsylvania
Philadelphia, Pennsylvania

Sarah J. Miller, DVM, DACVIM (Cardiology)
Staff Cardiologist
Southern California Veterinary Specialty Hospital
Irvine, California

Michael B. Mison, DVM, DACVS
Professor of Clinical Surgery
Department of Clinical Sciences and Advanced Medicine
University of Pennsylvania School of Veterinary Medicine
Philadelphia, Pennsylvania

Peter Moak, DVM
Assistant Professor
Department of Companion Animals
Atlantic Veterinary College
University of Prince Edward Island
Charlottetown, Prince Edward Island, Canada

Melanie Moore, BVM&S
Radiation Oncology Resident
Radiation Oncology
University of Missouri
Columbia, Missouri

Phillip A. Moore, DVM, DACVO
Professor of Ophthalmology
Department of Clinical Sciences
Auburn University College of Veterinary Medicine
Auburn, Alabama

Adam Mordecai, DVM, MS, DACVIM (SAIM)
Veterinary Medical Referral Service
Veterinary Specialty Center
Buffalo Grove, Illinois

Karen Moriello, DVM, DACVD
Clinical Professor of Dermatology
Department of Medical Sciences
University of Wisconsin-Madison School of Veterinary Medicine
Madison, Wisconsin

Helen Munro, BVMS, MRCVS
Honorary Fellow
Veterinary Pathology and Veterinary Clinical Studies
Royal (Dick) School of Veterinary Studies
University of Edinburgh
Edinburgh, Scotland, United Kingdom

Karen R. Muñana, DVM, MS, DACVIM (Neurology)
Professor of Neurology
Department of Clinical Sciences
North Carolina State University College of Veterinary Medicine
Raleigh, North Carolina

Laura A. Nafe, DVM, MS, DACVIM (SAIM)
Assistant Professor of Small Animal Internal Medicine
Department of Veterinary Clinical Sciences
Oklahoma State University Center for Veterinary Health Sciences
Stillwater, Oklahoma

Mirinda Nel van Schoor, BVSc, MMedVet (Med)
Specialist Physician
Department of Small Animal Medicine
Bakenkop Animal Clinic
Pretoria, South Africa

Stijn J.M. Niessen, DVM, PhD, DECVIM, FHEA, MRCVS
Professor of Internal Medicine in Veterinary Clinical Sciences
Royal Veterinary College
North Mymms, Hertfordshire;
Research Associate
Diabetes Research Group
Newcastle Medical School
Newcastle-upon-Tyne, Tyne and Wear;
Director, VetCT Telemedicine Hospital
Cambridge, Cambridgeshire, United Kingdom

Nicole C. Northrup, DVM, DACVIM (Oncology)
Zoey Bennett Professor of Oncology
Department of Small Animal Medicine and Surgery
University of Georgia College of Veterinary Medicine
Athens, Georgia

Dennis P. O'Brien, DVM, PhD, DACVIM (Neurology)
Chancellor's Chair in Comparative Neurology
Veterinary Medicine & Surgery
University of Missouri College of Veterinary Medicine
Columbia, Missouri

Mauria O'Brien, DVM, DACVECC
Criticalist
Portland Veterinary Emergency and Specialty Care
Portland, Maine;
Adjunct Clinical Associate Professor
Small Animal Emergency and Critical Care
University of Illinois, College of Veterinary Medicine
Urbana, Illinois

M. Lynne O'Sullivan, DVM, DVSc, DACVIM (Cardiology)
Professor
Department of Companion Animals
Atlantic Veterinary College
University of Prince Edward Island
Charlottetown, Prince Edward Island, Canada

Elizabeth O'Toole, Bsc, DVM, DvSc, DACVECC
Assistant Professor of Veterinary Emergency and Critical Care
Department of Clinical Sciences
Faculté de Médecine Vétérinaire
University of Montreal
St-Hyacinthe, Québec, Canada

Adesola Odunayo, DVM, MS, DACVECC
Clinical Associate Professor of Emergency and Critical Care
Department of Small Animal Clinical Sciences
University of Tennessee College of Veterinary Medicine
Knoxville, Tennessee

Natasha Olby, VetMB, PhD, DACVIM (Neurology)
Professor, Neurology and Neurosurgery
Dr. Kady M. Gjessing and Rihanna M. Davidson Distinguished Chair of Gerontology
Department of Clinical Sciences
North Carolina State University College of Veterinary Medicine
Raleigh, North Carolina

Maureen S. Oldach, DVM
Cardiology Resident
University of California-Davis School of Veterinary Medicine
Davis, California

Arthur I. Ortenburger, DVM, MS
Professor of Integrative Medicine
Atlantic Veterinary College
University of Prince Edward Island
Charlottetown, Prince Edward Island, Canada

João S. Orvalho, DVM, DACVIM (Cardiology)
Clinical Cardiology Specialist
University of California Veterinary Medical Center—San Diego
San Diego, California

Carl A. Osborne, DVM, PhD, DACVIM (Deceased)
Department of Veterinary Clinical Sciences
University of Minnesota College of Veterinary Medicine
St. Paul, Minnesota

Karen L. Overall, VMD, MA, PhD, DACVB
Senior Research Scientist
Department of Biology
University of Pennsylvania School of Veterinary Medicine
Philadelphia, Pennsylvania

LeeAnn Pack, DVM, DACVR
Diagnostic Imaging Specialist
Owner
Southland Vets, Inc.
Lake City, Arkansas

Nadia Pagé, DMV, MSc, DACVD
Staff Dermatologist
DMV Veterinary Center
Montréal, Québec, Canada

Manon Paradis, DMV, MVSc, DACVD
Professor of Dermatology
Department of Clinical Sciences
Faculté de Médecine Vétérinaire
University of Montreal
St-Hyacinthe, Québec, Canada

Rosa Maria Paramo-Ramirez, MVZ, PhD
Profesor Titular
Reproducción
Universidad Nacional Autónoma de México
Distrito Federal, Mexico

Romain Pariaut, DVM, DECVIM (Cardiology), DACVIM (Cardiology)
Associate Professor
Department of Clinical Sciences
Cornell University
Ithaca, New York

Adam P. Patterson, DVM, DACVD
Chief and Clinical Associate Professor of Dermatology
Department of Small Animal Clinical Sciences
Texas A&M University College of Veterinary Medicine
College Station, Texas

April Paul, DVM, DACVECC
Emergency and Critical Care Specialist
Emergency and Critical Care
Tufts VETS
Walpole, Massachusetts

Michael M. Pavletic, DVM, DACVS
Head of Surgical Services
Angell Animal Medical Center
Boston, Massachusetts

Paolo Pazzi, BVSc, Hons, MMedVet (Med), DECVIM-CA
Senior Lecturer
Companion Animal Clinical Studies
Onderstepoort, University of Pretoria
Pretoria, Gauteng, South Africa

Mayrim Lissette Perez-Gonzalez, DVM, DACVIM (SAIM)
Coral Springs Animal Hospital
Coral Springs, Florida

Jeffrey Person, DVM
Delton Veterinary Hospital
Edmonton, Alberta, Canada

Massimo Petazzoni, DVM
Clinica Veterinaria Milano Sud
Orthopedics
Peschiera Borromeo (Mi), Italy

Michael Peterson, DVM, MS
Associate Veterinarian
Reid Veterinary Hospital
Albany, Oregon

Polly B. Peterson, DVM, DACVIM (SAIM)
Staff Internal Medicine Specialist
Veterinary Specialty Center of Seattle
Lynnwood, Washington

Brenda Phillips, DVM, DACVIM (Oncology)
Medical Oncologist and Associate Medical Director
Veterinary Specialty Hospital
San Diego, California

Fredrick S. Pike, DVM, DACVS
Staff Surgeon, Medical Director
Surgery
Veterinary Specialty Hospital of San Diego
San Diego, California

Chantale L. Pinard, DVM, MSc, DACVO
Associate Professor
Department of Clinical Studies
Ontario Veterinary College
University of Guelph
Guelph, Ontario, Canada

Carlos R. F. Pinto, MedVet, PhD, DACT
Professor of Theriogenology
Department of Veterinary Clinical Sciences
Louisiana State University School of Veterinary Medicine
Baton Rouge, Louisiana

Caryn E. Plummer, DVM, DACVO
Associate Professor of Comparative Ophthalmology
Small and Large Animal Clinical Sciences
University of Florida College of Veterinary Medicine
Gainesville, Florida

Dan Polidoro, DVM, DACVS-SA
Surgeon
VCA San Francisco Veterinary Specialists
San Francisco, California

Barrak Michael Pressler, DVM, PhD, DACVIM (SAIM)
Small Animal Internal Medicine Veterinary Specialist
Northridge, California

Robert Prošek, DVM, MS, DECVIM-CA, DACVIM (Cardiology)
Adjunct Professor of Cardiology
University of Florida
Gainesville, Florida;
President
Cardiopulmonary Medicine and Interventional Therapy
Florida Veterinary Cardiology
Miami, Florida

David A. Puerto, DVM, DACVS
Chief of Surgery
Surgery
Center for Animal Referral and Emergency Services (CARES)
Langhorne, Pennsylvania

Gary Puglia, DVM, DACVECC
Department Head
Emergency and Critical Care
Center for Animal Referral and Emergency Services (CARES)
Langhorne, Pennsylvania

MaryAnn Radlinsky, DVM, MS, DACVS
General Surgeon
VetMed
Phoenix, Arizona

Gregg Rapoport, DVM, DACVIM (Cardiology)
Clinical Associate Professor of Cardiology
Department of Small Animal Medicine and Surgery
University of Georgia College of Veterinary Medicine
Athens, Georgia

Kenneth Rassnick, DVM, DACVIM (Oncology)
Director, Oncology Consultation Service
Veterinary Medical Center of Central New York
Syracuse, New York;
Director, Oncology Consultation Service
VCA Colonial Animal Hospital
Ithaca, New York

Rachel Reed, DVM
Veterinary Anesthesiologist
Large Animal Clinical Sciences
University of Georgia College of Veterinary Medicine
Athens, Georgia

Adam Reiss, DVM, DACVECC
Staff Veterinarian
Southern Oregon Veterinary Specialty Center
Medford, Oregon

Alexander M. Reiter, DVM, Dr. med. vet., DAVDC, DEVDC
Professor of Dentistry and Oral Surgery
Department of Clinical Sciences and Advanced Medicine
University of Pennsylvania School of Veterinary Medicine
Philadelphia, Pennsylvania

Meghan Respess, DVM, DACVECC
Medical Director and Staff Criticalist
Critical Care
BluePearl Veterinary Partners
Brooklyn, New York

Jaylyn Rhinehart, DVM, MS, DACVIM (Cardiology)
Assistant Professor
Department of Veterinary Clinical Sciences
The Ohio State University College of Veterinary Medicine
Columbus, Ohio

Keith Richter, DVM, MSEL, DACVIM (SAIM)
Co-Founder/Board Member
Ethos Veterinary Health
San Diego, California

Valeria Rickard, DVM
Chief of Staff
North Oatlands Animal Hospital & Reproduction Center
Leesburg, Virginia

Marcella D. Ridgway, VMD, MS, DACVIM (SAIM)
Clinical Professor of Small Animal Internal Medicine
Department of Veterinary Clinical Medicine
University of Illinois College of Veterinary Medicine
Urbana, Illinois

Sarah Bevin Rippy, DVM
Medical Oncology Resident
Oncology
University of Missouri
Columbia, Missouri

Carlos O. Rodriguez Jr., DVM, PhD, DACVIM (Oncology)
Staff Oncologist
Veterinary Specialists of North Texas
Fort Worth, Texas

Erin Rogers, DVM
Veterinary Internal Medicine Resident
MedVet New Orleans
Metairie, Louisiana

Patricia L. Rose, DVM, MS, DACVR
Staff Radiologist
MedVet Akron
Akron, Ohio

Desiree D. Rosselli, DVM, DACVS-SA
Surgeon
Department of Surgery
VCA West Lost Angeles Animal Hospital
Los Angeles, California

Lois Roth-Johnson, DVM, PhD, DACVP
President
Dual Boarded, Inc
Needham Heights, Massachusetts

Angela Royal, DVM, MS, DACVP
Assistant Clinical Professor
Veterinary Medical Diagnostic Laboratory
University of Missouri College of Veterinary Medicine
Columbia, Missouri

Elizabeth Rozanski, DVM, DACVIM (SAIM), DACVECC
Associate Professor
Department of Clinical Sciences
Cummings School of Veterinary Medicine at Tufts University
Grafton, Massachusetts

Jacob A. Rubin, DVM, DACVS-SA
Staff Surgeon
Maine Veterinary Medical Center
Scarborough, Maine

Kirk Ryan, DVM, DACVIM (SAIM)
Associate Professor
Department of Veterinary Clinical Sciences
Louisiana State University School of Veterinary Medicine
Baton Rouge, Louisiana

Pascale Salah, Dr. vet. med., DACVIM (Oncology)
University of Pennsylvania
School of Veterinary Medicine
Ryan Veterinary Hospital
Philadelphia, Pennsylvania

Andrew E. Sams, DVM, MS, DACVS
Orthopaedics and Arthroscopic Surgery
The Sams Clinic
Mill Valley, California

Sherry Lynn Sanderson, DVM, PhD, DACVIM (SAIM), DACVN
Associate Professor
Department of Veterinary Biosciences and Diagnostic Imaging
University of Georgia College of Veterinary Medicine
Athens, Georgia

Lynne S. Sandmeyer, DVM, DVSc, DACVO
Professor
Department of Small Animal Clinical Sciences
Western College of Veterinary Medicine
University of Saskatchewan
Saskatoon, Saskatchewan, Canada

John S. Sapienza, DVM, DACVO
Chair, Department of Ophthalmology
Long Island Veterinary Specialists
Plainview, New York

Suresh Sathya, BVSc, MVSc, MVetSc, DACVS-SA
Staff Surgeon
Surgery Service
VCA Guardian Veterinary Centre
Edmonton, Alberta, Canada

Frédéric Sauvé, DMV, MSc, DES, DACVD
Assistant Professor
Department of Clinical Sciences
Faculté de Médecine Vétérinaire
University of Montreal
St-Hyacinthe, Quebec, Canada

Christine Savidge, DVM, DACVIM (SAIM)
Assistant Professor
Department of Companion Animals
Atlantic Veterinary College
University of Prince Edward Island
Charlottetown, Prince Edward Island, Canada

Brian A. Scansen, DVM, MS, DACVIM (Cardiology)
Associate Professor
Department of Clinical Sciences
Colorado State University
College of Veterinary Medicine and Biomedical Sciences
Fort Collins, Colorado

Michael Schaer, DVM, DACVIM (SAIM), DACVECC
Professor Emeritus
Adjunct Professor, Emergency and Critical Care Medicine
University of Florida College of Veterinary Medicine
Gainesville, Florida

Mary Schell, DVM, DABT, DABVT
Senior Toxicologist
Animal Poison Control Center
ASPCA Animal Poison Control Center
Urbana, Illinois

Patricia A. Schenck, DVM, PhD
Consultant
DeWitt, Michigan

Amy Schnelle, DVM, MS, DACVP
Clinical Assistant Professor
Clinical Pathology
University of Illinois
College of Veterinary Medicine
Urbana, Illinois

Diana M. Schropp, DVM, DACVECC
Associate Veterinarian
Department of Emergency and Critical Care
Southern Oregon Specialty Center
Medford, Oregon

Erin M. Scott, VMD, DACVO
Assistant Professor
Department of Small Animal Clinical Sciences
Texas A&M College of Veterinary Medicine & Biomedical Sciences
College Station, Texas

Katherine D. Scott, DVM, DACVIM (SAIM)
Staff Internal Medicine Specialist
VCA Alameda East Veterinary Hospital
Denver, Colorado

Clare M. Scully, DVM, MA, MS, DACT
Associate Professor of Food Animal Health Maintenance
Department of Veterinary Clinical Sciences
Louisiana State University School of Veterinary Medicine
Baton Rouge, Louisiana

Kersti Seksel, BVSc (Hons), MRCVS, MA (Hons), FANZCVS, DACVB, DECAWBM
Adjunct Associate Professor
School of Animal and Veterinary Sciences
Charles Sturt University
Wagga Wagga, New South Wales, Australia;
Registered Specialist
Behavioural Medicine
Sydney Animal Behaviour Service
Sydney, New South Wales, Australia;
Registered Specialist
Behavioural Medicine
Animal Referral Hospital
Sydney, New South Wales, Australia

Rance K. Sellon, DVM, PhD, DACVIM (Oncology, SAIM)
Associate Professor
Department of Veterinary Clinical Sciences
Washington State University College of Veterinary Medicine
Pullman, Washington

Kim A. Selting, DVM, MS, DACVIM (Oncology), DACVR (Radiation Oncology)
Associate Professor
Department of Veterinary Clinical Medicine
University of Illinois College of Veterinary Medicine
Urbana, Illinois

Claire R. Sharp, BVMS, MS, DACVECC
Senior Lecturer in Veterinary Emergency and Critical Care
School of Veterinary Medicine
College of Science, Health, Engineering, and Education
Murdoch University
Murdoch, Western Australia

Scott Shaw, DVM, DACVECC
Specialty Regional Medical Director
VCA Inc
Oxford, Massachusetts

Andy Shores, DVM, MS, PhD, DACVIM (Neurology)
Clinical Professor and Section Chief, Neurology/Neurosurgery
Department of Clinical Sciences
Mississippi State University College of Veterinary Medicine and Veterinary Specialty Center
Mississippi State, Mississippi

Brian Skorobohach, DVM, DACVO
Ophthalmology Service
Calgary Animal Referral & Emergency Centre
Calgary, Alberta, Canada

Meg M. Sleeper, VMD, DACVIM (Cardiology)
Clinical Professor of Cardiology
Department of Small Animal Clinical Sciences
University of Florida College of Veterinary Medicine
Gainesville, Florida

Pascale M. Y. Smets, DVM, PhD, DECVIM-SA
Companion Animal Clinic
Faculty of Veterinary Medicine—Ghent University
Ghent, Belgium

Frances O. Smith, DVM, PhD, DACT
President
Orthopedic Foundation for Animals, Inc.
Columbia, Missouri;
Owner
Smith Veterinary Hospital, Inc.
Burnsville, Minnesota

Karla Smith, DVM
Consulting Veterinarian in Clinical Toxicology
ASPCA Animal Poison Control Center
Urbana, Illinois

Savannah Smith, RVT
Internal Medicine Technician
Small Animal Internal Medicine
University of Missouri College of Veterinary Medicine
Columbia, Missouri

Saralyn Smith-Carr, DVM, PhD, DACVIM (SAIM)
Associate Professor of Small Animal Internal Medicine
Department of Clinical Sciences
Auburn University College of Veterinary Medicine
Auburn, Alabama

Elizabeth Snead, BSc, DVM, MSc, DACVIM (SAIM)
Professor
Department of Small Animal Clinical Sciences
Western College of Veterinary Medicine
University of Saskatchewan
Saskatoon, Saskatchewan, Canada

Brandy R. Sobczak, DVM
Consulting Veterinarian in Clinical Toxicology
ASPCA Animal Poison Control Center
Urbana, Illinois

Maria M. Soltero-Rivera, DVM, DAVDC
Veterinary Specialist and Co-Medical Director
Department of Dentistry and Oral Surgery
VCA San Francisco Veterinary Specialists
San Francisco, California;
Adjunct Assistant Professor of Dentistry and Oral Surgery
Department of Clinical Sciences and Advanced Medicine
University of Pennsylvania School of Veterinary Medicine
Philadelphia, Pennsylvania

Mary Somerville, DVM, DACVS
Staff Surgeon
VCA-Animal Specialty and Emergency Center
Los Angeles, California

Ivan Sosa, DVM, DACVIM (Cardiology)
Veterinary Cardiologist
Massachusetts Veterinary Referral Hospital
Ethos Veterinary Health
Woburn, Massachusetts

Jörg M. Steiner, Dr. med. vet., PhD, DACVIM (SAIM), DECVIM-CA, AGAF
Dr. Mark Morris Chair in Small Animal Gastroenterology and Nutrition
Professor and Director, Gastrointestinal Laboratory
Department of Small Animal Clinical Sciences
Texas A&M University College of Veterinary Medicine & Biomedical Sciences
College Station, Texas

Rebecca L. Stepien, DVM, MS, DACVIM (Cardiology)
Clinical Professor of Cardiology
Department of Medical Sciences
University of Wisconsin School of Veterinary Medicine;
Clinical Cardiologist
UW Veterinary Care
Madison, Wisconsin

Joshua A. Stern, DVM, PhD, DACVIM (Cardiology)
Associate Professor of Cardiology
Department of Medicine & Epidemiology
University of California-Davis School of Veterinary Medicine
Davis, California

Laura Stern, DVM, DAVBT
Senior Toxicologist
ASPCA Animal Poison Control Center
Urbana, Illinois

Michael Stone, DVM, DACVIM (SAIM)
Clinical Associate Professor
Department of Clinical Sciences
Cummings School of Veterinary Medicine at Tufts University
Grafton, Massachusetts;
Ultrasonographer
Veterinary Internal Medicine Mobile Specialists
Woodstock, Connecticut

Elizabeth Streeter, DVM, DACVECC
Veterinarian
Critical Care
Iowa Veterinary Referral Center
Des Moines, Iowa

Keith Nelson Strickland, DVM, DACVIM (Cardiology)
Owner, President, Consultant
Veterinary Cardiac Consultations, LLC
Baton Rouge, Louisiana

Beverly K. Sturges, DVM, MS, MaS, DACVIM (Neurology)
Professor of Neurology/Neurosurgery
University of California-Davis School of Veterinary Medicine
Davis, California

Jan Suchodolski, MedVet, Dr. med. vet, PhD, DACVM
Associate Professor
Department of Small Animal Clinical Sciences;
Associate Director
GI Laboratory
Texas A&M University College of Veterinary Medicine & Biomedical Sciences
College Station, Texas

Lauren Sullivan, DVM, MS, DACVECC
Associate Professor
Department of Clinical Sciences
Colorado State University
College of Veterinary Medicine and Biomedical Sciences
Fort Collins, Colorado

Elizabeth A. Swanson, DVM, MS, DACVS-SA
Assistant Professor of Small Animal Surgery
Department of Clinical Sciences
Mississippi State University College of Veterinary Medicine
Mississippi State, Mississippi

Simon Swift, MA, VetMB, CertSAC, DECVIM-CA (Cardiology), MRCVS
Clinical Associate Professor of Cardiology
Medical Director and Service Chief, Cardiology
Department of Small Animal Clinical Sciences
University of Florida College of Veterinary Medicine
Gainesville, Florida

Graham Swinney, BVSc (Hons), DVCS, FANZCVS
Internal Medicine Consultant
IDEXX Laboratories
Sydney, New South Wales, Australia

Jane E. Sykes, BVSc (Hons), PhD, DACVIM (SAIM)
Professor of Medicine & Epidemiology
University of California-Davis School of Veterinary Medicine
Davis, California

Joseph Taboada, DVM, DACVIM (SAIM)
Professor, Small Animal Internal Medicine
Associate Dean, Academic Affairs
Louisiana State University School of Veterinary Medicine
Baton Rouge, Louisiana

Lauren Talarico, BS, DVM, DACVIM (Neurology)
Neurology/Neurosurgery
VCA SouthPaws Veterinary Specialty and Emergency Center
Fairfax, Virginia

Deborah J. Tate, RVT, VTS (Oncology)
Senior Veterinary Technician
University of Missouri College of Veterinary Medicine
Columbia Missouri

Susan M. Taylor, DVM, DACVIM (SAIM)
Professor Emeritus
Department of Small Animal Clinical Sciences
University of Saskatchewan
Saskatoon, Saskatchewan, Canada

Karen M. Tefft, DVM, MVSc, DACVIM (SAIM)
Clinical Assistant Professor
Department of Clinical Sciences
North Carolina State University College of Veterinary Medicine
Raleigh, North Carolina

William B. Thomas, DVM, MS, DACVIM (Neurology)
Professor, Neurology and Neurosurgery
Department of Small Animal Clinical Sciences
University of Tennessee College of Veterinary Medicine
Knoxville, Tennessee

John M. Thomason, DVM, MS, DACVIM (SAIM)
Associate Professor of Small Animal Internal Medicine
Mississippi State University College of Veterinary Medicine
Mississippi State, Mississippi

Stephanie A. Thomovsky, DVM, MS, DACVIM (Neurology), CCRP
Clinical Associate Professor Neurology and Neurosurgery
Department of Veterinary Clinical Sciences
Purdue University College of Veterinary Medicine
West Lafayette, Indiana

Mark S. Thompson, DVM, DABVP
Medical Director
Brevard Animal Hospital
Brevard, North Carolina

Karen M. Tobias, DVM, MS, DACVS
Professor of Small Animal Surgery
Department of Small Animal Clinical Sciences
University of Tennessee College of Veterinary Medicine
Knoxville, Tennessee

M. Katherine Tolbert, DVM, PhD, DACVIM (SAIM)
Clinical Associate Professor
Department of Small Animal Clinical Sciences
Texas A&M University College of Veterinary Medicine
College Station, Texas

Danna M. Torre, DVM, DACVECC
Emergency and Critical Care Veterinarian
Department of Emergency and Critical Care
Veterinary Specialty and Emergency Center
Philadelphia, Pennsylvania

Sandra P. Tou, DVM, DACVIM (Cardiology, SAIM)
Clinical Assistant Professor
Department of Small Animal Clinical Sciences
North Carolina State University College of Veterinary Medicine
Raleigh, North Carolina

Renee Tourdot, DVM
Consulting Veterinarian in Clinical Toxicology
ASPCA Animal Poison Control Center
Urbana, Illinois

H. Nicole Trenholme, DVM
Resident, Department of Anesthesia and Analgesia
Department of Emergency and Critical Care
University of Georgia College of Veterinary Medicine
Athens, Georgia

Nicholas J. Trout, VetMB, MA, MRCVS, DACVS, DECVS
Staff Surgeon
Surgery Department
Angell Animal Medical Center
Boston, Massachusetts

Mark Troxel, DVM, DACVIM (Neurology)
Staff Neurologist/Neurosurgeon
Neurology
Massachusetts Veterinary Referral Hospital
Woburn, Massachusetts;
CEO and Founder
Neuro Pet Vet, LLC
Andover, Massachusetts

Julie E. Trzil, DVM, MS, DACVIM (SAIM)
Internist
Internal Medicine Department
IndyVet Emergency and Specialty Hospital
Indianapolis, Indiana

David C. Twedt, DVM, DACVIM (SAIM)
Professor
Department of Clinical Sciences
Colorado State University
College of Veterinary Medicine and Biomedical Sciences
Fort Collins, Colorado

Shelly Vaden, DVM, PhD, DACVIM (SAIM)
Professor, Internal Medicine
Department of Clinical Sciences
North Carolina State University College of Veterinary Medicine
Raleigh, North Carolina

Beth A. Valentine, DVM, PhD, DACVP
Emeritus Professor of Anatomic Pathology
Department of Biomedical Sciences
Oregon State University
Carlson College of Veterinary Medicine
Corvallis, Oregon

Lucien V. Vallone, DVM, DACVO
Clinical Assistant Professor
Department of Small Animal Clinical Sciences
Texas A&M University College of Veterinary Medicine
College Station, Texas

Megan van Eeden, DVM
Resident in Small Animal Internal Medicine
University of Missouri College of Veterinary Medicine
Columbia, Missouri

Adronie Verbrugghe, DVM, PhD, DECVCN
Associate Professor
Department of Clinical Studies
Ontario Veterinary College, University of Guelph
Guelph, Ontario, Canada

Leen Verhaert, DVM, DEVDC
Practice Assistant
Small Animal Department
Ghent University Faculty of Veterinary Medicine
Ghent, Belgium;
Owner
Dier en Tand BVBA
Duffel, Belgium

Aida I. Vientós-Plotts, DVM
Clinical Instructor
Department of Small Animal Internal Medicine
University of Missouri College of Veterinary Medicine
Columbia, Missouri

Lenin A. Villamizar-Martinez, DVM, MS, PhD
Assistant Professor of Veterinary Dentistry and Oral Surgery
Department of Clinical Sciences
North Carolina State University College of Veterinary Medicine
Raleigh, North Carolina

Cecilia Villaverde, BVSc, PhD, DACVN, DECVCN
Founder and Consultant
Expert Pet Nutrition
Fermoy, County Cork, Ireland

Jordan P. Vitt, DVM, DACVIM (Cardiology)
Clinical Assistant Professor
Department of Veterinary Clinical Medicine
University of Illinois College of Veterinary Medicine
Urbana, Illinois

Annemarie M. W. Y. Voorbij, DVM, PhD, DECVIM-SA
Department of Clinical Sciences of Companion Animals
Utrecht University, Faculty of Veterinary Medicine
Utrecht, The Netherlands

Lori S. Waddell, DVM, DACVECC
Clinical Professor of Critical Care
Department of Clinical Studies & Advanced Medicine
University of Pennsylvania School of Veterinary Medicine
Philadelphia, Pennsylvania

Stephen Waisglass, DVM, CertSAD, DACVD
Veterinary Dermatologist
Veterinary Emergency Clinic and Referral Centre
Toronto, Ontario, Canada;
Veterinary Dermatologist
VCA 404 Veterinary Hospital Referral Centre
Newmarket, Ontario, Canada;
Adjunct Professor
Department of Clinical Studies
Ontario Veterinary College
Guelph, Ontario, Canada

Don Waldron, DVM, DACVS
Blacksburg, Virginia

Allison Wara, DVM, DACVN
Veterinary Clinical Nutritionist
Royal Canin Canada
Guelph, Ontario, Canada

Kirsten Waratuke, DVM, DABT
Toxicologist
ASPCA Animal Poison Control Center
Urbana, Illinois

Cynthia R. Ward, VMD, PhD, DACVIM (SAIM)
Meigs Distinguished Teaching Professor
Small Animal Medicine and Surgery
University of Georgia College of Veterinary Medicine
Athens, Georgia

Jennifer Wardlaw, DVM, MS, DACVS-SA
Owner, Chief Surgeon
Gateway Veterinary Surgery
St. Louis, Missouri;
Adjunct Faculty
Mississippi State University
College of Veterinary Medicine
Mississippi State, Mississippi

Aubrey Webb, DVM, PhD
Owner/Operator
CullenWebb Animal Eye Specialists
Riverview, New Brunswick, Canada

Craig B. Webb, DVM, PhD, DACVIM (SAIM)
Professor
Department of Clinical Sciences
Colorado State University
College of Veterinary Medicine and Biomedical Sciences
Fort Collins, Colorado

Cynthia R. L. Webster, DVM, DACVIM (SAIM)
Professor of Clinical Sciences
Cummings School of Veterinary Medicine at Tufts University
Grafton, Massachusetts

J. Scott Weese, DVM, DVSc, DACVIM (LAIM)
Professor
Pathobiology
Ontario Veterinary College, University of Guelph
Guelph, Ontario, Canada

Colette Wegenast, DVM
Consulting Veterinarian in Clinical Toxicology
ASPCA Animal Poison Control Center
Urbana, Illinois

Claire M. Weigand, DVM, DACVIM (SAIM)
Chief of Internal Medicine
Internal Medicine Department
Veterinary Emergency & Specialty Hospital
South Deerfield, Massachusetts

Kristin Welch, DVM, DACVECC
Chief of Emergency Medicine
Charleston Veterinary Referral Center
Charleston, South Carolina

Jocelyn Wellington, DVM, DACVD
Veterinary Dermatologist
Private Practice
Animal Dermatology Services
London, Ontario, Canada

Aaron Wey, DVM, DACVIM (Cardiology)
Medical Director
Cardiology
Upstate Veterinary Specialties, PLLC
Latham, New York

Richard Wheeler, DVM, DACT
Faculty
Department of Clinical Sciences
Colorado State University
College of Veterinary Medicine and Biomedical Sciences
Fort Collins, Colorado;
Poudre River Veterinary Clinic
Fort Collins, Colorado

Megan Whelan, DVM, DACVECC, CVA
Department of Emergency and Critical Care Medicine
Angell Animal Medical Center
Boston, Massachusetts

David A. Wilkie, DVM, MS, DACVO
Professor Emeritus, Veterinary Clinical Sciences
The Ohio State University College of Veterinary Medicine
Columbus, Ohio

Michael D. Willard, DVM, MS, DACVIM (SAIM)
Senior Professor and Professor Emeritus of Small Animal Clinical Sciences
Department of Small Animal Clinical Sciences
Texas A&M University College of Veterinary Medicine & Biomedical Sciences
College Station, Texas

Laurel E. Williams, DVM, DACVIM (Oncology)
Adjunct Professor
Department of Clinical Sciences
North Carolina State University College of Veterinary Medicine
Raleigh, North Carolina;
Clinical Oncologist
Veterinary Specialty Hospital of the Carolinas
Cary, North Carolina

Kathryn Winger, DVM, DACVIM (Neurology)
Assistant Professor of Neurology/Neurosurgery
Department of Small Animal Clinical Sciences
Michigan State University
East Lansing, Michigan

Tina Wismer, DVM, MS, DABVT, DABT
Medical Director
ASPCA Animal Poison Control Center
Urbana, Illinois

Wendy Wolfson, DVM
Assistant Professor of Shelter Medicine
Louisiana State University School of Veterinary Medicine
Baton Rouge, Louisiana

Michelle Woodward, DVM, MS, DACVD
Assistant Professor of Dermatology
Veterinary Clinical Sciences
Louisiana State University School of Veterinary Medicine
Baton Rouge, Louisiana

Kathy Wright, DVM, DACVIM (Cardiology, SAIM)
Cardiologist
MedVet Medical and Cancer Centers for Pets
Cincinnati, Ohio

Eleas M. Wu, DVM, DACT
Theriogenology Resident
Oregon State University
Carlson College of Veterinary Medicine
Corvallis, Oregon

Panagiotis G. Xenoulis, DVM, Dr. med. vet., PhD
Assistant Professor of Small Animal Medicine
Clinic of Medicine
University of Thessaly, Faculty of Veterinary Medicine
Kartditsa, Greece;
Adjunct Assistant Professor of Small Animal Internal Medicine
Department of Small Animal Clinical Sciences
Texas A&M University
College of Veterinary Medicine & Biomedical Sciences
College Station, Texas;
Chief of Medicine
Animal Medical Center of Athens
Athens, Greece

Aisha Young, DVM, MVSc, DACVR
Lecturer in Diagnostic Imaging
University of Melbourne Faculty of Veterinary and Agricultural Sciences
Werribee, Victoria, Australia

Danielle M. Zwueste, DVM, DACVIM (Neurology)
Assistant Professor
Department of Small Animal Clinical Sciences
Western College of Veterinary Medicine
Saskatoon, Saskatchewan, Canada

Cynthia Ruth Webster, DVM, DACVIM (SAIM)
Professor of Clinical Sciences
Cummings School of Veterinary Medicine at Tufts University
Grafton, Massachusetts

J. Scott Weese, DVM, DVSc, DACVIM (LAIM)
Professor
Pathobiology
Ontario Veterinary College
University of Guelph
Guelph, Ontario, Canada

Colette Wegenast, DVM
Consulting Veterinarian in Clinical Toxicology
ASPCA Animal Poison Control Center
Urbana, Illinois

Claire M. Weigand, DVM, DACVIM (SAIM)
Chief of Internal Medicine
Internal Medicine Department
Veterinary Emergency & Specialty Hospital
South Deerfield, Massachusetts

Kristin Welch, DVM, DACVECC
Chief of Emergency Medicine
Charleston Veterinary Referral Center
Charleston, South Carolina

Jocelyn Wellington, DVM, DACVD
Veterinary Dermatologist
Private Practice
Animal Dermatology Services
London, Ontario, Canada

Aaron Wey, DVM, DACVIM (Cardiology)
Medical Director
Cardiology
Upstate Veterinary Specialties PLLC
Latham, New York

Richard Wheeler, DVM, DACT
Faculty
Department of Clinical Sciences
Colorado State University
College of Veterinary Medicine and Biomedical Sciences
Fort Collins, Colorado
Poudre River Veterinary Clinic
Fort Collins, Colorado

Megan Whelan, DVM, DACVECC, CVA
Department of Emergency and Critical Care Medicine
Angell Animal Medical Center
Boston, Massachusetts

David A. Wilkie, DVM, MS, DACVO
Professor Emeritus, Veterinary Clinical Sciences
The Ohio State University
College of Veterinary Medicine
Columbus, Ohio

Michael D. Willard, DVM, MS, DACVIM (SAIM)
Senior Professor and Professor Emeritus of Small Animal Clinical Sciences
Department of Small Animal Clinical Sciences
Texas A&M University College of Veterinary Medicine & Biomedical Sciences
College Station, Texas

Laurel E. Williams, DVM, DACVIM (Oncology)
Adjunct Professor
Department of Clinical Sciences
North Carolina State University
College of Veterinary Medicine
Raleigh, North Carolina
Clinical Oncologist
Veterinary Specialty Hospital of the Carolinas
Cary, North Carolina

Kathryn Winger, DVM, DACVIM (Neurology)
Assistant Professor of Neurology/Neurosurgery
Department of Small Animal Clinical Sciences
Michigan State University
East Lansing, Michigan

Tina Wismer, DVM, MS, DABVT, DABT
Medical Director
ASPCA Animal Poison Control Center
Urbana, Illinois

Wendy Wolfson, DVM
Assistant Professor of Shelter Medicine
Louisiana State University School of Veterinary Medicine
Baton Rouge, Louisiana

Michelle Woodward, DVM, MS, DACVD
Assistant Professor of Dermatology
Veterinary Clinical Sciences
Louisiana State University School of Veterinary Medicine
Baton Rouge, Louisiana

Kathy Wright, DVM, DACVIM (Cardiology, SAIM)
Cardiologist
MedVet Medical and Cancer Centers for Pets
Cincinnati, Ohio

Eileen M. Wu, DVM, DACT
Theriogenology Resident
Oregon State University
Carlson College of Veterinary Medicine
Corvallis, Oregon

Panagiotis G. Xenoulis, DVM, Dr. med. vet., PhD
Assistant Professor of Small Animal Medicine
Clinic of Medicine
University of Thessaly, Faculty of Veterinary Medicine
Karditsa, Greece
Adjunct Assistant Professor of Small Animal Internal Medicine
Department of Small Animal Clinical Sciences
Texas A&M University
College of Veterinary Medicine & Biomedical Sciences
College Station, Texas
Chief of Medicine
Animal Medical Center of Athens
Athens, Greece

Astra Young, DVM, MVSc, DACVR
Lecturer in Diagnostic Imaging
University of Melbourne Faculty of Veterinary and Agricultural Sciences
Werribee, Victoria, Australia

Danielle M. Zwueste, DVM, DACVIM (Neurology)
Assistant Professor
Department of Small Animal Clinical Sciences
Western College of Veterinary Medicine
Saskatoon, Saskatchewan, Canada

Preface

With this fourth edition, the *Clinical Veterinary Advisor* enters its 15th year. What a journey so far! Its existence, and endurance, are a testimony to the veterinarians, veterinary students, technicians, and many others who have given it their genuine support. The positive comments, suggestions for improvements, and identification of errors fell on our receptive ears, and we have benefited greatly from this input. A glance back at the first, purple-cover edition shows how much ground we have covered—and the first edition was already a point of real pride. The subsequent editions, including this fourth one, would not have been possible without the enthusiasm we received from the readers who put this text to work in improving their day-to-day practice of veterinary medicine.

What makes this edition better? By far the most impactful change has been the joint involvement of the two of us. Dr. Leah Cohn is a clinician, researcher, and teacher with a specialty in small animal internal medicine. Her extensive work in infectious diseases, in respiratory medicine, and in urology makes her a well-rounded specialist and, to many of us, the internist's internist. She has mentored literally thousands of veterinarians, both general practitioners and specialists. Leah has spearheaded this edition after being the Nephrology and Urology editor since the inaugural edition. It was my (Côté's) dearest wish that she would take the reins of the *Advisor,* and I am eternally grateful to Leah for having done it so well. Her insights have made this the very best edition to date, and by far. The credit for recruiting, organizing, reviewing, persisting, and troubleshooting, from the very beginning of this edition, belongs with Leah. Likewise, all of this edition's innovations and improvements exist thanks to her.

As always, finding ways to improve on the last edition but not increase the book's physical size has been a tremendous challenge.

- Existing chapters have been comprehensively updated and edited to reflect changes in best practices. Once again, the foremost principle was to anticipate what a reader might be looking for when reaching for this book, and to make sure that was at the core of every item in this edition.
- The portion of the text devoted to Diseases and Disorders includes 35 new chapters on such clinically relevant topics as idiopathic hypercalcemia of cats, movement disorders, incidentally detected heart murmurs, food-related hyperadrenocorticism, and postoperative hemorrhage of sighthounds. These chapters, like everything else in the book, had to clear the bar of being current, clinically important, and written simply and with utmost accuracy.
- We have added 43 newly described procedures to the text, and all procedures are notated with a level of difficulty. Those with "one diamond" are described in enough detail that a veterinarian should be able to open the book and complete the task, such as performing a fecal transplant or administering a lipid emulsification infusion for intoxications. At the other extreme, "three diamond" procedures provide the practitioner with the kind of "need-to-know" information that will facilitate client conversations before referral for more specialized care, such as the placement of a subcutaneous ureteral bypass device. The "two diamond" techniques are very doable but might take a bit of practice with a more experienced colleague for a typical veterinarian.
- An entire section has been expanded. The Differential Diagnosis section is now Differentials, Lists, and Mnemonics, to acknowledge that the material includes much more than just differential diagnoses. Indeed, it includes useful lists like important hepatotoxins, blood types prevalence, antimicrobial spectrum of disinfectants, and much more. Entirely new to this edition are mnemonics: memory-helping devices that present useful information in the most compact way possible.
- New chapters have been added to all sections of the book. This edition provides practical information on laboratory tests such as symmetric dimethylarginine (SDMA) and Factor Xa inhibition. Likewise, there are new algorithms, including a step-by-step approach to treatment of hypernatremia with examples of mathematical calculations to help you choose the most appropriate fluid plan.
- A terrific aspect of practical and user-friendly material, we hope, is the creation of more than 35 new client consent templates. These simple documents describe routinely performed procedures, such as feline and canine neuter, dental prophylaxis and extraction, and general anesthesia in complete yet simple layperson's terms. The purpose is to inform the client about the planned procedure, and importantly, each document concludes with a statement of release of liability for clients to sign signifying that they understand the procedure and the foreseeable risks. These client consent templates go beyond the collection of Client Information Sheets that have been in the Advisor since its first edition and continue to grow (now 200, in both English and Spanish). The client consent templates expand the Advisor's mandate, which is to inform readers with practical material in an efficient way, into this new area that we are not aware of being covered in other textbooks.
- Finally, new videos and a revamped drug formulary are included, with bonus information in the online edition such as a generic to brand-name synonym cross reference for those times that you can remember the name "Prozac" but "fluoxetine" just won't come to mind.

The *Advisor* continues to include both a hard copy textbook and an electronic platform. The purpose is to appeal to readers who are resolutely print-friendly—those of us who remember the approximate position of a fact or photograph on a page and quickly flip through the book to find it—as well as to all of us who benefit from the electronic medium: searching, storing, etc. The electronic edition is comprehensive and contains not only all the material in the print book but many additional bonus chapters, lists, and algorithms.

From the first edition to this fourth, the *Clinical Veterinary Advisor* has been a labor of love. We love helping pets and their people.

While we have received great feedback on the *Advisor* through the years, one comment that stands out is that the *Advisor* works like a Swiss Army knife. The metaphor is a tremendous compliment: other books and resources may have individual strengths that are superior—a better blade, a better screwdriver—but the *Advisor* aims to bring the essentials into one reliable and portable instrument. This continues to be our goal: to provide you with a ready resource to provide practical guidance for the care of pets and their people. We thank you in advance for your comments, corrections, and general input.

Leah Cohn
Etienne Côté
4thclinicalvetadvisor@gmail.com

With love and deep gratitude to my family. This includes my parents, Hans and Esther Cofer Cohn, of beloved memory. They supported my dream of helping animals from the age of 12 as they arranged for me to "shadow" our family veterinarian and then proceeded to drop me off and pick me up from that veterinary practice day after day until I turned 16 and could drive myself. It also includes my always supportive husband, Dewayne Davis, who has sacrificed for me to follow my dreams, and put up with me spending every evening of the last 2 years with a computer in my lap editing chapters. And of course, I dedicate this book too to my most important "creations", Laura and Eli Davis. — Leah Cohn

To Jen and Hélène, who make it all worth it. — Etienne Côté

Acknowledgments

Our most profound thanks go to the many authors and section editors who have contributed to this textbook. The authors come from academia, private practice, industry, and nonprofit groups. The author list includes both a "who's who" of established and internationally recognized experts, as well as up-and-coming young veterinarians. Whether it was creating a brand-new chapter "from scratch", or revising previous chapters to keep them current, the ways that these authors created succinct yet comprehensive and accurate manuscripts is truly impressive. Likewise, we owe a tremendous debt to the section editors; from choosing the most important areas within their expertise to include in the text, to selecting excellent authors, to making sure that the submissions are easily understood, practical, and focused, the section editors made sure that each area provided the most important and readily useful information possible. We offer you our undying thanks. We also want to acknowledge the authors and section editors of prior editions, who established the solid platform on which this new edition was developed. Your past work is responsible for the strong reputation that this book enjoys today.

The team at Elsevier has been supportive of this textbook since the first edition, and that support has allowed the text to improve with each subsequent edition. We thank Penny Rudolph for her work championing prior editions and on starting this current edition, as well as her successor Jennifer Catando and her outstanding team. An undertaking as massive as the creation of this book takes a talented team with many participants along the way. It was our incredible great fortune to have Jennifer Shreiner on board as Senior Content Development Specialist to help craft a mass of individual submissions into an organized text. Jennifer was instantaneously responsive to authors and editors and solved any problems in real time with grace and expertise. We were also very lucky to be joined by Jodi Willard as the Senior Project Manager. Jodi took the baton at Production and worked with her team to turn a huge manuscript into an actual textbook. Jennifer's and Jodi's work exceeded any reasonable expectation and turned the bearable into the enjoyable.

We have many others to acknowledge. We have been blessed to learn from some of the greatest teachers ever in veterinary medicine. While there are more of those teachers than we can name, a few deserve a special thank you: Steve Ettinger, Ed Feldman, Ed Breitschwerdt, Al Legendre, Bob DeNovo, Jane Armstrong, and Susan Bunch. We both also owe a huge debt to many colleagues that have supported each of us along the way. Again, there are more names than are reasonable to include here, but there are a few that simply must be acknowledged. Leah is grateful for the support of Drs. John Dodam, Carol Reinero, Amy DeClue, Marie Kerl, Joe Kornegay, and Carolyn Henry. Etienne thanks Lynne O'Sullivan, Elaine Reveler, Deepmala Agarwal, Christine Savidge, Peter Foley, Stephanie Hamilton, Heather Gunn McQuillan, Erin Anderson, Jonathan Lichtenberger, Linda Fineman, Laura Garrett, Shannon Murray, and Brian Wagner. We both would like to acknowledge the many talented, dedicated, caring students, interns, residents, and technicians we have had the pleasure to work with and help teach throughout our careers. It is all of you that inspired the creation of this book, and that motivate us to find better ways to help you help animals.

And speaking of animals, we have both been blessed to love animals that have made our lives better. If we named them all, the list would rival the word count of the longest chapter. But we just have to put out there in the world our gratitude and love for Fuzzy Face, Timkin, Hammer, Woof, BK, Halley, Reba, Betsy, Friend, Daisy, Bruno, Fogo, Nina, Baloo, and Olive.

Contents

SECTION I Diseases and Disorders: By Discipline

DENTISTRY/ORAL SURGERY
Alexander M. Reiter

DERMATOLOGY
Manon Paradis

SECTION II **Procedures and Techniques**

SECTION III Differentials, Lists, and Mnemonics

SECTION IV **Laboratory Tests**

SECTION V Clinical Algorithms

SECTION VI Drug Compendium

Index, 1511

Client Education Sheets

The following client education sheets can be found on the companion website, *www.expertconsult.com.*

SECTION I

Diseases and Disorders

EDITORS

Ellen N. Behrend
VMD, PhD, DACVIM (SAIM)
Endocrinology

Benjamin M. Brainard
VMD, DACVAA, DACVECC
Emergency and Critical Care

Leah A. Cohn
DVM, PhD, DACVIM (SAIM)
Chief Concerns
Nephrology/Urology
Other Topics

Jonathan E. Fogle
DVM, PhD, DACVIM (SAIM)
Hematologic / Immunologic Disease

Megan Grobman
DVM, MS, DACVIM (SAIM)
Respiratory Disease

Diane V. H. Hendrix
DVM, DACVO
Ophthalmology

Michelle A. Kutzler
DVM, PhD, DACT
Theriogenology

Jennifer A. Larsen
DVM, PhD, DACVN
Nutrition

Kathleen Linn
DVM, MS, DACVS
Orthopedics

Karen R. Muñana
DVM, MS, DACVIM (Neurology)
Neurology

Karen L. Overall
VMD, MA, PhD, DACVB
Behavior

Manon Paradis
DMV, MVSc, DACVD
Dermatology

Kenneth Rassnick
DVM, DACVIM (Oncology)
Oncology

Alexander M. Reiter
DVM, Dr. med. vet., DAVDC, DEVDC
Dentistry / Oral Surgery

Keith Richter
DVM, MSEL, DACVIM (SAIM)
Hepatobiliary / Pancreatic Disease

Rance K. Sellon
DVM, PhD, DACVIM (Oncology, SAIM)
Gastroenterology

Meg M. Sleeper
VMD, DACVIM (Cardiology)
Cardiology

Elizabeth A. Swanson
DVM, MS, DACVS-SA
Soft-Tissue Surgery

Joseph Taboada
DVM, DACVIM (SAIM)
Infectious Diseases

Tina Wismer
DVM, MS, DABVT, DABT
Toxicology

This section, Diseases and Disorders, aims to summarize the most important clinical entities in small-animal practice. These entities include specific disease syndromes and general clinical findings.

The following pages summarize several hundred of the most frequently encountered diseases and disorders. Over 100 more, which are encountered less frequently but are well recognized in veterinary practice and are equally complete and up to date, are accessible online in this same format at www.ExpertConsult.com.

BASIC INFORMATION

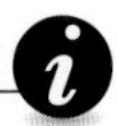

Definition

A brief explanation of the meaning of this disease or disorder

Synonyms

Where appropriate, other terms used interchangeably to name this disease or disorder

Epidemiology

SPECIES, AGE, SEX

The typical signalment of affected individuals

GENETICS, BREED PREDISPOSITION

Information regarding possible hereditary factors

RISK FACTORS

Elements that might predispose a patient to this disease or disorder

CONTAGION AND ZOONOSIS

Important information regarding infectious spread of certain diseases

GEOGRAPHY AND SEASONALITY

Features that would help to raise or lower the clinician's index of suspicion for a disease or disorder, based on environment and timing of occurrence

ASSOCIATED DISORDERS

Entities that often occur simultaneously with this disease or disorder

Clinical Presentation

DISEASE FORMS/SUBTYPES

If applicable, the different variants of a disease a clinician should consider

HISTORY, CHIEF COMPLAINT

The information provided by the owner (history), together with the primary reason for seeking veterinary attention (chief complaint)

PHYSICAL EXAM FINDINGS

The relevant abnormalities—or, if important, relevant normal findings—associated with the disease/disorder

Etiology and Pathophysiology

The mechanisms and pathways according to which the disease or disorder begins and then evolves

DIAGNOSIS

Diagnostic Overview

This segment is a brief summary that states what is appropriate to achieve a functional clinical diagnosis in most cases of the disorder. The goal of the Diagnostic Overview is to give direction to the reader/practitioner for applying the information provided subsequently. The result is diagnostic guidance, rather than just a list of possible diagnostic tests.

Differential Diagnosis

Other diseases or disorders that may mimic the one under discussion. When appropriate, the reader may be directed to concise lists of differentials in Section III of the text.

Initial Database

A summary of basic clinical tests that are appropriate when this disease/disorder might be present. These are largely tests that should be accessible in most outpatient clinics or facilities.

Advanced or Confirmatory Testing

Diagnostic tests that are performed if the initial database is insufficient for establishing the diagnosis. Some of these tests may be performed easily in any clinic or hospital, whereas others may require referral to a specialty center.

TREATMENT

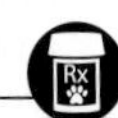

Treatment Overview

Like the Diagnostic Overview, this section summarizes the goals and priorities of treatment. The purpose is to offer guidance in the application of treatment information.

Acute General Treatment

Those forms of treatment that are instituted promptly, either because treatment is simple or because of immediate need

Chronic Treatment

When necessary, ongoing treatment typically provided at home

Nutrition/Diet

Alterations in food intake or food type that may assist in treatment

Behavior/Exercise

Information pertaining to deliberate changes in physical activity (increase, decrease, or new) and any forms of treatment related to behavioral modifications

Drug Interactions

Relevant information regarding incompatibility of medications commonly used in the treatment of the disease/disorder. This section by necessity is perhaps one of the least comprehensive; the reader is advised to seek information from clinical pharmacology sources to assist in identifying potential or real problems.

Possible Complications

Selected, recognized problems that may occur as a result of the disease process alone or as a complication of treatment

Recommended Monitoring

Methods the practitioner should use for ensuring that treatment and/or resolution of the disease or disorder is proceeding as expected

PROGNOSIS & OUTCOME

The expected evolution of the disease or disorder, with or without treatment.

PEARLS & CONSIDERATIONS

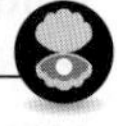

Comments

Single items of counterintuitive observations, pitfalls to avoid, and other important points that don't readily fit into other categories

Prevention

Methods to avoid recurrence or reduce occurrence of new cases

Technician Tips

This segment provides information relevant to nursing care and the role of the veterinary technician in managing cases of this disease/disorder.

Client Education

This section points out key features of the disease or disorder that can improve the client's understanding of the disorder or patient care.

SUGGESTED READING

Every disease and disorder has at least one recommended bibliographic source for additional consultation. In most cases, there are others in the online version of this book at www.ExpertConsult.com.

RELATED CLIENT EDUCATION SHEETS

In many chapters, the practitioner is directed to useful client information handouts available from the online edition of the text. This includes information regarding specific disorders, a variety of "How To" sheets that help explain at-home care, as well as documents designed to both provide a simplified explanation of commonly performed procedures and to serve as a printable form that can be signed by the client to document informed consent.

Abortion, Spontaneous (Dog)

BASIC INFORMATION

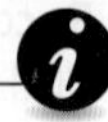

Definition

The expulsion of one or more fetuses before full-term pregnancy is uncommon; in the dog, resorption is more common.

Synonyms

Fetal loss, pregnancy wastage, miscarriage

Epidemiology

SPECIES, AGE, SEX

Sexually mature, intact, female dog

GENETICS, BREED PREDISPOSITION

- Inbreeding (inbreeding coefficient > 0.25): early embryonic death, conceptus resorption
- Brachiocephalic breeds (high-risk pregnancy)

RISK FACTORS

- Advanced maternal age
- History of previous pregnancy loss (e.g., recurrent hypoluteoidism)
- Malnutrition (pregnancy ketosis)
- Endocrinopathies (hypothyroidism, hypoluteoidism, diabetes mellitus, hyperadrenocorticism)
- Infections (e.g., *Brucella canis, Listeria monocytogenes, Streptococcus canis* [Lancefield groups C, L, and M], *Escherichia coli, Campylobacter* sp., *Leptospira* sp., *Salmonella* sp., *Mycoplasma, Chlamydia* sp., canine herpesvirus 1 [CHV-1], canine parvovirus 1 [minute virus of canines], bluetongue virus, canine distemper virus, canine adenovirus [infectious hepatitis], *Leishmania infantum, Toxoplasma gondii, Borrelia burgdorferi, Ehrlichia* spp., *Anaplasma* spp.)
- Unsolicited treatment with an endocrine disruptor, embryotoxic or teratogenic compounds (e.g., itraconazole, griseofulvin, plant toxins, insecticides, corticosteroids, polyester textiles)
  - The risk to the fetus is a result of the ability of a drug or toxin to reach the fetal circulation and produce toxic effects in the fetus. Special awareness is necessary during the organogenesis period (i.e., until day 20 of pregnancy in dogs and cats).
- Inadequate vaccination or deworming programs

CONTAGION AND ZOONOSIS

- *B. canis* is zoonotic.
  - Venereal transmission is significant in the dog. Contact with infected canine blood and vaginal secretions is important for human infection.
- *Salmonella* sp. and *Leptospira* sp. also have zoonotic potential.
- CHV-1 and minute virus of canines: transmission occurs through direct aerosol contact or contact with aborted fetuses and/or placentas. Male-to-female venereal contact is not a significant means of transmission.

GEOGRAPHY AND SEASONALITY

- Canine brucellosis: endemic in parts of North and South America and China
  - Although previously eradicated in Europe, sporadic cases have been reported since 2011.
- CHV-1: worldwide; serologic prevalence of 60%-80%
- Tick-borne diseases in spring and summer

ASSOCIATED DISORDERS

Vaginal discharge, depression, lethargy

Clinical Presentation

HISTORY, CHIEF COMPLAINT

- Pregnant bitch whelps prematurely with live or dead pups, or no pups are born at term.
- Abnormal vulvar discharge (bloody, purulent) during pregnancy, fever, or signs of abdominal pain may be reported by owner.
- Usually abortion is unnoticed by the owner because the dam may consume the fetuses and aborted tissues.
- Death of one or more fetuses may occur, whereas the remainder may continue to develop normally.
- Late-term abortions (between gestational days 45 and 59) are typical of *B. canis*.

PHYSICAL EXAM FINDINGS

- Often unremarkable
- Vulvar discharge that is purulent, hemorrhagic, greenish, blackish, or malodorous may indicate pregnancy complications that could lead to abortion. Normal vulvar discharge in pregnant bitches is clear to mucoid or pink-tinged and odorless.
- In late-term abortion, abdominal contractions, and expulsion of one or several fetuses may be observed.

Etiology and Pathophysiology

- Canine pregnancy requires normal luteal function throughout its duration.
  - Inadequate luteal function (hypoluteoidism) may cause resorption or abortion at any stage but generally occurs between days 25-35 post breeding.
  - Any toxin or hormone that induces endogenous release of prostaglandin F-2 alpha (PGF2a) and subsequent luteolysis may cause abortion, including bacterial toxins (e.g., coliforms, *Staphylococcus* sp.) and adrenergic agonists (e.g., phenylephrine).
- Fetal survival requires normal placental function and placental relaxin production.
  - Circulating relaxin concentration increases from day 26 and is detectable by relaxin assays from day 30 after mating.
  - Relaxin declines rapidly after the death of all fetuses but may remain elevated for some days.
- Pathogens that influence placental function (e.g., herpesvirus placentitis) may cause abortion.
- Cases of unexplained pregnancy loss or abortion may be caused by an inadequate uterine environment and not a primary infection.
- In dogs, fetal resorption is more common than abortion.
- Fetal mummification occurs when the fetus dies during the last third of pregnancy (i.e., after day 45-50) in a noninfected uterine environment after skeletal calcification has taken place.
- Fetal death due to infectious and noninfectious causes may give different clues. Infections often show characteristic gross microscopic lesions that reveal the causative agent (typically herpesvirus). The noninfectious causes may be more difficult to elucidate due to the variety of mechanisms involved (e.g., toxins, hypoluteoidism).

DIAGNOSIS

Diagnostic Overview

- Pregnancy diagnosis (pp. 816 and 819)
- Abortion should be suspected when the pregnancy is previously confirmed and the bitch later presents nonpregnant or expelled fetuses have been observed.
- A diagnostic approach is outlined on p. 1396.

Differential Diagnosis

- Pseudocyesis (overt false pregnancy)
  - Abdominal ultrasound examination after day 25 to confirm pregnancy status
- Vaginal discharge due to vaginitis or metritis (pyometra)
  - Abdominal ultrasound recommended
- Induced abortion (p. 819)

Initial Database

- Serologic testing and/or polymerase chain reaction (PCR) of affected dam
  - *B. canis*
  - CHV-1 (p. 466)
- Virus or bacterial isolation from microbial cultures of fetuses, placenta, milk, or vaginal secretions
  - For *B. canis*, blood culture with bacteriologic isolation provides a definitive diagnosis 5 weeks after exposure, but repeated samples may be necessary.
  - For acute CHV-1 infections, viral isolation from infected tissues is possible for 2-3 weeks.
- Necropsy of fetus (e.g., subcapsular hemorrhages in the kidneys are pathognomonic for CHV-1) and visual inspection of placenta

- Histologic examination of fetal organs, liver, spleen, thymus, kidneys, adrenals, intestines, stomach, heart, lung, thymus, and brain
- Serum progesterone level of dam must be > 2 ng/mL (6 nmol/L) to sustain pregnancy.
  - Concentrations below this threshold for more than 48 hours are diagnostic of hypoluteoidism.
  - Low progesterone level may also occur secondary to fetal death. Other causes of fetal death (e.g., genetic) should be ruled out.
- Thyroid hormone analyses: Subclinical hypothyroidism may be aggravated to a clinically significant disease during periods of stress (e.g., pregnancy) (p. 525).
- Routine laboratory testing: CBC and serum biochemistry profile
  - Normal hematocrit values in pregnant bitches are lower (30%-35%) than in nonpregnant bitches in diestrus (45%-55%) because of an increase in plasma volume.
  - Mild, mature neutrophilia is normal in pregnant bitches, but pronounced neutrophilia, immature neutrophils, or monocytosis is abnormal.

Advanced or Confirmatory Testing

- Ultrasonography may reveal fetal death (absence of a fetal heartbeat or movement) before onset of abortion.
- Contact diagnostic laboratories for further recommendations for specific pathogens.
- Toxicology of organs and/or blood is needed when a specific toxin or drug is suspected.

TREATMENT

Treatment Overview

- Acute supportive care of the bitch (e.g., intensive treatment of an infection) is the main aim of treatment since the prognosis for saving the current pregnancy is poor.
- *B. canis* infection
- With hypoluteoidism, progesterone supplementation may be attempted to prevent abortion of remaining fetuses. This preemptive approach has been effective in bitches that have aborted from hypoluteoidism in previous pregnancies.

Acute General Treatment

- Supportive: intravenous fluids (e.g., lactated Ringer's solution) if fever is present
- Broad-spectrum antibiotics safe for use during pregnancy: empirical pending culture and sensitivity results (if clinically feasible). For specific antimicrobial treatment of brucellosis, see web chapter.
  - Amoxicillin (22 mg/kg PO q 8h)
  - Pivampicillin (30 mg/kg PO q 12h)
  - Cephalexin or cefadroxil (20 mg PO q 8-12h)
  - Enrofloxacin (5 mg/kg SQ, IM, or PO q 24h) recommended for *B. canis* but may be teratogenic.
  - Trimethoprim/sulfadiazine (15 mg/kg PO q 12h) may be teratogenic.

Chronic Treatment

- Hormone replacement with confirmed cases of hypoluteoidism should be discontinued at least 2 days before expected term (i.e., 62-63 days after the luteinizing hormone surge) to allow for normal parturition. Hormone replacement options include
  - Progesterone in oil 2 mg/kg IM q 48h
  - Altrenogest 0.09 mg/kg PO q 24h
  - Micronized progesterone (Prometrium 10 mg/kg PO q 24h; or Utrogestan 5 mg/kg PO q 8h)
- If antibiotics are used in *B. canis*–infected dogs, antibiotic treatment should be continued for at least 4 weeks, based on culture and sensitivity results and clinical state.

Nutrition/Diet

A good-quality maintenance diet is recommended for bitches with lost pregnancies (p. 816). Puppy food should be continued for bitches undergoing treatment with remaining live fetuses.

Behavior/Exercise

Controlled physical activity is recommended during pregnancy. Avoid exposure to new dogs, extensive travel, or abrupt changes in the dam's environment.

Drug Interactions

Glucocorticoids are unpredictably abortifacient drugs in dogs.

Possible Complications

For hypoluteoidism, hormone replacement therapy is recommended only if the whelping date is known, as failure to discontinue supplementation at the appropriate time may cause prolonged gestation, fetal death, and lactation failure. In addition, supplementation with progesterone analogs (i.e., altrenogest) before sexual differentiation of the fetus (before day 45) is not recommended because of potential masculinization of female fetuses.

Recommended Monitoring

- If suspicious of impending abortion, serum progesterone concentrations should be monitored weekly. Frequent monitoring of fetal viability with abdominal ultrasonography can be valuable.
- If abnormal vaginal discharge is observed during gestation, abdominal ultrasonography should be used to assess fetal viability, and supportive therapy should be initiated.

PROGNOSIS & OUTCOME

- Prognosis is poor for maintaining pregnancy once signs of impending abortion occur.
- Bitches with hypoluteoidism may experience recurrent abortion.
- For causes of abortion other than hypoluteoidism usually there are no problems in subsequent pregnancies (exceptions: *B. canis* and occasionally recrudescent herpesvirus infections).

PEARLS & CONSIDERATIONS

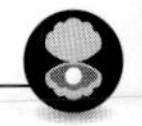

Comments

- Abortion is uncommon in the bitch; embryonic death with fetal resorption or mummification is more common.
- Most cases of canine abortion go unnoticed by the owner as the bitch may consume the aborted tissues.
- Infectious agents, notably viruses (CHV-1) or specific bacteria (*B. canis*), are the most common causes of canine abortion.
- The diagnosis of abortion should prompt a search for an underlying cause.

Prevention

- A CHV-1 vaccine (i.e., Eurican Herpes 205) is available in Europe. Vaccination should be given 1 month before anticipated estrus, followed by vaccination within 8 days after mating. If titers are below 1:128 at mid-pregnancy, a third vaccination may be given 10 days before parturition.
- Isolate pregnant bitches from showing or performing dogs during pregnancy, especially if herpesvirus or brucellosis is endemic in the area.
- Maintain an adequate vaccination and deworming program.
- Bitches with hypoluteoidism may experience recurrent abortion, and mating of these increases risk.
- Breeding dogs should be screened for *B. canis* and, if positive, should not be bred.

Technician Tips

An understanding of normal pregnancy, preventative measures for breeding animals, and pregnancy emergencies that require veterinary attention is essential. Ability to recognize abnormal vaginal discharge, signs of discomfort in pregnant females, and high-risk pregnancies is also important.

Client Education

- Pregnancy diagnosis should be made in bitches at day 25-30 after breeding using abdominal ultrasonography or a serum relaxin test (pp. 816 and 1378).
- Regular medical evaluation of breeding dogs with appropriate vaccinations and regular deworming
- Genetic counseling to avoid inbreeding
- Screen breeding pair for brucellosis.

SUGGESTED READING

Lamm CG, et al: Clinical approach to abortion, stillborn, and neonatal death in dogs and cats. Vet Clin North Am Small Anim Pract 42:501-513, 2012.

AUTHOR: Wenche K. Farstad, DVM, Dr. scient., PhD, DECAR
EDITOR: Michelle A. Kutzler, DVM, PhD, DACT

Abscess, Cat Bite

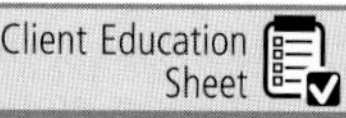

BASIC INFORMATION

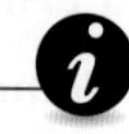

Definition

Focal pocket of purulent material located in the subcutaneous tissue of a cat due to a bite wound from another cat

Epidemiology

SPECIES, AGE, SEX

Cats of any age and either sex (more common in male cats)

RISK FACTORS

- Intact male
- Outdoor cat
- Multi-cat household

CONTAGION AND ZOONOSIS

- Feline immunodeficiency virus (FIV): transmission is mainly via bite wounds.
- Humans can develop severe cellulitis from cat bite wounds.

GEOGRAPHY AND SEASONALITY

Greater occurrence during warmer months (roaming cats)

ASSOCIATED DISORDERS

- Severe cellulitis
- Skin necrosis
- Osteomyelitis

Clinical Presentation

HISTORY, CHIEF COMPLAINT

- Painful swelling
- Crusted, dried discharge interpreted as matted hair
- Lethargy, inappetence

PHYSICAL EXAM FINDINGS

- Palpation: abscess may be well-circumscribed or broad-based and difficult to identify (e.g., cellulitis)
- Fever, dehydration, depression
- Draining tract with purulent material
- Open wound with presence of necrotic tissue
- Swollen and/or painful subcutis (focal or regional)

Etiology and Pathophysiology

- The bite punctures or lacerates skin and underlying tissue.
- Bacteria from oral cavity, hair, skin, and surrounding environment are injected into the subcutaneous tissue.
  - *Pasteurella multocida, Streptococcus,* and *Staphylococcus* spp. are most common.
  - Anaerobes
- Associated problems include cellulitis, draining tract, necrosis of overlying skin and osteomyelitis of underlying bone (rare). Fistula formation from bite perforation of hollow organ can occur (e.g., rectum).

DIAGNOSIS

Diagnostic Overview

Diagnosis relies on history, physical exam findings, and results of aspirate cytology. Additional testing is aimed at identifying the extent and complications of the abscess and injury.

Differential Diagnosis

Depends on the site of abscess

- Foreign body abscess
- Penetrating foreign body
- Anal sac abscess
- Salivary mucocele

Initial Database

- Complete blood count: normal, or changes consistent with sepsis
- Radiographs: if distal extremity; osteomyelitis possible
- FIV testing: indicated for all cats with bite wounds, since this is the main route of transmission for FIV (p. 325).
- Fine-needle aspiration and cytologic evaluation of abscess contents: to confirm septic inflammation if clinical features alone are ambiguous

Advanced or Confirmatory Testing

- Bacterial culture and susceptibility: often unnecessary with adequate surgical drainage and an otherwise stable patient; considered if the patient is systemically ill (other than fever) and/or fails to respond to treatment
- Consider feline leukemia virus serologic testing if not already performed.

TREATMENT

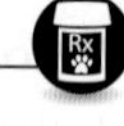

Treatment Overview

Drainage of the abscess and antibiotic therapy are the cornerstones of treatment and are successful in the vast majority of cases.

Acute General Treatment

- Surgically lance and drain abscess, flush with sterile saline or lactated Ringer's solution, and establish ongoing drainage. If necrotic tissue present, debride the wound.
- Antibiotic therapy is typically initiated.
  - Cephalexin 22 mg/kg PO q 12h, *or*
  - Cefovecin 8 mg/kg SQ once, *or*
  - Amoxicillin ± clavulanic acid 10-20 mg/kg PO q 12h
- Resolution of an abscess should occur within 5 days of effective therapy.
- Castration or ovariohysterectomy may decrease roaming and aggression.

Possible Complications

- Progressing cellulitis and necrosis of tissue due to inadequate debridement or improper antibiotic use (p. 907)
- Dehiscence of surgically closed wound
  - Avoid primary closure of an infected wound
  - Inadequate wound debridement
- Non-healing wound
  - High incidence in the axillary and inguinal regions (pocket wounds)
  - Biopsy and culture and susceptibility should be performed (mycobacteria, L-form bacteria may complicate wound healing).
  - Consider surgical referral of cats with pocket wounds.

PROGNOSIS & OUTCOME

- Excellent if proper therapy provided
- Guarded if cellulitis or tissue necrosis develops and/or a non-healing wound develops

PEARLS & CONSIDERATIONS

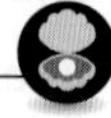

Comments

Do not close bite wounds primarily. Allow them to heal by second intention.

Technician Tips

Perform a wide clip and sterile prep before the abscess is lanced and drained.

SUGGESTED READING

Norsworthy GD, et al: The feline patient, ed 4, Ames, IA, 2011, Wiley-Blackwell, pp 44-45.

AUTHOR: Otto I. Lanz, DVM, DACVS
EDITOR: Elizabeth A. Swanson, DVM, MS, DACVS

Abscess, Lung

Client Education Sheet

BASIC INFORMATION

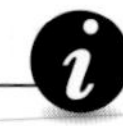

Definition

A localized collection of exudate due to suppuration of lung tissue, resulting in pulmonary cavitation

Synonym

Pulmonary abscess

Epidemiology

SPECIES, AGE, SEX

Dog and cat (more common), any age, either sex

GENETICS, BREED PREDISPOSITION

May be more common in hunting dogs due to field work

RISK FACTORS

Foreign body inhalation

GEOGRAPHY AND SEASONALITY

Inhalation of plant foreign body (e.g., grass awn) in endemic area (p. 398)

ASSOCIATED DISORDERS

Hypertrophic osteopathy (p. 508)

- Reported in dogs with chronic pulmonary abscessation
- Causes slowly progressive lameness
- May be associated with pyothorax that develops secondary to the lung abscess
- May be associated with spontaneous pneumothorax

Clinical Presentation

HISTORY, CHIEF COMPLAINT

- Chronic, progressive respiratory signs: cough, increased respiratory effort
- Acute dyspnea or respiratory decompensation: rupture of abscess resulting in pneumothorax or pyothorax
- Nonspecific signs of illness (anorexia, weight loss) with fever

PHYSICAL EXAM FINDINGS

- Poor body condition
- Fever may be present, but absence does not rule out the diagnosis.
- Thoracic auscultation
  - ± Loud bronchovesicular sounds or crackles
  - Muffled heart/lung sounds if pyothorax or pneumothorax
- Tachypnea or dyspnea

Etiology and Pathophysiology

- Foreign body migration
- Pneumonia (primary bacterial, fungal, aspiration)
- Parasitic infestation (*Paragonimus*)
- Primary pulmonary neoplasia

DIAGNOSIS

Diagnostic Overview

The diagnosis is suggested based on patient signalment, history, and physical examination findings. Confirmation requires 1) thoracic radiographs to demonstrate the pulmonary mass and 2) ultrasound to help differentiate abscess from neoplasia. Computed tomography (CT) scanning may be necessary to help confirm the diagnosis, determine extent of disease, and direct surgical intervention. Foreign bodies may be located in sites distant from the abscess and can be diagnosed with CT.

Differential Diagnosis

Other possible masses in the pulmonary parenchyma:

- Neoplasia
- Cyst
- Granuloma
- Parasitic nodules

Initial Database

- Complete blood count: possible neutrophilic leukocytosis with or without a left shift; anemia (usually mild, nonregenerative) possible with chronic abscessation
- Survey thoracic radiographs
  - Mass within pulmonary parenchyma; cavitation/gas in the lesion is pathognomonic.
  - Consolidated lung lobe may result from chronic abscessation.
  - ± Pneumothorax
  - Pleural effusion (if pyothorax)
- Analysis of pleural effusion, if present (pp. 1164 and 1343)
  - Cytologic evaluation
  - Aerobic and anaerobic bacterial culture and susceptibility testing

Advanced or Confirmatory Testing

CT scan

- Assess involvement of other intrathoracic structures; superior visualization compared to radiographs, especially when pleural effusion is present.
  - Additional pulmonary involvement
  - Mediastinal abscess
  - Pleural involvement
  - Presence of foreign material and migration to distant sites
- Assess if lesion is amenable to surgical resection.
- Possibly identify cause of abscess.
- Rule out other causes of pulmonary mass.

TREATMENT

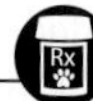

Treatment Overview

Surgical resection of the affected lung lobe(s) and culture-directed, long-term antimicrobial therapy generally is the treatment of choice.

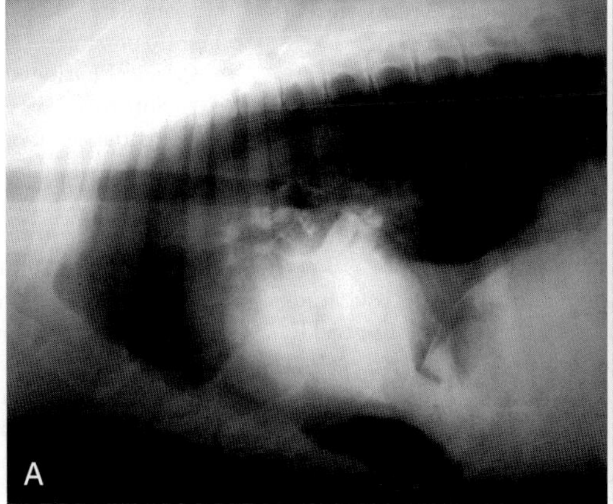

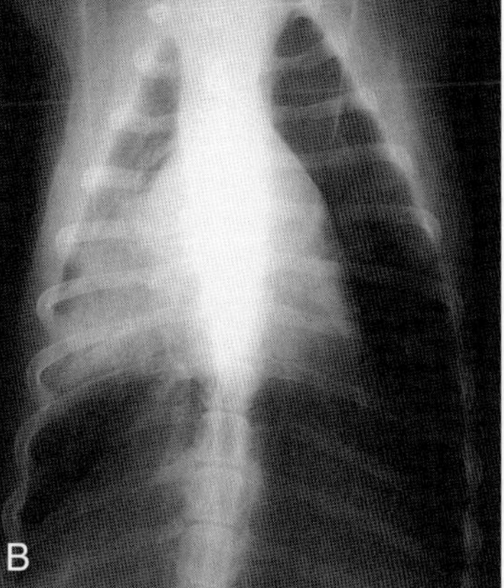

ABSCESS, LUNG Thorax of a dog with a lung abscess. **A,** Lateral radiograph shows that the abscessed lung area is the right middle lobe, which overlies the cardiac silhouette in this projection. **B,** In the dorsoventral thoracic view, opacities of the right middle lobe suggest extensive consolidation consistent with lung abscess. (Courtesy Dr. Richard Walshaw.)

Acute and Chronic Treatment

- Correction of fluid and electrolyte deficits
- Respiratory system support if needed
  - Oxygen supplementation (p. 1146)
  - Thoracocentesis (p. 1164) may be required if associated with pneumothorax or pyothorax.
- Antimicrobial therapy
  - Empirical therapy active against aerobic and anaerobic bacteria: second-generation cephalosporin (e.g., cefoxitin 22 mg/kg IV q 6h), amoxicillin (± clavulanic acid) 10-20 mg/kg PO q 12h
  - Definitive antimicrobial therapy should be based on results of aerobic and anaerobic bacterial culture and sensitivity testing (minimum treatment duration: 4 weeks).
- Thoracotomy for removal of affected lung lobe and treatment of pyothorax, if present (p. 857)

Possible Complications

Depends on cause

- Chronic pneumonia
- Abscesses in other lung lobes
- Failure to resolve associated pyothorax (e.g., failure to entirely remove inciting cause, such as foreign body that migrated outside the removed lung lobe or resected tissue)
- Care must be taken during surgical manipulation of the affected lung to avoid exudate entrance into other airways and the endotracheal tube.

Recommended Monitoring

Survey thoracic radiographs

- At completion of antibiotic therapy
- Periodically (q 3 months initially)

PROGNOSIS & OUTCOME

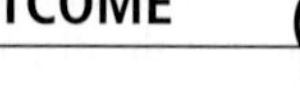

Depends on the cause

- If associated with sepsis and severe systemic illness: guarded to poor
- If an otherwise stable patient: fair, provided complete excision is possible
- Non-neoplastic abscessation is associated with a better prognosis than neoplastic abscess.

PEARLS & CONSIDERATIONS

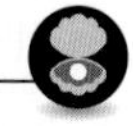

Comments

- Important to determine the underlying cause for optimal treatment.
- Medical treatment is needed to stabilize the patient. Ideally, antimicrobial choice is based on culture and susceptibility testing as early in the course of disease as possible.
- Surgical removal of the affected lobe is required to obtain definitive diagnosis and to remove the source of chronic infection.

Technician Tips

Knowledge of and experience in working with thoracostomy tubes is important in the postoperative management of patients who have undergone a thoracotomy.

SUGGESTED READING

Monnet E: Lungs. In Johnston SA, et al, editors: Veterinary surgery: small animal, ed 2, St. Louis, 2017, Elsevier, pp 1983-1999.

AUTHOR: MaryAnn G. Radlinsky, DVM, MS, DACVS
EDITOR: Elizabeth A. Swanson, DVM, MS, DACVS

Abscess, Oral

Client Education Sheet

BASIC INFORMATION

Definition

Abscess that develops in the soft tissues caudodorsal to the pharynx and dorsal or lateral to the esophagus

Epidemiology

SPECIES, AGE, SEX

- Most common in young dogs and cats
- No sex predisposition

RISK FACTORS

- Stick chewing
- Playing fetch with sticks
- Feeding chicken bones
- Fish hook or sewing needle ingestion
- Bite wound

CONTAGION AND ZOONOSIS

If from a bite wound of unknown origin, transmission of rabies from a wild animal should be considered.

Clinical Presentation

HISTORY, CHIEF COMPLAINT

- History of risk factors (see above) is common.
- Nonspecific complaints: lethargy, inappetence
- Dysphagia
- Ptyalism
- Reluctance to move head and neck
- Pain on opening of the mouth
- Pawing at the mouth

PHYSICAL EXAM FINDINGS

- Fever ±
- Depression or lethargy
- Ptyalism
- Halitosis
- Dyspnea
- Painful on manipulation of head and neck or when opening the mouth
- Punctures or granulomatous lesions on oral mucosa
- Palpable swelling caudal to the mandible
- Draining tract in the cranial cervical region

Etiology and Pathophysiology

- Penetrating trauma contaminates the retropharyngeal area with bacteria.
- Rapid healing of the pharyngeal tissue leads to a walled-off abscess that develops quickly.
- May be presence of foreign body

DIAGNOSIS

Diagnostic Overview

Diagnosis is based on patient signalment, history, and physical examination. Confirmation requires demonstration that the soft tissue mass in the neck is an abscess. Ultrasound examination with cytologic analysis of fine-needle aspirates strengthens the diagnosis.

Differential Diagnosis

- Inflammation/cellulitis
- Lymphadenopathy
- Neoplasia (lymphoma, metastatic disease, carotid body tumor)
- Pharyngeal salivary mucocele

Initial Database

- Complete blood count: leukocytosis, left shift possible
- Cervical radiographs
  - Soft tissue mass in the pharyngeal region
  - Ventral deviation of the larynx or esophagus
  - Radiopaque foreign body
- Thoracic radiographs
  - Check for thoracic involvement
- Cervical ultrasound
  - Identify the foreign body or abscess.
  - Obtain ultrasound-guided aspirate for cytology.
- Bacterial culture and susceptibility
  - Aerobic and anaerobic cultures (*Actinomyces* spp., *Nocardia* spp.)

Advanced or Confirmatory Testing

- Contrast radiology: if a draining tract is present, to identify foreign body and extent of abscess

- Contrast CT or MRI: to identify foreign body and extent of lesion

TREATMENT

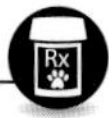

Treatment Overview

To resolve abscess and prevent recurrence, it is necessary to explore, debride, and lavage the abscess cavity; remove all foreign material; provide postoperative drainage; allow the pharyngeal wound to heal; and provide appropriate antibiotic therapy and nutritional support.

Acute General Treatment

- Oropharyngeal exam under general anesthesia
  - Identify the puncture site.
  - Identify alternative causes of retropharyngeal swelling (e.g., pharyngeal salivary mucocele, tonsillar tumor).
- Endoscopic examination of the penetration site, if possible, to identify and remove any foreign body
- Surgical exploration, debridement, and lavage of the abscess
  - Foreign body may no longer be present.
  - May be difficult to remove the entire abscess because of close proximity to vital structures in the head and neck
- Postoperative drainage
  - Closed-suction drain if entire abscess excised. Allow abscess to drain and heal by second intention if unable to excise entire abscess.
  - Open drainage decreases likelihood of formation of secondary abscess pockets.
- Bacterial culture and susceptibility
  - Use broad-spectrum antibiotics (e.g., amoxicillin-clavulanic acid) until definitive culture results are obtained. Presence of *Actinomyces* spp. and/or *Nocardia* spp. necessitates antibiotic therapy for 2-3 months.

Chronic Treatment

- Open wound management
  - Appropriate bandaging is difficult in this area of the body.
  - May require the use of tie-over bandages or vacuum-assisted closure therapy
- Percutaneous endoscopic gastrostomy tube or esophagostomy tube (pp. 1107 and 1109)
  - Indicated to bypass the oropharynx for healing purposes and to provide medication and nutritional feeding

Possible Complications

- Recurrence of the abscess or reformation of a draining tract
  - Failure to remove a foreign body
  - Primary closure of abscess can lead to dehiscence
- Extension of the abscess into the thoracic cavity (pyothorax) and/or mediastinum

Recommended Monitoring

- Patient should be rechecked for bandage changes.
- Evaluate the surgical site in 10-14 days for wound healing.
- Remove feeding tube once the pharynx has healed.

PROGNOSIS & OUTCOME

Good if the foreign body is removed and adequate surgical drainage is provided

PEARLS & CONSIDERATIONS

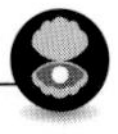

Comments

Primary closure of the wound should not be performed without providing drainage; allow drain site to heal by second intention.

Technician Tips

Familiarity with closed-suction drain management and bandaging techniques, including tie-over bandages, is imperative for postoperative care.

Client Education

Avoid letting dogs chew or play with sticks that could lead to penetration of the pharyngeal region.

SUGGESTED READING

Doran IP, et al: Acute oropharyngeal and esophageal stick injury in forty-one dogs. Vet Surg 37:781-785, 2008.

EDITOR: Elizabeth A. Swanson, DVM, MS, DACVS
AUTHOR: Otto I. Lanz, DVM, DACVS

Abscess, Periapical (Tooth Root)

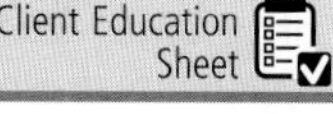

BASIC INFORMATION

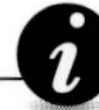

Definition

Suppurative process of the periapical region of a tooth, which is a relatively common disorder of dogs and cats

Synonyms

Periradicular abscess, tooth root abscess

Epidemiology

SPECIES, AGE, SEX

No species, age, or sex predisposition

RISK FACTORS

- Dental trauma (infective, mechanical, thermal, chemical)
- Endodontic and periapical disease
- Periodontal disease

ASSOCIATED DISORDERS

Tooth fractures (p. 980), tooth displacement injuries, and periodontal disease (p. 776)

Clinical Presentation

DISEASE FORMS/SUBTYPES

- Acute
- Chronic (more common)
- Acute abscesses may over time become chronic; exacerbated chronic abscesses may take on features of acute abscesses.

HISTORY, CHIEF COMPLAINT

- Visible swelling due to the physical presence of the abscess
- Owner notices discolored or fractured tooth.
- With acute abscess, owner may notice anorexia or a reluctance to eat.

PHYSICAL EXAM FINDINGS

- Fever, regional lymphadenopathy, maxillofacial swelling, intraoral or extraoral draining tracts are possible.
- Acute periapical abscess: affected tooth is very painful and slightly extruded from its alveolar socket; localized swelling or cellulitis may be present (e.g., maxillofacial swelling with or without draining tracts); regional lymphadenitis; fever
- Chronic periapical abscess: generally presents with no clinical signs (essentially a mild, well-circumscribed area of suppuration).
- Others (appearing variably in acute or chronic abscesses)
  - Fractures and/or discolored tooth crowns
  - Severe periodontal disease
  - Draining tracts (often at mucogingival junction intraorally or at skin covering the face and jaws extraorally)

Etiology and Pathophysiology

- The primary cause is dental trauma, resulting in irreversible pulpitis and pulp necrosis.
- If untreated, the inflammatory reaction spreads to involve the periapical region.
- A number of different tissue reactions (granuloma, cyst, abscess) may occur around the apex of the involved tooth.
- Periapical lesions do not represent distinct entities. In most cases, there is a subtle transformation from one type of lesion to another.

- The periapical abscess may develop directly as a result of pulp necrosis but more commonly originates from a periapical granuloma or cyst.

DIAGNOSIS

Diagnostic Overview

An acute periapical abscess should be suspected when a patient presents with fever, regional lymphadenitis, facial swelling, or intraoral or extraoral draining tracts. A chronic periapical abscess should be suspected when a patient presents with facial swelling or draining tracts. Confirmation requires meticulous oral examination under general anesthesia to identify teeth with pulpal lesions and dental radiography to assess the periapical status of affected teeth.

Differential Diagnosis

- Periapical granuloma: periapical bone lysis; accumulation of mononuclear inflammatory cells, fibroblasts, and collagen
- Periapical (radicular) cyst: periapical bone lysis; bone walls covered by cystic epithelium
- Osteomyelitis: diffuse, regional bone lysis; inflammation of bone and bone marrow

Initial Database

- Complete blood count, serum chemistry panel, urinalysis: preoperative and usually unremarkable (± leukocytosis)
- Meticulous oral examination under general anesthesia to identify teeth with pulpal lesions (fractured teeth, often with pulp exposure; discolored teeth; caries; drainage tracts) (p. 1140)

Advanced or Confirmatory Testing

- Dental radiography to assess periapical status of affected teeth (variable radiographic appearance depending on whether acute or chronic process)
  - Acute abscess (arising directly from a necrotic pulp) may show only mild widening of apical periodontal space.
  - Chronic abscess is associated with bone destruction (i.e., periapical lucency) around the apex of the tooth; resorption of the most apical portion of the tooth root may be present; the width of the root canals of affected teeth may be wider compared to the root canals of unaffected contralateral teeth.

TREATMENT

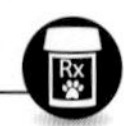

Treatment Overview

The goal of treatment (extraction or endodontic treatment of the affected tooth) is to achieve drainage and remove the cause of the inflammatory reaction.

Acute General Treatment

- Extraction or endodontic therapy (total pulpectomy and root canal filling)
- Endodontic therapy may need to be staged (i.e., performed in several sessions).
- Concurrent systemic antibiotic treatment (e.g., 2 weeks of amoxicillin/clavulanic acid 13.75 mg/kg PO q 12h or clindamycin, 5.5 mg/kg PO q 12h) is indicated if fever and/or regional lymphadenopathy exist, the associated swelling is diffuse, or cellulitis occurs.
- The use of systemic antibiotics alone is NOT appropriate treatment.
- Analgesic treatment with nonsteroidal antiinflammatory drugs (e.g., in dogs: meloxicam 0.2 mg/kg PO q 24h; or carprofen 2.2 mg/kg PO q 12h)

Chronic Treatment

- Extraction or endodontic therapy
- Monitor teeth at risk for pulpal disease (e.g., uncomplicated crown fractures).

Drug Interactions

Adverse reactions to systemic antibiotics and/or analgesics

Possible Complications

- Incomplete extraction
- Endodontic: incomplete removal of pulp, substandard obturation, and restoration

Recommended Monitoring

- Physical examination
- Radiographic evaluation to confirm healing

PROGNOSIS & OUTCOME

Excellent if therapeutic goals (drainage and removal of cause of inflammation) are achieved

PEARLS & CONSIDERATIONS

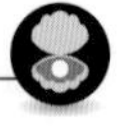

Comments

- Chronic abscess is more common than acute.
- An abscess associated with a draining tract usually causes less discomfort.
- Draining tracts commonly occur at the mucogingival junction on the labial or buccal aspect of the tooth.
- An acute periapical abscess with systemic signs and diffuse swelling (cellulitis) is a true emergency.
- If extraoral, the draining tract of an abscessed maxillary fourth premolar tooth in a dog usually is situated in the cheek skin at the level of the medial canthus of the eye, while the same location can be related to abscessed maxillary canine or fourth premolar teeth in the cat.

Prevention

- Minimize the risk of dental trauma.
- Monitor (clinically and radiographically) teeth that have been subjected to trauma

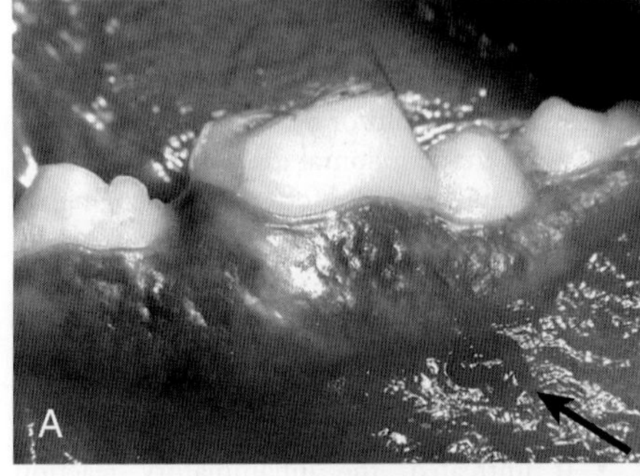

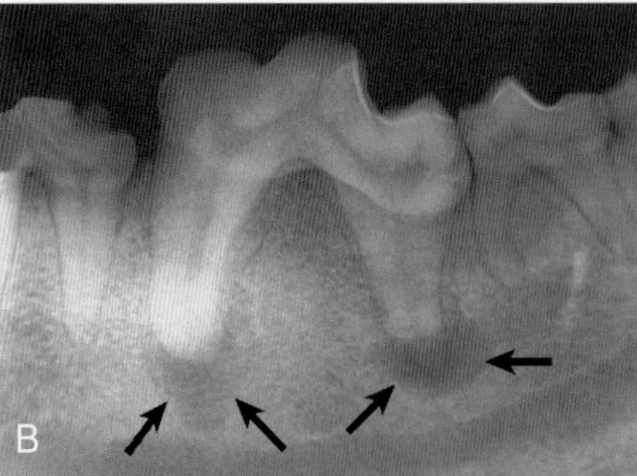

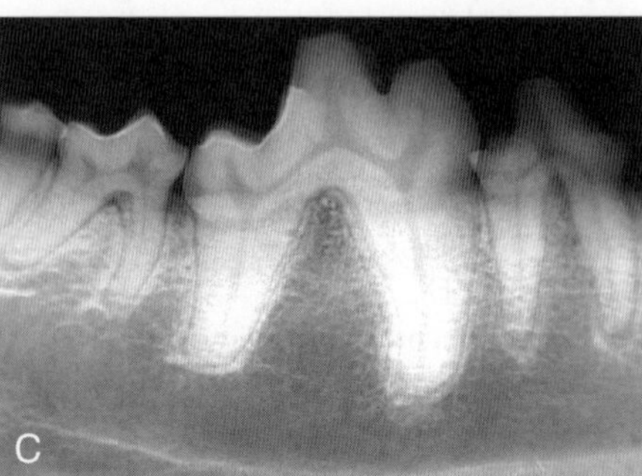

ABSCESS, PERIAPICAL (TOOTH ROOT) A, Left mandibular first molar periapical abscess: clinical picture of left mandibular first molar. Cusps of tooth are fractured or worn, producing pulp exposure. A draining tract is visible at the mucogingival junction near the distal root of this tooth *(arrow)*. **B,** Radiograph of the left mandibular first molar periapical abscess same patient. Cusps of tooth are fractured or worn with pulp exposure. Radiolucencies apparent around apices of both roots *(arrows)*. **C,** Normal appearance of periodontal and periapical tissues of the right mandibular first molar for comparison. Although cusps of this tooth appear fractured or worn (uncomplicated crown fractures [i.e., without pulp exposure]), there is no evidence of periodontal pocket formation or periapical radiolucency, which would suggest abscessation. (Copyright Dr. Alexander M. Reiter, University of Pennsylvania.)

and may develop periapical pathology (e.g., uncomplicated crown fracture).
- Perform prompt treatment (extraction or endodontic therapy) of teeth that have pulpal disease (e.g., complicated crown fracture).

Technician Tips

- Dental radiography is paramount for the evaluation of periapical disease.
- Learn how to obtain dental radiographs to assist the veterinarian in patient management.

Client Education

- Explain the pathophysiology of pulpal and periapical disease.
- Train owners to examine the oral cavity and look for abnormal teeth.

SUGGESTED READINGS

Reiter AM, et al: Periodontal and endodontic disease. In Bojrab MJ, Monnet E, editors: Mechanisms of disease in small animal surgery, ed 3, Jackson, WY, 2010, Teton NewMedia, pp 125-128.

AUTHOR & EDITOR: Alexander M. Reiter, DVM, Dr. med. vet, DAVDC, DEVDC

Abuse

BASIC INFORMATION

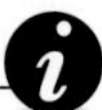

Definition

- Physical abuse: actions such as kicking, punching, beating, burning, microwaving, drowning, asphyxiation, and administration of drugs or poisons
- Sexual abuse: any use of an animal for sexual gratification
- Emotional abuse: threatening behavior
- Neglect: failure to provide the basic physical and/or emotional necessities of life (e.g., food, shelter, veterinary attention)

Synonyms

Battered pet syndrome, non-accidental injury, physical abuse

Epidemiology

SPECIES, AGE, SEX

Young male dogs and young cats are particularly at risk.

GENETICS, BREED PREDISPOSITION

Crossbred dogs, Staffordshire bull terriers, and domestic short-haired cats are at increased risk in the United Kingdom, but this may represent favoring of particular breeds by owners of low socioeconomic status.

RISK FACTORS

There is an association between animal abuse, domestic violence, and child abuse. Links within the community (e.g., social workers, police, child protection teams, animal welfare organizations) are highly advantageous for addressing the public health aspects of abuse. Interagency collaboration is effective and helps to reduce stress on the veterinarian.

Clinical Presentation

DISEASE FORMS/SUBTYPES

A variant of abuse is fabricated or induced illness.

- Factitious illness by proxy
- Munchausen syndrome by proxy
  - Uncommon
  - Involves invention or falsification of illness in animal by owner, motivation being attention seeking by owner
  - May involve repetitive injury

HISTORY, CHIEF COMPLAINT

Crucial to note that none of the following features alone is diagnostic. A combination raises suspicion, and the combination varies.

- History supplied is inconsistent with the injury. Usually, the injury is too severe to fit the history. Owner's explanation to account for the pet's injuries merits attention by its lack of plausibility (e.g., animal with severe burns "sat too close to the radiator" or "lay too close to the fire"; animal with fractures "fell down the stairs," "fell off the sofa," "fell from child's arms," or "fell off the bed").
- Discrepant history (e.g., person presenting the animal may change his/her story, history may differ from person to person)
- Particular person implicated (e.g., partner, child, even self-admission)
- Repetitive injury (i.e., animal presented more than once with injuries and/or different ages of injury are identified). All body systems may be involved, but fractures are important.
- Previous injury or death of another animal in the same home, particularly when unexplained
- Lack of history of a motor vehicle accident or any possible accident to explain injury
- The behavior of the owner causes concern (e.g., implausible, aggressive, embarrassed, obviously discomfited, lack of concern for the animal).
- The behavior of the animal causes concern (e.g., animal shows fear of owner, happier when hospitalized away from owner).
- Family violence known or suspected
- When obtaining the history of a case where abuse is on the differential diagnosis, some points are essential:
  - It is important to be objective and avoid jumping to conclusions.
  - It is necessary to remain polite and calm and avoid being confrontational.
  - If the decision is made to discuss concerns with the client, it can be helpful to present those concerns nonconfrontationally along the lines of the following: "It's difficult for me to match Spot's injuries with what you are saying. Is there anything else you'd like to tell me?"
  - It is important to ensure that clinical notes are comprehensive and thorough and that they are retained because of potential legal ramifications. Relying on memory can be problematic because it may be some time before the case goes to court.

PHYSICAL EXAM FINDINGS

Wide spectrum of possible injuries

- Superficial injuries are common: bruising of head, thorax, abdomen, and limbs; scleral/conjunctival hemorrhages. Shaving of the hair can reveal bruising, even in animals with very dark coats. Bruising is likely to be present over bony structures such as ribs or vertebrae but may be absent in the (soft) abdominal wall. Necropsy examination of suspected fatal cases must include thorough examination of all subcutaneous areas for bruising.
- Fractures and locomotor injuries: The most common fractures involve the skull, ribs, and femurs, although other bones may be involved.
- Physical signs of internal thoracoabdominal injuries: rupture of major organs (liver, kidney, spleen, urinary bladder); intrapulmonary hemorrhage; rupture of bowel uncommon
- Sexual abuse injuries involve the genitalia and/or the anal or rectal area. Both sexes may be abused.

Etiology and Pathophysiology

- Owner-associated risk factors for the animal include domestic abuse, alcoholism, substance abuse, and mental illness.
- Some authors suggest that animal abuse is more common in areas of social deprivation, but this is largely anecdotal, and abuse does occur in affluent groups.

DIAGNOSIS

Diagnostic Overview

A diagnosis of physical abuse is suspected when an animal suffers a series of injuries for which no satisfactory explanation is offered and/or the history does not fit the injuries.

Differential Diagnosis

- Naturally occurring conditions such as skeletal disorders (e.g., metabolic bone disease) and blood dyscrasias causing bruises

- Motor vehicle accidents/hit by car: History helps to differentiate (e.g., is the animal ever allowed out or is always kept in house?), as does physical exam (animals hit by cars often have tattered nails, skin abrasions, and dirt in the haircoat).

Initial Database

- Much of the diagnostic information in cases of abuse is obtained from the history and physical exam.
- Ancillary diagnostic tests depend on the specific details of each case.
  - Radiographic examination, particularly for fractures; fractures of differing ages may be found
  - Necropsy of fatal cases. Radiographic examination can also be helpful in fatal cases before necropsy.

TREATMENT

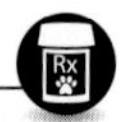

Acute General Treatment

As dictated by nature and extent of injuries

PROGNOSIS & OUTCOME

- Depends on the severity of the abuse. Fatal cases occur.
- Can be poor with fabricated or induced illness (Munchausen's syndrome by proxy) if the pet remains with the owner

PEARLS & CONSIDERATIONS

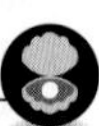

Comments

- No single injury or group of injuries, when divorced from the circumstances surrounding a suspect case, can be considered to conclusively indicate physical abuse.
- More than one type of abuse may be present at the same time. For example, physically abused animals may also suffer neglect from malnourishment or from lack of veterinary treatment for naturally occurring illness.
- When contact with the perpetrator of abuse ceases (e.g., when the animal is hospitalized), no further injuries occur.
- Considerable knowledge is available on injuries specifically associated with child abuse. Further research on equivalent animal abuse injuries is needed. The medical experience of child abuse injuries provides a useful starting point for researchers.
- It is highly desirable that an experienced veterinary pathologist, preferably one with forensic experience, perform a necropsy of fatal suspected abuse cases.
- Injury from sexual abuse may be absent. Common sense dictates that injury depends on animal size and the actual type of sex act, which can be variable.
- It is not the veterinarian's remit to prove abuse. That is the responsibility of the courts. The veterinarian's responsibility is limited to provision of veterinary evidence to the court.
- In so doing, it may be reassuring to be aware that investigation of an abuse case is multidisciplinary (e.g., animal welfare organizations, police) and that there may be lay witnesses of the abuse.
- The veterinarian may feel that in some cases there are extenuating circumstances with regard to the person perpetrating the abuse (e.g., emotional problems, other personal difficulties) (see Etiology and Pathophysiology section). These feelings may influence the veterinarian's decision to report a case. These circumstances are not the veterinarian's responsibility, nor does he or she have the relevant expertise to judge them. In the United Kingdom the law courts consider these circumstances.
- Each veterinary practice needs to consider its own procedures in relation to this difficult area. It is advisable to have a practice policy available for guidance. All staff members need to be familiar with this policy, which should undergo regular review.
- The law varies from country to country and within countries. Currently, reporting systems for dealing with child abuse cases are in place in many countries but in general have not been developed for animal abuse cases. Advice may be available from an animal welfare organization or veterinary association.
- In some circumstances, the veterinarian may feel that the welfare of the animal is so severely compromised that client confidentiality should be breached. In the United Kingdom, this is fully recognized in the comprehensive Royal College of Veterinary Surgeons Guide to Professional Conduct. The veterinarian is advised in the first instance to attempt to discuss concerns with the client. In cases where this would not be appropriate or the client's reaction increases rather than allays concerns, the veterinarian should consider whether the circumstances are sufficiently serious to justify disclosing the client's information without consent. Appropriate contact details are listed in this guide. Advice with contact details is also given on the reporting concerns about child abuse or domestic violence to appropriate authorities, regardless of whether animal abuse is present.

Technician Tips

Clients who have an abused pet may be more comfortable speaking about this situation with a technician rather than the attending veterinarian. The technician should listen neutrally and without passing judgment. Since repeat offenses are common, it is in the best interest of animals for the technician to share this information with the veterinarian afterward and to document it in the medical record.

SUGGESTED READING

Tong LJ: Identifying non-accidental injury cases in veterinary practice. Br Vet Assoc Pract 38:59-68, 2016.

AUTHOR: Helen M. C. Munro, BVMS, MRCVS
EDITOR: Leah A. Cohn, DVM, PhD, DACVIM

Acetaminophen Toxicosis

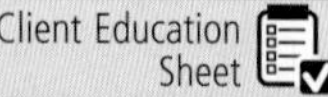

BASIC INFORMATION

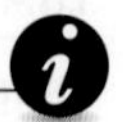

Definition

An acute toxicosis from accidental ingestion or owner administration that may result in hepatotoxicity, methemoglobinemia, and rarely keratoconjunctivitis sicca (KCS)

Synonyms

Tylenol, APAP, paracetamol, nonaspirin pain reliever

Epidemiology

SPECIES, AGE, SEX

- Cats are more sensitive than dogs.
- All breeds, ages, and sexes are susceptible.

RISK FACTORS

- Access to the medication
- Owner unaware of species sensitivity to acetaminophen
- Patients with pre-existing liver issues

GEOGRAPHY AND SEASONALITY

Toxicosis is common year-round, but more cases are reported during winter months coinciding with cold and flu season and increased human use of over-the-counter (OTC) pain relievers.

Clinical Presentation

HISTORY, CHIEF COMPLAINT

- Most common is witnessed or suspected exposure

- History of progressive lethargy, anorexia, vomiting, icterus, muddy or cyanotic mucous membrane color, tachypnea, dyspnea, weakness, or paw and facial edema

PHYSICAL EXAM FINDINGS

- Most often unremarkable if early in the clinical course
- Lethargy, depression
- Chocolate-colored mucous membranes (methemoglobinemia)
- Facial and/or paw edema (more common in cats)
- Tachypnea, dyspnea
- Tachycardia
- Icterus
- Vomiting
- KCS (rare) (p. 568)

Etiology and Pathophysiology

- When normal biotransformation pathways for detoxification (glucuronidation and sulfation) are overwhelmed, an oxidative metabolite (i.e., *N*-acetyl-*p*-benzoquinone imine [NAPQI]) is formed and binds to cellular macromolecules leading to cellular necrosis. If NAPQI is conjugated with glutathione, it is detoxified.
- Another metabolite, para-aminophenol (PAP), may be responsible for development of methemoglobinemia through oxidative damage.

DIAGNOSIS

Diagnostic Overview

Because exposure is usually witnessed or suspected, determining dose and risk are important. If there is doubt regarding recent exposure, acetaminophen concentrations (from a human hospital) should be considered, although this test is not sensitive enough for cats. Assess liver enzymes and methemoglobin for suspected intoxication.

Differential Diagnosis

- Hepatic injury: xylitol, aflatoxin, blue-green algae, cycad palms (e.g., *Cycas revoluta*, *Zamia furfuracea*), hepatotoxic mushrooms, salicylates
- Methemoglobinemia: benzocaine (Cetacaine) in cats, naphthalene, nitrites, chlorates, phenol, *Allium* sp., skunk spray
- Swollen face/paws: insect bite or sting, cutaneous adverse drug reaction

Initial Database

- CBC: often unremarkable in initial stages
  - Heinz body anemia may occur after methemoglobinemia
- Serum biochemical profile: often unremarkable in initial stages
  - Progressive increase in liver enzymes (alanine aminotransferase [ALT], alkaline phosphatase [ALP]) until hepatic function declines, then decreases in blood urea nitrogen (BUN), cholesterol, and albumin with increasing total bilirubin. Initial increases are typically seen within 24-36 hours of ingestion.
- Spot test for methemoglobinemia: Place one drop of blood on absorbent white paper from affected patient and compare to one drop of blood from unaffected patient. If affected patient's blood appears brown in comparison, there is a likely diagnosis of methemoglobinemia.

Advanced or Confirmatory Testing

- Acetaminophen levels at human hospital for dogs (ideally run 4 hours after exposure)
- Methemoglobin levels (not readily available)
- Schirmer tear test if suspect KCS
- Centrilobular liver necrosis and congestion on histopathology

TREATMENT

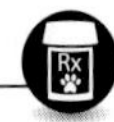

Treatment Overview

After exposure but before signs occur, decontamination with emesis and activated charcoal is important. Liver protectant and antioxidant, *N*-acetylcysteine, is advised to prevent and treat liver injury and may help with methemoglobinemia.

Acute General Treatment

- Decontamination, typically most beneficial within 2 hours of ingestion (only if asymptomatic)
  - Induction of emesis (p. 1188): Apomorphine 0.03 mg/kg IV or 0.04 mg/kg IM or conjunctivally (canine)
  - Activated charcoal (p. 1087) 1-2 g/kg PO with sorbitol, one dose
- Liver protectant or antioxidant
  - *N*-acetylcysteine (Mucomyst) 140 mg/kg loading dose (or 280 mg/kg in large overdoses), followed by 70 mg/kg every 6 hours for 7-17 doses. Oral and intravenous (IV) formulations are available. Dilute to 5% before giving (dextrose if PO, replacement fluids if IV). If giving orally, must wait 2-3 hours after administration of activated charcoal. May give IV *N*-acetylcysteine concurrently with activated charcoal.
  - *S*-adenosylmethionine (SAMe) 18-20 mg/kg PO q 24h for 2 weeks can be used instead of *N*-acetylcysteine if liver issues are expected but no methemoglobinemia occurred or after methemoglobinemia has resolved.
  - Ascorbic acid (helps reduce methemoglobin to hemoglobin, but efficacy is questionable): 30 mg/kg q 6-12h PO or SQ
  - Cimetidine (inhibitor of cytochrome P450) is no longer recommended; its inhibition of microsomal enzymes is considered too slow to be of benefit in dogs. In cats, cimetidine is contraindicated because it inhibits *N*-acetyltransferase 1 (NAT1), which can decrease the conversion of PAP to acetaminophen, putting patients at higher risk for methemoglobinemia.
- Supportive care
  - Oxygen (p. 1146)
  - Fluid therapy to maintain hydration and electrolyte balance
  - Blood transfusion may be needed if hemolytic anemia develops (p. 1169).

Chronic Treatment

- Ophthalmic cyclosporine until KCS resolves (typically 4-6 weeks)
- Continue SAMe until liver enzymes return to normal.

Behavior/Exercise

Restricted activity during treatment

Drug Interactions

Drugs that induce hepatic microsomal systems (e.g., phenobarbital) may increase acetaminophen toxicity due to increased formation of hepatotoxic metabolites.

Possible Complications

KCS, chronic liver disease

Recommended Monitoring

- Monitoring liver enzymes or function tests every 24 hours for initial 48 hours after exposure or until liver injury resolves
- Monitoring for evidence of methemoglobinemia in first 12 hours after exposure, followed by hemolytic anemia for 72 hours after exposure
- Monitor Schirmer tear test for evidence of KCS during initial 72 hours after exposure

PROGNOSIS & OUTCOME

- With prompt and aggressive care, prognosis is usually good.
- Methemoglobinemia and significant liver injury worsen prognosis, as does underlying health issues, particularly those involving the liver.

PEARLS & CONSIDERATIONS

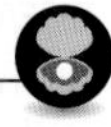

Comments

- Owners may use brand names as generic terms for OTC pain relievers. Verify active ingredient and strength of what the owner thinks was ingested.
- Emesis is not likely to be beneficial for feline patients because acetaminophen is absorbed very quickly (peak plasma level of 10-30 minutes). Activated charcoal may be beneficial if given within 30 minutes of exposure.
- Glucocorticoids and antihistamines will have no effect on paw and facial edema because they are not due to an allergic reaction.

Technician Tips

Check for other active ingredients in products because acetaminophen can be combined with other medications such as opioids, dextromethorphan, pseudoephedrine, or phenylephrine.

Client Education

- Owners should be aware that OTC pain relievers might not be safe for pets. They should always contact a veterinary professional before administration of any OTC medications.
- Phenazopyridine (Pyridium) is metabolized into acetaminophen and an aniline dye.

SUGGESTED READING

Sellon RK: Acetaminophen. In Peterson ME, Talcott PE, editors: Small animal toxicology, ed 3, St. Louis, 2013, Elsevier.

AUTHOR: Kirsten Waratuke, DVM, DABT
EDITOR: Tina Wismer, DVM, MS, DABVT, DABT

Achilles Tendon Injury

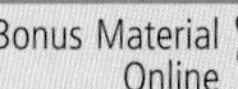
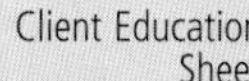
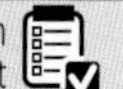

Bonus Material Online Client Education Sheet

BASIC INFORMATION

Definition

- The common calcanean or Achilles tendon is composed of three tendons inserting on the calcaneus: the gastrocnemius tendon; the combined tendon of biceps femoris, semitendinosus, and gracilis; and the superficial digital flexor (SDF) tendon.
- Injuries include lacerations, acute ruptures, and chronic rupture due to tendon degeneration.

Synonyms

Achilles mechanism failure, common calcanean tendon rupture, Achilles tendinopathy, dropped hock

Epidemiology

SPECIES, AGE, SEX

- Mature dogs; working or racing breeds
- Cats; females > males

GENETICS, BREED PREDISPOSITION

Labrador retrievers and Doberman pinschers appear to be overrepresented for tendon rupture.

RISK FACTORS

Overuse in active, large-breed dogs

Clinical Presentation

DISEASE FORMS/SUBTYPES

Insertional avulsion, chronic tendinopathy, avulsion of gastrocnemius origin from the femur, musculotendinous ruptures, midsubstance tendon lacerations and tears

HISTORY, CHIEF COMPLAINT

May present as an acute injury or as a chronic progressive lameness with tendinopathies

PHYSICAL EXAM FINDINGS

Variable lameness, palpable gap or swelling within tendon, plantigrade stance, dropped hock (excessive tarsal flexion during stance), excessive toe flexion (with ruptured gastrocnemius, intact SDF tendon)

Etiology and Pathophysiology

- Acute lesions caused by trauma, overload; repetitive stresses can lead to chronic degenerative changes.
- Gaps in tendon fill with fibrous tissue, causing gait/stance change due to excessive tendon length

DIAGNOSIS

Diagnostic Overview

Diagnosis is confirmed by results of physical, radiographic, and ultrasonographic examinations.

Differential Diagnosis

- Fracture of the calcaneus
- Tarsal hyperflexion injury
- Distal tibia/fibula fractures

Initial Database

- Lameness examination (p. 1143), palpation of Achilles tendon, simultaneous flexion/extension of stifle and hock joints
- Mediolateral and caudocranial radiographic projections of stifle and hock
- Ultrasonography of common calcaneal tendon complex
- CBC and chemistry panel based on signalment and nature of injury; usually unremarkable with tendon injury alone

Advanced or Confirmatory Testing

Magnetic resonance imaging (p. 1132) provides superior detail; canine normals have not yet been established.

TREATMENT

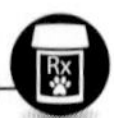

Treatment Overview

Therapeutic goals are to restore normal length and strength of the common calcaneal tendon.

Acute General Treatment

- Tendinopathies without calcaneal avulsion can be treated with immobilization in extension (cast, splint, calcaneotibial screw, external skeletal fixation, or orthotic) for 2-4 weeks, followed by controlled weight bearing for a further 2 weeks.
- Avulsed heads of gastrocnemius muscle repaired with wire/heavy suture around fabella and into the distal femur
- Acute midsubstance tears of each tendon are anastomosed using three-loop pulley, Bunnell, or locking-loop pattern.
- Tendons avulsed from tuber calcanei are reattached by Krackow or locking loop suture passed through bone tunnels.

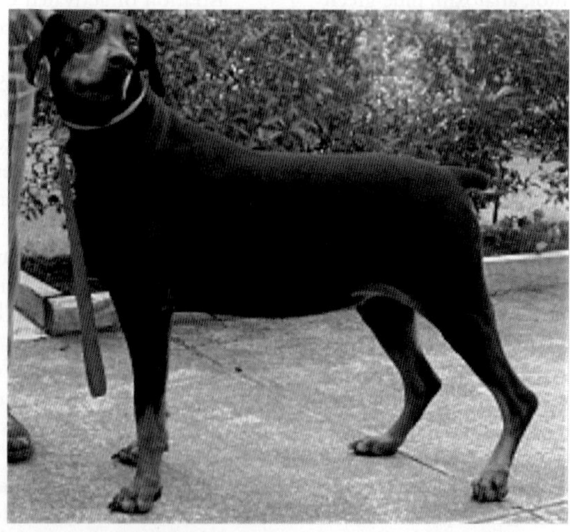

ACHILLES TENDON INJURY Doberman showing classic stance of a chronic Achilles tendinopathy injury. Note the left stifle extension, hock flexion, and digit flexion; also note overconditioning (body condition score 8/9).

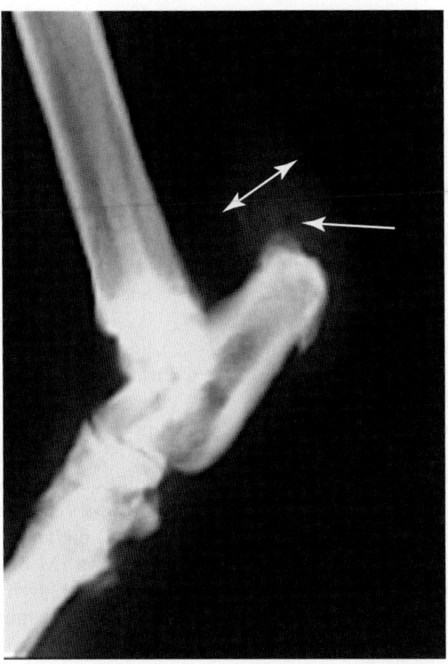

ACHILLES TENDON INJURY Radiograph showing thickening of distal tendon *(double-headed arrow)* and enthesophyte formation *(single-headed arrow)*.

- Avulsions of tuber calcanei bone fragments are stabilized with small pins and tension band wiring.
- All repairs are initially supported by an external fixator, internal bone screw, splint, or cast with the hock in extension.

Chronic Treatment

- Injection of platelet-rich plasma (PRP) into the affected area of the tendon under ultrasound guidance may help stimulate healing in chronic tendinopathy cases.
- Chronic tendinopathies with calcaneal avulsions are debrided and reattached by Krackow suture passed through bone tunnels followed by immobilization.
- For chronic tendon disruptions, fibrous scar is debrided, and tendon ends are reapposed. Fascial or synthetic mesh grafts, tendon transposition, and muscle-lengthening procedures have been used to span tendon gaps. Adjunctive support with the hock in extension is also required.

Possible Complications

- Repair failure
- Infection
- Morbidity with cast, splint, or fixator

Recommended Monitoring

- Weekly examination of limb to reduce problems associated with cast, splint, or fixator
- Removal of external support or screw 4-6 weeks after surgery
- Controlled exercise and rehabilitation for 3 months to avoid reinjury

PROGNOSIS & OUTCOME

- Good to excellent (≈80% success rate) with appropriate early treatment and postoperative care
- Fair for chronic or repeat injuries
- Poor with nonsurgical treatments

PEARLS & CONSIDERATIONS

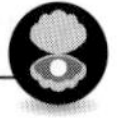

Comments

- Protect tendon repairs during the first 2-4 weeks after surgery; gradual, progressive loading is needed thereafter for optimal return of tendon strength.
- Controlled exercise and rehabilitation enhance recovery of tendon strength and may reduce adhesion formation.
- Tendinopathies can be bilateral.

Technician Tips

During bandage/splint changes, it is essential to prevent flexion of the hock as this reduces the risk of damage to the repair. Splints need to maintain the hock in extension during the first few weeks after surgery to minimize the risk of lengthening of the Achilles mechanism.

SUGGESTED READING

King M, et al: Achilles tendon rupture in dogs. Compend Contin Educ Pract Vet 25:613–620, 2003.

AUTHOR: Peter Gilbert, BVSc, MVetSc, MANZCVS, DACVS
EDITOR: Kathleen Linn, DVM, MS, DACVS

Acid or Alkali (Corrosives) Toxicosis

BASIC INFORMATION

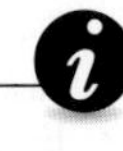

Definition

Exposure, usually by ingestion, to one of a number of household or commercial products containing acids (e.g., acetic, hydrochloric, sulfuric, nitric, phosphoric acid), alkalies (e.g., sodium or potassium carbonate, sodium hydroxide, ammonium hydroxide, potassium permanganate), or free halogens (e.g., chlorine, iodine, or bromine) in quantities sufficient to cause corrosive damage to tissues or produce systemic toxicosis

Epidemiology

SPECIES, AGE, SEX

- All dogs and cats are vulnerable, but dogs are more often affected.
- If contaminated, cats can ingest these toxicants from grooming their hair coat.

RISK FACTORS

Access to household or commercial products, including alkaline batteries, antirust compounds, toilet bowl cleaners, drain openers, and bleaches

Clinical Presentation

DISEASE FORMS/SUBTYPES

- Acids can cause localized coagulative necrosis and superficial burns (perforation less likely).
- Alkalies can cause deeper, penetrating (liquefactive) lesions by solubilizing the mucous membranes (perforation more likely compared to acids).

HISTORY, CHIEF COMPLAINT

- Exposure usually by accidental ingestion, skin or eye contact, or inhalation (rare)

- Evidence/history of exposure to a household cleaning product
- Salivation, protrusion of tongue (common in cats), vomiting (within a few minutes to hours of exposure) may be noted by owners.

PHYSICAL EXAM FINDINGS

- Oral ulcers (lips, gingiva, tongue)
  - Initially, corrosive burns appear milky white or gray, then become black.
- Dysphagia
- Hypersalivation/excessive licking
- Protrusion of tongue/swelling
- Corrosive burns on the skin
- Signs of pain (abdominal or generalized)
- Vomiting, diarrhea
- Lethargy
- Hyperthermia
- Anorexia
- Signs indicating esophageal perforation (rare), such as discomfort when swallowing, or signs of mediastinitis or of sepsis
- Corneal ulcer, blepharitis (ocular exposures)
- If concurrent laryngeal swelling, stridor and/or respiratory distress

Etiology and Pathophysiology

Sources:

- Common household products that contain acids include antirust compounds, gun barrel cleaning fluids, some toilet cleaning liquids, automobile batteries, and swimming pool cleaning agents.
- Alkali-containing products include drain cleaner, laundry products, automatic dishwasher detergents, many toilet bowl cleaners, alkaline batteries, and radiator cleaning agents.

Mechanism of toxicosis:

- Acids and similar corrosive agents cause rapid coagulative necrosis, resulting in pain. Mucosal penetration or perforation is rare.
- Concentrated alkali solutions can penetrate the mucous membranes by dissolving the lipoprotein matrix of cell membranes and destroying nerve endings. They can induce deep, penetrating lesions, including liquefactive necrosis and vascular hemolysis. Perforation is more likely compared to acids.

DIAGNOSIS

Diagnostic Overview

History of exposure to a product containing acid or alkali is the cornerstone of diagnosis and is supported by typical physical exam findings: any combination of hypersalivation, excessive licking, protrusion of tongue, lethargy, hyperthermia, vomiting, and oral lesions (ulcers).

Differential Diagnosis

- Uremic stomatitis
- Liquid potpourri toxicosis
- Cationic detergent exposure (similar to alkaline burns)
- Calicivirus (cats)
- Foreign body obstruction (intractable vomiting)
- Viral or bacterial gastroenteritis
- Garbage toxicosis

Initial Database

- CBC (stress leukocytosis possible)
- Serum biochemistry profile: electrolyte changes due to vomiting, dehydration are possible
- Urinalysis: usually unremarkable
- Thoracic radiographs: indicated if coughing, dyspnea, or fever of unknown origin. May show evidence of pleural effusion (rare; due to esophageal rupture) and/or aspiration pneumonia
- Abdominal radiographs: may show evidence of peritonitis if perforation has occurred

Advanced or Confirmatory Testing

- Abdominal ultrasound if peritonitis is suspected on physical exam or radiographically
- Upper gastrointestinal endoscopy to evaluate mucosal damage or to assess esophageal or gastric perforation, using great care to avoid causing a perforation of damaged tissue; perform within 24 hours of exposure to minimize risk for perforations.

TREATMENT

Treatment Overview

With oral exposure, immediately dilute with water or milk to protect the gastrointestinal (GI) mucosa. With dermal or ocular exposure, wash the exposed area or flush eyes with tepid water for 20 to 30 minutes. Follow up with evaluation and treatment as needed. Whether to hospitalize the patient depends on the amount of toxic exposure, extent of lesions, time course (if only minutes to 2 hours since exposure, full extent of lesions may not be apparent), and owner's emotional/financial/logistical concerns.

Acute General Treatment

- Decontamination of patient (p. 1087)
  - Dermal: Flush exposed area with water for 20 to 30 minutes. For severe burns, surgical debridement may be necessary.
  - Ocular: Flush eyes with tepid tap water (or isotonic saline) for 20 to 30 minutes. Stain the cornea with fluorescein to assess for corneal ulcers (p. 209).
  - Oral exposure: Immediately dilute with milk or water. Chemical neutralization with weak acid or alkali is contraindicated. This can cause an exothermic reaction and more thermal injuries.
  - Induction of vomiting: *contraindicated* (can cause more damage)
  - Activated charcoal: *contraindicated* (ineffective against caustic agents)
  - Gastric lavage: *contraindicated* (risk of perforation)
  - Inhalation (rare): In case of inhalation exposure, move animal to fresh air.
  - If esophageal perforation is suspected, do not allow food or water until the extent of injury is evaluated.
- Protect GI mucosa
  - Proton pump inhibitor (preferred over H2-antagonist)
    - Omeprazole, dogs/cats: 0.5-1 mg/kg PO q 12h
    - Pantoprazole, dogs/cats: 0.7-1 mg/kg IV q 24h; before oral therapy
  - H2-receptor antagonist
    - Famotidine, dogs/cats: 0.5-1 mg/kg PO, SQ, IM, IV q 12h
  - Sucralfate, dogs: 0.5-1 g PO q 8-12h; cats: 0.25-0.5 g PO q 8-12h; administer as a liquid
- Ensure patent airway if respiratory noise or effort apparent (p. 1166)
- Supportive care
  - IV crystalloid fluids (e.g., lactated Ringer's solution) for rehydration or maintenance
  - Broad-spectrum antibiotics (e.g., ampicillin 22 mg/kg IV q 8h plus enrofloxacin 5 mg/kg IM or diluted 1 : 1 with sterile saline and given slowly IV q 12h [5 mg/kg q 24h maximum in cats]) if GI mucosal integrity is compromised and/or secondary infection is identified
  - Glucocorticoids (controversial); may help prevent esophageal stricture due to esophagitis but may delay healing and predispose to infection; concurrent broad-spectrum antibiotic use is of unproven benefit. If used, dexamethasone 0.05-0.1 mg/kg IV or IM or prednisolone 0.5-1 mg/kg PO; q 12h for no more than 3 to 5 days.
  - Manage pain: opiates (e.g., buprenorphine 0.005-0.02 mg/kg IM, IV, or SQ; or fentanyl transdermal patch)
  - Antiemetics: maropitant 1 mg/kg SQ or IV or 2 mg/kg PO q 24h for 5 days
  - Nutrition/dietary therapeutics
    - Severe oral ulcerations may cause dysphagia; give liquid food only for several days.

Nutrition/Diet

Temporary feeding tube placement (esophagostomy, p. 1106) if oral lesions; gastrostomy (percutaneous endoscopic gastrostomy [PEG] for esophageal lesions, p. 1109) can help meet the patient's nutritional needs if he/she is not eating due to mucosal lesions (visual inspection for oral lesions; endoscopic observation for esophageal lesions).

Possible Complications

- Aspiration pneumonitis/pneumonia
- Esophageal perforation and mediastinitis; gastric/enteric perforation and peritonitis
- Esophageal stricture
- Upper airway obstruction if laryngeal edema/inflammation

Recommended Monitoring

- Acutely: blood pressure, respiratory effort, monitor for shock, body temperature
- Chronically: thoracic radiographs, CBC (for evidence of esophageal rupture and mediastinitis or aspiration pneumonia possibly due to esophageal stricture)

PROGNOSIS & OUTCOME

- Good to excellent if animal is treated immediately after exposure
- Poor in patients in hypovolemic shock or if esophageal or stomach perforation occurs

PEARLS & CONSIDERATIONS

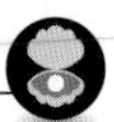

Comments

- Alkaline products with a pH of 12.5 can cause esophageal ulcers; products with a pH of 14 can cause acute esophageal perforation and chronic stricture formation.
- Most household cleaning agents are complex mixtures of chemicals. The clinician must carefully determine the most toxic ingredient and hazard resulting from exposure; consultation with a poison control center is advised.

Prevention

Keep household cleaning products out of reach of pets.

Technician Tips

As with any intoxication, identifying the toxic substance helps significantly with treatment accuracy, monitoring for complications, and prognostication. An owner who calls on the telephone because of possible or certain intoxication should be told to bring the container of what was ingested for identification (label) along with the pet as soon as possible.

Client Education

Store household products appropriately out of reach of pets.

SUGGESTED READING

Gwaltney-Brant SM: Miscellaneous indoor toxicants. In Peterson ME, Talcott PA, editors: Small animal toxicology, ed 3, St. Louis, 2013, Elsevier Saunders, pp 291-308.

AUTHOR: Mary Schell, DVM, DABT, DABVT
EDITOR: Tina Wismer, DVM, MS, DABVT, DABT

Acne

Client Education Sheet

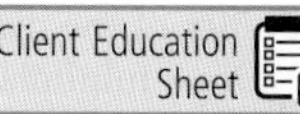

BASIC INFORMATION

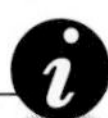

Definition

- Canine acne is a common chronic inflammatory disorder of the chin and lips of young dogs, characterized by deep folliculitis and furunculosis.
- Feline acne is a relatively common idiopathic disorder of follicular cornification.

Epidemiology

SPECIES, AGE, SEX

- Canine acne is more common in young dogs of short-coated breeds.
- Feline acne can develop at any age.

GENETICS, BREED PREDISPOSITION

Large, short-coated dog breeds appear predisposed: boxers, Doberman pinschers, English bulldogs, Great Danes, Weimaraners, mastiffs, rottweilers, and German short-haired pointers

Clinical Presentation

HISTORY, CHIEF COMPLAINT

- Skin lesions are restricted to the chin area, sometimes involving the lips.
- Lesions may be an incidental finding during routine examination.

PHYSICAL EXAM FINDINGS

- Canine acne: early lesions consist of erythematous papules. Lesions can progress to pustules, bullae, or occasional ulcerated draining tracts with serosanguineous discharge on the chin or muzzle.
- Feline acne: asymptomatic comedones on the chin and occasionally the lips. Lesions can evolve to papules, pustules, crusts, and alopecia. Furunculosis and cellulitis can be seen with secondary bacterial infection. Severely affected skin can be edematous, thickened, and scarred. Infected lesions may be pruritic. Regional lymphadenopathy can develop.

Etiology and Pathophysiology

- Unknown cause
- Bacterial involvement is secondary.
- Canine acne can be triggered by local trauma, and genetic predisposition has been suggested.
- Feline acne could be aggravated by poor grooming habits, underlying predisposition to seborrhea, production of abnormal sebum, hair cycle influences, stress, viruses, and immunosuppression.

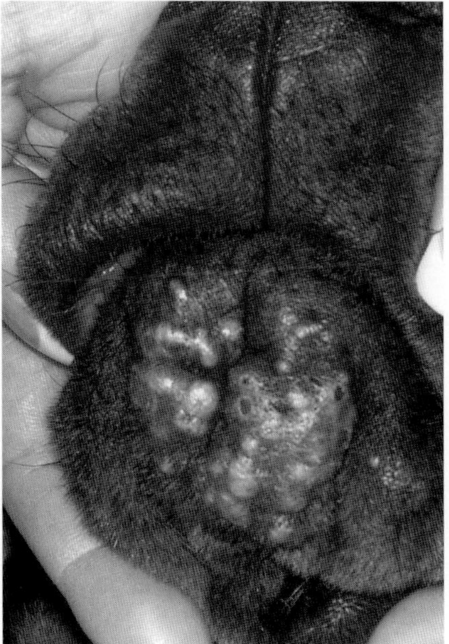

ACNE: CANINE Papular dermatitis with alopecia on the chin of a dog with acne. (Courtesy Dr. Nadia Pagé.)

DIAGNOSIS

Diagnostic Overview

The diagnosis is suspected based on the history and the distribution and aspect of the skin lesions.

Differential Diagnosis

- Demodicosis
- Dermatophytosis
- *Malassezia pachydermatis* dermatitis
- Eosinophilic granuloma (feline)
- Early juvenile cellulitis (canine)
- Contact dermatitis
- Sebaceous gland or other localized skin tumors

Initial Database

- Cytologic evaluation (pustules or exudates): suppurative inflammation and phagocytosed bacteria when secondary infection occurs
- *M. pachydermatis* occasionally can be found (cats).
- Skin scrapings to rule out demodicosis (p. 1091)

Advanced or Confirmatory Testing

- Dermatohistopathologic evaluation of skin biopsy (rarely necessary): follicular hyperkeratosis and dilation, perifolliculitis, folliculitis and/or furunculosis, and cellulitis; bacterial culture and sensitivity test may be needed if unresponsive to appropriate empirical antibiotic therapy
- Fungal culture in dermatophyte testing medium if dermatophytosis is suspected

TREATMENT

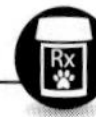

Treatment Overview

Treatment consists of elimination of secondary bacterial infection, if present, and control of recurrence.

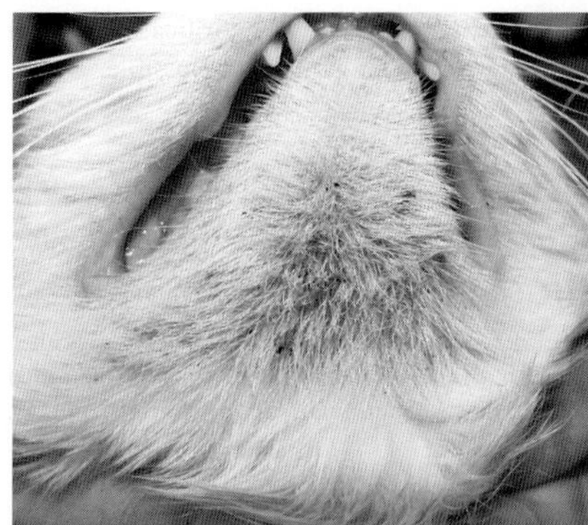

ACNE: FELINE Comedones (blackheads) on the chin of a cat with uncomplicated acne. (Courtesy Dr. Manon Paradis.)

Acute General Treatment

- Choice of treatment will depend on the severity of the disease.
  - Dogs: minimize trauma to the chin.
  - Cats: clipping the affected area can increase efficacy of topical treatment.

Topical treatment:

- Mild lesions can be controlled with application of benzoyl peroxide shampoo or gel (2.5%) q 24h until resolution, then 1-2 times per week as needed. Chlorhexidine shampoo or wipes can also be useful in secondarily infected lesions (dogs).
- Phytosphingosine-containing products (Douxo Seborrhea Spot-on) applied twice weekly can sometimes be useful in cats.
- Mupirocin or fusidic acid ointments or creams may be applied q 12-24h until resolution (3-4 weeks). These medications may be considered initially or if there is a lack of response to treatment with the above options.
- In cats, tretinoin 0.01%-0.025% cream or lotion may be used in refractory cases q 1-3 days for 4 weeks, then as needed.
- Glucocorticoid creams may temporarily be needed to reduce inflammation once secondary bacterial infection has been eliminated.
- Others: sulfur-salicylic acid shampoos, 0.75% metronidazole gel, other topical medications containing clindamycin, erythromycin, or tetracycline (cats)

Systemic treatment:

- In more severe cases, secondary bacterial infection can be treated with appropriate systemic antibiotics for 3-6 weeks. Good empirical choices include cephalexin 22 mg/kg PO q 8h or 30 mg/kg q 12h (dogs) and clavulanic acid–potentiated amoxicillin 13.75-25 mg/kg PO q 12h (cats, dogs). In cats hard to pill, cefovecin 8 mg/kg SQ q 2 weeks can be considered.
- Refractory feline cases may benefit from systemic isotretinoin (2 mg/kg PO q 24h; CAUTION: severe teratogenicity in animals and humans); in responsive cases, improvement should be seen in 1 month.

Chronic Treatment

For recurring lesions, topical medication can be used as needed for long-term therapy.

Possible Complications

- Localized irritation with topical preparations containing benzoyl peroxide or tretinoin
- Nephrotoxicity due to ingestion of the excipient polyethylene base in mupirocin ointment is unlikely with use of small amounts of the product on a localized skin area. The product should not be licked for 5-10 minutes after treatment.
- Chronic topical corticosteroids can cause adrenal suppression and local skin atrophy.
- Oral isotretinoin can induce side effects of diarrhea, anorexia, vomiting, conjunctivitis, increased liver enzyme levels, hypertriglyceridemia, and hypercholesterolemia. It is teratogenic. With chronic use, skeletal abnormalities are a concern. It can possibly be harmful in cases of accidental human ingestion.

Recommended Monitoring

With oral isotretinoin therapy: pretreatment measurement of tear production, CBC, chemistry profile, and urinalysis. Repeat monitoring every 1-2 months.

PROGNOSIS & OUTCOME

- Canine acne carries a good prognosis, with many dogs achieving a permanent cure. Some dogs require lifelong topical therapy.
- Feline acne also has a good prognosis, but lifelong intermittent or continuous therapy is often needed.
- In severe cases, active lesions can resolve with scarring.

PEARLS & CONSIDERATIONS

Comments

- Owners should avoid expressing the lesions because of possible internal rupture of the hair follicles, inducing local inflammation.
- Benzoyl peroxide–containing medications can bleach carpets and fabrics.
- When not secondarily infected, feline acne is a cosmetic disease that does not affect the cat's quality of life. It can be left untreated.

Technician Tips

The owners should be instructed to stop the topical treatment and contact the medical team if the patient develops worsened local irritation.

SUGGESTED READING

Miller WH Jr, et al: Bacterial skin diseases. In Muller & Kirk's Small animal dermatology, ed 7, St. Louis, 2013, Elsevier Mosby, p 201.

AUTHOR: Nadia Pagé, DMV, MSc, DACVD
EDITOR: Manon Paradis, DMV, MVSc, DACVD

Acral Lick Dermatitis

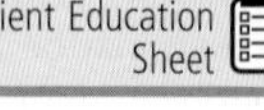

BASIC INFORMATION

Definition

- Multifactorial condition characterized by a firm, ulcerative, or alopecic cutaneous plaque induced by excessive, compulsive licking of the lower portion of a limb
- Acral (Greek: *akron*, "extremity"): pertaining to the extremities of peripheral body parts

Synonym

Lick granuloma

Epidemiology

SPECIES, AGE, SEX

Dogs, adult

GENETICS, BREED PREDISPOSITION

- Predisposed breeds: Doberman pinscher, Labrador retriever, Great Dane, Irish setter, golden retriever, German shepherd

RISK FACTORS

Underlying conditions include allergic disease and bacterial infection.

Clinical Presentation

HISTORY, CHIEF COMPLAINT

- Excessive, compulsive licking at a focal area on a distal limb, resulting in a firm, alopecic, eroded or ulcerated plaque or nodule.
- Occasional history of trauma or joint disease in the affected area

PHYSICAL EXAM FINDINGS

- Usually only a single lesion is noted. Most common sites include dorsal carpus, metacarpus, or metatarsus.

- A firm, erythematous, alopecic, eroded or ulcerated plaque or nodule is typical. Saliva staining of the surrounding hair, purulent oozing tracts, and dependent edema may also occur.
- The presence of multiple lesions is usually associated with an underlying skin disorder (e.g., atopic dermatitis, food hypersensitivity, pyoderma).

Etiology and Pathophysiology

- It was previously believed that most cases of acral lick dermatitis (ALD) were of psychogenic origin. Currently, it is thought that most cases are an organic disease (e.g., hypersensitivity skin disease, pyoderma, joint disease, hypothyroidism, neoplasia), and even in the few cases where a psychogenic cause was the instigating factor, secondary bacterial infection is common in these lesions.
- Lesion development is normally associated with chronic licking of the affected area. Chronic licking elicits a deep inflammatory response, leading to the development of an erosive plaque and frequent secondary deep bacterial infection.
- After initiation of the lesion, constant licking perpetuates the problem.
- In some cases, no organic cause can be identified. In these individuals, obsessive-compulsive behavior associated with boredom and separation anxiety is important.

DIAGNOSIS

Diagnostic Overview

Diagnosis is based on history and physical exam. The diagnostic plan must include tests to rule out underlying causes of chronic licking and self-mutilation. Diagnostic procedures are selected based in large part on the dog's signalment, the presence of other dermatologic signs, and response to previous treatments.

Differential Diagnosis

- Demodicosis (affected individuals normally have more widespread skin lesions)
- Fungal infection (dermatophytosis, deep mycosis)
- Hypersensitivity disorders (food, flea, environmental; affected dogs have more widespread skin lesions)
- Pyoderma (localized or generalized)
- Foreign body granuloma (historic information)
- Previous trauma (history of injury)
- Degenerative joint disease
- Neoplasia (histiocytoma, mastocytoma)
- Pressure point granuloma or pyoderma
- Calcinosis circumscripta
- Acral mutilation due to a sensory neuropathy
- Behavioral; boredom, separation anxiety (rule out organic skin disease)

Initial Database

- Clean the surface of the lesion, and then squeeze firmly until drops of seropurulent or serohemorrhagic exudate appear on the surface. This material can be collected for cytologic examination and bacterial culture.
- Fine-needle aspiration of skin for cytologic evaluation (to rule out neoplasia)
- Skin scrapings (to rule out demodicosis) (p. 1091)
- Fungal culture (to rule out dermatophytosis and deep mycosis)

Advanced or Confirmatory Testing

- Radiographic evaluation of chronic lesions may reveal a secondary periosteal reaction. Underlying joint disease may be identified.
- Skin biopsy (to rule out or confirm deep bacterial or fungal infections and neoplasia)
- Bacterial cultures may be obtained from an aseptically acquired biopsy punch specimen.
- Behavioral consultation (p. 1063)

TREATMENT

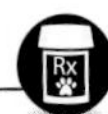

Treatment Overview

- Eliminate secondary infection and inflammation.
- Control behavioral factors (more effective after inflammation and secondary infection are controlled).
- It is critical that the patient not be allowed to lick the affected area once treatment commences.

Acute General Treatment

Choice of treatment will depend on the cause and severity of the condition:

- Systemic antibiotic therapy
    - Start with a course of antibiotic selected according to bacterial culture and sensitivity results (pending results, can use cephalexin) if a bacterial infection is confirmed or suspected. Prolonged antibiotic therapy (up to 6 months) may dramatically improve long-standing lesions and resolve licking. Continue treatment 3 weeks beyond regression of the lesion.
- Topical application q 8-12h of analgesic, steroidal, or bad-tasting medications (e.g., 8 mL of fluocinolone with DMSO (Synotic) mixed with 3 mL of flunixin meglumine (Banamine) *or* capsaicin (Zostrix). Their sole use is often disappointing.
- Intralesional triamcinolone acetonide (Vetalog) or methylprednisolone acetate (Depo-Medrol) injected directly into the lesion
- Physical restraint (Elizabethan collar, bandaging, casts, muzzle) is often essential.
- Surgical excision usually should not be attempted because of difficulties with closure and a high incidence of wound breakdown.
- CO_2 laser resurfacing may be beneficial in refractory, or multidrug-resistant infections.

Chronic Treatment

When dealing with a true psychogenic acral lick dermatitis:

- Endorphin blocker; naltrexone (2 mg/kg PO q 12-24h) *or*
- Endorphin substitute: hydrocodone (0.25 mg/kg PO q 8h)
- Behavior-modifying drugs: clomipramine (1-3 mg/kg PO q 24h), fluoxetine (1 mg/kg PO q 24h), or amitriptyline (1-3 mg/kg PO q 12h)

Drug Interactions

Do not concurrently use drugs with central nervous system depressant activity (e.g., antihistamines, clomipramine, amitriptyline, fluoxetine).

PROGNOSIS & OUTCOME

Guarded prognosis. Therapy must focus on organic dermatologic nature of the condition as well as behavioral factors involved.

PEARLS & CONSIDERATIONS

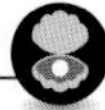

Comments

- Acral lick dermatitis remains one of the most challenging and frustrating problems seen by specialists and general practitioners.

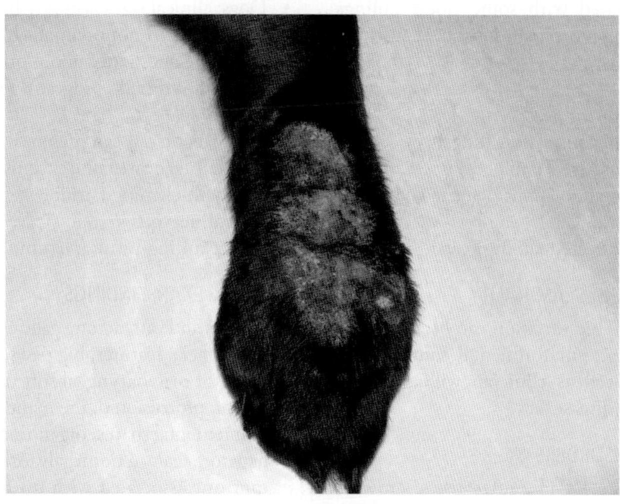

ACRAL LICK DERMATITIS Acral lick dermatitis on the dorsal carpus and metacarpus of a Labrador retriever. (Copyright Dr. Manon Paradis.)

- Infection should be suspected in all acral lick lesions, especially when the surface is ulcerated. Oral antibiotics are one of the most important treatments of acral lick dermatitis.
  - In one study, deep bacterial infection was present in 94% of the lesions, with 48% of cases yielding multidrug-resistant bacteria.
- Behavioral component is often secondary. Investigate potential for underlying skin disease and treat accordingly. One of the common causes of treatment failure in acral lick dermatitis is the inability to identify primary or perpetuating factors.

Technician Tips

Patients may lick and chew intensely at the lesion if it is uncovered even briefly, causing severe tissue damage. Close monitoring of bandages and Elizabethan collars are essential.

Client Education

Behavioral modification

SUGGESTED READING

Miller WH Jr, et al: Muller & Kirk's Small animal dermatology, ed 7, St. Louis, 2013, Elsevier Saunders, pp 205, 650-653.

AUTHOR & EDITOR: Manon Paradis, DMV, MVSc, DACVD

Acromegaly

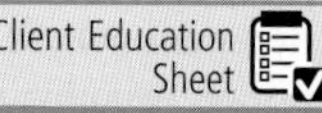

BASIC INFORMATION

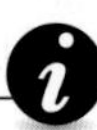

Definition

The clinical consequences of exposure to excess endogenous growth hormone (GH)

Synonym

Hypersomatotropism is often used as a synonym, although strictly speaking, it refers to excess endogenous GH alone and not its consequences.

Epidemiology

SPECIES, AGE, SEX

- Cats: middle-aged/older (mean, 10 years; range, 2-17 years); male predominance
- Prevalence among cats is higher than previously recognized, ranging from 1 in 6 to 1 in 3 diabetic cats. Nondiabetic cats can have acromegaly.
- Dogs: older, unspayed females overrepresented due to diestrus-induced GH production

GENETICS, BREED PREDISPOSITION

- No breed predisposition proven; Maine coon cats might be overrepresented.
- A polymorphism in the *AIP* gene has been associated with some cases; siblings with the polymorphism have been affected simultaneously.

RISK FACTORS

- Progestin administration (dogs)
- Being an unspayed female (dogs)
- Environmental organohalogenated contaminant exposure (cats)
- Having an affected sibling (cats)

GEOGRAPHY AND SEASONALITY

In cats, geographic variation can be associated with cause (e.g., environmental contaminant exposure) as well as clinician willingness to screen for the disease.

ASSOCIATED DISORDERS

- Chronic excess GH causes tissue growth, eventually resulting in myriad changes in various body systems (see below).
- GH-induced insulin resistance often (cats), although not always (dogs, some cats), leads to diabetes mellitus

Clinical Presentation

DISEASE FORMS/SUBTYPES

- Cats: excessive GH secretion by an adenoma of somatotrophs of the pituitary gland
- Dogs: almost always secondary to progestin-induced GH production and secretion by the mammary glands
  - Endogenous progesterone elevation (i.e., diestrus, pregnancy) or progestin administration (e.g., for estrus suppression) can induce mammary hyperplasia.
  - Can occur due to GH secretion by malignant or benign mammary tumors
  - Rarely due to GH-secreting pituitary adenomas

HISTORY, CHIEF COMPLAINT

- In diabetic acromegalic patients
  - Polyuria, polydipsia, polyphagia (sometimes extreme polyphagia)
  - Weight gain with good or poor diabetic control
  - Other complaints related to diabetes mellitus (p. 251)
- Dogs: clinical signs typically begin 3-5 weeks after estrus in nonpregnant bitches; owners should be questioned about prior administration of a synthetic progestin (e.g., megestrol acetate).
- Nondiabetic cats can present with myocardial thickening/heart failure, signs due to upper airway thickening (stridor/stertor), or rarely, central nervous system (CNS) signs due to an expanding pituitary tumor.

PHYSICAL EXAM FINDINGS

- In dogs and cats, acromegalic changes include broad facial features, big paws, diffuse thickening of oropharyngeal soft tissues, stridor/stertor, protrusion of the mandible, widening of interdental spaces, organomegaly (palpable hepatomegaly, renomegaly, or splenomegaly, murmur associated with cardiomegaly).
- Approximately 75% of cats have no phenotypic features specific to acromegaly.
- Cats: A minority presents with CNS signs due to an expanding tumor or with heart failure due to myocardial changes.
- Dogs may develop skin folds around the head, neck, and extremities.

Etiology and Pathophysiology

- In cats and rarely in dogs, the excess GH secretion is due to a tumor (usually adenoma) of the pars distalis of the anterior pituitary (somatotrophs).
- In dogs, disease stems from progesterone-induced GH secretion by mammary tissue. The progesterone may be endogenous (diestrus) or exogenous.
- Effects of GH are the same, whether secreted from the pituitary or mammary tissue.
- Chronic GH excess has catabolic and anabolic effects. GH results in elevation of liver-derived insulin-like growth factor 1 (IGF-1).
- Anabolic effects are almost entirely mediated by IGF-1, which causes proliferation of bone, cartilage, soft tissues, and viscera.
- Catabolic effects: GH stimulates hepatic gluconeogenesis and promotes lipolysis. Insulin antagonism occurs due to a decrease in insulin receptors and postreceptor antagonism. Diabetes mellitus usually results.

DIAGNOSIS

Diagnostic Overview

- Serum IGF-1 measurement is an effective screening tool in cats and dogs.
- Given the high prevalence of acromegaly among diabetic cats, screening of newly diagnosed diabetic cats is advocated by the author.
  - If IGF-1 is above the reference range, it is 95% certain the disease is present.
  - IGF-1 can be falsely low (≈10% of cats) in untreated or newly insulin-treated diabetic cats (IGF-1 production requires sufficient insulin); re-test 6 weeks after initiation of insulin therapy if suspicion for acromegaly remains.
- Screening for acromegaly should be considered in nondiabetic cats with cardiac

hypertrophy, polyphagic cats, and cats with unexplained inspiratory noise, among other presentations due to GH excess.
- Cats: intracranial imaging (CT or MRI) can further increase the certainty of the diagnosis, although absence of a visible pituitary mass does not rule out the possibility of acromegaly.

Differential Diagnosis

Differentials for insulin antagonism/resistance:
- Hyperadrenocorticism (p. 485)
- Infection
- Drugs (e.g., glucocorticoids, progestins)
- Hyperthyroidism (cats, p. 503)
- Hypothyroidism (dogs, p. 525)
- Chronic pancreatitis (cats, p. 740)
- Obesity (p. 700)
- Diabetes management problems with insulin type, storage, or administration (p. 251)

Differential for physical examination changes mimicking acromegaly:
- Primary hypothyroidism (dogs, p. 525)

Differentials for elevated IGF-1 (rare):
- GH and IGF-1 concentrations may be elevated in hypothyroid dogs. Measurement of total thyroxine (T_4), free T_4, and canine thyroid-stimulating hormone (cTSH) concentrations can be used to exclude primary hypothyroidism.
- IGF-1 can be elevated in diabetic cats without acromegaly (<5% of cases)

Differentials for myocardial thickening:
- Hypertrophic cardiomyopathy (primary HCM, p. 505)
- Systemic hypertension (p. 501)

Initial Database

- Determine if diabetes mellitus is present (fasting blood glucose, urine glucose, fructosamine); if diabetes is known to be present but uncontrolled, consider serial blood glucose assessment and revisit management with owner, including appropriate insulin storage.
- In nondiabetic and diabetic cases: serum IGF-1 measurement
- Abdominal imaging may be normal or hepatomegaly and renomegaly may be seen.

Advanced or Confirmatory Testing

- In cats, intracranial imaging (CT or MRI) of the pituitary gland can help establish whether the pituitary is enlarged or a mass is present; absence of enlargement does not exclude the disease.
- Cats and dogs: GH can be measured, but it is difficult to find a suitable laboratory with a validated assay.

TREATMENT

Treatment Overview

- Treatment is ideally aimed at removing the cause.
- Dogs: cessation of progestogen administration or neutering
- Cats (and rare dogs with a pituitary tumor): removal of the pituitary tumor or inhibition of tumoral GH secretion
- Dogs and cats: conservative treatment entails merely attending to the consequences of GH excess (including diabetes mellitus); this is suboptimal and above options yield better clinical results and quality of life.

Acute General Treatment

- Diabetic pets require treatment for the diabetes (p. 251).
- Dogs with diestrus-associated acromegaly could be treated temporarily with aglepristone, a progesterone receptor blocker (10 mg/kg/month), pending neutering or cessation of (the effects of) progestogen treatment.
- Cats presented in congestive heart failure should be treated accordingly (p. 408).

Chronic Treatment

- In cats, best results seen with hypophysectomy
  - Diabetes mellitus resolves in 85% of acromegalic, diabetic cats after surgery.
  - Availability is limited in the United States.
- In cats, the somatostatin analog pasireotide effectively inhibits GH secretion (short-acting form: 0.03 mg/kg q 12-24h; long-acting formulation 8 mg/kg/month or lowest effective dose)
  - Does not usually shrink tumor
  - Has been associated with diabetic remission in 1 of 4 cases
  - Currently very expensive
- Rarely, cats are responsive to the cheaper alternative cabergoline (5-15 mcg/kg/day).
- Radiotherapy can shrink a pituitary tumor and improve diabetic control.
  - Efficacy and timing of effect are unpredictable.
  - Multiple anesthetics episodes are necessary, and hormones never normalize.
- If the inciting cause is not removed, treat the consequences as best as possible.
  - Treating diabetes mellitus in cats can be frustrating, eventually requiring high insulin dosages.
  - Quality of life of treated cats should be monitored closely; appetite is not a good measure given the GH-driven polyphagia.

Nutrition/Diet

- Cats: if concurrently diabetic, use a low carbohydrate diet

Possible Complications

- Cats: if treated with high insulin dosages, hypoglycemia can occur due to pulsatile GH secretion by the pituitary tumor; monitoring of home blood glucose can screen for overdose. Owners should be instructed on how to deal with hypoglycemia effectively.
- Radiotherapy complications include damage to local tissues and hypopituitarism.
- With hypophysectomy, hypocortisolemia, and hypothyroidism; ongoing supplementation for both is necessary postoperatively.

Recommended Monitoring

- Serum IGF-1 should normalize with effective treatment.
- Diabetes mellitus should be monitored as for any diabetic patient (p. 251).

PROGNOSIS & OUTCOME

- Cats and dogs: if inciting cause is eliminated at an early stage, life span and quality of life can be normalized.
- If acromegaly has been present for a long time, some physical changes can cause significant morbidity (e.g., cardiac hypertrophy, narrowed airways, pancreatopathy/pancreatitis).
- Cats: myocardial changes are reversible with hypophysectomy.
- Cats: diabetes mellitus resolves in 85% of hypophysectomy-treated patients and 25% of pasireotide-treated patients

PEARLS & CONSIDERATIONS

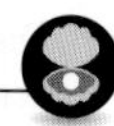

Comments

- Understanding of acromegaly/hypersomatotropism in cats is rapidly changing; among humans, most acromegalic patients are not diabetic. Increasingly, nondiabetic cats are recognized as suffering from acromegaly. Clinicians are therefore encouraged to keep an open mind about the exact presentation of feline acromegaly.
- If a cat or dog is treated for its diabetes only, regular quality of life assessments should be conducted, ideally using standardized assessment surveys (diabetes apps are available).
- Weight gain in the face of poorly controlled diabetes mellitus is highly suggestive of acromegaly.

Prevention

- In dogs, spaying and avoidance of exogenous progestin administration

Technician Tips

- Quality of life of diabetic, acromegalic cats can be improved by teaching the owners to perform home blood glucose monitoring and by conducting regular quality of life assessments.
- A pet diabetes app is available for free download onto smartphones and tablets from Android (http://bit.ly/1q3jCV5) and iPhone App stores (http://apple.co/203OoK2).

SUGGESTED READINGS

Niessen SJM, et al: Hypersomatotropism, acromegaly, and hyperadrenocorticism and feline diabetes mellitus. Vet Clin North Am Small Anim Pract 43:319-350, 2013.

AUTHOR: Stijn J.M. Niessen, DVM, PhD, DECVIM
EDITOR: Ellen N. Behrend, VMD, PhD, DACVIM

Actinomycosis and Nocardiosis

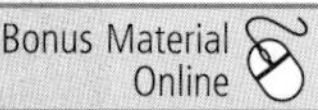

BASIC INFORMATION

Definition

Infection with *Actinomyces* or *Nocardia*, gram-positive, branching, filamentous bacteria

Epidemiology

SPECIES, AGE, SEX

- Cats and dogs of any age and either sex
- Middle-aged or older, male cats and large-breed, male dogs may be predisposed.

RISK FACTORS

- Outdoor cats that fight with other cats
- Dogs kept outdoors or used for hunting
- Important risk factors include
  - Immunosuppressive drug therapy
  - Infection with feline retroviruses
  - Animal fight injuries
  - Concurrent chronic illness
- Disseminated nocardiosis, including central nervous system (CNS) infection, reported in dogs treated with cyclosporine

CONTAGION AND ZOONOSIS

- Not highly contagious during casual contact but may be transmitted through bites, scratches, or contact of exudate with broken skin
- Caution while handling infected animals or exudate is warranted. Standard barrier precautions are recommended.
- Immunosuppressed people are at increased risk.

ASSOCIATED DISORDERS

- *Actinomyces* and *Nocardia* spp. have been isolated from pyothorax exudate in dogs and cats.
- *Actinomyces* and *Nocardia* spp. may be components of polymicrobial infections, particularly those caused by bite wounds, migrating foreign material, or other penetrating injuries.

Clinical Presentation

DISEASE FORMS/SUBTYPES

- Deep cutaneous and subcutaneous infections: most common in dogs
- Pyothorax, pneumonia
- Disseminated/systemic infections (often involving the skin but bone, CNS, and other anatomic sites may be affected)

HISTORY, CHIEF COMPLAINT

- Nonspecific clinical signs: fever, lethargy, inappetance, weight loss
- Cutaneous infections: history of a chronic non-healing wound with exudate or an indolent spreading infection is typical.
- Signs related to the site of infection (e.g., coughing, tachypnea, and dyspnea with thoracic infections)

PHYSICAL EXAM FINDINGS

- Systemic signs (see above)
- Cutaneous infections
  - Cervicofacial region is most commonly affected (up to 50% of cases in dogs).
  - Inflammation, marked exudate production, draining tracts, local extension
  - Skin lesions may develop into SQ abscess and may be masslike and painful.
- Pyothorax, pneumonia: systemic and respiratory signs
- Disseminated infection
  - Skin lesions often present (see above)
  - Neurologic deficits possible (by direct CNS infection or extension of vertebral osteomyelitis)
  - Ophthalmic changes if ocular infection

Etiology and Pathophysiology

- *Nocardia* spp. are aerobes commonly present in soil, detritus, and organic debris. *Actinomyces* spp. are anaerobic or microaerophilic organisms present in the normal oropharyngeal flora of cats, dogs, and people.
- *Nocardia* and *Actinomyces* infections may be transmitted by physical trauma and penetrating injuries (bites, scratches, and migrating foreign material).
- Pyothorax results from direct inoculation of organisms into the pleural space from bite wounds or other penetrating trauma. Pneumonia develops from inhalation of organisms and/or contaminated foreign material. Putatively, multinodular pulmonary infections may result from hematogenous spread.
- Abdominal abscesses, peritonitis, and internal organ infections are associated with disseminated disease or direct inoculation of the peritoneal cavity.
- Copious exudate inhibits phagocytosis and impairs antibiotic distribution and activity.
- Sulfur granules are grossly visible yellow, tan, or pale, 1-2 mm concretions of bacteria and exudate that are highly characteristic of but not pathognomonic for actinomycosis or nocardiosis.
- *Actinomyces* infections are often present as a co-infection with other bacteria (e.g., oral flora).
- *Nocardia* spp. are facultative, intracellular pathogens that may flourish in animals with impaired cell-mediated immunity.
- The risk of dissemination of infection increases with chronicity, compromised immune status, and when adequate therapy is delayed.

DIAGNOSIS

Diagnostic Overview

Actinomycosis or nocardiosis should be considered when a highly exudative infection is present, particularly in cases of pyothorax or deep cutaneous infection. Suspicion is enhanced by the presence of sulfur granules and confirmed by identification of filamentous organisms cytologically, histopathologically, or on culture.

Differential Diagnosis

- Uncomplicated abscesses and other deep pyodermas
- Neoplasia
- (Pyo-)granulomatous diseases (e.g., fungal, *Pythium* or *Lagenidium*, mycobacterial)
- Sterile nodular panniculitis

Initial Database

- Evaluate exudate grossly for the presence of sulfur granules, recalling that these granules may or may not be present.
- Cytologic evaluation (Diff-Quik, Wright-Giemsa, and/or Gram stains) of lesions or exudate may reliably demonstrate filamentous organisms.
- Aerobic culture is typically successful in isolating *Nocardia* spp.
- *Actinomyces* spp. are more fastidious, and overgrowth of co-infecting organisms may obscure the diagnosis.

Advanced or Confirmatory Testing

- Positive acid-fast staining of filamentous organisms (cytology or biopsy) supports a *Nocardia* diagnosis, but negative staining cannot be used to differentiate actinomycosis from nocardiosis.
- Histopathologic evaluation of tissue is used to rule out other disorders. In actinomycosis/nocardiosis, histology may confirm pyogranulomatous inflammation, with or without a fibrous capsule and/or filamentous organisms.

TREATMENT

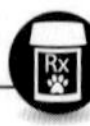

Treatment Overview

- Reduction of exudate by surgical intervention is advocated when practical.
- Clinical improvement is often detectable within 2 weeks. Duration of therapy depends on clinical response (a common treatment period is 6-12 weeks, but up to 12 months may be required).
- Prolonged antibiotic therapy should be based on results of culture and susceptibility testing.
- Some species of *Nocardia* (e.g., *N. farcinica*) are highly resistant to antibiotic treatment and justify a more intensive or combination drug treatment.

Acute and Chronic Treatment

- *Actinomyces* spp. are usually susceptible to penicillin V (40 mg/kg PO q 8h) and its derivatives or clindamycin (11-30 mg/kg PO q 12h).

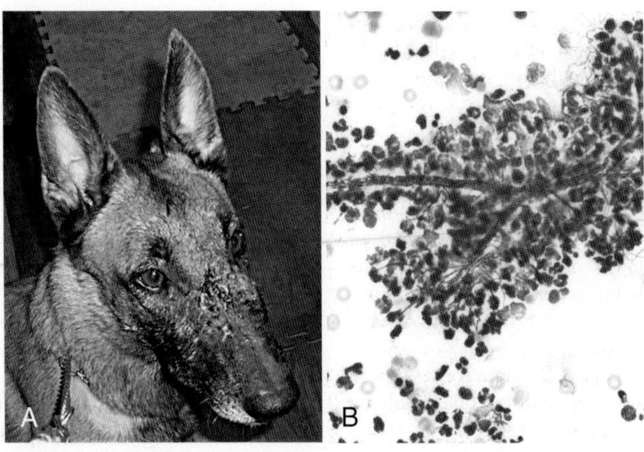

ACTINOMYCOSIS A, Ulcerative draining wound spreading across the muzzle of a 3-year-old Belgian Malinois with cervico-facial actinomycosis. **B,** Aspirates from a maxillary mass on the dog in panel **A** (50× magnification, Wright-Giemsa stain). Note the branching filamentous bacteria surrounded by inflammatory cells.

- *Nocardia* spp. are usually sensitive to sulfonamides (e.g., trimethoprim-sulfa 30-45 mg/kg PO q 12h). Successful treatment of nocardiosis has been reported with many antibiotics, including ampicillin, amikacin and erythromycin.

Possible Complications

When using sulfonamide antibiotics, monitoring of adverse effects such as anemia, leukopenia, keratoconjunctivitis sicca (dry eye), cutaneous drug eruptions, hepatopathy, and polyarthritis is indicated. Long-term sulfonamide treatment may increase the risk of these complications.

PROGNOSIS & OUTCOME

- *Actinomyces* infections have a more favorable prognosis compared to *Nocardia* infections.
- Localized infections may respond well to treatment. Disseminated disease carries a poor prognosis.
- Individual patient factors, such as immunosuppression, may impact prognosis.
- Recurrence may occur in some cases despite clinically apparent resolution and appropriate therapy.
- Relapse may occur if the duration of treatment is inadequate or if appropriate treatment is delayed or interrupted. Incomplete surgical excision may contribute to indolent infections.

PEARLS & CONSIDERATIONS

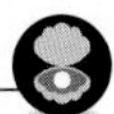

Comments

Culture and histopathologic analysis of tissue are gold standard diagnostic tests, but simple cytologic examination is a practical and high-yield test. Often, filamentous organisms may be cytologically apparent when culture or biopsy is inconclusive.

Technician Tips

Standard barrier precautions, such as a protective gown and gloves, should be worn while handling animals with draining lesions to protect against zoonosis and to prevent contamination of the skin.

SUGGESTED READING

Sykes J: Actinomycosis and nocardiosis. In Greene CE, editor: Infectious diseases of the dog and cat, ed 4, St. Louis, 2012, Elsevier Saunders, pp 484-495.

AUTHOR: Kirk Ryan, DVM, DACVIM
EDITOR: Joseph Taboada, DVM, DACVIM

Acute Abdomen

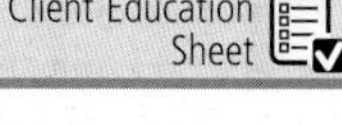

BASIC INFORMATION

Definition

A sudden onset of abdominal pain

Epidemiology

SPECIES, AGE, SEX

Dogs more commonly affected than cats

GENETICS, BREED PREDISPOSITION

Gastric dilation/volvulus (GDV) typically affects large-breed, deep-chested dogs. Pancreatitis is common in middle-aged, small- to medium-sized dogs.

RISK FACTORS

- Dietary indiscretion may result in pancreatitis or gastrointestinal (GI) foreign body.
- Previous abdominal surgery for intestinal foreign body or other conditions can increase the chance of subsequent obstruction through intestinal injury or adhesions.
- Infectious disease that can cause GI hypermotility (e.g., canine parvovirus) may predispose to intussusception.

CONTAGION AND ZOONOSIS

Certain infectious causes (e.g., canine parvovirus) can be highly contagious.

ASSOCIATED DISORDERS

Depends on severity and nature of underlying disorder. May include hypovolemia, hemorrhage, dehydration, sepsis, or hypoalbuminemia. Systemic complications may prove life-threatening.

Clinical Presentation

HISTORY, CHIEF COMPLAINT

- Evidence of abdominal pain
- Collapse
- Vomiting, including hemoptysis
- Diarrhea: small or large bowel (p. 1215)
- GI bleeding: melena (duodenal/jejunal) or hematochezia (colonic/rectal)
- Weight loss
- Anorexia
- History of dietary indiscretion
- History of medications that affect GI mucosal integrity (e.g., nonsteroidal antiinflammatory drugs [NSAIDs])
- History of incomplete or absent vaccinations (e.g., for canine parvovirus)

PHYSICAL EXAM FINDINGS

- Signs of abdominal pain
  - Tense abdomen, praying position, vocalizing
  - Limited accuracy: stoic patients may hide signs of pain; fearful patients may tense the abdomen even in absence of pain.
- Collapse/weakness
- Perfusion abnormalities (e.g., tachycardia, poor pulse quality, pale or hyperemic mucous membranes)
- Dehydration may coexist with hypovolemia (e.g., dry mucous membranes, skin tenting, enophthalmos)

Etiology and Pathophysiology

Causes can be categorized according to organ system and treatment approach:

- GI
  - Surgical: obstruction (e.g., foreign body, intussusception, neoplasia); GDV; perforation (e.g., ruptured gastric/duodenal

ulcer); strangulation (e.g., through a hernia); mesenteric volvulus; colonic torsion
  - Medical: gastroenteritis/dietary indiscretion; hemorrhage/ulceration; infectious (parvovirus, parasites)
- Liver
  - Surgical: neoplasia; abscess; bile peritonitis
  - Medical: acute hepatic injury (leptospirosis, ascending portal infection, severe intoxication), certain forms of neoplasia
- Pancreas
  - Surgical: neoplasia, abscess
  - Medical: pancreatitis (surgery seldom recommended for pancreatitis)
- Spleen
  - Surgical: neoplasia, torsion, trauma, abscess
- Urogenital
  - Surgical: pyometra, urolithiasis, trauma, ureteral obstruction, prostatic infection, neoplasia, uterine torsion, testicular torsion
  - Medical: pyelonephritis, urethral obstruction, urolithiasis, neoplasia
- Adrenal
  - Surgical: carcinoma, pheochromocytoma
- Generalized peritoneal disease
  - Surgical: septic peritonitis (e.g., ruptured viscus, bite wounds), chemical peritonitis (e.g., uroabdomen)
  - Medical: neoplasia (e.g., carcinomatosis)
- Systemic disorders
  - Medical: hemorrhage, thromboembolism, congestive heart failure, hypoalbuminemia, vasculitis

Pathophysiology:
- Abdominal pain is due to stimulation of nociceptors in the abdominal organs and peritoneum.
- Hemodynamic instability is a common sequela to acute abdomen (e.g., hemoabdomen, septic peritonitis) due to fluid loss. Vasodilation associated with systemic inflammatory response syndrome may also be present. Prompt resuscitation with intravenous fluids with or without vasopressors is a priority even before definitive diagnosis or therapy is recommended.

DIAGNOSIS

Diagnostic Overview
- The key decision regarding patients with an acute abdomen is whether emergent surgical intervention is required.
- History, physical examination, baseline laboratory data (including cytologic and laboratory analysis of peritoneal fluids), and diagnostic imaging findings all aid in reaching this important decision.
- A diagnostic approach to peritonitis is outlined on p. 1439.

Differential Diagnosis
- Chronic abdominal disorder with acute exacerbation
- Tension/abdominal guarding on exam in anxious patient
- Referred or apparent abdominal pain due to spinal pain (e.g., intervertebral disc disease [IVDD], discospondylitis, trauma)

Initial Database
- Packed cell volume (PCV)/total plasma protein (TPP) or total solids (TS): may identify anemia or hemoconcentration
  - Low TPP/TS in face of a normal or elevated PCV is concerning for acute blood loss but may also reflect hypoproteinemia from vasculitis, hepatic disease, or other cause.
- Lactate: elevated blood lactate concentration usually reflects hypoperfusion due to volume depletion or distributive shock.
- CBC and blood smear evaluation: leukocytosis or leukopenia, thrombocytopenia, anemia, erythrocytosis possible
  - Thrombocytosis may be identified in cases of chronic GI hemorrhage.
  - The presence of band neutrophils (left shift) is compatible with severe inflammation or infection.
- Serum biochemistry analysis: hypoproteinemia, azotemia, electrolyte derangements, liver enzyme elevations, hyperbilirubinemia, glucose abnormalities possible
- Urinalysis: pyuria, bacteruria, crystalluria possible. Avoid cystocentesis if pyometra suspected or if coagulopathy likely.
- Abdominal radiographs: evaluate for radiopaque foreign bodies, obstructive intestinal gas patterns, organ enlargement, or displacements (double bubble sign with GDV, large fluid-filled uterus) and loss of detail seen with abdominal effusion. Free peritoneal gas in the absence of recent abdominal surgery can be seen in cases of a ruptured viscus, anaerobic infection, or after penetrating trauma.
  - Right lateral and ventrodorsal projections preferred; horizontal beam radiography may be helpful to confirm pneumoperitoneum; pneumocolon may be helpful to distinguish different bowel segments
- Abdominal ultrasound: evaluate for abdominal effusion, GI obstruction, or the presence of foreign material, intra-abdominal masses, abscesses; evaluation of the biliary tract, pancreas, and urogenital system (operator dependent)
  - Ultrasound can aid with abdominocentesis or fine-needle aspiration of masses or organ parenchyma.
- Computed tomography: may be a more sensitive abdominal imaging modality, especially in large-breed or deep-chested dogs
- Abdominocentesis (pp. 1056 and 1343): analysis of effusion may aid rapid identification of underlying problem by assessing fluid characteristics (e.g., PCV/TP, concentrations of glucose, lactate, potassium, creatinine, and total bilirubin) and cytology (e.g., intracellular bacteria in neutrophils consistent with septic effusion)
  - High effusion creatinine (at least 2× peripheral) and/or potassium concentrations (1.4× peripheral in dogs, 1.9× peripheral in cats) is consistent with uroabdomen.
  - Intra-abdominal source of sepsis is likely if the peripheral glucose concentration is 20 mg/dL (1.1 mmol/L) ≥ the abdominal glucose concentration and if the blood lactate concentration is ≤ 2 mmol/L above the abdominal fluid lactate concentration.
- Point-of-care canine-specific pancreatic lipases tests have a high false-positive rate for dogs with signs of acute abdomen. A negative test result likely rules out the presence of pancreatitis, but a positive test result requires further diagnostics to confirm or refute its presence (e.g., imaging). Feline-specific pancreatic lipase testing is also available.

Advanced or Confirmatory Testing
- Fine-needle aspirates or biopsies of lesions (pp. 1064 and 1112)
- Platelet count, hemostatic tests (p. 1325) (prothrombin time, activated partial thromboplastin time, activated clotting time), buccal mucosal bleeding time (p. 1076), and thromboelastography are indicated to better characterize hemorrhagic conditions if a focal source for hemoperitoneum is not identified.

TREATMENT

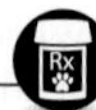

Treatment Overview
- Rapidly assess if patient has surgical or nonsurgical disease.
- Definitive treatment is based on underlying cause (e.g., ovariohysterectomy for pyometra, splenectomy for bleeding splenic mass).
- The main goals of emergent care are to optimize tissue perfusion by restoring and maintaining blood volume by means of resuscitation with fluids and/or blood products with or without the use of vasopressors and positive inotropes.

Acute General Treatment
- Cardiovascular support: intravenous fluid therapy is the mainstay of therapy in hypotensive and hypovolemic patients or those with extensive third-space losses.
  - Isotonic crystalloids are typically used, but hypertonic saline, synthetic colloids, albumin and blood products may also be considered, depending on the underlying disease and based on assessment (and reassessment) of perfusion parameters, lactate concentration, urine output, and blood pressure.
  - Patients with persistent hypoperfusion or hypotension refractory to adequate fluid resuscitation may require treatment with a vasopressor and/or positive inotropic support (p. 907).
- Pain management: opioids usually are first-line therapy; adjunctive analgesia may be provided with ketamine, lidocaine, and dexmedetomidine (if the patient is cardiovascularly stable) by constant-rate infusion and local/regional analgesia. Constant-rate

infusions are preferred to intermittent dosing due to the ability to better balance analgesia with possible adverse effects.

- Antibiotics: early administration of antibiotics in patients with sepsis or septic shock may improve outcome (p. 907)
- Exploratory laparotomy is indicated in the presence of
  - Intracellular bacteria seen in neutrophils in sample effusions (diagnostic for abdominal sepsis)
  - Obstructive GI disease (e.g., foreign body)
  - GDV
  - Bleeding intra-abdominal neoplasm
  - Pyometra
  - Uroabdomen (if a urinary catheter or other diversion device can be placed, surgery does not need to be emergent) (p. 1012)
  - Other abdominal sepsis (e.g., prostatic abscess)

Nutrition/Diet

Protracted inappetence likely contributes to overall morbidity. Early enteral feeding is ideal (e.g., voluntary intake, nasoesophageal or nasogastric feeding tube, esophagostomy tube), but parenteral nutrition may be necessary in some patients (pp. 1106 and 1107).

Drug Interactions

Potentially nephrotoxic medications (e.g., aminoglycosides, NSAIDs) should be avoided in patients with evidence of renal dysfunction or volume depletion.

Possible Complications

- Potentially high mortality rate is associated with many causes of acute abdominal pain (e.g., septic peritonitis, hemoabdomen) if not treated appropriately and promptly.
- Dehiscence of GI surgical sites is possible, usually 3-5 days postoperatively. Risk factors include hypoalbuminemia, peritonitis, and/or compromised intestinal viability.
- Risk of systemic inflammatory response syndrome, sepsis, hemostatic dysfunction (e.g., disseminated intravascular coagulation [DIC]), and multiple organ dysfunction/failure depending on underlying cause (p. 665)

Recommended Monitoring

Perfusion parameters (heart rate, pulse quality, mucous membrane color, capillary refill time), mentation, respiratory rate, temperature, urine output, PCV/TPP or TS, lactate, blood pressure and electrolyte levels are monitored frequently pending clinical improvement.

PROGNOSIS & OUTCOME

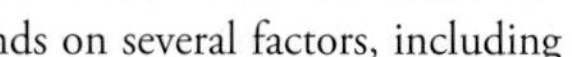

Depends on several factors, including

- Underlying disorder (i.e., reversible disease process or not)
- Stage of the underlying disorder (earlier presentation usually associated with improved chance of success)
- Client and individual factors (e.g., financial and emotional stress)
- If shock is present, earlier hemodynamic optimization is associated with improved outcome

PEARLS & CONSIDERATIONS

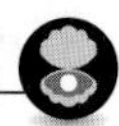

Comments

- Rapid identification of surgical disease is key to success.
- Pyometra should be considered in any intact female.

Technician Tips

- Severely volume-depleted patients may not always have free abdominal effusion evident initially. Recheck after fluid resuscitation and hourly during resuscitation.

SUGGESTED READING

Beal MW: Approach to acute abdomen. Vet Clin Small Anim 35:375-396, 2005.

AUTHOR: Alex Lynch, MRCVS, DACVECC
EDITOR: Benjamin M. Brainard, VMD, DACVAA, DACVECC

Acute Kidney Injury

BASIC INFORMATION

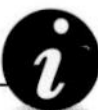

Definition

Abrupt decline of glomerular filtration rate results in an accumulation of nitrogenous waste products and inability to maintain normal fluid balance. Although acute kidney injury (AKI) is uncommon overall, it is a common result of exposure to nephrotoxicants or infectious agents or after kidney injury.

Synonyms

Acute renal failure (ARF), acute kidney failure, anuric/oliguric renal failure

Epidemiology

SPECIES, AGE, SEX

Both dogs and cats are susceptible. Often, animals with AKI are younger than those with chronic kidney disease (CKD).

GENETICS, BREED PREDISPOSITION

Large-breed dogs

RISK FACTORS

- Free-roaming pets
- Nephrotoxins
  - Ethylene glycol
  - Plants (e.g., Easter lily, raisins, grapes)
  - Heavy metals
  - Hypervitaminosis D (e.g., cholecalciferol-containing rodenticides, pharmaceuticals)
  - Drugs (e.g., aminoglycosides, amphotericin B, cisplatin, sulfonamides, tetracyclines, nonsteroidal antiinflammatory drugs, angiotensin-converting enzyme [ACE] inhibitors)
  - Diet-associated nephrotoxicity (melamine/cyanuric acid)
  - Pigmenturia (hemoglobinuria, myoglobinuria)
  - Radiographic contrast agents
- Ischemia: hypotension, trauma, shock, sepsis, systemic inflammatory response syndrome, hypoadrenocorticism, congestive heart failure, temperature extremes, prolonged anesthesia, anaphylaxis
- Infection
  - Dogs: leptospirosis, pyelonephritis, borreliosis, Rocky mountain spotted fever (*Rickettsia rickettsii*)
  - Cats: pyelonephritis, feline infectious peritonitis
- Other: thromboembolic disease, hypercalcemia, transfusion reaction, vasculitis, envenomation, trauma, urinary tract obstruction, renal lymphoma (cats > dogs)

CONTAGION AND ZOONOSIS

Dogs: leptospirosis is contagious and zoonotic with exposure to urine. Lyme disease and Rocky Mountain spotted fever are not directly contagious but require a tick vector.

ASSOCIATED DISORDERS

Uremia, pulmonary edema, uremic encephalopathy, acute lung injury, hypertension, hyperkalemia with bradyarrhythmia

Clinical Presentation

DISEASE FORMS/SUBTYPES

- Oliguric/anuric AKI
  - Anuria: urine production < 0.1 mL/kg/h
  - Oliguria: urine production < 0.5 mL/kg/h
- Polyuric AKI
  - Polyuria: urine production > 2 mL/kg/h

HISTORY, CHIEF COMPLAINT

Some or all may be present:

- Lethargy, depression
- Vomiting, anorexia
- Collapse
- Abdominal/general discomfort

- Renomegaly
- Recent-onset polydipsia, polyuria
- Absent urination (no urine production and no attempts to urinate)
- Multiple animals in same household developing AKI is consistent with toxin exposure, especially diet associated

PHYSICAL EXAM FINDINGS

- Common
  - Dehydration, halitosis, oral cavity debris/secretions, ptyalism, normal-sized/enlarged kidneys
- May also include
  - Small bladder
  - Abdominal/renal pain
  - Oral (uremic) mucosal ulcerations
  - Tachycardia, tachypnea

Etiology and Pathophysiology

- Renal injury initiated by various causes (e.g., ischemia, toxicant, infection)
- Renal response causes extension of insult through four mechanisms:
  - Impaired glomerular filtration by reduced ultrafiltration coefficient
  - Tubular obstruction (cellular casts, protein, hemoglobin, crystals)
  - Tubular backleak of ultrafiltrate
  - Intrarenal vasoconstriction
- Injury leads to failure of renal excretory, regulatory, and endocrine functions, with resultant uremia.

DIAGNOSIS

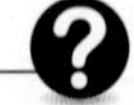

Diagnostic Overview

AKI is suspected when a previously healthy animal suddenly develops uremic signs and is found to have azotemia and isosthenuria, possibly accompanied by a change in urine output. Often, a risk factor for AKI can be identified. A typical approach to diagnosis and treatment is outlined on p. 1398.

Differential Diagnosis

- Azotemia differential diagnosis
  - Prerenal azotemia* (dehydration, gastrointestinal bleeding)
  - Renal failure (acute or chronic or acute-on-chronic failure)
  - Postrenal azotemia (urinary tract obstruction, urinary tract rupture)

Initial Database

- CBC: anemia (which often characterizes CKD) typically is absent; other changes related to cause of AKI (e.g., leptospirosis can be associated with neutrophilia and/or thrombocytopenia) may be identified
- Serum biochemical profile: azotemia is a consistent finding (elevated blood urea nitrogen, creatinine, phosphorus), hyperkalemia occurs with oliguria/anuria, metabolic acidosis is common, and hypocalcemia (e.g., ethylene glycol–induced AKI) or hypercalcemia (e.g., cholecalciferol-containing rodenticides) is sometimes noted.
- Urinalysis: isosthenuria (consistent finding), tubular casts (common), calcium oxalate monohydrate crystalluria (associated with ethylene glycol toxicity), pyuria (associated with pyelonephritis), ± proteinuria, ± hematuria, ± bacteriuria
- Abdominal radiographs: renomegaly often present (contrasts with small kidneys often identified with CKD)
- Abdominal ultrasound: renomegaly, renal pelvic dilation in association with pyelonephritis, alterations in renal parenchymal echogenicity often identified, loss of corticomedullary distinction often identified; hyperechoic cortices (associated with ethylene glycol toxicity but also seen in some healthy cats)
- Electrocardiogram (ECG, p. 1096): altered by pronounced hyperkalemia (bradycardia [more common in dogs than cats], absent P waves, wide QRS complexes)
- Measurement of urine output: assess after complete rehydration. Although polyuric AKI can occur, the classic presentation is oliguria or anuria. In contrast, chronic kidney failure is associated with normal or excessive volumes of urine.

Advanced or Confirmatory Testing

- Ethylene glycol testing (positive within 24 hours of toxin ingestion in dogs, false-positive after propylene glycol administration). Cats commonly have false-negative ethylene glycol test results (p. 314).
- Comparison of measured osmolality with calculated osmolality (osmole gap; measured osmolality > 10 mOsm/L above calculated osmolality suggests ethylene glycol toxicity)
- Serologic testing or polymerase chain reaction: leptospirosis (acute and convalescent titers), Lyme borreliosis, others. Unless another cause of AKI is highly suspected, all dogs with AKI should be tested for leptospirosis (p. 583).
- Adrenocorticotropic hormone stimulation test: to rule out hypoadrenocorticism, especially with hyperkalemia/hyponatremia (p. 512)
- Renal biopsy: can provide etiologic information
- Glomerular filtration rate: seldom required

TREATMENT

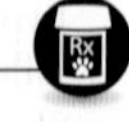

Treatment Overview

Animals with AKI require intensive therapy, monitoring, and nursing care. Initial rehydration and appropriate vascular volume expansion are imperative. Death is most often associated with respiratory failure due to acute lung injury or pulmonary edema from fluid overload, neurologic compromise from uremic encephalopathy or cerebrovascular accident, or fatal arrhythmia due to hyperkalemia. Hospitalization of survivors is typically required for days to weeks, and treatment is expensive. Animals that recover from AKI may have CKD.

Acute General Treatment

Isotonic crystalloid fluid therapy:

- Resolve dehydration within the first 6-12 hours.
  - Percent dehydration (expressed as a decimal [e.g., 10% = 0.1]) × body weight (kg) = deficit (liters)
- Compensate for estimated ongoing losses (e.g., vomiting, panting).
- Provide maintenance fluids (45-60 mL/kg/d).
  - Promote diuresis by increasing fluid rate above maintenance once dehydration is resolved. Practically, twice maintenance rates are usually appropriate, assuming polyuria has been confirmed and is ongoing and overhydration is avoided.
  - In oliguric/anuric animals, maintenance fluid rates may be excessive; monitor for overhydration.
- Avoid overhydration.
  - Respiratory rate and effort q 1-4h
  - Body weight q 6-12h
    - Weight loss represents fluid loss or muscle wasting.
    - Weight gain in hydrated animal implies fluid retention (i.e., overhydration).
  - Closed-system indwelling urinary catheter facilitates early recognition of polyuria, oliguria, or anuria in the hydrated animal.
  - If oliguria/anuria documented, discontinue maintenance fluid therapy, and institute "ins-and-outs" fluid therapy to maintain appropriate hydration.
    - Even if anuric, provide 20 mL/kg/d crystalloid fluid (i.e., insensible losses).
    - Measure and record urine volume q 1-4h. Add that volume of intravenous crystalloid to insensible loss for the next 1-4 hours.
    - Continue until oliguria/anuria resolves.
- Promote urine production with drugs if urine production remains < 1 mL/kg/h despite appropriate rehydration/fluid therapy.
  - Furosemide 2-6 mg/kg IV bolus. If oliguria persists, repeat bolus. If urine production > 1 mL/kg/h after bolus therapy, institute constant rate infusion (0.25-1 mg/kg/h).
  - Mannitol 250-500 mg/kg IV once. CAUTION: increased vascular volume may result in pulmonary edema if overhydrated.
  - Dopamine: not recommended
- If oliguria or anuria persists despite therapy, institute hemodialysis or peritoneal dialysis, or euthanize.

Address acid-base and electrolyte disorders:

- If potassium > 7 mEq/L: treat hyperkalemia (p. 495).
- If pH < 7.1, institute sodium bicarbonate therapy.
  - Calculate bicarbonate deficit ([0.3] × [BW kg] × [base deficit]).

*Occasionally, prerenal azotemia and isosthenuria occur simultaneously without kidney disease (e.g., hypoadrenocorticism, aggressive diuretic use, diabetes insipidus). Recognition of these conditions is imperative to avoid overdiagnosis of kidney failure.

- Administer ½ of the deficit in intravenous fluids over 6 hours.

Monitor blood pressure (p. 1065).
- Maintain mean arterial pressure > 60 mm Hg, systolic > 80 mm Hg.
- Systemic hypertension (systolic pressure > 170 mm Hg) can accompany AKI. Persistent hypertension should be addressed medically (amlodipine 0.1-0.5 mg/kg q 24h) (p. 501).

Medical therapy to decrease gastric acidity (see Drug Interactions):
- Omeprazole 0.5-1.5 mg/kg PO q 12-24h; efficacy delayed (days), *or*
- Famotidine 0.5-1 mg/kg PO, IM, IV q 12-24h

Antiemetic therapy as necessary:
- Maropitant 1-2 mg/kg SQ, IM, IV, or PO q 24h, *or*
- Metoclopramide 0.1-0.5 mg/kg PO, IM, SQ q 6-8h or 0.01-0.02 mg/kg/h IV constant rate infusion, *or*
- Dolasetron 0.5 mg/kg PO, IV, SQ q 24h, *or*
- Ondansetron 0.5-1 mg/kg IV q 8h

Specific therapy for underlying disorders:
- Leptospirosis (p. 583)
  - If another explanation for AKI is not evident, treat for leptospirosis pending diagnostic results.
- Ethylene glycol (p. 1416)

Discontinue nephrotoxic drugs and foodstuffs.

Chronic Treatment

- Manage underlying cause of renal failure.
- Maintain fluid balance throughout recovery period (6-8 weeks).
  - Intravenous (IV) fluids continued until the animal is producing urine, drinking, maintaining hydration
  - Wean IV fluids gradually (at least 2-3 days). Subcutaneous fluid administration may be continued for a period after IV fluids are halted.
  - Duration of hospitalization expected to take days to weeks
- For owners considering peritoneal dialysis or hemodialysis for persistently oliguric animals, facilitate early referral, and avoid jugular venipuncture to preserve vascular access for a dialysis catheter.
- Treat CKD if necessary (pp. 167 and 169).

Nutrition/Diet

- Protein and phosphorus restriction are ideal, but not at the expense of appetite/palatability.
- Cats and dogs that are anorexic from AKI can develop food aversions if a diet change is attempted before appetite returning; therefore, it may be more prudent to institute long-term, renal-type diet after resolution of uremic complications.
- Anorexia is common in AKI (p. 67).
  - If vomiting is rare/absent and anorexia is prolonged, consider enteral tube feeding.
  - If vomiting is intractable, consider parenteral nutrition.

Drug Interactions

- Drugs that are renally excreted (e.g., H2-receptor antagonists) may require dose reduction or increased dosing interval.
- If furosemide or metoclopramide is added to crystalloid fluids for constant-rate administration, the bag should be protected from light.
- Metoclopramide is incompatible with calcium-containing crystalloid fluids (e.g., Plasma-Lyte 148, Normosol-R).

Possible Complications

- Failure to produce urine
- Overhydration, systemic or pulmonary edema
- Hypertension
- Severe metabolic acidosis
- Electrolyte disorders, including hyperkalemia and cardiac dysrhythmia
- CKD
- Acute lung injury (uremic pneumonitis)
- Uremic encephalitis

Recommended Monitoring

- Until azotemia is resolving, urine output is > 1 mg/kg/h, and animal is drinking voluntarily
  - Body weight q 6-12h
  - Blood pressure q 24h
  - Serum blood urea nitrogen/creatinine q 24-48h
  - Electrolytes (Na^+, K^+, Cl^-), acid-base status, and blood pressure q 6-24h
  - Packed cell volume and total protein q 24h
  - Measure urine output
    - Indwelling urinary catheters predispose to urinary infection and should not be left in place longer than necessary.
    - Maintain good aseptic technique with catheters.
    - Closed, sterile urine collection systems and catheters should be cleaned daily and changed frequently (p. 1182).
    - Remove catheter after urine output has been appropriate for > 24 hours.
- Convalescent serologic evaluation as appropriate (e.g., leptospirosis)
- As uremic signs abate, reduce monitoring frequency.
- Body weight, serum chemistry, and packed cell volume are monitored often (at least every third day) until azotemia resolves or plateaus.
- With residual azotemia, long-term monitoring should proceed as for CKD.

PROGNOSIS & OUTCOME

- Short term: poor (60% mortality rate for all causes of AKI; >90% mortality for ethylene glycol intoxication)
- If animal survives short term (6-8 weeks), long-term prognosis can be good.
- Renal failure may become chronic or may resolve. Animals with resolved AKI may develop chronic kidney failure later in life.

PEARLS & CONSIDERATIONS

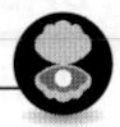

Comments

- Differentiating acute from chronic renal failure is essential for treatment and prognostication.
- Because of the zoonotic importance of leptospirosis, use barrier protection (e.g., gloves) when handling urine from all dogs with AKI.
- Renal biopsy no longer routinely recommended before dialysis.

Prevention

- If considering drugs with nephrotoxic potential, ensure hydration first, and monitor renal function.
- Educate owners regarding nephrotoxins.
- Formulate vaccination programs considering regional prevalence of infectious causes of AKI.

Technician Tips

- During initial telephone triage for vomiting or suddenly ill animals, remember that AKI can occur in animals of any age at any time. Inquire about potential exposure to toxins (antifreeze, raisins, grapes, Easter lilies) or drugs that can cause kidney damage. If exposure might have occurred, these animals should be seen immediately.
- For hospitalized animals with AKI, monitoring urine production for decreased and increased volumes is crucial.
- Use of barrier nursing protocols (e.g., gloves, face shield), minimizing contact with urine, and regular cleaning and disinfection can minimize risk of staff exposure to zoonotic infection (e.g., leptospirosis).
- Monitoring animals with AKI for respiratory rate and effort is critical.

Client Education

- Educate clients regarding nephrotoxins.
- Treatment of AKI may be costly, and recovery may require at least 6-8 weeks.
- Lifelong therapy of CKD may be required for surviving animals.

SUGGESTED READING

Langston C: Acute kidney injury. In Ettinger SJ, Feldman EC, Cote E, editors: Textbook of veterinary internal medicine, ed 8, St. Louis, 2016, Elsevier, pp 1919-1934.

AUTHOR: Marie E. Kerl, DVM, MPH, DACVECC, DACVIM
EDITOR: Leah A. Cohn, DVM, PhD, DACVIM

Acute Moist Dermatitis

Client Education Sheet 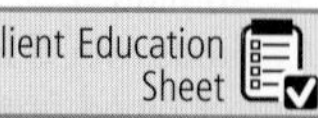

BASIC INFORMATION

Definition

A common, acute, and rapidly progressive exudative dermatitis associated with self-trauma from an underlying pruritic or painful condition

Synonyms

Hot spot, moist eczema, pyotraumatic dermatitis

Epidemiology

SPECIES, AGE, SEX

Acute moist dermatitis is most common in dogs < 4 years old and rarely diagnosed in cats.

GENETICS, BREED PREDISPOSITION

Any breed, but golden retrievers, Labrador retrievers, Saint Bernards, and German shepherds are overrepresented.

RISK FACTORS

Hot, humid weather is a risk factor. Dense-coated, long-haired breeds have increased risk. Other factors associated with acute moist dermatitis include allergy (flea, atopic dermatitis, adverse food reaction, contact), ectoparasites, insect bites, otitis externa, anal sac disease, excess moisture (e.g., swimming), unkempt coat, and painful musculoskeletal disease (recumbency).

Clinical Presentation

HISTORY, CHIEF COMPLAINT

- Acute onset of well-demarcated red, moist, and alopecic area that exudes serum and becomes matted with hair, especially at the periphery
- Lesion is often intensely pruritic, very painful, and often enlarges rapidly (minutes-hours).

PHYSICAL EXAM FINDINGS

- Various sizes of erosive to ulcerative lesion exuding serum
- Erythematous margins sharply demarcate lesion from surrounding normal skin.
- Erythematous papules at periphery of lesion suggest deep pyoderma.
- Lesions most frequently found on face, neck, dorsal lumbosacral area, and lateral thighs.
- Single lesion in one body region more is common than multiple lesions.

Etiology and Pathophysiology

- Any factor that initiates an itch-scratch cycle may predispose to acute moist dermatitis.
- Pyotraumatic lesions may become secondarily infected, leading to pyotraumatic folliculitis.

DIAGNOSIS

Diagnostic Overview

The diagnosis is almost entirely based on the history and characteristic skin lesion.

Differential Diagnosis

- Demodicosis
- Dermatophytosis
- Pyoderma
- Calcinosis cutis

Initial Database

- Skin scrapes: negative for mites (p. 1091)
- Impression of cytologic examination: bacterial colonization

Advanced or Confirmatory Testing

Skin biopsy: indicated only in poorly responsive or recurrent lesions

TREATMENT

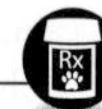

Treatment Overview

- Clip and cleanse lesions; sedation and analgesia is often required.
- Control inflammation and pruritus.
- Identify and control or resolve underlying causes.

Acute General Treatment

- Sedation or general anesthesia is warranted in some cases (when patient shows signs of intense pain at rest or often during initial approach to clipping of hair or cleansing of lesion) (see the back inside cover).
- Clip hair from lesions to allow cleaning and easier topical treatment.
- Gently but thoroughly flush area with an antiseptic solution such as diluted chlorhexidine solution to remove exudate and crusts.
- Topical therapy: often sole therapy warranted with small lesions. Apply astringent (2% aluminum acetate solution) topically q 8-12h for 3-7 days; more extensive or painful lesions benefit from topical glucocorticoid cream or combination steroid/antibiotic topical cream or gel applied q 12h for 5-7 days.
- Systemic glucocorticoids (e.g., prednisone 0.5-1 mg/kg PO q 24h): recommended for extensive or very painful lesions; treatment duration depends on severity of lesion but typically is 5-10 days.
- Nonsteroidal antiinflammatory drugs (e.g., meloxicam 0.1 mg/kg PO q 24h for 3-5 days): alternative for pain management; do not administer in conjunction with systemic glucocorticoids

Oclacitinib (0.4-0.6 mg/kg q 12h for 5-7 days

- Systemic antibiotics (e.g., cephalexin 22-30 mg/kg PO q 12h for minimum of 21 days): indicated if erythematous papules are noted at periphery of lesion

Recommended Monitoring

Re-evaluation in 5-7 days is recommended for extensive lesion or if lesion is not resolving with appropriate therapy.

PROGNOSIS & OUTCOME

- Most lesions respond rapidly and completely to topical and/or systemic therapy.
- Acute moist dermatitis will recur if predisposing causes have not been eliminated or controlled.

PEARLS & CONSIDERATIONS

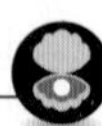

Comments

- Whenever an acute moist dermatitis lesion responds poorly to appropriate therapy or relapses quickly, an alternative diagnosis should be considered. Skin biopsy may be indicated.
- Papules and pustules surrounding an acute moist dermatitis lesion (satellite lesions) may indicate a primary follicular infection (pyotraumatic bacterial folliculitis and furunculosis), where the dog traumatizes the skin in the area of a pre-existing bacterial infection.

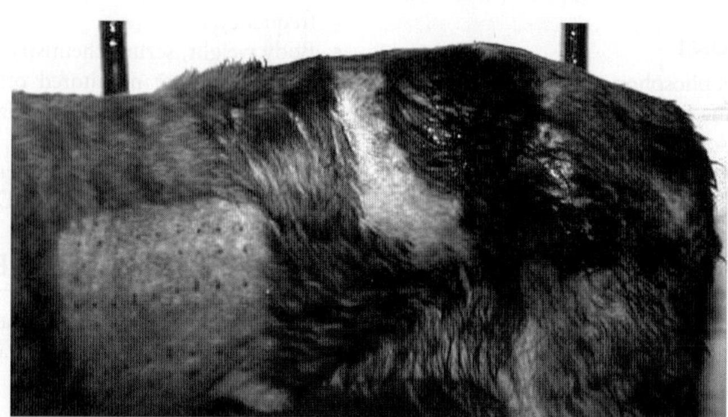

ACUTE MOIST DERMATITIS Acute moist dermatitis *(center)* in a dog with atopic dermatitis. The lateral thorax was clipped for intradermal skin testing *(lower left)*. (Courtesy Dr. Jocelyn Wellington.)

Technician Tips

These lesions can be among the most painful of any seen in practice. Be sure to minimize pain by ensuring that antiseptic lavage solutions are at body temperature before use and that clipper blades do not overheat if hair clipping is extensive.

Client Education

To minimize the owner's shock, inform clients on the patient's admission that the erosive lesion may be quite extensive once the matted hair is removed. Clipping the coat short in long-haired breeds that swim frequently during the warm weather months reduces the potential for acute moist dermatitis. Investigating and controlling or eliminating the underlying disease is critical to reduce/prevent recurrent acute moist dermatitis.

SUGGESTED READING

Holm BR, et al: A prospective study of clinical findings, treatment and histopathology of 44 cases of pyotraumatic dermatitis. Vet Dermatol 15(6):369–376, 2004.

AUTHOR: Jocelyn Wellington, DVM, DACVD
EDITOR: Manon Paradis, DMV, MVSc, DACVD

Acute Respiratory Distress Syndrome

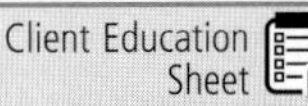

BASIC INFORMATION

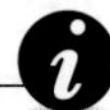

Definition

Acute respiratory distress syndrome (ARDS) refers to the development of noncardiogenic pulmonary edema as an inflammatory response to severe illness or injury.

Synonyms

Adult respiratory distress syndrome, ARDS, shock lung

Epidemiology

SPECIES, AGE, SEX

Any critically ill dog may be affected; it is unclear if cats can develop ARDS.

RISK FACTORS

Severe critical illness or injury

ASSOCIATED DISORDERS

Although ARDS may be associated with other disorders, common associations include sepsis and septic shock, polytrauma, neoplasia, and pancreatitis.

Clinical Presentation

DISEASE FORMS/SUBTYPES

- ARDS may be classified as mild, moderate, or severe. Broadly, all types of ARDS represent lung injury occurring within 1 week of a clinical insult, with progression to respiratory distress. Bilateral pulmonary infiltrates must be demonstrated by thoracic imaging (computed tomography [CT] or radiographs), without evidence of heart failure. Hypoxemia, when being supported by at least 5 cm H_2O positive end-expiratory pressure (PEEP), must be present.
- In human medicine, an ARDS definition task force developed a set of Berlin definitions; these replaced the term *acute lung injury* with the term *mild ARDS*. Subtyping is less well defined in veterinary medicine. A PaO_2/FIO_2 ratio characterizes ARDS as
  - Mild ARDS: 201-300 mm Hg (≤ 39.9 kPa)
  - Moderate ARDS: 101-200 mm Hg (≤ 26.6 kPa)
  - Severe ARDS: ≤ 100 mm Hg (≤ 13.3 kPa)
- Pulmonary ARDS may develop as a result of a direct pulmonary insult such as pneumonia or pulmonary contusion.
- Extrapulmonary ARDS may develop in a critically ill or injured dog as part of the multiple organ dysfunction syndrome when the initial insult was outside the lung (e.g., septic abdomen).
- A short-term ARDS-like syndrome that develops after blood transfusion is recognized in human medicine as transfusion-related acute lung injury (TRALI, p. 989).

HISTORY, CHIEF COMPLAINT

- Reflects the initial presenting complaint; while hospitalized, the dog does not improve as predicted or develops progressive tachypnea and respiratory distress over hours to days.
- ARDS usually is a condition that develops in hospitalized dogs.

PHYSICAL EXAM FINDINGS

Exam findings reflect ARDS and the underlying insult or nonrespiratory complications of the insult (e.g., evidence of polytrauma; petechial hemorrhage due to sepsis-related disseminated intravascular coagulation).

- Increased respiratory rate and effort
- Loud bronchovesicular sounds or crackles on thoracic auscultation
- Orthopnea
- Cyanosis if advanced

Etiology and Pathophysiology

- A pulmonary or extrapulmonary insult results in severe systemic inflammation.
- Cytokines and other proinflammatory products cause vasculitis, and when diffuse alveolar damage occurs, a protein-rich noncardiogenic pulmonary edema is the result.
- Pulmonary edema results in ventilation-perfusion (V-Q) mismatch and severe hypoxemia.
- Three stages of ARDS have been described: exudative, proliferative, and fibrotic. Surviving patients proceed through each stage. The actual time course for each stage in dogs is not known. However, the clinician should anticipate that recovery from ARDS requires weeks.
- ARDS in people is considered a clinical diagnosis not requiring histopathology. The criteria for diagnosis include
  - Underlying event (e.g., severe trauma/sepsis)
  - Diffuse bilateral pulmonary infiltrates on thoracic radiographs
  - Hypoxemia (PaO_2/FIO_2 ratio of < 300)
  - Decreased pulmonary compliance (stiff lungs)
  - Absence of heart failure (normal pulmonary capillary wedge pressure)
- Equivalent criteria have not been validated for veterinary patients.

DIAGNOSIS

Diagnostic Overview

ARDS usually is a composite diagnosis. Dyspnea in a systemically ill or traumatized patient with pulmonary interstitial to alveolar markings on thoracic radiographs, when congestive heart failure, pulmonary thromboembolism (PTE), and pneumonia are effectively ruled out as the sole issue, have a working diagnosis of ARDS. Benefits of diagnostic testing must be weighed against risks, and the certainty of diagnosis may be established only retrospectively with response to treatment or histopathology.

Differential Diagnosis

- Pneumonia
- Volume overload or congestive heart failure/cardiogenic pulmonary edema
- PTE

Initial Database

Thoracic radiographs to identify infiltrates and exclude other causes of respiratory distress

- Cardiogenic pulmonary edema typically predominates in a perihilar and right caudal pulmonary distribution, but when severe, it may not be clearly regional (p. 408).

- Pneumonia (p. 795), especially if by aspiration (p. 793), affects cranioventral lung regions most severely.
- PTE produces variable radiographic findings and is suspected (over noncardiogenic pulmonary edema or ARDS) when respiratory distress is disproportionately severe compared to radiographic lung appearance (p. 842).
- Pleural space disease is usually easily differentiated from noncardiogenic pulmonary edema or ARDS on radiographs (lung retraction).
- Any of these disorders may, if severe, produce pulmonary markings that are indistinguishable from noncardiogenic pulmonary edema or ARDS.

Arterial blood gas analysis: the stress accompanying collection of an arterial blood sample may outweigh the benefits with severe dyspnea (p. 1058). If a reliable pulse oximeter measure is available, it may be used to estimate PaO_2.

- Calculation of the PaO_2/FIO_2 ratio can characterize the stage of ARDS. PaO_2 is measured on an arterial blood gas sample; FIO_2 is the fraction of inspired oxygen (room air = 0.21; 40% oxygen = 0.4; 100% oxygen = 1).
  - Normal ratio > 475
  - ARDS < 300
  - Example: dog receiving 40% O_2 with measured PaO_2 of 60 mm Hg = 60/0.4 = 150

If available, the protein content of expectorated pulmonary edema fluid/foam may be evaluated on a refractometer.

- Pulmonary edema from noncardiac sources such as ARDS has a protein content at least 75% that of serum, whereas cardiogenic pulmonary edema has a protein content ≈30% that of serum.

Other tests as indicated by primary disease process (e.g., coagulation profile if possibility of pulmonary hemorrhage)

Advanced or Confirmatory Testing

- CT of lungs: superior resolution compared with radiographs but limited availability and requires sedation or anesthesia. If patient is anesthetized for mechanical ventilation, CT scanning is preferred. The level of PEEP is important (usually 5-10 cm H_2O), and motion (tachypnea) should be prevented. CT angiography may provide evidence to support the presence of PTE.
- Echocardiography (p. 1094) to exclude cardiac dysfunction or PTE (by evaluating for right-sided heart enlargement and tricuspid regurgitant flow indicating pulmonary hypertension)
- Transtracheal wash or bronchoalveolar lavage (pp. 1073 and 1074) with cytologic evaluation and culture to exclude infection or neoplasia

TREATMENT

Treatment Overview

Intubation and ventilation should be implemented if respiratory distress lasts for > 1 hour or is worsening, if $SpO_2 < 89\%$ despite supplemental oxygen (p. 1146), or in the presence of hypoventilation that may indicate respiratory fatigue (e.g., $PCO_2 > 65$ mm Hg).

Specific goals:

- Treatment of the underlying disorder and, if necessary, positive-pressure ventilation are the cornerstones of management of ARDS.
- No specific therapy for ARDS; limited tidal volumes during mechanical ventilation may mitigate ventilator-associated pulmonary injury and barotrauma.
- Provide support for the damaged lung parenchyma to permit healing.

Acute General Treatment

- Optimize oxygenation; mechanical ventilation with positive end-expiratory pressure (p. 1185); may require referral.
- Low tidal volumes (5-10 mL/kg) with an attempt to limit barotrauma are recommended.
- May result in increased $PaCO_2$ (permissive hypercarbia)
- Other supportive measures:
  - Antibiotics (e.g., ampicillin 22 mg/kg IV q 8h, with or without enrofloxacin 10 mg/kg IV diluted in sterile saline and given slowly IV q 24h [5 mg/kg q 24h in cats])
  - Surgery, if indicated, for primary disease
- Diuretics are not directly indicated, although every effort should be made to prevent volume overload.
  - If it is unclear whether volume overload is present, 2 mg/kg furosemide IV may be administered q 6h. If respiratory character improves in < 24 hours and radiographic markings improve in < 48 hours after diuretic treatment, cardiogenic pulmonary edema was more likely than ARDS.
- Colloids are not indicated for acute lung injury or ARDS. The altered permeability of the capillary-alveolar membrane may allow synthetic colloids to cross into the pulmonary parenchyma and worsen gas exchange.

Chronic Treatment

Empiric glucocorticoid use (prednisone 0.5-1 mg/kg PO q 24h) during recovery phase to delay/prevent pulmonary fibrosis; this therapy is unsupported by objective evidence

Possible Complications

- Failure of other organ systems
- Chronic pulmonary insufficiency
- Death from respiratory failure

Recommended Monitoring

Affected patients need intensive nursing care.

- Ventilation parameters, including airway pressures
- Oxygen saturation (and ideally, arterial blood gas analysis)
- Blood pressure (direct arterial is ideal)
- Continuous electrocardiographic monitoring
- Urine output

PROGNOSIS & OUTCOME

Guarded to grave. Survival after ARDS is possible but rare. Multiple organ failure, progressive hypoxemia, circulatory collapse, and ongoing costs associated with intensive care limit survival of affected dogs.

PEARLS & CONSIDERATIONS

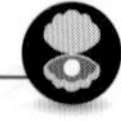

Comments

Accuracy in diagnosis: identify and treat causes of hospital-acquired respiratory distress that are more commonly responsive (better prognosis):

- Pneumonia
- PTE
- Volume overload/congestive heart failure

Prevention

Early identification of patients at risk (i.e., those with severe systemic inflammation from any cause) and implementation of intensive supportive care:

- Prevent sepsis from progressing to septic shock.
- Aggressive treatment for severely injured patients

Technician Tips

ARDS is one of the disorders that requires the greatest degree of monitoring and supportive care (see Recommended Monitoring above).

Client Education

ARDS is a severe disease associated with critical illness. Successful treatment requires committed clients with adequate emotional and financial resources (e.g., pet insurance).

SUGGESTED READING

Wilkins P, et al: Acute lung injury and acute respiratory distress syndromes in veterinary medicine: consensus definitions: The Dorothy Russell Havemeyer Working Group on ALI and ARDS in Veterinary Medicine. J Vet Emerg Crit Care 17:333-339, 2007.

AUTHOR: Elizabeth Rozanski, DVM, DACVIM, DACVECC
EDITOR: Benjamin M. Brainard, VMD, DACVAA, DACVECC

Adenocarcinoma, Anal Sac

Client Education Sheet

BASIC INFORMATION

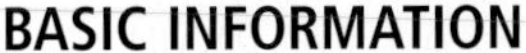
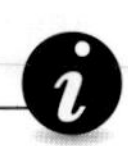

Definition
Malignant neoplasm arising from apocrine glands of the anal sac

Synonyms
Apocrine gland adenocarcinoma, apocrine gland anal sac adenocarcinoma (AGASA or AGASACA)

Epidemiology
SPECIES, AGE, SEX

Tumors occur more frequently in dogs than cats, typically in older animals (median age, 9-11 years and 12 years, respectively). There is no sex predisposition.

GENETICS, BREED PREDISPOSITION

Spaniel breeds, particularly English cocker spaniels

RISK FACTORS

Neutering may increase risk, particularly for male dogs.

ASSOCIATED DISORDERS

Paraneoplastic hypercalcemia occurs in approximately 50% of dogs with anal sac adenocarcinoma.

Clinical Presentation
HISTORY, CHIEF COMPLAINT

- Perineal irritation manifested by licking/biting at region, scooting, bleeding
- Dyschezia or tenesmus ± stranguria, especially with sublumbar lymphadenopathy
- If hypercalcemia present: polyuria, polydipsia, vomiting, poor appetite, weakness
- 40% of tumors are found incidentally on routine physical exam.

PHYSICAL EXAM FINDINGS

- Rectal exam reveals a mass in the region of the anal gland ± palpable sublumbar lymph node enlargement.
- Palpable caudal abdominal mass effect in cases of moderate to severe sublumbar lymph node enlargement
- Large tumors may be visible perineally.
- Tumors may be bilateral.

Etiology and Pathophysiology
- Anal sac apocrine gland adenocarcinoma tumors arise from the apocrine glands of the walls of the anal sacs.
- Tumors are locally invasive and have a high rate of metastasis to local lymph nodes (iliac, sacral, and sublumbar nodes) and distant sites in the body, most frequently the lungs, liver, spleen, and bone.
- Paraneoplastic hypercalcemia occurs in up to 50% of dogs with anal sac adenocarcinoma due to tumoral production of parathormone-related peptide (parathyroid hormone–related protein [PTHrP]).

DIAGNOSIS

Diagnostic Overview
Diagnosis is based on physical exam (visualization or palpation of a perineal mass) and history (tenesmus, dyschezia, signs of hypercalcemia).

- Fine-needle aspirate cytology is useful for differentiating neoplastic from inflammatory processes.
- Confirmation of the diagnosis requires histopathology.

Differential Diagnosis
- Other tumors of the anal sac (e.g., squamous cell carcinoma, melanoma)
- Perianal adenoma or adenocarcinoma
- Perineal hernia
- Anal sac abscess
- Other cutaneous neoplasia
- Perineal fistula

Initial Database
- CBC, serum chemistry profile, urinalysis, ± ionized calcium
- Thoracic radiographs or thoracic CT scan
- Abdominal ultrasound or CT scan

Advanced or Confirmatory Testing
- Fine-needle aspirate cytology of affected anal sac
- Incisional biopsy for larger tumors to aid in planning definitive surgical resection
- Abdominal CT or MRI, including the perineal region for clinical staging and surgical and/or radiation therapy planning

TREATMENT

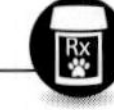

Treatment Overview
The goals of treatment are to

- Provide adequate locoregional control of disease
- Palliate clinical signs associated with the primary tumor, regional metastases, and/or hypercalcemia

Acute General Treatment
- Surgical excision of the primary tumor is recommended along with removal of enlarged regional lymph nodes, especially when causing obstruction of the pelvic canal or in cases of concurrent hypercalcemia.
  - Approximately one-half of the anal sphincter can be removed without the development of fecal incontinence.
  - Recurrence rates are 20%-50% with surgery alone.
  - Postoperative hypocalcemia can occur in previously hypercalcemic patients; careful monitoring of serum calcium levels in the immediate postoperative period is required.
- Radiation therapy
- Various chemotherapeutic agents have been investigated for adjuvant and palliative management of anal sac adenocarcinoma in dogs, including carboplatin, cisplatin, actinomycin-D, mitoxantrone, melphalan, and toceranib phosphate (Palladia), but the role of adjuvant chemotherapy in the treatment of anal sac adenocarcinoma remains poorly defined.
- Hypercalcemia should resolve on surgical removal of the primary tumor, but it may persist if widespread metastases are present.
- In dogs with advanced disease, palliative use of chemotherapy or radiation therapy may be indicated.

Chronic Treatment
- If metastases cause persistent hypercalcemia, additional therapy may be necessary (p. 491).

Possible Complications
- Postoperative complications include tenesmus, hematochezia, fecal incontinence, incisional dehiscence, incontinence, rectal prolapse, perirectal abscess, and stenosis.
- Acute radiation complications include erythema and dry or moist desquamation of perineal skin and mild to moderate colitis.
- Late radiation effects include rectal fibrosis or stricture and chronic diarrhea.
- Hypocalcemia (p. 515) can occur postoperatively in patients with hypercalcemia before surgical excision of their tumors.

PROGNOSIS & OUTCOME

- Approximate median survival times for dogs treated with surgery, radiation therapy, or chemotherapy alone are 7-9, 21, and 7 months, respectively.
- The longest reported median survival time for anal sac adenocarcinoma is 31.4 months with a combined therapy of surgery, definitive radiation therapy, and mitoxantrone chemotherapy
- Negative prognostic factors include hypercalcemia, primary tumor size > 10 cm, and pulmonary metastases.
- The presence of iliac lymphadenopathy is an inconsistent negative prognostic factor.
- Information on the outcome in cats is lacking; however, a multimodal treatment approach appears warranted.

PEARLS & CONSIDERATIONS

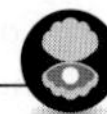

Comments
- Many anal sac tumors are diagnosed incidentally on physical exam. A rectal exam is

an essential component to a complete wellness exam.
- Sometimes, dogs are presented for signs of polyuria/polydipsia without an owner observation of rectal disease.

Technician Tips
- Owners can confuse stranguria with tenesmus. Although both may be seen with anal gland adenocarcinoma, the latter is more frequently observed. Careful inquiry as owner's observations can aid in differentiating between the two signs.

SUGGESTED READING

Turek M, et al: Perianal tumors. In Withrow S, Vail D, Page R, editors: Small animal clinical oncology, ed 5, St. Louis, 2013, Saunders, pp 423-431.

AUTHOR: Joanne L. Intile, DVM, MS, DACVIM
EDITOR: Kenneth M. Rassnick, DVM, DACVIM

Adenocarcinoma, Intestinal/Colonic

Client Education Sheet 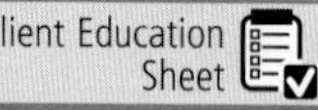

BASIC INFORMATION 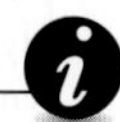

Definition
Malignant tumor arising from gastrointestinal (GI) tract epithelium

Epidemiology
SPECIES, AGE, SEX

Intestinal adenocarcinoma is rare in dogs and cats, accounting for 1% of tumors in necropsied cats and 0.1% of tumors in dogs. Colorectal adenocarcinoma is slightly more common than intestinal.
- Mean age of cats with small intestinal adenocarcinoma is 11 years; colorectal tumors in cats occur at a mean age of 16 years.
- Mean age of dogs with intestinal and colorectal adenocarcinomas is 9 years.

GENETICS, BREED PREDISPOSITION
- Intestinal adenocarcinoma is most common in boxers, collies, poodles, West Highland white terriers, German shepherds, and Doberman pinschers, and Siamese cats (70% of feline small intestinal adenocarcinomas occur in Siamese).
- Shar-peis may have increased incidence of intestinal adenocarcinoma.
- In dogs, colorectal tumors are most common in collies and German shepherds.

ASSOCIATED DISORDERS
- Intestinal obstruction
- Melena
- Hematochezia
- Anemia

Clinical Presentation
HISTORY, CHIEF COMPLAINT
- Clinical signs depend on lesion location: intermittent vomiting, hematemesis, anorexia, dehydration, melena, hematochezia, diarrhea, signs of intestinal obstruction or peritonitis, abdominal distention from peritoneal effusion due to carcinomatosis.
- Colorectal adenocarcinomas cause hematochezia, tenesmus, and dyschezia.
- Slowly progressive, non-obstructive tumors may cause anorexia, weight loss, and iron-deficiency anemia.

PHYSICAL EXAM FINDINGS
- Palpable abdominal mass
- Palpable mass and/or bleeding on rectal examination
- Abdominal effusion from carcinomatosis or peritonitis
- Signs of anemia
- Poor body condition

Etiology and Pathophysiology
Genetic predisposition is likely.

DIAGNOSIS 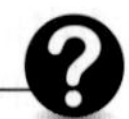

Diagnostic Overview
The diagnosis is suspected in patients with GI signs that fail to respond to conservative therapy, evidence of an intestinal mass, or both. Diagnostic imaging is essential for identifying a lesion, although results vary. Lesions must be sampled for histopathology or cytology to confirm the diagnosis.

Differential Diagnosis
Depends on lesion location and signs:
- Foreign body
- Intussusception
- Infectious enteropathy, chronic parasitism
- Inflammatory bowel disease
- Alimentary lymphoma
- Alimentary mast cell tumor in cats
- Colorectal polyps, adenomas
- Smooth muscle tumors (leiomyoma, leiomyosarcoma, GI stromal tumor)

Initial Database
- CBC results often are nonspecific: neutrophilia; regenerative, nonregenerative, or microcytic anemia secondary to blood loss
- Serum biochemistry panel: elevation of alkaline phosphatase, hypoalbuminemia/hypoproteinemia possible, increased blood urea nitrogen (BUN) if GI bleeding
- Urinalysis: usually unremarkable
- Thoracic radiographs for metastasis
- Abdominal radiographs may demonstrate signs of intestinal obstruction, mass effect, or may be noncontributory.
- Positive contrast GI study or barium enema may reveal mass or annular constrictive lesion.
- Ultrasonography can define primary mass and lymphadenomegaly or suggest organ metastasis and may guide fine-needle aspiration (p. 1112).

Advanced or Confirmatory Testing
Endoscopic or surgical biopsy, or aspiration cytology, is required for definitive diagnosis. Choice of approach depends on location of the lesion; colonoscopy is preferred over surgery for colonic neoplasia, but endoscopy (p. 1098) may be nondiagnostic for jejunal lesions (unable to reach the lesion).

TREATMENT 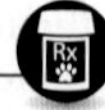

Treatment Overview
Surgical resection is the preferred treatment for intestinal and colonic adenocarcinoma. Additional measures such as chemotherapy or radiation therapy may be warranted, and consultation with an oncologist is recommended.

Acute General Treatment
General supportive care includes
- Rehydration and restoring electrolyte homeostasis
- Managing anemia with transfusions and hematinics as indicated
- Antibiotic and emergency management for peritonitis (p. 779)
- Analgesics for pain in obstructive lesions or peritonitis
- Promotility agents are contraindicated in obstructive disease.

Chronic Treatment
- Curative therapy for nonmetastatic intestinal and colonic adenocarcinoma is complete surgical excision.
- Even with metastatic disease or carcinomatosis, survival times are extended by surgical resection of obstructive lesions in cats with intestinal adenocarcinoma.
- Radiation therapy may be palliative or curative for nonresectable colonic lesions.
- Chemotherapy is usually unsuccessful, but therapy with nonsteroidal antiinflammatory drugs, doxorubicin, platinum agents, and antimetabolites (gemcitabine, fluorouracil)

may be attempted for nonresectable or metastatic, or carcinomatosis.

- Toceranib may be helpful for maintenance to limit blood vessel ingrowth to tumor sites.
- Intraluminal stent placement may be palliative in cats with colonic obstruction.

Possible Complications

- Surgical wound dehiscence with secondary peritonitis, pneumoperitoneum
- Chemotherapy-induced neutropenia predisposes to infection.
- Chemotherapy-induced thrombocytopenia may increase tumor hemorrhage.
- Chemotherapy may result in perforation of transmural lesions.

Recommended Monitoring

If primary lesion can be successfully resected, abdominal ultrasonography for metastasis or recurrence and thoracic radiographs are indicated periodically.

PROGNOSIS & OUTCOME

Prognosis depends on

- Histologic type and grade of the primary lesion: low-grade lesions or carcinoma *in situ* may be completely resected.
- Annular constrictive lesions are particularly aggressive.
- Potential for curative resection depends on tumor size and location.
- Metastatic disease and carcinomatosis are incurable and have a poor prognosis.
- In one study, cats with colonic adenocarcinoma treated with subtotal colectomies and carboplatin had mild toxicity with a median survival time of 269 days.

PEARLS & CONSIDERATIONS

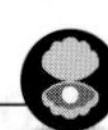

Comments

- The small intestine contains more than 90% of the GI epithelial cell population but is associated with only 10% of all GI malignancies.
- In cats, the large intestine is the most common location for intestinal adenocarcinoma, and adenocarcinoma is the most common tumor occurring in the large intestine.

Technician Tips

- These patients are very ill; observe for signs of hypotension and abdominal effusion that can indicate intestinal perforation.

SUGGESTED READING

Risseto K, et al: Recent trends in feline intestinal neoplasia: an epidemiologic study of 1,129 cases in the veterinary medical database from 1964 to 2004. J Am Anim Hosp Assoc 47:28, 2010.

AUTHOR: Barbara E. Kitchell, DVM, PhD, DACVIM
EDITOR: Rance K. Sellon, DVM, PhD, DACVIM

Adenoma/Adenocarcinoma, Perianal

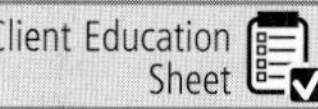

BASIC INFORMATION

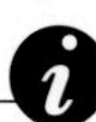

Definition

Neoplastic proliferation of the hormone-dependent, nonsecretory perianal sebaceous glands, which are located circumferentially within the skin surrounding the anus and skin along the caudal half of the body

Synonyms

Hepatoid tumor, circumanal gland tumor

Epidemiology

SPECIES, AGE, SEX

- Perianal adenoma: older, intact male and ovariohysterectomized female dogs
- Perianal adenocarcinoma: uncommon in dogs; average age is 11 years

GENETICS, BREED PREDISPOSITION

- Perianal adenoma: Alaskan malamute, beagle, bulldog, cocker spaniel, Siberian husky, Samoyed, shih tzu
- Perianal adenocarcinoma: German shepherd, Arctic breeds (Samoyed, Alaskan malamute, Siberian husky)

RISK FACTORS

- Perianal adenoma: sexually intact males, ovariohysterectomized female dogs (estrogen suppresses tumor growth), hyperadrenocorticism with associated excess testosterone secretion
- Perianal adenocarcinoma: neutered and intact males and females

ASSOCIATED DISORDERS

Hyperadrenocorticism, hyperandrogenism

Clinical Presentation

HISTORY, CHIEF COMPLAINT

- Perianal adenoma: slow-growing, nonpainful mass/masses in perineal region. Ulceration and infection can occur, but tumors usually remain freely movable.
- Perianal adenocarcinoma: rapidly growing, firm, fixed, ulcerated mass/masses in perineal region. Obstipation and dyschezia can occur with larger tumors or with metastasis to sublumbar lymph nodes
- Perianal adenomas and adenocarcinomas can occur anywhere along the haired skin of the caudal half of the body

PHYSICAL EXAM FINDINGS

- Cutaneous mass in the perineal region. The masses tend to be well circumscribed, superficial, and may be finely lobulated or cauliflower-like in appearance.
- ± Ulceration
- ± Diffuse skin thickening
- Differentiation from anal sac disorders and perineal hernia:
    - Visual inspection, as described previously
    - Rectal palpation: perianal adenomas are palpably superficial (cutaneous) and not associated with the anal sacs; the pelvic diaphragm is intact and without herniation.

Etiology and Pathophysiology

- Perianal glands are nonsecretory sebaceous glands.
- Perianal glands adenoma growth is stimulated by androgens and suppressed by estrogens.
- Hyperfunction of the zona reticularis of the adrenal gland results in elevated androgen levels regardless of neuter status.

DIAGNOSIS

Diagnostic Overview

The diagnosis of a perianal adenoma is suspected in an intact male dog presenting with a cutaneous growth along the perineal region. Confirmation requires histopathology, although lesions often regress in male dogs after neutering.

Differential Diagnosis

- Anal sac tumor (e.g., adenocarcinoma, squamous cell carcinoma, melanoma)
- Anal sac abscess
- Other cutaneous neoplasia
- Perineal hernia
- Perianal fistula

Initial Database

- CBC, serum chemistry panel, and urinalysis to evaluate for indications of hyperadrenocorticism; especially important in neutered dogs with perianal adenomas
- Fine-needle aspirate cytology: the morphology of perianal gland tissue resembles hepatocytes. Cells are arranged in clusters. There is abundant cytoplasm and a round, centrally located nucleus usually exhibiting a single, large nucleolus. Cellular pleomorphism varies and is inconsistently associated with malignancy.

Advanced or Confirmatory Testing

- Tissue biopsy is required to distinguish benign from malignant disease, with

invasiveness into surrounding tissue being the strongest characteristic of malignancy.
- Immunohistochemical markers of proliferation (e.g., proliferating cell nuclear antigen [PCNA]) are more strongly expressed in malignant tumors.
- Confirmatory testing for hyperadrenocorticism, if applicable (p. 485)

TREATMENT

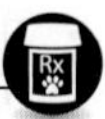

Treatment Overview

The goals of treatment are to control the tumor and eliminate the source of androgens.

Acute General Treatment

- Perianal adenoma: neutering intact male dogs results in full or partial tumor regression. Tumors can also be resected marginally at the time of the neuter to obtain tissue for biopsy.
- Marginal resection and cryosurgery may decrease the chance of tumor recurrence.
- Wide surgical resection is indicated for malignant adenocarcinoma.
- Wide resection may also be helpful in cases of persistent or recurrent adenoma tumors.
- Radiation therapy can be used for larger tumors or for those that do not regress after neutering. Radiation therapy can be used to reduce regrowth after incomplete excision. Preoperative radiation therapy may afford the ability to perform a less aggressive initial surgery.
- In dogs with concurrent hyperadrenocorticism, control of that disease may be essential for tumor control (p. 485).

Chronic Treatment

Recurrent perianal tumors can occur in intact dogs or dogs with hyperadrenocorticism. The treatment options remain the same as for dogs initially presenting with a tumor.

Possible Complications

- Postoperative complications include tenesmus, hematochezia, fecal incontinence, incisional dehiscence, rectal prolapse, perirectal abscess, and stenosis.
- Acute radiation complications include erythema and dry or moist desquamation of perineal skin, and mild to moderate colitis.
- Late radiation effects include rectal fibrosis or stricture and chronic diarrhea.

PROGNOSIS & OUTCOME

- Perianal adenomas: good (recurrence rate < 10%)
- Perianal adenocarcinomas: early, complete excision of small tumors can be curative. The metastatic rate at the time of diagnosis is 15%, but this rate may increase late in the course of disease.
- Tumor stage predicts outcome for adenocarcinoma:
  - Tumors < 5 cm; no distant metastasis: median survival, 24 months
  - Tumors > 5 cm in diameter; no distant metastasis: median survival, 12 months
  - If local or distant metastasis: median survival, 7 months

PEARLS & CONSIDERATIONS

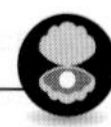

Comments

- Neutering can result in complete or partial tumor regression of perianal adenoma.
- Dogs with persistent or recurrent adenomas are candidates for more aggressive surgery and/or radiation therapy.
- Cats do not have perianal sebaceous glands; therefore, perianal adenoma or adenocarcinoma is not a clinically recognized entity in this species.

Prevention

Early neutering of male dogs is preventative for perianal adenoma.

Technician Tips

- Tumors in the perineal region cause irritation, and pets can show signs of licking, scooting, and tenesmus.
- Perianal adenocarcinomas cannot be grossly differentiated from perianal adenomas.

SUGGESTED READING

Turek M, et al: Perianal tumors. In Withrow S, Vail D, and Page R, editors: Small animal clinical oncology, ed. 5, St. Louis, 2013, Saunders, pp 423-431.

AUTHOR: Joanne L. Intile, DVM, MS, DACVIM
EDITOR: Kenneth M. Rassnick, DVM, DACVIM

Adhesives and Glues Toxicosis

BASIC INFORMATION

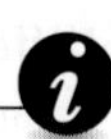

Definition

Adverse physical effects caused by oral, ocular, aural, or dermal exposure to common household adhesives, including super glue, expandable polyurethane glue, and white glue

Epidemiology

SPECIES, AGE, SEX

All animals of all ages and both sexes are susceptible; exposure is more common in dogs. Dermal exposure in cats can result in clinically significant oral exposure (grooming).

RISK FACTORS

Availability of common household adhesives in pet's environment

Clinical Presentation

HISTORY, CHIEF COMPLAINT

- Accidental exposure to adhesives
- Hypersalivation, retching/gagging, vomiting, anorexia, lethargy after oral exposure (super glue, polyurethane, white glue)

PHYSICAL EXAM FINDINGS

- Tissue adhesions after ocular or dermal exposure to super glues
- Presence of dried adhesive on the animal (skin, paws, fur, teeth, eyes, ears)
- Abdominal distention/discomfort (polyurethane/expandable-glue ingestion)
- Blepharospasm, epiphora, conjunctivitis, or keratitis with ocular exposure
- Hypersalivation, lethargy, anorexia with oral exposure (all adhesives)

Etiology and Pathophysiology

Super glues:
- Contain ethyl-2-cyanoacrylate 60% to 100% and poly(methylmethacrylate) 2% to 30%
- Super glues (cyanoacrylates) cause rapid adhesion of body structures on contact. These glues are usually mildly irritating to the mucous membranes.

Expandable polyurethane glue, industrial strength wood glue:
- Contain diphenylmethane diisocyanate and polymethylene polyphenyl isocyanate in various concentrations
- Ingestion of expandable polyurethane glues (containing isocyanates) is detrimental due to space-occupying properties; can form an expanding gastric foreign body. This is more likely to occur in dogs that chew the bottle of glue. These glues are usually mildly irritating. Expansion of glue is exothermic and damage to gastrointestinal (GI) mucosa can occur. The resulting foreign body is also rough and can traumatize the GI mucosa during peristaltic contractions.

White glues: contain polyvinyl acetate in various concentrations. They are mildly irritating to the mucous membranes but are not expandable.

DIAGNOSIS

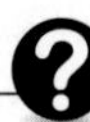

Diagnostic Overview

- For all glues: history and physical exam findings key to diagnosis; no confirmatory laboratory test exists.
- Super glue, white glue: diagnosis is based on observed or suspected exposure and/or presence of glue on the skin or mucous membranes and mild GI irritation signs.

- Expandable polyurethane glue, industrial strength wood glue: diagnosis is based on observed or suspected exposure, presence of glue on the skin or mucous membranes, and/or abdominal distention. Radiographs or endoscopy can help confirm the presence of the solidified expandable glue in the stomach.

Differential Diagnosis

- Other foreign body injury or ingestions (e.g., plastic, woods, metals)
- Other causes of vomiting (e.g., dietary indiscretion, viral gastroenteritis)
- Exposure to corrosives, detergents, bleaches, irritants

Initial Database

- Abdominal radiographs 12-24 hours after ingesting polyurethane glue typically indicate a large, mottled density resembling kibble in the stomach.
- CBC (± inflammatory leukogram), serum biochemistry profile, urinalysis: typically unremarkable
- Fluorescein staining to identify corneal ulcers (p. 1137)

Advanced or Confirmatory Testing

Endoscopy (p. 1098) may help determine the size of foreign body (polyurethane glue) and also evaluate esophageal and gastric mucosal damage (irritation, ulcers, perforation); rarely useful for removing foreign material (too friable, too large).

TREATMENT

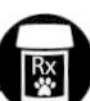

Treatment Overview

Treatment is aimed at separating adhered tissues if needed, assessing tissue damage, and supportive care for super and white glue (nonexpandable). For the polyurethane glues (expandable), gastrostomy to remove the gastric foreign body is necessary if glue concretion is too large to pass spontaneously.

Acute General Treatment

Super glue:

- Oral: adhered tissues typically separate spontaneously in 1-4 days. If necessary, separate tissues under general anesthesia. Apply margarine, mineral oil, or petroleum jelly, wait 15-30 minutes; gently peel or roll adherent tissues until separation. Do not pull adherent planes of tissue directly apart, due to high tensile strength of the bond. Expandable foreign body is not expected from ingestion of white or super glue (cyanoacrylates).
- Aural: Glue may bond to tympanum. Repeatedly applying 3% hydrogen peroxide (preferred) or acetone on cotton balls may loosen the bond to allow slow extraction of the glue cast. Lavage external ear canal with sterile water afterward.
- Ocular: rinse eye with 0.9% saline or water for 15 minutes. If the cornea is adhered to lids or lashes, may need to separate under general anesthesia as for oral exposure. If the lids or lashes are adhered to themselves, forced separation is often not needed. Assess the cornea for damage and treat abrasions with ophthalmic antibiotics and mydriatics (p. 209).
- Dermal: as for oral treatment

Polyurethane adhesives:

- Oral: manually remove glue from oral cavity. Emesis is not recommended due to concern for esophageal foreign body. Charcoal is not effective.
- Perform gastrotomy if concretion (gastric foreign body) is present.
- Sucralfate and acid-reducing drugs advised if GI signs are present and/or foreign body is removed:
  - Sucralfate, dogs: 0.5-1 g PO q 8-12h; cats: 0.25-0.5 g PO q 8-12h.
  - Famotidine, dogs/cats: 0.5 mg/kg PO, SQ, IM, IV q 12-24h; *or*
  - Omeprazole, dogs/cats: 0.5-1 mg/kg PO q 24h; *or*
  - Pantoprazole, dogs/cats: 0.7-1 mg/kg IV over 15 minutes q 24h.

Postoperative care:

- Administer broad-spectrum antibiotics after gastrotomy if evidence of contamination or infection (p. 384).
- Metoclopramide 0.4 mg/kg SQ q 8h for 1-2 days; or maropitant 1 mg/kg SQ q 24h or 2 mg/kg PO q 24h for up to 5 days. Contraindication to antiemetics: ongoing/unresolved GI tract obstruction
- Restrict food and water intake for first 12-24 hours after surgery.
- Postoperative pain control (e.g., fentanyl 3-6 mcg/kg/h IV infusion or hydromorphone 0.1-0.2 mg/kg IM, IV, or SQ q 2-6h)
- IV fluids as needed
- Dermal, ocular, aural: treat as for super glues.

White glue or other glues:

- Most exposures do not need extensive treatment because signs are usually mild and self-limited. Treat mild to moderate GI irritation supportively. Gastric foreign body is not expected.

Nutrition/Diet

A high-fiber diet may facilitate passage of the remnants of dried/expanded glue through the digestive tract.

Possible Complications

Stomach rupture and peritonitis possible (rare) with oral exposure to large volumes of expandable glue.

Recommended Monitoring

- Routine postoperative monitoring if gastrotomy performed (polyurethane glues)
- Physical observation of healing and resolution

PROGNOSIS & OUTCOME

- Super glues, white glue: very good in all situations unless extensive corneal or tympanic membrane damage occurs (super glue)
- Polyurethane glue: good in uncomplicated cases of gastric foreign body removal
- Polyurethane glue: guarded to poor if stomach rupture, torsion, or peritonitis has occurred

PEARLS & CONSIDERATIONS

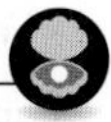

Comments

- General negative effects are as follows: super glues, binding of tissues; polyurethane glues, expansion to form GI foreign body; white glues, minimal.
- After the ingestion of expandable polyurethane glue (isocyanates), it is vital to verify the presence of a foreign body before performing a gastrostomy.
- Dried, already polymerized polyurethane glue (isocyanates) ingested does not expand further in the stomach.
- Expandable gastric foreign body is not expected from super glue or white glue ingestion.

Prevention

Keep adhesives out of reach of pets.

Technician Tips

Do not induce vomiting with exposure to any adhesives. It is usually unnecessary with super glue and white glue; with expanding polyurethane adhesives, it can be detrimental (glue can form a concretion in the esophagus).

SUGGESTED READING

Fitzgerald KT, et al: Polyurethane adhesive ingestion. Top Companion Anim Med 28(1):28-31, 2013.

AUTHOR: Cristine Hayes, DVM, DABT, DABVT
EDITOR: Tina Wismer, DVM, MS, DABT, DABVT

Adrenal Mass, Incidental

Client Education Sheet 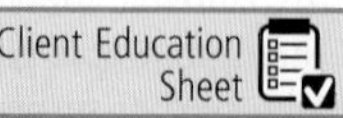

BASIC INFORMATION

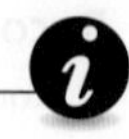

Definition

Adrenal mass discovered inadvertently during abdominal imaging (typically ultrasound) performed for any reason other than suspected adrenal disease

Synonym

Incidentaloma

Epidemiology

SPECIES, AGE, SEX

- Dogs: incidence estimated at 4%. Affected dogs typically > 9 years old and midsized to large breed.
- Cats: incidence and signalment unknown.

GENETICS, BREED PREDISPOSITION

Breed predisposition varies with type of mass.

Clinical Presentation

DISEASE FORMS/SUBTYPES

- An adrenal tumor should be suspected when there is loss of the typical adrenal gland shape (regardless of size), asymmetry in shape and size between affected and contralateral adrenal glands, or infiltration of vasculature or surrounding soft tissues.
- May be functional (i.e., secrete a hormone) or nonfunctional. Functional types include
  - Cortisol-secreting (p. 485)
  - Sex hormone–secreting (p. 490)
  - Aldosterone-secreting
  - Pheochromocytoma (p. 785)
- May be benign or malignant. May be primary to the adrenal gland or a metastatic lesion

HISTORY, CHIEF COMPLAINT

- By definition, these tumors are an incidental finding.
- Nonfunctional: usually no clinical signs. Rarely cause ascites or pelvic limb edema due to vena cava invasion; patient presents for enlarged abdomen or limb swelling.
- Functional: questioning may reveal signs consistent with hypercortisolemia, excess sex hormones, hyperaldosteronism, or pheochromocytoma.

PHYSICAL EXAM FINDINGS

- Nonfunctional: rarely, palpable adrenal mass
- Functional: may have findings consistent with hypercortisolemia, excess sex hormones, hyperaldosteronism, or pheochromocytoma

Etiology and Pathophysiology

- Of primary adrenal tumors, 75% are adrenocortical.
- Nonfunctional: rarely, manifestations occur due to invasion of vena cava or adjacent organs.
- Functional: clinical syndrome dependent on hormone produced.
  - Hyperadrenocorticism
  - Occult hyperadrenocorticism
  - Primary hyperaldosteronism
  - Pheochromocytoma

DIAGNOSIS

Diagnostic Overview

Definitive diagnosis of mass type requires biopsy or surgical removal and histopathology. Determination of functionality requires biochemical testing. Factors that determine the aggressiveness of the diagnostic approach include original reason for performing abdominal imaging, the severity of concurrent problems, patient age, likelihood the mass is functional and/or malignant, size and invasiveness of the mass, and the client's desires.

Differential Diagnosis

- Tumor
  - Adrenocortical adenoma or carcinoma
  - Pheochromocytoma
  - Lipoma/myelolipoma
  - Metastasis from elsewhere; pulmonary, mammary, prostatic, gastric, and pancreatic carcinomas and melanoma most likely
- Nontumorous mass
  - Abscess
  - Granuloma
  - Hematoma
  - Nodular hyperplasia

Initial Database

- Repeat abdominal ultrasound to ensure the mass is a consistent finding.
- Review history and physical exam for evidence of functionality (i.e., signs suggesting hyperadrenocorticism, excess sex hormones, hyperaldosteronism, or pheochromocytoma)
- Nonfunctional tumor
  - CBC, biochemical profile, urinalysis, and blood pressure often unremarkable
  - Thoracic radiographs usually normal; adrenal tumors rarely metastasize to lungs
- Functional tumor: see chapters on hyperadrenocorticism, occult hyperadrenocorticism, pheochromocytoma, and hyperaldosteronism (pp. 485, 490, and 785) for information related to expected findings.
  - CBC, biochemical profile and urinalysis
  - Thoracic radiographs
  - Blood pressure
- Abdominal radiographs
  - Occasionally, mass evident cranial to the kidneys
  - May contain mineralization whether benign or malignant; diffuse, ill-defined mineralization usually associated with adrenal neoplasia, but discrete, well-marginated mineralization typical of benign lesion
- Abdominal ultrasound
  - Evaluate gland shape, asymmetry between glands and invasion of surrounding tissues.
  - Echogenicity varies.
  - Findings suggesting malignancy are any tumoral diameter > 2 cm, evidence of metastasis, or invasion into surrounding tissues and/or vena cava.
  - Atrophy of contralateral adrenal gland suggests tumor is secreting cortisol or hormone with glucocorticoid activity.

Advanced or Confirmatory Testing

- Functionality can be determined by various tests:
  - For cortisol-secreting tumor, low-dose dexamethasone suppression test preferred (p. 1360)
  - For sex-hormone-secreting tumor, ACTH stimulation test with measurement of sex hormones (p. 1300)
  - For aldosterone-secreting tumor, measurement of aldosterone likely sufficient (p. 1303)
  - For pheochromocytoma, measurement of blood pressure and potentially urinary catecholamines
- Abdominal computed tomography (CT)
  - Poor glandular demarcation, irregular contrast-enhancement, and a nonhomogeneous texture suggest malignancy.
  - Vascular invasion can be determined with high but not perfect accuracy.
- Cytology
  - Skill is required to perform ultrasound-guided aspirates of adrenal gland tumors.
  - Aspirates not recommended if systemic blood pressure is significantly elevated.
  - Cytology has 90%-100% accuracy for differentiating cortical from medullary origin; not reliable for distinguishing benign from malignant

TREATMENT

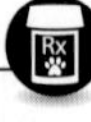

Treatment Overview

The same factors that determine the aggressiveness of the diagnostic approach affect the aggressiveness of the therapeutic approach. Medical and surgical options exist; if the mass is believed to be benign and nonfunctional, monitoring is sufficient.

Acute and Chronic Treatment

- If the mass is suspected to be malignant, adrenalectomy is preferred.
  - Medical therapy may be indicated prior to surgical intervention (pp. 35 and 785).
- If adrenalectomy is not indicated or not an option (e.g., metastatic disease, severe comorbid disease, very advanced age) and

yet clinical signs related to a functional mass develop with time or are recognized retrospectively, lifelong medical therapy can be instituted.
- Mitotane is the only true chemotherapeutic option and is effective for adrenocortical tumors only.
- Trilostane is used in cats with cortisol-secreting tumors.

Possible Complications

- Adrenalectomy should be undertaken only by experienced surgeons in a hospital with a well-equipped intensive care unit (ICU) and 24-hour observation and care.
- Postoperative complications include pancreatitis, pulmonary thromboembolism, acute renal failure, septic peritonitis, hypoadrenocorticism, hypotension, cardiac arrhythmias, and cardiac arrest.
- Mortality rate for adrenalectomy is approximately 10%-25%.

Recommended Monitoring

- A conservative approach (i.e., monitoring) is indicated if
  - No suggestion of malignancy is found
  - Tumor is < 2 cm in diameter
  - Functional tumor is not suggested by clinical signs or routine blood and urine tests
- Initial monthly ultrasound is recommended to determine the rate of mass growth and changes in the adrenal gland appearance.
  - If the mass has not increased in size after 3 months, repeat ultrasound q 3 months.
  - If the mass enlarges, changes in appearance, compresses, or infiltrates surrounding blood vessels or soft tissues or if clinical signs suggesting tumor functionality develop, consider adrenalectomy.

PROGNOSIS & OUTCOME

- Prognosis varies with type of tumor and therapy; survival can be months to years.
- Benign tumor: excellent to good
- Functional tumors: see relevant chapter
- Malignancy, larger tumor size, vena cava thrombosis, and presence of metastases associated with shorter survival

PEARLS & CONSIDERATIONS

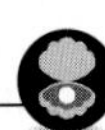

Comments

- Subtle clinical signs of functionality may become apparent with careful questioning of owner.
- An aggressive diagnostic or therapeutic approach is not always warranted.

Technician Tips

Functional adrenal test samples may require special handling; instructions should be read before obtaining a sample.

Client Education

Determining functionality of an adrenal tumor can be challenging. However, knowledge of functionality is crucial for preoperative and postoperative management or successful medical therapy.

SUGGESTED READING

Cook AK, et al: Clinical findings in dogs with incidental adrenal gland lesions determined by ultrasonography: 151 cases (2007-2010). J Am Vet Med Assoc 244:1181-1185, 2014.

AUTHOR & EDITOR: Ellen N. Behrend, VMD, PhD, DACVIM

Adrenocortical Neoplasia

Video Available  Client Education Sheet 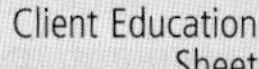 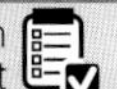

BASIC INFORMATION

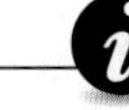

Definition

Tumors of the adrenal cortex that can be benign or malignant; they may also be nonfunctional or functional (e.g., secrete cortisol, sex hormones, or aldosterone). These can include incidentally identified adrenal tumors. Adrenal medullary neoplasia is discussed separately (p. 785).

Synonyms

- Adrenocortical carcinoma or adenoma
- Adrenal-dependent hyperadrenocorticism (p. 485)
- Hyperaldosteronism
- Incidental adrenal tumor or "incidentaloma" (p. 34)

Epidemiology

SPECIES, AGE, SEX

- Cortisol-secreting adrenocortical tumors
  - Dogs: > 9 years old
  - Cats: median 12.3 years old
- Aldosterone-secreting tumors: cats > 10 years old
- Incidentaloma: middle-aged to older dogs and cats

ASSOCIATED DISORDERS

- Hyperadrenocorticism (HAC) (p. 485)
- Hyperaldosteronism

Clinical Presentation

DISEASE FORMS/SUBTYPES

- Functional: secrete cortisol, sex hormones or aldosterone
- Nonfunctional

HISTORY, CHIEF COMPLAINT

- If functional, clinical signs depend on hormone(s) being secreted.
- If nonfunctional, often have normal physical examination; can also present for nonspecific signs related to space-occupying lesion (e.g., anorexia)

PHYSICAL EXAM FINDINGS

- If functional, findings depend on hormone(s) secreted.
- If nonfunctional, examination often normal; can have findings related to vena cava invasion (e.g., ascites)
- An abdominal mass may be palpable.

Etiology and Pathophysiology

- HAC is due to an adrenocortical tumor in approximately 15% of dogs and 20% of cats (p. 485).
  - Half are adenomas and half carcinomas.
  - Autonomous production of cortisol (usually) or a progestin (e.g., progesterone, 17-hydroxy-progesterone) inhibits ACTH production, resulting in atrophy of the contralateral adrenal cortex.
  - Cortisol excess causes clinical signs of HAC.
- Hyperaldosteronism is usually due to a unilateral adenoma or carcinoma.
  - Clinical signs are due to aldosterone excess causing hypokalemia and hypertension.
- On occasion, other hormones may be secreted.
  - Cortisol intermediates (e.g., desoxycorticosterone) causes clinical signs of HAC.
  - Androgens cause signs consistent with male behavior (e.g., roaming, spraying, growth of penile barbs in male cats).

DIAGNOSIS

Diagnostic Overview

- Most dogs with functional adrenocortical neoplasia have clinical signs consistent with

Cushing's syndrome, and diagnostics are directed toward confirming HAC.

- Occasionally, a patient presents with clinical signs consistent with both HAC and pheochromocytoma (e.g., polyuria/polydipsia [PU/PD] and mild to moderate hypertension). Differentiating the two is necessary for appropriate treatment.
- Alternatively, an adrenal mass may be identified in a patient with no reported clinical signs. After careful questioning of the owner, if clinical signs are not reported, additional diagnostics may not be necessary depending on the size of the mass (p. 34).
- Most cats with adrenocortical neoplasia have hyperaldosteronism, but some have HAC or an incidentaloma causing no clinical signs. Clinical signs usually direct the appropriate diagnostic path.
- The rest of the diagnostic and treatment section covers cortisol- and sex hormone–secreting adrenocortical neoplasia; see Hyperaldosteronism for more information on the diagnosis and treatment of aldosterone-secreting tumors.

Differential Diagnosis

- Pheochromocytoma
- Nodular hyperplasia associated with pituitary-dependent HAC (PDH)
- Metastatic neoplasia
- Granuloma

Initial Database

- Complete blood count, serum biochemistry, urinalysis, urine culture
  - If functional, results depend on hormone being secreted; findings often consistent with HAC
  - If nonfunctional, usually normal
- Thoracic radiographs
  - Pulmonary metastasis may be seen.
  - Pulmonary or hepatic metastasis occurs in about 10% of dogs with cortisol-producing adrenal adenocarcinoma.
- Abdominal radiographs
  - If cortisol-secreting, may see hepatomegaly
  - Mass may be visible cranial to kidneys.
  - Mineralization of adrenal tumor occurs in 50% of affected dogs; presence of mineralization does not help determine if benign or malignant.
  - Adrenal mineralization can occur in cats without adrenal disease.
- Abdominal ultrasound
  - Typically tumor is unilateral; bilateral adrenal tumors (adrenocortical and/or pheochromocytoma) occur rarely (see *Video*).
  - Patients with adrenal-dependent HAC can have an enlarged, hypoechoic liver, hepatic metastasis, and one large adrenal gland (>8 mm thickness) accompanied by an atrophied contralateral adrenal gland. If the contralateral gland is not atrophied (<5 mm) in a patient with confirmed HAC, consider the possibility that the mass is a hyperplastic nodule due to PDH.
  - Invasion of the vena cava or kidney may be visualized, but it is not apparent in some cases even if present.
- Blood pressure: often mildly to moderately increased with HAC; may be more severely increased (>220 mm Hg) in dogs with a pheochromocytoma.

Advanced or Confirmatory Testing

- To confirm and differentiate the cause of HAC, ACTH stimulation test, urine cortisol/creatinine ratio, low-dose dexamethasone suppression test, and/or endogenous ACTH concentration can be performed (p. 485).
- To help screen for pheochromocytoma, urine normetanephrine/creatinine ratio (p. 785)
- CT or MRI of the abdomen (p. 1132)
  - To confirm presence of the tumor and to assess invasion of adjacent structures
  - Recommended before adrenalectomy
- Histopathology is required after adrenalectomy to differentiate mass type.
  - Histopathology can help determine if adenoma or carcinoma, but differentiation can be difficult. Local tissue/blood vessel invasion and metastases are evidence of malignancy.
  - Functionality cannot be determined on histopathology; appropriate testing preoperatively is required.

TREATMENT

Treatment Overview

- Adrenalectomy is the preferred and most definitive treatment, but it has up to a 20% mortality rate and should be performed by a specialist in a 24-hour facility for postoperative monitoring.
- Dogs with tumors larger than 5 cm and/or that invade the vena cava or kidney have a worse prognosis.
- Medical treatment with trilostane (dogs and cats) or mitotane (dogs) is recommended in nonsurgical candidates (patients with metastasis, invasive tumors, comorbidities, or unwilling owners) if it is a functional tumor.

Acute General Treatment

Adrenalectomy

- If a tumor is cortisol-secreting, stabilization with trilostane (1-1.5 mg/kg PO q 12h, with food) is recommended for 3-4 weeks before surgery to decrease the risk of thromboembolism and dehiscence.
  - An ACTH stimulation test should be performed 10-14 days into therapy (p. 1300). Goal is to have post-ACTH cortisol concentration between 2 and 6 mcg/dL.

Chronic Treatment

Adrenalectomy

- Laparoscopic adrenalectomy is associated with fewer complications, less postoperative pain, and shorter hospitalization time than laparotomy.
- If the tumor is cortisol-secreting, glucocorticoids should be administered during and 3-6 months after surgery.
  - Dexamethasone 0.1 mg/kg is given over 6 hours intraoperatively and then tapered to 0.05 mg/kg q 12h until prednisone is tolerated.
  - Prednisone is started at 0.2-0.4 mg/kg q 12h and then tapered to 0.1 mg/kg SID over 3-6 months. Increase dose if lethargy or gastrointestinal signs noted.
  - Prednisone can be discontinued when post ACTH stimulation test cortisol concentration (performed at least 12 hours after prednisone) is > 5 mcg/dL.
- If bilateral adrenalectomy is performed, lifelong glucocorticoid and mineralocorticoid supplementation is necessary (p. 512)

Medical therapy

- Use only trilostane in cats.
- Mitotane (*o,p'*-DDD) can be used as when treating PDH or at higher doses as a chemotherapeutic agent to ablate all adrenocortical tissue (p. 485).
  - Adrenocortical tumors are more resistant to mitotane, and higher doses and longer induction periods are typically needed than when treating PDH.
  - Some dogs cannot tolerate the high doses required, especially when trying to ablate adrenocortical tissue.
- Trilostane 1-1.5 mg/kg q 12h or 2-3 mg/kg q 24h with food. Monitor and adjust dose as with PDH (p. 485).
- Treatment with mitotane and trilostane yields similar survival times in dogs when mitotane is not dosed for ablation.

Drug Interactions

- Do not give trilostane concurrently with ketoconazole because this can lead to excessive cortisol suppression and hypoadrenocorticism.
- Trilostane is more likely to cause hyperkalemia when given with angiotensin-converting enzyme inhibitors; monitor electrolytes closely.

Possible Complications

Postoperative complications

- Hemorrhage
- Thromboembolism
- Pancreatitis
- Acute kidney injury

Medical complications

- Hypoadrenocorticism

Recommended Monitoring

- After adrenalectomy, perform an ACTH stimulation test 2-4 weeks after the patient is clinically normal on 0.1 mg/kg/day of prednisone and monthly thereafter if needed. Prednisone can be discontinued after the post-stimulation cortisol is > 5 mcg/dL.

- Thoracic radiographs and abdominal ultrasound q 2-3 months to check for metastasis.

PROGNOSIS & OUTCOME

- Adrenalectomy: up to 20% mortality rate; 2-4 year median survival if patient survives the perioperative period.
- Medical therapy
  - Approximately 1 year without metastatic disease
  - Approximately 2 months with metastatic disease
  - No difference in survival between mitotane or trilostane, if PDH-type protocol used for mitotane

PEARLS & CONSIDERATIONS

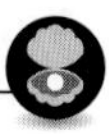

Comments

- Most surgeons require abdominal CT before adrenalectomy.
- Cats particularly benefit from preoperative stabilization with trilostane to decrease skin fragility and improve wound healing.
- Adrenalectomy should be performed by a board-certified surgeon in a facility with 24-hour monitoring.

Technician Tips

- If medical treatment is elected, make sure the owners understand that
  - If mitotane is used for treatment, the owners must contact the clinic and return for an ACTH stimulation test at the first sign of decreased water intake or appetite.
  - Treatment is for life.

SUGGESTED READING

Arenas C, et al: Long-term survival of dogs with adrenal-dependent hyperadrenocorticism: a comparison between mitotane and twice daily trilostane treatment. J Vet Intern Med 28:473-480, 2014.

AUTHOR: Patty Lathan, VMD, MS, DAVCIM
EDITOR: Ellen N. Behrend, VMD, PhD, DACVIM

Adulterated Diets

BASIC INFORMATION

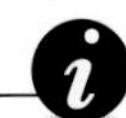

Definition

Food containing a deleterious or toxic substance in sufficient concentration to cause illness (uncommon)

Synonym

Food-borne illness

Epidemiology

SPECIES, AGE, SEX

Any dog or cat, but young, old, physiologically stressed, or immune-compromised animals are more susceptible.

CONTAGION AND ZOONOSIS

If adulterant is a pathogenic microbe (e.g., *Salmonella* spp.), potential exists for spread to other animals and people from contact with diet or infected biological material.

Clinical Presentation

DISEASE FORMS/SUBTYPES

Depends on specific etiological agent.

HISTORY, CHIEF COMPLAINT

Frequently causes vomiting and/or diarrhea. Other common complaints are food refusal/anorexia, lethargy, polydipsia/polyuria, anuria, jaundice, seizures, coma, or death. History often includes feeding a new product or new package of regularly used product within 1-30 days of illness.

PHYSICAL EXAM FINDINGS

Depends on specific etiologic agent

Etiology and Pathophysiology

Multiple possibilities; common ones include these:

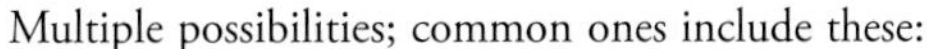

Etiologic Agent	Source	Associated Pathophysiology
Mycotoxins		
Aflatoxin	Corn, peanuts	Anorexia, icterus, ascites, hemorrhage, pale yellow-to-orange liver, edematous gallbladder, hepatic fibrosis (chronic)
Deoxynivalenol	Grains	Anorexia, weight loss, vomiting
Tremorgenic mycotoxins (e.g., penitrem A, roquefortine, verruculogen)	Moldy food	Fine muscle tremors, ataxia, seizures, prostration, polyuria, polydipsia
Enterotoxigenic bacteria (e.g., *Salmonella*, certain *E. coli* strains, *Clostridium*, *Staphylococcus*)	Contaminated or spoiled food	Vomiting, diarrhea, abdominal pain, distention, dehydration, gastrointestinal stasis to hyperactivity. *C. botulinum* produces progressive ascending flaccid paralysis
Metals		
Nutritive (e.g., zinc, selenium, copper, iodine)	Over formulation	Depends on specific metal
Non-nutritive (e.g., lead, mercury, cadmium)	Contaminant	Depends on specific metal
Vitamin D	Overformulation	Anorexia, lethargy, vomiting, diarrhea, hypercalcemia, soft tissue calcification, renal failure
Vitamin A	Overformulation	Anorexia, lethargy, weight loss, skin thickening and peeling, bone malformation, hemorrhage, decreased liver and kidney function
Pesticides	Contaminant	Depends on specific pesticide
Melamine + cyanuric acid	Contaminant	Kidney failure

DIAGNOSIS

Diagnostic Overview

Animals have usually eaten or refused food within a day of becoming clinically ill, implicating the food as a possible cause of illness. Definitive proof that illness was caused by the food requires: 1) clinical and pathophysiologic findings consistent with a specific substance or class of substances; 2) detecting the substance in the food at concentrations sufficient to produce observed clinical and pathophysiologic findings; and 3) in some instances, detecting the same substance or a metabolite in a sample from the animal.

Differential Diagnosis

- Depends on specific cause and pathophysiology

Initial Database

- Thorough, complete history, including all foods and products fed to the animal during the past 2-4 weeks; any husbandry conditions or activities allowing potential exposure to other etiologic agents capable of producing similar clinical presentations
- Minimum database: physical examination, complete blood count, complete biochemical profile, urinalysis

Advanced or Confirmatory Testing

Detection of suspected substance in food the animal was eating before illness. Detection assays should be validated for the substance in food. Identical microbial pathogens should be confirmed in food and biological samples from the animal. Check with laboratory for specific tests and preferred sample preparation. If food must be preserved before identifying appropriate laboratories and tests, it is usually best to double-bag in self-sealing plastic bags and freeze. Product label should also be saved.

TREATMENT

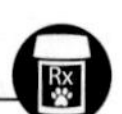

Treatment Overview

Change food to remove causative agent; stabilize critical physiologic functions; if definitive cause established, administer specific therapy as indicated.

Acute General Treatment

General supportive care

Chronic Treatment

Depends on initial outcome and residual compromise to physiological functions

Nutrition/Diet

If the patient's normal diet is a suspected cause, change the food. Select new diet based on status of major organ functions and on supportive treatment goals.

Behavior/Exercise

Prevent access to extraneous sources if cause is determined to be from environmental exposure.

Possible Complications

Chronic deficits to major organ system function (e.g., renal, hepatic, endocrine) are possible.

PROGNOSIS & OUTCOME

Grave prognosis for aflatoxicosis. Prognosis for other conditions varies by extent and duration of exposure to etiologic agent, organ compromise, and treatment response.

PEARLS & CONSIDERATIONS

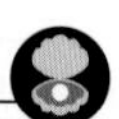

Comments

- Food is generally easy to implicate, but rarely confirmed as the cause when necessary diagnostics are performed. Before investing in testing food for adulterants, it is prudent to eliminate more common and likely differentials using the history and pathophysiologic results.
- Report suspected cases of food-borne illness to the state's FDA Consumer Complaint Coordinator (http://www.fda.gov/Safety/ReportaProblem/ConsumerComplaintCoordinators/default.htm)

Technician Tips

Ask about all foodstuffs, including treats or table scraps.

Client Education

- Product label should be kept as long as product from a package is being fed. Label contains key information (e.g., lot codes, best-by dates, manufacturing location) to allow follow-up sampling.
- Report a pet food product complaint electronically through the Safety Reporting Portal (https://www.safetyreporting.hhs.gov) or call your state's FDA Consumer Complaint Coordinators (https://www.fda.gov/Safety/ReportaProblem/ConsumerComplaintCoordinators/default.htm).

SUGGESTED READING

National Research Council (NRC). 2005. Mineral tolerance of animals revised, Washington, D.C.: National Academy Press.

AUTHOR: William J. Burkholder, DVM, PhD, DACVN
EDITOR: Jennifer A. Larsen, DVM, PhD, DACVN

Aggression, Cat

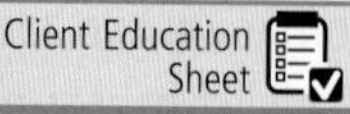

BASIC INFORMATION

Definition

Feline aggression can be a threat, challenge, or attack directed toward one or more individuals and can be intraspecific (between cats) or interspecific (between different species).

Epidemiology

SPECIES, AGE, SEX

Onset commonly occurs at social maturity (2-4 years of age) but can be seen at any age. Aggression is seldom recognized as a problem in kittens because they are assumed to be playing.

RISK FACTORS

- Underlying anxiety disorder
- Hand rearing (failure to learn social rules from other cats)
- Feral kittens
- Lack of exposure to humans between 2-7 weeks of age (this is a critical sensitive period of feline development when cats learn about other species)
- *In utero* and perinatal malnutrition
- Intracranial disease (e.g., toxoplasmosis, ischemic encephalopathy, intracranial neoplasia, rabies), hepatic encephalopathy, lead poisoning, arthritis, sensory deficits, hyperthyroidism, epilepsy, feline lower urinary tract disease, or any source of pain
- Medications such ketamine and glucocorticoids have been implicated.
- Feline elimination disorders may be associated with unresolved intercat aggression between cats in the same household.

CONTAGION AND ZOONOSIS

Bite or scratch wounds, pathogen transmission through bites or scratches (e.g., cat-scratch disease, retrovirus)

GEOGRAPHY AND SEASONALITY

Aggression between intact cats may be more apparent during the breeding season, but the extent to which seasonality affects aggression in neutered cats is unknown.

Clinical Presentation

DISEASE FORMS/SUBTYPES

May be passive (covert) or active (overt) and involve a threat, challenge, or an actual attack

- Passive aggression may involve behaviors such as staring, sitting in doorways, or blocking access; owners may not recognize this as aggression.
- Active aggression is usually more obvious: hissing, spitting, growling, actual fighting, and biting.

HISTORY, CHIEF COMPLAINT

- Sudden onset of aggression between two or more cats in a household or aggression to humans (owners or visitors). Aggression to humans may be redirected aggression.
- Cats may stalk and bite owners when they move or attempt to approach/handle cat (overt aggression). A cat may also block access

to areas (passive aggression). History should include a description and photos/videos of the physical location, body posture, vocal and physical signals, and the behavior sequences involved so that these can be used in management and prevention.
- Aggression may be associated with limited resources (e.g., food, litter boxes, beds).

PHYSICAL EXAM FINDINGS

Signs may be
- Visual (changes in body posture, piloerection)
- Auditory (hissing, spitting)
- Olfactory (spraying, scratching, or rubbing areas rich in sebaceous glands that secrete pheromones: chin, head, cheeks, tail base, and whisker area)
- Tactile (may involve use of teeth and/or claws)
- General exam usually unremarkable but medical disorders should be ruled out

Etiology and Pathophysiology
- The hypothalamus and amygdala are involved in defense and aggression.
- Monoamines and androgenic steroids act as modulators of offensive and defensive aggressive behaviors.

DIAGNOSIS

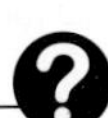

Diagnostic Overview
The diagnosis is based on a history of passive or active aggressive incidents directed toward other cats or people.

Initial Database
- CBC, serum biochemistry profile, urinalysis, diagnostic imaging: to rule out contributing medical factors and before prescribing medication
- A lead II electrocardiogram may identify cats with cardiac conduction disturbances (QT prolongation) that can increase risk of adverse cardiac reactions to medications (rare).

Advanced or Confirmatory Testing
- Diary of incidents (time, location) to establish frequency, duration, and intensity
- Video of the cat's interactions with other cats or people
- Video of the cat(s) when no people are home to assess social relationships of cats

TREATMENT

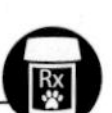

Treatment Overview
- In-house intercat aggression: aim is for the cats to tolerate each other's proximity by reducing the stress response, underlying arousal, and anxiety
- Intercat aggression to non-household cats: aim is to provide owners with management strategies
- Aggression directed toward owners: aim is to help the owners manage the cat's behavior and risk by providing treatment and management strategies
- Aggression directed to household visitors: aim is to provide owners with management strategies
- Cases that do not improve or resolve within a month or when the aggressive behaviors escalate should be referred to a veterinary behavior specialist

Acute General Treatment
- Any highly aroused cat should not be approached even to calm or reassure it because of potential hypothalamic *kindling*. The cat should be left alone until calm (at least 24-48 hours).
- Aggressive cats should be separated so they can hear and smell but not see each other for a minimum of 3 days.
- All situations that provoke aggression (e.g., petting) should be avoided. If the aggression to people is severe, the cat should be moved to another room using heavy blankets for protection; provided with food, water, and a litter tray and leave for 24-48 hours.

Chronic Treatment
In-house intercat aggression
- Each cat should separately be rotated around the house for at least 2 weeks until its scent is present in all rooms.
- While separated, feed and play with each cat during a predictable time each day. Offer favorite treats 5-6 times/day.
- Gradually reintroduce the cats to each other as one would a new cat. The aim is to create positive associations between cats, and feeding at a distance in each other's presence may help.
  - Cats must be very slowly reintroduced only after they can be fed treats in each other's presence. At first, cats should be in the same room during treat or meal times, possibly in cages or on harnesses at a distance from each other (e.g., at opposite ends of a large room). The cats must be completely calm in each other's presence, which may take weeks.
  - If no hissing or spitting occurs and each cat eats the food, the harnessed/caged cats are very gradually brought closer and closer to each other over a period of days and meals. This may take weeks to months.
  - One cat at a time is unharnessed/uncaged to explore. If no aggression occurs, the other cat is released while the first is restrained/confined.
  - If no signs of aggression occur, both cats can interact with supervision.
  - Reintroduction must be very gradual.
  - Caution is urged to avoid overzealous use of crates/cages. Clients often attempt to use cages in the hope that the cats accept each other's presence by continual exposure (flooding). Flooding is almost always traumatic and may result in permanent damage.
  - After cats are successfully reintroduced, provide separate food/water bowls, bedding, litter trays at a distance from each other.
  - Not all cats can be reintroduced; some must forever live separately.
- Anxiolytic medication may also be needed to treat one or both cats.
  - Blood tests before starting medication; auscultation possibly with an electrocardiogram for cats given tricyclic antidepressants (TCAs), selective serotonin reuptake inhibitors (SSRIs), or serotonin antagonist and reuptake inhibitors (SARIs)
  - TCAs: amitriptyline (0.5-1 mg/kg PO q 24h; average 5-10 mg/CAT PO q 24h) (up to q 12h) or clomipramine (0.5 mg/kg PO q 24h)
  - SSRIs: fluoxetine (0.5 mg/kg PO q 24h), paroxetine (0.5 mg/kg PO q 24h) or sertraline (0.5 mg/kg PO q 24h) for one or both cats
  - SARI: trazodone (0.5 mg/kg; ≈2.5-3.0 mg/CAT, PO q 12h) may be useful for one or both cats
  - Benzodiazepines such as alprazolam (0.0125-0.025 mg/kg PO q 12h), oxazepam (0.2-0.5 mg/kg PO q 12h), diazepam (0.2-0.4 mg/kg PO q 12h; ≈1-2 mg/CAT PO q 12h) may be helpful for victims.
  - Buspirone (0.5-1 mg/kg PO q 8-24h) may be helpful for cats that require more social confidence with the other cat.
  - Some medications may take up to 6-8 weeks to affect neurochemical and neuromolecular change; treatment for 6-12 months or more is often necessary (then wean gradually under veterinary supervision).

Intercat aggression involving non-household cats
- Contact between cats should be discontinued, even if this means confinement without visual contact.
- Outdoor enclosures should be avoided; they prevent tactile contact but may allow other social interaction that may cause the cats to become highly aroused.
- Anxiolytic medication may be needed to treat the cat(s) within the household, as above.

Aggression toward the owner
- It is important to identify and avoid all provocative situations (e.g., approaching, petting).
- Owners should initiate behavior modification in which the cat is rewarded for calm behavior.
  - The cat is taught to come or sit at the owner's request and rewarded with a treat.
  - If the cat solicits attention, the cat should be asked to sit and be rewarded. If the cat does not sit, the owner should walk away.
- Desensitization and counter-conditioning to handling and moving can be attempted slowly using rewards for acceptable behavior.
- No physical punishment should be used. It will exacerbate the problem, increase the underlying anxiety, and increase the risk for injury.

- Antianxiety medication may also be needed, as above.

Aggression toward human visitors

- Identify and then avoid all situations that may be provocative (e.g., approaching, petting). It is safest to confine the cat to another room when visitors are present.
  - If the owners wish to desensitize and counter-condition the cat to novel people, they can do so as above. When the cat is able to respond to the owners in all situations, visitors can be incorporated into this behavior modification plan if they will follow the instructions (e.g., treat the cat when it responds to the verbal/visual cue to sit or come).
  - Clicker or target training may facilitate behavior modification without touching the cat.

Behavior/Exercise

- Provision of physical and mental stimulation is important. For redirecting aggressive behaviors from people, toys suspended from poles such as cat dancers are useful.
- For indoor cats, provision of vertical (three-dimensional) space and places to hide (e.g., boxes) can be useful. All climbing spaces should have at least two entry/exit points so one cat cannot block escape routes.
- If urine spraying is part of the presenting complaint, appropriate management measures should be undertaken (p. 533).

Drug Interactions

TCAs and SSRIs should not be used together or with monoamine oxidase inhibitors such as selegiline (p. 1281).

Possible Complications

- Increased anxiety or arousal with some medications initially; benzodiazepines can disinhibit aggression
- Diazepam has been associated with hepatotoxicosis; most affected cats were overweight. Diazepam has a long $t_{1/2}$ in cats.

Recommended Monitoring

Follow-up examination 4-6 weeks after initial consultation to monitor progress with behavior modification/management strategies

PROGNOSIS & OUTCOME

The behavior can usually be successfully managed with owner education and compliance.

PEARLS & CONSIDERATIONS

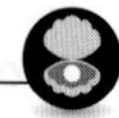

Comments

- Avoid punishment of aggression. It will worsen aggression and underlying anxiety and increase risk of injury.
- Clients should videotape the environment and the cats; this is a good educational tool for clients to understand feline body language and space use.
- Clients should concentrate on understanding the individual cat's needs rather than incorrectly labeling the cat's behaviors as spiteful or vindictive.

Prevention

Aggressive or anxious cats should not be bred. Kittens should be socialized.

Technician Tips

Educate owners of kittens regarding normal feline behavior and provide information about cat social environments as part of the first kitten visit. Kitten classes should be encouraged.

Client Education

- Attendance at kitten classes can help owners understand normal feline behavior, and it allows cats the opportunity to socialize.
- Owners should be cautioned about the risks of abruptly stopping medications.

SUGGESTED READINGS

Ahola MK, et al: Early weaning increases aggression and stereotypic behaviour in cats. Nature Sci Reports 7:10412, 2017

AUTHOR: Kersti Seksel, BVSc (Hons), MRCVS. MA (Hons), FANZCVS, DACVB, DECAWBM
EDITOR: Karen L. Overall, VMD, MA, PhD, DACVB

Aggression, Dog

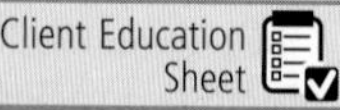

BASIC INFORMATION

Definition

An appropriate or inappropriate threat or challenge that is ultimately resolved by combat or deference

Synonyms

Aggression should not be equated with dog bites because a bite/puncture may result from normal grasping behavior using the mouth, and most pathologic/problematic aggression does not include biting.

Epidemiology

SPECIES, AGE, SEX

- Any age and either sex
- Pathological aggression often appears by end of sexual maturity (6-9 months) through social maturity (12-36 months)
- Impulse-control (formerly *dominance*, sometimes *conflict*) aggression: 90% male; in females, often very young (8 weeks old).

GENETICS, BREED PREDISPOSITION

- Impulse-control aggression affects any breed, but often in the United States, English springer spaniels (bench), Dalmatians; in the United Kingdom, English cocker spaniels, golden retrievers, and others
- Fear aggression affects any breed, but often border collies, German shepherds
- No one breed is at greater risk for bites to humans. Breed-specific legislation (BSL) has consistently failed to decrease dog bites; more effective approaches involve identifying/treating problem dogs and educating children/adults about normal dog behavior and signaling and supervising children when in the presence of a dog.

RISK FACTORS

- Genetic liability (largest risk factor)
- Dogs that are chained are overrepresented in dog bite statistics.
- Dog parks (dogs unknown to each other; clients may erroneously see interaction as a form of treatment for fearful or aggressive dogs)
- Misconceptions may worsen the problem. Clients are often mistakenly advised to "dominate" the dog or to be "alpha." These terms and their usage are based in profound misunderstandings of canine behavior, and this approach must not be used because it threatens dogs and increases risk.
- Puppy mill/commercially bred dogs may be more at risk for some forms of aggression, including food-related aggression.

CONTAGION AND ZOONOSIS

- Risk of physical trauma and of zoonosis (rabies, others) with bite wounds
- Bite wound characteristics reflect human response to the bite and movement, not the bite alone.
  - Boys 5-9 years old: highest risk for bites; dog is usually known to them
- Physical punishment (by humans) in response to canine aggression will almost always increase the risk to humans and worsen the condition.

ASSOCIATED DISORDERS

- Coexistence of more than one form of aggression or other behavioral disorders is common.
- Obtaining an accurate diagnosis of type of aggression is essential to help identify triggers.

Clinical Presentation

DISEASE FORMS/SUBTYPES

Victim/target (e.g., human directed vs. animal directed) approach is limited; prefer functional approach (see below)

Five commonly encountered types of pathologic aggression:

- Impulse-control/aggression: can involve dog's growling, baring teeth, staring, and/or biting, especially in response to certain human behaviors (e.g., staring at dog, reaching toward or over dog, punishment).
- Fear aggression: characterized by dog's trembling; growling, barking, or snapping while backing up; cowering; possibly biting from behind and running away. The fearful dog, even when aggressive, is signaling a desire to increase its distance from the target of aggression.
- Interdog aggression: characterized by dog making threats, staring, and challenges that are not normal and occur despite the response of the dog receiving these signals. Usually male-male or female-female. May be neuter-responsive in males that fight with non-household members. Not all aggressive behaviors that dogs exhibit toward each other are pathologic (consult veterinarian/behaviorist).
- Protective/territorial aggression: characterized by dog's barking, growling, snarling, biting to protect stationary (e.g., house) or mobile (e.g., car) property. Worse with discrete boundaries (e.g., fence). Not aggressive away from territory. May be normal and/or encouraged.
- Food-related aggression: characterized by growling when eating if approached (even from far away), biting if food/treat is thought to be threatened. This does not include mild grumbling that can occur between dogs as part of normal canine behavior. This is the most easily managed of these pathologic aggressions.

HISTORY, CHIEF COMPLAINT

- Early signs are often not noticed by clients and must be specifically screened for by veterinarians.
- Biting, growling, snarling, lip lifting, snapping, staring, and body posturing (e.g., blocking of access) are common early signs of aggression.
- Abuse, neglect, or lack of socialization seldom factor into histories of true pathologic aggression, with the exception of food-related aggression that may have hormonal and epigenetic associations with heightened reactivity/arousal.

PHYSICAL EXAM FINDINGS

Exam is almost always unremarkable, barring dog bite wounds in interdog aggression.

Etiology and Pathophysiology

Dogs with impulse-control aggression may have abnormal levels of cerebrospinal neurochemical metabolites and may excrete metabolites of excitatory neurotransmitters in their urine.

- Amygdala, caudate nuclei, and frontal cortex implicated in the cognitive component involving when and how to react

DIAGNOSIS

Diagnostic Overview

The diagnosis is entirely based on history and pattern of aggressive behavior; a complete history is necessary to identify features that optimize treatment and prognosis.

Differential Diagnosis

Primary neurologic disease (encephalitis, adverse medication reaction). Brain mass/neoplasm is an uncommon cause for aggression.

Initial Database

CBC, serum biochemistry profile, and urinalysis to rule out underlying medical conditions and contraindications for psychotropic medication. Generally unremarkable

Advanced or Confirmatory Testing

A video recording of the dog's behavior can provide essential information to distinguish between forms of aggression. Provocative testing leads to false-positives and enhanced risk.

TREATMENT

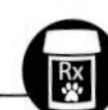

Treatment Overview

Treatment goals:

- Abort the exhibition of aggressive behaviors to render the dog safer and prevent the dog from learning to be more aggressive.
- Enhance public/familial safety and emotional bonds with the dog.
- Alleviate or prevent anxiety underlying the aggression.
- Render the dog happier by meeting its needs; this may mean that there are certain circumstances in which these patients should never be placed.
- Aggression involves a set of rules that allows the dog to cope with what it perceives to be an uncertain world and is ideally suited to treatment by substituting a more humane set of rules that helps make the world more predictable to the dog.

Acute General Treatment

- The key to keeping clients and dogs safe is to avoid all known provocative circumstances, even if humans must alter their behavior (applies to all forms of aggression). If the dog becomes reactive, ignore/avoid/contain it until the situation calms.
- Physical punishment/threats/discipline are strictly contraindicated—they intensify pathologic aggression.
- The trigger in impulse-control aggression is about the dog's perception of or response to humans who exhibit any type of action associated with control (e.g., reaching for the dog). Instead of reaching for the dog, clients can learn to call the dog to them and teach the dog, with positive reinforcement, to offer behaviors that are appropriate (e.g., teaching the dog to lift its head/neck for a collar to be slipped on).
- For fear aggression, the dog should feel protected. Do not continue to expose the dog to the feared trigger, thinking the dog will "get used to it"; usually, the dog will only suffer and become worse.
- For interdog aggression, separate the dogs when not supervised. A video of the dogs when they are not fighting reveals body postures and signals indicating which dog is the aggressor; this dog must be prevented from actively or passively threatening other dogs.
- For food-related aggression, if the food over which the dog is aggressive is a food toy (e.g., treat cube, rawhide), remove it from the dog's repertoire. If the dog is aggressive over meals, feed the dog separately behind a locked door, and do not take the food dish until the dog is out of the room and otherwise focused. If children are in the household, dogs and children must always eat separately.
- Do not kennel, crate, tie, chain, or put aggressive dogs in a run if they can be approached and harassed or if it makes them more reactive.
- If the client is thinking of euthanizing the dog or is afraid of living with the dog, consider boarding the dog for a week so the client can make an informed, nonimpulsive decision. The vast majority of these dogs improve dramatically when clients understand triggers for biting.

Chronic Treatment

- Dogs should be taught to sit and relax while making eye contact with the clients as a preferred default/substitute behavior when the dog encounters a situation about which it is anxious or unsure.
- Systematic desensitization can be used if the triggers can be safely identified and manipulated.
- Head collars can be used indoors/outdoors, allowing a dog's mouth to be humanely closed while behavior is redirected in a way that mimics normal dog signaling.
- More specific behavior modification designed to teach the dog to trust the client and take cues about the appropriateness of their behavior should be coupled with medications:
  - Amitriptyline (tricyclic antidepressant [TCA]): 1-2 mg/kg PO q 12h × 30 days to start, *or*
  - Fluoxetine (selective serotonin reuptake inhibitor [SSRI]): 1 mg/kg PO q 24h × 60 days to start, *or*
  - Clomipramine (TCA): up to 3 mg/kg PO q 12h × 60 days
  - Combinations of lower doses of amitriptyline and fluoxetine (synergistic)
  - Benzodiazepines are thought to disinhibit such dogs, but they actually only disinhibit inhibited aggressions, an effect

that worsens with the sedative effects of the medication. For some dogs who are globally anxious, the panicolytic medication alprazolam (0.02-0.04 mg/kg PO q 4-6h prn) may help calm reactivity while helping the dogs focus more on cognitive aspects of behavior modification.
- Gabapentin (10-20 mg/kg PO q 8-12h) affects regions of the GABA receptor and may dampen aggressive outbursts.

Nutrition/Diet

Polyunsaturated fatty acids (1200-1500 mg/DOG PO q 24h) may aid neurochemical recovery from aggressive events.

Drug Interactions

SSRIs and TCAs should not be used with monoamine oxidase inhibitors (e.g., amitraz, selegiline) due to enhancement of shared side effects (e.g., sedation, serotonin syndrome) (p. 1281).

Possible Complications

Failure to improve can be due to overly rapid behavior modifications, discordant approaches in the household, or history of choke chain, pinch collar, electronic/e-collar "corrections" (dog perceives clients as a threat). Forceful corrections of any kind (including those shown on popular TV dog training shows) should never be used with aggressive dogs; these types of corrections make the dog worse and put the client at risk.

Recommended Monitoring

- Frequent (weekly) contact with clients
- All instructions, including warnings, must be in writing and understood by the clients.

PROGNOSIS & OUTCOME

- The best prognosticators for canine aggression are 1) the client's determination to help the dog and 2) his/her ability to provide a predictable environment in which the dog can improve.
- Clients who accept that the dog has a problem anxiety and choose to protect the dog find that the dog improves simply because it is no longer being constantly stimulated to react.
- Understanding that the dog has a problem anxiety can alter client expectations. Through some complex interaction of human and canine behaviors, if clients avoid specific triggers for the dog, the dog can improve sufficiently for many clients.
- Clients who are afraid of the dog often have trouble with treatment (behavior modification).
- Clients with chaotic households have trouble protecting the dog and preventing the dog from being a risk to others.
- Clients who commit to treating the dog for the dog's sake typically see improvement, regardless of the diagnosis or level of aggression.
- With appropriate treatment (often including medication, perhaps lifelong), the vast majority of these dogs improve to the extent that it is hard to tell they had a behavior problem. Early intervention is easiest and best.
- Many dogs benefit from lifelong restriction to certain physical or social situations.

PEARLS & CONSIDERATIONS

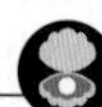

Comments

- Shock collars have no place in the treatment of any behavioral condition. They always exacerbate anxiety, even if they may suppress some behavioral signs. Their determined use by clients with aggressive dogs should prompt the suspicion of physical abuse (animal or human) in the household.
- The widely held belief that pathologic aggression in dogs stems from abusive handling in the past is entirely unsubstantiated. Abused dogs may also have problem aggressions, but aggression in response to abuse is sufficiently contextual that new environments may improve the lives of most abused dogs.
- Early deprivation in commercially bred dogs can lead to heightened reactivity that worsens aggression.

Prevention

- Humane training methods teach clients to read and understand dog signaling, a skill that leads to early detection of problematic behavior.
- Head collars and no-pull harnesses make it possible to raise even the most rambunctious dog to be relatively calm. All puppies should be fitted with these at their first appointment instead of neck collars.

Technician Tips

Technicians should calmly assess dogs' arousal levels beginning in puppyhood by emphasizing early skills (calm, settle, sit) and flag any early reactivity as requiring monitoring/treatment.

Client Education

- Consistency is key because it makes the world a more predictable place. Predictability lessens anxiety in a dog.
- Forceful training, training by compulsion, and training that involves physical restraint has no place in modern treatments of aggression. The Pet Professional Guild (www.petprofessionalguild.com) can direct clients to trainers who are trained and skilled in using only positive methods that enhance learning.
- With respect to impulse-control aggression, clients must understand that struggling with the dog will make the dog more dangerous. Treating these dogs is not about being their master; it is about treating their anxiety.
- With respect to interdog aggression, clients must understand that the dog they see being overtly aggressive may not have been the instigator. This is a complicated diagnosis. Quick fixes that are implied by simplistic recommendations ("reinforce the alpha dog") almost always worsen the condition.

SUGGESTED READING

Arata S, et al: "Reactivity to Stimuli" is a temperamental factor contributing to canine aggression. PLoS One 9:e100767, 2014.

AUTHOR & EDITOR: Karen L. Overall, VMD, MA, PhD, DACVB

Albuterol Toxicosis

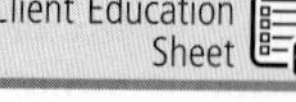

BASIC INFORMATION

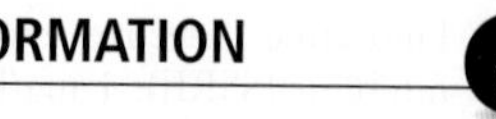

Definition

Albuterol is a primarily beta-2 adrenergic receptor agonist bronchodilator used for treating acute asthma and bronchospasm in humans, dogs, cats, and horses. Toxicosis can occur from inappropriate overdosing or pets chewing/biting into inhalers or vials used for nebulization.

Synonyms

Salbutamol; common brand names: Proventil (Merck); Ventolin (GSK), Combivent Respimat (Boehringer Ingelheim) in combination with the anticholinergic ipratropium

Epidemiology

SPECIES, AGE, SEX

All species, ages, breeds, and both sexes are susceptible. Dogs are more commonly exposed.

GENETICS, BREED PREDISPOSITION

Greyhounds may be more susceptible to severe cardiac arrhythmias compared with other dog breeds.

RISK FACTORS

- Pre-existing cardiac disease, systemic hypertension
- Patients taking tricyclic antidepressants or monoamine oxidase inhibitors

Clinical Presentation

HISTORY, CHIEF COMPLAINT

- Direct observation or evidence of exposure (chewed inhaler)
- Acute onset of panting, vomiting, anxiety, tremors, weakness, lethargy

PHYSICAL EXAM FINDINGS

- Tachycardia +/− arrhythmia
- Tachypnea
- Agitation, tremors, weakness

Etiology and Pathophysiology

- Albuterol is available in the form of inhalers (aerosolized powder or liquid), syrups, injectables, and tablets (prompt release and extended release).
- At therapeutic doses: albuterol binds to beta-2 receptors on the surface of bronchial smooth muscles. Cyclic adenosine monophosphate (cAMP) increases, leading to relaxation of bronchial muscle cells and bronchodilation.
- In overdoses, beta-2 receptor selectivity is lost, resulting in excessive beta-1 and beta-2 activity.
  - Beta-2 effects: hypotension, reflex sinus tachycardia, arrhythmias; tremors from stimulation of receptors in skeletal muscles; vomiting; intracellular shifting of potassium and phosphorus secondary to increased adenosine triphosphate enzymes (ATPases), and respiratory alkalosis from panting
  - Beta-1 effects and catecholamine release: positive inotropic effects on the heart, tachycardia, hypertension, restlessness, anxiety
  - Arrhythmias can also occur from secondary myocardial damage and hypokalemia. Aerosolized inhalers often contain hydrocarbons as the propellant, which can sensitize the myocardium and increase risk for arrhythmias.
  - Hypokalemia and prolonged tachycardia are often the causes for weakness.

DIAGNOSIS

Diagnostic Overview

Evidence of exposure (therapeutic or accidental) and presence of characteristic clinical signs (panting, tachycardia) establish the clinical diagnosis. Hypokalemia and/or hypophosphatemia offer further support.

Differential Diagnosis

- Toxicologic: pseudoephedrine, amphetamines, selective serotonin reuptake inhibitors (p. 1281), calcium channel blockers, cardiac glycosides
- Non-toxicologic: hypovolemic shock, cardiogenic shock, septic shock, neoplasia

Initial Database

- Complete blood count (CBC), serum biochemistry profile: mild to severe/critical hypokalemia is common; hypophosphatemia is possible.
- Blood pressure: hypo- or hypertension possible
- Electrocardiogram (ECG): premature ventricular complexes/ventricular tachycardia common

Advanced or Confirmatory Testing

Monitoring cardiac troponin-I concentration may be helpful to assess myocardial damage.

TREATMENT

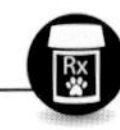

Treatment Overview

- Manage tachycardia with beta blockade (if required based on rapid sinus tachycardia) and/or correction of hypokalemia (if ventricular tachycardia).
  - Potassium supplementation may be needed, but avoid rebound hyperkalemia from over-supplementation: monitor and adjust (p. 516).
- Monitor for and manage arrhythmias (p. 1033).
- Manage tremors/stimulatory signs, if present, with benzodiazepines (p. 994).
- Decontamination (emesis and activated charcoal) is not indicated with ingestions of liquids, syrups, or inhalation forms of albuterol due to its rapid absorption. Consider emesis with 3% hydrogen peroxide or apomorphine in asymptomatic dogs that have ingested tablets (p. 1188) and are asymptomatic.
- Intravenous (IV) fluid support; adjust fluid rate cautiously in patients that already have cardiac arrhythmias or hypertension.

Acute General Treatment

- Propranolol (if normotensive) 0.02 mg/kg IV. If hypertensive, use esmolol: loading dose of 0.25-0.5 mg/kg (250-500 mcg/kg) slow IV over 2-5 minutes, followed by a constant rate infusion (CRI) of 10-200 mcg/kg/min.
- Correct hypokalemia (p. 516).
  - Hypokalemia favors ventricular arrhythmias and makes the myocardium refractory to lidocaine and other class I antiarrhythmics.
  - Correction of hypokalemia improves/resolves ventricular arrhythmias while also helping reduce or eliminate muscular weakness and lethargy.
- Lidocaine (for ventricular arrhythmia, only if normokalemic, p. 1457): 2-8 mg/kg slow IV over 1-2 min, followed by a CRI of 25-80 mcg/kg/min
- Potassium chloride (if potassium is < 3 mEq/L)
- Potassium phosphate (if potassium is < 3 mEq/L and phosphorus is < 1 mg/dL): 0.01-0.06 mmol/kg/h IV mixed in saline or dextrose
- For agitation/anxiety: diazepam 0.5 mg/kg IV or midazolam 0.2-0.4 mg/kg IV or IM

Drug Interactions

Propranolol: do not use if the patient is hypertensive. It could worsen the effects by blocking beta-2 receptors responsible for vasodilation, resulting in alpha-receptor dominance and vasoconstriction.

Possible Complications

- Ventricular premature complexes (VPCs), myocardial ischemia/damage or fibrosis
- Kidney injury from prolonged hypotension or hypertension
- Rebound hyperkalemia from excessive potassium supplementation
- Thermal injury to tissues from puncturing pressurized inhalers

Recommended Monitoring

- Heart rate, blood pressure, ECG
- Monitor for tremors, seizures, weakness
- Serum potassium and phosphorus levels

PROGNOSIS & OUTCOME

- Excellent with prompt and correct treatment of cardiac arrhythmias
- Development of arrhythmias and cardiac damage is more common with delayed treatment and could worsen prognosis.

PEARLS & CONSIDERATIONS

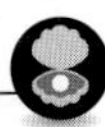

Comments

- All albuterol exposures should be taken seriously, and the patient should be evaluated quickly.
- Signs can develop even if the prescriptions are old/expired or from exposures to seemingly empty inhalers.
- Dogs biting into the inhaler can often receive a large dose of albuterol orally at once when pressured aerosol inhalers are punctured, leading to rapid onset of clinical signs within minutes to a few hours.
- Clinical signs and hypokalemia/hypophosphatemia associated with albuterol toxicosis may take 12-48 hours before completely returning to normal.
- Profound muscle weakness or collapse in dogs seen within a few hours of albuterol exposure correlates well with severe hypokalemia. Muscle weakness resolves when fluids are supplemented with potassium chloride or potassium phosphate.

Prevention

- Keep medications out of reach of pets.
- Properly dose animals that are being treated with albuterol.

Technician Tips

- Monitor the ECG and know how to recognize cardiac arrhythmias.
- Ask the client if the albuterol inhaler punctured by the dog was used or relatively new.

Client Education

- If pets are symptomatic, have them seen by a veterinary staff immediately.
- Teach proper dosing if owners are administering albuterol to patients at home to avoid overdosing.

SUGGESTED READING

Mensching D, et al: Breathe with ease when managing beta-2 agonist inhaler toxicoses in dogs. Vet Med June:369-373, 2007.

AUTHOR: Brandy R. Sobczak, DVM
EDITOR: Tina Wismer, DVM, MS, DABVT, DABT

Alopecia X

Bonus Material Online

BASIC INFORMATION

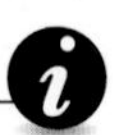

Definition

Acquired, progressive, noninflammatory alopecia of unknown cause seen typically in double-coat and dense-undercoat dogs and miniature poodles. Myriad names, etiopathogeneses, diagnostic procedures, and therapeutic modalities have been proposed, with varied validity and outcomes.

Synonyms

Hair cycle arrest, congenital adrenal hyperplasia, growth hormone–responsive alopecia, hyposomatotropism of the adult dog, pseudo-Cushing's, follicular dysplasia of Nordic breeds, follicular growth dysfunction of plush-coated breeds, black skin disease of Pomeranians, castration-responsive alopecia, coat funk in Alaskan malamutes

Epidemiology

SPECIES, AGE, SEX

- Dogs, both sexes, intact or neutered
- Onset at 1-10 years of age
- Breeds at greater risk include Pomeranian, chow chow, keeshond, Samoyed, Alaskan malamute, Siberian husky, and miniature and toy poodles.

Clinical Presentation

HISTORY, CHIEF COMPLAINT

Patients are generally presented because of owner-observed hair loss.

PHYSICAL EXAM FINDINGS

- Often starts with gradual loss of primary hairs progressing to complete alopecia of the neck, tail, perineum, and caudal thighs.
- Partial to complete alopecia of the entire trunk and tail, sparing the head and forelimbs, eventually develops.
- Hyperpigmentation is common.
- Scaling and superficial pyoderma are occasionally noted.
- No systemic signs of illness

Etiology and Pathophysiology

- Etiopathogenesis of this condition is unknown.
- Previous hypotheses such as growth hormone deficiency or hydroxylase-21 abnormality have been abandoned.
- Current popular hypotheses include a genetic predisposition to local follicular receptor dysregulation.

DIAGNOSIS

Diagnostic Overview

The diagnosis of alopecia X is by exclusion of other alopecic disorders.

Differential Diagnosis

- Endocrinopathies (hypothyroidism, hyperadrenocorticism, hyperestrogenism)
- Sebaceous adenitis
- Other follicular dysplasias

Initial Database

- History and physical examination findings
- Ruling out other differentials (may require CBC, serum chemistry panel, urinalysis, thyroid and adrenal function evaluation)

Advanced or Confirmatory Testing

- Skin biopsies are generally recommended to seek characteristic changes and rule out common differential diagnoses, notably sebaceous adenitis.
  - Histopathologic analysis typically reveals nonspecific changes of endocrinopathy. Excessive trichilemmal keratinization (flame follicles) seen in many cases of alopecia X is suggestive but not pathognomonic of this disorder.
- Sex hormone panels (baseline and post adrenocorticotropic hormone stimulation) have been recommended in the past, but usefulness has recently been questioned.

TREATMENT

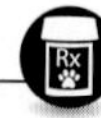

Treatment Overview

The therapeutic approach is highly empirical. Numerous treatment modalities have been proposed; none is always effective.

Acute General Treatment

- Neutering of intact dogs may induce permanent or temporary hair regrowth in ≈50%-75% of cases.

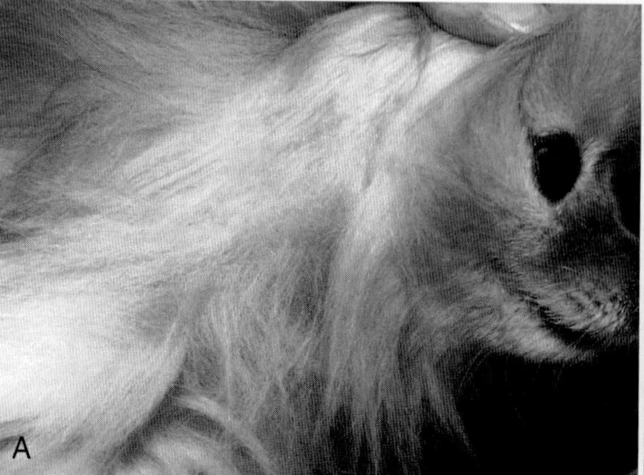

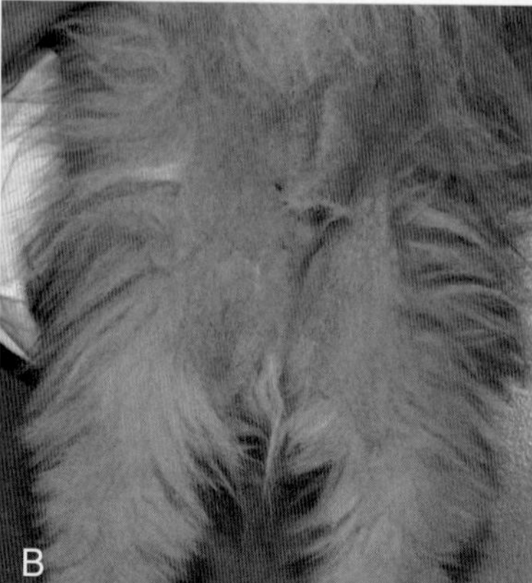

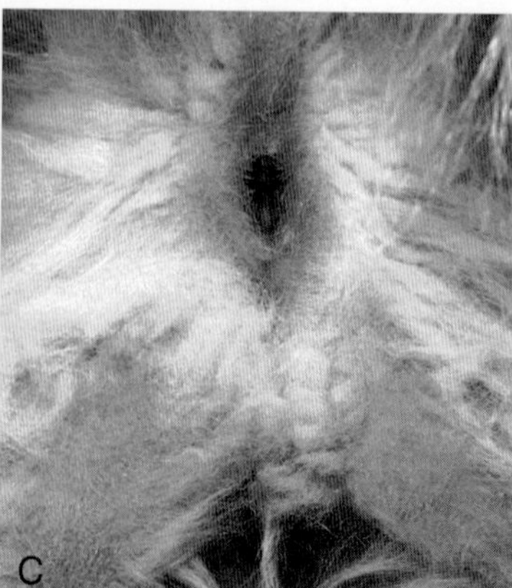

ALOPECIA X Alopecia X in 4-year-old, castrated male Pomeranian. Note alopecia affecting the neck (**A**), abdomen (**B**), and caudal thighs (**C**). (Copyright Dr. Manon Paradis.)

- Melatonin (3-6 mg/DOG PO q 8-12h for 3-4 months) is the first-line treatment for dogs with alopecia X if neutering was ineffective or the alopecia initially occurred after neutering or recurred after neutering. Partial to complete hair regrowth occurs in ≈30%-40% of cases, and treatment is very safe.
- Other therapeutic modalities can include
  - Mitotane (induction with 25 mg/kg q 24h or 25-50 mg/kg 2-3 times weekly has been suggested) is effective in ≈50% of cases. However, the risk of side effects (e.g., hypoadrenocorticism) should be carefully considered, and close monitoring is essential; *or*
  - Trilostane promotes hair regrowth in 90% of affected Pomeranians and miniature poodles.
  - Deslorelin implants appear effective only in intact male dogs.
  - Superficial mechanical skin trauma applied with microneedling device may induce hair regrowth in some dogs.

PROGNOSIS & OUTCOME

- Alopecia X is a purely cosmetic disorder. Proceeding without treatment is therefore a valid option.
- The progression of hair loss varies. Some dogs retain hair (puppy coat appearance) on the trunk for years; others become completely alopecic over the trunk within months.
- Hair regrowth is unpredictable with any of the current therapies and may not last lifelong.

PEARLS & CONSIDERATIONS

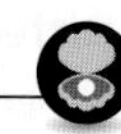

Comments

One of the unique features associated with alopecia X is hair regrowth at a site of skin trauma such as a biopsy or surgery site.

Technician Tips

Avoid unnecessary hair clipping because it may never grow back in dogs with alopecia X.

SUGGESTED READING

Paradis M: An approach to symmetrical alopecia in the dog. In Jackson H, et al, editors: BSAVA manual of canine and feline dermatology, ed 3, Gloucester, UK, 2012, BSAVA, pp 91-102.

AUTHOR & EDITOR: **Manon Paradis, DMV, MVSc, DACVD**

Alopecia, Cat

Bonus Material Online

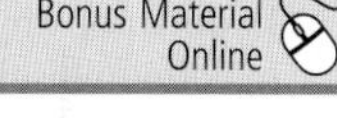

BASIC INFORMATION

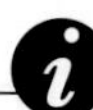

Definition

Hair loss in normally haired regions (alopecia) is a common dermatologic condition and may be congenital or acquired.

Epidemiology

SPECIES, AGE, SEX

- Congenital: young
- Acquired
  - Food allergy (dermatologic adverse food reactions): any age
  - Parasitic: any age
  - Dermatophytosis: any age
  - Atopic dermatitis (environmental allergies): young adult
  - Endocrine tumor: middle-aged to older

GENETICS, BREED PREDISPOSITION

- Alopecia universalis: Sphinx
- Hereditary hypotrichosis: Siamese, Devon rex, Burmese
- Follicular dysplasia: Cornish rex
- Dermatophytosis: Persian

RISK FACTORS

Multi-cat households/catteries; cats that venture outdoors; exotic breeds

CONTAGION AND ZOONOSIS

Some parasitic (e.g., fleas, cheyletiellosis) and fungal diseases (e.g., *Microsporum canis*) are both zoonotic and contagious. *Demodex gatoi* is contagious to other cats.

GEOGRAPHY AND SEASONALITY

Parasites have seasonal and geographic variations (e.g., fleas prefer warmer weather, increased humidity).

Clinical Presentation

DISEASE FORMS/SUBTYPES

- Congenital
- Acquired (pruritic, infectious, parasitic, behavioral, systemic)

HISTORY, CHIEF COMPLAINT

- Chief complaint: hair loss; overgrooming (not always noted by owners)
- Hyperthyroid cats may be polyphagic, underweight, and have an anxious disposition.
- Hypothyroid cats may be lethargic and obese.

PHYSICAL EXAM FINDINGS

- Hair loss, often bilaterally symmetrical
- Alopecia, self-induced secondary to pruritus:
  - Alopecia/barbering of ventrum, dorsum, antebrachia, and hindlimbs are common. Crusted papules (miliary dermatitis) raises index of suspicion. Excoriations secondary to the self-trauma may be noted.
- Alopecia, self-induced or not, secondary to a nonpruritic cause
  - Endocrine: variable amount of scaling; coat may appear dull and dry
    - Hyperadrenocorticism (rare in cats): thin skin, pendulous abdomen, and 50% of patients may experience skin fragility syndrome (skin tears easily with gentle traction)
    - Hypothyroidism (spontaneous is rare, iatrogenic secondary to treatment of hyperthyroidism more common); poor hair regrowth at pressure points, alopecia at neck, thorax, abdomen
  - Paraneoplastic (e.g., pancreatic neoplasia, hepatosplenic/bile duct tumors, colonic carcinoma): ventral abdominal alopecia and thin, shiny skin. Face, limbs, and footpads also may be affected.
  - Anal sac disorders: ventral abdominal alopecia, hair loss at the base of the tail
  - Cystitis/gastrointestinal disease: ventral abdominal alopecia
  - Dermatophytosis: variably pruritic. Patient may present with alopecia, scaling, miliary dermatitis, erythematosquamous macules, or patches.
  - Behavioral: "barbered" hairs with no primary lesions. Head and neck usually unaffected.

Etiology and Pathophysiology

- Pruritus: overgrooming
- Genetic: malformation/absence of hairs
- Fungal: mycotic destruction of hair shaft
- Endocrine: telogenization of hair follicles
- Medical: self-trauma secondary to discomfort (cystitis, gastrointestinal, anal sac disorder)
- Paraneoplastic alopecia: unknown
- Behavioral: compulsion, anxiety

DIAGNOSIS

Diagnostic Overview

First determine whether the cat is pulling the hair out or it is falling out spontaneously. If this is unclear, placement of an Elizabethan collar for several weeks can help to elucidate. If the hair is falling out, fungal culture, skin scrapings, skin biopsy, CBC, serum biochemical profile, and urinalysis are indicated. If the cause of the hair loss is self-trauma, a stepwise approach is taken to identify the cause among the multitude of possibilities. Many cases are multifactorial.

Differential Diagnosis

Congenital (all nonpruritic):

- Alopecia universalis (affected individuals born without hair)
- Hereditary hypotrichosis (affected individuals born with a thin hair coat progressing to alopecia)
- Follicular dysplasia (ongoing hair thinning progressing to alopecia)

Acquired:

- Pruritic
  - Parasitic (flea, *D. gatoi, Cheyletiella, Otodectes, Notoedres, Sarcoptes* [rare in cats], *Trombicula, Felicola subrostratus*)
  - Fungal (e.g., *M. canis*)
  - Food allergy
  - Atopic dermatitis
- Nonpruritic:
  - Fungal
  - Telogen/anagen effluvium
  - Feline degenerative mural folliculitis
  - Inflammatory bowel disease
  - Cystitis
  - Anal sacculitis
  - Endocrinopathy (hyperthyroidism; hypothyroidism: iatrogenic, spontaneous [very rare]; hyperadrenocorticism: iatrogenic, acquired [rare])
  - Neoplasia (cutaneous T-cell lymphoma, paraneoplastic syndrome, thymoma, hypereosinophilic syndrome)
  - Behavioral: compulsive, anxiety
  - Neurologic: hyperesthesia
  - See algorithm for feline alopecia (p. 1401).

Initial Database

- Comprehensive ectoparasite examination (flea combing, skin scrapings, trichograms)
  - Trichography: examination of hair tips to determine whether hair loss is self-inflicted (fractured hair shafts)
- Fungal culture (in-house dermatophyte test medium or external lab) (pp. 247 and 1091)
- Anal sac expression (anal sac disease may elicit excessive self-grooming; monitor long-term response to anal sac expression)

Advanced or Confirmatory Testing

Tests are selected based on information gathered to date and feasibility of testing with each case.

- CBC: eosinophilia may support a diagnosis of a hypersensitivity/parasites.
- Fecal evaluation may reveal an external parasite such as a flea, *Demodex*, or *Cheyletiella*.
- Serum biochemical profile: metabolic disease
- Urinalysis: metabolic disease, ventral abdominal alopecia (cystitis)
- Thyroid hormone evaluation
- An 8-12 week strict elimination dietary trial
- Response to steroid therapy is supportive of a pruritic cause.
- Intradermal and/or serum allergy testing is supportive but not conclusive that hair loss is due to environmental allergies. A negative test result does not eliminate the possibility.
- Feline leukemia virus and feline immunodeficiency virus testing (should be performed before cyclosporine use)
- Abdominal ultrasound/thoracic and abdominal radiographs (paraneoplastic, thymoma)
- Histopathologic evaluation of skin biopsies may be helpful in the diagnosis of endocrinopathy, neoplasia, paraneoplastic syndrome, mural folliculitis, and follicular dysplasia. Findings consistent with normal skin support a behavioral diagnosis but are not pathognomonic; behavioral cause (psychogenic alopecia) is a diagnosis of exclusion.

TREATMENT

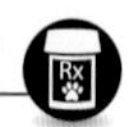

Treatment Overview

Correct underlying cause of alopecia.

Acute and Chronic Treatment

- Depends on underlying cause
- Specific parasiticide or broad-spectrum antiparasitic therapy:
  - Ectoparasiticide response trial (broad-spectrum parasiticide for 6-8 weeks, +/− fluralaner or lime sulfur dips for *D. gatoi*)
  - Express anal sacs (if ventral abdominal/tail head alopecia)
  - Elizabethan collar to differentiate self-trauma from hair loss

PROGNOSIS & OUTCOME

Uncomplicated disorders carry a better prognosis for control (atopic dermatitis) and possibly cure (fungal, parasitic, food allergy), but many cases can involve more than one cause. In these cases, the prognosis depends on the completeness of diagnostic testing and on client and patient compliance.

PEARLS & CONSIDERATIONS

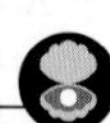

Comments

- A normal skin biopsy does not rule out pruritus as a cause of self-trauma.
- A large percentage of cats that self-traumatize have multiple, concurrent causes, emphasizing the need for a complete workup.
- Food allergy should be ruled out in all nonseasonally pruritic patients.
- Absence of parasites on physical examination does not preclude their presence. Perform empirical parasiticide therapeutic trials.

Technician Tips

Skin scrapes performed in regions difficult to groom (back of neck) may increase likelihood of finding *D. gatoi.*

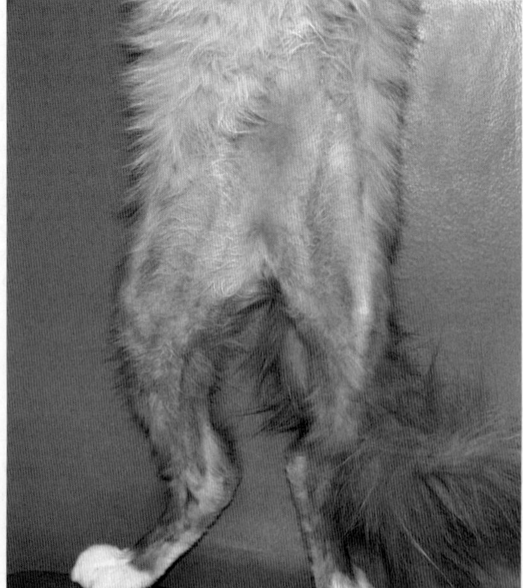

ALOPECIA, FELINE Self-induced alopecia on the abdomen due to intense pruritus in a 4-year-old Birman cat with *Demodex gatoi* infestation. (Copyright Dr. Manon Paradis.)

SUGGESTED READING

Mecklenburg L, et al: Hair loss disorders in domestic animals. Ames, IA, 2009, Wiley-Blackwell.

AUTHOR: Stephen Waisglass, DVM, DACVD
EDITOR: Manon Paradis, DMV, MVSc, DACVD

Alopecia, Dog

BASIC INFORMATION

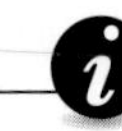

Definition

Complete or partial loss or absence of hair in areas where it is normally present. Alopecia can be localized, multifocal, or generalized.

Synonyms

Excessive shedding, hair loss, hypotrichosis

Epidemiology

SPECIES, AGE, SEX

Common; signalment depends on cause. Age of onset is clinically important.

GENETICS, BREED PREDISPOSITION

Breed predispositions exist for many causes of alopecia:

- Alopecia X (p. 44): plush-coated dogs (e.g., Pomeranian), arctic breeds, miniature poodle
- Breed-specific follicular dysplasia (p. 344): Chesapeake Bay and curly-coated retrievers, Portuguese water dog, Irish water spaniel
- Color dilution alopecia (CDA): blue or fawn Doberman pinscher, others
- Pattern alopecia: Boston terrier, dachshund
- Canine (recurrent) flank alopecia (p. 869): boxer, English bulldog, others
- Congenital hypotrichosis is normal in certain breeds (e.g., Chinese crested)
- Post-rabies vaccination panniculitis and alopecia: miniature poodle, other small dogs

CONTAGION AND ZOONOSIS

- Dermatophytosis
- Ectoparasites, including *Sarcoptes*, *Cheyletiella*, and fleas

GEOGRAPHY AND SEASONALITY

Seasonal: canine (recurrent) flank alopecia, self-inflicted alopecia due to atopic dermatitis or flea bite hypersensitivity

ASSOCIATED DISORDERS

- Hypothyroidism: lethargy, obesity
- Hyperadrenocorticism: Cushing's syndrome
- Sertoli cell tumor: male feminization
- Bacterial folliculitis or *Malassezia* dermatitis: often associated with underlying hypersensitivity dermatitis

Clinical Presentation

DISEASE FORMS/SUBTYPES

- Congenital or acquired
- Generalized or localized/multifocal
- Inflammatory or non-inflammatory

HISTORY, CHIEF COMPLAINT

- Determine age of onset and progression
- Question degree of pruritus
- Question other clinical signs (e.g., polyuria/polydipsia)
- Ask about recent pregnancy, serious illness, anesthesia (causes of telogen effluvium), vaccination (post-rabies vaccination panniculitis), drug administration (e.g., topical corticosteroid)

PHYSICAL EXAM FINDINGS

- Is alopecia diffuse or localized/multifocal? Symmetrical? Location?
- Is the hair absent (e.g., endocrine disease), broken (e.g., self-trauma), or miniaturized (e.g., pattern alopecia)?
- Does hair epilate easily (e.g., folliculitis)?
- Is there skin inflammation, skin lesions, or pruritus?
- Are there follicular casts (e.g., sebaceous adenitis, demodicosis)?
- What color is the hair (e.g., CDA)?
- Is the skin thickness normal (e.g., reduced: hyperadrenocorticism; increased: inflammatory conditions)?
- Is there evidence of endocrine disease (e.g., obesity, muscle atrophy) or other abnormal findings such as lymph node enlargement (e.g., pyoderma, leishmaniasis)?

Etiology and Pathophysiology

The mechanism of hair loss varies with the underlying cause:

- New hair failing to grow when old hairs are lost (e.g., endocrine)
- Inflammation in or around hair follicles (e.g., alopecia areata, sebaceous adenitis, infectious folliculitis with staphylococci, dermatophytes, or *Demodex*)
- Breakage of hair due to trauma (e.g., pruritus), structural hair defects (e.g., CDA), or direct infection (e.g., dermatophytosis)
- Dysplasia of hair follicles
- Diminution of hair follicle size (pattern alopecia)
- Ischemia (e.g., post-rabies vaccination panniculitis, dermatomyositis)
- Telogen effluvium (defluxion): synchronous arrest of the hair cycle caused by drugs, pregnancy, or other stressors
- Anagen effluvium (defluxion): sudden interruption of anagen resulting in an abnormal hair shaft and hair loss within days, not well documented in dogs

DIAGNOSIS

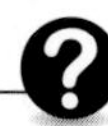

Diagnostic Overview

The distribution of alopecia and the degree of inflammation are helpful for prioritizing differential diagnoses and selecting diagnostic tests (p. 1091).

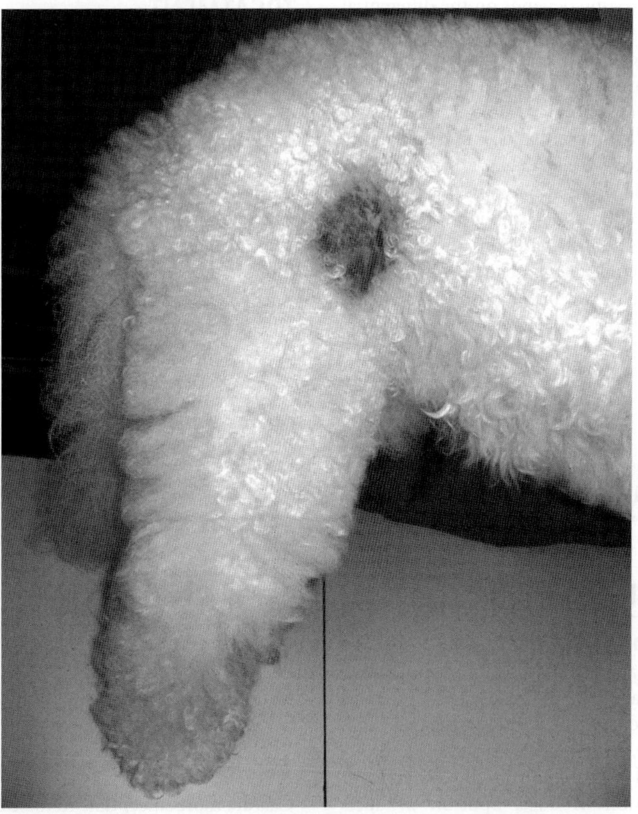

ALOPECIA, CANINE Post-rabies vaccination panniculitis and alopecia in a Bichon frisé.

Differential Diagnosis

Symmetrical or diffuse alopecia with minimal inflammation:

- Ectodermal defect or "normal" alopecic breed
- Hyperadrenocorticism (including iatrogenic)
- Hypothyroidism
- Hyperestrogenism (Sertoli cell tumor or other cause)
- Alopecia X
- Canine (recurrent) flank alopecia
- CDA
- Breed-specific follicular dysplasia
- Post-clipping alopecia
- Pattern alopecia
- Telogen (or anagen) effluvium
- Pituitary dwarfism

Symmetrical or diffuse alopecia with inflammation:

- Sebaceous adenitis
- Leishmaniasis

Localized or multifocal alopecia:

- Bacterial (staphylococcal folliculitis): most common cause in dogs
- Demodicosis
- Dermatophytosis
- *Malassezia* dermatitis
- Hypersensitivity dermatitis
- Pruritic ectoparasite infestation
- Immune-mediated diseases (alopecia areata, pseudopelade, post-rabies vaccination panniculitis and alopecia, dermatomyositis)
- Other: epitheliotropic lymphoma, traction alopecia

See algorithm for canine alopecia (p. 1400).

Initial Database

Appropriate testing depends on the differential diagnoses.

- Symmetrical/diffuse alopecia with minimal inflammation:
  - Trichography (microscopic examination of forcefully plucked hairs) can help identify demodicosis, CDA, black hair follicular dysplasia, dermatophytosis, telogen and anagen effluvium. Although trichography is useful in some conditions, the proportion of anagen to telogen hairs is highly breed dependent. Except in nonshedding breeds (e.g., poodles), telogen hairs predominate.
  - Skin scrapings
  - Minimum database: CBC, chemistry profile, urinalysis
  - Thyroid testing
- Localized, multifocal, or inflammatory alopecia:
  - Skin scrapings and other ectoparasite detection techniques
  - Wood's lamp examination and fungal culture for dermatophytes
  - Skin cytologic examination for bacteria and *Malassezia*
  - Trichography can help confirm traumatic hair fracture (self-trauma) or find *Demodex* mites, louse or *Cheyletiella* ova, and dermatophyte-infected hairs.

Advanced or Confirmatory Testing

- Symmetrical/diffuse alopecia with minimal inflammation:
  - Skin biopsies
  - ACTH stimulation, low-dose dexamethasone suppression, or urine cortisol/creatinine ratio
  - Adrenal reproductive hormone panel is not commonly used.
  - Abdominal radiography/ultrasonography
  - Response to time (e.g., telogen effluvium) or empirical therapy (e.g., melatonin)
- Localized, multifocal, or inflammatory alopecia:
  - Skin biopsies
  - Response to empirical therapy (e.g., treatment for infection if bacterial folliculitis is suspected)

TREATMENT

Treatment Overview

Correct underlying cause of alopecia.

PROGNOSIS & OUTCOME

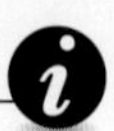

- The prognosis for alopecia is good if the underlying cause of hair loss is identified and treated and if hair follicles are still present.
- Extensive scarring and chronic ischemia limit hair regrowth.

PEARLS & CONSIDERATIONS

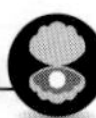

Comments

- Skin biopsies for alopecia: draw a fine, dark marker line along the direction of hair growth, and center the biopsy over it. Ask the laboratory to section the biopsy along this line to obtain longitudinal sections of the hair follicles. Collect several biopsies, and sample the most alopecic areas, partially alopecic areas, and normal skin.
- In dogs, multifocal alopecia with concurrent inflammation is most commonly caused by bacterial folliculitis. Treat appropriately for bacterial folliculitis, then re-evaluate.
- Skin scrapings are appropriate in almost all cases.
- Consider alopecia X in healthy, plush-coated or Arctic-breed dogs exhibiting truncal alopecia.
- Melatonin (3-6 mg/DOG PO q 12h for 3-4 months) is a safe and variably effective supplement to stimulate hair regrowth in the treatment of various noninflammatory alopecic disorders.
- Cyclosporine's ability to stimulate hair growth makes it useful for inflammatory, alopecic diseases such as sebaceous adenitis.

Technician Tips

- Trichography (p. 1091) can be used in evaluating alopecic dogs, but normal anagen/telogen ratios are not established for most breeds. The test is most useful for finding ectoparasites (particularly *Demodex* and louse ova), identifying hair shaft fracture, and finding large melanin clumps causing hair shaft distortion in color-dilution alopecia and black hair follicular dysplasia.
- Clients often ask about excessive shedding. It is truly only excessive if alopecia results.

SUGGESTED READING

Paradis M: An approach to symmetrical alopecia in the dog. In Jackson H, et al, editors: BSAVA Manual of canine and feline dermatology, ed 3, Gloucester, UK, 2012, BSAVA, pp 91-102.

AUTHOR: Kinga Gortel, DVM, MS, DACVD
EDITOR: Manon Paradis, DMV, MVSc, DACVD

Amitraz Toxicosis

BASIC INFORMATION

Definition

Amitraz is an acaricide that is an alpha-2 adrenergic agonist. It is used for control of mite, lice, and tick infestations in dogs and several large-animal species. Amitraz-impregnated collars and dips are available for tick prevention in dogs. Spot-on products were historically available. Toxicosis is characterized by sedation, ataxia, bradycardia, and hyperglycemia.

Synonym

Mitaban toxicosis

Epidemiology

SPECIES, AGE, SEX

Cats are more susceptible to toxic effects relative to dogs, but amitraz-containing products are more commonly used on dogs. Young, geriatric, and small patients may also have increased sensitivity.

GENETICS, BREED PREDISPOSITION

No specific breed predispositions are known.

RISK FACTORS

Topical exposure to large-animal formulations or incorrectly diluted small-animal products may result in clinical signs. Mild effects also have been reported in patients with topical exposure to correct dosages. Animals with inflamed or broken skin are more at risk. Ingestion of portions of amitraz-impregnated collars may cause significant toxic effects.

GEOGRAPHY AND SEASONALITY

Increased frequency of amitraz toxicosis may correlate with warm seasons and locations in which the environmental tick burden is higher.

Clinical Presentation

HISTORY, CHIEF COMPLAINT

Chief presenting complaint is often significant lethargy, depression, and/or ataxia. Pet owners may also identify ptyalism, vomiting/diarrhea, mydriasis, and hypothermia.

PHYSICAL EXAM FINDINGS

Mild cases due to topical exposure may display only mild lethargy and depression. More severe cases can display hypothermia, hypotension, bradycardia, vomiting, diarrhea, ileus, coma, and seizures.

Etiology and Pathophysiology

- Amitraz is an alpha-2 adrenergic agonist, and clinical signs and physiologic effects generally stem from central nervous system (CNS) effects, including subsequent effects on the cardiovascular and gastrointestinal (GI) systems.
- Amitraz is also a weak inhibitor of monoamine oxidase (MAO) activity in the CNS.

DIAGNOSIS

Diagnostic Overview

Amitraz toxicosis is suspected due to the combination of clinical signs and a history of exposure or potential exposure to amitraz-containing products. Sources report LD50 (lethal doses capable of killing 50% of test animals) of 100 mg/kg in dogs, although mild clinical signs have been reported with topical exposure at therapeutic dosages.

Differential Diagnosis

- Other toxicants
  - Opioids/narcotics
  - Alcohols (ethanol, methanol)
  - Marijuana
  - Muscle relaxants such as baclofen
  - Benzodiazepines
  - Barbiturates
  - Antidepressant and anxiolytic medications
  - Ivermectin
  - Botulism
  - Tick paralysis
- Systemic diseases/conditions
  - CNS disease or trauma
  - Hepatoencephalopathy
  - Sepsis, especially secondary to significant GI disease/perforation
  - Myasthenia gravis
  - Addisonian/hypoadrenocortical crisis

Initial Database

Temperature, pulse, respiratory rate, blood pressure, and electrocardiogram should be included in initial assessment. Specific clinicopathologic changes definitive for amitraz toxicosis have not been identified. Hyperglycemia may result from inhibition of insulin release. Electrolyte alterations may be due to vomiting and/or diarrhea, and azotemia may be present if the patient is dehydrated (correlate with urine specific gravity before fluid therapy to help exclude renal insufficiency/failure, Addisonian crisis, etc.). CBC abnormalities are absent or nonspecific.

Advanced or Confirmatory Testing

Radiographic imaging may reveal the collar buckle in ingestion cases, but collar fragments may not be visible. Upper GI endoscopy may identify ingested collar segments. Laboratory testing for amitraz is inconsistently available through diagnostic laboratories, and turnaround time may preclude utility in the emergency setting.

TREATMENT

Treatment Overview

In topical exposures, removal of the product via bathing with dish soap is an important step in resolution of signs. However, this step should be delayed until the patient is clinically stable, and care must be taken to ensure adequate thermoregulation during and after bathing. In ingestion cases, passage or removal of the collar segments is important for permanent resolution of clinical signs, but endoscopic or surgical intervention may be limited by patient clinical status.

Acute General Treatment

Reversal of the alpha-2 adrenergic agonist effects by administration of atipamezole (preferred) or yohimbine is expected to result in significant improvement in clinical signs, although repeated dosing may be necessary. Signs may persist for several days, particularly if waiting for ingested collar segments to pass. Intravenous fluid support is recommended in hypotensive patients, but diuresis does not speed the elimination of amitraz from the body. Amitraz adsorbs to activated charcoal, but the alpha-2 agonist effects may result in ileus, prolonging passage and elimination of the activated charcoal.

Chronic Treatment

If the patient survives the topical or ingestion exposure, long-term effects are generally not expected.

Drug Interactions

Patients receiving or concurrently exposed to MAO inhibitors or selective serotonin reuptake inhibitors (SSRIs) may display more severe effects due to compounded effects.

Possible Complications

Foreign body obstruction associated with collar ingestion

Recommended Monitoring

Ongoing monitoring of temperature, pulse, respirations, and blood pressure is recommended. Monitoring of blood glucose concentration may be helpful, but administration of insulin for hyperglycemia is not generally recommended.

PROGNOSIS & OUTCOME

For mildly to moderately affected patients, particularly those with topical exposures, prognosis is good, with no expected long-term ill effects. In patients with high-dose exposures, prognosis is guarded, particularly in case of ingestion that may exceed the LD50.

PEARLS & CONSIDERATIONS

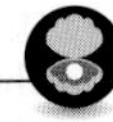

Comments

Although clinical signs can be significant, many cases of amitraz toxicosis have a positive outcome.

Prevention

Prevent pet access to loose collars and removed collar segments. The use of amitraz-containing products on cats, toy dogs, young or geriatric animals should be avoided if possible.

Technician Tips

Due to the reduced ability to thermoregulate, patient body temperature should be monitored. Warming or cooling devices should be used with care and close supervision. Bathing of patients with topical exposure and compromised thermoregulation should be done with caution and delayed until the patient is stabilized. Continued monitoring of the pet's temperature after bathing (i.e., during drying period) is important.

Client Education

Pet owners using amitraz-impregnated collars for tick prevention should be thoroughly educated about the risk of ingestion to pets and children.

SUGGESTED READING

Andrade SF, et al: The comparative efficacy of yohimbine and atipamezole to treat amitraz intoxication in dogs. Vet Hum Toxicol 45:124-127, 2003.

AUTHOR: Amy Schnelle, DVM, MS, DACVP
EDITOR: Tina Wismer DVM, MS, DABVT, DABT

Amphetamine Toxicosis

Client Education Sheet 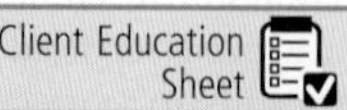

BASIC INFORMATION 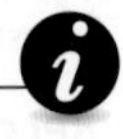

Definition

Amphetamines result in central nervous system (CNS) and cardiovascular (CV) stimulation. Toxicosis is typically caused by ingestion of prescription attention deficit disorder/attention deficit hyperactivity disorder (ADD/ADHD) medication or illicit drugs (e.g., methamphetamine, ecstasy [MDMA]).

Epidemiology

SPECIES, AGE, SEX

Dogs and young animals are overrepresented because they are more likely to ingest nonfood items.

RISK FACTORS

- Presence of amphetamines in the household
- The drugs are often prescribed to children, who may be more likely to leave them out where pets can get to them.

GEOGRAPHY AND SEASONALITY

An increase in exposures is reported in the fall, when children are going back to school.

Clinical Presentation

DISEASE FORMS/SUBTYPES

Ingestion of extended-release prescription medications can have a delayed onset of clinical signs.

HISTORY, CHIEF COMPLAINT

- Ingestion of prescription medication or illicit drugs
- Acute onset of CNS and CV stimulation; head bobbing and circling is common with large ingestions.

PHYSICAL EXAM FINDINGS

- Head bobbing, circling
- Hyperactivity or agitation
- Hyperthermia
- Tachyarrhythmias, tachycardia, or reflex bradycardia
- Hypertension
- Mydriasis
- Hyperesthesia
- Tremors, seizures
- Coma

Etiology and Pathophysiology

- Amphetamines stimulate the release of catecholamines, resulting in an increase in norepinephrine, dopamine, and serotonin and inhibiting monoamine oxidase.
- Increased catecholamine release and inhibition of reuptake results in vasoconstriction with hypertension, tachycardia, and CNS stimulation. Cardiac output is typically not affected due to reflex bradycardia.
- Rhabdomyolysis from increased motor activity can cause myoglobinuria with secondary kidney injury (p. 1367).
- Increased muscular activity can cause hyperthermia with secondary complications (p. 421).

DIAGNOSIS 

Diagnostic Overview

Although confirmatory tests exist, diagnosis is typically based on evidence of exposure to amphetamines and/or consistent clinical signs.

Differential Diagnosis

Toxins: 5-Hydroxytryptophan; pseudoephedrine, phenylephrine, ephedrine; nicotine; albuterol; cocaine; phenylpropanolamine; caffeine or other methylxanthines (chocolate); guarana

Initial Database

- CBC, serum chemistry profile, and urinalysis: nonspecific; possible findings include myoglobinuria, azotemia due to acute kidney injury, hypoglycemia, or thrombocytopenia if hyperthermia leads to secondary coagulopathy
- Coagulation profile: if coagulopathy is suspected
- Acid base status: metabolic acidosis and compensatory respiratory alkalosis is common.

Advanced or Confirmatory Testing

Human point-of-care urine multidrug test or gas chromatography and mass spectrometry analysis on urine or plasma can be used to confirm exposure.

TREATMENT

Treatment Overview

Decontaminate asymptomatic patients. After signs occur, treatment is symptomatic and supportive. Acepromazine is the mainstay of treatment for clinical signs of CNS stimulation and often at least partially controls the signs of CV stimulation. Administration of intravenous (IV) fluids is indicated for thermoregulation, renal protection, and CV support.

Acute General Treatment

- Decontamination
  - Emesis (p. 1188): asymptomatic patients with a recent exposure (typically less than 30 minutes with prompt-release product, up to 2 hours with extended-release product)
  - Activated charcoal 1 g/kg PO with sorbitol or other cathartic for asymptomatic patients with recent exposure (monitor for hypernatremia)
- Control of CNS stimulation
  - Acepromazine 0.05-1 mg/kg IV, titrate to effect, give prn, *or*
  - Chlorpromazine 0.5 mg/kg IV, titrate to effect
  - Cyproheptadine: dogs: 1.1 mg/kg; cats: 2-4 mg/CAT PO or crushed in saline and given rectally for signs of serotonin syndrome
  - Minimize sensory stimuli
- Thermoregulation
  - Control stimulatory signs
  - Fans, cool towels, IV crystalloid fluids prn
- Cardiac arrhythmias
  - Sinus tachycardia in a calm pet
    - Propranolol 0.02-0.06 mg/kg IV, titrate slowly to effect, *or*
    - Esmolol 25-200 mcg/kg/minute CRI
  - Ventricular tachyarrhythmias
    - Lidocaine 1-4 mg/kg IV, followed by CRI of 25-80 mcg/kg/min CRI, if needed
- Antiepileptics
  - Diazepam 0.5-2 mg/kg IV; benzodiazepines can be used for seizure control but should be avoided for other uses because it can worsen the stimulatory signs, *or*
  - Phenobarbital 3-4 mg/kg IV, *or*
  - Gas anesthesia or propofol: refractory seizures
- Generalized muscle tremors
  - Methocarbamol 55-220 mg/kg slow IV to effect
- Fluid diuresis
- Vomiting, nausea
  - Maropitant 1 mg/kg SQ q 24h
  - Ondansetron 0.1-0.3 mg/kg IV q 8-12h

Drug Interactions

Benzodiazepines can worsen clinical signs of agitation and disorientation but can be used for seizures if needed.

Possible Complications

Acute kidney injury; hyperthermia; coagulopathy; hypernatremia from activated charcoal use

Recommended Monitoring

Frequent monitoring of mentation, heart rate and rhythm (ECG), body temperature, blood pressure, hydration status, acid-base status

PROGNOSIS & OUTCOME 

Prognosis is generally good with prompt and aggressive treatment. Severe hyperthermia and seizures are indicators of a worse prognosis.

PEARLS & CONSIDERATIONS 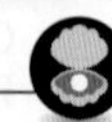

Comments

- Acepromazine is the mainstay of treatment. Failure to control stimulatory signs is often a direct result of conservative dosing of acepromazine.

- Patients can have significant insensible water loss and may require aggressive fluid administration. Fluid ins and outs can help estimate hydration status, especially because amphetamines are renally excreted. Excretion of amphetamines is decreased with alkaline urine.
- Signs can last up to 72 hours. Discharge pets only after > 8 hours free from any stimulatory signs.
- Cats may become more withdrawn and stare, rather than becoming hyperactive. Given the typical amount of stress that cats experience when hospitalized, response to acepromazine may be very helpful in differentiating a cat that is showing clinical signs of toxicosis from one that is showing stress of hospitalization. If a very low dose of acepromazine (0.01-0.02 mg/kg IV) resolves the clinical signs, they are not likely due to toxicosis.

Prevention

Keep all medications out of pet's reach, including keeping children's backpacks in a closet or hung on a high hook.

Technician Tips

- Keep affected animals in a dark and quiet environment. Minimizing stimulation often decreases the amount of sedatives needed.
- Body temperature should be monitored closely because hyperthermia can lead to seizures and coagulopathy.

Client Education

- Keep all medications out of the reach of pets.
- Make sure children know ADHD/ADD medications can harm their pets.

SUGGESTED READING

Stern LA, et al: Management of attention deficit disorder/attention deficit hyperactivity disorder drug intoxication in dogs and cats. Vet Clin of N Am: Small Anim Pract 42:279-288, 2012.

AUTHOR: Laura Stern, DVM, DABVT
EDITOR: Tina Wismer, DVM, MS, DABVT, DABT

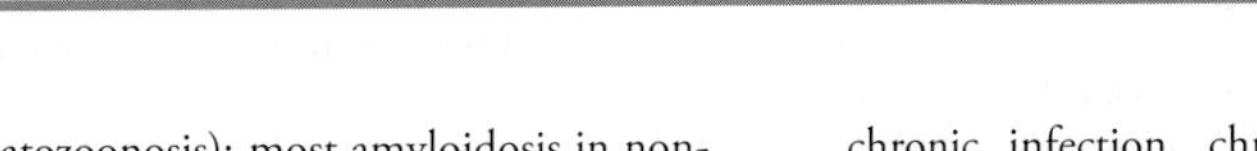

Amyloidosis

Client Education Sheet

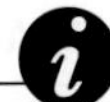

BASIC INFORMATION

Definition

Amyloidosis is the pathologic deposition of polymerized proteins in a beta-pleated sheet conformation; it disrupts function of involved organs, most often the kidneys.

Epidemiology

SPECIES, AGE, SEX

Uncommon in dogs; rare in cats. Middle-aged to older dogs (median age at diagnosis, 9 years) and cats; Chinese Shar-peis present at a younger age (median age at diagnosis, 4.5 years)

GENETICS, BREED PREDISPOSITION

- Dogs: Chinese Shar-peis (renal and hepatic amyloidosis), English foxhounds; any breed may be affected by reactive/secondary form
- Cats: Abyssinians (renal amyloidosis), Siamese/oriental cats (systemic amyloidosis)

RISK FACTORS

Chronic inflammatory/infectious/neoplastic diseases predispose to reactive amyloidosis.

ASSOCIATED DISORDERS

- Protein-losing nephropathy (PLN) ± nephrotic syndrome
- Chronic kidney disease (CKD) and renal failure
- Other organ dysfunction depends on sites of amyloid deposition.
- In Chinese Shar-peis: swollen hock syndrome, familial Shar-pei fever

Clinical Presentation

DISEASE FORMS/SUBTYPES

- Reactive amyloidosis occurs secondary to chronic inflammatory diseases (e.g., hepatozoonosis); most amyloidosis in nonpredisposed breeds is reactive.
- Dogs:
    - Reactive amyloid deposition causes glomerular disease with PLN and variable progression to renal failure.
    - Amyloidosis in Chinese Shar-peis: variable proteinuria; renal failure possible without PLN
        - History may include intermittent fever and inflammatory, nonerosive polyarthritis.
        - Hepatic amyloidosis with or without renal amyloidosis may also occur.
- Cats: amyloid deposition can occur without clinical signs.
    - Abyssinians: glomerular and/or medullary amyloid deposition with variable severity of proteinuria; renal failure may develop without PLN.
    - Siamese/oriental cats: systemic amyloid deposition; clinical signs depend on organs affected.

HISTORY, CHIEF COMPLAINT

- Clinical signs frequently absent until late in disease
- Chinese Shar-peis may be intermittently febrile and/or lame from a young age.
- Siamese or oriental cats may present with life-threatening intraabdominal hemorrhage due to liver lobe fracture secondary to massive hepatic deposition of amyloid.
- Clinical signs of uremia (p. 169) are common.
- Clinical signs of nephrotic syndrome (e.g., edema/ascites [pp. 79 and 284]) and/or concurrent hypercoagulability (e.g., pulmonary thromboembolism [p. 842]) may be noted.
- For reactive amyloidosis, clinical signs may be attributable to an underlying process (e.g., chronic infection, chronic inflammatory disease, myeloma).

PHYSICAL EXAM FINDINGS

- Often unremarkable; mild enlargement of involved organs is possible.
- For reactive amyloidosis, abnormalities depend on underlying inflammatory process.
- Chinese Shar-peis may have fever, joint effusion, and arthralgia (especially distal joints).
- If nephrotic syndrome is present (p. 691)
    - Ascites, edema, or effusion
    - Variable kidney size
    - Evidence of thromboembolism
    - Evidence of hypertension (e.g., choroidopathy, central nervous system [CNS] signs)
- Rarely, cats with systemic amyloidosis develop hepatic rupture and acute hemoabdomen.
- Pulmonary, cardiac, dermal, or CNS amyloid deposition and resultant organ dysfunction occur rarely.

Etiology and Pathophysiology

- Proteins with beta-pleated sheet conformation accumulate within extracellular spaces, leading to organ dysfunction.
    - Glomeruli are the most common site of accumulation in dogs other than Shar-peis, leading to proteinuria.
    - Deposition within the renal medulla, liver, and other organs may occur with or without glomerular involvement.
- Reactive amyloidosis is most common.
    - Deposited protein is amyloid protein A, a fragment of serum amyloid A (SAA).
    - SAA increases with systemic inflammation.
    - Evidence suggests a dysregulated inflammatory response leads to amyloid deposition.

- Immunoglobulin light chain–associated amyloidosis is rare.
  - Associated with multiple myeloma, some lymphomas, and plasma cell tumors

DIAGNOSIS

Diagnostic Overview

Definitive diagnosis of amyloidosis requires biopsy of an affected organ (usually kidney). Presumptive diagnosis is appropriate for Chinese Shar-peis with history of fever and/or joint pain.

Differential Diagnosis

- Proteinuria: see p. 1272.
- Other differential diagnoses depend on organ involvement (e.g., hepatomegaly [p. 456]).

Initial Database

- CBC: unremarkable or reflective of underlying inflammatory process
- Chemistry profile: unremarkable or reflective of underlying disease until amyloidosis is advanced. Most dogs with renal amyloidosis eventually develop hypoalbuminemia and may develop findings typical of nephrotic syndrome (p. 691) and/or CKD (pp. 167 and 169). Azotemia can occur without proteinuria in Chinese Shar-pei dogs and cats. Chinese Shar-pei dogs are less likely to develop nephrotic syndrome than dogs with reactive amyloidosis and are more likely to be azotemic at time of diagnosis.
- Urinalysis: proteinuria secondary to glomerular amyloid deposition. Ability to concentrate urine is compromised as kidney damage progresses.
- Arterial blood pressure: systemic hypertension common
- Urine protein/creatinine (UPC) ratio: often dramatically increased in non–Chinese Shar-pei dogs; variably increased in Chinese Shar-peis and cats
- Imaging: kidneys and liver may be mildly enlarged and hyperechoic on ultrasonographic examination. Rarely, hemoabdomen and hepatic fracture identified in Oriental cats with hepatic amyloid deposition.

Advanced or Confirmatory Testing

- Biopsy is required for definitive diagnosis. Histologic findings:
  - Hematoxylin and eosin stain: homogeneous eosinophilic material within affected organs, particularly the glomerular mesangium
  - Congo red stain: apple-green birefringence when viewed under polarized light
  - Amyloid deposition in Chinese Shar-peis and Abyssinian cats may be limited to the renal medulla, and biopsy may not be diagnostic (renal biopsies should contain only cortex).
  - Because other organs can be affected, biopsy can confirm amyloid outside of the kidney. Hepatic biopsy may be preferred when there is clinicopathologic evidence of liver dysfunction.
- Additional testing may be indicated to identify underlying inflammatory/infectious/neoplastic disease.

TREATMENT

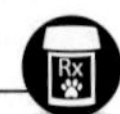

Treatment Overview

Prognosis is guarded to poor unless an underlying disease is identified and corrected. Nonspecific therapies include reduction of proteinuria and treatment of renal failure and its consequences. Efficacy of specific treatments for amyloidosis is unknown.

Acute General Treatment

- Stabilization and treatment of uremic crisis if present
- General therapy for PLN: see Glomerulonephritis (p. 390)
- Treatment of complications: see Acute Kidney Injury (p. 23); Chronic Kidney Disease, Occult (p. 167); Chronic Kidney Disease, Overt (p. 169); Nephrotic Syndrome (p. 691); Pulmonary Thromboembolism (p. 842); Systemic Hypertension (p. 501)
- Acute hemoabdomen (p. 430) in cats with hepatic rupture requires abdominal exploratory and supportive care (e.g., transfusion).

Chronic Treatment

- Management/resolution of any concurrent inflammatory diseases
- Continued management of PLN and chronic kidney disease
- Dimethyl sulfoxide may slow or prevent progression of amyloidosis: 300 mg/kg PO q 24h, or dilute 90% solution 1 : 4 in sterile water and administer 20-80 mg/kg SQ 3 times/week. Owners should wear gloves when administering. SQ injections may cause local irritation. Treatment is lifelong.
- Colchicine should be administered to Chinese Shar-peis at earliest diagnosis, regardless of disease severity or presence of proteinuria: 0.01-0.03 mg/kg PO q 24h. If vomiting/diarrhea develop, decrease dose temporarily. Treatment is lifelong.
- Prednisone and other antiinflammatory medications are of no known benefit.

Nutrition/Diet

Renal diets are appropriate for affected animals.

Recommended Monitoring

UPC ratio, urinalysis, serum albumin and creatinine, blood pressure, body weight, and body condition score should be monitored weekly to monthly initially. After patients are stable, recheck every 3-6 months unless therapy or condition changes.

PROGNOSIS & OUTCOME

- Guarded to grave despite treatment. Median survival of dogs with renal amyloidosis is 5 days from time of diagnosis, with only 20% of dogs surviving ≥ 30 days.
  - Survival is negatively associated with serum creatinine concentration. Azotemic dogs often rapidly progress to uremic crisis.
- Prognosis may be improved (with occasional reported resolution) if concurrent diseases are identified and successfully treated.
- Early colchicine therapy (before onset of renal failure) for Chinese Shar-pei dogs can greatly improve prognosis.

PEARLS & CONSIDERATIONS

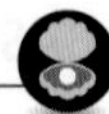

Comments

- Differentiation of amyloidosis from other causes of PLN requires biopsy. Histologic diagnosis allows tailored therapy and prognosis.
- Amyloidosis is primarily a renal cortical disease in dogs other than Chinese Shar-peis.
- Chinese Shar-peis with consistent clinical signs (recurrent lameness and fever with or without proteinuria and azotemia) can be presumptively diagnosed with amyloidosis even without biopsy.
- Substantial amyloid deposition may be present despite normal blood urea nitrogen, creatinine, and urine-specific gravity values.

Prevention

Affected animals should not be bred.

SUGGESTED READING

Segev G, et al: Renal amyloidosis in dogs: a retrospective study of 91 cases with comparison of the disease between shar-pei and non-shar-pei dogs. J Vet Intern Med 26:259-268, 2012.

AUTHOR: Barrak M. Pressler, DVM, PhD, DACVIM; Leah A. Cohn, DVM, PhD, DACVIM
EDITOR: Leah A. Cohn, DVM, PhD, DACVIM

Anal Sac Diseases

Client Education Sheet

BASIC INFORMATION

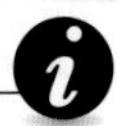

Definition

Diseases of the anal sacs, the most clinically important of which are impaction, inflammatory/infectious, or neoplastic (primarily adenocarcinoma). Information on neoplastic anal sac disease can be found on (p. 29).

Synonyms

Anal sacculitis, anal sac impaction, anal sac abscess, adenocarcinoma of the apocrine glands of the anal sac

Epidemiology

SPECIES, AGE, SEX

Dogs are affected with anal sac disease more often than cats. There is no sex predisposition to inflammatory anal sac disease.

GENETICS, BREED PREDISPOSITION

Small-breed dogs that typically weigh < 15 kg may be at increased risk for impaction. Miniature and toy poodles, Chihuahuas, American cocker spaniels, and English springer spaniels have been singled out as at-risk breeds. Increased risk of infection in Siamese cats has been suggested.

RISK FACTORS

Obesity; diarrhea or chronic soft stools (impaction); seborrheic disorders (impaction); routine expression of anal sacs in normal dogs has been suggested to pose a risk of inadvertent anal sac trauma and recurrent anal sac disease.

Clinical Presentation

DISEASE FORMS/SUBTYPES

Clinical features may reflect those of the primary anal sac disease or distant/systemic consequences of anal sac neoplasia (p. 29).

HISTORY, CHIEF COMPLAINT

Most affected animals present with one or more of the following:

- Scooting
- Licking or chewing at perianal region
- Reluctance to sit or lift tail
- Tenesmus or painful defecation
- Fresh blood on stool
- Others possible with anal sac neoplasia

PHYSICAL EXAM FINDINGS

Physical examination abnormalities are typically limited to the perianal region:

- Anal sac distention
- Pain during rectal examination
- Bloody anal sac contents
- Loss of hair, redness, perianal swelling and pain in tissues overlying anal sac (abscess)
- Draining tract (abscess)
- Fever (abscess)
- Anal sac mass
- Others possible with anal sac neoplasia

Etiology and Pathophysiology

The underlying cause of impaction and inflammatory/infectious anal sac disease is unknown. Some speculated causes include retention of anal sac secretions or abnormal composition of secretions leading to bacterial colonization and inflammation or impaction. Experimental models that occlude the anal sac duct or establish infection have not consistently reproduced features of the clinical disease.

DIAGNOSIS

Diagnostic Overview

The diagnosis of anal sac disease is based primarily on clinical signs and physical examination findings of anal sac distention, pain or discomfort, or a mass during examination of the anal sacs.

Differential Diagnosis

- Other causes of tenesmus or hematochezia
  - Acute or chronic colitis
  - Rectal masses
  - Perianal fistula
- Other causes of perianal pruritus and inflammation
  - Allergic skin disease
  - Food allergy
  - Flea allergy dermatitis
  - Parasitic skin disease
  - Perianal pyoderma
  - Tail fold or perivulvar dermatitis

Initial Database

Results of a CBC, biochemical profile, and urinalysis are nonspecific. In severe cases, there can be an inflammatory leukogram.

Advanced or Confirmatory Testing

- There are no specific cytologic features that suggest the diagnosis. Clinically normal dogs can have intracellular and extracellular bacteria and leukocytes in anal sac secretions. In conjunction with clinical signs, large numbers of intracellular bacteria and erythrocytes seen on cytologic examination of anal sac contents support a diagnosis of anal sac infection.
- Skin scrapes, diet trials, or other skin-specific approaches may be needed in patients with clinical signs that persist after treatment of anal sac disease or that have obvious features of dermatoses.

TREATMENT

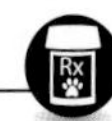

Treatment Overview

Treatment is largely directed at expressing anal sac contents (impaction) and treating infection (sacculitis or abscess).

Acute General Treatment

- Anal sac impaction: expression of anal sac contents is often sufficient to alleviate clinical signs, although recurrence is not unusual. Sedation and lavage of anal sacs with saline may be needed in some animals to soften secretions for easier expression.
- Anal sacculitis: typical approach to treatment is expression of anal sac followed by infusion of antibiotic/glucocorticoid-containing ointments (otic or ophthalmic products) through the anal sac duct into the anal sac. Lavage of anal sacs, perhaps with ceruminolytic agents, may be helpful in severe cases.
- Anal sac abscess: therapy as described for anal sacculitis and also systemically administered antimicrobials, typically those with a gram-positive spectrum such as beta-lactams (e.g., cephalosporins, amoxicillin-clavulanic acid), or clindamycin. Drainage (lance and lavage) may be needed in some. Antibiotics often continued for 2-3 weeks to the point of no further signs of infection.

Chronic Treatment

Patients with recurrent anal sac impaction or infection may be candidates for anal sacculectomy or anal sac marsupialization to achieve long-term resolution of disease.

Nutrition/Diet

Some clinicians advocate adding fiber to the diet or changing diets in patients with soft/loose stools to produce a stool quality that promotes emptying of anal sacs during defecation, but the role of diet in management of anal sac disease has not been explored.

Possible Complications

Potential complications of anal sac surgery include fecal incontinence or fistulas if the anal sac is incompletely resected.

Recommended Monitoring

Clinical signs; serial microscopic examination of anal sac secretions to document decreasing intracellular bacterial numbers and erythrocytes may be considered, but is not routinely done.

PROGNOSIS & OUTCOME

The prognosis for most patients with anal sac disease is good to excellent with treatment. Persistence of clinical signs can provoke investigation into other causes of colonic or perianal skin disease.

PEARLS & CONSIDERATIONS

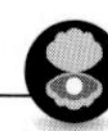

Comments

Rectal examinations should be performed as a part of routine physical examinations on dogs for early detection of anal sac masses.

Technician Tips

- Curved-tip syringes facilitate infusion of anal sacs with antibiotic-containing preparations. Some patients need sedation for effective expression and treatment of anal sac disease.
- Avoid overly aggressive manipulation of the anal sacs while emptying the contents.

Client Education

- Although uncomfortable, inflammatory anal sac disease is not usually a major health threat.
- Persistent clinical signs may indicate an unrelated disorder.
- Anal sac masses, even small ones, should not be ignored.

SUGGESTED READINGS

Muse R: Diseases of the anal sac. In Bonagura JD, et al, editors: Current veterinary therapy XIV, St. Louis, 2009, Saunders Elsevier.

AUTHOR & EDITOR: Rance K. Sellon, DVM, PhD, DACVIM

Anaphylaxis

BASIC INFORMATION

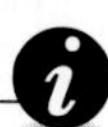

Definition

An acute hypersensitivity reaction results in the generalized release of inflammatory mediators from basophils and mast cells. This life-threatening systemic allergic reaction can result in cardiovascular collapse, respiratory distress, and death.

- Urticaria: cutaneous manifestation of anaphylaxis, consisting of pruritic wheals
- Angioedema: nonpainful cutaneous and visceral edema (regional or generalized) that is one of the hallmarks of anaphylaxis

Synonyms

Allergic reaction, anaphylactic reaction/shock, type I hypersensitivity, urticaria (hives)

Epidemiology

SPECIES, AGE, SEX

Most species; no age or sex predisposition

GENETICS, BREED PREDISPOSITION

Boxers and pit bulls are most often affected with urticaria.

RISK FACTORS

- Previous exposure to an antigen or hapten (molecules that attach to cells, conferring antigenicity) suspected to cause anaphylaxis increases risk, but previous exposure is not always recognized.
- Can be triggered by a number of medications (e.g., hormones, antibiotics, chemotherapeutic agents, parasiticides, human albumin, vaccines), antigens (e.g., heartworms, bee sting), or mast cell tumor degranulation

GEOGRAPHY AND SEASONALITY

- Summer or warm weather for insect-related anaphylaxis
- Geographic areas where mosquitos that carry heartworm are present

Clinical Presentation

DISEASE FORMS/SUBTYPES

- Anaphylactic reactions occur because of the interaction of an antigen or hapten with an antibody molecule (immunoglobulin E [IgE]) that has been formed from a previous exposure.
- Reactions occurring without previous exposure were historically referred to as anaphylactoid reactions but more recently have been grouped with anaphylactic reactions because their clinical presentation is identical.

HISTORY, CHIEF COMPLAINT

- Recent exposure to an inciting antigen or hapten (e.g., vaccine, medication, food ingredient, heartworm)
- Agitation
- Vomiting/diarrhea
- Hypersalivation
- Respiratory distress
- Collapse
- For urticaria, severe pruritus
- For angioedema, swelling

PHYSICAL EXAM FINDINGS

- Wheals, facial angioedema
- Weakness or acute collapse
- Mentation changes: depression or excitation
- Evidence of hypoperfusion (pale mucous membranes, prolonged capillary refill time, poor to nonexistent pulse quality)
- Tachycardia
- Dyspnea (cats)
- Coma
- Death

Etiology and Pathophysiology

Anaphylactic reactions:

- Initial exposure to an antigen results in the production of specific IgE antibody.
- Subsequent re-exposure to the antigen results in the binding of the antigen to IgE on the surface of basophils in circulation and mast cells in tissues.
- Activated basophils and mast cells release granules containing primary mediators of anaphylaxis: histamine, heparin, proteases, and chemotactic factors.
- Activation of the arachidonic acid cascade results in release of secondary mediators, including leukotrienes, prostaglandins, thromboxanes, and platelet-activating factor.
- Cytokine synthesis also occurs, contributing to the inflammatory response.

Alternatively, in animals without previous exposure to the antigen:

- Exposure to the antigen or hapten results in activation of the complement cascade, leading to production of anaphylatoxins (C3a and C5a), which cause activation of mast cells and basophils and release of primary mediators not involving an antibody response.
- Mast cells can also be stimulated directly.

Activation, synthesis, and release of inflammatory mediators result in peripheral vasodilation, increased vascular permeability, hypotension, bronchospasm, laryngeal edema, increased airway secretion production, intestinal hypermotility, cardiac arrhythmias, stimulation of pain receptors, and pruritus.

DIAGNOSIS

Diagnostic Overview

The diagnosis is based on history and physical exam findings alone. It is essential that treatment for anaphylaxis be instituted before extensive diagnostic testing because the prompt initiation of treatment is a primary determinant of survival.

Differential Diagnosis

- Dermatologic disease
- Cardiorespiratory disease (severe cases)
  - Shock (hypovolemic, cardiogenic, septic)
  - Pulmonary edema
  - Cardiac arrhythmias
  - Feline asthma
- Acute gastrointestinal disease

Initial Database

- Blood pressure: monitor for hypotension
- CBC, serum chemistry, urinalysis: generally unremarkable, may have decreased platelet count
- Thoracic radiographs: to rule out pulmonary disease if respiratory distress or tachypnea is present
- Heartworm testing: antigen (dogs) or antigen and antibody (cats)

- Coagulation testing may reveal hypocoagulability

Advanced or Confirmatory Testing

- Abdominal ultrasound may reveal a halo sign around the gallbladder.
- Animals with chronic heartworm disease may have pulmonary artery or cardiac abnormalities visible on survey thoracic radiographs.

TREATMENT

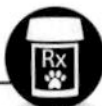

Treatment Overview

- Cardiovascular and respiratory support
- Antagonize inflammatory mediators
- Support coagulation
- Block further release of inflammatory mediators.
- Remove causative agent.

Acute General Treatment

Emergency treatment should be instituted based on history and physical examination and before extensive diagnostic testing in severe cases (patients with dyspnea, hemodynamic instability, or depression/coma). Treatment is cardiovascular support with intravenous (IV) fluid therapy and epinephrine or other pressor support as necessary. Mild reactions, including urticarial alone, require less intensive intervention.

Cardiovascular support:

- IV catheter placement, facilitated techniques, or cut-down procedure may be necessary
- If cardiovascular instability is present, then epinephrine to treat hypotension, bronchoconstriction, and block release of inflammatory mediators
  - Epinephrine: 0.01-0.02 mg/kg IV (IM for less severe cases), *or*
  - Epinephrine 0.02-0.2 mg/kg intratracheal administration in intubated patients
  - Vasopressin 0.5-2 U IV bolus repeated up to 3 times as needed in refractory cases
  - Isotonic crystalloids 20-30 mL/kg IV bolus, repeated as required after reassessment
  - Fresh-frozen plasma used to treat coagulopathy can also provide intravascular volume support

Establish airway patency:

- With upper airway obstruction or apnea due to severe laryngeal edema:
  - Endotracheal intubation
  - Tracheostomy (p. 1166)
- Oxygen therapy if evidence of hypoxemia (p. 1146)
- Bronchodilation if bronchospasm persists despite epinephrine administration
  - Aminophylline: dog: 5-10 mg/kg IM or slow IV; cat: 5 mg/kg IM or slow IV
  - Terbutaline 0.01 mg/kg IM/IV
  - Inhaled albuterol 1-2 puffs from metered dose inhaler per 5-10 kg of patient weight (p. 1122)

Chronic Treatment

May be instituted instead of acute treatment if a patient is showing only mild clinical signs and is hemodynamically stable (common). In general, treatment of anaphylaxis is complete within 24-72 hours of presentation. In some animals with severe shock, chronic care is focused on treatments of shock sequelae (e.g., gastrointestinal injury, coagulopathy).

- Glucocorticoid therapy to block release of secondary mediators:
  - Dexamethasone sodium phosphate 0.1-0.2 mg/kg IV once
  - Some animals require a short (2-3 day) course of prednisone 0.25-0.5 mg/kg PO q 24h
- Antihistamine therapy:
  - H1-blocker: diphenhydramine 1-2 mg/kg IM, SQ, PO q 8h for 24-48h
  - H2-blocker: famotidine 0.5-1 mg/kg IV, IM, SQ, PO q 12h

Nutrition/Diet

Avoid dietary triggers. Severe food allergies are rare in dogs and cats in contrast to people, for whom peanuts and other life-threatening food allergies are reported more regularly.

Drug Interactions

- Epinephrine, aminophylline, and terbutaline may be arrhythmogenic. Use caution when used together.
- Chronic glucocorticoid therapy is contraindicated in patients receiving nonsteroidal antiinflammatory drug (NSAID) therapy.

Possible Complications

- Cardiac arrhythmias
- Consumptive coagulopathy
- Organ dysfunction

Recommended Monitoring

- For mild cases (skin reaction only), monitoring at home for recurrence
- For severe cases
  - Frequent monitoring should be continued for 24-48 hours after reaction.
  - Heart rate, respiratory rate, respiratory effort, pulse rate, pulse quality, mentation, mucous membrane color, capillary refill time, temperature, urine output
  - Blood pressure
  - Electrocardiogram
  - Pulse oximetry or arterial blood gases
  - Packed cell volume and total solids
  - Serum biochemistry analysis
  - Coagulation testing

PROGNOSIS & OUTCOME

Immediate recognition and prompt intervention are the keys for a successful outcome. Anaphylaxis can result in death within 1 minute of exposure to the inciting agent in severe cases, but with prompt appropriate treatment, prognosis is good.

PEARLS & CONSIDERATIONS

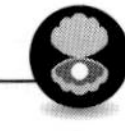

Comments

- Anaphylaxis does not always involve a previous exposure and sensitization.
- Anaphylaxis should be suspected in patients with unexplained acute cardiovascular and respiratory collapse.
- Fluid therapy and epinephrine are the first lines of treatment for severe anaphylaxis.

Prevention

- Administer IV medications slowly.
- Be aware of and use caution with medications known to be associated with anaphylaxis.
- For patients with a history of anaphylaxis, pretreatment with antihistamines and glucocorticoids may be useful in blunting the inflammatory response when re-exposure is unavoidable.
- Avoid revaccination of pets with a history of a severe reaction.

Technician Tips

Prompt recognition of anaphylaxis with initiation of treatment is key to a successful outcome.

Client Education

- Be familiar with your pet's medical history, and alert your veterinarian of medications your pet has received, previous blood product transfusions, and previous allergic reactions.
- A pediatric EpiPen may be prescribed for animals with prior life-threatening reactions.

SUGGESTED READING

Shmuel DL, et al: Anaphylaxis in dogs and cats. J Vet Emerg Crit Care 23:377-394. 2013.

AUTHOR: Gareth J. Buckley, MA, VetMB, DACVECC
EDITOR: Benjamin M. Brainard, VMD, DACVAA, DACVECC

Anemia, Aplastic

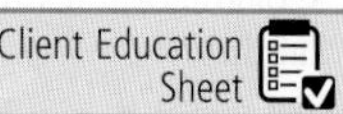

BASIC INFORMATION

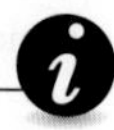

Definition

A bone marrow disorder that causes a bicytopenia or pancytopenia in the blood and a hypocellular bone marrow with a majority of the hematopoietic space replaced by adipose tissue. Disorders with a pancytopenia and a normocellular or hypercellular bone marrow are not considered to be aplastic anemia.

Synonym

Aplastic pancytopenia

Epidemiology

SPECIES, AGE, SEX

Dogs and cats of any age and either sex

RISK FACTORS

- Cats: young, outdoor, male cats with roaming and fighting behavior
  - Feline leukemia virus (FeLV)– and feline immunodeficiency virus (FIV)–positive cats

CONTAGION AND ZOONOSIS

- Retroviral infections, parvovirus

Associated Disorders

- Fever associated with secondary infection; bleeding associated with thrombocytopenia

Clinical Presentation

DISEASE FORMS/SUBTYPES

- Acute: destruction of progenitor and proliferative cells in the bone marrow within 2 weeks of marrow injury. Neutropenia develops 5-6 days and thrombocytopenia develops 8-10 days after marrow insult. Due to the long erythrocyte life span, anemia is usually absent or mild.
- Chronic: injury to all hematopoietic stem cells creates a moderate to marked pancytopenia.

HISTORY, CHIEF COMPLAINT

- Acute: neutropenia (lethargy, inappetence, fever), thrombocytopenia (hemorrhage)
- Chronic: same as acute plus signs of anemia (weakness, tachypnea, collapse)

PHYSICAL EXAM FINDINGS

- Acute: fever, petechia, hemorrhage
- Chronic: same as acute plus pale mucous membranes, tachycardia, systolic heart murmur

Etiology and Pathophysiology

- Decreased or absent stem or progenitor cell proliferation
- Potential causes:
  - Infectious: *Ehrlichia* spp, parvovirus, FeLV and FIV
  - Drug-associated: estrogen (dogs), cancer chemotherapeutic agents, sulfa drugs, phenylbutazone, thiacetarsemide (dogs), griseofulvin (cats), methimazole (cats), albendazole, quinidine
  - Toxins: aflatoxin B_1
  - Total-body irradiation
  - Starvation (cats)
  - Idiopathic
- Fever develops secondary to opportunistic infection during neutropenia, and bleeding develops during times of thrombocytopenia.

DIAGNOSIS

Diagnostic Overview

Cytopenias are commonly observed on a CBC, but a definitive diagnosis of aplastic anemia requires histopathologic examination of the bone marrow. A thorough history should include exposure to drugs, toxins, chemicals, and infectious agents, especially 2-3 weeks before development of clinical signs.

Differential Diagnosis

- Myelodysplasia (p. 671)
- Neoplasia: myelophthisis, leukemia (pp. 586 and 588)
- Myelofibrosis
- Myelonecrosis

Initial Database

- CBC:
  - Acute: granulocytopenia (neutropenia, eosinopenia) and thrombocytopenia occur first, and a nonregenerative anemia may be absent or mild.
  - Chronic: moderate to marked granulocytopenia, thrombocytopenia, and nonregenerative anemia
- Blood smear evaluation:
  - No consistent abnormalities with aplastic anemia, but a blood smear evaluation can identify other causes
- Serum biochemistry and urinalysis:
  - Can help identify an underlying disorder or secondary complication (e.g., azotemia due to pyelonephritis)
- Cats: FeLV and FIV serologic testing

Advanced or Confirmatory Testing

- A definitive diagnosis of aplastic anemia requires a bone marrow biopsy (p. 1068).
- A bone marrow aspirate allows identification of individual cells, but a core biopsy assesses marrow cellularity and architecture.
  - Core biopsy: in aplastic anemia, hematopoietic cells constitute 0%-25% of the marrow (50% in healthy marrow), with the remainder of the marrow space replaced with adipose tissue.
  - Acute: stem cells repopulate the marrow within 10-14 days after the cessation of marrow injury, and cell lines may recover within 21 days.
  - Chronic: marrow repopulation is uncertain, and recovery may require months.
- Infectious disease serologic testing: *Ehrlichia canis*, parvovirus as appropriate

TREATMENT

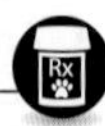

Treatment Overview

There is no specific treatment for aplastic anemia in dogs or cats, but supportive therapy for neutropenia (broad-spectrum antibiotics) and transfusions for anemia are essential until the bone marrow recovers.

Acute General Treatment

- Discontinue all medications or chemicals associated with the development of aplastic anemia.
- Treat any identified underlying cause.
- Broad-spectrum antibiotics: for signs of infection or prophylactically if neutrophil count < 500-1000/mcL
- Transfusions (p. 1169)
  - Anemia with clinical signs: whole blood or packed red blood cells
  - Thrombocytopenia and actively bleeding: fresh whole blood or platelet concentrate, generally reserved for life-threatening hemorrhage
  - Donors should be universal or have the same blood type as the recipient.
  - Cross-match before each transfusion because repeat transfusions are often required

Chronic Treatment

- Bone marrow transplantation may be the superior treatment option but is not currently feasible.
- Immunosuppressive therapy is commonly used to treat aplastic anemia but may not be effective at enhancing the marrow recovery.
  - Prednisolone 2 mg/kg PO q 24h (large-breed dogs, 40 mg/m²/day)
  - Cyclosporine 5 mg/kg PO q 12h (pharmacodynamics monitoring recommended)
  - Azathioprine 2 mg/kg PO q 24h (dogs only)
  - Mycophenolate mofetil 5-10 mg/kg PO q 12h
- The therapeutic benefits of hematopoietic growth factors, erythropoietin, and granulocyte colony-stimulating factor in dogs and cats with aplastic anemia are unknown.

Behavior/Exercise

Limit exposure of neutropenic dogs to other animals.

Possible Complications

- Secondary infections/sepsis due to neutropenia and/or immunosuppressive therapy
- Adverse drug effects (p. 60)
- Transfusion reactions (p. 989)

Recommended Monitoring

- Repeat CBC at least weekly (depending on severity of signs) until full recovery.
- On recovery, CBCs should be monitored monthly for an additional 3 months.

PROGNOSIS & OUTCOME

- Depends on underlying cause
  - Acute: good to guarded; often reversible within 2-3 weeks after resolution of marrow insult
  - Chronic and idiopathic: guarded to poor; less responsive to therapy with long recovery times (months)
- Young dogs may be more likely to recover or respond to immunosuppressive therapy.
- Most cats die or are euthanized within 1 month of diagnosis, but some cats can survive for years despite pancytopenia.

PEARLS & CONSIDERATIONS

Comments

Early recognition of aplastic anemia may improve the chance of marrow recovery.

Prevention

- CBCs should be monitored regularly in animals receiving medications associated with the development of aplastic anemia.
- For cats, minimize the risk of exposure to FeLV and FIV (pp. 325 and 329).

Technician Tips

- Individuals handling a severely neutropenic patient should wear protective gear (gloves, mask, gown, hair and shoe covers) to prevent transmission of infectious agents to the patient.
- Severely thrombocytopenic patients are prone to bleeding, and minimal, gentle handling can reduce the risk of hemorrhage.
- Monitor patients closely during transfusion for early recognition of adverse reactions.

SUGGESTED READING

Weiss DJ: Aplastic anemia. In Weiss DJ, et al, editors: Schalm's Veterinary hematology, ed 6, Ames, IA, 2010, Blackwell, pp 256-260.

AUTHOR: John M. Thomason, DVM, MS, DACVIM
EDITOR: Jonathan E. Fogle, DVM, PhD, DACVIM

Anemia, Blood Loss

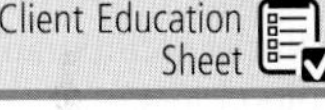

BASIC INFORMATION

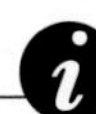

Definition

A decrease in total red blood cell (RBC) mass secondary to loss of RBCs from the vascular space

Synonym

Hemorrhagic anemia

Epidemiology

SPECIES, AGE, SEX

Varies depending on underlying cause

RISK FACTORS

Neoplasia, gastrointestinal (GI) ulcers, thrombocytopenia, coagulopathy, heavy parasite load (e.g., fleas, hookworms)

Clinical Presentation

HISTORY, CHIEF COMPLAINT

- Weakness, lethargy, collapse, anorexia, exercise intolerance
- Trauma
- Abdominal distention, melena, epistaxis, hematuria
- Pica may be noted with chronic anemia.

PHYSICAL EXAM FINDINGS

Varies with severity and duration:

- Pallor
- Weakness, exercise intolerance; collapse or syncope
- Tachycardia, tachypnea, bounding pulses
- Heart murmur: systolic, left-sided, and generally soft (<III/VI)
- Melena on rectal exam
- Hemorrhage from surgery, trauma, or underlying cause
- Hemoabdomen
- Petechiae, ecchymoses: suggestive of underlying bleeding disorder

Etiology and Pathophysiology

- Acute blood loss
  - Trauma
  - Surgery
  - Bleeding neoplasm (especially hemangiosarcoma)
  - GI ulcer
  - Bleeding disorder (thrombocytopenia, anticoagulant rodenticide toxicosis, hemophilia)
- Chronic blood loss/iron-deficiency anemia
  - GI bleeding most common: neoplasia, hookworms, GI ulcers
  - Less common: heavy flea infestation, urinary tract hemorrhage
  - Iatrogenic (overuse of blood donors or frequent phlebotomy)
  - Iron-deficiency anemia from chronic external bleeding:
    - Iron depletion leads to decreased synthesis of hemoglobin and delayed RBC maturation. RBCs are less deformable, with accelerated lysis.
    - Young animals at increased risk, due to decreased iron storage

DIAGNOSIS

Diagnostic Overview

The diagnosis of hemorrhagic anemia is suspected in patients with pale mucous membranes, weakness, and tachycardia/tachypnea, often with a history of surgery, trauma, or melena or with an abdominal fluid wave. Confirmation requires a CBC demonstrating a decreased hematocrit with evidence of red cell regeneration (reticulocytosis, anisocytosis, polychromasia) in the absence of hemolysis. The cause may be apparent from history and physical exam alone or may require additional testing.

Differential Diagnosis

- Differentiate from hemolytic anemia (pp. 59 and 60).
- Blood loss anemia is typically characterized by decreased plasma total protein (TP) without autoagglutination, spherocytosis, hyperbilirubinemia/-uria, or hemoglobinemia/-uria.

Initial Database

- Packed cell volume (PCV)/TP: with acute blood loss, there is initially little change in PCV because of concurrent loss of plasma with RBCs. Over hours, redistribution of fluid occurs, resulting in lowered PCV and TP.
- CBC/blood smear (p. 1327):
  - Normocytic, normochromic RBCs initially
  - Reticulocytosis 3-5 days after acute loss; hypochromic macrocytosis and polychromasia
  - Microcytosis, increased red cell distribution width and hypochromasia suggest chronic blood loss/iron-deficiency anemia
  - The platelet count is usually normal, but it can be mildly decreased due to consumption or increased with chronic bleeding. Severe thrombocytopenia may be the cause of blood loss.
  - Schistocytes are possible with hemangiosarcoma or other splenic mass.
- Serum biochemistry panel: panhypoproteinemia may be present if there has been external blood loss.

- +/− Abdominocentesis (p. 1056) if fluid wave (caution if bleeding disorder): hemoabdomen secondary to trauma, splenic disease (e.g., hemangiosarcoma), bleeding disorder
- +/− Coagulation panel and buccal mucosal bleeding time (p. 1076) to rule out a hemostatic defect
- +/− Thoracic radiographs: neoplasia, pulmonary hemorrhage, hemorrhagic pleural effusion
- +/− Abdominal radiographs, ultrasound, endoscopy: neoplasia, GI ulceration
- Fecal flotation/fecal occult blood
- Urinalysis to rule in/rule out hematuria and urinary tract blood loss

Advanced or Confirmatory Testing

Uncommonly required:

- Iron-deficiency anemia
  - Low serum iron concentration, low serum ferritin concentration, and low transferrin saturation (<20%) (p. 1355)
  - Bone marrow: erythroid hyperplasia; Prussian blue stain: absence of iron particles in dogs
- Nuclear scintigraphy may confirm occult GI blood loss.
- Cystoscopy may be used to localize the source of hematuria.

TREATMENT

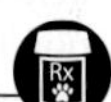

Treatment Overview

The mainstays of treatment are to control active hemorrhage if present, restore circulating blood volume (with fluid resuscitation and/or blood transfusion) if decreased, and correct the underlying cause.

Acute General Treatment

- Acute blood loss
  - IV fluids: crystalloids +/− colloids to correct hypovolemia
  - If signs of hypoxemia (weakness, tachycardia, tachypnea), consider transfusion: packed RBCs (6-10 mL/kg) are the best option if available, or use whole blood (10-20 mL/kg).
  - Autotransfusion if severe hemorrhage in a body cavity and no contamination with bacteria or neoplastic cells. Requires aseptic collection and a blood filter.
  - If a coagulopathy is present, correct with vitamin K_1, 1-5 mg/kg SQ q 24h, +/− fresh-frozen plasma (6-10 mL/kg), +/− cryoprecipitate (1 unit/10 kg IV) depending on severity and cause (p. 1169).
- Chronic blood loss
  - Transfusion if severe (p. 1169)
  - Treatment of underlying cause (may involve GI protectants, dewormer, surgery for intestinal tumor, etc.)

Chronic Treatment

Chronic blood loss/iron-deficiency anemia: replace iron with iron dextran 10-20 mg/kg IM or ferrous sulfate 100-300 mg/DOG/day or 50-100 mg/CAT/day PO

Possible Complications

- Massive blood loss: hypoxemia, hypovolemic shock, death
- Transfusion reactions (p. 989)
  - Dogs: determine blood type before transfusion to ensure blood type compatibility. If recipient is not typed, donor should be negative for DEA-1.1. All dogs that have previously received a transfusion should have a cross-match before transfusion.
  - Cats: possess naturally occurring antibodies against the blood type antigen they lack (alloantibodies). All cats must be typed or cross-matched before any transfusions.
- Adverse drug reactions: iron dextran: injection site pain, anaphylactic reaction; ferrous sulfate: vomiting, diarrhea, dark stools

Recommended Monitoring

- Acute blood loss
  - Monitor PCV/TP q 12h initially; monitor heart rate, respiratory rate, blood pressure, mucous membrane color, and capillary refill time.
  - Polymerized bovine hemoglobin (Oxyglobin, if the product is available) increases oxygen-carrying capacity without increasing PCV; need to monitor blood hemoglobin concentration
- Chronic blood loss
  - Monitor CBC every 1-4 weeks if clinically stable.
- Reticulocytosis may be the first sign of response.

PROGNOSIS & OUTCOME

- Good with blood loss secondary to trauma or surgery after hemorrhage is controlled and cardiovascular status is stabilized
- Excellent with parasites and appropriate treatment
- Fair with various bleeding disorders, depending on severity of and ability to control blood loss
- Fair with GI ulcers after underlying disease treated
- Guarded to grave with neoplasia; short-term response with surgery with or without additional chemotherapy, depending on tumor type and extent

PEARLS & CONSIDERATIONS

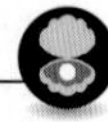

Comments

- In acute blood loss, PCV is not a good indicator of patient status. Indicators of perfusion (pulse quality, capillary refill time, blood pressure, and blood lactate) are more important in acute situations.
- Decision to transfuse a patient should be based on clinical signs rather than PCV alone. For example, a patient with massive, rapid blood loss may require transfusion despite PCV = 25%, whereas slow blood loss may elicit compensatory responses that limit clinical signs despite PCV = 15%. However, at a PCV < 12%, virtually all patients show clinical signs and require a transfusion.
- If a patient has signs consistent with acute blood loss (low PCV/TP), without an identifiable source, GI blood loss should be suspected. There may be extensive GI blood loss before melena, hematemesis, or hematochezia is noted.
- Do not treat iron-deficiency anemia without searching for an underlying cause of blood loss.

Prevention

Concurrent use of corticosteroids and nonsteroidal antiinflammatory drugs (NSAIDs) is contraindicated (GI ulceration, blood loss).

Technician Tips

In addition to mucous membrane color, capillary refill time, and heart and respiratory rates, a patient's mentation and pulse strength are important (and often overlooked) indicators of the severity of anemia and are useful for monitoring.

Client Education

Stress importance of follow-up for chronic/iron-deficiency anemia.

SUGGESTED READING

Giger U: Anemia. In Silverstein D, et al., editors: Small animal critical care medicine, St. Louis, 2009, Saunders, 518-523.

AUTHOR: Alicia K. Henderson, DVM, DACVIM
EDITOR: Jonathan E. Fogle, DVM, PhD, DACVIM

Anemia, Hemolytic

Client Education Sheet 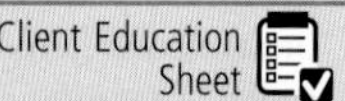

BASIC INFORMATION

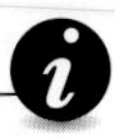

Definition

Decrease in red blood cell (RBC) mass due to destruction or shortened life span of RBCs. Immune-mediated hemolytic anemia (IMHA) is the most common cause and is discussed as a separate topic (p. 60).

Epidemiology

SPECIES, AGE, SEX

Any dog or cat

- Neonatal isoerythrolysis: neonatal kittens
- Inherited RBC defects: 6 months to 3 years of age, dogs > cats
- Caval syndrome: dogs
- Toxins: cats more susceptible, but dogs more likely exposed

GENETICS, BREED PREDISPOSITION

- Inherited RBC defects:
  - Phosphofructokinase (PFK) deficiency: English springer spaniels, rarely cocker spaniels
  - Pyruvate kinase (PK) deficiency: basenjis, beagles, West Highland white terriers, Cairn terriers, miniature poodles, toy Eskimos, dachshunds, Chihuahuas, pugs; Abyssinian, Somali, Bengal, Maine coon, and other pure-breed cats
  - Feline porphyria (rare): Siamese, domestic short hairs
- Infectious:
  - Babesiosis: greyhounds and pit bulls overrepresented
- Histiocytic neoplasia: Bernese mountain dogs, flat-coated retrievers, golden retrievers, rottweilers

RISK FACTORS

Oxidative damage (cats at increased risk); ectoparasites or endoparasites; hypophosphatemia

GEOGRAPHY AND SEASONALITY

Cytauxzoonosis: Southeast, Midwest, and mid-Atlantic United States, South America

Clinical Presentation

DISEASE FORMS/SUBTYPES

- Intravascular: direct RBC lysis within vasculature results in hemoglobinemia/-uria and icterus.
- Extravascular: RBCs are phagocytosed by the mononuclear phagocytic system, resulting in splenomegaly, hepatomegaly, and bilirubinemia/-uria.
- Intravascular and extravascular hemolysis can occur simultaneously.

HISTORY, CHIEF COMPLAINT

- Anorexia, weakness, exercise intolerance, collapse/syncope
- Signalment, known risk factors may provide clues (e.g., neonatal kitten from breed with high prevalence of B blood type, young English Springer spaniel with hemolytic crisis after exercise, cat with history of acetaminophen administration)
- Signs related to concurrent disease (e.g., diabetic ketoacidosis in animal with hemolysis from hypophosphatemia)

PHYSICAL EXAM FINDINGS

- Pallor, weakness, lethargy, tachycardia, tachypnea
- Icterus
- Hepatosplenomegaly
- Fever and lymphadenopathy are less common
- Murmur: systolic, soft (grade II/VI or less), left-sided
- Cyanosis if methemoglobinemia is present

Etiology and Pathophysiology

See Causes of Hemolysis (p. 1198).

- Immune-mediated anemia (p. 60)
- Intoxication:
  - Most but not all toxins that cause hemolysis do so by oxidative damage to RBCs.
  - Oxidant damage causes Heinz body formation or methemoglobinemia, with decreased RBC life span and decreased delivery of oxygen to tissues, respectively.
  - Heinz bodies make RBCs prone to intravascular lysis or phagocytosis. Heinz bodies are considered an absolute marker of oxidative RBC injury in dogs, less so in cats (present in 10%-50% of healthy cats).
  - Methemoglobinemia, suspected with cyanosis or brown-colored blood, does not affect RBC life span or induce hemolysis; it decreases the oxygen-carrying capacity of RBCs.
  - Oxidant RBC injury can cause Heinz bodies, methemoglobinemia, or both; Heinz bodies are more routinely identified first (blood smear).
- Infectious organisms: can infect RBCs directly and cause hemolysis or can trigger secondary RBC destruction. See Hemotropic Mycoplasmosis (p. 438), Babesiosis (p. 105), and Cytauxzoonosis (p. 235).
- Microangiopathic: hemangiosarcoma, disseminated intravascular coagulopathy (DIC), hepatic/splenic disease, heartworm disease (i.e., caudal caval syndrome), vasculitis
  - Fragmentation of RBCs by abnormal vascular structures or narrowing of vessels
- Hypophosphatemia: complication of ketoacidotic diabetes mellitus, hepatic lipidosis, refeeding syndrome, phosphate-binding antacids (p. 1241)
  - Usually with serum phosphorus < 1.5 mg/dL (<0.48 mmol/L)
  - Depletion of erythrocyte adenosine triphosphate (ATP), diphosphoglycerate (DPG), and reduced glutathione; decreased RBC deformability, increased osmotic fragility, and susceptibility to oxidative injury
- Hereditary erythrocyte defects:
  - PK deficiency: glycolytic enzyme deficiency, causing decreased ATP, leading to osmotic fragility. Anemia typically not manifested until early adulthood.
  - PFK deficiency: glycolytic enzyme deficiency, causing decreased 2,3-DPG; results in increased intracellular pH and RBC fragility in alkaline conditions such as hyperventilation during exercise
  - Feline porphyria: deficiency of uroporphyrinogen III cosynthetase; decreased production of hemoglobin
- Feline neonatal isoerythrolysis (p. 686): type B queens with anti-A alloantibodies in colostrum destroy RBCs in kittens with type A blood.
- Miscellaneous causes: incompatible blood transfusion, hemolytic uremic syndrome, hypotonic fluid administration, others (p. 1198)

DIAGNOSIS

Diagnostic Overview

Hemolytic anemia is suspected in a patient with anemia, no evidence of blood loss, and typically, evidence of RBC regeneration. Signalment, history, and physical examination can provide direction for diagnostic testing, but RBC morphology abnormalities are often key to determining cause of hemolysis.

Differential Diagnosis

- Blood-loss anemia (p. 57); bleeding may be overt or occult.
- Anemia due to decreased RBC production. May be RBC specific (e.g., chronic kidney disease, pure red cell aplasia) or may be part of pancytopenia (e.g., bone marrow disorders)

Initial Database

- CBC/blood smear:
  - Decreased hematocrit, RBC count, and hemoglobin
  - Evidence of regeneration:
    - Absolute reticulocytes > 60,000/microL
    - Macrocytosis, hypochromasia
    - Regeneration may not be evident for 3-5 days (until bone marrow responds)
  - Morphology: anisocytosis, polychromasia, Heinz bodies, schistocytes (microangiopathy), parasites. If spherocytes are present, suspect IMHA.
- Serum biochemistry panel and urinalysis: hyperbilirubinemia/-uria if severe acute

hemolysis. Hemoglobinemia/-uria with intravascular hemolysis. Total protein normal unless separate protein-losing disorder is occurring concurrently or anemia is from blood loss, not hemolysis. Rule out hypophosphatemia.
- Slide agglutination (and if negative, Coombs' test) to rule out IMHA
- Fecal floatation and heartworm serology: rule out parasites (e.g., hookworms, heartworm)
- Coagulation panel to assess for DIC (if thrombocytopenia or evidence of hemostatic defect on exam)
- Radiographs to rule out metallic gastrointestinal foreign body (zinc); ultrasound for neoplasia or splenic abnormalities (e.g., torsion, hemangiosarcoma), echocardiogram for caval syndrome

Advanced or Confirmatory Testing
- Polymerase chain reaction (PCR) and/or serologic testing for *Mycoplasma* (especially cats), *Babesia* (especially pit bull or greyhound)
- DNA tests for PK/PFK deficiency; porphyrins in urine and RBCs for porphyria
- Bone marrow aspiration: not indicated if regenerative; erythroid hyperplasia

TREATMENT

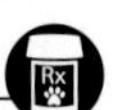

Treatment Overview
Treatment consists of stabilizing the patient with fluid support and blood transfusions (as needed, based on clinical signs), followed by specific therapy to resolve the underlying cause of hemolysis.

Acute General Treatment
- If severe, may require transfusion: packed RBCs (6-10 mL/kg IV) or whole blood (10-20 mL/kg IV) (p. 1169)
- Intoxication:
  - Zinc foreign body: remove by endoscopy/surgery (p. 1098)
  - Acetaminophen: *N*-acetylcysteine diluted in saline at 140 mg/kg IV, then 70 mg/kg q 6h × 6 doses (p. 10)
- Hypophosphatemia: potassium phosphate 0.01-0.06 mmol/kg/hr IV until normal
- Infection: see Hemotropic Mycoplasma, Babesiosis, and Cytauxzoonosis (pp. 105, 235, and 438)

Chronic Treatment
- Avoid excitement/exercise with PFK deficiency.
- Prednisolone and splenectomy in canine and feline PK deficiency

Possible Complications
- Hypercoagulation/pulmonary thromboembolism
- Transfusion reactions (p. 989)
  - Dogs: blood typing should be performed before transfusion. If recipient is not typed, donor should be negative for DEA-1.1. Previously transfused dogs require a cross-match before transfusion.
  - Cats: have naturally occurring alloantibodies. Fatal transfusion reactions can occur if transfusion is given arbitrarily, and cats must be typed and cross-matched before any transfusions.

Recommended Monitoring
During hospitalization, monitor packed cell volume (PCV) every 12-24 hours initially and monitor heart rate, respiratory rate, mucous membrane color, and capillary refill time (CRT) frequently to determine need for repeat transfusion.

PROGNOSIS & OUTCOME

- If cause of hemolysis is resolved, prognosis is good after patient is stabilized.
- Some causes of hemolysis carry a poor prognosis: cytauxzoonosis, isoerythrolysis, canine PK deficiency, hemangiosarcoma, DIC.

PEARLS & CONSIDERATIONS

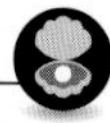

Comments
- Decision to transfuse should be based on clinical signs rather than PCV alone. However, when PCV is < 12%, patients generally decompensate and require transfusion.
- Although IMHA is the most common cause of hemolysis in dogs, other causes of hemolysis should be considered, especially in young or old dogs.

Prevention
Ectoparasite and heartworm prophylaxis; avoid breeding pets with congenital defects; avoid breeding type B queens to type A toms.

Technician Tips
In addition to mucous membrane color, capillary refill time, and heart and respiratory rates, mentation and pulse strength are external indicators of severity of anemia and are very useful for patient monitoring.

Client Education
- Counsel clients on causes of oxidative damage and that acetaminophen should especially be avoided.
- Counsel owners and breeders on heritable defects to avoid breeding of affected dogs.

SUGGESTED READING

Owen JL, et al: Hemolytic anemia in dogs and cats due to erythrocyte enzyme deficiencies. Vet Clin North Am Small Anim Pract 42:73-84, 2012.

EDITOR: Jonathan E. Fogle, DVM, PhD, DACVIM
AUTHOR: Alicia K. Henderson, DVM, DACVIM

Anemia, Immune-Mediated Hemolytic

Bonus Material Online

Client Education Sheet

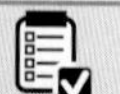

BASIC INFORMATION

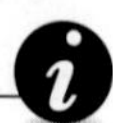

Definition
Immune-mediated hemolytic anemia (IMHA) is a common cause of anemia in dogs. IMHA results from increased destruction or phagocytosis of red blood cells (RBCs) that have been coated with immunoglobulin (Ig), complement (c′), or both. IMHA can be classified as primary (idiopathic) or secondary (identifiable underlying cause).

Synonyms
- Autoimmune hemolytic anemia
- Pure red cell aplasia (PRCA, p. 63): considered an IMHA variant in which RBC precursors in the bone marrow are destroyed
- Evans syndrome occurs when IMHA develops with concurrent immune-mediated thrombocytopenia (IMTP, p. 972).

Epidemiology
SPECIES, AGE, SEX
- More common in dogs
- Dogs: 1-13 years old (mean, 6 years); females slightly overrepresented
- Cats: 0.5-9 years old; most are ≤ 3 years old; males may be overrepresented

GENETICS, BREED PREDISPOSITION
Cocker spaniel, shih tzu, Bichon frisé, old English sheepdog, collie, miniature schnauzer, Maltese, Labrador retriever, poodle, dachshund, beagle, English springer spaniel, and Jack Russell terrier are overrepresented.

RISK FACTORS
- In dogs, IMHA is most often a primary or idiopathic condition. Infection and neoplasia are the most common causes of secondary IMHA.
- In cats, IMHA is most commonly a secondary condition with *Mycoplasma haemofelis* infections, feline leukemia virus (FeLV), feline immunodeficiency virus (FIV), and lymphoma being the most common underlying causes.
- Recent vaccination is suggested as a trigger of IMHA in some cases (dogs, cats).

- Anecdotal reports in dogs suggest previous drug administration (e.g., beta-lactam and sulfa antibiotics) may cause a secondary IMHA.

GEOGRAPHY AND SEASONALITY

In dogs, increased incidence in the spring (40% of cases in May and June)

ASSOCIATED DISORDERS

- Thromboembolism and pulmonary thromboembolism (PTE) (very common)
- Disseminated intravascular coagulopathy (DIC)
- Thrombocytopenia (<50,000/microL) occurs in one-third to one-half of cases (Evans syndrome).

Clinical Presentation

DISEASE FORMS/SUBTYPES

- *Primary (idiopathic)* IMHA: Immunoglobulins attach to antigens or components of the RBC membrane, causing extravascular hemolysis, intravascular hemolysis, intravascular RBC agglutination, and/or activation of the c′ cascade.
- *Secondary* IMHA: RBCs are destroyed as innocent bystanders in an immune reaction against antigens or foreign proteins attached to the cell membrane.
- *Extravascular* hemolysis: Immunoglobulin or c′-coated RBCs are selectively destroyed by macrophages in the spleen and liver.
- *Intravascular* hemolysis: c′-mediated RBC membrane damage causes cell rupture.

HISTORY, CHIEF COMPLAINT

- Signs of anemia: tachycardia, tachypnea, dyspnea, lethargy, progressive weakness, collapse
- Inappetence, anorexia
- Vomiting, diarrhea
- Discolored urine (bilirubinuria or hemoglobinuria)
- Icterus
- Respiratory distress with acute PTE (p. 842)

PHYSICAL EXAM FINDINGS

- Pale mucous membranes
- Tachycardia
- Tachypnea
- Bounding pulses
- Icterus
- Heart murmur (systolic, left base)
- Hepatomegaly and/or splenomegaly
- If Evans syndrome or DIC, possible petechiae and/or ecchymosis

Etiology and Pathophysiology

- Extravascular hemolysis
  - Commonly occurs in the spleen (occasionally liver).
  - Immunoglobulin (Ig), mainly IgG, attach to RBC and cause phagocytosis; minimal c′-mediated cell membrane damage
  - Partial erythrophagocytosis can cause spherocytes, a hallmark of IMHA.
  - Splenomegaly from active phagocytosis and extramedullary hematopoiesis
- Intravascular hemolysis
  - Binding of IgM and IgG immunoglobulins to the RBC membrane activates the c′ cascade, causing direct damage to the cell membrane with influx of extracellular fluid and cell rupture.
- Potential causes of secondary IMHA in dogs
  - Infectious (ehrlichiosis, babesiosis, anaplasmosis, leptospirosis, dirofilariasis)
  - Neoplasia (lymphoma, histiocytic sarcoma)
  - Drugs (trimethoprim-sulfonamide, penicillin, cephalosporin).
- Autoagglutination (antibody-mediated RBC clumping), hallmark of IMHA, primarily occurs with IgM coating of RBCs.
- Moderate to marked leukocytosis with a neutrophilic left shift is common in dogs. This neutrophilia is likely due to an increased release of cells from the bone marrow during a strong erythroid response and/or cytokine response to systemic inflammation and/or necrosis.
- Hyperbilirubinemia is associated with hemolysis (most common) and decreased hepatic clearance of bilirubin.
- Elevated serum liver enzymes (especially alanine transaminase [ALT]) suggest hypoxic hepatocellular injury.
- Moderate to marked thrombocytopenia could be due to Evans syndrome or early DIC.
- Dogs with IMHA are hypercoagulable and at risk for thromboembolism. Increased liver values, decreased platelet count, and decreased antithrombin activity are associated with thromboembolism in dogs with IMHA.
- Reticulocytosis is more common in dogs at the time of diagnosis than in cats.
  - Absence of reticulocytes: inadequate time for bone marrow response (3-5 days), and/or immune-mediated destruction of RBC precursors

DIAGNOSIS

Diagnostic Overview

The diagnosis is supported by findings of anemia, hemolysis (hemoglobinemia or hemoglobinuria), evidence of antibodies directed against RBC (autoagglutination, spherocytosis, or positive Coombs' test), and response to immunosuppressive therapy. No finding is pathognomonic for primary IMHA, and causes of secondary IMHA must be investigated as relevant (e.g., retroviral testing of cats, vector-borne disease testing based on geography).

Differential Diagnosis

Anemia:

- Other hemolytic anemias (p. 59)
- Hemorrhage (p. 433)
- Bone marrow disorder, chronic disease

Icterus (p. 528)

Initial Database

- CBC with microscopic blood smear evaluation
  - Decreased hematocrit (HCT), packed cell volume (PCV), RBC count, hemoglobin
  - Mild to marked thrombocytopenia
  - Approximately 50% of dogs with IMHA have a nonregenerative or poorly regenerative anemia at diagnosis.
  - Hallmarks of IMHA: spherocytosis (79% of dogs), autoagglutination (42%-66%), polychromasia (90%), or some combination of these clinical findings in 96% of IMHA dogs.
  - Moderate to marked leukocytosis with a neutrophilic left shift and/or nucleated RBCs.
  - RBC parasites: *Babesia* spp (dog), *M. haemofelis* (cat), others
- Serum biochemistry
  - Elevated total bilirubin, liver enzymes (ALT, alkaline phosphatase [ALP]), sometimes blood urea nitrogen (BUN)
  - Artifactual hypophosphatemia (interference from hyperbilirubinemia)
  - Normal total protein with anemia is consistent with hemolysis.
- Urinalysis
  - Bilirubinuria and/or hemoglobinuria
  - If pyuria or bacteriuria is present, perform bacterial culture and sensitivity.
- In cats, FeLV and FIV serologic tests
- Saline agglutination test (slide autoagglutination)
  - Mix 1 drop of anticoagulated whole blood with 1 drop of saline on a microscope slide.
  - If enough antibodies are present on the cell membrane, RBC agglutination can be identified grossly and microscopically.
- Coomb's test (p. 1328), also known as direct antiglobulin/antigen test (DAT): perform if no visible autoagglutination
  - Direct Coombs' test detects antibodies attached to RBCs.
  - The sensitivity in IMHA is 60%-89%. A negative Coombs' test result does not exclude a diagnosis of IMHA.
- Coagulation assessment
  - DIC (p. 269)
  - Hypercoagulability: increased D-dimers and/or fibrin degradation products (FDPs), decreased fibrinogen, decreased antithrombin
- Abdominal radiographs
  - Evaluate spleen and liver size.
  - Identify an underlying cause for secondary IMHA.
  - Identify metallic (zinc) gastrointestinal foreign bodies as a cause of non–immune-mediated hemolysis.
- Abdominal ultrasonography
  - Identify an underlying cause (neoplasia) of secondary IMHA.
- Thoracic radiographs
  - Usually unremarkable; marked pulmonary interstitial pattern, patchy alveolar opacities, and mild pleural effusion might be associated with a PTE.

Advanced or Confirmatory Testing

- Serologic and/or polymerase chain reaction (PCR) tests for
  - Dogs: dirofilariasis, ehrlichiosis, babesiosis, anaplasmosis, Lyme, leptospirosis
  - Cats: hemotropic mycoplasmosis (PCR)

TREATMENT

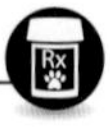

Treatment Overview

Therapy consists of immune suppression, supportive care (improving or maintaining perfusion and normal tissue oxygenation), and anticoagulant therapy. For secondary IMHA, the cause should be addressed.

Acute General Treatment

- Transfusion therapy
  - Maintenance of tissue oxygenation is the most important supportive therapy for severely anemic patients.
  - Need indicated by clinical signs (e.g., tachypnea, dyspnea, tachycardia, bounding pulses, weakness, collapse) rather than numeric value of PCV.
  - Transfusion products: packed RBCs or whole blood
- Immunosuppressive therapy
  - Glucocorticoids (cornerstone of IMHA therapy): prednisone (2 mg/kg PO q 24h or divided q 12h; for large-breed dogs, 40 mg/m^2/day) or dexamethasone sodium phosphate (0.15-0.25 mg/kg IV q 24h)
  - When glucocorticoids fail to maintain remission or produce unacceptable side effects, additional immunosuppressive therapy should be administered.
  - Cyclosporine 5 mg/kg PO q 12h
  - Human immunoglobulin 0.5-1.5 g/kg IV infused over 6-12 hours, up to 3 doses may increase risk of thromboembolism.
- Antithrombotic therapy
  - Anticoagulant therapy: low-molecular-weight heparin (dalteparin 150 IU/kg SQ q 8-12h or enoxaparin 0.8-1 mg/kg SQ q 6-8h) or unfractionated heparin (150-300 IU/kg SQ q 6-8h or CRI 10-25 IU/kg/h). The use of unfractionated heparin requires titration to prolong the activated partial thromboplastin time (aPTT) to 1.5-3 × baseline values or monitor anti-factor Xa activity.
  - Antiplatelet therapy: clopidogrel (1-2 mg/kg PO q 24h), or (less preferred) low-dose aspirin (1-2 mg/kg PO q 24h [dogs]) if platelet count > 50,000/microL.
- Additional supportive care
  - Intravenous crystalloid fluids to support renal blood flow, especially in cases with intravascular hemolysis
  - Oxygen supplementation provides little benefit for most anemic patients but might be beneficial for patients with PTEs.
  - Gastric protectant: omeprazole (1 mg/kg PO q 12h)

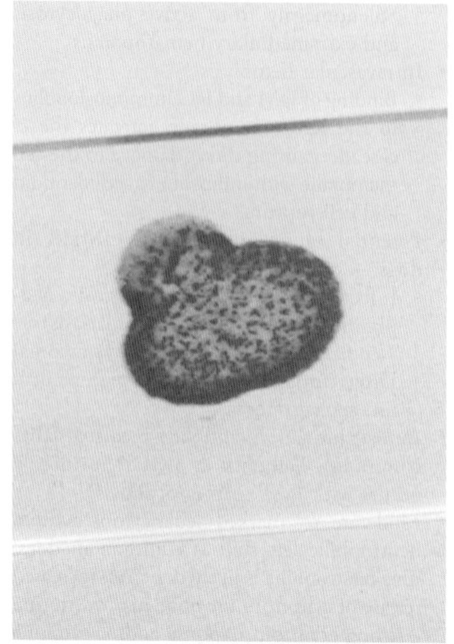

ANEMIA, IMMUNE-MEDIATED HEMOLYTIC Positive slide agglutination test (macroagglutination/clumping of cells) from a dog with primary IMHA. The test is performed with a drop of anticoagulated blood mixed with a drop of saline.

- For secondary IMHA, treatment of the underlying cause is essential and can reduce the need for and duration of additional therapy.

Chronic Treatment

- Continue immunosuppression with glucocorticoids until well-established disease remission (often ≥ 6 months)
- If single agent glucocorticoids fail to maintain remission or produce unacceptable side effects, adjunctive immunosuppressive medications may be required.
  - Cyclosporine 5 mg/kg PO q 12h; pharmacodynamic (or pharmacokinetic) monitoring is recommended.
  - Azathioprine 2 mg/kg PO q 24h initial dose (dogs only)
  - Mycophenolate mofetil 10 mg/kg PO q 12h
  - Leflunomide 2-4 mg/kg PO q 24h (dogs)
  - Adjunctive immunosuppressive therapies can be used as acute therapy, but the onset of action may be delayed by weeks (azathioprine, mycophenolate mofetil, and leflunomide).
  - Cyclophosphamide is *not* recommended.
- After the PCV stabilizes, taper the medication dosage by 15%-25% every 2-4 weeks for 4-8 months. Glucocorticoid tapering can occur more quickly if an adjunctive immunosuppressive agent is used. After glucocorticoid dose is < 1 mg/kg/day, consider switch to every other day dosing before additional taper.
- Thromboprophylaxis: Continue short-term anticoagulant therapy (low-molecular-weight heparin or unfractionated heparin) tapered over 10-14 days. Continue long-term antiplatelet therapy with clopidogrel or low-dose aspirin. Taper antithrombotic medications when immunosuppression and PCV are stable.

Possible Complications

- Thromboembolism (PTE, portal vein or splenic thrombosis)
  - Avoid jugular intravenous catheters.
- Secondary infections due to immunosuppressive therapy
- Adverse drug side effects
  - Glucocorticoids: polyuria/polydipsia, polyphagia, gastrointestinal ulceration, weakness, panting
  - Cyclosporine: vomiting, diarrhea, decreased appetite, gingival hyperplasia
  - Azathioprine: myelosuppression, hepatopathy, pancreatitis
  - Mycophenolate: diarrhea, decreased appetite
  - Leflunomide: decreased appetite
- Antithrombotic therapy: excessive or inadvertent hemorrhage
- Transfusion reactions (p. 989)

Recommended Monitoring

- During acute crisis, mentation and respiratory effort should be assessed frequently. PCV should be assessed q 8-12h initially, then q 12-24h while hospitalized.
- The PCV stabilizes in most dogs 4-6 days after starting immunosuppressive therapy.
- After discharge, PCV should be monitored weekly for the first month.
- PCV should be evaluated before any dose reduction during taper and 1 week after the change in drug dose to detect a relapse.

PROGNOSIS & OUTCOME

- Overall mortality rate for primary canine IMHA is estimated to be 20%-70%.
- Negative prognostic indicators include nonregenerative anemia, thromboembolism, persistent autoagglutination, thrombocytopenia, leukocytosis with a left shift, and hyperbilirubinemia.
- Approximately 20% of dogs experienced a clinical relapse within 1 year after cessation of therapy, perhaps related to inadequate treatment duration.
- Thromboembolism is a major complication, and dogs receiving antithrombotic therapy have improved outcomes.
- Cats with primary IMHA have a lower overall mortality rate, possibly due to a lower incidence of thromboembolism.

PEARLS & CONSIDERATIONS

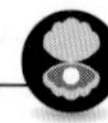

Comments

- Spherocytes may develop after transfusion; a diagnostic blood smear should be evaluated before transfusion.
- Dogs with IMHA die from anemia or thromboembolism.

  - RBC transfusion is an essential therapy in severe IMHA cases.
  - Antithrombotic therapy is important for the prevention of thromboembolism.
- In dogs, mild primary IMHA may respond to immunosuppression with only a glucocorticoid.
- Adjunctive immunosuppressive medications may improve immunosuppression and allow for an accelerated reduction in glucocorticoids to minimize side effects but could increase the risk of secondary infections.
- Non–immune-mediated hemolytic anemia may present with signs similar to IMHA, including hemolysis, icterus, and regenerative anemia. (p. 59).
- Pit bull dogs should be screened by serology and PCR for *Babesia gibsoni* as soon as hemolysis is recognized (p. 105).

Technician Tips

Thromboembolism can develop unexpectedly (often during recovery from the initial crisis), and signs of respiratory effort, collapse, or abdominal distention warrant prompt evaluation.

Client Education

- Clearly describe the side effects associated with high-dose glucocorticoid therapy.
- After immunosuppressive therapy is stopped, monitor the patient's PCV for early signs of relapse.
- If the development of IMHA was associated with a recent vaccination, discretion should be used for future vaccinations.

SUGGESTED READINGS

Swann JW, et al: Systemic review of evidence relating to the treatment of immune-mediated hemolytic anemia in dogs. J Vet Intern Med 27:1-9, 2013.

AUTHOR: John M. Thomason, DVM, MS, DACVIM
EDITOR: Jonathan E. Fogle, DVM, PhD, DACVIM

Anemia, Nonregenerative, and Pure Red Cell Aplasia

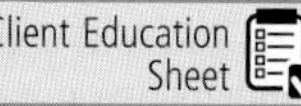

BASIC INFORMATION

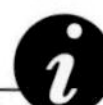

Definition

A decrease in red blood cell (RBC) mass, hematocrit (HCT), or hemoglobin lacking an appropriate compensatory, regenerative response (absence of reticulocytosis). Pure red cell aplasia (PRCA) is a type of nonregenerative anemia that is associated with marked depletion or absence of erythroid precursor cells in the bone marrow, without affecting leukocyte and platelet precursor cells.

Epidemiology

SPECIES, AGE, SEX

- Nonregenerative anemia
  - Dogs and cats of any age or either sex
  - Depends on underlying cause
- PRCA
  - Dogs: middle-aged, both sexes (females may be overrepresented)
  - Cats: young (<3 years old), both sexes

GENETICS, BREED PREDISPOSITION

Congenital cobalamin deficiency: giant schnauzer, border collie, Shar-pei, beagle, Australian shepherd

RISK FACTORS

- Nonregenerative anemia: chronic kidney disease (CKD), cobalamin deficiency disorders, many chronic systemic or inflammatory illnesses
- PRCA: cats: feline leukemia virus (FeLV; p. 329) and feline immunodeficiency virus (FIV; p. 325) positive

CONTAGION AND ZOONOSIS

Feline retroviral infection

Clinical Presentation

HISTORY, CHIEF COMPLAINT

Signs develop over weeks to months and can include lethargy, weakness, exercise intolerance, collapse, and tachypnea.

PHYSICAL EXAM FINDINGS

Pale mucous membranes, tachycardia, tachypnea, systolic heart murmur, weakness. Perform rectal exam to check for melena.

Etiology and Pathophysiology

- Nonregenerative anemia
  - Delay in regeneration: insufficient time to stimulate regeneration (2-5 days)
  - Anemia of chronic disease: several mechanisms: infections (FeLV, FIV, ehrlichiosis, *Anaplasma*, parvovirus), nonseptic inflammation, neoplasia, chronic liver disease, hypoadrenocorticism, hypothyroidism
  - Bone marrow disorders: immune-mediated (immune-mediated hemolytic anemia [IMHA], PRCA), FeLV, neoplasia (leukemia, lymphoma, myelophthisis), myelofibrosis, myelodysplastic syndrome, aplastic anemia; often part of bicytopenia or pancytopenia.
  - Lack of factors needed for effective erythropoiesis or hemoglobin synthesis: deficiencies in erythropoietin (CKD), iron (often due to gastrointestinal [GI] bleeding), folate, cobalamin
  - Drug-induced dyscrasia: chemotherapeutic agents, estrogenic compounds
- PRCA
  - Primary: immune-mediated
  - Secondary: parvovirus (dogs), FeLV positive (cats)

DIAGNOSIS

Diagnostic Overview

Anemia confirmed with a complete blood count (CBC) or packed cell volume (PCV), but a diagnosis of a nonregenerative anemia requires a corrected or absolute reticulocyte count. Diagnostic investigation of systemic, underlying causes of anemia should be initiated before performing a bone marrow aspirate/biopsy. A bone marrow aspirate is necessary to diagnose PRCA and is indicated when a persistent nonregenerative anemia exists without an identifiable underlying cause.

Differential Diagnosis

Acute hemorrhage or erythrocyte destruction with insufficient time for reticulocytosis (3-5 days)

Initial Database

- CBC: severity of anemia, changes in erythrocyte indices
  - PRCA, dogs and cats: marked normocytic, normochromic anemia. Leukocyte and platelet counts are within normal limits or slightly above reference intervals.
- Reticulocyte count: corrected count: < 1%, absolute count: < 60,000/mcL
  - PRCA, dogs and cats: corrected count: commonly ≤ 0.1%, absolute count: commonly ≤ 10,000/mcL
- Blood smear: abnormal cell morphology, basophilic stippling (lead poisoning), spherocytosis (IMHA)
  - PRCA, dogs and cats: no consistent abnormalities (occasional spherocytes or microcytes)
- Serum biochemistry and urinalysis: detect underlying disorders (e.g., CKD)
  - Normal total serum proteins and bilirubin (pp. 57 and 59)
  - Nonregenerative anemia and PRCA: no consistent abnormalities
- Cats: FeLV and FIV serologic testing; ± FeLV PCR

Advanced or Confirmatory Testing

- Diagnostic tests to identify primary or underlying systemic disorders as clinically indicated (e.g., thoracic radiographs, abdominal ultrasound) before performing bone marrow aspirate/ biopsy
- Bone marrow aspirate or core biopsy (p. 1068): cellularity, myeloid-to-erythroid

(M/E) ratio, completeness and orderliness of maturation, presence of abnormal cells
- PRCA: a bone marrow aspirate/biopsy is required to make a diagnosis. The aspirate reveals no or very few precursor cells, with a M/E ratio > 75 : 1 (normal: 1 : 1 to 2 : 1). Lymphocytosis is common in cats and occasionally seen in dogs.
- Special tests on marrow may be indicated (e.g., immunofluorescent antibody test for FeLV)

- Coombs' test (p. 1328)
  - PRCA: Dogs are usually negative, and approximately 50% of cats are positive.

TREATMENT

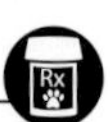

Treatment Overview

Therapy for nonregenerative anemias consists of supportive care (improve oxygen-carrying capacity, transfusion) and treatment of the primary or underlying cause. It is essential to determine the primary cause of the anemia to initiate effective, appropriate therapy. The cornerstone of therapy for PRCA is immunosuppressive therapy, particularly corticosteroids.

Acute General Treatment

Transfusion is typically indicated if HCT is ≤ 15% and/or the patient has developed clinical signs due to the severity of anemia. Packed red blood cells (pRBCs) from a universal donor is the blood product of choice.

Chronic Treatment

- Treat underlying disorders.
- Anemia of chronic inflammatory disease resolves with treatment of the underlying cause.
- Immune-mediated nonregenerative anemia and PRCA require immunosuppressive therapy.
  - Prednisolone 2-4 mg/kg PO q 24h (large-breed dogs, 40 mg/m^2/day). After the PCV stabilizes, taper the medication by 15%-25% every 2-4 weeks.
- If inadequate response with prednisolone alone, consider other immunosuppressive medications (p. 60):
  - Azathioprine 2 mg/kg PO q 24h, tapering to 0.5-1 mg/kg PO q 48h (dogs only)
  - Cyclosporine microemulsion (Atopica, Neoral) 5 mg/kg PO q 12h; pharmacodynamic monitoring recommended
  - Mycophenolate mofetil 5-10 mg/kg PO q 12h
- PRCA may require long-term (months) of immunosuppressive therapy before response to therapy is noticed.
- Repeat transfusions may be necessary; cross match first.

Possible Complications

- Secondary infections due to immunosuppressive therapy
- Adverse drug effects
  - Prednisolone: polyuria/polydipsia, polyphagia, GI ulceration, weakness
  - Azathioprine: myelosuppression, hepatopathy
  - Cyclosporine: vomiting, diarrhea, decreased appetite
  - Mycophenolate: diarrhea
- Transfusion reactions (p. 989)

Recommended Monitoring

Repeat PCV every 1-2 weeks until it increases or the patient develops clinical signs of anemia. After the PCV begins to increase, monitor every 2-4 weeks until normal and stable. The PCV should be re-evaluated before any dose reduction and 1-2 weeks after a reduction to detect relapse.

PROGNOSIS & OUTCOME

Depends on primary disorder

PEARLS & CONSIDERATIONS

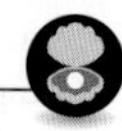

Comments

- With acute anemia of any cause, 3-5 days are required to detect reticulocytosis.
- Anemia of inflammatory disease is usually mild (PCV > 25%).
- Chronic nonregenerative anemias often result in a gradual onset of clinical signs due to compensation, even if the anemia itself is quite severe.
- Bone marrow evaluation is needed to distinguish PRCA from other nonregenerative anemias.
- Over half of cats with primary IMHA anemia present with nonregenerative anemia.

Technician Tips

- Inspect blood units before infusion; discolored, hemolyzed, or expired units should be discarded.
- Monitor patients closely during the transfusion and use a checklist to ensure careful patient monitoring and early recognition of potential reactions.

SUGGESTED READINGS

Abrams-Ogg A: Non-regenerative anemia. In Ettinger SJ, et al, editors: Textbook of veterinary internal medicine, ed 7, St. Louis, 2010, Saunders Elsevier, pp 788-797.

AUTHOR: John M. Thomason, DVM, MS, DACVIM
EDITOR: Jonathan E. Fogle, DVM, PhD, DACVIM

Anesthetic-Related Complications

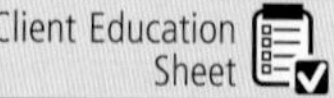

BASIC INFORMATION

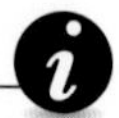

Definition

Complications occurring in the peri-anesthetic period attributed to an anesthetic cause

Epidemiology

SPECIES, AGE, SEX

Any species/age/sex

GENETICS, BREED PREDISPOSITION

- Sighthounds may have delayed recovery from barbiturates, propofol, or alfaxalone.
- Herding breeds may have exaggerated effects of drugs, including acepromazine and torphanol.
- Boxers of European descent may have an adverse reaction to acepromazine, characterized by bradycardia and collapse.
- Brachycephalic breeds may be difficult to intubate and have difficulty breathing after extubation due to airway swelling or edema.

RISK FACTORS

Increased risk:

- Extremes of age (neonates, geriatrics)
- Coexisting disease (ASA status ≥ 3), especially cardiovascular and pulmonary disease
- Emergency anesthesia
- Prolonged anesthetic duration
- Small size (cats < 2 kg; dogs < 5 kg)
- Anesthetic monitoring not used

ASSOCIATED DISORDERS

Respiratory arrest, cardiac arrest, hypotension

Clinical Presentation

DISEASE FORMS/SUBTYPES

- Respiratory complications
- Cardiovascular complications
- Equipment failure
- Anesthetic overdose
- Anaphylaxis
- Hyperthermia, hypothermia
- Prolonged anesthetic recovery

HISTORY, CHIEF COMPLAINT

- Pre-anesthetic/anesthetic
  - Apnea/hypoventilation/dyspnea
  - Pallor/cyanosis
  - Bradycardia/tachycardia/arrhythmias
  - Hypotension/hypertension
  - Hypothermia/hyperthermia

PHYSICAL EXAM FINDINGS

See History, Chief Complaint section.

Etiology and Pathophysiology

Respiratory complications:

- Anesthetic agents cause respiratory depression and sometimes apnea. Patient positioning can lead to atelectasis of dependent lung lobes. Tight restraint may cause hypoventilation.
- Equipment malfunction can lead to rebreathing of CO_2, delivery of a hypoxic gas mixture, or failure of anesthetic gas delivery.
- Tracheal tears lead to pneumothorax, pneumomediastinum, and/or subcutaneous emphysema.
- Closure of the pop-off valve or administration of positive-pressure ventilation with excessive airway pressure can result in barotrauma and pneumothorax.

Cardiovascular complications:

- Many anesthetic agents cause cardiovascular effects, including bradycardia, arrhythmias, vasodilation, and hypotension.
- Surgical manipulation of the heart and thoracic structures can cause arrhythmias.
- Hemorrhage secondary to surgery decreases cardiac output.
- Patients with pre-existing cardiovascular disease may be more susceptible.

Neurologic complications:

- Patients with pre-existing intracranial disease are susceptible to the consequences of increased intracranial pressure associated with hypercapnia, hypoxemia, and/or hypertension.
- Blindness has occurred in cats after use of a mouth gag due to maxillary artery occlusion.

Musculoskeletal complications:

- Propofol and alfaxalone occasionally cause myoclonus.

Thermoregulation:

- Anesthetic agents depress the thermoregulatory system. Hypothermia can cause alterations in coagulation, increased wound infection rates, reduced metabolic rate, decreased anesthetic requirements, arrhythmias, and death.
- Hyperthermia can occur in cats receiving mu-agonist opioids.
- Hyperthermia and burns may result from overzealous heat support (p. 138).
- Malignant hyperthermia is a rare complication of inhalants.

DIAGNOSIS

Diagnostic Overview

A physical exam should be performed to identify the body systems affected and direct diagnostics.

Differential Diagnosis

- Surgically-induced respiratory/cardiovascular complications (e.g., pneumothorax, hemorrhage, vagal reflexes)
- Progression of primary disease (e.g., sepsis, hemorrhage, traumatic brain injury)
- Neurologic dysfunction due to surgical manipulation
- Failure or misinterpretation of monitors
- Anesthesia machine malfunction

Initial Database

- Heart rate and rhythm; pulse palpation
- Blood pressure
- Mucous membrane color, capillary refill time (CRT), packed cell volume (PCV), and total solids (TS)
- Anesthetic depth
- Body temperature
- Respiratory rate and effort, auscult for normal lung sounds bilaterally; evaluate capnogram and end-tidal CO_2 ($ETCO_2$)
- Hemoglobin saturation by pulse oximetry; consider arterial blood gas to assess hypoxemia
- Evaluate anesthetic equipment, ensure proper functionality

TREATMENT

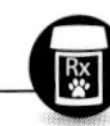

Treatment Overview

Support oxygen delivery to tissues through cardiovascular and respiratory stability. Identify and eliminate cause of complication. Physiologic abnormalities should be managed as soon as possible.

Acute General Treatment

Apnea/hypoventilation, cyanosis, pallor:

- Manual positive-pressure ventilation should be provided in the presence of apnea or hypoventilation; subjectively assess compliance of the patient's lungs while providing manual breaths. A sudden increased resistance to delivering a breath could indicate pneumothorax or airway obstruction.
- Administer 100% oxygen.
- Assess patient's cardiovascular status; rule out cardiac arrest.
- Lighten anesthetic plane if too deep.
- If an anesthesia machine malfunction is suspected, disconnect patient from the anesthetic circuit and administer breaths using an Ambu bag.
- Ensure that the endotracheal tube is placed correctly and at the correct depth.
- Consider reversal of drugs that can contribute to hypoventilation.

Tachypnea:

- Adjust anesthetic plane if indicated.
- Perform thoracocentesis (p. 1164) if pneumothorax is suspected.
- Ensure normothermia.

Bradycardia:

- Assess airway equipment and anesthesia machine, ensuring proper function (e.g., pop-off valve open).
- Identify possible causes of vagal stimulation.
- If hypotension is identified, heart rate is unacceptably low, or heart rate is rapidly falling, administer atropine (0.02-0.04 mg/kg IV) or glycopyrrolate (0.01-0.02 mg/kg IV).
- Consider reversal of drugs associated with bradycardia (alpha-2 agonists, opioids).
- Ensure normothermia.

Tachycardia:

- Ensure adequate depth of anesthesia.
- Ensure adequate analgesia.
- For ventricular tachycardia (heart rate > 180 bpm with ventricular complexes), consider lidocaine 2 mg/kg IV, followed by continuous IV infusion of 30-50 mcg/kg/min.
- If tachycardia is due to hypovolemia (p. 911), consider IV bolus of isotonic crystalloid fluids (5-10 mL/kg or more, as indicated by serial reassessment).

Hypotension:

- Lighten anesthetic plane if too deep.
- If also bradycardic, administer atropine (0.01-0.04 mg/kg IV) or glycopyrrolate (0.01 mg/kg IV).
- If the patient is hypovolemic, administer a bolus of isotonic crystalloid replacement solution (5-10 mL/kg IV) unless the patient is unable to tolerate a fluid bolus (e.g., due to cardiac disease).
- Consider partial intravenous anesthesia with opioids and tranquilizers to reduce inhalant requirement.
- For refractory hypotension, consider the use of positive inotropes and vasopressors.

Hypothermia warming strategies (p. 523):

- Blankets to prevent radiant heat loss
- Avoid contact with cold surfaces.
- Increase room temperature.
- Avoid cold lavage/scrub solutions.
- Forced air warming devices
- Circulating warm water blankets
- Heating pads designed for use with veterinary patients
- Radiant heat support by ceramic or infrared warmers

Neurologic complications:

- For continued sedation/obtundation, reverse anesthetic agents.
- Provide supportive care, including manual ventilation until patient can appropriately ventilate, oxygen supplementation, heat support, fluid therapy, etc.
- Measure blood pressure, PCV/total protein (TP), blood glucose and correct as necessary

Possible Complications

- Hypotension or hypoxemia can damage vital organs.
- Hypothermia can lead to anesthetic overdose, increased infection rates, arrhythmias, cardiac arrest.
- Hypercapnia, hypoxemia, or severe hypertension can lead to increased intracranial pressure, especially in patients with pre-existing intracranial disease.
- Prolonged recovery from anesthesia is a common sequela of anesthetic overdose, decreased metabolic rate, hypothermia, hypoglycemia, and hypotension.

Recommended Monitoring

- Heart rate and rhythm by electrocardiogram (ECG); pulse rate and quality
- Blood pressure, CRT
- Pulse oximetry, mucous membrane color
- Capnography; respiratory rate and effort
- Body temperature
- Arterial blood gas
- Serial PCV/TP and blood glucose concentrations

PROGNOSIS & OUTCOME

- Depends on the severity and duration of the complication.
- Most carry a good prognosis for full recovery if rapidly recognized and addressed.

PEARLS & CONSIDERATIONS

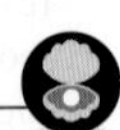

Comments

- Most anesthetic complications are easily prevented by diligent monitoring and anesthetic checklists to ensure correct procedures and machine function.
- Anesthetists should be familiar and comfortable with anesthetic drugs, procedures, equipment, and monitoring devices.
- Death associated with anesthesia frequently occurs in the postoperative period. Patient monitoring should continue throughout recovery.

Prevention

- Anesthetic plans catered to individual patients in consideration of signalment, coexisting disease, and procedure.
- Maintenance of high quality, correctly functioning anesthetic equipment.

Technician Tips

Careful observation of patients during and immediately after anesthesia can avert complications.

SUGGESTED READING

Matthews N, et al: Factors associated with anesthetic-related death in dogs and cats in primary care veterinary hospitals. JAVMA 250:655-665, 2017.

AUTHOR: Rachel A. Reed, DVM, DACVAA
EDITOR: Benjamin M. Brainard, VMD, DACVAA, DACVECC

Angular Limb Deformities

Bonus Material Online 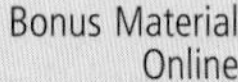 Client Education Sheet 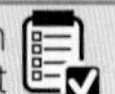

BASIC INFORMATION

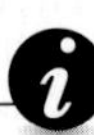

Definition

Abnormal growth of a limb due to premature closure of a physis (growth plate). Most commonly occurs in the forelimb, with radial or ulnar physeal closures. Rarely affects the hindlimb, with premature closure of a tibial physis.

Synonyms

Premature closure of radial, ulnar, or tibial physis; radius curvus; carpus valgus

Epidemiology

SPECIES, AGE, SEX

Primarily young dogs (<1 year old); uncommon in cats

RISK FACTORS

- Trauma to limb and physis
- Some chondrodystrophic breeds may be predisposed.

Clinical Presentation

HISTORY, CHIEF COMPLAINT

- Trauma to the limb 3-4 weeks before deformity begins
- Often, dog is presented when the limb begins to appear deformed.

PHYSICAL EXAM FINDINGS

- Lameness of affected limb, with pain on palpation of carpus or elbow
- The limb may appear shortened or have an angular deviation.

Etiology and Pathophysiology

- Premature closure of the distal ulnar physis is the most common physeal injury, likely due to the conical shape of this physis in dogs.
  - Because of the paired bone system, cessation of growth in the ulna causes cranial bowing, external rotation, and valgus deformity of the radius as it continues to grow. Elbow and carpal incongruities can also occur.
- Asymmetrical closure of the distal radial physis can cause an angular deformity similar to closure of the ulnar physis.
- Symmetrical closure of either radial physis often leads to radial shortening and elbow incongruity but no angular deformity.

DIAGNOSIS

Diagnostic Overview

Premature closure of a physis is suspected in a young dog with a shortened or angularly deformed limb and confirmed on radiographs when compared to the normal limb.

Differential Diagnosis

- Malunion of a fracture
- Ligamentous or tendinous damage at the elbow or carpus
- Retained cartilaginous core of the ulna

Initial Database

- CBC and serum chemistry panel: no abnormal findings expected
- Mediolateral and craniocaudal elbow-to-carpus radiographs of the affected and contralateral limb to assess location and degree of deformation

Advanced or Confirmatory Testing

- CT is helpful for further defining the limb deformation and joint congruency.
- CT images can be used to produce three-dimensional, life-sized, stereolithographic models for surgical planning.

TREATMENT

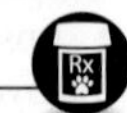

Treatment Overview

Surgical treatment aims to restore joint congruity, normalize limb length, and correct angular and rotational deformities. In immature dogs, additional aims are to restore unrestricted growth of affected bones and prevent joint incongruities from developing.

Acute General Treatment

- Ulnar ostectomy: used in an immature dog with premature closure of the ulnar physis to restore radial growth potential
  - A fat graft placed in the ostectomy prevents premature bone union.
- Distraction osteogenesis (by circular external fixation): used for treating premature closure of the distal radius
  - This allows for limb lengthening and correction of angular deformities.
- Corrective radial wedge or dome osteotomy (stabilized with a T-plate, circular or linear external fixation, in combination with an ulnar osteotomy or ostectomy): performed in mature dogs for acute correction of angular and rotational deformities and to restore joint congruity
- Proximal ulnar osteotomy: permits correction of elbow incongruities

Chronic Treatment

- In the postoperative period, a soft, padded bandage or metasplint may be placed to protect the limb. The bandage or splint is often applied for 2-4 weeks.
- Physical rehabilitation to reduce risk of complications

Behavior/Exercise

Exercise restriction for at least 6 weeks until radiographs confirm bone healing

Possible Complications

- External fixation may have premature loosening of the fixation pins or pin tract infection.
- Inappropriate amount of surgical correction may result in persistent valgus.

- Distal radial plating may result in decreased antebrachiocarpal joint range of motion.
- Distraction osteogenesis may lead to flexor tendon contracture.

Recommended Monitoring

- Suture removal and recheck 2 weeks after surgery
- Radiographs at 4 to 6 weeks to evaluate bone healing

PROGNOSIS & OUTCOME

- Guarded after ulnar ostectomy alone. Often an additional surgical procedure is necessary at skeletal maturity to correct the angular deformity.
- Good after definitive corrective osteotomy if the amount of correction is adequate.

PEARLS & CONSIDERATIONS

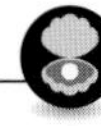

Comments

- Stereolithographic models produced from CT scan images may be used to preplan surgical correction.
- Corrective osteotomy is performed at the point of maximum deformity to provide optimal realignment of the articular surfaces and appropriate limb alignment.
  - The deformity may be localized and quantified using the center of rotation of angulation (CORA) method.
- If there is distal radial head subluxation with minimal radial shortening, proximal ulnar ostectomy can shorten the ulna and restore elbow congruity.
- During ulnar ostectomy in growing dogs, periosteum must be removed at the ostectomy site to prevent union before radial growth is complete.
- Pes varus is a rare condition associated with asymmetrical distal tibial physeal closure in dachshunds.

Technician Tips

Radiographs should include the elbow and carpus on the same image to allow accurate assessment of angular changes.

SUGGESTED READING

Fox DJ. Radius and ulna. In Tobias KM, Johnston SA, editors: Veterinary surgery small animal, St. Louis, 2012, Elsevier Saunders, pp 764-777.

AUTHOR: Raviv J. Balfour, DVM, DACVS
EDITOR: Kathleen Linn, DVM, MS, DACVS

Anorexia

BASIC INFORMATION

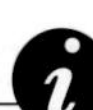

Definition

Anorexia is defined as lack or loss of appetite. Hyporexia is defined as a reduction of appetite rather than a total loss. Dysrexia is defined as a change in food preferences.

Synonyms

Inappetence, decreased appetite, loss of appetite

Epidemiology

SPECIES, AGE, SEX

- Dogs or cats of any age and either sex
- Cats seem to develop food aversion more often than dogs.

Clinical Presentation

HISTORY, CHIEF COMPLAINT

Anorexia/hyporexia is extremely common as a part of many systemic or gastrointestinal (GI) illnesses. Occasionally, owners may report reduced appetite in a seemingly healthy pet.

- Differentiate between lack of appetite versus inability to eat due to oropharyngeal or neurologic disease (pseudoanorexia).
- Obtain a complete medical history, including whether vomiting has occurred. Nausea is a common cause of anorexia/hyporexia.
  - For cats especially, food aversions often develop if they associate a particular food with illness, nausea, or pain.
- Obtain a complete dietary history, including recent changes in the type of diet fed.
- Obtain an environmental history. Stressful environmental changes or warm weather may reduce appetite, or placement of food may make eating difficult (e.g., cats with arthritis may be reluctant to jump onto counters to reach food; another animal in the home may prevent feeding by the patient).
- Inquire about new medications or supplements that may affect appetite.
- Inquire about other recent behavioral changes.

PHYSICAL EXAM FINDINGS

Findings on physical exam depend largely on the underlying cause of anorexia. Examination may be normal, especially if reduced appetite is due to food aversions or other psychological cause.

- Abdominal pain or discomfort may be recognized.
- Patients with chronic anorexia or hyporexia may present with weight loss or cachexia.
- Careful oropharyngeal examination is mandatory and may reveal severe periodontal disease, oropharyngeal foreign bodies, or oral tumors that explain reluctance to eat.
- An orthopedic and neurologic exam is recommended. Arthritis or other painful conditions may make animals less likely to seek food, and central nervous system (CNS) disease may affect appetite.

Etiology and Pathophysiology

- Appetite is regulated by a coordinated interplay of GI, metabolic, and sensory systems that affect the satiety and hunger centers.
- CNS factors
  - Control of hunger and satiety are mainly regulated by the hypothalamus. Within the hypothalamus, there is an interaction between orexigenic neurons (expressing neuropeptide Y/agouti–related protein) and anorexigenic neurons (expressing pro-opiomelanocortic cocaine/amphetamine–related transcript).
  - Peripheral signals modulate the activity of these neurons, including stimulation of orexigenic neurons (ghrelin stimulation) and anorexic neurons (leptin and insulin stimulation).
- GI factors
  - Gastric and intestinal distention and ileus decrease appetite.
  - GI hormones that decrease appetite include cholecystokinin (CCK), pancreatic polypeptide, peptide YY, glucagon-like peptide-1 (GLP-1), and oxyntomodulin.
- Other factors
  - Nausea (any GI or non-GI cause)
  - Pain
  - Dietary changes
  - Environmental stress
  - Palatability issues, including anosmia
  - Endocrine factors: thyroid and adrenal dysfunction impact appetite
  - Systemic disease

DIAGNOSIS

Diagnostic Overview

There is a litany of causes for reduced appetite. The first step is to differentiate between pseudoanorexia (inability to eat) and true anorexia. History and physical examination combined with minimal laboratory data is often sufficient to determine the cause for anorexia. Imaging studies are frequently helpful, and occasionally advanced diagnostics (e.g., endoscopy, CT scan) are required.

Differential Diagnosis

Inability to eat (pseudoanorexia):

- Painful apprehension or mastication
  - Dental disease
  - Mandibular fractures
  - Oral or retrobulbar neoplasia/foreign bodies
  - Masticatory myositis and polymyositis
- Oropharyngeal dysphagia
  - Oropharyngeal mass
  - Cricopharyngeal achalasia
  - Inflammatory myopathies, peripheral neuropathies, neoplasia
- Trigeminal neuritis
  - Painful swallowing (odynophagia) and esophageal disorders
  - Difficulty reaching food (e.g., arthritis, neuromuscular disease)

Initial Database

- Pseudoanorexia: observation of the animal eating and drinking. If suspect pseudoanorexia
  - Complete oropharyngeal exam under anesthesia (pp. 1125 and 1140).
  - Neurologic examination (p. 1136)
  - Dental radiographs or a head CT scan may be necessary to further evaluate the oronasal cavity.
  - Thoracic radiographs and endoscopy (p. 1098) to evaluate obstructions and esophagitis
  - Fluoroscopic studies are required to assess pharyngeal and esophageal function and motility.
- True anorexia
  - History and examination may provide explanation without need for further investigation. For example, a young cat recently obtained from a shelter presenting with fever, oral ulcers, and ocular and nasal discharge is likely inappetent due to viral upper respiratory infection and may not require further testing.
  - CBC, serum chemistry profile, and urinalysis often clarify the reason for anorexia (e.g., azotemia, ketoacidotic diabetes mellitus, hepatopathy).
  - Abdominal imaging studies are often useful (e.g., rule out GI obstruction, abdominal mass effect, echogenic changes in and around the pancreas suggestive of pancreatitis).

Advanced or Confirmatory Testing

Additional testing is based on results of initial investigations.

TREATMENT

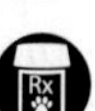

Treatment Overview

The most important aspect of treatment is to identify and address the underlying cause for inappetence.

- Assisted feeding is often recommended when nutritional intake is less than resting energy requirements (RER) = 70 (body weigh $kg^{0.75}$) for 3-5 days.
  - Enteral feeding is indicated for animals with sufficient GI function that are able to hold food down without vomiting.
  - Parenteral feeding is reserved for patients with severe GI dysfunction or uncontrollable vomiting.
- Nutritional support is key in the management of critically ill patients. Protein and calorie malnutrition leads to decreased immune competence and delayed healing.
- Cats have a higher protein requirement than dogs and become protein malnourished quickly when anorexic.
- Overconditioned cats are at risk for hepatic lipidosis when anorexic for any reason for more than a few days.

Acute General Treatment

- Maintain fluid and electrolyte balances; isotonic crystalloid fluids with potassium supplementation, as deemed necessary.
- Address pain, if present.
- Judicious use of antiemetic drugs in animals with nausea or vomiting
  - Maropitant citrate 1 mg/kg SQ q 24h IV over 1-2 minutes. Acts at the emetic center as a neurokinin-1 receptor antagonist. Can be continued at 2 mg/kg PO if necessary.
  - Ondansetron 0.5-1 mg/kg IV q 12h (dog), 0.1-1 mg/kg IV, IM (cat); 5-HT3 receptor antagonist
  - Metoclopramide 0.2-0.5 mg/kg IM, SQ, or IV constant rate infusion at a rate of 0.01-0.09 mg/kg/h. It has antiemetic properties and improves gastric motility.
- Pharmacologic appetite stimulation is not always appropriate, such as in critically ill or severely malnourished patients.
  - Mirtazapine 1.88 mg/CAT PO q 24h (q 48h in cats with chronic kidney disease) and 3.75-30 mg/DOG (depending on dog size) PO q 24h; tetracyclic antidepressant, serotonin receptor antagonist
  - Capromorelin 3 mg/kg PO q 24h in dogs; selective ghrelin receptor agonist
  - Cyproheptadine 1-4 mg/CAT PO q 8-24h in cats; serotonin antagonist
- Nutritional support therapy
  - Provide a palatable food; warming the food may be helpful (p. 1199).
  - Enteral nutrition by nasoesophageal, esophagostomy, or gastrostomy tube can maintain intestinal structure and function (pp. 1106, 1107, and 1109).
  - Parenteral nutrition is reserved for patients that cannot tolerate enteral nutrition (p. 1148).
  - Nutritional support can prevent further loss of lean body tissue in the acute stages of illness.

Chronic Treatment

The objective is to provide necessary nutrients and calories until the patient consumes an adequate amount of food. Esophagostomy and gastrostomy tubes can be used for extended periods of time.

Nutrition/Diet

- Use a conservative energy estimate to avoid overfeeding critically ill patients. Calculation using the RER without "illness factors" is preferred. This energy estimate can be increased by 25% if the patient continues to lose weight (p. 1077).
- Individualized nutritional assessment is important to identify factors that can affect the nutritional plan.

Possible Complications

- The pharmacokinetics and side effects of pharmacologic appetite stimulants must be considered.
- Overfeeding can lead to hyperglycemia (parenteral) or regurgitation, vomiting, and diarrhea.
- Refeeding syndrome is possible after prolonged anorexia.

Recommended Monitoring

Monitor body weight, albumin, triglycerides, electrolytes. and glucose. In patients with enteral feeding, the stoma should be cleaned periodically. Catheters used for parenteral nutrition should be monitored regularly to detect problems early (e.g., vasculitis, malposition).

PROGNOSIS & OUTCOME

Loss of appetite is a symptom, and prognosis depends on the underlying disease.

PEARLS & CONSIDERATIONS

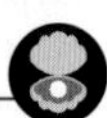

Comments

- Treatment of nausea and pain, if present, are crucial to regain appetite.
- Prolonged anorexia/hyporexia is distressing to pet owners; they may opt for euthanasia sooner than necessary if the pet does not willingly eat.
- Early enteral nutrition in dogs with critical illness has a positive impact on survival. However, overfeeding can lead to severe metabolic and GI complications and is associated with the development of hyperglycemia.
- Pharmacologic appetite stimulation is not recommended in critically ill patients and is generally not effective.
- Cats (and dogs) will not eat if they are unable to smell food. Anosmia can cause anorexia.

Technician Tips

- Creating a comfortable environment increases the likelihood of a patient eating. Increasing the palatability of the meal offered can be achieved by feeding a diet with a higher moisture or increased content of fat and protein. Adding a sweet flavor can increase palatability of food for dogs but not cats.
- Food aversion can occur readily in cats when eating or the smell of food is associated with being nauseous or painful. Avoid leaving food in the cage of nauseous or painful cats.

Client Education

- Increased food palatability and food options
- Identify weight loss and signs of nausea or pain
- Inspect the entry site for feeding tubes daily for inflammation or excessive discharge. Keep the tube as clean as possible.

SUGGESTED READING

Agnew W, et al: Pharmacological appetite stimulation: rational choices in the inappetent cat. J Fel Med Surg 16:749-756, 2014.

AUTHOR: Silvia Funes Sebastián, DVM, MS, DACVIM
EDITOR: Leah A. Cohn, DVM, PhD, DACVIM

Anticoagulant Rodenticide Toxicosis

Client Education Sheet 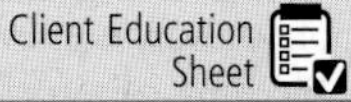

BASIC INFORMATION

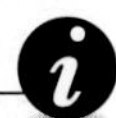

Definition

Anticoagulant rodenticides are designed to kill rats, mice, and other rodents by internal bleeding. Toxicosis in small animals generally manifests 4-7 days after consuming the bait and is characterized by generalized hemorrhage, pale mucous membranes, hematomas, anorexia, lethargy, swollen joints, melena/hematochezia, dyspnea, weakness, or sudden death. Anticoagulant toxicosis ranks among the more commonly reported poisonings in dogs but is uncommon in cats.

Synonyms

Because formulations for rodenticides can change, always attempt to identify the active ingredient by packaging or U.S. Environmental Protection Agency (EPA) registration number.

Agent Name	Selected Trade Names
Warfarin	Anchor Rat and Mouse Bait, Cat-in-a-Bag
Pindone	Purina Rat Kill Soluble, Eaton's AC Formula 50
Diphacinone	Assassin Rodenticide Bait, Exterminator's Choice
Difethialone	D-Cease, Generations, D-Con Rat and Mouse Bait
Brodifacoum	D-Con Mouse Prufe II, Havoc, Jaguar, Final Blox
Bromadiolone	Boot Hill, Hawk, Just One Bite

Epidemiology

SPECIES, AGE, SEX

All are susceptible; young and elderly animals are more sensitive.

RISK FACTORS

- Underlying hepatic disease can enhance toxic effects.
- A high-fat diet enhances anticoagulant absorption.
- Prolonged treatment with sulfonamides can enhance toxicity by reducing the synthesis of vitamin K_1.
- Secondary (relay) toxicosis may occur in dogs or cats that eat poisoned rodents (e.g., barn cats).
- Transfer across placenta and into milk is thought to occur.

GEOGRAPHY AND SEASONALITY

Poisoning is more common in fall and winter months but possible any time of year.

Clinical Presentation

HISTORY, CHIEF COMPLAINT

- Often, there is no history of exposure.
- History or evidence of exposure (e.g., colored bait appearing in stool) several days before onset of signs
- Initial clinical signs are often vague.
  - Lethargy, exercise intolerance, anorexia, dyspnea, coughing, lameness, swollen joints
- Sudden death with no reported clinical signs is possible.

PHYSICAL EXAM FINDINGS

- Pale mucous membranes
- Tachycardia, dyspnea, harsh lung sounds
  - Pulmonary hemorrhage
  - Hemorrhagic pleural effusion
  - Mediastinal hemorrhage
  - Airway hematoma: upper respiratory sounds
  - Hypovolemic shock
- Weakness, exercise intolerance
- Subcutaneous masses (subcutaneous or intradermal hematomas)
- Oozing or bleeding at venipuncture sites or wounds
- Lameness, swollen joints
- Epistaxis
- Exophthalmos (retrobulbar hemorrhage)
- Petechiae, ecchymoses
- Frank bleeding from the mouth, rectum (rare); melena
- Paralysis or seizures if bleeding into spinal canal or brain

Etiology and Pathophysiology

Source:

- First-generation warfarin anticoagulants
  - Warfarin products list 4-hydroxycoumarin in active ingredients.
- Second-generation anticoagulants
  - Brodifacoum, bromadiolone, diphacinone, difenacoum
  - Second-generation anticoagulants are generally more toxic and longer acting than first-generation anticoagulants, resulting in more persistent effects.
- Indanediones
  - Indanedione products (pindone, chlorophacinone, difethialone) list 1,3 indanedione in active ingredients.
  - Chlorophacinone and difethialone are considered second-generation anticoagulants.
- Many generics and trade names. Some companies market products with the same trade name but different active ingredients. In the United States, second-generation anticoagulants and loose pellets are being removed from the market.
- Concentrations of active ingredients range from 0.0025% (difethialone) to 0.005% (most others), whereas warfarin-containing baits often have concentrations of 0.025%.

Mechanism of toxicosis:

- Anticoagulants block activation of vitamin K–dependent clotting factors by inhibiting vitamin K_1 epoxide reductase, which results in inability of vitamin K to be recycled to its active form.
  - Affected clotting factors include II, VII, IX, and X, altering the extrinsic, intrinsic, and common pathways.
    - Factor VII has the shortest half-life; therefore, the extrinsic pathway is affected first in anticoagulant rodenticide toxicosis, and prothrombin time (PT) is elevated before activated partial thromboplastin time (aPTT).
    - The resulting vitamin K_1 deficiency is responsible for coagulopathy and is the basis for treatment with vitamin K_1.
  - Coagulation factors already present degrade naturally and are used up slowly. Therefore, clinical signs are not expected for 4-7 days after ingestion.

DIAGNOSIS

Diagnostic Overview

Anticoagulant rodenticide toxicosis is possible in patients presenting with vague, nonspecific signs such as lethargy or dyspnea. Suspicion increases with history of exposure, evidence of internal or external hemorrhage, or failure of blood to clot at venipuncture sites. Confirmation is achieved with a combination of active bleeding, markedly increased PT, and lack of other explanations for bleeding. Absolute confirmation may include analysis of stomach contents, feces, blood/serum, liver, or kidney for the presence of anticoagulants, but this is rarely performed or necessary in clinical cases.

Differential Diagnosis

Toxicologic:

- Accidental ingestion of warfarin-based anticoagulant human medications (rare), toxins causing severe hepatic necrosis (xylitol [dogs], blue-green algae, sago palm, aflatoxin)

Spontaneous, nontoxicologic:

- Bleeding disorders due to liver disease, hemophilia, thrombocytopenia, disseminated intravascular coagulation
- Differentiation is often straightforward based on signalment, history, physical examination, and routine laboratory tests.

Initial Database

- CBC
  - Regenerative anemia may be present due to bleeding.
  - Mild to moderate thrombocytopenia may occur (50,000-150,000/mL).
- Serum chemistry panel (no specific changes expected)
- Coagulation panel
  - PT and aPTT increase before hemorrhage occurs, and elevation persists during clinical signs.
    - PT increases first and is more sensitive than aPTT for anticoagulant rodenticide toxicosis.
  - Proteins induced by vitamin K_1 absence or antagonism (PIVKA) will be elevated.
    - Test not as widely available
  - Increased PT or PIVKA value three or more times higher than normal is supportive of anticoagulant rodenticide toxicosis.
  - Prior administration of vitamin K_1 can attenuate PT prolongation.
  - No change expected if exposure was witnessed in preceding 24 hours; test still done for baseline PT value.
- Radiographs may reveal thoracic or abdominal effusions or pulmonary infiltrate. Tracheal narrowing or soft-tissue opacity may be present due to airway hematoma.

Advanced or Confirmatory Testing

- Results are generally not received in time to impact treatment but can be important in medicolegal cases.
- Stomach contents, blood, or serum may be analyzed for anticoagulants by a veterinary or other diagnostic laboratory.
- Necropsy samples include serum, liver, and kidney.

TREATMENT

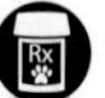

Treatment Overview

Patients showing overt signs due to toxicosis may require treatment on several levels simultaneously, depending on abnormalities identified:

- Vascular volume support if bleeding has caused hypovolemia (blood transfusions, intravenous [IV] crystalloids/colloids)
- Respiratory support (airway hematoma, mediastinal hemorrhage, pleural effusion, pulmonary hemorrhage)
- Vitamin K_1 is antidotal, plus plasma transfusion (active clotting factors) if severe signs.
- Early decontamination (induction of vomiting, activated charcoal administration); not indicated if signs are apparent as exposure would have been days earlier
- If ingestion was recent (<24 hours), no clinical signs should be apparent and decontamination of the patient is appropriate.

Acute General Treatment

Decontamination of the patient (p. 1087) and monitoring of patients without overt clinical signs:

- Induction of vomiting (p. 1188), followed by administration of activated charcoal (1-2 g/kg) and a cathartic (use labeled doses for commercial products)
- Monitor PT, aPTT, or PIVKA at baseline, 48 hours, and 72 hours. If the 72-hour PT/PIVKA is normal, no additional treatment is needed.
- Because coagulopathy develops over several days, an injection of vitamin K_1 on the day of bait ingestion is NOT necessary.
- If PT or PIVKA increases, start vitamin K_1 1.5-2.5 mg/kg PO q 12h or 3-5 mg/kg q 24h.
  - The injectable formulation of vitamin K_1 may be used orally for very small animals (e.g., nursing puppies or kittens).
  - Continue treatment for 14-30 days, depending on the specific anticoagulant.
  - PT or PIVKA should be checked 48 hours after the last dose of vitamin K_1.
    - If PT or PIVKA is elevated 48 hours after last dose (16-32 days after exposure), resume vitamin K_1 treatment for 1 more week, and then remeasure PT or PIVKA 48 hours after last dose. Some animals require vitamin K_1 treatment for 30-50 days.
    - After the PT or PIVKA is normal at 48 hours, discontinue vitamin K_1 therapy.

Treatment of hemorrhaging animals:

- Decontamination of the patient is contraindicated.
- Blood transfusions to replace lost red cell mass if indicated (p. 1169)
- Frozen or fresh-frozen plasma transfusions to provide clotting factors immediately (p. 1169)
- Vitamin K_1 2.5 mg/kg PO q 8-12h
- With hemorrhagic pleural effusion causing severe dyspnea, thoracocentesis may be necessary (p. 1164). Removed blood can be given back to the patient to increase oxygen carrying capacity, but this blood has no clotting factors, and those need to be replaced by whole blood or fresh/fresh-frozen plasma transfusion.
- Supportive care (as needed)
  - Intravenous fluids
  - Oxygen supplementation
  - Thermoregulation
  - Cage rest

Chronic Treatment

- Vitamin K_1 treatment may be required for many weeks in cases involving large amounts of ingested bait and/or ingestion of long-acting anticoagulants.
- Physical activity modifications
  - Confine animals and limit exercise while monitoring PT or PIVKA after recent ingestions or during vitamin K_1 therapy, even if animal "feels normal."
  - Cage rest is essential for animals exhibiting coagulopathy.

Nutrition/Diet

Administer vitamin K_1 with high-fat food (e.g., canned dog/cat food, peanut butter, cheese) to enhance vitamin absorption.

Drug Interactions

Anticoagulants are highly protein bound. Concurrent use of highly protein-bound drugs such as corticosteroids or nonsteroidal antiinflammatory drugs may increase anticoagulant toxicity.

Possible Complications

- Retrobulbar hemorrhage: temporary blindness
- Permanent neurologic dysfunction if bleeding occurs in the central nervous system (CNS)

Recommended Monitoring

Clinical signs, PT, hematocrit

PROGNOSIS & OUTCOME

- Excellent if animal is presented before clinical signs develop. Most animals respond very well to vitamin K_1 therapy.
- Prognosis guarded to poor if animal bleeds into chest or CNS

PEARLS & CONSIDERATIONS

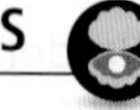

Comments

- New EPA regulations restrict sales of pelleted bait products and replace them with block forms in a tamper-resistant station. Only chlorophacinone and diphacinone are available for the consumer market. Agricultural and professional use products may still contain second-generation anticoagulant rodenticides.
  - Many homes continue to have older packaging and pelleted baits available.
- Brodifacoum is among the most toxic of the anticoagulants; the LD50 for dogs is 0.2-4 mg/kg.
  - Animals can develop toxicosis after ingestion of one-tenth of the LD50.
  - Animals ingesting a dose > 0.02 mg/kg should be decontaminated and monitored.

For example, decontamination is recommended if a 20-lb (9-kg) dog eats approximately 5 g (1 tsp) of 0.005% brodifacoum.
- Animals can ingest subtoxic doses over several days, developing cumulative toxicosis.
- Anticoagulants can cause fetal loss at doses that are not toxic to the dam.
- Vitamin K_1 injection (even when given SQ) can cause anaphylaxis in some animals.
- Injectable vitamin K_1 has no advantage over oral vitamin K_1 therapy (both have similar bioavailability).
- Vitamin K_1 comes as injectable (2 or 10 mg/mL), 5-mg tablets (human), 25-mg capsules (veterinary), or 25- and 50-mg chewable tablets (veterinary).

Prevention

- Keep all baits out of the reach of pets. Rodents may drag packages within reach of pets.
- Baits are attractive to pets. Remove the bait from the animal's environment.

Technician Tips

The color and form (e.g., bar, pellet, tracking powder) do not differentiate brands or active ingredients. The packaging lists active ingredients and the EPA registration number that can be used to determine the class of rodenticide and the specific treatment required.

SUGGESTED READING

Murphy MJ, et al: Anticoagulant rodenticides. In Peterson ME, et al, editors: Small animal toxicology, ed 3, St. Louis, 2013, Saunders Elsevier, pp 435-445.

AUTHOR: Sharon M. Gwaltney-Brant, DVM, PhD, DABVT, DABT
EDITOR: Tina Wismer DVM, MS, DABVT, DABT

Antidepressant (SSRI/SNRI) Drug Toxicosis

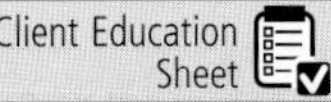

BASIC INFORMATION

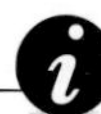

Definition

Toxicosis secondary to ingestion of a selective serotonin reuptake inhibitor (SSRI) or a serotonin and norepinephrine reuptake inhibitor (SNRI). Toxicosis is characterized by sedation, ataxia, disorientation, and with increasing doses, agitation, vocalization, tremors, and cardiovascular signs. SSRIs include citalopram, escitalopram, fluoxetine, fluvoxamine, paroxetine, sertraline, vilazodone, and vortioxetine. SNRIs include desvenlafaxine, duloxetine, levomilnacipran, milnacipran, sibutramine, and venlafaxine.

Synonym

Serotonin syndrome

Epidemiology

SPECIES, AGE, SEX

All species are susceptible.

RISK FACTORS

Household members prescribed these medications

Clinical Presentation

HISTORY, CHIEF COMPLAINT

- History of exposure, evidence of chewed bottles
- Sedation and ataxia *or*
- Agitation, vocalization, and tremors
- Vomiting, hypersalivation, diarrhea

PHYSICAL EXAM FINDINGS

- As above
- Dilated pupils, nystagmus, blindness
- Hyperthermia
- Tachycardia, hypotension

Etiology and Pathophysiology

- SSRIs are antidepressants that inhibit reuptake of serotonin. Serotonin is a monoamine neurotransmitter involved with sensorimotor function. Excessive stimulation leads to serotonin syndrome, which is characterized by autonomic disturbances (hypertension, tachycardia), neuromuscular dysfunction (tremor), and altered mental state (agitation, disorientation).
- SNRIs inhibit the reuptake of serotonin and norepinephrine. Both serotonin syndrome and more severe cardiovascular signs may occur.

DIAGNOSIS

Diagnostic Overview

Diagnosis is usually based on a history of ingestion and clinical signs. Blood levels can be obtained for some of the medications, but they are not clinically relevant or timely. Venlafaxine can give a false-positive result for phencyclidine (PCP) on over-the-counter urine drug screens.

Differential Diagnosis

- Toxicologic: 5-hydroxytryptophan (5-HTP), anticholinergics, antihistamines, ethylene glycol, hops, lead, monoamine oxidase inhibitors, metaldehyde, tricyclic antidepressants
- Non-toxicologic: heat stroke, malignant hyperthermia, meningitis (e.g., rabies, distemper, meningitis of unknown cause), neoplasia

Initial Database

- No direct effects on liver or kidneys are expected, but tremors and hyperthermia can lead to alterations in renal and coagulation values.
- Blood gases in symptomatic cases (metabolic acidosis)

TREATMENT

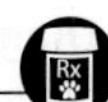

Treatment Overview

Decontaminate asymptomatic animals with emesis and activated charcoal if indicated. Provide supportive care to symptomatic patients to control tremors, body temperature, and cardiovascular signs.

Acute General Treatment

- Emesis (p. 1188) if asymptomatic
- Activated charcoal (p. 1087) if asymptomatic (not indicated if all pills quickly removed through emesis)
- Cyproheptadine is a nonselective serotonin antagonist and can help reduce serotonergic signs. Dogs: 1.1 mg/kg PO or rectally, can repeat once in 4-6 hours if still symptomatic. Cats: 2-4 mg/CAT PO
- Intravenous (IV) fluids to help regulate body temperature and blood pressure. Fluids also help protect kidneys from secondary damage from myoglobinuria due to rhabdomyolysis.
- If hyperthermia occurs, fans, alcohol sprays, etc.
- For agitation: acepromazine 0.05 mg/kg IV or IM, titrate to effect as needed; *or* chlorpromazine 0.5 mg/kg IV, IM or SQ, titrate up as needed
- For tachycardia: propranolol 0.02-0.06 mg/kg IV, titrate up as needed
- For tremors: methocarbamol 50-100 mg/kg IV, titrate up as needed
- For seizures: diazepam 0.5-2 mg/kg IV *or* phenobarbital 3-4 mg/kg IV
- Consider intralipids (p. 1127) in cases with severe signs

Drug Interactions

Avoid other SSRI or SNRI medications (e.g., tramadol, ondansetron) (p. 1281).

Possible Complications

- Hyperthermia: see Heatstroke (p. 421).
- Rhabdomyolysis: see Acute Kidney Injury (p. 23).

Recommended Monitoring

Closely monitor heart rate, body temperature, blood pressure, and urine color.

PROGNOSIS & OUTCOME

- Prognosis is good in most cases (signs abate in most cases in 12-24 hours, up to 72 hours for extended-release formulations).
- Prognosis worsens if kidney injury or hyperthermia occur.

PEARLS & CONSIDERATIONS

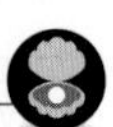

Comments

Low doses of these medications cause depressive signs that usually do not need medical intervention. Higher doses cause stimulatory signs that need to be treated.

Prevention

- Keep medications out of the reach of pets.
- Do not store human and veterinary medications together.

Technician Tips

Closely monitor vital signs.

Client Education

Take pills over the sink so that if a pill is dropped, pets cannot ingest it from the floor.

SUGGESTED READING

Bloom FE: Neurotransmission and the central nervous system. In Brunton LL, et al, editors: Goodman & Gilman's the pharmacological basis of therapeutics, ed 11, New York, 2006, McGraw-Hill Professional, pp 317-340.

AUTHOR & EDITOR: Tina Wismer, DVM, MS, DABVT, DABT

Antidepressant (Tricyclic) Drug Toxicosis

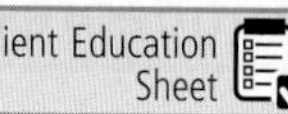

Client Education Sheet

BASIC INFORMATION

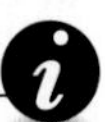

Definition

Tricyclic antidepressant (TCA) toxicosis is caused by accidental ingestion or inadvertent overdose of this class of drug, resulting in gastrointestinal (GI), central nervous system (CNS), and cardiovascular signs. In fatal cases, conduction disturbances (cardiovascular toxicosis) are the main cause of death.

Synonyms

TCAs: amitriptyline (Elavil), amoxapine, clomipramine (Clomicalm), desipramine, doxepin (Adapin), imipramine (Tofranil), maprotiline, nortriptyline, protriptyline, trimipramine

Epidemiology

SPECIES, AGE, SEX

All pets are at risk if they have access to these medications. Younger animals, and dogs > cats, are more likely to be exposed because of their chewing or inquisitive natures.

RISK FACTORS

TCAs are commonly available prescription medications in a household. Dogs are at increased risk for a large exposure because they tend to chew on the bottles/containers. Cats may ingest a dropped tablet.

Clinical Presentation

DISEASE FORMS/SUBTYPES

Mild signs (sedation, lethargy, vomiting) at low dosages and severe signs (tremors, hyperactivity, cardiac arrhythmias, seizures) at high doses

HISTORY, CHIEF COMPLAINT

- History of exposure or use of a TCA
- Lethargy, sedation, vomiting, and ataxia within 30 minutes to a few hours of acute exposure
- Agitation, tremors, seizures, cardiac arrhythmias (usually indicate severe toxicosis)

PHYSICAL EXAM FINDINGS

- Initial findings include lethargy, vomiting, and ataxia.
- Later, any combination of disorientation, tremors, hyperactivity, coma, seizures
- Hypotension, tachycardia or bradycardia, and other cardiac arrhythmias, mydriasis, dyspnea, ileus, urinary retention, acidosis, hyperthermia, and dyspnea due to pulmonary edema may occur. Body temperature and respiratory rate should be recorded at presentation and monitored carefully.

Etiology and Pathophysiology

Source:

- TCAs are used in humans to treat a variety of disorders; used in dogs for pituitary-dependent hyperadrenocorticism, cognitive dysfunction, aggression, fear/anxiety disorders, and obsessive-compulsive disorder; and used in cats for urine spraying and anxiety disorders.

Mechanism of toxicosis:

- TCAs inhibit sodium channels in the myocardium, which slows ventricular depolarization. Their neurologic effects are thought to be due to inhibition of the reuptake of the neurotransmitters dopamine, norepinephrine, and serotonin in the CNS and through blocking acetylcholine at the neuronal synapses. They also have antihistaminic, anticholinergic, and alpha-adrenergic blocking effects.

DIAGNOSIS

Diagnostic Overview

Diagnosis is facilitated with a history of use of a TCA in the household or known accidental overdose together with GI, CNS, or cardiovascular effects within 30 minutes to several hours after the exposure.

Differential Diagnosis

- Toxicology rule outs: amphetamines, methylxanthines, pseudoephedrine, cocaine, herbal preparations containing ma huang or guarana root, quinidine, propranolol, albuterol, digoxin
- Non-toxicology rule outs: hyperkalemia, cardiomyopathy, other primary cardiac diseases, epilepsy

Initial Database

- Neurologic exam (p. 1136)
- Electrocardiogram (p. 1094) if tachycardia or arrhythmia on physical exam
- Arterial blood pressure (p. 1065)
- Blood gas (acid-base status)

Advanced or Confirmatory Testing

TCAs can be detected in serum, plasma, whole blood, and urine; assay not readily available and not useful for clinical cases. Contact a diagnostic laboratory or a human hospital for additional information.

TREATMENT

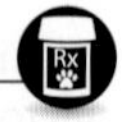

Treatment Overview

- First stabilize the patient by managing any critical neurologic or cardiovascular effects. Once stabilized, consider decontamination (emesis and activated charcoal).
- Hospitalization may be required for > 24 hours for supportive care.

Acute General Treatment

- Stabilization: initially, may include managing seizures or severe hyperactivity with diazepam, IV fluids for hypotension, and managing significant cardiac arrhythmias. Avoid atropine (use only preanesthetic dose 0.01-0.02 mg/kg IV if necessary) for bradycardia because it may add to the anticholinergic effects of TCAs. Oxygen therapy for dyspneic patients.

- Decontamination of the patient (p. 1087) after stabilization. For patients without clinical signs on presentation, measurement of heart rate, rhythm, and blood pressure should precede decontamination. Consider emesis induction (apomorphine or 3% hydrogen peroxide in dogs, xylazine or dexmedetomidine in cats) if the exposure occurred < 1 hour earlier. With large exposures, activated charcoal and/or gastric lavage may be considered.
- Multiple doses of activated charcoal (q 6-8h) may be indicated because of enterohepatic recirculation of TCAs. GI absorption of the TCA may be prolonged because of anticholinergic activity (paralytic ileus).
- Duration of treatment: initially monitor the patient for a minimum of 6 hours for CNS and cardiac effects if no signs were present at admission. If signs develop, treatment may be necessary for 1-2 days or more.
- Maintain cardiovascular function and adequate blood pressure.
- Manage vomiting with maropitant 1 mg/kg SQ q 24h or metoclopramide 0.2-0.5 mg/kg PO, SQ, or IM q 6-8h.
- Monitor for acidosis. Increased blood pH has improved prognosis in dogs experimentally poisoned by TCAs. Correct acidosis with sodium bicarbonate. Acid-base monitoring is ideal (in the absence of monitoring, can give sodium bicarbonate at a dose of 2-3 mEq/kg IV slowly over 15-30 minutes).
- Supportive care: fluid diuresis with IV fluids
- Thermoregulation: maintain body temperature within normal range
- Diazepam (0.2-0.5 mg/kg IV) can be used to treat agitation.
- Cyproheptadine (dogs: 1.1 mg/kg PO or per rectum; cats: 2-4 mg total) can be used for serotonin syndrome (hyperthermia, agitation, nervousness), especially if diazepam is not effective.
- Severely affected animals: monitor for an additional 24 hours after cessation of signs for the development of pulmonary edema, coagulation disorders, and pancreatitis.

Drug Interactions

Concurrent use of other sedatives, anticholinergics, antihistamines, sympathomimetics, or highly protein-bound drugs can interact with the functioning of TCAs.

Possible Complications

Possible CNS damage from severe seizures or myocardial problems (i.e., congestive heart failure) from cardiac tachyarrhythmias

Recommended Monitoring

- CNS effects (seizures), heart rate, blood pressure, electrocardiogram (cardiac arrhythmias), GI motility (ileus), acid-base status (acidosis), respirations +/− thoracic radiographs (pulmonary edema)
- Although there are no direct blood or organ effects, monitor CBC and serum biochemistry profile in severely affected animals. Secondary conditions such as disseminated intravascular coagulation, pancreatitis, and renal effects secondary to rhabdomyolysis from severe tremors can occur.

PROGNOSIS & OUTCOME

TCAs have a narrow margin of safety. Good prognosis if treated early and intensively. Poor prognosis if severe cardiac arrhythmias or seizures develop.

PEARLS & CONSIDERATIONS

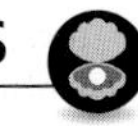

Comments

- Therapeutic dosages of various TCAs in animals range between 1 and 4 mg/kg. Mild adverse effects (sedation, lethargy) can be seen at the recommended dosage and may not require any treatment.
- Acute exposure of > 15-20 mg/kg can be potentially lethal.
- Delayed gastric emptying (paralytic ileus) sometimes can prolong toxicity.

Prevention

Clients should be instructed to keep all medications in a tightly secured place to prevent pets from chewing on the containers.

Technician Tips

Several TCAs are used off label in cats and dogs. Clomicalm is an approved veterinary product for separation anxiety in dogs.

Client Education

Discuss adverse effects with the owner when prescribing TCAs for pets.

SUGGESTED READING

Volmer PA: Tricyclic antidepressants. In Peterson ME, et al, editors: Small animal toxicology, ed 3, St. Louis, 2013, Saunders, pp 328-330.

AUTHOR: Camille DeClementi, VMD, DABT, DABVT
EDITOR: Tina Wismer, DVM, MS, DABVT, DABT

Antihistamines/Cold Medications Toxicosis

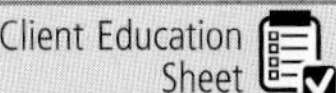

BASIC INFORMATION

Definition

Toxicosis in pets caused by accidental acute ingestion or overdose of human cold medications (CMs) containing (depending on the purpose) antihistamines, decongestants, analgesics, cough suppressants, or expectorants

Synonyms

- First-generation antihistamines: chlorpheniramine, dimenhydrinate, diphenhydramine, promethazine, meclizine, hydroxyzine
  - Sedating because they can cross the blood-brain barrier
- Second-generation antihistamines: loratadine, cetirizine, fexofenadine
  - Nonsedating because they do not cross the blood-brain barrier at therapeutic doses

Epidemiology

SPECIES, AGE, SEX

All dogs and cats susceptible

RISK FACTORS

- Availability of the medications in the pet's environment or accidental overdose given by the owner
- Pre-existing liver disease may prolong elimination and therefore duration of clinical signs.

GEOGRAPHY AND SEASONALITY

Seasonal human use of these drugs makes toxicosis from CMs more likely during the winter, and toxicosis from antihistamines may be more frequent in spring.

Clinical Presentation

HISTORY, CHIEF COMPLAINT

History or evidence of exposure:

- Antihistamines: lethargy, sedation, mydriasis within a few hours, or agitation, hyperactivity, vocalization, seizures (rare), nervousness (paradoxical reaction), vomiting, diarrhea
- Dextromethorphan: sedation or agitation, ataxia, panting, facial edema

PHYSICAL EXAM FINDINGS

- Antihistamines: central nervous system (CNS) depression, anticholinergic effects (dry mouth, tachycardia, mydriasis, hyperthermia, hypertension or hypotension, seizures,

urinary retention) from first-generation antihistamines; rare with second-generation drugs
  - Higher doses of antihistamines may have stimulatory CNS effects (excitation, agitation, hyperactivity), particularly in young animals. Hyperthermia may be identified.
- Dextromethorphan: as above; at high doses, disorientation, hallucination, stimulatory, and dissociative effects; facial edema

Etiology and Pathophysiology

- Antihistamines: H1-receptor antagonists are quickly absorbed orally; delayed gut emptying following anticholinergic effects of antihistamines may delay absorption.
- Dextromethorphan: a non-addicting opioid, acts centrally by elevating cough threshold. It also has dopamine receptor blocking activity and serotonin agonist activity at higher doses.

DIAGNOSIS

Diagnostic Overview

The diagnosis is suspected based on history/evidence of ingestion of antihistamine and/or CM and presence of gastrointestinal (GI), CNS, or cardiovascular signs within a few hours.

Differential Diagnosis

- Rule out other toxicoses that can cause CNS depression, including marijuana, opiates, antidepressants, benzodiazepines, ethylene glycol, and ivermectin.
- Paradoxical reactions from antihistamines can be confused with CNS stimulants such as amphetamines, pseudoephedrine, ephedrine, cocaine, and methylxanthines.

Initial Database

- CBC, serum biochemistry profile: no significant changes expected
- Heart rate and blood pressure (p. 1065): increased initially, reduced later
- Electrocardiogram (ECG): if arrhythmia suspected (p. 1096)

Advanced or Confirmatory Testing

Some antihistamines and their metabolites can be measured in serum and urine (human hospital). This can help confirm exposure but is not helpful clinically.

TREATMENT

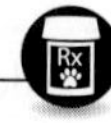

Treatment Overview

Decontamination of patient if asymptomatic (induce emesis and give activated charcoal); control CNS, GI signs, hyperthermia, cardiovascular effects, and provide supportive care as needed.

Acute General Treatment

Decontamination of patient (any high-dose CM) (p. 1087)

- Emesis in patients not showing any clinical signs; most effective when used within 1 hour of exposure
- Activated charcoal 1-2 g/kg PO mixed with a cathartic, if dose is high enough that severe signs are expected
- Gastric lavage (p. 1117) for life-threatening doses if inducing emesis is not safe, followed by activated charcoal

Control CNS signs (antihistamines, dextromethorphan):

- Diazepam 0.5-1 mg/kg IV for CNS excitation. Note: give slowly IV over 1-2 minutes; can aggravate CNS excitation if given rapidly
- Acepromazine 0.05-0.1 mg/kg IM or IV for agitation (avoid if patient hypotensive)
- Cardiovascular effects: beta-blocker (e.g., propranolol 0.02-0.06 mg/kg IV; generally start low and repeat as needed, with continuous ECG monitoring) for persistent sinus tachycardia
- Vasopressors may be indicated for severe hypotension that does not respond to fluids. Epinephrine is contraindicated, as it may worsen hypotension.
- Control vomiting: maropitant 1 mg/kg SQ q 24h
- Thermoregulation: cooling fans (hyperthermia) or heat source (hypothermia) prn
- Supportive care: IV crystalloid fluids prn
- Serotonin syndrome (p. 1281): cyproheptadine 1.1 mg/kg PO or per rectum; q 6-8h for disorientation, agitation in dextromethorphan overdose

Behavior/Exercise

Limit or confine animals with neurologic effects to prevent injury.

Recommended Monitoring

Body temperature, heart rate and blood pressure, hydration status

PROGNOSIS & OUTCOME

- Good with prompt decontamination and control of CNS and cardiovascular effects
- Guarded with poorly controlled seizures

PEARLS & CONSIDERATIONS

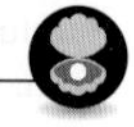

Comments

- A CM may contain one active ingredient or many.
- Antihistamines used therapeutically in dogs and cats can cause mild sedation at the recommended dose that does not require treatment. They also possess some antiemetic effects.
- Depending on the dose, presence of decongestants (pseudoephedrine) (p. 240), acetaminophen (p. 10), ibuprofen (p. 695), or other painkiller may pose a higher risk for the patient. These medications are usually present at much higher concentrations compared with antihistamines, cough suppressants, or expectorants.
- Stimulatory CNS effects from antihistamines can be treated with diazepam and patient kept in a semi-dark room for a few hours.

Prevention

Keep all medications in closed cabinets or drawers, not on countertops.

Technician Tips

Check label to ascertain whether dealing with one or multiple active ingredients.

Client Education

Consult with a veterinarian before giving any over-the-counter medications to your animal.

SUGGESTED READING

Christie J: Antitussives and expectorants. In Hovda L, editor. Blackwell's 5 minute veterinary consult: small animal toxicology, ed 2, Ames, IA, 2016, Wiley, pp 313-319.

AUTHOR: Laura Stern, DVM, DABVT
EDITOR: Tina Wismer, DVM, MS, DABVT, DABT

Aortic Thromboembolism, Feline

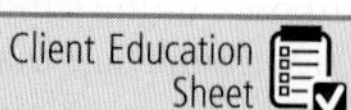

BASIC INFORMATION

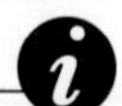

Definition

- Thromboembolism is a well-recognized syndrome caused by occlusion of a systemic artery (typically the aortic trifurcation) by an embolus that has dislodged from the site of thrombus formation (typically the left side of the heart) and the associated clinical sequelae.
- *Thrombus* refers to a concretion of cells and blood constituents (clot) in a discrete location in the circulation.
- *Embolus* refers to a thrombus or thrombus fragment that has traveled through the circulation and obstructs a vessel in an organ or tissue.
- Thrombi (and subsequent emboli) are most commonly a sterile matrix of fibrin, platelets, and associated red and white blood cells, but tumor or septic emboli are occasionally the cause of thromboembolic disease.

Synonyms

Feline aortic thromboembolism (FATE), saddle thrombus, arterial thromboembolism

Epidemiology

SPECIES, AGE, SEX

Feline, all ages of adults reported, male predisposition

GENETICS AND BREED PREDISPOSITION

None beyond predispositions for specific underlying heart diseases

RISK FACTORS

- Heart disease (hypertrophic cardiomyopathy, restrictive cardiomyopathy, unclassified cardiomyopathy, dilated cardiomyopathy, congenital cardiac disorders)
- Spontaneous contrast in the left atrium or left ventricle (echocardiographically)
- Pulmonary or other neoplasia

Clinical Presentation

DISEASE FORMS/SUBTYPES

- Saddle thrombus: total or partial occlusion of the distal aortic trifurcation
- Brachial artery embolus (single forelimb affected)
- Visceral artery thromboembolism (renal artery, mesenteric artery): less common, may accompany saddle thrombus

HISTORY, CHIEF COMPLAINT

- History of heart disease or physical exam findings of cardiac disease (murmur, arrhythmia) is common.
  - A pre-existing heart murmur is less commonly noted in the history of cats with restrictive and unclassified cardiomyopathy.
- Saddle thrombus: peracute onset of pain and paresis/paralysis of hindlimbs
- Brachial artery thrombus: sudden onset of lameness or disuse of a forelimb, may or may not be painful
- Visceral thromboemboli: acute onset abdominal pain, vomiting, and lethargy

PHYSICAL EXAM FINDINGS

Saddle thrombus:

- Pain (often appears excruciating, with vocalization and panting) and varying degrees of paralysis of the hindlimbs
- Typically absence of femoral pulses
  - Incomplete forms may have unilateral loss of femoral pulse or a differential in the femoral pulse strength.
- Firm, painful quadriceps and gastrocnemius musculature
- Hypothermia (via rectal thermometer) is common.
- Footpads are cyanotic and cool to the touch; nail beds are cyanotic.
- Dyspnea is common; diagnostic testing must distinguish between pain and congestive heart failure (CHF) as the cause.

Brachial artery embolus: various degrees of forelimb paralysis (typically paw knuckled under); absence of brachial pulse, footpad cyanotic and cool to the touch; may or may not be visibly painful.

Etiology and Pathophysiology

- Thromboembolism is positively correlated with increasing left atrial size, suggesting blood stasis in the atrium as a predisposing cause for thrombus formation.
- Hypercoagulability exists in some cats with cardiomyopathy and atrial enlargement with coexisting spontaneous echocardiographic contrast, atrial thrombi, or an existing thromboembolus but not in cats with left atrial enlargement alone.
- Less common causes include primary tumor emboli and sterile emboli related to pulmonary neoplasia.

DIAGNOSIS

Diagnostic Overview

The diagnosis is generally apparent from the physical examination findings alone.

Differential Diagnosis

- Trauma (pelvic fractures, femoral fractures, spinal injury)
- Primary neurologic disease (spinal infarction, intervertebral disc disease, spinal neoplasia, trauma)
- Severe systemic hypotension

Initial Database

- CBC, biochemical profile, urinalysis: commonly noted abnormalities include hyperglycemia, elevations in alanine aminotransferase (ALT) and aspartate aminotransferase (AST), hypocalcemia, and various degrees of azotemia (suggests concomitant renal infarction)
- Thyroid hormone analysis (if ≥ 6 years old)
- Feline leukemia, feline immunodeficiency serology (if at risk for these diseases; not a direct contributor to FATE)
- Full coagulation profile (prothrombin time [PT], activated partial thromboplastin time [aPTT], and platelet count)
  - Decreased PT and/or aPTT: no correlation with whether a cat is in a procoagulant state but often useful as baseline for monitoring therapy.
- Full-body radiographs
  - Thorax: signs of congestive heart failure (pulmonary edema, pleural effusion), signs of cardiac disease (cardiac chamber enlargement), evidence of pulmonary neoplasia
  - Spine: fractures, neoplasia (differential diagnosis)
- Echocardiography (once stable) to diagnose associated cardiac disease, evaluate for intracardiac thrombi, and spontaneous echocardiographic contrast (p. 1094)
- Electrocardiography (once stable) (p. 1096)
- Blood pressure determinations (p. 1065)

Advanced or Confirmatory Testing

- Abdominal ultrasound: may be helpful in identifying extent of vessel occlusion and coexisting abdominal organ infarction, particularly if the diagnosis is unclear or if signs suggest visceral infarction.
- Nonselective angiography: can confirm extent of vessel occlusion and associated visceral artery occlusion; rarely done.
- Computed tomography/magnetic resonance imaging: provides detailed information about the extent of vascular occlusions but requires general anesthesia, which is problematic in these unstable patients; rarely done.

TREATMENT

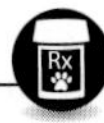

Treatment Overview

- Treatment is mainly supportive, including pain management; the efficacy of thrombolytic and antithrombotic/antiplatelet treatments in the acute stage is not established.
- Supportive care (pain control, maintain hydration, treat associated CHF [p. 408], maintain electrolyte balance and renal perfusion, applying warm water bottles to hindlimbs)
- Clot dissolution: the goal of thrombolytic therapy is attempted (tissue plasminogen activator, streptokinase). Rarely attempted, but best performed by experienced specialist as soon as possible.
- Preventing extension of the thromboembolus: antithrombotic and antiplatelet therapy
- Prevention of additional thromboembolic episodes

Acute General Treatment

- Pain management (hydromorphone 0.1-0.2 mg/kg SQ or IV q 4-8h, or morphine 0.05-0.2 mg/kg SQ q 6-8h, or buprenorphine 0.01-0.015 mg/kg SQ or IV q 6-12h, or butorphanol 0.1-0.4 mg/kg SQ or IV q 2-4h)
- Diuretics, if CHF present (furosemide 1-4 mg/kg SQ or IV q 4-12h)
- Vasodilators: if blood pressure is adequate, may help collateral circulation in the hind legs (hydralazine 0.5-1 mg/kg PO q 12h, acepromazine 0.025-0.05 mg/kg SQ q 12-24h); angiotensin-converting enzyme inhibitors (enalapril, benazepril) usually avoided in the acute setting due to potential coexisting renal infarctions
- Oxygen therapy (p. 1146): if CHF, dyspnea
- Fluid therapy: conservative crystalloid therapy is typically administered in patients in the absence of fulminant CHF.

Chronic Treatment

- Aimed at treatment for the underlying condition (treatment of heart disease, removal of primary lung tumor) and prevention of repeated thromboembolic episodes
- Anticoagulant therapy
  - Rivaroxaban 2.5 mg/CAT PO q 24h is being evaluated as an alternative to clopidogrel 18.75 mg/CAT PO q 24h for prevention of recurrent episodes of FATE *or*
  - Warfarin 0.25 mL of 1 mg/mL suspension initially administered per cat q 24h, dose

titrated q 5-7 days to maintain a PT or international normalized ratio of 1.5 to 2 times upper limit of normal. Ideally, patients are initially anticoagulated with heparin 150 U/kg SQ q 8h and have a 48-hour heparin-warfarin overlap
  - Warfarin therapy has not been investigated sufficiently to analyze safety or efficacy in feline patients, *or*
  - Low-molecular-weight heparin (LMWH) (e.g., dalteparin 100 IU/kg SQ q 12-24h); LMWH may not be efficacious at these doses.
- Antiplatelet therapy
  - Clopidogrel (18.75 mg PO/CAT q 24h) has been shown in a prospective, double-blind, placebo-controlled trial to be associated with longer survival times after an initial thromboembolic event compared to aspirin therapy.
  - Aspirin (dosages range from 5 mg PO/CAT every 72 hours to 81 mg/CAT every 48 hours). Typically administered at 20-25 mg q 48h. Usually administered to patients who do not tolerate clopidogrel (vomiting, refusal); sometimes administered concurrently with clopidogrel

Drug Interactions

Multiple drug interactions reported for warfarin (see drug formularies in Section VI for detailed list)

Possible Complications

- Disease complications: gangrenous necrosis of a hindlimb; self-mutilation of the limb; visceral occlusions leading to organ infarction, organ failure, and death; cardiac arrhythmias; repeat thromboembolic episodes
- Thrombolytic therapy: hemorrhagic complications, acute reperfusion syndromes (hyperkalemia, acidosis, death)
- Anticoagulant therapy: bleeding complications
- Antiplatelet therapy: bleeding complications
- Diuretic therapy: volume contraction, azotemia
- Vasodilator therapy: hypovolemia, decompensation of renal function
- Fluid therapy: volume overload, CHF

Recommended Monitoring

- Frequent physical examination
- Daily renal, electrolyte, and coagulation profile monitoring during hospitalization
- Continuous ECG (arrhythmias common) during hospitalization

PROGNOSIS & OUTCOME

- Guarded prognosis: 33%-50% rate of discharge from the hospital, high chance of repeat thromboembolic episodes
- Prognosis more favorable for partial or forelimb emboli (75% rate of discharge from the hospital)
- Grave prognosis with visceral artery occlusions
- Body temperature at admission appears to be positively correlated with prognosis: more favorable if temperature > 98.9°F (37.2°C)

PEARLS & CONSIDERATIONS

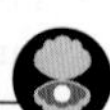

Comments

- Although much anecdotal discussion exists, there have been no studies proving that any preventive measures decrease the likelihood of suffering a thromboembolic event. Clopidogrel is the sole agent that has been shown to significantly increase long-term survival of cats who have survived an initial thromboembolic event.
- Intermittent claudication (lameness) may signal that a patient is at high risk for aortic thromboembolism and should prompt a discussion about preventive therapy.
- Dogs are also susceptible to thromboembolic disease, but the cause and consequences differ from those of feline saddle thrombus.

Prevention

- Treatment of associated cardiac disease
- Use of antiplatelet agents in patients at risk for thromboembolic disease

Technician Tips

- Supportive care and excellent nursing care is paramount to successful outcome.
- The patient should be kept warm and dry. Monitoring of urination is important, and bladder expression may be necessary.
- Managing clinician should be alerted of clinical deterioration suggesting possible intraabdominal infarction (progressive lethargy, vomiting).

Client Education

- All cats with cardiac disease are presumed to be at risk for thromboembolic complications.
- Cats with increasing amounts of left atrial enlargement with spontaneous contrast and/or an intracardiac thrombus are at high risk for thromboembolism.
- Risk/benefit discussion of preventive measures
- Patients who have had a thromboembolic event are at very high risk for recurrent events.
- Prognosis should be discussed for short- and longer-term outcomes.

SUGGESTED READING

Smith SA, et al: Arterial thromboembolism in cats: acute crisis in 127 cases (1992-2001) and long-term management with low-dose aspirin in 24 cases. J Vet Intern Med 17:73-83, 2003.

AUTHOR: Nancy J. Laste, DVM, DACVIM
EDITOR: Meg M Sleeper VMD, DACVIM

Arrhythmogenic Right Ventricular Cardiomyopathy, Dog

Bonus Material Online   Client Education Sheet

BASIC INFORMATION

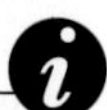

Definition

Adult-onset inherited cardiomyopathy, primarily affecting boxer dogs, is classically characterized by ventricular arrhythmias. A proportion of dogs experience supraventricular arrhythmias, and rarely some dogs demonstrate chamber dilation accompanied by left ventricular (LV) systolic dysfunction. Dogs may have an asymptomatic life or develop symptomatic ventricular arrhythmias (syncope, sudden death) or rarely have left-sided or biventricular congestive heart failure (if myocardial systolic dysfunction is present).

Synonyms

Arrhythmogenic right ventricular cardiomyopathy (ARVC), boxer cardiomyopathy, arrhythmogenic cardiomyopathy (AC), arrhythmogenic right ventricular dysplasia, familial ventricular arrhythmia (FVA) of boxers

Epidemiology

SPECIES, AGE, SEX

- ARVC is an adult-onset familial disease of boxer dogs.
- Age-related penetrance and expression dictates that the disease is more frequent and more severe with advanced age.
- The disease usually affects dogs > 3 years of age.
- Males and females are equally represented.

GENETICS, BREED PREDISPOSITION

- Boxer dogs have an identified genetic basis of disease, characterized by an autosomal dominant deletion mutation in the striatin gene with incomplete and age-related penetrance.
  - Approximately 70% of dogs with the mutation will develop some form of the disease (variable severity).
  - Those homozygous positive for the striatin mutation may have a more severe form

with higher numbers of arrhythmias and are more likely to develop structural heart disease (type III ARVC, dilated cardiomyopathy [DCM]–like phenotype)
  - ARVC is occasionally reported in dogs free of the striatin mutation, suggesting at least one other cause of this disease.
- Bulldogs have a genetic predisposition to a similar disease that usually involves structural change to the heart, including dilation of the right and/or left ventricle in addition to arrhythmias. A causative genetic mutation has not yet been identified.

RISK FACTORS

- Because it is an inherited cardiomyopathy, familial history is the most important risk factor.
- Positive genetic test status for the striatin mutation, particularly homozygous status, indicates clear risk.
- Increased age is also associated with higher risk for disease.

Clinical Presentation

DISEASE FORMS/SUBTYPES

- Type I (occult or concealed) is characterized by ventricular arrhythmias without clinical signs.
- Type II (overt) is characterized by ventricular arrhythmias with clinical signs (e.g., syncope).
- Type III (myocardial dysfunction) is characterized by ventricular and/or supraventricular arrhythmias and cardiac dilation with systolic dysfunction. This form resembles DCM, and dogs may have clinical signs of left or biventricular congestive heart failure (CHF) and/or syncope. Prognosis is significantly worse than for types I and II.

HISTORY, CHIEF COMPLAINT

- Type I patients may be diagnosed during breed screening or because an arrhythmia was incidentally identified on examination.
- Type II patients present for evaluation of clinical signs relatable to a ventricular tachyarrhythmia, most commonly syncope or presyncope (collapse, weakness, or transient ataxia). The first clinical sign may be sudden death.
- Type III patients present for evaluation of clinical signs related to a tachyarrhythmia, including syncope or presyncope, or may present with signs related to left or biventricular CHF, including cough, respiratory distress, increased respiratory rate, exercise intolerance, abdominal distention (ascites), and weakness.

PHYSICAL EXAM FINDINGS

- In types I and II, physical examination may be normal.
  - Possible physical exam findings include an auscultable arrhythmia with post-extrasystolic pauses and possible pulse deficits.
- In type III, possible findings include the following:
  - S_3 gallop sound
  - Hypokinetic pulse quality
  - Auscultable arrhythmia, which may be represented as persistent tachycardia or intermittent premature beats with post-extrasystolic pauses and possible pulse deficits
  - Left apical systolic heart murmur due to annular stretch and secondary mitral regurgitation, which is not to be confused with left basilar ejection murmurs present in many healthy boxers and boxers with aortic or subvalvular aortic stenosis
  - Possible signs of left-sided CHF, including fine pulmonary crackles, increased respiratory effort or rate
  - Possible signs of right-sided CHF, including a palpable abdominal fluid wave (ascites), jugular venous pulsation/distention, positive hepatojugular reflux

Etiology and Pathophysiology

- The hallmark histopathologic lesions include fibrofatty infiltration of the right ventricle and myocytolysis, which may spread more broadly in some cases to include the atria and left ventricle. The events that lead to the observed myocardial change are unclear. These changes explain the characteristic right-sided ventricular premature complexes (VPCs) noted on the electrocardiogram (ECG) (predominantly upright in lead II).
- A deletion mutation in the striatin gene, which codes for a desmosomal protein, has been implicated in this disease. This mutation leads to disruption of cardiac desmosomes and may trigger loss of normal cell-to-cell adhesion.
- ARVC is also associated with calstabin 2 deficiency and alterations in beta-catenin. Calstabin 2 is an important regulator of the ryanodine receptor in the myocardium and helps prevent calcium leakage from the sarcoplasmic reticulum; without it, calcium leakage can potentiate arrhythmias seen in this disease. Beta-catenin alterations suggest possible involvement of the canonical Wnt pathway, a driver of adipocyte differentiation.
- A similar disease that is also referred to as ARVC has been described in cats, bulldogs, and several other breeds of dogs, and it usually involves dilation of the right and sometimes left ventricles in addition to arrhythmias.

DIAGNOSIS

Diagnostic Overview

- No single antemortem diagnostic test is confirmatory; ARVC is a presumptive diagnosis based on findings of ventricular arrhythmias (most commonly right sided or upright in lead II) with exclusion of other causes of ventricular arrhythmias.
- Diagnosis is strongly supported by positive genetic testing (heterozygote or homozygote for the striatin mutation).
- Diagnosis is also supported by a family history of the disease and the presence of supraventricular or ventricular arrhythmias.
- 24-hour ambulatory ECG results showing > 300 single VPCs or complex ventricular arrhythmias in boxers are consistent with a diagnosis and particularly important for breed screening.
- 24-hour ambulatory ECG results showing 50-300 single VPCs in boxers is equivocal for a diagnosis of ARVC.
- 24-hour ambulatory ECG results showing < 50 single VPCs is considered normal in the boxer.

Differential Diagnosis

- Type I: consider all causes of ventricular arrhythmias, including the following:
  - Metabolic disturbance: endocrinopathy, acid-base derangements, immune-mediated disease or inflammation, neoplasia, and electrolyte derangements (commonly hypercalcemia, hypokalemia, and hypomagnesemia)
  - Underlying cardiac disease: acquired valvular disease, congenital cardiac disease, other cardiomyopathy, cardiac neoplasia, or myocarditis
  - Abdominal disease: abdominal neoplasia, splenic or hepatic disease, gastric dilation/volvulus, and peritonitis
  - Autonomic imbalance: stress/pain or a pathologic increase in sympathetic tone (e.g., pheochromocytoma)
  - Drugs/toxins: digoxin, methylxanthines, oleander, catecholamines, and chemotherapeutics (most commonly doxorubicin)
- Type II: consider all causes of ventricular arrhythmias as described for type I and all causes of episodic weakness/syncope, including the following:
  - Causes of syncope: neurocardiogenic (reflex-mediated) syncope, poor cardiac output (DCM, severe mitral valve regurgitation), congenital heart disease, bradyarrhythmias, tachyarrhythmias, and pulmonary hypertension (which is unlikely in the boxer)
  - Episodic weakness that may be mistaken for syncope (e.g., hypoglycemia, splenic tumor hemorrhage)
  - Seizure disorder
  - Narcolepsy (rare)
- Type III: consider all causes of a dilated cardiomyopathy phenotype and CHF.
  - Primary structural cardiac disease with resultant cardiac dilatation and systolic dysfunction (e.g., acquired valvular disease, congenital cardiac lesions)
  - Myocarditis
  - Severe systemic disease (e.g., sepsis) with resultant systolic dysfunction
  - Hypothyroid cardiomyopathy
  - Nutritional cardiomyopathy (taurine-deficient or carnitine-deficient DCM)

Initial Database

- Documentation of ventricular arrhythmia on ECG in the absence of the above comorbidities supports ARVC in boxers. VPCs are

typically positive in lead II, consistent with a right-ventricular origin.
- A 24-hour ambulatory ECG (Holter monitor) is recommended in animals without malignant arrhythmias (animals requiring immediate treatment based on initial ECG).
- Thoracic radiographs are usually normal but may show LV enlargement with possible signs of left/biventricular CHF if the patient has type III disease. Thoracic radiographs may be useful to rule out structural heart disease as a source of ventricular arrhythmias.
- Echocardiogram
  - Echocardiogram is generally normal in types I and II, although prolonged tachycardia can cause transient systolic dysfunction from myocardial stunning.
  - LV and/or right ventricular dilation with persistent systolic dysfunction despite tachyarrhythmia control is consistent with type III ARVC (DCM phenotype).
- CBC, chemistry, and urinalysis are generally normal but may be useful to rule out metabolic- or electrolyte-related causes of ventricular arrhythmias.

Advanced or Confirmatory Testing

- The genetic test for the striatin mutation can be helpful for supporting a diagnosis of ARVC and may be helpful in providing prognostic information.
  - Animals that test positive homozygous for the striatin mutation are more likely to be affected by type III disease; monitoring with annual Holter and echocardiogram is recommended. These animals also more commonly demonstrate severe ventricular arrhythmias, and genetic testing may help guide reevaluation schedules and influence the choice and dose of antiarrhythmic therapies.
  - Animals that test heterozygous positive may or may not demonstrate signs of the disease and should be monitored annually with Holter and/or echocardiogram after the age of 3 years.
  - Boxer dogs without the mutation should still be screened by Holter because some dogs with ARVC have been identified that do not test positive for the striatin mutation.
- Cardiac troponin I may be supportive of and correlate with severity of disease but is not sensitive or specific for diagnosis of the ARVC.
- Postmortem histopathology demonstrates myocytolysis with fibrofatty infiltration in the right ventricle (and/or the left ventricle). The degree of myocytolysis and fibrofatty infiltration is related to disease severity.

TREATMENT

Treatment Overview

- Treatment is not necessary for all dogs with ventricular arrhythmias secondary to suspected ARVC, and the decision to treat should be based on the severity of the arrhythmia.
- Ideally, treatment should be based on Holter results; however, dogs with clinical signs that have frequent ventricular arrhythmias on baseline ECG should be treated immediately.
- In general, treatment indications include the following:
  - Clinical signs (e.g., syncopal dogs) with ventricular arrhythmias or those demonstrating hemodynamic compromise
  - Ventricular tachycardia on Holter or baseline ECG
  - R on T complexes, particularly if frequent or in ventricular runs
  - Frequent multiform VPCs
- Goals of treatment
  - Reduced frequency of clinical signs related to the arrhythmia
  - Decreased arrhythmia complexity, including fewer R on T complexes, fewer ventricular couplets/triplets/runs, elimination of multiform complexes, and slower rates of ventricular arrhythmias
  - Reduction of the absolute number of ventricular arrhythmias by > 85% on subsequent 24-hour Holter monitoring reports

Acute General Treatment

- Dogs with R on T ventricular complexes, frequent couplets/triplets or ventricular tachycardia runs should be treated emergently with lidocaine at a 2 mg/kg IV dose; this bolus may be repeated up to 4 times, with 3-5 minutes between boluses, or until the patient shows signs of nausea/vomiting (the first sign of toxicity).
- Initial boluses should be followed by a lidocaine continuous rate infusion (CRI) at 25-80 mcg/kg/min, titrated to effect and reduced if signs of toxicity occur (nausea/vomiting or neurologic signs).
- Begin concurrent oral therapy (see below).

Chronic Treatment

- Sotalol 1.5-3 mg/kg PO q 12h and/or mexiletine 5-6 mg/kg PO q 8h
  - Typically begin with sotalol monotherapy (low side effect profile, q 12h administration). Mexiletine is more likely to cause gastrointestinal (GI) side effects, but combination therapy is occasionally necessary and more effective than either drug alone.
- Atenolol 1-1.5 mg/kg PO q 12h may also be used if arrhythmia control is not attained with sotalol or mexiletine. This medication should *not* be used in a patient with CHF or severe systolic dysfunction.
- Amiodarone is not commonly used due to high side effect profile, but it is occasionally necessary to treat refractory arrhythmias.
- Fish oil (780 mg EPA and 497 mg DHA) PO q 24h as an adjunct to sotalol/mexiletine has been shown to decrease the number of daily VPCs.
- Dogs with CHF should be treated with standard CHF therapy, including pimobendan, furosemide, angiotensin-converting enzyme (ACE) inhibitor, and spironolactone (pp. 408 and 409).

Drug Interactions

Antiarrhythmic drugs carry proarrhythmic risks, particularly when used in combination. When possible, reevaluation of Holter monitoring is indicated 2-4 weeks after initiation of therapy.

Possible Complications

Due to the potential for antiarrhythmic drugs to be proarrhythmic, patients may rarely develop worsening clinical signs, including more frequent or severe syncopal episodes and sudden death. This underscores the importance of monitoring antiarrhythmic therapy.

Recommended Monitoring

- Holter monitors are used to assess arrhythmia frequency and severity and to judge response to therapy. Frequency of monitoring depends on severity of disease.
  - Type I dogs that are not receiving treatment should receive annual Holter monitoring.
  - Type II dogs and type I dogs that are receiving treatment should be monitored at least annually by Holter monitors, but more frequent monitoring may be indicated by clinical severity.
- Annual echocardiogram should be used to monitor for development of type III disease, which can develop as a progression of type I or II disease. This is of particular concern in dogs that are homozygous for the striatin mutation.
  - Monitoring for CHF in type III dogs should include evaluation of periodic thoracic radiographs (for pulmonary edema) assessment for cavitary fluid (ascites/pleural effusion), blood pressure measurement, and renal function monitoring in patients receiving ACE inhibitor or diuretic therapy.
  - Owners should be trained to monitor resting respiratory rate at home because trending increases in respiratory rate or persistent elevations > 35 breaths per minute while sleeping indicate possible development of CHF.

PROGNOSIS & OUTCOME

- Dogs are at risk of sudden cardiac death.
- Types I and II ARVC patients have a similar survival to non-ARVC boxers, with a reported median survival time of 11 years. However, successful treatment results in reduced clinical signs in affected dogs (e.g., collapse, syncope).
- Type III ARVC patients have a worse prognosis and greater risk for sudden death. Average survival time after a diagnosis of concurrent CHF is approximately 6-9 months.

PEARLS & CONSIDERATIONS

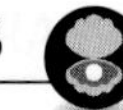

Comments

- ARVC is a diagnosis of exclusion. Presumptive diagnosis is made based on signalment and right-sided VPCs (complexes that are upright in lead II) after other causes of ventricular arrhythmias have been ruled out.
- Genetic testing can support a diagnosis of ARVC and has important prognostic value because homozygous positive dogs have a more severe disease type.
- Not all dogs with ARVC require treatment, and many that do will live normal lives on ventricular antiarrhythmic drugs as long as clinical signs (e.g., syncope) are controlled.
- There are no clear guidelines on when to treat dogs with ARVC, but the decision of whether or not to treat should be primarily based on the presence of clinical signs and evidence of malignant ventricular tachyarrhythmias on baseline or 24-hour Holter ECG.
- There is a broad spectrum of disease severity, with type III dogs having the worst prognosis. Dogs with severe ventricular arrhythmias on ECG are at high risk for sudden death.

Prevention

All breeding boxers should be tested for the mutation. Dogs that test homozygous positive for the striatin mutation can be detected before they display characteristics of the disease and should not be bred. Avoidance of breeding striatin mutation heterozygous positive dogs to each other will gradually reduce the disease prevalence while preserving genetic diversity within the boxer breed.

Technician Tips

- Because the morphology of the VPCs is helpful when establishing a diagnosis of ARVC, proper ECG electrode placement and patient positioning (right lateral recumbency) are important when evaluating a dog with suspected ARVC.
- Genetic testing may be performed by whole blood sample (EDTA) or buccal swab. If buccal swabs are used, ensure that the patient has not eaten for 60 minutes before swabbing to avoid contamination with food proteins.

SUGGESTED READING

Meurs KM, et al: Natural history of arrhythmogenic right ventricular cardiomyopathy in the boxer dog: a prospective study. J Vet Intern Med 28:1214-1220, 2014.

AUTHORS: Joshua A. Stern, DVM, PhD, DACVIM; Maureen Oldach, DVM
EDITOR: Meg M. Sleeper, VMD, DACVIM

Ascites

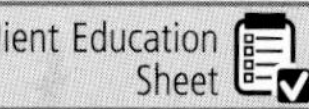
Client Education Sheet

BASIC INFORMATION

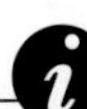

Definition

Accumulation of transudate effusion within the abdominal cavity

Synonyms

Abdominal or peritoneal effusion can be used to refer to any fluid (transudates or exudates) accumulation in the abdominal cavity

Epidemiology

SPECIES, AGE, SEX

Depends on underlying disease process

GENETICS, BREED PREDISPOSITION

- Lymphangiectasia (p. 600)
- Protein-losing nephropathy (p. 390)

RISK FACTORS

Vector-borne infections (e.g., heartworm, Lyme)

GEOGRAPHY AND SEASONALITY

Heartworm common in southeastern United States

ASSOCIATED DISORDERS

Abdominal distention, increased respiratory effort, tachypnea, hyporexia

Clinical Presentation

HISTORY, CHIEF COMPLAINT

Abdominal distention may be the primary complaint, with insidious or acute onset. If ascites is secondary to right-sided heart failure, presenting complaints may also include

- Syncope
- Exercise intolerance
- Cough
- Hyporexia or anorexia

If ascites is secondary to gastrointestinal or hepatic disease, presenting complaints may also include

- Diarrhea
- Vomiting
- Hyporexia or anorexia

PHYSICAL EXAM FINDINGS

- Abdominal distention
- Palpable fluid wave
- Tachypnea ± respiratory effort due to pressure on diaphragm
- Heart murmur and jugular distention if right-sided heart failure
- Muffled heart sounds if cardiac tamponade
- Icterus possible if cirrhotic liver disease

Etiology and Pathophysiology

Ascites can occur secondary to a number of underlying disease conditions associated with

- Increased hydrostatic pressure: portal hypertension
  - Cirrhotic liver disease
  - Budd-Chiari syndrome: obstruction of hepatic venous outflow
  - Right-sided heart failure
    - Caval syndrome
    - Cardiac tamponade
- Decreased oncotic pressure: hypoalbuminemia
  - Liver failure
  - Protein-losing enteropathy
  - Protein-losing nephropathy
- Increased vascular permeability
  - Vasculitis
- Transudate related to portal hypertension or vasculitis often has a higher protein (modified transudate)

DIAGNOSIS

Diagnostic Overview

Abdominocentesis with fluid analysis and cytology are required to determine fluid type (transudate or modified transudate vs. exudate). Other tests are aimed at determining the cause of ascites, with the choice of test determined by history and examination findings.

Differential Diagnosis

See Abdominal Distention (p. 1192).

Initial Database

- Abdominocentesis: clear fluid with low protein, low cellularity (pp. 1056 and 1343)
- CBC: normal, anemia of inflammatory disease, or suggestive of infection/inflammation (e.g., eosinophilia with heartworm infection)
- Serum biochemistry: albumin < 1.5 g/dL identifies low oncotic pressure
  - Cirrhotic liver disease/liver failure: may demonstrate high or normal alanine aminotransferase (ALT), alkaline phosphatase (ALP), gamma-glutamyltransferase (GGT), bilirubin; low cholesterol, blood urea nitrogen (BUN), glucose
  - Protein-losing nephropathy: may demonstrate high cholesterol, BUN, creatinine, phosphorous
  - Protein-losing enteropathy: may demonstrate low globulins, cholesterol
- Urinalysis: proteinuria suggests protein-losing nephropathy
- Thoracic radiographs: rule out right-sided cardiomegaly, globoid heart due to tamponade, enlarged pulmonary arteries due to heartworm, and pleural effusion

- Abdominal radiographs: limited utility due to lack of serosal detail
- Abdominal ultrasonography: evaluate hepatic and renal parenchyma

Advanced or Confirmatory Testing

Guided by initial findings

- If evidence of hypoalbuminemia and concurrent hyperglobulinemia, intestinal biopsies may be indicated to determine cause of protein-losing enteropathy (p. 600).
- If hypoalbuminemia and proteinuria, urine protein: creatinine ratio (p. 1391) indicated
- If murmur, jugular pulses, or cardiovascular abnormalities detected, echocardiogram (p. 1094) and heartworm antigen test (p. 1350) indicated

TREATMENT

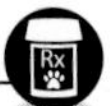

Treatment Overview

Depends on underlying cause

Acute General Treatment

If abdominal distention due to fluid accumulation is severe enough to compromise respiration, therapeutic abdominocentesis or adominal drainage may be indicated (p. 1056).

Chronic Treatment

Treatment aimed at underlying disorder

Nutrition/Diet

Protein-losing enteropathy, protein-losing nephropathy, and cardiac disease have unique nutritional requirements.

Recommended Monitoring

Resting respiratory rate, body weight; abdominal circumference can be used to estimate change in volume of ascites fluid.

PROGNOSIS & OUTCOME

Variable depending on cause

PEARLS & CONSIDERATIONS

Comments

- Excessive fluid drainage may promote further effusion and dehydration.
- Lasix has no role in management of ascites unless due to heart failure.

Prevention

Ectoparasite and endoparasite prophylaxis

Technician Tips

- Animals with severe ascites may have difficulty breathing, especially when restrained while lying on their side or back (e.g., during abdominal ultrasound).
- Avoid blind cystocentesis in animals with ascites.

SUGGESTED READING

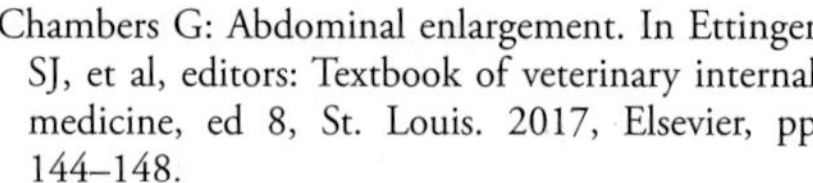

Chambers G: Abdominal enlargement. In Ettinger SJ, et al, editors: Textbook of veterinary internal medicine, ed 8, St. Louis. 2017, Elsevier, pp 144–148.

AUTHOR: Aida I. Vientós-Plotts, DVM
EDITOR: Leah A. Cohn, DVM, PhD, DACVIM

Aseptic Necrosis of the Femoral Head

Client Education Sheet

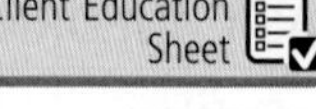

BASIC INFORMATION

Definition

A painful hip condition caused by interruption of blood supply to the proximal femoral epiphysis, producing bone necrosis and collapse of the articular cartilage and eventually hip osteoarthritis. The problem is unilateral in about 80% of cases.

Synonyms

Legg-Calvé-Perthes (LCP) disease, Legg-Perthes disease, Perthes disease, avascular or aseptic necrosis of the femoral head

Epidemiology

SPECIES, AGE, SEX

- Small-breed dogs
- Mean age of onset of clinical signs is 7 months, with a range of 3-11 months.
- This disease has not been reported in cats.

GENETICS, BREED PREDISPOSITION

- Autosomal recessive trait in West Highland white and Manchester terriers, miniature poodles
- Other commonly affected breeds include Yorkshire, Lakeland, and cairn terriers; miniature pinschers; toy poodles; Australian shepherds; Chihuahuas; dachshunds; Lhasa apsos; pugs.

Clinical Presentation

HISTORY, CHIEF COMPLAINT

Slowly progressing or acute onset of hip pain/lameness during the first year of life

PHYSICAL EXAM FINDINGS

- Pain on extension and flexion of the affected hip joint(s)
- Affected limb may be non–weight-bearing
- Muscle atrophy in the affected limb(s)
- Crepitus unusual but may be present in dogs that have developed degenerative joint disease

Etiology and Pathophysiology

- Cause and pathogenesis are unknown.
- The primary lesion appears to be ischemic injury causing necrosis of the bone of the femoral capital epiphysis.
- Dead bone trabeculae collapse, forming hollow spaces that cause loss of support to overlying articular cartilage. Trabeculae that form in their place are abnormally thin and unable to support normal loads.
- Subsequent weight bearing causes collapse of the femoral head and deformation of the cartilage, leading to development of osteoarthritis.

DIAGNOSIS

Diagnostic Overview

Signalment, physical findings, and radiographic confirmation make the diagnosis.

Differential Diagnosis

- Capital physeal or femoral neck fractures
- Hip dysplasia
- Coxofemoral luxation
- Septic arthritis of the hip
- Other causes of rear limb lameness (e.g., patellar luxation, stifle injury)

Initial Database

- Physical examination of affected and unaffected hind limb, with special emphasis on the hip joints
- Hip radiographs (lateral and ventrodorsal projections)
  - Early stage: femoral head lucency
  - Later stages: femoral head deformity and degenerative changes in the hip

Advanced or Confirmatory Testing

Computed tomography, magnetic resonance imaging, nuclear scintigraphy: not routinely required but could be useful when radiographic changes are not yet apparent

TREATMENT

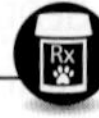

Treatment Overview

Treatment is aimed at restoration of normal, pain-free activity.

Acute General Treatment

- Medical management (analgesics, exercise modification; one report of successful use of an Ehmer sling): return to pain-free function in about 25% of cases
- Surgical intervention
  - Femoral head and neck excision (FHNE) or femoral head ostectomy (FHO) is the most common treatment.
  - Total hip replacement (THR)

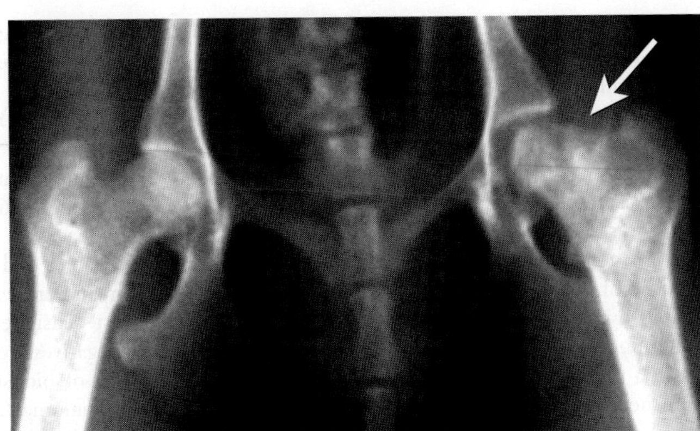

ASEPTIC NECROSIS OF THE FEMORAL HEAD Ventrodorsal view of the coxofemoral joints of a 10-month-old pug with left hindlimb lameness and hip joint pain. Note the bone deformation of the left femoral head *(arrow)* compared with the normal right joint.

Chronic Treatment

- The same surgical options can be used in chronic cases, but postoperative recovery may be less satisfactory due to learned behavior (avoidance of use of the affected leg) or chronic muscle atrophy.
- If surgery is not done or lameness resolves incompletely, one of the following nonsteroidal antiinflammatory drugs (NSAIDs) can be given on an intermittent or (if necessary) daily basis:
  - Carprofen 2.2 mg/kg PO q 12h *or* 4.4 mg/kg PO q 24h; *or*
  - Deracoxib 1-2 mg/kg PO q 24h; *or*
  - Meloxicam 0.1 mg/kg PO q 24h

Nutrition/Diet

- Aim to maintain normal body condition.
- Dietary supplements do not appear to be helpful.

Drug Interactions

- Concurrent administration of glucocorticosteroids and NSAIDs can result in severe gastrointestinal irritation, ulceration, and perforation.
- Chronic NSAID treatment can exacerbate liver or renal dysfunction.

Possible Complications

- Pain due to inadequate removal of the femoral neck in FHNE
- Poor limb usage from inadequate physical rehabilitation after FHNE

Recommended Monitoring

- Postoperative radiographs to evaluate FHNE osteotomy
- Monthly physical examinations to evaluate limb function until normal

PROGNOSIS & OUTCOME

- Lameness resolves in > 80% of cases after FHNE or THR.
- Lameness resolves in < 25% of cases with medical treatment alone.

PEARLS & CONSIDERATIONS

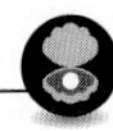

Comments

- Radiographic changes are subtle early in the course of the disease; serial radiography may be helpful in diagnosis.
- Physical rehabilitation is important for obtaining the best results after FHNE. Range-of-motion exercises, swimming, and limited weight-bearing exercises help create a nonpainful pseudoarthrosis with an adequate range of motion.
- Continued lameness after FHNE is usually due to a femoral neck remnant and often resolves if this remnant is removed.
- Chronic femoral capital physeal fractures (in cats and dogs) can be confused with aseptic necrosis on radiographs, but the cause is different.

Technician Tips

- Postoperative radiographs should include an extended-limb ventrodorsal view and a frog-leg view with femurs pulled cranially (parallel to the spine) to highlight femoral neck remnants.
- Leash-controlled walking and range-of-motion exercises should be started immediately after surgery to encourage normal limb use.

Client Education

- Breeders of dogs at risk should be warned that this condition is heritable. Affected animals should be removed from the breeding pool.
- For postoperative care at home, provide client with client education sheet: How to Perform Range-of-Motion Exercises (www.ExpertConsult.com).

SUGGESTED READING

Towle Millard HA, et al: Miscellaneous orthopedic conditions. In Johnston SA, et al, editors: Veterinary surgery: small animal, St. Louis, 2018, Elsevier, p 1309.

Reproduced from the third edition in modified form.

THIRD EDITION AUTHORS: D. Michael Tillson, DVM, MS, DACVS; Katrin Saile, DVM, MS, DACVS
AUTHOR & EDITOR: Kathleen Linn, DVM, MS, DACVS

Aspergillosis

Bonus Material Online

BASIC INFORMATION

Definition

Regional or disseminated infection with the opportunistic hyphal fungus *Aspergillus* spp

Epidemiology

SPECIES, AGE, SEX

Dogs more commonly affected than cats; often middle-aged adults

GENETICS, BREED PREDISPOSITION

- Systemic aspergillosis: German shepherd dogs overrepresented
- Sinonasal aspergillosis: medium- to large-breed, dolichocephalic dogs overrepresented. Conversely, brachycephalic cat breeds (e.g., Persian) are predisposed to upper respiratory aspergillosis (sinonasal or sino-orbital).

RISK FACTORS

- Systemic/disseminated: immunosuppression, primary immune deficiencies
- Sinonasal: other primary nasal disease, immunoglobulin A deficiency, prolonged antibiotic use, nasal conformation

CONTAGION AND ZOONOSIS

Aspergillosis is an opportunistic infection; it is not zoonotic or contagious.

ASSOCIATED DISORDERS

- Systemic: discospondylitis
- Sinonasal: chronic rhinitis; fungal sinusitis

Clinical Presentation

DISEASE FORMS/SUBTYPES

- Systemic
- Sinonasal
- Sino-orbital (cats)

HISTORY, CHIEF COMPLAINT

Systemic:

- Nonspecific signs predominate (e.g., lethargy, inappetence, decreased activity).
- Signs may have been present and slowly progressive for weeks to months.
- Acute signs related to discospondylitis (e.g., acute paresis/paralysis) occur in some cases.

Sinonasal:

- Chronic nasal discharge, sneezing, epistaxis, depigmentation of nares

Sino-orbital (cats):

- Facial/ocular deformity along with nasal signs

PHYSICAL EXAM FINDINGS

Systemic:

- Signs of ill thrift (lethargy, weight loss, poor haircoat, dehydration)
- Spinal pain during deep palpation
- Firm/hard limb swelling with adjacent cutaneous draining tracts may be present.
- Signs of uveitis (e.g., conjunctival redness, photophobia) are possible and may occur before other signs.

Sino-nasal:

- Nasal discharge is common, generally mucopurulent ± blood
- Evidence of nasal pain
- Depigmentation/ulceration of the ventral nares (the path of nasal discharge) is common.
- Epistaxis (unilateral or bilateral)
- Nasal airflow often sounds congested/obstructed due to nasal discharge but may be clearer sounding than normal if no discharge is present and extensive turbinate destruction has occurred.

Sino-orbital:

- In cats, an invasive sino-orbital form accounts for 65% of upper respiratory aspergillosis
- Massive facial and ocular deformity are typical, with inability to retropulse involved eye

Etiology and Pathophysiology

- Systemic: *Aspergillus terreus* most common
- Sinonasal: *Aspergillus fumigatus* most common
- *Aspergillus* fungi are normal environmental organisms that often are found incidentally on the skin and mucosa of dogs. Their presence alone does not indicate infection.
- *Aspergillus* fungi are routinely inhaled, ingested, and inoculated during normal activities and are eradicated by the host, especially by cell-mediated immune mechanisms.
- With systemic aspergillosis, multiplication and proliferation of *Aspergillus* spp occurs when the patient fails to eradicate the organism, typically after routine exposure by inhalation.
  - Systemic aspergillosis requires management of the mycosis and identification and management of any underlying immunodeficiency.
- With sinonasal aspergillosis, the role of immunocompromise is unclear.
  - Affected dogs generally do not have any evidence of systemic illness or immunocompromise.
  - Impaired lymphocyte blastogenesis may be a cause or a result of infection.
  - A dominant helper T-cell type 1 (T_H1)–regulated, cell-mediated immune response has been identified.
- Mutual exclusion: sinonasal aspergillosis is not suspected to lead to disseminated aspergillosis, and disseminated aspergillosis essentially never causes signs of nasal disease.

DIAGNOSIS

Diagnostic Overview

- For systemic aspergillosis, the diagnosis is suspected in a German shepherd (other breeds sometimes affected) with chronic weight loss, neurologic deficits, and radiographic evidence of bony lesions or discospondylitis. Although serologic testing can be helpful, confirmation ideally based on cytology or histopathologic evaluation of affected organs.
- For sinonasal aspergillosis, the diagnosis is suspected in a dolichocephalic or mesaticephalic breed with nasal discharge, epistaxis, and/or depigmentation of the nares. Although serologic testing can be helpful, confirmation requires demonstration of fungal hyphae on samples of nasal tissue with supportive diagnostic imaging findings.

Differential Diagnosis

- Systemic: other opportunistic mycoses, bacterial discospondylitis, vertebral or other bone neoplasm
- Sinonasal: nasal neoplasia, other fungal or bacterial rhinitis, foreign body, bleeding disorder (if epistaxis) (p. 1255)

Initial Database

- CBC, serum biochemistry panel: mature neutrophilia/stress leukogram common for systemic disease but nonspecific. Rule out thrombocytopenia as cause of epistaxis.
- Systemic
  - Urinalysis may show fungal hyphae.
  - Radiographs of the spine may reveal evidence of discospondylitis (vertebral endplate lysis).
  - Radiographs of bony swellings can reveal lytic-proliferative lesions.
  - Abdominal ultrasound is indicated to identify visceral fungal granulomas, lymphadenomegaly.
- Sinonasal
  - Swabs of nasal exudates are not useful; generally identify secondary bacterial infection only, and when *Aspergillus* is present, it may only be a contaminant.

Advanced or Confirmatory Testing

Systemic:

- Fine-needle aspirates of enlarged lymph nodes, affected intervertebral discs, or bone lesions may show hyphae.
- Serologic testing variable, and many tests are unreliable. Serum and urine galactomannan assays are most sensitive, but false-positives and false-negatives are possible.
- Histologic evaluation of biopsied tissue is diagnostic (fungal granulomas). If a clinical suspicion of aspergillosis exists at the time of biopsy, a portion of the specimen should also be submitted for fungal culture. Laboratory culture is needed to differentiate *Aspergillus* spp from *Penicillium* spp and from other saprophytic infections such as *Mucorales* or *Alternaria* spp.

Sinonasal:

- Diagnosis is confirmed when fungal hyphae can be demonstrated histologically within nasal tissue and/or when at least two of the following criteria are fulfilled: positive serum titer for *A. fumigatus*, positive *Aspergillus* fungal culture, visible fungal plaques on rhinoscopy, and supportive imaging (radiographic/CT) findings.
- Imaging: CT is the modality of choice (greater resolution than radiographs, good bone detail, unlike MRI). Typical findings are nasal turbinate loss, intranasal fluid opacity (exudates), and possibly fluid opacity in the frontal sinuses.
- Nasal radiographs show regional or diffuse, asymmetrical turbinate loss and increase (due to intranasal exudate) or decrease (if scant exudate and loss of turbinate and overlying mucosa) of soft-tissue/fluid opacity. A drawback is the difficulty in determining whether soft-tissue/fluid opacity in the nasal passages is due to discharge (fluid) or mass (e.g., neoplasm).
- Rhinoscopy (p. 1159) is the preferred method for direct observation and sampling. An abnormally vast, cavernous nasal cavity is common (turbinate loss). Fungal plaques or granulomas may be observed directly. Microscopic identification of *Aspergillus* from a macroscopically visible intranasal or intrasinus colony is considered pathognomonic. Both left and right nasal cavities are examined because findings often are asymmetrical.
- Rhinotomy is highly invasive, and surgical exploration offers little or no advantage over rhinoscopy in patients with nasal aspergillosis.
- *Aspergillus* serologic results (agar gel immunodiffusion [AGID], ELISA) vary, and titers cannot be used as a sole diagnostic test for nasal aspergillosis. Galactomannan antigen ELISA useful for systemic disease is insensitive for sinonasal or sino-orbital disease.
- Fungal culture results that demonstrate *Aspergillus* from samples not involving a macroscopic fungal colony are equivocal and

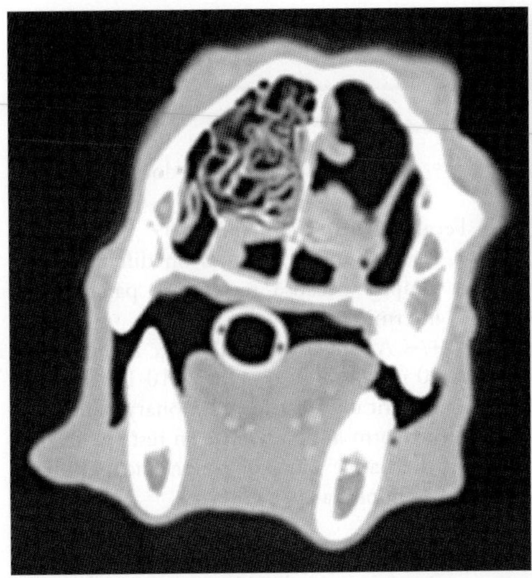

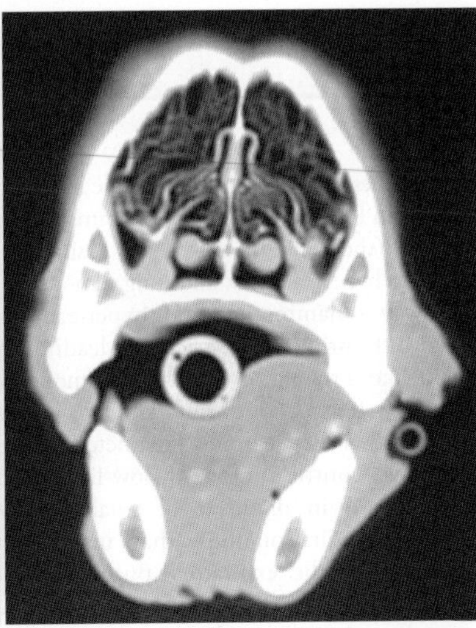

ASPERGILLOSIS Computed tomographic image of the nasal cavities of two dogs. The dog on the left has nasal aspergillosis; there is asymmetrical loss of turbinates. The dog on the right is normal (for comparison). (Courtesy Robert O'Brien, DVM, DACVR, University of Illinois.)

must be supported by additional tests to make the diagnosis.

TREATMENT

Treatment Overview

For systemic aspergillosis, treatment consists of long-term systemic antifungal medication and supportive care. For sinonasal aspergillosis, treatment is usually locally administered antifungal medications. No ideal treatment has been identified for feline sino-orbital disease.

Acute and Chronic Treatment

Systemic:

- Voriconazole is the treatment of choice and associated with improved survival in people. A loading dose of 6 mg/kg PO q 12h is given for 2 days, followed by a maintenance dose of 3-4 mg/kg PO q 12h for several months after complete resolution of clinical signs. Often cost prohibitive in veterinary patients.
- *A. terreus* is resistant to amphotericin B, and this drug is no longer recommended for treatment of systemic disease from *A. terreus* in people.
- Alternative: itraconazole 5 mg/kg PO q 12h indefinitely and often lifelong. Monitor for liver adverse effects. Absorption enhanced substantially by administering with food.

Sinonasal:

- Endoscopic/nonsurgical intranasal clotrimazole or enilconazole infusion is the treatment of choice, provided the cribriform plate is intact (as assessed on CT).
- Debridement of the nasal passages/sinuses (by trephination if necessary) improves outcome of topical treatment.
- Refractory cases or those with damage to the cribriform plate can be treated with long-term posaconazole (5 mg/kg q 12h) and terbinafine (30 mg/kg q 12h).

Possible Complications

- Intractable infection
- Voriconazole can cause adverse neurologic events in cats and dose-related visual disturbances and photophobia in people. Anaphylactoid reactions have been reported after intravenous administration in people. This is a very new drug to veterinary medicine, and little is known about side effects in dogs.
- Resistance to azoles, the first line of treatment, is an emerging concern and appears to be due to long-term treatment as well as extended use in agriculture.

Recommended Monitoring

Evolution/resolution of clinical signs; serial titers are not useful.

PROGNOSIS & OUTCOME

Systemic:

- The prognosis is almost universally poor, although some dogs may obtain palliation. The induction of long-term clinical remission with oral itraconazole was reported in four dogs.
- Many affected dogs are euthanized at the time of conclusive diagnosis because of the extent of lesions and underlying deficiencies in immunity.

Canine sinonasal: fair to good

- Clinical signs resolve with a single treatment in 65% of dogs, and 87% of dogs with a total of one or more treatments.
- A lesser extent of radiographic lesions is associated with a better prognosis.

Feline sino-orbital: poor prognosis

PEARLS & CONSIDERATIONS

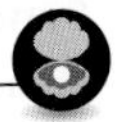

Comments

- For sinonasal aspergillosis, nasal discharge ceases (permanently) in most dogs within 2 weeks of treatment. Occasional recurrence of nasal signs due to secondary bacterial rhinitis is possible due to destruction of nasal turbinates.
- The frontal sinuses should be imaged in any patient suspected of having nasal aspergillosis.
- Polymerase chain reaction (PCR) is becoming more common to establish a diagnosis in people and may become more available in veterinary medicine in the future.
- Combination therapy with echinocandins (antifungal agents that act on the cell wall) plus azoles is currently being studied in people.
- The recent discovery that *A. fumigatus* has a sexual reproductive cycle may offer future treatment options as the genetic basis of the pathogenicity is elucidated.
- Although nasal turbinates may have the potential to regrow, there is limited information in veterinary medicine and no follow-up studies aimed at assessing this question.

Technician Tips

CT can be done with minimum to no sedation if the VetMousetrap is used (for small dogs and cats).

Client Education

Diagnosis of aspergillosis is complex but important because diagnostic tests help determine the likelihood of success.

SUGGESTED READING

Stewart J, et al: Treatment of refractory sino-nasal aspergillosis with posaconazole and terbinafine in 10 dogs. J Small Anim Pract 58:504-509, 2017.

AUTHOR: Maureen A. McMichael, DVM, DACVECC
EDITOR: Joseph Taboada, DVM, DACVIM

Asthma, Feline

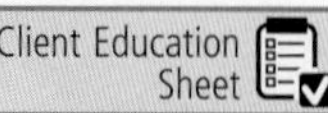

BASIC INFORMATION

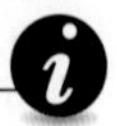

Definition

A syndrome triggered by allergen-specific activation of immune cells culminating in cough, wheeze, and/or respiratory distress, eosinophilic inflammation of airways, bronchoconstriction, and structural pulmonary changes

Synonyms

Feline allergic asthma, feline allergic bronchitis, feline eosinophilic bronchitis

Epidemiology

SPECIES, AGE, SEX

Typically young to middle-aged at onset; either sex

GENETICS, BREED PREDISPOSITION

Possible breed predisposition in Siamese cats

GEOGRAPHY AND SEASONALITY

Seasonality depends on the allergen (e.g., indoor allergens, year-round; outdoor allergens may be seasonal).

ASSOCIATED DISORDERS

Secondary bacterial infections of the lower airways

Clinical Presentation

DISEASE FORMS/SUBTYPES

- Acute, life-threatening disease (status asthmaticus)
- Chronic persistent signs
- Waxing and waning signs
  - Note: airway inflammation persists in the absence of clinical signs.

HISTORY, CHIEF COMPLAINT

Cough (which owners may interpret as unsuccessful attempts to vomit a hairball), wheeze, tachypnea, respiratory distress

PHYSICAL EXAM FINDINGS

- Cough, may be inducible with tracheal palpation
- Expiratory wheezes sometimes audible with or without a stethoscope
- Respiratory distress, often with a prominent expiratory component (expiratory push)
- Tachypnea
- Paradoxic breathing (chest and abdomen move in opposition)
- Increased bronchovesicular sounds
- Physical exam may be normal between episodes.

Etiology and Pathophysiology

- Sensitization to aeroallergens activates type 2 helper T cells (T_H2), leading to production of proinflammatory cytokines.
- Cytokines promote allergen-specific immunoglobulin E (IgE) production, inflammatory cell influx (the hallmark cell is the eosinophil), airway hyperreactivity, and lung remodeling.
- Airway inflammation and hyperreactivity provoke bronchoconstriction, leading to cough and respiratory difficulty. Remodeling changes (e.g., smooth muscle hypertrophy) can further reduce luminal diameter of small airways, contributing to airflow limitation.
- Reduction in diameter of small airways impairs expiration more than inspiration, leading to the expiratory push observed during physical examination and air trapping on thoracic radiographs.

DIAGNOSIS

Diagnostic Overview

Asthma is suspected in cats exhibiting cough, wheeze, and/or respiratory distress when other causes of cardiac or respiratory disease have been excluded. Airway eosinophilia in conjunction with a favorable response to therapy supports the diagnosis.

Differential Diagnosis

Physical examination findings (cough, wheeze, respiratory distress):

- Pleural effusion (any cause; e.g., chylothorax, pyothorax, transudate associated with heart failure)
- Cardiogenic or noncardiogenic pulmonary edema
- Pneumonia (infectious, aspiration, foreign body)
- Neoplasia
- Interstitial lung disease
- Laryngeal disease (musical noises are loudest over the larynx; characterized by inspiratory distress)

Radiographic findings:

- Chronic bronchitis
- Lung worms
- Heartworm-associated respiratory disease (HARD)
- *Toxocara cati* larval migration

Initial Database

Thoracic radiographs:

- Bronchial or bronchointerstitial pattern
- Lung hyperinflation (air trapping)
  - Expanded lung fields
  - Increased radiolucency of lung fields
  - Flattened diaphragm
  - Increased distance between the caudal cardiac silhouette and diaphragm on the lateral view
- Lung lobe collapse (usually right middle lobe)
- May be unremarkable

CBC:

- Eosinophilia: compatible with allergic or parasitic disease
  - Absence of eosinophilia does not rule out asthma.

Fecal analysis (Baermann test):

- Perform multiple times on different stool samples because respiratory parasites are intermittently shed.
- +/− Antiparasitic trial (e.g., fenbendazole 50 mg/kg PO q 24h × 10-14 days) to empirically treat for pulmonary parasites

Heartworm antibody/antigen test (p. 415):

- Alternative cause of cough and peripheral eosinophilia

Advanced or Confirmatory Testing

- Respiratory wash with cytologic analysis and culture
  - Collected by blind bronchoalveolar lavage (BAL) through an endotracheal tube or by bronchoscopy (pp. 1073 and 1074)
  - Submit a portion of the wash sample for culture to exclude secondary bacterial infection and another for *Mycoplasma* spp polymerase chain reaction (PCR).
  - Cytology demonstrates increased percentages of eosinophils (>16%) in BAL fluid with asthma and increased percentages of neutrophils (>7%) with chronic bronchitis.
    - Reference ranges for BAL fluid cell differentials are controversial.
    - Coexistence of eosinophilic and neutrophilic inflammation suggests chronic asthmatic bronchitis (long-standing asthma-associated inflammation can promote concurrent chronic bronchitis with neutrophilic inflammation) or secondary bacterial infection (may also see degenerate neutrophils).
- Serum allergen-specific IgE testing may help determine which aeroallergens contribute to clinical signs or are triggers for status asthmaticus, potentially helping guide environmental management.
- Thoracic CT may provide details of airways and interstitium (including vasculature) that could help differentiate asthma from parasitic disorders (e.g., HARD, *Toxocara cati*).
- Pulmonary function testing with bronchoprovocation: limited availability; mainly a research tool
- Serum vitamin D concentration may be determined in refractory cases.
  - Although unproven in cats, human asthmatics with vitamin D deficiency respond to supplementation with improved symptoms and quality of life.

TREATMENT

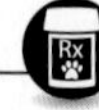

Treatment Overview

In an acute crisis, rapid stabilization of respiratory function with oxygen and bronchodilators is critical. Chronic therapy consists of minimizing exposure to environmental allergens and irritants, suppressing inflammation, and alleviating bronchoconstriction as needed. A recommended treatment approach and protocol are provided on p. 1403.

Acute General Treatment

Cats may be well at the time of presentation or in crisis. When in crisis,

- Minimize handling and stress.
- Administer oxygen (p. 1146).
- Bronchodilators, parenteral
  - Terbutaline 0.01-0.04 mg/kg SQ or IM q 4-8h prn
  - In severe cases, epinephrine 0.1 mg/CAT SQ, IM, or IV may be beneficial.
    - Hypoxemia can cause epinephrine to be arrhythmogenic, and oxygen should be administered concurrently.
    - Contraindicated in cats with heart disease or systemic hypertension
- Bronchodilators by nebulization or metered-dose inhalers (p. 1134):
  - Albuterol 0.5% solution for nebulization: give 0.1-0.25 mL diluted in 2 mL sterile saline through a nebulizer q 4h.
  - Metered-dose inhalants (MDI) are delivered by using a spacer with a face mask designed for cats. Albuterol 17-g inhalant: 1-2 actuations (puffs) into the spacer while the cat takes ≈10 breaths can be repeated q 30 minutes if necessary for 1-4 hours.
- Glucocorticoids, parenteral:
  - Prednisolone sodium succinate (1-2 mg/kg slowly IV) or dexamethasone (0.2-0.3 mg/kg IV or IM)
  - Inhaled glucocorticoids do not work fast enough to be of benefit in acute treatment.

Chronic Treatment

Glucocorticoids:

- Critical to reduce airway inflammation that leads to airway hyper-responsiveness and remodeling
- Oral glucocorticoids preferred initially: prednisolone 2 mg/kg PO q 24h
- Metered-dose inhaled glucocorticoids ideal for long-term maintenance because systemic glucocorticoid effects are reduced: fluticasone 110-220 mcg q 12h administered into spacer while the cat takes ≈10 breaths (p. 1134)
  - Train owners to count breaths, not seconds, as cats may breath hold when the mask is initially placed over the muzzle.
  - Overlap oral and inhaled steroids because it can take up to 2 weeks for inhaled steroids to effectively blunt airway inflammation.
  - Other inhalant steroids (e.g., flunisolide, budesonide) may have efficacy.
- Repositol injectable glucocorticoids often appear to lose efficacy over time and must be given more and more frequently.

Bronchodilators: oral route ideal for routine chronic therapy (if required)

- Terbutaline 0.625 mg/CAT PO q 12h, *or*
- Theophylline 25 mg/kg PO q 24h, *or*
- Aminophylline 4-5 mg/kg PO q 8h
- For cats requiring only occasional bronchodilator use, albuterol MDI (as for acute treatment) is acceptable.
- Chronic use of racemic aerosolized albuterol exacerbates airway eosinophilia; levalbuterol (*R*-albuterol) is a better alternative for inhalant albuterol if administered more than 2-3 times weekly.
- Owners can be taught to give terbutaline 0.01-0.04 mg/kg SQ to cats that develop status asthmaticus at home.

Antibiotics:

- If secondary bacterial infection (uncommon) is documented based on cytologic evidence and culture and susceptibility, an appropriate antibiotic can be administered.
- Alternatively, if response to glucocorticoids is suboptimal, a short course of a broad-spectrum antibiotic that penetrates into bronchial secretions and bronchial epithelium may be tried (e.g., doxycycline 5 mg/kg PO q 12h; azithromycin 10 mg/kg PO q 24h).

Cyclosporine (5 mg/kg PO q 12h to start):

- May be considered in cats refractory to other medications, or cats with concurrent diseases that prevent treatment with glucocorticoids (e.g., diabetes mellitus, heart disease)
- Therapeutic blood monitoring is strongly recommended (p. 1333).
- Cyclosporine has been evaluated only in an experimental model of asthma.

Tyrosine kinase inhibitors (masitinib 50 mg/CAT PO q 24h): currently unavailable

- May reduce airflow limitation and airway eosinophilia
- Consider only in severe refractory cases or if concurrent diseases prevent treatment with glucocorticoids.
- Masitinib has been evaluated in an experimental model of asthma; severe proteinuria is common and dose limiting. Toceranib may have similar effects but has not been evaluated.

Mesenchymal stem cell therapy (adipose derived):

- Intravenous stem cell therapy was found to have a delayed treatment effect in cats with experimentally induced asthma, reducing inflammation 9 months after treatment.
- Early intervention reduced airway remodeling in experimentally induced asthma.

No benefit has been demonstrated in experimental models of feline asthma for cysteinyl leukotriene antagonists (e.g., zafirlukast), antiserotonergic agents, (cyproheptadine), neurokinin-1 receptor antagonists (e.g., maropitant), or second-generation H1-receptor antagonists (e.g., cetirizine to control eosinophilic airway inflammation).

Nutrition/Diet

Omega-3 polyunsaturated fatty acids and luteolin as adjunctive treatment may improve airflow limitation but are not suitable as monotherapy because they do not blunt airway inflammation.

Behavior/Exercise

- Ideally, remove the allergen triggering clinical signs.
  - In practice, this is difficult or impossible to do.
  - Serum allergen-specific IgE testing and intradermal skin testing are options for determining specific allergens to minimize/avoid.
- Minimize exposure to airborne irritants (e.g., dusts, smoke, aerosols).
- HEPA-type air filters for cats spending a considerable amount of time indoors, especially if IgE reactivity to indoor allergens can be documented

Drug Interactions

Do not give propranolol or other nonspecific beta-adrenergic blockers to asthmatics; these drugs can exacerbate bronchoconstriction.

Possible Complications

- Long-term oral glucocorticoids can predispose to development of diabetes mellitus and exacerbation of heart disease in some cats.
- Theophyllines have a low therapeutic index, and dosages should be based on lean body weight. They are relatively contraindicated in patients with hypertension, hyperthyroidism, and cardiac disease. The sustained-release oral formulations of theophylline (currently unavailable) are not designed for absorption by the gastrointestinal tracts of small animals, and variable assimilation of the drug (underabsorption or overabsorption) is possible. Manifestations of toxicosis include tachycardia and behavior changes such as agitation and anxiety (similar to theobromine toxicosis).
- Masitinib (and other tyrosine kinase inhibitors) can cause marked proteinuria in cats, which may be reversible with early detection and discontinuation of the drug.

Recommended Monitoring

- Clinical signs at home
  - Persistence or exacerbation of clinical signs implies poor control.
  - Absence of clinical signs does not imply resolution of airway inflammation and cannot be assumed to reflect good control.
- Physical examination and thoracic radiographs if initially abnormal.
- If response is poor, BAL fluid cytologic re-evaluation to recognize subclinical airway inflammation and check for secondary infection

PROGNOSIS & OUTCOME

- Prognosis can range from grave to good, depending on the number and severity of status asthmaticus episodes and response to acute and chronic management. Prognosis also depends on the magnitude of irreversible structural changes in the lung.

- If respiratory distress is a manifestation of disease, sudden death can occur before veterinary intervention. Owners can be trained to administer injections of a bronchodilator or MDI albuterol until veterinary intervention.
- For cats presenting with cough but not distress and if inflammation is controlled with glucocorticoids and environmental modulation, prognosis is good to excellent.
- If inflammation is not well controlled, lung damage can occur and lead to airflow limitation, in which case the prognosis is guarded to fair.

PEARLS & CONSIDERATIONS

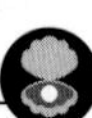

Comments

- Bronchodilators should not be given as monotherapy because they do not suppress airway inflammation; chronic airway inflammation leads to structural changes and permanent damage.
- Novel drug therapies evaluated have not been shown to be more effective at reducing airway eosinophilia and bronchoconstriction than traditional therapy.
- Allergen-specific immunotherapy (ASIT; allergy shots) modulates the immune response to induce tolerance to allergen or alter the immune response so that it is less damaging. ASIT reduced inflammation and altered immune responses in an experimental model of feline asthma and may one day prove to be a useful therapeutic strategy.

Technician Tips

- Monitor respiratory rate and effort for early detection of an asthmatic crisis.
- Minimize stress and avoid inhaled irritants (e.g., cat litter, aerosols) in asthmatic cats.
- Oxygen supplementation and bronchodilators are necessary during episodes of respiratory distress.

Client Education

- Keeping a record of when clinical signs occur can help establish the seasonality to allergen exposure.
- Teach owner how to administer emergency bronchodilator at home.

SUGGESTED READING

Trzil JE, et al: Update on feline asthma. Vet Clin North Am Small Anim Pract 44:91-105, 2014.

AUTHOR: Laura A. Nafe, DVM, MS, DACVIM
EDITOR: Megan Grobman, DVM, MS, DACVIM

Ataxia

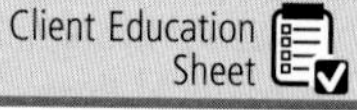

Client Education Sheet

BASIC INFORMATION

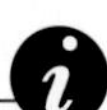

Definition

Failure of muscular coordination; a sign of sensory dysfunction in the nervous system seen commonly in animals with neurologic disease

Epidemiology

SPECIES, AGE, SEX

Depends on the underlying cause

GENETICS, BREED PREDISPOSITION

Depends on underlying cause: small, chondrodystrophic dogs (intervertebral disc disease [IVDD]); young, large-breed, nonchondrodystrophic dogs and miniature schnauzers (fibrocartilaginous embolism); Great Danes and Doberman pinschers (cervical stenotic myelopathy); German shepherds and boxers (degenerative myelopathy)

Clinical Presentation

DISEASE FORMS/SUBTYPES

- *Proprioceptive (sensory) ataxia*: dysfunction of the proprioceptive pathways in any or all of the spinal cord, brainstem, or cerebrum. The appearance is that of a patient's failure to perceive where its limbs are in space.
- *Vestibular ataxia*: dysfunction of the peripheral vestibular system in the inner ear or the central vestibular system in the medulla. The appearance is that of a patient with loss of balance/disequilibrium.
- *Cerebellar ataxia:* results from diseases affecting the cerebellum. The appearance is that of loss of fine motor control despite normal initiation of movements. Patients may have hypermetria, tremors, and truncal sway but are not paretic.

HISTORY, CHIEF COMPLAINT

- Onset: peracute to chronic/insidious, depending on cause
- Hyperesthesia may be associated with proprioceptive ataxia.
- "Walking as if intoxicated" may be reported.
- Owners of animals with acute onset of vestibular ataxia often think their animal is seizuring.
- History of otitis externa (vestibular ataxia)
- Recent therapy with metronidazole or aminoglycosides (vestibular ataxia)

PHYSICAL EXAM FINDINGS

Some or all findings may be present.

Proprioceptive ataxia:

- Generally accompanied by paresis
- Base-wide stance
- Circumduction, abduction, and crossing over of the limbs
- Delayed limb protraction with an elongated stride
- Mild hypermetria
- Standing on the dorsum of the paw; "knuckling over"
- Ulceration of the dorsal aspect of the paw and wear of the claws
- With cervical lesions, there may be only pelvic limb ataxia, or forelimbs may show a stiff/short-stride ("two-engine") gait

Vestibular ataxia:

- The hallmark of vestibular ataxia is a head tilt, with the ventral ear indicating the side of the lesion. Rarely, the head tilt may be directed away from the lesion in paradoxical vestibular syndrome.
- The trunk may lean, fall, or drift toward the side of the lesion, causing patients to press against a wall.
- Ipsilateral positional ventral strabismus (ventral deviation of the globe when the examiner lifts the head)
- Ipsilateral limb flexion and contralateral limb extension may be noted.
- Paresis and proprioceptive deficits are not a component of peripheral vestibular disease but may be seen with central vestibular disease.
- With peripheral vestibular disease, nystagmus is horizontal or rotary, with the fast phase away from the lesion, and it does not change with different head positions.
- In central vestibular disease, nystagmus may be horizontal, rotary, or vertical or may change direction with different head positions.
- Mentation may be depressed with central vestibular disease.
- Patients should be examined for positional nystagmus while rolled on their backs because resting nystagmus is often absent in chronic vestibular conditions.
- Postural reactions are usually normal with peripheral vestibular disease and delayed with central vestibular disease, although with severe peripheral disease, patients may not correct a knuckled paw despite normal proprioception.
- Bilateral peripheral vestibular disease (most commonly an idiopathic feline condition) causes a crouched posture with wide head excursions bilaterally, absent physiologic nystagmus without the presence of head tilt, resting nystagmus, or postural deficits.

Cerebellar ataxia:

- Broad-based stance
- Dysmetria, hypermetria, spasticity (abnormal, excessive, stiff movement of the limbs, respectively)

- Intention tremor (i.e., tremor precipitated by the onset of voluntary movement, such as responding to a command)
- Preservation of strength and postural reactions
- Ipsilateral absent menace response possible with cerebellar disease
- Head tilt away from the lesion in paradoxical vestibular syndrome
- Opisthotonos with normal/anxious mentation, thoracic limb extensor rigidity, and pelvic limb flexion with acute severe lesions (decerebellate rigidity)

Etiology and Pathophysiology

Proprioceptive ataxia:
- IVDD
- Cervical spondylomyelopathy/wobbler syndrome
- Degenerative myelopathy
- Congenital malformations (spina bifida, syringomyelia)
- Intraarachnoid diverticula
- Fibrocartilaginous emboli
- Neoplasia
- Myelitis
- Trauma

Vestibular ataxia:
- Idiopathic peripheral vestibular disease (old dog, any age cat)
- Otitis media/interna
- Vascular event
- Encephalitis
- Neoplasia
- Inflammatory polyp (cat, middle ear)
- Hypothyroidism (older dog)
- Chiari-like malformation (caudal occipital malformation syndrome)
- Polyneuropathy
- Toxic (e.g., aminoglycosides, metronidazole), especially topical (ear medication) with disrupted tympanum
- Thiamine deficiency (cats)

Cerebellar ataxia:
- Abiotrophy
- Atrophy/hypoplasia (*in utero* panleukopenia infection in cats, herpesvirus in dogs, others)
- Infectious (feline infectious peritonitis, distemper)
- Inflammatory (meningoencephalitis: granulomatous, steroid-responsive, necrotizing)
- Neoplasia
- Caudal occipital malformation syndrome (Chiari-like malformation)
- Vascular event

Additional details on the causes of ataxia are provided on p. 1201.

DIAGNOSIS

Diagnostic Overview

Diagnosis and initial evaluation of ataxia depends on performing a careful neurologic exam to demonstrate neurologic deficits that localize the lesion to a specific region of the nervous system.

Differential Diagnosis

- Orthopedic disease (e.g., ruptured cranial cruciate ligament, hip dysplasia)
- Weakness (metabolic, neuromuscular)

Initial Database

- Complete physical and neurologic examination (p. 1136), including fundic (p. 1137) and otoscopic exam (p. 1144) to precisely localize the lesion and guide further diagnostics
- CBC, serum chemistry, urinalysis, thyroid profile to rule out systemic causes

Advanced or Confirmatory Testing

- Imaging modalities (radiography, MRI [p. 1132], CT, myelography)
- Cerebrospinal fluid analysis (pp. 1080 and 1323) essential for the diagnosis of inflammatory disorders
- Electrodiagnostics (e.g., brainstem auditory evoked response) for vestibular diseases and suspected brainstem disease
- Serum and cerebrospinal fluid titers for infectious diseases

TREATMENT

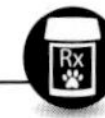

Treatment Overview

Identify and eliminate the underlying cause; referral to a veterinary neurologist is often indicated.

Behavior/Exercise

- To prevent falling, access to stairs should be restricted for ataxic patients. Specifically, descending stairs can exacerbate the signs of vestibular ataxia.
- In patients being treated conservatively for suspected disc extrusion, strict cage confinement is recommended for 4 weeks (p. 555).
- In patients who knuckle when they walk, booties should be used for preventing trauma.

Possible Complications

- Trauma resulting from falls associated with ataxia
- Anorexia and dehydration due to incapacitation or nausea
- Respiratory dysfunction with severe cervical spinal cord lesions

Recommended Monitoring

Follow-up exam and serial diagnostic studies as directed by the patient's clinical progression

PROGNOSIS & OUTCOME

- Depends on the underlying cause
- In general, diseases with an acute onset have a more favorable prognosis than those with a chronic course.

PEARLS & CONSIDERATIONS

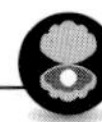

Comments

- Accurate identification and characterization of ataxia are the most important aspects of neurologic localization.
- Diffuse lower motor neuron disease causes weakness but not ataxia; affected animals have a short-stride gait, but careful examination reveals that although they may not have the strength to appropriately place their limbs, they are aware of the position of the limbs in space.
- When examining an abnormal gait, pay attention to whether you can predict where the patient will place the paw next (orthopedic) or not (ataxia).

Technician Tips

Animals with vestibular dysfunction prefer to lie/be restrained on the side to which the head tilts.

SUGGESTED READING

de Lahunta A, et al: Veterinary neuroanatomy and clinical neurology, ed 4, St. Louis, 2015, Saunders.

AUTHOR: Greg Kilburn, DVM, DACVIM
EDITOR: Leah A. Cohn, DVM, PhD, DACVIM

Atlantoaxial Instability

Bonus Material Online 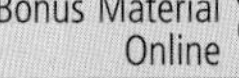 Client Education Sheet 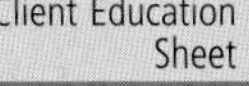 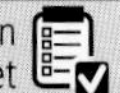

BASIC INFORMATION

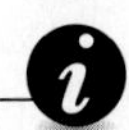

Definition

Atlantoaxial instability (AAI) is an abnormal range of motion occurring between the atlas (C1) and the axis (C2), resulting in subluxation of C2 relative to C1 and injury to the cranial cervical spinal cord and sometimes the caudal brainstem. It is most often caused by congenital malformation of the C1-C2 vertebrae and their associated ligaments, trauma, or a combination of both.

Synonyms

Atlantoaxial subluxation, atlantoaxial malformation

Epidemiology

SPECIES, AGE, SEX

- Congenital form: toy and small breeds of dogs, usually ≤ 1 year of age
- Traumatic form: large-breed dogs (rare), toy/small-breed dogs, cats (rare)

GENETICS, BREED PREDISPOSITION

All toy/small breeds are predisposed: Yorkshire terriers, miniature and toy poodles, Chihuahuas, Pomeranians, Pekinese overrepresented; also in Cavalier King Charles spaniels

ASSOCIATED DISORDERS

Other congenital anomalies: syringohydromyelia, hydrocephalus, Chiari-like malformation, vertebral anomalies

Clinical Presentation

HISTORY, CHIEF COMPLAINT

- Variable onset of disease that can present with acute, chronic, or intermittent signs.
- Cervical pain is a consistent presenting complaint. Ataxia, difficulty walking, or inability to ambulate can be the chief complaint, depending on the severity of associated spinal cord injury.
- Seizure-like activity or "passing out" is occasionally reported.

PHYSICAL EXAM FINDINGS

Range of neurologic deficits:

- Cervical pain alone
- Cervical myelopathy (C1-C5) with varying degrees of generalized ataxia and tetraparesis
- Stiff, slightly extended head and neck carriage
- Tetraplegia and hypoventilation (rare) in severely affected animals

Etiology and Pathophysiology

- Causes
  - Congenital malformation of the atlas (C1) and/or axis (C2), with associated malarticulation
  - Abnormal development of the dens of C2, including agenesis, hypoplasia, and dorsal angulation and/or malformation; absence; or laxity of the ligaments that normally secure the dens onto the ventral aspect of the C1 vertebral canal (transverse, dorsal atlantoaxial, and/or alar ligaments).
  - Cervical trauma or hyperflexion injury resulting in C2/dens fracture and/or ligamentous rupture
- Any of the above can result in AAI, allowing C2 to subluxate dorsally relative to C1, especially when the neck is ventroflexed. This action causes the dens and cranial aspect of C2 to traumatize the cranial cervical spinal cord, resulting in contusive and compressive injury.
- Associated edema, inflammation +/− hemorrhage can further injure the spinal cord and extend into the caudal brainstem.

DIAGNOSIS

Diagnostic Overview

A tentative diagnosis is based on signalment, history, and clinical signs. Confirmation requires diagnostic imaging.

Differential Diagnosis

- Intervertebral disc disease (C2-C5)
- Vertebral column trauma (C1-C5)
- Meningitis/myelitis: infectious or noninfectious (e.g., granulomatous meningoencephalomyelitis)
- Other congenital anomalies affecting the cervicomedullary junction
- Vertebral column neoplasia (C1-C5)
- Discospondylitis (C2-C5)

Initial Database

- CBC/serum biochemical profile/urinalysis: generally unremarkable (pre-anesthesia)
- Plain radiography under general anesthesia (preferred) or heavy sedation because perfectly positioned images are required to make the diagnosis.
  - Lateral vertebral column radiographic findings
    - Widened space between dorsal aspect of C1 and C2
    - Dorsally displaced dens/cranial body of C2
  - Oblique views
    - If needed to visualize the dens (C2)
  - Stressed views
    - If needed to determine "instability"
    - NOTE: Use *extreme caution* whenever moving the atlantoaxial (AA) joint under anesthesia; use dorsiflexion rather than ventroflexion to demonstrate instability to prevent further spinal cord injury.
  - Ventrodorsal views
    - If needed to determine dens hypoplasia or agenesis
    - For surgical planning

Advanced or Confirmatory Testing

- Plain radiographs usually sufficient to diagnose the problem
- Advanced imaging (MRI [p. 1132] or CT) often useful to rule out other regional differential diagnoses that can be coincident with AAI, such as Chiari-like malformation or syringomyelia.
- NOTE: If surgery is performed for AAI, nontitanium metallic implants prevent future MR/CT imaging of this anatomic region.

TREATMENT

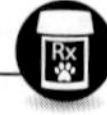

Treatment Overview

- AA joint reduction and stabilization
- Treatment of associated spinal cord injury

Acute General Treatment

- Immobilization of the cervical spine with the AA joint positioned in relative extension
  - Soft, supportive, comfortable bandage extending from the temporomandibular joint (TMJ) to the caudal cervical region. A Styrofoam coffee cup, cut open from top to bottom with the bottom removed, can be gently wrapped around the neck, from just behind the ears (level of TMJ) to the caudal cervical region and secured with a strip of tape.
- Cage confinement
- Pain medication +/− antiinflammatory medication
- Ventilation therapy (p. 1185) if respiratory compromise

Chronic Treatment

Surgical repair: AA joint reduction and stabilization

- Indications
  - Most adult dogs; puppies with marked instability
  - Any dog with recurrent neurologic signs
  - Dorsally angulated dens

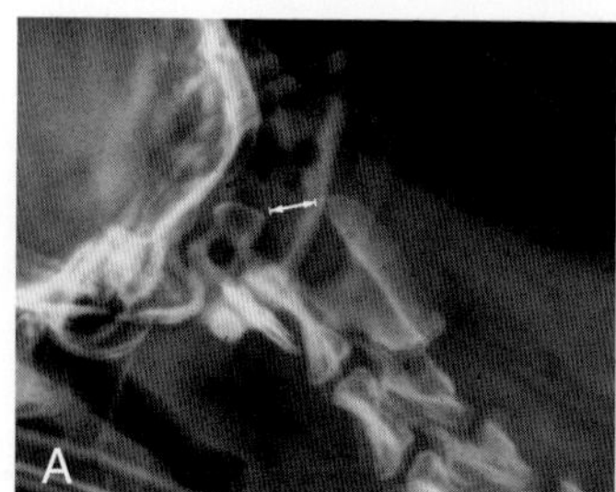

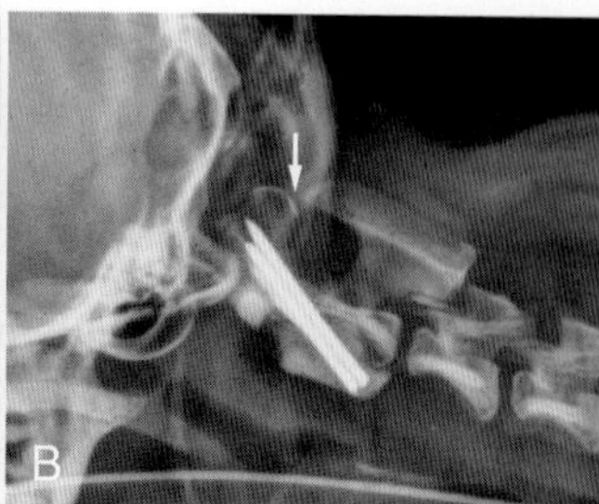

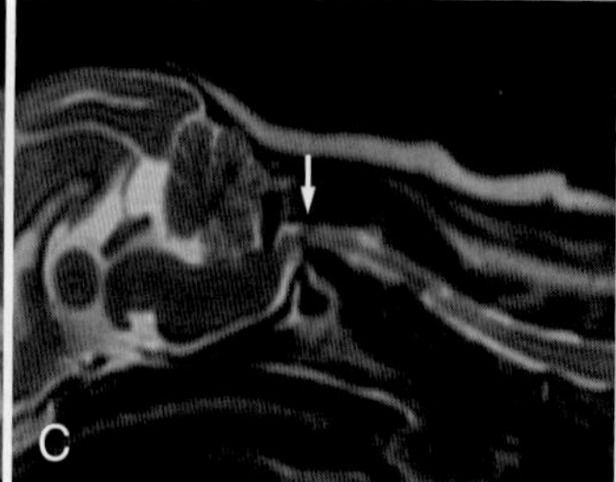

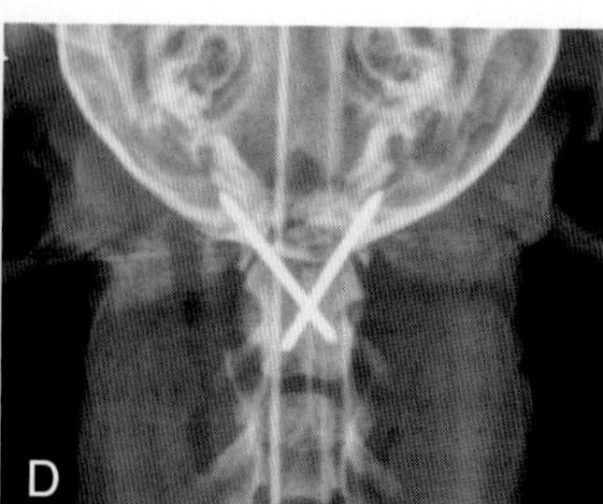

ATLANTOAXIAL INSTABILITY Diagnosis of atlantoaxial instability in a 1-kg Yorkshire terrier. **A, C,** Plain lateral radiographs and midsagittal T2-weighted MR image, neutral view, shows increased space between the dorsal lamina of C1 and C2 *(arrows)*. On the MRI, the dens can be seen compressing the spinal cord. **B, D,** With neck extension, the subluxation reduces *(arrow)*. C1-C2 transarticular pins provide stabilization and promote arthrodesis of the joint.

- Surgical stabilization: various implants used to achieve AA joint immobility
  - Ventral techniques provide superior fixation. Advantages: immediate relief of pain, definitive and long-term resolution of instability through promotion of AA joint arthrodesis. Disadvantages: more technically demanding, high-risk complications.
  - Dorsal repair techniques immobilize the joint variably. The primary advantage is less demanding surgical technique(s). However, there is a higher rate of repair failure and recurrence of disease.

Nonsurgical management:

- Indications
  - Toy breed puppies (<1 year) with good motor function whose bones are too small or too soft to hold implants well; recommend surgical repair in these patients at skeletal maturity, sooner if ambulation is not regained within a few weeks
  - Client is unable or unwilling to pursue surgical repair.
- Recommendations
  - Soft, padded bandage (as above) with cage confinement for 4-8 weeks
  - Pain medication as needed
  - No neck leads; use harness only
  - Change of lifestyle to avoid risky activities (see below)

Behavior/Exercise

Surgically treated patients:

- Avoid sudden or extreme neck flexion, neck leads, play with other dogs, and similar activities for 6 weeks postoperatively, and then gradually resume normal activity.

Nonsurgical approach:

- Avoid behaviors promoting acute neck flexion (e.g., jumping off bed, play with other dogs, tug-of-war).
- May benefit from intermittent use of supportive bandage prn

Possible Complications

Surgical:

- Iatrogenic spinal cord/brainstem injury causing paralysis or death
- Implant infection or failure
- Vertebral fracture and associated complications

Nonsurgical:

- Persistent instability and pain
- Recurrent neurologic signs
- Complications of chronic supportive bandaging

PROGNOSIS & OUTCOME

Surgical:

- Good to excellent prognosis if preoperative motor function is good and surgical repair results in good AA joint reduction and eventual arthrodesis
- Guarded prognosis if minimal preoperative motor function and/or respiratory compromise is present

Nonsurgical:

- Fair prognosis if
  - Dog < 8 months
  - Mild to moderate subluxation/instability
  - Acute onset with no prior occurrence
  - Neurologic signs are mild to moderate
  - Rapid resolution of signs with treatment
- Poor prognosis if
  - Marked subluxation/instability
  - Chronic or recurrent neurologic signs
  - Severe neurologic deficits (respiratory compromise, marked tetraparesis)

PEARLS & CONSIDERATIONS

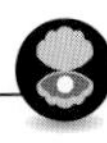

Comments

- Surgical repair of AAI using a ventral technique is the treatment of choice in all dogs except young puppies ≤ 1 kg. Nonsurgical treatment is used in these patients until the dog becomes skeletally mature and surgical repair is feasible. Maintain them in a supportive bandage until surgical repair is performed.
- Minimalist bandaging (see above) is usually effective, better tolerated, and associated with far fewer complications than large, heavy splints and orthotics due to the small size of most AAI patients. It also allows the client to check the bandage daily and keep it clean and dry.

Technician Tips

- Dogs with AAI require constant, gentle attention when handling to avoid acute cervical flexion.
- Take special care during intubation and manipulation under sedation/anesthesia to avoid flexion of the neck. It is best to keep the neck bandaged in mild extension until ready to position for surgery. Once under anesthesia, gently taping the patient to a backboard, with neck in extension is recommended in clinical settings where the patient is transported by gurney or undergoing advanced imaging procedures.
- Meticulous bandage care required

Client Education

- Most dogs develop clinical signs of AAI after minor trauma from routine activities (e.g., jumping off the sofa, playing with other dogs) or traumatic events.
- Nonsurgical treatment must be accompanied by change in lifestyle to avoid activities predisposing to neck trauma; no neck leads should be used (indefinitely).
- Ventral surgical repair effects the best long-term outcome.

SUGGESTED READING

Slanina MC: Atlantoaxial instability. Vet Clin Small Anim 46:265-275, 2016.

AUTHOR: Beverly K. Sturges, DVM, MS, MAS, DACVIM
EDITOR: Karen R. Muñana, DVM, MS, DACVIM (Neurology)

Atonic or Hypotonic Urinary Bladder

BASIC INFORMATION

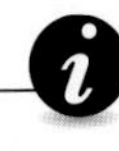

Definition

Absent or incomplete detrusor muscle (bladder wall) contraction

Synonyms

Bladder atony, bladder overdistention, lower motor neuron (LMN) bladder

Epidemiology

SPECIES, AGE, SEX

Dog or cat, any age, either sex

RISK FACTORS

Spinal cord injury/disease, peripheral nervous system disorders (including dysautonomia), urine retention, pelvic injuries

GEOGRAPHY AND SEASONALITY

Dysautonomia

ASSOCIATED DISORDERS

- Cystitis, bacterial (p. 232)
- Incontinence, urinary (p. 538)

Clinical Presentation

DISEASE FORMS/SUBTYPES

- Detrusor atony/hypotonia with sphincter atonia/hypotonia (LMN bladder)
- Detrusor atony/hypotonia with normal or hypertonic sphincter tone
  - Neurogenic: upper motor neuron (UMN) bladder
  - Non-neurogenic: as a result of bladder overdistention from any cause

HISTORY, CHIEF COMPLAINT

- Absent/weak attempts to void
- Leakage or dribbling of urine
- Associated signs of neurologic dysfunction unrelated to micturition (e.g., paresis)

PHYSICAL EXAM FINDINGS

- Distended bladder is characteristic.
- Large volume of residual urine
- Bladder expression may be easy or difficult (depending on sphincter tone, obstruction).
  - LMN (sacral lesion or peripheral nervous system): flaccid bladder, anus, tail
  - UMN (suprasacral lesion): turgid bladder, perineal tone intact
  - Detrusor muscle atony (primary muscle): flaccid bladder, perineal tone intact

Etiology and Pathophysiology

- LMN dysfunction disrupts parasympathetic control of detrusor muscle (p. 871).
  - Intramural bladder weakness, causing inability to contract and empty normally and completely
  - Lesions in sacral spinal cord, sacral nerves, or pelvic plexus
  - Internal urethral sphincter tone may be retained because sympathetic innervation (hypogastric nerve) is not affected by sacral spinal cord lesions.
- Severe UMN lesions (L7 to pons) may lead to loss of voluntary micturition and resultant bladder overdistention.
  - Disinhibition of sympathetic innervation may increase urethral sphincter tone.
- Non-neurogenic bladder atony results from urethral outflow obstruction or pelvic disease (i.e., pain, fractures).
  - Bladder overdistention disrupts tight junctions between detrusor smooth muscle fibers.
  - Disruption inhibits the wave of excitation between myofibers, resulting in a flaccid bladder.

DIAGNOSIS

Diagnostic Overview

Bladder atony is often secondary to an underlying condition affecting function of the urinary bladder and causing urine retention. Diagnosis begins with confirmation of the historical problem and is based on determining the localization (neurogenic versus non-neurogenic) of the primary disease. The physical and neurologic examinations can inform an anatomic or neurologic differential diagnosis.

Differential Diagnosis

- Hypotonia from LMN disease
  - Sacral spinal cord, cauda equina, or nerve root lesions
    - Degenerative: intervertebral disc herniation, degenerative lumbosacral stenosis
    - Anomalous: vertebral malformation
    - Neoplasia, including extradural (primary bone, metastatic [prostatic carcinoma, lymphoma]), intradural extramedullary (meningioma, nerve sheath tumor), and intramedullary (oligodendroglioma, astrocytoma, ependymoma, metastatic [lymphoma, hemangiosarcoma])
    - Infectious: discospondylitis
    - Traumatic: vertebral fracture/luxation, traction spinal cord injury (tail pull/avulsion)
    - Vascular: thromboembolic disease, fibrocartilaginous emboli
  - Peripheral nervous system disease
    - Neuropathy
    - Dysautonomia
    - Myopathy
    - Neuromuscular junction
      - Myasthenia gravis
      - Botulism
- Hypotonia from overdistention
  - Neurogenic
    - UMN lesions (suprasacral: L7 to pons)
  - Non-neurogenic
    - Inability to ambulate or posture for urination, leading to urine retention (e.g., pain, pelvic fracture, inflammation, confinement/behavior)
    - Urethral obstruction causing overdistention (e.g., calculi, intraluminal or extraluminal mass)
    - Infiltrative diseases (inflammatory, neoplasm)

Initial Database

- Residual urine volume increased (normal, < 0.2-0.4 mL/kg in dogs, or < 10 mL in dogs and < 2 mL in cats). Urinary bladder catheterization may allow detection of urethral obstruction.
- Rectal examination
  - Anal tone
    - LMN lesion: decreased or absent
    - UMN or non-neurogenic lesion: present
  - Urethra/prostate: possible obstruction, mass effect
- Neurologic examination and neuroanatomic localization
  - Complete neurologic examination (p. 1136), including perineal and bulbocavernosus reflex, tail tone, and sensory testing
    - UMN lesion (usually T3 to L3): sacral reflexes intact
    - LMN lesion (L7 to coccygeal region; peripheral nerves): decreased or absent reflexes
- Routine blood tests
  - CBC: unremarkable
  - Serum biochemistry profile: unremarkable (with urethral obstruction, may reflect postrenal azotemia, hyperkalemia)
  - Urinalysis, urine culture, and susceptibility: secondary urinary tract infection (UTI) common
- Abdominal radiography: distended bladder; possible evidence of vertebral, pelvic, prostatic disease, or urethral calculi

Advanced or Confirmatory Testing

- Neurodiagnostic testing
  - Electromyography (see www.ExpertConsult.com): denervation potentials indicate peripheral nerve (e.g., pudendal and sciatic nerves) disease
  - Nerve conduction studies (see www.ExpertConsult.com): decreased conduction velocity and abnormal waveform of sciatic nerve indicate neuropathy (e.g., cauda equina, peripheral nerve)
  - Somatosensory evoked response testing: monitors afferent pathways of spinal cord
  - Cross-sectional imaging:
    - MRI: provides detail of neural and surrounding tissues
    - CT: provides detail of spinal column
- Contrast radiography
  - Retrograde urethrography (p. 1181): evaluate for obstructive patterns
- Abdominal ultrasonography may reveal non-neurogenic cause for urine retention (e.g., mass).
- Cystoscopy and urethroscopy (p. 1085): identifies masses causing urethral obstruction
- Urodynamic testing
  - Cystometry: determine bladder contractile function
  - Urethral pressure profile: evaluate urethral tone
  - Leak point pressure measurement: evaluate urethral resistance

TREATMENT

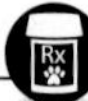

Treatment Overview

Management of bladder atony is contingent on treating the underlying condition. Bladder emptying is important in restoring bladder wall function. Empirical pharmacologic therapy is begun at the low end of the dosage range and adjusted based on observed response. UTI is a common sequela to urine retention and may be difficult to eliminate while bladder function remains defective.

Acute General Treatment

- Urinary bladder catheterization
  - Indwelling urinary catheter (closed-collection system)
  - Intermittent catheterization has a lower risk of inducing UTI than indwelling catheters.
- Urethral sphincter relaxation
  - Smooth muscle relaxation (alpha-antagonists)
    - Prazosin: dogs: 1 mg/15 kg PO q 8-12h; cats: 0.25-0.5 mg/CAT PO q 12-24h. Side effects: hypotension, mild sedation. Contraindications: see phenoxybenzamine.
    - Phenoxybenzamine: dogs: 5-15 mg/DOG PO q 12-24h; cats: 1.25-5 mg/CAT PO q 12h. Onset of action takes up to 4 days. Side effects: hypotension, tachycardia, increased intraocular pressure. Contraindications: cardiovascular disease, glaucoma, kidney disease. Brand-name product (Dibenzyline 10-mg capsules) is cost-prohibitive; USP-grade powder for compounding is more cost-effective.

- Striated (skeletal) muscle relaxation
  - Diazepam: dogs: 2-10 mg/DOG PO q 8h; cats: 2-5 mg/CAT PO q 8h (use with caution) or 0.2-0.5 mg/kg IV as needed. Centrally acting muscle relaxant. Side effects: sedation, excitation, idiosyncratic hepatic necrosis in cats.
  - Methocarbamol: dogs: 15-20 mg/kg PO q 8h; cats: initial dose 33 mg/kg PO q 8h, then 20 mg/kg PO q 8h. Centrally acting muscle relaxant. Side effects: weakness, sedation, lethargy, vomiting.
- Detrusor muscle contraction
  - Bethanechol (parasympathomimetic): dogs: 5-25 mg/DOG PO q 8h; cats: 1.25-5 mg/CAT PO q 8h. Side effects: ptyalism, vomiting, diarrhea, bronchoconstriction. Contraindications: urethral or gastrointestinal obstruction.
  - Cisapride (prokinetic; enhances acetylcholine release): dogs: 0.5 mg/kg PO q 8h; cats: 1.25-5 mg/CAT PO q 8-12h. Side effects: diarrhea, abdominal pain.

Chronic Treatment

- Resolution of underlying disorder
- Long-term supportive drug therapy
- Maintain a small or empty bladder (intermittent catheterization may be required).

Drug Interactions

- Bethanechol minimally effective if tight junctions completely disrupted or when nerves have been avulsed or transected
- Bethanechol may enhance urethral sphincter tone, and it is important to treat with alpha-antagonist (e.g., phenoxybenzamine, prazosin) before starting bethanechol.

Possible Complications

- Bladder wall fibrosis and permanent bladder hypotonia
- Recurrent UTI

Recommended Monitoring

- Frequently monitor voiding activity (provide opportunity to urinate).
- Monitor residual urine volume during catheterization procedures. If residual volume normalizes, catheterization is no longer required.
- Periodic urinalysis ± urine culture; initially every several weeks

PROGNOSIS & OUTCOME

- Good if cause is non-neurogenic
- Guarded for sacral spinal cord lesions
- Poor for dysautonomia, nerve root avulsion, nerve transection, or severe sacral spinal cord injury (especially with loss of nociception)

PEARLS & CONSIDERATIONS

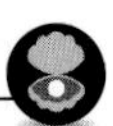

Comments

Expedient and early management of an overdistended bladder is crucial for resolution and prevention of bladder wall fibrosis.

Prevention

- Successful management depends on identification and treatment of underlying disorder.
- Monitoring voiding is important for postoperative neurosurgical and orthopedic patients.

Technician Tips

- To reduce risks for UTI, aseptic protocols (cleanse external catheter and genital areas; change collection bag) should be instituted in patients requiring urinary catheterization.
- Secondary urine overflow increases risks for urine scald and decubitus ulceration. The patient should be kept clean and dry on a padded surface with frequent (q 4h) rotation if recumbent.

Client Education

- If signs persist, the client will need instructions for intermittent bladder catheterization.
- The client should be educated to differentiate urine overflow from voluntary micturition.

SUGGESTED READING

Byron JK. Micturition disorders. Vet Clin Small Anim 45:769-782, 2015.

AUTHOR: Joan R. Coates, DVM, MS, DACVIM
EDITOR: Leah A. Cohn, DVM, PhD, DACVIM

Atopic Dermatitis

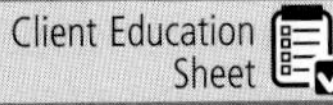

BASIC INFORMATION

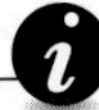

Definition

An inflammatory and pruritic cutaneous hypersensitivity disorder most commonly associated with immunoglobulin E (IgE) antibodies to environmental allergens with genetic predisposition

Epidemiology

SPECIES, AGE, SEX

Dogs and cats: age of onset 4 months to 7 years, typically between 6 months and 3 years

GENETICS, BREED PREDISPOSITION

- Breeds at risk may vary with geographic region and breed popularity.
- Dogs: Boston terrier, boxer, Chinese Shar-pei, Dalmatian, fox terrier, French and English bulldogs, golden and Labrador retrievers, pug, shih tzu, West Highland white terrier, Yorkshire terrier, and many others.
- Cats: no breed predispositions have been demonstrated.

RISK FACTORS

- Dogs: genotype influencing the skin barrier function and immune response, certain breeds are more at risk
- Environmental factors (e.g., regular bathing, born during the pollen season)

GEOGRAPHY AND SEASONALITY

- There is marked geographic variation in specific allergen exposure.
- Depending on exposure to sensitizing allergens and the pruritic threshold, the clinical signs may be seasonal or nonseasonal.
- Majority of patients with seasonal signs exhibit perennial signs over a 1- to 4-year period.

ASSOCIATED DISORDERS

- Concurrent flea allergy dermatitis (more prevalent in flea-endemic areas)
- Concurrent adverse cutaneous food reactions (up to 25% in cats and 30% in dogs)
- Secondary infections with bacteria and yeast are common (especially dogs).
- Otitis externa (common in dogs, rare in cats)
- Hyperhidrosis (sweating)
- Conjunctivitis (20%-60% of dogs)
- Rhinitis (6.7% of dogs)
- Feline asthma (rare)

Clinical Presentation

HISTORY, CHIEF COMPLAINT

- Pruritus is the dominant chief complaint.
- May be presented for pruritic recurrent skin infection (without significant pruritus between episodes of skin infection).
- Other clinical signs may mimic any type of pruritic dermatoses, particularly adverse cutaneous food reactions (p. 345).

PHYSICAL EXAM FINDINGS

Dogs:

- Pruritus (scratching, licking, chewing, rubbing, scooting, head shaking), initially with mild or no visible lesions
- Possible primary erythema (macules or small papules)
- Areas most commonly affected include muzzle, periocular region, ears, flexor aspect of elbows, carpal and tarsal joints, interdigital spaces, axillary and inguinal areas, ventrum, and perianal area.
- Different phenotypes exist (e.g., dorsum commonly affected in Chinese Shar-peis and Labrador retrievers; urticaria is common in boxers).
- Secondary skin lesions: excoriations, alopecia, hyperpigmentation, lichenification, crusting
- Saliva staining of hair may be noted.
- Secondary bacterial and yeast infections of skin and ears, and acute moist dermatitis (hot spots) may also be noted (pp. 247 and 851).

Cats:

- Pruritus (including excessive grooming) rapidly leading to excoriation, especially face, pinnae, and neck
- Papulocrustous (miliary) dermatitis: especially dorsum
- Eosinophilic granuloma complex lesions: indolent ulcer (upper lip), eosinophilic plaque (mainly ventral abdomen), eosinophilic granuloma (p. 300).
- Self-induced alopecia: more or less symmetrical (especially abdomen, medial thighs, front limbs, rump)

Etiology and Pathophysiology

- Atopic dermatitis is a genetically programmed, multifactorial, allergic skin disease in which the patient becomes sensitized to environmental allergens.
- Atopic animals are thought to have a defective epidermal barrier function (aggravated by numerous factors such as the diet, microbial exposure, stress, climate, exposure to skin irritant) and polarization toward a type 2 helper T lymphocyte (T_H2) immunologic response (resulting in high levels of IgE).
- Predisposed patients percutaneously absorb allergens that provoke the production of allergen-specific IgE.
- Inhalation or ingestion of allergen may be of lesser significance.
- After a sensitization phase, epidermal Langerhans cells capture allergens with antigen-specific IgE, provoking a storm of cytokine and chemokine release from keratinocytes, mast cells, and infiltrating eosinophils, neutrophils, allergen-specific T_H2 lymphocytes, and dermal dendritic cells.
- Dogs and cats are most commonly sensitized to house dust and storage mites, molds, pollens, and danders.
- *Malassezia* antigens may represent major allergens, but staphylococcal antigens are not currently proven to have a role. Both *Staphylococcus* spp and *Malassezia* spp frequently cause severe disease exacerbation through secondary infection.
- The role of food allergens as possible triggers for atopic dermatitis is currently accepted.

DIAGNOSIS

Diagnostic Overview

The diagnosis of atopic dermatitis is based on history, physical examination, and ruling out other causes of a similar presentation. Although a different set of clinical criteria have been proposed in dogs to help support a diagnosis of atopic dermatitis (the latest one being the Favrot criteria), there is common agreement that the diagnosis should not be based exclusively on any set of criteria.

Differential Diagnosis

- Ectoparasites: *Sarcoptes*, *Demodex* (especially *D. gatoi* and *D. injai*), *Cheyletiella*, *Notoedres*, *Otodectes*, *Trombicula*, fleas, lice
- Bacterial infections: especially *Staphylococcus pseudintermedius*
- Fungal infections: *Malassezia*, dermatophytosis
- Other hypersensitivities: fleas, food, contact, drug
- Behavioral disorders: feline psychogenic alopecia (rare)
- Neoplasia: epitheliotropic lymphoma

Initial Database

- The minimum database for a pruritic patient should include a complete history and physical examination and a thorough dermatologic examination for ectoparasites, bacteria, and yeast.
- An initial dermatologic database (p. 1091)
  - Skin scrapings
  - Trichography
  - Skin and ear cytologic examination
  - +/– Fungal culture in cats

Advanced or Confirmatory Testing

Testing for allergen-specific IgE (allergy testing)

- Should be performed only when the diagnosis of atopic dermatitis is supported by history, clinical presentation, dermatologic findings, and ruling out other differential diagnoses
- Allergy tests do not diagnose allergy; they only document sensitization, which may have no clinical significance.
- Allergy testing is available as an intradermal test performed by veterinary dermatologists or as a blood test (serologic testing offered by numerous commercial laboratories). Regardless of method, test results must be reviewed in light of allergen exposure and the patient's history.
- *Intradermal testing*: considered gold standard, but animals must be clipped and sedated.
- *Serologic testing:* false-positives are common but more convenient and less affected by antipruritic therapies. No clinical correlation associated with the number and magnitude of positive reactions.
- Poor correlation between intradermal and serologic testing; none of them is standardized. It is probable that the most appropriate information for avoidance and allergen-specific immunotherapy (ASIT) would be gathered by performing both types of testing on every patient, but this may not always be practical.
- Mite infestations *(Sarcoptes*, *Notoedres*, *Otodectes*, *Cheyletiella)* cause cross-reactions with house dust and storage mite antigens, often resulting in false-positive reactions in intradermal and blood testing. These infestations should be treated and allergy testing postponed for 3-4 months if possible.
- Annual vaccinations can cause increased levels of allergen-specific IgE for up to 3 weeks.
- In geographic areas with well-defined, pronounced pollen and mold seasons, allergy testing is best performed at season's end or within 2 months after the peak allergy season.
- Drug therapy can suppress allergy test results.
  - Withdraw oral, topical, and long-acting injectable glucocorticoids for 2-3, 2, and 4-8 weeks, respectively. This applies to intradermal and serologic testing.
  - Withdraw antihistamines and omega-6/omega-3 fatty acid–containing supplements and diets at least 7 days before intradermal testing.
  - Cyclosporine does not appear to affect allergy test results. However, withdrawal for days to weeks might be considered if administered for a number of months.
  - Oclacitinib and lokivetmab (Apoquel and Cytopoint) do not appear to interfere with results of intradermal or serologic testing.
  - Avoid acepromazine, oxymorphone, and morphine if sedating the patient for intradermal testing.

TREATMENT

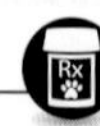

Treatment Overview

- Atopic dermatitis is almost always a lifelong problem, and the goal is to eliminate or minimize allergen exposure while maintaining the pet's comfort and homeostasis of the skin.
- Appropriate clinical protocol depends on the seasonality of the problem, distribution and severity of lesions, concurrent health issues, patient and client compliance, and cost and availability of therapy. It typically requires adjustment over time.
- Allergen avoidance is ideal but rarely possible.
- Although ASIT is the sole therapy inducing immune tolerance to the offending allergens, additional antipruritic therapy is often required.
- Secondary yeast and bacterial infections should be controlled by appropriate therapy before any attempt is made to further control pruritus.
- Antiparasitic preventives should be administered to avoid pruritic parasitic infestation.

Acute and Chronic Treatment

Because of the multifactorial nature of atopic dermatitis, the best therapeutic approach often involves combinations of multiple modalities (topical/systemic and short-term/long-term) individualized for each patient.

Corticosteroids:

- Highly and rapidly effective for controlling pruritus associated with environmental allergies (short-term and long-term use)
- May be administered orally or topically (if pruritus is localized)
- Although topicals are considered safer, they can cause local and systemic adverse effects (skin absorption).
- Dogs: prednisone or prednisolone at an initial daily dose of 0.5-1 mg/kg/day before weaning to an alternate-day schedule is the first choice glucocorticoid for atopic dermatitis.
- Cats: prednisolone at an initial daily dose 1-2 mg/kg/day or dexamethasone 0.1-0.2 mg/kg/day, then q 48-72h, respectively.

Cyclosporine:

- Cyclosporine is an effective, slow-acting (2-3 weeks) calcineurin inhibitor and potent immunomodulatory agent.
- Microemulsion type (Atopica): 5 mg/kg (dog) or 7 mg/kg (cat) PO q 24h
- Between 50% and 65 % of dogs will have a satisfactory reduction in pruritus. About half of dogs that benefit from daily cyclosporine will continue to do well on alternate-day therapy.
- Treatment is expensive, especially for medium- or large-breed dogs.
- Vomiting is the most common side effect, although gingival hyperplasia, hypertrichosis, and secondary infections (viral, bacterial) have been noted.
- Cats that have a negative *Toxoplasma* titer should be confined indoors.

Oclacitinib:

- Oclacitinib (Apoquel), a fast-acting Janus kinase inhibitor, blocks the action of some proinflammatory and pruritogenic cytokines, especially interleukin-31 (IL-31).
- Dogs: 0.4-0.6 mg/kg PO q 12h for up to 14 days and then administered q 24h
- A flare-up of clinical signs may be noticed when reduced to once daily.
- About 70% of dogs experience a reduction in pruritus of at least 50% (useful for short-term and/or long-term management).
- Not approved for use in cats nor dogs younger than 12 months
- Adverse reactions are uncommon; leukopenia is reported.

Lokivetmab:

- Leukivetmab (Cytopoint), a caninized monoclonal antibody (mAb) that targets canine IL-31, is a safe and very effective therapy for controlling clinical signs associated with atopic dermatitis.
- Dogs: 2 mg/kg SQ every 4-8 weeks. DO NOT USE IN CATS.
- No specific adverse events have been reported with its use nor when administered concomitantly with other drugs (antibiotics, antifungals, and allergy medications).

Antihistamines:

- Not to be used as sole therapy in severe cases nor in acute phase
- Limited benefit; may alleviate pruritus in 20%-30% of cases
- Responses are unpredictable; several compounds should be given in 2-week trials.
- May be used in combination with other therapies
- Side effects include drowsiness, lethargy, and nervousness. Reducing the frequency of administration and dose may minimize these effects.
- Oral antihistamines that may have some benefit for dogs include hydroxyzine 2.2 mg/kg PO q 8-12h, diphenhydramine 2.2 mg/kg PO q 8-12h, chlorpheniramine 0.4 mg/kg q 8-12h, amitriptyline 1 mg/kg PO q 12h
- Antihistamines that may be useful in cats include chlorpheniramine 2 to 4 mg/CAT q 12h, amitriptyline 0.5-1 mg/kg PO q 12h.

Essential fatty acids (EFAs):

- No clear evidence supporting real benefit of supplementing with EFA, but can be part of long-term management
- May alleviate pruritus in 10%-20% of cases. They are given for 4-12-week trials, usually not as sole therapy.
- Omega-3 EFA in oral capsule form as a supplement (eicosapentaenoic acid 30-40 mg/kg/day) or in food may theoretically help manage pruritus by decreasing the production of proinflammatory mediators.

Topical antipruritic therapy:

- A cool bath has an antipruritic effect from the cooling effect of evaporation and rehydrating the skin.
- Mild cleansing or moisturizing (e.g., colloidal oatmeal) shampoos +/− conditioners may be beneficial.
- Spot-on or spray barrier-restoring products (e.g., ceramides, phytosphingosine) are of undetermined benefit.
- Topical glucocorticoids (Cortavance, Genesis) are useful for focal areas of pruritus and to prevent flare-ups.
- Topical 0.1% tacrolimus (Protopic), a calcineurin inhibitor, is useful for focal areas of pruritus. The U.S. Food and Drug Administration (FDA) has issued a public health advisory warning of a potential cancer risk. If used, apply short-term or intermittently.
- Physical barriers (e.g., Elizabethan collar, T-shirts, bodysuits, boots) may be helpful in preventing self-trauma and secondary infections

ASIT:

- Subcutaneous or oral (sublingual immunotherapy) administration of a gradually increasing dose of allergens that produced positive reactions on allergy testing, are present in the patient's environment, and are consistent with the patient's allergy season.
- Beneficial in approximately 70% of cases
- ASIT is usually considered to treat atopic dermatitis if there is a long allergy season or nonseasonal pruritus, when antipruritic therapy does not provide sufficient relief, or when allergy medications are contraindicated.
- Response to therapy is individualized; may be seen as early as 1 month or may take up to a year.
- Maintenance treatments are given as often as needed to maintain the response (usually every 1-3 weeks), and usually therapy is lifelong. Sublingual immunotherapy is administered 6 days a week.

Drug Interactions

Drugs that inhibit cytochrome P450 enzymes (azoles, macrolides, avermectins, corticosteroids) will increase cyclosporine blood levels.

PROGNOSIS & OUTCOME

- With environmental allergy, it is imperative that clients understand that the allergy is likely to affect the pet (and owners) for life.
- With good client compliance and individualized therapy, > 90% of cases can be satisfactorily managed, particularly with the recent availability of effective systemic antipruritic therapies.

PEARLS & CONSIDERATIONS

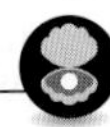

Comments

- Canine atopic-like dermatitis is a similar disease in which IgE cannot be detected (negative results for serology and intradermal tests).
- Hypoallergenic diet may be helpful in some atopic patients.
- Topical and/or systemic antipruritic therapy should be part of the therapy, at least initially, when ASIT is indicated.
- Routine follow-up examinations, including physical examination, CBC, chemistry profile, and urinalysis, are recommended every 6-12 months for dogs on long-term therapy, especially a corticosteroid.
- Canine atopic dermatitis has a strong genetic component, and affected dogs should not be used for breeding.

Technician Tips

- Client counseling is very important before starting treatment; unrealistic expectations and lack of understanding are causes of client dissatisfaction.
- The regular use of topical antimicrobials (shampoos or sprays) and regular baths may help control microbial overgrowth and wash out allergens caught by hairs.

SUGGESTED READING

Hensel P, et al: Canine atopic dermatitis: detailed guidelines for diagnosis and allergen identification. BMC Vet Res 11:196-209, 2015.

AUTHOR: Frédéric Sauvé, DMV, MSc, DES, DACVD
EDITOR: Manon Paradis, DMV, MVSc, DACVD

Atrial Fibrillation

Bonus Material Online Client Education Sheet 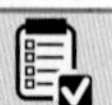

BASIC INFORMATION

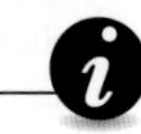

Definition

Atrial fibrillation is a supraventricular arrhythmia characterized by a rapid, irregular rhythm.

Synonym

A fib

Epidemiology

SPECIES, AGE, SEX

- Atrial fibrillation (AF) is the most common clinically significant arrhythmia in dogs, but cats are rarely affected.
- Incidence low in dogs < 2 years old, increases with age
- Giant breed dogs develop AF earlier in life, small breeds later in life.
- Males are overrepresented (60%-75%); females have later onset with longer survival.

GENETICS, BREED PREDISPOSITION

AF is most common in giant and large-breed dogs; small-breed dogs have a low susceptibility to AF.

- Highest predisposition in Irish wolfhound (IWH), Great Dane, Newfoundland, mastiff, St. Bernard, Doberman, and Bouvier des Flandres
- In IWHs, multiple genetic loci are responsible for inherited dilated cardiomyopathy (DCM) (affecting 9.5%) and AF (affecting 80.5% of those with DCM).
- In Dobermans, mutation in *PDK4* (NCSU DCM1) and NCSU DCM2 can lead to DCM; AF is often associated with end-stage DCM.

RISK FACTORS

- Structural heart disease resulting in atrial fibrosis and atrial enlargement predisposes to AF.
  - DCM
  - Chronic atrioventricular (AV) valvular heart disease
  - Congenital heart diseases (e.g., left-to-right shunting patent ductus arteriosus)
  - Infiltrative disease (e.g., cardiac neoplasia)
- Gastrointestinal disease
- Hypothyroidism
- Hypoadrenocorticism
- Mechanical irritation of the myocardium (e.g., pericardiocentesis, cardiac catheterization)
- Drugs (especially anesthetic drugs, opiates)
- Inherently large hearts in giant-breed dogs predispose to AF, even when no overt structural cardiac disease is present (lone fibrillation).
- Cats with hypertrophic, restrictive, or dilated cardiomyopathy and secondary atrial enlargement are predisposed.

Clinical Presentation

DISEASE FORMS/SUBTYPES

- Chronic AF: associated with atrial dilation and structural heart disease
- Paroxysmal AF: may terminate when underlying systemic disease is corrected
- Primary (lone) AF: occurs without an identifiable cause or structural heart disease in giant breeds

HISTORY, CHIEF COMPLAINT

- AF may be an incidental finding.
- Weakness, exercise intolerance, anorexia are common
- May show signs of congestive heart failure (CHF): dyspnea, ascites, cough
- Syncope (rare)

PHYSICAL EXAM FINDINGS

- Irregularly irregular rhythm (as opposed to a regularly irregular rhythm, as in sinus arrhythmia)
- Heart rate (HR) is usually rapid (up to 250 beats/min), particularly if structural heart disease is present.
- Variable pulse strength with pulse deficits
- Signs associated with underlying heart disease or concurrent CHF: murmur, dyspnea, pulmonary crackles, and/or ascites

Etiology and Pathophysiology

- Atrial pathology and/or increased atrial size predisposes to AF
- Atrial stretch, fibrosis, or altered autonomic tone, as occurs during CHF, predisposes to atrial premature contractions (APCs)
  - Atrial stretch is associated with increased dispersion of refractoriness and altered electrical propagation.
  - APCs originating from abnormal atrial tissue or from pulmonary veins can trigger onset of reentry arrhythmias.
  - Multiple, simultaneous reentrant wavelets create continuous chaotic electrical activity.
- The atrial activity in AF is irregular and usually exceeds 400 beats/min.
  - The AV node filters many of these impulses, resulting in an irregular, rapid ventricular response.
- Hemodynamic compromise may occur as the result of loss of the atrial kick.
  - Suboptimal ventricular filling, especially at high rates, can decrease cardiac output up to 30%.
  - AF can trigger onset or recurrence of CHF by decreased cardiac output and tachycardia.

DIAGNOSIS

Diagnostic Overview

AF is suspected based on auscultation of a rapid, irregularly irregular heart rhythm that is typically accompanied by pulse deficits. An electrocardiogram (ECG) confirms the diagnosis.

Differential Diagnosis

On the ECG, AF should be differentiated from

- Baseline artifact (poor grounding, purring, shivering movement): ventricular rate is not irregularly irregular, P waves appear if interference is corrected.
- Atrial flutter: atrial activity shows regular sawtooth pattern instead of irregular F waves. R-R intervals may show regularity, even if variable conduction across AV node (e.g., 2:1, 3:1, 4:1)
- Atrial tachycardia: has distinct P′ waves at PP intervals of up to 300 beats/min. If P′ waves are hiding in preceding T waves, try vagal maneuver to slow down rate.
- Wide QRS tachycardia: can be true ventricular tachycardia; rhythm may be irregular, similar to AF, but QRS is wide and bizarre, sometimes polymorphic versus AF with a ventricular conduction disturbance (bundle branch block), which can mimic ventricular tachycardia
- Atrial standstill: the R-R intervals are usually regular, and rate is slow (escape rhythm) versus AF with low-voltage or invisible F-wave oscillations may appear as if there is absence of atrial activation.

Initial Database

ECG is the gold standard for diagnosis. Auscultation raises suspicion of AF but is not a definitive test. ECG features of AF:

- An irregularly irregular ventricular rhythm (irregular RR intervals with no predictable pattern)
  - At very fast rates, the irregularity is harder to appreciate.
- The ventricular rate is typically fast but may be normal.
- Narrow QRS complexes (but QRS complexes may appear wide due to concurrent ventricular conduction disturbance [bundle branch block])
- No distinct P waves (in any leads)
- +/− F waves (low-voltage oscillations of various amplitudes) visible during diastolic interval
- Vagal maneuver may decrease the ventricular rate and aid in the diagnosis of AF by revealing definitive lack of P waves
- Thoracic radiography and echocardiography aid in diagnosing underlying cardiac disease and CHF.

Advanced or Confirmatory Testing

Ventricular rate during AF is influenced by autonomic tone; stressful situations such as hospital visits typically elevate the ventricular rate excessively. To verify if a dog has chronically

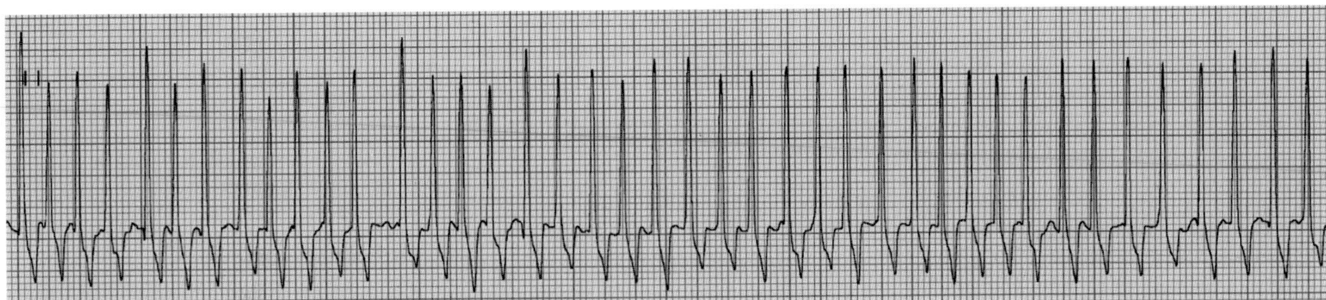

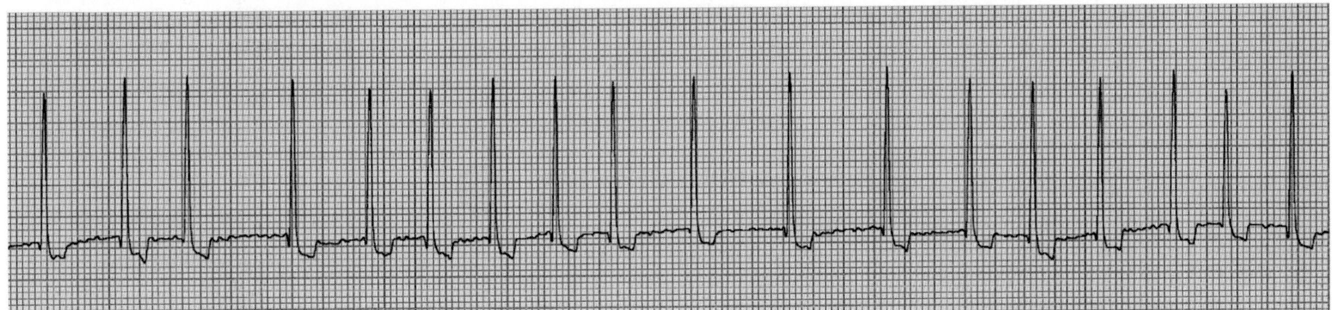

ATRIAL FIBRILLATION A, Lead II ECG showing atrial fibrillation with a rapid ventricular response rate (290-300 bpm) in a dog with CHF. Note the narrow QRS complexes and irregular R-R intervals (often less apparent at rapid ventricular rates). 25 mm/sec. **B,** Lead II ECG showing atrial fibrillation in the same dog 2 weeks after appropriate treatment for CHF, including diltiazem and digoxin. The ventricular response rate is 120-130 bpm, and the irregularity of the R-R intervals and lack of P waves can be seen easily. 25 mm/sec.

elevated HR, a 24-hour ambulatory ECG (Holter) recording in the home environment is recommended (p. 1120).

TREATMENT

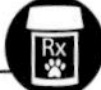

Treatment Overview

Goal of treatment of AF is to reduce long-term effects of uncontrolled tachycardia on myocardial function. Aims are either

- Restore and maintain sinus rhythm with electric or pharmacologic cardioversion (rhythm control). Most dogs fail pharmacologic cardioversion or do not maintain sinus rhythm for very long after electric cardioversion because of advanced myocardial pathology.
- Control the ventricular rate by slowing conduction across the AV node with antiarrhythmic drugs (rate control), allowing AF to persist but at a reduced HR. Target HR on an in-hospital ECG with rate control therapy should be less than 150 beats/min, or on Holter, a 24-hour mean HR should be less than 125 beats/min.

Acute General Treatment

- For unstable dogs (overt weakness, syncope, or CHF) with HR > 250 beats/min, consider the calcium channel blocker (CCB) diltiazem IV bolus (0.1-0.25 mg/kg IV up to 3 times) and/or constant rate infusion (2-6 mcg/kg/min).
  - If impaired systolic function is suspected (e.g., DCM), monitor blood pressure during infusion of CCB because of the negative inotropic effects (choose lowest dose and titrate upward based on response).
  - Simultaneously treat CHF, if present, because cardiac decompensation contributes to high sympathetic tone and fast ventricular response (p. 408).
- For acute onset of vagally mediated AF (e.g., under anesthesia/opioid administration) attempt cardioversion using IV lidocaine as a rapid bolus at 2-3 mg/kg over 5 seconds. Repeat up to 3 times, not to exceed 8 mg/kg.
- Electrical cardioversion or pharmacologic cardioversion (with amiodarone) may be attempted by a cardiologist. There is limited success in restoring normal sinus rhythm long term with these techniques in veterinary patients.

Chronic Treatment

For rate control, CCB, digoxin, and beta-blockers are used alone or in combination. Combination therapy of diltiazem with digoxin controls ventricular rate better than monotherapy.

- Diltiazem extended-release (Dilacor-XR, Cardizem-CD): 2.5-3.5 mg/kg PO q 12h (dog), 30-60 mg/dose PO q 12-24h (cat) *or* diltiazem modified release: diltiazem CD 2-3 mg/kg PO q 8h (dog). Effect on HR occurs within a few hours of oral dosing. Only mild effects on contractility when given at prescribed doses
- Atenolol: 0.5-2 mg/kg q 12-24h; start at a low dose and titrate up as needed; use caution in dogs with poor systolic function or in heart failure
- Digoxin
  - Dog: 0.003-0.004 mg/kg PO q 12h (or 0.11 mg/m^2 q 12 h). Not to exceed 0.25 mg q 12h
  - Cat: 0.03125 mg (one quarter of 0.125-mg tablet)/CAT PO q 48-72h
- In patients with AF and significant concurrent ventricular arrhythmias, sotalol (1-2 mg/kg PO q 12h) may be used cautiously for rate control and suppression of ventricular arrhythmias. Sotalol can also be combined with digoxin.
- Cats with AF usually have structural heart disease and require anticoagulation (p. 505); dogs typically do not require anticoagulation.

Drug Interactions

- Simultaneous administration of digoxin with amiodarone or quinidine can increase digoxin serum concentrations and potentially cause digoxin toxicosis.
- CCB should not be combined with beta-blockers for rate control because excessive AV block, hypotension, and reduced cardiac contractility may ensue.

Possible Complications

- CCB
  - Overdose causes excessive AV block (pauses); clinical signs include weakness, lethargy, or fainting.
  - Without clinical signs (listed above), pauses noted during sleep on a 24-hour Holter should not be a reason to lower the dose of rate control medication.
  - Intravenous CCB may cause transient hypotension and reduced contractility; start with very low dose and monitor arterial blood pressure. Titrate to effect. Stop infusion if hypotension is evident.

- Beta-blocker: same as CCB
  - Not recommended in dogs with acute decompensated CHF
  - When discontinuing chronic beta-blocker therapy, taper over several days to avoid risk of catecholamine-mediated arrhythmias.
- Digoxin
  - Signs of digoxin toxicity include lethargy, inappetance, vomiting/diarrhea. Occasionally, proarrhythmic effects are seen (first-degree AV block, ventricular arrhythmias). Elimination half-life in dog: 14-56 hours; if digoxin toxicity is suspected, stop digoxin for several days, and then start up again at a lower dose. Consider reducing the dose of digoxin in the presence of cachexia, ascites or obesity, hypoproteinemia, hypokalemia, hypothyroidism, renal dysfunction.

Recommended Monitoring

- To determine efficacy of pharmacologic rate control therapy, repeat ECG or ideally a 24-hour Holter in the home environment 5-7 days after starting oral medications.
- To avoid toxicity, digoxin serum concentrations should be measured 5-7 days after starting digoxin therapy at trough levels (6-8 hours after pilling). Ideal trough level should be 0.5-1.0 ng/mL.

PROGNOSIS & OUTCOME

CHF is a major risk factor for development of AF and vice versa. The combination of AF and CHF carries a worse prognosis than either alone. Mortality of dogs with AF is associated with the HR. Median survival of dogs under rate control therapy achieving a mean 24-hour average HR < 125 beats/min was 2.8 years, but for dogs with a mean 24-hour HR ≥ 125 beats/min, it was only 3.75 months. Dogs without underlying disease have a better prognosis; median survival for lone AF is 3.3 years.

PEARLS & CONSIDERATIONS

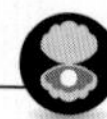

Comments

If AF and acute decompensated CHF (especially pulmonary edema) are present simultaneously, treatment of CHF (e.g., diuretics, pimobendan) must be instituted at the same time as rate control therapy. Either abnormality is very difficult to resolve while the other is present (rapid HR and CHF).

Prevention

Dogs with AF from breeds with a known genetic predisposition (e.g., IWH) should be excluded from breeding programs, even if no overt structural heart disease is identified.

Technician Tips

Counting the HR by auscultation is usually inaccurate in AF when the rate is > 180 beats/min. Obtain an ECG to confirm the diagnosis and to get an accurate HR assessment.

SUGGESTED READING

Pedro B, et al: Retrospective evaluation of the effect of heart rate on survival in dogs with atrial fibrillation. J Vet Intern Med 32(1):86-92, 2018.

AUTHOR: Anna R. M. Gelzer, DMV, PhD, DACVIM, DECVIM
EDITOR: Meg M. Sleeper, VMD, DACVIM

Atrial Premature Complexes and Atrial Tachycardia

BASIC INFORMATION

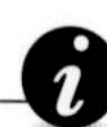

Definition

- Atrial premature complex (APC): a premature beat originating from ectopic focus in the atria
- Atrial tachycardia (AT): a rapid, regular rhythm originating from a focus in the atria other than the sinus node (three or more consecutive APCs are considered AT)
- Supraventricular tachycardia (SVT): originates from the atria or the atrioventricular (AV) junction (includes AT and AV junctional tachycardia)
  - This definition may also be considered to include atrial fibrillation and atrial flutter, which are discussed in a separate section (p. 94).

Synonyms

Premature atrial or supraventricular complex, contraction, or impulse

Epidemiology

SPECIES, AGE, SEX

Occasional APCs can be a normal occurrence in very old dogs.

GENETICS, BREED PREDISPOSITION

An orthodromic reciprocating tachycardia (antegrade conduction through the AV node and retrograde back to the atria by a bypass tract) has been identified in Labrador retrievers.

RISK FACTORS

Cardiac diseases, especially those causing atrial enlargement:

- Chronic myxomatous/degenerative valvular heart disease
- Dilated, hypertrophic, or restrictive cardiomyopathy
- Congenital heart disease
- Atrial tumors such as hemangiosarcoma

Noncardiac disease:

- Increased sympathetic tone
- Hyperthyroidism
- Sepsis
- Electrolyte and acid-base abnormalities (i.e., hypokalemia)
- Hypoxemia
- Anemia

Drugs:

- Digoxin toxicity (may produce AT with AV block)
- Sympathomimetic agents
- Anesthetic agents

Ventricular pre-excitation:

- Wolff-Parkinson-White syndrome

Clinical Presentation

DISEASE FORMS/SUBTYPES

- Isolated APCs
- AT, SVT: paroxysmal (noncontinuous bursts of at least three APCs in a row) or sustained (continuous)

HISTORY, CHIEF COMPLAINT

- May be an incidental finding in a patient without clinical signs
- Syncope or weakness are possible with rapid tachycardias
- Patient may have dyspnea related to congestive heart failure (CHF).
- SVTs may rarely precipitate sudden death if resultant myocardial ischemia leads to ventricular tachycardia or fibrillation or if antiarrhythmic medications used in treatment have a proarrhythmic effect.

PHYSICAL EXAM FINDINGS

- An irregular heart rhythm is ausculted with early beats.
  - When beats are very premature, pulse deficits are also noted.
  - It is not possible to determine whether a premature beat is an APC or a ventricular premature complex (VPC) on physical examination alone.
- A burst or bursts of a rapid, regular rhythm can be ausculted with paroxysmal AT/SVT or can be sustained with continuous AT/SVT.

Etiology and Pathophysiology

- Hemodynamic effects of atrial tachyarrhythmias depend on the underlying disease, ventricular rate, and whether the patient is at rest or exercising.
  - Excessively rapid ventricular rates reduce cardiac output, systemic blood pressure, and coronary artery perfusion secondary to the shortened diastolic interval.
- Sustained or frequently recurrent ATs may lead to tachycardia-induced cardiomyopathy,

which may be reversible with appropriate treatment.

DIAGNOSIS

Diagnostic Overview

Initial suspicion is usually based on auscultation of premature beats or a rapid heart rate. Definitive diagnosis is made based on the electrocardiogram (ECG).

Differential Diagnosis

- AT must be differentiated from sinus tachycardia; sinus tachycardia is usually an appropriate physiologic tachycardia in response to pain or anxiety.
- Uncommonly, atrial arrhythmias may coexist with aberrant conduction/bundle branch block, producing wide QRS complexes and causing APCs and AT to appear similar to VPCs and ventricular tachycardia, respectively. With APCs and AT/SVT, a P′ wave precedes each QRS complex at a repeatable interval (sometimes buried in preceding T wave).

Initial Database

ECG (APCs):

- A P′ wave represents premature atrial depolarization. Its ectopic origin (outside the sinoatrial node) means it propagates differently through the atria than a sinus-origin impulse, and P′ waves are therefore of different shape and occur sooner (prematurely) compared to the expected normal P waves.
- The complete heartbeat (P′-QRS-T) occurs earlier than the next expected sinus beat.
- P′ waves may not be visible if the rate is so fast that they are buried in the preceding T wave or they are isoelectric in that lead (examine other ECG leads).
- QRS complexes typically are narrow and positive in lead II, like the patient's sinus QRS complexes.
- APCs are usually followed by a noncompensatory pause; the ectopic atrial impulse resets the sinus node, such that the R-R interval of two normal sinus complexes enclosing the APC is less than the R-R intervals of three consecutive sinus complexes.

ECG (AT):

- Three or more APCs in a row; regular or slightly irregular rhythm
- P′ waves are present but may be hidden or superimposed on preceding T waves.
- The onset and termination at AT is usually sudden (paroxysmal) and does not speed up or slow down.
- The P′R interval is usually constant.
- Narrow QRS complexes (rarely, can be wide with coexisting bundle branch block or aberrant conduction)
- At extremely rapid atrial rates, there may be varying degrees of AV block (i.e., nonconducted P′ waves due to refractoriness of the AV node).

ECG (AV junctional tachycardia):

- Negative P′ waves in lead II
- Difficult to distinguish from AT

Vagal maneuver:

- May suddenly terminate atrial and junctional tachycardias or slow rate to aid in diagnosis
- Should have no effect on ventricular tachycardia

Thoracic radiography and echocardiography: may be used in diagnosing underlying cardiac disease or concurrent CHF.

Advanced or Confirmatory Testing

Electrophysiologic studies: may be used for determining the underlying mechanism of arrhythmia. Not widely available.

TREATMENT

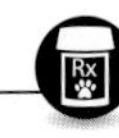

Treatment Overview

- Always correct underlying cause or contributing factors first (e.g., CHF/hypoxemia, hypokalemia, acidosis, hypovolemia).
- Return hemodynamic stability, especially with continuous rapid AT; isolated, infrequent APCs do not cause hemodynamic instability, and no specific treatment is required.
- Conversion of the arrhythmia to sinus rhythm is not always possible, especially with atrial enlargement (substrate for arrhythmia recurrence/persistence).
- Control the ventricular response rate if too rapid.
  - Target rate is achieved with drugs that slow AV node conduction to optimize the ventricular rate.
  - Target rate varies with the underlying cardiac disease.
  - Intravenous (IV) treatment if extremely rapid rate and/or causing clinical signs (e.g., severe anxiety, syncope)
  - Oral medications to reduce long-term effect of uncontrolled tachycardia on myocardial function

Acute General Treatment

- AT/SVT producing sustained ventricular rates > 250 beats/min in dogs often severely compromises diastolic ventricular filling and can be considered critical; IV antiarrhythmics to decrease ventricular rate are warranted. Patients should have an IV catheter and continuous ECG monitoring during drug administration.
- Perform vagal maneuver first. Some ATs/SVTs terminate with ocular pressure or carotid sinus massage. If not, judicious IV drugs are warranted.
- Calcium channel blockers: commonly used as first-choice agents:
  - Diltiazem: 0.05 mg/kg IV over 1-2 min, repeat prn to total dose of 0.75 mg/kg, *or*
  - Verapamil: 0.05 mg/kg IV q 5-10 min up to total dose of 0.15 mg/kg, or 2-10 micrograms/kg/min constant rate infusion
- Beta-blockers:
  - Esmolol: 0.05-0.5 mg/kg slow IV; can follow with 0.05-0.1 mg/kg/min constant rate infusion if needed, *or*
  - Propranolol: 0.02 mg/kg IV slowly over 2-3 minutes, titrate dose up to effect (to maximum of 0.1 mg/kg)

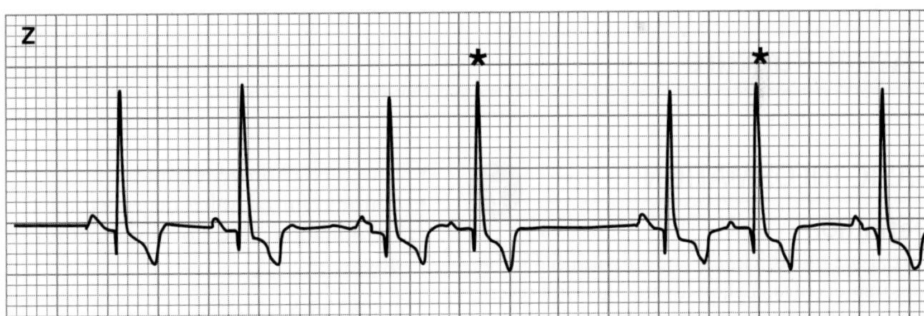

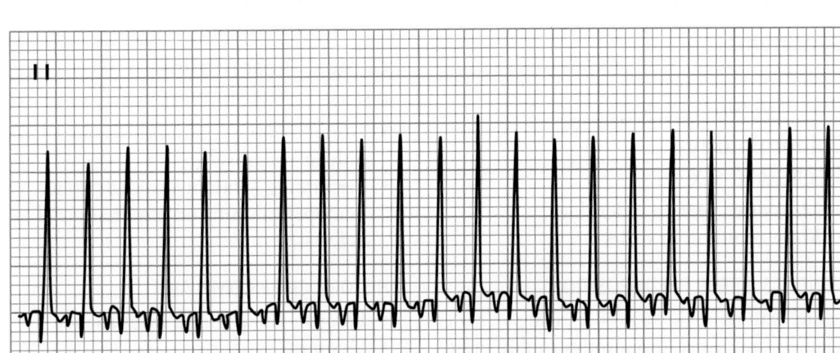

ATRIAL PREMATURE COMPLEXES A, Lead II ECG showing atrial premature complexes *(asterisks)* in a dog with respiratory sinus arrhythmia. A P′ wave initiates a heartbeat that is premature but with a QRS complex that is of the same shape as the sinus QRS complexes (25 mm/sec). **B**, Atrial/supraventricular tachycardia lead II ECG showing a rapid, narrow-complex, monomorphic (QRS complexes all of the same shape) tachycardia. The heart rate is 330 beats/min. A supraventricular tachycardia is diagnosed on the basis of the narrow, upright QRS complexes in this lead II tracing (25 mm/sec).

Chronic Treatment

Calcium channel blockers:

- Diltiazem (Cardizem): 0.5-2 mg/kg (titrated to maximum of 4 mg/kg) PO q 8h (dog), 7.5 mg/dose PO q 8-12h (cat)
- Diltiazem-sustained release (Dilacor-XL, Cardizem-CD): 1.5-6 mg/kg PO q 12-24h (dog), 30-60 mg/dose PO q 12-24h (cat)
- Verapamil: 0.5-3 mg/kg PO q 8h (dog)

Beta-blockers:

- Atenolol (start low, titrate to effect): 0.5-1 mg/kg PO q 12-24h or start at 6.25-12.5 mg q 12-24h and up-titrate to effect (dog); 6.25-12.5 mg/dose PO q 12-24h (cat)

Digoxin: 0.005-0.01 mg/kg PO q 12h, not to exceed 0.25 mg PO q 12h (or 0.00425 mg/kg q 12h for elixir) (dog); 0.03125 mg/dose (one quarter of 0.125-mg tablet) PO q 48-72h (cat)

Combination therapy is sometimes necessary (see Drug Interactions).

Drug Interactions

- Simultaneous administration of digoxin with verapamil, amiodarone, or quinidine can increase digoxin serum concentrations and potentially cause digoxin toxicosis.
- There are many potential drug interactions associated with digoxin, and the patient's complete medication regimen should be reviewed.
- It is generally not recommended to use calcium channel blockers in conjunction with beta-blockers due to combined negative effects on blood pressure and contractility.

Possible Complications

- Calcium channel blockers, beta-blockers: much more likely to cause complications with IV use. Use repeated small doses with monitoring instead of single large dose.
    - Negative inotropism (especially verapamil and beta-adrenergic blockers) (use with caution with left ventricular systolic dysfunction)
    - Hypotension (lesser risk with beta-blockers compared to calcium channel blockers)
    - Severe bradycardia or asystole
    - Gastrointestinal (GI) signs with oral calcium channel blockers
- Chronic beta-blocker therapy should not be abruptly discontinued (risk of excessive catecholamine-mediated tachycardia).
- Digoxin
    - GI signs related to toxicity (anorexia, vomiting, diarrhea)
    - AV block, other arrhythmias

Recommended Monitoring

- Serial ECGs
- Digoxin: measure trough (6-8 hours after dose) digoxin serum level 7-10 days after starting therapy or adjusting dose

PROGNOSIS & OUTCOME

Depends on underlying cause and cardiac disease

PEARLS & CONSIDERATIONS

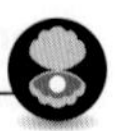

Comments

The absence of a P′ wave cannot always differentiate a VPC from an APC. The P′ wave before an APC may be superimposed (hidden) in the preceding complex. Additionally, if a VPC is only mildly premature a sinus P wave may be identified.

Technician Tips

APCs are differentiated from ventricular premature complexes on ECG based on a narrow QRS appearance, which is similar to the normal sinus beats.

SUGGESTED READING

Tilley LP: Analysis of common canine cardiac arrhythmias. In Tilley LP, editor: Essentials of canine and feline electrocardiography, Philadelphia, 1992, Lippincott Williams & Wilkins, pp 127-207.

AUTHOR: Rebecca L. Malakoff, DVM, DACVIM
EDITOR: Meg M Sleeper, VMD, DACVIM

Atrial Rupture

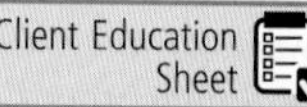

BASIC INFORMATION

Definition

Partial- or full-thickness endomyocardial splitting that occurs occasionally in dogs with severe mitral valve disease, marked left atrial enlargement, and elevated left atrial pressure

Synonyms

Endomyocardial split of the left atrium, left atrial tear, left atrial split

Epidemiology

SPECIES, AGE, SEX

- Most often seen in older dogs
- More common in males

GENETICS, BREED PREDISPOSITION

More common in Cavalier King Charles spaniels and other chondrodystrophic breeds such as cocker spaniels, dachshunds, and miniature poodles

RISK FACTORS

- Left atrial enlargement due to long-standing mitral regurgitation
- Ruptured chordae tendineae
- Chronic mitral valve degeneration (mitral regurgitation due to myxomatous valve disease)

ASSOCIATED DISORDERS

- Congestive heart failure
- Hemopericardium

Clinical Presentation

DISEASE FORMS/SUBTYPES

- Nonperforating endocardial splits are found only at necropsy.
- Perforating endomyocardial splits cause hemopericardium or acquired atrial septal defects.

HISTORY, CHIEF COMPLAINT

- Long-standing mitral insufficiency
- Dyspnea
- Acute collapse

PHYSICAL EXAM FINDINGS

- Nonspecific acute collapse
- Tachycardia
- Weak pulses
- Pale mucous membranes
- Loud systolic murmur at left apex
- If hemopericardium is present, there may be signs of cardiac tamponade (p. 773).

Etiology and Pathophysiology

- Left atrial rupture is caused by increased wall tension associated with marked left atrial enlargement and elevated left atrial pressure.
- These changes usually are due to chronic mitral valve disease with valve incompetence and coexisting endocardial degeneration, but endocardial splitting also may occur in young dogs with patent ductus arteriosus and marked left atrial enlargement.
- Multiple splits are usually present, and a deep endomyocardial split may fully perforate the left atrial wall, resulting in hemopericardium or an acquired atrial septal defect, depending on its location.
- Healed, endothelialized splits are often present in dogs with fresh thrombus-covered splits.
- Dogs with acquired atrial septal defects usually have otherwise healed splits.

DIAGNOSIS

Diagnostic Overview

Left atrial rupture is suspected when an old dog of a predisposed breed with mitral regurgitation and significant cardiomegaly has sudden collapse and signs of hypotensive or cardiogenic shock. A working clinical diagnosis is established with echocardiography that demonstrates pericardial effusion and a blood clot adjacent to the left atrium in a patient with a perforating split. In patients with acquired atrial septal defect, Doppler echocardiography reveals left-to-right blood flow through the split-induced atrial septal defect.

Differential Diagnosis

- Other myocardial disease
- Atrial neoplasm
- Neoplastic pericardial effusion
- Idiopathic pericardial effusion
- Congenital atrial septal defect

Initial Database

- Auscultation to identify loud systolic murmur in mitral valve area; occasionally, the murmur may be very soft if severe tamponade and/or hypotension is/are present.
- Thoracic radiographs to detect large, globoid cardiac silhouette plus left atrial enlargement
- Electrocardiogram to identify arrhythmias such as atrial premature beats or atrial fibrillation and conduction abnormalities such as wide, notched P waves.

ADVANCED OR CONFIRMATORY TESTING

- Two-dimensional (2D) echocardiography to detect pericardial effusion (hemopericardium) and a laminar blood clot, usually near the left atrium in the long-axis view when epicardial perforation has occurred
- Color Doppler echocardiography of atrial septum to detect left-to-right shunt when atrial septal perforation has occurred

TREATMENT

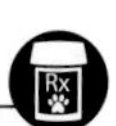

Treatment Overview

- Treatment depends on the location and depth of the rupture. Nonperforating (partial) left atrial ruptures usually cannot be confirmed antemortem; treatment consists of standard therapy for congestive heart failure.
- Acquired atrial septal defects are endomyocardial ruptures of the interatrial septum. These may relieve left heart failure signs (dyspnea) but are eventually followed by right heart failure signs (ascites), and periodic abdominocentesis may be required in addition to optimal diuretic therapy.
- Epicardial perforations causing survivable hemopericardium usually are small and located in the caudal wall of the left atrium near the left atrial appendage. Therapy includes partial pericardiocentesis if there is significant tamponade (CAUTION: in some patients, the epicardial clot dislodges, and hemorrhage becomes brisk, requiring urgent surgical intervention or euthanasia), vasodilators, and surgical closure of the perforation site.

Acute General Treatment

- Therapy for acute severe congestive heart failure (p. 408)
- Pericardiocentesis (p. 1150) may be considered when there is hemopericardium and significant tamponade; the owner should be warned that intractable atrial hemorrhage is possible, and a plan (including whether to proceed to thoracotomy and code designation in the case of cardiac arrest) should be finalized before beginning the procedure.
- Thoracotomy and suture closure of epicardial perforation

Chronic Treatment

As appropriate for advanced myxomatous mitral valve disease (p. 409); may include

- Furosemide 1-2 mg/kg PO q 12h, adjusted as needed, if congestive heart failure is present
- Pimobendan 0.25 mg/kg PO q 12h if congestive heart failure is present
- Enalapril 0.5 mg/kg PO q 12h if congestive heart failure is present
- Amlodipine 0.05-0.2 mg/kg PO q 12-24h if more vasodilator effect is needed
- Surgical creation of an atrial septal defect to decompress the left atrium
- Circumferential suture of the mitral annulus to reduce mitral regurgitation

Possible Complications

- Additional atrial hemorrhage
- Death if intractable atrial hemorrhage causes critical cardiac tamponade

Recommended Monitoring

Periodic radiographs or echocardiogram to monitor atrial size and hemopericardium

PROGNOSIS & OUTCOME

- Generally poor, but some dogs have survived with intensive vasodilator therapy.
- Survival has been observed for several months if an atrial septal defect develops.

PEARLS & CONSIDERATIONS

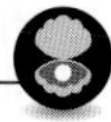

Comments

- The chief radiographic signs are marked enlargement of the cardiac silhouette and a large left atrium.
- The chief echocardiographic signs are pericardial effusion and a blood clot near the left atrium. Hemopericardium due to other causes typically is chronic in nature, larger in volume, and is not associated with a blood clot at this site.
- If the animal is hemodynamically stable and a blood clot is on the left atrium, there is merit in not removing the hemopericardium so that counterpressure is maintained on the left atrium until vasodilator therapy can be initiated and/or preparations can be made for surgery.
- Acquired atrial septal defects are small, and detection with Doppler echocardiography may require searching the dorsocaudal aspect of the right atrium.

Technician Tips

- Dogs at greatest risk of atrial rupture are those with degenerative valve disease (i.e., small-breed dogs), which are generally less likely to develop idiopathic or neoplastic pericardial effusion.
- In a small-breed dog with a murmur typical of mitral regurgitation, presenting with signs typical of pericardial effusion and cardiac tamponade, keep atrial rupture on the differential list.

Client Education

Avoid stress and hyperactivity. Teach owner to monitor respiratory rate at home to detect progressive congestive heart failure.

SUGGESTED READING

Buchanan JW: Spontaneous left atrial rupture in dogs. Adv Exp Med Biol 22:315-324, 1972.

AUTHOR: James W. Buchanan, DVM, M Med Sci, DACVIM
EDITOR: Meg M. Sleeper, VMD, DACVIM

Atrial Standstill

BASIC INFORMATION

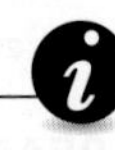

Definition

Cardiac arrhythmia with total absence of depolarization of the atria, despite normal sinoatrial (SA node) impulse formation. The two main causes are hyperkalemia (temporary) and atrial myopathy (permanent).

Synonyms

Atrial paralysis, silent atrium

Epidemiology

SPECIES, AGE, SEX

Dogs and cats: any age, either sex

RISK FACTORS

Diseases that can cause hyperkalemia (pp. 495 and 1235) and therefore atrial standstill include

- Hypoadrenocorticism
- Urethral obstruction
- Urinary bladder rupture
- Acute renal failure
- Iatrogenic (improper addition of KCl to intravenous [IV] fluids; direct IV administration of undiluted KCl or potassium penicillin)
- Muscle necrosis (reperfusion injury, massive trauma)

Clinical Presentation

DISEASE FORMS/SUBTYPES

- Hyperkalemia-induced (generally, $K^+ \geq$ 7.0 mEq/L)
- Atrial myopathy-induced
- Quinidine or digitalis toxicosis–induced
- Hypoxemia/hypothermia/myocardial infarction–induced

HISTORY, CHIEF COMPLAINT

- Hyperkalemia induced: generally reflective of underlying disorder (e.g., lethargy, inappetence, vomiting in dogs with hypoadrenocorticism)
- Atrial myopathy induced: exercise intolerance, lethargy, weakness, possibly syncope or congestive heart failure
- Quinidine or digitalis toxicosis induced: drug history, systemic signs (e.g., vomiting, inappetence common)
- May be an incidental finding on electrocardiogram (ECG)

PHYSICAL EXAM FINDINGS

- Bradycardia is a suggestive finding.
  - Typical ventricular rate = 40-100 beats/min in dogs with atrial standstill.
  - In cats, bradycardia may be present; however, cats with severe, life-threatening hyperkalemia causing atrial standstill may still have heart rate > 200 beats/min.
- Other signs depend on the inciting cause (e.g., markedly enlarged urinary bladder with urethral obstruction).

Etiology and Pathophysiology

- Atrial myopathy–associated atrial standstill
  - Atrial stretch and replacement of atrial myocytes with fibrous tissue, disrupting myocyte-to-myocyte conduction of electrical impulses through the atria
  - Typically, the ventricular depolarization is initiated at the atrioventricular (AV) junction (junctional escape rhythm).
  - Most commonly occurs in cats with marked atrial enlargement due to cardiomyopathy; sporadic cases occur in dogs and cats without atrial enlargement (normokalemic).
  - Atrial standstill is typically permanent.
- Hyperkalemia causing atrial standstill
  - Rising serum potassium concentrations decrease the transmembrane concentration gradient of cardiomyocytes, slowing repolarization (phases 1-4 of depolarization).
  - High serum potassium concentrations slow or may totally inhibit cardiac sodium channels and attendant phase 0 depolarization.
  - Atrial myocardium is exquisitely sensitive to the paralytic effects of hyperkalemia, much more so than ventricular myocardium. SA nodal tissue is most resistant.
  - The heartbeat originates from the SA node, travels normally through the atria along the internodal pathways, and reaches the AV node normally but fails to depolarize the surrounding atrial tissue along the way (sinoventricular rhythm). No P waves are seen on the ECG.
  - Atrial standstill caused by hyperkalemia is reversible with normalization of serum potassium.

DIAGNOSIS

Diagnostic Overview

The diagnosis is suspected when a patient is bradycardic, hyperkalemic, or both. The ECG (multiple leads) is confirmatory.

Differential Diagnosis

Bradycardia on physical examination:

- Second-degree AV block
- Third-degree AV block
- Sinus bradycardia/sinus arrhythmia
- Sick sinus syndrome/sinus node dysfunction

Initial Database

- ECG is the gold standard of clinical diagnosis.
  - P waves absent in all ECG leads
  - Regular rhythm (constant R-R interval)
  - Heart rate: bradycardia (dogs: typically < 100 beats/min) or any heart rate (cats: 120-260 beats/min in most cases, but possibly < 80-100 beats/min if terminally ill)
  - ECG must display multiple leads (e.g., not just lead II) to make a diagnosis of atrial standstill. Otherwise, P waves may be isoelectric in one lead, which may give the impression of atrial standstill on single-lead ECGs of patients in normal sinus rhythm.
- Serum electrolyte panel
  - Serum potassium concentration is an essential test in every patient with atrial standstill. Hyperkalemia severe enough to produce atrial standstill is a medical emergency.
  - Absence of hyperkalemia in a patient with atrial standstill provides the diagnosis of atrial myopathy (by exclusion).
- Digoxin level (if relevant, given the patient's medication/exposure history)

Advanced or Confirmatory Testing

- Thoracic radiographs and echocardiography: atrial structure should be evaluated if atrial standstill coexists with normokalemia. Atrial contractility may be inherently reduced with atrial myopathy.
- Serum ionized calcium level: should be evaluated in cats with atrial standstill secondary to urethral obstruction–related hyperkalemia. Hypocalcemia is commonly present and may be arrhythmogenic.

TREATMENT

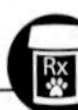

Treatment Overview

Identify cause, and reverse it if possible.

Acute General Treatment

Depends on cause:

- Treatment for hyperkalemia if present (p. 495)
- Treatment for atrial myopathy–associated atrial standstill involves treatment of the underlying cardiac disorder as indicated, regardless of atrial standstill. If overt clinical signs (e.g., exercise intolerance, syncope, congestive heart failure) occur despite treatment for the underlying heart problem, pacemaker implantation may be necessary.
- Treatment for digitalis toxicosis involves supportive care with adjusted antiarrhythmics and temporary pacing if necessary.

PROGNOSIS & OUTCOME

- Hyperkalemia-associated atrial standstill: immediate prognosis is guarded. Successful management of hyperkalemia and its inciting cause often results in a good long-term prognosis.
- Atrial myopathy–associated atrial standstill: guarded prognosis, specifically depends on degree of atrial enlargement and severity of clinical signs

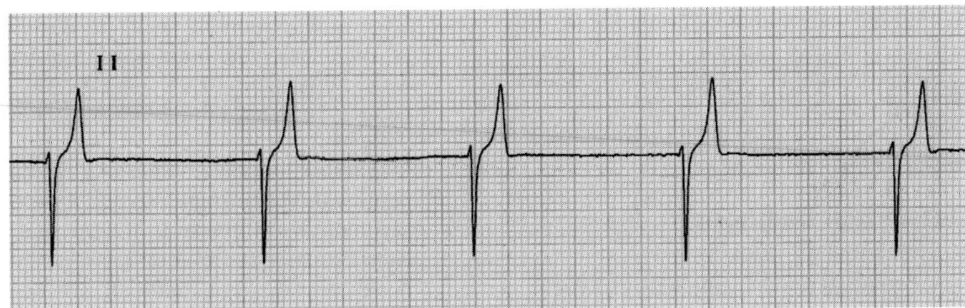

ATRIAL STANDSTILL Electrocardiogram of a young Australian blue heeler dog with atrial standstill and right-sided congestive heart failure. Cause is atrial myopathy, based on a normal serum potassium level. Patient responded well to permanent pacemaker implantation. Rhythm is regular (constant R-R interval), consistent with a junctional escape rhythm. No P waves are seen in this lead II tracing, nor were they present in any other lead. 50 mm/sec, 1 cm/mV.

- Digitalis toxicosis–associated atrial standstill: prognosis depends on severity of intoxication and underlying cardiac disease

PEARLS & CONSIDERATIONS

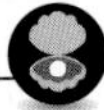

Comments

- Atrial standstill in hyperkalemic patients is a harbinger of life-threatening arrhythmias. Failure to note atrial standstill (loss of P waves on ECG) in patients with hyperkalemia may allow hyperkalemia to worsen, leading to cardiac arrest.
- Artifactual hyperkalemia is common in dogs and cats: platelets release potassium *in vitro* when activated (e.g., blood clotting in a red-top tube). Artifact is ruled out by measuring potassium on blood from a heparinized (green-top) tube.
- In cats, tachycardia (or normal heart rate) does not rule out atrial standstill, but in dogs, atrial standstill almost always causes bradycardia.

Technician Tips

- Mix potassium chloride thoroughly when injecting into IV fluid bags to avoid settling (and direct IV infusion of high KCl concentrations from the bottom of the bag).
- Supplemental potassium must never be given faster than 0.5 mEq/kg/h.

SUGGESTED READING

Nakamura RK, et al: Adult-onset nemaline myopathy in a dog presenting with persistent atrial standstill and primary hypothyroidism. J Small Anim Pract 53:357-360, 2012.

AUTHOR: Mandi Kleman, DVM, DACVIM
EDITOR: Meg M. Sleeper, VMD, DACVIM

Atrioventricular Block

BASIC INFORMATION

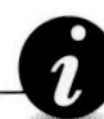

Definition

Subclassification: first-, second-, and third-degree atrioventricular (AV) block

- First-degree block: delayed conduction from the sinoatrial (SA) node through the AV junction (AV node and bundle of His) to the ventricles; electrocardiographically manifested as prolongation of the PQ interval (PR interval if no Q wave present)
- Second-degree block: intermittent failure of transmission of SA nodal impulses through AV junction; some P waves not followed by a QRS
- Third-degree block: persistent blockage of SA nodal impulses through the AV junction; P waves occur regularly and at a normal or elevated sinus rate; QRSs also occur regularly but independently and at a slower escape rate.
    - QRS morphology may be wide and bizarre (dogs > cats) or narrow and normal in appearance (cats > dogs).

Synonyms

- For AV block: heart block
- For Mobitz type I second-degree AV block (see below): Wenckebach phenomenon
- For third-degree AV block: complete heart block

Epidemiology

SPECIES, AGE, SEX

- First-degree block: cats and dogs of any age
- Second-degree block: dogs > cats
- Third-degree block: cats and dogs of any age; more common in older animals

GENETICS, BREED PREDISPOSITION

- First- and second-degree AV block: common in cocker spaniels, dachshunds, and brachycephalic dog breeds
- Second-, third-degree AV block: secondary to His bundle stenosis in pugs

ASSOCIATED DISORDERS

- Reported association between Lyme disease and third-degree AV block in dogs and people
- Mobitz type I second-degree AV block usually associated with increased vagal tone; often occurs concurrently with respiratory sinus arrhythmia and/or sinus bradycardia
- Third-degree AV block reported in association with hypertrophic cardiomyopathy in cats and as possible complication for some dogs with myxomatous mitral valve degeneration

Clinical Presentation

DISEASE FORMS/SUBTYPES

- Second-degree AV block subclassified into Mobitz types I and II: for impulses conducted through the AV junction, the PQ interval is variable (Mobitz type I) or is fixed (Mobitz type II).
    - Classic Mobitz type I second-degree AV block includes progressively prolonged PQ interval preceding nonconducted (blocked) P wave (Wenckebach phenomenon)
- Mobitz type II second-degree AV block more often pathologic and unrelated to vagal tone
    - Further described by the ratio of P waves to QRS complexes (e.g., 5:4)
    - High-grade/advanced second-degree AV block: two or more consecutive nonconducted P waves (P/QRS ratio of 3:1 or higher)

HISTORY, CHIEF COMPLAINT

- First-degree AV block: incidental finding on electrocardiogram (ECG); clinical signs relate to underlying condition, if any
- Second-degree AV block
    - Mobitz type I: as for first-degree AV block
    - Mobitz type II: if bradycardia is present, episodic or persistent signs of low cardiac output (e.g., lethargy, weakness, syncope) or congestive heart failure (CHF) (e.g., dyspnea, abdominal distention) are common
    - Third-degree AV block: episodic or persistent signs of low cardiac output or CHF; cats often show no clinical signs, likely due to a more rapid ventricular escape rhythm compared to dogs

PHYSICAL EXAM FINDINGS

- First-degree AV block: unremarkable
- Second-degree AV block: heart rate typically normal or decreased; cardiac rhythm regularly irregular with skipped beats (no ventricular contraction when block occurs); femoral pulse strength typically normal; may be supranormal for beats following pauses due to increased ventricular filling; no pulse deficits (i.e., every ventricular contraction generates a pulse); for Mobitz type II only, signs of low cardiac output and/or CHF may be present
- Third-degree AV block: bradycardia (heart rate typically < 50/min in dogs, < 140/min in cats); intermittent prominent jugular pulse (cannon *a* wave) caused by right atrial contraction against closed tricuspid valve; intermittent prominent first heart sound (bruit de cannon) due to dissociation between atrial and ventricular contraction; other findings referable to low cardiac output or CHF if present

Etiology and Pathophysiology

Etiology:

- First-degree AV block
  - May occur as normal variation (manifestation of prevailing vagal tone)
  - Iatrogenic: medications that slow AV nodal conduction (e.g., digoxin, beta-adrenergic antagonists, calcium channel antagonists, opioids)
  - Diseases that increase vagal tone (e.g., respiratory, gastrointestinal, and intracranial central nervous system disorders)
  - Less commonly: primary cardiomyopathies, idiopathic AV nodal fibrosis, infiltrative myocardial disease, myocardial infarction
- Second-degree AV block
  - As for first-degree AV block
  - May occur seconds to minutes after intravenous (IV) atropine or glycopyrrolate (transient)
- Third-degree AV block
  - Pathologic conditions as listed for first- and second-degree AV block

Pathophysiology:

- Above causes may produce slowing (first-degree AV block) or blockage (second- and third-degree AV block) of electrical impulse conduction by the specialized cardiac myocytes of the AV junction.
- In third-degree AV block, ventricular depolarization (and contraction) results from an escape rhythm generated by pacemaker cells in the more distal part of the AV junction (His bundle) or in the ventricles.
- Result is faster atrial rate (P waves per minute) and slower ventricular rate (QRS complexes per minute) occurring independently of one another.

DIAGNOSIS

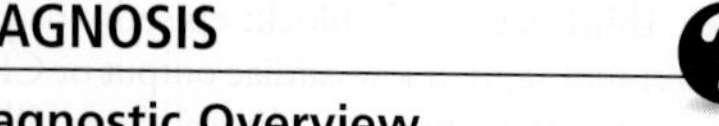

Diagnostic Overview

All types of AV block require ECG for diagnosis. On a normal ECG, each P wave is followed by a QRS complex at a species-specific normal interval. The PQ interval (or PR interval) encompasses atrial depolarization (P-wave duration) and conduction through the AV node (PR segment), normally ≤ 0.13 second in dogs or ≤ 0.09 second in cats.

Differential Diagnosis

- First-degree AV block
  - Artifact (e.g., changing paper speed)
- Second-degree AV block
  - Auscultatory: pronounced respiratory sinus arrhythmia (common), sinoatrial arrest or block (uncommon)
  - ECG: third-degree AV block, rhythmic motion artifact (e.g., purring, shivering)
- Third-degree AV block
  - Historical: other causes of syncope (e.g., tachyarrhythmias, structural heart disease, pulmonary hypertension, intracranial disease, metabolic disease) (p. 953)
  - Auscultatory: Other bradyarrhythmias (e.g., sinus bradycardia, persistent atrial standstill, high-grade second-degree AV block)

Initial Database

- First-degree AV block
  - ECG: PQ or PR interval > 0.13 second in dogs, > 0.09 second in cats
  - Additional testing as pertains to underlying/concurrent condition, if any
- Second-degree AV block
  - ECG: some P waves not followed by QRS complexes, resulting in a faster atrial rate than ventricular rate; also to rule out other arrhythmias
  - Echocardiogram: rule out structural intracardiac causes; incidental finding of other abnormalities is common (e.g., myxomatous AV valve disease) and not always related
  - Thoracic radiographs: rule out CHF
  - CBC, serum biochemistry profile, and urinalysis: unremarkable unless concurrent conditions
- Third-degree AV block
  - ECG: unrelated faster atrial rate (P waves) and slower ventricular rate (QRS complexes)
    - Escape rhythm (QRS complexes) may appear wide and bizarre or normal (presumably arising from the ventricles or lower AV junction, respectively)
    - Rate: typically 25-50 beats/min in dogs, 70-140 beats/min in cats
    - Also rule out other arrhythmias
  - Echocardiogram, thoracic radiographs, and minimum laboratory database as for second-degree AV block

Advanced or Confirmatory Testing

Atropine response test (0.04 mg/kg IV, SQ [longer response time])

- For second-degree AV block, Mobitz type II (or Mobitz type I if accompanied by sinus bradycardia and vague clinical signs)
- To differentiate between physiologic and pathologic causes
  - Complete response: total resolution of AV block and heart rate increases by ≥ 50% (typically resulting in sinus tachycardia), suggesting physiologic, not pathologic
  - Incomplete response: some AV block persists, and/or heart rate increases < 50%
  - Incomplete response may indicate individual variation (normal) or structural AV nodal disease (e.g., fibrosis); syncope decreases in a small minority of these patients when treated with oral medications (see below), but most require pacemaker implantation.
- Limited accuracy; Holter or cardiac event monitoring (p. 1120) obtained at the time of clinical event/collapse is superior for confirming a pathologic arrhythmia

TREATMENT

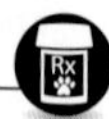

Treatment Overview

For second- and third-degree AV block, goals are to restore normal cardiac output and resolve CHF if present. When clinical signs are present (typically syncope), pacemaker implantation is almost always necessary.

Acute General Treatment

- For first-degree and Mobitz type I second-degree AV block: no specific therapy required
- For all cases of high-grade second-degree AV block causing clinical signs and all cases of third-degree AV block:
  - Standard therapy for CHF if applicable (p. 408)
  - IV positive chronotropes (e.g., isoproterenol 0.04-0.08 mcg/kg/min IV infusion): temporary support (e.g., before pacemaker implantation) but often ineffective, particularly with third-degree AV block
  - Temporary and/or permanent artificial pacemaker implantation

Chronic Treatment

- Indicated for high-grade Mobitz type II second-degree AV block and all cases of third-degree AV block
- Oral positive chronotropes (e.g., propantheline 0.5-1 mg/kg PO q 8h, terbutaline 0.2 mg/kg PO q 8-12h, or theophylline 5-10 mg/kg PO q 8-12h) may be used but generally inadequate
- Permanent pacemaker implantation

Possible Complications

- Mobitz type II second-degree AV block may progress to third-degree AV block.
- Patients requiring pacemaker implantation are at risk for sudden death before implantation.
- Patients with high-grade Mobitz type II second-degree AV block or third-degree AV block are at risk for developing CHF

Recommended Monitoring

- First-degree AV block: no specific monitoring necessary

First-degree

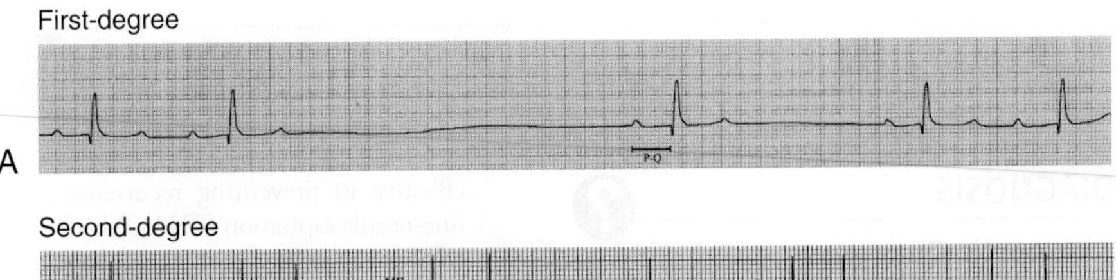

A

Second-degree

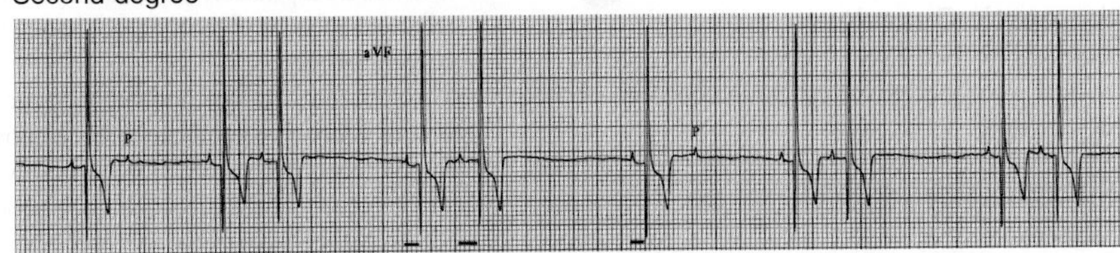

B

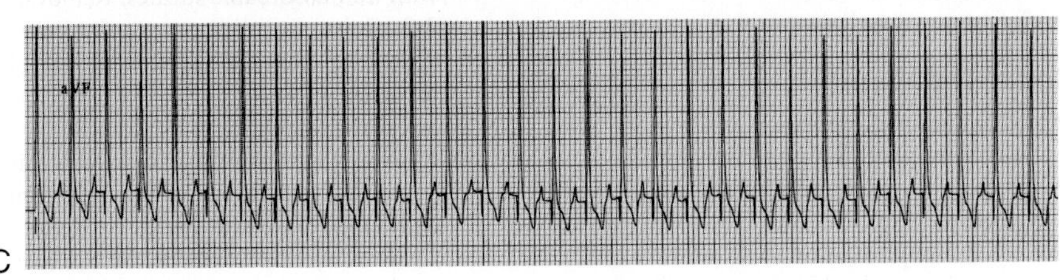

C

Third-degree

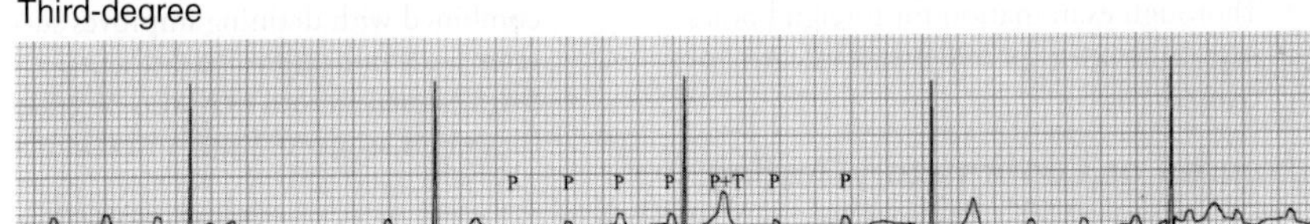

D

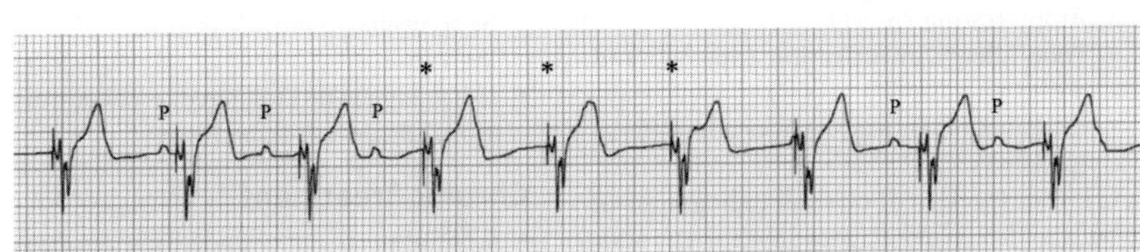

E

ATRIOVENTRICULAR BLOCK A, First-degree AV block in a 5-year-old German shepherd with severe inflammatory bowel disease. PQ interval is prolonged at 0.20 second; upper limit of normal in dogs = 0.13 second. Lead II, 50 mm/sec. **B, C,** Mobitz type I second-degree AV block in an 11-year-old cocker spaniel evaluated for lethargy. Note two nonconducted P waves and *solid lines* marking variable PQ intervals. Positive response to atropine (ECG recorded 30 minutes after atropine 0.04 mg/kg) (**C**). Heart rate has increased from 70/min to 230/min, and AV block has resolved, suggesting that AV block is physiologic in this patient and not responsible for lethargy. Lead aVF, 25 mm/sec. **D, E,** Third-degree AV block in a 2-year-old Irish spaniel with syncope before and after permanent jugular transvenous pacemaker implementation. Admission (**D**): note atrial rhythm (P waves, 190/min) and unrelated ventricular rhythm (QRS complexes, 40/min). One P wave is superimposed on a T wave (P + T). After pacemaker implantation (**E**): ventricular-paced rhythm at a rate of 90/min. Note that unrelated, nonconducted P waves can still be seen. Pacemaker spikes *(asterisks)* precede each QRS complex. Lead aVF, 25 mm/sec.

- Second-degree AV block, Mobitz type I: consider periodic ECGs to ensure no progression
- Second-degree AV block, Mobitz type II: without pacemaker implantation, periodic ECGs (e.g., every few months or as dictated by clinical signs)

PROGNOSIS & OUTCOME

- First-degree AV block: excellent (no implications as sole entity)
- Second-degree AV block, Mobitz type I: excellent (similar to first-degree AV block)
- Mobitz type II second-degree AV block, no overt clinical signs: fair to good
- High-grade Mobitz type II second-degree AV block and/or overt clinical signs present: guarded to poor without treatment, but generally good to excellent with permanent pacemaker implantation
- Third-degree AV block: poor without treatment; generally good to excellent with permanent pacemaker implantation (better without CHF)
- After pacemaker placement (mainly in dogs with third-degree AV block), clinical signs resolve in 92% of dogs and 1-, 3-, and 5-year survival rates = 86%, 65%, and 39%, respectively.

PEARLS & CONSIDERATIONS

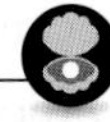

Comments

- First-degree AV block does not cause clinical signs; it serves as clue that an underlying cardiac or systemic problem may (or may not) be present (i.e., new first-degree AV block may be indicator of drug toxicosis if a patient is receiving a drug that delays AV nodal conduction (e.g., digoxin).
- Mobitz type I second-degree AV block rarely causes clinical signs and does not predict degeneration to Mobitz type II second-degree AV block or third-degree AV block.
- For AV block requiring pacemaker implantation, ventricular antiarrhythmic agents are contraindicated until artificial pacing is established due to potential for suppression of ventricular escape foci.
- Therapy for CHF can usually be tapered or discontinued after pacemaker implantation.
- Clinical signs may be subtle (e.g., progressive lethargy) and most apparent retrospectively after pacemaker implantation.

Technician Tips

- For patients with a previously implanted pacemaker, any recurrence of clinical signs referable to bradycardia (e.g., weakness, collapse) should prompt suspicion for pacemaker malfunction and/or dislodgement and warrants immediate re-evaluation.
- Patients with pacemakers should never have blood drawn from the jugular veins (risk of permanently damaging pacemaker lead).

SUGGESTED READING

Johnson MS, et al: Results of pacemaker implantation in 104 dogs. J Small Anim Pract 48:4-11, 2007.

AUTHOR: Gregg Rapoport, DVM, DACVIM
EDITOR: Meg M. Sleeper, VMD, DACVIM

Aural Hematoma

Client Education Sheet 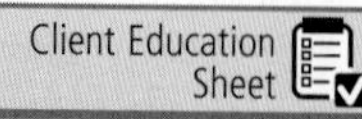

BASIC INFORMATION

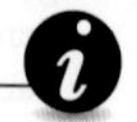

Definition

A collection of blood, typically fluctuant/fluid-filled, within the split cartilage plate of the ear or on the concave surface of the ear pinna

Epidemiology

SPECIES, AGE, SEX

Dogs and cats; it is the seventh most commonly treated surgical condition in small animal practice.

GENETICS, BREED PREDISPOSITION

Dogs with pendulous pinnae may be at increased risk of rupturing capillaries during self-trauma.

RISK FACTORS

- Otitis externa
- Pinna trauma

CONTAGION AND ZOONOSIS

Parasitic infestation (*Otodectes* spp)

GEOGRAPHY AND SEASONALITY

- Geographic distribution of parasitic causes of otitis externa
- Associated with seasonal incidence of otitis externa: warmer weather (humidity, swimming), atopic disease

Clinical Presentation

HISTORY, CHIEF COMPLAINT

- Head shaking or scratching ears
- Acute or chronic otitis externa
- Generalized dermatologic problems

PHYSICAL EXAM FINDINGS

- Characteristic soft, fluid-filled, or fluctuant swelling on concave surface of pinna
  - Swelling may become firm and cauliflower-like as fibrosis develops.
  - Usually not painful
- Otitis externa
  - Evidence of parasitic infestation/bacterial or yeast infection
  - Evidence of other causes (excessively hairy ear canals, structural anomaly)
- Generalized dermatologic problem

Etiology and Pathophysiology

- Aural hematomas are most often caused by self-trauma (head shaking or scratching) to the pinna secondary to otitis externa.
- Shearing forces fracture the cartilage and cause rupture of epithelial and intrachondral blood vessels with subsequent hemorrhage and hematoma formation into the resulting dead space.

DIAGNOSIS

Diagnostic Overview

Diagnosis is based on highly characteristic physical examination findings and history of otitis externa.

Differential Diagnosis

- Abscess
- Seroma
- Soft-tissue neoplasia

Initial Database

- CBC, serum biochemistry profile, and urinalysis: generally unremarkable
- Otic examination under anesthesia (p. 1144)
  - Samples of exudate are collected for microscopic examination (bacteria, yeast, parasites) and culture/susceptibility testing
  - Thorough examination for foreign bodies (e.g., grass awn [p. 398]) and integrity of tympana

Advanced or Confirmatory Testing

- Workup to determine cause of generalized dermatologic problem
  - Thyroid profile (pp. 525 and 1386)
  - Atopy testing (p. 91)
  - Food allergy investigation (pp. 345 and 347)
  - Examination for parasite infestations (fleas) (p. 1091)
- CT scan (preferred) or skull radiographs of bulla to detect and diagnose concurrent otitis media

TREATMENT

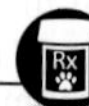

Treatment Overview

Successful resolution of the aural hematoma depends on 1) complete evacuation and ongoing drainage with stabilization of the pinna until adhesion formation and 2) control/elimination of the inciting cause.

Acute General Treatment

- Surgical treatment is most successful.
  - Incisional method, using longitudinal, S-shaped, or elliptical incision. The incision is made through the inner concave skin layer and is extended through the cartilage, if necessary, to reach the hematoma. The hematoma is completely evacuated. To prevent deformations and cauliflower ear, full-thickness mattress sutures are placed through the pinna parallel to the incision over Penrose drains or intravenous (IV) tubing to avoid pressure necrosis. Healing of the incision occurs by second intention.
  - Temporary insertion of a closed suction drainage system can be effective, allowing controlled scar formation. This is more effective in preventing recurrence than fine-needle aspiration (FNA). May be less effective if significant scar tissue has already formed.
  - Through-and-through indwelling Penrose drains. A proximal and distal incision over the hematoma is made and flushed with sterile saline. The Penrose drain is placed through the hematoma site and secured with non-absorbable sutures. Removal in 2-3 weeks.
  - CO_2 laser drainage has been successfully reported.
- Medical treatment
  - FNA of the hematoma: invariably ineffective long term. Should be performed daily until adhesions form.
  - Oral or injectable corticosteroids (dexamethasone 0.2 to 0.5 mg/kg IV q 24h) combined with draining improves success rates with nonsurgical treatments.
  - Intralesional steroid may also be effective (dexamethasone 0.2 mg intralesional q 24h × 5 days)
- Pinna is ideally bandaged to head to prevent further trauma and allow tissue adhesion to occur (2-3 weeks). However, ear canals must be accessible to provide treatment of underlying cause.
- If bandage is not tolerated, e-collar must be worn to prevent scratching.

Chronic Treatment

- Control/treatment of underlying dermatologic problem is imperative to limit recurrence.
- Affected patients should have regular otic examinations with cleaning if necessary.
- General anesthesia (or heavy sedation) is usually necessary.
  - To allow thorough examination and cleaning
  - To provide analgesia
  - To minimize iatrogenic damage to the ear canal

Possible Complications

- Recurrence of the hematoma due to inadequate/ineffective treatment and failure to identify or control underlying cause
- Associated with treatment
  - Incisional technique
    - Insufficient incision size may lead to premature closure, hematoma recurrence.
    - Incorrect orientation of incision and inadvertent ligation of an auricular artery may cause regional necrosis.
  - Closed suction drain: premature removal by patient
  - Passive drainage: premature removal of Penrose drains
  - FNA technique: failure to remove all fluid prevents tissue adhesion
  - Corticosteroids: side effects of these drugs.

- With any of the above techniques, failure to adequately immobilize pinna to allow tissue adhesion and healing to occur results in recurrence.

Recommended Monitoring

- Appropriate regular otic examination and cleaning
- Re-evaluation to ensure that underlying cause of otitis externa is being adequately controlled/treated

PROGNOSIS & OUTCOME

- Prognosis is good to excellent with appropriate treatment of the hematoma and management of the underlying dermatologic problem.
- Recurrence is likely if underlying cause is not managed appropriately.

PEARLS & CONSIDERATIONS

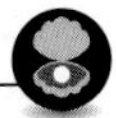

Comments

- Evacuation of the contents of the hematoma, establishment of drainage, and prevention of pinna deformation are necessary for successful treatment of aural hematomas.
- Aural hematomas are caused by trauma to the pinna, most often due to head shaking or vigorous scratching by the animal.
- Always examine the complete external canals of both ears.
- To remove the bandage, cut it along the ventral midline of the dog's neck to avoid cutting the pinna lying reflected on the dorsal head.

Prevention

Determination of the underlying cause of the head shaking or scratching is essential to prevent recurrence.

Technician Tips

- Maintaining the pinna securely bandaged to the head can be a challenge. Regular bandage changes are necessary to evaluate healing, clean the ear, and make sure the pinna is securely held in place. The client may need considerable assistance with bandage maintenance.
- To remove the bandage, cut it along the ventral midline of the dog's neck to avoid cutting the pinna lying reflected (within the bandage) on the dorsal head.

Client Education

- Evacuation of the contents of the hematoma, establishment of drainage, and prevention of pinna deformation are necessary for successful treatment of aural hematomas.
- Aural hematomas are caused by underlying trauma to the ear pinna, most often due to head shaking or vigorous scratching by the animal.

SUGGESTED READING

Bacon NJ: Pinna and external ear canal. In Johnston SA, et al, editors: Veterinary surgery: small animal, ed 2, St. Louis, 2018, Elsevier, pp 2310-2327.

AUTHOR: Lindsey M. Kurach, DVM, DACVS
EDITOR: Elizabeth A. Swanson, DVM, MS, DACVS

Babesiosis

BASIC INFORMATION

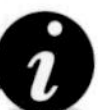

Definition

Canine babesiosis is a tick-borne disease caused by a hemoprotozoan parasite that infects red blood cells of dogs, causing hemolytic anemia and thrombocytopenia. Two primary species have been identified: *Babesia canis* (large *Babesia*) and *Babesia gibsoni* (small *Babesia*).

Synonyms

- Babesiosis: piroplasmosis
- *Babesia/Theileria annae: Babesia microti*–like parasite
- *Babesia gibsoni: B. gibsoni* (Asian genotype)
- *Babesia conradae:* may be referred to as *B. gibsoni* (U.S. genotype)
- *Babesia canis* subspecies: three subspecies of *B. canis* have been proposed: *B. canis vogeli, B. canis canis,* and *B. canis rossi.* Some have suggested they represent three species of *Babesia.*
- *Babesia "coco":* Large, unnamed *Babesia* sp in North America

Epidemiology

SPECIES, AGE, SEX

Dogs of any age and either sex

GENETICS, BREED PREDISPOSITION

- American pit bull terriers (APBTs) and Tosa Inus at increased risk for *B. gibsoni*
- Greyhounds at increased risk for *B. canis vogeli*

RISK FACTORS

- Dog fights (particularly bites by an APBT)
- Tick infestation
- Blood transfusion
- Shared needles or surgical instruments
- Vertical transmission (infected dam)

CONTAGION AND ZOONOSIS

- Transmission is through blood contamination or arthropod infestation (*Rhipicephalus, Haemaphysalis,* or *Dermacentor* spp).
- Canine babesiosis is not a documented zoonotic disease; *B. microti* is a small *Babesia* infecting human red blood cells. Canine species of *Babesia* causing infections in humans have not been well documented.

GEOGRAPHY AND SEASONALITY

- Because babesiosis can be acute or chronic, it can be diagnosed at any time of year.
- Small *Babesia* spp
    - *B. gibsoni* was once limited to Asia but now has a worldwide distribution.
    - *B. microti*—like: Spain and North America
    - *B. conradae:* southern California
- Large *Babesia* spp
    - *B. canis vogeli:* worldwide
    - *B. canis canis:* Europe
    - *B. canis rossi:* Africa

One of the novel large *Babesia* sp has been diagnosed in the United States and the other in the United Kingdom.

ASSOCIATED DISORDERS

- Some patients with babesiosis have been concurrently diagnosed with other tick-borne diseases.
- The novel large *Babesia* sp identified in United States (coco) has been primarily diagnosed in dogs that have previously undergone splenectomy or are undergoing chemotherapy.

Clinical Presentation

DISEASE FORMS/SUBTYPES

Babesiosis can cause severe, life-threatening disease in some dogs; others show few or no outward clinical signs. *B. microti*–like infections are commonly associated with azotemia and proteinuria.

HISTORY, CHIEF COMPLAINT

Owners may observe weakness, lethargy, anorexia, pallor, icterus, or discolored urine (bilirubinuria or hemoglobinuria). Other historical findings may include tick exposure, recent blood transfusion, or recent dog fight (especially with an APBT).

PHYSICAL EXAM FINDINGS

Pallor and splenomegaly, +/− lymphadenopathy, fever, petechiae, or icterus may occur

Etiology and Pathophysiology

- Sporozoites in tick salivary glands transmitted to dog during feeding (requires 2-3 days)
- Sporozoites enter red blood cells (RBCs), where they become merozoites and undergo asexual reproduction.
- Intravascular and extravascular hemolysis occurs.
- Secondary immune-mediated destruction of RBCs and platelets may occur.
- Azotemia and proteinuria are presumed to be secondary to glomerulonephritis and are most commonly seen with *B. annae* infections but are recognized with increasing frequency in association with other *Babesia* spp.

DIAGNOSIS

Diagnostic Overview

Most dogs with babesiosis have one or more of the following abnormalities: thrombocytopenia, anemia, hyperglobulinemia, and/or splenomegaly. Polymerase chain reaction (PCR) assays have become the primary means of accurately diagnosing *Babesia* infections; however, serologic testing can help make a presumptive diagnosis of babesiosis in cases with low numbers of circulating parasites.

Differential Diagnosis

- Immune-mediated hemolytic anemia
- Immune-mediated thrombocytopenia
- Zinc toxicosis
- Splenic torsion
- Ehrlichiosis
- Leptospirosis
- Heartworm disease with caval syndrome
- Neoplasia: lymphoma or hemangiosarcoma

Initial Database

One or more of the following may be identified in dogs with babesiosis:

- Regenerative anemia: important to note that not all dogs with *Babesia* infections have anemia
- Thrombocytopenia: the most common hematologic abnormality in dogs with babesiosis; platelet counts can be as low as < 5000 platelets/mcL.
- Blood smear: identification of *Babesia* organisms (an erythrocyte is ≈8 microns in diameter) (figure at www.ExpertConsult.com)
    - Small babesiosis: 1-3 micron signet ring forms
    - Large babesiosis: 3-6 micron single or paired teardrop forms, but other more ameboid forms can predominate
- Serum bilirubin: may be increased
- Hyperglobulinemia: a polyclonal gammopathy is frequently detected
- Urinalysis: +/− bilirubinuria, hemoglobinuria or proteinuria
- Coombs' test: positive in up to 85% of cases
- Protein losing nephropathy: has been the primary finding in some cases

Advanced or Confirmatory Testing

- PCR test: only way to determine species or subspecies and is more sensitive than blood smear
    - False-positive, false-negative results recognized
    - Tests vary between laboratories.
    - Not always able to detect all species (check with laboratory about sensitivity and specificity)
- IFA test > 1:64 is considered positive.
    - Cannot differentiate species
    - False-negative results can occur with acute or peracute disease or severe immunosuppression.

TREATMENT

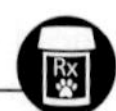

Treatment Overview

It may not be possible to completely eradicate the parasite in all cases, but clinical signs usually improve with supportive care and antiparasitic therapy. The treatment of choice depends on which *Babesia* species is identified. Currently, most data are available for treatment of *B. canis* and *B. gibsoni*.

Acute General Treatment

- Supportive treatment may require blood transfusion (p. 1169) for animals that are anemic.
- Intravenous (IV) fluids may be required in animals that are febrile and dehydrated.
- Imidocarb diproprionate 6.6 mg/kg IM once, repeat in 7-14 days. Pretreatment with atropine (0.02-0.04 mg/kg IM or SQ 30 minutes before imidocarb injection) may reduce cholinergic side effects. Imidocarb appears to reduce morbidity and mortality for nearly all *Babesia* spp but is not effective for the clearance of *B. gibsoni*. It is the treatment of choice for *B. canis vogeli*.
- Atovaquone 13.5 mg/kg PO q 8h with fatty meal for 10 days plus azithromycin 10 mg/kg PO q 24h for 10 days is the treatment of choice for *B. gibsoni*. Results in elimination or reduction of the parasite below the limit of detection of PCR testing in ≈82% of cases. Resistance to atovaquone has been identified.
- Clindamycin 25 mg/kg PO q 12h for 14 days as a single agent has been associated with clinical improvement but not clearance of *B. gibsoni*.
- A combination of clindamycin 25 mg/kg PO q 12h, metronidazole 15 mg/kg PO q 12h, and doxycycline 5 mg/kg PO q 12h has been associated with elimination or reduction of the parasite below the limit of detection of PCR testing. A well-defined treatment course has not been established, with treatment times ranging from 24-92 days.
- Concurrent immune suppression should be avoided whenever possible because it may reduce the ability to clear the infection with antiprotozoal drugs.

Chronic Treatment

- Vector control: topical, oral or wearable acaricides
- Dogs with positive *Babesia* titers or PCR should never be used as blood donors, even after treatment.

Possible Complications

Prolonged immunosuppressive therapy before specific antibabesial treatment can worsen outcome and should not be used in sick, hospitalized dogs.

Recommended Monitoring

- Monitor hematocrit and platelet count daily until improvement is seen and then every 1-3 weeks until anemia and thrombocytopenia resolve.
- PCR should be negative 60 and 90 days after treatment if the parasite has been successfully eradicated.

PROGNOSIS & OUTCOME

- Good prognosis with early diagnosis and treatment; prognosis worsens if treatment preceded by immunosuppressive therapy
- Animals may remain subclinically infected for life.
- Severely anemic animals may die without supportive care such as blood transfusions or hemoglobin-based oxygen-carrying solutions.

PEARLS & CONSIDERATIONS

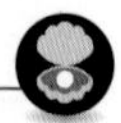

Comments

- New *Babesia* species are being identified through molecular techniques.
- *Babesia* spp can be transmitted vertically and should be considered in puppies with weakness and pallor.

Prevention

- Effective tick control is likely to reduce the risk of infection.
- Screening blood donors for *Babesia* infections can reduce the chances of iatrogenic infections.
- Screen breeding bitches of at-risk breeds.
- Avoid blood transmission via transfusion from infected or previously infected dogs or blood-contaminated instruments (e.g., shared needles).

Technician Tips

The characteristic features of *Babesia* make them identifiable on a blood smear, but they are often found in low numbers

Client Education

In highly endemic areas, use a topical/oral acaricide plus a repellent tick collar.

SUGGESTED READING

Birkenheuer AJ, et al: Double-blind placebo controlled trial evaluating the efficacy of an atovaquone azithromycin combination therapy for chronic *Babesia gibsoni* infections. J Vet Intern Med 18:494-498, 2004.

AUTHOR: Adam J. Birkenheuer, DVM, PhD, DACVIM
EDITOR: Joseph Taboada, DVM, DACVIM

Back Pain

Client Education Sheet

BASIC INFORMATION

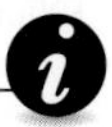

Definition

Pain localized to the thoracolumbar spinal column

Synonyms

Spinal hyperesthesia or hyperpathia

Epidemiology

SPECIES, AGE, SEX

Depends on the underlying cause

- Dogs: middle-aged adults (type I intervertebral disc disease [IVDD], acute noncompressive nucleus pulposus extrusion [ANNPE]), older adults (type II IVDD, neoplasia)
- Cats: older adults (neoplasia), males > females (aortic thromboembolism)

GENETICS, BREED PREDISPOSITION

Dogs*:* chondrodystrophic breeds (type I IVDD)

RISK FACTORS

Cats*:* thromboembolism associated with cardiomyopathy

Clinical Presentation

HISTORY, CHIEF COMPLAINT

Vocalization, reluctance to movement or activity, pain elicited if patient touched or moved

PHYSICAL EXAM FINDINGS

- Hunched posture (kyphosis), pain elicited on epaxial palpation; ataxia, paresis, or paralysis; heat or swelling in epaxial region; splinting and pain on abdominal palpation
- Fever, if back pain is associated with infection (e.g., discospondylitis)
- Heart murmur, diminished femoral pulses, cyanosis of toenails if back pain is associated with aortic thromboembolism

Etiology and Pathophysiology

- Neurogenic: compression, inflammation, or traumatic disruption of spinal cord, spinal roots, spinal nerves, dorsal root ganglia, or meninges
- Vertebral column: trauma, inflammation, or lysis of vertebral bone, intervertebral discs, or articular facets
- Epaxial muscle: inflammation, abscessation, ischemia, or trauma

DIAGNOSIS

Diagnostic Overview

Back pain often presents nonspecific physical signs (or absence of any observable deficits). Careful palpation and thorough neurologic and orthopedic examinations are used for eliciting and, if possible, localizing signs of back pain. Diagnostic imaging and specific techniques then help to elucidate the source of the pain.

Differential Diagnosis

- Spinal, orthopedic
- Spinal, neurologic
- Vascular
- Other (abdominal, limb, cutaneous, anxiety)

For a detailed differential diagnosis, see p. 1202.

Initial Database

- Neurologic and orthopedic exams (pp. 1136 and 1143)
- CBC, serum biochemistry profile, urinalysis: often unremarkable unless systemic disease or infection present
- Radiographs: bone lysis or proliferation (neoplasia, osteomyelitis), vertebral fracture or luxation (trauma), intervertebral disc mineralization, disc space narrowing, wedging or displacement (IVDD, ANNPE), vertebral endplate lysis or proliferation (discospondylitis), articular facet sclerosis and malformation, spondylosis. Radiographs may be unremarkable.

Advanced or Confirmatory Testing

Selection is based on history, clinical signs, and results of initial database:

- Cerebrospinal fluid tap (pp. 1080 and 1323): cytologic evaluation, culture, serologic testing for immunoglobulin A (IgA) or infectious agents
- Computed tomography (CT) allows three-dimensional assessment of the vertebral column; particularly useful for spinal trauma or neoplasia; CT myelography is very sensitive for evaluating spinal cord compression
- Magnetic resonance imaging (MRI) (p. 1132) has greater sensitivity than CT for spinal cord lesions without the need for myelography and offers better evaluation of spinal cord parenchyma.
- Myelogram: identify and discern among extradural compression (IVDD), intradural/extramedullary lesion (meningioma), and intramedullary lesion (other neoplasia or cord swelling, such as due to ischemic myelopathy). Often augmented by CT or replaced by MRI when available
- Urine culture (discospondylitis)
- Blood culture and sensitivity (discospondylitis, osteomyelitis, bacterial meningitis) (p. 1333)
- Needle aspirate of intervertebral disc (discospondylitis)
- Serologic titers: *Brucella canis* (discospondylitis), rickettsial diseases (polyarthritis, meningitis)
- Arthrocentesis (p. 1059): cytology (polyarthritis), culture (septic polyarthritis or meningitis)
- Serum protein electrophoresis and bone marrow if suspect multiple myeloma (p. 663)
- Biopsy of vertebral bone (neoplasia, osteomyelitis)

TREATMENT

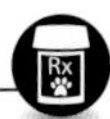

Treatment Overview

- Elimination of infectious or noninfectious paraspinal inflammatory causes
- Elimination of any compressive lesion on spinal cord or nerve roots
- Stabilization of vertebral column

Acute General Treatment

Address the underlying cause.

Chronic Treatment

- Degenerative joint disease may require persistent or recurrent nonsteroidal antiinflammatory drug (NSAID) administration. See Hip Dysplasia section (p. 469) for medication options.
- Chronic IVDD or immune-mediated disease may require intermittent or persistent corticosteroid treatment.
- Antibiotic therapy for discospondylitis (p. 266) or vertebral osteomyelitis continued for 6 weeks beyond resolution of clinical signs

Drug Interactions

Glucocorticoids and NSAIDs must not be administered concurrently because of the risk of severe gastrointestinal ulceration.

Possible Complications

- Worsening or recurrence of signs
- Progression of spinal cord lesions
- Myelomalacia
- Valvular endocarditis, for infectious conditions

Recommended Monitoring

- Repeat physical and neurologic examination within 12-24 hours of treatment.
- Follow-up examination and radiographs as needed

PROGNOSIS & OUTCOME

Depends on underlying cause

PEARLS & CONSIDERATIONS

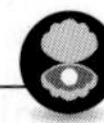

Comments

- Localization of pain requires thorough physical and neurologic examination.

- Acute back pain with neurologic deficits may represent a surgical emergency and should be evaluated immediately.
- Perceived back pain may actually be abdominal or kidney pain; use care when isolating source of pain on examination.

Technician Tips

- Avoid injury. Examination of painful patients may require analgesia and restraint, although opioids can alter exam findings.
- Exercise caution with examination if back pain may be associated with spinal instability, such as fracture or luxation.

Client Education

- Owner should monitor for recurrence of signs.
- Acute worsening of signs warrants emergency evaluation and treatment.

SUGGESTED READING

Lorenz MD, et al: Handbook of veterinary neurology, St. Louis, 2012, Saunders, pp 413-431.

AUTHOR: Peter Moak, DVM
EDITOR: Leah A. Cohn, DVM, PhD, DACVIM

Baclofen and Other Centrally Acting Muscle Relaxants Toxicosis

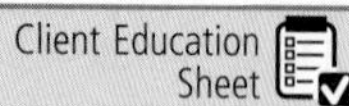

BASIC INFORMATION

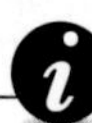

Definition

Syndrome developing after the ingestion of one of several centrally acting skeletal muscle relaxants (SMRs) and characterized mainly by central nervous system (CNS) depression

Synonyms

Generic Name	Trade Names
Baclofen	Lioresal, Kemstro
Carisoprodol	Soma
Chlorphenesin carbamate	Maolate
Chlorzoxazone	Parafon Forte
Cyclobenzaprine	Flexeril
Guaifenesin	Gecolate
Metaxalone	Skelaxin
Methocarbamol	Robaxin, Robaxin-V
Orphenadrine	Norflex
Tizanidine	Zanaflex

Drugs	Chief Complaints
Baclofen	Onset of signs within 15 minutes to 7 hours after ingestion Dogs: vomiting, ataxia, hypersalivation, depression, vocalization, disorientation or agitation, recumbency, coma, seizure Cats: vomiting, depression, ataxia, weakness, hypothermia, recumbency, coma, mydriasis, diarrhea
Cyclobenzaprine	Onset within 30 minutes to several hours Depression, ataxia, vomiting, weakness, mydriasis, tachycardia, vocalization, agitation, tremors, seizures
Orphenadrine	Onset within 30 minutes to several hours Weakness, vomiting, tachycardia, agitation, seizures
Tizanidine	Onset within 30 minutes to 4 hours Lethargy, somnolence, bradycardia, hypotension, recumbency, weakness, vocalization, urinary retention, collapse, coma
Other SMRs: carisoprodol, chlorphenesin carbamate, chlorzoxazone, metaxalone, methocarbamol, guaifenesin	Stupor, hypotension, coma, respiratory depression, seizures (rare)

Epidemiology

SPECIES, AGE, SEX

All species susceptible; dogs more likely because of indiscriminate eating habits

RISK FACTORS

- Availability of muscle relaxants in the animal's environment
- Many people taking skeletal muscle relaxants for spasticity disorders (e.g., multiple sclerosis) also take other medications, increasing the risk for multiple drug exposures by pets.

Clinical Presentation

HISTORY, CHIEF COMPLAINT

History of exposure to muscle relaxants or presence of drugs in environment (see Table)

PHYSICAL EXAM FINDINGS

Baclofen

- As above (see Table)
- Hypothermia (if recumbent), hyperthermia (if seizing)
- Hypertension or hypotension
- Tachycardia or bradycardia
- Hypoventilation
- Miosis (dogs) or mydriasis (cats)
- Muscular hypotonia, weakness

Cyclobenzaprine and orphenadrine

- Depression or agitation, hyperesthesia (cats), vocalization
- Miosis (dogs) or mydriasis (cats), nystagmus (occasional, dog and cat)
- Muscle weakness, tremors, fasciculation
- Panting
- Tachycardia or bradycardia
- Hyperthermia

Tizanidine

- Depression, weakness, ataxia
- Hypotension, bradycardia
- Pale mucous membranes, prolonged capillary refill time
- Hypothermia

Other SMRs

- Depression, somnolence, weakness
- Hypoventilation, cyanosis
- Tachycardia, hypotension
- Hypothermia (if recumbent), hyperthermia (if seizing)

Etiology and Pathophysiology

Source:

- Most centrally acting SMRs are used for controlling spasticity in humans with neuromuscular disorders. May also be prescribed for relief of musculoskeletal pain.

Mechanism of toxicosis:

- Baclofen: mimics gamma-aminobutyric acid (GABA) in the spinal cord, blocking excitatory responses to sensory input and causing flaccid paralysis. Seizures may be due to interference with GABA release from

presynaptic neurons, resulting in excessive postsynaptic nerve firing.
- Cyclobenzaprine: structurally and functionally related to tricyclic antidepressants. Skeletal muscle relaxation may be related to sedative effects and inhibition of brainstem and spinal cord gamma and alpha motor neurons. In overdose situations, anticholinergic and antihistaminic effects become exaggerated.
- Tizanidine's mechanism of action is like that of xylazine and clonidine. It stimulates alpha-adrenoreceptors in the brainstem, causing decreased vascular resistance, heart rate, and blood pressure. At therapeutic levels, skeletal muscle effects predominate, but in overdose situations, pronounced cardiovascular effects occur.
- Orphenadrine has pronounced anticholinergic and antihistaminic effects.
- Chlorphenesin carbamate, guaifenesin, and methocarbamol may act by blocking nerve impulse transmission within the brainstem, spinal cord, and subcortical levels of the brain. Some skeletal muscle relaxant effect is due to sedation.
- Carisoprodol causes skeletal muscle relaxation by depression of postsynaptic spinal reflexes. Some skeletal muscle relaxant effect is due to sedation.
- Chlorzoxazone and metaxalone have no direct effect on skeletal muscles; muscle relaxant properties are likely due to sedative effects.

DIAGNOSIS

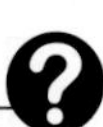

Diagnostic Overview

Diagnosis is based on history of exposure or presence of drugs in animal's environment along with appropriate clinical signs (e.g., ataxia, depression, coma, vocalization).

Differential Diagnosis

Toxicologic:
- Other CNS depressants: barbiturates, benzodiazepines, opioids, avermectins, ethylene glycol, tick paralysis, botulinum toxin, ionophore ingestion (dogs)
- Other causes of seizures: amphetamines, ethylene glycol, metaldehyde, strychnine, methylxanthines, zinc phosphide, tricyclic antidepressants, serotonergic drugs

Non-toxicologic, spontaneous:
- Spinal trauma, CNS trauma
- Polyradiculoneuritis, tick paralysis
- Organic brain disease (e.g., neoplasia, inflammation)

Initial Database

- CBC, serum biochemistry profile: minimal alterations expected from SMR (identify pre-existing liver or kidney dysfunction that may interfere with drug elimination)
  - Orphenadrine overdose in humans has been associated with hypokalemia, hypoglycemia, liver enzyme elevations, and bleeding disorders.

Advanced or Confirmatory Testing

- Baclofen, carisoprodol, chlorzoxazone, cyclobenzaprine, guaifenesin, and methocarbamol levels can be determined in urine and/ or serum; presence will confirm exposure.
  - Turnaround time may limit usefulness in dealing with an acute intoxication.
  - Cyclobenzaprine results in a positive serum or urine assay result for amitriptyline.

TREATMENT

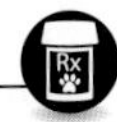

Treatment Overview

Treatment is aimed at early decontamination of asymptomatic patients (emesis induction; administration of activated charcoal) and supportive care to address overt signs when they are present.

Acute General Treatment

- Stabilize the patient.
  - Maintain respiration: endotracheal intubation and positive-pressure mechanical ventilatory support may be required.
  - Control seizures: diazepam 0.5-1 mg/kg slow IV to effect; propofol or isoflurane may be considered in cases refractory to diazepam (induce, keep anesthetized 5-10 minutes, then recover). Barbiturates should be considered a last resort because their use may result in exacerbation of CNS depression; diazepam is also generally useful for managing agitation.
- Manage cardiovascular abnormalities: most arrhythmias and blood pressure irregularities resolve during supportive care. Nitroprusside constant-rate IV infusion (1-2 mcg/kg/min [dogs] or 0.5 mcg/kg/min [cats], increased incrementally q 3-5 minutes until blood pressure is reduced to < 180 mm Hg systolic) has been successfully used to manage baclofen-induced hypertension in dogs.
- Atropine is contraindicated in the management of bradycardia due to orphenadrine or cyclobenzaprine toxicosis because it exacerbates anticholinergic effects.
- Supportive care
  - Fluid diuresis: for hypotension/hypovolemia and to promote urine formation; may enhance excretion of baclofen
  - Atipamezole (50 mcg/kg, give one-fourth to one-third of dose IV, remainder IM) or yohimbine (0.25 mg/kg slow IV) can be helpful to reverse hypotension from tizanidine.
  - Cyproheptadine (1.1 mg/kg PO or PR; can repeat once if needed) may be helpful in reducing vocalization in dogs.
  - Thermoregulation is essential, especially in comatose or recumbent animals.
- Decontamination of patient (p. 1087)
  - Induction of emesis is contraindicated in animals showing overt clinical signs.
  - Induce emesis (p. 1188): because of the potential for rapid onset of clinical signs, induction of emesis is best done under veterinary supervision.
  - Gastric lavage (p. 1117): consider for large ingestions (many tablets); protect airway with cuffed endotracheal tube.
  - Activated charcoal 1-2 g/kg PO or dose according to packaging label for commercial products. Repeated doses of activated charcoal (q 8h with a cathartic for 24h) are recommended for cyclobenzaprine and orphenadrine if signs persist; single doses are recommended for the remaining SMRs.
- Anecdotally, intravenous lipid solutions have hastened recovery of dogs with baclofen toxicosis (p. 1127).

Chronic Treatment

Ventilatory support (p. 1185) may be required for several days (particularly with baclofen).

Nutrition/Diet

For patients requiring long-term ventilatory support, feeding tubes or parenteral nutrition may be considered (pp. 1107 and 1148).

Drug Interactions

Use caution when administering drugs to agitated animals.

Recommended Monitoring

Respiratory rate and rhythm, heart rate, blood pressure, body temperature, blood gases, serum electrolytes, hydration status, fluid ins/outs

PROGNOSIS & OUTCOME

- Signs can persist for hours to days, depending on the SMR involved and the dose ingested.
- Most patients with mild to moderate signs receiving prompt and appropriate veterinary attention have excellent prognoses.
- Patients exhibiting respiratory depression requiring ventilatory support, seizures, or coma more guarded prognosis

PEARLS & CONSIDERATIONS

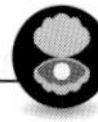

Comments

- Because the primary effect of these drugs is CNS depression, when treating animals showing paradoxical excitation, it is important to use the lowest sedative dose necessary to relieve the stimulation to avoid oversedation after the agitation has resolved.
- Baclofen, cyclobenzaprine, and tizanidine have narrow margins of safety, and significant (potentially life-threatening) signs can be seen at low doses.
  - Baclofen: doses > 1 mg/kg can cause signs; doses ≥ 8 mg/kg can be fatal to dogs.
  - Cyclobenzaprine: doses of 0.07 mg/kg have resulted in clinical signs in dogs.
  - Tizanidine: doses of 0.05 mg/kg have been associated with clinical signs in dogs, with hypotension occurring at doses as low as 0.08 mg/kg.
- Muscle relaxants methocarbamol, guaifenesin, and chlorphenesin carbamate have large margins of safety, and overdoses rarely cause life-threatening problems.

Prevention

Keep medications out of reach of pets.

Technician Tips

- Be prepared for paradoxical excitement (vocalization, paddling) when a sedative is given to patients with SMR intoxication. Be sure doors are closed to prevent escape, have the patient on a surface clear of sharp or breakable objects, and take precautions to avoid being injured.
- Regurgitation/aspiration is a common complication in comatose and recumbent animals with SMR toxicosis. Leave the endotracheal tube in an appropriate amount of time and keep the head of the patient lower than the chest to reduce the risk of aspiration.

Client Education

- When taking medication, do so in a room away from pets with the door closed to prevent pets from ingesting an accidentally dropped tablet.
- Never administer human medications to pets without first consulting a veterinarian.

SUGGESTED READING

Gwaltney-Brant SM: Skeletal muscle relaxants. In Plumlee KH, editor: Clinical veterinary toxicology, St. Louis, 2004, Mosby, p 324.

AUTHOR: Sharon M. Gwaltney-Brant, DVM, PhD, DABVT, DABT
EDITOR: Tina Wismer, DVM, MS, DABVT, DABT

Barking, Excessive

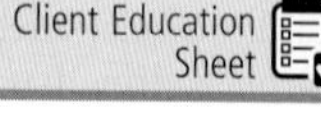

BASIC INFORMATION

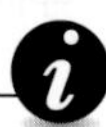

Definition

A normal amount of barking that is deemed unacceptable to humans or a pathologic amount of barking as part of an anxiety or other behavioral disorder

Epidemiology

SPECIES, AGE, SEX

- Dogs of any age and either sex
- Puppy vocalizations: more often associated with care-seeking behaviors
- Adult vocalizations: more often associated with care-giving behaviors, social interaction, cohesion

RISK FACTORS

In breeds that have been selected for specific vocalization behaviors, such vocalizations may become more annoying to clients and/or their neighbors but be normal.

CONTAGION AND ZOONOSIS

Naive/newly added puppies or adults may learn barking by observation.

GEOGRAPHY AND SEASONALITY

Dogs kept outdoors, especially if confined and not walked, are more likely to use barking to communicate with other dogs in the vicinity.

ASSOCIATED DISORDERS

Barking may be a nonspecific sign in any anxiety-based disorder, including separation anxiety, aggression, obsessive-compulsive disorder (OCD), and noise, storm, and social phobias.

Clinical Presentation

HISTORY, CHIEF COMPLAINT

- Excessive barking is noted by client or from neighbor complaints.
- Barking can appear indiscriminate or in response to external stimuli. Barking associated with an anxiety disorder may be accompanied by hypervigilant behavior (continuous monitoring of the social and physical environments). In these cases, dogs may scan at windows, along fences, and at doors. Clients may also describe the patient as unable to relax.
- Determining whether barking occurs in the owner's absence (e.g., associated with separation anxiety) or whether it ends with the owner's inadvertently rewarding the behavior, as with a treat to silence the dog (i.e., learned behavior) is important.

PHYSICAL EXAM FINDINGS

- Generally unremarkable
- Acute excessive barking may lead to inflammation of the vocal cords and surrounding tissue.
- Rarely, a source of pain or other physical abnormality can be identified as a trigger for excessive barking.

Etiology and Pathophysiology

- Barking may be used for making contact with others (including when reuniting after being apart); to signal alarm, concern, or distress; and to solicit information from other dogs (depending on pitch, tone, frequency, and pattern).
- Spectrographic analysis of canine barks shows that their structure varies predictably according to context; barks likely can be divided into contextual subtypes and are thought to convey complex information to canine and human listeners.
- Studies support the observation that people can distinguish between barks and can correctly identify the context in which a bark was given.
- Barking can also be a sign of an anxiety disorder, including OCD (p. 701).

DIAGNOSIS

Diagnostic Overview

The diagnosis is made based on history. The context in which the barking occurs determines whether the behavior is normal but inconvenient or indicative of a mood disorder.

Differential Diagnosis

- Normal barking, especially alarm barking by watch and guard dogs selected to alert by barking, reactive barking in terrier and hound breeds, and working barking in some herding breeds. These barking behaviors can be modified with humane training and are typically context-appropriate, although inconvenient or undesirable for some clients.
- Learned behavior: barking that elicits a response/reward from the client (e.g., the dog barks and it is let out or petted to calm it down)
- Separation anxiety
- Thunderstorm phobia
- Noise phobia
- OCD

Change in vocalization is described on p. 1039.

Initial Database

Minimum database: complete blood count, serum chemistry profile, and urinalysis to rule out underlying contraindications for psychotropic medication, if their use is warranted. Other laboratory or imaging procedures should address any physical exam abnormalities.

Advanced or Confirmatory Testing

Learned behaviors are ruled out if they are extinguished by complete removal of the reward. Extinction is a gradual waning in occurrence of a behavior in the absence of a reward. The longer the behavior has been ongoing, reinforced, and/or rewarded, the longer it will take to extinguish it.

TREATMENT

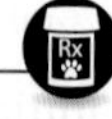

Treatment Overview

The goal is to treat the disorder or modify the normal behavior based on accurate identification of cause.

Acute and Chronic Treatment

- If barking is within the normal behavioral repertoire, given triggers, and context, the dog can be taught when (reward good

barking) and when not to bark (ignore bad barking), coupling both to words used only in those situations.
  - When the dog barks in a context that annoys the owner, redirecting the dog to an incompatible behavior (e.g., catching a toy with the mouth, playing tug) stops barking and rewards an alternative behavior. The offered alternative behavior must be of higher value to the dog.
- If barking is pathologic, the anxiety state that leads to the abnormal vocalization must be treated.
  - Identify triggers and limit exposure to them whenever possible.
  - When barking occurs, redirect the dog's attention and activity to alternative behaviors (play, relaxation) and reward for compliance; use a leash or head collar if necessary; reward all decreases in barking in response to triggers.
  - A neutral stimulus (noise, bouncing ball/toy) may be used for interrupting the behavior, followed by positive engagement in a different, non–barking-related behavior that can be rewarded.
  - Treatment with psychotropic medication is appropriate only if barking is a manifestation of a behavioral disorder (e.g., anxiety); consider referral to a behavior specialist.
  - Punishment, yelling, and use of shock collars should be avoided. Aversive responses serve only to increase rather than decrease arousal and may exacerbate the barking behavior.
- Dogs should be taught to relax while making eye contact with the clients as a preferred default/substitute behavior when the dog encounters a situation about which it is anxious or unsure.
- Systematic desensitization can be used if the triggers can be identified and manipulated (e.g., Pet Tutor [https://smartanimaltraining.com/]).
- An alternative alert should be taught so the dog still signals information (e.g., sitting in a designated spot or in front of the clients).

Drug Interactions

- Amitriptyline, fluoxetine, and clomipramine should not be used with monoamine oxidase inhibitors (e.g., amitraz, selegiline). Combinations of different classes of psychotropic medications at lowered doses are usually safe other than the potential for sedation, in which case dosages can be adjusted downward.
- Fluoxetine, paroxetine, and possibly sertraline, if given with tramadol, may increase the risk of serotonin syndrome (p. 1281). If coadministration is necessary, start both at reduced dosages, titrate each to effect, and monitor for serotonin syndrome.

Possible Complications

Clients who attempt behavior modification too quickly (e.g., rewarding sitting even when the dog is distressed instead of working on relaxation), with force, or inconsistently (in a multi-person household) may experience slow or no progress. Leash, choke chain, or pinch collar corrections are contraindicated; they can damage the esophagus, trachea, larynx, and adjacent structures.

Recommended Monitoring

Frequent follow-up with clients (at least weekly) is helpful. Medications should be monitored for cardiac, renal, or hepatic side effects (uncommon) or sedation (more common).

PROGNOSIS & OUTCOME

- For species-appropriate but inconvenient barking, prognosis is very good to excellent when owners understand the diagnosis.
- For pathologic barking, prognosis ranges from fair to very good, depending on severity and chronicity of disorder.
- Both are influenced by client compliance, environmental circumstances, and response to psychotropic medication in the case of pathologic barking.

PEARLS & CONSIDERATIONS

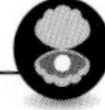

Comments

Shock collars have no place in the treatment of any behavioral condition. They always exacerbate anxiety, even if they may suppress some aspects of behavioral signs; the behavior of dogs trained with a shock collar changes even outside the context of the training environment (display of signs of anxiety). Assessment for the potential risk of physical abuse of pets, spouses, and children should be made in any case in which owners insist on their use.

Prevention

Early intervention is key. When dogs are added to the home, education of the dog about what level of barking is acceptable to the client should be instituted on the first episode of unwanted barking.

Technician Tips

- Verbal reprimands serve no useful purpose. If a dog is barking excessively in the hospital, changing stimuli (e.g., moving the dog to an area with less/more activity or different animals in surroundings) is far better.
- Dogs may bark or whine in a hospital setting due to anxiety and the stress of being in an unfamiliar and overwhelming environment in addition to the physical distress of illness/injury. These vocalizations should *not* be ignored; distress has a negative effect on the immune system and healing. Evaluate the patient's body language so that the need for analgesics, short-term anxiolytics (e.g., benzodiazepines), or sedatives is not ignored.
- Reactive barking in the examination room should trigger a conversation with the owner to inquire what other situations provoke a similar reaction.

Client Education

- Yelling at a dog to be quiet will increase arousal and is therefore counterproductive.
- Clients can teach their dog the level of alarm barking they can tolerate by calmly taking the barking dog away from the trigger (using a leash if necessary), asking for an alternative behavior (sitting while looking at the client in a relaxed fashion), and then rewarding the quiet response.
- Clients can also thank their dog for barking when the barking is appropriate (e.g., someone is in the driveway) and then reward them for stopping, which the dog will do when he or she looks at the client in response to the client's praise.

SUGGESTED READING

Pongrácz P, et al: Barking in family dogs: an ethological approach. Vet J 183:141-147, 2010.

AUTHOR: Soraya V. Juarbe-Diaz, DVM, DACVB
EDITOR: Karen L. Overall, VMD, MA, PhD, DACVB

Bartonellosis

BASIC INFORMATION

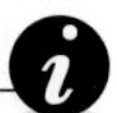

Definition

Bartonellosis is infection with any of a number of different species of intracellular, fastidious gram-negative bacteria in the genus *Bartonella.* These bacteria are transmitted by hematophagous insects. Of more than 36 known species, at least 17 are pathogenic.

Synonyms

- Cat-scratch disease (common disease consequence of human infection with *Bartonella henselae,* resulting in self-limiting lymphadenomegaly ± fever and malaise)

- Bacillary angiomatosis (rare subdermal disease consequence of human infection with *B. henselae* or *Bartonella quintana*)
- Peliosis hepatis (rare vascular condition of the liver with several causes, including *B. henselae* infection)

Epidemiology

SPECIES, AGE, SEX

- Dogs and cats of either sex and any age, although bacteremia with some *Bartonella* spp seems to be more common in young and old animals
- Cats are the reservoir host for *B. henselae*, *Bartonella clarridgeiae*, and *Bartonella koehlerae*.
- Wild canids and dogs are the reservoir hosts for *Bartonella vinsonii* subsp *berkhoffii*, *Bartonella rochalimae*, and *Candidatus Bartonella merieuxii*.
- Numerous other *Bartonella* spp exist in other reservoir hosts, and accidental infection can occur in dogs or cats.

RISK FACTORS

- Exposure to and lack of protection from hematophagous insects such as fleas, ticks, and biting flies increase risk of infection.
- Immunosuppression or co-infection increase risk of illness associated with *Bartonella* infection.

CONTAGION AND ZOONOSIS

- These pathogens are transmitted primarily through exposure to insect vectors or their waste (e.g., flea frass).
- Each *Bartonella* species is associated with one or more adapted reservoir host. Although easily transmitted from one such adapted host to another, overt disease in the adapted species is uncommon.
- Disease is more likely when *Bartonella* infect a nonadapted or accidental host. Although many *Bartonella* spp can cause zoonotic infection, the best known infections associated with dogs and cats are listed in the table.

GEOGRAPHY AND SEASONALITY

Worldwide; especially common where vectors are likely (often warm climates)

ASSOCIATED DISORDERS

Numerous manifestations of acute or chronic infection are possible.

Clinical Presentation

DISEASE FORMS/SUBTYPES

- The complete spectrum of illness associated with bartonellosis is not understood. Although some disease manifestations are clearly associated with infection (e.g., endocarditis), other illnesses have been recognized in infected animals, but a causal relationship has not been established.
- *B. henselae* in cats is most often a subclinical infection of primary importance as a zoonotic pathogen (i.e., cat-scratch disease).
    - Uveitis, infertility, abortion, and stillbirth are described in experimentally infected cats.
    - Fever, endocarditis, and myocarditis are described in naturally infected cats.
    - Osteomyelitis, stomatitis suggested to be caused by bartonellosis
- *B. vinsonii* subsp *berkhoffii* is best understood as a cause of blood culture–negative endocarditis in dogs. Other possible manifestations include
    - Endocarditis, myocarditis, arrhythmia
    - Bacillary angiomatosis
    - Granulomatous hepatitis, splenitis, and lymphadenitis
    - Panniculitis
    - Polyarthritis
    - Rhinitis
    - Meningoencephalitis
    - Vasculitis (cutaneous)
    - Uveitis and chorioretinitis
    - Immune-mediated blood disorders (e.g., immune-mediated hemolytic anemia)
    - Thromboembolism

HISTORY, CHIEF COMPLAINT

- Because the types of illness caused by infection are diverse and not well characterized, the history of infected animals is also quite varied.
- *B. henselae* in cats: most often, no clinical signs. Occasionally, nonspecific signs of anorexia, lethargy, weakness, or ocular abnormalities noticed. Abortion or stillbirths may occur.
- *B. vinsonii* subspecies *berkhoffii* in dogs: infection is often subclinical. Illness is usually accompanied by nonspecific signs that can include lethargy, exercise intolerance, weight loss, collapse, sudden death (p. 294).

PHYSICAL EXAM FINDINGS

- *B. henselae* in cats: usually unremarkable. Possible abnormalities include
    - Fever
    - Ocular abnormalities suggestive of uveitis (p. 1023)
    - Heart murmur
    - Cardiac arrhythmia
    - Lymphadenomegaly
    - Stomatitis (usually in cats co-infected with feline immunodeficiency virus)
- *B. vinsonii* subsp *berkhoffii* in dogs: possible abnormalities include
    - Heart murmur
    - Fever
    - Arrhythmia
    - Evidence of congestive heart failure (CHF) (p. 408)
    - Lymphadenomegaly
    - Splenomegaly/hepatomegaly
    - Lameness
    - Uveitis

Etiology and Pathophysiology

- *Bartonella* spp are relatively newly recognized pathogens, with new species and new disease manifestations still being described on a frequent basis.
- Organisms are passed from one animal to another by hematophagous insects such as fleas, ticks, lice, keds, biting flies, and perhaps others.
- Pathogens may be passed in the excrement of the vectors, as appears to be the case for *B. henselae*, and potentially through saliva by ticks or sand flies.
- In the adapted reservoir host, the organisms exist in red blood cells (RBCs) and vascular endothelial cells for long periods. The organisms also gain access to mononuclear and other cell types. Because the bacteria escape immune control, they are often described as *stealth pathogens*. The location of the pathogen in RBCs is ideal for transmitting the bacterium to naïve vector insects.
- Because the bacteria are well adapted to the reservoir host, diseases may not occur at all or may be delayed in onset. Chronic bacteremia is often detected by polymerase chain reaction (PCR) assays or blood culture in seemingly healthy reservoir hosts. Although overt illness is not common in the infected reservoir host, long-term infection may exact a biological toll on the host that predisposes to disease at some point in life. Immune suppression or other stressors make illness in the reservoir more likely.
    - Endocarditis, myocarditis, and vascular pathology may be consequences of infection.
    - Immune-mediated (e.g., glomerulonephritis) and autoimmune (e.g., immune-mediated hemolytic anemia) disease may be manifestations of infection.
- When nonadapted animals become infected, disease is more likely to occur than in adapted hosts. Nevertheless, subclinical infections are also well documented in nonadapted hosts.

DIAGNOSIS

Diagnostic Overview

Bartonellosis should be considered in the differential diagnosis for a number of disorders, especially when another cause is not identified; if there has been a history of exposure to insect vectors; if an underlying immunodeficiency or immunosuppression is recognized; or if the animal fails to improve with standard care.

It can be challenging to prove that bartonellosis is the cause of clinical disease. There are no specific suggestive findings on routine laboratory testing or imaging studies. The bacterium is too small to see on microscopic evaluation of the blood smear or in most instances tissue histopathology. Culture of the organisms from blood is possible in the reservoir host, but infection in the reservoir does not prove disease causation and may be common in a given population and therefore incidental to an illness. Culture from the nonadapted host, on the other hand, is extremely challenging. Serologic testing is often positive in a predisposed population (i.e., those exposed to insect vectors) and is sometimes negative despite infection in animals with bartonellosis. Specialized PCR performed after culture in an insect growth media is the preferred test method but is still prone to false-negative results, especially when only a single sample is tested.

Differential Diagnosis

- The differential diagnosis list is broad and varies with the disease manifestation.
- Consider co-infection with other vector transmitted pathogens.
- Consider routine bacterial endocarditis (p. 294).

Initial Database

- CBC, serum chemistry profile, urinalysis: variable depending on manifestation; can be entirely normal
  - May recognize thrombocytopenia, anemia, monocytosis, or eosinophilia
  - With liver involvement, liver enzymes can be increased
- Imaging studies: variable depending on manifestation. With endocarditis, evidence of cardiomegaly and CHF is possible.
- Retroviral and hemotropic *Mycoplasma* testing (cats) to rule out concurrent infection
- Other tests as indicated by history and examination (e.g., with suspected endocarditis, echocardiogram and routine blood culture are indicated)

Advanced or Confirmatory Testing

- Serologic tests: extremely poor sensitivity to detect infection
  - Only 50% of dogs infected with *B. vinsonii* subsp *berkhoffii* and 25% of dogs infected with *B. henselae* are seropositive.
  - A single positive titer demonstrates prior infection but cannot prove disease causation.
  - A fourfold increase in titer over 2-3 weeks can confirm acute infection.
- Culture of organisms from blood, another bodily fluid, or tissue:
  - Positive culture is often possible from infected reservoir host
  - Culture is rarely positive from accidental host
- Routine PCR: poor sensitivity
- PCR after enrichment in insect growth media: improved sensitivity
  - Blood/fluid/tissue is first cultured in insect-based liquid culture media (*Bartonella* alpha Proteobacteria growth medium [BAPGM]) for ≥ 7 days.
  - PCR assay applied to amplify *Bartonella* from media
  - Galaxy Diagnostics, Inc. (contact@galaxydx.com, Morrisville, NC)
  - Optimal results with fresh-frozen tissue or three blood samples collected at different times

TREATMENT

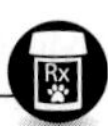

Treatment Overview

An optimal protocol for treatment of bartonellosis has not been established. *Bartonella* spp can develop rapid antimicrobial resistance to macrolides. Supportive care for the specific manifestation of disease is important. Usually, long-term treatment with a combination of antibiotics is recommended to combat infection, but it is unlikely to produce complete microbiological cure.

Acute General Treatment

- Usually, a combination of a fluoroquinolone and tetracycline is recommended for 4-12 weeks.
  - For stable animals, start with only one antimicrobial drug and then add the second several days to 1 week later. This is to avoid the rare but potentially serious complication of a Jarisch-Herxheimer–like reaction. This reaction, presumably due to bacterial death and cytokine release by the host, usually begins 4 to 7 days after therapy is begun and results in fever, lethargy, and vomiting.
  - Enrofloxacin 10 mg/kg PO q 24h (dogs) or pradofloxacin 7.5-10 mg/kg PO q 24h (cats)
  - Doxycycline or minocycline 10 mg/kg PO q 12h (dogs) or 8.8 mg/kg q 24h (cats); note the dose required is higher than that required to treat other vector-borne infections such as ehrlichiosis.
- In animals with life-threatening manifestations such as endocarditis and associated heart failure, initial additional use of aminoglycoside antibiotics has been suggested (e.g., amikacin 15-30 mg/kg IV, IM, or SQ q 24h for 7-10 days [dog] or 10-14 mg/kg IV, IM, or SQ q 24h [cat])
- Due to rapid antibacterial resistance, the use of azithromycin is no longer recommended.
- Address specific disorders as appropriate; for example
  - Endocarditis (p. 294)
  - CHF (p. 408)
  - Uveitis (p. 1023)

Possible Complications

- Jarisch-Herxheimer–like reaction 4-7 days after initiation of therapy
- Tetracycline drugs can cause esophageal irritation and stricture; follow tablet/capsule with food or water. Compounded liquid tetracyclines have a short shelf life.
- Treatment failure

Recommended Monitoring

- Clinical response to treatment
- For animals that were seropositive before treatment, repeat titers at 1 month and 6 months after treatment may be informative (resolution of antibody response is a good prognostic indicator, but an unchanged titer may suggest additional antimicrobial therapy is warranted).
- For seronegative animals, consider repeating serology 2-3 weeks after starting antibiotics to document seroreactivity and support for clinical diagnosis.
- Ideally, BAPGM enrichment PCR is repeated 2 and 6 weeks after completion of therapy.

PROGNOSIS & OUTCOME

Varies; prognosis for endocarditis is guarded, but other manifestations may respond well to treatment. Recurrent or persistent infection is possible with any species or disease manifestation.

PEARLS & CONSIDERATIONS

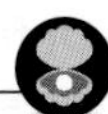

Comments

- Currently, there is a steep learning curve regarding bartonellosis in animals and humans, with new species and vectors recognized routinely. Similarly, new potential disease manifestations related to these infections are recognized on a frequent basis. If bartonellosis is suspected, it is worth consultation with a veterinary internal medicine or microbiology specialist for the most up-to-date information.
- In areas with high flea burdens, seroprevalence of *Bartonella* spp in cats can be > 90%, with bacteremia rates of > 50%.
- Seroprevalence rates for *Bartonella* spp in dogs vary, but risk is higher for free-roaming male dogs living in rural areas.
- *B. henselae* bacteria remain viable in flea feces for at least 9 days.
- Humans become infected by inoculation of flea feces when cats (or dogs) scratch or bite; the best way to avoid zoonotic infection is strict flea control.
- There is no benefit to serologic testing of a cat for *Bartonella* spp before adoption.
- There is no benefit to antimicrobial treatment of a healthy, seropositive cat because 1) it is

Select *Bartonella* Species and Reservoir Host

Bartonella Species	Reservoir Host	Potential Vectors	Accidental Hosts
B. clarridgeiae	Cats	Fleas, ticks	Humans, dogs
B. henselae	Cats, dogs	Fleas, ticks	Humans, dogs
B. koehlerae	Cats, gerbils	Fleas	Humans
Candidatus B. merieuxii	Dogs	Fleas	
B. rochalimae	Dogs	Sandflies	Humans
B. vinsonii subsp *berkhoffii*	Coyotes, dogs, foxes	Ticks	Humans

Adapted from Breitschwerdt EB: Bartonellosis, One Health and all creatures great and small. Vet Dermatol 28:96-e21, 2017.

not certain the pathogen can be eliminated by treatment, and 2) even if the cat is bacteremic, zoonosis is not transmitted to people in the absence of fleas.

Prevention

Strict prevention of ectoparasites (fleas, ticks); avoid allowing animals to roam

Technician Tips

- People diagnosed with cat-scratch disease need not get rid of the cat. Instead, strict flea control is warranted.
- Veterinarians and veterinary technicians are at a higher risk than the general population for *Bartonella* spp infection. Animals that have fleas should be treated for fleas (e.g., nitenpyram) before hospitalization.
- Needlestick transmission of *B. henselae* and *B. vinsonii* subsp *berkhoffii* have been documented in veterinary workers.

Client Education

Strict flea control is the best way to avoid zoonotic infection with *Bartonella* spp.

SUGGESTED READING

Breitschwerdt EB: Bartonellosis, one health and all creatures great and small. Vet Dermatol 28:96-e21, 2017.

AUTHOR: Leah A. Cohn, DVM, PhD, DACVIM
EDITOR: Joseph Taboada, DVM, DACVIM

Bee and Other Insect Stings

BASIC INFORMATION

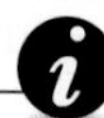

Definition

Stings from insects such as bees, wasps, and hornets. Spider envenomation is discussed separately (p. 928).

Epidemiology

SPECIES, AGE, SEX

More likely to occur in young, inquisitive animals. Cats may be more tolerant than dogs to many insect toxins.

GENETICS, BREED PREDISPOSITION

Boxers and pit bulls seem especially prone to insect hypersensitivity.

GEOGRAPHY AND SEASONALITY

Bee stings are more common during warm weather when insects are active.

Clinical Presentation

HISTORY, CHIEF COMPLAINT

For bees, wasps, hornets (order Hymenoptera), usually, sting is unwitnessed. Instead, animals present for clinical signs associated with allergic reaction (p. 54). Severity of signs will depend on the type of venom, location of the sting, number of stings, and sensitivity of the animal receiving the sting.

PHYSICAL EXAM FINDINGS

- Bees, wasps, hornets
  - Local reaction associated with an immunologic response is the most common finding. This may include a swollen head/face or diffuse urticaria. Cases with severe facial swelling can develop upper airway obstruction and respiratory distress.
  - Less commonly, an animal may develop anaphylaxis, usually within 15 minutes of sting (p. 54). Anaphylaxis in dogs manifests as vomiting, defecation, urination, muscular weakness, collapse, respiratory depression, or seizures. Cats often show signs of pruritus, dyspnea, salivation, incoordination, and collapse.
  - Animals with massive envenomation may show signs of acute respiratory distress syndrome (p. 27) or disseminated intravascular coagulation (p. 1218).

Etiology and Pathophysiology

- Most systemic signs result from an immunoglobulin E (IgE)–mediated allergic reaction (p. 1238).
- Bee stings result in the loss of the stinger, which remains in the victim, and the venom sac (if attached) will continue to administer venom (apitoxin).
  - Melittin is a major component of apitoxin, and with phospholipase A_2, it results in altered cell permeability, prostaglandin production, and cell death. Other components include histamine and hyaluronidase, which support inflammation and tissue damage.
- Wasps can sting multiple times and inject a small amount of venom at each sting.
  - Venom contains histamine, hyaluronidase, phospholipase, and other small peptides. The venom also contains acetylcholine, which contributes to pain.
- A small number of dogs and cats may develop anaphylaxis.

DIAGNOSIS

Diagnostic Overview

The diagnosis is frequently presumptive and based on clinical signs and history of possible exposure. Stings are seldom witnessed by pet owners.

Differential Diagnosis

- Cellulitis
- Peripheral edema
- Other causes of allergy or anaphylaxis

Initial Database

- Packed cell volume
- Serum total protein
- Blood glucose
- Blood urea nitrogen/creatinine

Advanced or Confirmatory Testing

Rarely required except in cases of anaphylaxis (p. 54)

TREATMENT

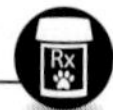

Treatment Overview

Provide relief of discomfort, address hypersensitivity reaction

Acute General Treatment

Facial edema/urticaria:

- Remove stinger if present. Use fine forceps/tweezers or a flat object (e.g., dull side of a scalpel blade), taking care not to press on the stinger's sac (if present).
- Diphenhydramine 1-2 mg/kg IM
- Dexamethasone sodium phosphate 0.2 mg/kg IM or slow IV

Anaphylaxis may require diphenhydramine and dexamethasone, as well as one or more of the following treatments, according to escalating degree of severity of the reaction:

- Intravenous isotonic crystalloid fluids (up to 45-90 mL/kg IV, given incrementally)
- Epinephrine 0.01 mg/kg IV

Behavior/Exercise

Animals should be leash-walked or supervised when outside to avoid re-exposure.

Recommended Monitoring

Animals with facial swelling or urticaria should be monitored for 20-30 minutes to ensure clinical signs are not progressing.

PROGNOSIS & OUTCOME

Most animals with insect bites and stings have an excellent prognosis. Animals with severe systemic signs have a more guarded short-term prognosis as dictated by the severity of signs.

PEARLS & CONSIDERATIONS

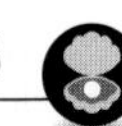

Prevention

Avoid insects and spiders and the places where hives have been identified.

Technician Tips

Animals with facial edema of unknown origin should have the face and lips examined for the presence of a stinger.

SUGGESTED READING

Fitzgerald KT, et al: Hymenoptera stings. Clin Tech Small Anim Pract 21:194-204, 2006.

AUTHOR: Scott P. Shaw, DVM, DACVECC
EDITOR: Benjamin M. Brainard, VMD, DACVAA, DACVECC

Behavioral Problems, Miscellaneous

BASIC INFORMATION

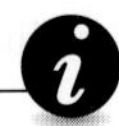

Definition

Species-typical, normal behaviors that may inconvenience clients

Dogs:

- Coprophagy (p. 204)
- Digging
- Mounting/humping
- Roaming
- Fence running/scratching

Cats:

- Scratching of furnishings
- Late-night activity
- Climbing on counters

Pathologic behavior disorders (e.g., phobias, separation anxiety) are dealt with in other chapters.

Epidemiology

SPECIES, AGE, SEX

Younger animals more likely to exhibit exploratory and play behaviors that may irritate clients; intact males: roaming

GENETICS, BREED PREDISPOSITION

- Hounds and northern dog breeds (e.g., husky, malamute, Samoyed) may look more readily for opportunities to roam.
- Highly active breeds or individuals with inadequate stimulation and exercise to satisfy their behavioral and cognitive needs may look for substitute behaviors that may be intolerable to owners.

RISK FACTORS

Management practices fail to provide enrichment (mental and physical) or fail to establish a humane rule structure that meets a pet's physical, social, developmental, behavioral, and cognitive needs:

- Lack of adequate cognitive stimulation
- Lengthy daily confinement for dogs (e.g., > 8 hours per day)
- Lack of interactive toys
- Lack of basic training
- Inadequate exercise
- Inadequate social exposure/interaction
- Shelter pets may not have access to stimulation and may lack appropriate behaviors to deal with this deficit.

CONTAGION AND ZOONOSIS

Social facilitation may occur in multiple-pet households, fostering these behaviors. In social facilitation, the behaviors of one individual in a group stimulate others to similar behaviors.

ASSOCIATED DISORDERS

Obsessive-compulsive disorders (p. 701)

Clinical Presentation

DISEASE FORMS/SUBTYPES

Bouts of behaviors that can be interrupted and appear to occur only opportunistically may be normal but annoying behaviors or management-related behavior problems. If the behaviors cannot be easily interrupted or the animal is constantly seeking ways to perform them, a more serious disorder should be suspected (e.g., obsessive-compulsive disorder).

HISTORY, CHIEF COMPLAINT

- Behavior that is annoying (e.g., cat walking on counters) or disgusting (e.g., dog rolling in feces) to the client but not threatening or dangerous
- Obtain a complete description of the behaviors and the context in which they occur. Cell phone cameras allow videorecording of the patient engaging in the problematic behaviors.
- Context is critical for assessing whether the behaviors are species-typical ones that can be redirected or managed while still meeting the animal's needs.
  - For example, a cat's scratching at an inanimate object (e.g., furniture) is normal behavior and can be redirected, but scratching at humans or other cats may represent aggression.

PHYSICAL EXAM FINDINGS

Usually unremarkable

Etiology and Pathophysiology

- Clients must understand that animals do not perform these behaviors out of spite or jealousy. Attention seeking is commonly involved, but the key to managing these problems is having clients comprehend the significance of the behaviors in terms of normal dog and cat behavior.
- Most of these behaviors are normal behaviors in context, intensity, and frequency, at least at first.
- If behaviors become increasingly abnormal, their context, intensity, and frequency will change, as will the animal's focus, interactions with humans and other animals, and daily time budget.
- Effective behavior modification: positive behaviors are encouraged and repeated when they result in a pleasurable outcome. This repetition leads to learning at the neurochemical level, where new proteins at synapses are made. These more efficient neuronal connections increase the likelihood that the dog or cat will continue with the behavior. Early identification and intervention maximizes odds of positive outcomes.

DIAGNOSIS

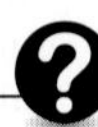

Diagnostic Overview

Many nuisance behaviors fall within the species' normal behavioral repertoire. A problem exists when their expression is undesirable to owners and should not be considered a sign of abnormal behavior. The history is diagnostic; the behavior's context determines whether the behavior is normal but inconvenient or indicates a true disorder.

Differential Diagnosis

- If any of the signs are excessive, repetitive, and performed to the exclusion of other comfort, social, and maintenance behaviors, an anxiety disorder such as obsessive-compulsive disorder (p. 701) must be considered.
- Late-night activity in middle-aged to older cats that is new and uncharacteristic based on the pattern of previous nocturnal behavior could be a sign of feline cognitive dysfunction (p. 188).
- Hyperthyroidism should be ruled out whenever an adult cat's activity level increases uncharacteristically.

Initial Database

- CBC, serum biochemistry profile, urinalysis, ± T_4 (cats): generally unremarkable
- Ingestion of feces or other nonnutritive items: fecal flotation, serum cobalamin level, trypsin-like immunoreactivity (p. 317)

TREATMENT

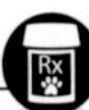

Treatment Overview

Provide an acceptable outlet for the unmet behavioral, cognitive, and species-typical needs that lead the pet to engage in the behavior the client finds objectionable.

Acute General Treatment

- Increase activity through exercise and interactive play with humans or dogs/cats. Play with compatible conspecifics (animals of the same species), particularly for dogs, usually provides more effective exercise with greater aerobic and psychologic scope than does play with humans.
- Environmental modification should be used for preventing access to or limiting the repetition of the undesirable behavior and to foster alternative, acceptable behaviors.

Chronic Treatment

- Behavior modification can provide outlets or encourage substitute behaviors that allow acceptable expression of the individual's mental and social needs. Depending on the problem, this may consist of exercise, goal-oriented activities (obedience, agility, tracking, coursing training for dogs, treibball; interactive predatory play for cats). Rewards—verbal, physical (e.g., petting or stroking), and food—should be given for all spontaneous and calm behaviors (e.g., chewing on chew-toys, clawing on provided surfaces, digging in a sandbox provided for this purpose, pouncing on cat toys).
- Attention-seeking behaviors such as jumping or playful whining or biting need to be ignored completely. Elimination of the reward (i.e., attention) can extinguish the behavior only if the client is consistent in not responding.
- In mild cases, devices that interrupt the behavior with an aversive stimulus can be useful early in the course of the problem only if the animal is not afraid of the stimulus and only if the behavior can be redirected toward an appropriate outlet.
- Examples of aversive but not harmful or fear-inducing disruptive stimuli include inverted plastic carpet runners (spike side up), static electricity mats for surfaces the client wants to be off-limits to the pet, and pressurized air blasts triggered by motion-detector sensors. Note that some animals will be afraid of these stimuli. If this is the case, the devices should not be used. The purpose of a disruptive stimulus is to stop the behavior in a way that encourages the animal to seek information and engage in an alternative behavior that can be rewarded. If the animal is afraid, it cannot do this.

Possible Complications

Poor client compliance can lead conversely to continued self-reinforcement, worsening of the problem, and deterioration of the pet-client relationship. A cornerstone of treatment is owner understanding of the basis for the behavior and the intention of the proposed treatment.

Recommended Monitoring

- Frequent follow-up improves client compliance.
- Demonstrations that show clients new ways to interact with their pet are essential.
- Dedicate these tasks to one staff member to enhance continuity, consistency in advice and follow-up. Clients feel that their veterinarians care more about them under these conditions.

PROGNOSIS & OUTCOME

- Excellent if the clients understand the pets' needs and are willing and able to meet them
- Poor if clients have unrealistic expectations, consider pets recyclable, feel guilty about discussing the issue with their veterinarian, or are unwilling or unable to meet their pets' needs

PEARLS & CONSIDERATIONS

Comments

- Annoyance behaviors that are extreme and interfere with normal physical and social functioning are characteristic of obsessive-compulsive disorder and other anxiety-related conditions. This does not mean that performing these miscellaneous behaviors will lead to obsessive-compulsive disorders. It does mean that the nonspecific signs and complaints can be similar and clients should not dismiss unusual behaviors out of hand as just "bratty" behaviors without having them evaluated first. Referral to a veterinary behaviorist may be very helpful in such situations.
- Relinquishment and euthanasia are frequent sequelae to behaviors clients find undesirable, whether or not the behaviors were the pet's fault. The effect of this pattern on veterinary economics and veterinary staff morale is huge and often preventable.
- This is a quality-of-life issue for pets.

Prevention

Puppy and kitten classes, basic obedience and agility training, and understanding of basic behavioral, physical, and social needs of dogs and cats can help prevent behaviors from becoming problems.

Technician Tips

Start a conversation by asking the owner if the pet is making the "naughty or nice Santa's list." If you don't ask, they won't tell.

Client Education

Keep a loaning library of books, newsletters, and videos covering basic behaviors of dogs and cats and a list of trainers and facilities that hospital staff members have verified to use humane training techniques. This provides the atmosphere of caring that makes it easier for clients to get the help they need. A useful source of video and other training and behavioral material can be found at https://drsophiayin.com/.

SUGGESTED READING

Yin S: How to behave so your dog behaves, Neptune, NJ, 2010, TFH Publications.

AUTHOR: Soraya V. Juarbe-Diaz, DVM, DACVB
EDITOR: Karen L. Overall, VMD, MA, PhD, DACVB

Benzodiazepine Toxicosis

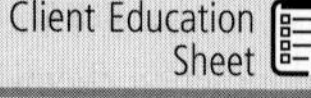

BASIC INFORMATION

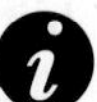

Definition

Iatrogenic overdose or accidental ingestion of benzodiazepines such as diazepam (Valium), alprazolam (Xanax), lorazepam (Ativan), or midazolam (Versed)

Epidemiology

SPECIES, AGE, SEX

- Any age, sex, or species is potentially susceptible because this class of medication is frequently used or prescribed for humans and animals and is commonly available in many homes.
- Repeated oral dosing of diazepam in cats has been associated with hepatic necrosis.

RISK FACTORS

Cats with underlying liver disease may be at higher risk for developing hepatic necrosis with oral diazepam dosing.

Clinical Presentation

DISEASE FORMS/SUBTYPES

Veterinary patients generally tolerate benzodiazepines better, on a mg/kg basis, than human patients.

HISTORY, CHIEF COMPLAINT

Accidental overdose in a hospital setting or evidence of ingestion at home (e.g., scattered pills, chewed bottle, and/or symptomatic pet)

PHYSICAL EXAM FINDINGS

- Frequent: central nervous system (CNS) depression, sedation, ataxia, and weakness
- Common: hypotension, bradycardia, and hypothermia
- Possible: paradoxical excitation (e.g., tachycardia, agitation, vocalization); more common in cats
- Rare: respiratory depression, coma
- Reported in cats with oral diazepam use: hepatic necrosis (idiosyncratic, cause unknown)

Etiology and Pathophysiology

- Benzodiazepines are commonly prescribed as sedatives, muscle relaxants, and anxiolytics. They are also frequently used for acute management of tremors and seizures.
- They are available in an injectable form as well as in various milligram strengths of tablets and rectal gels.
- Benzodiazepines increase gamma-aminobutyric acid (GABA) activity. Because GABA is an inhibitory neurotransmitter, it promotes generalized muscle relaxation and CNS depression.
- Benzodiazepines are metabolized in the liver. The active metabolites are conjugated through glucuronidation (cats have limited capabilities for this). Excretion is through the kidneys.

DIAGNOSIS

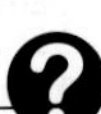

Diagnostic Overview

Evidence of exposure at home or in hospital setting or the presence of clinical signs such as sedation, ataxia, weakness, or in some cases, paradoxical excitement (e.g., vocalization, agitation, tachycardia) can suggest the diagnosis. Over-the-counter (OTC) urine tests can be used for a quick confirmation but are not validated in animals.

Differential Diagnosis

- Sedative effects: opioids, barbiturates, phenothiazines, cannabis, alcohols (ethanol, methanol, ethylene glycol), antidepressants, other anxiolytics
- Stimulatory effects: methylxanthines, amphetamines, selective serotonin reuptake inhibitors (SSRIs)

Initial Database

- No serum biochemical changes expected with acute overdose. Chemistry panel may reveal underlying renal or hepatic impairment that can affect elimination and prolong clinical signs.
    - Increase in liver enzymes and/or bilirubin in cats that develop hepatic necrosis
- Prolonged or unmanaged severe clinical signs (especially hypotension) may lead to biochemical sequelae.

Advanced or Confirmatory Testing

- OTC illicit drug urine tests may be of benefit. False-positives may occur with sertraline or with some nonsteroidal antiinflammatory drugs (NSAIDs) (e.g., oxaprozin, ibuprofen); false-negatives could occur because these screens do not detect all benzodiazepines.
- Diagnostic laboratory can confirm exposure but blood concentrations are not clinically relevant.

TREATMENT

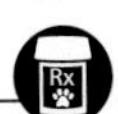

Treatment Overview

Symptomatic and supportive care is usually all that is needed. Flumazenil can be given if signs are severe.

Acute General Treatment

- Emesis can be attempted in asymptomatic pets within 15-30 minutes of tablet ingestion (p. 1188).
- Pets with mild sedation or ataxia can be monitored at home.
- Activated charcoal is rarely needed.
- Intravenous fluids can be used for hypotension. Forced diuresis is not required.
- Monitor body temperature. Use active warming as needed.
- Flumazenil 0.01 mg/kg IV, repeat in 1 to 3 hours if needed: is a direct antagonist and may be used if severe CNS, cardiovascular, or respiratory depression develops.
    - Use with caution because there could be potential risk for arrhythmias or seizures.
- Acepromazine 0.02 mg/kg IV: has been successfully used to manage paradoxical excitation. Do not treat stimulatory signs with a benzodiazepine.
- Diphenhydramine 1 to 2 mg/kg IM: can be used for extrapyramidal signs (muscle spasms, leg jerking) or dyskinesia (paddling, vocalization).

Chronic Treatment

Cats with acute liver disease should be managed with intravenous fluid, antioxidants, and other supportive care as needed (p. 442).

Behavior/Exercise

If monitoring at home for mild ataxia, it is safest to confine to prevent injury.

Drug Interactions

Barbiturates, other benzodiazepines, opioids, antidepressants, and any other sedatives may increase CNS and respiratory depression.

Recommended Monitoring

Monitor heart rate, blood pressure, body temperature while symptomatic

PROGNOSIS & OUTCOME

Generally a good prognosis; veterinary patients have a higher tolerance to benzodiazepines than humans.

PEARLS & CONSIDERATIONS

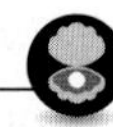

Comments

- Cats and young dogs are overrepresented in paradoxical CNS excitation reactions
- For pregnant and lactating animals: single acute exposures do not likely pose significant risks to the fetus.

Prevention

Keep medications out of reach of pets.

Technician Tips

Have the owner bring the bottle with them to verify the drug, milligram strength, and number of tablets ingested and to determine if at risk for foreign body from any missing portions of the pill vial.

Client Education

Do not administer benzodiazepines to pets without discussing with veterinarian.

SUGGESTED READING

Volmer PA: Recreational drugs. In Peterson ME, et al, editors: Small animal toxicology, ed 3, St. Louis, 2013, Elsevier, pp 309-334.

AUTHOR: Ginger Watts Brown, DVM
EDITOR: Tina Wismer, DVM, MS, DABVT, DABT

Bile Duct Obstruction, Extrahepatic

Client Education Sheet 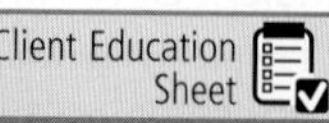

BASIC INFORMATION

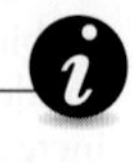

Definition

Obstruction of the extrahepatic bile duct system

Synonym

Extrahepatic bile duct obstruction, EHBDO, biliary obstruction

Epidemiology

SPECIES, AGE, SEX

- Dogs (middle-aged to older adults): gallbladder (GB) mucocele, pancreatitis; less commonly, neoplasia
- Cats (middle-aged to older adults): neoplasia

RISK FACTORS

- Dogs: pancreatitis, hyperadrenocorticism, hypothyroidism, neoplasia
- Cats: pancreatitis, cholangitis/cholangiohepatitis, inflammatory bowel disease, eosinophilic sclerosing fibroplasia, neoplasia

ASSOCIATED DISORDERS

Dogs:

- Cholecystitis
- GB mucocele
- Hypercoagulability (in contrast to hypocoagulability, as previously believed)

Dogs and cats:

- Cholangitis/cholangiohepatitis
- Cholelithiasis
- Bile peritonitis
- Neoplasia

Clinical Presentation

HISTORY, CHIEF COMPLAINT

- Dogs: anorexia, lethargy, vomiting, diarrhea
- Cats: anorexia, lethargy, weight loss, vomiting

PHYSICAL EXAM FINDINGS

- Dogs: icterus, fever, tachycardia, ± abdominal pain
- Cats: icterus, dehydration, fever or hypothermia

Etiology and Pathophysiology

Dogs:

- Pancreatitis: pancreatic swelling compresses common bile duct (p. 742)
- Mucocele: biliary sludge or gelatinous mucous obstruct biliary outflow (p. 374)
- Cholelithiasis: choleliths (stones) obstructing biliary outflow; cause poorly understood (p. 162)

Cats:

- Extrahepatic biliary obstruction often associated with a triad of diseases: cholangitis, pancreatitis, and inflammatory bowel disease (pp. 160, 543 and 740)
  - Common opening of the pancreatic and common bile ducts into the duodenum and the increased duodenal bacterial content may predispose cats to ascending cholangitis and pancreatitis after vomiting associated with inflammatory bowel disease.

Dogs and cats:

- Other possible causes include neoplasia, stricture in biliary system, duodenal obstruction by a foreign body, diaphragmatic hernia, and parasitic infection.
- Lack of bile entering intestinal tract
  - Decreases absorption of fat and fat-soluble vitamins, notably vitamin K: potential coagulopathy. May also result in increased absorption of endotoxin from the gut. Paradoxically, dogs with EHBDO recently have been shown to be hypercoagulable.

DIAGNOSIS

Diagnostic Overview

The diagnosis is suspected based on presenting history and physical examination findings. Confirmation requires demonstration by abdominal ultrasound exam that the icterus is caused by an obstructed common bile duct.

Differential Diagnosis

Hyperbilirubinemia (p. 528):

- Rule out hemolysis (pp. 59 and 60)
- Rule out hepatic disease (pp. 174, 442, 452, and 458)

Initial Database

- CBC
  - Possible mild anemia (unless concurrent gastrointestinal ulceration). In contrast, hyperbilirubinemia/icterus caused by hemolysis generally produces moderate to marked anemia.
  - Inflammatory leukogram
- Serum biochemistry profile
  - Increased bilirubin concentration
  - Increased liver enzyme concentrations (proportional alkaline phosphatase [ALP] > alanine aminotransferase [ALT])
  - Possible increased amylase and lipase concentrations
  - Hypokalemia
- Urinalysis: bilirubinuria is common in both species, but mild bilirubinuria is also normal in healthy dogs.
- Survey abdominal radiographs
  - Cranial abdominal detail may be decreased in cases with biliary leakage and peritonitis.
  - May delineate radiopaque choleliths
- Survey thoracic radiographs: rule out metastatic disease if neoplasia is suspected.

Advanced or Confirmatory Testing

- Abdominal ultrasound examination
  - Normal diameter of common bile duct in dogs and cats: 3-4 mm
  - Common bile duct dilation signifying obstruction: > 5 mm in cats, varies in dogs
  - Stellate or kiwi fruit pattern if GB mucocele
  - Visible contraction of the GB is not expected in healthy or diseased states
- Peritoneal fluid analysis obtained during abdominal ultrasound examination (p. 1343)
  - Elevated bilirubin concentration: bile peritonitis
  - Cytologic analysis and microbiological (aerobic and anaerobic) culture and sensitivity testing: septic peritonitis
- Coagulation profile (p. 1325)
- Thromboelastography

TREATMENT

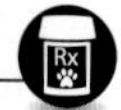

Treatment Overview

Patients require surgical correction of the problem along with appropriate intensive and supportive postoperative care. A crucial exception is transient biliary obstruction caused by acute pancreatitis, which often improves with medical therapy alone.

Acute General Treatment

- Rehydration by intravenous administration of balanced electrolyte solution
- Parenteral antibiotics effective against gram-negative bacteria and anaerobes:
  - Empirical therapy
    - Cefoxitin 30 mg/kg IV q 2h perioperatively, then q 6h (dogs and cats), *or*
    - Metronidazole 7.5-15 mg/kg IV q 12h with
    - Enrofloxacin 2.5-5 mg/kg IV q 12h (dogs only)
    - Ampicillin 22 mg/kg IV q 6-8h can be added to cefoxitin to add gram-positive coverage
  - Specific long-term therapy based on culture and sensitivity test results
- Sometimes, fresh-frozen plasma may be beneficial
  - Hypoproteinemia
  - Coagulopathy
- Vitamin K administration: 2.5 mg/kg SQ q 12h × 3-5 days, then once weekly
- Surgical intervention for relief of extrahepatic biliary obstruction
  - Duodenotomy and retrograde and antegrade flushing of biliary system: all cases
  - Common bile duct stenting: if temporary or dynamic obstruction likely (i.e., pancreatitis) and severe persistent hyperbilirubinemia
  - Cholecystoduodenostomy/jejunostomy: if advanced or permanent obstruction
  - Tube cholecystostomy
  - Cholecystectomy: for GB mucoceles, cholecystolithiasis, or if GB wall is devitalized

- Choledochotomy: for removal of stones that are lodged in the common bile duct
  - High risk of dehiscence
- Bile duct resection and anastomosis: for stricture or damage/trauma – *only* if bile duct is distended
  - High risk of dehiscence
- Gastrointestinal biopsies: association of biliary disease with inflammatory bowel disease and possibly eosinophilic sclerosing fibroplasia in cats
- Ultrasound-guided centesis of the GB in dogs with pancreatitis-associated biliary obstruction can relieve GB luminal pressure. There is an inherent risk of leakage from the centesis site.

Chronic Treatment

Maintain bile flow using ursodeoxycholic acid 10-15 mg/kg PO q 24h after relief of obstruction (biliary obstruction relative contraindication).

Nutrition/Diet

Provide enteral feeding at surgery or if anorexia persists afterward (e.g., esophagostomy tube [p. 1106], gastrostomy tube [p. 1109]).

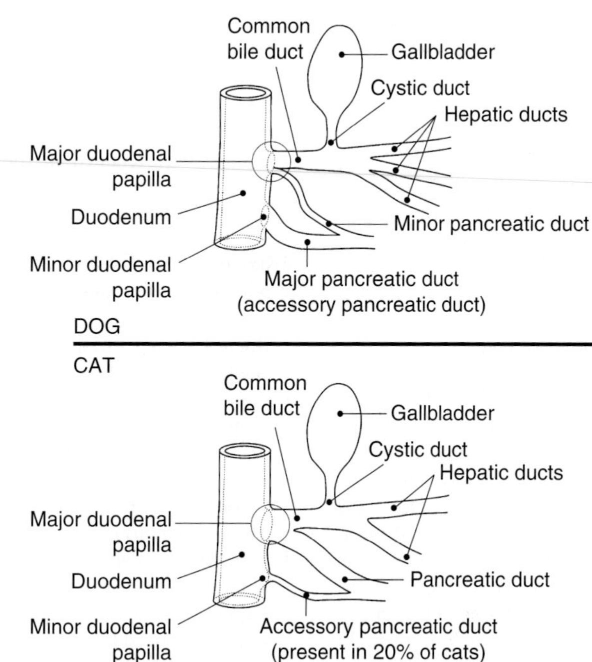

BILE DUCT OBSTRUCTION Comparative anatomy of the canine and feline biliary systems. (Courtesy Glenda Clements-Smith.)

Possible Complications

- Ongoing pancreatitis, bile leakage, peritonitis, endotoxemia, sepsis, death
- Duodenotomy and retrograde flushing of bile duct may lead to pancreatitis.

Recommended Monitoring

- Clinical and laboratory parameters assessing perfusion, including capillary refill time, pulse rate and quality, blood pressure, urine output, arterial pH, and lactate concentrations
- Respiratory function
- Serum liver enzyme and bilirubin concentrations
- Coagulation profile, hematocrit and total solids

PROGNOSIS & OUTCOME

- Poor if biliary obstruction is associated with neoplasia: 100% mortality rate for cats
- Guarded if biliary obstruction is associated with non-neoplastic causes in cats
- Guarded to fair if biliary obstruction is associated with non-neoplastic causes in dogs

PEARLS & CONSIDERATIONS

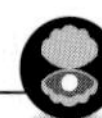

Comments

- Pancreatitis, which is the most common cause of biliary obstruction in dogs, typically resolves with medical treatment; surgery is avoided whenever possible.
- Given the association of biliary obstructive disease in cats with cholangitis/cholangiohepatitis and inflammatory bowel disease, a liver biopsy and culture, bile culture, and small-intestinal biopsies must be obtained at the time of surgery in this species. A convenient site for duodenal biopsy is the edge of the duodenotomy performed to cannulate the duodenal papilla(e) or to perform a cholecystoduodenostomy.
- In assessing hyperbilirubinemia, total bilirubin concentration is important. Conjugated versus unconjugated bilirubin is not linked to the source of hyperbilirubinemia in dogs and cats as it is in humans.

Technician Tips

Diagnostic imaging is vital for evaluating animals with suspected biliary obstruction. Plain radiographs can visualize cholecystoliths; ultrasound visualizes mucoceles and masses associated with obstruction.

SUGGESTED READING

Baker SG, et al: Choledochotomy and primary repair of extrahepatic biliary duct rupture in seven dogs and two cats. J Small Anim Pract 52:32-37, 2011.

AUTHOR: David Holt, BVSc, DACVS
EDITOR: Elizabeth A. Swanson, DVM, MS, DACVS

Bilious Vomiting Syndrome

BASIC INFORMATION

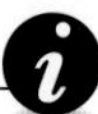

Definition

Suspected motility disorder resulting in vomiting of bile, often in the morning after a long period with an empty stomach

Synonyms

Gastroduodenal reflux, reflux gastritis syndrome, idiopathic gastric hypomotility

Epidemiology

SPECIES, AGE, SEX

Uncommon in dogs and rare in cats. Middle-aged, neutered male, mix-breed dogs are predisposed.

RISK FACTORS

Once-daily feeding; diseases causing delayed gastric emptying could predispose to bilious vomiting syndrome. This includes nearly any gastrointestinal disease (e.g., outflow obstructions, gastritis, gastric ulcers, neoplasia, inflammatory bowel disease, gastric dilation/volvulus, surgery), pancreatitis, or other diseases that induce defective gastric propulsion and/or bile reflux.

Clinical Presentation

DISEASE FORMS/SUBTYPES

Bilious vomiting syndrome is seen as vomiting of bile in otherwise healthy animals. If the patient is unwell or severely affected, other underlying disease should be suspected first.

HISTORY, CHIEF COMPLAINT

- Intermittent vomiting of bile (85%), often in the morning (60%)
- Abdominal pain, nausea, hyporexia/anorexia, and weight loss may also be seen.

PHYSICAL EXAM FINDINGS

- Often unremarkable
- Some dogs may have ptyalism, borborygmus, and cranial abdominal pain.

Etiology and Pathophysiology

Bilious vomiting syndrome is caused by abnormal gastroduodenal motility and reflux of bile into the gastric lumen, resulting in gastric mucosal irritation and vomiting. Decreased gastric motility may result in decreased intragastric pressure, leading to gastroduodenal reflux. There may also be changes to the gastrointestinal "housekeeping complex"/migratory motor complex secondary to overnight fasting.

DIAGNOSIS

Diagnostic Overview

Bilious vomiting syndrome is a diagnosis of exclusion and diagnostics are aimed at ruling out underlying diseases.

Differential Diagnosis

- Gastric outflow obstruction: foreign body, pyloric stenosis, neoplasia, polyp, intussusception, motility disorder
- Parasitism
- Gastrointestinal inflammation: gastritis, gastroenteritis, pancreatitis, colitis, others
- Dietary hypersensitivity or intolerance
- Metabolic disease: renal disease, hepatobiliary disease, hypokalemia, hypocalcemia, hypoadrenocorticism
- Drugs/toxicity: anticholinergics, narcotics, nonsteroidal antiinflammatory drugs (NSAIDs), other drugs
- Nervous inhibition: trauma, pain, stress

Initial Database

- CBC, serum biochemistry, and urinalysis: usually unremarkable. Hypokalemia, hypochloremia, and metabolic alkalosis with or without aciduria would suggest gastric or proximal duodenal obstruction.
- Total T_4 and feline immunodeficiency virus (FIV)/feline leukemia virus (FeLV) testing should be considered for the initial database in appropriate cats
- Fecal flotation
- Abdominal radiographs: usually unremarkable. Evaluate for evidence of obstruction and other pathology. Gastric outflow obstruction or hypomotility is likely if gastric contents are retained in the stomach for longer than 8 hours and especially beyond 12-16 hours postprandially

Advanced or Confirmatory Testing

- Abdominal ultrasound: evaluation of gastric/intestinal wall thickness, wall layering and discrete masses. Intraluminal masses/foreign bodies can be difficult to assess.
- Contrast radiography (barium study): can evaluate gastric emptying, gastrointestinal obstructions, and mural lesions. Gastric emptying time varies with different food consistencies and between dogs (p. 1172).
- Fluoroscopy: usually unremarkable
- Scintigraphy: considered the most accurate determination of gastric emptying but requires radioactive isotopes and has limited availability outside a referral setting. Gastric emptying time is 100-180 minutes.
- Gastroduodenoscopy and biopsies (p. 1098): rule out inflammatory diseases, parasites, foreign bodies, and structural abnormalities in the stomach and proximal duodenum. Motility cannot be reliably assessed during anesthesia. Barium or sucralfate administration interferes with endoscopic visualization.
- Wireless motility capsule: measures pH, temperature, and pressure as capsules traverse the gastrointestinal tract. Gastric emptying time: 6-15 hours
- ACTH stimulation test: rule out hypoadrenocorticism (p. 512)

TREATMENT

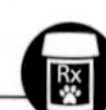

Treatment Overview

Nutritional and medical management are mainstays of therapy.

Acute General Treatment

Treat underlying diseases, dehydration, or metabolic derangements if identified.

Chronic Treatment

- Altered feeding schedule (see Nutrition/Diet)
- Prokinetics: if anatomic/structural disease has been ruled out, prokinetics can be instituted. Treatment trials of at least 7-10 days are recommended before trying another prokinetic.
  - Metoclopramide 0.2-0.5 mg/kg PO or SQ q 8h was associated with the best outcome in a retrospective study, *or*
  - Cisapride 0.1-0.5 mg/kg q 8-24h has limited availability, *or*
  - Erythromycin 0.5-1 mg/kg PO q 8-12h between meals, *or*
  - Ranitidine 1-2 mg/kg PO or SQ q 8-12h
- Gastroprotectants
  - Omeprazole 1 mg/kg PO q 12-24h preferred, *or*
  - Famotidine 0.5-1 mg/kg SQ or PO q 12-24h

Nutrition/Diet

- Frequent meals: 3-6 times daily to minimize the time with an empty stomach; feed right before bedtime and first thing in the morning.
- To facilitate gastric emptying, a semiliquid, low-fat, and low-fiber diet can be used (e.g., commercial intestinal diets blended with water and equal volume of rice)
- Some dogs may benefit from a hypoallergenic or novel protein diet trial. These dogs may have food hypersensitivity/intolerance.

PROGNOSIS & OUTCOME

Good to excellent with dietary +/− medical therapy

PEARLS & CONSIDERATIONS

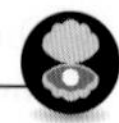

Comments

If the patient is severely affected (weight loss, electrolyte abnormalities, marked lethargy or abdominal pain, or signs of hypovolemia) or does not improve with medical management, further diagnostics should be pursued to rule out underlying disease.

Technician Tips

Weigh the patient frequently because weight loss can indicate another underlying disease.

Client Education

Trials with different drugs or diets may be necessary to resolve clinical signs in some dogs, and patience and perseverance may be needed during the initial treatment period.

SUGGESTED READING

Ferguson L, et al: Bilious vomiting syndrome in dogs: retrospective study of 20 cases (2002-2012). J Am Anim Hosp Assoc 52:3, 2016.

AUTHOR: Janne G. Lyngby, DVM, DACVIM
EDITOR: Rance K. Sellon DVM, PhD, DACVIM

Blastomycosis

Bonus Material Online Client Education Sheet

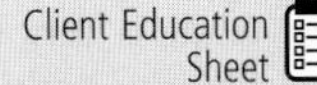

BASIC INFORMATION

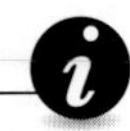

Definition

Systemic mycotic infection caused by the dimorphic fungus *Blastomyces dermatitidis*, affecting many mammalian species, including humans, dogs, and cats

Epidemiology

SPECIES, AGE, SEX

- Occurs most often in dogs, less commonly in cats
- Often occurs in young, large-breed, male dogs; dogs 2 to 4 years of age are overrepresented

GENETICS, BREED PREDISPOSITION

Sporting and working breed dogs are at increased risk.

RISK FACTORS

- Outdoor, roaming dogs in endemic areas living within 400 meters of water are at increased risk.
- Exposure to sandy, acidic soil disrupted by construction involving earth moving or excavation

CONTAGION AND ZOONOSIS

- Common-source exposure is possible, but true zoonosis is rare because yeast form is too large to be inhaled. Exception remains inoculation of the organism (e.g., needlestick injuries, cut during necropsy of infected animal).
- Risk of aerosolization and possible transmission from culture samples

GEOGRAPHY AND SEASONALITY

- *B. dermatitidis* is found in North America, Africa, and Central America. Endemic areas include the Mississippi, Missouri, Tennessee, Ohio, and St. Lawrence River valleys; mid-Atlantic states; northern California, Pacific Northwest, and the Canadian provinces of Alberta, Manitoba, Ontario, Quebec, and Saskatchewan.
- No seasonal distribution in the United States
- The specific location of the fungus in soil is unknown; the fungal colonies are not grossly visible and are difficult to isolate from the environment.
- A microfocus model for the ecology of *B. dermatitidis* suggests that environmental pockets of fungal growth occur when a suitable combination of soil type and moisture is present. Rain, physical disruption of soil, or both may promote release of spores.
- Proximity of the face to soil increases likelihood of inhalation/infection.

Clinical Presentation

DISEASE FORMS/SUBTYPES

Disseminated disease is most common (two-thirds of cases). The pulmonary form of the disease accounts for one-third of cases. Cutaneous, ocular, and osseous forms also are reported.

HISTORY, CHIEF COMPLAINT

Any combination of anorexia, weight loss, cough, dyspnea, exercise intolerance, ocular changes, lameness, skin lesions, and neurologic signs is possible.

PHYSICAL EXAM FINDINGS

Clinical signs depend on organ systems affected:

- Fever, lethargy, emaciation, lymphadenomegaly
- Pulmonary involvement: harsh lung sounds; cough; dyspnea at rest
- Ocular changes: signs of uveitis (p. 1023), chorioretinitis with retinal detachment, endophthalmitis, corneal edema, glaucoma
- Skin lesions (nasal planum, face, nail beds): subcutaneous abscesses, ulcerated draining lesions, or granulomatous proliferative lesions. Large abscesses are more common in cats than in dogs.
- Bone involvement: lameness due to fungal osteomyelitis, paronychial inflammation
- Neurologic signs may include abnormal mentation, paresis, vestibular ataxia, cranial nerve deficits, and decreased to absent postural responses.

Etiology and Pathophysiology

- *B. dermatitidis* is a dimorphic fungus that exists in the mycelial form in the soil and as a yeast in tissues.
  - The mycelial form grows in warm, moist, sandy soil rich in organic matter, especially in manure-enriched soil, and produces conidia that are released into the air. Soil disruption exposes organisms from deep within the soil.
- The route of infection is by inhalation of mycelial spores that enter the terminal airways from the environment.
- At body temperature, the conidia become yeasts and establish an infection in the lungs that may then spread throughout the body by blood and lymphatics.
- Organisms cause a pyogranulomatous inflammation with a predilection for the skin, eyes, bones, lymph nodes, subcutaneous tissues, mouth, nares, brain, mammary tissues, prostate, and testes.
- Cats are less commonly infected but develop a similar spectrum of lesions as dogs and may also have pharyngeal lesions. Central nervous system (CNS) involvement is more common in cats.

DIAGNOSIS

Diagnostic Overview

Most often, characteristic lesions on thoracic radiographs of a patient that has been in an endemic area alert the clinician to the possibility of fungal infection. Identification of organisms by cytology or histopathology is ideal. A urine antigen test for blastomycosis is more sensitive than serologic testing.

Differential Diagnosis

- Pulmonary form: metastatic neoplasia; bacterial or viral pneumonia, interstitial lung disease
- Bone form: bacterial osteomyelitis, primary or metastatic bone tumors
- Cutaneous form: bacterial, fungal, parasitic, autoimmune dermatitis
- Other systemic mycoses

Initial Database

CBC:

- Mild normocytic, normochromic anemia
- Moderate leukocytosis (17,000-30,000 white blood cells/mcL), left shift, lymphopenia

Serum biochemistry panel:

- Hyperglobulinemia
- Hypoalbuminemia
- Hypercalcemia (occasionally)

Thoracic radiographs:

- Diffuse, nodular interstitial and bronchointerstitial lung patterns common
- Solitary to multiple nodules may be seen.
- Tracheobronchial lymphadenopathy seen less often than with histoplasmosis
- Less commonly: pleural effusion, pneumomediastinum
- Radiographs of bones: osteolytic or periosteal proliferation with soft-tissue swelling

Advanced or Confirmatory Testing

- Identification of the organism in more than half of the cases by cytologic examination of lymph node aspirates, draining exudates, skin impression smears, or vitreous aspirates
  - A thick-walled, broad-based budding yeast is characteristic of *Blastomyces.*
- Lung aspirates (p. 1113) often identify the organism. Tracheal wash is less sensitive than a lung aspirate, but sensitivity may be increased by bronchoalveolar lavage (pp. 1073 and 1074).
- Urine *Blastomyces* antigen test has > 90% sensitivity and is the preferred approach when organisms are not found. The *Blastomyces* urine antigen test is done by MiraVista Labs (Indianapolis, IN, www.miravistalabs.com/veterinary-testing/blastomycosis/). A negative antigen test does not exclude infection; cross-reactivity with *Histoplasma* is seen (p. 1365).

- Agar gel immunodiffusion test: a positive test result is very specific, but the test is not sensitive early in the disease process (p. 1314).

TREATMENT

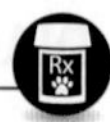

Treatment Overview

Itraconazole is considered the treatment of choice, but fluconazole may be more cost-effective despite longer treatment duration. Dogs with neurologic disease should be treated with amphotericin B.

Acute and Chronic Treatment

- General supportive care to include supplemental oxygen (p. 1146) to dyspneic patients. Dyspnea is considered a negative prognostic factor.
  - Dogs with dyspnea may require short-term glucocorticoid therapy (predniso[lo]ne 0.5 mg/kg q 12h × 5-7 days) to reduce pulmonary inflammation. Glucocorticoids should not be used before antifungal therapy is begun.
- Antifungal drugs
  - Itraconazole is considered the drug of choice in most cases.
  - Fluconazole, although requiring longer treatment times, is usually more cost-effective in dogs.
  - Amphotericin B may be superior in severe disease and in dogs with neurologic involvement.
- Itraconazole
  - Dogs: 5 mg/kg q 12h PO for 3 days, then 5 mg/kg PO q 24h for at least 60 days and for 30 days after all evidence of disease has resolved. Give capsules with canned food for maximal absorption. Brand-name itraconazole is preferred, but generic itraconazole can be effective; poor absorption can occur with compounded itraconazole. Itraconazole is expensive in large dogs.
  - Cats: 5 mg/kg PO q 12h. The pellets from the capsules can be mixed with palatable food for ease of administration. Oral liquid formulation is available (10 mg/mL) and has higher bioavailability.
- Fluconazole
  - Dogs: 10 mg/kg PO q 24h for a minimum of 4-6 months
  - Cats: 50 mg/CAT PO q 24h
- Amphotericin B (IV)
  - Dogs: 0.5 mg/kg IV in 5% dextrose 3 times/week at evenly spaced intervals. A cumulative dose of amphotericin B of at least 9 mg/kg is usually required. Therapy is continued until signs have resolved or until nephrotoxicity occurs, at which time treatment can be changed to itraconazole.
  - Cats: 0.25 mg/kg IV 3 times/week. Monitor closely for nephrotoxicosis.
  - Nephrotoxicity is the main side effect. Ensure animals are adequately hydrated before infusion. Monitor blood urea nitrogen (BUN) and creatinine during treatment and stop if > 50% increase in either parameter.
- Lipid-complexed amphotericin B
  - Dogs, cats: 1-2 mg/kg IV 3 times weekly. Higher cumulative doses can be achieved because less nephrotoxic.

Drug Interactions

Itraconazole should not be administered with drugs that inhibit cytochrome P450, such as some anticoagulants.

Possible Complications

- Itraconazole may cause hepatotoxicosis and anorexia in dogs and cats. Itraconazole at doses of 10 mg/kg/d may produce vasculitis, with ulcerative skin lesions that may resemble lesions of blastomycosis.
- Nephrotoxicity with amphotericin B
- Lung disease often worsens initially with treatment due to inflammation from dying organisms. Glucocorticoid therapy can be lifesaving in dyspneic dogs but should be given only after starting antifungal drugs.

Recommended Monitoring

- Liver enzyme activities should be monitored every 2-4 weeks during treatment in animals treated with itraconazole and measured if the patient develops anorexia.
- Perform thoracic radiographs monthly to assess response to treatment in dogs with pulmonary involvement. Median time to resolution of radiographic signs ≈6 months. Improvement typically continues even after discontinuing treatment.
- Following urine antigen concentrations is useful in predicting when treatment can be discontinued and for documenting relapse.

PROGNOSIS & OUTCOME

- The mortality rate is ≈20%.
- 50%-75% of dogs can be cured with the initial course of treatment.
- Animals with severe lung involvement (dyspnea) or CNS involvement have a guarded prognosis. Most deaths occur in the first week after presentation, despite treatment.
- More than 1500 bands/microL on CBC may be a poor prognostic indicator.
- Recurrence of blastomycosis occurs in 20%-25% of treated dogs in a few months to a year after completion of treatment. Most dogs with recurrence are cured when given another course of treatment.
- Eyes that have anterior uveitis usually become glaucomatous and blind. Retinal lesions are more likely to be cured. Blind eyes should be enucleated because they can harbor organisms.

PEARLS & CONSIDERATIONS

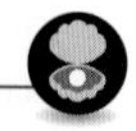

Comments

- Early recognition is critical for successful treatment. Comprehensive diagnostic testing should be done initially in suspect cases.
- Obtaining a travel history when dogs have signs suspicious of blastomycosis is an important step for raising or lowering the disease on the differential diagnosis.

Prevention

Restrict activity in endemic areas, particularly lakes, creeks, and heavily shaded areas with moist soil in endemic areas.

Technician Tips

- Although the disease is infectious (acquired by inhalation), it is not transmitted by inhalation from an infected patient to other animals or humans. Most zoonotic infections are acquired by needlestick injuries after fine-needle aspiration (FNA). Care should be taken when handling needles. Specifically, needles should not be recapped after FNA.
- Never culture a lesion or exudate if it could harbor *Blastomyces*; the spores aerosolize from culture medium and are highly infectious.

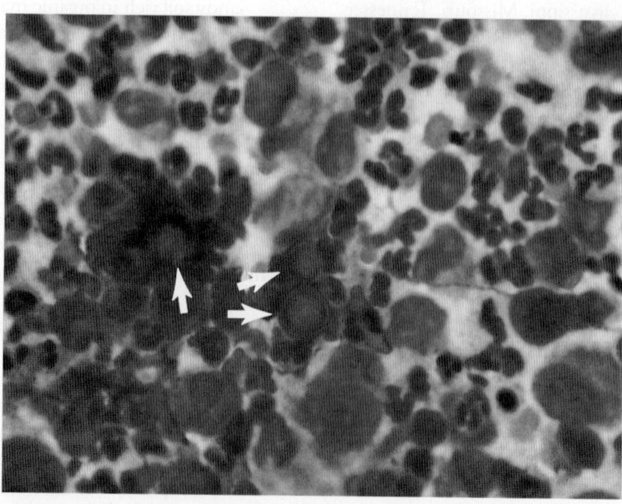

BLASTOMYCOSIS Cytologic evaluation of a fine-needle aspiration from a patient with blastomycosis. The cytologic diagnosis is made based on the thick-walled, basophilic, spherical *B. dermatitidis (arrows)*. The intense inflammatory infiltrate surrounding the yeasts is typical.

- Bandages contaminated with exudates should be disposed of as infectious waste (incinerated), but the likelihood of aerosolization is low because of the specific conditions *Blastomyces* organisms require to grow.

Client Education

- Long-term treatment is necessary.
- Can be fatal despite treatment

- Yeast form found in animal tissues is not directly transmissible.
- Can be transmitted by penetrating wounds

SUGGESTED READING

Dedeaux, AM, et al: Blastomycosis and histoplasmosis. In Ettinger SJ, et al, editors: The textbook of veterinary internal medicine, ed 8, St. Louis, 2017, Saunders, pp 1027-1035.

AUTHORS: Andrea Dedeaux, DVM; Joseph Taboada, DVM, DACVIM
EDITOR: Joseph Taboada, DVM, DACVIM

Blindness

Client Education Sheet

BASIC INFORMATION

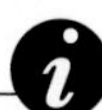

Definition

Loss of vision

Synonyms

Blindness due to central nervous system disorders is also called amaurosis or central blindness.

Epidemiology

SPECIES, AGE, SEX

Dogs and cats, any age, either sex

GENETICS, BREED PREDISPOSITION

Depends on causative disorder

RISK FACTORS

- Age: older animals may be predisposed to blindness associated with optic chiasmal neoplasia (p. 559), cataracts (p. 147), and retinal detachment (p. 885).
- Outdoor access may predispose to infectious diseases and/or toxins associated with blindness.

Clinical Presentation

DISEASE FORMS/SUBTYPES

- Unilateral or bilateral
- Sudden or progressive
- Red eye blindness: associated with visible conjunctival redness on physical exam
  - Glaucoma (p. 387), severe uveitis (p. 1023), cataracts (p. 147), lens luxation (p. 581), complex corneal ulceration (p. 209), orbital disease (p. 716)
- Non–red, non–inflamed eye blindness: no conjunctival or scleral redness is observed in the blind eye(s)
  - Prechiasmal/chiasmal blindness; lesion affecting retina, optic nerve, optic chiasm
  - Postchiasmal/cortical blindness; lesion affecting optic tracts, lateral geniculate nucleus (LGN), optic radiations, or visual cortex of the cerebrum

HISTORY, CHIEF COMPLAINT

- Depends on the cause, whether the blindness is unilateral or bilateral, and sudden or progressive in onset
- In cases of sudden blindness, some or all of the following may be reported:
  - Disorientation
  - Suddenly starts bumping into objects
  - Inability to find food bowl, toys
  - Lethargy, anxiety
- In cases of progressive blindness, some or all of the following may be reported:
  - Occasionally bumping into objects in own environment
  - Frequently bumping into objects in unfamiliar environments
  - Vision deficits in dim light and/or darkness (e.g., progressive retinal atrophy [PRA])
  - Patients may be lethargic and/or anxious but generally adjust and compensate better with more slowly progressive vision loss.

PHYSICAL EXAM FINDINGS

- See Neurologic Examination (p. 1136) and Ophthalmologic Examination (p. 1137).
- Red eye blindness (p. 870)
- Non–red eye blindness
  - Prechiasmal/chiasmal lesion
    - Menace response (blink in response to hand motion toward the eye) absent
    - Dazzle reflex (blink in response to a bright light) decreased (i.e., sluggish) or absent
    - Pupil(s) dilated +/− fixed/unresponsive
    - Pupillary light response (PLR) decreased (i.e., sluggish and incomplete) or absent. *Consensual PLR* refers to reaction of contralateral eye when ipsilateral eye is illuminated (e.g., absent consensual PLR of the right pupil in response to light shone into the left eye).
    - ± Anisocoria (asymmetry between the size of the pupils)
  - Postchiasmal/cortical lesion
    - Menace response variable depending on localization and severity of lesion
    - If a unilateral lesion is present
      - Menace response is absent or decreased in the contralateral eye
        - Small percentage of contralateral nasal/medial visual field may be preserved due to undecussated (those not crossed over) lateral optic nerve fibers
      - Menace response is usually present in the ipsilateral eye.
        - Menace response may be absent in the nasal visual field due to loss of the small percentage of lateral undecussated fibers.
    - Menace response absent in both eyes in bilateral/diffuse optic tract, lateral geniculate nucleus, optic radiation, or visual cortical lesions
    - Pupil size and PLRs are normal with central disease because PLR fibers separate from the vision pathway just before the LGN.
      - Exceptions: a concurrent iris disorder exists
    - Subtle anisocoria may occur with optic tract lesions before the LGN (i.e., contralateral pupil more dilated).
    - Dazzle reflex(es) normal (dazzle reflex does not involve the visual cortex)

Etiology and Pathophysiology

Red eye blindness: the lesion is ocular or intraocular:

- Opacity of the ocular media (e.g., cornea, aqueous humor, lens, vitreous) in cases of corneal edema/ulceration/pigmentation, uveitis, cataract and vitreal debris or hemorrhage
- Retinal degeneration with or without detachment and optic nerve atrophy in glaucoma
- Retinal detachment in cases of chorioretinitis

Non–red eye blindness:

- Prechiasmal/chiasmal lesion: lies along the retina–optic nerve–optic chiasm pathway
  - Retinal diseases (pp. 883 and 885)
  - Optic nerve lesions (e.g., congenital optic nerve hypoplasia, inflammation), neoplasia (e.g., meningioma), or atrophy (e.g., glaucoma, trauma)
  - Optic chiasmal lesions (e.g., neoplasia, abscess)
- Postchiasmal/cortical lesion: affects the optic tract and/or radiations to and including the visual (occipital) cerebral cortex
  - Encephalitis (extension to bilateral optic tracts through cerebrospinal fluid)
  - Cerebral edema
  - Cerebral infectious, inflammatory, neoplastic, or traumatic disease

DIAGNOSIS

Diagnostic Overview

Lesion localization is the cornerstone of accurate diagnosis and treatment. Complete cranial nerve and general neurologic exams are an essential first diagnostic step. If the cause of blindness is not readily apparent, referral of affected patients to a veterinary ophthalmologist is advised. Early diagnosis is key to determining whether return of vision with therapy is possible.

Differential Diagnosis

Red eye blindness:
- May be confused with disorientation due to causes other than blindness (p. 268) and concurrent non–vision-threatening causes of red eye, including conjunctivitis, episcleritis, and corneal disease (p. 870)

Non–red, non–inflamed eye blindness:
- May be confused with disorientation due to causes other than blindness

Unilateral versus bilateral:
- Unilateral: ocular trauma, complex corneal ulceration, lens luxation, cataract, severe uveitis, retinal detachment, subretinal hemorrhage, glaucoma, cerebral lesions (optic radiation/visual occipital cortex)
- Bilateral: cataracts, retinal detachment, subretinal hemorrhage, severe uveitis, glaucoma, optic neuritis, optic chiasm lesions, sudden acquired retinal degeneration, progressive retinal degeneration/atrophy, diffuse cerebral/visual cortex disease

Initial Database

The essential first step for lesion localization is to perform a complete neurologic exam (p. 1136) and ophthalmic exam (p. 1137).
- Important neuro-ophthalmic findings in a blind patient
  - Normal PLRs: lesion is usually postchiasmal/cortical (with a non–red, non–inflamed eye blindness) or due to opacity of ocular media
  - Sluggish, incomplete/absent PLR and dilated pupil: lesion involves retina, optic nerve, optic chiasm (causes bilateral blindness), or optic tract, or a separate, primary lesion of the pupil is present.
  - Chromatic PLR testing
    - Absent red light/positive blue light PLR: lesion involves photoreceptors (e.g., PRA, sudden acquired retinal degeneration [SARD], retinal detachment)
    - Absent red and blue light PLR: lesion involves optic nerve (e.g., optic neuritis)
- Important elements of the ophthalmic exam in a blind patient
  - Intraocular pressure assessment
  - Exam of anterior segment
    - Evaluate for opacity of the cornea, aqueous humor, lens, or vitreous
  - Posterior segment/fundic exam after pharmacologic pupil dilation (1% tropicamide)
    - Pharmacologic pupil dilation is contraindicated with glaucoma.
    - Evaluate optic nerve (size, shape, color).
    - Evaluate tapetum for brightness and/or color changes (hyperreflective/bright with retinal degeneration and/or certain forms of retinal detachment; hyporeflective/dull gray to pigmented with subretinal inflammation, certain forms of retinal detachment).
    - Evaluate nontapetal fundus (located ventrally and typically pigmented) for whitish or gray discoloration (e.g., edema, inflammatory exudate, depigmentation from active or past inflammation or retinal detachment) or hemorrhages.
    - Evaluate vasculature of retina (should see small arteries and larger veins coming from the optic disk and coursing peripherally), and look for changes in vessel direction to indicate detachment or attenuation (thinning) to indicate degeneration.
- CBC, serum chemistry profile, urinalysis to assess systemic status
- Blood pressure measurement with retinal hemorrhage and/or detachment

Advanced or Confirmatory Testing

- Thoracic radiographs (screen for neoplasia or systemic infectious disease if intraocular mass or uveitis, chorioretinitis are noted and/or if optic neuritis is suspected)
- Serologic titers for infectious diseases if presence in/travel to endemic area: rickettsial diseases (particularly if intraocular hemorrhage is noted), systemic mycoses (particularly if chorioretinal lesions with uveitis and/or optic neuritis are detected), borreliosis (if history of tick exposure + uveitis), bartonellosis (if history of flea exposure + uveitis), and toxoplasmosis (if history of rodent exposure + chorioretinal lesions)
- Aspiration of enlarged lymph nodes for cytologic evaluation
- Ocular ultrasonography if opacity of ocular media precludes fundic exam
- Histopathologic evaluation in cases when eye is blind and painful and enucleation is advised
- Referral is advisable for all cases of blindness of undetermined cause for additional evaluation, including one or more of the following:
  - Electroretinography to assess retinal function
  - Cerebrospinal fluid tap
  - Advanced imaging (computed tomography or magnetic resonance imaging)
  - Vitreous centesis with cytology, culture, titers

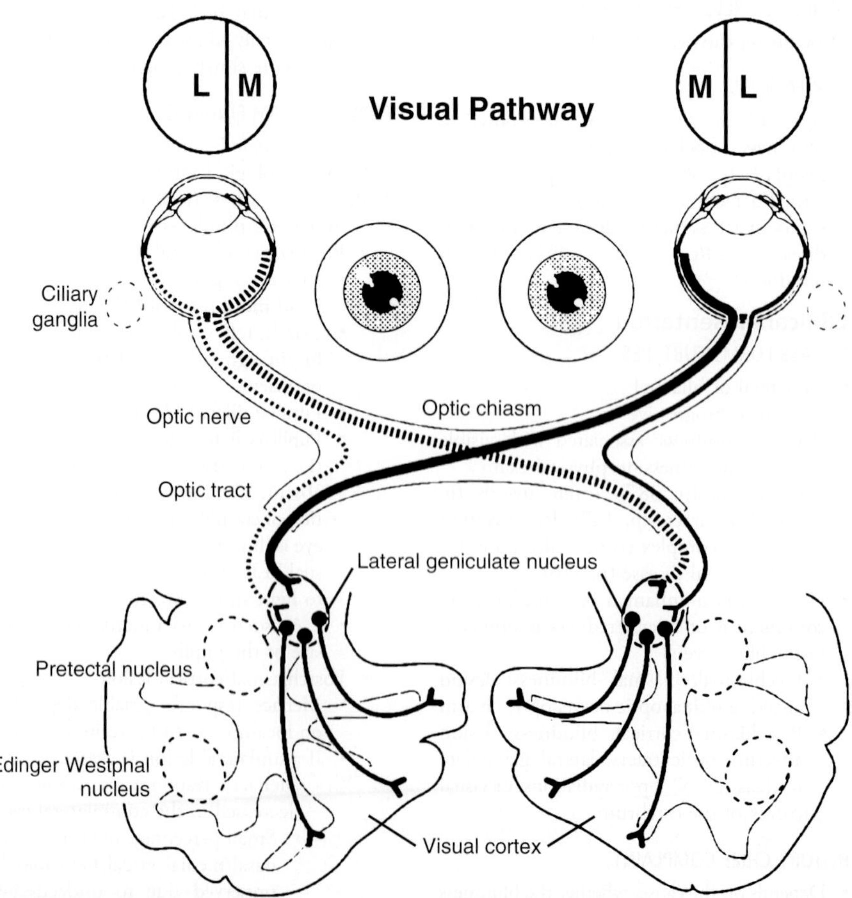

BLINDNESS Anatomy of visual pathway from the eye to the visual cortex of the cerebrum. *Circles* adjacent to the visual pathway title indicate visual fields. *L*, Lateral; *M*, medial.

TREATMENT

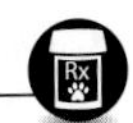

Treatment Overview

- Treatment is directed at addressing underlying cause of blindness such as hypertensive retinopathy, uveitis, cataracts.
- Administration of empirical therapy is usually not recommended until a tentative or final diagnosis has been reached.
  - Administration of systemic corticosteroids prematurely may preclude diagnosis of neoplasia and some inflammatory disorders and may exacerbate systemic infectious diseases.

Acute General Treatment

Depends on underlying cause

Chronic Treatment

- Manage underlying conditions such as chronic renal failure, systemic hypertension, systemic infectious disease.
- Systemic mycoses and immune-mediated disorders typically require long-term therapy.
- Treat primary cause of blindness when possible (e.g., refer for surgery of mature cataracts).

Recommended Monitoring

- Monitor for return of vision, PLR, dazzle reflex after commencing therapy.
- Serial fundic exam

PROGNOSIS & OUTCOME

- Depends on underlying cause
- Restoration of vision after acute vision loss may be possible after rapid diagnosis of underlying condition and intensive appropriate therapy.
- In many cases, blindness is irreversible, and long-term management aims to provide comfort if pain is likely (e.g., glaucoma).

PEARLS & CONSIDERATIONS

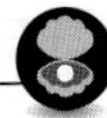

Comments

- Assessment of the direct and consensual PLRs and dazzle reflexes is imperative in evaluation of blindness.
  - Absence of the PLR and/or dazzle reflex is a poor prognostic indicator because minimal retinal function is required to retain these reflexes.
- The PLR and dazzle reflexes do not involve the visual cortex so are normal with central blindness caused by optic radiation and cortical lesions.
- A PLR depends only on *quantity* of light; vision depends on *quality* of light; therefore, the PLR should remain intact despite opacity of the ocular media (e.g., cataract) if there is no concurrent retinal or optic nerve damage.

Technician Tips

Blind patients may appear to be aware of their surroundings. Be sure to mark cages to alert staff to blind status when handling the animal, and ideally, place blind patients in a floor-level cage to avoid falls from an open cage door.

Client Education

Provide client with education sheet: "How to Change the Environment for a Pet That Is Blind."

SUGGESTED READING

Plummer C: Diagnosing acute blindness in dogs. Todays Vet Pract 6:18-23, 2016.

AUTHOR: Anne J. Gemensky-Metzler, DVM, MS, DACVO

EDITOR: Diane V. H. Hendrix, DVM, DACVO

Bordetellosis

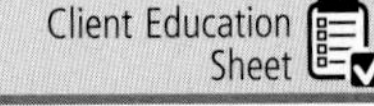

BASIC INFORMATION

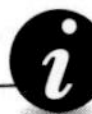

Definition

Diseases caused by *Bordetella bronchiseptica*, a highly contagious, aerobic, gram-negative coccobacillus that is a primary respiratory pathogen for dogs and cats; commonly causes acute or chronic respiratory disease or subclinical infections

Synonyms

B. bronchiseptica is considered a contributing agent in the acute canine infectious respiratory disease (CIRD) syndrome, also known as infectious tracheobronchitis or kennel cough.

Epidemiology

SPECIES, AGE, SEX

- Dogs, cats, and many other domestic and wild animal species
- Young animals more susceptible to disease, especially severe disease (i.e., pneumonia)

RISK FACTORS

- Exposure to other animals with respiratory infection
- Housed in crowded conditions (shelters, boarding kennels, breeding facilities)
- Lack of vaccination

CONTAGION AND ZOONOSIS

- *B. bronchiseptica* is highly contagious: animal-to-animal contact, aerosol, or fomites. Infected animals shed the organism in nasal and oropharyngeal secretions for 3 months or longer after infection. Infection can be transmitted between species.
- *B. bronchiseptica* is a rare cause of zoonotic disease. Human infection (respiratory disease, pleuritis, meningitis, peritonitis, pancreatic abscess) can occur opportunistically in infants or immunocompromised people.
- *B. bronchiseptica* can be isolated from the upper respiratory tract in
  - Up to 10% of healthy household dogs and 5%-11% of healthy household cats
  - Up to 78% of dogs and up to 44% of cats with acute respiratory infections
  - 19.5% of asymptomatic dogs and 24% of asymptomatic cats in U.S. animal shelters

GEOGRAPHY AND SEASONALITY

Worldwide distribution, year-round

ASSOCIATED DISORDERS

Bordetellosis is commonly part of a disease complex that often includes co-infections with canine parainfluenza, canine adenovirus-2, canine distemper, *Mycoplasma* spp, and/or *Streptococcus* spp in dogs and feline rhinotracheitis (feline herpesvirus), feline calicivirus, and other pathogens in cats (pp. 987 and 1006).

Clinical Presentation

DISEASE FORMS/SUBTYPES

Bordetellosis in small animals typically causes a syndrome of tracheobronchitis but may cause bronchopneumonia.

HISTORY, CHIEF COMPLAINT

- History typically includes exposure to multiple non-housemate animals several days before onset of coughing.
- Chief complaint in dogs is usually acute-onset, nonproductive hacking cough, including bouts of severe coughing that result in terminal retch.
- Chief complaint in cats is most often sneezing, oculonasal discharge, and cough.
- Severe or complicated cases may have signs of pneumonia (p. 795), including respiratory distress.

PHYSICAL EXAM FINDINGS

- Spontaneous or inducible cough (nonspecific)
- ± Conjunctivitis
- ± Nasal or ocular discharge
- ± Submandibular lymphadenopathy

- ± Mild to moderate fever, tachypnea and increased lung sounds (pneumonia) in severe cases

Etiology and Pathophysiology

- The organism colonizes the nasal and tracheal respiratory epithelium and can establish persistent, often subclinical infections.
- Infection occurs by contact of the organism with the upper airway and adherence to the respiratory epithelium by direct binding to cilia, inducing ciliary stasis and reducing mucociliary escalator clearance of bacteria and other particulate matter from the airways.
- Airway colonization induces an inflammatory response and increased mucus production.
- *Bordetella* spp produce multiple factors that allow them to persist chronically and predispose the host to secondary infections.

DIAGNOSIS

Diagnostic Overview

Bordetellosis often is a clinical diagnosis, and because many infections are mild and self-limited, the urgency of establishing a definitive diagnosis of bordetellosis is low. Treatment is usually based only on clinical signs of upper respiratory infection.

Differential Diagnosis

Dogs:

- Other agents of infectious tracheobronchitis (p. 987)
- Chronic bronchitis
- Collapsing trachea
- Traumatic tracheitis
- Airway foreign body
- Mechanical or chemical airway irritant
- Other causes of pneumonia: infectious, aspiration

Cats:

- Other upper respiratory infections/agents (p. 1006)
- Other causes of pneumonia

Initial Database

- CBC: often unremarkable; neutrophilia with left shift or toxic neutrophils may be seen with pneumonia
- Thoracic radiographs: indicated with signs of systemic illness (e.g., fever, anorexia) or respiratory distress. Usually unremarkable; interstitial to alveolar infiltrates with pneumonia

Advanced or Confirmatory Testing

- Bacterial culture and susceptibility (C&S): many healthy animals harbor *B. bronchiseptica*.
  - Nasal or oropharyngeal swabs for bacterial culture: should be plated on selective medium to decrease overgrowth by other respiratory flora
  - Transtracheal wash or bronchoalveolar lavage (BAL) (p. 1073) if pneumonia or lower airway disease suspected. Can confirm infection, provide susceptibility, and test for secondary pathogens.
- Serologic testing not helpful; many healthy animals have positive titers
- Polymerase chain reaction (PCR) techniques may be applied to nasal or pharyngeal swabs, transtracheal wash, or BAL fluid samples. Often, PCR is part of a multi-pathogen panel testing for several agents of CIRD. Some assays can differentiate *Bordetella* species. Quantitative PCR of BAL samples is reported to be the most sensitive means of confirming infection.

TREATMENT

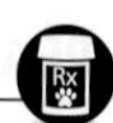

Treatment Overview

Treatment is largely supportive care ± antimicrobial drugs. Cough suppressants can help break the cough cycle but are contraindicated in cases with pneumonia or productive cough. Unless intensive treatment required (i.e., pneumonia), outpatient treatment best to reduce nosocomial risk.

Acute General Treatment

Antimicrobials:

- Antimicrobials are not always necessary. Typical upper respiratory infection is self-limited, and antimicrobials have not been shown to shorten the course of illness or reduce period of shedding.
- Antimicrobials are indicated for dogs with fever, lethargy, inappetence, or mucopurulent nasal discharge and for dogs with evidence of pneumonia.
- *Bordetella* spp show high level of antimicrobial resistance; should treat based on C&S
- Pending C&S for outpatient treatment
  - Doxycycline 5 mg/kg PO q 12h or minocycline 5-12 mg/kg PO q 12h for 7-10 days is the traditional antimicrobial of choice (most *Bordetella* isolates are susceptible) *or*
  - Amoxicillin-clavulanate 12.5-25 mg/kg PO q 12h; resistance common and ineffective for possible concurrent *Mycoplasma* *or*
  - Trimethoprim-sulfonamide 15-30 mg/kg PO q 12h; resistance common *or*
  - Pradofloxacin suspension 7.5 mg/kg PO q 24h (cats)
- Pending C&S for animals with pneumonia
  - Enrofloxacin 5-20 mg/kg IM, IV q 24h (dogs), 5 mg/kg q 24h (cats)
  - Gentamicin 9-14 mg/kg IV q 24h (dogs), 5-8 mg/kg (cats)

Antitussives:

- For suppression of dry, nonproductive cough in milder cases (animal is otherwise well); titrate dose to reduce cough without causing sedation.
  - Butorphanol 0.5-1 mg/kg PO q 8-12h *or*
  - Hydrocodone 0.22-0.5 mg/kg PO q 8-12h (dogs)
- *Contraindicated* with pneumonia or productive cough

Bronchodilators:

- May be indicated in patients with pneumonia

Nebulization therapy (p. 1134):

- Nebulization with sterile saline may help hydrate airway secretions and facilitate clearance, but patient must have adequate systemic hydration.
- Nebulization with antibiotic solutions (gentamicin, enrofloxacin, kanamycin, or polymyxin B) has been suggested for refractory cases to reduce *Bordetella* populations in the trachea and bronchi, but dose delivery to airways is unpredictable.

Glucocorticoids (controversial):

- Antiinflammatory doses administered short term may reduce cough (e.g., prednisolone 0.5 mg/kg PO q 12-24h for 3-5 days)
- Does not shorten course of disease
- May exacerbate disease in immunocompromised animals
- Do not use in cases with severe/complicated disease.

Adequate systemic hydration very important to facilitate clearance of respiratory secretions.

Behavior/Exercise

Exercise may exacerbate coughing during acute infection.

Drug Interactions

Reduce dose of trimethoprim-sulfonamide, and avoid gentamicin in patients with renal disease. Tetracyclines may cause discoloration of dental enamel in young animals, although less likely with doxycycline than other types.

Possible Complications

- Pneumonia may develop secondary to *Bordetella*-induced impairment of respiratory defenses.
- Dental or bone staining (in very young animals) or gastrointestinal (GI) side effects may occur with doxycycline or minocycline; avoid in neonates or pregnant dogs, and follow every dose with an oral bolus of tap water or morsel of food to reduce risk of drug-associated esophagitis and stricture. Tetracyclines may cause fever in cats.
- Sulfonamides may induce keratoconjunctivitis sicca, hypersensitivity reactions, crystalluria, renal tubule obstruction, polyarthritis, hepatic inflammation, and GI signs.

Recommended Monitoring

- Mild to moderate: clinical response
- Pneumonia (p. 795)

PROGNOSIS & OUTCOME

- Disease is usually self-limited; uncomplicated cases resolve within approximately 2 weeks.
- Severe (potentially fatal) pneumonia may occur in young or debilitated animals.

PEARLS & CONSIDERATIONS

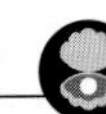

Comments

- Shedding of organisms may continue for > 3 months after resolution of clinical signs. Transmission of infection to other animals and immunocompromised people may continue during that time, warranting suitable precautions.
- *B. bronchiseptica* is the evolutionary progenitor of *B. pertussis*, a human-specific pathogen that is the causative agent of whooping cough.

Prevention

- Limit transmission by quarantine of new animals and isolation of infected animals.
- Decrease stress, overcrowding, and provide adequate hygiene and care.
- Disinfect cages and other surfaces (1:32 dilute bleach solution).
- Vaccination
  - Injectable, intranasal (IN), and oral vaccines are available for dogs; intranasal for cats. Comparative efficacy of vaccine types is not well defined, but IN vaccination has some advantages (rapid onset of protection, mimics natural route of exposure at mucosal surface). Mild cough and/or nasal discharge can occur after IN vaccination.
  - Effective in reducing infection rate and severity of clinical signs
  - Vaccinate at least 5 days before anticipated exposure (boarding) if possible.
  - Some IN vaccines may be used as early as 2 weeks of age.
  - Animals receiving modified live vaccines shed bacteria that may cause infection ± disease in susceptible animals and humans.
- Natural immunity lasts at least 6 months after infection.

Technician Tips

Caution is warranted when preparing a vaccine: erroneous SQ injection of intranasal vaccine in dogs has caused severe acute hepatic injury.

Client Education

Highly contagious disease. Care should be taken to avoid coughing dogs at dog parks, pet stores, and other areas where dogs may congregate.

SUGGESTED READING

Ford RB: Canine infectious respiratory disease. In Greene CE, editor: Infectious diseases of the dog and cat, ed 4, Philadelphia, 2012, Saunders, pp 55-65.

AUTHOR: Marcella D. Ridgway, VMD, MS, DACVIM
EDITOR: Joseph Taboada, DVM, DACVIM

Botulism

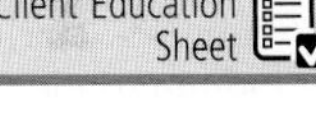

BASIC INFORMATION

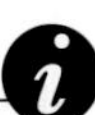

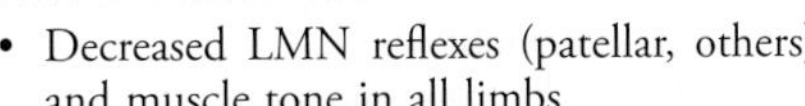

Definition

An acute, rapidly progressive generalized lower motor neuron (LMN) paralytic disorder caused by ingestion of *Clostridium botulinum* exotoxin

Epidemiology

SPECIES, AGE, SEX

Any breed dog, either sex. Cats appear highly resistant to botulism (no natural cases reported).

RISK FACTORS

Contaminated food/carrion ingestion

ASSOCIATED DISORDERS

Aspiration pneumonia, ventilatory failure (respiratory arrest)

Clinical Presentation

DISEASE FORMS/SUBTYPES

There are seven antigenically identified types of botulinum neurotoxins, all with similar neurotoxic effects. Dogs: type C; large animals: type B; humans: types A, B, F.

HISTORY, CHIEF COMPLAINT

- LMN paresis/paralysis that is often ascending
  - Begins as weakness in the pelvic limbs and can progress to quadriplegia
- History of ingestion of carrion or other source of anaerobic bacterial contamination
  - The incubation period after ingestion ranges from hours to 6 days.
  - Botulism is especially likely if multiple animals are affected.

PHYSICAL EXAM FINDINGS

- Decreased LMN reflexes (patellar, others) and muscle tone in all limbs
- Cranial nerve abnormalities (decreased/absent palpebral and menace, decreased jaw tone and gag, mydriasis, voice change)
- Level of consciousness maintained, pain perception preserved
- In severely affected animals, decreased abdominal and intercostal muscle tone can require ventilation or lead to death from ventilatory failure.
- Tail wag is maintained.
- Parasympathetic dysfunction can also be observed (heart rate changes, regurgitation due to megaesophagus).

Etiology and Pathophysiology

- *C. botulinum* is a gram-positive, saprophytic, spore-forming bacterial rod in soil.
- Clinical signs develop after ingestion of preformed toxin; it enters the gastrointestinal (GI) lymphatics and is transported to the neuromuscular junction (NMJ) of cholinergic nerves.
- A metalloprotease (botulinal toxin) prevents the presynaptic release of acetylcholine at the NMJ. Toxin binding is quick, irreversible, and independent of temperature and neural activity.
- The severity of signs varies with the amount of toxin ingested and individual susceptibility.
- Blocked release of acetylcholine from the presynaptic membrane causes symmetrical, ascending LMN paresis/paralysis.
- Duration of illness in dogs: 14-24 days

DIAGNOSIS

Diagnostic Overview

The diagnosis is based on a history suggestive of toxin ingestion and the resultant clinical signs. Toxin identification may be undertaken to confirm the diagnosis, but treatment, which is supportive and may be urgently required, is initiated based on neurologic deficits and history.

Differential Diagnosis

- Early tick paralysis
- Early polyradiculoneuritis
- Rabies

Initial Database

- CBC, serum biochemical analysis, and urinalysis: usually normal
- Assess oxygenation: pulse oximetry or arterial blood gas analysis (p. 1058)
- Neurologic examination (p. 1136) consistent with diffuse LMN dysfunction
- Thoracic and abdominal radiographs may occasionally reveal megaesophagus (with or without signs of aspiration pneumonia) and carrion skeletal remains in the GI tract, but radiographic abnormalities are not required to make the diagnosis of botulism.

Advanced or Confirmatory Testing

- Confirmatory diagnosis is based on finding the toxin in serum, feces, vomitus, or food samples.
- Preferred method of toxin identification is the mouse neutralization test.
- Other *in vitro* tests (radioimmunoassay, passive hemagglutination, enzyme-linked

immunosorbent assay, and polymerase chain reaction) exist but have not replaced the mouse test.
- Electrophysiologic testing
  - Marked reduction in muscle action potential amplitude evoked by electrical stimulation of the motor nerve
  - Normal or only mildly reduced nerve conduction velocities
  - Normal electromyography

TREATMENT

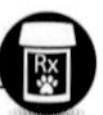

Treatment Overview

Treatment consists principally of supportive care during spontaneous recovery.

Acute General Treatment

- Antitoxin (type specific) must be administered before the botulinal toxin binds to receptors at the myoneural junction.
  - Type C polyvalent antitoxin (dog) 10,000-15,000 IU/DOG IV or IM, 2 doses given 4 hours apart
  - Anaphylaxis (p. 54) is a potential risk; intradermal skin testing (inject 0.1-0.2 mL intradermally and assess for wheal 30 minutes later) is recommended before administration.
  - Antitoxin may be effective to prevent further toxin binding if ongoing intestinal absorption/circulation.
- Antibiotic use is debated; penicillin and metronidazole have been given to reduce potential intestinal growth of *C. botulinum*, but disease occurs due to ingestion of preformed toxin.
- Antibiotics if secondary infection (e.g., aspiration pneumonia)
- Hypoxemia due to hypoventilation characterized by low PaO2 and high PaCO2 warrants referral for respiratory (i.e., ventilator) support (p. 1185).

Chronic Treatment

Long-term physical rehabilitation, frequent turning, and soft bedding are essential.

Nutrition/Diet

Important to meet energy requirements through balanced nutrition (esophagostomy tube or percutaneous endoscopic gastrostomy [PEG] tube) if the patient is not able to eat voluntarily (pp. 1106 and 1109)

Behavior/Exercise

Passive range-of-motion exercises as well as hydrotherapy in the recovery phase of the disease

Drug Interactions

Avoid aminoglycosides (associated with neuromuscular blockade).

Possible Complications

- Aspiration pneumonia
- Decubital ulcers
- Muscle atrophy and fibrosis
- Ventilatory failure

Recommended Monitoring

- Respiratory rate and character +/− pulse oximetry or blood gas; temperature and pulse
- Chest radiographs
- Serial neurologic examinations

PROGNOSIS & OUTCOME

- Good to guarded
- Recovery usually occurs 2-3 weeks after regrowth of terminal motor branches; depends on severity of signs and complications
- Complete recovery can occur spontaneously in moderately affected animals.

PEARLS & CONSIDERATIONS

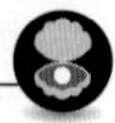

Comments

- The index of suspicion for botulism increases markedly if more than one animal is affected simultaneously.
- Referral may be necessary if long-term supportive care and ventilatory support are needed.

Prevention

- Avoid carrion/spoiled food.
- Thorough cooking of foods
  - Botulinal toxin is destroyed by heating to 176°F (80°C) for 30 minutes or 212°F (100°C) for 10 minutes.

Technician Tips

- Respiratory watch: monitor for signs of distress or increased effort.
- Recumbency care is essential.

Client Education

- Do not allow pets to roam.
- If your pet is suspected of eating carrion, seek immediate veterinary care.
- Full recovery may or may not occur, and there may be permanent neurologic impairment.

SUGGESTED READING

Barsanti JA. Botulism. In Greene CE, editor: Infectious diseases of the dog and cat, ed 4, St. Louis, 2012, Elsevier, pp 416-422.

AUTHOR: Karen L. Kline, DVM, MS, DACVIM
EDITOR: Karen R. Muñana, DVM, MS, DACVIM

Brachycephalic Airway Syndrome

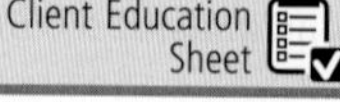

BASIC INFORMATION

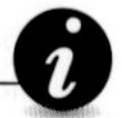

Definition

Narrowing of the upper airway secondary to selective breeding of aesthetic traits; anatomic and functional abnormalities of the upper airway found in brachycephalic (short-nosed) dogs

Synonyms

- Brachycephalic obstructive airway syndrome (BOAS)
- Brachycephalic airway syndrome (BAS)
- Brachycephalic syndrome

Epidemiology

SPECIES, AGE, SEX

- Most commonly found in dogs but can occur in selected breeds of cats. Age at presentation varies with severity of anatomic abnormalities.
  - < 6 months of age: signs are usually related only to stenotic nares

GENETICS, BREED PREDISPOSITION

- Inherently genetic condition: breeds that are affected include shih tzus, pugs, French bulldogs, English bulldogs, Pekingeses, Boston terriers, Cavalier King Charles spaniels.
- Cats that are affected include Himalayans, Persians, and British shorthairs.
- By definition, Chihuahuas and Yorkshire terriers are considered brachycephalic, although they seem to be less clinically affected.

RISK FACTORS

- Obesity can exacerbate clinical signs.
- Heat and exercise can exacerbate clinical signs.

GEOGRAPHY AND SEASONALITY

Signs of respiratory compromise or distress may worsen in hot weather.

ASSOCIATED DISORDERS

- Gastrointestinal (GI) disorders (e.g., esophagitis, hiatal hernia)
  - BAS patients often have signs of GI disease (regurgitation, vomiting)
  - High likelihood of esophageal or gastric ulceration
  - Severity of GI disease may be correlated to severity of respiratory signs
- Pharyngeal collapse, laryngeal collapse
- Urethral prolapse
- Chemodectoma
- Macroglossia
- Aspiration pneumonia
- Epidermoid cyst

Clinical Presentation

DISEASE FORMS/SUBTYPES

- Subclinical: mildly stertorous breathing or mild exercise intolerance may be present from early in life. Patients continue to have physiologic changes that can cause progression to clinical disease later in life.
- Clinical: patients have active clinical signs that adversely affect quality of life.

HISTORY, CHIEF COMPLAINT

- Stertor (heavy snoring) is the most common complaint, with stridor (high pitched) less common.
- Exercise intolerance, cyanosis, or collapse
- Insomnia
- Owners may notice inability to get comfortable after exercise.
- Occasional regurgitation may be present secondary to hiatal hernia or gastric ulcerations.
    - Acute onset of severe dyspnea may occur secondary to aspiration pneumonia.
    - Must rule out noncardiogenic edema secondary to obstructive episode

PHYSICAL EXAM FINDINGS

- Flat face with stenotic nares (common but not uniformly present)
- Stertor or sometimes stridor; increased inspiratory sounds
- Increased bronchovesicular sounds if concurrent pneumonia or noncardiogenic edema (± crackles), or bronchitis (± wheeze)
- If in respiratory distress: cyanosis, labored breathing, collapse, hyperthermia
- ± "Puffing out" of thoracic inlet during respiration (due to lung lobe herniation)
- Examination of the soft palate and laryngeal ventricles should take place after heavy sedation (p. 1125).

Etiology and Pathophysiology

- Selective breeding has led to rostrocaudal shortening of the skull and nasal passages in these breeds.
- Redundant pharyngeal soft tissues contribute to increased airway resistance and various degrees of obstruction of the nasal passages and pharynx during inspiration.
- To achieve appropriate oxygenation, increased force is necessary to pull air in. The excessive negative pressure causes inflammation, edema, and weakening of the components of the upper airway (larynx, pharyngeal wall, soft palate).
- This also contributes to an increase in intraabdominal pressure, leading to possible herniation (lung lobe herniation, hiatal hernia, urethral prolapse).
- Primary anatomic components of BAS (any/all may be present)
    - Stenotic nares
    - Elongated soft palate (caudal to tip of epiglottis)
    - Hypoplastic trachea (tracheal diameter/thoracic inlet ratio < 0.15) (p. 521)
    - Caudal aberrant nasal turbinates (nasal turbinates obstructing nasopharynx)
- Secondary airway changes can develop due to increased airway resistance.
    - Laryngeal collapse (grade I, laryngeal saccule eversion; grade II, cuneiform process collapse; grade III, corniculate process collapse)
    - Pharyngeal collapse
    - Tracheal collapse
    - Everted tonsils

DIAGNOSIS

Diagnostic Overview

Initial diagnostics for BAS should identify concurrent disease processes that can complicate surgical correction. Thoracic radiographs can identify pulmonary disease that may hinder ability to compensate under general anesthesia and are necessary to identify hypoplastic trachea. Acute onset of clinical signs in a middle-aged to older individual should raise concern about other conditions exacerbating clinical signs.

Differential Diagnosis

- Upper airway mass (neoplasia/polyp, granuloma, abscess, epidermoid cyst, pharyngeal sialocele)
- Laryngeal collapse
- Pharyngeal collapse
- Cervical or laryngeal trauma
- Laryngeal paralysis
- Laryngeal neoplasia
- Rhinitis

Initial Database

- Complete blood count may identify mild polycythemia. Chemistry panel may show mild increase in TCO_2 or mild decrease in HCO_3^-.
- Thoracic radiographs usually identify hypoplastic trachea but should be performed to evaluate pulmonary disease.
    - Ratio of trachea diameter to thoracic inlet < 0.15 consistent with hypoplastic trachea
    - Bulldogs typically have a smaller ratio of < 0.12.

Advanced or Confirmatory Testing

- Sedated upper airway examination using a rapid-acting induction agent (e.g., alfaxalone 1-3 mg/kg slowly IV to effect or propofol 1-6 mg/kg IV to effect)
    - Confirmation of elongated soft palate and eversion of laryngeal ventricles
    - Palate should not extend past the caudal pole of the tonsil and should barely make contact with an upright epiglottis. (Keep head and tongue in a natural position to best evaluate.)
    - Also evaluate for everted tonsils, redundant or hyperplastic pharyngeal soft tissues, advanced stages of laryngeal collapse
    - Clinician should be prepared to intubate/ventilate if necessary
- Arterial blood gas analysis often identifies hypercapnia and hypoxemia (p. 1315).
- Older animals (>7 years) that have previously compensated throughout life should receive advanced imaging.
    - Advanced nasal imaging (CT) may identify caudal aberrant turbinates or intranasal epidermoid cysts.
    - Fluoroscopy may be necessary to diagnose pharyngeal collapse.
    - Retroflex pharyngostomy to identify +/− treat caudal aberrant nasal turbinates

TREATMENT

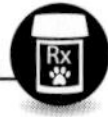

Treatment Overview

Treatment consists of addressing surgically correctable abnormalities that can functionally open the upper airway. Ideally, this should occur as young as possible, before development of secondary affects that occur due to chronic negative pressure in the upper airway.

Acute General Treatment

- If dyspnea is severe on presentation or during hospitalization
    - Minimize patient anxiety with sedatives (e.g., butorphanol 0.3 mg/kg, acepromazine 0.01-0.2 mg/kg).
    - Administer glucocorticoids to reduce airway inflammation and swelling (dexamethasone SP 0.1-0.5 mg/kg).
    - Supplement oxygen with placement in oxygen cage/tent (p. 1146)
    - Orotracheal intubation or tracheostomy (p. 1166) if necessary
- Once stabilized, relieve upper airway obstruction by surgical correction.
- Stenotic nares
    - Lateral or vertical alarplasty
    - Trader's technique
- Elongated soft palate
    - Shorten excessive palatal tissue
    - Landmarks are caudal pole of the laryngeal tonsils and tip of the epiglottis in an upright position when the tongue is in its normal position.
    - Sharp excision of soft palate requires suturing of palatal mucosa. Extra care should be made to appose the cut edges of the nasoesophageal and oropharyngeal palatal mucosa.
    - CO_2 laser and cautery excision can cause granulation tissue when not sutured (not recommended).
- Tonsillar eversion
    - Excise tonsils if obstructing airway
- Everted laryngeal saccules
    - Excision should be performed very carefully so as to not cause too much trauma ventrally with scissors or scalpel blade. CO_2 laser should be used only with guarded endotracheal tube.
    - If not everted and just effacing tissue, may decide not to treat
- Laryngeal collapse
    - Only surgically correct if impairing ventilation
    - Partial arytenoidectomy may also be useful
    - Permanent tracheostomy

- Pharyngeal collapse
    - No treatment currently available
- Caudal aberrant nasal turbinates
    - New treatments are being explored, such as laser ablation of aberrant turbinates.

Chronic Treatment

Treatment of underlying GI disease may improve outcome. Surgical correction of hiatal hernia may be necessary if medical management does not improve clinical signs (p. 468).

Nutrition/Diet

Maintain lean body weight (p. 1077).

Behavior/Exercise

- Patients should avoid hot environments because they have limited ability for thermoregulation.
- Avoid strenuous exercise, especially during warm weather.

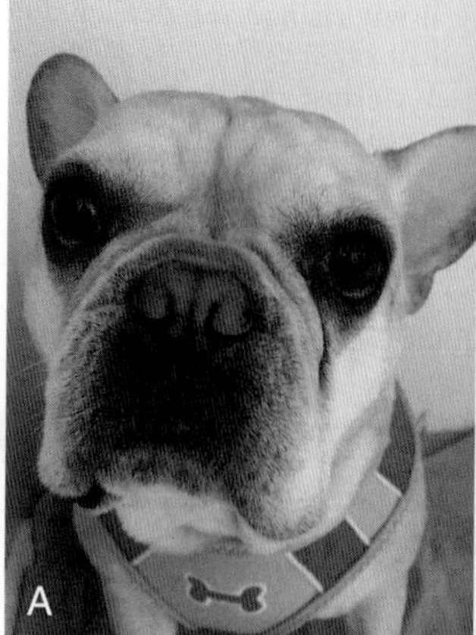

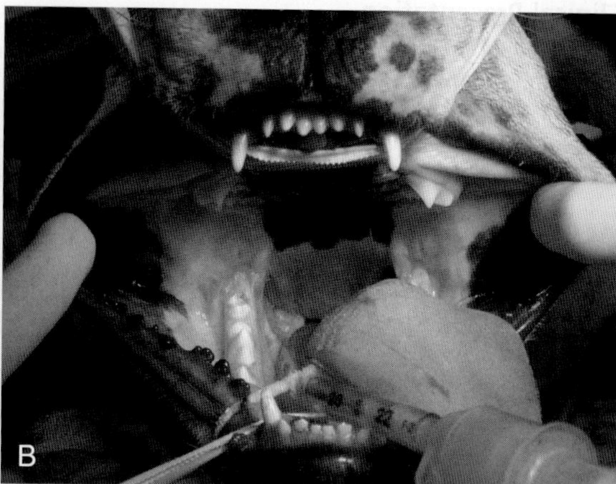

BRACHYCEPHALIC AIRWAY SYNDROME A, French bulldog with severe stenotic nares. **B,** Sedated airway examination of an English bulldog; note that the soft palate extends and obscures the larynx.

Possible Complications

- Hyperthermia
- Noncardiogenic pulmonary edema (pp. 27 and 836)
    - Can cause persistence of hypoxemia and cyanosis even after obstruction has been corrected
- Aspiration pneumonia
- Oronasal reflux if excessive shortening of soft palate
    - Do not excise rostral to the caudal pole of the tonsillar crypt.
- Upper airway obstruction secondary to inflammation
    - Be prepared to perform temporary tracheostomy in cases of soft palate resection or laryngeal sacculectomy (p. 1166).

Recommended Monitoring

- Postoperative monitoring should minimally include respiratory rate and effort, oxygenation, mucous membrane color, mentation, and evidence of regurgitation/vomiting.
- Monitor for recurrence of clinical signs, which may indicate progression of or degeneration of upper airway disease (laryngeal collapse, pharyngeal collapse). Additional sedated airway exam may show excessive granulation tissue on soft palate or inappropriate resection.

PROGNOSIS & OUTCOME

- Prognosis depends on secondary effects of the chronic negative airway pressure. Correction after 2 years of age has been shown to have worse prognosis.
- Presence of laryngeal collapse associated with a worse prognosis due to limited surgical corrections

PEARLS & CONSIDERATIONS

Comments

- Early decision and surgical correction may reduce the secondary clinical signs caused by chronic negative inspiratory pressure. Correction at the time of early neuter is often ideal.
- Severe dyspnea should be treated with sedation and oxygen therapy; may need endotracheal intubation
- Use caution with sedation in brachycephalic patients, who may be predisposed to upper airway obstruction. If sedation is necessary, oxygen supplementation is necessary to prevent hypoxemia.
- Endotracheal tube should be sized smaller than expected for patient size.
- Identification of features such as pharyngeal collapse and caudal aberrant turbinates may help to better elucidate prognosis.

Prevention

BAS is a genetically inherited disease. Until such a time as public perceptions of extreme flat faces in certain breeds are undesirable, breeding practices are unlikely to change.

Technician Tips

- Hospitalized patients with BAS require intensive preoperative and postoperative care and constant monitoring. Respiratory obstruction is a potential problem at any time. Technicians caring for these patients perioperatively should be familiar with and comfortable performing:
    - Orotracheal intubation in a brachycephalic dog
    - Oxygen administration
    - Tracheostomy care

Client Education

- Discuss breed-associated heritability of brachycephalic conditions.
- Syndrome is progressive and may cause clinical signs later in life. Clients should limit activities that exacerbate clinical signs and should avoid obesity, high ambient temperatures, and stress.
- Early surgical intervention may result in best long-term outcome.

SUGGESTED READING

Dupré G, et al: Brachycephalic syndrome. Vet Clin North Am Small Anim Pract 46:691-707, 2016.

AUTHOR: Jacob A. Rubin DVM, DACVS
EDITOR: Elizabeth A. Swanson DVM, MS, DACVS

Bromethalin Toxicosis

BASIC INFORMATION

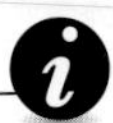

Definition

A neurotoxic syndrome results from exposure to bromethalin-based rodenticides. Incidence of exposure is increasing in the United States as the second-generation anticoagulant rodenticides have been removed from the market and replaced with bromethalin baits.

Synonym

N-methyl-2,4-dinitro-*N*-(2,4,5-tribromophenyl)-6-(trifluoromethyl) benzenamine

Epidemiology

SPECIES, AGE, SEX

- Exposure is more common in dogs, although cats are more sensitive to the toxin.
- Juveniles are believed to be more sensitive.

RISK FACTORS

- Indiscriminant eating habits
- Placement of rodenticide in an area accessible to pets

CONTAGION AND ZOONOSIS

Relay toxicosis (toxicity after ingesting poisoned rodents) is not expected.

GEOGRAPHY AND SEASONALITY

Exposure is common all year long, but an increase in cases is seen in the fall and winter.

Clinical Presentation

DISEASE FORMS/SUBTYPES

Clinical signs and their onset are dose dependent for dogs:

- Paralytic syndrome (delayed-onset syndrome): characterized by decreased conscious proprioception, paresis, ataxia, and depression. More common after an exposure below the LD50 (2.4-5.6 mg/kg for dogs). Signs develop 24-86 hours after the exposure.
- Convulsant syndrome (acute-onset syndrome): characterized by hyperesthesia, hyperthermia, tremors, and seizures. Generally seen in dogs ingesting close to or more than the LD50. Signs develop 4-24 hours after exposure.
- Cats more commonly develop a paralytic syndrome regardless of the amount of bait ingested.

HISTORY, CHIEF COMPLAINT

- Witnessed or evidenced exposure to bromethalin-based rodenticide
- Acute onset of progressive central nervous system (CNS) signs
- Potentially, bait in stool

PHYSICAL EXAM FINDINGS

- With very recent exposure, patient is clinically normal.
- Symptomatic animals show neurologic deficits: depression, ataxia, paresis, hyperesthesia, tremors, seizures, stupor, and coma
- Less common findings: anisocoria, positional nystagmus, Schiff-Sherrington posture, extensor rigidity, opisthotonus, loss of vocalization

Etiology and Pathophysiology

- Bromethalin's metabolite, desmethylbromethalin, uncouples oxidative phosphorylation in neuronal mitochondria, resulting in depletion of ATP synthesis.
- Loss of ATP impairs sodium-potassium ion pumps. Sodium and fluid accumulate within the myelin sheaths, resulting in impaired nerve conduction.
- Elevated intracranial pressure contributes to CNS dysfunction.

DIAGNOSIS

Diagnostic Overview

Diagnosis largely depends on history consistent with exposure to bromethalin-based rodenticide. Owner may notice color of bait passing in stool. There are no clinically relevant tests available.

Differential Diagnosis

- Toxic: metaldehyde, strychnine, zinc phosphide, ethylene glycol, tremorgenic mycotoxins, hypernatremia, 5-fluorouracil, lamotrigine, macadamia nut, opioids, benzodiazepines, serotonergic medications, muscle relaxants, avermectins
- Nontoxic: traumatic brain injury, infectious or inflammatory encephalomyelitis, neoplasia, myasthenia gravis, tick paralysis, botulism, polyradiculoneuritis

Initial Database

- Affected patients show no clinically relevant changes on CBC, serum chemistry, or urinalysis.
- Cerebrospinal fluid (CSF) analysis will be normal or may show mild inflammatory changes.

Advanced or Confirmatory Testing

- Histopathologic lesions of brain and spinal cord consist of spongiosis of the white matter with minimal inflammatory response.
- Gas chromatography can be used to detect bromethalin in frozen samples of kidney, fat, liver, brain, or stomach contents.

TREATMENT

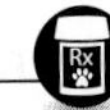

Treatment Overview

In the unaffected patient with a recent exposure, treatment is focused on thorough decontamination. In the symptomatic patient, treatment is focused on reducing edema in the CNS and managing the symptoms.

Acute General Treatment

- Animals exposed < 4 hours before presentation should have emesis induced (p. 1188).
  - This should be followed with 0-6 doses of activated charcoal, depending on the total dosage of bromethalin ingested (p. 1087).
- Symptomatic patients
  - Mannitol 1 g/kg IV, then 0.5 g/kg IV q 6h and furosemide 2.5-4.5 mg/kg PO q 6-8h or 0.5 mg/kg/h IV CRI to reduce CNS edema. Patients receiving diuretics should be administered intravenous (IV) balanced crystalloid fluids and monitored for complications associated with diuretic use.
  - Dexamethasone SP 2 mg/kg IV may also help with cerebral edema.
  - Unfortunately, the edema is within the myelin sheaths, and these therapies are unlikely to be efficacious.
- Control seizures with anticonvulsants such as diazepam 0.5-2 mg/kg IV, levetiracetam 20-60 mg/kg IV, or barbiturates. Patients in status epilepticus or with refractory seizures may require general anesthesia.
- Tremors should be treated with methocarbamol 50-150 mg/kg IV, titrate up as needed; if exceeding 330 mg/kg/day monitor respiratory effort
- Metoclopramide 1-2 mg/kg/day CRI and/or enemas may be helpful for animals with ileus.
- The use of intralipid emulsion remains controversial and is not considered to be part of the standard of care at this time (lipids can increase absorption of some toxins, and it is unknown if this happens with bromethalin).
- Because the prognosis is extremely poor after severe symptoms are recognized, humane euthanasia is a reasonable consideration.

Possible Complications

- Iatrogenic hypernatremia can occur with use of activated charcoal. Clinical hypernatremia can mimic the symptoms of bromethalin toxicosis. Monitor serum sodium levels frequently and provide parenteral and oral fluids to patients receiving activated charcoal.
- Use antiemetics to help prevent vomiting and aspiration in symptomatic patients.
- Neurologic deficits in symptomatic animals may be permanent because of neuronal demyelination and vacuolization.

Recommended Monitoring

- Serum sodium if giving multiple doses of activated charcoal
- Neurologic status over days to weeks

PROGNOSIS & OUTCOME

- Good prognosis for patients with a recent exposure that are promptly and properly decontaminated
- Fair prognosis for patients that ingested a dose below the LD50 and have mild signs. Signs may resolve over the course of days to weeks, or they may progress.
- Grave prognosis for patients with severe signs of seizures, tremors, or coma

PEARLS & CONSIDERATIONS

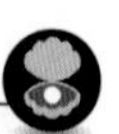

Comments

- Identification of the ingredient and concentration should be taken directly from the packaging whenever possible. The U.S. Environmental Protection Agency (EPA) registration number can be used to accurately identify the bait. Clinicians should be wary of identifications made from Internet searches as packages that look similar in appearance may contain bait with different active ingredients.
- Rodenticides that contain 0.01% bromethalin contain 0.1 mg/g bromethalin. There are 2.84 mg of bromethalin in each ounce of 0.01% bait. The LD50 for dogs is 2.4 to 5.6 mg/kg.
- Patients that develop CNS signs while receiving activated charcoal should have hypernatremia ruled out before starting other treatments.

Prevention

Place rodenticides in areas inaccessible to pets.

Technician Tips

An accurate history is vital for successful treatment of bromethalin ingestions. Determine the exact identification of the bait, the worst-case scenario amount ingested, and when the exposure occurred. Encourage clients to retrieve bait packaging and investigate for remaining bait when necessary.

Decontamination Recommendations for Bromethalin Ingestion

Dose Ingested (mg/kg)	Time Since Exposure	Treatment
Dogs		
0.1-0.49	<4	Emesis or 1 dose AC
	>4	1 dose AC
0.5-0.75	<4	Emesis + AC q 8h for 24h (3 doses total)
	>4	AC q 8h for 24h (3 doses total)
>0.75	<4	Emesis + AC q 8h for 48h (6 doses total)
	>4	AC q 8h for 48h (6 doses total)
Cats		
0.05-0.1	<4	Emesis or 1 dose AC
	>4	1 dose AC
0.1-0.3	<4	Emesis + AC q 8h for 24h (3 doses total)
	>4	AC q 8h for 24h (3 doses total)
>0.3	<4	Emesis + AC q 8h for 48h (6 doses total)
	>4	AC q 8h for 48h (6 doses total)

AC, Activated charcoal.
Data from ASPCA: APCC's decontamination recommendations for bromethalin ingestion. https://www.aspcapro.org/sites/default/files/0903toxbrief_0.pdf.

Client Education

- Place rodenticides in areas inaccessible to pets; pet-resistant bait stations are not completely pet-proof.
- Keep all packaging from rodenticides so it can be referenced if needed.

SUGGESTED READING

Tourdot R: The decontamination dilemma: bromethalin ingestion. Todays Vet Pract Jan/Feb:95-100, 2017.

AUTHOR: Renee Tourdot, DVM
EDITOR: Tina Wismer, DVM, MS, DABVT, DABT

Bronchiectasis

Bonus Material Online
Client Education Sheet

BASIC INFORMATION

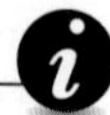

Definition

Irreversible, pathologic dilation of airways due to destruction of elastic and muscular components of airway walls

Epidemiology

SPECIES, AGE, SEX

- Dogs > cats; cats frequently subclinical
- Young if associated with congenital abnormalities (rare)
- Older (i.e., dogs > 10 years have an increased risk) if associated with chronic inflammation (e.g., chronic bronchitis, eosinophilic bronchopneumopathy), infection, or neoplasia
- In dogs, either sex equally affected; male cats may be overrepresented

GENETICS, BREED PREDISPOSITION

American cocker spaniel, West Highland white terrier, miniature and standard poodles, Siberian husky, Alaskan malamute, English springer spaniel, and beagle may have an increased risk.

RISK FACTORS

- Congenital defects (e.g., primary ciliary dyskinesia, immunodeficiency diseases)
- Acquired diseases
  - Chronic bronchitis (p. 136)
  - Eosinophilic bronchitis/eosinophilic bronchopneumopathy (p. 298)
  - Bronchopneumonia (p. 795)
  - Immunosuppressive states
  - Neoplasia

ASSOCIATED DISORDERS

Bronchopneumonia

Clinical Presentation

DISEASE FORMS/SUBTYPES

- Focal, multifocal, and diffuse distribution
- Cylindrical, saccular, and cystic forms

HISTORY, CHIEF COMPLAINT

- Incidental radiographic finding in the absence of clinical signs (especially in cats), *or*
- Cough
- Tachypnea

- Respiratory distress
- Other signs that reflect underlying disease (e.g., nasal discharge with ciliary dyskinesia)

PHYSICAL EXAM FINDINGS

- Cough may be inducible on tracheal palpation, but an inducible cough is not specific for bronchiectasis.
- Other findings may reflect underlying disease (e.g., fever with bacterial pneumonia).

Etiology and Pathophysiology

- Predisposing conditions lead to cycles of damage to the bronchial epithelium and/or its cilia, inflammation, impairment of mucociliary function, and secondary infection.
- Cellular damage, inflammation, and infection perpetuate the cycle of airway wall destruction, leading to bronchiectasis.

DIAGNOSIS

Diagnostic Overview

Diagnosis is usually accomplished by survey thoracic radiographs; CT and/or histopathology may be necessary to detect subtle lesions. A diagnosis of bronchiectasis warrants a thorough diagnostic evaluation (including bronchoscopy and bronchoalveolar lavage [BAL]) to identify underlying/concurrent diseases.

Differential Diagnosis

See Cough (p. 1209) and Respiratory Distress (p. 879).

- Other airway diseases (e.g., chronic bronchitis, eosinophilic bronchitis, secondary bacterial bronchitis, obstructive airway disease)
- Pneumonia (infectious, aspiration, foreign body)
- Neoplasia
- Pulmonary thromboembolism (PTE)
- Cardiogenic/noncardiogenic pulmonary edema
- Pleural effusion
- Pneumothorax
- Interstitial lung disease (e.g., pulmonary fibrosis)

Initial Database

CBC: neutrophilia +/− band neutrophils may support underlying infection; peripheral eosinophilia may be present with eosinophilic bronchitis

Thoracic radiographs:

- Bronchiectasis has a pathognomonic radiographic appearance
  - Cylindrical: most common (70% of canine cases); dilated bronchi with nontapering ends
  - Saccular: cluster of grapes appearance to airways (advanced disease)
  - Cystic: rounded ends of very small bronchi (end stage of saccular form)
- Spatial classification
  - Focal, multifocal, or diffuse distribution
  - In dogs, multiple lung lobes are affected in 89% of cases; right cranial lung lobe overrepresented (93%), although this may be an overestimate because the right cranial bronchus is more visible on lateral radiographs.
- Evidence of concurrent/underlying pulmonary disease is frequently present.
- Radiographs may be unremarkable in the early stages of disease, although they are important to evaluate for other causes of cough and respiratory distress.

Advanced or Confirmatory Testing

- CT is highly sensitive and may help detect subtle lesions, especially in cats. Bronchoarterial ratio > 2.0 in dogs is consistent with bronchiectasis in most cases.
- Bronchoscopy and BAL (for cytology and culture) may identify underlying/concurrent diseases (p. 1074). Depending on accessibility of the airway affected, distortion and dilation of the airway is recognized. Often, hyperemia, edema, airway excessive secretions, or inspissated mucus and debris may be recognized.
- Specialized functional and immunologic studies such as mucociliary scintigraphy, CCDC39 mutation in Old English sheepdogs with suspected primary ciliary dyskinesia, immunoglobulin A (IgA) concentration, and others may be needed to evaluate patients for suspected congenital disease.
- Other tests, as guided by preliminary information (e.g., Baermann fecal exam, serologic tests for specific pathogens)
- Lung biopsy is sometimes needed to identify underlying/concurrent disease.

TREATMENT

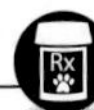

Treatment Overview

Any recognized cause of inflammation should be addressed directly, if possible (e.g., chronic bronchitis, infection). Bronchiectasis is irreversible except focal disease treated by lung lobectomy. Long-term management focuses on decreasing inflammation, enhancing mucociliary clearance, and appropriate treatment for secondary infections.

Acute General Treatment

Address underlying illness and secondary complications (e.g., bacterial bronchopneumonia).

Chronic Treatment

- Humidification or nebulization enhances mucociliary function by increasing water content of the mucociliary blanket.
- Treat recurrent secondary bacterial infections if present, ideally based on culture and sensitivity with an antibiotic that penetrates the blood-bronchus barrier (e.g., tetracyclines, fluoroquinolones).
- Glucocorticoids
  - If inflammation minimal and bronchiectasis is secondary to resolved pneumonia or obstructive disease, glucocorticoids may not be indicated.
  - If secondary to noninfectious inflammatory disease (e.g., chronic bronchitis), long-term, low-dose glucocorticoids often will be needed.
  - Oral (e.g., prednisone 0.5 mg/kg q 24h) initially to control inflammation
  - Continuation of glucocorticoids is based on the underlying disease contributing to bronchiectasis.
  - Metered-dose inhalant glucocorticoids (e.g., fluticasone: empirically start at 110 to 220 mcg per actuation, one puff using a spacer q 12h, tapering slowly to the lowest effective dose) may minimize systemic long-term side effects (pp. 136 and 1122).
- If bronchiectasis is confined to a single lung lobe (e.g., due to prior bacterial pneumonia or obstruction from bronchial tumor or foreign body), lung lobectomy may be curative.
  - A CT scan should be performed before lung lobectomy to assess for occult areas of bronchiectasis and structural changes in other lung lobes.
- Bronchodilators are unlikely to be helpful.
- Cough suppressants are *contraindicated* because they impair mucociliary clearance.

Behavior/Exercise

Minimize exposure to irritants (dust, smoke, and aerosols); HEPA-type air filters may be helpful.

Possible Complications

- Glucocorticoids may impair immunologic clearance of secondary infection. Bronchiectasis itself is associated with impaired mucociliary function, which also predisposes to bacterial infections.
- Frequent use of antibiotics may lead to development of bacterial resistance. With recurrent pneumonia/bacterial infections, culture and sensitivity should guide antibiotic therapy.

Recommended Monitoring

- Clinical signs at home
- Physical examination and repeat thoracic radiography, as warranted by signs or q 6-12 months
- Repeated airway cytology and cultures, as indicated

PROGNOSIS & OUTCOME

- If bronchiectasis is focal, lung lobectomy may be curative.
- Diffuse bronchiectasis cannot be cured and must be treated chronically by balancing antibiotics for secondary infections and antiinflammatory doses of glucocorticoids (if inflammation is present). In the absence of life-threatening infection or serious underlying disease (e.g., neoplasia), long-term survival is possible.

PEARLS & CONSIDERATIONS

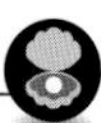

Comments

- Bronchiectasis is generally secondary to an underlying condition, although the primary disease (e.g., bacterial pneumonia) may have resolved by the time of evaluation.
- Management of secondary bacterial infections should be based on culture and sensitivity to minimize antibiotic resistance.

Prevention

The best means of preventing bronchiectasis is early identification and treatment of diseases that predispose to its development (e.g., inflammation, infection).

Technician Tips

- When preparing for respiratory washes, use solutions without bacteriostatic additives. If possible, prewarm solutions in a 37°C incubator (or suitable alternative).
- Before performing a lavage in a cat, administer a bronchodilator. Provide supplemental oxygen before and after the procedure.

Client Education

Owners must understand that bronchiectasis is not curable (unless focal disease can be resolved by lobectomy). In patients with multifocal or diffuse disease, recurrent secondary bacterial infections are common and can be life-threatening.

SUGGESTED READING

Hawkins EC, et al: Demographic, clinical, and radiographic features of bronchiectasis in dogs: 316 cases (1988-2000). J Am Vet Med Assoc 223:1628-1635, 2003.

AUTHORS: Laura A. Nafe, DVM, MS, DACVIM
EDITOR: Megan Grobman, DVM, MS, DACVIM

Bronchiolar and Pulmonary Neoplasia

Client Education Sheet 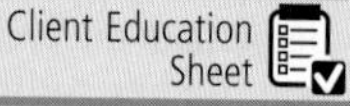

BASIC INFORMATION

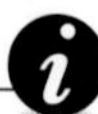

Definition

Malignant growth in the pulmonary parenchyma that may be primary (bronchiolar or alveolar) or metastatic

Synonyms

Lung cancer, pulmonary neoplasia, metastatic pulmonary neoplasia, pulmonary metastasis

Epidemiology

SPECIES, AGE, SEX

- Dogs and cats of either sex
- Mean age: dogs, 11 years; cats, 12-13 years

GENETICS, BREED PREDISPOSITION

Breeds that may be overrepresented are boxers, Doberman pinschers, Australian shepherds, Irish setters, Bernese mountain dogs and, among cats, possibly Persians.

RISK FACTORS

Dogs with primary lung cancer have increased anthracosis (accumulation of carbon within the bronchial mucosa and pulmonary parenchyma) compared to normal dogs, suggesting exposure to pollution may play a role in lung cancer development.

ASSOCIATED DISORDERS

Hypertrophic osteopathy

Clinical Presentation

DISEASE FORMS/SUBTYPES

Malignant neoplasia:

- Bronchoalveolar carcinoma (most common primary lung tumor in dogs)
- Adenocarcinoma (most common primary lung tumor in cats)
- Adenosquamous cell carcinoma
- Squamous cell carcinoma
- Histiocytic sarcoma
- Lymphoma
- Metastatic tumors to lungs

HISTORY, CHIEF COMPLAINT

- Often an incidental finding
- Respiratory signs are common (e.g., respiratory distress, cough, tachypnea, hemoptysis).
- Weight loss is sometimes recognized, as are lethargy and hyporexia.
- In cats, vomiting and diarrhea often noted
- Lameness is occasionally noted.
  - Cats: pulmonary adenocarcinoma or squamous cell carcinoma can metastasize to the digits
  - Dogs: hypertrophic osteopathy

PHYSICAL EXAM FINDINGS

- Usually no findings specific for pulmonary tumors
- Auscultation might reveal
  - Increased bronchovesicular sounds
  - Decreased heart and lungs sounds ventrally if pleural effusion present
  - Decreased lung sounds over an area of large mass
- Neurologic abnormalities (metastasis to central nervous system [CNS])
- Poor body condition
- Lameness (hypertrophic osteopathy, digital metastasis)
- Distant primary tumor may be recognized anywhere on the body with metastatic lung cancer.

Etiology and Pathophysiology

- Continual unregulated cellular proliferation
- Experimentally, smoking and inhaled plutonium increased occurrence in dogs

DIAGNOSIS

Diagnostic Overview

Primary lung cancer is often incidentally found on screening radiographs or found on thoracic radiographs performed for workup of coughing as solitary or multiple pulmonary masses. Approximately 30% of cats also have pleural effusion. Definitive diagnosis requires cell sampling.

Differential Diagnosis

- Granuloma (e.g., fungal pneumonia)
- Abscess
- Hematoma
- Lung lobe torsion
- Pulmonary parasites
- Pulmonary eosinophilic infiltrates
- Lymphoid granulomatosis
- Fluid or blood filled bulla

Initial Database

- Complete blood count (CBC), chemistry panel, urinalysis: often unremarkable
- Thoracic radiographs: large solitary or multiple pulmonary masses
  - Solitary, well-defined nodule more likely to be primary lung cancer
  - Nodular interstitial pattern more likely to be metastatic cancer. Often, nodules vary in size.
  - Histiocytic sarcomas often large mass/entire lobe with internal air bronchogram
  - Lymphoma has a varied appearance, including alveolar, nodular, or unstructured interstitial patterns; bronchial infiltrates; or masses.
- Abdominal imaging (radiographs, ultrasound, or CT): with primary lung tumors, abdominal imaging often normal. With metastatic lung cancers, abdominal imaging sometimes identifies a primary tumor.
  - If a tumor is recognized in the abdomen or limbs, fine-needle aspirate for cytology can provide a likely diagnosis for metastatic lung disease.

Advanced or Confirmatory Testing

- Thoracic CT scan: more sensitive than radiography for assessing number/size of pulmonary masses, tracheobronchial lymph node size, and may help plan surgery

- Cytology: may be nondiagnostic but often provides diagnostic sample
  - Transthoracic needle aspiration of peripheral lesions (p. 1112): results are improved with imaging guidance and larger masses
  - Bronchoalveolar lavage (pp. 1073 and 1074)
- Biopsy
  - If primary lung cancer is suspected, lobectomy can be diagnostic and therapeutic.
  - If primary lung cancer is not suspected and cytology is nondiagnostic, biopsy can provide information necessary for treatment.

TREATMENT

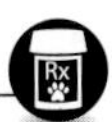

Treatment Overview

Treatment is specific to the type of tumor, and a definitive diagnosis is critical.

Acute General Treatment

Supportive care as indicated: thoracocentesis if pleural effusion or pneumothorax present and impairing respiration (p. 1164), oxygen supplementation (p. 1146) as needed

Chronic Treatment

- For solitary lung mass, surgery is the treatment of choice using partial or complete lung lobectomies, depending on mass size and location within the lung lobe. Biopsy of hilar lymph nodes is also recommended for prognostic information.
- Chemotherapy for treatment of primary lung cancer is not well studied in dogs or cats. Vinorelbine reaches higher concentrations in lung tissue than plasma in people, and 2 of 7 dogs with bulky tumors responded to treatment in one study. Platinum-based drugs may also be considered. Chemotherapy after incomplete surgical resection or in dogs or cats with lymph node metastasis is not well studied.
- Pulmonary metastasis carries guarded to poor prognosis; consultation with a veterinary oncologist is recommended.
- Lymphoma treatment is described on pp. 607 and 609.

Recommended Monitoring

- Thoracic radiographs every 2-3 months for the first year postoperatively.
- If treating bulky disease with chemotherapy, monitoring thoracic radiographs regularly (every 6-8 weeks) is recommended. Monitoring CBC for cytopenia is also indicated. Other monitoring depends on chemotherapy drug used.

PROGNOSIS & OUTCOME

- Dogs treated with surgery for primary lung cancer
  - No clinical signs at diagnosis (median survival 545 vs. 240 days)
  - No metastasis to lymph nodes (median survival 15 vs. 1-2 months)

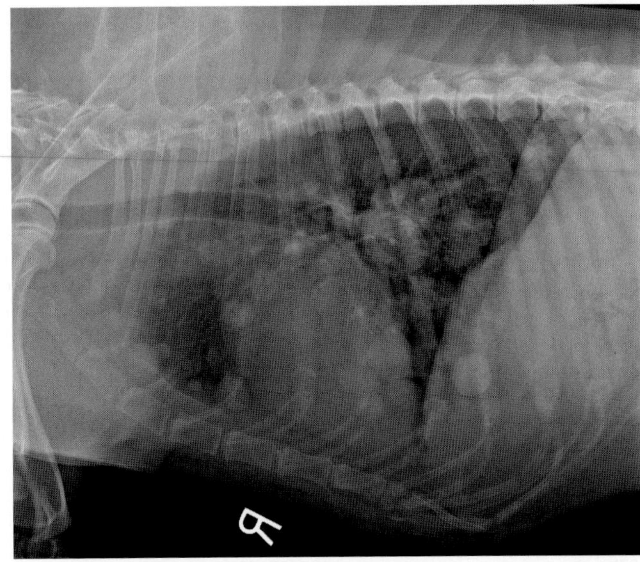

BRONCHIOLAR AND PULMONARY NEOPLASIA Lateral radiographs of metastatic osteosarcoma to the lungs.

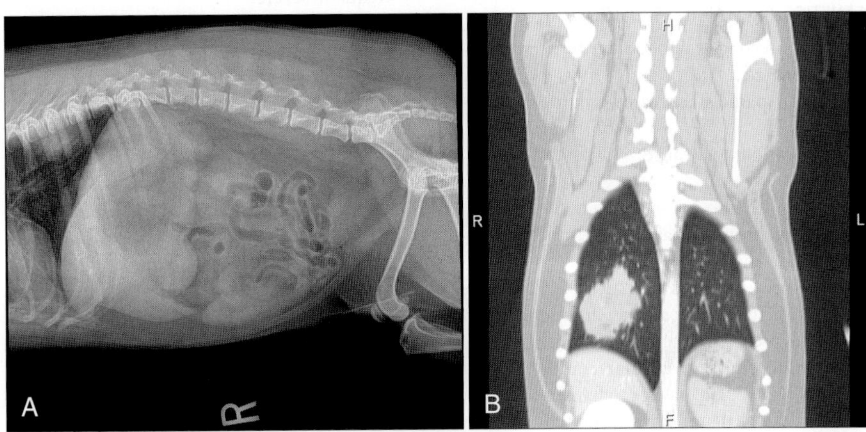

BRONCHIOLAR AND PULMONARY NEOPLASIA A, Primary lung tumor found incidentally on abdominal radiographs for an unrelated problem. **B,** CT scan for surgical planning in the same dog.

  - Histologic grade: median survival for well differentiated, 790 days; moderately differentiated, 251 days; poorly differentiated, 5 days
- Cats treated with surgery for primary lung cancer
  - Histologic grade: median survival for well differentiated, 23 months; poorly differentiated, 2.5 months
- Metastatic lung cancer: guarded to poor prognosis

PEARLS & CONSIDERATIONS

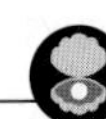

Comments

- A diagnosis of pulmonary neoplasia cannot be made with thoracic imaging alone. Cellular confirmation is necessary because some disorders that closely mimic cancer carry a good prognosis (e.g., eosinophilic bronchopneumopathy, parasitic granuloma).
- Early intervention is best; once a pulmonary mass is found, full staging and evaluation for surgery should be discussed with clients.

Technician Tips

- Thoracic radiographs should include all lung fields and the entire diaphragm.
- Three views (right and left lateral, ventrodorsal) are best for evaluation.
- Imaging the thorax alone rather than thorax and abdomen will allow for the best technique.

SUGGESTED READING

Polton GA, et al: Impact of primary tumour stage on survival in dogs with solitary lung tumors. J Small Anim Pract 49:66-71, 2008.

AUTHOR: Sandra M. Bechtel, DVM, DACVIM
EDITOR: Megan Grobman, DVM, MS, DACVIM

Bronchitis, Chronic

Bonus Material Online 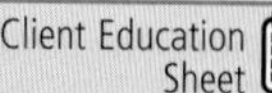 Client Education Sheet 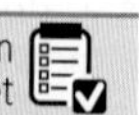

BASIC INFORMATION

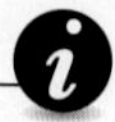

Definition

Chronic bronchitis (CB) is an inflammatory disease of the airways characterized by sterile suppurative inflammation and cough lasting ≥ 2 months in the absence of other identifiable causes.

Synonyms

Chronic cough, canine asthma (inaccurate), feline asthma (inaccurate), chronic obstructive pulmonary disease (COPD), chronic asthmatic bronchitis

Epidemiology

SPECIES, AGE, SEX

- Dogs: middle aged to older
- Cats: any age, but generally older than 1 year, rare geriatric onset

GENETICS, BREED PREDISPOSITION

- Small-breed dogs (poodles, terriers) overrepresented
- Cocker spaniels: increased risk for bronchiectasis
- No clear genetic cause

RISK FACTORS

- Obesity, bronchomalacia, and tracheal collapse are thought to play a role.
- Exposure to irritants such as cigarette smoke is intuitively a risk. Although further studies are needed, epigenetic changes have been identified in cellular components of bronchoalveolar lavage (BAL) fluid in dogs exposed to environmental tobacco smoke.
- Prior infectious respiratory disease (as a puppy or a community-acquired pneumonia) may trigger later bronchitis.
- Chronic microaspiration (e.g., laryngeal paralysis, gastroesophageal reflux disease) may also contribute.
- ± Chronic rhinitis (expert opinion rather than evidence based)
- Aspirated foreign material
- Asthma: chronic allergic inflammation leading to airway damage and CB (chronic allergic asthma [p. 84])

CONTAGION AND ZOONOSIS

Although CB is not due to infection, it is necessary to exclude infectious cases of chronic cough.

GEOGRAPHY AND SEASONALITY

Possibly more severe in warmer/humid months, but this is not universally reported

ASSOCIATED DISORDERS

- Some dogs with tracheal collapse will also develop CB, making it occasionally challenging to determine whether cough is from lower airway disease or tracheal collapse. In many cases of mild to moderate tracheal collapse, there is also a component of CB.
- Small-breed dogs are also predisposed to mitral valve disease, which can develop concurrently with CB. Both disorders can cause cough.
- Chronic rhinitis in some dogs (p. 890)
- Syncope (seen with high vagal tone)
- Pulmonary hypertension (p. 838)
- Bronchomalacia
- Emphysema (rare)

Clinical Presentation

DISEASE FORMS/SUBTYPES

- Unless there are comorbid conditions, most affected pets seem well other than cough. Coughing varies from mild/occasional to frequent/severe.
- Mild: daily cough, minimal other signs
- Moderate to severe: frequent and/or severe cough impacts patient and owner's quality of life
  - Sometimes, exercise intolerance noted
- In cats, bronchitis may be clinically indistinguishable from asthma (p. 84). Allergic asthma is defined by reversible bronchoconstriction, eosinophilic airway inflammation, with evidence of airway remodeling. Airway cytology (airway eosinophilia vs. neutrophilia) can help distinguish these two conditions. Pulmonary parasites and feline heartworm infection can cause a similar clinical appearance and are also characterized by eosinophilic airway lavage.

HISTORY, CHIEF COMPLAINT

- By definition, cough is the chief complaint. Many dogs have a gradual, progressive disease course. Sometimes, a historical precipitating insult can be identified (e.g., cough persists long after resolution of infectious airway disease). Respiratory distress is rare in the absence of comorbid conditions (e.g., bronchiectasis with pneumonia, airway collapse, congestive heart failure).
- Cats may present with wheeze or cough. Clients sometimes mistake cough in cats for hairballs, although no trichobezoar is found after the episode.

PHYSICAL EXAM FINDINGS

Dogs:

- Often overconditioned (body condition score > 6/9)
- Increased tracheal sensitivity on palpation (inducible cough): nonspecific finding
- ± Wheezes or crackles on lung auscultation
  - Wheezes (often expiratory): suggest narrowing of the airways. Acute reversible bronchoconstriction, as is characteristic of feline asthma, is uncommon in dogs with airway disease. Airway narrowing in dogs is usually due to airway exudate or architectural remodeling.
  - Crackles (often inspiratory): often best appreciated after a cough (post-tussive crackles) and suggest concurrent pulmonary edema, fibrosis, or secondary pneumonia
- Severely affected dogs may have a marked expiratory push, occasionally with abdominal muscular hypertrophy or "heave" line. Typically seen with concurrent small airway collapse/bronchomalacia
- Concurrent soft (grade 2 or 3) systolic apical murmur is common.
- Sinus arrhythmia: normal variant in dogs, commonly seen in CB due to increased vagal tone

Cats:

- Cats with bronchitis typically lack the acute airflow limitation seen in asthmatic cats (status asthmaticus) except in cases of chronic asthmatic bronchitis.
- Rarely, emphysema may result in respiratory distress that is weakly responsive to bronchodilators.
- ± Crackles and wheezes on auscultation: see above

Etiology and Pathophysiology

- Causation is unknown but speculated to be secondary to a previous insult (often unknown) that sets up cycle of chronic inflammation.
- Inflammation results in airway hypertrophy/malacia, airflow limitation, excessive mucus production, and cough.
- Cough precipitates further inflammation.
- Airway hyperreactivity (bronchospasm) may occur in cats, although this is more commonly seen in asthma (p. 84).
- Asthma versus bronchitis in cats: are immunologically distinct processes. Asthma is presumed to be allergically mediated (T_H2 lymphocyte driven), and bronchitis is thought to be due to a previous airway insult. Because chronic allergic inflammation can lead to airway damage, there is some overlap between these two conditions (chronic asthmatic bronchitis).

DIAGNOSIS

Diagnostic Overview

The diagnosis of CB depends on recognition of chronic cough and airway inflammation when no other cause for these can be identified. The goal of diagnostic testing is to exclude other conditions that are more specifically treatable (e.g., infectious tracheobronchitis [p. 987]) or potentially life-threatening (e.g., congestive heart failure [p. 408]). Thoracic radiographs and cytology of airway secretions (nonseptic, degenerative neutrophilic inflammation) support the diagnosis. Attempts should be made to exclude pathogenic bacteria, fungi, parasites, or other relevant causes of cough (e.g., heart failure if murmur is recognized).

Differential Diagnosis

- Cough (p. 217)
- Key differential diagnoses include tracheal collapse (dogs), congestive heart failure (dogs), pneumonia, interstitial lung disease/pulmonary fibrosis, lung tumor, and asthma (cat).

Initial Database

- CBC/chemistry profile/urinalysis: typically unremarkable
- Heartworm testing: antigen (dog), antigen and antibody (cats). In Europe or Newfoundland, Canada, consider testing for *Angiostrongylus vasorum*.
- Fecal examination (Baermann fecal floatation); insensitive due to intermittent fecal shedding
- Thoracic radiographs
    - Bronchiolar pattern characteristic (e.g., "donuts and tramlines")
    - Bronchiectasis may be present in chronic disease.
    - Hyperinflation may be seen in cats with concurrent asthma.
    - Examine for evidence of comorbid disease (e.g., left atrial enlargement) or alternative diagnosis (e.g., lung tumors).

Advanced or Confirmatory Testing

- Echocardiography (p. 1094): indicated if cardiac examination is abnormal (e.g., murmur) or if radiographs identify abnormalities of the cardiac silhouette or blood vessels. Can also be used to identify pulmonary hypertension (p. 838) in animals with evidence of airway remodeling.
- Bronchoscopy (p. 1074): irregular mucosal surface, often thick, rough, or granular in appearance. Hyperemia and excessive mucus accumulation often appreciated. Bronchiectasis is sometimes recognized.
- Airway lavage (cytology and culture)
    - Bronchoscopic airway lavage: advantage of airway visualization, as above (figure at www.ExpertConsult.com)
    - Blind bronchoalveolar lavage (p. 1073)
    - Transtracheal wash
    - > 10% nondegenerative neutrophils on cytology
    - Eosinophilic inflammation suggests an alternative diagnosis (e.g., parasites, allergic asthma).
    - Diagnosis of CB cannot be confirmed if there are degenerative neutrophils with a positive bacterial culture (must rule out infection before diagnosis of CB).
    - Consider polymerase chain reaction (PCR) assay for *Mycoplasma* spp.
- Computed tomography: more sensitive than radiographs, with far greater airway/pulmonary detail; not routinely indicated

TREATMENT

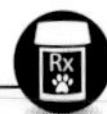

Treatment Overview

Treatment is directed at limiting airway inflammation, controlling cough, and treating any comorbid condition (including secondary infection). Weight loss is crucial in overweight or obese dogs. Cats and rarely dogs may benefit from bronchodilator therapy.

Acute General Treatment

Animals with CB are managed as outpatients and seldom require acute or emergent care. Disease exacerbations can occur from secondary infection or comorbid disease, and re-evaluation is appropriate. Importantly, because mitral valve disease is a common finding in dogs with CB, some patients eventually develop concurrent congestive heart failure.

Chronic Treatment

- Glucocorticoids (oral or inhaled): mainstay of therapy for CB
    - Prednisone or prednisolone (preferred for cats): starting dose 1-2 mg/kg PO q 24h. If cough improves, taper by ≈25% q 3 weeks to the lowest possible dose to control cough.
    - Fluticasone 110-222 mcg/puff, one puff q 12h by face mask (e.g., AeroDawg, AeroKat). Inhaled steroids have a delayed onset of efficacy, and are not more effective than oral steroids. However, they minimize systemic effects. Recommended starting with oral steroids before transitioning to inhaled.
- Cough suppressants (e.g., hydrocodone, butorphanol, diphenoxylate): antitussive therapy is controversial because it may mask poor disease control, allowing airway inflammation and remodeling to progress. Antitussives may be recommended in patients with concurrent collapsing trachea contributing to chronic cough (p. 194) or if quality of life is compromised by cough despite appropriate medical therapy.
- Antibiotics: as needed for secondary pneumonia (ideally based on culture and susceptibility) or during acute exacerbation of cough (e.g., doxycycline, azithromycin)
- Bronchodilators: very little evidence of efficacy for dogs with CB but likely more useful for cats (p. 84)
- Additional proposed therapies (limited experience)
    - Maropitant: small clinical trial supported efficacy
    - Gabapentin
    - Fish oil supplementation
- Eliminate environmental irritants
- Address pulmonary hypertension, if present (p. 838).

Nutrition/Diet

Maintain a lean body weight (p. 1077).

Behavior/Exercise

Encourage moderate exercise for weight control, but avoid outdoor exercise during high heat and humidity.

Drug Interactions

- Theophylline or aminophylline levels may be increased by the concurrent administration of fluoroquinolone antibiotics.
- Prednisone can contribute to weight gain, which can worsen clinical signs.

Possible Complications

- Pulmonary hypertension
- Secondary pneumonia
- Bronchomalacia: airway collapse secondary to chronic inflammation
- Although rare, spontaneous pneumothorax may develop associated with chronic cough.

Recommended Monitoring

- Body condition, weight gain, cough frequency/severity
- Physical examination and thoracic radiographs if clinical signs worsen or q 6-12 months
- ± Pulmonary hypertension check (echocardiogram)

PROGNOSIS & OUTCOME

- CB is managed rather than cured.
- Mild to moderately affected dogs: good prognosis for disease control
- Severely affected: severity of cough, exercise intolerance, secondary complications (e.g., bronchomalacia, secondary pneumonia) sometimes result in euthanasia (quality of life considerations).

PEARLS & CONSIDERATIONS

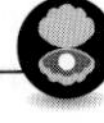

Comments

- If apparent exacerbation of cough is recognized in dogs, especially if animal is tachycardic, rule out heart failure (p. 408).
- Inflammatory airway disease is usually recognized in younger cats. Maintain suspicion of an alternate diagnosis in cats > 12 years.

Prevention

It seems prudent to avoid exposure to tobacco smoke and pollution.

Technician Tips

Technicians should work closely with owners to ensure treatment compliance and to teach them how to use inhalers. Supporting pet owners who deal with this frustrating condition is vital.

Client Education

- Canine CB is a progressive, incurable disease, and exacerbations occur periodically. The goal of therapy is to minimize cough to improve the quality of life for pet and owner. Cough may not resolve completely.

- Avoid exposure to dogs with infectious respiratory diseases (e.g., infectious tracheobronchitis), and maintain vaccination for these contagious infections.
- Do not allow the pet to become overweight on glucocorticoid therapy.

SUGGESTED READING

Rozanski E: Canine chronic bronchitis. Vet Clin North Am Small Anim Pract 44(1):107-116, 2014.

AUTHOR: Elizabeth Rozanski, DVM, DACVIM, DACVECC
EDITOR: Megan Grobman, DVM, MS, DACVIM

Burns

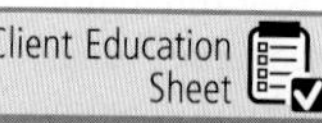

BASIC INFORMATION

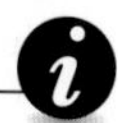

Definition

- *Burns* result from exposure to flame, extreme heat, scalding, inhalation, and chemical or electrical trauma.
- *Eschar:* a thick, coagulated crust or slough that develops as a result of a burn
- *Compartmentalization:* a condition associated with third- and fourth-degree burns in which swelling within tissue compartments creates strictures that can decrease thoracic wall motion (leading to hypoventilation) or cause ischemic injury to limbs

Epidemiology

SPECIES, AGE, SEX

All animals are susceptible to burn injury.

RISK FACTORS

Temperature and duration of exposure contribute to the degree of thermal injury. Common causes of companion animal burns include heating pads, hot water bottles, fire, exhaust systems, and hot pipes. Scalding water can also produce severe burns. Debilitating comorbid conditions increase risk for fatal complications.

ASSOCIATED DISORDERS

Bacterial infections, smoke inhalation, carbon monoxide poisoning

Clinical Presentation

DISEASE FORMS/SUBTYPES

First-degree (superficial) burns:
- Affect the epidermis
- Typically thickened, erythematous, and desquamated
- Typically painful

Second-degree (deep, partial-thickness) burns:
- Affect the superficial layers of dermis
- Typically edematous and erythematous
- Typically wet and very painful

Third- and fourth-degree burns:
- Affect the superficial layers of dermis (third degree) and subcutaneous layers, tendon, and bone (fourth degree)
- Typically waxy and leathery in appearance
- Typically less painful than first- or second-degree burns
- Third- and fourth-degree burns carry a greater risk of wound sepsis, coagulation disorders, limb ischemia, or compression severe enough to cause ventilatory compromise or abdominal problems.

Electrical burns (p. 292):
- High-voltage burns: associated with compartmental syndromes and ischemia
- Low-voltage burns: seldom associated with complications

Chemical or tar burns:
- Usually involve the superficial dermis layers and may be delayed in appearance by 3-4 days after contact

HISTORY, CHIEF COMPLAINT

- Burn event may or may not have been witnessed. With acts of malicious intent, history may be unknown.
- Recent anesthetic procedures should prompt suspicion of heating blanket or heating lamp burn.

PHYSICAL EXAM FINDINGS

- Physical examination findings depend on the location and extent of the burn.
- Burns from contact may not initially be apparent until rapid skin and hair loss occur 2-3 days later (e.g., chemical burns, heating pads), although the animal may be inexplicably painful when the area is touched.
- Thermal burn resulting from a heating blanket or lamp will present as a defined injury reflective of the size and positioning of the animal during recumbency. For 2-4 days, skin is firm but not ulcerated, making delayed identification common.
- Animals with extensive burns may present in hypotensive shock or with hypothermia.
- The presence of singed whiskers or burn debris in the mouth is strongly suggestive of inhalation (p. 919).
- Respiratory distress can occur rapidly from pharyngeal and laryngeal edema, progressive upper airway obstruction, pulmonary edema, inhalation of burn debris, or carbon monoxide toxicity.
- Corneal ulceration may be present (p. 209). Repeat fluorescein stain 24 hours after admission if negative initially to rule out corneal trauma.
- Neurologic signs (seizures, loss of consciousness, ataxia [p. 1136]) can result from carbon monoxide or cyanide intoxication immediately or after a delay.

Etiology and Pathophysiology

- Localized wound inflammation results in release of inflammatory mediators and capillary leakage, causing extravasation of fluid.
- If systemic inflammation or vasculitis occurs, fluid losses may be severe and result in hypotension or cardiac collapse.
- Due to large volume of dead tissue, impaired blood supply, and impaired antimicrobial delivery, large burn areas are at high risk for infection. Initial organisms are normal flora, including gram-positive cocci, but in 3-5 days, gram-negative bacteria colonize the wound. Debridement and topical antibiotics are essential to treatment.
- Sepsis may result from wound infection, nosocomial infection due to the presence of multiple invasive catheters, or pneumonia.
- Systemic inflammation may result in coagulopathy, including disseminated intravascular coagulopathy.
- Inhalation injury (p. 919)

DIAGNOSIS

Diagnostic Overview

Often, history suggests or is conclusive for thermal injury; attempt to ascertain time from and duration of injury. Determining the severity of the burn and appropriate treatment course requires examination of the lesion, including underlying and surrounding normal tissue. The full extent of burns may not be apparent immediately after the injury. Diagnostic testing for related disorders (e.g., smoke inhalation) is applied on a case-by-case basis.

Differential Diagnosis

- Severe bacterial pyoderma
- Severe drug eruption
- Toxic epidermal necrolysis

Initial Database

- CBC, including a manual platelet count: thrombocytopenia is common.
- Serum biochemistry profile: hypoalbuminemia and electrolyte disturbances are common.
- Urinalysis
- Coagulation profile (p. 1325)
- Survey radiographs: thoracic radiographs for all thermal burn patients and other areas as

indicated by examination. Radiographic changes in the lungs may progress after injury.
- Baseline aerobic wound culture to allow targeted antibiotic therapy.
- Co-oximetry (if available) to measure carboxyhemoglobin concentrations. Pulse oximetry and arterial blood gas analysis may provide falsely elevated oxygen levels after carbon monoxide exposure.

Advanced or Confirmatory Testing

- Central nervous system imaging (CT, MRI) for unexplained alteration in mentation
- If pneumonia is suspected, airway lavage for appropriate antibiotic selection, assuming patient is stable (p. 1073)

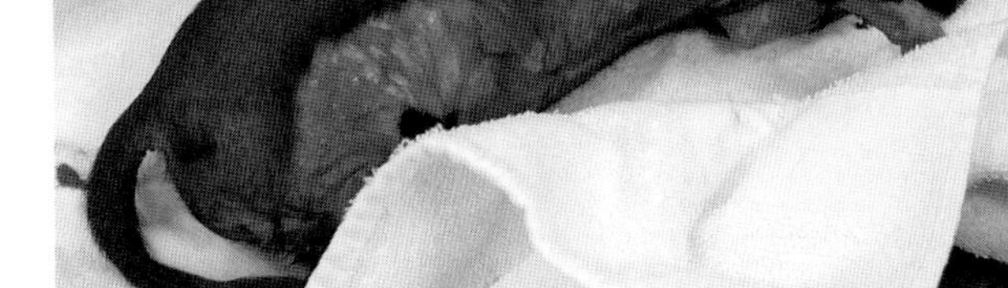

BURNS A puppy with severe burns after being placed in hot water.

TREATMENT

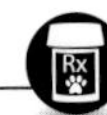

Treatment Overview

Goals are to maintain a patent airway and oxygenation, support arterial blood pressure and plasma oncotic pressure, maintain adequate urine production, and manage wounds to prevent tissue loss and reduce risk of infection or septic complications. Intravenous fluids, broad-spectrum antimicrobials, and in some cases, supplemental oxygen are cornerstones of treatment.

Acute General Treatment

- Rapidly cooling burns within 20 minutes of injury is beneficial to prevent ongoing tissue damage. Continuous lavage with cold (15°C) tap water for 20 minutes is recommended. Avoid ice.
- Support respiratory function
  - Oxygen supplementation for patients with carbon monoxide poisoning from smoke inhalation (pp. 919 and 1146)
  - Maintain airway patency in presence of pharyngeal or laryngeal edema (intubation if necessary) (p. 1166).
  - Mechanical ventilation (p. 1185) may be required for management of direct lung injury from inhalation of carbon debris, aspiration pneumonia, or pulmonary edema.
- Intensive intravenous (IV) fluid resuscitation with crystalloid fluids during the initial 8-12 hours after injury to maintain adequate mean arterial blood pressure and urine production at 1-2 mL/kg/h. Avoid overhydration and complications secondary to edema (subcutaneous, pulmonary, cerebral) formation.
- Systemic inflammation and leaky vessels may result in protein loss and severe hypoalbuminemia.
  - Judicious use of IV synthetic colloids (e.g., Hetastarch 20 mL/kg/24h, Vetstarch 20-40 mL/kg/24h) to maintain colloid oncotic pressure and mean arterial blood pressure. Avoid synthetic colloids if there is kidney dysfunction or thrombocytopenia (platelet count < 75,000/mcL).
  - Canine or human albumin may be transfused for oncotic pressure. Human albumin has been associated with severe anaphylaxis and death in some dogs.
  - Stored or fresh-frozen plasma may be considered in patients in need of colloid support who cannot receive synthetic colloids or for secondary coagulopathy (fresh-frozen plasma) (p. 1169).
- Oil-based wound dressings (e.g., Vaseline-impregnated gauze) should be avoided.
- Third- and fourth-degree burns may require early escharotomy (debridement) or fasciotomy to limit wound sepsis and compartmentalization.
- Broad-spectrum antimicrobial coverage if evidence of pneumonia until culture results are available (e.g., ampicillin 22 mg/kg IV q 8h plus enrofloxacin 10 mg/kg IV q 24h, or 5 mg/kg IV q 24h in cats).
- First- and second-degree burn wounds may require little debridement; application of antimicrobial topical creams (silver sulfadiazine or 0.5% silver nitrate) is recommended.

Chronic Treatment

- Small eschars should be debrided for primary closure early during wound care.
- Large eschars not amenable to primary closure should be debrided, allowed to form granulation tissue, and grafted. Vacuum-assisted wound closure (VAC) has been used successfully for large burn wounds. Moist wound care should be used with open wound management (e.g., manuka honey and nonadherent dressings). Avoid wet-to-dry dressings, which can delay formation of granulation tissue.
- Extensive/deep burns involving the limbs should be debrided to avoid limb ischemia and treated with variations of splinting to avoid contracture.

Nutrition/Diet

Severe burns cause increased metabolic demand and significant protein losses; early enteral nutrition should be instituted. In critically ill patients, nasoesophageal or nasogastric feeding tubes are indicated (p. 1107). Concurrent partial parenteral nutrition can be administered to achieve full energy requirements.

Behavior/Exercise

- For third- and fourth-degree burns, especially when involving tissues affected by motion (e.g., limbs, axilla, inguinal region, flank), strict rest for 3-4 weeks may be necessary.
- Physical therapy or hydrotherapy may be beneficial to patients with large body surface regions affected.

Possible Complications

Wound infection, pneumonia, nosocomial infection, sepsis, limb ischemia from wound contracture, coagulopathy

Recommended Monitoring

- Close initial monitoring of vital parameters
- Arterial blood pressure
- Quantification of urine production
- Oxygen saturation (or ideally co-oximetry)
- Serial CBC, serum biochemistry profile, coagulation tests

PROGNOSIS & OUTCOME

- Outcome is generally good for first- and second-degree burns and guarded for third- and fourth-degree burns.
- Prognosis is guarded to poor for moderate to severe inhalation injury.
- Prognosis relies on response to fluid resuscitation in severe burn injury. Prognosis improves with appropriate and successful wound management and worsens with development of complications.

PEARLS & CONSIDERATIONS

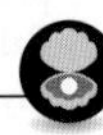

Comments

- Third- and fourth-degree burns and/or inhalational injuries are best treated in a tertiary care facility with 24-hour intensive

care management and surgeons skilled in surgical burn management, including skin grafting.
- Severe eschars causing constriction of ventilatory muscles or limb ischemia require early debridement and primary wound closure or grafting to limit wound infection and reduce the risk of compartmentalization.
- Respiratory distress in a patient with evidence of smoke inhalation (e.g., burned whiskers) may be due to pharyngeal or laryngeal edema and warrants intubation to obtain and maintain airway patency.

Prevention

- Use circulating warm water/air blankets for patient warmth, not electric heating blankets or hot water bottles, especially during diagnostic imaging with MRI.
- Duration of time in contact with the warming device influences the extent of injury; therefore, the patient or warming device should be repositioned frequently.

Technician Tips

- Always place a towel or blanket between a patient and a warming device.
- Rotate the patient and location of the warming device frequently.

SUGGESTED READING

Vaughn L, et al: Severe burn injury, burn shock, and smoke inhalation in small animals. Part 2. Diagnosis, therapy, complications and prognosis. J Vet Emerg Crit Care 22(2):187-200, 2012.

AUTHOR: Kristin Welch, DVM, DACVECC
EDITOR: Benjamin M. Brainard, VMD, DACVAA, DACVECC

Calcium Channel Blocker Drug Toxicosis

Client Education Sheet 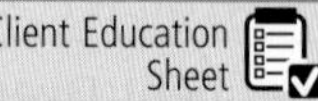

BASIC INFORMATION

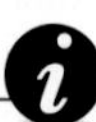

Definition

Calcium channel blocker (CCB) drugs are commonly used for the treatment of hypertension and tachyarrhythmias in human and veterinary medicine. Adverse effects at therapeutic dose or with overdose result in hypotension and bradycardia or tachycardia, weakness, ataxia, and inappetence within 30 minutes to 12 hours after ingestion.

Epidemiology

SPECIES, AGE, SEX

All animals are susceptible. Exposure is more common in dogs.

RISK FACTORS

- Pre-existing renal or cardiovascular disease may predispose to signs.
- Hepatic disease may reduce metabolism and elimination of CCBs.

Clinical Presentation

DISEASE FORMS/SUBTYPES

Sustained/controlled/extended/delayed-release preparations may delay onset of signs (6-12 hours), whereas immediate-release preparations can cause signs within 30 minutes.

HISTORY, CHIEF COMPLAINT

- History of suspected or observed exposure
- Weakness, depression, ataxia, vomiting possible

PHYSICAL EXAM FINDINGS

- Hypotension and bradycardia are common; reflex tachycardia possible if hypotension predominates (dihydropyridine CCBs)
- Pale mucous membranes
- Hypothermia possible (due to hypotension)
- Depression, ataxia, seizures, or coma possible
- Respiratory distress possible (pulmonary edema)

Etiology and Pathophysiology

Source:
- Prescription medication (human or veterinary)
- Dihydropyridine-type CCBs (e.g., amlodipine, nifedipine): effects are confined to vascular smooth muscle. They are used for treating hypertension.
- Nondihydropyridine-type CCBs (e.g., diltiazem, verapamil) have greater potency in cardiac muscle and cardiac nodal tissues than in the vasculature. They are used for treating arrhythmias and hypertrophic heart diseases.

Mechanism of toxicosis:
- CCBs close L-type calcium channels by binding to their alpha-1c subunits. Decreased calcium influx results in vasodilation (dihydropyridine type) or a decrease in myocardial contractility and electrical impulse conduction at the sinoatrial (SA) and atrioventricular (AV) nodes (nondihydropyridine type).
- CCBs decrease pancreatic insulin secretion, resulting in hyperglycemia.
- CCBs may cause noncardiogenic pulmonary edema (mechanism unknown).

DIAGNOSIS

Diagnostic Overview

The diagnosis is suspected based on observation or evidence of ingestion (chewed container) along with physical exam findings of hypotension and/or bradycardia. Confirmation with plasma drug levels is uncommonly performed, and treatment generally should be initiated without such results.

Differential Diagnosis

Toxicologic:
- Beta-adrenergic receptor antagonists overdose (propranolol, metoprolol), alpha-adrenergic receptor agonists (imidazoline-type decongestants), cardiac glycosides (e.g., digoxin, cardiac glycoside–containing plants, *Bufo* toad), antidepressant, organophosphate, and carbamate insecticides toxicoses

Spontaneous, non-toxicologic:
- Primary cardiac disease, systemic illness causing hypotension

Initial Database

- Arterial blood pressure (BP): hypotension (p. 1065)
- Electrocardiogram (ECG) (p. 1096)
  - Sinus bradycardia, AV block with verapamil or diltiazem
  - Sinus tachycardia with dihydropyridines
- Serum chemistry profile: hyperglycemia, hypokalemia, hypophosphatemia, hypomagnesemia possible
- Acid-base status: lactic acidosis possible

Advanced or Confirmatory Testing

Plasma CCB levels may be measured at a human hospital for confirmation of exposure. Therapeutic monitoring to assess response to treatment is not useful for animals.

TREATMENT

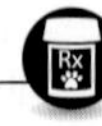

Treatment Overview

Treatment consists of decontamination (emesis and charcoal administration), stabilizing the cardiovascular system, and maintaining tissue perfusion by maintaining adequate BP. Continuous monitoring in a veterinary facility for 12-24 hours or longer after ingestion is recommended because signs can be delayed, especially with extended-release formulations.

Acute General Treatment

Decontamination (p. 1087):
- Emesis for a recent ingestion or an animal showing no overt signs of toxicosis (p. 1188)
- Activated charcoal 1-2 g/kg (or labeled dosage) with a cathartic PO; repeat one-half of the original dose q 6h for large ingestions or extended-release preparations

- Gastric lavage: if large number of tablets, which can form concretions

Fluid therapy:

- Fluid rate should be guided by BP monitoring; avoid volume overload (iatrogenic pulmonary edema)

Treatment of hypotension:

- Intravenous (IV) crystalloid fluids
- Colloids (Hetastarch, VetStarch) for persistent hypotension despite IV crystalloid fluids (dosage adjusted based on response):
    - Dogs: initial 5 mL/kg IV bolus over 15-30 minutes, followed by 15 mL/kg/day IV constant rate infusion (CRI)
    - Cats: 10 mL/kg/day IV CRI
- Calcium chloride or calcium gluconate for refractory hypotension; monitor continuous ECG, and discontinue if bradycardia worsens (p. 515)
    - Calcium chloride (10% solution; 27.2 mg Ca/mL): 0.1-0.5 mL/kg slow IV bolus or CRI of 0.01 mL/kg/h (5 mg/kg/h), *or*
    - Calcium gluconate (10% solution; 9.3 mg Ca/mL): 50-150 mg/kg (0.5-1.5 mL/kg) slow IV over 5 minutes to effect or CRI of 5 mg/kg/h (0.05 mL/kg/h)
- Insulin administered with dextrose to maintain euglycemia may be considered for refractory hypotension; can improve cardiac inotropy and decrease capillary vascular resistance
    - Regular insulin 1 U/kg bolus followed by 0.1-10 U/kg/h IV CRI along with 7%-20% dextrose IV. Blood glucose and potassium should be monitored frequently. Effect may be seen in 30-45 minutes.
- If hypotension persists after crystalloids, Hetastarch, insulin/dextrose and calcium supplementation, dopamine 1-20 mcg/kg/min IV CRI titrated to response may be used, provided the patient is volume-expanded/well hydrated.

Sequestration of toxin:

- Consider using 20% intravenous lipid emulsion (ILE) solution (p. 1127).

Severe bradycardia/AV block:

- Atropine 0.02-0.04 mg/kg IV, SQ, or IM; repeat as needed *or*
- Isoproterenol 0.02-0.4 mcg/kg/min IV (quick rule of thumb: dilute 1 mg in 500 mL 5% dextrose and infuse at 0.5 to 1 mL/min IV to effect) *or*
- Temporary cardiac pacing

Control seizures (p. 903):

- Diazepam 0.5-1 mg/kg IV or pentobarbital 3-15 mg/kg IV slowly to effect
- Supplement potassium if serum potassium < 3 mEq/L (p. 516)

Drug Interactions

- CCBs increase blood levels of propranolol and digoxin.
- Propranolol, ketoconazole, and itraconazole reduce clearance, thereby increasing CCB levels.
- Cimetidine and phenobarbital will increase bioavailability of CCBs.

Possible Complications

- Pulmonary edema
- Renal insufficiency due to decreased renal perfusion

Recommended Monitoring

- BP
- ECG
- Serum chemistry panel, especially renal parameters and electrolytes
- Respiration (rate, lung sounds, pulse oximetry)
- Mentation

PROGNOSIS & OUTCOME

- Prognosis is generally good with prompt treatment. Refractory hypotension, severe hyperglycemia, and pulmonary edema may convey a guarded prognosis.
- After recovery, long-term effects are uncommon. Organ dysfunction secondary to sustained hypotension is possible, such as myocardial ischemia or chronic kidney disease.

PEARLS & CONSIDERATIONS

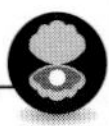

Comments

- Many preparations of CCBs are sustained-, controlled-, extended-, or delayed-release medications, which may substantially lengthen the onset and duration of signs.
- Bezoar formation is possible with ingestion of large quantities of sustained/controlled/extended/delayed-release preparations, especially nifedipine.
- Signs of toxicosis can occur at veterinary therapeutic doses of CCBs. These medications have a narrow margin of safety.
- Noncardiogenic pulmonary edema is possible as a toxic effect; fluid overload should be avoided.

Prevention

Owners should keep all medications out of reach of pets.

Technician Tips

It is important to know whether the CCB involved in the intoxication is regular or extended-release medication.

Client Education

Owners should be made aware of possible adverse effects when patients are prescribed CCBs.

SUGGESTED READING

Hayes CL, et al: Calcium channel blocker toxicity in dogs and cats. Vet Clin North Am Small Anim Pract 42:263-277, 2012.

AUTHOR: Cristine Hayes, DVM, DABT, DABVT
EDITOR: Tina Wismer, DVM, MS, DABT, DABVT

Calicivirus, Feline

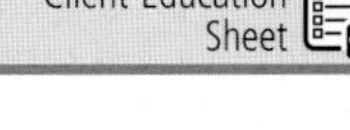

BASIC INFORMATION

Definition

Widespread, highly contagious, single-stranded RNA virus of cats

Synonyms

FCV, feline upper respiratory tract disease (FCV is a single contributing pathogen to URTD), limping kitten syndrome, febrile limping syndrome, virulent systemic feline calicivirus (VS-FCV)

Epidemiology

SPECIES, AGE, SEX

- Acute oral/respiratory disease and febrile limping syndromes more likely in kittens or young cats
- VS-FCV more severe in adult cats

RISK FACTORS

- Crowding
- Multi-cat households, colonies, and shelters
- Poor husbandry practices (e.g., poor sanitation)
- Stress
- Immunosuppression
- Other upper respiratory pathogens

CONTAGION AND ZOONOSIS

Highly contagious but not zoonotic

GEOGRAPHY AND SEASONALITY

Worldwide distribution

ASSOCIATED DISORDERS

- Chronic ulceroproliferative and lymphoplasmacytic stomatitis
- Faucitis
- Ulcerative glossitis
- Pyrexia
- Lameness (transient)
- Systemic illness (see VS-FCV entries)
- Implicated in feline lower urinary tract disease and enteritis (role not well established)
- Respiratory distress (rare)
- Other respiratory pathogens (p. 1006)

Clinical Presentation

DISEASE FORMS/SUBTYPES

- Subclinical infection
- Acute oral/respiratory tract disease
- Chronic stomatitis
    - FCV isolated from most cats with chronic ulceroproliferative and lymphoplasmacytic stomatitis
- Limping syndrome
- VS-FCV (rare but occurs in outbreaks)

HISTORY, CHIEF COMPLAINT

History and clinical signs depends on infecting strain, age, and disease form. Common complaints:

- Inappetence/anorexia
- Ocular/nasal discharge
- Sneezing
- Drooling
- Halitosis
- Lameness

PHYSICAL EXAM FINDINGS

- Subclinical infection: none
- Acute oral/respiratory tract disease: acute onset of sneezing, serous nasal discharge, oral ulcers, epiphora, blepharospasm, fever, inappetence, ± ptyalism
- Chronic stomatitis: ulcerative or proliferative faucitis/stomatitis
- Limping syndrome: transient fever and lameness, typically follows acute oral/respiratory disease or vaccination with modified live FCV vaccine
- VS-FCV: severe acute oral/upper respiratory signs (see above), fever (often > 105°F), cutaneous edema (head and limbs), cutaneous ulcerations (nose, lips, footpads, ears, periocular), icterus (hepatic necrosis, pancreatitis), respiratory distress (pulmonary edema [pp. 836 and 879]), petechial or ecchymotic hemorrhage (from disseminated intravascular coagulation)

Etiology and Pathophysiology

- Highly variable and rapidly evolving single-stranded RNA virus with multiple subtypes
    - Single serotype despite antigenic variability
- Transmission: oral and nasal secretions by fomites or direct contact; aerosol transmission (minor)
    - Non-enveloped virus; resistant to environmental stressors (e.g., light, temperature) and disinfectants (e.g., quaternary ammonium compounds); persists ≥ 1 month in cool dry environment
- Incubation 2-10 days, replication in the oropharynx. VS-FCV tissue tropism may be wider than for non-VS-FCV.
- Shedding occurs primarily during acute disease but may persist up to years after recovery. Some cats are lifelong shedders.
- Prevalence is proportional to the number of cohabitating cats (10% in single-cat households, 40% in shelters, 90% in some colonies)
- VS-FVC: disease is sporadically reported in the United States and Europe.

DIAGNOSIS

Diagnostic Overview

Often a clinical diagnosis without confirmatory testing. Specific positive tests for FCV infection should be interpreted in light of presentation because the carrier state is common.

Differential Diagnosis

- Other upper respiratory pathogens (p. 1006)
- Corneal injury/trauma
- Caustic chemical exposure (e.g., liquid potpourri, acids or alkali)
- Electrical burns
- Periodontal disease
- Eosinophilic granuloma
- Oral ulcers (p. 1002)

Initial Database

- Oral examination: identify ulcerations, proliferative changes, periodontal disease
- Feline leukemia (FeLV) and feline immunodeficiency virus (FIV) testing (note: maternal immunity can cause false-positive FIV test result in kittens < 6 months)
- Ocular fluorescein staining
- CBC/serum biochemical profile/urinalysis (not routinely performed): unremarkable
    - In cases of pneumonia and VS-FCV: inflammatory leukogram, thrombocytopenia, anemia, and changes consistent with multiple organ dysfunction

Advanced or Confirmatory Testing

Viral identification usually only necessary for epidemiologic purposes (e.g., shelter or cattery outbreak)

- Virus and antigen detection
    - Reverse transcription polymerase chain reaction (RT-PCR): conjunctival/oropharyngeal swabs: false-negatives due to varied viral genome, markers for VS-FCV unavailable
    - Viral isolation: conjunctival, nasal, oropharyngeal swabs, less sensitive to virus variability than RT-PCR. False-negatives due to low viral burden and viral deactivation. Collecting conjunctiva and oropharyngeal swabs may maximize yield.
- Antibody detection: ELISA
    - Prevalence is high due to frequent natural infection and vaccination.
    - Not clinically useful for diagnosis
- Thoracic radiographs: usually unremarkable; pneumonia/pulmonary edema in severe disease

TREATMENT

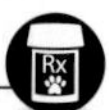

Treatment Overview

Treat as outpatient wherever possible to prevent nosocomial infection. Supportive care is sufficient for most patients with mild to moderate disease. Outbreaks usually resolve by 2 months with appropriate control measures.

Acute General Treatment

- Acute oral/respiratory tract disease: symptomatic and supportive care (rehydration, pain management, nutritional support (e.g., appetite stimulants), clear nasal secretions, nebulization)
    - Syringe feeding is not recommended to avoid food aversion.
    - Treat corneal ulceration if present (p. 209).
    - Buprenorphine 0.01-0.03 mg/kg q 8-12h IM, IV, PO if analgesia warranted
- Limping syndrome: usually self-limited, but analgesia should be considered
- VS-FCV: aggressive supportive care, antibiotics, consider antiviral therapy
    - Extremely contagious; strict isolation with barrier protection vital
    - Judicious use of fluids due to edema
    - Address organ dysfunction, coagulopathy
    - Antivirals: feline interferon omega inhibits replication of FCV *in vitro. In vivo* studies are lacking. Most veterinary antivirals inhibit replication of DNA or retroviruses.

Chronic Treatment

- Relapses are uncommon, although re-infection with new disease subtypes is possible.
- Chronic stomatitis (p. 943): Clinical trials are lacking. Potentially, antibiotics, dental prophylaxis, glucocorticoids ± immunomodulatory drugs, whole mouth extractions, interferon omega (systemic/intralesional)

Nutrition/Diet

Feeding tubes may be required for patients with protracted anorexia or chronic stomatitis (pp. 1106 and 1107).

Drug Interactions

Avoid combining nonsteroidal antiinflammatory drugs and glucocorticoids.

Possible Complications

- Hepatic lipidosis (prolonged anorexia)
- Viral or secondary bacterial pneumonia (p. 795)
- Death from VS-FCV or severe disease

Recommended Monitoring

Clinical signs

PROGNOSIS & OUTCOME

- Good for acute oral/respiratory tract disease and limping syndrome

- Chronic stomatitis: variably persistent clinical signs
- VS-FCV: guarded prognosis, mortality rate up to 67%

PEARLS & CONSIDERATIONS

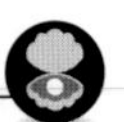

Comments

Fomites (including hospital personnel) are important factors in spread of disease.

Prevention

- Vaccination: FCV is a core vaccine and protects against acute oral/respiratory signs.
  - Modified live and killed (SQ and intranasal) vaccines are available.
  - Vaccination does not prevent infection or shedding.
  - Does not protect against all strains
  - Follow American Association of Feline Practitioners/American Veterinary Medical Association vaccination guidelines, including booster vaccinations
- Proper cleaning and husbandry practices
  - FCV is resistant to most disinfectants. Bleach (5% sodium hypochlorite) diluted to 1 part bleach to 32 parts tap water is effective.
- Shelters: identify causative pathogen in an URTD outbreak. Isolate affected cats, and vaccinate newcomers as soon as possible.

Technician Tips

Precautions should be taken for all cats showing signs of upper respiratory infection to prevent an outbreak.

Client Education

Educate clients on proper husbandry and vaccination practices for their specific environment (e.g., home, shelter, cattery).

SUGGESTED READING

Radford A, et al: Feline calicivirus infection: ABCD guidelines on prevention and management. J Feline Med Surg 11:556-564, 2009.

AUTHOR & EDITOR: **Megan Grobman, DVM, MS, DACVIM**

Cardiotoxic Plants

Bonus Material Online 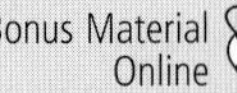
Client Education Sheet 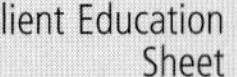 

BASIC INFORMATION

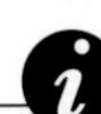

Definition

Toxicosis occurring as a result of ingestion of plants that produce substances harmful to the heart

Epidemiology

SPECIES, AGE, SEX

Dogs are more likely to be affected than cats; all ages and breeds

RISK FACTORS

Plants or flower bouquets in pet's environment. Pre-existing cardiac disease may increase risk.

GEOGRAPHY AND SEASONALITY

Toxicosis occurs throughout the year but is more likely to occur in spring and summer months (outdoor exposures).

Clinical Presentation

HISTORY, CHIEF COMPLAINT

- History or evidence of exposure (witnessed ingestion, chewed plant, or plant material present in the vomitus)
- Cardiac glycosides: onset of clinical signs within 2-8 hours of ingestion: salivation, vomiting, lethargy, depression, hypoglycemia, and ataxia. With severe intoxications, convulsions and death are possible.
- Grayanotoxins: signs occur within 6 hours of ingestion: lethargy, salivation, vomiting, signs of abdominal pain, ataxia, lateral recumbency, and seizures are possible.
- Yew (*Taxus* spp)

PHYSICAL EXAM FINDINGS

- Cardiac glycoside–containing plants: pale mucous membranes, weak pulses, tachypnea, bradycardia, or paroxysmal tachycardias
- Grayanotoxin-containing plants: tachycardia, tachypnea, hyperthermia, vomiting, lethargy, hypotension, and bradycardia; diarrhea is uncommon

Etiology and Pathophysiology

Source:

- Present in nature, landscaping, house plants, and floral arrangements
- Common cardiac glycoside–containing plants: *Asclepias* spp (some): milkweed; *Convallaria majalis*: lily of the valley; *Digitalis purpurea*: foxglove; *Hellebore* spp; *Kalanchoe* spp; *Nerium oleander*: oleander; *Thevetia nerifolia*: yellow oleander; *Thevetia peruviana*: yellow oleander
- Common grayanotoxin-containing plants: *Rhododendron* spp: rhododendron, azalea, rosebay; *Kalmia* spp: laurels; *Pieris* spp: Japanese pieris, mountain pieris; *Leucothoe* spp: black laurel

Mechanism of toxicosis:

- Cardiac glycosides
  - Inhibition of Na^+/K^+-ATPase pump in the myocardial cell
  - Result: decreased intracellular potassium, increased intracellular sodium. Intracellular sodium is exchanged for calcium, raising intracellular calcium levels. Excessive extracellular potassium may depress cardiac contractility.
  - Effects noted include atrioventricular (AV) block due to progressive interference with cardiac electrical conduction and increased vagal tone; decrease in normal resting membrane potential; decreased myocardial cell pacemaker activity, leading (in severe toxicoses) to malignant cardiac arrhythmias (ventricular) or asystole.
- Grayanotoxins: bind to sodium channels, slowing their opening and closing and decreasing their ion selectivity (maintain state of depolarization). Results are similar to cardiac glycosides. Many cells are affected, especially excitable cells (neurologic, cardiac, muscle cells).

DIAGNOSIS

Diagnostic Overview

Diagnosis is based on history of exposure and the presence of gastrointestinal (GI) and cardiac signs. Plant material present in pet's environment, vomitus, or lavage fluid may also help in arriving at a diagnosis. Serum digoxin levels are confirmatory for cardiac glycoside plants (cross-reactivity with cardiac glycosides); turnaround time limits utility in critical cases, but in cases that are less severe, the test is helpful for identifying exposure and to prevent future re-exposure.

Differential Diagnosis

Toxicologic:

- *Bufo* toad ingestion
- Digoxin overdose
- Antiarrhythmic medication ingestion

Spontaneous, non-toxicologic:

- Primary cardiac disease
- Systemic illness causing ventricular arrhythmias
- Gastroenteritis

Initial Database

- CBC: no significant changes expected
- Serum biochemistry panel: hyperkalemia possible; hypokalemia markedly worsens the toxic effects (including making the heart refractory to antiarrhythmics such as lidocaine and procainamide) and needs to be corrected if present (p. 516).
- Blood glucose: hypoglycemia has been reported secondary to oleander intoxication.

- Electrocardiogram (ECG) (p. 1096) to identify cardiac arrhythmias
  - A combination of first- or second-degree AV block with the possibility of exposure to an incriminating plant and compatible clinical signs is highly suggestive of the clinical diagnosis of glycoside plant cardiotoxicosis.
  - Ventricular or atrial arrhythmias of virtually any type are possible.
  - The most common ECG changes include first-, second-, or even third-degree AV block; ventricular arrhythmias; and ST-segment changes.
- Blood pressure (p. 1065): hypotension possible

Advanced or Confirmatory Testing

- Serum digoxin levels (cardiac glycoside–containing plants). Any detectable amount in a patient not receiving digoxin pharmaceutically confirms the diagnosis. Test can be performed at a local human hospital or veterinary diagnostic laboratory.
- Presence of oleandrin in GI contents and body fluids can confirm exposure to oleander (available in some veterinary diagnostic laboratories).

TREATMENT

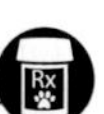

Treatment Overview

Treatment is aimed at management of severe cardiac arrhythmias and systemic disturbances (e.g., dehydration, hypoglycemia) and early decontamination of the patient (emesis induction and administration of activated charcoal). An intravenous (IV) antidote (Digibind) exists for cardiac glycosides, but it is often cost-prohibitive.

Acute General Treatment

- Decontamination of patient (p. 1087)
  - Emesis induction if recent ingestion (p. 1188) and asymptomatic
  - Activated charcoal (if asymptomatic): after emesis or if a few hours have elapsed after exposure, 1-2 g/kg with a cathartic such as 70% sorbitol 3 mL/kg PO
- Treat cardiac arrhythmias
  - Bradyarrhythmias in a normotensive patient: atropine 0.02-0.04 mg/kg IV, repeat as needed
  - Ventricular arrhythmias (p. 1033)
  - Digoxin immune Fab (Digibind) may be used for treating refractory cardiac arrhythmias or severe hyperkalemia in cardiac glycoside toxicosis.
  - Temporary cardiac pacing if profound bradycardia unresponsive to atropine
- Supportive care
  - IV fluids as needed; avoid calcium-containing fluids (e.g., lactated Ringer's solution) unless hypocalcemia
  - Dextrose (bolus or CRI) as needed to correct hypoglycemia (p. 552)
  - Correct acid-base status and electrolytes (notably hyperkalemia or hypokalemia [pp. 495 and 516]) as needed.
  - Control seizures with a benzodiazepine if needed (e.g., diazepam 0.5-1 mg/kg IV) (p. 903)
  - Control severe vomiting with metoclopramide 0.1-0.4 mg/kg PO, SQ, or IM q 6h or maropitant 1 mg/kg SQ q 24h or 2 mg/kg PO q 24h after GI obstruction is ruled out.

Possible Complications

Permanent cardiac damage

Recommended Monitoring

ECG, electrolytes, blood pressure, heart rate, pulse, ± glucose

PROGNOSIS & OUTCOME

- Cardiac glycosides: animals with moderate to severe cardiovascular signs have a guarded prognosis; even with intensive supportive care, serious intoxications may require several days of in-hospital treatment.
- Animals with only GI signs but no subsequent cardiovascular signs have a good prognosis.
- Prognosis is generally good with grayanotoxin-containing plants.

PEARLS & CONSIDERATIONS

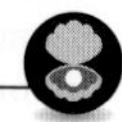

Comments

- Domesticated grayanotoxin plants, such as those sold in nurseries, appear to be less toxic than their wild counterparts and mainly cause GI signs.
- Cardiac glycosides are bitter tasting; however, when leaves dry, sugar is released, and the leaves may be more attractive for ingestion.
- Cardiotoxicity of these plants is arrhythmogenic; structural heart disease (e.g., valve disease) is not caused by these plants.

Prevention

Advise clients to keep plants or flower bouquets out of pet's environment.

Technician Tips

If unsure of type of plant/flower, consult with a plant nursery or floral shop.

Client Education

Client should be made aware of toxic plants in the pet's environment.

SUGGESTED READING

Page C, et al: Hypoglycemia associated with oleander toxicity in a dog. J Med Toxicol 11:141-143, 2015.

AUTHOR: Eric Dunayer, VMD, MS, DABT, DABVT
EDITOR: Tina Wismer, DVM, MS, DABVT, DABT

Carpal Flexural Deformity of Puppies

Bonus Material Online Client Education Sheet

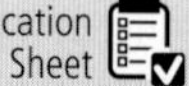

BASIC INFORMATION

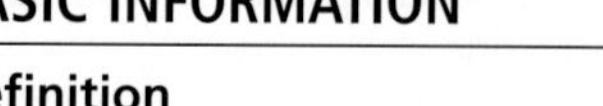

Definition

Carpal flexural deformity (CFD) is an uncommon musculotendinous disorder producing transient flexion of the carpus and supination of the manus in young animals.

Synonyms

Flexural deformity, contracture of the flexor tendon, flexion syndrome, carpal hyperflexion, carpal laxity syndrome, carpal hyperflexion syndrome

Epidemiology

SPECIES, AGE, SEX

Generally affects medium-, large-, and giant-breed puppies between 6 and 16 weeks of age. CFD has been described in a kitten.

GENETICS, BREED PREDISPOSITION

Multiple affected littermates have been reported for Doberman pinschers and shar-peis, suggesting familial predisposition.

RISK FACTORS

Affected puppies come from breeds that typically stand with fairly straight (almost 180°) carpi.

Clinical Presentation

HISTORY, CHIEF COMPLAINT

- Lameness and/or visible carpal deformity
- The onset is acute, with a possible sudden worsening after a few days.
- CFD is usually bilateral, although each forelimb may be involved at a different time

Diseases and Disorders

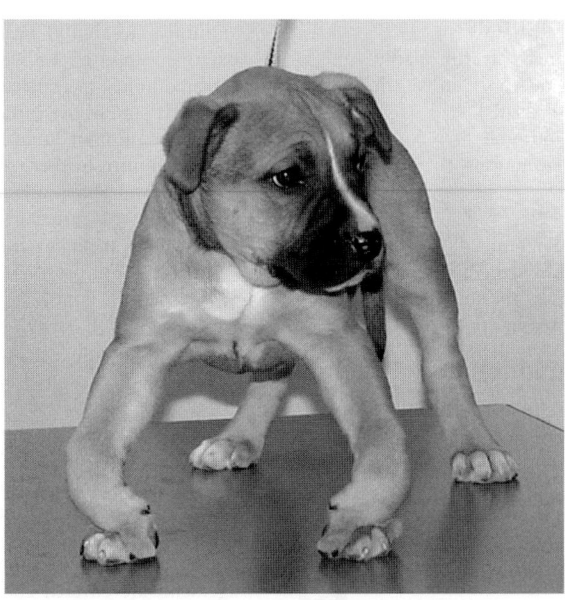

CARPAL FLEXURAL DEFORMITY Severe procurvatum and varus deformity at all levels of the carpus.

and with varied severity. Severely affected puppies may stumble when walking.

PHYSICAL EXAM FINDINGS

- Characteristic appearance: carpal hyperflexion and varus deviation/supination of the manus, sometimes with weight bearing on the lateropalmar surfaces of the digits
- Lameness of varied severity; often worsens with exercise. In severe cases, affected animals tend to lean on the lateral surfaces of the digits.
- In mild cases, carpal deviation may be evoked by wheelbarrowing the puppy.
- Carpal effusion and crepitus are absent. Manipulation of the carpus does not cause pain. The carpus can usually be extended, albeit with some difficulty and with increased tension within the flexor tendons.

Etiology and Pathophysiology

- Flexor carpi ulnaris (FCU) muscle contracture produces the deformity, but its cause is unknown.
- One possibility is lack of synchrony between growth of the radius/ulna and the FCU.
- Affected FCU muscle contains more type I fibers than normal; this may predispose to the condition.

DIAGNOSIS

Diagnostic Overview

Diagnosis is based on signalment, history, and physical findings; radiographs are normal.

Differential Diagnosis

Distal radius and ulna deformities (p. 66); ligamentous injury or bone deformity within the carpus

Initial Database

Radiographs of the antebrachium and carpus: bones, growth plates, and level of mineralization should be normal.

TREATMENT

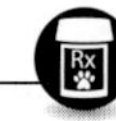

Treatment Overview

The disease is self-limited, and conservative therapy is appropriate.

Acute and Chronic Treatment

- Enforced rest and exercise have been recommended, with similar results.
- Refractory cases might benefit from a bandage extending from the elbow to the paw and with the limb in normal stance position, maintained for 1 to several weeks.

Nutrition/Diet

Provide a balanced diet; avoid caloric excess and mineral/vitamin supplementation.

PROGNOSIS & OUTCOME

Even in severe cases, improvement occurs within a few days to 2 weeks, and recovery is complete by the second to fourth week.

PEARLS & CONSIDERATIONS

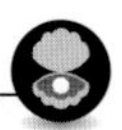

Comments

- Tenotomy of one or both heads of the tendon of the FCU is therapeutic excess, even in severely affected animals.
- The disorder is remarkable by the contrast between the severity of the deformity apparent on physical exam and the benign, self-resolving course of the disease process.

Technician Tips

Reserve bandaging for cases in which improvement has not occurred within 2 weeks. In such cases, check every 5-7 days to reduce risk of carpal hyperextension.

SUGGESTED READING

Çetinkaya MA, et al: Carpal laxity syndrome in forty-three puppies. Vet Comp Orthop Traumatol 20:126-130, 2007.

AUTHOR: Massimo Petazzoni, MV
EDITOR: Kathleen Linn, DVM, MS, DACVS

Carpal Trauma/Breakdown

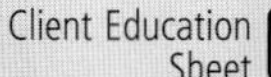

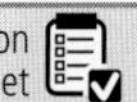

Client Education Sheet

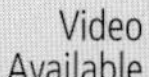

Video Available

BASIC INFORMATION

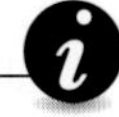

Definition

Carpal trauma includes ligamentous (sprain), fibrocartilaginous (hyperextension), fracture, and shearing injuries.

Synonyms

Palmar carpal breakdown, carpal hyperextension

Epidemiology

SPECIES, AGE, SEX

Dogs > cats; usually adult animals

GENETICS, BREED PREDISPOSITION

- Racing greyhounds: radial and accessory carpal bone fractures
- Boxers: radial carpal bone fracture

RISK FACTORS

Racing, agility, or other intense activities; distal forelimb trauma; obesity; erosive polyarthropathy

Clinical Presentation

DISEASE FORMS/SUBTYPES

- Sprains
- Fractures

- Shearing/degloving wounds
- Coaptation-related injuries

HISTORY, CHIEF COMPLAINT

- Forelimb trauma, especially falling/jumping injuries
- Lameness
- Slowing/drifting wide on racetrack turns

PHYSICAL EXAM FINDINGS

- Lameness (see *Video*).
- Carpal swelling
- Pain/crepitation during palpation
- Open wounds
- Instability characterized by palmigrade or hyperextended carpal stance
- Mediolateral instability

Etiology and Pathophysiology

- In pets, hyperextension or ligament injuries are more common than fractures.
- Erosive polyarthropathies can lead to carpal ligament injury or hyperextension.
- Incomplete fusion of centers of ossification of the radial carpal bone may predispose this bone to fractures.
- In racing animals, fractures usually involve the accessory carpal bone. Track animals racing counterclockwise are predisposed to right-sided injuries (80%).

DIAGNOSIS

Diagnostic Overview

Diagnosis of carpal pathology is mainly based on physical and radiographic examinations.

Differential Diagnosis

- Immune-mediated polyarthropathy
- Infectious (Lyme borreliosis, rickettsial diseases, septic arthritis)
- Carpal laxity syndrome
- Flexor tendon lacerations

Initial Database

- Orthogonal radiographs of the distal limb
- CBC and serum biochemistry panel
- Electrocardiography and thoracic radiography (if massive trauma has occurred)

Advanced or Confirmatory Testing

- Oblique radiographic views and/or CT to outline nondisplaced fractures
- Stress radiography (mediolateral view with carpus forced into hyperextension, and dorsopalmar views with medial/lateral stress applied) for localizing level of instability

TREATMENT

Treatment Overview

The goal of therapy is to re-establish normal anatomy and restore pain-free function:

- Ligamentous injuries: re-establishment of carpal support with ligament repair, arthrodesis, or external coaptation in some cases.
- Fractures: anatomic reduction and stabilization
- Shearing injuries: wound management, and surgical stabilization if needed

Acute General Treatment

- Minimally displaced nonarticular fractures, grade I (no instability), and most grade II (minimal instability) ligament sprains are externally splinted 4-8 weeks.
- Luxated joints, intraarticular fractures, and grade III sprains are initially supported in a modified Robert Jones bandage or splint (p. 1161) until further treatment.
  - Hyperextension injuries are managed with partial or pancarpal arthrodesis.
  - Collateral ligament injuries are usually replaced with prosthetic sutures.
  - Radial carpal bone luxation is treated with reduction and screw fixation; pancarpal arthrodesis may be indicated for comminuted or chronic fractures.
  - Accessory carpal bone fractures are treated with lag-screw fixation or external coaptation for comminuted fractures.
- Small radial and accessory carpal bone fractures have good outcomes with surgical excision.
- Shearing injuries, after initial wound management, are covered and supported until definitive treatment.
  - Gentle wound lavage using saline, lactated Ringer's or dilute chlorhexidine solutions.
  - Wounds are debrided and bandaged until definitive stabilization is done; honey or sugar application may be useful with highly contaminated wounds.
  - Wounds with healthy granulation tissue and early epithelialization can be sutured or covered with a nonadherent dressing and allowed to heal by second intention.

Chronic Treatment

- Some surgical repairs require 4-12 weeks of external coaptation and exercise restriction.
- Chronic fractures and instabilities with resultant osteoarthritis are treated with carpal arthrodesis.

Possible Complications

- Reduction/implant failure
- Delayed/failed arthrodesis
- Wound infection
- Coaptation-related morbidity
- Degenerative joint disease

Recommended Monitoring

- Lameness evaluation 1-3 months after injury and treatment
- Serial radiographic studies to evaluate fracture healing or progression of arthrodesis

PROGNOSIS & OUTCOME

- Good to excellent for noncompeting dogs
- Varies for athletic dogs needing to return to preinjury competition levels
- Severe shearing injuries with neurovascular compromise may necessitate limb amputation.

PEARLS & CONSIDERATIONS

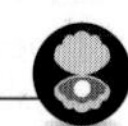

Comments

- Complete palmar carpal breakdown/hyperextension requires arthrodesis.

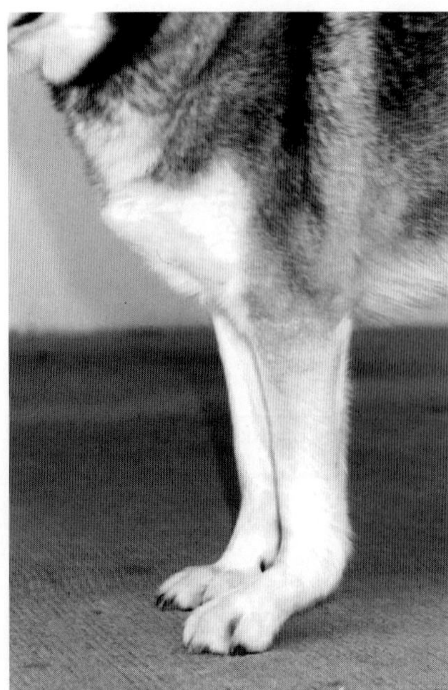

CARPAL HYPEREXTENSION Mature malamute with left palmar carpal hyperextension. (Courtesy Dr. Joseph Harari)

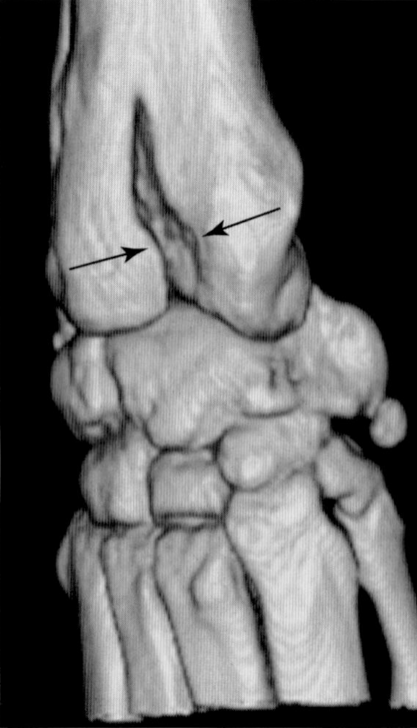

CARPAL TRAUMA/BREAKDOWN Oblique view, three-dimensional CT reconstruction demonstrates a distal radial articular fracture *(arrows)* that could not be seen on orthogonal radiographs.

- The use of orthotics has shown promise (11/14 cases back to full function) in managing mediolateral instabilities. They can also be used to support hyperextension injuries if surgery is not possible.
- Intraarticular fractures treated conservatively rarely heal with osseous bridging, leading to degenerative joint disease.
- Consider CT if a fracture is still suspected despite normal radiographs.
- Partial carpal arthrodesis can promote a return to most preinjury activities, but some loss in range of motion (flexion) is to be expected.
- In racing greyhounds, treatment of radial carpal or accessory carpal bone fractures with lag-screw fixation (preferred) or fragment excision can provide a return to competitive performance.

Technician Tips

After case evaluation, prepare for modified Robert Jones bandaging with/without splinting and wound management if applicable.

SUGGESTED READING

Kapatkin AS, et al : Carpus, metacarpus, and digits. In Tobias KM, et al, editors: Veterinary surgery small animal, St. Louis, 2012, Elsevier, pp 789-798.

AUTHOR: Louis Huneault, DMV, MSc, DES, DACVS
EDITOR: Kathleen Linn, DVM, MS, DACVS

Cataracts

Client Education Sheet 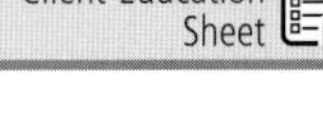

BASIC INFORMATION 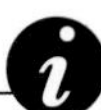

Definition

Any opacity, regardless of size, of the ocular lens or its capsule is called a *cataract*. A cataract results from a change in the lens protein composition or lens fiber arrangement, and it is one of the most common canine ocular abnormalities.

Epidemiology

SPECIES, AGE, SEX

- Dogs and cats
- Age of onset depends on breed and cause.
- Cataracts affect 16.8% of mixed-breed dogs ages 7-15+ years.

GENETICS, BREED PREDISPOSITION

- In dogs, most cataracts have an inherited component; the most common mode of inheritance is autosomal recessive.
- Highest prevalence in dogs: smooth fox terrier, Havanese, Bichon frisé, Boston terrier, poodles (toy, miniature, standard), silky terrier, American cocker spaniel, and miniature schnauzer
- Canine cataracts can also occur secondary to diabetes mellitus, which has a genetic predisposition in some breeds.
- Presumed congenital feline cataracts: Persian, Birman, Himalayan, and domestic shorthair

RISK FACTORS

See Etiology and Pathophysiology below.

Clinical Presentation

DISEASE FORMS/SUBTYPES

Cataracts are classified by age at onset, location, severity, and cause.

- Age at onset
  - Congenital (present at birth)
  - Juvenile (few months to 6 years)
  - Senile (>6 years)
- Location
  - Capsule (anterior/posterior)
  - Cortex (anterior/posterior or equatorial)
  - Nucleus: nuclear cataracts are always congenital, but not all congenital cataracts are nuclear.
- Severity
  - Incipient: <10% of retinal examination obstructed
  - Immature: early, 10%-50% of retinal examination obstructed; late, 50%-99% of retinal examination obstructed
  - Mature: 100% of retinal examination obstructed
  - Hypermature: liquefaction/resorption with associated lens-induced uveitis (p. 1023)
  - Morgagnian (cortex has liquefied and the nucleus falls ventrally in the capsule)

HISTORY, CHIEF COMPLAINT

- Vision disturbance
- Cloudy white pupil
- Pain, redness, epiphora may be noted if the cataract results in secondary anterior uveitis.
- The chief complaint may reflect a systemic cause of cataracts (e.g., polyuria/polydipsia, weight loss with diabetes mellitus).

PHYSICAL EXAM FINDINGS

- Opacity of the lens (unilateral or bilateral) with any or all of the following:
  - Anterior uveitis (p. 1023)
  - Glaucoma (p. 387)
  - Lens subluxation/luxation (p. 581)
  - Retinal degeneration, retinal detachment (pp. 883 and 885)
  - Systemic abnormalities may be present when cataracts are caused by a generalized disorder (e.g., weight loss with diabetes mellitus).

Etiology and Pathophysiology

Regardless of the cause, all cataracts occur through a change in the lens protein composition or lens fiber arrangement.

- Inherited
- Diabetes mellitus: increased blood glucose results in diffusion of glucose into the lens, overwhelming standard lens metabolism, causing excess glucose to be shunted to the sorbitol pathway, which forms polyols and subsequently osmotically draws water into the lens, causing opacification (dogs). All dogs with diabetes mellitus develop cataracts: 50% by 170 days and 80% by 470 days after the onset of diabetes mellitus.
- Secondary to intraocular disease: uveitis, glaucoma, intraocular neoplasia, retinal degeneration/detachment, lens luxation
- Trauma to lens: blunt or penetrating
- Age related
- Nutritional: in puppies and kittens fed milk replacer. Proposed mechanism is amino acid deficiency, such as arginine, at crucial stage during lens development
- Hypocalcemia
- Radiation therapy/injury when primary beam near or on globe
- Medications (e.g., long-term oral ketoconazole; mostly in young, large-breed dogs given higher doses [6-13.9 mg/kg/day])
- Toxins (e.g., dinitrophenol, diazoxide)
- Electric shock

Not all cataracts are progressive. Cataracts can progress to become hypermature and result in lens-induced uveitis and increased risk of vitreal degeneration, retinal detachment, and secondary glaucoma.

DIAGNOSIS 

Diagnostic Overview

The diagnosis of cataract is suspected based on observation of a cloudy pupil in an animal that may be visually compromised. It is confirmed by the finding of a lens opacity after complete dilation of the pupil using a short-acting mydriatic (1% tropicamide).

Differential Diagnosis

- Nuclear/lenticular sclerosis: normal aging change; seen in all animals ≥ 7 years old; does not cause vision loss; center of lens becomes opalescent to hazy, but tapetal reflection (usually yellow greenish) is still

visible, versus cataracts, which obstruct this reflection.
- Hyperlipidemia may result in lipid aqueous flare. This will obstruct the ability to see the iris and pupil. Most common in the miniature schnauzer.
- Diseases causing diffuse corneal edema (bluish white opacity of the *cornea*, not in pupil, may obstruct ability to see the pupil), including glaucoma, anterior uveitis, and corneal endothelial degeneration or dystrophy
- Diseases causing secondary cataracts
  - Retinal degeneration or detachment
  - Anterior uveitis (cataracts typically incomplete if due to inflammation; uveitis may also occur secondary to cataracts; if cataracts occupying large extent of lens in predisposed breed, assume lens-induced uveitis) (p. 1023)
  - Lens luxation (p. 581)

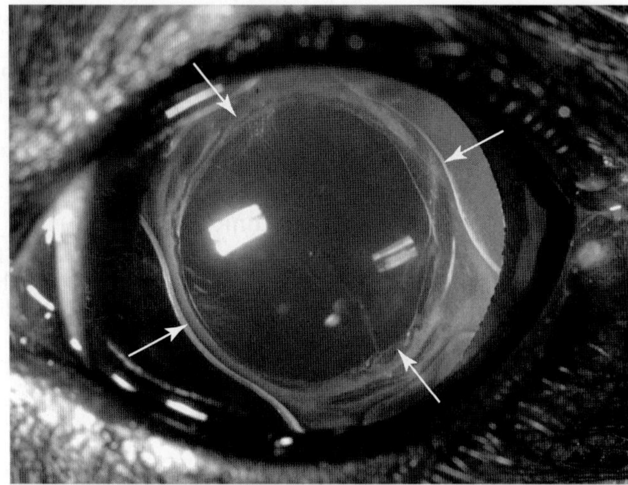

CATARACTS Canine eye 6 months after cataract surgery and foldable, acrylic intraocular lens implantation. The pupil has been dilated, and the lens implant *(arrows)* is centered within the pupil.

Initial Database

- Complete ophthalmic examination (p. 1137), including
  - Menace response, maze test, dazzle reflex
  - Evaluation of pupil size, symmetry, and pupillary light reflexes
  - Intraocular pressure (IOP): rule out glaucoma (>20-25 mm Hg)
  - After IOP assessment (assuming normal result), dilate pupil with 1% tropicamide
  - Penlight, transilluminator, or monocular slit lamp (Heine) to characterize the cataract, evaluate for concurrent uveitis
  - Fundic (posterior segment) examination
- Blood and urine glucose determination (dogs primarily)

Advanced or Confirmatory Testing

- CBC, serum biochemistry profile, and urinalysis to rule out systemic metabolic disease (e.g., diabetes mellitus, hypocalcemia) as cause of cataracts and/or to assess patient before considering referral for possible cataract surgery
- Ocular ultrasound if the cataract is immature or worse in severity and precludes accurate evaluation of the posterior segment of the eye
- Electroretinogram to assess retinal function (routinely conducted by veterinary ophthalmologists before cataract surgery)

TREATMENT

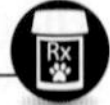

Treatment Overview

- Incipient and nonprogressive early immature cataracts do not require immediate treatment, but must be monitored for progression.
- Progressive immature, mature, and hypermature cataracts are treated to
  - Restore vision (i.e., cataract surgery)
  - Prevent secondary sequelae of cataracts: uveitis, glaucoma, and retinal detachment. When compared to surgically treated eyes, eyes managed with topical antiinflammatories alone have 4 times greater failure rate and eyes left untreated have a 255 times greater failure rate.
  - Referral to a veterinary ophthalmologist will help in triage, diagnosis, and treatment of cataracts.

Acute General Treatment

- Treat or prevent associated secondary uveitis with topical mydriatics and antiinflammatories (p. 1023).
- Treat secondary glaucoma accordingly (p. 387).
- Referral for cataract surgery if cataract is vision threatening and animal systemically stable (e.g., diabetes mellitus is controlled).
  - Cataract surgery requires preliminary ocular ultrasound and electroretinogram that indicate the posterior segment of the eye is normal.
  - Phacoemulsification (ultrasonic lens fragmentation) to remove the cataract
    - Followed by implantation of an artificial intraocular lens (IOL) to restore emmetropia (normal vision, neither far-sighted nor near-sighted)
    - Without an IOL implant, animals are 14 diopters hyperopic (far-sighted) with little useful vision.

Chronic Treatment

- After cataract surgery, treat as directed by the veterinary ophthalmologist.
  - Topical antibiotics and antiinflammatories
  - Exercise restriction/Elizabethan collar: 2 weeks
  - Antiinflammatory therapy may be continued in a decreasing fashion for months or, in some cases (diabetics), indefinitely.
  - Frequent re-evaluation of IOL position, IOP, Schirmer tear test (diabetics especially), retinal examination, and inflammation control
- If cataract surgery is not an option
  - Monitor cataracts for progression, and treat prophylactically for secondary uveitis with topical antiinflammatories long term.
  - Use IOP-lowering drugs in combination with antiinflammatories if secondary glaucoma develops.
  - Enucleation or evisceration and intrascleral prosthesis for end-stage, blind, painful globes

Drug Interactions

Corticosteroids (topical ophthalmic or especially oral) may interfere with management of diabetes mellitus.

Possible Complications

- Without cataract surgery, the following can occur: uveitis, glaucoma, lens luxation, retinal detachment, blindness. The risk of these is significantly decreased with administration of long-term topical antiinflammatories.
- After cataract surgery, the following can occur: uveitis, glaucoma, corneal ulceration, surgical wound/incisional dehiscence, intraocular infection, retinal detachment, IOL displacement, lens capsule fibrosis (lessened by the use of new foldable, acrylic IOL implants), corneal endothelial degeneration and secondary corneal edema, keratoconjunctivitis sicca (KCS).
- Dogs with diabetes mellitus are at increased risk for chronic uveitis, KCS, facial nerve palsy, Horner's syndrome, corneal ulceration, retinal detachment secondary to systemic hypertension, and retinal petechiae resulting from diabetic retinopathy.

Recommended Monitoring

- Without cataract surgery, monitor for cataract progression and secondary complications (see Possible Complications above) q 2-4 months or more or less frequently, depending on the extent of cataract, rate of cataract development, and presence or absence of associated ocular complications.
- After cataract surgery, monitor according to veterinary ophthalmologist's recommendations; generally, involves re-evaluations

at postoperative weeks 2, 8, and 20, and long-term follow-up q 6-12 months for life.

PROGNOSIS & OUTCOME

- Rate of cataract progression variable depending on cause and location of the cataract and age of the animal.
- Success of cataract surgery (i.e., phacoemulsification), as determined by a positive visual outcome, is 90%-95%.
- Success is increased with early referral (i.e., before animal is blind) and surgery and with diligent postoperative monitoring and treatment.

PEARLS & CONSIDERATIONS

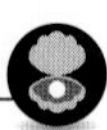

Comments

- Early referral and prompt surgical intervention before the onset of hypermaturity and lens-induced uveitis can result in a more successful outcome.
- Animals affected with cataracts, regardless of the severity, should not be used for breeding unless it is known specifically that the cataract is of nongenetic origin.

Prevention

- Ophthalmic screening of animals used for breeding by a board-certified veterinary ophthalmologist and registration through the Eye Certification Registry (http://www.offa.org/) helps remove affected animals from the breeding population.
- Prompt treatment of intraocular inflammation will decrease the likelihood of secondary cataracts.
- Early diagnosis and proper management of diabetes mellitus can delay cataract formation, but even the most well-managed diabetics still develop cataracts. Once present, cataracts caused by diabetes mellitus are irreversible and will not resorb, even with good diabetic control.
- In the future, use of aldose reductase inhibitors and antioxidants may have a role in the delay and prevention of cataracts.

Technician Tips

Clients often confuse lenticular sclerosis, a normal aging change, with cataracts. Lenticular sclerosis occurs in all dogs and cats over 6 years of age, is bilateral and symmetrical, and does not interfere with vision.

Client Education

- It is essential that clients understand that not all cataracts are progressive.
- If a cataract is progressive, the client must decide about surgery.
- Although surgery is associated with some risks, opting against surgery is associated with greater risk of lens-induced uveitis, secondary glaucoma, retinal detachment, and ocular pain.
- Animals undergoing cataract removal surgery that do not receive an intraocular lens implant have vision that, in human equivalence, is worse than 20/400 and corresponds to being legally blind.

SUGGESTED READING

Davidson MG, et al: Diseases of the lens and cataract formation. In Gelatt KN, editor: Veterinary ophthalmology, ed 4, Ames, IA, 2007, Blackwell, pp 859-887.

AUTHOR: David A. Wilkie, DVM, MS, DACVO
EDITOR: Diane V. H. Hendrix, DVM, DACVO

Cervical Spondylomyelopathy

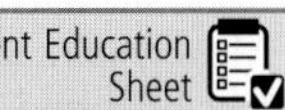

BASIC INFORMATION

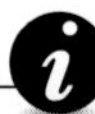

Definition

Cervical spondylomyelopathy (CSM) is a common disease of the cervical vertebral column of large- and giant-breed dogs that is characterized by compression of the cervical spinal cord and nerve roots caused by osseous and/or disc-associated lesions.

Synonyms

CSM, wobbler syndrome, caudal cervical spondylomyelopathy (CCSM), cervical malformation/malarticulation syndrome, cervical vertebral instability, disc-associated cervical spondylomyelopathy (DA-CSM)

Epidemiology

SPECIES, AGE, SEX

- Large-breed dogs (e.g., Dobermans with the disc-associated form of CSM): usually > 3 years of age, mean age of 7 years
- Giant-breed dogs (e.g., Great Danes with the osseous form of CSM): usually younger, with a mean age of 3.5 years, although early and late presentations are occasionally seen
- Males and females are affected, with a male predisposition in giant breeds.

GENETICS, BREED PREDISPOSITION

Doberman pinschers and Great Danes are overrepresented; ≈5% of Dobermans and Great Danes are affected. A genetic basis exists in Dobermans, with an autosomal dominant (with variable penetrance) mode of inheritance proposed.

RISK FACTORS

Genetics; body conformation and fast growth rate have been proposed but not confirmed.

ASSOCIATED DISORDERS

Dilated cardiomyopathy, hypothyroidism, and von Willebrand disease are common in Dobermans and Great Danes. Because these diseases can affect outcome, screening for them is recommended.

Clinical Presentation

DISEASE FORMS/SUBTYPES

CSM can be divided into two forms: disc- and osseous-associated

- Disc-associated compression: dogs are born with relative vertebral canal stenosis, which is complicated later in life by intervertebral disc protrusion. Thickening of the ligamentum flavum can occur.
- Osseous-associated compression: osseous malformation and osteoarthritic changes can compress the spinal cord dorsally, dorsolaterally, or laterally.

HISTORY, CHIEF COMPLAINT

- Chronic, progressive history of gait changes (weakness and ataxia) is typical. Acute or acute-on-chronic presentations are occasionally seen.
- This weak, uncoordinated gait is seen primarily in the pelvic limbs but can also affect the thoracic limbs.

PHYSICAL EXAM FINDINGS

- Gait changes are characterized by proprioceptive ataxia and paresis (weakness) that are more obvious in the pelvic limbs with lesions in the caudal cervical spine (C5-6, C6-7).
- Proprioceptive positioning deficits are usually present but may not be observed in dogs with chronic ataxia.
- Dogs can present non-ambulatory.
- Extensor muscle tone is commonly increased in all four limbs. Patellar reflexes are normal or increased. Flexor (withdrawal) reflex may be decreased in the thoracic limbs due to increased extensor tone or involvement of the C6-8 spinal cord segments.
- Neck pain can be detected on spinal palpation, mainly in large-breed dogs.

Etiology and Pathophysiology

- CSM is a congenital disease. Affected dogs are born with vertebral canal stenosis, which can become more severe later in life secondary to vertebral malformation, intervertebral disc protrusions, and/or ligamentous hypertrophy.
- Static (direct and constant) and dynamic (movement-related) compressions are seen with disc- and osseous-associated forms of the disease.

DIAGNOSIS

Diagnostic Overview

CSM should be suspected when a young giant-breed dog or a middle-aged large-breed dog is presented for ataxia and weakness. The neurologic examination (p. 1136) should confirm gait changes in all four limbs. Survey radiographs ruling out other diseases with or without radiographic changes suggesting CSM support the presumptive diagnosis. Definitive diagnosis requires magnetic resonance imaging (MRI) or myelography with or without computed tomography (CT).

Differential Diagnosis

- Intervertebral disc disease
- Neoplasia
- Spinal cord cysts (arachnoid or synovial)
- Discospondylitis or vertebral osteomyelitis
- Trauma
- Meningomyelitis

Initial Database

- CBC, serum biochemistry profile, urinalysis: generally unremarkable
- Cervical radiographs: mainly useful to rule out differentials such as neoplasia and discospondylitis. Radiographs can reveal vertebral canal stenosis secondary to vertebral body malformation or articular facet proliferation.
- Myelography: useful to confirm the diagnosis when CT and MRI are unavailable
- CT: must be combined with myelography to determine sites and directions of compression
- MRI (p. 1132): best diagnostic modality because it is safe and allows assessment of the spinal cord parenchyma. Kinematic MRI, mainly extension views, can reveal lesions not seen with neutral positioning.

TREATMENT

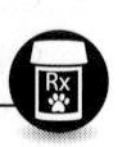

Treatment Overview

- Medical treatment can provide improvement or stabilization of neurologic status. Surgical treatment offers the best chance for complete neurologic recovery, but depending on the chronicity and severity of the lesions, it may lead only to partial improvement or stabilization.
- Surgical procedures for CSM can be grouped into three categories: decompressive (ventral slot, dorsal laminectomy), distraction/stabilization (pin or screws and polymethylmethacrylate), or disc arthroplasty. The number and direction of compressions should dictate the choice of surgical procedure.
- It is important to consider comorbidities when deciding on the type of treatment.

Acute General Treatment

- Exercise restriction
- Glucocorticoids: dose and route depends on the severity of neurologic status.
  - Severe (non-ambulatory) cases: dexamethasone 0.25 mg/kg IV (once only)
  - Mild presentations: low-dose oral prednisone therapy (e.g., 0.5-1 mg/kg PO q 12h), progressively tapering

Chronic Treatment

- Chronic treatment with prednisone 0.5-1.0 mg/kg PO q 12h, progressively tapering every 5-7 days to the lowest effective dose every 48 hours, or nonsteroidal antiinflammatory drugs (NSAIDs)
- Glucocorticoids and NSAIDs should never be coadministered.
- Gastrointestinal protectants such as omeprazole should be administered to dogs on chronic glucocorticoid therapy.

Behavior/Exercise

Dogs with CSM should have exercise restriction and should always wear a body harness rather than a neck collar.

Possible Complications

- Non-ambulatory tetraparesis with lesion progression
- Severe cervical pain
- Glucocorticoid-related complications if used long term (e.g., iatrogenic hyperadrenocorticism, gastric ulcers)

PROGNOSIS & OUTCOME

- Surgical treatment leads to improvement in ≈80% of patients.
- Approximately 50% patients improve with medical treatment (restricted activity +/− glucocorticoids or NSAIDs), and 25% remain stable.
- Long-term prognosis is less favorable. Many dogs deteriorate ≈3 years after diagnosis, independent of method of treatment.

PEARLS & CONSIDERATIONS

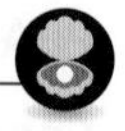

Comments

The large number (28) of reported surgical techniques for CSM indicates that the ideal treatment is still unknown.

Technician Tips

- Affected patients are often large, heavy dogs that require assistance. Self-protection to minimize the risk of human back injuries is essential.
- The patient's neck pain can be significant, and the neck should be handled gently; use a harness if the patient is ambulatory.

Client Education

- Avoid breeding dogs with CSM.
- Neck leashes are strongly contraindicated; use a body harness after the diagnosis.

SUGGESTED READING

da Costa RC: Cervical spondylomyelopathy (wobbler syndrome). Vet Clin North Am Small Anim Pract 40:881-913, 2010.

AUTHOR: Ronaldo C. da Costa, DMV, MSc, PhD, DACVIM
EDITOR: Karen R. Muñana, DVM, DACVIM

Chagas' Disease

Client Education Sheet 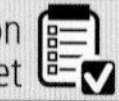 Bonus Material Online 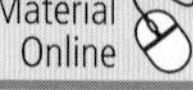

BASIC INFORMATION

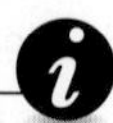

Definition

Canine Chagas' disease is a relatively rare zoonosis caused by the vector-borne hemoprotozoan parasite, *Trypanosoma cruzi*. It has a tropism for cardiomyocytes, resulting in myocarditis with arrhythmias and myocardial failure.

Synonyms

American trypanosomiasis, chagasic myocarditis

Epidemiology

SPECIES, AGE, SEX

Young dogs (<1 year of age) develop a more severe form of the acute stage of the disease, which is often rapidly progressive and fatal.

RISK FACTORS

Hunting dogs may be at increased risk because of more frequent exposure to the vector and reservoir hosts, but house dogs can be infected.

CONTAGION AND ZOONOSIS

Vector-borne transmission by triatomines, also known as kissing bugs: *Triatoma gerstaeckeri, Triatoma protracta, Triatoma sanguisuga* in the United States, occurs in humans and dogs. Blood-borne transmission possible during handling of blood samples from infected dogs; however, risk is low.

GEOGRAPHY AND SEASONALITY

In the United States, most canine cases occur in Texas and other southern states. Chagas' disease is a major human health problem in South America, Mexico, and Central America.

Clinical Presentation

DISEASE FORMS/SUBTYPES

The disease occurs in three phases:

- Acute phase: 0-4 weeks after inoculation; peak at 2 weeks. In younger dogs, usually lethargy, fever, and generalized lymphadenopathy. Less commonly, acute myocarditis with severe bradyarrhythmia/tachyarrhythmia and risk of sudden death. Absence of clinical signs common in older dogs. *T. cruzi* present in peripheral blood.
- Indeterminate (latent) phase: lasts months to years. Absence of clinical signs and electrocardiographic (ECG) abnormalities
- Chronic phase: late complications in some infected dogs, with myocardial failure and recurrence of arrhythmias, resulting in congestive heart failure (CHF) and risk of sudden death

HISTORY, CHIEF COMPLAINT

History of travel to/residence in southernmost United States, Mexico, or Central or South America. Detection of arrhythmias, lethargy, syncope, and/or CHF

PHYSICAL EXAM FINDINGS

- Acute phase: may be normal in adult dog; irregular cardiac rhythm and pulse deficits; peripheral lymphadenopathy; occasionally fever
- Indeterminate phase: normal physical examination
- Chronic phase: bradyarrhythmia or tachyarrhythmia with/without pulse deficits, weak pulses, soft systolic heart murmur, dyspnea and tachypnea, abdominal distention from ascites/hepatomegaly, jugular distention

Etiology and Pathophysiology

- Trypomastigotes (circulating flagellated form) are deposited in the vector's feces at the insect's bite site and enter the bloodstream through the infected bite. Alternatively, direct ingestion of infected triatomine bug or of an infected reservoir host (e.g., armadillo, opossum, raccoon, mouse, squirrel, rat). Blood transfusion–mediated and transplacental and transmammary transmission also occur.
- Trypomastigotes enter monocytes and macrophages in cardiac and skeletal tissue (possibly nervous tissue) and transform into amastigotes (nonflagellated form) and then multiply rapidly, leading to cell rupture and causing clinical signs.
- The amastigotes transform back to trypomastigotes before cell rupture. Rising parasitemia occurs, peaking at 2-3 weeks after inoculation and decreasing by 4 weeks after inoculation. Signs of acute myocarditis are possible during this period.
- Latent stage starts 4 weeks after inoculation.
- Late complications (months to years after infection) from inflammatory reaction induced by *T. cruzi* include myocardial necrosis/fibrosis, local coronary spasm, and possible autoimmune progression.
- Myocardial lesions lead to systolic dysfunction (dilated cardiomyopathy) and/or CHF, severe bradyarrhythmias (advanced second-degree or third-degree atrioventricular [AV] block), and ventricular tachyarrhythmias.
- Protective immunity does not develop.

DIAGNOSIS

Diagnostic Overview

The disease is suspected when hunting dogs that are kept outside develop myocardial failure and/or complex cardiac arrhythmias (brady-/tachyarrhythmias) when living in or traveling to endemic areas. Higher suspicion is justified if the breed is not predisposed to primary cardiac diseases. Markedly increased cardiac troponin I blood level confirms myocarditis with ongoing cardiomyocyte death. Trypomastigotes may be detected in blood samples during the acute phase. Confirmation requires a Chagas' titer.

Differential Diagnosis

- Dilated cardiomyopathy (idiopathic) (p. 263)
- Other causes of myocarditis (p. 675)
- Other causes of right heart failure (p. 409)
- Other causes of AV block (p. 101)
- Other causes of ventricular tachycardia (p. 1033)

Initial Database

- Serum biochemistry profile: liver enzymes may show mild to moderate elevation
- CBC: lymphocytosis is common
- Blood smear or buffy coat (better) stained with Giemsa or Wright stain (acute phase only): definitive diagnosis if organism is seen (trypomastigotes, flagellate organisms are 2-3 times as long as the diameter of erythrocytes). Can also examine lymph node aspirates, ascitic or pleural fluid.
- ECG: expect ventricular premature complexes/ventricular tachycardia or second-/third-degree AV block
- Thoracic radiographs: cardiomegaly with or without evidence of CHF (e.g., pulmonary edema) can occur
- Holter monitoring (24-hour ambulatory ECG [p. 1120]) if severe arrhythmias on ECG and syncope
- Echocardiography (p. 1094): to identify chamber dilation and poor systolic function, if present
- Serum cardiac troponin I concentration: high (acute phase only); not specific for chagasic myocarditis

Advanced or Confirmatory Testing

- Cytologic identification of trypomastigotes during acute phase
- Chagas' titer in dogs suspected of chagasic myocarditis. Titer is typically positive by 3 weeks after infection and persists throughout the life of the animal. Cross-reactivity with antibodies to *Leishmania*
- Serologic testing
  - Indirect fluorescent antibody test (offered by Texas A&M Veterinary Medical Lab [http://tvmdl.tamu.edu/] and IDEXX [www.idexx.com])
  - ELISA
  - Radioimmunoprecipitation
- Polymerase chain reaction (PCR): high specificity but low sensitivity in chronic cases
- Histopathologic identification of amastigotes in myocardium at necropsy

TREATMENT

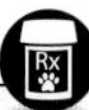

Treatment Overview

Supportive treatment for arrhythmias and CHF is recommended. There is no effective treatment to eliminate the organism. Therapeutic goals:

- Palliation of clinical signs caused by CHF and/or arrhythmias

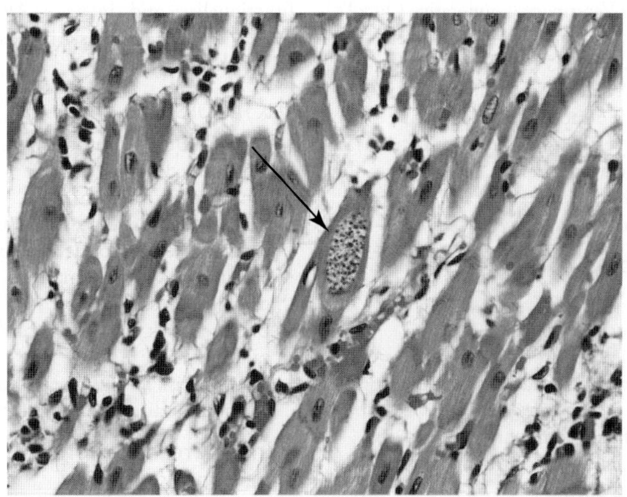

CHAGAS' DISEASE Protozoal pseudocyst containing many amastigotes within a cardiomyocyte *(arrow)* from a 5-month-old dog who died of Chagas' disease (40× magnification, hematoxylin-eosin stain).

- Prevention of progressive ventricular systolic dysfunction (nonspecific cardioprotective therapies)
- Control of the organism (elimination of infection is not considered possible)

Acute General Treatment

- See Heart Failure, Acute/Decompensated (p. 408)
- See Atrioventricular Block (p. 101)
- See Ventricular Arrhythmias (pp. 1033 and 1457)
- Benznidazole 7 mg/kg PO q 12h for 60 days or nifurtimox may be useful in the acute stage, but these drugs are not approved by the U.S. Food and Drug Administration (FDA) and are therefore extremely difficult to obtain. They may not eliminate long-term effects of the disease and have clinically significant side effects.
- Glucocorticoids: antiinflammatory dose (prednisone 0.5-1 mg/kg PO q 12-24h) sometimes used
- Ketoconazole, albaconazole 1.5 mg/kg PO q 24h for 60-90 days and allopurinol have been investigated, but proof of benefit is lacking.

Possible Complications

Refractory CHF and/or cardiac arrhythmias may occur during the acute phase in young dogs and puppies and as late complications months to years after infection.

Recommended Monitoring

- Monitor for arrhythmias by Holter recording q 6-12 months.
- Monitor for signs of systolic dysfunction by echocardiography q 6-12 months.

PROGNOSIS & OUTCOME

- High risk of sudden death if severe ventricular arrhythmias during the acute phase
- Dogs that survive the acute phase may be free of clinical signs for months to years. Some dogs never develop late complications of the disease.
- Young dogs (<1 year of age), puppies typically are at higher risk for overt signs of CHF and/or severe ventricular arrhythmias.
- After clinical signs develop, appropriate palliative therapy may prolong life. Dogs with clinical signs of CHF or severe arrhythmias have a guarded long-term prognosis, but appropriate palliative therapy can prolong their lives by months to a few years.

PEARLS & CONSIDERATIONS

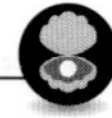

Comments

Chagas disease is a regional cause of myocarditis, which is likely underdiagnosed.

Prevention

- Limit exposure to the vector by upgrading housing, using insecticides, limiting ingestion of raw reservoir hosts, and otherwise limiting contact between dogs and reservoir hosts.
- Deltamethrin-treated collars may be effective at repelling triatomine insects.
- Blood donors should be screened.
- Breeding bitches in endemic/high-risk areas should also be screened to prevent transplacental and transmammary infection.

Technician Tips

Blood specimens in veterinary practice often are handled with less care than in human medical settings. In areas where Chagas' disease is endemic, blood specimens and products from infected animals should be handled with caution by all staff (zoonosis).

SUGGESTED READING

Barr SC: Canine Chagas' disease (American trypanosomiasis) in North America. Vet Clin North Am Small Anim Pract 39:1055-1064, 2009.

AUTHOR: Romain Pariaut, DVM, DACVIM, DECVIM
EDITOR: Joseph Taboada, DVM, DACVIM

Chemotherapy: Adverse Events

Bonus Material Online 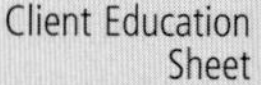 Client Education Sheet 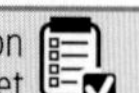

BASIC INFORMATION

Definition

Chemotherapy is well tolerated by most patients, but adverse effects (AEs) are possible due to actions of the drugs or idiosyncratic reactions. The Veterinary Cooperative Oncology Group common terminology criteria for adverse events (VCOG-CTCAE, v1.1, https://onlinelibrary.wiley.com/doi/full/10.1111/vco.283#vco283-sec-0002-title) define AEs according to established standard criteria. Most are mild to moderate and manageable with supportive therapy. Alterations in treatment protocols/dosing may be required.

Epidemiology

SPECIES, AGE, SEX

AEs in cats but not dogs:

- Doxorubicin: nephrotoxicity
- Temozolomide: pleural/pericardial effusion

Drugs not to be used in cats:

- Cisplatin: fatal pulmonary edema
- 5-Fluorouracil: fatal central nervous system necrosis and edema

AEs in dogs but not cats:

- Cyclophosphamide: hemorrhagic cystitis
- Doxorubicin: cardiotoxicosis

Cats (vs. dogs) have reduced risk of L-asparaginase allergic reaction and lomustine hepatotoxicity

GENETICS, BREED PREDISPOSITION

MDR1/ABCB1-Δ mutations decrease permeability glycoprotein (P-glycoprotein) functionality and increase AEs with substrates. A list of at-risk breeds is available (p. 638).

RISK FACTORS

- *MDR1/ABCB1-Δ* mutation
- Small-breed dogs (<10 kg)
- Illness at time of treatment
- Pre-existing gastrointestinal (GI), renal, or hepatic disease, especially if dysfunction
- Significant bone marrow infiltration: myelosuppression
- Breeds at risk for dilated cardiomyopathy: cardiotoxicity
- Breeds at risk for pulmonary fibrosis, chronic pulmonary disease: pulmonary fibrosis

Clinical Presentation

DISEASE FORMS/SUBTYPES

Adverse reactions during administration:

- Allergic reactions (L-asparaginase, doxorubicin, taxanes)
- Extravasation injury (vinca alkaloids, doxorubicin, carboplatin [undiluted], dacarbazine, mechlorethamine, cisplatin, rabacfosadine, actinomycin D)
- Acute vomiting: common (cisplatin, dacarbazine); less common (doxorubicin, cyclophosphamide, mechlorethamine, procarbazine)

Delayed adverse reactions:

- GI: common (doxorubicin, MOPP [mechlorethamine, vincristine, procarbazine, prednisone], toceranib, cisplatin, dacarbazine); less common (vinca alkaloids, cyclophosphamide, mitoxantrone, carboplatin, actinomycin D, rabacfosadine)
- Myelosuppression: common (lomustine, carboplatin); possible (doxorubicin, mitoxantrone, cyclophosphamide, vinca alkaloids, dacarbazine, toceranib, rabacfosadine)

Unique adverse reactions:

- Paralytic ileus (vincristine)
- Hemorrhagic colitis (doxorubicin)
- Pancreatitis (toceranib)
- Cardiotoxicosis (doxorubicin)
- Hemorrhagic cystitis (cyclophosphamide, ifosfamide)
- Nephrotoxicosis (cisplatin; uncommon: doxorubicin [cats], toceranib)

- Hepatotoxicosis (lomustine, toceranib, vinorelbine, rabacfosadine, rare idiosyncratic reactions with others)
- Nonspecific muscle pain (toceranib)
- Pulmonary fibrosis (rabacfosadine, rare: some alkylating agents)
- Dermatologic toxicosis (rabacfosadine)

HISTORY, CHIEF COMPLAINT

- Chemotherapeutic agent administered within appropriate time frame to expect AE
- Presenting/historical signs vary with AEs
  - Allergic: facial swelling, erythema, urticaria, vomiting, or collapse during/within hours of treatment
  - Extravasation injury: irritation at infusion site hours to 14 days after chemotherapy
  - GI toxicosis: vomiting, diarrhea, lethargy, anorexia, 2-5 days after chemotherapy
  - Myelosuppression: usually none; possible: lethargy, inappetence, typically 7-14 days after chemotherapy
  - Ileus: inappetence, lethargy, abdominal discomfort, vomiting, constipation
  - Cardiotoxicosis: often none; possible: exercise intolerance, tachypnea, weakness, collapse
  - Hemorrhagic cystitis: stranguria, pollakiuria, hematuria, incontinence
  - Nephrotoxicosis: often none; possible: polyuria and polydipsia (PU/PD), lethargy, inappetence
  - Hepatotoxicosis: often none; possible: lethargy, inappetence, vomiting, diarrhea, icterus
  - Dermatoxicosis: otitis, pruritic alopecic lesions, dorsal distribution
  - Pulmonary fibrosis: exercise intolerance, dyspnea, tachypnea, cough

PHYSICAL EXAM FINDINGS

- Allergic reactions during/within hours of treatment (p. 54)
- Extravasation injury: irritation at site hours to 14 days after treatment, can progress to slough of skin and subcutis
- Cardiotoxicosis: often none; possible arrhythmia, tachycardia, pulse deficits, new murmur, tachypnea, dyspnea (p. 408)
- Nephrotoxicosis: often none; possible weight loss, dehydration
- Hepatotoxicosis: often none; possible weight loss, icterus
- Dermatoxicosis: otitis, alopecic pinnae, pruritic alopecia, ulcerations, excoriations on dorsum; possibly painful
- Pulmonary fibrosis: dyspnea, tachypnea, cyanosis, syncope, possible crackles

Etiology and Pathophysiology

- Allergic reactions: L-asparaginase: type I hypersensitivity; doxorubicin: mast cell degranulation
- Extravasation injury: multiple mechanisms
- Acute vomiting: chemoreceptor trigger zone irritation
- GI toxicosis: epithelial injury
- Myelosuppression/febrile neutropenia: injury to proliferating hematopoietic cells. Severe neutropenia can allow opportunistic infection, usually by gram-negative GI flora.
- Cardiotoxicosis: doxorubicin: multiple; reactive oxygen species and toxic metabolites cause intracellular damage, apoptosis, and myocardial cell death; irreversible dilated cardiomyopathy (DCM) weeks-months after treatment; typically in dogs at cumulative doses ≥ 180-240 mg/m^2.
- Hemorrhagic cystitis: cyclophosphamide metabolite injures urothelium
- Nephrotoxicosis: cisplatin: tubular injury, decreased glomerular filtration rate; toceranib: renal protein loss, azotemia, hypertension due to glomerular and tubular epithelium effects
- Hepatotoxicosis: lomustine: hepatocellular and ductal epithelial injury with inflammation and cholestasis, eventually cirrhosis
- Toceranib AE: tyrosine kinase inhibition

DIAGNOSIS

Diagnostic Overview

AEs of chemotherapy are suspected based on characteristic signs and timing after the drugs are administered, and diagnosis is supported by resolution and lack of recurrence with dose delay, reduction, or substitution.

Differential Diagnosis

Exacerbation of neoplastic disease, paraneoplastic syndromes, unrelated diseases

Initial Database

- CBC +/− serum biochemistry profile, urinalysis
- Additional tests determined by history, exam, and preliminary diagnostic results

TREATMENT

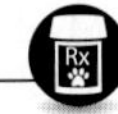

Treatment Overview

Goals are resolution of AEs and prevention of complications.

Acute General Treatment

AEs during administration:

- First step: discontinue administration.
- Allergic reactions: diphenhydramine 2 mg/kg IM and dexamethasone sodium phosphate (SP) 0.2-0.5 mg/kg IV. If indicated, intravenous fluids 90 mL/kg/h (dog, initial bolus of 30 mL/kg) or 50 mL/kg/h (cat, initial bolus of 15 mL/kg); if severe, epinephrine 0.1 mL/kg of 1 : 10,000 or 0.01 mL/kg of 1 : 1000 solution IV
- Extravasation injury: aspirate back before removing catheter. *Cold* compress for all drugs (except for vinca alkaloids [warm]) 10 minutes q 6h for 72 hours. There is limited information about antidotes/treatments. For vinca alkaloids, infuse 1 mL 1% hyaluronidase SQ at extravasation site for each mL leaked. For doxorubicin, administer dexrazoxane 400-600 mg/m^2 IV in a different vein within 3 hours of extravasation; repeat at 24 and 48 hours. For dacarbazine or mechlorethamine, inject 5 mL of 0.16 M sodium thiosulfate (4 mL sodium thiosulfate 10% solution with 6 mL sterile water for injection) divided between the displaced IV catheter and in pincushion fashion into extravasation site. Repeat hours later. E-collar, wound management as needed
- Acute vomiting: stop administration; antiemetic therapy (see below); IV fluid support if indicated

Delayed AEs:

- GI: usually resolves in 2-3 days
  - Patient normal, decreased appetite: maropitant citrate 1-2 mg/kg (dog), 1 mg/kg (cat) PO q 24h, tempting food. For cats, mirtazapine 3.75 mg/CAT q 72h. Capromelin is new alternative appetite stimulant for dogs and cats. If mild vomiting, antiemetic, NPO, then water and bland diet trial (pp. 67, 1040, and 1199)
  - Patient normal, mild diarrhea: bland diet, consider metronidazole 15 mg/kg PO q 12h for colitis
  - Patient lethargic, vomiting/diarrhea persistent or watery/bloody: hospitalize for supportive care:
    - Intravenous fluids
    - Antiemetic (e.g., maropitant citrate 1 mg/kg IV q 24h; if refractory, add ondansetron 0.5-1 mg/kg IV slowly q 12h [dog] or 0.1-0.5 mg/kg IV slowly q 6-12h [cat]); for vincristine-induced ileus, metoclopramide 1.1-2.2 mg/kg/day IV CRI.
    - Gastric acid reduction: pantoprazole 1 mg/kg IV slowly q 12-24h
    - Antibiotic therapy if bloody vomit/diarrhea, neutropenia, fever
    - Nutritional support
- Myelosuppression: usually none required; counts normalize within 2-3 days (potentially prolonged with carboplatin and lomustine [cats]).
  - If neutrophil count < 1000 cells/mcL, prophylactic antibiotics for 3-7 days (dogs only): enrofloxacin 10 mg/kg PO q 24h or amoxicillin/clavulanate 20 mg/kg PO q 12h or sulfadiazine-trimethoprim 15 mg/kg PO q 12h
  - If febrile/ill, hospitalize for intravenous fluids and antibiotics. Empirical treatment: ampicillin or ampicillin/sulbactam 22 mg/kg IV q 8h, with enrofloxacin 5 mg/kg (cats) or 10 mg/kg (dogs), dilute and give slowly IV q 24h

Unique AEs:

- Cardiotoxicosis: discontinue doxorubicin; manage cardiac disease (pp. 263, 408, and 1033)
- Hemorrhagic cystitis: often self-limiting (weeks-months); permanent damage possible. Treat bacterial cystitis, if present; antiinflammatory (nonsteroidal or prednisolone), analgesic (gabapentin 10 mg/kg q 8-12h or an opioid); consult with oncologist if refractory
- Nephrotoxicosis: discontinue drug. If uremia, oliguria, and/or anuria (p. 23). Proteinuria: may need to discontinue drug; angiotensin-converting enzyme (ACE) inhibitor (e.g., benazepril 0.5 mg/kg q 12-24h), renal diet,

omega-3 fatty acids control hypertension (p. 501)
- Hepatotoxicosis: discontinue drug; treat acute liver injury (p. 442)
- Muscle pain: treatment break, nonsteroidal antiinflammatory, +/− gabapentin 10 mg/kg q 8-12h or opioid
- Dermatologic toxicity: treatment break, symptomatic treatment, pain medications, prednisone (if antiinflammatory needed), antibiotics (if needed for secondary infection)
- Pulmonary fibrosis: supportive care, poor prognosis
- For toceranib AEs, treatment can usually be resumed with dose reduction.

Chronic Treatment

Cardiotoxicosis, chronic bone marrow injury, nephrotoxicosis, and hepatotoxicosis may require ongoing therapy.

Drug Interactions

Veterinarians administering chemotherapy should know possible interactions with other drugs.

Recommended Monitoring

- CBC at expected neutrophil nadir with first administration of a drug (typically 7 days after treatment, weekly for carboplatin and lomustine [in cats]). CBC before administration of myelosuppressive drugs, monthly for toceranib, q 2 months for chronic drugs (chlorambucil, melphalan)
- Serum biochemistry profile and urinalysis q 6 months, initially q 4 weeks for toceranib (renal/urinary parameters). Liver enzymes every other dose for lomustine. Creatinine every dose of cisplatin.

PROGNOSIS & OUTCOME

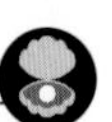

Most patients recover. Cardiotoxicosis, chronic bone marrow injury, nephrotoxicosis, and hepatotoxicosis generally do not resolve but may improve or stabilize.

PEARLS & CONSIDERATIONS

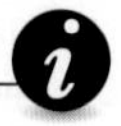

Comments

- Double-check dosage calculations, route of administration, and patient's history, weight, and diagnostics before prescribing/administering chemotherapy.
- Test breeds at risk for *MDR1/ABCB1-Δ* mutation.

Prevention

Allergic reactions:
- L-Asparaginase: if received L-asparaginase previously, premedicate with diphenhydramine 2 mg/kg IM 20 minutes before administration. Monitor patient 30-60 minutes after treatment. If allergic reaction, patient should not receive L-asparaginase again.
- Doxorubicin: administer slowly (10-20 minutes). If reaction, premedicate with diphenhydramine (as above) ± dexamethasone SP 0.5 mg/kg SQ, and administer slower.

Extravasation injury:
- Administer chemotherapy only through an IV catheter placed perfectly on first attempt in a vein not punctured within 24 hours. Sedate patient if needed.
- Flush catheter with 3-5 mL of 0.9% NaCl before and after administration. Monitor site for swelling during treatment. Do not administer with a pump.

Acute vomiting:
- Administer chemotherapy slowly; pretreat with maropitant 1 mg/kg SQ 1 hour before treatment.

GI toxicosis:
- If patient hospitalized with GI toxicosis, reduce next dose by 10%-20%.
- History of GI toxicosis: prophylactic maropitant 2 mg/kg PO (dog) or 1 mg/kg PO (cat) q 24h with that drug
- Avoid nonsteroidal antiinflammatory drugs (NSAIDs) or prednisone on same day as toceranib.

Myelosuppression/febrile neutropenia:
- CBC before myelosuppressive chemotherapy. Do not treat if < 1500 neutrophils/mcL or < 100,000 platelets/mcL. Consider cause of low platelet count. If suspect chronic bone marrow injury or patient receiving lomustine, recommend consultation with oncologist.
- CBC at neutrophil nadir after first dose of each myelosuppressive drug; if neutrophil count < 1000 cells/mcL, reduce next dose of that drug by 10%-20%.
- If overdose, recombinant human granulocyte colony-stimulating factor (rhG-CSF) 5 mcg/kg q 24h SQ × 3-5 days starting 24 hours after treatment. Monitor CBCs daily; start antibiotic prophylaxis when neutrophils < 1000/mcL.

Cardiotoxicosis (doxorubicin):
- Pretreatment cardiac evaluation for breeds at risk for DCM and dogs with heart murmurs, arrhythmias, or cardiomegaly
- Limit cumulative dose to < 180-240 mg/m^2; substitute noncardiotoxic agent after 150 mg/m^2 (most commonly, mitoxantrone) (pp. 607 and 609).

Hemorrhagic cystitis (cyclophosphamide):
- Concurrent furosemide 2 mg/kg, same route as cyclophosphamide, ad lib water, frequent opportunities to urinate

Nephrotoxicosis/hepatotoxicosis:
- Serum biochemistry profiles and urinalyses as in monitoring section; urine protein/creatinine ratio if proteinuria with receptor tyrosine kinase (RTK) inhibitors. *S*-adenosylmethionine (SAMe) to prevent lomustine hepatotoxicity

Technician Tips

- Technicians administering chemotherapy must be familiar with AEs that can occur during administration and how to prevent, recognize, and manage them.
- It is important to quickly report extravasation of drug and any AEs observed.
- For each treatment, record the date, drug, dose, and site of administration.
- Signs of serious AEs may be subtle (e.g., lethargy, inappetence). It is important to educate clients to communicate with the veterinary team if AEs are suspected.

Client Education

Clients should be provided with information that allows them to recognize AEs of each drug and instructs them to seek veterinary care promptly.

SUGGESTED READING

Gustafson DL, et al: Cancer chemotherapy. In Withrow SJ, et al, editors: Small animal clinical oncology, ed 5, St. Louis, 2013, Saunders, pp 157-179.

AUTHOR: Nicole C. Northrup, DVM, DACVIM
EDITOR: Kenneth M. Rassnick, DVM, DACVIM

Cheyletiellosis

BASIC INFORMATION

Definition

A highly contagious, zoonotic skin disease of dogs, cats, and rabbits caused by the surface-living mite, *Cheyletiella* spp

Synonym

Walking dandruff

Epidemiology

SPECIES, AGE, SEX

Young animals are more frequently affected.

GENETICS, BREED PREDISPOSITION

Long-haired cats appear to be more commonly affected.

RISK FACTORS

Animal shelters, breeding establishments, and boarding/grooming facilities: increased risk

CONTAGION AND ZOONOSIS

- *Cheyletiella* spp mites are very contagious and not host specific; they transfer readily among dogs, cats, and rabbits.
- Cheyletiellosis is a zoonotic disease; humans are at risk if exposed to an infested pet (whether or not overt clinical signs are present in the pet).

Clinical Presentation

HISTORY, CHIEF COMPLAINT

Reason for presentation can be any combination of scaling, pruritus, or zoonosis.

PHYSICAL EXAM FINDINGS

- Scaling ("dandruff") noted primarily over the dorsum and neck *and/or*
- Mild to intense pruritus or overgrooming in cats *and/or*
- Dorsal erythema, papules, and crusting noted occasionally, particularly in cats ("miliary dermatitis")
- Among the exfoliated epidermal cells, *Cheyletiella* mites can be seen moving, hence the name "walking dandruff." The term should not be overinterpreted; the mites are much smaller than skin scales, and a pet has to be very still to enable the clinician to see the subtle movement of mites carrying scales and/or the mites themselves.
- Some pets not noted by the owner to have clinical signs are presented for evaluation because of suspected zoonotic lesions in a human in contact with the animal.

Etiology and Pathophysiology

- *Cheyletiella* is a relatively large mite (0.4 mm) with prominent hooklike mouth parts. It lives on the skin surface and feeds on surface debris and exudates. These mites form pseudotunnels in the surface keratin.
- The mite eggs, smaller than lice eggs, are loosely attached to hair shafts.
- The entire life cycle is completed on the host within ≈3 weeks.
- Although adult mites may survive in the environment for 10 days, eggs are shed into the environment with the pet's hair and may be an important source of reinfestation beyond those 10 days.

DIAGNOSIS

Diagnostic Overview

The diagnosis is suspected from the history and clinical signs, potentially including zoonotic lesions in humans. Demonstration of mites or eggs under the microscope is confirmatory.

Differential Diagnosis

- In dogs, differential diagnosis (DDx) depends on the clinical presentation.
  - If only scaling is present, DDx includes ectoparasites (e.g., fleas, lice, *Demodex*), intestinal parasitism, poor nutrition, cornification disorders (e.g., ichthyosis, sebaceous adenitis).
  - If pruritus is present, DDx includes ectoparasites (e.g., lice, fleas, scabies), hypersensitivities (e.g., flea bites, atopic dermatitis, food), pyoderma, and fungal infections (e.g., *Malassezia*, dermatophytosis).
- In cats, DDx includes dermatophytosis, ectoparasites (e.g., lice, flea infestation, otodectic mange), and hypersensitivities (e.g., flea bites, food, environmental).
- In humans, the pruritic erythematous papular eruption (papular urticaria) induced by a hypersensitivity reaction to *Cheyletiella* mites is often indistinguishable from other zoonotic (e.g., fleas, *Sarcoptes* spp, *Dermanyssus* spp) or nonzoonotic (e.g., harvest mites, straw itch mites, bedbugs) arthropod bite reactions.

Initial Database

- Confirmation relies on collecting and identifying the mite or its eggs. Occasionally they may be difficult to recover, especially in adult cats, because of cats' grooming habits.
- Mites and eggs can be harvested using adhesive acetate tape (transparent Scotch tape) preparations, superficial skin scrapings, flea combing, fecal flotation, or by collecting scales dislodged when rubbing/petting the animal's back.
- The epidermal debris is examined directly with a magnifying lens or is put on a glass slide, mixed with mineral oil, covered with a cover slip, and examined with a microscope at low power.

Advanced or Confirmatory Testing

Therapeutic trials with reliable acaricides are essential to confirm or rule out cheyletiellosis in pruritic or scaling animals with negative samplings, as well as when a human in contact has a pruritic papular eruption evocative of skin lesions caused by zoonotic arthropod bite reactions.

TREATMENT

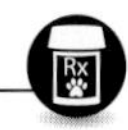

Treatment Overview

- The goal of treatment is to thoroughly eradicate the mites. All affected and in-contact animals should be treated with an appropriate acaricide regardless of presence or absence of clinical signs.
- All suspected cheyletiellosis cases should be treated even if the parasite has not been isolated.
- Environmental treatment may be required in severe cases.
- Traditional topical acaricides (lime sulfur, amitraz, organophosphates) have been largely replaced by off-label macrocyclic lactones.

Acute General Treatment

- Selamectin (Revolution/Stronghold) and moxidectin/imidacloprid (Advantage Multi/Advocate) are not approved for the treatment of cheyletiellosis but appear effective when applied topically every 2-4 weeks for 2 months.
- Off-label ivermectin remains a treatment option in cats and can still be a therapeutic alternative in dogs but should never be used in collies or related breeds carrying the *MDR1/ABCB1-Δ* mutation (p. 638). The injectable product (Ivomec 1% injection for cattle and swine) is usually given (0.3 mg/kg q 7 days PO or q 14 days SQ for 6-8 weeks). The 0.5% alcohol-based pour-on ivermectin formulation (Ivomec Pour-On for cattle) is also effective and practical when applied topically to the interscapular skin (0.5 mg/kg q 14 days for 3-4 treatments).
- Milbemycin oxime (Interceptor), albeit more expensive, is also effective (2 mg/kg PO q 3-7 days for 6-9 doses).
  - Although not documented, isoxazoline drugs are also likely to be effective.

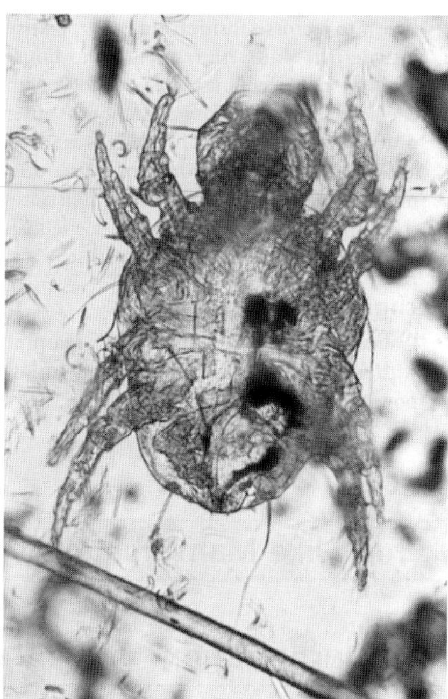

CHEYLETIELLOSIS Microscopic view of adult *Cheyletiella* mite. (Copyright Dr. Manon Paradis.)

Possible Complications

In collies and other herding breeds, the *MDR1/ABCB1-Δ* mutation can cause intoxication with commonly recommended dosages of ivermectin or other off-label macrocyclic lactones (p. 638).

PROGNOSIS & OUTCOME

- Prognosis with appropriate treatment is excellent.
- In humans, the zoonotic infestation is transient, with resolution of the pruritic papular eruption when the mites are eradicated from the animals.

PEARLS & CONSIDERATIONS

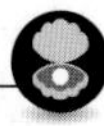

Comments

- Infested animals may show no clinical signs.
- Cheyletiellosis is possible even if there is only one animal with clinical signs among a household full of pets without any clinical signs.

- Due to cross-sensitization, a positive intradermal skin test result for the house dust mite is seen in ≈50% of dogs with cheyletiellosis. Within a few months after mite eradication, all clinical signs resolve, and intradermal reactions to house dust mites are generally negative. This illustrates the importance of ruling out cheyletiellosis before testing for atopic dermatitis.

Technician Tips

- Collect scales from exam table and examine with a magnifying glass or microscope at low power.
- Cheyletiellosis has zoonotic potential. Try to limit direct contact with the affected animal.
- Hospital environment should be decontaminated.

Client Education

Humans transiently infected with *Cheyletiella* spp mites may develop an uncomfortable, pruritic papular eruption, especially on the arms, trunk, and buttocks. This should spontaneously resolve within 3 weeks when the mites are eradicated from the animals and the environment. Persistent symptoms should prompt the person to consult with a physician.

SUGGESTED READING

Miller WH Jr, et al: Muller & Kirk's Small animal dermatology, ed 7, St. Louis, 2013, Saunders, pp 300-303.

AUTHOR & EDITOR: **Manon Paradis, DMV, MVSc, DACVD**

Chiari-like Malformation

Client Education Sheet 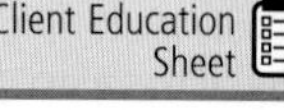

BASIC INFORMATION

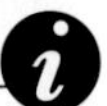

Definition

A congenital condition characterized by decreased volume of the caudal fossa of the skull relative to the brain parenchyma, with herniation of cerebellum through the foramen magnum and subsequent crowding of the cervicomedullary junction

Synonyms

Chiari-like malformation (CLM), caudal occipital malformation syndrome (COMS), occipital bone hypoplasia, Chiari type 1 malformation, occipital malformation

Epidemiology

Affects dogs (less often, cats) of either sex. Age of onset for clinical signs varies. Age of affected dogs ranges from 6 months to 3 years, although it has been appreciated in older dogs.

- Cavalier King Charles spaniel
  - Most commonly affected breed
  - Evidence of heritability; mode of inheritance not yet established but thought to be epistatic (influenced by many loci)
- Documented primarily in small breeds: Brussels griffon, Chihuahua, Yorkshire terrier, Maltese terrier, toy/miniature poodle, pug, shih tzu, Pomeranian, Boston terrier, French bulldog, Pekingese, Havanese, papillon, Staffordshire terrier, miniature Dachshund, and miniature pinscher.
- Cats: reports in domestic short hair, Persian

ASSOCIATED DISORDERS

- Syringomyelia (SM), also called *syrinx*, is a fluid-filled cavity within the spinal cord. Theories have been proposed as to why syrinxes occur in patients with CLM but none confirmed. A syrinx can occur in the absence of CLM or in conjunction with another disease process affecting the spinal cord (e.g., neoplasia, vertebral fractures).
- Malformations that can occur in association or concurrently with CLM: hydrocephalus or intracranial arachnoid cyst
- Primary secretory otitis media (PSOM): a condition of Cavalier King Charles spaniels in which mucus accumulates within the middle ear causing partial or complete hearing loss. Some patients will have concurrent vestibular signs such as a head tilt or resting nystagmus, and others are clinically unaffected.

Clinical Presentation

HISTORY, CHIEF COMPLAINT

- Early on, clinical signs can be intermittent and tend to occur during times of excitement or stress.
- Patients present with a variety of clinical manifestations.
  - Most common presenting sign is cervical pain; can manifest as phantom scratching of the neck region.
  - Neurologic signs localizing to a cervical myelopathy and/or cerebellovestibular system are also frequently seen.

PHYSICAL EXAM FINDINGS

- General physical examination is usually normal.
- Neurologic examination usually indicates a cervical myelopathy (i.e., upper motor neuron deficits in all four limbs), cerebellovestibular dysfunction (head tilt, resting nystagmus, circling, loss of balance, cerebellar/vestibular ataxia, intention tremor, loss of menace response despite normal vision), or both.
- Hallmarks for CLM are hyperesthesia (pain) and/or paresthesia (abnormal sensations) in the head/neck region. Back pain has also been documented.
- Clinical signs such as scoliosis, weakness/collapse, deafness, and seizures have been appreciated.

Etiology and Pathophysiology

- Current theory: developmental abnormality of the occipital bone resulting in intracranial overcrowding within the caudal fossa. Overcrowding results in cerebellar herniation and compression of the cervicomedullary junction, which can lead to abnormal cerebrospinal fluid (CSF) dynamics and subsequent SM in the spinal cord.
- Over time, the meninges can hypertrophy at the cervicomedullary junction, leading to exacerbation of syrinx formation.

DIAGNOSIS

Diagnostic Overview

A diagnosis of CLM is strongly suspected based on the patient's breed and presenting clinical signs. To ascertain an accurate diagnosis and rule out other differentials, MRI of the head and neck and CSF analysis are indicated. To fully evaluate extent of disease in the central nervous system, multiplanar (axial, sagittal, and dorsal) MRI of the head, cervical, thoracic, and lumbar spinal cord is recommended.

Differential Diagnosis

- Intervertebral disc disease (IVDD)
- Meningoencephalitis
- Vertebral anomalies
- Primary secretory otitis media

Initial Database

- Neurologic examination (p. 1136)
- CBC, chemistry panel, and urinalysis usually normal.
- Survey radiographs of cervical spine: to screen for other differentials (IVDD, vertebral anomalies)

Advanced or Confirmatory Testing

- Diagnosis of CLM is based on MRI findings of caudal cerebellar herniation, bony compression of caudal cerebellum, medullary kinking, and SM; midsagittal T2-weighted MR image of most importance (p. 1132)
- CSF analysis is often performed to rule out concurrent inflammatory brain or spinal cord disease (pp. 1080 and 1323).

Diseases and Disorders

- CT can also be used to evaluate for CLM when MRI is not available; imaging modality is limited in its ability to obtain detailed information about brain and spinal cord parenchyma.
- Brainstem auditory evoked response (BAER) can be performed to evaluate hearing. Hearing pathways can become adversely affected in CLM.

TREATMENT

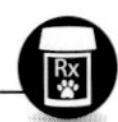

Treatment Overview

The therapeutic goal is to halt disease progression and achieve improvement or resolution of clinical signs of neurologic dysfunction. This can be achieved using conservative medical therapy or surgical intervention. Surgical intervention has been typically reserved for young patients that are severely affected and older patients that have failed medical management.

Acute General Treatment

- Most respond favorably to glucocorticoid therapy (prednisone 0.5 mg/kg PO q 12h, then taper).
- Decrease CSF production: omeprazole (0.5-1.5 mg/kg PO q 12-24h). Acetazolamide and methazolamide can be used as adjunct therapy for short periods.
- Analgesia
  - For acute or chronic pain: tramadol 4-10 mg/kg PO q 8-12h or codeine 0.5-2 mg/kg PO q 8-12h
  - For scratching or chronic pain: gabapentin 10-20 mg/kg PO q 8-12h. In refractory cases, amantadine 3-5 mg/kg PO q 24h and/or pregabalin 2-4 mg/kg PO q 8-12h can be administered.
- Patients that respond poorly to conservative medical therapy may require surgical intervention.

Chronic Treatment

Surgical decompression (foramen magnum decompression) may be necessary in severe or medically refractory cases.

Possible Complications

- Adverse effects of long-term glucocorticoid administration
- Medical complications: continued neurologic decline despite therapy; neurologic signs can become refractory to continued medical therapy
- Surgical complications: intraoperative death, postoperative worsening of neurologic status or continued neurologic decline, and/or possible need for re-operation at surgical site due to formation of excessive fibrous tissue

Recommended Monitoring

Postoperative in hospital monitoring for 3-5 days.

PROGNOSIS & OUTCOME

- Most patients improve with medical therapy, but clinical signs often do not resolve. Some patients will have disease progression despite medical therapy.
- Surgical therapy has been reported to have an 81% success rate, but recurrence of clinical signs can necessitate repeat surgery in 8%-47% of cases.

PEARLS & CONSIDERATIONS

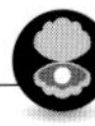

Comments

MRI findings do not correlate with patient clinical signs. Patients can have significant MRI findings with minimal neurologic deficits and vice versa.

Prevention

Breeders should be advised to access online resources for current guidelines on breeding and MRI screening (www.veterinary-neurologist.co.uk/Syringomyelia/).

Technician Tips

- CLM is a heritable disease that is associated with high morbidity.
- Neurologic signs usually consist of cervical pain and discomfort. Care should be taken during physical restraint because some of these patients are sensitive to normal touch.

Client Education

- SM is a potential slowly progressive sequela of CLM. It is thought to be due to an alteration in CSF flow dynamics, structural compression/obstruction, or a combination of both.
- It has been proposed that surgical intervention may be necessary to achieve resolution of SM, although more scientific research is needed to confirm this.
- To date, there has not been a documented surgical technique that has consistently led to resolution of SM. Veterinary specialists can offer their recommendations based on scientific research, experience, and expertise.

SUGGESTED READING

Marino DJ, et al: Chiari-like malformation and syringomyelia: a handbook for veterinary professionals, The Canine Chiari Institute (website). http://caninechiariinstitute.org/index.php/doctor-center/dvm-guide-chiari/.

AUTHOR: Joshua Gehrke, DVM, DACVIM
EDITOR: Karen R. Muñana, DVM, MS, DACVIM

Chlamydiosis

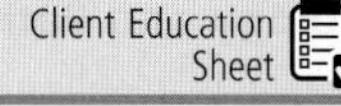

BASIC INFORMATION

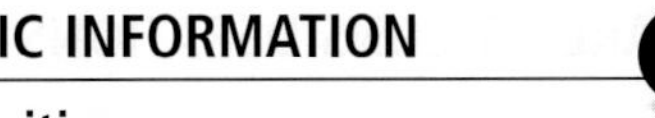

Definition

A bacterial infection associated with acute, chronic, or recurrent conjunctivitis and occasionally signs of mild upper respiratory infection such as sneezing and nasal discharge. The primary pathogen implicated is *Chlamydia felis* (formerly *Chlamydia psittaci* and *Chlamydophila felis*).

Synonym

Feline pneumonitis (outdated)

Epidemiology

SPECIES, AGE, SEX

C. felis has been positively correlated with conjunctivitis and upper respiratory tract disease in cats of either sex. The prevalence of *C. felis* ranges from 10%-30% in cats with clinical signs. Most cats with *C. felis* are < 5 years of age, but it is common for affected cats to be < 1 year old.

Non-*C. felis* infections have been reported:

- *Chlamydia pneumoniae*: cats >2 years
- *Neochlamydia hartmannellae*: 30% in cats <1 year and 54% in cats > 10 years

RISK FACTORS

Primarily young age; multi-cat households; higher incidence in stray/outside cats

CONTAGION AND ZOONOSIS

- Highly contagious and spread by direct contact with ocular discharge or respiratory tract secretions, by aerosol, or through contact with fomites
- Zoonosis is rare but reported for *C. felis* with a confirmed case of conjunctivitis in an immunocompromised human; other reports likely related to a cross-reaction between *C.*

felis with other *Chlamydia* spp or *Bartonella* spp
- *C. pneumoniae* is a pathogen associated in humans with community-acquired pneumonia, atherosclerosis, and conjunctivitis and has been identified in cats with conjunctivitis.
- Cat owners who are immunocompromised should limit direct contact with infected cats, observe good hygienic practices, and obtain prompt treatment of affected cats.

GEOGRAPHY AND SEASONALITY

Worldwide

ASSOCIATED DISORDERS

Co-infections with feline herpesvirus 1 (FHV-1), feline calicivirus, and *Mycoplasma felis* are common and increase severity of clinical disease.

Clinical Presentation

HISTORY, CHIEF COMPLAINT

- Ocular discharge or redness
- Conjunctivitis: often unilateral initially and later becomes bilateral
- Occasionally decreased appetite
- Sneezing
- Nasal discharge

PHYSICAL EXAM FINDINGS

- Ocular discharge: serous or mucopurulent
- Blepharospasm
- Conjunctival hyperemia
- Chemosis
- Conjunctival hyperemia
- Nasal discharge: serous, mucoid or mucopurulent
- Keratitis/corneal ulceration
  - Rare, often related to a co-infection (e.g., FHV-1)
  - Other chlamydial species: *Parachlamydia acanthamoebae* and *N. hartmannellae* reported in cats with keratitis, corneal ulceration, and conjunctivitis (clinical relevance unclear, DNA also identified in normal cats)
- Transient fever
- Weight loss
- Inappetence
- Vaginal discharge

Etiology and Pathophysiology

- *C. felis* is an obligate intracellular bacterium that is similar in structure to gram-negative bacteria.
- Two forms: an infectious extracellular elementary body form that infects the epithelium of ocular, respiratory, gastrointestinal, and genitourinary systems; a noninfectious, intracellular reticulate body form that replicates inside the cytoplasm of epithelial cells
- Reticulate bodies divide within a cytoplasmic vacuole (inclusions) and are released from the host epithelial cell as elementary bodies.
- Systemic disease; organisms are shed from the conjunctiva, vagina, and rectum
- Appearance of conjunctivitis typically parallels clinical shedding; shedding may continue after signs resolve.
- Transmission is by direct contact with respiratory secretions or ocular discharge; aerosol, or contact with fomites.
- Incubation period is 3-5 days, and infection may persist for months.

DIAGNOSIS

Diagnostic Overview

Diagnosis is suspected based on history and clinical findings from examination. Rule out that the conjunctivitis is not secondary to an intraocular disease process (e.g., uveitis, glaucoma) (p. 199).

Differential Diagnosis

Infectious causes:
- FHV-1
- Feline calicivirus
- *Bordetella bronchiseptica*
- *Mycoplasma* spp
- *Cryptococcus* spp
- *Aspergillus* spp
- *Histoplasmosis* spp

Noninfectious causes:
- Neoplasia (e.g., squamous cell carcinoma, lymphoma)
- Nasopharyngeal polyps
- Dental disease
- Congenital eyelid malformation
- Palate defects
- Local irritants (e.g., chemical, contact allergy, topical eye preparations)
- Trauma
- Foreign body
- Immune-mediated/inflammatory (e.g., eosinophilic keratoconjunctivitis)
- Keratoconjunctivitis sicca

Initial Database

- Conjunctival cytology to evaluate for intracytoplasmic basophilic inclusions (reticulate bodies) using Giemsa stain
  - Low sensitivity and specificity for early stages of infection
  - Topical eye preparations can create cytoplasmic inclusions resulting in misdiagnosis.
  - Suppurative inflammation on conjunctival cytology is common with *C. felis*.

Advanced or Confirmatory Testing

- Polymerase chain reaction (PCR) and real-time PCR: high sensitivity and specificity; varies by laboratory. Assays specific for *C. felis* may miss other chlamydial species. Conjunctival swabs recommended
- ELISA antigen test kits: sensitivity and specificity varies and is lower than other testing options available
- Cell culture: requires special transport media so primarily research tool, low sensitivity
- Serology: not widely available or considered useful

TREATMENT

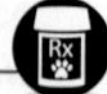

Treatment Overview

The cornerstone of treatment is antibiotic therapy (doxycycline) along with supportive care. In multi-cat households, all contact cats should be treated and good hygienic practices followed.

Acute General Treatment

- Due to the systemic nature of the disease, systemic therapy has shown superior efficacy to topical therapy alone.
- Treat all cats in the household simultaneously.
- Doxycycline 10 mg/kg PO q 24h or minocycline 5-12 mg/kg PO q 12h for at least 4 weeks
- Alternative is pradofloxacin 5 mg/kg PO q 24h
- Azithromycin ineffective in clearing infection compared to doxycycline
- A 4-week course of amoxicillin-clavulanic acid (12.5 mg/kg PO q 12h) may also eliminate *C. felis*.

Chronic Treatment

Ocular infections initially respond to topical treatment, but recurrence has been documented without systemic therapy. Treatment should be continued for 2 weeks after resolution of clinical signs.

Possible Complications

- Risk of discoloration of the teeth in kittens if tetracyclines are used in the last 2-3 weeks of pregnancy or for kittens in the first few months of life. Little evidence for this complication with doxycycline
- Esophagitis reported with the administration of doxycycline tablets. If tablets are administered, they should be followed by a water bolus by syringe. Administration of doxycycline liquid oral suspension minimizes the risk of esophagitis; compounded suspensions may have a short shelf life.
- Enrofloxacin can be effective but has been associated with retinal toxicity and blindness in cats and is not recommended.

PROGNOSIS & OUTCOME

- Excellent in households with low numbers of cats
- Fair in cattery situations; recurrence with large numbers of cats and poor compliance
- All cats in the household/cattery must be treated with the full course of antimicrobials and proper hygiene and quarantine maintained.

PEARLS & CONSIDERATIONS

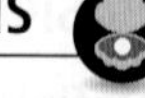

Comments

C. felis has been associated with lameness and reproductive disorders in experimental infections.

Prevention

- Environmental hygiene in catteries and disinfection with a 1 : 32 solution of bleach in tap water; detergent may be added. Other disinfectants (accelerated hydrogen peroxide and potassium peroxymonosulfate) also effective

- Modified live and inactivated cell culture vaccines are available; do not prevent infection but reduce the severity of clinical signs
- Vaccines are not considered core but are recommended in situations in which a large number of cats will be housed together (catteries).
- Vaccines should be used with caution in immunocompromised cats; use only inactivated vaccines. Lethargy, fever, anorexia, and limb soreness may occur 1-3 weeks after vaccination.

Technician Tips

Close contact is required for cat-to-cat transmission. Cats with suspected infection should be singly housed to limit transmission. Decontaminate contact surfaces/cages between uses.

SUGGESTED READING

Sykes, JE. Chlamydial Infections. In Sykes JE, editor: Canine and feline infectious diseases, St. Louis, 2014, Elsevier, pp 326-333.

AUTHOR: Renee T. Carter, DVM, DACVO
EDITOR: Joseph Taboada, DVM, DACVIM

Chocolate Toxicosis

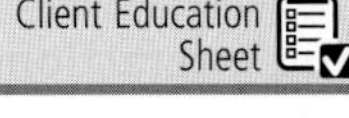

BASIC INFORMATION

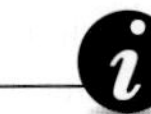

Definition

Chocolate toxicosis refers to the acute onset of stimulatory signs that occur in a dose-dependent manner after ingesting chocolate containing naturally occurring alkaloids referred to as methylxanthines. Theobromine and caffeine are the methylxanthines of concern in chocolate.

Synonym

Methylxanthine toxicosis

Epidemiology

SPECIES, AGE, SEX

Dogs far more often affected than cats

GEOGRAPHY AND SEASONALITY

Major holidays (Easter, Christmas, Valentine's Day, Halloween) result in increased opportunity for intoxication due to increased presence of chocolate in homes.

Clinical Presentation

DISEASE FORMS/SUBTYPES

Signs are typically dose dependent

- <20 mg/kg of methylxanthines: gastrointestinal (GI) upset, polydipsia, and pancreatitis
- 20-40 mg/kg of methylxanthines: above plus hyperactivity
- 40-50 mg/kg of methylxanthines: above plus cardiotoxicity
- >60 mg/kg of methylxanthines: above plus tremors and seizures

HISTORY, CHIEF COMPLAINT

Owners will typically report an exposure to chocolate. Pets will often be polydipsic and may vomit before presentation, with chocolate evident in the vomitus. Signs can progress to hyperactivity, tachycardia, tremors, and seizures.

PHYSICAL EXAM FINDINGS

- Tachycardia
- Tense, often distended abdomen
- Hypersalivation
- Hyperactivity
- Dehydration
- Cardiac arrhythmias (sinus tachycardia, premature ventricular contractions, ventricular tachycardia)
- Hyperthermia
- Tremors, seizure

Etiology and Pathophysiology

- Proposed mechanism of action
  - Competitive inhibition of cellular adenosine receptors: cerebral cortical stimulation, seizures, diuresis, increased myocardial contraction, and smooth muscle relaxation
  - Caffeine: stimulates synthesis and release of catecholamines, especially norepinephrine

DIAGNOSIS

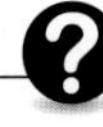

Diagnostic Overview

A tentative diagnosis is made based on history (or other evidence of exposure to chocolate such as chocolate in vomitus), compatible clinical signs, or both. There are no clinically relevant confirmatory tests.

Differential Diagnosis

- Toxic: caffeine, theophylline, aminophylline, guarana, 5-hydroxytryptophan, pseudoephedrine, phenylephrine, amphetamines, albuterol, cocaine, phenylpropanolamine, antihistamines, metaldehyde, serotonergic medications (antidepressants)
- Nontoxic: vomiting, arrhythmia (p. 1284), hypersalivation (p. 1274)

Initial Database

- Packed cell volume (PCV)/total solids (TS): ± evidence of hemoconcentration due to dehydration
- Serum chemistry profile
  - Blood glucose: ± hyperglycemia
  - Electrolytes: risk of hypernatremia, especially if activated charcoal is given
- Electrocardiogram (ECG [p. 1096]): sinus tachycardia, rarely ventricular dysrhythmias
- Blood pressure (p. 1065): hypertension possible
- Abdominal imaging: if persistent GI signs or abdominal pain, to rule out other differential diagnoses

Advanced or Confirmatory Testing

Methylxanthine levels in serum, plasma, stomach contents, and urine are not helpful for treatment and are seldom measured.

TREATMENT

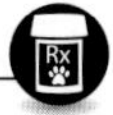

Treatment Overview

Decontamination can be considered in asymptomatic patients up to 8 hours after exposure and is extremely effective in reducing the risk of clinical signs. After signs are present, treatment involves adequate fluid administration for cardiovascular support and to prevent dehydration, the use of sedatives to control central nervous system (CNS) stimulation, antiarrhythmics for cardiac dysrhythmias, and supportive care for GI upset.

Acute General Treatment

- Decontamination of patient (p. 1087):
  - Emesis (p. 1087): up to 8 hours after exposure in asymptomatic dogs.
  - Activated charcoal 1-2 g/kg PO once, with sorbitol or other cathartic: chocolate will increase the risk of hypernatremia from activated charcoal. Monitor for hypernatremia and associated signs (tremor, ataxia, seizures). Benefit must outweigh the risk of hypernatremia; give only if over a lethal dose of chocolate.
  - Urinary catheter: caffeine may be reabsorbed through the bladder wall. High doses may warrant placement of a urinary catheter to help decrease this reabsorption and increase caffeine elimination.
- CNS stimulation
  - Acepromazine 0.025-0.05 mg/kg IV, titrate up as needed, for hyperactivity
  - Methocarbamol 55-100 mg/kg slow IV to effect for tremors
  - Diazepam 0.5-2 mg/kg IV *or* midazolam 0.1-0.5 mg/kg IV for hyperactivity, tremors, and seizures
  - Barbiturates, gas anesthesia for seizures refractory to benzodiazepines
- Cardiac arrhythmias
  - Beta-blockers for significant sinus tachycardia in calm patients

- Propranolol 0.02-0.06 mg/kg slow IV to effect
- Esmolol loading dose 0.05-0.1 mg/kg IV bolus over 1-2 minutes followed by a constant rate infusion (CRI) of 10-200 mcg/kg/min
  - Ventricular tachyarrhythmias
    - Lidocaine (dog) 1-4 mg/kg IV, then 30-50 mcg/min prn
- Fluid diuresis
- Vomiting, nausea
  - Maropitant 1 mg/kg SQ q 24h *or*
  - Ondansetron 0.5-1 mg/kg IV q 8-12h

Nutrition/Diet

Bland diet in pets with GI upset

Drug Interactions

Erythromycin, glucocorticoids, and cimetidine decrease methylxanthine clearance rate

Possible Complications

Pancreatitis, catecholamine depletion, hypernatremia, hyperglycemia, ketoacidosis in diabetic patients

Recommended Monitoring

ECG, heart rate, blood pressure, mentation, fluid ins and outs

PROGNOSIS & OUTCOME

- Prognosis is generally good, especially with successful and timely decontamination.
- Prognosis is guarded with large exposures or with seizures.

Approximate Methylxanthine Content of Selected Products

Type of Chocolate	Caffeine (mg/oz)	Theobromine (mg/oz)	Total Methylxanthines (mg/oz)
White chocolate	0.25	0.85	1.1
Milk chocolate	58	6	64
Dark chocolate*	138	22	160
Unsweetened baking chocolate	393	47	440
Cocoa powder	737	70	807

*If the percent cacao of a dark chocolate is known, the methylxanthine content can be more accurately estimated by using this formula: methylxanthines (mg/oz) = 400 × % cacao (reported as a decimal).

PEARLS & CONSIDERATIONS

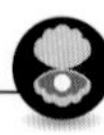

Comments

- Emesis is often extremely effective in decontaminating asymptomatic pets and can be effective up to 6-8 hours after exposure. Onset of clinical signs can be delayed up to 12 hours for pets ingesting a large amount of chocolate due to the formation of a bezoar in the stomach.
- Patients with underlying diabetes mellitus are at increased risk of hyperglycemia, pancreatitis, and ketoacidosis.
- LD50 for theobromine in dogs is 250-500 mg/kg; for cats, 200 mg/kg

Prevention

Keep chocolate away from pets.

Technician Tips

- Methylxanthines are excreted in the urine. They and their metabolites can be reabsorbed in the urinary tract. Patients with large exposures should have a urinary catheter or be walked frequently to keep the bladder empty.
- Patients with chocolate ingestion can require a high rate of fluids due to losses and osmotic pull of fluids into the GI tract. Fluid ins and outs should be monitored to help ensure adequate hydration.

Client Education

The darker the chocolate, the higher the risk of poisoning.

SUGGESTED READING

Dolder LK: Methylxanthines: caffeine, theobromine, theophylline. In Peterson ME, et al, editors: Small animal toxicology, ed 3, St. Louis, 2013, Elsevier, pp 647-652.

AUTHOR: Laura Stern, DVM, DABVT
EDITOR: Tina Wismer, DVM, MS, DABVT, DABT

Cholangitis, Feline

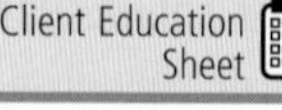

BASIC INFORMATION

Definition

- Cholangitis: inflammation centers on the bile ducts; it may or may not extend into the hepatic parenchyma.
- Several distinct forms of cholangitis are included within a single umbrella term (see below).
- Cholangitis is one of the most common feline hepatobiliary disorders.

Synonyms

- Feline inflammatory liver disease
- Cholangitis or cholangiohepatitis
- Acute and chronic neutrophilic cholangitis: suppurative cholangitis
- Chronic lymphocytic cholangitis: lymphocytic portal hepatitis

Epidemiology

SPECIES, AGE, SEX

- Any breed, either sex. Persians overrepresented in United Kingdom, Norwegian Forest cats in Netherlands
- Although affected cats range in age from < 1 to > 16 years old, most are middle-aged.

RISK FACTORS

Extrahepatic biliary obstruction, inflammatory bowel disease (IBD), pancreatitis, cholestatic disease, cholelithiasis, bacterial infection or splenic abscess, feline infectious peritonitis (FIP), toxoplasmosis, immunodeficiencies, choledochal stent placement, drugs (diazepam, tetracyclines, others)

CONTAGION AND ZOONOSIS

Not contagious or zoonotic

ASSOCIATED DISORDERS

Triaditis is the term used for describing the combination of cholangitis with IBD and pancreatitis. IBD or pancreatitis occurs in 50%-85% of the cases of cholangitis, with both present in up to 40% of cholangitis patients. Cholangitis can also be associated with hepatic lipidosis, or secondary to a variety of other diseases/conditions (see Risk Factors).

Clinical Presentation

DISEASE FORMS/SUBTYPES

- On the basis of histopathologic findings, four distinct forms of cholangitis exist as defined by the World Small Animal Veterinary Association Liver Diseases and Pathology Standardization Research Group:
  - Neutrophilic, acute or chronic
  - Lymphocytic

- Liver fluke infestation associated
- Destructive
- The different forms present with a similar clinical picture (history, initial presentation, chief complaint, cause, progression, and outcome).
- Progressive lymphocytic cholangitis is a form seen predominantly in Europe in young cats presenting with ascites, icterus, and hyperglobulinemia.
  - Some pathologists classify this as low-grade (well-differentiated) lymphoma.
- Lymphocytic portal hepatitis is a separate entity confined to portal triads and is often an incidental finding in older cats.

HISTORY, CHIEF COMPLAINT

- Patients with the neutrophilic form of cholangitis usually present with an acute onset of illness: anorexia, fever, and vomiting in an icteric cat with abdominal discomfort.
- Patients with the lymphocytic form of cholangitis may present with a more chronic condition with nonspecific signs (including weight loss and chronic or intermittent vomiting and anorexia); a subset of patients may present with acute signs.
- Patients with concurrent IBD (p. 543) and pancreatitis (p. 740) (i.e., triaditis) may present with a wide variety of signs and various degrees of severity, depending on the severity of inflammation in these other organs.
- Patients with neutrophilic or lymphocytic forms are usually icteric, and a few may have ascites.
- Patients with the chronic (typically lymphocytic) condition may rarely be polyphagic, although usually they are presented for lethargy, anorexia, vomiting, and weight loss.

PHYSICAL EXAM FINDINGS

- Neutrophilic cholangitis: fever, dehydration, and icterus are common; there may be signs of abdominal discomfort with palpation or ptyalism.
- Lymphocytic cholangitis: findings range from minimal physical exam abnormalities to icterus with weight loss. Hepatomegaly on abdominal palpation in ≈50% of cases.

Etiology and Pathophysiology

- Bacterial infection (*Escherichia coli, Streptococcus, Clostridium, Salmonella* serovar Typhimurium, *Enterococcus faecium*, other enteric organisms, anaerobes); ascending infection of the biliary tract (acute neutrophilic cholangitis)
- In association with other infections (e.g., toxoplasmosis, FIP)
- Immune-mediated disorder (chronic lymphocytic cholangitis)
- Extrahepatic bile duct obstruction
- Secondary or concurrent pancreatitis, especially with the suppurative form; pancreatic and bile ducts enter duodenum through a common opening in the cat
- IBD

DIAGNOSIS

Diagnostic Overview

Lethargy and anorexia in a cat with elevated liver enzymes is consistent with cholangitis and with several other hepatobiliary disorders. The diagnosis is confirmed histologically on liver biopsy.

Differential Diagnosis

- Hepatic lipidosis
- Hepatic neoplasia (especially lymphoma)
- Extrahepatic bile duct obstruction
- Pancreatitis
- IBD
- Other systemic infections (e.g., cytauxzoonosis, tularemia)
- FIP
- Sepsis

Initial Database

CBC: the following are variably present:

- Leukocytosis; neutrophilia with a left shift and/or toxic neutrophils
- Lymphopenia
- Mild nonregenerative anemia with poikilocytes and/or Heinz bodies

Serum biochemistry panel:

- Elevated liver enzyme activities (alanine aminotransferase, alkaline phosphatase, aspartate aminotransferase) in the majority of cases
- Elevated serum total bilirubin
- Hyperglobulinemia
- Hyperglycemia, azotemia, electrolyte abnormalities

Other:

- Increased serum bile acids concentrations (redundant test in an icteric cat)
- High feline pancreatic lipase immunoreactivity (fPLI) with pancreatitis
- Low serum cobalamin concentration with severe IBD
- Clotting time abnormalities (prothrombin time, activated partial thromboplastin time) or portal vein thrombus (PVT)
- Hepatomegaly (radiographs)

Advanced or Confirmatory Testing

- Abdominal ultrasound: the following abnormalities are variably present:
  - Hepatic parenchyma: nonspecific changes in echogenicity
  - Gallbladder distention, cholelithiasis, biliary sludge, thickened gallbladder wall
  - Cystic and common bile duct dilation and tortuosity
  - Evidence of pancreatic or intestinal inflammation
  - Ascites (lymphocytic cholangitis; high protein level, low cellularity)
- Fine-needle aspiration (FNA) of the liver
  - Be cognizant of clotting abnormalities before FNA or biopsy.
  - Inflammatory cell infiltration but difficult to distinguish whether from hepatic or peripheral blood origin
  - Hepatocellular vacuolation (nonspecific: concurrent lipidosis is possible)
  - Bacterial culture and sensitivity of liver is low yield
  - Although minimally invasive, liver FNA is frequently nondiagnostic or inaccurate
- Percutaneous ultrasound-guided cholecystocentesis
  - Minimally invasive; cytology, culture and sensitivity for bacterial isolates
  - Higher yield (up to 40%) and preferred culture sample over liver FNA
  - *E. coli* is the most common isolate; other enteric organisms possible
- Liver biopsy (wedge or ultrasound-guided core [p. 1064]): as above for FNA plus
  - Periportal hepatocellular necrosis, bile duct dilation and proliferation (neutrophilic)
  - Periductal fibrosis, diminished bile duct number, and sclerosing cholangitis (lymphocytic)
- Laparoscopy (p. 1128):
  - Ability to obtain multiple biopsy samples from different lobes
  - Can visualize and biopsy the pancreas
  - Safest biopsy method
- Laparotomy: as above for laparoscopy
  - Assess biliary system for extrahepatic biliary obstruction
  - Feeding tube placement possible

TREATMENT

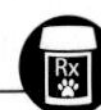

Treatment Overview

In addition to supportive care and specific treatment, the treatment plan must address concurrent conditions (frequent) for optimal patient outcomes.

Acute General Treatment

- Treatment should be tailored to the individual patient.
- Crystalloid fluids (e.g., Normosol, lactated Ringer's solution) with potassium supplementation
- Antibiotics (based on culture and sensitivity when possible) for all forms of cholangitis
  - Amoxicillin-clavulanate 15-20 mg/kg PO q 12h, 6-8 weeks, *or*
  - Amoxicillin 10-20 mg/kg PO q 12h, *or*
  - Cephalexin or cefadroxil 22 mg/kg PO q 8h, *or*
  - Pradofloxacin 7.5 mg/kg PO q 24h (preferred over enrofloxacin in cats for anaerobic efficacy and improved safety)
  - Vancomycin has been reported for one case of multidrug-resistant *Enterococcus faecium.*
- Ursodeoxycholic acid 10-15 mg/kg PO q 24h for choleresis, unless physical obstruction to gallbladder outflow exists
- Vitamin K_1 5 mg/CAT PO q 24h in cases of coagulation abnormalities
- Surgery for extrahepatic biliary obstruction
- Necessary treatments for associated conditions (especially pancreatitis, IBD, hepatic lipidosis)

Chronic Treatment

- Long-term management highly depends on an accurate diagnosis and requires

histopathologic analysis of a liver biopsy. Continue supportive medications (see below) for 3-6 months.
- Continue antibiotics (see above) 3-6 months if neutrophilic cholangitis
- Prednisolone (for chronic neutrophilic or lymphocytic cholangitis) 2 mg/kg q 12h initially, gradual taper over 2-4 months
- Cobalamin 250 mcg SQ weekly for 6 weeks, then every 30 days if cobalamin deficient
- Refractory cases of lymphocytic cholangitis may require chemotherapeutics or aggressive immunosuppression: methotrexate 0.13 mg/CAT PO q 8h for 3 doses at 7-day intervals, if tolerated, cyclosporine 3-5 mg/kg PO q 12h, or chlorambucil 2 mg (total dose) PO q 48h for 2-4 weeks, then taper; or if < 4 kg, 2 mg (total dose) q 72h
- Vitamin E (alpha-tocopherol acetate 10-30 IU/kg) for all forms of cholangitis
- *S*-adenosylmethionine 20 mg/kg PO q 24h (enteric-coated tablet) for all forms of cholangitis
- Ursodeoxycholic acid (see above)
- Continued treatment of concurrent conditions such as pancreatitis and/or IBD
- Treatment for ascites if present: spironolactone 2 mg/kg PO q 12-24h ± hydrochlorothiazide 0.5-2 mg/kg PO q 12h; angiotensin-converting enzyme inhibitors: enalapril 0.5 mg/kg PO q 12-24h; salt restriction
- For biliary cirrhosis (sclerosing cholangitis), consider pulsatile therapy with methotrexate 0.13 mg/CAT PO q 8h for 3 doses at 7-day intervals if tolerated, being cognizant of potential adverse side effects (gastrointestinal, hepatic, renal, bone marrow toxicoses).

Nutrition/Diet

- Route determined by clinical condition
- Protein restriction in cats is problematic because they are strict carnivores; should be avoided unless there is clear evidence of hepatic encephalopathy (rare)
- Consider supplementation with L-carnitine 250 mg/CAT PO q 24h; taurine 250-500 mg/CAT PO q 24h; thiamine (B_1) 50-100 mg PO q 24h for 3 days

Possible Complications

- Hepatic lipidosis with prolonged anorexia or inadequate nutritional support
- Diabetes mellitus with glucocorticoid treatment of lymphocytic form or treatment of IBD
- Advanced fibrosis/cirrhosis
- Progression of acute to chronic disease
- Necrotizing cholecystitis, choleliths
- Portal vein thrombosis

Recommended Monitoring

- Hepatic enzyme activity and total bilirubin concentration (at 2-week intervals until stable, then monthly)
- Clotting times if abnormalities are present initially or to monitor vitamin K_1 therapy
- Consider repeat bile acids measurement to monitor liver function.

PROGNOSIS & OUTCOME

- Acute neutrophilic cholangitis may be a single curable event, or it may recur (especially if antibiotic therapy is curtailed prematurely), but the prognosis is generally good with timely diagnosis and appropriate treatment.
- Lymphocytic cholangitis is a chronic condition but carries a fair to good prognosis with long-term therapy.
- Concurrent pancreatitis and/or IBD may affect the prognosis negatively.

PEARLS & CONSIDERATIONS

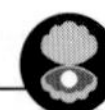

Comments

- Feline cholangitis is a constellation of clinical signs, biochemical abnormalities, and structural derangements. The cause may be unclear initially, and determining whether an infectious process is a contributing factor has a critical bearing on treatment decisions. Following the appropriate and sufficient diagnostic steps in the workup of a cat with inflammatory liver disease is critical for therapeutic success.
- Acute cholangitis is often infectious in nature (and therefore treated initially with antibiotics), whereas chronic neutrophilic or lymphocytic cholangitis may have an immune-mediated basis (and therefore are treated with immunosuppressive drugs).

Prevention

Treat contributing or concurrent conditions such as chronic pancreatitis or IBD.

Technician Tips

- Nutritional support is a crucial component of supportive care in these cats.
- The ability to medicate these cats may be compromised, and consideration should be given to placement of an esophagostomy tube (p. 1106) to help the owner administer nutrition and medications. Pretreat with vitamin K_1 (3 doses) before esophagostomy tube placement if a coagulopathy is present.

Client Education

- Vigilant monitoring is important for early detection in the presence of anorexia, lethargy, vomiting, or abdominal discomfort because suppurative cholangiohepatitis may recur.
- Compliance with medication administration may be a lifelong commitment.
- Proper nutritional support is critical.

SUGGESTED READING

Boland L, et al: Feline cholangitis. Vet Clin North Am Small Anim Pract 47:703-724, 2017.

AUTHOR: Craig B. Webb, DVM, PhD, DACVIM
EDITOR: Keith P. Richter, DVM, MSEL, DACVIM

Chole(cysto)lithiasis

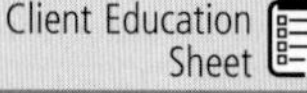

BASIC INFORMATION

Definition

Formation of stones in the extrahepatic bile duct system (choleliths) and/or specifically in the gallbladder (cholecystoliths)

Synonym

Gallstones

Epidemiology

SPECIES, AGE, SEX

- Dogs*:* older, small-breed, spayed females appear to be predisposed.
- Cats*:* middle-aged to older adults

ASSOCIATED DISORDERS

Cats:

- In some cats, possible association with cholangitis, pancreatitis, inflammatory bowel disease (i.e., triaditis)

Dogs:

- Cholecystitis
- Gallbladder perforation
- Bile peritonitis due to gallbladder rupture
- Biliary adenocarcinoma (rare)

Clinical Presentation

DISEASE FORMS/SUBTYPES

- Cholelithiasis without specific clinical signs
  - Incidental finding on abdominal radiographs or ultrasound performed for another reason

- Cholelithiasis associated with clinical signs
  - Gastrointestinal disease
  - Biliary obstruction
  - Peritonitis when cholelithiasis is associated with biliary disruption/rupture

HISTORY, CHIEF COMPLAINT

- Generally nonspecific: malaise and gastrointestinal signs predominate
- Dogs: vomiting, anorexia, lethargy, weakness, polydipsia, polyuria, weight loss
- Cats: vomiting, dehydration, anorexia, lethargy
- NOTE: choleliths may be an incidental finding in dogs and cats and may not be associated with any clinical signs.

PHYSICAL EXAM FINDINGS

- Icterus is common when cholelithiasis is associated with cholangitis, cholecystitis, gallbladder obstruction, or gallbladder rupture and bile peritonitis.
- Fever may be noted in dogs in association with infection and/or bile peritonitis.
- Signs of abdominal pain are not consistently noted, even when biliary obstruction is present.

Etiology and Pathophysiology

- Cause is poorly understood
- In dogs and cats, most choleliths consist mainly of calcium rather than cholesterol (as seen in humans).
- Choleliths may obstruct the extrahepatic biliary system (p. 118).
- Hypercoagulability has been documented in dogs with extrahepatic biliary obstructions by using thromboelastography.
- Decreased bile secretion into the intestine may result in decreased binding of endotoxin, predisposing to endotoxemia.
- Cholelithiasis has been associated with concurrent cholecystitis and gallbladder rupture, resulting in bile peritonitis (pp. 118 and 779).

DIAGNOSIS

Diagnostic Overview

Diagnosis of this problem generally requires diagnostic imaging. Abdominal ultrasonography is the best diagnostic method.

Differential Diagnosis

Cholelithiasis with extrahepatic biliary obstruction and jaundice (p. 528):

- Hemolysis (i.e., prehepatic icterus) (pp. 59 and 60)
- Hepatic disease (i.e., hepatic icterus) (pp. 172, 442, 452, 458, 543, and 740)
- Biliary obstruction or rupture (i.e., post-hepatic icterus): pancreatitis, mucocele, biliary rupture, cholangitis, neoplasia, stricture, foreign body obstruction in the duodenum, diaphragmatic hernia
- Cholelithiasis without biliary obstruction: often incidental finding for any issue prompting abdominal imaging studies

Initial Database

- CBC: often normal; possible anemia, although usually mild; inflammatory leukogram
- Serum biochemistry profile: increased liver enzymes (proportional alkaline phosphatase [ALP] > alanine aminotransferase [ALT]), increased bilirubin with obstruction; ± increased amylase and lipase concentrations; ± hypokalemia
- Survey abdominal radiographs: may delineate radiopaque choleliths
- Survey thoracic radiographs: rule out metastatic disease if neoplasia is suspected.

Advanced or Confirmatory Testing

Abdominal ultrasound examination:

- Common bile duct dilation
  - Further delineate choleliths
  - Normal diameter of common bile duct in dogs and cats: 3-4 mm
  - Common bile duct dilation signifying obstruction: > 5 mm in cats, varies in dogs
- Evaluate gallbladder in dogs with concurrent cholecystitis
  - Wall thickness
  - Contents: choleliths, mucocele
  - Presence of attached omentum: indicates rupture
  - Surrounding fluid: indicates severe inflammation or rupture
- Evaluate intestine for increased wall thickness and loss of layering associated with neoplasia or inflammatory bowel disease.
- Obtain and perform analysis of peritoneal fluid (pp. 1056 and 1343)
  - Bilirubin concentration (elevated: bile peritonitis)
  - Cytologic examination and microbiologic culture and sensitivity testing: septic peritonitis
- Coagulation profile (p. 1325), thromboelastography

TREATMENT

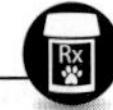

Treatment Overview

- If the choleliths are an incidental finding, no treatment is required. The patient should be monitored for development of clinical signs associated with cholelithiasis.
- If signs of biliary stasis, disruption, or obstruction are noted, patient stabilization and surgical intervention are necessary.

Acute General Treatment

- Rehydration by intravenous administration of balanced electrolyte solution
- Normalization of serum electrolyte concentrations
- Parenteral antibiotics effective against gram-negative bacteria and anaerobes
  - Empirical therapy
    - Cefoxitin 30 mg/kg IV q 4-6h perioperatively, then q 6h (dogs and cats), *or*
    - Metronidazole 7.5-15 mg/kg IV q 12h *with*
    - Enrofloxacin 5-15 mg/kg (dogs; 5 mg/kg for cats) q 24h IV
    - Add ampicillin 22 mg/kg IV q 6-8h to cefoxitin for gram-positive coverage (dogs and cats)
  - Specific long-term therapy based on culture and sensitivity test results
- Possible administration of fresh-frozen plasma (if hypoproteinemia, coagulopathy)
- Vitamin K administration
- Removal of choleliths/relief of extrahepatic biliary obstruction
- Duodenotomy and retrograde flushing of the biliary system
- Choledochotomy for removal of one or two large choleliths
- Cholecystectomy
  - Results in the best long-term prognosis if all stones are removed and biliary system is patent
- Common bile duct stenting
- Cholecystoduodenostomy/jejunostomy
- Tube cholecystostomy
- Treatment of bile peritonitis if biliary disruption has occurred (p. 779)

Chronic Treatment

Maintain bile flow using ursodeoxycholic acid 10-15 mg/kg PO q 24h; contraindicated while gallbladder obstruction is present

Nutrition/Diet

Provide access for enteral feeding if patient is anorexic (pp. 1106, 1107, and 1109).

- Gastrostomy/jejunostomy tubes may be placed intraoperatively.

Possible Complications

Recurrence of cholelithiasis, bile leakage, pancreatitis, peritonitis, endotoxemia, sepsis, death

Recommended Monitoring

- If clinical signs were/are present
  - Clinical and laboratory parameters assessing perfusion, including capillary refill time, pulse rate and quality, blood pressure, urine output, arterial pH, and lactate concentrations
  - Respiratory function
  - Serum liver enzymes and bilirubin concentrations
  - Coagulation profile
- If incidental finding
  - Physical exam and serum biochemistry profile every 6 months

PROGNOSIS & OUTCOME

- Fair in clinically ill animals if all choleliths removed and a cholecystectomy is performed
- Guarded if cholelithiasis is associated with biliary leakage and aseptic bile peritonitis
- Poor for patients with septic bile peritonitis
- Open prognosis for patients without clinical signs (incidental finding)

PEARLS & CONSIDERATIONS

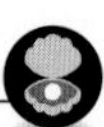

Comments

- Although cholelithiasis is common in people, it is uncommon in pets.
- In cats, liver biopsy and culture, bile culture, and small intestinal biopsies should be obtained at the time of surgery because of the association of biliary obstructive disease (cholelithiasis) with cholangitis/cholangiohepatitis and inflammatory bowel disease.
- The role, if any for ursodeoxycholic acid in dogs or cats with incidentally discovered cholelithiasis but with no evidence of illness remains to be determined. Some clinicians favor treatment in the hope that it might reduce the risk of later illness or obstruction.
- Biliary surgery should be performed by experienced surgeon.

Technician Tips

Chole(cysto)liths may be an incidental finding on abdominal radiographs taken to investigate another problem.

SUGGESTED READING

Kanemoto H, et al: Intrahepatic cholelithiasis in dogs and cats: a case series. Can Vet J 58:971-973, 2017.

AUTHOR: David Holt, BVSc, DACVS
EDITOR: Elizabeth A. Swanson, DVM, MS, DACVS

Cholecalciferol and Vitamin D_3 Analog Toxicosis

Client Education Sheet

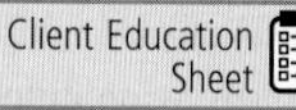

BASIC INFORMATION

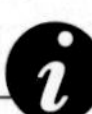

Definition

Cholecalciferol (vitamin D_3) and its synthetic analogs are used as dietary supplements, topical medications for psoriasis, and as rodenticides. Toxicosis is characterized by hypercalcemia, hyperphosphatemia, soft-tissue mineralization, and renal failure.

Synonyms

- Cholecalciferol = vitamin D_3
- Ergocalciferol = vitamin D_2
- Calcitriol = 1,25-dihydrocholecalciferol
- Calcipotriene, calcipotriol (Dovonex, Taclonex) = 1,25-dihydrocholecalciferol analog
- Tacalcitol = 1,24-dihydrocholecalciferol analog

Epidemiology

SPECIES, AGE, SEX

All species are susceptible; dogs more likely to be involved

RISK FACTORS

- Juveniles and animals with pre-existing renal disease are more at risk.
- Presence of vitamin D or its analogs in pet's environment

CONTAGION AND ZOONOSIS

Secondary (i.e., relay) toxicosis (consumption of prey that has ingested cholecalciferol) has not been reported.

GEOGRAPHY AND SEASONALITY

Rodenticide intoxication incidence increases in fall and winter.

Clinical Presentation

HISTORY, CHIEF COMPLAINT

- History of ingestion of vitamin D or its analogs (source: dietary supplements, topical human medications, or rodenticides)
- Anorexia, vomiting, lethargy within 12-24 hours after ingestion
- Polyuria/polydipsia (PU/PD) within 24-72 hours, followed by oliguria/anuria

PHYSICAL EXAM FINDINGS

- Depression, lethargy, weakness
- Vomiting (possibly with blood), diarrhea (melena rare)
- Dehydration
- Cardiac arrhythmias (rare, usually bradycardia)
- Dyspnea (rare)
- Seizures (rare)

Etiology and Pathophysiology

- Vitamin D and its analogs increase intestinal absorption of calcium (Ca), stimulate resorption of Ca from bone, and decrease renal excretion of Ca. This results in hypercalcemia and hyperphosphatemia.
- Unregulated increases in Ca and phosphorous (PO_4) lead to soft-tissue mineralization (especially kidneys, myocardium, large blood vessels, and gastrointestinal [GI] tract) and secondary renal failure.

DIAGNOSIS

Diagnostic Overview

Diagnosis is based on history of exposure, compatible clinical signs, and characteristic laboratory findings. Hypercalcemia and hyperphosphatemia occur in all clinically important cases. Extreme hypercalcemia in a previously healthy young animal should increase suspicion for intoxication.

Differential Diagnosis

Hypercalcemia (pp. 491 and 1232)

Initial Database

- CBC, serum biochemistry profile
  - Baseline if possible (<8 hours after exposure)
  - Monitor Ca, PO_4, blood urea nitrogen (BUN), creatinine q 24h for at least 4 days or longer if animal becomes symptomatic.
  - If serum product of Ca (mg/dL) × PO_4 (mg/dL) is rising (>60), therapy is required (risk of soft-tissue mineralization occurs when Ca × PO_4 > 60-70). Because young animals may have Ca × PO_4 that normally exceeds 60, monitor trends.
- Urinalysis: isosthenuria or hyposthenuria are common (p. 1390)
- Radiographs: soft-tissue mineralization

Advanced or Confirmatory Testing

- Serum 25-hydroxycholecalciferol levels will be elevated with cholecalciferol toxicosis but will not detect calcipotriene. Due to turnaround time, testing is not usually clinically relevant.
- Serum parathyroid hormone (PTH) or parathyroid hormone–related peptide (PTHrP) are sometimes measured to help distinguish between differential diagnoses. With toxicosis, PTH levels are low and PTHrP undetectable (pp. 491 and 1370).
- Histopathologic evidence of tissue mineralization (kidney, aorta, GI mucosa, lungs, heart)
  - Total wet weight Ca may be elevated in kidneys (300-1000 ppm [normal, 100-150 ppm])

TREATMENT

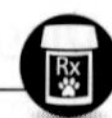

Treatment Overview

- Soon after exposure, prevent absorption to decrease the risk of clinical signs.
- When Ca and PO_4 are elevated, treatment is aimed at lowering these values to prevent soft-tissue mineralization by promoting calciuresis and reducing PO_4 absorption. Management of renal complications is also necessary.
- Complicated cases may need to be managed for days to weeks, and referral to a 24-hour care facility is optimal.

Acute General Treatment

Treatment needed if confirmed cholecalciferol ingestion > 0.1 mg/kg *or* calcipotriene > 10 mcg/kg.

- Emesis if < 1 hour since ingestion (up to 4 hours with rodent baits) (p. 1188)

- One dose of activated charcoal (1-2 g/kg) with cathartic, followed by cholestyramine 300 mg/kg PO q 8h for 4 days. Cholestyramine is a resin that binds bile acids and disrupts the enterohepatic recirculation of vitamin D.
- If Ca is increasing, promote calciuresis: 0.9% NaCl IV (adjust rates as needed); furosemide 2.5-4.5 mg/kg PO, IM, or IV q 6-8h; prednisolone 1-2 mg/kg/day PO divided
- Hyperphosphatemia: aluminum (or magnesium) hydroxide 30-90 mg/kg/day PO divided
- If still hypercalcemic after all of the above: pamidronate 1.3-2 mg/kg IV over 2 hours; repeat in 3-7 days if needed (caution in juveniles)
- Address acute kidney injury (p. 23).

Chronic Treatment

Several days to weeks of oral therapy may be needed until Ca normalizes.

Nutrition/Diet

With anorexia, use of feeding tubes may be indicated (p. 1106). Use diet low in Ca and PO_4, such as a renal diet.

Drug Interactions

Avoid Ca-containing fluids.

Possible Complications

- Calcification of soft tissues (irreversible): chronic kidney disease, arrhythmias, aneurysms
- Pulmonary edema (mineralization and leakage of pulmonary vessels)

Recommended Monitoring

Follow serum Ca, PO_4, BUN, and creatinine levels daily, then weekly until they remain normal without medical support. If no elevations by day 4, therapy can be stopped.

PROGNOSIS & OUTCOME

- Good prognosis if animal is decontaminated and treated before persistent hypercalcemia and soft-tissue mineralization occurs.
- Prognosis is poor to guarded with prolonged elevations in Ca, leading to soft-tissue mineralization. Tissue calcification is not reversible and can lead to chronic GI or renal issues and potentially rupture of great vessels (aneurysm).

PEARLS & CONSIDERATIONS

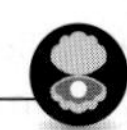

Comments

- 1 IU of vitamin D_3 = 0.000025 mg
- Prescription strength vitamin D is available in 50,000 IU (1.25 mg).

Prevention

Prevent pet access to all vitamin D or analog-containing products.

Technician Tips

Many times, anorexia or vomiting is the first indication that the serum Ca is increasing.

Client Education

Pet proofing is important for medications and rodenticides.

SUGGESTED READING

Rumbeiha WK: Cholecalciferol. In Peterson ME, et al, editors: Small animal toxicology, ed 3, St. Louis, 2013, Saunders, pp 489-498.

AUTHOR & EDITOR: Tina Wismer, DVM, MS, DABVT, DABT

Chondrosarcoma

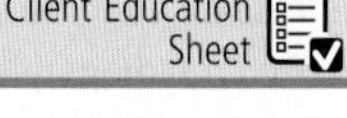

BASIC INFORMATION

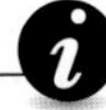

Definition

Chondrosarcoma (CSA) is a malignant mesenchymal tumor that produces chondroid and fibrillar matrix but never osteoid.

Epidemiology

SPECIES, AGE, SEX

- In dogs, CSA is the second most common primary bone tumor, accounting for 5%-10% of all primary bone tumors.
  - Median age is about 8 years (reported range, 1-15 years).
  - There is no sex predisposition.
- In cats, primary bone tumors are uncommon, and CSA is third in incidence behind osteosarcoma and fibrosarcoma. CSA also can occur in the soft tissues at sites of previous vaccinations (p. 550).

GENETICS, BREED PREDISPOSITION

- CSA is most common in medium- to large-breed dogs weighing 20-40 kg.
- Mixed-breed dogs, golden retrievers, boxers, and German shepherd dogs are overrepresented.

Clinical Presentation

DISEASE FORMS/SUBTYPES

- Most CSAs arise from flat bones: 30% occur in the nasal cavity, accounting for 15% of all nasal tumors, and 20% of CSAs arise from the ribs, accounting for 30%-40% of all primary rib tumors.
- Of CSAs, 20% arise from the appendicular skeleton, often but not always at sites where osteosarcoma typically occurs. CSA accounts for only 3%-5% of all primary bone tumors in the appendicular skeleton.
- Other reported sites include facial bones, skull, vertebrae, pelvis, digits, and os penis.
- Rarely, CSA can arise in soft-tissue (extraskeletal) sites, including the larynx and trachea.

HISTORY, CHIEF COMPLAINT

- Patients often present with a visible mass at the affected site. Additional clinical signs vary with the site of involvement.
- Nasal CSA usually is associated with unilateral or bilateral epistaxis. Other clinical signs include sneezing, mucopurulent discharge, respiratory effort, and swelling over the nasal cavity.
- Appendicular CSA usually is associated with lameness.

PHYSICAL EXAM FINDINGS

- Findings for CSA will depend on the anatomic location. Often, but not always, a firm to hard mass will be palpable.
- Patients with nasal CSA often have reduced airflow through the nares, and hemorrhagic discharge might be present. More advanced tumors may be associated with a visible mass effect (externally or orally). The ipsilateral eye may not retropulse or may be exophthalmic.
- Rib CSA most commonly arises near the costochondral junction. Any rib can be affected.
- Patients with appendicular and digital CSA are variably lame, ranging from minimal to non–weight-bearing.

Etiology and Pathophysiology

The cause is largely unknown. Osteochondromatosis (multiple cartilaginous exostoses) lesions can undergo malignant transformation to CSA or, less commonly, osteosarcoma.

DIAGNOSIS

Diagnostic Overview

CSA is not the most common primary bone tumor, but it still should be considered as a differential when an aggressive bone lesion is identified, especially when the lesion involves the rib or nasal cavity. Histopathology is required for definitive diagnosis.

Differential Diagnosis

General differential diagnoses for aggressive bone lesions:

- Other primary bone tumors: osteosarcoma, fibrosarcoma, hemangiosarcoma

- Metastatic bone tumors: transitional cell, prostatic, mammary, thyroid, anal sac apocrine gland carcinomas
- Tumors that locally invade adjacent bone: nasal carcinoma; oral tumors (squamous cell carcinoma, melanoma, fibrosarcoma, ameloblastoma), synovial cell sarcoma, histiocytic sarcoma, digital tumors (squamous cell carcinoma, melanoma)
- Hematopoietic tumors: myeloma, lymphoma. Radiographic lesions typically are purely lytic.
- Bacterial or fungal osteomyelitis

Additional differentials for epistaxis (p. 1221)

Initial Database

- Radiographic imaging of the primary tumor
  - The aggressive bone changes associated with CSA are the same as those seen with osteosarcoma (p. 726).
  - Nasal neoplasia is most often associated with soft-tissue opacity in the nasal cavity and/or frontal sinuses, as well as destruction of the turbinates, nasal septum, vomer, or surrounding palatine, maxillary, and/or frontal bones.
  - Primary rib tumors often can be distinguished from tumors originating from the lung by the presence of an extrapleural sign, characterized by a smoothly marginated indentation of the lung that tapers gradually at the junction of the thoracic wall.
- After a radiographic or histologic diagnosis, patients should be completely staged with a CBC, chemistry panel, urinalysis, and three-view thoracic radiographs.

Advanced or Confirmatory Testing

- For axial tumors, CT imaging is recommended to more accurately stage local disease and help with planning surgery and/or radiation therapy. CT imaging can be done in place of radiographic studies.
  - For nasal tumors, CT is superior to radiographs for detecting soft-tissue opacity within the nasal cavity and surrounding sinuses, bony destruction, and extension through the cribriform plate into the brain.
  - If a patient is undergoing CT, concurrent imaging of the lungs is recommended as a more sensitive way to screen for pulmonary metastasis.
- For accessible tumors, fine-needle aspiration (FNA) for cytologic evaluation is a minimally invasive procedure that can help support a diagnosis of CSA.
  - FNA can be considered for lesions with associated bony cortical destruction. Ultrasound guidance can be used to aid sample collection.
  - Alkaline phosphatase cytochemical analysis on FNA samples is recommended. Alkaline phosphatase is a highly sensitive and fairly specific marker for osteosarcoma, and a positive result would make a diagnosis of CSA less likely.
- Histopathologic evaluation is required to confirm the diagnosis of CSA.
  - For nasal tumors and large, nonresectable tumors, an incisional biopsy is recommended. For resectable tumors, an incisional biopsy is not contraindicated, but it is reasonable to surgically remove all local disease, with biopsy submission after surgery.

TREATMENT

Treatment Overview

Nasal CSA, like most other nasal tumors, is most effectively treated with radiation therapy (RT). For CSAs arising in other locations, surgery is indicated whenever possible. Palliative therapy, which focuses on controlling pain and other associated clinical signs, is recommended for advanced-stage tumors or when definitive therapy is declined.

Acute General Treatment

- Treatment of nasal CSA (p. 680)
- The treatment of choice for rib CSA is wide surgical resection. Multiple ribs and/or underlying lung may need to be removed. Prosthetic mesh may be needed for thoracic wall closure, and diaphragmatic advancement techniques may be necessary for caudal thoracic tumors.
  - Adjuvant RT is recommended if excision is incomplete, but there is little information regarding efficacy.
- The treatment of choice for appendicular CSA is amputation. Limb-sparing techniques can be considered for tumors arising from the distal radius, distal ulna, or proximal femur.
- For CSA arising from other sites, wide surgical excision is recommended whenever possible. When excision is incomplete, adjuvant RT may help improve local control, but there is limited information regarding efficacy. Stereotactic RT has not been evaluated for CSA. However, based on experience with osteosarcoma (p. 726), it should be considered for nonresectable CSA.
- There is no information regarding the efficacy of chemotherapy for the treatment of CSA; it is not routinely recommended.
- Palliative care is indicated for patients with advanced local disease or visible metastasis and when owners decline definitive therapy.
  - Nonsteroidal antiinflammatory drug (NSAID) choices include aspirin 10-25 mg/kg PO q 8-24h; carprofen 2 mg/kg PO q 12h; deracoxib 1-2 mg/kg PO q 24h, may use 3-4 mg/kg PO q 24h for first 7 days only; meloxicam 0.1 mg/kg PO q 24h; or firocoxib 5 mg/kg PO q 24h.
  - Other oral analgesic drugs include acetaminophen with codeine (never in cats) (Tylenol #4 = 300 mg acetaminophen, 60 mg codeine) 0.5-2 mg/kg PO q 6-8h, with dosing based on codeine; tramadol 2-5 mg/kg PO q 6-12h; gabapentin 10-15 mg/kg PO q 8-12h; amantadine 3-5 mg/kg PO q 24h.
  - Pamidronate (1-2 mg/kg diluted in saline IV over 2 hours) and zoledronate (0.1 mg/kg diluted in saline IV over 15 minutes) are bisphosphonates that increase bone mineral density and can reduce the pain associated with bone tumors. They have been studied most thoroughly for the treatment of osteosarcoma (p. 726).
  - Palliative RT effectively controls the pain associated with bone tumors. Most information regarding efficacy is from the treatment of osteosarcoma, but similar benefits are seen in patients with CSA.
  - Patients with pulmonary metastasis or nasal congestion often benefit from anti-inflammatory doses of oral glucocorticoids such as prednisone 0.5-1 mg/kg PO q 24h (do not combine with NSAIDs).

Recommended Monitoring

Patients should be evaluated every 2-3 months with a physical examination. Thoracic radiographs should be performed every 4-6 months. Imaging of the site of the primary tumor may be indicated, depending on location, completeness of excision, and clinical signs.

PROGNOSIS & OUTCOME

Nasal CSA: distant metastasis is uncommon.

- With conventional RT, median survival is ≈15 months. Patients with nasal CSA are 3.3 times less likely to have local recurrence than are patients with nasal carcinomas.
- For patients with nasal tumors in general, extension into the frontal sinuses and/or erosion through the bones of the nasal passage is associated with a 2.3-fold increase in risk of local recurrence. Unilateral versus bilateral involvement is not a significant prognostic factor.
- There is limited information regarding prognosis with stereotactic RT, but it likely is similar or better compared to conventional RT.
- With palliative care alone, survival times are ≈3 months.

Non-nasal CSA:

- 15%-30% develop metastatic disease (lungs most common).
- With aggressive surgery, median survival is > 3 years, and many dogs will enjoy long-term local control. However, depending on tumor location and completeness of excision, up to 40% will develop local recurrence.
- With palliative care alone, survival times of > 1 year are still possible depending on tumor location, patient clinical signs and comfort, and rate of tumor growth.

PEARLS & CONSIDERATIONS

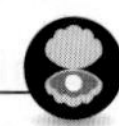

Comments

Chondroblastic osteosarcoma can resemble CSA on small biopsy samples. Whenever possible, always submit the entire lesion for histopathologic evaluation.

Technician Tips

When CSA is suspected, use caution when positioning the patient for radiographs to minimize pain and risk of pathologic fracture.

SUGGESTED READING

Waltman SS, et al: Clinical outcome of nonnasal chondrosarcoma in dogs: thirty-one cases (1986-2003). Vet Surg 36:266-271, 2007.

AUTHOR: Dennis B. Bailey, DVM, DACVIM
EDITOR: Kenneth M. Rassnick, DVM, DACVIM

Chronic Kidney Disease, Occult (Asymptomatic)

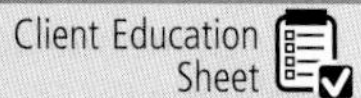

BASIC INFORMATION

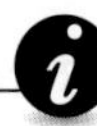

Definition

- Chronic kidney disease (CKD): an abnormality in renal structure or function existing for longer than 3 months
- International Renal Interest Society (IRIS) staging system for CKD: classification scheme for canine and feline CKD based on serum creatinine and symmetric dimethylarginine (SDMA), with substages for proteinuria and blood pressure (BP):
    - At risk: creatinine < 1.4 mg/dL (<124 mmol/mL), dogs; < 1.6 mg/dL (<141 mmol/mL), cats. SDMA ≤ 14 mcg/dL, dogs and cats. History suggests increased risk of CKD (e.g., exposure to nephrotoxic drugs, breed, old age)
    - Stage I: creatinine < 1.4 mg/dL (<124 mmol/mL), dogs; < 1.6 mg/dL (<141 mmol/mL), cats. SDMA > 14 mcg/dL, dogs and cats. Nonazotemic. Some other renal abnormality present (e.g., inadequate concentrating ability without identifiable nonrenal cause; abnormal renal palpation, and/or abnormal renal imaging findings; persistent proteinuria of renal origin; abnormal renal biopsy results; progressively increasing creatinine concentration)
    - Stage II: creatinine 1.4-2 mg/dL (124-177 mmol/mL), dogs; 1.6-2.8 mg/dL (141-248 mmol/mL), cats. Mild renal azotemia (lower end of the range lies within the reference range for many labs, but the insensitivity of creatinine as a screening test means that animals with creatinine values close to the upper end of the reference range often have excretory failure). Clinical signs usually absent
    - Stage III: creatinine 2.1-5 mg/dL (186-442 mmol/mL), dogs; 2.9-5 mg/dL (256-442 mmol/mL), cats. Moderate renal azotemia. Systemic clinical signs often present.
    - Stage IV: creatinine > 5 mg/dL (>442 mmol/mL), dogs and cats. Severe renal azotemia. Systemic clinical signs usually present
- Occult CKD: CKD in which no clinical signs are present. Usually corresponds to IRIS stage I or II but has been documented in stages III and IV.
- CKD causing overt clinical signs (p. 169)

Synonyms

- Subclinical CKD, latent CKD, preclinical CKD, renal insufficiency
- The terms *kidney failure* and *chronic renal failure* are no longer preferred for use.

Epidemiology

SPECIES, AGE, SEX

- CKD is one of the most common geriatric diseases of cats.
- Canine CKD occurs less frequently, but manifests in geriatric patients and juvenile patients (congenital CKD).

GENETICS, BREED PREDISPOSITION

- Multiple studies have not identified a breed predisposition in cats, but reports do exist of increased frequency in Maine coon, Abyssinian, Siamese, Russian Blue, Burmese, and Ragdoll cats.
- Familial nephropathies may lead to early-onset CKD and are reported in numerous breeds of dogs and cats (p. 169).

RISK FACTORS

Advanced age, prior episode of acute kidney injury (including nephrotoxic exposure, obstructive disease, or infectious disease), familial/breed disposition

ASSOCIATED DISORDERS

Cardiovascular disease (e.g., systemic hypertension in cats and dogs), endocrinopathies (e.g., hyperthyroidism and hyperaldosteronism in cats, renal secondary hyperparathyroidism in cats and dogs), and urinary tract infections (UTIs)

Clinical Presentation

HISTORY, CHIEF COMPLAINT

Occult CKD is usually detected incidentally by routine geriatric or pre-anesthetic screening or during investigation of unrelated illness.

PHYSICAL EXAM FINDINGS

Frequently no abnormal findings. Small or irregular kidneys may be palpated.

Etiology and Pathophysiology

- CKD is the result of a variety of insults to the kidney. If the glomerulus is irreversibly damaged, the associated tubule will degenerate, and vice versa.
- Histopathologic renal lesions consist primarily of inflammatory infiltrates in the tubulointerstitium, in the glomeruli, or in both simultaneously. Concurrent fibrosis is usually present to various degrees. Additional findings include tubular atrophy and glomerular sclerosis or senescence.
- As nephrons are lost, the remaining nephrons hypertrophy. Although initially adaptive, glomerular hypertension damages the nephron, leading to further nephron loss. After a certain amount of damage has been sustained (generally when creatinine > 3.5 mg/dL [>309 mmol/mL]), kidney disease may be progressive despite resolution of the initiating cause.
- The specific cause of CKD is often undetermined.
    - Tubulointerstitial nephritis: most common cause in cats
    - Glomerular disease: most common cause in dogs
    - Other demonstrable causes: amyloidosis, renal dysplasia, polycystic kidney disease, lymphoma, chronic pyelonephritis, obstructing nephroliths or ureteroliths, vasculitis, infarction, and sequelae to acute kidney injury with incomplete resolution
    - Obstructive nephropathy from previous or current ureterolithiasis is increasingly recognized in cats.

DIAGNOSIS

Diagnostic Overview

CKD may be diagnosed based on structural (e.g., nephrolithiasis, renal size/shape changes, polycystic disease) or functional (e.g., proteinuria, azotemia, inadequately concentrated urine) abnormalities.

Differential Diagnosis

Azotemia:

- Increased blood urea nitrogen (BUN) from extrarenal factors (e.g., high-protein diet, gastrointestinal bleeding)

- Hemodynamic azotemia (e.g., dehydration, hypotension) typically distinguished from CKD by urine specific gravity (concentrated with hemodynamic azotemia, inadequately concentrated with CKD).
- Intrinsic azotemia with inadequately concentrated urine may be due to kidney disease (most commonly) or to dehydration (i.e., hemodynamic azotemia) combined with extrarenal impairment of urine concentration.
  - Drug therapy (e.g., diuretics, glucocorticoids)
  - Osmotic diuresis (e.g., diabetes mellitus)
  - Impaired medullary concentration gradient (e.g., hypoadrenocorticism, portosystemic shunting)
  - Central diabetes insipidus
  - Nephrogenic diabetes insipidus (e.g., hypercalcemia, pyometra, pyelonephritis)
- Postrenal azotemia (e.g., urinary obstruction, rupture) is generally differentiated from kidney disease by dysuria or imaging and biochemical findings consistent with uroperitoneum, respectively.

Initial Database

- CBC: usually unremarkable; occasionally mild anemia
- Serum biochemistry profile: azotemia, hyperphosphatemia, hypokalemia, metabolic acidosis, and hypercholesterolemia occur to various degrees.
- Urinalysis: frequently isosthenuric or minimally concentrated specific gravity (dogs < 1.030; cats < 1.035). Active sediment may indicate UTI. Proteinuria should be quantified by urine protein/creatinine ratio.
- Urine culture may be indicated to rule out infection.
- Symmetric dimethylarginine (SDMA): this relatively new blood test may detect CKD earlier than creatinine and is less affected by loss of lean body mass. If occult CKD is suspected but creatinine is normal, SDMA may be useful (p. 1381).
- Thyroid hormone assay (elderly cats): rule out hyperthyroidism as concurrent disorder.
  - Some of the clinical signs of hyperthyroidism (particularly polyuria and polydipsia) can mimic those of CKD.
  - Correction of hyperthyroidism can exacerbate azotemia.
  - In cats that have both hyperthyroidism and CKD, treatment emphasis is placed on the disease most responsible for clinical signs (p. 503).
- BP (p. 1065): hypertension (systolic BP > 160-179 mm Hg, diastolic BP > 95-119 mm Hg) present in 20% of cats with CKD; may cause end-organ damage (especially heart, eyes, central nervous system, kidneys).
- Abdominal radiographs and/or ultrasound: may further elucidate cause of or factors contributing to CKD (e.g., obstructing or partially obstructing nephroliths or ureteroliths, renal neoplasia, polycystic disease, perinephric pseudocysts). Alterations of shape, size, and echogenicity of kidneys are common.

Advanced or Confirmatory Testing

- Urine protein/creatinine ratio: pathologic proteinuria (urine protein/creatinine [UPC] ratio > 0.5 [dogs], > 0.2-0.4 [cats]; urinary sediment is inactive, and culture is negative) provides prognostic information as well as a therapeutic target.
- Glomerular filtration rate (GFR) measurement: can confirm inadequate GFR, particularly when azotemia is absent or cause of impaired urine concentration is unclear. Iohexol clearance, creatinine clearance, and nuclear scintigraphy are most commonly used.
- CKD in cats may complicate the diagnosis of concurrent hyperthyroidism by suppressing total thyroxine. Additional thyroid testing may be warranted if total thyroxine (T_4) value is normal but hyperthyroidism suspected clinically (p. 503).

TREATMENT

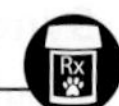

Treatment Overview

The treatment goal is to slow progression of kidney disease.

Acute General Treatment

Because patients are asymptomatic, acute treatment is not needed.

Chronic Treatment

- For patients with proteinuria, renin-angiotensin-aldosterone system (RAAS) inhibition (e.g., angiotensin-converting enzyme [ACE] inhibition, angiotensin receptor blockade) reduces proteinuria in cats and dogs and slows progression of kidney disease in dogs (enalapril or benazepril 0.25-0.5 mg/kg PO q 12-24h initially) (pp. 51 and 390).
- As kidney disease progresses, animals may decompensate (show overt signs caused by CKD). For specific therapeutic recommendations, see p. 169.

Nutrition/Diet

- Diets specifically formulated for dogs and cats with kidney disease slow progression of CKD:
  - The level of kidney dysfunction at which a renal diet should be introduced is controversial. It may be best to transition to a renal diet that is palatable to the patient when renal disease is occult or mild, rather than waiting until the animal is overtly ill (uremic).
  - The low-solute characteristics of most renal diets may reduce the urine volume modestly in some patients with polyuria.
  - There are many different brands of renal diet, and acceptance of different formulations varies with the individual patient.
  - Homemade renal diets may also be used but should be formulated by a board-certified veterinary nutritionist.
  - Maintaining adequate caloric intake and avoiding protein malnutrition is paramount.
- A gradual (over several weeks) and methodical introduction to the renal diet often results in a higher compliance rate.

Drug Interactions

- Nephrotoxic drugs (e.g., aminoglycosides) or drug combinations (e.g., nonsteroidal antiinflammatory drugs [NSAIDs] plus ACE inhibitors) should be avoided whenever possible, and if a nephrotoxic drug is used, clients should be counseled to discontinue if signs of illness become manifest.
- Dosage adjustment of most drugs is unnecessary at this stage of CKD.
- Phosphate binders can interfere with absorption of orally administered medications, especially antibiotics and fat-soluble vitamins.

Recommended Monitoring

- Stable patients with incidental CKD should be monitored every 3-6 months.
- Evaluations should include body weight, CBC (or at least packed cell volume), serum biochemistry profile with electrolytes, and BP measurement.
- Clinical manifestations of hypokalemia, hyperphosphatemia, anemia, and hypertension may not occur until they result in severe clinical manifestations; early interventions can be based on detection by routine screening.
- Urinalysis +/− urine protein/creatinine ratio every 6-12 months.
- Urine culture should be performed if suspicion of lower or upper urinary tract infection exists.

PROGNOSIS & OUTCOME

- Some animals with incidental CKD may remain stable and free of clinical signs for years, but others progress more rapidly.
- There are no reliable predictors of the rate of progression of kidney disease, except perhaps the presence of proteinuria (as quantified by UPC) and body condition score (for dogs).

PEARLS & CONSIDERATIONS

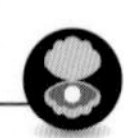

Comments

- Occult CKD may progress slowly or rapidly; the course of progression cannot be predicted. Advanced age, higher plasma creatinine and phosphorus levels, and proteinuria generally are associated with more rapid progression. As with rate of progression, survival time is highly varied and likely influenced by owners' decisions for euthanasia at various stages of disease.
- If anesthesia or potentially nephrotoxic drugs (e.g., ACE inhibitors) must be used, ensure adequate hydration and monitor carefully for deterioration in renal function.

Technician Tips

The technician can help clients develop a plan for a gradual transition from a maintenance diet to a renal diet.

Client Education

Animals with occult CKD should be promptly presented to a veterinarian for signs of clinical illness because they may be less able to cope with extrarenal disorders, especially those that predispose to dehydration. For instance, vomiting from any cause may lead to dehydration, which may worsen renal function, leading to exacerbation of all extrarenal clinical signs, as well as manifestations of uremia. Prompt fluid therapy (IV or SQ, depending on severity and underlying illness) may be required to interrupt this cycle.

SUGGESTED READING

Quimby JM: Update on medical management of clinical manifestations of chronic kidney disease. Vet Clin North Am Small Anim Pract 46:1163-1181, 2016.

AUTHORS: Catherine E. Langston, DVM, DACVIM; Adam Eatroff, DVM, DACVIM
EDITOR: Leah A. Cohn, DVM, PhD, DACVIM

Chronic Kidney Disease, Overt (Symptomatic)

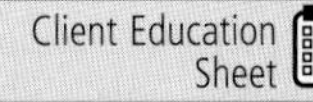

BASIC INFORMATION

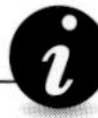

Definition

- Chronic kidney disease (CKD): an abnormality in renal structure or function existing for longer than 3 months
- International Renal Interest Society (IRIS) staging system for CKD: classification scheme for canine and feline CKD based on serum creatinine, with substages for proteinuria and blood pressure (p. 167)
- Overt CKD: CKD that manifests clinical signs, most commonly secondary to uremia. Usually corresponds to IRIS stage III or IV, but clinical signs occasionally are present in stages I and II.
- Azotemia is an increased concentration of blood urea nitrogen and/or creatinine. Uremia is the constellation of clinical signs associated with excretory renal failure (i.e., not all azotemic animals are uremic).
- Occult CKD: incidentally discovered, not producing overt signs (p. 167)

Synonyms

- Clinical CKD, decompensated CKD, symptomatic CKD, uremic CKD
- *Kidney failure* and *chronic renal failure* are no longer preferred terms.

Epidemiology

SPECIES, AGE, SEX

- CKD is one of the most common geriatric diseases of cats, but it can occur in cats of any age.
- Canine CKD occurs less frequently but manifests in both geriatric and juvenile patients (e.g., congenital renal disease).

GENETICS, BREED PREDISPOSITION

- Multiple studies have not identified a breed predisposition in cats, but reports exist of increased frequency in Maine coon, Abyssinian, Siamese, Russian blue, Burmese, and Ragdoll cats.
- Familial nephropathies may lead to early-onset CKD. Familial nephropathies reported in Abyssinian cats, Persian cats, Siamese cats, Oriental cats, Alaskan malamutes, basenjis, beagles, Bedlington terriers, Bernese mountain dogs, boxers, Brittany spaniels, bull terriers, bullmastiffs, cairn terriers, chow chows, cocker spaniels, Dalmatians, Doberman pinschers, Dutch kooikers, English foxhounds, English springer spaniels, German shepherds, golden retrievers, keeshonds, Lhasa apsos, miniature schnauzers, navostas, Newfoundlands, Norwegian elkhounds, Pembroke Welsh corgis, rottweilers, Samoyeds, Shar-peis, shih tzus, soft-coated Wheaten terriers, standard poodles, and West Highland white terriers.

RISK FACTORS

Advanced age, prior episode of acute kidney injury (including nephrotoxic exposure, obstructive disease, or infection), familial/breed disposition

ASSOCIATED DISORDERS

In addition to disorders that occur concurrently with occult CKD (p. 167), comorbidities that occur in overt CKD include anemia, dehydration, electrolyte disorders, metabolic acidosis, ulcers (gastric or oral), vomiting, and weight loss/malnutrition.

Clinical Presentation

DISEASE FORMS/SUBTYPES

- Incidentally diagnosed in apparently healthy animals (occult CKD, typically IRIS stages I or II)
- Overtly ill (symptomatic) but stable patients (managed as outpatients)
- Decompensated patients (require hospitalization until stabilized)

HISTORY, CHIEF COMPLAINT

Some or all may be present.

- Polyuria/polydipsia (very common)
- Anorexia
- Weight loss
- Lethargy
- Halitosis
- Vomiting occurs in decompensated (uremic) animals.
- Altered consciousness (general dullness) in decompensated (uremic) animals
- Seizures (seen rarely; end-stage uremia)
- Abnormal hemostasis (rarely spontaneous bleeding; increased risk of bleeding with invasive procedures)

PHYSICAL EXAM FINDINGS

Some or all may be present.

- Signs of dehydration
- Kidney palpation: small, irregular kidneys (common) or large kidney (rare)
  - In cats, renal asymmetry is common after obstructive nephropathy or chronic ascending pyelonephritis.
  - Typically not painful on kidney palpation unless an acute insult is concurrent with CKD
- Uremic halitosis
- Oral ulceration (with severe azotemia)
- Poor haircoat
- Poor body/muscle condition
- Mucous membrane pallor (if anemic)
- Heart murmur or gallop rhythm (cats)

Etiology and Pathophysiology

See Chronic Kidney Disease, Occult (p. 167).

DIAGNOSIS

Diagnostic Overview

CKD may be diagnosed based on gross structural (e.g., nephrolithiasis, renal size/shape changes, polycystic disease) or functional (e.g., proteinuria, azotemia, persistent isosthenuria) abnormalities. Azotemia is always present if there are clinical signs of uremia.

Differential Diagnosis

Chronic kidney disease, occult (p. 167)

- Hemodynamic (i.e., prerenal) azotemia
- Azotemia with inadequately concentrated urine
  - CKD
  - Hemodynamic azotemia with extrarenal impairment of urine concentration (e.g., diuretics, hypoadrenocorticism, osmotic diuresis, diabetes insipidus)
- Postrenal azotemia (e.g., urinary obstruction, rupture)

Initial Database

- Assess hydration: azotemia may be exacerbated by dehydration. Hemodynamic azotemia may completely resolve with intravenous fluid therapy.
- CBC: nonregenerative anemia (due to erythropoietin deficiency, gastrointestinal [GI] bleeding, anemia of chronic disease, or a combination); severity varies.
- Serum biochemistry profile: azotemia, hyperphosphatemia, hypokalemia or hyperkalemia (rare), total hypercalcemia or ionized hypocalcemia (clinical signs of abnormal calcium concentrations are rare in the absence of concurrent diseases), hypercholesterolemia, and metabolic acidosis
- Urinalysis: usually isosthenuric (1.008-1.012) or minimally concentrated specific gravity (dogs: 1.013-1.030; cats: 1.013-1.035). Active sediment may indicate urinary tract infection (UTI). Proteinuria with inactive sediment exam should be quantified by urine protein/creatinine ratio.
- Urine culture: indicated with active sediment to investigate for pyelonephritis. Subclinical bacteruria can occur in cats with CKD
- Thyroid hormone assay (elderly cats): rule out hyperthyroidism as concurrent disorder (p. 503)
- Blood pressure (BP [p. 1065]): hypertension (systolic BP > 160-179 mm Hg, diastolic BP > 95-119 mm Hg) often identified; may cause end-organ damage (especially heart, eyes, central nervous system, kidneys)
- Abdominal radiographs and/or ultrasound: may further elucidate cause of or factors contributing to CKD (e.g., partially obstructing nephroliths or ureteroliths, renal neoplasia, cystic disease, perinephric pseudocysts, pyelectasia). Alterations of shape, size, and echogenicity of kidneys are common.

Advanced or Confirmatory Testing

- Glomerular filtration rate (GFR) measurement: not useful when azotemia is present
- Urine protein/creatinine ratio: pathologic proteinuria (urine protein/creatinine [UPC] ratio > 0.5 in dogs, > 0.2-0.4 in cats; urinary sediment is inactive, and culture is negative) provides prognostic information and a therapeutic target.
- Renal biopsy: indicated primarily with renomegaly (rule out lymphoma, feline infectious peritonitis, amyloidosis), persistent proteinuria, or in cases for which CKD cannot be otherwise distinguished from acute kidney injury.
- Although CKD in cats may complicate the diagnosis of concurrent hyperthyroidism by suppressing total thyroxine (T_4) value, advanced testing for hyperthyroidism is usually withheld until the patient's clinical signs have been addressed. Thyroid scintigraphy or combined measurement of free T_4 with total T_4 +/− thyroid-stimulating hormone is indicated to increase sensitivity of diagnosis for hyperthyroidism if total T_4 is normal but hyperthyroidism suspected.

TREATMENT

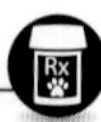

Treatment Overview

The goals of treatment are to alleviate clinical signs associated with uremia and slow progression of kidney disease. A global approach to diagnosis and treatment is outlined on p. 1406.

Acute General Treatment

Compensated state: see Chronic Treatment
Decompensated state (uremia; dehydrated, anorexic, vomiting)

- Hospitalization is ideal because oral therapies often poorly tolerated.
- Fluid therapy
  - Restoration of effective fluid volume over 4-12 hours is usually appropriate.
    - Replacement intravenous (IV) crystalloid fluid therapy (e.g., lactated Ringer's solution, Plasmalyte, 0.9% saline) should be based on the patient's presenting fluid deficit, as well as ongoing assessment of hydration status and acid-base/electrolyte status.
    - Fluid rate: replacement of dehydration (percent dehydration written as a decimal [e.g., 10% = 0.1] × kg body weight = liters deficit) plus ongoing losses (estimated volume of polyuria, vomiting) plus maintenance needs
  - Maintain intravascular volume.
    - Rate highly variable depending on degree of polyuria, extrarenal losses, and voluntary intake; 60-75 mL/kg/day is an appropriate starting point. Rate should be adjusted from this point based on acute changes in body weight and acid-base/electrolyte status.
    - Potassium supplementation of fluids based on electrolyte measurement (do not exceed 0.5 mEq/kg/h [p. 516])
- Vomiting or anorexia
  - Persistent nausea/vomiting
    - Maropitant 1 mg/kg SQ or IV *or* 2 mg/kg PO q 24h for 5 days; approved for use in cats
    - Ondansetron 0.1-0.5 mg/kg IV or SQ q 8-12h; dolasetron 0.6-1 mg/kg IV or SQ q 12-24h
    - Metoclopramide 0.2-0.4 mg/kg SQ q 6h *or* 0.04-0.08 mg/kg/h as constant-rate infusion
  - Address stomach ulcers (rare but may contribute to anemia due to GI blood loss)
    - Proton pump inhibitors (e.g., omeprazole 0.7 mg/kg PO q 24h *or* pantoprazole 1 mg/kg IV q 24h)
    - Histamine blockers (e.g., famotidine 0.2-0.5 mg/kg IV, SQ, PO q 24h) but less effective acid suppression than proton pump inhibitors
    - Sucralfate 0.25-1.0 g (total dose) PO q 8h until signs resolve
  - Other treatments described for chronic therapy may be applicable (see Chronic Treatment section). Injectable forms are used until oral medications are tolerated.
  - Parenteral antimicrobial therapy should be instituted if infection is present until oral administration of drugs is tolerated. Avoid nephrotoxic drugs.

Chronic Treatment

- Goals are delay of progression and optimization of quality of life (p. 167).
- Additional therapies may be used, depending on presence of particular uremic signs.
  - Nausea/vomiting (see Acute General Treatment above)
  - Hyperphosphatemia: dietary restriction ± phosphate binders (must be given with food to prevent absorption of phosphorus)
    - Aluminum hydroxide or aluminum carbonate 30-90 mg/kg/day PO with food, divided and administered with meals; dose titrated based on serum phosphorus concentration
    - Calcium acetate 60-90 mg/kg/day PO with food; hypercalcemia is a possible side effect
    - Chitosan (Epakitin) 1 g/5 kg twice daily with food; contains calcium carbonate
    - Lanthanum carbonate 30-90 mg/kg/day PO with food
    - Niacinamide 25-100 mg/kg PO q 12h, may promote gut excretion of phosphorus
  - Hypokalemia (more likely in cats than dogs)
    - Potassium gluconate 2 mEq per 4.5 kg PO per day
    - Potassium citrate 75 mg/kg PO q 12h
  - Acidosis: consider treatment if total CO_2 < 16 mEq/L or pH < 7.2
    - Potassium citrate 75 mg/kg PO q 12h (also addresses hypokalemia)
    - Sodium bicarbonate 10 mg/kg PO q 8-12h
  - Anemia
    - Transfusion based on clinical need
    - Darbepoetin (Aranesp) 6.25 mcg/CAT; dogs 1 mcg/kg up to 25 mcg SQ q 7 days until hematocrit rises; then q 14-21 days to maintain low-normal hematocrit. Risk of pure red cell aplasia from cross-reactive antibodies appears lower with darbepoetin compared to human recombinant erythropoietin (Epogen, Procrit).
    - Iron dextran 5-10 mg/kg IM q 2-4 weeks. Necessary to restore deficient iron stores for effective use of darbepoetin or erythropoietin, especially if red blood cell transfusion (excellent source of bioavailable iron) not administered. Risk of acute hypersensitivity reaction exists.
  - Systemic hypertension: calcium channel blockers recommended. If proteinuria is present or calcium channel blocker is

insufficient, add angiotensin-converting enzyme (ACE) inhibitor (p. 501).
    - Chronic dehydration: SQ fluid administration. Dose is empirical, based on subjective assessment of the patient's well-being, hydration status, and presence of other disorders (e.g., cardiac disease). Typically for cats without heart problems, 100-150 mL isotonic replacement fluid (e.g., lactated Ringer's solution) SQ q 24-72h. Avoid giving glucose solutions SQ.
    - Proteinuria: ACE inhibition (e.g., benazepril) or angiotensin receptor antagonists (e.g., telmisartan) may reduce proteinuria and convey renoprotection. These drugs must be discontinued if dehydration or hyperkalemia occurs (p. 167).
    - Management of renal secondary hyperparathyroidism
- Renal transplantation may be appropriate for some cats. May be preceded by hemodialysis. The highest likelihood of a successful outcome occurs in mildly to moderately azotemic cats without concurrent illness or infection. Availability and success of renal transplantation is extremely limited for dogs.
- Chronic hemodialysis is costly and has limited availability but can improve quality of life significantly in dogs without comorbidities (typically not recommended for cats).

Nutrition/Diet

A restricted-quantity but high-quality protein and restricted-phosphorus diet (i.e., renal diet) slows progression of CKD and decreases severity of clinical uremia.

- Acceptance of diet changes can be problematic, particularly in uremic patients.
- Maintaining adequate caloric intake to avoid weight loss takes precedence over nutrient composition of the diet.
- Renal diets should be introduced when uremia (illness) is minimized and clinical signs optimally controlled.
- Nutritional support occasionally requires appetite stimulation.
    - Mirtazapine 1.88 mg/dose PO q 48-72h (cats); 0.6 mg/kg PO q 24-48h (dogs)
    - Capromorelin, a new ghrelin receptor agonist, may be useful but experience very limited
- Assisted feeding by an esophagostomy or gastrostomy tube is often necessary to meet caloric needs in cases of advanced (stage IV) CKD.

Drug Interactions

- Phosphate binders can interfere with absorption of orally administered medications, especially antibiotics and fat-soluble vitamins.
- Sucralfate works best in an acid environment and, if used, should be given at least 30 minutes before antacid therapy if possible.
- Nephrotoxic drugs (e.g., aminoglycosides) or drug combinations (e.g., nonsteroidal antiinflammatory drugs [NSAIDs] plus ACE inhibitors) should be avoided whenever possible.
- Drugs that undergo renal elimination may need adjustment in dose strength or frequency in animals with CKD.

Possible Complications

- Anorexia, vomiting, hyperphosphatemia, hypokalemia, acidosis, anemia, and hypertension are common sequelae of CKD.
- Volume overload (pleural effusion, pulmonary edema, dyspnea, or peripheral fluid accumulation) is a concern at high rates of fluid administration, particularly in anemic animals or those with concurrent heart disease.
- Platelet dysfunction in CKD increases risks of bleeding (gingival, GI, bruising, bleeding after invasive procedures).
- ACE inhibition can result in exacerbated azotemia/uremia and hyperkalemia when administered in volume-depleted or anorexic patients.

Recommended Monitoring

- Routine recheck, including physical exam, weight, CBC (or packed cell volume), and biochemistry panel. Frequency depends on disease severity:
    - Stage I-II: recheck every 3-6 months
    - Stage III: recheck every 2-3 months
    - Stage IV: recheck monthly
- Urinalysis +/− urine protein/creatinine ratio +/− urine culture should be performed at least twice each year.
- Blood pressure measurement at least every 3 months or 1 week after antihypertensive drug dose adjustments.
- Changes in clinical signs should prompt a recheck, regardless of predetermined schedule.

PROGNOSIS & OUTCOME

- Longevity is difficult to predict in an individual patient, with a range of days to years.
- Median survival times are approximately
    - 3 years in cats; 1 year in dogs with stage II CKD
    - 2 years in cats; 6 months in dogs with stage III CKD
    - 1 month in cats; 3 months in dogs with stage IV CKD

PEARLS & CONSIDERATIONS

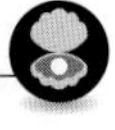

Comments

- Therapeutic measures are seldom begun all at once, but instead added as appropriate during disease progression.
- Renal biopsy is rarely informative in cats with CKD (the inciting cause is rarely identified, unless neoplasia or feline infectious peritonitis is present).
- At an early stage of decompensation, renal transplant can be considered for otherwise healthy cats.

Technician Tips

Technicians can be invaluable for teaching owners how to administer subcutaneous fluids. They can also help to emphasize the importance of allowing the animal a constant source of fresh water. The technician can help clients develop a plan for a gradual transition from a maintenance diet to a renal diet.

Client Education

- CKD is a terminal condition in which treatments are aimed primarily at improving the quality of life and delaying the progression of disease.
- For pets with advanced CKD, the owners should be provided with realistic expectations for costs and inconvenience associated with potential treatments and prognosis.
- With successful renal transplantation in cats, intensive lifelong medication and frequent rechecks are required, but quality of life can be excellent.

SUGGESTED READING

Polzin DJ: Chronic kidney disease. In Ettinger SJ, et al, editors: Textbook of veterinary internal medicine, ed 8, St. Louis, 2017, Elsevier, 1938-1959.

AUTHORS: Catherine E. Langston, DVM, DACVIM; Adam Eatroff, DVM, DACVIM
EDITOR: Leah A. Cohn, DVM, PhD, DACVIM

Chylothorax

Client Education Sheet 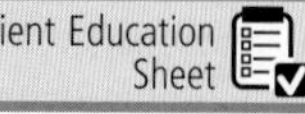

BASIC INFORMATION

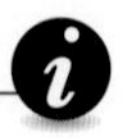

Definition

Accumulation of fluid with a high triglyceride concentration (chyle) within the pleural space

Epidemiology

SPECIES, AGE, SEX

Cats and dogs; some diseases associated with chylothorax are more common in middle-aged to older patients.

GENETICS, BREED PREDISPOSITION

Possible breed predispositions include Afghan hounds and Shiba inu dogs and purebred cats, especially Asian breeds.

RISK FACTORS

- Thoracic trauma
- Intestinal or generalized lymphangiectasia
- Congestive heart failure (CHF); cats > dogs
  - Hyperthyroidism (cats)
- Thoracic neoplasia/granulomas
- Thoracic surgery (damage to the left brachiocephalic vein)
- Pulmonary/caval thrombosis
- Heartworm disease (HWD)
- Pericardial disease
- Peritoneopericardial diaphragmatic hernia (PPDH)
- Cardiac disease (e.g., double-chamber right ventricle, tricuspid dysplasia, cardiomyopathy)

ASSOCIATED DISORDERS

Fibrosing pleuritis

Clinical Presentation

HISTORY, CHIEF COMPLAINT

- Respiratory distress/increased respiratory effort
- Lethargy, anorexia, weight loss, exercise intolerance
- History of thoracic trauma/surgery
- Some animals, especially cats, may show minimal clinical signs until effusion volume is quite large.

PHYSICAL EXAM FINDINGS

- Respiratory: tachypnea, increased inspiratory effort, shallow respirations, restrictive or generalized paradoxical breathing pattern, ± coughing
  - Severely affected patients may demonstrate orthopnea, open-mouth breathing, and/or cyanosis.
- Thoracic auscultation
  - Muffled ventral heart/lung sounds
  - Murmurs or arrhythmias (heart disease)
  - Displacement of point of maximal intensity of heartbeat (mass effect)
  - Increased bronchovesicular lung sounds dorsally
  - Thoracic percussion: hyporesonance ventrally
  - Abnormalities can be very subtle in cats.
- Jugular vein distention/pulsation may be present in animals with CHF or pericardial disease.
  - Large-volume pleural effusions can cause increased central venous pressure (CVP) and jugular venous distention/pulsation.
  - Radiation of a normal carotid pulse through the overlying jugular vein should not be misinterpreted as jugular pulsation.
- Peripheral lymphadenopathy with some causes of intrathoracic neoplasia
- ± Peritoneal effusion
- Decreased cranial thoracic compressibility (cats) if associated with mediastinal mass or pleural effusion
- Fever is uncommon

Etiology and Pathophysiology

- Chyle is formed from lymphatic drainage of the gastrointestinal tract and mesentery (composed of chylomicra, electrolytes, fat-soluble vitamins, proteins, and lymphocytes), and collected in the cisterna chyli. The sole outflow of the cisterna chyli is the thoracic duct (TD), a single or paired structure that courses dorsally though the thorax and empties into the cranial vena cava.
- Impaired or disrupted lymphatic drainage
  - Traumatic rupture of the TD
  - Neoplasia: mediastinal, thoracic wall, or any affecting TD (e.g., lymphangiosarcoma)
  - Thoracic lymphangiectasia (± intestinal lymphangiectasia)
  - Fungal granulomas
  - Congenital abnormalities of the TD
- Increased CVP (TD empties into cranial vena cava)
  - CHF (right sided in dogs, left or right sided in cats)
  - Pericardial disease: pericardial effusion, restrictive pericardial disease, PPDH
  - Pulmonary thromboembolism
  - HWD
  - Cranial vena caval thrombosis: may be associated with implantation of a device (e.g., pacemaker lead) in either jugular vein.
- Chylothorax has occurred in a small number of dogs after lung-lobe torsion correction.
  - Chylothorax and lung-lobe torsion are often concurrent disorders, and it is often unclear which was the primary abnormality.
- Often, the cause of chylothorax cannot be determined (idiopathic).

DIAGNOSIS

Diagnostic Overview

Patients typically present with signs suggesting pleural space disease. Effusion is confirmed by imaging (radiographs/ultrasonography) or thoracocentesis. A diagnosis of chylothorax is achieved by fluid analysis and comparison of serum and fluid triglyceride levels. Attempts should be made to identify underlying disorders.

Differential Diagnosis

- Other causes of pleural effusion
  - Hypoalbuminemia
  - CHF
  - Intrathoracic neoplasia
  - Lung-lobe torsion
  - Pyothorax
  - Pseudochylothorax
  - Hemothorax
  - Feline infectious peritonitis (FIP) in cats
- Pneumothorax
- Pulmonary parenchymal disease

Initial Database

- Thoracic radiographs: pulmonary parenchymal, mediastinal, or cardiac disease more likely to be identified after thoracocentesis.
  - Interlobar fissure lines
  - Reduced visualization of the heart, especially on dorsoventral views
  - Retraction of lung margins from the thoracic wall, with an interposed fluid opacity
  - Blunting of lung margins at the costophrenic angles
  - Increased opacity dorsal to the sternum on lateral views, with rounding of the lung margins ventrally
  - The diaphragm is often obscured.
  - Widened mediastinum
  - Avoid ventrodorsal views: increases the risk of respiratory distress
  - Atelectatic lung lobes may give a false impression of lung masses.
  - Fibrosing/constrictive pleuritis secondary to chronic chylothorax may prevent complete re-expansion after drainage and can cause many of the same radiographic abnormalities seen with pleural fluid.
- Thoracic ultrasonography: detect pulmonary or mediastinal masses/lesions, lymphadenopathy, pulmonary consolidation, and lung-lobe torsion and confirm presence of effusion if in doubt.
  - If the patient is stable, ultrasound is ideally performed before effusion is completely removed to provide an acoustic window.
  - Thoracic ultrasound can detect small-volume effusions, guide thoracocentesis if fluid is compartmentalized, and guide fine-needle aspiration of masses (p. 1113) or other lesions.
- Thoracocentesis (p. 1164): chyle is often grossly white/pink and opaque and remains so after centrifugation.
  - Animals on low-fat diets may lack characteristic color and opacity.
  - Chyle may be classified as a modified transudate (<3000-5000 nucleated cells/

microL, total protein > 2.5 g/dL) or a nonseptic exudate (>5000 nucleated cells/microL, total protein > 2.5 g/dL) (p. 1343).
  - Predominant cell type: early chylothorax: small lymphocytes; chronic chylothorax: nondegenerate neutrophils ± macrophages
- CBC: ± lymphopenia; changes are rarely specific
- Serum biochemistry profile: hypocalcemia, hypocholesterolemia, and hypoalbuminemia/hypoproteinemia are possible especially with concurrent lymphangiectasia.
- Urinalysis: unremarkable
- Heartworm antigen test (± antibody test in cats): rule out infection
- Feline retroviral testing: rule out infection
- Thyroid testing (all cats > 5 years)

Advanced or Confirmatory Testing

- Echocardiography (p. 1094) to assess for myocardial, valvular, or pericardial disease
- Biochemical analysis of pleural fluid: compared to serum concentrations, increased pleural fluid triglyceride and decreased pleural fluid cholesterol concentrations are consistent with chylous effusion (p. 1343)
  - Pleural/serum triglyceride ratios > 10-20:1 are common.
  - Pseudochylous effusions (rare): effusion cholesterol concentration > serum cholesterol concentration, and effusion triglyceride concentration < the serum triglyceride concentration
  - In fasted/anorexic animals, pleural fluid may have a reduced triglyceride concentration and lack milky appearance. Consider checking postprandial effusion and serum triglyceride concentrations.
- CT ± lymphangiogram or MRI (p. 1132) may aid assessment of structural abnormalities in the thoracic cavity.
  - Percutaneous popliteal lymphangiograms have been performed.

TREATMENT

Treatment Overview

Treatment goals: alleviate respiratory distress when present and treat an underlying cause when possible

Acute General Treatment

- Oxygen if respiratory distress (p. 1146)
- Thoracocentesis (p. 1164) is the initial therapy of choice.
  - Complete drainage is unnecessary to relieve/improve clinical signs and may be hazardous.
  - Fibrosing pleuritis limits the degree of lung expansion. Re-expansion pulmonary edema may occur with complete drainage, particularly if disease is chronic (p. 836).

Chronic Treatment

- Specific treatment of any identified underlying disease (e.g., CHF, HWD) may resolve chylothorax.
- Traumatic chylothorax can resolve spontaneously with only supportive care.
- Intermittent thoracocentesis, as respiratory signs dictate
  - If frequent thoracocentesis is performed, monitor serum electrolytes; hyponatremia, and hyperkalemia can occur.
  - If fluid accumulation is rapid, thoracostomy tubes may be required.
- Medical management (idiopathic chylothorax)
  - Low-fat diet (commercial or homemade): Suggested to reduce the flow of chyle, but effect of diet has been questioned. Medium-chain triglyceride supplementation no longer recommended
  - Rutin (250-500 mg/CAT or 50 mg/kg PO q 8-12h): used for treating lymphedema in humans and has been used in feline chylothorax with limited success and no documented adverse effects.
  - Octreotide (somatostatin analog): thought to reduce fluid flow through the TD. Neither efficacy nor dose established; range from 1-20 mcg/kg SQ, IM q 6-8h
- Surgery: optimal timing for surgery is undetermined, but delaying surgical intervention increases the risk of fibrosis pleuritis. Because medical management of idiopathic chylothorax has a guarded prognosis, surgical intervention has been suggested as the initial treatment of choice. Surgical options include TD ligation alone, TD ligation combined with pericardectomy or other procedures, and/or cisterna chyli ablation.

TD ligation:

- Ligation of the TD and its branches, often in combination with lymphangiography (TD rupture rarely detected). Used as sole procedure, reported rate of resolution for dogs 53%, for cats 20%-53%
  - Intercostal or transdiaphragmatic approach most common or less often by median sternotomy
  - Lymphangiography repeated after ligation to ensure all branches have been ligated
  - Thoracoscopic TD ligation combined with mesenteric lymphangiography has been described.

TD ligation combined with other procedures:

- TD ligation with pericardectomy:
  - A thickened pericardium may increase right-sided venous pressures, impeding drainage of chyle.
  - Reported success rates approach 100% for dogs and 80% for cats.
  - The addition of omentalization to pericardectomy does not appear to improve outcome.
  - TD ligation and pericardial window placement or pericardectomy can be performed less invasively with video-assisted thoracoscopic surgery.
- Omentalization: exploits the large surface area and lymph-draining capability of the omentum.
- Placement of a PleuralPort device: owners can drain the effusion at home using a Huber needle placed into a subcutaneous drainage hub.
- Active pleuroperitoneal or pleurovenous drainage techniques: disadvantages include cost, thrombosis, catheter obstruction, air embolism, venous occlusion, sepsis, abdominal distention (if pleuroperitoneal), and potential lack of owner compliance.
- Pleurodesis and passive pleuroperitoneal drainage: not recommended
- Cisterna chyli ablation combined with TD ligation has been described as superior to TD ligation alone. Cisterna chyli and TD glue embolization has been reported in two dogs with refractory chylothorax.

Possible Complications

- Incomplete resolution of chylothorax can occur with any treatment technique.
  - Nonchylus effusions may develop in some patients.
- Surgical and anesthetic risks
- Fibrosing pleuritic: pleural thickening by fibrous tissue that restricts normal lung expansion
- Re-expansion pulmonary edema, electrolyte disorders associate with thoracocentesis

Recommended Monitoring

- Clinical signs
- Thoracic radiographs to assess pleural fluid accumulation/resolution
- Postoperative patients should also be monitored for reaccumulation of fluid.

PROGNOSIS & OUTCOME

- Rarely, spontaneous resolution is reported. Resolution is more likely if an underlying disease can be corrected or after traumatic TD rupture.
- For patients with idiopathic chylothorax or thoracic lymphangiectasia, TD ligation combined with pericardectomy and/or cisterna chyli ablation appears to offer the best results. Early surgical referral is warranted.
- After fibrosing pleuritis has developed, the prognosis worsens regardless of treatment.

PEARLS & CONSIDERATIONS

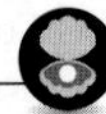

Comments

- Cats with pleural effusion are fragile and must be handled carefully (e.g., during restraint); the degree of resting dyspnea may be surprisingly mild with large pleural effusions in this species.
- Long-standing chylous effusion can lead to fibrotic pleural disease, an irreversible cause of respiratory impairment.
- Repeated thoracocentesis is not a viable long-term solution due to fibrosing pleuritis that interferes with pulmonary expansion; fibrosis also leads to fluid pockets, making draining far more difficult.

Technician Tips

- Animals with pleural effusions can be very fragile and susceptible to stress with

handling. Therefore, minimal handling is important.
- Supplemental oxygen is helpful in a dyspneic patient with pleural effusion.
- Avoid dorsal recumbency for radiographs in animals with pleural effusions.
- Supplies for emergency thoracocentesis: clippers, skin preparation materials, a butterfly needle or needle with an extension set, 3-way stopcock, and syringes
- Complications of thoracocentesis: pneumothorax and hemothorax. Monitor for tachypnea/increased respiratory effort after pleural drainage and alert clinician if identified.

Client Education

Chylothorax can be a frustrating disease and requires diagnostic assessment to identify treatable underlying causes.

SUGGESTED READING

McAnulty JF: Prospective comparison of cisterna chyli ablation to pericardectomy for treatment of spontaneously occurring idiopathic chylothorax in the dog. Vet Surg 40:926-934, 2011.

AUTHOR: Graham Swinney, BVSc, DVCS
EDITORS: Megan Grobman, DVM, MS, DACVIM

Cirrhotic/Fibrosing Liver Disease

Client Education Sheet 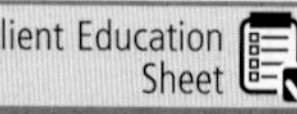

BASIC INFORMATION 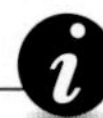

Definition

- Fibrosis: replacement of hepatic parenchyma with extracellular matrix (ECM), collagen, and connective tissue
- Cirrhosis: diffuse hepatic fibrosis with concurrent formation of regenerative nodules that results in irreversible loss of normal hepatic architecture
- Sometimes a sequella to *chronic hepatitis*, this disorder is being recognized with increasing frequency in a variety of breeds.

Epidemiology

SPECIES, AGE, SEX

- Incidence is highest in middle-aged to older dogs (>7 years) with chronic liver disease.
- Middle-aged cats with chronic cholangitis may suffer from biliary cirrhosis.
- Copper storage hepatopathy (≈1-5 years) and idiopathic hepatic fibrosis (<2 years) occur in younger dogs.

GENETICS, BREED PREDISPOSITION

- Doberman pinschers, cocker spaniels, Scottish terriers, Labrador retrievers, and English springer spaniels have a familial predisposition to idiopathic chronic hepatitis (pp. 450 and 452).
- Copper storage disease is inherited in Bedlington terriers, West Highland white terriers, Labrador retrievers, and Dalmatians (p. 458).
- German shepherds and standard poodles develop juvenile idiopathic hepatic fibrosis.

RISK FACTORS

Idiopathic chronic hepatitis (formerly chronic active hepatitis) in dogs, excess hepatic copper or iron storage, extrahepatic biliary obstruction, drug administration (phenobarbital, others) (p. 1231)

ASSOCIATED DISORDERS

- Portal hypertension, ascites, hepatic encephalopathy (HE), coagulopathies, urolithiasis, acquired portosystemic shunts, gastric ulceration, portal vein thrombosis, fat malabsorption and steatorrhea, hypoglycemia, and hypoalbuminemia may result from fibrosing liver disease.
- Rare occurrence of pulmonary edema (hypoalbuminemia), chronic kidney disease/uremia (hepatorenal syndrome), or transient erythropoietic protoporphyria.

Clinical Presentation

HISTORY, CHIEF COMPLAINT

- Chronic condition of varied severity that usually includes lethargy, anorexia, and weight loss
- Vomiting, diarrhea, melena, and polyuria/polydipsia also frequently are part of the history.
- Owners occasionally note jaundiced color of sclera or skin.
- Owners may report abdominal distention from ascites as weight gain, even as the patient loses muscle mass.
- Neurologic signs can occur as a manifestation of HE (p. 440).

PHYSICAL EXAM FINDINGS

- May be unremarkable except for weight loss and muscle wasting
- Icterus occurs commonly.
- Ascites and evidence of coagulopathy in advanced cases
- Microhepatica may be present (dogs), although cats with biliary cirrhosis may have large livers.
- Manifestations of cerebral dysfunction (depression, stupor, others) due to HE

Etiology and Pathophysiology

- ECM deposition (fibrosis) is stimulated by inflammatory mediators and cytokines, which activate hepatic stellate cells to produce collagen (congenital or idiopathic).
- Chronic fibrosis and regenerative nodule formation results in cirrhosis. Chronic progressive collagen deposition irreversibly destroys normal hepatic architecture.
- Normal hepatic blood flow and bile flow are disrupted, perpetuating hepatocellular injury.
- Any chronic inflammatory hepatic condition may be responsible, although a specific cause is not often identified (i.e., idiopathic).
- Possible underlying causes include cholangitis (cats), copper storage disease and high-copper diets in predisposed breeds (dogs), drugs and/or toxins (aflatoxin, anticonvulsants, azole antifungals, timethoprim-sulfadiazine), immune-mediated disease, leptospirosis, canine infectious hepatitis virus, hypoxia, extrahepatic biliary obstruction, a single episode of massive hepatic necrosis (i.e., postnecrotic cirrhosis), or *COMMD1* deficiency (which leads to hepatic copper accumulation and chronic hepatitis).
- Hepatic vascular resistance may increase, resulting in portal hypertension, ascites, acquired portosystemic shunts, and encephalopathy.

DIAGNOSIS 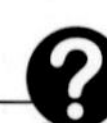

Diagnostic Overview

Although plasma markers of this condition are being developed (transforming growth factor beta-1, others), histopathologic analysis of a liver biopsy specimen remains central to the diagnosis. It is particularly important to look for excess copper accumulation as a treatable cause of progressive hepatic lesions.

Differential Diagnosis

- Idiopathic chronic hepatitis (dogs)
- Ductal plate abnormalities
- Congenital hepatic fibrosis
- Cholangitis (cats)
- Noncirrhotic portal hypertension
- Biliary duct obstruction
- Pancreatitis
- Hepatic neoplasia (primary or metastatic)
- Exposure to hepatotoxic drugs or toxins
- Feline infectious peritonitis, toxoplasmosis
- Chronic fibrosing pancreatitis
- Congenital portosystemic shunt
- Hepatic lipidosis (cats)

Initial Database

- CBC
  - Nonregenerative anemia (normocytic, normochromic, or microcytic)
  - Acanthocytes (cats)

- Serum biochemistry panel
  - Elevated hepatic enzyme activities (alkaline phosphatase, alanine aminotransferase, aspartate aminotransferase, gamma-glutamyl transferase) typical
  - Hyperbilirubinemia (depending on stage)
  - Low blood urea nitrogen (BUN) (variable)
  - Hypoalbuminemia and hyperglobulinemia (variable)
  - Hypocholesterolemia (variable)
  - Hypoglycemia (variable)
  - Electrolyte abnormalities (hypokalemia, hyponatremia)
- Urinalysis
  - Isosthenuria
  - Ammonium biurate crystalluria (variable)

Advanced or Confirmatory Testing

- Abdominocentesis and fluid analysis of ascites (pp. 1056 and 1343): pure transudate (hypoalbuminemia) or modified transudate (portal hypertension)
- Coagulation studies: prolonged activated clotting time (ACT), partial thromboplastin time (PT), activated partial thromboplastin time (aPTT), fibrinogen concentration, proteins induced by vitamin K antagonism or absence (PIVKA), buccal mucosal bleeding time, and thromboelastography (TEG). It has not been shown that any of these studies will help predict bleeding after hepatic biopsy.
- Serum bile acids: elevated (fasting and postprandial). Bile acids are abnormal (and therefore an unnecessary test) in cases where the total bilirubin concentration is elevated.
- Radiographs: small liver (dogs), large liver (cats), loss of abdominal detail
- Abdominal ultrasound
  - Nodular hyperechoic/mixed echogenicity of hepatic parenchyma with abdominal effusion
  - +/− Acquired portosystemic shunt(s)
  - +/− Ascites
- Laparoscopy or laparotomy
  - Small, firm, irregular liver
- Liver biopsy (p. 1128) for histopathologic analysis: confirmatory
  - Fibrosis: inflammatory (bridging) or noninflammatory (sinusoidal, triads). Request reticulin and Masson's trichrome stains (or Sirius Red stain).
  - Cirrhosis, nodular regeneration, loss of normal hepatic architecture
  - NOTE: suspicion of cirrhotic/fibrosing liver disease should prompt the consideration of wedge biopsy of the liver rather than ultrasound-guided needle-core biopsy because biopsies from a firm, severely fibrotic liver often yield small pieces of fragmented tissue, and it may be difficult to penetrate the liver safely with needle-core biopsy instruments, especially if ascites is present. Needle-core biopsies are often inaccurate in cirrhotic livers.

TREATMENT

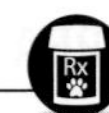

Treatment Overview

Very few treatment options are proven to directly impact the progression of this condition unless a specific cause (e.g., copper accumulation, drug-induced condition) can be targeted. Fortunately, very few of the myriad of potentially beneficial nonspecific treatments (e.g., antioxidants, liver protectants) are thought to have significant adverse effects.

Acute General Treatment

- Intravenous fluids (balanced electrolyte solution) as needed
  - Avoid 0.9% NaCl with ascites and hypoalbuminemia
  - Avoid lactate if hepatic failure
  - Potassium (20-40 mEq/L or more, based on serum potassium concentration) and dextrose (2.5%-5%) supplementation may be necessary.
  - Dextrans, hetastarch, or plasma transfusion for oncotic pressure support. Plasma advantages include presence of albumin (contributes positively to protein balance), presence of clotting factors, and persistence in circulation (vs. protein-losing enteropathy or nephropathy, in which the transfused proteins may be lost quickly).
- Therapeutic abdominocentesis when necessary (i.e., respiratory compromise, significant abdominal discomfort)

Chronic Treatment

See HE (p. 440).

- Antibiotics
  - Specific to infectious agent if identified as underlying cause (rarely in dogs)
  - For signs of hepatic encephalopathy, consider
    - Metronidazole 10-15 mg/kg PO q 12h, *or*
    - Amoxicillin-clavulanate 12-25 mg/kg PO q 12h, *or*
    - Ampicillin 20-40 mg/kg PO q 8h, *or*
    - Neomycin 20 mg/kg PO q 8h
- Antiinflammatory: with histopathologic confirmation of chronic noninfectious inflammation, consider prednisolone 1-2 mg/kg PO q 24-48h (taper if possible) and/or azathioprine 2 mg/kg PO q 24h initially, tapered to 1 mg/kg. Other immunosuppressive agents used for chronic hepatitis are discussed on p. 452.
- Antifibrotic: colchicine 0.03 mg/kg PO q 24h, although no published data support its use or clearly demonstrate a beneficial effect; veterinary data regarding safety and efficacy are lacking at present. Telmisartan 0.5-1 mg/kg PO q 12h and phosphatidylcholine 20-70 mg/kg/day PO decrease stellate cell activation and may be beneficial. Prednisone (antiinflammatory) and D-penicillamine (copper chelator) 10-15 mg/kg PO q 12h also have weak antifibrotic properties.
- Lactulose 0.25-0.5 mL/kg PO q 8h (titrated to achieve loose fecal consistency) with cleansing and/or retention enemas (povidone-iodine diluted 1:10 with tap water or lactulose diluted 1:3 with tap water) to decrease ammonia production/absorption in cases of HE. Generally, patients with advanced disease requiring this level of therapy have a grave prognosis.
- Ursodiol 10-15 mg/kg PO q 24h as a choleretic in cases of cholestasis
- Alpha-tocopherol (vitamin E) 200-600 IU PO q 24h, *S*-adenosylmethionine 20 mg/kg PO q 24h, and milk thistle/silymarin (optimal dose unknown) may act as hepatoprotective antioxidants.
- Spironolactone 1-2 mg/kg PO q 12h or furosemide 1-2 mg/kg PO q 12h in cases of ascites
- Vitamin K_1 1-2 mg/kg SQ or IM if overt clinical bleeding is identified or if PT or aPTT are prolonged > 2 × normal
- Sucralfate 1 g/25 kg PO q 8-12h, omeprazole 1 mg/kg PO q 12h as gastrointestinal ulcer therapy

Nutrition/Diet

- Most commercial geriatric, liver, or renal diets are appropriate. Copper restriction appropriate for copper-associated hepatic disease (p. 459)
- Adjust protein consumption in the face of HE (decreased/optimal quantity, replace meat proteins with dairy and/or vegetable protein). Protein restriction is not warranted in the absence of encephalopathy.
- Fermentable fiber in cases of HE
- Water-soluble vitamin supplementation
- Avoid mineral supplements containing copper.

Drug Interactions

- Animals with hepatic failure are anesthetic risks. Barbiturates should be avoided, and benzodiazepines should be used with care. Isoflurane or sevoflurane are the gas anesthetics of choice. Propofol, although hepatically metabolized, may be administered to effect (usually requiring a small fraction of normal dosages) for controlling seizures due to HE.
- Lidocaine, theophylline, propranolol, captopril, and tetracyclines should be avoided.
- Diuretics may worsen HE, promote dehydration or metabolic alkalosis, and should be used only in otherwise stable patients for the long-term delay of return of ascites.
- Glucocorticoids should be avoided in animals with active infection, may precipitate hepatic failure and/or gastric ulceration, and cause sodium retention (may use dexamethasone [no mineralocorticoid activity] as an alternative to prednisone).
- Nonsteroidal anti-inflammatory drugs may exacerbate gastrointestinal ulceration.
- Avoid medications that rely solely or predominantly on hepatic metabolism for effectiveness or clearance.

Possible Complications

HE, septicemia, hemorrhage/coagulopathy, disseminated intravascular coagulation

Recommended Monitoring

Body weight, abdominal girth, liver enzymes, albumin, BUN, and bile acids should be monitored on a monthly basis.

PROGNOSIS & OUTCOME

- In one report, 94% of dogs with hepatic fibrosis/cirrhosis were dead within 1 week of diagnosis.
- Dogs with idiopathic hepatic fibrosis/cirrhosis have been reported to survive for up to 6 years, and intensive therapy may extend survival, although the prognosis is usually very poor with advanced disease.
- Histopathologic findings may be helpful as a prognostic indicator.
- Patients that are anorectic, demonstrate clinical signs of HE, have coagulopathy (prolonged PT, aPTT, or thrombocytopenia), ascites, hypoglobulinemia, or histologically severe changes (cirrhosis, advanced fibrosis) usually have a poor prognosis.

PEARLS & CONSIDERATIONS

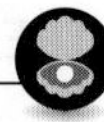

Comments

- Hepatic fibrosis and cirrhotic changes indicate a progressive, terminal condition that is often not recognized or apparent until the patient is in an advanced stage of disease. An underlying cause is not often identified, making specific therapy impossible. A histopathologic diagnosis is essential in cases of suspected hepatic fibrosis/cirrhosis.
- Even with severe cirrhotic/fibrosing liver disease, patients may have little active liver inflammation and therefore can have normal or near-normal serum liver enzyme activities.
  - Bile acids (especially postprandial) are much more sensitive for assessment of hepatic function.

Prevention

- Early testing of animals with breed predispositions (e.g., Bedlington terriers; genetic test available) may lead to early intervention.
- Avoid oversupplementation with copper-containing products and high-copper diets in predisposed breeds.
- Use hepatotoxic drugs with caution and monitor during use (e.g., phenobarbital).

Technician Tips

- Pursuing a liver biopsy (histopathology; copper, zinc, and iron quantification) and gallbladder aspiration (cytology and culture) may identify treatable abnormalities (e.g., copper accumulation)
- Although clotting times are not directly correlated to post-biopsy bleeding, most clinicians will measure clotting parameters in preparation for a biopsy procedure.

Client Education

Even extremely small amounts of meat protein (e.g., one small meat-based treat) may precipitate severe signs of HE in susceptible patients.

SUGGESTED READING

Favier RP, et al: A retrospective study of oral prednisolone treatment in canine chronic hepatitis. Vet Q 33:113-120, 2013.

AUTHOR: Craig B. Webb, DVM, PhD, DACVIM
EDITOR: Keith P. Richter, DVM, MSEL, DACVIM

Claw Disorders

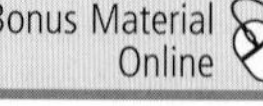

BASIC INFORMATION

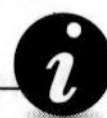

Definition

In dogs and cats, the term *claw* is more appropriate than *nail.*

- Onychodystrophy: claw malformation
- Onychogryphosis: hypertrophic claw with abnormal curvature
- Onycholysis: separation of claw from underlying corium
- Onychomadesis: sloughing of claw
- Onychomycosis: fungal infection of claw
- Onychorrhexis: brittle claws tending to split or break
- Paronychia: inflammation of soft tissue around claw
- Symmetric lupoid onychodystrophy/onychitis (SLO): lupus-like condition that causes sloughing (onychomadesis) and subsequent onychodystrophy of multiple claws on all paws

Epidemiology

SPECIES, AGE, SEX

Most claw conditions have no specific age or sex predispositions other than those listed here:

- SLO: in dogs 3-8 years old; rare in cats
- Subungual squamous cell carcinoma (SCC): in older dogs
- Subungual melanomas: in older dogs; rare in cats
- Onychomycosis: *Malassezia* infection common but dermatophytosis rare in dogs and cats

GENETICS, BREED PREDISPOSITION

- SLO: often noted in German shepherds, Gordon setters, miniature poodles, schnauzers, and rottweilers
- Subungual SCC: seen in large breeds (75% of cases) and in breeds with a black coat (66% of cases), such as in the black Labrador retriever and black poodle

RISK FACTORS

Non-neoplastic claw disorders: immunosuppression, feline leukemia virus (FeLV) infection, vascular insult, trauma, improper trimming/care of claws, diabetes mellitus

ASSOCIATED DISORDERS

- In cats and dogs: hyperadrenocorticism, diabetes mellitus, hypothyroidism, dermatomyositis, arteriovenous fistula, cold-agglutinin disease, drug reaction, vaccine reaction, vasculitis, trauma, leishmaniasis, food allergy
- In cats only: hyperthyroidism, primary pulmonary bronchiolar adenocarcinoma (lung-digit syndrome), pulmonary SCC, cutaneous SCC with metastasis

Clinical Presentation

HISTORY, CHIEF COMPLAINT

Pruritus of affected digit(s), signs of pain/lameness, misshaped claws, claw sloughing, or a swollen toe or a mass seen during claw trim. A single paw or multiple paws can be involved. The claw disorder can be part of a more generalized skin condition.

PHYSICAL EXAM FINDINGS

- Bacterial claw infections
  - One or many affected digits
  - Paronychia, toe swelling, purulent discharge, possible separation of claw, and pain
  - Regional lymphadenopathy, with fever and possible osteomyelitis
  - Other clinical signs of immunocompromising conditions
- Onychomycosis
  - Dermatophytic claw infections result in paronychia with minimal pain, irritation, or pruritus. Typically, only one or two affected digits with friable and misshapen claws are seen on the same paw. Usually accompanied by focal or multifocal skin lesions

- A notable brown line on the claws (consisting of a waxy discharge or stain) is a clue for *Malassezia* overgrowth and is typically associated with moist interdigital dermatitis, paronychia, and pruritus and other areas of cutaneous involvement such as body folds (p. 614).
- SLO
  - Onychomadesis starts with a single abnormal claw on two or more paws; within 2-9 weeks, all claws on all four paws are affected.
  - Regrowth of short, misshapen, dry, soft, brittle, and crumbling claws
  - Paronychia is uncommon unless a secondary bacterial infection is present.
- Subungual SCC
  - Single, swollen, painful toe with paronychia and associated erosive/ulcerative dermatitis and often loss of the claw
  - Multiple digits can be affected over time in black Labradors, black standard poodles, giant schnauzers, and rottweilers.
- Subungual melanoma
  - Solitary, well-circumscribed, dome-shaped, firm, wartlike growth at claw base
  - Varies in size: 0.5-10 cm in diameter
  - Possibly pigmented or nonpigmented and ulcerated

Etiology and Pathophysiology

- Bacterial claw infection
  - Infection is secondary (e.g., trauma if one or two claws are infected; if many claws are infected, consider hypothyroidism, hyperadrenocorticism, immune-mediated condition [pemphigus, vasculitis or SLO]).
  - *Staphylococcus pseudintermedius* is the most common bacterium isolated.
  - Leishmaniasis should be considered in endemic areas (the Mediterranean, limited areas in the United States).
- Onychomycosis
  - *Microsporum canis* in cats
  - *Trichophyton mentagrophytes* in dogs
  - *Malassezia* spp in dogs and cats
  - *Microsporum gypseum* and candidiasis (yeast) less common
- SLO: currently regarded as an idiopathic condition. It may be a clinical manifestation of many different diseases or an immune-mediated condition itself. Current emphasis is to look for potential underlying conditions, including hypersensitivity disorders (drug, food, environmental allergens) and hormonal and metabolic abnormalities before committing a pet to lifelong therapy.
- Subungual SCC
  - Neoplasm generally originating from the germinal epithelium of the claw
  - Reverse also possible (metastasis from a primary pulmonary neoplasm/carcinoma to toe), a sequence that is more common in cats than in dogs
- Subungual melanoma: malignant proliferation of melanocytes involving the claw beds in older dogs

DIAGNOSIS

Diagnostic Overview

The diagnosis originates with observation of claw abnormalities on physical exam. Complementary testing is selected based on history, remainder of exam (especially whether one or several claws is/are affected and skin involvement distant to claws), and results of the initial database.

Differential Diagnosis

- Single claw affected
  - Trauma-induced condition
  - Neoplasia (subungual SCC, subungual melanoma, high-grade mast cell tumors, inverted squamous papilloma, fibrosarcoma, neurofibrosarcoma, eccrine carcinoma, osteosarcoma, subungual keratoacanthoma)
- Multiple claw involvement
  - SLO
  - Immune-mediated diseases (pemphigus complex, bullous pemphigoid, drug eruption, vasculitis, cold-agglutinin disease, dermatomyositis)
  - Metabolic disease (hypothyroidism, hyperadrenocorticism, feline hyperthyroidism) (rare)
  - Primary pulmonary bronchiolar adenocarcinoma, pulmonary SCC, and cutaneous SCC with metastasis to digits in cats

Initial Database

- Cytologic examination of claw exudates
  - Suppurative or pyogranulomatous inflammation with engulfed bacteria: consistent with bacterial claw infection
  - Broad-based budding yeast consistent with *Malassezia* infection (p. 614)
  - Evidence of acantholytic cells: indicative of pemphigus
  - Round cell tumor cells: consistent with melanoma
- Fungal culture (Dermatophyte Test Medium) of claw trimmings and surrounding hair
  - Indicated if a single claw/claw bed is involved (p. 247)
  - Contact laboratory to determine if polymerase chain reaction (PCR) ringworm testing is suitable for claw samples
- CBC, serum biochemistry profile, urinalysis
  - Evidence of systemic conditions (diabetes mellitus, hyperadrenocorticism, systemic lupus erythematosus [SLE])
- Thyroid profile
  - Indicated if multiple claws are affected and other consistent clinical signs are present. Hypothyroidism (in dogs) and hyperthyroidism (in cats with onychogryphosis) are rare concurrent/causative conditions.

Advanced or Confirmatory Testing

- Bacterial culture and sensitivity: often *S. pseudintermedius*
- Biopsy for histopathologic exam and special stains
  - Usually by a toe amputation; longitudinal claw and ungula bed excision may be complex and painful.
  - SLO: hydropic and lichenoid interface dermatitis
  - Rule out other immune-mediated (pemphigus, bullous pemphigoid) and neoplastic conditions.
  - Identify fungal hyphae and arthrospores or bacterial organisms.
  - About 10% of melanomas (identified by histologic examination) behave aggressively.
- Radiographs
  - Rule out osteomyelitis with bacterial claw disease.
  - Bony lysis of third phalanx (P3) and tissue swelling due to neoplasia, particularly with subungual SCC
  - Thoracic radiographs: metastasis check
- Antinuclear antibody (ANA) test to rule in the possibility of SLE
- FeLV/feline immunodeficiency virus (FIV) serology
- Fine-needle lymph node aspiration if SCC or melanoma is suspected

TREATMENT

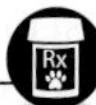

Treatment Overview

The goal of treatment is to achieve permanent cure or control of the disease. Sometimes, palliative management is the only option (e.g., SLO).

Acute General Treatment

- Claw fracture or avulsion: the clinician should trim or file (using a Dremel tool) any fractured claws, using sedation, analgesia, local/general anesthesia as necessary. Remove loose claws, and bandage foot. In severe conditions or patients with suspected neoplasia, P3 amputation may be necessary; submit it for histopathology.
- Bacterial claw infections
  - Antibiotic therapy for 2 weeks beyond clinical resolution: cephalosporin (e.g., cephalexin 30 mg/kg PO q 12h), amoxicillin-clavulanate 22 mg/kg PO q 12h, or potentiated sulfonamide (e.g., trimethoprim-sulfadiazine 15-30 mg/kg PO q 12h).
  - Topical creams/ointments: silver sulfadiazine
  - Paw scrubs: 2%-4% chlorhexidine topical soaks q 12-24h for 7 days beyond clinical resolution
- Onychomycosis
  - Ketoconazole 10 mg/kg PO q 24h, itraconazole 5-10 mg/kg PO q 24h, fluconazole 5 mg/kg PO q 24h, or terbinafine 10-40 mg/kg PO q 24h given with food for maximal absorption unless using liquid azoles
  - Long-term antifungal/anti-yeast treatment on a daily or pulse basis (6 months or longer), such as 3 days on and 4 days off (ketoconazole) or 1 week on and 1 week off (itraconazole)

- Dermatophytosis: treatment continued 1-3 months beyond complete claw regrowth and a negative repeat fungal culture from claw trimmings
- *Malassezia*: treatment continued 2-4 weeks beyond clinical resolution
- Topical antifungal products include chlorhexidine, miconazole, clotrimazole, terbinafine, enilconazole, or lime sulfur.

- SLO
  - Prednisone/prednisolone 2-4 mg/kg PO q 24h induction to halt inflammation/pain; weaning based on a favorable response
- Subungual SCC
  - Post-staging amputation of the affected digit to the proximal interphalangeal level
  - SCC is locally invasive and metastasis rate is low; no need for chemotherapy or radiation therapy
- Subungual melanoma
  - Radical surgical excision of malignant and benign-appearing areas to achieve tumor-free margins
  - Follow-up chemotherapy, immunotherapy, or radiation therapy (p. 644)

Chronic Treatment

SLO: various combinations of these treatments are used based on individual response and tolerance:

- Omega-3 fatty acids 36 mg/kg PO q 24h and omega-6 fatty acids 500-1000 mg PO q 24h for a minimum of 3 months, then as maintenance therapy
- Vitamin E 10-20 IU/kg PO q 8-12h for a minimum of 3 months or longer if improved
- Biotin 5 mg/kg PO q 24h for a minimum of 3 months or longer if improved
- Elimination diet for 8-12 weeks to rule out adverse food reaction as a trigger
- Tetracycline and niacinamide 500 mg of each for dogs > 10 kg; 250 mg of each for dogs < 10 kg PO q 8h until improvement (2-3 months), then taper the medication monthly. Doxycycline 5-10 mg/kg PO q 12h or minocycline (anecdotally) 10-25 mg/kg PO q 12h may be substituted for tetracycline.
- Pentoxifylline 10-30 mg/kg PO q 8-12h until resolution of lesions, then taper the medication monthly.
- Cyclosporine 5 mg/kg PO q 12-24h (Atopica, Neoral) until resolved, then taper to lowest frequency that controls relapse of clinical signs
- Azathioprine 1.5-2.2 mg/kg q 24-48h (dogs only) as a glucocorticoid-sparing agent
- Onychectomy (P3 amputation) as a last resort

Nutrition/Diet

Commercial diets enriched with fatty acids may help improve the integrity of the claw.

PROGNOSIS & OUTCOME

- Bacterial claw infections
  - Generally good for complete resolution
  - Response may be influenced by any underlying cause.
- Onychomycosis
  - Prognosis is good to guarded because of incomplete resolution in dermatophytic onychomycosis. May require P3 amputation or pulse antifungal therapy for life
  - Prognosis for *Malassezia* infection is good if underlying cause is addressed.
  - Response may be influenced by any underlying cause.
- SLO
  - Chronic and recurrent problem if not treated
  - Clinical improvement is usually seen within 3 to 4 months; if not, change therapies.
  - Claw regrowth is good, although claws may be slightly deformed or friable.
  - Refractory cases may require P3 amputation.
- Subungual SCC
  - Locally invasive with low metastatic potential: regional node or distant metastasis in < 30% of cases
  - The 1- and 2-year survival rates are 95% and 75%, respectively, if SCC is subungual.
- Subungual melanomas
  - Good if localized; poor if metastasized. About 50% of dogs die because of distant metastasis.

PEARLS & CONSIDERATIONS

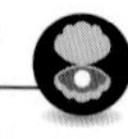

Comments

- When re-evaluating the claws, look for normalization of growth patterns at the base of the claw; growth of a new claw will take weeks (roughly 1 mm/week).
- With SLO, taper immunomodulatory medications gradually, and treat for several months beyond clinical resolution.

Prevention

Routine claw care will result in early detection of claw disorders.

Technician Tips

Shortening claws using a claw file or Dremel tool tends to be more readily accepted by pets with fragile claws.

Client Education

Use patience—claws grow slowly.

SUGGESTED READING

Miller WH, et al: Diseases of eyelids, claws, anal sacs, and ears. In Muller & Kirk's Small animal dermatology, ed 7, St. Louis, 2013, Elsevier Saunders, pp 724-733.

AUTHOR: Adam P. Patterson, DVM, DACVD
EDITOR: Manon Paradis, DMV, MVSc, DACVD

Cleaning Products Toxicosis

BASIC INFORMATION

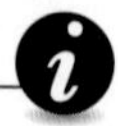

Definition

Accidental exposure (dermal, oral, or ocular) of pets to household cleaning products, including soaps, detergents, bleaches, and disinfectants. Bleaches are discussed in greater detail on p. 13.

Epidemiology

SPECIES, AGE, SEX

- Dogs more commonly involved than cats
- Cats more sensitive to cationic detergents, phenol (due to poor glucuronidation), and pine oil–containing products

Clinical Presentation

HISTORY, CHIEF COMPLAINT

- Observed or suspected exposure to a household cleaning product
- Onset of signs can be rapid (minutes to a few hours) or delayed by 6-12 hours.

PHYSICAL EXAM FINDINGS

- Hypersalivation, vomiting, diarrhea, oral ulcers (phenol, cationic detergents), lethargy, depression, hyperthermia
- Respiratory depression, dyspnea (cats), abnormal respiratory sounds, aspiration (pine oil)
- Ocular exposure: corneal ulcer, conjunctivitis/blepharitis (phenol, pine oil, cationic detergents)
- Distinct smells: bleach, pine oil

Etiology and Pathophysiology

Source:

- Soaps are salts of fatty acids made by the reaction of alkali with fatty acids.
- Detergents are surfactants in combination with inorganic ingredients such as phosphates, silicates, or carbonates. They are classified as nonionic, anionic, cationic, or zwitterionic according to their charge present in solution. The classification depends on the active ingredient.

- Nonionic detergents: hand dishwashing detergent, some shampoos, many low-sudsing laundry products; alkyl ethoxylate, alkyl phenoxy polyethoxy ethanol, polyethylene glycol stearates
- Anionic detergents: laundry detergents, electric dishwashing detergents, some shampoos, solvent/detergent degreasers; alkyl sodium sulfonates, alkyl sodium sulfates, dioctyl sodium sulfosuccinates, sodium lauryl sulfates, tetrapropylene benzene sulfonate
- Cationic detergents (quaternary ammonium compounds): fabric softeners, liquid potpourri, germicides, sanitizers; benzethonium chloride, benzalkonium chloride, alkyl dimethyl 3,4-dichlorobenzene, cetylpyridinium chloride
- Zwitterionic detergents: most shampoos, bath products, and nonirritant toiletries

- Disinfectants are chemicals applied on inanimate objects to inhibit or kill microorganisms (e.g., quaternary ammonium compounds [cationic detergents], phenols, pine oils, bleaches, alcohols).

Mechanism of toxicosis:

- Depending on dosage and concentration, soaps, anionic, nonionic, and zwitterionic detergents, and chlorine bleaches are mildly irritating to the mucous membranes. Oral or cutaneous burns are rare. Laundry pods have an increased risk of aspiration pneumonia.
- Homemade soaps/laundry detergents and alkaline anionic detergents (e.g., electric dishwashing detergents) can cause more severe oral lesions.
- Inhalation of chlorine fumes can cause pulmonary irritation, coughing, and if severe, dyspnea and noncardiogenic pulmonary edema.
- Quaternary ammonium compounds are structurally similar to decamethonium (neuromuscular blocking agent) and hexamethonium (ganglionic blocking agent). The systemic effects may resemble organophosphate insecticide toxicosis (p. 718). They also cause corrosive damage to skin and oral mucosa.
- Phenol (1%-5%) can cause oral or dermal burns, respiratory stimulation, and alkalosis followed by metabolic acidosis.
- Pine oil disinfectants are irritating to the mucous membranes.

DIAGNOSIS

Diagnostic Overview

Diagnosis is considered based on suspicion or evidence of exposure to a cleaning product and the presence of oral/dermal ulcers, hypersalivation, vomiting, excessive licking motions, and/or diarrhea.

Differential Diagnosis

- Corrosives toxicosis (alkali, acids)
- Uremia (oral ulcers)
- Acute vomiting

Initial Database

- CBC: leukocytosis (cationic detergents, phenol); methemoglobinemia (phenol)
- Serum biochemistry profile: electrolyte changes (from severe vomiting or dehydration; cationic detergents, phenols); hepatic or renal failure (phenol)
- Urinalysis: unremarkable unless renal failure
- Fluorescein staining for corneal ulcers (cationic detergents, phenol)
- Abdominal imaging (radiographs, ultrasound): to rule out other causes of acute severe vomiting
- Thoracic radiographs if respiratory signs are present; may show evidence of aspiration pneumonia and/or noncardiogenic pulmonary edema

Advanced or Confirmatory Testing

Endoscopic examination of esophagus to rule out perforation within 12-24 hours (cationic detergents, phenol)

TREATMENT

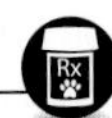

Treatment Overview

- Emesis induction is *contraindicated* in most types of cleaning liquid intoxications because vomiting risks further esophageal injury or aspiration; also, many patients spontaneously vomit.
- Dilution by administration of oral liquid, such as milk or water
- Prophylactic protection of gastrointestinal (GI) mucosa
- Supportive therapy based on clinical signs

Acute General Treatment

Decontamination of patient (p. 1087):

- Oral dilution: milk (preferred) or water. Approximately 0.25-0.5 cup (125-250 mL) for a 14-kg (30-lb) dog and 1-2 tablespoons (5-10 mL) for a 5-kg (11-lb) cat
- Emesis induction (p. 1188) is rarely needed. For use in cases of toxicosis with soaps (usually bar soaps) or detergents (other than cationic), perform within 2 hours only if very large amounts have been ingested. *Do not induce vomiting for alkaline anionic detergents, cationic detergents, phenol, or pine oils.*
- Dermal: wash exposed area (cationic detergents, phenol) with water for 20-30 minutes.
- Ocular: flush eyes with tepid tap water (or saline) for 20-30 minutes. Fluorescein stain to assess for corneal ulcers

Protect GI mucosa (for cationic detergents, phenol in dogs and cats):

- Omeprazole 0.5-2 mg/kg PO q 24h, *or*
- Pantoprazole 0.7-1 mg/kg IV over 15 minutes q 24h
- Sucralfate 0.5-1 g PO q 8-12h (dogs); 0.25-0.5 g PO q 8-12h (cats)

Control vomiting:

- Maropitant (Cerenia) 1 mg/kg SQ or 2 mg/kg PO q 24h, *or*
- Ondansetron 0.1-0.3 mg/kg IV q 8-12h, *or*
- Dolasetron mesylate 0.6 mg/kg IV q 24h

Broad-spectrum antibiotics if caustic burns and/or secondary infection present:

- Ampicillin 22 mg/kg IV q 8h plus enrofloxacin 5 mg/kg IM or diluted 1 : 1 with sterile saline and given slowly IV q 12h (5 mg/kg q 24h in cats), *or*
- Amoxicillin-clavulanate 12.5 mg/kg PO q 12h (dogs); 62.5 mg/CAT PO q 12h (cats) until signs resolve

Supportive care:

- Crystalloid intravenous fluids for rehydration
- Manage pain (caustic burns): opiates (fentanyl patch, buprenorphine 0.01-0.03 mg/kg IM, IV, SQ q 6-8h, or butorphanol 0.1-1 mg/kg IM, IV, or SQ q 6-12h).
- Rarely, ventilation required for respiratory manifestations (p. 1185)

Nutrition/Diet

- Watery slurry or soft mashed food while visible mucosal erosions are present
- Feeding tube (pp. 1106 and 1109) if anorexia is prolonged

Recommended Monitoring

- CBC, serum chemistry profile: electrolyte changes and other effects of vomiting
- Monitor oral cavity, perioral skin for caustic burns (cationic detergents, phenol) to determine when to introduce solid food.
- Pulse oximetry, thoracic radiography if aspiration (pine oils, laundry pods)

PROGNOSIS & OUTCOME

- Excellent with soaps, detergents (other than cationic), and household bleaches
- Good to guarded if pulmonary edema develops or if caustic burns are present (cationic detergents, phenols in cats)

PEARLS & CONSIDERATIONS

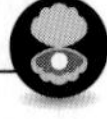

Comments

Soaps, detergents (other than cationic), and household bleaches have a low order of toxicity and can be treated by immediate dilution (oral administration of milk or water). Exposure to cationic detergents, phenol, and alkaline anionic detergents can lead to oral ulcers/burns and systemic effects (ataxia, weakness, seizures).

Prevention

Keep household cleaning products out of reach of pets.

Technician Tips

- Rapid oral dilution with milk or water will limit the extent of signs.
- Emesis induction and activated charcoal administration are typically *not* recommended.
- Ingestion of laundry pods often results in vomiting and aspiration pneumonia.

- Advise owner to bring label or container (tightly sealed, and out of reach of pet or children) to assist in identifying active ingredients/toxins.

SUGGESTED READING

Gwaltney-Brant SM: Miscellaneous indoor toxicants. In Peterson ME, et al, editors: Small animal toxicology, ed 3, St. Louis, 2013, Saunders, pp 291-298.

AUTHOR: Cristine Hayes, DVM, DABT, DABVT
EDITOR: Tina Wismer, DVM, MS, DABVT, DABT

Cleft Palate and Acquired Palate Defects

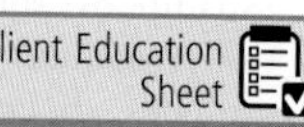

BASIC INFORMATION

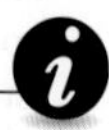

Definition

- Cleft palate: congenital (present at birth) defect of the hard and/or soft palate
- Acquired palate defect: acquired (after birth) defect of the hard and/or soft palate

Synonyms

Harelip, cleft lip: defect of the primary palate present at birth

Epidemiology

SPECIES, AGE, SEX

- Dogs and cats of either sex
- Incidence for congenital defects higher in brachycephalic dogs and Siamese cats
- Nursing difficulties noted in puppies and kittens soon after birth
- Cats after high-rise or motor-vehicle trauma

GENETICS, BREED PREDISPOSITION

Inherited as autosomal recessive or irregularly dominant genes

RISK FACTORS

See Etiology and Pathophysiology below.

ASSOCIATED DISORDERS

- Aspiration pneumonia
- Sneezing, nasal discharge, chronic rhinitis

Clinical Presentation

DISEASE FORMS/SUBTYPES

The upper lip and most rostral hard palate supported by the palatine processes of the incisive bones constitute the *primary palate.* The hard palate that is supported by the palatine processes of the maxillae and the horizontal laminae of the palatine bones and the soft palate constitute the *secondary palate.*

- Primary palate defects: unilateral, midline, or bilateral; unilateral defects are more often found on left side.
- Secondary palate defects
  - Midline cleft of hard and soft palate or soft palate only
  - Unilateral cleft of soft palate
  - Hypoplasia of soft palate
- Acquired palate defects can be located anywhere on the hard or soft palate.

HISTORY, CHIEF COMPLAINT

- Primary palate defects
  - Lip defects only: owner may note physical appearance.
  - Most rostral hard palate defects: mild nasal congestion, sneezing, and discharge
- Secondary palate defects: failure to create negative pressure for nursing, nasal discharge (drainage of milk from the nares during or after nursing), coughing, gagging, sneezing, nasal reflux, rhinitis, tonsillitis, laryngotracheitis, aspiration pneumonia, poor weight gain, and general unthriftiness
- Acquired palate defects
  - Signs depend on the size and location of the defect; the larger the defect, the more likely is it that clinical signs are present. Small rostral defects may not cause clinical signs beyond nasal discharge from local rhinitis.
  - Owners often report a causative event.

PHYSICAL EXAM FINDINGS

Congenital clefts:

- Small stature
- Nasal discharge, sneezing
- Auscultation: dyspnea, increased lung sounds, wheezing, or crackles (aspiration pneumonia)
- Oral examination (pp. 1125 and 1140)
  - Primary palate defects: harelip only (unilateral, midline, or bilateral lip defect); rostral hard palate defect only (unilateral or bilateral); or defects of the lip and most rostral hard palate; can also be associated with abnormalities of the secondary palate
  - Secondary palate defects: midline hard palate cleft can usually be visualized, but soft palate defect may be difficult to evaluate without chemical restraint.

Etiology and Pathophysiology

Congenital clefts:

Etiology:

- Hormonal: gestational glucocorticoid administration
- Infectious: viral induced
- Mechanical: intrauterine trauma
- Metabolic
- Nutritional
- Toxic: secondary to drug, viral toxins
- Hereditary: autosomal recessive or irregularly dominant genes; growth of palatine bones in the fetus may compete with growth of the skull, especially in broad-skulled (brachycephalic) dogs, to achieve normal closure of the palatine plates.

Pathophysiology:

- Defects of the primary and secondary palate result from a *failure of fusion* of paired (and one unpaired) structures during development.

Acquired palate defects:

- Causes include chronic infections (e.g., severe periodontal disease, osteomyelitis/osteonecrosis), trauma (e.g., high-rise syndrome, motor-vehicle trauma, electric cord injury, projectile trauma, animal bites, foreign body penetration, pressure wounds secondary to malocclusion), neoplasms, and surgical and radiation therapy.

DIAGNOSIS

Diagnostic Overview

Clinical signs are suggestive of the disorder (classically, milk discharge from nostrils in a nursing puppy or kitten; water and food discharge from nostrils in an adult animal), or the defect is identified as an incidental finding during routine examination. In either situation, complete assessment is done under sedation or anesthesia.

Differential Diagnosis

Defects due to severe periodontitis (oronasal fistula [p. 720])

Initial Database

- CBC, serum biochemistry panel, urinalysis: assessment of unthrifty patients
- Thoracic radiographs: evaluation of possible aspiration pneumonia

Advanced or Confirmatory Testing

Oral examination under general anesthesia: define extent of secondary palate defects (p. 1140)

TREATMENT

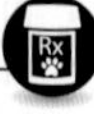

Treatment Overview

Essential elements:

- Treat and resolve aspiration pneumonia before surgery.
- Nutritional support (transoral tube feeding) until the patient with congenital cleft palate is of adequate age and health for surgery
- Consider postponing definitive repair for several weeks in the case of extensive tissue damage resulting from thermal/electric burns, gunshot trauma, or infection/inflammation or when teeth needed to be extracted at the planned site of surgery.
- Complete closure of palate defects

Acute General Treatment

Treat aspiration pneumonia, if present (p. 793).

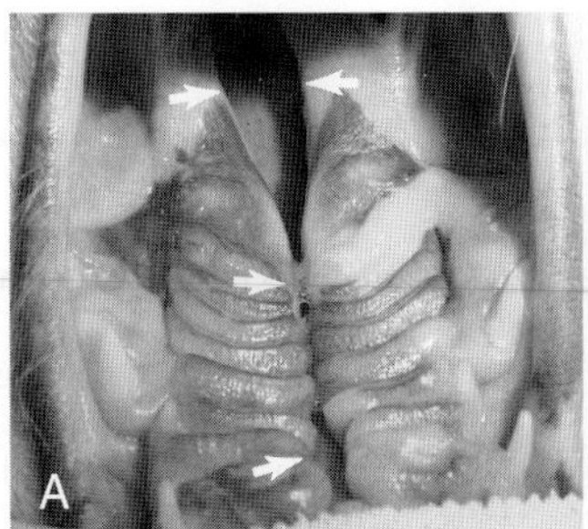

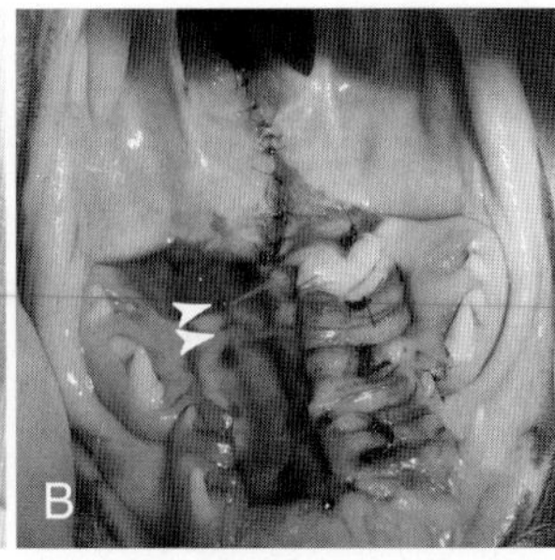

CLEFT PALATE A, Congenital cleft palate. This 14-week-old dog is under general anesthesia and in dorsal recumbency; rostral is toward the bottom of the image. A congenital defect of the secondary palate (midline cleft of the hard and soft palate) is seen *(arrows)*. **B,** Repaired congenital cleft palate. The hard palate defect was repaired using the overlapping flap technique; note the exposed major and accessory palatine arteries *(arrowheads)*. The donor area is left to granulate and epithelialize. The soft palate defect was repaired using the medially positioned flap technique. (Copyright Dr. Alexander M. Reiter, University of Pennsylvania.)

Chronic Treatment

Repair of primary palate defects:
- Cleft of most rostral hard palate: reconstructed by creating overlapping flaps of oral (and nasal) tissue or advancement, rotation, and transposition flaps harvested from oral tissue only; removal of one or more incisors and canine tooth on the affected side facilitates flap management.
- Cleft lip: reconstructive cutaneous surgery to provide symmetry (elective)

Repair of secondary palate defects:
- Midline hard palate cleft: overlapping flaps (preferred technique); medially positioned flaps or unilateral rotation (single pedicle) flaps may be used; the harvested mucoperiosteal flaps must be supplied by major palatine arteries; exposed bone is left to granulate and epithelialize.
- Midline soft palate cleft: medially positioned flaps (with at least a two-layer closure) or overlapping flaps
- Unilateral soft palate cleft: tonsillectomy at affected side, followed by creation and suturing of two nasopharyngeal and two oropharyngeal flaps
- Soft palate hypoplasia: bilateral tonsillectomy, followed by bilateral creation and suturing of two nasopharyngeal and two oropharyngeal flaps

Repair of acquired palate defects (depending on size and location):
- Defect in dental arch (p. 720)
- Smaller, round to oval, middle to caudal hard palate defect: split palatal U-flap with rotation flaps that must contain viable major palatine arteries (original technique with two equally long rotation flaps or modified technique with two unequally long rotation flaps)
- Larger palate defects (any location): labial- or buccal-based, overlapping advancement, rotation, or transposition flaps; local axial pattern flaps based on the major palatine and infraorbital arteries; distant axial pattern flaps based on the angularis oris, caudal auricular, or superficial cervical arteries; free tissue transfer with auricular cartilage or microvascular composite grafts; flexible bone membrane
- Nonsurgical closure of hard palate defects by using prosthetic devices (palatal obturators made of synthetic resin, silicone, or titanium) that are removable or attached to teeth

Ancillary care:
- Pain control: maxillary nerve block (0.5% bupivacaine hydrochloride) intraoperatively followed by opioids (e.g., hydromorphone 0.1-0.2 mg/kg IV or IM as needed up to q 2-4h) and postoperative opioid medication (butorphanol 0.2-0.4 mg/kg PO q 6-12h) or nonsteroidal antiinflammatories (e.g., carprofen 2 mg/kg PO q 12h) for 4-7 days
- Antibiotics: not required unless existing aspiration pneumonia
- Wound management: oral application of dilute chlorhexidine solution or gel for 4 weeks; Elizabethan collar to prevent pawing at surgical site

Nutrition/Diet

Preoperatively in congenital cleft patients:
- Transoral tube feeding with milk replacer or other suitable diet (e.g., Hill's a/d) until 3-4 months of age
  - Supplies nutritional needs
  - Minimizes rhinitis
  - Allows patient to mature: anesthetic purposes, greater strength of palatal tissues, more working room in the oral cavity and oropharynx to effect repair

Postoperatively:
- Soft food, no chewing toys/treats for 4 weeks; esophagostomy or gastrostomy tubes to bypass the oral cavity are rarely needed.

Possible Complications

Dehiscence causes:
- Excess tension if inadequate mobilization of tissue for closure
- Flap necrosis if major palatine artery or wound edges are compromised during surgery
- Tongue movements, chewing on hard material, self-trauma (consider e-collar, postoperative tube feeding)

Recommended Monitoring

Re-examination in 2 weeks for removal of skin sutures at lips

PROGNOSIS & OUTCOME

- Multiple procedures may be required to close a palate defect. Follow-up surgeries should not be attempted before healing (granulation and epithelialization) of all tissues involved (6-8 weeks).
- Poor prognosis for congenital soft palate hypoplasia (restoration of a pharyngeal sphincteric ring and normal swallowing function may not be achieved)
- Guarded prognosis for secondary palate defects without surgical repair (risk of aspiration)

PEARLS & CONSIDERATIONS

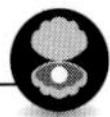

Comments

The best chance of success is with the first surgical procedure. Avoid electrocoagulation for hemostasis, handle flaps as carefully as possible, and avoid creating closure that is under tension. Referral to an experienced oral surgeon is recommended.

Prevention

- Selective breeding
- Avoid gestational glucocorticoid administration and other insult during pregnancy (see Etiology and Pathophysiology above).

Technician Tips

Technicians caring for patients with congenital cleft palate preoperatively and postoperatively should be skilled in correct tube-feeding technique and feeding tube care (pp. 1106 and 1107).

Client Education

Management of patients with congenital cleft palate requires intensive nursing care at home for 2-4 months until surgery can be performed. Owners should be warned that multiple procedures might be required to completely close a congenital or acquired palate defect.

SUGGESTED READING

Reiter AM, et al: Palate surgery. In Tobias KM, et al, editors: Veterinary surgery: small animal, St. Louis, 2012, Elsevier, pp 1707-1717.

AUTHOR & EDITOR: Alexander M. Reiter, DVM, Dr. med. vet., DAVDC, DEVDC

Clostridial Enterocolitis

Client Education Sheet 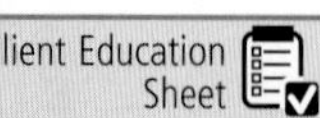

BASIC INFORMATION 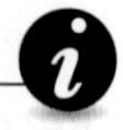

Definition

Clostridial enterocolitis or clostridial enterotoxicosis is an intestinal disease that causes diarrhea in dogs and cats and is suspected to be caused by *Clostridium perfringens*. It typically causes large-intestinal diarrhea, which may be acute and self-limited, or chronic. *C. perfringens* may be associated with antibiotic-responsive diarrhea.

Synonyms

Acute nosocomial colitis, canine nosocomial diarrhea, clostridia-associated diarrhea

Epidemiology

SPECIES, AGE, SEX

Dogs are more commonly affected than cats. Acute disease can occur in any age animal, whereas chronic disease occurs more commonly in middle-aged to older animals.

RISK FACTORS

Any stressors to the gastrointestinal (GI) tract, abrupt dietary change, chronic antibiotic use or underlying GI disease

CONTAGION AND ZOONOSIS

May be contagious; zoonotic potential unknown

ASSOCIATED DISORDERS

May be associated with other enteric diseases, including parvovirus (p. 760), inflammatory bowel disease (p. 543), or acute hemorrhagic diarrhea syndrome (p. 259)

Clinical Presentation

DISEASE FORMS/SUBTYPES

C. perfringens type A

HISTORY, CHIEF COMPLAINT

Some or all may be present.

- Large-intestinal diarrhea is most common. Small volumes of feces, increased frequency of defecation, and straining are common, and mucus and/or fresh blood may be visualized in the feces. Vomiting and flatulence may be present in some patients. Many patients show no clinical signs other than diarrhea.
- A small number of patients may also have small-bowel diarrhea marked by large volumes of watery feces and abdominal discomfort.
- The majority of patients are not systemically ill but have GI signs due to Clostridia or concurrent disease.

PHYSICAL EXAM FINDINGS

- Findings are nonspecific and relate to large-intestinal diarrhea. There may be abdominal discomfort during palpation. There may also be signs of pain, along with blood and mucus, during digital rectal examination. Signs of systemic illness are uncommon.
- Acute nosocomial diarrhea associated with *C. perfringens* is often seen 1-5 days after boarding or kenneling. This syndrome appears to be self-limited and responds well to supportive care. Typically, clinical signs last 5-7 days.
- Chronic cases often have intermittent clinical signs that may recur every 4-6 weeks.

Etiology and Pathophysiology

- *C. perfringens* is an anaerobic, spore-forming, gram-positive bacillus that is also found in healthy dogs and cats.
- Sporulation of toxigenic strains causes release of enterotoxin A. This enterotoxin can cause mucosal damage and fluid secretion in the colon.
- Other factors must also be involved. Enterotoxin-related damage cannot be the sole explanation for this disorder because enterotoxin has been identified in the feces of normal animals.

DIAGNOSIS 

Diagnostic Overview

Definitive diagnosis is challenging. The diagnosis may be supported with fecal bacterial cultures, but in most cases, the transient nature of the illness means that a definitive diagnosis is neither achieved nor clinically necessary. *C. perfringens* may be cultured from healthy animals. The disease often presents as an antibiotic-responsive diarrhea, but response is not sufficient for a diagnosis.

Differential Diagnosis

- All causes of large-intestinal diarrhea, both primary GI and systemic/nonprimary GI forms, need to be considered (pp. 1213 and 1215).
  - Primary GI disease includes parasites, inflammatory bowel disease, neoplasia, fungal disease, idiopathic colitis, and histiocytic ulcerative colitis.
  - Systemic/extraintestinal causes of acute diarrhea include pancreatitis, anxiety/nervousness, other intraabdominal disorders, and intoxications (e.g., organophosphates).

Initial Database

Fecal analysis is very important in all cases of large-bowel diarrhea and may yield important clues to the problem, even if the diagnosis is elusive.

- CBC, biochemical profile, urinalysis, fecal flotation: generally unremarkable
- Fecal ELISA to rule out *Giardia* or other pathogens
- Fecal smear with new methylene blue, Wright or Diff-Quick stain for safety-pin–appearing spores; numbers do not correlate with clinical disease
- Rectal scraping for cytologic evaluation to rule out histoplasmosis, lymphoma or other neoplasia, histiocytic ulcerative colitis (p. 1157)

Advanced or Confirmatory Testing

- Abdominal radiographs or ultrasound are often normal but can help rule out extra-gastrointestinal diseases.
- Colonoscopy is rarely indicated to diagnose this condition but, in severe cases, may be necessary to rule out other causes of colitis:
  - Mucosal hyperemia or ulceration is typical.
  - Histopathologic evaluation of biopsies may indicate neutrophilic colitis, the presence of other inflammatory bowel disease, or may be normal.
- Sporulating clostridial organisms, which have the appearance of safety pins, may be seen on fecal cytology (3-5 organisms/field on oil immersion). However, the presence of these organisms does not confirm that *Clostridium* is the primary cause of the clinical disease.
- Anaerobic fecal cultures will typically identify high concentrations of *C. perfringens*.
- Other available diagnostic tests include ELISA enterotoxin assays and polymerase chain reaction (PCR) enterotoxin genotyping.

TREATMENT 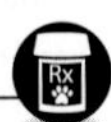

Treatment Overview

Therapeutic goals are to provide supportive care and eliminate large-bowel diarrhea. Most can be treated as outpatients, but patients that are systemically ill, dehydrated, or have electrolyte abnormalities should be hospitalized. Supportive care should be directed toward correcting volume deficits, correcting electrolyte disturbances, and reducing intestinal discomfort (including vomiting) so the patient will be more comfortable and eat.

Acute General Treatment

- Treatment with intravenous crystalloid solutions to correct volume deficits is very important. In severe cases, colloids may also be used to complement crystalloid therapy.
- The use of antimicrobials is generally beneficial. Options include amoxicillin or ampicillin 20 mg/kg PO q 8h, clindamycin 10-20 mg/kg PO q 12h, tylosin 5-10 mg/kg PO q 12h, or metronidazole 15-20 mg/kg PO q 12h for 5-7 days.. Parenteral antibiotics with anaerobic bactericidal activity (e.g., ampicillin 20 mg/kg IV q 6-8h) are indicated if the patient is systemically ill.

Chronic Treatment

- Long-term antimicrobial therapy may be required along with dietary management.

- In some cases, antibiotic therapy may be discontinued as long as the high-fiber diet is maintained.
- Probiotics may also be useful.
- Anecdotally, fecal transplant (p. 1105) has had some success in otherwise healthy dogs. It should be attempted only after other causes of disease have been ruled out and standard treatments have failed.

Nutrition/Diet

High-fiber diets reduce clinical signs and speed recovery.

Recommended Monitoring

Based on the presence or absence of diarrhea and signs of systemic illness

PROGNOSIS & OUTCOME

The prognosis depends on the presenting condition of the patient. In most cases, the prognosis is excellent. Prognosis may also be related to underlying disease if *Clostridium* is a secondary condition.

PEARLS & CONSIDERATIONS

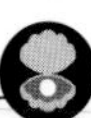

Comments

- There is no gold standard on how to treat this disease; treatment is customized based on specific abnormalities identified on physical exam and diagnostic testing.
- There is still some question about whether Koch's postulates have been fulfilled regarding causality of *C. perfringens* and this form of enteritis.

Prevention

- Environmental exposure is a risk factor.
- High-fiber diets may promote enteral health and be preventive.

Technician Tips

- Clinical signs related to systemic illness, such as dehydration and fever, should be noted.
- Supportive care and hygiene are the most important aspects of patient management.

Client Education

In most cases, signs associated with this disease subside with supportive care, but some patients may be chronically affected.

SUGGESTED READING

Weese JS, et al: The roles of *Clostridium difficile* and enterotoxigenic *Clostridium perfringens* in diarrhea in dogs. J Vet Intern Med 15:374-378, 2001.

AUTHOR: Steven L. Marks, BVSc, MS, DACVIM
EDITOR: Rance K. Sellon, DVM, PhD, DACVIM

Cobalamin Deficiency

BASIC INFORMATION

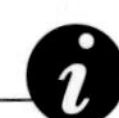

Definition

A reduced serum concentration of the B vitamin cobalamin is usually secondary to insufficient intestinal uptake due to malnutrition/malabsorption.

Synonym

Vitamin B_{12} deficiency, Imerslund-Gräsbeck syndrome (congenital form)

Epidemiology

SPECIES, AGE, SEX

- Acquired form: dogs and cats (mean age for cats: 7 years)
- Congenital form: young kittens and puppies (6-12 weeks old)

GENETICS, BREED PREDISPOSITION

Chinese Shar-pei, giant schnauzer, beagle, Border collie, Australian shepherd

RISK FACTORS

- In theory, a pure vegetarian diet may cause cobalamin deficiency (reported in humans); unlikely in dogs and cats eating commercial pet food
- Surgical resection of the ileum (main site of cobalamin absorption)
- Exocrine pancreatic insufficiency (EPI): in dogs and cats, the pancreas is a major source of intrinsic factor, which is necessary for ileal absorption of cobalamin.
- Severe and chronic small-intestinal disease may damage ileal cobalamin receptors.

Clinical Presentation

DISEASE FORMS/SUBTYPES

- Congenital (rare): defect in receptors for uptake
- Secondary (common): caused by EPI, intestinal dysbiosis (small intestinal bacterial overgrowth [SIBO]/antibiotic-responsive diarrhea [ARD]), chronic enteropathies (e.g., inflammatory bowel disease [IBD], lymphoma, histoplasmosis), any form of chronic malabsorption/malnutrition; interference with ileal cobalamin uptake

HISTORY, CHIEF COMPLAINT

- Congenital form: gastrointestinal (GI) disorders, failure to thrive, hematologic and biochemical abnormalities, proteinuria, seizures
- Acquired form: clinical signs of GI disease most common

PHYSICAL EXAM FINDINGS

- Most dogs and cats with cobalamin deficiency show only clinical signs of GI disease (chronic diarrhea, vomiting, weight loss, poor body condition), depending on the underlying cause.
- Neurologic signs have been reported occasionally in dogs and cats with selective cobalamin deficiency (i.e., hyperammonemic encephalopathy, organic acidemia).
- Neutropenia and anemia (usually normocytic) are usually features of the congenital form and occur rarely in acquired disease.

Etiology and Pathophysiology

- Cobalamin (vitamin B_{12}) is a water-soluble vitamin produced exclusively by microorganisms. Animals are unable to synthesize cobalamin and depend on nutritional sources. Cobalamin is an important cofactor for a variety of biochemical reactions (e.g., amino acid metabolism, DNA synthesis).
- Dietary cobalamin binds to intrinsic factor, which in dogs and especially in cats is mainly produced in the pancreas, serving as a transporter for absorption at the distal small intestine.

DIAGNOSIS

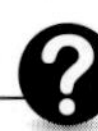

Diagnostic Overview

Cobalamin deficiency is usually suspected as a possible secondary complication of GI disease or exocrine pancreatic insufficiency. Measurement of serum cobalamin levels is the clinical diagnostic test of choice.

Differential Diagnosis

- Chronic GI disease: IBD, intestinal dysbiosis/SIBO/ARD, intestinal lymphoma, histoplasmosis
- EPI

Initial Database

CBC, serum biochemistry profile: to rule out other systemic disease

- With congenital disease: normocytic nonregenerative anemia/pernicious anemia, neutropenia
- Panhypoproteinemia often identified with maldigestion/malabsorption

Advanced or Confirmatory Testing

- Measurement of serum cobalamin
    - Reference range established at the GI Laboratory at Texas A&M University

- Dogs: 251-908 ng/L, cats: 290-1500 ng/L
- Other laboratories may have different reference ranges.
- Measurement of methylmalonic acid (MMA) in serum or urine: not routinely available
  - Increased serum or urinary MMA indicates cobalamin deficiency at the cellular level.
- Serum trypsin-like immunoreactivity to rule out EPI
- Serum folate to rule out SIBO/ARD

TREATMENT

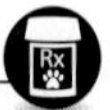

Treatment Overview

The goal is to correct cobalamin deficiency at the cellular level and correct clinical signs (i.e., GI, hematologic, immunologic, and neurologic).

Chronic Treatment

Repeated high doses of cobalamin by parenteral administration or daily oral supplementation are necessary; lifelong parenteral dosing is mandatory for patients with congenital cobalamin deficiency because they cannot absorb orally administered cobalamin.

- Cyanocobalamin is the preferred form, but hydroxycobalamin can also be used.

Recommended empirical parenteral dosing schedule of cyanocobalamin:

- 150-250 mcg per injection in cats; 250-1200 mcg per injection in dogs
- Dose every 7 days for 6 weeks, then one dose after 30 days, and retesting 30 days after the last dose

Recommended empirical oral dosing schedule of cyanocobalamin:

- 250 mcg in cats and 250-1000 mcg in dogs, depending on the size of the patient
- Daily oral administration for total of 12 weeks and recheck serum cobalamin concentration 1 week after the last dose.

If the underlying disease process has resolved and cobalamin body stores have been replenished, serum cobalamin concentration should be supranormal at the time of re-evaluation.

- If serum cobalamin concentration is in the normal range, cobalamin supplementation should be continued at least monthly (parenteral) or daily (oral).
- If serum cobalamin concentration at the time of recheck is subnormal, further investigation is required to identify the underlying disease process. Cobalamin supplementation should be continued weekly or biweekly (parenteral) or daily (oral). Dogs or cats with chronic disease often require lifelong therapy to maintain appropriate cobalamin levels.

Possible Complications

Cobalamin is nontoxic and can be administered in large doses with minimal risk of side effects.

Recommended Monitoring

- Depending on the underlying cause of cobalamin deficiency and the clinical signs, measure serum cobalamin concentration every few months.
- In animals with the congenital form, more frequent checks may be necessary until an optimal dose regimen has been established.

PROGNOSIS & OUTCOME

- In the congenital form, the response to parenteral cyanocobalamin is usually excellent, leading to reversal of clinical abnormalities.
- In the acquired form, prognosis depends on the underlying disease.
  - Usually excellent in animals with EPI in combination with pancreatic enzyme replacement therapy
  - Hypocobalaminemia has been associated with a poor outcome in dogs with severe chronic enteropathies.

PEARLS & CONSIDERATIONS

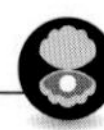

Comments

- Patients with severe cobalamin deficiency often do not respond to therapy of the underlying GI disorder until cobalamin is supplemented.
- Monitoring of serum cobalamin in geriatric cats is recommended as part of routine evaluation because they may become deficient due to decreased ability to absorb B_{12}.
- A study has shown that cats with chronic GI disease and cobalamin deficiency unresponsive to previous therapy responded with weight gain quickly after beginning cobalamin supplementation.
- Cobalamin deficiency on a cellular level may occur even when serum cobalamin concentration is at the low end of the normal range (<350 ng/L); parenteral or oral cobalamin supplementation should be considered for these patients.

Technician Tip

Multivitamin preparations contain an insufficient amount of cobalamin and are not recommended for supplementation.

SUGGESTED READING

Toresson L, et al: Oral cobalamin supplementation in dogs with chronic enteropathies and hypocobalaminemia. J Vet Intern Med 30:101, 2016.

AUTHOR: Jan S. Suchodolski, MedVet, Dr. Med. Vet., PhD, DACVM
EDITOR: Rance K. Sellon, DVM, PhD, DACVIM

Coccidioidomycosis

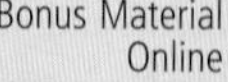

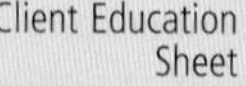

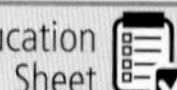

BASIC INFORMATION

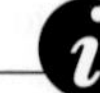

Definition

A respiratory or systemic fungal infection caused by *Coccidioides immitis* or *Coccidioides posadasii;* occurs predominantly in the southwestern United States

Synonyms

San Joaquin Valley fever, valley fever

Epidemiology

SPECIES, AGE, SEX

Young adult, male, medium- to large-breed outdoor dogs are more commonly infected. Cats are less frequently diagnosed with coccidioidomycosis and often have severe disseminated disease at the time of diagnosis.

RISK FACTORS

- Amount of roaming space > 1 acre
- Walking in the desert (in endemic areas, a decreased risk has been associated with walking preferentially on sidewalks)
- Being predominantly outdoors during the day
- Travel to Arizona, New Mexico, west Texas, or the central valley of California
- Young adult age
- Digging behavior
- ± Immunosuppression
- A retrospective study suggested that Hungarian Vizslas, Dalmatians, Weimaraners, greyhounds, English pointers, bull terriers, Brittany spaniels, and boxers might be at increased risk when compared with the hospital background population.

CONTAGION AND ZOONOSIS

- Coccidioidomycosis occurs in humans, who can become infected from the same environmental source as animals.
- Direct transmission from infected animals to humans is unlikely because the spherule phase (present at body temperature) is not transmitted by aerosol. Transmission of *Coccidioides* to a human from a cat bite has been reported.
- Conversion of the yeast phase to the mycelial phase, which produces infectious spores (arthroconidia) that can be inhaled, could occur on stored necropsy specimens, old bandages, tissue specimens, or instruments; such material should be dealt with safely and immediately (e.g., disinfected/autoclaved).

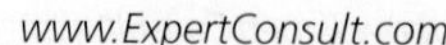

- The mycelial/hyphal form of *Coccidioides,* which grows *in vitro* and in nature is highly infectious by the aerosol route; cultures are a significant risk to laboratory personnel and should be performed only in well-equipped microbiology laboratories with trained personnel.

GEOGRAPHY AND SEASONALITY

- Coccidioidomycosis occurs mainly in the southwestern United States, including the central valley of California *(Coccidioides immitis);* southern regions of Arizona, Nevada, Utah, and New Mexico; and western Texas *(Coccidioides posadasii).* Disease has also emerged in south-central Washington state. To a lesser extent, it occurs in regions of Mexico and Central and South America (particularly Venezuela). Having lived in or traveled through these regions up to several years before the onset of illness is almost always a component of the history.
- Because the disease is acquired through inhalation of airborne spores, the incidence increases after soil disturbance (dust storms, earthquakes, construction).

Clinical Presentation

HISTORY, CHIEF COMPLAINT

- Chronic cough (pulmonary or hilar lymph node involvement) may be dry and harsh or moist and productive. Severe pulmonary involvement may be associated with respiratory distress.
- Other presenting complaints include inappetence, weight loss, lethargy, lameness, cutaneous masses with or without draining tracts, signs of head or neck pain, signs of vision loss, or neurologic signs such as seizures and ataxia. Dogs with pericardial involvement may present with signs of right-sided heart failure or restrictive pericarditis.
- Skin lesions are uncommon and usually a manifestation of disseminated disease rather than a primary localized infection.

PHYSICAL EXAM FINDINGS

Harsh breath sounds, cough, dyspnea, and tachypnea are common. Systemic signs may include fever, lethargy, and weakness. Lameness may be noted ± firm swellings over long bones. Cutaneous masses with or without draining tracts may be present. Other findings include lymphadenopathy, cranial and cervical hyperesthesia, ascites, and signs of uveitis, focal chorioretinitis, or panophthalmitis.

Etiology and Pathophysiology

- *Coccidioides* spp are dimorphic fungi; they exhibit different forms in tissues and in the environment.
  - The mycelial form exists in soil and produces arthroconidia that are dispersed by wind and other disruption of the soil and easily inhaled.
  - Inhalation of 10 or fewer arthroconidia is sufficient to cause infection that produces clinical signs.
  - After inhalation, arthroconidia enter the pulmonary alveoli and cause subpleural lesions.
  - After infection of the respiratory system, the fungus changes morphology, forming spherules containing endospores in tissue. The spherule releases endospores that can disseminate after phagocytosis and form new spherules. This, together with the pyogranulomatous inflammatory response, results in clinical illness.
  - The incubation period from the time of inhalation to the appearance of respiratory signs is typically 1-3 weeks, but sometimes months. In some cases, infection may be present for years before causing overt signs. Immune-complex glomerulonephritis has been described in some dogs with chronic coccidioidomycosis.
- Disease may remain localized to the respiratory tract or become systemic with dissemination to lymph nodes, bones, eyes, skin, pericardium, spleen, liver, kidney, testes, and central nervous system (CNS).
- As in humans, many animals develop transient, subclinical infections, and some may recover from localized respiratory illness without developing disseminated disease and without therapy.
  - Approximately 28% of dogs living in an endemic region develop antibodies to *Coccidioides* spp by the age of 2 years, but only about 6% develop clinical infection.

DIAGNOSIS

Diagnostic Overview

A definitive diagnosis of coccidioidomycosis is made by cytologic or histologic visualization of the organism in tissues. If the organism cannot be identified, the diagnosis is based on compatible presentation and results of serologic tests.

Differential Diagnosis

- Cough (p. 1209)
- Bone lesions: bacterial osteomyelitis, other fungal infections, bone neoplasia
- Skin lesions: draining tracts due to other systemic mycoses, nocardia, actinomycosis, or mycobacterial infections, bony lesions such as infected sequestra, abscesses due to bite wounds or other penetrating injuries, or neoplasia
- Ocular lesions: other systemic infectious illnesses and immune-mediated diseases

Initial Database

- CBC may reveal an inflammatory leukogram with a monocytosis and a mild nonregenerative anemia.
- Hypoalbuminemia (almost all cases) and hyperglobulinemia (≈50% of cases) are common. Hypercalcemia has not been described in dogs or cats with coccidioidomycosis but does occur in people.
- Urinalysis is usually unremarkable, but some dogs may have proteinuria.
- Thoracic radiographs are frequently abnormal and are indicated for any suspect patient.
  - Common findings include a diffuse interstitial or nodular interstitial pattern and hilar lymphadenopathy, which may be profound.
  - Alveolar infiltrates, miliary interstitial patterns, or nodules with or without pleural effusion or evidence of pericardial effusion may be seen.
  - Spontaneous pneumothorax has been described.
- Radiographs of long bones may reveal mixed proliferative and lytic lesions, typically located distally on long bones (distal diaphysis, metaphysis, epiphysis). Biopsy or cytology is necessary for a definitive diagnosis.
- Magnetic resonance imaging of the CNS often reveals single focal lesions that may be extraaxial or intraaxial. Typically, lesions have indistinct borders and vary in signal intensities and the degree of contrast enhancement.

Advanced or Confirmatory Testing

- Coccidioidomycosis can be definitively diagnosed by cytologic examination of exudates, sputum, or aspirates or by histopathologic examination of tissue.
  - Spherules are large (1-10 times the diameter of a red blood cell), round structures with a distinct cell wall typically surrounded by neutrophils and macrophages.
  - Transtracheal washes and lymph node aspirates are often falsely negative. Cytologic evaluation of fluid from draining tracts or of pleural effusion is more likely to yield organisms, which appear on Romanowsky stains (e.g., Diff-Quik) as sometimes crinkled, deeply basophilic structures.
  - Organisms can be difficult to find histopathologically but when present are readily identified by their distinct morphology. In lesions with low numbers of organisms, periodic acid–Schiff and silver stains may assist in identification of spherules.
- Several canine and feline serologic tests are available for immunoglobulin M (IgM) and IgG. Serologic tests may be positive in subclinically infected dogs. The agar gel immunodiffusion assay (AGID), which detects IgM and IgG, is most commonly used.
  - A positive IgM titer (tube precipitin antigens) can be noted within 2 weeks of exposure (i.e., during or just after the incubation period) and may last 4-6 weeks.
  - A positive IgG titer (complement fixation [CF] antigens) indicates exposure or infection. The magnitude of the titer is considered important, higher titers (≥1 : 64) are most consistent with clinical disease. Titers ≤ 4 may be consistent with previous exposure and recovery.
  - IgG titer is expected to decrease slowly but may not reach zero with successful treatment.
  - Positive IgG titers from dogs living in endemic areas are more likely due to exposure than from active infection.

- Negative serologic tests of dogs infected with *Coccidioides* spp are uncommon but can occur.
- An antigen diagnostic test that identifies *Coccidioides* spp galactomannan antigen in serum and urine is available. The test shows cross-reactivity with *Histoplasma capsulatum* and *Blastomyces dermatitidis* and has low sensitivity. It may be helpful in antibody-seronegative coccidioidomycosis.
- Polymerase chain reaction (PCR) testing: not yet widely applied to this disease in dogs and cats

TREATMENT

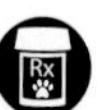

Treatment Overview

Antifungal therapy (itraconazole, fluconazole, or ketoconazole) is most commonly employed. Itraconazole and fluconazole have fewer adverse effects and greater bioavailability than ketoconazole. Fluconazole is the treatment of choice for CNS or ocular involvement. Amphotericin B may be required for treatment of severe disseminated disease.

Acute General Treatment

- Supportive care for systemic illness and respiratory distress as warranted
  - Oxygen supplementation (p. 1146)
  - Treatment of systemic hypotension
- Mild respiratory cases may resolve without treatment, but antifungal therapy is often instituted to avoid dissemination. Avoid broad-spectrum antibiotics and immunosuppressive medications.
- Azole antifungal drugs: if using generic azole preparations, obtain only from a reliable source. Liver enzyme activities ± serum drug levels should be monitored periodically during therapy.
  - Fluconazole 5-10 mg/kg PO q 12h (dogs); 10 mg/kg PO q 12h (25-50 mg/CAT PO q 12-24h) (cats). Penetrates better than itraconazole into the eye, prostate, and CNS tissues
  - Itraconazole 5 mg/kg PO q 12h for 1 week, then 5 mg/kg PO q 24h thereafter (dogs); 3-5 mg/kg q 12h for 1 week, then 5 mg/kg PO q 24h thereafter (cats). Name brand is costly, but compounded formulations may not be efficacious. Unless significant inflammation is present, it may not penetrate the eye and CNS. Capsules should be administered with food but the solution can be administered on an empty stomach. Serum drug concentrations may be needed to confirm bioavailability.
  - Ketoconazole 5-10 mg/kg PO q 12h; variably effective depending on absorption. Least costly; may produce adverse hepatic effects or vomiting/inappetence. Serum drug concentrations may be needed to confirm bioavailability. Ketoconazole is poorly tolerated by cats.
  - Other azoles such as voriconazole or posaconazole could be considered for dogs that fail to respond to treatment with itraconazole or fluconazole.
- Deoxycholate amphotericin B 0.5 mg/kg IV on a Monday-Wednesday-Friday basis, given over 4-6 hours in 5% dextrose for 1 month barring nephrotoxicosis (dogs); 0.25 mg/kg (cats). Can be used in patients that are not responding to or do not tolerate azoles (e.g., anorexia, vomiting, hepatic dysfunction). Adverse effects include nephrotoxicosis and perivascular irritation/sloughing. Renal parameters should be assessed before each dose. Lipid forms of amphotericin B (e.g., 1-3 mg/kg IV, given on a Monday-Wednesday-Friday basis over 1-2 hours [dogs]; 1 mg/kg IV [cats]) are less nephrotoxic but more expensive.
- Surgical treatment by subtotal pericardectomy and epicardial excision has been used successfully for relief of right-sided heart failure in dogs with effusive-constrictive pericarditis.

Chronic Treatment

- The decision to stop antifungal therapy should be based on resolution of clinical signs, radiographic lesions, and serologic titers. Therapy should continue for at least 2 months beyond resolution of clinical signs and radiographic abnormalities, which may be > 12 months with disseminated disease (especially if there is bone involvement). Depending on the severity of disseminated disease and the immune competence of the patient, treatment may be lifelong.
- Rising titers suggest an inadequate response to therapy, although decreasing titers are not necessarily predictive of a good response.

Drug Interactions

- Some patients receiving azole drugs can develop liver dysfunction, vomiting or diarrhea, thrombocytopenia, and skin reactions.
- Compatibility of other medications with antifungal agents should be investigated before use.
- Caution should be taken in patients receiving *o,p'*-DDD, warfarin, digoxin, phenobarbital, phenytoin, methylprednisolone, or cyclosporine because azole drugs may raise serum levels of these medications substantially.

Possible Complications

If clinically significant respiratory signs are left untreated, systemic spread of illness may occur.

PROGNOSIS & OUTCOME

- Prognosis for patients with disease limited to the respiratory tract is fair to good.
- Patients with disseminated disease have a guarded to poor prognosis for full recovery, depending on the severity of disease and degree of dissemination.
- Patients with CNS involvement have a poor prognosis.

PEARLS & CONSIDERATIONS

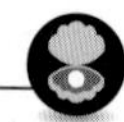

Comments

- Radiographic changes cannot distinguish bony neoplasia from fungal osteomyelitis; biopsy is required.
- Fungal culture of *Coccidioides* should not be attempted in a veterinary practice because the mycelial form that produces arthroconidia in culture is highly infectious.

Prevention

To minimize the risk of infection in endemic areas, keep animals away from desert soil and locations where soil is disrupted (e.g., construction sites), and discourage digging.

Technician Tips

- Bandages used for covering cutaneous draining tracts for prolonged periods have the potential to become infectious to humans if the lesion is due to *Coccidioides* infection. Bandages should be avoided in such situations, or if indispensable, they should be changed on a daily basis and disinfected or destroyed (autoclaved) immediately when removed.
- If a needlestick injury occurs (e.g., during fine-needle aspiration of affected tissues), medical advice should be sought immediately.

SUGGESTED READING

Sykes JE: Coccidioidomycosis. In Sykes JE, editor: Canine and feline infectious diseases, St. Louis, 2014, Elsevier, pp 613-623.

AUTHORS: Jane E. Sykes, BVSc, PhD, DACVIM; Sharon M. Dial, DVM, PhD, DACVP
EDITOR: Joseph Taboada, DVM, DACVIM

Coccidiosis, Intestinal

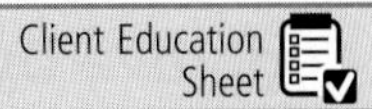

BASIC INFORMATION

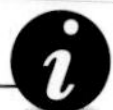

Definition

A diarrheal disease caused by intestinal tract infection with Apicomplexan parasites in the genus *Cystoisospora*

Synonym

Isospora

Epidemiology

SPECIES, AGE, SEX

- Dogs and cats
- Generally very young animals or animals that are immunosuppressed

RISK FACTORS

- Recent weaning or overcrowded conditions
- Immunosuppression
- Co-infection with other intestinal organisms

CONTAGION AND ZOONOSIS

Cystoisospora spp are host specific and do not infect people.

GEOGRAPHY AND SEASONALITY

Worldwide distribution, present year round

Clinical Presentation

HISTORY, CHIEF COMPLAINT

- Vomiting
- Diarrhea with or without blood; often foul smelling, pasty, and semiformed to liquid
- Inappetence

PHYSICAL EXAM FINDINGS

- Weight loss (or poor growth)
- Dehydration
- Possible abdominal discomfort

Etiology and Pathophysiology

- Intestinal coccidiosis in cats is caused by *Cystoisospora felis* and *Cystoisospora rivolta*. Intestinal coccidiosis in dogs is caused by *Cystoisospora canis, Cystoisospora ohioensis, Cystoisospora neorivolta*, and *Cystoisospora burrowsi.*
- Infection follows ingestion of sporulated oocysts; sporozoites infect intestinal epithelial cells.
- Intestinal damage is caused by rupture of infected host cells lining the small intestinal villi. Villous atrophy and villous erosions occur secondary to parasite multiplication.

DIAGNOSIS

Diagnostic Overview

Diagnosis is suspected in pups or kittens with diarrhea. Diagnosis is confirmed by finding oocysts on routine fecal flotation examination in the presence of appropriate clinical findings.

Differential Diagnosis

- Viral diarrhea: parvovirus, coronavirus, rotavirus
- Bacterial diarrhea: *Clostridium, Campylobacter, Salmonella enteritides*
- Other gastrointestinal parasites
- Dietary indiscretion

Initial Database

- Fecal flotation examination and demonstration of characteristic oocysts. False-negative results are uncommon, but erratic shedding of oocysts can necessitate repeat examinations.
- Presence of oocysts in immunocompetent adult animals is most likely incidental.
- Parvovirus ELISA is indicated for affected puppies and kittens with severe diarrhea to investigate concurrent parvoviral enteritis and panleukopenia, respectively.
- Kittens (>4 months) should be tested for feline leukemia virus or feline immunodeficiency virus.
- Rarely, regenerative anemia may develop from excessive intestinal blood loss from heavy parasite burdens.

TREATMENT

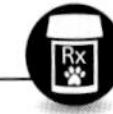

Treatment Overview

Goals of treatment are remission of diarrhea and cessation of oocyst shedding.

Acute General Treatment

Drug of choice: sulfadimethoxine (Albon oral suspension 5%):

- 50-60 mg/kg PO q 24h for 5-20 days
- To prevent dehydration, adequate water intake must be maintained during treatment.
- Supportive care includes fluids; providing a warm, dry environment; and a high-quality, highly digestible diet.

Off-label:

- Ponazuril (Marquis) 20 mg/kg PO twice, 1-7 days apart, or 50 mg/kg PO once
- A combination of sulfadimethoxine with ormetoprim (Primor) 55 mg/kg PO q 24h (for up to 21 days) is also effective.
- Amprolium (Corid) 300-400 mg/DOSE PO q 24h for 5 days in dogs, with the lower dosage recommended for puppies; 60-100 mg/DOSE PO q 24h for 5 days in cats. Amprolium is bitter, and care should be taken that the dose is ingested and not spit out.

Nutrition/Diet

Highly digestible diets with the addition of a probiotic has been helpful in shortening the duration of diarrhea and the length of shedding in young kittens in two separate studies in an animal shelter environment.

Drug Interactions

Sulfonamides with cyclosporin, ACE inhibitors, warfarin

Recommended Monitoring

Adult animals with documented coccidiosis should be evaluated for other causes of intestinal disease (e.g., inflammatory bowel disease, lymphoma) or immunocompromise (e.g., hyperadrenocorticism).

PROGNOSIS & OUTCOME

Good to excellent; most animals respond readily to treatment.

PEARLS & CONSIDERATIONS

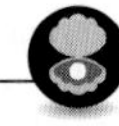

Comments

- It is virtually impossible to prevent exposure to coccidia in dogs and cats.
- Clinical disease often develops around weaning or after other stressful events such as shipping or rehoming.
- The strategic use of newer anticoccidials (ponazuril) at times when animals are likely to develop coccidiosis may become common practice in the future. An example of a strategic treatment would be administration of ponazuril a few days before (or at) weaning.

Prevention

Coccidiosis tends to be a problem in unsanitary environments.

- Prompt removal of feces is important.
- Do not allow fecal contamination of food and water bowls.
- Treatment of dams and queens before parturition can decrease prevalence.
- Cockroaches and flies may serve as mechanical vectors of oocysts.

Technician Tips

- Oocysts are very resistant and can survive freezing temperatures and environmental conditions for many months.
- Cages and fomites should be disinfected with steam cleaning, boiling water, or 10% ammonia solution.

SUGGESTED READING

Litster AL, et al: Use of ponazuril paste to treat coccidiosis in shelter-housed cats and dogs. Vet Parasitol 202:319-325, 2014.

AUTHOR: Katherine D. Scott, DVM, DACVIM
EDITOR: Rance K. Sellon, DVM, PhD, DACVIM

Cognitive Dysfunction

Bonus Material Online 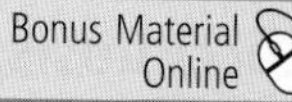

BASIC INFORMATION

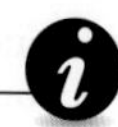

Definition

The decline in behavioral condition with advanced age, in the absence of causative physical or medical conditions

Synonyms

Senility, cognitive dysfunction syndrome (CDS), brain aging

Epidemiology

SPECIES, AGE, SEX

- Cats: typically > 10 years old
- Dogs: typically > 6 years old (large breeds), > 12 years (small breeds)

GENETICS, BREED PREDISPOSITION

Dogs and cats, like humans, may have susceptibility genes for the development of lesions associated with clinical cognitive syndromes. The understanding of tauopathies that exists for human medicine does not currently exist for veterinary medicine.

ASSOCIATED DISORDERS

Concurrent anxiety-related conditions are common.

Clinical Presentation

HISTORY, CHIEF COMPLAINT

- Disorientation (confusion at doors/accessways), changes in social and interactive behavior (becoming needier or, conversely, more aloof), changes in locomotor (nonfunctional repetitive movement) and sleep cycle (disrupted sleep cycles and Diehl behaviors) behaviors, and loss of housetraining
- In early cognitive dysfunction, animals may have only slightly altered sleep cycles and appear more anxious.

PHYSICAL EXAM FINDINGS

- May be unremarkable
- Possible abnormalities include worn claws or acute superficial erosions of the nasal planum if trapped in corners or if exhibiting ritualistic locomotor behavior.
- Weight loss (from excessive locomotion and/or inappetence due to anxiety)
- When examined on video, the behaviors exhibited by an animal with CDS often seem without purpose; in extreme cases, animals appear to be moving as if they cannot stop or staring blankly.
- Frank mentation changes may be apparent when asked to solve problems/puzzles or orient. Physical aging affects speed, not accuracy, of problem/puzzle solving. Cognitive dysfunction affects accuracy and interest.
- May have testable changes in response to olfactory stimuli that would have caused a response earlier in life.

Etiology and Pathophysiology

- Dogs, like humans, develop amyloid plaques in the brain, the density of which appears to roughly correlate with the level of impairment.
- Unlike humans, dogs/cats/rodents do not appear to develop neurofibrillary tangles associated with the tauopathy Alzheimer's disease.
- Cats and dogs experience a decrease in brain cortical mass and a relative increase in ventricular volume with aging. These changes may be more extreme in patients with cognitive dysfunction.

DIAGNOSIS

Diagnostic Overview

Cognitive dysfunction is an insidious-onset, slowly progressive disorder that is almost always suspected based on history and signalment (geriatric patient). Emphasizing problem solving and cognitive tests, including the emphasis on nosework, offers an opportunity for diagnostic insight. Routine tests are indicated to identify confounding systemic metabolic abnormalities, if any. Confirmation using brain imaging and cerebrospinal fluid (CSF) analysis is undertaken only if the clinical picture suggests a different disorder is possible (e.g., cranial nerve or other deficits are more consistent with a disorder other than cognitive dysfunction). Nonspecific brain shrinkage is the absence of other notable lesions on MRI and may be linked to cognitive changes.

Differential Diagnosis

- Generalized anxiety disorder
- Anxiety: usually transient; associated with changes in physical capabilities (e.g., diminished or changing sensory or locomotor capabilities)
- Separation anxiety: old-age onset
- Panic disorder
- Attention-seeking behavior
- Meningoencephalitis
- Hepatic encephalopathy
- Brain neoplasia
- Hyperthyroidism (cat), hypothyroidism (dog)

Initial Database

- CBC, serum biochemistry profile, and urinalysis: generally unremarkable
- Neurologic examination (p. 1136): generally unremarkable
- Thyroid profile: rule out hyperthyroidism (cats) or hypothyroidism (dogs)
- Starting at middle age, screening for deficits should occur at every visit.

Advanced or Confirmatory Testing

- If neurologic signs are present, a full neurologic evaluation, including CSF analysis (pp. 1080 and 1323) and brain CT or MRI (p. 1132) may be indicated. If MRI shows only increased ventricle size and all other laboratory and physical findings are unremarkable, a presumptive diagnosis of cognitive dysfunction may be made.
- Activity monitors may show changes in patterns of recent activity (more starting and stopping, more ritualized behaviors) and altered sleep patterns.

TREATMENT

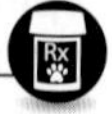

Treatment Overview

Goals of treatment are a decrease in the rate at which the animal appears to mentally fail and relieving pain and distress associated with changes in physical and mental status. Early intervention (e.g., nutritional/nutraceutical support to combat effects of reactive oxygen species (ROS), routine aerobic exercise and cognitive and olfactory stimulation) may have a protective effect as for humans and mice. All treatment modalities (behavioral, nutritional, medication, environmental) should be used concurrently.

Acute General Treatment

- Avoid exposure to stimuli known to cause distress.
- Early rewarding of any normal, preferred, or good interactive or elimination behaviors and encouraging normal locomotion
- There should be absolutely no punishment—physical, verbal, deprivational, or mental—for any undesirable behavior that occurs as a result of this condition. Such actions will render the patient more anxious.
- Protect the patient from wanderings or odd behaviors while keeping it comfortable. The latter may involve containing it in an area with an absorbent surface when left alone.
- Mental stimulation in the early stages is important and may delay clinical progression. Treat balls, food toys, games involving puzzle solving, safe exercise, interactive tasks (e.g., "get the mouse," "bring the ball"), and olfactory stimulation are useful.
- Omega-3 fatty acids (1500-2000 mg/day) may aid in protection from neurocytotoxic damage.

Chronic Treatment

- Physically and mentally stimulating exercises, such as swimming, massage, range-of-motion exercises
- Encourage relaxation.
- If loss of housetraining occurs, ensure that the animal is taken out frequently and reward as for a young pup; if needed, clip and diaper dog to decrease client and dog distress.
- Encourage re-establishment of daily cycles by feeding at regular hours and at least a few hours before bedtime, and administer

a benzodiazepine (alprazolam, clonazepam) before bed if needed.
- Protect the pet from accidents (e.g., falling into the swimming pool, falling down stairs).
- The monoamine oxidase inhibitor selegiline (Anipryl) 0.5 mg/kg PO q 24h (may double dose after 1 month if ineffective) is the drug of choice and is licensed for use for the treatment of canine cognitive dysfunction in the United States.
- Memantine 0.3-0.5 mg/kg PO q 12h, an NMDA receptor antagonist, may help some dogs.
- Vasodilators may be helpful.
- All concomitant anxiety-related conditions must be treated with relevant medications.

Nutrition/Diet

- Dietary supplements may slow progression (e.g., Senilife, Novifit [SAM-e], omega-3 fatty acids).
- Diets using ketones as energy sources (medium-chain triglycerides: Purina EN, Purina Neurocare) may protect and/or improve neurologic/cognitive function, and those containing antioxidants or compounds constituent for neuronal membrane maintenance and mitochondrial cofactors may decrease the rate of cognitive dysfunction progression, improve behavioral function, and have a protective effect or improve cognitive function (Hill's B/D [Brain Diet], Royal Canin's CALM Diet).
- In the United Kingdom, nutraceutical food additives are available and have been shown to improve function in dogs with cognitive changes (e.g., Aktivait).

Possible Complications

Any concurrent, untreated anxiety-related or behavioral conditions generally worsen with age and render the signs of cognitive dysfunction worse. These anxiety conditions should be treated. In other species, there is some evidence that treatment with antianxiety medications (e.g., selective serotonin reuptake inhibitors [SSRI], tricyclic antidepressants [TCAs]) and antiinflammatories may help delay cognitive aging.

Recommended Monitoring

- Examination, CBC, serum chemistry profile, urinalysis, ± thyroid profile as needed and at least q 6-12 months if medications
- Any ongoing medical condition could worsen an older animal's anxiety and make the signs of cognitive dysfunction appear to worsen.

PROGNOSIS & OUTCOME

- The course is inexorable, but with diet, range-of-motion and aerobic exercise, and appropriate cognitive stimulation, patients in the early stages can have years of quality life.
- Prognosis is improved by early diagnosis; comprehensive treatment, including preventive treatment with antioxidants and cognitive stimulation in middle age; and client compliance.

PEARLS & CONSIDERATIONS

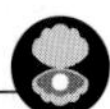

Comments

- If the clients videotape the animal early in the development of the condition, they will be better able to monitor changes, assess treatment, and make quality-of-life decisions.
- Clients often are made the saddest by the feeling that they are losing their emotional and intellectual connection with their pet. Treatment must acknowledge this concern and address it when possible.
- Other cats or dogs in the household can often help calm these patients and help them with activities they may now find challenging.

Prevention

- Diets rich in antioxidants/polyunsaturated fatty acids (1200-1500 mg/day) may decrease risk.
- Mental and physical activity is essential and may have a much larger role to play than originally thought. For cats and dogs, olfactory stimulation is likely coupled with cognition, and some mental stimulation should involve work for food, food puzzles, food games, or some mental exercise that involves olfaction (e.g., nosework).
- Asking cats and dogs for responses throughout the day (e.g., come with, up, down, left, right, high fives) and coupling find-it games with aerobic scope can benefit most dogs and cats.

Technician Tips

These patients may require extra care/handling, especially when known to the hospital staff for many years. It is a common mistake of veterinarians and technicians to assume a pet can behave the same as always when he/she ages, and being aware of such potential changes can help prevent injury.

Client Education

- Clients must understand that problematic behaviors attendant with cognitive dysfunction are not willful acts of disobedience.
- Treatment of this condition is an ongoing process and will continue for the life of the pet. Relapses may occur with treatment discontinuation or added stressors.

SUGGESTED READING

Bellows J, et al: Common physical and functional changes associated with aging in dogs. J Am Vet Med Assoc 246:67-75, 2015.

AUTHOR & EDITOR: Karen L. Overall, VMD, MA, PhD, DACVB

Colitis, Acute

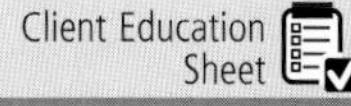

BASIC INFORMATION

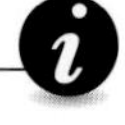

Definition

A common disorder characterized by sudden onset (<72 hours) of colonic inflammation (large-bowel diarrhea and straining to defecate), manifesting with diarrhea that is typically mild, of small volume, and contains mucus and/or fresh blood (p. 257). Systemic signs of illness are generally absent.

Synonym

Stress colitis

Epidemiology

SPECIES, AGE, SEX

Predominantly seen in young dogs and cats (<1 year old) as a consequence of parasitism, bacterial enteropathogens, or dietary indiscretion

RISK FACTORS

Age (predominantly young animals), recently kenneled animals, dietary factors, free-roaming pets, gastrointestinal tract parasitism

CONTAGION AND ZOONOSIS

Helminth parasites (*Trichuris* spp), protozoa (*Giardia* spp, *Tritrichomonas* spp), and bacteria (*Campylobacter* spp, *Clostridium* spp, enterotoxigenic *Escherichia coli*, *Salmonella* spp) have potential for contagion, common-source infection, and/or zoonosis.

Clinical Presentation

HISTORY, CHIEF COMPLAINT

Large-bowel diarrhea, which is characterized by tenesmus (straining), increased frequency of defecation, mucoid feces, and fresh (red) blood

PHYSICAL EXAM FINDINGS

Generally well fleshed without systemic signs (e.g., unthriftiness or weight loss) of illness. Rectal examination fails to reveal significant abnormalities except the character of feces.

Etiology and Pathophysiology

- Parasites: helminth and protozoa
- Dietary causes: gluttony, spoiled food, dietary indiscretion with ingestion of foreign or abrasive materials (e.g., cat litter, rocks, indigestible materials such as hair in long-haired cats)
- Specific bacterial pathogens may cause colonic inflammation by invasion or enterotoxin production.

DIAGNOSIS

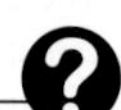

Diagnostic Overview

Acute colitis rarely requires extensive diagnostic evaluation. A thorough history, physical examination, routine fecal examination for nematode or protozoal parasites, and fecal/rectal smears for cytologic evaluation are indicated.

Differential Diagnosis

Other causes of diarrhea (p. 1213)

Initial Database

- Physical examination: abdominal palpation and digital rectal examination with collection of feces
- Fecal examination for nematode and protozoal parasites. Both fecal flotations and direct fecal smears should be performed. Multiple (three) zinc sulfate flotation tests using fresh feces may be required for identification of *Giardia* spp trophozoites.
- Commercial ELISA kits are sensitive for the detection of *Giardia* antigen.
- Rectal cytology (p. 1157) may show evidence of bacterial pathogens (e.g., vegetative spores of *Clostridia*) or increased numbers of fecal leukocytes indicative of acute mucosal inflammation.

Advanced or Confirmatory Testing

Generally not indicated. Animals that fail to respond to empirical therapy (see below) require confirmatory testing (e.g., fecal cultures, polymerase chain reaction [PCR], other assays) for suspected bacterial or protozoal pathogens.

TREATMENT

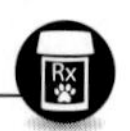

Treatment Overview

Initial management of animals with acute colitis is nonspecific and supportive. In most instances, signs are self-limited and/or respond readily to empirical therapy.

Acute General Treatment

- Treat for suspected nematode and protozoan parasites using appropriate broad-spectrum anthelmintics or antiprotozoal medications (e.g., fenbendazole 50 mg/kg PO q 24h for 3 days).
- Avoid the use of antibiotics in animals, except those with confirmed bacterial causes of their gastrointestinal signs. Empirical use of commercial probiotics (FortiFlora, Prostora Max) for 3-5 days may facilitate clinical recovery, although clinical trial data supporting their use are limited.

Nutrition/Diet

- Feed a bland or mixed-fiber diet (commercial or homemade), giving small volumes at increasingly frequent intervals for 3-5 days.
- Avoid all treats and dietary supplements (except probiotics) during the dietary trial period.
- If using a bland diet, add fiber (small amounts of soluble fiber such as psyllium mucilloid, 1 teaspoon/10 kg at each feeding) to the diet to reduce tenesmus and facilitate colonic epithelial repair. Fiber supplements should be avoided in animals with small-bowel–type diarrhea.

Recommended Monitoring

Have clients communicate their pet's progress after 48-72 hours of therapy.

PROGNOSIS & OUTCOME

Generally excellent for full recovery

PEARLS & CONSIDERATIONS

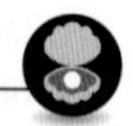

Comments

In general practice, acute colitis is a common complaint that is very responsive to supportive therapy. Elimination of infectious and parasitic causes is the key to treating acute colitis.

Prevention

- Prophylactic deworming
- Avoid dietary indiscretion.
- Avoid allowing pets to roam freely.
- In cats with recurrent colitis due to hair, frequent brushing, administration of hairball laxatives, or removing excess hair (shaving) may be indicated to control signs.

Technician Tips

Always perform multiple fecal examinations to exclude parasitism as a cause of colitis.

Client Education

Monitor for failure to respond to empirical treatments.

SUGGESTED READING

Bybee SN, et al: Effect of the probiotic *Enterococcus faecium* SF68 on presence of diarrhea in cats and dogs housed in an animal shelter. J Vet Intern Med 25:856, 2011.

AUTHOR: Albert E. Jergens, DVM, MS, PhD, DACVIM
EDITOR: Rance K. Sellon, DVM, PhD, DACVIM

Colitis, Chronic

Bonus Material Online 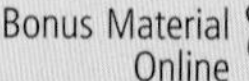 Client Education Sheet 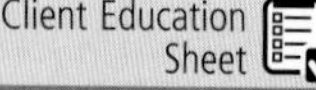

BASIC INFORMATION

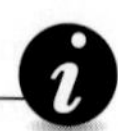

Definition

A common cause of persistent (>3 weeks' duration) signs of colonic inflammation characterized by large-bowel diarrhea with tenesmus, dyschezia, and increased frequency of defecation. Feces often contain mucus and/or fresh blood. Systemic signs attributable to nutrient malabsorption (e.g., weight loss) are uncommon.

Epidemiology

SPECIES, AGE, SEX

More common in middle-aged and older dogs and cats as a consequence of infiltrative mucosal disorders (e.g., inflammatory bowel disease [IBD], neoplasia). Infectious disorders (e.g., *Trichuris vulpis*, gastrointestinal [GI] histoplasmosis, *Tritrichomonas foetus*) may be seen in younger animals (less common).

GENETICS, BREED PREDISPOSITION

Boxers, French bulldogs, and possibly German shepherds are predisposed to granulomatous colitis (GC [p. 395]). German shepherds and purebred cats are at increased risk for lymphocytic-plasmacytic enterocolitis.

CONTAGION AND ZOONOSIS

Some bacterial enteropathogens (e.g., *Clostridium perfringens,* potentially contagious) may cause chronic colitis if not detected early. Some helminth parasites (*Trichuris* spp, potentially contagious) and protozoa (*Giardia* spp, potentially zoonotic; *Tritrichomonas* spp, potentially contagious) also may cause persistent signs of colitis in pets.

GEOGRAPHY AND SEASONALITY

Midwestern and southern United States for GI histoplasmosis

ASSOCIATED DISORDERS

Colonic motility disorders (e.g., irritable bowel syndrome in dogs and colonic constipation/obstipation in cats) may mimic mucosal inflammation and cause signs of large-bowel diarrhea with tenesmus. These diseases are due to functional disturbances in colonic motility and have no significant contribution from inflammatory/structural disease.

Clinical Presentation

DISEASE FORMS/SUBTYPES

- Diet-responsive disorders (p. 347): includes food intolerance (nonimmunologically mediated) and dietary sensitivity (immunologically mediated). Food-responsive causes of GI signs, including large-bowel diarrhea, are common in dogs and cats.
- Infectious disorders: includes selected nematode/protozoal parasites, bacteria, and fungal organisms (especially GI histoplasmosis). *T. foetus* may cause chronic intermittent colitis in young cats.
- Infiltrative mucosal diseases: includes fungal, idiopathic benign (e.g., IBD), and malignant (e.g., mucosal neoplasia) diseases

HISTORY, CHIEF COMPLAINT

Persistent large-bowel diarrhea, which is characterized by tenesmus (straining to defecate), increased frequency of defecation, mucoid feces, and fresh blood (p. 1215). Some disorders (e.g., IBD, GI histoplasmosis, GI lymphoma) may affect the small intestine as well, causing mixed large- and small-bowel signs.

PHYSICAL EXAM FINDINGS

- The animal is often well fleshed without systemic signs (e.g., unthriftiness, weight loss) of illness unless the small bowel is also affected. Fungal disease, severe IBD, and colorectal neoplasia may cause weight loss, fever, alterations in appetite, and peripheral/mesenteric lymphadenopathy.
- Rectal examination: evaluate the character of the feces, obtain fecal samples for parasitic examination, procure exfoliative cytologic specimens, and evaluate the rectum for mucosal abnormalities, possible mass lesions, and sublumbar lymphadenomegaly.

Etiology and Pathophysiology

- Large-bowel diarrhea is characterized by increased amounts of mucus because of the large numbers of mucus-secreting goblet cells in the colon.
- Hematochezia indicates severe mucosal disruption of the distal colon and rectum.
- Parasites, including helminths and protozoa: *T. vulpis* (dogs), *T. foetus* (cats), *Giardia lamblia* (dogs, cats)
- Dietary causes: incriminating antigens or dietary ingredients (nonimmunologic)
- Specific bacterial pathogens: cause colonic inflammation by invasion or enterotoxin production. Adherent/invasive *E. coli* (AIEC) is a recently recognized enteropathogen associated with GC.
- Infiltrative mucosal disorders: benign, malignant, or infectious (e.g., fungal)

DIAGNOSIS

Diagnostic Overview

Diagnoses of many causes of chronic colitis will require histologic evaluation of mucosal biopsy specimens.

Differential Diagnosis

- Specific causes: see Etiology and Pathophysiology above.
- Occasionally, patients with rectal diseases (e.g., perineal hernia, perianal fistula, diverticula, rectal polyps or masses) will present with signs of large-bowel disease. These are generally distinguished by digital examination and careful inspection; normal perineal and rectal structure on examination more strongly suggests large-bowel disease in such cases.
- Colonic motility disorders can be mistaken for colitis, but motility disorders are not associated with inflammation.

Initial Database

- Physical examination: abdominal palpation and digital rectal examination, with collection of feces
- Fecal examination for nematode and protozoal parasites. Fecal flotations and fecal smears should be performed. Multiple (three) zinc sulfate flotation tests using fresh feces may be required for identification of *Giardia* spp trophozoites (p. 386).
    - Commercial ELISA kits are also sensitive for the detection of *Giardia* antigen.
- Rectal cytology may demonstrate evidence of bacterial pathogens (e.g., vegetative spores of *Clostridia*) or increased numbers of fecal leukocytes indicative of mucosal inflammation. Exfoliative cytology (e.g., rectal scrape using a uterine curette or a curette of the same type used for bone graft harvesting [p. 1157]) is also a useful tool for confirming the presence of *Histoplasma* organisms contained within colonic macrophages.
- Polymerase chain reaction (PCR) for detection of *T. foetus* infection (p. 997)
- Abdominal imaging (survey radiographs, pneumocolonography, ultrasonography) may identify fecal impaction, mass lesions, bowel wall thickening, and/or evidence of significant mesenteric lymphadenomegaly. Generally, ultrasonography is a poor screening tool for colonic disease because of the obstructive effect of air in the colonic lumen on the ultrasound beam and because colonic wall thickness is difficult to standardize.

Advanced or Confirmatory Testing

- Colonoscopy with procurement of multiple mucosal biopsy specimens may be required to diagnose infiltrative diseases. Collection of biopsy specimens from all colonic regions (full colonoscopy) will allow neoplasia to be ruled out and differentiation between the different types of colonic inflammation.
- Fluorescence *in situ* hybridization (FISH) performed on colonic biopsy samples from dogs with GC confirms the presence of AIEC.
- Urine antigen testing for histoplasmosis (p. 1365)
- Colonic biopsies should not be obtained by laparotomy because the bacterial content of the colon and attendant risk of bacterial peritonitis after biopsy of a diseased colon are markedly greater than with small intestinal biopsies.

TREATMENT

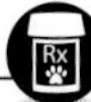

Treatment Overview

Treatment is based on the specific definitive diagnosis because empirical therapies are often inadequate or deleterious (e.g., use of glucocorticoids in animals with GI histoplasmosis).

Chronic Treatment

- Treatment for suspected nematode and protozoan parasites is often warranted before completing expensive or invasive diagnostic testing, even if fecal exams are negative for parasites. Use appropriate broad-spectrum anthelmintics or antiprotozoal (e.g., fenbendazole 50 mg/kg PO q 24h for 3-5 days) medications. Confirm efficacy of therapy with repeat follow-up fecal examinations or, if no parasites were identified, response to therapy.
- Feed an appropriate diet to animals with dietary-responsive disorders and IBD. This may range from a hypoallergenic/hydrolysate diet, to a highly digestible diet, or to a homemade diet. Reduction in the quantity of dietary antigens will assist in reducing mucosal inflammation with these disorders. Other animals with colitis, but not requiring a specific antigen-restricted diet, will benefit from being fed a low-fat, fiber-enriched commercial ration.
- Avoid all treats and supplements containing protein or flavors during the dietary trial period.
- Use diets with added soluble or mixed fiber, or add small to moderate amounts of soluble fiber to the diet to reduce tenesmus and facilitate colonic epithelial repair.
- Use antibiotics only in animals with confirmed bacterial causes (e.g., colonization with enteropathogenic bacteria) of clinical signs. Antimicrobials used in this fashion are

best chosen based on susceptibility testing to the incriminating pathogen. Exceptions are animals with GC, which responds to oral fluoroquinolone therapy (enrofloxacin 10 mg/kg PO q 24h), and tylosin-responsive diarrheas.
- Tylosin-responsive diarrhea has been reported in large-breed dogs that respond rapidly to oral tylosin dosed at 25 mg/kg PO for 2 weeks.
- Glucocorticoids (e.g., prednisone or prednisolone 1 mg/kg PO q 12h for dogs; 1-2 mg/kg PO q 12h for cats) are first-choice immunosuppressive drugs for therapy of colonic IBD. For dogs showing adverse effects or when there is a need for long-term steroid therapy, consider the use of budesonide 1-3 mg/DOG PO q 24h for IBD.
- Drugs effective against GI histoplasmosis (p. 476), if diagnosis confirmed.
- Treatment for colonic neoplasia (pp. 30 and 604), if diagnosis confirmed.
- Probiotics (multiple commercial products available) may serve a useful adjunct role to drug therapy to reduce inflammation in animals with chronic colitis. Multi-strain probiotics have shown efficacy in clinical trials.

Nutrition/Diet

- Appropriate dietary management may include elimination, fiber-supplemented, or low-residue diets. The remission of signs due to food-responsive causes for chronic colitis requires feeding an elimination (intact protein or hydrolysate) diet for 3-4 weeks in dogs and 1-2 weeks in cats.
- Soluble fiber supplementation is an important component of therapy because these dietary additives bind colonic irritants, normalize dysmotility, and promote colonic epithelial repair and renewal (by beneficial short-chain fatty acid [butyrate] production).
- Prebiotics (i.e., soluble fiber, fructooligosaccharides) may also promote beneficial populations of mucosa-associated bacteria to reduce inflammation.

Possible Complications

- Cure is not possible with colonic IBD, but the prognosis for control of signs is good with effective therapy.
- Animals treated with amphotericin B for GI histoplasmosis are at risk for drug-induced renal disease.
- Myelosuppression may occur with chemotherapy drugs for malignant colonic neoplasia.

Recommended Monitoring

Ideally, animals responsive to elimination diets (e.g., those having diet-responsive causes of chronic colitis) should be returned to their normal (incriminating) diet to see if large-bowel signs recrudesce. This is impractical in most instances.

PROGNOSIS & OUTCOME

The prognosis varies with the underlying cause from good (e.g., tylosin-responsive or diet-responsive disorders when the inciting dietary constituent is removed) to poor (e.g., some colonic neoplasia).

PEARLS & CONSIDERATIONS

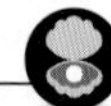

Comments

- Major causes of chronic colitis include dietary, infectious, and infiltrative disorders.
- Most animals with chronic signs of large-intestinal disease will require a thorough diagnostic evaluation to rule out the various causes of colonic inflammation. Prophylactic deworming and dietary trials with an elimination diet and/or soluble fiber supplementation are easy and cost-effective empirical therapies to offer clients before more extensive diagnostic testing.
- Colonoscopy with mucosal biopsy is imperative for diagnosis of most forms of chronic colitis that fail rational empirical therapies. Endoscopic standards for GI biopsy collection have been published.
- Perform FISH on colon biopsies obtained from dogs at risk for GC.

Prevention

- Prophylactic deworming
- Avoid dietary indiscretion.
- Perform dietary trials.

Technician Tips

- If in an endemic area for histoplasmosis, perform rectal scrape for collection of cytologic specimens, which may have macrophages laden with budding yeasts.
- Always administer an oral colonic lavage prep (e.g., GoLYTELY or others) prior to colonoscopy. This will expedite the procedure and enhance diagnostic yield from mucosal biopsies.

Client Education

- Diet trials must be extremely strict to yield useful information.
- Dietary modification to a diet suitable for colonic disease may be required for the life of the pet.

SUGGESTED READING

Cassmann E, et al: Alterations of the ileal and colonic mucosal microbiota in canine chronic enteropathies. PLoS One 11:e0147321, 2016.

AUTHOR: Albert E. Jergens, DVM, MS, PhD, DACVIM
EDITOR: Rance K. Sellon, DVM, PhD, DACVIM

Collapse

Client Education Sheet 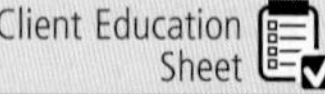

BASIC INFORMATION

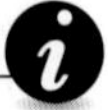

Definition

Loss of the ability to support weight and ambulate; may be transient and may include altered consciousness

Epidemiology

SPECIES, AGE, SEX

- Dogs, cats
- Age predisposition depends on disorder causing collapse.

GENETICS, BREED PREDISPOSITION

- Inherited neurologic disorders causing collapse during strenuous exercise occur in Labrador retrievers (exercise-induced collapse [EIC] [p. 316]) and border collies (border collie collapse [BCC]).
- Inherited myopathies causing progressive muscle atrophy, weakness, and collapse occur rarely in young dogs and cats.
- Partial seizures causing episodes of collapse with no loss of consciousness are common in dogs (especially Labrador retrievers) with inherited epilepsy.
- Boxers with arrhythmogenic right ventricular cardiomyopathy often collapse during syncopal episodes.
- Ruptured splenic hemangiosarcoma is a common cause of collapse in large-breed dogs.

Clinical Presentation

HISTORY, CHIEF COMPLAINT

Depends on underlying cause. In animals with recurrent historical collapse but no abnormal physical findings, it is very important to get a good description or video of a collapse episode to guide the diagnostic approach. Important information:

- Whether collapse occurred acutely or progressed over time
- Whether systemic abnormalities were noticed before, during, or after collapse
- Duration of collapse
- Mentation/consciousness, muscle tone, mucous membrane color, and respiratory pattern during the episode of collapse

- Activity, events preceding collapse (e.g., possible triggers)

PHYSICAL EXAM FINDINGS

Findings depend on underlying cause. A normal physical examination is common in animals presented for historical episodes of collapse. In contrast, animals presented to a veterinarian during collapse often have physical findings that help determine the best diagnostic approach. Findings that may directly assist diagnosis:

- Pallor, hypotension, ascites, abdominal mass (e.g., acute hemoabdomen)
- Tachycardia, weak femoral pulses, muffled heart sounds (e.g., cardiac tamponade)
- Tachycardia, bradycardia, irregular pulses (e.g., arrhythmia causing syncope)
- Inspiratory or expiratory dyspnea, cough (e.g., primary respiratory disorder)
- Neurologic exam abnormalities localizing disease to the brain, spinal cord, peripheral nerves, or neuromuscular junction
- Muscle weakness and muscle atrophy
- Fever, muscle pain, joint pain, bone pain, neck pain

Etiology and Pathophysiology

Collapse is caused by any condition that disrupts the ability of the animal to remain upright and walk. The pathophysiologic mechanism is specific to each cause (see Differential Diagnosis, below) (p. 1206).

DIAGNOSIS

Diagnostic Overview

Most animals presented while collapsed have a signalment and historical and physical findings that will clearly guide the most direct diagnostic approach. Animals examined because of one or more episodes of historical collapse with no physical abnormalities should undergo routine screening bloodwork, thoracic radiographs, and a complete neurologic examination; if no abnormalities are revealed, the patient may be hospitalized for observation or the owner can be asked to videorecord episodes at home.

Differential Diagnosis

- Metabolic/endocrine: anemia, shock, sepsis, anaphylaxis, hypoglycemia, hypokalemia, hypocalcemia, hypoadrenocorticism, hypothyroidism, heat stroke
- Cardiovascular: arrhythmia, congestive heart failure, cardiac tamponade, arterial thromboembolism, pulmonary hypertension, congenital right to left shunt
- Respiratory: brachycephalic upper airway obstruction, pharyngeal or laryngeal mass or foreign body, laryngeal paralysis, tracheal collapse, asthma, pneumonia, pulmonary edema, pleural effusion, lung-lobe torsion
- Partial seizures: idiopathic epilepsy, brain disease
- Spinal cord: trauma, hemorrhage, fibrocartilaginous embolism, intervertebral disc extrusion, neoplasia, meningitis/myelitis, wobblers
- Brain/cranial nerves: hemorrhage, infarct, neoplasia, encephalitis, hydrocephalus, geriatric canine vestibular syndrome, intoxications
- Neuromuscular/musculoskeletal: myasthenia gravis, polyradiculoneuritis, tick paralysis, botulism, polyarthritis, polyneuropathy, polymyositis
- EIC: suspect based on signalment, normal physical examination, and typical clinical features of collapse. Differentiate from other episodic disorders such as hypoglycemia, hypoadrenocorticism, cardiac arrhythmia, epilepsy.
- For greater detail, see Collapse in Section 3 (p. 1206).

Initial Database

- CBC, serum biochemical profile, urinalysis
- Neurologic exam (p. 1136), orthopedic exam (p. 1143)
- Electrocardiogram (p. 1096), blood pressure (p. 1065)
- Thoracic radiographs

Advanced or Confirmatory Testing

As dictated by history, features of collapse, physical findings, and initial test results:

- Echocardiogram (p. 1094); if unremarkable, consider Holter monitor or event monitor (p. 1120) if episodic collapse
- Abdominal ultrasound
- ACTH stimulation test if hypoadrenocorticism suspected
- Sequential blood glucose measurements
- Pharyngeal, laryngeal, and tracheal endoscopy if signs of respiratory obstruction; arterial blood gas if hypoxemia suspected
- Advanced imaging (MRI) if spinal cord or brain disease suspected (p. 1132)
- Anticholinesterase response test if myasthenia gravis suspected (p. 668): neostigmine (0.01 mg/kg) plus atropine (0.02 mg/kg)
- Electrodiagnostics and muscle/nerve biopsy if muscle or peripheral nerve disease suspected
- Arthrocentesis (p. 1059) if polyarthritis suspected
- DNA testing for EIC and for some congenital muscle diseases

TREATMENT

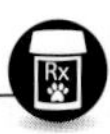

Treatment Overview

Correct acute/life-threatening disturbances (severe biochemical or electrolyte abnormalities, severe anemia, hypotension, body temperature abnormalities). Address underlying problem.

Acute General Treatment

Emergency treatment as indicated based on initial physical and laboratory findings: intravenous fluids, oxygen supplementation, blood transfusion (anemia), dextrose (hypoglycemia), calcium (hypocalcemia), dexamethasone (hypoadrenal crisis), anticonvulsants (seizures), antibiotics (sepsis), diuretics (heart failure), antiarrhythmic medications, pericardiocentesis (cardiac tamponade)

Chronic Treatment

Depends on underlying disease process

PROGNOSIS & OUTCOME

Variable, depending on underlying disease process

PEARLS & CONSIDERATIONS

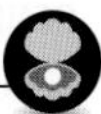

Comments

- The most common causes of episodic collapse with no other historical abnormalities and a normal physical examination between episodes are idiopathic epilepsy, cardiac arrhythmia, pulmonary hypertension, and EIC (in Labrador retrievers).
- Hemoabdomen and hypovolemic shock secondary to mass rupture and cardiac tamponade are common causes of collapse that can be suspected based on physical examination.
- Detection of hypoglycemia in pets with insulinoma may be optimal within 15 minutes of eating a meal.

Technician Tips

- A good description of collapse episodes is essential for identifying possible causes in animals that are normal between episodes.
- Activity preceding collapse and mentation, respiratory pattern, posture, muscle tone in each limb during collapse, and behavior after collapse can be important diagnostic clues.

SUGGESTED READING

Cosford KM, et al Exercise intolerance in retrievers. Vet Med 105:64-74, 2010.

AUTHOR: Susan M. Taylor, DVM, DACVIM
EDITOR: Leah A. Cohn, DVM, PhD, DACVIM

Collapsing Trachea

Bonus Material Online   Client Education Sheet

BASIC INFORMATION

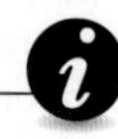

Definition

Progressive weakening of the tracheal cartilages with dorsoventral flattening of tracheal rings and prolapse of the tracheal membrane (TM) into the lumen resulting in cough and airflow limitation

Synonyms

Collapsing trachea, tracheal collapse (TC), tracheomalacia

Epidemiology

SPECIES, AGE, SEX

- Small- and toy-breed dogs; rarely reported in large-breed dogs and cats
- Considered a disease of middle-aged dogs, although 25% of affected dogs show clinical signs by 6 months of age
- No sex predisposition

GENETICS, BREED PREDISPOSITION

- Yorkshire terriers: one-third to two-thirds of reported cases
- Toy and miniature poodles, Maltese, Chihuahua, and Pomeranian
- Congenital disorder suspected

RISK FACTORS

Conditions leading to exacerbations of clinical signs

- Inhalation of airway irritants
- Obesity
- Respiratory tract infection
- Tracheal intubation
- Stress/excitement
- Increased environmental temperatures/humidity

ASSOCIATED DISORDERS

- Laryngeal paralysis (p. 574)
- Chronic bronchitis (p. 136)
- Bronchomalacia (45%-83% of dogs with tracheal collapse)
- Pneumonia secondary to impaired tracheobronchial clearing mechanisms
- Hyperthermia
- Respiratory distress (p. 879)
- Syncope
- Hepatomegaly (significance unclear)
- Pharyngeal collapse
- Mitral valve endocardiosis

Clinical Presentation

DISEASE FORMS/SUBTYPES

- Can involve the extrathoracic and/or intrathoracic trachea. Common at the thoracic inlet, TC often occurs in more than one location. Collapse of the large bronchi also common
- Grades of TC
  - I: minor protrusion of TM into airway lumen, < 25% reduction in diameter; generally not associated with clinical signs
  - II: 50% reduction in airway lumen, tracheal rings elongated and mildly flattened
  - III: 75% reduction in airway lumen, tracheal rings markedly flattened
  - IV: >90% reduction in airway lumen, severely flattened tracheal rings, possibly with dorsal deviation of ventral tracheal surface; often associated with severe clinical signs

HISTORY, CHIEF COMPLAINT

- Chronic paroxysms of a loud, honking cough (goose honking) ± terminal gag/retch
  - Signs may worsen with excitement, heat, eating/drinking, or exercise
- Clinical signs are often progressive.
- Cyanosis, respiratory distress, or syncope in severely affected animals

PHYSICAL EXAM FINDINGS

- Cough elicited with tracheal palpation
  - Nonspecific: dogs with other respiratory disorders, (e.g., pulmonary edema), and clinically normal dogs may have elicitable cough
  - Occasionally, tracheal shape abnormalities palpable
- Extrathoracic TC: wheezes may be ausculted over the cervical trachea.
  - ± Increased effort on inspiration
- Intrathoracic TC: tracheal snap may be ausculted due to dynamic opening and collapse of large airways (sound due to airway opening during inspiration).
  - ± Increased effort on expiration
- Although not related to TC directly, many affected dogs are obese, demonstrate systolic mitral murmurs, and/or have palpable hepatomegaly.

Etiology and Pathophysiology

The cause is unknown and likely multifactorial. Suggested mechanisms:

- Congenital
  - Failure of chondrogenesis
- Acquired
  - Secondary to chronic small airway disease
  - Cartilage degeneration
  - Trauma
  - Loss of innervation of the trachealis dorsalis muscle
- Disease is exacerbated/perpetuated by a cycle of chronic inflammation worsened by chronic cough.

DIAGNOSIS

Diagnostic Overview

TC is suspected in at-risk breeds with characteristic history and exam findings; confirmation requires assessment of the trachea with radiographs, fluoroscopy, or bronchoscopy.

Differential Diagnosis

- Cough (pp. 217 and 1209)
- Other causes of syncope (p. 953) or collapse (p. 1206)

Initial Database

- CBC/serum biochemical profile/urinalysis: unremarkable or increased liver enzymes
- Heartworm antigen: rule out heartworm disease
- Radiographs: inspiratory (cervical collapse) and expiratory (thoracic collapse) views are necessary. Both false-positive and false-negative interpretations occur.
  - Minimum of three thoracic views to assess for comorbid conditions (e.g., pneumonia)
  - May underestimate degree of collapse or miss dynamic collapse

Advanced or Confirmatory Testing

- Fluoroscopy: noninvasive and helpful in identifying dynamic collapse in real time; an elicited cough may improve detection and can help grade collapse severity
- Bronchoscopy: assesses location and severity of collapse and allows collection of airway wash samples to rule out concurrent infectious/inflammatory conditions
  - Requires anesthesia and intubation that can precipitate respiratory decompensation in severely affected patients.

TREATMENT

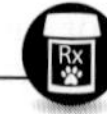

Treatment Overview

Medical management includes antitussives, weight management, environmental modification, and treatment of comorbid conditions. Other therapies (e.g., antiinflammatories, antibiotics, +/– bronchodilators) can be added if initial response is inadequate or during exacerbation in signs. In severe cases nonresponsive to medical management, tracheal stents can be placed to alleviate airway obstruction.

Acute General Treatment

- Oxygen support (p. 1146), sedation, external cooling, and cough suppressants may be necessary in an acute crisis (pp. 879 and 574).
  - Antitussive: butorphanol 0.02-0.1 mg/kg SQ q 4-6h
  - Low-dose acepromazine 0.05-0.1 mg/kg IM, maximum of 3 mg/DOG for sedation in cases of severe TC-related coughing. Some authors have reported excessive sedation at this dose, preferring 0.01-0.03 mg/kg IM or IV.
- Intubation may be required for dogs in respiratory distress, ideally followed by immediate stent placement.

Chronic Treatment

- Medical management: most (71%-93%) dogs respond well
- Maintain ideal/lean body condition score (BCS, 4-5/9)
- Avoid environmental triggers (e.g., inhaled irritants, excessive excitement, hot/humid environments, neck leads [harnesses preferred])
- Antitussives: reduce clinical signs and tracheal inflammation
  - Hydrocodone 0.22 mg/kg PO q 6-12h, *or*
  - Butorphanol 0.55-1 mg/kg PO q 8-12h
  - Alternatives: maropitant 2 mg/kg q 48h; Lomotil 0·2-0·5 mg/kg PO q 12h
- Antiinflammatory prednisone (short course): decrease laryngeal/tracheal inflammation
  - Prednisone 0.5-1 mg/kg PO q 24h tapered and discontinued after 5-7 days
- Manage comorbid conditions (e.g., chronic bronchitis [p. 136])
  - Consider empiric short course of antimicrobial appropriate for airway infection (e.g., doxycycline 5 mg/kg PO q 12h for 7 days)
- Bronchodilators: controversial; has not been critically evaluated in dogs with TC. Consider as a trial in refractory patients (withdraw if there is no improvement).
  - Beta-2 agonists: terbutaline (total amount per dose): small dogs, 0.625-1.25 mg PO q 12h; medium dogs, 1.25-2.5 mg PO q 12h; large dogs, 2.5-5 mg PO q 12h; *or* albuterol 0.05 mg/kg PO q 8h
  - Methylxanthines. extended-release theophylline 10 mg/kg PO q 12h; not all products have equivalent bioavailability. Consider switching bronchodilators if no improvement. Certain animals may develop toxicosis at doses that are well tolerated by others.
- Tracheal stents: salvage procedure (failed medical management or respiratory distress). Consult with specialist in internal medicine, surgery, or interventional radiology.
  - Surgical implantation of external prosthetic rings: generally limited to cervical trachea
  - Intraluminal stents: cervical or thoracic collapse, placed with endoscopic or fluoroscopic guidance. Relieves obstruction to airflow but not necessarily cough

Behavior/Exercise

Weight loss with controlled exercise regimens and dietary management improves clinical signs in many dogs.

Possible Complications

- Acute upper airway obstruction and death
- Cough suppressants: sedation
- Stents: stent migration, stent fracture, exuberant granulation tissue, tracheitis, cough
  - Coughing increases risk of stent fracture; antitussives are frequently needed after stenting.

Recommended Monitoring

Clinical signs

PROGNOSIS & OUTCOME

- Despite improvement with treatment, many dogs show some degree of persistent clinical signs. Prognosis for cure is poor because TC is irreversible and progressive, but prognosis for survival is good.
- Dogs with severe clinical signs (e.g., cyanosis, syncope) have a guarded prognosis that may improve with stent placement.

PEARLS & CONSIDERATIONS

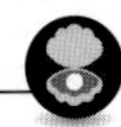

Comments

Hydrocodone cough suppressants can be difficult to obtain. Many are combined with other medications (acetaminophen, guaifenesin, and various antihistamines) that may not be safe or routinely recommended. Controlled drug status limits refill options.

Prevention

Do not be breed affected dogs.

Technician Tips

When performing radiographs to evaluate for TC, obtain inspiratory and expiratory films, including the cervical and thoracic trachea.

Client Education

For most dogs, tracheal collapse is managed with weight control, antitussives, and periodic administration of antiinflammatory drugs.

SUGGESTED READING

Tappin SW: Canine tracheal collapse. J Small Anim Pract 57:9-17, 2016.

AUTHOR: Laura Ridge Cousins, DVM, MS, DACVIM
EDITOR: Megan Grobman, DVM, MS, DACVIM

Color Disorders of the Skin and Haircoat

BASIC INFORMATION

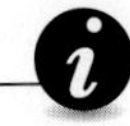

Definition

Very common spectrum of innate or acquired pigmentary abnormalities of the skin or hair

Synonyms

- Hyperpigmentation, melanoderma, melanotrichia
- Hypopigmentation, depigmentation, leukoderma, leukotrichia, achromotrichia, poliosis

Epidemiology

SPECIES, AGE, SEX

Although some conditions are present at birth (e.g., albinism), most are acquired.

GENETICS, BREED PREDISPOSITION

Hyperpigmentation:

- Recurrent flank alopecia: boxer, English bulldog, Airedale terrier
- Papillomavirus-associated plaques: pug, miniature schnauzer, Shar-pei

Hypopigmentation:

- Vitiligo: rottweiler, Belgian shepherd, Siamese cat, others
- Idiopathic acquired nasal hypopigmentation ("snow nose"): Labrador and golden retrievers, Siberian husky
- Waardenburg-Klein syndrome: white cats, Dalmatian, bull terrier, others
- Premature graying: golden and Labrador retrievers, Irish setter
- Dermatomyositis: Shetland sheepdog, collie
- Color dilution alopecia: blue or fawn Doberman pinscher and many others
- Canine cyclic hematopoiesis: collie (gray collie syndrome, rare)
- Chédiak-Higashi syndrome: Persian cat (rare)

RISK FACTORS

Various, including heredity

CONTAGION AND ZOONOSIS

Hyperpigmentation: dermatophytosis and *Sarcoptes scabiei* are zoonotic.

GEOGRAPHY AND SEASONALITY

- Snow nose: decreased nasal pigmentation during winter months
- Recurrent flank alopecia: can be seasonal
- Leishmaniasis: highly varied geographic distribution

ASSOCIATED DISORDERS

- Postinflammatory hyperpigmentation or hypopigmentation: many (see Differential Diagnosis below)
- Waardenburg-Klein syndrome: blue eyes, deafness
- Uveodermatologic syndrome: uveitis, blindness
- Dermatomyositis: myositis possible
- Chédiak-Higashi syndrome: immunologic deficiency

- Canine cyclic hematopoiesis: usually lethal before age 6 months

Clinical Presentation

HISTORY, CHIEF COMPLAINT

Question owners about sun exposure, changes in health, and inflammation (e.g., pruritus).

PHYSICAL EXAM FINDINGS

- Note distribution of color change: where on body; affecting skin and/or hair? Examine skin for lesions and evidence of inflammation (e.g., erythema, lichenification).
- Certain physical abnormalities are associated with specific pigmentation disorders (see Associated Disorders above).

Etiology and Pathophysiology

Normal pigmentation is a highly complex process under the influence of numerous genetic and acquired factors. Both depigmentation and hyperpigmentation can result from inflammatory and noninflammatory conditions.

DIAGNOSIS

Diagnostic Overview

Causes of color disorders of dogs and cats are myriad. Some are visually distinctive.

Differential Diagnosis

Acquired hyperpigmentation:

- Postinflammatory: very common in dogs but not cats; can occur with any chronic inflammatory process but particularly common with hypersensitivity disorders, *Malassezia* infection, demodicosis, and pyoderma. In cats, skin hyperpigmentation it is most often seen with dermatophytosis. Inflammation can also darken hair color (melanotrichia) in dogs and in Siamese and Himalayan cats.
- Hormone associated: hyperadrenocorticism, hypothyroidism, hyperestrogenism
- Neoplasia: feline Bowen disease, other pigmented tumors
- Acanthosis nigricans in dachshunds: localized to axillae; a reaction pattern with multiple causes. Friction, infection, hypersensitivity are more likely than a primary genetic form.
- Others include alopecia X, recurrent flank alopecia, sun exposure, drug therapy induced, papillomavirus-associated plaques, trauma, and burns.

Acquired hypopigmentation:

- Postinflammatory: less common than hyperpigmentation but pyoderma, dermatomyositis, leishmaniasis, and other inflammatory conditions can cause depigmentation in affected areas (usually haired skin). On the nasal planum, consider discoid lupus erythematosus and pemphigus erythematosus, pemphigus foliaceus, uveodermatologic syndrome, and other immune-mediated diseases.

Other causes are less common.

- Neoplasia: particularly epitheliotropic lymphoma, which can cause striking leukotrichia and leukoderma.
- Vitiligo: multifactorial, with genetic cause likely in some cases. Symmetrical depigmentation of hair, skin, and mucosa in patches, most often on the face (including nose and lips). Affected skin usually looks otherwise normal. Affects dogs, Siamese cats
- Nasal hypopigmentation: noninflammatory conditions include "snow nose," in which partial symmetrical depigmentation of the nasal planum occurs, usually in winter
- Nutrition (e.g., reddish-brown coat in black cats due to tyrosine deficiency)
- Lightening of the coat can occur with excessive exposure to chlorinated water, sunlight, or in hair cycle arrest (e.g., endocrine disease). Dark coats can become red or blond.
- Others: drug-induced changes, burns or cold injuries, scars

Genetic hyperpigmentation or hypopigmentation:

- Hypopigmentation: color dilution alopecia, oculocutaneous albinism, Waardenburg-Klein syndrome, piebaldism, canine cyclic hematopoiesis, Chédiak-Higashi syndrome, "Dudley nose"
- Hyperpigmentation: lentigo (e.g., orange cats)

Initial Database

May include (p. 1091)

- Skin scrapings
- Skin cytologic examination
- Skin biopsies: required in many cases, particularly with hypopigmentation
- Trichography (microscopic examination of plucked hairs, useful for assessing color dilution alopecia)
- CBC, serum biochemistry profile, urinalysis

Advanced or Confirmatory Testing

Additional testing for specific diseases:

- Endocrine testing (hyperadrenocorticism, hypothyroidism)
- Ocular examination (uveodermatologic syndrome)
- Dermatophyte examination: Wood's light, fungal culture
- Muscle evaluation (dermatomyositis)
- Auditory evaluation (Waardenburg-Klein syndrome)
- Serologic testing for deep fungal infections, leishmaniasis

TREATMENT

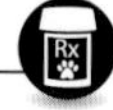

Treatment Overview

The goal is to restore normal pigmentation to skin and hair. Treatment is not always indicated.

Chronic Treatment

Depends on underlying cause:

- Many conditions do not require or respond to treatment.
- Inflammation, endocrinopathy, or neoplasia may be treatable.
- Uveodermatologic syndrome requires aggressive therapy to save vision.
- Reduce sun exposure in hypopigmented dogs.

PROGNOSIS & OUTCOME

- Good prognosis for cases of acquired color change if the underlying condition can be controlled; prognosis varies for other conditions.
- Improvement may be very slow for all conditions.

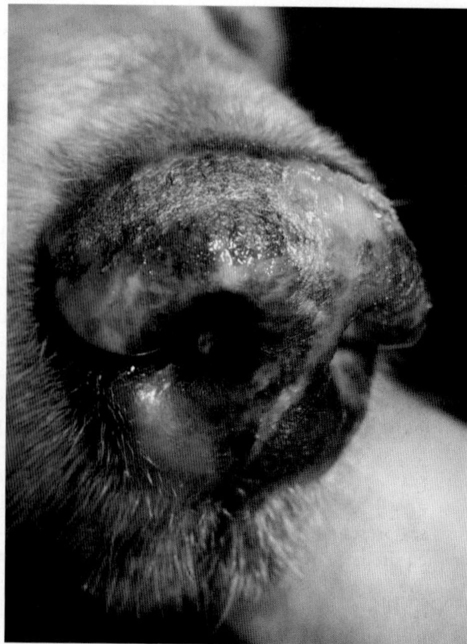

COLOR DISORDERS OF THE SKIN AND HAIRCOAT Depigmentation of the nasal planum and leukotrichia in a golden retriever with epitheliotropic lymphoma.

PEARLS & CONSIDERATIONS

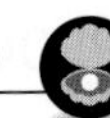

Comments

- When examining the nasal planum, look for changes in the surface architecture. Inflammatory and infiltrative processes (e.g., discoid lupus erythematosus) cause a loss of the normal cobblestone architecture. Conversely, processes with little or no inflammation (e.g., vitiligo, snow nose) spare the normal surface pattern.
- Ventral depigmentation of the nasal planum in dogs with nasal discharge may be associated with aspergillosis.
- Lattice-like hyperpigmentation is common with hypersensitivity dermatoses.
- Hyperpigmentation of the follicular ostia is common with demodicosis.
- The best sites to biopsy the nasal planum (or other mucocutaneous junction) exhibiting depigmentation are gray, partially depigmented areas.

Technician Tips

Abundant small, oval melanin granules can be seen in epithelial cells from surface cytologic examination of hyperpigmented skin. Although they can be mistaken for bacteria, they are distinctly brown rather than blue/purple on a Diff-Quik preparation.

SUGGESTED READING

Pigmentary abnormalities. In Miller WH, et al, editors: Muller & Kirk's Small animal dermatology, ed 7, St. Louis, 2013, Mosby, pp 618-629.

AUTHOR: Kinga Gortel, DVM, MS, DACVD
EDITOR: Manon Paradis, DMV, MVSc, DACVD

Coma and Stupor

Client Education Sheet 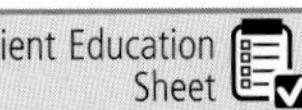

BASIC INFORMATION

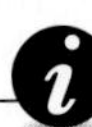

Definition

A state of unconsciousness unresponsive to stimuli; an uncommon but well-recognized neurologic emergency

Epidemiology

RISK FACTORS

- Any condition that increases intracranial pressure (ICP)
- Older animals: neoplasia, cardiovascular, urinary disorders
- Younger animals: trauma, infection, toxins
- Traumatic brain injury most common cause in dogs and cats

CONTAGION AND ZOONOSIS

Consider rabies

Clinical Presentation

DISEASE FORMS/SUBTYPES

- Prognosis is generally worse in descending order
  - Obtunded: conscious state with mild to moderate reduction in alertness
  - Stupor: unconscious state that requires strong stimuli (usually noxious; toe pinch) to evoke a response (often reduced)
  - Coma: unconscious state unresponsive to all stimuli

HISTORY, CHIEF COMPLAINT

- Acute onset or rapid deterioration: consider toxin, trauma, rapidly bleeding tumor, or embolism/infarction
- Chronic slow progression: consider tumor, metabolic disease, or encephalitis

PHYSICAL EXAM FINDINGS

- Recumbent with no response
- May present in shock
- Neurologic exam (p. 1136): focus on level of consciousness (response to toe pinch and loud noise), pupillary size and light reflexes, ability to elicit physiologic nystagmus, limb rigidity, and respiratory patterns to determine prognosis.

Etiology and Pathophysiology

- There are two general causes of unconsciousness:
  - Diffuse cerebral cortical injury
  - Interruption of the ascending reticular activating system located in the brainstem
- Diffuse cortical injury generally carries a better prognosis than brainstem injury.
- Brainstem (midbrain, medulla) injury suspected based on
  - Deficits in pupillary light response or pupil size: midbrain (assuming exam reveals no evidence of ocular or optic nerve lesion)
  - Inability to elicit normal physiologic nystagmus: medulla (assuming no evidence of middle/inner ear abnormality on exam)
  - Limb rigidity: medulla (assuming no spinal cord or neuromuscular signs)
  - Respiration abnormalities: medulla or midbrain (barring primary airway/lung lesion)
    - Kussmaul (rapid, deep, labored breathing, associated with diabetic coma)
    - Cheyne-Stokes (abnormal breathing pattern with alternating periods of apnea and deep, rapid breathing; the cycle begins with slow, shallow breaths that gradually increase in depth and rate and are then followed by a period of apnea)

DIAGNOSIS

Diagnostic Overview

Suspected in any recumbent animal with no response on initial physical examination and stimulation. Confirmed after a neurologic examination that identifies the patient as recumbent and unresponsive to all stimuli (including noxious stimuli).

Differential Diagnosis

- Intracranial: acute/rapidly progressive (e.g., trauma, hemorrhage)
- Intracranial: chronic/slowly progressive (e.g., tumor, abscess)
- Infectious
- Systemic disease
- See Coma, Section 3 (p. 1206) for detailed differential diagnosis.

Initial Database

Laboratory tests:

- CBC (infection or thrombocytopenia)
- Serum biochemistry panel (metabolic disorders)
- Urinalysis
  - Glucose, ketones (diabetes mellitus/ketoacidosis)
  - Calcium oxalate monohydrate crystals (ethylene glycol intoxication)
  - Ammonium biurate crystals (portosystemic shunt)
  - Low urine specific gravity (USG)/casts (renal disease [consider other causes of low USG])
- Prothrombin time/partial thromboplastin time or activated clotting time (coagulopathies)
- Serum bile acids (liver failure)
- Arterial blood gas analysis (hypoxemia, hypercarbia); alternative, SpO_2 and capnography

Imaging, as suggested by history and examination:

- Thoracic radiographs (metastatic lesions, trauma, or infections)
- Skull radiographs (trauma/skull fractures)

Arterial blood pressure (p. 1065)

Advanced or Confirmatory Testing

Magnetic resonance imaging (p. 1132) or computed tomography followed by cerebrospinal fluid analysis (pp. 1080 and 1323): after systemic disease is eliminated

TREATMENT

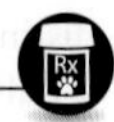

Treatment Overview

Coma has numerous causes. Initial therapy should focus on stabilization of the cardiovascular (perfusion), respiratory (oxygenation and ventilation), and neurologic (cerebral oxygen delivery and ICP) systems, followed by specific therapy tailored to the underlying cause.

Acute General Treatment

Airway and breathing:

- Endotracheal intubation assists ventilation and protects the airways (comatose patients cannot swallow; salivary secretions, regurgitation, and vomiting may cause airway obstruction and aspiration pneumonia). Avoid inducing cough, which increases ICP.
- Provide supplemental oxygen (maintain PaO_2 > 60 mm Hg, SaO_2 > 90%) (p. 1146).
  - CAUTION: nasal oxygen lines can induce sneezing, which increases ICP.
- Ensure ventilation (maintain PCO_2 between 35 and 45 mm Hg).

Circulation:

- Place intravenous catheter (avoid jugular veins if ICP elevated).
- Correct hypovolemia.
  - Fluid choice is controversial.
    - Crystalloids usually sufficient. Administer ¼ shock dose (15 mL/kg in dogs; 10 mL/kg in cats) rapidly intravenous (IV); repeat as needed for cardiovascular stability.
    - Hypertonic saline (5%-7.5% at 4-6 mL/kg over 10 minutes) may decrease ICP while improving perfusion. Avoid in hyperosmolar syndromes, hyponatremia, heart failure, and marked dehydration.
  - Avoid overhydration.
- Provide maintenance fluids, and replace ongoing fluid losses.
- With cardiac disease or hyperosmolar syndromes, administer any fluids cautiously.

Address (i.e., reduce) ICP:

- In comatose patient, assume ICP elevated until proved otherwise.
- Elevate head 20-30 degrees.
- Avoid pressure on jugular veins.
- Give mannitol (0.5-2 g/kg IV over 20-30 minutes) if diagnosis is unconfirmed or patient shows neurologic deterioration.
- Avoid mannitol in dehydrated, hypovolemic patients and when underlying cardiac disease or hyperosmolar states are present.
- Hypertonic saline (5%-7.5% at 4-6 mL/kg over 10 minutes) may be advantageous for traumatic brain injury. Can be repeated. Sodium concentration should be monitored (aim for 10-15 mEq/L above upper reference value).

Supportive care:

- Control seizures (p. 903):
  - Diazepam 0.5-1 mg/kg IV; can repeat twice in 15 minutes. If ineffective, use constant-rate infusion or different drug, *or*
  - Phenobarbital 2-15 mg/kg slow IV bolus (monitor respiration), *or*
  - Propofol (if severe hepatopathy/hepatic coma) 1-6 mg/kg IV bolus, can repeat or switch to constant-rate infusion (monitor respiration)
  - Levetiracetam 20-30 mg/kg IV, may repeat
- Treat hypoglycemia with 0.5 g/kg IV dextrose (p. 552).
  - Dilute 1 mL/kg of 50% dextrose in 3 × volume of 0.9% saline for slow IV administration to avoid injury due to hyperosmolar fluid infusion (e.g., for 2 kg dog, dilute 2 mL of 50% saline in 6 mL saline).
  - Avoid hyperglycemia.
- Glucocorticoids (e.g., methylprednisolone sodium succinate 30 mg/kg IV initial dose, then according to standard protocols, or dexamethasone 0.1 mg/kg IV) may be beneficial (neoplasia) or harmful (trauma).
  - Try to confirm diagnosis before giving glucocorticoids.
  - If life-threatening deterioration occurs before the diagnosis is confirmed, rapid-acting intravenous glucocorticoids can be administered for suspected neoplasia or encephalitis.

Specific therapy: see specific diseases.

Possible Complications

- Hypotension
- Hypothermia
- Brain herniation
- Cardiac arrhythmias
- Hypoventilation
- Aspiration pneumonia
- Seizures

Recommended Monitoring

Rapid deterioration possible: monitor until stable and improving.

- Neurologic examination every 30-60 minutes
- Continuous electrocardiogram
- Blood pressure every 30-60 minutes (systolic: > 90 mm Hg but < 180 mm Hg; mean, > 60 mm Hg but < 140 mm Hg)
- Blood gases ($PaCO_2$ and PaO_2) every 60 minutes or capnography and pulse oximetry continuously
- Blood glucose and electrolytes as needed

PROGNOSIS & OUTCOME

- Varies with underlying disease
- Generally guarded until diagnosis confirmed
- Declines as level of consciousness decreases
- Worse with systemic complications
- Unresponsive pupils, decerebrate rigidity, abnormal respiratory patterns, and loss of physiologic nystagmus carry a grave prognosis.
- Miotic responsive pupils suggest cortical lesions and a better prognosis.
- Hypoglycemia due to insulin overdose has a good prognosis.
- Can use modified Glasgow coma scale for prognosis in dogs with head trauma (p. 404).
- Failure to improve over 5-7 days warrants poor prognosis.

PEARLS & CONSIDERATIONS

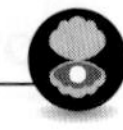

Comments

- Animals that display decerebrate rigidity are also comatose.
- Cranial nerve reflexes (depending on location of the lesion) and spinal reflexes are often present.
- Bradycardia with concurrent hypertension suggests elevated ICP.
- Can use caloric test to evaluate nystagmus (infusion of warm or cold water into the ear canal normally results in nystagmus).
- Administration of lidocaine during intubation (0.75 mg/kg IV) may suppress gag and cough reflexes, which would otherwise increase ICP.

Technician Tips

- Physical therapy, turning to change recumbencies, lubrication of the eyes, and moistening the mouth every 4 hours are important elements of support for comatose patients.
- A urinary catheter assists with monitoring urine output and preventing urine scald.

Client Education

- Full neurologic recovery can take weeks to months.
- Long-term neurologic deficits and seizures can occur.

SUGGESTED READING

Parratt CA, et al. Retrospective characterization of coma and stupor in dogs and cats presenting to a multicenter out-of-hours service (2012-2015):386 animals. J Vet Emerg Crit Care 28, 2018. https://doi.org/10.1111/vec.12772.

AUTHOR: Søren R. Boysen, DVM, DACVECC
EDITOR: Leah A. Cohn, DVM, PhD, DACVIM

Conjunctivitis, Cats

Client Education Sheet 

BASIC INFORMATION 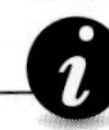

Definition

Inflammation of the mucous membranes (conjunctiva) surrounding the eye

Epidemiology

SPECIES, AGE, SEX

Both sexes and all ages can be affected. *Chlamydia felis* usually occurs in cats < 1 year old and is uncommon > 5 years old.

GENETICS, BREED PREDISPOSITION

C. felis appears to be more prevalent among purebred cats, but this may be biased by exposure in catteries.

RISK FACTORS

- Densely populated environments (shelters, rescues, catteries, multi-cat households) predispose to infectious causes.
- UV light may contribute to lipogranulomatous conjunctivitis because cases usually occur in light-colored cats (white, orange).

CONTAGION AND ZOONOSIS

- Many of the common causes are infectious and can spread from cat to cat (feline herpesvirus 1 [FHV-1], *C. felis,* feline calicivirus [FCV]).
- *C. felis* has a low potential for zoonosis, with immunocompromised people at highest risk.
- *Thelazia* spp infect humans by the vector fly but not through contact with infected cats.

GEOGRAPHY AND SEASONALITY

- *Thelazia callipaeda* (Europe, Asia) and *Thelazia californiensis* (western United States) infections may be seasonal because they involve a fly intermediate host (*Musca* spp, *Fannia* spp, *Phortica variegata, Amiota* spp).
- Allergic conjunctivitis (rare in cats) may have a seasonal component.

ASSOCIATED DISORDERS

- Symblepharon, keratitis, and corneal ulceration with FHV-1
- Some cats with lipogranulomatous conjunctivitis are concurrently diagnosed with squamous cell carcinoma of the eyelid skin adjacent to the conjunctival lesions.

Clinical Presentation

DISEASE FORMS/SUBTYPES

- Acute versus chronic
- Primary disease versus recrudescent disease (FHV-1)
- Primary versus secondary causes

HISTORY, CHIEF COMPLAINT

- Blepharospasm
- Ocular discharge
- "Red eye"
- Swelling around the eye
- May be unilateral or bilateral
- May be acute or chronic/intermittent
- +/− Systemic signs (sneezing, anorexia, lethargy)

PHYSICAL EXAM FINDINGS

- Blepharospasm
- Ocular discharge (serous to mucopurulent, mild to severe)
- Chemosis (especially *C. felis*)
- Hyperemia
- +/− Keratitis or corneal ulceration, depending on cause (FHV-1, entropion, rarely distichia)
- Whitish/yellow palpebral conjunctival nodules near eyelid margin (lipogranulomatous conjunctivitis)
- Other ocular disease (entropion, orbital disease, distichiasis, glaucoma, anterior uveitis)
- Sneezing, nasal discharge (FHV-1, less commonly *C. felis*)
- Lymphadenopathy (*C. felis,* infectious or neoplastic causes of uveitis)
- Fever (*C. felis,* FCV, infectious or inflammatory causes of uveitis)
- Oral ulceration (FCV)

Etiology and Pathophysiology

Conjunctivitis is often what causes a diseased eye to appear red and can have primary causes or occur secondary to numerous other ocular diseases.

Primary causes:

- Infectious
  - Viral: FHV-1, FCV
  - Bacterial: *C. felis,* +/− *Mycoplasma felis,* +/− *Mycoplasma gatae*
- Parasitic: *T. callipaeda, T. californiensis* (nematodes of conjunctival sac), *Cuterebra* spp
- Immune-mediated
  - Allergic conjunctivitis (rare in cats)
  - Proliferative keratoconjunctivitis (eosinophilic)
- Inflammatory
  - Lipogranulomatous conjunctivitis
- Trauma
- Chemical burn
- Environmental irritants (e.g., smoke, sand)
- Foreign bodies
- Therapeutic radiation

Secondary to other ocular disease:

- Corneal ulceration
- Entropion
- Distichiasis (rare)
- Tear film abnormalities (keratoconjunctivitis sicca, qualitative disorders)
- Uveitis
- Glaucoma
- Orbital disease
- Blepharitis

DIAGNOSIS

Diagnostic Overview

A complete ophthalmic exam is essential because numerous ocular disorders can cause secondary conjunctivitis. Most cases of chronic conjunctivitis are treated empirically based on history and exam because they are likely due to FHV-1 (for which diagnostics are unreliable) or *C. felis* (which can be treated empirically).

Differential Diagnosis

Episcleral injection is engorgement of the scleral blood vessels. It causes periocular redness and occurs secondary to ophthalmic diseases such as uveitis, glaucoma, and orbital disease.

Initial Database

Complete ophthalmic examination (p. 1137):

- Schirmer tear test (normal > 15 mm/minute in dogs, varies in cats)
  - Can be artificially decreased in cats due to stress
- Fluorescein dye application
- Intraocular pressure (normal: 10-20 mm Hg)
- Examination of the eyelid margin and palpebral conjunctiva with magnification and a good light source
- Examination of the cornea
- Fundic examination

Advanced or Confirmatory Testing

- Polymerase chain reaction (PCR) testing: recommended for *C. felis* and *Mycoplasma,* unreliable for FHV-1 (p. 464)
- Conjunctival cytology: diagnostic for proliferative keratoconjunctivitis (eosinophilic) (p. 568), rarely can see inclusion bodies with *C. felis* and *Mycoplasma*
- Conjunctival cultures and biopsy are rarely used. *Mycoplasma* and *C. felis* are difficult to culture. The conjunctiva of normal cats is not sterile, and *Mycoplasma* can be cultured from asymptomatic cats. Asymptomatic shedding of *C. felis* can occur. Histopathology confirms lipogranulomatous conjunctivitis but is not routinely done because exam findings are characteristic.

TREATMENT 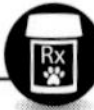

Treatment Overview

Treatments depend on the underlying cause. The goals of treatment are to relieve clinical signs and prevent spread of disease.

Acute General Treatment

- FHV-1: For conjunctivitis secondary to FHV-1 without keratitis, antiviral therapy is usually not warranted unless the cat is immunocompromised and the conjunctivitis severe or chronic (p. 464).
- FCV: (p. 141)

- *C. felis*
  - Topical treatment with oxytetracyline with or without polymyxin B q 6h for 2 weeks past resolution of clinical signs is most commonly used but may not eliminate shedding, which could be important in multiple cat households.
  - Doxycycline 10 mg/kg PO q 24h × 4 weeks or amoxicillin-clavulanic acid 13.75 mg/kg PO q 12h × 4 weeks is recommended to eliminate shedding. Continue for 2 weeks past clinical signs. Caution with tetracyclines in young cats; follow doxycycline tablets with water to minimize esophageal stricture formation.
  - If topical oxytetracycline is not available and systemic treatment is not elected, topical ophthalmic erythromycin is also effective in resolving clinical signs but must be used 2 weeks past resolution of clinical signs.
- *Thelazia* spp: manual removal of worms with forceps after topical anesthetic alone or follow with single dose of any of the following: ivermectin SQ at 0.2 mg/kg, milbemycin oxime 2 mg/kg PO, topical 2.5% moxidectin
- *Cuterebra* spp: manual removal of larvae after topical anesthetic, topical antibiotic +/− antiinflammatory prn
- Proliferative keratoconjunctivitis (eosinophilic)
- Allergic conjunctivitis: topical corticosteroids (Neopolydex, prednisolone acetate) and/or topical antihistamines (Ketotifen) q 6-24h prn based on severity; consider systemic management (p. 91)
- Lipogranulomatous conjunctivitis: surgical resection of nodules if causing irritation
- Foreign bodies and chemical/environmental irritants: manual removal of foreign body or elimination of irritant and topical lubricant, antibiotic, and/or antibiotic-corticosteroid q 6-24h prn
- For secondary causes, treat the underlying ophthalmic disorder.

Chronic Treatment

- Antivirals may be useful for chronic conjunctivitis caused by FHV-1, especially in cats that are immunosuppressed (p. 464).
- Proliferative keratoconjunctivitis often requires chronic treatment with topical corticosteroids or immunosuppressives.

Nutrition/Diet

Oral lysine may be beneficial in some cats with chronic conjunctivitis secondary to FHV-1 (p. 464).

Possible Complications

- Topical and oral corticosteroids can cause FHV-1 recrudescence.
- Topical corticosteroids must be avoided when corneal ulceration is present.
- A shortened topical or systemic antibiotic course may allow recrudescence of *C. felis.* Topical treatment or shorter systemic course may lead to persistent shedding. The possible complications and difficulties with oral treatment must be weighed against the possible complication of shedding. This is more of a concern in multi-cat housing.

Recommended Monitoring

Phone or email communication with owners can be useful for managing chronic FHV-1 cases to minimize stress from frequent exams.

PROGNOSIS & OUTCOME

Most acute cases completely resolve with proper treatment. Chronic conjunctivitis can be a frustrating, lifelong, intermittent problem that may not resolve with treatment, especially if due to FHV-1.

PEARLS & CONSIDERATIONS

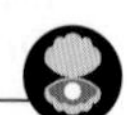

Comments

- Most cases are infectious and suspected to be due to recrudescent FHV-1.
- *C. felis* typically starts unilaterally and becomes bilateral within 2 weeks.
- Keratitis is common with FHV-1 and rare with *C. felis.*
- The role of *Mycoplasma* is controversial because it can be present on the conjunctiva of asymptomatic cats and experimental infection requires immunosuppression. However, treatment is the same as that for *C. felis.*
- *C. felis* and *Mycoplasma* inclusions are often confused with medication blue bodies and melanin granules on cytology.
- Enrofloxacin can be used to treat *C. felis* but is not recommended due to potential drug-induced retinal degeneration.
- Pradofloxacin 5 mg/kg, q 24h for 42 consecutive days has been studied, and although clinical improvements were seen, the presence of *C. felis* DNA was still positive based on PCR.
- Ophthalmic antibiotics have rarely been associated with anaphylaxis in cats and should be used only when indicated.
- Topical or systemic corticosteroids should be avoided in cases of feline conjunctivitis unless a specific diagnosis such as proliferative keratoconjunctivitis (eosinophilic) has been made. Unlike dogs, most feline cases are infectious.

Prevention

- Environmental and behavioral modifications to decrease stress may minimize FHV-1 flares.
- Vaccination for *C. felis* may help in environments with high prevalence.
- Fly prevention may prevent *Thelazia* spp.
- Minimize UV exposure for light cats for lipogranulomatous conjunctivitis.

Technician Tips

- Wear gloves and wash hands when restraining cats with conjunctivitis due to the possible but rare zoonotic potential of *C. felis* and to prevent spread to other cats.
- Owners disagree about whether ophthalmic solutions or ointments are easiest to apply. Compliance may increase if given their preferred formulation.

Client Education

- Medicating cats can be difficult, especially chronically or multiple times per day. A technician demonstrating how to properly administer ophthalmic medications to the cat during the appointment may be helpful.
- Call or return if signs worsen to rule out development of a corneal ulcer or topical medication hypersensitivities.

SUGGESTED READING

Maggs DJ: Conjunctiva. In Maggs DJ, et al, editors: Slatter's Fundamentals of veterinary ophthalmology, ed 5, St. Louis, 2013, Saunders.

RELATED CLIENT EDUCATION SHEET

How to Administer Eye Medications

AUTHOR: Sony Kuhn, DVM, DACVO
EDITOR: Diane V. H. Hendrix, DVM, DACVO

Conjunctivitis, Dogs

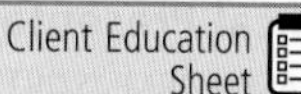

Client Education Sheet

BASIC INFORMATION

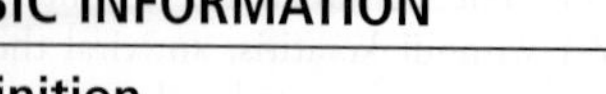

Definition

Conjunctivitis refers to inflammation of the conjunctiva. The conjunctiva lines the inside of the eyelids (palpebral conjunctiva) and forms the conjunctival fornix as it reflects back at the level of the orbital rim onto the surface of the globe to become the bulbar conjunctiva. The conjunctiva also lines the palpebral and bulbar surface of the nictitating membrane. The conjunctiva plays an important role in maintaining ocular health through the conjunctiva-associated lymphoid tissue (CALT) and through goblet cells, which provide the mucin layer of the precorneal tear film. Conjunctivitis is common in dogs as an isolated problem and in conjunction with a wide array of other ophthalmic conditions and some systemic diseases.

Synonym

Pink eye

Epidemiology

SPECIES, AGE, SEX

No sex predisposition. Young dogs are predisposed to follicular conjunctivitis.

GENETICS, BREED PREDISPOSITION

Breed predisposition:

- Deep conjunctival pockets (deep medial canthal pocket syndrome): dolichocephalic breeds
- Ectropion, entropion, or other conformational abnormalities of the eyelids: bulldogs, cocker spaniels (p. 296)
- Keratoconjunctivitis sicca (KCS) (p. 568)
- Pannus: German shepherds (p. 748)
- Atopy (p. 91)

RISK FACTORS

- Outdoor activities (environmental allergens, parasitic)
- Contact with chemicals or irritants (including ophthalmic drugs such as neomycin or pilocarpine)
- Unvaccinated dogs, contact with dogs infected with canine herpesvirus 1 (CHV-1) and canine distemper virus

CONTAGION AND ZOONOSIS

Most cases of conjunctivitis in dogs are not contagious. Selected cases may be contagious, including viral conjunctivitis (CHV-1, canine distemper virus, canine adenovirus 1 and 2 [CAV-1, CAV-2])

ASSOCIATED DISORDERS

KCS, qualitative tear film deficiency, blepharitis, uveitis, glaucoma, pannus, atopy, eyelid abnormalities (entropion, ectropion, trichiasis, ectopic cilia), orbital inflammation

Clinical Presentation

DISEASE FORMS/SUBTYPES

- Unilateral or bilateral
- Acute versus chronic
- Primary: follicular, immune-mediated (pannus), bacterial (rare), parasitic
- Secondary: associated with other ocular (e.g., KCS) or systemic disorders (atopy, distemper)

HISTORY, CHIEF COMPLAINT

- Mucoid or mucopurulent ocular discharge
- "Red eye"
- Painful eye
- Ocular rubbing/pruritus

PHYSICAL EXAM FINDINGS

- Conjunctival hyperemia
- Mucoid or mucopurulent ocular discharge (may be pronounced)
- +/− Chemosis
- +/− Blepharospasm
- +/− Elevated nictitating membrane
- +/− Lymphoid follicles (typically most numerous in the conjunctival fornix or bulbar surface of the nictitating membrane)
- +/− Conjunctival petechiae or ulcerations (CHV-1)
- +/− Other signs of ocular disease such as pigmentary keratitis, entropion, trichiasis, etc.

Etiology and Pathophysiology

Primary:

- Environmental or mechanical irritation
- Follicular conjunctivitis
- Allergies (atopy, food allergy, contact allergy) are also a common cause of conjunctivitis; conjunctivitis is reported in 60% of dogs with atopic dermatitis.
- Immune-mediated: pannus
- Infectious primary conjunctivitis in dogs is rare but may include viral infection (CHV-1), or parasitic infection (*Onchocerca lupi, Thelazia*).
    - Bacterial conjunctivitis is typically associated with other conditions such as KCS.

Secondary:

- Other ocular causes of red eye:
    - Adnexal abnormalities
    - Tear film disorders
    - Corneal ulceration
    - Keratitis
    - Glaucoma
    - Uveitis
- Conjunctivitis secondary to systemic infection is rare but may include viral infection (canine distemper virus, CAV-1, CAV-2), bacterial infection (rickettsial, periocular, or retrobulbar cellulitis), or parasitic infection (*Leishmania*).
- Neoplastic causes are rare: lymphosarcoma is the most common.
- Systemic noninfectious diseases such as systemic histiocytosis or ligneous conjunctivitis associated with a plasminogen deficiency are rare.

DIAGNOSIS

Diagnostic Overview

Diagnostics should center on determining whether there is an ocular cause for the conjunctivitis.

Differential Diagnosis

Conjunctivitis must be differentiated from other causes of red eye:

- Anterior uveitis
- Glaucoma
- KCS
- Corneal ulceration
- Keratitis
- Episcleritis/scleritis
- Orbital disease

Initial Database

Complete ophthalmic exam (p. 1137):

- Schirmer tear test (normal > 15 mm/min in dogs)
- Tonometry (normal is > 15 mm Hg and < 25 mm Hg)
- Fluorescein dye application
- Complete exam of the eyelids, anterior segment, and posterior segment of both eyes
- Physical exam and history to evaluate for concurrent systemic disease

Advanced or Confirmatory Testing

- Conjunctival biopsy and histopathologic evaluation may be indicated in unusual or persistent cases.
- Conjunctival cytology
- Bacterial or fungal culture (rarely rewarding)
- Polymerase chain reaction (PCR) assay or serology for infectious diseases based on history and systemic signs

TREATMENT

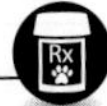

Therapeutic Overview

Determining the underlying cause of conjunctivitis is critical to direct therapy. Goals of treatment are to alleviate ocular discomfort, eliminate or ameliorate the underlying cause (e.g., establish normal tear production with lacrimomimetic therapy in cases of KCS, address atopy with systemic medications/food trial), and eliminate underlying infection if present.

Acute General Treatment

Allergic, follicular, immune-mediated, or environmental conjunctivitis:

- Topical steroid or steroid/antibiotic combinations (e.g., neomycin, polymyxin, dexamethasone or plain dexamethasone 0.1% solution or ointment) q 6-8h until the symptoms resolve, and then taper
- Limit exposure to irritants such as dust, wind, smoke, or contact irritants
- Elizabethan collar may be required to limit self-trauma
- Irrigate the conjunctival fornices with saline q 12h to remove ocular discharge, allergens, and irritants; long-term irrigation indicated for dogs with medial canthal pocket syndrome in conjunction with prn topical steroids
- Address underlying allergies.

Conjunctivitis secondary to an underlying cause:

- Treat the associated ocular condition (e.g., topical cyclosporine or tacrolimus for KCS).
- Treat underlying infection or neoplasia
- Topical antiviral therapy is indicated for CHV-1; idoxuridine 0.1% or trifluridine 1% solutions 6-8 times daily for 48 hours, then 4 times daily; cidofovir 0.5% solution q 12h all for 1 week past resolution
- *O. lupi* is treated with medical therapy (melarsomine IM, tetracycline antibiotics PO, ivermectin SQ or PO) +/− surgical removal of the nematodes; *Thelazia* infections may be treated with manual removal of the nematodes and anthelmintics.

Chronic Treatment

- Lifelong therapy is indicated for most cases of KCS and pannus.

- Allergic conjunctivitis may require long-term systemic therapy and/or the intermittent use of topical steroids.
  - Dogs with medial canthal pocket syndrome typically require intermittent or maintenance topical steroids.

PROGNOSIS & OUTCOME

Most cases of isolated conjunctivitis due to mechanical irritation or allergies resolve with topical corticosteroid therapy. However, recurrences are common, and ongoing or intermittent therapy may be indicated.

PEARLS & CONSIDERATIONS

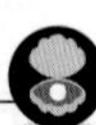

Comments

- Conjunctival hyperemia can be differentiated from episcleral injection (usually associated with intraocular diseases such as glaucoma or uveitis) by noting that conjunctival vessels have a small diameter and branching pattern versus the larger diameter, nonbranching episcleral vessels. Conjunctival vessels are also mobile and will blanch after the topical application of phenylephrine or epinephrine; episcleral vessels are nonmobile and do not blanch quickly after the application of topical phenylephrine or epinephrine.
- Do not forget to check Schirmer tear test values when evaluating dogs for conjunctivitis.
- Avoid topical corticosteroids in cases of corneal ulceration.
- Systemic steroids can cause recrudescence of CHV-1 infection.

Technician Tips

A Schirmer tear test, tonometry, and fluorescein staining should be done on any dog evaluated for a red eye.

SUGGESTED READING

Hendrix DVH. Diseases and surgery of the canine conjunctiva and nictitating membrane. In Gelatt KN, et al, editors: Veterinary ophthalmology, ed 5, Ames, Iowa, 2013, Wiley-Blackwell, pp 945-975.

AUTHOR: Nancy Johnstone McLean, DVM, DACVO
EDITOR: Diane V. H. Hendrix, DVM, DACVO

Constipation/Obstipation and Megacolon

Client Education Sheet

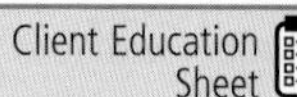

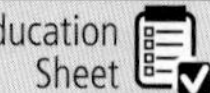

BASIC INFORMATION

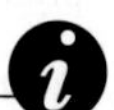

Definition

- Constipation: infrequent or difficult evacuation of feces; does not imply loss of function
- Obstipation: intractable constipation
- Megacolon: persistent dilation of the large intestine associated with chronic constipation or obstipation; may occur secondary to idiopathic loss of colon function. Dilated megacolon implies permanent disruption of colonic structure and loss of colonic function.

Epidemiology

SPECIES, AGE, SEX

Constipation: dogs and cats. Obstipation/megacolon may be more common in middle-aged, male, domestic short-haired or long-haired or Siamese cats. Megacolon is rarely reported in dogs.

GENETICS, BREED PREDISPOSITION

Manx cats may be predisposed to neurogenic megacolon. Congenital segmental aganglionosis (Hirschsprung disease in humans) has been documented in only one kitten.

RISK FACTORS

- Intrinsic dysfunction that prevents passage of feces: spinal cord/spinal nerve disease or trauma, dysautonomia
- Mechanical obstruction that prevents passage of feces: pelvic fracture, colonic stricture or neoplasia, extraluminal mass or stricture compressing colon, rectoanal stricture, colonic foreign body
- A bony diet and low levels of exercise may predispose dogs to megacolon.

ASSOCIATED DISORDERS

Perineal hernia may be the cause or result of constipation and megacolon.

Clinical Presentation

DISEASE FORMS/SUBTYPES

- Hypertrophic megacolon: develops as a consequence of obstructive lesions and may be reversible with early therapy.
- Dilated megacolon: end stage of colonic dysfunction (idiopathic or untreated hypertrophic megacolon) and may be poorly responsive to treatment

HISTORY, CHIEF COMPLAINT

- Reduced, absent, or painful defecation is typical.
- Fecal balls are often very hard if passed; occasionally, watery diarrhea may be passed around fecal concretion.
- Prolonged constipation will result in anorexia, lethargy, weight loss, or vomiting (may be projectile).

PHYSICAL EXAM FINDINGS

- Poor body condition
- Dehydration
- Colon distended with hard feces on abdominal palpation; signs of abdominal pain may be present
- Perineal irritation/ulceration
- Rectal exam (usually requires sedation in cats): hard feces, ± pelvic narrowing, ± stricture or mass palpated, ± perineal hernia

Etiology and Pathophysiology

- Prolonged retention of feces in colon due to functional (neurogenic) or mechanical obstruction
- Inflammation can be associated with constipation (perianal fistula, proctitis, anal sac abscess, or perianal bite wounds).
- Water absorption from feces in colon results in concretion that is difficult or impossible to pass (common in cats with chronic kidney disease or diabetes mellitus).
- Neurogenic dysfunction from dysautonomia (autonomic system failure), trauma to pelvic or hypogastric nerves (pelvic fracture), neoplasia of spinal cord, or caudal spinal cord diseases (e.g., lumbosacral disease, lumbosacral stenosis/cauda equina syndrome, Manx cat sacral deformities)
- Prolonged distention of colon causes irreversible changes in colonic smooth muscles and nerves.
- Retained bacterial toxins may be absorbed, resulting in endotoxemia and anorexia, lethargy, and/or vomiting.

DIAGNOSIS

Diagnostic Overview

The diagnosis of constipation is based on a history of difficult, reduced, or absent defecation and finding firm feces in the colon on abdominal palpation. Some underlying causes can be determined by physical examination and abdominal radiography.

Differential Diagnosis

Reversible causes of constipation:

- Dehydration, electrolyte disorders, inflammatory diseases of the anorectum
- Drug administration (opioids, anticholinergics)
- Environmental changes (inactivity, litter box changes)

Any risk factors causing mechanical obstruction

Initial Database

- CBC: unremarkable or leukocytosis (mature neutrophilia/stress leukogram), occasionally anemia
- Serum biochemistry profile: unremarkable or azotemia (associated with dehydration or concurrent chronic kidney disease), hypokalemia, hypercalcemia
- Urinalysis: no specific changes. Isosthenuria with azotemia if chronic kidney disease
- Abdominal radiographs
  - Feces-distended colon. Ratio of maximal diameter of colon to length of fifth lumbar vertebra > 1.48 defines megacolon in cats. Ratio of maximal diameter of colon to length of seventh lumbar vertebra > 1.5 defines megacolon in dogs.
  - Underlying cause of initial colonic distention/fecal retention may be evident (pelvic fractures, evidence of spinal trauma [vertebral fracture/luxation], extraluminal compressive mass, foreign material in colon).

Advanced or Confirmatory Testing

- Ultrasonography identifies suspected extraluminal masses. Poor utility for intraluminal visualization because even minute amounts of colonic gas block ultrasound waves
- Barium enema defines strictures or intraluminal masses.
- Endoscopy identifies colorectal neoplasia, stricture, inflammatory lesions, sacculations and diverticula, and other conditions.
- Evaluation of animals with suspected neurologic impairment may include cerebrospinal fluid analysis (pp. 1080 and 1323), CT/MRI scanning of distal spinal cord and cauda equina region (p. 1132), myelogram, and electrophysiologic studies (electromyography).
- Diagnosis of dysautonomia, a rare cause of megacolon, is based on finding other systemic evidence of the disease (megaesophagus, mydriasis, decreased lacrimation, prolapsed nictitans, and bradycardia).

TREATMENT

Treatment Overview

Mild to moderate constipation is usually successfully treated with a combination of enemas, laxatives, colonic prokinetic agents, and diet modification. Patients with severe constipation often also require intravenous fluid therapy and manual extraction of feces under anesthesia. Subtotal colectomy is necessary for patients with end-stage megacolon. See p. 1407 for a recommended treatment approach and protocol.

Acute General Treatment

- Fluid therapy for dehydration to assist in constipation relief through rehydration of the colonic mucosa
- Enemas and careful manual extraction of feces if obstipated. In most cats, sedation or anesthesia will be required. Multiple procedures over a day or two may be needed in the most severely obstipated/impacted cats to prevent additional injury or rupture of the diseased colon.
- Warm water enemas (5-10 mL/kg water) using a 12-14 Fr, well-lubricated, red rubber catheter are usually well tolerated (p. 1099). Higher volumes of water must be used with caution because they may cause vomiting (and aspiration).
- Enemas should not contain soaps or other irritants; lactulose or mineral oil can be used.
- Enemas containing sodium phosphate (e.g., Fleet) are *contraindicated* in cats and small dogs because they can cause severe hyperphosphatemia, hypocalcemia, and death.
- Broad-spectrum antibiotics (e.g., ampicillin sulbactam 22 mg/kg IV q 6-8h and enrofloxacin 5-10 mg/kg diluted 1 : 1 in saline and given slowly IV q 24h [dogs] or cefoxitin 10-30 mg/kg q 8h [cats]) are indicated if signs of endotoxemia or fever are noted.

Chronic Treatment

- Medical therapy includes stool softeners or laxatives (e.g., polyethylene glycol PEG 3350 [Miralax] ⅛ - ¼ teaspoon [0.6-1.3 mL] powder/CAT PO q 12h, or lactulose 0.25-0.5 mL/kg PO q 8-12h, or docusate sodium/dioctyl sulfosuccinate 50 mg/CAT PO q 12-24h) and prokinetics (cisapride 0.1-1 mg/kg PO q 8-12h or 2.5-5 mg/CAT PO q 8-12h). Polyethylene glycol is easier to use than lactulose (not sticky). The dosage for any of these is titrated to produce a soft to semiformed stool.
- Bulk-forming laxatives (cellulose, psyllium) will not be effective in cats prone to dehydration or in cats with poor colonic muscle function because their mechanism of action is similar to high-fiber diets.
- Stimulant laxatives (e.g., bisacodyl, castor oil, cascara) should not be used for relieving constipation but are best used as a preventive in cats that still have normal colonic function.
- Prokinetic therapy may assist smooth-muscle function in cats with recurrent constipation or obstipation. The most effective drugs are the serotonergic agonists (cisapride, prucalopride [available in Europe, Canada, and Israel]).
- Correct underlying cause when present: remove masses or strictures causing obstruction to outflow, or correct pelvic fractures obstructing outflow with pelvic osteotomy.
- Subtotal colectomy (with or without preservation of the ileocolic valve) may be indicated if lack of response to medical treatment or pelvic fracture malunion > 6 months from onset of obstipation.

Nutrition/Diet

- Control recurrent constipation with high-fiber/low-residue diet; prescription diets specifically designed to meet this need are available.
- High-fiber diets induce colonic contraction and are useful when the patient still has a functional colon and is well hydrated. Avoid high-fiber diets in patients that are prone to dehydration (high-fiber content can exacerbate colonic mucosal dehydration).
- Low-residue diets are often best used in patients with chronic recurrent obstipation or true megacolon because they reduce the amount of material reaching the colon and make it easier to maintain a soft stool.

Possible Complications

- Medical treatment: perforation secondary to trauma from enemas and evacuation of feces; gentle manipulation, and being patient (do not be in a hurry to remove the concretion) are essential.
- Subtotal colectomy: leakage, dehiscence, and peritonitis; chronic diarrhea (may be associated with bacterial overgrowth from loss of ileocolic sphincter); recurrent constipation; stricture

Recommended Monitoring

- For cats undergoing medical management, close observation of fecal passage by the owner is essential for prevention of severe recurrent constipation.
- After subtotal colectomy, monitor
  - Hydration
  - Appetite
  - Temperature, blood glucose, abdominal pain (signs of leakage or dehiscence of anastomosis)

PROGNOSIS & OUTCOME

- Fair prognosis with medical management. Recurrent constipation requiring repeated enemas and manual evacuation is common.
- Good to excellent prognosis in cats with subtotal colectomy. Owner needs to be aware that stools are usually soft and the frequency of defecation is increased for 2 to 3 months after surgery. Occasionally, diarrhea is a persistent, long-term problem.
  - Guarded to fair after subtotal colectomy in dogs. Because of species differences in rectal blood supply, there is a greater risk of rectocolic anastomosis site dehiscence in dogs. Persistent diarrhea/soft stool is more common in dogs, depending on how much colon is resected.
- Guarded prognosis with pelvic osteotomy/hemipelvectomy for pelvic fracture malunion; correction of obstruction may not resolve megacolon and constipation.

PEARLS & CONSIDERATIONS

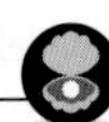

Comments

- Correction of pelvic malunion by pelvic osteotomy/hemipelvectomy if > 6 months from onset of signs of obstipation will most likely result in recurrence of obstipation and the need for subtotal colectomy.
- Do not perform enema immediately before surgery for megacolon. It is more difficult

to control contamination of the abdomen with liquid feces during surgery.

Prevention

Early repair of pelvic fractures can prevent obstruction of pelvic canal. Pelvic canal narrowing > 45% carries a high risk of constipation.

Technician Tips

Avoid colon perforation during enemas by using a well-lubricated red rubber catheter that is passed gently and slowly (see Acute General Treatment above).

Client Education

Warn owners that diarrhea can be severe after subtotal colectomy. Diarrhea/soft stools are usually persistent in dogs but usually resolves in cats within 8 weeks. If the cecum is removed during surgery, consider treatment for bacterial overgrowth if diarrhea persists for more than 8 weeks.

SUGGESTED READING

Byers CG, et al: Feline idiopathic megacolon. Compend Contin Educ Vet 28:658-665, 2006.

AUTHOR: Lori Ludwig, VMD, MS, DACVS
EDITOR: Elizabeth A. Swanson, DVM, MS, DACVS

Coprophagia

BASIC INFORMATION

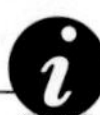

Definition

The consumption of fecal matter, involving the patient's own stools and/or those produced by other animals

Epidemiology

SPECIES, AGE, SEX

- Ubiquitous behavior among domestic dogs
- Associated with exploratory behavior in puppies
- Normal component of husbandry in nursing bitches and queens during early lactation
- Otherwise rare in cats

RISK FACTORS

- Conditions associated with maldigestion/malabsorption
- Polyphagia
- Central nervous system (CNS) disturbances that result in pica
- Insufficient social interaction and environmental enrichment
- Thiamin deficiency

CONTAGION AND ZOONOSIS

Increased risk of gastrointestinal (GI) parasitism (e.g., hookworms, roundworms)

GEOGRAPHY AND SEASONALITY

Recognized year-round, although weather patterns may impact exposure and accessibility of stool, and temperature may alter the appeal. Frozen stool is particularly alluring for some dogs.

ASSOCIATED DISORDERS

- Behavioral conditions (pica, anxiety, attention seeking)
- GI disturbances
- Malnutrition

Clinical Presentation

DISEASE FORMS/SUBTYPES

- Autocoprophagy: ingestion of own feces
- Allocoprophagy: ingestion of another animal's feces

HISTORY, CHIEF COMPLAINT

Owners typically report recurrent episodes of stool consumption, including the pet's own feces and/or those belonging to another animal.

PHYSICAL EXAM FINDINGS

- Typically unremarkable unless associated with a GI cause
- Halitosis may be noted.

Etiology and Pathophysiology

- Although distressing for pet owners, coprophagy is a common and typically normal behavior among dogs.
- Specific attributes of stool, such as odor, texture, and taste, may have a unique appeal.

DIAGNOSIS

Diagnostic Overview

The diagnosis is based on history and is typically reported by owners.

Differential Diagnosis

- Primary GI disease (exocrine pancreatic insufficiency [EPI], malabsorptive conditions)
- Behavioral conditions (pica, anxiety, attention-seeking)

Initial Database

- Physical examination
- Fecal flotation
- A thorough history should be obtained, including diet, appetite, fecal score, environment, and behavioral patterns.
- If a primary medical disturbance is suspected, CBC, serum biochemistry panel, and urinalysis should be performed ± other tests based on clinical indication (e.g., trypsin-like immunoreactivity [TLI]).

TREATMENT

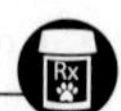

Treatment Overview

- If a primary disorder is present (e.g., EPI), appropriate medical therapies should be directed to the cause.
- Dietary supplements or substances applied directly to the stool itself to alter taste and texture have unreliable efficacy.
- Although coprophagy can be offensive and distressing to many owners, it is a normal behavior in dogs. Treatment strategies directed toward behavioral modification are recommended but often unsuccessful.

Acute General Treatment

- Minimize access to feces by establishing appropriate hygiene in the pet's environment.
- Employ the use of a head collar or basket muzzle to deter negative behavior on walks.
- Ensure prompt removal of feces after defecation.
- Prevent access to litter boxes in the household. The installation of a baby gate may be useful to act as a physical barrier.
- Reward desirable behaviors with praise and affection.
- Consider the use of a remote-controlled citronella collar to discourage the behavior.
- Avoid inadvertently reinforcing the behavior in attention-seeking cases.

Nutrition/Diet

- Ensure the pet is receiving a complete and balanced diet that is life stage and species appropriate.
- Address abnormalities in body condition score (BCS); aim for a BCS of 4-5/9 on a 9-point scale.

Behavior/Exercise

- Ensure adequate exercise and environmental enrichment to reduce boredom.
- Address predisposing factors such as compulsive behaviors.

PROGNOSIS & OUTCOME

Behavior is likely to continue if client compliance toward prevention, supervision, and environmental management is poor.

PEARLS & CONSIDERATIONS

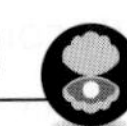

Comments

Coprophagy may be initiated and perpetuated by competitive behaviors between animals in a shared environment. In these instances, treatment should be focused on management of group dynamics, particularly around food.

Prevention

- Supervision and redirection of negative behaviors must be emphasized.
- Access to feces in the pet's environment should be vigilantly monitored and removed.

Technician Tips

- Patients with this behavior should be kept on a monthly parasite prevention schedule, a complete and balanced diet, and receive daily physical activity and social interactions.
- Technicians should also monitor patients over time for signs indicating GI disturbances, including weight loss, changes in appetite, and vomiting, so that potential medical causes are not overlooked in lieu of an otherwise normal behavior.

Client Education

- Stools may be particularly appealing for some dogs, and the behavior can be highly self-rewarding.
- For dogs that lack social stimulation, coprophagy may be perpetuated by the reward of attention when the behavior results in a response by the owner.

SUGGESTED READING

Horwitz DF, et al: Coprophagia. In Horwitz DF, et al, editors: Canine and feline behavior, Ames, IA, 2007, Blackwell, p 236.

AUTHOR: Allison Wara, DVM, DACVN
EDITOR: Leah A. Cohn, DVM, PhD, DACVIM

Corneal Lipid Infiltrates

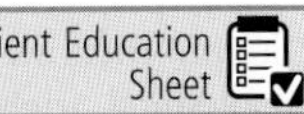

BASIC INFORMATION

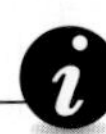

Definition

The accumulation of lipid (mostly unesterified cholesterol and phospholipids) in the corneal stroma is a feature shared by three distinct disorders:

- Corneal dystrophy: common primary hereditary condition with bilateral and mostly symmetrical lipid deposits in the central cornea; not associated with underlying systemic or ocular disease
- Corneal degeneration: acquired degenerative condition with unilateral or bilateral lipid or calcium deposits in any region of the cornea; associated current or previous local ocular inflammation and corneal vascularization
- Lipid keratopathy: rare acquired condition with bilateral lipid deposits in the peripheral cornea; associated with systemic diseases that cause hyperlipidemia

Synonyms

- Corneal dystrophy, corneal epithelial dystrophy, corneal stromal dystrophy, corneal crystalline stromal dystrophy
- Lipid keratopathy, corneal lipidosis, corneal arcus, arcus lipoides corneae

Epidemiology

SPECIES, AGE, SEX

- Corneal lipid infiltrates are common in dogs and rare in cats.
- Corneal dystrophy usually develops in young adult dogs.

GENETICS, BREED PREDISPOSITION

Breeds most commonly affected with corneal dystrophy include the Cavalier King Charles spaniel, Alaskan malamute, Siberian husky, Samoyed, rough collie, beagle, Airedale terrier, and Shetland sheepdog.

ASSOCIATED DISORDERS

- Corneal dystrophy: none
- Corneal degeneration: any pathologic condition that causes chronic corneal vascularization such as keratitis, episcleritis, uveitis, limbal neoplasia (melanoma), pannus, and ocular trauma
- Lipid keratopathy: any systemic disease that causes hyperlipidemia, such as primary hyperlipidemia, hypothyroidism, diabetes mellitus, hyperadrenocorticism, chronic pancreatitis, and liver disease

Clinical Presentation

DISEASE FORMS/SUBTYPES

Corneal dystrophy, corneal degeneration, and lipid keratopathy are most commonly differentiated by clinical findings seen on ophthalmic exam (see Physical Exam Findings below).

HISTORY, CHIEF COMPLAINT

White corneal opacity

PHYSICAL EXAM FINDINGS

Corneal lipid infiltrates appear as well-demarcated, refractile, crystalline white-gray opacities in the superficial stroma.

- Corneal dystrophy: bilateral and nearly symmetrical circular, oval, or ringlike lipid deposits in the central cornea. Lesions are not painful and stain negative with fluorescein. Appearance varies somewhat between breeds.
- Corneal degeneration: unilateral or bilateral, varied shapes of lipid deposits in any location of the cornea. Often associated with corneal vascularization. May also be associated with corneal ulceration, pigmentation, or fibrosis.
- Lipid keratopathy: usually bilateral lipid deposits in the shape of an arc in the peripheral cornea with a band of clear cornea between the deposits and the limbus. Lesions are not painful, fluorescein negative, and variably associated with vascularization.

Etiology and Pathophysiology

- Corneal dystrophy: heritable with unknown pathogenesis; possible local metabolic defect in corneal fibroblasts
- Corneal degeneration: acquired secondary to local pathologic changes in the cornea
- Lipid keratopathy: acquired secondary to hyperlipidemia; likely deposited by perilimbal blood vessels

DIAGNOSIS

Diagnostic Overview

Complete ophthalmic exam with magnification and a bright focal light source is recommended to evaluate corneal lipid infiltrates. Determination of the type of lipid disorder is important for diagnostic and therapeutic recommendations and prognosis.

Differential Diagnosis

White corneal opacities:

- Calcium/mineral deposits (matt chalky white; often difficult to differentiate from lipid)
- Fibrosis/scarring (dull, gray-white, and wispy; does not retain fluorescein stain)
- Inflammatory/infectious infiltrate (yellow-white and fluffy)
- Edema (light blue-gray and hazy)
- Florida spots, Florida keratopathy: benign, usually multifocal corneal opacities in dogs and cats from tropical regions

Initial Database

- Complete ophthalmic exam (p. 1137)
  - Schirmer tear test: should be normal unless corneal degeneration is associated with keratoconjunctivitis sicca (<15 mm/min)
  - Fluorescein stain: should be negative unless corneal degeneration is associated with ulcerative keratitis (positive)

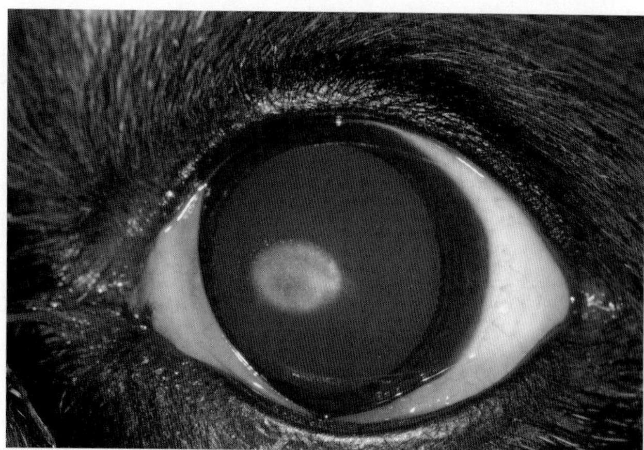

CORNEAL DYSTROPHY Note the oval, white, glittery area in the axial cornea in this Cavalier King Charles spaniel. (Courtesy Diane Hendrix, DVM, University of Tennessee.)

- Serum chemistry panel (including fasting cholesterol, triglycerides if lipid keratopathy is suspected)
  - Corneal dystrophy: normal
  - Corneal degeneration: normal
  - Lipid keratopathy: hyperlipidemia

Advanced or Confirmatory Testing

- Referral to a veterinary ophthalmologist for confirmation by slit-lamp biomicroscopy
- Thyroid panel, adrenal function evaluation if indicated

TREATMENT

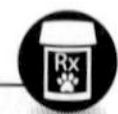

Treatment Overview

Goals of treatment:

- Minimize further lipid infiltration if possible.
- Manage any underlying systemic disease.

Acute General Treatment

- Corneal dystrophy: none required
- Corneal degeneration: address underlying ocular disease
  - If calcium component is present, topical application of disodium EDTA in an ophthalmic preparation (0.4%-3.75% q 6-8h) can be used in an attempt to chelate the mineral.
- Lipid keratopathy: address underlying systemic disease

Chronic Treatment

In rare instances dense lipid deposits can cause visual deficits. Referral to a veterinary ophthalmologist for surgical removal by a superficial keratectomy is possible. Deposits may re-form after surgery.

Nutrition/Diet

Low-fat diets are recommended in cases of hyperlipidemia (lipid keratopathy). Dietary restrictions are noted anecdotally to decrease or control lipid infiltrates due to corneal dystrophy or corneal degeneration in some dogs.

Drug Interactions

Long-term use of topical corticosteroids may cause or exacerbate corneal lipid infiltrates, a condition known as corticosteroid keratopathy.

Recommended Monitoring

Corneal degeneration and lipid keratopathy require management of ocular and systemic diseases, respectively.

PROGNOSIS & OUTCOME

Good. Corneal dystrophy may be slowly progressive but rarely interferes with vision. Corneal degeneration and lipid keratopathy may resolve or remain static if underlying conditions are treated.

PEARLS & CONSIDERATIONS

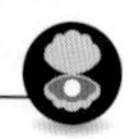

Comments

Corneal dystrophy is the most common condition causing corneal lipid infiltrates in dogs. Clients planning to breed dogs with this condition should be informed that it is a heritable trait and Orthopedic Foundation for Animals (OFA) eye evaluations are recommended.

Technician Tips

Lipid deposits in the cornea are usually not painful and fluorescein negative. If the patient has ocular pain or corneal ulceration, additional evaluation to identify the underlying ocular disease and topical ophthalmic medications are likely required.

Client Education

Corneal dystrophy is a heritable trait, and dogs used for breeding should be evaluated by an ophthalmologist for disease conformation and recommendations.

SUGGESTED READING

Crispin S: Ocular lipid deposition and hyperlipoproteinemia. Prog Retin Eye Res 21:169-224, 2002.

AUTHOR: Erin M. Scott, VMD, DACVO
EDITOR: Diane V. H. Hendrix, DVM, DACVO

Corneal Pigmentation

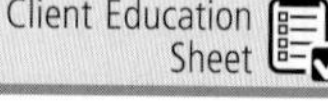

BASIC INFORMATION

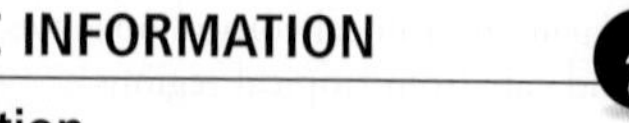

Definition

Brown to black discoloration of the cornea, usually due to the presence of melanin

Epidemiology

SPECIES, AGE, SEX

- Dogs: pigmentary keratitis: brachycephalic breeds, especially pug breed; pannus (chronic superficial keratitis) (p. 748): large-breed dogs, especially German shepherd breed
- Cats: corneal sequestrum (p. 208): primarily brachycephalic breeds

Clinical Presentation

HISTORY, CHIEF COMPLAINT

- Brown discoloration of cornea
- Concurrently: redness of the conjunctiva, ocular discharge, ocular pain, reduced vision

PHYSICAL EXAM FINDINGS

- Brown or black discoloration of the corneal epithelium, stroma, or endothelium
- Extensive pigmentation may cause reduced or absent menace response.
- Other findings will vary depending on the underlying cause.

Etiology and Pathophysiology

- Epithelial and stromal pigmentation
  - Melanin is produced in the cornea by melanocytes in response to chronic corneal irritation from desiccation (p. 568), mechanical trauma, or secondary to chronic inflammation in response

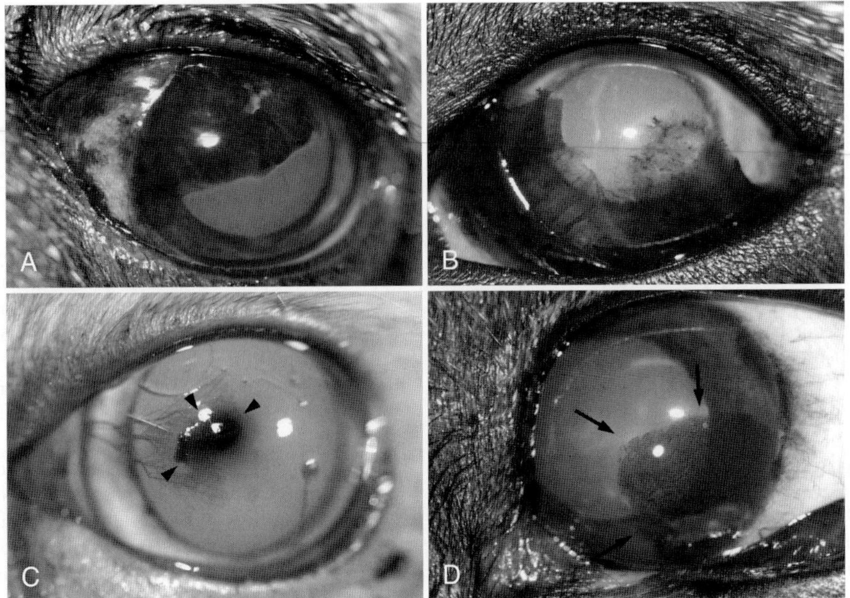

CORNEAL PIGMENTATION Causes of corneal pigmentation. **A**, Pigmentary keratitis in a pug dog. **B**, Chronic superficial keratitis (pannus) in a German shepherd dog. **C**, Corneal sequestrum in a Persian cat. **D**, Endothelial pigmentation in a mixed-breed dog.

to corneal ulceration, degeneration, or corneal antigen.

- Endothelial pigmentation
  - Adherence of melanin or melanin-containing cells, usually arising from the anterior uvea, to the endothelium
- Stromal infiltration at the limbus as extension of a melanin-containing neoplasm
- Protrusion of pigmented iris through a corneal defect (p. 209)
- Corneal sequestrum (p. 208):
  - Associated with chronic irritation
  - The central/paracentral corneal stroma becomes necrotic, brown-stained, and the overlying epithelium is usually disrupted.

DIAGNOSIS

Diagnostic Overview

The diagnosis is apparent on physical examination. Species and breed are also important considerations.

Differential Diagnosis

- Epithelial and stromal pigmentation
  - Pigmentary keratitis: large palpebral fissure, lagophthalmos (incomplete closure of the eyelids), trichiasis (entropion, nasal folds, aberrant dermis at medial canthus)
  - Exposure keratitis: buphthalmos (chronic glaucoma), neuroparalytic keratitis (cranial nerve VII lesion)
  - Keratoconjunctivitis sicca (KCS) (p. 568)
  - Pannus (chronic superficial keratitis) (p. 748): dogs
  - Limbal melanocytoma (NOTE: Melanomas of the limbus in dogs and cats are almost always benign and therefore are appropriately called melanocytomas [p. 559])
  - Invasive anterior uveal melanoma/ melanocytoma
  - Protrusion of iris tissue through corneal defect (i.e., iris prolapse [p. 209])
  - Corneal sequestrum (cats): brown foreign material (p. 208)
  - Dermoid: congenital presence of abnormal epithelial tissue
- Endothelial pigmentation: persistent pupillary membrane (iris to cornea), anterior synechia, uveal melanoma/melanocytoma, rupture of pigmented uveal cyst [p. 1023])

Initial Database

- Neuro-ophthalmic exam (p. 1136): evaluate palpebral reflexes and completeness of eyelid closure.
- Ophthalmic exam (p. 1137): evaluate for abnormalities of eyelids and aberrant cilia, iris abnormalities, uveal cysts.
  - Schirmer tear test (STT): values < 10 mm/min and clinical signs consistent with keratoconjunctivitis
  - Fluorescein staining: positive if corneal ulceration is present. Fluorescein uptake usually occurs only around the edge of a corneal sequestrum.
  - Tonometry: elevated intraocular pressure (>25 mm Hg) in glaucoma (can rise with uveal melanoma/melanocytoma and uveal cysts)

TREATMENT

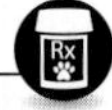

Treatment Overview

The goals of treatment are to address the underlying cause, halt progression, reduce pigmentation, and reduce ocular discomfort.

Acute and Chronic Treatment

Treatment will vary depending on the underlying cause.

Recommended Monitoring

Recheck at regular intervals (every 4-6 months or more frequently depending on the cause).

PROGNOSIS & OUTCOME

Prognosis and outcome vary, depending on the underlying cause.

PEARLS & CONSIDERATIONS

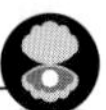

Comments

Ocular examination is an essential part of the routine physical examination because corneal pigmentation may go unnoticed by owners until it is so extensive it compromises vision.

Technician Tips

Digital photography aids in monitoring progression of lesions and response to therapy.

SUGGESTED READING

Morreale RJ: Corneal diagnostic procedures. Clin Tech Small Anim Pract 18:145-151, 2003.

AUTHOR: Lynne S. Sandmeyer, DVM, DVSc, DACVO
EDITOR: Diane V. H. Hendrix, DVM, DACVO

Corneal Sequestration, Cats

Client Education Sheet 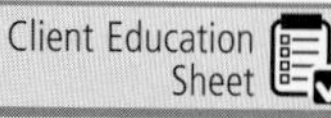

BASIC INFORMATION 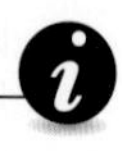

Definition

Corneal sequestration is a disease unique to cats, characterized by an area of necrotic cornea that is variably pigmented.

Synonyms

Corneal mummification, corneal necrosis, corneal sequestrum, corneal nigrum, necrotizing keratitis

Epidemiology

SPECIES, AGE, SEX

Cats of any age; average age of 5 years in retrospective studies

GENETICS, BREED PREDISPOSITION

All breeds, but Persian, Himalayan, and Burmese appear predisposed.

RISK FACTORS

- Feline herpesvirus type 1 (FHV-1 [p. 464]), particularly in domestic short hairs and long hairs
- Any corneal insult
- Brachycephalic cats are predisposed.
- Grid keratotomy performed for nonhealing/ indolent corneal ulcers in cats.

Clinical Presentation

HISTORY, CHIEF COMPLAINT

- Black spot on eye
- Blepharospasm
- Ocular discharge
- "Red eye"

PHYSICAL EXAM FINDINGS

- Circular to oval pigmented lesion in central to paracentral cornea is pathognomonic.
- Pigmentation varies from subtle tan discoloration of cornea to a dense, black, opaque lesion.
- Lesion may form a slightly raised, irregular corneal plaque.
- Corneal neovascularization or granulation tissue with chronicity
- Variable corneal edema and inflammation surrounding sequestrum
- A rim of loose, edematous corneal epithelium may develop around the sequestrum.
- Depth of corneal involvement (i.e., extent of lesion) is difficult to ascertain because sequestra are often opaque.

Etiology and Pathophysiology

- Associated fundamental problems are 1) pain, 2) obstruction of vision, and 3) cosmetic appearance.
- Chronic corneal irritation, such as that found with entropion and/or lagophthalmos (incomplete closure of the eyelids), is a common feature.
- FHV-1 ulceration is linked to sequestrum formation, particularly in nonbrachycephalic cats (p. 464).
- Tear film deficiencies (e.g., keratoconjunctivitis sicca, qualitative tear film abnormalities) have been reported in cats with sequestra.
- Source of pigment unknown; cats with sequestra may have pigmented tears. Contact lenses placed in cats with sequestra (see Acute General Treatment below) often become discolored.

DIAGNOSIS 

Diagnostic Overview

The diagnosis is based on physical appearance of the lesion.

Differential Diagnosis

Corneal rupture with iris prolapse (should have dyscoric/misshapen pupil and uveitis if this has occurred)

Initial Database

- Complete ophthalmic exam (p. 1137) to assess for underlying causes of corneal irritation
- Fluorescein dye application (sequestrum itself often does not retain fluorescein dye; there may be positive fluorescein dye retention around the sequestrum)

Advanced or Confirmatory Testing

- Consider testing for FHV-1 (p. 464) if there is a chronic history of ocular disease.
- Tear film break-up time (p. 1137)

TREATMENT 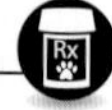

Treatment Overview

Treatment goals:

- Completely remove the sequestrum and prevent recurrence.
- Eliminate ocular pain.
- Minimize corneal scarring.

Acute General Treatment

- Prophylactic topical antibiotic therapy (ointment or solution formulation), such as oxytetracycline/polymyxin B, ciprofloxacin, or neomycin/polymyxin/gramicidin q 6-8h, particularly if fluorescein-positive
- If sequestrum appears small and superficial and eye is comfortable, observation is a treatment option:
  - Sequestrum may slough, resulting in minimal scarring; however, sequestra can take months to years to slough. Corneal rupture may occur if sequestrum is deep.
- If sequestrum is chronic, large, or eye is painful, keratectomy is indicated (sequestrum excision using a corneal dissector; generally a referable procedure)
  - No postoperative pigmented corneal tissue should remain; a contact lens may be placed for protection for 2 weeks.
  - Very deep sequestra may require conjunctival or frozen donor corneal grafting.

Chronic Treatment

Treat underlying contributing factors/causes, such as entropion or lagophthalmos (p. 296) and FHV-1 (p. 464).

Possible Complications

- Recurrence of the sequestrum after surgery
- If the sequestrum is allowed to slough, descemetocele formation or corneal rupture is possible (p. 209).

Recommended Monitoring

- If the lesion is not treated surgically, owners should monitor carefully for sequestrum sloughing, and return to the veterinarian immediately after the sequestrum sloughs

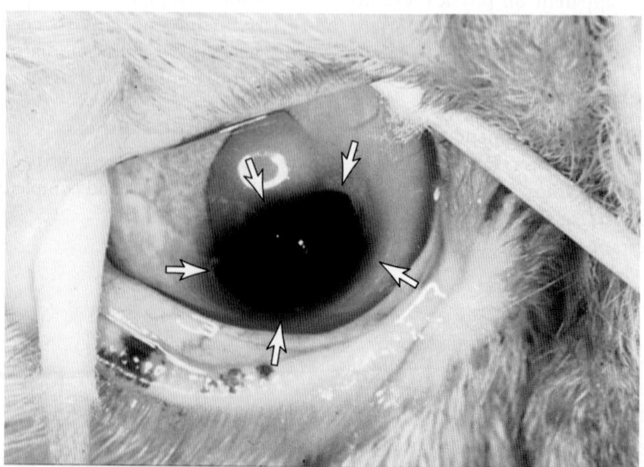

CORNEAL SEQUESTRATION Corneal sequestrum in a cat *(arrows)*. Note its dark appearance and paracentral location.

to avoid complications from deep corneal defects.

- At the time of sequestrum sloughing, initiation of prophylactic topical antibiotic treatment (see Acute General Treatment) is indicated, and referral for further evaluation (with or without surgical treatment) should be considered.
- Surgical treatment: usually several rechecks at 1- to 2-week intervals until defect is epithelialized

PROGNOSIS & OUTCOME

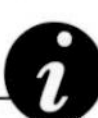

Good, but recurrence is possible

PEARLS & CONSIDERATIONS

Comments

Avoid topical corticosteroid use because this may induce herpetic stromal keratitis if FHV-1 is an underlying cause.

Technician Tips

Avoid pressure on globe when handling an affected cat after the sequestrum sloughs.

Client Education

Recurrence is possible, as is involvement of the contralateral eye.

SUGGESTED READING

Featherstone HM, et al: Feline corneal sequestra: a review of 64 cases (80 eyes) from 1993 to 2000. Vet Ophthalmol 7:213-227, 2004.

AUTHOR: Ellison Bentley, DVM, DACVO
EDITOR: Diane V. H. Hendrix, DVM, DACVO

Corneal Ulceration

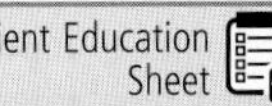

Client Education Sheet

BASIC INFORMATION

Definition

Loss of corneal epithelium with or without loss of varying amounts of the underlying corneal stroma. A common condition, there are three main categories:

- *Simple* corneal ulcer: an acute loss of epithelial layers of the cornea due to trauma; usually not infected
- *Complex* corneal ulcer: an acute or chronic loss of epithelial and/or stromal layers of the cornea due to trauma and/or infection
- *Indolent/refractory* corneal ulcer: a superficial ulcer resulting from failure of epithelial adhesion to the corneal basement membrane and stroma

Synonyms

Corneal abrasion/erosion, ulcerative keratitis, keratomalacia, spontaneous chronic corneal epithelial defects (SCCED)

Epidemiology

SPECIES, AGE, SEX

- Simple/complex ulcers: dogs and cats of any age or sex
- Indolent/refractory ulcers: middle-aged to older dogs

GENETICS, BREED PREDISPOSITION

- Simple/complex ulcers: any breed; brachycephalic breeds (dogs and cats) are predisposed
- Indolent/refractory ulcers: dogs: any breed; boxers are predisposed

RISK FACTORS

- Keratoconjunctivitis sicca (KCS [p. 568])
- Brachycephalic conformation
- Eyelid conformational abnormalities (pp. 273 and 296)
- Feline herpesvirus type 1 (FHV-1) (p. 464)

CONTAGION AND ZOONOSIS

FHV-1 keratoconjunctivitis is contagious among cats.

Clinical Presentation

DISEASE FORMS/SUBTYPES

Three main categories of corneal ulceration:

- Simple corneal ulcer
- Complex corneal ulcer
  - Stromal ulcer (loss of varying amounts of the corneal stroma)
  - Keratomalacia/melting ulcer (softening and necrosis of the cornea, often associated with infection)
  - Descemetocele (loss of all stromal layers down to Descemet's membrane [basement membrane of the corneal endothelium] and endothelium)
  - Ruptured ulcer/iris prolapse (perforation of the cornea)
- Indolent/refractory corneal ulcer

HISTORY, CHIEF COMPLAINT

- Variable onset, from acute to insidious/chronic
- ± History of trauma
- Ocular pain (squinting and/or rubbing at eye)
- Cloudiness to surface of eye
- "Red eye"
- Ocular discharge (watery, mucoid, or mucopurulent)
- Occasionally, upper respiratory signs in cats (p. 1006)

PHYSICAL EXAM FINDINGS

Simple and indolent corneal ulcers: any or all of the following may be present:

- Blepharospasm (squinting)
- Conjunctival hyperemia (enlarged vessels) ± swelling
- Third eyelid elevation
- Ocular discharge, often serous
- Corneal edema, usually focal
- Obvious defect in corneal epithelium
- Fluorescein dye retention in corneal stroma
- Miotic (small) pupil (reflex uveitis [p. 1023])
- Aqueous flare

Complex corneal ulcer: any or all of the above *and* one or more of the following:

- Mucopurulent ocular discharge
- Diffuse corneal edema
- Corneal blood vessels (p. 212); indicative of chronicity
- Corneal white-yellow cellular infiltrate (inflammatory cells ± microorganisms)
- Corneal stromal defect (i.e., crater appearance to affected cornea)
- Keratomalacia/melting (severe edema, a soft gelatinous ± bulging appearance to the affected stroma, and/or stromal loss)
- Hypopyon (p. 522)

Descemetocele: any or all of the above *and* the following:

- Fluorescein-negative clear center of a deep stromal ulcer (Descemet's membrane is hydrophobic and does not retain fluid or fluorescein stain)

Ruptured corneal ulcer: any or all of the above *and* one or more of the following:

- Copious ocular discharge with fibrin and/or blood (p. 511) in the anterior chamber
- Visible tan-brown-black iris prolapse (iris filling the corneal defect) and/or tan-yellow fibrin clot within ulcer
- Shallow anterior chamber
- Dyscoria (abnormal pupil shape)
- Visible anterior synechia (iris adhesion) to the ulcerated area

Indolent ulcer: any or all findings of a simple ulcer *and* the following:

- Rim of loose epithelium
- Halo of fainter fluorescein uptake around stained ulcer
- Minimal to moderate pain

- ± Corneal vascularization (slow to vascularize)
- Not infected

Etiology and Pathophysiology

- Trauma
- Ocular foreign body
- Tear film abnormalities
  - Keratoconjunctivitis sicca
  - Mucin and/or lipid deficiency (i.e., qualitative tear film deficiency)
- Eyelid conformational abnormalities
  - Entropion/ectropion
  - Distichiasis/ectopic cilia/trichiasis
  - Lagophthalmos (incomplete closure of the eyelids, usually in brachycephalics)
- Neurologic disorders (e.g., facial nerve paralysis [cranial nerve VII lesion]; corneal denervation [cranial nerve V lesion])
- FHV-1 infection
- Corneal sequestration: cats (p. 208)
- Simple corneal ulcers may progress to complex or ruptured corneal ulcers secondary to bacterial infection or sterile inflammation.
- Indolent ulcers result from a primary defect of corneal epithelial adhesion to the underlying corneal basement membrane and stroma.

DIAGNOSIS

Diagnostic Overview

- Corneal ulceration is suspected based on history, and the cornerstone of diagnosis is a complete ophthalmic examination, including tear testing and fluorescein staining and assessment of the cornea for edema, vessels, pigment, cellular infiltrate, fibrosis, and epithelial and stromal defects.
- Goals of the ophthalmic exam are to 1) confirm that an ulcer is present (versus healed defects), 2) determine if there is an underlying cause, 3) determine whether the ulcer is acute or chronic (consider history and presence/length of corneal vessels), 4) determine the depth of the ulcer (and risk of perforation), and 5) determine whether the ulcer may be infected (presence of cellular infiltrate, marked pain, uveitis, stromal loss).
- When infection is suspected, corneal culture and susceptibility and cytologic examination are indicated for appropriate antimicrobial therapy.

Differential Diagnosis

- Corneal facet (re-epithelialized stromal ulcer)
- Corneal dystrophy, degeneration or scarring
- Proliferative/eosinophilic keratoconjunctivitis (cats)
- Anterior uveitis
- Horner's syndrome

Initial Database

Neurologic (p. 1136) and ophthalmic (p. 1137) examinations:

- Cranial nerve examination: menace response, pupillary light reflexes, palpebral and corneal reflexes
- Corneal culture and sensitivity: ideally, sample obtained before Schirmer tear test (STT) and topical anesthesia
- STT: normal > 15 mm/min in dogs, variable in cats
- Fluorescein dye application: stains exposed stroma to confirm and demarcate ulcer
- Corneal cytologic evaluation: assess for evidence of infection, such as neutrophils, bacteria (gram-positive cocci, gram-negative rods), and/or fungal hyphae. Identification of microorganisms can direct initial choice of therapy.
- Intraocular pressure to rule out glaucoma (recommended for any form of red eye)

Advanced or Confirmatory Testing

- Keratectomy sample for corneal histopathologic evaluation
- Corneal swab and/or keratectomy sample for polymerase chain reaction (PCR) assay (FHV-1, bacterial, fungal)

TREATMENT

Treatment Overview

Goals of treatment:

- Treat any underlying cause
- Prevent progressive loss of corneal stroma and corneal rupture.
- Eliminate ocular pain.
- Prevent or eliminate corneal infection.
- Promote corneal epithelialization.
- Minimize corneal scarring.

Acute General Treatment

Simple corneal ulcer:

- Broad-spectrum topical antibiotic solution or ointment (e.g., triple antibiotic or oxytetracycline/Polymyxin B) q 6h
  - Gentamicin is a poor first choice because of its narrow spectrum for primarily gram-negative bacteria (ocular flora is primarily gram-positive bacteria).
- Topical atropine 1% ophthalmic solution or ointment q 12-48h
- ± Systemic nonsteroidal antiinflammatory drug (NSAID)

Complex corneal ulcer: any or all of the above *and* one or more of the following (treatment frequency decreases as improvement is seen):

- Anticollagenase therapy is indicated if keratomalacia/melting/stromal loss detected
  - Autogenous serum q 1-4h (prepared by obtaining a sample of a healthy dog's blood, coagulating and centrifuging and using the supernatant [serum] topically for its antiprotease, anticollagenase properties) *and/or*
  - Oxytetracycline/polymyxin B (Terramycin) ointment topically q 4-6h or oral doxycycline 10 mg/kg q 12-24h
- Topical fluoroquinolone antibiotic (e.g., ciprofloxacin, ofloxacin, or levofloxacin q 4-6h) for improved corneal penetration and spectrum of activity. Use at increased frequency (q 2h for 12-24h) for keratomalacia/melting/stromal ulcer. Alternatively, cefazolin 33 mg/mL in artificial tears *and* ophthalmic tobramycin can be used for broad-spectrum activity at same frequency as above.
- ± Topical antifungal agent q 4-6h (e.g., natamycin, voriconazole, miconazole) if fungal keratitis is implicated by corneal cytologic evaluation and/or culture (fungal keratitis is rare in cats and dogs)
- Hospitalization of animals with deep or rapidly progressive ulcers for frequent medical treatments and monitoring
- ± Structural surgical repair (i.e., keratectomy to remove the diseased cornea with placement of a graft: conjunctival, corneal); referral procedure is advisable if
  - Stromal loss continues despite aggressive appropriate medical management
  - Ulcer exceeds 50% stromal depth or is ruptured

Indolent/refractory ulcer:

- Application of topical ophthalmic anesthetic (e.g., proparacaine 0.5% solution) with or without sedation or general anesthesia (depending on the temperament of the dog)

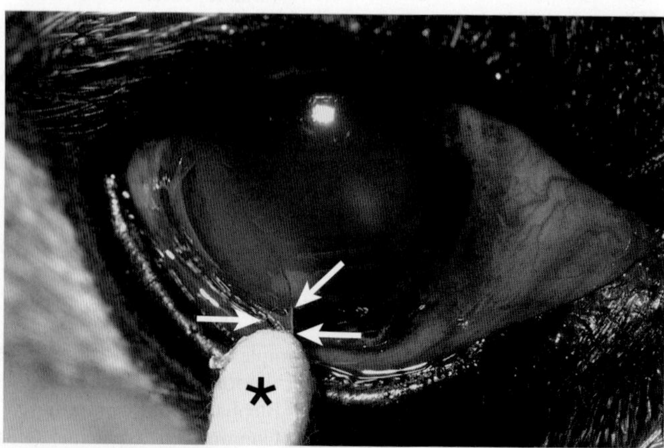

CORNEAL ULCERATION Debridement of an indolent corneal ulcer of the right eye in a dog. Note the lip of nonadherent corneal epithelium *(arrows)* attached to the sterile cotton-tipped applicator *(asterisk)*.

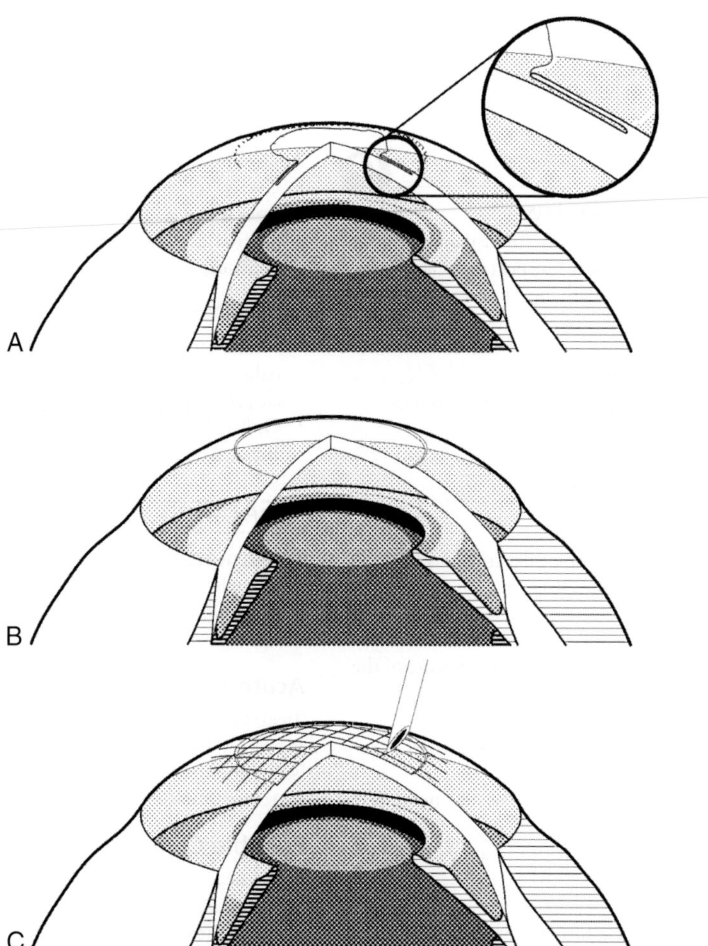

CORNEAL ULCERATION Grid keratotomy. **A,** Indolent ulcer with corneal epithelial flaps (at time of presentation). **B,** After topical anesthesia and debridement. **C,** Performing the grid keratotomy.

- Debridement of all loose corneal epithelium with dry, sterile, cotton-tipped applicators
- Perform one of the following procedures to promote epithelialization
  - Grid keratotomy with the beveled edge of a 25-gauge needle held at a 45-degree angle (or tangential) to the cornea
    - Gentle vertical and horizontal scratches every 0.5 mm over ulcerated area just into the normal epithelium and just through basement membrane into superficial stroma (grid lines should be barely visible)
    - Contraindicated in cats (may predispose to sequestrum formation)
  - Diamond burr (Algerbrush II) debridement of the ulcerated area
    - Use a fine or medium 2.5- or 3.5-mm round polishing bur.
    - Apply very slight pressure with rotating bur using even, circular movement across ulcer and normal epithelial margins.
- Oxytetracycline/polymyxin B (Terramycin) ointment (promotes corneal epithelialization) q 6-8h
- Atropine 1% ophthalmic solution or ointment q 24-72h
- ± Systemic NSAID (e.g., carprofen)
- ± Application of a bandage soft contact lens to improve comfort and minimize mechanical forces of eyelids on migrating corneal epithelium
- Placement of an Elizabethan collar to prevent dog from rubbing eye

Chronic Treatment

- Treat underlying cause if present.
- Adjust antimicrobial therapy as directed by culture and susceptibility results and/or lack of improvement.
- Change to a topical antibiotic with expanded-spectrum and/or improved corneal penetration (e.g., fluoroquinolone).
- FHV-1 ulcer: additional, specific antiviral treatments (p. 464); avoid topical neomycin in cats due to possible hypersensitivity. Erythromycin or oxytetracycline-polymyxin B (Terramycin) ointment is usually well tolerated.

Possible Complications

Corneal perforation, corneal scarring, corneal pigmentation, permanent corneal stromal defect (i.e., facet), corneal sequestration (cats), vision impairment/loss are possible.

Recommended Monitoring

- Evaluate for epithelialization (healing) or progressive loss of corneal stromal layers.
- Repeat corneal cytologic evaluation and/or culture to monitor response to antimicrobial therapy, especially if progressive stromal loss occurs despite current therapies.
- STT: repeat after ulcer is healed to rule out KCS as initiating cause.

PROGNOSIS & OUTCOME

- Simple: most heal with minimal scarring within 5-10 days with appropriate treatment.
- Indolent: most heal with minimal scarring within 2-3 weeks with appropriate treatment.
- Complex: healing may take 2-8 weeks, and substantial corneal scarring is expected.

PEARLS & CONSIDERATIONS

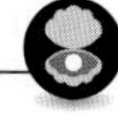

Comments

- Topical corticosteroids are contraindicated with ulceration; they delay healing and promote infection and keratomalacia/melting.
- Referral to a veterinary ophthalmologist is recommended if ulcer progresses despite appropriate medical management and/or if ulcer exceeds 50% stromal depth or is ruptured because surgical repair is usually required.
- Any simple corneal ulcer that does not heal in 5-10 days should be considered a complex or indolent/refractory ulcer, and underlying causes such as infection, foreign body, ectopic cilia, and distichia must be ruled out.

Prevention

Avoid or treat underlying cause(s).

Technician Tips

To prevent rupture or expulsion of aqueous humor due to increased intraocular pressure, avoid excessive restraint or jugular pressure in patients diagnosed with a descemetocele or corneal rupture.

Client Education

- Simple corneal ulcers may become complex; topical antibiotic treatment and regular follow-up to assess ulcer healing are crucial.
- Indolent corneal ulcers may recur in the same eye or occur in the opposite eye.
- The patient's eye is frequently more uncomfortable for 24-48 hours after epithelial debridement and multiple grid keratotomy or diamond burr debridement have been performed to treat an indolent corneal ulcer.

SUGGESTED READING

Maggs DJ: Cornea and sclera-corneal ulcers and erosions in all species. In Maggs DJ, et al, editors: Slatter's Fundamentals of veterinary ophthalmology, ed 5, St. Louis, 2013, Saunders, pp 195-211.

AUTHOR: Anne J. Gemensky-Metzler, DVM, MS, DACVO
EDITOR: Diane V. H. Hendrix, DVM, DACVO

Corneal Vascularization

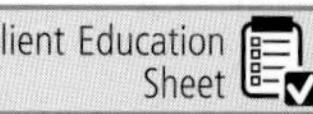

BASIC INFORMATION

Definition
The presence of blood vessels in the cornea

Synonyms
Corneal neovascularization, vascularized keratitis

Epidemiology
SPECIES, AGE, SEX

Varies, depending on underlying cause

ASSOCIATED DISORDERS

Corneal ulceration, irritation, desiccation, uveitis, glaucoma, pannus (chronic superficial keratitis), keratoconjunctivitis: eosinophilic, cats, episcleritis, or scleritis

Clinical Presentation
HISTORY, CHIEF COMPLAINT

Some or all may be present:
- History
  - Ocular trauma
  - Chronic ophthalmic disorder (e.g., keratoconjunctivitis sicca [KCS], indolent corneal ulcer, pannus, eosinophilic keratoconjunctivitis in cats)
- Chief complaint
  - Reddish discoloration of the eye
  - Signs of ocular pain (e.g., blepharospasm, rubbing eye, temperament change)

PHYSICAL EXAM FINDINGS
- Focal to diffuse red discoloration of the superficial or deep cornea
- New corneal vessels enter stroma at the limbus:
  - May give the affected cornea a reddish haze
  - Vessels are leaky and cause surrounding corneal edema (bluish haze).
- Other findings vary, depending on the cause.

Etiology and Pathophysiology
Blood vessel ingrowth occurs:
- As a response to injury of the corneal epithelium or stroma as a normal component of healing
  - Neutrophils, which enter the cornea from the tear film and the limbus, are important sources for angioblast and fibroblast growth factors.
  - There is a 7-10 day delay before the ingrowth of corneal blood vessels at the limbus is easily visible.
  - Ingrowth then occurs at a rate of approximately 1 mm/day.
- As part of an ocular immune-mediated inflammatory response
- Secondary to disease of adjacent ocular tissues, including uveitis, episcleritis, scleritis, and glaucoma and others

DIAGNOSIS

Diagnostic Overview
Diagnosis is made on careful visual inspection of the corneal surface. Important features for pinpointing the underlying cause and treatment approach include the location and pattern of vascularization, and evaluation for other concurrent ocular disease.

Differential Diagnosis
Corneal injury or inflammation:
- Corneal ulceration (p. 209)
- Chemical irritation
- Mechanical irritation
  - Distichiasis/ectopic cilia/trichiasis (p. 273)
  - Entropion (p. 296)
- Exposure
  - Large palpebral fissure
  - Lagophthalmos (incomplete closure of the eyelids)
  - Ectropion
  - Buphthalmos (chronic glaucoma)
  - Exophthalmos
- Neuroparalytic keratitis (cranial nerve VII lesion)
- Neurotrophic keratitis (cranial nerve V lesion)
- KCS (p. 568)
- Qualitative tear film abnormalities
- Pannus (dogs) (p. 748)
- Eosinophilic keratoconjunctivitis in cats
- Corneal degeneration (corneal lipid infiltrates [p. 205])

Adjacent ocular disease:
- Uveitis (p. 1023)
- Episcleritis/scleritis (p. 304)
- Orbital disease (p. 716)
- Glaucoma (p. 387)

Initial Database
- Neuro-ophthalmic exam (p. 1136): evaluate palpebral reflexes and completeness of eyelid closure
- Ophthalmic exam (p. 1137): evaluate for abnormalities mentioned above

TREATMENT

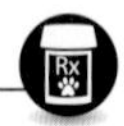

Treatment Overview
The goals of treatment are to address the underlying cause, halt progression, and reduce ocular discomfort.

Acute and Chronic Treatment
Treatment will vary depending on the underlying cause. Treatment of the vascularization itself is rarely indicated. After the underlying cause is treated, the vessels will recede.

Possible Complications
- Corneal vascularization may precede pigmentation and scarring.
- Vascularization is often part of normal healing and, in general, should not be suppressed.
- Intracorneal stromal hemorrhage is uncommon; however, risk of this increases with certain ocular and systemic diseases.

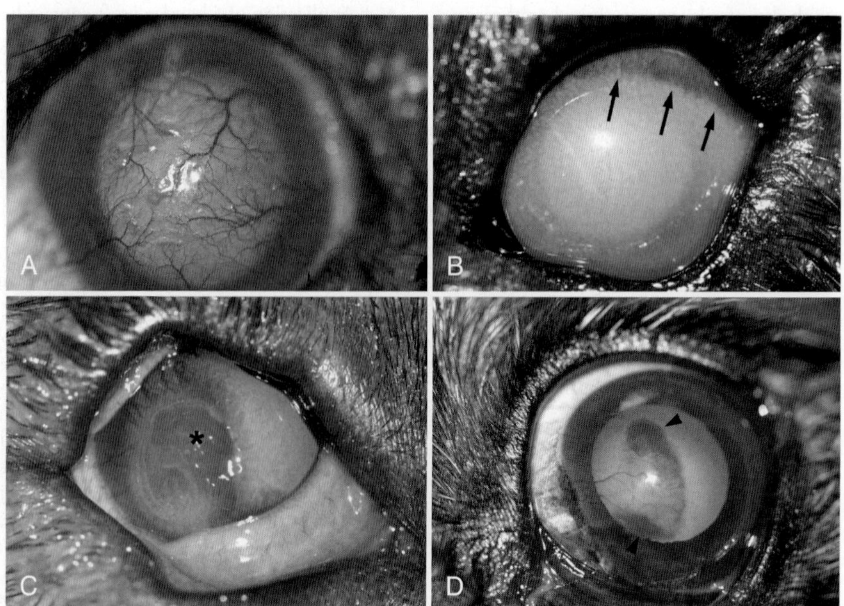

CORNEAL VASCULARIZATION A, Superficial vascularization secondary to keratoconjunctivitis sicca (note branching blood vessels). **B,** Deep vascularization secondary to uveitis (note the straight brush-border appearance of deep vessels). **C,** Vascularization and raised granulation tissue *(star)* due to chronic irritation caused by entropion. **D,** Superficial vascularization with intracorneal stromal hemorrhage *(arrowheads)*.

PROGNOSIS & OUTCOME

- Prognosis and outcome vary, depending on the underlying cause.
- In corneal injury, corneal vascularization denotes progression toward healing and is therefore a positive sign, provided the underlying problem can be controlled or eliminated.

PEARLS & CONSIDERATIONS

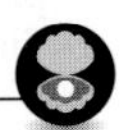

Comments

It may be useful to distinguish between superficial and deep vascularization:

- Superficial vascularization occurs in response to superficial corneal or external ocular disease.
  - Superficial blood vessels arise from the conjunctiva, cross the limbus, are bright red, and branch frequently.
- Deep vascularization occurs in response to deep corneal or intraocular disease.
  - Deep blood vessels arise from the ciliary circulation, disappear at the limbus, and appear darker red and straight.

Technician Tips

Digital photography is a simple but useful tool for monitoring progression and response to therapy.

SUGGESTED READING

Violette NP, et al: Intracorneal stromal hemorrhage in dogs and its associations with ocular and systemic disease: 39 cases. Vet Ophthalmol 20:27-33, 2017.

AUTHOR: Lynne S. Sandmeyer, DVM, DVSc, DACVO
EDITOR: Diane V. H. Hendrix, DVM, DACVO

Corneal/Scleral Trauma

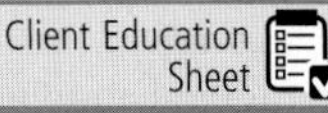

BASIC INFORMATION

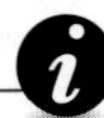

Definition

Ocular injury secondary to blunt or sharp trauma. *Penetrating* infers partial-thickness injury; *perforating* infers full-thickness injury. *Simple* wounds involve only the cornea or sclera; *complicated* wounds involve multiple ocular structures.

Epidemiology

SPECIES, AGE, SEX

Dogs more frequently than cats, but any breed, either sex

RISK FACTORS

- Young, active animals
- Hunting animals
- Interanimal fighting
- Dog's head out the window while car is in motion
- Existing visual impairment may predispose

Clinical Presentation

HISTORY, CHIEF COMPLAINT

- Owner may or may not observe trauma or causal event.
- Dog might have run through dense or dry vegetation just before onset of clinical signs.
- Acute onset of any or all of the following:
  - Blepharospasm
  - Ocular discharge
  - Blood or fluid coming from eye
  - Swelling around the eye (e.g., eyelids; conjunctiva)
  - Cloudy eye

PHYSICAL EXAM FINDINGS

- Signs of pain on ophthalmic exam (p. 1137) manifested by blepharospasm and resistance to exam
- Linear, V-shaped, or stellate corneal lesion of acute onset accompanied by any or all of the following:
  - Hyphema and/or subconjunctival hemorrhage
  - Corneal edema with or without cellular infiltrate
    - Uveal prolapse: appears as pigmented structure in damaged cornea or sclera; associated with dyscoria (misshapen pupil) and/or fibrin and hyphema
  - Foreign body embedded in cornea or perforating cornea
  - Signs of uveitis, particularly with perforating trauma (p. 1023)
  - Fibrin, light tan to yellow, in cornea may fill perforation; may be associated with blood
  - Yellowish/whitish lens material in anterior chamber and cataract if lens is damaged
  - Shallow anterior chamber if wound actively leaking
- Thorough exam of the entire conjunctival sac is necessary to identify any retained foreign material. Sedation, general anesthesia, or referral may be required in difficult cases or if this procedure is unfamiliar to the practitioner.
- Subconjunctival hemorrhage and hyphema should alert clinician to possibility of posterior scleral rupture if no anterior segment lesions are present, particularly if accompanied by very low intraocular pressure (<10 mm Hg).

Etiology and Pathophysiology

- Variable; usually traumatic (sharp or blunt) in origin
- Foreign body may be retained in laceration.

DIAGNOSIS

Diagnostic Overview

History and exam suggest the diagnosis; an ophthalmic exam helps define whether the cornea and/or sclera has/have been damaged. If so, the exam should also determine whether the lesion is partial or full thickness (affects prognosis).

Differential Diagnosis

If traumatic event not witnessed, consider other causes:

- Corneal ulceration
- Uveitis
- Hyphema

Initial Database

- Assess vision: menace response, dazzle reflex, direct and consensual pupillary light reflexes (p. 1137)
- Cytologic evaluation and aerobic culture and sensitivity of wound
- CBC, serum biochemistry profile, urinalysis for preanesthetic purposes if surgery necessary

Advanced or Confirmatory Testing

- Consider ocular ultrasound exam to determine extent of intraocular involvement, presence of intraocular foreign body, or posterior globe rupture.
- Orbital radiographs or CT to determine presence or path of foreign body if suspected
- Seidel test to determine if cornea or scleral wound is sealed: apply dry fluorescein strip carefully to surface of wound to cover surface with stain; leaking aqueous appears as a green rivulet.

TREATMENT

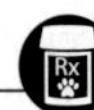

Treatment Overview

Goals of treatment:

- Remove foreign bodies if present.
- Repair lacerations that penetrate > 50% of the thickness of the corneal stroma or perforate the cornea or sclera.
- Eliminate infection.
- Control intraocular inflammation.

Acute General Treatment

- Do not put pressure on the globe until the possibility of rupture is eliminated.
- Elizabethan collar to prevent self-trauma
- For small, nonperforating or very small, sealed perforating wounds without uveal prolapse, consider conservative therapy.
  - Topical antibiotic solution (e.g., neomycin/polymyxin/gramicidin, gentamicin or tobramycin and cefazolin, or ciprofloxacin) q 6h
  - Add broad-spectrum systemic antibiotics if perforating (e.g., amoxicillin-clavulanate 13.75 mg/kg PO q 12h; base long-term choice on culture and sensitivity).
  - Systemic antiinflammatory therapy with nonsteroidal antiinflammatories (e.g., carprofen 2 mg/kg PO q 12h or meloxicam 0.1 mg/kg PO q 24h) or antiinflammatory doses of prednisone (e.g., 0.5-1 mg/kg PO q 24h)
  - Topical atropine 1% solution q 6-24h if significant uveitis (p. 1023)
- Perforating or deep, large, or gaping penetrating wounds and wounds with uveal prolapse require primary surgical repair (referable procedure) involving
  - Replacement of viable uveal tissue or resection of nonviable uveal tissue
  - Irrigation and reinflation of anterior chamber
  - Repair of cornea with appropriate-size suture material (8-0 to 10-0)
  - Careful inspection of lens; if lens rupture is noted, lens may need to be removed by phacoemulsification

Chronic Treatment

- Monitor and treat for uveitis and wound dehiscence.
- Consider changing antibiotics if indicated by culture and sensitivity results.

Drug Interactions

Do not use topical ophthalmic ointments if globe rupture is suspected.

Possible Complications

- Retinal detachment
- Cataracts
- Chronic uveitis
- Glaucoma
- Endophthalmitis (inflammation of the uveal tract and anterior and posterior compartments of the eye with or without infection)
- Loss of vision and eye
- Cats may develop posttraumatic ocular sarcomas years after the original injury, particularly if lens involved.

Recommended Monitoring

- Re-evaluate in 24-48 hours to ensure wounds are sealed, inflammation is improving, and there are no signs of infection.
- Frequency of exam depends on response to therapy.

PROGNOSIS & OUTCOME

- Intuitively, small, shallow penetrating wounds of the cornea or lacerations involving only the cornea have a good prognosis, whereas complicated, perforating wounds with uveal and/or lens involvement have a poorer prognosis for vision.
- Wounds involving sclera or sclera and uvea have a grave prognosis for vision.
- Blunt trauma usually has a grave prognosis for vision, particularly if extensive hyphema is present.
- Negative menace response and negative dazzle and pupillary light reflexes at initial exam of a patient with corneal or scleral trauma indicate grave prognosis for vision.

PEARLS & CONSIDERATIONS

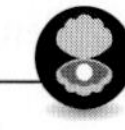

Comments

- Consider sedation to keep patient calm and prevent self-trauma.
- Elizabethan collar to prevent self-trauma

Prevention

- Animals should be monitored when introduced to new environment with other animals.
- Dogs should not be allowed to ride in cars with head out of window.

Technician Tips

Avoid pressure on neck and eye when handling affected animal.

Client Education

Discuss the possibility of long-term complications that could lead to loss of vision and loss of an eye.

SUGGESTED READING

Miller PE: Ocular emergencies. In Maggs DJ, et al, editors: Slatter's Fundamentals of veterinary ophthalmology, ed 4, Philadelphia, 2008, Saunders, p 419.

AUTHOR: Ellison Bentley, DVM, DACVO
EDITOR: Diane V. H. Hendrix, DVM, DACVO

Cornification Disorders

Bonus Material Online

Client Education Sheet

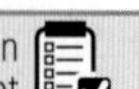

BASIC INFORMATION

Definition

A well-recognized class of scaling or greasy skin disorders resulting from primary (usually hereditary) or secondary (acquired) defects in epidermal maturation, desquamation, or sebum production

Synonyms

- Keratinization defects/disorders
- Keratoseborrheic disorders
- Many disorders were formerly grouped under the heading *seborrhea*, but this term was nonspecific and inaccurate and is now obsolete.

Epidemiology

SPECIES, AGE, SEX

- Primary (hereditary) causes: early in life for many conditions; diagnosed by ruling out secondary disorders
- Secondary (acquired): any age; usually adult animals (majority of cases)

GENETICS, BREED PREDISPOSITION

- Primary idiopathic seborrhea: cocker spaniel, West Highland white terrier, basset hound, Shar-pei, dachshund, Doberman pinscher, English springer spaniel, German shepherd, Irish setter, Labrador retriever
- Primary hereditary seborrhea oleosa: Persian, Himalayan, and exotic short-haired cats
- Vitamin A–responsive dermatosis: cocker spaniel, Labrador retriever, miniature schnauzer, Gordon setters
- Zinc-responsive dermatosis: Alaskan Malamute, Siberian Husky, Samoyed, Pharaoh hounds
- Lethal acrodermatitis: bull terrier
- Sebaceous adenitis (p. 901): standard poodle, Akita, others
- Ichthyosis: golden retriever, American bulldog, Jack Russell terrier, Norfolk terrier (autosomal recessive)

CONTAGION AND ZOONOSIS

Most are not contagious, but parasitic and fungal causes have contagious and zoonotic potential.

GEOGRAPHY AND SEASONALITY

Scaling (formerly called seborrhea sicca) is more common in the winter (low environmental humidity).

ASSOCIATED DISORDERS

Primary cornification disorders may be associated with ceruminous otitis externa.

Clinical Presentation

DISEASE FORMS/SUBTYPES

- Primary cornification disorders (usually hereditary and incurable) or secondary (acquired, usually curable)
- Generalized or localized

HISTORY, CHIEF COMPLAINT

Owners generally present pets for evaluation of an unpleasant-appearing, usually scaly or waxy haircoat or coat with a foul, rancid odor.

PHYSICAL EXAM FINDINGS

- Primary cornification disorders: various degrees of alopecia and dry scale that may be focal, multifocal, or generalized over the trunk. Animals may present with large hyperkeratotic patches of adherent scale. Follicular casts (waxy debris surrounding hair shafts), fronds (clumps of hairs stuck together like a paintbrush), or severe dandruff with large flakes may be noted.
- Localized cornification disorders
  - Nasal parakeratosis of the Labrador retriever: restricted to the nasal planum
  - Nasodigital hyperkeratosis: restricted to nasal planum and digital pads
  - Ear margin dermatosis: alopecia and scaling of distal pinnal margins, possibly associated with fissures
  - Feline acne: comedones on the chin +/− lips; papules, pustules, erosion, crust, and pruritus if secondarily infected
  - Tail gland hyperplasia
- Secondary cornification disorders: general physical findings depend on underlying cause. Cutaneous findings include a dull (or waxy) coat with various combinations of alopecia, scaling, crusting, collarettes, and excoriations secondary to self-trauma and pyoderma.

Etiology and Pathophysiology

- Cornification encompasses all the processes that lead to the formation of the stratum corneum. This includes keratinization and formation of the lipid-rich intercellular domain that binds corneocytes to maintain a relatively impermeable barrier.
- Disorders of cornification are due to a defective cornification process or excessive proliferation and/or defective desquamation (retention hyperkeratosis). Any alteration in epidermal turnover times, maturation processes, and/or desquamation or trans-epidermal water loss lead to scaling.
- Other considerations include abnormal apocrine or sebaceous glandular secretions (in volume or quality).

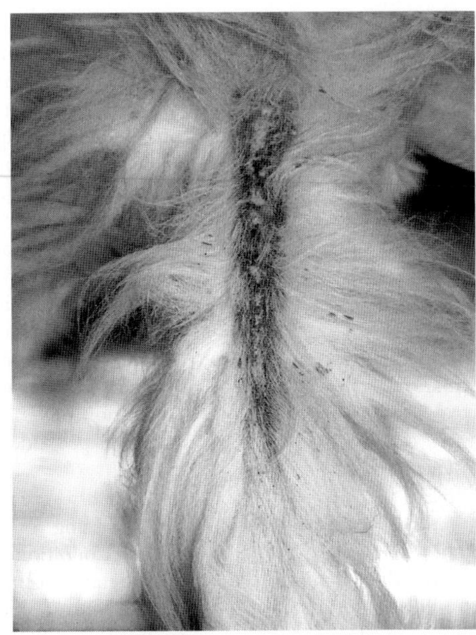

CORNIFICATION DISORDERS Stud tail in a Persian cat. (Copyright Dr. Manon Paradis.)

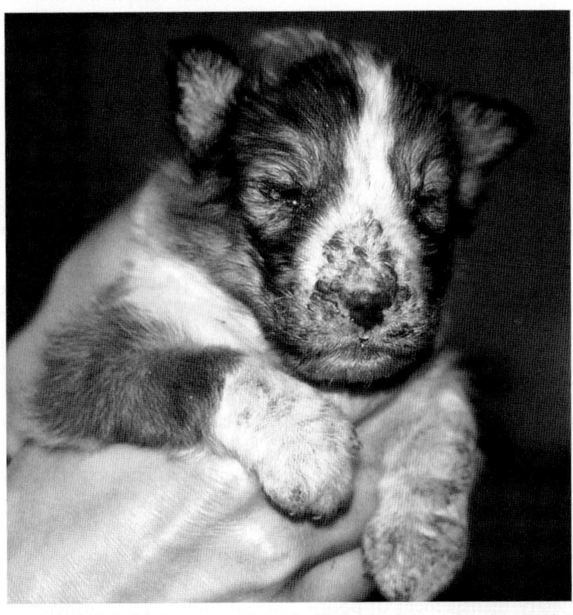

CORNIFICATION DISORDERS Ichthyosis in a 5-week-old Shetland sheepdog. (Copyright Dr. Manon Paradis.)

DIAGNOSIS

Diagnostic Overview

Scale formation is a common response of the skin to any insult. It is critical to evaluate the patient for underlying causes—particularly the roles parasitic and microbial dermatitis may be playing if any—before pursuing other causes.

Differential Diagnosis

Secondary cornification disorders; underlying causes include

- Microbial: pyoderma, *Malassezia*, dermatophytosis, leishmaniasis
- Parasitic: flea infestation, cheyletiellosis, sarcoptic mange, pediculosis, and demodicosis (including *Demodex injai*, the long-bodied *Demodex* mite that has been associated with a greasy seborrheic dermatosis, especially in adult terriers)
- Endocrinopathy: hypothyroidism, hyperadrenocorticism, hyperestrogenism (e.g., Sertoli cell tumor)
- Allergic: environmental, dermatologic adverse food reaction (food allergy)
- Management deficiencies: low environmental humidity, inappropriate topical therapy or frequency, nutritionally inadequate diet (especially if high in phytates and fiber, low in fatty acids)
- Metabolic disease (especially liver disease)

- Immune-mediated disease: pemphigus foliaceus, systemic or cutaneous lupus erythematosus, adverse drug reaction
- Neoplasia: cutaneous epitheliotropic lymphoma, exfoliative dermatitis associated with thymoma in cats

Primary cornification disorders: usually genetically determined; may be multifocal and generalized or localized:

- Multifocal and generalized
  - Idiopathic primary seborrhea (dogs)
  - Hereditary seborrhea oleosa (cats)
  - Vitamin A–responsive dermatosis
  - Zinc-responsive dermatosis
  - Sebaceous adenitis
  - Epidermal dysplasia
  - Schnauzer comedo syndrome
  - Sebaceous gland dysplasia
  - Canine ichthyosis
- Localized
  - Nasal parakeratosis of the Labrador retriever (autosomal recessive)
  - Footpad hyperkeratosis in dogues de Bordeaux and Irish terrier
  - Feline acne
  - Stud tail
  - Ear margin dermatosis

Initial Database

- Comprehensive evaluation for ectoparasites (skin scrapings, flea combing, acetate tape preparations, fecal evaluation, ectoparasiticide response trial)
- Skin cytologic examination (to rule out bacterial and yeast involvement) (p. 1091)
- Fungal culture (dermatophytosis)
- CBC, serum biochemical profile, urinalysis (as appropriate, to look for evidence of underlying disease)

Advanced or Confirmatory Testing

- Skin biopsy: useful for many disorders after infectious and parasitic causes have been ruled out
- Elimination diet trial to rule out food allergy (if pruritic)
- Intradermal and serum allergy testing for atopic dermatitis (if pruritic)
- Response to dietary management (if poor-quality diet)
- Thyroid function testing
- Adrenal function testing
- Genetic tests available for carriers of American bulldog ichthyosis and golden retriever ichthyosis

TREATMENT

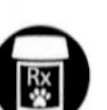

Treatment Overview

The goal of treatment is to address the underlying cause specifically if possible. In primary conditions, it is important to control secondary microbial dermatitis while controlling the amount of scale produced.

Acute General Treatment

- Systemic and/or topical antimicrobial treatment as needed (pp. 247, 614, and 851)
- Essential fatty acid (EFA) oral supplementation (omega-3 and omega-6); rarely provides complete control of scaling but may be beneficial as adjunctive therapy
- Topical therapy: clipping of haircoat may benefit topical therapy
  - Topical veterinary antiseborrheic products, including those containing phytosphingosine, essential oils, or a ceramide-fatty acid spot-on, may be of benefit.
  - Greasy, scaly skin in dogs can be degreased using products containing benzoyl peroxide, or selenium sulfide (not in cats). These products should be followed with a conditioner. NOTE: Shampoos containing benzoyl peroxide are drying and bleach fabric.
  - Mild, dry scaling may respond to moisturizing or hypoallergenic shampoos. Conditioners containing lipids or humectants (agents that help the skin to retain moisture) are beneficial.

Chronic Treatment

Generalized disease:

- Primary idiopathic seborrhea: topical therapy as already described; EFA supplementation; antibiotics administered as already described. Consider retinoids: acitretin (Soriatane) 0.5-1 mg/kg PO q 24h or cyclosporine 5 mg/kg PO q 24h.
- Vitamin A–responsive dermatosis: topical therapy and antibiotics as already described; vitamin A 625-800 IU/kg PO q 24h; usually 10,000 IU PO q 24h, lifelong, for the average cocker spaniel. Dosages up to 1200 IU/kg PO q 24h are reported to be safe. Improvement is noted by 3-8 weeks.
- Zinc-responsive dermatosis: zinc supplementation is recommended at 2-3 mg/kg elemental zinc PO q 24h.
- Sebaceous gland dysplasia: antiseborrheic shampoos followed by conditioners, fatty acid supplementation, vitamin A, and 50% propylene glycol spray may aid in control.
- Schnauzer comedo syndrome: benzoyl peroxide shampoos help the condition by follicular flushing. Systemic or topical antimicrobial treatments to control bacterial folliculitis. In some cases, retinoids such as isotretinoin (Accutane) 1 mg/kg PO q 24h or divided q 12h may be helpful but can be costly. Wean to alternate-day therapy after 4 weeks if a favorable response is noted.
- Canine ichthyosis: antiseborrheic shampoos and a topical spray conditioner containing propylene glycol and humectants can be useful. Try isotretinoin (Accutane 1-3 mg/kg PO q 24h for 8-12 weeks, decreasing to alternate-day therapy if effective) in more severe cases.
- Sebaceous adenitis (p. 901)

Localized disease:

- Feline acne (p. 15)
- Ear margin dermatosis: local use of an antiseborrheic shampoo q 24-48h. If inflammation is moderate, topical glucocorticoid such as 0.5%-1% hydrocortisone may reduce inflammation. In severe cases, a more potent topical glucocorticoid or a short course of oral prednisone 1 mg/kg PO q 24h may be indicated.
- Nasal and digital hyperkeratosis: moisturize affected area with water or wet dressings, and then apply petrolatum jelly. More severely affected animals may benefit from topical application of an ointment containing salicylic acid and urea, or 50%-75% propylene glycol, or 0.025% or 0.01% tretinoin gel (Retin-A).

Drug Interactions

Cyclosporine: concurrent use of cyclosporine with other permeability (P)-glycoprotein inhibitors or substrates can increase blood cyclosporine levels. This may be beneficial (e.g., lowers the dose of cyclosporine required by one-half when administered with ketoconazole) but can also increase the potential for toxicosis.

Possible Complications

- High fatty acid treatment may increase the potential for gastrointestinal (GI) disturbance or pancreatitis.
- Retinoids: keratoconjunctivitis sicca, conjunctivitis, pruritus, hyperactivity, stiffness, mucocutaneous junction erythema, vomiting, diarrhea, teratogenicity, elevated liver enzymes
- Cyclosporine: diarrhea, vomiting, anorexia, gingival hyperplasia, gingivitis, papillomatosis, renal effects, monitor animals for tumors

Recommended Monitoring

- Vitamin A, retinoids: monitor liver enzymes and tear production.
- Cyclosporine: physical examination (tumor, infection, gingival hyperplasia), urea, creatinine, urinalysis, and liver enzymes; blood pressure. Check trough serum cyclosporine levels if adverse reactions are noted or there is a poor clinical response (p. 1333).

PROGNOSIS & OUTCOME

Primary causes often require lifelong therapy; secondary syndromes usually recover with correction or control of underlying cause.

PEARLS & CONSIDERATIONS

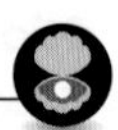

Comments

- Control secondary microbial dermatitis, and evaluate thoroughly for other underlying secondary causes before diagnosing a primary seborrheic syndrome.
- The term *seborrhea* as a diagnosis should be limited to the breed-specific diseases (e.g., idiopathic primary seborrhea of cocker spaniel, primary hereditary seborrhea oleosa of Persian cats). Use other descriptive terms such as *scaling, exfoliation, crusting, greasiness, malodor* to characterize skin changes rather than the nonspecific term *seborrhea*.
- Many dermatologists doubt that idiopathic primary seborrhea is a true entity in dogs.

Prevention

Animals affected with primary (genetically determined) cornification disorders should not be used for breeding.

Technician Tips

Regarding baths:

- Most medicated dog shampoos do not lather well.
- Contact time is important (should be left on the dog for at least 5 minutes before rinsing).
- Use enough shampoo to cover the dog without overdoing it.

Client Education

Explain the concept of control versus cure.

SUGGESTED READING

Miller WH Jr, et al: Muller & Kirk's Small animal dermatology, ed 7, St. Louis, 2013, Saunders, pp 630-646.

AUTHOR: Stephen Waisglass, DVM, CertSAD, DACVD
EDITOR: Manon Paradis, DMV, MVSc, DACVD

Cough

Client Education Sheet

BASIC INFORMATION

Definition

Respiratory protective mechanism characterized by inhalation followed by forceful expulsion of air from the lungs and airways against a closed glottis. Cough is distinct from a throat clear/expiration reflex, in which inhalation is absent.

Epidemiology

SPECIES, AGE, SEX

All animals cough; predispositions exist for some of the disorders that cause excessive cough.

RISK FACTORS

May be precipitated by factors related to underlying disease process:

- Infection: exposure to bacterial, viral, fungal, protozoal, or parasitic pathogens
- Irritant/allergen exposure: asthma, chronic bronchitis
- Aspiration pneumonia: dysphagia, regurgitation, vomiting, recent anesthesia
- Impaired respiratory protective mechanisms: ciliary dyskinesia, bronchiectasis, laryngeal paralysis
- Degenerative processes: collapsing trachea, bronchomalacia
- Heart disease: left-sided congestive heart failure (CHF), compression of bronchi by enlarged atria

CONTAGION AND ZOONOSIS

Pathogens of tracheobronchitis (pp. 271, 545, and 987) are highly contagious; rarely, *Bordetella bronchiseptica* infects immunosuppressed people.

GEOGRAPHY AND SEASONALITY

Infectious agents, including parasites (e.g., *Dirofilaria immitis*) and fungal organisms (e.g., *Histoplasma capsulatum, Blastomyces dermatitidis, Coccidioides immitis*) endemic to certain areas

Clinical Presentation

DISEASE FORMS/SUBTYPES

Cough is a nonspecific respiratory protective mechanism, but when excessive, it serves as a marker of disease. Coughing may or may not be accompanied by respiratory distress (p. 879).

HISTORY, CHIEF COMPLAINT

Owner description of cough is subjective. For example, cough in cats is frequently mistaken for vomiting or hairballs.

- Duration: time course varies with underlying cause (e.g., infectious tracheobronchitis [acute], chronic bronchitis [chronic])
  - Acute ≤ 3 weeks
  - Subacute 3-8 weeks
  - Chronic ≥ 8 weeks
- Character
  - Productive versus nonproductive/wet versus dry: considerable overlap and does not routinely provide discriminating information
  - Harsh versus soft: harsh cough tends to be associated with airway disorders, and soft cough is often associated with parenchymal lung disease, although overlap occurs
  - Hemoptysis: infectious/inflammatory, trauma, neoplasia, foreign bodies, coagulopathic, and thromboembolic disorders; warrants prompt investigation
  - Repetitive swallow/changes in appetite: suggest reflux or postnasal drip
  - Honking character typical of collapsing trachea but not specific
- Exposure history
  - Indoor: cigarette smoke, molds, wood burning stoves, deodorants, cleaners, and aerosols
  - Outdoor: boarding kennels, grooming facilities, dog parks, and general exposure to other animals

PHYSICAL EXAM FINDINGS

- Changes in respiratory effort, if present, may be helpful in localizing disease (p. 879).
- Concurrent nasal and ocular discharge suggests an infectious process; use biosecurity precautions (p. 987).
- Inducible cough on tracheal palpation does not definitively localize disease to the large airways. (e.g., cough may be induced in patients with pulmonary parenchymal disease and in clinically normal patients)
- Tracheal/laryngeal auscultation
  - Can help differentiate referred upper airway noises from lower airway or pulmonary sounds on thoracic auscultation
  - Stridor, stertor, tracheal snap/click may be appreciated in animals with laryngeal paralysis, nasopharyngeal disease, or collapsing trachea, respectively.
- Pulmonary auscultation
  - Crackles (often inspiratory) suggest edema, pneumonia, contusions, or fibrosis.
  - Crackles often heard best immediately after a cough (post-tussive crackle).
  - Wheezes (often expiratory) suggest airway narrowing (e.g., bronchoconstriction, exudate).
  - Dull lung sounds may be noted with an intrathoracic mass effect.
  - Muffled heart and lung sounds suggest pleural space disease.
- Cardiac auscultation
  - Tachycardia is more typical of heart disease while sinus arrhythmia more typical of lung/thoracic disease
  - Cardiac causes of cough are very unlikely in dogs with neither a murmur nor arrhythmia
  - Cats with CHF may or may not have a heart murmur.
  - Characteristics of a heart murmur may suggest a type of heart disease (p. 414).
  - Murmurs may be coincidental and not related to the cause of cough.
- Complete physical exam can provide clues. For example, cachexia is often due to neoplasia, CHF, or chronic infection (e.g., fungal pneumonia).

Etiology and Pathophysiology

- See Cough, Section 3 (p. 1209).
- Cough is a somatosensory reflex arc involving visceral sensation triggered by receptors in the mucosa of the pharynx, trachea, and large airways, followed by a reflex motor response intended to expel secretions or material from the airways.
- Most often, coughing is associated with disorders of the airways, lungs, or heart. Less commonly, pleural disease, gastroesophageal reflux, or drugs cause coughing.

- Cough is a marker of disease control in the case of chronic inflammatory disease (e.g., asthma).
- Cough may result in progressive disease through the perpetuation of inflammation (e.g., collapsing trachea).

DIAGNOSIS

Diagnostic Overview

Signalment, history, and physical examination are often adequate to formulate a likely differential diagnosis list and guide further tests, but thoracic radiographs are almost always indicated.

Differential Diagnosis

See Cough, Section 3 (p. 1209).

Initial Database

- Thoracic radiographs: a minimum of three-view thoracic radiographs obtained on inspiration is standard (p. 1155)
  - If collapsing trachea suspected, include cervical trachea, and obtain inspiratory and expiratory imaging.
  - Assess size of cardiac silhouette, pulmonary vasculature
  - Assess airway diameter, deviation, or compression
  - Assess pulmonary parenchymal pattern (e.g., alveolar, unstructured or nodular interstitial)
  - Assess pleural space (e.g., effusion, pneumothorax, diaphragmatic hernia)
- Heartworm testing (pp. 415 and 418)
- Retroviral testing (cats)
- Fecal sedimentation (Baermann) or flotation for respiratory parasites
- CBC/serum biochemical profile/urinalysis: normal or reflects cause of cough

Advanced or Confirmatory Testing

Choice of tests guided by prior findings. Commonly used tests:

- Laryngeal function examination (p. 574)
- Plasma N-terminal pro-B-type natriuretic peptide (NT-pro-BNP) (p. 1369): cardiac disease
- Echocardiography (p. 1094): CHF, pulmonary hypertension
- Respiratory fluoroscopy: dynamic airway collapse/obstruction (e.g., tracheal collapse, mainstem bronchial collapse, epiglottic retroversion)
- Thoracic CT: more detail than thoracic radiographs, quick assessment of all thoracic structures
- Bronchoscopy with bronchoalveolar lavage for culture and cytology (p. 1073)
- Bronchoalveolar lavage, blind or transtracheal wash (p. 1073)
- Fine-needle aspiration (p. 1113): mass lesion, heavy infiltrates
- Lung biopsy: diagnosis of interstitial lung disease (p. 553)
- Infectious disease testing, as appropriate

TREATMENT

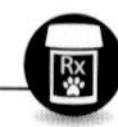

Treatment Overview

Treatment depends on underlying cause of cough

Acute General Treatment

If cough accompanied by respiratory distress, oxygen supplementation (p. 1146) and possibly other intervention may be required (p. 879)

Chronic Treatment

Varies with the underlying disease process. Cough suppressants should be avoided in cases of cardiogenic cough, infectious/inflammatory cough, and when the patient has evidence of systemic illness. Animals with degenerative disorders (e.g., collapsing trachea) may benefit from cough suppression (e.g., butorphanol 0.25-1 mg/kg PO q 8-24h; hydrocodone 0.25 mg/kg PO q 6-24h)

Recommended Monitoring

Often, acute, uncomplicated cough without evidence of systemic illness resolves in 7-10 days. Failure to resolve or systemic illness warrants investigation.

PROGNOSIS & OUTCOME

Depends on underlying disease process

PEARLS & CONSIDERATIONS

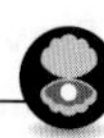

Comments

- Treatments for some disorders causing cough may be contraindicated in others (e.g., cough suppressants should not be used with bacterial pneumonia).
- Gastroesophageal reflux can cause cough. For dogs with chronic cough but otherwise in good health for whom more serious causes of cough have been ruled out, a trial course of omeprazole 1 mg/kg PO q 12h 30 minutes before meals may be warranted.
- Ironically, angiotensin-converting enzyme (ACE) inhibitors that are often used to treat heart disease cause cough in humans. This has not been reported in dogs or cats.

Prevention

Dogs and cats should be kept on heartworm prophylaxis.

Technician Tips

Ask about the regular use of heartworm prevention in all coughing pets.

Client Education

- Cough suppression is not beneficial, and may be harmful for many causes of cough.
- Resting respiratory rates may be performed at home to monitor for disease progression.

SUGGESTED READING

Lappin MR, et al: Antimicrobial use guidelines for treatment of respiratory tract disease in dogs and cats: antimicrobial guidelines working group of the International Society for Companion Animal Infectious Diseases. J Vet Intern Med 31:2. 2017.

RELATED CLIENT EDUCATION SHEETS

How to Count Respirations and Monitor Respiratory Effort
How to Deal With Incessant Coughing
How to Provide Home Respiratory Therapy (Humidification, Nebulization, Coupage)

AUTHOR: Megan Grobman, DVM, MS, DACVIM
EDITOR: Leah A. Cohn, DVM, PhD, DACVIM

Cranial Cruciate Ligament Injury

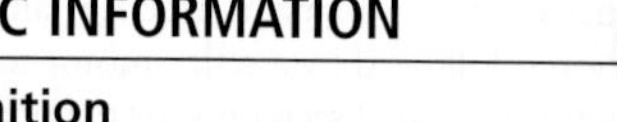

Video Available 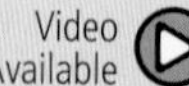 Bonus Material Online 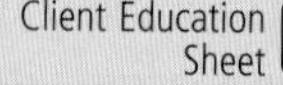 Client Education Sheet 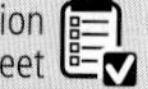

BASIC INFORMATION

Definition

Partial or complete tearing of the cranial cruciate ligament (CrCL), causing stifle instability; a very common condition in dogs and an uncommon condition in cats. Isolated caudal cruciate ligament tears are rare. Multiple ligamentous disruptions of the stifle are uncommon traumatic injuries of dogs and cats.

Synonyms

- Anterior cruciate ligament (ACL) rupture
- For multiple ligamentous disruption: stifle derangement, stifle luxation

Epidemiology

SPECIES, AGE, SEX

Seen in dogs and less frequently in cats of all ages

GENETICS, BREED PREDISPOSITION

- Dogs: especially common in rottweilers, Labrador retrievers, Newfoundlands,

Staffordshire terriers, but all dog sizes are affected.

- Genetic predisposition has been demonstrated in Newfoundlands, Labrador retrievers, and boxers.

RISK FACTORS

- Hyperadrenocorticism, autoimmune disease, cutaneous asthenia
- Obesity
- Ovary removal

ASSOCIATED DISORDERS

- Meniscal injury (usually medial) very commonly accompanies CrCL rupture.
- Patellar luxation
- Osteoarthritis
- Immune-mediated arthritis

Clinical Presentation

DISEASE FORMS/SUBTYPES

- Traumatic CrCL tears
- Degenerative CrCL tears
- Avulsion of the insertion of the CrCL: immature dogs
- Isolated caudal cruciate ligament tears (rare)
- Multiple ligamentous injury

HISTORY, CHIEF COMPLAINT

- Variable lameness of one or both hindlimbs; onset acute or progressive
- Lameness may worsen with exercise and improve with rest.

PHYSICAL EXAM FINDINGS

- Unilateral or bilateral hindlimb lameness: affected limb may be held up in acute injuries but will be weight bearing with more chronic affliction, although affected limb is still off-weighted when the animal is standing (see *Video*).
- Affected stifles are externally rotated and more flexed than normal when walking.
- Stifle joint effusion and thickening of joint capsule is often most pronounced over medial aspect of proximal tibia (medial buttress formation).
- Asymmetrical sitting position with one stifle abducted
- Cranial drawer sign and cranial tibial thrust (see Initial Database below) may or may not be elicited.
- Meniscal clicking may be present during joint manipulation.
- With caudal cruciate rupture, the tibia can be caudally displaced relative to the femur (caudal drawer sign).
- With multiple ligamentous injury, the cranial and caudal drawer sign as well as mediolateral instability can be elicited; stifle may be obviously luxated.

Etiology and Pathophysiology

- Biomechanical instability of the stifle joint results from an imbalance of forces necessary to control the cranial tibial thrust, excessive internal rotation, and hyperextension of the stifle usually limited by an intact cranial cruciate ligament.
- In dogs, CrCL rupture is usually due to degeneration rather than direct trauma. The cause of this degeneration is unknown: conformation problems, collagen abnormalities, abnormalities in ligament homeostasis, and immune disease may play a role.
- In cats and in both species with multiple ligamentous injury, direct trauma is usually the cause.

DIAGNOSIS

Diagnostic Overview

Presence of the characteristic hindlimb lameness combined with evidence of stifle effusion on physical examination and radiographs suggests CrCL disease. Absence of pain on manipulation, of cranial drawer sign, or of cranial tibial thrust does *not* rule out cranial cruciate rupture as the source of the lameness.

Differential Diagnosis

- Patellar luxation
- Lumbosacral disease
- Hip dysplasia or osteoarthritis
- Iliopsoas strain
- Bone/joint neoplasia
- Osteochondrosis of the lateral femoral condyle
- Inflammatory arthritis
- Caudal cruciate or collateral ligament injury (uncommon)
- Long digital extensor tendon avulsion (uncommon)
- Isolated meniscal injury (boxers almost exclusively)

Initial Database

- Palpation of stifle joints for instability (may require sedation)
  - Cranial drawer sign: manual cranial displacement of tibia relative to femur

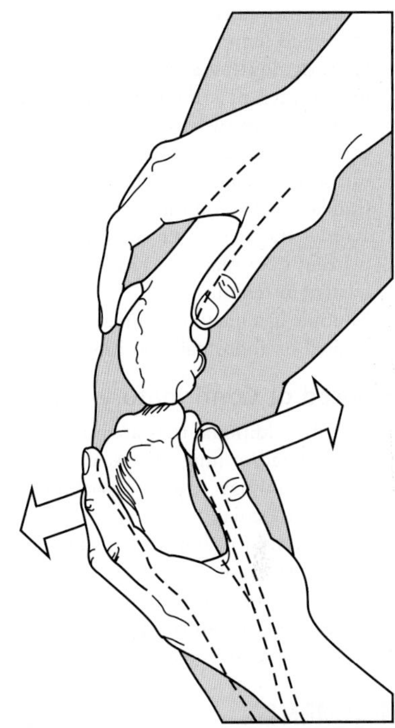

CRANIAL CRUCIATE LIGAMENT INJURY Palpation of the stifle joint for cranial drawer motion of the tibia relative to the femur with cranial cruciate ligament insufficiency.

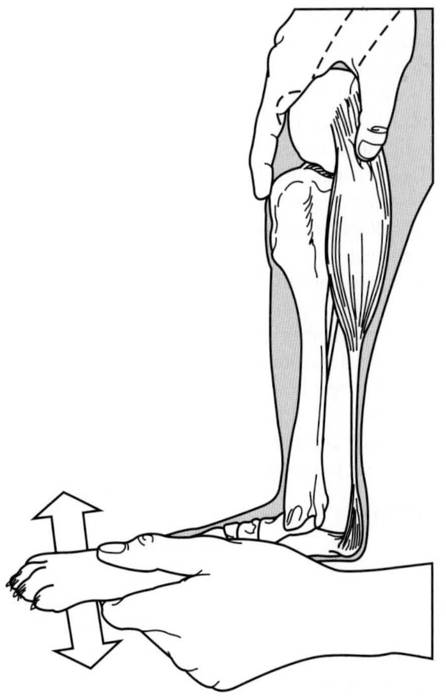

CRANIAL CRUCIATE LIGAMENT INJURY Palpation of the stifle joint using tibial compression test for cranial cruciate ligament injury. With cranial cruciate ligament injury, flexion of the hock causes cranial displacement of the tibia.

   - Tibial compression test: cranial movement of tibial tuberosity as hock is flexed
- Lateral and craniocaudal stifle radiographs
   - Medium-sized to large dogs: joint effusion almost always is present; degenerative changes evident after 3 weeks
   - Small dogs, and cats: joint effusion may be minimal; tibia often cranially displaced relative to femur (static drawer)
   - Growing dogs: an avulsed bone fragment may be seen near the CrCL insertion.
   - Measurements such as tibial plateau slope angle are made for planning when an osteotomy technique is chosen for repair.
   - Caudal cruciate rupture: there may be an avulsed fragment over the caudal tibial plateau; tibia may be caudally displaced relative to femur.
   - Multiple ligamentous injuries: stifle often luxated or abnormally positioned

Advanced or Confirmatory Testing

Occasionally, additional tests are warranted:
- Rickettsial and/or fungal titers, as indicated by other findings (e.g., polyarthropathy, thrombocytopenia)
- Arthrocentesis to eliminate inflammatory arthritides as causes (p. 1059)
- Arthroscopy or arthrotomy, the most common way to confirm diagnosis
- Magnetic resonance imaging (see p. 1132)

TREATMENT

Treatment Overview

- Medical management (including physical rehabilitation and weight control) has about a 60% success rate for return to normal activities; surgical management (by most techniques) has an 85%-90% success rate.
- Surgical management usually involves inspection (and debridement or release if necessary) of menisci, combined with a stabilization technique. Stabilization techniques involve creation of a prosthetic ligament to mimic the function of the CrCL or a change (usually by osteotomy) in the geometry of the stifle so there is minimal cranial tibial translation when the limb is bearing weight.
- Success rates are similar for prosthetic ligament and osteotomy (tibial plateau leveling osteotomy [TPLO], tibial tuberosity advancement [TTA], triple tibial osteotomy [TTO]) repairs. Return to full weight bearing is usually faster with osteotomy techniques. Cats and small dogs are most commonly treated with prosthetic ligament techniques.

Acute General Treatment

Medical management:
- Physical rehabilitation
   - Controlled leash walks
   - Sit-to-stand exercises
   - Swimming, water treadmill work
- Nonsteroidal antiinflammatory drugs (NSAIDs):
   - Carprofen (dogs) 2 mg/kg PO q 12h, *or*
   - Robenacoxib 1-2 mg/kg PO q 24h (up to 6 days' use for cats), *or*
   - Deracoxib (dogs) 1-2 mg/kg PO q 24h (may use 3-4 mg/kg PO q 24h for first 7 days only), *or*
   - Meloxicam 0.1 mg/kg PO q 24h, *or*
   - Tepoxalin 10 mg/kg PO q 24h

Surgical stabilization of the stifle (CrCL tear): many variations exist for all of these techniques:
- Intra-articular patellar tendon, fascial, or hamstring graft: aims to replace missing CrCL's function
- Extracapsular suture stabilization (femoral condyle or fabella to tibia): limits cranial motion and internal rotation. There are a number of variations on this theme.
- TPLO and cranial closing wedge osteotomy: neutralizes cranial tibial thrust by changing tibial plateau angle and transferring stress from the absent CrCL to the intact caudal cruciate ligament
- TTA: neutralizes cranial tibial thrust by making the pull of the patellar tendon perpendicular to the tibial plateau when the stifle is bearing weight
- Pinning or wiring to reattach ligament insertion can be done in young dogs with large avulsion fragments.
- Proximal tibial epiphysiodesis: in dogs ≤ 5 months of age, a screw can be placed across the cranial aspect of the tibial physis to progressively decrease tibial plateau angle as the dog grows.

Treatment of meniscal injury:
- Removal of the torn portion of the meniscus
- Medial meniscal release (has an effect similar to meniscectomy, sometimes done prophylactically)

Treatment of caudal cruciate injury:
- In almost all cases, conservative therapy suffices for return to full function.
- Suture or fascial imbrication can be used in persistently lame dogs.

Treatment of multiple ligamentous injury:
- Debride torn menisci.
- Extracapsular sutures to replace function of caudal cruciate, medial (occasionally lateral) collateral, and cranial cruciate ligaments
- In cats, a transarticular pin can be used to stabilize the stifle for 10-21 days, after which the pin is removed, and fibrosis holds things in place.

Chronic Treatment

- Management includes the same treatments as in acute cases, but long-term medical management of osteoarthritis may be required. Success rates are similar for surgical treatment of acute and chronic cranial cruciate injuries, with or without meniscal tears.
   - NSAIDs as listed previously
   - Physical rehabilitation
   - Disease-modifying osteoarthritis agents may be helpful:
      - Polysulfated glycosaminoglycan 5 mg/kg IM once weekly × 4-6 weeks, *or*
      - Pentosan polysulfate 3 mg/kg SQ once weekly, *or*
      - Oral formulations (glucosamine, chondroitin sulfate, avocado soy unsaponifiables): according to formulation/labeled instructions
- Intra-articular injection of mesenchymal stem cells and/or platelet-rich plasma may decrease pain.
- For animals with end-stage osteoarthritis (rare with cruciate disease), total stifle replacement can be considered.

Nutrition/Diet

Weight control helps alleviate lameness due to osteoarthritis (p. 1077).

Behavior/Exercise

Most dogs and cats can return to full function after recovery from surgical treatment of cruciate disease.

Possible Complications

Medical management:
- Gastrointestinal, hepatic, renal, or other systemic reactions from NSAID therapy
- Continued lameness; progression of degenerative joint disease

Surgical management:
- Postoperative meniscal tears
- Suture breakage, stretch, or slippage
- Infection
- Fracture or implant failure
- Progression of degenerative joint disease

Recommended Monitoring

- Weight loss, exercise levels (rehabilitation), and clinical signs as dictated by the patient.
- Basic laboratory monitoring of patients on NSAID therapy.
- Radiographic monitoring of healing of osteotomies (usually at 6-8 and 10-12 weeks after surgery) and of any repair if clinical signs worsen

PROGNOSIS & OUTCOME

- Long-term function for patients that have undergone a reconstructive procedure is good. Published assessments of most techniques in the past 25 years describe improvement in 80%-90% of dogs after surgery, regardless of methodology.
- Prognosis after surgery is not affected by whether meniscectomy has been necessary or by degree of osteoarthritis evident on preoperative radiographs.
- The majority of dogs with caudal cruciate ligament tears return to full function with medical therapy.
- Prognosis for surgically treated multiple ligamentous injury is similarly good; about 80% of animals return to previous level of performance.
- Postoperative rehabilitation is critical for full recovery.

PEARLS & CONSIDERATIONS

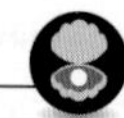

Comments

- Bilateral lameness may be difficult to recognize and is often confused with neurologic disease.
- Injury of the contralateral cranial cruciate ligament occurs in 40%-50% of canine

patients. No measures have been identified to prevent this from occurring.
- Consider consultation and referral with an orthopedic surgeon; selection of the best procedure continues to be controversial among specialists.

Prevention

- No reliable preventive measures have been identified. Because several recent studies have implicated ovariohysterectomy as a risk factor for CrCL rupture, this may be a point to discuss with owners of puppies intended for high-performance work.
- Maintaining lean body weight may be beneficial.

Technician Tips

Most dogs should be partially weight bearing on the operated limb by the end of the first postoperative day. Dogs who have had epidural analgesia for stifle surgery may require bladder expression for up to 24 hours.

SUGGESTED READING

Kowaleski MP, et al: Stifle joint. In Johnston SA, et al, editors: Veterinary surgery: small animal, ed 2, St. Louis, 2018, Elsevier, pp 1079-1141.

AUTHOR & EDITOR: **Kathleen Linn, DVM, MS, DACVS**

Cranial Vena Cava Syndrome

Client Education Sheet 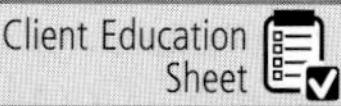

BASIC INFORMATION 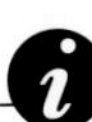

Definition

Cranial vena cava syndrome is an uncommon sequela to extraluminal compression, invasion, or intraluminal obstruction of the cranial vena cava (CrVC). Obstruction of the CrVC results in pitting edema of the head, neck, and forelimbs.

Synonyms

Caval syndrome, precaval syndrome, superior vena caval syndrome

Epidemiology

SPECIES, AGE, SEX

Depends on underlying cause

RISK FACTORS

- Jugular catheters
- Cranial mediastinal neoplasia (e.g., thymoma, lymphoma, carcinoma, aortic body tumors, pleural mesothelioma)
- Hypercoagulable conditions (e.g., sepsis, immune-mediated hemolytic anemia, protein-losing nephropathies, glucocorticoid excess, neoplasia, pancreatitis)
- Mycoses leading to the formation of granulomas (e.g., blastomycosis, cryptococcosis)
- Transvenous pacemaker implantation

CONTAGION AND ZOONOSIS

Fungal granulomas causing CrVC syndrome may be caused by organisms that can also infect humans *(Blastomyces dermatitidis, Cryptococcus neoformans)*, but they would be common-source infections, not zoonoses.

GEOGRAPHY AND SEASONALITY

Infectious causes (e.g., blastomycosis, cryptococcosis) are more prevalent in certain geographic areas.

Clinical Presentation

HISTORY, CHIEF COMPLAINT

- Head, neck, and forelimb swelling
- Additional clinical signs depend on underlying cause.

PHYSICAL EXAM FINDINGS

- Symmetrical, nonpainful pitting edema of head, neck, and forelimbs
- Dyspnea, tachypnea, muffled heart/lung sounds (if pleural effusion present)
- Weakness, tachycardia, arrhythmias, muffled heart sounds (if pericardial effusion present)
- ± Jugular venous distention
- ± Engorgement of conjunctival and scleral vessels
- Additional physical exam findings depend on underlying cause.

Etiology and Pathophysiology

- Extraluminal compression, invasion, or intraluminal obstruction of the CrVC causes impaired venous return from the cranial portion of the body. This leads to interstitial fluid accumulation, resulting in edema of the head, neck, and forelimbs.
- The most common causes include mediastinal neoplasia, fungal granulomas, CrvC thrombosis (e.g., secondary to hypercoagulable states, tumor emboli, jugular catheters), and transvenous pacemaker implantation.

DIAGNOSIS 

Diagnostic Overview

The physical exam findings (pitting edema of the head and forelimbs) are highly suggestive of the diagnosis. Diagnostic tests such as thoracic radiographs, advanced imaging, cytologic evaluation of masses and effusions, and histopathologic examination of tissue specimens are used in sequential steps to confirm the diagnosis and identify the underlying cause.

Differential Diagnosis

For head and neck swelling:
- Angioedema (e.g., vaccine reaction, insect-bite hypersensitivity)
- Generalized peripheral edema (e.g., secondary to hypoalbuminemia, vasculitis, right-sided congestive heart failure)
- Acute blunt trauma to head/neck
- Subcutaneous emphysema
- Lymphangiosarcoma of the head and neck
- Myxedema (e.g., secondary to hypothyroidism)
- Foreign body around neck (e.g., elastic band)
- Salivary mucocele (cervical)
- Jugular vein thrombosis or mass
- Abscessation or cellulitis
- Snake bite

Initial Database

To help determine underlying cause:
- CBC
- Serum biochemistry profile
- Urinalysis
- Feline leukemia and feline immunodeficiency virus tests (to help evaluate for lymphoma in cats)
- Thoracic radiographs (to identify cranial mediastinal masses, pleural and/or pericardial effusion)

Advanced or Confirmatory Testing

- Thoracic ultrasonography (to visualize emboli or tumor compression/invasion of cranial vena cava)
- Nonselective angiography, venography (to identify CrVC filling defects, localize site of obstruction, highlight collateral circulation)
- CT or MRI (p. 1132)
    - CT-angiography has been used to diagnose acquired collateral venous pathways in a dog with CrvC.
- Echocardiography (p. 1094); (to identify pericardial effusion or masses at the level of the terminal CrVC)
- Fine-needle aspiration or biopsy of thoracic masses
- Additional testing as indicated by suspected underlying cause (e.g., *Blastomyces* urine antigen test if *Blastomyces* granuloma suspected)
- Thromboelastography (TEG) can be used to assess hypercoagulable state and aid in guidance of thromboprohylaxis or thrombolytic therapy.

TREATMENT 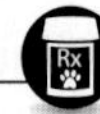

Treatment Overview

Treatment is directed toward removing the obstructive lesion from CrVC and treating the inciting cause.

Acute General Treatment

- Mediastinal masses: depending on tumor type, treatment may include surgery, chemotherapy, or radiation therapy (alone or in combination).
- Fungal granulomas: systemic antifungal drugs (e.g., itraconazole, fluconazole), depending on type of mycosis
- CrVC thrombosis
  - Treat underlying cause.
  - Remove jugular catheters if present.
  - ± Anticoagulants (e.g., heparin): efficacy unproven
  - ± Thrombolytic agents (e.g., streptokinase, tissue plasminogen activator): efficacy controversial; may result in life-threatening hemorrhage
  - ± Balloon venoplasty
- ± Diuretics (to minimize edema formation): efficacy limited

Chronic Treatment

Directed to improving/resolving underlying disease

Possible Complications

Thrombolytic agents may result in life-threatening hemorrhage. Careful monitoring and titration of treatment are essential.

PROGNOSIS & OUTCOME

- Prognosis depends on severity of underlying illness; presence of CrVC syndrome does not appear to confer a worse prognosis than that of the underlying disorder alone.
- Head, neck, and forelimb edema may abate if CrVC obstruction is removed and/or if adequate collateral circulation develops.

PEARLS & CONSIDERATIONS

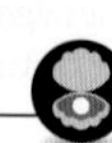

Comments

- Although similarly named, heartworm caval syndrome is an entirely different clinical entity involving right-sided heart failure, hemolysis, and hemoglobinuria as a consequence of severe heartworm disease (p. 418).
- If presentation is unusual, consider intercurrent disease (fungal and neoplastic).
- Human medicine offers promising alternatives to the current therapies available in veterinary medicine.
  - Surgical bypass of the CrVC obstruction
  - Endovascular therapy—a combination of
    - Stent placement at the level of vascular obstruction
    - ± Anticoagulants

Prevention

- Avoid jugular catheters in hypercoagulable patients.
- Consider prophylactic anticoagulant therapy in patients with hypercoagulable disorders.
- If thrombolysis is successful, the use of antiplatelet therapy (e.g., clopidogrel) to reduce vascular re-occlusion because of residual thrombus or endothelial injury is recommended.

Technician Tips

Monitoring plans will depend on underlying disease process and therapy chosen.

SUGGESTED READING

Ricciardi M et al: Acquired collateral venous pathways in a dog with cranial vena cava obstruction. J Vet Med Sci 79(11):1772-1775, 2017.

AUTHOR: Lyndsay Nichole Kubicek, DVM, DACVR
EDITOR: Meg M. Sleeper, VMD, DACVIM

Cricopharyngeal Achalasia/Dysphagia

Client Education Sheet 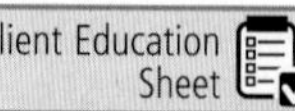

BASIC INFORMATION

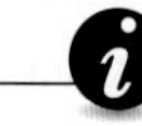

Definition

A rare condition representing failure of the upper esophageal sphincter (cricopharyngeus muscle) to relax (achalasia) or asynchrony between contraction of pharyngeal muscles and relaxation of the cricopharyngeus muscle (dysphagia)

Synonyms

Cricopharyngeal dysphagia, cricopharyngeal asynchrony

Epidemiology

SPECIES, AGE, SEX

- Spaniel dogs overrepresented (springer, cocker)
- Often congenital; most cases present when young, usually on weaning but may be up to 1 year of age
- Rarely diagnosed in older animals or in conjunction with other conditions, including hypothyroidism

Clinical Presentation

HISTORY, CHIEF COMPLAINT

- Clinical signs often begin at the time of weaning on introducing solid food.
- Signs include gagging, retching, regurgitating food, coughing, and nasal reflux. Repeated attempts to swallow may be seen with careful observation during eating.
- Dogs are often thin and in poor body condition because of ineffective food intake and may lose weight despite an increased appetite.

PHYSICAL EXAM FINDINGS

- Patients are usually thin, may be smaller in stature compared to littermates.
- The dog should be observed while eating; repeated ineffective attempts to swallow suggest cricopharyngeal achalasia.
- Observation of respiratory effort and thoracic auscultation may suggest the presence of aspiration pneumonia (p. 793).

Etiology and Pathophysiology

- Cricopharyngeal achalasia results from failure of relaxation of the cricopharyngeus muscle, preventing food bolus movement into the proximal esophagus.
- The cricopharyngeus muscle contracts during normal activity. When a bolus, formed by pharyngeal muscular activity, is pushed caudally by the base of the tongue, the cricopharyngeus muscle relaxes, allowing passage of the bolus into the upper esophagus.
- Asynchronous cricopharyngeal relaxation results in repeated caudal movement of a bolus against the persistently contracted cricopharyngeal muscle. Boluses may eventually reach the upper esophagus, may be regurgitated, or may be aspirated into the trachea.

DIAGNOSIS

Diagnostic Overview

The history of successful prehension of food but inability to swallow is highly suggestive. Confirmation is obtained with fluoroscopic evaluation of the oropharyngeal and esophageal processing of liquids and solids. Clinical signs and static imaging (even with contrast) may not differentiate oral, pharyngeal, and cricopharyngeal disorders. A correct diagnosis is imperative before surgical treatment to avoid worsening of clinical signs and aspiration pneumonia.

Differential Diagnosis

- Pharyngeal dysfunction usually results in the inability to form a food bolus.
- Oral dysfunction interferes with prehension
- Oropharyngeal or proximal esophageal obstruction by mass or foreign body apparent radiographically, on sedated oropharyngeal exam, or endoscopically

Initial Database

- Abnormalities in CBC and chemistries as a result of malnutrition or aspiration pneumonia or age-related findings typical of puppies
- Thoracic radiographs to rule out megaesophagus or aspiration pneumonia

Advanced or Confirmatory Testing

A definitive diagnosis is made with fluoroscopy of the pharynx and esophagus when the patient is offered food mixed with barium (p. 1062).

- A bolus is formed, but repeated attempts at caudal movement of the bolus beyond the upper esophageal sphincter result in little or no entry of barium into the esophagus. Barium may enter the nasopharynx or the trachea.
    - The bolus forms normally, pharyngeal contractions repeatedly propel the bolus caudally, but the cricopharyngeus muscle rarely relaxes to allow the entry of barium into the esophagus.
- When barium does enter the esophagus, esophageal motility should be carefully evaluated before considering surgical correction of the condition. Decreased esophageal motility or megaesophagus are contraindications to surgical therapy.
- Standing fluoroscopy is preferred to recumbent imaging if appropriate equipment is available.

TREATMENT

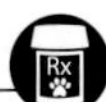

Treatment Overview

- Surgical correction of the disease is the treatment of choice; however, medical management of aspiration pneumonia is important for preoperative stabilization.
- The goal of surgical treatment (myotomy/myectomy of the cricopharyngeal muscle) is to allow unimpaired passage of food boluses from the pharynx into the esophagus without tracheal contamination.

Acute and Chronic Treatment

- Treatment of complications before anesthesia (e.g., aspiration pneumonia, undernourishment)
- Cricopharyngeal myotomy or myectomy is most common. Thyropharyngeal myectomy also is suggested by some surgeons. Referral to a veterinary soft-tissue surgeon is recommended.

Nutrition/Diet

- Preoperatively, esophagostomy tube (p. 1106) or gastrostomy tube (p. 1109) placement may be required to meet nutritional requirements, normalize body condition, and decrease aspiration of food.
- Postoperatively, the patient is fed canned food in the form of easily swallowed round portions. The diet is returned to normal over a period of 1 month.

Possible Complications

- Clinical signs can recur due to inadequate or imprecise muscular excision or fibrosis of the myectomy/myotomy site. Reoperation on the contralateral side of the cricopharyngeus muscle may be performed if necessary.
- Surgery with concurrent esophageal dysfunction is relatively contraindicated because it may result in reflux of esophageal contents into the caudal pharynx and tracheal aspiration.

PROGNOSIS & OUTCOME

- The prognosis for cricopharyngeal achalasia is good if the correct diagnosis is made, precise surgery performed, and there is no concurrent pharyngeal or esophageal dysfunction.
- Recurrence of clinical signs or aspiration pneumonia has been reported in 0 of 6 and 8 of 14 patients in two different studies.

PEARLS & CONSIDERATIONS

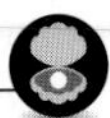

Comments

- Interpretation of swallowing imaging studies is complex; consultation with a radiologist is recommended.
- Aggressively treat severe malnutrition and/or aspiration pneumonia before surgical intervention to decrease the morbidity and mortality of anesthesia and surgery.
- Seriously consider whether cricopharyngeal myectomy should be done in patients with esophageal motility disorders because aspiration pneumonia is likely after surgery.
- Cricopharyngeal achalasia must be differentiated from pharyngeal dysfunction because operation on the latter will worsen clinical signs.
- Closely monitor patients after surgery and consider reoperation if clinical signs recur.

Technician Tips

- Avoid force feeding.
- Notify veterinarian of any signs that could indicate aspiration pneumonia (e.g., lethargy, fever, hyporexia, tachypnea, coughing)

SUGGESTED READING

Warnock JJ, et al: Surgical management of cricopharyngeal dysphagia in dogs: 14 cases (1989–2001). J Am Vet Med Assoc 223:1462-1468, 2003.

AUTHOR: MaryAnn G. Radlinsky, DVM, MS, DACVS
EDITOR: Elizabeth A. Swanson, DVM, MS, DACVS

Cryptococcosis

BASIC INFORMATION

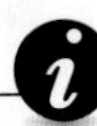

Definition

Fungal infection of people and animals. Most common systemic fungal infection of cats

Epidemiology

SPECIES, AGE, SEX

Cats, dogs, and ferrets of any age, but young adult cats and dogs are predisposed.

GENETICS, BREED PREDISPOSITION

American cocker spaniel, German shepherd, Doberman pinscher, Great Dane are predisposed; Siamese, Birman, and Ragdoll cats are predisposed in Australian studies.

RISK FACTORS

Immunosuppression is an important risk factor in humans but does not appear to be a significant risk factor in cats and dogs.

CONTAGION AND ZOONOSIS

Infections occur after environmental exposure. Human infection associated with immunosuppression but is not considered zoonotic.

GEOGRAPHY AND SEASONALITY

Cryptococcus neoformans: Worldwide
Cryptococcus gattii: subtropics, British Columbia, and Pacific Northwest of United States

ASSOCIATED DISORDERS

Cats with concurrent retroviral infections do not respond as well to treatment.

Clinical Presentation

DISEASE FORMS/SUBTYPES

Sinonasal infection most common in cats; systemic infection most common in dogs; central nervous system (CNS) and ocular infections occur frequently in both species; otitis externa and skin ulcers can occur.

HISTORY, CHIEF COMPLAINT

Chronic infection in cats usually causing mild lethargy and anorexia with moderate to severe rhinosinusitis. Dogs usually have more severe systemic signs with absent/minimal rhinosinusitis. Neurologic signs sometimes noted, as are dermal ulcers, vomiting, and diarrhea.

PHYSICAL EXAM FINDINGS

Cats:

- Upper respiratory tract signs predominate. Swelling or ulcerated mass over the bridge of the nose is common. Stertor or stridor may occur with pharyngeal/nasopharyngeal involvement. Dyspnea from pleural or lower airway involvement is less common. Submandibular lymphadenopathy is often seen.
- Fundic exam often reveals granulomatous chorioretinitis, retinal hemorrhage, retinal detachment, and/or evidence of optic neuritis.
- Cutaneous or subcutaneous masses/nodules or ulcerated lesions may be noted. Ulcers on footpads may result in lameness.
- CNS signs are usually subtle in cats.

Dogs:

- Systemic involvement with findings that depend on significance of organ system involvement.
- Ocular, CNS, and cutaneous signs are common.
- Fundic exam as in cats.
- Severe lethargy and anorexia or obtunded state may be noted.
- Upper respiratory tract signs less common in dogs.
- Cutaneous and subcutaneous masses and ulcerated lesions may be noted.

Etiology and Pathophysiology

- Caused by a dimorphic fungus of the genus *Cryptococcus*
- Filamentous form in the environment produces basidiospores that are inhaled and form encapsulated yeast in nasal cavity or lung tissue before disseminating by hematogenous route.
- *C. neoformans* and *C. gattii* cause the majority of infections in cats, dogs, and humans, but at least 19 species have been implicated.
- Pigeons are considered an important vector; organisms can survive up to 2 years in pigeon roosts and droppings.

DIAGNOSIS

Diagnostic Overview

- In patients with systemic signs, CBC, serum chemistry panel, urinalysis, and diagnostic imaging (thoracic radiographs, abdominal ultrasound) will usually be the first steps.
- If nasal involvement is obvious or cutaneous nodules or ulcers are apparent, samples (swabs, fine-needle aspirates, impression smears, biopsy) should be collected for cytology, culture, and/or histopathology.
- Serologic testing for cryptococcal antigen is an inexpensive and a sensitive and specific test that should be performed early in the workup if cytology has not revealed cryptococcal organisms.
- CNS signs should result in neurologic exam with cross-sectional imaging based on neurolocalization. Cerebrospinal fluid (CSF) tap often reveals organisms, but complications may be seen after CSF tap due to increased intracranial pressure.
- Anterior uveitis and granulomatous chorioretinitis should increase suspicion for fungal infection.

Differential Diagnosis

- Nasal discharge (p. 1255); nasal deformity makes neoplasia the primary differential diagnosis
- CNS
  - Infectious: many, including feline infectious peritonitis, toxoplasmosis, rabies, canine distemper, rabies, ehrlichiosis, Rocky Mountain spotted fever
  - Noninfectious: granulomatous meningoencephalitis, neoplasia
- Cutaneous: abscesses, autoimmune skin disease, neoplastic disease
- Other systemic fungal disease (dogs)

Initial Database

- Ocular exam may reveal anterior uveitis and posterior segment changes (granulomatous chorioretinitis, retinal detachment, optic neuritis, retinal hemorrhage, and exophthalmos).
- CBC, serum chemistry panel, and urinalysis: usually minimal change. Normocytic, normochromic nonregenerative anemia is common. Mild leukocytosis with neutrophilia and monocytosis is often seen with eosinophilia likely in cats and a left shift occasionally seen in dogs. Mild serum chemistry panel changes reflect organ system involvement. Occasionally, *Cryptococcus* organisms are found in urine sediment.
- Thoracic radiographs are usually normal; sternal or hilar lymphadenopathy or focal increases in pulmonary parenchymal opacity may be noted in dogs. Rare pleural effusion
- Abdominal ultrasound is usually normal in cats but may reveal mild ascites, lymphadenopathy, focal/multifocal thickening of the stomach and intestines, and/or masses associated with spleen, kidney, or pancreas in dogs.

Advanced or Confirmatory Testing

- Cytology of aspirates of nodules, smears of nasal discharge, body fluids, or impression smears from ulcerated skin lesions may reveal cryptococcal organisms in 60%-80% of cases. Diff-Quik, Romanowsky-type, and Gram stains can be used to demonstrate round yeast organisms with a large mucopolysaccharide capsule. Granulomatous or pyogranulomatous inflammation is typical.
- Serologic testing has the advantages of being inexpensive, highly sensitive and specific, and noninvasive. Latex agglutination assays detect capsular antigen and can be used on serum or CSF. Serum antigen titers are usually very high, but even low titers may indicate active infection. Titers can be used to follow treatment because they decrease significantly in successfully treated animals.
- Fungal culture and/or histopathology may be needed to confirm diagnosis in some cases. Fungal sensitivity testing can be performed when the organism is cultured.
- Cross-sectional imaging is not usually necessary but may increase suspicion of fungal infection when multifocal mass lesions in the CNS or evidence of meningoencephalitis is noted. MRI may reveal meningeal enhancement along with single or multifocal contrast-enhancing mass lesions that tend to be hyperintense on T2-weighted images and hypointense on T1-weighted images. In cats and dogs with sinonasal disease, nasal mass lesions or fluid opacification are common on CT, with contrast-enhancing mass lesions often associated with lysis of the nasal septum and cribriform plate.

TREATMENT

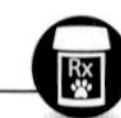

Treatment Overview

Long-term treatment which azole antifungal drugs such as fluconazole or itraconazole is effective in many infected patients. Surgical cytoreduction may improve treatment success if masses can be easily removed.

Acute General Treatment

- Although the most effective therapy is likely amphotericin B in combination with 5-flucytosine (cats) or fluconazole (dogs), most patients can initially be treated with azole monotherapy or a combination of an azole and terbinafine.
- Itraconazole 5-10 mg/kg PO q 24h or fluconazole 10 mg/kg PO q 12h are the azoles of first choice. Fluconazole penetrates the blood-brain and blood-ocular barriers better than itraconazole and is excreted through the urinary tract, but studies in humans indicate equal efficacy in CNS infection.

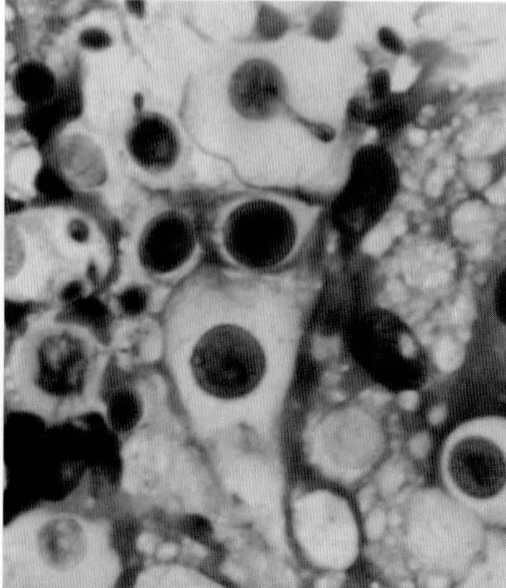

CRYPTOCOCCOSIS Cytology shows capsulate yeasts with narrow-neck budding and prominent unstained region surrounding each yeast (corresponding to capsule) from the Diff-Quik–stained smear. (Courtesy Professor Richard Malik, University of Sydney, Sydney, Australia.)

- Surgical removal of large granulomas may improve response to treatment.
- Posaconazole has proved effective in humans with resistant infections and is affordable in cats.
- Antiinflammatory doses of glucocorticoids may be necessary in patients with significant CNS signs for the first 3-5 days of treatment.

Chronic Treatment

Treatment with azoles should be continued until all signs of infection have disappeared and titers are negative. This usually takes months to over a year, and some patients will need to be treated for life. A fourfold to fivefold drop in titer is indicative of a response to treatment.

Recommended Monitoring

- Liver enzymes (alanine aminotransferase [ALT], aspartate aminotransferase [AST], alkaline phosphatase [ALP]) should be monitored monthly while on azole antifungals.
- Antigen titers should be monitored monthly and then every 3-6 months after treatment is discontinued because the titers usually increase before clinical signs associated with relapse.

PROGNOSIS & OUTCOME

- Prognosis for resolution of clinical signs is good in cats with *C. neoformans* nasal infection, guarded in dogs with systemic infection.
- Prognosis is worse when CNS disease is present in any species.
- Approximately 75% of cats respond completely, although relapse is possible even years after treatment has been discontinued.
- Cats with retroviral infections do not respond as well to treatment (data for itraconazole).

PEARLS & CONSIDERATIONS

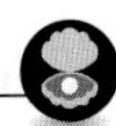

Comments

Cryptococcosis is the most common fungal infection of cats, most often causing clinical signs associated with chronic nasal disease.

Prevention

Avoid areas with pigeon droppings.

Technician Tips

The subtle deformation of the muzzle or face of an early lesion of cryptococcosis may first be noticed by a member of the technical staff and is an important observation to bring to the attention of the attending veterinarian.

SUGGESTED READING

Taboada J: Cryptococcosis. In Ettinger SJ, et al, editors: Textbook of veterinary internal medicine, ed 8, St. Louis, 2017, Elsevier, pp 1019-1023.

AUTHOR & EDITOR: Joseph Taboada, DVM, DACVIM

Cryptosporidiosis

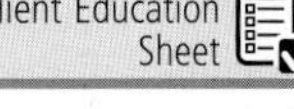

BASIC INFORMATION

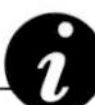

Definition

A sporadic gastroenterocolitis caused by *Cryptosporidium* spp, a ubiquitous coccidian parasite

Epidemiology

SPECIES, AGE, SEX

Cats of any age or sex can be affected. In dogs, clinical disease is almost entirely confined to puppies < 6 months old and immunocompromised, young adult dogs.

RISK FACTORS

- Immunosuppression due to concurrent viral infection (e.g., feline leukemia virus [FeLV], feline immunodeficiency virus [FIV], canine distemper virus [CDV])
- Overcrowded and stressful conditions (e.g., humane shelters, catteries) raise prevalence of infection because oocysts shed in feces are highly infective.
- Presence of other gastrointestinal (GI) parasites (*Giardia* sp, *Toxocara cati*) or, in adult cats, severe intestinal disease (e.g., inflammatory bowel disease, lymphoma)
- Feeding undercooked home diets

CONTAGION AND ZOONOSIS

- Transmission occurs through a fecal-oral route, usually by consuming contaminated water or food.
- Cats with formed stool or diarrhea can potentially transmit organism, but parasite most often is found in dogs with diarrhea.
- Zoonotic risk from dogs and cats is minimal because most organisms are host adapted. Immunocompromised humans should be cautioned to not handle strays or pets from high-risk environments before screening for oocyst shedding.

GEOGRAPHY AND SEASONALITY

Worldwide; prevalence of *Cryptosporidium* species varies by geographic location.

Clinical Presentation

DISEASE FORMS/SUBTYPES

Subclinical; mild to moderate diarrhea; severe protein-losing enteropathy

HISTORY, CHIEF COMPLAINT

- Chronic small-bowel diarrhea (p. 1215) is the main clinical sign initially.
- Vomiting is less likely.
- Tenesmus, hematochezia, and weight loss may occur in long-standing infections.

PHYSICAL EXAM FINDINGS

Many *Cryptosporidium*-infected cats appear well. In cats with severe diarrhea, gas and fluid-filled intestinal loops can be found during abdominal palpation. Cats with chronic disease may appear thin, unthrifty, and undernourished. Fever usually does not occur.

Etiology and Pathophysiology

- Natural infections of *Cryptosporidium parvum, Cryptosporidium felis, Cryptosporidium muris, and Cryptosporidium rynae* have been found in cats. Infections with *C. parvum, C. canis,* and *Cryptosporidium meleagridis* have been documented in dogs.
- Oocysts found in feces may be shed intermittently during diarrhea or in the absence of clinical signs. The incidence of shedding from carriers (not showing signs) is low.
- Infection occurs without invasion into intestinal epithelium.
- Clinical disease is postulated to result from alterations of normal flora by the parasite and later influx of inflammatory cells into the intestinal epithelium, leading to villous atrophy, secretory diarrhea, and malabsorption.
- The terminal ileum usually has the highest parasite load.

DIAGNOSIS

Diagnostic Overview

Routine screening specifically for *Cryptosporidium* is a low-yield procedure given current techniques and the low prevalence of shedding, but testing should be considered in animals with compatible clinical signs and/or for immunocompromised pets or owners. More than one method of parasite identification may be necessary to rule out infection in highly suspect animals with clinical disease.

Differential Diagnosis

- Causes of gastroenterocolitis that prevail in overcrowded conditions: *Giardia* spp,

Cystoisospora spp, *Tritrichomonas foetus*, *Toxoplasma gondii*, *Entamoeba histolytica*
- Other causes of diarrhea and weight loss: inflammatory bowel disease, GI lymphoma, hyperthyroidism, others (p. 1213)

Initial Database

- Complete fecal examination consisting of direct smear, Sheather's solution flotation, and $ZnSO_4$ analysis is recommended for cats with diarrhea.
  - *Cryptosporidium* oocysts are small but may be identified by light microscopy at 100× power using any of these techniques. False-negative results are common.
  - Multiple fecal samplings improve the likelihood of finding oocysts.
  - Phase microscopy on unstained preparations from a Sheather's fecal float may offer a greater chance of finding the oocyst but still may yield negative results.
  - Microscopic identification of oocysts may require submission of feces to a commercial laboratory for acid-fast staining (modified Ziehl-Neelsen or Kinyoun technique) or antigen detection by immunologic methods (direct immunofluorescence assay [DFA]), enzyme immunoassay [EIA]).
  - Use of multiple methods of testing during clinical disease is recommended.
- CBC, serum biochemistry profile, urinalysis, total T_4, abdominal imaging: if diarrhea and weight loss are present (rule out other disorders)
- FeLV and FIV ELISA (cats)

Advanced or Confirmatory Testing

- Fecal specimens submitted to commercial laboratories should be sent in 38% formaldehyde (100% formalin) solution added at a 1:10 dilution to kill oocysts but still allow detection. The oocysts are detected after centrifugation using DFA or acid-fast stain.
- A DFA kit is available (Merifluor) that detects *Cryptosporidia* and *Giardia* oocysts but requires an incubation chamber and fluorescent microscope for use.
- Available EIA test kits specific for fecal antigen in humans and rodents are difficult to use, and acid-fast stain may be just as effective for dogs and cats.
- A feline serum cryptosporidial immunoglobulin G (IgG) enzyme-linked immunosorbent assay (ELISA) is available and highly correlates with exposure with parasite but not necessarily with active infection.
- Polymerase chain reaction (PCR) tests for detecting cryptosporidial nucleic acids in feces are very sensitive (false-positives occur) and are recommended only for oocyst molecular typing.
- Intestinal biopsy may not confirm infection and is not cost effective. Necropsy samples should be taken within hours after death because postmortem autolysis can prevent confirmation.

TREATMENT

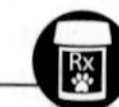

Treatment Overview

The overall goals of treatment are to cure the infection, resolve clinical signs, and prevent further oocyst shedding. High numbers of oocysts may still be shed after completion of a course of therapy with resolution of clinical signs. Treatment should persist in an attempt to stop fecal shedding of oocysts.

Acute General Treatment

- Parenteral fluid therapy to correct hypovolemia, electrolyte imbalances, and acid-base disturbances if present
- Antiprotozoal and antibiotic agents are effective.
  - Azithromycin 7-15 mg/kg PO q 12h for 5-7 days, current drug of choice for human cryptosporidiosis. Studies in cats have not been performed, but efficacy would be expected.
  - Paromomycin 125-165 mg/kg PO q 12h for 5 days was the traditional drug of choice, but because of side effects, has fallen from favor
  - Tylosin 11 mg/kg PO q 12h for 28 days, helpful in treatment of diarrhea only
  - Nitazoxanide successfully used in human infections, but dosage for cats and dogs unknown

Chronic Treatment

Treatment of concurrent intestinal dysbiosis/antibiotic-responsive enteritis/small-intestinal bacterial overgrowth (e.g., metronidazole 10-15 mg/kg PO q 12-24h for 5-7 days) (p. 260) may be beneficial in addition to treatment for *Cryptosporidium*.

Nutrition/Diet

Feeding a highly digestible diet is recommended in addition to pharmacotherapy in cats with severe clinical signs of chronic infection.

Possible Complications

Chronic infection: intestinal intussusception or lymphangiectasia is possible.

Recommended Monitoring

- Fecal analysis is recommended after treatment to determine whether oocyst shedding is still occurring.
- Another fecal analysis may be required if diarrhea persists and/or recurs after treatment.
- Animals with chronic infection should be re-evaluated at frequent intervals to assess progress.

PROGNOSIS & OUTCOME

Prognosis is good with treatment in cats that do not have FeLV/FIV infection. Prognosis is guarded with protein-losing enteropathy and weight loss.

PEARLS & CONSIDERATIONS

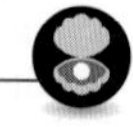

Comments

- This disease occurs predominantly in immunocompromised cats.
- Disease has also been reported in young puppies secondary to immunocompromise from other diseases.
- Glucocorticoids and other immunosuppressive agents should be avoided until infection is resolved.

Prevention

- This is a disease that is prevalent in overcrowded and unsanitary conditions, and reducing environmental contamination with improved sanitation is an important aspect of prevention.
- Although 5% ammonia will kill parasites, it requires 18 hours of contact for effect. Higher concentrations of ammonia are required if contact time is shortened. *Cryptosporidium* is resistant to 5.25% sodium hypochlorite (commercial bleach).

Technician Tips

- *Cryptosporidium* oocysts are yeastlike in appearance when evaluated on a wet mount.
- The cysts are about 4-6 microns in diameter (one-half of the diameter of a red blood cell), and oil immersion must be used to detect.

Client Education

- Potential for zoonosis
- Caution with immunosuppressed individuals and young children (greatest potential for infection)

SUGGESTED READING

Scorza V, et al: Cryptosporidiosis and cyclosporiasis. In Greene CE, editor: Infectious diseases of the dog and cat, ed 4, St. Louis, 2012, Saunders, pp 840-851.

AUTHOR: Saralyn Smith-Carr, DVM, PhD, DACVIM
EDITOR: Rance K. Sellon, DVM, PhD, DACVIM

Cutaneous Adverse Drug Reaction

BASIC INFORMATION

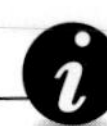

Definition

Development of cutaneous or mucocutaneous lesions after drug administration (topical, oral, inhalation, or injectable). The lesions may be limited to the cutaneous/mucocutaneous areas or may be part of a systemic reaction. These uncommon reactions can be predictable (pharmacologic) or unpredictable (idiosyncratic).

Synonyms

Drug eruption, drug allergy

Epidemiology

SPECIES, AGE, SEX

The incidence of cutaneous adverse drug reactions (CADRs) in dogs and cats with skin diseases has been reported as 2% and 1.6%, respectively. It is likely that many cases of CADR go unrecognized and unreported.

GENETICS, BREED PREDISPOSITION

No clear breed predisposition

RISK FACTORS

The number of drugs administered, a concomitant infection suppressing the immune system, or other immunosuppressive state might increase the risk of developing a CADR. Metabolic or enzymatic dysfunctions may predispose to a CADR.

Clinical Presentation

HISTORY, CHIEF COMPLAINT

- History of drug administration
- The chief complaint is variable because of the wide spectrum of clinical signs.

PHYSICAL EXAM FINDINGS

Several clinical presentations have been described:

- Erythroderma/exfoliative dermatitis: localized or diffuse erythema that can lead to scales, crusts, and alopecia
- Urticaria/angioedema: edematous papules and wheals or hives; variable erythema and pruritus. Angioedema is usually localized to head and face.
- Maculopapular eruptions: usually erythematous, pruritic or not
- Pruritus: localized or widespread, can lead to self-induced lesions
- Autoimmune-like (pemphigus-like, pemphigoid reactions, lupus-like reactions): clinical presentation varies from pustules and crusts to vesicles, bullae, and ulcers, depending on the autoimmune dermatosis mimicked.
- Erythema multiforme (EM) and Stevens-Johnson syndrome/toxic epidermal necrolysis (SJS/TEN): spectra of diseases manifested by an acute reaction pattern of skin and mucous membranes. EM is characterized by erythematous maculopapules and flat or raised annular or polycyclic lesions, with minimal epidermal detachment. SJS/TEN involves widespread erythema, blistering, and severe epidermal detachment.
- Fixed reactions: well-demarcated erythematous lesions sometimes associated with blistering and necrosis
- Injection-site reactions: local reaction characterized by alopecia, inflammation, necrosis, or ulceration
- Vasculitis: purpura, necrosis, and punctate ulcers, especially localized over extremities, pressure points, and oral mucosa; may be painful (p. 1031)
- Sweet and Wells syndromes: characterized by a neutrophilic and eosinophilic dermatitis, respectively. Erythema, plaques, nodules; may be painful
- Contact dermatitis: edema, erythema, papules, and vesicles localized in the area of direct contact with the offending drug. Secondary lesions may develop with chronicity.

Etiology and Pathophysiology

- Although some drugs are more frequently associated with drug reactions (e.g., sulfonamides), any drug might cause a CADR.
- CADR may be immediate after first administration, after weeks to months of administration without prior apparent reaction, or a few days after the drug is discontinued.
- The predictable (pharmacologic) reactions are related to the pharmacologic actions of the drugs and are more common. They are associated with the dose, the pharmacologic side effects/toxicity, or drug interactions and resolve when the drugs are discontinued.
- The unpredictable (idiosyncratic) reactions are usually considered immunologically mediated. They can also be associated with individual genetic differences in the metabolism of drugs, leading to inappropriate generation or accumulation of toxic metabolites (e.g., *MDR1/ABCB1-Δ* gene mutation [p. 638] in collies and other herding breeds).

DIAGNOSIS

Diagnostic Overview

- The key elements necessary for identifying a CADR are a thorough history, including drug administration and appropriate timing for the development of skin eruptions; a lack of alternative explanations for the lesions; and dechallenge, with resolution of skin lesions within 1-2 weeks. Rechallenging with the suspected drug confirms the diagnosis but is generally not recommended.
- A human drug scoring system has been evaluated in veterinary dermatology. It has variable sensitivity (0%-50%) and specificity (53%-100%). It should not be used for confirming the diagnosis.

Differential Diagnosis

- Erythroderma/exfoliative dermatitis: epitheliotropic lymphoma
- Urticaria/angioedema, maculopapular eruptions, pruritus: hypersensitivity disorders, ectoparasitosis, superficial bacterial or fungal infection, and mast cell tumor
- Autoimmune skin diseases: spontaneous autoimmune disease not related to drugs (more common)
- EM and SJS/TEN: superficial and deep infection (bacterial and fungal), urticaria, autoimmune skin diseases, burns, ulcerative stomatitis, and epitheliotropic lymphoma
- Fixed reactions: contact dermatitis, hypersensitivity disorders, pyoderma, and fungal infection
- Injection-site reactions: traction alopecia, hypersensitivity disorders, pyoderma, dermatophytosis, alopecia areata, and neoplasia
- Vasculitis: urticaria, autoimmune skin diseases, EM, SJS/TEN, disseminated intravascular coagulation, coagulopathy, frostbite, and neoplasia
- Contact dermatitis: ectoparasites, hypersensitivity disorders, bacterial overgrowth, superficial fungal infection

Initial Database

- History of drug administration before onset of skin lesions (at least 7 days before development of skin lesions if never administered before)
- Routine dermatologic diagnostics (skin scrapings, skin cytology, skin biopsy, fungal culture) based on differential diagnosis
- Although a wide range of histologic patterns exists in CADR, skin biopsies can help confirm the diagnosis or exclude differential diagnoses.

Advanced or Confirmatory Testing

- Suspected vasculitis: rickettsial titers, if other clinical signs suggestive
- Suspected systemic lupus erythematosus: antinuclear antibody test
- Cats: feline immunodeficiency virus (FIV)/feline leukemia virus (FeLV) serology

TREATMENT

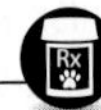

Treatment Overview

Stop the pharmacologic or immunologic reactions causing the drug eruption.

Acute General Treatment

- Discontinue use of the offending medication and other chemically related medications.
- Supportive care as needed (e.g., fluid therapy, nutritional support, analgesics, antipruritic therapy, wound care)

- Consider short-term glucocorticoid or immunosuppressive therapy if severe pruritus or immune-mediated dermatosis exists and concurrent infection is absent.
- Immunomodulatory therapy can be beneficial for EM, SJS/TEN, injection-site reactions, or vasculitis.

PROGNOSIS & OUTCOME

Good, unless internal organs are affected or there is extensive epidermal necrosis

PEARLS & CONSIDERATIONS

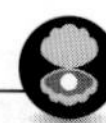

Comments

- Avoid future use of the offending medication or chemically related drugs.
- Hospitalization may be indicated.

Technician Tips

If ulcers/wounds are present, they should be kept clean and protected from potential self-mutilation.

SUGGESTED READING

Miller WH, et al: Muller & Kirk's Small animal dermatology, ed 7, St. Louis, 2013, Saunders, pp 466-472.

AUTHOR: Frédéric Sauvé, DMV, MSc, DES, DACVD
EDITOR: Manon Paradis, DMV, MVSc, DACVD

Cutaneous Lupus Erythematosus

BASIC INFORMATION

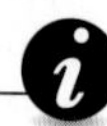

Definition

- Cutaneous lupus erythematosus (CLE) is a chronic, inflammatory, autoimmune skin disease with a broad spectrum of clinical manifestations and a variable course. None of the five forms described to date progress to systemic lupus erythematosus (SLE).
  - Discoid lupus erythematosus (DLE) is a relatively benign skin disease with no systemic involvement. A generalized form of DLE (GDLE) has been characterized.
  - Mucocutaneous lupus erythematosus (MCLE) manifests as chronic juxtamucosal erosive lesions.
  - Two other forms, exfoliative cutaneous lupus erythematosus (ECLE) and vesicular cutaneous lupus erythematosus (VCLE), can be debilitating and potentially fatal.

Epidemiology

SPECIES, AGE, SEX

- Uncommon in dogs; rare in cats
- Adults (DLE and VCLE); female/male ratio = 2.4 : 1 (VCLE)

GENETICS, BREED PREDISPOSITION

Breeds include German shepherd (MCLE), Siberian Husky, Brittany spaniel, collies, and Australian herding breeds (DLE); German short-haired pointer (ECLE); rough collie and Shetland sheepdog (VCLE).

RISK FACTORS

Breed, exposure to ultraviolet (UV) light

GEOGRAPHY AND SEASONALITY

More common in summer months and sunny climates

Clinical Presentation

HISTORY, CHIEF COMPLAINT

Lesions on the nasal planum +/− bridge of the nose (DLE), multifocal to generalized (GDLE), urogenital or perianal (MCLE), generalized scaling (ECLE), or ulcerative skin lesions of the axillae and groin (VCLE)

PHYSICAL EXAM FINDINGS

- DLE: usually localized to the nasal planum (unhaired, rostral surface of the nose). Less commonly, lip folds, oral cavity, periocular area, pinnae, genitalia, and rarely distal limbs
  - Erythema, depigmentation, and scaling of the nasal planum with or without involvement of the bridge of the nose. Early depigmentation manifests as a change in color from normal black to gray/white; there is a change in surface texture of the nasal planum from the normal, rough, cobblestone-like appearance to a smooth, shiny surface.
  - Scaling and crusting may be present at the junction between nasal planum and haired skin. Dogs with DLE are otherwise healthy.
- GDLE: generalized multifocal, annular (discoid) to polycyclic plaques with pigment changes, erythematous margin, adherent scaling, follicular plugging, and central alopecia
- MCLE: erosions and ulcers in the perigenital, perianal regions. Affects dogs most commonly in mid-adulthood
- ECLE: initially there is scaling on the face, pinnae, and dorsum, progressing to a more generalized distribution. Peripheral lymphadenopathy and fever may be present.
- VCLE: characteristic lesions include annular, polycyclic, and serpiginous ulcerations distributed over sparsely haired areas of the body, specifically the ventral abdomen, axilla, groin, and concave aspects of the pinna.

Etiology and Pathophysiology

- Pathogenesis is thought to involve autoreactive T cells that stimulate B cells to produce antibodies to a number of nuclear proteins.
- UV light may initiate the process of expression in photosensitive individuals (50% of cases).
- Antibodies are deposited in the basement membrane, and epidermal basal layer cells are subsequently damaged. This results in subepidermal vesicle formation and immune complex deposition in the basement membrane zone.

DIAGNOSIS

Diagnostic Overview

A strong suspicion exists on physical examination alone. The differential diagnosis varies according to the type of CLE. Biopsy for histopathologic evaluation is the confirmatory test of choice.

Differential Diagnosis

- Bacterial infection: mucocutaneous pyoderma (DLE), staphylococcal folliculitis
- Immune-mediated diseases: systemic lupus erythematosus, pemphigus foliaceus and erythematosus
- Drug reaction, uveodermatologic syndrome
- Vitiligo
- Neoplasia: squamous cell carcinoma, epitheliotropic lymphoma (DLE)
- Trauma
- Dermatophytosis
- Demodicosis
- Dermatomyositis (collie and Shetland sheepdog)
- Nasal parakeratosis in Labrador retriever (DLE)

Initial Database

- Deep skin scrapings (p. 1091)
- Skin cytology (impression smear)
- Dermatophyte culture
- Routine CBC, serum biochemistry profile, and urinalysis: generally unremarkable
- Serum antinuclear antibody test: usually negative (helps rule out SLE)

Advanced or Confirmatory Testing

- Biopsy (under general anesthesia for DLE) for histopathologic evaluation, which is the gold standard for diagnosis. The typical lesional patterns are a lymphocyte-rich interface dermatitis along the dermoepidermal junction,

hair follicles, and adnexal glands in conjunction with hydropic degeneration and apoptosis in the basal cell layer in DLE
- Focal immunoglobulin G (IgG) deposition in the basement membrane zone for MCLE (immunohistochemistry)
- Hyperkeratosis and lymphocytic interface dermatitis in ECLE; and a lymphocyte-rich interface dermatitis and folliculitis with vesiculation at the dermal-epidermal junction in VCLE
- Immunohistochemistry may be required.
- Biopsy for fungal and bacterial culture (DLE)

TREATMENT

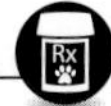

Treatment Overview

Control and resolution of existing lesions are the goals of treatment. More than one therapeutic modality may be necessary. Typically, secondary/concurrent infections are treated first if present, and immunosuppression is the cornerstone of treatment.

Acute General Treatment

DLE:
- Routine antibiotic therapy (e.g., cephalexin 22-30 mg/kg PO q 8-12h for 30 days) to rule out mucocutaneous pyoderma
- If no or only partial improvement is noticed, a potent topical glucocorticoid (e.g., betamethasone or 0.1% amcinonide) can be used. Switch to a low-potency product (e.g., 1% hydrocortisone cream) after a favorable response is noted. If long-term topical glucocorticoid is not an option, the following treatment can be attempted.
- Topical tacrolimus, 0.1% ointment (Protopic) q 12h initially, wean based on a favorable response
- Vitamin E 400-800 IU/day
- Essential fatty acids (n3 EFA, eicosapentaenoic acid) 30 mg/kg PO q 24h
- Tetracycline and niacinamide: dogs > 10 kg, 500 mg (<10 kg, 250 mg) of each drug PO q 8h. May take 6-8 weeks to produce improvement. If good response, wean gradually (several weeks). Doxycycline 5-10 mg/kg PO q 24h as an alternative to tetracycline
- In refractory cases, systemic glucocorticoids: prednisone 1.7-2 mg/kg/d PO initially, then wean based on a favorable response. Concomitant azathioprine 1-2 mg/kg PO q 24-48h while administering prednisone

GDLE:
- Lesions respond to a variety of treatments, including cyclosporine, hydroxychloroquine, topical tacrolimus, and oral tetracycline/niacinamide

MCLE: as for DLE

ECLE and VCLE:
- Oral immunosuppressive doses of prednisone 1.7-2 mg/kg are the first choice, with appropriate antibiotic therapy (p. 851).
- Cyclosporine 5-10 mg/kg q 24h
- Azathioprine 1-2 mg/kg, q 24-48h or cyclosporine 5 mg/kg PO q 12h may be added if lesions persist. Some form of combination therapy will likely be required in most cases.
- Hydroxychloroquine 5 mg/kg q 24h. Assess retinal function (possibly toxic).

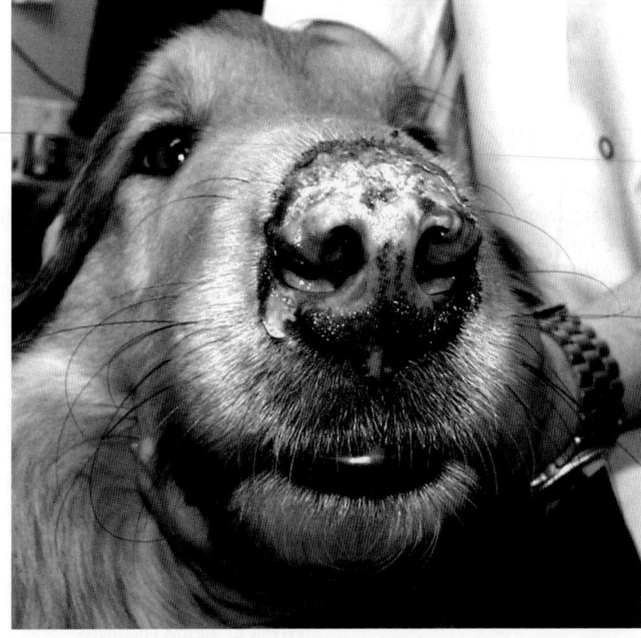

CUTANEOUS LUPUS ERYTHEMATOSUS Discoid lupus erythematosus in a collie. Note the depigmentation, erosion, and crusting of the nasal planum. (Copyright Dr. Manon Paradis.)

Chronic Treatment

- Avoid intense sunlight (e.g., 8 AM-5 PM).
- Topical sunscreens if sunlight exposure is unavoidable
- Bilateral rotational nasal flaps for refractory cases (DLE)

Possible Complications

- Nasal cartilage erosion and arteriole hemorrhage (DLE)
- Squamous cell carcinoma (DLE)
- Septicemia (VCLE)
- Iatrogenic hyperadrenocorticism with chronic glucocorticoid use

Recommended Monitoring

- Routine CBC and serum biochemistry profiles if using azathioprine. Initially assessed q 14 days, reducing to q 3 months when condition is stable
- High-dose glucocorticoids are rarely required, but appropriate serum biochemistry profiles and urinalysis should be used in such cases.
- With chronic use of intermediate- or long-acting topical glucocorticoid application, adrenal function should be monitored.

PROGNOSIS & OUTCOME

- DLE and GDLE: good, but may require chronic therapy
- MCLE: good but relapses are common with tapering therapy
- VCLE: guarded
- ECLE: poor

PEARLS & CONSIDERATIONS

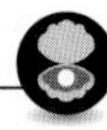

Comments

- Dogs with DLE typically feel and act well; the disorder is usually confined to the nasal planum.
- Depigmentation on the inner surfaces of the nostrils accompanied by nasal discharge suggests an intranasal problem (e.g., nasal aspergillosis) rather than DLE.
- In the past, many cases of mucocutaneous pyoderma and nasal parakeratosis have been wrongly diagnosed as DLE.
- Oral antibiotic trial is required before skin biopsies of the nasal planum, particularly in German shepherd dogs.

Technician Tips

Dogs may quickly lick topical medications applied to the rostral nose, reducing their efficacy (and causing systemic absorption). Application of a thin film of topical creams or liquids to the nasal planum (using gloves with immunosuppressant drugs such as tacrolimus) should be followed by distraction of the patient, feeding of a small treat, or other measures to reduce the likelihood of immediately licking away the medication.

Client Education

- Avoid intense ultraviolet light.
- Use sunscreen.

SUGGESTED READING

Olivry T, et al. Cutaneous lupus erythematosus in dogs: a comprehensive review. BMC Vet Res 14:132-150, 2018.

AUTHOR: Michael Hannigan, BVMS
EDITOR: Manon Paradis, DMV, MVSc, DACVD

Cutaneous Neoplasia

Bonus Material Online 

BASIC INFORMATION

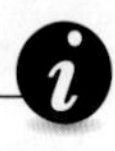

Definition

Benign or malignant tumor arising from cells within the skin and adnexa. The most common cutaneous neoplasms in dogs are, in descending order of frequency, lipoma, sebaceous gland hyperplasia/adenoma, mast cell tumor, histiocytoma, and papilloma. In cats, basal cell tumors are the most common, followed by squamous cell carcinoma, mast cell tumor, and fibrosarcoma. Squamous cell carcinoma (p. 939) and mast cell tumor (canine [p. 634] and feline [p. 632]) are discussed separately.

Synonyms

- Basal cell tumor: basal cell epithelioma
- Infundibular keratinizing acanthoma: keratoacanthoma, intracutaneous cornifying epithelioma

Epidemiology

SPECIES, AGE, SEX

- Dogs: 30% of all tumors arise within the skin.
- Cats: 20% of all tumors arise within the skin.
- Median age for cutaneous neoplasia is 10.5 years for dogs and 12 years for cats.
- Predisposition for histiocytoma in young dogs

GENETICS, BREED PREDISPOSITION

- Canine breeds with highest incidence of skin tumors include the boxer, Scottish terrier, bullmastiff, Weimaraner, Kerry blue terrier, and Norwegian elkhound.
- Shar-peis tend to develop mast cell tumors at a younger age (mean, 4 years).
- Feline breeds with highest incidence are Siamese and Persian.
- Infundibular keratinizing acanthoma: generalized form may have a hereditary basis in Norwegian elkhound and keeshond. German shepherds and Old English sheepdogs also develop the generalized form.

RISK FACTORS

- Basal cell carcinoma: a strong correlation in humans exists between exposure to ultraviolet light and tumor development. This association has not been established in dogs and cats.
- Cutaneous hemangioma/hemangiosarcoma: short-coated dogs with nonpigmented skin in sun-exposed areas such as the glabrous (hairless) skin of the ventral abdomen and white cats are at higher risk.

Clinical Presentation

DISEASE FORMS/SUBTYPES

- Basal cell tumors: benign or malignant (basal cell carcinoma) tumors arising from the pluripotential basal epithelial cells in the epidermis and adnexa
- Hemangioma/hemangiosarcoma: benign or malignant neoplasms arising from endothelial cells of blood vessels
- Histiocytoma: benign neoplasm that arises from epidermal Langerhans cells
- Infundibular keratinizing acanthoma: benign neoplasms of hair follicle origin
- Trichoepithelioma: benign neoplasms that arise from keratinocytes that differentiate toward all three segments of the hair follicle
- Sebaceous gland hyperplasia/adenoma: epithelial growths arising from sebocytes

HISTORY, CHIEF COMPLAINT

Solitary to multiple cutaneous masses

PHYSICAL EXAM FINDINGS

- Basal cell tumor: solitary, well-circumscribed, firm to cystic, alopecic, commonly ulcerated, often pigmented mass, typically located on the head, neck, shoulders, or thorax. In cats, malignant lesions also can occur on the nasal planum and eyelids.
- Cutaneous hemangioma/hemangiosarcoma: dermal or subcutaneous, solitary or multiple, oval masses or red to dark red plaques, usually located along the limbs and ventral abdomen. In cats, bluish to reddish black nodules to plaques
- Histiocytoma: solitary, well-circumscribed, firm, erythematous, intradermal nodule found most frequently on the head, limbs, and thorax. Fast growing but benign. Occasionally observed as multiple cutaneous nodules or plaques
- Infundibular keratinizing acanthoma: most commonly found on the back, neck, thorax, and limbs. Well-circumscribed dermal or subcutaneous masses with a pore opening to the skin surface; pore usually consists of a keratin plug; not metastatic
- Trichoepithelioma: usually solitary, solid or cystic, elevated, round, and well circumscribed; frequently becomes ulcerated and alopecic
- Sebaceous gland tumors: solitary or multiple, raised, wartlike to smooth, may ulcerate; most commonly found on limbs, trunk, eyelids, head

Etiology and Pathophysiology

- Neoplastic transformation relies on changes in specific growth-regulating genes.
- Principal growth-regulating genes include
  - Oncogenes that code for proteins that increase growth
  - Tumor-suppressor genes that decrease proliferation and differentiation

DIAGNOSIS

Diagnostic Overview

The only way to distinguish benign neoplasms from malignant neoplasms and non-neoplastic proliferative skin disease is histopathologic examination of biopsy tissue samples. Malignant lesions typically show sudden onset, rapid invasive growth, infiltration, +/− metastasis.

Differential Diagnosis

- Bacterial and fungal granulomas
- Abscesses
- Sterile granuloma
- Pyogranuloma syndrome
- Sterile nodular panniculitis

Initial Database

- CBC, serum biochemistry profile, urinalysis (if indicated): assess systemic abnormalities
- Cytologic exam (fine-needle aspiration):
  - Basal cell tumor: small, round to cuboidal epithelial cells arranged in groups or ribbons. Basal cell carcinomas are difficult to differentiate cytologically from benign lesions.
  - Histiocytoma: sheets of round cells with a pale blue cytoplasm and variable sizes and shapes of the nuclei; variable numbers of neutrophils and lymphocytes, depending on stage of growth and involution
  - Sebaceous gland hyperplasia: clusters of lipid sebocytes
- Histopathologic exam (biopsy)

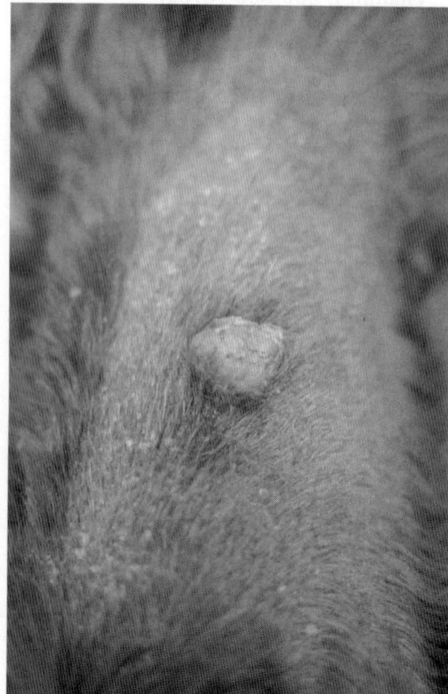

CUTANEOUS NEOPLASIA Sebaceous adenoma along the dorsal tail of a 7-year-old Labrador retriever. (Copyright Dr. Ed Jazic.)

- Basal cell tumor: well-circumscribed, symmetrical proliferation of basal epithelial cells that has a broad zone of connection to the overlying epidermis
- Basal cell carcinoma: circumscribed, irregular dermal mass comprising multiple epithelial cell aggregates embedded in a fibrous stroma that may extend into the underlying subcutis
- Hemangioma: proliferation of blood-filled vascular spaces lined by single layers of well-differentiated endothelial cells
- Hemangiosarcoma: invasive proliferation of atypical endothelial cells with areas of vascular space formation
- Histiocytoma: uniform sheets and cords of histiocytes infiltrating the dermis and subcutis; characteristic high mitotic index
- Infundibular keratinizing acanthoma: keratin-filled crypt in the dermis that has an opening to the skin surface

Advanced or Confirmatory Testing

Abdominal and cardiac ultrasonography to determine whether hemangiosarcoma lesions are primary or metastatic

TREATMENT

Treatment Overview

Treatment typically should be localized for local disease. Systemic attack on cancer should be reserved for generalized disease or disease in which local therapy alone is not likely to be curative. Treatment options include surgery, chemotherapy, radiation therapy, cryosurgery, electrosurgery, immunotherapy, and combinations thereof or observation.

Acute General Treatment

- Basal cell tumor: surgical excision is curative.
- Hemangioma: surgical excision, cryotherapy, or electrosurgery is usually curative.
- Hemangiosarcoma: aggressive surgical excision is treatment of choice; complete excision of subcutaneous tumor is difficult.
- Histiocytoma: spontaneous remission may occur within 3 months. Surgical excision is curative for lesions that do not regress.
- Infundibular keratinizing acanthoma: may resolve spontaneously. Surgical excision, cryosurgery, and observation without treatment are also options.
- Trichoepithelioma: surgical excision, cryosurgery, electrosurgery, or observation without treatment
- Sebaceous gland hyperplasia/adenoma: surgical excision, cryotherapy, or observation without treatment. May recur after surgery. Sebaceous gland carcinomas rarely metastasize.

Chronic Treatment

Hemangiosarcoma: see chemotherapy protocols and outcomes (p. 424).

Possible Complications

Hemangiosarcoma: local recurrence and metastasis are common in dogs; metastasis is rare in cats.

PROGNOSIS & OUTCOME

- Excised basal cell tumor and trichoepithelioma: generally very good
- Intradermal hemangiosarcoma: excellent
- Subcutaneous hemangiosarcoma: poor
- Excised solitary histiocytoma: excellent

PEARLS & CONSIDERATIONS

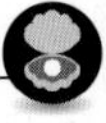

Comments

- The most effective way to separate benign neoplasms from malignant neoplasms and non-neoplastic proliferative skin disease is histopathologic examination of biopsied tissue.
- The key to successful management is an accurate diagnosis.
- Cytologic evaluation of smears may provide valuable information about the cell type.
- Immunohistochemistry has markedly improved the ability to determine progenitor cells for many skin neoplasms, with a positive impact on treatment selection and on prognostication in some cases.

Technician Tips

Fine-needle aspirates of subcutaneous masses cannot reliably be interpreted without a microscope. The water-droplet appearance on a glass slide of classic adipose tissue is also observed with mast cell tumors and other malignant tissues, not just lipomas. Routine staining and microscopic assessment are essential.

SUGGESTED READING

Miller WH Jr, et al: Muller & Kirk's Small animal dermatology, ed 7, St. Louis, 2013, Saunders, pp 774-843.

AUTHOR: Edward Jazic, DVM, DACVD
EDITOR: Manon Paradis, DMV, MVSc, DACVD

Cyanosis

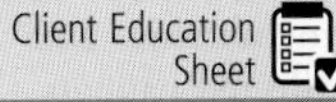

BASIC INFORMATION

Definition

A bluish or grayish discoloration of the mucous membranes or skin due to hypoxemia

Synonyms

Oxidized hemoglobin: oxygenated hemoglobin
Reduced hemoglobin: deoxygenated hemoglobin

Epidemiology

SPECIES, AGE, SEX

Dogs and cats of any age and either sex

GENETICS, BREED PREDISPOSITION

Predispositions for underlying causes of hypoxemia (e.g., idiopathic pulmonary fibrosis in West Highland white and Staffordshire terriers)

Clinical Presentation

DISEASE FORMS/SUBTYPES

- Generalized (central) cyanosis: all mucous membranes have a bluish tinge.
- Differential cyanosis: cyanosis of the caudal but not cranial half of the body; associated with Eisenmenger's syndrome (e.g., reverse patent ductus arteriosus) (p. 764)
- Regional (peripheral) cyanosis: localized hypoxia (e.g., vessel obstruction such as tourniquet's effect on a limb, thromboembolism [p. 74]) (not discussed further)

HISTORY, CHIEF COMPLAINT

- Exercise intolerance
- Respiratory distress
- Collapse
- Hindlimb collapse (e.g., unexplained periods of sitting during walks) in cases of differential cyanosis
- Syncope
- Visible cyanosis noted by owner

PHYSICAL EXAM FINDINGS

- By definition, cyanosis. Check oral mucous membranes and vaginal/preputial mucous membranes for differential cyanosis.
- Mild to severe dyspnea correlates with severity of the underlying problem.
  - An exception is right-to-left shunting heart disease, which may cause pronounced cyanosis even in a patient with minimal dyspnea.
  - Pattern of respiratory distress may suggest disease localization (e.g., inspiratory distress suggests upper airway obstruction).
  - Thoracic auscultation may suggest disease localization (e.g., crackles suggest pulmonary parenchymal disease, muffled lungs suggest pleural space disease).

 - Other findings depend on cause (e.g., flail chest, paralysis causing hypoventilation)
 - Heart murmur, gallop sound, arrhythmia, or pulse abnormalities possible with some cardiac causes
- Stunted growth if congenital cardiac shunts

Etiology and Pathophysiology

- Etiology (p. 231)
- Deoxygenated (reduced) hemoglobin is blue, whereas oxygenated (oxidized) hemoglobin is red.
- Cyanosis appears when the amount of deoxygenated hemoglobin increases in the blood.
 - The deep blue color of a deoxygenated hemoglobin molecule overwhelms the red color of an oxygenated hemoglobin molecule.
 - In a patient with a normal hematocrit, cyanosis is clinically apparent when the blood concentration of deoxygenated hemoglobin is > 5 g/dL (normal total blood hemoglobin concentration: 12.4-19.1 g/dL [dog], 8.5-14.4 g/dL [cat]).
- When cyanosis is observed, severe hypoxemia exists. In a patient with a normal hematocrit, cyanosis becomes apparent when PaO_2 < 50 mm Hg, which corresponds to SaO_2 ≈ 80% (normal PaO_2 = 90-100 mm Hg when breathing room air; normal SaO_2 > 95%).
- The *absolute* amount of deoxygenated hemoglobin determines the presence of cyanosis, not the proportion of total hemoglobin that is deoxygenated. In anemic patients, severe hypoxemia is needed to observe cyanosis, if at all. Conversely, animals with erythrocytosis can be cyanotic with proportionally less reduced hemoglobin or even under normal conditions.
- Carboxyhemoglobin, which is elevated in carbon monoxide poisoning, confers a cherry-colored flush to the skin and mucous membranes and may mask cyanosis in affected patients.

DIAGNOSIS

Diagnostic Overview

Cyanosis is recognized on physical exam. Beyond a history to suggest recent causes (e.g., smoke inhalation), a CBC (including examination of whole blood for methemoglobinemia, if relevant) and thoracic radiographs are usually of highest priority. A diagnostic approach is outlined on p. 1408.

Differential Diagnosis

- Methemoglobinemia from oxidative injury to red blood cells (e.g., acetaminophen toxicosis in cats) or congenital disorders
 - Methemoglobin gives a muddy color to the mucous membranes, which may be indistinguishable from cyanosis.
 - Gross appearance of the blood helps differentiate methemoglobinemia from cyanosis. A drop of blood is applied to a white paper towel. With cyanosis, dark blue blood becomes redder with exposure to oxygen, but the brown blood of methemoglobinemia remains dark.
- Normal pigmentation/melanin: differentiation involves evaluation of other, nonpigmented mucous membranes or measurement of an arterial blood gas sample for oxygen content.
- Normal pink mucous membranes: observed in certain lighting conditions (e.g., fluorescent lights) may falsely appear cyanotic.

Initial Database

- Thoracic and lateral cervical radiographs: identify airway or lung structural lesions
- CBC: clues indicating underlying disease or erythrocytosis due to chronic hypoxemia
- Arterial blood gas: confirm hypoxemia
- Echocardiography: identify cardiac shunts or other cardiac disease
- Oral and pharyngeal exam if upper airway dyspnea or apnea: identify and correct obstruction

TREATMENT

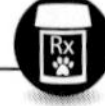

Treatment Overview

Correct critical hypoxemia and address cause.

Acute General Treatment

Oxygen supplementation (p. 1146): although usually beneficial, minimal/no response expected with right-to-left shunts

Chronic Treatment

Address underlying cause

Possible Complications

Worsening hypoxemia leading to respiratory arrest

Recommended Monitoring

Observation of respiratory effort, mucous membrane color, pulse oximetry

PROGNOSIS & OUTCOME

- Short term: guarded, because of hypoxemia
- Long term: varies widely, depending on underlying cause

PEARLS & CONSIDERATIONS

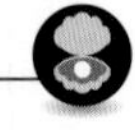

Comments

- Cyanosis depends on the absolute amount of deoxygenated hemoglobin in the circulation. Animals with hypoperfusion (e.g., shock) or anemia are less cyanotic despite severe hypoxemia, whereas animals with erythrocytosis may show cyanosis with minimal hypoxemia.
- A patient with marked cyanosis and minimal dyspnea should be suspected of having right-left shunting or methemoglobinemia.

Technician Tips

- Pulse oximetry and/or arterial blood gas measurements help quantify response to treatment but are not a replacement for careful observation of respiratory effort.
- Cyanotic patients are at risk for respiratory arrest with stress; avoid excessive restraint, dorsal positioning.

SUGGESTED READING

Tidholm A: Cyanosis. In Ettinger SJ, et al, editors: Textbook of veterinary internal medicine, ed 8, St. Louis, 2017, Elsevier, pp 210-213.

AUTHORS: Shauna Blois, DVM, DVSc, DACVIM; Etienne Côté, DVM, DACVIM
EDITOR: Leah A. Cohn, DVM, PhD, DACVIM

Cystitis, Bacterial

Client Education Sheet

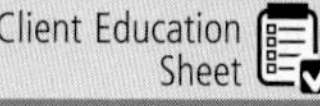

BASIC INFORMATION

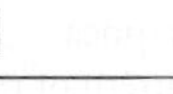

Definition

Bacterial infection of the urinary bladder, a disorder that is very common in dogs and less common in cats

Synonym

Lower urinary tract infection (UTI)

Epidemiology

SPECIES, AGE, SEX

- Dogs affected more often than cats
- Females affected more often than males

RISK FACTORS

- Bladder disease, including cystic calculi and neoplasia
- Congenital or acquired structural defects of the lower urinary tract
- Conditions causing formation of dilute urine, including diabetes mellitus and hyperadrenocorticism

- Immunosuppressive drug therapy, including glucocorticoids
- Disorders of micturition, including urine retention (physical or functional causes), urinary incontinence, and vulvar (or rarely, preputial) conformational abnormalities
- Bacteremia
- Prostatitis, vaginitis, pyometra, pyelonephritis
- Urinary catheterization, especially indwelling catheters
- Perineal urethrostomy

CONTAGION AND ZOONOSIS

Occasionally, clonally identical strains of uropathogenic *Escherichia coli* are transmitted between human and animal members of a household.

ASSOCIATED DISORDERS

Struvite urolithiasis, pyelonephritis, emphysematous cystitis, prostatitis

Clinical Presentation

DISEASE FORMS/SUBTYPES

- Uncomplicated: first infection in the absence of structural or functional host defects
- Complicated: infection in a dog with structural or functional defects (see Risk Factors above), in any cat, or any recurrent or refractory UTI
- Recurrent: repeated infections with the same (relapse) or different (reinfection) species of bacteria
- Refractory: persistent infection with the same bacteria despite antibiotic treatment
- Subclinical bacteriuria: positive bacterial urine culture for an animal with no clinical evidence of infection

HISTORY, CHIEF COMPLAINT

- Signs encountered most commonly include
  - Pollakiuria
  - Stranguria/dysuria
  - Hematuria
  - Inappropriate elimination
  - Malodorous urine
  - Perivulvar dermatitis
- If clinical signs absent, subclinical bacteriuria is a more appropriate diagnosis than cystitis/UTI; treatment generally not required.

PHYSICAL EXAM FINDINGS

- Usually unremarkable
- Occasionally: findings related to associated illness or condition (e.g., findings suggestive of endocrine disorder, urolithiasis, prostatitis)
- Rarely
  - Painful bladder
  - Palpably thickened urethra on rectal exam (concurrent urethritis)

Etiology and Pathophysiology

- Infecting bacteria usually ascend through the urethra to the bladder, but hematogenous infection or infection from pyelonephritis is possible.
- Bacterial virulence factors influence likelihood of infection. Flora adapted for preputial and vaginal environments are protective from uropathogenic infection.
- Multiple physical (e.g., intact uroepithelium, voiding action of urination, urethral pressure and length), chemical (e.g., urine osmolality, urea content, pH), and immunologic host defenses protect from infection. Disruption or defects in these defenses predispose to infection.
- The most common pathogens are *E. coli, Staphylococcus, Proteus, Enterococcus, Klebsiella, Streptococcus, Enterobacter,* and *Pseudomonas.* Only ≈20% of infections involve more than one species.
- Bacterial resistance to antibiotics can be problematic. Resistance may be inherent or may result from genetic transfer of resistance factors or from mutation and selection pressures.

DIAGNOSIS

Diagnostic Overview

In animals with signs of dysuria, cystitis is often recognized on urinalysis (obtained by cystocentesis, catheter, or midstream catch) as bacteriuria and pyuria. Urine culture and susceptibility are indicated for all complicated UTIs. Absence of bacteriuria cannot rule out UTI, especially when urine is poorly concentrated.

Differential Diagnosis

- Urolithiasis
- Prostatitis
- Lower urinary tract neoplasia (e.g., transitional cell carcinoma)
- Feline lower urinary tract signs/disease; interstitial cystitis
- Obstructive uropathy

Initial Database

- CBC and serum biochemistry profile: unnecessary for uncomplicated cystitis; may reflect predisposing illness or condition in complicated infections
- Urinalysis: bacteriuria, pyuria, hematuria, and/or proteinuria. Sample should be obtained by midstream catch (clean perineum first), clean catheterization, or cystocentesis (ideal unless bladder cancer or coagulopathy suspected).
  - May reflect predisposing illness or condition (e.g., crystals, glucosuria)
  - Sediment exam may be inactive despite infection, especially with diabetes mellitus, hyperadrenocorticism, or other conditions causing dilute urine.
  - Leukocyte squares on urine dipstick are notoriously inaccurate.
- Gram stain of urine sediment
- Urine culture/susceptibility
  - Samples should be collected by clean catheterization or cystocentesis (ideal unless bladder neoplasia or bleeding disorder suspected). Bacterial number should be quantified to distinguish contamination ($<10^3$ bacteria/mL) from infection.
  - Although preferred, culture is not necessary for first occurrence of uncomplicated cystitis.
  - Culture/sensitivity should always be obtained from complicated UTI.
  - An inactive sediment does not eliminate the need for culture and sensitivity when UTI is suspected because many concurrent disorders produce dilute urine, limit leukocyte responses in the urine, or both, producing a negative microscopic sediment exam despite active cystitis.

Advanced or Confirmatory Testing

Reserved for complicated UTI, primarily with the intention of identifying risk factors:

- Abdominal radiographs: radiopaque uroliths, prostatomegaly, rarely emphysematous cystitis

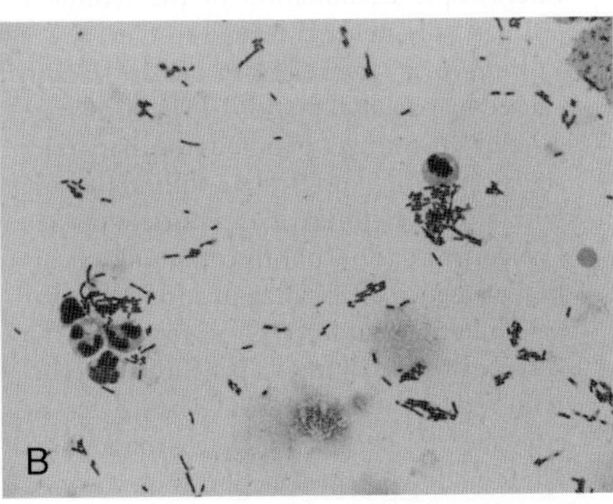

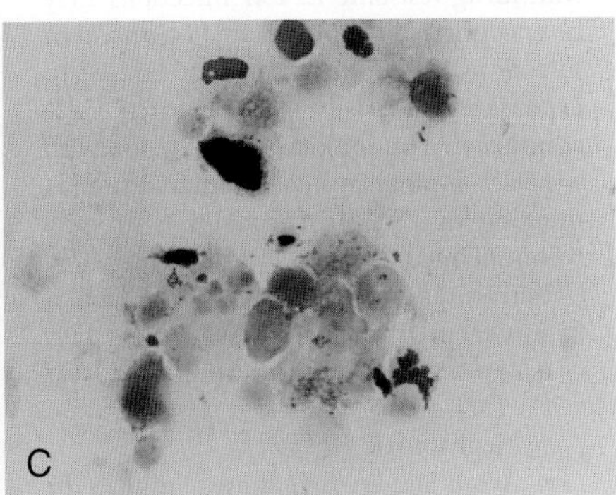

CYSTITIS, BACTERIAL Urinalysis for dogs with bacterial cystitis often demonstrates white blood cells (**A**) and bacteria: rods (**B**) and/or cocci (**C**). Gram stain can inform the initial antimicrobial choice while awaiting results of culture and susceptibility.

- Abdominal ultrasound: identify radiolucent uroliths, thickened bladder wall or mass, evidence of pyelonephritis or prostatic disease
- Urinary contrast studies: identify radiolucent uroliths, bladder mass, evidence of pyelonephritis, urethral abnormalities

TREATMENT

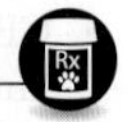

Treatment Overview

Most uncomplicated UTIs respond readily to a short course of antimicrobial drugs. Complicated UTI may be very difficult to cure.

Acute General Treatment

Antibiotic choices appropriate for empirical treatment of uncomplicated infection or pending culture/sensitivity results in complicated infection:

- Gram-positive infections: amoxicillin 15-20 mg/kg PO q 8 -12h
- Gram-negative infections: amoxicillin or trimethoprim-sulfadiazine (TMS) 15-30 mg/kg q 12h. Although often effective, fluoroquinolones reserved for UTI resistant to amoxicillin or TMS
- Cefovecin 8 mg/kg SQ once has been used off-label with good success (*Enterococcus* spp and *Pseudomonas* spp will be resistant).
- Avoid antimicrobials with hepatic or gastrointestinal rather than renal elimination (e.g., tetracyclines).

Chronic Treatment

- Predisposing illnesses or conditions should be addressed.
- Duration of antibiotic therapy
  - Uncomplicated: 5-7 days; shorter courses may be adequate
  - Complicated: optimum duration unknown; historically, 4 weeks or more suggested but shorter courses (5-10 days) likely adequate
- Antibiotic therapy is adjusted based on *in vitro* susceptibility results while considering cost-effectiveness, potential adverse reactions, and the likelihood of developing resistance. Fluoroquinolones are often useful for complicated infection. Enrofloxacin 5-20 mg/kg PO q 24h (dogs); pradofloxacin 3-5 (tablet) or 5-7.5 (suspension) mg/kg PO q 24h (cats)
- Multidrug-resistant *E. coli* infections may be encountered in complicated or persistent infections. Susceptibility may be limited to expensive, potentially toxic, or parenterally administered antibiotics. Consultation with specialist in small animal internal medicine, microbiology, or pharmacology is strongly recommended:
  - Nitrofurantoin 4.4-5 mg/kg PO q 8h
  - Amikacin 15-30 mg/kg SQ (or IV, IM) q 24h or gentamicin 2-6 mg/kg SQ (or IV, IM) q 24h
    - Nephrotoxic
    - Avoid use in dehydrated animals or those with compromised renal function.
  - Meropenem 8.5 mg/kg SQ (or IV) q 8-12h
  - Fosfomycin tromethamine may be useful for *E. coli* UTI: 40 mg/kg PO q 12h for 3 days
- Other therapies may be used to reduce recurrence (see Prevention below).

Possible Complications

- Emphysematous cystitis: rare complication resulting in gas formation in bladder wall; most often identified in diabetic animals
- Pyelonephritis: vesicoureteral junction usually prevents bacterial ascension to kidneys
- Urolithiasis: struvite
- Adverse reactions to antibiotics are possible (e.g., TMS may cause keratoconjunctivitis sicca, gentamicin is nephrotoxic, enrofloxacin is detrimental to cartilage in growing dogs and, in high doses, may irreversibly damage the feline retina).

Recommended Monitoring

- For uncomplicated infection, monitoring clinical signs is adequate.
- For complicated infection, urinalysis may be repeated 7-10 days after completion of therapy. Even if bacteriuria persists, in the absence of clinical signs, additional antimicrobials are likely unnecessary. If signs persist, repeat culture.
- Periodic urine culture is no longer routinely recommended for animals with risk factors for UTI but without lower urinary signs.

PROGNOSIS & OUTCOME

- Prognosis for uncomplicated infection is excellent.
- Prognosis for complicated infection depends on ability to correct predisposing illness or condition.

PEARLS & CONSIDERATIONS

Comments

- Any bacterial cystitis in a male dog should be viewed as a complicated infection with potential for prostatic involvement.
- Struvite crystalluria in dogs is most commonly due to bacterial UTI or delayed microscopic examination of the sediment and virtually never is related to diet.
- Lower urinary tract signs in cats are seldom caused by bacterial cystitis (<5% of cats age 10 years or younger with lower urinary tract signs), making empirical antibiotic therapy without urine culture inappropriate in cats.
- Concurrent pyelonephritis commonly occurs in the absence of classic signs such as lumbar pain, intermittent fever, or neutrophilia. The absence of these signs in a patient with recurrent bacterial cystitis should not defer an evaluation for pyelonephritis (e.g., abdominal ultrasound) when pyelonephritis is otherwise suspected (e.g., azotemia).
- Many antibiotics are present in high concentration in the urine as a result of renal excretion:
  - Disk diffusion assays of sensitivity usually evaluate expected serum drug concentration, and sensitivity of a uropathogen *in vivo* may be greater than that predicted *in vitro*.
  - If expected urine concentration of antibiotic exceeds minimum inhibitory concentration by four times, the antibiotic should be effective.
- Persistent bacterial cystitis usually results from inappropriate choice of antibiotic or inadequate dose/duration of administration, emergence of bacterial resistance to the chosen antibiotic, or failure to correct underlying illness or condition allowing infection to occur.
- Subclinical bacteriuria is increasingly recognized in animals. Antimicrobial therapy is generally not needed in such cases and may do more harm than good.

Prevention

- Correction of predisposing illness or conditions is the most effective strategy to prevent infection.
- For animals in which predisposing factors cannot be corrected and recurrent infections are problematic, urinary antiseptics may be warranted:
  - Antiseptics (dogs): methenamine mandelate 10 mg/kg PO q 6-8h or methenamine hippurate 500 mg PO q 12h. Both effective in acidic urine; may require addition of ammonium chloride as acidifying agent (60-100 mg/kg q 12h). CAUTION: urinary acidification may precipitate formation of certain uroliths.
  - Alternative (unproven) therapies: cranberry juice concentrate, probiotics (oral or vaginal), D-mannose, *Coleus forskohlii* (herb), antiseptic instillation (e.g., Tricide-Neo)

Technician Tips

- When collecting midstream sample for urinalysis, first clip long hair and clean perineum.
- Urine culture is best collected by cystocentesis unless bleeding disorder or bladder neoplasia is suspected.

Client Education

Resolution of signs of dysuria is the most important piece of information to assess effective therapy. Owners should be vigilant in observation of related clinical signs.

SUGGESTED READING

Olin SJ, et al: Urinary tract infections: treatment/comparative therapeutics. Vet Clin North Am Small Anim Pract 45:721-746, 2015.

AUTHOR & EDITOR: Leah A. Cohn, DVM, PhD, DACVIM

Cytauxzoonosis

Bonus Material Online

BASIC INFORMATION

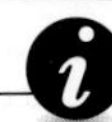

Definition

Cytauxzoon felis is a protozoal organism transmitted by ticks that causes potentially fatal illness in domestic cats.

Epidemiology

SPECIES, AGE, SEX

C. felis infects only domestic and wild cats, with no age or sex predisposition.

RISK FACTORS

Outdoor cats with tick exposure in endemic areas are at risk. Specific risk factors include urban-edge habitats and close proximity to wooded or unmanaged areas. It is common for multiple cats from the same household or neighborhood to become infected.

CONTAGION AND ZOONOSIS

Requires tick vector for transmission

GEOGRAPHY AND SEASONALITY

C. felis infection has been reported in the south central and southeastern United States, but its range appears to be expanding north and east, corresponding to changes in distribution of the tick *Amblyomma americanum*. Most cases occur between March and September, with a peak incidence between March and June and a second wave of infections occurring in August and September.

Clinical Presentation

DISEASE FORMS/SUBTYPES

- Acute cytauxzoonosis (classic severe illness)
- Chronic carrier state (cats recovered from illness or even discovered with incidental erythroparasitemia)

HISTORY, CHIEF COMPLAINT

Clinical signs are acute and nonspecific and include acute onset of anorexia, lethargy, dyspnea, icterus, and pallor. Cats may be reported to seem as if in pain.

PHYSICAL EXAM FINDINGS

- Affected cats are usually febrile (103°F-107°F [39.4°C-41.7°C]), but hypothermia is seen in moribund cats. Icterus and/or pallor are common, as is elevation of the nictitans.
- Abdominal palpation reveals splenomegaly and hepatomegaly.
- Tachypnea, tachycardia, altered mentation, vocalization, seizures, and coma can be seen in the later stages of disease.
- Most cases exhibit a rapid course, with death occurring within 1 week of onset of signs if left untreated.

Etiology and Pathophysiology

- The natural host is thought to be the eastern bobcat *(Lynx rufus rufus)*, which develops a mild or subclinical infection compared to the rapidly progressive and usually fatal disease seen in domestic cats.
- The organism is transmitted by *A. americanum* (suspected predominant vector) or *Dermacentor variabilis* ticks during feeding.
- Sporozoites released from the tick salivary glands infect macrophages.
- Asexual reproduction occurs within the host macrophage during the schizogenous phase, causing infected cells to grow to enormous size (≥250 microns in diameter). These schizont-laden macrophages then occlude arterioles, venules, and capillaries, causing organ failure and clinical illness.
- When the schizonts rupture, merozoites are released to infect erythrocytes. Merozoites are minimally pathogenic but may cause initial hemolysis.
- Healthy, recovered cats can harbor erythrocyte piroplasms for years; they can transmit the pathogen to ticks during feeding.

DIAGNOSIS

Diagnostic Overview

Early diagnosis through blood smear examination or aspiration of lymph nodes, spleen, or bone marrow is indicated when a clinical suspicion exists. Although most often diagnosed by microscopic identification of piroplasms in red blood cells (RBCs), illness can occur before appearance of piroplasms, and piroplasms may be seen in low number in chronic carriers. Identification of schizont-laden macrophage on the feathered edge of a blood smear or by cytology of fine-needle aspirates is pathognomonic for disease.

Differential Diagnosis

- Toxoplasmosis
- Cholangitis/cholangiohepatitis
- Pancreatitis
- Hemotropic *Mycoplasma* infection
- Feline infectious peritonitis
- Immune-mediated hemolytic anemia
- Feline leukemia virus infection
- Feline immunodeficiency virus
- Tularemia
- Virulent systemic calicivirus
- Feline panleukopenia virus

Initial Database

Blood smear: pleomorphic (round, oval, anaplasmoid, bipolar [binucleated], or rod-shaped) organism; the round and oval piroplasm forms are most common (0.8-2.2 microns in diameter; typical erythrocyte diameter ≈8 microns). Infected macrophages may occasionally be seen on the feathered edge and may be mistaken for platelet clumps at low power.

- If cytauxzoonosis is suspected but not immediately detected by examination of a blood smear, tissue aspirates of lymph node, liver, and spleen are indicated to identify infected macrophages. These cells range in size from 15-250 microns in diameter, typically have a large distinct nucleolus, and their cytoplasm is filled with numerous small (1-2 micron) basophilic particles (i.e., developing merozoites).
- CBC: pancytopenia (normocytic, normochromic, nonregenerative anemia, leukopenia, and thrombocytopenia) is the classic finding, but monocytopenias or bicytopenias may occur.
- Serum biochemistry profile: elevated liver enzymes (frequently lower than expected for the degree of hyperbilirubinemia), hyperbilirubinemia (mild to moderate), and hyperglycemia are the most common findings.
- Urinalysis reveals bilirubinuria.
- Imaging studies do not contribute directly to the diagnosis.
  - Abdominal imaging: splenomegaly and hepatomegaly common
  - Thoracic radiographs: ± pleural effusion, pulmonary infiltrates
- Coagulation testing may be consistent with disseminated intravascular coagulation (DIC) (p. 269).

Advanced or Confirmatory Testing

- Polymerase chain reaction (PCR) testing can confirm infection before appearance of schizonts or piroplasms but will also be positive in chronic carriers.
- Necropsy with histopathology can confirm the diagnosis and is usually how cytauxzoonosis is first recognized in regions that were previously considered nonendemic.

TREATMENT

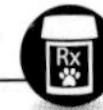

Treatment Overview

New treatments with antiprotozoal therapy have proved effective along with supportive care in this disease, which was previously considered universally fatal. Because the disease progression is very rapid, specific treatment should be instituted immediately in suspected cases.

Acute General Treatment

- Minimal stress and handling is recommended; early placement of nasogastric tube (p. 1107) may facilitate administration of medication and nutrition with less stress.
- Crystalloid fluids: to correct dehydration, restore intravascular volume, and maintain perfusion
- In anemic animals, oxygen delivery to tissues must be restored with a transfusion (p. 1169) of whole blood (20 mL/kg IV administered over 4 hours) or packed RBCs (20 mL/kg IV administered over 4 hours) (p. 1169).

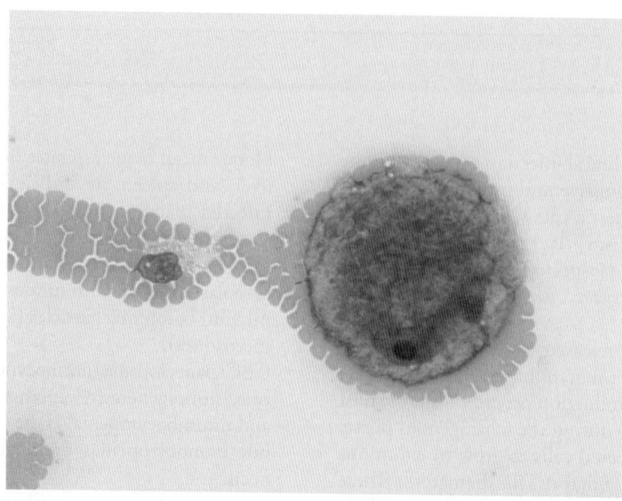

CYTAUXZOONOSIS A large schizont-laden mononuclear cell surrounded by red blood cells. Although identification of schizonts on the blood smear is uncommon, it is pathognomonic for active cytauxzoonosis. (Courtesy Dr. Leah A. Cohn, University of Missouri, Columbia.)

- Some clinicians treat/prevent DIC with heparin 100-300 IU/kg SQ q 8h or 18 IU/kg/h IV constant-rate infusion (CRI).
- Animals with respiratory compromise may require supplemental oxygen (p. 1146) or thoracocentesis if pleural effusion is identified (p. 1164).
- Antiprotozoal therapy should be started immediately. Options include
  - Atovaquone 15 mg/kg PO q 8h administered with a fatty meal for 10 days combined with azithromycin 10 mg/kg PO q 24h for 10 days is the treatment of choice and is associated with survival rates of approximately 65%. Atovaquone absorption in most mammals is increased by coadministration with a fatty meal (facilitated by feeding tube).
  - Imidocarb dipropionate (Imizol) 3-5 mg/kg IM then repeated in 7-14 days. Pretreat with atropine 0.04 mg/kg SQ to minimize cholinergic side effects. Survival with imidocarb treatment ≈25% although some claim higher success rates.
  - Diminazene aceturate (Ganaseg) 2 mg/kg IM repeated in 7 days. A small case series showed this to be a promising treatment, but it is not approved by the U.S. Food and Drug Administration (FDA) or available in the United States.
- Doxycycline 5 mg/kg PO q 12-24h × 14 days may be considered as treatment for co-infection with other tick-borne pathogens.
- Analgesia is recommended.
  - Buprenorphine 0.01-0.02 mg/kg SQ, IM, or IV q 6-12h prn
  - Meloxicam (given only after rehydration in nonazotemic patients) 0.1 mg/kg PO q 24h can also reduce fever.

Chronic Treatment

Some cats that survive illness remain chronically infected but do not exhibit clinical signs of illness. Because no treatments have been demonstrated to consistently clear the carrier phase, recovered cats should be kept indoors.

Nutrition/Diet

Most patients are anorexic; nasogastric tube facilitates enteral nutrition during acute illness.

PROGNOSIS & OUTCOME

- With early diagnosis and treatment (atovaquone and azithromycin), survival rates are ≈65%.
- Even with early diagnosis and treatment, some cats that survive infection develop severe clinical disease that lasts for 5-7 days.
- Progressive hemolysis (presumably associated with antibody production against parasite antigens) is common after several days of treatment and may require treatment with blood products, but immune suppression has not been required in the author's hospital.
- All clinical, hematologic, and biochemical abnormalities resolve in 4-6 weeks.
- Chronic infection does not appear to be associated with decreased life span.
- Recurrent severe infections appear extremely rare in surviving animals, suggesting some degree of protective immunity.
- Without treatment, death usually occurs within 1 week of clinical illness.
- Hypothermia, icterus, severe anemia, and seizures warrant a poor prognosis.

PEARLS & CONSIDERATIONS

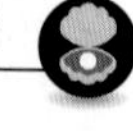

Comments

- The likelihood of survival varies regionally. In some areas, incidental discovery of erythroparasitemia is common (indicating that the cat survived acute infection), and in other areas, survival is rare even with aggressive treatment.
- In the author's hospital, suppression of fever is not necessary and may be associated with a worsened prognosis.

Prevention

In endemic areas, an effective acaricide and tick repellent should be used to prevent exposure to ticks. Because infections have occurred despite acaricide treatment, keeping cats indoors is strongly recommended.

Technician Tips

Atovaquone is very viscous and therefore difficult to accurately dose. Fill the dosing syringe a few minutes before administration to allow the drug to settle in order to be sure that the entire dose is present (the thick drug can coat the sides of the syringe causing inadvertent underdosage).

Client Education

Outdoor cats in areas where bobcats roam are at risk for this deadly disease.

SUGGESTED READING

Cohn LA, et al: Efficacy of atovaquone and azithromycin or imidocarb dipropionate in cats with acute cytauxzoonosis. J Vet Intern Med 25:55-60, 2011.

AUTHORS: Adam J. Birkenheuer, DVM, PhD, DACVIM; Leah A. Cohn, DVM, PhD, DACVIM
EDITOR: Joseph Taboada, DVM, DACVIM

Deafness

Client Education Sheet

BASIC INFORMATION

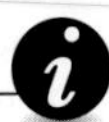

Definition

- *Deafness:* the inability to hear
- *Sensorineural deafness* results from an abnormality in the inner ear and/or vestibulocochlear nerve and/or the auditory pathways in the brain.
- *Conduction deafness* results from a lesion in the outer ear and/or tympanum and/or middle ear.

Epidemiology

SPECIES, AGE, SEX

Dogs and cats, any age, either sex

GENETICS, BREED PREDISPOSITION

- Cats with white haircoats and blue irides are commonly affected by congenital deafness.
- Dogs with white, piebald, spotted, merle, or dapple haircoats are predisposed to congenital deafness.
- Sensorineural deafness is also seen in breeds not related to coat colors (e.g., Doberman pinscher, Rhodesian ridgeback).
- Juvenile/adult onset, inherited sensorineural deafness: Rhodesian ridgebacks, working lines of border collies
- Breeds with presumed inherited conditions involving the conduction portion of the ear (external and middle ears) are predisposed to developing hearing loss (e.g., Cavalier King Charles spaniels with secretory otitis media) (p. 728).

RISK FACTORS

- Old age
- Repeated exposure to loud noises
- Breeds of cats or dogs susceptible to otitis externa and/or otitis media
- Exposure to systemic or topical ototoxic drugs, such as aminoglycosides, erythromycin, loop diuretics, cisplatin, nitrogen mustard, or topical chlorhexidine antiseptic. Topical drugs are potentially more ototoxic if the tympanum is not intact.

ASSOCIATED DISORDERS

- Otitis externa and/or media
- External or middle ear canal neoplasia
- Nasopharyngeal polyps (cats)

Clinical Presentation

DISEASE FORMS/SUBTYPES

- Congenital, juvenile, or adult-onset
- Inherited or noninherited
- Sensorineural, conduction, or mixed

HISTORY, CHIEF COMPLAINT

- Animals with bilateral congenital or adult-onset deafness
  - Overly aggressive with other puppies in a litter (congenital deafness)
  - Nonresponsive to auditory stimuli (certain frequencies/magnitudes)
  - Difficult to obedience train or adult loss of responsiveness to auditory commands
  - Tendency to startle when approached
  - Increased tendency to sleep
  - Not aroused from sleep with auditory stimuli
- Diagnosis of unilateral deafness is not possible with behavioral markers alone, and electrodiagnostic evaluation is required.

PHYSICAL EXAM FINDINGS

- Animals with normal hearing may not respond to loud sounds in the clinical setting; behavioral response to auditory stimuli alone is unreliable for evaluating deafness.
- Animals with peripheral sensorineural deafness typically have no abnormal physical exam findings.
- Animals with acquired conduction deafness may have one or all of the following clinical signs:
  - Abnormal aural exam
  - Head tilt
  - Facial droop
  - Horner's syndrome
  - Head shaking
  - Neurogenic keratoconjunctivitis sicca
  - Signs of pain on ear manipulation
- Animals with deafness resulting from diseases affecting the vestibulocochlear nerve or central auditory pathways will typically demonstrate other concurrent neurologic signs.

Etiology and Pathophysiology

- Acquired conduction deafness resulting from otitis externa/media
  - Impaired conduction of sound waves to the tympanum from debris, cerumen, or pus in the external ear canal
  - Impaired sound wave transduction to otic ossicles due to stiffened, fibrotic, or ruptured tympanum
  - Impaired mechanoelectrical transduction due to otic ossicle sclerosis
- Acquired conduction deafness from external or middle ear masses
  - Obstruction of sound waves to the tympanum
  - Destruction of middle ear structures
- Presbycusis (senile deafness)
  - Degeneration of the neural components of the inner ear
  - ± Stiffening of the tympanum
  - ± Ankylosis of otic ossicles
- Loud noise exposure
  - Damage to inner ear hair cells and/or ossicles and/or tympanum
- Congenital hereditary deafness associated with coat color
  - Abnormal migration of neural crest cells (precursor to melanocytes) to the inner ear (thought to provide nourishment to inner ear); associated with sacculocochlear-type degeneration

DIAGNOSIS

Diagnostic Overview

Bilateral complete deafness is apparent from lack of response to loud noises; diagnostic evaluation should consider history, neurologic exam, and otoscopic exam. Unilateral or partial bilateral deafness may be apparent only on auditory testing and is generally of interest for prevention (breeding).

Differential Diagnosis

- Primary behavioral/psychological disorder
- Canine cognitive dysfunction syndrome (geriatric dogs)

Initial Database

- Distant and proximal physical exams
- Neurologic exam (p. 1136)
- Thorough aural exam (p. 1144)

Advanced or Confirmatory Testing

Brainstem auditory evoked response/potential (BAER or BAEP) testing using air- or bone-conducting stimuli.

TREATMENT

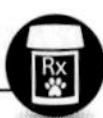

Treatment Overview

- Prevent hearing loss from developing or progressing.
- Improve hearing ability.

Acute General Treatment

- No treatment for congenital inherited sensorineural deafness; careful selection of breeding animals by using only nondeaf animals for breeding (perform BAER tests on untested adults and all puppies considered high risk based on breed or color).
- No practical treatments for animals with sensorineural deafness. Custom-fit hearing aids are offered by some specialty practices (consult with neurologist or audiologist).
- For acquired conduction deafness, treat the underlying cause of the disease.
- Use ototoxic drugs with caution or not at all (topically) if the tympanum is not known to be intact.

Recommended Monitoring

Repeated BAER testing to monitor response to therapy in animals with incomplete deafness

PROGNOSIS & OUTCOME

- Inherited sensorineural deafness and deafness resulting from degeneration of inner ear is permanent.
- Various prognoses for animals with conduction deafness (depends on chronicity and/or severity of the disease)

PEARLS & CONSIDERATIONS

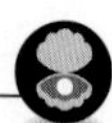

Comments

- For coat color–related deafness, unilaterally deaf animals are as likely as bilaterally deaf animals to produce deaf offspring.
- Animals with bilateral deafness require special care:
  - Keeping animals on leash, especially when near traffic
  - Obedience training using hand signals
  - To minimize the risk of bite injury, prevent children from startling the animal.
- Animals with presbycusis may have concurrent cognitive decline, accounting for behavioral changes.

Prevention

- Use nondeaf animals for breeding.
- For predisposed breeds: use animals with nonblue irides for breeding.

Technician Tips

Approach deaf dogs calmly and with caution, especially if the animal has concurrent vision impairment or is looking away.

Client Education

For dog breeders:

- Coat color–related deafness is a multifactorial genetic condition and is not easily eliminated from particular breeds.
- Breeding unilaterally or bilaterally deaf animals together increases the incidence of deafness in the offspring; conversely, the incidence of deafness decreases when two hearing dogs are bred together.
- Breeding two hearing dogs together can still produce unilaterally or bilaterally deaf puppies (for inherited deafness).
- Avoid producing animals homozygous for the merle gene.
- Congenital sensorineural deafness and vestibular disease affecting Doberman pinschers is an autosomal recessive trait. Try to breed affected animals and known carriers to noncarriers or unaffected animals (a commercially available genetic test is pending).

For pet owners:

- See Client Education Sheet: How to Change the Environment for a Pet That Is Deaf.
- Recommend Susan Cope Becker's book, *Living with a Deaf Dog* (Cincinnati, 1997, Susan Cope Becker).

SUGGESTED READING

Strain GM: Deafness in dogs and cats: information on deafness prevalence, causes and management for owners, breeders and researchers (website). www.lsu.edu/deafness/deaf.htm.

AUTHOR: Aubrey A. Webb, DVM, PhD
EDITOR: Leah A. Cohn, DVM, PhD, DACVIM

Deciduous Teeth, Persistent (Retained)

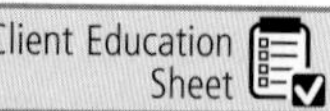

BASIC INFORMATION

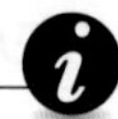

Definition

Deciduous teeth that failed to exfoliate

Synonym

- Retained deciduous teeth
- *Retained* refers to failure to erupt or emerge through the gingival surface; *persistent* is more accurate because it refers to failure to exfoliate (i.e., shed) the deciduous tooth.

Epidemiology

SPECIES, AGE, SEX

Dogs and cats. Permanent dentition eruption schedules dictate when a deciduous tooth is considered persistent. Use table cautiously; breed and individual variation can be significant (± 1-2 months):

Permanent Dentition Eruption Times in Dogs and Cats

Teeth	Dogs	Cats
Incisors	3-5 months	3-4 months
Canines	4-6 months	4-5 months
Premolars	4-6 months	4-6 months
Molars	5-7 months	4-5 months

GENETICS, BREED PREDISPOSITION

High prevalence among toy-breed dogs (Yorkshire terriers, miniature poodles, Pomeranians) suggests inheritance.

Clinical Presentation

DISEASE FORMS/SUBTYPES

As a result of persistence of deciduous teeth:

- Periodontal disease
- Malocclusion
- Malposition, retarded eruption, impaction of permanent teeth
- Palatal/labial trauma

HISTORY, CHIEF COMPLAINT

- Teeth appear too numerous or are angled abnormally.
- A large percentage of persistent deciduous teeth are found on physical examination of adolescent dogs and cats presented for neutering.

PHYSICAL EXAM FINDINGS

- A narrower deciduous tooth is observed alongside an erupting or fully erupted permanent tooth.
- The deciduous canine and incisor teeth are most commonly affected, although persistent deciduous premolars do occur.
- There are no deciduous molars or first premolars.

Etiology and Pathophysiology

- Commonly reported causes
  - Lack of permanent successors
  - Dentoalveolar ankylosis of deciduous teeth
  - Failure of the erupting permanent crown to apply pressure to the deciduous tooth root
  - Hormonal abnormalities affecting growth or metabolism
- Pathophysiologically important information includes
  - Persistent deciduous teeth may result in malpositioned permanent teeth.
  - Permanent mandibular incisors, canines, and premolars erupt lingual (i.e., toward the tongue) to persistent deciduous teeth; lingually deviated permanent mandibular canine teeth may cause palatal trauma.
  - Permanent maxillary incisors and premolars erupt palatal (i.e., toward the palate) to persistent deciduous teeth.
  - Permanent maxillary fourth premolars erupt buccal/labial (i.e., toward the cheek/lip) and distal (i.e., away from the midline of the dental arch) to persistent deciduous teeth.
  - Permanent maxillary canine teeth erupt mesial (i.e., toward the midline of the dental arch) to persistent deciduous teeth.
  - Food, debris, plaque, and calculus accumulating on and between deciduous and permanent teeth may cause periodontal disease even in young animals.

DIAGNOSIS

Diagnostic Overview

Physical examination is highly suggestive; presence of a deciduous tooth in a dog or cat with otherwise permanent dentition. Dental radiography is indicated before intervention.

Differential Diagnosis

- Missing, malformed, malpositioned or unerupted permanent tooth

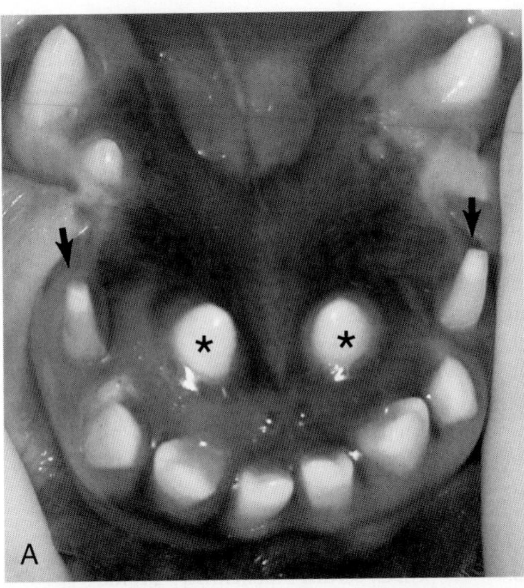

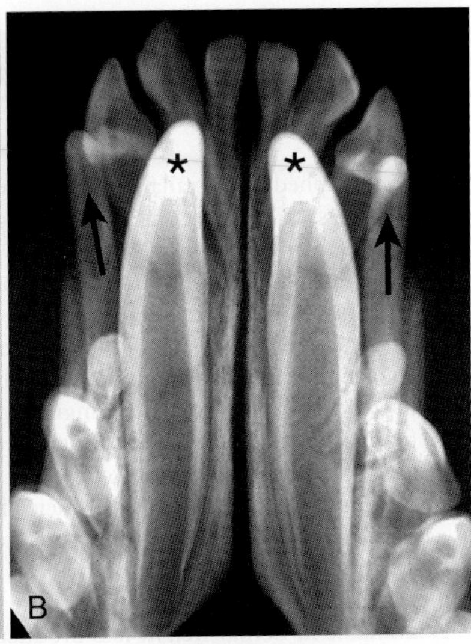

DECIDUOUS TEETH, PERSISTENT A, Bilateral persistent deciduous mandibular canine teeth in a dog *(arrows)*, causing permanent canines *(asterisks)* to be displaced lingually. **B,** Radiograph of lower jaw of same dog. Persistent deciduous canine teeth *(arrows)* block normal eruption pathway of permanent successors *(asterisks)*. Radiograph arranged in labial mounting; rostral is toward top of image, patient's left is on right of image. (Copyright Dr. Alexander M. Reiter, University of Pennsylvania.)

- Supernumerary permanent tooth
- Malocclusion

Initial Database

- CBC, serum chemistry panel, urinalysis: preoperative, generally unremarkable
- Full-mouth dental radiographs: evaluate root structures, confirm and document presence of healthy permanent teeth

Advanced or Confirmatory Testing

Hormone levels if metabolic/endocrine disease is suspected

TREATMENT

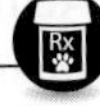

Treatment Overview

Extraction is indicated in virtually all cases (exception: no equivalent permanent tooth) to alleviate dental crowding, soft-tissue trauma, and/or dental interlock, prevent periodontal disease, prevent malpositioning of permanent teeth and malocclusion, and correct existing malocclusion.

Acute General Treatment

- No treatment is needed for uncrowded, healthy persistent deciduous teeth that have no permanent counterpart.
- Extraction of all other persistent deciduous teeth is advised.
- Closed and open extraction techniques are acceptable, depending on tooth to be extracted and degree of root resorption.
  - Closed extraction for mobile teeth
  - Open extraction by creation of a mucoperiosteal flap and alveolar bone removal for solid teeth with complete root structures
  - Slow, steady pressure with a dental elevator is key for inducing periodontal ligament fatigue and successful extraction.
  - Be sure to keep all instrumentation away from the erupting permanent tooth.
- Extraction sites should be closed using rapidly absorbable synthetic suture material while avoiding placing sutures directly over an erupting tooth.
- Postoperative dental radiographs are recommended to ensure complete extraction, evaluate surrounding structures for damage, and provide documentation.
- Antibiotics are not usually necessary after extraction.
- Pain management: intraoperative nerve block (0.5% bupivacaine hydrochloride 0.2-0.3 mL near middle mental, inferior alveolar, infraorbital, or maxillary nerve), followed by oral nonsteroidal antiinflammatory medication (e.g., carprofen 2 mg/kg PO q 12h) for 2-3 days postoperatively.

Possible Complications

- Root fracture and retained root tips, leading to infection of the permanent tooth
- Retarded eruption, malpositioning, and/or mechanical damage to the permanent tooth
- Accidental extraction of permanent tooth

Recommended Monitoring

- Examination in 1-2 weeks to evaluate extraction sites
- Examination in 4-6 weeks to evaluate occlusion if necessary; if abnormalities persist, therapeutic recommendations are offered.

PROGNOSIS & OUTCOME

Excellent for regional healing and reduction of risk of periodontal disease

PEARLS & CONSIDERATIONS

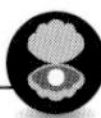

Comments

- Early extraction (5-7 months of age) of persistent deciduous teeth is key to success.
- Deciduous teeth have a thin dentinal layer and long, spindly roots. They are difficult to extract and break easily. The first rule is to *go slowly!*

Prevention

Selective breeding

Technician Tips

- One tooth in one place at one time is the general rule of thumb.
- If deciduous and permanent teeth of the same type are occupying the same space, the deciduous tooth is persistent.

Client Education

Genetic counseling

SUGGESTED READING

Tsugawa AJ, et al: Extraction of canine teeth in dogs. In Verstraete FJM, et al, editors: Oral and maxillofacial surgery in dogs and cats. Philadelphia, 2012, Saunders, p 121-129.

AUTHOR & EDITOR: Alexander M. Reiter, DVM, Dr. med. vet., DAVDC, DEVDC

Decongestant Toxicosis

Client Education Sheet 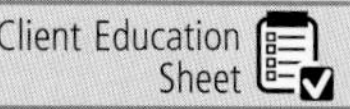

BASIC INFORMATION

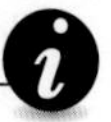

Definition

Common decongestants are pseudoephedrine, ephedrine, phenylephrine, and imidazoline derivatives (oxymetazoline, naphazoline, tetrahydrozoline, xylometazoline). They are active ingredients in over-the-counter (OTC) human medications used for the treatment of cold, flu, sinusitis, and allergies. Toxicosis from other active ingredients is discussed separately (pp. 10, 73, and 695).

Epidemiology

SPECIES, AGE, SEX

All species, breeds, and both sexes are susceptible; dogs are more likely to be involved, based on their predisposition for dietary indiscretion.

RISK FACTORS

Pre-existing cardiac disease, systemic hypertension, and seizure disorders may exacerbate signs of toxicosis.

Clinical Presentation

HISTORY, CHIEF COMPLAINT

- Direct observation or indirect evidence of exposure
- Pseudoephedrine/ephedrine: rapid onset (within 15-30 minutes with immediate-release products; 2-12 hours with extended-release medications) of agitation, hyperactivity, restlessness, panting, mydriasis, shaking, circling, or head bobbing
- Phenylephrine: less likely to result in systemic clinical effects because of enterohepatic degradation by monoamine oxidases and resultant poor bioavailability (38%); mild hyperactivity, pacing, shaking possible within 1-2 hours of exposure
- Imidazoline decongestants: rapid onset (within 60 minutes; not expected after 3-4 hours) of vomiting, weakness, collapse

PHYSICAL EXAM FINDINGS

- Pseudoephedrine/ephedrine: as above plus hyperemia, hyperthermia, hypertension, tachycardia, or reflex bradycardia
- Phenylephrine: as above plus tachycardia, possible panting, shaking
- Imidazoline: as above plus bradycardia, hypotension, prolonged capillary refill time

Etiology and Pathophysiology

Source:

- Toxicosis can occur when animals accidentally ingest OTC medications or are mistakenly given the medication.
- Decongestants stimulate alpha-adrenergic receptors, resulting in vasoconstriction of arterioles in the nasal passages, improving airflow.
    - Pseudoephedrine: available as a hydrochloride or sulfate salt, as a single ingredient immediate-release (30-mg or 60-mg regular tablet), or extended-release (120 mg as 12-hour tablet or 240 mg as 24-hour tablet), or as a liquid (varying concentrations). It is commonly available in combination with other ingredients (cough suppressants, antihistamines, acetaminophen, ibuprofen).
    - Ephedrine: found in products marketed for asthma, colds, and allergies; most products contain less than 65 mg
    - Ma huang (herbal form of ephedra) is available in herbal weight loss products.
    - Phenylephrine: oral preparations (mostly 5- to 15-mg immediate-release tablets or 10- to 40-mg sustained-release tablets), nasal sprays (0.125%-1%), or eye drops (0.1-10%). It is available in combination with other medications (antihistamines, cough suppressants, pain killers).
    - Imidazoline decongestant: oxymetazoline, tetrahydrozoline, naphazoline, and xylometazoline. These are available as nasal and ophthalmic solutions of various concentrations (0.01%-0.1%).

Mechanism of toxicosis:

- Adverse effects are dose dependent and reflect excessive stimulation of the adrenergic nervous system.
- With pseudoephedrine, the release of norepinephrine increases the potential for central nervous system (CNS) stimulation. Ingestion of > 3 mg/kg in an otherwise healthy dog typically warrants decontamination of the patient and close monitoring.
- Ingested phenylephrine is less likely to result in systemic clinical signs due to first-pass effect, resulting in poor bioavailability.
- With imidazoline decongestants, overdoses cause excess stimulation of central alpha-2 receptors, which results in hypotension. The margin of safety is very narrow with these agents, and ingestion of even a small amount can result in toxicosis.

DIAGNOSIS

Diagnostic Overview

Diagnosis is based on a combination of evidence of exposure along with presence of clinical signs. OTC urine drug-test kits can detect pseudoephedrine, or it can be detected in plasma at a diagnostic laboratory (can help retrospectively determine exposure).

Differential Diagnosis

Toxicologic:

- Pseudoephedrine/ephedrine/phenylephrine: amphetamines, antihistamines, cocaine, metaldehyde, methylxanthines, phenylpropanolamine, strychnine, 5-hydroxytryptophan, antidepressants
- Imidazoline: alcohols, amitraz, barbiturates, benzodiazepines, calcium channel blockers, clonidine, essential oils, dexmedetomidine, xylazine

Non-toxicologic:

- Pseudoephedrine/phenylephrine: pheochromocytoma, renal disease, intracranial disease
- Imidazoline: hypoadrenocorticism, advanced cardiovascular disease/cardiogenic shock, sepsis, hypovolemic shock, trauma

Initial Database

- CBC, serum biochemistry profile
- Blood pressure (Blood Pressure Measurement; see p. 1065): high or low
- Electrocardiogram (ECG): heart rate high or low (p. 1096), arrhythmia

Advanced or Confirmatory Testing

Urine drug screening with OTC test kit (optional, most diagnostic for pseudoephedrine)

TREATMENT

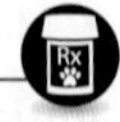

Treatment Overview

Treatment is indicated based on clinical suspicion (history and physical examination), without urine test confirmation. Treatment may consist of decontamination (emesis and administration of activated charcoal) if clinical signs are absent or management of cardiovascular and CNS aberrations and thermoregulation if clinical signs are present.

Acute General Treatment

Decontamination of patient (p. 1087):

- Pseudoephedrine/ephedrine/phenylephrine
    - Induction of emesis (p. 1188) if asymptomatic and within 1 hour of ingestion of immediate-release products (2 hours if extended-release product)
    - Activated charcoal (1-2 g/kg PO; use lowest labeled dose for commercial products)
- Imidazoline decongestants
    - Due to the rapid onset of signs after imidazoline decongestant ingestion, emesis and charcoal are generally not recommended.

Specific treatment:

- Pseudoephedrine/ephedrine/phenylephrine
    - Control CNS excitation. Phenothiazines are drugs of choice: acepromazine 0.05-0.15 mg/kg IV or IM, repeat as needed; useful for mild hypertension and CNS stimulatory signs or chlorpromazine 0.05-0.5 mg/kg IV
    - Control tachycardia (assess ECG): if sinus tachycardia, reduction of CNS excitation may be sufficient (see above). If severe, persistent sinus tachycardia (e.g., >180

beats/min in dogs, >260 beats/min in cats), consider propranolol 0.02-0.06 mg/kg IV only if normotensive, repeat as needed. If also hypertensive, avoid propranolol (use esmolol 0.2-0.5 mg/kg IV or 10-200 mcg/kg/min IV)
  - If ventricular tachycardia (p. 1033)
- Imidazoline decongestants
  - Atipamezole 50 mcg/kg (¼ of the dose IV and the rest IM); may be repeated as needed for life-threatening hypotension and bradycardia, *or*
  - Yohimbine 0.1 mg/kg IV; repeat in 2-3 hours if needed. Use if atipamezole is not available.

Supportive care for all decongestant exposures causing overt clinical signs:
- Intravenous fluids
- Thermoregulation: cool fluids, external cooling measures as needed
- Keep the patient calm, and reduce external stimuli (quiet surroundings).

Drug Interactions

- Diazepam may be contraindicated; paradoxical response (when given at high doses or when given too fast) may add to stimulatory signs from pseudoephedrine/ephedrine/phenylephrine.
- Propranolol: contraindicated if systemic hypertension is present (blockade of beta-2 receptors in vessels may cause vasoconstriction, worsening hypertension)
- Atropine: contraindicated for reflex bradycardia due to hypertension

Possible Complications

- Disseminated intravascular coagulation (DIC) due to hyperthermia
- Permanent brain damage from prolonged stimulation/seizures
- Acute kidney injury from systemic hypotension or hypertension and/or rhabdomyolysis

Recommended Monitoring

Heart rate/rhythm, blood pressure, temperature, mentation, serum biochemistry profile with electrolytes, acid-base status

PROGNOSIS & OUTCOME

Generally favorable with prompt presentation and appropriate care. Presence of prolonged hyperthermia or DIC carries a guarded/poor prognosis. Pseudoephedrine exposures > 10 mg/kg are potentially lethal without treatment.

PEARLS & CONSIDERATIONS

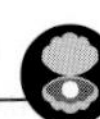

Comments

- The use and availability of pseudoephedrine in several U.S. states has been restricted because of use in illegal amphetamine synthesis. Pseudoephedrine is being replaced by phenylephrine.
- Other agents (nonsteroidal antiinflammatory drugs [p. 695], antihistamines [p. 73], cough suppressants [p. 73], acetaminophen [p. 10]) may also cause toxicosis if a combination product was ingested; be sure to monitor and treat accordingly.
- The signs of pseudoephedrine toxicosis are very similar to amphetamine toxicosis in dogs and cats.
- Several weight-loss OTC products contain various levels of ma huang, a natural source of ephedrine.

Prevention

- Keep medications out of animal's reach.
- Instruct owners that when purchasing OTC antihistamines for pets, they need to read labels carefully and avoid products that contain pseudoephedrine.

Technician Tips

The OTC availability of these medications may give owners the wrong impression that they are harmless. Any casual mention by an owner of this type of medication is worth discussing with the veterinarian, especially if physical signs compatible with toxicosis are present.

Client Education

- Never administer OTC medications to pets without consulting a veterinarian, and purchase medications with only the specific active ingredient that has been recommended by a veterinarian.
- Prevent all pets from access to human medications.

SUGGESTED READING

Wegenast C: Toxicology brief: phenylephrine ingestion in dogs: What's the harm? Vet Med 107(11):476, 2012.

AUTHOR: Brandy R. Sobczak, DVM
EDITOR: Tina Wismer, DVM, MS, DABVT, DABT

Degenerative Myelopathy

Bonus Material Online   Client Education Sheet

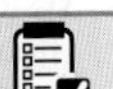

BASIC INFORMATION

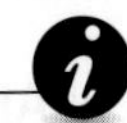

Definition

Canine degenerative myelopathy (DM) is an inherited, adult-onset central nervous system (CNS) degenerative disease, most severely affecting the thoracolumbar spinal cord.

Synonyms

Canine degenerative radiculomyelopathy, German shepherd dog myelopathy

Epidemiology

SPECIES, AGE, SEX

Canine; age at onset approximately 8-14 years; mean age: 9 years in large dogs, 11 years in Pembroke Welsh corgis

GENETICS, BREED PREDISPOSITION

- Presumed autosomal recessive mutation in the canine superoxide dismutase-1 gene *(SOD1)*
- The genetic mutation is similar to some forms of human amyotrophic lateral sclerosis (Lou Gehrig disease)
- Breed predisposition: purebred and mixed-breed dogs—American Eskimo dog, Australian shepherd, Bernese mountain dog, bloodhound, borzoi, boxer, Cardigan Welsh corgi, Cavalier King Charles spaniel, Czechoslovakian wolfdog, Chesapeake Bay retriever, collie (rough coat), English Springer spaniel, German shepherd dog, golden retriever, Hovawart, Kerry Blue terrier, Labrador retriever, Nova Scotia duck tolling retriever, Pembroke Welsh corgi, poodle (miniature), poodle (standard), pug, Rhodesian ridgeback, Shetland sheepdog, Siberian Husky, soft-coated wheaten terrier, wire-haired fox terrier

Clinical Presentation

HISTORY, CHIEF COMPLAINT

- Progressive weakness of pelvic limbs
- Initially, affected dogs drag the claws and show general proprioceptive ataxia in pelvic limbs.
- Difficulty jumping
- The disease results in a progressive paraparesis to paraplegia within 12 months of onset of clinical signs.

PHYSICAL EXAM FINDINDINGS

Early disease: upper motor neuron (UMN) signs in pelvic limbs:

- Asymmetrical truncal general proprioceptive ataxia
- UMN spastic paraparesis (long stride length)
- Postural reaction deficits (e.g., toe dragging, absent proprioceptive placement [paw replacement])
- Spinal reflexes present or exaggerated
- Absence of paraspinal hyperesthesia

Late disease: lower motor neuron (LMN) signs and spread to thoracic limbs:

- Paraplegia and LMN signs develop in pelvic limbs; then weakness and neurogenic muscle atrophy spread to thoracic limbs.
- Widespread muscle atrophy and wasting
- Flaccid tetraparesis
- Urinary and fecal incontinence
- End stage: swallowing and respiratory dysfunction

Etiology and Pathophysiology

Cause: mutation in the *SOD1* gene, resulting in a toxic gain of function

- Misfolding of the SOD protein causes abnormal accumulations of aggregates in the neuron.
- Dogs homozygous for the mutation are at risk for DM.
- Neuropathologic lesion distribution in the CNS involves axons and myelin in all funiculi of the spinal cord, notably the dorsal funiculus and dorsal portion of the lateral funiculus of the thoracolumbar spinal cord.
- Neurons in affected dogs contain cytoplasmic aggregates that stain with anti-SOD1 antibodies and show loss in terminal disease.
- Some studies have shown degenerative changes in some neurons of the brainstem.
- Dogs with chronic DM develop muscle atrophy consistent with denervation. Peripheral nerve lesions are consistent with an axonopathy and secondary demyelination.
- The clinical spectrum of DM has now been broadened to include the UMN and LMN systems and is considered a multisystem disease involving central and peripheral axons.

DIAGNOSIS

Diagnostic Overview

The diagnosis of DM is based on exclusion of other spinal cord disorders that mimic it. The genetic test may assist with interpretation of clinical signs and diagnostic testing toward a presumptive diagnosis of DM.

Differential Diagnosis

Other spinal cord disorders mimic signs of DM:

- Intervertebral disc disease: Hansen type II
  - The Pembroke Welsh corgi is a chondrodystrophic breed that is also prone to Hansen type I intervertebral disc disease
- Inflammatory disease of the spinal cord: myelitis
- Spinal cord neoplasia
- Degenerative lumbosacral stenosis
- Cervical spondylomyelopathy
- Other coexisting orthopedic diseases and spinal cord disorders

Initial Database

- Neurologic exam (p. 1136)
  - See Physical Exam Findings above for clinical findings.
    - Nonpainful progressive myelopathy
  - Neuroanatomic localization: initial disease stage—UMN signs (T3 to L3 spinal cord segments); later disease stage involves LMN signs to the pelvic and thoracic limbs; terminal stage—generalized LMN signs to include brainstem signs
- Clinical pathologic tests: generally unremarkable
- Thoracic radiography
  - Screening for metastatic neoplasia (CNS neoplasia, differential diagnosis)
- Survey spinal radiography
- Genetic testing
  - A direct mutation test for a susceptibility gene is available through the Orthopedic Foundation for Animals (www.offa.org) and other genetic testing companies. For diagnostic purposes, a blood sample can be submitted through the Animal Molecular Genetic Diseases Laboratory at the University of Missouri (www.caninegeneticdiseases.net).
  - Dogs that are homozygous for the mutation *are at risk for* DM, but not all at-risk dogs will develop DM. Some dogs that are heterozygous for the mutation have developed DM.
  - For recessive diseases, the results are expressed as follows:
    - Normal: homozygous for the normal gene
    - Carrier: heterozygous, with one copy each of the normal and mutated gene
    - At risk: homozygous for the mutated gene

Advanced or Confirmatory Testing

- Clinical working diagnosis is based on ruling out other diseases that cause progressive myelopathy.
- Cerebrospinal fluid analysis (pp. 1080 and 1323): may show increased protein concentration.
- Electrophysiologic testing
  - Electromyography and nerve conduction studies
  - Used for ruling out other neuropathic disorders
  - In later disease stage, dogs with DM show evidence of peripheral axonopathy and secondary demyelination.
- Cross-sectional imaging: no evidence of a compressive myelopathy
  - CT combined with myelography
  - MRI (p. 1132)
- Definitive diagnosis is determined only by postmortem histopathologic examination of the spinal cord and peripheral nervous system.

TREATMENT

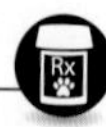

Treatment Overview

There are no proven effective therapies for DM. Supportive and palliative care are provided to maintain quality of life.

Acute and Chronic Treatment

Exercise, vitamin supplementation (B_{12}, E, and C), and protease inhibitors (aminocaproic acid) have been advocated as potential therapies, although efficacy of medical therapy still remains to be proven.

- Ongoing clinical trials are testing therapeutic strategies for canine DM.
- Encourage exercise and physical rehabilitation in ambulatory dogs to slow onset of disuse muscle atrophy.
- When the dog becomes nonambulatory, keep on a well-padded surface.
- Monitor for urinary and fecal incontinence.
  - Basic nursing care and hygiene if incontinence occurs to prevent the onset of urine scald, infected decubital ulcers, or similar skin lesions
- Monitor for decubital ulcers in dogs with generalized muscle atrophy.
- Assistive walking devices enable ambulation support and improve quality of life.

Possible Complications

- Urinary tract infection; see bacterial cystitis (p. 232)
- Decubital ulcer formation

Recommended Monitoring

- Monitor for secondary urinary tract infection.
- Monitor for proper nursing care.

PROGNOSIS & OUTCOME

- Long-term prognosis is considered poor.
- Dogs often lose their ability to ambulate in the pelvic limbs within 12 months from onset of signs.
- The disease eventually will progress to affect the thoracic limbs and swallowing function.
- Owners of large dogs often will elect for euthanasia when their dog needs ambulatory assistance.

PEARLS & CONSIDERATIONS

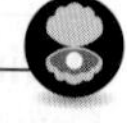

Comments

- Lack of paraspinal hyperesthesia is a key clinical feature of DM.
- A suspected diagnosis is based on exclusion of other spinal cord disorders.

Technician Tips

- Physical rehabilitation using light exercise may improve the patient's quality of life.
- Caution must be used when rehabilitation—especially therapeutic exercise—is considered because these dogs can be exhausted easily. Inducing fatigue in already diseased muscle can potentially hasten the disease process.

- Closely monitor the patient for urine scald and decubitus ulceration when the disease progresses to LMN involvement.

Client Education

- Meticulous nursing care is essential for the recumbent patient.
    - Keep patient clean and dry to prevent urine scald.
    - Keep patient on a protective surface (optimize padding, traction, and ease of cleaning).
- Sling support or a cart can assist with patient mobility.
- Physical rehabilitation using range-of-motion and isometric exercises will help maintain joint flexibility and muscle strength.
- It is important to realize the emotional support an individual or family can provide to maintain quality of life for a companion animal. As a DM-affected dog progresses through the disease stages, the dog's owner encounters the challenges of at-home management and providing appropriate daily care for the pet.

SUGGESTED READING

Coates JR, et al: Canine degenerative myelopathy. Vet Clin North Am Small Anim 40:929-950, 2010.

AUTHOR: Joan R. Coates, DVM, MS, DACVIM
EDITOR: Karen R. Muñana, DVM, MS, DACVIM

Dehydration

BASIC INFORMATION

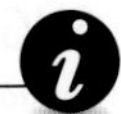

Definition

Clinical state in which fluid losses (sensible loss [renal] and insensible loss [normal daily gastrointestinal, respiratory]) exceed fluid intake

Synonyms

Decreased circulating blood volume, negative fluid balance

Epidemiology

SPECIES, AGE, SEX

All animals are susceptible to dehydration, depending on the underlying disease process. Due to a high ratio of body surface area to volume, smaller animals (<10 kg) are more prone to dehydration.

RISK FACTORS

- Diseases and toxins that affect appetite, decrease water consumption, and hamper renal and intestinal conservation of water; poor vascular integrity
- Infectious diseases (e.g., parvoviral enteritis, coccidiosis); metabolic disturbances secondary to chronic kidney disease, hypoadrenocorticism, gastrointestinal disease, and other disorders with systemic effects; endocrinopathies (e.g., diabetes mellitus, diabetes insipidus); and intoxications (e.g., ethylene glycol)

CONTAGION AND ZOONOSIS

Some of the diseases that cause dehydration (e.g., parvoviral enteritis, leptospirosis) are contagious to other pets and/or have zoonotic potential.

GEOGRAPHY AND SEASONALITY

- Hotter weather in the summer may make a sick animal become dehydrated more rapidly.
- Frozen water bowls in the winter may cause pets to become dehydrated.

Clinical Presentation

DISEASE FORMS/SUBTYPES

Hypertonic, isotonic, or hypotonic dehydration

HISTORY, CHIEF COMPLAINT

Anorexia, vomiting, diarrhea, lethargy, weakness, panting, and signs related to underlying disease

PHYSICAL EXAM FINDINGS

- Lethargy, dry/tacky mucous membranes, tachycardia, poor pulse quality, skin tenting, sunken eyes/enophthalmos, and weight loss.
- The approximate level of dehydration is estimated based on the following physical exam findings: 5% = dry/tacky mucous membranes; 6%-8% = dry mucous membranes and delayed skin tent test; 10%-12% = hypovolemic shock
    - Signs of shock include all of the above plus bilaterally symmetrical enophthalmos, tachycardia (dogs), weakness, slow capillary refill time, poor pulse, and lethargy or obtundation.

Etiology and Pathophysiology

- Causes: see Risk Factors above
- Mechanism: regardless of cause, dehydration results in a decrease in circulating blood volume, which directly affects perfusion and oxygen delivery to essential tissues/organs. Mild cases may be clinically insignificant, but in moderate or severe dehydration, the metabolic processes in hypoperfused tissues must rely on anaerobic pathways to produce adenosine triphosphate, which is a less efficient process. A byproduct of anaerobic metabolic pathways is lactic acid, which accumulates in states of decreased perfusion and results in metabolic acidosis.

DIAGNOSIS

Diagnostic Overview

Because dehydration is unlikely to be a primary problem, a diagnostic search for an underlying cause is always warranted. Simply the history and physical exam often provides an explanation for dehydration.

Differential Diagnosis

- Skin tent: old age, thin/emaciated body condition (false increase), obesity (false decrease)
- Tacky mucous membranes: oral mucous membranes may be tacky due to panting; nausea with hypersalivation or recent water consumption can obscure recognition of tacky membranes.

Initial Database

- CBC, serum biochemical profile, urinalysis, fecal exam, ± imaging studies to look for cause
- Depending on degree and on comorbid disease, dehydration can cause increased packed cell volume (PCV), increased total solids, increased albumin, increased blood urea nitrogen (BUN) ± creatinine, increased sodium, concentrated urine (>1.040 dog; > 1.050 cat).

Advanced or Confirmatory Testing

Diagnostics are dictated by initial diagnostic information and case evolution.

TREATMENT

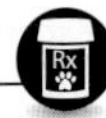

Treatment Overview

- Fluid replacement
- Correction of electrolyte abnormalities
- Treatment of underlying disease

Acute General Treatment

Fluid replacement with an isotonic crystalloid such as lactated Ringer's solution, Normosol-R, or 0.9% sodium chloride

- Maintenance rate and dehydration replacement must be calculated.
- Dehydration volume is delivered over ≈24-48 hours and is added to maintenance rates.
    - Shock and severe dehydration often require more rapid correction.
    - Initial bolus administration of crystalloid fluids (initial bolus of 20 mL/kg, repeated as required and not to exceed 90 mL/kg/h in dogs or 60 mL/kg/h in cats) may be appropriate
- Maintenance rate = 40 mL/kg/24 hours for large dogs (>10 kg), 60 mL/kg/24 hours for cats and small dogs (<10 kg)

- Dehydration replacement volume (mL) = % dehydration as a decimal (e.g., 10% is 0.1) × body weight in kg × 1000
- Adjustment of fluid rate and frequent, close monitoring of respiratory rate and comfort if heart disease, renal disease, or systemic hypertension is present
- Electrolyte replacement
    - Do not supplement potassium at a rate of > 0.5 mEq/kg/h (p. 516).
    - Do not raise or lower serum sodium at a rate of > 1 mEq/L/h (pp. 498 and 518).

Nutrition/Diet

If vomiting absent, access to water for oral intake recommended

Drug Interactions

Do not add sodium bicarbonate to calcium-containing fluids (precipitation reaction).

Possible Complications

- Overhydration/volume overload: increased respiratory rate, chemosis, serous nasal discharge, subcutaneous and distal limb edema, pulmonary edema, pleural or peritoneal effusion, hemodilution, cerebral edema, peripheral edema
    - Monitor more closely if heart or kidney disease

Recommended Monitoring

Body weight, respiratory rate, urine output, heart rate, pulse quality, capillary refill time, skin turgor, blood pressure, PCV/total solids, BUN, creatinine

PROGNOSIS & OUTCOME

- Dehydration can be addressed by fluid administration.
- Prognosis depends on cause.

PEARLS & CONSIDERATIONS

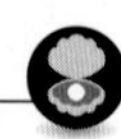

Comments

- Urine output and change in body weight are among the easiest and most accurate ways to gauge the level of hydration.
- Absent vomiting, oral rehydration (nasoesophageal tube) is ideal for animal with marked heart disease.
- Subcutaneous fluids are poorly absorbed from animals with marked dehydration.
- For severe dehydration (>8%), recheck electrolyte (sodium, potassium, chloride, and phosphorus) imbalances and acid-base status frequently (every 4-8 hours) during the first 24 hours of therapy to ensure treatment goals are being achieved.
- Consider colloidal therapy (plasma, albumin, hetastarch) if hypoalbuminemia is present.

Technician Tips

- Assessing hydration status by skin turgor alone can be misleading, especially in elderly or cachectic patients (false impression of dehydration).
- The conjunctival mucous membranes are often most reliable (barring ocular disease) because oral mucous membranes are prone to drying (open-mouth breathing/panting in dogs) or coating with mucus (vomiting).

Client Education

Anorexic animals or those with vomiting and diarrhea (especially very young or very old) can become dehydrated quickly and should be examined by a veterinarian as soon as possible.

SUGGESTED READING

Rudloff E, et al: Fluid resuscitation and the trauma patient. Vet Clin North Am Small Anim Pract 38(3):645-652, 2008.

AUTHOR: Adam J. Reiss, DVM, DACVECC
EDITOR: Leah A. Cohn, DVM, PhD, DACVIM

Demodicosis

Client Education Sheet 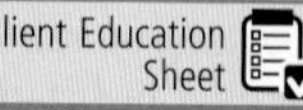

BASIC INFORMATION

Definition

An inflammatory skin disease associated with excessive proliferation of *Demodex* mites.

Synonym

Demodectic mange

Epidemiology

SPECIES, AGE, SEX

- Canine demodicosis caused by *Demodex canis* is most common in young dogs.
- Feline demodicosis can affect cats of any age; *Demodex gatoi* has a highly regional distribution.

GENETICS, BREED PREDISPOSITION

- Dogs with juvenile-onset generalized demodicosis and their first-degree relatives should not be bred. A hereditary predisposition exists.
- Purebred dogs are predisposed, with short-coated breeds overrepresented (e.g., pit bull–type dogs).

RISK FACTORS

- Juvenile onset: most likely results from temporary immunodeficiency
- Adult onset: often immunosuppressive diseases or treatments

CONTAGION AND ZOONOSIS

Demodex mites are host specific, and demodicosis is not typically contagious for immunocompetent animals. However, *D. gatoi* is contagious to healthy, in-contact cats.

GEOGRAPHY AND SEASONALITY

D. gatoi is common in the southeastern United States but apparently rare worldwide.

ASSOCIATED DISORDERS

Canine generalized demodicosis is very frequently complicated by pyoderma, which can be deep and severe.

Clinical Presentation

DISEASE FORMS/SUBTYPES

Canine:

- Localized (*D. canis*): one to several small areas of alopecia, often on the face and forelegs, typically starting at 3-6 months of age
- Generalized (*D. canis*): affects an entire body region, completely involves two or more paws, or presents with more than six lesions. Usually more severe skin lesions and secondary pyoderma and multiple lesions present at onset. Classification of localized versus generalized requires clinical judgment.
    - Juvenile-onset generalized demodicosis begins at < 18 months of age.
    - Adult-onset generalized demodicosis often appears at > 4 years of age.
- Other
    - *Demodex injai:* a much longer follicular mite than *D. canis*, present in low numbers. Associated with pruritus and greasy skin and haircoat on the dorsal trunk and face (over-represented in terrier breeds).
    - A short-bodied *Demodex* mite sometimes found on skin scrapings is likely a morphologic variant of *D. canis*.

Feline:

- *Demodex cati:* rare, often associated with immunosuppression in adult cats
- *D. gatoi:* regionally common, pruritic, contagious. Very different condition from that caused by other canine and feline *Demodex* mites
- A third unnamed species of mite has been reported in cats.

HISTORY, CHIEF COMPLAINT

- Chief complaint in canine demodicosis is hair loss, with variable pruritus and other skin lesions. Pruritus is common if pyoderma is present.
- Pruritus is a major feature of *D. gatoi* infestation in cats and frequently of *D. injai* infestation in dogs.

- In adult-onset demodicosis, signs caused by underlying disease (e.g., hyperadrenocorticism) or by immunosuppressive treatment can be present.

PHYSICAL EXAM FINDINGS

Canine:
- Localized demodicosis: several small areas of patchy alopecia, mild erythema, scaling, and variable hyperpigmentation on the face or forelimbs
- Generalized demodicosis: lesions can be similar but are usually more severe, extensive, and complicated by pyoderma. Comedones, papules, pustules, follicular casts, crusts, edema, and deep folliculitis/furunculosis are common. Hyperpigmentation of follicular ostia is suggestive. Peripheral lymphadenopathy, pain, pruritus, and malaise may also be present. In adult-onset cases, physical changes associated with underlying disease (e.g., hyperadrenocorticism, neoplasia) may be found.
- *D. injai:* greasy skin and pruritus on dorsal trunk (or face)

Feline:
- *D. cati:* patchy alopecia and scaling or ceruminous otitis
- *D. gatoi:* symmetrical, self-induced truncal alopecia

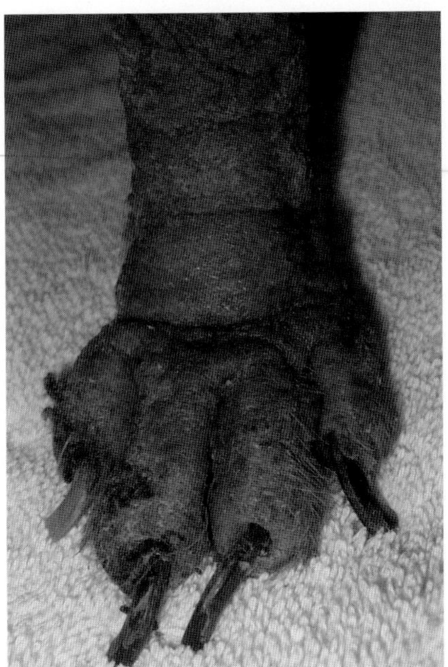

DEMODICOSIS Pododemodicosis resembles many other conditions. Skin scrapings and trichograms should be collected in dogs of any age presenting with pedal lesions.

Etiology and Pathophysiology
- The immunologic defect leading to canine demodicosis is poorly understood.
- In adult dogs, consider underlying cause, including corticosteroid administration (common), spontaneous hyperadrenocorticism, hypothyroidism, leishmaniasis, neoplasia, and immunosuppressive treatments.
- Poor nutrition, estrus, parturition, and stress can contribute.

DIAGNOSIS

Diagnostic Overview
In most cases, canine demodicosis is a straightforward diagnosis as long as skin scrapings are not overlooked. The diagnosis rests on finding mites in affected skin. Although *D. canis* is a normal skin inhabitant, it is rare to find mites unless they are causing disease.

Differential Diagnosis
Uncomplicated demodicosis resembles other skin disorders:
- Dogs: bacterial folliculitis, dermatophytosis, dermatomyositis, pemphigus foliaceus and other immune-mediated diseases, sebaceous adenitis
- Cats: hypersensitivity disorders and other ectoparasites *(D. gatoi)*, psychogenic (symmetrical) alopecia *(D. gatoi)*, dermatophytosis *(D. cati)*, otodectic acariasis *(D. cati)*

Initial Database
- Deep skin scrapings from at least three sites for follicular-dwelling *Demodex* mites (p. 1091)
    - Squeeze skin to extrude mites from hair follicles immediately before and/or during scraping; scrape until mild capillary bleeding is seen.
    - Subjective assessments of mite numbers (0-4+) and the proportion of live mites and juvenile mites/eggs are important for baseline and subsequent monitoring of therapy.
- In sensitive areas, trichography (microscopic examination of 50-100 hairs forcefully plucked using forceps or hemostats) is an easier but less sensitive method. If the trichogram is negative, consider sedation for scrapings in these areas.
- Acetate tape impressions with skin squeezing are an alternate technique but less often used.

Advanced or Confirmatory Testing
- Be sure to collect deep skin scrapings and trichograms before performing biopsies because histopathologic evaluation usually is not necessary to diagnose demodicosis. Skin biopsies may be needed to find mites when extensive scarring is present (e.g., feet).
- In adult-onset demodicosis cases, recommend diagnostic workup for internal disease as deemed appropriate (e.g., CBC, chemistry profile, urinalysis, imaging, screening tests for endocrinopathies, FeLV/FIV evaluation).
- In pruritic cats with *D. gatoi* infestation, mites are easy to miss because the cat removes them by licking.
    - Less pruritic housemate cats and fecal flotations can yield the mites.
    - In geographic areas where *D. gatoi* is endemic: if broad superficial skin scrapings, acetate tape preparations, and fecal flotation are negative, treatment trials have been used.

TREATMENT

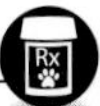

Treatment Overview
- Treatment of canine demodicosis has been revolutionized by the use of the isoxazoline drugs: fluralaner (Bravecto), afoxolaner (NexGard), sarolaner (Simparica), and lotilaner (Credelio).
- Generalized demodicosis requires miticidal therapy, but most cases of canine localized demodicosis resolve without treatment.
- Treat for underlying or concurrent disease, or discontinue immunosuppressive therapy in adult patients.
- Treatment of secondary pyoderma is essential for reducing pruritus and restoring normal skin appearance. Unless deep or severe pyoderma is present, antibacterial shampoo therapy is often sufficient, and systemic antibiotics are not needed if effective miticidal therapy is given.
- Cure is achieved when there has been no relapse for at least 1 year after treatment completion.

Acute and Chronic Treatment
- Localized demodicosis does not require treatment. The rationale for not treating these mild cases is that their resolution indicates adequate immune function (and has positive implications if the dog is to be used for breeding).
- Therapy for generalized canine demodicosis is continued for several months. All treatments should continue for at least 1 month after two consecutive sets of skin scrapings are negative.
- Response to therapy is monitored by clinical improvement and skin scrapings approximately every 4 weeks.
- Isoxazoline drugs likely represent the safest and most effective therapy. One report of successful treatment with extralabel oral fluralaner for *D. gatoi;* the licensed topical product may also be effective. The use of other treatments, including macrocyclic lactones, is becoming less common.

Options for treating canine demodicosis:
- Oral isoxazoline drugs
    - Extralabel use for this condition: very convenient with an excellent safety profile when used as labeled. Note that minimum age for some products is 6 months.
    - Sufficient published and anecdotal evidence exists to recommend the use of these drugs as first-line therapy for canine generalized demodicosis. Studies of *D. injai* are lacking.
    - Rapid clinical and microscopic improvement is expected. Negative skin scrapings are attained quite rapidly; typically mite numbers are dramatically reduced at 1 month and negative at 2 months.

- The fluralaner, sarolaner, and lotilaner studies have dosed the drugs approximately as per the label (every 12 weeks (fluralaner) and every 28-30 days (lotilaner and sarolaner), respectively. In the afoxolaner study, dogs were treated on days 0, 14, 28, and 56; subsequent anecdotal experience suggests that afoxolaner is effective given monthly as per the label.

- Oral ivermectin (e.g., 10 mg/mL bovine injectable solution)
  - Extralabel use in dogs: the best studied of the oral macrocyclic lactones but now largely replaced by isoxazoline drugs
  - Effective at 0.3-0.6 mg/kg PO q 24h, recommend to incrementally increase to full dose (e.g., over 7-10 days)
  - Absolutely contraindicated in certain dogs (see Possible Complications below)
  - Extralabel use in cats; likely effective for *D. cati.* Dosing information is scant.
- Topical moxidectin with imidacloprid (Advantage Multi, Advocate)
  - Labeled for dogs with demodicosis in some countries (not United States)
  - Monthly topical application (as labeled in many countries) is likely insufficient.
  - Weekly administration (extralabel in many countries) can be effective but less rapid than isoxazoline drugs
- Amitraz dips
  - Approved for dogs in the United States and Canada but rarely used due to adverse effects. Additional references should be consulted if treatment is considered.
- If deep or severe pyoderma present: systemic antistaphylococcal antibiotic therapy: empirical (e.g., cephalexin 22-30 mg/kg PO q 12h) or based on bacterial culture if resistance is suspected
- Weekly benzoyl peroxide or chlorhexidine shampooing
- In adult-onset cases, treat the underlying disease.

Options for treating feline demodicosis:

- There is little information regarding the treatment of cats; all treatments are extralabel. For *D. cati*, daily oral ivermectin or weekly lime sulfur dips have been used. For *D. gatoi*, weekly topical imidacloprid and moxidectin or weekly lime sulfur dips have been used with variable results.
- The efficacy of the feline topical fluralaner formulation for any species of feline *Demodex* is not known, but anecdotal reports are encouraging. Consult the current literature for more information on this newly available product.

Possible Complications

- Macrocyclic lactones (ivermectin, oral moxidectin, doramectin, milbemycin [p. 566]): monitor carefully for neurotoxicity, and educate clients about potential signs.
- In general, these drugs should be avoided in dogs homozygous for the *MDR1/ABCB1-Δ* gene mutation (p. 638). Dogs at risk for carrying this mutation, including herding breeds, some sighthounds, and their crosses, should be tested before the drugs are administered.
- Isoxazoline class drugs have rarely been associated with neurologic adverse reactions, including muscle tremors, ataxia, or seizures.

Recommended Monitoring

Skin scrapings typically are performed every 4 weeks during therapy at the same sites that were previously positive for mites. Score the approximate number of mites, the proportion of live mites, the proportion of adults versus immature mites, and the number of eggs at each visit. Adjust therapy if parameters are not improving. Continue therapy for 1 month after two consecutive scrapings are obtained.

PROGNOSIS & OUTCOME

- The prognosis for localized juvenile-onset demodicosis is excellent. The prognosis for generalized juvenile-onset cases is good, but a small proportion requires long-term treatment.
- In adult-onset demodicosis, the prognosis for cure is guarded but mite populations can usually be controlled with ongoing parasiticidal therapy.

PEARLS & CONSIDERATIONS

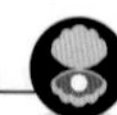

Comments

- *D. canis* mites are usually easy to find by skin scraping in affected animals. However, this test is sometimes skipped. Treatment trials are no substitute for skin scrapings, which should always be part of the dermatology minimum database.
- If only one mite is found on scrapings from a dog, scrape more sites.
- Consult the current literature for further information regarding the treatment of demodicosis using fluralaner or other isoxazolines in cats.
- Hair plucks (trichography) are an alternate way of looking for *Demodex* in dogs.
- Skin scrape greasy terriers, particularly on the dorsal trunk, to look for *D. injai*. It can be difficult to find because its numbers are low.
- Hyperpigmented follicular ostia in dogs should increase the suspicion of demodicosis.
- In *D. gatoi*–endemic areas, treatment trials are sometimes part of the workup for pruritic cats.
- Check labels for minimum age, which is 6 months for some products.
- Cats treated with inhaled glucocorticoids may develop infection only in areas where the face mask is used (i.e., chin, muzzle).

Technician Tips

- Finding dead mites, or just mite segments, is still considered a positive scraping.
- Skin scrapings should examine all scraped material.
- Use a coverslip and increase contrast (e.g., by lowering the microscope condenser); examine the slides under the 4× or 10× objective.
- *Demodex* mite eggs are fusiform (spindle shaped) and important to record because they indicate an actively reproducing population.
- Some isoxazoline drugs must be administered with food; be sure to instruct clients if this is the case with the product dispensed.

SUGGESTED READING

Miller WH Jr, et al: Muller & Kirk's Small animal dermatology, ed 7, St. Louis, 2013, Saunders, pp 304-315.

AUTHOR: Kinga Gortel, DVM, MS, DACVD
EDITOR: Manon Paradis, DMV, MVSc, DACVD

Dermatophytosis

Bonus Material Online 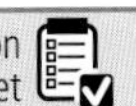 Client Education Sheet

BASIC INFORMATION

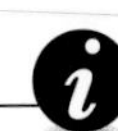

Definition

A superficial fungal disease of the keratin of hair, skin, or claws

Synonyms

Ringworm

Epidemiology

SPECIES, AGE, SEX

Cats and dogs of either sex and any age

GENETICS, BREED PREDISPOSITION

Persian, Himalayan, and Rex cats and Yorkshire and Jack Russell terriers are overrepresented.

RISK FACTORS

- Seropositive feline immunodeficiency virus (FIV) or feline leukemia virus (FeLV) status in cats alone does not increase risk of disease.
- Hunting and working dogs are at increased risk for disease and kerion reactions.
- Physiologic stress from concurrent illness, poor nutrition, endoparasitism or ectoparasitism, neoplasia, poor husbandry, overcrowding in conjunction with microtrauma to skin, and concurrent spore exposure are major risk factors for adult animals.
- Group housing in shelters, rescue agencies, pet stores coupled with exposure and the risk of microtrauma to the skin increase prevalence.

CONTAGION AND ZOONOSIS

- Dermatophytosis is a low-level zoonotic disease; infection in people causes skin lesions and is curable.
- Most common complication of *Microsporum canis* infections in immunocompromised people is possible prolonged treatment time.
- Disease is transmitted by direct contact between an infected animal to another susceptible animal or person.
- Infection from contaminated environments is a commonly cited risk factor, but there is only one documented case; mechanical carriage of spores on the hair is a confounder for environmental contamination.
- *M. canis* is not part of the normal fungal flora and isolation indicates true infection or mechanical carriage, but mechanical carriage is not infection, and the term *carriers* should not be used.
- Refer humans (clients or staff) to medical doctors for consultation regarding treatment of their lesions.

GEOGRAPHY AND SEASONALITY

Disease prevalence is higher in warmer tropical or subtropical geographic regions, particularly in locales with large stray animal populations.

Clinical Presentation

DISEASE FORMS/SUBTYPES

- *Subclinical infection:* incubation period from contact with spores to invasion of skin and hair is ≈7 days, and these early lesions are easily missed in dogs or cats.
- *Kerion:* an uncommon, overly exuberant immunologic/inflammatory response leading to thickened plaquelike to smooth, nodular growths or masses; more common with *Trichophyton* infections
- *Mycetoma or pseudomycetoma:* rare pyogranulomatous draining nodules from deeper extension of infection in an immunocompromised host; more common in Persian cats

HISTORY, CHIEF COMPLAINT

Skin lesions seen in newly acquired pet. Owner may also have skin lesions.

PHYSICAL EXAM FINDINGS

- Focal to multifocal areas of hair loss, scaling, crusting, hyperpigmentation, with or without erythema and variable pruritus. Lesions tend to be asymmetrical and can mimic pyotraumatic dermatitis (dogs) or eosinophilic lesions (cats).
- Early lesions are most commonly found in thinly haired areas (face) and on extremities.
- Uncommon: pustular lesions or lesions that resemble pemphigus

Etiology and Pathophysiology

- Causes: *M. canis*, *Microsporum gypseum*, and *Trichophyton* spp. *M. canis* is more commonly involved. Feline infections with *Trichophyton* are common in winter and/or in cats from farms.
- Arthrospores attach within 2 hours of contact and start invading and germinating in skin in 6-8 hours.
- Infection requires spore exposure, microtrauma, and moisture for successful establishment. Active infection with shedding of spores can occur within 7 days, as documented by biopsy, Wood's lamp examination, direct examination, and fungal culture.
- Dermatophytosis is a self-curing disease in healthy animals, and most infections resolve without treatment in 28-100 days. Recovery is associated with development of a strong cell-mediated immunity (CMI); lack of development of CMI results in persistent infection until a treatment intervention.

DIAGNOSIS

Diagnostic Overview

Diagnosis is based on clinical signs and use of complementary tests (see below). No one test is considered the gold standard.

Differential Diagnosis

- In dogs, rule out superficial staphylococcal pyoderma and demodicosis.
- In cats, rule out flea allergy and mite infestations. Other allergies should be considered along with other causes of generalized scaling and pruritus. Common disease in kittens but uncommon in adult cats

Initial Database

- Careful dermatologic examination in room light, followed by Wood's lamp examination. This is a highly useful tool for identification of lesions not visible in room light.

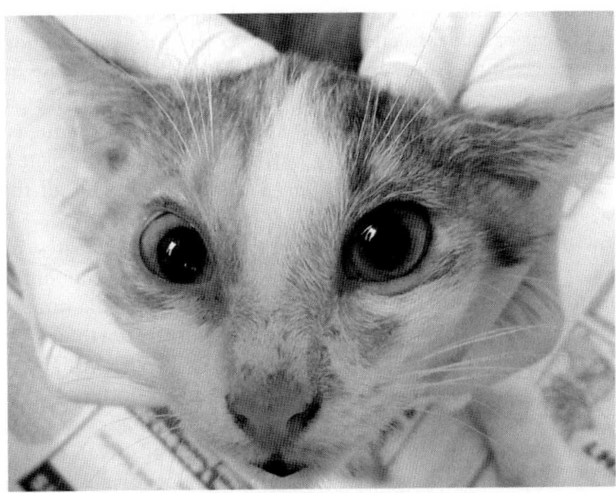

DERMATOPHYTOSIS Ambient white light examination of an affected cat shows periocular moist dermatitis and erythema bilaterally, extending to the left lateral bridge of the nose. Under white light, lesions suggest simple upper respiratory tract infection. (Copyright Alana Canupp.)

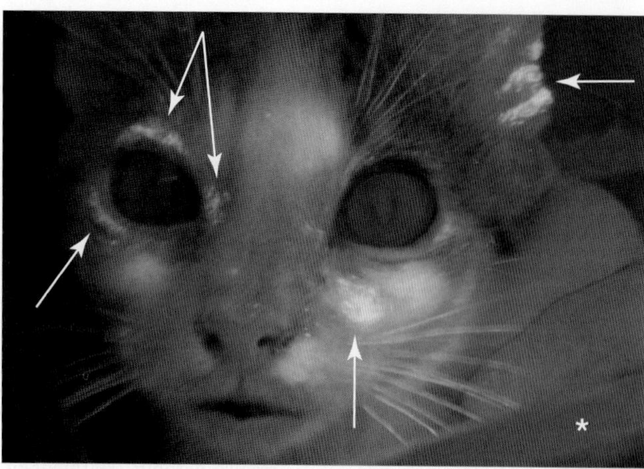

DERMATOPHYTOSIS Same cat. Wood's lamp shows extent of facial lesions and fluorescence of dermatophytosis lesions not observed in white light *(arrows)*. One fluorescent tube of the Wood's lamp is visible diagonally at the bottom of the image *(asterisk)*. (Copyright Alana Canupp.)

- Commonly overlooked infection sites include paws, periocular area, ear and inside the bell of the ear, tail, ventrum, and axilla.
- Wood's lamp examination
  - *M. canis* is the only veterinary pathogen of clinical significance that glows when exposed to 320-400 nm ultraviolet (UV) light. Positive fluorescence is apple green and is found only on the hair shaft. It is due to a fungal metabolite (produced while the hair is growing) that is very stable; hair samples have remained Wood's lamp positive for >18 years. Fluorescence is an inherent property of *M. canis*. Evidence-based review showed that in untreated animals, 91%-100% of *M. canis* lesions fluoresced.
  - Use Wood's lamp with built-in magnification. Do not use a black lamp.
  - Wood's lamps *do not* need to be warmed up.
  - Do allow several minutes for examiner's eyes to adapt to low light.
  - Hold Wood's lamp close to skin (2-4 cm), and move slowly, starting at the head. This is important to minimize distracting fluorescence from scales and debris on the coat and maximize seeing lesions.
  - Only the hair shaft fluoresces, never the crusts or nails. Newly infected hairs are very short and often obscured by crusts (lift crusts as needed). The target color is apple green; blue fluorescence of scale and dull yellow fluorescence of excessive sebum (chin, tail) should not be mistaken for dermatophytosis. If in doubt, examine hair bulb by plucking hair or strip a lesion with clear acetate tape to collect sample.
- Direct examination
  - More than 85% of dermatophyte infections (*M. canis, M. gypseum, Trichophyton spp*) can be confirmed by direct examination of combined skin scraping and hair plucking.
  - Using mineral oil, gently scrape hairs from lesion margins and center of lesion. Pluck Wood's lamp–positive hairs in the direction of growth, transfer to glass microscope slide, add mineral oil and a coverslip, and examine. Do not use clearing agents. Infected hairs are easily seen, even under a 10× objective because they are wider and pale. If there is any confusion or hairs cannot be found, holding the Wood's lamp over the slide can reveal glowing hairs.
  - Microscopically, ectothrix spores appear as numerous, refractile, spindle-shaped bodies in cuffs around the hair shaft.
- Fungal culture
  - Use soft-bristled toothbrush, and focus on collecting specimen from the lesion(s). Comb target sites 20 times or until hairs are visibly trapped in the bristles. Wrap head of toothbrush in plastic bag, and place entire toothbrush into a second bag.
  - The optimal fungal culture medium is one that can be easily inoculated with a toothbrush; small plates used in human laboratories, glass jars, or "diagnosis by color" products are not recommended.
  - Inoculate the plate by stabbing the bristles in the medium; if agar is seen on the bristles the technique is adequate. *Do not* overinoculate the plate because it inhibits sporulation, and all that will be seen is hyphae.
  - Always place plates in plastic bags to prevent cross-contamination and infestation with media mites.
  - Optimal growth and sporulation occurs at 80°F (28°C); light conditions do not matter. Fourteen days is adequate for holding plates for untreated animals (99% positive) and treated animals (98% positive). Examine the plates *daily* for growth. Look for a whitish, fluffy to powdery colony, with a red color change in the medium *at the same time* that the colony is first visible. NOTE: Color change in the medium may be delayed 24-48 hours in specimens from treated animals. Dermatophyte colonies are never black, gray, green, or multicolored.
  - All suspect colonies must be microscopically confirmed using lactophenol cotton blue stain or methylene blue. It is helpful to make the mount and allow it sit for 10-15 minutes before examination, which helps highlight the macroconidia.

Advanced or Confirmatory Testing

Skin biopsy is not needed for routine diagnosis, and if dermatophytosis is identified, the presentation was likely atypical. Polymerase chain reaction (PCR) testing is highly specific and highly sensitive. It is important to submit adequate amounts of hairs and crusts for testing but only from the lesion site.

TREATMENT

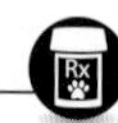

Treatment Overview

This disease will spontaneously resolve without treatment, but treatment is recommended to shorten the course of infection and minimize transmission to other animals and people. Both topical and systemic therapy are used together.

Acute General Treatment

Reasonable confinement:

- Reasonably confine pet to a room that is easily cleaned but that still allows for activity and exercise. This disease is most common in animals during critical socialization periods, and human contact and socialization are necessary to prevent lifelong behavioral problems. Confinement is primarily done to minimize the areas that need cleaning.
- It is *not* acceptable to cage or crate animals for the duration of treatment.

Cleaning:

- Primary reason for cleaning is not to prevent disease transmission but rather to minimize false-positive fungal cultures or PCR tests.
- Change bedding daily. Laundry can be decontaminated by washing in domestic washing machine on long wash cycle. Avoid overloading the machine. Bleach and hot water were no more effective than cold water without bleach.
- Mechanically remove shed hairs and debris daily using disposable dust cloths or washable floor dusters.
- Wipe contaminated surfaces daily with a one-step ready-to-use bathroom cleaner labeled as efficacious against *Trichophyton mentagrophytes*.
- Twice weekly, wash target surfaces with soap and detergent, rinse, and dry. Area should be visibly clean. Most surfaces can be decontaminated with aggressive washing with a detergent. Judiciously use a ready to use bathroom disinfectant (see above) to kill spores on surfaces.

- AVOID the use of bleach; it has no detergency effect, has not been shown to be more effective than other disinfectants, is readily inactivated after dilution, and when exposed to light, is an irritant and damages surfaces. It is an animal and human health risk and irritant.
- Carpets can be decontaminated by steam cleaning or two washings with a beater-brush carpet shampooer.
- Important to stress to owners that spores do not multiply in the environment and do not invade homes like mildew or black mold. Spores in the environment are dormant and are not alive.
- Furnace filters are excellent at trapping spores and hairs and do not spread spores throughout the home.

Pet-Focused Treatment

Topical therapy:

- Topical therapy is equally important as systemic therapy. It is the only way to disinfect the haircoat and kill infective spores on hairs.
- Comb haircoat before application to remove loose hairs.
- Apply topical therapy twice per week to the whole body, being sure to soak hairs and the skin.
- Rinses
  - Lime sulfur solution: $\frac{1}{16}$ dilution (8 ounces in 1 gallon of tap water; 30 mL in 480 mL of tap water). Use lukewarm water, and be sure to soak the skin and hair; do not rinse. Towel dry. In some countries, agricultural products are used. They are labeled 23% calcium polysulfide or 23% sulfur sulfide, which is equivalent to a 76.9% lime sulfur solution. The same dilution ($\frac{1}{16}$) is therefore required to obtain the same solution dilution.
  - Enilconazole topical solution 0.2% (dilute per label instructions); in cats, prevent grooming with Elizabethan collar until dry.
- Shampoos
  - Use combination of chlorhexidine + miconazole, chlorhexidine + ketoconazole, or chlorhexidine + climbazole. Dilute 1 : 4 before application, and shampoo for at least 3-5 minutes. Disadvantage is that this does not have residual activity.
- Mousse
  - Leave-on climbazole mousse can be used in patients that cannot be wetted (e.g., animals with bandages or upper respiratory infections).
- Concurrent focal therapy
  - Use concurrent focal topical therapy for hard-to-treat areas that are often nidus of residual infection. Apply miconazole vaginal cream 2% to lesions in hard to treat areas such as the face and periocular area. For ears, use miconazole- or ketoconazole-containing ear rinse to disinfect hairs in bell of ear. Apply daily.

Systemic Therapy

- Terbinafine has the lowest minimum inhibitory concentration (MIC) against dermatophytes. It is the drug of choice for dogs and an alternative to itraconazole for cats.
- Terbinafine 30-40 mg/kg PO q 24h or week on/week off until cured
- Itraconazole 5 mg/kg PO q 24h, week on/week off (i.e., 7 days of treatment, 7 days without until mycologic cure) is the systemic drug of choice for cats. Cost limits its use in dogs. Pulse therapy works because the drug accumulates in hair and skin. Do not use compounded formulations of this product in cats or dogs.
- Ketoconazole 5-10 mg/kg PO q 24h is an option for dogs but has higher MIC than terbinafine or itraconazole. Avoid use in cats due to gastrointestinal intolerance.
- Fluconazole has poor antifungal efficacy against dermatophytes and highest MIC compared to itraconazole, terbinafine, ketoconazole, or griseofulvin.
- Griseofulvin is less effective than itraconazole and terbinafine and is no longer recommended for use.
- Lufenuron is not effective for treatment or prevention in cats.

Recommended Monitoring

- Animals responding to therapy show rapid clinical cure, some as early as 1-2 weeks after starting therapy.
- Monitor *M. canis* infections using a Wood's lamp. Any evidence of fluorescence on the hair shaft makes the animal high risk for still being infected. Glowing hair tips are often seen in cured animals and represent residual pigmentation.
- PCR can be used to determine mycologic cure, but it detects viable and nonviable fungal DNA. Wash animal in shampoo before testing to remove residual fungal DNA. A negative test result indicates mycologic cure; a positive test may be from nonviable DNA.
- If using fungal cultures, perform weekly or start when Wood's lamp examinations are negative. Monitor the number of colony-forming units per plate. Recovery is associated with fewer colony-forming units on the plate. Both cure and poor treatment compliance are best identified this way.
- Weekly fungal cultures are cost-effective; the first and second negative cultures can be detected sooner than with q 2 week or q 4 week intervals.

PROGNOSIS & OUTCOME

- Prognosis is good, even for cats with long hair.
- Terbinafine and itraconazole are well tolerated. Most animals achieve cure in 4-8 weeks.
- Cats or dogs that do not achieve a cure usually have an underlying medical problem causing immunosuppression.

PEARLS & CONSIDERATIONS

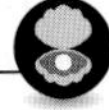

Comments

- Clipping of the haircoat is not needed unless the coat is so matted that topical therapy cannot be applied adequately.
- Combing the animal's coat with a flea comb to remove broken hairs and decrease infective load is an effective alternative to clipping.

Prevention

- Include room light and Wood's lamp examinations as part of the examination of all new pets. Perform fungal cultures for high-risk individuals. Use topical therapy pending results when infection suspected.
- Catteries should routinely quarantine cats pending fungal culture results for all new additions or cats returning to the facility.

Technician Tips

Create a positive control for the Wood's lamp examination by pressing clear acetate tape to a glowing lesion and then mounting it on a glass slide. Seal edges with fingernail polish.

SUGGESTED READING

Moriello KA, et al: Diagnosis and treatment of dermatophytosis in dogs and cats. Clinical consensus guidelines for the World Association of Veterinary Dermatology. Vet Dermatol 28:266-303, 2017.

AUTHOR: Karen Moriello, DVM, DACVD
EDITOR: Manon Paradis, DMV, MVSc, DACVD

Diabetes Insipidus

Client Education Sheet 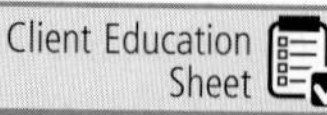

BASIC INFORMATION

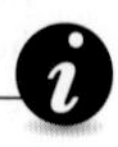

Definition

Inadequate urine-concentrating ability due to insufficient antidiuretic hormone (ADH; i.e., vasopressin) secretion (central diabetes insipidus [CDI]) or action (nephrogenic diabetes insipidus [NDI])

Epidemiology

SPECIES, AGE, SEX

- Affects dogs and cats
- No breed, sex, or age predisposition

Clinical Presentation

DISEASE FORMS/SUBTYPES

- CDI: hypothalamic/pituitary gland disorder
- NDI: disorder at the renal level

HISTORY, CHIEF COMPLAINT

- The major manifestations are polyuria (PU) and polydipsia (PD). The PU may result in hypovolemia.
- Stupor, disorientation, ataxia, and seizures possible when a large neoplasm in the area of the pituitary is the underlying cause or when insufficient drinking has resulted in (life-threatening) hypertonic encephalopathy.

PHYSICAL EXAM FINDINGS

- Usually normal
- Dehydration may be noted if the animal has not had free access to water.
- Neurologic abnormalities (e.g., stupor, disorientation, ataxia) possible with severe hypernatremia or with CDI due to hypothalamic/pituitary mass lesion

Etiology and Pathophysiology

- Normal daily water consumption < 100 mL/kg/d for dogs and < 250 mL/d for cats
- ADH is released by the neurohypophysis (i.e., posterior pituitary) in response to increased plasma osmolality and, to a lesser degree, to reduced blood volume.
- ADH binds to vasopressin-2 receptors in the renal distal tubules and collecting ducts. Activation of these receptors results in insertion of water channels (aquaporins) in the luminal membrane of the tubular cells, leading to increased water absorption from the lumen of the ducts into the renal interstitium. The end result is concentrated urine. Water resorption also depends on the osmotic gradient of the renal interstitium.
- CDI results from a lack of hypothalamic production or release of ADH secondary to immune-mediated destruction of ADH-producing neurons, cerebral trauma (head injury), intracranial neoplasia (often a pituitary tumor), or other hypothalamic/pituitary lesions. In dogs, hyperadrenocorticism may also result in reduced ADH secretion. Animals without a discernible underlying cause are classified as having idiopathic CDI.
- In NDI, the kidneys are unable to concentrate urine despite adequate circulating levels of ADH. Frequently, the cause of inadequate ADH action remains unknown (i.e., idiopathic NDI). NDI may also be a consequence of other disorders (i.e., secondary NDI).
  - *Escherichia coli* endotoxins (e.g., pyometra, pyelonephritis) and hypercalcemia may interfere with the renal action of ADH.
  - In dogs, glucocorticoids (endogenous hypercortisolism or therapeutic administration) and mineralocorticoids (hyperaldosteronism) interfere with the renal action of ADH.
- Congenital NDI and congenital CDI are rare.

DIAGNOSIS

Diagnostic Overview

The diagnostic approach to diabetes insipidus is directed at ruling out metabolic, endocrine, or other causes of PU/PD by using a CBC, routine biochemistry profile (including plasma osmolality), urinalysis, urine culture, and test(s) for adrenal gland disorders. After other differential diagnoses are excluded, differentiation of CDI from NDI or primary PD requires serial measurements of urine osmolality (Uosm), a trial therapy with exogenous ADH, and eventually, a water deprivation test.

Differential Diagnosis

Other causes of PU/PD (pp. 812, 1271, and 1442)

Initial Database

- CBC: usually normal; mild hemoconcentration may be seen if the animal is dehydrated
- Serum biochemical profile: usually no abnormalities except for slight hypernatremia and elevated plasma osmolality in cases of inadequate replenishment of excreted water
- Urinalysis: usually hyposthenuria to isosthenuria (urine specific gravity [USG] < 1.013, often < 1.008) but may be higher in cases of partial CDI or NDI
- Other tests to rule out causes of secondary NDI include urine culture, *Leptospira* serology, abdominal ultrasonography, and testing for hyperadrenocorticism (p. 485).

Advanced or Confirmatory Testing

- Random plasma osmolality: a large overlap exists among CDI, NDI, and primary PD. Plasma osmolality < 280 mOsm/kg suggests primary PD.
- Serial measurements of urine osmolality and trial therapy with exogenous ADH
  - The owner should collect urine samples q 2h (q 4h during the night) for 24 hours. If Uosm in one of these samples is > 1000 mOsm/kg (USG > 1.030), primary PD is diagnosed. If all samples have Uosm < 1000 mOsm/kg (USG < 1.030), a vasopressin analog (desmopressin acetate [DDAVP]) is administered for 5 days: one drop of an intranasal solution (100 mcg/mL) is administered by the owner in the conjunctival sac q 8h. During the last day of DDAVP administration, the owner should collect another series of urine samples as before. If Uosm remains < 1000 mOsm/kg in these samples, CDI is very unlikely, and the patient has primary PD or NDI instead.
- Water deprivation test
  - Used for differentiating NDI from primary PD (i.e., after CDI has been excluded)
  - Should not be performed if azotemia or dehydration is present
  - The patient must be monitored throughout the test.
  - Procedure
    - Fast the patient for 12 hours before the test.
    - At the start of water deprivation, empty the patient's bladder, and determine the patient's body weight, plasma osmolality, and USG or preferably Uosm.
    - Withhold water and monitor clinical demeanor, body weight (after emptying bladder), and USG (or Uosm) q 2h. After a urine sample has been collected, the bladder must be emptied.
    - The test is stopped when 5% of body weight has been lost, USG increases to > 1.030 or Uosm to > 1000 mOsm/kg, USG or Uosm do not increase for > 6 hours, or the pet becomes clinically dehydrated or depressed.
    - Slowly reintroduce water when the test is completed.
  - Interpretation
    - USG or Uosm in patients with primary PD should slowly increase to > 1.030 or > 1000 mOsm/kg, respectively.
    - Patients with NDI will show little or no increase in USG or Uosm.
  - Possible complications of the test: hypernatremia/hypertonic dehydration (irritability, weakness, ataxia, stupor, coma)
- CT or MRI (p. 1132) of the hypothalamic/pituitary area can be used to determine whether a cranial mass is the cause of CDI.
- Endogenous creatinine or iohexol clearance testing or nuclear scintigraphy to estimate glomerular filtration rate may be used to rule out renal insufficiency.

TREATMENT

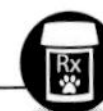

Treatment Overview

Therapy is aimed at improving patient and owner quality of life through reduction or resolution of PU/PD. Treatment is expected to be lifelong unless an underlying cause can be identified and resolved.

Acute General Treatment

None generally required

Chronic Treatment

- The treatment of choice for CDI is exogenous ADH administration (DDAVP as tablets [0.1 mg/DOG PO q 8h or 0.025-0.05 mg/CAT q 8-12h; increase dose if no response within 1 week] or intranasal drops administered into the conjunctival sac [1 drop/patient q 8-12h]). Patients with NDI are usually unresponsive to DDAVP therapy.
- For NDI, thiazide diuretics (hydrochlorothiazide 2-4 mg/kg PO q 12h) with a low-sodium diet to reduce total-body sodium concentration. This increases renal sodium and water resorption and reduces urine volume, albeit often without a significant change in Uosm.
- If PU/PD is not disruptive to the owners and the animal has free access to water and a place to urinate, treatment may not be required.

Possible Complications

- Cellular overhydration can occur in patients that consume large volumes of water shortly after receiving DDAVP because of a decreased ability to excrete the free water after DDAVP reaches therapeutic effect. Neurologic signs (ataxia, depression, tremors, seizures) can occur as a consequence of cerebral edema. It is recommended that pets not have free access to water immediately after each dose.
- Mild conjunctival irritation can occur with topical ocular DDAVP.
- Thiazide diuretics may cause hypokalemia.
- Untreated animals can become dehydrated, hypovolemic, and hyperosmolar very quickly if denied access to water or in cases of vomiting/regurgitation.

Recommended Monitoring

- Clinical response should be monitored in patients receiving DDAVP therapy.
- Serum electrolytes should be periodically monitored if thiazide diuretics are used.

PROGNOSIS & OUTCOME

- In patients with idiopathic CDI, clinical signs generally resolve completely with DDAVP therapy, and patients can have a normal life expectancy. Lifelong treatment is not feasible for some pet owners due to the expense of DDAVP.
- CDI secondary to an intracranial neoplasm has a guarded prognosis because progressive neurologic signs may develop in the ensuing months.
- The PU/PD of primary NDI is often difficult to manage medically and is therefore associated with a guarded prognosis.

PEARLS & CONSIDERATIONS

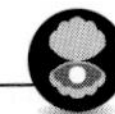

Comments

- Hypercortisolism is a likely differential in a patient that initially responds to exogenous DDAVP therapy but later has recurrence of PU/PD.
- Because they are highly correlated, USG measurements by refractometry can be used in place of Uosm. However, Uosm measurements are preferred because homeostatic mechanisms maintaining water and electrolyte balance are related to osmolality. Moreover, in approximately 15% of samples, USG is not a correct reflection of Uosm.
- Complete emptying of the bladder after a urine sample has been collected is essential during a water deprivation test because the decision about whether to continue the test depends on a correct determination of urine concentration during the previous period. When urine volume is small, catheterization may be needed to obtain a sample and to ascertain that the bladder is emptied. In cats, the use of an indwelling urinary catheter may be necessary.
- Head trauma can result in transient CDI that resolves on its own.

Technician Tips

The water deprivation test requires extremely diligent monitoring for the entire duration of the test. Without it, there is a very real risk of progressive, life-threatening dehydration in these patients.

Client Education

Patients with diabetes insipidus must always have free access to water.

SUGGESTED READING

Meij BP, et al: Hypothalamus-pituitary system. In Rijnberk A, et al, editors: Clinical endocrinology of dogs and cats, ed 2, Hannover, Germany, 2010, Schlütersche, pp 13-54.

AUTHOR: **Hans S. Kooistra, DVM, PhD, DECVIM**
EDITOR: **Ellen N. Behrend, VMD, PhD, DACVIM**

Diabetes Mellitus

Bonus Material Online  Client Education Sheet

BASIC INFORMATION

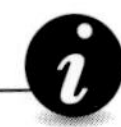

Definition

Project Agreeing Language in Veterinary Endocrinology (ALIVE), endorsed by the European Society of Veterinary Endocrinology and Society for Comparative Endocrinology, defines diabetes mellitus (DM) as follows:

- A complex syndrome identified by the presence of pathologic hyperglycemia
- Best seen not as one disease but rather as a consequence of one or more primary disease processes
- Many factors can contribute to development of DM, including patient genetics, presence of pancreatic disease, or conditions causing insulin resistance.
- Classification of DM in small animals according to cause is recommended, as is done for diabetic people.
- The final stage in DM development is a relative or absolute deficiency of insulin production by pancreatic beta cells.
- Clinical signs result from a combination of insufficient insulin action in the body and the resulting hyperglycemia and hyperlipidemia.

Epidemiology

SPECIES, AGE, SEX

- Cats: middle-aged to older (>6 years); male neutered cats may be overrepresented
- Dogs: middle-aged to older (>6 years); no sex predisposition (except diestrus- or pregnancy-related DM)
  - Occasionally seen in animals < 1 year of age (juvenile DM)

GENETICS, BREED PREDISPOSITION

Cats:

- Any cat can develop DM.
- Tonkinese, Norwegian Forest, and Burmese cats are predisposed compared with crossbred cats.
- Melanocortin-4 receptor gene *(MC4R)* implicated in susceptibility to DM

Dogs:

- Any dog can develop DM.
- Various breeds are associated with increased risk of DM (e.g., terriers, Samoyed, miniature schnauzer); others have a decreased risk (e.g., boxer, German shepherd).

- Susceptibility may be associated with immune response genes.

RISK FACTORS

- Cats: odds of developing DM increase with body weight > 4 kg, when cats are overweight or obese, with glucocorticoid or progestogen administration, and with hypersomatotropism/acromegaly (p. 17) or hyperadrenocorticism (p. 485)
- Dogs: unspayed female dogs at risk for diestrus-induced DM; dogs with hyperadrenocorticism and pancreatitis also at risk

GEOGRAPHY AND SEASONALITY

Canine DM occurs year-round but is more frequently diagnosed at the end of winter.

ASSOCIATED DISORDERS

- Primary disease processes underlying the DM (see etiologic classification below)
- Diabetic ketoacidosis (DKA), mostly with untreated DM or when concurrent disease is present (p. 254)
- Diabetic neuropathy (mostly cats) (p. 808)
- Diabetic cataracts (dogs) (p. 147)
- Exocrine pancreatic insufficiency (mostly with canine juvenile DM) (p. 317)
- Urinary tract infections (dogs and cats) (p. 232)

Clinical Presentation

DISEASE FORMS/SUBTYPES

Project ALIVE recommends the following etiologic classification; an individual can have concurrent underlying causes.

Insulin-deficient DM (beta-cell-related disorders):

- Reduced insulin secretion due to
  - Beta cell destruction related to immune-mediated disease, exocrine pancreatic disease, other causes such as toxicity (diazoxide) or idiopathic causes
  - Beta cell death (apoptosis) from glucotoxicity, lipotoxicity, other or idiopathic causes
  - Beta cell aplasia/abiotrophy/hypoplasia
- Production of defective insulin

Insulin-resistant DM (target-organ disorders):

- Endocrine influences
  - Growth hormone: hypersecretion (i.e., acromegaly) from pituitary or mammary origin (p. 17) or exogenous administration. Hypothyroidism can increase growth hormone production.
  - Steroids: glucocorticoids from hypersecretion (i.e., hyperadrenocorticism [p. 485]) or exogenous administration; progesterone/progestins from secretion (i.e., pregnancy or, in dogs, diestrus) or exogenous administration
  - Catecholamines
  - Thyroid hormone (i.e., hyperthyroidism [p. 503])
- Obesity
- Drugs
  - Thiazide diuretics
  - Beta-adrenergic agonists
- Inflammatory mediators
- Disorders of insulin receptor and intracellular signaling

HISTORY, CHIEF COMPLAINT

- Common complaints of uncomplicated DM include polyuria, polydipsia, polyphagia, and/or weight loss.
  - Blindness (dogs) or gait changes (cats) may reflect complications of DM.
- Owners should be questioned about previous or current medical conditions, including administration of diabetogenic drugs.
- DKA presents with inappetence or anorexia, vomiting, signs of weakness and dehydration, and/or hypovolemia (p. 254).
- With the exception of DKA, DM does not cause inappetence; inappetence without DKA suggests presence of a concurrent disease.
- Underlying disease process(es) causing DM can result in additional clinical signs (e.g., acromegaly can cause heart failure, hyperadrenocorticism could cause dermatologic changes, pancreatitis could cause inappetance and abdominal pain).
- History and physical exam findings are not pathognomonic for DM; other common clinical conditions should be considered (e.g., hyperthyroidism, chronic kidney disease).

PHYSICAL EXAM FINDINGS

- Depending on duration of illness and underlying or concurrent disease processes, pet may be overweight/obese or underweight/emaciated at initial presentation.
- Diabetic neuropathy in some cats and rare in dogs, including plantigrade posture
- Approximately 80% of dogs suffer from diabetic cataracts within 1 year of diagnosis.
- The underlying disease process causing the DM can result in a variety of additional physical exam findings.

Etiology and Pathophysiology

- Consider the ALIVE etiologic classification of DM at time of diagnosis.
- Type of DM dictates best diagnostic and treatment practice.

DIAGNOSIS

Diagnostic Overview

- Step 1: establish whether the clinical signs are compatible with DM
- Step 2: documentation of pathologic hyperglycemia
- Step 3: exclusion of other diseases/phenomena that could lead to hyperglycemia
- Step 4: establish type of DM

Differential Diagnosis

- Stress hyperglycemia (more frequent in cats, possible in dogs) (p. 1235)
- Other causes of polyuria/polydipsia (p. 812); top differentials to consider:
  - Hyperadrenocorticism (not normally associated with weight loss if occurs without DM)
  - Hyperthyroidism (cats)
  - Chronic kidney disease (not normally associated with increased appetite)
- Other causes of polyphagia (p. 809) and weight loss (p. 1047)

Initial Database

- CBC, biochemical profile and urinalysis to evaluate for DM and concurrent disease
- Per Project ALIVE, DM defined by
  - In dogs, persistently increased fasting (minimum, 8 hours) hyperglycemia (blood glucose [BG] > 144 mg/dL) *or* a single measurement of hyperglycemia with concurrent glucosuria and/or elevated concentrations of glycated blood proteins and compatible clinical signs of DM with no other plausible cause
  - In cats, one or more measurements of hyperglycemia (BG > 126 mg/dL) and an elevated concentration of glycated blood proteins
- A glycated protein concentration within the reference interval does not rule out DM. Diagnosis of DM can be achieved by demonstration of persistent or worsening hyperglycemia and/or glucosuria on follow-up.
- Most commonly measured glycated proteins
  - Fructosamine; reflects average BG concentrations over the prior 1-3 weeks (p. 1345)
  - Glycosylated hemoglobin: reflects average BG concentrations over previous 2-3 months (cats) and 3-4 months (dogs) (p. 1349)

Advanced or Confirmatory Testing

- Given the diverse nature of underlying and concurrent diseases causing DM, the following screening tests should be considered:
  - Serum IGF-1 for acromegaly (cats)
  - Serum feline pancreatic lipase immunoreactivity (fPLI) or canine pancreatic lipase immunoreactivity (cPLI) and abdominal ultrasound (for pancreatitis)
  - Urine analysis, sediment, and culture (urinary tract infections are common in diabetic pets)
- Screening for other diseases depends on level of suspicion, as well as on a discussion with the owner about costs and relevance of diseases.

TREATMENT

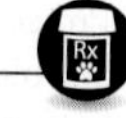

Treatment Overview

Main treatment goals:

- Resolution of clinical signs of DM along with improvement of pet's and owner's quality of life (QoL)
- Avoiding complications (hypoglycemia, DKA); cataracts are difficult to prevent

Considerations in achieving these goals:

- Treat the underlying condition causing the DM whenever possible.
- Clinical signs improve or resolve after BG is maintained < 270 mg/dL most of the time.

- Owner understanding of disease and good communication between owners and the health care team are essential.
- Remission can be achieved in a proportion of diabetic cats (approximately 30% in a general population, 80% of acromegaly-induced diabetics).
- No unbiased evidence exists proving that protocols that aim for euglycemia are superior to traditional control protocols in cats.

Acute General Treatment

- Address the underlying or associated disease and/or risk factors as soon as possible.
- DM should be treated as soon as possible with exogenous insulin injections and an appropriate dietary regimen in stable patients with preserved appetite.
- An insulin preparation should be chosen that is legal to be used in the relevant country and is long acting.
  - Protamine zinc insulin (ProZinc), glargine (Lantus), and detemir (Levemir) have proved to be equally successful for use in cats.
  - Porcine lente insulin (Caninsulin, Vetsulin) and detemir (Levemir) have proved useful in dogs.
  - NPH insulin often proves to be short-acting for dogs and especially for cats.
- For most insulin types (exception: detemir) a safe starting dose is 0.25-0.5 units/kg (dog) or 1 unit/CAT SQ q 12h.
- Insulin response is highly variable among patients; most insulin types need to be used twice daily in most patients.
- Occasionally, insulin administration before feeding (up to 1 hour) can prove beneficial by matching insulin peak activity with post-prandial hyperglycemia, especially in dogs.
- Immediate treatment goals should be that owner and pet become familiar with insulin injections and that owners can monitor clinical signs.
- In general, oral hypoglycemic drugs (sulfonylureas such as glipizide) should be considered only in cats, and they uncommonly prove successful; acarbose can be used in combination with insulin in dogs or cats but is seldom helpful.
- If DKA or hyperosmolar syndrome is present, hospitalize and treat accordingly (p. 254)

Chronic Treatment

- After insulin is started, the animal is sent home.
- Unless hypoglycemia occurs, insulin dose changes should not occur quickly, leaving 7-10 days between each dose change.
- If hypoglycemia is present at any time, insulin dose must be decreased.
- Consider introducing the owner to home blood glucose monitoring (HBGM).
- Support from the veterinary and nursing team is essential, especially in the beginning.
- Various monitoring methods exist, all with advantages and disadvantages; an individualized monitoring regimen should be discussed with the owner.
- The clinical picture should always lead a treatment decision.
- Using a clinical scoring system for the clinical signs standardizes communication between owner and medical team.

Nutrition/Diet

- Cats ideally should be transitioned to a low-carbohydrate (<7% of metabolizable energy), wet diet.
- For dogs, diet should be changed only if obesity or comorbidity needs to be addressed.
- Dogs and cats should be given a palatable diet that is eaten reliably in an amount aimed at an ideal body condition.
- Should ideally be fed two meals of one-half their daily caloric requirement (unless overweight/obese) roughly 12 hours apart. Graze feeding can be continued if preferred by patient.

Behavior/Exercise

Exercise levels are best kept constant, resulting in reliable and predictable insulin need. Exercise should be increased for overweight/obese animals.

Possible Complications

- Diabetic ketoacidosis (p. 254) or hyperosmolar syndrome
- Insulin use can cause hypoglycemia; to avoid this
  - Use a conservative starting dose.
  - Avoid rapid dose increases.
  - Avoid BG values close to the hypoglycemic range.
  - Periodically screen for possible hypoglycemia when there are no diabetic signs (e.g., absence of morning glucosuria indicates possible hypoglycemia).
  - Ensure good owner education/communication.

Recommended Monitoring

- Various methods are available.
- Clinical picture is the most important monitoring tool (consider using scoring system).
- Various apps are available to enable communication and structured recording of relevant information.
- Choice of glycemic monitoring tool depends on owner and pet factors.
- Glycemic indicators can be used on their own or in combination:
  - Serial blood glucose curve (usually q 2h for 12 hours)
  - Glycated proteins (fructosamine, glycosylated hemoglobin)
  - Urine glucose: useful to screen for remission (if urine does not contain glucose); not to be used to increase insulin dose
  - Continuous subcutaneous glucose monitoring systems (e.g., Freestyle Libre, Guardian, Dexcom)
  - All above parameters can be influenced by nondiabetic factors such as stress and day-to-day variation; they should *always* be interpreted with caution and in light of the clinical picture.

PROGNOSIS & OUTCOME

- DM can be treated effectively in most cases, provided clinician, nurse/technician, and owner work as a team.
- Remission is possible in cats, especially if an underlying condition is present that can be controlled/cured. Remission is rare in dogs except for pregnancy/progesterone-related DM.

PEARLS & CONSIDERATIONS

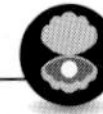

Comments

The veterinary team should acknowledge the impact of the daily treatment regimen on the pet and owner. A validated QoL tool (i.e., DIAQoL-pet) can be used to investigate and monitor impact.

Prevention

Prevent diabetogenic risk factors (see ALIVE etiologic classification of DM).

Technician Tips

- Regular recording of body weight and body condition score (9-point scale) is essential.
- To measure QoL of diabetic pets and their owners, use the DIAQoL-pet by the Royal Veterinary College Pet Diabetes App. It also serves as a tool to communicate clinical data. (Android: http://bit.ly/1q3jCV5 and iPhone: http://apple.co/203OoK2).

Client Education

Evidence-based information and pet diabetes videos can be found on Facebook (www.facebook.com/RVC.Diabetic.Remission.Clinic).

SUGGESTED READING

Gilor C, et al: What's in a name? Classification of diabetes mellitus in veterinary medicine and why it matters. J Vet Intern Med 30(4):927-940, 2016.

AUTHOR: Stijn J.M. Niessen, DVM, PhD, DECVIM, FHEA
EDITOR: Ellen N. Behrend, VMD, PhD, DACVIM

Diabetic Ketoacidosis

Client Education Sheet 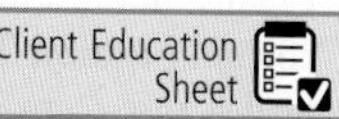

BASIC INFORMATION

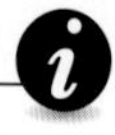

Definition

A serious, often life-threatening form of diabetes mellitus (DM), diabetic ketoacidosis (DKA) is characterized by hyperglycemia, glucosuria, ketonemia/ketonuria, and metabolic acidosis.

Synonym

DKA

Epidemiology

SPECIES, AGE, SEX

Most commonly, dogs and cats are middle-aged or older, with a median age of 8 years for dogs and 9 years for cats (p. 251).

GENETICS, BREED PREDISPOSITION

Siamese and Abyssinian cats may have an increased risk for DKA.

RISK FACTORS

Uncontrolled or undiagnosed DM

ASSOCIATED DISORDERS

Concurrent disorders occur in approximately 70% of dogs and 55%-90% of cats. Most common ones:

- Dogs: urinary tract infection (p. 232), acute pancreatitis (p. 742), hyperadrenocorticism (p. 490)
- Cats: hepatic lipidosis (p. 444), acute pancreatitis (p. 740), chronic renal failure (p. 169), cholangiohepatitis (p. 160), neoplasia

Clinical Presentation

HISTORY, CHIEF COMPLAINT

- Patients may present with clinical signs related to uncontrolled DM, DKA, and/or a concurrent disease.
- History is variable due to the progressive nature of DKA. Signs include those typical of uncomplicated DM as well as the DKA (e.g., anorexia, vomiting).
- Most common clinical signs:
  - Polyuria/polydipsia
  - Lethargy or depression
  - Anorexia
  - Vomiting
  - Weight loss
- Clinical signs related to the DKA typically progress quickly.

PHYSICAL EXAM FINDINGS

- Physical exam findings can vary in severity. Potential findings related to DKA:
  - Dehydration
  - Abdominal pain
  - Decreased mentation
  - Lateral recumbency
  - Hepatomegaly
  - Tachypnea
  - An acetone odor of the breath
- Cats are more likely to be subjectively underweight, and dogs are more likely to be overweight.
- Physical exam findings related to DM (e.g., cataracts in dogs) or to the concurrent disease may be noted.

Etiology and Pathophysiology

- In dogs and cats with DM, there is a lack of insulin or resistance to insulin.
- Without insulin, hyperglycemia develops, leading to osmotic diuresis and the classic clinical signs of DM: polyuria, polydipsia, polyphagia, and weight loss.
- Without glucose as an energy source for cells, fat cells are broken down, releasing free fatty acids. The liver converts free fatty acids to triglycerides and ketone bodies (i.e., acetoacetic acid, beta-hydroxybutyric acid, acetone).
- Typically, a concurrent illness leads to an increase in secretion and blood concentrations of stress hormones glucagon, epinephrine, cortisol, and growth hormone, which counteract the actions of insulin further.
- The stress hormones stimulate lipolysis, gluconeogenesis, and glycogenolysis, leading to a worsening hyperglycemia and continued formation of ketone bodies.
- A state of ketosis and acidosis develops as ketone bodies continue to accumulate and saturate the body's buffering systems.

DIAGNOSIS

Diagnostic Overview

Diagnosis is based on documentation of hyperglycemia, glucosuria, ketonuria/ketonemia, and metabolic acidosis. Routine blood tests will identify hyperglycemia. Ketones can be detected by a urine dipstick using urine or serum as the sample. A quantitative value can be obtained using a handheld ketone meter. Ideally, acidosis should be confirmed by identification of metabolic acidosis by blood gas measurement (p. 1315). If this is not possible, a low bicarbonate concentration or an elevated anion gap measurement on a blood chemistry profile helps support the diagnosis.

Differential Diagnosis

- Hyperglycemic hyperosmolar syndrome
- Diabetic ketosis without acidosis

Initial Database

- A CBC, serum biochemical profile, and urinalysis with bacterial culture and sensitivity tests should be performed. Ideally, blood gases should also be measured.
- CBC: nonspecific changes are seen.
  - Nonregenerative anemia (50% of dogs)
  - Leukocytosis +/− left shift
  - +/− Thrombocytosis
- Chemistry profile: hyperglycemia is always present. Other typical findings:
  - Hypokalemia
  - Hypophosphatemia; 50% of dogs and 65% of cats
  - Hypomagnesemia
  - Hyponatremia: may be pseudohyponatremia secondary to hyperglycemia; for every 100 mg/dL increase in glucose concentration, sodium concentration decreases 1.6 mEq/L.
  - Elevated liver enzyme activities
  - Azotemia, prerenal and renal; more common in cats
- Urine analysis
  - Glucosuria (p. 1227)
  - Ketonuria; standard test does not detect beta-hydroxybutyrate (p. 1355)
  - Possible pyuria
- Urine culture; should always be performed in patients with DKA regardless of urine sediment exam findings
- Thoracic and abdominal radiographs
  - Hepatomegaly
  - +/− Free abdominal fluid; if present, most likely secondary to neoplasia or pancreatitis
- Abdominal ultrasound is useful to diagnose concurrent disease processes (e.g., pancreatitis).

Advanced or Confirmatory Testing

- Serum ketones
  - Requires a handheld ketone meter
  - Chance of DKA is low if serum ketones ≤ 2.8 mmol/L in dogs and ≤ 2.55 mmol/L in cats.
- Endocrine testing
  - Hyperadrenocorticism and hypothyroidism can occur in dogs with DKA.
  - To test for hyperadrenocorticism, an ACTH stimulation test should be performed (p. 485) if clinically indicated.
  - To test for hypothyroidism (p. 525), a thyroid panel may be performed if clinically indicated.
- Abdominal fluid analysis (p. 1343); may be supportive of pancreatitis or help diagnose neoplasia.
- Fine-needle aspirate +/− biopsy of liver
  - Aspirates may confirm hepatic lipidosis (cats) or neoplasia (dogs and cats).
  - A biopsy may be required to diagnosis cholangiohepatitis (p. 160).
  - If infectious cholangiohepatitis is suspected, aerobic and anaerobic cultures of bile are recommended (p. 1112).

TREATMENT

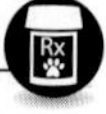

Treatment Overview

Patients with diabetic ketosis but not acidosis are typically stable and do not present with signs such as vomiting, anorexia, or lethargy. They may have a small amount of ketones in their urine and/or serum. These patients may be treated with long-acting insulin. The following discussion pertains to patients with DKA. Intravenous fluid therapy is the mainstay of treatment. Restoration of perfusion and hydration should begin as soon as possible.

Acute General Treatment

- Address perfusion deficits immediately with a 10-20 mL/kg IV bolus of an isotonic crystalloid such as Normosol-R, lactated Ringer's solution, or 0.9% NaCl. Reassess perfusion parameters immediately after bolus and at 15-minute intervals until stable. Repeat bolus therapy as necessary.
- Continue intravenous fluid therapy with an isotonic crystalloid at a rate calculated to include maintenance, dehydration deficit, and ongoing losses. Correct the dehydration over 6-12 hours, or slower if cardiac disease is present. To calculate the dehydration deficit, use this formula: percentage dehydration (as a decimal) × body weight (kg) × 1000 mL/kg.
- Adjust fluid rate to maintenance plus ongoing losses after correction of dehydration. Reassess hydration at least q 12h.
- Electrolyte supplementation is also crucial.
  - Correct hypokalemia with potassium chloride supplementation (p. 495).
  - Dilute potassium chloride in the crystalloid solution being given intravenously, using the table below.
  - The final rate should not exceed 0.5 mEq/kg/h. If initial serum potassium concentration is normal, assume it will drop with fluid and insulin therapy, and begin potassium supplementation with 20 mEq/L.
  - Recheck potassium q 4-12h initially, depending on severity.

Serum Potassium	mEq KCl Added per 1 L of Fluid
3.5-5	20
3.0-3.4	30
2.5-2.9	40
2.0-2.4	60
<2.0	80

  - Correct hypophosphatemia if serum concentration is < 1.5 mg/dL with potassium phosphate 0.01-0.12 mM/kg/h IV. Take into account the potassium contained in potassium phosphate (4.4 mEq/mL) when calculating total potassium requirements to avoid oversupplementation. A simple way to do this is to calculate total potassium requirement and give one-half as potassium phosphate and one-half as potassium chloride.
  - Correct hypomagnesemia if serum concentration is < 1.2 mg/dL; use magnesium sulfate 0.5-1 mEq/kg/day added to intravenous fluids.
  - Monitor electrolytes at least q 12h or more frequently, depending on severity of imbalance.
- Insulin therapy is necessary to decrease blood glucose concentration and stop the formation of ketone bodies. The goal is a blood glucose level of 100-250 mg/dL. Use regular, short-acting insulin in the acute treatment phase. Give as an intravenous constant-rate infusion (CRI), adjusted based on patient glucose concentration, or as intermittent intramuscular doses. Start insulin only *after* initial rehydration and correction of electrolytes have been started.
  - For an insulin CRI: add 1 U/kg (cat) or 2 U/kg (dog) regular insulin to a 250-mL bag of 0.9% NaCl.
  - Measure blood glucose concentration q 1-2h, and adjust insulin rate depending on blood glucose.
  - When the blood glucose concentration drops below 250 mg/dL, dextrose supplementation is necessary to avoid hypoglycemia.

Blood Glucose Level (mg/dL)	Insulin CRI	Percent Dextrose in Fluids
>250	10 mL/h	None
200-250	7 mL/h	2.5%
150-200	5 mL/h	2.5%
100-150	5 mL/h	5%
<100	None	5%

- The intramuscular protocol is less labor intensive. Give 0.25 U/kg IM q 4h. The insulin dose and dextrose concentration should be adjusted based on blood glucose concentration as for the CRI protocol.
- Consider glargine insulin in cats; give 0.25 U/kg SQ q 12h in addition to 1 U IM up to q 6h if the blood glucose level is > 250 mg/dL. This protocol allows owners to use the same vial of insulin at home as in the hospital.
- Treat any concurrent disease process specifically, if possible; otherwise treat supportively.
- Sodium bicarbonate supplementation is rarely warranted because acid-base abnormalities typically resolve with other therapies.

Chronic Treatment

- After the patient is alert, eating, and drinking; blood glucose is relatively controlled; and ketosis has resolved, start a long-acting insulin (p. 251).
- If using a CRI, it should be stopped for approximately 4 hours before beginning maintenance insulin therapy.

Nutrition/Diet

- If the patient is anorectic in the hospital, place a short-term feeding tube such as a nasoesophageal or nasogastric tube to facilitate nutrition (p. 1107). Forced oral feeding is not recommended.
- Once eating, dietary recommendations are the same as for chronic therapy of DM (p. 251).

Drug Interactions

- Insulin should be given through a dedicated IV catheter to avoid an inadvertent bolus.
- Because insulin may adhere to the administration set, run ≈50 mL of insulin-saline solution through the tubing (i.e., waste 50 mL) before use.

Possible Complications

- Hypoglycemia secondary to insulin overdose or lack of dextrose supplementation: monitor blood glucose q 1-4h to avoid.
- Electrolyte deficiencies: monitor electrolytes q 4-12h, depending on severity. Supplement aggressively based on bloodwork findings. Potassium supplementation should not exceed 0.5 mEq/kg/h.
- Hemolytic anemia can occur due to hypophosphatemia (serum phosphorus < 1.5 mEq/L).
- Rarely, neurologic signs occur from rapid decreases in sodium and glucose. Monitor blood glucose q 1-4h and sodium q 4-12h to ensure a slow, gradual drop in both. The goal is a drop in blood glucose concentration < 50-100 mg/dL/h.

Recommended Monitoring

- Aggressive monitoring is necessary during the acute phase of therapy for DKA. Severe cases require 24-hour care.
  - Monitor blood glucose concentration q 1-4h.
  - Monitor electrolyte concentrations, including sodium, potassium, phosphorus, and magnesium, q 4-12h.
  - Monitor serum or urine ketones q 24h.
  - Monitor hydration status, including body weight, q 6-12h.
  - Depending on severity of clinical signs and concurrent disease processes, consider monitoring of blood pressure, electrocardiogram, pulse oximetry, packed cell volume, and urine output.

PROGNOSIS & OUTCOME

- The majority of dogs (≈70%) and cats (≈60%) survive to discharge.
- In dogs, concurrent hyperadrenocorticism is associated with a worse prognosis, as are low calcium (total or ionized) concentrations, anemia, and low venous pH at presentation.
- In cats, poor outcome is associated with azotemia and hyperbilirubinemia at presentation.

PEARLS & CONSIDERATIONS

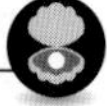

Comments

- Patients often require high rates of fluid for rehydration and maintenance of hydration.
- If urine cannot be obtained due to dehydration, use serum to test for ketones.

Technician Tips

- To facilitate frequent blood draws, place a sampling catheter in a central or peripheral vein.
- Patients require intensive monitoring of mentation, fluid balance, pain, and other health parameters.

SUGGESTED READING

Koenig A: Endocrine emergencies in dogs and cats. Vet Clin Small Anim 43:869-897, 2013.

AUTHOR: Lenore Bacek, DVM, MS, DACVECC
EDITOR: Ellen N. Behrend, VMD, PhD, DACVIM

Diaphragmatic Hernia

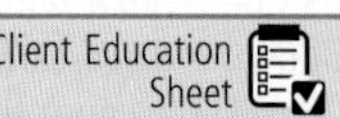

BASIC INFORMATION

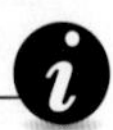

Definition

Disruption of the continuity of the diaphragm such that abdominal organs can shift into the thoracic cavity

Synonyms

Pleuroperitoneal hernia (peritoneopericardial diaphragmatic hernias are covered separately on p. 778)

Epidemiology

SPECIES, AGE, SEX

- Dogs and cats
- Congenital: rare; many affected animals die soon after birth
- Traumatic: most common in male dogs 1-3 years old

RISK FACTORS

- Trauma is the most common cause of diaphragmatic hernia (DH).
- *Hit by car* (HBC) is the most common cause of trauma resulting in DH.

ASSOCIATED DISORDERS

- Incarceration, obstruction, and strangulation of abdominal viscera
- Hepatic venous stasis, biliary tract obstruction, icterus, and ascites secondary to herniation of the liver
- Pleural effusion (hemothorax, chylothorax, bile pleuritis, pneumothorax) can complicate hernias.
- Musculoskeletal, pulmonary, cardiac, hematologic, or neurologic abnormalities secondary to trauma

Clinical Presentation

DISEASE FORMS/SUBTYPES

- Congenital pleuroperitoneal hernia: animals often die at birth or soon after from severe respiratory deficiency.
- Traumatic DH: clinical course can be acute or chronic.

HISTORY, CHIEF COMPLAINT

- Acute
  - History of recent trauma
  - Shock
  - Respiratory distress
- Chronic: can be an incidental finding (typically radiographic) in a well animal. Potential signs:
  - Dyspnea or tachypnea
  - Exercise intolerance
  - Anorexia
  - Depression
  - Vomiting
  - Dysphagia
  - Diarrhea
  - Constipation
  - Weight loss
  - Cough
  - Difficulty in lying down
  - Abdominal distention
- Some animals are clinically normal, and the hernia is an incidental (typically radiographic) finding.

PHYSICAL EXAM FINDINGS

- Signs of hypovolemic shock (p. 911)
- Dyspnea and/or tachypnea: respiratory effort is inspiratory or paradoxical
- Pale or cyanotic mucous membranes
- Cardiac arrhythmias (e.g., tachycardia, ventricular premature contractions)
- Muffled heart and lung sounds ventrally
- Borborygmi on thoracic auscultation
- Hyporesonance on chest wall percussion (pleural effusion)
- Hyperresonance on chest wall percussion (gastric tympany)
- Tucked-up or empty appearance/feel of the abdomen
- Abdominal distention with fluid wave if ascites

Etiology and Pathophysiology

Congenital:

- Defect in the dorsolateral part of the diaphragm
- The intermediate part of the left lumbar muscle of the crus may be absent, or the defect may be more extensive, with both crura and parts of the central tendon missing.

Traumatic:

- Direct
  - Thoracoabdominal stab and gunshot wounds
  - Iatrogenic injury (e.g., thoracocentesis)
- Indirect
  - HBC most common; other blunt abdominal trauma can also cause DH.
  - An abrupt increase in intraabdominal pressure with an open glottis results in a large pleuroperitoneal pressure gradient.
    - The diaphragm tears at its weakest points; usually the muscular portions (diaphragmatic costal muscles).
    - The location and size of the tear depend on the position of the animal on impact and the location of the viscera.
    - Viscera malpositioned in the thoracic cavity can suffer ischemic injury from alterations in blood flow.
    - Venous congestion of entrapped liver lobes can lead to pleural or abdominal effusion.
  - Clinical signs reflect respiratory dysfunction secondary to loss of diaphragmatic integrity, pleural effusion, or displacement of pulmonary parenchyma.
  - Signs may also reflect dysfunction of displaced abdominal viscera.

DIAGNOSIS

Diagnostic Overview

The diagnosis is usually established by demonstrating a loss of diaphragmatic integrity by thoracic or abdominal imaging, particularly in patients with evidence of pleural space disease after trauma.

Differential Diagnosis

- Peritoneopericardial DH (p. 778)
- Other causes of pleural or peritoneal effusion
- Pneumothorax
- Pneumonia
- Other causes of abdominal distention or ascites

Initial Database

- CBC, biochemistry panel, urinalysis: varies, depending on chronicity, severity, hypoxemia, and organs displaced into the thorax
- Thoracic radiographs may show
  - Loss of the diaphragmatic line
  - Loss of cardiac silhouette
  - Dorsal displacement of lungs
  - Pleural effusion
  - Presence of gas-filled viscera (stomach or intestines) in the thoracic cavity
- Thoracocentesis if large volume of pleural effusion obscures diagnostic thoracic radiographs
- Abdominal radiographs may show absence or cranial displacement of normal abdominal viscera.

Advanced or Confirmatory Testing

- Ultrasonography may demonstrate a rent in the diaphragm with organ herniation or abnormally positioned viscera.
- Positive-contrast celiography may demonstrate contrast medium in the pleural cavity, absence of a normal liver lobe outline, and incomplete visualization of the abdominal surface of the diaphragm.
- Contrast radiography of the intestinal tract may show barium-filled stomach or intestine in the thoracic cavity.
- Cross-sectional imaging (CT or MRI) may be helpful.
- In some animals, the diagnosis is confirmed during exploratory surgery.

TREATMENT

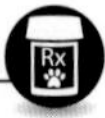

Treatment Overview

- Stabilize patient.
- Resolve respiratory distress.
- Return the abdominal organs to the abdominal cavity.
- Repair the diaphragmatic defect.

Acute General Treatment

- Oxygen administered by face mask, nasal cannula, or oxygen cage if dyspnea or hypoxemia (p. 1146)
- Fluid therapy as needed to stabilize cardiovascular status (particularly for acute trauma)
- Thoracocentesis if needed (p. 1164)
- Position the patient in sternal recumbency with the head elevated above the rear limbs (forelimbs elevated) if tolerated.

Chronic Treatment

Surgical treatment:

- DHs are often repaired through a midline celiotomy. A median sternotomy may be required for additional exposure. A ninth intercostal lateral thoracotomy provides exposure of herniated organs and diaphragmatic tears if the side is known.
- Return the abdominal organs to the abdominal cavity.
  - Excise the falciform ligament to improve exposure.
  - The diaphragmatic defect can be enlarged if necessary to reposition organs that have become swollen/congested or that have developed adhesions.
  - Serosal adhesions < 2 weeks old consist primarily of fibrin and can be gently broken down digitally.
- Close the diaphragmatic defect by standard herniorrhaphy, abdominal muscle flaps, porcine small-intestinal submucosal patches (Vet BioSIS), or synthetic material (Silastic sheeting).
  - Use 3-0 to 0 USP absorbable synthetic monofilament suture material for primary herniorrhaphy.
- Remove air and fluid from the pleural cavity after closing the diaphragmatic defect. A thoracostomy tube may be indicated.
- Explore the entire abdominal cavity for associated injuries if DH caused by trauma.

Possible Complications

- Re-expansion pulmonary edema can follow rapid lung re-expansion perioperatively (p. 836).
- Hypoventilation or hypoxia due to pain, pneumothorax, hemothorax, or tight bandages
- Abdominal compartment syndrome (increased intraperitoneal pressures) can occur with chronic hernias.

Recommended Monitoring

- Vital signs
- Perfusion parameters
- Respiratory patterns
- Pain

PROGNOSIS & OUTCOME

- Prognosis is good if the animal survives the early postoperative period (12-24 hours).
- Oxygen dependence preoperatively and postoperatively were associated with an increased mortality.
- Increased duration of anesthesia and surgery were associated with an increased mortality.
- Animals with concurrent orthopedic and soft-tissue injuries had 7.3 times greater odds of mortality.

PEARLS & CONSIDERATIONS

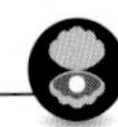

Comments

- Physical examination may be normal in some animals.
  - DH can be an incidental finding.
- The radiographic diagnosis of DH can be challenging.
  - Ultrasonography may be more useful in making the diagnosis, especially if moderate to severe pleural effusion is present.
- Delay surgery until the patient's condition has stabilized.
- Perform surgery as soon as possible if the stomach has herniated into the thoracic cavity.

Prevention

Routine use of leashes or fenced confinement to avoid HBC injuries

Technician Tips

- To stabilize the patient while prepping for surgery, evacuate pleural fluid just after anesthetic induction (p. 1164).
- Extra towels, wedge pillow, or something to prop/elevate the cranial half of the body while prepping for surgery may help move abdominal contents out of the thoracic cavity and improve respiratory function.

Client Education

Patients with DH usually have a history of trauma, but failure to perform radiographic examination of the thorax often delays diagnosis.

SUGGESTED READING

Hunt G, et al: Diaphragmatic hernias. In Tobias K, et al, editors: Veterinary small animal surgery, St. Louis, 2012, Saunders, pp 1380-1390.

AUTHOR: Michael B. Mison, DVM, DACVS
EDITOR: Megan Grobman, DVM, MS, DACVIM

Diarrhea, Acute

Client Education Sheet

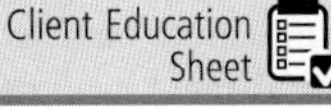

BASIC INFORMATION

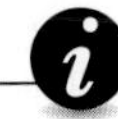

Definition

An increase in frequency of defecation, stool fluidity, and/or fecal volume that is sudden in onset and of < 2 weeks' duration

Epidemiology

SPECIES, AGE, SEX

Dogs and cats, any age, both sexes

RISK FACTORS

- Environment: overcrowding, poor sanitation, immune compromise (infectious causes)
- Unsupervised activity/dietary indiscretion, stress/increased shedding of infectious organisms, confluence of animals from varied geographic areas such as dog/cat shows (greater exposure to variety of pathogens)
- Raw diets: salmonellosis, *Escherichia coli* infection (especially young or immunocompromised patients)

CONTAGION AND ZOONOSIS

Potential zoonoses (others possible): *Ancylostoma caninum* (cutaneous larval migrans), *Balantidium coli*, *Campylobacter* spp, *Clostridium difficile*, *Cryptosporidium parvum*, *Echinococcus* spp, *Entamoeba histolytica*, *E. coli*, *Giardia* spp, *Pentatrichomonas hominis*, *Salmonella* spp, *Shigella* spp, *Toxocara* spp (visceral and ocular larval migrans), *Toxoplasma gondii*, *Yersinia enterocolitica*

Clinical Presentation

DISEASE FORMS/SUBTYPES

Small-intestinal (SI) diarrhea, large-intestinal (LI) diarrhea, or both

HISTORY, CHIEF COMPLAINT

- Loose stool and/or fecal incontinence
- May be markedly depressed, anorexic, and ill or may simply have diarrhea
- Source of the pet, vaccination, anthelmintic and dietary history, environment, recent medications, and recent stressful episode may help identify trigger factors.
- Determine whether other household pets or owners are similarly affected (contagion/zoonosis).
- Differentiate SI diarrhea from LI (p. 1215); can be mixed.

PHYSICAL EXAM FINDINGS

- Infections/intoxications more likely if depressed and dehydrated

- Mucous membrane color
  - Brick red/injected: sepsis, hemorrhagic gastroenteritis (p. 259)
  - Pallor: hypoperfusion/shock/pain versus anemia (gastrointestinal [GI] blood loss)
- Dehydration (caveat: nauseated animal may have moist mucous membranes despite dehydration)
- Signs of shock/sepsis (e.g., fever, tachycardia [cats: bradycardia more common], tachypnea, cool extremities [variable])
- Posture as sign of abdominal pain: "dog-praying" position/arched back
- Abdominal palpation ±
  - Evidence of pain
  - Thickened, fluid or gas-filled bowel (inflammation, neoplasia)
  - Mass effect (obstruction, foreign body)
  - Lymphadenomegaly (neoplasia, inflammation, infection)
  - Urinary bladder size (with respect to hydration status and renal function)
- Perineum: external erythema
- Rectal palpation: perineal hernia, anal sac disorders, and perianal fistulas may mimic signs of LI disease (e.g., pain, tenesmus, hematochezia).
- Observe animal defecating (tenesmus, dyschezia, character of feces)

Etiology and Pathophysiology

- Abnormal transmucosal movement of water and solute
  - Osmotic (decreased solute absorption), secretory (hypersecretion of ions), exudative (increased permeability), abnormal motility
- More than one mechanism possible, depending on underlying cause

DIAGNOSIS

Diagnostic Overview

The extensive list of causes can be narrowed substantially based on a thorough history and examination. Fecal examinations (fresh sample) are indicated in all cases. A large proportion of acute diarrhea cases are self-resolving and do not warrant further testing. Additional diagnostics are indicated if the patient is systemically ill, a zoonotic concern exists, the history or physical exam suggests a nontransient cause, or recurrent or prolonged episodes occur.

Differential Diagnosis

See Diarrhea, Section 3 (p. 1213) for detailed differential diagnoses.

- Dietary (e.g., new food, dietary indiscretion)
- Infectious (viral, bacterial, parasitic; less often, fungal, algal)
- Inflammatory (e.g., enteritis, pancreatitis)
- Toxins/medications

Initial Database

Fecal examinations: typically, a minimum of three samples or until a positive result is found

- Cytology (fresh saline smears)
- Flotation
- Parasite antigen test (more sensitive)

Advanced or Confirmatory Testing

- As dictated by clinical suspicion
- Consider CBC, serum biochemical profile, urinalysis, infectious disease testing, especially if depressed, dehydrated, or febrile (e.g., canine parvoviral antigen ELISA).
- Abdominal radiographs, ± contrast radiography, and/or ultrasonography if obstruction or mass lesion suspected

TREATMENT

Treatment Overview

- Many cases of acute diarrhea in otherwise normal dogs and cats are transient and self-resolving.
- Palliative treatment for comfort (e.g., antidiarrheal medications, bland diet, probiotics) is often a good option for benign acute diarrhea caused by spontaneous or temporary disorders, such as dietary indiscretion.
- Acute diarrhea can be instigated by disorders that will not resolve spontaneously or are contagious/zoonotic. For these, the cause must be identified and addressed.
- Additional diagnostic testing and treatment are warranted if the patient is markedly ill, there is failure to respond to empirical treatment within 24-48 hours, or the patient's condition deteriorates.
- Acute diarrhea may lead to volume depletion that requires parenteral fluid therapy: maintenance ± dehydration ± ongoing loss (pp. 259 and 760).
- It is important to have an established hospital protocol to prevent infectious transmission to other patients or hospital personnel when dealing with pets with diarrhea.

Acute General Treatment

- A bland, easily digestible diet; anthelmintic treatment (if parasites are suspected or identified); and/or probiotics are common first-line, general treatments for mild acute diarrhea. The author has had good luck using adsorbents (e.g., zeolite compounds).
- Antidiarrheal drugs may be considered as nonspecific treatment for 24-48 hours in animals that are systemically well: kaolin and pectin 1-2 mL/kg PO q 8-12h; bismuth subsalicylate 0.1-1 mg/kg PO q 8-12h. Neither is recommended in cats (decreased ability to metabolize salicylates).
- Motility modifiers (e.g., loperamide 0.1-0.2 mg/kg PO q 8-12h) may be considered *only* for intractable diarrhea and if an infectious cause has been excluded. Use judiciously and for no longer than 3 days.

Drug Interactions

Anticholinergics are contraindicated with obstruction and/or sepsis.

Possible Complications

- Dehydration
- Sepsis/endotoxemia
- Development of intussusception/other intestinal accident

PROGNOSIS & OUTCOME

- Dietary indiscretion: often benign and self-resolving
- Parasitic diseases: generally good, barring obstruction
- Infectious, endocrine causes, intoxications, mechanical obstruction and hemorrhagic gastroenteritis: potentially life-threatening

PEARLS & CONSIDERATIONS

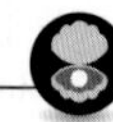

Comments

Do not use antibiotics indiscriminately; alters microbiome, promotes bacterial resistance

Technician Tips

Proper hygiene vital: avoids contagion/zoonoses (handwashing between patients, gloves when cleaning patients with diarrhea, avoid human food in clinic areas, strict isolation for suspected infection such as parvovirus)

Client Education

- Feeding raw diets is discouraged.
- Proper hygiene is essential (especially with raw diets): frequent handwashing, regular cleaning of food bowls/bedding/litter boxes

SUGGESTED READING

Marks SL: Diarrhea. In Washabau RJ, et al, editors: Canine and feline gastroenterology, St. Louis, 2013, Saunders, pp 99-108.

AUTHOR: Lisa Carioto, DVM, DVSc, DACVIM
EDITOR: Leah A. Cohn, DVM, PhD, DACVIM

Diarrhea, Acute Hemorrhagic

BASIC INFORMATION

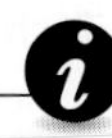

Definition

Acute, profuse hematemesis and hemorrhagic diarrhea accompanied by hypovolemia; may progress to circulatory collapse, multiple organ dysfunction, and death

Synonym

Hemorrhagic gastroenteritis (HGE)

Epidemiology

SPECIES, AGE, SEX

Dogs, usually young (mean, 5 years old)

GENETICS, BREED PREDISPOSITION

Acute hemorrhagic diarrhea syndrome (AHDS) can occur in any breed; small dogs may be predisposed.

CONTAGION AND ZOONOSIS

Does not appear to be contagious

GEOGRAPHY AND SEASONALITY

More prevalent in urban dogs

Clinical Presentation

HISTORY, CHIEF COMPLAINT

- Anorexia and lethargy initially
- Acute onset of vomiting that may be profuse and contain fresh blood
- Acute onset of diarrhea that may become grossly bloody; consistency varies from watery to jelly-like.

PHYSICAL EXAM FINDINGS

- Depressed but afebrile
- Markers of perfusion: heart rate, pulse quality, gum color, capillary refill time (CRT) initially normal. As fluid is lost into the gastrointestinal (GI) tract, signs of hypovolemia, characterized by pallor, slow CRT, and tachycardia, quickly develop.
- Skin turgor may not reflect the full extent of fluid losses.
- Patients may be moribund at presentation if veterinary attention is delayed.
- Abdominal palpation reveals fluid-filled bowel loops with nonlocalized discomfort.
- Rectal examination: fresh dark blood or strawberry jelly–like feces

Etiology and Pathophysiology

- A novel pore-forming toxin (NetF) from type A *Clostridium perfringens* is the probable cause of AHDS/HGE.
- GI permeability increases markedly, with extravasation of fluid, proteins, and red blood cells into the intestinal lumen.
- Although vomiting (often with hematemesis) is expected, the stomach is grossly and microscopically unaffected.
- Loss of plasma water, electrolytes, and protein can be extreme. Packed cell volume (PCV) rises rapidly and often exceeds 65% (due to hemoconcentration).
- If untreated, hypovolemic shock and death can occur.

DIAGNOSIS

Diagnostic Overview

A presumptive diagnosis is made based on history and evidence of hemoconcentration (PCV > 65%). Dogs with AHDS/HGE can die unless the disorder is recognized quickly and treated intensively. It is important to rule out other possibilities, but treatment should not be delayed while diagnostics are performed.

Differential Diagnosis

- Infectious gastroenteritis: viral (parvovirus) or bacterial (*Salmonella, Clostridium difficile,* salmon poisoning [*Neorickettsia helminthoeca*] in endemic regions)
- Dietary indiscretion, toxicity
- Hypoadrenocorticism
- Intestinal volvulus, partial obstruction, or intussusception
- Other causes of hypovolemic or endotoxic shock (e.g., intestinal perforation, peritonitis)
- Necrotizing pancreatitis
- Coagulopathy

Initial Database

- PCV is often > 65%; total solids are low or borderline normal.
- CBC: stress leukogram; immature neutrophils or mild toxic change may be noted; modest thrombocytopenia is common.
- Serum biochemistry profile: increased blood urea nitrogen (BUN) level and alanine aminotransferase activity are expected; hypokalemia and panhypoproteinemia are common; metabolic acidosis may be severe.
- Urinalysis: unremarkable; high specific gravity expected in response to hypovolemia
- Coagulation profile: usually normal initially; may show prolongations if disseminated intravascular coagulation (DIC) develops
- Fecal evaluation (centrifuged flotation and saline preparation): no pathogens noted
- Fecal stained microscopic exam: increased numbers of red cells, some white cells
- Fecal ELISA for parvovirus (if neonate or unvaccinated): negative
- Canine pancreas-specific lipase immunoassay (cPLI): not consistent with pancreatitis
- Abdominal radiographs: fluid- and gas-filled small-intestinal loops; colon may be empty
- Colloid oncotic pressure (COP): usually normal at presentation but then declines
- +/− Serum cortisol > 2 mcg/dL (>55 nmol/L) excludes hypoadrenocorticism.

TREATMENT

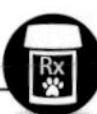

Treatment Overview

- Quickly restore and maintain an effective circulating blood volume.
- Provide appropriate colloid support and crystalloid fluid replacement.
- Anticipate complications of hypovolemia and widespread intestinal mucosal compromise.

Acute and Chronic Treatment

- Initiate fluid resuscitation with IV fluid therapy (p. 911).
  - Colloids (e.g., Hetastarch, Vetstarch) should be started immediately in hypovolemic patients. Administer 5 mL/kg over 20 minutes if the patient is substantially hypovolemic; otherwise, begin a continuous-rate infusion of 1 mL/kg/h; total daily dose should not exceed 20 mL/kg.
  - Crystalloid fluids should be administered concurrently. Replacement-type fluids (e.g., Normosol-R, lactated Ringer's solution, Plasmalyte 148, 0.9% NaCl) should be used. If necessary, calculate a shock dose of crystalloids (90 mL/kg), and give one-third of this amount as a bolus over 20 minutes. Do not administer Normosol-R rapidly because this fluid contains acetate and may cause refractory hypotension.
  - Estimate lost volume (by % body weight) and aim to replace over 6-12 hours.
  - Continue fluids as needed to replace ongoing losses and meet maintenance requirements.
  - If available, use COP measurement to guide colloid administration.
- Electrolyte disturbances are common: hypokalemia (p. 516) should be addressed specifically; changes in sodium and chloride should self-correct with standard fluid therapy.
- Antibiotics are of questionable benefit (despite evidence of an underlying Clostridial cause) unless the clinical assessment suggests sepsis. If so, provide broad-spectrum coverage (e.g., ampicillin 30 mg/kg IV q 8h and enrofloxacin 10 mg/kg slow IV q 24h).
- Antiemetics should be administered to control vomiting.
  - Maropitant 1 mg/kg SQ q 24h (patient must be > 8 weeks old), *or*
  - Metoclopramide 1.1-2.2 mg/kg/24 hours given IV as constant-rate infusion)
- Gastric acid suppressing drugs are not specifically indicated but may reduce the risk of esophagitis in patients with sustained emesis.
  - Pantoprazole 0.7 mg/kg IV q 24h or famotidine 0.5 mg/kg IV or SQ q 12-24h
- Probiotics/prebiotics may hasten recovery, but evidence to support their use is limited.

Nutrition/Diet

- Withhold water until vomiting is adequately controlled, and then offer small amounts every 1-2 hours.
- Food should be offered as soon as vomiting is reduced. Easily digestible diets (e.g., boiled white rice with cottage cheese, low-fat turkey breast) may be beneficial initially because gastric emptying times are shorter.

Drug Interactions

- Maropitant is protein bound and may affect metabolism of other highly protein-bound drugs such as nonsteroidal antiinflammatories and anticonvulsants.
- Metoclopramide interacts with numerous drugs; avoid concurrent use of sedatives, tranquilizers, and narcotics. It is also incompatible with many antibiotics (including ampicillin), and infusion must be discontinued while other medications are administered.

Possible Complications

- Can progress to hypovolemic shock, DIC, and death if not treated appropriately
- Esophagitis may occur if vomiting is persistent.
- Obtunded patients are vulnerable to aspiration pneumonia.
- Translocation of bacteria across the compromised intestinal mucosa may cause sepsis.

Recommended Monitoring

- Monitor vital parameters (temperature, heart rate, mucous membranes, CRT, pulse quality, blood pressure [p. 1065]) and ongoing fluid losses every 2 hours.
- Initially, check hematocrit and total solids every 4-6 hours and glucose, BUN, and electrolytes every 6-8 hours.
- COP should be checked every 6-8 hours or as needed to guide decisions about colloid therapy.

PROGNOSIS & OUTCOME

- Recovery is usually rapid and complete over 1-2 days; severely affected dogs may require supportive therapy for several days before return of normal GI function.
- Condition can progress quickly to multiple organ dysfunction syndrome, DIC, and death.
- About 10% of affected dogs may die despite therapy.

PEARLS & CONSIDERATIONS

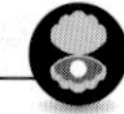

Comments

- The diagnostic hallmark for AHDS/HGE is a markedly elevated hematocrit with normal to slightly low total protein level.
- Colloid support is often essential and should not be overlooked.
- Exclude hypoadrenocorticism in high-risk breeds (pp. 512 and 1300).

Technician Tips

- Patient status can change quickly; careful attention to markers of perfusion (e.g., CRT, pulse rate and quality, mental status, urine output) is essential.
- Diarrhea can be profuse; wrapping the tail and shaving the hind end may improve patient cleanliness and comfort.

Client Education

Approximately 10%-15% of dogs will have repeated episodes of AHDS/HGE.

SUGGESTED READING

Mazzaferro E, et al: Fluid therapy for emergent small animal patients: crystalloids, colloids and albumin products. Vet Clin North Am Small Anim Pract 43:721-734, 2013.

AUTHOR: Audrey K. Cook, BVM&S, DACVIM, DECVIM, DABVP
EDITOR: Rance K. Sellon, DVM, PhD, DACVIM

Diarrhea, Antibiotic-Responsive/Small-Intestinal Dysbiosis

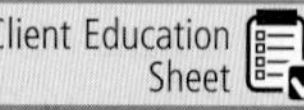

BASIC INFORMATION

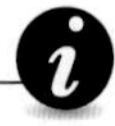

Definition

Any diarrhea demonstrating responsiveness to or resolution with antibiotic therapy. Antibiotic-responsive diarrhea (ARD) and small-intestinal bacterial overgrowth (SIBO), the previously used term, are likely due to increased numbers and/or changes in the composition of small-intestinal bacteria, with associated clinical signs. ARD and SIBO may be used interchangeably; however, because historically used cutoff values for small-intestinal bacterial counts are inadequate, the preferred terms are *antibiotic-responsive diarrhea* or *small-intestinal dysbiosis* (SID).

Synonyms

Antibiotic-responsive enteropathy (ARE), tylosin-responsive diarrhea (TRD), small intestinal dysbiosis (SID)

Epidemiology

SPECIES, AGE, SEX

Dogs and cats, either sex. Young animals predominate, but all ages are represented.

GENETICS, BREED PREDISPOSITION

Beagles, German shepherds (immunoglobulin A [IgA] dysregulation/deficiency suspected but not confirmed)

RISK FACTORS

Factors that allow dysregulation and/or overgrowth of small-intestinal bacteria include underlying immunologic gastrointestinal (GI) disease, exocrine pancreatic insufficiency (EPI), or other causes of maldigestion/malabsorption, achlorhydria (primary or iatrogenic), intestinal motility disorders (including those related to endocrinopathy), obstructive GI disease, and the creation of blind intestinal loops after GI surgery, all resulting in changes in the microbiota. Antibiotic-induced dysbiosis has recently been recognized. In most animals, the microbiota recovers within a few weeks after cessation of antibiotic administration, but some animals may have prolonged dysbiosis, potentially causing signs of intestinal disease.

CONTAGION AND ZOONOSIS

Possible if ARD is caused by infectious agents with zoonotic potential (e.g., *Salmonella* spp, *Campylobacter* spp)

Clinical Presentation

DISEASE FORMS/SUBTYPES

- Primary or idiopathic ARD, in which no underlying functional abnormality or disease is identified (rare)
  - Likely encompasses several different disorders
  - A more general microbial overgrowth and/or imbalance is associated with diarrhea, and antibiotic responsiveness is usually favorable.
- Secondary ARD occurs as a complication of other underlying primary GI disease, such as
  - Chronic enteropathy, such as food-responsive diarrhea or idiopathic inflammatory bowel disease (IBD)
  - EPI (common)

HISTORY, CHIEF COMPLAINT

Small-bowel diarrhea, with variable severity (p. 1215) and weight loss, poor body condition, borborygmus, flatulence, steatorrhea, vomiting (due to underlying GI disease)

PHYSICAL EXAM FINDINGS

No physical examination findings are diagnostic of ARD; nonspecific small-bowel diarrhea ± weight loss

Etiology and Pathophysiology

- Bacterial counts in the small intestine can reach > 10^9 colony-forming units (CFU)/mL for aerobic and anaerobic bacteria in clinically healthy dogs. Normal dogs have a mix of aerobic and anaerobic bacteria (*E. coli, Streptococcus, Clostridium, Fusobacterium, Bacteroides*).

- Cats appear to have higher bacterial counts (10^5-10^8 CFU/mL), and anaerobic bacteria (*Bacteroides*, *Fusobacterium*, *Eubacterium*) predominate.
- In the normal host, overgrowth of normal flora or pathogens is prevented by protective mechanisms such as gastric acid secretion, intestinal motility (peristalsis and interdigestive migrating complexes), pancreatic and bile antimicrobial secretions (enzymes, immunoglobulins), and local enteric immunoglobulin production. Disruptions in these protective mechanisms can predispose to ARD.
- The pathophysiologic mechanism of ARD is thought to involve intraluminal effects of proliferating bacteria, damage to mucosal enterocytes, injury to brush border enzymes and carrier proteins, secretion of enterotoxins, deconjugation of bile acids, hydroxylation of fatty acids, decreased mucin production, bacterial competition for nutrients and vitamins (i.e., cobalamin), and increased mucosal permeability.
- The net result is intermittent small-bowel diarrhea with or without weight loss and variable vomiting, anorexia, and malnutrition due to malabsorption of fats, carbohydrates, proteins, and fat-soluble vitamins.

DIAGNOSIS

Diagnostic Overview

Most cases of ARD are diagnosed empirically, based on a response to a course of oral antibiotics implemented when other common causes of diarrhea have been ruled out.

Differential Diagnosis

See Diarrhea, Section 3 (p. 1213).
- Intestinal parasitism (helminthiasis, giardiasis)
- Dietary intolerance/hypersensitivity
- IBD
- Intestinal lymphoma
- EPI
- Intestinal obstruction: stricture, intussusception, neoplasia, foreign body (may cause secondary ARD)
- Motility disorders
- Surgical causes: bypass procedures, ileocolic valve resection

Initial Database

- Fecal flotation and direct smear to rule out parasites
- Results of CBC, biochemistry panel, and urinalysis are usually nonspecific; hypoproteinemia may suggest protein-losing enteropathy.
- Abdominal radiography and/or ultrasonography may show underlying obstructive disease or neoplasia.

Advanced or Confirmatory Testing

- Increased serum folate concentrations or decreased serum cobalamin concentrations lack sensitivity and specificity. Specificity increases if serum levels of both vitamins are altered and EPI has been ruled out.
- Serum trypsin-like immunoreactivity to rule out EPI
- Rectal scrape (p. 1157) cytology to rule out other causes of diarrhea
- Endoscopic mucosal biopsies demonstrate minimal inflammatory infiltrates/changes in primary ARD; in secondary ARD, GI biopsies may demonstrate the underlying primary disease.
- Fecal culture: rarely helpful except for the isolated case of *Salmonella* or *Campylobacter* infection. Duodenal juice culture is of no diagnostic use.
- Dysbiosis index (dogs only)
  - The fecal dysbiosis index (DI) is a polymerase chain reaction (PCR)–based assay that quantifies the abundances of major bacterial groups in fecal samples and summarizes them in a single number.
  - A DI below 0 indicates a normal fecal microbiota; a DI above 2 indicates dysbiosis due to chronic enteropathy or EPI. A DI between 0 and 2 is equivocal.
  - Due to microbiota differences along the intestine, evaluation of the fecal DI may not accurately reflect microbiota changes in the small intestine. Concurrent evaluation of serum concentration of cobalamin/folate with assessment of the fecal dysbiosis index may help in the diagnosis of dysbiosis.

TREATMENT

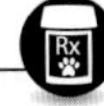

Treatment Overview

Resolution of diarrhea with appropriate antibiotic therapy

Acute General Treatment

- Identify and treat underlying contributory disorders (e.g., EPI, IBD).
- Fenbendazole 50 mg/kg PO q 24h for 3-5 days should be considered for occult parasitism before antibiotic therapy.
- Unless specifically directed by fecal culture, antibiotic choices include
  - Tylosin 10-25 mg/kg PO q 12h for up to 6 weeks, *or*
  - Metronidazole 10-15 mg/kg PO q 12h for up to 2 weeks, *or*
  - Enrofloxacin 5-10 mg/kg PO q 24h (only for *E. coli*–associated histiocytic ulcerative colitis)
- Parenteral or oral B_{12} supplementation to normalize serum levels (p. 183)
- Low-fat, highly digestible diet
- Prebiotic therapy: fructo-oligosaccharides may stimulate normal microbiota
- Dietary fiber: increase, decrease, or change in type (soluble vs. insoluble) to alter microbiota

Chronic Treatment

- Some animals have recurrent signs when antibiotic treatment ends. Long-term, low-dose antibiotic therapy (tylosin) may be required, although only when underlying causes have definitively been addressed. The combination of tylosin therapy with diet modification has been useful in dogs with ARD (i.e., TRD). Tylosin can be empirically tapered to 10-25 mg/kg PO q 24h for long-term therapy.
- Recognize underlying contributory disorders that may be associated with ARD/SIBO and may require other treatment.

Nutrition/Diet

Highly digestible, low-fat diets are recommended and may reduce food-related (due to intolerance or poor nutrient digestibility) causes of dysbiosis.

Drug Interactions

Metronidazole is a radiation sensitizer in animals undergoing concurrent radiation therapy.

Possible Complications

Central nervous system signs occur with high-dose metronidazole (do not exceed 30 mg/kg/d, and do not exceed 2 weeks of treatment at this dose).

Recommended Monitoring

Monitor for recurrence of diarrhea after therapy.

PROGNOSIS & OUTCOME

Usually excellent; may require chronic treatment, especially if underlying GI disease is present and ARD is secondary

PEARLS & CONSIDERATIONS

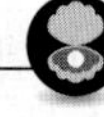

Comments

- Primary (idiopathic) ARD is rare; always evaluate for underlying GI tract disease.
- Decreased intestinal motility is probably an important cause of ARD; in addition to GI tract disease, consider endocrine (hypothyroidism, diabetes mellitus, hypoadrenocorticism) and neurologic causes.
- German shepherd dogs are likely predisposed to ARD due to EPI (p. 317).
- Enzyme replacement for EPI may not be efficacious until antibiotic therapy is instituted.
- Histiocytic ulcerative colitis (large-bowel disease) is an antibiotic-responsive diarrhea in dogs suspected to be secondary to invasive and adherent *E. coli* strains (p. 395).

Technician Tips

- Long-term antibiosis may be required for therapeutic success, but recent data suggest that chronic antibiotic use may be a risk factor for various metabolic disorders due to the negative impacts on colonic microbiota.
- Slow tapering of the tylosin dose over time appears to reduce relapse rate of clinical signs.

Client Education

Long-term antibiotic therapy may be required. In addition to antibiotic therapy, long-term diet control (low-fat, highly digestible) may be beneficial.

SUGGESTED READING

Suchodolski JS: Diagnosis and interpretation of intestinal dysbiosis in dogs and cats. Vet J 215:30-37, 2016.

AUTHOR: Jan S. Suchodolski, MedVet, Dr. med. vet., PhD, DACVM
EDITOR: Rance K. Sellon, DVM, PhD, DACVIM

Diarrhea, Chronic

Client Education Sheet 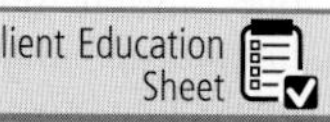

BASIC INFORMATION

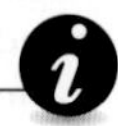

Definition

A persistent (>2-3 weeks) or episodic increase in frequency of defecation, stool fluidity, and/or fecal volume (increased water content or fecal solids)

Epidemiology

SPECIES, AGE, SEX

Any animal can be affected

CONTAGION AND ZOONOSIS

See Diarrhea, Acute, Section 1 (p. 257).

Clinical Presentation

DISEASE FORMS/SUBTYPES

Small-intestinal (SI) diarrhea versus large-intestinal (LI) diarrhea (p. 1215) or mixed

- Further characterized as maldigestion or malabsorption disorders
- Malabsorption further divided into non–protein-losing enteropathies versus protein-losing enteropathies (PLE)

HISTORY, CHIEF COMPLAINT

- Signalment, when/where the pet was acquired, vaccinations, medications, anthelmintic use, dietary and travel history, environment, including other animals, and progression of clinical signs may help identify triggering factors.
- Discrimination between LI and SI causes will influence the differential diagnosis; many affected animals have a combination of both (p. 1215).

PHYSICAL EXAM FINDINGS

- May appear healthy or may be systemically ill (e.g., vomiting, depression, weakness, lethargy, dehydration)
- Pale mucous membranes: chronic GI blood loss, anemia of chronic illness/inflammation
- Emaciation, dull haircoat suggest malnutrition, chronic malabsorption (fatty acids, protein, vitamins), neoplasia, PLE.
- Fever: inflammation, infection, neoplasia
- Dyspnea with decreased lung/heart sounds (pleural effusion), distended abdomen (ascites), peripheral edema: suggest PLE
- Abdominal palpation may reveal a mass (foreign body, neoplasm, granuloma, abscess, lymphadenomegaly), thickened bowel (inflammation, neoplasia), aggregated bowel loops (mass, adhesions), sausage-shaped intestinal loop (foreign body, intussusception), pain (inflammation, obstruction, ischemia, gas), or gas/fluid distention (ileus, fluid, obstruction).
- Rectal palpation (mandatory unless intractably painful): mass (polyp, neoplasm, granuloma), circumferential narrowing (stricture, spasm, neoplasm), irregular mucosa (colitis, polyp, neoplasm, perineal fistula)
- Observe defecation: tenesmus, dyschezia, character of feces
- Cats: check for thyroid nodule

Etiology and Pathophysiology

Small intestine:

- Decreased fluid and electrolyte absorption
- Incomplete nutrient absorption (fats/carbohydrates)
- Increased fluid and electrolyte secretion

Large intestine:

- Decreased fluid and electrolyte absorption
- Secretion of fluid and electrolytes
- Failure of reservoir function

DIAGNOSIS

Diagnostic Overview

The list of causes is exhaustive. It is most important to obtain a thorough history and to consider the pet's environment and diet before embarking on tests that may be unwarranted. Every animal should have a rectal exam, fecal flotation test, and a direct smear performed on fresh fecal samples.

Differential Diagnosis

See Diarrhea, Section 3 (p. 1213), for detailed differential diagnoses.

Initial Database

Fecal examinations:

- Cytology (fresh saline smears): ova, larvae, certain bacteria/protozoa
  - Identification of *Campylobacter* alone is insufficient to make a diagnosis; many are nonpathogenic.
  - Iodine stain: enhances visualization of *Giardia* trophozoites
  - Low sensitivity for certain parasites (e.g., *Tritrichomonas foetus*)
- Flotation/zinc sulfate centrifugation (*Giardia* cysts)
- Gram stain
- ELISA: *Giardia* and *Cryptosporidium*-specific antigen; hookworm, roundworm, and whipworm antigen tests (more sensitive replacement for flotation)
- Routine minimum database: CBC, serum biochemical profile, urinalysis (specific gravity)
- Cats: retroviral serology, serum thyroxine level (>5 years old)

Advanced or Confirmatory Testing

Testing is guided by prior findings. If initial testing is unremarkable and animal is stable or financial constraints prohibit additional testing, empirical trial therapy is a reasonable next step.

- Pursue clues such as hypoalbuminemia (p. 1239) identified on initial testing.
- Abdominal imaging
  - Radiographs: survey, ± contrast radiography
  - Ultrasonography: mass, thickened bowel, loss of GI wall detail, evaluation of other abdominal organs
- Baseline cortisol/adrenocorticotropic hormone stimulation test (p. 512)
- Trypsin-like immunoreactivity (species-specific test) (p. 317)
- Serum cobalamin (vitamin B_{12}), folate (pp. 1325 and 1344)
- Pancreatic lipase immunoreactivity (species-specific PLI) test (pp. 740 and 742)
- Infectious disease testing, as appropriate
  - Fecal cultures (*E. coli*, *Salmonella* spp, *C. jejuni*, *Clostridium* spp, *Yersinia enterocolitica*): controversial; many of these bacteria are commensal organisms; see specific organisms/disorders
  - Molecular techniques (e.g., PCR): often offered as GI or diarrhea panels for multiple pathogens
  - Specific tests, such as histoplasmosis urine antigen testing (p. 1365)
- Occult blood: may reflect chronic blood loss; false-positives possible with meat-based diets.
- Gastroduodenoscopy and colonoscopy (≈30% of dogs with colitis vomit)
- Exploratory laparotomy: full-thickness biopsies (biopsy even if no gross lesions)

TREATMENT

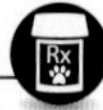

Treatment Overview

The goal of treatment is correction of the underlying cause. For otherwise stable animals, empirical therapy may be used as a diagnostic trial if initial testing results were unremarkable. Unsuccessful trial should prompt a change of course (diagnostic or therapeutic).

Acute and Chronic Treatment

Depends on underlying cause. Empirical therapy often includes anthelmintics, dietary trials, probiotics/prebiotics, antimicrobials (metronidazole, tylosin, enrofloxacin [boxer, French bulldog colitis]), cobalamin, immunomodulators, or antiinflammatories.

- Anthelmintic (e.g., fenbendazole 50 mg/kg PO q 24h × 3 days, repeated 3 weeks later)
- Elimination/hypoallergenic diet trial (p. 347)
- Probiotics/prebiotics (p. 260)
- Cobalamin supplementation (p. 183)
- Antimicrobials (see specific organism). Possible immunomodulating and antiinflammatory activities (metronidazole and tylosin)
- Immunosuppressive agents best if histologically proven inflammatory bowel disease (p. 543)

Nutrition/Diet

Consultation with a veterinary nutritionist may be beneficial, especially if there are comorbidities with additional nutritional implications.

- Small, frequent meals (3-6 times/day)
- Elimination diet: novel protein source or hydrolyzed protein diet as sole food source (avoid chewable medications); at least 2-3 weeks
- Pancreatitis/EPI/lymphangiectasia/PLE: highly digestible and low-fat diet
- Colitis: high soluble fiber

Possible Complications

- Excessive protein loss: peripheral edema, cavity effusions
- Pancreatic enzyme supplementation (EPI): buccal mucosal irritation
- Iatrogenic hyperadrenocorticism; use minimum effective glucocorticoid dose

Recommended Monitoring

Body weight, body condition score, fecal consistency, serum protein/albumin concentrations, CBC (immunosuppressive agents)

PROGNOSIS & OUTCOME

Depends on underlying cause, response to treatment, owner compliance, and individual variation

PEARLS & CONSIDERATIONS

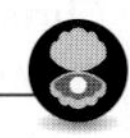

Comments

Avoid indiscriminant use of antibiotics because they alter microbiome and promote emergence of resistance bacteria.

Technician Tips

Proper hygiene is vital to avoid contagion/zoonoses (handwashing between patients, gloves when cleaning a patient with diarrhea, avoid human food in clinic).

Client Education

Treatment for some causes of diarrhea can be frustrating. Client communication is essential to avoid unrealistic expectations/disappointment.

SUGGESTED READING

Marks SL: Diarrhea. In Washabau RJ, et al, editors: Canine and feline gastroenterology, St. Louis, 2013, Saunders, pp 99-108.

AUTHOR: Lisa Carioto, DVM, DVSc, DACVIM
EDITOR: Leah A. Cohn, DVM, PhD, DACVIM

Dilated Cardiomyopathy

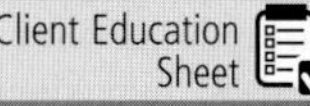

Client Education Sheet

BASIC INFORMATION

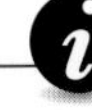

Definition

Dilated cardiomyopathy (DCM) is a myocardial systolic dysfunction disorder (primary or secondary) leading to phenotypic ventricular dilation (left > right ventricle), diastolic dysfunction, and atrial enlargement and causing congestive heart failure (CHF), arrhythmias, or both.

Synonyms

- Primary: idiopathic DCM
- Secondary: nutritional cardiomyopathy, toxic cardiomyopathy, end-stage myocarditis

Epidemiology

SPECIES, AGE, SEX

Dogs:

- Adult onset most common; (4-10 years of age)
- Early onset
  - Standard schnauzer (1-2 years)
  - Portuguese water dog (2-32 weeks)
  - Toy Manchester terrier (10-58 weeks)

Cats:

- Adult onset (2-16 years; median, 9.5 years)

GENETICS, BREED PREDISPOSITION

Dogs:

- Large-breed dogs (>20 kg) overrepresented: Doberman pinscher, Irish wolfhound, Great Dane, Newfoundland, Scottish deerhound, boxer, Afghan hound, Old English sheepdog, Dalmatian
  - Size exceptions are American and English cocker spaniels.
- Doberman pinschers: lifetime risk of 58.2% with an autosomal dominant pattern
  - Two mutations identified in affected Dobermans: *PDK4* and *DCM2*
  - Each mutation can independently lead to development of DCM.
  - Dogs affected with both mutations are 30 times more likely to develop DCM.
- Great Danes: 25% prevalence
  - X-linked, recessive; males (affected) > females (carriers)
- Golden retriever (Duchenne muscular dystrophy, rare)
  - X-linked
- Boxers: arrhythmogenic right ventricular cardiomyopathy (p. 76)
  - Autosomal dominant
- Portuguese water dog: autosomal recessive
- Irish wolfhound (sex-specific alleles); male > female

Cats: reported overrepresentation in Persian, domestic shorthair and long hair, Abyssinian, Birman, Burmese, Siamese cats

RISK FACTORS

Dogs:

- Idiopathic
  - Large breed dogs (>20 kg)
- Nutritional
  - A DCM phenotype has been associated with certain grain-free diets.
- Toxic: doxorubicin (and other anthracycline chemotherapeutic agents); low incidence
  - Cumulative doses > 180 mg/m^2 at greatest risk
  - Dogs can be affected at lower doses; screening before treatment is recommended

Cats:

- Taurine-deficient diets
- End-stage restrictive cardiomyopathy (RCM) and hypertrophic cardiomyopathy (HCM) can result in a DCM phenotype.
- Idiopathic DCM is rare in the cat.

CONTAGION AND ZOONOSIS

- Myocarditis is a secondary cause of phenotypic DCM.
- Usually a rare cause of systolic dysfunction, but a DCM phenotype can occur at end stage of myocarditis.
- Arrhythmias are more common than systolic dysfunction (p. 675).

GEOGRAPHY AND SEASONALITY

See Myocarditis, Section 1 (p. 675).

ASSOCIATED DISORDERS

Congestive heart failure, arrhythmia

Clinical Presentation

DISEASE FORMS/SUBTYPES

- Occult DCM: asymptomatic with systolic dysfunction and/or ventricular dilation based on echocardiography and/or the presence of ventricular arrhythmias.
- Symptomatic
  - Arrhythmias
    - Ventricular arrhythmias (most common in boxers, Doberman pinschers)
    - Atrial fibrillation (most common in the giant breeds)
  - CHF: left > right sided; biventricular possible
  - Sudden cardiac death (first sign in 35% of dogs)

HISTORY, CHIEF COMPLAINT

- Occult DCM: asymptomatic, diagnosed during screening examination or incidental finding
- Cardiac arrhythmias: lethargy, collapse/syncope, weakness, precipitation of CHF (e.g., atrial fibrillation)
- CHF: dyspnea, tachypnea, coughing, abdominal distention (biventricular failure or arrhythmia induced), lethargy, restlessness, weight loss

PHYSICAL EXAM FINDINGS

- Auscultation: soft murmur 1/6 to 3/6 left or right apical systolic, gallop heart sound, arrhythmia
- Pulses: hypokinetic femoral pulses, pulse deficits with premature beats or atrial fibrillation
- Findings in CHF: tachypnea, weakness, cachexia, pale/cyanotic mucous membranes
  - Left-sided CHF: pulmonary crackles/rales, muffled lung sounds with pleural effusion
  - Right-sided CHF: abdominal distention, jugular pulses/distention, muffled heart and lung sounds with pleural effusion, ventral subcutaneous (pitting) edema (rare)

Etiology and Pathophysiology

- Causes of DCM
  - Inherited cardiomyopathy (in many breeds, DCM that was previously thought to be idiopathic has been recognized to have a genetic influence)
  - Infectious myocarditis
  - Nutritional deficiency
  - Toxicity: doxorubicin cardiotoxicity
  - Other: tachycardia induced, hypothyroidism
  - Idiopathic: an underlying cause is not identified
- Primary myocardial systolic dysfunction leads to reduced cardiac output, followed by activation of various neurohormonal and cytokine pathways to support blood pressure (BP) and organ perfusion. This leads to short-term stability but long-term myocardial remodeling and enlargement (p. 408).
- The clinical stages of symptomatic DCM are characterized by two distinct outcomes:
  - CHF: 1-year survival rate < 10%
  - Sudden cardiac death: presumptive malignant ventricular arrhythmias

DIAGNOSIS

Diagnostic Overview

- Diagnosis includes disease confirmation in animals with clinical abnormalities and diagnostic screening in well dogs of commonly affected breeds; well cats are not routinely screened for DCM.
- Echocardiography is the current standard for diagnosis of systolic dysfunction, with or without dilation. DCM also causes ventricular arrhythmias that can result in sudden cardiac death. Gold standard screening includes an echocardiogram (p. 1094) and Holter monitoring (24-hour ECG) (p. 1120).
- Radiographs are indicated for patients with clinical signs referable to the respiratory system (tachypnea, dyspnea). CHF should be considered if left atrial and/or ventricular enlargement, pulmonary venous congestion, and/or pulmonary edema are noted.

Differential Diagnosis

- Respiratory distress (p. 1219)
- Collapse (p. 192)
- Pleural or abdominal effusion (pp. 79 and 791)

Initial Database

- Echocardiogram (see Advanced or Confirmatory Testing)
- Holter monitor (see Advanced or Confirmatory Testing)
- +/− N-terminal pro-B-type natriuretic peptide (NT-pro-BNP)
  - >500 pmol/L: echocardiogram recommended
- Screening recommendations vary by breed.
  - Doberman pinschers: for breeding animals, yearly echocardiography and 24-hour Holter monitoring is recommended.
    - Prevalence increases with age
    - Ventricular premature complexes (VPCs): only abnormality noted in 37% of occult DCM cases

Diagnosis of symptomatic animals:

- CBC usually normal
- Biochemistry panel: usually normal
  - Decreased total protein: if presence of large volume effusion (pleural or abdominal)
  - Prerenal azotemia from poor cardiac perfusion
  - Elevated alanine aminotransferase (ALT): mild, if present
  - Electrolytes: especially important in patients with arrhythmias. In particular, hypokalemia and/or hypomagnesemia can exacerbate arrhythmias and/or reduce efficacy of antiarrhythmic agents.
- BP
  - Normal to low: systolic ≤ 100 mm Hg with myocardial failure
- Radiographs
  - Thoracic: cardiomegaly, pulmonary venous distention, perihilar pulmonary edema, or pleural effusion
  - Occult DCM: often unremarkable (poor screening tool)
- ECG
  - Normal sinus rhythm does not rule out presence of ventricular or atrial arrhythmias and does not rule out DCM. May note atrial premature contractions (APCs), VPCs, atrial fibrillation, ventricular tachycardia
  - One VPC on a 5-min ECG strongly warrants further examination for DCM in Doberman pinschers.
- Effusion analysis
  - Modified transudate consistent with CHF (nucleated cell count < 2500/mcL, total protein < 4.0 g/dL); chylous effusion possible
  - Biventricular heart failure or severe tachyarrhythmias (e.g., atrial fibrillation) may cause pleural and abdominal effusion.
  - Presence of only pleural effusion is unusual presentation for CHF.
- Echocardiogram: required for definitive diagnosis of DCM; not required for initiating therapy

Advanced or Confirmatory Testing

- Echocardiogram: ventricular and atrial dilation (left > right), reduced myocardial systolic function (decreased fractional shortening [%] and ejection fraction [%])
  - LV internal diameter in diastole: > 49 mm; > 99% specific for DCM in Dobermans
  - LV internal diameter in systole: > 40 mm; > 99% specific for DCM in Dobermans
  - End-diastolic volume index > 95 mL/m^2; 96% specific for DCM in Dobermans
  - End-systolic volume index > 55 mL/m^2; 94% specific for DCM in Dobermans
  - Doppler: functional mitral regurgitation common
- Holter monitoring
  - Diagnostic for DCM in Dobermans
    - >100 VPCs/24 hours
    - >50 VPCs/24 hours on two consecutive Holters 6 months apart
- Additional case-specific testing
  - Taurine concentration
    - Deficiency if < 45-50 nmol/mL (plasma) or < 250 nmol/mL (whole blood)
  - Cardiac troponin I
    - >0.34 ng/mL in combination with LV enlargement suggests an increased risk of sudden cardiac death
  - Infectious disease testing (e.g., Chagas titer, Lyme titer)

TREATMENT

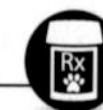

Treatment Overview

- Asymptomatic: treatment is aimed at prolonging the preclinical period.
- Symptomatic: treatment is aimed at relieving clinical symptoms associated with CHF (pulmonary edema and/or effusion), life-threatening ventricular arrhythmias, and significant supraventricular arrhythmias.

Acute General Treatment

Goal is to alleviate overt clinical signs and/or control life-threatening arrhythmias.

Symptomatic:

- CHF (p. 408)
  - Oxygen supplementation (p. 1146)
  - Furosemide 2-4 mg/kg IV or IM bolus for severe distress, additional boluses prn
    - Authors' bolus 2 mg/kg IV q 1-2h until respiratory rate has decreased by half of initial presentation or until < 40 breaths/min
    - Cats: 1-2 mg/kg IV bolus, followed by 1 mg/kg boluses q 2-6h; cats do not tolerate high doses of diuretic therapy
  - Pimobendan 0.2-0.3 mg/kg PO q 8-12h in hospital
  - Minimize stress: sedation prn
    - Butorphanol 0.2-0.4 mg/kg IV or IM
    - Acepromazine 0.005 mg/kg IV or IM, only if systolic BP > 100 mm Hg
  - Dobutamine: fulminant CHF or cardiogenic shock
    - Monitoring: ECG for arrhythmias and BP for systemic hypertension
    - Dogs: 2.5-15 mcg/kg/min
  - Increase by 2.5 mcg/kg/min increments q 15-30 minutes to effect. If VPCs noted or heart rate (HR) increases > 10%, decrease to previous rate.
    - Cats: 1-10 mcg/kg/min. Use with caution because may cause seizures
  - Effusion
    - Prompt thoracocentesis (p. 1164) and/or abdominocentesis (p. 1056) indicated for large volume effusions to alleviate patient discomfort
- Arrhythmias: acute treatment indicated for life-threatening and hemodynamically significant arrhythmias (pp. 94, 96, and 1033)

Chronic Treatment

Goal is to alleviate clinical signs while avoiding iatrogenic side effects from medications. If a patient is tolerating medications, the authors do not recommend dose reduction, with the exception of using the lowest dose of diuretics (i.e., furosemide) that controls clinical signs.

Asymptomatic:

- Echocardiogram
  - Normal indices: no treatment
  - Evidence of systolic dysfunction (the PROTECT study demonstrated that pimobendan prolonged the time to onset of clinical signs and extended survival in Dobermans with occult DCM)
    - Pimobendan 0.2-0.25 mg/kg PO q 12h
- Holter or ECG: see Arrhythmias section below and other sources (pp. 94, 96, and 1033)

Symptomatic:

- CHF (p. 409)
  - Lasix 2 mg/kg PO q 12h
  - Pimobendan 0.2-0.25 mg/kg PO q 12h
  - Angiotensin-converting enzyme (ACE) inhibitor 0.25-0.5 mg/kg PO q 12h
    - Delay starting if patient anorexic or azotemic
  - Spironolactone 1-2 mg/kg PO q 12h
    - Start at recheck if tolerating other medications
  - Beta-blockers are contraindicated in CHF and not recommended
  - Potassium supplementation prn
    - 2 mEq per 4.5 kg PO q 12h

Arrhythmias:

- Ventricular
  - Holter or ECG: treatment with ventricular antiarrhythmic agents does not reduce the risk of fatal arrhythmias, and these agents may be proarrhythmic. However, treatment is generally recommended if couplets, triplets, paroxysms/bursts/salvos, or runs of ventricular tachycardia are very closely coupled (e.g., R on T).
  - Chronic medical management
    - Sotalol 1-2 mg/kg PO q12h (authors' preference)
    - Mexiletine 4-8 mg/kg PO q 8h (may be combined with sotalol prn)
    - Amiodarone 10-20 mg/kg PO q 24h for 7-10 days, then reduce to 3-15 mg/kg PO q 24-48h (for refractory arrhythmias, discontinue sotalol)
- Supraventricular (e.g., atrial fibrillation, flutter, or supraventricular tachycardia)
  - Treatment is aimed at HR control.
  - HR > 160 beats/min in hospital
    - Goal of treatment: HR < 160 beats/min in hospital
    - Diltiazem XR (12-hour release formulation) 2-4 mg/kg PO q 12h (authors' preference)
    - Digoxin 0.001-0.005 mg/kg PO q 12h (0.003 mg/kg PO q 12h is authors' preference); combined with diltiazem if HR not adequately controlled
    - Amiodarone 10-20 mg/kg PO q 24h for 7-10 days, then reduce to 3-15 mg/kg PO q 24-48h; combined with diltiazem if HR not adequately controlled
  - Cardioversion not routinely performed in CHF patients

Nutrition/Diet

Diet changes should be implemented after CHF is controlled:

- Diet should not be changed at expense of patient appetite.
- Ensure adequate protein intake.
- Avoid grain-free boutique diets.
- Eliminate high-sodium treats.
  - Sodium-restricted commercial diets (Royal Canin Early Cardiac, Hill's g/d or h/d) or balanced home-cooked meals
- Omega-3 fatty acids may improve appetite and reduce cardiac cachexia
  - Dog: eicosapentaenoic acid (EPA) 40 mg/kg PO q 24h and docosahexaenoic acid (DHA) 25 mg/kg PO q 24h

When indicated on a case by case basis:

- Taurine supplementation
  - Cats: 250 mg/CAT PO q 12h
  - Dogs: 500 mg/DOG PO q 12h
- L-carnitine supplementation
  - Dogs: 110 mg/kg PO q 12h in boxers and American cocker spaniels
- Appetite stimulants: prn
  - Dogs: mirtazapine 0.6 mg/kg PO q 24h; cyproheptadine 0.2 mg/kg PO q 24h; or capromorelin 3 mg/kg PO q 24h
  - Cats: mirtazapine 3.75 mg/CAT PO q 72h or cyproheptadine 2 mg/CAT q 12h

Behavior/Exercise

- Absolute rest during treatment of CHF or life-threatening arrhythmias
- After CHF is resolved, slowly increase activity to normal levels.
- Always allow patient to take breaks or stop exercising when tired.

Drug Interactions

- Dobutamine and furosemide precipitate (requires two catheters)
- Amiodarone will increase serum digoxin levels
- Hypokalemia, hypercalcemia, renal dysfunction, and hypothyroidism will predispose to digitalis intoxication (reduce dose of digoxin)

Possible Complications

- Renal insufficiency due to low cardiac output and/or overzealous diuresis
- Mild to moderate azotemia often occurs with diuretic therapy.
  - Ensure patient is on lowest diuretic dose that controls CHF.
  - Consider reducing ACE inhibitor dose.
  - Mild azotemia is tolerable if patient clinically normal
- Sudden death due to arrhythmias

Recommended Monitoring

- Renal/electrolyte panel 5-7 days after starting or changing medications (diuretics, ACE inhibitors)
- Thoracic radiographs, ECG, BP, depending on clinical exam
- Holter monitor: 1-4 weeks after starting or adjusting antiarrhythmic medication
- Echocardiography: if significant or unexpected change in patient's condition
- Serum digoxin level: 1 week after starting therapy, 6-8 hours after pill
  - Therapeutic range: 0.8-1.8 ng/mL

PROGNOSIS & OUTCOME

- Asymptomatic (occult DCM): pimobendan significantly prolongs the onset of clinical signs.
  - Doberman pinschers and Irish wolfhounds
  - Effect in other breeds and cats has not been evaluated at this stage.
- Symptomatic (CHF or syncope)
  - Pimobendan, furosemide, and an ACE inhibitor confer the best long-term prognosis.
  - Prognosis is influenced by response to treatment, underlying cause, owner compliance, and tolerance of medications.
  - Atrial fibrillation confers a shorter median survival time.

- Doberman pinschers, Irish wolfhounds, and Great Danes
  - Poor median survival time after onset of CHF
- Portuguese water dogs and other juvenile-onset DCM dogs have a grave prognosis.
- Cats with DCM not caused by taurine deficiency have a grave prognosis.

PEARLS & CONSIDERATIONS

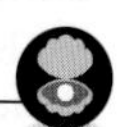

Comments

- Screening is key to best long-term prognosis.
  - Doberman pinschers: begin screening at 2-3 years of age
- Murmurs, gallops, or arrhythmias in a predisposed, asymptomatic dog warrant full cardiac screening.
  - Soft murmurs do not rule out significant disease (e.g., functional mitral regurgitation from severe dilation)
- Ventricular arrhythmias in the absence of echocardiographic changes are common.
- Do not discontinue antiarrhythmic therapy before consultation with a specialist.
- Radiographic heart size is an insensitive marker for DCM, but radiography is gold standard for CHF diagnosis.
- Do not delay CHF treatment in lieu of an echocardiogram.
- In mild azotemia, reduce ACE inhibitor frequency or dose before adjusting diuretics.
- Supplement potassium when in low-normal range if patients are hyporexic or increasing diuretic dose.
- Low fractional shortening (%) common in normal large-breed dogs; high false-positive DCM diagnosis with inexperienced scanners

Prevention

Patients predisposed should be screened at an early age with an echocardiogram and Holter monitor. Consider NT-pro-BNP in cases with financial constraints; if elevated, full screening is recommended. Any VPCs noted on 5-minute ECG strongly predicts DCM, and full screening is recommended.

Technician Tips

- IV catheters, volume received, and administration lines should be checked hourly if patients are on continuous-rate infusions (CRIs) to ensure adequate dosing and patency.
- Furosemide is light sensitive, and if being administered by CRI, administration lines and syringes should be covered.

Client Education

- Monitor breathing rates at home daily for patients with a history of CHF and weekly for patients with occult DCM.
  - Performed at rest (sleeping): normal < 30 breaths/min
- Reinforce importance of annual screening.
- Reinforce prevalence of sudden death in asymptomatic and symptomatic DCM.
- Establish early discussions about quality-of-life and end-of-life decisions after CHF.

SUGGESTED READING

Stern JA, et al: Myocardial disease: canine. In Ettinger SJ, et al, editors: Textbook of veterinary internal medicine, ed 8, St. Louis, 2017, Elsevier.

AUTHORS: Ryan C. Fries, DVM, DACVIM; Jordan P. Vitt, DVM, DACVIM
EDITOR: Meg M. Sleeper, VMD, DACVIM

Discospondylitis

Client Education Sheet 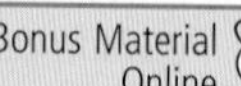 Bonus Material Online 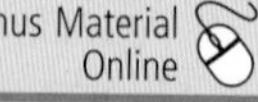

BASIC INFORMATION

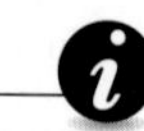

Definition

Inflammation of the intervertebral disc and adjacent vertebral endplates due to a bacterial or, less often, fungal infection

Epidemiology

SPECIES, AGE, SEX

- Most commonly reported in large-breed, middle-aged to older dogs. Males outnumber females 2:1.
  - *Brucella canis* more common in sexually intact dogs
- Although risk appears to increase with age, it has been reported in juvenile dogs (<6 months of age).
- Rare in cats; typically associated with local trauma such as a bite wound

GENETICS, BREED PREDISPOSITION

- Predisposed breeds include German shepherd dogs, Great Danes, boxers, rottweilers, Doberman pinschers, bullmastiffs, and English bulldogs.
- German shepherd dogs and Rhodesian ridgebacks are overrepresented for fungal infections.

RISK FACTORS

- Immunosuppression
- Among juveniles, recent history of blunt force trauma, bite wounds, or previous parvovirus infection

CONTAGION AND ZOONOSIS

B. canis poses a zoonotic risk and is a reportable disease

GEOGRAPHY AND SEASONALITY

Prevalence of causative agents varies geographically.

Clinical Presentation

HISTORY, CHIEF COMPLAINT

- Varied course of disease; usually chronic and progressive over weeks to months
- Spinal hyperesthesia is the most common chief complaint, present in > 80% of cases
- Systemic signs can include pyrexia, lethargy, weakness, stiffness/lameness, anorexia, weight loss, and dull mentation.

PHYSICAL EXAM FINDINGS

- Most cases have hyperesthesia on paravertebral palpation.
- Neurologic signs can develop from secondary compressive lesions; the dura is usually an effective barrier to prevent extension of infection into the spinal cord itself. Neurologic signs occur in nearly half of cases and reflect localization of the lesion, ranging from proprioceptive deficits to paralysis.
- Worsening neurologic grade correlates with an increase in the number of sites of infection and the degree of spinal cord compression.
- ± Fever
- Other findings relate to additional sites of infection, if present (e.g., murmur due to endocarditis)

Etiology and Pathophysiology

- Hematogenous spread to the vertebral endplates (with extension into the disc space); less commonly, direct inoculation of the intervertebral disc
- Most common bacterial isolate is coagulase-positive *Staphylococcus* spp. Others include coagulase-negative *Staphylococcus* spp, *Streptococcus* spp, gram-negative aerobes (*Escherichia coli*, *B. canis*), and fungal agents (*Aspergillus*, *Paecilomyces*, *Candida*).
- Source of infection is often elusive; proposed sites include the urogenital tract, oral cavity, respiratory tract, endocardium, and skin.
- Local extension from migrating foreign material, penetrating wounds, or surgical site infection is possible.

DIAGNOSIS

Diagnostic Overview

Diagnosis is primarily based on radiographic findings. Occult cases are possible; if radiographs are inconclusive, advanced imaging is indicated. If neurologic signs are present, advanced imaging is useful to detect spinal cord compression.

Differential Diagnosis

- Intervertebral disc herniation
- Spinal trauma
- Meningitis/myelitis
- Spinal neoplasia

- Myositis
- Polyarthritis

Initial Database

- Complete blood count can reveal mild to moderate neutrophilia; serum biochemistry abnormalities can include hypoalbuminemia and hyperglobulinemia.
- Urine culture: positive in roughly one-third of cases. Fungal hyphae may be seen in urine sediment or identified on routine urine culture.
- Blood cultures increase the likelihood of a positive culture result to two-thirds of cases.
- *B. canis* testing should be performed in endemic areas, regardless of patient's reproductive status (p. 1319).
- Galactomannan antigen assay: very sensitive for diagnosis of disseminated aspergillosis. (p. 1309)
- Radiographs remain the mainstay of diagnosis. A delay of up to 6 weeks between the onset of signs and radiographic changes is possible; serial radiographs may be of benefit if the index of suspicion for discospondylitis is high. Characteristic findings include
  - Loss of definition/irregularity of endplate margins
  - Lysis and sclerosis of the adjacent endplates and vertebral bodies
  - In early disease, the vertebral bodies can appear shorter and the disc spaces wider as destruction occurs. In juvenile dogs, early signs more commonly include disc space narrowing and subluxation.
  - With chronic disease, collapse of the disc space and fusion of the adjacent vertebral bodies can occur.
  - Periosteal new bone formation on the ventral and lateral aspects of affected vertebrae
  - The lumbosacral space is most commonly affected. Majority of dogs have lesions in the thoracolumbar spine. Cervical lesions are present in < 20% of cases.
  - Up to 40% of cases have multifocal disease; it is recommended that survey radiographs of the entire vertebral column be obtained.
- Radiographic changes must be distinguished from spondylosis deformans and vertebral neoplasia.
  - Spondylosis deformans is characterized by smooth, regular new bone formation ventrally, and discospondylitis causes irregular bony lysis.
  - Bony lysis is centered over the vertebral body and remains confined to one vertebra for most neoplastic diseases, but discospondylitis involves two adjacent vertebral endplates.

Advanced or Confirmatory Testing

- Ultrasonography can have clinical applicability early in the course of disease because characteristic sonographic findings can appear before radiographic changes.
- CT and MRI (p. 1132): increase the diagnostic yield and should be considered when neurologic signs are present.
- Cerebrospinal fluid analysis (pp. 1080 and 1323): findings generally are nonspecific; elevated protein is most commonly reported abnormality, and pleocytosis is rare.
- Echocardiogram and abdominal ultrasound: used to evaluate for underlying/concurrent systemic disease (e.g., endocarditis, abdominal abscess or lymphadenomegaly)
- Percutaneous disc aspirates and culture or surgical biopsy: typically reserved for patients that are not responding to medical therapy or when a clear diagnosis cannot be reached with imaging alone.

TREATMENT

Treatment Overview

Treatment is initiated with broad-spectrum antibiotics, ideally based on culture and sensitivity results (blood, aspirate from disc space, or less ideally, urine). Antimicrobial therapy should be continued until clinical and radiographic resolution is documented, typically a minimum of 6 months.

Acute General Treatment

- If culture and sensitivity is not available, first-line therapy often involves first-generation cephalosporins or beta-lactamase–resistant penicillins, as treatment for coagulase-positive *Staphylococcus.*
- Resolution of spinal hyperesthesia generally occurs within 3-5 days of appropriate antimicrobial therapy. Pain control can be achieved with nonsteroidal antiinflammatory drugs (NSAIDs).
- Antimicrobial therapy should be continued for at least 4-6 weeks after radiographic changes become static.
- If no improvement after 1 week, consider additional diagnostics or adding a second antimicrobial agent (fluoroquinolone or aminoglycoside).
- For patients with severe illness, initiate therapy with intravenous antimicrobials (24-48 hours).
- *Aspergillus* spp are intrinsically resistant to fluconazole; multiple antifungal drugs (itraconazole or voriconazole ± amphotericin B) may be needed for the treatment of fungal discospondylitis (p. 81).
- *B. canis*: tetracyclines (doxycycline or minocycline) for a minimum of 1-2 months in combination with aminoglycosides (streptomycin or gentamicin) for the first 1-2 weeks of treatment. Recently, the use of enrofloxacin has been described.
  - Brucellosis cannot be cured, and zoonotic risk must be considered before opting for treatment.
- Surgical decompression may be warranted if neurologic deficits are severe due to significant spinal cord compression and signs do not resolve with appropriate antibiotic therapy. Spinal stabilization is often required if surgery is performed.

Chronic Treatment

Physical rehabilitation therapy can help maximize recovery for patients with severe neurologic deficits.

Behavior/Exercise

Exercise restriction advised during the initial 4-6 weeks of therapy.

Drug Interactions

Some of the drugs that may be considered are nephrotoxic (e.g., amphotericin B, aminoglycosides).

Possible Complications

- Secondary pathologic vertebral fracture and subluxation
- Epidural abscessation/empyema
- If neurologic progression is documented, advanced imaging is recommended.

Recommended Monitoring

- Serial radiographs every 4-6 weeks or sooner if the clinical signs worsen.
- Treatment is continued until there is clinical and radiographic evidence of disease resolution. In adult dogs, radiographic progression can occur for up to 9 weeks after the initiation of therapy, even in patients showing a good clinical response. In dogs < 1 year of age, radiographic improvement correlates well

Organism	Antimicrobial Agent	Dosage
Staphylococcus spp	Cefazolin	22 mg/kg IV q 8h
	Cephalexin	25-30 mg/kg PO q 8h
	Ampicillin-sulbactam	20 mg/kg IV q 8h
	Amoxicillin-clavulanate	20-25 mg/kg PO q 12h
Streptococcus spp	Amoxicillin	22 mg/kg PO q 12h
Escherichia coli	Enrofloxacin	5 mg/kg PO q 12h
	Cephalexin	25-30 mg/kg PO q 8h
	Amoxicillin-clavulanate	20-25 mg/kg PO q 12h
Brucella canis	Doxycycline	10-15 mg/kg PO q 12h
	Streptomycin	20 mg/kg IM q 24h
	Gentamicin sulfate	9-14 mg/kg IV, IM, SQ q 24h
	Enrofloxacin	5 mg/kg PO q 12h
Aspergillus	Itraconazole	5 mg/kg PO q 12-24h
	Voriconazole	5 mg/kg PO q 12h
	Amphotericin B	Formulations vary

with clinical improvement. Radiographic signs of healing:
- Absence or smoothing of the lytic focus
- Bridging spondylosis/new bone formation

- Antimicrobials can be discontinued 4-6 weeks after there is no evidence of ongoing lysis.
- Recheck radiographs 1-2 months after discontinuation of therapy.

PROGNOSIS & OUTCOME

- Bacterial discospondylitis: good to excellent prognosis. Patients with pronounced neurologic deficits often have a more protracted recovery but can still have a functional outcome.
- Fungal discospondylitis carries a poor prognosis and may require lifelong treatment.
- The prognosis for *B. canis* infection is guarded. Poor response to therapy is likely due to the intracellular nature of the organism and periodic bacteremia. Relapses are common. Euthanasia of affected individuals may be the best way to achieve control in group populations and to avoid zoonosis.

PEARLS & CONSIDERATIONS

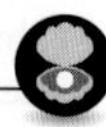

Comments

- Discospondylitis should be considered as a differential diagnosis for puppies with back pain, especially those with a recent history of trauma or systemic infection. Radiographic findings can differ in juveniles compared to adults.
- Multiple organism infections are possible, including mixed bacterial and fungal infections. Although cultures help guide therapy, the bacterial organisms identified in urine cultures may not be those present in the disc space.

Technician Tips

- A complete study of the vertebral column involves five lateral radiographs and five orthogonal projections. Positioning devices should be used to ensure the spine is parallel to the tabletop. Sedation is often required.
- Due to its zoonotic potential, care should be taken while handling patients (handwashing, gloves, minimizing exposure to urine) until *B. canis* has been ruled out.

Client Education

Discospondylitis can be a life-threatening illness. Compliance with medication administration and follow-up is essential to ensure a positive outcome.

SUGGESTED READING

Burkert BA, et al: Signalment and clinical features of discospondylitis in dogs: 513 cases (1980-2001). J Am Vet Med Assoc 227:268-275, 2005.

AUTHOR: Kathryn Winger, DVM, DACVIM
EDITOR: Karen R. Muñana, DVM, MS, DACVIM

Disorientation/Confusion

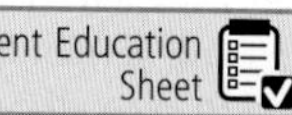

BASIC INFORMATION

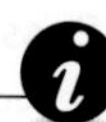

Definition

An inappropriate state of confusion with respect to time and/or place and/or identity characterized by atypical and/or inappropriate behaviors to a given stimuli or environmental condition (e.g., pacing, wandering aimlessly, not responding to being called by name in a normal-hearing patient, escalating separation anxiety)

Epidemiology

SPECIES, AGE, SEX

Dogs and cats, any age or sex

GENETICS, BREED PREDISPOSITION

- Brachycephalic and dome-headed breeds are prone to congenital hydrocephalus (p. 481).
- Breeds predisposed to inherited inborn errors of metabolism (e.g., various lysosomal storage diseases)
- Breeds predisposed to various diseases resulting in metabolic derangements (e.g., portosystemic shunts resulting in hepatic encephalopathy [p. 814])
- Breeds of animals predisposed to epilepsy (i.e., disorientation/confusion during the postictal period [p. 301])
- Breeds predisposed to blindness (e.g., sudden acquired retinal degeneration [p. 883])

RISK FACTORS

- Old age: canine and feline cognitive dysfunction syndrome (p. 188)
- Access to psychoactive drugs or potentially neurotoxic substances
- Pre-existing liver or kidney disease, diabetes mellitus, hypothyroidism, or other diseases causing osmotic, electrolyte, and/or acid-base disturbances

Clinical Presentation

HISTORY, CHIEF COMPLAINT

Can be acute or insidious in onset. Acute presentations often associated with trauma, ingestion of toxic substances with central nervous system (CNS) effects, encephalopathy, or metabolic illness.

- Barring history or suggestion of observed trauma or intoxication, owners may describe any combination of the following signs:
  - Not responding to being called by name
  - Wandering aimlessly
  - Seemingly getting stuck in corners of home
  - Behaving unaware or forgetful of surroundings or of owner/family members
  - Urinating or defecating in inappropriate places
  - Not behaving in anticipatory manner with regard to daily routines (e.g., not being excited to be fed at usual time)
- Obtain clear, concise description of primary complaint, and ask questions about
  - Vision or hearing changes
  - Potential access to toxins or psychotropic drugs
  - Signs associated with metabolic disturbances (e.g., alterations in thirst, appetite, gastrointestinal/urologic behaviors)
  - History of recent trauma
  - History of seizures (animals can be disoriented during the postictal period)

PHYSICAL EXAM FINDINGS

- Physical exam findings depend on the cause (see specific diseases).
- For accurate treatment and prognosis, it is important to identify the cause of disorientation:
  - Primary brain origin (e.g., canine or feline cognitive dysfunction syndrome, congenital hydrocephalus, brain neoplasia)
  - Secondary to some other cause (e.g., trauma, various metabolic encephalopathies, various toxicities)
  - Resulting from visual impairment: may note mydriasis in normal ambient lighting (p. 123)
  - Resulting from hearing impairment (p. 237)
  - Benign behavioral origin

Etiology and Pathophysiology

- Disorientation can result when a disease affects the cerebrum.
- Pathophysiologic explanation of altered frontal and temporal lobe function varies with each disease but may include
  - Alterations in neuronal metabolism (e.g., hypoglycemia, hypothyroidism, hypocalcemia)
  - Accumulation of neurotoxic substances (e.g., hepatic encephalopathy)
  - Chronic oxidative stress in the brain, leading to neurodegeneration (e.g., canine and feline cognitive dysfunction syndrome)
  - Alterations in brain neurotransmitters (e.g., hepatic encephalopathy, epilepsy)

- Alterations in neuronal excitability (e.g., electrolyte disturbances)
- Direct mechanical damage (head trauma)
- Animals can become disoriented despite normal cerebral function when they are blind and/or deaf.

DIAGNOSIS

Diagnostic Overview

The history and physical exam provide essential clues to investigate this nonspecific chief complaint. A neurologic exam is indicated in all cases, as are routine laboratory tests to investigate metabolic causes.

Differential Diagnosis

- Differential diagnosis for disorientation
  - Psychological (e.g., stereotypies)
  - Vision impairment
  - Hearing impairment
  - Primary (e.g., head trauma) or secondary (e.g., hepatic encephalopathy) disease affecting the brain

Initial Database

- Age of onset
  - NOTE: diagnosis of age-related cognitive dysfunction is one of exclusion in elderly patients; therefore, first consider other diseases resulting in disorientation.
- Complete neurologic exam (p. 1136)
- Complete ophthalmic exam (p. 1137)
- CBC, serum biochemistry, urinalysis: recognize underlying systemic condition and preanesthetic evaluation (if needed)

Advanced or Confirmatory Testing

- Clinical laboratory diagnostic tests for endocrinopathies, liver function tests, toxicology screen, as suggested by clinical information
- Tests of vision: scotopic and photopic maze testing/obstacle course, electroretinogram
- Tests of hearing: auditory stimulus, brainstem auditory evoked response testing.
- CT or MRI (p. 1132) of brain
- Cerebrospinal fluid (p. 1080) cytologic analysis with biochemical ± serologic testing as indicated by case findings

TREATMENT

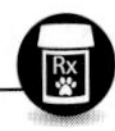

Treatment Overview

Treat the underlying cause of disorientation when possible.

Acute General Treatment

Acute treatment varies according to the cause.

Chronic Treatment

Animals with incurable disorientation (e.g., age-related cognitive dysfunction) may need special care:

- Confine within a yard or home to prevent wandering away
- Take animal outside to urinate/defecate more frequently if dog is inappropriately urinating/defecating in the house
- Selegiline hydrochloride 0.5-1 mg/kg PO q 24h is FDA approved for canine cognitive dysfunction but benefit may be minor.

Nutrition/Diet

- Several diets have been formulated for dogs with cognitive dysfunction (e.g., Hill's Prescription Diet b/d, Purina Bright Mind).
- Several nutraceutical supplements are marketed for the same condition (e.g., Senilife, Ceva Animal Health; ProNeurozone, Animal Health Options; Neutricks, Novifit [SAMe], Virbac) or for reducing neurodegeneration (e.g., NeuroConnex, Animal Necessity).
- Further study of the efficacy of these therapies is warranted.

PROGNOSIS & OUTCOME

Prognosis depends on the cause.

PEARLS & CONSIDERATIONS

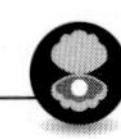

Comments

- Up to 75% of dogs 7 years or older will demonstrate at least one clinical sign consistent with canine cognitive dysfunction syndrome.
- Approximately 25% of cats 11-14 years of age and more than 50% of cats older than 15 years of age will demonstrate cognitive decline.
- Animals with clinical signs of disorientation related to vision or hearing loss will commonly adapt to their surroundings and have a good quality of life, provided they are not used for tasks requiring these senses and if their home environment does not change drastically (e.g., moving furniture frequently).
- Selegiline may be associated with adverse effects and drug interactions.

Technician Tips

- For any patient with disorientation/confusion always be cognizant of potential infectious zoonotic disease (e.g., rabies) and handle accordingly.
- Exercise caution as disorientated/confused animals may become aggressive.

Client Education

When applicable, provide client with client education sheets: "How to Change the Environment for a Pet That Is Blind" and "How to Change the Environment for a Pet That Is Deaf."

SUGGESTED READING

ASPCA Poison Control Center: Information and links pertaining to toxicologic information on various plants and drugs (websites). www.aspca.org/pet-care/animal-poison-control/.

AUTHOR: Aubrey A. Webb, DVM, PhD
EDITOR: Leah A. Cohn, DVM, PhD, DACVIM

Disseminated Intravascular Coagulation

BASIC INFORMATION

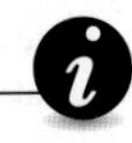

Definition

An acquired syndrome in which coagulation is abnormally and inappropriately activated, with widespread fibrin deposition in the microvasculature. Depletion of platelets and coagulation factors can result in overt hemorrhage.

Epidemiology

SPECIES, AGE, SEX

- Dogs of any age, breed, or sex
- Infrequently identified in cats

RISK FACTORS

Primary disorders that may lead to disseminated intravascular coagulation (DIC) are infectious, inflammatory, neoplastic, or traumatic.

ASSOCIATED DISORDERS

DIC is a secondary condition developing from an underlying primary disease (see Risk Factors above and Disease Forms below).

Clinical Presentation

DISEASE FORMS/SUBTYPES

- Acute DIC: associated with fulminant diseases (e.g., sepsis, anaphylaxis, heatstroke, pancreatitis, envenomation)
- Chronic DIC: secondary to solid tumors and hematopoietic neoplasia; common in dogs with hemangiosarcoma

HISTORY, CHIEF COMPLAINT

Typically reflect the primary disease (see above); signs of DIC are nonspecific and may be indistinguishable from signs of the underlying disorder.

PHYSICAL EXAM FINDINGS

- Varies and depends on primary disease and extent of thrombosis or factor depletion and spontaneous/exaggerated hemorrhage.

- Any of the following may be apparent: collapse, pallor, tachycardia, tachypnea, petechiae, ecchymoses, melena, epistaxis, icterus

Etiology and Pathophysiology

- Two major pathways initiate DIC
  - Systemic inflammatory response with cytokine and coagulation cascade activation (e.g., sepsis, polytrauma)
  - Release of procoagulant stimuli into the vascular space initiates widespread activation of coagulation (e.g., hemangiosarcoma, mammary carcinoma).
- Systemic fibrin deposition is insufficiently balanced by opposing anticoagulant mechanisms.
  - Antithrombin depletion from consumption, degradation, and suppressed synthesis
  - Protein C system: downregulated by proinflammatory cytokines
- Fibrinolysis is concomitantly suppressed.
  - High plasminogen activator inhibitor levels impair fibrinolysis.
- Subsequent depletion of coagulation factors and prolongation of coagulation times or clinical hemorrhage
- Consumption of platelets and subsequent thrombocytopenia
- Local thrombosis contributes to acidosis, ischemia, organ dysfunction, and tissue necrosis, which can perpetuate the syndrome.

DIAGNOSIS

Diagnostic Overview

No single laboratory test is diagnostic for DIC. Early diagnosis of the thrombotic phase is especially challenging and requires an elevated index of suspicion. Nonspecific physical exam abnormalities (see above), especially together with a documented recent decrease in platelet count and/or altered coagulation parameters in a patient with a recognized risk factor, suggest the possibility of DIC. After clinical hemorrhage occurs, DIC is likely advanced to the overt hemorrhagic phase and more difficult to treat effectively.

Differential Diagnosis

- Hemorrhagic DIC
  - Anticoagulant rodenticides
  - Severe primary thrombocytopenia
  - Inherited or acquired platelet dysfunction (thrombocytopathia)
  - Dextran or hetastarch administration (prolonged clotting times)
  - Liver failure
- Thrombotic DIC: organ failure or pulmonary thromboembolism (PTE) from cardiac disease, heartworm disease, tumor emboli, or hypercoagulability associated with antithrombin loss

Initial Database

- CBC, platelet count, blood smear
  - Thrombocytopenia typical
  - Schistocytes, keratocytes, or acanthocytes (fragmented red blood cells) from shredding by intravascular fibrin strands or microangiopathic hemolysis
- Serum biochemistry profile, urinalysis: evidence of underlying disease; effects of thromboembolism (renal, hepatic)
- Chest and abdominal radiographs or ultrasound: evidence of underlying disease and/or thromboembolism, hemorrhage
- Coagulation testing: prolonged prothrombin time (PT), and/or prolonged activated partial thromboplastin times (aPTT), decreased fibrinogen (p. 1325)
- D-dimer or fibrin/fibrinogen degradation product (FDP) concentration: typically increased (pp. 1334 and 1342)
- Antithrombin activity: typically decreased (p. 1309)

Advanced or Confirmatory Testing

- Reduced protein C or protein S activity
- High concentration of thrombin to antithrombin complexes
- A scoring system has been developed for dogs (Wiinberg et al., 2010).
- Thromboelastrography or thromboelastometry may help diagnose occult or chronic DIC or identify hypercoagulability.

TREATMENT

Treatment Overview

DIC is a secondary condition arising from a serious underlying disorder. Treatment involves control of thromboembolism or hemorrhage (whichever predominates) and management of the primary disorder.

Acute General Treatment

- Always treat the primary condition.
- Support adequate perfusion with intravenous fluids as needed.
- Oxygen therapy if indicated (pulmonary disease including PTE) (p. 1146)
- Red blood cell transfusion in anemic patients (p. 1169)
- Fresh-frozen plasma (FFP) transfusion if fibrinogen and clotting factor depletion causes hemorrhage or if fibrinogen-deficient patients require surgery (p. 1169). Repeated doses of FFP may be needed (10-15 mL/kg IV q 8-12h).
- Heparin should be considered if dyspnea from PTE or organ failure from thrombosis occurs (p. 842).
  - Regular unfractionated heparin (UFH) 100-200 U/kg SQ q 8h or 15-25 U/kg/h IV continuous rate infusion
  - Low-molecular-weight heparin: dalteparin (Fragmin) 100 IU/kg SQ q 12h or enoxaparin (Lovenox) 1-1.5 mg/kg SQ q 12h

Chronic Treatment

DIC is always secondary, and treatment should be directed toward the primary condition.

Drug Interactions

Avoid heparin, hetastarch, and dextrans, and platelet inhibitors (e.g., aspirin, clopidogrel) when coagulation times are prolonged due to severe factor and fibrinogen depletion or if there is severe thrombocytopenia.

Possible Complications

- PTE
- Thromboembolism (kidney, brain, pelvic limbs, liver, portal vein)
- Hemorrhage (+/− anemia, hypovolemia)
- Organ dysfunction and death

Recommended Monitoring

- Serial platelet counts and coagulation times every 24-48 hours
- Monitor organ function and tissue oxygenation.
- For heparin treatment, monitor for signs of hemorrhage, falling platelet count, or excessive prolongation of *in vitro* clotting time (UFH therapy).
- A target prolongation of aPTT to 1.5-2 times baseline is evidence of UFH high-dose anticoagulant effect.
- UFH and low-molecular-weight heparins can be monitored by inhibition of factor Xa. In humans, the target range of anti-Xa activity = 0.3-0.7 U/mL (UFH) and for low-molecular-weight heparin = 0.5-1.0 U/mL.

PROGNOSIS & OUTCOME

- Depends on the underlying condition and extent of thromboembolism or hemorrhage
- Fulminant or hemorrhagic DIC carries a poor to grave prognosis.

PEARLS & CONSIDERATIONS

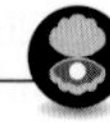

Comments

- Laboratory diagnostics are insensitive for identifying early DIC.
- Development of DIC contributes to the morbidity and mortality of the primary disease.
- Treatment is challenging and no gold standard approach is known.
- Treatment becomes less rewarding late in the disease process.
- Having an early suspicion that DIC may develop is important for selecting appropriate diagnostic tests and for monitoring the patient.

Prevention

Critical factors in preventing or ameliorating DIC are specific and aggressive corrections of the primary disease.

Technician Tips

- If DIC is suspected, avoid jugular phlebotomy.
- When collecting blood samples from very ill dogs, consider collecting a citrate sample for coagulation testing such as PT, aPTT, or D-dimer.

Client Education

Development of DIC represents a severe complication of many systemic diseases.

SUGGESTED READING

Stokol T: Laboratory diagnosis of disseminated intravascular coagulation in dogs and cats: the past, the present and the future. Vet Clin Small Anim 42(1):189-202, 2012.

AUTHOR: Jonathan F. Bach, DVM, DACVIM, DACVECC
EDITOR: Jonathan E. Fogle, DVM, PhD, DACVIM

Distemper, Canine

Client Education Sheet 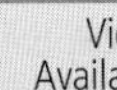 Video Available 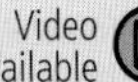

BASIC INFORMATION 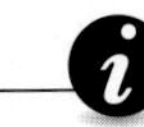

Definition

Viral disease caused by a morbillivirus of the family Paramyxoviridae. Clinical disease includes mild to severe systemic illness with high morbidity and variable mortality (mortality often related to central nervous system [CNS] infection).

Synonyms

Distemper, hardpad disease

Epidemiology

SPECIES, AGE, SEX

- Dogs, especially urban or suburban dogs between 3 and 6 months of age
- Other susceptible species include additional members of the order Canidae (e.g., coyote, wolf, fox), ferrets, mink, skunk, raccoon, sea mammals, and selected members of the order Felidae (e.g., lions, tigers).

GENETICS, BREED PREDISPOSITION

More common, and higher mortality rates, in dolichocephalic versus brachycephalic breeds

RISK FACTORS

Exposure to infected animals, inadequate vaccination, immunocompromise, and transplacental transmission

CONTAGION AND ZOONOSIS

Highly contagious (aerosol route common) between infected and susceptible individuals; not zoonotic

GEOGRAPHY AND SEASONALITY

Worldwide distribution

ASSOCIATED DISORDERS

- Hyperkeratosis of the footpads (hardpad disease)
- Ocular signs (anterior uveitis, optic neuritis, retinal degeneration, keratoconjunctivitis) can develop with systemic disease or as a sequela.
- Postencephalitic epilepsy
- Myoclonus
- Persistent anosmia (loss of sense of smell) possible in recovered patients

Clinical Presentation

DISEASE FORMS/SUBTYPES

- Subclinical to mild disease is probably most common, but systemic/generalized form is the most recognized.
- Generalized distemper manifests initially as a respiratory infection followed by gastrointestinal (GI) signs and often CNS signs; CNS signs may manifest concomitant with or after resolution of respiratory and GI signs.
- Old-dog encephalitis (ODE), a rare and chronic form of panencephalitis, likely results from an inflammatory reaction associated with persistent canine distemper virus (CDV) infection of the CNS gray matter. Signs can include ataxia, compulsive movements such as head pressing or continual pacing, and uncoordinated hypermetric gait. Systemic signs are not associated with this form.
- Chronic relapsing demyelinating encephalomyelitis is a persistent, spontaneous CDV infection.
- Inclusion-body polioencephalitis is a variant of the disease that can occur after vaccination and manifests only as a CNS disease. The pathogenesis is similar to that of ODE.

HISTORY, CHIEF COMPLAINT

With the generalized form of the disease, initial presentation typically includes one or more of the following: lethargy, ocular and nasal discharge (serous or mucopurulent), cough, inappetence, vomiting, and diarrhea. A patient with a more advanced form of the disease often has a history of neurologic signs (e.g., seizures, ataxia, myoclonus).

PHYSICAL EXAM FINDINGS

- Systemic disease: as above; fever, ocular signs (keratitis, conjunctivitis, uveitis), loud breath sounds on auscultation, dehydration, cachexia, poor haircoat. Dental abnormalities (dental enamel hypoplasia, tooth impaction, oligodontia) in dogs that survive neonatal infections.
- Neurologic disease: signs indicate encephalitis or encephalomyelitis (seizures, vestibular signs, cerebellar signs/hypermetria, paresis). Seizures commonly manifest as chewing-gum seizures (vigorous repetitive opening and closing of the mouth) but can be generalized. Hyperesthesia attributable to viral meningitis is uncommon. Myoclonus (rhythmic twitching of the head, neck, or one or more limbs) occurs as the disease progresses and is very suggestive of canine distemper (see *Video*). Optic neuritis and chorioretinitis can be observed.
- Systemic and neurologic signs are not always present at the same time. Often, neurologic disease occurs 1-3 weeks after recovery from systemic signs, but the two forms can coincide. Rarely, the neurologic signs will occur weeks to months later.

Etiology and Pathophysiology

- Certain strains of CDV are more virulent and neurotropic.
- Shedding of the virus begins by the seventh day after infection and may continue for up to 90 days.
- Shedding is primarily aerosol; the virus can also be recovered from urine, feces, nasal and ocular secretions, and skin.
- After initial exposure, CDV replicates in the upper respiratory epithelial tissue macrophages. Macrophages are carried by the local lymphatics to the tonsils and retropharyngeal and bronchial lymph nodes. Here, the virus multiplies and disseminates systemically in mononuclear cells, creating an initial fever and leukopenia 3-6 days after exposure. Lymphopenia is associated with viral damage to T and B lymphocytes.
- Viremia occurs by the ninth day after infection as the virus spreads hematogenously to epithelial tissues and the CNS. Occurrence of viremia depends on host humoral and cell-mediated immunity. Infection of epithelial tissue correlates with shedding of the virus and occurs through all epithelial secretions, even in animals with subclinical infections.
    - Dogs with adequate humoral and cell-mediated immunity clear the virus by day 14.
    - Dogs with an intermediate level of immunity have infection of epithelial tissues by day 14. Clinical signs that develop eventually resolve if the antibody titer increases and the virus is cleared from most tissues. Some virus may persist in footpads and CNS.
    - In dogs with poor immunity, virus spreads to many tissues by day 14, including skin, endocrine glands, exocrine glands, and epithelial cells of the GI tract, the respiratory system, and the genitourinary tract.
- Clinical signs are often severe. Secondary bacterial infections are common; although this advances morbidity, studies indicate it does not increase mortality.

- CNS infection occurs hematogenously through infected mononuclear cells that cross the blood-brain barrier or anterograde through the olfactory nerve. CDV enters the CNS through meningeal perivascular spaces, choroid plexus, and ventricular ependymal cells. Acute CDV encephalomyelitis occurs early in the course of the disease of young and immune-deficient dogs, causing a polioencephalomyelitis.
- Full recovery from CDV illness in young animals is uncommon but likely produces lifelong immunity.
- Transplacental infections can result in abortions or stillbirths. Puppies that survive transplacental infections can develop neurologic signs by 6 weeks of age and often have lifelong immunodeficiency.
- Some dogs will continue to shed the virus for up to 2 months after infection.

DIAGNOSIS

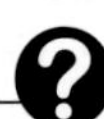

Diagnostic Overview

A presumptive diagnosis in a young, unvaccinated dog is based on presentation of clinical signs that include oculonasal discharge, vomiting, and/or diarrhea with or without a recent onset of neurologic signs. Older dogs can initially present with signs consistent with infectious tracheobronchitis. Clinical confirmation typically comes from a blood sample submitted for immunofluorescent antibody testing of white blood cells or anti-CDV antibody titers in cerebrospinal fluid (CSF).

Differential Diagnosis

- Canine infectious tracheobronchitis
- Canine parvoviral enteritis
- Other CNS diseases of young to middle-aged dogs

Initial Database

- CBC: absolute lymphopenia; rarely, CDV inclusions are identified in lymphocytes, monocytes, neutrophils, or erythrocytes
- Serum biochemistry profile and urinalysis: varies and nonspecific
- Thoracic radiographs: interstitial pattern in early phases; evidence of bronchopneumonia in later stages with secondary bacterial infection

Advanced or Confirmatory Testing

- Serum antibody testing: elevated serum immunoglobulin M (IgM) titers in unvaccinated dogs confirm recent exposure or current infection (p. 1321).
- CSF (pp. 1080 and 1323)
    - Elevated CSF protein and lymphocytic pleocytosis are typical.
    - Presence of CSF antibody titers to CDV is confirmatory when there is no blood contamination of the sample.
    - With potential blood contamination of the CSF sample, paired samples of CSF and serum are tested for CDV and canine parvovirus (CPV) antibody titers; because CPV does not cross the blood-brain barrier, a CDV/CPV ratio that is higher in CSF than in blood suggests CDV infection.
    - Severely immunosuppressed patients or those with the noninflammatory demyelinating form of CDV may have normal CSF, often with low CSF protein (<5 mg/dL).
- Fluorescent antibody testing
    - Cytologic smears from buffy coat, tonsillar or conjunctival epithelial scrapings, CSF, bone marrow, urine sediment
    - More rewarding on conjunctival scrapings early in course of the disease
- Polymerase chain reaction (PCR) test for CDV: whole blood, serum, CSF
- Airway lavage (p. 1073) for cytology and for culture and susceptibility of secondary bacterial pathogens if indicated by worsening pneumonia.
- Postmortem testing: immunofluorescent techniques for frozen samples of tonsils, lymph nodes, GI epithelium, spleen, urinary bladder, brain

TREATMENT

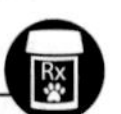

Treatment Overview

Treatment includes supportive care, antibiotics to control secondary bacterial infection, and anticonvulsants to control seizures. There is no medication to eradicate the virus. Suspected or confirmed cases must be kept in isolation to prevent spread of this highly contagious virus.

Acute General Treatment

- Broad-spectrum antibiotics (parenterally initially) such as ampicillin 22 mg/kg IV q 8h or other parenteral antibiotic therapy for secondary bacterial infections
- Nebulization and coupage if pneumonia is apparent radiographically
- Antiemetics (e.g., maropitant 1 mg/kg SQ or 2 mg/kg PO q 24h; dolasetron 0.3-0.6 mg/kg IV or SQ q 12-24h; or metoclopramide 0.2-0.4 mg/kg SQ q 8h), antidiarrheals (e.g., loperamide 0.1-0.2 mg/kg PO up to q 8h), and GI protectants (e.g., omeprazole 1.0 mg/kg PO q 24h) as needed.
- IV fluid resuscitation to correct dehydration and electrolyte disturbances
- Diazepam or midazolam 0.5 mg/kg IV or 1 mg/kg per rectum prn up to four times in 2 hours if acute seizure control is needed
    - Levetiracetam injectable 30 mg/kg q 8h if necessary for continued seizure control

Chronic Treatment

- Anticonvulsant therapy (levetiracetam 30 mg/kg PO q 8h or phenobarbital 2-4 mg/kg PO q 12h) for seizure control. Sodium valproate 60-100 mg/kg PO q 8h can be considered in early stages of myoclonus but is ineffective in later stages.
- The use of glucocorticoids is controversial. Antiinflammatory doses are considered useful to combat optic neuritis. Immune-suppressive doses are sometimes advocated for acute inflammatory CDV encephalitis in older dogs without systemic disease. Glucocorticoids are advocated in the treatment of ODE and vaccine-induced CDV, tapered to the lowest effective dose. They are *contraindicated* for systemic disease with mucosal (respiratory, ocular, GI) signs and any evidence of secondary bacterial infections or if CSF analysis shows no signs of inflammation and very low total protein (≤5 mg/dL).

Possible Complications

- Recovery from systemic signs of the disease may precede development of neurologic signs weeks to months later.
- A possible link has been noted between rheumatoid arthritis and CDV.

PROGNOSIS & OUTCOME

- Development of CNS signs is the most important negative prognostic factor.
- Dogs with adequate immunity do not develop clinical signs and clear the virus within 14 days after infection. The incidence of late-onset CNS signs in these dogs is low.
- Dogs with inadequate immunity develop mild to severe systemic signs and frequently develop CNS signs.

PEARLS & CONSIDERATIONS

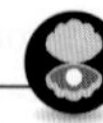

Comments

- CDV has a worldwide distribution and most commonly affects puppies and young, unvaccinated adults.
- Unvaccinated puppies exposed to an infected dog in the waiting room of a veterinary hospital should be vaccinated at that time and usually develop sufficient immunity before the virulent virus produces systemic signs.
- Weimaraners may have an unusual susceptibility to vaccination (see below).

Prevention

- Routine vaccination with a modified live canine distemper (ML-CDV) vaccine is indicated in puppies (every 3-4 weeks, beginning at 6 weeks and ending at 16 weeks). A booster vaccine is given 1 year later and then periodically (every 3 years).
- Vaccination usually confers adequate immunity. Immunocompromised dogs or dogs exposed to a large amount of a highly virulent CDV strain can still develop disease.
- Serum titers correlate well with level of protection and a titer of ≥ 32 has been considered protective (may vary among laboratories and from one individual to the next).
- Vaccine-induced infections are rare and produce only CNS signs.
- Complications from the vaccine are rare but can include hypertrophic osteodystrophy (HOD) and juvenile cellulitis. Clinical signs usually develop within 10 days of vaccination

(range, 4-21 days) and have been associated with all ML-CDV vaccine strains.
- Weimaraners are the most frequently affected breed, and some evidence suggests there are familial tendencies. A glucocorticoid-responsive neutrophilic meningitis/arteritis has also been described in this breed in association with ML-CDV vaccination. The use of a recombinant CDV vaccine in young Weimaraners instead of ML-CDV is suggested. Additional vaccinations in Weimaraners after 1 year of age have not shown the same problems.
- Recombinant CDV vaccines are currently available and have shown efficacy comparable to ML-CDV vaccines.

Technician Tips

- Affected dogs should be isolated from other hospitalized patients, and gowns and gloves should be worn by personnel when handling these patients to prevent transmission of disease to other dogs.
- Transmission by fomites can be devastating; be sure that nebulization equipment and other objects are thoroughly disinfected before and after each use.
- In the environment, CDV is very sensitive to UV light, heat, and drying.

Client Education

- Vaccination of young dogs is essential.
- Dogs with CDV infections that survive should be isolated from healthy dogs for at least 2 weeks after cessation of signs. Some dogs will continue to shed the virus for up to 2 months after infection.

SUGGESTED READING

Greene CE, et al: Canine distemper. In Greene CE, editor: Infectious diseases of the dog and cat, ed 4, St. Louis, 2012, Saunders, pp 25-42.

AUTHOR: Andy Shores, DVM, MS, PhD, DACVIM
EDITOR: Joseph Taboada, DVM, DACVIM

Distichiasis/Ectopic Cilia/Trichiasis

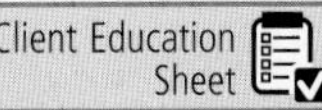

BASIC INFORMATION

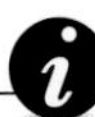

Definition

- Distichiasis: abnormal cilia emerging from the meibomian gland openings on the eyelid margins of the upper and lower eyelids.
- Ectopic cilia: aberrant individual cilia that arise from the meibomian glands and grow through the palpebral conjunctiva toward the cornea.
- Trichiasis: cilia or hairs that arise from normal facial/eyelid skin that are directed toward the conjunctiva/cornea.

Synonyms

Aberrant cilia, abnormal eyelashes

Epidemiology

SPECIES, AGE, SEX

- Common in dogs, rare in cats
- Can occur at any age, but most often in young dogs

GENETICS, BREED PREDISPOSITION

- Distichiasis: seen in many breeds of dogs, especially shih tzus, poodles, golden retrievers, cocker spaniels, and English bulldogs
- Ectopic cilia: any breed is susceptible but common in boxers and shih tzus
- Trichiasis
  - Congenital condition seen in English cocker spaniels and in brachycephalic small breeds with prominent nasal folds (e.g., Pekingese, pug) and eyelid coloboma (agenesis)
  - Acquired condition seen in breeds with redundant dorsal skin folds (English bulldogs, Shar-pei, chow chow, bloodhound, Saint Bernard)
  - Medial canthal trichiasis: trichiasis of the caruncle is common in brachycephalic breeds

RISK FACTORS

Conformation:
- Brachycephalic: nasal folds
- Redundant dorsal skin folds

ASSOCIATED DISORDERS

- Conjunctivitis
- Ulcerative keratitis (p. 209)
- Nonulcerative keratitis (pp. 206 and 212)

Clinical Presentation

HISTORY, CHIEF COMPLAINT

Distichiasis:
- Generally does not produce clinical signs unless hairs are coarse or numerous
- Epiphora and blepharospasm are seen if ocular irritation is present.

Ectopic cilia:
- Acute signs of severe blepharospasm and epiphora
- Superficial corneal ulceration usually just dorsal to axial; may be chronic, acute, or recurring

Trichiasis:
- Epiphora and blepharospasm

PHYSICAL EXAM FINDINGS

Distichiasis:
- Single to multiple cilia along the upper/lower eyelid margins
- Epiphora, mild conjunctivitis, and nonulcerative keratitis are observed if cilia are causing mild ocular irritation; blepharospasm, ulcerative keratitis, +/− entropion (secondary/spastic) in severe cases.

Ectopic cilia:
- Commonly observed at the 12-o'clock position (center upper eyelid)
- Observed emanating through the palpebral conjunctiva 4-6 mm caudal to the eyelid margin
- Acute blepharospasm and epiphora are typical.
- Ulcerative keratitis often presents as an oval that follows the path of eyelid movement.

Trichiasis:
- Congenital: cilia or hair that contacts the cornea; often located on the medial third of the lower eyelid
- Medial canthal: hairs are identified at the medial eyelid margin and within the caruncle, which is aberrant dermis at the canthus; corneal pigmentation is often present on the nasal cornea
- Trichiasis is a common finding associated with agenesis of the lateral two-thirds of the upper eyelid in cats.
  - Signs of ocular irritation, such as epiphora and blepharospasm, if mild
  - Keratitis (ulcerative and nonulcerative) if severe

Etiology and Pathophysiology

- Meibomian glands may spontaneously develop distichiasis or ectopic cilia if the glands become metaplastic.
- Distichiasis
  - Originates from metaplastic meibomian glands and develop secondary to chronic inflammation (meibomitis), emerging through meibomian gland openings located along the lid margin.
  - May or may not contact corneal surface
- Ectopic cilia
  - Originate from metaplastic meibomian glands, emerging through the palpebral conjunctiva of the upper eyelid
  - Always contact the corneal surface
  - Can occur at any age of the pet's life
- Trichiasis
  - Normal hairs that are abnormally directed toward the corneal surface
  - Congenital trichiasis of the upper eyelid can be bilateral or unilateral.
  - Acquired trichiasis is associated with redundant skin folds that result in ptosis.

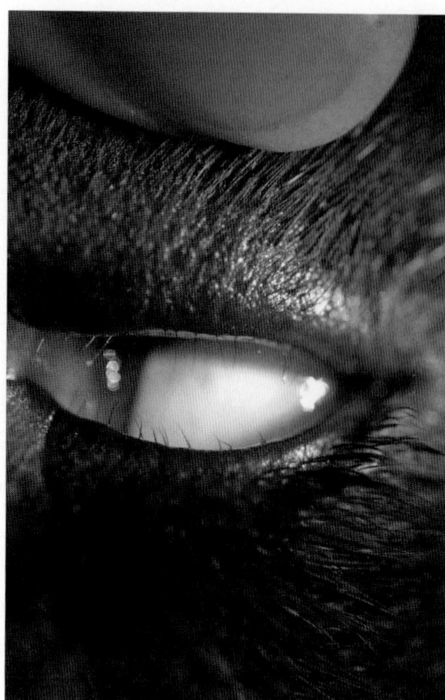

DISTICHIASIS/ECTOPIC CILIA/TRICHIASIS Distichiasis in a dog. Note the numerous long, aberrant hairs along the upper and lower eyelid margins and arising from the meibomian gland ducts. These hairs were an incidental finding, and because they caused no clinical signs, no treatment was warranted.

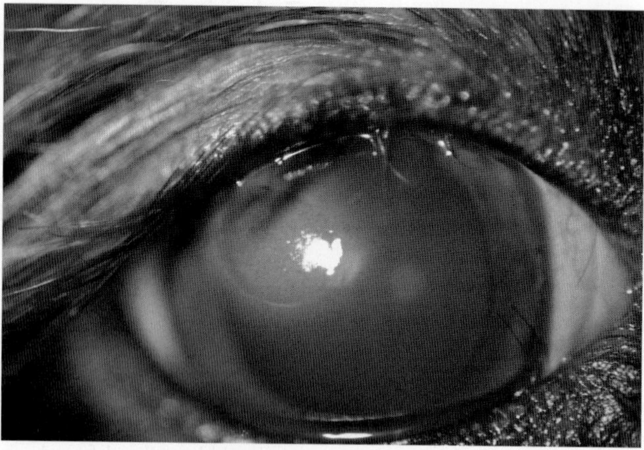

DISTICHIASIS/ECTOPIC CILIA/TRICHIASIS Distichiasis in a dog. Note the clusters of aberrant hairs located along the upper and lower eyelid margins and arising from the meibomian ducts. These hairs were the cause of a superficial corneal ulcer and required surgical removal.

(see Genetics and Breed Predisposition above)
  - Older dogs develop acquired trichiasis secondary to ptosis and entropion that results from loss of muscle tone and orbital fat
  - Trichiasis is most commonly seen with entropion, prominent nasal folds, and medial canthal hairs (eyelids and caruncle).

DIAGNOSIS

Diagnostic Overview

- Distichiasis should be suspected on identifying conjunctivitis or ulcerative and/or nonulcerative keratitis. Distichiae are confirmed when adventitious lashes are observed originating from the meibomian glands (no magnification necessary in most cases).
- Ectopic cilia should be suspected in dogs with acute blepharospasm and epiphora with signs of focal ulcerative and/or nonulcerative keratitis; confirmation requires magnification to identify cilia emerging from the palpebral conjunctiva.
- Trichiasis should be suspected in dogs with conjunctivitis or ulcerative and/or nonulcerative keratitis when normal eyelid/facial hair is directed toward and contacts the conjunctiva or corneal surface.

Differential Diagnosis

- Trichomegaly (excessively long eyelashes)
- Other causes of blepharospasm, including corneal ulceration, conjunctivitis, uveitis, epiphora
- Entropion

Initial Database

Complete ophthalmic exam (p. 1137):

- Schirmer tear test (normal > 15 mm/min in dogs, varies in cats)
- Fluorescein dye application
- Intraocular pressure (normal: 10-20 mm Hg)
- Examination of the eyelid margin and palpebral conjunctiva with magnification and a good light source
- Examination of the cornea

Advanced or Confirmatory Testing

Examination with 5× to 10× magnification is often required to visualize ectopic cilia. Ectopic cilia are often the same color as the haircoat. The conjunctiva may be pigmented adjacent to the cilia or mucus may be trapped by the cilia.

TREATMENT

Treatment Overview

The goals of treatment are to eliminate the ocular irritation to determine whether distichiasis, trichiasis, or ectopic cilia is responsible for the clinical signs of ocular disease and to remove the offending cilia or direct the cilia away from the globe. Distichiasis and/or trichiasis without signs of ocular irritation do not require treatment. Depending on complexity of condition and number of offending hairs or cilia, consider referral to veterinary ophthalmologist.

Acute General Treatment

Distichiasis:

- Usually does not produce clinical signs, and no treatment is required.
- Hairs regrow in 4-5 weeks with mechanical epilation/plucking, but this may be done to determine significance of distichiae in corneal irritation or disease.
- If clinical signs are present, consider treatment (under general anesthesia)
  - Before removal, manual expression of the meibomian glands is attempted; this pushes hidden hairs from the glands.
  - Cryotherapy along the palpebral surface of the meibomian glands using a double freeze/thaw cycle is effective for large numbers of distichiae.
  - Electrolysis is useful for single or low numbers of cilia; tedious procedure with increased risk of tissue damage.
  - Carbon dioxide laser removal is tedious, with increased risk of tissue damage
  - Resection from the conjunctival surface; effective for single or multiple cilia
  - Eyelid splitting techniques: not recommended; risk for postoperative eyelid deformities and regrowth of hairs

Ectopic cilia:

- Usually requires surgical treatment
- En bloc resection of aberrant cilia, including associated conjunctiva and meibomian gland with a scalpel blade or 2-3 mm biopsy punch; allow to heal by second intention
- Surgical removal is usually successful, but new cilia or regrowth is possible.

Trichiasis

- Conservative management may be effective for minor ocular irritation.
  - Clip hairs short to prevent ocular contact.
- Variable surgical therapies, depending on location of trichiasis
  - Medial canthal trichiasis may be corrected by permanent medial canthoplasty (pocket or Wyman techniques) or cryotherapy.
  - Nasal fold trichiasis may require resection of prominent nasal folds.
  - Trichiasis associated with ptosis (drooping upper eyelid) may be corrected by a Stades procedure.
  - Trichiasis associated with eyelid agenesis in cats may be corrected by cryotherapy until kitten is older for permanent surgery (e.g., rotational flap).

Chronic Treatment

For recurrence, repeat treatment may be required.

Possible Complications

- The most common complication for all conditions is recurrence.
- Postoperative eyelid scarring ± entropion

- Repeated cryotherapy can lead to qualitative tear film abnormalities secondary to meibomian gland damage.

Recommended Monitoring

Owners should monitor postoperatively for signs of recurrent ocular irritation, which may indicate regrowth of offending hair(s).

PROGNOSIS & OUTCOME

Generally good prognosis; however, recurrence is possible regardless of treatment.

PEARLS & CONSIDERATIONS

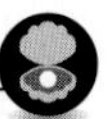

Comments

- Distichiasis and trichiasis are among the most common eyelid abnormalities.
- Goal is not simply to diagnose distichiasis or trichiasis, but to determine whether abnormal hairs are causing ocular irritation. This finding will help determine if treatment is necessary.
- Keratitis in a vertical pattern that follows the path of upper eyelid movement should raise suspicion of an ectopic cilium in the upper eyelid.
- Magnification is needed commonly to identify ectopic cilia. Without magnification, the diagnosis should not be ruled out based on absence of visualization.
- Ectopic cilia and distichiae will regrow in 4-5 weeks with mechanical epilation/plucking.
- No single treatment guarantees permanent resolution of distichiasis, ectopic cilia, or trichiasis.

Prevention

Avoid breeding affected or closely related dogs.

Technician Tips

Distichiasis, ectopic cilia, and/or trichiasis should be considered as a possible cause for every dog that presents with a corneal ulcer. Closely evaluate the eyelid margin (distichiasis), palpebral conjunctiva over the meibomian glands (ectopic cilia), and corneal surface for signs of irritation caused by trichiasis due to entropion, nasal folds, or eyelid coloboma.

Client Education

- Distichiasis or trichiasis does not necessarily require treatment.
- Animals with distichiasis, ectopic cilia, or trichiasis should be monitored for signs of ocular irritation.
- Recurrence is possible regardless of treatment.

SUGGESTED READING

Maggs DJ: The eyelids. In Maggs DJ, editor: Slatter's Fundamentals of veterinary ophthalmology, ed 5, St. Louis, 2013, Elsevier.

RELATED CLIENT EDUCATION SHEETS

How to Assemble and Use an Elizabethan Collar

AUTHOR: Shannon D. Boveland, DVM, DACVO
EDITOR: Diane V. H. Hendrix, DVM, DACVO

Drowning

BASIC INFORMATION

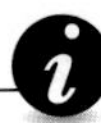

Definition

Potentially fatal disorder characterized by asphyxia and possible progression to dysfunction of multiple organ systems due to submersion in a liquid medium (typically water)

Epidemiology

SPECIES, AGE, SEX

Dogs and cats of either sex and any age; cats rarely venture into water but could accidentally fall into water or could be drowned maliciously.

GENETICS, BREED PREDISPOSITION

Some dogs are innately better swimmers (e.g., retrievers compared to bulldogs), which may improve their ability to swim to safety but may also increase the risk of venturing into unsafe waters.

RISK FACTORS

- Pre-existing disorders (orthopedic injury, neurologic dysfunction, visual deficits, respiratory abnormality) can predispose an animal to fall into water or become submerged.
- Lack of adequate supervision: similar to small children, dogs should be supervised when swimming or near access to water.

GEOGRAPHY AND SEASONALITY

Late autumn and early spring, when ponds and lakes begin to freeze: increased risk of falling through the ice

ASSOCIATED DISORDERS

Acute respiratory distress syndrome (ARDS [p. 27])
Water intoxication
Hypernatremia, if accompanied by salt water ingestion (p. 498)

Clinical Presentation

DISEASE FORMS/SUBTYPES

Aspiration of fresh versus salt water

HISTORY, CHIEF COMPLAINT

There is almost always a known submersion incident. If possible, it is helpful to obtain information regarding factors with potential prognostic importance (extrapolated from human medicine):

- Circumstances surrounding submersion (severe internal injuries worsen prognosis)
- Duration of submersion (prognosis worsens with increased time)
- Tonicity and temperature of the water (prognosis better with fresh/ice water)
- Apnea after rescue (prognosis better with spontaneous breathing)
- Immediate neurologic condition after rescue (prognosis worse with poor condition)

PHYSICAL EXAM FINDINGS

Depends on severity but may include wet fur, collapse, dyspnea, tachypnea, tachycardia, bradycardia, cyanosis, hypoperfusion, hypothermia, increased bronchovesicular breath sounds, or cardiac or respiratory arrest.

Etiology and Pathophysiology

- Pulmonary, fresh water: affects the surface-tension properties of pulmonary surfactant (surfactant washout), leading to alveolar instability, the possibility of noncardiogenic pulmonary edema, and altered ventilation/perfusion ratio. Because of the hypotonicity of fresh water, aspirated fluid is generally quickly absorbed into the circulation. If enough fluid is absorbed, hyponatremia causes hemolysis and altered mentation (p. 518).
- Pulmonary, salt water: elicits fluid influx into the pulmonary parenchyma (osmotic gradient) and alveolar flooding; fluid volume shift may be great enough to cause hypovolemia.
- Cardiovascular effects: elevated systemic and pulmonary vascular resistance, cardiac arrhythmias, and cardiac arrest are primarily due to hypoxemia. In humans, they are positively related to the length of anoxic insult and negatively related to the effects of hypothermia and effectiveness of resuscitation.
- Hepatocellular: hepatic ischemia (hypoxemia, hypoperfusion) causes direct hepatic injury and lobar necrosis.
- Hematologic: hypoxemia, vascular stasis, and acid-base disturbances predispose animals to development of disseminated intravascular coagulation.
- Acute kidney injury: renal hypoxia contributes to tubular cell death.

- Neurologic effects: ischemia leads to an elevation in extracellular central nervous system tissue glutamate concentration, which is thought to be directly related to neuronal damage. Cerebral ischemia and hypoxia can lead to irreversible neurologic dysfunction.
- About 90% of drowning victims aspirate fluid into the lungs; in 10%, drowning is associated with laryngospasm and inhalation against a closed glottis, causing noncardiogenic pulmonary edema without aspiration of water.

DIAGNOSIS

Diagnostic Overview

Known history of recent submersion is generally sufficient to make the diagnosis.

Differential Diagnosis

In the absence of witnessed drowning, other causes of acute respiratory distress should be considered, including pulmonary contusions, pneumonia, and pulmonary edema.

Initial Database

- Arterial blood gas analysis (p. 1058); hypoxemia variable with degree of aspiration/noncardiogenic pulmonary edema; metabolic acidosis possible and appears detrimental to prognosis
- Pulse oximetry: low SpO_2
- Electrocardiogram (p. 1096): ventricular arrhythmias possible
- CBC, serum biochemistry profile, urinalysis: increased liver enzymes, possibly hypoproteinemia, hyper/hyponatremia, azotemia
- Thoracic radiographs (pulmonary infiltrates of various locations and types)
- Blood pressure (monitor for hypotension [p. 1065])

Advanced or Confirmatory Testing

Bronchoalveolar lavage (p. 1073) or transtracheal wash if warranted by clinical suspicion of pulmonary infection; not required for diagnosis of drowning

TREATMENT

Treatment Overview

- Improve ventilation (goal: $PaCO_2$ = 30-40 mm Hg or less).
- Ensure adequate blood oxygen saturation (SpO_2 > 95%, PaO_2 > 80 mm Hg).
- Maintain appropriate intravascular volume and tissue perfusion (*mean* arterial blood pressure > 60-80 mm Hg, central venous pressure = 2-5 cm H_2O, urine production > 1-2 mL/kg/h).
- Correct electrolyte imbalances or severe acidosis (e.g., if pH < 7.1).
- Referral for therapeutic ventilation may be warranted early in the course of disease and should be considered for animals with severe respiratory distress (SpO_2 < 92%, PaO_2 < 80 mm Hg) despite oxygen supplementation.

Acute General Treatment

- Regain spontaneous ventilation and circulation (p. 1077).
- Oxygen supplementation (p. 1146)
- IV fluid administration as indicated to support blood pressure and urine output
- Mechanical ventilation with positive end-expiratory pressure as indicated (p. 1185)
- Abdominal thrust or gravitational drainage offers *no* advantage and may increase complications such as regurgitation and aspiration and delaying adequate treatment.
- Antibiotic therapy is not indicated unless clinical and radiographic evidence of pulmonary infection. Ongoing antibiotic use should be based on culture and sensitivity results.
- Glucocorticoid therapy was once suggested but has failed to demonstrate any therapeutic advantage in large studies and may predispose patients to infection.

Possible Complications

- In addition to being risk factors that led to the incident, pre-existing problems such as respiratory disease, heart disease, and seizure disorders may complicate resuscitation.
- Infrequently, grossly contaminated water can cause lower airway obstruction (particulate matter) or pulmonary infection.
- Uncommonly, renal function can become compromised due to decreased renal perfusion, hypoxemia, or severe hemoglobinuria.
- Cerebral hypoxia, cerebral hypoperfusion, or carbon dioxide narcosis can cause varying degrees of neurologic impairment but are rarely permanent.

Recommended Monitoring

- Thoracic auscultation, respiratory rate and effort
- Arterial or venous blood gas analysis
- Urine output
- Serial neurologic evaluation and modified Glasgow coma score designation (p. 404)
- Hematocrit, electrolyte concentrations
- Electrocardiogram

PROGNOSIS & OUTCOME

- Most near-drowning animals are markedly improved within 24 hours. Failure to rapidly improve is associated with a grave prognosis, as is persistent hypoxemia.
- By extrapolation from human medicine, the need for cardiopulmonary resuscitation on presentation, blood pH < 7.0, and apnea or coma are poor prognostic indicators.
- Similar to human beings, submersion for > 25 minutes, resuscitation for > 25 minutes, cardiac arrest at time of presentation, and lack of return of purposeful movements within 24 hours of the incident are associated with severe neurologic deficits or death.

PEARLS & CONSIDERATIONS

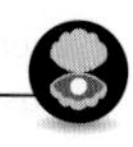

Comments

Abdominal thrust and gravitational pull (suspended upside down) offer no benefits and may increase complications.

Prevention

- Outdoor supervision
- Avoidance of swimming by dogs with disorders causing episodic lack of control (seizures, syncope) or dogs with permanent tracheostomies
- Some surgeons advise limiting swimming by retrievers after arytenoid lateralization surgery due to increased risk of aspirating.
- Precautionary poolside safety measures such as pool covers and gated pool areas
- Boating safety measures: flotation devices; keeping animals in boat cabin, on boat floor, or away from railings
- Avoid semifrozen lakes, ponds, or rivers.

Technician Tips

- Early placement of an arterial catheter allows rapid, accurate, serial interpretation of pulmonary gas exchange. Intermittent SpO_2 measurement requires the oxygen cage to be open for longer periods, can be difficult to interpret in a panting animal, and does not give information pertaining to changes in acid-base status or PCO_2.
- A urinary catheter and closed collection set allows frequent, accurate calculation of urine output and may aid in nursing care.
- Many dogs presented on emergency for drowning have pre-existing visual, neurologic, musculoskeletal, or other deficits that predisposed them to the incident. It is important to be aware of these pre-existing deficits when monitoring recovery to avoid misinterpreting the long-standing condition as a complication of drowning.

SUGGESTED READING

Goldcamp CE: Canine drowning. Compend Contin Educ Vet 30(6):340-352, 2008.

AUTHOR: Geoff Heffner, DVM, DACVECC
EDITOR: Benjamin M. Brainard, VMD, DACVAA, DACVECC

Dysphagia

Client Education Sheet

BASIC INFORMATION

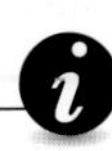

Definition

Difficulty swallowing

Synonyms

Oral, pharyngeal, and esophageal dysphagia; regurgitation

Epidemiology

SPECIES, AGE, SEX

- Dogs > cats
- Congenital abnormalities: young animals (onset often at birth or weaning)
- Acquired abnormalities: middle-aged or older animals

GENETICS, BREED PREDISPOSITION

Depends on underlying disease process:

- Oral dysphagia: severe periodontal disease (anecdotally more common in small-breed dogs), trigeminal neuritis (golden retrievers), stomatitis (cats)
- Pharyngeal dysphagia: cricopharyngeal achalasia (golden retrievers, cocker and springer spaniels, toy breeds)
- Esophageal dysphagia: regurgitation (p. 873), hiatal hernia (brachycephalic breeds, Chinese Shar-pei)

RISK FACTORS

- Reflux (gastroesophageal and/or extraesophageal reflux)
- Dietary indiscretion
- Feline immunodeficiency virus (FIV), feline leukemia virus (FeLV)
- Myasthenia gravis (MG)
- Megaesophagus
- Periodontal disease
- Recent anesthesia
- Neuropathy/myopathy
- Endocrine disease: hypoadrenocortisolism, hypothyroidism
- Sialocele
- Lymphadenopathy
- Central nervous system (CNS) disorders, cranial nerve deficits
- Rabies
- Toxicity: tetanus, botulism, lead, thallium
- Dysautonomia
- Brachycephalic airway syndrome

CONTAGION AND ZOONOSIS

Rabies in animals with unknown vaccination history

ASSOCIATED DISORDERS

- Aspiration pneumonia (p. 793)
- Weight loss/cachexia
- Dehydration
- Halitosis
- Ptyalism (p. 833)

Clinical Presentation

DISEASE FORMS/SUBTYPES

Disease variants:

- Anatomic location: oral, pharyngeal, or esophageal dysphagia; a large number of dogs may have abnormalities in more than one location
- Cause: obstruction (mechanical or functional) or pain

HISTORY, CHIEF COMPLAINT

- Varies with underlying cause and location of defect
- Presenting complaints may include weight loss, regurgitation, coughing, gagging, halitosis, and ptyalism.
- Ravenous appetite or anorexia may be reported.
- Clients often mistake regurgitation for vomiting, warranting careful questioning.

PHYSICAL EXAM FINDINGS

General:

- Weight loss/poor body condition
- Increased respiratory effort, tachypnea, and cough may be appreciated with aspiration.

Specific physical examination findings depend on localization, severity, and underlying cause:

- Oral dysphagia: difficulty with mastication, bolus formation, or prehension
  - Clinical observations: dropping food, chewing on one side of the mouth, ptyalism, halitosis, signs consistent with cranial nerve (CN) dysfunction (V, VII, IX, XII)
  - Oral disease may be obvious (e.g., severe dental or periodontal disease, mass).
- Pharyngeal dysphagia: inability to propel the food bolus from the base of the tongue through the upper esophageal sphincter.
  - Clinical observations: exaggerated/repetitive swallows, gagging, ptyalism, halitosis, signs consistent with CN dysfunction (V, IX, X, XI)
- Esophageal dysphagia: regurgitation (p. 873) is the hallmark feature of esophageal dysphagia.
  - Clinical observation: esophageal bulge, regurgitation, halitosis, ptyalism, signs consistent with CN X or diffuse autonomic dysfunction

Etiology and Pathophysiology

- Dysphagia may occur secondary to pain or functional or mechanical defect of any of the three swallow phases (oral, pharyngeal, esophageal).
- Oral
  - Mechanical: oral masses (neoplasia, abscess, granuloma), foreign body (FB), lymphadenopathy, sialocele, hematoma, cleft palate, facial/oral trauma
  - Functional: depressed consciousness, CN deficits (V, VII, IX, XII), trigeminal neuritis, masticatory muscle myositis
  - Pain: pain secondary to periodontal disease, retrobulbar abscess, trauma, stomatitis, or temporomandibular joint (TMJ) disease
- Pharyngeal
  - Mechanical: pharyngeal masses (neoplasia, abscess, granuloma, tonsillar enlargement), FB, pharyngeal swelling, cricopharyngeal achalasia
  - Functional: CN deficits (V, IX, X, XI), cricopharyngeal asynchrony, rabies, CNS (brainstem) disease, MG, toxicity (botulism, tetanus), polymyositis, polyneuritis
  - Pain: pharyngitis, stomatitis
- Esophageal (p. 873)

DIAGNOSIS

Diagnostic Overview

Dysphagia describes any defect in the swallow mechanism and is therefore nonspecific. A combination of signalment, clinical course, observation during feeding, and physical exam findings can help localize the lesion. Specific testing can be tailored as appropriate.

Differential Diagnosis

- Vomiting
- Regurgitation (p. 873)
- Expectoration
- Ptyalism

Initial Database

- Oral/oropharyngeal examination (may require sedation [pp. 1125 and 1140])
- CBC/serum biochemical profile/urinalysis: usually nonspecific changes; inflammatory leukogram may be seen with aspiration pneumonia, changes consistent with endocrine disorders (hypoadrenocortisolism, hypothyroidism), increased creatine kinase with diffuse myositis
- Radiographs (dental, cervical, thoracic): a minimum of three thoracic radiographic views is recommended to assess concurrent aspiration pneumonia. Abdominal compression may be applied to evaluate for sliding hiatal hernia.

Advanced or Confirmatory Testing

- Videofluoroscopic swallow study (VFSS): necessary for the characterization of pharyngeal and esophageal dysfunction.
- Manometry: characterization of esophageal dysfunction (not widely available)
- ACTH stimulation test (hypoadrenocortisolism [p. 512])
- Thyroid function testing (hypothyroidism [p. 525])

- Acetylcholine receptor antibody testing (MG [p. 668])
- Type 2M muscle antibody serology (masticatory muscle myositis [p. 637])
- Electromyography to assess for neuromuscular disorders
- Muscle and nerve biopsies
- MRI (p. 1132), CT
- Cerebrospinal fluid analysis (CSF [pp. 1080 and 1323])

TREATMENT

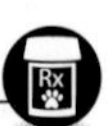

Treatment Overview

- Treatment is location and disease specific.
- Maintain good body condition with adequate caloric intake and minimizing risk of aspiration pneumonia through appropriate feeding practices.

Acute General Treatment

Patients may present in acute crisis secondary to aspiration pneumonia (p. 793).

Nutrition/Diet

- Ensure adequate nutrition; if oral feeding is inadequate esophagostomy or gastrostomy tubes may be considered (pp. 1106 and 1109).
- There is no ideal dietary consistency. Controlled trials with food items of different consistencies are recommended on a case-by-case basis.
- Upright feeding may benefit animals with esophageal dysphagia (p. 642).

Possible Complications

Aspiration pneumonia, weight loss

Recommended Monitoring

- Body weight/condition
- Hydration status
- Respiratory rates to monitor for possible aspiration events
- Frequent thoracic radiographs of asymptomatic animals are not recommended.

PROGNOSIS & OUTCOME

Prognosis depends on the underlying disease process. Long-term prognosis is poor for those who cannot maintain body condition or those with recurrent aspiration events.

PEARLS & CONSIDERATIONS

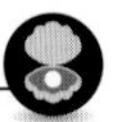

Comments

Dysphagia is a nonspecific descriptor for a number of different disease processes. Localizing/identifying the underlying disease process is critical for determining further diagnostics and treatment.

Technician Tips

Animals with dysphagia are at risk for aspiration events. Force feeding should be avoided.

Client Education

Clients should be instructed to monitor respiratory rates at home as well as to monitor for weight loss in patients with dysphagia.

SUGGESTED READING

Pollard R: Imaging evaluation of dogs and cats with dysphagia. ISRN Vet Sci 2012. https://www.hindawi.com/journals/isrn/2012/238505/.

AUTHOR: Megan Grobman, DVM, MS, DACVIM
EDITOR: Leah A. Cohn, DVM, PhD, DACVIM

Dystocia

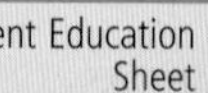

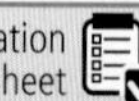

Client Education Sheet

BASIC INFORMATION

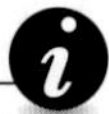

Definition

Difficulty giving birth by vaginal delivery, resulting in morbidity or mortality for the dam, fetus, or neonate

Epidemiology

SPECIES, AGE, SEX

Dogs > cats; older > younger

GENETICS, BREED PREDISPOSITION

- Higher incidence in brachycephalic and hydrocephalic breeds
- Some purebred lines and service dog colonies have a higher than breed average incidence of dystocia, suggesting heritability.
- Breed, parity (number of previous litters), and litter size can influence gestational length by no more than 1-2 days. Fetal overgrowth can result from prolonged gestation. Large litters tend to have shorter gestations.

RISK FACTORS

- Large litters (secondary uterine inertia)
- Poor prepartum condition of the dam
- Obese dam
- Small litters with resultant oversized fetuses
- Breed conformation, metabolic abnormalities (pregnancy diabetes, pregnancy toxemia, pre-eclampsia), vaginal canal abnormalities (undetected strictures, vaginal hyperplasia, vulvar edema), pelvic abnormalities (healed fractures with reduction in pelvic canal), and abdominal wall defects (hernias) can predispose a dam to dystocia.
- A previous uncomplicated cesarean section does not predispose a bitch to dystocia.

ASSOCIATED DISORDERS

Hypocalcemia, hypoglycemia, hypovolemia, systemic inflammatory reaction, sepsis, postpartum metritis, fading puppy/kitten syndrome

Clinical Presentation

DISEASE FORMS/SUBTYPES

Dystocia can be categorized as resulting from maternal causes or fetal causes, but it most commonly results from a combination of both.

HISTORY, CHIEF COMPLAINT

A client's perception that labor is not initiated or progressing as expected, most commonly due to the following:

- Failure of labor to begin at perceived due date
- Excessive time between stages of labor. Stage I labor normally lasts no more than 12-24 hours; stage II, 8 hours (depending on litter size); and stage III, 12-24 hours.
- Time between sequential deliveries of neonates: normally, deliveries should be within 1 hour of one another.
- Stillbirths or weak neonates should prompt evaluation for dystocia.

The clinician must quickly obtain a careful reproductive history:

- Gestational length (canine) is determined by previous ovulation timing (day of LH surge or the initial rise in progesterone is day 0; normal gestation is 64-66 days). The first day of diestrus (the first-day vaginal cytology is < 50% superficial cells) is 56-58 days before normal parturition. If no ovulation timing was performed, establishing the first day of behavioral diestrus (refusing the male) can approximate the first day of diestrus. Breeding dates (58-72 days before delivery) are not specific and do not correlate closely with gestational length. See alternative ultrasonographic methods for determining whether pregnancy is term (below).
- For the queen, the mean gestation is 65-66 days from a breeding with adequate coital contact to cause the LH surge.
- Previous eutocia or dystocia
- General medical history, including diet and medications/supplements and what, if any, therapeutics have already been administered for dystocia

PHYSICAL EXAM FINDINGS

- Physical exam may be unremarkable; normal physical exam findings do not rule out dystocia.
- Typically, dams in stage I labor (uterine contractions) or stage II labor (uterine and abdominal contractions) are euthermic, mildly agitated, trembling, mildly hyperpneic, and nesting. Mild hypothermia associated with luteolysis at term can be prodromal to labor.
- Abnormal physical findings include moderate to severe pain, atypical vulvar discharge (green, malodorous, frankly hemorrhagic), a fetus or fetal membranes remaining in the birth canal (i.e., presence of a fetus caudal to the cervix, which may be palpable over the brim of the pelvis or may be partially protruding out of the vulva), muscle tremors, tetany, fatigue/weakness, persistent vomiting, and protracted tenesmus (abdominal efforts).
  - Uteroverdin (green vaginal discharge) indicates placental separation and underscores the need for veterinary medical or surgical intervention if fetal delivery is not prompt.
  - Malodorous discharge suggests fetal death and necrosis or metritis.
  - Inappropriately voluminous hemorrhage should prompt evaluation for uterine or vaginal trauma (torsion, tear) requiring surgical exploration or abnormal placental site coagulation (coagulopathy).
- Protracted muscle tremors, tetany, repeated vomiting, or marked fatigue suggest metabolic abnormalities (hypoglycemia, hypocalcemia, ketosis) or exhaustion.
- Protracted tenesmus suggests an obstruction or uterine inertia.

Etiology and Pathophysiology

Normal labor proceeds through three stages:

- Stage I labor begins with the progressive increase in the frequency and strength of myometrial contractions. Typically, luteolysis (progesterone < 2 ng/mL) and the associated temperature drop occur 12-24 hours before stage I labor begins.
- Stage II labor begins when abdominal efforts (tenesmus) coincide with myometrial contractions, resulting in the delivery of a neonate through the birth canal. Strong abdominal contractions do not mean myometrial contractions are present or adequate.
- Stage III labor consists of the delivery of the placenta.
- Dams typically progress through stage I labor in 12-24 hours and then alternate between stages II and III until all fetuses and placentae are delivered. Placentae normally may be delivered with the neonate or separately and often are consumed quickly, making correct counting difficult.

Common causes of dystocia:

- Maternal dystocia: primary (no myometrial contractions occur) or secondary (myometrial contractions falter) uterine inertia, birth canal (strictures) or abdominal wall (hernias) defects, severe vulvar edema, lack of lubrication in the birth canal, uterine torsion or tear, metabolic derangements
- Fetal dystocia: oversized, malformed (anasarca), malpositioned, malpostured fetus
- Combined maternal/fetal dystocia: mismatch of birth canal size versus fetal size
- Cranial and caudal (breech in humans) presentations in dogs and cats are normal.

DIAGNOSIS

Diagnostic Overview

A correct diagnosis of dystocia depends on taking an accurate history and performing an appropriate physical exam in a timely manner.

Differential Diagnosis

- Normal labor; usually stage I
- Misinformation about gestational length (see History, Chief Complaint), in which case, lack of labor is then normal
- Previous ultrasound measurements (days 25-50 of gestation) can be helpful in determining gestational age when ovulation timing data are not available. Ultrasound evaluation of intestinal motility or renal architecture as indicators of term gestation are not accurate in dogs or cats. Radiography of a pregnant bitch at term should show mineralization of fetal dentition.
- Completion of labor, client misinformation about litter size

Initial Database

- Minimally, hematocrit and total protein (mild decreases expected due to hemodilution), blood glucose (decreased with prolonged labor), serum electrolytes, and ionized calcium (hypocalcemia possible with prolonged labor) should be evaluated. Urine can be checked for glucose/ketones (indicating prenatal diabetes or malnourishment).
- Vaginal digital and/or vaginoscopic (p. 1184) exam to determine if a vaginal obstruction exists. In the dog, the cervix (assessing for dilation) and cranial vagina (assessing for obstruction) are beyond the reach of the human finger.
- Abdominal ultrasound or fetal Doppler evaluation to assess fetal viability (normal fetal heart rate > 200 beats/min; stress causes fetal bradycardia).
- Abdominal radiograph to evaluate litter size, relative fetal size, appearance, and position.

Advanced or Confirmatory Testing

- Uterine monitoring (tocodynamometry) to assess presence, strength, and frequency of contractions.
- Canine and feline uterine monitors are available for short- or long-term lease through Veterinary Perinatal Services (www.whelpwise.com).
- Tocodynamometry is the only method of confirming uterine inertia, differentiating primary from secondary inertia, or directly evaluating the quality of uterine contractions and response to medical therapy.

TREATMENT

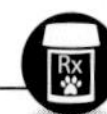

Treatment Overview

Therapeutic goals:

- Facilitate delivery of viable neonates, with minimal morbidity to the dam.
- Avoid unnecessary surgical intervention by timely diagnosis and medical intervention.
- Differentiate cases requiring surgical versus medical intervention. Surgery is warranted if
  - Refractory (unresponsive) uterine inertia
  - Fetal distress and suboptimal response to medical management
  - Intractable pain in bitch or queen
  - Obvious mismatch of fetal-maternal birth canal size
  - Birth canal abnormalities, such as strictures or pelvic stenosis that cannot be remedied

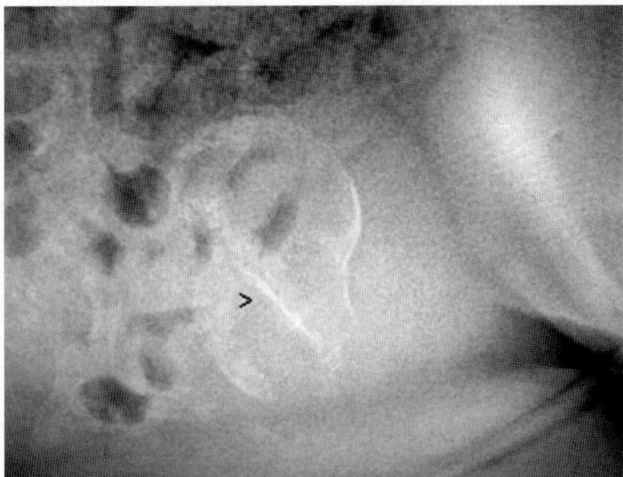

DYSTOCIA Lateral abdominal radiograph shows the skull of term canine fetus. *Arrow* indicates mineralized fetal dentition.

Formulas for Predicting Gestational Age and Days Before Parturition

Gestational Age in Dogs (± 3 Days)*	Gestational Age in Cats (± 2 Days)*
Less Than 40 Days†	
GA = (6 × GSD) + 20	CRL = 0.2423 × GA − 4.2165
GA = (3 × CRL) + 27	
Greater Than 40 Days†	
GA = (15 × HD) + 20	GA = 25 × HD + 3
GA = (7 × BD) + 29	GA = 11 × BD + 21
GA = (6 × HD) + (3 × BD) + 30	
Days Before Parturition‡	
DBP = 65 − GA	DBP = 61 − GA

*Gestational age (GA) is based on days after the luteinizing hormone (LH) surge in the dog and days after breeding in the cat.
†Gestational sac diameter (GSD), crown-rump length (CRL), head diameter (HD), and body diameter (BD) measurements are in centimeters.
‡Number of days before parturition (DBP) is based on 65 ± 1 days after the LH surge in the dog and 61 days after breeding in the cat.
Modified from Nyland TG, et al: Small animal diagnostic ultrasound, ed 2, Philadelphia, 2002, Saunders.

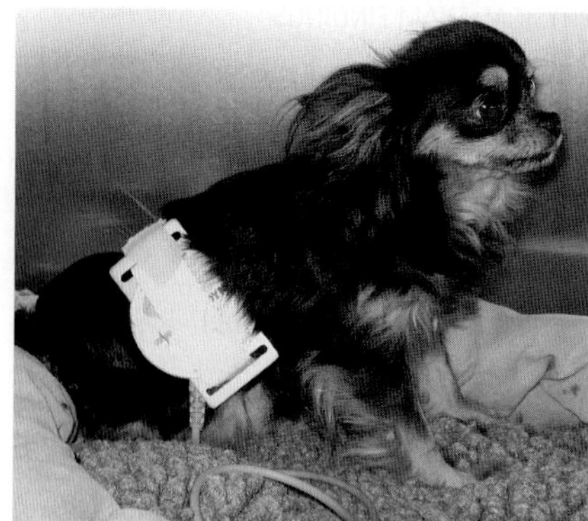
DYSTOCIA Uterine contractions are being recorded from this prepartum bitch using veterinary tocodynamometry.

- Minimize fetal stress; neonatal death (fading puppy/kitten) during the first week of life is related to stress during labor and the immediate postpartum period.
- Avoid fetal or maternal mortality.
- Preserve the reproductive capacity of a valuable dam.
- Ovariohysterectomy at the time of cesarean section is not advised unless indicated by the condition of the uterus (necrotic, hemorrhagic) because surgery/anesthesia is prolonged, hypovolemia is exacerbated, and lactation without estrogen can be problematic.

Acute General Treatment

- Supportive: intravenous (IV) balanced electrolyte solution with 5% dextrose if appropriate (dam is often hypovolemic, dehydrated, or hypoglycemic)
- Evaluate indications for medical therapy (p. 1415).
  - Without tocodynamometry, evaluation of fetal heart rates before and after administration of calcium gluconate and oxytocin is important. Worsening bradycardia dictates surgical intervention.
- Calcium: calcium gluconate 10% solution (≈10 g/100 mL solution, or 0.465 mEq Ca^{2+}/mL)
  - Give first (before oxytocin); even if eucalcemic (see below)
  - Given SQ at 1 mL/4.5 kg (10 lb) body weight as indicated by the strength of uterine contractions, usually not more frequently than every 4-6 hours during the second stage of labor. CAUTION: large volumes of calcium gluconate given subcutaneously may cause local irritation or even skin necrosis; doses > 6 mL should be divided. More concentrated forms of calcium gluconate are not advised.
  - Intravenous use: generally unnecessary unless systemic signs of severe hypocalcemia are present; see Hypocalcemia, (p. 515) for signs of hypocalcemia and intravenous calcium gluconate doses.
  - Although most dams are eucalcemic, the benefit of calcium administration on myometrial contractility is still seen, suggesting a cellular or subcellular effect.
- Oxytocin
  - Give 10-15 minutes after administration of calcium if delivery has not occurred.
  - The administration of oxytocin increases the frequency of uterine contractions, whereas the administration of calcium increases their strength.
  - Oxytocin (10 USP units/mL) is most effective at mini doses: start with 0.25 units/dose SQ or IM to a maximal dose of 4 units per bitch or 1 unit per queen. IV oxytocin is not advised in the bitch or queen.
  - The frequency of oxytocin administration is dictated by the labor pattern, and it is generally not given more frequently than every 30-60 minutes.
  - Uterine contractions compromise placental blood flow and cause fetal hypoxia. Excessive contractions (due to uterine hypertonicity, overdosage of oxytocin, obstruction) can compromise fetal survival. Uterine relaxation between contractions allows normal placental blood flow to resume.
  - Absolute contraindications to oxytocin therapy: fetal obstruction in any part of the uterus or birth canal, uterine torsion, uterine laceration or rupture.
- Persistence of a fetus in the birth canal beyond 5-10 minutes warrants assisted delivery.
  - Placental separation and the potential for fetal hypoxemia are likely.
  - CAUTION: Traction applied to a fetus retained in the birth canal must be very gentle to avoid fetal trauma.
  - Traction is advised only if the veterinarian can position his/her fingers around the fetal shoulders or hips for gentle traction in a downward direction along the plane of the vagina and vestibule.
  - Lubrication delivered by a red rubber catheter and water-soluble lubricant jelly can be helpful.
  - Elevation of the bitch's forequarters can assist in manipulation of the fetus in the birth canal.

Chronic Treatment

Medical therapy for dystocia, based on the administration of calcium gluconate and oxytocin, can be directed and tailored based on the results of tocodynamometry.

Drug Interactions

Calcium is given before oxytocin in most cases, improving contractile strength before increasing frequency of contractions.

Possible Complications

- Hypercalcemia-induced arrhythmias can result if calcium gluconate is given intravenously at too rapid a rate.
- Fetal hypoxia secondary to placental compression during uterine contractions induced by parenteral oxytocin administration, particularly if given inappropriately (e.g., too early in labor, when fetal obstruction is present, if uterine torsion is present, too frequently) or at excessive doses
- Uterine rupture, with fetal and maternal morbidity and mortality if ecbolic agents (oxytocin) are given excessively, inappropriately (too early in labor, when fetal obstruction is present, if uterine torsion is present, too frequently, too rapidly), or when the uterine wall is compromised or torn

Recommended Monitoring

- Progression of labor with viable neonates delivered
- Using real-time transabdominal ultrasonography or a fetal Doppler, fetal heart rates should be > 180-200 beats/min with only transient decelerations.
- Sustained fetal heart rates < 180 beats/min are associated with fetal distress.
- Continued uterine monitoring using tocodynamometry, showing continuation and progression of appropriate contractile strength and frequency

PROGNOSIS & OUTCOME

Fair to good with timely intervention and appropriate monitoring

PEARLS & CONSIDERATIONS

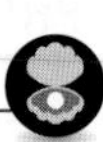

Comments

Obstruction of the birth canal, regardless of cause (fetal malposition, fetal-dam size mismatch, or anatomic defects of dam), must be ruled out by vaginal palpation or vaginoscopy. Obstruction of the birth canal is an indication for cesarean section and an absolute contraindication for treatment with oxytocin.

Prevention

- Complete prebreeding evaluation of the bitch, including a vaginal exam
- Prepartum abdominal radiography to estimate fetal number and relative size in comparison to the dam (best after 55 days' gestation)

Technician Tips

- Hospitalization in a secluded but closely monitored area of the clinic during labor is ideal, decreasing stress to the dam.
- Neonates should be allowed to nurse immediately after delivery; direct supervision of new or postanesthesia dams is important to ensure normal maternal instincts are present and smothering of neonates is prevented. Neonates should then be moved into a warm box until the next nursing or discharge to the owner. Weigh neonates before and after nursing to ensure colostrum has been ingested.

Client Education

Discuss proper perinatal husbandry, accurate gestational length interpretation based on ovulation timing, and prompt recognition of dystocia.

SUGGESTED READING

Davidson AP: Clinical conditions of the bitch and queen. In Nelson RW, et al, editors: Small animal internal medicine, ed 5, St. Louis, 2014, Elsevier, pp 915-950.

AUTHOR: Autumn P. Davidson, DVM, MS, DACVIM
EDITOR: Michelle A. Kutzler, DVM, PhD, DACT

Eclampsia

Client Education Sheet

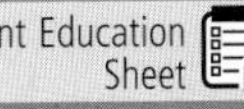

BASIC INFORMATION

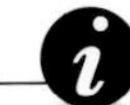

Definition

Acute onset hypocalcemia occurring during late pregnancy or early lactation

Synonyms

Milk fever, puerperal tetany

Epidemiology

SPECIES, AGE, SEX

- Dogs: younger bitches
- Cats: rare in queens

GENETICS, BREED PREDISPOSITION

More frequent in toy and small breed dogs

RISK FACTORS

- Young dogs of low parity (parity and age do not seem to be risk factors for the queen)
- Poor perinatal nutrition
- Calcium supplementation during pregnancy
- Large litter size

ASSOCIATED DISORDERS

- Hypomagnesemia
- Hypoglycemia
- Hyperthermia

Clinical Presentation

DISEASE FORMS/SUBTYPES

Queens may be more prone to hypothermia and exhibit a flaccid paralysis rather than hyperexcitability.

HISTORY, CHIEF COMPLAINT

- Bitches typically present during the first 3 weeks of lactation but they may also be seen during late pregnancy or parturition.
- Queens typically present in late pregnancy.

PHYSICAL EXAM FINDINGS

- Clinical signs are related to hypocalcemia and progress rapidly if left untreated (p. 515).
- Early signs include anorexia, depression, and agitation.
- Signs progress to include facial pruritus, panting, weakness, and muscle fasciculation.
- Later signs are more severe and include salivation, stiffness, and tonic-clonic muscle spasms, which may progress to epileptiform seizures in the bitch.
  - Flaccid paralysis may be seen in the queen.
- Hyperthermia and dysrhythmias may also be seen in the bitch.
- Hypothermia may occur in the queen.

Etiology and Pathophysiology

- Eclampsia occurs when serum ionized calcium is < 0.8 nmol/L or total serum calcium concentration is < 7 mg/dL.

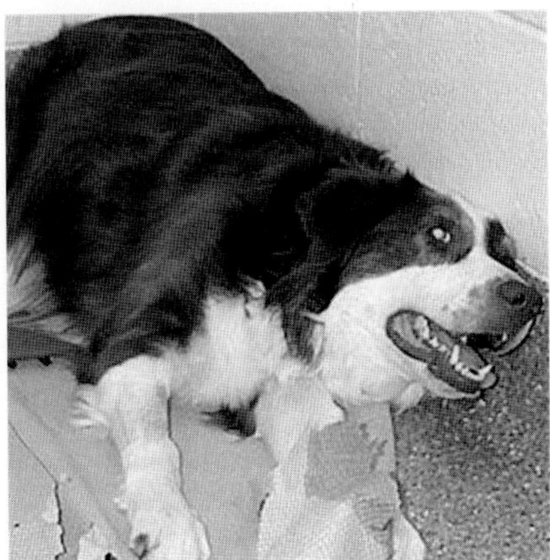

ECLAMPSIA Aberrant behavior in a Brittany bitch with eclampsia. (Courtesy www.PetPlace.com.)

- Peripheral nerve cells are more permeable to sodium when extracellular calcium levels are low.
- Calcium ions are also important for microvascular tone and maintenance of arterial pressure.
- Eclampsia is thought to occur due to the metabolic imbalance between the high calcium demands of fetal skeletal development and lactation and the intake from diet, intestinal absorption, and bone resorption.
- Exogenous calcium supplementation may contribute to hypocalcemia due to parathyroid atrophy.
- Alkalosis may decrease ionized calcium levels and cause signs of eclampsia even when serum total calcium concentrations are normal.

DIAGNOSIS

Diagnostic Overview

A provisional diagnosis of eclampsia is based on the presenting clinical signs of hypocalcemia during late pregnancy or early lactation and a rapid response to intravenous calcium supplementation. Low serum calcium concentration confirms the diagnosis.

Differential Diagnosis

- Hypocalcemia of other cause (p. 1239)
- Neuromuscular disease (e.g., tetanus, rabies)
- Hypoglycemia

Initial Database

- Total serum calcium concentration < 7 mg/dL (<1.74 mmol/L) or ionized serum calcium ≤ 0.8 mmol/L is the biochemical finding of eclampsia.

- Blood glucose and magnesium should also be evaluated because they are frequently abnormal.

TREATMENT

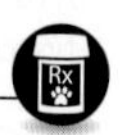

Treatment Overview

Initial treatment is aimed at reversing the clinical signs of hypocalcemia by administering intravenous (IV) calcium while simultaneously monitoring for dysrhythmia or bradycardia. Response to treatment occurs within 10-15 minutes. Secondary clinical signs (e.g., hyperthermia, hypothermia) and comorbid abnormalities (e.g., hypoglycemia, hypomagnesemia) should be concurrently managed as needed.

Acute General Treatment

- Slow IV administration of 0.5-1.5 mL/kg 10% calcium gluconate over 10-30 minutes to effect while simultaneously auscultating the heart for dysrhythmia or bradycardia; calcium is cardiotoxic.
  - Calcium administration should be stopped immediately if any cardiac abnormalities are noted on auscultation. Calcium administration may be restarted, although at a slower rate and only after normal cardiac rhythm is established.
  - Electrocardiographic (ECG) monitoring may be used (see Recommended Monitoring below) in place of auscultation.
- Refractory cases should be evaluated/treated for hypomagnesemia and hypoglycemia. Repeated IV doses of calcium gluconate given as required.
- After clinical signs are resolved, the equivalent amount of calcium gluconate given as an initial IV dose may be administered over the subsequent 24-48 hours diluted 1 : 1 with saline and administered subcutaneously.
- Body temperature should be monitored and hyperthermia (bitch) or hypothermia (queen) treated appropriately.

Chronic Treatment

- Neonates should be prevented from nursing for 12-24 hours and permanently removed if clinical signs of hypocalcemia recur when nursing recommences.
- Cabergoline 5 mcg/kg PO q 24h for 7 days may be used to stop lactation.
- Dams should be maintained on a high-quality commercial food approved for use during lactation and supplemented with oral calcium.
- An appropriate daily calcium supplement for the queen is 50-100 mg/kg/day, and for the bitch, it is 25-50 mg/kg/day divided into 3 or 4 daily doses for the duration of lactation.
- Vitamin D_3 is not recommended due to the transient nature of lactation, the lag time needed for a response, and the potential for hypercalcemia.

Nutrition/Diet

- All pregnant females should be maintained on a growth diet and transitioned to ad libitum feeding of a diet suitable for lactation in the postpartum period.
- Supplemental feeding of neonates with a milk replacer early in lactation may help reduce lactation demands on the dam, especially if the litter size is large.
- Calcium supplementation is not recommended during pregnancy because it alters parathyroid function and may increase the risk of hypocalcemia.

Drug Interactions

Oral calcium supplements may interfere with absorption of other medications.

Possible Complications

Intravenous calcium administration can induce fatal bradycardia or dysrhythmia.

Recommended Monitoring

ECG monitoring for bradycardia and shortening of the QT interval may be used instead of auscultation as a marker of calcium-induced cardiac toxicity when administering IV calcium gluconate.

PROGNOSIS & OUTCOME

Excellent short-term prognosis for recovery with immediate treatment, with a long-term risk of recurrence.

PEARLS & CONSIDERATIONS

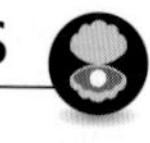

Comments

Magnesium supplementation may be beneficial for dams with refractory clinical signs.

Prevention

- Adequate nutrition can minimize the risk of eclampsia but is not necessarily preventative.
- Do not administer calcium supplements during pregnancy.

Technician Tips

Calcium gluconate is the only calcium preparation that should be administered intravenously or diluted and administered subcutaneously.

Client Education

- Eclampsia may recur during subsequent pregnancies.
- Calcium supplementation during pregnancy should be avoided because it may increase the risk of eclampsia.
- Optimal perinatal and lactation nutrition is important for minimizing eclampsia risk.

SUGGESTED READING

Drobatz KJ, et al: Eclampsia in dogs: 31 cases (1991-1998). J Am Vet Med Assoc 217(2):216-219, 2000.

AUTHOR: Sophie A. Grundy, BVSc, MANZCVS, DACVIM
EDITOR: Michelle A. Kutzler, DVM, PhD, DACT

Ectopic Ureter

Client Education Sheet 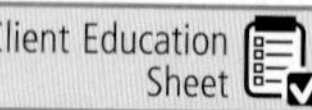

BASIC INFORMATION

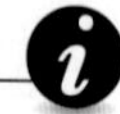

Definition

A congenital abnormality in which the ureteral orifice is located anywhere distal to the normal trigone location, typically causing urinary incontinence in young dogs

Synonym

Ureteral ectopia

Epidemiology

SPECIES, AGE, SEX

- Young female dogs (median age at diagnosis, 10 months)
- Prevalence among male dogs is likely underestimated due to lack of incontinence presumably because of urethral length and external urethral sphincter (median age of diagnosis, 24 months).

GENETICS, BREED PREDISPOSITION

Labrador retriever, Siberian husky, golden retriever, Newfoundland, English bulldog, West Highland white terrier, fox terrier, Skye terrier, Entlebucher mountain dog, and miniature and toy poodles are overrepresented.

ASSOCIATED DISORDERS

- Other urinary tract anomalies: urethral sphincter mechanism incompetence, pelvic bladder, ureterocele, hydroureter, hydronephrosis, and renal agenesis or dysplasia
- Concurrent urinary tract infections are common.

Clinical Presentation

DISEASE FORMS/SUBTYPES

- Unilateral or bilateral
- Extramural or intramural
  - Extramural ureter: bypasses the urinary bladder and inserts at a distal location (urethra, vagina, or vestibule in females and ductus deferens in males)
  - Intramural ureter (more common): enters the bladder in the normal

dorsolateral location but then tunnels through the submucosa of the bladder and opens distal to the normal trigone location. Amenable to cystoscopic laser ablation

HISTORY, CHIEF COMPLAINT

- Urinary incontinence, intermittent or continuous
- Recurrent urinary tract infections (typically causing pollakiuria, stranguria, and/or hematuria)

PHYSICAL EXAM FINDINGS

- Moist or urine-stained hair in the perivulvar/preputial region
- Urinary incontinence may be noted during physical exam.
- Dermatitis due to urine scalding
- Small or moderately sized bladder on palpation (typically small)
- Vulvovaginal stricture or persistent hymen palpated on digital vaginal exam
- Vulvovaginitis

Etiology and Pathophysiology

- Ectopic ureters are the result of dysembryogenesis of the ureteral bud of the mesonephric duct.
- The deviation of the ureteral bud from the normal position determines the location of the ectopic opening.

DIAGNOSIS

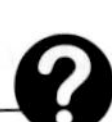

Diagnostic Overview

Ectopic ureters should be suspected in any young dog with urinary incontinence. Confirmation requires advanced imaging (abdominal ultrasound, excretory urography, contrast-enhanced CT, or transurethral cystoscopy).

Differential Diagnosis

Differential diagnosis for urinary incontinence:

- Ureterocele
- Pelvic bladder
- Urge incontinence (e.g., urinary tract infection, urolithiasis)
- Urethral sphincter mechanism incompetence
- Vaginal abnormality (e.g., vaginal stricture)
- Neurologic disorders
- Congenital urethral incompetence or hypoplasia

Initial Database

Urinalysis (may be normal):

- Pyuria
- Hematuria
- Bacteriuria

Abdominal radiographs (often normal):

- Provide information regarding the size, shape, and location of the kidneys and bladder
- Small bladder size
- Pelvic bladder
- Mainly used to rule out cystolithiasis and identify structural abnormalities associated with the kidneys, ureter (if visible), and bladder

Advanced or Confirmatory Testing

Abdominal ultrasound (may be normal):

- Hydroureter
- Hydronephrosis
- Ureterocele
- May see abnormal location of ureteral orifice
- Evidence of cystitis if secondary urinary tract infection

Excretory urography (EU) with survey radiographs (p. 1101):

- Identify location of ureteral opening distal to the trigone of the bladder
- Ureteral dilation (>0.09 times the length of the L2 vertebrae)
  - Most commonly associated with intramural ureters that open into the urethra or vagina
  - Due to intermittent or partial urinary obstruction and/or secondary to a urinary tract infection
- Lateral, ventrodorsal, and oblique views are necessary to identify the distal segment of nondilated ureters.
- Inability to consistently identify ectopic ureter may be due to ureteral peristalsis, poor renal excretion of contrast, or superimposition of other structures.
- Diagnostic accuracy improves if combined with pneumocystography.

Contrast-enhanced CT scan (EU with CT):

- Sensitive and specific method for diagnosis and characterization of ectopic ureters (e.g., exact location of ureteral orifice, identifying multiple openings)

Transurethral cystoscopy (p. 1085):

- Direct visualization of the lower urinary tract using a rigid or flexible endoscope
- Identification of ectopic ureteral openings, but may be difficult to confirm intramural nature of ureter with cystoscopy alone (CT or fluoroscopy may be useful for this)
- Allows for identification of other congenital structural abnormalities of the lower urinary tract involving the bladder, vagina, vestibule, and urethra
- Commonly paired with CT or performed alone by a skilled cystoscopist

Urodynamic evaluation:

- Determination of the urethral pressure profile may be useful in gaining information regarding function of the urethra in patients with urinary incontinence.
- Used to help predict continued postoperative urinary incontinence in patients with ectopic ureter
- Limited availability

TREATMENT

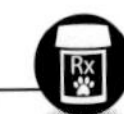

Treatment Overview

The treatment goal for patients with ectopic ureters consists of correcting the abnormal urethral orifice to resolve or reduce urinary incontinence. This requires open surgical correction or laser ablation by transurethral cystoscopy.

Acute General Treatment

- Appropriate treatment of concurrent urinary tract infection (if present) is important before surgery.
- Surgical technique used depends on the location and morphology of the ectopic ureter. Surgical techniques commonly performed:
  - Ureteral reimplantation with ligation of the distal ureter (extramural ectopic ureters)
  - Neoureterostomy and urethra-trigone reconstruction (intramural ectopic ureters)
  - Nephroureterectomy: removal of a nonfunctional kidney and associated ureter; considered a salvage procedure. Important to determine renal function in the contralateral kidney is normal
- Cystoscopic-guided laser ablation
  - Laser ablation of the wall between the urethral lumen and the intramural ureteral lumen is practical only for patients with intramural ectopic ureters.
  - Can be an effective, minimally invasive technique for correction of intramural ectopic ureters
  - Performed using a holmium:YAG or diode laser
  - Limited availability

Chronic Treatment

Management of concurrent urethral sphincter mechanism incompetence, if present (p. 1011)

Possible Complications

- Hydroureter and hydronephrosis due to obstruction postoperatively
- Persistent urinary incontinence: most common complication after surgical repair of ectopic ureters (40%-70% of patients)
- Recurrent urinary tract infections

Recommended Monitoring

Routine monitoring for urinary tract infections

PROGNOSIS & OUTCOME

- Prognosis with surgical repair or laser ablation of ectopic ureter(s) is good if there is no evidence of renal dysfunction before surgery.
- Prognosis for return of urinary continence without specific therapy for urethral sphincter incompetence is poor, with up to 70% of dogs remaining incontinent postoperatively. Most dogs will improve with medical management for urethral sphincter mechanism incompetence.

PEARLS & CONSIDERATIONS

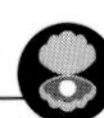

Comments

- Ectopic ureter(s) should be suspected in any young dog with urinary incontinence.
- Although surgery is often successful for surgical correction of ectopic ureters, 40%-70%

of dogs will still have urinary incontinence after surgical correction due to concurrent urethral sphincter mechanism incompetence.

Technician Tips

Immediate postoperative monitoring should focus on urine production and fluid volume status because signs of reduced urine production and fluid overload may indicate possible urinary tract obstruction.

Client Education

Understanding that a large percentage of dogs with ectopic ureters continue to have urinary incontinence after repair of the ectopic ureter(s) is important when discussing surgery and postoperative expectations with clients.

SUGGESTED READING

Davidson AP, et al: Diagnosis and management of urinary ectopia. Vet Clin North Am Small Anim Pract 44:343-353, 2014.

AUTHOR: Laura A. Nafe, DVM, MS, DACVIM
EDITOR: Leah A. Cohn, DVM, PhD, DACVIM

Edema, Subcutaneous

BASIC INFORMATION

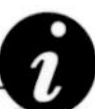

Definition

Local or generalized swelling from excessive fluid accumulation in the interstitial tissue spaces under the skin. Normally, only a small amount of fluid leaks from vessels into the interstitium, and it is removed by lymphatic vessels.

Synonyms

Peripheral edema (edema of the head, neck, torso, and/or limbs), anasarca (generalized, massive subcutaneous [SQ] edema)

Epidemiology

SPECIES, AGE, SEX

Dogs and cats: any age, either sex

RISK FACTORS

Severe hypoproteinemia, right-sided congestive heart failure (CHF), inflammation, vasculitis, extensive trauma or heat, lymphatic malformation, acquired venous or lymphatic obstruction (e.g., tumor, granuloma)

Clinical Presentation

HISTORY, CHIEF COMPLAINT

Regional swelling (e.g., one limb, both hind limbs, head) or a diffusely swollen appearance, most commonly in dependent areas (e.g., sternum, distal limbs, scrotum)

PHYSICAL EXAM FINDINGS

- Local or diffuse thickening of SQ tissues
  - Most commonly, edema pits. Digital pressure exerted on edematous skin may leave a depression (i.e., pit) for several seconds after the pressure is released, when fluid accumulation is interstitial rather than intracellular.
  - Although uncommon, swelling may be painful or warm if associated with infection.
  - Sometimes associated with ascites (e.g., hypoalbuminemia, right-sided CHF)
- The hock with its lateral saphenous vein, the gastrocnemius tendons, and the bony prominence of the mandible are useful to evaluate for SQ edema because these areas are consistently well-defined, even in obese animals. With edema, these areas are less defined and overlying skin has a thickened, jelly-like appearance.
- Edema tends to accumulate where gravity draws it, where lymphatic obstruction or insufficiency is greatest, or a combination of both. The pattern of edema distribution varies.
- Additional physical abnormalities depend on underlying cause of edema.

Etiology and Pathophysiology

More fluid leaves the capillaries than enters:

- Increased vascular hydrostatic pressure
  - Right-sided CHF
  - Impaired venous flow (e.g., mediastinal or abdominal mass)
  - Iatrogenic fluid overload
  - Excessive fluid retention (e.g., anuric kidney failure)
- Decreased plasma oncotic pressure
  - Hypoalbuminemia: increased loss or decreased production (p. 1239)
- Increased vascular permeability
  - Allergic response (histamine release)
  - Acute inflammation
  - Burn injury
  - Envenomation

Normal volume of interstitial fluid not reabsorbed by the lymphatic system:

- Lymphatic obstruction (usually localized)
  - Neoplasia
  - Inflammation
  - Trauma
  - Congenital (lymphedema)

DIAGNOSIS

Diagnostic Overview

- SQ edema is identified on physical exam (readily if severe, with difficulty if mild).
- Diffuse edema, or edema in disparate locations, suggests systemic disturbance. Regional edema (e.g., head/neck, single limb) suggests regional disease.
- Acute edema is more likely related to causes such as allergy, envenomation, or thermal

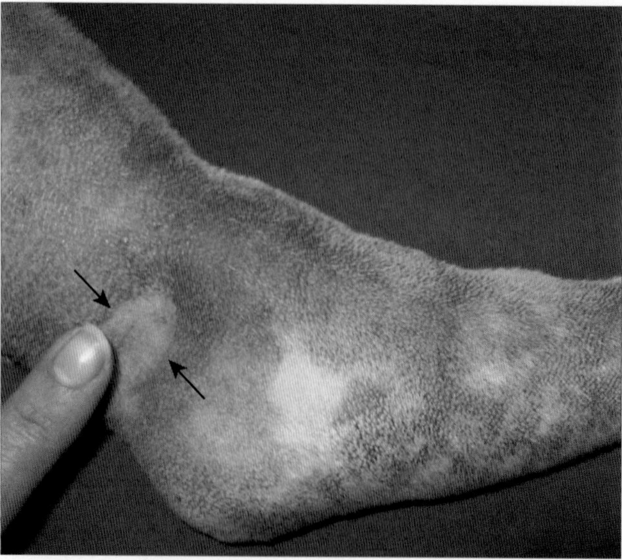

EDEMA, SUBCUTANEOUS Subcutaneous edema in the tarsal region of a dog. In this image, the clinician just removed her index finger after applying digital pressure for several seconds, revealing the depression or pit *(arrows)* that characterizes pitting edema.

injury that may be apparent based on history and exam. Persistent edema should be further investigated.
- Serum albumin should be assessed, and if severe hypoalbuminemia is present, the cause should be cause pursued (pp. 600 and 174).
- Imaging studies are often warranted (especially if albumin is normal).

Differential Diagnosis

Myxedema (p. 503) may be confused with SQ edema.

Initial Database

- Complete blood count: depends on cause; low total solids with severe hypoalbuminemia
- Serum biochemistry profile: evaluate for hypoalbuminemia
- Urinalysis: rule out pathologic proteinuria

Advanced or Confirmatory Testing

Specific testing is guided by results of history, exam, and screening tests:
- Thoracic radiographs often warranted
  - If right-sided CHF suspected from exam (or echocardiography)
  - Rule out cranial mediastinal mass as cause of head/neck or forelimb edema.
  - Rule out metastatic neoplasia.
- Abdominal imaging (radiographs, ultrasound) for hind limb edema
- Special studies such as lymphangiogram, CT, MRI (p. 1132), or PET/CT may be useful.

TREATMENT

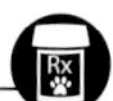

Treatment Overview

Management of SQ edema is typically nonemergent and is targeted toward treatment of the underlying condition, with therapy to restore vascular-extravascular fluid balance as needed.

Acute General Treatment

- Patients with severe decrease in oncotic pressure may benefit from oncotic support, especially if fluid therapy is necessary.
  - Synthetic colloids (hydroxyethyl starches, dextrans): Hetastarch (6% hydroxyethyl starch 130/0.4 in 0.9% sodium chloride); typical dose 1-2 mL/kg/h; adverse reactions may include coagulopathy, volume overload, kidney injury.
  - Human (HSA) or canine serum albumin (CSA): CSA is more expensive than HSA but may be safer (HSA can cause life-threatening immune-mediated reaction). Dose in grams = 10 × desired albumin concentration (g/dL) − patient albumin concentration (g/dL) × patient weight (kg) × 0.3
  - Canine plasma transfusion: large volumes required to increase colloid oncotic pressure; 45 mL/kg of plasma required to raise albumin 1 g/dL

PROGNOSIS & OUTCOME

Depends on cause. Lymphedema is usually congenital or neoplastic in origin, can be very challenging to manage long term, and is often incurable.

PEARLS & CONSIDERATIONS

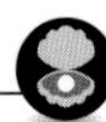

Comments

- Pitting edema represents interstitial fluid accumulation, whereas nonpitting edema is formed by intracellular swelling (e.g., wheal).
- Acute edema in a single limb may be due to injury or envenomation; shaving sometimes reveals a bite wound or injury not identified on exam of haired skin.
- Dogs tend to suffer snake bites on the nose/head, and cats suffer bites on a front limb; these bites cause local edema.
- Persistent edema in a single limb may be related to neoplastic obstruction to venous or lymphatic return. For example, hemangiosarcoma in the musculature of the thigh in large breed dogs may cause edema in a single limb.
- Myxedema due to hypothyroidism is nonpitting and often associated with hypothermia and marked lethargy to stupor or coma.

Technician Tips

Gentle physical manipulations (e.g., massage), barring pain, skin fragility, or a fractious patient, can be beneficial. Adequate movement (traction in cage flooring, walks outside for dogs) is also important for supporting normal lymphatic flow and reducing edema.

SUGGESTED READING

Mathews KA: Monitoring fluid therapy and complications of fluid therapy. In DiBartola SP, editor: Fluid, electrolyte, and acid-base disorders in small animal practice, ed 4, St. Louis, 2012, Saunders, pp 386-404.

AUTHOR: Mandi Kleman, DVM, DACVIM
EDITOR: Leah A. Cohn, DVM, PhD, DACVIM

Ehrlichiosis, Monocytic

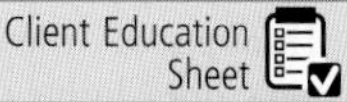

BASIC INFORMATION

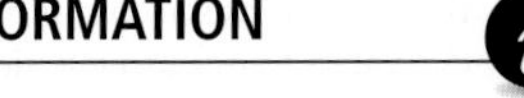

Definition

Canine monocytic ehrlichiosis (CME) is a common tick-borne disease caused by infection with *Ehrlichia canis* (dogs; rarely cats) or *Ehrlichia chaffeensis* (humans, dogs).

Synonyms

Human monocytic ehrlichiosis (HME), canine and human monocytotropic ehrlichiosis, tropical canine pancytopenia (old terminology), ehrlichiosis

Epidemiology

SPECIES, AGE, SEX

Dogs (common), cats (rare); no known age or sex predisposition

GENETICS, BREED PREDISPOSITION

German shepherd dogs are predisposed to severe clinical disease; suspect deficient cell-mediated immunity.

RISK FACTORS

Lack of adequate tick prevention and the risk of tick exposure (e.g., geographic location, outdoor activities)

CONTAGION AND ZOONOSIS

- Most infections occur by inoculation from a tick bite; inadvertent inoculation with blood from an infected animal is less likely. Direct transmission from dog to human has never been confirmed.
- *E. canis* is a canine disease, but a human infection was documented in South America.
- *E. chaffeensis* was originally recognized as a human pathogen, but it can infect dogs.

GEOGRAPHY AND SEASONALITY

- *E. canis*: worldwide distribution, with highest prevalence in tropical climates (South America, Caribbean) and subtropical climates (southern United States)
  - Acute infection: usually in warmer months, when brown dog tick activity is highest
  - Chronic form: occurs at any time of year
- *E. chaffeensis*: central, southeastern, and eastern United States, from Florida to Maine
  - Most clinical cases occur from early spring to mid-summer, when lone star tick activity is highest.

ASSOCIATED DISORDERS

- Co-infection with other tick-borne pathogens
  - Brown dog tick (vector for *E. canis*): *Anaplasma platys, Babesia canis, Rickettsia rickettsii, Hepatozoon canis*
  - Lone star tick (vector for *E. chaffeensis*): *Ehrlichia ewingii* (found in Panola Mountain State Park, GA), *Cytauxzoon felis* (cats), *Francisella tularensis*, ± *R. rickettsii*

Clinical Presentation

DISEASE FORMS/SUBTYPES

The incubation period is 1-3 weeks after tick inoculation, after which three phases of infection can occur:

- Acute phase (lasts 1-4 weeks): dogs show clinical signs but recover. Untreated animals recover spontaneously but progress to the subclinical phase and are carriers of the agent; treated dogs clear the organism. Host and pathogen factors influence severity of acute illness.
- Subclinical phase (lasts months to many years): no clinical signs; some dogs remain in this subclinical state for life, whereas others progress to the chronic phase.
- Chronic phase: various manifestations of clinical disease (well documented for *E. canis*, likely for *E. chaffeensis* in dogs)

HISTORY, CHIEF COMPLAINT

- Infection is often recognized in healthy dogs by screening tests.
- With illness, the most common complaints are nonspecific: lethargy, anorexia, weight loss, bleeding tendencies.
- Additional signs during the chronic phase may be related to anemia (e.g., weakness, collapse), neurologic signs, or renal disease (e.g., polyuria/polydipsia).
- Because clinical manifestations occur weeks to years after tick inoculation, a history of tick exposure is variable.

PHYSICAL EXAM FINDINGS

- Throughout the subclinical phase and sometimes during the acute or chronic disease phases, exam findings are unremarkable.
- If abnormalities are present during illness (i.e., acute or chronic phase), common findings include fever (especially in acute phase), lymphadenopathy, splenomegaly, epistaxis, and petechiae.
- Other potential abnormalities include pallor, ocular hemorrhage, lameness, and neurologic signs.

Etiology and Pathophysiology

- *E. canis* is transmitted by the brown dog tick (*Rhipicephalus sanguineus*) and *E. chaffeensis* by the lone star tick (*Amblyomma americanum*).
- Because transovarial transmission in these ticks has not been demonstrated, the tick must acquire the infection at the larval or nymph state from a mammalian reservoir host.
- After attaching to a susceptible dog for as little as 3 hours, the tick transmits the organism in its saliva.
- After inoculation, the organism invades lymphocytes and monocytes/macrophages, multiplies intracellularly, and forms membrane-bound vacuoles or morulae that contain several individual bacteria. A positive antibody titer is first detected 7-28 days after inoculation.
- During the acute phase of infection, few organisms may be found in circulating monocytes and lymphocytes, and the spleen is thought to harbor the infection.
- During the subclinical phase, immune stimulation results in seropositive diagnostic test results, even though the animal is not overtly ill.
- During the chronic phase of infection, direct damage done by the organism and damage resulting from the host's immune response can cause several clinical and hematologic abnormalities, notably severe bone marrow suppression and pancytopenia (often fatal).
- CME is a multisystemic disease with many clinical manifestations due to the presence of organisms in various tissues and the host's immune response. Host response to newly exposed or altered antigens can worsen clinical signs directly and by the formation and deposition of immune complexes in glomeruli, synovial membranes, and meninges (causing nephropathies, arthropathies, and neuropathies, respectively).

DIAGNOSIS

Diagnostic Overview

Dogs with consistent clinical findings and thrombocytopenia should be suspected of having CME and/or other related vector-borne agents and should be tested accordingly, regardless of known tick exposure. Confirmation of infection requires finding morulae in circulating monocytic cells (rare), a positive point-of-care or laboratory based serologic test, or polymerase chain reaction (PCR) analysis.

Differential Diagnosis

- Co-infection with other tick-borne organisms: other *Ehrlichia* spp, *Anaplasma* spp, *Bartonella* spp, *Rickettsia* spp, *Borrelia* spp
- Immune-mediated causes of peripheral cytopenias, polyarthritis, meningitis, and glomerulonephritis
- Large, granular lymphoid leukemia: like CME, it can be associated with high peripheral granular lymphocytosis (6000-17,000 cells/mcL).
- Multiple myeloma: like CME, it can be associated with monoclonal or biclonal gammopathy and bone marrow plasmacytosis, as well as thrombocytopenia.

Initial Database

- CBC, serum biochemical profile, urinalysis: during subclinical phase, routine laboratory tests are unremarkable. Cytopenias and hyperglobulinemia are hallmarks of clinical infection.
  - Thrombocytopenia (from immune-mediated destruction, sequestration, or decreased production): 90% of cases
  - Anemia (as a result of hemorrhage, anemia of chronic inflammatory disease, or bone marrow suppression)
  - Neutropenia or neutrophilia
  - Lymphocyte count variable; marked granular lymphocytosis is common with chronic CME and must be distinguished from a lymphoid leukemia.
  - Identification of morulae in mononuclear cells is rare but strongly supports the diagnosis.
  - Hyperglobulinemia, typically a polyclonal gammopathy; monoclonal gammopathy can occur with chronic CME, and this finding along with bone marrow plasmacytosis must not lead to a misdiagnosis of multiple myeloma.
  - Nonspecific increases in liver enzyme activities and blood urea nitrogen (BUN) and hypoalbuminemia are common.
  - Proteinuria is possible in the chronic phase due to glomerulonephritis.
- Point-of-care serologic tests: SNAP 4Dx Plus detects antibodies to *E. canis*, *E. chaffeensis*, and *E. ewingii*; WITNESS *Ehrlichia* detects antibodies to *E. canis*.
  - Excellent for routine screening and supportive evidence for chronic infection
  - In acute infections, antibody levels may not be detectable: if point-of-care test result is negative in a case with signs suggesting CME, PCR is recommended.
  - The SNAP antibody reaction does not distinguish between the three *Ehrlichia* species, but geographic region and clinical presentation can help determine which infection is more likely. Although CME can cause acute or chronic illness (which may have very different types of presentation), *E. ewingii* usually causes acute polyarthropathy or neurologic signs (p. 393).
  - It is crucial to remember that in areas endemic for any of the *Ehrlichia* spp, a positive antibody test result does not prove that ehrlichiosis accounts for the observed clinical signs in a given patient. The animal could be in the subclinical phase of CME (or recovered from prior infection with another species of *Ehrlichia*) and therefore antibody positive, but the current disease may be caused by something entirely unrelated to the infection.

Advanced or Confirmatory Testing

- Buffy coat smears: enhanced detection of morulae in circulating mononuclear cells compared to regular blood smears; still uncommon findings, except in animals with acute disease
  - Finding morulae in monocytic cells confirms the dog as having *E. canis* or *E. chaffeensis*.

- Lymph node aspirates: cytologic evaluation rarely may demonstrate morulae in lymphocytes.
- Advanced serologic testing: IFA tests for detecting serum antibodies to *E. canis* and *E. chaffeensis*
  - A reciprocal titer ≥ 64 with clinical signs is recommended to confirm a diagnosis. However, titers may initially be negative in acute cases. Therefore, a ≥ fourfold rise between acute and convalescent titers (2-4 weeks apart) is ideal for serologic confirmation of acute infection. Titers are not expected to rise during chronic infection.
- PCR analysis can detect and distinguish between *E. canis* and *E. chaffeensis* DNA in blood.
  - PCR is much more sensitive than microscopic evaluation for detecting organisms in acutely infected dogs. However, animals that are chronically infected or are subclinical carriers may be seropositive and PCR negative due to low numbers of circulating organisms.
  - A negative PCR result can never be used to rule out ehrlichiosis.

TREATMENT

Treatment Overview

- In a patient with a positive *Ehrlichia* serologic result, a CBC, serum biochemistry profile, and urinalysis should be evaluated along with physical exam findings.
  - In many dogs, the positive screening result (e.g., positive SNAP 4Dx Plus) is an incidental finding (no clinical signs of CME) and laboratory results are unremarkable. Treatment in such cases may not be necessary; the potential benefit must be weighed against the risk of overtreatment (test may be positive due to exposure but not active disease). Whether treated or not, seropositive dogs should be monitored annually (CBC, biochemistry profile, urinalysis), and any relevant abnormalities would warrant treatment.
  - A SNAP-positive animal with relevant clinical signs and laboratory abnormalities (e.g., thrombocytopenia, hyperglobulinemia) compatible with CME should receive a 4-week course of doxycycline or minocycline.
  - Due to genetic predisposition to CME, any German shepherd with a positive SNAP test result should be treated regardless of laboratory findings.
  - Partial responders or animals that relapse after completion of doxycycline therapy should be tested for other vector-borne agents, particularly *Bartonella* spp or *Babesia* spp, which are poorly responsive or nonresponsive to doxycycline.

Acute General Treatment

- Doxycycline or minocycline 5-10 mg/kg PO q 12h × 28 days is the treatment of choice.
  - In acute infection, this results in rapid (24-48 hours) resolution of clinical signs.
  - In chronic infection, illness may not respond quickly, or damage may be irreparable (e.g., pancytopenia may not resolve).
  - Extended treatment (4 weeks) is recommended but may or may not eradicate the organism.
- Imidocarb dipropionate or enrofloxacin are *not* effective.
- Glucocorticoids can be used judiciously at antiinflammatory or immunosuppressive dosages if a course of antimicrobial therapy has failed to relieve immune-mediated cytopenias, glomerulopathies, meningitis, or arthropathies.

Chronic Treatment

- Most chronic cases of CME respond to the treatment regimen described above, but recovery from some manifestations of disease (e.g., pancytopenia, glomerulonephritis) may be slow or may not occur.
- Animals that develop severe pancytopenia may require supportive care (e.g., blood transfusions [p. 1169]).
  - No proven benefit of bone marrow stimulants (erythropoietin, granulocyte colony-stimulating factor)
- Animals with other complications may require specific supportive care (e.g., severe neutropenia can cause secondary bacterial infection; glomerulonephritis can respond to standard therapy [p. 390]).

Drug Interactions

Vomiting and drug-induced esophagitis are possible with doxycycline. Risk reduced by giving it with meals and giving water after medicating

Possible Complications

- Anemia (bleeding tendencies from severe thrombocytopenia; bone marrow suppression)
- Thrombocytopenia (immune-mediated destruction of platelets, splenic sequestration of platelets, bone marrow suppression)
- Severe neutropenia (bone marrow suppression or, less likely, immune-mediated destruction)
- Bone marrow aplasia is a severe life-threatening complication of CME.
- Protein-losing glomerulonephropathy (limited number of dogs with CME)
- Co-infections with other vector-borne agents can result in more severe clinical manifestations and/or poor response to antimicrobial therapy.

Recommended Monitoring

- Periodic CBCs until cytopenias resolve
- Serum biochemical profiles to monitor disease progression by resolution of abnormalities
- Urinalysis to monitor status of glomerular disease by presence/magnitude of proteinuria

PROGNOSIS & OUTCOME

- The prognosis for complete recovery is good for animals with acute infections or mild chronic disease. Clinical improvement is typically noted within 24-48 hours from the initiation of therapy.
- Severe cases of CME with bleeding disorders have guarded prognosis, with up to a 25% mortality.
- Severely pancytopenic patients have poor prognosis, with mortality rates near 100%.

PEARLS & CONSIDERATIONS

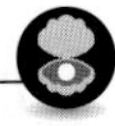

Comments

- Animals that are febrile, lethargic, and thrombocytopenic should be tested for vector-borne agents such as *E. canis* and *E. chaffeensis*.
- *E. canis* infections in the United States are often less virulent than infections in other parts of the world during the acute and chronic phases of illness.
- Many animals that become infected do not develop clinical signs or have transient clinical disease such that therapy is not initiated during the acute phase of infection. These animals often progress to subclinically infected, chronic carriers. They will test positive on screening assays but appear clinically healthy.
- The two *Ehrlichia* spp that cause zoonotic disease (*E. chaffeensis* and *E. ewingii*) are much more prevalent in the canine population than is *E. canis* in areas of the United States where the lone star tick is found. In a large serosurvey in lone star-endemic areas, dogs were positive for *E. canis* (0.8%), *E. chaffeensis* (2.8%), and *E. ewingii* (5.1%).

Prevention

- Regular use of acaricides for dogs, even using combinations of products for those with heavy tick exposure
- Physical tick screening and removal immediately after activity in tick-bearing areas

Technician Tips

- Medical hygiene precautions are important; blood from acutely infected animals has the potential to spread infection if inadvertently inoculated by contaminated needles.
- Seropositive animals or animals previously infected with any tick-borne disease should not be used as blood donors.
- Gloves should be used when removing ticks from dogs and cats.

Client Education

- A positive blood test result may indicate a risk for common-source exposure of other dogs or of humans.
- Tick prevention is critical in subclinically infected, seropositive animals.
  - Additional exposure to other tick-borne agents increases the likelihood for the development of clinical manifestations.
  - Subclinically or clinically infected dogs are potential reservoirs for ehrlichial

organisms because ticks may extract the organism from the dog during the feeding process, This can increase the pathogen burden in the tick population in the dog's environment.

SUGGESTED READING

Harrus S: Perspectives on the pathogenesis and treatment of canine monocytic ehrlichiosis *(Ehrlichia canis)*. Vet J 204:239-240, 2015.

AUTHOR: A. Rick Alleman, DVM, PhD
EDITOR: Joseph Taboada, DVM, DACVIM

Elbow Dysplasia

Bonus Material Online 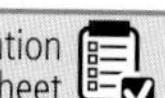 Client Education Sheet

BASIC INFORMATION

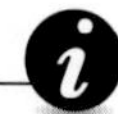

Definition

A common group of developmental disorders, including fragmented medial coronoid process (FCP; also called medial compartment disease), ununited anconeal process (UAP), osteochondritis dissecans (OCD), and elbow incongruity (uneven radial head and medial coronoid surfaces) that cause degenerative joint disease in the elbow

Epidemiology

SPECIES, AGE, SEX

- Primarily in dogs 6-9 months of age
- Manifested in older dogs as secondary degenerative joint disease

GENETICS, BREED PREDISPOSITION

Elbow dysplasia is hereditary but is also associated with rapid growth and high-energy diet.

- UAP is found primarily in German shepherds, basset hounds, and Saint Bernards.
- FCP and OCD affect primarily retriever breeds, Bernese mountain dogs, and rottweilers.
- Other affected breeds include Newfoundlands, mastiffs, Australian shepherds, and increasingly, smaller breeds.

Clinical Presentation

DISEASE FORMS/SUBTYPES

- FCP is a separation of the medial aspect of the coronoid process from the ulna; the coronoid process may also be abnormal without being fragmented.
- UAP is a failure of the anconeal process to fuse to the ulna.
- OCD is an abnormality of endochondral ossification causing separation of cartilage from the medial aspect of the humeral condyle (p. 723).

HISTORY, CHIEF COMPLAINT

- History of lameness of one or both forelimbs, often worse after exercise
- Reluctance to play or take long walks

PHYSICAL EXAM FINDINGS

- Lameness of one or both forelimbs
- Pain on manipulation of the elbow, especially on extension
- If osteoarthrosis is advanced, crepitation or effusion may be palpable along with decreased flexion to the joint.

Etiology and Pathophysiology

- OCD occurs when there is a failure of endochondral ossification, which leads to cartilage thickening and fissure formation.
- Joint incongruity, leading to increased pressure on the anconeus, may contribute to UAP.
- UAP may also be a form of osteochondrosis with abnormal thickened cartilage, leading to failure of unification.
- The underlying pathophysiology of FCP is unknown but is thought to result from elbow incongruity or a form of osteochondrosis.
  - Incongruity of the joint, especially an increase in length of the ulna in relation to the radius, can increase load on the medial aspect of the coronoid process, leading to fissuring and fragmentation.
  - Osteochondrosis may lead to a delay in ossification of the coronoid region and subject the joint to fragmentation when bearing weight.

DIAGNOSIS

Diagnostic Overview

Radiography is the standard means of diagnosing elbow dysplasia. However, canine elbow dysplasia can be present without radiographic signs, and advanced imaging (nuclear scintigraphy, ultrasonography, CT, and MRI) or arthroscopy may help diagnose subtle lesions.

Differential Diagnosis

- Panosteitis
- OCD of the shoulder
- Elbow luxation

Initial Database

- CBC, serum chemistry panel: generally unremarkable (preanesthetic)
- Mediolateral, craniocaudal, and flexed lateral radiographs of both elbows
  - An oblique craniocaudal view with the elbow flexed 30° and rotated medially 15° may help to assess the medial coronoid process.
  - The flexed lateral is the best radiographic view to identify UAP.
  - OCD lesions are seen on the medial aspect of the humeral condyle, primarily on the craniocaudal view.
  - Elbow congruity is best assessed on the mediolateral view, with the beam centered on the elbow joint.

Advanced or Confirmatory Testing

- A bone scan can be used for localizing the lameness if a complete orthopedic exam and radiographs are inconclusive.
- CT or MRI (p. 1132) can be used for characterizing and delineating the elbow lesion.
  - CT is recommended on all elbows with radiographic evidence of UAP because a

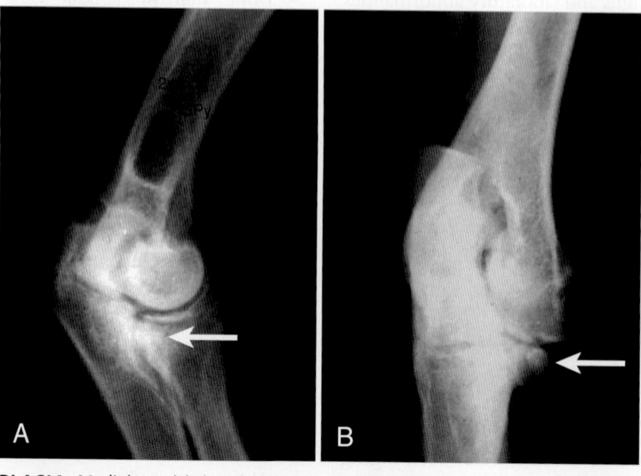

ELBOW DYSPLASIA Mediolateral (**A**) and craniocaudal (**B**) projections of a canine elbow with fragmented medial coronoid process *(arrows)*. (Courtesy Dr. J. Harari; reproduced with permission.)

large percentage of patients have concurrent coronoid disease.
  - CT evaluation of both elbows is useful in the diagnosis of coronoid disease to differentiate fragmentation, fissuring, and chondromalacia of the medial coronoid process.
- Arthroscopy is more sensitive than CT for cartilage lesions and can be used for diagnosis and treatment.
- Arthrocentesis (p. 1059) can be performed to rule out other causes of joint effusion.

TREATMENT

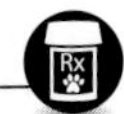

Treatment Overview

In persistently lame dogs with elbow dysplasia, surgical treatment involves removal of the FCP, OCD, or UAP fragment, which often improves limb function. In dogs with elbow incongruity, surgery to improve congruity usually lessens lameness and may slow progression of osteoarthritis; nevertheless, degenerative joint disease progresses in most cases.

Acute General Treatment

- Elbow arthroscopy by a medial portal is used for treatment of FCP and OCD and to assess elbow incongruity.
  - The FCP is identified and removed with grasping forceps or a motorized shaver.
  - Curettage or removal of the medial coronoid process by a subtotal coronoid ostectomy can be used when fissuring or chondromalacia is present without gross fragmentation.
  - OCD lesion is identified and the cartilage flap removed. A motorized shaver is used for removing fragments and to treat the underlying subchondral bone. Osteochondral autograft transfer as well as a synthetic allograft transfer system may be used as a treatment option for OCD lesions.
- A sliding humeral osteotomy has been proposed to redistribute forces from the medial to the lateral compartment of the elbow, thereby decreasing pain associated with medial coronoid disease.
- In skeletally mature dogs, a UAP is often surgically removed by a lateral approach.
- In skeletally immature dogs, ulnar osteotomy may be used to reduce pressure on the anconeal process and allow bony or fibrous union of the fragment.
  - This may be used simultaneously with lag screw fixation of the anconeal process. Lag screw fixation causes compression of the anconeal process to the ulna and leads to bone fusion.
- If elbow incongruity exists, ulnar osteotomy or ulnar ostectomy can be done to help equalize lengths of the ulna and radius; some surgeons stabilize the osteotomy with an intramedullary pin.
- Partial or total elbow replacement or elbow arthrodesis may be performed in dogs with moderate to severe elbow osteoarthritis secondary to elbow dysplasia.

Chronic Treatment

- Medical therapy, alone or after surgery (if osteoarthritis is present), can include nonsteroidal antiinflammatory drugs (NSAIDs) and chondroprotective/joint fluid modifying agents (pp. 469 and 721).
- Physical therapy may be useful to maintain range of motion in the elbow joint.
- Intraarticular injection of autologous adipose-derived mesenchymal stem cells or platelet-rich plasma (PRP) may be useful in alleviating clinical signs associated with osteoarthritis.
  - Anecdotes suggest some efficacy for alternative pain control modalities such as acupuncture (p. 1056), but there is no proof of efficacy.

Nutrition/Diet

- Prescription joint diets may help ameliorate signs of elbow osteoarthritis.
  - High levels of omega-3 fatty acids to maintain a healthy joint environment
  - Controlled calorie content to help maintain healthy weight

Possible Complications

Continued lameness, postoperative infection, implant failure if performing lag screw fixation

Recommended Monitoring

- Suture removal and recheck at 2 postoperative weeks
- Repeat radiographs at 6 postoperative weeks if an ulnar osteotomy, lag screw fixation of the anconeal process, sliding humeral osteotomy, or partial/total elbow replacement was performed.

PROGNOSIS & OUTCOME

- Surgery will help alleviate lameness for OCD, FCP, and UAP, but most affected dogs will continue to have progressive degenerative joint disease and need medical therapy.
- Medical treatment consisting of weight control, exercise restriction, NSAIDs, and polysulfated glycosaminoglycan therapy is reported to have an outcome similar to surgical treatment of OCD and FCP.

PEARLS & CONSIDERATIONS

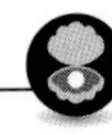

Comments

- Clinical signs of FCP may not correlate with radiographic evidence of disease.
  - Initial radiographic change is mild osteophytosis on the anconeal process.
  - Some dogs may show mild or no radiographic changes but be profoundly lame; MRI, CT, or arthroscopy is needed for diagnosis.
  - Conversely, some dogs are not lame but have radiographic evidence of degenerative joint disease.
  - Treatment is directed toward the patient, not the radiograph.
- Lameness may not be evident if bilateral forelimb disease is present.
- Because of the prevalence of bilateral disease, both elbows may undergo arthroscopy with one anesthetic episode if clinically indicated.
- The anconeal process does not fuse until 5 months of age (7 months in bassets) and cannot be diagnosed radiographically as ununited before that time.
- When manipulating the elbow to check for pain, avoid movement of the shoulder, which may obscure localization of the discomfort.

Technician Tips

Sedation of the animal for radiographs allows better positioning and quality of the images.

Client Education

Because of the hereditary component of elbow dysplasia, affected dogs should not be used for breeding.

SUGGESTED READING

Griffon DJ. Surgical diseases of the elbow. In Tobias KM, Johnston SA. Veterinary surgery small animal, St. Louis, 2012, Saunders, pp 733-751.

AUTHOR: Raviv J. Balfour, DVM, DACVS
EDITOR: Kathleen Linn, DVM, MS, DACVS

Elbow Hygroma

BASIC INFORMATION

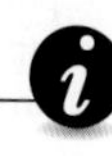

Definition

Soft-tissue swelling on lateral elbow containing serum that is located between skin and bony prominence (olecranon)

Epidemiology

SPECIES, AGE, SEX

- Short-haired large/giant dog breeds
- Usually younger than 2 years of age

RISK FACTORS

- Lying on hard surfaces
- Thin skin and small amount of subcutaneous fat
- Pressure coupled with inflammation from repetitive trauma leads to edema and fibrous tissue formation.
- Associated orthopedic disorders
  - Hip dysplasia
  - Bilateral cranial cruciate ligament disease (chronic partial tears)

Clinical Presentation

HISTORY, CHIEF COMPLAINT

- Gradual enlargement of a fluid-filled swelling over the lateral aspect of the olecranon
- Hygromas may become infected or may ulcerate, open, and drain.

PHYSICAL EXAM FINDINGS

- Fluid-filled swelling located on the lateral aspect of the olecranon
- May be unilateral or bilateral

Etiology and Pathophysiology

- Repetitive pressure or trauma to the elbow leads to accumulation of serum in the subcutaneous tissues
- Chronic lesions lead to thickening of skin, subcutaneous fibrous tissue development

DIAGNOSIS

Diagnostic Overview

Diagnostics are aimed at differentiating between a normal elbow callus, hygroma, abscess (infected hygroma), or a neoplastic lesion, as treatments differ for each problem. It is important to determine if orthopedic disease is present that may necessitate additional therapy to help offload the elbows.

Differential Diagnosis

- Abscess
- Neoplasia

Initial Database

- CBC, serum biochemistry and urinalysis: usually unremarkable
- Fine-needle aspirate (FNA)
  - Cytology: rule out neoplasia
  - Culture and sensitivity: if abscess is suspected
- Radiographs
  - Affected elbow to rule out underlying orthopedic disease, such as fracture or degenerative joint disease
  - Pelvis and stifle: rule out degenerative joint disease (hip dysplasia and chronic cruciate ligament disease)

TREATMENT

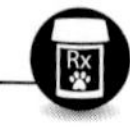

Treatment Overview

Goals are to decrease continued trauma and provide protection of the hygroma to allow healing of the fibrous tissues.

Acute and Chronic Treatment

- Treat or correct underlying orthopedic disease.
- Drainage with Penrose drains or closed suction drains can be successful, but recurrence rates are high.
- Avoid excisional surgery: hygroma resection with primary surgical closure is difficult, recurrence rates are high, and complications (dehiscence, infection) are common.
- Adjustable padded neoprene/polyester elbow sleeves are available. Long-term use is possible. Commercially available foam pipe insulation material has been used effectively.
- Bandaging to protect area is difficult.
- Provide padded bedding.

Possible Complications

- Recurrence
- Infection
  - Repeated needle drainage
  - Surgical intervention
- Chronic non-healing wound
  - Infected hygroma
  - Surgical wound dehiscence
  - Continued trauma to the hygroma

Recommended Monitoring

- Observe the affected elbow for evidence of
  - Recurrence
  - Infection of the overlying skin
  - Necrosis of the overlying skin
- Monitor for signs of underlying orthopedic disease.

PROGNOSIS & OUTCOME

Good with proper conservative management

PEARLS & CONSIDERATIONS

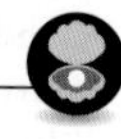

Comments

- Do not attempt surgical intervention or surgical excision of an elbow hygroma.
  - Complications are serious, common, and may become chronic after excisional surgery.
  - If surgery is considered as a last resort, refer to a veterinary soft-tissue surgical specialist.
- Injections with glucocorticoids are contraindicated and should not be used.
- A thorough orthopedic evaluation (p. 1143) should be performed in all cases.
  - Especially for evidence of hip dysplasia or chronic cranial cruciate ligament disease
- Best treatment of an elbow hygroma is for the patient to wear proper padded elbow sleeves and to pad the bedding/environment.
  - The pressure point must be off-loaded for healing.

Prevention

- Large dogs should be restricted from lying on hard surfaces.
  - Especially if there are already orthopedic problems
- Proper bedding for dogs
- Proper treatment of orthopedic diseases in large-breed dogs

Technician Tips

- Commercial products are available for the prevention and treatment of elbow hygromas.
- Familiarity with the foam pipe insulation bandage is greatly helpful for management of elbow hygromas and elbow wounds.

Client Education

It is much easier to prevent than to treat elbow hygromas.

SUGGESTED READING

Pavletic MM: Use of commercially available foam pipe insulation as a protective device for wounds over the elbow joint area in five dogs. J Am Vet Med Assoc 239(9):1225-1231, 2011.

AUTHOR: Otto I. Lanz, DVM, DACVS
EDITOR: Elizabeth A. Swanson, DVM, MS, DACVS

Elbow Luxation

Client Education Sheet

BASIC INFORMATION

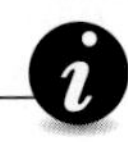

Definition

Dislocation between brachium (humerus) and antebrachium (radius and ulna)

Synonym

Elbow dislocation

Epidemiology

SPECIES, AGE, SEX

- Uncommon in dogs; rare in cats
- Any breed, age, or sex for traumatic luxations
- Juvenile dogs for congenital luxations

GENETICS, BREED PREDISPOSITION

- Congenital luxations generally are more common in small breeds of dogs, but radial head luxation specifically occurs more frequently in larger breeds.
- Suspected hereditary predisposition
- Chondrodystrophic breeds are prone to asynchronous growth between radius and ulna, resulting in subluxation.

RISK FACTORS

Forelimb trauma

ASSOCIATED DISORDERS

Some forms of congenital luxation may be associated with more generalized joint laxity syndromes.

Clinical Presentation

DISEASE FORMS/SUBTYPES

- Traumatic
- Congenital, complete
- Congenital, partial (radial head luxation only)

HISTORY, CHIEF COMPLAINT

- Forelimb trauma secondary to motor vehicle accident, fall, or rough play/fighting
- Spontaneous
- Lameness/deformity in young dog

PHYSICAL EXAM FINDINGS

- Traumatic: non–weight-bearing lameness with antebrachium and paw abducted, elbow flexed, and severe elbow swelling and pain
- Congenital: partial weight-bearing lameness and joint thickening; discomfort during range-of-motion maneuvers

Etiology and Pathophysiology

- Majority of traumatic luxations are lateral (proximal radius/ulna are lateral to distal humerus).
- Medial luxations are associated with severe soft-tissue derangements.
- Traumatic injuries may cause avulsion fracture(s) of collateral ligament(s).
- Congenital/developmental luxations and subluxations may be associated with asynchronous growth of the radius and ulna.

DIAGNOSIS

Diagnostic Overview

Diagnosis is based on history, physical exam, and radiographs (sedated patient) of the affected limb to include carpus, elbow, and shoulder joints.

Differential Diagnosis

- Distal humeral fracture
- Monteggia fracture (cranial displacement of radial head and proximal ulna fracture)
- Elbow neoplasia

Initial Database

- Craniocaudal and mediolateral radiographs of the elbow
- Survey radiographs for other traumatic injuries, especially thoracic cavity
- Radiographs of the contralateral elbow in patients with congenital or developmental luxations
- Assess for neurologic injury; check for limb withdrawal and pain sensation.

Advanced or Confirmatory Testing

CT scan useful to detect small articular lesions or fractures

TREATMENT

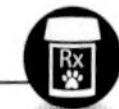

Treatment Overview

Goal of therapy is to achieve anatomic reduction of joint surfaces so normal joint mobility is restored, with eventual return to full weight bearing and elimination of discomfort.

Acute General Treatment

- Traumatic elbow luxations are best managed by early closed reduction before muscle contraction makes manipulations difficult (p. 1158).
- Patient must be anesthetized for reduction.
- Concurrent injuries may result in postponement of anesthesia and early reduction.
- If closed reduction is not achieved, open reduction and reconstruction of the collateral ligaments are indicated.
- If open reduction is needed, the limb should be bandaged to reduce patient discomfort and tissue swelling before surgery.
- Use of a modified transarticular external fixator instead of a splint can maintain joint stability, and it is in place for 3-4 weeks after reduction and/or surgery.
- Appropriate analgesics should be administered.
- Congenital luxations are less amenable to closed reduction, which is best attempted at 4 months of age or younger.
- Congenital luxations may require osteotomies or ostectomies for treatment.
- Surgical intervention for congenital luxations may slow progression of osteoarthritis. However, some dogs with radial head luxation do well with conservative management.

Chronic Treatment

- Immobilization with elbow bandaged in extension for 1-2 weeks
- Initially, a heavy padded bandage (or more rigid splint; spica splints preferred for open reductions and those with severe collateral ligament damage), with gradual reduction in bandage thickness/stiffness as swelling subsides and stability increases
- Gentle, passive range-of-motion (flexion/extension) physiotherapy instituted after bandage removal
- Continued use of analgesic/antiinflammatory agents as needed for patient comfort

Possible Complications

- Recurrent luxation/instability: most common complication
- Articular cartilage damage and secondary osteoarthritis
- Reduced range of motion from pericapsular fibrosis
- Chronic lameness

Recommended Monitoring

- Postreduction radiographs to confirm restoration of joint congruency
- Weekly bandage check/change until removal
- Lameness evaluations 2, 4, and 8 weeks after surgery; radiographs at 2 weeks and at 6-8 weeks if open reduction/implants

PROGNOSIS & OUTCOME

- Most dogs and cats with properly treated traumatic luxations will return to normal or near-normal function.
- Chronic fibrosis will result in a permanently thickened elbow.
- More guarded prognosis for congenital/developmental luxations
- Severe complications/failures might necessitate salvage surgery (arthrodesis, total joint arthroplasty, or amputation).

PEARLS & CONSIDERATIONS

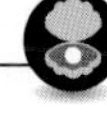

Comments

- Early diagnosis is critical for promoting successful closed reduction.
- Closed reduction for a lateral luxation is achieved by flexing elbow (moves anconeal process caudally), followed by abduction of the antebrachium, with the paw flexed (moves anconeal process medially, attempting to hook anconeal process medial to lateral epicondylar crest of the humerus), followed by adduction and pronation of the antebrachium (attempting to snap the radial head medially to its proper location under the capitulum of the humerus as the anconeal process acts as a fulcrum).
- Can consider temporary pharmacologic paralysis of the patient (requires ventilation

of patient for gas exchange) to achieve greater muscle relaxation to facilitate reduction maneuvers

Technician Tips

Patients should be checked weekly to detect secondary wounds that may result from bandage/splint contact.

Client Education

- Bandage/splint care
- Controlled activity (kennel/leash)
- Passive range-of-motion physiotherapy after removal
- Neuter dogs with congenital luxations because of potential heritability.

SUGGESTED READING

Griffon DJ: Surgical diseases of the elbow. In Tobias KM, et al, editors: Veterinary surgery small animal. St. Louis, 2012, Elsevier, pp 725-732.

AUTHOR: Mary E. Somerville, DVM, DACVS
EDITOR: Kathleen Linn, DVM, MS, DACVS

Electrocution

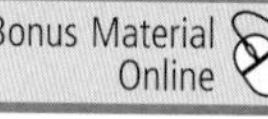

BASIC INFORMATION

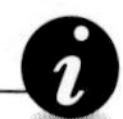

Definition

The passage of electricity through tissue, resulting in electrophysiologic disruption of the tissue

Epidemiology

SPECIES, AGE, SEX

Most common in young cats and dogs (5 weeks to 1.5 years of age), with no sex predisposition

RISK FACTORS

Young age and environmental access

GEOGRAPHY AND SEASONALITY

Seasonal associations: Christmas holidays (decorative holiday lights); possibly late spring to early autumn, when owners are more likely to operate corded electrical devices (e.g., fans)

ASSOCIATED DISORDERS

Noncardiogenic pulmonary edema, cardiac arrhythmias, oral burns, and seizures

Clinical Presentation

DISEASE FORMS/SUBTYPES

- High-voltage injury versus low-voltage injury, based on the nature and intensity of the current. The most severe injuries are caused by high-current, high-voltage discharge and result in a worse clinical outcome.
- Electrical sources can produce energy levels that range from relatively low (e.g., 9-volt battery) to intermediate (e.g., household outlets) to very high (e.g., electrical metal utility cover). Household current is the most common exposure.

HISTORY, CHIEF COMPLAINT

Sometimes witnessed; other times the owner reports sudden onset of dyspnea, collapse, or dysphagia. Owner finds chewed wires/bite marks on electrical cords.

PHYSICAL EXAM FINDINGS

- Oral burns to the tongue, palate, and commissures of the lips; ptyalism
- Respiratory problems: dyspnea (harsh lung sounds, upper airway edema), cyanosis, coughing
- Cardiac problems: arrhythmias (ventricular fibrillation), asystole
- Neurologic abnormalities: loss of consciousness, focal muscle tremors, seizures

Etiology and Pathophysiology

- Electricity (usually 60 Hz of alternating current and 120 volts in most households in North and much of South America; in most of the rest of the world, it is usually 50-60 Hz alternating current and 220 volts) disrupts the electrophysiologic activity of tissue, causing muscle spasms, ventricular arrhythmias, and vasomotor changes in the central nervous system, resulting in acute pulmonary edema. The electrical energy is also transformed into heat, which can cause coagulation of tissue proteins. Sudden death may result from these processes.
- Electrocution is almost always accidental, typically from a young pet chewing on an electrical cord.

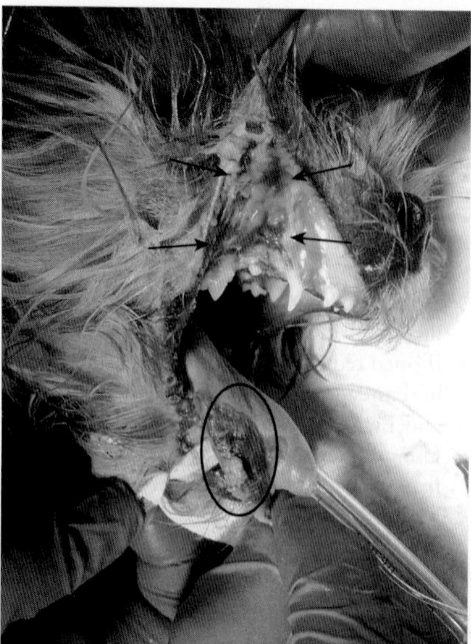

ELECTROCUTION Electrical cord injury in a Yorkshire terrier puppy. Note the extensive, circumscribed sloughing of the tongue *(oval)* and linear necrotic lesion of the lateral canthus of the lips *(arrows)*. (Courtesy Dr. Gareth Buckley, University of Florida Veterinary Teaching Hospital.)

DIAGNOSIS

Diagnostic Overview

If unwitnessed, the diagnosis is suspected in a young pet with characteristic oral burns and dyspnea. Thoracic radiographs classically show noncardiogenic pulmonary edema (interstitial/alveolar pattern with a caudodorsal distribution [p. 836]).

Differential Diagnosis

Chemical or thermal burns, exposure to fire, smoke inhalation, other causes of respiratory distress

Initial Database

Initial database requirements depend on the severity of injury. In some cases, if the animal has no physical exam abnormalities, no testing is required. In other cases, if the pet is dyspneic or pulmonary crackles are ausculted, chest radiographs are warranted. For severely affected animals, CBC, serum biochemistry profile, coagulation profile, and urinalysis are warranted.

Advanced or Confirmatory Testing

Pulse oximetry or arterial blood gas analysis may be useful to document hypoxemia. However, in young or small animals, the stress of arterial blood sample collection should be weighed against the potential benefits.

TREATMENT

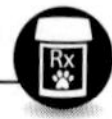

Treatment Overview

Treatment mainly consists of supportive care, but the degree of intervention depends on severity. Burns should be cleaned; if severe, surgical debridement is indicated after the patient is stable. Noncardiogenic pulmonary edema is treated with supplemental oxygen administration. If severe or if pharyngeal edema is present, intubation and mechanical ventilation may be necessary.

Acute General Treatment

Noncardiogenic pulmonary edema is treated with rest and supplemental oxygen (pp. 836

and 1146). The most severe cases may require mechanical ventilation (p. 1185).

Chronic Treatment

Treat burns with antibiotics, wound cleaning, surgical debridement, and closure, as needed. Soft food can be fed or a feeding tube used if burns are in the mouth. Puppies will commonly eat despite severe oral injury.

Nutrition/Diet

Offer soft or blenderized food. If oral burns are severe and the patient will not eat, enteral nutrition may be instituted by placement of a nasoesophageal (p. 1107) or esophagostomy (p. 1106) tube.

Possible Complications

Infection of non-healing burns, acute respiratory distress syndrome. A rare but possible long-term complication is cataract formation.

Recommended Monitoring

Respiratory rate and effort (± assessment of oxygenation) should be monitored frequently until stabilized. Healing of burns also should be monitored.

PROGNOSIS & OUTCOME

Depends on the degree of pulmonary edema. Overall survival appears to be greater for cats than dogs. Critical period is the first 24-48 hours after electrical shock; if the animal survives this period, it will likely survive to discharge with minimal or no permanent aftereffects.

PEARLS & CONSIDERATIONS

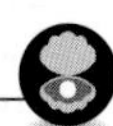

Comments

Noncardiogenic pulmonary edema can be difficult to treat. Treatment is symptomatic, with no specific recommendations.

Prevention

When left unobserved, puppies and kittens should be crated or otherwise confined so access to electrical cords can be avoided.

Technician Tips

When administering treatments, stress should be minimized, and treatments should be conducted in a stepwise manner.

Client Education

Education about re-exposure and removal of damaged or faulty electrical cords

SUGGESTED READING

Mann FA: Electrical and lightning injuries. In Silverstein DC, et al, editors: Small animal critical care medicine, St. Louis, 2009, Saunders, p 687.

AUTHOR: Megan Whelan, DVM, DACVECC, CVA
EDITOR: Benjamin M. Brainard, VMD, DACVAA, DACVECC

Encephalopathy, Vascular

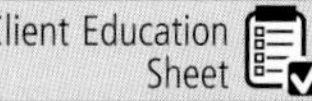

BASIC INFORMATION

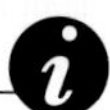

Definition

Brain dysfunction resulting from a disease process that compromises its blood supply; categorized as ischemic (due to occlusion of a vessel) or hemorrhagic (due to rupture of vasculature). It can involve a focal region or the entire brain. Clinical signs correlate to the neuroanatomic area that is affected (forebrain, cerebellum, brainstem).

Synonyms

Stroke, infarction, vascular event, cerebrovascular accident

Epidemiology

SPECIES, AGE, SEX

Any species, age, or sex can be affected.

GENETICS, BREED PREDISPOSITION

Greyhounds and Cavalier King Charles spaniels are overrepresented in ischemic cerebrovascular disease.

RISK FACTORS

- Focal ischemic events can be associated with hypertension or a hypercoagulable state. Diseases that can cause a hypercoagulable state include hyperadrenocorticism, renal disease (particularly protein-losing nephropathy), and neoplasia.
- Hemorrhagic infarcts can be seen in association with diseases that induce a hypocoagulable state, such as liver failure, sepsis, immune-mediated thrombocytopenia, and disseminated intravascular coagulation.
- Global cerebral hypoxia is most commonly seen with adverse anesthetic events or after resuscitation from cardiopulmonary arrest.

GEOGRAPHY AND SEASONALITY

- Some cases of feline ischemic vascular events in North America have been linked to intracranial migration of *Cuterebra* larva.
- *Angiostrongylus vasorum*, a parasite of the European mainland and Atlantic Canada, can induce marked coagulation abnormalities that result in intracranial hemorrhage in dogs.

Clinical Presentation

DISEASE FORMS/SUBTYPES

- Cerebrovascular accidents are ischemic or hemorrhagic in nature; ischemic events are more common.
- Ischemic events are further classified as lacunar or territorial infarctions, depending on the size of the vessel involved.
- Global ischemia occurs infrequently and is usually associated with an adverse anesthetic event.

HISTORY, CHIEF COMPLAINT

The chief complaint will vary depending on the region of the brain affected, but clinical signs are characteristically peracute to acute in onset and nonprogressive after 24 hours. Common presenting signs include seizures, behavioral changes, circling, falling, or difficulty walking.

PHYSICAL EXAM FINDINGS

- General physical examination findings can be unremarkable or reveal abnormalities in another organ system that can suggest a predisposing disease.
- Neurologic examination findings will vary depending on the part of the brain affected.
  - Cerebellum: hypermetria, head tilt, ataxia, and intention tremors
  - Forebrain: circling, seizures, changes in vision, proprioceptive deficits, and rarely, vestibular signs

Etiology and Pathophysiology

- Ischemia to brain tissue causes decreased oxygen delivery and impairs energy metabolism, leading to neurologic dysfunction.
- Dysfunction can range from mild (with reversible signs) to severe (causing brain necrosis).

DIAGNOSIS

Diagnostic Overview

Vascular encephalopathy should be considered in animals with a peracute onset of nonprogressive signs of brain dysfunction. Definitive diagnosis is based on findings from MRI of the brain. Animals with a cerebrovascular accident should be screened thoroughly for a predisposing disease. If an underlying cause is recognized, appropriate treatment can help prevent recurrence.

Differential Diagnosis

- Neoplasia
- Inflammatory disease, sterile or infectious
- Trauma

Initial Database

- CBC, serum biochemistry profile: evaluate for underlying disease, thrombocytopenia
- Urinalysis by cystocentesis: screen for proteinuria
  - Urine protein to creatinine ratio: if proteinuria present to confirm protein-losing nephropathy
- Serial blood pressure measurements: systolic pressure greater than 180 mm Hg in the presence of neurologic signs supportive of hypertensive encephalopathy
- Funduscopic examination: evaluate for hemorrhage or tortuous vessels
- Thoracic radiographs: screen for cardiovascular disease and metastatic neoplasia
- Abdominal ultrasound, if indicated
- Testing for adrenal and thyroid disease, if indicated

Advanced or Confirmatory Testing

- Thromboelastography (TEG): evaluate for hypercoagulability
- Coagulation profile (prothrombin time/partial thromboplastin time): evaluate for hypocoagulability
- MRI of brain (p. 1132): diagnostic test of choice
  - Diffusion-weighted imaging to confirm ischemia
  - Gradient recalled echo sequences to evaluate for hemorrhage
- Cerebrospinal fluid analysis (p. 1323): may be normal or show mild, nonspecific changes

TREATMENT

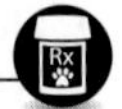

Treatment Overview

There is no definitive treatment for brain infarction other than supportive care. If an underlying disease is identified, treatment of that condition is recommended to prevent recurrence.

Acute General Treatment

- Anticonvulsant therapy should be instituted in an animal that presents with seizures. Therapy should be continued for a minimum of 3-6 months and can then potentially be tapered if no further seizures are noted.
- For vestibular signs: maropitant 1 mg/kg SQ q 24h (dog) or 2 mg/kg PO q 24h for up to 5 days; 1 mg/kg SQ or PO q 24h for up to 5 days (cat), or meclizine 25 mg PO q 24h (dog); 12.5 mg PO q 24h (cat) is recommended to treat nausea and ptyalism.

Chronic Treatment

Treat any underlying condition.

Possible Complications

- Aspiration pneumonia associated with recumbency or vestibular dysfunction
- Recurrence of vascular event

Recommended Monitoring

- Serial neurologic examinations
- Serial blood pressure measurements if hypertensive

PROGNOSIS & OUTCOME

The prognosis for focal cerebrovascular accidents in dogs and cats is generally good. Global ischemic events carry a more guarded prognosis.

PEARLS & CONSIDERATIONS

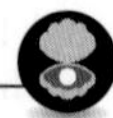

Comments

Although previously thought to be uncommon, cerebrovascular disease is a well-recognized cause of brain dysfunction in dogs and cats, and increases in frequency with age.

Prevention

Appropriate treatment of underlying disease is important to prevent further cerebrovascular accidents. For some hypercoagulable states, chronic use of platelet antagonists or anticoagulants may be indicated.

Technician Tips

Recovery from a cerebrovascular accident should be slow and steady. Worsening signs call for reevaluation of the diagnosis.

Client Education

Strokes tend to have a much better prognosis for dogs and cats than humans. In most cases, recovery can be expected to occur over the course of several weeks.

SUGGESTED READING

Garosi LS: Cerebrovascular disease in dogs and cats. Vet Clin North Am Small Anim Pract 40:65-79, 2010.

AUTHOR: Sheila Carrera-Justiz, DVM, DACVIM
EDITOR: Karen R. Muñana, DVM, MS, DACVIM

Endocarditis, Infective

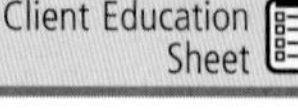

BASIC INFORMATION

Definition

Endocarditis is inflammation of the endocardium (inner surface) of the heart. *Infective endocarditis* (IE) is a microbial infection of the endocardium, involving the valve leaflets, chordae tendineae, and/or mural surfaces. *Vegetative endocarditis* describes the formation of small masses (vegetations) composed of platelets, fibrin, microorganisms, and inflammatory cells at the site of infection. Endocarditis (term and disease) is unrelated to the most common form of chronic valvular heart disease in dogs, myxomatous/degenerative valve disease or *endocardiosis.*

Epidemiology

SPECIES, AGE, SEX

- Uncommon in dogs, rare in cats
- Middle-aged to older, large-breed, male dogs are most commonly affected.

RISK FACTORS

- Conditions causing endothelial damage can lead to colonization of affected tissue by circulating bacteria.
  - Dogs with congenital subaortic stenosis (SAS) are predisposed to IE, presumably due to valvular endothelial damage by turbulent blood flow. Sporadic cases of IE have been reported with other forms of congenital heart disease.
  - Endocardial trauma (e.g., heart surgery, interventional cardiac catheterization)
- Bacteremia: possible sources include intravenous catheters, discospondylitis, prostatitis, periodontal disease, pneumonia, and pyoderma.
- Immune suppression may be a factor.

GEOGRAPHY AND SEASONALITY

IE is recognized more frequently in warmer climates (e.g., southern and western United States).

Clinical Presentation

DISEASE FORMS/SUBTYPES

Endocarditis can be classified based on mode of presentation (acute, subacute, or chronic) or according to location.

HISTORY, CHIEF COMPLAINT

- Nonspecific signs such as lethargy, weakness, weight loss, and anorexia
- History of fever is common.
- Reluctance to move (back pain, polyarthritis)
- Intermittent lameness (muscle embolization, polyarthritis)

PHYSICAL EXAM FINDINGS

Most patients diagnosed with IE have a heart murmur:

- Auscultation may reveal a new murmur or worsening of a known murmur (change in intensity, quality, timing, or duration). Some animals with IE have a pre-existing heart murmur (e.g., from SAS). The presence of a diastolic murmur in a systemically ill animal dramatically raises the index of suspicion for IE.

- Respiratory abnormalities (e.g., tachypnea, dyspnea, cough) when congestive heart failure (CHF) is present
- Musculoskeletal abnormalities (e.g., lameness, joint pain/stiffness)
- Neurologic abnormalities (e.g., ataxia)

Etiology and Pathophysiology

- The left-sided heart valves (aortic and/or mitral) are affected most commonly in canine and feline IE.
- *Staphylococcus* spp, *Streptococcus* spp, and *Escherichia coli* are the most common isolates. Less commonly isolated pathogens include *Pseudomonas, Proteus, Erysipelothrix, Enterobacter, Pasteurella*, and *Corynebacterium.*
- *Bartonella* spp is a common cause of culture-negative IE and appears to have tropism for the aortic valve.
- Anaerobic bacteria (e.g., *Bacteroides*) are uncommon.

DIAGNOSIS

Diagnostic Overview

The diagnosis of IE is based on a constellation of clinical, microbiologic, and echocardiographic findings. The modified Duke criteria, which represent the cornerstone of diagnosis of human IE, have been adapted for veterinary use. Definitive IE is based on the presence of 2 major criteria or histopathologic confirmation. Possible IE is based on positive echocardiographic findings and 1 minor criterion, 1 major and 3 minor criteria, or 5 minor criteria. The following criteria have been suggested for the diagnosis of IE in dogs:

- Major criteria: positive echocardiogram (vegetative/oscillating lesion; erosive lesion; valve/mural abscess), new valvular insufficiency and/or aortic insufficiency, positive blood culture (≥ 2 positive blood cultures isolating a typical organism or > 3 positive blood cultures with common skin contaminant)
- Minor criteria: fever, medium-sized to large dog (>15 kg), SAS, thromboembolic disease, immune-mediated disease (e.g., polyarthritis; glomerulonephritis), positive blood culture not meeting major criteria, *Bartonella* titer or positive PCR using BAPGM (i.e., *Bartonella* alpha-Proteobacteria growth medium; Galaxy Diagnostics, Morrisville, NC)

Differential Diagnosis

- Other systemic illness with nonspecific complaints (e.g., fever, inappetence, weight loss, lameness)
- IE should be considered in any patient with fever of unknown origin, especially in the presence of a heart murmur.

Initial Database

- CBC and serum biochemical changes are not specific. Anemia, leukocytosis (neutrophilia and monocytosis), thrombocytopenia, hypoalbuminemia, and azotemia are common.
- Urinalysis may reveal pyuria, hematuria, and proteinuria. Bacteruria may be present. Urine should be submitted for aerobic bacterial culture.
- Thoracic radiographs may show evidence of CHF.
- Echocardiography may show an independently oscillating mass associated with a heart valve or adjacent structures; independently oscillating means that movements of the mass are distinct and different from those of the valve. Valve thickening from myxomatous/degenerative valvular disease can complicate echocardiographic interpretation. Some animals have mural endocarditis without valvular involvement.

Advanced or Confirmatory Testing

- Three separate blood samples (5-10 mL each, patient size permitting), obtained aseptically by separate venipunctures at least 30-60 minutes apart, should be submitted for aerobic and anaerobic culture.
  - In acutely ill patients, three blood cultures 5-10 minutes apart are adequate.
  - Common causes of culture-negative IE are previous antibiotic therapy and infection by fastidious microorganisms.
- Identification of *Bartonella* spp typically requires PCR and culture using BAPGM.
  - *Bartonella* serologic testing is useful to identify antibody titers.
- PCR amplification of 16S ribosomal bacterial DNA used in conjunction with standard blood cultures increases the likelihood of bacterial isolation.
- An electrocardiogram to identify any arrhythmia or conduction disturbance (e.g., atrioventricular block), increasing the suspicion of perivalvular extension
- Arthrocentesis (p. 1059) with joint fluid analysis and culture in dogs exhibiting lameness
- Urine protein/creatinine (UPC) ratio in dogs with proteinuria

TREATMENT

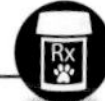

Treatment Overview

- Provide effective antibiotic therapy to minimize valve damage.
- Manage complications (e.g., CHF, thromboembolism, polyarthritis).
- Surgical valve repair or replacement, considered in human IE cases, is not practical in veterinary medicine.

Acute General Treatment

- Hospitalization and aggressive treatment with parenteral antibiotics for 1-2 weeks is ideal after blood cultures are obtained. Antibiotic therapy can be completed on an outpatient basis using oral antibiotics.
- Antibiotic selection should be based on results of blood culture and susceptibility profile if possible. Pending culture results or in cases of culture-negative IE, empirical antibiotic therapy is warranted.
- Empirical IV antibiotic therapy in dogs may include a combination of an extended-spectrum penicillin (e.g., ampicillin with sulbactam 22 mg/kg IV q 8h), with a fluoroquinolone (e.g., enrofloxacin 5 mg/kg IV q12h) or aminoglycoside (e.g., amikacin). Amikacin may be preferable against *Bartonella*, but requires monitoring for nephrotoxicity.
- Treatment of CHF if indicated (p. 408).
- Anticoagulation does not appear to diminish the risk of bacterial embolization in humans and should be considered on a case-by-case basis.

Chronic Treatment

- Oral antibiotic therapy is generally continued for 6-10 weeks and is based on culture and sensitivity results. In culture-negative cases, empirical oral therapy may include an extended-spectrum penicillin (e.g., amoxicillin with clavulanic acid 14 mg/kg PO q 12h), fluoroquinolone (e.g., enrofloxacin 10 mg/kg PO q 24h) and doxycycline 5 mg/kg PO q 12h. Repeat blood and urine cultures (and potentially 16S PCR) are ideal after starting antibiotic therapy and again 1-2 weeks after stopping antibiotics. Long-term therapy may be warranted in dogs with recurrent clinical and/or persistent diagnostic abnormalities.
- Repeat echocardiograms to monitor the size/appearance of vegetative lesion(s), severity of valvular regurgitation, and extent of cardiac chamber dilation.
- Treatment of chronic CHF if indicated (p. 409).

Possible Complications

- CHF
- Kidney injury (glomerulonephritis/protein-losing nephropathy, chronic kidney disease, or both) and/or neurologic complications, secondary to embolic events and organ (various) infarction
- Immune-mediated disease (e.g., glomerulonephritis, polyarthritis)
- Sudden death, due to malignant arrhythmia and/or infarction caused by embolization

PROGNOSIS & OUTCOME

- Overall prognosis is guarded to grave due to the possibilities of embolic complications and CHF. Long-term survival is possible in the absence of CHF or severe neurologic complications.
- CHF (pulmonary edema) is common, resulting from volume overload caused by severe aortic insufficiency and/or severe mitral regurgitation.
- Prognosis appears to vary, depending on the valve affected; aortic valve IE is often associated with a grave prognosis (days to weeks, especially grave in the presence of CHF or severe neurologic signs); longer survival is more typical of mitral valve IE as long as

CHF or severe neurologic complications are not present initially.
- Recurrence or treatment failure is likely with inadequate duration of therapy, inappropriate antibiotic selection, or owner nonadherence to prescribed treatment.
- Despite optimal therapy and monitoring, cure rates for IE do not appear promising for dogs, and CHF or other serious or fatal complications are common.

PEARLS & CONSIDERATIONS

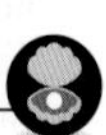

Comments

- Although IE and myxomatous/degenerative valve endocardiosis can cause valve thickening and heart murmurs, the two conditions typically differ dramatically in patient signalment, history, murmur duration, location, quality, timing, and clinical presentation.
- A high index of suspicion is justified for any animal with fever (or history of fever) and a new murmur, particularly a diastolic murmur. Diastolic murmurs are typically soft, blowing, decrescendo, and best heard at the left heart base.
- Identification of an independently oscillating mass (vegetation), along with suggestive clinical signs, is consistent with IE.
- Culture-negative IE is common in veterinary medicine, often warranting empirical antibiotic therapy.

Prevention

- Animals with SAS, implanted cardiac devices (e.g., transvenous pacemakers), and other conditions potentially causing endothelial damage should receive routine antibiotic prophylaxis for all procedures that are likely to induce transient bacteremia. By extrapolation from the current American Heart Association Guidelines, recommended antibiotic prophylaxis consists of a single oral or IV antibiotic dose (e.g., cefazolin 22 mg/kg IV) before the start of the procedure.
- Year-round use of ectoparastie prevention should reduce the risk of bartonellosis.

Technician Tips

- Animals with IE are usually very ill, and symptoms of sepsis are common.
- IE is an important cause of diastolic heart murmur.

SUGGESTED READING

MacDonald K: Infective endocarditis in dogs: diagnosis and therapy. Vet Clin North Am 40:665-684, 2010.

AUTHORS: Sandra P. Tou, DVM, DACVIM; Bruce W. Keene, DVM, MSc, DACVIM
EDITOR: Meg M. Sleeper VMD, DACVIM

Entropion/Ectropion

Client Education Sheet 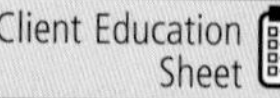 Bonus Material Online 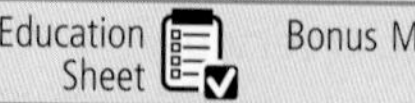

BASIC INFORMATION

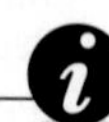

Definition

- Entropion is inversion of part of or the entire eyelid margin toward the globe; it can be developmental or acquired.
- Ectropion is eversion of part of or the entire eyelid margin away from the globe; it can be developmental or acquired.

Synonyms

Inrolled eyelid (entropion); everted eyelid (ectropion)

Epidemiology

SPECIES, AGE, SEX

Entropion:
- Common in dogs; rare in cats
- Can occur at any age; developmental entropion usually occurs in dogs < 1 year of age
- Can occur at any age in cats but usually older cats

Ectropion:
- Dogs (variable ages depending on the cause)

GENETICS, BREED PREDISPOSITION

- Developmental (conformational) entropion:
  - Lateral entropion: English bulldog, chow chow, Shar-pei, Saint Bernard, boxer, rottweiler, pointers, spaniels, and all retrievers
  - Medial canthal entropion: miniature and toy poodles, English bulldog, Cavalier King Charles spaniel, Maltese, and brachycephalic breeds, including Pekingese, pug and shih tzu; brachycephalic cats
  - Genetics not fully understood; most likely polygenic but could be inherited as a dominant trait with incomplete penetrance or a recessive trait
- Developmental ectropion: bloodhound, Saint Bernard, Great Dane, bullmastiff, Newfoundland, and some spaniel breeds
- Combination entropion-ectropion affecting the same lid: bloodhound, Saint Bernard, and English bulldog

RISK FACTORS

- Developmental entropion and ectropion: breed predispositions
- Acquired entropion
  - Conditions that stimulate blepharospasm (e.g., corneal ulceration)
  - Eyelid trauma
  - Blepharitis
  - Older age and associated loss of orbital fat (especially cats)
  - Phthisis bulbi (p. 705)
  - Enophthalmos
- Acquired ectropion
  - Eyelid trauma
  - Blepharitis
  - Old age and associated loss of orbicularis oculi muscle tone
  - Facial nerve paralysis

ASSOCIATED DISORDERS

- Conjunctivitis
- Keratitis (ulcerative and nonulcerative)
- See Risk Factors above

Clinical Presentation

DISEASE FORMS/SUBTYPES

- Developmental: secondary to abnormal or poor conformation, may be congenital, juvenile, or senile (entropion and ectropion)
- Spastic (entropion)
- Cicatricial (entropion and ectropion)

HISTORY, CHIEF COMPLAINT

Entropion:
- Ocular discharge
- Blepharospasm
- Red eye
- Visible inrolling of eyelid
- ± Vision impairment in severe cases

Ectropion:
- Ocular discharge
- Red eye
- Droopy/long lower eyelid

PHYSICAL EXAM FINDINGS

Entropion:
- Inversion of the eyelid and any of the following:
  - Conjunctivitis (pp. 199 and 200)
  - Epiphora, mucoid or mucopurulent ocular discharge
  - Blepharospasm
  - Protrusion of the third eyelid
  - Nonulcerative keratitis (pp. 206 and 212)
  - Ulcerative keratitis (p. 209)
  - Corneal sequestration in cats (p. 208)
  - Enophthalmos secondary to atrophy of retrobulbar fat in cats

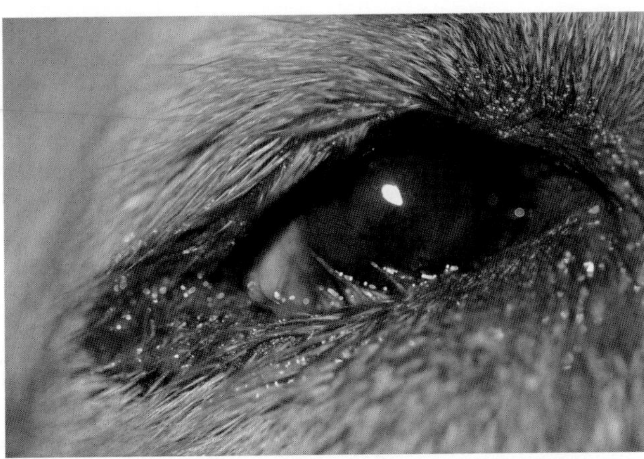

ENTROPION/ECTROPION Entropion of the ventral lateral eyelid of the right eye in a dog. Note the facial hairs (trichiasis) rubbing on the lateral corneal surface, causing corneal pigmentation and fibrosis (keratitis), with mild ocular discharge adhered to the facial hairs.

Ectropion:
- Eversion of the lower eyelid and some or all of the following:
  - Conjunctivitis
  - Keratitis
  - Lagophthalmos (incomplete closure of the eyelids)

Etiology and Pathophysiology

Dogs:
- Developmental entropion (conformational)
  - Can be congenital or juvenile in onset
  - Related to abnormal skull and palpebral fissure (eyelid opening) conformation
  - Associated with misdirection of the lateral canthal ligament in mesaticephalic (intermediate facial somatotype; neither brachycephalic nor dolichocephalic) breeds
  - Associated with ptosis and weight from excessive dorsal skinfolds: upper eyelid entropion
  - Associated with microblepharon (small eyelids)
- Acquired entropion
  - Decreased orbital support (decreased orbital mass, phthisis bulbi, or retractor bulbi muscle contraction) predisposes to loss of lid support (involutional entropion)
  - Secondary to blepharospasm and enopthalmus from pain (spastic entropion)
  - Secondary to scarring and contraction of the eyelid from a previous eyelid injury and/or inflammation (cicatricial entropion)
- Developmental ectropion
  - Mild ectropion is a desired feature in some breeds (i.e., hounds).
  - Related to abnormal skull and palpebral fissure confirmation
  - Associated with laxity of the palpebral fissure related to macroblepharon
- Acquired ectropion
  - Transient ectropion results from the laxity of the eyelid from relaxation or following excessive exercise in breeds with long lower eyelids.
  - Scarring and contraction of the eyelid from a previous eyelid injury and/or inflammation
  - Facial nerve paralysis

Cats:
- Developmental entropion (rare)
  - Medial canthal entropion in brachycephalic breeds
- Acquired entropion
  - Decreased orbital support associated with loss of orbital and periorbital fat predisposes to loss of eyelid support (usually older cats) (involutional entropion)
  - Secondary to blepharospasm, related to conjunctival and corneal irritation (spastic)
  - Associated with scarring and contraction from chronic conjunctival and/or eyelid inflammation (cicatricial)

DIAGNOSIS

Diagnostic Overview

The diagnosis of entropion is based on the presence of ocular irritation (epiphora, conjunctivitis, or keratitis) and is confirmed by identification of abnormal lid confirmation (inversion of part of or the entire eyelid). Ectropion is diagnosed on physical exam: eversion of the lower eyelid. For both disorders, an ophthalmic exam is indicated to identify lesions caused by the eyelid malformation and determine the cause of eyelid malformation.

Differential Diagnosis

Entropion:
- Usually diagnosed on clinical exam; must be differentiated from
  - Distichiasis: one or more cilia emerge from the meibomian glands instead of the normal peripheral lid margin.
  - Trichiasis: normal eyelid or facial hair directed toward and contacting the conjunctiva or cornea

Ectropion:
- Usually diagnosed based on clinical exam: apparent even before handling the patient

Initial Database

Complete ophthalmic exam (p. 1137):
- Schirmer tear test (normal > 15 mm after 1 minute in dogs, varies in cats)
- Fluorescein dye application
- Intraocular pressures
- Careful examination of confirmation of eyelid margins, conjunctiva, and cornea

Advanced or Confirmatory Testing

- Varies, depending on underlying cause of entropion and/or ectropion
- With entropion, apply topical anesthetic (e.g., proparacaine 0.5%) to evaluate degree of spastic entropion (i.e., entropion secondary to ocular pain) vs. developmental entropion. Spastic entropion secondary to painful ocular disease such as ulcerative keratitis temporarily resolves or decreases in severity within a few minutes of application. Many dogs with developmental entropion will also have a spastic component.
- Examine animal in a relaxed state to determine extent of entropion and/or ectropion and to select most appropriate corrective surgical procedure; restraining the animal or manipulation of the head during examination can increase the severity of blepharospasm and exaggerate the degree of entropion.

TREATMENT

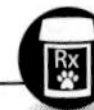

Treatment Overview

- Treatment goals for entropion include resolution of underlying painful ocular disorders (e.g., conjunctivitis, keratitis) for spastic entropion and surgical repair for developmental (conformational) entropion.
- Treatment goals for ectropion are to restore normal lid conformation only if severe and predisposing to chronic ocular irritation and keratitis. Mild ectropion is normal for many large-breed dogs.

Acute General Treatment

Entropion:
- Treat underlying condition(s).
- Temporary correction in puppies until adult conformation reached (developmental entropion in puppies) or until underlying condition resolved (spastic entropion)
  - Roll eyelids away from eye by placing temporary tacking (vertical mattress sutures) or temporary tarsorrhaphy sutures to prevent chronic ocular pain and blepharospasm and to prevent or treat corneal ulceration, pigmentation, vascularization, and scarring.
  - If successful, condition may not require permanent repair.
- Permanent surgical correction once adult confirmation is reached and no underlying condition (see Chronic Treatment)

Chronic Treatment

Chronic entropion in mature animals requires surgery to evert the eyelid margin. Procedures

other than the modified Hotz-Celsus are rarely done and may require referral. The amount of skin to be removed must be determined before sedation or anesthesia.
- Cases of mild entropion
  - Consider modified Hotz-Celsus procedure (involves elliptical skin incision adjacent to the eyelid margin).
- Lateral canthal entropion
  - Creation or cutting of the lateral canthal ligament (modified Wyman's lateral canthoplasty or lateral canthal tenotomy, respectively)
  - Modified Hotz-Celsus and eyelid-shortening procedures may be required.
- Medial canthal entropion
  - Medial canthoplasty procedure (e.g., pocket flap or Wyman technique)
  - Localized modified Hotz-Celsus procedure
- Ptosis and upper eyelid entropion
  - Stades procedure to evert upper eyelid margin

Ectropion:
- Surgery rarely needed unless severe or if concurrent entropion is present
- Cases of severe ectropion: consider modified Kuhnt-Szymanowski technique (lid-shortening technique)
- Cicatricial (scar-induced) ectropion: V-Y blepharoplasty may be used.

Possible Complications
- Temporary tacking sutures may pull through the skin, requiring repeat procedure(s) until animal is mature or until underlying condition is resolved.
- Undercorrection or overcorrection of entropion
- Correction of subclinical ectropion predisposes to entropion.
- Surgical correction of spastic entropion leads to ectropion.

Recommended Monitoring
- Leave temporary tacking sutures or temporary tarsorrhaphy in place until adult conformation is reached or for 2-3 weeks, until concurrent ocular disease resolves.
- Permanent entropion and/or ectropion repairs require suture removal approximately 10-14 days after surgery if nonabsorbable suture is used. Absorbable polyglactin 910 (Vicryl or Vicryl Rapide) is excellent for this use because it becomes soft when wet and does not require removal.

PROGNOSIS & OUTCOME

- Prognosis for restoring normal eyelid confirmation is good.
- Recurrence of entropion is possible, depending on underlying cause and surgical treatment.

PEARLS & CONSIDERATIONS

Comments
- Treat any concurrent ocular disease before surgically addressing entropion.
- Determination of whether the entropion is spastic or developmental is paramount when determining the course of treatment (tacking vs. surgical).
- No single surgical procedure is effective for correction of all forms of entropion and/or ectropion (see Chronic Treatment above).
- The modified Hotz-Celsus can be used on any area of the lid for entropion, and its size and shape vary with the location and severity of the entropion.
- Surgical overcorrection of entropion could result in ectropion; therefore, err on the side of caution. Future surgical correction of undercorrection is much easier to manage.
- Correction of naturally occurring ectropion is rarely needed unless it is severe or occurs in conjunction with entropion on the same eyelid.

Prevention
Avoid breeding affected or closely related dogs with developmental entropion or clinically significant developmental ectropion.

Technician Tips
Any animal that has entropion should have a Schirmer tear test and fluorescein stain done.

Client Education
If the initial repair is ineffective or the disease progresses, additional surgical procedures may be required. Many large-breed dogs with ectropion develop conjunctivitis, but that alone does not warrant surgery. Some kennel clubs prohibit showing of dogs that have had cosmetic surgeries.

SUGGESTED READING

Maggs DJ: The eyelids. In Maggs DJ, editor: Slatter's fundamentals of veterinary ophthalmology, ed 5, St. Louis, 2013, Elsevier.

RELATED CLIENT EDUCATION SHEETS

How to Administer Eye Medications
How to Assemble and Use an Elizabethan Collar

AUTHOR: Shannon D. Boveland, DVM, DACVO
EDITOR: Diane V. H. Hendrix, DVM, DACVO

Eosinophilic Bronchopneumopathy

Client Education Sheet

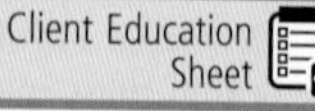

BASIC INFORMATION

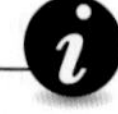

Definition
Idiopathic eosinophilic inflammation of airways, interstitium, and sometimes alveoli and/or nasal cavities. The disease is well recognized, but uncommon.

Synonyms
Eosinophilic pneumonia, pulmonary infiltrates with eosinophils (PIE), canine idiopathic eosinophilic bronchopneumopathy (EBP; the most current term), eosinophilic bronchitis

Epidemiology
SPECIES, AGE, SEX
- Dogs of either sex and any age
- Young to middle-aged adults predisposed
- No strict corresponding disease in cats; EBP is distinct from feline asthma

GENETICS, BREED PREDISPOSITION

Any breed; Siberian Huskies and Alaskan Malamutes may be predisposed.

Clinical Presentation
HISTORY, CHIEF COMPLAINT
- Most common: chronic cough poorly responsive to antimicrobials. Cough may be intermittent, frequent, or persistent and is often accompanied by a terminal gag/retch. Severe, productive coughing can occur, with expectoration of thick respiratory secretions, gagging, and/or retching.
- Nasal discharge (serous or mucopurulent)
- Exercise intolerance
- Depression and weight loss are absent
- Pruritus (rare)

PHYSICAL EXAM FINDINGS
- Cough and retch
- Crackles, wheezes, and increased bronchovesicular sounds
  - Auscultation may be normal
- Tachypnea/dyspnea
- Fever (rare)
- Bronchospastic reactions, such as expiratory dyspnea and wheezes (rare)

Etiology and Pathophysiology
- A hypersensitivity reaction is suspected as the main pathophysiologic process.
- The precipitating cause is rarely identified.

DIAGNOSIS

Diagnostic Overview

Clinical presentation is similar to other causes of chronic cough. Peripheral eosinophilia may be seen on a CBC, and nonspecific bronchointerstitial changes and peribronchial infiltrates are commonly seen on thoracic radiographs. Clinical diagnosis rests on identifying sterile eosinophilic airway inflammation by respiratory cytology and exclusion of other eosinophilic diseases.

Differential Diagnosis

Other diseases associated with eosinophilic respiratory inflammation:

- Respiratory parasites (*Oslerus osleri*, *Filaroides hirthi*, *Eucoleus aerophilus* [formerly *Capillaria*], *Crenosoma vulpis*, *Paragonimus kellicotti*, and others)
- Chronic respiratory infection (bacterial, fungal)
- Pulmonary neoplasia (primary or metastatic)
- Vascular parasites (*Angiostrongylus vasorum*, *Dirofilaria immitis* (heartworm) infections
- Eosinophilic granulomatosis (nodular pulmonary disease on radiographs)
- Hypereosinophilic syndrome
- Eosinophilic leukemia

Initial Database

- CBC
  - Inflammatory leukogram
  - Occasional peripheral eosinophilia (50%-60%)
- Serum biochemical profile and urinalysis results are usually unremarkable.
- Thoracic radiographs: bronchial/peribronchiolar patterns; increases in interstitial markings and occasionally alveolar patterns. Lobar consolidation, bronchiectasis, and/or miliary pattern in severe cases
- Fecal examinations (flotation, sedimentation techniques [Baermann]) are negative for parasites and ova. Repeat fecal examinations in suspect cases due to intermittent shedding. Empiric treatment with an appropriate anthelmintic may also be considered.
- Heartworm and *Angiostrongylus* blood tests are negative.

Advanced or Confirmatory Testing

- Respiratory washes/brush cytology shows a mix of neutrophils and eosinophils with increased total cell numbers in wash samples. Infectious agents, neoplastic cells, or evidence of respiratory parasites are absent.
- Bronchoscopic (p. 1074) abnormalities
  - Abundant green to yellow-green mucus is commonly found in airways.
  - Airway mucosa may appear reddened, thickened, nodular, or polypoid; airway collapse may be evident during expiration. Bronchiectasis may be observed in severe and chronic disease.
- A positive standard bacterial culture of respiratory washes reflects a secondary bacterial infection, and clinical signs persist despite antimicrobial therapy.
- *Crenosoma* and *Angiostrongylus* polymerase chain reaction (PCR) detection in respiratory washes is negative.
- CT: Various lesions reported; increased peribronchial cuffing, bronchiectasis, mucous plugging, and pulmonary nodules
- Intradermal skin testing (not routinely performed): positive tests do not necessarily indicate the allergen identified is responsible for disease. Test before starting glucocorticoids.

TREATMENT

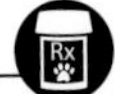

Treatment Overview

Glucocorticoids are needed to resolve eosinophilic inflammation and associated clinical signs.

Acute General Treatment

Glucocorticoids (e.g., prednisone 0.5-1 mg/kg PO q 12h)

Chronic Treatment

Glucocorticoids on a slowly tapering (weeks to months) schedule are often needed for control of clinical signs:

- Clinical signs are likely to recur if glucocorticoids are administered inconsistently or if tapering occurs too quickly.
- Low-dose glucocorticoid therapy may be needed indefinitely for some animals. Administer the lowest dose q 24-48h to control clinical signs.
- Inhaled steroid therapy (IST) (e.g., fluticasone 40-250 mcg q 12h) is well tolerated and allows a reduction of oral glucocorticoid dosage in steroid-dependent animals; long-term IST alone does not allow optimal management in all affected dogs.

Possible Complications

- Side effects of oral glucocorticoid therapy (e.g., polyuria, polydipsia, polyphagia) are expected in treated animals.
- Long-term inhalation fluticasone therapy may induce inhibition of pituitary-adrenal axis but rarely signs of hypercortisolemia.
- Untreated or inadequately treated patients may develop bronchiectasis (an irreversible airway change) (p. 132).
- Acute severe bronchoconstriction has been described after bronchoalveolar lavage (rare).

Recommended Monitoring

- Clinical signs
- Thoracic radiographs

PROGNOSIS & OUTCOME

- Prognosis is generally good. Some animals can be completely weaned from glucocorticoids.
- Excessively rapid cessation of glucocorticoids may provoke a relapse of clinical signs.

PEARLS & CONSIDERATIONS

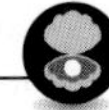

Comments

The beneficial role of hyposensitization against antigens identified by allergy testing has not been documented.

Technician Tips

Eosinophils are easily recognized with rapid staining methods. If sputum is expectorated (productive retch), it can be used to make slides for cytologic review.

Client Education

Clients should understand the importance of consistent treatment with glucocorticoids. Dogs being treated should be regularly monitored to adjust therapy and because infection with parasites or bacteria can always occur.

SUGGESTED READING

Clercx C, et al: Canine eosinophilic bronchopneumopathy. Vet Clin North Am Small Anim Pract 37:917-935, 2007.

AUTHOR: Cécile Clercx, DVM, PhD, DECVIM
EDITOR: Megan Grobman, DVM, MS, DACVIM

Eosinophilic Granuloma Complex

Client Education Sheet 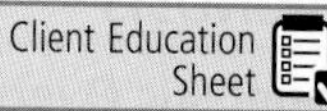

BASIC INFORMATION

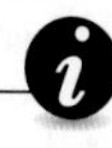

Definition

- Cats: group of distinct cutaneous or oral reaction patterns with eosinophilic infiltrate
- Dogs: rare disease process characterized by single or multiple ulcerated lesions in oral cavity

Synonyms

Feline eosinophilic skin diseases, indolent ulcer, eosinophilic plaque, rodent ulcer

Epidemiology

SPECIES, AGE, SEX

More common in cats than dogs. Lesions are more common in young animals.

GENETICS, BREED PREDISPOSITION

- Cats: no breed predisposition
- Dogs: Siberian Huskies, Alaskan Malamutes, Cavalier King Charles spaniels (CKCS) appear to be predisposed.

CONTAGION AND ZOONOSIS

Multiple cases in multi-cat households and experimental transmission from one area of a cat to another suggest an infectious or allergic cause.

GEOGRAPHY AND SEASONALITY

Worldwide; warm weather seasonality may be observed.

ASSOCIATED DISORDERS

Miliary dermatitis or symmetrical alopecia may be noted concurrently in cats.

Clinical Presentation

DISEASE FORMS/SUBTYPES

Three distinct clinical presentations in cats:

- Eosinophilic granuloma (formerly called collagenolytic granuloma, linear granuloma)
- Indolent ulcer (synonyms: eosinophilic ulcer, rodent ulcer)
- Eosinophilic plaque

HISTORY, CHIEF COMPLAINT

Lesions may be insidious in onset.

- Skin lesions associated with pruritus, pain
- Oral lesions associated with dysphagia, ptyalism, halitosis, inappetence

PHYSICAL EXAM FINDINGS

Three major forms in cats (all three forms may be observed in the same patient):

- Eosinophilic granuloma
  - Erythematous, alopecic, raised, linear skin lesions on lateral thorax, lateral shoulder, or caudal aspect of thighs; variable pruritus and pain
  - Nodules in oral cavity (dorsal and lateral tongue surfaces, hard and soft palate, glossopharyngeal folds) or at chin; surface often is speckled with small, dense white areas.
- Indolent ulcer
  - Well-demarcated ulcer (raised edges surround a pink-yellow ulcerated surface) on the upper lip (midline or adjacent to the maxillary canine tooth); may also affect the philtrum; nonpruritic, apparently painless
- Eosinophilic plaque
  - Erythematous, raised plaquelike skin lesions, commonly on the ventral abdomen, perianal region, and medial thighs; variable pruritus and pain

Two major forms in dogs:

- Single or multiple (often confluent) ulcerated lesions on soft palate and lateral pharyngeal mucosa, especially in CKCS
- Firm, raised, yellowish to brownish pink, irregular, ulcerated lesions with well-demarcated edges on lateral or ventral tongue surfaces or lingual frenulum; especially in Siberian Huskies and Alaskan Malamutes

Etiology and Pathophysiology

- Generally regarded as different reaction patterns to underlying antigenic stimulation (hypersensitivity reaction), most commonly arthropods (fleas, mosquitoes), food, and contact or environmental (house dust mites, pollens) allergies
- Other reported causes include viral and bacterial infections, chronic trauma, poor oral hygiene, genetic heritable eosinophilic dysregulation, and immune-mediated reaction.

DIAGNOSIS

Diagnostic Overview

The diagnosis is primarily visual and is confirmed by biopsy.

Differential Diagnosis

- Eosinophilic granuloma and plaque: cutaneous lymphoma, mast cell tumor, squamous

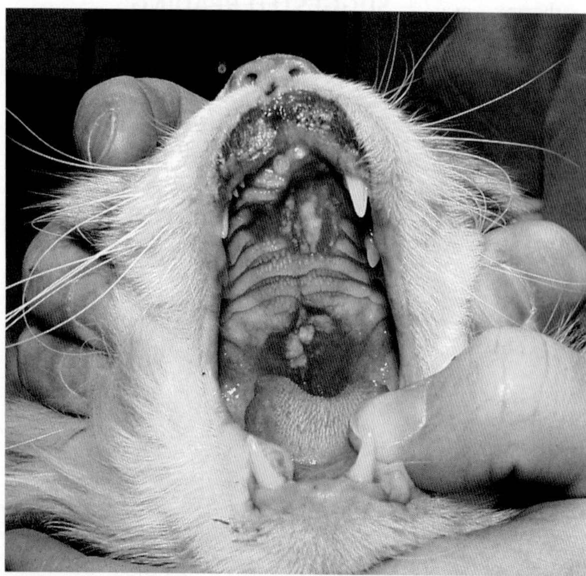

EOSINOPHILIC GRANULOMA COMPLEX Eosinophilic ulcer of the upper lip and eosinophilic granuloma on the palate of a cat. (Copyright Dr. Manon Paradis.)

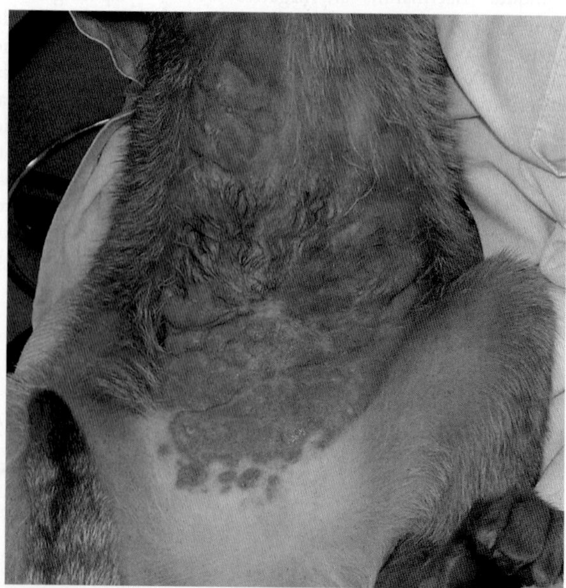

EOSINOPHILIC GRANULOMA COMPLEX Eosinophilic plaque on the abdomen of a cat. (Copyright Dr. Frédéric Sauvé.)

cell carcinoma, demodicosis, dermatophytosis, bacterial pyoderma, mycobacterial infection
- Indolent ulcer: squamous cell carcinoma; herpesvirus, calicivirus, feline leukemia virus (FeLV), or *Cryptococcus* infections
- Lip/oral cavity lesions: squamous cell carcinoma, fibrosarcoma, focal inflammation due to a foreign body, trauma, or an infectious agent

Initial Database

- Microscopic exam of plucked hair (trichography [p. 1091]), acetate tape preparation, skin scraping, and flea-combing samples to rule out ectoparasites; alternatively, an improvement after appropriate empirical ectoparasiticidal therapy also supports parasitosis.
- Cytologic exam of the surface of lesions may reveal large numbers of eosinophils and bacterial or *Malassezia* overgrowth.
- Mild to moderate eosinophilia may occasionally be noted on CBC (rare in cats and inconsistent in dogs with oral lesions).
- Feline immunodeficiency virus/FeLV testing

Advanced or Confirmatory Testing

- Skin biopsies reveal a superficial to deep to interstitial to diffuse predominantly eosinophilic dermal infiltrate +/− flame figures (collagen fibers surrounded by eosinophilic material).
- Oral biopsy is indicated to rule out neoplasia such as squamous cell carcinoma and fibrosarcoma and to establish a diagnosis.
- Adverse food reaction: improvement with 8-10 weeks of elimination diet trial; relapse on challenge

TREATMENT

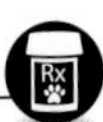

Treatment Overview

- Treatment of choice consists of early and aggressive glucocorticoid therapy.
- Treat secondary infection and underlying cause where appropriate.
- Surgical excision and laser therapy can be attempted for single oral lesions.

Acute General Treatment

- Oral glucocorticoids: prednisolone or prednisone 1-2 mg/kg PO q 12h initially, then taper to lowest effective dose. Prednisolone is a superior choice in cats (unpredictable absorption or metabolism of prednisone).
- Injectable glucocorticoids (cats): methylprednisolone 4 mg/kg (maximum, 20 mg, Depo-Medrol) can be given up to 2-3 times, 2 weeks apart. This should not be a standard therapy. Adverse reactions include congestive heart failure, diabetes mellitus, secondary infection, and iatrogenic hyperadrenocorticism
- Oral clavulanic acid–potentiated amoxicillin q 12h for 3 weeks has been shown to significantly decrease size of eosinophilic cutaneous plaques in cats.
- Oral cyclosporine (Atopica) approved for the treatment of allergic dermatitis in cats at a dosage of 7 mg/kg PO q 24h initially, then taper to q 48-72h based on clinical response. Main side effects include vomiting, diarrhea, weight loss, decreased appetite, and lethargy.
- Off-label use of oclacitinib (Apoquel) at a dosage of 0.4-0.6 mg/kg PO q 12h for up to 14 days and q 24h thereafter may be effective in some cases.

Chronic Treatment

- Rigorous flea control program if fleas are present or suspected.
- Allergen-specific immunotherapy (hyposensitization) for treatment of atopic dermatitis based on results of intradermal test and/or aeroallergen-specific immunoglobulin E serum test

Nutrition/Diet

Strict hypoallergenic diet in proven cases of adverse food reaction

Possible Complications

- Inadequate initial therapy may result in refractory lesions.
- Oronasal communication may result after surgical excision of palatal lesions.

PROGNOSIS & OUTCOME

Good

PEARLS & CONSIDERATIONS

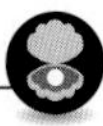

Comments

- Feline eosinophilic granuloma complex is not a specific diagnosis. A primary underlying cause is likely and should be investigated.
- Squamous cell carcinoma and eosinophilic granuloma of the tongue and sublingual tissues can clinically appear very similar. Biopsy and histopathologic exam are essential to obtain an accurate diagnosis.

Prevention

If an underlying allergic cause can be determined and controlled, the problem can be prevented from reoccurring.

Technician Tips

Explain how to institute a rigorous program of flea control.

Client Education

- Because skin lesions tend to wax and wane, reoccurrence is unpredictable (sometimes seasonal).
- Because glucocorticoids mask the problem rather than eliminating it, efforts should be made to identify the cause.
- Cats can (rarely) outgrow the disease over time.

SUGGESTED READING

Buckley L, et al: Feline eosinophilic granuloma complex(ities): some clinical clarification. J Feline Med Surg 14:471-481, 2012.

AUTHOR: Vincent E. Defalque, DVM, DACVD
EDITOR: Manon Paradis, DMV, MVSc, DACVD

Epilepsy, Idiopathic

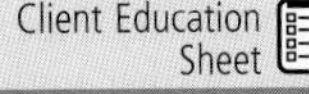

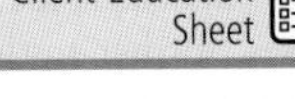

BASIC INFORMATION

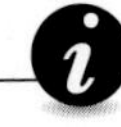

Definition

A syndrome characterized by chronic recurrent seizures for which there is no identifiable cause other than a suspected genetic origin

Synonyms

- Primary epilepsy
- Genetic epilepsy: used when genetic factors are known to play a major role
- Status epilepticus: one seizure lasting more than 5 minutes or two or more seizures in which there is incomplete recovery of consciousness
- Cluster seizures (i.e., *serial* or *acute repetitive seizures*): two or more isolated seizures occurring within 24 hours

Epidemiology

SPECIES, AGE, SEX

- Dogs: common (≈0.75% prevalence in general population), 6 months to 6 years old, slightly more common in males
- Cats: less common than in dogs, but not rare, 1-5 years old, no sex predisposition

GENETICS, BREED PREDISPOSITION

A genetic basis is known or suspected in many breeds, although in most cases, the precise genetic mutation has not been identified. Any breed of dog, including mixed breeds, can be affected.

Clinical Presentation

HISTORY, CHIEF COMPLAINT

- Two or more unprovoked seizures occurring > 24 hours apart
- Most common are generalized tonic-clonic seizures characterized by loss of consciousness

and sustained contraction of all muscles (tonic phase) followed by rhythmic muscle contractions, especially of the limbs and masticatory muscles (clonic phase). Autonomic discharge (salivation, urination, defecation) can also occur.
- Also possible are milder, generalized, tonic-clonic seizures in which consciousness is maintained and focal seizures in which only part of the body is involved (e.g., fly-biting movements).
- The animal is normal during the interictal period (between seizures, after recovery), and owners do not report evidence of ongoing neurologic deficits.

PHYSICAL EXAM FINDINGS

- Normal unless examined immediately after a seizure, when temporary postictal deficits are possible, including generalized ataxia, abnormal behavior, and blindness
- Persistent neurologic deficits such as hemiparesis, abnormal behavior, or visual deficits are inconsistent with idiopathic epilepsy and suggest an underlying structural brain lesion (p. 1136).
- A fundic exam (p. 1137) may show uveal, retinal, or optic disk diseases associated with an underlying cause of seizures. These include optic neuritis, feline infectious peritonitis, toxoplasmosis/neosporosis, systemic mycoses, rickettsial diseases, systemic hypertension, lymphoma, and metastatic neoplasia.

Etiology and Pathophysiology

Theories include inborn abnormalities in neuronal excitability, neurotransmitter, and receptor function.

DIAGNOSIS

Diagnostic Overview

- Idiopathic epilepsy is a clinical diagnosis based on the typical age of onset, lack of persistent neurologic deficits, and exclusion of other potential causes of seizures based on diagnostic testing.
- A presumptive diagnosis of idiopathic epilepsy may be made when the patient's signalment and history are consistent with epilepsy and the physical and neurologic exam findings and initial database results are normal. In such cases, further testing should be pursued if there is deterioration in neurologic status or failure to respond to medication.

Differential Diagnosis

- Metabolic disorders: hepatic encephalopathy (including portosystemic shunt), hypoglycemia, polycythemia, hypocalcemia
- Toxins: lead, ethylene glycol, organophosphate, carbamate, metaldehyde
- Brain malformations: hydrocephalus, lissencephaly
- Inherited degenerative diseases such as lysosomal storage diseases
- Encephalitis: immune-mediated encephalitis, distemper, tick-borne infections, fungal encephalitis, *Neospora caninum, Toxoplasma gondii*, feline infectious peritonitis
- Neoplasia: primary or metastatic brain tumor
- Vascular lesions: infarct, hemorrhage
- Head injury
- Consider nonepileptic episodes such as syncope, episodic movement disorders (e.g., myoclonus), narcolepsy, exercise-induced weakness, vestibular dysfunction, and episodes of pain.

Initial Database

- CBC: unremarkable; nucleated red blood cells and/or basophilic stippling suggest lead toxicosis; acanthocytes suggest hepatic disease as cause of seizures
- Serum chemistry profile, urinalysis: unremarkable. Can identify metabolic causes of seizures (e.g., hypoglycemia, hepatic encephalopathy, hypocalcemia, azotemia). Fasting hypercholesterolemia may suggest hypothyroidism and attendant central nervous system effects if hyperlipidemia is severe. Hyperglobulinemia in cats raises the possibility of feline infectious peritonitis–based encephalitis as the cause of seizures rather than idiopathic epilepsy.
- Serum bile acids (preprandial and postprandial)
  - Substantial elevation of either or both suggests hepatic encephalopathy (portosystemic shunt, cirrhotic/fibrosing liver disease, other).
  - Moderate elevations in bile acids may occur soon after a seizure of any cause. In these cases, recheck bile acids 2-4 weeks later to see whether the abnormality persists.
- Pursue alternative cause of seizure, as appropriate (e.g., blood lead concentration if potential exposure or basophilic stippling of red cells).

Advanced or Confirmatory Testing

- Brain CT or MRI (p. 1132), and cerebrospinal fluid (CSF) analysis (pp. 1080 and 1323) are indicated in the following patients presenting with seizures and no identifiable systemic cause: onset < 6 months or > 6 years of age, persistent neurologic deficits, an initial onset of status epilepticus/cluster seizures, and cats. Results of these tests are normal with idiopathic epilepsy.
- Electroencephalography (EEG) may show seizure activity but is insensitive and nonspecific with respect to cause.

TREATMENT

Treatment Overview

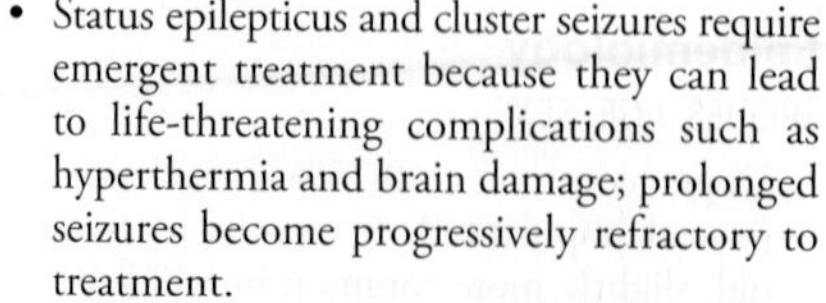

- Status epilepticus and cluster seizures require emergent treatment because they can lead to life-threatening complications such as hyperthermia and brain damage; prolonged seizures become progressively refractory to treatment.
- Long-term treatment with antiseizure drugs is started if seizures are severe and/or frequent.
- Daily antiseizure medication is not indicated in patients with a single seizure, seizures caused by a transient condition (e.g., acute intoxication), or isolated seizures separated by a long period.
- Daily antiseizure medication is indicated in patients with more than one isolated seizure per month, clusters of multiple seizures per day or status epilepticus, or a clear pattern of increasing frequency or severity of seizures.

Acute General Treatment

- To stop an active seizure: diazepam 0.5-1 mg/kg or midazolam 0.1-0.5 mg/kg IV to effect
- If the seizure does not stop with three doses of diazepam, administer
  - Levetiracetam 20-60 mg/kg IV over several minutes; if effective, repeat as needed (typically q 8-12h) *or*
  - Propofol 1-8 mg/kg IV to effect, followed by continuous infusion at 0.1 mg/kg/min titrated to effect
- If the seizure stops with the above therapy but recurs soon after, options, include
  - Load with phenobarbital 12-24 mg/kg slow IV, IM, or PO single dose, followed by maintenance doses of 2-3 mg/kg slow IV, IM, or PO q 12h, *or*
  - Diazepam or midazolam continuous-rate infusion: 0.5-1 mg/kg/h in 2.5% dextrose plus 0.45% saline. Titrate based on seizure control and sedation.

Chronic Treatment

- Options for ongoing therapy in dogs include phenobarbital, zonisamide, levetiracetam, imepitoin, and bromide. Initial therapy in cats is phenobarbital.
  - Phenobarbital
    - Initial dose: 2-3 mg/kg PO q 12h (dog, cat) subsequently adjusted based on clinical effects and therapeutic monitoring
    - Steady-state serum concentrations are reached about 10-14 days after starting therapy or changing the dose.
    - Common side effects: polyuria/polyphagia, sedation, ataxia
  - Zonisamide 10 mg/kg PO q 12h (dog); or 5-10 mg/kg PO q 24h (cat)
    - Side effects include ataxia, sedation, and inappetance.
    - Hepatopathy and erythema multiforme are rare idiosyncratic adverse effects.
  - Levetiracetam
    - Immediate-release formulation: 20 mg/kg PO q 8h (dog, cat)
    - Extended-release formulation: 30 mg/kg PO q12h (dog). Do not crush or divide tablet.
    - Minimal side effects (ataxia)
  - Imepitoin (not currently available in North America)
    - 10 mg/kg PO q 12h (dog) initial dose. Dosages may be increased after 1 week in 50%-100% increments to a maximum of 30 mg/kg q 12h.

- Mild, transient side effects (hyperactivity, ataxia)
  - Potassium bromide
    - Initial dose: 20-30 mg/kg PO q 24h with food (dog), subsequently changed based on clinical effects and therapeutic monitoring
    - Cats: do not use because of substantial risk of pneumonitis
    - Steady-state serum concentrations are reached 2-3 months after starting therapy or changing the dose.
    - For more rapid control of seizures in dogs with frequent, severe seizures, administer a loading dose of 50-66 mg/kg PO q 6-8h × 48 hours.
    - Common side effects are polyuria/polyphagia, sedation, and ataxia.
- If seizures are not adequately controlled despite target serum concentrations of the first drug, add a second drug while continuing the first drug. If the seizures become well controlled, it may be possible to gradually wean the first drug.
- Other drugs to consider for add-on therapy when seizures are not controlled with initial drug
  - Gabapentin 100-300 mg/dose PO q 8h (dog, cat)
  - Felbamate 15-45 mg/kg PO q 8h (dog)
  - Pregabalin 2-4 mg/kg PO, q 12h (dog). Start at low end of dose to minimize sedation.
  - Topiramate 5-10 mg/kg PO q 8-12h (dog). Start at low end of dose to minimize side effects (sedation and ataxia).
- A ketogenic medium-chain triglyceride diet can improve seizure control in dogs already being treated with antiseizure drugs.
- For dogs that suffer clusters of multiple seizures despite daily medication, at-home administration of diazepam per rectum can decrease the need for emergency veterinary care. The client administers 2 mg/kg of parenteral diazepam solution per rectum using a syringe and urinary catheter or teat cannula, repeated for a maximum total of 3 doses within 24 hours. Because diazepam adheres to plastic, do not store in a syringe. Diazepam suppositories are not well absorbed in dogs.

Drug Interactions

- Phenobarbital increases clearance of levetiracetam and zonisamide and can decrease the effect of other drugs, such as chloramphenicol, glucocorticoids, doxycycline, propranolol, and metronidazole. Other depressants and chloramphenicol can increase the effect of phenobarbital.
- Bromide: higher chloride intake increases bromide elimination, which increases the dosage requirement; lower chloride decreases bromide elimination.

Possible Complications

- Phenobarbital-induced hepatotoxicosis
  - Minimized by avoiding serum concentrations > 35 mcg/mL
  - Evidence of hepatotoxicosis: increases in bile acid concentrations; proportionally larger increases of alanine aminotransferase (ALT) compared to alkaline phosphatase (ALP); icterus, weight loss, ascites if very severe and advanced
  - Potentially reversible if phenobarbital is stopped early enough
  - Elevations in ALP and, to a lesser degree, ALT are common in dogs taking phenobarbital and do not indicate or predict clinically significant liver disease or the need to withdraw the drug.
- Phenobarbital rarely causes hematologic abnormalities, including neutropenia, anemia, and thrombocytopenia; the drug must be stopped if these abnormalities occur.
- Bromide increases the risk of pancreatitis and may be associated with megaesophagus.

Recommended Monitoring

Phenobarbital (p. 1372):
- Measure serum concentrations 14 days after starting therapy or changing dose, when seizures are not adequately controlled, when signs of dose-related toxicosis occur, and every 6-12 months.
- Blood sample is obtained immediately before the next dose is due (trough serum level), 8-12 hours after preceding dose was given.
- Blood should *not* be drawn into serum separator tubes because the separator material may artifactually reduce phenobarbital concentrations *in vitro*.
- Target range: 20-35 mcg/mL (85-150 mmol/L)

Bromide (p. 1319):
- Measure serum concentrations 1 month and 3-4 months after starting therapy or changing dose, when seizures are not adequately controlled, when signs of dose-related toxicity occur, and every 6-12 months.
- Because of the drug's extremely long elimination half-life, blood samples need not be drawn a certain number of hours after dosing.
- Target range: 1-2 mg/mL (100-200 mg/dL; 1000-2000 mcg/mL) when used concurrently with phenobarbital and 2-3 mg/mL (200-300 mg/dL; 2000-3000 mcg/mL) when used as monotherapy

PROGNOSIS & OUTCOME

- About 70% of dogs with idiopathic epilepsy can be adequately treated with phenobarbital and/or bromide and enjoy a good quality of life.
- In general, dogs with idiopathic epilepsy have a normal life span. However, some dogs with recurrent episodes of status epilepticus requiring emergency treatment have a decreased expected life span (≈8 years vs. ≈11 years).

PEARLS & CONSIDERATIONS

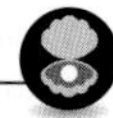

Comments

- A common cause of poor seizure control is failure to reach target serum concentrations before switching to a second drug.
- Referral to a neurologist is considered if the diagnosis is uncertain or the seizures are not adequately controlled within 3 months.

Prevention

- Animals with idiopathic epilepsy should not be bred because of potential genetic factors.
- Females should be spayed because estrus tends to increase seizures.

Technician Tips

Have clients bring all medications to their pet's appointment to check dosages and compliance.

Client Education

Client education is vital. The client must understand the goal of treatment, potential side effects, and need for periodic monitoring and dose adjustment. The client must agree that the benefits of treatment outweigh the side effects and must not alter treatment without consulting the attending veterinarian.

SUGGESTED READING

Thomas WB, et al: Seizures and narcolepsy. In Dewey CW, et al, editors: A practical guide to canine and feline neurology, ed 3, Ames, IA, 2016, Wiley-Blackwell, pp 249–268.

AUTHOR: William B. Thomas, DVM, MS, DACVIM
EDITOR: Karen R. Muñana, DVM, MS, DACVIM

Episcleritis/Scleritis

Bonus Material Online  Client Education Sheet

BASIC INFORMATION

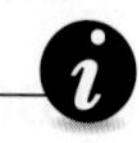

Definition

- Episcleritis: focal or diffuse inflammation of the episclera, a thin, collagenous, and vascular membrane that makes up the superficial layer of the sclera
- Scleritis: inflammation and thickening of the anterior and posterior sclera, involving the cornea, uvea, and retina in advanced cases

Synonyms

Collie granuloma, fibrous histiocytoma, necrotizing scleritis, nodular fasciitis, proliferative keratoconjunctivitis, limbal granuloma, nodular granulomatous episcleritis/episclerokeratitis (NGE), non-necrotizing deep scleritis, non-necrotizing superficial scleritis

Epidemiology

SPECIES, AGE, SEX

Dogs; no age or sex predisposition

GENETICS, BREED PREDISPOSITION

Spaniel breeds, especially American cocker spaniel (episcleritis, scleritis), collie, Shetland sheepdog

Clinical Presentation

DISEASE FORMS/SUBTYPES

- Episcleritis: primary (simple, nodular) or secondary
- Scleritis: necrotizing granulomatous or non-necrotizing granulomatous

HISTORY, CHIEF COMPLAINT

Episcleritis:
- Pinkish-red growth on eye (nodular)
- Red eye (diffuse)
- Typically painless

Scleritis:
- Signs of ocular pain noted by owner: photophobia, blepharospasm, excessive tearing, engorged scleral vessels, ink-tan colored sector lesions near the limbus

PHYSICAL EXAM FINDINGS

Episcleritis:
- Conjunctival hyperemia
- Engorgement of episcleral vessels
- Thickening of episclera (partial or diffuse)
- With nodular forms, multiple or single, raised, pinkish-red mass(es) may be apparent at limbus; typically bilateral
- ± Perilimbal keratitis with corneal vascularization and edema (e.g., nodular granulomatous episclerokeratitis)

Scleritis:
- Conjunctival hyperemia
- Engorgement of episcleral vessels
- Typically bilateral, mildly elevated, red lesions in the anterior sclera
- Peripheral corneal vascularization and edema
- Nongranulomatous anterior uveitis (p. 1023)

Advanced scleritis: presence of signs of scleritis and any or all of the following:
- Stromal keratitis
- Inflammation of the vitreous
- Secondary glaucoma (p. 387)
- Retinochoroidal degeneration (p. 883)
- Cystic/bullus retinal detachment (p. 885)
- Scleral thinning, which may cause subconjunctival iris prolapse or staphyloma

Etiology and Pathophysiology

Episcleritis/scleritis:
- Often idiopathic; immune-mediated disease
- Association with positive *Toxoplasma* titers has been found.

Episcleritis, primary:
- Simple (uncommon): not associated with systemic disease; usually responsive to therapy; often self-limited
- Nodular (common): proposed pathogenesis of nodular granulomatous episcleritis involves production of inflammatory mediators by T lymphocytes and subsequent chemotaxis of histiocytes.

Episcleritis, secondary:
- Develops as a result of inflammation extending to episclera from severe intraocular diseases, including panophthalmitis/endophthalmitis, chronic glaucoma, or ocular trauma

Scleritis, non-necrotizing granulomatous:
- Characterized by infiltration of lymphocytes, plasma cells, and macrophages
- Granulomatous response seen in cornea with corneal extension
- ± Secondary uveitis
- Damaged sclera replaced by fibrous tissue and/or cystic spaces, causing scleral thinning after several episodes

Scleritis, necrotizing granulomatous (rare):
- Aggressive disease causing necrosis of scleral collagen
- Typically affects anterior and posterior segments of the eye
- Commonly associated with secondary uveitis, glaucoma, and retinal detachment
- *Ehrlichia canis* infection reported in certain cases

DIAGNOSIS

Diagnostic Overview

Episcleritis/scleritis should be strongly suspected on the clinical appearance of the affected globe(s), ruling out other causes of red eye, and response to treatment. If the ocular disease does not respond to medical therapy as expected, episcleral biopsy (usually referrable procedure) for a histologic diagnosis is warranted.

Differential Diagnosis

- Nodular episcleritis; other pinkish, raised lesions
  - Neoplasia
    - Conjunctival neoplasia (e.g., mast cell tumor; hemangiosarcoma; histiocytoma)
    - Extension of intraocular tumor
- Granuloma (e.g., foreign body; parasitic: *Onchocerca* spp)
- Granulation tissue
- Diffuse episcleritis/scleritis; other causes of red eye
  - Conjunctivitis
  - Glaucoma
  - Uveitis

Initial Database

- Complete ophthalmic examination (p. 1137), including
  - Schirmer tear test (normal > 15 mm in 1 minute for dogs)
  - Fluorescein dye application
  - Intraocular pressures (normal > 15 mm Hg and < 25 mm Hg)
  - Examination of the anterior and posterior segments of the eye
- Cytologic examination of nodular lesion; may help differentiate neoplasia from inflammation (see Differential Diagnosis above)

Advanced or Confirmatory Testing

- Episcleral biopsy and histopathologic evaluation (nodular granulomatous episcleritis characterized by histiocytes, plasma cells, lymphocytes, and fibroblasts)
- Serologic titers for infectious diseases if supportive systemic signs (e.g., *T. gondii; E. canis*)
- Laboratory testing: canine rheumatoid factor, antinuclear antibody, lupus erythematosus cell identification negative in most cases
- Ocular ultrasound if ocular media opaque, compromising evaluation of deeper ocular structures; useful for ruling out concurrent ocular abnormalities (i.e., retinal detachment)

TREATMENT

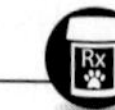

Treatment Overview

Many forms of episcleritis respond well to topical corticosteroid application, tapered gradually to the lowest effective frequency. Therapeutic goals are to promote regression of disease, eliminate ocular pain, and keep disease in remission with maintenance therapy. Treatment of NGE and scleritis often requires topical and systemic therapies, including oral prednisone ± azathioprine.

Acute General Treatment

To be implemented only if fluorescein staining has ruled out corneal ulceration:
- Topical corticosteroids (e.g., 0.1% dexamethasone solution or ointment or 1% prednisolone acetate) q 6-8h for 2-3 weeks, then gradually tapered

- ± Topical cyclosporine 0.2%-2% q 12h, used in addition to corticosteroids in refractory cases.

Chronic Treatment

NGE and scleritis often require topical (see Acute General Treatment above) and systemic therapy(ies):

- Prednisone 1-2 mg/kg PO q 24h until clinical improvement, then gradually tapered over 3-4 weeks until maintenance dose reached
- ± Azathioprine 1.5-2 mg/kg PO q 24h until clinical improvement, then gradually tapered to as low a dose as possible (e.g., 0.75-1 mg/kg PO q 24h, then q 48h, then once weekly for maintenance)
- Oral cyclosporine 5 mg/kg PO q 24h for 30 days, then 5 mg/kg PO q 48h or 2.5 mg/kg q 24h
- Options if medical management ineffective
  - Cryosurgery
  - Surgical excision

Alternative medical treatment includes tetracycline (doxycycline 10 mg/kg PO q 24h), with or without niacinamide 125 mg/DOG PO q 8h for dogs < 5 kg, 250 mg/DOG PO q 8h for dogs 5-10 kg, or 500 mg/DOG PO q 8h for dogs > 10 kg); clinical response may take 1-2 months; occasional gastrointestinal side effects from niacinamide

Possible Complications

- Chronic ocular pain
- Uveitis
- Secondary glaucoma
- Blindness
- Azathioprine may cause severe life-threatening myelosuppression; potentially hepatotoxic

Recommended Monitoring

- Monitor for regression of disease every 2-3 weeks until clinical signs resolve, then as needed depending on response to therapy.
- In animals receiving azathioprine therapy, CBC and liver enzymes should be assessed every 1-2 weeks for the first 2 months, then regularly (e.g., monthly) once clinically stable.

PROGNOSIS & OUTCOME

- Varies, depending on underlying condition and cause
- Episcleritis: prognosis usually good
- Relapse possible

PEARLS & CONSIDERATIONS

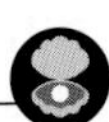

Comments

Lifelong treatment is typically required.

Technician Tips

Some ophthalmic drugs have virtually identical names for formulations with and without corticosteroids. This similarity presents a risk of using the wrong drug. Before topical application, it is extremely useful for technicians to carefully read the label of the tube/vial and identify whether it contains corticosteroids and to check the medical record for consistency. Substitution error (especially administering corticosteroids when they are contraindicated) can be devastating and has been made by veterinarians, technicians, and clients.

SUGGESTED READING

Grahn BH, et al: Canine episcleritis, nodular episclerokeratitis, scleritis and necrotic scleritis. Vet Clin North Am Small Anim Pract 38:291-308, 2008.

AUTHOR: Ursula M. Dietrich, Dr.med.vet., DACVO, DECVO, MRCVS
EDITOR: Diane V. H. Hendrix, DVM, DACVO

Epistaxis

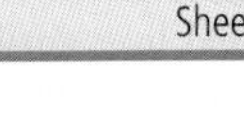

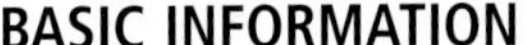

BASIC INFORMATION

Definition

Bleeding from the nasal cavity

Synonym

Hemorrhagic nasal discharge, nosebleed

Epidemiology

SPECIES, AGE, SEX

Dogs more commonly affected than cats; depends on underlying cause:

- Young, purebred animals: hereditary coagulopathies
- Young to middle-aged animals: infectious diseases, trauma, immune-mediated diseases
- Older animals: neoplasia

GENETICS AND BREED PREDISPOSITION

- Platelet disorders: otter hounds, basset hounds, others
- von Willebrand disease: many breeds (p. 1043)
- Hemophilia: German shepherds, Kerry blue terrier, others (p. 431)
- Nasal lesions
  - Aspergillosis: German shepherd, dolichocephalic breeds (p. 81)
  - Neoplasia: dolichocephalic breeds (p. 680)

RISK FACTORS

- See Genetics and Breed Predisposition
- Exposure to ticks
- Exposure to anticoagulant drugs or toxins
- Systemic hypertension

CONTAGION AND ZOONOSIS

- Vector transmitted infection: canine leishmaniasis, rickettsial infection
- Fungal infections (transmission potential minimal)

GEOGRAPHY AND SEASONALITY

Areas where leishmaniasis, rickettsial diseases are endemic

Clinical Presentation

HISTORY, CHIEF COMPLAINT

Some or all may be present:

- Nasal hemorrhage: usually acute
- Sneezing
- Pawing at mouth and/or nose
- With bleeding disorder: hematochezia, melena, hematuria, or hemorrhage
- Systemic signs (e.g., lethargy, anorexia) common with systemic causes of epistaxis
- Central nervous system (CNS) deficits possible with tumor invasion, bleeding disorder, hyperviscosity, or systemic hypertension

PHYSICAL EXAM FINDINGS

- Nasal hemorrhage, alone or mixed with mucopurulent discharge
- Melena: from swallowing blood, or associated with concurrent gastrointestinal bleeding
- With intranasal disease (neoplasia, sinonasal aspergillosis): mucopurulent nasal discharge, nasal deformation, regional lymphadenopathy, obstruction of airflow, nasal depigmentation (p. 678)
- With bleeding disorder: petechiae, ecchymosis, hematomas, hematochezia, melena, and hematuria (p. 433)
- Fundic changes possible if bleeding disorder, hyperviscosity, systemic hypertension

Etiology and Pathophysiology

Epistaxis occurs secondary to other disease. Intranasal disease is more common than systemic disease as a cause of epistaxis in dogs and cats in North America.

DIAGNOSIS

Diagnostic Overview

Diagnostic testing to rule out systemic causes (e.g., hemostatic disorder) is indicated first because it is less invasive. If none, evaluation of the nasal cavities consists of diagnostic imaging and biopsies.

Differential Diagnosis

Nasal disease:
- Neoplasia, trauma, foreign body, fungal disease, inflammatory rhinitis, others

Bleeding disorder:
- Thrombocytopenia, thrombocytopathia, von Willebrand disease, or coagulation factor defect

Systemic disease:
- Hyperviscosity: multiple myeloma, ehrlichiosis, erythrocytosis, leishmaniasis
- Vasculitis: immune-mediated, rickettsial diseases
- Systemic hypertension (severe)

Initial Database

CBC:
- Anemia if sufficient hemorrhage has occurred
- Thrombocytopenia: may be cause of bleeding (if severe) or associated with other disease (e.g., ehrlichiosis)
- Neutrophilia: infection, ± neoplasia
- Pancytopenia: bone marrow disease

Urinalysis:
- Usually normal
- Hematuria (bleeding disorder); isosthenuria and/or proteinuria with renal failure (systemic hypertension, uremic thrombocytopathy)

Serum biochemistry profile:
- Hypoproteinemia if sufficient hemorrhage has occurred
- Elevated urea with normal creatinine: gastrointestinal bleeding
- Hyperglobulinemia: ehrlichiosis, leishmaniasis, multiple myeloma
- Elevated liver enzymes and total bilirubin: severe hepatic disease causing coagulopathy

Blood pressure: rule out severe hypertension (p. 1065) as contributor to epistaxis or hypotension as result of hemorrhage

Advanced or Confirmatory Testing

Other laboratory tests:
- Coagulation profile: prolonged times with coagulation factor defects; normal with thrombocytopenia and thrombopathia
- Platelet function testing (buccal mucosal bleeding time, von Willebrand factor analysis)
- Infectious disease testing: as indicated by geography for *Ehrlichia, Rickettsia, Leishmania*

Diagnostic imaging:
- Thoracic radiographs: metastatic neoplasia
- Nasal radiographic series: open mouth and frontal sinus views
- CT scan: more sensitive than radiographs for nasal diseases

Other diagnostic procedures:
- Rhinoscopy (p. 1159), nasal flush, nasal biopsy often indicated for suspected intranasal disease, removing foreign bodies
- Cytologic and histopathologic examination of nasal tissue
- Fungal, ± bacterial culture
- Bone marrow aspiration and cytology (± core biopsy) with pancytopenia

TREATMENT

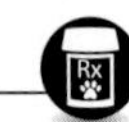

Treatment Overview

- Stop hemorrhage
- Treat primary cause

Acute General Treatment

For persistent, voluminous epistaxis:
- Cage rest ± sedation (e.g., opioids; avoid hypotension)
- Ice packs, pressure to muzzle
- Topical epinephrine (1 : 100,000): 2-4 drops or soaked gauze intranasal tamponade
- Whole blood or packed red blood cell (pRBC) transfusion may be needed with severe anemia (p. 1169).
- In refractory cases, general anesthesia to gauze pack nasal passages may be necessary; carotid artery ligation for life-threatening arterial epistaxis
- Although unproven, topical intranasal application or oral administration of Yunnan Baiyao, a hemostatic powdered herbal mixture, has been reported to help reduce hemorrhage from various causes.

Chronic Treatment

Appropriate treatment for bleeding disorder, systemic illness, or intranasal disease

Possible Complications

Anemia, collapse

Recommended Monitoring

- Serial packed cell volume (PCV) and total protein (TP), as needed to assess severity of hemorrhage
- Monitor clinical signs
- Monitor underlying disorder as appropriate

PROGNOSIS & OUTCOME

Depends on cause

PEARLS & CONSIDERATIONS

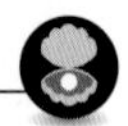

Comments

- Remember that epistaxis may indicate a systemic bleeding disorder; use caution with venipuncture (prefer peripheral vein to jugular for compression) and cystocentesis.
- Systemic causes (e.g., bleeding disorder) can present as acute unilateral epistaxis.
- Rule out systemic diseases and bleeding disorders before focusing on nasal disease, especially if acute onset.
- Recurrent bouts of epistaxis, especially if associated with mucopurulent discharge, typically signals intranasal disease.

Technician Tips

- Monitor for pallor, hypotension that indicate severe or worsening anemia and hypovolemia
- Petechiation, ecchymoses, other sites of bleeding indicative of bleeding disorders

Client Education

Monitor for recurrence of presenting signs.

SUGGESTED READING

Bissett SA, et al: Prevalence, clinical features, and causes of epistaxis in dogs: 176 cases (1996-2001). J Am Vet Med Assoc 231:1843-1850, 2007.

AUTHOR: Shauna Blois, DVM, DVSc, DACVIM
EDITOR: Leah A. Cohn, DVM, PhD, DACVIM

Epulides

Client Education Sheet

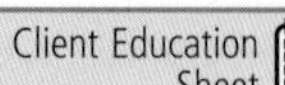

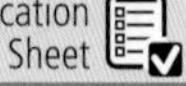

BASIC INFORMATION

Definition

- *Epulis* (plural *epulides*) is a nonspecific clinical descriptive term referring to a local, exophytic growth on the gingiva (e.g., focal fibrous hyperplasia, peripheral odontogenic fibroma, acanthomatous ameloblastoma, nonodontogenic tumors).
- This chapter focuses on peripheral odontogenic fibroma, giant cell granuloma, and acanthomatous ameloblastoma, which are all benign tumors (i.e., do not metastasize). Peripheral odontogenic fibromas and giant cell granulomas do not invade bone, but acanthomatous ameloblastomas are locally invasive.

Synonyms

- *Peripheral odontogenic fibroma* replaces the terms *fibromatous* (or *fibrous*) *epulis* and *ossifying epulis*. Fibromatous epulis is distinguished from ossifying epulis by containing less bone or dental hard tissue within the tumor's soft tissue. Another synonym is *periodontal ligament tumor*.

- *Giant cell granuloma* has also been called *giant cell tumor* or *giant cell epulis.*
- *Acanthomatous ameloblastoma* replaces the terms *acanthomatous epulis* and *adamantinoma.*

Epidemiology

SPECIES, AGE, SEX

Dogs:

- Prevalence: common (except giant cell granuloma, which is rare)
- Distribution: peripheral odontogenic fibroma ≈80%, acanthomatous ameloblastoma ≈18%, and giant cell granuloma ≈2%
- Breed: acanthomatous ameloblastoma more commonly diagnosed in Shetland sheepdogs
- Age: unknown for giant cell granuloma; dogs with peripheral odontogenic fibroma usually > 5 years old; dogs with acanthomatous ameloblastoma usually > 7 years old (but can affect dogs as young as 1 year of age)
- Sex: conflicting results; female dogs more often affected than males with acanthomatous ameloblastoma, male dogs more often affected than females with peripheral odontogenic fibroma and giant cell granuloma

Cats:

- Prevalence: uncommon
- Distribution: peripheral odontogenic fibroma ≈63%, giant cell granuloma ≈29%, and acanthomatous ameloblastoma ≈8%
- Breed: no predisposition reported
- Age: cats with single peripheral odontogenic fibroma and giant cell granuloma usually > 7 years old; acanthomatous ameloblastoma and multiple feline epulides particularly in young-adult cats
- Sex: no predisposition reported

ASSOCIATED DISORDERS

Oral tumors, benign (p. 711). Hypercalcemia of malignancy has been reported in some dogs with acanthomatous ameloblastomas (increased serum concentrations of ionized calcium, total calcium, and parathyroid hormone–related peptide).

Clinical Presentation

DISEASE FORMS/SUBTYPES

- Peripheral odontogenic fibroma
  - Slow growth; gingiva-like
  - Fibroblast is main component in mass
  - Slow recurrence after incomplete excision
  - Multiple feline epulides may not originate from the periodontal ligament but may represent reactive lesions arising from the periosteum.
- Giant cell granuloma
  - Rapid growth; inflammatory and ulcerative changes
  - Multinucleated giant cell is main component in mass; osteoid and woven bone formation
  - Rapid recurrence after incomplete excision
- Acanthomatous ameloblastoma
  - Rapid growth; cauliflower-like
  - Basal cell is main component in mass

HISTORY, CHIEF COMPLAINT

- Gingival mass noticed by owner or at routine oral examination
- Clinical complaints mostly absent with peripheral odontogenic fibromas; dysphagia, increased salivation, bloody oral discharge, and halitosis occasionally reported with giant cell granulomas and acanthomatous ameloblastomas

PHYSICAL EXAM FINDINGS

- Peripheral odontogenic fibroma
  - Firm, rarely ulcerated gingival mass that measures 0.5-3 cm in diameter
  - Located near canine, premolar, and molar teeth (less commonly in the incisor tooth area) and variably fixed to the gum line
  - Covered by oral epithelium; ulceration infrequent
- Giant cell granuloma
  - Soft, reddish purple
  - Ulcerated and inflamed
- Acanthomatous ameloblastoma
  - Cauliflower-like, red, ulcerated, easily bleeding gingival mass that measures 0.5-10 cm in diameter
  - Most commonly located in the rostral lower jaw near incisor and canine teeth; less often in the rostral upper jaw (incisor and canine tooth area), caudal lower jaw (near first molar), and caudal upper jaw (near fourth premolar)

Etiology and Pathophysiology

- Peripheral odontogenic fibroma
  - Mixed or mesenchymal (depending on literature studied) odontogenic tumor
  - Arising from cells in the periodontal ligament
- Giant cell granuloma: considered to be a variant of the peripheral odontogenic fibroma in which extensive ulceration and inflammation result in strongly increased osteoclastic activity, but the real origin remains unknown
- Acanthomatous ameloblastoma
  - Epithelial odontogenic tumor
  - Debatable whether arising from epithelial rests of Malassez in periodontal ligament (intraosseous/central ameloblastoma) or epithelial rests of Serres in gingival connective tissue (extraosseous/peripheral ameloblastoma)

DIAGNOSIS

Diagnostic Overview

Diagnosis requires staging, including oral examination under anesthesia, thoracic radiographs, regional diagnostic imaging (dental radiographs, computed tomography), lymph node palpation and aspiration, and biopsy of the gingival mass.

Differential Diagnosis

Dogs:

- Gingival hyperplasia (often generalized)
- Pyogenic granuloma (uncommon; usually developing on gingiva/alveolar mucosa caudobuccal to the mandibular first molar in cats)
- Dentigerous cyst (around crown of an unerupted tooth)
- Odontoma (not a neoplastic lesion, but a hamartoma, which is an accumulation of normal cells in an abnormal manner)
- Viral papillomatosis (usually in puppies or immunocompromised adults)
- Plasmacytoma (usually solitary, pink-red, well circumscribed)
- Osteoma (slow-growing)
- Malignant melanoma (most common malignant oral tumor)
- Squamous cell carcinoma (second most common oral malignant tumor)
- Fibrosarcoma (third most common malignant tumor)
- Peripheral nerve sheath tumor (along major nerves)
- Osteosarcoma (usually osteolytic type; variant: multilobular tumor of bone)
- Lymphoma (also look for lesions on skin around mouth and nasal plane, bilateral enlargement of tonsils and regional lymph nodes)
- Amyloid-producing odontogenic tumor (rare)

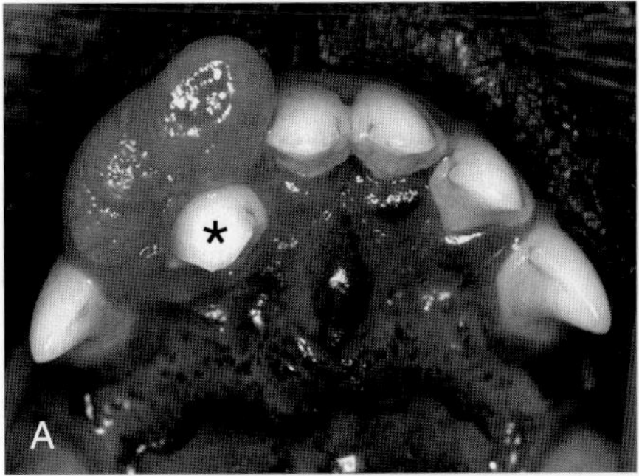

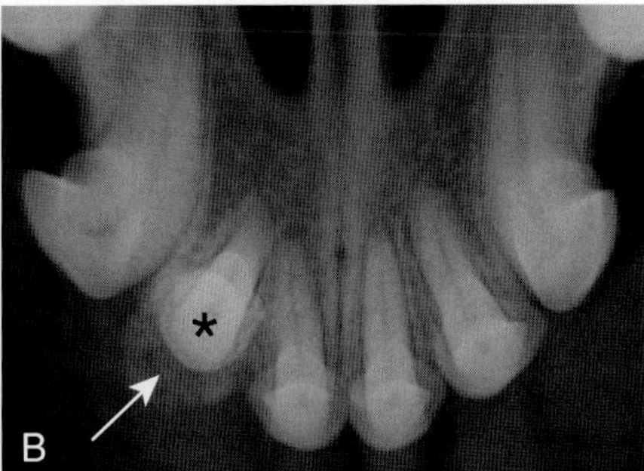

EPULIDES A, Rostral upper jaw in a dog with peripheral odontogenic fibroma. Note smooth-surfaced and minimally ulcerated/inflamed gingival mass associated with palatally displaced right maxillary second incisor *(asterisk)*. **B,** Dental radiograph of rostral upper jaw in same patient (radiograph arranged in labial mounting; rostral toward bottom of image, and patient's right side is on left of image). Note displaced right maxillary second incisor *(asterisk)* and hard tissue *(arrow)* within tumor's soft-tissue shadow. (Copyright Dr. Alexander M. Reiter, University of Pennsylvania.)

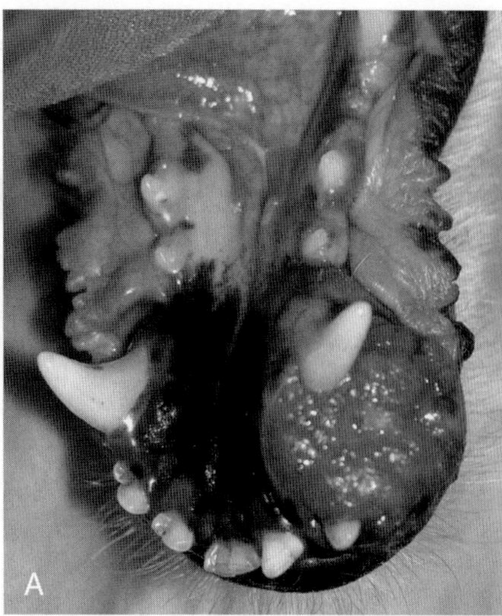

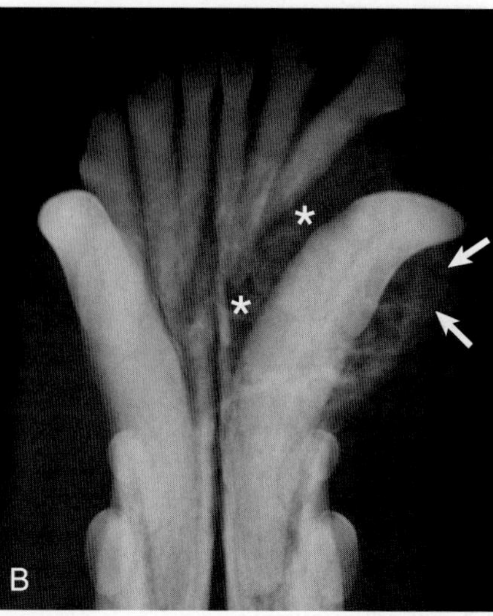

EPULIDES A, Rostral lower jaw in a Shetland sheepdog with acanthomatous ameloblastoma. Note red, cauliflower-like, and easily bleeding mass located between left mandibular third incisor and canine tooth. **B**, Dental radiograph of rostral lower jaw in same patient (radiograph arranged in labial mounting; rostral toward the top of image, and patient's left side is on right of image). Note displacement of involved teeth, lysis of alveolar bone *(asterisks)*, and sunburst pattern at left lateral mandibular border *(arrows)*. (Copyright Dr. Alexander M. Reiter, University of Pennsylvania.)

- Erythema multiforme (also look for lesions on skin)
- Autoimmune diseases (bullous pemphigoid, lupus erythematosus)
- Eosinophilic granuloma (usually on soft palate and lateral edges of the tongue)

Cats:

- Gingival hyperplasia, osteoma, plasmacytoma
- Squamous cell carcinoma (most common malignant oral tumor)
- Fibrosarcoma (second most common oral malignant tumor)
- Feline inductive odontogenic tumor (rare)
- Amyloid-producing odontogenic tumor (rare)
- Eosinophilic granuloma (usually on upper lip, tongue, sublingual tissues, and palate)

Initial Database

- Physical examination, CBC, serum biochemistry profile
- Dental and head radiographs:
  - Peripheral odontogenic fibromas: not invasive; radiographic changes to alveolar bone unlikely
  - Acanthomatous ameloblastomas: invasive; changes to alveolar bone visible on dental radiographs
- CT: superior to radiography, particularly for maxillary and caudally located mandibular lesions
- Biopsy
  - Cytologic techniques less diagnostic; biopsy for histopathologic examination the only definitive test to establish an accurate diagnosis
  - Excisional biopsy for small lesions during initial oral examination may be curative.
  - Incisional biopsy for larger lesions to determine tumor type will allow the clinician to properly plan for future definitive surgery.

Advanced or Confirmatory Testing

CT is valuable to determine local disease extension and bony invasion in dogs with maxillary or caudal mandibular acanthomatous ameloblastoma. This facilitates achieving wide surgical margins and allows for radiation therapy planning.

TREATMENT

Treatment Overview

The primary goal of treatment is complete tumor removal with minimal functional and cosmetic compromise.

Acute General Treatment

- Surgery: conservative and radical
  - Peripheral odontogenic fibroma: gingival excision with conservative margins, extraction of the associated tooth (or teeth in case pinpointing the lesion to one tooth is difficult), and curettage of the alveolar socket(s) to remove the periodontal ligament; local excision without tooth extraction and socket curettage is rarely curative (recurrence is likely because these tumors arise from cells in the periodontal ligament).
  - Acanthomatous ameloblastoma: mandibulectomy and maxillectomy with at least 1-cm margins (depending on location of the tumor)
- Radiation therapy: considered for nonresectable masses, incomplete resections, and recurrent tumors; options include conventional radiation therapy and stereotactic radiosurgery (SRS), such as CyberKnife SRS, which is associated with high conformality, submillimeter accuracy, fewer treatments required (usually three), and fewer side effects.
  - Peripheral odontogenic fibroma: effective but rarely required, as surgical resection typically results in complete cure
  - Acanthomatous ameloblastoma: effective, with tumor control achieved in about 90% of dogs, especially for smaller tumors; larger tumors (>4 cm) are more likely to recur (only about 30% tumor control); higher radiation doses may be required to improve control rates.
  - Acute and late side effects can occur, most notably radiation-induced tumors (many years after radiation therapy in about 3.5%-12.5% of dogs with acanthomatous ameloblastoma) and bone necrosis.
- Cryosurgery: causes cellular death after controlled freezing and thawing of the tumor
  - Best for low-grade tumors < 2 cm in diameter and adherent to or minimally invasive into one cortex; tumor should first be debulked and biopsied, followed by cryosurgery applied to underlying bone.
  - Inadequate for tumors with extensive fixation to or invasion into bone; full-thickness freezing of maxillofacial bones (e.g., maxilla, mandible) can lead to bone necrosis, bone fracture, or oronasal fistula
  - Despite maintenance of the bony framework and preservation of oral function, recurrence is more common than with surgical excision.

Nutrition/Diet

Soft food and avoidance of chew treats/toys for 2 weeks after tooth extraction or radical resection (mandibulectomy, maxillectomy)

Possible Complications

- Wound dehiscence
- Incomplete resection and tumor recurrence
- Bone necrosis after cryosurgery or radiation therapy

Recommended Monitoring

- Clinical re-examination at 2 weeks, 6 and 12 months, and then once yearly after definitive treatment
- Radiographic re-examination (for acanthomatous ameloblastoma) once yearly

PROGNOSIS & OUTCOME

- Peripheral odontogenic fibroma and giant cell granuloma: excellent prognosis (after complete gingival resection, tooth extraction, and curettage of the alveolus); cats with multiple fibromas may have higher recurrence rates.
- Acanthomatous ameloblastoma: excellent prognosis (after mandibulectomy and maxillectomy procedures when clean histopathologic margins can be accomplished); smaller tumors and rostral location are positive prognostic factors because these masses are detected earlier and are easier to remove; postoperative radiation therapy may occasionally be required for tumor control.

PEARLS & CONSIDERATIONS

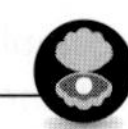

Comments

- Because peripheral odontogenic fibromas and giant cell granulomas arise from the periodontal ligament, excision limited to the gingiva will be inadequate, resulting in tumor recurrence. Gingival excision, extraction of the involved tooth, and curettage of the alveolar sockets to remove any remaining periodontal ligament will usually be curative.
- Aggressive surgical excision (mandibulectomy, maxillectomy) is usually curative in dogs with acanthomatous ameloblastoma.
- Radiation therapy offers excellent long-term control for treatment of acanthomatous ameloblastoma, but malignant tumor development in the irradiated area several years later has been reported.

Prevention

- Early tumor detection (daily home oral hygiene and oral examination at every patient visit)

Technician Tips

When you identify a gingival swelling/mass during oral examination and dental cleaning procedures, notify the veterinarian so that a diagnosis and treatment plan can be formulated.

SUGGESTED READING

Fiani N, et al: Clinicopathologic characterization of odontogenic tumors and focal fibrous hyperplasia in dogs: 152 cases (1995-2005). J Am Vet Med Assoc 238:495-500, 2011.

AUTHORS: Sue N. Ettinger, DVM, DACVIM; Alexander M. Reiter, DVM, Dr. med. vet., DAVDC, DEVDC
EDITOR: Alexander M. Reiter, DVM, Dr. med. vet., DAVDC, DEVDC

Esophageal Perforation/Rupture

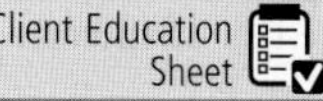
Client Education Sheet

BASIC INFORMATION

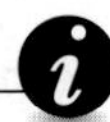

Definition

A full-thickness defect in the esophagus with leakage of esophageal contents into the cervical tissues, mediastinum, and potentially the pleural space (pp. 312 and 351)

Epidemiology

SPECIES, AGE, SEX

- No age or sex predisposition
- Perforation has been reported in more dogs than cats (attributed to the less discriminating feeding behavior of dogs)

GENETICS, BREED PREDISPOSITION

Eighty-six percent of esophageal foreign bodies are reported in dogs weighing < 12 kg (26 lb).

RISK FACTORS

- Foreign body ingestion (p. 351) by dogs weighing < 10 kg: foreign bodies present for 3 days and bone foreign bodies in the esophagus are risk factors for complications of endoscopic foreign body retrieval. Esophageal perforation is more common than gastric.
- Balloon dilation of esophageal strictures (p. 310)
- General anesthesia with secondary esophageal damage

ASSOCIATED DISORDERS

- Mediastinal abscess
- Pneumothorax
- Pyothorax
- Bronchoesophageal fistula
- Esophageal diverticulum

Clinical Presentation

HISTORY, CHIEF COMPLAINT

History may include
- Retching, regurgitation, vomiting, ptyalism, anorexia
- Coughing, dyspnea
- Restlessness, weight loss, pain
- Cervical swelling, subcutaneous emphysema

PHYSICAL EXAM FINDINGS

The duration of clinical signs associated with esophageal perforation is reported to be longer than with esophageal foreign body alone. Physical findings may include
- Fever
- Subcutaneous emphysema
- Rapid shallow respiration consistent with pneumothorax or pyothorax
- Moist rales on auscultation, if aspiration pneumonia is present
- Dehydration

Etiology and Pathophysiology

- Sharp edges of a foreign body may lacerate the esophagus and, rarely, the great vessels.
- Large foreign bodies can result in pressure necrosis of the esophageal wall; the greatest damage is usually associated with pressure points of the foreign body against the esophageal wall.
- The most common site of foreign body lodgment is the distal esophagus just cranial to the gastroesophageal junction; other sites are the heart base, thoracic inlet, and less often, the cervical esophagus.
- Esophageal perforation can be caused by esophageal trauma or balloon dilation of esophageal strictures.
- Full-thickness necrosis of the esophagus has been reported in a dog due to concurrent use of an esophageal electrocardiogram probe and an electrosurgical unit. Maintenance of the unit and handpieces to avoid fluid contact and corrosion and avoiding use of the devices concurrently during surgery are recommended to avoid the complication.
- Significant esophageal damage secondary to general anesthesia for elective procedures has been reported in two cats.

DIAGNOSIS

Diagnostic Overview

Esophageal perforation can be difficult to diagnose. Cervical and thoracic radiographs and contrast esophagram and/or esophagoscopy are required to confirm the diagnosis of perforation and the location of the lesion.

Differential Diagnosis

- Megaesophagus
- Hiatal hernia or gastroesophageal intussusception
- Intrinsic or extrinsic esophageal masses
- Neoplasia
- Parasite infestation
- Esophagitis
- Esophageal diverticulum
- Vascular ring anomaly
- Abnormal pharyngeal or esophageal motility

Initial Database

CBC:
- Neutrophilic leukocytosis
- More immature neutrophils are present with a perforated esophagus than with esophageal foreign body alone.

Diagnostic imaging:
- Survey cervical and thoracic radiographs may demonstrate esophageal foreign body (radiopaque bone common), air within the periesophageal tissues, pneumomediastinum, pneumothorax, pleural effusion/pyothorax, and/or increased lung density with concurrent aspiration pneumonia
- Contrast esophagram (p. 1062) should be performed with water-soluble contrast if perforation is suspected; the procedure has a false-negative rate of 14.5%.

Esophagoscopy:
- Performed with care; do not create or worsen pneumothorax or cause esophageal rupture.
- Evaluate integrity and viability of esophagus, and identify site of perforation.
- Possible foreign body removal

Analysis of pleural effusion, if present (p. 1164): cytologic analysis of fluid and bacterial culture and susceptibility testing (aerobic and anaerobic)

TREATMENT

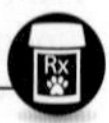

Treatment Overview

Treatment approach depends on the location of the perforation and the severity of associated problems. Surgical intervention other than abscess drainage may or may not be indicated for cervical perforation, but it is required for all thoracic perforations to avoid life-threatening consequences associated with leakage of contents (e.g., pyothorax). Nutritional support that bypasses the damaged esophagus is essential after medical or surgical management, as is medical management of esophagitis to reduce the risk of stricture formation.

Acute General Treatment

- Correction of fluid and electrolyte deficits
- Antimicrobial therapy
  - Empiric therapy using an antibiotic with a broad spectrum of aerobic activity, such as cefazolin 22 mg/kg IV q 6h or ampicillin-sulbactam 30 mg/kg IV q 8h
  - Definitive antimicrobial therapy should be based on results of microbiologic culture and susceptibility testing of pleural fluid and/or mediastinal abscess
- Surgical intervention
  - Removal of foreign body if underlying cause
  - Repair of perforation: primary closure +/− resection and anastomosis
  - Debridement and lavage if mediastinal abscess, pyothorax
- Treatment of esophagitis
  - H2 antagonists (e.g., famotidine 0.5 mg/kg IV q 12-24h) or preferably, antisecretory agents (e.g., omeprazole 0.7 mg/kg by feeding tube q 24h or pantoprazole 1 mg/kg IV q 12-24h) to decrease gastric acid production
  - Motility agents (metoclopramide 0.2-0.5 mg/kg SQ or PO q 6-12h or cisapride 0.1-1 mg/kg PO q 8-12h) to promote normal gastroesophageal sphincter tone (reduce gastroesophageal reflux and esophagitis) and gastric emptying
- Nutritional support until esophagus has healed and normal function has returned: percutaneous endoscopic gastrostomy (PEG) feeding tube (p. 1109) to bypass esophagus, typically for 10-14 days

Chronic Treatment

Treatment of pyothorax (p. 857): long-term antibiotic therapy, based on accurate identification of organism(s) involved. Up to 3 months of therapy may be required.

Possible Complications

- Dehiscence of esophageal repair causing recurrent leakage
- Esophageal diverticulum formation secondary to the presence of a foreign body
- Esophageal stricture formation secondary to damage caused by foreign body, surgical technique, or esophagitis

Recommended Monitoring

- If PEG tube has been placed, removal may be possible in 10-14 days; 7-10 day minimum required before removal to allow proper adhesion of the stomach to the abdominal wall
- Ensure that normal esophageal function returns. Esophageal stricture, if it occurs, usually becomes clinically apparent 3-4 weeks after injury (increasing problem of regurgitation).

PROGNOSIS & OUTCOME

Prognosis associated with esophageal perforation is guarded due to multiple possible complications and is specifically influenced by the presence or absence of

- Mediastinitis/mediastinal abscess formation
- Development of pyothorax
- Development of esophageal stricture

PEARLS & CONSIDERATIONS

Comments

Endoscopic evaluation and removal of esophageal foreign bodies must be performed carefully, with special attention paid to the patient's ventilatory pattern, oxygen saturation, heart rate, and blood pressure. Insufflation of the esophagus with air in the presence of a perforation can lead to tension pneumothorax and acute cardiopulmonary compromise of anesthetized patients.

Prevention

Do not let dogs and cats eat foreign objects that have the potential to become lodged in the esophagus.

Technician Tips

- Post-treatment nutritional support by PEG tube feeding is necessary for these patients while the esophagus heals.
  - Be familiar with PEG tube use and how to educate clients on use of the tube.
  - Ensure that patient is receiving correct amount of food and water.
- Knowledge of and experience in working with thoracostomy tubes is important in those patients who have undergone thoracotomy.

SUGGESTED READING

Gianella P, et al: Oesophageal and gastric endoscopic foreign body removal: complications and follow-up of 102 dogs. J Small Anim Pract 50:649-654, 2009.

AUTHOR: MaryAnn G. Radlinsky, DVM, MS, DACVS
EDITOR: Elizabeth A. Swanson, DVM, MS, DACVS

Esophageal Stricture (Benign)

Bonus Material Online | Client Education Sheet

BASIC INFORMATION

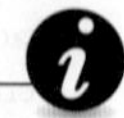

Definition

Scar tissue that forms after deep esophageal injury (esophagitis with inflammation extending into submucosal and muscular layers) (pp. 312 and 642)

Epidemiology

SPECIES, AGE, SEX

Strictures due to foreign bodies and anesthesia-associated acid reflux are more common in dogs, and strictures secondary to esophagitis caused by pills composed of caustic agents are more common in cats.

RISK FACTORS

- Gastroesophageal reflux during anesthesia
- Dogs: esophageal foreign objects that cause deep, circumferential ulceration
- Cats: administration of medications not followed with water or food (capsules or uncoated tablets are the most common medications that lodge and cause esophagitis or stricture)

ASSOCIATED DISORDERS

- Esophagitis (common)
- Esophageal foreign bodies (common)

Clinical Presentation

HISTORY, CHIEF COMPLAINT

- Regurgitation is the classic presenting sign. Distinguish from vomiting: regurgitation classically involves no prodromal signs, no active retching, no bile or digested blood.
- Difficulty swallowing or pain associated with swallowing (repeated swallowing efforts)
- Ptyalism/hypersalivation
- Inappetence
- Lethargy (primarily if there is severe, concomitant esophagitis)
- Weight loss (if the condition is long-standing)

- Cough, increased respiratory rate or effort may be seen if the patient has concurrent aspiration pneumonia (p. 793).

PHYSICAL EXAM FINDINGS

- Typically normal if acute
- Weight loss if chronic
- Ptyalism or gagging
- Coughing, fever, or increased bronchovesicular sounds if aspiration pneumonia has occurred

Etiology and Pathophysiology

- Acid reflux during anesthesia is the most important cause of benign strictures in dogs. Although infrequent, it is very important.
- Drug-induced esophagitis (especially doxycycline and clindamycin) is important in cats.
- Esophageal foreign bodies and esophagitis secondary to chronic persistent vomiting may also be responsible.
- Infrequently, benign esophageal stricture follows esophageal *Pythium* spp infection or prior esophageal surgery (e.g., to remove foreign bodies, masses).
- Esophageal stricture formation requires substantial esophageal injury (usually chemical or mechanical) causing inflammation extending to the submucosal or muscular layers. Subsequent normal repair processes include formation of fibrous connective tissue, which narrows or closes the esophageal lumen.

DIAGNOSIS

Diagnostic Overview

- Regurgitation is an indication for thoracic radiographs. If no abnormality is seen, barium contrast radiography or esophagoscopy is then warranted.
- A barium contrast esophagram can be diagnostic, but fluoroscopy or, better still, use of barium-impregnated food may be necessary.
- Benign strictures are usually obvious during esophagoscopy unless 1) the patient is large and the stricture relatively minor, or 2) the stricture is so close to the lower esophageal sphincter that it is mistaken for being part of the sphincter.

Differential Diagnosis

Regurgitation:

- Esophagitis
- Esophageal foreign body
- Esophageal mass (granuloma, parasites, neoplasia)
- Esophageal motility disorders (megaesophagus, congenital or acquired)
- Esophageal diverticulum
- Persistent right aortic arch
- Gastroesophageal reflux during anesthesia (history of anesthesia is important)
- Gagging/dysphagia
- Oropharyngeal, nasopharyngeal disease

Initial Database

- CBC, serum chemistry panel, urinalysis results likely normal; changes are nonspecific
  - Inflammatory leukogram possible if aspiration pneumonia
  - Dehydration possible if stricture is severe
- Thoracic/abdominal radiographs are indicated in regurgitating patients.
  - Plain thoracic radiographs may be normal but may document air/food cranial to the stricture or demonstrate pulmonary changes due to aspiration pneumonia.
  - Abdominal radiographs are usually unremarkable.

Advanced or Confirmatory Testing

- Esophagoscopy (p. 1098) is the test of choice for diagnosing esophageal strictures, esophagitis, and other anatomic esophageal abnormalities. Endoscopy can also be used for dilation of the stricture (ballooning or bougienage).
- Contrast radiographs may reveal strictures or esophageal motility defects. Liquid or paste barium may pass through a stricture so quickly that diagnosis is impossible without fluoroscopy; using contrast-impregnated food is much more sensitive. Contrast imaging may diagnose multiple strictures when the endoscope cannot pass through the first stricture (p. 1062).
- Fluoroscopy is often needed to identify lower esophageal sphincter defects causing reflux.
- Abdominal ultrasound rarely finds abdominal causes of gastroesophageal reflux (e.g., large hepatic masses putting pressure on the stomach).

TREATMENT

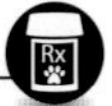

Treatment Overview

Therapeutic goals are to remove the obstruction, protect esophageal mucosa from additional injury, and eliminate the cause of the injury. Return to normal anatomy is not always possible, in which case being able to maintain nutrition and minimize regurgitation by feeding soft diets is considered a success.

Acute General Treatment

- Resolution of the cause of the stricture (e.g., acid reflux, persistent vomiting, foreign body) and treatment of esophagitis if present (p. 312)
- If the stricture is mild (soft foods pass through the stricture site with minimal clinical signs, and no weight loss occurs), management may be attempted by dietary modification (feeding soft or liquid foods in frequent, small meals).
- Strictures refractory to conservative dietary management require dilation. If this is not possible, a gastric feeding tube must be placed to allow maintenance of hydration and nutrition (p. 1109).
- Dilation can be accomplished by ballooning or esophageal bougienage.
- Balloon dilation entails passing an inflatable balloon catheter into the stricture site and inflating it to tear/break down the scar tissue and increase the esophageal luminal diameter.
- Bougienage involves passing rigid dilators of gradually increasing size through the stricture site.
- Both methods require concurrent endoscopic or fluoroscopic guidance to perform the procedure accurately and safely and identify complications (e.g., esophageal tear) early.
- Intralesional injection of glucocorticoids, topical application of mitomycin C, 3- or 4-quadrant nicking of the stricture before dilation, insertion of a stent, and/or use of a balloon-esophagostomy tube may help reduce the chance of stricture recurrence after the dilation procedure; however, no technique is uniformly successful.
- Lifelong dietary management may be necessary in some patients.
- Patients with any residual stricture will be at increased risk for esophageal foreign body.

Chronic Treatment

- Animals with severe strictures often require many dilations to achieve an esophageal opening sufficiently large to accommodate liquid or gruel diets.
- Patients with esophagitis due to gastroesophageal reflux often require long-term therapy (proton pump inhibitors, prokinetics).

Nutrition/Diet

May need a softened or gruel-like diet if stricture cannot be resolved. Occasionally, gastrostomy tube feeding may be required.

Possible Complications

- The main catastrophic complication of stricture dilation is esophageal rupture or perforation. Severe hemorrhage rarely occurs but can be life-threatening.
- Stricture recurrence often occurs if the dilation procedure is too aggressive and produces excessive inflammation.
- Aspiration pneumonia is possible if the patient continues to regurgitate or does not have well-controlled dietary management (e.g., dog gets into the garbage or is allowed to eat foods that will not pass).

PROGNOSIS & OUTCOME

- The prognosis for mild strictures is good.
- The prognosis for severe strictures, especially those that are several centimeters long and requiring multiple dilations is guarded.
- If the patient can be managed on softened diets with minimal to no regurgitation, treatment is considered successful. Complete resolution of severe strictures may fail, and these patients must be maintained on softened, semiliquid to liquid diets, or even with the use of feeding tubes.

PEARLS & CONSIDERATIONS

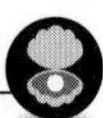

Comments

Esophageal strictures should be referred as soon as possible to specialists who have extensive experience with them. Do not attempt to dilate a stricture unless one has the equipment and substantial experience.

Prevention

- Animals should be fasted before general anesthesia to reduce risk of reflux.
- Position anesthetized patients to reduce risk of gastroesophageal reflux and inflate endotracheal tube cuff appropriately.
- Patients should receive food or water after administration of oral medications to prevent capsules or tablets from lodging in the esophagus (especially cats).
- Prevent animals from eating bones, rocks, fish hooks, and other foreign objects.
- Routine administration of a proton pump inhibitor and a gastric prokinetic before anesthetic procedures is controversial but may lessen the frequency of anesthesia-associated gastroesophageal reflux. If perianesthesia gastroesophageal reflux is suspected, the esophagus should immediately be washed out with water and antacid therapy begun.

Technician Tips

- Watch closely for any evidence of anesthesia-associated reflux.
- Always give cats fluid or food after administering pills.

Client Education

- It is important to give water after administration of oral medications.
- If any evidence of esophageal dysfunction or dysphagia is noted after an anesthetic procedure, notify the veterinarian at once.
- Long-term management of patients with partially resolved strictures requires strict, lifelong dietary management.

SUGGESTED READING

Bissett SA, et al: Risk factors and outcome of bougienage for treatment of benign esophageal strictures in dogs and cats: 28 cases (1995-2004). J Am Vet Med Assoc 235:844-850, 2009.

AUTHOR: Michael D. Willard, DVM, MS, DACVIM
EDITOR: Rance K. Sellon, DVM, PhD, DACVIM

Esophagitis

Bonus Material Online 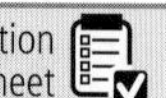 Client Education Sheet

BASIC INFORMATION

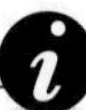

Definition

Acute or chronic inflammation of the esophagus, classically secondary to gastric acid (often due to reflux or persistent vomiting), foreign bodies, or medications

Synonyms

Gastroesophageal reflux, reflux esophagitis

Epidemiology

SPECIES, AGE, SEX

Dogs and cats of any age and either sex

GENETICS, BREED PREDISPOSITION

Brachycephalic dogs may be prone to hiatal hernia, which can cause reflux esophagitis.

RISK FACTORS

- General anesthesia, even of short duration
  - Most commonly reported cause of reflux esophagitis in the dog and cat
- Hiatal hernia or other causes of lower esophageal sphincter (LES) dysfunction
- Esophageal foreign body
- Oral medications (e.g., tetracyclines, ciprofloxacin, nonsteroidal antiinflammatory drugs [NSAIDs]) given without being followed by food or water administration
- Persistent vomiting
- Gastric hyperacidity (e.g., gastrinoma)
- *Pythium insidiosum* infection
- Large cranial abdominal masses (e.g., primary hepatic tumors) that displace the stomach dorsally

ASSOCIATED DISORDERS

Benign esophageal strictures, especially secondary to severe anesthesia-associated reflux (p. 310)

Clinical Presentation

HISTORY, CHIEF COMPLAINT

- Mild esophagitis may be subclinical.
- Clinical signs may include
  - Increased swallowing motions, ptyalism
  - Inappetence, hyporexia, and/or odynophagia (discomfort when swallowing) due to pain
  - Regurgitation (mild to severe) or vomiting
  - Reluctance to move or lie down
  - Cats may vocalize after eating as an indication of esophageal pain.
- Affected patients may have a history that reveals risk factors (see Risk Factors above).

PHYSICAL EXAM FINDINGS

May be normal; abnormalities may include

- Thin body condition
- Dehydration
- Ptyalism
- Pharyngitis, stomatitis, and/or glossitis
- Cranial abdominal/thoracic discomfort
  - Hunched-up appearance
  - Guarding or pain on palpation

Etiology and Pathophysiology

Etiology:

- Premedications (atropine, benzodiazepines, phenothiazines, opioids) and anesthetic induction agents may decrease LES tone, allowing gastroesophageal reflux.
- Anatomic abnormalities (e.g., hiatal hernia) can increase risk of reflux esophagitis.
- Because of their pH or osmolarity, ingested medications or chemicals can damage the esophagus if retained in the esophagus for long periods.

Pathophysiology:

- Esophageal mucosal contact with low-pH gastric fluid, pepsin, trypsin, bile salts, and/or alkaline fluid or with caustic agents (e.g., detergents, alkalis, acids) causes mucosal damage and inflammation sometimes extending to the deeper layers of the esophagus.
- Volume, frequency, and duration of contact of noxious material with the esophagus affect the severity of esophageal damage.
- Hypersensitivity might (?) predispose to eosinophilic esophagitis.

DIAGNOSIS

Diagnostic Overview

Diagnosis can be suspected based on a suggestive history (dysphagia after anesthesia or protracted vomiting) or response to treatment, but other diseases may respond to therapy for esophagitis. Esophagitis can be easily confirmed by direct endoscopic visualization. Biopsy is

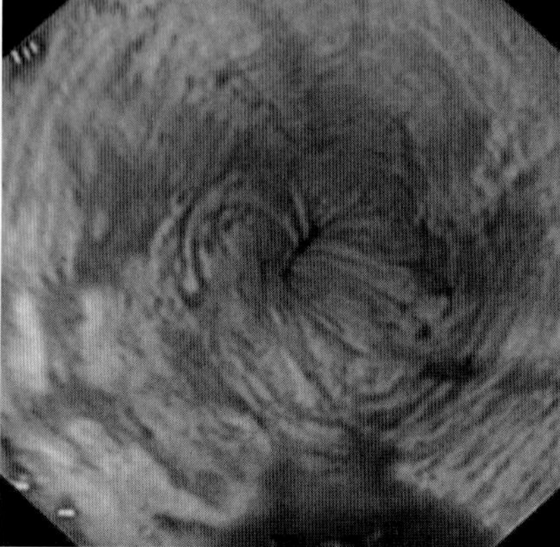

ESOPHAGITIS Endoscopic view of a patient with esophagitis. Note the longitudinal, darker, patchy areas indicative of inflammation and mucosal erosion. Fluid pooling is apparent at the bottom of the image.

Diseases and Disorders

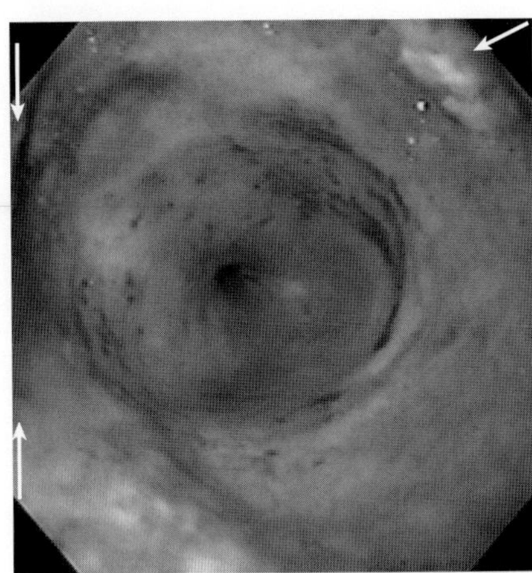

ESOPHAGITIS Endoscopic view of a patient with ulcerative esophagitis demonstrating multifocal areas of hemorrhage and hyperemia. Ulcers are apparent as deep depressions in the esophageal wall on the left edge of the image *(arrows)* and at the 1-o'clock position *(single arrow)*. Mucosal hemorrhages are also evident as darker, thin, circumferential streaks and pinpoint lesions on or near the gastroesophageal sphincter. Bleeding and/or hyperemia is not due to endoscopy in normal dogs because the stratified squamous epithelium of the esophageal mucosa is relatively tough.

necessary to diagnose eosinophilic esophagitis (rare).

Differential Diagnosis

- Esophageal foreign body: odynophagia (pain on swallowing) and/or regurgitation
- Megaesophagus: regurgitation
- Vomiting
- Neoplasia or mass lesions (esophageal intra or extralumenal; extraesophageal): regurgitation
- Vascular ring anomaly: regurgitation
- Hiatal hernia: regurgitation
- Gastroesophageal intussusception (rare)
- Thermal esophageal damage (e.g., tube feeding with excessively hot liquids [rare])

Initial Database

- CBC, serum biochemistry profile, urinalysis: results often normal
- Survey thoracic radiographs are seldom diagnostic but might show esophageal dilation.
- Contrast esophagram sometimes demonstrates retention of barium on the esophageal mucosa, mucosal ulceration or hyperplasia, or decreased esophageal motility.

Advanced or Confirmatory Testing

- Esophagoscopy (p. 1098) allows definitive diagnosis, exclusion of other disorders, and evaluation of extent and severity.
  - Flexible endoscopic biopsy of canine esophageal mucosa is extremely difficult in most animals but occasionally reveals organisms such as yeast *(Candida)* or eosinophilic infiltrate.
  - Biopsy may be important in cats with chronic inflammation at the LES, which may not be grossly obvious.
- Fluoroscopy often needed to detect LES dysfunction not due to hiatal hernia

TREATMENT

Treatment Overview

Goals of therapy are to protect the esophageal mucosa from further damage, decrease the amount and frequency of reflux, and eliminate acid from reflux.

Acute General Treatment

- Lessen or eliminate gastric acid secretion.
  - Currently available H2-receptor antagonists are ineffective and not recommended.
  - Proton pump inhibitors (e.g., omeprazole 1-2 mg/kg PO q 12h): most effective class of drugs; requires 2-5 days to reach maximal efficacy, but immediate effects are superior to H2-receptor antagonists
- Minimize reflux by increasing LES tone and keeping stomach empty.
- Prokinetic drugs (metoclopramide 0.2-0.5 mg/kg PO or SQ q 8h; cisapride 0.1-0.25 mg/kg PO q 8-12h; erythromycin 0.5-1.0 mg/kg PO or IV q 8h; ranitidine 2.2-4.4 mg/kg PO or IV q 8-12h).
- Sucralfate suspension (0.25-1 g/PATIENT PO q 8h)
  - Especially helpful to reduce discomfort if patient is painful
- A 4% viscous lidocaine or 2% lidocaine jelly at 4-5 mL/kg PO q 6h for severe pain

Chronic Treatment

- Treat until esophagitis resolves.
- Indefinite prokinetic and antacid therapy may be needed when chronic lower esophageal dysfunction does not resolve and is not amenable to surgical resolution.

Nutrition/Diet

- Feed a moderate- to high-protein, low-fat diet, which increases lower esophageal tone and encourages gastric emptying.
- Rarely, need to place gastrostomy tube to ensure nutrition and ability to medicate anorexic patients that regurgitate everything given orally (p. 1109).

Possible Complications

Esophageal stricture formation

Recommended Monitoring

- Normal eating without dysphagia, ptyalism, or regurgitation usually implies resolution.
- Inappetence, dysphagia, ptyalism, or regurgitation necessitates re-examination for stricture or persistent inflammation.
- Strictures may cause regurgitation beginning days to 4 weeks after injury.

PROGNOSIS & OUTCOME

- If inflammation is not severe, is recognized early and treated appropriately, and the inciting cause can be controlled, prognosis is usually good.
- Prognosis is guarded if the cause cannot be resolved, esophagitis is severe, or patient develops severe esophageal strictures.

PEARLS & CONSIDERATIONS

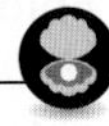

Comments

- Prevent prolonged contact of medication with esophageal mucosa by administering water (e.g., 5-10 mL by syringe) after any tablet or capsule given without food.
- Consider reflux esophagitis in patients showing ptyalism, inappetence, or regurgitation shortly after anesthesia.

Prevention

- Fast animals before general anesthesia.
- Routine preanesthetic use of proton pump inhibitors and prokinetic drugs will probably decrease (not eliminate) the incidence/severity of anesthesia-associated gastroesophageal reflux.
- Esophageal lavage and suction is helpful in patients that are known to have regurgitated during anesthesia.

Technician Tips

If a dog or cat shows any signs of dysphagia, ptyalism, or regurgitation after anesthesia, notify the clinician immediately.

Client Education

Administer water (e.g., 5-10 mL by syringe trickled in the cheek pouch) after any tablet or capsule given without food.

SUGGESTED READING

Zacuto AC, et al: The influence of esomeprazole and cisapride on gastroesophageal reflux during anesthesia in dogs. J Vet Intern Med 26:518-525, 2012.

AUTHOR: Michael D. Willard, DVM, MS, DACVIM
EDITOR: Rance K. Sellon DVM, PhD, DACVIM

Ethylene Glycol Intoxication

BASIC INFORMATION

Definition

Ethylene glycol (EG) intoxication manifests as peracute-onset, marked central nervous system (CNS) depression and progressive, dose-related metabolic acidosis and acute kidney injury (AKI).

Synonyms

- EG poisoning, radiator antifreeze poisoning
- Ethylene glycol: 1,2-ethanediolmonoethylene glycol, glycol alcohol, CAS 107-21-1

Epidemiology

SPECIES, AGE, SEX

- All animals are susceptible.
- Cats are extremely sensitive to EG intoxication.
- Dogs are more commonly exposed than cats. Intact young male dogs may be more likely to be involved.

RISK FACTORS

- Pets living outdoors or having access to EG sources (e.g., garages)
- Freezing temperatures provide increased opportunity, especially when water sources are limited (frozen), and antifreeze remains in the liquid state because of its low freezing point.
- In hot climates, cars may overheat and leak engine coolant (i.e., antifreeze).
- Engine leak is the most common source of exposure in pets, and a home garage is the most common exposure location.
- Malicious poisoning is encountered on occasion.

GEOGRAPHY AND SEASONALITY

- EG poisoning occurs year round; it is no longer a seasonal problem.
- Colder climate zones are overrepresented, but exposure can occur anywhere. Summer automobile radiator flushing is considered routine maintenance.

Clinical Presentation

HISTORY, CHIEF COMPLAINT

- Indirect evidence of exposure
  - Pet being near an automobile garage or work area
  - Roaming free in areas suspected or known to have EG sources
- Classic "drunken sailor" behavior (stupor, narcosis, ataxia, falling, nausea) may be noted within 1-2 hours of ingestion.
- Stupor phase gradually subsides over several hours.
  - Stupor phase may go unnoticed, especially in outdoor pets
  - Owner may note the pet is "getting better."
  - Patient is quiet, depressed, polydipsic, and polyuric
- Patient gradually shows more weakness, depression, ataxia, anorexia, and tachypnea/dyspnea as AKI and oliguria/anuria occur 24-72 hours after ingestion.

PHYSICAL EXAM FINDINGS

- CNS depression, generalized weakness, hyporeflexia, hypothermia, slow capillary refill time (CRT), tachycardia, vomiting
- Urinary bladder may be empty on palpation.
- Patient may have already progressed beyond the initial drunken phase, potentially delaying or confusing the clinical picture.
  - Overt signs of AKI (oliguria/anuria, anorexia, vomiting, renomegaly with signs of renal pain) typically begin 24-72 hours after ingestion.
- In severe intoxications, seizures, nystagmus, and tremors may occur in the first few hours after ingestion (grave prognosis).

Etiology and Pathophysiology

- Lethal dose of 95% ethylene glycol: 4.4 mL/kg (dog), 1.4 mL/kg (cat)
- Rapid oral absorption of EG
  - Blood levels detectable in < 30 minutes
  - Initial CNS depression and narcosis, vasodilation, and hypotension with reflex tachycardia, diuretic effect
- Metabolism involves hepatic alcohol dehydrogenase oxidation of EG to the aldehyde (glycoaldehyde), a saturable, rate-limiting step.
  - Metabolic progression can be interrupted at this point with fomepizole or ethanol.
- Glycoaldehyde is very toxic but quickly converts to glycolic acid.
- Glycolic acid (30%-45% of metabolite load) is fairly stable and further oxidizes to glyoxylic acid, which then converts to oxalic acid, glycine, formate, hippurate, CO_2, and other compounds.
- Aldehyde and acid load create a high–anion-gap metabolic acidosis.
- Metabolites inhibit the citric acid cycle and substrate level phosphorylation, depress serotonin and pyruvate metabolism, and alter CNS amine levels.
- Secondary lactate accumulation, hypoperfusion, and calcium oxalate crystal formation and precipitation in microvasculature and renal tubules occur.

DIAGNOSIS

Diagnostic Overview

A high index of suspicion should exist based on history alone (e.g., owner saw pet licking or in the same room as fluorescent green liquid). Treatment must be implemented early—before kidney injury and possibly before definitive diagnostic confirmation in many cases. The diagnosis is more straightforward, but the prognosis is worse > 12-24 hours after ingestion, when overt clinical signs are more prominent. A typical approach to diagnosis and treatment is outlined on p. 1416.

Differential Diagnosis

- Acute CNS depression, ataxia, acidosis, or AKI: encephalitis, cranial trauma, intracranial neoplasia, diabetic ketoacidosis; or intoxication with barbiturates, aspirin, methanol, ethanol, isopropanol, propylene glycol, glycol ethers, vitamin D_3, *Lilium* and *Hemerocallis* spp (cats), nonsteroidal antiinflammatory drugs, grapes, or raisins
- AKI (p. 23)

Initial Database

- Kacey Diagnostics Ethylene Glycol Veterinary Test Strips (www.kaceydiagnostics.com/Toxicology.html or 828-685-3569): quantitative test for dogs and cats; false-positives for alcohols, including methanol and xylitol
- VetSpec Ethylene Glycol Qualitative Reagent Test Kit (www.catacheminc.com/brochures/Ethylene-Glycol-Flyer.pdf or 203-262-0330): qualitative test for dogs and cats; false-positives for propylene glycol, glycerol, diethylene glycol (or other *cis*-1,2 diols), and sorbitol
- Serum biochemistry panel and electrolytes (especially Ca^{2+}, Mg^{2+}, K^+, and P): azotemia, hyperphosphatemia, hyperkalemia with oliguria/anuria, ± hypocalcemia, ± hyperglycemia
- Acid-base: blood pH, PCO_2, PO_2, serum bicarbonate; metabolic acidosis common ± compensatory respiratory alkalosis
- Urinalysis: specific gravity, crystals, glucose, cellular debris, granular casts
  - As for any cause of acute anuric kidney injury, specific gravity is not necessarily isosthenuric
  - Calcium oxalate monohydrate crystals (picket fence boards, flattened hexagon shapes: ⬡) can be observed 3-18 hours after EG ingestion and are much more specific for ethylene glycol intoxication than calcium oxalate dihydrate crystals (Maltese cross or square envelope appearance: ⊠), which can occur from nutritional or laboratory artifactual causes as well as EG intoxication; only about 40% of cases have crystals.
- Fluids: measure total input and output; body weight
- Optional Wood's lamp examination (detects fluorescein dye in antifreeze); scan of muzzle, paws, vomitus, urine (excretes < 3-6 hours in humans) for fluorescence that subjectively supports exposure

Advanced or Confirmatory Testing

- EG and glycolic acid levels (serum, urine); requires STAT turnaround time to benefit

early diagnosis in determining treatment approach
- Serum osmolality; requires colloid osmometer
  - Normal osmole gap: 5-10 mOsm/kg (dogs and cats). Osmole gap = measured osmolality − calculated osmolality; measured osmolality is obtained with a colloid osmometer, and calculated osmolality is obtained from the following equation using values from the serum biochemistry profile: 2 × ([Na^+] + [K^+]) + BUN (mg/dL)/2.8 + glucose (mg/dL)/18.
  - >20 mOsm/kg strongly suggests EG intoxication; parallels EG blood level; significant increase within 1 hour of exposure
- Anion gap (calculated from serum biochemistry profile: ([Na^+] + [K^+]) − ([Cl^-] + [HCO_3^-])
  - Normal anion gap: 10-25 mEq/L (dogs and cats)
  - >25 mEq/L can occur with EG intoxication
  - May note change by 3 hours but may require 6 hours; is therefore less preferred as an early diagnostic tool
- Ultrasound: increased renal cortical echogenicity at 4-6 hours; late in the course, halo sign indicative of anuria and grave prognosis
  - Many normal, healthy cats have diffuse hyperechogenicity of renal cortices (avoid overinterpretation).
- Renal calcium level in postmortem tissue sample

TREATMENT

Treatment Overview
- EG toxicosis is a medical emergency. Due to rapid progression and irreversibility of renal lesions, any patient suspected of consuming EG should be tested and treated unless/until exposure has been ruled out.
- The greatest window of opportunity for intervention is < 8-12 hours after exposure in dogs, < 2 hours after exposure in cats.
- Empirical treatment with fomepizole or ethanol is indicated if the index of suspicion is high and a confirmatory test is not immediately available.
- Emesis induction and administration of activated charcoal can be considered in asymptomatic cases presented within 1 hour of exposure. Confirmed cases should receive fomepizole or ethanol and be hospitalized for management of acid-base abnormalities, fluid diuresis for renal protection, and supportive care.

Acute General Treatment
- Induction of vomiting (pp. 1087 and 1188): helpful within 30-60 minutes; indicated if patient is a good risk. Some clinicians precede this by very rapidly feeding a tasty meal to provide a substrate for the vomiting if the pet has an otherwise empty stomach.
- Activated charcoal 1-2 g/kg PO once: binds poorly but may be given if asymptomatic; will make EG tests false-positive.
- Interrupt conversion to toxic metabolites with fomepizole (4-MP, 4-methylpyrazole)
  - Dog: 20 mg/kg slow IV infusion (15-20 minutes), 15 mg/kg slow IV at 12 and 24h, 5 mg/kg IV at 36h
  - Cats < 3 hours after ingestion: 125 mg/kg slow IV infusion (15-30 minutes), 31.25 mg/kg at 12, 24, 36h
  - Must be compounded as Antizol-Vet is no longer commercially available
- *Or* interrupt conversion to toxic metabolites with 7% ethanol solution in 5% dextrose or 0.9% saline
  - Commonly, Everclear (190 proof, or 95% ethanol) or plain vodka (80 proof, or 40% ethanol) is used as ethanol source (divide the proof by 2 to get the ethanol percentage).
  - To make a bag of fluids plus ethanol for infusion: (7%/ethanol %) × mL of fluids = mL of ethanol. For example, if using vodka (7%/40%) × 1000 mL = 175 mL. Therefore, remove 175 mL of dextrose/saline from a 1-L bag, and add 175 mL of vodka.
  - Loading dose: 8.6 mL/kg slow IV of the solution
  - Maintenance dose: 1.43-2.86 mL/kg/h constant-rate infusion (CRI) to effect
  - Duration of infusion: approximately 48 hours (5-7 times the half-life of EG)
  - Dogs treated with ethanol starting at 3 hours after ingestion of EG excrete 80% of EG intact.
- Hemodialysis (more effective) or peritoneal dialysis while on ethanol or fomepizole. Immediate dialysis of any patient showing clinical signs of intoxication tends to increase the survival rate.
- Crystalloids: high infusion rates required to correct severe dehydration and hypoperfusion. Must use great caution in case oliguria/anuria develops to avoid overhydration (p. 23)
- Acid-base and fluid volume management is critical to survival.
  - Sodium bicarbonate as needed for metabolic acidosis
- Provide cofactors for metabolism of toxic compounds
  - Pyridoxine 1-2 mg/kg IV q 6h
  - Thiamine 50 mg slow IV q 6h
- For animal with oliguria/anuria, euthanasia is a reasonable consideration.

Chronic Treatment
Dialysis to allow regeneration of damaged tubular basement membrane; recovery may take many weeks

Possible Complications
- Complications of AKI, including acute respiratory distress syndrome, pulmonary edema, seizures, and death
- Chronic renal compromise; depends on degree of insult and response to intensive treatment

Recommended Monitoring
Intensive early monitoring of respiratory rate, electrolytes, acid-base status, renal function (BUN, creatinine), and urine production (ins and outs). If clinical signs of AKI develop, best to refer to 24-hour care facility, ideally with ability to perform dialysis.

PROGNOSIS & OUTCOME

- Dogs: fair to good with intensive intervention within 8-12 hours of ingestion; prognosis worsens if clinical signs of AKI are apparent at presentation and/or a large dose was ingested.
- Cats: guarded to poor in any animal showing clinical signs; intensive intervention (interruption of metabolism with high doses of fomepizole, dialysis, acid-base management) within 3 hours of exposure can prove successful.

PEARLS & CONSIDERATIONS

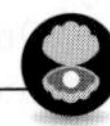

Comments
- Progression of irreversible, life-threatening effects from EG is rapid (hours), and evaluation and treatment are urgent, even in animals without overt clinical signs.
- "Safe antifreeze" contains propylene glycol, which is less toxic compared to EG; much less risk of renal injury. Dogs need to ingest three or four times more propylene glycol than EG to develop clinical signs.
- Use of injectable medications (diazepam), or commercial preparations of activated charcoal before using EG test kits can give a false-positive result due to their propylene glycol, glycerol, and/or sorbitol content.

Prevention
Keep animals indoors and not in the garage, especially in freezing temperatures (frozen water sources but antifreeze remains as liquid).

Technician Tips
- Human hospital laboratory may be able to detect and quantify EG.
- Antifreeze (EG) usually is fluorescent green, viscous (like light syrup), and has no volatile odor; windshield washer fluid (not EG) is translucent blue, pungent (volatile odor), and nonviscous (like water).

Client Education
- Lock antifreeze containers away from chewing dogs.
- Use cat litter to clean up spills and leaks.
- About 1 tsp (5 mL) of EG is potentially lethal to an adult cat.

SUGGESTED READING

Thrall MA, et al: Ethylene glycol. In Peterson ME, et al, editors: Small animal toxicology, ed 3, St. Louis, 2013, Saunders Elsevier, pp 551-567.

AUTHOR & EDITOR: Tina Wismer, DVM, MS, DABVT, DABT

Exercise-Induced Collapse in Labrador Retrievers

Client Education Sheet 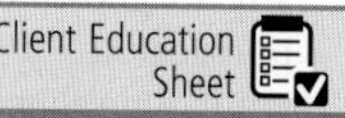

BASIC INFORMATION 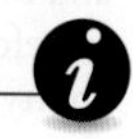

Definition

Exercise-induced collapse (EIC) of Labrador retriever dogs is a common, breed-associated, inherited neurologic disorder causing weakness and inability to stand and walk during or after strenuous physical activity.

Epidemiology

SPECIES, AGE, SEX

Dogs of either sex. Signs typically first occur at 9-18 months of age.

GENETICS, BREED PREDISPOSITION

Autosomal-recessive inheritance of dynamin 1 gene *(DNM1)* mutation

- Only dogs homozygous for the *DNM1* mutation are susceptible to collapse.
- The mutation and associated collapse are common in Labrador retrievers (approximately 7% homozygous/affected, 38% heterozygous/carriers).
- The condition also occurs in Boykin spaniel, curly coated retriever, Old English sheepdog, Chesapeake Bay retriever; rarely in Bouvier des Flandres, German wirehaired pointer, Welsh corgi, and cocker spaniel

RISK FACTORS

- Homozygosity for the *DNM1* mutation
- Hot weather, high level of excitement: most likely to trigger collapse

Clinical Presentation

HISTORY, CHIEF COMPLAINT

Affected dogs typically are normal except for episodes of collapse. After participating in strenuous exercise for 5-15 minutes, dogs develop pelvic limb weakness, ataxia, and inability to support weight. Dogs often continue to run while dragging the pelvic limbs. This may progress to include all four limbs. Collapse lasts 5-30 minutes. Dogs appear clinically normal after recovery.

PHYSICAL EXAM FINDINGS

During collapse, muscles are flaccid, and the patellar reflex is absent. Body temperature is high (average 41.7°C [107.1°F]), but this is normal for exercising Labradors. No cardiac, respiratory, or mentation abnormalities. After dogs recover, physical and neurologic examination findings are normal.

Etiology and Pathophysiology

Affected dogs are homozygous for a mutation in DMN1, a protein in the brain and spinal cord that is important for repackaging neurotransmitters into synaptic vesicles for release during high-level neurologic stimulation (during exercise, excitement, and increased body temperature).

DIAGNOSIS

Diagnostic Overview

Diagnosis is suspected based on breed predisposition and typical episodes of collapse in an otherwise normal dog. Confirmation is obtained with a DNA test.

Differential Diagnosis

- Cardiac arrhythmias, hypoglycemia, glucocorticoid deficiency, and epilepsy can cause nonpainful episodes of collapse in otherwise healthy dogs.
- Dogs with collapse due to heat stroke are mentally abnormal and do not experience rapid spontaneous recovery.
- EIC is the most common reason for exercise-induced collapse in otherwise healthy Labrador retrievers.
- When collapse episodes are not typical for EIC, partial seizures due to epilepsy may be more likely.

Initial Database

- CBC, biochemistry profile, urinalysis
- Thoracic radiographs
- Neurologic and orthopedic exams (pp. 1136 and 1143)

Advanced or Confirmatory Testing

DNA test for the *DMN1* gene mutation: specimen can be sterile cheek swab/sterile applicator (purchase kit at pharmacy), whole blood (1-3 mL in lavender-top EDTA tube), dewclaws from puppies (place in plain glass red-top tube), or semen (1 straw or 0.5 mL in plain glass red-top tube). University of Minnesota College of Veterinary Medicine Veterinary Diagnostic Laboratory website: https://www.vdl.umn.edu/services-fees/canine-neuromuscular-eic

TREATMENT 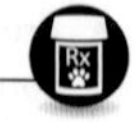

Treatment Overview

Treatment is nonspecific and supportive when an episode occurs.

Acute General Treatment

- Stop activity at the first sign of abnormal gait.
- Cool collapsed dogs (fan, vaporized water on body, isopropyl alcohol to footpads, cool water enemas if severe hyperthermia) (p. 421).
- No treatment except avoiding participation in exciting trigger activities, which consistently reduces or eliminates the occurrence of collapse in affected dogs.

Possible Complications

Rarely, affected dogs die during collapse. Cause of death is unknown; hyperthermia, respiratory muscle weakness, or *DMN1* effects on the brain are possible mechanisms. No causative lesion has been found at necropsy.

PROGNOSIS & OUTCOME 

Excellent prognosis for a normal life if participation in trigger activities can be limited

PEARLS & CONSIDERATIONS 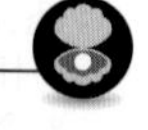

Comments

- EIC is the diagnosis until proven otherwise for a healthy Labrador retriever with an episode of pelvic limb collapse during exercise that recovers completely by the time the dog is examined by a veterinarian.
- The tendency of affected dogs to collapse does not change over time, and affected dogs do not develop other associated signs as they age.

Prevention

- Collapse episodes can be prevented by limiting participation in trigger activities (high-excitement, strenuous activity).
- EIC status should be determined for all Labradors before breeding. The high prevalence of the mutation in this breed makes it unreasonable to try to eliminate all affected and carrier dogs from the population, but genetic testing makes it possible to avoid producing affected puppies.

Technician Tips

Death during EIC collapse is rare and may be due to hyperthermia in affected dogs. In a collapsed dog, ensure that nothing is obstructing ventilation, to facilitate the main source of heat dissipation (panting).

Client Education

Limit participation in trigger activities by dogs homozygous for *DMN1*. Halt activity and cool dog if the onset of an abnormal gait is apparent during exercise.

SUGGESTED READING

Furrow E, et al: Relationship between dynamin-1 mutation status and phenotype in 109 Labrador retrievers with recurrent collapse during exercise. J Am Vet Med Assoc 242:786-791, 2013.

AUTHOR: Susan M. Taylor, DVM, DACVIM
EDITOR: Leah A. Cohn, DVM, PhD, DACVIM

Exocrine Pancreatic Insufficiency

Client Education Sheet

BASIC INFORMATION

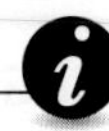

Definition

A syndrome caused by insufficient secretion of pancreatic digestive enzymes by the exocrine pancreas

Epidemiology

SPECIES, AGE, SEX

Occurs more commonly in dogs than in cats. In dogs belonging to breeds that are affected by pancreatic acinar atrophy (PAA), exocrine pancreatic insufficiency (EPI) is most commonly diagnosed in young adults. In other dog breeds and cats, EPI can occur at any age.

GENETICS, BREED PREDISPOSITION

In some dog breeds (i.e., German shepherds, rough-coated collies, and Eurasians), EPI is considered to be hereditary. A simple autosomal-recessive inheritance, until recently suspected to be the mode of inheritance in the German shepherd dog, has now been disproven. There is no known breed predisposition in cats. See Etiology below regarding PAA.

RISK FACTORS

- Chronic pancreatitis can lead to destruction of exocrine pancreatic tissue and EPI.
- Rarely, pancreatic adenocarcinoma or abdominal surgery can lead to obstruction of the pancreatic duct, causing lack of pancreatic enzyme secretion into the small intestines.

ASSOCIATED DISORDERS

Many canine and feline patients with EPI have other gastrointestinal disorders. Dogs with EPI commonly have secondary small-intestinal dysbiosis (formerly known as small-intestinal bacterial overgrowth or antibiotic-responsive diarrhea [p. 260]); other dogs and cats can have concurrent idiopathic inflammatory bowel disease (p. 543).

Clinical Presentation

HISTORY, CHIEF COMPLAINT

- Weight loss is the most common clinical sign in dogs and cats.
- Loose stools and less commonly diarrhea
- Ravenous appetite
  - Unlike dogs, approximately 40% of cats with EPI can have decreased appetite.

PHYSICAL EXAM FINDINGS

- Poor body condition (NOTE: due to timely diagnosis in dogs, emaciated patients are rare.)
- Poor haircoat and sometimes in cats, greasy soiling of the haircoat, especially in the perianal area

Etiology and Pathophysiology

- Approximately 50% of dogs with EPI have PAA, a condition that is mostly seen in German shepherds, rough-coated collies, and Eurasians.
- In the vast majority of the remainder of dogs and in almost all cats, EPI is due to chronic pancreatitis.
- Other potential but rare causes of EPI include obstruction of the pancreatic duct by a pancreatic adenocarcinoma or abdominal surgery, pancreatic aplasia, or pancreatic hypoplasia.
- Decreased secretion of pancreatic digestive enzymes leads to lack of these enzymes in the small intestine, which leads to maldigestion and associated clinical signs.
- Secondary cobalamin deficiency is very common in dogs and occurs in almost all cats with EPI.
- In patients with EPI due to chronic pancreatitis, pancreatic inflammation may also lead to destruction of islets of Langerhans and cause concurrent diabetes mellitus.

DIAGNOSIS

Diagnostic Overview

The most reliable diagnostic test for EPI for dogs and cats is serum trypsin-like immunoreactivity (TLI) concentration, which is measured by species-specific assays.

Differential Diagnosis

- Primary small-intestinal disease (e.g., inflammatory or infiltrative bowel disease)
- Other secondary causes of chronic diarrhea and weight loss (e.g., hepatic failure, chronic kidney disease, hypoadrenocorticism, hypothyroidism [dogs], hyperthyroidism [cats], other less common causes)

Initial Database

- CBC, serum chemistry profile, and urinalysis results are usually within normal limits.
- Imaging studies are usually unremarkable.

Advanced or Confirmatory Testing

- Serum TLI is the test of choice for a diagnosis of EPI in dogs and cats.
  - A severely decreased serum TLI concentration is diagnostic of EPI.
    - In dogs: ≤ 2.5 mcg/L (cTLI; reference interval, 5.7-45.2 mcg/L)
    - In cats: ≤ 8.0 mcg/L (fTLI; reference interval, 12-82 mcg/L)
  - Some patients may have a serum TLI concentration in the questionable range (>2.5 but <5.7 mcg/L [dog]; >8.0 but <12.0 mcg/L [cat]).
    - These patients most likely have chronic small-intestinal disease and should be evaluated accordingly and then retested 4-6 weeks later.
- If no other disease process can be identified, trial therapy may be helpful.
- Other diagnostic tests are much less reliable and should *not* be used for the diagnosis of EPI in dogs or cats:
  - Fecal proteolytic activity is recommended only for species for which a TLI assay is not available (e.g., ferrets).
  - Measurement of fecal elastase concentration is available only for dogs and only in Europe. A positive test result is not specific for EPI and must be confirmed with a decreased cTLI concentration.
- Serum cobalamin concentration should be assayed because > 80% of dogs and virtually all cats will be cobalamin deficient and therefore require oral or parenteral supplementation.

TREATMENT

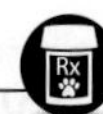

Treatment Overview

- Pancreatic enzyme replacement is crucial.
- Cobalamin can be supplemented parenterally or orally if cobalamin deficiency is present.

Acute General Treatment

- Oral enzyme replacement therapy
  - Starting dose: 1 tsp/10 kg body weight with each meal
  - Tablets and capsules are not as effective as powder.
  - Premixing the pancreatic enzymes with the diet is not necessary.
- Oral or parenteral cobalamin supplementation if the patient is cobalamin deficient
  - Oral supplementation: 250 mcg (cats and small dogs) to 1500 mcg (giant-breed dogs) daily for 90 days, then re-evaluate 2 weeks after last dose
  - Parenteral supplementation: 250 mcg (cats and small dogs) to 1500 mcg (giant-breed dogs) weekly for 6 weeks with one more dose a month later and re-evaluation a month after that

Chronic Treatment

- Oral enzyme replacement therapy
  - After patients have fully responded and returned to their ideal body weight, the amount of enzyme supplement can be decreased to the lowest effective dose, titrated based on stool quality and body condition score or weight.
- Oral antibiotic therapy (e.g., tylosin 25 mg/kg PO q 12h for 6 weeks) and cobalamin supplementation in patients that do not respond to enzyme replacement therapy alone.
- Insulin therapy if patient has concurrent diabetes mellitus (p. 251)

Nutrition/Diet

- Dietary fat restriction is not recommended.
- Several studies in dogs have failed to show any impact of diet on therapeutic response.

- A premium, highly digestible maintenance diet is sufficient.

Possible Complications

Enzyme supplementation can lead to oral bleeding in ≈10%-20% of patients:

- Oral bleeding will stop in most of these patients after a reduction of the dose.
- Patients rarely develop bleeding diathesis due to vitamin K deficiency, which must be treated with vitamin K supplementation.

Recommended Monitoring

Body weight and fecal quality

PROGNOSIS & OUTCOME

Most patients with EPI respond to therapy and have a normal life.

PEARLS & CONSIDERATIONS

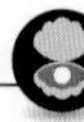

Comments

- Some patients may not respond to enzyme replacement therapy and cobalamin supplementation alone.
  - Many of these patients have concurrent small-intestinal disease (i.e., small-intestinal dysbiosis and/or inflammatory bowel disease).
  - If concurrent disease cannot be identified, gastric acid inhibition can be tried (omeprazole 0.7-1.0 mg/kg PO q 12h has been most useful).
- Fresh-frozen raw pancreas can also be used for enzyme replacement therapy (1-2 oz [30-60 g] of ground raw pancreas equals about 1 tsp of powdered pancreatic extract).

Technician Tips

Serum TLI assays are species specific, and submitting a serum sample with the incorrect species designation can lead to a false diagnosis of EPI.

SUGGESTED READING

Steiner JM: Exocrine pancreas. In Steiner JM, editor: Small animal gastroenterology, Hannover, Germany, 2008, Schlütersche Verlagsgesellschaft, pp 283-306.

AUTHOR: Jörg M. Steiner, Dr. med. vet., PhD, DACVIM, DECVIM, AGAF
EDITOR: Keith P. Richter, DVM, MSEL, DACVIM

Eyelid Defects: Trauma, Masses

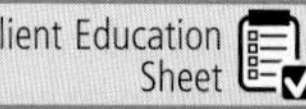

BASIC INFORMATION

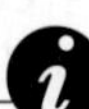

Definition

Eyelid trauma is associated with any injury to the eyelid predisposing to inflammation or laceration. Eyelid masses are very common and are associated with neoplastic or inflammatory conditions.

Synonyms

- Chalazion: hordeolum, meibomian gland cyst
- Meibomian glands: tarsal glands, palpebral glands

Epidemiology

SPECIES, AGE, SEX

- Dogs and cats
- Eyelid trauma may occur at any age.
- Eyelid mass: average age 9-10 years (eyelid neoplasia, dogs) but depends on type of mass

GENETICS, BREED PREDISPOSITION

- Eyelid trauma: more common in young animals, outdoor animals, and sporting breeds of dogs
- Eyelid mass (dogs): more common in American cocker spaniel, boxer, poodle, golden retriever, Labrador retriever, English springer spaniel, beagle, collie, Siberian Husky, and English setter

RISK FACTORS

Excessive sunlight and white hair in the periocular region predispose to squamous cell carcinoma (SCC), the most common eyelid neoplasm in cats.

ASSOCIATED DISORDERS

Eyelid trauma:

- Corneal/scleral trauma
- Uveitis

Eyelid mass:

- Blepharitis (eyelid inflammation)
- Conjunctivitis
- Corneal ulceration

Clinical Presentation

HISTORY, CHIEF COMPLAINT

Eyelid trauma:

- Witnessed traumatic event
- Swollen eyelid(s) (blepharedema)
- ± Eyelid laceration

Eyelid mass:

- Growth on eyelid and/or eyelid margin
- Persistent or intermittent bleeding of eyelid
- Signs of ocular pain if mass is large and causing conjunctival and/or corneal irritation
- Ocular discharge

PHYSICAL EXAM FINDINGS

Eyelid trauma (some or all of the following):

- Blepharedema
- Eyelid laceration (partial or full thickness)
- Blepharospasm
- Ocular discharge/hemorrhage
- Conjunctival hyperemia/edema (chemosis)
- Keratitis (ulcerative or nonulcerative)

Eyelid mass (some or all of the following):

- Mass located along eyelid margin or adjacent to margin of eyelid
- Size, location, and appearance vary with type of mass
  - Neoplasm associated with the meibomian gland appears as an irregular, raised, variably sized mass ± pigment on the eyelid margin that may extend into the eyelid.
  - SCC appears as an erosive, ulcerated mass along the eyelid, often near the medial canthus.
  - Chalazion (meibomian gland cyst) is a smooth, raised, yellow to white mass on the palpebral conjunctiva associated with the meibomian gland.
- Ocular discharge, blepharospasm, conjunctivitis, keratitis if mass irritating the eye
- Eyelid hemorrhage
- Lagophthalmos (incomplete closure of the eyelids)

Etiology and Pathophysiology

- Eyelid trauma is generally associated with blunt trauma, fight with other animal, penetration by sharp objects, or self-mutilation (pawing at eye).
- Eyelid mass (neoplastic)
  - Common in dogs; most are benign.
  - Rare in cats; most are SCC (malignant) or mast cell tumors.
  - Similar to those of the skin; arise from epithelial, mesenchymal, and melanogenic cells
  - In dogs, 82% of eyelid neoplasms are sebaceous adenomas, papillomas, or melanomas.
  - Sebaceous gland tumors (sebaceous adenoma, sebaceous epithelioma, and sebaceous adenocarcinoma) arise from the meibomian glands.
- Focal eyelid inflammation: a chalazion is a pyogranuloma associated with retained meibomian gland secretions.

DIAGNOSIS

Diagnostic Overview

- The diagnosis of eyelid trauma is suspected based on the presence of blepharedema and/or acute blepharitis with or without ocular discharge/hemorrhage.
- The diagnosis of an eyelid mass is suspected based on the presentation of a mass-type lesion or swelling adjacent to or along the

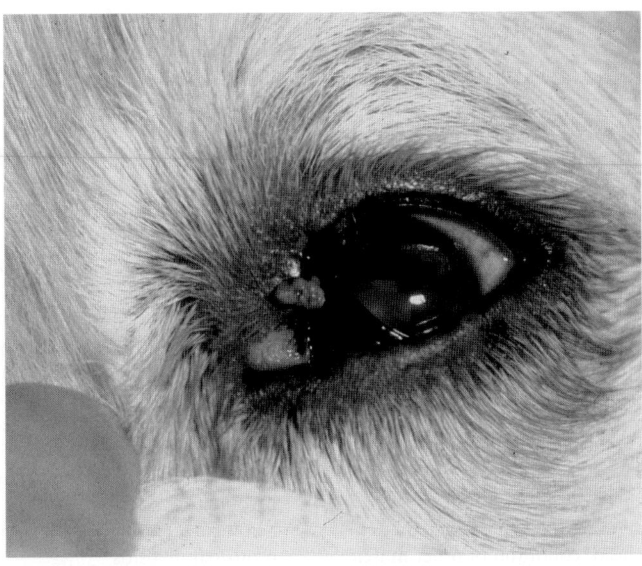

EYELID DEFECTS Eyelid mass. (Courtesy Dr. Phillip A. Moore, Auburn University.)

lid margin; confirmation of the nature of the mass requires cytologic and/or histopathologic assessment.

Differential Diagnosis

Eyelid swelling:

- Anaphylaxis
- Conjunctival/subpalpebral foreign body

Initial Database

Complete ophthalmic examination (p. 1137):

- Schirmer tear test
- Fluorescein dye application evaluating for corneal ulceration secondary to trauma
- Intraocular pressures
- Examination of periocular (e.g., conjunctiva) and intraocular structures, especially if trauma suspected
- Examination of eyelid margin for extent of laceration or extent and point of origin of mass

Advanced or Confirmatory Testing

- Fine-needle aspiration and cytologic evaluation of eyelid masses
- Histopathologic evaluation of all surgically removed eyelid masses

TREATMENT

Treatment Overview

Treatment goals are to restore normal eyelid conformation, eliminate ocular irritation, and prevent recurrence of eyelid mass. Treatment for an eyelid mass should be initiated early in the course of the disease to ensure normal eyelid conformation.

Acute General Treatment

Eyelid trauma:

- Laceration requires primary/surgical closure of wound.
- If full-thickness laceration, close in two layers (conjunctiva/deep stroma, then skin) starting at eyelid margin with a figure-eight suture to ensure accurate apposition of eyelid margin.
  - No suture should penetrate the palpebral conjunctiva and contact the cornea.

Eyelid mass (neoplastic):

- Surgical removal
  - If involves eyelid margin and ≤ ⅓ length of eyelid, remove by a full-thickness V-shaped or house-shaped excision
  - Close in two layers (see above).
  - Eyelid margin mass > ⅓ eyelid length requires a plasty procedure to ensure proper eyelid length (i.e., H-plasty, semicircular flap, or lip-to-eyelid rotational graft). Consider referral to ophthalmologist or surgeon.
- Cryosurgery with curettage
  - Useful for benign eyelid mass in older animals
  - May be performed under sedation
  - Recurrence rate higher with cryotherapy than with full-thickness excision
  - May also be effective for small SCC in cats

Eyelid mass (chalazion):

- Medical therapy with neomycin-polymyxin-dexamethasone ophthalmic ointment q 8h in combination with warm compresses several times a day may be attempted initially.
- Surgical treatment if no response to medical therapy
  - Scalpel incision of overlying palpebral conjunctiva with curettage; heals by second intention
- Topical antibiotic/corticosteroid (e.g., neomycin-polymyxin-dexamethasone suspension or ointment) q 8h for 7 days after surgery; corticosteroid contraindicated if cornea is not intact.

Possible Complications

- Poor apposition of eyelid margin results in cicatrix (scar) formation, predisposing to entropion or ectropion, or step to eyelid margin, resulting in corneal irritation and ulceration.
- Improperly placed sutures at the eyelid margin can predispose to corneal ulceration.
- Local regrowth of eyelid mass if mass not completely removed

Recommended Monitoring

Re-evaluate apposition of eyelid margin, and remove skin sutures 10 days after surgery.

PROGNOSIS & OUTCOME

- Eyelid laceration: prognosis good if apposition of eyelid margin is achieved.
- Removal of eyelid neoplasm: dogs, prognosis good, majority are benign; cats, prognosis guarded, majority are malignant.
- Local recurrence is possible if an eyelid mass is not completely excised.

PEARLS & CONSIDERATIONS

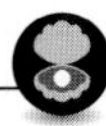

Comments

- Eyelid lacerations are treated surgically as an emergency, not as open wounds, to prevent eyelid scarring, contraction, and distortion of the eyelid margin.
- Eyelid masses should be removed early to prevent the need for plasty procedures.

Prevention

Limit actinic radiation (sunlight) exposure in white cats to decrease the potential for SCC.

Technician Tips

Dogs that have had eyelid surgery should wear an Elizabethan collar until the sutures are removed.

Client Education

Recurrence is possible after the removal of any eyelid mass.

SUGGESTED READING

Maggs DJ: Eyelids. In Maggs DL, et al, editors: Slatter's Fundamentals of veterinary ophthalmology, ed 5, St. Louis, 2013, Elsevier, p 110.

AUTHOR: Phillip A. Moore, DVM, DACVO
EDITOR: Diane V. H. Hendrix, DVM, DACVO

Facial Muscle Wasting

Client Education Sheet 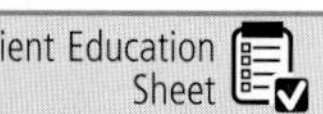

BASIC INFORMATION

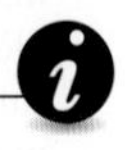

Definition

Atrophy of the muscles of mastication, primarily temporal and masseter muscles

Synonym

Masticatory muscle atrophy

Epidemiology

SPECIES, AGE, SEX

Dogs (most commonly) and cats (rarely), any age, any sex; with muscular dystrophy (MD), only males affected

GENETICS, BREED PREDISPOSITION

- German shepherds, retrievers, Doberman pinschers, spaniels: masticatory myositis (MM [p. 637])
- Shetland sheepdogs, rough- and smooth-coated collies: dermatomyositis (DM)
- German shepherds, other large breeds: idiopathic polymyositis (IP)
- Large-breed dogs: glucocorticoid-induced muscle atrophy
- Congenital myopathies
  - Labrador retrievers: centronuclear myopathy (CM) and X-linked myotubular myopathy
- MDs
  - Golden retrievers, Labrador retrievers, German short-haired pointer, and Cavalier King Charles spaniels: dystrophin mutations
  - Boston terriers, cocker spaniels, and Chihuahuas: sarcoglycan deficiency
  - Brittany spaniel, springer and spaniel mixed-breed dog, and cats: laminin alpha-2 deficiency
  - Sphinx and Devon rex cats: alpha-dystroglycan deficiency
- Bassett hounds: temporomandibular joint (TMJ) dysplasia

ASSOCIATED DISORDERS

- Submandibular and prescapular lymphadenopathy (p. 598)
- Generalized muscle atrophy

Clinical Presentation

HISTORY, CHIEF COMPLAINT

- Detailed history, including previous bouts of painful mastication or chronic glucocorticoid use
  - Chronic daily glucocorticoid administration may cause facial muscle wasting.
- History may reflect abnormalities isolated to facial musculature or generalized myopathy.
  - Facial
    - Prominence of external occipital protuberance
    - Difficulty or inability to prehend food (less common)
    - Weakness (decreased jaw tone) or masticatory muscle fibrosis (increased jaw tone or trismus [inability to open the mouth])
    - Painful mastication and crying while chewing: MM, TMJ dysplasia
  - Generalized
    - Concomitant mild to severe weakness, exacerbated by exercise; generalized muscle atrophy
    - Bunny hopping gait progressing to a more stilted gait with a plantigrade stance: MD

PHYSICAL EXAM FINDINGS

- Full physical exam, paying particular attention to the head, condition of other muscle groups, and skin
- Bilateral atrophy of the temporal and masseter muscles; skull-like appearance of the head
  - Dogs with MM can show salivation, dysphagia, and difficulty in opening the mouth, progressing to trismus.
  - Dogs with DM can show generalized muscle atrophy, skin lesions, decreased jaw tone, facial nerve paralysis, stiff gait, dysphagia, and regurgitation.
- Enophthalmos, with third eyelid protrusion and small palpebral fissure due to dramatic loss of retrobulbar muscular support (p. 716)
- Unilateral temporal muscle atrophy: ipsilateral denervation of the mandibular branch of the trigeminal nerve

Etiology and Pathophysiology

- Developmental
- Neuropathy
- Infectious
- Immune mediated
- Iatrogenic
- Metabolic
- Neoplastic
- Disuse atrophy

DIAGNOSIS

Diagnostic Overview

Specific diagnosis is often made histopathologically, with the exception of serologic titers for infectious causes or for the detection of antibodies against type 2M muscle fibers.

Differential Diagnosis

See Etiology above and a complete differential list (p. 1222).

Initial Database

- CBC usually normal by the time the muscles are atrophied
- Serum biochemistry profile
  - Elevated muscle enzyme levels (creatine kinase and aspartate aminotransferase): IP, MM, DM, MD, CM
  - Hyperglobulinemia: IP

Advanced or Confirmatory Testing

- Muscle biopsies and histopathology:
  - Immunohistochemistry shows lack of dystrophin (MD).
  - High proportion of centralized myofiber nuclei (CM)
  - Antibodies against type 2 myofibers on frozen sections of muscle (MM)
  - Myofiber necrosis with mononuclear cell infiltrates, atrophy, and fibrosis (DM)
  - Multifocal necrosis and phagocytosis of type 1 and type 2 myofibers (IP)
- Circulating serum antibodies against type 2 myofiber muscle fibers: MM
- Serologic titers for *Toxoplasma* and *Neospora:* protozoal myositis
- DNA-based tests are available for some neuromuscular diseases: DM, CM
- Electromyography is more useful in determining neurologic rather than muscular cause of the atrophy.

TREATMENT

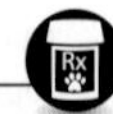

Treatment Overview

- Treatment depends on the underlying cause and may include glucocorticoid therapy to halt the process of muscle inflammation or appropriate antibiotics or antiprotozoal therapy for infectious myositis.
- Glucocorticoid therapy
  - Masticatory myositis (p. 637)
  - Idiopathic polymyositis: prednisone 1-2 mg/kg PO q 12h × 14 days, then tapering over at least 4 weeks to 12 months or longer
  - DM (varied response)
- Upright feeding of dogs with megaesophagus

Possible Complications

Glucocorticoid side effects

Recommended Monitoring

Monitor for glucocorticoid side effects, and taper the dose, depending on muscle condition and function.

PROGNOSIS & OUTCOME

Varies, depending on the underlying cause; process is reversible provided no extensive fibrosis

PEARLS & CONSIDERATIONS

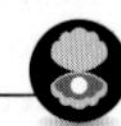

Comments

- Facial muscle atrophy is a common feature of many emaciating conditions in which there is also generalized loss of lean body mass.
- Generalized muscle atrophy is often first noticed in the facial muscles, especially in long-haired breeds.

- Only trigeminal nerve abnormalities, MM, and anomalies of the TMJs are strictly confined to facial muscle atrophy.

Technician Tips

- Masseter muscle atrophy may lead to trismus; a jaw should never be forced open, even under anesthesia.
- To maintain daily nutritional requirements, dogs with trismus often lick liquid gruel, but additional feeding strategies (e.g., esophagostomy tube [p. 1106]) may be required.

Client Education

Early evaluation provides the best chance of response.

SUGGESTED READING

Taylor SM: Disorders of muscle. In Nelson RW, et al, editors: Small animal internal medicine, ed 5, St. Louis, 2013, Mosby, pp 1090-1102.

AUTHOR: Paolo Pazzi, BVSc, MMedVet, DECVIM-CA
EDITOR: Leah A. Cohn, DVM, PhD, DACVIM

Facial Nerve Paralysis, Idiopathic

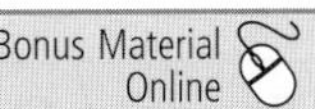

BASIC INFORMATION

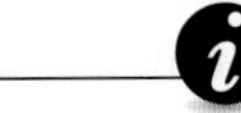

Definition

Acute lower motor neuron paresis or paralysis of unknown cause affecting one or both facial nerves

Epidemiology

SPECIES, AGE, SEX

Affects adult dogs (>5 years of age)

GENETICS, BREED PREDISPOSITION

No genetic link known; cocker spaniels overrepresented

ASSOCIATED DISORDERS

Keratoconjunctivitis sicca (KCS) +/− secondary corneal ulceration, oral ulcerations, idiopathic vestibular disease

Clinical Presentation

HISTORY, CHIEF COMPLAINT

Acute-onset paresis to paralysis of one or both facial nerves manifesting as

- Inability to blink
- Inability to hold food or water in the mouth
- Excessive drooling from one or both sides of the mouth

PHYSICAL EXAM FINDINGS

- Decreased to absent palpebral reflex(es)
- Decreased to absent menace response(s)
- Decreased movement of the facial muscles unilaterally or bilaterally when stimulated (trigeminofacial reflex)
- KCS and possible secondary corneal ulceration
- Drooping lip(s) and/or ears
- Decreased to absent contraction of the lateral commissure(s) of the mouth is most evident when panting. In chronically affected patients, contraction of the commissure(s) is/are observed.
- Increased drooling secondary to lip weakness
- Ulceration of the mucosa at the lateral commissure of the mouth associated with collection of food in this area, secondary to lip weakness

Etiology and Pathophysiology

- Pathogenesis unknown
- Resembles Bell's palsy in humans, which has been linked to a viral infection
- Histopathologic studies reveal demyelination and axonal loss.

DIAGNOSIS

Diagnosis Overview

The diagnosis is based on clinical history and findings from complete neurologic exam. This is a diagnosis of exclusion; other causes of facial nerve dysfunction must be ruled out.

Differential Diagnosis

- Metabolic disease: hypothyroidism
- Infectious/inflammatory disease: noninfectious neuritis versus infectious neuritis, otitis media/interna or primary secretory otitis media
- Trauma: causes hemorrhage into the tympanic bulla and secondary inflammation of the facial nerve
- Toxin: otic toxins
- Neoplasia: affecting the nerve itself (peripheral nerve sheath tumor versus lymphoma) or the tympanic bulla (adenocarcinoma versus polyp)

Initial Database

- Neurologic exam (p. 1136)
- Otic exam: to rule out otitis media/interna (p. 1144)
- CBC, biochemistry panel: unremarkable
- Thyroid testing: normal
- Schirmer tear test: reduced tear production associated with facial nerve deficits (p. 1137)

Advanced or Confirmatory Testing

- MRI (p. 1132): contrast enhancement of affected facial nerve(s) can be observed. Normal facial nerves do not enhance.
    - Speed and completeness of recovery is proportional to the percentage of the nerve that enhances on MRI. Dogs recovered complete function at 8 weeks when one section of the nerve showed enhancement; dogs showed partial resolution of neurologic function at 6 months when three or four sections of the nerve showed enhancement; complete recovery was seen at 4 weeks when no enhancement was observed.
- Electromyogram can show evidence of denervation (spontaneous activity) when musculature innervated by the facial nerve is examined.

TREATMENT

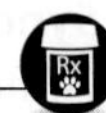

Treatment Overview

There is no specific treatment to improve the function of the facial nerve, although there is some evidence that acupuncture can speed recovery and even lead to complete resolution of clinical signs. KCS should be treated to avoid exposure keratitis.

Acute General Treatment

Treatment for KCS includes frequent corneal lubrication. Topical antibiotics can be used to treat corneal ulceration (pp. 209 and 568).

Possible Complications

Recurrent corneal ulceration if paresis/paralysis does not resolve

PROGNOSIS & OUTCOME

Complete or partial resolution takes weeks to months. Some evidence that degree of contrast enhancement on MRI determines likelihood of full recovery and expected timeline of recovery (see Advanced or Confirmatory Testing above).

PEARLS & CONSIDERATIONS

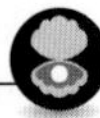

Comments

Daily cleaning of the oral commissures after meals is recommended. Food caught in weak lip muscles can lead to oral ulceration. Ocular assessment is important to ensure signs of corneal ulceration (blepharospasm, aversion to head palpation, discomfort) are not present.

Technician Tips

Assess corneal appearance for signs of ulceration, and liberally apply topical lubricant to the affected eye(s).

Client Education

- Instruct owners to assess for blepharospasm or corneal opacities at home. If observed, owners should seek veterinary care immediately.
- Owners should clean the lip commissures after meals.

SUGGESTED READING

Dewey CW, et al: Disorders of the peripheral nervous system: mononeuropathies and polyneuropathies. In Dewey CW, et al, editors: Practical guide to canine and feline neurology, ed 3, Ames, IA, 2016, John Wiley & Sons, pp 453-454.

AUTHOR: Stephanie A. Thomovsky, DVM, MS, DACVIM, CCRP
EDITOR: Karen R. Muñana, DVM, MS, DACVIM

Fanconi Syndrome

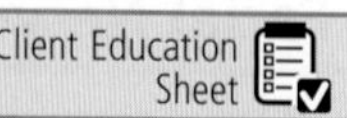

BASIC INFORMATION

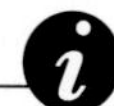

Definition

Uncommon constellation of renal tubular reabsorptive defects (including glucose, ketones, amino acids, phosphates, bicarbonate, calcium, and potassium) accompanied by renal tubular acidosis and isosthenuria or hyposthenuria

Synonym

Proximal renal tubular impairment/acidosis

Epidemiology

SPECIES, AGE, SEX

- Inherited and acquired forms in dogs; anecdotal reports in cats
- No sex predisposition
- Inherited forms: glucosuria, aminoaciduria, phosphaturia, and renal sodium loss are first documented when dogs are adults.

GENETICS, BREED PREDISPOSITION

- Inherited in basenji dogs, affecting 10%-30% of basenjis in the United States; mode of inheritance unknown
- Other breeds (not necessarily inherited): border terriers, Norwegian elkhounds
- West Highland white terriers and single cases among Clumber spaniel, Cardigan Welsh corgi with hepatic copper storage disease can have a reversible Fanconi syndrome, with or without copper accumulation in renal proximal tubular cells (similar to Wilson disease in humans). Anecdotally, renal involvement can be seen in any breed with copper storage disease (p. 458).

RISK FACTORS

- Copper storage hepatopathy
- Ingestion of contaminated jerky treats
- Renal tubular injury (e.g., *Leptospira* spp infection, nephrotoxic insult [see Etiology below]).
- Hypoparathyroidism (causality unconfirmed)
- Chlorambucil (cats)

CONTAGION AND ZOONOSIS

Leptospira spp can cause Fanconi syndrome.

ASSOCIATED DISORDERS

- Polyuria and polydipsia
- Metabolic acidosis
- Electrolyte abnormalities
- Renal tubular acidosis
- Acute kidney injury (AKI) or chronic kidney disease (CKD)
- Urinary tract infection (UTI)
- Skeletal disease is uncommon in dogs (rickets common in children with Fanconi syndrome).
- Urolithiasis
- Gastrointestinal disturbances (with any cause of Fanconi syndrome but especially common with jerky treat intoxication)
- Systemic manifestations of leptospirosis

Clinical Presentation

DISEASE FORMS/SUBTYPES

- Tubular reabsorptive defects can vary among individual dogs.
- Acquired: signs associated with primary disease (e.g., copper hepatopathy, leptospirosis) may dominate clinical presentation.
- Hereditary: dogs typically appear well until middle age or older.
  - Fanconi syndrome may be discovered incidentally during routine health screens.

HISTORY, CHIEF COMPLAINT

Complaints may be absent; some or all may be present:

- Polyuria, polydipsia
- Weight loss, muscular weakness
- Poor haircoat
- Gastrointestinal signs (vomiting, diarrhea, anorexia)

PHYSICAL EXAM FINDINGS

Exam may be normal; some or all may be present plus those listed above:

- Dehydration
- Uremic halitosis
- Oral ulceration with severe azotemia
- Poor body/muscle condition
- Mucous membrane pallor if anemic
- Muscle weakness if hypokalemic/hypophosphatemic

Etiology and Pathophysiology

- Inherited disease: pathophysiology not fully elucidated
- Acquired disease has been associated with heavy metal intoxication (lead, copper, mercury, organomercurials), copper storage hepatopathy, maleic acid, Lysol, drugs (e.g., tetracycline, gentamicin, cephalosporins, cisplatin, salicylate, zonisamide, chlorambucil), amyloidosis, hyperglobulinemia, hyperparathyroidism, vitamin D deficiency, hypokalemia, interstitial nephritis, glomerulonephritis associated with antibodies to glomerular basement membrane, leptospirosis, and renal transplantation.
- Starting in 2007, a form of acquired Fanconi syndrome has been recognized in dogs and putatively associated with ingestion of jerky treats. This form of AKI varies in presentation (glucosuria not always present) and can wax and wane in severity. Gastrointestinal signs may overshadow manifestations of renal disease (e.g., polyuria or uremia).
- Defects: primarily proximal tubular resorptive function
  - Renal glucosuria: defective transport mechanism allows glucosuria even when blood glucose concentration is below transport maximum (≥180-220 mg/dL [10-12.2 mmol/L]).
  - Aminoaciduria: generalized or selective (specific carrier molecules for acidic, basic, and neutral amino acids). Some dogs have cystinuria with minor defects in resorption of methionine, glycine, and dibasic amino acids.
  - Phosphate reabsorption defect (proximal tubule); if severe, can cause hypophosphatemia
  - Hyperchloremic metabolic acidosis possible
  - Hypokalemia possible (kaliuresis is exacerbated with primary bicarbonaturia or supplementation alkali)
- Dogs with Fanconi syndrome are resistant to antidiuretic hormone, creating a form of nephrogenic diabetes insipidus (DI).

Before onset of azotemia, hyposthenuria is frequently documented.

DIAGNOSIS

Diagnostic Overview

Presence of glucosuria +/– ketonuria in the absence of hyperglycemia is a hallmark of Fanconi syndrome, but other tubular defects (proteinuria and aminoaciduria, increased fractional excretion of electrolytes) can also occur.

Differential Diagnosis

- Diabetes mellitus
- Primary renal glucosuria (e.g., glucosuria without aminoaciduria)
- Nephrogenic or central DI
- Renal tubular acidosis (distal or mixed)
- AKI or CKD (all causes should be considered)

Initial Database

- Urinalysis
    - Hyposthenuria, isosthenuria, or minimally concentrated urine (dogs < 1.030; cats < 1.035)
    - Glucosuria is common.
    - Proteinuria is common but mild.
    - Ketonuria is common.
    - Secondary UTI is common (p. 232).
- CBC: anemia occurs late in disease course (with kidney failure).
- Serum biochemistry profile
    - Normoglycemia is typical (despite glucosuria).
    - Hypophosphatemia (may be offset to normophosphatemia if renal failure)
    - Hypokalemia is common.
    - Hyperchloremic metabolic acidosis
        - Venous blood gas preferred to measurement of PCO_2 for confirmation of metabolic acidosis.
    - Azotemia (late finding)

Advanced or Confirmatory Testing

- In a basenji with glucosuria and normoglycemia, no further confirmation is necessary.
- For other breeds
    - Urinary amino acids
        - Cyanide nitroprusside–based array for cystinuria
        - Urine organic/amino acid excretion (http://research.vet.upenn.edu/penngen)
    - Fractional excretion of electrolytes: $(U_x/S_x) \times (S_{cr}/U_{cr}) \times 100$, where U_x is urine concentration of electrolyte, S_x is serum concentration of electrolyte, S_{cr} is serum creatinine, and U_{cr} is urine creatinine
        - Elevated fractional excretion values are expected.
    - Heavy metal testing, if indicated
    - *Leptospira* spp serologic testing, if indicated

TREATMENT

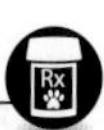

Treatment Overview

A treatment protocol known as the Gonto protocol is used by many owners of affected basenji dogs. The protocol, which is used to replace substances excreted in excess in the urine, has not been compared to other (potentially simpler) protocols to determine whether it improves survival or quality of life. At a minimum, electrolyte and acid-base deficiencies should be corrected, and supportive care for uremia (if present) should be provided.

Acute General Treatment

- If patient is experiencing a uremic crisis (e.g., dehydrated, anorexic, vomiting), hospitalization is appropriate for management, including intravenous fluid therapy (p. 169).
- Electrolyte supplementation as needed
- Address acid-base disorders as appropriate.
- Discontinue potentially nephrotoxic drugs (e.g., aminoglycosides) and eliminate exposure to ingested nephrotoxins (e.g., jerky treats).
- For severe gastrointestinal signs associated with jerky treat ingestion, hospitalization for intravenous fluid therapy and appropriate care for acute gastroenteropathy should be prioritized.

Chronic Treatment

Use the Gonto protocol (https://basenjirescue.org/Fanconi/Fanconi-Protocol-2015.pdf):

- Acidemia: oral sodium bicarbonate is titrated to keep venous pH within reference range. Starting dose 1-10 mEq/kg/day PO in divided doses q 8-12h, increased based on venous blood gas analyses performed q 3-5 days. Doses may exceed 11 mEq/kg/day.
- Hypokalemia: 5-15 mEq K^+/DOG PO total daily dose. Potassium gluconate, potassium citrate
- Treat underlying disease associated with acquired Fanconi syndrome as appropriate (e.g., chelation for copper storage hepatopathy).

Nutrition/Diet

See Gonto protocol:

- Vitamin and mineral replacement: daily canine multivitamin (e.g., Pet-Tab Plus), Pet-Cal (calcium, phosphorus, vitamin D supplement), and weekly human multivitamin with trace minerals (i.e., Centrum) have been advocated for dogs with polyuria and polydipsia. Do not give Pet-Cal if dog is azotemic because it will exacerbate hyperphosphatemia, hypercalcemia, and soft-tissue mineralization.
- Some owners provide amino acid replacement: starting at 1 Amino Fuel tablet (1000 mg) per week.

Possible Complications

- Neurologic signs (seizures, ataxia, dementia, or central blindness) of unknown cause occur in ≈20% of dogs.
- Manipulation of electrolyte and acid-base balance can lead to overcorrection of deficiencies if the disease is dynamic.

Recommended Monitoring

- Recheck serum biochemistry profile 8-10 weeks (and venous blood gas no more than 1 week) after starting therapy.
- CBC and serum biochemistry profile q 4-6 months in stable patients and a venous blood gas analysis should be performed as indicated (typically 1 week after adjustments and every 2-3 months) for titration of electrolyte, alkali, and nutritional supplementation.
- Culture urine if indicated.

PROGNOSIS & OUTCOME

- For basenji dogs, life span is not substantially reduced from normal (median survival time, 5.25 years from diagnosis). End-stage CKD is the most common cause of death (40%).
- In other breeds, prognosis depends on ability to address underlying cause. Fanconi syndrome may be transient, depending on the underlying cause.

PEARLS & CONSIDERATIONS

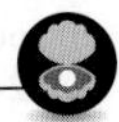

Comments

Consumption of chicken jerky treats (especially those manufactured in China) has been linked to illness, notably Fanconi syndrome, in thousands of dogs over the past several years. A specific cause (e.g., pathogen, chemical) responsible for the illness has not been identified. Owners should be cautioned against feeding these treats.

Prevention

This is an inherited disease in basenji dogs. Dogs with this disease should not be bred, although late onset of disease (3-8 years) complicates reproductive planning.

Technician Tips

A careful diet history may reveal consumption of jerky treats. Many clients are unaware of the association with kidney disease and may have trouble determining the source of the ingredients used in treats.

SUGGESTED READING

Kerl ME: Renal tubular diseases. In Ettinger SJ, et al, editors: Textbook of veterinary internal medicine, ed 8, St. Louis, 2017, Elsevier, 1972-1977.

AUTHORS: Catherine E. Langston, DVM, DACVIM; Adam Eatroff, DVM, DACVIM
EDITOR: Leah A. Cohn, DVM, PhD, DACVIM

Fear Due to Veterinary Visits/Treatments

BASIC INFORMATION

Definition

Extremely common iatrogenic condition in which the veterinary staff, facilities, and/or any veterinary experiences engender fear and behavioral distress in the patient

Epidemiology

SPECIES, AGE, SEX

- Fear is very common in dogs and even more so in cats. Estimates are that 60% of pets of either sex may be affected.
- More common in dogs > 2 years of age and may worsen with exposure

GENETICS, BREED PREDISPOSITION

Possibly worse in breeds with familial behavioral concerns associated with social anxieties (e.g., Bernese mountain dogs: generalized anxiety disorder), fear (e.g., German shepherd dogs), phobias (e.g., German shepherd dogs, Australian shepherds, border collies: noise phobia), and/ or panic (many herding and coursing breeds)

RISK FACTORS

- Social maturity: occurs most often at age 12-18 (up to 36) months in dogs, 24-48 months in cats
- Dogs/cats that appear developmentally delayed and/or overly fearful within their first few months of life may be more susceptible to this form of learned fear.
- Possibly worse for those with pre-existing fear conditions, lack of exposure to veterinary clinics, and/or pathology-associated pain.

CONTAGION AND ZOONOSIS

Affected animals may bite veterinary professionals.

ASSOCIATED DISORDERS

- Generalized anxiety disorder
- Noise phobia
- Fear (generalized or specific)
- Fear aggression

Clinical Presentation

HISTORY, CHIEF COMPLAINT

Clients recognize that their pets "do not like to go to the vet." Physical and behavioral signs of stress, distress, and anxiety are generally recognized but ignored because they are considered normal for veterinary patients, especially for cats.

PHYSICAL EXAM FINDINGS

Physical exam findings are those associated with the physical and behavioral signs of stress, distress, and anxiety:

- Salivation and/or clear nasal discharge
- Shaking/tremor
- Mydriasis
- Yawning/licking lips
- Scratching
- Increased shedding /exfoliation of dry skin
- Tucking tail
- Panting, tachypnea, tachycardia, hyperthermia
- Hyperemia
- Social withdrawal (unwilling to interact); particularly cats (may not come out of crate)
- Physical freezing and rigidity
- Avoidance of stimulus (e.g., metal table, smell of alcohol, nonslip flooring)
- Vocalization, including whining, barking, growling, hissing, whimpering
- Escape behaviors
- Grabbing with mouth or paws
- Chewing through restraints (e.g., leads)
- Hiding, crouching, low body posture
- Increased or decreased sensitivity to pain
- Increased or decreased reactivity to touch or approach
- Exacerbation of any cardiac, respiratory, or skeletal condition that may be comorbid

Etiology and Pathophysiology

- Exposure to stimuli and environments that animals feel are worrisome, threatening, or uncertain and from which they cannot escape, despite signaling their need to do so. Regardless of whether humans feel the environment is not threatening, what matters is the patient's perception.
- The pathophysiologic mechanism is as for any condition involving behavioral stress, distress, and/or anxiety and appears to be rooted in neurochemical encoding in the amygdala.
- Rodent studies show that fear is most easily erased in very young animals whose brains are still developing. After this period (undefined for cats and dogs), perineuronal nets protect memories of fear from modification. This is why it is so important not to learn to fear.

DIAGNOSIS

Diagnostic Overview

The diagnosis is made based on visual observation of signs of stress, distress, and/or anxiety in association with veterinary visits. Because this problem is highly prevalent, it is often downplayed or ignored.

Differential Diagnosis

All signs of this iatrogenic condition are shared by other behavioral conditions and by many physical conditions, including various neuropathies and toxicoses. The key to assigning a cause is to ask whether the signs are manifested only under conditions involving veterinary care.

Initial Database

- No testing is required to make the diagnosis.
- Many laboratory test results can be skewed by the condition:
  - Altered lymphocyte/neutrophil ratios and leukocytosis (stress leukogram)
  - Increased serum cortisol concentration
  - Hyperglycemia (especially cats)
  - Increased serum creatine kinase concentration
  - Increased hematocrit due to splenic pooling

TREATMENT

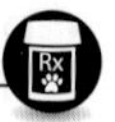

Treatment Overview

- Treatment should focus on ameliorating signs of stress, distress, or anxiety and preventing them from worsening through learning. This means specific triggers must be identified and addressed for the patient population as a whole (some hospitals are scarier than others) and for each animal as an individual.
- A list of triggers of stress, distress, or anxiety should be compiled at each visit and long-term and short-term plans made for how to address the triggers (e.g., replace slippery tile flooring with nonslip flooring; use yoga mats for scales/exams; vaccinate outside while dog is watching other dogs; use high-quality treats to reward less fearful behaviors and to assess distress threshold).

Acute and Chronic Treatment

- Avoid environments or behaviors that provoke the patient (e.g., if patients are resistant to getting on the table, let them sit on the floor; if they slip on the table, give them a nonslip mat).
- If the patient continues to manifest distress, consider panicolytic medications
  - Alprazolam: dogs, 0.01-0.1 mg/kg [likely most effective range: 0.02-0.04 mg/kg] PO q 4-6h prn; cats, 0.0125-0.025 mg/kg PO q 12-24h. CAUTION: some published sources mistakenly recommend a tenfold higher dose.
  - Lorazepam: dogs, 0.5-1.0 mg/kg PO q 12-24h; cats, 0.5-1.0 mg/kg PO q 12-24h
  - Dexmedetomidine (Sileo), extra-label use; dogs, 125 mcg/m^2 oral transmucosal gel q 2h prn up to 5 doses
  - Gabapentin: dogs, 10-20 mg/kg PO q 8-12h; cats, 3-5 mg/kg PO q 12-24h
  - Trazodone: dogs, 2-20 mg/kg PO q 12-24h; cats, 7-17 mg/kg (typically 25 or 50 mg/CAT) PO q 24h
- Medications are best used as a preventive; consider rescheduling non-emergent visits until premedication can be affected.
  - Benzodiazepines (BZD), Sileo, trazodone, gabapentin can be given 2 hours before the visit/event and repeated 30 minutes beforehand, if needed.
  - Clonidine (dogs: 0.01 mg/kg PO q 12-24h, increased stepwise up to 0.05 mg/kg

PO q 12-24h, maximum dose 0.9 mg/day), gabapentin, trazodone, and benzodiazepines can be given q 8-12 h for 2-3 days before visit.

- Have all staff work to reward the dog for calm and comfortable behaviors.
- Integrate certified, no-force trainers (www.petprofessionalguild.com) with extensive experience in behavior modification into the practice.
- Treatment of phobias (p. 787) and separation anxiety (p. 905) as needed

Behavior/Exercise

- Well-pet veterinary visits should be enjoyable for the pet. Interventional veterinary visits should be nonthreatening, calming, and as stress-free as possible.
- Because patients learn fear as they age, early appointments should involve treats, play, and massage before anything threatening (e.g., vaccination) is attempted. Puppy and kitten visits should be longer to allow positive interactions with staff and to explore the hospital.
- On-site puppy/kitten and young dog manners classes are an excellent vehicle for these exposures.
- Environments should be friendly to animals. This means that practices should attempt to do the following:
    - Modulate noise (e.g., acoustic tiles, Plexiglas cage doors/walls) when possible. Consider Mutt Muffs (www.muttmuffs.com) or ear plugs for hospitalized/anesthetized animals.
    - Modulate the visual environment (e.g., movable barriers, flexible and non-harsh lighting). Consider Doggles (www.doggles.com), Thunder/Calming caps (www.thundershirt.com), or eye shades as needed, especially on anesthetic recovery. Provide hiding and perching boxes/containers for caged cats.
    - Modulate the olfactory environment by allowing animals to have T-shirts or gloves worn by their humans with them in cages and during manipulations or anesthetic inductions. Rinse common areas with plain water. Use peroxide compounds instead of bleach when appropriate (bleach solutions ≤ 1%, well rinsed and aired after use).
    - Change tactile environments with nonskid flooring, yoga mats, and covering tables and scales with nonslip surfaces.
    - Use treats to reward good behaviors, and teach animals to participate in the exam process by offering body parts.

Possible Complications

- These animals are at risk for inadequate veterinary care (making physical illness more likely and more severe), relinquishment, or even euthanasia.
- Human injury may result from fearful veterinary patients.

Recommended Monitoring

Screen each animal at every visit for behavioral concerns manifested at home or during examinations/interventions.

PROGNOSIS & OUTCOME

Varies, depending in part on recognition and subsequent modification of approach to address the problem

PEARLS & CONSIDERATIONS

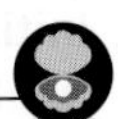

Comments

- Iatrogenic fear conditioned by veterinary care may trigger otherwise latent pathologic behavioral conditions.
- Positive trainers can help teach dogs to get on scales and tables and offer body parts for exam.
- Fear manifestations are commonly cited as reasons for relinquishment, euthanasia, or avoidance of veterinary visits.
- Everyone can recognize the signs associated with this condition. Only when we find it unacceptable to scare patients will we stop doing it.

Prevention

- This condition is completely preventable. Routine behavioral assessments help to identify fear early, when it responds fastest to redress, possibly with a specialist's help.
- Kittens and puppies should be exposed to pleasant interactions with people, animals, and environments between 2-9 weeks and 3-16 weeks of age, respectively. Any profoundly fearful reactions during this period should trigger a behavioral consult and inform the quality and quantity of future interactions/exposure.
- Use topical lidocaine or lidocaine/prilocaine before venipuncture, vaccines, intravenous catheters, and anal sac expression. Effect takes about 10 minutes for well-vascularized areas for most patients.

Technician Tips

- Technicians, particularly those with an interest in behavior modification, can improve patients' lives.
    - Become comfortable with examining cats in carriers using towels, use of towel wraps for cats and smaller dogs, use of examination bags for cats and small dogs, and the use of head collars and no-pull harnesses.
    - Learn to trim toenails and draw blood without restraint.
    - Teach dogs and cats to offer body parts for examination.
    - Modify the environment according to the pet's needs.
    - Do not pull or shake cats out of carriers.
- If feeding is allowed, use high-quality treats to repeatedly test stress levels during visit; stressed animals may refuse treats.
- Many practices have one or a few technicians who are adept at deciphering and acting appropriately on cues of stress; much can be learned by example from these individuals.

Client Education

- Clients should be taught it is not normal for pets to fear veterinary visits.
- There are programs intended to help veterinary professionals decrease fear. Cat Friendly Practice information can be found at http://www.catvets.com/cfp/cfp. Fear-Free Certification information can be found at https://fearfreepets.com/courses/fear-free-certification-program/.

SUGGESTED READINGS

Döring D, et al: Fear-related behaviour of dogs in veterinary practice. Vet J 182:38-43, 2009.

AUTHOR & EDITOR: **Karen L. Overall, VMD, MA, PhD, DACVB**

Feline Immunodeficiency Virus Infection

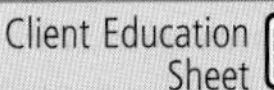

BASIC INFORMATION

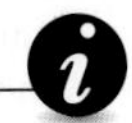

Definition

Common viral infection of cats that can result in immunosuppression after a long latent stage

Epidemiology

SPECIES, AGE, SEX

- Feline immunodeficiency virus (FIV) and related viruses are able to infect all Felidae.
- Male cats are about twice as likely to be infected as female cats, and adult cats are more commonly infected than kittens.
- Adult, male, sexually intact, free-roaming cats (fighting cats) are at higher risk for infection.

RISK FACTORS

Free roaming and fighting/biting behavior

CONTAGION AND ZOONOSIS

- Transmissible through saliva and blood, most commonly through bite wounds and mating. Experimentally, also *in utero* or via milk but uncommon under natural circumstances
- Environmental contamination is no concern because virus is infectious only for minutes outside the cat and highly sensitive to desiccation, disinfectants, and heat.
- Not zoonotic

GEOGRAPHY AND SEASONALITY

Common worldwide, with a higher prevalence in regions with larger numbers of free-roaming cats (e.g., Italy, Japan, Thailand); prevalence in the United States ≈2%-3%

ASSOCIATED DISORDERS

- FIV infection–induced immunosuppression
- Increasing susceptibility to chronic secondary infections, neoplasia, and stomatitis

Clinical Presentation

DISEASE FORMS/SUBTYPES

Clinical presentation in FIV-infected cats is rarely caused by FIV itself. Clinical signs usually are the result of secondary diseases such as infections or tumors. In most FIV-infected cats, there are no clinical signs, and the infection is an incidental or serendipitous finding.

HISTORY, CHIEF COMPLAINT

- Most commonly discovered incidentally during routine screening or when evaluating a cat for other illness
- Clinical manifestations are usually associated with secondary infections, neoplasia (e.g., lymphoma), or FIV-associated neurologic disorders (rare).

PHYSICAL EXAM FINDINGS

- Commonly unremarkable
- Gingivostomatitis (most common abnormality, if any exist)
- Findings related to secondary infection or neoplasia
- Rarely, central nervous system (CNS) signs, such as behavioral changes, seizures, and paresis

Etiology and Pathophysiology

- Lentivirus (RNA virus) of the family Retroviridae that causes life-long infection with no cure
- Several subtypes in different geographic regions worldwide, based on sequence differences in the *env* gene; not differentiated by routine testing
- Much less pathogenic than human immunodeficiency virus (HIV) infection or feline leukemia virus (FeLV) infection
- Several stages after experimental FIV infection, similar to HIV infection, including an acute phase (lasting days to weeks), a clinically asymptomatic (latent) phase of various durations (usually many years), and a terminal phase sometimes called feline acquired immunodeficiency syndrome (feline AIDS). Stages are not recognized in natural infection.
- Clinical recovery even in cats in moribund condition with severe immunosuppression and secondary infections is possible with appropriate care.

DIAGNOSIS

Diagnostic Overview

Usually by detection of FIV-specific antibodies with ELISA or similar tests:

- Negative results are highly reliable (in an area with low prevalence); positive results need confirmation because false-positive results are possible.
- Vaccination-induced and maternal antibodies can interfere with results of some tests.

Differential Diagnosis

Other immunosuppressive conditions, such as FeLV infection

Initial Database

Routine laboratory tests: CBC, serum chemistry panel, urinalysis

- Usually unremarkable in the latent stage; in later stages, sometimes lymphopenia (because FIV replication occurs mainly in lymphocytes and macrophages) or hyperglobulinemia (because of an immune-mediated response)
- For exclusion of other (secondary or unrelated) diseases

As screening tests of choice, point-of-care ELISA or other immunochromatography tests (using a similar technique) for detecting FIV antibodies in blood

- Presence of FIV antibody considered consistent with infection because a cat, once infected, never clears the infection.
- Two exceptions in which an uninfected cat has antibodies (false-positives):
  - FIV vaccination (some tests, such as SNAP and VetScan, are positive in vaccinated cats; vaccination will cause no interference with tests that contain gp40 as the capture antigen, such as Anigen and Witness, if vaccination has occurred more than 6 months before testing)
  - Presence of maternal antibodies (if queen is infected or vaccinated) detected up to 6 months of age
- One exception in which an infected cat has no antibodies (false-negatives):
  - Acute infection (up to 8 weeks are required for antibody production)

Advanced or Confirmatory Testing

Western blot (detection of antibodies):

- Confirmatory test of choice for antibody detection
- Higher sensitivity and specificity than ELISA and related tests

Polymerase chain reaction (PCR) test (detection of proviral DNA):

- Useful if cat vaccinated or vaccination history unknown (can confirm infection if positive)
- However, false-negatives are common (up to 50% false-negative results); test requires meticulous lab conditions to avoid false-positive results.

TREATMENT

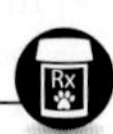

Treatment Overview

Lifestyle management is the cornerstone of treatment and prevention. Indoor-only lifestyle is highly recommended, to minimize risk of secondary infections. For cats with no clinical signs, no treatment is required. For cats with secondary infections, comprehensive treatment is required. In FIV-infected cats with gingivostomatitis or neurologic signs, antiviral treatment can be considered.

Acute and Chronic Treatment

Treatment in healthy FIV-infected patients

- No treatment necessary, but strict indoor-only lifestyle is strongly suggested (protect patient and other cats).
- Routine ectoparasite control and deworming suggested
- Core vaccinations are not recommended for indoor-only FIV-infected cats.

Treatment if clinical signs present:

- Identify and aggressively treat underlying diseases (FIV alone is usually not responsible for the clinical signs).

Treatment of FIV-infected cats with gingivostomatitis:

- Glucocorticoids are *not* recommended.
- If concurrent feline calicivirus (FCV) infection, local oromucosal treatment with feline interferon-omega (1×10^6 IU/cat q 24h)
- If no FCV infection or interferon-omega not effective, treatment trial with azidothymidine (AZT) 5-10 mg/kg PO q 12h plus antibiotics. In addition, trial with lactoferrin 40 mg/kg q 24h applied topically to the oral mucosa.
- If insufficient improvement, removal of all teeth (usually in two sessions; total removal of all tooth roots must be confirmed by radiographs)

Treatment of FIV-infected cats with neurologic signs:

- Identification and treatment of any underlying diseases causing the neurologic signs
- If no underlying disease identified (and the neurologic signs are assumed to be caused by FIV directly), treatment with AZT 5-10 mg/kg PO q 12h

Treatment of FIV-infected cats with recurring infections

- Intensive treatment of recurring infections (e.g., long-term antibiotics after culture and sensitivity)
- Measure quantitative virus load by reverse transcription PCR (RT-PCR) or $CD4^+$ and $CD8^+$ cell counts. If virus load is high or $CD4^+$ cell counts low, treatment with antivirals (e.g., plerixafor 0.5 mg/kg SQ q 12h or AZT 5-10 mg/kg PO q 12h) should be considered; treatment has been associated

with improvement in clinical signs and quality of life in cats with stomatitis and neurologic signs.

Nutrition/Diet

Avoid raw meat, milk, or eggs to reduce risk of secondary infections through food-borne pathogens.

Behavior/Exercise

Strict indoors-only lifestyle is the most important life-prolonging advice to reduce exposure of the FIV-infected cat to other secondary infections and to prevent contagion with FIV to other cats.

Drug Interactions

- Avoid immunosuppressive drugs whenever possible.
- Griseofulvin (e.g., for dermatophyte infections) should be avoided because of risk of severe neutropenia.

Possible Complications

Reversible nonregenerative anemia is an adverse effect of AZT.

Recommended Monitoring

Regular monitoring for evidence of secondary infections, neoplasia, or progression of FIV infection. Recheck veterinary visits every 6 months are recommended.

PROGNOSIS & OUTCOME

Prognosis is good with well-managed veterinary care. FIV-infected cats can have excellent quality of life for many years with no reduction in survival time. FIV infection is not in itself a reason for euthanasia.

PEARLS & CONSIDERATIONS

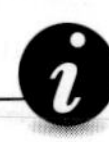

Comments

- The FIV status of all cats should be known, independent of age.
  - If cat < 6 months old is found to be FIV antibody-positive, retesting should be performed when > 6 months old because positive results in cats less than 6 months of age are commonly caused by maternal antibodies.
  - In vaccinated cats, Anigen and Witness are more specific than SNAP and VetScan for detection of infection.
- FIV infection is not a reason for euthanasia; infected cats can live many years with excellent quality of life. However, diagnosis should result in indoor-only lifestyle and more frequent veterinary monitoring.
  - Core vaccinations are not recommended in indoor-only, FIV-infected cats. Vaccination recommended only for FIV-infected cats at high risk (e.g., open multi-cat households, outdoor access).

Prevention

- FIV vaccination is controversial. FIV incidence is relatively low in household pets, and infection can be prevented (without vaccination) by preventing FIV-negative cats from interacting with FIV-positive, unfamiliar and unowned cats.
- FIV vaccination can interfere with some routine testing methods.
- FIV vaccines contain adjuvants and can be associated with the development of injection-site sarcomas (p. 550).
- For high-risk cats with a known FIV-negative status, FIV vaccination might be considered.

Technician Tips

- The FIV status of every cat should be known.
- FIV is infective only for minutes outside the cat and is susceptible to all disinfectants, including common soap. Simple precautions and routine cleaning procedures prevent transmission in the hospital.
- House FIV-infected cats in individual animal cages and never in an infectious disease ward with cats that have contagious diseases (e.g., upper respiratory infections).

Client Education

- Every cat should be tested for FIV.
- Benefits of neutering cats should be emphasized.

SUGGESTED READING

Hartmann K: Management of feline retrovirus-infected cats. In Bonagura JD, et al, editors: Kirk's current veterinary therapy XV, St. Louis, 2014, Elsevier, pp 1275-1283.

AUTHOR: Katrin Hartmann, Dr.med.vet., Dr.habil., DECVIM
EDITOR: Joseph Taboada, DVM, DACVIM

Feline Infectious Peritonitis

Video Available 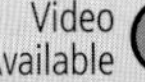 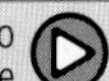 Client Education Sheet 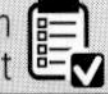

BASIC INFORMATION

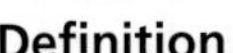

Definition

Fatal disease of cats often characterized by body cavity effusions, neurologic signs, or uveitis. It is caused by a common feline coronavirus (FCoV) that, in cats with feline infectious peritonitis (FIP), has spontaneously mutated from a benign, minimally pathogenic virus to an aggressive, lethal virus.

Epidemiology

SPECIES, AGE, SEX

FIP can occur in all Felidae family members. Young cats during postweaning periods are most susceptible (peak age, 3 months to 2 years), but cats of all ages can be affected.

GENETICS, BREED PREDISPOSITION

- More common in purebred cats, mainly because of living in multi-cat environments
- Genetic predisposition likely: littermates of kitten with FIP are four times more likely to develop FIP than other kittens in the same environment.

RISK FACTORS

All factors leading to increased FCoV replication in the intestines increase the risk that the mutation takes place and FIP develops.

- Living in multi-cat households (e.g., catteries, shelters, pet-hoarding environments)
- Stress (e.g., vaccinations, elective surgery, rehoming)
- Immunosuppression (e.g., feline immunodeficiency virus [FIV] infection, feline leukemia virus [FeLV] infection, glucocorticoid treatment)
- Young age

CONTAGION AND ZOONOSIS

- FCoV mainly transmitted by fecal-oral route
- FCoV infection widespread and ubiquitous in multi-cat environments
- Horizontal transmission (cat to cat) of FIP or the mutated virus does not occur under natural circumstances. The ability of the virus to mutate inside the cat determines whether FCoV infection remains innocuous or develops into FIP.

GEOGRAPHY AND SEASONALITY

FCoV infection and FIP occur worldwide.

ASSOCIATED DISORDERS

Usually no clinical signs in FCoV infection but occasionally mild diarrhea; clinical signs of FIP after mutation of FCoV

Clinical Presentation

DISEASE FORMS/SUBTYPES

- Historically, differentiation of two clinical forms of FIP: dry form (non-effusive) and wet form (effusive). Distinction is inaccurate

because every cat with body cavity effusion also has microgranulomas. A cat with the dry form will commonly develop effusion later.
- Important to detect effusion for diagnostic purposes. Tests performed on the effusion much more helpful diagnostically than tests on blood

HISTORY, CHIEF COMPLAINT

- Commonly nonspecific signs, including lethargy, inappetence, and weight loss
- Persistent fever, nonresponsive to antibiotics
- Abdominal distention in cats with ascites
- Dyspnea in cats with pleural effusion or pulmonary granuloma
- Other complaints are related to site of granulomas (e.g., central nervous system [CNS] signs, icterus diarrhea)

PHYSICAL EXAM FINDINGS

- Abdominal effusion: abdominal distention, sometimes with a palpable fluid wave
- Pleural effusion: dyspnea, muffled heart and lung sounds
- Organomegaly or abdominal masses sometimes palpable (e.g., enlarged mesenteric lymph nodes, nodules in other organs, intestinal thickening, irregular kidneys)
- Icterus may be noted due to liver involvement but can also be caused by interference of tumor necrosis factor-alpha with bilirubin transport (i.e., icterus with no hemolysis, biliary obstruction, or increase in liver enzymes)
- Encephalitis: ataxia, personality changes, nystagmus, or seizures
- Uveitis: change in iris color, hyphema, aqueous flare, keratic precipitates, vitreous clouding, vascular cuffing, manifesting as gray lines parallel to retinal vessels
- Unusual presentations include skin fragility syndrome and other skin lesions, orchitis, and priapism.

Etiology and Pathophysiology

- Benign FCoV replicates in enterocytes. If a mutation takes place in the spike protein of the FCoV, virus loses its ability to replicate in enterocytes, making it unlikely that mutated virus would be transmitted to other cats.
- The mutated virus is taken up by macrophages and distributed throughout the body. A second mutation is potentially necessary to enable the virus to effectively replicate in macrophages.
  - Replication of the mutated FCoV in macrophages is the key event in the pathogenesis of FIP.
  - The virus within macrophages initiates the ultimately fatal immune-mediated reaction to virus.
- Signs caused by granulomatous lesions in target organs (CNS, eyes, and parenchymatous organs) and vasculitis leading to fluid accumulation in body cavities

DIAGNOSIS

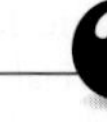

Diagnostic Overview

Definitive diagnosis is achieved only through immunohistochemistry staining of FCoV antigen in macrophages of tissues with typical histopathologic lesions that have to be obtained through laparotomy, laparoscopy, or post mortem. Less invasive diagnostic methods with relatively high specificity include polymerase chain reaction (PCR) specific for mutations in the spike gene and detection of FCoV antigen in macrophages by immunofluorescence or immunocytology of effusions or other fluids. *In vivo* diagnosis for cats without effusion is much more difficult.

Differential Diagnosis

- Body cavity effusions: neoplasia, cholangiohepatitis, pancreatitis, bacterial peritonitis, pyothorax, chylothorax, diaphragmatic hernia, cardiomyopathies
- Uveitis: toxoplasmosis, FIV infection, systemic mycoses (p. 1023)
- Multifocal neurologic lesions: toxoplasmosis, bacterial meningoencephalitis, metabolic, and toxic CNS diseases
- Hyperglobulinemia: multiple myeloma, heartworm disease, FIV infection, severe inflammatory conditions

Initial Database

Thoracic and abdominal radiographs:
- Pleural effusion, ascites (in case of effusion)

Abdominal ultrasound:
- Ascites, abdominal masses, lymphadenopathy

CBC (can be normal or nonspecific changes):
- Lymphopenia, neutrophilia without left shift (stress leukogram)
- Mild nonregenerative anemia of chronic inflammation

Serum biochemistry profile (can be normal):
- Hyperglobulinemia (and low albumin/globulin ratio)
- Increased bilirubin, often with normal liver enzyme activity

Serum protein electrophoresis (not necessary if values of albumin and total protein are available):
- Polyclonal gammopathy

Fluid analysis (ascites, pleural effusion, pericardial effusion):
- Clear, viscous, straw-colored fluid
- Analysis (p. 1343): nonseptic exudate with protein > 3.5 mg/dL (35 g/L) (often much higher), total cell count increased but relatively mildly (e.g., 2000/mcL) for an exudate (lower than in bacterial serositis), mainly macrophages and nondegenerate neutrophils

Rivalta test for cats with effusion (addition of 1 drop effusion to water-acetic acid mixture, watching for coagulation (lava lamp look); sensitivity 91%, specificity 65%) (see *Video*)
- If negative, FIP extremely unlikely
- If positive, FIP likely (but false-positives with lymphoma, bacterial serositis)

Cerebrospinal fluid (CSF) analysis (pp. 1080 and 1323). CAUTION: patient can be at increased risk for cerebellar/medullary herniation.
- Can be unremarkable
- High protein content (>20 mg/dL, often markedly higher) and cell count (>5 cells/mcL, often much higher; mononuclear pleocytosis with some neutrophils)

Computed tomography or magnetic resonance imaging of the brain: hydrocephalus common if CNS involvement, multifocal granuloma

Advanced or Confirmatory Testing

Immunohistochemistry staining of FCoV antigen in macrophages of tissues with typical histopathologic lesions:
- Gold standard of diagnosis
- Only way to definitively diagnose FIP
- Requires histopathology of tissue samples obtained through laparotomy, laparoscopy, or post mortem.

Mutation PCR:
- Most specific noninvasive method for diagnosis
- PCR detects specific mutations in the spike protein that leads to FIP-inducing FCoV pathotypes.
- High specificity (96%) and moderate sensitivity (69%) for effusion; not useful for blood due to very low sensitivity

Detection of FCoV antigen in macrophages by immunofluorescence or immunocytology staining:
- Second best method to diagnose FIP
- Can be done on effusion, CSF, aqueous humor, and lymph node aspirates; not useful for blood
- Relatively high specificity (72%) and sensitivity (85%) for effusion; some false-positive test results occur, which limits the utility.

FCoV antibody detection:
- Very limited usefulness because presence of antibodies indicates only exposure to a coronavirus (including FIP vaccine virus), not FIP
- Most cats with FCoV antibodies never develop FIP.
- About 10% of cats with FIP have no serum antibodies, especially in terminal stages. A negative antibody test does not rule out FIP.

Conventional PCR for detecting any FCoV:
- False-positive results and false-negative results for blood PCR are common because cats with benign enteric FCoV infection also can have viremia and cats with FIP often lack viremia.
- For effusion, PCR more specific and sensitive but still not diagnostic for FIP

TREATMENT

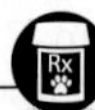

Treatment Overview

FIP is an incurable disease. Treatment goals are to prolong life and provide comfort and supportive/palliative care.

Acute General Treatment

- In cats with effusion, thoracocentesis (p. 1164) or abdominocentesis (p. 1056) should be performed as needed, especially in cats with dyspnea.
- Oxygen therapy (p. 1146) should be provided to cats with dyspnea.
- Cornerstone of treatment for quality of life and prolonging life is immunosuppression (e.g., with glucocorticoids), but this does not help all cats.

Chronic Treatment

Treatment options include antiviral drugs, immunomodulating drugs, immunosuppression, and supportive therapy. Most drugs tested in placebo-controlled, double-blind studies fail to show efficacy. For some drugs (e.g., antivirals), adverse effects limit their utility.

- Antiviral drugs
  - Proteinase inhibitors and nucleoside analogues: promising results in cats with experimentally induced and naturally occurring FIP but not on the market yet
  - Ribavirin: *contraindicated* because severely toxic in cats
- Immunomodulating drugs
  - Human interferon-alpha 30 U/CAT PO q 24h on alternating weeks; no controlled studies to show efficacy; few to no adverse effects
  - Feline interferon-omega: no efficacy in a placebo-controlled, double-blind study
  - Polyprenyl Immunostimulant: effective in a case series to prolong life of three cats with FIP without effusion; some effect in an uncontrolled trial in cats without effusion, but controlled studies are missing
- Immunosuppression (can prolong life of some cats up to 2 years after diagnosis)
  - In cats with effusion: dexamethasone 1 mg/kg q 24h intraperitoneally or intrathoracically (after removal of the effusion) as long as effusion is present, then followed by prednisolone 2 mg/kg PO q 24h, which may be reduced after the cat is stable for a few months
  - In cats without effusion: prednisolone 2 mg/kg PO q 24h, which may be reduced after the cat is stable for a few months but should be continued at a lower dose lifelong
- Supportive therapy as indicated by clinical condition
  - Ocular therapy (e.g., uveitis)
  - Broad-spectrum antibiotics to control secondary bacterial infections

Nutrition/Diet

Nutritional support, including warming of food, offering multiple types of dry and moist food, and hand feeding if ill cats are unwilling to eat, is important in supportive care (p. 1199).

PROGNOSIS & OUTCOME

- Very poor prognosis irrespective of treatment
- Median survival time in cats after diagnosis is 8 days.
- Some (few) cats live longer with immunosuppressive treatment; survival up to 2 years after diagnosis has been observed.

PEARLS & CONSIDERATIONS

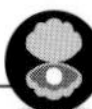

Comments

There is no FIP test. Presence of FCoV antibodies indicates only exposure to a coronavirus, which may be pathogenic (and FIP causing) or benign. Antibody detection has close to zero value in the diagnosis of FIP but can be used in the management of multi-cat households or before considering vaccination.

Prevention

Intranasal FIP vaccination:

- Controversy concerning efficacy: discrepant results from experimental studies and nonconvincing efficacy in few field trials
- Safe because no systemic spread of the vaccine virus and no antibody-dependent enhancement observed (and therefore increased susceptibility against FIP) in field trials
- Generally not recommended due to lack of efficacy
- If used, limit to cats that have not been exposed to FCoV beforehand and therefore have no antibodies.

Prevention of FIP in multi-cat households:

- Minimizing risk of FCoV transmission through reduction of infection pressure, identifying permanent/high-virus excreters, reducing the number of FCoV excreters, maintaining small groups of cats and high levels of hygiene, breeding of resistant cats
- Controlling the development of FIP through reduction of predisposing factors: stress due to overcrowding, new surroundings, high noise level, other illnesses

Technician Tips

- FIP is not a contagious infection because the mutated virus is not transmitted from cat to cat. There is no need to handle a patient with FIP as infective and no supplemental precautions required.
- Cats with FIP shed no (or less) FCoV than cats without FIP from the same environment.

Client Education

- Select new cats from a reputable breeder with low numbers of cats.
- Catteries should select cats with no FCoV antibodies. Healthy antibody-negative cats are not infected with FCoV and not at risk to develop FIP.

SUGGESTED READING

Hartmann K: Coronavirus infections (canine and feline), including infectious peritonitis. In Ettinger SJ, et al, editors: Textbook of veterinary internal medicine, ed 8, St. Louis, 2017, Elsevier, pp 983-996.

AUTHOR: Katrin Hartmann, Dr.med.vet., Dr.habil., DECVIM
EDITOR: Joseph Taboada, DVM, DACVIM

Feline Leukemia Virus Infection

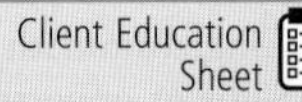

BASIC INFORMATION

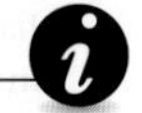

Definition

Viral infection of cats that can result in immunosuppression, myelosuppression, and neoplasia

Epidemiology

SPECIES, AGE, SEX

- Mainly domestic cats; feline leukemia virus (FeLV) rarely found in wild felids
- Young cats (<1 year old) more likely to become progressively infected

GENETICS, BREED PREDISPOSITION

No genetic or breed predisposition

RISK FACTORS

Free-roaming cats are more likely to be infected.

CONTAGION AND ZOONOSIS

- Transmission most commonly occurs through saliva during grooming, playing, and sharing food or water bowls, but also possible through biting, transplacentally, or blood transfusions. Often transmitted from queen to kittens
- Environmental contamination is not a concern because virus is infectious only for minutes outside the cat and highly sensitive to desiccation, disinfectants, and heat.
- Not zoonotic

GEOGRAPHY AND SEASONALITY

Worldwide, nonseasonal. Prevalence has decreased globally (currently ≈2%-3% in the United States) as a result of testing programs and vaccination.

ASSOCIATED DISORDERS

Immunosuppression caused by FeLV results in secondary infections (e.g., bacterial, fungal, protozoal), neoplasia (mainly lymphoma), myelosuppression, and less common conditions such as neurologic disorders, infertility, and fading kitten syndrome.

Clinical Presentation

DISEASE FORMS/SUBTYPES

- Clinical presentation in FeLV-infected cats is usually associated with secondary diseases, such as infections, myelosuppression, or neoplasia.
- As a result of the common use of screening serology, infection is often detected in healthy cats.
- Three major FeLV subgroups: A, B, and C. Subgroup A occurs in all infected cats. Subgroups B and C develop *de novo* from mutations or recombinations of subtype A genome with host DNA in a FeLV-A-infected cat. Subtype B is common and associated with neoplasia. Subgroup C is rare and associated with nonregenerative anemia.

HISTORY, CHIEF COMPLAINT

- FeLV infection can be diagnosed incidentally during yearly or routine new-cat screening. Due to the long subclinical phase, even cats with progressive FeLV infection are often recognized before clinical signs develop.
- Progressive infection eventually leads to clinical signs months to years after infection.
- Signs due to secondary infections (e.g., nasal or ocular discharge) or nonspecific signs attributable to anemia or cancer, such as weakness, lethargy, or inappetence, should prompt veterinary consultation.
- FeLV is sometimes responsible for abortion and infertility in infected queens
- Fading kitten syndrome can occur in newborn kittens that die within the first weeks of life
- Various other signs can occasionally occur as a result of infection (e.g., urinary incontinence, ocular abnormalities).

PHYSICAL EXAM FINDINGS

During subclinical phase, exam is unremarkable, but with illness, may recognize

- General findings
  - Lymphadenopathy
  - Gingivostomatitis
  - Signs of opportunistic infection (due to immunosuppression)
- Lymphoma-associated signs
  - Dyspnea due to mediastinal lymphoma and pleural effusion
  - Diarrhea due to gastrointestinal (GI) lymphoma
  - Vomiting (GI lymphoma or uremia from renal lymphoma)
  - Icterus (hepatic lymphoma)
- Myelosuppression-associated signs
  - Pallor due to nonregenerative anemia; anemia-related heart murmur, tachycardia, or tachypnea
  - Hemorrhage due to thrombocytopenia
- Neurologic deficits (due to FeLV-associated neuropathy)

Etiology and Pathophysiology

- Oncornavirus (RNA virus) of the family Retroviridae
- Once established, lifelong infection with no cure
- Three possible outcomes of FeLV infection:
  - Abortive infection: result of good immune response. These cats develop antibodies but are FeLV antigen-negative (ELISA negative) and provirus-negative (polymerase chain reaction [PCR] negative). Cats with abortive infection are healthy, not contagious, and have lifelong protection from new infection.
  - Regressive infection: if less effective immune response, regressive infection develops. These cats are antigen-negative (or only positive during transient viremia for a short period) but provirus-positive on PCR. They also have antibodies. In regressively infected cats, provirus is integrated into the cellular genome of the cat, but no virus is actively produced. They do not transmit the virus (except through blood transfusions), but infection can be reactivated after immunosuppression. If this occurs, they can become antigen positive and can develop FeLV-associated diseases. They are usually asymptomatic, but rarely, regressive infection itself can result in conditions in which the integrated provirus causes the problem (e.g., neoplasia, myelosuppression).
  - Progressive infection: progressive infection develops if there is an ineffective immune response. These cats are antigen- and provirus-positive (i.e., ELISA and PCR positive) and usually have no detectable antibodies. They will likely develop FeLV-associated diseases.

DIAGNOSIS

Diagnostic Overview

- Progressive FeLV infection is usually diagnosed by detection of FeLV antigen by ELISA or other immunochromatography tests (using a similar technique).
  - Negative results are highly reliable to rule out progressive infection in an area with low prevalence.
  - Positive results need confirmation because false-positive results are possible.
- Diagnosis of regressive FeLV infection through PCR (in blood) to detect integrated FeLV provirus in an ELISA-negative cat.
- Diagnosis of abortive FeLV infection is through detection of antibodies in FeLV antigen-negative, PCR-negative cats. Rarely performed in clinical setting at present

Differential Diagnosis

- Other immunosuppressive conditions, such as feline immunodeficiency virus (FIV) infection
- Other causes of clinical signs (e.g., anemia, neurologic signs).

Initial Database

Routine diagnostic testing:

- CBC, serum biochemistry panel, urinalysis
  - Initial database to rule out other illnesses or infections; changes are not specific to FeLV infection, and results often normal in FeLV-infected cats.
  - CBC in cats with myelosuppression can show mild to marked abnormalities, including nonregenerative anemia, neutropenia, thrombocytopenia, or pancytopenia.
  - Serum biochemistry profile and urinalysis are usually normal or reveal nonspecific changes.
- Radiographs and ultrasound
  - Thoracic or abdominal radiographs and abdominal ultrasound (including fine-needle aspiration of mass lesions for cytologic evaluation [p. 1112]) are performed to diagnose FeLV-associated neoplasia. A mediastinal mass with pleural effusion on thoracic radiographs is suggestive of thymic lymphoma.

As screening tests of choice to detect progressive infection, fast point-of-care ELISA or other immunochromatography tests (using a similar technique) are used for detecting free FeLV antigen in blood. Immunofluorescence assay (IFA) is sometimes used for detecting intracellular FeLV antigen in neutrophils and platelets in blood smears or bone marrow.

- Diagnosis of progressive FeLV infection (antigen-positive, provirus-positive cats)
  - For detection of FeLV antigen, ELISA is more sensitive and detects infection earlier than IFA. ELISA is the diagnostic test of choice for general screening.
  - Saliva- or tear-based antigen tests are not recommended (poor sensitivity due to intermittent shedding).
  - Do not pool blood from multiple kittens for testing (inaccurate results).
- Diagnosis of regressive FeLV infection (antigen-negative, provirus-positive cats)
  - PCR to detect the integrated provirus (FeLV DNA) on whole blood is the test of choice
  - Very sensitive and specific
  - Can also be used as a confirmatory test for positive antigen test results
- Diagnosis of abortive FeLV infection (antigen-negative, provirus-negative, but antibody-positive cats)
  - Detection of abortive infection requires detection of antibodies (test not widely available).
  - Detecting antibodies can help predict whether a cat is protected from new infection.
  - Can be used as an additional screening test to decide if it is necessary to vaccinate a cat.

Advanced or Confirmatory Testing

- No gold standard available
- PCR can be used to confirm results of positive antigen tests.

TREATMENT

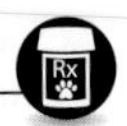

Treatment Overview

Lifestyle management is the cornerstone of treatment and prevention. Indoor-only lifestyle is highly recommended, reducing risk of secondary infections. In progressively infected cats with no clinical signs, no other treatment is required. Supportive care includes comprehensive treatment of secondary infections, treatment of neoplasia, blood transfusion, and other therapy as needed. When overt clinical signs are present, antiviral treatment (e.g., feline interferon-omega, azidothymidine [AZT]) might be beneficial.

Acute General Treatment

Intensive treatment should be given for recognized disorders, such as antibiotic therapy for secondary bacterial infections or blood transfusion for life-threatening anemia (p. 1169).

Chronic Treatment

- If no clinical signs are present, no treatment is necessary. Strict indoor-only lifestyle and good preventative health care (e.g., parasite control, vaccinations) are recommended.
- If clinical signs are present
  - Identify any underlying diseases. FeLV alone might not be responsible for the clinical signs (e.g., secondary infections might be present).
  - Underlying diseases should be treated aggressively (e.g., bactericidal antimicrobials for bacterial infection).

Treatment of FeLV-infected cats with lymphoma:

- Chemotherapy (p. 607)
- Owners should be informed about more guarded prognosis.

Treatment of FeLV-infected cats with anemia:

- Blood transfusions recommended if anemia is severe (p. 1169).
- Treatment trial with erythropoietin (100 IU/kg SQ q 48h)
- If no effect, consider glucocorticoid treatment (anemia in FeLV-infected cats can have an immune-mediated origin, and some cats respond to immunosuppressive therapy).

Treatment of FeLV-infected cats with neurologic signs:

- First identify and then treat any underlying diseases (e.g., lymphoma) causing the neurologic signs.
- If no underlying disease is identified (and the neurologic signs are assumed to be caused by FeLV directly), treat with AZT 5 mg/kg PO q 12h.

Treatment of FeLV-infected cats with recurrent infections:

- Intensive treatment of recurring infections (e.g., long-term antibiotics after culture and sensitivity)
- Treatment trial with immunomodulators (e.g., feline interferon-omega 1×10^6 IU/kg SQ once weekly).

Nutrition/Diet

No raw meat, milk, or eggs to avoid secondary infections through food-borne pathogens

Behavior/Exercise

Strict indoor-only lifestyle is important life-prolonging advice to reduce exposure of the FeLV-infected cat to other infections and to prevent transmission of FeLV to other cats.

Drug Interactions

Avoid immunosuppressive or myelosuppressive drugs whenever possible.

Possible Complications

Reversible nonregenerative anemia is an adverse effect of AZT.

Recommended Monitoring

- Regular monitoring for evidence of secondary infectious diseases, neoplasia, or progression of infection
- Recheck veterinary visits with CBC every 6 months

PROGNOSIS & OUTCOME

- Abortive infection: excellent prognosis; cats are protected lifelong and do not develop clinical signs.
- Regressive infection: good prognosis; cats rarely develop clinical signs (due to lymphoma or myelosuppression) or reactivate their infection (≈10 % of cats).
- Progressive infection: good to fair prognosis if recognized before the onset of clinical signs and with good veterinary care
  - Historic findings for a median life span of 3 years are likely outdated. Nowadays normal longevity is possible, although FeLV-associated syndromes require treatment.
  - Prognosis for cats that develop leukemia or myelosuppression is guarded to poor. Cats with FeLV-associated lymphoma still can experience remission and an improved quality of life with chemotherapy.
  - Cats with severe myelosuppression (e.g., anemia) sometimes respond to therapy.

PEARLS & CONSIDERATIONS

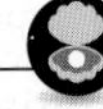

Comments

- The FeLV status of all cats should be known, and every cat should be tested independent of age. Progressive FeLV infection can be detected from birth onward by antigen testing.
- Even progressive FeLV infection is not a reason for euthanasia because the cats can live several years with a good quality of life. However, the diagnosis has certain implications.
  - Strict indoor-only lifestyle
  - More intense veterinary care
  - Vaccination programs to prevent common serious infectious diseases should be maintained; revaccination on a more frequent basis (e.g., q 6 months) is recommended given these cats' immunoincompetence.

Prevention

- Vaccination against FeLV is efficacious in cats at risk for exposure to the virus, but level of protection is not sufficient in cats with very high infectious pressure (e.g., naive cat living with FeLV-shedding cats).
- FeLV vaccine can be associated with development of injection-site sarcomas in cats (p. 550). Only cats at risk should be vaccinated (e.g., not cats that live entirely indoors). Vaccinate against FeLV distally in the hindlimb or tail to allow amputation for removal of injection-site sarcomas if they occur. Vaccines without adjuvants should be used.
- Cats used for blood donation should be screened by PCR as well as ELISA.

Technician Tips

- The FeLV status of every cat should be known.
- FeLV is infective only for minutes outside the cat and is susceptible to all disinfectants, including common soap. Simple precautions and routine cleaning procedures prevent transmission in the hospital.
- House FeLV-infected cats in individual animal cages and never in an infectious disease ward with cats with contagious diseases (e.g., upper respiratory infections).

Client Education

- Every cat should be tested for FeLV; a progressively FeLV-infected cat can live for many years as an indoor pet with regular veterinary care.
- Importance of neutering cats should be emphasized.

SUGGESTED READING

Hartmann K, et al: Feline leukemia virus infection. In Ettinger SJ, et al, editors: Textbook of veterinary internal medicine, ed 8, St. Louis, 2017, Elsevier, pp 978-983.

AUTHOR: Katrin Hartmann, Dr.med.vet., Dr.habil., DECVIM
EDITOR: Joseph Taboada, DVM, DACVIM

Feline Lower Urinary Tract Signs, Idiopathic

Client Education Sheet 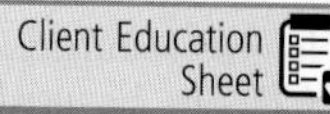

BASIC INFORMATION

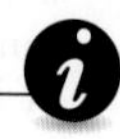

Definition

Lower urinary tract signs (LUTS) include stranguria, hematuria, dysuria (difficult or painful urination), pollakiuria (frequent passage of small amounts of urine), and periuria (urination in inappropriate locations). These signs can occur with lower urinary tract disease (LUTD) of any cause. Idiopathic feline LUTD is the most common cause of LUTS and is a diagnosis of exclusion (see Differential Diagnosis below).

Synonyms

Feline lower urinary tract disease (FLUTD), feline idiopathic cystitis (FIC), feline urologic syndrome (FUS)

Epidemiology

SPECIES, AGE, SEX

Cats of either sex, any age. Male cats develop lower urinary tract obstruction more than female cats (narrow penile urethra).

GENETICS, BREED PREDISPOSITION

Persians and long-haired cats may be at increased risk and Siamese at reduced risk. Familial factors (e.g., quality of maternal care) may play a role.

RISK FACTORS

Identified risk factors vary between studies but often include stress (e.g., changes in feeding, litter boxes, human and animal family members, owner schedule), neutering, indoor housing, increased weight, decreased activity, multi-cat households, and season/geographic climatic variation (spring in the Northeastern United States).

ASSOCIATED DISORDERS

Cats with LUTS may be at increased risk for separation anxiety disorder and other behavioral abnormalities (fear, nervousness, aggression), and obesity. Urethral obstruction may occur in male cats with LUTS.

Clinical Presentation

HISTORY, CHIEF COMPLAINT

- Abrupt onset of LUTS in an otherwise healthy, young adult cat (usually 2-6 years old at first occurrence)
- Often, affected cats are housed entirely indoors and are neutered.
- Male cats with obstructive LUTD have unproductive stranguria and may vocalize, vomit, and become progressively depressed/obtunded.

PHYSICAL EXAM FINDINGS

- Often anxious, may be aggressive or shy
- Bladder typically small and difficult to palpate (unobstructed)
  - Bladder may be large, painful, turgid, and inexpressible (obstructed)

Etiology and Pathophysiology

- The cause is not known, although a subset of patients appear to have a congenital disorder of the stress-response system that results in persistent sensitization of the system and reduced adrenocortical function. The sensitivity may be unmasked by cat-perceived threats in the environment, such as conflict with other animals, and impoverished environments.
- The enhanced sympathetic drive may reduce epithelial tight-junction integrity, resulting in increased exposure of afferent neurons to environmental stimuli. When this occurs in the bladder of a cat with an activated stress-response system, LUTS may result.
- The imbalance between the sympathetic nervous system and hypothalamic-pituitary adrenal axis that occurs in some affected cats may result in impaired blood flow and release of inflammatory mediators that cause lower urinary tract edema, smooth muscle spasm, and pain.
- Neurohormonal alterations may occur alone or in combination with physical obstruction of the urinary tract by a cystolith or urethral plug that precipitates lower urinary obstruction.

DIAGNOSIS

Diagnostic Overview

The diagnosis is suspected based on signalment, history, and physical exam. Urinalysis with sediment exam plus culture and susceptibility can help rule out urinary tract infection, and imaging studies can rule out urolithiasis. Additional diagnostic tests are warranted in cats with atypical presentations, persistent or frequent episodes of LUTS, or urethral obstruction.

Differential Diagnosis

- Urolithiasis
- Behavioral disorder (e.g., territorial marking [p. 533])
- Urinary tract infection
- Anatomic urinary tract defect (notably vesicourachal diverticula)
- Bladder neoplasia (uncommon; transitional cell carcinoma most often identified tumor type)

Initial Database

- Urinalysis with sediment exam will often reveal hematuria, hypersthenuria (urine specific gravity > 1.035), proteinuria, +/− crystalluria.
- Urine culture and susceptibility: infection is rare in studies of FLUTD in the United States but seems more common in European studies.
- For cats with a typical first-time presentation and without urinary obstruction, no additional diagnostic tests may be required.

Advanced or Confirmatory Testing

For cats with complicated initial presentations or recurrent episodes, diagnostic testing is aimed at ruling out the most common alternative diagnosis. With idiopathic LUTS, no abnormalities are expected.

- Radiography of the entire lower urinary tract (including the distal urethra) to identify radiopaque stones
- CBC, biochemical analysis, and serologic testing for feline leukemia virus and feline immunodeficiency virus
- Other lower urinary tract imaging (e.g., ultrasonography, double-contrast cystography) or cystoscopy is rarely indicated.
- A comprehensive history and investigation of the cat's environment is warranted in cats with recurrent episodes to better understand provocative events and make recommendations regarding environmental enrichment (EE).

TREATMENT

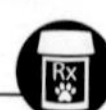

Treatment Overview

Long-term treatment focuses on stress reduction through owner education and EE. With lower urinary tract obstruction, prompt attention is required to manage the associated metabolic derangements and re-establish urine flow because urethral obstruction is a life-threatening condition. A step-by-step approach to treatment is provided on p. 1417.

Acute General Treatment

If the cat is obstructed, relief of the obstruction (p. 1176), re-establishment of urine flow and correction of fluid, electrolyte, and acid-base imbalances are of prime importance.

- Establish intravenous (IV) access and provide appropriate analgesia.
- Perform serum biochemical profile, CBC, and urinalysis. Although all can provide useful information, serum potassium concentration is of the utmost importance for cats with urethral obstruction. Point-of-care venous blood gas, electrolyte, and acid-base profiles generally include potassium concentrations and can provide results in a timely fashion.
- Resuscitate moribund cats with IV fluids, and correct serious electrolyte and acid-base disturbances before sedation or anesthesia for placement of a urinary catheter.
  - Obtain an electrocardiogram (ECG) of all systemically ill cats with urethral obstruction. Cardiotoxic effects of severe hyperkalemia may need to be addressed

even before laboratory values for serum potassium (K^+) return if arrhythmias are present (p. 495).
- Consider decompressing the bladder by cystocentesis before attempting to pass a urinary (urethral) catheter (p. 1009).
- Several methods are described for urethral obstruction relief. A widely used technique is detailed on p. 1009.
- Manage cats medically unless recurrent obstructions occur. For most, analgesics and appropriate fluid therapy are indicated. Evidence is lacking for alpha-blocking drugs (e.g., phenoxybenzamine, prazosin).
- Monitor urine output frequently in very ill cats. Postobstructive diuresis (>2 mL/kg/h) may occur shortly after relief of obstruction and rehydration. During this period, it is essential to give sufficient IV fluids to replace the volume lost as urine. The diuresis declines by 2-5 days.

- The role of glucocorticoids (e.g., prednisone) and nonsteroidal antiinflammatory drugs (e.g., aspirin, meloxicam) remains poorly defined, and none of these drugs has been shown to be an effective treatment for acute LUTS. Nonsteroidal antiinflammatory drugs are absolutely contraindicated in the presence of azotemia due to the risk of nephrotoxicity.

Chronic Treatment

- Step 1: EE/multimodal environmental modification (MEMO)
  - Provide at least one food bowl, one water bowl, and one litter box per cat plus one. Locate these resources in quiet places where the cat is not startled during use.
  - Provide opportunities for the cat to hide safely and explore its environment. Placing perches at windows so the cat can look outside and structures the cat can climb on seem to be important parts of EE.
  - Safe outdoor spaces (e.g., fenced enclosures) provide excellent EE opportunities.
  - Provide a regularly scheduled time for petting, play, and/or trick teaching, working toward at least 10 minutes each day.
  - Identify and resolve intercat conflict to the extent possible.
  - If ineffective, proceed to step 2.
- Step 2: step 1 plus consider use of pheromones (Feliway). If ineffective, proceed to step 3.
- Step 3: steps 1 and 2 plus consider use of a tricyclic antidepressant (TCA) agent (e.g., clomipramine or amitriptyline) or selective serotonin reuptake inhibitor (SSRI; such as fluoxetine) at the lowest effective dose possible. These drugs should be used only after steps 1 and 2 have been implemented and the cat is so severely affected he/she continues to have recurrences. Conclusive results regarding the efficacy of behavior-modifying drugs are lacking.
- Perineal urethrostomy may be needed in severe recurrent obstructive cases.
  - This surgery increases the risks of bacterial urinary tract infections, and postoperative strictures are a potential complication.
  - Clients should be made aware that this surgery does not correct the underlying problem, and recurrent episodes of urolithiasis and LUTS still can occur.

Drugs Commonly Used for Cats With LUTS

Drug*	Dosage	Potential Side Effects
Acute Analgesic		
Butorphanol (Torbugesic)	0.2-0.4 mg/kg IV, IM, SQ q 2-8h (IV: use lower end of dose range; not an ideal choice due to short duration of analgesia)	Sedation
Buprenorphine (Buprenex)	0.01-0.02 mg/kg IM, IV, or SQ q 8-12h; 0.015 mg/kg PO or sublingual/transmucosal q 8-12h (anecdotal)	
Methadone	0.1-0.3 mg/kg IM, IV q 4-6h	Sedation
Fentanyl CRI or patch (Duragesic)	1-5 mcg/kg/h CRI or 25 mcg/h patch	Respiratory depression, bradycardia
Bladder/Urethral Contractility		
Acepromazine (PromAce)	0.01-0.05 mg/kg SQ q 8h, 2.5 mg/CAT PO	Sedation, hypotension
Prazosin (Minipress)	0.5 mg/CAT PO q 12h	Hypotension
Phenoxybenzamine (Dibenzyline)	2.5 mg/CAT PO q 12h	Hypotension
Bethanechol (Urecholine)	2.5-5 mg/CAT PO q 12h	Salivation, vomiting, diarrhea
Chronic Analgesic/Anxiolytic		
Clomipramine (Anafranil)	0.5 mg/kg PO q 24h	Sedation, anticholinergic effects
Amitriptyline (Elavil)	5-12.5 mg/CAT PO q 12-24h	Sedation, weight gain, urine retention; urolith formation
Fluoxetine hydrochloride	0.5-1 mg/kg PO q 24h	Decreased food intake

*These are all off-label uses.

Nutrition/Diet

- Dietary therapy may be indicated if uroliths or crystals are identified and depends on the type of urolith.
- Glycosaminoglycan (GAG) supplementation has been suggested, but its efficacy remains unproved in cats.

Possible Complications

- When introducing EE, offer changes to the cat (e.g., new food in a separate bowl rather than in place of the familiar diet) to avoid precipitating a threat response. Make changes the client wants to make, if possible, to secure support and adherence to the EE effort. Make changes sequentially.
- When TCA or SSRI drugs are being used and the decision is made to discontinue them, they should be tapered slowly over at least 2 weeks to avoid adverse reactions.

Recommended Monitoring

Liver and kidney function should be assessed before use of TCAs and at least annually for young animals if therapy is extended.

PROGNOSIS & OUTCOME

Most cases of idiopathic, nonobstructive, feline LUTS are self-limited, usually resolving in 5-10 days. However, recurrent episodes, including urinary tract obstruction, occur with variable frequency. Overall prognosis depends on the cat, client, and environment:

- Cat
  - Genetic predisposition
  - Duration of the problem
  - Frequency of occurrences
  - Number of areas and different types of surfaces soiled
- Client
  - Ability to identify modifiable causes
  - Strength of bond with affected cat
  - Willingness to pay for treatment
  - Amount of time to devote to solution
  - Willingness to accept and use medications
- Environment
  - Number of cats in the household
  - Number of affected cats
  - Practicality of allowing limited outdoor access
  - Ability to rearrange the environment

PEARLS & CONSIDERATIONS

Comments

EE often is sufficient to suppress clinical signs and should be discussed with all owners of cats exclusively housed indoors.

Prevention

EE recommendations should be provided to all owners of indoor cats, not just those with a clinical problem.

Technician Tips

A great deal of effort should be made to help clients understand EE for indoor cats and appropriate litter box management.

Client Education

Client-oriented information is available at www.indoorcat.org.

SUGGESTED READING

Buffington CAT: Idiopathic cystitis in domestic cats—beyond the lower urinary tract. J Vet Intern Med 25:784-796, 2011.

AUTHOR: Claire R. Sharp, BVMS, MS, DACVECC
EDITOR: Leah A. Cohn, DVM, PhD, DACVIM

Fever of Unknown Origin

Client Education Sheet 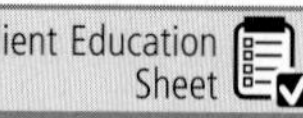

BASIC INFORMATION 

Definition

- Fever is defined as an elevated body temperature (>103°F [>39.5°C]) due to an altered hypothalamic set point.
- Fever of unknown origin (FUO) is defined in human medicine as an illness of at least 3 weeks' duration with a fever, for which a cause is not identified after 3 hospitalized days or outpatient visits. Veterinary equivalents are adaptations of this definition.
- Temperatures consistently > 105°F (>40.6°C) are uncommon in FUO, and temperatures > 106°F (>41.1°C) are more common with nonfebrile hyperthermia (p. 421).

Synonyms

- Pyrexia
- Fever is a subset of hyperthermia, not a synonym. Nonfebrile hyperthermia (e.g., high body temperature due to physical exertion, heat stroke, muscle fasciculations) does not involve alterations in the hypothalamic set point and is not treated with antipyretic drugs.

Epidemiology

SPECIES, AGE, SEX

- Any age, breed, or sex
- Young patients are more likely to have infectious causes.
- Middle-aged patients are more likely to have noninfectious inflammatory diseases, including immune-mediated disorders.
- Older patients are more likely to have neoplastic causes.

GENETICS, BREED PREDISPOSITION

- Shar-pei: possible cytokine abnormality
- Gray collie: cyclic hematopoiesis
- Irish setter: leukocyte adhesion deficiency
- Weimaraner: neutrophil function defect
- Blue Persian: Chédiak-Higashi syndrome

RISK FACTORS

- Immunosuppression or immunodeficiency
- Exposure to infectious agents or vectors
- Travel to endemic areas of disease

CONTAGION AND ZOONOSIS

Risk varies, depending on underlying cause

GEOGRAPHY AND SEASONALITY

Some regions are endemic for particular infectious diseases. See specific individual topics.

ASSOCIATED DISORDERS

Temperatures > 106°F (>41.1°C) may cause multiple organ dysfunction (p. 665), disseminated intravascular coagulation (p. 269), and death.

Clinical Presentation

HISTORY, CHIEF COMPLAINT

Depends on underlying cause but often is associated with nonspecific clinical signs such as lethargy, depression, and anorexia. Individual and environmental influences may raise the body temperature of normal, healthy patients and must be considered when interpreting a patient's temperature, but elevated temperature over days to weeks is most often caused by true fever.

PHYSICAL EXAM FINDINGS

A thorough physical exam of all patients with FUO must include rectal palpation (dog), fundic, oral, orthopedic, and neurologic exams, meticulous examination of the skin, and thoracic auscultation.

- Depression/lethargy
- Tachycardia
- Tachypnea/hyperpnea
- Dehydration
- Lymphadenopathy with infectious or neoplastic disease
- Neck or back pain or central signs with meningitis, meningoencephalitis, discospondylitis
- Joint pain or swelling with monoarthritis or polyarthritis
- Heart murmur may indicate endocarditis, especially if new in onset and/or diastolic.
- Chorioretinitis or uveitis with infectious disease (p. 1137)
- Localized swelling and/or pain with cellulitis or abscesses

Etiology and Pathophysiology

Pathophysiology:

- Fever occurs when the hypothalamic set point is raised.
- Inflammation and/or pathogens increase the hypothalamic set point by causing the release of endogenous pyrogens such as interleukin-1 or exogenous pyrogens such as lipopolysaccharides (LPSs) and other bacterial endotoxins.

DIAGNOSIS

Diagnostic Overview

FUO is not a disease diagnosis, but the result of disease. Use of the term FUO is justified when an elevated body temperature has been documented on several occasions (typically over several days) in the absence of confounding factors such as anxiety or warm ambient temperatures.

Differential Diagnosis

- A detailed differential diagnosis of FUO is provided on p. 1223.
- Rule out nonfebrile causes of an elevated body temperature.

Initial Database

- CBC (with blood smear evaluation), serum biochemistry profile, urinalysis: results vary with organ system involvement and disease causation.
- Urine bacterial culture and sensitivity should be performed in all cases of FUO, even if urine sediment is inactive.
- Feline leukemia virus antigen and feline immunodeficiency virus antibody testing should be done for all cats.
- Thoracic and abdominal radiographs, abdominal ultrasound: results vary with organ system involvement.

Advanced or Confirmatory Testing

Further laboratory testing depends on history, physical exam findings, and minimal database results.

- Laboratory tests
  - Blood cultures: to detect bacteremia associated with discospondylitis, endocarditis, or other foci of bacterial infection. A negative culture result does not rule out bacteremia.
  - Cytology and cultures of bile, cerebrospinal fluid (CSF) or synovial fluid, as indicated
  - Cytology of aspirates from lymph nodes or affected organs
  - Serologic tests: antibody titers or antigen tests for specific infectious agents. If infectious disease is suspected and initial titers are negative, repeat in 2-4 weeks.

  - *Brucella canis* screening test, if appropriate
  - Polymerase chain reaction (PCR) testing for specific infectious agents
  - Immune tests: antinuclear antibody test if systemic lupus erythematosus is suspected; Coombs' test if immune-mediated hemolytic anemia is suspected but cannot be confirmed otherwise; serum protein electrophoresis if hyperglobulinemic
- Imaging
  - Abdominal ultrasound: examine for evidence of pyelonephritis, prostatitis, or pyometra; identify ± aspirate enlarged abdominal organs or masses.
  - Echocardiogram: identify vegetative valvular lesions of endocarditis.
  - Spinal long bone and joint radiographs: examine for evidence of discospondylitis, osteomyelitis, periosteal proliferation, erosive arthritis, hypertrophic osteodystrophy, panosteitis.
  - CT/MRI (p. 1132)
- Diagnostic procedures
  - Arthrocentesis (p. 1059): polyarthritis
  - Bone marrow aspirates and/or biopsy (p. 1064): if CBC changes suggest bone marrow involvement
  - CSF tap (p. 1080): if neurologic signs (± fundic exam) suggest meningoencephalitis or meningitis
  - Muscle biopsy: hepatozoonosis
  - Abdominocentesis (p. 1056): peritonitis and pancreatitis
  - Transtracheal wash or bronchoalveolar lavage: if respiratory involvement (p. 1073)
  - Laparoscopy, thoracoscopy, or exploratory surgery for biopsies, as appropriate

TREATMENT

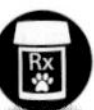

Treatment Overview

- The goal in all cases of FUO is to obtain a specific diagnosis and treat accordingly.
- A therapeutic trial should be initiated only when a specific diagnosis cannot be ascertained.

Acute General Treatment

- Intravenous crystalloid fluid therapy at 1.5-2 times maintenance for fevers > 103.5°F (>39.7°C)
- Mechanical cooling methods such as cool water baths or fans for fevers > 106°F (>41.1°C)
- Antipyretic agents (e.g., nonsteroidal anti-inflammatory drugs [NSAIDs] given only when the patient is fully hydrated) may be considered for fevers > 106°F (>41.1°C) that do not respond to fluids and cooling.
  - Antipyretics can mask the effects of other therapies and can be associated with adverse effects such as gastrointestinal ulceration and hepatic and/or renal toxicosis.

Chronic Treatment

Antibiotic trials:

- Broad-spectrum antibiotic therapy may be initiated after all culture specimens have been collected. Therapy should be based on the agents most likely present, their known antibiotic sensitivity, and the organ or system affected.
- If no response is seen after 72 hours, an antibiotic with a different spectrum of activity may be chosen; however, the clinician should first re-evaluate whether bacterial infection is the underlying cause.
- Commonly used empirical antibiotics include amoxicillin-clavulanate 10-20 mg/kg PO q 8-12h and enrofloxacin 5-10 mg/kg (dog), 5 mg/kg (cat) PO q 24h; if anaerobic infection is suspected, metronidazole 10-15 mg/kg PO q 12h or clindamycin 5-15 mg/kg PO q 8-12h; if tick-borne disease is suspected, doxycycline 10 mg/kg PO q 24h or 5 mg/kg PO q 12h.

Antifungal trials:

- In areas where systemic mycoses are endemic, antifungal agents may be used in patients with typical signs of fungal infection.
- The response to antifungal therapy may take days to weeks.
- Examples: itraconazole 5-10 mg/kg PO q 24h or 5 mg/kg PO q 12h; fluconazole 5-15 mg/kg PO q 12-24h

Glucocorticoid trials:

- Used when immune-mediated disease is suspected
- Should be used only after infectious disease has been reasonably ruled out
- A dramatic response (fever reduction, striking improvement in systemic signs) should be seen in 24-48 hours, but glucocorticoids can reduce fever initially even when they do not effectively treat the underlying disease (e.g., infectious disease).
- Examples: prednis(ol)one 1 mg/kg PO q 12h or dexamethasone 0.2 mg/kg IV q 24h; dosages for long-term use are adjusted based on the specific underlying cause.

Drug Interactions

Avoid the use of NSAIDs in combination with glucocorticoids.

Possible Complications

- Drug therapy trials without a definitive diagnosis may interfere with future diagnosis (e.g., antibiotic use may impair culture) and exacerbate an undiagnosed condition that may become life-threatening (e.g., glucocorticoids may worsen fungal infection).
- Glucocorticoids may lead to immunosuppression or may mask clinical signs due to their antiinflammatory effects.

Recommended Monitoring

Monitor temperature at least q 8h. Response to trial therapy may be nonspecific or coincidental, and monitoring should continue for a sufficient time to confirm that resolution of the fever can be attributed to selected therapy.

PROGNOSIS & OUTCOME

Depends on specific cause

PEARLS & CONSIDERATIONS

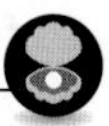

Comments

- Infectious disease, immune-mediated conditions, and neoplasia account for > 75% of FUO cases.
- With comprehensive diagnostic testing, usually only 10% of FUO cases are considered idiopathic.
- Immune-mediated polyarthritis will frequently *not* be associated with detectable joint swelling. Arthrocentesis is indicated in all FUO cases where no underlying cause has been identified, even absent a history of lameness.
- Lymphoma, leukemia, myeloma, and hepatic neoplasia are particularly common causes of fever in association with cancer.
- Drug fevers may occur at any time after initiation of drug therapy, even after weeks or months. Careful drug history is warranted, as is a trial discontinuation of drugs.

Prevention

- Ectoparasite prevention may reduce risk of vector-borne disease transmission.
- Indoor pets are less likely to be exposed to vector-borne diseases.
- Vaccination against specific disease agents for at-risk pets
- Yearly retroviral testing ± vaccination in high-risk cats
- Routine screening of geriatric pets to facilitate early diagnosis and treatment of cancer

Technician Tips

- Fever may wax and wane in a patient with FUO.
- Patients receiving a glucocorticoid trial should be closely monitored because of the risk of exacerbating an infectious disease.
- It is important that owners understand that not all fevers are due to infection and not all infections respond to antibiotic treatment.

Client Education

- Animals may serve as sentinels for infections or transmit some infections to humans.
- Investigation of FUO can be time consuming and costly.

SUGGESTED READING

Lunn KF: Fever of unknown origin: a systematic approach to diagnosis. Compend Contin Educ Vet 23:976-992, 2001.

AUTHOR: Karen M. Tefft, DVM, MVSc, DACVIM
EDITOR: Leah A. Cohn, DVM, PhD, DACVIM

Fibrocartilaginous Embolism

Client Education Sheet 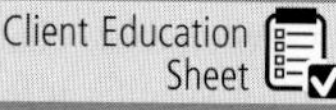

BASIC INFORMATION

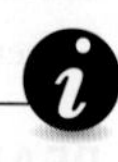

Definition

An ischemic vascular event of the spinal cord caused by fibrocartilaginous material occluding an intraparenchymal spinal cord vessel

Synonyms

Fibrocartilaginous embolism (FCE), fibrocartilaginous embolic myelopathy (FCEM), ischemic myelopathy

Epidemiology

SPECIES, AGE, SEX

- Young to middle-aged dogs (median age, 5 years)
- Middle-aged to older cats

GENETICS, BREED PREDISPOSITION

- Mostly large- to giant-breed dogs
- Reported in small-breed dogs: miniature schnauzers appear to be predisposed
- Juvenile, male Irish wolfhounds (<13 weeks old)
- Domestic short-hair cats

Clinical Presentation

HISTORY, CHIEF COMPLAINT

FCEM has a peracute onset of neurologic dysfunction localizable to the site of spinal cord injury with no history of blunt trauma. Physical activity and/or vocalization can be associated with the onset of signs. It typically has nonprogressive neurologic signs, although progression of signs can occur over the first 24 hours.

PHYSICAL EXAM FINDINGS

On neurologic exam, the deficits depend on the location of spinal cord injury, and signs are often lateralized or asymmetric. T3-L3 myelopathy is the most common localization in dogs and cervical myelopathy in cats. Affected animals are usually not painful on vertebral palpation, although pain can be elicited in some instances for up to 24 hours after the onset of signs. The reminder of the physical exam is usually unremarkable.

Etiology and Pathophysiology

- FCEM is caused by the embolization of fibrocartilaginous material into the spinal cord vasculature, causing ischemic damage to the spinal cord parenchyma.
- The fibrocartilaginous material is thought to arise from the nucleus pulposus of the intervertebral disc.
- The mechanism by which the fibrocartilaginous material enters the spinal cord vasculature is unknown.

DIAGNOSIS

Diagnostic Overview

To definitively diagnose FCEM, histopathology of affected spinal cord segments must be performed. An antemortem clinical diagnosis can be made based on presenting signs and the elimination of other causes of an acute-onset, nonpainful (vertebra palpation), nonprogressive, focal myelopathy. CBC, serum chemistry, and urinalysis should be performed to exclude systemic causes for thrombi or emboli. MRI is the diagnostic test of choice to support a clinical diagnosis of FCEM due to its ability to visualize lesions within the spinal cord parenchyma. Cerebral spinal fluid (CSF) analysis should be performed to eliminate inflammatory causes. A presumptive diagnosis can be made without imaging and CSF analysis based on the clinical presentation and lack of progression. However, advanced diagnostics allow for a more tailored treatment regimen.

Differential Diagnosis

- More likely differentials (similar history and clinical signs)
  - Acute noncompressive nucleus pulposus extrusion (ANNPE) (p. 930)
  - A thrombus or other emboli (parasitic, bacterial, neoplastic, fat) causing an ischemic myelopathy
  - Intraparenchymal hemorrhage (coagulopathy)
- Less likely differentials (unlikely to have a similar history and clinical signs)
  - Intervertebral disc extrusion or protrusion
  - Spinal cord or vertebral neoplasia
  - Infectious or immune-mediated myelitis
  - Vertebral trauma
  - Discospondylitis with secondary spinal cord compression or myelitis

Initial Database

- CBC, serum chemistry, and urinalysis: typically unremarkable; useful to evaluate systemic causes of hemorrhage, thrombi, or emboli
- Blood pressure: evaluate for hypertension
- Survey vertebral radiographs: unremarkable; should be considered in patients with an unknown history to screen for vertebral fractures

Advanced or Confirmatory Testing

- MRI: evidence of T2 hyperintensity in spinal cord parenchyma, possible spinal cord swelling; rule out compressive myelopathy (p. 1132)
- Other imaging modalities such as myelography and CT show only nonspecific changes such as spinal cord swelling with FCEM but can eliminate other differential diagnoses.
- CSF analysis: can be normal or show a mild increase in nucleated cell count and/or elevation in protein concentrations; useful in excluding myelitis

TREATMENT

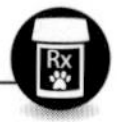

Treatment Overview

The mainstay of therapy for FCEM is nursing care, recumbency care, and rehabilitation. Surgery is not indicated because FCEM does not cause spinal cord compression. Affected animals often improve without the administration of glucocorticoids. If advanced imaging is not available, the clinical suspicion of FCEM can be supported by observing neurologic improvement over time in a patient that has not been administered glucocorticoids.

Acute General Treatment

- Therapy targeted at maintaining spinal cord perfusion (maintaining blood pressure) should be administered in the acute phase to try to minimize secondary spinal cord injury.
  - Scientifically proven neuroprotective therapy is not available, but such agents may be available in the future.
- Bladder management is imperative for paraplegic animals that can be assumed to have lost the ability to voluntarily urinate (manual expression, intermittent bladder catheterization, or an indwelling urinary catheter).
- Ventilator support may be necessary for animals with hypoventilation associated with severe tetraparesis or tetraplegia (p. 1185).

Chronic Treatment

- Recumbency care
  - Animals should be housed on dry, clean bedding that is routinely checked.
  - The skin should be closely monitored for signs of urine scalding.
  - Provide adequate padding, and turn animals from side to side every 6-8 hours to prevent pressure sores and reduce the risk of pneumonia.
- Bladder management
  - Bladder management should be continued until the patient regains pelvic limb motor function and is able to completely evacuate its bladder.
  - Animals with spinal cord injury requiring bladder management are predisposed to urinary tract infections.
- Physical rehabilitation
  - Strict cage confinement is not recommended for animals with a clinical diagnosis of FCEM. Physical rehabilitation is essential to prevent muscle atrophy

and restricted joint mobility. Physical rehabilitation can also help maximize a functional recovery.

- If a presumptive diagnosis of FCEM is made on clinical suspicion alone, restricted activity for 4-6 weeks with controlled exercise is recommended. If other differentials have not been excluded, care must be taken to minimize the risk of further spinal cord injury (e.g., further disc extrusion in an animal with intervertebral disc disease).
- Physical rehabilitation should be performed at home by the owners and augmented by sessions at a certified veterinary physical rehabilitation facility.

Behavior/Exercise

Physical rehabilitation is important.

Possible Complications

- Decubital ulcers
  - Ensure adequate recumbency care.
  - Initiate wound management if skin ulceration is noted.
- Pneumonia
  - Ensure proper recumbency care.
  - Monitor appetite, respiratory rate, and body temperature.
  - Perform thoracic radiograph if there is clinical suspicion of pneumonia.
- Urinary tract infection (p. 232)
  - Monitor for hematuria, pollakiuria, stranguria.
  - Perform urinalysis and urine culture.
  - Treat based on culture and sensitivity results.
- Muscle atrophy and loss of joint range of motion
  - Ensure proper physical rehabilitation is provided.

Recommended Monitoring

Serial neurologic exams (q 1-2 weeks) to monitor for recovery of function

PROGNOSIS & OUTCOME

- The prognosis for FCEM varies based on the neurologic status at presentation and extent of the spinal cord injury.
- Prognosis for dogs and cats with intact nociception (deep pain perception) at presentation is generally good to excellent. These animals often return to an ambulatory neurologic status within 2-3 weeks but can have persistent neurologic deficits such as urinary incontinence, fecal incontinence, pelvic limb ataxia, and/or toe scuffing.
- As with any type of spinal cord injury, animals that lack nociception have a poor prognosis.
- Animals with lower motor neuron signs (involvement of an intumescence) can have a more guarded prognosis or more prolonged recovery.
- MRI and CSF analysis findings can provide information regarding prognosis.

PEARLS & CONSIDERATIONS

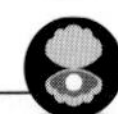

Comments

- There should be strong clinical suspicion of FCEM when a dog presents with a peracute onset of nonprogressive signs of myelopathy and is not painful on vertebral palpation.
- An animal with FCEM will show evidence of improvement, often over a few days, without the administration of glucocorticoids. For cases in which there is clinical suspicion of FCEM but advanced diagnostics cannot be pursued, valuable information can be obtained by monitoring for clinical improvement without initiating glucocorticoid therapy. Improvement of neurologic status with glucocorticoids is very nonspecific and does not help to eliminate potential differential diagnoses.

Technician Tips

Nursing care is the mainstay of therapy for patients with FCEM. Patients with FCEM can take weeks to recover, and day-to-day improvement can be minimal in the hospital. These cases require a great deal of work but can be very rewarding.

Client Education

Clients should be informed of the commitment necessary to care for non-ambulatory patients at home. Realistic expectations about the recovery of a patient with FCEM should be discussed with clients so that owners do not give up prematurely. Animals with FCEM can return to a great quality of life as a functional pet but may not return to normal.

SUGGESTED READING

Bartholomew K, et al: Clinical characteristics of canine fibrocartilaginous embolic myelopathy (FCE): a systemic review of 393 cases (1973-2013). Vet Rec 179:650, 2016.

AUTHOR: Hillary Greatting, DVM, MS, DACVIM, CCRT
EDITOR: Karen R. Muñana, DVM, MS, DACVIM

Fibrosarcoma

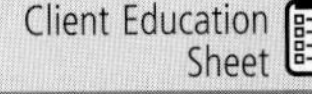

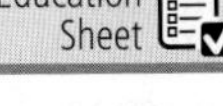

Client Education Sheet

BASIC INFORMATION

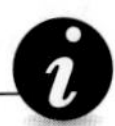

Definition

A common, primary, malignant neoplasm of fibrous tissue. Fibrosarcoma is most common in the skin, subcutis, and oral cavity but can occur anywhere, including the spleen.

Epidemiology

SPECIES, AGE, SEX

Fibrosarcomas are more common in middle-aged to older dogs and cats. Injection-site sarcomas are discussed separately (p. 550).

Clinical Presentation

DISEASE FORMS/SUBTYPES

- The most common form of fibrosarcoma in dogs is a solitary mass, typically found on the head, limbs, or oral cavity.
- Sarcomas that are histologically low grade but biologically high grade (malignant behavior) are an uncommon variant of fibrosarcoma found in the maxilla and mandible in large-breed dogs.

HISTORY, CHIEF COMPLAINT

Most animals present with a progressive mass noticed by the owner or clinical signs related to the location of the tumor (e.g., oral or splenic tumor).

PHYSICAL EXAM FINDINGS

- Fibrosarcoma often appears as a firm, palpable mass in the subcutis or deep tissues; it is occasionally hairless or ulcerated. Oral fibrosarcomas often appear as smooth, round masses. On the hard palate, fibrosarcomas are frequently flat and ulcerated.
- Regional lymphadenopathy may be present secondary to inflammation or (rarely) lymph node metastasis.
- Dogs with a splenic fibrosarcoma may present with an abdominal mass, pain, or enlargement.

Etiology and Pathophysiology

- Fibrosarcomas are spontaneously occurring tumors in most cases in dogs.
- Prior irradiation and metal implants have been implicated as causes of fibrosarcoma. There are cases of fibrosarcoma in cats developing at sites of microchips and surgical sponges.
- Specific dysfunction caused by fibrosarcomas depends on the location of the primary tumor.

DIAGNOSIS

Diagnostic Overview

Definitive diagnosis can be confirmed only histopathologically, although additional tests such as diagnostic imaging are often helpful in defining the extent of the tumor, especially for oral fibrosarcomas.

Differential Diagnosis

- Other soft-tissue sarcomas
- Other skin and subcutaneous tumors (e.g., mast cell tumors [p. 628])
- Other oral tumors (e.g., epulis, melanoma, squamous cell carcinoma)
- Benign or non-neoplastic masses
  - Benign tumor (e.g., lipoma)
  - Abscess, granuloma

Initial Database

- Fine-needle aspiration and cytologic evaluation may help identify the tumor type before other diagnostics are considered.
- Three-view thoracic radiographs to rule out pulmonary metastases
- Radiographs of the affected area may reveal involvement of underlying bone.
- Abdominal ultrasound to identify splenic tumors and rule out metastasis
- Fine-needle aspiration and cytologic exam of the regional/draining lymph node to assess for metastasis

Advanced or Confirmatory Testing

- Biopsy of mass
  - Histopathologic confirmation of fibrosarcoma
  - Special immunohistochemical stains may be necessary to differentiate fibrosarcoma from other soft-tissue sarcomas, especially poorly differentiated tumors.
- CT or MRI (p. 1132) may be necessary to delineate the local extent of the tumor and to plan for surgery or radiation therapy.
- Histopathologic grade of the tumor is necessary for determining the prognosis and treatment of most soft-tissue sarcomas (p. 927).

TREATMENT

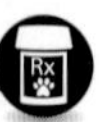

Treatment Overview

- Definitive treatment is based on complete eradication of the primary tumor whenever possible.
- Because metastasis is uncommon, additional treatment such as chemotherapy is rarely used but could be considered for high-grade tumors or tumors that have already metastasized.
- Palliative treatment options, such as palliative irradiation, may help control pain or discomfort in patients with advanced tumors or in patients when definitive treatment cannot be tolerated.
- Palliative irradiation or metronomic chemotherapy (daily low doses of chemotherapy) may help control the local tumor for significant periods.
- Marginal tumor excision with intralesional chemotherapy beads can result in long-term control and may be considered as an alternative to radiation for some cases.

Acute and Chronic Treatment

- Aggressive surgical resection, radiation therapy, and/or chemotherapy may be used for treatment of fibrosarcoma (p. 1451).
- Chemotherapy may be indicated for tumors of the spleen or high-grade tumors.

Possible Complications

Complications of treatment for fibrosarcomas depend on the types of treatments and the location of the primary tumor.

Recommended Monitoring

After appropriate local treatment, regular follow-up exams are indicated to monitor for recurrence and metastasis. High-grade tumors may require more frequent monitoring for metastases during and after chemotherapy administration.

- Dogs that are likely to develop metastasis (splenic tumors, high-grade tumors) should be monitored closely (q 2-3 months) with a physical exam, lymph node palpation, and thoracic radiographs.
- Dogs with low- or intermediate-grade tumors that have adequate local treatment should have physical exams q 2-3 months or more frequently, depending on risk of side effects from treatment. Thoracic radiographs could be done less frequently (6 months and 1 year after therapy).

PROGNOSIS & OUTCOME

- A combination of radiation therapy and surgery has resulted in long-term tumor control in 86% of dogs with fibrosarcoma in peripheral sites and 54% of fibrosarcomas from all sites, including the oral cavity.
- Radiation therapy alone has resulted in 1-year tumor control rates of only 33% and therefore is not typically recommended for fibrosarcomas. However, this statistic may underestimate efficacy because it is derived from studies that used suboptimal radiation dose schedules.
- In certain situations where surgery is not indicated (e.g., nonresectable tumors or metastatic disease), radiation therapy may be used to provide some degree of tumor control.
- Prognosis is excellent for low- to intermediate-grade fibrosarcomas with appropriate local treatment. This includes surgical resection with clean histopathologic margins or incomplete resection combined with radiation therapy.
- Palliative radiation after incomplete tumor excision has resulted in tumor control in 65% of dogs with soft-tissue sarcomas at 5 years.
- Metronomic chemotherapy using cyclophosphamide and piroxicam has been shown to result in tumor control for a median of more than 400 days after incomplete tumor excision of soft-tissue sarcomas.
- Information is limited regarding prognosis for high-grade fibrosarcomas, but it is considered to be guarded based on the increased likelihood for metastases.
- Dogs with splenic fibrosarcomas are more likely to develop metastases and therefore have a poor prognosis.

PEARLS & CONSIDERATIONS

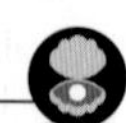

Comments

Many animals with fibrosarcoma are successfully treated with wide surgical excision of the tumor. Animals with tumors that are difficult to treat in this manner (e.g., oral sarcomas, grade 3 sarcomas, nonresectable tumors) should be referred for consultation with a specialist (surgeon, oncologist, or radiation oncologist) to develop a multimodality treatment approach.

Technician Tips

All masses in dogs and cats, even slow-growing ones, should be aspirated to rule out malignant tumors.

Client Education

Pet owners can be educated to monitor their pets for the occurrence of tissue masses such as fibrosarcomas. Early detection and treatment may allow for less aggressive treatments with fewer side effects.

SUGGESTED READING

Liptak JM, et al: Soft tissue sarcomas. In Withrow SJ, et al, editors: Small animal clinical oncology, Philadelphia, 2013, Saunders, pp 356-380.

AUTHOR: John Farrelly, DVM, MS, DACVIM, DACVR
EDITOR: Kenneth M. Rassnick, DVM, DACVIM

5-Fluorouracil Toxicosis

BASIC INFORMATION

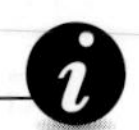

Definition

Adverse effects caused by exposure to 5-fluorouracil (5-FU), a pyrimidine analog–type antineoplastic, antimetabolite drug used for palliative management of certain carcinomas and solar keratoses in humans and occasionally in dogs

Synonyms

Common brand names: Efudex, Fluoroplex, Adracil, and Carac. Generic: 2,4-dioxo-5-fluoropyrimidine; 5-fluoro-2,4(1H,3H)-pyrimidinedione

Epidemiology

SPECIES, AGE, SEX

No age, breed, or sex predisposition. Exposure occurs more often in dogs than cats. Central nervous system (CNS) signs more common in dogs and cats than in people. Cats are more sensitive than dogs, and use of 5-FU in cats is contraindicated.

RISK FACTORS

- Pre-existing liver or kidney dysfunction can increase risk of toxicosis.
- Presence of 5-FU in a pet's environment

Clinical Presentation

HISTORY, CHIEF COMPLAINT

- History of exposure to product containing 5-FU
- Clinical signs begin within 30 minutes to 5 hours of exposure.
- Vomiting, hypersalivation, lethargy, vocalization, diarrhea, tremors, ataxia, seizures
- Some animals show vomiting progressing quickly to seizures; others have tremors and seizures without vomiting.

PHYSICAL EXAM FINDINGS

- Seizures (often status epilepticus)
- Vomiting (with or without blood)
- Diarrhea (with or without blood)
- Tremors
- Lethargy
- Ataxia
- Cardiac arrhythmias (all kinds)
- Respiratory depression

Etiology and Pathophysiology

Source:

- 5-FU or similar agents are available for use as injections, topical creams (0.5%-5%) or lotions (1%-5%), and capecitabine (prodrug of fluorouracil) is available as tablets. Flucytosine is an antifungal agent that is converted to 5-FU.
- Toxicosis occurs after ingestion of products containing 5-FU and occasionally secondary to repeated use in dogs.

Mechanism of toxicosis:

- 5-FU inhibits RNA processing and function and DNA synthesis and repair, inhibiting cell division. Actively dividing cells (bone marrow stem cells, intestinal crypt cells) are most affected.
- Neurotoxicosis may occur by production of fluorocitrate, which limits cellular energy production by interfering with the Krebs cycle.

DIAGNOSIS

Diagnostic Overview

History of exposure within 5 hours of onset of compatible clinical signs is sufficient to make a clinical diagnosis.

Differential Diagnosis

Diseases or intoxications that could cause vomiting (p. 1040) and/or seizures (pp. 301 and 903)

Initial Database

- Serum biochemistry profile: ± elevated liver enzymes ± hypokalemia due to severe gastrointestinal (GI) signs (i.e., vomiting, diarrhea)
- CBC with differential (baseline, monitor q 24-72 hours for 20 days); initial leukocytosis followed by leukopenia, pancytopenia in 5-20 days. Hematocrit increased due to dehydration, then decreased due to GI bleeding
- Blood gas analysis if severe systemic signs
- Urinalysis

Advanced or Confirmatory Testing

- Analysis of 5-FU and its metabolites in plasma is possible but not readily available.
- Necropsy lesions: hemorrhagic colitis, GI mucosal ulceration (throughout), stomatitis, myocardial ischemia, pulmonary edema, hepatic and renal congestion

TREATMENT

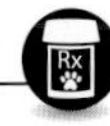

Treatment Overview

Stabilize the patient first; control seizures and vomiting, and provide supportive care.

Acute General Treatment

Decontamination of asymptomatic patient (p. 1087):

- Because of rapid onset of signs, emesis induction and administration of activated charcoal is often not possible.
- Hemodialysis, peritoneal dialysis, or intravenous (IV) fluid diuresis may enhance elimination.

Manage vomiting:

- Maropitant 1 mg/kg SQ q 24h for up to 5 consecutive days
- Do not use metoclopramide (contraindicated with GI hemorrhage and seizure disorder).

GI protection

- Sucralfate 0.5 (small dog, cats) to 1 g (large dog) PO q 8h
- Omeprazole 0.5-1 mg/kg PO q 24h or famotidine 0.5-1 mg/kg IV or PO q 12-24h

Manage tremors and seizures (p. 903).

- Seizures are rarely controlled with diazepam alone (dogs: 1-2 mg/kg IV; cats: 0.5-1 mg/kg IV). If seizures persist after diazepam therapy, give phenobarbital IV bolus 2-5 mg/kg (can be repeated at 20-minute intervals up to two times). May then add phenobarbital IV infusion (2-10 mg/h IV, titrated to effect) to diazepam, *or*
- Pentobarbital 3-15 mg/kg IV slowly to effect, *or*
- Propofol 4-6 mg/kg IV or as continuous IV infusion 0.1-0.6 mg/kg/min, *or*
- Gas anesthesia

Supportive care:

- Intravenous fluids
- Thermoregulation
- Ventilatory support as needed (p. 1185)
- Maintain normal acid-base status and electrolyte balance.
- Manage pain.
  - Buprenorphine 0.005-0.05 mg/kg, IM, IV q 4-8h, *or* fentanyl patch
- Broad-spectrum antibiotics to prevent secondary infection from bacterial translocation
- For neutropenia: filgrastim (Neupogen) 4-6 mcg/kg SQ

Chronic Treatment

Intensive supportive care may be needed for days/weeks, especially if myelosuppression occurs.

Nutrition/Diet

- Bland diet while GI signs present
- Tube feeding if prolonged anorexia is present (p. 1106)

Drug Interactions

Metronidazole may increase toxicity of 5-FU by reducing clearance. Use of hydrochlorothiazide and leucovorin can increase risk of myelosuppression; leucovorin can also increase GI toxicosis risk.

Possible Complications

- CNS complications due to direct effect or secondary to severe seizures
- Hyperthermia due to seizures, tremor
- Myelosuppression (in 5-20 days)

Recommended Monitoring

- Heart rate, blood pressure, body temperature
- Respiratory rate and character
- CBC, serum biochemistry profile
- Blood gases

PROGNOSIS & OUTCOME

Guarded to poor; mortality rate is high among symptomatic dogs. Out of 72 intoxication cases, 35 dogs died, and 11 were euthanized.

PEARLS & CONSIDERATIONS

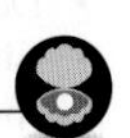

Comments

- Severe signs or death can result from 5-FU toxicosis; early decontamination when possible and immediate, intensive treatment are essential; owners should be advised of the seriousness of exposure to 5-FU.
- Estimated toxic dose in dogs is 8.6 mg/kg PO. Minimum lethal dose in dogs is 20 mg/kg PO. If a 70-lb (32-kg) dog ingests 1 tablespoon (15 g) from a tube containing 5% 5-FU, the dose of 5-FU for the dog is approximately 23 mg/kg, a potentially lethal dose.

Prevention

Keep medications out of pets' reach.

Technician Tips

- Because of the rapid onset of signs, decontamination is often not possible.
- Protect the airway because animals often present with vomiting and seizures.

Client Education

5-FU toxicosis in pets can be life-threatening.

SUGGESTED READING

Friedenberg SG, et al: Successful treatment of a dog with massive 5-fluorouracil toxicosis. J Vet Emerg Crit Care 23:643-647, 2013.

AUTHOR: Judy K. Holding, DVM, RN
EDITOR: Tina Wismer, DVM, MS, DABVT, DABT

Flail Chest

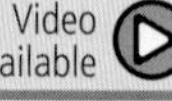

BASIC INFORMATION

Definition

Multiple fractures of adjacent ribs resulting in asynchronous motion of the chest wall during breathing

Synonyms

Flail segment, multiple rib fractures

Epidemiology

SPECIES, AGE, SEX

Any animal, but young, roaming, intact males are at increased risk for trauma

RISK FACTORS

Roaming behavior; intact males

ASSOCIATED DISORDERS

Pulmonary contusions; subcutaneous emphysema; pneumothorax; diaphragmatic hernia, other consequences of trauma (e.g., fractures)

Clinical Presentation

HISTORY, CHIEF COMPLAINT

Traumatic event; respiratory distress

PHYSICAL EXAM FINDINGS

- Paradoxical chest wall movement of flail segment while breathing (see *Video*)
  - Injured chest wall moves inward during inspiration and outward during expiration.
  - May not see obvious puncture or open wounds
- Respiratory distress (i.e., dyspnea) and tachypnea, with or without:
  - Dull lung sounds due to pleural effusion or pneumothorax
  - Crackles secondary to pulmonary contusions
- ± Subcutaneous emphysema
- ± Signs of shock (e.g., pale gums, weak pulses, tachycardia, tachypnea)
- ± Traumatic injuries (e.g., bite wounds, lacerations, limb fractures, head trauma)

Etiology and Pathophysiology

- To become a flail segment, adjacent ribs must have at least two fractures, which allows a segment of two or more ribs to move independently.
- Unstable flail segment causes pain and impairs ventilation.
- Hypoventilation, with or without contusions or pneumothorax, causes hypoxemia.

DIAGNOSIS

Diagnostic Overview

Flail chest can be recognized on physical examination, but thoracic radiographs define the flail segment and help rule out other pulmonary or pleural disorders.

Differential Diagnosis

- Pseudoflail chest: direct communication with the thoracic cavity causing the skin to move paradoxically during breathing with no true flail segment
- Intercostal muscle damage

Initial Database

- Thoracic radiographs
  - Obtain orthogonal views, including right and left lateral. Ventrodorsal (VD) view may be very stressful; consider dorsoventral (DV) view instead to improve patient comfort and tolerance of radiographic positioning.
  - Identify concurrent pulmonary or pleural space injury.
  - Contraindicated in unstable patients; delay until stabilized
- Pulse oximetry
  - Hypoxemia common ($SpO_2 < 95\%$)
  - May be difficult to obtain accurate reading if in respiratory distress or shock
- CBC, serum chemistry profile, lactate, and urinalysis can help assess other consequences of traumatic injury

Advanced or Confirmatory Testing

Arterial blood gas (p. 1058)

- Confirmation of hypoxemia ($PaO_2 < 80$ mm Hg) and hypoventilation ($PCO_2 > 50$ mm Hg)

Thoracic CT

- More sensitive for detection of rib fractures than radiographs
- Requires heavy sedation or anesthesia

TREATMENT

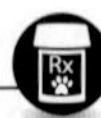

Treatment Overview

Goals are to stabilize hemodynamic status of traumatized patient, optimize oxygenation and ventilation, and provide analgesia.

Acute General Treatment

- Prevent excessive movement of flail segment
  - If tolerant, place patient on treatment table with flail segment side down, which reduces excessive movement of flail segment and improves patient comfort.
  - Soft, padded bandages or chest wraps can restrict chest wall movement if too tight.
- Pain control
  - Opioids: all opioids may cause respiratory depression at higher doses.
    - Fentanyl 2-5 mcg/kg IV bolus, then 2-5 mcg/kg/h IV CRI
    - Hydromorphone 0.05-0.1 mg/kg IV, IM, SQ q 4-6h
    - Buprenorphine 0.005-0.02 mg/kg IV, IM, SQ q 6-8h
    - Methadone 0.05-0.5 mg/kg IV, IM, SQ q 4-8h
    - Consider multimodal analgesia for severe pain (fentanyl-lidocaine-ketamine or morphine-lidocaine-ketamine)
  - Intercostal nerve blocks
    - Dogs: bupivacaine 1-2 mg/kg or lidocaine 1-4 mg/kg q 6h; cats sensitive to toxic effects: use one-half of dog dose

- Inject at the caudal aspect of the rib and dorsally (near head of rib) above fracture. Do not give IV.
- Block two adjacent intercostal spaces cranial and caudal to fractured ribs.
- Mild sedation may be necessary to reduce patient anxiety and stress.
  - Butorphanol 0.2-0.4 mg/kg IV, IM is a good sedative; may partially reverse effects of other opioids
  - Midazolam or diazepam 0.2-0.5 mg/kg IV, IM; use in conjunction with opioids
- Oxygen supplementation (p. 1146)
- Manage concurrent intrathoracic disease
  - Thoracocentesis if needed for pneumothorax (p. 1164)
  - Recurrent pneumothorax may require thoracostomy tube or exploratory thoracotomy.
- Mechanical ventilation (p. 1185)
  - If unresponsive to oxygen supplementation and pain control
  - Indications for ventilation: severe hypoxemia despite oxygen supplementation ($PaO_2 < 60$ mm Hg, $SpO_2 < 90\%$), severe hypoventilation despite above therapies ($PaCO_2 > 60$ mm Hg), excessive respiratory effort with impending muscle fatigue
  - Caution using excess positive-pressure ventilation if concurrent pneumothorax
- Surgery: rarely necessary
  - Consider repair of flail segment if exploratory thoracotomy or extensive surgical wound management required.
  - Other indications: open chest wounds, fractures causing continued damage to underlying structures, unable to control pain, mechanical ventilation required
  - Fracture stabilization: percutaneous sutures passed around rib fragments of the flail segment and attached to an external fixation device or splint. Internal fixation with cerclage wires are an option if patient undergoing thoracotomy or if open fractures present.

Behavior/Exercise

Cage rest for 4-6 weeks after injury

Recommended Monitoring

- Close monitoring of respiratory rate and effort
- Treat shock and concurrent injuries.
  - ECG: arrhythmias from traumatic myocarditis, shock, hypoxemia (p. 1094)
  - Blood pressure: hypertension from pain; hypotension from hypovolemia, shock (p. 1065)
- Recumbency care if patient unable to move due to pain or other injuries

PROGNOSIS & OUTCOME

Good if prompt, intensive supportive care provided and no major concurrent injuries

PEARLS & CONSIDERATIONS

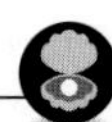

Comments

Underlying pulmonary damage and pain are the primary causes of respiratory dysfunction

Prevention

- Keep animals on leash or confined.
- Prevent interactions between aggressive large dogs and small dogs and cats.

Technician Tips

- Provide flow-by oxygen immediately.
- If open chest wounds, quickly cover the injury.
- Placing the animal in lateral recumbency with the flail segment down may help initial stabilization.

SUGGESTED READING

Olsen D, et al: Clinical management of flail chest in dogs and cats: a retrospective study of 24 cases (1989-1999). J Am Anim Hosp Assoc 38:315-320, 2002.

AUTHOR: Selena L. Lane, DVM, DACVECC
EDITOR: Benjamin M. Brainard, VMD, DACVAA, DACVECC

Flatulence and Borborygmi

BASIC INFORMATION

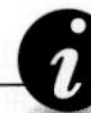

Definition

- Flatulence is the excessive passage of gastrointestinal (GI) gas (i.e., flatus) through the rectum and anus.
- The primary components of flatus include five odorless gases (O_2, N_2, H_2, CO_2, and CH_4); the characteristic odor is attributed to trace gases (sulfur-containing compounds).
- Borborygmus refers to the gurgling sounds that result from intestinal fluid and gas movement.

Epidemiology

SPECIES, AGE, SEX

- Common in dogs of any age and sex
- Infrequent in cats

GENETICS, BREED PREDISPOSITION

Aerophagia, a potential risk factor for flatulence, is more common in brachycephalic dogs.

RISK FACTORS

- Abrupt dietary changes
- Inactivity and indoor confinement
- GI disorders
- Deficiency in lactase activity
- Diets enhanced in soluble or rapidly fermentable fibers
- Diets containing high concentrations of nonabsorbable oligosaccharides, fructose, or resistant starches
- Conditions or behaviors which promote aerophagia (e.g., rapid food consumption, stenotic nares, elongated soft palate)

ASSOCIATED DISORDERS

- Conditions that cause maldigestion/malabsorption are often associated with excessive flatus and borborygmus because of increased bacterial fermentation in the large intestine.
- May be seen concurrently with other clinical signs suggestive of GI disease (nausea, vomiting, diarrhea)

Clinical Presentation

DISEASE FORMS/SUBTYPES

- Flatulence and borborygmus may occur concurrently or independently, often accompanied by belching.
- Occurs nocturnally and diurnally

HISTORY, CHIEF COMPLAINT

- Owners report excessive flatus and/or audible abdominal rumbling.
- Onset of clinical signs may be associated with dietary changes.
- Unless precipitated by underlying GI disease, patient history is otherwise unremarkable.

PHYSICAL EXAM FINDINGS

- Typically unremarkable
- Abdominal palpation may elicit gas production.
- Abdominal distention and/or discomfort may be present.

Etiology and Pathophysiology

Four mechanisms contribute to the entry of gas into the digestive tract:

- Aerophagia (O_2 and N_2)
- Interaction between bicarbonate ions and acid (CO_2)
- Diffusion from circulation (CO_2, N_2, and O_2)
- Bacterial fermentation (CO_2, H_2, CH_4, and sulfur-containing gases)

Three mechanisms contribute to removal of gases from the digestive tract:

- Diffusion into circulation
- Bacterial consumption
- Convection out the esophagus (eructation) or anus (flatus)

The overall quantity, composition, and frequency of gases liberated into the environment are a function of the net flow of these mechanisms.

DIAGNOSIS

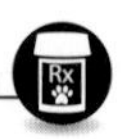

Diagnostic Overview

These clinical signs are typically reported by the owner, but attempts should be made to identify predisposing conditions, such as acute dietary changes.

Differential Diagnosis

- Dietary indiscretion
- Competitive or compulsive feeding behaviors
- Diseases that cause maldigestion/malabsorption: exocrine pancreatic insufficiency, inflammatory bowel disease, intestinal dysbiosis, lymphangiectasia, food hypersensitivity

Initial Database

- Obtain a thorough dietary history, including basal diet (formulation, amount, frequency, duration of use), treats, snacks, human foods, supplements, and feeding behaviors.
- Document current medications (antibiotic use may affect host microflora, resulting in flatulence).
- Determine activity level, exercise regimen, and environment.
- Laboratory testing (e.g., fecal exam, serum biochemical profile, folate/cobalamin) is not necessary unless an underlying intestinal condition is suspected.

TREATMENT

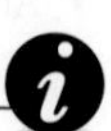

Treatment Overview

Treatment is generally aimed at controlling aerophagia, decreasing consumption of substrates that contribute to gas production, and increasing physical activity.

Acute General Treatment

- When associated with GI disease, prompt treatment directed toward the cause is the priority.
- Short-term use of bismuth subsalicylate or zinc acetate may provide patient relief.
- Nonabsorbable antibiotics (neomycin) have been shown to reduce flatulence in dogs, but routine use in otherwise healthy animals is not advised.
- Pharmacologic treatments such as activated charcoal and simethicone have limited benefits.

Chronic Treatment

- Management of primary small-intestinal disease may require lifelong therapy.
- Dietary changes (see below)
- Physical activity (see below)

Nutrition/Diet

- Highly digestible (low-fiber) diets which reduce substrate availability for large-intestinal bacterial fermentation may be useful.
- High-fiber foods, especially soluble/fermentable (pectins, guar gum) and mixed fibers (psyllium, beet pulp), should be minimized.
  - Aim for a diet with ≤ 5% fiber on a dry matter basis.
- Ammonia and volatile amines may contribute to excessive gas production, and excessive intake of dietary protein should be avoided. Nonleguminous protein sources are preferred over leguminous ones.
- Abstain from offering sulfur-containing vegetables (e.g., broccoli, cauliflower).
- Reduce access to garbage and litter boxes to reduce the risk of dietary indiscretion.
- If a food hypersensitivity is suspected, transition to a highly digestible novel protein or hydrolyzed protein diet. Trial and error may be necessary to determine the feeding strategy that is best tolerated for the individual.
- Minimize treats, snacks, and table foods, particularly those that contain lactose.
- Minimize stress associated with feeding, including competitive behaviors. Allow predisposed individuals to consume meals in solitude and in a quiet environment.
- Modify feeding practices: smaller, more frequent volumes may be helpful.

Behavior/Exercise

- Maintain a consistent exercise regimen.
- Provide outdoor walks within 30 minutes of meals to encourage gas transit and regular defecation patterns.

PROGNOSIS & OUTCOME

When dietary modifications and physical activity are implemented, prognosis is typically favorable.

PEARLS & CONSIDERATIONS

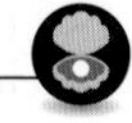

Comments

When pursuing a diet change, a gradual transition period (7-10 days) is generally recommended to avoid GI upset and potential exacerbation of the problem.

Technician Tips

Clinical signs often require dietary modifications that are best identified by trial and error. Technicians caring for animals with flatulence should encourage follow up communications with the owner to help guide future decisions.

SUGGESTED READING

Roudebush P, et al: Flatulence. In Hand MS, et al, editors: Small animal clinical nutrition, ed 5, Topeka, KS, 2010. Mark Morris Institute.

AUTHOR: Allison Wara, DVM, DACVN
EDITORS: Leah A. Cohn, DVM, PhD, DACVIM; Mark Thompson, DVM

Flea Bite Allergy

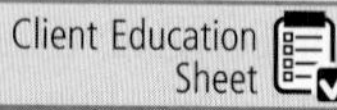

BASIC INFORMATION

Definition

Development of hypersensitivity reaction(s) and subsequent pruritic skin lesions in response to exposure to flea salivary antigens is very common in flea-endemic regions. It must be differentiated from flea infestation alone, where fleas are present on the animal or in the environment, but the animal does not develop clinical signs of skin disease.

Synonyms

Flea allergy dermatitis (FAD), flea bite hypersensitivity

Epidemiology

SPECIES, AGE, SEX

- Dogs: any age but typically older than 1 year of age; onset is most common in 3- to 5-year-olds
- Cats: no age predisposition reported

GENETICS, BREED PREDISPOSITION

Dogs and cats: no breed predisposition reported

RISK FACTORS

- Dogs: intermittent flea exposure may increase risk.
- Atopic patients are at greater risk for flea bite allergy.

GEOGRAPHY AND SEASONALITY

- Diagnosed worldwide wherever fleas are found

- Seasonal in climates with cold winters
- Continuous in indoor infestations or warm, humid climates

ASSOCIATED DISORDERS

- Infestation with *Dipylidium caninum*
- Gastric trichobezoars (hairballs) associated with excessive grooming
- Secondary bacterial pyoderma

Clinical Presentation

DISEASE FORMS/SUBTYPES

Canine flea bite allergy:
- Pruritic papular dermatitis
- Acute moist dermatitis (hot spot)
- Fibropruritic nodules in chronic cases

Feline flea bite allergy:
- Pruritic papulocrustous dermatitis (miliary dermatitis)
- Symmetrical, self-induced alopecia
- Eosinophilic granuloma complex

HISTORY, CHIEF COMPLAINT

- Dogs: acute onset of moderate to severe pruritus and hair loss and malodor in longer-standing cases. Clients may report live fleas on their pet or experience flea bites themselves.
- Cats: hair loss, pruritus, excessive grooming, vomiting hairballs, or small, crusted papules are noted under the haircoat. Lip ulcers, raised plaques, or granulomas may be noted. Fleas are less commonly observed than in dogs.

PHYSICAL EXAM FINDINGS

Dogs:
- Papulocrustous lesions, varying degrees of alopecia, erythema, and excoriations. Most commonly affected regions are dorsal lumbosacral region, tailhead, and caudomedial thighs. Ventral abdomen, especially near the umbilical area, flanks, neck, and feet may also be affected.
- Well-demarcated, moist, erythematous, exudative skin lesions with alopecia
- Lichenification, lattice pattern hyperpigmentation, scaling
- Poor body condition, weight loss, worn incisor teeth
- ± Fleas, flea excreta (flea dirt)

Cats:
- Self-inflicted, symmetrical hair loss on the ventral abdomen, lateral flanks, and caudomedial thighs
- Erythematous, crusted papules around the neck and on the lumbosacral region (miliary dermatitis)
- Lesions consistent with eosinophilic granuloma complex (indolent ulcer, eosinophilic plaque, eosinophilic granuloma)
- Excoriations, crusts
- Weight loss, poor body condition, peripheral lymphadenopathy
- Uncommonly, fleas, flea excreta (flea dirt)

Etiology and Pathophysiology

- Repeated exposure to flea salivary polypeptides, histamine-like compounds, enzymes, and amino acids induces development of various hypersensitivity reactions (p. 1238).
  - Type I (immediate/anaphylactic) hypersensitivity (dogs, cats)
  - Cutaneous basophil hypersensitivity (dogs)
  - Type IV (delayed/cell-mediated) hypersensitivity (dogs, cats)
  - Late-phase, IgE-mediated reactions (dogs)
- Hypersensitivity reactions, particularly intermittent, may become more intense and be triggered with progressively less antigen (flea saliva).

DIAGNOSIS

Diagnostic Overview

The diagnosis of flea bite allergy is based almost entirely on history and physical exam findings. Even in the absence of live fleas or flea excreta, physical signs as described warrant empirical antiflea treatment before or while pursuing advanced diagnostic testing for other causes of pruritus.

Differential Diagnosis

Dogs, cats:
- Other hypersensitivities (atopic dermatitis, foods, intestinal parasites, drugs)
- Ectoparasitic dermatoses
- Bacterial folliculitis

Dogs:
- *Malassezia* dermatitis

Cats:
- Dermatophytosis
- Anal sac disease (excessive grooming of ventral abdomen, lateral flanks, and caudomedial thighs)

Initial Database

History, physical exam findings ± observation of fleas or flea excreta

Advanced or Confirmatory Testing

- Intradermal testing with 1 : 1000 w/v aqueous solution of whole flea antigen
- ELISA serologic allergen screening for flea saliva antigens: accuracy varies, does not document delayed hypersensitivity reactions
- Response to flea eradication: considered by many to be the most definitive test

TREATMENT

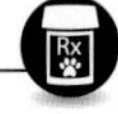

Treatment Overview

In flea infestation, the goals of treatment are focused on eradication of the flea population from the animal and its environment (i.e., integrated flea management). In flea bite allergy, the goals of treatment also include providing rapid relief of the clinical signs and discomfort.

Acute General Treatment

Antiinflammatory therapy:
- Dogs: prednisone/prednisolone 1 mg/kg PO q 24h for 5-7 days, then taper; may also use hydrocortisone aceponate spray topically once daily as monotherapy or in addition to oral predniso(lo)ne, *or* use oclacitinib 0.4-0.6 mg/kg PO q 12h for 7-14 days, then once daily
- Cats: prednisolone 2.2 mg/kg PO q 24h for 5-7 days, then taper. If daily oral drug administration is not possible, may substitute methylprednisolone injectable 5 mg/kg or 20 mg/CAT IM or SQ; however, there are multiple risks with use (e.g., diabetes mellitus, iatrogenic hyperadrenocorticism, congestive heart failure).

Topical flea adulticide: several options (NOTE: product types and names may change):
- Permethrin sprays/spot applications (e.g., Active-3, numerous others)
- Imidacloprid (e.g., Advantage, Advantage-Multi, Advantix for dogs; Seresto collar)
- Fipronil (e.g., Frontline, Catego for cats, others)
- Selamectin (e.g., Revolution)
- Indoxacarb (e.g., Activyl)
- Spinetoram (e.g., Cheristin for cats)
- Fluralaner (Bravecto for cats)
- Dinotefuran, permethrin, pyriproxyfen (e.g., Vectra 3D) for dogs, Vectra without permethrin for cats

Oral flea adulticide:
- Nitenpyram (Capstar)
- Spinosad (e.g., Comfortis, Trifexis) for dogs
- Isoxazoline class drugs for dogs: afoxolaner (NexGard), fluralaner (Bravecto), sarolaner (Simparica), lotilaner (Credelio)

Specific therapy for any secondary infections (p. 851)

Chronic Treatment

Integrated flea management is essential for eradication of the problem:
- Ongoing use of flea adulticide
- Insect growth regulators: methoprene, pyriproxyfen, others. NOTE: some products are formulated for spraying the patient; others are for treating the environment.
- Insect development inhibitors: lufenuron oral, monthly or semiannual injectable (cats)
- Environmental control may be required for flea infestation.
  - Identify "point sources" of infestation.
  - Cleaning or frequent vacuuming
  - Organic debris removal outdoors
  - Use of an approved insect growth regulator premise spray
- Immunotherapy is experimental at this time.

Possible Complications

- Neurotoxicosis with the use of pyrethrins, permethrins in cats (p. 858); isoxazoline compounds
- Diabetes mellitus, iatrogenic hyperadrenocorticism (glucocorticoids, especially sustained-release injections)

Recommended Monitoring

Routine flea combing

PROGNOSIS & OUTCOME

Good with long-term management

PEARLS & CONSIDERATIONS

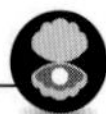

Comments

- Clients may not recognize excessive grooming as a manifestation of pruritus.
- Trichograms (microscopic exam of hair plucks) showing broken ends of hair shafts confirm self-induced alopecia.
- Excessive grooming decreases live flea population.

Prevention

- Avoidance of flea bites prevents disease recurrence in flea-allergic patients.
- Continued integrated flea control is mandatory.

Technician Tips

- Clients are frequently in denial, and compliance with a treatment plan may be poor.
- Challenge the clients to follow through with the treatment plan and disprove the diagnosis.

Client Education

- Progressive disease unless fleas are eradicated
- Preventable, not curable, disease
- Treatment of all in-contact pets is mandatory.

SUGGESTED READING

Merck Veterinary Manual: Flea and flea allergy dermatitis (website). http://www.merckvetmanual.com/integumentary-system/fleas-and-flea-allergy-dermatitis/flea-allergy-dermatitis/.

AUTHOR: Stephanie R. Bruner, DVM, DACVD
EDITOR: Manon Paradis, DMV, MVSc, DACVD

Follicular Dysplasia, Dog

BASIC INFORMATION

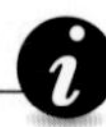

Definition

Group of noninflammatory disorders of the haircoat that result in hair loss and altered coat quality. Genetic predisposition for abnormal follicular development has been noted in specific breeds.

Epidemiology

SPECIES, AGE, SEX

- Dogs, both sexes, intact or neutered
- Color dilution alopecia (CDA) and black hair follicular dysplasia (BHFD) are disorders of early onset (usually < 1 year of age).
- Non–color-linked follicular dysplasias usually start during adulthood.

GENETICS, BREED PREDISPOSITION

CDA: several breeds with dilute coat colors such as blue Doberman pinscher, Yorkshire terrier, and Chihuahua

Clinical Presentation

DISEASE FORMS/SUBTYPES

Color-linked follicular dysplasia:

- CDA and BHFD

Non–color-linked follicular dysplasias:

- Canine recurrent flank alopecia (p. 47)
- Alopecia X (p. 44)
- Follicular dysplasia of specific breeds (e.g., Portuguese water dog, red and black Doberman, Irish water spaniel, Chesapeake Bay retriever, curly coated retriever, Pont Audemer spaniel dog)

HISTORY, CHIEF COMPLAINT

Dogs born with a normal haircoat are presented because of gradual thinning of the haircoat.

PHYSICAL EXAM FINDINGS

- CDA: alopecia, involving exclusively hair follicles in the areas with diluted coat color, starting at an early age and progressing at a variable rate during the first 2-3 years of age. These dogs are prone to follicular plugging and secondary recurrent bacterial folliculitis that can aggravate the hair loss and may cause pruritus.
- BHFD: same as CDA but affecting only area of black-haired coat.

Etiology and Pathophysiology

- Follicular dysplasia can be divided histologically into categories in which the hair cycle is abnormal (canine recurrent flank alopecia, alopecia X) and those in which there are abnormalities in the process of melanization of the pilosebaceous units (CDA, BHFD).
- All known forms of follicular dysplasia appear to be genetically determined. Irish water spaniel, Chesapeake Bay retriever, curly coated retriever, and Pont Audemer spaniel may share a pathogenesis since they are genetically related breeds.
- In CDA, an inherited autosomal recessive disorder of melanosome transportation has been demonstrated. The dilution is required for the development of CDA, but not all diluted coats progress to alopecia.

DIAGNOSIS

Diagnostic Overview

The diagnosis is suspected from history, clinical findings, breed predisposition, and in some cases, an early onset of color-linked alopecia (CDA, BHFD).

Differential Diagnosis

- Endocrinopathies (hypothyroidism, hyperadrenocorticism, hyperestrogenism)
- Infectious process (pyoderma, demodicosis, dermatophytosis) in some clinical presentations

Initial Database

Trichogram: large melanin clumps along the hair shaft, causing distortion and fracture of the hair in cases of CDA and BHFD

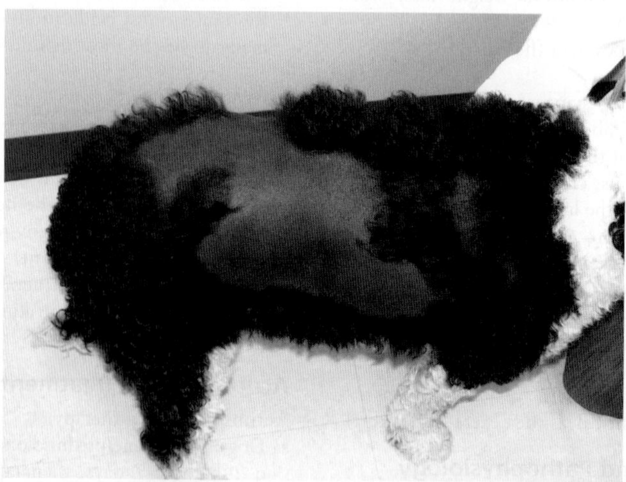

FOLLICULAR DYSPLASIA, CANINE Follicular dysplasia in a Portuguese water dog. Note the area of alopecia and hyperpigmentation and lack of inflammation of the skin. (Copyright Dr. Manon Paradis.)

Advanced or Confirmatory Testing

- Skin biopsy and histopathologic evaluation: dilated and cystic hair follicles with melanin clumping in follicular basal cells, hair bulbs, hair shafts, follicular lumen in CDA and BHFD
- Any diagnostic procedure necessary to rule out other differential diagnoses (p. 1091)

TREATMENT

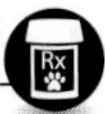

Treatment Overview

The main goals are to attempt hair regrowth and control secondary bacterial folliculitis, which is commonly seen in CDA.

Acute General Treatment

Anecdotal evidence exists for the efficacy of melatonin (3-6 mg/DOG PO q 8-12h for 1-2 months) to stimulate hair growth in CDA.

PROGNOSIS & OUTCOME

- These entities are incurable, genetically based dermatoses.
- Affected dogs are otherwise healthy, with the exception of secondary pyoderma in CDA.

PEARLS & CONSIDERATIONS

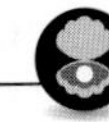

Comments

- The early onset, color link (CDA, BHFD), and/or breed predisposition make the diagnosis straightforward in many cases.
- The main impact of these disorders is cosmetic rather than medical, unless secondary infection or sunburn occurs.

Technical Tips

Discuss sun protection with owners of dogs suffering alopecia, particularly if skin is lightly pigmented.

SUGGESTED READING

Cerundolo R, et al: Breed specific hair-cycle abnormalities. In Mecklenburg L, et al, editors: Hair loss disorders in domestic animals, Ames, IA, 2009, Wiley-Blackwell, pp 169-175.

AUTHOR & EDITOR: Manon Paradis, DMV, MVSc, DACVD

Food Allergy, Dermatologic

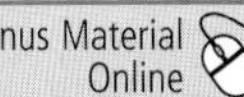
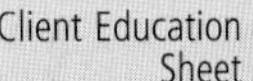
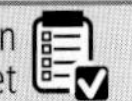

Bonus Material Online Client Education Sheet

BASIC INFORMATION

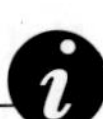

Definition

A well-recognized, abnormal response to an ingested food or food additive that produces clinical signs affecting the skin, most commonly pruritus

Synonyms

The preferred term is *cutaneous adverse food reaction* (CAFR). The terms *food allergy* or *food hypersensitivity* are often incorrectly used synonymously with *adverse food reaction*. These terms more accurately refer specifically to the subcategory of adverse food reactions that have an immunologic basis. The term *food intolerance*, also encompassed within CAFR, is reserved for the subcategory of adverse food reactions without an immunologic basis and includes metabolic food reactions, food poisoning, food idiosyncrasies, and pharmacologic reactions to food.

Epidemiology

SPECIES, AGE, SEX

- Dogs: age of onset from 4 months to 14 years (mean, 2.2 years; 77% develop signs by 3 years)
- Cats: from 6 months to 12 years (mean, 4 years; 52% develop signs by 3 years)

GENETICS, BREED PREDISPOSITION

Dogs and cats: no strong breed predisposition

RISK FACTORS

Risk factors include certain foods or food ingredients, poorly digestible proteins, any disease that increases intestinal mucosal permeability, selective immunoglobulin A (IgA) deficiency, age (<1 year), and concurrent allergic disease.

GEOGRAPHY AND SEASONALITY

Nonseasonal

ASSOCIATED DISORDERS

- 20%-30% of cases may have concurrent atopic dermatitis or flea allergy dermatitis.
- 20%-25% of cases may have concurrent gastrointestinal (GI) signs (e.g., vomiting, diarrhea, flatulence).
- Secondary skin infections with bacteria and yeast are common.

Clinical Presentation

HISTORY, CHIEF COMPLAINT

- The chief complaint is nonseasonal pruritus, recurrent pyoderma, or otitis externa.
- There may be a history of a poor response to glucocorticoid therapy.
- Adverse food reactions with an immunologic component usually develop after prolonged exposure to a food allergen, whereas food intolerance may occur after a single exposure because immune mechanisms are not involved.

PHYSICAL EXAM FINDINGS

- No specific pattern of skin lesions exists.
- Dogs
  - Lesion/pruritus distribution: feet, face, ears, axillae, perianal region, inguinal region, and rump
  - There may be pruritus without lesions or lesions secondary to infections and pruritus such as papules, pustules, erythema, excoriations, lichenification, alopecia, scales, crust, and acute moist pyotraumatic dermatitis.
  - Rare primary lesions, such as urticaria, or angioedema may occur.
- Cats
  - Lesion/pruritus distribution: often centered on the head and neck but may be generalized
  - Manifestations may consist of generalized pruritus without lesions; miliary dermatitis; pruritus with self-trauma centered around the head, neck, and ears; self-induced alopecia; or lesions of the eosinophilic granuloma complex.

Etiology and Pathophysiology

- A variety of causes are proposed.
- The majority are attributed to food allergies; however, immunologic tests are rarely performed to confirm this suspicion.
- Common food allergens in dogs include beef, dairy products, chicken, wheat, and lamb.
- Common food allergens in cats include beef, fish, and chicken.
- Food allergies are thought to be the result of primarily a type I hypersensitivity reaction, although type III and IV reactions have also been proposed.
- Several host defenses exist to prevent absorption of intact allergens from the GI tract, including effective digestion, intestinal peristalsis, an intact intestinal mucous layer, tight junctions between mucosal cells, and mucosal IgA. The small amounts of food proteins that do cross the intestinal mucosa activate suppressor T cells and stimulate an immune response in the gut-associated lymphoid tissue that leads to tolerance. A defect in any of these defense mechanisms may lead to sensitization of the immune system and development of a food allergy.

- Some foods, such as scombroid fish (tuna, mackerel, skipjack, and bonito), contain vasoactive amines such as histamine and cadaverine, which may cause a direct pharmacologic effect resulting in CAFR.

DIAGNOSIS

Diagnostic Overview

- The majority of the cases are clinically identical to environmental allergies in dogs and cats.
- It can be definitively diagnosed only by completing a strict elimination diet trial, including challenge at trial end.
- Multiple differentials, most commonly secondary bacterial or yeast infections of the skin and ears, should be identified and resolved before determining the need for a diet trial.
- Environmental allergies are a diagnosis of exclusion that cannot be ruled out by *in vitro* testing.

Differential Diagnosis

- Ectoparasites (*Sarcoptes*, *Demodex* [uncommonly], *Cheyletiella*, *Notoedres*, *Otodectes*, fleas, lice, *Trombicula*, and *Pelodera*)
- Secondary cutaneous bacterial or yeast infections
- Other hypersensitivity disorders (environmental allergens, flea bite, other ectoparasites, intestinal parasite, contact, drug)
- Dermatophytosis (ringworm)
- Behavioral disorders (feline psychogenic alopecia, flank sucking, tail-biting, self-nursing)
- Neoplasia (mast cell tumor, epitheliotropic lymphoma)

Initial Database

- Skin cytology: to investigate the presence of microbial (bacteria, yeast) infection. Ears, interdigital, and intertriginous regions are commonly affected. The contribution of a confirmed secondary microbial infection to clinical signs is determined by assessing the patient's response to appropriate antimicrobial therapy.
- Skin scrapings: deep focal skin scrapes should be used for detecting *Demodex canis*, whereas broad superficial scrapes may be more beneficial in detecting *Sarcoptes*, *Cheyletiella*, and *Demodex gatoi* (cats). NOTE: *Sarcoptes*, *Cheyletiella*, and *D. gatoi* mites may not be detected on all skin scrapings; they require a trial course of appropriate therapy to be fully ruled out when the index of suspicion for infection is high. See specific chapters for details.
- Examination for fleas/flea comb: presence of fleas, flea dirt, or tapeworms raises the index of suspicion for flea allergy dermatitis, but this differential should be fully ruled out by treatment with appropriate adulticidal flea control

Advanced or Confirmatory Testing

- Elimination diet: resolution of clinical signs after an elimination diet trial is the only useful test for confirming the diagnosis of CAFR.
  - Novel or hydrolyzed protein diet (NOTE: approximately 50% of patients may show some exacerbation of signs on exposure to hydrolyzed versions of proteins to which they are allergic.)
  - Offer home-cooked or prescription source (¾ of tested nonprescription soy-free diets contained detectable soy protein and were therefore inappropriate to rule out CARF).
  - During diet trial, no other food, treats, flavored medications or toothpaste, rawhides, and other items are allowed.
  - Duration of at least 8 weeks (90% of dogs or cats achieve complete remission by this point)
- Dietary challenge is a necessary step to confirm the diagnosis. The original diet is fed back to the animal for 10-14 days. In most cases of true CAFR, there is an exacerbation in pruritus within 3-7 days, but it may take up to 14 days.
  - Return to elimination diet until pruritus is under control again.
  - Individual ingredients may be reintroduced one at a time for 14 days each to determine which ingredients caused the adverse reaction.
  - In most cases, only one or two substances are the cause of the adverse reaction.
- Serologic and skin tests correlate poorly with the true offending allergen and are not recommended at this time.
- Salivary or hair antigen tests have become popular but are unvalidated and cannot be recommended. Studies suggest poor correlation with presence or absence of CARF and poor ability to accurately detect the offending allergen in known food-allergic patients.

TREATMENT

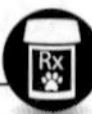

Treatment Overview

- Identification and avoidance of the offending food
- Identification and treatment of secondary infections

Acute General Treatment

- Manage any secondary microbial infections with appropriate antimicrobial therapy. Topical therapy (e.g., chlorhexidine or azole antifungal shampoos, sprays, wipes) should be used preferentially when patient and owner compliance allows.
- Systemic or topical antipruritic therapy, such as oral antihistamines or topical oatmeal-based shampoos, may be necessary initially to control self-trauma. Corticosteroid or oclacitinib use should be avoided when possible because it may mask other conditions and make it more difficult to assess response to the elimination diet trial. In cases of marked pruritus, corticosteroids or oclacitinib may be necessary initially (e.g., prednisolone 0.5-1 mg/kg PO q 24h × 1-2 weeks maximum to avoid masking effect of elimination diet).

Nutrition/Diet

The patient should be maintained on a balanced home-cooked or commercial (hypoallergenic) diet that avoids the offending food, or provocative testing with individual ingredients may be used for determining which dietary components can be tolerated. A thorough dietary history can help in choosing ingredients to avoid. Consultation with a veterinary nutritionist may be useful if home cooking is preferred over commercial hypoallergenic diets (p. 479).

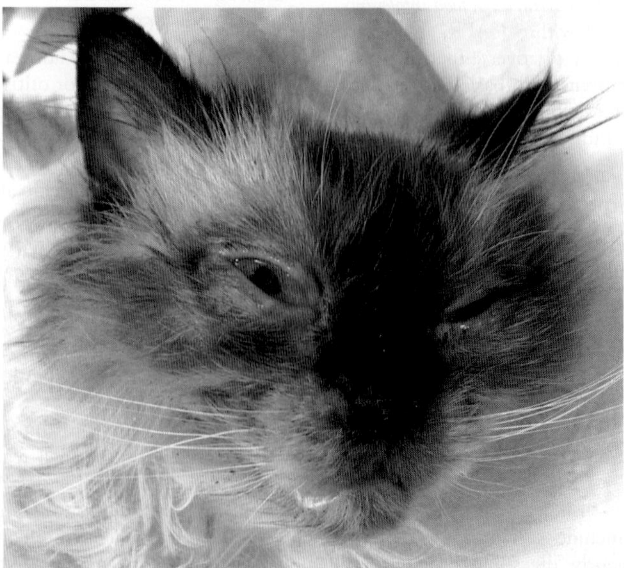

FOOD ALLERGY, DERMATOLOGIC Facial erythema and excoriation in a Himalayan cat with food allergy. (Copyright Dr. Manon Paradis.)

PROGNOSIS & OUTCOME

The prognosis is excellent with avoidance of offending foods.

PEARLS & CONSIDERATIONS

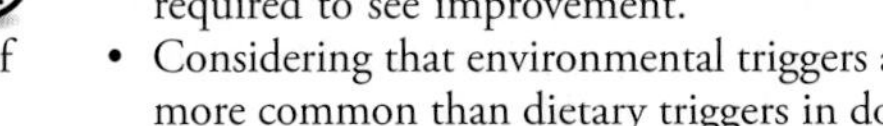

Comments

- The first step when dealing with any suspected CAFR is to make sure other causes of pruritus such as bacterial and yeast infection and ectoparasites have been ruled out.
- In some cases, a single elimination trial may be insufficient, and a second elimination trial using an alternative prescription novel protein or hydrolyzed protein diet or a novel-protein home-cooked diet may be required to see improvement.
- Considering that environmental triggers are more common than dietary triggers in dogs with allergy, it is important to inform the owner that approximately 70%-80% of dogs do not show appreciable reduction in pruritus during the food trial. Doing so may help avoid owner frustration and ensure better compliance.

Technician Tips

- Label the patient's file in a readily identifiable manner so that inappropriate treats or diets are not fed if the patient is in hospital.
- Technicians have an important role in informing/educating clients on the feeding changes and need for strict food control during the elimination diet trial. Many owners do not understand that "just one treat" may invalidate the entire process, and hearing this reinforced by the technician can be extremely valuable.

SUGGESTED READING

Miller WH Jr, et al: Muller & Kirk's Small animal dermatology, ed 7, St. Louis, 2013, Saunders, pp 397-405.

AUTHOR: Andrew Lowe, DVM, MSc, DACVD
EDITOR: Manon Paradis, DMV, MVSc, DACVD

Food Allergy, Gastrointestinal

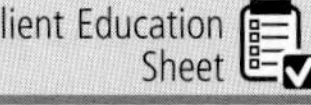

BASIC INFORMATION

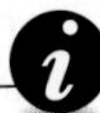

Definition

Food allergy and food intolerance are repeatable adverse reactions to specific dietary components that respond to exclusion of the causative agent. Food allergy is immune mediated, whereas food intolerance is not.

Synonyms

Dietary/food hypersensitivity, food-responsive enteropathy/diarrhea, adverse reaction to food

Epidemiology

SPECIES, AGE, SEX

- Dogs and cats: no sex predisposition
- Wide age range but tends to occur in younger animals (median, ≈3 years in dogs; onset of signs at < 1 year in 33%-51% of dogs)

GENETICS, BREED PREDISPOSITION

- Any breed, but German shepherd, Labrador retriever, Wheaten terrier, and Shar-pei are frequently cited.
- Genetic predisposition can play a role in development of food allergy.
  - Irish setters may develop a familial gluten-sensitive enteropathy.

RISK FACTORS

- Increased intestinal permeability (e.g., intestinal inflammation)
- Immunoglobulin A (IgA) deficiency and other immune dysregulations (speculative)
- Allergic disease (e.g., atopic dermatitis)

GEOGRAPHY AND SEASONALITY

Usually nonseasonal because the provocative antigen(s) is part of the normal diet

ASSOCIATED DISORDERS

- Gastrointestinal (GI): any disorder leading to decreased protein digestibility, defective mucosal barrier, defective oral tolerance, or increased mucosal permeability
- Dermatologic: dermatologic food allergy (p. 345), atopic dermatitis (p. 91)

Clinical Presentation

HISTORY, CHIEF COMPLAINT

- Signs can include vomiting, weight loss, intermittent abdominal pain, soft feces, diarrhea (often predominantly large bowel), borborygmus, flatulence, increased frequency of defecation (>3 times/day), perianal pruritus, and recurrent anal sacculitis.
- Concurrent pruritus and cutaneous signs raise index of suspicion.
- The allergen(s) typically has/have been ingested for months to years before signs develop.
- Signs may be intermittent due to factors such as frequency and amount of allergen(s) consumed and allergic threshold.

PHYSICAL EXAM FINDINGS

- Systemic: thin body condition, weight loss, lethargy
- GI specific (see History above): patients often have a lower canine chronic enteropathy clinical activity index (CCECAI).
- Skin: pruritus (face, neck, ears, ventral trunk, feet, perianal), otitis externa, urticaria, or angioedema; in cats, self-inflicted alopecia or miliary dermatitis may be observed.

Etiology and Pathophysiology

- Mechanisms unknown but genetic (e.g., immune dysregulation) and environmental (e.g., intestinal microbiota) factors are suspected to play a role.
- Antigen is typically a protein or glycoprotein of sufficient size to induce an immune reaction (in humans, typically 10-70 kD).
- Most common antigens incriminated include beef, dairy, chicken, egg, wheat, lamb, and soy (dogs); beef, dairy, fish, lamb, chicken, and barley/wheat (cats).
- Patient factors (e.g., compromised digestive function, defective oral tolerance, increased mucosal permeability) play a role in inciting an inappropriate immune response to an innocuous food.

DIAGNOSIS

Diagnostic Overview

Diagnosis is based on a positive response to an elimination food trial. An accurate diagnosis requires 1) proper elimination diet selection of a hydrolyzed protein diet or a diet that is truly novel to that patient (complete dietary history to ensure all ingredients previously ingested are eliminated during the trial); 2) strict dietary compliance during the trial; and 3) no concurrent confounding factors (e.g., antibiotics, glucocorticoids). For stable animals with chronic GI signs, diet trial is often warranted before undertaking more invasive tests such as intestinal biopsy.

Differential Diagnosis

- Any primary disorder of the GI tract (e.g., parasitism, exocrine pancreatic insufficiency, protein-losing enteropathy, antibiotic-responsive enteropathy, steroid-responsive enteropathy, inflammatory bowel disease, GI lymphoma, other infiltrative disease)
- Extraintestinal disorders manifesting with GI signs (e.g., hypoadrenocorticism, hyperthyroidism, liver, pancreatic disease)

Initial Database

- Dietary history
  - Thoroughly evaluate the diet, including regular food, treats, human foods and scraps, flavored medications, foods used to hide medication, supplements, and anything else ingested; read all ingredient labels.
- CBC: often unremarkable

- Serum biochemistry profile: nonspecific changes; low serum albumin concentration associated with poorer outcome
- Serum cobalamin, folate, and trypsin-like immunoreactivity (TLI): results variable but TLI expected to be normal
- Urinalysis: nonspecific; proteinuria possible with chronic inflammatory disease
- Fecal flotation and smear: rule out parasitism
- Feline immunodeficiency virus/feline leukemia virus testing
- T_4/thyroid profile (cats > 5 years)

Advanced or Confirmatory Testing

Elimination food trial is diagnostic and therapeutic.

- Diet containing a limited number of novel, highly digestible ingredients (hydrolyzed or novel protein and novel carbohydrate as based on diet history). Avoid ingredients that may cause a nonimmunologic reaction (e.g., vasoactive amines, lactose). Select a commercial or complete and balanced home-cooked diet (consult with veterinary nutritionist).
- Feed diet exclusively for at least 4 weeks. GI signs due exclusively to food allergy often improve within a few days to 2 weeks. Partial response after 4 weeks warrants continuing the trial longer.
- Must have strict adherence to prescribed diet and protocol (recommend owner keep a diary to record all ingested foods and clinical signs).
- Partial resolution of clinical signs with recrudescence on provocation testing suggests food allergy as one component of the underlying disease process.
- No improvement in GI signs despite appropriate diet selection and strict adherence to protocol makes food allergy unlikely. However, a second diet trial using a different novel protein/carbohydrate, a different hydrolyzed diet, or a different home-cooked recipe may be considered.

After a positive response to elimination diet, provocation (challenge) testing confirms the diagnosis and determines the inciting antigen(s):

- One food or individual ingredient is introduced at a time while feeding the elimination diet.
- Adverse GI reaction typically occurs within days, and the patient may react to more than one food ingredient.

If no improvement to an appropriately conducted elimination diet trial, consider additional diagnostic testing to rule out other causes of chronic enteropathy:

- Abdominal imaging, endoscopic or surgical biopsies, serum bile acids
  - GI biopsies from patients with food allergy or inflammatory bowel disease (IBD) may reveal nonspecific increases in lymphocytes, plasma cells, or eosinophils in the lamina propria; confirmation of food allergy requires favorable response to dietary modification.
- Intradermal skin or serum allergen testing are not reliable for diagnosis of food hypersensitivity.

TREATMENT

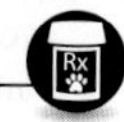

Treatment Overview

The goal of treatment is to control or abolish clinical signs.

Acute and Chronic Treatment

- Elimination of the provocative dietary component(s) as determined by elimination diet trial and subsequent provocation testing
- Most owners prefer a commercial diet. Must be sustainable for months to years.

Nutrition/Diet

- See Advanced or Confirmatory Testing above for proper selection of elimination diet and testing protocol.
- Long-term control of clinical signs may be possible by feeding a complete and balanced diet that avoids ingredients that elicit an allergic response in that patient.
- Be sure all treats, flavorings, and supplements also avoid the offending antigens.

Possible Complications

- Inappetence, weight loss
- Nutritional-related problems if an incomplete or imbalanced diet is fed
- Patient may develop a hypersensitivity to the previously tolerated intact novel protein in the future.

Recommended Monitoring

- If clinical improvement occurs during the elimination diet trial, a diagnosis of food sensitivity is confirmed by recurrence of clinical signs after reintroduction of the offending allergen (provocative challenge).
- If the patient develops a hypersensitivity to a previously tolerated intact novel protein, repeat the elimination diet trial with a new novel or hydrolyzed diet.

PROGNOSIS & OUTCOME

Good long-term prognosis if offending foods or ingredients are identified and eliminated from the diet.

PEARLS & CONSIDERATIONS

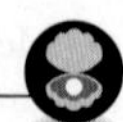

Comments

- Food hypersensitivity should be a differential diagnosis for all animals presenting with chronic GI signs. Many patients can have a long-term positive response to diet as the first-line treatment for chronic enteropathy.
- Over-the-counter novel or limited-ingredient diets are not suitable for a diagnostic elimination trial due to the possibility of cross-contamination with food antigens during manufacturing.
- Many owners cannot provide a complete diet history if they have used multiple foods; in these situations, hydrolyzed diets may offer an advantage over novel allergen diets.
- It can be difficult for owners to complete a strict food trial, but this should be encouraged because pets with food sensitivity have a good prognosis and can be successfully managed with an appropriate diet.
- Using a food diary during the elimination trial helps the owner monitor clinical response and compliance.

Technician Tips

- Recommend gradual transition to a new food. Mix more of the new elimination diet food with less of the old food over a period of at least 7 days.
- An alternative method for transitioning involves offering a small amount of the new food side by side with the old food in identical dishes and increasing the amount of new food while decreasing the amount of the old food over the transition period.

Client Education

- Strict adherence to the elimination diet trial protocol is critical.
  - Human food sources, treats, flavored medications, supplements, and food from other sources (e.g., multi-pet households, pet with unsupervised outdoor access) must be eliminated.
  - Stress that a single violation with a small amount of food during the trial can reactivate hypersensitivity.
- Provide a handout listing all items the animal cannot ingest during the food trial to be read by all household members.
- Contact the owner during the first week of the food trial to check that the elimination diet has been started, provide support, and address any questions.

SUGGESTED READING

Dandrieux JRS: Inflammatory bowel disease versus chronic enteropathy in dogs: are they one and the same? J Small Anim Pract 57:589-599, 2016.

AUTHOR: Laura Eirmann, DVM, DACVN
EDITOR: Rance K. Sellon, DVM, PhD, DACVIM

Diseases and Disorders

Food, Adverse Reaction (Nonallergic)

Client Education Sheet

BASIC INFORMATION

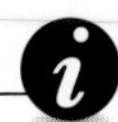

Definition

Adverse reaction to an ingested food or food additive due to nonimmunologic mechanisms (vs. immunologically based reactions [pp. 345 and 347])

Synonyms

Food intolerance, food poisoning or toxicity, lactose intolerance, food idiosyncrasy

Epidemiology

SPECIES, AGE, SEX

Dogs and cats: no age, sex, or breed predisposition

RISK FACTORS

- Food contaminated with microorganisms or toxic metabolites
- Specific foods or additives (e.g., onions, chocolate, propylene glycol in cats)
- Preformed vasoactive amines (e.g., histamine) in food such as spoiled fish
- Dairy products
- Dietary indiscretion (gluttony, pica)

CONTAGION AND ZOONOSIS

Food contaminant may be zoonotic (e.g., *Salmonella, Listeria*)

ASSOCIATED DISORDERS

- Lactose intolerance
- Food-responsive enteropathy
- Dietary hypersensitivity
- Inflammatory bowel disease

Clinical Presentation

HISTORY, CHIEF COMPLAINT

Clinical signs, which can occur on initial exposure, include vomiting, diarrhea, decreased appetite or anorexia, abdominal pain, abdominal distention, soft feces, excessive flatulence, increased frequency of defecation

PHYSICAL EXAM FINDINGS

Evidence of diarrhea (small or large bowel), vomiting, abdominal distention or discomfort, dehydration, rarely urticaria or angioedema (secondary to vasoactive amines)

Etiology and Pathophysiology

Diet-induced reaction (occurs in most individuals if sufficient quantity is consumed):

- Food poisoning: consumption of raw or improperly cooked/stored food contaminated with pathogenic microorganisms or their toxic metabolites (e.g., aflatoxin)
- Food toxicosis (e.g., onions, chocolate, xylitol, propylene glycol in cats)
- Dietary indiscretion: consumption of unusual or spoiled foods (e.g., scavenging garbage), consumption of too much food (gluttony), or eating nonfood substances (pica)
- Pharmacologic reactions such as ingestion of vasoactive amines (e.g., histamine) in food such as spoiled scombroid fish

Patient-induced reaction (unpredictable, individualistic response upon ingestion of a specific food item):

- Metabolic food reaction such as lactose intolerance due to lactase deficiency; difficult to differentiate from true allergic reaction to proteins in milk because clinical signs may be identical and both respond to dietary elimination
- Idiosyncratic adverse reactions to food or additives (e.g., food colorings, preservatives, emulsifying agents, thickeners): occur infrequently and unpredictably and are not apparently dose related; offending agent may be suspected based on repeated exposures and elimination of other triggers

DIAGNOSIS

Diagnostic Overview

Adverse food reaction is suspected on the basis of diet history and clinical signs, often but not always occurring as a result of acute dietary alterations. Diagnosis is often retrospective, with resolution of clinical signs as a result of proper diet. In contrast to dietary hypersensitivity (food allergy), the response to the change in food is usually more rapid (often within days). If no clinical improvement occurs within 2 weeks, the diagnosis should be questioned.

Differential Diagnosis

- Any primary disorder of the gastrointestinal (GI) tract (e.g., inflammatory bowel disease, parasitism, protein-losing enteropathy, antibiotic-responsive enteropathy, infiltrative disease)
- Food hypersensitivity
- Non-GI disorders manifesting with GI signs (e.g., hypoadrenocorticism, hyperthyroidism)

Initial Database

- CBC, serum biochemistry profile, urinalysis: normal, or nonspecific changes
- Fecal flotation: rule out parasitic causes of GI signs

Advanced or Confirmatory Testing

Further testing may be used to identify other disorders with similar signs or for identifying inciting causes (differential diagnosis).

- Proper nutrition/elimination food trial
- Abdominal radiography and ultrasonography: rule out other causes of vomiting and diarrhea (e.g., intestinal obstruction, intestinal mass)
- Endoscopy with biopsy and histopathologic evaluation of GI mucosa (p. 1098): mucosa may be normal or show increases in lamina propria lymphocytes or plasma cells

TREATMENT

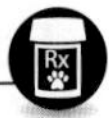

Treatment Overview

Treat episodes of dietary indiscretion with supportive care.

Acute General Treatment

- Nonspecific supportive care is based on clinical signs (e.g., parenteral fluid administration for dehydration).
- Clinical signs of GI disease usually resolve within 2 days to 2 weeks on a diet that does not contain the offending substance.

Nutrition/Diet

- Maintain strict avoidance of offending foods or ingredients.
- Find an appropriate commercial or a complete and balanced homemade diet for long-term maintenance and ensure proper handling and storage of food.
- Control episodes of gluttony and pica.

Possible Complications

Certain types of food poisoning and toxicities can cause serious and life-threatening disease.

PROGNOSIS & OUTCOME

Good prognosis if offending foods or ingredients are eliminated from the diet

PEARLS & CONSIDERATIONS

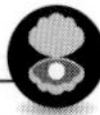

Comments

- Report suspected food-related adverse reactions to the manufacturer and the U.S. Food and Drug Administration (FDA) or state feed control official (p. 37).
- Maintain detailed medical records; instruct the owner to save food samples and package labels when a food-related adverse event is suspected.

Prevention

- Avoid exposure to contaminated food, food toxins, dairy products, and dietary sources of vasoactive amines.
- For recurrent adverse reactions to food, a food diary can help monitor clinical response and compliance.
- Be alert to and notify clients of recalls on pet foods or treats.

Technician Tips

Thorough diet history is essential. Human food sources, snacks, treats, and food for other animals in the household can trigger this type of adverse reaction. Ask if a new food item or new package of current food has been recently fed.

SUGGESTED READING

Roudebush P, et al: Adverse reactions to food. In Hand MS, et al, editors: Small animal clinical nutrition, ed 5, Topeka, KS, 2010, Mark Morris Institute, pp 609-635.

AUTHOR: Laura Eirmann, DVM, DACVN
EDITOR: Rance K. Sellon, DVM, PhD, DACVIM

Footpad Disorders

BASIC INFORMATION

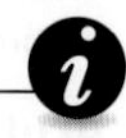

Definition

The pathologic condition involves the footpad skin. The most common causes are trauma, contact dermatitis, cornification defects, pigmentation disorders, autoimmune disease, secondary bacterial infection, and self-trauma. Pododermatitis and phalangeal disorders are discussed on p. 799.

Synonym

Paw pad disorders

Epidemiology

SPECIES, AGE, SEX

- Dogs and cats: although uncommon, footpad diseases are more frequently seen in cats in comparison to dogs, while interdigital lesions are more common in dogs (p. 799).
- Dogs < 1 year old: hereditary footpad hyperkeratosis, collagen disorder of the footpads of German shepherds, familial vasculopathies, acrodermatitis, junctional and dystrophic epidermolysis bullosa, and acral mutilation syndrome
- Older dogs: superficial necrolytic dermatitis (SND), epitheliotropic lymphoma, nasodigital hyperkeratosis

GENETICS, BREED PREDISPOSITION

- Vitiligo: Siamese cats, Belgian sheepdogs, rottweilers, Doberman pinschers, others
- Footpad hyperkeratosis: Irish terriers, dogues de Bordeaux, Kerry blue terriers, Labrador and golden retrievers
- Collagen disorders of the footpads: German shepherds
- Familial vasculopathy: German shepherds and Jack Russell terriers
- Acral mutilation syndrome: German shorthaired and English pointers, English springer spaniels, and French spaniels
- Dermatomyositis: Beauceron shepherd dogs
- Uveodermatologic syndrome: Akitas, Alaskan Malamutes, Siberian Huskies, Australian shepherds, and others
- Zinc-responsive dermatosis: Alaskan Malamutes, Siberian Huskies, bull terriers
- Systemic lupus erythematosus (SLE): collies, Shetland sheepdogs, German shepherds
- Wartlike lesions or corns on footpads: greyhounds, sighthounds

RISK FACTORS

- Lacerations/trauma: outdoor activities, roaming
- Footpad calcinosis cutis: renal failure
- SND: hepatopathy or glucagon-producing pancreatic tumor

GEOGRAPHY AND SEASONALITY

Leishmaniasis in endemic areas

ASSOCIATED DISORDERS

- SLE: systemic signs, depending on the organs involved
- Feline paraneoplastic alopecia: pancreatic or bile duct carcinoma
- Xanthomatosis: can be associated with diabetes mellitus, presumed hereditary hyperlipoproteinemia in cats
- Feline plasma cell pododermatitis: possible concurrent feline immunodeficiency virus (FIV) infection, immune-mediated glomerulonephritis or renal amyloidosis, plasma cell stomatitis, nasal swelling
- Uveodermatologic syndrome: granulomatous uveitis
- Cutaneous horns in cats: possible concurrent feline leukemia virus (FeLV) infection

Clinical Presentation

HISTORY, CHIEF COMPLAINT

Skin lesions are located on one or multiple footpads. Self-trauma and lameness may be observed. Paw involvement may also be part of a more generalized condition. With footpad lacerations, owner-observed bleeding often is the first sign.

PHYSICAL EXAM FINDINGS

- Number of paws affected: lesions on multiple paws (see Associated Disorders above) versus on one paw (neoplasia, trauma, infection)
- Depending on the disease, several changes can be present on the footpads
  - Swelling and inflammation
  - Hyperkeratosis
  - Cracking and fissuring
  - Ulcers
  - Hypopigmentation or hyperpigmentation
  - Draining tracts
  - Change in footpad texture
  - Signs of pain on walking or during handling of the paw(s)

Etiology and Pathophysiology

Footpad lesions can arise from various pathomechanisms:

- Direct trauma
- Contact with an irritant or corrosive substance
- Development of antibodies or activated lymphocytes against normal body constituents (autoimmune diseases) or against inciting antigens (drugs, bacteria, viruses), causing tissue damage
- Altered process of cornification resulting in hyperkeratosis
- Defective melanin production or a destruction of melanocytes leads to pigment disorders. A disorder at the dermoepidermal junction level can result in hypopigmentation.
- Hereditary sensitive neuropathy in acral mutilation syndrome
- In addition to primary causes, self-trauma and secondary bacterial infection can result in footpad lesions.

DIAGNOSIS

Diagnostic Overview

The diagnosis will be based on a dermatologic exam and on complementary testing, which will vary depending on the possible differential diagnosis.

Differential Diagnosis

- Environmental: trauma, irritant contact dermatitis, calcinosis cutis caused by percutaneous penetration of calcium salts, and thallium toxicosis
- Hereditary: see Genetics and Breed Predisposition above.
- Allergic or immune mediated
  - Dogs: pemphigus foliaceus, SLE, vasculitis, toxic epidermal necrolysis, erythema multiforme, cryoglobulinemia and cryofibrinogenemia, bullous pemphigoid, epidermolysis bullosa acquisita, uveodermatologic syndrome, and drug reactions
  - Cats: eosinophilic granuloma complex, pemphigus foliaceus, SLE, erythema multiforme, toxic epidermal necrolysis, vasculitis, cryoglobulinemia and cryofibrinogenemia, drug reactions, and plasma cell pododermatitis
- Nutritional: zinc-responsive dermatosis, xanthomatosis associated with feeding high-fat foods

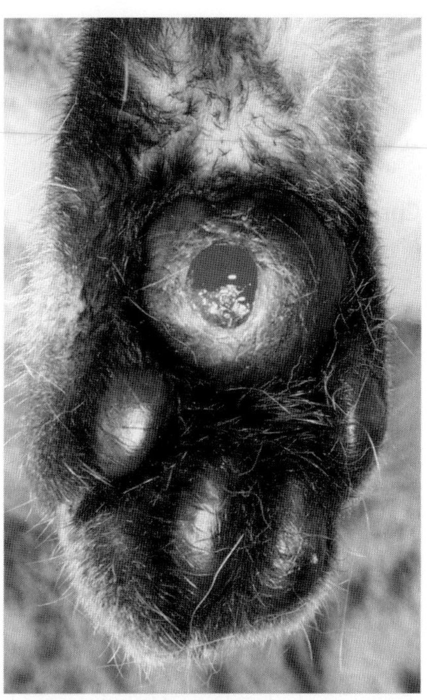

FOOTPAD DISORDERS Swollen, ulcerated footpad in a cat with plasma cell pododermatitis.

- Endocrine/metabolic: SND (dogs), footpad calcinosis cutis (often associated with chronic kidney disease), paraneoplastic alopecia (cats), xanthomatosis (when associated with diabetes mellitus or presumed feline hereditary hyperlipoproteinemia)
- Neoplastic: epitheliotropic cutaneous lymphoma, squamous cell carcinoma, fibrosarcoma, mast cell tumor, others
- Infectious: canine distemper, cowpox virus or calicivirus infection in cats, subcutaneous or systemic mycotic infections, canine papillomatosis, and hookworm and *Pelodera* dermatitis
- Miscellaneous: noninflammatory hypomelanosis (vitiligo), cutaneous horns, idiopathic nasodigital hyperkeratosis, split paw pad disease, and sterile granuloma/pyogranuloma syndrome

Initial Database

- History and general exam are important in the diagnostic process.
- Cytology of exudates: bacteria, inflammatory cells, acantholytic keratinocytes (pemphigus), and fungal organisms

Advanced or Confirmatory Testing

- Skin biopsies for histopathology
- CBC/biochemistry panel/urinalysis: results variable, depending on cause
- Thoracic/abdominal imaging, if relevant, to confirm systemic disease (e.g., SND) or to stage tumors
- Endocrine tests and serology, depending on suspected disease
- Coombs' test: cryoglobulinemia/cryofibrinogenemia
- Antinuclear antibody test (ANA): positive for most patients with SLE

TREATMENT

Treatment Overview

The goal of treatment is to reach permanent cure or control of the disease, but sometimes, palliative treatment is the only option (e.g., malignancy).

Acute General Treatment

Depends on the cause of the lesion and possible secondary infection

- Foot soaks or bandages sometimes useful
  - Hyperkeratotic lesions: warm water foot soaks for 5-10 minutes, followed by application of a softening agent (e.g., petroleum jelly). This can be messy.
  - For more severe hyperkeratosis, daily foot soaks in 50% propylene glycol. Improvement is expected within a few days. Lifelong maintenance therapy (1-2 times weekly as needed) is often required.
- Surgery can be considered for some diseases: closure of uncontaminated sharp lacerations, excision of cutaneous horns and tumors, surgical debridement of devitalized tissues
- Medication varies, depending on underlying cause.

PROGNOSIS & OUTCOME

Will vary according to the disease; generally good with localized lesions, reversible causes, and dedicated owners and guarded to poor with progressive systemic illness

PEARLS & CONSIDERATIONS

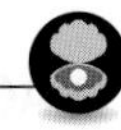

Comments

- Successful therapy is based on identifying the underlying cause.
- Skin biopsies are often needed for the diagnosis of footpad disorders.

Prevention

Advise against breeding of animals with hereditary diseases.

Technician Tips

Patients with footpad lesions can be painful and reluctant to walk. Care should be taken when walking them.

SUGGESTED READING

Miller WH Jr, et al: Muller & Kirk's Small animal dermatology, ed 7, St. Louis, 2013, Elsevier.

AUTHOR: Nadia Pagé, DMV, MSc, DACVD
EDITOR: Manon Paradis, DMV, MVSc, DACVD

Foreign Body, Esophageal

Client Education Sheet

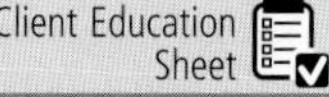

BASIC INFORMATION

Definition

Any object that lodges in the esophagus

Epidemiology

SPECIES, AGE, SEX

Dogs (more commonly) and cats of any age, either sex

GENETICS, BREED PREDISPOSITION

Smaller dogs seem to be affected more commonly.

RISK FACTORS

Feeding bones, carelessness when fishing (exposing hook/lure to dog)

ASSOCIATED DISORDERS

- Some degree of esophagitis is expected with any foreign body present for more than a day.
- Esophageal perforation can occur within 3-5 days in some cases and cause septic mediastinitis, pyothorax, and/or pneumothorax.

Clinical Presentation

DISEASE FORMS/SUBTYPES

- Nonpenetrating foreign objects: main concerns are malnutrition, esophagitis potentially leading to stricture, and aspiration pneumonia.
- Penetrating foreign objects: main concerns are mediastinitis, pyothorax, esophagitis, aspiration, and pneumonia.

HISTORY, CHIEF COMPLAINT

- Acute regurgitation is suggestive.
  - Distinguish acute vomiting (prodromal signs, active abdominal contractions leading to expulsion of food, bile or digested blood in expelled material) from acute regurgitation (no prodromal signs, passive expulsion of food from the mouth, no bile or digested blood in expelled material).
- Anorexia and ptyalism can occur.
- Some patients can drink and retain water but will not attempt to eat solid food; some exhibit pain when swallowing, and if they eat solid food it is often promptly regurgitated.
- Lethargy, anorexia, fever, and/or dyspnea are possible if perforation occurs.

- Rarely, pressure of foreign object on trachea causes coughing or choking.

PHYSICAL EXAM FINDINGS

- Ptyalism occasionally noticed
- Dysphagia or gagging seen rarely
- Dyspnea/fever sometimes seen secondary to perforation, mediastinitis/pleuritis, and/or aspiration pneumonia
- Rarely, can palpate the foreign object in the cervical esophagus

Etiology and Pathophysiology

- Bones are the most common foreign body in dogs.
- Other common foreign objects include food, fishhooks, rawhide treats, and dental chew toys.
- Hairballs are important in cats.

DIAGNOSIS

Diagnostic Overview

History is important; ask whether the patient swallowed anything immediately before clinical signs began or if it frequently chews or mouths objects (i.e. has a propensity to foreign body ingestion). Plain cervical and thoracic radiographs are the tests of choice and are confirmatory in almost all cases (assuming good radiographic technique); esophagoscopy is always confirmatory and is usually therapeutic.

Differential Diagnosis

Regurgitation:

- Esophagitis
- Megaesophagus (acquired [idiopathic or secondary to systemic disease] or congenital)
- Esophageal mass
- Esophageal stricture
- Vascular ring anomaly

Initial Database

- CBC and serum biochemistry panel to prepare for anesthesia
- Plain thoracic radiographs
  - Differentiate esophageal foreign body from megaesophagus (often generalized dilation as opposed to esophageal dilation associated with foreign body, which can be seen cranial to the foreign body) and other thoracic masses.
  - Almost all foreign objects can be seen with good-quality films, but radiolucent objects (e.g., poultry bones, rawhide) may require excellent technique. Three views may be needed to see some foreign objects.
  - Concurrent pneumothorax, pneumomediastinum, or pleural effusion is suggestive of esophageal perforation.
  - Esophageal foreign objects can radiographically resemble pulmonary or mediastinal lesions.
  - Assess for complications: aspiration pneumonia and/or evidence of perforation (mediastinal widening, pleural effusion suggesting mediastinitis or pleuritis/pyothorax, respectively)
- Contrast esophageal radiographs
  - Rarely needed and may obscure visualization during esophagoscopy; it is typically better to do esophagoscopy if plain radiographs are not diagnostic but foreign body is strongly suspected.
  - Risk of aspiration of contrast material or leakage of contrast into the mediastinum: use iodide-based contrast instead of barium

Advanced or Confirmatory Testing

Esophagoscopy (p. 1098): always provides a definitive diagnosis

TREATMENT

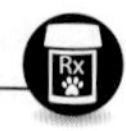

Treatment Overview

Remove the foreign object and resolve complications (e.g., esophagitis or perforation with resulting pleural/mediastinal sepsis).

Acute General Treatment

- Esophageal foreign objects should be removed as soon as the patient is an acceptable anesthetic candidate to reduce chance of esophageal perforation.
- Esophagoscopy to remove foreign object and determine degree of esophagitis (p. 1098)
  - If foreign object cannot be removed, attempt to push into the stomach for surgical removal or dissolution (bone).
- A Foley catheter can be used for objects without sharp edges (place balloon behind foreign object, inflate balloon, then pull the catheter out so that the balloon draws the foreign object orad and out). A lubricated Foley catheter can be used to open lower esophageal sphincter when pushing object into stomach.
- Surgery if esophagoscopy is unsuccessful at removing the foreign object
- Prokinetics (e.g., metoclopramide 0.2-0.4 mg/kg IM, SQ, or PO q 8h) and/or antacid (omeprazole 1-2 mg/kg PO q 12h or pantoprazole 1 mg/kg IV q 12h) to treat esophagitis (p. 312). Do not give antacids if bone has been pushed into the stomach because gastric acid is needed to dissolve the bone.
- Appropriate treatment of aspiration pneumonia, pleuritis/mediastinitis, if present

Chronic Treatment

Mechanical dilation of strictures, if necessary (p. 310)

Nutrition/Diet

Place gastrostomy feeding tube (p. 1109) if esophagitis is so severe that the patient cannot or will not eat.

Possible Complications

- Stricture (cicatrix) causing partial or complete esophageal obstruction
- Esophageal perforation causing septic pleuritis/mediastinitis (p. 857) or uncommonly bronchoesophageal fistula
- Insufflation of air during esophagoscopy can cause tension pneumothorax if there is a perforation and/or gastric dilation if the scope cannot be advanced into the stomach to remove air.
- Severe bleeding is uncommon (and rarely life-threatening) but possible when manipulating/removing foreign object.

Recommended Monitoring

Be sure patient is able to eat without regurgitation within 1-2 days of foreign body removal. If regurgitation occurs after several days, evaluate for possible stricture.

PROGNOSIS & OUTCOME

- Good if there is no perforation and esophagitis is not severe
- Good to guarded if severe, near-circumferential esophagitis is likely to cause stricture
- Guarded to poor if severe septic mediastinitis or pleuritis from perforation

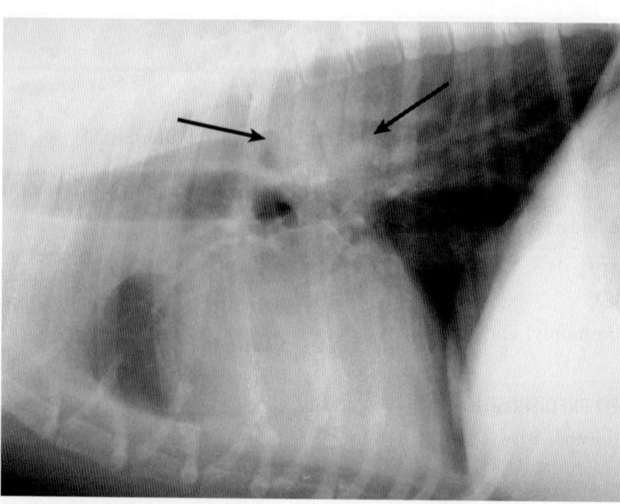

FOREIGN BODY, ESOPHAGEAL Lateral thoracic radiograph of a dog. A soft-tissue-opacity foreign object is apparent in the esophagus, dorsal and caudal to the carina *(arrows)*. Gas in the esophagus cranial and caudal to the foreign body helps make the diagnosis apparent without administration of contrast material.

PEARLS & CONSIDERATIONS

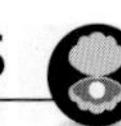

Comments

- Rigid endoscopes are more effective than flexible scopes in removing foreign objects, but most rigid scopes are only 25-35 cm long, limiting their usefulness in larger patients.
- If a contrast esophagram is required, use a water-soluble iodide-based contrast agent; do not use barium.

Prevention

- Avoid feeding bones.
- Be careful about allowing dogs to chew rawhides.
- Use caution when dogs are around baited fish hooks/lures.

Technician Tips

Technicians involved in postoperative care of these patients should be familiar with use and maintenance of feeding tubes (especially gastrostomy).

SUGGESTED READING

Thompson HC, et al: Esophageal foreign bodies in dogs: 34 cases (2004-2009). J Vet Emerg Med Crit Care (San Antonio) 22:253-261, 2012.

AUTHOR: Michael D. Willard, DVM, MS, DACVIM
EDITOR: Rance K. Sellon, DVM, PhD, DACVIM

Foreign Body, Linear Gastrointestinal

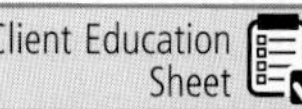

BASIC INFORMATION

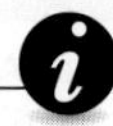

Definition

A common disorder involving ingestion of a linear object that lodges in the proximal alimentary system (under the tongue or at the pylorus) and causes plication of intestines distally, along the length of the object

Synonym

String foreign body

Epidemiology

SPECIES, AGE, SEX

- Young animals are more likely to ingest foreign objects.
- A linear foreign body is more common in cats than dogs, but dogs tend to be older than affected cats.
- Cats frequently present with string or thread ingestion, and dogs ingest fabric such as clothing or carpet.

RISK FACTORS

Some animals are more prone to ingesting foreign objects than others (individual behavior), irrespective of age.

GEOGRAPHY AND SEASONALITY

December to January: ingestion of Christmas tree icicles (long, thin strips of foil-like plastic), tinsel, or ribbons

Clinical Presentation

HISTORY, CHIEF COMPLAINT

- Owners may witness object ingestion.
- String may be visualized protruding from the anus.
- Clinical signs vary with duration of foreign body ingestion, degree of gastrointestinal (GI) compromise, as well as presence of a partial or complete obstruction.
- Vomiting, anorexia, ptyalism, depression, and weight loss (if chronic) are typical.

PHYSICAL EXAM FINDINGS

- Thorough exam at the base of the tongue should be performed to inspect for anchored foreign material.
  - Complete exam may require sedation or general anesthesia.
  - In cats, elevation of the base of the tongue is best accomplished by opening the mouth by depressing the lower jaw using an index fingernail for pressure on the lower incisors. The thumb of the same hand is then used for externally pressing upward (dorsally) in the intermandibular space.
- Painful and bunched intestines may be detected on abdominal palpation.
- Dehydration, depression, or shock; with complete obstruction or peritonitis

Etiology and Pathophysiology

- Anchoring of ingested linear material around base of tongue, at the pylorus, or in the proximal intestinal tract
  - Without an anchor point, ingested linear foreign bodies may pass through the GI tract without complication.
- Peristalsis results in plication of intestines along the length of the fixed material, and obstruction of intestinal tract results.
- Due to peristalsis, continued sawing action of the foreign material along the mesenteric border may result in intestinal erosion and perforation and the development of septic peritonitis (p. 779).
  - Perforation is more likely in dogs than in cats.
- Concurrent presence of an intussusception (p. 561) is possible.

DIAGNOSIS

Diagnostic Overview

Any history of vomiting or anorexia in a dog or cat should prompt an inspection of the base of the tongue during the physical exam; a circumferential erosive lesion containing the foreign body is pathognomonic. If no such finding is apparent, diagnostic imaging is indicated in all young animals presenting with vomiting, anorexia, abdominal pain, or a history of foreign body ingestion. Plain abdominal radiography is often sufficient for a diagnosis, but occasionally, the disorder is confirmed only during abdominal exploratory surgery.

Differential Diagnosis

- All other causes of intestinal obstruction, such as neoplasia, intussusception, granuloma, stricture, adhesions, or volvulus
- Ileus

Initial Database

- CBC: normal or shows evidence of inflammation/sepsis due to peritonitis
- Serum chemistry profile
  - Hypokalemia associated with vomiting, anorexia
  - Hypoglycemia associated with peritonitis
  - Azotemia associated with dehydration
  - Hyponatremia may be more commonly seen in dogs with linear foreign bodies than in those with discrete foreign bodies.
- Urinalysis: unremarkable
- Abdominal radiographs
  - Characteristic findings include plication of intestines with or without eccentric, teardrop-shaped, or "comma-shaped" intraluminal gas bubbles.
  - Dogs may be more likely than cats to have characteristic radiographic findings, allowing the diagnosis of linear foreign body to be made radiographically.
  - Free gas in the abdomen (seen caudal to the dorsal aspect of the diaphragm on lateral views as gas bubbles not associated with intestinal loops or on a cross-table view in lateral recumbence) indicates GI perforation.
- Abdominocentesis (p. 1056) with fluid evaluation is indicated if peritonitis is suspected.

Advanced or Confirmatory Testing

- Contrast radiography (p. 1172) or abdominal ultrasound may be used if survey radiographic findings are inconclusive.
- Abdominal ultrasound (limited efficacy when gas or barium is present in the intestine)
  - May document a tortuous path of the proximal intestine as well as presence of an intraluminal linear object
  - May document associated disorders such as an intussusception or peritonitis
- Noniodinated contrast material is often recommended for upper GI radiographic

contrast series because up to 16% of cats and 41% of dogs may have perforation of the intestinal tract.
   - The advantage of iodine (resorbed from the peritoneal cavity if perforation exists, unlike barium) must be weighed against its reduced degree of contrast, foul taste (compliance), and the access to any spilled barium at the time of laparotomy because surgical intervention is indicated if perforation is confirmed.

TREATMENT

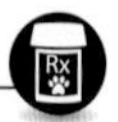

Treatment Overview

Rehydration and rapid surgical intervention are recommended. Specific treatment goals:
- Correct dehydration and electrolyte imbalances.
- Remove obstructing foreign body.
   - Although conservative treatment in the cat has been reported, the high likelihood of perforation and the associated morbidity of peritonitis dictate that these cases be treated as surgical emergencies.
   - Conservative treatment is *not* described for the dog because of the high risk of developing peritonitis.

Acute General Treatment

- Intravenous fluid therapy with electrolyte (potassium) supplementation according to need
- Prophylactic antibiotics
   - Cefazolin 22 mg/kg IV q 90 minutes during the perioperative period
- Surgical intervention includes thorough inspection of the entire intestinal tract for evidence of perforation.
- If the linear foreign body is fixed around the base of the tongue, it should be cut at this point.
- Foreign material is removed through a single or multiple enterotomies.
- Gastrotomy is performed to remove any foreign material trapped in the stomach, particularly at the pylorus.
- Single enterotomy removal using a red rubber catheter has been reported when no intestinal perforations are present.
   - This technique involves a single duodenal enterotomy with attachment of a red rubber catheter to the linear object. The enterotomy is closed, and the catheter with attached object is advanced distally until removed from rectum.
- If any necrosis, perforation, or intussusception of the intestines is present, a resection and anastomosis should be performed.
- Omentum or serosal patch may be placed to reinforce suture line.
- Change gloves and surgical instruments before copious abdominal lavage and closure.

Chronic Treatment

Postoperative considerations:
- Continue rehydration and daily electrolyte monitoring.

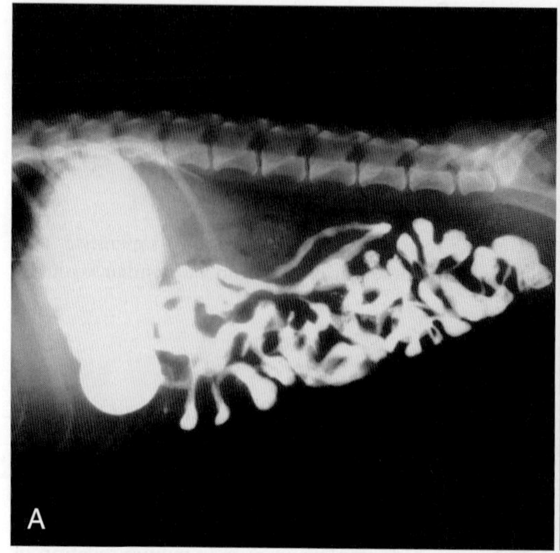

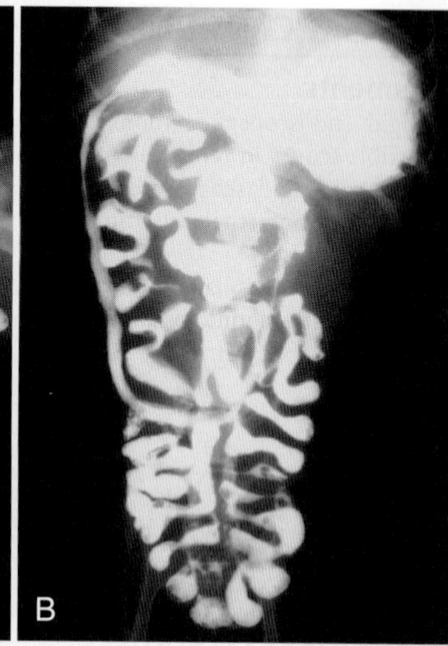

FOREIGN BODY, LINEAR GASTROINTESTINAL Lateral (**A**) and ventrodorsal (**B**) radiographic projections of upper gastrointestinal (UGI) barium study. Patient had a gastrointestinal linear foreign body. Characteristic teardrop-shaped appearance of small-intestinal segments is apparent. (Courtesy Dr. Richard Walshaw.)

- Nothing per os 6-12 hours after enterotomy, 12 hours after resection and anastomosis
- Administer GI protectants or antiemetics as needed.

Nutrition/Diet

Feeding tube placement (typically esophageal [p. 1106]) at the time of surgery should be considered in animals with anorexia, marked weight loss, hypoalbuminemia, or evidence of intestinal perforation or peritonitis.

Possible Complications

- Dehiscence; animals should be monitored in hospital for 48-72 hours postoperatively for signs of peritonitis. Risk factors include presence of preoperative peritonitis, serum albumin concentration < 2.5 g/dL (<25 mg/mL), and presence of a foreign body (vs. neoplastic disease).
- Ileus
- Short bowel syndrome; unlikely if < 70% of small intestine resected
- Stricture
- Recurrence

Recommended Monitoring

The following parameters should be monitored q 6-12h until discharge from hospital:
- Body temperature, heart rate, and respiratory rate
- Blood glucose, electrolytes, hematocrit, and total solids
- Presence of abdominal pain

PROGNOSIS & OUTCOME

- Delay in surgical intervention may increase risk of perforation and peritonitis.
- Presence of peritonitis or free abdominal gas on radiographs is associated with increased rate of mortality among dogs.
- Dogs that require surgery for linear foreign bodies may be more ill at presentation and will be more likely to have peritonitis or require a resection and anastomosis than dogs with nonlinear foreign bodies. Higher costs and a longer length of hospitalization should be anticipated.
- Morbidity and mortality are 50% higher for dogs than cats.

PEARLS & CONSIDERATIONS

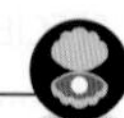

Comments

- Do not put forceful traction on the linear object before or during surgery; this may cause iatrogenic laceration of the mesenteric border of the small intestine.
- Consider placing a feeding tube (p. 1106) intraoperatively, as based on nutritional status, degree of patient debilitation, or anticipated postoperative anorexia.

Technician Tips

A history of prior foreign body ingestion can aid the diagnosis. Client education to prevent repeat offenders is vital.

Client Education

Owners should be educated to restrict access to linear material in general and especially after a confirmed episode. Behavioral preference for playing with and swallowing these materials means that without owner vigilance, the risk of recurrence is high.

SUGGESTED READING

Hobday MM, et al: Linear versus non-linear gastrointestinal foreign bodies in 499 dogs: clinical presentation, management and short-term outcome. J Small Anim Pract 55:560-565, 2014.

AUTHOR: Janet Kovak McClaran, DVM, DACVS, DECVS, MRCVS
EDITOR: Elizabeth A. Swanson, DVM, MS, DACVS

Foreign Body, Respiratory Tract

Client Education Sheet 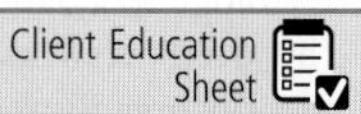

BASIC INFORMATION

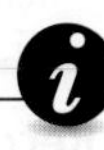

Definition

Inhaled, penetrating, or migrating objects that cause obstruction, inflammation, or secondary infection of the respiratory tract

Synonyms

Migrating foreign body (FB), nasal FB, tracheal/bronchial FB

Epidemiology

SPECIES, AGE, SEX

Dogs and cats of either sex, may be more prevalent in young animals

GEOGRAPHY AND SEASONALITY

May be more common during hunting season or in areas with oat/cereal fields or grass awns (foxtails)

ASSOCIATED DISORDERS

- Chronic intranasal FB: aspergillosis (p. 81) or bacterial rhinitis
- Intratracheal FB: focal tracheal stenosis (granuloma)
- Bronchial FB: lobar pneumonia
- If laryngeal or tracheal obstruction: noncardiogenic pulmonary edema (p. 836)
- If penetration of esophageal FB through bronchus: bronchoesophageal fistulas
- If FB migration into or through pleural space: pyothorax (p. 857)

Clinical Presentation

DISEASE FORMS/SUBTYPES

- Rhinitis
- Tracheitis/bronchitis or tracheobronchial obstruction
- Pyothorax (empyema)
- Pneumonia
- Pneumothorax

HISTORY, CHIEF COMPLAINT

- Nasal FB: nasal discharge (p. 678), acute sneezing, pawing at face, or other signs of discomfort
- Nasopharyngeal FB: stertor, sneezing, reverse sneezing, halitosis with chronicity
- Tracheal/bronchial FB: acute cough +/− respiratory distress, chronic cough, halitosis, hemoptysis, retching/vomiting possible, exercise intolerance or cyanosis if severe obstruction, temporary or recurring response to antibiotics in some chronic cases
- Intrathoracic FB: anorexia, lethargy, weight loss, fever, increased respiratory effort/tachypnea, poor performance

PHYSICAL EXAM FINDINGS

Nasal FB:

- Assessment of decreased air movement through one nostril
  - Occlude nostrils one at a time, and listen closely for airflow or watch for movement of an object (e.g., wisp of cotton, pet's hair) held in the path of airflow.
  - Hold a chilled glass microscope slide in front of the nostrils, and observe for fogging.
  - Aspergillosis may erode turbinates and negate FB obstruction of airflow.
- Nasal discharge: unilateral, mucopurulent ± blood tinge initially. It may be bilateral in cats, or with chronic erosion of nasal septum (p. 1255).
- Possible ocular discharge

Nasopharyngeal FB:

- Stertor
- Halitosis
- Reverse sneezing
- Acute onset of vomiting, retching, or gagging

Tracheal/bronchial FB:

- Cough
- Tachypnea
- Increased respiratory noise: stridor; high-frequency wheeze with partial obstruction (auscult trachea with stethoscope to localize to trachea)
- Dyspnea (inspiratory and/or expiratory); proportionate to obstruction
- Cyanosis, collapse, or sudden death with severe obstruction

Intrathoracic FB: as for pyothorax (p. 857)

Etiology and Pathophysiology

- Inhalation is the most common path of FB entry for dogs.
  - Plant material (e.g., seeds, awns, grass, depending on region) most common; may migrate into pleural space (pp. 797 and 857).
  - Other common FBs: stones, teeth, bone fragments, food
- Nasopharyngeal FB is usually a bone in dogs.
- In cats, FBs often lodge at nasal choanae after flipping up over soft palate.
- Sharp esophageal or gastric foreign bodies may migrate into lungs or pleural space.
- Local inflammatory reaction and contamination may result in secondary bacterial or fungal infection.

DIAGNOSIS

Diagnostic Overview

Respiratory FB is suspected based on acute onset of clinical signs or chronic focal disease that can be responsive to antibiotics on a recurring basis. Confirmation can be made by radiographs (e.g., radiodense bone fragments in airway), but endoscopy is often required. Migrating intrathoracic grass awns should be suspected in sporting/hunting breeds with a history of cough and fever that have focal pulmonary opacities, pleural effusion, and pleural thickening seen on radiographs or CT.

Differential Diagnosis

- Nasal FB (p. 1255)
- Nasopharyngeal FB: polyp, granuloma, neoplasia, rhinitis
- Tracheal/bronchial FB: laryngeal paralysis, collapsing trachea, elongated soft palate, trauma, neoplasia, infection
- Lung or intrapleural FB: bronchopneumonia, pyothorax from trauma or systemic disease, pneumothorax, neoplasia.

Initial Database

- CBC
  - Neutrophilic leukocytosis ± left shift and toxic neutrophils, with pyothorax, secondary bronchopneumonia, or severe secondary rhinitis
  - Eosinophilia possible with tracheobronchial grass awns
- Serum biochemistry profile and urinalysis often unremarkable
  - With pyothorax, may find hypoalbuminemia, hypoglycemia, or proteinuria.
- Coagulation profile (hemoptysis, epistaxis): unremarkable
- Radiographs: findings other than radiopaque FB may include
  - Nasal FB: increased intranasal soft-tissue opacity, local turbinate destruction (chronic)
  - Tracheal FB: increased airway soft-tissue/fluid opacity on cervical or thoracic films, noncardiogenic pulmonary edema if severe obstruction
  - Bronchial FB: ill-defined peribronchial radiopacity, or
  - Lung or bronchial FB: lung consolidation with secondary bronchopneumonia, pneumothorax
  - Intrapleural FB
    - Focal pulmonary interstitial to alveolar opacities, most common in caudal or accessory lobes
    - Pleural effusion, pleural thickening
    - Collapsed lung lobes
    - Spontaneous pneumothorax may occur with penetrating or migrating thoracic foreign bodies.
- Pyothorax: inflammatory exudates (degenerate neutrophils ± bacteria) on cytology of pleural fluid obtained by thoracocentesis (p. 1164). Macrophages and plasma cells increase with chronicity.
  - Commonly cultured organisms: obligate anaerobes (e.g., *Fusobacterium*), *Nocardia asteroides*, *Actinomyces* in dogs, *Pasteurella multocida* in cats

Advanced or Confirmatory Testing

- Intranasal FB may be visible with anterior rigid scope or posterior flexible scope, although nasal discharge may obscure view. Nasal flushing removes discharge to improve visualization and may flush out FB.

- Cytologic evaluation/culture of nasal cavity (by deep nasal swab or tissue biopsy) to identify organisms associated with secondary rhinitis. Culture of nasal secretions is not recommended.
- Nasal CT: mucosal thickening, focal bone thickening and destruction; may not differentiate FB rhinitis from nasal aspergillosis. Small and/or soft-tissue density FB seldom identified on CT.
- Nasopharyngeal FB may be visible in anesthetized patients by soft palate retraction during oropharyngeal exam (p. 1125) or retroflexed nasopharyngoscopy.
- Bronchoscopy (p. 1074) is generally diagnostic for tracheal foreign bodies and some bronchial foreign bodies (may be obscured by mucopurulent exudates or beyond the reach of endoscope).
  - Airway lavage: neutrophilia ± bacteria on cytology for tracheobronchial FB
  - Neutrophils are often degenerative when associated with bacterial infection.

TREATMENT

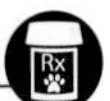

Treatment Overview

Remove FB, and treat secondary infections. Animals in respiratory distress from obstruction may require immediate anesthesia and FB retrieval.

Acute General Treatment

- Oxygen supplementation (p. 1146) if needed
- Sedation if extremely stressed (i.e., anxiety is contributing to dyspnea)
  - Acepromazine (0.1-0.5 mg total dose IM or IV) or dexmedetomidine if not systemically ill
  - Butorphanol 0.2-0.4 mg/kg IV may be given additionally q 2-4h as needed
- Rehydrate as needed.
- Thoracocentesis if respiratory compromise from pleural effusion or pneumothorax (p. 1164)
- Immediate anesthesia and FB removal if trachea severely obstructed
  - Distal tracheostomy (p. 1166) may be needed for short-term airway management.
- If possible, nonsurgical (often endoscopic) removal of nasal, laryngeal, tracheal, and some bronchial FBs
  - Nasal FB sometimes removed during retrograde or antegrade lavage/flush
  - Tracheal FB in cats removed with custom-made, 24-inch grasping forceps under fluoroscopic guidance. Successful retrieval with tracheobronchoscopy and alligator forceps through scope channel in 83% of cats
  - Some tracheal FBs removed with vacuum suction or passage of balloon (Fogarty) catheter beyond the FB and then inflation and retraction of balloon
- Rhinotomy (dorsal or ventral), tracheotomy, bronchotomy, or lung lobectomy for nonretrievable intraluminal FB
  - Lobectomy for lung lobe consolidation, bronchopneumonia, or bronchoesophageal fistula; histopathologic evaluation and culture (aerobic and anaerobic) of excised tissue
- For pyothorax or bronchopneumonia, broad-spectrum antibiotics
- For pyothorax, bilateral large diameter thoracostomy tubes or thoracotomy (median sternotomy for generalized disease) and thoracic lavage/drainage (p. 857)
  - If tubes, lavage with sterile, lukewarm isotonic fluids (20 mL/kg) q 12h for 5-7 days
- Surgical exploration if intrathoracic mass, radiographic evidence of pulmonary or mediastinal lesions, pneumothorax, *Actinomyces*, or no improvement with medical therapy

Chronic Treatment

- Antibiotics for secondary infections, based on culture/sensitivity
  - Amoxicillin or amoxicillin plus clavulanic acid 12.5-20 mg/kg PO q 12h for obligate anaerobes, *Pasteurella* spp, *Actinomyces* spp
  - Trimethoprim sulfa 10-15 mg/kg PO q 12h (possibly higher but may increase risk of adverse effects), or amikacin for *Nocardia* spp
  - For pyothorax, antibiotics are administered for 1-2 months.
- Bronchodilators (theophylline, terbutaline, or inhaled albuterol) for 3-5 days after endoscopic removal of bronchial foreign bodies, particularly in cats.

Possible Complications

- Inability to oxygenate during endoscopy or surgery
- Worsening of obstruction with flushing, FB manipulation, or endoscopic trauma (mucosal swelling)
- Noncardiogenic pulmonary edema may develop within hours after FB removal.
- Pulmonary abscess or recurrent pyothorax if migrating FB remains or inappropriate antibiotics used
- Chronic rhinitis possible if turbinates are removed during rhinotomy
- Tracheal rupture or tear

Recommended Monitoring

- Tracheal/bronchial/lung/thoracic FB: repeat radiographs or endoscopy if clinical signs recur.
- Pyothorax or pneumonia: repeat radiographs 1 week after discontinuing antibiotics or if clinical signs recur.

PROGNOSIS & OUTCOME

- Outcome is excellent if patient survives FB extraction and secondary infections are treated appropriately.
  - Bronchopulmonary abscess develops with FB migration if tracheobronchial grass awn is present for more than 2 weeks.
- Complication and mortality rates are higher with chronicity.
- Endoscopy is successful in removing 76%-84% of tracheobronchial FBs.
  - Tracheobronchial plant material can fragment, requiring multiple endoscopic episodes for complete removal.

PEARLS & CONSIDERATIONS

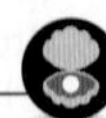

Comments

- Some nasal FBs can be removed with vigorous flushing.
- Right bronchial systems are more likely to be affected by inhaled bronchial FBs because of direct tracheobronchial path; however, 21% of affected dogs have more than one tracheobronchial FB.
- If sulfur granules or branching, filamentous, gram-positive rods suggestive of *Actinomyces* infection are seen during cytologic

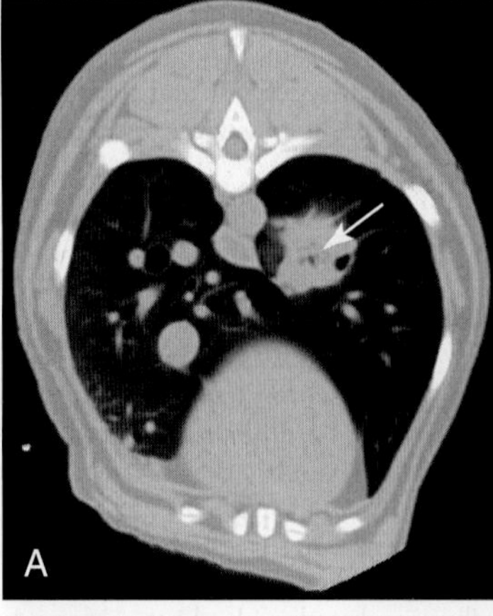

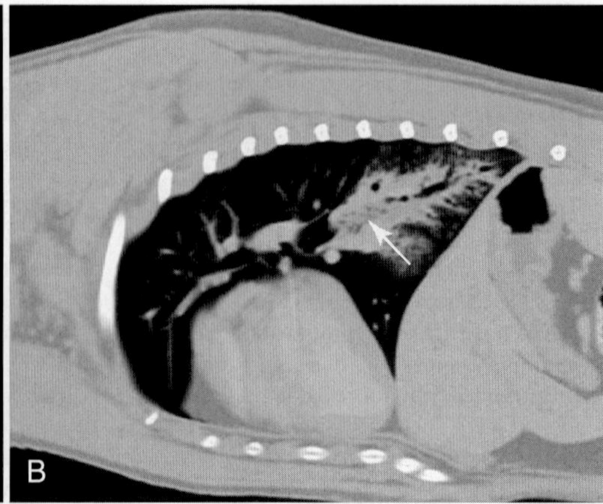

FOREIGN BODY, RESPIRATORY TRACT CT scan of a 3-year-old, intact, male Siberian Husky–cross dog with chronic cough. On axial (**A**) and sagittal reconstruction (**B**), there is a suggestion of an intrabronchial foreign body *(arrows)*. There is substantial peribronchiolar and alveolar infiltrate. A large piece of wheat was removed bronchoscopically.

examination of pleural fluid, consider long-term (4-6 weeks) antibiotic treatment.
- *Cuterebra* larvae may be tracheal FBs, especially in cats.

Technician Tips

- During rhinoscopy for FBs, fluids exit the nares and nasopharynx; therefore, the endotracheal tube should be in place with the cuff properly inflated. Pack the oropharynx with laparotomy sponges.
- Teeth and pieces of dental calculus may become tracheal or bronchial foreign bodies if not removed from the mouth after dental cleaning.
- Intubation and endoscopy may inadvertently force tracheal foreign bodies toward the tracheal bifurcation or into the bronchi. Affected animals may require an emergency thoracotomy and intubation of the distal trachea or bronchus through the thoracotomy site; materials should be available for clipping, prepping, and thoracotomy.

Client Education

- Acute cough in high-performance sporting dogs during hunting or harvest season may indicate tracheobronchial FB.
- Provide indestructible bones and toys that are appropriately sized for the dog.

SUGGESTED READING

Tenwolde AC, et al: The role of bronchoscopy in foreign body removal in dogs and cats: 37 cases (2000-2008). J Vet Intern Med 24:1063-1068, 2010.

AUTHOR: Karen M. Tobias, DVM, MS, DACVS
EDITOR: Megan Grobman, DVM, MS, DACVIM

Fractures, Abnormal Healing

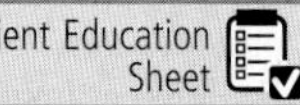
Client Education Sheet

BASIC INFORMATION

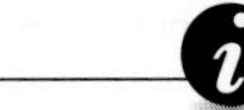

Definition

- Delayed union: bone healing progressing at a slower rate than anticipated
- Nonunion: failure to achieve bony union of a fracture
- Malunion: fracture healing with abnormal bone/limb alignment and/or abnormal function

Epidemiology

SPECIES, AGE, SEX

Older patients may take longer to heal.

GENETICS, BREED PREDISPOSITION

- Toy-breed dogs have increased incidence of avascular nonunion with radius/ulna and possibly metacarpal/metatarsal fractures.
- Feline tibial fractures may be at greater risk for nonunion than those in dogs.

Clinical Presentation

DISEASE FORMS/SUBTYPES

Delayed union: failure of fractures to heal within the expected period (usually about 16 weeks in adult dogs and cats, but this varies with the animal's age and health as well as with the nature of the fracture). Delayed unions are differentiated from normal healing and nonunions using sequential radiographs and a timeline from the initial injury.

Nonunions are divided into categories to help guide treatment:
- Viable (vascular; hypertrophic and oligotrophic)
  - Usually result from fracture instability
  - Associated with nonbridging callus. The biological environment is generally adequate for fracture healing; union is achieved by neutralization of uncontrolled fracture forces.
- Nonviable (avascular or atrophic)
  - Usually result from poor blood supply combined with fracture instability
  - Minimal or no callus formation present; fracture gap may be increased; bone fragment edges may be sclerotic or tapered
  - To achieve union, the fracture must be rigidly stabilized, blood supply must be improved, and osteogenesis stimulated.
- Nonunions of either type may form pseudarthroses; the fracture ends cease healing activities and instead form a false joint that may include joint-like fluid within a surrounding capsule.

Malunion: fracture has healed but with shortening, angulation, or rotational malalignment of the fragments.

HISTORY, CHIEF COMPLAINT

- Continued lameness after fracture stabilization
- Abnormal limb angulation
- Decreased muscle mass of the affected limb

PHYSICAL EXAM FINDINGS

- Lameness
- Muscle atrophy
- Crepitus or obvious instability of the affected bone
- Palpably excessive callus formation in the face of physical instability
- Limited range of joint motion or discomfort on manipulation of the affected limb
- Draining tracts or evidence of inflammation over the fracture site suggests osteomyelitis.

Etiology and Pathophysiology

Fracture environment, the patient's ability to heal, and decisions about case management affect fracture healing. Several factors can impede bone healing:
- Infection
- Excessive fracture gap or bone loss
- Inadequate fracture stabilization: motion at the fracture site shears off blood supply and prevents progression of healing from fibrous tissue to bone
- Poor vascular supply to the fracture site
  - Disruption of soft tissues during initial trauma or surgery
  - Placement of implants that impede blood supply to the bone
- Inadequate fracture reduction; interposition of soft tissue in the fracture gap

Other factors can influence normal bone healing:
- Polytrauma
- Pre-existing metabolic diseases or other catabolic conditions

DIAGNOSIS

Diagnostic Overview

- Diagnosis of delayed or nonunion requires a complete patient history and timeline since injury. The ultimate diagnosis is based on physical exam and comparison of sequential radiographs.
- Clinical findings include decreased limb usage, sudden changes in limb usage, and increased bone pain; fracture stability is unaffected unless implant failure has occurred.
- Delayed unions and nonunions are normally identified during routine follow-up exams by lack of radiographic evidence of bone healing (blurring of fracture lines, increased fracture gap opacity, callus formation) at a time when healing would be expected.
- Malunions are often first noted in animals that have changed owners, recently been adopted, or found as strays. They may or may not cause lameness.

Differential Diagnosis

Nonunion/delayed union differential diagnoses:
- Normal healing for that individual
- Infection
- Neoplasia

Malunion differential diagnoses:
- Congenital or breed-associated bone malformations (e.g., dwarfism, chondrodystrophic breeds)

- Abnormal bone growth secondary to soft-tissue abnormalities
- Osteoproliferative diseases and neoplasia causing bone deformity

Initial Database

Radiographs: good-quality orthogonal views are essential. Radiographic union may lag behind clinical union, especially for fractures involving metacarpal and metatarsal bones in both species and radii in cats. Fracture stability and limb function must be assessed every time radiographs are taken.

- For growing animals, radiographs are commonly taken 3-6 weeks after fracture repair and thereafter at 3-4 week intervals until healing is documented. For most fractures, union is expected within 3-12 weeks after fracture stabilization, depending on the patient's age.
- For adult animals, radiographs are commonly taken 6-8 weeks after fracture repair and thereafter at monthly intervals until healing is documented. For most fractures, union is expected by 16-18 weeks after fracture stabilization.
- With delayed/nonunion, there is lack of progression or no bony healing over a period of months. The time to union also is influenced by the type of fracture fixation used for stabilizing the fracture. Bones stabilized with less rigid implants (e.g., casts, intramedullary pins) normally produce more callus and are radiographically healed sooner than with more rigid types of fixation (e.g., dynamic compression plating).
- With malunion, shortening or angulation of a bone may be evident. Torsional malunions cause internal or external rotation of joints.

Advanced or Confirmatory Testing

- Aerobic and anaerobic culture of the bone by fine-needle aspiration if infection is suspected
- Scintigraphy can be used to evaluate the fracture site for activity.
- CT or MRI (p. 1132) may aid in making the diagnosis and in monitoring healing. Three-dimensional (3D) reconstructive techniques may aid in diagnosis and in treatment planning.

TREATMENT

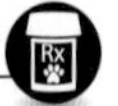

Treatment Overview

The goal of treatment for delayed union or nonunion is to achieve fracture union. This requires accurate diagnosis of the underlying factors that resulted in impaired fracture healing.

Acute General Treatment

Treatment for a *delayed union* is aimed at augmenting or continuing the original therapeutic plan, unless the original plan was inadequate (e.g., external coaptation) for the fracture type.

- If implant stability and blood supply to the fracture site are adequate, patience and regular radiographic monitoring are warranted.
- If the implants are stable but a poor biological environment exists, healing can be promoted by injection of bone marrow, autogenous cancellous bone grafting, or commercially available substrates containing bone morphogenetic proteins (BMPs).
- Medical or nutritional disorders that could negatively impact bone healing should be addressed.

Treatment for a *nonunion* requires eliminating factors that negatively affect healing and replacing them with factors that promote healing. The goal is to correct mechanical or biological inadequacies and jumpstart the process of fracture healing.

- Identify the reason(s) for the nonunion:
  - Mechanical: motion at the fracture site
  - Biological: excessive fracture gap, necrotic bone, infection, poor vascularity
- Improve the fracture environment:
  - Culture for infection, and treat it if present.
  - Remove loose/broken implants.
  - Viable nonunions: removal of excessive callus is not required but may allow better plate contouring. Debridement of fracture ends and bone grafting is usually not necessary.
  - Atrophic nonunions: debride fibrous tissue and fracture ends until some bleeding is evident from the bone. This provides mesenchymal cells and promotes ingrowth of vascular supply. It also provides better fracture apposition and allows compression of the fracture site. Add autogenous cancellous bone graft or other substances to promote bone healing.
- Rigid fixation is essential:
  - Bone plate (DCP or locking) stabilization is considered the fixation method of choice; plate/rod combination, external skeletal fixation, and interlocking nail are alternatives.
  - Circular and linear fixators may be used by experienced surgeons to lengthen limbs or transport bone across a gap by distraction osteogenesis.
- Bone grafting is critical for successful treatment of atrophic nonunions to fill in defects, promote osteogenesis, and hasten healing time.
- Aggressive physical therapy is appropriate for the recovery period.

Many *malunions* do not require treatment; those that do are addressed with corrective osteotomy (referral to an orthopedic specialist is recommended).

Nutrition/Diet

A high-quality, species-specific diet should be adequate to promote bone healing. Use of excessive supplements or high-caloric diets can be detrimental.

Possible Complications

- Failure of nonunions to heal despite intervention
- Cancellous bone graft donor site morbidity: pain or (rarely) iatrogenic fracture
- Implant failure, bone healing problems, or soft-tissue morbidity at corrective osteotomy sites

Recommended Monitoring

- Monthly follow-up radiographs until union is documented
- Limb use and fracture site stability should be assessed monthly until union occurs.
- If infection was detected, cultures should be taken 6 weeks after antibiotic therapy was instituted.

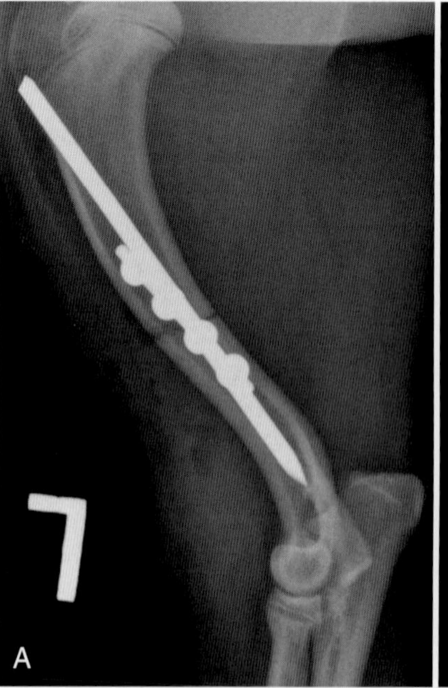

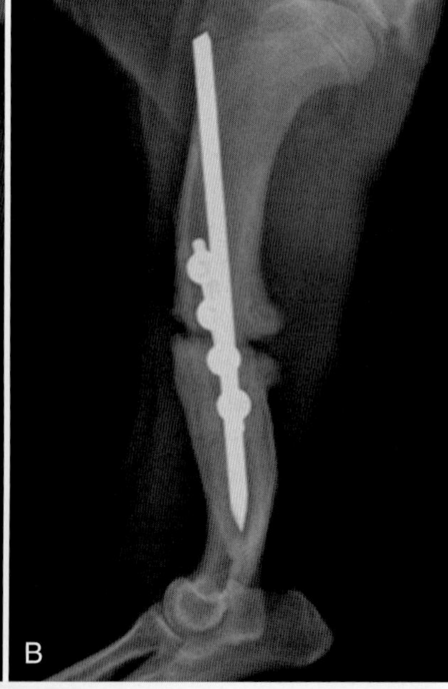

FRACTURES, ABNORMAL HEALING Delayed union. **A**, Midshaft humeral fracture after surgical stabilization. **B**, Same fracture at 8 weeks' re-examination. The radiographic interpretation is a delayed union. There is a moderate amount of callus formation, widening of the fracture gap, and increased intramedullary opacity. If the radiographic appearance is the same at 12-16 weeks, the diagnosis is changed to a nonunion. (Courtesy Dr. John Hathcock, Auburn University.)

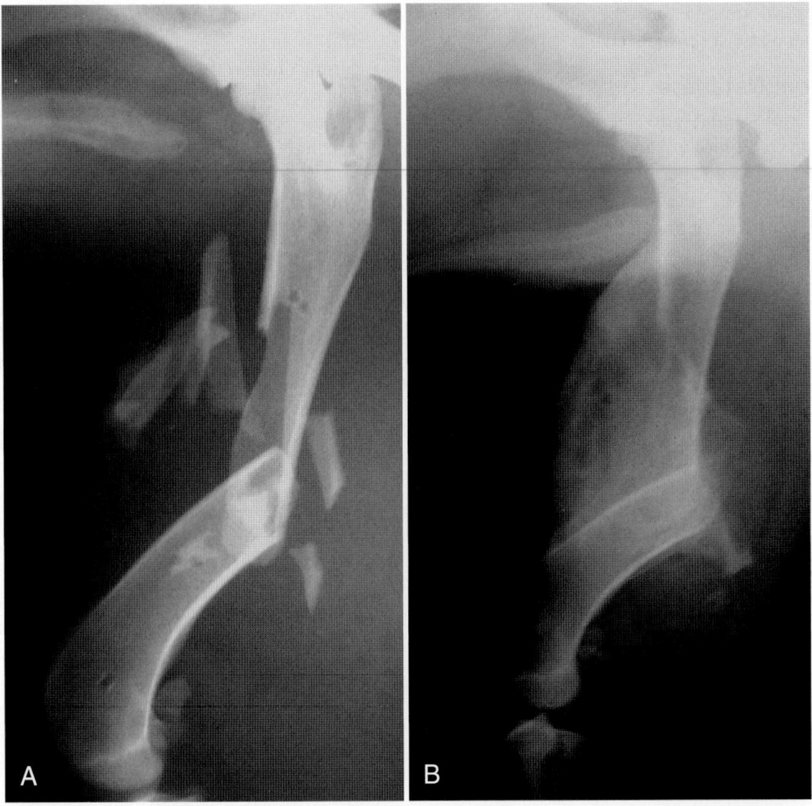

FRACTURES, ABNORMAL HEALING Malunion. **A,** Lateral radiograph of a comminuted femoral fracture. **B,** Fracture healed as a malunion. Note lack of long-bone alignment and excessive callus formation. Opacity and smooth surface of fracture callus indicate a chronic malunion. (Courtesy Dr. John Hathcock, Auburn University.)

PROGNOSIS & OUTCOME

- Delayed unions and viable nonunions have a generally positive prognosis if the underlying conditions causing the delay in healing can be resolved.
- Nonviable nonunions have a guarded prognosis for healing.
- Malunions have a varied prognosis.
  - If the limb is functional but shortened, the animal likely can adapt by decreasing joint angles to compensate.
  - If limb function is impaired, reconstructive procedures may be required to permit normal ambulation.
  - If joint angles are compromised by the malunion, there is risk of degenerative joint disease and osteoarthritis.

PEARLS & CONSIDERATIONS

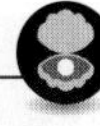

Comments

- Use of glucocorticoids may have a negative effect on bone healing.
- When a comminuted fracture is being repaired, all bone fragments should be retained unless they are contaminated; removing them increases the likelihood of nonunion.
- Delayed unions and nonunions are often associated with poor decision making or technical failures on the part of the intervening surgeon. Patient factors and owner compliance are less common reasons for nonunions.

Technician Tips

Fracture healing can be difficult to assess due to superimposition of metal implants. Oblique views can be a helpful addition to the normal orthogonal views.

Client Education

- Postoperative care instructions require communication (spoken and written) between the surgeon(s) and owner. There needs to be a clear understanding of expectations and follow-up requirements.
- Clients need to understand they are an important part of this process from the beginning, and that compliance with postoperative instructions for exercise restriction, follow-up exams, appropriate physical therapy, and consistent administration of all medications is critical to achieving a successful outcome.
- Owners of animals with a fracture malunion must understand restorative orthopedic procedures are not always effective, and complications can arise that affect bone healing or limb function.

SUGGESTED READING

Kraus KH, et al: Delayed unions, nonunions and malunions. In Johnston SA, et al, editors: Veterinary surgery: small animal, St. Louis, 2018, Elsevier, pp 752-761.

Reproduced from the third edition in modified form.

THIRD EDITION AUTHORS: D. Michael Tillson, DVM, MS, DACVS; Katrin Saile, DVM, MS, DACVS
AUTHOR AND EDITOR: Kathleen Linn, DVM, MS, DACVS

Fractures of the Femur

Client Education Sheet

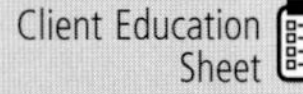

BASIC INFORMATION

Definition

Fractures of the femur can be classified as proximal (capital physis, femoral head or neck, trochanter), midshaft (diaphyseal), or distal (supracondylar, condylar).

Synonyms

Capital (head) physeal fracture, slipped capital epiphysis or physis

Epidemiology

SPECIES, AGE, SEX

Any dog or cat; castrated male cats between 1 and 2 years of age especially prone to capital physeal fractures (a.k.a., femoral physeal dysplasia)

RISK FACTORS

- Trauma to the caudal trunk or hindlimbs
- Prepubertal castration may predispose male cats to capital physeal fracture.

Clinical Presentation

HISTORY, CHIEF COMPLAINT

- Trauma to the caudal trunk/limb
  - Motor vehicle accident
  - High-velocity impact
  - Falls
- Femoral capital physeal fractures in cats may occur without a history of trauma.
- Acute lameness

PHYSICAL EXAM FINDINGS

- Lameness of affected limb
- Swelling, bruising, or shortening of limb
- Crepitation/pain at hip/stifle joint
- Loss of sensation to medial (femoral nerve) or lateral (sciatic nerve) digits due to regional swelling, bruising, and transient peripheral nerve dysfunction
- There may be evidence of trauma to other parts of the body, or even signs of shock.

Etiology and Pathophysiology

- Most common (45%) long-bone fracture
- Concurrent injuries to abdominal wall or organs, pelvis, and lumbar spine are common.
- Capital physeal fracture (immature animals) disrupts ascending vessels and compromises healing.
- Extensive hemorrhage with midshaft fractures contributes to shock.

DIAGNOSIS

Diagnostic Overview

Diagnosis is based on a history of trauma and on typically severe to non–weight-bearing hindlimb lameness, proximal limb pain, soft-tissue swelling, and discoloration. Plain radiography is confirmatory.

Differential Diagnosis

- Coxofemoral luxation (radiography can elucidate the lesion)
- Acetabular/pelvic fracture (radiography can elucidate the lesion)
- Bone neoplasia and pathologic fracture (radiography can elucidate the lesion)
- Spinal trauma: bilateral hindlimb paresis/paralysis, abnormal reflexes

Initial Database

- Craniocaudal and lateral radiographs of affected hindlimb and pelvis ± lumbar spine
- Abdominal and thoracic radiographs if whole-body trauma
- Evaluation of medial/lateral sensations of digits
- Comprehensive neurologic exam (p. 1136) to evaluate for spinal trauma
- CBC, serum biochemistry panel, and urinalysis to assess anesthetic risk; see American Society of Anesthesiologists classification (p. 1196)

Advanced or Confirmatory Testing

Ultrasound-guided aspirate or biopsy if pathologic fracture suspected radiographically

TREATMENT

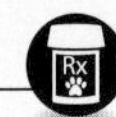

Treatment Overview

The goals of therapy are restoration of limb function and alignment and reconstruction of damaged articular surfaces. Major trauma may cause comorbid conditions that require emergent therapy (e.g., hemorrhage, shock [p. 433 and 911])

Acute General Treatment

- External coaptation (e.g., casts, splints [p. 1161]) is usually ineffective and carries a high likelihood of inducing complications.
- Fractures involving a joint require accurate reconstruction.
- Midshaft fractures are stabilized with bone plate/screws, external fixator, interlocking nail, intramedullary pins/cerclage, or plate/rod.
- Supracondylar fractures are repaired with lag screws, pins, condylar plates, or locking plates.
- Trochanteric fractures are repaired with pin and tension-band wiring or lag screws to counteract pull of gluteal muscles.
- Femoral neck and capital physeal fractures are repaired with multiple small pins or lag screw(s).
- Femoral head and neck excision (FHNE; also known as femoral head ostectomy [FHO]) can be performed for neck and capital physeal fractures in cats and small dogs.
- Total hip replacement may be considered for certain fractures of the femoral head and/or neck.

Chronic Treatment

- Restricted activity until radiographs at 4-6 weeks to assess healing
- Radiograph early for suspected complications based on clinical signs of recurrent lameness, fever, limb swelling, peri-incisional draining tracts
- FHNE for failed proximal repairs

Possible Complications

- Malunion (especially external rotation of the hip with shaft fractures), nonunion (inadequate fixation) (p. 357)
- Degenerative joint disease (articular fractures)
- Sciatic nerve damage (with retrograde intramedullary pin placement)
- Decreased hip motion with femoral head and neck excision
- Implant failure
- Infection

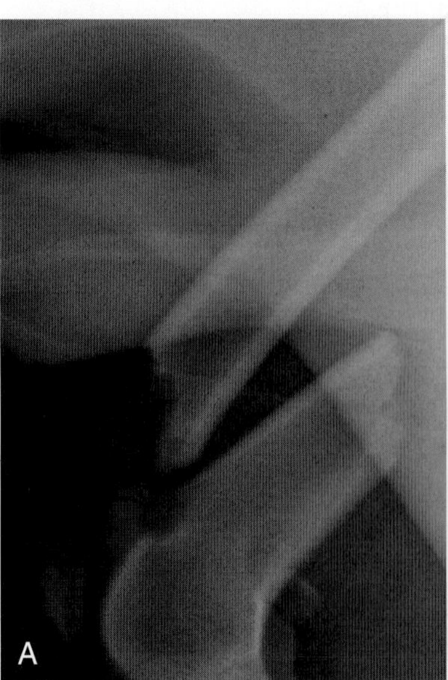

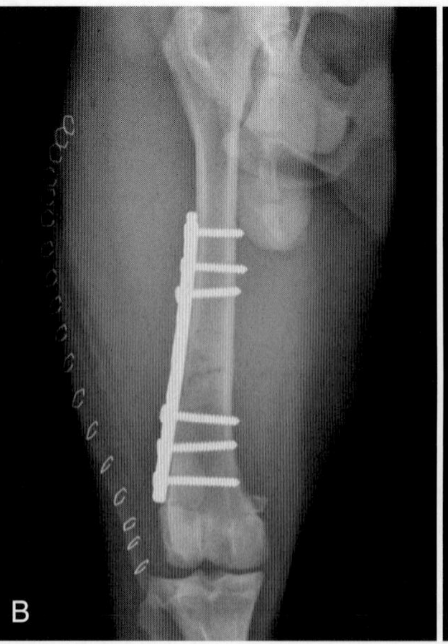

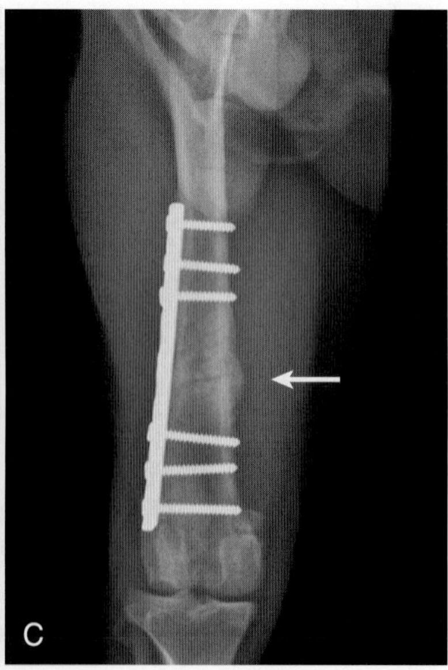

FRACTURES OF THE FEMUR **A**, Lateral view of transverse, distal-third femoral fracture in an 18-month-old, male boxer weighing 20 kg. **B**, Postoperative ventrodorsal radiograph of femoral fracture stabilized by a bone plate and screws applied to lateral aspect of bone. **C**, One-month follow-up radiograph illustrating normal endosteal healing of the fracture, along with a periosteal callus *(arrow)* on medial aspect of bone.

- Patellar luxation (medial or lateral) with distal femur fractures that heal with varus or valgus
- Quadriceps contracture and inability to flex the stifle (young animals with midshaft and distal femoral fractures)
- Limb shortening

Recommended Monitoring

- Lameness evaluation every 4 weeks for 2-3 months; expect gradual gait improvement.
- Evaluate patients with distal fractures 2 weeks after surgery to assess stifle mobility and avoid restrictive fibrosis.
- Radiographs every 4-6 weeks to evaluate fracture healing (1-3 months based on patient age) and implant stability; initiate physical rehabilitation and controlled activity based on normal imaging findings.

PROGNOSIS & OUTCOME

- Based on severity of injury and presence or absence of complications (e.g., nerve damage, infection)
- Neuropraxia (temporary nerve damage): may need 2-12 weeks to assess for functional recovery
- Good to excellent for nonarticular lesions treated with appropriate surgical intervention
- Quadriceps contracture/tie-down requires physical therapy or surgical intervention.

PEARLS & CONSIDERATIONS

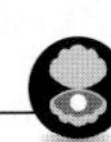

Comments

- Additional orthopedic injuries of the same or other limbs are common.
- Initial proprioceptive deficits of the affected limb can be due to pain, shock, and fracture edema rather than spinal injury.

Technician Tips

Recheck exams should include evaluation for pain or dysfunction due to implants or contracture because early recognition and therapy can prevent or minimize long-term mobility complications.

SUGGESTED READING

Guiot LP, et al: Fractures of the femur. In Johnston SA, et al, editors; Veterinary surgery: small animal, St Louis, 2018, Elsevier, pp 1019-1071.

AUTHOR: Mary E. Somerville, DVM, DACVS
EDITOR: Kathleen Linn, DVM, MS, DACVS

Fractures of the Humerus

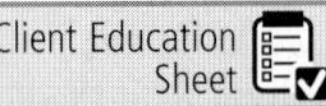

BASIC INFORMATION

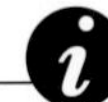
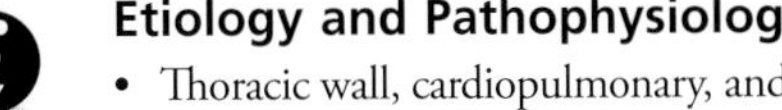

Definition

Humeral fractures commonly involve the proximal physis, greater tubercle, metaphysis, diaphysis, supracondylar region, or condyle.

Epidemiology

SPECIES, AGE, SEX

Traumatic fractures can occur in dogs and cats of any age or sex. Pathologic fractures are more likely in older animals.

GENETICS, BREED PREDISPOSITION

Spaniel breeds have a higher incidence of condylar fractures, in many cases secondary to incomplete ossification of the humeral condyle (IOHC). French bulldogs also may be predisposed to condylar fractures.

RISK FACTORS

- Forelimb trauma from gunshot injuries, falls, or motor vehicle accidents
- Focal bone lesions (e.g., bone neoplasm) or diffuse bone disease (e.g., nutritional, metabolic, or inherited) in cases of pathologic fractures

Clinical Presentation

HISTORY, CHIEF COMPLAINT

- Severe trauma to the forelimb
- Acute lameness after a fall
- Acute lameness with minimal or no trauma (condylar fractures in spaniels, pathologic fracture)

PHYSICAL EXAM FINDINGS

Non–weight-bearing lameness with swelling, pain, instability of the humerus; forelimb often held with paw knuckled under

Etiology and Pathophysiology

- Thoracic wall, cardiopulmonary, and brachial plexus injuries may exist.
- Most fractures involve the middle- or distal-third segments.
- Condylar fractures involve the lateral portion more frequently than the medial; can be due to incomplete ossification.
- Humeral fractures not caused by severe trauma may be pathologic fractures; these fractures are difficult to treat and may heal very slowly or not at all.

DIAGNOSIS

Diagnostic Overview

Humeral fracture is suspected with acute non–weight-bearing lameness in a forelimb and confirmed with radiographs.

Differential Diagnosis

- Brachial plexus injury
- Neoplastic bone disease
- Elbow or shoulder luxation
- Cervical spinal cord disease (e.g., disc herniation, tumor)

Initial Database

- CBC and serum biochemistry panel if indicated, such as prior to anesthesia
- Mediolateral and craniocaudal radiographs of the bone
- Electrocardiogram and thoracic radiography to evaluate for myocarditis or pneumothorax secondary to trauma
- Establish presence of deep and superficial pain perception and voluntary motor function in the limb to assess nerve function.

Advanced or Confirmatory Testing

CT or MRI (p. 1132) can be used for evaluating bone if a pathologic fracture secondary to neoplasia is suspected.

TREATMENT

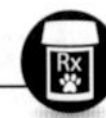

Treatment Overview

Humeral fractures require stabilization to restore joint congruency (with articular fractures) and limb function. If the fracture is displaced or comminuted, external coaptation is often unsuccessful, and surgical stabilization is warranted.

Acute General Treatment

- In young animals, minimally displaced fractures that do not involve a joint may be treated with a spica splint. The splint should remain until there is radiographic evidence of fracture healing.
- Most humeral fractures require surgical treatment with open reduction and internal/external fixation:
  - Proximal physeal and metaphyseal fractures: stabilized with divergent pins or screws
  - Greater tubercle fractures: tension-band wiring or screw stabilization
  - Diaphyseal fractures: stabilized with bone plate, plate/rod, interlocking nail, intermedullary (IM) pin/cerclage or external skeletal fixation (ESF); minimally invasive plate osteosynthesis (MIPO) may be used.
  - Supracondylar fractures: stabilized with pinning, plate, plate/rod fixation, or ESF
  - Condylar fractures: stabilized with a transcondylar lag screw and an antirotational

pin, screw or plate across the metaphyseal part of the fracture

Chronic Treatment

- A carpal flexion bandage may be placed to prevent weight bearing for the first 2-3 weeks (p. 1161).
- A spica bandage can also be used for limiting postoperative forelimb motion.
- Exercise restriction until radiographs confirm good fracture healing
- Elbow range-of-motion exercises multiple times daily maintain joint mobility.

Possible Complications

- Iatrogenic damage to the radial nerve with mid-diaphyseal fracture repair
- Degenerative joint disease with condylar fractures
- Infection
- Implant failure

Recommended Monitoring

- Suture removal and exam at 2 postoperative weeks
- Physical and radiographic exams at 4-6 and 8-10 postoperative weeks to evaluate limb function and bone healing (p. 357)

PROGNOSIS & OUTCOME

- Good to excellent with proper bone realignment, joint congruency, healing, and rehabilitation, along with minimal trauma occurring to soft-tissue structures (nerves, vessels, muscles)
- Guarded to poor with pathologic humeral fractures; healing is delayed or clinically nonexistent, pain often persists, and surgical repair is difficult or contraindicated (leading to amputation or euthanasia).

PEARLS & CONSIDERATIONS

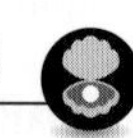

Comments

- Patients with cardiopulmonary injury should be hemodynamically stabilized before surgery/anesthesia.
- Olecranon osteotomy can improve exposure/reduction of a supracondylar or bicondylar fracture.
- Condylar fractures are difficult to identify on a single lateral radiograph.
- A disproportionately mild degree of trauma as a cause for humeral fracture should prompt suspicion of a pathologic fracture or IOHC.
- IOHC is often bilateral; evaluate the opposite humerus with a CT scan or a radiograph when treating condylar fractures in susceptible breeds.

Prevention

- Lag screw stabilization of an incompletely ossified condyle may decrease chances of fracture.
- Placement of autogenous bone graft in addition to the lag screw may increase the chance of achieving ossification of the condyle and decrease the surgical complication rate.

Technician Tips

Assess for concurrent trauma, especially cardiopulmonary, and give oxygen supplementation (p. 1146) or other stabilization therapy as necessary.

Client Education

Emphasize the importance of exercise restriction and bandage care. Provide client with applicable client education sheets.

SUGGESTED READING

DeCamp CE, et al: Brinker, Piermattei, and Flo's handbook of small animal orthopedics and fracture repair, ed. 5, St. Louis, 2016, Elsevier, pp 298-326.

AUTHOR: Raviv J. Balfour, DVM, DACVS
EDITOR: Kathleen Linn, DVM, MS, DACVS

Fractures of the Mandible and Maxilla

Client Education Sheet 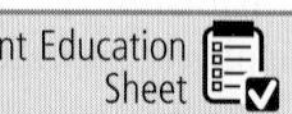

BASIC INFORMATION

Definition

- Mandibular fractures can involve the horizontal body or vertical ramus of the mandible; separation of the mandibular symphysis also can occur.
- Maxillary fractures can involve the incisive, nasal, frontal, maxillary, palatine, zygomatic, or temporal bones.

Synonyms

Jaw fractures, maxillofacial fractures

Epidemiology

SPECIES, AGE, SEX

- Traumatic jaw fractures are more likely to occur in younger animals; pathologic jaw fractures are more likely in older animals.
- Mandibular fractures are more common than maxillary fractures.
- In dogs, areas near the mandibular canine and caudal cheek teeth are more often involved.
- In cats, the region of the mandibular symphysis and the condylar process are typically involved.

GENETICS, BREED PREDISPOSITION

Mandibular fractures in dogs occur more often in smaller breeds.

RISK FACTORS

- Traumatic fracture: vehicular trauma, bites, kicks, hits, high-rise falls, gunshots, and secondary to tooth extraction
- Pathologic fracture: advanced periodontitis, neoplasia, metabolic disease

ASSOCIATED DISORDERS

Tooth fractures (p. 980), tooth displacement injuries, temporomandibular joint luxation, high-rise syndrome, craniofacial and soft-tissue injuries to structures of the head

Clinical Presentation

HISTORY, CHIEF COMPLAINT

- Head trauma
- Malocclusion
- Recent dental procedure
- Oral/nasal bleeding
- Dropped lower jaw
- Difficulty closing or opening the mouth

PHYSICAL EXAM FINDINGS

Malocclusion, difficulty closing or opening the mouth, swelling, bruising of face/oral cavity, tongue extrusion, nasal bleeding, stertor, dysphagia, oral bleeding, blood-tinged saliva, drooling, crepitus, palpable or visible fracture lines, emphysema, pain

Etiology and Pathophysiology

- Symphyseal separation/perisymphyseal fracture: most common mandibular injury in cats
- The most common sites for mandibular fracture in dogs are the areas near the last premolar (fourth premolar) and first and second molars, followed by the area just caudal to the canine tooth.
- Concurrent injuries to the head, thorax, or both are common and may require urgent treatment and delay surgical repair of maxillary/mandibular fractures.
- Surgical repair should avoid damage to the mandibular canal, which contains the inferior alveolar nerve, artery and vein, and the infraorbital canal, containing infraorbital neurovascular structures.
- In small dogs, tooth roots often reach into the ventral mandibular cortex and leave little bone farther ventrally.
- Favorable versus unfavorable mandibular fractures
  - Favorable mandibular fracture: oblique fracture line running in a rostroventral direction; relatively stable (muscle forces hold fracture segments in apposition)
  - Unfavorable mandibular fracture: oblique fracture line running in a caudoventral direction; unstable (muscle forces lead to displacement of fracture segments)

DIAGNOSIS

Diagnostic Overview

The diagnosis is suspected based on history and physical examination; the fracture may be grossly apparent or may be subtle. Radiography under general anesthesia is often confirmatory and is indicated in all cases to determine optimal treatment. Nutritional support can be important if the patient cannot prehend and swallow food, and esophagostomy tube placement may be performed under general anesthesia before or immediately after jaw fracture management.

Differential Diagnosis

- Trigeminal neuritis/neuropathy/mandibular neurapraxia (cranial nerve V)
- Temporomandibular joint luxation
- Open-mouth jaw locking
- Primary dental/periodontal disease
- Neoplasia
- Foreign body

Initial Database

- CBC/serum chemistry panel: generally unremarkable
- Head radiographs of stable, sedated patient can provide limited information.
- Open-mouth, oblique, lateral, and ventrodorsal views, and intraoral dental radiographs are preferred, and general anesthesia is usually necessary.
- Thoracic/abdominal radiographs to delineate other traumatic lesions
- Cranial nerve examination

Advanced or Confirmatory Testing

CT provides high resolution for maxillary and caudal mandibular fractures (but a proper diagnosis can be obtained without CT in most cases).

TREATMENT

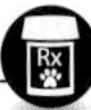

Treatment Overview

Acutely, all patients should receive adequate analgesia (systemic and/or local). Immediate fracture stabilization can be achieved with application of a custom-made muzzle. Long-term goals are to provide fracture reduction and fixation to restore dental occlusion and oral functions.

Acute General Treatment

- Teeth may need to be removed to allow proper occlusion or closure of soft-tissue defects.
- Mandibular body
  - Muzzling in stable or minimally displaced fracture: muzzle should be flexible (nylon or white cotton hospital-type tape) and be sufficiently snug to immobilize fracture while still allowing the patient to drink water and lick liquid food. Favorable mandibular fractures in animals < 6-8 months old often do not require treatment other than suturing of torn soft tissues and placing a tape muzzle for 2-3 weeks.
  - Interdental wiring and intraoral composite splint (preferred noninvasive technique of jaw fracture repair)
  - Intraosseous/interfragmentary wiring
  - Circumferential wire for symphyseal separation/perisymphyseal fracture
  - External skeletal fixation
  - Bone plating
- Mandibular ramus
  - Fractures rarely require any particular treatment beyond muzzling (snug tape muzzle through which the patient can still eat/drink) or modified labial button technique (sutures attach buttons on the left and right upper lips to a button on the chin).
  - If the mandible is displaced, resulting in malocclusion, treatment is required; noninvasive techniques first (interarch splinting such as composite bridge between maxillary and mandibular canine teeth) before considering placing intraosseous wires or bone plates.
  - Condylar process fractures may require condylectomy if there is progressive difficulty in opening the mouth (temporomandibular joint ankylosis).
- Maxilla
  - Interdental wiring and intraoral composite splint, intraosseous wiring, bone plating
  - Midline palatal separation: primary (surgical) soft-tissue closure if no tension; interquadrant splinting (wire-reinforced composite splint) if severe distraction
- Adjunctive treatment: broad-spectrum antibiotic therapy (e.g., amoxicillin-clavulanate 13.75 mg/kg PO q 12h) for 1-2 weeks with open/contaminated fractures

Chronic Treatment

- Teeth causing mild malocclusion can be surgically reduced (without pulp exposure) or extracted.
- Tape muzzles and sutures through labial buttons are removed in 2-6 weeks, composite bridges in 5-8 weeks.
- Partial mandibulectomy possible for chronic nonunions
- Oronasal fistulas (p. 720) may need secondary or delayed closure.
- Adjunctive treatment: oral instillation of dilute (0.12%) chlorhexidine solution or gel for 2-4 weeks; brushing of teeth and intraoral splints

Nutrition/Diet

Provide nutritional support during healing. Blenderize food into liquid slurry, or place

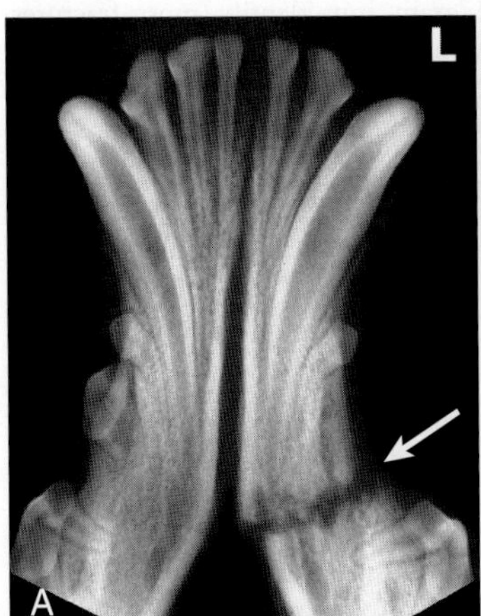

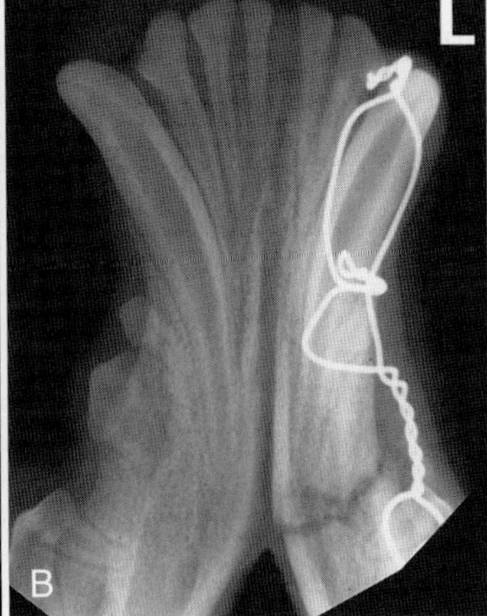

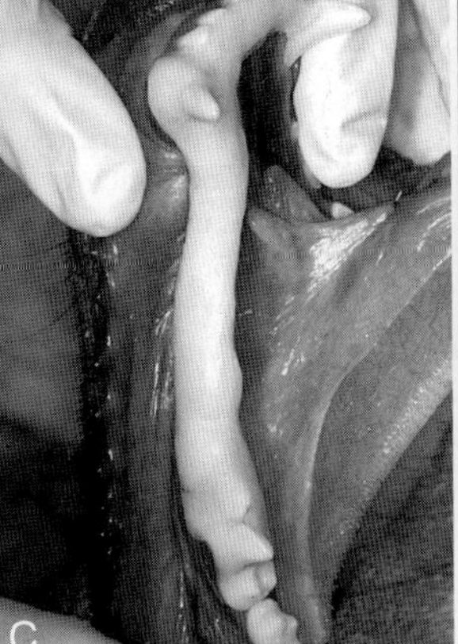

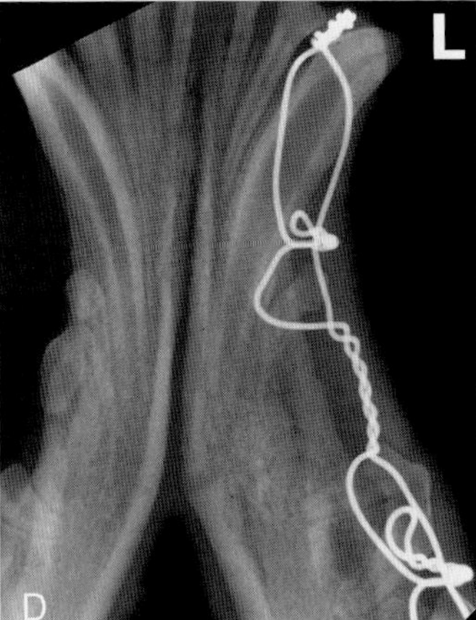

FRACTURES OF THE MANDIBLE AND MAXILLA **A**, An 8-month-old dog presented for evaluation and treatment of a left mandibular fracture between the first and third premolar *(arrow)*. The second premolar is missing. Radiograph is arranged in labial mounting; rostral is toward top of image, and patient's left is on right of image. **B**, Intraoperative radiograph. Fracture was first reduced with interdental wiring. **C**, Open-mouth view of same patient; rostral is to top. An intraoral splint was then fabricated to cover the wire and tooth crowns. **D**, A 5-week re-examination. Fracture site healed nicely; splint and wire were removed, and root canal therapy of nonvital left mandibular canine tooth was performed (not shown). (Copyright Dr. Alexander M. Reiter, University of Pennsylvania.)

esophagostomy tube (p. 1106) while patient is under general anesthesia.

Possible Complications

- Malocclusion
- Damage to dental structures
- Soft-tissue infection
- Osteomyelitis/sequestrum
- Implant failure
- Tongue and other soft-tissue trauma from exposed wires or plates
- Delayed union, nonunion
- Oronasal fistula
- Temporomandibular joint ankylosis
- Local pyoderma due to muzzle or buttons (transient)
- Malnutrition (very uncommon)

Recommended Monitoring

- Body weight (monitor adequate nutrition)
- Recheck at postoperative 2 weeks; remove skin sutures
- Radiographs at 5-8 weeks and 6 months to evaluate bone healing
- Interdental wires, intraoral splints, and external fixators are removed after fracture healing (5-8 weeks). Bone implants may be left in place if soft-tissue damage and osseous abnormalities are absent.
- Teeth in fracture lines require radiographic monitoring in 6-12 months to determine pulp vitality.

PROGNOSIS & OUTCOME

- Good to excellent if proper occlusion is established
- Fractures with tooth loss and severe periodontitis may heal slowly and by fibrous union only.

PEARLS & CONSIDERATIONS

Comments

- Teeth in the fracture line should be preserved whenever possible because they contribute to stability and alignment; they should be removed if severely loose, fractured, or diseased.
- Administration of inhaled anesthetics by pharyngostomy or temporary tracheostomy can aid with proper bone/teeth alignment during surgery.
- An esophagostomy feeding tube can reduce stress on repair(s), aid healing, and provide nutrition.
- Plates must have exact bone contour, or malocclusion will result.
- Minimally displaced maxillary fractures and fractures of the mandibular ramus may not require surgery beyond soft-tissue closure.
- The mandible is a curved and small bone, containing neurovascular structures in its mandibular canal. Intramedullary pinning is inappropriate because it does not provide rotational stability and causes damage to nerves and vessels that supply teeth and lips.

Technician Tips

- Technicians should learn how to fabricate tape muzzles in cats and dogs and be able to give instructions to pet owners on the appropriate management of the patient at home.
- Patients with tape muzzles or composite bridges between maxillary and mandibular canine teeth may have compromised thermoregulation and should not be outdoors on warm or hot days. Restriction in mouth opening also bears the risk of aspiration in the regurgitating or vomiting patient.
- Tape muzzles may be removed during drinking and eating and put back in place after feeding is completed to reduce the possibility of local pyoderma from a soiled muzzle. Multiple copies of the original muzzle can be fabricated so that the owner can replace an old one with a new one.

SUGGESTED READING

Reiter AM, et al: Trauma-associated musculoskeletal injuries of the head. In Drobatz K, et al, editors: Manual of trauma management in the dog and cat. Ames, IA, Wiley-Blackwell, 2011, pp 255-278.

AUTHOR & EDITOR: Alexander M. Reiter, DVM, Dr.med.vet., DAVDC, DEVDC

Fractures of the Metacarpus and Metatarsus

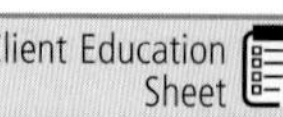

BASIC INFORMATION

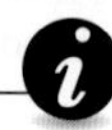

Definition

Metacarpal and metatarsal fractures account for 5% of long-bone fractures and may involve the proximal base, body, or distal head of the bone.

Synonym

Fracture of the paw

Epidemiology

SPECIES, AGE, SEX

Young, male, athletic dogs are at greater risk due to increased muscle mass and later physeal closure.

RISK FACTORS

- Direct trauma
- Repetitive stress from racing counterclockwise (greyhounds) causes fatigue fractures of the right medial and left lateral metacarpals. Poor training and nutritional deficiencies increase the risk.

ASSOCIATED DISORDERS

- Carpal hyperextension (damage to the palmar carpometacarpal ligaments)
- High-rise syndrome (falls from high places causing multiple injuries)
- Shearing and degloving injuries (usually due to vehicular trauma)

Clinical Presentation

HISTORY, CHIEF COMPLAINT

- Acute lameness
- Poor racing performance with episodic lameness

PHYSICAL EXAM FINDINGS

- Pain, swelling, and crepitus of the affected paw
- Joint effusion, palpable dorsally, with intraarticular fractures
- Valgus (lateral) or varus (medial) displacement with fractures near the collateral ligament insertion on metacarpus (MC)/metatarsus (MT) II or V
- Luxation of the phalanx with distal condylar fractures

Etiology and Pathophysiology

The central bones (MC/MT III and IV) are the major weight bearers, and these fractures cause marked lameness and loss of structural integrity.

DIAGNOSIS

Diagnostic Overview

Physical exam can identify most fractures. Radiographs are used for defining the extent of injury and determining the best method of repair.

Differential Diagnosis

- Joint luxation
- Sesamoid bone fracture, stress periostitis
- Cellulitis or foreign body

Initial Database

- Lateral and craniocaudal radiographs
- Oblique and stress radiographs if complex fractures or collateral ligament damage
- CBC, serum biochemistry panel, and urinalysis to assess anesthetic risk; see American Society of Anesthesiologists classification (p. 1196)

Advanced or Confirmatory Testing

Thermography, bone scintigraphy, or CT imaging for suspected fractures not apparent radiographically

TREATMENT

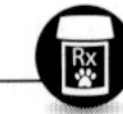

Treatment Overview

Choice of external coaptation versus internal fixation depends on the fracture type and patient size and activity. However, reported outcomes for surgery and external coaptation are similar, regardless of the number of bones fractured.

Acute General Treatment

- A fitted cast or molded palmer splint provides more support than a preformed splint, especially if multiple bones are fractured.
- Surgical repair affords greater fracture stability but risks disrupting the local blood supply. A minimally invasive approach is recommended whenever possible. Indications include
    - Proximal or distal fractures with joint instability or articular involvement, using lag screws or tension-band wire or intramedullary/external skeletal fixator constructs
    - Shaft fractures involving the central weight-bearing bones, using small plates, slot IM or dowel pins, or external fixators
    - In most cases, a molded splint or cast is applied postoperatively for added support.

Chronic Treatment

These fractures often heal without the abundant callus seen with other fractures. Exercise is restricted for several weeks after radiographic confirmation of bony union.

- If a splint, cast, or external fixator is the primary method of fixation, it can be removed after clinical union (average 6-8 weeks in younger animals, longer in older animals).
- Splints used to supplement internal fixation may be removed in 3-4 weeks.
- Bone plates and intramedullary pins penetrating the proximal or distal cortex should be removed after healing. Bone screws, wires, and toggled intramedullary pins usually can be left in place.

Possible Complications

- Unstable or highly comminuted fractures are at risk for delayed union, malunion, and synostoses.
- Nonunions are uncommon but may result from inadequate stabilization, infection, or inadequate blood supply.
- Intraarticular fractures or incorrect pin placement can damage the articular cartilage and interfere with joint motion, resulting in degenerative joint disease and chronic lameness.

Recommended Monitoring

When external coaptation is used alone:

- Regular splint checks/changes
- Recheck radiographs post-reduction and then every 3-4 weeks until union has occurred

With surgical repair:

- Regular splint checks/changes until coaptation is removed.
- Recheck radiographs after surgery and then every 4-6 weeks until union has occurred.

PROGNOSIS & OUTCOME

- Good for most MC and MT fractures, regardless of the number of bones fractured or the treatment modality selected
- Guarded for fractures with varus or valgus instability or severe articular damage

PEARLS & CONSIDERATIONS

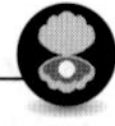

Comments

Splints and bandages require thorough client education and diligent monitoring to prevent iatrogenic skin injury.

Technician Tips

Follow-up radiographs should replicate the initial post-reduction positioning and technique to best monitor fracture healing.

SUGGESTED READING

DeCamp CE, et al: Fractures and other orthopedic conditions of the carpus, metacarpus, and phalanges. In DeCamp CE, editor: Brinker, Piermattei, and Flo's Handbook of small animal orthopedics and fracture treatment, ed 5, St. Louis, 2015, Elsevier, pp 418-425.

AUTHOR: Elizabeth J. Laing, DVM, DVSc, DACVS
EDITOR: Kathleen Linn, DVM, MS, DACVS

Fractures of the Pelvis

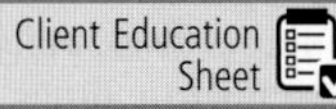

BASIC INFORMATION

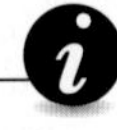

Definition

Pelvic fractures include ilial, ischial, pubic, and acetabular fractures; sacroiliac luxation and sacral fractures are also often included.

Epidemiology

SPECIES, AGE, SEX

Active, outdoor, sexually intact, roaming animals are most likely to be injured by motor vehicles. Dogs lying in driveways may be inadvertently run over.

RISK FACTORS

- Motor vehicle trauma and falling injuries (e.g., high-rise apartment buildings)
- Racing greyhounds are prone to spontaneous stress acetabular fractures.

ASSOCIATED DISORDERS

Multisystemic polytrauma: concurrent orthopedic, thoracic, urologic, and neurologic injuries

Clinical Presentation

DISEASE FORMS/SUBTYPES

- Blunt force trauma: all animals
- Racing injury (acetabular fracture) in greyhounds

HISTORY, CHIEF COMPLAINT

Severe hindlimb trauma from motor vehicle accident or fall, inability to walk with one or both hindlimbs, pain

PHYSICAL EXAM FINDINGS

- Lameness in one or both pelvic limbs; possibly non-ambulatory
- Palpable crepitus and/or pain on manipulation of rear leg(s)
- Palpable deformity of the pelvic canal during rectal exam
- Contusion (bruising) of skin overlying site(s) of injury

Etiology and Pathophysiology

- Very common sequela to blunt force injury caused by vehicular trauma
- Normal boxlike pelvic structure accounts for frequency of injuries affecting two or more sites in the pelvis.
- Concurrent injuries are common.
- Direct blows to the greater trochanter of the femur may cause an isolated impaction fracture of the adjacent acetabulum, with displacement of the femoral head through the medial acetabular wall into the pelvic canal.

DIAGNOSIS

Diagnostic Overview

Diagnosis is based on history and results of physical and radiographic exams.

Differential Diagnosis

- Spinal fracture/luxation and spinal cord injury
- Long-bone fracture in pelvic limb
- Coxofemoral luxation(s)
- Concurrent orthopedic and soft-tissue injuries

Initial Database

- Thoracic and abdominal radiographs; abdominal ultrasonography (p. 1102) for visceral and abdominal wall injuries
- Neurologic exam (p. 1136)
- CBC, serum biochemistry panel, and urinalysis to assess anesthetic risk; see American Society of Anesthesiologists classification (p. 1196)
- Electrocardiogram to identify dysrhythmia due to traumatic myocarditis

Advanced or Confirmatory Testing

- Multiple-view radiographs—lateral, oblique lateral(s), ventrodorsal—for assessment of the two hemipelves, sacroiliac joint, sacrum, tail, and distal lumbar spine. Narcotic sedation/general anesthesia usually required.
- CT to assess extent of injuries, identify sacral and acetabular fractures, and for surgical planning (especially complex sacral fractures)
- If indicated, imaging studies of urinary tract to identify tears in ureter(s), urinary bladder, or urethra

TREATMENT

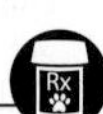

Treatment Overview

Treatment must focus on hemodynamic stabilization after trauma and pain control. Goals next include restoration of normal ambulation and pelvic canal diameter as well as prevention of secondary nerve injuries from unstable or misaligned bone fragments.

Acute General Treatment

- Intravenous fluids to treat hypovolemia (p. 911)
- Analgesia compatible with other systemic injuries (e.g., opioids, nonsteroidal antiinflammatory drugs [NSAIDs])
- Ensure patent/continuous urinary conduit
- Delay surgery until patient is adequately stabilized.
- Injuries affecting the transmission of weight-bearing forces from the limb to the spine usually require surgery.
  - Acetabular fractures are usually stabilized with plate/screws or pins/wires/screws embedded in polymethylmethacrylate bone cement.
- Iliac fractures are usually stabilized with plate(s)/screws.
- Sacroiliac and sacral body injuries are usually stabilized with screws/pins.
- External skeletal fixators are sometimes employed for stabilization.
- Patient size, degree of displacement, inherent stability, risk of secondary nerve injuries, and presence of other injuries help determine which injuries should be managed surgically versus conservatively (cage rest).

Chronic Treatment

- Confinement, sling support, and controlled activity for 1-2 months, analgesics as needed
- Monitor for delayed signs of abdominal trauma (e.g., biliary disruption/leakage, delayed manifestations of lower urinary tract rupture) and cardiac complications (myocarditis/ventricular dysrhythmia).
- Protection of paw(s) if knuckling from sciatic neurapraxia

Behavior/Exercise

Cage rest initially, with slow return to controlled activity

Possible Complications

- Malunions (especially acetabular in cats) resulting in pelvic canal compromise, with secondary constipation/megacolon or dystocia
- Malunions or callus formation resulting in sciatic nerve impingement or entrapment, with neuropraxia
- Urethral damage or rupture
- Coxofemoral osteoarthritis (acetabular fractures)
- Persistent neurologic deficits
- Persistent lameness or gait alteration
- Iatrogenic sciatic nerve injury during surgical manipulations
- Ventral abdominal hernia secondary to prepubic tendon avulsion or displaced pubic fracture
- Constipation

Recommended Monitoring

- Periodic radiographs to assess fracture healing
- Periodic clinical exams, including rectal palpation to assess improvement/resolution, function, and comfort
- Electromyography as needed in patients with peripheral nerve injuries/dysfunction

PROGNOSIS & OUTCOME

- Increased risk for prolonged or persistent disability with fractures of the acetabulum or fractures associated with nerve injuries
- Improved prognosis for return to function when injuries that involve the sacrum, sacroiliac joint, ilium, or acetabulum are treated with anatomic reduction and rigid fixation of bone fragments
- Intensive nursing care is involved for most patients and includes padded rest area, cleanliness after eliminations, pain management, nutrition, and physical therapy.

PEARLS & CONSIDERATIONS

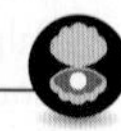

Comments

- Look for secondary injuries to the pelvic girdle (sacroiliac joints, sacral wings, and sacral body) with any diagnosis of pelvic fracture. Use oblique radiographic views to isolate the hemipelvis. Always get at least two orthogonal radiographic views to avoid missing fractures where the bone ends overlap on one view.
- Acetabular fractures require accurate reconstruction of the articular surface to reduce the risk of osteoarthritis. Controversy exists about whether fractures that involve only the caudal third of the acetabular articular surface require surgical treatment, but in general, all acetabular fractures would have a better prognosis with accurate anatomic reduction and stabilization.
- If acetabular repair cannot be achieved or if disabling osteoarthritis develops, a salvage surgery (hip replacement or femoral head/neck excision) can produce a functional result.

Prevention

- Reduce free roaming by use of leashes, fences, neutering. Use window screens to prevent falls from open windows.
- Counsel clients to always use precautions when backing up on driveways and in garages.

Technician Tips

- A disproportionately high pain response or development of knuckling may signal development of sciatic nerve entrapment.
- Monitor urination and watch for hematuria because it can indicate bladder trauma.
- Sling support on walks can improve patient comfort; variations on regular sling structure may be needed to accommodate pubic or ischial symphysis disruptions.

Client Education

- Proper confinement/activity restriction is needed during healing and recovery.
- Many pets with conservatively treated acetabular fractures return to good function, but if pain persists, hip salvage procedures may be needed.

SUGGESTED READING

DeCamp CE, editor: Brinker, Piermattei, and Flo's Handbook of small animal orthopedics and fracture repair, ed 5, Philadelphia, 2015, Elsevier, pp 395-421.

AUTHOR: Suresh Sathya, BVSc, MVSc, MVetSc, DACVS-SA
EDITOR: Kathleen Linn, DVM, MS, DACVS

Fractures of the Radius and Ulna

Client Education Sheet

BASIC INFORMATION

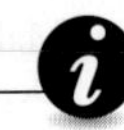

Definition

- Fractures of the radius involve the head, shaft, or medial styloid process.
- Fractures of the ulna involve the olecranon, shaft, or lateral styloid process.

Epidemiology

SPECIES, AGE, SEX

Dogs and cats of either sex at any age

RISK FACTORS

Forelimb trauma; toy-breed dogs especially susceptible

Clinical Presentation

HISTORY, CHIEF COMPLAINT

Trauma from motor vehicle/firearm accidents, falls, and fights causing forelimb lameness

PHYSICAL EXAM FINDINGS

Variable degrees of lameness, bone instability, soft-tissue swelling, bruising, and open wounds associated with an antebrachial injury

Etiology and Pathophysiology

- Almost 20% of fractures in dogs and cats involve the radius and ulna.
- The radius is the primary weight-bearing bone and is the most often stabilized; conversely, ulnar fractures can realign during repair of the radius and heal *in situ.*
- The radius and ulna are a paired bone system connected by annular, collateral, and interosseous ligaments. Growth plate trauma and disturbed growth in either bone causes forelimb deformation (p. 66).
- Diminished vascularity in the distal aspect of the bones in small and toy breeds impairs bone healing.

DIAGNOSIS

Diagnostic Overview

In most cases, the diagnosis is obvious on physical exam. Radiographs are confirmatory and help guide treatment decisions.

Differential Diagnosis

- Elbow luxations
- Antebrachial cellulitis
- Humeral condyle fractures
- Carpal luxations and fractures
- Radial nerve or brachial plexus injury

Initial Database

- CBC, serum biochemistry panel, urinalysis, electrocardiogram, and thoracic radiography to assess anesthetic risk; see American Society of Anesthesiologists classification (p. 1196).
- Standard craniocaudal and mediolateral radiographic projections of forelimb

TREATMENT

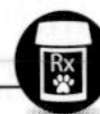

Treatment Overview

- Initial bandage and caudal splint support are useful in reducing patient morbidity (p. 1161).
- Goals of treatment:
    - Anatomic or functional realignment of fractures to maintain elbow and carpus congruency and parallelism
    - Tension-band stabilization (pins and wires or bone plate/screws) of olecranon fractures to neutralize distraction by the triceps muscles
    - Tension-band pinning/wiring or screw fixation of styloid process fractures to provide collateral ligament support

Acute General Treatment

- First aid: heavy bandage to limit soft-tissue swelling, reduce bone fragment motion, provide limb support, and cover open wounds
- Lavage and debridement of open, contaminated lesions; microbial culture and sensitivity assay not routinely recommended unless infection is evident.
- Antibiotic (therapeutic or prophylactic), analgesic, and nonsteroidal antiinflammatory therapies as indicated
- Radial shaft fractures are stabilized with bone plate/screws applied cranially or external skeletal fixation (ESF) with transfixation pins angled craniocaudally (type 1a or 1b) or applied mediolaterally (type 2).
- Fresh autogenous cancellous bone graft or commercially available allograft should be used for enhancing fracture healing.
- Ulnar fractures can be stabilized with an intramedullary pin or bone plate/screws.
- Proximal ulnar fracture(s) with cranial displacement of the radial head (Monteggia fracture) requires ulnar fracture repair, reduction of the radial luxation, and suturing of the annular ligament.
- Casting of radius/ulna fractures can be recommended only for minimally displaced, stable lesions in young, non–small-breed dogs and cats.

Chronic Treatment

After surgical intervention: bandage support, sometimes with caudal splint placement, and controlled exercise until radiographic and clinical evidence of bone union

Possible Complications

- Implant failure, stress protection (osteopenia), and cold conduction with the use of bone plate and screws for stabilization of radial fractures
- Pin tract sepsis and instability with ESF pins and frames
- Poor healing of distal radial and ulnar fractures in small or toy breeds
- Nonunion, delayed union, or malunion secondary to intramedullary pinning of the radius

Recommended Monitoring

Clinical and radiographic evaluations 4-6 and 10-12 weeks after surgery (p. 357)

PROGNOSIS & OUTCOME

- Bone plates/screws and ESF yield the most consistent clinical recoveries and return of limb function.
- External coaptation (casts or splints) is effective for minimally displaced fractures in young, healthy patients.
- Intramedullary pinning of the radius causes malunions and carpal joint damage and is rarely indicated.

PEARLS & CONSIDERATIONS

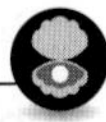

Comments

- Irreparable proximal or distal lesions of the radius and ulna may require arthrodesis of the adjacent joint (elbow or carpus) to salvage the limb, or limb amputation.
- ESF can be used in a minimally invasive or closed approach to preserve the soft tissues during a biological surgical approach.
- Patients with ESF require more intensive postoperative care than those treated with a bone plate/screws.
- Infrequently, plate removal is required after bone union in dogs that are lame due to cold conduction or have radiographic evidence of osteopenia under the implant.
- Toy-breed dogs with distal radial/ulnar fractures often have unsatisfactory healing without surgical intervention (i.e., plating).

Technician Tips

Surgery patients can be placed in lateral recumbency for a craniomedial (down limb) or craniolateral (upper limb) approach to the fractured bone(s).

SUGGESTED READING

DeCamp CE, et al: Brinker, Piermattei, and Flo's Handbook of small animal orthopedics and fracture repair, ed 5, St. Louis, 2015, Elsevier, pp 366-388.

AUTHOR: Joseph Harari, DVM, MS, DACVS
EDITOR: Kathleen Linn, DVM, MS, DACVS

Fractures of the Scapula

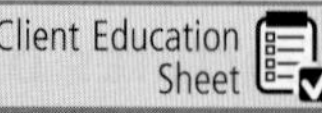

BASIC INFORMATION

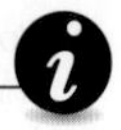

Definition

Scapular fractures involve the spine, body, neck, or glenoid regions of the bone.

Epidemiology

SPECIES, AGE, SEX

Dogs and cats, either sex and any age

RISK FACTORS

Trauma to the proximal forelimb

Clinical Presentation

HISTORY, CHIEF COMPLAINT

Forelimb trauma secondary to motor vehicle/firearm accidents, falls, bites, or other injury

PHYSICAL EXAM FINDINGS

- Variable degrees of lameness
- Swelling, bruising, open wounds around scapula
- Pain on palpation of shoulder joint

Etiology and Pathophysiology

- Uncommon fractures, representing 0.5%-2.5% of all fractures treated at referral hospitals
- Can be associated with regional injury to cervicothoracic spine, thoracic structures (pulmonary contusions, pneumothorax), and brachial plexus
- Extensive medial and lateral musculature provides support and extraosseous vascularity to fractured bone segments.
- Fractures are classified based on location: body, spine, neck, and glenoid *or* stable/unstable extraarticular versus intraarticular lesions.

DIAGNOSIS

Diagnostic Overview

Radiography is necessary for diagnosis. Sedation or general anesthesia may be required to obtain diagnostic images because positioning is key for highlighting certain fractures.

Differential Diagnosis

- Shoulder luxation
- Dorsal displacement of the scapula

Initial Database

- Mediolateral and ventrodorsal radiographic projections of proximal aspect of limb
- CBC, serum biochemistry panel, and urinalysis to assess anesthetic risk; see American Society of Anesthesiologists classification (p. 1196).
- Electrocardiogram (p. 1096) and thoracic radiography for complications of thoracic trauma

Advanced or Confirmatory Testing

Computerized tomography (CT) delineates occult lesions.

TREATMENT

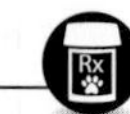

Treatment Overview

Treatment goals are fracture stabilization for bone healing and maintenance of glenoid (joint) congruency.

Acute General Treatment

- Minimally displaced, nonarticular fractures can be stabilized for 1 month with external bandage support such as a Velpeau sling or spica splint (p. 1161).
- Severely displaced spine or body fractures are stabilized with orthopedic wire or bone plate/screws.
- Neck fractures are stabilized with small pins or bone plate/screws.
- Glenoid fractures require alignment of joint surface and are stabilized with screws or pins.
- Avulsions of the acromion process or supraglenoid tubercle require tension-band wiring to counteract distraction by the deltoideus and biceps muscles, respectively.

Chronic Treatment

- Bandage support for 4-6 weeks for comminuted lesions and tenuous fixations
- Controlled ambulation and passive flexion/extension exercises to maintain muscle tone and joint motion for 6 weeks until radiography confirms bone healing

Possible Complications

- Suprascapular nerve damage with neck fracture or surgical repair
- Malalignment of fractured bone segments
- Degenerative joint disease with glenoid fractures
- Infection
- Implant failure

Recommended Monitoring

- Lameness evaluation 1-3 months after injury and treatment
- Radiography at 6-10 weeks to evaluate fracture healing

PROGNOSIS & OUTCOME

- Based on severity of injury
- Good to excellent for nonarticular lesions

PEARLS & CONSIDERATIONS

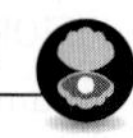

Comments

- Scapular fractures can be missed if lameness is mild or ambulation is not evaluated at hospital admission (e.g., patient is carried in).
- Fractures are often identified during thoracic radiography of trauma patients.
- Suprascapular nerve damage is characterized by atrophy of supraspinatus and infraspinatus muscles.
- Scapular fractures tend to heal well because of abundant periosseous vascularity and cancellous bone supply distally.

Technician Tips

Skin at the edges of Velpeau slings should be watched carefully for rub sores.

SUGGESTED READING

Johnson AL: Scapular fractures. In Fossum TW, editor: Small animal surgery, ed 4, St. Louis, 2013, Mosby, p 1122.

AUTHOR: Joseph Harari, DVM, MS, DACVS
EDITOR: Kathleen Linn, DVM, MS, DACVS

Fractures of the Spine/Luxations of the Spine

Client Education Sheet 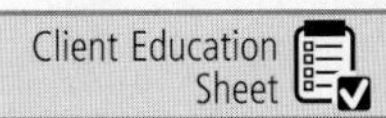

BASIC INFORMATION

Definition

Disorders primarily due to trauma that cause spinal instability, spinal cord damage, or spinal nerve damage

Epidemiology

SPECIES, AGE, SEX

Any dog or cat but most commonly younger animals

RISK FACTORS

- Trauma
- Focal or diffuse bone demineralization due to vertebral column neoplasia (primary or secondary)
- Infection
- Chronic phosphorus and calcium imbalances
- Osteoporosis
- Nutritional secondary hyperparathyroidism
- Diffuse idiopathic skeletal hyperostosis

Clinical Presentation

HISTORY, CHIEF COMPLAINT

- Trauma (most commonly vehicular trauma, less frequently falls, bite, or gunshot wounds)
- Spinal pain, swelling, or deformity
- Weakness or inability to stand/walk

PHYSICAL EXAM FINDINGS

- Signs of hypovolemic/hypotensive shock in acute trauma patients (pp. 477 and 911)
- Guarding of neck, arched back, spinal hyperpathia and/or deformation
- Crepitus, excessive spinal movement in unstable fractures
- Neurologic deficits (p. 1136) depend on localization and severity of lesion (proprioceptive, motor, or sensory deficits); monoparesis, paraparesis, or tetraparesis; upper motor neuron (UMN) or lower motor neuron (LMN) signs; loss of central recognition of pain; areflexia; ipsilateral Horner's syndrome; enlarged UMN or LMN bladder
- Spinal reflexes for fractures involving spinal cord segments:
  - C1-C5: UMN to the forelimbs and hindlimbs
  - C6-T2: LMN to the forelimbs and UMN to the hindlimbs
  - T3-L3: Normoreflexia to the forelimbs and UMN to the hindlimbs
  - L4-S3: Normoreflexia to the forelimbs and LMN to the hindlimbs

Etiology and Pathophysiology

- Traumatic vertebral fractures result from forces causing spinal hyperextension, hyperflexion, compression, and/or rotation.
- Fractures occur most commonly at the craniocervical, cervicothoracic, thoracolumbar, and lumbosacral junctions.
- A decrease in spinal canal diameter may cause mechanical injury to nervous tissue.
- Secondary pathophysiologic events include ischemia, hemorrhage, alteration in blood flow to the spinal cord, and edema. These secondary effects are often more harmful than the initial mechanical injury.

DIAGNOSIS

Diagnostic Overview

Spinal fractures are most commonly suspected due to history of trauma associated with spinal hyperpathia, deformation, and/or neurologic deficits associated with myelopathy. Confirmation requires diagnostic imaging (spinal radiography, CT, and/or MRI).

Differential Diagnosis

Intervertebral disc disease, meningomyelitis, discospondylitis, vertebral osteomyelitis, congenital malformations, spinal neoplasia

Initial Database

- CBC, serum chemistry, urinalysis, thoracic and abdominal radiographs: assess for concomitant injuries or pre-existing conditions
- Spinal survey radiographs to detect discontinuity and fracture lines of vertebral column, malalignment or narrowing of intervertebral space, and/or articular facets
- For cooperative patients, initial radiographs could be taken without sedation or anesthesia.

Advanced or Confirmatory Testing

- Spinal radiographs of anesthetized, stable patients permit more accurate positioning and characterization of lesions (e.g., for surgical planning). Care must be taken to avoid iatrogenic exacerbation of injury when handling the anesthetized patient.
- CT or myelography: used to exclude compression of spinal cord by herniated disc material or bone fragments
- MRI (p. 1132): superior for imaging surrounding/stabilizing soft-tissue structures and spinal cord; CT may be better for imaging bone abnormalities.

TREATMENT

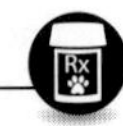

Treatment Overview

Initial treatment frequently requires stabilization of patients in shock. External coaptation may be needed for temporary and definitive fracture stabilization. Pain management and physical rehabilitation are critical for recovery. Evaluation by a neurologic or orthopedic specialist is strongly recommended.

Acute General Treatment

- Initial medical management:
  - Shock treatment in trauma patients
  - Tape thoracolumbar fracture patients to rigid board or stabilize on a *vacuum*-activated *surgical positioning* system, and apply neck brace to patients with cervical fractures to minimize further spinal cord damage. Sedate fractious or agitated patients.
  - Pain management with opiates or nonsteroidal antiinflammatory drugs (NSAIDs)
- Definitive treatment:
  - Choice between nonsurgical (strict confinement, neck or back brace, and pain management) and surgical management (spinal cord and nerve root decompression, fracture reduction, and subsequent stabilization with implants) is based on initial neurologic status, serial re-evaluations, spinal stability, and presence of concurrent injuries.
  - Unstable injuries include lamina, pedicle, dorsal spinous process, and articular facet fractures, and supraspinous/interspinous ligament tears.
  - Stable injuries include disc protrusion, ventral longitudinal ligament rupture, and avulsion of ventral vertebral body.
- Nonsurgical management for patients with mild neurologic signs (pain, proprioceptive and motor deficits) and/or stable fractures that respond to medical management
- Surgery for patients with more severe neurologic signs (uncontrollable pain, minimal motor function, paresis or plegia), for unstable fractures or lesions not improving with medical management
  - Stabilization with internal implants, pins, wires, plates, or screws; implants may be embedded in methylmethacrylate for additional stabilization
  - External fixators have been used less frequently.

Chronic Treatment

- Supportive care: appropriate bedding to reduce pressure sores, providing traction for patients, bladder expression in patients without bladder control
- Wheelchairs for patients with loss of limb function

Nutrition/Diet

- Food and water need to be placed near immobilized patients.
- Hand feeding in upright position for tetraplegic patients

Behavior/Exercise

- Strict crate rest and short, controlled leash walks until radiographic evidence of healing
- Physical rehabilitation: assisted standing and walking, aquatherapy, gait and proprioceptive training

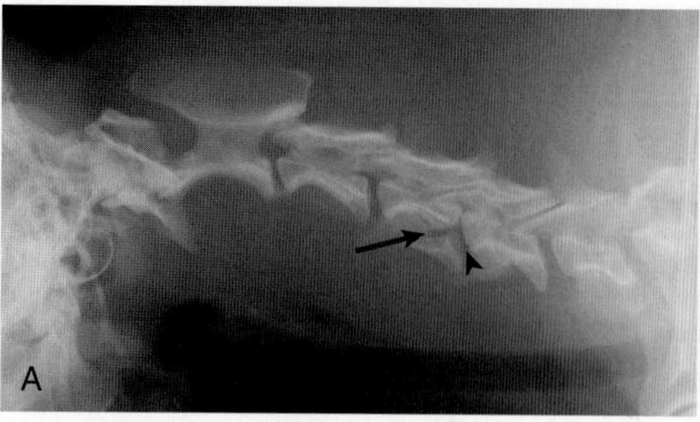

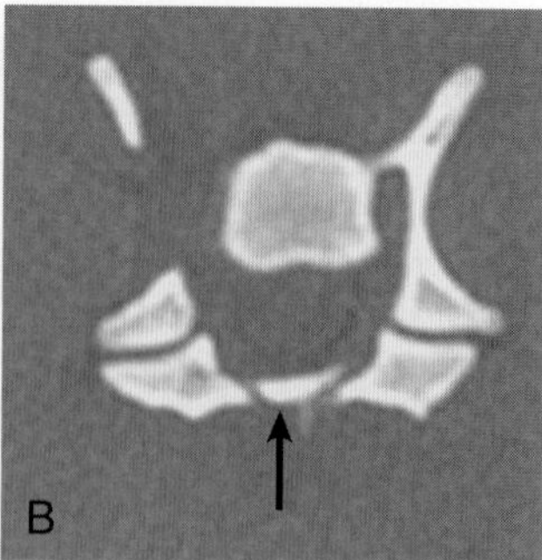

FRACTURES OF THE SPINE/LUXATIONS OF THE SPINE Radiograph of a canine cervical spine. **A,** Lateral view showing an oblique C4 vertebral body fracture through caudal endplate *(arrow)* with ventral displacement. Intervertebral disc space at C4-C5 is collapsed *(arrowhead)*. **B,** Transverse CT view (dorsal at bottom of the image) of the C4 vertebra showing a laminar fragment compressing the spinal cord *(arrow)*. This lesion could not be detected with cervical radiographs.

Drug Interactions

Do not give steroidal and NSAID medications simultaneously, and avoid NSAIDs until animal is well hydrated and shock is resolved.

Possible Complications

- Respiratory arrest due to cervical fractures
- Hemorrhage
- Neurologic deterioration
- Myelomalacia
- Infection, including urinary tract infection
- Implant failure

Recommended Monitoring

- Serial neurologic evaluations
- Respiratory monitoring with cervical fractures and trauma patients

PROGNOSIS & OUTCOME

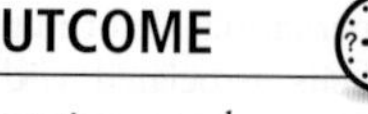

- Patients with pain sensation: good prognosis for functional recovery
- Patients with loss of pain sensation: fair to guarded prognosis
- Severed spinal cord or areflexia: grave prognosis
- Perioperative mortality for surgical stabilization of cervical vertebral fractures is up to 36%. Nonsurgical treatment often provides reasonable outcome.

PEARLS & CONSIDERATIONS

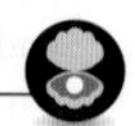

Comments

- Up to 20% of patients with traumatic spinal fractures have a second fracture.
- Radiographs may not reflect maximal spinal displacement. Neurologic evaluation is often more helpful than radiographic evaluation for prognosis.
- Radiographs have moderate sensitivity for spinal fractures and subluxations and low negative predictive values for canal narrowing or fragments within canal.

Technician Tips

When admitting a patient with spinal injury, provide safe transport of patient on rigid board or vacuum-activated surgical positioning system from car into the clinic and prevent owners from carrying patient by themselves.

Client Education

Care for paralyzed patients is laborious. It can take months until improvement is observed, and return to function cannot be guaranteed. Depending on severity of injury, euthanasia may be a reasonable option.

SUGGESTED READING

Weh M, et al: Vertebral fractures, luxations, and subluxations. In Johnston SA, et al, editors: Veterinary surgery: small animal, ed 2, St. Louis, 2018, Elsevier, pp 529-548.

AUTHOR: Susanne K. Lauer, Dr.med.vet., DACVS, DECVS, DACVSMR
EDITOR: Kathleen Linn, DVM, MS, DACVS

Fractures of the Tibia and Fibula

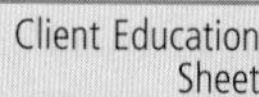
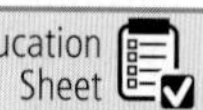

BASIC INFORMATION

Definition

Fractures of the tibia and fibula account for 20% of long-bone fractures and include avulsion of the tibial tuberosity, separation of the proximal or distal tibial physis, tibial shaft fractures, and fractures of the medial or lateral malleolus.

Epidemiology

SPECIES, AGE, SEX

Tuberosity avulsions and physeal fractures occur in immature animals.

RISK FACTORS

- Direct trauma
- Muscle contraction causing avulsion fractures
- Torsional athletic injuries
- Bone tumors or metabolic bone disease
- Complication of cranial cruciate ligament repair (tibial plateau leveling osteotomy [TPLO] or tibial tuberosity advancement [TTA])

Clinical Presentation

HISTORY, CHIEF COMPLAINT

Acute lameness

PHYSICAL EXAM FINDINGS

- Pain, swelling, and crepitus at the fracture site
- Stifle effusion with proximal physeal or tuberosity avulsion fractures
- Tarsocrural (hock) instability with malleolar fractures

Etiology and Pathophysiology

- Because of sparse soft-tissue coverage, tibial fractures are often open.
- Most fibular fractures occur with tibial fractures and are not repaired unless stability of the stifle or hock is compromised.

DIAGNOSIS

Diagnostic Overview

History and physical examination can identify most fractures. Radiographs are used to confirm the diagnosis and determine the best method for repair.

Differential Diagnosis

- Osteochondrosis of the tibial tuberosity
- Primary or metastatic bone neoplasia
- Stifle or hock luxation

Initial Database

- Craniocaudal and lateral radiographs, including the stifle and hock
- Stress radiography if a nondisplaced malleolar fracture is suspected
- CBC, serum biochemistry panel, and urinalysis to assess anesthetic risk; see American Society of Anesthesiologists classification (p. 1196).

Advanced or Confirmatory Testing

- Radiographs of the contralateral leg to differentiate traumatic physeal separation from a normal open physis (growth plate) in immature patients
- Bone biopsy for suspected pathologic fracture

TREATMENT

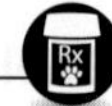

Treatment Overview

Tibial fractures require stabilization for optimal healing. The method of repair should maintain normal limb length and joint alignment without compromising future bone growth, and must take into account the nature of the fracture, patient size, and activity level.

Acute General Treatment

- External coaptation (casting or splinting (p. 1161) for compliant animals
  - Minimally displaced tibial physeal fractures: for adequate stabilization, the support must extend above the distal femur and immobilize the stifle.
  - Reducible and stable tibial shaft and malleolar fractures: if the fibula is intact, it provides additional stability by acting as an internal splint.
- Open reduction and internal fixation (ORIF)
  - Tibial tuberosity avulsions: repair with pin/tension band to counter quadriceps muscle distraction.
  - Displaced or unstable proximal tibial or distal malleolar fractures: repair with cross pins, bone screws, or a buttress plate.
  - Proximal fibular fractures: stabilize the proximal fragment with a bone screw or pin/tension band to preserve the insertion of the lateral collateral ligament.
  - Complex tibial fractures; diaphyseal fractures requiring rigid support: treatment options include intramedullary pinning, interlocking nails, bone plates, and external fixators.
- Minimally invasive plate osteosynthesis (MIPO)
  - A bone plate may be applied as an extramedullary splint, providing bone alignment without disturbing the fracture site. By preserving soft-tissue attachments and blood supply to the fracture bed, healing time may be shorter than with more invasive techniques.
  - Adding an intramedullary rod strengthens the repair.

Chronic Treatment

- Casts, splints, and external fixators are removed after radiographs confirm bony union.
  - Average healing occurs in 6-12 weeks, with younger patients healing more quickly.
  - Exercise restriction should be continued another few weeks.
- Implants used in physeal fractures may cause premature physeal closure and should be removed as soon as possible after union.
- Other implants are removed only if they cause problems such as cold intolerance or soft-tissue and joint irritation.

Possible Complications

- Delayed unions or nonunions
- Osteomyelitis
- Patellar luxation following poorly reduced tibial tuberosity fractures
- Degenerative joint disease, especially if there are intraarticular fractures or implants
- Growth disturbances causing limb shortening or angular limb deformity

Recommended Monitoring

Casts and splints require frequent monitoring and, in immature animals, adjustment as the patient grows. Regular physical and radiographic examinations should be done in all cases until clinical recovery.

PROGNOSIS & OUTCOME

Most fractures in young, healthy patients heal quickly and without complications, provided good patient and owner compliance. Complex injuries in older patients heal more slowly, with increased risk of complications. Repair of pathologic fractures may provide palliative relief, but the long-term prognosis depends on the underlying disease.

PEARLS & CONSIDERATIONS

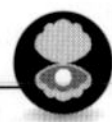

Comments

- To avoid iatrogenic stifle damage, normograde intramedullary pinning of the tibia is preferred over retrograde pinning.
- Proximal tibial physeal fractures can be radiographically subtle. If left untreated, the epiphyseal fragment can progressively displace caudodistally, leading to an excessive tibial plateau slope that may predispose the stifle to cranial cruciate ligament rupture.

Technician Tips

- Splints and bandages require thorough client education and diligent monitoring to prevent iatrogenic skin injury.
- Follow-up radiographs should replicate the initial post-reduction positioning and technique. It is usually safer to radiograph the bone through the splint than to risk loss of stability with premature splint removal.

SUGGESTED READING

DeCamp CE, et al: Fractures of the tibia and fibula. In DeCamp CE, et al, editors: Brinker, Piermattei, and Flo's Handbook of small animal orthopedics and fracture treatment, ed 5, St. Louis, 2016, Elsevier, pp 670-706.

AUTHOR: Elizabeth J. Laing, DVM, DVSc, DACVS
EDITOR: Kathleen Linn, DVM, MS, DACVS

Frostbite

BASIC INFORMATION

Definition

Tissue damage caused by exposure to cold agents or temperatures; effects may be reversible with rewarming or may be irreversible due to necrosis. Hypothermia is discussed in greater detail on p. 523.

Synonym

Hypothermic injury

Epidemiology

SPECIES, AGE, SEX

- Any animal exposed to cold environmental temperatures, especially if the body temperature falls < 34°C (<93°F). Young animals outdoors or those in poor body condition are at greater risk.
- Affected tissues often include the tail, testicles, and pinnae.

GENETICS, BREED PREDISPOSITION

Hairless or short-haired breeds of dogs and cats are predisposed.

RISK FACTORS

Low ambient temperatures

GEOGRAPHY AND SEASONALITY

Winter months in temperate to cold climates

ASSOCIATED DISORDERS

Hypothermia

Clinical Presentation

HISTORY, CHIEF COMPLAINT

- History of exposure to cold temperatures or agents
- Lesions visible to the owner depend on the time course since cold injury.
- Animals may be presented for evaluation of acute injury (e.g., vehicular trauma) and white, waxy skin, or injury may not be noticed until later stages when tissue is sloughing.

PHYSICAL EXAM FINDINGS

- Depends on extent of exposed body parts
  - Mild cold injury to the extremities (toe tips, ear tips, tail tip) may go undetected.
  - Very extensive regional cold injury may be evident as a frozen limb or other severe cold injury.
- Acutely affected animals have pale areas of skin that are cool to the touch, with or without freezing of deeper tissues. Cyanosis may be evident.
- Sensation in affected body parts may be decreased or hyperesthetic.
- As the affected area thaws, the tissue may become reddened and swollen:
  - Depending on the extent of affected tissue, the thawing process may be associated with intense pain.

- Affected skin may blister.
- Days after the frostbite has occurred, the tissues may appear shrunken and discolored and may begin to slough if necrotic. Days to weeks after injury, alopecia and sloughing may occur.

Etiology and Pathophysiology

- Cold induces vasoconstriction to affected tissue, endothelial damage, and thrombosis.
- Freezing results in crystallization of extracellular fluid and damages cell membranes, causing a fluid shift from the cell to the extracellular space. The change in electrolyte concentration in the cell leads to change in cellular proteins.
- Lack of nutrients and direct cellular damage result in local tissue damage.

DIAGNOSIS

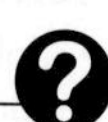

Diagnostic Overview

The diagnosis is based on history of exposure to cold and physical exam findings. Patients may be prone to frostbite if debilitated by pre-existing disorders, and diagnostic testing for these comorbidities may be indicated by the history and physical exam.

Differential Diagnosis

Burn injuries may appear similar.

Initial Database

- Arterial blood pressure if signs of systemic illness (p. 1065)
- Quick assessment tests: packed cell volume, total solids, blood glucose, blood urea (Azostix)
    - Hyperglycemia (blood glucose concentration > 300 mg/mL [>16.6 mmol/L]) possible
- Routine laboratory evaluation if systemic illness is suspected
- Imaging and further evaluation as dictated by other disorders or injuries (e.g., frostbite caused by cold exposure after the patient was hit by a car)

TREATMENT

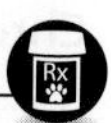

Treatment Overview

Prevent further damage to tissues from continued cold exposure or self-trauma and secondary infection by using aseptic technique in handling wounds. Allow damaged tissue to declare itself before extensive debridement or amputation.

Acute General Treatment

- Ensure hemodynamic stability first (e.g., mean arterial blood pressure > 65 mm Hg)
    - Profound bradycardia due to hypothermia may be present.
- If patient is severely hypothermic (<94°F [<34.4°C]), external heat supplementation can cause peripheral vasodilation and predispose to hypotension, even if patients appear to be hemodynamically stable on presentation.
- Central warming techniques may be beneficial (p. 523).
- Immerse affected areas if possible in warm (102°F-104°F [39°C-40°C]) water. Avoid warmer temperatures that may potentiate tissue injury.
- Dry affected areas, and apply sterile, light, noncompressive bandages over wounds (p. 909).
- Consider antioxidant agents and free radical scavengers (e.g., lidocaine 50 mcg/kg/min IV, *N*-acetylcysteine 70 mg/kg IV, q 6h) if there is risk of reperfusion injury.
- Consider Doppler ultrasound and comparison of paired regional and systemic blood glucose concentrations to screen patients for local tissue thrombosis. Angiography can be conducted if considering fibrinolytic or anticoagulant therapy unless contraindicated. Angiography may also help define the overall arterial blood supply to the affected region.
- Analgesia (e.g., using opioid analgesics) should be provided.
- Debride infected wounds or sloughing tissue. Some tissue may not be immediately identified as viable. Leave questionable tissue intact until more definitive assessment can be made.

Chronic Treatment

- Assess necrotic tissue conservatively.
    - Do not amputate or debride large areas early on in the healing process unless signs of infection or sepsis are present.
- Tissue damaged by frostbite will likely be more susceptible to cold injury in the future.
- Prevent further cold exposure.

PROGNOSIS & OUTCOME

- Varies, depending on amount of tissue affected
    - Extremities (ear tips, toes, tail tip) may slough or require amputation without affecting quality of life or longevity.
    - More substantial frostbite (e.g., limbs) carries a greater risk of systemic complications such as infection and therefore a more guarded prognosis.
- Hypothermia may complicate frostbite and alter the prognosis, depending on severity.

PEARLS & CONSIDERATIONS

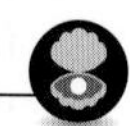

Comments

In some hypothermic animals, neurologic status cannot be ascertained until confounding variables (e.g., hypotension, hypothermia) have been corrected. Caution is advised regarding prognostication early in the course of hospitalization.

Prevention

Bring animals indoors during periods of very low ambient temperature.

Technician Tips

Wear gloves when handling frostbitten regions to reduce the risk of infecting the patient.

SUGGESTED READING

Swaim SF: Trauma to the skin and subcutaneous tissues of dogs and cats. Vet Clin North Am Small Anim Pract 10:599-618, 1980.

AUTHOR: Geoff Heffner, DVM, DACVECC
EDITOR: Benjamin M. Brainard, VMD, DACVAA, DACVECC

Fungal Infections, Opportunistic

Bonus Material Online 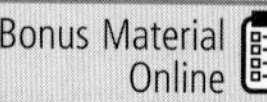

BASIC INFORMATION

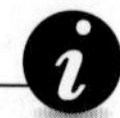

Definition

Infection of cutaneous tissues occurs with saprophytic fungal organisms found in the environment (soil). These organisms lack distinct morphologic characteristics that allow identification to the genus and species level based on cytologic or histopathologic exam alone. Instead, they are typically broken down into categories based on the presence of fungal melanin in cell walls. *Phaeohyphomycosis* refers to infection with pigmented hyphae or yeastlike cells, whereas the term *hyalohyphomycosis* is used to describe infections with clear or hyaline hyphae (excluding the genera *Aspergillus* or *Penicillium* or the class Zygomycetes).

Epidemiology

SPECIES, AGE, SEX

Dogs are most commonly affected. This is likely due to the increased incidence of immune-mediated disease and treatment with immunosuppressive therapy in this species.

RISK FACTORS

- Exposure to outdoors
- Use of cyclosporine or other immunosuppressive therapies
- Risk may increase with each additional immunosuppressive drug added

CONTAGION AND ZOONOSIS

Infection is contracted through contact with organisms in the environment. No animal-to-animal or animal-to-human transmission has been reported.

GEOGRAPHY AND SEASONALITY

Worldwide

ASSOCIATED DISORDERS

Seen in animals on immunosuppressive therapy, often for immune-mediated disease requiring multiple immunosuppressive agents; especially if cyclosporine is being used

Clinical Presentation

DISEASE FORMS/SUBTYPES

- Phaeohyphomycosis: cutaneous nodules or draining lesions generally present on the digits, paw pads, and skin of immunocompromised dogs and cats. Although these lesions are typically locally invasive, dissemination to regional lymph nodes, bone, and beyond have been reported.
- Hyalohyphomycosis: typically, patients have ulcerative, draining skin lesions. Dissemination has been noted to lymph node, bone, kidney, heart, pericardium, and liver. Systemic spread appears to occur more often with hyalohyphomycosis than phaeohyphomycosis.

HISTORY, CHIEF COMPLAINT

New-onset skin lesions usually occur in dogs and cats receiving combination immunosuppressive therapy (especially protocols involving cyclosporine). Bone involvement may lead to lameness as a presenting complaint. With disseminated infection, weight loss, lethargy, or other signs may be reported.

PHYSICAL EXAM FINDINGS

- Multifocal cutaneous lesions commonly occur on the digits and may be grossly pigmented.
- Lymphadenomegaly
- Other findings possible if infection is disseminated (e.g., lameness, hepatomegaly)

Etiology and Pathophysiology

- Causative agents are soil saprophytes and typically do not cause disease unless host defenses are diminished.
- Organisms are transmitted by cutaneous inoculation from the environment.
- Disease typically remains locally invasive, but spread to the regional lymph nodes and other sites has been reported.

DIAGNOSIS

Diagnostic Overview

Fungal culture is ideal, but not always performed because these infections are sometimes not considered at the time of initial sample collection.

Differential Diagnosis

- Neoplasia
- Actinomycosis
- Nocardiosis
- Pythiosis/lagenidiosis
- Sporotrichiosis
- Blastomycosis
- Histoplasmosis
- Cryptococcosis
- Aspergillosis
- Chronic foreign body granulomas

Initial Database

- Cytology of skin lesions, lymph nodes, or other affected tissues reveals irregular, poorly septate fungal hyphae or yeastlike organisms with associated pyogranulomatous inflammation. Fungal melanin can be visualized as brown or green pigmentation of organisms on Wright-Giemsa–stained slides. The absence of pigmentation on cytology does not exclude a diagnosis of phaeohyphomycosis.
- Fungal culture: ideal to submit fresh tissue instead of swabs for culture, and it is recommended to use a laboratory with experience in molecular identification when morphologic features alone are unable to provide definitive identification of fungal organisms to genus and species level, such as the Clinical Bacteriology and Mycology Laboratory at the University of Tennessee College of Veterinary Medicine (https://vetmed.tennessee.edu/vmc/dls/bacteriology/Pages/default.aspx). Culture results should always be interpreted in light of cytologic or histopathologic results because the soil saprophytes can be common laboratory contaminants.

Advanced or Confirmatory Testing

Histopathology shows thick-walled, irregularly septate hyphae or yeastlike cells with associated pyogranulomatous inflammation. Fontana-Mason stain can be used to evaluate fungal melanin.

TREATMENT

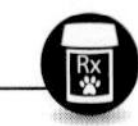

Treatment Overview

Treatment usually begins by reducing or discontinuing immunosuppressive therapy. Unfortunately, most immunosuppressed animals have multifocal disease, precluding surgical removal of dermal lesions. Systemic medical therapy with azole antifungals is typically recommended for at least 6 months or 2 months after resolution of the lesion.

Acute General Treatment

- Lesions may resolve with discontinuation of immunosuppressive therapy alone; however, oral azole therapy is typically also recommended, especially in cases where immunosuppressive drug therapy cannot be altered.
- Itraconazole 10 mg/kg/day PO is the treatment of choice (innovator formulated or generic itraconazole). Compounded formulations should not be used due to poor oral bioavailability.
- Use of newer-generation azoles, such as posaconazole and voriconazole, may be warranted in cases that fail to respond to itraconazole therapy or if there is dissemination. Patients with disseminated disease may also benefit from treatment with amphotericin B along with an oral azole.
- Terbinafine may increase efficacy if used in conjunction with azole antifungals.

Possible Complications

- Systemic dissemination can occur, especially if immunocompetence is not restored.
- Itraconazole at high doses may cause vasculitis and ulcerative skin lesions.
- Itraconazole can cause hepatopathy.
- Amphotericin B is nephrotoxic.

Recommended Monitoring

Liver enzymes should be monitored monthly when treating with azole antifungals because increased activity may indicate hepatotoxicity. If amphotericin is used, urinalysis and serum chemistry profile must be closely monitored to minimize nephrotoxicity.

PROGNOSIS & OUTCOME

Prognosis is good if immunosuppressive drug therapy can be altered and lesions are dermal. Patients with disseminated disease have a guarded to poor prognosis.

PEARLS & CONSIDERATIONS

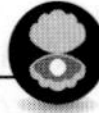

Comments

Predisposition to opportunistic fungal infection is often related to iatrogenic immunosuppression. When iatrogenic causes are not apparent, evaluation for predisposing systemic disease (e.g., neoplasia, endocrinopathy, other infections) is warranted.

Prevention

Avoid excessive or long-term immunosuppression (especially with cyclosporine) in dogs and cats to prevent development of these infections.

Technician Tips

Check the digits and paws of all patients receiving immunosuppressive drug therapy.

SUGGESTED READING

Grooters AM: Miscellaneous fungal diseases. In Sykes JE, editor: Canine and feline infectious diseases, ed 1, St. Louis, 2014, Saunders, pp 660-663.

AUTHOR: Andrea Dedeaux, DVM, DACVIM
EDITOR: Joseph Taboada, DVM, DACVIM

Gallbladder Mucocele

Video Available 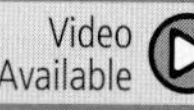 Client Education Sheet

BASIC INFORMATION 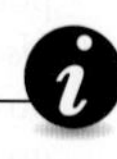

Definition

An accumulation of bile-laden mucus within the gallbladder (GB). Histologic exam of the GB wall shows cystic mucinous hyperplasia. GB mucocele is the most common reason for biliary surgery in dogs.

Synonyms

Kiwi gallbladder, cystic mucinous hyperplasia of the gallbladder

Epidemiology

SPECIES, AGE, SEX

Older, small or medium-sized dogs; no sex predisposition reported; one feline case reported

GENETICS, BREED PREDISPOSITION

Cocker spaniels, Shetland sheepdogs, border terriers, and miniature schnauzers are predisposed. An insertion mutation in the *ABCB4* gene was suggested as an underlying cause, but it has not been verified by additional studies.

RISK FACTORS

Hyperadrenocorticism (spontaneous or iatrogenic), hypothyroidism, imidacloprid use

ASSOCIATED DISORDERS

Bile peritonitis with secondary septic peritonitis, extrahepatic biliary obstruction

Clinical Presentation

HISTORY, CHIEF COMPLAINT

- May be an incidental finding on abdominal ultrasonography (US)
- Clinically affected patients often vomit, along with inappetence, and lethargy
- Other complaints include weight loss, diarrhea, ptyalism, and polyuria/polydipsia.

PHYSICAL EXAM FINDINGS

Abdominal pain, ascites, tachypnea, tachycardia, fever, and icterus are all possible in advanced cases.

Etiology and Pathophysiology

- Likely triggered by production of abnormal gel-forming mucins by the GB epithelium; this changes the physical and functional properties of GB mucus.
- Cystic mucinous hyperplasia of GB epithelium is probably a response to abnormal mucus production.
- Abnormal mucins result in accumulation of mucus and inspissated bile.
- The association between biliary sludge and mucocele formation is unclear.
- Pressure necrosis of the GB wall may result in rupture.

DIAGNOSIS 

Diagnostic Overview

- GB mucocele can be an incidental finding or responsible for the presenting complaint.
- Abdominal US is the standard diagnostic tool. GB contents in nonruptured cases are hyperechoic and non–gravity dependent, with a classic stellate pattern (hence the terms *kiwi* or *starfish* GB).
- GB rupture may be associated with focal or generalized peritonitis, indicated by fluid around the GB (+/− elsewhere in the abdomen) and inflammation of adjacent structures.

Differential Diagnosis

For vomiting with elevated liver enzyme activities +/− icterus:

- Pancreatitis
- Acute hepatotoxicosis
- Cholecystitis (acute, chronic, or necrotizing)
- Cholelithiasis
- Acute or chronic hepatitis

For hyperechoic GB contents on US:

- GB sludge (gravity dependent, unlike GB mucocele)

Initial Database

- CBC: neutrophilic leukocytosis with monocytosis if clinical signs present
- Serum biochemistry profile: elevated alanine aminotransferase (ALT), alkaline phosphatase (ALP), aspartate aminotransferase (AST), and gamma-glutamyltransferase (GGT) activities. Serum bilirubin concentration is high in most clinically ill patients. Hypercholesterolemia, hyperglobulinemia, and hypoalbuminemia may be noted.
- Urinalysis: generally unremarkable; bilirubinuria possible (nonspecific)
- Abdominal radiography: generally unremarkable. In cases with GB rupture, decreased serosal detail may be noted.
- Abdominal US: characteristic stellate/striated intraluminal GB contents (see *Video*); subjective GB distention can be noted. The GB wall should be assessed for integrity.
- After GB rupture, free abdominal fluid may be seen; the fluid should be analyzed for evidence of sepsis and/or bile peritonitis. Concurrent pancreatitis and inflammation of adjacent structures may be noted. In rare cases, the mucocele may be free in the abdominal cavity.

Advanced or Confirmatory Testing

- At surgery, GB contents are solid and rubbery or semiliquid, with lumps of organized mucus.
- Histopathologic exam of the GB wall confirms cystic mucinous hyperplasia.

TREATMENT 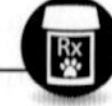

Treatment Overview

- Surgical intervention is indicated in sick dogs, with cholecystectomy generally considered the treatment of choice.
- Prophylactic laparoscopic or open surgical cholecystectomy may be considered in stable patients without evidence of GB rupture or peritonitis.
- Medical therapy can be considered in patients with minimal clinical compromise and no evidence of GB wall compromise.
- Dogs should be screened for underlying endocrinopathy and treated as indicated.

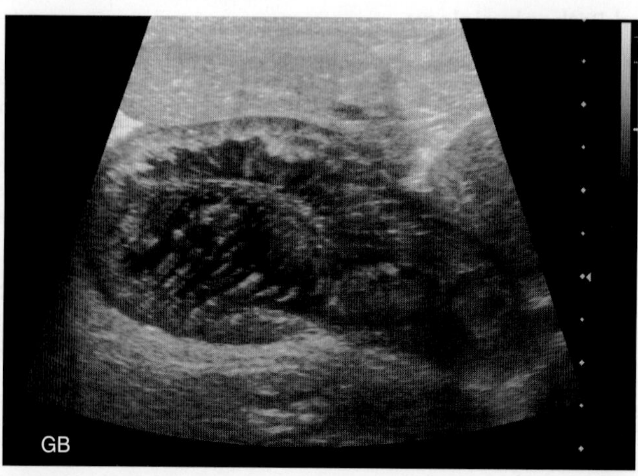

GALLBLADDER MUCOCELE Ultrasonographic image of a gallbladder mucocele. Note the classic kiwi appearance.

Acute General Treatment

- Immediate laparotomy is indicated for cases of suspected GB rupture. Affected patients are often hemodynamically unstable and require intensive perioperative supportive care.
- Initial presurgical therapy generally includes fluid therapy, broad-spectrum intravenous antibiotics, antiemetics, and analgesics.
- Cholecystectomy is the treatment of choice.
- During surgery, confirmation of patency of the common BD is imperative. Gastrointestinal and hepatic biopsies should be considered.
- Samples of GB wall and/or intraluminal contents should be collected for aerobic and anaerobic culture.
- Consider placing an esophagostomy tube to facilitate postoperative nutritional support (p. 1106).

Chronic Treatment

Nonsurgical resolution of GB mucocele has been reported using ursodiol 7.5 mg/kg PO q 12h, low-fat diet (<2 g/100 kcal), and management of concurrent endocrinopathies.

Nutrition/Diet

Low-fat diets are advised as part of chronic management and in the postoperative period. Many dogs eventually tolerate standard diets after cholecystectomy.

Possible Complications

- Postoperative complications include pancreatitis, peritonitis, sepsis, and disseminated intravascular coagulation.
- Obstruction of the common bile duct has been reported; patency must be confirmed during surgery.
- Patients managed medically may fail to respond as expected, with subsequent GB obstruction, necrosis, or other sequelae.

Recommended Monitoring

Serial US q 3 months is essential for patients managed medically. Failure to resolve mucocele may be indication for surgical intervention in well dogs.

PROGNOSIS & OUTCOME

- Perioperative mortality rate is approximately 25%.
- The long-term prognosis for postoperative patients surviving to release from hospital is good.
- Studies differ regarding impact of GB rupture on mortality rates in dogs treated by cholecystectomy.
- Diffuse bile peritonitis carries a guarded to grave prognosis.

PEARLS & CONSIDERATIONS

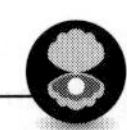

Comments

- Mucocele rupture does not preclude a successful outcome.
- Always confirm patency of the common BD after cholecystectomy.
- Identify and manage underlying endocrine disorders (e.g., hypothyroidism, hyperadrenocorticism) in patients treated medically.
- Consider elective cholecystectomy if medical management is unsuccessful after 6 months.

Technician Tips

- Postoperative hypotension and hyperlactatemia are associated with poor outcome after cholecystectomy.
- Low-fat diets should be offered in the postoperative period.

SUGGESTED READING

Malek S, et al: Clinical findings and prognostic factors for dogs undergoing cholecystectomy for gallbladder mucocele. Vet Surg 42:418-426, 2013.

AUTHOR: Audrey K. Cook, BVM&S, DACVIM, DECVIM, DABVP
EDITOR: Keith P. Richter, DVM, MSEL, DACVIM

Gallbladder Rupture

Client Education Sheet

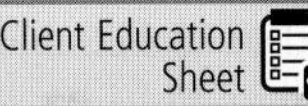

BASIC INFORMATION

Definition

Loss of gallbladder wall integrity

Epidemiology

SPECIES, AGE, SEX

Dogs:

- Trauma: younger (mean, 2.8 years)
- Intrinsic gallbladder disease: middle- to older-aged dogs (mean, 8.1 years)

Cats: uncommon

GENETICS, BREED PREDISPOSITION

Shetland sheepdogs and possibly cocker spaniels are overrepresented.

ASSOCIATED DISORDERS

Dogs:

- Cholelithiasis, cholecystitis, bile peritonitis, sepsis
- Gallbladder mucocele (p. 374)
- Gallbladder infarction
- Hypothyroidism and hyperadrenocorticism may predispose a subset of dogs to gallbladder infarction/rupture.

Clinical Presentation

DISEASE FORMS/SUBTYPES

- Gallbladder infarction/necrotizing cholecystitis:
  - Without rupture
  - With hepatic and omental adhesions and possibly fistulas to other abdominal structures
  - With gallbladder perforation and diffuse peritonitis
- Gallbladder perforation associated with penetrating trauma and subsequent bile peritonitis

HISTORY, CHIEF COMPLAINT

- Nonspecific signs: vomiting, anorexia, weakness, polydipsia, polyuria, weight loss. Can be chronic (duration from onset of signs to presentation: up to 1 month; mean, 12 days)
- Some owners may notice icterus, discolored urine (bilirubinuria)

PHYSICAL EXAM FINDINGS

- Icterus: very common (77% of bile peritonitis cases)
- Abdominal distention: common (65% of bile peritonitis cases), may be subtle
- Signs of abdominal pain
- Pyrexia
- Shock

Etiology and Pathophysiology

- Causes of gallbladder rupture
  - Necrotizing cholecystitis
  - Gallbladder infarction
  - Abdominal trauma: penetrating or blunt
  - Inadequate choleresis due to excessively thick bile, mucocele, defective gallbladder contractility, and/or altered outflow
  - Bile duct obstruction: rare
- Gallbladder rupture may result in development of septic or nonseptic peritonitis (p. 779).
- Lack of bile secretion into the intestine results in lack of digestion and absorption of fat and fat-soluble vitamins, most importantly vitamin K (coagulopathy).

DIAGNOSIS

Diagnostic Overview

The diagnosis is suspected based on nonspecific history and physical exam finding of icterus

+/− abdominal signs. Confirmation requires abdominal ultrasound exam and peritoneal fluid analysis.

Differential Diagnosis

Icterus: (p. 1243)
- Prehepatic: hemolysis
- Hepatic diseases
- Extrahepatic biliary obstruction: choleliths, pancreatitis, cholangitis, neoplasia, stricture, gallbladder mucocele
- Biliary leakage from other parts of the biliary system (traumatic rupture of the common or hepatic bile ducts)

Abdominal distention (if icterus not apparent) (p. 1192):
- Septic peritonitis: gastrointestinal perforation, penetrating trauma
- Uroabdomen
- Hemoabdomen: ruptured mass/viscus, bleeding disorder
- Abdominal organ dilation/enlargement: gastric dilation/volvulus, mesenteric volvulus, splenic torsion, overeating, hyperadrenocorticism
- Intraabdominal abscess: severe pancreatitis, hepatic abscess, ruptured prostatic abscess, ruptured pyometra
- Portal hypertension
- Congestive heart failure (right-sided)

Initial Database

CBC:
- Inflammatory leukogram
- Degenerative left shift with toxic changes (septic bile peritonitis)

Serum biochemistry profile:
- Elevated bilirubin concentration (virtually all cases)
- Elevated liver enzyme concentrations (virtually all cases)
- Hypokalemia

Survey abdominal radiographs:
- Increased opacity/loss of detail in anterior abdomen
- Cholelithiasis (in dogs, 14%-48% are radiopaque)
- Generalized loss of abdominal detail/fluid (bile peritonitis)

Advanced or Confirmatory Testing

Abdominal ultrasound exam:
- Evaluate gallbladder wall thickness and integrity (cholecystitis), contents (choleliths, mucocele), presence of attached omentum, and surrounding fluid, suggesting bile peritonitis or unrelated (e.g., other differential diagnoses)

Peritoneal fluid analysis (obtained during abdominal ultrasound exam):
- Bilirubin concentration: more than twice that of serum bilirubin is diagnostic of bile peritonitis
- Cytologic evaluation and bacterial culture and sensitivity testing (aerobic and anaerobic): possible septic peritonitis

Coagulation profile:
- Prothrombin time is first to be abnormal with vitamin K deficiency/malabsorption.
- Thromboelastography and D-dimers (p. 1334) to identify hypercoagulable state

TREATMENT

Treatment Overview

Treatment consists of patient stabilization followed by surgical exploration of the abdomen, with removal of the ruptured gallbladder and treatment of associated bile peritonitis. Adjunctive pain control is important.

Acute General Treatment

- Rehydration: intravenous administration of balanced electrolyte solution
  - Normalization of serum electrolyte concentrations
- Parenteral antibiotics effective against gram-negative bacteria and anaerobes based on culture and susceptibility results. Initial options for empirical therapy:
  - Cefoxitin 30 mg/kg IV q 2h perioperatively, then q 6h (dogs and cats) and add ampicillin 22 mg/kg IV q 6-8h for gram-positive coverage, *or*
  - Metronidazole 7.5-15 mg/kg IV q 12h *with* enrofloxacin 5 mg/kg q 12h or 10-15 mg/kg IV q 24h for dogs (maximum 5 mg/kg/day for cats due to retinopathy risk); use small-animal enrofloxacin preparation, diluted and given slowly.
- Possible administration of fresh-frozen plasma for coagulopathy (also provides minimal colloid support) (p. 1169)
- Vitamin K 2.5 mg/kg SQ q 12h × 3 days, then weekly
- Exploratory laparotomy after animal is stabilized:
  - Cholecystectomy
  - Ensure patency and integrity of biliary system.
  - Aerobic and anaerobic microbiologic culture of peritoneal fluid
  - Treatment of bile peritonitis: consider open peritoneal drainage

Chronic Treatment

Maintenance of bile flow: ursodeoxycholic acid 10-15 mg/kg PO q 24h; give only after biliary obstruction is definitively ruled out/corrected

Nutrition/Diet

Nutritional support by placement of feeding tube if indicated (pp. 1106, 1107, and 1109):
- Gastrostomy/jejunostomy tubes may be placed intraoperatively.

Possible Complications

- Ongoing/recurrent bile leakage
- Failure to resolve septic bile peritonitis
  - Endotoxemia
  - Sepsis
- Biliary obstruction
  - Recurrence of cholelithiasis
- Pancreatitis
- Hypercoagulability with possible pulmonary thromboembolism

Recommended Monitoring

- Frequent initial assessment of clinical and laboratory parameters: respiratory rate/effort, perfusion (including capillary refill time), pulse rate and quality, blood pressure, urine output, arterial pH, and lactate concentrations
- Serum liver enzymes and bilirubin concentrations
- Coagulation profile including D-dimer levels, thromboelastography

PROGNOSIS & OUTCOME

- Guarded to fair in animals with aseptic bile peritonitis
- Poor to guarded in animals with septic bile peritonitis

PEARLS & CONSIDERATIONS

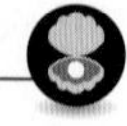

Comments

In dogs and cats with bile peritonitis:
- Peripheral white blood cell count is significantly lower in survivors (mean, 20,608/mcL) compared with nonsurvivors (mean, 35,715/mcL).
- The immature neutrophil count is significantly lower in survivors (mean, 686/mcL) than in nonsurvivors (mean, 4852/mcL).

Technician Tips

Change in respiratory rate or effort can be an early sign of pulmonary thromboembolism. Do not assume it is due to pain alone.

SUGGESTED READING

Crews LJ, et al: Clinical, ultrasonographic, and laboratory findings associated with gallbladder disease and rupture in dogs: 45 cases (1997-2007). J Am Vet Med Assoc 234:359-366, 2009.

AUTHOR: David Holt, BVSc, DACVS
EDITOR: Elizabeth A. Swanson, DVM, MS, DACVS

Gastric Dilation/Volvulus

Client Education Sheet 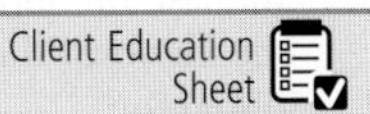

BASIC INFORMATION

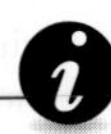

Definition

Rotation of the stomach on its mesenteric axis is associated with gastric distention and well recognized in large- and giant-breed dogs.

Synonyms

Bloat, gastric torsion, GDV

Epidemiology

SPECIES, AGE, SEX

Risk of gastric dilation/volvulus (GDV) increases with age; rarely reported in small dogs or cats

GENETICS, BREED PREDISPOSITION

- Large- and giant-breed dogs
- Great Dane, German shepherd, Weimaraner, Saint Bernard, Gordon setter, Irish setter, Doberman pinscher, Old English sheepdog, and standard poodle are overrepresented.
- Having a first-degree relative with GDV confers an increased risk.

RISK FACTORS

Increased risk may be associated with

- Narrow and deep thoracic cavity
- Stress
- Fearful temperament
- Being underweight
- Nutritional risk factors include once-daily feeding, feeding dry dog food, rapid ingestion of food, consumption of large volumes of food, and eating from a raised feeding bowl.
- Conflicting reports regarding risk associated with prior splenectomy

GEOGRAPHY AND SEASONALITY

Possible increased incidence in the months of November, December, and January (United States)

ASSOCIATED DISORDERS

- Inflammatory bowel disease
- Gastric foreign body or mass
- Hypovolemic shock
- Cardiac arrhythmias

Clinical Presentation

HISTORY, CHIEF COMPLAINT

- Acute onset abdominal distention
- Abdominal pain
- Restlessness
- Ptyalism
- Retching or vomiting (nonproductive with volvulus)
- Acute collapse

PHYSICAL EXAM FINDINGS

- Abdominal distention and tympany
  - Simultaneous auscultation and percussion of the abdomen may reveal a tympanic sound, indicating a taut, gas-filled stomach.
- Splenomegaly
- Clinical signs of hypovolemic shock: weak pulses, tachycardia, pale mucous membranes, prolonged capillary refill time, dyspnea

Etiology and Pathophysiology

- In most cases, the pylorus moves ventrally and from right to left; the rotation may be 90°-360°.
- Gastric dilation occurs secondary to failure of eructation and pyloric outflow obstruction. Dilation can occur before or after gastric rotation.
- The distended stomach results in caudal vena cava and portal vein compression, causing decreased venous return to the heart.
- Decreased venous return results in decreased cardiac output, decreased arterial blood pressure, and myocardial ischemia.
- Myocardial ischemia causes cardiac arrhythmias.
- In the case of volvulus, increased intraluminal gastric pressure, portal hypertension, and avulsion of the short gastric vessels compromise blood flow to the gastric wall. Gastric necrosis and perforation can result. Breakdown of gastrointestinal mucosa allows bacterial translocation.
- Portal vein compression/hypertension causes sequestration of splanchnic blood and decreased ability to clear gram-negative endotoxins.
- Endotoxemia further potentiates hypotension and decreased cardiac output.
- Pressure on the diaphragm, decreased lung perfusion, and decreased lung compliance cause respiratory dysfunction and exacerbate tissue hypoxia.

DIAGNOSIS

Diagnostic Overview

GDV should be suspected in large- or giant-breed dogs presenting with an acute history of a distended or painful abdomen, often with preceding or concurrent attempts at vomiting. Physical exam usually reveals a tympanic abdomen and often signs of shock. Treatment for shock is initiated before confirming the diagnosis with radiography.

Differential Diagnosis

- Gastric bloat associated with overeating
- Mesenteric volvulus
- Splenic torsion
- Diaphragmatic hernia with stomach herniation

Initial Database

- Abdominal radiographs
  - Right lateral view is preferred.
  - Shows gas-filled pylorus cranial and dorsal to the fundus (Popeye sign, C sign, or double bubble)
  - Free abdominal air suggests gastric perforation.
- Quick assessment tests
  - Packed cell volume/total solids (PCV/TS): often increased due to hypovolemia
  - Serum electrolyte and glucose concentrations: +/− hypokalemia and hypoglycemia
  - Acid-base analysis: metabolic acidosis due to lactic acidosis is frequently present.
- Coagulation panel and platelet count: thrombocytopenia, increased prothrombin time/activated partial thromboplastin time/fibrinogen concentration and/or fibrin degradation product concentration associated with disseminated intravascular coagulation (DIC)
- Electrocardiogram (ECG [p. 1094]): ventricular arrhythmias are common.

Advanced or Confirmatory Testing

- Definitive diagnosis confirmed at surgery
- Plasma lactate concentration: may assist in determining prognosis. In dogs, a cutoff of 7.4 mmol/L at admission correctly predicts presence or absence of gastric necrosis with 82% accuracy and survival versus euthanasia/death with 88% accuracy.

TREATMENT

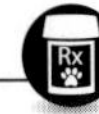

Treatment Overview

The initial therapeutic goal is to manage hypovolemia with intravenous (IV) fluids and to decompress the stomach to re-establish systemic and gastric perfusion. Definitive treatment involves surgery to correct the position of the stomach, remove devitalized tissue, and perform a gastropexy to prevent recurrence.

Acute General Treatment

- Place large-bore IV catheters in both cephalic veins or cephalic and jugular veins, and infuse isotonic crystalloids at an initial dose of 20 mL/kg as fast as possible to effect (lowered heart rate, raised blood pressure). Additional doses can be given if needed. Colloids can be administered in combination with crystalloids at 5-20 mL/kg over 15-30 minutes. For severe shock, hypertonic saline can be administered at 4 mL/kg over 10-15 minutes, followed by crystalloids (p. 911).
- Administer parenteral prophylactic antibiotics (e.g., cefoxitin 30 mg/kg IV perioperatively, then q 6h).
- Decompress the stomach by orogastric intubation (p. 1117).
- If orogastric intubation is not possible and patient has visible abdominal distention with a radiographically confirmed GDV, perform percutaneous trocarization of the stomach:
  - Aseptically clip and prepare an area on the dorsolateral abdomen, just caudal to

the last rib and ventral to the hypaxial muscles over the region of most obvious distention.
  ◦ Using a large-bore needle or needle-styleted catheter (e.g., 16 or 14 gauge) directed ventrally and slightly cranially, penetrate all layers of the body wall and stomach. When successful, the procedure should produce a hissing sound associated with a release of fetid-smelling gas through the needle.
- Immediate surgery to derotate the stomach and return it to a normal position
  ◦ Placing traction on the pylorus and elevating it while putting downward (dorsal) pressure on the fundus aids derotation in a counterclockwise direction (most but not all cases are rotated clockwise).
  ◦ Evaluate stomach and spleen for irreversible vascular compromise and necrosis.
  ◦ Perform partial or complete splenectomy if splenic necrosis, infarction, or torsion. Perform resection of necrotic areas of stomach.
  ◦ Perform gastropexy of pyloric antrum to the right body wall.
- Medical treatment alone (repeated intubation, trocarization) has been uniformly ineffective and is not recommended.

Chronic Treatment

- Postoperative potassium supplementation if hypokalemic (do not exceed 0.5 mEq/kg/h IV [p. 516]).
- If ventricular arrhythmias are noted on the electrocardiogram (ECG [p. 1033])
  ◦ Is hypokalemia present? If so, institute potassium replacement immediately. Ventricular arrhythmias are refractory to treatment with lidocaine, procainamide, and other antiarrhythmics when hypokalemia is present.
  ◦ Hypomagnesemia may also predispose patient to ventricular arrhythmias.
  ◦ Is anemia, hypoxemia, or acidosis present? Many ventricular arrhythmias resolve spontaneously if systemic abnormalities are corrected.
  ◦ Is the heart rate rapid (>160 beats/min) or the pulse weak despite addressing the systemic abnormalities? If so, consider treatment with lidocaine (p. 1457). If arrhythmia and tachycardia continue for days, treat with oral sotalol 0.5-2 mg/kg q 12h.
- Treat peritonitis (p. 779) if gastric perforation has occurred (fluids, antibiotics, abdominal lavage ± drainage).
- Treat gastric ulceration: proton pump inhibitors (omeprazole 0.7-1 mg/kg PO q 12-24h or pantoprazole 0.7 mg/kg IV q 24h) with or without H2-receptor antagonists (famotidine 0.5-1 mg/kg IV, IM, SQ, or PO q 12-24h, *or* ranitidine 0.5-2 mg/kg IV, IM, SQ, or PO q 8-12h) and sucralfate slurry (0.5-1 g/dose PO q 6-8h)
- Use drugs that increase gastric motility (e.g., metoclopramide 0.2-0.4 mg/kg PO, SQ, or IM q 8h or 1-2 mg/kg/d IV as a continuous infusion, *or* cisapride 0.1-0.5 mg/kg PO q 8h) if recurrent bloating occurs after gastropexy, without evidence of gastric outflow obstruction.
- Pain management is important (e.g., fentanyl 3-5 mcg/kg/h), but nonsteroidal antiinflammatory drugs are contraindicated.

Nutrition/Diet

- Enteral/oral feeding can begin the day after surgery if the patient is not vomiting.
- Several recommendations are made to prevent gastric bloat after discharge or to prevent GDV in dogs that have not had a gastropexy:
  ◦ Divide feedings into several small meals each day.
  ◦ Do not feed dry kibble.
  ◦ Avoid stress during feeding.
  ◦ Avoid heavy activity immediately after eating or drinking.
  ◦ Do not elevate feeding bowl during eating.
  ◦ Regular moderate activity outside may decrease risk.

Possible Complications

- Cardiac arrhythmias
- Reperfusion injury
- Gastric necrosis, perforation, and peritonitis can occur if devitalized gastric tissue is not excised.
- Gastric ulceration
- Esophagitis and regurgitation
- Gastroparesis and ileus
- DIC
- Aspiration pneumonia
- Acute kidney injury
- Recurrence of dilation
- Recurrence of volvulus if gastropexy is not performed properly

Recommended Monitoring

- ECG: ventricular arrhythmias common within 36 hours of surgery
- Blood pressure (p. 1065)
- Serum chemistry and electrolyte concentrations: correct hypokalemia, hypoglycemia
- PCV/TS: hemoconcentration indicates need for increased fluid therapy. Anemia can occur from bleeding of torn short gastric vessels.
- Physical parameters: mucous membrane color, capillary refill, pulse quality, heart rate, temperature, respiratory effort, lung auscultation, abdominal distention, bruising

PROGNOSIS & OUTCOME

- GDV patients treated surgically have ≈15% mortality rate.
- Gastric necrosis and need for gastric resection or splenectomy with or without partial gastrectomy are associated with increased mortality rate.
- Increased risk of death if
  ◦ Clinical signs are present for > 6 hours before exam
  ◦ Hypothermia is present
  ◦ Hypotension is present
  ◦ Peritonitis is present
  ◦ DIC is present
  ◦ Preoperative arrhythmias are present
- Serum lactate level in dogs with GDV (see above)
  ◦ 99% survival if < 6 mmol/L at presentation
  ◦ Initial values may not be as predictive as lack of improvement in values after

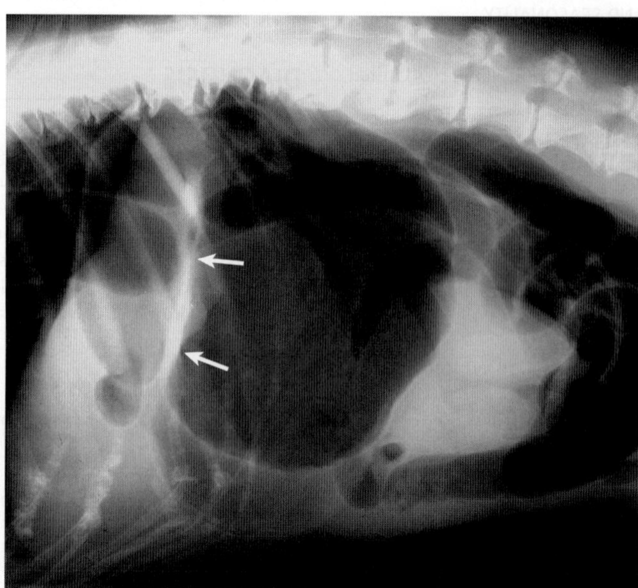

GASTRIC DILATION/VOLVULUS Lateral abdominal radiograph of a dog with gastric dilation/volvulus. Characteristic septation *(arrows)* of the gastric shadow is seen. A displaced, gas-filled antrum is cranial to the *arrows* (left on this image), whereas a gas-filled fundus is caudal (*arrows* are within it). A gas-filled esophagus and evidence of ileus in the form of distended, gas-filled small intestine can be seen. (Courtesy Dr. Richard Walshaw.)

treatment. Decreased survival is associated with lactate > 6.4 mmol/L, absolute change < 4 mmol/L, or a percentage change < 42.5% of the original value or with < 50% decrease in lactate within 12 hours of presentation.

PEARLS & CONSIDERATIONS

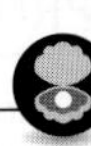

Comments

- Begin fluid resuscitation before abdominal radiography.
- Do not assume the stomach is not rotated just because a stomach tube can be passed.
- Assess suspect areas of stomach for viability 10-15 minutes after derotation by palpation, evaluating blood flow, and stomach wall color. If stomach wall is green or gray or the wall is thin on palpation, the area needs to be resected.
- Ventricular arrhythmia indicates the need to evaluate for hypokalemia, hypomagnesemia, anemia, hypoxemia, pain, or acidosis that must be corrected for the arrhythmia to resolve.

Prevention

- See Nutrition/Diet above.
- Do not breed dogs with history of GDV.
- Prophylactic gastropexy is recommended in breeds at high risk for GDV.
  - Performed during ovariohysterectomy or as an elective procedure
  - Commonly performed by laparoscopy

Technician Tips

- Place large-bore catheters in cephalic or jugular veins immediately for fluid therapy.
- Monitor for pulse deficits and rapid heart rate with weak pulses.

SUGGESTED READING

Beck JJ, et al: Risk factors associated with short-term outcome and development of perioperative complications in dogs undergoing surgery because of gastric dilatation-volvulus: 166 cases (1992-2003). J Am Vet Med Assoc 229:1934-1939, 2006.

AUTHOR: Lori Ludwig, VMD, MS, DACVS
EDITOR: Elizabeth A. Swanson, DVM, MS, DACVS

Gastric Neoplasia

Client Education Sheet 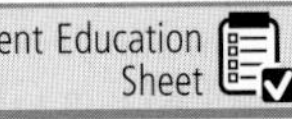

BASIC INFORMATION

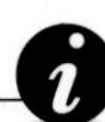

Definition

Benign or malignant tumors of epithelial, lymphoid, or mesenchymal origin affect gastric function, are often painful, and may cause secondary systemic effects such as electrolyte disturbances, anemia, and weight loss.

Synonyms

Gastric adenocarcinoma, gastric adenoma, gastric polyps (benign), gastric carcinoma, gastric extramedullary plasmacytoma, gastric lymphoma (p. 604), gastrointestinal stromal tumor (GIST), leiomyoma, leiomyosarcoma, scirrhous carcinoma

Epidemiology

SPECIES, AGE, SEX

- In dogs, gastric tumors account for < 1% of all malignancies.
  - Median age for adenocarcinoma is 10 years.
  - Median age for leiomyomas and GIST is 11 years.
- In cats > 7 years old, gastric tumors are most commonly lymphoma.

GENETICS, BREED PREDISPOSITION

- Gastric adenocarcinomas: rough collies, Staffordshire terriers, Belgian shepherds, chow chows (may be familial)
- Leiomyoma and GIST: German shepherds

RISK FACTORS

Gastric adenocarcinomas:

- Chronic nitrosamine exposure experimentally
- Association of gastric carcinoma and lymphoma with chronic inflammation from *Helicobacter pylori* infection in people; suspected in companion animals

CONTAGION AND ZOONOSIS

- *Helicobacter* spp organisms are often found in normal dogs and cats, but pathologic importance is not firmly established.
- Zoonotic potential exists for *H. pylori*, but prevalence in animals is low.

ASSOCIATED DISORDERS

Gastric lymphoma in cats is generally not associated with retroviral infection (e.g., feline leukemia virus, feline immunodeficiency virus).

Clinical Presentation

HISTORY, CHIEF COMPLAINT

- Chronic vomiting
- Hematemesis/melena
- Anorexia, weight loss
- Depression and lethargy
- Pain or restlessness

PHYSICAL EXAM FINDINGS

Physical exam may be normal or include some or all of the following:

- Poor body condition (e.g., body condition score < 4/9)
- Pale mucous membranes, other signs of anemia (e.g., tachycardia)
- Abdominal mass
- Abdominal pain

Etiology and Pathophysiology

- Chronic vomiting may result in weight loss and electrolyte imbalance.
- Anemia secondary to chronic gastrointestinal (GI) bleeding may be hypochromic or microcytic due to iron depletion.
- Panhypoproteinemia due to GI blood loss
- Hypoglycemia may occur secondary to insulin-like growth factor 2 release from smooth muscle tumors.
- GISTs are associated with activating mutations of the *KIT* receptor tyrosine kinase oncogene.

DIAGNOSIS

Diagnostic Overview

The diagnosis is suspected when signs of GI disease fail to respond to conservative management and/or are accompanied by systemic disturbances (e.g., weight loss). Radiographs and ultrasound may help localize the lesion; confirmation requires cytology or histopathology.

Differential Diagnosis

Any GI or systemic cause of chronic vomiting may mimic gastric neoplasia (p. 1294):

- Gastric foreign body
- Gastric ulceration
- Granulomatous gastritis
- Infiltrative (inflammatory, infectious, neoplastic) small intestinal disease
- Chronic pancreatitis
- Systemic disease associated with chronic vomiting (e.g., renal, hepatic, hypoadrenocorticism)

Initial Database

- CBC, serum chemistry panel with electrolytes, urinalysis: frequently normal or nonspecific changes secondary to GI electrolyte or blood losses (e.g., nonregenerative anemia, increased blood urea nitrogen with normal creatinine, hypochloremia)
- Three-view thoracic radiographs (metastasis)
- Abdominal ultrasound: assess gastric wall changes often not seen on routine radiographs and rule out other causes of vomiting (e.g., pancreatitis, liver disease); GIST more likely associated with abdominal effusion
- Positive contrast gastrogram (p. 1172): assess for outflow obstruction; does not differentiate

neoplasia from other infiltrative diseases such as pythiosis
- Ultrasound-guided fine-needle aspiration cytology (p. 1112): if a gastric wall abnormality or lymphadenomegaly is present. Lymphoma readily exfoliates; GIST or gastric muscle tumors do not.

Advanced or Confirmatory Testing

- Endoscopic biopsy (p. 1098): for some patients, histopathologic diagnosis is essential for treatment and prognosis. Endoscopy effectively samples mucosal tissue but may be inadequate for tumors in the muscular or serosal layers, requiring surgical biopsy.
- Surgical biopsy: exploratory surgery provides opportunity for diagnosis and treatment (surgical removal of the affected region).
- Diagnosis is confirmed by cytology or biopsy with histopathology, and for some tumors, immunohistochemical (IHC) markers to better define tumor type. Common IHC assessment of gastric tumors includes:
  - Immunohistochemical stains for expression of KIT in GIST
  - Cytokeratin, vimentin immunohistochemistry for undifferentiated tumors
  - Immunophenotyping for lymphoma

TREATMENT

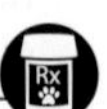

Treatment Overview

Benign gastric lesions and early-diagnosed, low-grade malignancy may be cured surgically. Other surgical goals are to relieve gastric obstruction or remove tumors for clinical palliation. Chemotherapy is potentially helpful in prolonging survival, although malignant gastric tumors are typically incurable.

Acute General Treatment

- Antiemetics: maropitant 1 mg/kg PO, SQ or dolasetron 0.3 mg/kg q 12-24h IV, SQ; metoclopramide should be avoided if obstruction is suspected.
- Gastroprotectants: omeprazole 1 mg/kg PO q 12-24h favored over famotidine 0.5-1 mg/kg IV, PO q 12h
- Rehydration with intravenous fluids, if indicated
- Antibiotics for *Helicobacter* infection, if indicated
- Blood transfusion and hematinic therapy for nonregenerative iron-deficiency anemia, if indicated
- Analgesics as indicated by clinical signs

Chronic Treatment

- Gastric tumor resection often results in motility disorders.
  - May require motility modifiers: metoclopramide 0.2-0.5 mg/kg IV, PO q 6-8h or cisapride 0.5 mg/kg q 8-12h PO
- Chronic antiemetic therapy may be required.
- Chemotherapy with doxorubicin, platinum agents, or antimetabolites may prove helpful.
- Systemic chemotherapy for gastric lymphoma provides remission and prolonged survival (p. 604).
- Receptor tyrosine kinase inhibitor (toceranib 2.5-2.75 mg/kg PO q 48h or M, W, F) for GIST with *KIT* gene mutation requires gastric acid reduction with omeprazole (preferred) or famotidine.

Nutrition/Diet

- Diet modification to easily-digested, high-energy content food
- Parenteral alimentation if the patient has not eaten for > 3 days or is unable or unwilling to eat after surgery

Possible Complications

- Surgical wound dehiscence with secondary peritonitis, pneumoperitoneum
- Chemotherapy-induced neutropenia can predispose to infection; thrombocytopenia can increase gastric hemorrhage.
- Chemotherapy may result in perforation of transmural lesions.

Recommended Monitoring

- Postoperative thoracic radiographs and abdominal ultrasound for recurrence or metastasis every 1-2 months for 1 year
- Monitor CBC for recovery from nonregenerative anemia or chemotherapy-induced myelosuppression.
- Monitor for signs of dissemination of alimentary lymphoma.

PROGNOSIS & OUTCOME

- Favorable for benign lesions (polyps, adenomas, leiomyomas), although complete resection of mesenchymal tumors is unlikely
- Poor for adenocarcinoma, carcinoma, GIST, especially when metastatic
  - These dogs generally do not live beyond 6 months, even with therapy.
- Guarded to fair for focal mass presentation of lymphoma
- Guarded for diffuse or multicentric alimentary lymphoma because lesions typically regress slowly and may have an indolent course but are ultimately incurable

PEARLS & CONSIDERATIONS

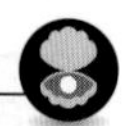

Comments

- Gastric carcinoma is associated with early lymphatic spread. Lymph nodes detected on ultrasound can be aspirated for diagnosis and prognosis.
- Gastric carcinomas may overexpress cyclooxygenase-2; nonsteroidal antiinflammatory drugs (piroxicam 0.3 mg/kg PO q 24h) may be palliative.
- Scirrhous carcinoma is rapidly fatal.

Technician Tips

Monitor for signs of hypotension and abdominal effusion that may indicate gastric perforation.

SUGGESTED READING

Frost D, et al: Gastrointestinal stromal tumors and leiomyomas in the dog: a histopathologic, immunohistochemical and molecular genetic study of 50 cases. Vet Pathol 40:42, 2003.

AUTHOR: Barbara E. Kitchell, DVM, PhD, DACVIM
EDITOR: Rance K. Sellon DVM, PhD, DACVIM

Gastric Ulcers

Client Education Sheet

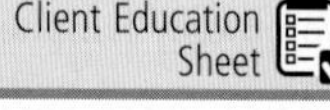

BASIC INFORMATION

Definition

Disruption of the gastric mucosa as a result of coagulative necrosis that breaches the mucosal layer and exposes the submucosa or deeper layers of the stomach wall

Epidemiology

SPECIES, AGE, SEX

Dogs and cats of any age and either sex

RISK FACTORS

- Iatrogenic: administration of cyclooxygenase (COX) inhibitors, other nonsteroidal antiinflammatory drugs (NSAIDs), or corticosteroids
- Hypergastrinemia (e.g., gastrinoma, chronic kidney disease)
- Hyperhistaminemia (high-grade mast cell tumors)
- Severe hypovolemia or ischemia (shock)
- Extremes of exercise (e.g., racing sled dogs, explosive detection)

Clinical Presentation

HISTORY, CHIEF COMPLAINT

- Vomiting, hematemesis, and melena are common complaints.
- Inappetence or anorexia and hypersalivation can be seen.
- Acute encephalopathic signs (e.g., stupor, seizures, or drooling in cats) may be observed in patients with concurrent severe liver disease.

PHYSICAL EXAM FINDINGS

Generally nonspecific and may be normal:

- ± Pain on abdominal palpation or pain manifested as a praying position
- ± Evidence of anemia (e.g., pale mucous membranes, tachycardia)
- ± Melena on rectal exam
- Signs of shock (p. 911) possible with severe bleeding or gastric perforation
- Evidence of septic peritonitis (p. 779) possible with gastric perforation

Etiology and Pathophysiology

- See causes of gastrointestinal (GI) ulceration (p. 1225).
- Primary gastroduodenal diseases (e.g., toxins or foreign bodies, chronic gastritis, inflammatory bowel disease, neoplasia [lymphoma, adenocarcinoma, leiomyosarcoma, GI stromal tumor, gastrinoma], pyloric outflow obstruction)
- Gastric hyperacidity disorders (e.g., gastrinomas, hypergastrinemia due to drugs, mast cell tumors)
- Drug-induced ulcers (e.g., COX inhibitors, other NSAIDs, corticosteroids)
- Exercise-induced ulcers theorized to occur from prolonged hyperthermia during exercise that increases gastric paracellular permeability to acid, resulting in mucosal damage.
- Other metabolic, endocrine, or systemic causes (e.g., pancreatitis, disseminated intravascular coagulation, hypoadrenocorticism, chronic kidney disease, liver failure, hypovolemic/septic shock, neurologic diseases [especially intervertebral disc disease])
- The causes of ulceration are similar to those of gastritis and erosion, but for unknown reasons, the reparative mechanisms of the mucosa are overwhelmed, resulting in deep indolent lesions.
- Ulcer healing starts as necrotic mucosa sloughs and granulation tissue fills the ulcer. Mucus and bicarbonate are secreted by the neighboring mucosa to protect the ulcer. Granulation tissue eventually organizes, a connective tissue bed develops, and epithelial tissues slide across the surface to re-epithelialize it. Glandular structures are the last to repopulate the denuded area.
- Reduced gastric acid secretion facilitates healing by decreasing tissue damage from acid and by decreasing further damage from pepsin, which is less active at higher pH.

DIAGNOSIS

Diagnostic Overview

Gastric ulceration should be suspected in patients with any signs of GI disturbance that persist or worsen beyond the degree expected for the primary diagnosis. There may be a history of receiving ulcerogenic medications or other known risk factors for ulcer. In many mild cases, diagnosis is only presumptive (response to antiulcer medications); a definitive diagnosis requires endoscopy or laparotomy, particularly if severe or associated with gastric perforation and peritonitis.

Differential Diagnosis

- Acute vomiting (p. 1293)
- Hematemesis
  - Coagulopathies or platelet disorders (decreased number or function)
  - Ingested blood (nasopharyngeal, oral, esophageal, or pulmonary bleeding)
  - Acute hemorrhagic diarrhea syndrome
  - Any cause of severe GI erosion
- Melena (p. 644)
- Abdominal pain (p. 21)

Initial Database

- Rectal exam to assess presence of melena; not always found
- CBC, serum biochemistry profile, urinalysis: important to identify underlying cause of gastric ulceration and especially important if hematemesis or melena is present
  - CBC may show anemia (variably regenerative if acute, depending on the time between onset of bleeding and time of testing; nonregenerative in the setting of underlying chronic disease; in dogs with iron deficiency from chronic blood loss may be microcytic, hypochromic, and either regenerative or nonregenerative), neutrophilia (± left shift if associated with perforation), hypoproteinemia, or mild thrombocytopenia (rarely less than 75,000/mcL) or thrombocytosis.
  - Serum biochemistry profile may or may not show a high blood urea nitrogen (BUN)/creatinine ratio or identify conditions associated with ulcers (e.g., kidney disease).
  - Urinalysis: essential for differentiating BUN elevation due to kidney disease (urine specific gravity [USG] = 1.008-1.020) from BUN elevation due to prerenal causes (USG > 1.035) or GI bleeding (any USG).
- Fecal occult blood test has limited utility.
  - *O*-tolidine–based tests are significantly more specific (0/108 false-positive results in healthy dogs) than guaiac-based tests (64/108 false-positive results in same dogs).
- Imaging studies
  - Plain radiographs cannot confirm gastric ulceration. If perforation has occurred, loss of detail (suggesting peritonitis or free abdominal fluid) or free peritoneal gas may be present.
  - Contrast radiographs (p. 1172) may identify a mucosal filling defect.
  - Ultrasonography may show focal gastric wall thickening, loss of normal layering, a wall defect or crater, fluid accumulation in the stomach, and diminished gastric motility. In animals with perforation, there may be evidence of free abdominal fluid.
  - CT scan may be more sensitive than radiographs or ultrasonography.

Advanced or Confirmatory Testing

- Serum gastrin levels may help diagnose gastrinoma, but the animal should not be receiving acid-suppressing drugs at the time of testing.
- If gastric perforation is suspected and no free gas is seen in the abdomen on imaging, abdominocentesis (p. 1056) is indicated. Ultrasound can guide sampling of even small amounts of free fluid sufficient for cytological evaluation. Cytological evaluation may show only neutrophilic inflammation with no evident cause in up to 44% of cases. Peritoneal lavage may be needed to obtain samples if fluid accumulation is scant.
- Gastroscopy (p. 1098): preferred for confirmation of gastric ulcer and tissue sampling; can identify or confirm perforation and need for immediate surgical intervention
  - A solitary ulcer in an otherwise normal stomach should raise suspicion of gastric neoplasia, especially if the edges and surrounding mucosa are thickened.
  - NSAID-induced ulcers can be solitary, but the surrounding mucosa is usually not normal because of generalized mucosal disease (gastritis and other erosions are common).
  - Multiple, diffuse, small ulcers can be seen with NSAIDs, uremia, liver disease, high-grade mast cell tumor, and gastrinoma.
  - Biopsies should be obtained from the ulcer periphery to avoid perforation. Repeated biopsies from the same site may improve the likelihood of identifying neoplasia. In some cases, endoscopic biopsies are inadequate for diagnosis (neoplastic tissue is deeper than superficial mucosal tissues sampled with endoscopic biopsies), and laparotomy is required for full-thickness biopsies.

TREATMENT

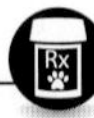

Treatment Overview

Goals are to remove the primary cause and promote healing. For animals with massive bleed or perforation, stabilization must be the first priority.

Acute General Treatment

Supportive care:

- Intravenous fluids, antibiotics, antiemetics, and opioid analgesics may be required for the patient with severe vomiting that has resulted in dehydration and electrolyte disturbances.
- Blood transfusion for the patient with severe anemia as a result of massive bleeding

Surgery:

- Surgical resection is indicated when the ulcer appears deeply penetrating (volcano crater appearance), is bleeding continuously, has perforated, or is large and fails to heal.
- Surgical exploration may identify the cause (neoplasia) and allow resection of the mass/ulcer.

Medical:

- Proton pump inhibitor (PPI): recommended as *best choice for acid reduction* in dogs and cats; multiple studies support PPIs as superior to H2-blockers in reducing gastric acidity. Dosing every 12 hours is preferred, and options include
  - Omeprazole 0.5-2.5 mg/kg PO q 12h; available in 10-, 20-, 40-mg tablets
  - Esomeprazole (Nexium) 0.5-1.5 mg/kg PO q 12h
  - Lansoprazole (Prevacid) 1 mg/kg IV or PO q 12h
  - Pantoprazole (Protonix) 0.5 mg/kg IV q 12h; 0.7-1 mg/kg PO q 12h
  - Rabeprazole (Aciphex) 0.7-1 mg/kg PO q 24h
- H2-blockers: famotidine 0.5-1 mg/kg PO, IV, or SQ q 12h is the preferred H2-blocker, although inferior to PPIs in acid reduction. Cimetidine requires q 8h dosing and inhibits hepatic cytochrome P450 activity. These drugs are inferior to PPI for treatment of gastric ulcer.
- Prostaglandin E_2 inhibitor: drug of choice for reducing NSAID-induced ulcers, although efficacy for NSAIDs other than aspirin has not been demonstrated; no evidence for efficacy in the treatment of gastric ulceration; not for use in cats or pregnant females
  - Misoprostol 3-5 mcg/kg PO q 8h
- Sucralfate: mucosal protectant; as oral suspension, or dissolved in 6-10 mL tap water if tablet; inferior to PPIs; not affected by other acid-reducing therapy
  - Dogs: 0.5-1 g/dose PO q 8h
  - Cats: 0.25 g/dose PO q 8h
- Antiemetics as needed to control emesis
  - Maropitant 1 mg/kg SQ or IV q 24h; may provide visceral analgesia. The author has safely used up to 2 mg/kg SQ or IV q 12h for intractable vomiting associated with severe gastric disease.
  - Metoclopramide 0.2-0.4 mg/kg PO or SQ q 8h; also 1-2 mg/kg/24 hours as a CRI
  - Dolasetron 0.3 mg/kg IV q 12-24h

Chronic Treatment

- Duration of antacid treatment varies. If the underlying cause can be removed, 2 weeks of antacid therapy may be sufficient. In dogs or cats with co-morbidities, 4 weeks or longer may be needed. If treated more than 3-4 weeks, tapering of antacids may be required to prevent rebound hyperacidity. Longer duration or indefinite use may be necessary if the underlying cause cannot be corrected.
- Misoprostol is indicated for preventing ulcers in dogs that need to be on NSAIDs (e.g., osteoarthritis) but are prone to developing ulcers.

Drug Interactions

- Co-administration of sucralfate may alter the absorption of some drugs (e.g., levothyroxine, antifungals, ciprofloxacin).

Possible Complications

The most important complications of gastric ulceration are blood-loss anemia (can be severe, requiring transfusions) and perforation resulting in septic peritonitis and shock.

Recommended Monitoring

In dogs or cats with acute hematemesis, the packed cell volume/total protein must be monitored to determine if a blood transfusion or surgical intervention is needed. Anemia may not be immediately apparent with peracute bleeding.

PROGNOSIS & OUTCOME

The prognosis for most gastric ulcers is good unless the underlying cause is not identified or cannot be corrected.

PEARLS & CONSIDERATIONS

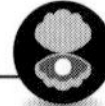

Comments

- Careful endoscopic evaluation of the lesser curvature of the stomach is critical for identification of gastric adenocarcinoma.
- Patients with GI bleeding often have BUN elevations with normal creatinine levels, concentrated urine, and normal renal function. A BUN/creatinine ratio > 30 suggests GI bleeding.
- Combining acid-suppressing therapies provides no additional benefit in ulcer healing.
- PPIs (e.g., omeprazole) are the most effective drugs for reducing acid secretion. H2-blockers are much less potent, and of the group, only famotidine has been shown in dogs to adequately decrease gastric acidity.

Prevention

- Careful administration of NSAIDs or use of NSAIDs with COX-2 selective properties to minimize the risk of ulceration
- NSAIDs and corticosteroids should not be co-administered unless using low-dose aspirin (0.5 mg/kg/d) or physiologic doses of glucocorticoids.
- Allow for a sufficient wash-out period (48-72 hours) when changing NSAIDs or after/beginning glucocorticoid administration.

Technician Tip

- Always verify NSAID dosing with the client and make certain the pet is not receiving any other NSAID or corticosteroid.

Client Education

- Advise clients of the potential dangers of NSAID use, and provide them with signs to watch for that may indicate gastritis or ulcer formation.
- Advise clients about the potential dangers of over-the-counter NSAIDs in dogs and cats because some of the most potent ulcerogenic drugs in dogs are ibuprofen, regular aspirin, and naproxen.
- Advise clients about the risk of potentially life-threatening complications from any over-the-counter NSAID given to cats.

SUGGESTED READING

Fitzgerald E, et al: Clinical findings and results of diagnostic imaging in 82 dogs with gastrointestinal ulceration. J Small Anim Pract 58:211-218, 2017.

AUTHOR: Kenneth R. Harkin, DVM, DACVIM
EDITOR: Rance K. Sellon, DVM, PhD, DACVIM

Gastroenteritis: Acute, Nonspecific

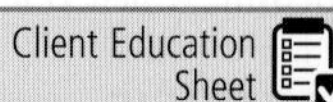

BASIC INFORMATION

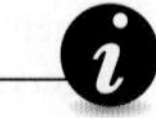

Definition

Very common disorder characterized by sudden onset of vomiting and/or diarrhea that may be accompanied by anorexia and evidence of abdominal discomfort. Generally self-limited, although supportive care may be necessary in severe cases

Synonyms

Acute gastritis, dietary indiscretion, acute enteritis

Epidemiology

SPECIES, AGE, SEX

Dogs are more often affected because of less discriminatory dietary behaviors.

RISK FACTORS

Poor supervision; access to garbage or other inappropriate items

CONTAGION AND ZOONOSIS

By definition, nonspecific gastroenteritis is not contagious. Infectious causes of acute vomiting and diarrhea must always be considered and excluded before making this diagnosis.

ASSOCIATED DISORDERS

In severe cases: dehydration, hypokalemia, metabolic acidosis

Clinical Presentation

HISTORY, CHIEF COMPLAINT

- Acute onset of vomiting and/or diarrhea
  - Vomitus may contain food or foreign material.
  - Diarrhea may be accompanied by mucus, urgency, and tenesmus.
- Anorexia, lethargy, and mild abdominal discomfort may be noted.
- Owner may report recent dietary indiscretion.

PHYSICAL EXAM FINDINGS

- Normal vital parameters (temperature, heart rate, respiratory rate, pulse quality, blood pressure) in most cases
- Possible dehydration in more severe cases
- Mild nonlocalized abdominal discomfort may be noted.
- Mucoid stool may be noted on rectal exam.

Etiology and Pathophysiology

- Specific cause is often not determined.
- Vomiting is likely due to direct gastric irritation or dysmotility.
- Diarrhea is likely due to irritation, dysmotility, or dysregulation of normal intestinal microbial populations.
- Diagnosis is usually based on history, absence of an identifiable cause of gastrointestinal (GI) signs, and prompt response to supportive therapy.
- Often associated with dietary indiscretion (e.g., ingestion of garbage, nontoxic plants, spoiled food)

DIAGNOSIS

Diagnostic Overview

This is a diagnosis of exclusion; pursue other differentials as appropriate. If clinical signs persist for more than 48 hours, further diagnostic testing is strongly indicated.

Differential Diagnosis

Other causes of vomiting and diarrhea (pp. 1213 and 1293)

- Infection: parasitic, bacterial, viral, protozoal
- GI obstruction
- Drug or toxin ingestion
- Systemic disease (e.g., pancreatitis, acute hepatic injury, kidney disease, hypoadrenocorticism)

Initial Database

- Extensive diagnostics usually are unnecessary if physical exam and hydration status are unremarkable.
- CBC: stress leukogram is expected in canine patients; erythrocytosis may be noted if the patient is dehydrated.
- Serum biochemistry profile: hypokalemia common; metabolic acidosis common; mild azotemia may be evident if patient is substantially dehydrated.
- Urinalysis: nonspecific; if dehydrated, concentrated urine specific gravity expected.
- Fecal evaluation (centrifuged flotation and saline preparation): no pathogens noted
- Radiographs: generally unremarkable; ileus may be apparent
- ± Pancreatic lipase immunoreactivity (if high-risk breed, other risk factors): within normal range
- ± Fecal ELISA for parvovirus (if young and/or questionable vaccination status): negative
- ± Fecal antigen test for *Giardia*: negative
- ± Serum cortisol: > 2 mcg/dL (>55 nmol/L) expected and excludes hypoadrenocorticism

TREATMENT

Treatment Overview

Provide supportive care; select appropriate therapies based on physical exam and clinical evaluation. If animal is not improved within 48 hours, additional diagnostic testing is indicated.

Acute General Treatment

- Small quantities of water or an oral electrolyte solution may be offered if vomiting is infrequent.
- Subcutaneous crystalloids may be used for small animals with mild hydration deficits.
- Intravenous fluids are required if patient is moderately dehydrated or hypovolemic.
- Antiemetics should be administered, provided GI obstruction has been ruled out.
  - Maropitant 1 mg/kg SQ q 24h or 2 mg/kg PO q 24h is an effective first choice (dogs > 8 weeks old; cats > 16 weeks old).
  - Metoclopramide 0.2-0.5 mg/kg SQ or PO q 6-8h must be given frequently or provided as a constant-rate infusion of 1-2 mg/kg/day.
- Gastric acid–reducing drugs may reduce the risk of esophagitis and are always appropriate if hematemesis is noted.
  - Omeprazole 0.7-1.5 mg/kg PO q 12h
  - Pantoprazole 0.7-1 mg/kg slow IV q 24h
- Protectants/adsorbents provide little clinical benefit. Products containing salicylate should be avoided in cats.
- Opiate antidiarrheals (e.g., loperamide) decrease GI motility and secretion and should be used with caution in dogs because they may cause constipation and depression (avoid in cats).
- Antibiotics are not indicated and may contribute to intestinal dysbiosis.
- Probiotics +/− prebiotics are unlikely to significantly hasten recovery.

Nutrition/Diet

Food should be provided as soon as the patient is interested in eating. Easily digestible diets (e.g., boiled white rice with cottage cheese or low-fat turkey breast, commercially available highly digestible enteric diets) may be beneficial in vomiting patients because gastric emptying times are shorter.

Drug Interactions

- Maropitant is protein bound and may affect metabolism of other highly protein-bound drugs such as nonsteroidal antiinflammatories and anticonvulsants.
- Metoclopramide interacts with numerous drugs; avoid concurrent use of sedatives, tranquilizers, and narcotics.

Possible Complications

- Esophagitis may be prevented by acid-reducing drugs.
- Aspiration pneumonia is more likely in depressed or sedated patients.
- Intussusception is uncommon but more likely in young dogs.

Recommended Monitoring

- Hydration status
- Temperature, pulse, respiratory rate
- Volume of fluid losses

PROGNOSIS & OUTCOME

Prognosis is excellent. This disorder usually resolves within 48 hours of onset.

PEARLS & CONSIDERATIONS

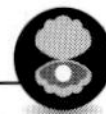

Comments

- Animals with marked dehydration, hypovolemia, depression, melena, substantial hematemesis, or overt abdominal pain require prompt diagnostic evaluation and treatment (often including hospitalization).
- GI obstruction should be excluded (e.g., abdominal radiographs) before administration of antiemetics.

Prevention

Prevent access to garbage or spoiled food.

Technician Tips

- Encourage food intake by warming and offering frequently (p. 1199).
- Maropitant SQ may be painful; chilling the injectable formulation may reduce patient discomfort.

Client Education

- Signs should resolve within 48 hours. Further veterinary care should be sought if vomiting or diarrhea persists.
- Neonates, geriatric animals, and those with pre-existing disorders are more prone to dehydration and may need more aggressive fluid support.

SUGGESTED READING

Gallagher A: Vomiting and regurgitation. In Ettinger SJ, et al, editors: Textbook of veterinary internal medicine, ed 8, St. Louis, 2017, Saunders, pp 158-164.

AUTHOR: Audrey K. Cook, BVM&S, DACVIM, DECVIM, DABVP
EDITOR: Rance K. Sellon, DVM, PhD, DACVIM

Gastrointestinal Obstruction

Bonus Material Online

Client Education Sheet 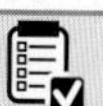

BASIC INFORMATION

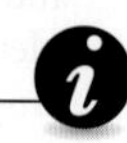

Definition

Common disorder caused by a foreign object or mass that partially or completely occludes the pylorus or intestinal lumen. Obstructions caused by gastric dilation and volvulus (p. 377), mesenteric volvulus (p. 649), linear foreign bodies (p. 353), and intussusception (p. 561) are discussed separately.

Synonyms

Intraluminal obstruction, intestinal blockage

Epidemiology

SPECIES, AGE, SEX

Gastrointestinal (GI) obstruction can occur in dogs or cats of either sex. Foreign body obstruction is more common in dogs, likely related to their behaviors (e.g., chewing rawhides, bones, toys). Younger animals are more likely to ingest foreign material, and older animals are more likely to have a neoplastic obstruction.

RISK FACTORS

- Younger animals are at greater risk for dietary indiscretion and therefore foreign body ingestion.
- Some animals are more prone to ingesting foreign objects than others (individual behavior), irrespective of age.
- Older animals are at greater risk for neoplasia.

ASSOCIATED DISORDERS

Animals with diseases that cause pica are more at risk for foreign object ingestion.

Clinical Presentation

HISTORY, CHIEF COMPLAINT

- Vomiting, anorexia, and depression are common primary complaints.
- Severity of clinical signs varies, depending on duration and location of obstruction.
- Proximal and complete obstructions are associated with more severe clinical signs of illness.
- History of being unable to hold down water is very suspicious for GI obstruction.
- Distal or partial obstructions may be associated with vague and chronic signs such as intermittent vomiting, anorexia, weight loss, or diarrhea. When associated with GI obstruction, diarrhea is usually scant and not profuse.
- Intermittent obstruction of the pylorus by gastric foreign bodies results in intermittent clinical signs.

PHYSICAL EXAM FINDINGS

- Abdominal splinting or signs of pain on palpation may be noted.
- Mass or foreign object may be identified with careful palpation.
- Dehydration, depression, or shock; with proximal and complete obstructions

Etiology and Pathophysiology

Causes of GI tract obstruction:

- Foreign body
- Mass
- Intussusception
- Linear foreign body
- Trichobezoar
- Volvulus or torsion
- Stricture or adhesion

Mechanism:

- Physical obstruction of the intestinal lumen causes mechanical ileus, and fluid and gas accumulation proximal to the obstruction.
- Duodenal and proximal jejunal obstruction is often associated with acute and severe signs.
- Persistent vomiting and loss of gastric secretions associated with proximal obstructions may lead to electrolyte imbalances (hypochloremic metabolic alkalosis).
- Lymphatic and capillary stasis causes intestinal wall edema.
- Impaired intestinal mucosal barrier allows bacterial translocation, potentially resulting in endotoxemia, sepsis, or rarely, septic peritonitis without intestinal necrosis or perforation.
- High intraluminal pressure causes intestinal wall ischemia that may progress to necrosis and peritonitis.

DIAGNOSIS

Diagnostic Overview

The diagnosis is suspected based on history and physical exam, is supported by imaging (radiographic and/or ultrasonographic) findings, and is confirmed by endoscopy or surgery. Diagnostic imaging should be considered in any young animal that presents with vomiting, anorexia, or a painful abdomen or has a history of foreign body ingestion.

Differential Diagnosis

- Vomiting (pp. 1293 and 1294)
- Functional ileus
  - Infectious disease of the GI tract (parvoviral or coronaviral enteritis)
  - Intoxication
  - Dysautonomia

Initial Database

CBC, serum biochemistry profile, and urinalysis:

- Evidence of dehydration (e.g., blood urea nitrogen, creatinine elevations with urine specific gravity > 1.030; hemoconcentration/elevated packed cell volume)
- Electrolyte imbalances
  - Hypochloremia occurs in 51% of cases and is the most common abnormality.
  - Hypokalemia: 25%
  - Hyponatremia: 20% (occurs more commonly with linear than discrete foreign bodies)
- Metabolic alkalosis with proximal obstruction; metabolic acidosis with hypoperfusion, sepsis secondary to peritonitis, or other systemic effects

Abdominal radiographs: often the most informative test. Urgent consultation with a radiologist can be helpful:

- Radiopaque foreign objects may be visualized.
- Fluid- or gas-distended intestinal loops
- Pathologic dilation of intestinal loops: small-bowel lumen should not exceed the diameter of twice the width of a rib or be greater than 1.6 times the height of the fifth lumbar vertebra.
- Radiographs that demonstrate a foreign body must be recent (minutes or hours before induction of general anesthesia or, better still, retaken just after induction) if surgery is planned. A gastric or duodenal foreign body can be displaced into the esophagus during anesthetic induction, and an intestinal foreign body might have been defecated since the original radiographs were taken.

Thoracic radiographs: older animals with suspected neoplasia to look for metastasis

Advanced or Confirmatory Testing

Contrast radiographs:

- Barium sulfate suspension for upper GI study unless perforation suspected (p. 1172)
  - If perforation suspected, consider using nonionic iodinated contrast medium or other diagnostic techniques (abdominocentesis, peritoneal lavage).
- Barium enema
  - For assessing an obstructive pattern in the distal intestine
  - For differentiating small bowel from large bowel if it is not clear whether a gas-filled viscus is a pathologically distended segment of small intestine or the normal colon

Abdominocentesis (p. 1056) and fluid analysis (p. 1343)

- If perforation/peritonitis suspected

Abdominal ultrasound:

- Site of obstruction may be visualized.
- Identification of small amounts of free abdominal fluid
- Localization of free fluid for accurate centesis
- Ultrasonographic evidence of the intestinal diameter enlargement of the jejunum > 1.5 cm suggests an obstruction. Ultrasonography was definitive for obstruction in 97% of dogs (compared with 70% accuracy on radiographs) in a recent study.

Diagnostic peritoneal lavage:

- If peritonitis is suspected but centesis is unrewarding

- Limited efficacy, largely replaced by ultrasound-guided centesis

Upper GI endoscopy (p. 1098) for suspected gastric foreign body can be diagnostic and allow retrieval of foreign material.

TREATMENT

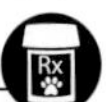

Treatment Overview

Rehydration and rapid surgical intervention are recommended in any patient with intestinal obstruction, and endoscopy can be used in place of surgery for some gastric obstructions. Correct dehydration and electrolyte abnormalities with intravenous fluid administration. Exploratory laparotomy is indicated to relieve the obstruction.

Acute General Treatment

- Exploratory laparotomy for foreign body retrieval or mass resection
  - Some gastric foreign bodies can be removed by endoscopy (p. 1098).
- An enterotomy may suffice for acute foreign body removal; if intestinal viability is questionable, resection and anastomosis are warranted.
- Wide-margin (4-8 cm) resection and anastomosis should be performed if neoplastic disease is suspected based on the gross appearance of the lesion. In this case, lymph node and liver biopsies also are indicated.
- Omentum or serosal patch may be placed to reinforce suture line.
- Change gloves and surgical instruments before abdominal lavage and closure to minimize contamination.
- Administer prophylactic antibiotics (cefazolin 22 mg/kg IV q 90 minutes during the perioperative period).
- Obtain gastric, small-intestinal, and liver biopsies, even if all appear grossly normal. Biopsy any abnormal-looking organ. Future course of illness may evolve in such a way as to make these specimens essential for diagnosis.

Chronic Treatment

Postoperative considerations:

- Continue rehydration and daily electrolyte monitoring. Treat accordingly (especially hypokalemia arising from dilution [IV fluids] and anorexia).
- With proper technique and no contamination in straightforward cases, postoperative antibiotics are not necessary and may mask signs of dehiscence and peritonitis.
- Nothing by mouth (NPO) 6-12 hours after enterotomy, 12 hours after resection and anastomosis
- Administer GI protectants as needed: pantoprazole 0.7 mg/kg IV q 24h
- Administer antiemetics as needed (contraindicated before resolution of obstruction).
  - Maropitant 1 mg/kg SQ q 24h
  - Dolasetron 0.5 mg/kg IV, SQ q 24h
  - Metoclopramide 0.2-0.4 mg/kg PO, SQ, or IM q 6h (antiemetic and prokinetic)

Nutrition/Diet

Feeding tube placement (p. 1106) at the time of surgery should be considered in animals with marked weight loss, hypoalbuminemia, or evidence of peritonitis. If anorexia persists postoperatively, syringe feeding, feeding tubes, or total parenteral nutrition may be considered.

Possible Complications

- Dehiscence: highest risk at 3-5 days postoperatively. Animals should be monitored in hospital for 48-72 hours in the postoperative period for signs of peritonitis. Risk factors include preoperative peritonitis, serum albumin concentration < 2.5 g/dL, and presence of a foreign body (vs. neoplastic disease).
- Ileus
- Short-bowel syndrome: unlikely if less than 70% of small intestine resected
- Stricture
- Recurrence

Recommended Monitoring

- The following parameters should be monitored daily until discharge from hospital: body temperature, blood glucose, electrolytes, abdominal pain
- The patient should be eating and not vomiting. If anorexia or vomiting persists after surgery, consider performing abdominocentesis and CBC to evaluate for possible development of peritonitis.

PROGNOSIS & OUTCOME

- A good prognosis may be expected for acute disease, and animals with preoperative debilitation or shock should be given a more guarded prognosis.
- Prognosis for neoplastic disease depends on histopathologic grade, evidence of metastasis, and completeness of surgical excision. Lymphoma (p. 604) and adenocarcinoma (p. 30) are the most frequently encountered intestinal tumors.

PEARLS & CONSIDERATIONS

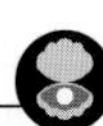

Comments

Consider placing an intraoperative feeding tube (esophagostomy, gastrostomy, or gastrojejunostomy tube [p. 1106]) in these patients based on preoperative nutritional status, degree of patient debilitation, or anticipated postoperative anorexia.

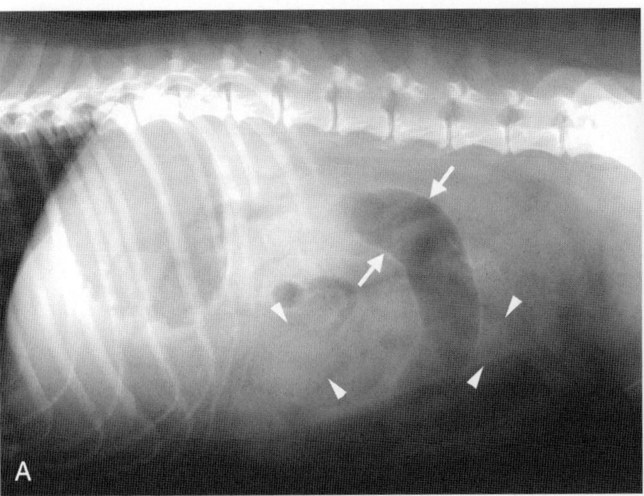

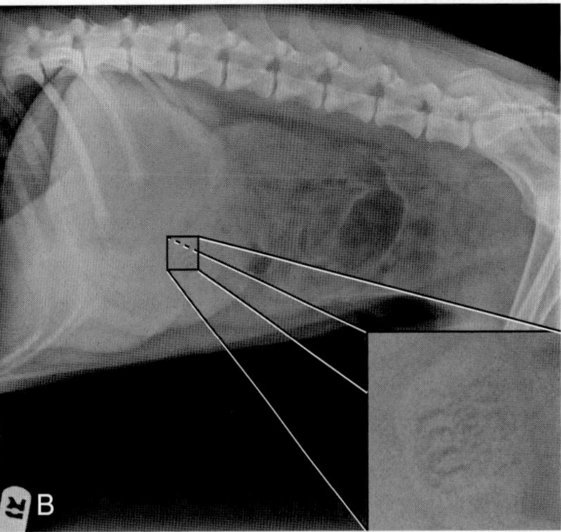

GASTROINTESTINAL OBSTRUCTION Radiographic lateral views of small-intestinal obstruction in two patients. **A,** In this dog, a small-intestinal segment is markedly distended with gas *(arrows),* and another is markedly distended with fluid/soft tissue *(arrowheads).* **B,** The 5-year-old Labrador dog has several loops of gas-distended intestine. *Inset,* Exploratory laparotomy revealed a mid-jejunal obstruction caused by a foreign body (corn cob). (**A,** Courtesy Dr. Richard Walshaw; **B,** Courtesy Dr. Patricia Rose.)

Prevention

Basket muzzles may be considered for dogs that present multiple times for GI obstruction due to foreign body ingestion.

Technician Tips

Intestinal obstruction patients may be in a critical state and require intensive care. Technicians treating and caring for these patients should be alert to any changes in animal's vital parameters, bodily eliminations, attitude, or perceived pain.

SUGGESTED READING

Hobday MM, et al: Linear versus non-linear gastrointestinal foreign bodies in 499 dogs: clinical presentation, management and short-term outcome. J Small Anim Pract 55:560-565, 2014.

AUTHOR: Janet Kovak McClaran, DVM, DACVS, DECVS
EDITOR: Elizabeth A. Swanson, DVM, MS, DACVS

Giardiasis

Bonus Material Online 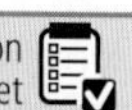 Client Education Sheet

BASIC INFORMATION 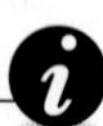

Definition

Giardia duodenalis is a flagellate protozoan intestinal parasite of humans and animals. Clinical disease usually appears as acute small-bowel diarrhea but can vary, with some animals showing chronic small-bowel or acute or chronic large-bowel diarrhea.

Synonyms

Giardia duodenalis, Giardia lamblia, Giardia intestinalis

Epidemiology

SPECIES, AGE, SEX

Infection can affect humans and domestic animals and is most common in younger animals.

RISK FACTORS

Immunodeficient adults, young animals, and animals confined in large, crowded groups are at increased risk.

CONTAGION AND ZOONOSIS

Various genotypes differ in host range. Species-specific genotypes are the most commonly encountered in dogs and cats. Of the genotypes found in dogs (A, B, C, D) and cats (A, F), several (A, B) also infect humans, and the potential for zoonotic exposure to people from pets therefore exists.

Clinical Presentation

HISTORY, CHIEF COMPLAINT

- Infections are usually subclinical.
- If diarrhea results, it can be acute and short lived, intermittent, or chronic.
- Steatorrhea or weight loss may be observed.
- Excessive fecal mucus is often observed in clinically affected cats.
- Emesis, fever, and anorexia may occur but are not typical.

PHYSICAL EXAM FINDINGS

No specific abnormalities

Etiology and Pathophysiology

- The *Giardia* life cycle is direct. Cysts are ingested and excyst in the duodenum, with each cyst producing two motile trophozoites that replicate in the lumen of the small intestine. Before being shed in feces, the trophozoite encysts. On excretion, the cysts are immediately infective to another host. Cysts can survive for days to weeks in a cool, moist environment.
- Autoinfection from fecal material adhered to the haircoat or cysts in drinking water/ environment is possible. Reinfection is probable in catteries and kennels because of environmental contamination.
- Trophozoites cause sloughing of intestinal epithelial cells and blunting of intestinal villi, resulting in a reduction in absorptive surface area, causing malabsorption.
- Abnormalities in cellular and humoral immunity likely predispose individuals to clinical infection.

DIAGNOSIS 

Diagnostic Overview

The diagnosis is made by the detection of cysts, trophozoites, or antigen in feces.

Differential Diagnosis

- Other intestinal parasitoses
- Idiopathic inflammatory bowel disease
- Maldigestion secondary to pancreatic exocrine insufficiency
- Neoplastic intestinal disease (e.g., lymphoma)
- Infectious intestinal disease (viral, bacterial, fungal)
- Food intolerance or dietary indiscretion (acute cases)

Initial Database

- Direct saline fecal smear: can detect viable, motile trophozoites
  - Trophozoites may predominate in diarrheic feces but due to their fragile nature are usually detected only in fresh samples (feces examined within 20 minutes of defecation).
  - Positive result is definitive; negative result does not rule out infection.
- Zinc sulfate centrifugal fecal flotation (ZSCF): detection of cysts. Due to intermittent fecal cyst shedding, sensitivity is increased by examining two or three fecal

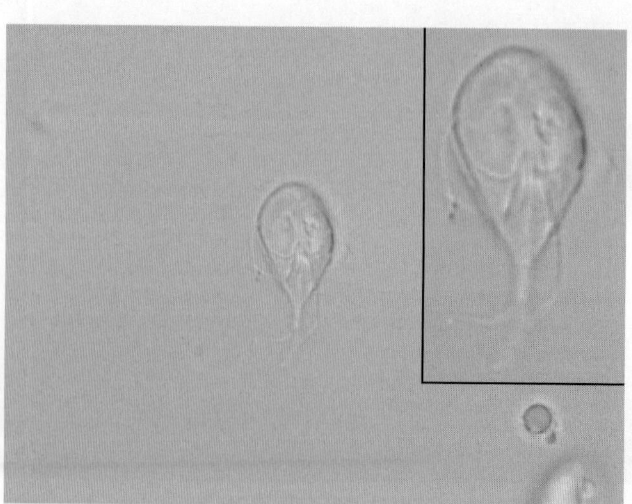

GIARDIASIS A *Giardia duodenalis* trophozoite detected on a direct saline fecal smear (typical appearance with 40× objective (*inset,* 100× oil objective). Trophozoites are teardrop shaped with two nuclei and eight flagella and are 12-17 × 7-10 microns. Motile trophozoites have a typical falling-leaf movement and are easily kept in the microscopic field of view.

samples obtained over 3-5 days. If samples are shipped for testing, they should be maintained at 4°C. Lack of centrifugation and/or use of sugar or one of the other salts as flotation media can greatly decrease the detection sensitivity for *Giardia* cysts.

Advanced or Confirmatory Testing

- ELISA kits to identify fecal *Giardia* antigens. Fresh, frozen, or formalin-preserved feces are suitable. Sensitivity of one ELISA is similar to that of two or three fecal samples tested using ZSCF.
  - ELISA available as point-of-care test (SNAP Giardia Test)
- Direct immunofluorescent testing for *Giardia* cysts in feces. Samples should be preserved in 10% formalin (1 part feces to 3 parts formalin) before being shipped to the laboratory.

TREATMENT

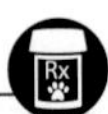

Treatment Overview

Treatment goals are to eliminate clinical signs of *Giardia* infection, including diarrhea and weight loss, and eliminate shedding of infective cysts.

Acute General Treatment

- Fenbendazole 50 mg/kg PO q 24h for 3-10 days (dogs and cats), *or*
- Febantel-pyrantel-praziquantel: dose according to febantel content (febantel dosage 37.8 mg/kg PO q 24h for 3-5 days [dogs, cats])
- Metronidazole 15-25 mg/kg PO q 12-24h for 5-7 days (dogs and cats). Use as second choice; less effective than fenbendazole, *or*
- Ronidazole 30-50 mg/kg PO q 12h for 7 days (tried on a limited number of dogs)

Chronic Treatment

- Heightened efforts for sanitation/hygiene, use of quaternary ammonium disinfectants, and bathing animals are important in preventing reinfection.
- The contention that *Giardia* vaccination can reduce shedding in chronically infected dogs is unsupported.

Possible Complications

Albendazole: myelosuppression, hepatotoxicosis (especially in cats) and suspected teratogen. Not recommended.

PROGNOSIS & OUTCOME

Prognosis is usually good; clinical signs resolve in most individuals, but recurrent clinical signs due to persistent infection/reinfection may occur in some animals.

PEARLS & CONSIDERATIONS

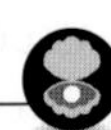

Comments

- Empirical fenbendazole treatment is recommended in dogs with diarrhea to address *Giardia* and occult whipworm infection as possible underlying causes.
- *Giardia*-ELISA kits have limited usefulness for post-treatment diagnostic surveillance because of prolonged persistent antigen shedding, even in animals with resolution of clinical signs and no detectable cysts on ZSCF.

Prevention

The *Giardia* vaccine appears to be ineffective in prevention of infection.

Technician Tips

Standard laboratory safety measures should be observed in the handling of animals and fecal samples.

SUGGESTED READING

Payne PA, et al: The biology and control of *Giardia* spp. and *Tritrichomonas foetus*. Vet Clin North Am Small Anim Pract 39(6):993-1007, 2009.

AUTHOR: Gary A. Conboy, DVM, PhD, DACVM
EDITOR: Rance K. Sellon DVM, PhD, DACVIM

Glaucoma

Bonus Material Online 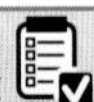 Client Education Sheet

BASIC INFORMATION

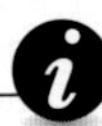

Definition

- Glaucomas are a group of diseases characterized by visual impairment and blindness from damage to the retina and optic nerve caused by increased intraocular pressure (IOP).
- Glaucoma may be the result of primary eye disease (i.e., abnormalities of the drainage/iridocorneal angle [primary glaucoma]), secondary to other eye diseases (secondary glaucoma), or less commonly, congenital anomalies of the anterior segment of the eye (congenital glaucoma).
- Dogs in North America have a 0.9% prevalence of primary glaucoma and an 0.8% prevalence of secondary glaucomas.

Synonyms

Ocular hypertension, buphthalmos, megaloglobus (enlargement of the globe secondary to elevated IOP)

Epidemiology

SPECIES, AGE, SEX

- Dogs and cats: age of onset depends on underlying cause
- Primary glaucoma
  - Typically middle-aged to older dogs (3-12 years; average, 8 years); rare in cats
  - In some breeds of dogs, primary glaucoma occurs more frequently in females.
- Secondary glaucoma due to
  - Lens luxation: usually affects young to middle-aged dogs (3-7 years); older cats
  - Intraocular neoplasia: usually older animals (>7 years)
  - Anterior uveitis: any age
- Congenital glaucoma
  - Young animals; elevation in IOP develops soon after birth

GENETICS, BREED PREDISPOSITION

Primary glaucoma:

- Commonly affected breeds include American cocker spaniel, basset hound, chow chow, Shar-pei, Boston terrier, Siberian Husky, and miniature poodle.
- Primary open-angle glaucoma is inherited in the beagle as an autosomal recessive trait.
- Primary closed-angle glaucoma in the Welsh springer spaniel and Great Dane appears to be inherited as an autosomal dominant trait with varied expression.
- Cats: Siamese, Burmese, and Persian breeds may have inherited primary glaucoma.

Secondary glaucoma:

- Lens luxation: terrier breeds
- Pigmentary uveitis: golden retrievers, cairn terriers
- Lens induced uveitis: miniature schnauzer

RISK FACTORS

Primary glaucoma:

- Abnormalities of the iridocorneal angle (often called *pectinate ligament dysplasia* or *goniodysgenesis*) may narrow the opening to the sclerociliary cleft and increase the probability of glaucoma (dogs).

Secondary glaucoma:

- Anterior uveitis (p. 1023) due to
  - Cataract formation (common in dogs)
  - Systemic bacterial and mycotic diseases (dogs and cats)
  - Feline leukemia and feline immunodeficiency viruses (cats)
  - Idiopathic/immune-mediated uveitis (dogs and cats)
- Lens luxation (p. 581)
- Intraocular neoplasia (p. 559)
- Hyphema (p. 511)
- Uveal cysts in golden retrievers

ASSOCIATED DISORDERS

Secondary glaucoma may follow uveitis (intraocular inflammation), lens luxation, or intraocular neoplasia.

Clinical Presentation

DISEASE FORMS/SUBTYPES

Glaucoma may be classified by
- Cause: primary, secondary, or congenital
- Duration: acute (vision potential) versus chronic (typically blind, buphthalmic eye)

HISTORY, CHIEF COMPLAINT

Transient or constant red or cloudy eye with any or all of the following:
- Various evidence of pain (usually present when IOP > 40 mm Hg) manifesting as unwillingness to be handled around the face or head or blepharospasm
- Bumping into objects or other manifestations of visual impairment or blindness
- Increased reflection from eye (i.e., tapetal reflection from dilated pupil)
- Enlargement of the globe (buphthalmos)

PHYSICAL EXAM FINDINGS

Unilateral or bilateral ocular changes; initially unilateral with primary glaucoma:
- Corneal edema (typically diffuse)
- Episcleral injection (dilated and tortuous episcleral vessels)
- Dilated pupil and sluggish to absent pupillary light reflexes
- Possible lens subluxation/luxation (look for aphakic crescent)
- Variable optic nerve cupping and retinal degeneration
- Corneal stria (breaks in Descemet's membrane appearing as white lines within cornea; uncommon)

Etiology and Pathophysiology

- Impediment to aqueous humor outflow, causing elevated IOP
- Elevated IOP can damage the retina (retinal ganglion cells) and optic nerve head by reducing retinal, choroidal, and optic nerve head blood flow and axoplasmic flow in the optic nerve head.
- Onset and severity of these glaucomatous changes appear to be influenced by the duration and extent of the IOP elevation.
- About 50% of first eyes of dogs presented with the primary glaucomas are blind at initial ophthalmic exam.

DIAGNOSIS

Diagnostic Overview

A diagnosis of glaucoma should be considered for any case that presents for evaluation of red eye(s), particularly if the ocular hyperemia is accompanied by mydriasis and corneal edema and especially if it occurs in a predisposed breed. Elevated IOP on tonometric evaluation is confirmatory.

Differential Diagnosis

Glaucoma must be differentiated from other causes of red eye (p. 870).

Initial Database

Complete ophthalmic exam (p. 1137):
- Tonometry (measurement of IOP): most important diagnostic test
  - Applanation tonometry (e.g., Tono-Pen)
    - Rebound tonometry (e.g., TonoVet)
    - Schiøtz indentation tonometry (requires conversion of value from instrument to mm Hg using human calibration chart accompanying instrument or dog/cat calibration chart)
- Normal IOP values range from 15-25 mm Hg; > 25 mm Hg = glaucoma (dogs and cats).

Advanced or Confirmatory Testing

- Referral to veterinary ophthalmologist for
  - Additional or multiple tonometric measurements
  - Gonioscopy (direct observation of the iridocorneal angle)
  - Ophthalmoscopy of the ocular fundus
- Ocular ultrasound if ocular media are opaque and prevent evaluation of deeper ocular structures; helps rule out concurrent ocular abnormalities (i.e., lens luxation, lens capsule rupture, retinal detachment, intraocular masses)

TREATMENT

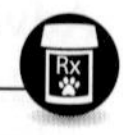

Treatment Overview

- In acute cases, it is critical that the IOP be lowered as soon as possible to maintain or restore vision. If tonometry is unavailable, glaucoma suspects should be referred to a veterinary ophthalmologist (as an emergency) for IOP measurement.
- Early surgical intervention may permit better and longer control of IOP; the clinician is urged to consider early referral, especially when vision in one eye has already been lost.
- Long-term treatment of glaucoma can be a frustrating endeavor because the disease tends to progress despite medical therapy. Diligent monitoring, regular reassessment of therapeutic success, and client education are critical.
- Therapeutic goals are to lower IOP of affected eye to maintain vision for as long as possible, eliminate ocular pain, and treat contralateral eye prophylactically with IOP-lowering drugs to delay the median time to onset of glaucoma from ≈6 months (untreated) to 30 months (with prophylactic treatment) (primary glaucoma).
- A step-by-step approach to treatment is shown on p. 1419.

Acute General Treatment

Medical:
- Regardless of the type of glaucoma, the following may be administered initially and then long term if indicated:
  - Topical beta-adrenergic antagonists (0.5% timolol or 0.5% betaxolol, usually q 8-12h; decreases pressure about 5-7 mm Hg), *and*

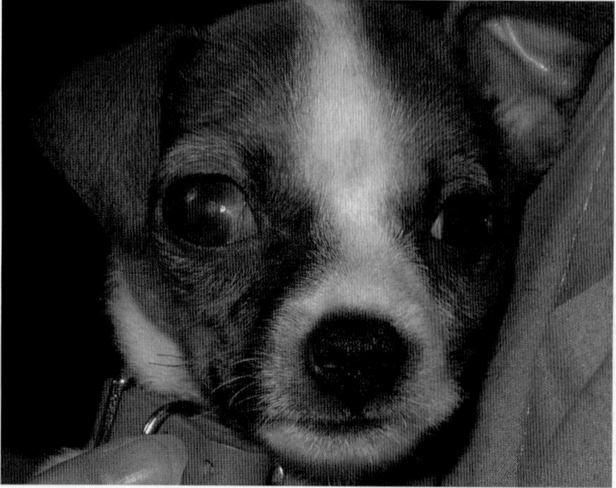

GLAUCOMA Congenital glaucoma in a terrier puppy. This occurred because of incomplete development of the iridocorneal drainage angle. Note the profound buphthalmia affecting the right eye. The globes of young animals are much more elastic than those of adults and therefore have a greater capacity for enlargement.

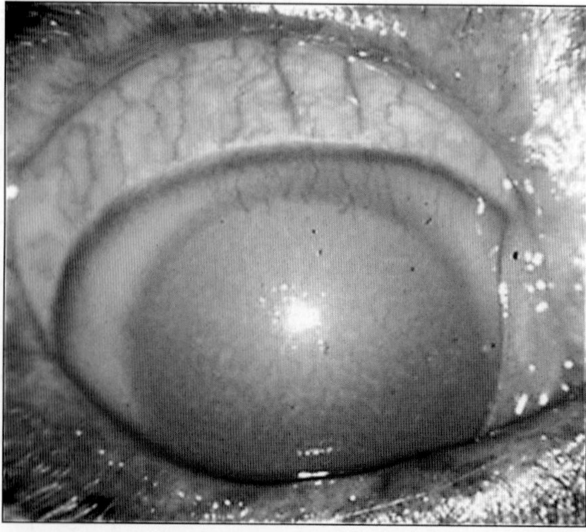

GLAUCOMA Acute congestive glaucoma in a mixed-breed dog. There is episcleral injection, diffuse corneal edema, and mydriasis.

- Topical carbonic anhydrase inhibitors (CAIs) (topical 2% dorzolamide or 1% brinzolamide q 8h, decreases pressure about 5-7 mm Hg)
- Topical dorzolamide/timolol combination (q 12h) can be administered rather than the individual products.

- Mannitol 1-2 g/kg IV over 20 minutes (usually greatly decreases pressure) to rapidly lower IOP (first effects in 1-2 hours; maximum effect in 4-6 hours; duration ≈8-10 hours) when there is a chance for return of vision (e.g., acute primary glaucoma)
- Topical prostaglandins (PGF analogs, 0.005% latanoprost, 0.03% bimatoprost, or 0.004% travoprost q 8-24h), usually greatly decrease pressure: used for primary glaucoma in dogs; not as effective in the feline glaucomas) may be used in the emergent case to promptly lower IOP; however, they should not be used in cases of lens luxation or instability or be used with caution when there is significant uveitis.
- Topical q 6h corticosteroids (prednisolone 1% or dexamethasone 0.1%) are indicated if anterior uveitis is also present with no corneal ulceration.

Chronic Treatment

Medical:

- Topical carbonic anhydrase inhibitors (2% dorzolamide or 1% brinzolamide q 8h)
- Topical beta-adrenergic antagonists or blockers (0.5% timolol or 0.5% betaxolol, usually q 8-12h)
- Topical prostaglandins (PGF analogs, 0.005% latanoprost, 0.03% bimatoprost, or 0.004% travoprost q 12-24h): used for primary glaucoma in dogs; not as effective in feline glaucomas
- ± Topical and/or systemic corticosteroids (prednisolone) (when anterior uveitis also present; taper to lowest effective dose)
- In all of the breed-related *primary glaucomas*, the disease continues to progress (even though IOP may be controlled), and often, combinations of several topical IOP-lowering drugs or surgery (see below) are eventually necessary.

Surgical:

- Anterior chamber shunts and laser cyclophotocoagulation are procedures offered by most veterinary ophthalmologists to prolong vision and prevent ocular pain. Laser cyclophotocoagulation may be performed with a transscleral approach or with the assistance of a microendoscope.
- Removal of the lens (referable procedure; glaucoma secondary to lens luxation) should be performed as soon as possible in cases of anterior lens displacement/luxation.
- End-stage blind and buphthalmic glaucomatous globes may be treated by
  - Enucleation
  - Evisceration and intrascleral prosthesis
  - Intravitreal gentamicin or cidofovir injection (dogs)
  - Enucleation or evisceration and implant surgeries should be followed with histopathologic exam of the removed tissue to help determine cause of glaucoma (i.e., primary vs. secondary) and prognosis for fellow eye.

Drug Interactions

- Topical beta-adrenergic blockers may lower heart rate and blood pressure and may cause bronchoconstriction in small-breed dogs and in cats.
- Systemic CAIs in dogs and cats are rarely used since the advent of topical CAIs because they may cause metabolic acidosis and electrolyte imbalances, as evidenced by depression (perhaps related to hypokalemia), and in dogs, vomiting and diarrhea that require drug cessation. Topical CAI preparations are rarely associated with these side effects.
- Topical prostaglandins often cause conjunctival hyperemia within minutes after instillation that gradually declines over an hour or so and miosis that persists with the IOP reduction.
- Mannitol, an osmotic diuretic, should be avoided in patients with heart disease (risk of fluid overload/iatrogenic pulmonary edema).

Possible Complications

With poor or inadequate control of IOP, any or all of the following may occur:

- Buphthalmos (p. 705) causing increased corneal exposure ± recurrent corneal ulceration/corneal vascularization/corneal pigmentation
- Lens luxation/subluxation
- Optic nerve and retinal degeneration
- Ocular, head pain
- Blindness

Recommended Monitoring

- Regular exams with tonometry (e.g., monthly after IOP control initially achieved) are necessary to monitor IOP (should be maintained at < 15 mm Hg) and maintain vision for as long as possible.
- As the glaucoma progresses, increased frequency and/or additional topical drugs to lower IOP are usually necessary.

PROGNOSIS & OUTCOME

- Prognosis is usually poor for the first eye presented with primary glaucoma in dogs because the disease is often advanced and refractory to medical therapy.
- Prognosis for the fellow eye is better, and prophylactic therapy with a beta-adrenergic blocker or prostaglandin can significantly delay the onset of glaucoma for up to 30 months.

PEARLS & CONSIDERATIONS

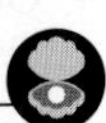

Comments

- Patients with dilated pupils, corneal edema, and conjunctival hyperemia require tonometry to estimate IOP.
- Clinical management of glaucoma is often difficult, and referral of these cases to a veterinary ophthalmologist is advised.
- Medical therapy of glaucoma is expensive and is often required long term.
- Buphthalmos indicates chronic glaucoma, whereas acute glaucoma, with its potentially better prognosis for vision, manifests with episcleral injection and almost never with buphthalmos.
- Treatment (e.g., evisceration and implant, enucleation) is generally indicated for permanently blind, persistently glaucomatous eyes to remove the source of chronic intense pain.
- Digital pressure (pressing on the eyes through closed eyelids) cannot be used to accurately assess IOP.

Prevention

The benefits of periodic tonometry in breeds and/or eyes at risk are unknown but should be considered. Anterior uveitis that is unrecognized or inadequately treated and controlled predisposes an eye to secondary glaucoma. Cataractous eyes should be examined regularly for evidence of lens-induced uveitis, and treatment should be initiated when signs appear to prevent or delay glaucoma.

Technician Tips

- Veterinary nurses and technicians should encourage clients to bring their pets in for evaluation promptly to rule out glaucoma if they complain of a bloodshot eye or acute visual disturbance.
- Restraint for animals undergoing tonometry is important. Care should be taken to avoid placing any pressure on the jugular veins or eyelids because excessive pressure in these areas may result in falsely elevated IOP measurements. Excessive struggling should be avoided as well because this may alter IOP readings.

Client Education

- Glaucoma is a chronic disease that requires regular and diligent therapy. Missed medication results in inadequate control of IOP, loss of sight, and pain.
- Primary glaucoma occurs in more than 20 dog breeds.
- Dogs with cataracts that are not surgical candidates require periodic eye exams and tonometry indefinitely because they are at increased risk for developing glaucoma.

SUGGESTED READING

Plummer CE, et al: The canine glaucomas. In Gelatt KN, editor: Veterinary ophthalmology, ed 5, Ames, IA, 2013, Wiley-Blackwell, pp 900-1142.

AUTHOR: Caryn E. Plummer, DVM, DACVO
EDITOR: Diane V. H. Hendrix, DVM, DACVO

Glomerulonephritis

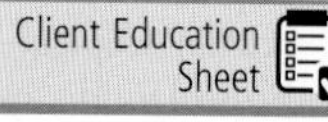

BASIC INFORMATION

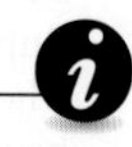

Definition

Glomerulonephritis (GN) is a common kidney disorder characterized by proteinuria due to immune complex deposition in the glomeruli and resultant inflammation. The condition is often idiopathic, but it can result from inflammatory, infectious, or neoplastic disease processes.

Epidemiology

SPECIES, AGE, SEX

Dogs > cats, with no sex predisposition; any age, but most are middle-aged or older

GENETICS, BREED PREDISPOSITION

Membranoproliferative GN:

- Bernese mountain dogs
- Labrador retrievers, golden retrievers, and Shetland sheepdogs with positive *Borrelia* titers
- Brittany spaniel (complement deficiency)

Proliferative and sclerosing GN:

- Soft-coated Wheaten terrier

RISK FACTORS

- Chronic bacterial infections (e.g., pyoderma, endocarditis, pyelonephritis, borreliosis, mycoplasmal polyarthritis)
- Fungal infection (e.g., coccidioidomycosis)
- Parasitic (e.g., heartworm disease)
- Rickettsial disease (e.g., ehrlichiosis)
- Protozoal infection (e.g., babesiosis, hepatozoonosis, leishmaniasis)
- Viral disease (e.g., feline immunodeficiency virus, feline leukemia virus, canine adenovirus)
- Neoplasia (e.g., mastocytosis, lymphoma, systemic histiocytosis)
- Immune-mediated disease (e.g., polyarthritis, systemic lupus erythematosus)
- Chronic inflammatory disease (e.g., inflammatory bowel disease, pancreatitis, cholangiohepatitis, thyroiditis)
- Glucocorticoid excess
- Trimethoprim-sulfadiazine therapy
- Congenital C3 (complement) deficiency
- Genetic predisposition

See further discussion on p. 1226.

CONTAGION AND ZOONOSIS

Some causes of secondary GN are zoonotic (e.g., leptospirosis, leishmaniasis).

GEOGRAPHY AND SEASONALITY

Several causes of secondary GN have specific geographic distributions (e.g., borreliosis in northeastern and north central United States).

ASSOCIATED DISORDERS

- Protein-losing nephropathy
- Nephrotic syndrome
- Chronic kidney disease (CKD)
- Systemic hypertension
- Hyperlipidemia
- Thromboembolic disease, including pulmonary thromboembolism
- Sideroblastic anemia

Clinical Presentation

DISEASE FORMS/SUBTYPES

Morphologic classification: histopathologic (correlates to therapy and prognosis not as well developed as in human nephrology)

- Membranoproliferative GN: common
  - Type I: mesangiocapillary GN associated with infectious disease; most common type
  - Type II: dense deposit disease
- Proliferative GN: rare

HISTORY, CHIEF COMPLAINT

Clinical signs may be absent. When signs are present, they may be due to uremia (p. 169), nephrotic syndrome (p. 691), or to the underlying disease responsible for GN:

- Vomiting (uremia or underlying disease)
- Lethargy (uremia or underlying disease)
- Anorexia (uremia or underlying disease)
- Weight loss (uremia, proteinuria, or underlying disease)
- Peripheral edema (hypoalbuminemia)
- Pendulous abdomen/ascites (hypoalbuminemia)
- Polyuria/polydipsia (CKD)
- Halitosis (uremia)
- Dyspnea/panting (pulmonary thromboembolism, ascites)
- Blindness (systemic hypertension)
- Signs associated with underlying infectious, inflammatory, or neoplastic disease

PHYSICAL EXAM FINDINGS

Clinical findings may be absent or may include

- Poor body condition
- Dehydration
- Poor haircoat
- Signs associated with hypoalbuminemia
  - Peripheral edema
  - Ascites (pure transudate)
  - Pleural effusion (rare)
- Signs associated with uremia
  - Oral ulceration
  - Halitosis (uremia)
- Pallor (due to anemia or poor perfusion if severe illness)
- Lipid corneal deposits
- Retinal hemorrhage/detachment (systemic hypertension)
- Kidneys may be normal sized or small.
- Other findings related to underlying disease

Etiology and Pathophysiology

- Immune complexes form or are trapped in glomeruli. Although GN is often a primary process (idiopathic), many diseases can provide the antigen to which antibody is produced, resulting in secondary immune complex formation.
- Glomerular immune complexes initiate an inflammatory cascade that damages the glomerulus, neutralizes glomerular endothelial electrical charge, and causes vasoconstriction and decreased glomerular filtration. The glomerulus responds to these insults with cellular proliferation.
- Albumin and similarly sized proteins are lost in urine and may result in hypoalbuminemia and the nephrotic syndrome. Eventually, tubular function is lost as well, resulting in azotemia and uremia.

DIAGNOSIS

Diagnostic Overview

The diagnosis is suspected based on the identification of proteinuria, an elevated urine protein/creatinine (UPC) ratio, and characteristic blood and imaging findings. Confirmation requires renal biopsy.

Differential Diagnosis

Proteinuria:

- Preglomerular (e.g., Bence Jones proteinuria, exercise, hemolysis, fever, seizure)
- Renal (glomerular causes of proteinuria typically result in greater proteinuria than nonglomerular causes)
  - GN
  - Amyloidosis
  - Glomerulosclerosis, including CKD
  - Familial glomerulonephropathy
  - Tubular
  - Interstitial nephritis
- Postglomerular (e.g., urinary tract infection, neoplasia, urolithiasis)

Initial Database

- Retinal exam: tortuous retinal vessels, retinal hemorrhages (acute or chronic), or retinal detachments can result from systemic hypertension.
- Blood pressure: systemic hypertension (repeatable systolic readings > 180 mm Hg in calm environment) is common (pp. 501 and 1065).
- CBC: often unremarkable; nonregenerative anemia (of chronic disease or due to CKD), leukocytosis (if inflammatory disease is present)
- Serum biochemical profile
  - Hypoalbuminemia with normal or increased globulin level
  - Hypercholesterolemia
  - Hypocalcemia (relative, due to hypoalbuminemia)
  - Azotemia, hyperphosphatemia, hyperamylasemia, metabolic acidosis (in advanced disease)

- Urinalysis: proteinuria, variable urine concentration, sometimes hematuria
  - Proteinuria must be interpreted in light of urine concentration and urine sediment exam.
  - Dipstick measure of proteinuria should be confirmed by sulfosalicylic acid (SSA) test or quantitative measures (e.g., UPC ratio [p. 1391]).
  - Significant proteinuria often precedes loss of urine concentrating ability or azotemia.
- Urine culture: indicated in all cases
- Thoracic radiographs: evidence of underlying disease (neoplasia, chronic infectious or inflammatory disease) or pulmonary thromboembolism occasionally identified
- Abdominal radiographs: often unremarkable. Kidneys may be small. May identify evidence of underlying disease (neoplasia, chronic infectious or inflammatory disease).
- Abdominal ultrasound: hyperechoic, small kidneys, decreased corticomedullary distinction, evidence of underlying disease (neoplasia, chronic infectious or inflammatory disease), or unremarkable

Advanced or Confirmatory Testing

- UPC ratio
  - Concurrent culture and sensitivity results must be negative to rule out bacterial infection as cause of elevated ratio.
  - Normal for dogs < 0.5; cats < 0.4. Most animals with GN (or amyloidosis) have ratios > 2.
- Microalbuminuria testing
  - Does not provide additional benefit in animals with elevated UPC. These assays detect very small quantities of urine albumin that would be missed on routine dipstick and are redundant when proteinuria has been identified.
- Renal biopsy is the only definitive means of diagnosis of GN, allowing morphologic classification of disease and identifying type and location of immunoglobulin. Cortical tissue is examined by light microscopy, immunofluorescence, and electron microscopy. Contact the International Veterinary Renal Pathology Service at The Ohio State University (Dr. Rachel Cianciolo's lab) or Texas A&M University (Drs. George Lees and Mary Nabity's lab).
- Determining serum antithrombin concentrations may help quantify risk of thromboembolic disease (<80% suggests increased risk).
- A variety of other tests may be indicated in a search for an underlying cause of GN. The choice of tests depends on history and physical exam, results of initial evaluation (CBC, serum biochemistry profile, imaging studies), geographic region, and environmental exposures. Common examples include
  - Serologic tests for heartworm, borreliosis, feline leukemia virus, feline immunodeficiency virus, *Ehrlichia canis,* coccidioidomycosis
  - Antinuclear antibody test
  - Arthrocentesis, echocardiography, bone marrow aspirate, thoracic radiographs
  - Adrenocorticotropic hormone stimulation or low-dose dexamethasone suppression test
  - Species-specific pancreatic lipase, trypsin-like immunoreactivity

TREATMENT

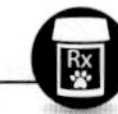

Treatment Overview

Treatment mainly consists of medications to decrease the degree of proteinuria. When appropriate, medications for the management of hypertension and thromboembolic disease are used. If the patient is in renal failure, supportive management is advised. A step-by-step approach to treatment is shown on p. 1420.

Acute and Chronic Treatment

- Address underlying disease conditions directly.
- If respirations are compromised by large-volume pleural effusion or severe ascites, centesis is indicated. Diuretic drugs are largely ineffective for rapid mobilization of body cavity fluid (p. 1164).
- Oxygen support may be required for animals with pulmonary thromboembolism (pp. 842 and 1146).
- Proteinuria reduction by angiotensin-converting enzyme (ACE) inhibitor treatment: for dogs, enalapril 0.5 mg/kg PO q 12-24h or benazepril 0.5 mg/kg PO q 24h, up to a maximum of 2 mg/kg/day
- If proteinuria persists (UPC > 1) despite ACE inhibitor use, consider angiotensin II receptor antagonists (e.g., telmisartan 1 mg/kg PO q 24 hours; can increase to maximum daily dose of 5 mg/kg) and/or aldosterone antagonist (spironolactone 1-2 mg/kg PO q 12h)
  - If UPC remains > 1 or is not reduced by one-half after single-agent ACE inhibitor or angiotensin II receptor blocker (ARB), consider cautious use of combined therapy. In humans but not dogs, combined therapy has been linked to higher incidences of kidney failure.
- If hypertension persists despite ACE inhibitor use, calcium channel blockers may be indicated (amlodipine 0.05-0.5 mg/kg PO q 24h [dogs]; 0.625 mg/CAT PO q 12-24h).
- Anticoagulant therapy can reduce the risk of thromboembolic disease. Unfractionated heparin is *not* effective because of loss of antithrombin.
  - Aspirin 0.5 mg/kg PO q 24h to q 12h (dog) or clopidogrel 2 mg/kg PO q 24h (dog)
  - Warfarin initial dose is 0.1-0.2 mg/kg PO q 24h.
    - Prothrombin time (PT) should be monitored and dose adjusted until PT = 1.5 to 2.5 times upper limit of normal range. Not generally recommended unless benefit outweighs risk (e.g., prior embolic event while on aspirin)
- Uremic animals may require fluid therapy (p. 169). Hypoalbuminemia may result in edema, in which case colloidal support may be necessary. Use cautiously.
  - Hetastarch 10-20 mL/kg/day IV
  - Dextrans: use with caution because of reported link to renal failure.
  - Large volumes of species-specific plasma or human albumin: expensive and short-lived effect (ongoing renal loss)
- Immunosuppressive treatment may be useful in up to 48% of protein-losing nephropathy cases (e.g., glucocorticoids, mycophenolate [p. 60])
  - Immunosuppression is best reserved for animals with biopsy-confirmed immune-mediated GN after the most likely underlying infectious causes have been ruled out. It can also be considered in rapidly progressing disease where biopsy is not indicated due to advanced state of disease.
- Clinical signs of uremia and electrolyte and acid-base disorders are addressed as for overt CKD (pp. 169 and 516).
- Dietary therapy: supplementation of polyunsaturated fatty acids and dietary protein restriction (i.e., renal diet)

Drug Interactions

- ACE inhibitors may cause hypotension when combined with diuretics or other vasodilators (rare but greater risk in hypovolemic/inappetent patient).
- ACE inhibitors may reduce proteinuria and ameliorate hypertension but may worsen azotemia, requiring monitoring of blood urea nitrogen (BUN) and creatinine during therapy.
- Nonsteroidal antiinflammatory agents may reduce efficacy of ACE inhibitors (avoid use).

Possible Complications

- Third-space retention of fluids
- Cachexia
- Worsening renal azotemia as a result of ACE inhibitor use (uncommon)
- Hypotension secondary to ACE inhibitor and calcium channel blocker
- Worsening of renal azotemia with dextran use
- Thromboembolic disease as a result of low antithrombin and/or protein C levels
- Bleeding tendency from aspirin, warfarin use
- Gastrointestinal ulceration as a result of azotemia or aspirin therapy
- Hyperkalemia due to ACE inhibitors and/or aldosterone antagonists

Recommended Monitoring

Stable animals are monitored every 3-4 months. Rechecks should be more frequent if treatment changes are made or when indicated by changing clinical signs.

- Physical exam
- UPC (ideally, pooled samples)
- Serum BUN/creatinine/phosphorus/potassium/albumin
- Blood pressure
- Urinalysis/culture

PROGNOSIS & OUTCOME

- Prognosis is best when an underlying disease can be identified and eliminated.
- When elimination of an underlying disease is not possible, survival is variable, but disease is usually progressive over months to 1-2 years.
- In dogs, prognosis for GN in general is better than for renal amyloidosis.
- Prognosis is worse when azotemia and/or uremia present at diagnosis
- Prognosis is worse for cats than dogs.
- Prognosis is poor for dogs where GN is associated with borreliosis.

PEARLS & CONSIDERATIONS

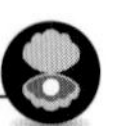

Comments

- Investigation of potential underlying diseases can become expensive. Clinical judgment should guide the choice of ancillary tests for each animal.
- After protein-losing nephropathy is identified, renal biopsy is useful as a prognostic tool and may influence choice to use immunosuppressive therapy. In one retrospective study of 733 renal biopsies, 48% demonstrated immune complex glomerulonephritis.

Prevention

- Ectoparasite prophylaxis
- Heartworm prophylaxis

Technician Tips

- When presenting for recheck exams, advise owners to not allow dogs to urinate just before the appointment.
- Pooled aliquots of approximately equal volume from three urine samples (stored in freezer or refrigerator) best for repeat UPC measurement.

Client Education

- Diligent rechecks are very important for adjusting medications and identifying complications early.
- Finding an underlying disease process may mean a better prognosis for the pet.

SUGGESTED READING

IRIS Canine GN Study Group, Diagnosis Subgroup: Consensus recommendations for the diagnostic investigation of dogs with suspected glomerular disease. J Vet Intern Med 27(suppl 1):S19-S26, 2013.

AUTHOR: Anne M. Dalby, DVM, DACVIM
EDITOR: Leah A. Cohn, DVM, PhD, DACVIM

Glyphosate Herbicide Toxicosis

BASIC INFORMATION

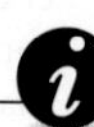

Definition

Acute intoxication with glyphosate, a common household and agricultural herbicide. Glyphosate is a phosphangoglycine-type of nonselective herbicide available as ready-to-use or concentrates for residential and agricultural use. Toxicosis can occur after oral and dermal (walk through recently treated weeds) exposures and is characterized by gastrointestinal (GI) signs.

Synonyms

N-(phosphonomethyl)glycine, weed and grass killer, Roundup

Epidemiology

SPECIES, AGE, SEX

All dogs and cats are at risk, but dogs with history of indiscriminate eating habits may be more likely to be exposed.

RISK FACTORS

- Dogs and cats that are outside while owners are gardening
- Patients with history of GI disorders may be at higher risk for signs.

GEOGRAPHY AND SEASONALITY

Toxicosis is more likely during warmer months of the year (spring/summer), when herbicides are more likely to be used.

Clinical Presentation

DISEASE FORMS/SUBTYPES

- Most cases involve ready-to-use products; signs are acute in nature, begin < 2 hours after exposure, and are restricted to mild hypersalivation and vomiting.
- The surfactants (soaps) in the concentrated products can cause oral irritation and potentially cause ulcers.

HISTORY, CHIEF COMPLAINT

- Known exposure or potential access to product
- Sudden-onset vomiting, hypersalivation, or oral ulceration

PHYSICAL EXAM FINDINGS

- Vomiting
- Hypersalivation
- Oral ulceration (for high–surfactant containing concentrate product)
- Dehydration is possible with more severe signs

Etiology and Pathophysiology

- These products are sprayed on plants, wetting the surface. Animals can be exposed to the liquid product (e.g., chewing the bottle), by skin contact with wet plant leaves, or by consuming recently treated plant material.
- Glyphosate kills plants by disrupting the metabolic pathway (shikimic acid pathway) that produces folates and several amino acids. This pathway is not present in animals.
- In animals, glyphosate has a wide margin of safety; toxicity often is related to inactive ingredient (surfactants) or other herbicides found in the product
- Surfactants lead to mucosal irritation or, in high concentrations, mucosal ulceration.

DIAGNOSIS

Diagnostic Overview

There are no specific tests for diagnosing glyphosate toxicity. Typically, diagnosis is based on evidence of exposure or potential access to product and clinical signs.

Differential Diagnosis

- Other causes of oral ulceration (p. 1002)
  - Alkaline battery
  - Caustic cleaning agents (acids, alkalis)
  - Cationic detergents
- Any potential cause of gastritis (e.g., viral, bacterial, dietary indiscretion)

Initial Database

- Specific lab tests are not needed in most patients.
- Monitor electrolytes in patients that have more than mild vomiting or diarrhea.
- Other tests may be indicated to rule out other causes of GI signs or oral ulcers if exposure to the herbicide is unconfirmed.

Advanced or Confirmatory Testing

Serum and urine glyphosate concentrations can be measured. Assays are not readily available and are unlikely to aid in patient treatment.

TREATMENT

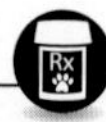

Treatment Overview

Signs are typically mild and self-limited. Dilution soon after exposure is helpful. If

GI signs are seen, care is symptomatic and supportive.

Acute General Treatment

- Because signs are mild and self-limited for the majority of patients, limited treatment is warranted.
- Oral exposure: dilution with water or milk (2-6 mL/kg PO) after recent exposure
- Antiemetic and fluid therapy if vomiting is more than mild
  - Maropitant 1 mg/kg SQ (or 2 mg/kg PO q 24h)
- GI protectants if caustic injury is noted
  - Omeprazole 0.5-1 mg/kg PO q 12h
  - Sucralfate 250-500 mg for small dogs and cats, 1 g for large dogs q 6-12h, should be crushed and suspended in water
- Dermal exposure: bath with liquid hand dishwashing detergent

Nutrition/Diet

Withhold food and water until vomiting under control

Recommended Monitoring

Most commonly monitored at home for mild GI signs (vomiting, diarrhea). If concentrate product was involved or product with high surfactant concentration was ingested, monitor for oral ulceration.

PROGNOSIS & OUTCOME

Inadvertent or small ingestions rarely cause serious toxicity, and prognosis is generally excellent. If product is a concentrate, it may have a higher surfactant concentration that can cause oral ulceration or more significant GI signs.

PEARLS & CONSIDERATIONS

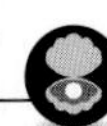

Comments

- Onset of signs, if signs occur, is generally rapid (within 1 hour of exposure).
- Products with surfactant concentrations of 18% or higher are more likely to cause mucosal irritation and ulceration.

Prevention

Do not allow pets in treated areas until they are dry.

Technician Tips

- Very commonly used herbicide in the United States
- Toxicity is typically mild; if a pet owner is concerned about exposure to a nonconcentrated product, it is usually adequate for them to bathe (if dermal exposure) and monitor pet at home.

Client Education

- Owners should be advised to keep pets out of area where herbicide is used until the sprayed plants are dry.
- Plants may be more palatable after being treated.

SUGGESTED READING

Talcott PA: Miscellaneous herbicides, fungicides and nematocides. In Peterson ME, editors: Small animal toxicology, ed 3, St. Louis, 2013, Elsevier, pp 401-408.

AUTHOR: Kirsten Waratuke, DVM, DABT
EDITOR: Tina Wismer, DVM, MS, DABVT, DABT

Granulocytic Anaplasmosis and Ehrlichiosis

Bonus Material Online 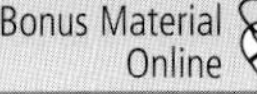 Client Education Sheet 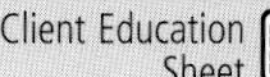 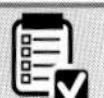

BASIC INFORMATION

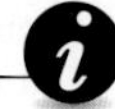

Definition

Common tick-borne diseases caused by infection with intracellular rickettsial bacteria *Anaplasma phagocytophilum* or *Ehrlichia ewingii*

Synonyms

- *E. ewingii*: granulocytic ehrlichiosis
- *A. phagocytophilum*: granulocytic anaplasmosis (*Ehrlichia equi* is outdated nomenclature)

Epidemiology

SPECIES, AGE, SEX

- *A. phagocytophilum*: dogs and cats
- *E. ewingii*: dogs

GENETICS, BREED PREDISPOSITION

Golden retrievers and Labrador retrievers may be overrepresented.

RISK FACTORS

Risk of tick exposure and lack of adequate tick prevention

CONTAGION AND ZOONOSIS

Animals and humans may be infected from tick bites, but there is no evidence of direct transmission.

GEOGRAPHY AND SEASONALITY

- *A. phagocytophilum:* northeastern United States, Wisconsin, Minnesota, California (reflecting prevalence of deer tick)
- *E. ewingii:* southeastern and south central United States, with apparent northern expansion (reflecting prevalence of lone star tick)

ASSOCIATED DISORDERS

Co-infection with other tick-borne pathogens, such as *Borrelia burgdorferi, Bartonella* spp (deer tick); *Ehrlichia chaffeensis*, Panola Mountain *Ehrlichia, Rickettsia rickettsii* (lone star tick)

Clinical Presentation

DISEASE FORMS/SUBTYPES

- Acute infections: clinical cases of canine granulocytic anaplasmosis and ehrlichiosis
- Chronic infections: persistent subclinical infection is well documented; unclear if clinical signs ever develop in chronically infected animals

HISTORY, CHIEF COMPLAINT

- Clinical signs are most likely in warm months when ticks are active. There may or may not be a recognized tick bite 1-3 weeks before illness, but environmental tick exposure is commonly recognized (e.g., animal spends time outdoors).
- For both pathogens, common complaints include lethargy, anorexia, and lameness or reluctance to walk (associated with polyarthropathy).
  - Less common complaints include gastrointestinal signs (*A. phagocytophilum*) or signs of meningitis or vestibular disease (*A. phagocytophilum, E. ewingii*)
- Clinical signs are not usually associated with chronic infection with either organism.

PHYSICAL EXAM FINDINGS

Infection can be present without any illness. When illness occurs:

- Fever is the most common physical exam finding.
- Pain or swelling in multiple joints; particularly common in carpi and stifles
- Lymphadenopathy (mild) and splenomegaly
- Hemorrhage, epistaxis, melena, or petechiae possible but uncommon
- Rarely, neurologic signs (e.g., proprioception deficits, vestibular signs)

Etiology and Pathophysiology

- *A. phagocytophilum* and *E. ewingii* are indistinguishable when identified in circulating neutrophils or synovial fluid granulocytes.

- Most infected animals remain well but can develop a chronic carrier state (either pathogen).
- The reason that some animals develop clinical disease is uncertain and may depend on the immune status of the animal and complicating co-infections with other vector-borne agents.
- *A. phagocytophilum* is transmitted by the deer tick (*Ixodes scapularis, Ixodes pacificus, Ixodes ricinus*), and *E. ewingii* is transmitted by the lone star tick (*Amblyomma americanum*).
- After inoculation, the organism invades granulocytes and multiplies in membrane-bound vacuoles, forming morulae that contain several individual bacteria.
- Organisms are found in circulating granulocytes, granulocytes in synovial fluid, and in various tissues, including liver and spleen.

DIAGNOSIS

Diagnostic Overview

The diagnosis is suspected in any dog with a febrile lameness (or other findings listed above) that lives in or has recently traveled to an endemic area. Confirmation of infection requires finding morulae in granulocytic cells, serologic evidence of infection, or polymerase chain reaction (PCR) analysis.

Differential Diagnosis

- Because many tick-borne/vector-borne agents can result in similar clinical findings, ticks can be simultaneously infected with multiple agents, and pets often have multiple ectoparasites simultaneously, other tick-borne disease should be considered in the differential diagnosis, including but not limited to other *Ehrlichia* spp, *Anaplasma* spp, *Bartonella* spp, and *Rickettsia* spp.
- Other causes of polyarthritis (pp. 803 and 1270)

Initial Database

- CBC
  - Thrombocytopenia is the most common abnormality (up to 90% of ill animals).
  - Mild anemia possible, particularly in dogs with evidence of hemorrhage
  - Initial, transient neutropenia; then normal neutrophil count or neutrophilia
  - Morulae may or may not be identified in neutrophils.
  - Lymphocyte counts vary; a reactive lymphocyte population is common.
- Serum biochemical profile: nonspecific findings; increases in liver enzyme (alanine aminotransferase, alkaline phosphatase) activities may occur. Transient hypoalbuminemia possible in dogs with acute *A. phagocytophilum* infection.
- Radiographs of affected joints: soft-tissue swelling from nonerosive polyarthritis
- Arthrocentesis (p. 1059): with polyarthritis, the synovial fluid contains increased numbers of neutrophils. Morulae can be seen in granulocyte cytoplasm in some cases, depending on stage of infection and the microscopist's skill.

Advanced or Confirmatory Testing

- Microscopic analysis: buffy coat smears prepared from peripheral blood can enhance the probability of identifying morulae in circulating granulocytes.
- Serologic testing
  - Negative serology result can occur in acute infection because antibody production takes time.
  - Positive antibody test result does not prove disease causation and must be interpreted in light of other clinical findings.
  - The in-clinic ELISA, SNAP 4Dx Plus, can detect antibodies to *E. ewingii, Ehrlichia canis, E. chaffeensis, A. phagocytophilum,* and *Anaplasma platys.*
  - IFA tests run by diagnostic laboratories detect antibodies in patient serum and provide a numeric titer. Ideally, serologic confirmation is based on a ≥ fourfold rise in titer between acute and convalescent serum samples taken 2-4 weeks apart, although a single titer ≥ 64 in an animal with suggestive clinical signs is strongly supportive.
- PCR analysis (anticoagulated blood, synovial fluid) performed at commercial labs can detect and distinguish between *A. phagocytophilum* and *E. ewingii.*
  - PCR is much more sensitive in detecting organisms than microscopic evaluation.
  - Those chronically infected or subclinical carriers may be seropositive and PCR negative due to the low numbers of circulating organisms.
  - Even a single dose of appropriate antibiotic can result in a negative PCR test.

TREATMENT

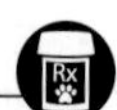

Treatment Overview

Doxycycline is the treatment of choice and often results in rapid (24-48 hours) resolution of clinical signs. Prolonged treatment is usually prescribed to attempt to eradicate the infection, but the efficacy of this treatment regimen for eliminating the organism has been questioned.

Acute and Chronic Treatment

- Doxycycline or minocycline 5-10 mg/kg PO q 12h for 28 days
- Nonsteroidal antiinflammatory drugs or antiinflammatory doses of glucocorticoids can be used judiciously in the initial period to relieve clinical signs of joint disease.
- Animals with an incomplete response or relapse should be tested for other vector-borne agents, particularly those that respond poorly to doxycycline (e.g., *Bartonella* spp).

Drug Interactions

Some dogs are sensitive to the gastrointestinal side effects (nausea and vomiting) associated with doxycycline. To avoid these side effects, oral doxycycline should be given with meals.

Possible Complications

Co-infections with other tick-borne/vector-borne agents can result in more severe clinical manifestations and/or poor response to antimicrobial therapy.

Recommended Monitoring

- Clinical response to treatment
- To confirm infection if initially serology negative, perform convalescent titers in ≈3 weeks.

PROGNOSIS & OUTCOME

The prognosis for recovery from acute *A. phagocytophilum* or *E. ewingii* infection is excellent, but the organism may not be cleared entirely.

PEARLS & CONSIDERATIONS

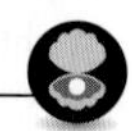

Comments

- In endemic areas, veterinarians often treat based on clinical presentation (polyarthropathy, fever, thrombocytopenia) with or without laboratory confirmation.
- Although illness due to these infections is remarkably similar and appearance of morulae is identical, there is only minor overlap in the geographic area where these infections are recognized.
- A positive *Anaplasma* serologic test on the SNAP 4Dx Plus in an area where *E. ewingii* infection is more likely than *A. phagocytophilum* may be due to *A. platys. A. platys* causes cyclic canine thrombocytopenia, but in the United States, clinical bleeding from the infection rarely occurs.
- Most animals that become inoculated with either agent do not develop clinical signs or have clinical disease that is transient and self-limited. These animals often have positive results on screening assays such as SNAP 4Dx Plus but are clinically healthy.
- Repeat infection/illness has not been known to occur with either of these agents.

Prevention

Tick control: routine use of ascaricides and careful examination of the skin and haircoat after any activity that carries the risk of tick exposure

Technician Tips

- It is best to use a smaller-gauge needle and an easily compressible vein (cephalic or saphenous, not jugular) and apply prolonged pressure after venipuncture in animals with severe thrombocytopenia.
- Blood from acutely infected animals has the potential to spread infection if inadvertently inoculated into another animal or person by contaminated needles.
- Seropositive animals or animals previously infected with either of these agents, or any

tick-borne disease, should not be used as blood donors.

Client Education

- There is essentially no risk of contracting these infections directly from a pet. However, people share the same environment with their pets, and they should also make efforts to reduce the risk of tick exposure to prevent tick-transmitted diseases for themselves and family members.
- Tick prevention remains important in previously/subclinically infected animals to avoid co-infections with other agents that may result in more severe clinical illness and to prevent transfer of pathogens from subclinical carriers to ticks. Allowing ticks to feed on infected dogs has the potential to increase the pathogen burden in the tick population.

SUGGESTED READING

Little SE: Ehrlichiosis and anaplasmosis in dogs and cats. Vet Clin North Am Small Anim Pract 40:1121-1140, 2010.

AUTHOR: A. Rick Alleman, DVM, PhD
EDITOR: Joseph Taboada, DVM, DACVIM

Granulomatous Enteritis/Colitis

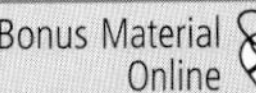

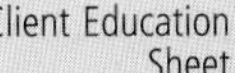

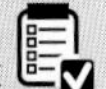

BASIC INFORMATION

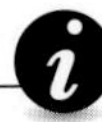

Definition

Uncommon cause of persistent (>3 weeks) signs of small-intestinal or, more often, colonic inflammation associated with mucosal infiltration of macrophages

- In the colon, the most common cause is mucosal invasive *Escherichia coli* infection (i.e., adherent/invasive *E. coli* [AIEC]). Affected animals have large-bowel diarrhea and systemic signs (fever, anorexia, weight loss).
- Other types of infections (e.g., algal, fungal, parasitic) can cause granulomatous inflammation in small or large bowel or in both segments.

Synonyms

Boxer colitis refers to the old inflammatory bowel disease (IBD) variant; *granulomatous colitis* (GC) is the contemporary term describing *E. coli* infection in boxers and French bulldogs.

Epidemiology

SPECIES, AGE, SEX

- Granulomatous enteritis is much more common in dogs than cats.
- GC seen with AIEC appears to be most prevalent in young male dogs.

GENETICS, BREED PREDISPOSITION

- Predisposition in boxers and French bulldogs is associated with defective clearance of intracellular bacteria and GC.
- Large-breed dogs are more commonly affected with systemic fungal infections.
- Hunting/sporting dogs more often infected with schistosomiasis (i.e., *Heterobilharzia*) and pythiosis.
- German shepherd, collies, and boxers overrepresented for protothecosis

GEOGRAPHY AND SEASONALITY

Geographic or seasonal influence important for several fungal, algal, and parasitic infections (see specific chapters for detail)

Clinical Presentation

DISEASE FORMS/SUBTYPES

- GC: associated with AIEC and characterized by mucosal infiltration with periodic acid–Schiff (PAS) stain–positive macrophages
- Other infectious causes of granulomatous enteritis
  - *Heterobilharzia americana*
  - *Histoplasma capsulatum* (p. 476)
  - *Pythium insidiosum* (p. 860)
  - *Prototheca* spp

HISTORY, CHIEF COMPLAINT

- GC: persistent large-bowel diarrhea, tenesmus (straining to defecate), increased frequency of defecation, mucoid feces, and fresh blood (p. 1215)
- Cachexia, anorexia, and weight loss are common with GC, in sharp contrast to other causes of colonic inflammation.
- Infectious causes of GC can be associated with small-intestinal gastrointestinal (GI) signs (e.g., vomiting, melena) or other organ signs (e.g., blindness, cutaneous lesions, central nervous system signs).

PHYSICAL EXAM FINDINGS

- Colonic mucosa may feel thickened or cobblestone-like on rectal palpation. Fresh blood or mucus may be recognized after palpation.
- Fever, cachexia, weight loss, and peripheral/mesenteric lymphadenomegaly are observed with infectious causes.
- Dogs with AIEC may not have mesenteric lymphadenomegaly.
- Other examination abnormalities can be related to pathogen infection of other tissues (e.g., uveitis, paresis, head tilt, ataxia with *Prototheca* spp infection; respiratory effort, peripheral lymphadenomegaly with histoplasmosis).

Etiology and Pathophysiology

- GC
  - Chronic enteropathy of boxers and French bulldogs, much less common than lymphocytic plasmacytic colitis seen in other breeds
  - Additional evidence suggests GC may not be IBD but rather a unique and specific form of infectious colitis (AIEC).
- Granulomatous enteritis
  - Mucosal disease caused by fungi, parasites, oomycetes, or algae
  - Can involve large and/or small bowel
  - Dissemination to other organs is common with systemic mycotic and algal infections.

DIAGNOSIS

Diagnostic Overview

The diagnosis may be suspected based on history of signs of chronic colitis and weight loss, prompting endoscopic or full-thickness intestinal biopsies (definitive confirmation).

Differential Diagnosis

Other differential diagnoses: severe colonic IBD, neoplasia (p. 604)

Initial Database

- CBC, serum biochemistry, and urinalysis: evaluate involvement of diverse organ systems.
- Fecal flotation and direct examination for GI parasites, including *Heterobilharzia*
- Exfoliative cytology (e.g., rectal scrape [p. 1157]) is easy and inexpensive and can sometimes confirm infection with *Histoplasma* or, less often, with *Prototheca* spp or *Pythium* in endemic regions.
- Urinary *Histoplasma* antigen (highly sensitive and specific assay [p. 1365]): simple noninvasive test for GI histoplasmosis
- Abdominal imaging (survey radiographs, contrast radiography, and/or ultrasonography): diffuse colonic wall thickening, loss of wall layering, and/or mesenteric lymphadenomegaly indicative of infiltrative mural disease, but these changes are not specific for any specific cause of colitis.

Advanced or Confirmatory Testing

- Depending on level of suspicion, other infectious disease testing may be appropriate:
  - Polymerase chain reaction (PCR) (tissue) or ELISA (serum): *Pythium* spp infection
  - Vitreocentesis may detect *Prototheca* spp organisms in animals with ocular lesions.
- Ultimately, diagnosis depends on finding PAS-positive macrophages or granulomatous inflammation with infectious organisms in intestinal biopsy specimens.
  - Endoscopy (p. 1098) or colonoscopy generally preferred
  - Avoid surgical full-thickness biopsy of colon whenever possible.
  - If AIEC suspected (i.e., boxer, French bulldog), submit mucosal biopsy sample for bacterial culture and susceptibility testing.
- Fluorescence *in situ* hybridization (FISH) performed on tissue sections confirms presence of AIEC in infected dogs.

TREATMENT

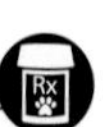

Treatment Overview

Treatment requires a specific definitive diagnosis determined by mucosal biopsy or other confirmatory testing.

Acute and Chronic Treatment

- Treat AIEC-associated GC with enrofloxacin 5 mg/kg PO q 24h for 6-8 weeks, alone or in combination with metronidazole or amoxicillin. Some dogs may respond to single drug therapy, but others may require combination therapy.
  - Extend treatment 14 days past resolution of signs because of severity of most *E. coli* infections. Resolution of GI signs generally correlates with eradication of mucosal bacteria.
  - Antimicrobial resistance is common among AIEC patients and impacts clinical response. Antimicrobial therapy is best guided by mucosal culture and susceptibility testing.
- For specific treatment guidelines, see chapters on histoplasmosis (p. 476), pythiosis (p. 860), protothecosis, or schistosomiasis.

Nutrition/Diet

- Feed a low-fat, fiber-enriched commercial diet. Fiber binds colonic irritants, normalizes dysmotility, and promotes colonic epithelial repair and renewal.
- If the animal will not eat a commercial fiber-containing diet, addition of fiber (small to moderate amounts of soluble fiber [e.g., psyllium mucilloid/Metamucil sprinkled on food: 1-2 teaspoons (5-10 mL dry)/10 kg body weight per feeding]) to the regular diet.
- In some instances, a restricted-antigen (e.g., elimination) diet may also be helpful because dogs may develop dietary sensitivity (p. 347).
- Dogs with small-intestinal involvement and protein-losing enteropathy are generally protein-calorie malnourished but may benefit from low-fat rations with high-quality, highly digestible protein sources. Assess cobalamin status in these patients, and supplement if deficient (p. 183).

Possible Complications

- Boxers with GC may require repeated intermittent or long-term therapy for remission of signs. If dogs fail to respond to enrofloxacin, consider antibiotic resistance as a strong possibility for treatment failure. Alternative drugs to consider are based on culture and susceptibility results. Alternatively, clinicians may try combination therapy using fluoroquinolones and other macrophage-penetrating antibiotics such as chloramphenicol, trimethoprim-sulfadiazine, or amikacin.
- Cure is often not possible in animals with pythiosis or protothecosis. These animals will likely die regardless of therapy.

Recommended Monitoring

Rechecks at 2-4 week intervals for animals with GC. Monitor clinical disease activity and body weight, and taper medications as GI signs resolve. Monitoring of other infectious diseases depends on presentation.

PROGNOSIS & OUTCOME

- GC carries a good short-term prognosis; long-term studies of full remission are lacking.
- Prognosis for schistosomiasis is good, and for GI histoplasmosis, fair to good with appropriate therapy.
- GC caused by *Pythium* spp and *Prototheca* spp carries a poor prognosis.

PEARLS & CONSIDERATIONS

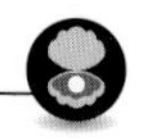

Comments

- Major causes of granulomatous enteritis are infectious organisms.
- Colonoscopy with mucosal biopsy is imperative for diagnosis in most instances. Ancillary testing (FISH) can identify mucosally invasive bacteria.
- A thorough diagnostic evaluation is warranted to rule out the varied causes of colonic inflammation.
- The disease formerly known as "boxer colitis" seems to be due to AIEC and should not be treated with immune suppression.

Technician Tips

- These animals can become dehydrated and quite debilitated. Fastidious nursing care and close monitoring are required.
- Careful fecal examination is necessary for all animals with chronic diarrhea.

Client Education

Dietary modification may be required for the life of the pet.

SUGGESTED READING

Craven M, et al: Granulomatous colitis of boxer dogs. Vet Clin North Am Small Anim Pract 41:433, 2011.

AUTHOR: Albert E. Jergens, DVM, MS, PhD, DACVIM
EDITOR: Rance K. Sellon, DVM, PhD, DACVIM

Grapes and Raisins Toxicosis

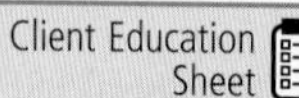

BASIC INFORMATION

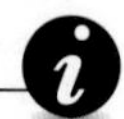

Definition

Acute kidney injury (AKI) after ingestion of grapes, raisins, or currants (*Vitis* spp)

Epidemiology

SPECIES, AGE, SEX

- Documented in dogs only
- Anecdotally reported in cats, ferrets
- No known age or sex predisposition; all breeds susceptible
- Ingestion of grapes or raisins does not consistently cause AKI in all dogs.

RISK FACTORS

Animals with pre-existing kidney disease may be at increased risk for AKI.

Clinical Presentation

HISTORY, CHIEF COMPLAINT

- Ingestion suspected or directly observed
- Evidence of grapes/raisins in vomitus or stool
- Most common signs are manifestations of uremia (AKI-induced oliguria/anuria): vomiting, lethargy, anorexia, diarrhea, decreased urine output, signs of abdominal pain, ataxia, and weakness (p. 23)
- Vomiting, lethargy, anorexia within 24 hours; vomiting is often seen within 12 hours after ingestion

PHYSICAL EXAM FINDINGS

- Dehydration, lethargy
- Signs of abdominal pain in some dogs
- ± Uremic ulcers, uremic odor to breath

Etiology and Pathophysiology

- Toxicity is poorly understood.
- Renal tubular necrosis is a consistent histopathologic finding.
  - Tubular basement membrane often remains intact, providing possibility for recovery.
  - Evidence of tubular regeneration may be present in some dogs.
- Mineralization of kidneys, gastric mucosa, myocardium, lungs, and blood vessels can occur.

DIAGNOSIS

Diagnostic Overview

Diagnosis of grape/raisin toxicosis is suspected based on suspicion/evidence of exposure, presence of grapes/raisins in the vomitus/stool, and the onset of vomiting, anorexia, lethargy, diarrhea, decreased urine output, ataxia or weakness, or a combination of these. Azotemia and other serum biochemical changes consistent with AKI are seen in 1-3 days.

Differential Diagnosis

Rule out other causes of AKI (p. 23):

- Leptospirosis
- Ethylene glycol toxicosis
- Bacterial pyelonephritis
- Lily toxicosis in cats
- Iatrogenic/medication nephrotoxicosis (e.g., aminoglycoside antibiotics)
- Renal thromboembolism (usually accompanied by thromboembolism of other aortic branches)

Initial Database

- Serum chemistry profile within 24-72 hours
  - Azotemia; creatinine may rise before blood urea nitrogen (BUN)
  - Hyperphosphatemia
  - Hypercalcemia
  - Elevated total calcium × phosphorus product (Ca × P): > 60 when both are measured in mg/dL, present when enough time has passed and ingestion was substantial
- Urinalysis before fluid therapy may reveal
  - Urine specific gravity typically isosthenuric but may be minimally concentrated if acute anuria
  - Glucosuria
  - Proteinuria
  - Cylindruria (casts)
- Abdominal radiographs; abnormalities uncommon (renomegaly, metastatic mineralization)
- Ultrasonography to assess kidneys and pancreas

Advanced or Confirmatory Testing

- Specific testing may be helpful to rule out differential diagnosis (e.g., polymerase chain reaction [PCR] or serology for leptospirosis; test kit or measured osmole gap for ethylene glycol intoxication)
- Renal biopsy may help determine prognosis.

TREATMENT

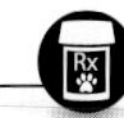

Treatment Overview

- If patient has eaten a substantial quantity of grapes (e.g., > 5 grapes in an 8-kg dog) or raisins (>0.03 oz/kg [>0.85 g/kg]), decontamination is justified to reduce the risk of permanent renal damage.
- Decontamination (induction of vomiting and administration of activated charcoal) aims to decrease absorption in early ingestions, when no clinical signs are apparent.
- When clinical signs are present, treatment consists of fluid diuresis, nutritional support, vomiting and seizure control, and management of AKI (p. 23) as needed.
- Urine production should be > 0.5 mL/kg/h; oliguria is urine production < 0.5 mL/kg/h, and anuria is < 0.1 mL/kg/h.

Acute General Treatment

- Decontamination of patient (p. 1087)
  - Emesis is useful 6-12 hours after exposure (p. 1188).
  - Activated charcoal 1-2 g/kg PO is useful up to 12-24 hours after exposure.
- Fluid diuresis
  - Intravenous fluid diuresis for 48 hours in patients not yet showing clinical signs may prevent AKI.
  - Treat signs of AKI as needed (p. 23). For concurrent hypercalcemia, consider using 0.9% normal saline.
- Manage vomiting.
  - Maropitant 1 mg/kg SQ (or 2 mg/kg PO) q 24h up to 5 consecutive days, *or*
  - Metoclopramide 0.2-0.4 mg/kg q 6h PO, SQ, or IM or 1-2 mg/kg/d constant-rate infusion (CRI)
- Treat anuria/oliguria.
  - Correct dehydration first.
  - Mannitol 0.25-0.5 g/kg IV over 3-5 minutes or as IV CRI 2-5 mL/min of 5%-10% mannitol in lactated Ringer's solution
  - Furosemide 2-4 mg/kg IV up to 6 mg/kg if needed (if oliguria/anuria persists) q 8h
  - Hemodialysis or peritoneal dialysis may be useful in some cases.

Chronic Treatment

Ongoing supportive care is based on severity, response to treatments, individual's sensitivity, and extent of permanent renal injury (pp. 167 and 169).

Possible Complications

- Uremia-related neurologic (seizures, ataxia) or respiratory (acute respiratory distress syndrome) signs
- Metastatic mineralization (renal, cardiac, vascular, pulmonary)
- Pancreatitis

Recommended Monitoring

- Baseline BUN, creatinine, total calcium, phosphorus, Ca × P, potassium, total protein, hematocrit: daily at first, then as needed
- Urine output: hourly at first
- Signs of overhydration (respiratory character/effort, body weight)
- Acid-base status

PROGNOSIS & OUTCOME

- In two separate studies, approximately 50% of dogs with clinical signs of grape/raisin toxicosis recovered with treatment, and the remainder died or were euthanized.
- Oliguria/anuria, ataxia, and weakness indicate a poor prognosis.
- Higher serum total calcium concentration and Ca × P indicate a poor prognosis.

PEARLS & CONSIDERATIONS

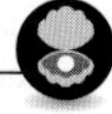

Comments

- The toxic dosage may be low. AKI has occurred after ingestion of 0.013 oz/lb (0.85 g/kg) of raisins or 5 grapes in an 8.2-kg dog.
- Raisins are 4.5 times more concentrated than grapes on an ounce-per-ounce basis.
- Not all dogs that ingest raisins or grapes develop AKI.
- AKI has occurred with ingestion of raisins in baked goods.
- Patients with AKI may need treatment for days to weeks.

Prevention

Keep raisins and grapes out of dogs' reach.

Technician Tips

Decontamination with induction of vomiting can be effective up to 12 hours and administration of charcoal up to 24 hours after exposure.

Client Education

- Do not feed grapes or raisins to dogs.
- Treatment may be extensive and expensive and is associated with a guarded prognosis after signs are present.
- Zante currants are *Vitis* sp (grapes) and can be toxic; real currants are *Ribes* sp and are nontoxic.

SUGGESTED READING

Eubig PA, et al: Acute renal failure in dogs after the ingestion of grapes or raisins: a retrospective evaluation of 43 dogs (1992-2002). J Vet Intern Med 19:663-674, 2005.

AUTHOR: Cristine Hayes, DVM, DABT, DABVT
EDITOR: Tina Wismer, DVM, DABT, DABVT, MS

Grass Awn Migration

Client Education Sheet Bonus Material Online 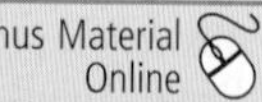

BASIC INFORMATION 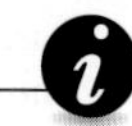

Definition

Grass awns are bristles growing from the spikelets of certain grasses. They may penetrate the skin and body orifices of dogs and cats, causing abscesses, granulomas, or draining tracts anywhere in the body.

Epidemiology

SPECIES, AGE, SEX

Most common in young, active dogs; rare in cats

GENETICS, BREED PREDISPOSITION

Increased prevalence in hunting and working breeds (spaniels, retrievers, terriers)

RISK FACTORS

Hunting and working dogs are at risk due to increased exposure to plants in the field while exercising and open-mouth breathing. Longer haircoats may increase risk.

GEOGRAPHY AND SEASONALITY

- *Hordeum glaucum, Hordeum leporinum,* and *Hordeum jubatum* (foxtails) in the western United States; barley grass awn (*Stripa* and *Setaria* spp) in the southern United States; wild oat grass awn (*Avena* spp) in Australia and Europe
- Spring and summer for grass awn penetration
- Long latent period means affected animals may be presented at any time of the year.

ASSOCIATED DISORDERS

Secondary bacterial infection (*Streptococcus* spp, *Actinomyces* spp, *Nocardia* spp) is common, causing chronic, suppurative tissue reaction +/− granuloma formation.

Clinical Presentation

DISEASE FORMS/SUBTYPES

- Numerous, depending on site of penetration and course of tissue migration
- Grass awns enter skin, subcutaneous tissue, and body recesses, including the external ear canal, conjunctival fornix, nasal cavity and sinuses, and oral cavity. They often migrate, following the path of least resistance along tissue planes, blood vessels, and nerves, and causing disease in locations distant from the entry point. Animals may have clinical signs of thoracic, abdominal, or rarely, intracranial disease from grass awns that have migrated.
- Less common disease forms include fibrotic iliopsoas myopathy, pseudoaneurysm of the celiac artery, and retrobulbar abscess.

HISTORY, CHIEF COMPLAINT

- Outdoor activity in area where grass awns are endemic
- Clinical signs are referable to affected body system
- Signs may improve with antimicrobial therapy and then recur or worsen after discontinuation.

PHYSICAL EXAM FINDINGS

Depend on location and migration path of the grass awn:

- Subcutaneous tissue (very common): palpable soft-tissue mass +/− draining tract, regional lymphadenopathy, fever; interdigital spaces are especially commonly affected in dogs
- Ear canal (unilateral or bilateral): head shaking (may cause aural hematoma), otic exudate, otitis externa. An otoscopic exam is warranted in any animal suspected of having a grass awn foreign body, even in the absence of signs.
- Oral cavity: gagging, pawing at mouth, often lodged in tonsillar crypt
- Nasal cavity: sneezing (often violent and persistent), nasal discharge
- Lungs: tachypnea/dyspnea, decreased lung sounds
- Pericardium (pericardial effusion): muffled heart sounds, tachycardia, weak pulse, ascites
- Abdomen: lethargy, fever, signs of abdominal pain, palpable abdominal mass
- Retroperitoneal space/sublumbar musculature: fever, back pain, flank swelling +/− draining tracts, myelopathy (neurologic deficits such as paresis/paralysis)

Etiology and Pathophysiology

Grass awns penetrate the skin, interdigital spaces, and the ear canal, causing inflammation, abscessation, and draining tracts. Thoracic or peritoneal cavity migration:

- Penetration of the thoracic or abdominal body wall
- Grass awns may be inhaled into the trachea, move along bronchi, and migrate through the lung to the pleural space.
- Grass awns may be ingested and migrate through the esophageal wall, penetrating intrathoracic viscera.
- Intrathoracic grass awns may continue to migrate along the diaphragmatic margins into the retroperitoneal space and along the sublumbar musculature.
- Retrograde migration of grass awns from the urethral opening may result in lower urinary tract signs and may act as a nidus for cystolithiasis.

DIAGNOSIS 

Diagnostic Overview

Diagnosis is suspected based on geographic risk, outdoor exposure, and appropriate clinical signs ranging from highly suggestive to vague and nonspecific. Confirmation is by direct visualization of the awn.

Differential Diagnosis

- Subcutaneous tissue: bacterial abscess, neoplasia
- Ear canal: otitis externa, atopic dermatitis, neoplasia, otitis media
- Thorax: other causes of pneumonia (bacterial, viral, fungal, and parasitic); other causes of pleural effusion (neoplastic, infectious, sterile inflammatory, cardiogenic); other causes of pericardial effusion (neoplastic, infectious, inflammatory)
- Abdomen: mass lesions and lymphadenopathy may occur secondary to neoplastic, inflammatory, and infectious disease processes. Cystolithiasis is most commonly caused by urinary tract infection or a metabolic abnormality.
- Retroperitoneal space/sublumbar musculature: neoplastic, inflammatory/infectious causes of retroperitoneal masses
- Cranium: neoplastic, immune-mediated, and infectious diseases (e.g., bacterial, viral, protozoal, fungal)

Initial Database

- CBC: inflammatory leukogram with left shift +/− toxic neutrophils +/− mild anemia of chronic disease are possible; may be unremarkable during or immediately after antibiotic therapy
- Serum biochemistry profile: no specific changes
- Radiographs of affected area: to evaluate for other lesions that could produce similar signs (e.g., osteomyelitis as cause of draining tract, rather than grass awn) and to evaluate

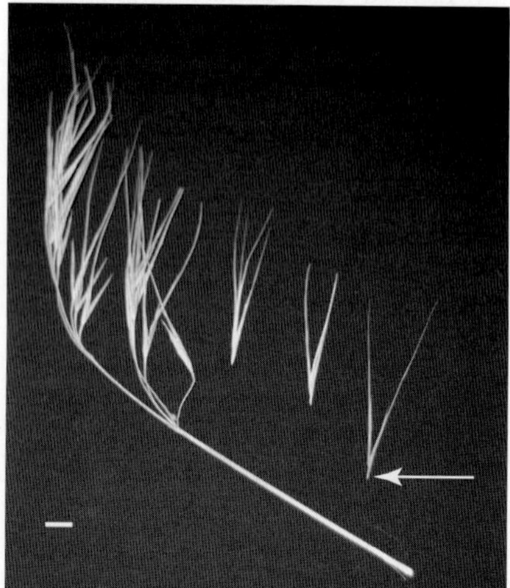

GRASS AWN MIGRATION Dried foxtails *(Hordeum jubatum)* from California. The awns break free (three shown) from the stem and penetrate skin with the sharp point first *(arrow)*. They then may burrow into tissue. Bar = 1 cm. (Courtesy Etienne Côté, DVM, DACVIM.)

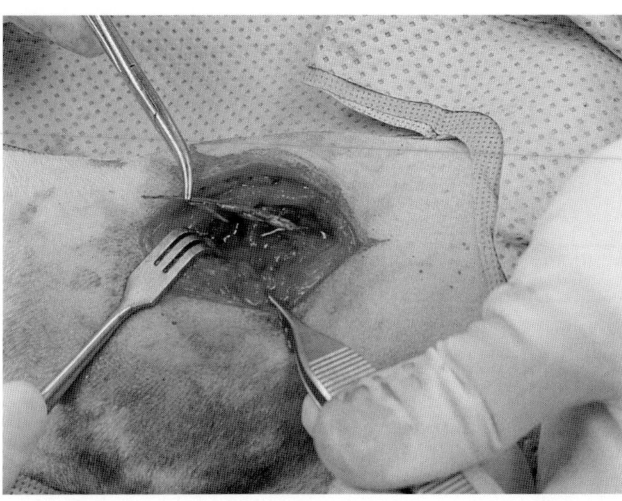

GRASS AWN MIGRATION A firm, 4-cm mass located on the ventral neck just left of midline was consistent with an abscess on aspiration. A large grass awn was found within the mass on surgical exploration.

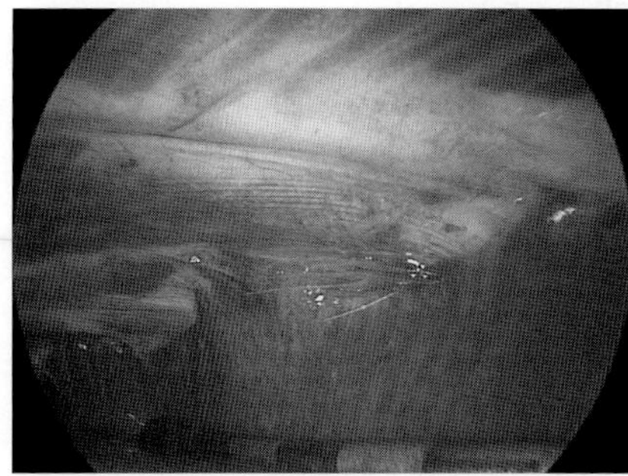

GRASS AWN MIGRATION A grass awn can be seen within the pleural cavity. The grass awn migrated through the lung parenchyma. After awns have passed through the lung, they can often be found embedded in the angle between the thoracic wall and the diaphragmatic insertion.

extent of lesions (e.g., pulmonary infiltrates with inhaled grass awns). Grass awns are radiolucent.
- Fine-needle aspiration of soft-tissue swelling/mass: exudate; bacterial culture, and susceptibility testing are indicated. Cytology of regional lymph nodes: reactive (p. 1112)

Advanced or Confirmatory Testing

- Rhinoscopy, vaginoscopy if signs suggest these locations
- High-resolution ultrasonography by an experienced operator can allow a definitive diagnosis in 82% of acute cases with nonspecific clinical signs. Hallmark feature is a hyperechoic spindle- or fork-shaped structure.
- CT: identify affected thoracic and/or abdominal structures; may allow visualization of the foreign body or contrast-enhanced tract
- Fistulography can be helpful in identifying the course of the grass awn in some cases (variable effectiveness).
- Surgical exploration and tissue resection may be required to confirm the diagnosis. All excised tissues should be submitted for histopathologic exam after resection. Expected result: pyogranulomatous inflammation +/− remnants of plant debris.
- Culture growth of *Actinomyces* spp or *Nocardia* spp suggest concurrent infection with organic plant material.

TREATMENT

Treatment Overview

Definitive treatment is removal of the grass awn(s) and antibiotic therapy.

Acute General Treatment

- Patients with respiratory or cardiac distress or with severe neurologic disease should be stabilized before pursuing extraction of the grass awn.
- Removal of grass awns can be performed under ultrasonographic or endoscopic guidance or may require surgical exploration and resection.
- Concurrent bacterial infections should be treated with appropriate antimicrobials. *Actinomyces* spp generally are susceptible to penicillins, whereas *Nocardia* spp are susceptible to potentiated sulfonamides.
- Initiate broad-spectrum antibiotic therapy while awaiting culture and sensitivity results; a suitable empirical choice in this situation is amoxicillin/clavulanic acid 13.75 mg/kg PO q 12h.

Chronic Treatment

Treatment may be needed again if not all awns could be identified and removed and/or if the animal is exposed to additional grass awns.

Possible Complications

- The migratory nature and small size of grass awns makes localization and complete resection by exploratory surgery difficult.
- Clinical management is most difficult when the grass awn has migrated intrathoracically, intracranially, or into the sublumbar region.
- Recurrence of clinical signs after grass awn removal is common because small remnants may not be apparent or additional grass awns may be present in other areas of the body.

PROGNOSIS & OUTCOME

- Initially, a guarded prognosis is warranted in most cases because additional grass awns may exist elsewhere in the body and because detection of grass awns (for removal) may be exceedingly challenging.
- Superficially located grass awns causing acute signs have a good to excellent prognosis if all grass awns are removed and infection is treated appropriately.
- In chronic cases, if all grass awns are not removed during surgery or in cases where grass awns are located in the abdominal cavity, thoracic cavity, epaxial musculature, or intracranially, worsening clinical signs and/or a need for repeated surgeries can be expected.

PEARLS & CONSIDERATIONS

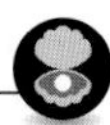

Comments

- For subcutaneous foreign bodies that lie deep within tissue, the authors mark the abnormal tissue surrounding the foreign material with methylene blue under ultrasound guidance before surgery. This makes abnormal tissue, draining tracts, and foreign material easier to identify during surgical dissection.
- En bloc resection of tissue is often indicated, especially in chronic cases when the grass awn has decomposed to smaller fragments, making it challenging to identify the foreign plant material.
- In regions where grass awns are indigenous, all dogs with a chief complaint of head-shaking and/or aural hematoma should have a meticulous otoscopic exam (sedated if necessary) to identify and remove any otic grass awn foreign body.
  - Similarly, all dogs suspected of atopic dermatitis based on chewing of the paws should have a careful exam of the interdigital spaces.

Prevention

- Dogs and cats in geographic areas where grass awns are indigenous should not exercise in environments containing plant awns.
- Animals should be inspected after outdoor activities, and all plant debris, including grass awns and burs, should be removed from interdigital spaces and fur to minimize risk of penetration through the skin.

Technician Tips

Counseling owners to examine their dogs for grass awns in the fur during the spring and summer may help to reduce the chance of foxtail penetration at common sites such as the interdigital spaces.

Client Education

Be aware that several grass awns often penetrate, and removal of one does not guarantee cure. Prevention is strongly recommended to avoid future recurrence.

SUGGESTED READING

Shultz RM, et al: Radiographic, computed tomographic, and ultrasonographic findings with migrating intrathoracic grass awns in dogs and cats. Vet Radiol Ultrasound 49:249-255, 2008.

AUTHORS: Krista N. Adamovich, DVM, DACVS; Philipp D. Mayhew, BVM&S, DACVS
EDITOR: Elizabeth A. Swanson, DVM, MS, DACVS

Gunshot Wounds

Client Education Sheet 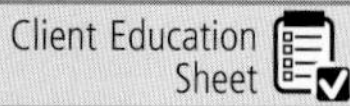

BASIC INFORMATION

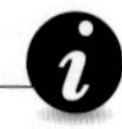

Definition

A type of projectile injury involving handguns, air-powered weapons, shotguns, or rifles

Epidemiology

SPECIES, AGE, SEX

- Dogs and cats of any age
- Male (intact) dogs may be overrepresented.

RISK FACTORS

- Unsupervised roaming; especially night and early morning hours
- Dogs threatening the public or law enforcement officers
- Stray dogs in rural areas (e.g., deliberately shot if considered a nuisance or potential threat to livestock)
- During hunting season, dogs may be shot mistakenly as game or maliciously for sport.
- Guard dogs, police dogs, and hunting dogs are at risk for being shot during work.

GEOGRAPHY AND SEASONALITY

- Higher-crime urban neighborhoods
- Rural areas: shotgun and rifle injuries more common
- Air-powered weapons: more likely in residential or rural areas

Clinical Presentation

DISEASE FORMS/SUBTYPES

Subtypes:

- Pellet and BB guns (air-powered projectiles)
- Handguns
- Rifles
- Shotguns

HISTORY, CHIEF COMPLAINT

- Pets may present with respiratory distress, internal hemorrhage, neurologic injury, or musculoskeletal injuries (fracture).
- Pets with abdominal gunshot wounds may present with life-threatening peritonitis, especially with delayed presentation or treatment.
- Wounds may escape notice or be mistaken for bite wounds, especially if event was not witnessed.
- Dogs and cats with extensive blood loss present in shock (p. 911).
- Patient may present in pain; minor cases may present with little evidence of overt discomfort.

PHYSICAL EXAM FINDINGS

- Open wounds
  - Circular, oval, or angular cutaneous entry wounds with solitary projectiles, often smaller than the projectile
  - Cutaneous burns/lesions if firearm muzzle was at close range
  - There may be no exit wound if the projectile is retained; low-velocity projectiles are more likely to be retained than high-velocity projectiles.
  - Exit wounds are frequently larger and irregular in shape. Bullet deformation and secondary projectiles (bone shards) increase exit wound size. Wounds may appear smaller if swelling present.
  - At close range, shotgun injuries can cause extensive destruction of the skin and underlying tissues.
  - Low-velocity BBs and pellets (air powered) create small entry wounds. Because of their low mass and comparatively low velocity, many of these projectiles are retained (no exit wound).
- Internal injuries
  - Clinical signs are commensurate with tissues impacted and the severity of trauma (orthopedic, spinal, ocular, gastrointestinal, pulmonary involvement).
  - Elastic tissues (lung, muscle) can stretch, partially dissipating the kinetic energy of the projectile. Inelastic organs, such as the liver (low collagen content), may show massive tissue destruction from a high-velocity rifle round compared with a low-velocity bullet.
  - Abdominal gunshot wounds have a high probability for peritonitis (gastrointestinal tract penetration).

Etiology and Pathophysiology

- Bullets may have an outer metallic jacket to control the shape or expansion of the bullet as it impacts a target.
  - Hollow points mushroom on impact.
  - Frangible bullets break apart on impact.
  - Military-style full metal jacket bullets are designed to minimize deformation.
- Projectiles can lodge and then migrate through the respiratory tract, urogenital tract, gastrointestinal tract, cardiovascular system, and fascial planes.
- Shotgun pellets expand in a conical pattern; they are particularly destructive within 10 meters of the muzzle. Shotguns also may fire slugs for larger game.
- Most handguns are low-velocity weapons with less destructive capability. Larger-caliber handguns are capable of extensive tissue destruction.
- High-velocity rifles cause tremendous soft-tissue and bone destruction by producing shock waves in the tissues.

DIAGNOSIS

Diagnostic Overview

- Bullets, BBs, and pellets may be an incidental finding on radiographs, causing confusion when evaluating an acutely ill or injured patient; acute gunshot wounds have an entry wound.
- Gunshot wounds are commonly mistaken for bite wounds and vehicular trauma.
- Radiographs are an important tool for assessing evidence of a retained projectile.

Differential Diagnosis

Other penetrating objects (e.g., sticks, pointed metallic objects) can create a skin opening that mimics a bullet wound.

Initial Database

- CBC, serum chemistry profile, blood typing, and urinalysis for massive soft-tissue wounds or wounds that penetrate the abdomen or thorax
- Radiographs (two-view minimum) for the body region shot, based on bullet retention or entry/exit wound locations. In a gunshot wound with no evidence of exit, additional views may be needed to locate a retained projectile.
- Focused assessment by sonography for triage of the abdomen (AFAST) and/or thorax (TFAST) can be helpful (p. 1102).

Advanced or Confirmatory Testing

- Ultrasonography, abdominocentesis (p. 1056), fluid analysis, cytology, Gram stains, and culture and susceptibility (aerobic and anaerobic) to confirm peritonitis
- Thoracocentesis (p. 1164) can be lifesaving and diagnostic for patients with pneumothorax or hemothorax; aerobic and anaerobic cultures if infection is suspected

TREATMENT

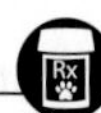

Treatment Overview

A team effort by doctors and technical support is necessary to efficiently stabilize critically injured patients.

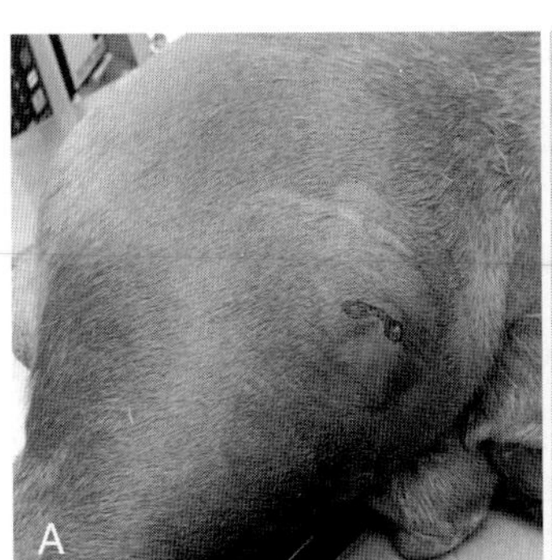

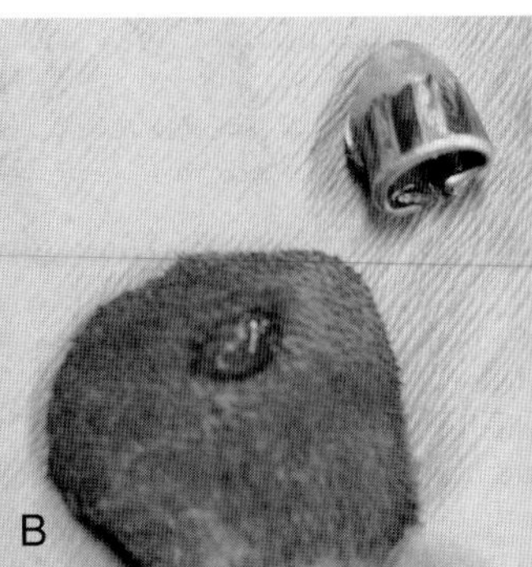

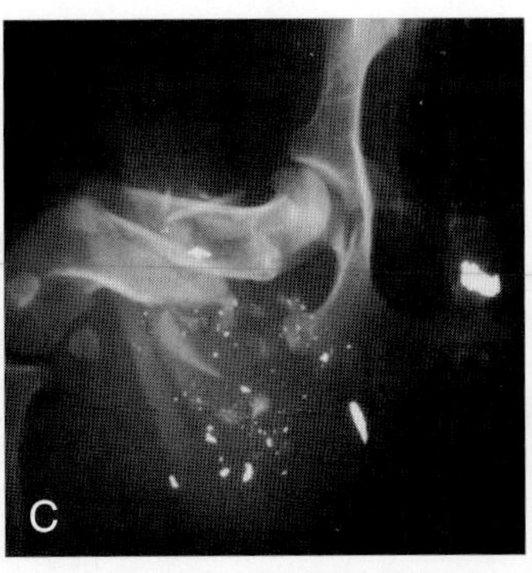

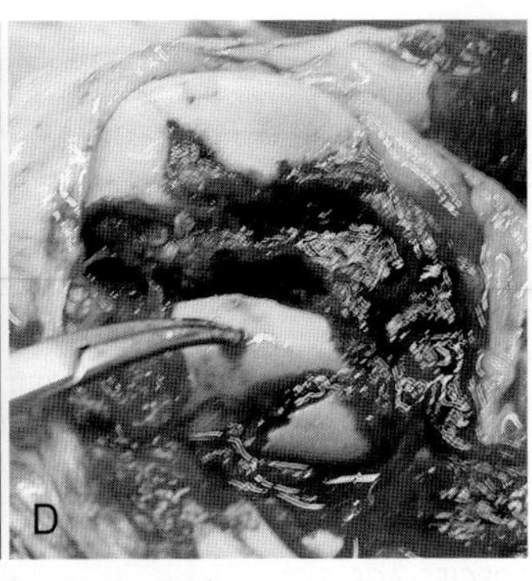

GUNSHOT WOUNDS A, Large retriever cross with gunshot wounds to the right thigh. Note the entry wound proximal to the right stifle and extensive soft-tissue swelling. **B**, A 9-mm round *(above)* and the entry wound of the dog in **A** *(below)*. Note the smaller diameter of the skin wound compared with the bullet. **C**, Hunting rifle round, shattering the femur of a different dog. Note the bone and projectile fragments, creating secondary projectiles within the wound and enhancing soft-tissue trauma. **D**, Handgun round shattered the humeral joint of a different dog. Amputation was performed as a result of the extensive trauma.

- Control visible blood loss.
- Maintain an established airway, and ensure satisfactory breathing.
- Place one or more intravenous lines for fluid support.
- Address life-threatening injuries and overlapping medical crises.
- Initiate pain therapy to reduce patient discomfort and stress.
- Initiate wound care and a plan for long-term management of the injuries.

Acute General Treatment

- Control external hemorrhage by external compression, tourniquets, ligatures, and vascular clips. Wear gloves to prevent bacterial contamination and protect from blood-borne disease.
- Intravenous fluid support (crystalloids, colloids, hypertonic saline, whole blood products)
- Establish and maintain respiratory system: intubation, emergency tracheostomy, thoracic tube placement (e.g., hemothorax, pneumothorax) if indicated
- Morphine, methadone, hydromorphone, butorphanol, and buprenorphine can be used to manage pain. Care must be taken not to mask or compromise the patient's status.
- A muzzle or Elizabethan collar may be used to protect attendants from being bitten by the anxious or painful patient.
- Clip, clean, and pressure lavage (35-mL syringe and an 18-gauge needle) the external wound; the wound may require enlargement to prevent entrapment of lavage fluids. Apply protective dressings to the individual wounds.
- Initiate broad-spectrum intravenous antibiotics (e.g., cefazolin 22 mg/kg IV q 6h) in the seriously injured patient.
- Not all critical patients can be fully stabilized before surgery (i.e., cases with massive hemorrhage).
- Perform wound exploration under general anesthesia for detailed wound exam, debridement, and definitive repair.
- Explore all acute abdominal gunshot wounds by celiotomy because of the high risk of peritonitis secondary to bowel penetration. All organs must be inspected closely for concomitant trauma.

Chronic Treatment

- Prolonged open wound management (e.g., serial debridement, multiple dressing applications) may be needed for contaminated or necrotic injuries.
- Peritonitis may require prolonged wound drainage (open abdomen, closed-suction drain systems, sump drains), abdominal lavage, and possible re-exploration.
- Problematic soft-tissue wounds, including extensive skin loss, may require reconstructive surgery.
- With extensive orthopedic trauma (reparable), closed-suction drains can be used for controlling dead space. Pain can be reduced by placing lidocaine infusion catheters, by temporary lidocaine infusion into the tubing for a closed-suction drain system (Jackson-Pratt drains), or by local nerve blocks and epidural blocks using preservative-free 0.5% bupivacaine.

Possible Complications

- Eyes are vulnerable to projectile wounds, with blindness and eye loss possible.
- Paresis or paralysis may result from spinal cord trauma.
- Infection is a concern in gunshot wounds with extensive tissue destruction.
- Patients generally are at low risk for lead poisoning, except for lead in joints (should be removed).
- Delayed or nonhealing wounds

Recommended Monitoring

Vital signs in critical injuries

PROGNOSIS & OUTCOME

- Determined by extent of injury and subsequent treatment
- Prompt stabilization and definitive medical/surgical intervention can reduce the risk of life-threatening infection and improve the rate of survival and positive long-term outcome.
- Gunshot wounds to the brain, spinal cord, and abdomen normally carry a worse prognosis.

PEARLS & CONSIDERATIONS

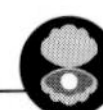

Comments

- Due to potential legal ramifications of gunshot wounds, records must be detailed and accurate; all conversations should be detailed, complete, and noted in the medical record. Photographs of the injuries (entry, exit, tissue trauma inflicted) are useful evidence in court, along with supporting radiographs.
- A board-certified veterinary pathologist is best used to conduct detailed postmortem exam of deceased animals.
- It is critically important to transfer bullets and bullet fragments only to a qualified law enforcement officer. Handle bullets gently (no metal forceps; wrap in tissue paper, and place in labeled, sealed container) should they be used as evidence in court.

Technician Tips

Follow the "chain of custody" for projectiles removed from patients. Maintain a written record of individuals who controlled this item of evidence for presentation to a court of law. Keep projectile in a secured area to prevent tampering. In legal cases, do not return projectile to the owner even if requested.

SUGGESTED READING

Pavletic MM: Atlas of small animal wound management and reconstructive surgery, ed 4, Ames, IA, 2018, Wiley-Blackwell.

AUTHOR: Michael M. Pavletic, DVM, DACVS
EDITOR: Elizabeth A. Swanson, DVM, MS, DACVS

Halitosis

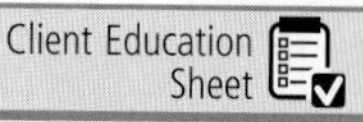

BASIC INFORMATION

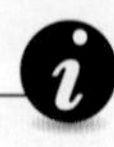

Definition

An offensive odor emanating from the oral cavity, which may arise from intraoral or extraoral causes

Epidemiology

SPECIES, AGE, SEX

Any species, age, and either sex may be affected.

RISK FACTORS

Dental disease (e.g., periodontal disease, caries), oral mucosal diseases (e.g., ulcerative stomatitis), oral tumors, foreign bodies, hyposalivation, dental appliances (e.g., splints, orthodontic devices), gastrointestinal (GI) diseases, respiratory diseases, metabolic diseases, perioral skin diseases, diet, certain medications. Although halitosis has multifactorial origins, the source in > 90% of cases is the oral cavity.

Clinical Presentation

HISTORY, CHIEF COMPLAINT

Important components of the history include diet, treats, toys, home oral hygiene, professional oral care, pertinent medical history, and medications. Bad breath is a common complaint for patient presentation.

PHYSICAL EXAM FINDINGS

- Most intraoral disorders that cause halitosis are apparent on oral exam. Extraoral causes may be identified with additional diagnostics.
- Distinguishing between nasal and oral odor is important. Smell emanating only from the nose can indicate nasal disease (e.g., nasal tumor), and combined nasal and oral odor may indicate a communication between the cavities (i.e., oronasal fistula).
- Physical exam findings depend on the underlying disease process. For example, rare but possible oral manifestations of leptospirosis (depending on the serovar) include halitosis, petechiae, oral hemorrhages, ulceration, glossitis with necrosis, and sloughing of the tongue.
- Evidence of periodontal disease may be noted, including gingivitis, gingival recession, root exposure, tooth mobility, and accumulation of plaque and calculus. Odorous, volatile sulfur compounds are produced by bacteria associated with periodontal disease. Stomatitis or oral masses may also be found. Close attention should be paid to the sublingual region in cats and the oropharynx in dogs for the presence of tumors or foreign bodies.
- Visual inspection of the prepuce/vulva and palpation of the anal sacs is important because licking of these areas or their secretions is a recognized cause of halitosis in dogs and cats.

Etiology and Pathophysiology

Intraoral causes:

- Plaque and calculus accumulation, gingivitis, periodontitis, stomatitis
- Cheilitis, lip fold pyoderma
- Osteomyelitis, osteonecrosis
- Oral tumors, particularly those that outgrow their blood supply and become necrotic (e.g., malignant melanoma, osteosarcoma)
- Foreign bodies, oral implants
- Oronasal communications

Extraoral causes: see Differential Diagnosis below.

DIAGNOSIS

Diagnostic Overview

Physical exam helps differentiate intraoral from extraoral causes; further diagnostic tests are selected accordingly.

Differential Diagnosis

The DAMNIT scheme can be used as a guide to differential diagnosis:

- *D*evelopmental, *d*egenerative: congenital and acquired palate defects/oronasal communications
- *A*utoimmune, *a*natomic, *a*llergic: pemphigus vulgaris, bullous pemphigoid, systemic lupus erythematosus, erythema multiforme, drug eruption; mouth breathing associated with brachycephalic head conformation
- *M*etabolic, *m*echanical: diabetic ketoacidosis, uremia, hepatic dysfunction causing hyperammonemia, retention of food debris and/or saliva
- *N*utritional, *n*eoplastic: gastroesophageal reflux; oral, pharyngeal, esophageal, gastric neoplasia; dietary indiscretion/consumption of spoiled food
- *I*nfectious, *i*nflammatory, or *i*diopathic: dental plaque/calculus (oral bacteria), periodontal disease (gingivitis and periodontitis), gingival hyperplasia, contact mucositis and contact mucosal ulceration, stomatitis; leptospirosis; local and systemic fungal diseases; cheilitis and lip fold pyoderma; bronchitis, pneumonia; infection with feline leukemia virus (FeLV), feline immunodeficiency virus (FIV), feline calicivirus (FCV), or feline herpesvirus (FHV)
- *T*oxic, *t*raumatic: toxic epidermal necrolysis, trauma from malocclusion, tooth fracture, jaw fracture, non-healing oral wounds, oral foreign body, chemical or electric burns

Initial Database

Sensory evaluation and complete physical exam (including oral exam in the conscious patient)

Advanced or Confirmatory Testing

- CBC, chemistry panel, urinalysis: if history and physical exam suggest an extraoral cause (e.g., rule out azotemia, diabetic ketoacidosis) or prior to anesthesia
- Viral testing: FeLV, FIV, +/− calicivirus in cats
- General anesthesia, oral exam, and biopsy of suspicious lesions
- Case-specific advanced diagnostics centered on the mouth and upper airway when an intraoral cause is suspected (e.g., dental radiography, CT, thoracic radiographs for metastasis screening of suspected oral neoplasms) and systemic evaluations when an extraoral diagnosis is suspected
- Organoleptic measurements and a halimeter can be used to detect the most common causative agents of oral malodor (i.e., hydrogen sulfide, methyl mercaptan, and dimethyl sulfide).

TREATMENT

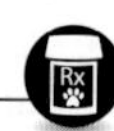

Treatment Overview

The goal of treatment is to control halitosis by addressing its underlying causes. For intraoral causes, primary treatment is often followed by preventive care. For extraoral causes, treatment of the underlying disorder is the basis of therapy.

Acute General Treatment

Improve oral hygiene by professional dental cleaning and periodontal therapy, with specific attention to treatment of oral disease associated with halitosis (e.g., extraction of teeth with severe periodontitis). Specific treatment for halitosis caused by extraoral disorders is directed toward the underlying disorder.

Chronic Treatment

- Maintain a healthy periodontium by routine home oral hygiene (daily toothbrushing; application of chlorhexidine products to teeth and gums; use of diets, treats, and chew toys that help control plaque and calculus accumulation) to maintain oral health between regularly scheduled professional dental cleanings and periodontal therapy.
- An oral topical gel with essential oils and polyphenolic antioxidants applied twice daily after an initial professional dental cleaning decreased oral malodor in dogs.
- Control underlying diseases that are extraoral causes of halitosis.

Nutrition/Diet

Home oral hygiene products, diets, treats, and toys proved to control plaque and calculus accumulation (see the Veterinary Oral Health Council website: http://vohc.org/)

Recommended Monitoring

Follow-up as indicated for routine management of underlying intraoral or extraoral cause

PROGNOSIS & OUTCOME

Depends on the ability to eliminate underlying cause:
- Fair to good prognosis: active disorders that respond to treatment and can be controlled with ongoing care (e.g., periodontitis, gingival hyperplasia, stomatitis); intraoral/extraoral causes that can be eliminated, cured, or controlled (e.g., foreign bodies, excised oral tumors, controlled diabetes)
- Guarded prognosis: aggressive or nonresectable oral neoplasia; uncontrolled, advanced, or untreatable systemic diseases. The severity of the causative problem may make halitosis difficult to control

PEARLS & CONSIDERATIONS

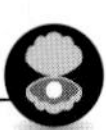

Comments

- Halitosis is a leading concern of pet owners because it can negatively affect the relationship with their beloved pet. A nonmalodorous oral cavity improves the human-animal bond as well as the pet's health and well-being.
- Volatile sulfur compounds produced by bacteria, even at low concentrations, may be toxic to periodontal tissues and play a role in the pathogenesis of periodontal disease.

Prevention

- Plaque accumulation on teeth, a major cause of halitosis, can easily be prevented by daily home oral hygiene and yearly professional dental cleaning and periodontal therapy.
- Other intraoral causes of halitosis can be recognized early by means of home oral exam by the owner and professional oral exam by the veterinarian during wellness visits.

Technician Tips

Technicians are on the front line of identifying oral disorders, including halitosis, in at least two important ways: bringing oral abnormalities to the attention of the clinician and demonstrating proper home oral hygiene techniques to the owner.

Client Education

- The oral cavity can be easily assessed by most owners.
- Halitosis is obvious, abnormal, and requires appropriate veterinary intervention.
- Home oral hygiene is important to general health. Proper brushing techniques should be demonstrated to owners and importance of daily maintenance stressed.

SUGGESTED READING

Milella L: The negative effects of volatile sulphur compounds. J Vet Dent 32:99-102, 2015.

AUTHOR: Maria M. Soltero-Rivera, DVM, DAVDC
EDITOR: Alexander M. Reiter, DVM, Dr.med.vet., DAVDC, DEVDC

Head Tilt

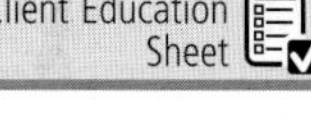

BASIC INFORMATION

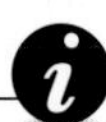

Definition

A postural abnormality resulting from the unilateral loss of antigravity muscular tone in the cervical region. The head tilt may be to the right or to the left (referred to according to which side of the patient's head is deviated ventrally) along the long axis of the body.

Epidemiology

SPECIES, AGE, SEX

Dog or cat, any age, either sex. Idiopathic vestibular disease typically occurs in dogs > 5 years; no age predisposition in cats

GENETICS, BREED PREDISPOSITION

Congenital vestibular disease (uncommon) in the Doberman pinscher, cocker spaniel, beagle, Akita, German shepherd (dogs) and Siamese, Tonkinese, and Burmese (cats)

RISK FACTORS

Otitis externa

CONTAGION AND ZOONOSIS

Canine distemper is highly contagious; cryptococcosis and feline infectious peritonitis is less so.

GEOGRAPHY AND SEASONALITY

Idiopathic vestibular disease in cats may predominate in late summer/early fall.

ASSOCIATED DISORDERS

- Other vestibular signs: nystagmus, ataxia, circling, vomiting. With central vestibular disease, ipsilateral cranial nerve (CN) deficits, ipsilateral conscious proprioceptive (CP) deficits, and mentation changes can occur.
- Concurrent Horner's syndrome can occur (usually indicates peripheral vestibular disease).
- Concurrent facial nerve paralysis suggests concurrent middle ear disease (idiopathic or central vestibular disease still possible).
- Concurrent otitis externa (increased risk of otitis media/interna)

Clinical Presentation

DISEASE FORMS/SUBTYPES

- Peripheral vestibular disease (middle/inner ear lesion)
- Central vestibular disease (brain lesion)

HISTORY, CHIEF COMPLAINT

Acute onset of head tilt is common.
- Owners may report other vestibular signs.
- Idiopathic vestibular disease is typically of acute onset and static (not progressive).

PHYSICAL EXAM FINDINGS

- Head tilt associated with peripheral vestibular disease (one or more may be present)
  - Head tilt (ipsilateral)
  - Nystagmus (p. 698)
  - Circling (ipsilateral)
  - Ataxia +/− falling
  - Facial nerve paresis
- Head tilt associated with central vestibular disease (one or more may be present)
  - Head tilt (ipsilateral to lesion, except with paradoxical vestibular disease)
  - Nystagmus
  - Circling (ipsilateral to lesion, except with paradoxical vestibular disease)
  - Ataxia
  - Proprioceptive deficits (always ipsilateral to lesion, even with paradoxical vestibular disease)
  - CN deficits V through XII possible (always ipsilateral to lesion, even with paradoxical vestibular disease)
  - Mentation changes
  - Bradycardia
- Otitis externa increases likelihood of otitis media/interna but does not rule out other causes.

Etiology and Pathophysiology

- Peripheral vestibular disease: infection (otitis media/interna), idiopathic, otopharyngeal polyps (young cats), neoplasia, hypothyroidism (rare cause of head tilt), trauma, after middle ear surgery or external ear cleaning (if tympanum is not intact), intoxication (e.g., aminoglycoside antibiotics, cleaning solutions), congenital/hereditary
- Central vestibular disease: neoplasia, idiopathic, vascular (hemorrhagic or ischemic infarction), hypothyroidism (uncommon cause of head tilt), inflammation (granulomatous meningoencephalitis, necrotizing meningoencephalitis), infection (bacterial, viral, fungal, protozoal or central extension of otitis media/interna), trauma, congenital/developmental, thiamine deficiency (cats)

DIAGNOSIS

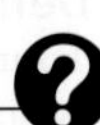

Diagnostic Overview

A head tilt indicates vestibular dysfunction. A complete neurologic exam can help differentiate peripheral from central vestibular disease.

However, the earliest stages of central vestibular disease may produce signs that mimic those of peripheral vestibular disease.

Differential Diagnosis

Torticollis (nose pointed to one side but ears parallel) can be mistaken for head tilt (one ear lower with head rotated on median plane).

Initial Database

- CBC, serum chemistry profile, and urinalysis: usually unremarkable
- Otoscopic exam (p. 1144):
  - Otitis externa, polyp, blood (head trauma) possible
  - Ruptured tympanic membrane or fluid in the middle ear possible
- Tympanic bulla radiographs (limited benefit)

Advanced or Confirmatory Testing

- Serum thyroid panels if hypothyroidism suspected (dogs)
- CT scan: excellent for detailed imaging of inner ear but often poor at evaluating the brain
- MRI (p. 1132): superior soft-tissue resolution and is the preferred imaging modality for the brain but not bony structures
- Cerebrospinal fluid (CSF) analysis (pp. 1080 and 1323) if deficits suggest intracranial disease or to evaluate for central extension of otitis media/interna
- Myringotomy (piercing of the tympanic membrane to collect exudate for cytologic evaluation and bacterial culture) if otitis media/interna is present
- Infectious disease serum titers considered in light of MRI/CSF results and environmental risk factors
- Brainstem auditory evoked response (BAER) testing can help localize vestibular disease.

TREATMENT

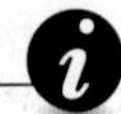

Treatment Overview

- Supportive care
- Treat primary cause when possible.

Acute General Treatment

Acute vestibular signs:

- Supportive care
- Consider maropitant 1 mg/kg SQ or 2 mg/kg PO q 24h as needed for up to 5 days as an antiemetic. Prolonged use of vestibular suppressants (antiemetic drugs, antihistamines, sedatives) can delay vestibular compensation/recovery.
- If evidence of increased intracranial pressure: mannitol 0.5 g/kg slow IV over 20 minutes
- Begin treatment of underlying cause if known.

Chronic Treatment

- Antibacterial therapy (based on culture and susceptibility) is required for several months to treat bacterial otitis media/interna due to poor blood supply to the tympanic cavity and osteomyelitis.
- Neoplasms causing head tilts are often not easily surgically accessible. Neoplasms at the foramen magnum or outer margin of the cerebellum may be surgically pursued; others may be amenable to radiation therapy or palliative treatment (e.g., glucocorticoids).

Behavior/Exercise

Limit exposure to situations that pose a risk of trauma (e.g., vehicular traffic, top of staircase) during vestibular disturbance.

PROGNOSIS & OUTCOME

- Idiopathic vestibular disease: excellent prognosis; recurrence possible. Head tilt often improves but may not fully resolve.
- Vascular disease: often good prognosis
- Otitis media/interna: typically good prognosis. Head tilt may remain.
- Otopharyngeal polyps: recurrence rate of 30%-40% with traction removal, 8% when removal is combined with bulla osteotomy
- Neoplasia: prognosis is guarded to poor, depending on cause, ability to treat, and response to therapy. Initial improvement is common with glucocorticoid treatment.

PEARLS & CONSIDERATIONS

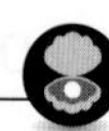

Comments

- Otitis media/interna is the most common cause of peripheral vestibular disease.
- Idiopathic vestibular disease is the second most common cause of peripheral vestibular disease in dogs.
- Vestibular compensation (improvement) can occur with diseases other than idiopathic and vascular.
- Idiopathic vestibular disease is a diagnosis of exclusion.
- Concurrent facial nerve paralysis suggests peripheral vestibular disease. Occasionally, idiopathic facial nerve paralysis and idiopathic vestibular disease occur together.
- Central vestibular disease often, but not always, produces intracranial signs.
- An insidious, progressive history often indicates a cause other than idiopathic vestibular disease.
- Occasionally, pain (head or neck) results in a head posture change that mimics a head tilt.

Technician Tips

Use caution when cleaning the external ear canals. If the tympanic membrane is not intact, most cleaning solutions and antibiotics can cause damage.

Client Education

- Owners need to know that idiopathic vestibular disease usually resolves with time.
- A nightlight can be of benefit and increase comfort in patients with vestibular disease of any kind. An abnormal sense of balance compromises proprioception, and the patient relies more on eyesight.

SUGGESTED READING

Rossmeisl JH: Vestibular disease in dogs and cats. Vet Clin North Am Small Anim Pract 40:81-100, 2010.

AUTHOR: James Lavely, DVM, DACVIM
EDITOR: Leah A. Cohn, DVM, PhD DACVIM

Head Trauma

BASIC INFORMATION

Definition

Traumatic injury resulting in damage to the skull, soft tissues of the head, intracranial structures, or some combination of these. It is important to distinguish brain injury from head trauma.

Synonyms

Traumatic brain injury (TBI), intracranial injury, facial trauma

Epidemiology

SPECIES, AGE, SEX

Animals of any age or breed; young animals may be overrepresented

RISK FACTORS

Free-roaming or unsupervised activity

ASSOCIATED DISORDERS

Traumatic injuries affecting other body systems

Clinical Presentation

DISEASE FORMS/SUBTYPES

Blunt or penetrating (e.g., bite wound, arrow)

HISTORY, CHIEF COMPLAINT

- History of traumatic event
- Owners may report loss of consciousness, inappropriate behavior, or seizure activity.

PHYSICAL EXAM FINDINGS

- Signs of hypovolemic shock (e.g., tachycardia, hypotension, pale mucous membranes [p. 911]) may be present.
- Neurologic exam (p. 1136); indicators of intracranial injury:
  - Anisocoria, abnormal pupil reactivity (excluding ocular trauma): dilated, unresponsive pupils (in the absence of ocular trauma or atropine) indicate severe neurologic injury and a poor prognosis.
  - Diminished or absent oculocephalic (doll's eye) reflex
  - Postural reaction deficits (may be due to spinal injury [p. 930]: note remainder of neurologic findings)
  - Diminished or altered consciousness (may be due to shock; note remainder of physical exam)
- Skull fractures may be palpable.
- Respiratory, musculoskeletal, and other body systems may show signs of traumatic injury.
  - Hemorrhage may be visible in ear canal, eyes (episcleral or hyphema), or epistaxis.

Etiology and Pathophysiology

- Cerebral blood flow (CBF) is mainly determined by blood pressure (BP). Autoregulation maintains blood flow to the brain over a range of blood pressures (60-160 mm Hg) but is lost when systolic arterial BP < 50 mm Hg or after brain injury (at which time arterial BP is directly correlated to blood flow to the brain).
- Cerebral perfusion pressure (CPP = mean arterial pressure [MAP] − intracranial pressure [ICP]) is used for estimating CBF. As ICP rises or MAP decreases, cerebral perfusion decreases.
- Trauma can result in primary (at the time of incident due to direct neuronal damage and hemorrhage) or secondary (hours or days after the incident due to energy depletion, free radical generation, cytokine release) injury to the brain. Treatment aims to prevent or limit secondary injury.

DIAGNOSIS

Diagnostic Overview

Diagnosis is based on a history of trauma with physical signs of intracranial injury. Complete neurologic evaluation is essential for establishing the treatment plan and prognosis. Concurrent injuries affecting other body systems are common and should be evaluated as part of the diagnostic plan.

Differential Diagnosis

- Rule out other causes of intracranial disease (e.g., neoplasia, infectious, inflammatory, congenital), especially when trauma is not witnessed.
- Animals with hypotensive shock may manifest altered consciousness without neurologic damage. Repeat full neurologic assessment after initial stabilization has been completed.
- Metabolic diseases (e.g., hypoglycemia, liver disease) may also affect neurologic exam and should be considered as differentials if no traumatic event is reported or if the history is uncertain.

Initial Database

Baseline tests (packed cell volume/total solids [PCV/TP], blood glucose, blood urea nitrogen); initial assessment of some metabolic causes of altered mentation:

- Consider transfusion if necessary (p. 1169) to support oxygen delivery to tissues.
- Avoid hyperglycemia.
- If azotemia or dehydration is present, diuretics should be used with caution if at all; maintaining normotension is paramount.

Blood pressure (p. 1065):

- Identify and correct systemic hypotension.
- Systemic hypertension may be a result of elevated ICP or a consequence of pain or anxiety.

Blood gas or pulse oximetry:

- Identify hypoxemia (e.g., PaO_2 < 80 mm Hg, SpO_2 < 95% when breathing room air), and provide supplemental oxygen p. 1146.
- Identify and correct hypoventilation ($PaCO_2$ > 50 mm Hg).

Heart rate/electrocardiogram (p. 1096):

- Sinus tachycardia common with hypovolemia or pain; ventricular arrhythmias possible (p. 1033)
- Bradycardia may be seen with elevated ICP; a rapid onset of bradycardia with hypertension (Cushing's response) portends brain herniation.

Advanced or Confirmatory Testing

- Radiographs
  - May be useful in identifying skull fractures
  - Of limited value in the overall assessment of intracranial injury
- CT
  - Comatose/obtunded patients may be imaged without anesthesia.
  - Evaluate for skull fractures, hemorrhage, or other injuries.
- MRI (p. 1132)
  - May be helpful in detecting subtle lesions and provide prognostic guidance
- ICP monitoring
  - Useful for directing therapies; may have prognostic significance
  - Infrequently used in veterinary medicine; requires specific skills and advanced care

TREATMENT

Treatment Overview

Treatment is aimed at ensuring adequate cerebral perfusion and decreasing ICP. Important goals include maintaining adequate systemic BP and systemic oxygenation (oxygen delivery to tissues). A global approach to diagnosis and treatment is outlined on p. 1421.

Acute General Treatment

Maintain mean arterial BP > 60 mm Hg (generally signifies that systolic BP > 90 mm Hg): manage by titration of intravenous fluids. Options:

- Isotonic crystalloids: (10-20 mL/kg IV) exact dose is titrated to BP; do not over-resuscitate
  - Avoid fluids with excessive free water (maintenance fluids, 5% dextrose in water, 0.45% saline).
- Hypertonic saline (7.5%) 2-4 mL/kg IV slowly; provides rapid volume expansion
  - Decreases ICP as effectively as mannitol
- Colloids (e.g., hetastarch, pentastarch 5 mL/kg IV bolus, maximum of 20-40 mL/kg/day, depending on product). Oncotic effect draws free water into the vasculature and provides intravascular volume with limited fluid administration volumes.

Decrease intracranial pressure:

- Mannitol 0.5-1 g/kg IV q 6-8h; limit to three bolus injections/24-hour period. Osmotic diuretic with free radical–scavenging properties decreases blood viscosity, increases cerebral blood flow.
  - Diuresis may decrease blood volume and BP (ensure adequate BP and volume status before administration).
  - May result in reverse osmotic shift. In areas of hemorrhage, mannitol may leak into interstitium, worsening cerebral edema. The effects of mannitol on lowering ICP may outweigh these potential effects on damaged areas.
  - May be combined with furosemide 2 mg/kg in emergency situations or when needed for other therapy (e.g., pulmonary edema)
- Hypertonic saline (7%) 2-4 mL/kg IV: hypertonic crystalloid fluid with antiinflammatory and free radical–scavenging properties.
  - ICP lowering drug of choice in hypotensive patients (does not result in diuresis)
  - May be combined with colloid for volume expansion effects

Maintain adequate oxygenation:

- Supplemental oxygen as needed (p. 1146)
  - Sneezing increases ICP, and oxygen cages are preferable to nasal cannulas, if available.
- Ensure adequate oxygen-carrying capacity (hematocrit/hemoglobin) and delivery (adequate cardiac output).
- Elevate head by placing patient on a ramp raised 15°-25° from the ground, which promotes venous drainage from the cerebrum and may help to decrease ICP.
- Kinks in the neck can obstruct jugular venous drainage from the brain, and use of a ramp is important.

Miscellaneous therapies:

- Surgery
  - Craniotomy: removal of hematomas, control of hemorrhage with depressed skull fractures, or for removal of penetrating objects

 - Substantial decrease in ICP (15% with craniotomy, additional 65% reduction with durotomy); superior in this effect compared with any medical therapy
- Hyperventilation ($PaCO_2$ < 30 mm Hg)
 - Emergency therapy: lowers arterial CO_2. Resultant vasoconstriction decreases cerebral perfusion pressure and decreases ICP. However, decreased perfusion to brain parenchyma may have deleterious consequences.
 - Current recommendation: ventilate patient such that $PaCO_2$ = 30-35 mm Hg.
- Hypothermia
 - Reduces cerebral metabolic rate, decreasing cerebral perfusion by reflex vasoconstriction, and consequently decreases ICP
 - May also limit secondary brain injury by limiting neuroexcitatory activities and suppression of local inflammatory response
 - Can result in coagulation abnormalities, cardiac disturbances, and hypotension
 - Moderate hypothermia (90°F-91.4°F [32°C-33°C]) has been efficacious in human trials and animal models of brain injury; clinical veterinary use is uncertain.
- Glucocorticoids: contraindicated in treatment of head injury

Nutrition/Diet

Supplemental nutrition may be needed in severely compromised patients.

- Enteral route preferred if possible/safe (pp. 1106 and 1107); prevent sneezing during tube placement
- Parenteral nutrition (p. 1148) may be needed in patients at risk for aspiration pneumonia.

Behavior/Exercise

- Animals with severe neurologic deficits may be recumbent with limited mobility.
- Range-of-motion exercises and physical rehabilitation may be beneficial for these patients.

Possible Complications

- Infection (aspiration pneumonia, nosocomial infection)
- Seizures
- Kidney injury, oliguria/anuria, uremia
- Persistent neurologic deficits

Recommended Monitoring

- Assess neurologic status.
 - Repeated examination may aid in evaluating the efficacy of therapy.
 - Imaging (CT or MRI) may be helpful in assessing injury.
 - Therapy to decrease ICP if indicated
- Monitor oxygenation (arterial blood gas/pulse oximetry).
- Ensure adequate BP.

PROGNOSIS & OUTCOME

- Prognosis depends on severity and type of injury.

Modified Glasgow Coma Scale

Exam Findings*	Score
Motor Activity	
Normal gait, normal spinal reflexes	6
Hemiparesis, tetraparesis, or decerebrate rigidity	5
Recumbent, intermittent extensor rigidity	4
Recumbent, constant extensor rigidity	3
Recumbent, constant extensor rigidity with opisthotonos	2
Recumbent, hypotonia of muscles, depressed or absent spinal reflexes	1
Brainstem Reflexes	
Normal pupillary light reflexes and oculocephalic reflexes	6
Slow pupillary light reflexes and normal to reduced oculocephalic reflexes	5
Bilateral unresponsive miosis with normal to reduced oculocephalic reflexes	4
Pinpoint pupils with reduced to absent oculocephalic reflexes	3
Unilateral unresponsive mydriasis with reduced to absent oculocephalic reflexes	2
Bilateral unresponsive mydriasis with reduced to absent oculocephalic reflexes	1
Level of Consciousness	
Occasional periods of alertness, responsive to environment	6
Depression or delirium, capable of responding to environment but response may be inappropriate	5
Stupor, responsive to visual stimuli	4
Stupor, responsive to auditory stimuli	3
Stupor, responsive only to repeated noxious stimuli	2
Coma, unresponsive to repeated noxious stimuli	1
Total score	
Assessment of Prognosis	
Good	15-18
Guarded	9-14
Grave	3-8

*The modified Glasgow coma scale is based on the neurologic exam findings for the categories of motor activity, brainstem reflexes, and level of consciousness. Entries in each category are scored 1-6, with 1 indicating more severe dysfunction. The three category scores are summed for the total score, which is interpreted as shown to establish the prognosis.

 - Fair to good with minor, nonprogressive injury
 - Severely injured animals have poorer short-term recovery rates and may have longer rehabilitation/recovery periods if they survive.
- Modified Glasgow coma scale (MGCS) has been used for scoring injury severity in cases of head trauma and has been correlated with outcome.

PEARLS & CONSIDERATIONS

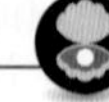

Comments

- Head trauma is a common and serious injury in dogs and cats.
- Clinicians must recognize the signs of progressive neurologic injury.
 - The MGCS may be helpful as a monitoring tool.

Technician Tips

Diligent monitoring and nursing care are important for an optimal outcome.

- Even subtle changes in neurologic assessment can be important and should be brought up with the veterinarian.
- Comprehensive nursing care is important to prevent complications such as nosocomial infection or aspiration pneumonia.
- Avoid jugular compression or jugular venipuncture in head trauma patients.

Client Education

- Clients must be informed of the potential for long recovery periods for severely injured animals.
- Clients should also be made aware of the need for intensive treatment and monitoring of animals with head injury.
- The MGCS may be helpful in quantitating injury severity to provide the client with a prognosis.

SUGGESTED READING

DiFazio J, et al: Updates in the management of the small animal patient with neurologic trauma. Vet Clin North Am Small Anim Pract 43:915-940, 2013.

AUTHOR: Elizabeth M. Streeter, DVM, DACVECC
EDITOR: Benjamin M. Brainard, VMD, DACVAA, DACVECC

Heart Base Tumor

Client Education Sheet 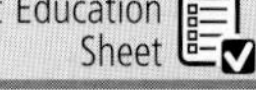

BASIC INFORMATION

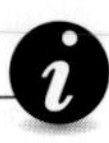

Definition

Heart base tumor is a general term describing a cardiac neoplasm of any type located at the base of the heart, often in association with the ascending aorta but without right atrial involvement.

Synonyms

Chemoreceptor cell tumor, chemodectoma, aortic body tumor, nonchromaffin paraganglioma

Epidemiology

SPECIES, AGE, SEX

- Dogs: second most common cardiac tumor (after hemangiosarcoma), mean age of 10 years (range, 5-15 years), males may be overrepresented
- Cats: reported but rare

GENETICS, BREED PREDISPOSITION

Brachycephalic breeds (English bulldogs, boxers, Boston terriers) are predisposed.

RISK FACTORS

Chronic hypoxemia may be a contributing factor.

ASSOCIATED DISORDERS

Pericardial effusion, right-sided congestive heart failure (CHF), cardiac tamponade

Clinical Presentation

DISEASE FORMS/SUBTYPES

- Most commonly causes clinical signs due to pericardial effusion and cardiac tamponade
- May be an incidental finding

HISTORY, CHIEF COMPLAINT

- Acute collapse/syncope
- Lethargy/exercise intolerance
- Abdominal distention
- Anorexia/inappetence
- Cough or tachypnea/dyspnea

PHYSICAL EXAM FINDINGS

- Findings associated with pericardial effusion (tachycardia, weak peripheral pulses, and muffled heart sounds)
- Findings consistent with right-sided CHF (ascites, hepatomegaly, jugular distention/pulsation)
- ± Tachypnea/dyspnea

Etiology and Pathophysiology

- Chemodectoma
  - Tumor of specialized neuroepithelial cells in the adventitia of the aortic arch; majority of heart base tumors in dogs
  - Typically benign and slow growing but may be very large at the time of diagnosis; occasionally locally invasive and uncommonly metastatic
- Ectopic thyroid carcinoma
  - 5%-10% of heart base tumors in dogs; usually nonfunctional
  - Risk of metastasis increases with tumor size
- Mesothelioma may rarely form a mass lesion at the heart base (dogs).
- Regardless of type, heart base tumors typically result in pericardial effusion, causing cardiac tamponade and right-sided CHF.
- Large masses may cause clinically significant compression of cardiac structures and great vessels, inhibiting inflow or outflow.

DIAGNOSIS

Diagnostic Overview

The diagnosis is most often made with echocardiographic identification of a mass at the heart base. Although a presumptive diagnosis of chemodectoma is often based on echocardiographic appearance, definitive diagnosis of the tumor type requires histopathologic evaluation.

Differential Diagnosis

- Other intrapericardial tumors (hemangiosarcoma, mesothelioma, lymphoma, rare primary cardiac tumors, metastatic tumors)
- Other causes of pericardial effusion (p. 773)

Initial Database

- Echocardiography (p. 1094): diagnostic test of choice. Heart base tumors typically originate from the ascending aorta, most commonly the left cranial aspect, and lie between the aorta and the main pulmonary artery. They are usually homogeneous with smooth margins. Presence and severity of pericardial effusion is also assessed.
- Thoracic radiographs: enlarged or globoid cardiac silhouette in most, but not all, cases of cardiac tamponade (80%). A soft-tissue mass effect at the heart base may cause dorsal and lateral deviation of the trachea.
- Electrocardiogram (p. 1096): sinus tachycardia, low-amplitude QRS complexes, and/or electrical alternans with pericardial effusion.
- CBC, serum biochemistry profile, and urinalysis: often unremarkable

Advanced or Confirmatory Testing

- Cytologic evaluation and pH of the pericardial effusion are not generally useful. Heart base tumors typically do not exfoliate cells, reactive mesothelial cells mimic malignant cells, and there is much overlap in pH between pericardial effusions from various causes.
- Histopathologic evaluation of the tumor allows a definitive diagnosis of tumor type. Requires surgical biopsy and often does not alter treatment plan
- CT and/or MRI may provide additional anatomic information for surgical or radiation therapy planning.

TREATMENT

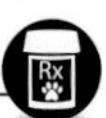

Treatment Overview

Treatment is generally aimed at removal of pericardial fluid when cardiac tamponade occurs and eliminating recurrent effusion. When a heart base tumor is an incidental finding, no treatment may be necessary initially.

Acute General Treatment

- Pericardiocentesis (p. 1150) is essential for cardiac tamponade but may not be necessary if only mild effusion is present and not causing hemodynamic effects.
- Diuretics are contraindicated in acute treatment of cardiac tamponade.

Chronic Treatment

- Repeated pericardiocentesis as needed for recurrent pericardial effusion
- Diuretics to delay effusion recurrence are controversial.
- Pericardiectomy alone is an effective palliative treatment for recurrent pericardial effusion. Less-invasive alternatives to surgical pericardiectomy include thoracoscopic pericardiectomy and percutaneous balloon pericardiotomy.
- Complete surgical resection is rarely possible due to high vascularity of the tumor and close association with great vessels.
- Radiation therapy has been reported to reduce tumor size, but long-term benefit is unknown.
- Chemotherapy with toceranib phosphate (Palladia, Zoetis) may provide clinical benefit in some cases, but controlled efficacy data are lacking.

Possible Complications

- Pericardiocentesis-related (p. 1150)
- Surgical complications related to pericardiectomy; surgical resection carries substantial risks.
- Because most heart base tumors are benign, metastasis is uncommon.

Recommended Monitoring

- Follow-up exams and echocardiography to assess for recurrent pericardial effusion and tumor progression
- Thoracic radiographs and abdominal ultrasound for tumor staging

PROGNOSIS & OUTCOME

- Guarded to fair without pericardiectomy
- Pericardiectomy alone improves survival time considerably (median survival, 730 vs. 42 days).

PEARLS & CONSIDERATIONS

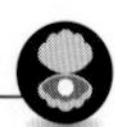

Comments

- Characteristic echocardiographic findings lead to the presumptive diagnosis of a heart base tumor, which typically has a better prognosis than other cardiac tumors such as hemangiosarcoma.
- Cytologic and biochemical evaluations of pericardial fluid are unreliable.

Technician Tips

Intravenous fluid boluses may be used to stabilize a patient with cardiac tamponade until pericardiocentesis can be performed.

Client Education

- Pericardiocentesis and pericardiectomy are palliative and not curative.
- Pericardiectomy can likely lead to longer survival time with fewer clinical signs in the interim.

SUGGESTED READING

Ehrhart N, et al: Analysis of factors affecting survival in dogs with aortic body tumors. Vet Surg 31:44-48, 2002.

AUTHOR: Herbert W. Maisenbacher, III, VMD, DACVIM
EDITOR: Meg M. Sleeper, VMD, DACVIM

Heart Failure, Acute/Decompensated

Client Education Sheet 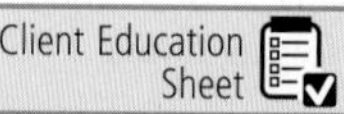

BASIC INFORMATION

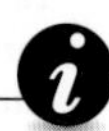

Definition

Acute (or decompensated) heart failure (HF) is characterized by the sudden onset of clinical signs associated with pulmonary edema or cavitary effusions due to heart disease. Acute/decompensated HF is a common cause of respiratory distress and usually results from worsening cardiac performance in patients with chronic heart disease.

Synonyms

Acute congestive heart failure (CHF), decompensated heart disease, overt heart failure

Epidemiology

SPECIES, AGE, SEX

Signalment reflects predispositions for the causative heart disorder:

- Geriatric small-breed dogs: chronic mitral/tricuspid regurgitation (myxomatous valve disease)
- Cats: hypertrophic cardiomyopathy (HCM)

GENETICS, BREED PREDISPOSITION

- Dilated cardiomyopathy (DCM): Doberman pinschers, Great Danes, Irish wolfhounds, and other large- and giant-breed dogs
- Mitral/tricuspid myxomatous valve disease: Cavalier King Charles spaniels, dachshunds, many others
- HCM: inherited in Maine coon cats and in Ragdoll cats; it is possible that feline HCM is a genetic disease.

RISK FACTORS

- In patients with underlying heart disease
  - Dietary sodium excess
  - Acute intravascular volume load (e.g., parenteral fluids)
  - Possibly corticosteroids (cats)
  - Possibly ketamine/tiletamine (cats)
- Electrocardiographic, echocardiographic variables: predictive of likelihood of future HF or sudden, unexpected death in Doberman pinschers with DCM

Clinical Presentation

DISEASE FORMS/SUBTYPES

- Left-sided HF results in pulmonary edema.
- Right-sided HF causes ascites and sometimes concurrent pleural effusion.
- In cats, pleural effusion may result from left- and/or right-sided heart disease.

HISTORY, CHIEF COMPLAINT

- Respiratory signs predominate. Specifically, the characteristic manifestations include tachypnea, dyspnea, and, in the dog, cough. HF seldom causes coughing in cats.
- Clients may report that the patient appears to be uncomfortable, restless, or unwilling to lie down.

PHYSICAL EXAM FINDINGS

- Tachycardia is a relatively consistent, although nonspecific, finding in dogs with HF. Heart rates of cats with acute HF differ little from heart rates of healthy cats. Some cats with acute HF have bradycardia.
- In dogs, respiratory sinus arrhythmia makes a diagnosis of acute HF virtually untenable; other explanations for the clinical signs should be considered.
- In patients with pulmonary edema, tachypnea and respiratory distress are usually apparent during physical examination. Loud lung sounds or crackles may be ausculted.
- Dogs with acute HF due to myxomatous valve disease have a cardiac murmur; usually the murmur is loud (≥III/VI).
- An audible, low-frequency third or fourth heart sound—a gallop—reflects high atrial pressures and reduced ventricular compliance. Relatively specific marker of acute HF in dogs.

Etiology and Pathophysiology

- Congestive signs result when high venous pressures cause the development of edema or cavitary effusions.
- In dogs, HF that results primarily from systolic dysfunction—impaired ventricular emptying—is most common.
- HF in cats usually results from diseases that impair ventricular filling (diastolic dysfunction).
- HF is associated with neuroendocrine activation that temporarily maintains perfusion pressure and cardiac output through vasoconstriction and increases in heart rate and contractility.
- In patients with systolic dysfunction, systemic vascular resistance rises disproportionately, causing a detrimental increase in afterload; this explains the beneficial effect of vasodilators.

DIAGNOSIS

Diagnostic Overview

HF is a clinical or radiographic diagnosis:

- Left HF is defined by the presence of radiographic pulmonary opacities in association with left atrial enlargement.
- Right HF is defined by the finding of ascites in association with jugular venous distention and/or evidence of right atrial/right ventricular enlargement from imaging studies.

Differential Diagnosis

Other causes of respiratory distress and/or cough (pp. 217, 879, 1209, and 1219).

Initial Database

- Thoracic radiographs
  - Dogs: cardiac silhouette enlarged with distinct left atrial enlargement. Pulmonary edema may result in interstitial or alveolar densities. Patients with valvular disease may develop perihilar densities but focal edema—often affecting the right caudal lung lobe—is common. In patients with DCM, pulmonary edema may have a similar appearance, although acute decompensation may result in diffusely distributed but patchy alveolar densities.
  - Cats: cardiac silhouette is generally enlarged, but specific chamber enlargement is less distinct than in dogs.

Pulmonary edema typically has a diffuse but patchy distribution. Pleural effusion may be present and may be the primary manifestation of congestion.
- Electrocardiography (ECG) is indicated when arrhythmias complicate the presentation.
- Serum biochemistry profile and urinalysis: in all cases, preferably before initiating treatment

Advanced or Confirmatory Testing

- Echocardiography defines the causative disorder.
- Supraphysiologic concentrations of circulating NT-pro-BNP reflect elevated ventricular wall tension and are a diagnostic marker of HF (p. 1369).
  - Evaluation of serum NT-pro-BNP concentrations may help to distinguish dyspnea caused by HF from dyspnea due to primary respiratory tract disease.

TREATMENT

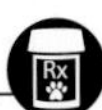

Treatment Overview

The goal of treatment is to restore ventilatory function by eliminating lung edema or pleural effusion and, in some cases, to improve cardiac performance.

Acute General Treatment

- Rest
- Judicious/minimal restraint and other measures for reducing anxiety are essential.
- Furosemide: diuretic of choice in acute HF. Dose and dosage interval are best determined by clinical response.
  - Initially: relatively high dose of 2-4 mg/kg IV, IM. If no evidence of effect (reduction in respiratory rate/improved effort), this dose can be repeated in 45-60 minutes.
  - If respiratory rate and effort decrease: 1-2 mg/kg IV or IM q 1-6h until respirations normalize
  - The effect of furosemide is rapid but short lived; low doses at short intervals are preferred.
  - Constant-rate infusion of furosemide is an alternative to frequent bolus administration, but advantages in veterinary patients are uncertain; dosage = total projected daily dosage of furosemide divided by 24 as the hourly rate of the infusion.
  - In general, cats require lower doses than dogs.
- Supplementary oxygen (p. 1146)
- Morphine 0.05-0.3 mg/kg SQ, IM, or IV or acepromazine 0.01-0.03 mg/kg IM or IV can be considered for dogs that are anxious due to respiratory distress.
- Thoracocentesis (p. 1164) if physical or radiographic findings indicate that pleural effusion is likely responsible for respiratory distress
- Patients with systolic dysfunction and evidence of diminished cardiac output at rest may benefit from intravenous administration of nitroprusside 0.5-15 mcg/kg/min and/or dobutamine 2-15 mcg/kg/min constant-rate infusion. Careful monitoring is required.
- Dogs with acute/decompensated HF due to valvular disease or dilated cardiomyopathy benefit from administration of the inodilator pimobendan 0.25 mg/kg PO q 12h. The use of pimobendan in acute (or decompensated) HF has not been systematically evaluated.
- IV or SQ fluid administration is generally contraindicated unless used as a vehicle for the administration of drugs or electrolytes.

Chronic Treatment

See the chapter on Chronic Heart Failure (p. 409).

Possible Complications

- Hypovolemia/impaired renal perfusion due to excessive diuresis
- Hypotension
- Electrolyte abnormalities due to diuretic use.

Recommended Monitoring

- Frequent monitoring of vital signs (especially respiratory rate), mucous membranes, body weight
- ECG if arrhythmias
- Flow-directed (Swan-Ganz) pulmonary artery catheterization and/or arterial cannula can be considered for hemodynamic monitoring of severely affected dogs admitted to an intensive care unit; rarely performed and benefit uncertain.

PROGNOSIS & OUTCOME

- Most patients presented for first treatment of acute HF respond promptly to conservative therapy consisting of rest, supplemental oxygen, and furosemide.
- Despite favorable initial response, HF is generally associated with a poor long-term prognosis unless the causative disorder is curable.

PEARLS & CONSIDERATIONS

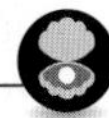

Comments

- Although ancillary therapy, including vasodilators and inotropes, may speed recovery from acute HF, most patients that are destined to recover respond to conservative management.
- Response to empirical therapy is diagnostically useful. When treatment is based on a presumptive diagnosis, failure to respond to diuretic therapy suggests the possibility that clinical signs are due to primary respiratory tract disease or that the patient has refractory HF.

Technician Tips

Teaching the owners to count resting respiratory rate is a helpful way to monitor for recurrence of CHF.

Client Education

Chronic medical therapy is generally required even after apparent recovery.

SUGGESTED READING

Atkins C, et al: ACVIM consensus statement: guidelines for the diagnosis and treatment of canine chronic valvular heart disease. J Vet Intern Med 23:1142-1150, 2009.

AUTHOR: Jonathan A. Abbott, DVM, DACVIM
EDITOR: Meg M. Sleeper, VMD, DACVIM

Heart Failure, Chronic

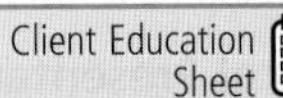

Client Education Sheet

BASIC INFORMATION

Definition

- Heart failure (HF) is a syndrome that results from impaired filling or emptying of the heart, typically manifesting with cardiogenic edema or effusion.
- A new classification system can be applied to HF in small-animal practice. In this schema, patients with HF are staged as follows:
  - Stage A: patients at risk for HF (no overt or occult signs of heart disease)
  - Stage B: patients that have structural heart disease but have not developed HF
    - In the setting of canine myxomatous valvular disease, stage B1 defines patients with mitral regurgitation but without cardiac chamber enlargement. Stage B2 refers to mitral regurgitation associated with chamber enlargement.
  - Stage C: patients that have *or previously have had* clinical signs of HF
  - Stage D: patients with refractory HF
- The term *chronic HF* is used as a synonym for stage C HF as described above. Urgent therapy of acute or decompensated HF is addressed on p. 408.

Synonym

Congestive heart failure (CHF)

Epidemiology

SPECIES, AGE, SEX

HF is a syndrome that can result from practically any cardiac disease; signalment reflects predispositions for the causative disorder:

- Geriatric small-breed dogs: chronic mitral and tricuspid regurgitation due to myxomatous valve disease
- Adult large- and giant-breed dogs: dilated cardiomyopathy (DCM)
- Cats: hypertrophic cardiomyopathy (HCM; males > females), restrictive/unclassified cardiomyopathy

GENETICS, BREED PREDISPOSITION

- DCM: canine DCM is generally familial. Doberman pinschers, Great Danes, Irish wolfhounds, and other large- and giant-breed dogs. A genetic mutation associated with the development of DCM in Doberman pinschers has been identified.
- Mitral and tricuspid regurgitation due to myxomatous valve disease: geriatric small-breed dogs, including Cavalier King Charles spaniels, dachshunds, and many others
- HCM: inherited in Maine coon cats and Ragdoll cats. It is possible that feline HCM in other breeds, and in mix-breeds, has a genetic basis.

RISK FACTORS

- Electrocardiographic and echocardiographic variables that predict the development of stage C HF in Doberman pinschers have been described. Elevated serum B-type natriuretic peptide (BNP) concentration identifies Doberman pinschers at risk for HF with high specificity but relatively low sensitivity.
- In Irish wolfhounds and other giant-breed dogs, atrial fibrillation sometimes precedes the development of HF.
- In small-breed dogs, a murmur caused by myxomatous mitral degeneration is a risk factor for development of HF, but there is great interindividual variability in the rate at which valvular disease progresses.
- Supraphysiologic BNP concentration and left atrial enlargement independently predict the onset of stage C HF in dogs with myxomatous valve disease.
- In cats, echocardiographically evident left atrial enlargement is associated with the development of HF.

Clinical Presentation

DISEASE FORMS/SUBTYPES

- Left-sided HF results in pulmonary edema.
- Right-sided HF causes ascites and sometimes concurrent pleural effusion.
- In cats, pleural effusion results from left-sided, right-sided, or biventricular HF; ascites is uncommon.

HISTORY, CHIEF COMPLAINT

Clinical signs such as respiratory distress generally improve or resolve with initial treatment, but signs such as progressive abdominal distention, syncope, lethargy, and weight loss may persist. Patients with chronic HF are subject to additional episodes of acute/decompensated HF.

PHYSICAL EXAM FINDINGS

- Patients with HF due to mitral/tricuspid myxomatous valve disease have a cardiac murmur; usually the murmur is loud, and its intensity is generally not affected by treatment.
- An audible third or fourth heart sound—a gallop—reflects high atrial pressures and reduced ventricular compliance. In dogs, it is a relatively specific marker of HF.

Etiology and Pathophysiology

- Congestive signs result when high venous pressures cause the development of edema or cavitary effusions.
- In dogs, HF that results primarily from systolic dysfunction (impaired ventricular emptying) is most common.
- HF in cats usually results from diseases that impair ventricular filling; diastolic ventricular (filling) pressures are abnormally high when ventricular volume is normal or small.
- A high filling pressure is reflected upstream to the venous circulation, resulting in edema or pleural effusion.
- HF is associated with neuroendocrine activation: specifically, impaired cardiac performance leads to increased activity of the renin-angiotensin-aldosterone system (RAAS) and the adrenergic nervous system (ANS).
- Angiotensin II (ATII) is the biologically active product of a biochemical cascade for which the final step is catalyzed by angiotensin-converting enzyme (ACE).
- ATII is a vasoconstrictor, but it also stimulates the release of aldosterone, augments activity of the ANS, and acts as a cardiomyotrophic factor.
- Activation of the RAAS and ANS serves to temporarily maintain perfusion pressure and cardiac output.
- Vasoconstriction increases vascular resistance so that blood pressure is maintained when cardiac output is subnormal. In patients with mitral/tricuspid myxomatous valve disease or DCM, vascular resistance is high, causing a detrimental increase in afterload; this partly explains the beneficial effect of vasodilators.

DIAGNOSIS

Diagnostic Overview

Chronic HF occurs when acute/decompensated HF is treated successfully, but the underlying cause cannot be cured. Clinical features of chronic HF can include a history of acute/decompensated HF, with partial or complete resolution of signs with treatment but persistence of the underlying cardiac disease.

Differential Diagnosis

Other causes of respiratory distress, cough, abdominal distention, lethargy, inappetence, and weight loss (cardiac cachexia)

Initial Database

- Thoracic radiography
  - When other clinical findings are compatible, left atrial enlargement with pulmonary opacities is diagnostic for left-sided HF.
  - With diuretic treatment of decompensated HF, clinical improvement is usually rapid (minutes to hours), but radiographic resolution of pulmonary infiltrates may take 24 hours or more.
  - Cats commonly develop pleural effusion in association with left-sided cardiac disease.
- Electrocardiography (ECG) is indicated when arrhythmias complicate the presentation. Atrial fibrillation is commonly associated with HF in large-breed dogs, but tachyarrhythmia of virtually any type may complicate the presentation of HF (pp. 94 and 1033).
- Noninvasive estimation of systemic blood pressure using Doppler or the oscillometric method should be considered. The finding of systemic hypertension (SH) provides evidence of concurrent disease; SH may complicate HF, but it is not a result of HF. However, documented SH should be treated because untreated SH may accelerate the progression of the primary cardiac disorder.
- Serum biochemistry profiles provide useful ancillary information and are important in monitoring the effects of therapy (especially renal and electrolyte effects).

Advanced or Confirmatory Testing

- BNP is released by cardiomyocytes in response to increases in ventricular filling pressures; elevated circulating BNP is a marker of the HF state.
- Echocardiography generally provides the diagnosis of the underlying cardiac disorder. Echocardiography is complementary to physical exam and thoracic radiography but does not replace them.

TREATMENT

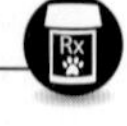

Treatment Overview

- Increase in quality and duration of life is the goal.
- Although individual patient characteristics must be taken into account, polytherapy consisting of furosemide, an ACE inhibitor, and pimobendan has become standard treatment for management of stage C HF in dogs.
- There is uncertainty regarding optimal therapy for cats with HF resulting from diastolic dysfunction; furosemide and an ACE inhibitor are widely used.

Chronic Treatment

- Diuretics: furosemide is the most effective agent for management of congestive signs.
  - In dogs, a dose of 1-2 mg/kg PO q 12h is often initially adequate when given concurrently with ancillary agents such as ACE inhibitors and pimobendan. Cats

with HF generally require lower initial doses: 0.5-2 mg/kg PO q 12-24h.
  - Furosemide is used first, but the progressive nature of the HF state generally requires adjustment of doses. If clinical signs suggest diuretic resistance or electrolyte derangements are documented, other diuretics such as hydrochlorothiazide 2-4 mg/kg PO q 12h or spironolactone 1-2 mg/kg PO q 12h (dog) can be added. Doing so allows for synergistic diuretic action; different diuretics act in different parts of the nephron, which may minimize the negative effects of long-term (weeks or more) administration of high doses of a single diuretic (e.g., > 3-4 mg/kg q 8-12h of furosemide).
  - For patients with advanced disease and refractory HF, the use of torsemide 0.1-0.2 mg/kg q 12-24h can be considered as an *alternative* to furosemide.
  - Diuretic dose should be determined by clinical response; the optimal dose is the lowest one that eliminates congestive signs.
  - Excessive diuretic administration may decrease renal perfusion, create electrolyte imbalances, and contribute to potentially harmful neuroendocrine activation.
  - Most patients require lifelong diuretic administration; progression of the underlying disorder generally necessitates increases in furosemide dose and/or the use of additional diuretics.
  - Furosemide administration sometimes can be tapered or temporarily discontinued in cats with HCM.
- ACE inhibitors partially blunt the effects of RAAS activation and reduce afterload.
  - ACE inhibition has proven benefits for patients with chronic HF caused by systolic dysfunction. Preliminary evidence suggests a benefit for patients with chronic HF caused by diastolic dysfunction (e.g., cats with HF caused by HCM or restrictive/unclassified cardiomyopathy).
  - Of the ACE inhibitors, veterinary experience is greatest with enalapril 0.5 mg/kg PO q 12-24h (dog), benazepril 0.25-0.5 mg/kg PO q 24h (dog), 0.5-1 mg/kg PO q 24h (cat), and ramipril 0.125 mg/kg PO q 24h (dog), 0.5 mg/kg PO q 24h (cat).
- Digoxin
  - 0.22 mg/m^2 PO q 12h (dog); 0.03125 mg/CAT PO q 48h
  - Important in management of patients with supraventricular tachycardia, in particular atrial fibrillation.
- Pimobendan 0.1-0.3 mg/kg PO q 12h administered when stomach is empty is a phosphodiesterase inhibitor that acts as an inodilator. It is indicated for the treatment of dogs that have developed advanced stage B2 or stage C HF due to valvular disease or DCM.
  - Pimobendan decreased mortality rates compared with benazepril in patients with HF due to valvular disease. The evidence that pimobendan decreases mortality rates among Doberman pinschers with stage C HF due to DCM is strong.
  - Adverse effects associated with the administration of pimobendan are apparently uncommon, although there is some evidence that the drug may harm patients with mild subclinical valvular disease. Use of this drug should be reserved for dogs with stage C mitral valve degeneration and for dogs with stage B2 mitral valve degeneration that meet the inclusion criteria of the EPIC clinical trial (see inclusion criteria under Prevention below). A proarrhythmic effect is possible but appears uncommon, if it even exists in dogs.
- Spironolactone 1-2 mg/kg PO q 12h (dog)
  - In chronic HF, excess aldosterone may contribute to the development of myocardial fibrosis.
  - Spironolactone is an aldosterone antagonist, which may limit the detrimental effects of hyperaldosteronemia; careful monitoring of electrolytes is advised.
  - Minimal diuretic efficacy as monotherapy in the dog
  - Severe facial dermatitis was identified in 30% of Maine coon cats receiving spironolactone, and caution should therefore be used in cats.
- Cautious addition of amlodipine 0.0625-0.25 mg/kg PO q 24h (dog), 0.125 mg/kg-0.25 mg/kg PO q 24h (cat) to conventional therapy can be considered for patients with refractory HF caused by systolic dysfunction or for those in which SH complicates the clinical presentation. Blood pressure monitoring is essential (p. 1065).
- Beta-blockers (BBs): despite experimental evidence to support the use of BBs in dogs with DCM or advanced mitral/tricuspid valve disease a benefit has not been supported by clinical experience. These medications must be added very carefully for dogs and cats with chronic HF.
  - BBs are never started before a patient's pulmonary edema has resolved.
- Moderate dietary sodium restriction generally is indicated. If palatable to the patient, low-sodium diets may reduce diuretic requirements.

Nutrition/Diet

Moderate sodium restriction, adequate protein and energy content, and palatability are important attributes of an optimal diet for HF patients.

Possible Complications

- The cardiorenal syndrome, a decrease in renal function in patients with cardiac dysfunction, reflects the complex cardiovascular-renal interactions characteristic of HF. Azotemia is associated with declining cardiac performance and diuretic administration, but the cause of azotemia in HF is multifactorial and has been incompletely defined.
  - When azotemia is encountered in patients receiving furosemide and ACE inhibitors, *furosemide* is first decreased by 50%, provided the patient is free of congestive signs. If the creatinine does not decrease, diuretic therapy is discontinued, provided congestive signs are not evident. Only if this is unsuccessful is the ACE inhibitor discontinued.
  - There are unfortunately few alternatives for patients that develop clinical signs specifically due to azotemia when congestive signs are present concurrently; this may reflect medically intractable HF. However, caution must be exercised because overinterpretation of radiographs or abnormal lung sounds (e.g., pulmonary rales/crackles due to interstitial lung fibrosis, not edema) can lead to inappropriately high diuretic doses, volume depletion, and azotemia.

Recommended Monitoring

- Serum urea, creatinine, and electrolytes
- When applicable, serum digoxin concentration
- A resting, at-home respiratory rate in excess of 35 breaths/min is associated with pulmonary edema in dogs treated for chronic HF.

PROGNOSIS & OUTCOME

Despite a favorable initial response, HF is generally associated with a poor long-term prognosis unless the causative disorder is curable. With current medical therapy, survival of 6 months or more is a reasonable expectation, but longevity is determined by numerous factors, including the causative disease.

PEARLS & CONSIDERATIONS

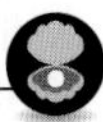

Comments

- When the causative disorder is not curable, chronic HF is a progressive and terminal syndrome. Attempts to identify a correctable cause are therefore important. Some patients with DCM respond to supplementation with nutraceuticals such as taurine and L-carnitine.
- For sodium content of dog and cat foods, see http://vet.tufts.edu/heartsmart/diet/reduced_sodium_diet.html.

Prevention

- In patients with clinically silent DCM, the onset of HF may be delayed by the administration of cardiac medications (p. 263).
  - A clinical trial has provided evidence that administration of pimobendan to Doberman pinschers with subclinical echocardiographic evidence of DCM delays the onset of stage C HF.
- Recently published data provided evidence that pimobendan, relative to placebo, delays the onset of pulmonary edema in canine patients with radiographically and echocardiographically demonstrated cardiac enlargement resulting from subclinical

(asymptomatic) mitral valve regurgitation. Relevant inclusion criteria for the trial that demonstrated this effect were a vertebral heart sum > 10.5, an echocardiographic left atrial–aortic ratio > 1.6, and left ventricular enlargement.
- ACE inhibition may have a positive effect on the time to development of stage C HF in canine patients with left atrial enlargement due to mitral valve regurgitation.
- Evidence that medical therapy slows the progression of HCM is lacking.

Technician Tips
Teaching owners to keep a log of their pet's resting respiratory rates can allow early detection of HF decompensation so that medications can be adjusted and hopefully hospitalization for acute HF can be avoided.

Client Education
Management of the veterinary patient with chronic HF requires careful monitoring and relatively frequent adjustment of medical therapy (see client education sheet: How to Count Respirations and Monitor Respiratory Effort)

SUGGESTED READING
Atkins C, et al: ACVIM consensus statement. Guidelines for the diagnosis and treatment of canine chronic valvular heart disease. J Vet Intern Med 23:1142-1150, 2009.

AUTHOR: Jonathan A. Abbott, DVM, DACVIM
EDITOR: Meg M. Sleeper, VMD, DACVIM

Heart Murmur, Incidental Finding

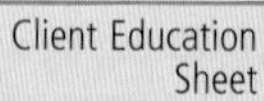

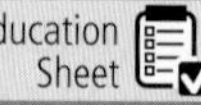

BASIC INFORMATION

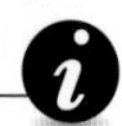

Definition
A heart murmur that is detected in the process of an examination that was not initially directed at the cardiovascular system

Synonym
Asymptomatic heart murmur

Epidemiology
SPECIES, AGE, SEX

Any species, all ages, both sexes

GENETICS, BREED PREDISPOSITION

Predispositions mirror those of the causative cardiac diseases (pp. 263, 505, 657, 658, 764, 844, and 948).

RISK FACTORS
- Structural heart disease
- Anemia
- Youth

Clinical Presentation
HISTORY, CHIEF COMPLAINT
- By definition: identified in patients that are presented for noncardiovascular concerns, such as annual wellness exams, noncardiac medical concerns, or preanesthetic evaluation.
- Although no historical signs are associated with the murmur, misleading or overlapping signs are common, including cough, exercise intolerance, and others, which can be caused by unrelated comorbidities.

PHYSICAL EXAM FINDINGS
- Heart murmur (by definition), which is described according to timing, grade, and point of maximal intensity (p. 414)
- Auscultatory features of murmurs that are nonpathologic (see Differential Diagnosis below) classically meet the six S criteria, which are typically systolic, soft (grade 1-2/6), sensitive (prone to change in intensity with heart rate or body posture), short (midsystolic), single (unaccompanied by other abnormal sounds), and small (not widely radiating).

Etiology and Pathophysiology
- A heart murmur is caused by turbulent blood flow in the heart (p. 414).
- Identifying the timing, location, and intensity of the murmur may be straightforward or challenging; uncertainty favors pursuing diagnostic testing.
- The presence of a heart murmur does not warrant treatment. Rather, determining its cause (definitively or presumptively) can lead to an assessment of whether treatment is indicated.

DIAGNOSIS

Diagnostic Overview
First, an incidentally detected heart murmur is pursued through careful characterization of the murmur's timing, grade, and point of maximal intensity. Second, these characteristics, combined with the patient's signalment, may provide a strong suspicion of a likely underlying cause. If so and the veterinarian's tentative diagnosis is of a benign process, the client is satisfied with this opinion without confirmation, and the animal is not to be used for breeding nor subjected to cardiovascular stress, diagnostic testing is not essential. Otherwise, diagnostic testing should be pursued.

Differential Diagnosis
Murmurs may be nonpathologic (the heart is structurally normal) or pathologic (caused by a structural heart lesion):
- Nonpathologic (benign) murmurs are further described as *functional* if a plausible physiologic cause is detectable (e.g., anemia) or as *innocent* if no cardiac or extracardiac cause for the murmur can be identified.
- Pathologic murmurs can be caused by any cardiac disorder of any degree and do not automatically indicate a severe condition.

Initial Database
- Thoracic radiographs may be considered as the initial diagnostic test in small- to medium-breed dogs with systolic murmurs that are loudest over the mitral valve region.
- An echocardiogram should be considered for any adult animal with one or more of the following: uncertain or unusual murmur characteristics, murmur characteristics suggesting a form of heart disease that requires initiation of treatment, large-breed dog (auscultation and thoracic radiographs have low specificity for individual cardiac disorders), impending cardiovascular stress (e.g., plane travel, general anesthesia), breeding prospects, or owner who wishes to have confirmation of the cause of the murmur.
- An echocardiogram should be considered for puppies and kittens with a murmur that is grade 3/6 or louder, that is diastolic or continuous, that obscures the second (or both) heart sounds, that radiates to the carotid region or is loudest over the left apex or right hemithorax, or that is a direct relative of an animal with congenital heart disease.
- NT-pro-BNP testing in cats can raise or lower the likelihood of structural heart disease (notably cardiomyopathy) as the cause of the murmur.

TREATMENT

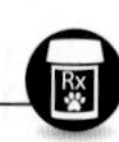

Treatment Overview
Because a murmur is a physical finding alone, no treatment is warranted.

Acute and Chronic Treatment
Initiation of treatment in the absence of a diagnosis is not appropriate. It can lead to administration of medications a patient does not need (or that are contraindicated), cause unnecessary expense, and cause adverse treatment effects.

Possible Complications

Overinterpretation or underinterpretation of incidentally detected heart murmurs can lead to failure to provide an accurate treatment plan and prognosis.

PROGNOSIS & OUTCOME

Because incidentally detected murmurs occur in animals without associated clinical signs, the prognosis is often fair to good. Many disorders are progressive, but some (notably patent ductus arteriosus) lend themselves to being cured. The exact prognosis therefore depends on establishing the underlying cause and its degree of severity.

PEARLS & CONSIDERATIONS

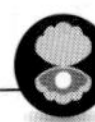

Comments

- 25%-69% of cats with heart murmurs have no detectable heart disease.
- Treatment of a heart murmur is never indicated. The murmur is a clue, and the cause to which the clue is pointing may or may not benefit from treatment.

Technician Tips

Cats routinely have heart murmurs that are heart-rate dependent or that can vary in intensity between anesthesia and being awake. These characteristics are typical of physiologic murmurs, but it is impossible to be certain of the murmur's cause (pathologic or nonpathologic) without an echocardiogram.

SUGGESTED READING

Côté E, et al: Management of incidentally-detected heart murmurs in dogs and cats. J Am Vet Med Assoc 246:1076, 2015.

AUTHOR: Etienne Côté, DVM, DACVIM
EDITOR: Meg M. Sleeper, VMD, DACVIM

Heart Murmur, Physiologic

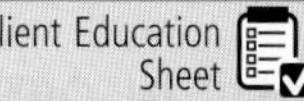

Client Education Sheet

BASIC INFORMATION

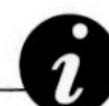

Definition

Heart murmurs not associated with cardiac disease

Synonyms

Innocent murmurs, flow murmurs, nonpathologic heart murmurs

Epidemiology

SPECIES, AGE, SEX

Physiologic heart murmurs are common in puppies and kittens, and these generally disappear by 4-6 months of age. Other causes for murmurs unrelated to heart disease can be detected at any age.

GENETICS, BREED PREDISPOSITION

- Hound dogs (e.g., greyhound, Italian greyhounds, salukis) and, in general, athletic dog breeds are particularly prone to developing physiologic heart murmurs.
- Boxer dogs

RISK FACTORS

- Athleticism
- Anemia
- Other high cardiac output conditions (anxiety, hyperthyroidism, fever)

ASSOCIATED DISORDERS

Commonly associated with severe anemia

Clinical Presentation

HISTORY, CHIEF COMPLAINT

- Physiologic murmurs in puppies/kittens or athletic dogs are found during routine checkups.
- Patients with murmurs caused by anemia or fever can show clinical signs associated to these underlying conditions.

PHYSICAL EXAM FINDINGS

- These murmurs are more easily auscultated over the left heart base, occur during systole, and are usually soft (<III/VI).
- Pale mucous membranes may be evident in patients with physiologic heart murmurs caused by anemia.
- Fever may cause a physiologic murmur.

Etiology and Pathophysiology

- The genesis of a murmur is affected by multiple factors; structural heart disease creates turbulence and/or increases blood velocity due to valvular leakage (regurgitation), abnormal shunts, or obstructive lesions (p. 414).
- Physiologic heart murmurs result from a relatively high cardiac output. It is hypothesized that young patients have a relatively high stroke volume for their great vessels, causing physiologic murmurs. As these patients grow, their great vessels enlarge and the murmur disappears, usually by 6 months of age.
- Changes in blood properties, such as its viscosity or density, can also lead to heart murmurs in normal hearts. In patients with anemia, the combination of decreased blood viscosity due to a low hematocrit and an increased stroke volume can result in a physiologic murmur.
- Greyhounds and other athletic hunting dogs may have a soft, basilar systolic murmur that is physiologic. An echocardiogram, which is necessary to rule out a pathologic cause for the murmur, may demonstrate transaortic velocities that are slightly increased but still in the normal range and a normal cardiac structure.
- Although boxer dogs are predisposed to subaortic stenosis (SAS), these dogs also have an increased prevalence of physiologic murmurs that are thought to be due to a relatively smaller left ventricular outflow tract without other changes consistent with SAS.
- Emotional stress also increases cardiac output and should be taken into consideration when auscultating and/or echoing these patients.

DIAGNOSIS

Diagnostic Overview

Physiologic heart murmurs cannot be diagnosed solely by auscultation, and an echocardiogram is necessary to rule out structural heart disease. However, the echocardiogram may be delayed if there is evidence supporting a cause for physiologic murmur (e.g., if severe anemia exists, echocardiogram may be postponed to see if resolution of anemia results in resolution of murmur).

Differential Diagnosis

Other causes of heart murmurs: congenital (pulmonic or subaortic stenosis, ventricular septal defects, atrioventricular valve stenosis), acquired (degenerative valvular disease, secondary valvular regurgitation due to dilated, hypertrophic, or restrictive cardiomyopathy, bacterial endocarditis).

Initial Database

- Echocardiogram
- Hematocrit

TREATMENT

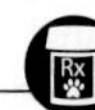

Treatment Overview

- No treatment is necessary for pediatric or athletic murmur.
- Patients with physiologic murmurs due to anemia or fever need treatment for the underlying systemic condition.

PROGNOSIS & OUTCOME

Physiologic murmurs do not affect health directly. If the murmur is caused by fever, anemia, or other systemic illness, prognosis depends on the underlying condition.

PEARLS & CONSIDERATIONS

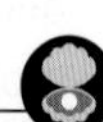

Comments

Murmurs that change significantly in character with changes in heart rate are more likely to be physiologic.

Technician Tips

When auscultating murmurs in anxious patients, it helps to wait until the patient is calm. Because stress increases cardiac output and this can be a reason for physiologic murmurs, a decrease in the intensity of the murmur as the patient settles is often noticed with physiologic murmurs.

Client Education

It is important to reiterate to owners that patients with physiologic heart murmurs, although they may be currently free of heart disease, can still develop acquired heart disease in the future.

SUGGESTED READING

Belanger MC: Innocent heart murmurs. In Ettinger SJ, et al, editors: Textbook of veterinary internal medicine, ed 7, St. Louis, 2010, Saunders.

AUTHOR: Ivan Sosa, DVM, DACVIM
EDITOR: Meg M. Sleeper, VMD, DACVIM

Heart Murmurs

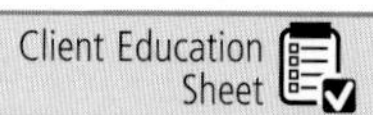

BASIC INFORMATION

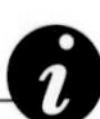

Definition

Normal blood flow in the circulatory system is laminar in nature and very quiet. When laminar flow through the heart is altered, turbulence develops, causing a sound that can be heard: a heart murmur. This can be likened to a slow-flowing, wide river undulating quietly back and forth; if suddenly an obstruction such as a large boulder is placed in the river, the quiet river becomes a noisy one as the water flows around the rock, creating turbulence.

Epidemiology

SPECIES, AGE, SEX

A heart murmur is a clinical sign that may develop in any animal. Pathologic murmurs caused by structural heart lesions generally increase in intensity with age and disease progression. Characteristics of functional or physiologic heart murmurs (p. 413) in young, growing dogs and cats:

- Soft (grade II/VI or less)
- Systolic
- Point of maximal intensity: left hemithorax or left parasternal region in kittens
- Abolished with an increase in heart rate or change in body position
- Usually disappear around 4 months of age
- Often eliminated by reduction in pressure of the stethoscope on the thoracic wall

GENETICS, BREED PREDISPOSITION

Many breeds are predisposed to specific congenital heart malformations that are associated with heart murmurs (e.g., patent ductus arteriosus [PDA], subaortic stenosis, pulmonic stenosis, ventricular septal defect, tricuspid dysplasia) and to adult-onset disorders, some of which have a heritable basis (e.g., myxomatous mitral valve disease, dilated cardiomyopathy). See specific chapters on the individual diseases for lists of at-risk breeds.

RISK FACTORS

- Heart murmurs may occur secondary to various noncardiac entities such as fever, anemia, hyperthyroidism, extreme thinness or obesity, and pregnancy.
- Some breeds of dogs and cats are more prone to physiologic murmurs, especially under stress circumstances, and diseases of the heart (myocardium, heart valves, endothelial lining of the heart) and the great vessels.
- Heart murmurs develop with congenital and acquired heart defects.
- Physiologic murmurs are unusual in adult dogs; this is a murmur present in the absence of any cardiac or systemic abnormalities. Dynamic right ventricular outflow turbulence (dRVOT) has been described in cats and is associated with obstruction to flow in the ventricle; clinical consequences may develop over time.
- Murmurs also may be identified in the veins and arteries under circumstances that cause nonlaminar flow, such as arteriovenous fistulas or extravascular partial obstructions.
- Systemic infection may cause bacterial endocarditis (p. 294).

Clinical Presentation

HISTORY, CHIEF COMPLAINT

- Heart murmurs may be detected during a routine exam in a patient that is otherwise well. The goal is to identify the cause of the murmur (may be highly suggestive based on signalment, history, and exam findings or may require diagnostic testing).
- Heart murmurs may be noted in a patient that is systemically ill (e.g., anemic). Ascertain whether the murmur can be explained by the systemic illness alone (see Risk Factors above) or an underlying heart problem is coexistent (e.g., endocarditis).
- Differentiate murmurs that are present but not causing a problem from those related to the clinical signs for which the animal is presented.
- Heart murmurs may be noted in patients with overt signs compatible with heart disease (e.g., dyspnea, exercise intolerance, collapse, signs of thromboembolism). The murmur is a clue that these generalized signs may be caused by a heart problem and that cardiac diagnostic testing is indicated.

PHYSICAL EXAM FINDINGS

- Murmurs should be identified during the physical exam process. Using the stethoscope, the dog's or cat's thorax is thoroughly auscultated using the diaphragm and then using the bell of the instrument. All four valve areas—mitral, tricuspid, pulmonic, and aortic regions—are ausculted, listening for abnormalities of the heart rate and rhythm, for alterations in the heart sounds, and most commonly, for a heart murmur. If a murmur exists, it must be identified with respect to timing, intensity, and musical tonality, as well as where it is heard loudest on the thorax (point of maximal intensity) and if the sounds spread to other parts of the thorax or into the jugular region of the neck. This is radiation of the murmur to another part of the thorax. Some stethoscopes are single head only. When gently placed on the thorax, they intensify the low frequency sounds, and when pressed more firmly, they bring out the entire range of heart sounds.
- Murmurs are described by their intensity. Using a grading system with a maximum of VI, I/VI is the least intense and barely heard; II/VI is soft but unmistakably heard; III/VI is easily distinguished; IV/VI is intense but without a palpable thrill; V/VI is loud, intense, and associated with a precordial vibration (thrill) on the thorax where it is auscultated; and VI/VI is so loud that it is heard with the stethoscope off the thorax and so intense that a thoracic thrill is present.
- The murmur is identified by when it occurs—in systole, diastole, or seamlessly through both of these physiologic periods

of the heart cycle (continuous). Murmurs are also described as being early, middle, or late (within systole or diastole) and are characterized by their musical quality or tone, such as high frequency, midrange, or low frequency. Although not always true, in some cardiac diseases the intensity of the murmur can correlate with the severity of the disease. Other cardiac diseases may not have a murmur, and the absence of a murmur does not rule out the presence of cardiac disease.

Etiology and Pathophysiology

- Systolic murmurs are associated with congenital conditions such as aortic stenosis, pulmonic stenosis, septal defects, atrioventricular valve dysplasia, tetralogy of Fallot, and other, less common congenital lesions.
- Acquired systolic murmurs are auscultated with mitral or tricuspid degenerative valvular heart disease (insufficiency), cardiomyopathies, anemia, fever, hyperthyroid disease, heartworm disease, endocarditis, and diastolic dysfunction syndromes.
- Diastolic murmurs in small-animal veterinary medicine are unusual but are associated with mitral stenosis, aortic valvular insufficiency, and pulmonic valvular insufficiency.
- Continuous murmurs are heard with PDA or atrioventricular vascular shunting lesions on the left thorax (PDA) or in the peripheral vascular system.

DIAGNOSIS

Diagnostic Overview

By definition, a heart murmur is detected during auscultation of the heart. Knowing the cause of the murmur is important for therapeutic and prognostic reasons, and the need for diagnostic testing is determined by the rest of the physical exam and discussion with the pet's owner regarding the advantages and drawbacks of performing such tests. A global approach to diagnosis and management is outlined on p. 1422.

Differential Diagnosis

Heart murmurs must be differentiated from breath sounds. In animals with particularly noisy breathing, respiratory distress, or anxiety, the breath sounds may be confused with heart murmurs because of the noise from the thorax or upper respiratory system during auscultation and physical exam.

Initial Database

Depends on the context in which the murmur is noted (see History, Chief Complaint above):

- Second opinion auscultation: to confirm or refute the presence of the murmur if unclear
- Thoracic radiographs: diagnostic test of choice for left-sided congestive heart failure (pulmonary edema)
  - Moderate and advanced states of heart disease can alter the shape and size of the cardiac silhouette in a way that is diagnostically useful.
  - Radiographs are very useful for establishing a baseline in dogs if myxomatous or degenerative mitral valve disease is the most likely cause of the murmur. Absence of cardiomegaly in these dogs suggests early disease and no justification for treatment (p. 658).
- Echocardiography: diagnostic test of choice for pinpointing the cardiac lesion responsible for the murmur
- CBC, serum chemistry panel, urinalysis, abdominal imaging: as indicated for possible concurrent systemic disorders
- Cardiac biomarkers (particularly NT-pro-BNP [p. 1369]): NT-pro-BNP level may have significance in correlating with the severity of cardiac disease. NT-pro-BNP testing may be useful to screen murmur significance in asymptomatic cats or for distinguishing respiratory signs caused by CHF from primary respiratory disease in the feline.

TREATMENT

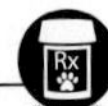

Treatment Overview

Treatment of heart murmurs is not an option. The veterinarian must first identify the murmur, then the cause of the murmur, and then make associations with the disease/condition present. A murmur does not mean the animal requires therapy. The intensity of the murmur usually is directly related to the severity of the disease; increased radiographic vertebral heart score together with a murmur is usually a good indication of the severity of the cardiac disease.

PROGNOSIS & OUTCOME

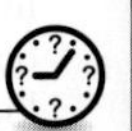

Highly variable depending on the underlying cause of the murmur. The prognosis of a patient with a heart murmur is influenced by the disorder causing the murmur, not by the murmur itself.

PEARLS & CONSIDERATIONS

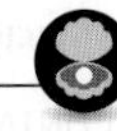

Comments

- For dogs that are panting, anxious, sniffing, or whining, closure of the mouth and intermittent occlusion of the dog's nostrils for 2-3 seconds at a time is useful for intermittently masking breath sounds that interfere with auscultation of the heart.
- For cats, the sound of running water or scruffing (lifting the skin of the nape of the neck) helps abolish purring.
- A systolic whoop is an uncommon but loud musical systolic murmur produced by resonance of the mitral valve. It may appear or disappear spontaneously and is not related to the presence or severity of any underlying heart problem, although further monitoring is indicated. Usually, dogs with systolic whoops ultimately develop murmurs associated with valvular heart disease over time.

Technician Tips

Optimal auscultation is done with the patient in a standing position. In recumbent patients, shifting of the heart may alter the perceived point of maximal intensity and alter intensity of the murmur.

SUGGESTED READING

Prosek R: Abnormal heart sounds and heart murmurs. In Ettinger SJ, et al, editors: Textbook of veterinary internal medicine, ed 8, St. Louis, 2017, Elsevier, pp 220-224.

AUTHOR: Stephen J. Ettinger, DVM, DACVIM
EDITOR: Meg M. Sleeper, VMD, DACVIM

Heartworm Disease, Cat

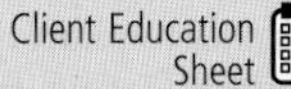

BASIC INFORMATION

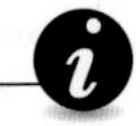

Definition

Heartworm disease (HWD) is the clinicopathologic manifestation of infestation with *Dirofilaria immitis*, an intravascular parasite that resides in the pulmonary arteries, the right side of the heart, and venae cavae. Infestation results in pneumonitis, pulmonary endarteritis, pulmonary thromboembolism (PTE), and uncommonly, pulmonary hypertension (PH) with/without cor pulmonale and rarely congestive heart failure (CHF).

Epidemiology

SPECIES, AGE, SEX

- Felids are atypical hosts for this canine parasite.
- There is no age predisposition.
- Male cats generally have an increased risk of exposure and have higher experimental infection rates and worm burdens than females.
- Prevalence of heartworm infection (HWI) in cats is estimated to be 5%-15% that of unprotected dogs in the same area.

RISK FACTORS

- Cats not receiving a heartworm preventive in endemic areas are at risk, with various individual risks determined by time spent outdoors, season of the year, and geographic location.
- Outdoor cats are predisposed, but indoor cats are also at risk (up to one-fourth of cats with HWI are reported to be indoor cats).
- Feline leukemia virus and feline immunodeficiency virus are not predisposing factors.

CONTAGION AND ZOONOSIS

Cats with mature HWI are rarely microfilaremic, and the likelihood of transmission to other cats, dogs, or humans is low (p. 418).

GEOGRAPHY AND SEASONALITY

- The prevalence of feline HWI correlates with that of dogs in the same geographic region (5%-15% that of dogs).
- Reported worldwide and is variously endemic in most parts of the United States
- Heartworm transmission is unlikely in regions or seasons where the ambient temperature does not average more than 65°F (>18°C) during a 30-day period.
- Prevalence: up to 14% in shelter cats and 9% in pet cats presented for cardiorespiratory signs (26% of these cats were heartworm antibody positive, indicating heartworm exposure and possible heartworm-associated respiratory disease [HARD]). In the United States, exposure rate is approximately 12%.
- Clinical signs associated with early infection typically occur in late fall and early winter.

ASSOCIATED DISORDERS

- Aberrant migration of larvae is thought to be more common in cats than in dogs (neurologic, dermatologic, ophthalmic, and peripheral thromboembolic complications).
- HARD: clinical (cough, wheeze, dyspnea) and pulmonary histopathologic findings associated with death of immature fifth-stage larvae in the pulmonary vasculature, with or without the presence of mature heartworms. Pulmonary thromboembolism may be due to dead worms (natural or pharmacologic death) or intravascular thrombi formed in response to the infection, resulting in vascular occlusion, rarely in infarction, and sometimes in acute respiratory death.
- Noncardiogenic pulmonary edema, often fulminant (sometimes with pulmonary thromboembolism), possibly represents acute respiratory distress syndrome (ARDS). This may result acutely after adult worm death or deterioration.
- Eosinophilic pneumonitis with cough, wheezing, dyspnea
- CHF (right-sided heart failure) is uncommon; signs include pleural effusion (hydrothorax or chylothorax) and/or ascites.
- *Wolbachia* sp: as for dogs (p. 418)

Clinical Presentation

DISEASE FORMS/SUBTYPES

- Clinical classification: 1) no clinical signs, 2) acute or peracute, and 3) chronic (most common)
- Most feline HWIs are occult infections, defined as an infection in which microfilariae are not detectable; microfilaremia in cats is uncommon (<20%), inconsistent, and transient.

HISTORY, CHIEF COMPLAINT

- About 28% of cats with HWI show no clinical signs of HWD.
- Chronic signs usually predominate (cough [38%]; dyspnea [48%], vomiting, anorexia, weight loss, lethargy, exercise intolerance, and rarely right-sided CHF).
- Acute signs include tachypnea/dyspnea secondary to PTE, severe pneumonitis, or ARDS. Sudden death in ≈10%.

PHYSICAL EXAM FINDINGS

- Usually nonspecific. There appears to be little correlation between the clinical signs, physical exam findings, and radiographic changes.
- Adventitial lung sounds may be heard.
- An audible heart murmur and/or gallop sound is uncommon, and CHF is rare. Jugular venous distention (often with pulsation), dyspnea, diminished lung sounds, and (rarely) ascites may be detected if CHF is present.

Etiology and Pathophysiology

- Female mosquitoes serve as intermediate hosts after feeding on microfilaremic dogs.
- Being an atypical host, cats have an inherent resistance.
  - Lower worm burdens (usually fewer than six, typically one to three)
  - Longer pre-patent period and shorter worm patency than in dogs
  - Higher frequency of amicrofilaremia or low microfilaria counts than in dogs
  - Shortened life span of adult heartworms (2-3 years, although some new information suggests that worms may live up to 4 years) compared with dogs
- Disease severity is determined in part by the number of adult heartworms and the host's response to live and dead, immature and mature heartworms.
  - Pulmonary response is more severe in cats compared with dogs. Clinical signs can be seen before maturation of the larvae (HARD)—or despite no worms reaching maturity (i.e., larvae are cleared)—and can be observed as early as 3 months after infection.
- Response of the pulmonary arteries, pulmonary parenchyma, airways, and air spaces
  - Eosinophilic infiltrates predominate.
  - Significant bronchointerstitial infiltrates decrease functional pulmonary volume.
  - Pulmonary arterial medial and intimal hypertrophy with or without thrombosis, often resulting in obliteration of the vascular lumen
  - Altered vascular permeability allows plasma leakage, producing noncardiogenic pulmonary edema (ARDS), which is typically fatal.
  - Chronic changes can result in diminished pulmonary function, hypoxemia, dyspnea, and cough.
- Acute or sudden death of affected cats is typically associated with adult worm death and resultant respiratory failure.
  - Lungs are considered to be the shock organ in cats.
  - Immune-mediated reaction to heartworm antigens produces bronchiolar and bronchial constriction, pulmonary congestion and interstitial edema, acute inflammatory interstitial disease, superficial pulmonary hemorrhage, and periarterial hemorrhage with subsequent fatal respiratory failure.
  - Heartworm embolism
    - Smaller feline pulmonary arterial tree with less collateral circulation is more susceptible to worm embolization with subsequent pulmonary infarction.
    - May contribute to episodes of dyspnea and/or sudden death

DIAGNOSIS

Diagnostic Overview

The diagnosis should be suspected when a cat in an endemic geographic area demonstrates signs of respiratory dysfunction or other systemic signs. Serum antibody and antigen testing, thoracic radiography, and echocardiography each may contribute to confirming the diagnosis, and the tests are selected in sequence depending on availability and cost.

Differential Diagnosis

- Cat with respiratory signs
  - Bronchitis or asthma
  - Lungworms (*Aelurostrongylus abstrusus*) and other nematodes (*Toxocara cati*)
  - *Paragonimus kellicotti* infection
  - Pleural effusions (pyothorax, hydrothorax, chylothorax, or neoplastic)
  - CHF due to cardiac disease
  - Neoplasia
  - Pneumonia (infectious or noninfectious)
  - Pneumothorax
- Cat with neurologic signs (brain or spinal cord)
  - Various inflammatory, ischemic, neoplastic, or degenerative diseases of central nervous system
- Cat with gastrointestinal (GI) signs, typically vomiting
  - Various systemic diseases such as neoplasia, hyperthyroidism, and renal failure or primary GI disease

Initial Database

- CBC, chemistry profile, urinalysis
  - Mild nonregenerative anemia or eosinophilia in about 33%
  - Basophilia is highly suggestive but rare.
  - Microalbuminuria and proteinuria secondary to glomerular disease possible
- Tracheal wash or bronchoalveolar lavage may contain eosinophils with or without the presence of peripheral eosinophilia (similar to allergic asthma or lungworms).
- Fecal exam for lung parasites (flotation, sedimentation, Baermann procedure)
- Imaging
  - Thoracic radiographs (findings depend on duration of infection and HWI severity).
    - Enlarged and sometimes tortuous, truncated caudal pulmonary arteries. Right heart enlargement, common in dogs, is unusual in cats.
    - Patchy mixed interstitial-alveolar pattern with perivascular infiltrates (primarily in caudal lung lobes)
    - Radiographic vascular findings may be transient.
    - Mimics asthma with bronchovascular pattern and possibly pulmonary hyperinflation (controversial)

Advanced or Confirmatory Testing

- The diagnosis of HWI/HWD in cats can be difficult and often requires an elevated index of suspicion and serial application of diagnostic tests.
- Microfilariae: most cats are amicrofilaremic. Filter and modified Knott's tests are preferred over wet direct blood smear. A positive result is uncommon but diagnostic.
- Heartworm antibody tests
  - Used in the detection of *exposure* to heartworms and possible HARD or mature HWI; does not prove ongoing infection
  - In addition to multiple send-off options, a point-of-care test is available (Solo Step, Heska, Loveland, CO).
  - Although used as a screening test, up to 14% of cats with mature HWI may be antibody negative. Approximately 2% of heartworm-infected, antibody-negative cats are heartworm antigen positive.
- Heartworm antigen tests (ELISA and immunochromatographic; assess for antigen elaborated by adult female heartworms) are specific, and some are semiquantitative. A positive result is diagnostic.
  - High number of false-negative results due to low female worm burdens, immature infections, and possibly immune complex (antigen-antibody) formation
  - A feline-specific antigen test has been marketed (adaptation of the canine test with reported 15% increase in sensitivity [IDEXX SNAP Feline Heartworm Antigen test, Westbrook, ME]).
  - Clinical signs can and often do occur *before* the presence of detectable heartworm antigen.
  - Heat treatment of serum dissociates immune complexes and appears to increase the sensitivity of antigen tests. Serum samples are heated to 103°C for 10 minutes, the resulting coagulum is centrifuged, and the supernatant is tested.
- Echocardiography (p. 1094)
  - Dilated pulmonary arteries
  - Parallel linear hyperechoic densities in pulmonary arteries, the right heart, and/or the venae cavae represent heartworms
  - Heartworms identified in 40% and 78% of naturally infected cats in two small studies
- Electrocardiography may demonstrate a right axis shift and/or atrial or ventricular arrhythmias in severe cases (uncommon).

TREATMENT

Treatment Overview

- Address complications.
- Prevent future infection.
- Aggressive adulticidal therapy is generally not recommended.
  - There is no role for melarsomine in cats.
  - A slow-kill approach has logic in that it protects from future infection and rids the cat of adult worms gradually.

Acute General Treatment

- Cats with HWD should receive HWI-preventive medication (see Chronic Treatment below); short-term corticosteroid therapy (prednisone 0.5-1 mg/kg PO q 24h) may be used for managing respiratory signs.
- Emergency therapy for acute dyspnea:
  - Oxygen therapy (oxygen cage at 40% O_2 or nasal insufflation at 50-100 mL/kg/min [p. 1146])
  - Cage rest
  - Corticosteroids (dexamethasone 0.125 to 0.5 mg IV or IM, repeat q 24h as necessary or prednisolone sodium phosphate or succinate 1 to 2 mg/kg IV q 24h)
  - Bronchodilator therapy (terbutaline 0.01 mg/kg SQ or IM, or aminophylline 2-5 mg/kg IV slow infusion over 30-60 min)
  - Antithrombotic therapy: aspirin (80 mg PO q 72h) is controversial. Clopidogrel recently was shown to be superior to aspirin as an antiplatelet agent in cats (18.75 mg/CAT PO q 24h).
- Worm extraction
  - Historically, mortality rates in one report (2 of 5 cats died) made this option unappealing, but the use of newer, less traumatic catheter devices such as micro-snare kits has proved successful in a small number of cases, likely due to reduced anaphylaxis from worm trauma.
- Microfilaricide therapy
  - No agent is currently approved by the U.S. Food and Drug Administration for the elimination of microfilaria.
  - The authors' recommendation for microfilaricidal therapy is to initiate macrolide prophylactic therapy at the time of diagnosis.

Chronic Treatment

Preventive therapy is a safe and effective option for the prevention of HWI in cats. Pretesting for antigen and/or microfilaria is considered unnecessary.

- Ivermectin (Heartgard for Cats): 25 mcg/kg PO monthly, *or*
- Selamectin (Revolution): 6-12 mg/kg topically monthly, *or*
- Imidacloprid-moxidectin (Advantage Multi): 10 mg/kg imidacloprid and 1 mg/kg moxidectin applied monthly

Chronic treatment of HWI:

- Continue one of the above preventatives
- Doxycycline 5 mg/kg PO q 12h × 4 weeks can be considered empirically. Precautions should be taken to avoid esophagitis.

CHF:

- As described on pp. 408 and 409.
- Sildenafil 1 mg/kg PO q 8h can be used empirically to reduce pulmonary hypertension.

Eosinophilic pneumonitis/HARD:

- Corticosteroids: prednisolone 0.5-1 mg/kg PO q 24h, tapering over 4 weeks; reinstitute as needed at lowest q 48h dosage that maintains the cat free of clinical signs
- For cats that can be tapered to alternate-day steroids, consider transition to fluticasone 110-220 mcg by metered-dose inhaler with spacer and face mask, 1 puff q 12h.
- Albuterol 90 mcg by metered-dose inhaler with spacer and face mask can be used at home in case of respiratory distress (1 puff every 30 minutes for up to 4 hours).

Possible Complications

Chronic corticosteroid therapy is diabetogenic in cats.

Recommended Monitoring

Every 6-12 months, if stable (perhaps only by telephone, if financial concerns)

PROGNOSIS & OUTCOME

- Fair for asymptomatic HWI
- Guarded for the remainder of non-CHF and non-ARDS patients
- Grave for ARDS
- Guarded for CHF; worm retrieval may help
- Overall, beyond day 1, the prognosis for cats with HWI is similar (median survival, 4.5 years) to that for hypertrophic cardiomyopathy (median survival, 6.5 years), which shares a median age at diagnosis of approximately 6 years.
- For most patients surviving the initial insult, median survival is much greater than 1 year. Acute decompensation and even death can occur, however, in any heartworm-infected cat, regardless of initial presentation.
- Studies suggest that some cats remain asymptomatic and self-cure, with the infection unrecognized.

PEARLS & CONSIDERATIONS

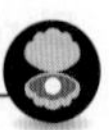

Comments

- Preventive therapy is indicated for cats in heartworm-endemic areas.
- Signs may be peracute, acute, chronic, or absent in cats with HWI.
- Most often, signs are respiratory.
- Consider HWI whenever feline bronchointerstitial disease is suspected.
- Cats that resist mature infection may still develop clinical signs produced by immature heartworms (HARD).
- Adulticide therapy is generally not recommended.
- Diagnosis may be difficult, requiring a high index of suspicion and multiple tests including antibody tests, antigen tests, thoracic radiography, and echocardiography.
- HWD is easily mistaken for feline asthma or lungworm infestations.

Technician Tips

Veterinary staff can help prevent HWI in cats by making sure that owners are aware that cats can contract this parasite and that definitive diagnosis and therapy are very difficult. Informative signs in the waiting or exam room(s) may be useful.

Client Education

- HWI is a preventable disease, and cats are susceptible.
- If dogs in the practice area receive a heartworm preventive, cats should also receive a heartworm preventive.
- Testing before initiation of macrocyclic lactone preventive is unnecessary in cats.
- Most preventives are broad-spectrum antiparasitic drugs.
- Importance of year-round preventives and yearly testing: issues of compliance

SUGGESTED READING

Atkins CE: Heartworm disease. In Ettinger SJ, et al, editors: Textbook of veterinary internal medicine, ed 8, St. Louis, 2017, Elsevier, 1316-1343.

AUTHORS: Keith Nelson Strickland, DVM, DACVIM; Marisa K. Ames, DVM, DACVIM
EDITOR: Meg M. Sleeper, VMD, DACVIM

Heartworm Disease, Dog

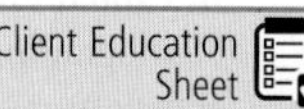

BASIC INFORMATION

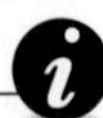

Definition

- Heartworm disease (HWD) is the clinicopathologic manifestation of infestation with *Dirofilaria immitis*, an intravascular parasite that resides in the pulmonary arteries and, less often, the right side of the heart and venae cavae. It results in pneumonitis, pulmonary endarteritis, pulmonary hypertension (PH), pulmonary thromboembolism (PTE), and/or cor pulmonale.
- An occult heartworm infection (HWI) is defined as an infection in which microfilariae are not detectable in blood.

Synonyms

Heartworm infection, dirofilariasis, dirofilariosis

Epidemiology

SPECIES, AGE, SEX

- Wild and domestic canids most commonly; lower prevalence in cats (p. 415)
- Most dogs are 3-6 years old when diagnosed although infection can occur at any age (uncommon in dogs < 1 year old).

GENETICS, BREED PREDISPOSITION

- Sporting breeds are predisposed.
- Caval syndrome occurs most commonly in spring and early summer in middle-aged males housed outdoors.

RISK FACTORS

- Lack of HWD-preventive drug administration in endemic areas. Dogs most often become infected in summer.
- Signalment and lifestyle: for example, male outdoor dogs are more likely to become infected than female indoor dogs due to vector exposure.

CONTAGION AND ZOONOSIS

Human infections are rare (typically with aberrant migration), not directly associated with a specific heartworm-infected pet, and usually innocuous.

GEOGRAPHY AND SEASONALITY

- Throughout the United States, especially within 150 miles of the Gulf of Mexico and Atlantic coastlines and along the Mississippi River and its tributaries
- Endemic in Australia, Japan, and some Mediterranean countries
- Heartworm transmission is unlikely in regions or seasons where the ambient temperature does not average more than 65°F (18°C) during a 30-day period.
- Prophylactic failures (often with presumed good client compliance) have been noted along the Mississippi River Delta. One explanation is macrolide resistance. Another explanation is occult lack of client compliance.

ASSOCIATED DISORDERS

- Aberrant migration of larvae can result in neurologic, dermatologic, and ophthalmic complications.
- Retrograde migration of part of the worm burden into the right atrium and cavae can result in heartworm caval syndrome (most common in highly endemic areas), a life-threatening complication involving entanglement of a worm mass in the tricuspid valve apparatus, causing intravascular hemolysis, an acute-onset murmur of tricuspid regurgitation, and signs of forward (hypoperfusion) and backward (congestive) heart failure.
- PTE may be due to dead worms (natural or pharmacologic death) or intravascular thrombi formed as a consequence of the infection.
- PH can occur secondary to pulmonary vascular disease and may result in congestive heart failure (CHF), hemoptysis, and exercise intolerance.
- CHF (due to PH or caval syndrome) with signs of right-sided heart failure (ascites and occasionally pleural effusion)
- Allergic pneumonitis (somewhat common) and eosinophilic granulomatosis (rare)
- Glomerulonephritis (virtually all dogs with HWI; typically mild)

Clinical Presentation

DISEASE FORMS/SUBTYPES

- Class 1: few or no overt clinical signs
- Class 2: moderate clinical signs
- Class 3: severe clinical signs
- Class 4: caval syndrome

HISTORY, CHIEF COMPLAINT

- Most dogs with HWI are in class 1 and show no clinical signs. HWI is detected as part of routine blood screening.
- When clinical signs exist, coughing is the most common complaint.
- Other complaints include exercise intolerance, weight loss, syncope or collapse, and manifestations of right-sided CHF induced by PH.
- Acute dyspnea secondary to PTE
- Chronic tachypnea/dyspnea due to PH

PHYSICAL EXAM FINDINGS

- Dogs without overt clinical signs evident to the owner usually have no abnormal physical exam findings.
- Spontaneous or inducible (tracheal palpation) cough possible
- A loud or split second (S_2) heart sound may be heard if PH is severe.

- Jugular venous distention (right heart failure) and pulsation with a right apical holosystolic murmur are indicative of tricuspid regurgitation due to chronic PH.
- Palpable fluid wave (ballottement) if abdominal distention (ascites) is noted.
- Discolored urine (hemoglobinuria), murmur of tricuspid regurgitation, tachypnea/dyspnea, collapse, and right-sided CHF and/or left-sided forward failure indicate caval syndrome.

Etiology and Pathophysiology

- Female mosquitoes serve as intermediate hosts after feeding on microfilaria-positive dogs.
- Microfilariae molt twice within the mosquito into L3 larvae and can infect another dog in 2-2.5 weeks during the warm months of summer.
- Patent infection (microfilaremia) occurs 6-7 months after inoculation of a susceptible host by infective (L3) larvae.
  - Occult (amicrofilaremic) infections exist during this prepatent period; other causes of occult infection include immune-mediated microfilarial destruction, unisex infections, acute high-dose or chronic macrolide prophylactic administration.
- Disease severity is determined in part by the duration of infection, number of adult heartworms, the host's response to live and dead heartworms, and amount of exercise. Some changes may be permanent.
- *Wolbachia* sp (an obligate intracellular, gram-negative bacterium) has a symbiotic relationship with *D. immitis* and possibly participates in the heartworm inflammatory response by releasing endotoxins and antigens associated with worm death.
  - *Wolbachia* spp are necessary for *D. immitis* reproduction.
  - Microfilariae produced in absence of *Wolbachia* sp do not become infective in the mosquito.
- Response of the pulmonary arteries
  - Damage from direct contact and other mechanisms (e.g., immune mediated, waste product release) to vessel intima
  - Villous proliferation of the intima and subintimal smooth muscle hypertrophy
  - PH: results from obstruction of blood flow (PTE) and reduced vascular compliance induced by endothelial and medial thickening and probably biological incompetence (failure of damaged vessels to respond to vasodilatory stimuli); results in dilated, often tortuous and truncated pulmonary arteries
- Response of the pulmonary parenchyma
  - Deposition of heartworm antigen in the microvasculature causes parenchymal immune/allergic reactions (periarterial edema and inflammation).
  - Corticosteroid-responsive allergic pneumonitis in 14% of HWIs
  - Severe chronic HWI causes irreversible pulmonary fibrosis with PH.
- Cardiac response
  - Right ventricular enlargement secondary to moderate-severe PH and subsequent tricuspid regurgitation and eventual myocardial failure
  - Right-sided CHF (ascites) in up to 50% of *severe* HWIs
- Systemic response
  - Renal: glomerulonephritis, proteinuria, infrequent hypoalbuminemia, and decreased antithrombin (increases pulmonary thromboembolic risk)

DIAGNOSIS

Diagnostic Overview

The diagnosis is made in one of two contexts: an incidental finding of a positive antigen test in an overtly healthy dog (more common) or overt clinical signs caused by infection-related secondary lesions. The antigen test is the confirmatory test of choice, and additional testing is indicated based on severity of physical signs and thoracic radiographic changes.

Differential Diagnosis

- Microfilaremia: *Acanthocheilonema* (formerly *Dipetalonema*) *reconditum* microfilariae are shorter, narrower, and have a blunted head compared with *D. immitis* microfilariae. *D. immitis* is < 6 microns in diameter (less than red blood cells [RBCs]), whereas *A. reconditum* is > 6 microns in diameter (approximately ≥ RBC diameter).
- Coughing: primary bronchointerstitial disease, collapsing trachea, infectious tracheobronchitis, pneumonia, left-sided CHF (p. 1209)
- PH: PTE (due to other causes); chronic pulmonary disease; cyanotic right-to-left shunting cardiac disease such as patent ductus arteriosus and ventricular septal defect with primary or secondary PH; and primary PH
- CHF (left sided [respiratory signs] or right sided [ascites or pleural effusion]): primary or secondary myocardial failure, chronic congenital or acquired valvular disease
- Pulmonary neoplasia (primary or metastatic), granulomatous or other infiltrative pulmonary disease

Initial Database

- CBC, serum biochemistry profile, urinalysis: eosinophilia and basophilia sometimes identified. Evidence of hemolysis and hemoglobinuria if class 4 (caval syndrome). Pathologic proteinuria common due to glomerulonephritis; may be reversible with treatment
- Electrocardiography (p. 1096) may demonstrate a right axis shift (prominent S waves in leads I, II, III, and V_3, indicating right ventricular enlargement) and/or atrial or ventricular arrhythmias in class 2 and 3 HWI.
- Thoracic radiographs (may be normal)
  - Dilated and sometimes tortuous, truncated pulmonary arteries
  - Patchy mixed interstitial-alveolar pattern with perivascular infiltrates demonstrated most frequently in caudal lung lobes
  - Right heart enlargement
  - Enlarged caudal vena cava if CHF is present or imminent
- Diagnostic workup may be abbreviated or even forgone if finances do not allow for young, clinically normal dogs, with attendant increases in risk. Workup may be even more detailed in instances of severe, complicated HWD.

Advanced or Confirmatory Testing

- Heartworm antigen tests (ELISA and immunochromatographic) are specific, sensitive, and some are semiquantitative.
  - False-negative results with low female worm burdens, immature infections, or rarely due to antigen-antibody complexes making antigen unavailable
    - Heat treatment of serum can improve sensitivity of ELISA test if false-negative suspected
  - False-positive results are rare but should be considered when positive results occur in areas of low heartworm incidence.
- Microfilaria: when used as a diagnostic test for HWI, filter and modified Knott's tests preferred over wet direct blood smear
  - Indicated to ascertain presence of microfilariae in dogs with HWI before institution of therapy; wet mount direct smear is adequate in this instance.
- Echocardiography (p. 1094) for moderate to severe HWI to assess PH and caval syndrome
  - Dilated pulmonary arteries
  - Parallel linear hyperechoic densities in pulmonary arteries (and sometimes the right heart and venae cavae) with large worm burdens
  - Right ventricular eccentric and concentric hypertrophy with flattened intraventricular septum in severe cases
  - High-velocity tricuspid regurgitation (TR) or pulmonic insufficiency on Doppler echocardiography with PH (TR Vmax > 3 m/s)

TREATMENT

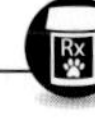

Treatment Overview

- Eliminate worm burden and microfilariae (if present).
  - Reduce risk of adverse events to adulticidal therapy.
- Address complications.
- Prevent future infection.

Acute General Treatment

Pulmonary thromboembolism:

- Oxygen therapy (oxygen cage at 40% O_2 or nasal insufflation at 50-100 mL/kg/min) (p. 1146)
- Cage rest
- Corticosteroids: prednisone 1 mg/kg PO q 24h for 7-10 days

- Antithrombotic therapy (aspirin or heparin) is not recommended. Caution should be used if corticosteroid and aspirin therapies are combined (not advised).

Allergic pneumonitis:
- Cage rest and corticosteroids (prednisone 1 mg/kg PO q 24h for 7-10 days)

Adulticide therapy:
- Melarsomine (immiticide)
  - Up to 98% efficacy after three doses; 50% of worm burden killed after a single dose
  - Plan A: melarsomine administered once at 2.5 mg/kg IM, followed by two injections at 2.5 mg/kg 24 hours apart, given 1-3 months later (authors' preference if owner finances allow)
  - Plan B: melarsomine administered as two 2.5 mg/kg IM injections given 24 hours apart
    - Plan A is the option recommended by the American Heartworm Society because Plan B results in reduced worm death (90% vs. 98%), and treatment success is generally less.
  - Strict adherence to manufacturer's instructions for intramuscular injection of arsenical agent
  - Consider corticosteroids (prednisone 1 mg/kg PO q 24h) or administration of a nonsteroidal antiinflammatory drug (NSAID) at manufacturer's recommended dosage at the time of IM injections to reduce injection-site inflammation.
  - Doxycycline 10 mg/kg PO q 12h should be administered for 1 month before the first treatment with melarsomine.
  - Exercise restriction for 4-6 weeks after melarsomine injections is extremely important.
- Macrolides as adulticides (i.e., slow kill)
  - Ivermectin and selamectin at preventive dosages have 40%-95% efficacy against young HWIs when administered continuously for 18 or 31 months, respectively. Moxidectin (Advantage Multi, Coraxis) also has adulticidal effects.
  - Milbemycin: modest adulticide activity
  - Pulmonary and vascular manifestations of HWI still result during macrolide adulticide therapy, especially if patient is active.
  - Ivermectin or moxidectam at preventive dosage with a 4-week course of doxycycline is reserved for cases in which financial constraints or concurrent medical problems prohibit melarsomine therapy. If this therapeutic approach is taken, perform a microfilarae test in 4 months to ensure that microfilariae are cleared.
  - Use of the two-dose method (plan B), eschewing pretreatment workup if necessary, is a better option than macrolide adulticidal therapy. In either instance, doxycycline therapy for 30 days before adulticidal therapy is recommended.

Worm embolectomy:
- Reserved for caval syndrome treatment
- Blind or fluoroscopically (or sonographically) guided surgical removal of heartworms from the venae cavae and right heart with alligator forceps, an endoscopic basket retrieval device, or loop snare device
- Avoid damaging the heartworms when extracting them because PTE and/or anaphylactoid reaction may result.

Microfilaricidal therapy:
- Current protocols using doxycycline with regular doses of macrocyclic lactones at preventative doses have essentially eliminated the need for post-adulticidal elimination of microfilariae. However, the clearance of microfilariae should be confirmed.
- Only imidacloprid-moxidectin (Advantage-Multi) is approved by the U.S. Food and Drug Administration for the elimination of microfilariae.
  - Milbemycin and imidacloprid-moxidectin are more rapidly microfilaricidal (adverse reactions in approximately 10% of cases) at the preventive dosage. Patients should be hospitalized, pre-treated, and observed for 8 hours for adverse reactions.
    - Shock, depression, hypothermia, and vomiting
    - Fluid and corticosteroid (dexamethasone 0.1-0.2 mg/kg IV) therapy, if severe
    - Diphenhydramine 2 mg/kg IM and dexamethasone 0.25 mg/kg IV may be administered prophylactically to prevent adverse reactions.

Chronic Treatment

- Preventive therapy
  - Prophylaxis should be administered in a timely manner (i.e., every 30 days or 6 months, depending on the product being used). Reliance on the concept of the so-called reachback effect is strongly discouraged. All are gradually microfilaricidal at preventive dosages except for milbemycin (rapidly microfilaricidal) and imidacloprid-moxidectin (approved as moderately rapid microfilaricide at preventive dosage).
  - Ivermectin/pyrantel (Heartgard Plus: ivermectin 6-12 mcg/kg, pyrantel 5 mg/kg PO monthly), *or*
  - Selamectin (Revolution): 6-12 mg/kg topically monthly, *or*
  - Milbemycin/spinosad (Trifexis: milbemycin 0.5-0.999 mg/kg, spinosad 30 mg/kg PO monthly), *or*
  - Moxidectin/imidacloprid topical (Advantage Multi; imidacloprid 10 mg/kg, moxidectin 2.5-6.8 mg/kg topical monthly) or moxidectin injectable (ProHeart 6 0.17 mg/kg SQ every 6 months)
    - Package insert states that injectable moxidectin should not be administered to heartworm-positive dogs.
- CHF (p. 409)
- PH (arterial) (p. 838)
  - Adulticidal therapy when deemed safe

Possible Complications

- Injection-site inflammation (adulticide)
- PTE

PROGNOSIS & OUTCOME

- Good in mild to moderate HWIs
- Fair to guarded in severe cases
- Poor to grave even with treatment in caval syndrome, severe PTE, and CHF

PEARLS & CONSIDERATIONS

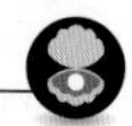

Comments

- Macrolide slow-kill adulticide method (using preventive drugs rather than melarsomine) does not prevent pathologic response and potentially permanent or life-threatening lesions from HWI. It also may contribute to the problem of resistance and is therefore not recommended unless melarsomine is contraindicated.
- Exercise restriction is an extremely important part of HWI therapy.
- Rarely, heartworm antigen testing may be negative due to antigen-antibody complex formation. If HWD is suspected despite negative antigen and microfilaria tests, commercial laboratories can heat treat serum for re-testing.
- The American Heartworm Society (www.heartwormsociety.org) is an excellent resource with up-to-date recommendations for diagnosis and treatment of HWD.

Technician Tip

Technicians play a key role in educating clients about the importance of heartworm prevention.

Client Education

- HWI is a preventable disease.
- Yearly testing is advised.
- For a client whose dog has just received adulticide treatment, provide a client education sheet: How to Care for a Dog After Heartworm Adulticide Treatment.
- Small pockets of resistance have been identified but are geographically restricted. All preventives are highly effective in the vast majority of instances.
- Most preventives are broad-spectrum antiparasitic drugs.
- Importance of year-round preventives
  - Adulticidal effect
  - Other parasiticidal effects
  - Reduced issues of compliance

SUGGESTED READING

Atkins CE: Canine and feline heartworm disease. In Ettinger SJ, et al, editors: Textbook of veterinary internal medicine, ed 8, Vol 1, St. Louis, 2017, Elsevier, pp 1316-1343.

AUTHORS: Keith Nelson Strickland, DVM, DACVIM; Marisa Ames, DVM, DACVIM
EDITOR: Meg M. Sleeper, VMD, DACVIM

Heat Stroke/Hyperthermia

BASIC INFORMATION

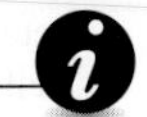

Definition

- Heat stroke is a life-threatening condition caused by extreme or prolonged hyperthermia.
- Hyperthermia is elevation of core body temperature.
- Hyperthermia can result from exposure to excessive environmental temperatures (i.e., nonexertional hyperthermia), excessive heat generation (i.e., caused by seizures, tremors, or exertion), or the inability to cool effectively (e.g., dogs with brachycephalic airway syndrome or laryngeal paralysis).
- Fever (increased temperature due to pyrogen exposure) is considered separately (p. 334).

Epidemiology

SPECIES, AGE, SEX

Dogs > cats; pediatric or geriatric animals are at higher risk.

GENETICS, BREED PREDISPOSITION

Increased likelihood:

- Brachycephalic dog breeds
- Obese patients
- Dark-colored and/or long-haired dogs exposed to direct sunlight

RISK FACTORS

Lack of acclimatization, poor access to shade or cool water

Excessive muscle activity:

- Status epilepticus
- Metaldehyde, permethrin, or garbage (mycotoxin) intoxication
- Hypocalcemic tetany

Excessive external heat/inadequate heat dissipation:

- Exposure to high ambient temperatures, including enclosure in small spaces such as clothes dryers or cars
  - Anxiety-related behaviors (e.g., pacing) associated with the realization of enclosure can worsen elevations in body temperature.
- Vigorous exercise
- Respiratory abnormalities (e.g., brachycephalic syndrome, laryngeal paralysis)
- Obesity

Other:

- Drugs such as phenothiazines, opioids (cats), inhalant anesthetics (malignant hyperthermia, most associated with halothane), amphetamines, serotonin syndrome
- Intoxications: macadamia nuts, hops
- Central nervous system lesions

GEOGRAPHY AND SEASONALITY

More common in early summer before heat acclimation occurs or on hot summer days (e.g., trapped in closed car)

ASSOCIATED DISORDERS

- Systemic inflammatory response syndrome (SIRS)
- Multiple organ dysfunction syndrome (MODS [p. 665])
- Disseminated intravascular coagulation (DIC [p. 269])

Clinical Presentation

HISTORY, CHIEF COMPLAINT

Although hyperthermia can be mild, heat stroke is a life-threatening emergency. Heat stroke is accompanied by changes in behavior and mentation (in contrast to simple hyperthermia or heat exhaustion).

- Hemodynamic and respiratory stabilization of the patient is a priority and may need to precede obtaining a complete history.
- Dogs generally present due to excessive panting or collapse or after being found overheated.
- Most commonly, animals present with a history of environmental exposure (e.g., outside on a hot day, left in a car) or recent strenuous physical activity (e.g., hunting, chasing, seizures).
- It is helpful to obtain information suggesting laryngeal paralysis (recent voice change, upper respiratory stridor), dysphagia, medications, or prior seizure history to identify underlying risk factors.

PHYSICAL EXAM FINDINGS

- Elevated rectal temperature
  - Heat stroke generally > 40°C (105.8°F); temperature at presentation may not reflect actual peak temperature if emergency cooling attempted by owner before arrival.
- Altered mental status
- Hyperemic mucous membranes
- Increased respiratory effort and loud upper airway sounds
- Petechiae
- Evidence of diarrhea and vomiting usually present

Etiology and Pathophysiology

- Elevation of core body temperature causes release of inflammatory cytokines, alters mitochondrial function, denatures proteins and enzymes, and leads to cell necrosis.
- Pulmonary: disruption of alveolar pneumocytes and pulmonary capillary beds leads to protein-rich fluid accumulation in the alveolar space, altering surfactant and inciting additional inflammation, which impairs gas exchange, increases shunt fraction, and reduces pulmonary compliance. This can lead to noncardiogenic pulmonary edema, severe hypoxemia, and acute respiratory distress syndrome (p. 27).
- Cardiovascular: hyperthermia, hypoperfusion, tachycardia, and acidosis result in ischemia and necrosis of cardiac myocytes and Purkinje fibers, leading to ventricular arrhythmias, conduction disturbances, and myocardial dysfunction.
- Hematologic: thermal injury of endothelial cells allows release of procoagulant factors, activates platelets, and activates complement and coagulation, causing a systemic inflammatory response and consumptive coagulopathy (e.g., DIC [p. 269]).
- Renal: acute kidney injury (AKI [p. 23]) results from direct thermal injury, microemboli, hypoxia, and hypoperfusion in addition to myoglobinuria caused by damaged muscles.
- Neurologic: excess inflammatory and endogenous cytokines and microemboli can result in cerebral edema and neuronal tissue death. Poor cerebral perfusion also contributes to these signs.
- Malignant hyperthermia is a rare heritable disorder involving rapid-onset hyperthermia, usually triggered by exposure to specific agents such as halothane or succinylcholine.

DIAGNOSIS

Diagnostic Overview

Heat stroke is easily recognized (markedly elevated body temperature, compatible history), and diagnostic efforts are aimed at identifying and monitoring secondary complications that occur in severe cases and an inciting cause if one is not evident from the history alone.

Differential Diagnosis

Fever, malignant hyperthermia (rare), exercise-induced collapse of Labrador retrievers (p. 192)

Initial Database

- Complete physical exam, including neurologic exam (p. 1136); obtundation is a negative prognostic indicator.
- CBC: common abnormalities include hemoconcentration (can be severe), circulating nucleated red blood cells (negative prognostic indicator) (68% of cases), thrombocytopenia (62% at admission, 83% during hospitalization), and neutrophilic leukocytosis (leukopenia sometimes identified).
- Serum biochemistry profile: elevated creatinine kinase activity from muscle damage, hypoglycemia (negative prognostic indicator) and elevated creatinine (negative prognostic indicator) concentrations (>50% of patients), increased liver enzymes
- Urinalysis: presence of urinary casts may indicate AKI, the presence of myoglobinuria may result in AKI if adequate diuresis is not established.
- Prothrombin time (PT) and activated partial thromboplastin time (aPTT) are frequently prolonged (negative prognostic indicators) in severely affected patients.

TREATMENT

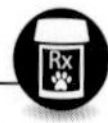

Treatment Overview

Mild hyperthermia requires no treatment beyond providing a cool environment. Heat stroke requires active cooling efforts, treatment of underlying disorders contributing to heat generation (e.g., control seizures in status epilepticus), aggressive supportive care, and careful monitoring for and management of complications such as DIC, AKI, sepsis, or cerebral edema.

Acute General Treatment

- For obtunded/comatose patients or those with upper airway obstruction, endotracheal intubation can improve gas exchange, facilitate oxygen supplementation (p. 1146), reduce the risk of aspiration pneumonia, and enable additional heat dissipation.
- Lukewarm (room temperature) intravenous (IV) fluids and cool water baths (avoid ice water, which causes peripheral vasoconstriction). Fans improve convective heat loss. Additional cooling techniques include infusion of the bladder with sterile, lukewarm fluid, or cold-water gastric lavage (using an orogastric tube in an endotracheally intubated patient), or enema.
- Active external cooling should be discontinued after the rectal temperature reaches 39.2°C-39.4°C (103°F-103.5°F) to reduce the risk of severe hypothermia. Rectal temperature monitoring is not reliable for patients who have received cool water enemas.
- Treat hypoglycemia (p. 552) if present.
- Mannitol 0.5-1 g/kg IV slowly over 15-20 minutes or 7% NaCl 1-3 mL/kg slow IV if increased intracranial pressure or cerebral edema is suspected.
- For seizures: diazepam 0.2-0.5 mg/kg IV, repeated up to 3 times; if ineffective, phenobarbital 2- 4 mg/kg IV q 30 minutes up to a total dose of 16 mg/kg or propofol continuous-rate infusion 2-6 mg/kg IV bolus, followed by 0.1-0.2 mg/kg/min. Some neurologists advocate levetiracetam (pp. 301 and 903).
- Ventricular arrhythmias (pp. 1033 and 1457) are treated if necessary.
- Fresh-frozen plasma (10-15 mL/kg) should be administered if coagulation times are prolonged and there is clinical evidence of bleeding (p. 1169).
- Broad-spectrum antibiotics such as cefazolin 22 mg/kg IV q 8h, enrofloxacin 5-20 mg/kg IV q 24h, maximum 5 mg/kg in cats, and metronidazole 10-15 mg/kg IV q 12h may be indicated because of venous pooling within the splanchnic circulation and risk for bacterial translocation.
- Gastrointestinal (GI) protectants such as pantoprazole 1 mg/kg, IV, q 12-24h; omeprazole (if no vomiting) 0.7 mg/kg PO q 12-24h DOG or 5 mg/CAT PO q 12-24h; sucralfate (if no vomiting) 250-1000 mg PO q 6-8h

Possible Complications

- DIC
- AKI (oliguria/anuria)
- GI sloughing/bacterial translocation/diarrhea/melena
- Acute hepatic injury
- MODS
- Cerebral edema/altered neurologic status
- Bone marrow dysfunction

Recommended Monitoring

- Frequent recheck of vital parameters until stable; serial neurologic evaluation
- Continuous electrocardiographic (ECG) monitoring for changes in heart rate or worsening arrhythmia (p. 1096)
- Blood pressure monitoring (goal: systolic > 100-120 mm Hg) and blood glucose assessment (goal: 80-140 mg/dL [4.4-7.8 mmol/L]) q 2-4h as clinically indicated) (p. 1065)
- Urine output (goal: > 1-2 mL/kg/h), serial rechecks of urinalysis, serum blood urea nitrogen (BUN) and creatinine
- Blood gas evaluation, as clinically indicated
- Recheck of coagulation times if initially prolonged or evidence of bleeding (pp. 433 and 1325)
- Recheck of platelet count

PROGNOSIS & OUTCOME

- The prognosis associated with heat stroke varies widely, depending on clinical severity at hospital admission. Animals recovering from heat stroke may be at increased risk for future heat stroke.
- Initial body temperature has NOT been correlated with outcome.
- The following have been associated with a poor prognosis:
  - Coagulopathy at admission (>150% prolonged PT or aPTT compared with the upper limit of the reference range)
  - Fibrinogen < 172 mg/dL or prolonged aPTT at 24 hours after presentation
  - Nucleated red blood cells > 18/100 white blood cells
  - Persistent hypoglycemia
  - Serum creatinine (>1.5 mg/dL [> 132.6 mmol/L]) after 24 hours
  - Seizures
  - Delayed admission
  - Obesity

PEARLS & CONSIDERATIONS

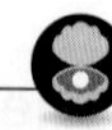

Comments

- Hyperthermia due to excitement or exercise does not require active cooling if the animal retains normal mentation and behavior.
- Self-cooling efforts (e.g., panting) cease with severe heat stroke; this should not confuse the diagnosis in an overheated animal with mentation changes suggesting heat stroke.
- Aggressive early cooling is warranted for heat stroke.
- Avoid overcorrection of body temperature and hypothermia.
- Multiple organ failure and DIC are common with heat stroke. The best chance of recovery involves 24-hour care with access to appropriate monitoring tools.

Prevention

Avoid exposing the animal to high ambient temperatures or prolonged physical activity.

Technician Tips

- Avoid jugular venipuncture until coagulation status can be ascertained.
- Avoid hypothermia by discontinuing active cooling when temperature reaches 39.2°C-39.4°C (103°F-103.5°F).
- Monitor for recurrent respiratory distress on extubation, particularly in animals with brachycephalic syndrome or laryngeal paralysis. Prolonged intubation, temporary tracheostomy (p. 1166), or definitive airway correction may be required.
- Placement of a urinary catheter and closed collection system enables frequent, accurate calculation of urine output and characterization of urine (color, turbidity).

Client Education

- Educate about the dangers of leaving pets in cars or prolonged exercise on hot days or if upper airway diseases exist.
- Clinical signs such as weakness and panting in hot weather may be an emergency; institute cooling measures, and consult a veterinarian.
- Dousing the animal with cool water before transport can initiate cooling in patients with heat-related illness (heat exhaustion or heat stroke).

SUGGESTED READING

Bruchim Y, et al: Heat stroke in dogs: a retrospective study of 54 cases (1999-2004) and analysis of risk factors for death. J Vet Intern Med 20(1):38-46, 2006.

AUTHOR: Geoff Heffner, DVM, DACVECC
EDITOR: Benjamin M. Brainard, VMD, DACVAA, DACVECC

Hemangiopericytoma

Client Education Sheet

BASIC INFORMATION

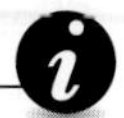

Definition

A common, locally invasive, slowly progressive tumor that occurs most commonly on the limbs; carries a fair to good prognosis with complete excision or incomplete excision combined with radiation therapy

Synonyms

Malignant schwannoma, neurofibrosarcoma, peripheral nerve sheath tumor

Epidemiology

SPECIES, AGE, SEX

Common in middle-aged to older dogs; rare in cats

GENETICS, BREED PREDISPOSITION

Large-breed dogs may be overrepresented.

Clinical Presentation

HISTORY, CHIEF COMPLAINT

Most animals are presented for evaluation of a progressively enlarging mass noticed by the owner. Pets with hemangiopericytoma in certain areas may be presented because of clinical signs related to the location of the tumor (e.g., limb tumors may result in lameness).

PHYSICAL EXAM FINDINGS

- Visible or palpable mass, more commonly on the limbs (any location on the limb)
- Mass is usually firm and fixed to underlying tissues. Occasionally, the mass can be hairless or ulcerated.
- Regional lymphadenopathy may be secondary to inflammation caused by the tumor or (rarely) lymph node metastasis.
- The remainder of the physical exam typically is unremarkable.

Etiology and Pathophysiology

- Hemangiopericytoma has some histologic features similar to the tumor of the same name in humans, but the actual cell of origin of this tumor is disputed.
- Hemangiopericytomas are spontaneously occurring in most cases in dogs.
- Disturbances caused by hemangiopericytomas depend on the location of the primary tumor and invasion into and destruction of surrounding normal structures.
- Hemangiopericytomas are typically slow growing and slow to metastasize. Over time, they can invade into surrounding soft-tissue structures.
- It is unclear whether hemangiopericytomas, schwannomas, and nerve sheath tumors are identical or related but distinct tumors. Immunohistochemical staining can differentiate some of these similar tumor types, but because they have similar biological behavior, differentiating the specific tumor type may not add useful information.

DIAGNOSIS

Diagnostic Overview

Definitive diagnosis can only be confirmed histopathologically, although additional tests such as diagnostic imaging (e.g., CT, MRI) are often helpful in defining the extent of the tumor.

Differential Diagnosis

- Other soft-tissue sarcomas
  - Fibrosarcoma
  - Malignant fibrous histiocytoma
  - Others
- Mast cell tumors
- Other skin and subcutaneous tumors (p. 628)
- Benign or non-neoplastic masses
  - Benign tumor (e.g., lipoma)
  - Abscess, granuloma
  - Elbow hygroma

Initial Database

- Fine-needle aspiration and cytologic evaluation may help identify the tumor type before other diagnostics
- Three-view thoracic radiographs to rule out pulmonary metastases
- Radiographs of the affected area may rarely reveal involvement of underlying bone.
- Fine-needle aspiration of draining lymph nodes helps rule out metastasis.

Advanced or Confirmatory Testing

- Biopsy and histopathologic evaluation of tissue is the diagnostic procedure of choice.
  - Biopsy is typically excisional, with removal of the entire tumor if possible or removal of the greatest feasible extent of the mass if not entirely resectable.
  - Incisional biopsy may be performed to obtain the diagnosis before treatment, especially when multiple treatment modalities may be necessary (e.g., preoperative radiation therapy).
  - Occasionally, special immunohistochemical stains may be necessary to differentiate hemangiopericytoma from other types of soft-tissue sarcomas, especially poorly differentiated tumors.
- CT or MRI may be necessary to delineate the local extent of the tumor and plan for surgery or radiation therapy.
- Histopathologic grade of the tumor is necessary for determining prognosis and treatment of most soft-tissue sarcomas (p. 927). Although most hemangiopericytomas are low to intermediate grade, high-grade tumors can occur and may be more likely to metastasize.

TREATMENT

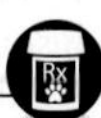

Treatment Overview

Definitive treatment is based on complete resection of the primary tumor whenever possible. Because metastasis is rare, additional treatment such as chemotherapy is rarely used but can be considered for high-grade tumors or tumors that have already metastasized. Palliative treatment options, such as palliative radiation therapy, may help control pain or discomfort in patients with advanced tumors or those for which definitive treatment is not an option. Palliative radiation therapy or metronomic chemotherapy (daily low doses of chemotherapy) may help control the local tumor for significant periods.

Acute and Chronic Treatment

- Aggressive surgical resection (aim: 3-cm gross margins but often not possible, especially on distal limb).
- Tumors that are incompletely resected or cannot be surgically resected (e.g., highly invasive or metastatic) may be treated with a combination of radiation therapy and surgery, which is associated with favorable long-term outcomes. Metronomic chemotherapy has been shown to slow progression of these tumors.
- Radiation therapy alone provides good long-term outcomes, although tumor control rates are higher with combined surgery and radiation therapy.
- Chemotherapy may be indicated for hemangiopericytomas that are high grade based on histologic features.

Possible Complications

Complications of treatment for hemangiopericytomas depend on types of treatments and location of primary tumor.

Recommended Monitoring

After appropriate local treatment of the primary tumor, routine follow-up exam is indicated to monitor for local recurrence and metastasis. High-grade tumors may require more frequent monitoring for metastases during and after chemotherapy administration.

- Dogs likely to develop metastasis (splenic tumors, high-grade tumors) should be monitored closely (q 2-3 months) with a physical exam, including lymph node palpation and thoracic radiographs.
- Dogs with low- or intermediate-grade tumors that have adequate treatment should have physical exams done q 2-3 months or more frequently, depending on risk of side effects from treatment. Thoracic radiographs can be done less frequently (6 months and 1 year after therapy).

PROGNOSIS & OUTCOME

Prognosis is excellent for most hemangiopericytomas with appropriate treatment. This includes complete surgical resection with clean histopathologic margins or incomplete resection combined with radiation therapy.

- Combined surgery with radiation therapy results in long-term tumor control in 86% of dogs with hemangiopericytoma. Median survival times for dogs treated this way are > 5 years, with 85% tumor free at 3 years.
- Radiation therapy alone has resulted in 1-year tumor control rates of up to 75% at higher doses. However, these studies used suboptimal radiation dose schedules. In certain situations in which surgery is not indicated, radiation therapy may be used for providing some degree of tumor control.
- Palliative radiation therapy after incomplete tumor excision resulted in tumor control in 65% of dogs with soft-tissue sarcomas at 5 years in one study.
- Metronomic chemotherapy using cyclophosphamide and piroxicam has been shown to result in tumor control for more than 400 days after incomplete tumor excision of soft-tissue sarcomas. Marginal tumor excision with intralesional chemotherapy beads can provide long-term control and may be considered as an alternative to radiation therapy for some cases.
- High-grade hemangiopericytoma is rare, and information is limited regarding prognosis.

PEARLS & CONSIDERATIONS

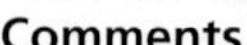

Comments

Despite uncertainty about the cell of origin for these tumors, hemangiopericytoma, peripheral nerve sheath tumor, schwannoma, and neurofibrosarcoma generally show the same biological behavior and should be treated in the same way.

Technician Tips

All masses in dogs and cats, even slow growing ones, should be aspirated to rule out malignant tumors.

Client Education

Pet owners can be educated to monitor their pets for the occurrence of masses under the skin and have the masses evaluated in a timely fashion. Early detection may allow easier treatment by surgery and may help avoid the need for radiation therapy.

SUGGESTED READING

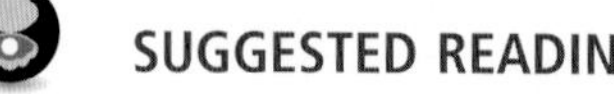

Liptak JM, et al: Soft tissue sarcomas. In Withrow SJ, et al, editors: Small animal clinical oncology, Philadelphia, 2013, Saunders, pp 356-380.

AUTHOR: **John Farrelly, DVM, MS, DACVIM, DACVR**
EDITOR: **Kenneth M. Rassnick, DVM, DACVIM**

Hemangiosarcoma

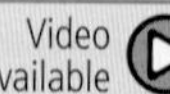

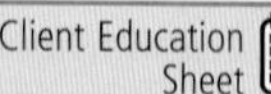

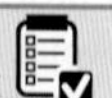

BASIC INFORMATION

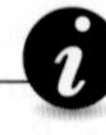

Definition

A malignant, highly metastatic tumor arising from vascular endothelial cells. Most commonly arises in the spleen, right auricle or right atrium, and skin or subcutaneous tissues.

Synonyms

Angiosarcoma, HSA, malignant hemangioendothelioma

Epidemiology

SPECIES, AGE, SEX

- Dogs: common
  - Cutaneous: adults, no sex predisposition
  - Noncutaneous: adults (median, 8 years), neutered animals may be at increased risk
- Cats: adults (median, 8 years), males > females; uncommon

GENETICS, BREED PREDISPOSITION

- Dogs
  - Cutaneous: no genetics known, although short-haired breeds are predisposed (e.g., whippets, pit bulls, Dalmatians)
  - Noncutaneous: genetic predisposition strongly suspected with evidence in golden retrievers (estimated 1 in 5 lifetime risk); German shepherds and other large breeds are overrepresented.
- Cats: specific breed predisposition known

RISK FACTORS

Dogs:

- Cutaneous: dermal hemangiosarcoma (HSA) arises on nonhaired skin and is associated with ultraviolet (UV) light exposure.
- Subcutaneous HSA arises in haired skin and is not associated with UV exposure.

ASSOCIATED DISORDERS

Dogs:

- Cutaneous
  - UV exposure may predispose to cutaneous hemangioma or squamous cell carcinoma.
- Noncutaneous
  - With splenic, hepatic, or right atrial/auricular appendage HSA, potentially life-threatening hemorrhage can occur. Occasionally, cutaneous or subcutaneous HSA lesions may be associated with significant bleeding.
  - Cardiac HSA is the most common reason for pericardial effusion. Pericardial effusion can result in potentially fatal cardiac tamponade.
  - Splenic, hepatic, and right atrial/auricular appendage HSA are associated with cardiac arrhythmias.
  - In any patient with HSA, disseminated intravascular coagulation (DIC) may arise because formation of abnormal (tumor-related) vascular channels triggers the coagulation cascade.

Clinical Presentation

DISEASE FORMS/SUBTYPES

Dogs:

- Cutaneous
  - Tends to arise on lightly haired areas (e.g., ventral abdomen). Tumors < 5 cm in diameter and confined to the dermis are classified as stage I. Tumors that are > 5 cm in diameter or invade subcutaneous or deeper tissues are classified as stage II.
- Noncutaneous
  - Splenic lesions are most common, followed by right atrial/auricular appendage. Primary HSA of the liver can occur, but most often, hepatic lesions are metastases from another site. HSA can arise anywhere.
  - Cardiac tamponade due to intrapericardial hemorrhage from the tumor site
  - Occasionally can be an incidental finding on physical exam (splenomegaly), abdominal ultrasound, or echocardiography

Cats:

- Subcutaneous and splenic lesions are most common, but HSA can arise anywhere in the body, including ocular structures, bone, gastrointestinal (GI) tract, and skin.

HISTORY, CHIEF COMPLAINT

Dogs:

- Cutaneous
  - History of extensive sunlight exposure; development of one or more cutaneous masses

- Noncutaneous
  - Often nonspecific complaints (e.g., mild exercise intolerance, mild decrease in appetite, weight loss) commonly attributed at first to old age, environmental change (weather) or other factors, but then culminating in subacute (days before presentation) or acute (hours before presentation) deterioration with lethargy, weakness, tachypnea, inappetence/anorexia, and/or abdominal distention
  - Acute onset of weakness or collapse is often mentioned and associated with tumor rupture and hemorrhage.
  - Collapse may be self-resolving by the time the patient is presented for veterinary attention, but physical signs of hemorrhage, abdominal mass, and/or arrhythmia persist.
  - Cardiac: overlap or combination of the following is possible:
    - Acute collapse with pallor; may have partially resolved over preceding hours or days
    - Vomiting is common (>50%) in dogs with pericardial effusion
    - General malaise, lethargy, anorexia, exercise intolerance
    - Visible abdominal distention

Cats:

- Cutaneous: bleeding from the mass in a patient that is otherwise well may be the chief complaint.
- Noncutaneous: typically, nonspecific signs such as inappetence/anorexia, weight loss, lethargy, and vomiting

PHYSICAL EXAM FINDINGS

Dogs:

- Cutaneous
  - Single or multiple cutaneous masses, typically on the ventral abdomen. Usually raised, hairless, smooth, and dark red, although they may also appear as polypoid, hairless lesions that are the same color as surrounding skin.
- Noncutaneous
  - Most often, findings are related to tumor rupture and hemorrhage into a body cavity. The most common physical findings include lethargy, pale mucous membranes, abdominal fluid wave, sinus tachycardia (reflex), and weak pulses.
  - A palpable intraabdominal mass is often present, and the masses should be palpated with great care to avoid further damaging fragile blood vessels on the surface of the neoplasm and inducing further hemorrhage.
  - Soft heart sounds, cardiac arrhythmia, and signs of circulatory failure may be present as a result of a ruptured abdominal HSA or a cardiac HSA and subsequent pericardial effusion, or both.
- In some cases, jugular distention, pulsus paradoxus, or positive hepatojugular reflux may be observed.

Cats:

- Cutaneous or subcutaneous lesions are typically readily identified on physical exam. Visceral disease is often evident on abdominal palpation. Other possible findings include pale mucous membranes and weak pulses.

Etiology and Pathophysiology

- Cutaneous HSA is associated with UV light exposure. Cutaneous HSA is less likely to metastasize and is not usually associated with underlying visceral disease/involvement; subcutaneous HSA may metastasize and may be a marker for underlying visceral disease/involvement.
- Malignant vascular endothelial cells form abnormal vascular channels.
- Microangiopathic disease (abnormal blood vessels in the neoplasm) results in platelet aggregation, erythrocyte morphology changes, and DIC.
- Tumor rupture leads to anemia, weakness, and inappetence/anorexia.
- Cardiac HSA is most often a right atrial/auricular infiltration of neoplastic cells that grow on the epicardial surface and ultimately cause rupture of superficial myocardial vessels of various sizes, triggering bleeding into the pericardial space. The result is cardiac tamponade when intrapericardial pressure exceeds right atrial and ventricular filling pressures.
- Metastatic disease occurs in the lungs, mesentery, and throughout the body.
- Death is often due to uncontrollable bleeding from tumor rupture.

DIAGNOSIS

Diagnostic Overview

HSA is typically first suspected when signs of hemodynamic compromise (most commonly due to hemoabdomen or cardiac tamponade) are associated with a mass lesion in an organ commonly affected by hemangiosarcoma. Less commonly, a mass may be found incidentally (e.g., on the skin, during routine abdominal palpation, during an abdominal ultrasound exam performed for another reason) or in the course of evaluation of a cardiac arrhythmia. Noninvasive tests do not confirm hemangiosarcoma, and a definitive diagnosis must be obtained through histopathologic exam of affected tissue.

Differential Diagnosis

Dogs:

- Cutaneous: hemangioma, soft-tissue sarcoma, mast cell tumor
- Splenic: splenic torsion, lymphoma, hemangioma, hematoma, extramedullary hematopoiesis, nodular regeneration, other sarcoma
- Hepatic: hepatocellular adenoma/adenocarcinoma, hematoma
- Cardiac: idiopathic benign pericardial effusion, other neoplasia (chemodectoma, mesothelioma, lymphoma), hemopericardium (atrial rupture, anticoagulant rodenticide intoxication), exudative/infectious pericarditis, congestive heart failure (right sided), peritoneopericardial diaphragmatic hernia, hydropericardium due to hypoalbuminemia, pericardial cysts, diseases that cause radiographic enlargement of the cardiac silhouette (e.g., dilated cardiomyopathy, severe atrioventricular endocardiosis/valvular heart disease)

Cats:

- Subcutaneous: abscess, other neoplasia such as injection-site sarcoma, fibrosarcoma
- Splenic: splenic mast cell tumor, lymphoma, nodular hyperplasia, other sarcoma

Initial Database

- Careful abdominal palpation, assessment for a fluid wave
- Auscult heart and check pulses (for quality and synchronicity); check for jugular pulse.
- Complete blood count, serum biochemistry profile, urinalysis, coagulation profile
  - Anemia (regenerative or nonregenerative, depending on acuity) and hypoproteinemia are common due to blood loss (e.g., abdominal hemorrhage)
  - Schistocytosis may occur as a result of microangiopathic damage of red blood cells traveling through abnormal vessels in the neoplasm.
  - Prolongation of prothrombin time (PT) and activated partial thromboplastin time (aPTT) may be secondary to aberrant procoagulant tissue factor expression on hemangiosarcoma tumor cells and DIC
- Thoracic and abdominal radiographs
  - Mass effect is commonly apparent on abdominal radiographs; detail may be obscured by abdominal effusion.
  - Pulmonary metastasis of HSA can involve hundreds to thousands of 1-2 mm nodules, which appear as pulmonary interstitial pattern.
  - Cardiac silhouette may be enlarged (globoid), indicating pericardial effusion, but lack of globoid cardiac silhouette does not rule out pericardial effusion.
  - Cardiac silhouette is rarely affected by presence of a mass lesion.
- Abdominal ultrasound if suspected splenic or hepatic involvement (abdominal effusion/distention, abdominal mass). Utility of ultrasound for patients with a palpable abdominal mass
  - Confirm presence of the mass, its organ of origin, and likelihood of resectability
  - Identify lesions suggesting metastasis
  - Identify abdominal fluid and guide needle abdominocentesis (if small volume)
  - Identify internal structure of mass, indicating feasibility of fine-needle aspiration/core biopsy (contraindicated if mixed echogenicity and high vascularity)
- Echocardiography (see *Video*)
  - Right atrial wall collapse (sail sign; the right atrial wall motion seen in pericardial tamponade resembles a sail flapping in the wind)

 - Diastolic collapse of right ventricular wall if severe tamponade
 - Tumor mass or blood clot from bleeding tumor may be seen bobbing in fluid adjacent to or involving a thickened (infiltrated) right atrial/auricular wall.
 - Diminished right atrium, right ventricle, left ventricle volume
 - Swinging motion of the heart within the anechoic pericardial fluid
 - Mass seen occasionally on/in the wall of the right atrium, especially at the right atrial/right ventricular junction or the right auricle; absence of mass does not exclude HSA because of limitations of imaging right auricle with routine (transthoracic) echocardiography.
 - Doppler evaluation of pulmonic flow shows large variation in beat-to-beat peak velocities.
- Electrocardiogram if an arrhythmia is found on physical exam and if splenic involvement, cardiac involvement, or recent hemorrhage is evident. Most common arrhythmias with cardiac HSA are ventricular arrhythmias, supraventricular tachycardia, atrioventricular block, and right bundle branch block.
- Fine-needle aspiration cytology of regional lymph node in patients with cutaneous HSA

Advanced or Confirmatory Testing

- Surgical biopsy for histopathologic evaluation is gold standard for diagnosis. With splenic HSA, the entire spleen should be submitted; some laboratories request it to be shipped chilled on ice (not frozen), whereas others request it be fixed in a 10 : 1 ratio of formalin/tumor for 24-48 hours, after which the fixed tissues can be sent to the laboratory in a small amount of formalin.
- Contrast ultrasonography may be helpful in assessing the nature of ultrasonographically identified splenic and hepatic nodules. Metastatic liver nodules have a hypoechoic appearance, in contrast to benign nodules, which are isoenhancing.
- Fine-needle aspiration cytology or cytologic evaluation of hemorrhagic fluids is rarely diagnostic. Aspiration cytology of visceral masses may result in hemorrhage and is not recommended in suspected noncutaneous HSA.

TREATMENT

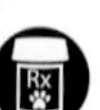

Treatment Overview

Therapeutic goals:

- Reduce tumor burden and prevent/minimize future hemorrhagic episodes.
- Relieve cardiac tamponade (palliative), if present.
- Control metastatic disease.
- Prolong survival.

Acute General Treatment

- Cutaneous (either species): surgery to remove tumor
- Noncutaneous (either species)
 - If evidence of recent or ongoing hemorrhage: IV fluids ± oxygen ± transfusion (p. 430)
 - Pericardiocentesis (p. 1150) if cardiac tamponade is present
 - Diuretics: contraindicated in acute pericardial effusion/cardiac tamponade

Chronic Treatment

- Cat and dog (cutaneous): surgery alone may be curative in most patients with dermal HSA. Margins should be at least 1-3 cm wide and one or more fascial planes deep.
- Cat and dog (noncutaneous and stage II cutaneous HSA)
 - Surgery to remove the tumor
 - Chemotherapy with a protocol of five doses of doxorubicin given every 3 weeks 30 mg/m^2 IV. Special handling requirements and potentially severe or life-threatening adverse patient effects exist with this chemotherapeutic drug; these concerns and rapid evolution of protocols warrant consultation with/referral to an oncologist.
 - Consider adjuvant radiation therapy for patients with incompletely excised subcutaneous stage II HSA.
 - Dog cardiac HSA: repeated pericardiocenteses or subtotal pericardectomy (usually performed after second event of tamponade). If possible, right auricular ablation ± chemotherapy (see Prognosis & Outcome below).
   - Yunnan Baiyao ± epsilon-aminocaproic acid have not been shown to 1) decrease the need for repeat pericardiocentesis or 2) prolong survival time in dogs with right atrial masses and pericardial effusion.

Possible Complications

- Disease complications
 - Metastasis, hemorrhage leading to hypovolemia and anemia, cardiac tamponade, DIC, death
- Chemotherapeutic complications
 - General chemotherapy toxicoses: myelosuppression, GI upset
 - Specific doxorubicin toxicoses: hypersensitivity during administration, perivascular sloughing with drug extravasation, cumulative myocardial toxicosis and heart failure (dogs), cumulative nephrotoxicosis (cats)

Recommended Monitoring

- Cat and dog (cutaneous): recheck physical exam every 3-4 months
- Cat and dog (noncutaneous): weekly complete blood count initially, thoracic radiographs every 1-2 months, abdominal ultrasound every 1-2 months
- Echocardiography 24 hours after pericardiocentesis; 1 week after pericardiocentesis, monthly thereafter

PROGNOSIS & OUTCOME

- Cat and dog (cutaneous): < 30% of patients with dermal (stage I) HSA develop metastases, and complete surgical excision is often curative.
- Dog and cat (noncutaneous and stage II cutaneous HSA)
 - Highly metastatic; with surgery alone, median survival is often 2-3 months. Despite occasional reports of several months' survival, survival to/beyond 1 year is very uncommon.
 - If all grossly detectable neoplastic tissue can be removed surgically, adjuvant chemotherapy may extend survival to a median time of 6 months.
 - If grossly apparent neoplastic tissue persists in postoperative period, median survival time approximates 2 months.
 - Adjuvant radiation therapy considered for patients with incompletely excised stage II cutaneous HSA, but there are limited data regarding benefit.
 - Right auricular ablation plus chemotherapy may prolong life (median survival for eight dogs with right auricular ablation alone: 42 days vs. eight other dogs with right auricular ablation plus chemotherapy: 175 days).

PEARLS & CONSIDERATIONS

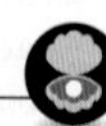

Comments

- Large size of a splenic mass as identified by exam or imaging does not imply greater chance of malignancy than smaller mass.
- Most often, HSA of the liver is due to metastatic disease because primary hepatic HSA is uncommon.
- Nodules of ectopic splenic tissue on the omentum and regenerative hepatic nodules are benign, dark red/brown tissue that must not be misinterpreted as HSA metastases during laparotomy in a patient with a splenic mass. Biopsy is advised to avoid misdiagnosis.
- Although rare in cats, this tumor has a similarly aggressive biological behavior.
- Fine-needle aspiration/cytologic evaluation and core biopsy are often unrewarding due to poor cellular yield and blood dilution, and both carry the real possibility of causing rupture of the tumor and potentially life-threatening hemorrhage. These procedures are therefore *contraindicated* for evaluation of masses when HSA is on the differential diagnosis list: masses of splenic, hepatic, renal, or cardiac origin that on ultrasound exam are of mixed echogenicity and may be highly vascularized based on color-flow Doppler assessment.
- Fine-needle aspiration and cytologic evaluation may be considered for evaluation of skin masses for which HSA is on the differential diagnosis list, but diagnostic yield is limited for the same reasons.

- Cutaneous HSA in dogs and cats has a less metastatic behavior, and surgical excision may be curative.
- In dogs with splenic HSA treated with chemotherapy, histologic grade (specifically, mitotic rate) may be associated with survival time. Further studies are warranted.
- Even with doxorubicin chemotherapy, reported survivals are short (median ≈6 months) in both species.
- The best chemotherapy protocol for the treatment of HSA remains unknown. Combining doxorubicin with cyclophosphamide is well tolerated and may provide longer survival times than doxorubicin alone. Adding vincristine to a doxorubicin and cyclophosphamide protocol is associated with more significant toxicosis than with doxorubicin and cyclophosphamide or doxorubicin alone.
- Alkylating agents such as lomustine and ifosfamide may prove to have activity against this disease; however, large studies documenting efficacy are lacking. Dogs treated with splenectomy, doxorubicin, and toceranib did not survive longer than dogs treated with splenectomy and doxorubicin.

Prevention

The development of cutaneous HSA is related to UV light exposure. Minimize sun exposure in animals with white or thin haircoats.

Technician Tips

Use safe chemotherapy practices (closed system).

Client Education

- Watch for recurrent signs associated with return of tamponade or other body cavity hemorrhage.
- Watch for signs of respiratory compromise associated with pulmonary metastasis.

SUGGESTED READING

Wendelburg KM, et al: Survival time of dogs with splenic hemangiosarcoma treated by splenectomy with or without adjuvant chemotherapy: 208 cases (2001-2012). J Am Vet Med Assoc 247:393-403, 2015.

AUTHOR: Ruthanne Chun, DVM, DACVIM
EDITOR: Kenneth M. Rassnick, DVM, DACVIM

Hematochezia

Client Education Sheet 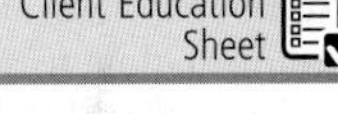

BASIC INFORMATION 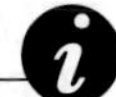

Definition

Frank, nondigested, bloody stool indicating bleeding from the lower gastrointestinal (GI) tract, such as the colon, rectum, anus, or anal sacs

Epidemiology

SPECIES, AGE, SEX

Depends on the cause

GENETICS, BREED PREDISPOSITION

Perianal fistulas: German shepherds

RISK FACTORS

Exposure to anticoagulant rodenticide or pathogens (e.g., parvovirus, pythiosis)

CONTAGION AND ZOONOSIS

Some causes have contagious or zoonotic potential (e.g., *Giardia*)

GEOGRAPHY AND SEASONALITY

Pythiosis most often identified in autumn; some infectious causes are geographically limited (e.g., histoplasmosis)

Clinical Presentation

DISEASE FORMS/SUBTYPES

Hematochezia may be due to disease of the distal GI tract or, less commonly, hemostatic disorders. GI disease may be primary (e.g., neoplasia, granulomatous colitis) or secondary (e.g., uremia, hypoadrenocorticism). Depending on specific cause, patients may present with chronic or stable disease (e.g., stress colitis, parasitism) or in an acute crisis (e.g., hemorrhagic diarrhea syndrome, mesenteric volvulus).

HISTORY, CHIEF COMPLAINT

- Colonic or rectal disease: may have tenesmus, frequent small-volume defecation, and mucoid or malodorous diarrhea
- Rectal or anal sac disease: may have a history of perineal licking and chewing, scooting, or painful defecation

PHYSICAL EXAM FINDINGS

- Confirm hematochezia and evaluate fecal consistency with digital rectal exam. Palpate for rectal masses, strictures, sublumbar lymphadenopathy, pain, thickened or roughened rectal mucosa, and anal sac disease. Inspect the perineal region visually.
  - Perianal fistulae, distal rectal mass/polyp, or ruptured anal sacs are often recognized by exam alone
- Patients with hematochezia induced by hemostatic disorders often bleed in additional locations (e.g., melena, petechiae, ecchymotic hemorrhages).

Etiology and Pathophysiology

Hematochezia is caused by a bleeding mucosal lesion in the distal GI tract or a hemostatic disorder.

DIAGNOSIS 

Diagnostic Overview

The history, physical exam findings, and initial diagnostic tests should provide clues about the cause of bleeding and guide additional diagnostic testing.

Differential Diagnosis

- GI tract causes include neoplasia, infectious organisms (e.g., *Histoplasma*, *Pythium*, *Prototheca*, *Tritrichomonas foetus*, *Giardia*, helminth infestations, parvovirus, circovirus, enteropathogenic bacterial infections), acute hemorrhagic diarrhea syndrome, granulomatous colitis, inflammatory bowel disease, pancreatitis, uremia, nonsteroidal antiinflammatory drug (NSAID) administration, hypoadrenocorticism, strictures, intussusceptions, perianal fistulas, stress colitis, ischemic or traumatic injury (e.g., heat stroke, volvulus), vascular malformations, and colorectal polyps.
- Hemostatic disorders (e.g., coagulopathies, thrombocytopenia) are less common.

Initial Database

Laboratory abnormalities depend on the cause and severity of bleeding.

- CBC
  - With acute bleeding, the CBC may be normal or a regenerative anemia may exist; reticulocyte count determines if anemia is regenerative.
  - Nonregenerative anemia and thrombocytosis suggests chronic GI bleeding.
  - Patients with acute hemorrhagic diarrhea syndrome may have an increased packed cell volume (PCV).
  - Severe thrombocytopenia (<30,000 platelets < 30,000/mcL platelets) may explain the cause of GI bleeding.
  - The total white blood cell count may be increased, normal, or decreased, depending on the underlying cause. A neutrophil count above 50,000/mcL should raise suspicion for infectious disease and/or GI perforation.
- Biochemical profile
  - Total protein may be at low end or below reference range. Animals with an infectious

or neoplastic cause of hematochezia may have a hyperglobulinemia.

- Centrifugation fecal flotation
  - Evaluate for helminths and *Giardia* cysts; empirical deworming is recommended if clinical suspicion exists.
- Activated partial thromboplastin time/prothrombin time
  - Performed as initial diagnostic test if clinical suspicion for hemostatic disorder exists.
- Abdominal radiographs/ultrasound: useful for identification of moderate to large colonic lesions unless in the pelvic canal
  - Thickened colon (inflammation, infection, neoplasia)
  - Lesions suggesting infection or neoplasia such as masses or lymphadenopathy
  - GI foreign bodies

Advanced or Confirmatory Testing

- Thoracic imaging: include in initial diagnostics if metastatic neoplasia or systemic infectious disease is suspected.
- Additional fecal testing, including fecal sedimentation, fecal wet mount, Baermann, and *Giardia* ELISA, should be considered to evaluate for GI parasites.
- Rectal scrape for cytologic interpretation may be useful if rectal mucosal abnormal on digital palpation (p. 1157).
- Specific infectious disease testing (e.g., *Histoplasma capsulatum* ELISA, enteropathogenic bacteria screening) recommended, depending on initial findings and the prevalence of enteropathogens in the practice area.
- Colonoscopy/proctoscopy can be used to identify and sample the source of GI bleeding.

TREATMENT

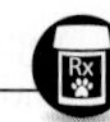

Treatment Overview

Successful treatment depends on the ability to identify and address the cause of bleeding.

Acute General Treatment

Treatment depends on suspected cause.

- Patients with severe blood loss or coagulopathies may need supportive measures such as intravenous fluids, blood transfusions, and correction of electrolyte disturbances.
- Sucralfate slurry or barium administered per rectum can be considered for patients with severe hematochezia, unless GI perforation is suspected.
- For stable animals with small amounts of blood, treatment with fenbendazole 50 mg/kg PO q 24h for 5 days may be attempted before more advanced diagnostic testing.

Chronic Treatment

Administration of iron dextran 5-10 mg/kg IM q 3-4 weeks may be indicated for patients with evidence of iron-deficiency anemia (e.g., microcytosis, nonregenerative anemia) from chronic blood loss.

Possible Complications

- If hematochezia is associated with GI ulceration, perforation and septic peritonitis are possible.
- Prolonged or severe hematochezia can cause severe blood-loss anemia necessitating blood transfusions.

Recommended Monitoring

Clinical signs of anemia (e.g., tachypnea, tachycardia, lethargy) and PCV/total solids (TS) monitored to assess severity of blood loss.

PROGNOSIS & OUTCOME

The prognosis for hematochezia is good if the underlying cause can be resolved. Other causes (e.g., metastatic neoplasia) may be life-threatening.

PEARLS & CONSIDERATIONS

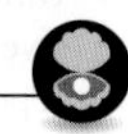

Comments

- Abdominal ultrasound can be excellent for identification of colonic masses except those in the pelvic canal.
- Distal rectal masses may be associated with additional masses orad, and colonoscopy is often warranted before removal.

Technician Tips

Advise clients to monitor for hematochezia when administering ulcerogenic drugs, platelet inhibitors, or anticoagulants to their pets.

SUGGESTED READING

Willard M: Hemorrhage (gastrointestinal). In Washabau R, et al, editors: Canine & feline gastroenterology, St. Louis, 2013, Saunders, pp 129-134.

RELATED CLIENT EDUCATION SHEETS

Consent to Perform Abdominal Ultrasound
Consent to Perform Endoscopy, Lower GI (Colonoscopy)
How to Collect a Fecal Sample

AUTHOR: M. Katherine Tolbert, DVM, PhD, DACVIM
EDITOR: Leah A. Cohn, DVM, PhD, DACVIM

Hematuria

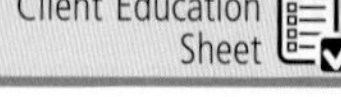

BASIC INFORMATION

Definition

The presence of blood (gross or microscopic) in the urine; encountered commonly in dogs and cats

Epidemiology

SPECIES, AGE, SEX

Dogs or cats of either sex and any age may develop hematuria for a variety of benign or pathologic reasons.

GENETICS, BREED PREDISPOSITION

Welsh corgi (renal telangiectasia), Abyssinian cats (glomerular disease), Scottish terrier (transitional cell carcinoma)

RISK FACTORS

- Acquired or hereditary bleeding disorders (e.g., rodenticide intoxication, thrombocytopenia, hemophilia)
- Upper or lower urinary tract trauma, neoplasia, infection, or inflammation
- Urolithiasis
- Renal insult (e.g., acute kidney injury, glomerulonephritis)
- Vascular malformation
- Urinary parasites (*Capillaria plica*, *Dioctophyma renale*)
- Cyclophosphamide administration
- Prostatitis
- Proestrus

CONTAGION AND ZOONOSIS

- Transmissible venereal tumor usually causes a mass effect but can cause hematuria.
- Some infections can result in thrombocytopenia and secondary hematuria.

Clinical Presentation

DISEASE FORMS/SUBTYPES

- Macroscopic hematuria: grossly discolored, bloody-appearing urine
- Microscopic hematuria: > 5 erythrocytes/high-power field without overt urine discoloration

HISTORY, CHIEF COMPLAINT

Gross hematuria may occur at initiation of urination, throughout urination, or at the end of urination.

- Initial hematuria: lower urinary tract or reproductive origin
- Total hematuria: origin anywhere along urinary/reproductive tract
- Terminal hematuria: upper urinary tract, bladder origin

Depending on causation, any of the following may be reported:

- Red, pink, or brown urine (macroscopic)
- Dysuria/stranguria (suggestive of lower urinary tract disorders)
- Pollakiuria (suggestive of lower urinary tract disorders)
- Bloody discharge from penis or vulva unassociated with urination (suggestive of genital origin)
- Abdominal pain
- Systemic signs (e.g., anorexia, vomiting) suggestive of upper urinary disorders, obstruction, or urinary tract rupture.

PHYSICAL EXAM FINDINGS

Depends on cause; findings may include

- Palpable renal/bladder/urethral mass
- Prostatomegaly
- Abdominal pain
- Bleeding unrelated to the urinary/genital tract (e.g., petechiae, ecchymoses, epistaxis), suggesting systemic bleeding disorder

Etiology and Pathophysiology

Causes of hematuria: p. 1229

- Primary (platelet) or secondary (coagulation factors) hemostatic defects or vasculitis may result in hematuria in the absence of urinary or reproductive disorders.
- Bleeding anywhere along the length of the urinary tract or from the reproductive tract may cause hematuria.
- A variety of inflammatory, infectious, neoplastic, traumatic, or toxic insults may result in hematuria. Traumatic cystocentesis can cause iatrogenic hematuria.
- Vascular malformations (e.g., telangiectasia) are a rare but important cause of marked hematuria.

DIAGNOSIS

Diagnostic Overview

In most cases, a presumptive diagnosis can be achieved on the basis of history, exam, urinalysis, and abdominal radiographs and/or ultrasound.

Differential Diagnosis

- Pigmenturia: p. 1216
- Hemoglobinuria
- Myoglobinuria

Initial Database

- History reviewed for drugs/toxins (e.g., cyclophosphamide, phenols) or iatrogenic procedures (e.g., cystocentesis) that may induce hematuria
  - If microscopic hematuria is observed after cystocentesis, later evaluation of a voided sample is warranted.
- If petechiae, ecchymosis, or bleeding from other sites is found on physical exam, evaluate coagulation.
- Rectal examination: prostate, intrapelvic urethra
- Digital vaginal exam/cytologic evaluation if vulvar bleeding
- Urinalysis: hematuria differentiated from hemoglobinuria, myoglobinuria, or pigmenturia (all of which discolor urine and may produce a positive blood result by urine dipstick) by presence of intact erythrocytes on microscopic exam (hematuria only)
  - Cystocentesis is avoided if coagulopathy, ascites, peritonitis, or neoplastic bladder disease is possible.
  - Urethral catheterization: detection of urethral calculi/mass, urine collection
  - Hematuria in samples obtained by catheterization or cystocentesis suggests origin is kidney(s), ureter(s), or bladder. Conversely, if red blood cells are absent from these samples but found in voided urine, source of bleeding is likely urethra or reproductive tract.
- CBC: thrombocytopenia suggests hemostatic defect; neutrophilia suggests upper urinary infection/inflammation; anemia may correlate to degree of blood loss.
- Serum biochemical profile: azotemia and hyperkalemia suggest renal disease or urinary obstruction/rupture.
- Urine culture is indicated if bacteria/pyuria detected.
- Abdominal radiographs: shape and size of kidneys, bladder, prostate evaluated. Radiopaque stones may be observed.
- Abdominal (urinary and genital) ultrasound: renal parenchyma, bladder wall and luminal content, prostate, uterus, and portions of ureters/urethra evaluated for masses/radiolucent stones.

Advanced or Confirmatory Testing

- If coagulopathy is suspected, platelet count, bleeding time, prothrombin time, activated partial thromboplastin time, and/or activated coagulation time indicated.
- Excretory urographic contrast studies (p. 1101) may delineate masses, stones, or tears in the urinary tract not previously identified.
- Cystoscopy (p. 1085) may identify source of bleeding from vagina, urethra, bladder, or either kidney/ureter.
- Diagnostic/traumatic catheterization when urethral/bladder mass detected allows cytologic evaluation
- Bladder tumor antigen test unreliable in the face of hematuria
- Consider biopsy of kidney, bladder, prostate, urethra as appropriate.

TREATMENT

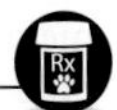

Treatment Overview

Treatment for hematuria depends entirely on the cause.

Acute and Chronic Treatment

- Coagulopathy is addressed directly.
- Traumatic injury may require supportive care alone or surgical intervention.
- Urinary calculi are treated by medical dissolution and/or mechanical removal, depending on type and location of stone.
- Urinary tract or reproductive infections are treated with appropriate antimicrobials.
- Neoplastic disease may require surgical intervention (e.g., unilateral renal carcinoma) or chemotherapy (e.g., transitional cell carcinoma).
- Drugs (e.g., cyclophosphamide, nonsteroidal antiinflammatory drugs) that might induce hematuria are disallowed.
- Rarely, renal hematuria may lead to blood loss sufficient to warrant transfusion.

Possible Complications

- Blood clots can lead to ureteral or urethral obstruction: rare.
- Anemia: rare

PROGNOSIS & OUTCOME

Depend on cause

PEARLS & CONSIDERATIONS

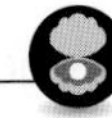

Comments

- Usually, hematuria is a sign of underlying disease rather than a primary disorder.
- Renal telangiectasia is an uncommon hereditary condition in Welsh corgi dogs, resulting in potentially profound renal bleeding due to vascular malformations. Diagnosis depends on biopsy, and organs other than the kidney may be involved.
- Benign essential hematuria is an uncommon disorder of young dogs in which no cause for profound, persistent hematuria can be identified. Often, it occurs unilaterally; interventional sclerotherapy or nephrectomy may be curative.

Technician Tips

Cystocentesis should not be performed on animals with hematuria until the clinician is reasonably certain that the animal 1) does not have a coagulopathy and 2) does not have a transitional cell carcinoma.

SUGGESTED READING

Francey T: Hematuria and other conditions causing discolored urine. In Ettinger SJ, et al, editors: Textbook of veterinary internal medicine, St. Louis, 2017, Elsevier, pp 190-193.

AUTHOR & EDITOR: Leah A. Cohn, DVM, PhD, DACVIM

Hemoabdomen

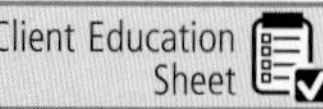

BASIC INFORMATION

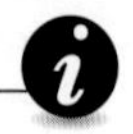

Definition

Hemoabdomen is characterized by the presence of free blood within the peritoneal cavity.

Synonym

Hemoperitoneum

Epidemiology

SPECIES, AGE, SEX

Dogs and cats of any age and either sex

GENETICS, BREED PREDISPOSITION

Young dogs are more likely to develop hemoabdomen secondary to trauma. Older, large-breed dogs without a history of trauma often develop hemoabdomen due to a ruptured splenic or hepatic mass such as hemangiosarcoma.

RISK FACTORS

Dogs that roam may ingest anticoagulant rodenticides or suffer trauma.

ASSOCIATED DISORDERS

Animals with intraabdominal hemangiosarcoma can develop pericardial effusion due to rupture of a concurrent right atrial hemangiosarcoma.

Clinical Presentation

HISTORY, CHIEF COMPLAINT

History can range from reports of acute collapse to mild lethargy. Some dogs are presented for evaluation of gastrointestinal signs such as vomiting or a distended abdomen. Many dogs have a history of weakness, collapse, or transient polyuria/polydipsia during the weeks before presentation. Presumptively, this indicates a prior episode of hemorrhage.

PHYSICAL EXAM FINDINGS

- Most physical exam findings are referable to blood loss and hemorrhagic shock and vary depending on the severity of shock. Animals may have pale mucous membranes, tachypnea, tachycardia, and weak or bounding pulses.
- An abdominal fluid wave may be detected.
- In some cases, a discrete abdominal mass may be palpable.
- Traumatic hemoabdomen may be supported by the presence of additional injuries.
- Coagulopathy is suggested by evidence of bleeding at other sites.

Etiology and Pathophysiology

- Hemoabdomen can be caused by trauma, rupture of diseased tissue/vessel, or coagulation disorders.
- In dogs without a history of trauma and a normal coagulation profile, hemangiosarcoma is the most likely cause, and the spleen is the most likely organ to bleed.
- Benign splenic hematomas account for a substantial proportion of canine splenic masses in general but comprise only 5%-10% of splenic masses seen in dogs with hemoabdomen.

DIAGNOSIS

Diagnostic Overview

The clinician should work to quickly rule in or rule out hemoabdomen (and/or pericardial effusion) in any middle-aged or older dog presenting with collapse and hypotension. Use of abdominal ultrasound provides the quickest diagnosis of free abdominal effusion and allows ultrasound-guided centesis.

Differential Diagnosis

Ascites (p. 79) or abdominal distention of another cause

Initial Database

- Packed cell volume (PCV) and serum total protein (TP); followed by CBC with manual platelet count. If bleeding is peracute, anemia may be mild or inapparent.
- Blood lactate concentration
- Coagulation testing (prothrombin time [PT], activated partial thromboplastin time [aPTT]): rule out coagulopathy as cause of hemoabdomen or as complication of disease (e.g., disseminated intravascular coagulation associated with hemangiosarcoma)
- Serum biochemical profile
- Abdominocentesis (p. 1056):
  - Nonclotting bloody effusion: if neoplasia or coagulopathy
  - Bloody effusion with clots: if trauma, or direct aspiration of an organ; rarely, with voluminous bleed from mass

Advanced or Confirmatory Testing

- Abdominal ultrasound may identify the source of hemorrhage in dogs with abdominal masses (p. 1102)
- Abdominal radiography may show mass effect, but effusion can obscure disease.
- Thoracic radiographs should be performed before surgery in dogs with an abdominal mass (to rule out metastasis).

TREATMENT

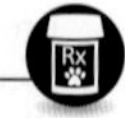

Treatment Overview

Dogs with hemoabdomen frequently present with hemorrhagic/hypovolemic shock. Once identified (poor pulse quality, cold extremities, mentation changes, very pale/white mucous membranes), obtain vascular access and begin fluid resuscitation with intravenous fluids and/or blood products as indicated. Initial treatment should be directed toward reversing cardiovascular instability. Further treatment should focus on preventing ongoing hemorrhage.

Acute General Treatment

- Intravenous fluids as indicated by the patient's cardiovascular status (p. 911)
- Blood transfusion (p. 1169) in patients with a PCV < 20%-25% that are hemodynamically unstable (e.g., concurrent hypotension, hemorrhagic shock, or rapid sustained ventricular arrhythmia)
  - Autotransfusion of the hemorrhagic effusion may be helpful for non-neoplastic, nonseptic hemoabdomen (e.g., coagulopathy, trauma).
- Patients with a coagulopathy should be treated with 15 mL/kg of fresh-frozen plasma, or 30 mL/kg of fresh whole blood if they are also anemic. Antifibrinolytic medications may be useful if hyperfibrinolysis is suspected (e.g., aminocaproic acid 50-100 mg/kg IV or PO q 8h).
- Emergent laparotomy is indicated in dogs with ongoing intraabdominal hemorrhage. Surgery should not be delayed to permit a dog to stabilize when the dominant concern is intraabdominal blood loss.
- Dogs with abdominal neoplasia benefit from surgical removal of the bleeding tumor although postoperative survival times may only range from weeks to months, depending on the nature of the neoplasm.
- Abdominal wrap to provide compression can be useful after an acute traumatic event resulting in hemoabdomen, but the animal's hemodynamic status and respiratory effort must be carefully monitored.

Chronic Treatment

Patients with neoplasia may benefit from chemotherapy.

Possible Complications

- Ongoing hemorrhage
- Some splenic or liver masses have metastasized by the time of laparotomy, and the masses may not be resectable.
- Severe ventricular arrhythmia may develop and may require antiarrhythmic therapy.

Recommended Monitoring

- Electrocardiographic (ECG) monitoring is indicated, especially in dogs with splenic disease, which are prone to ventricular arrhythmias.
- Frequent reassessment of the PCV and TP is warranted in the initial urgent setting.
- Recheck coagulation times after plasma transfusions.
- Specific long-term monitoring depends on cause.

PROGNOSIS & OUTCOME

- Prognosis depends on cause of hemoabdomen.
- Dogs with hemangiosarcoma have a poor prognosis, with an average survival of only

months with surgical treatment. Some dogs that stabilize without continued bleeding may be discharged home for palliative care.
- Dogs with splenic hematomas may be cured with splenectomy.
- Traumatic hemoabdomen or rodenticide-induced coagulopathy usually respond well to supportive nonsurgical management.

PEARLS & CONSIDERATIONS

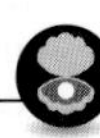

Comments

- In dogs with acute hemorrhage, the TP falls before the PCV falls.
- It is essential to submit large sections of spleen (preferably the entire spleen) for histopathologic analysis of splenic masses (p. 424).
- Benign splenic hematomas account for a large proportion of canine splenic masses, but only 5%-10% of the splenic masses in dogs with hemoabdomen.
- Hepatic fracture is an uncommon cause of hemoabdomen in cats with amyloidosis.

Prevention

- Keep pets confined or supervised to reduce the risk of trauma or intoxication.
- Any large-breed dog with collapse should be evaluated for possible hemoabdomen.
- IV catheter placement may be difficult in severe shock, and a cut-down or facilitated placement may be necessary.

SUGGESTED READING

Hammond TN, et al: Prevalence of hemangiosarcoma in anemic dogs with a splenic mass and hemoperitoneum requiring a transfusion: 71 cases (2003-2005). J Am Vet Med Assoc 232:553-558, 2008.

AUTHOR: Scott P. Shaw, DVM, DACVECC
EDITOR: Benjamin M. Brainard, VMD, DACVAA, DACVECC

Hemophilias and Other Hereditary Coagulation Factor Deficiencies

BASIC INFORMATION

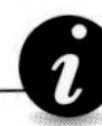

Definition

- Congenital hemostatic defects caused by mutations that impair the production of active clotting factors
- Hemophilia A, and factor XII deficiency in cats, are the most common of these conditions noted in general practice.
- *Bleeding diatheses* are defects causing failure of normal hemostatic processes (vs. bleeding due to defects in blood vessel integrity).
- Bleeding diatheses may be categorized as
  - Primary hemostatic defects (failure of platelet plug formation)
  - Secondary hemostatic defects, also called coagulopathies (failure of fibrin clot formation).
- Hemophilias and other factor deficiencies are classified as secondary hemostatic defects.

Synonyms

Specific defects are classified by the deficient factor. Alternate names in common use are shown below.

Hemophilias and Other Hereditary Coagulation-Factor Disorders

Deficient Factor	Alternate Name
Fibrinogen (factor I)	Dysfibrinogenemia, hypofibrinogenemia
Factor II	Prothrombin deficiency
Factor VII	Proconvertin or extrinsic factor deficiency
Factor VIII	Hemophilia A or classic hemophilia
Factor IX	Hemophilia B or Christmas disease
Factor X	Stuart-Prower deficiency
Factor XI	Hemophilia C
Factor XII	Hageman trait

Epidemiology

SPECIES, AGE, SEX

- Dogs and cats: severe bleeding disorders typically manifest by 6-12 months of age.
- Males almost exclusively affected in hemophilia A and B (factor VIII and factor IX deficiencies)
- Males and females equally affected in all other factor deficiencies

GENETICS, BREED PREDISPOSITION

- X-linked recessive inheritance pattern: hemophilias A and B
- Autosomal recessive (or incomplete dominant): all other factor deficiencies
- Breed predisposition
  - Dogs: hemophilia A, the most common hereditary coagulation defect, may develop in any purebred or mixed-breed dog. Mild to moderate forms of hemophilia A have been propagated in German shepherds and golden retrievers. Less common defects: factor VII deficiency in beagles, factor X deficiency in Jack Russell terriers, factor XI deficiency in Kerry blue terriers
  - Cats: hemophilia A and B occur in any breed and domestic cats. Factor XII deficiency is the most common hereditary factor deficiency in domestic and purebred cats. Combined deficiency of factors II, VII, IX, and X in Devon rex cats
  - Mutations causing factor deficiencies can arise in any breed.

Clinical Presentation

DISEASE FORMS/SUBTYPES

- Severe bleeding tendency: deficiencies of factors I, II, VIII, IX, and X
- Mild to moderate bleeding tendency: deficiencies of factors VII, XI, and some forms of factor VIII and IX deficiency
- No clinical signs: factor XII deficiency

HISTORY, CHIEF COMPLAINT

- Severe forms: spontaneous and recurrent hematomas, weakness, dyspnea from bleeding into body cavities, lameness from hemarthrosis, prolonged and potentially fatal bleeding from loss of deciduous teeth or minor wounds
- Mild forms: few spontaneous or severe bleeds, abnormal bleeding typically observed after surgical or traumatic injury

PHYSICAL EXAM FINDINGS

- Abnormal hemorrhage
  - Manifestations of hemorrhage into body cavities or potential spaces (hemarthrosis, hematoma, hemoabdomen, hemothorax, central nervous system hemorrhage)
  - Bleeding from traumatic/surgical wounds
  - Occasionally epistaxis or intraocular bleeds
  - In contrast to platelet disorders, factor deficiencies rarely cause petechiae or ecchymoses.
- Pallor (blood-loss anemia)

Etiology and Pathophysiology

- Specific factor deficiencies are caused by mutations in the corresponding coagulation factor genes.
- De novo mutations (mutations arising for the first time in a family member) occur most often in the factor VIII gene.
- Mutations causing mild to moderate clinical signs are more likely to become widely propagated in a breed or line.
- Although factor XII deficiency causes prolongation of the activated clotting time (ACT) and activated partial thromboplastin time (aPTT) coagulation screening tests, it does *not* cause a clinical bleeding tendency.

DIAGNOSIS

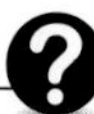

Diagnostic Overview

Relatively high prevalence of hemophilia warrants coagulation screening tests early in the diagnostic workup of males with spontaneous or unexpected hemorrhage.

Differential Diagnosis

- Acquired coagulation disorder (e.g., rodenticide intoxication, liver disease, disseminated intravascular coagulation)
- Thrombocytopenia
- Hereditary platelet function defect or von Willebrand disease
- Bleeding caused by tissue injury or infiltrative disorder
- Defect of fibrinolysis

Initial Database

- Thorough physical exam to define site(s) of hemorrhage. Hemorrhage from more than a single site suggests a hemostatic defect rather than blood loss from vessel injury.
- Baseline hematocrit and plasma protein
- Platelet count: usually normal unless prolonged hemorrhage (platelet loss)
- Point-of-care coagulation screening tests (*, markedly abnormal):
  - ACT: prolonged (factors I, II, VIII, IX, X, XI, and XII deficiencies) or normal (factor VII deficiency)
  - aPTT: prolonged (factors I, II, VIII, IX, X, XI*, and XII* deficiencies) or normal (factor VII deficiency)
  - Prothrombin time (PT): prolonged (factors I, II, VII, and X deficiencies) or normal (factors VIII, IX, XI, and XII deficiencies)
- Laboratory coagulation panel
  - aPTT, PT: as above
  - Fibrinogen: low (factor I deficiency), normal for others
  - Thrombin clotting time: prolonged (factor I deficiency), normal for others

Advanced or Confirmatory Testing

Definitive diagnosis based on identifying low levels of specific coagulation factors:

- Clottable fibrinogen (factor I)
- Coagulant activity assays (factors II through XII)

TREATMENT

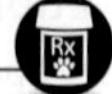

Treatment Overview

Patients with confirmed factor deficiencies but without clinical signs should receive a prophylactic transfusion before surgery. Patients with confirmed factor deficiencies who are actively bleeding may require repeated transfusions and, rarely, withdrawal of blood if compromising vital functions (e.g., large-volume pleural effusion). In both categories, avoid unnecessary surgery or invasive procedures.

Acute General Treatment

- Transfusion to supply hemostatic levels of the deficient factor (p. 1169)
  - Use of plasma components reduces risk of intravascular volume overload and red cell sensitization while maximizing factor replacement.
  - Fresh-frozen plasma (10-12 mL/kg IV):
    - Appropriate replacement therapy for deficiencies of fibrinogen and factors II through XI
  - Cryoprecipitate (unit dosage varies by supplier):
    - Replacement therapy for fibrinogen defects and factor VIII deficiency
  - Cryopoor plasma or cryosupernatant (10-12 mL/kg IV):
    - Replacement therapy for factors II, VII, IX, X, and XI deficiencies
- Replacement of red cells for severe blood-loss anemia
  - Fresh whole blood (12-20 mL/kg) or packed red cells (6-12 mL/kg)

Chronic Treatment

- Intermittent transfusion as needed to control hemorrhagic events
- Preoperative transfusion to prevent abnormal bleeding
- Avoidance of unnecessary invasive procedures

Behavior/Exercise

- Strenuous activity should be avoided to help limit intraarticular hemorrhage.
- Hemophilic cats should remain indoors; dogs should be supervised when outdoors.
- Owners must balance quality of life with reasonable exercise restriction.

Drug Interactions

Avoid drugs with anticoagulant or antiplatelet effects (e.g., nonsteroidal antiinflammatory drugs [NSAIDs], clopidogrel, sulfonamides, heparin, warfarin, plasma expanders, estrogens, cytotoxic drugs).

Possible Complications

- Red cell sensitization causing transfusion reactions
  - Transfuse plasma components when possible.
  - Feline transfusion: donor and recipient must be type matched for any transfusion.
  - Canine transfusion: perform crossmatch before second and subsequent transfusions.
- Development of inhibitory anti-factor antibodies (rare)

Recommended Monitoring

Confirmation of adequate factor replacement:

- Cessation of active bleeding
- Stabilization of hematocrit/plasma protein
- Resolution of lameness and hematoma

PROGNOSIS & OUTCOME

- Mild to moderate factor deficiencies: good quality of life possible; patient may require occasional transfusion.
- Severe factor deficiencies: fair to poor prognosis due to recurrent bleeding and dependence on repeated transfusion; acute fatal bleeds may occur.

PEARLS & CONSIDERATIONS

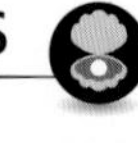

Comments

- Hemophilia A (factor VIII deficiency) is the primary rule out for abnormal bleeding in young male dogs and cats.
- Feline factor XII deficiency does not cause clinical bleeding; typically identified in workup for an acquired disease process.
- Platelet dysfunction is usually associated with petechiae or ecchymoses, while clotting factor dysfunction is associated with bleeding into spaces such as the abdomen, thorax, and joints.

Prevention

- Factor-deficient dogs and cats should never be used for breeding.
- Familial testing is indicated to identify asymptomatic carriers before breeding.

Technician Tips

- A blue-top tube (sodium citrate anticoagulant) must be adequately filled for coagulation screening tests.
- Avoid jugular venipuncture if abnormal hemostasis is apparent.

Client Education

Definitive diagnosis aids in determining prognosis, selecting appropriate transfusion therapy, and providing genetic counseling.

SUGGESTED READING

Cuoto CG: Disorders of hemostasis. In Cuoto CG, et al, editors: Small animal internal medicine, ed 5, St. Louis, 2014, Mosby, pp 1245-1247.

AUTHOR: Marjory B. Brooks, DVM, DACVIM
EDITOR: Jonathan E. Fogle, DVM, PhD, DACVIM

Hemorrhage

BASIC INFORMATION

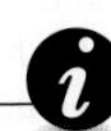

Definition

- The loss of blood from the vascular space into surrounding tissues or from body surfaces
- Clinical signs of hemorrhage result from one of two general mechanisms:
  - Blood loss from damaged or diseased blood vessels
  - Bleeding diatheses: defects causing failure of normal hemostatic processes

Epidemiology

SPECIES, AGE, SEX

Dogs and cats of all breeds and either sex may be affected, with specific predispositions depending on underlying cause. Blood vessel defects are acquired, whereas bleeding diatheses may be hereditary (e.g., von Willebrand disease) or acquired (e.g., coagulopathy of rodenticide poisoning).

GENETICS, BREED PREDISPOSITION

See chapters on hemophilias, von Willebrand disease, and platelet dysfunction (pp. 431 and 1043).

ASSOCIATED DISORDERS

- Blood vessel defects typically arise from
  - Traumatic or surgical injuries
  - Inflammatory or neoplastic conditions causing vessel erosion and infiltration
- Bleeding diatheses are classified as
  - Failure of platelet plug formation (primary hemostatic defects)
  - Failure of fibrin clot formation (secondary hemostatic defects = coagulopathies)
- Disease conditions such as hypertension, anemia, and hyperviscosity alter the normal flow properties of blood (hemorrheology) and are associated with microvascular hemorrhage.

Clinical Presentation

DISEASE FORMS/SUBTYPES

Subtype classification is based on

- Duration: acute versus chronic hemorrhage
- Location: focal or regional versus multiple anatomic sites
- Tissue or vessel involvement: capillary bleeding versus hemorrhage into joint space, body cavities
  - Primary hemostatic defects: failure of platelet plug formation (e.g., thrombocytopenia or platelet dysfunction) causes signs of hemorrhage involving capillaries and small vessels (arterioles, venules), clinically evident as petechiae, ecchymoses, bleeding from mucosal surfaces, and nonspecific bleeding from surgical and traumatic wounds
  - Secondary hemostatic defects: coagulopathies, failure of fibrin clot formation (e.g., coagulation factor deficiency) generally cause spontaneous hemorrhage into body cavities or potential spaces (i.e., pleural space or intramuscular tissue planes), resulting in hemothorax, hemoabdomen, hemarthrosis, hematoma formation, and nonspecific bleeding from surgical and traumatic wounds

HISTORY, CHIEF COMPLAINT

Depends on underlying cause. Frank hemorrhage, hematoma formation, and petechiae are obvious signs that prompt owners to seek veterinary care. Additional signs include pallor and collapse due to acute hemorrhagic shock or gradual onset of weakness due to chronic blood-loss anemia.

PHYSICAL EXAM FINDINGS

- Physical exam alone may differentiate vessel defects from systemic bleeding diatheses.
  - Frank hemorrhage due to traumatic or surgical blood vessel injury or vessel infiltration due to solid tumors or inflammatory mass lesions may be obvious on physical exam or by ancillary diagnostics (endoscopy, radiography).
  - Petechiae evident on cutaneous or mucosal surfaces or funduscopic exam indicate primary hemostatic defect.
  - Retinal hemorrhage and alterations of the normal retinal vasculature may result from abnormal blood flow (hemorrheologic defects such as systemic hypertension, hyperviscosity, anemia).
- Other signs are nonspecific (epistaxis, hematuria, melena, hematemesis, hemothorax, hemoabdomen).
- Hemorrhage from multiple anatomic sites and/or recurrent episodes suggest a bleeding diathesis rather than blood vessel defects.

Etiology and Pathophysiology

Bleeding diatheses:

- Acquired primary hemostatic defects
  - Thrombocytopenia is the most common bleeding diathesis.
  - Platelet dysfunction
- Hereditary primary hemostatic defects
  - Platelet dysfunction/thrombopathia
  - von Willebrand disease
- Acquired coagulopathies (secondary hemostatic defects)
  - Vitamin K deficiencies (anticoagulant rodenticide intoxication, biliary obstruction, chronic oral antibiotic administration, warfarin overdose, neonatal)
  - Hepatic synthetic failure (hepatic necrosis, atrophy, portosystemic shunts)
  - Consumptive coagulopathy (disseminated intravascular coagulation [DIC])
  - Acute coagulopathy of trauma/shock (hyperfibrinolytic coagulopathy)
  - Drug intoxications, envenomation, complication of heparin, hetastarch, dextran, fibrinolytic drug therapy
  - Dilutional coagulopathy: platelet and/or factor deficiency secondary to massive transfusion with stored blood products or high-volume fluid administration
- Hereditary coagulopathies (secondary hemostatic defects)
  - Hemophilia
  - Autosomal factor deficiencies
- Premature fibrinolysis (p. 435)
- Blood vessel defects: physical disruption (described above)

DIAGNOSIS

Diagnostic Overview

Vascular injury is by far the most common cause of hemorrhage. Begin with a thorough physical exam to identify a source of injury. If history and exam are inconsistent with injury, a prompt evaluation for hemostatic defects is warranted to avoid delays in treatment.

Differential Diagnosis

Blood vessel defect versus bleeding diathesis:

- Initial physical exam and imaging studies may define the site and cause of vessel defects.
- If a vessel defect cannot be defined on physical exam, blood pressure measurement and screening tests to rule out bleeding diatheses must be performed *before* performing invasive procedures.

Initial Database

- Thorough physical exam to define nature and location of hemorrhage
- Baseline hematocrit and plasma protein
- Platelet count (examine smear for platelet clumping; repeat sampling may be necessary)
- Blood pressure measurement (p. 1065)
  - Normal in calm setting, awake and resting patient, repeatable measures using Doppler: systolic < 180 mm Hg (dog, cat)
  - Hypertension and other cause(s) of hemorrhage may coexist.
- Coagulation screening tests: if evidence points to bleeding diathesis
  - Activated clotting time (ACT [p. 1300]):
    - Expected time to fibrin clot endpoint ≈120 seconds (dogs and cats)
    - Deficiencies of the intrinsic or common pathway factors cause prolongation of the ACT.
    - Normal in-house values should be established.
  - Activated partial thromboplastin time (aPTT [p. 1301])
    - The aPTT, like ACT, is sensitive to deficiencies of intrinsic or common pathway factors; however, aPTT is

generally a more specific and reproducible test than the ACT.
    - Long aPTT is seen in hereditary coagulopathies such as hemophilia and in combined factor deficiencies such as rodenticide intoxication and DIC.
    - Prolongation of aPTT to a target value of 1.5-2 times baseline is used for adjusting unfractionated heparin dosage.
    - Hemorrhage caused by blood vessel defects or primary hemostatic defects (platelet abnormalities) should not produce abnormal aPTT results.
  - Prothrombin time (PT [p. 1377])
    - Test is sensitive to deficiencies of extrinsic and common pathway factors.
    - Specific prolongation of PT is an indication of factor VII deficiency. Because factor VII is vitamin K dependent with short plasma half-life (3-6 hours), prolongation of PT develops in conditions causing vitamin K deficiency (e.g., anticoagulant rodenticide, severe hepatopathy).
    - The anticoagulant effect of warfarin and its dosage adjustments are based on prolongation of PT and its calculated derivative, the international normalized ratio (INR).
    - PIVKA (proteins induced by vitamin K absence or antagonism) testing performed using the Thrombotest assay and provides information equivalent to the PT.
    - The PT is usually normal with hemorrhage caused by blood vessel defects or primary hemostatic defects (platelet abnormalities).
  - Thrombin clotting time (TCT) and fibrinogen
    - Detect a lack of clottable fibrinogen
    - Long TCT and low fibrinogen develop in patients with severe hepatic insufficiency (due to synthetic failure) or dilutional coagulopathy and hemorrhagic DIC (due to depletion of fibrinogen).
    - Vitamin K deficiency does not prolong TCT or decrease fibrinogen values.
    - Hemorrhage caused by blood vessel defects or primary hemostatic defects (platelet abnormalities) should not produce abnormal TCT or fibrinogen results.
- Coagulopathies cause prolongation of one or more coagulation screening tests.
  - The pattern of abnormalities depends on which factor or groups of factors are deficient (p. 431).
  - Expected coagulation screening test results for common coagulopathies:
    - Vitamin K deficiencies: prolonged ACT, aPTT, and PT due to impaired activation of factors II, VII, IX, and X. Fibrinogen and TCT are normal.
    - Severe hepatic synthetic failure causes deficiencies of all factors and fibrinogen. ACT, aPTT, PT, and TCT are prolonged, and fibrinogen is low.
    - Hemorrhagic DIC typically results in depletion of all factors and fibrinogen. Mild to severe prolongation of clotting times and low fibrinogen levels accompany hemorrhagic DIC. In contrast, high fibrinogen level may accompany thrombotic DIC and other hypercoagulable syndromes.
    - Hemorrhage due to anticoagulant drug overdose or envenomation causes factor inhibition or fibrinogen depletion. All coagulation screening tests can detect severe drug overdose; however, aPTT and PT are preferentially sensitive to unfractionated heparin and warfarin levels, respectively.

Advanced or Confirmatory Testing

Based on results of initial database:

- Thrombocytopenia: rule out collection/laboratory artifact; may include bone marrow, spleen, and lymph node aspiration and cytologic review; serologic evaluation to detect evidence of pathogens; platelet-associated antibody testing
- Evaluation for platelet dysfunction
- Thromboelastography (TEG)
- Ancillary diagnostics to differentiate coagulopathies include specific coagulation factor analyses, determinations of antithrombin activity and fibrin breakdown products, and drug detection (i.e., heparin or warfarin levels).

TREATMENT

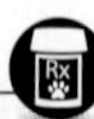

Treatment Overview

The two main goals are to control bleeding and stabilize the patient with one or more of the following: local wound care, supportive medical therapy, and/or transfusion therapy. It is important to collect pretreatment samples to perform screening and confirmatory tests. Additional information on treatment is available on p. 57.

Acute General Treatment

- Hemorrhagic/hypovolemic shock: volume replacement (intravenous fluid therapy [p. 911]), red cell replacement (p. 1169).
- Blood vessel injuries: control bleeding after visualization of the damaged vessels (physical exam, endoscopic exam, ultrasound exam, or surgical exploration).
- Bleeding diatheses: identify and correct the underlying cause of acquired bleeding diatheses; transfusion if needed to correct hereditary defects or pending response to medical management

Chronic Treatment

Depends on underlying cause of hemorrhage

Drug Interactions

Avoid drugs with anticoagulant or antiplatelet effects (e.g., nonsteroidal antiinflammatory drugs, clopidogrel, sulfonamides, heparin, warfarin, plasma expanders, estrogens, cytotoxic drugs).

HEMORRHAGE The coagulation cascade.

Possible Complications

- Uncontrolled hemorrhage and hemorrhagic shock are potentially fatal conditions.
- Chronic hemorrhage may result in iron-deficiency anemia, requiring iron supplementation for appropriate bone marrow response.

Recommended Monitoring

Resolution of hemorrhage is demonstrated by

- Cessation of bleeding
- Fading of petechiae, absence of development of new lesions
- Stabilization and normalization of hematocrit/plasma protein
- Correction of low platelet count and/or long clotting times

PROGNOSIS & OUTCOME

Depends on

- Initial stabilization and correction of hemorrhagic shock
- Ability to identify and correct vessel defect or cause of acquired bleeding diatheses
- Ability to diagnose and manage hereditary bleeding diatheses

PEARLS & CONSIDERATIONS

Comments

- Blood vessel injury or infiltration is by far the most common cause of hemorrhage.
- Screening for common bleeding diatheses by performing platelet count and ACT (or point-of-care aPTT and PT) is indicated early in the diagnostic workup of patients with hemorrhage.
- Anticoagulant rodenticide intoxication is a common acquired coagulopathy. Vitamin K therapy (vitamin K_1 2 mg/kg PO or SQ q 24h) and plasma transfusion (if severe hemorrhage) should be initiated pending results of coagulation screening, regardless of specific history of product ingestion (p. 69).
- Results of coagulation tests (PT, aPTT) that are below the normal range do not indicate hypercoagulability.

Technician Tips

Collect pre-treatment samples (1 EDTA and 1 citrate tube) before starting transfusion or vitamin K therapy.

SUGGESTED READING

Callan MB: Red blood cell transfusion in the dog and cat. In Weiss DJ, et al, editors: Schalm's Veterinary hematology, Ames, IA, 2010, Wiley-Blackwell, pp 738-743.

AUTHOR: Marjory B. Brooks, DVM, DACVIM
EDITOR: Jonathan E. Fogle, DVM, PhD, DACVIM

Hemorrhage, Postoperative, Sighthounds

BASIC INFORMATION

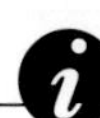

Definition

Local and systemic postoperative bleeding disorder that occurs in greyhound dogs 36-48 hours after surgery. Excessive bleeding may also occur after trauma.

Epidemiology

SPECIES, AGE, SEX

Any age or sex of greyhound dog may be affected after surgery or trauma.

GENETICS, BREED PREDISPOSITION

Greyhounds but may also occur in other sighthounds

Clinical Presentation

HISTORY, CHIEF COMPLAINT

Bruising or bleeding at site of surgery or trauma 36-48 hours after insult; may include hemoabdomen after laparotomy, including spay in females

PHYSICAL EXAM FINDINGS

Bruising at surgical site, bruising at venipuncture site, bleeding from surgical wound or tooth extraction, hemoabdomen, excessive bleeding at sites of trauma; rarely generalized petechiae and ecchymoses may develop.

Etiology and Pathophysiology

- Approximately 25%-30% of greyhounds develop postoperative bleeding 36-48 hours after routine gonadectomy.
  - After more invasive surgery (i.e., amputation), postoperative bleeding may occur in up to 66% of greyhounds.
  - Preoperatively, there are no significant differences between dogs who subsequently bleed and dogs who do not bleed in any of the following: platelet count, hematocrit, platelet function, von Willebrand factor (vWF), one-stage prothrombin time (OSPT), activated partial thromboplastin time (aPTT), fibrinogen (FIB), factor XIII, plasminogen, and D-dimer.
- Greyhounds with spontaneous bleeding also have normal platelet counts (for the breed), vWF, FIB, OSPT, and aPTT at the time of postoperative hemorrhage, making common bleeding disorders such as thrombocytopenia, platelet dysfunction, and clotting factor or vWF deficiencies unlikely causes of the bleeding.
  - Greyhounds with postoperative bleeding have altered thromboelastograph (TEG) values, including a smaller alpha angle and lower maximal amplitude (MA), indicative of hypocoagulability.
- The main hemostatic abnormality is the inability of the blood clot to strengthen postoperatively. Greyhounds that bleed have lower antiplasmin (AP) levels; AP is an important inhibitor of clot dissolution.
- Although there have been several studies of this disorder in retired racing greyhounds, it remains poorly understood in regard to cause and genetic influences.

DIAGNOSIS

Diagnostic Overview

Clinically, it can be a diagnosis of exclusion. Routine coagulation testing (OSPT, aPTT, platelet count) results are normal. There is no reliable test at present for preoperative diagnosis.

Differential Diagnosis

- Disseminated intravascular coagulation
- Immune-mediated thrombocytopenia
- Vasculitis
- von Willebrand disease

Initial Database

- Results of CBC (including platelet count) and serum biochemistry profile are normal in most patients.
  - Anemia and low plasma protein are possible with marked hemorrhage.
- Results of hemostasis assays are normal in most patients.

Advanced or Confirmatory Testing

- TEG may be helpful.
  - In normal individuals, the clot strength (MA) increases 24-48 hours after surgery from baseline as part of the reparative process. The relatively increased MA is within the reference interval for most patients. Affected bleeding greyhounds do not have an elevated MA.
  - Similarly, the alpha angle is increased 24-48 hours after surgery from baseline in normal dogs. A low alpha angle is supportive of the condition.

TREATMENT

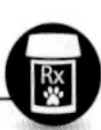

Treatment Overview

Prevention consists of perioperative administration of epsilon aminocaproic acid (EACA). In the absence of a confirmatory preoperative test, this treatment can be given to all greyhounds that are scheduled to undergo major surgery (e.g., laparotomy, castration, dental extraction, amputation).

Acute General Treatment

- EACA 500-1000 mg/GREYHOUND PO q 8h, starting the day of surgery and continuing for three days
  - This treatment protocol reduced the incidence of delayed postoperative bleeding from 30% to 10% after gonadectomy.
  - Alternative dose, 50-100 mg/kg PO, IV q 6-8h
- Fresh-frozen plasma is usually not necessary when using EACA, but it may be necessary in some cases.
- Blood products and supportive care if blood loss is extensive (very unlikely)
  - Management of postoperative bleeding, should it occur, is supportive (pp. 57 and 1169).
- Tranexamic acid 10 mg/kg IV bolus followed by 10 mg/kg/h IV constant-rate infusion over 3 hours is an alternative to EACA.
  - Published data on treatment efficacy are not available; it may induce vomiting.

Possible Complications

- Rarely can progress to disseminated bleeding associated with rhabdomyolysis and thrombocytopenia
- Hyperkalemia and azotemia can be associated with rhabdomyolysis.

Recommended Monitoring

Incisions should be monitored frequently for up to 3 days for the presence of excessive hemorrhage in all greyhound dogs.

PROGNOSIS & OUTCOME

- Excellent with treatment
- Greyhounds that bleed postoperatively are at risk for bleeding after subsequent surgeries.

PEARLS & CONSIDERATIONS

Comments

- Affected greyhounds bleed actively despite normal results on routine tests of hemostasis.
- This is not disseminated intravascular coagulation; there are no erythrocyte fragments or changes in hemostasis profiles.

Prevention

EACA 500-1000 mg/DOG PO q 8h, starting the day of surgery and continuing for 3 days

Technician Tips

- Look for bleeding/bruising around the surgical site as the earliest overt sign of this disorder.
- Help remind veterinarian to pretreat greyhound dogs before surgery.

SUGGESTED READING

Marin LM, et al: Epsilon aminocaproic acid for the prevention of delayed postoperative bleeding in retired racing greyhounds undergoing gonadectomy. Vet Surg 41:594-603, 2012.

AUTHOR: Jonathan Bach, DVM, DACVIM, DACVECC
EDITOR: Jonathan E. Fogle, DVM, PhD, DACVIM

Hemothorax

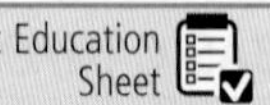

BASIC INFORMATION

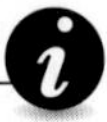

Definition

Any effusion within the pleural space with a hematocrit ≥ 25%-50% of peripheral blood. Hemorrhagic effusion is nonclotting except where hemorrhage is peracute.

Synonyms

Hemorrhagic pleural effusion, hemorrhagic pleuritis, hemorrhagic exudate

Epidemiology

SPECIES, AGE, SEX

Cats and dogs: age at presentation depends on cause:

- Young dogs: coagulopathy (e.g., anticoagulant rodenticide toxicity, inherited coagulopathy)
- Older dogs and cats: neoplastic (e.g., hemangiosarcoma, mesothelioma, pulmonary carcinoma)
- Young cats: mediastinal lymphoma (feline leukemia virus [FeLV] positive)

GENETICS, BREED PREDISPOSITION

- Dogs with congenital coagulopathies are predisposed.
- Siamese and oriental breeds (cats) with FeLV-related mediastinal lymphoma
- Lung lobe torsion (e.g., pugs; Afghan hounds; large-breed, deep-chested dogs)

RISK FACTORS

Common risk factors:

- Trauma (free-roaming animals at greater risk)
- Acquired coagulopathy (e.g., ingestion of anticoagulant rodenticides)
- Intrathoracic neoplasia
- Recent thoracic surgery

Less common risk factors:

- Thymic disease
- Lung lobe torsion
- Migrating foreign body
- Pulmonary abscess
- Fungal granuloma
- Congenital coagulopathy
- Pneumonia (e.g., canine influenza, *Streptococcus equi* subsp *zooepidemicus*)
- Parasitic disease (e.g., *Dirofilaria immitis, Angiostrongylus vasorum, Spirocerca lupi*)
- Diaphragmatic hernia
- Iatrogenic (e.g., central venous catheter placement, thoracentesis, pericardiocentesis)
- Ehlers-Danlos syndrome (cutaneous asthenia)
- Acute traumatic coagulopathy (ATC)
- Pleuritis

CONTAGION AND ZOONOSIS

- Canine influenza (p. 545)
- Feline leukemia virus (FeLV) (p. 329)

GEOGRAPHY AND SEASONALITY

- *A. vasorum*: prevalent in Europe and Newfoundland
- *S. lupi*: found in warmer climates with worldwide distribution

ASSOCIATED DISORDERS

- Anemia
- Respiratory distress (p. 879)
- Hypovolemic shock (p. 911)
- Primary or metastatic pulmonary neoplasia (p. 134)
- Pulmonary re-expansion injury

Clinical Presentation

DISEASE FORMS/SUBTYPES

Presentation and treatment are often specific to the underlying process. Anemia, weakness/collapse, and increased respiratory effort are common complaints.

HISTORY, CHIEF COMPLAINT

- Complaints due to pleural effusion (p. 791)
- Potential exposure to rodenticide/warfarin, a history of trauma, or prior thoracic surgery in some cases

PHYSICAL EXAM FINDINGS

- Respiratory distress (p. 879)
- Pleural effusion (p. 791)
- Hypovolemic shock (p. 911)
- Other injuries likely if due to trauma

Etiology and Pathophysiology

Hemothorax occurs as a result of a primary disease process. Determination of this cause is vital to appropriate therapy.

- Hemothorax (p. 1230)
- Trauma to the lung, heart, mediastinum, or great vessels
- Coagulopathic: hypocoagulable
  - *Toxic* (e.g., anticoagulant rodenticide toxicity)
  - *Acquired* (e.g., anticoagulants such as heparin, rivaroxaban), hepatic failure, disseminated intravascular coagulopathy (DIC), induced by anaphylaxis (e.g., heartworm disease)
  - *Congenital* (e.g., hyperfibrinolytic syndrome, hemophilia)
- Coagulopathic: hypercoagulable
  - Pulmonary thromboembolism (PTE)
- Neoplastic (primary or metastatic): pleural, mediastinal, pulmonary, ruptured abdominal neoplasm
- Infectious (e.g., viral, bacterial, parasitic, fungal) (see Risk Factors above)
- Iatrogenic (typically clotted blood with no erythrophagocytosis) (see Risk Factors above)
- Miscellaneous
  - Lung lobe torsion
  - Pancreatitis
  - Subpleural arteriovenous malformations
  - Aneurysms (aorta, pulmonary artery)
  - Pulmonary bulla rupture
  - Vascular rupture (Ehlers-Danlos syndrome)
  - Thymic brachial cyst
  - Thyroglossal cyst

DIAGNOSIS

Diagnostic Overview

Hemothorax is confirmed by thoracentesis with fluid analysis. After ensuring hemodynamic stability of the patient, evaluation can proceed and usually should include coagulation testing.

Differential Diagnosis

Pleural effusion (p. 791)

Initial Database

- Thoracic-focused assessment with sonographic evidence of trauma (TFAST [p. 1102]): hypoechoic fluid that may have a hyperechoic texture if highly cellular (similar to smoke appearance)
- Thoracocentesis (p. 1164): cage-side evaluation
  - Spun packed cell volume (PCV) > 25% of the animal's peripheral blood PCV
  - Unless peracute, effusion does not clot
  - Peracute hemorrhage (<1 hour) is very similar to peripheral blood
- CBC or initial peripheral blood PCV and total solids (TS)
  - May be normal in peracute period, followed by anemia
  - Total solids below reference range
  - Thrombocytopenia possible, depending on cause of hemothorax
- Blood pressure (p. 1065): if compensated, may be normotensive or could be hypotensive with massive hemorrhage
- Arterial blood gas (p. 1058): metabolic/lactic acidosis, hypoxemia, elevated alveolar to arterial gradient
- Coagulation testing (p. 1325): if hypocoagulable, expect
  - Prothrombin/partial thromboplastin time (PT/aPTT): prolonged (PT before aPTT if rodenticide intoxication)
  - Activated clotting time (ACT): prolonged with severe depletion of clotting factors
  - Thromboelastography (TEG): prolonged R time +/− smaller maximal amplitude (MA) with thrombocytopenia +/− normal to larger MA with anemia, hyperfibrinolysis with trauma/disseminated intravascular coagulation

Advanced or Confirmatory Testing

- Fluid analysis with cell count/cytology (p. 1343): erythrophagocytosis, no platelets +/− clumping of neoplastic cells +/− pink supernatant if spun down (hemolysis)
- Thoracic radiographs (preferably after therapeutic thoracocentesis): loss of detail due to remaining effusion, interstitial to alveolar pattern consistent with parenchymal hemorrhage +/− mass effect (pulmonary, mediastinal), depending on cause
- CT and thoracic ultrasound: if trauma and coagulopathy have been ruled out, necessary in 90% cases to confirm suspicion of neoplasia
  - If mass present, consider aspiration/biopsy (p. 1113)
- Anticoagulant rodenticide screening (spectrophotometry) to confirm rodenticide coagulopathy (rarely performed)

TREATMENT

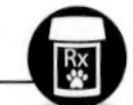

Treatment Overview

The therapeutic steps highly depend on the cause of hemothorax but generally include blood products, therapeutic thoracocentesis, and definitive therapy for the primary condition.

Acute General Treatment

- For every patient, immediately: oxygen supplementation (p. 1146), obtain intravenous access, and begin fluid resuscitation (if hypotensive [p. 911])
- If coagulopathic, administer frozen plasma (15 mL/kg IV over 4 hours)
- Thoracocentesis to remove enough volume to ease respiration (after any coagulopathy is addressed)
  - Not necessary or beneficial to remove all effusion
  - Generally, removal of 10 mL/kg adequate to improve clinical signs
- If anemic, administer blood products (p. 1169).
- Packed red blood cells (RBCs) or whole blood typical
- Unless due to neoplastic cause, autotransfusion allows RBCs in hemorrhagic fluid removed from the chest to be returned (through a blood filter) to the patient's peripheral circulation.

Chronic Treatment

After initial stabilization, further therapy and monitoring may be necessary.

- Serial TFAST scans to evaluate for recurrent/ongoing hemorrhage
  - If continued hemorrhage, may need to consider chest tube placement
- In anticoagulant rodenticide patients, vitamin K_1 2.5 mg/kg PO q 12h (p. 69)
- Refractory traumatic hemothorax
  - Evaluate for hyperfibrinolytic ATC with TEG and subsequent antifibrinolytic therapy (e.g., aminocaproic acid 50-100 mg/kg PO q 8h for 5 days) if present
  - If cannot identify underlying source of hemorrhage, may require thoracic exploratory surgery
- Neoplasia: palliative or definitive therapy, depending on type and location
- If patient has retained blood clots, consider fibrinolytic agent administration (humans).

Behavior/Exercise

The patient should be kept calm until definitive therapy is instituted. Gentle patient handling is necessary to minimize further hemorrhage.

Possible Complications

Numerous complications noted in human literature: retention of blood clots in the pleural space, pyothorax/empyema (1%-4% overall, 26.8% traumatic cases [humans]), and fibrothorax. Hemorrhage can recur/progress or may not be able to be removed safely.

Recommended Monitoring

Serially monitor heart and respiratory rates, respiratory effort as well as blood pressure, PCV, and TS. If tolerated, monitor pulse oximetry and/or arterial oxygenation. Serial TFAST exams are recommended to evaluate for recurrence or progression of hemorrhage.

PROGNOSIS & OUTCOME

- Highly depends on the underlying cause of hemothorax, with the best prognosis associated with rodenticide anticoagulant intoxication (98.6% survival) and self-limited or correctable causes of traumatic hemothorax.
- Prognosis for infectious causes depends on the response to supportive care and treatment of particular pathogen.
- Prognosis for neoplastic causes of hemothorax depends on the type of neoplasia: that for solitary primary pulmonary neoplasia amenable to surgery can be good with follow-up chemotherapy; mediastinal lymphoma cases have short survival times (days to months); and metastatic neoplasia/carcinomatosis

cases have poor to grave prognosis after a spontaneous hemorrhage occurs.

PEARLS & CONSIDERATIONS

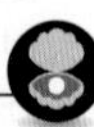

Comments

- For animal with cavitary bleeding due to anticoagulant rodenticide toxicity, quick administration of plasma is key.
- Therapeutic thoracocentesis is important for stabilizing a patient in respiratory distress; however, if the patient is coagulopathic, thoracocentesis can worsen bleeding. Treatment with plasma before thoracocentesis in these patients is usually appropriate.
- Attempts to remove all effusion can be harmful; remove only enough to improve respiration.

Prevention

- Prevent exposure to anticoagulant rodenticides.
- Do not allow animals to freely roam to reduce risk of trauma.
- Vaccinate cats in the household to minimize the exposure of other housemates to FeLV.
- Maintain year-round prevention against *D. immitis* in dogs and cats, and minimize stagnant water in their environment.

Technician Tips

- Gentle handling is necessary to minimize the risk of bleeding. Sternal recumbency can facilitate full lung expansion and minimize atelectasis.
- Hemorrhagic effusion can recur and become imminently life-threatening. Close monitoring of these patients is essential.
- Rechecking the PCV/TS in the fluid removed by means of a chest tube can provide valuable information on progress.

SUGGESTED READINGS

Nakamura RK, et al: Non-coagulopathic spontaneous hemothorax in dogs. J Vet Emerg Critical Care 18:292-297, 2008.

AUTHOR: H. Nicole Trenholme, DVM
EDITOR: Meghan Grobman, DVM, MS, DACVIM

Hemotropic Mycoplasmosis, Cat

BASIC INFORMATION

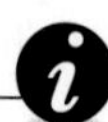

Definition

Hemotropic mycoplasmas (hemoplasmas) are bacteria that reside on the surface of erythrocytes and can mediate hemolytic anemia. *Mycoplasma haemofelis* is the most pathogenic species, and infection with this organism is most commonly associated with an extravascular hemolytic anemia. Two additional hemoplasma species, *Candidatus Mycoplasma turicensis* and *Candidatus Mycoplasma haemominutum*, have been reported in cats and are less pathogenic than *M. haemofelis* and associated with a mild (subclinical) to moderate anemia.

Synonyms

Haemobartonella felis (outdated), feline hemotropic (or hemotrophic) mycoplasmosis, feline infectious anemia

Epidemiology

SPECIES, AGE, SEX

Domestic and wild felids of any age and either sex

RISK FACTORS

- Male cats are more likely to be infected, potentially due to roaming and fighting behavior.
- Access to outdoors
- Young cats may be more likely to present with hemolysis.
- Retrovirus infection (feline immunodeficiency virus)
- Bloodsucking arthropods (fleas, ticks, and mosquitoes) suggested but unconfirmed as mode of transmission
- Biting and fighting activity (cat-bite abscess) may precede infection by a few weeks (potential mode of transmission)

CONTAGION AND ZOONOSIS

- Mode of transmission is unknown, but several methods of transmission have been suggested: bloodsucking arthropods (fleas, ticks, mosquitoes), cat fighting and biting activity, transplacental transmission and blood transfusions.
- The DNA of *M. haemofelis* has been detected in a person co-infected with HIV and *Bartonella henselae* from Brazil, and hemoplasma DNA from animal species have been detected in humans. Although the true zoonotic potential is unknown, caution is advised when handling infected blood and tissues.

GEOGRAPHY AND SEASONALITY

Worldwide

Clinical Presentation

DISEASE FORMS/SUBTYPES

- Acute, chronic, or subclinical
- Hemoplasma species involved impacts severity of illness.
- Presence and severity of clinical signs depend on anemia (severity and rate of development), concurrent disease, and immunosuppression.

HISTORY, CHIEF COMPLAINT

- Acute: weakness, lethargy, anorexia, weight loss, vomiting
  - Anemia: pale mucous membranes, tachypnea, tachycardia, collapse, acute neurologic signs, and sudden death
- Chronic: lethargy, anorexia, weight loss, mild to moderate clinical signs of anemia
- Subclinical: no reported clinical signs; more likely to occur with *Ca. M. turicensis* and *Ca. M. haemominutum* infections

PHYSICAL EXAM FINDINGS

- Acute: pale mucous membranes, fever, tachypnea, tachycardia, obtundation, weakness, splenomegaly, hemic cardiac murmur, icterus (uncommon)
- Chronic: pale mucous membranes, poor body condition, weakness, splenomegaly

Etiology and Pathophysiology

- Organisms reside on the surface of and possibly replicate within erythrocytes. The presence of these organisms cause extravascular hemolysis by immune-mediated destruction, erythrophagocytosis, and/or increased erythrocyte fragility.
- Three species of feline hemotropic mycoplasmas have been identified:
  - *M. haemofelis*: the most pathogenic species, causing hemolytic anemia in immunocompetent cats
  - *Ca. M. haemominutum*: identified in as many as one of five cats visiting veterinary hospitals and is usually associated with a subclinical or clinically insignificant hemolytic anemia
  - *Ca. M. turicensis*: usually associated with a subclinical or clinically insignificant hemolytic anemia
- Co-infection may occur with two or more of these species.
- The presence of large numbers of organisms identified on blood smear evaluation is associated with a dramatic decline in the hematocrit. Infected cats may recover from this bacteremic phase of infection, leading to a normalization of the hematocrit. At this phase of infection, it can be difficult to make a diagnosis based solely on blood smear exam because organisms occur in very low numbers. A carrier state may develop in

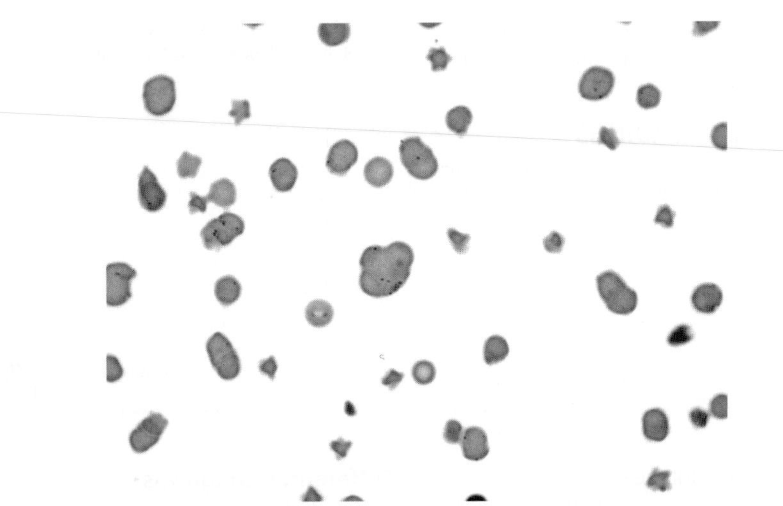

HEMOTROPIC MYCOPLASMOSIS, CAT Multiple coccoid epicellular *M. haemofelis* organisms are visible on this 100× magnification of a Wright-Giemsa–stained peripheral blood smear. (Courtesy Dr. John M. Thomason, Mississippi State University, Starkville, MS.)

some cats, especially cats infected with *Ca, M. haemominutum.*

DIAGNOSIS

Diagnostic Overview

Infection should be suspected when a cat is anemic, has an unexplained fever, or an organism is identified on the surface of erythrocytes during a blood smear evaluation. Hemotropic mycoplasmas cannot be cultured, and making a diagnosis depends on organism identification on blood smears (low sensitivity and specificity) or molecular diagnosis using polymerase chain reaction (PCR) assay. PCR assays are considered the gold standard for diagnosis, but results must be interpreted differently based on the hemoplasma species identified.

Differential Diagnosis

- Primary immune-mediated hemolytic anemia
- Heinz body anemia (e.g., acetaminophen intoxication, zinc intoxication, diabetic ketoacidosis, onion and garlic [including baby food] ingestion)
- Cytauxzoonosis
- Hereditary erythrocyte disorders (pyruvate kinase deficiency)
- Feline leukemia virus and feline immunodeficiency virus infections
- Hemorrhage

Initial Database

- Blood smear: visual identification of organism
  - Nonrefractile basophilic cocci, rods, or ring forms on the surface of erythrocytes
  - Organism identification is < 50% sensitive. *Ca. M. turicensis* may never be seen on blood smears.
  - Ideally, a thin, fresh blood smear should be made immediately after blood collection (without exposure to anticoagulants) and stained with a Romanowsky stain (e.g., Diff-Quik).
  - False-positive identifications are common due to confusion with Howell-Jolly bodies, Heinz bodies, stain precipitates, and refractile artifacts (p. 1327).
  - Performing an ear prick with immediate transfer of blood onto a microscope slide may improve the likelihood of cytologic identification of the organism.
- CBC: regenerative anemia, macrocytosis, normoblastosis, mild to moderate neutrophilia, and monocytosis are common. Thrombocytopenia is possible. In acute cases, the anemia may be nonregenerative.
- Serum biochemistry profile: usually unremarkable; hyperbilirubinemia uncommon despite hemolysis, occasional increases in the activities of alanine aminotransferase, alkaline phosphatase
- Urinalysis: usually unremarkable; occasionally bilirubinuria
- Abdominal imaging: usually unremarkable; diffuse, mild to marked splenomegaly possible
- Retrovirus testing: rule out co-infection

Advanced or Confirmatory Testing

- Hemoplasmas cannot be cultured.
- If a hemoplasma infection is suspected, blood should be submitted for PCR analysis. Contact the laboratory to determine which hemoplasma species are detected by the PCR assays. Cats positive for *Ca. M. turicensis* or *Ca. M. haemominutum* should still undergo a thorough diagnostic investigation to rule out alternative causes of anemia.

TREATMENT

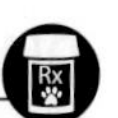

Treatment Overview

Doxycycline is the antimicrobial of choice, but pradofloxacin and enrofloxacin may also be effective. Antimicrobial therapy may lead to resolution of anemia for cats infected with *M. haemofelis,* but the organism may not be completely eliminated based on PCR analysis. Therapeutic goals should include resolution of anemia and elimination of acute clinical bacteremia.

Acute General Treatment

- Supportive care
  - Severe anemia: blood transfusion (p. 1169) or oxygen-carrying compounds
  - IV crystalloid fluid replacement as needed
- Doxycycline (drug of choice to reduce bacteremia; minocycline as alternative) 10 mg/kg PO q 24h for a minimum of 14 days
- Fluoroquinolones for a minimum of 14 days may be effective.
  - Pradofloxacin 5-10 mg/kg PO q 24h
  - Marbofloxacin 2.75-5.5 mg/kg PO q 24h
  - Enrofloxacin 5 mg/kg PO q 24h
- No antimicrobial therapy has been shown to completely eliminate a hemoplasma infection, and cats may remain PCR positive after treatment and resolution of clinical signs. Antimicrobial therapy is not recommended for cats that are not anemic and not demonstrating clinical signs.
- Glucocorticoids should be reserved for cats that do not respond to appropriate antimicrobial therapy, cats with a severe anemia, or when primary immune-mediated hemolytic anemia is possible.

Drug Interactions

- Doxycycline: esophagitis/esophageal strictures in cats. Oral doxycycline administration should be followed by a bolus of water or food to ensure passage of the medication into the stomach. Liquid formulations are less likely to cause esophagitis, but compounded liquid doxycycline has a very short shelf life.
- High doses of enrofloxacin may cause retinal degeneration and blindness in cats; do not exceed 5 mg/kg q 24h.

Recommended Monitoring

Packed cell volume, hematocrit, or CBC

PROGNOSIS & OUTCOME

Infections range in severity from subclinical to life-threatening, but a patient's prognosis is usually good with an accurate diagnosis, supportive care, and appropriate antibiotic therapy. During periods of stress or disease, infections may recrudesce.

PEARLS & CONSIDERATIONS

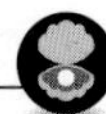

Comments

All cats used for blood donation should be tested by PCR for hemotropic *Mycoplasma* spp. Any cat that tests positive should not be used as a donor, even after completion of an antibiotic course.

Prevention

- Minimize the risk of exposure, and reduce outdoor time and contact with other felines, especially feral populations.

- Neuter outdoor male cats to decrease roaming and fighting behaviors.
- Provide effective flea and tick prevention.

Technician Tips

- Avoid needlestick injuries.
- After administering oral doxycycline, it is essential to give an adequate bolus of water by syringe or a small meal to ensure that the tablet has passed through the esophagus and into the stomach.

SUGGESTED READINGS

Sykes JE: Feline hemotropic mycoplasmas. Vet Clin North Am Small Anim Pract 40:1157-1170, 2010.

AUTHOR: John M. Thomason, DVM, MS, DACVIM
EDITOR: Joseph Taboada, DVM, DACVIM

Hepatic Encephalopathy

Client Education Sheet 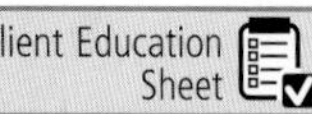

BASIC INFORMATION 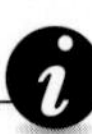

Definition

Hepatic encephalopathy (HE) is a reversible metabolic central nervous system (CNS) disturbance secondary to hepatic disease.

Epidemiology

SPECIES, AGE, SEX

- Dogs and cats
- Congenital hepatic vascular disease: young animal
- Acquired hepatic disease: middle-aged to older animal

GENETICS, BREED PREDISPOSITION

- Hepatic vascular disease: several breed predispositions (p. 814)
- Acquired liver disease (p. 174)

RISK FACTORS

- Type A: acute hepatic failure (pp. 442 and 1231)
- Type B: congenital portosystemic shunts (CPSS) and congenital urea cycle enzyme deficiency (rare)
- Type C: multiple acquired portosystemic shunts (MAPSS)
  - Cirrhosis and portal hypertension
  - Congenital vascular disease
    - Hepatic arteriovenous malformation
    - Portal vein atresia
    - Primary hypoplasia of the portal vein with portal hypertension
  - Ductal plate malformations

Clinical Presentation

HISTORY, CHIEF COMPLAINT

Signs of HE typically are episodic, involving three systems:

- Neurologic: diffuse cerebral disturbance: lethargy, altered behavior, ataxia, aimless wandering, head pressing, disorientation, seizures, blindness, stupor, coma, poor anesthesia tolerance/prolonged recovery
- Gastrointestinal (GI): vomiting, diarrhea, poor weight gain, ptyalism (cats)
- Urinary: polyuria and polydipsia; stranguria, pollakiuria, and/or hematuria (biurate urolithiasis)

PHYSICAL EXAM FINDINGS

- Signs of diffuse cerebral disease may be subclinical at the time of examination due to HE's episodic nature. Rarely, signs can be multifocal/lateralizing.
- Signs associated with underlying hepatopathy (e.g., icterus, ascites in acquired hepatic disease) or CPSS (e.g., small stature, copper-colored iris in cats)
- Type A HE: initial neuroexcitatory behavior (restlessness, agitation, seizures) progressing to neuroinhibitory states (depression, coma)
- Hepatic arteriovenous malformation: a continuous murmur may be auscultable on the cranioventral abdomen.

Etiology and Pathophysiology

Complex multifactorial cause:

- Associated with the accumulation of neurologic toxins, most likely of GI origin, that escape hepatic detoxification as a result of portal to systemic shunting of blood
- GI toxins derived primarily from bacterial metabolism of proteinaceous material
  - Ammonia generation in the colon
  - Endogenous benzodiazepine-like substances
- Alterations in inhibitory (gamma-aminobutyric acid) and excitatory (glutamate) neurotransmitter balance play a secondary role.
- Low-grade cerebral edema due to astrocyte detoxification of ammonia to glutamine may also play a role (portosystemic shunting).
- Low-grade systemic inflammation
- Pathophysiology of HE from acute liver failure is distinct from chronic HE: acute HE involves blood-brain barrier disturbances causing intracranial hypertension and cerebral edema and release of neurotoxic substances by the necrotic liver, which trigger a systemic inflammatory response; frequently complicated by neuroglycopenia.

DIAGNOSIS 

Diagnostic Overview

A tentative diagnosis is made when a patient with liver disease shows signs of neurologic dysfunction, other signs of encephalopathy are excluded, and there is response to treatment.

Differential Diagnosis

- Neurologic signs: hypoglycemia, hyponatremia or hypernatremia, lead toxicosis, congenital CNS malformation (e.g., hydrocephalus, storage disease), infectious or granulomatous meningoencephalitides, CNS neoplasia, nutritional (e.g., thiamine or cobalamin deficiency), uremic encephalopathy
- Chronic GI or lower urinary signs may mimic primary GI disease or suggest primary genitourinary or endocrine disorders.

Initial Database

- CBC: microcytosis, poikilocytosis (cats)
- Serum biochemistry profile
  - Hepatic vascular disease (p. 814)
  - Acquired hepatic disease (pp. 174 and 442)
- Urinalysis: isosthenuria common; ammonia biurate crystalluria, hematuria, pyuria, bacteriuria possible
- Prolongations of prothrombin time and activated prothrombin time common with liver failure

Advanced or Confirmatory Testing

Clinical pathology:

- Increased total serum bile acids: sensitive for the detection of congenital or acquired portosystemic shunting (2-hour postprandial sample more sensitive); not useful if icteric (p. 1312)
- Hyperammonemia: specific indicator of HE but can be normal even during overt HE. Ammonia tolerance test more sensitive to detect HE but may induce severe neurologic signs (p. 1305). Sample handling and assay conditions are critical; test not widely available.
- Abdominal effusion: pure or modified transudate with diseases that cause portal hypertension

Imaging:

- Abdominal ultrasound: reflective of the underlying disorder (pp. 452, 655, and 814)
- CT angiography: gold standard to look for single and multiple shunts

Histopathology (liver biopsy):

- Hepatic biopsy: same pattern of histologic changes (arteriolar proliferation, hepatic atrophy, attenuation of portal vasculature, lobular collapse) seen with all forms of hepatic disease associated with chronic hypoperfusion. Necroinflammatory changes with chronic hepatitis/fibrosis. Hepatic necrosis with acute liver failure. Dysplastic bile duct proliferation with ductal plate malformation.

- Urea cycle disorders diagnosed by enzyme activity in hepatic tissue.

TREATMENT

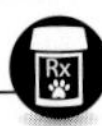

Treatment Overview

Goals of treatment are to lower levels of circulating neurotoxins by modulating GI protein metabolism, maintain optimal nutritional plane, and control precipitating factors.

Acute and Chronic Treatment

- Nothing per os if stupor or coma is present
- Medications that increase GI protein tolerance (first line of therapy)
  - Lactulose is drug of choice. Nonabsorbable disaccharide is broken down by colonic bacteria into short-chain fatty acids. Traps soluble ammonia (NH_3) as ammonium (NH_4^+), which is nonabsorbable and excreted in the feces. Alters bacterial metabolism so that less ammonia is generated
  - Lactulose is titrated from an initial dose of 0.5-1 mL/kg PO q 8-12h to a dose that produces 3-4 soft stools per day. If stupor or coma is present, may be given rectally in a retention enema (p. 1099)
  - Antibiotics alter bacterial metabolism, synergistic with lactulose
    - Metronidazole 7.5 mg/kg PO q 8-12h, low dose to avoid neurotoxicosis secondary to decreased hepatic metabolism, *or*
    - Neomycin 10-22 mg/kg PO q 12h; can be given orally or as a retention enema, *or*
    - Amoxicillin 22 mg/kg PO q 12h, *or*
    - Rifaximin 10 mg/kg PO q 12h; antibiotic of choice in humans with HE but limited veterinary experience
- Control seizure activity
  - Barbiturates (e.g., phenobarbital 6-10 mg/kg slow IV to effect); patient should be monitored closely for respiratory depression
  - Propofol is useful for controlling HE-induced status epilepticus. Because it is metabolized by the liver, small doses may be effective and may have a long duration of action. Maintain an anesthetized state for several hours before tapering and observe for recurrence. Monitor for apnea during use.
  - Cerebral edema is likely if seizures observed with acute liver failure; prognosis is grave (seizures often refractory to treatment).
    - Mannitol 0.5 g/kg IV over 10-15 minutes
    - *N*-acetylcysteine 140 mg/kg slow IV initially followed by 70 mg/kg as needed; may correct disturbances in microcirculation
    - Glucocorticoids of no benefit and may be detrimental
    - Hypoglycemia may require infusion of high concentrations of dextrose-containing solutions (monitor q 4h).
- Address fluid and electrolyte imbalances; avoid lactated solutions if acute liver failure; sodium-restricted fluids if ascites present; potassium, glucose, and B vitamins (especially thiamine and cobalamin in cats) supplementation as needed
- Control precipitating factors
  - Oral protein burden: GI hemorrhage, high-protein meals
  - Catabolic conditions: infection, dehydration, azotemia
  - Alkalosis with hypokalemia: increases renal ammonia production
  - Synergistic neural inhibition with sedatives, tranquilizers, or anesthetic agents; use these with caution if at all (e.g., diazepam)
  - Transfusion with stored blood products (high ammonia concentrations)
  - Constipation
  - Concurrent azotemia
- Correct underlying disorder if possible (e.g., surgical correction of CPSS after stabilization)

Nutrition/Diet

- Adequate calories to avoid catabolism of muscle (highly ammoniagenic; may make control of HE difficult)
- Modulation of protein content: high-quality protein derived preferably from plant and dairy products. Start with diet containing minimum daily protein requirements (cat: 6.5 g/100 kcal; dog: 5.1 g/100 kcal) in combination with medications to increase protein tolerance, and decrease protein only if necessary.
- Increase fiber content of diet.
- Vitamin supplementation: in cats, thiamine 50-100 mg/CAT PO q 24h; if associated coagulopathy, vitamin K 0.5 mg/kg SQ q 12h for 5-7 days initially parenterally, then once weekly
- Sodium restriction necessary only with ascites: 0.04-0.05 g/100 kcal

Drug Interactions

- Neuroinhibitory drugs (e.g., sedatives, anesthetics, and tranquilizers) should be used cautiously because they may potentiate the neuroinhibition of HE.
- Avoid drugs that depend heavily on hepatic metabolism and/or excretion if possible.

Recommended Monitoring

- Blood ammonia concentration
- Mentation and appetite at home
- Body weight and body condition score
- Serum albumin

PROGNOSIS & OUTCOME

Depends on nature of underlying liver disease causing HE:

- Hepatic vascular disease (PSS, microvascular dysplasia, arteriovenous malformation): signs often respond quickly and fully to appropriate drug and dietary intervention. Long-term prognosis depends on response to medical management or correction of the vascular defect.
- Acquired chronic hepatic disease: clinical signs of HE generally abate with proper intervention, but long-term prognosis depends on nature and severity of the underlying hepatic disorder. Patients with signs of severe HE due to acquired hepatic diseases generally have a very poor prognosis unless the underlying disease can be reversed.
- Acute liver failure: HE is more refractory to therapy, probably reflecting a more complex underlying cerebral lesion or process. Encephalopathy progressing to coma or stupor (grade 3-4) is considered a grave prognostic sign and is one of the criteria used for determining the need for liver transplantation in human patients.
- Ductal plate malformation: poor if portal hypertension and HE present

PEARLS & CONSIDERATIONS

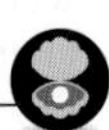

Comments

- Normal blood ammonia concentration does not rule out the presence of HE.
- Initial treatment of HE involves nonabsorbable disaccharides and antibiotics in combination with dietary protein modulation but not excessive protein restriction.
- Be aware of common comorbid conditions that can complicate control of HE, such as GI bleeding, dehydration, hypokalemia, azotemia, constipation, and alkalosis.
- HE accompanying acute liver failure differs from that accompanying congenital vascular disorders or chronic hepatic failure in that it involves the development of overt cerebral edema and an initial neuroexcitatory state often refractory to therapeutic intervention.
- Development of HE is determined by the amount of functional hepatic tissue and the presence of intrahepatic and extrahepatic shunting of blood away from the hepatic vascular system.

Technician Tips

- Note changes in mentation or the appearance of abnormal behavior because they may indicate increasing grade of HE.
- Avoid feeding high-protein meals and limit intake of snacks containing protein.
- Lactulose is expected to cause soft stools, although overt diarrhea warrants a decreased dose.

Client Education

HE is an episodic, chronic condition that can often be controlled with strict adherence to dietary modulation and drug therapy.

SUGGESTED READING

Lidbury JA, et al: Hepatic encephalopathy in dogs and cats. J Vet Emerg Crit Care 26:471-487, 2016.

AUTHOR: Cynthia R. L. Webster, DVM, DACVIM
EDITOR: Keith P. Richter, DVM, MSEL, DACVIM

Hepatic Injury, Acute

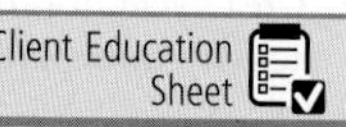

BASIC INFORMATION

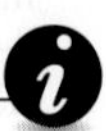

Definition

The lack of a consistent definition for acute hepatic/liver injury (ALI) and acute hepatic/liver failure (ALF) in veterinary medicine results in ambiguity in describing the disorders. Here, ALI indicates acute hepatocellular damage and necrosis with adequate hepatic function. ALF is a progression of ALI and occurs when at least 70%-80% of hepatic synthetic, excretory, and regulatory functions are compromised, particularly with development of hepatic encephalopathy (HE) and/or coagulopathy. In human literature, ALI/ALF occur in the absence of preexisting liver disease; however, this can be challenging to determine in dogs and cats.

Synonyms

Acute hepatic injury, acute or fulminant hepatic failure, acute liver failure

Epidemiology

SPECIES, AGE, SEX

- Dogs > cats
- Any age and sex
  - Younger and pregnant animals are most susceptible to aflatoxicosis.
  - Young or unvaccinated dogs of any age are at risk for canine adenovirus-1 and leptospirosis.
  - Hepatic cancers are more common in older animals.

RISK FACTORS

Drug administration, free-roaming animals, lack of vaccines, exposure to toxins

CONTAGION AND ZOONOSIS

Untreated dogs with leptospirosis pose a contagious/zoonotic risk because spirochetes are shed in the urine. Leptospirosis is most often contracted by contact with infected urine or urine-contaminated water or fomites (p. 583).

GEOGRAPHY AND SEASONALITY

- Southern United States and Hawaii: cycad palms toxicities (although plant may be ornamental indoor plant in any climate)
- Fungal hepatopathy: histoplasmosis in Mississippi and Ohio River valleys; coccidioidomycosis in southwestern United States
- Late summer to autumn: leptospirosis (can be any time), blue-green algae

ASSOCIATED DISORDERS

Gastrointestinal (GI) ulceration, acute kidney injury, coagulation disorders (e.g., disseminated intravascular coagulation [DIC]), central neurologic signs (due to hepatic encephalopathy [HE] or cerebral edema), cardiopulmonary diseases (e.g., aspiration pneumonia, congestive heart failure)

Clinical Presentation

DISEASE FORMS/SUBTYPES

Often difficult to distinguish between acute exacerbation of preexisting subclinical disease and acute injury

- Clinical signs and biochemical evidence of ALI/ALF in the absence of known preexisting liver disease
- Unexpected finding of increased serum liver enzyme activities and bilirubin concentration with minimal clinical signs

HISTORY, CHIEF COMPLAINT

- Common clinical signs (most common to least)
  - Lethargy
  - Inappetence / anorexia
  - Vomiting
  - Icterus
  - Dullness
  - Melena
- Less common clinical signs
  - Diarrhea
  - Hematuria
  - Neurologic abnormalities
  - Polydipsia/polyuria
  - Fever
  - Spontaneous bleeding and/or bruising
- Careful review of history for potential exposure to hepatotoxins is warranted (p. 1231). Clinical signs often develop within days after toxin exposure.

PHYSICAL EXAM FINDINGS

- Dehydration
- Icterus
- Ptyalism (more common in cats)
- Abdominal/hepatic pain
- Abdominal distention due to ascites and/or hepatomegaly
- Bluish discoloration of mucous membranes with acetaminophen-induced methemoglobinemia
- Melena with coagulopathy or GI hemorrhage
- Petechiae, ecchymoses with thrombocytopenia, and/or coagulopathies
- Other findings may be related to cause of hepatic injury (e.g., uremic breath, oral ulcers, tachypnea, conjunctivitis in dogs with leptospirosis)

Etiology and Pathophysiology

Normal liver function:

- Production of proteins, including albumin and coagulation factors
- Detoxification of blood by metabolizing ammonia and lactate
- Defense against GI bacterial invasion
- Major glucose reservoir in the form of glycogen and involved in gluconeogenesis
- Loss of at least 70%-80% of the normal hepatic synthetic, excretory, and regulatory functions defines liver failure.

Important causes of ALI/ALF:

- Hepatotoxins (p. 1231): sago palms, xylitol, aflatoxins, blue-green algae, *Amanita* mushrooms, heavy metals
- Adverse drug reactions: acetaminophen, azole antifungal drugs, methimazole, many others
- Infectious agents
  - Viral: infectious canine hepatitis, canine herpesvirus, coronavirus (feline infectious peritonitis), virulent feline calicivirus
  - Bacterial: leptospirosis, liver abscess, cholangitis/cholangiohepatitis, *Bartonella* spp, *Helicobacter canis*, *Clostridium piliforme*
  - Fungal: histoplasmosis, coccidioidomycosis
  - Parasitic: liver flukes; heartworm with caval syndrome
  - Protozoal: *Toxoplasma gondii*, *Neospora caninum*, *Babesia* spp, *Cytauxzoon felis*
  - Rickettsial: *Ehrlichia* spp, *Rickettsia rickettsiae*
- Inflammatory hepatopathies: hepatitis, cholangiohepatitis (p. 452)
- Breed-related hepatopathy: copper storage hepatopathy, other (pp. 459 and 450)
- Neoplasia (pp. 446 and 1230)
- Metabolic disease: feline hepatic lipidosis, acute pancreatitis, sepsis/endotoxemia, heat stroke, massive trauma
- Ischemia/hypoxic injury: surgical hypotension and hypoxia, liver lobe torsion, thromboembolic disease

DIAGNOSIS

Diagnostic Overview

Acute hepatopathy is typically suspected based on history and clinical findings, including basic laboratory data. Imaging studies are indicated and can help prioritize differential diagnoses. Ultimately, in most cases, hepatic cytology or histopathology is needed to confirm a diagnosis.

Differential Diagnosis

- Icterus (p. 528): consider prehepatic causes (hemolysis) and posthepatic (biliary obstruction or rupture) causes
- Pancreatitis
- Chronic hepatic disease: cholangiohepatitis (p. 160), chronic hepatitis (p. 452), hepatic cirrhosis (p. 174), breed related hepatopathy (pp. 450 and 459), hepatic cancer (p. 446)

Initial Database

- CBC: can be normal or may suggest infectious or inflammatory disorder. Leukocytosis ± left shift, anemia, and thrombocytopenia common
- Serum biochemical profile
  - Elevated transaminases and inducible liver enzymes (essentially always identified in ALI/ALF)
    - Increased activities of aspartate aminotransferase (AST), alkaline phosphatase (ALP), alanine aminotransferase (ALT), gamma-glutamyltransferase (GGT)
    - Increases in ALT and AST activities are sensitive indicators of acute liver damage.
    - Often proportional increase ALT > ALP
  - Hyperbilirubinemia (common with ALF)
  - Hypoalbuminemia (common with ALF)
  - Hypocholesterolemia (common with ALF)
  - Blood urea nitrogen decreased (ALF), increased (leptospirosis, dehydration), or normal
  - Hypoglycemia can be severe with *Amanita phalloides* and xylitol toxicities.
  - Electrolyte disorders possible
  - Other findings depend on cause (e.g., azotemia with leptospirosis)
- Urinalysis
  - Bilirubinuria (common)
  - Isosthenuric or minimally concentrated urine (common)
  - Glucosuria possible
  - Occasionally ammonium biurate crystalluria
- Serum bile acids (SBA) concentration (p. 1312): not indicated if animal is icteric (provides no additional information)
- Coagulation testing
  - ± Prolonged prothrombin time (PT) and activated partial thromboplastin time (aPTT)
  - ± Thrombocytopenia
  - D-dimers and fibrin degradation products can be increased with DIC
  - Coagulation abnormalities due to ALF are similar to DIC except for factor VIII, which is often increased in ALF and decreased in DIC.
- Abdominal radiography
  - Allows evaluation of liver size, although subjective
  - In many cases, radiographs unremarkable
- Ultrasound
  - Sensitive tool for evaluating hepatic parenchyma, biliary system, and vascular structures
  - Permits guided sampling of liver and peritoneal effusion and screening for post-hepatic causes of icterus
  - Can be normal despite ALI, with an overall accuracy for diffuse hepatic disease of < 40% in dogs and < 60% in cats

Advanced or Confirmatory Testing

Advanced testing is guided by results of initial database but often includes cytology and/or biopsy.

- Serum ammonia testing (p. 1305): difficulties with sample handling make this impractical in most settings, but hyperammonemia is a useful hepatic function test for icteric animals. Hyperammonemia is associated with an increased mortality rate.
- Infectious disease testing, as appropriate based on other findings (e.g., serology for leptospirosis if azotemia and ALI seen simultaneously)
- Hepatic cytology
  - Minimally invasive and relatively inexpensive
  - No information on architecture and small sample size limits diagnostic accuracy
  - Most useful with diffuse neoplasia (e.g., lymphoma), some infections, and suppurative hepatitis
- Hepatic histopathology
  - Percutaneous, laparoscopic, or surgical biopsy
  - Bacterial culture and copper quantification are beneficial.
  - Characterizes hepatic pathology and architecture
  - Can distinguish between chronic and acute disease and may provide specific diagnosis
  - Most common lesion with ALF is necrosis.
- Hepatic toxin testing (rarely used; clinical illness occurs days after toxin exposure)
  - Liquid chromatography mass spectrometry can be performed.
  - Can submit materials from the environment that may have caused toxicity (e.g., feed sample for aflatoxin testing, mushrooms)

TREATMENT

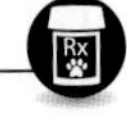

Treatment Overview

The majority of patients with ALF need hospitalization for IV fluids, supportive care, and additional specific therapy directed at the underlying (known or suspected) cause.

Acute General Treatment

- If an underlying cause of injury is known or suspected, specific treatment is warranted (e.g., doxycycline for suspect leptospirosis).
- Fluid resuscitation with intravenous fluid therapy is critically important, especially in hypovolemic and hypotensive patients.
  - Crystalloid solutions, such as Plasmalyte-A or 0.9% NaCl
  - Lactated Ringer's solution should be avoided because lactate buffer requires hepatic metabolism.
  - If hypotension persists despite correction of volume depletion, vasopressor therapy should be considered (p. 911).
- Colloidal solution (e.g., Hetastarch) should be considered in hypoalbuminemic patients unable to maintain adequate colloid osmotic pressure and intravascular volume.
- Fresh-frozen plasma (initial dose 10 mL/kg) indicated if prolonged PT and aPTT with clinical evidence of hemorrhage
- Correct electrolyte abnormalities (e.g., hypokalemia, hypoglycemia, hypophosphatemia, hypomagnesemia), if present.
- Address severe hypoglycemia, if present (p. 552).
- Antibiotics
  - Prophylactic antimicrobials have not been shown to improve outcome or survival.
  - Many dogs are treated for possible leptospirosis during the initial evaluation while screening for an underlying cause.
  - If suspicious of sepsis-induced ALI/ALF, empirical antimicrobial therapy should include broad-spectrum coverage for gram-positive and gram-negative bacteria.
- Address HE (p. 440): lactulose, neomycin, amoxicillin, flumazenil
  - Treat cerebral edema with mannitol 0.5-1 g/kg over 15-20 minutes IV or hypertonic saline 7.5% NaCl, 4 mL/kg IV.
- Supplements
  - Multiple hepatoprotective medications have been advocated for treatment of ALI/ALF patients (pp. 174 and 452).
  - Replacement of depleted glutathione stores using *N*-acetylcysteine (NAC) or *S*-adenylmethionine (SAMe) is indicated, particularly with acetaminophen toxicity
- Additional therapies
  - Vitamin K_1 0.5-1.5 mg/kg PO or SQ for 3 doses has been recommended by some for all ALF patients; others recommend only if patient is coagulopathic, hyperbilirubinemic, or if there is evidence of cholestasis.
  - Treat for possible GI ulceration. Proton-pump inhibitors (pantoprazole 1 mg/kg IV q 12h, omeprazole 1 mg/kg PO q 12h) are likely most effective.

Chronic Treatment

- Chronic therapy is typically directed at the cause of the ALI/ALF.
- Often, the inciting insult remains unknown. If the animal improves with supportive care, it can be discharged with ongoing supplements and hepatoprotective medications (e.g., SAMe, silybin [Denamarin]) as well as treatment for HE or GI ulcers, as needed.

Nutrition/Diet

- Small, frequent meals may help maintain blood glucose concentrations.

- Dietary therapy is based on concern for HE.
  - If no clinical signs of HE, provide a high-quality/digestible protein source (i.e., GI diets)
  - If concerned about HE, dietary protein should be limited; dogs, 15%-20%; cats, 30%-35% dry matter protein (liver or kidney diets)
- For patients with persistent inappetence, enteral feeding through feeding tubes should be considered (p. 1106)
- Parenteral nutrition required rarely for patients that cannot tolerate enteral feedings (p. 1148)

Drug Interactions

- Potentially hepatotoxic drugs should be avoided (particularly nonsteroidal antiinflammatory drugs [NSAIDs]).
- Consider dose reduction ± duration prolongation ± avoidance of drugs with hepatic metabolism (e.g., many chemotherapy and anesthetic drugs, maropitant)

Possible Complications

- HE
- Ascites
- Hypoglycemia
- GI ulceration
- Bleeding and/or bruising
- Pancreatitis
- Acute kidney injury
- Septicemia

Recommended Monitoring

- Monitor for mentation changes, signs of excessive fluid administration (e.g., tachypnea, edema), and presence of bruising.
- Frequent monitoring of pulse and respiratory rate, blood pressure, and body weight
- Daily to multiple times daily monitoring of electrolytes (potassium, sodium, phosphorus), glucose, lactate, packed cell volume, total solids
- Initially monitor liver enzymes and bilirubin at least every several days and periodically until normalized.

PROGNOSIS & OUTCOME

- Prognosis depends on the underlying cause and response to treatment; however, overall, ALF has a high mortality rate. Hypoalbuminemia, bleeding, and ascites are poor prognostic indicators.
- In dogs with aflatoxicosis, the mortality rate was 68%. Nonsurvivors had longer PT and aPTT and lower antithrombin concentrations at presentation compared with survivors.
- In dogs with cycad seed toxicosis, higher ALT and bilirubin concentrations at presentation were associated with a poor prognosis.
- Lower platelet counts at presentation may be associated with a poor prognosis and the development of DIC.
- In cats with hepatic lipidosis, negative prognostic indicators include anemia, hypokalemia, and older age.
- Dogs with rapidly treated leptospirosis have a good prognosis.

PEARLS & CONSIDERATIONS

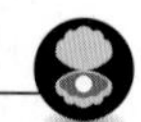

Comments

- Considering the good prognosis with rapid therapy and zoonotic concern with lack of therapy, treat for possible leptospirosis until proven otherwise.
- Always consider an adverse drug reaction as the cause of ALI/ALF because discontinuing the suspected drug can result in improved hepatic function.
- Keeping a list of potential hepatotoxins can be helpful to review with the pet's owner.

Prevention

Vaccinate for infectious diseases (e.g., infectious canine hepatitis, leptospirosis), and educate clients about hepatotoxins (e.g., xylitol, sago palm).

Technician Tips

- A thorough medical history, including any medication and herbal supplement exposures, is very important for pets with ALI/ALF because hepatotoxins are a common cause of injury but cannot be identified with typical testing.
- Zoonotic precautions, including barrier nursing, should be considered for any dog with possible leptospirosis. These dogs should not be allowed to void in common areas where other dogs could be exposed.

SUGGESTED READING

Weingarten M, et al: Acute liver failure in dogs and cats. J Vet Emerg Crit Care 25:4, 2015.

AUTHOR: Marnin A. Forman, DVM, DACVIM
EDITOR: Keith P. Richter, DVM, MSEL, DACVIM

Hepatic Lipidosis

Client Education Sheet 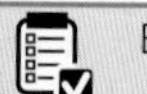 Bonus Material Online 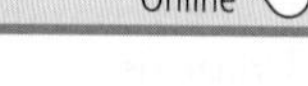

BASIC INFORMATION

Definition

Hepatic lipidosis (HL) is the accumulation of triglycerides in hepatocytes, resulting in intrahepatic cholestasis and liver failure. It is the most common hepatobiliary disease in cats.

Synonyms

Fatty liver disease, steatosis of the liver

Epidemiology

SPECIES, AGE, SEX

- Cats of any age, sex, or breed are susceptible.
  - Most often reported in middle-aged cats (median age, 7 years)
  - Females seem to be overrepresented.
- Rarely encountered in young dogs, especially toy breeds

RISK FACTORS

Most likely in obese cats, especially after sudden reduction in food intake

GEOGRAPHY AND SEASONALITY

High incidence in North America, Great Britain, Japan, and Western Europe; associated with the prevalence of obesity in cats from these regions

ASSOCIATED DISORDERS

Severe HL can result in gastrointestinal (GI) ulceration, hepatic encephalopathy, coagulation abnormalities, and acute kidney injury.

Clinical Presentation

DISEASE FORMS/SUBTYPES

- Primary HL: occurs when a previously healthy (usually overweight) cat does not have access to food or will not eat (e.g., food not palatable, stressful event)
- Secondary HL: occurs when a cat with systemic illness becomes anorexic as a consequence of underlying disease. Common causes include pancreatitis, acute or chronic kidney disease, GI diseases, cancer, cholangiohepatitis, diabetes mellitus, heart failure, or medications.

HISTORY, CHIEF COMPLAINT

- Anorexia and weight loss
- GI signs: constipation or diarrhea, vomiting
- Neurologic signs
  - Hepatic encephalopathy (p. 440): ataxia, somnolence, seizures, opisthotonus
  - Altered mentation, ptyalism common in cats with hepatic encephalopathy
  - Although rare, neurologic signs in dogs usually due to hypoglycemia

PHYSICAL EXAM FINDINGS

If HL is secondary to another disease process, additional exam findings are likely (e.g., thickened, ropey intestines with GI lymphoma or inflammatory bowel disease). Some findings are more directly linked to HL:

- Icterus
- Dehydration and weakness
- Hepatomegaly

- Cervical ventroflexion
- Ptyalism
- Poor hair coat

Etiology and Pathophysiology

- Hepatic lipidosis can develop rapidly (after 2-14 days of inappetence).
- Anorexia in cats results in a negative energy balance and deficiency of obligatory essential fatty acids (FAs), amino acids, and vitamins and is the primary initiating cause for HL.
- An imbalance develops between the influx of FAs, rate of hepatic FA oxidation for energy, and the dispersal of hepatic triglycerides by excretion of very low-density lipoproteins.
- Triglycerides primarily accumulate in the liver with HL; however, the exact metabolic abnormalities causing the accumulation are not completely understood.
- HL has been reported in young, toy-breed, anorexic puppies after development of hypoglycemia. Hypoglycemia develops due to inadequate glyconeogenesis to sustain their high basal metabolic energy requirements.

DIAGNOSIS

Diagnostic Overview

A presumptive diagnosis is based on the patient's presentation, clinicopathologic findings, and hepatic ultrasound, with diagnosis confirmed by hepatic cytology (or less commonly, histopathology). Confirmation is important because inflammatory or neoplastic hepatic disease can have a similar presentation. Because secondary HL is common, efforts should be made to identify an underlying disease process.

Differential Diagnosis

- Icterus (p. 1243)
- Inflammatory biliary or hepatopathies, including cholecystitis, cholangitis, and cholangiohepatitis
- Neoplasia (p. 1230)
- Hepatotoxins and adverse drug reactions (p. 1231)
- Infectious hepatopathy (p. 1230): feline infectious peritonitis, cholangitis, histoplasmosis, liver flukes, toxoplasmosis, cytauxzoonosis
- Ischemia/hypoxic injury, including surgical hypotension and hypoxia
- GI disorders: inflammatory bowel disease, intestinal neoplasia, foreign bodies
- Severe systemic or metabolic disorders: acute pancreatitis, sepsis, heat stroke, trauma

Initial Database

- CBC: low-grade, nonregenerative anemia and leukocytosis, neutrophilic left shift and/or thrombocytopenia, if present, are usually secondary to underlying disease.
- Serum biochemical profile
  - Increased serum alkaline phosphatase (ALP) activity is extremely common. A greater magnitude of increase in ALP compared with gamma-glutamyl transferase (GGT) is strongly suggestive of HL.
  - Hyperbilirubinemia is common.
  - Electrolyte abnormalities: hypokalemia, hypomagnesemia, and hypophosphatemia are common and prognostically significant.
  - Hyperglycemia due to insulin resistance is more likely than hypoglycemia due to liver failure in cats. Hypoglycemia is often recognized in young, toy-breed dogs with HL.
  - Mild hypoalbuminemia or low blood urea nitrogen (BUN) sometimes identified
- Urinalysis: bilirubinuria common, urine often minimally concentrated to isosthenuric, and biurate crystals sometimes found
- Coagulation abnormalities: prolonged prothrombin (PT) and activated partial thromboplastin times (aPTT) are common, as are clinical bleeding tendencies (45%-73%)
- Abdominal radiography: ± hepatomegaly (not specific for HL)
- Abnormal ultrasonography: diffuse hepatomegaly with a hyperechoic echogenicity compared with the falciform fat and normal echotexture. This is a highly sensitive finding, although it is important to note that healthy obese cats and cats with infiltrative liver disease can have similar hepatic ultrasound findings.
- Measurement of serum bile acids is not useful in icteric patients.
- Although technically difficult and not widely used, measurement of blood ammonia can support recognition of hepatic encephalopathy.

Advanced or Confirmatory Testing

- Hepatic cytology (p. 1112)
  - Least invasive and most cost-effective
  - Small sample size and lack of architectural detail limit diagnostic accuracy for many liver diseases, but cytology often adequate for HL.
  - Expect abnormal retention of lipids (macrovesicular or microvesicular steatosis) in > 80% of the hepatocytes.
  - Can rule out some neoplastic and infectious causes of hepatopathy
- Hepatic biopsy (p. 1128) permits a more accurate characterization of hepatic pathology but is often unnecessary.
  - On gross examination, liver is enlarged, diffusely pale yellow.
  - Many cats are at increased surgical risk (coagulopathy common); assay coagulation before biopsy, and prepare for transfusion if necessary.
  - Expect diffuse microvesicular or macrovesicular vacuolation within hepatocytes.

TREATMENT

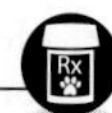

Treatment Overview

The cornerstone of treatment of HL is early nutrition with the goal of achieving a positive calorie balance. This usually involves the placement of an enteral feeding tube. As with all systemically ill cats, correction of hypoperfusion and electrolyte derangements is very important.

Acute General Treatment

- Nutritional therapy is crucial and usually requires a feeding tube.
- If an underlying cause of secondary HL is identified, treatment should be directed at it. Often, there is no quick fix for such disorders.
- Dehydration is common, and fluid resuscitation is important, especially in hypovolemic and hypotensive patients.
  - Balanced isotonic crystalloid infusion (0.9% NaCl or Plasmalyte-A) is recommended.
  - Avoid lactated Ringer's solution because it contains lactate as a buffer, which requires hepatic metabolism and may worsen hyperlactatemia.
  - Start with small-volume resuscitation (5-10 mL/kg IV bolus given over 30 minutes) in hypovolemic cats with serial assessment of hydration and perfusion.
  - Calculate correction of dehydration (% of body weight) + maintenance fluid requirements (40-60 mL/kg/d) ± ongoing losses (vomiting, diarrhea, polyuria; 2-6 mL/kg/h), and administer IV over 24 hours.
- Electrolyte abnormalities should be corrected before starting nutritional therapy.
- Additional therapies
  - Antiemetics often indicated. The following can be used alone or in combination.
    - Maropitant 1 mg/kg IV or SQ q 24h
    - Ondansetron 0.1-0.5 mg/kg IV q 8-12h
    - Metoclopramide 0.2-0.5 mg/kg PO, SQ, or IM q 6-8h or 0.01-0.09 mg/kg/h IV as a constant-rate infusion (CRI)
  - Consider treatment for GI ulceration (pantoprazole 1 mg/kg IV q 12h or omeprazole 1 mg/kg PO q 12h).
  - Vitamin K_1 0.5-1.5 mg/kg PO or SQ q 12h for 3-4 doses if a bleeding tendency is noted
- If necessary, address hepatic encephalopathy (p. 440).

Chronic Treatment

- Maintain tube feeding until appetite normalizes.
- In cats with secondary HL, chronic therapy is directed at the cause.

Nutrition/Diet

- Dietary therapy is essential in treating primary and secondary HL to reverse the negative energy balance and catabolic state.
- Ideally, initiate a nutrition plan the day of admission as soon as severe electrolyte abnormalities and hypoperfusion are addressed.
- If no clinical signs of HE, provide a diet that is high in protein (30%-40% of the metabolizable energy [ME]), moderate in lipids (approximately 50% of the ME) and reduced in carbohydrates (approximately 20% of the ME)
  - Most feline veterinary recovery diets meet these requirements.
  - Providing a diet with lower protein content (25% of the ME) was shown to attenuate but not ameliorate HL.

- Dietary therapy is modified based on concern for hepatic encephalopathy; if encephalopathic, reduce protein (e.g., liver or kidney diet appropriate).
- Small, frequent meals can be offered, but most patients have persistent inappetence. Almost always, tube feeding is required initially. Parenteral nutrition is rarely needed but is used in patients who do not tolerate enteral feedings (p. 1148).
  - Forced enteral feeding is typically ineffective and increases the risk of food aversions or aspiration.
  - Appetite stimulants are ineffective in the initial stages of HL.
  - Feeding tubes (nasoesophageal, esophageal, and gastric) permit administration of enteral nutrition, fluid, and medications. The decision on type of feeding tube to place depends on many factors, including patient stability, clinician experience, and cost.
  - A nasoesophageal feeding tube (5-8 Fr) is a logical first choice (ease of placement, low cost, noninvasive, no anesthesia required) (p. 1107).
  - For many cats, esophagostomy tube facilitates hospital discharge and at-home nutritional support after initial stabilization (p. 1106).
  - Daily calorie requirements can be calculated using the formula (resting energy requirements [RER] = 70 [body weight in kg]$^{0.75}$). Illness factors are not recommended due to the risk of overfeeding.
  - A percentage of RER is provided each day and divided over multiple feedings (4-8/d) or as a CRI. On the first day, 25%-33% of RER is provided, and a slow, incremental increase is given each day with a goal to reach full RER in 3-4 days.
  - Rapid caloric administration to an anorexic patient should be avoided to decrease the risk of refeeding syndrome and vomiting due to feeding volume intolerance.
- Nutritional supplements: multiple supplements have been advocated in treatment of cats with HL, but there is minimal to no documentation of efficacy.
  - L-carnitine 250-500 mg/CAT/d PO
  - *S*-adenosylmethionine 20 mg/kg/d PO, given at least 1 hour before meals
  - Vitamin B_{12} 250 mcg SQ once weekly for 6 weeks, then once q 2 weeks for 6 weeks, and then monthly
  - Taurine 250 mg total daily dose PO for 7-10 days

Drug Interactions

- Any potentially hepatotoxic drug should be avoided.
- Consider dose reduction ± duration prolongation ± avoidance of any drug with extensive hepatic metabolism

Possible Complications

- Hypophosphatemia due to refeeding
- Persistent vomiting leading to complications and ineffective nutritional support
- Anesthesia complications
- Enteral tube complications (e.g., infection, inappropriate placement)

Recommended Monitoring

- Serial serum chemistry profiles: there should be gradual improvement in liver parameters, usually over a 3-12 week period.
- Monitor for return of appetite.
  - Gradually taper enteral tube feeding as voluntary feeding resumes.
  - After the cat is eating voluntarily with no enteral tube feeding for 2 weeks, the tube can be removed.

PROGNOSIS & OUTCOME

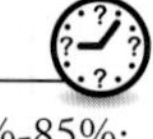

- Reported recovery rate of 80%-85%; prognosis is good assuming any underlying disorders are corrected and provided rapid nutritional support.
- Positive prognostic indicators include younger age and higher median serum potassium concentration and hematocrit.
- Negative prognostic factors indicators include anemia, hypoalbuminemia, hypokalemia, hypophosphatemia, and older age.

PEARLS & CONSIDERATIONS

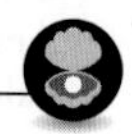

Comments

- HL is rare in dogs, but in a study of dogs with acute liver failure, HL was noted on histopathology of 41%.
- Begin enteral feeding through feeding tubes as early as possible in the treatment of all types (primary and secondary) of HL.

Prevention

Maintain ideal body condition. Although weight loss is encouraged for obese cats, dramatic, sudden calorie reduction should be avoided (pp. 700 and 1077).

Technician Tips

Become comfortable using and maintaining a variety of enteral feeding tubes.

Client Education

- Anorexia, especially in overweight cats, can cause HL in as a little as 2 days.
- Intensive veterinary care can result in a complete reversal of HL.

SUGGESTED READING

Valtolina C, et al: Feline hepatic lipidosis. Vet Clin North Am Small Anim Pract 47:683-702, 2017.

AUTHOR: Marnin A. Forman, DVM, DACVIM
EDITOR: Keith P. Richter, DVM, MSEL, DACVIM

Hepatic Neoplasia, Malignant

Client Education Sheet 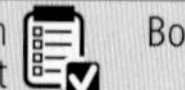 Bonus Material Online 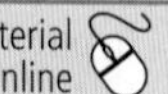

BASIC INFORMATION

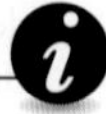

Definition

- Primary malignant neoplasm of the liver or biliary tract
- Epithelial origin: hepatocellular carcinoma (HCC) (most common), biliary carcinoma, carcinoid (neuroendocrine)
- Mesenchymal origin: hemangiosarcoma (most common mesenchymal tumor in cats) and leiomyosarcoma (most common in dogs), fibrosarcoma
- Hemolymphatic tumors: lymphoma (dogs, cats), histiocytic sarcoma (dogs, rare in cats), and myeloproliferative disorders (cats). Hepatic lymphoma and histiocytic sarcoma may be part of multicentric disease or the primary site.
- Metastatic hepatic neoplasia: hemangiosarcoma, mast cell tumor, islet cell carcinoma, pancreatic adenocarcinoma, intestinal adenocarcinoma, leiomyosarcoma, mammary carcinoma, transitional cell carcinoma, renal carcinoma, pheochromocytoma, and others. Metastatic tumors are more common in dogs, and primary tumors are more common in cats.

Synonyms

- Biliary adenoma: biliary cystadenoma in cats
- Biliary carcinoma: cholangiocarcinoma, cystadenocarcinoma

Epidemiology

SPECIES, AGE, SEX

- Primary hepatobiliary tumors are uncommon, accounting for less than 1.5% of all canine neoplasms and 1%-2.9% of all feline neoplasms.
- HCC accounts for more than one-half of hepatobiliary tumors in dogs; in cats, adenoma is more common than HCC.

- Feline primary hepatic neoplasms can be subdivided into benign and malignant hepatocellular tumors, cholangiocellular carcinomas, small cell carcinomas with hepatic progenitor cell characteristics, neuroendocrine carcinomas, and squamous cell carcinomas.
- Biliary carcinomas and adenomas are the most common primary hepatic tumors in cats. Biliary tumors account for 22%-41% of malignant liver tumors in dogs.
- Tumors occur primarily in older animals (average age, 10-12 years).

RISK FACTORS

- Potential causes in humans include cirrhosis, toxins, chemicals, parasites, viruses, and radioactive compounds.
- Biliary carcinoma in juvenile cats with feline leukemia virus infection
- Cirrhosis occurred in 7% of dogs with HCC in one study; it is therefore an unlikely contributor to development of HCC in dogs. There is no known viral association with primary hepatic neoplasia in dogs.

ASSOCIATED DISORDERS

- Paraneoplastic hypoglycemia is occasionally seen in dogs with HCC (up to 38% of cases) and less frequently in dogs with hepatocellular adenoma, leiomyosarcoma, or hemangiosarcoma. Serum insulin concentrations are normal to decreased.
- Paraneoplastic alopecia has been reported in cats with biliary carcinoma and HCC.
- Bile duct obstruction, clinically relevant coagulopathies, and hepatic encephalopathy (HE) are uncommon.
- Myasthenia gravis was associated with biliary carcinoma in one report.

Clinical Presentation

DISEASE FORMS/SUBTYPES

HCC: three gross morphologic subtypes:

- Massive HCC, defined as a large tumor affecting a single liver lobe, represents 53%-83% of cases. The nodular form occurs in 16%-25%, and the diffuse form occurs in 0%-19% of cases.
- Histopathologic and immunohistochemical exam of canine primary hepatic neoplasms can differentiate hepatocellular, cholangiocellular and neuroendocrine tumors in accordance with the most recent human classification system and may be predictive of biologic behavior.

Biliary carcinoma in dogs:

- Massive form occurs in 37%-46%, nodular in 0%-54%, and diffuse in 17%-54% of cases. Biliary carcinomas can also be extrahepatic within bile ducts or gallbladder.

Carcinoid:

- Usually intrahepatic, although can be extrahepatic in the gallbladder
- Nodular in 33%, diffuse in 67%

Sarcoma:

- Massive in 36%, nodular in 64%; diffuse form not reported

HISTORY, CHIEF COMPLAINT

Clinical signs are usually vague and nonspecific. Inappetence, lethargy, weight loss, polydipsia, polyuria, vomiting, and abdominal distention are the most common presenting complaints. Less frequent presenting problems are icterus, diarrhea, excessive bleeding, and signs of central nervous system (CNS) dysfunction (due to HE, hypoglycemia, or CNS metastases).

PHYSICAL EXAM FINDINGS

- The most common finding in dogs and cats with primary hepatic tumors is a palpable cranial abdominal mass or marked hepatomegaly.
- Ascites or hemoabdomen may also contribute to abdominal distention.
- Icterus, cachexia, weakness, and pale mucous membranes due to anemia are potential findings.
- Exam may be unremarkable.

Etiology and Pathophysiology

- Cause is unknown.
- The more common massive HCCs in dogs generally have a low potential for metastasis, with rates varying from 0%-37%. The less common nodular and diffuse HCCs have metastatic rates as high as 100%.
- Extrahepatic metastases occur more commonly with biliary carcinoma, with metastasis occurring in 67%-88% of dogs and cats.
- Metastasis is common for hepatic carcinoids.
- Metastatic rates of 86%-100% for hepatic sarcomas in dogs
- Metastatic patterns are to regional lymph nodes, peritoneum, and lungs, and can be widespread to other abdominal organs. Metastasis to bone marrow can occur with histiocytic sarcoma.

DIAGNOSIS

Diagnostic Overview

The diagnosis is typically based on the presence of a liver mass/masses that are palpated and/or identified on abdominal ultrasound exam. Confirmation is by cytologic or histopathologic exam of tissue specimens.

Differential Diagnosis

- Hepatic nodular hyperplasia (p. 449)
- Diffuse hepatomegaly (e.g., vacuolar hepatopathy, hepatic congestion, lipidosis)
- Hepatic nodular regeneration, cirrhosis
- Hepatobiliary cysts
- Hepatic abscess

Initial Database

- CBC: variable anemia, leukocytosis, and thrombocytosis. Pancytopenia may be seen with hemolymphatic malignancies that involve bone marrow and secondarily involve the liver.
- Coagulation profile: prolonged prothrombin times and activated partial thromboplastin times are not common (when coagulopathies occur, they are most common with hepatic hemangiosarcoma).
- Serum chemistry profile: mild to marked increases in activities of alanine aminotransferase (ALT), aspartate aminotransferase (AST), and alkaline phosphatase (ALP). ALP and ALT are more commonly elevated in primary hepatic tumors and AST more commonly elevated in metastatic tumors. Liver enzyme activities are normal in up to 50% of dogs with metastatic tumors. Hyperbilirubinemia (uncommon in dogs with primary hepatic neoplasia, more common in dogs with metastatic liver disease) occurs in one-third of cats with primary liver tumors. Other biochemical abnormalities may include hypoalbuminemia, hyperglobulinemia, and hypoglycemia.
- Serum bile acids concentration: elevated in 50%-75% of cases, often with mild magnitude of increase
- Abdominal radiographs: symmetrical or asymmetrical hepatomegaly, ascites, and caudolateral gastric displacement
- Three-view thoracic radiographs: evaluate for pulmonary metastasis, although this is an uncommon finding at the time of initial diagnosis.
- Abdominal ultrasound: very useful for evaluation of the liver when primary or metastatic hepatic neoplasia is suspected. However, there can be extensive variability and overlapping ultrasonographic appearance among neoplastic and non-neoplastic conditions. Caution is warranted when attempting to use ultrasound alone to diagnose hepatic lesions:
  - HCC usually appears as a focal hyperechoic or mixed echogenic mass.
  - Primary or metastatic neoplasia often appears as focal or multifocal hypoechoic or mixed echogenic lesions.
  - Target lesions, nodules or masses with a hypoechoic rim and a hyperechoic or isoechoic center, are often neoplastic, with a positive predictive value for malignancy of 74% for solitary lesions and 81% for multiple lesions.
  - Hyperplastic nodules are usually multifocal hyperechoic lesions, although hypoechoic or mixed echogenic lesions can occur.
  - The ultrasonographic appearance of hepatic lymphoma is quite variable, ranging from normal to mild, diffuse hyperechogenicity or hypoechogenicity, multifocal hypoechoic lesions, or mixed echogenic target lesions.
  - Contrast harmonic ultrasound can discriminate between benign and malignant nodules in the canine liver. This method requires ultrasound contrast media and contrast harmonic software. Results depend on operator experience with this modality.
  - The ultrasound exam should assess for feasibility of resection (relationship to vena cava, portal vein, and biliary tract).

Advanced or Confirmatory Testing

- An ultrasound-guided, percutaneous fine-needle aspirate for cytology can correctly diagnose neoplasia in up to 62% of patients with liver tumors. False-positive results also occur. Cytologic evaluation is most useful for the diagnosis of diffuse hemolymphatic tumors such as lymphoma, myeloproliferative disease, and mast cell tumors. There is low risk to the patient with fine-needle aspiration (p. 1112).
- Ultrasound-guided, percutaneous core-needle biopsy versus laparoscopic biopsy (p. 1128) for histopathologic evaluation of liver tissue (confirmatory)
  - Needle biopsies are generally accurate (80%), but because of the small size of biopsy samples, differentiation of nodular hyperplasia from primary hepatic neoplasia may be difficult.
  - Sometimes, a larger biopsy specimen obtained by laparoscopy or laparotomy is necessary. Laparoscopy enables larger biopsy samples and is useful for staging (observe peritoneal surface and lymph nodes for infiltration or other abnormalities). Intraoperative conversion from laparoscopy to laparotomy may become necessary, with neoplasia a risk factor for such conversion.
- Peritoneal fluid cytology in animals that have ascites may reveal neoplastic cells, especially in advanced cases, although often ascites is a modified transudate without exfoliation of neoplastic cells.
- Abdominal CT or MRI scan can be considered for lesion characterization and staging. MRI is possibly useful for differentiating benign from malignant focal hepatic lesions in dogs.

TREATMENT

Treatment Overview

- Surgical removal of the tumor for focal, solitary primary hepatic neoplasia such as HCC, hepatoma, primary hemangiosarcoma, and biliary carcinoma
- Chemotherapy for hepatic lymphoma, histiocytic sarcoma, and hepatic mast cell tumor
- Palliative therapy for metastatic hepatic cancer or nodular to diffuse primary hepatic neoplasia
- Consultation with or referral to an oncologist is recommended.

Acute General Treatment

- Supportive therapy for paraneoplastic hypoglycemia (p. 552), clinically relevant coagulopathies, or HE (p. 440)
- Liver lobectomy for primary hepatic tumors involving a single lobe
- Treatment options are very limited for nodular, diffuse, and metastatic liver neoplasia, and the treatment focus for these tumors is often palliative.

Chronic Treatment

- Chemotherapy for hepatic lymphoma, histiocytic sarcoma, mast cell tumor, myeloproliferative disease, and possibly as an adjuvant after surgery for hemangiosarcoma
- No radiation therapy protocols have been reported for hepatic tumors.
- Several chemotherapy drugs (carboplatin, gemcitabine, mitoxantrone, doxorubicin, 5-fluorouracil) have been used anecdotally for other hepatic neoplasms, although efficacy has not been proven. Given the poor response in humans with hepatobiliary cancer, it is unlikely that systemic chemotherapy with the currently available agents can play a major role in the treatment of hepatobiliary cancer in dogs and cats.
  - Chemoresistance may be due to expression of P-glycoprotein (MDR1), which is associated with multidrug resistance, and/or the detoxification enzymes contained in hepatocytes.
- Newer treatment modalities such as intra-arterial chemotherapy, transarterial chemoembolization (performed successfully in dogs and cats), percutaneous ethanol injection, and immunotherapeutic strategies may be applicable to veterinary patients. A novel treatment method for HCC in dogs using fractional excision with a Cavitron ultrasonic surgical aspirator has been described.

Possible Complications

- Hemorrhage is the most common surgical complication. Blood products should be available in the event a transfusion is necessary.
- Although not common, hypoglycemia is a potential transient complication of extensive partial hepatectomy.

Recommended Monitoring

After removal of primary liver tumors, follow-up abdominal ultrasound exams are recommended every 3 months for 2 years. Due to less common pulmonary metastasis, recommended frequency for repeat thoracic radiographs is variable, but semiannually for 2 years is suggested.

PROGNOSIS & OUTCOME

- For massive HCC treated by liver lobectomy, the prognosis is good with a complete excision, with median survival time of > 1460 days.
  - High serum ALT and AST activity is associated with decreased survival, and right-sided tumors have a worse intraoperative prognosis due to increased complication rate.
- In one study, lethargic dogs had a mortality risk 10.2 times that of nonlethargic dogs. Dogs that experienced anesthetic complications had a mortality risk 100 times that of dogs that did not.
- The prognosis for nodular or diffuse HCC is poor.
- Biliary carcinoma, hepatic carcinoids, and hepatic sarcomas have a poor prognosis because they are commonly nodular or diffuse and have high metastatic rates.
- Hepatic lymphoma has a variable prognosis that depends on the grade and response to chemotherapy. For dogs with primary hepatic lymphoma treated with chemotherapy, median survival is 63 days (2-402 days), though patients with complete response and normal serum bilirubin concentrations have improved survival.
- The liver is a common site of metastasis for a variety of canine cancers, and metastatic liver disease has a poor prognosis.

PEARLS & CONSIDERATIONS

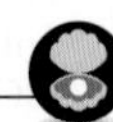

Comments

- The most common primary hepatobiliary tumor in dogs is a massive HCC. With liver lobectomy providing a complete excision of massive HCC, long-term survival or cure is common.
- The most common feline hepatobiliary tumors are bile duct carcinoma and biliary cystadenoma. Bile duct carcinoma has a high metastatic rate and a poor prognosis, whereas biliary cystadenoma is benign and generally has a good prognosis.
- Ultrasonography, CT, and MRI are useful modalities to preoperatively stage hepatobiliary tumors, but imaging modalities alone are insufficient to diagnose hepatobiliary tumors.
- Laparoscopy is a useful method to stage the abdominal cavity and obtain diagnostic specimens.
- Hepatobiliary tumors, with the exception of lymphoma and histiocytic sarcoma, are rarely responsive to chemotherapy.

Technician Tips

Intraoperative hemorrhage during liver lobectomy is common. All patients should have compatible blood products available before surgery. Increasing heart rate, decreasing blood pressure, decreasing packed cell volume/total solids, and decreasing body temperature can be suggestive of hemorrhage in the immediate postoperative period.

SUGGESTED READING

Withrow SJ: Cancer of the gastrointestinal tract: hepatobiliary tumors. In Withrow SJ, et al, editors: Small animal clinical oncology, ed 5, Philadelphia, 2013, Saunders, pp 405-412.

AUTHORS: Brenda Phillips, DVM, DACVIM; Steve Hill, DVM, MS, DACVIM
EDITOR: Keith P. Richter, DVM, MSEL, DACVIM

Hepatic Nodules, Benign

Client Education Sheet

BASIC INFORMATION

Definition

- Hepatic adenoma: benign neoplasia of hepatocytes
- Nodular hyperplasia: discrete accumulation of hyperplastic hepatocytes surrounded by normal hepatocytes
- Nodular regeneration: discrete accumulation of hyperplastic hepatocytes surrounded by abnormal hepatocellular parenchyma, particularly fibrotic changes

Synonyms

Nodular hyperplasia, hyperplastic nodules, nodular regeneration, regenerative nodules

Epidemiology

SPECIES, AGE, SEX

- Hepatic adenomas: rare tumors in dogs and cats; patients usually > 10 years old
- Nodular hyperplasia: common lesion in old dogs. Prevalence in dogs > 14 years old: 70%-100%
- Nodular regeneration: seen in middle-aged/older dogs with acquired parenchymal hepatic disease

GENETICS, BREED PREDISPOSITION

Nodular regeneration: breeds predisposed to chronic hepatitis (Doberman pinscher, cocker spaniel, Labrador retriever, English springer spaniel) and copper-storage hepatopathy (Bedlington terrier, West Highland white terrier, Labrador retriever, Dalmatian)

RISK FACTORS

Nodular regeneration: chronic hepatic disease

Clinical Presentation

HISTORY, CHIEF COMPLAINT

- Adenoma: incidental finding, no clinical signs; rarely, abdominal discomfort from rupture with hemoperitoneum, or abscessation causing signs of infection (p. 455)
- Nodular hyperplasia: incidental finding, no clinical signs, hepatic failure (rare)
- Nodular regeneration (pp. 174 and 452)

PHYSICAL EXAM FINDINGS

- Adenoma: rarely abdominal pain, inappetence, ascites; pallor (if ruptured)
- Nodular hyperplasia: normal exam
- Nodular regeneration (pp. 174 and 452)

Etiology and Pathophysiology

- Adenoma: unknown; may be associated with chronic inflammation or hepatotoxicosis
- Nodular hyperplasia: unknown; may be associated with nutritional factors or a result of focal areas of ischemia/thrombosis; not preneoplastic
- Nodular regeneration: compensatory response of the liver to chronic injury

DIAGNOSIS

Diagnostic Overview

- Hepatic adenoma and nodular hyperplasia are often encountered incidentally during abdominal ultrasound or surgery or during evaluation of serum liver enzyme elevations in healthy pets. Confirmation of the diagnosis requires histologic evaluation of a biopsy specimen. In animals with no overt clinical signs of hepatobiliary disease and normal or mildly elevated serum liver enzyme activities, a conservative approach consisting of monitoring for increases in serum liver enzymes ± increases in serum bile acids with periodic abdominal ultrasound examination may be pursued instead of a biopsy.
- Nodular regeneration often accompanies chronic fibrosing hepatopathies. Typically, the livers appear small and nodular on ultrasound, and serum liver enzymes and/or results of hepatic function tests (albumin, bilirubin, bile acids) are abnormal. Hepatic biopsy should be strongly considered in these cases.

Differential Diagnosis

- Adenoma: nodular hyperplasia, primary or metastatic hepatic neoplasia, hepatic abscess
- Nodular hyperplasia: primary or metastatic hepatic neoplasia, adenoma, nodular regeneration with cirrhosis, vacuolar hepatopathy, hepatic cysts
- Nodular regeneration: nodular hyperplasia, metastatic hepatic neoplasia, vacuolar hepatopathy

Initial Database

Hepatic adenoma:

- Serum chemistry: varied increases in serum liver enzyme activities
- CBC: usually normal; leukocytosis ± monocytosis if necrotic regions within adenomas, anemia if ruptures
- Total serum bile acids: usually normal
- Radiographs: cranial abdominal mass effect possible; rarely, gas pocket in necrotic region (abscess)
- Abdominal ultrasonography: solitary mass with variable echogenicity that may contain cystic cavities and/or blood- or gas-filled spaces. Ascites and hemoperitoneum are seen with rupture.

Nodular hyperplasia:

- Commonly associated with mild to moderate increases in serum alkaline phosphatase (ALP) activity; less commonly with mild increases in serum transaminases
- Total serum bile acids: usually normal
- Abdominal ultrasonography: single to multiple lesions with highly variable appearance; easily mistaken for primary or metastatic neoplasia or nodular regeneration

Nodular regeneration:

- Serum bile acids concentration: usually abnormal
- Other CBC, serum chemistry, and urinalysis findings (pp. 174 and 452)
- Abdominal ultrasonography: typically appears as one or more nodules that are most often hypoechoic but may be of mixed echogenicity or even rarely appear as target lesions

Advanced or Confirmatory Testing

- Hepatic histopathology differentiates the three conditions but often requires wedge biopsy (by laparoscopy or surgery) because adjacent hepatic tissue is necessary to make a definitive diagnosis.
- Fine-needle aspiration or single-needle biopsies of focal lesions may result in misdiagnosis of hepatic vacuolar hepatopathy.
- MRI (p. 1132) of focal hepatic masses may provide better discrimination of lesions (future direction).
- Preliminary studies with contrast-enhanced (harmonic) ultrasonography have shown some ability to discriminate benign from malignant nodules.

Specific:

- Adenoma
    - Well-circumscribed, expansive nodule of variable sizes containing hyperplastic but well-differentiated hepatocytes arranged in cords that are 1-2 cells thick with absent portal tracts
    - Surrounded by normal hepatic parenchyma
- Nodular hyperplasia
    - Well-circumscribed, expansive nodules usually < 3 cm in diameter, containing hyperplastic hepatocytes that often contain cytoplasmic vacuoles and are loosely organized into hepatic cords with discernible portal tracts
    - Nodules surrounded by normal hepatic parenchyma
    - Lipogranulomas are a common associated finding.
- Nodular regeneration
    - Similar histologic appearance to nodular hyperplasia, but surrounding hepatic parenchyma is abnormal, most often with mixed inflammation and fibrosis

TREATMENT

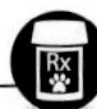

Treatment Overview

Not all focal lesions require treatment, even when hepatic enzyme increases are present. Treatment is required when there is ongoing inflammatory or cirrhotic hepatopathy.

Acute General Treatment

- Adenoma
    - No treatment necessary for healthy animal with small masses

- Surgical excision for large masses causing abdominal discomfort or for those associated with abscessation or hemorrhage
- Nodular hyperplasia
  - No treatment necessary
- Nodular regeneration
  - Treatment of the underlying disorder (pp. 174 and 452)

Recommended Monitoring

Sequential monitoring of serum liver enzyme activities and abdominal ultrasonography q 4-6 months

PROGNOSIS & OUTCOME

- Adenoma and nodular hyperplasia: excellent long-term prognosis
- Nodular regeneration (pp. 174 and 452)

PEARLS & CONSIDERATIONS

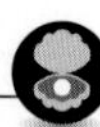

Comments

- Distinguishing nodular hyperplasia from more serious hepatopathies is important.
  - It is a common cause of increased serum ALP activity in older dogs.
  - The ultrasonographic appearance may mimic primary or metastatic hepatic neoplasia.
- Evaluation of coagulation profile is appropriate prior to liver biopsy (p. 1325).

Technician Tips

Watch patients for signs of bleeding such as pale mucous membranes, increased heart rate, or drop in packed cell volume/total solids (PCV/TS) after hepatic aspiration or biopsy.

SUGGESTED READING

Cullen J: Summary of the World Small Animal Veterinary Association standardization committee guide to classification of liver disease in dogs and cats. Vet Clin North Am Small Anim Pract 39:395-418, 2009.

AUTHOR: Cynthia R. L. Webster, DVM, DACVIM
EDITOR: Keith P. Richter, DVM, MSEL, DACVIM

Hepatitis (Chronic), Breed-Associated

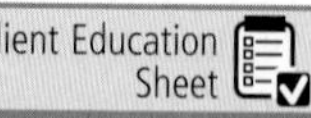

BASIC INFORMATION

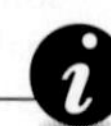

Definition

Progressive, chronic inflammatory liver disease (hepatitis) associated with certain breeds of dogs. American and English cocker spaniels, Doberman pinschers, and English springer spaniels are thought to have a breed-associated chronic hepatitis.

Synonyms

Cocker spaniel hepatitis, Doberman hepatitis, springer spaniel hepatitis, chronic hepatitis, chronic idiopathic hepatitis

Epidemiology

SPECIES, AGE, SEX

- In English and American cocker spaniels, the mean age at diagnosis is ≈5 years, and males are overrepresented.
- Doberman pinschers are identified between the ages of 2 and 10 years. Subclinical disease is reported to occur between 2-4 years of age, with clinical disease generally observed between 4-7 years of age, and females are markedly overrepresented.
- In English springer spaniels, the mean age at diagnosis is reported to be ≈4 years, and females are overrepresented.

GENETICS, BREED PREDISPOSITION

The high incidence of hepatitis in these breeds suggests a genetic predisposition, but the mode of genetic transmission is unknown. Likely, environmental factors also play a role. The prevalence of Doberman pincher hepatitis is reported to be 2%-20% in some European countries.

Clinical Presentation

DISEASE FORMS/SUBTYPES

- Subclinical hepatitis: no clinical signs but abnormal liver enzymes
- Clinical hepatitis: various clinical signs and abnormal liver enzymes
- Cirrhosis: advanced or end stage, demonstrating signs of liver failure

HISTORY, CHIEF COMPLAINT

- Dogs with subclinical hepatitis show no overt signs but can be identified through biochemical testing. Most have clinically silent disease until an advanced stage of chronic liver disease.
- Early signs of clinical hepatitis are vague and may be associated with intermittent gastrointestinal (GI) signs and weight loss.
- When clinical hepatitis progresses to liver failure, some or all of the following signs may occur:
  - Polydipsia, polyuria
  - Weight loss
  - Abdominal distention from ascites
  - Anorexia and vomiting
  - Altered mental status associated with hepatic encephalopathy (HE)

PHYSICAL EXAM FINDINGS

With clinical hepatitis some or all of the following may be found:

- Weight loss
- Icterus
- Ascites
- Signs of HE
- Hemorrhage

Etiology and Pathophysiology

- The cause of cocker spaniel, Doberman pinscher, and springer spaniel hepatitis is unknown. Complex genetic and environmental factors likely play a role. Copper accumulation is not a consistent feature in cocker and springer spaniels.
- Cocker spaniel hepatitis is thought to be associated with abnormal alpha-1 antitrypsin accumulation in hepatocytes when compared with other breeds. Whether alpha-1 antitrypsin is the cause or the result of the liver disease is unknown.
- Doberman pinscher hepatitis has been associated with copper accumulation in some but not all dogs. Impaired biliary excretion of hepatic copper was identified using copper radioisotope studies. Hepatic copper concentrations in affected dogs range from 1000-3000 mcg/g dry weight liver (normal < 400 mcg/g). Copper does not appear to accumulate with age, and copper chelation therapy improves the histology. There is evidence that the disease also has an immune component because of abnormal expression of major histocompatibility complex (MHC) class II antigens in hepatocytes, but the DLA class II complex can occur as a secondary phenomenon.
- In English springer spaniels, one study suggested DLA class II expression to be significantly associated with the risk of developing hepatitis. This suggests an immune component.

DIAGNOSIS

Diagnostic Overview

The combination of signalment (breed) and physical and/or biochemical evidence of hepatobiliary disease are strongly suggestive of the diagnosis; confirmation is obtained with a liver biopsy.

Differential Diagnosis

- Hepatic disease from other causes
- Nonhepatic conditions associated with abnormal liver enzyme activities, often referred to as nonspecific reactive hepatopathy

Initial Database

- Subclinical disease
  - Elevation in serum alanine aminotransferase (ALT), aspartate aminotransferase (AST), gamma-glutamyltransferase (GGT), and/or alkaline phosphatase (ALP) activity; ALT elevations are the most consistent laboratory change
- Clinical disease
  - Elevations in serum ALT, AST, GGT, ALP activities
  - Elevated serum bile acid concentrations in most; not useful in icteric animals
  - Hypoalbuminemia is common.
- Advanced disease
  - Elevation of serum total bilirubin concentration
  - Low serum albumin, blood urea nitrogen, and glucose concentrations
  - Prolonged clotting times

Advanced or Confirmatory Testing

- Abdominal radiographs: normal or microhepatica ± ascites (loss of serosal detail)
- Ultrasound: early hepatitis may be normal or have altered parenchymal echogenicity; with advanced hepatitis, there is microhepatica ± ascites ± vascular changes associated with portal hypertension. Acquired portosystemic shunts may be evident.
- Surgery or laparoscopy (p. 1128): varies from normal to small liver; micronodular or macronodular and fibrotic in advanced cirrhosis. Test coagulation first.
- Liver histopathology: subclinical disease is associated with mixed inflammation varying from mild-moderate to marked lymphoplasmacytic infiltrates and evidence of hepatocyte death (apoptosis or necrosis). Variable fibrosis, ductular response, and regenerative nodule formation occur as hepatitis progresses.
- Hepatic metal quantitative analysis: hepatic copper is usually normal in cocker and springer spaniels but often high in Doberman pinchers. Hepatic iron may be increased in all breeds and is thought to be secondary to chronic hepatic inflammation.

TREATMENT

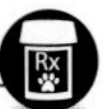

Treatment Overview

Goals of treatment are to slow progression of the inflammatory component, provide general supportive care, and treat complications of liver disease such as HE, ascites, GI ulceration, and nutritional imbalance. If abnormal hepatic copper is a component of the disease, specific therapy is required.

Acute General Treatment

- Crystalloid fluid support, as appropriate
- Treatment of HE, ascites, and GI ulceration (see Chronic Treatment below) (pp. 174, 380, and 440)
- Coagulopathies and sepsis are treated as they occur.

Chronic Treatment

- Anti-inflammatory or immunosuppressive therapy
  - Glucocorticoid therapy (prednisolone 1-2 mg/kg PO q 24-48h; maximum dose of 60 mg q 24h) may be beneficial in slowing inflammatory component of the liver disease. With clinical improvement, dose may be slowly tapered to 0.5 mg/kg q 48h. With ascites, dexamethasone 0.2 mg/kg PO q 24h should be used instead of prednisolone to avoid mineralocorticoid effect. Anecdotally, cocker spaniels have improved survival after prednisolone therapy. Springer spaniels are reported to have improved liver enzymes and prolonged survival with therapy.
  - Immunosuppressive therapy using cyclosporine 5 mg/kg q 12h followed by dose taper is reported to result in remission in many cases based on normalization of liver enzymes during therapy. With liver enzyme improvement, cyclosporine dose and frequency of administration can be tapered. Vomiting often transiently occurs as a side effect of the medication, and giving the drug with food or freezing the capsules before administration often resolves this. Gingival hyperplasia is sometimes observed. There are no reported studies evaluating other immunosuppressive drugs, although some authors recommend mycophenolate mofetil 10-15 mg/kg q 12h as the immunosuppressive drug of choice.
- Copper chelation using penicillamine 10-15 mg/kg q 12h may be required in some Doberman pinchers (p. 458). Treatment is generally for 4 months or longer based on repeated measurement of hepatic copper concentrations. Concentration of ALT often returns to normal if copper is removed and inflammation controlled.
- Palatability is important in advanced cases because adequate caloric intake is required. Feed a high-quality, moderate-protein diet in small, multiple feedings. Dietary protein restriction is necessary only when protein intolerance occurs (i.e., HE); milk and vegetable protein sources are better for avoiding HE than meat protein–based diets. Fermentable fiber may also be beneficial in controlling HE. Doberman pinschers with abnormal hepatic copper should be fed a low-copper diet (homemade formulated diet or veterinary therapeutic liver diets).
- Provide liver support with antioxidants (vitamin E 10 IU/kg PO q 24h; *S*-adenosylmethionine 20 mg/kg PO q 24h; and/or milk thistle [silybin complexed with phosphatidylcholine] 24-70 mg/kg PO q 24h). Combination antioxidants are available (e.g., Denamarin).
- Ursodeoxycholic acid 10-15 mg/kg PO q 24h is given for antioxidant activity, antiinflammatory effects, immunomodulating effects, and to promote choleresis.
- Antifibrotics (e.g., colchicine 0.03 mg/kg PO q 24h) have failed to prolong survival in humans, and few studies report their use in dogs. Angiotensin II receptor blockers have shown promise in inhibiting fibrosis in humans and may have an application in dogs (e.g., telmisartan 1 mg/kg PO q 12-24h), but veterinary studies on safety and efficacy are lacking. Phosphatidylcholine 20-70 mg/kg/d PO may also have antifibrotic effects.
- Advanced clinical hepatitis
  - Treatment for HE (p. 440): high-quality, limited-protein diet; lactulose 0.1-0.5 mL/kg PO q 12h, titrated to achieve loose fecal consistency; and/or intestinal antibiotics (metronidazole 7.5-10 mg/kg PO q 12h; amoxicillin-clavulanate 15 mg/kg q 12h, or 15 neomycin 20 mg/kg PO q 12h).
  - Ascites therapy: spironolactone 1 mg/kg PO q 12h or furosemide 0.5-2 mg/kg PO q 12h
  - Gastric ulceration: omeprazole 1 mg/kg PO q 12-24h and/or sucralfate 0.25-1 g PO q 8-12h.

Drug Interactions

- Avoid drugs that require hepatic metabolism or alter hepatic biotransformation (e.g., cimetidine).
- Glucocorticoids may cause sodium retention, promote GI ulceration, precipitate hepatic failure in advanced disease, and cause increased liver enzymes (making interpretation difficult).
- Penicillamine and zinc should not be given together because penicillamine chelates zinc.
- Diuretics may worsen HE, promote dehydration or metabolic alkalosis, and should be used only in otherwise stable patients for the long-term delay of return of ascites or for concurrent conditions (e.g., congestive heart failure).
- Nonsteroidal antiinflammatory drugs may exacerbate GI ulceration.

Possible Complications

- Glucocorticoids may precipitate ascites and HE and result in early death in advanced cases.
- Because von Willebrand disease is common in Doberman pinschers, von Willebrand factor, buccal mucosal bleeding time, or both should be evaluated before biopsy procedures.

Recommended Monitoring

- Young adult dogs of these breeds should have periodic liver enzymes measured as screening tests to help identify affected dogs early in the disease process.

- Routine CBC, serum biochemistry profile, and urinalysis to monitor disease progression, remission, or complications
- Serial liver biopsies may be helpful to monitor therapy (e.g., hepatic copper content).

PROGNOSIS & OUTCOME

- Diagnosis and appropriate therapy in subclinical cases may slow progression of disease.
- Clinical hepatitis with hypoalbuminemia and ascites denotes advanced disease, and the long-term prognosis is guarded. With early detection and therapy, a median survival time of 1 to several years has been reported.

PEARLS & CONSIDERATIONS

Comments

- The first abnormality observed in young, subclinical dogs is an increase in serum ALT activity. Unexplained elevated serum ALT activities in these breeds should be investigated.
- Diagnosis is confirmed with a liver biopsy; treatment and prognosis depend mainly on whether disease is subclinical (incidental finding, no clinical signs) or clinically overt (advanced signs of liver disease, including HE and portal hypertension).
- Copper reduction appears to be helpful in affected dogs.
- Many dogs are presented when the disease is advanced. The prognosis is poor at this stage.

Technician Tips

- Ensure patients intended for bile acid panel testing, abdominal imaging, and liver biopsy are fasted for 12 hours.
- After liver biopsy, the patient must be monitored closely for bleeding, including obtaining a packed cell volume/total solids (PCV/TS) evaluation at 3 and 6 hours after biopsy.

Client Education

- The incidence and genetic mode of inheritance are unknown. Affected dogs or related dogs should not be used for breeding.
- Screening laboratory testing of enzymes in young dogs can lead to an early diagnosis and may improve prognosis with therapy.

SUGGESTED READING

Poldervaart JH, et al. Primary hepatitis in dogs: a retrospective review (2002-2006). J Vet Intern Med 23:72-80, 2009.

AUTHOR: David C. Twedt, DVM, DACVIM
EDITOR: Keith P. Richter, DVM, MSEL, DACVIM

Hepatitis (Chronic, Idiopathic) of Dogs

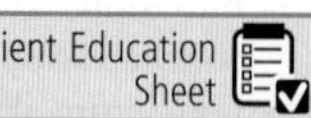

BASIC INFORMATION

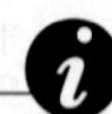

Definition

Chronic hepatitis is the most common canine liver disease when secondary reactive hepatopathies are excluded. It is a chronic, progressive hepatic disorder of unknown cause, characterized by parenchymal inflammation, hepatocyte death, and fibrosis that can ultimately progress to cirrhosis. In most cases, an underlying cause is never determined.

Synonyms

Chronic active hepatitis, chronic hepatitis/hepatopathy

Epidemiology

SPECIES, AGE, SEX

Commonly middle-aged dogs 3-10 years of age (mean, ≈7 years at time of presentation); females are overrepresented.

GENETICS, BREED PREDISPOSITION

- Breed predispositions: Labrador retriever, standard poodle, cocker spaniel, and springer spaniel.
- Breed-specific copper-associated chronic hepatitis (pp. 458 and 459) is observed in the Bedlington terrier, West Highland white terrier, Doberman pinscher, cocker spaniel, springer spaniel, Labrador retriever, Dalmatian, and Skye terrier.

RISK FACTORS

Drug therapy (including phenobarbital, possibly nonsteroidal antiinflammatory drugs [NSAIDs], and potentially any other drug), infectious diseases such as leptospirosis, toxin-induced hepatopathy, or other causes of acute hepatitis may eventually progress to chronic hepatitis. Diets high in copper may result in copper-associated hepatitis in susceptible dogs.

CONTAGION AND ZOONOSIS

Leptospirosis, leishmaniasis, canine adenovirus type 1, and canine acidophil cell hepatitis (suspected but poorly documented) are reportedly associated with chronic hepatitis and potentially are contagious (all) and zoonotic (leptospirosis, leishmaniasis).

ASSOCIATED DISORDERS

Hepatic inflammation can result from disorders such as pancreatitis, peritonitis, or inflammatory bowel disease. The type and character of inflammation in the liver is different from typical progressive idiopathic chronic hepatitis; in these disorders, the inflammation is usually mild, multifocal, or confined to the portal triads, and there is an absence of fibrosis. This is commonly referred to as a *secondary nonspecific reactive hepatopathy.*

Clinical Presentation

DISEASE FORMS/SUBTYPES

Chronic hepatitis is a progressive disease associated with several clinical stages:

- Subclinical hepatitis associated only with abnormal serum liver enzyme activities
- Clinical hepatitis associated with variable clinical signs
- Cirrhosis associated with advanced disease or hepatic failure

HISTORY, CHIEF COMPLAINT

Historic signs for clinical disease vary based on the extent of liver damage:

- Subclinical
  - None; often identified because of abnormal liver enzyme activity found on routine blood screen
- Clinical hepatitis
  - Lethargy
  - Vomiting
  - Anorexia
  - Weight loss
  - Diarrhea
  - Polyuria or polydipsia
- Cirrhosis/hepatic failure
  - Abdominal distention from ascites
  - Signs of neurologic dysfunction associated with hepatic encephalopathy (HE)
  - Bleeding or bruising due to coagulopathy
  - Anorexia, vomiting, and other signs of gastrointestinal (GI) ulceration

PHYSICAL EXAM FINDINGS

Physical findings vary with severity of disease:

- Subclinical: dogs appear normal
- Abnormal findings in clinically ill dogs (see History above)
  - Icterus
  - Poor body condition
  - Hepatic encephalopathy (p. 440)
  - Ascites (mainly in cirrhosis/hepatic failure [pp. 79 and 174])

Etiology and Pathophysiology

In an individual dog, the cause is usually unknown, but the following have potential roles:

- Infections: leptospirosis, canine adenovirus 1 (infectious canine hepatitis) infection, and possibly *Helicobacter* spp, *Bartonella* spp, *Leishmania* spp, or other infectious agents

- Immune-mediated mechanisms: poorly documented in the dog. Studies measuring liver-associated antibodies or cell-mediated responses in affected cases fail to determine if the response is primary or a secondary phenomenon. Expression of dog lymphocyte antigen (DLA) class II in some dogs suggests a role for the immune system in chronic hepatitis.
- Drug-associated: anticonvulsants, NSAIDs, trimethoprim-sulfadiazine, lomustine, or potentially almost any drug
- Copper-associated liver disease: defective copper metabolism or increased dietary copper intake
- Other conditions: aflatoxins, chemicals, or other environmental factors

DIAGNOSIS

Diagnostic Overview

The diagnosis is suspected in any dog with historical, physical, biochemical, or imaging-identified signs of hepatobiliary disease. Confirmation is achieved by histologic analysis of a liver biopsy specimen. Unexplained persistent abnormal liver enzyme activities should initiate investigation of possible chronic hepatitis.

Differential Diagnosis

- Acute hepatitis
- Hepatic neoplasia
- Pancreatitis
- Reactive hepatopathies secondary to systemic, metabolic, or GI disease
- Congenital portosystemic shunts (HE)
- Cholecystitis or extrahepatic bile duct obstruction (icterus)

Initial Database

- CBC: nonregenerative anemia, stress leukogram possible
- Serum biochemistry profile: increased liver enzyme activities, including alanine aminotransferase (ALT), aspartate aminotransferase (AST), alkaline phosphatase (ALP), and gamma-glutamyltransferase (GGT), are extremely common. In advanced disease, hyperbilirubinemia and decreased albumin, glucose, blood urea nitrogen, and/or cholesterol concentrations may occur. Hyperglobulinemia is often observed.
- Urinalysis: bilirubinuria, variable specific gravity, and sometimes ammonium biurate crystalluria associated with hyperammonemia
- Abdominal radiographs: normal or small liver ± signs of ascites in advanced disease (cirrhosis/hepatic failure)

Advanced or Confirmatory Testing

- Elevated serum bile acid concentrations suggesting altered hepatic function or portal shunting
- Elevated plasma ammonia concentrations or ammonia tolerance test (often associated with portosystemic shunting).
- Coagulation tests: prothrombin time (PT), activated partial thromboplastin time (aPTT; most common abnormality), thrombocytopenia, and proteins induced by vitamin K antagonism (PIVKA) may become abnormal in advanced disease. Thromboelastography (TEG) may demonstrate a hypercoagulable or hypocoagulable state.
- Abdominal ultrasonography: variable hepatic parenchymal changes. Microhepatica, nodular liver, and ascites occur in late-stage disease (cirrhosis/hepatic failure). Decreased portal flow and evidence of acquired shunt formation are seen with portal hypertension. Ultrasound findings may be normal or nonspecific, even in advanced disease.
- Ultrasound-directed fine-needle aspiration and cytology *cannot* accurately diagnose chronic hepatitis, but can identify some other causes of hepatic dysfunction (e.g., neoplasia).
- Serologic testing as indicated by geography or other clinical signs: potentially includes tests for leptospirosis, bartonellosis, leishmaniasis, and antinuclear antibody (ANA) titer for immune-mediated disease.
- Abdominocentesis (pp. 1056 and 1343) in patients with ascites demonstrates a pure or modified transudate.
- Surgery or laparoscopy (p. 1128): grossly, liver may appear normal (subclinical disease) or may be small, nodular, and fibrotic/firm (advanced disease).
- Liver biopsy and histopathologic evaluation
  - Assess coagulation before biopsy, and consider pre-biopsy plasma transfusion if indicated.
  - Large biopsies (obtained by laparoscopy or laparotomy) are preferred over needle-core biopsies because of superior diagnostic accuracy.
  - Obtain liver samples for quantitative copper and iron analysis and for culture and sensitivity.
  - Subclinical disease is associated with infiltration of mononuclear inflammatory cells into portal and parenchymal areas.
  - Clinical disease is associated with evidence of active hepatitis, with areas of piecemeal and bridging necrosis.
  - In cirrhosis, extensive fibrosis and nodular regeneration are also present.
  - Histochemical staining for copper and iron are often positive.
- Hepatic metal quantitative analysis: hepatic copper can accumulate secondary to the liver disease; concentrations often range from 600-1500 mcg/g dry weight liver (normal < 400 mcg/g). Values > 1000 mcg/g can be associated with a primary copper-associated hepatopathy (p. 458). Hepatic copper can also be determined with computer-assisted digital analysis of copper-stained hepatic biopsy specimens. Hepatic iron is often elevated > 1200 mcg/g dry weight and is thought to accumulate in macrophages from hepatic parenchymal death.

TREATMENT

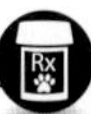

Treatment Overview

If an underlying cause can be identified, it should be addressed directly. Otherwise, treatment is aimed at halting/slowing progression of ongoing inflammation, providing optimal nutrition and hepatic support, and treating complications as they occur.

Acute General Treatment

Complications of chronic hepatitis should be treated as they occur. Commonly used treatments during acute management of idiopathic chronic hepatitis:

- Fluid therapy to correct deficits and electrolyte losses: supplemental dextrose 2.5%-5% is recommended; limit sodium with ascites (e.g., switch to low-sodium, isotonic maintenance fluid when patient is hydrated, such as Plasma-Lyte 56 plus 5% dextrose, with potassium supplementation).
- Dextrans, hetastarch, plasma, or albumin infusions if necessary to improve oncotic pressure during administration of IV crystalloid fluids
- Gastric ulceration (p. 380): omeprazole 0.7-1 mg/kg PO q 12-24h and sucralfate 0.5-1 g PO q 8h; avoid cimetidine because of hepatic metabolism
- HE treatment (p. 440): lactulose, antibiotics
- Coagulopathies are treated with fresh-frozen plasma or fresh whole blood (p. 1169) if there is evidence of overt bleeding and anemia. Stored blood should be avoided due to high ammonia concentrations.
- If ascites causes discomfort or respiratory compromise, treat with abdominocentesis (p. 1056). Diuretics are less effective and possibly associated with greater side effects in the acute stages of mobilizing ascitic fluid (see below).
- Sepsis (p. 907): if present, appropriate antibiotics immediately

Chronic Treatment

All therapy discussed below lacks critical scientific review in dogs but reflects the current consensus of a number of veterinary gastroenterologists:

- Antiinflammatory therapy using prednisolone 1-2 mg/kg PO q 24h; maximum dose 60 mg/day. Dosage is often tapered to 0.5 mg/kg q 24-48h after there is clinical improvement. Corticosteroids cause a secondary vacuolar (steroid) hepatopathy; monitoring of ALP is not helpful, but there should be a decline in serum bilirubin, ALT, and AST concentrations and often an increase in serum albumin concentration during effective treatment.
  - If ascites present, dexamethasone 0.2 mg/kg PO q 24-48h is used instead to avoid mineralocorticoid effect.
  - For corticosteroid-intolerant animals or for additional immunomodulation, azathioprine 2 mg/kg PO q 24h for 1 week, then q 48h, or mycophenolate mofetil

10-15 mg/kg q 12h can be given alone or in combination with glucocorticoids.
  - Cyclosporine (author's preference) 5 mg/kg q 12h, tapering to 5 mg/kg PO q 24h with improvement can be given for immunosuppression without the need for glucocorticoids and with potentially fewer side effects than azathioprine or mycophenolate.
  - Corticosteroids or immunosuppressive therapy appears to prolong survival or resolve hepatitis, although large case studies are lacking.
- Copper chelation if hepatic copper concentrations are > 600-1000 mcg/g dry liver weight (p. 458)
- If there is deficiency in advanced disease, zinc gluconate 2-3 mg/kg PO q 24h is indicated. Higher doses of zinc block intestinal copper absorption and could be considered after copper chelation therapy.
- Ursodeoxycholic acid 10-15 mg/kg PO q 24h is a hydrophilic bile acid that has immunomodulatory, antioxidant, hepatoprotective, and choleretic effects. Although widely used for canine hepatopathy, strong evidence of efficacy is lacking.
- Antioxidant therapy is used because oxidative damage is shown to occur in many dogs with hepatic disease. Selection of one or several antioxidants is suggested, including vitamin E 10 IU/kg PO q 24h, *S*-adenosylmethionine (SAMe) 20 mg/kg PO q 24h or q 48h, or milk thistle (silybin complexed with phosphatidylcholine) 24-70 mg/kg/day. Commercial products (e.g., Denamarin, Nutramax Laboratories) combine multiple antioxidants.
- Antibiotics are used to modify GI bacterial flora in HE, treat or reduce the incidence of secondary infection, or to treat a primary pathogen (e.g., *Leptospira*).
- The mainstay of antifibrotic therapy is reducing inflammation. Although colchicine 0.03 mg/kg PO q 24h inhibits collagen formation, few studies report its use in dogs, and human studies fail to show prolonged survival. Angiotensin-receptor blockers have shown promise in inhibiting fibrosis in humans and may have an application in dogs (e.g., telmisartan 0.5-1 mg/kg PO q 12h), although studies on safety and efficacy are lacking. Phosphatidylcholine 20-70 mg/kg/day PO may also have antifibrotic effects but has not been studied in this setting.
- Ascites
  - Medical treatment involves diuretics for long-term chronic management. Spironolactone 0.5-1 mg/kg PO q 12h is suggested as the initial diuretic. If ascites is not controlled, furosemide 0.5-2 mg/kg PO q 12h or combination of both drugs should be considered.
  - Abdominal drainage can be performed intermittently as needed for comfort when patients develop tense ascites (very large volumes of abdominal fluid). Caution is advised because abdominocentesis may result in hypovolemia and protein loss.

Nutrition/Diet

- Palatability is important in advanced cases because adequate caloric intake is crucial.
- Avoid protein restriction unless HE is present. Dietary protein content should represent 18%-22% of digestible kcal/day. Feed a high-quality, moderate-protein diet given in small multiple feedings. Milk and vegetable protein sources are more beneficial in HE than meat protein–based diets.
- Fermentable fiber may also be beneficial in controlling HE.
- Specialty veterinary hepatic diets are low in copper and prevent hepatic copper accumulation. These diets are also rich in antioxidants and other liver-support ingredients.

Drug Interactions

- Avoid drugs that require hepatic metabolism or alter hepatic biotransformation (e.g., cimetidine), and avoid drugs with known risk for hepatotoxicity (e.g., phenobarbital).
- Glucocorticoids may cause sodium retention, promote GI ulceration, or precipitate hepatic failure with advanced disease. Glucocorticoids also result in a vacuolar (steroid) hepatopathy, making laboratory evaluation of treatment response difficult.
- Penicillamine and zinc should not be given together; penicillamine can chelate zinc.
- Animals with hepatic failure are anesthetic risks. Barbiturates should be avoided, and benzodiazepines should be used with care. Isoflurane or sevoflurane are the gas anesthetics of choice. Propofol, although metabolized in the liver, is generally safe when administered to effect (usually requiring a small fraction of usual dosages).
- Lidocaine, theophylline, propranolol, captopril, and tetracyclines should be avoided.
- Diuretics may worsen HE, promote dehydration or metabolic alkalosis and should be used only in otherwise stable patients for the long-term delay of return of ascites or if necessary for concurrent conditions (e.g., congestive heart failure).
- NSAIDs may exacerbate GI ulceration.

Possible Complications

Ascites, HE, GI ulceration, sepsis, and disseminated intravascular coagulation are potential complications and are grave prognostic indicators.

Recommended Monitoring

- Monitor general condition, body weight, and behavior.
- Periodic evaluation of laboratory tests (CBC, serum biochemical profile)
- Follow-up liver biopsy provides the best means of evaluating treatment response for amount of ongoing inflammation and hepatic copper concentrations.

PROGNOSIS & OUTCOME

- Guarded to fair based on clinical signs at the time of diagnosis and extent of liver damage
- Early diagnosis and therapy can prolong survival, but limited studies are available on survival times (cirrhosis 1-2 months; chronic hepatitis several months to years).
- Most dogs are diagnosed when clinical signs occur, which are usually associated with more advanced hepatitis and a guarded prognosis.
- By the time liver failure manifests (e.g., ascites, HE, hypoalbuminemia), the prognosis is grave.

PEARLS & CONSIDERATIONS

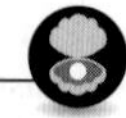

Comments

- The first clue to chronic hepatitis is unexplained abnormal serum liver enzyme activities (increased ALT is especially concerning).
- Because of the great reserve capacity of the liver, signs of liver failure do not occur until the disease is advanced.
- Immunomodulatory therapy in early stages of hepatitis may prolong survival.

Technician Tips

- Ensure patients intended for bile acid panel testing, abdominal imaging, and liver biopsy are fasted for 12 hours.
- After liver biopsy, the patient must be monitored closely for bleeding, including obtaining a packed cell volume/total solids (PCV/TS) evaluation 3 and 6 hours after biopsy.

Client Education

- A complete cure is unlikely.
- Medication is generally lifelong but may prolong quality of life and survival time.
- Repeat liver biopsies are recommended to monitor response to therapy.

SUGGESTED READING

Bexfield N: Canine idiopathic chronic hepatitis. Vet Clin North Am Small Anim Pract 47:645-663, 2017.

AUTHOR: David C. Twedt, DVM, DACVIM
EDITOR: Keith P. Richter, DVM, MSEL, DACVIM

Hepatobiliary Infections and Abscesses (Bacterial)

Client Education Sheet

BASIC INFORMATION

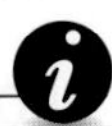

Definition

Bacterial hepatobiliary infections and hepatic abscesses are uncommon but potentially important infectious diseases in pets. *Cholangitis* refers to inflammation of intrahepatic bile ducts; *cholangiohepatitis* refers to inflammation of the bile ducts that has spread to adjacent hepatic tissues. Use of the term *cholangitis* for both conditions is recommended by the World Small Animal Veterinary Association (WSAVA) Liver Diseases and Pathology Standardization Group. Hepatic abscess characterizes areas of suppuration (microscopic or macroscopic) in the liver. Septic and aseptic forms of these inflammatory conditions occur, but this chapter deals only with bacterial infections other than leptospirosis (p. 583) and not with viral, fungal, protozoal, or parasitic hepatic infections.

Synonyms

Bacterial cholecystitis, bacterial cholangitis, bacterial cholangiohepatitis, choledochitis, emphysematous cholecystitis, neutrophilic cholangitis, suppurative cholangitis, hepatic microabscess, hepatic macroabscess

Epidemiology

SPECIES, AGE, SEX

- Hepatic abscess is uncommon in dogs and rare in cats.
- Bacterial cholangitis is more common in cats (p. 160) than dogs.
- Female dogs may be slighly predisposed; abscess is more likely in older animals.

RISK FACTORS

Although not proven, potential risk factors include an immunocompromised state, immunosuppressive drug therapy, trauma, extrahepatic infection, sepsis, biliary surgery, altered blood flow, and neoplasia.

ASSOCIATED DISORDERS

Pancreatitis, inflammatory bowel disease, feline triaditis, acute hepatitis, chronic hepatitis, hepatic neoplasia, cholelithiasis, biliary mucocele, sepsis, peritonitis, and coagulopathies

Clinical Presentation

HISTORY, CHIEF COMPLAINT

- Clinical signs are nonspecific and can be acute, chronic, or sometimes peracute (more likely with biliary or abcess rupture).
- Animals with hepatic abscess are more likely to have severe clinical illness, and those with cholangitis can have minimal signs of disease.
- Possible clinical signs include inappetence/anorexia, vomiting, diarrhea, lethargy, weight loss, pyrexia, polyuria, polydipsia, bleeding diathesis, hypersalivation, and icterus.

PHYSICAL EXAM FINDINGS

Depends on clinical presentation/disease severity and can be largely unremarkable or include the above findings plus abdominal discomfort, poor body condition, and depressed mentation. Sometimes, there may be evidence of systemic inflammatory response syndrome (SIRS) or other organ dysfunction (p. 665).

Etiology and Pathophysiology

- Bacteria can be found in the hepatobiliary tract without concurrent inflammation or illness but can also be associated with disease. In cats, 14% of hepatic cultures and 36% of biliary cultures are positive for bacterial growth, compared with 5% and 28% in dogs, respectively.
- Bacteria most commonly isolated include obligate anaerobes, Enterobacteriaceae, *Enterococcus*, *Streptococcus*, and *Staphylococcus* spp. Multiple isolates are found in ≈50% of dogs and 20% of cats. Emphasematous cholecystisis is usually associated with *Clostridium* or *Escherichia coli* infection.
- Bacteria usually invade the hepatobiliary tract by ascending from the gastrointestinal (GI) tract through the common bile duct or by the portal vein. The hepatic artery can also transport systemic bacteria to the liver.

DIAGNOSIS

Diagnostic Overview

Routine laboratory testing may raise suspicion, but confirmation of infection is obtained using advanced imaging with abdominal sonography and/or abdominal computed tomography with guided gallbladder and lesional aspiration, followed by cytology and culture.

Differential Diagnosis

- Icterus (pp. 528 and 1243)
- Acute abdomen (p. 21)
- Other causes of primary hepatobiliary disease (e.g., chronic hepatitis, gallbladder mucocele, feline infectious peritonitis)

Initial Database

- Complete blood count: varies; neutrophilic leukocytosis ± left shift ± lymphopenia ± anemia
- Serum biochemical panel
  - Usually, increased liver enzyme activities (alkaline phosphatase [ALP], alanine aminotransferase [ALT], aspartate aminotransferase [AST], gamma-glutamyltransferase [GGT])
  - Rarely, evidence of synthetic failure (i.e., hypoalbuminemia, hypoglycemia, low blood urea nitrogen [BUN], low cholesterol concentrations)
  - Sometimes, increased cholesterol and bilirubin concentrations (with extrahepatic biliary obstruction)
  - Electrolyte abnormalities may occur due to vomiting.
- Urinalysis: bilirubinuria common, crystalluria occasionally
- Bile acid testing (p. 1312): to assess function in anicteric patients
- Coagulation profile (p. 1325): before any surgical intervention or procedure
- Abdominal radiographs: can be unremarkable but hepatomegaly and cholelithiasis are sometimes recognized. In emphysematous cholecystitis, gas may be seen in region of the gallbladder. With hepatic abscess, may identify mass effect, abdominal effusion, or rarely, pneumoperitoneum with rupture.
- Abdominal ultrasonography: may recognize homogenous or heterogenous increase in echogenicity, prominent portal vasculuture, thickened/emphysematous gallbladder wall, distention of biliary tree, free abdominal fluid (peritonitis), or hypo/anechoic hepatic mass
  - Fine-needle aspirates for cytologic evaluation if there is suspicion of infection, even in a sonographically normal liver (p. 1112)
  - Degenerate neutrophils ± intracellular bacteria
  - Helps rule out other types of hepatic disease
- Testing for leptospirosis often indicated to rule out this zoonotic infection (p. 583)
- If abdominal effusion present, abdominocentesis with fluid analysis (pp. 1056 and 1343)

Advanced or Confirmatory Testing

- Percutaneous ultrasound-guided cholecystocentesis to rule out infection, and/or if there are ultrasonographic changes suggesting infection; submit for cytology, aerobic/anaerobic culture, and sensitivity.
  - Ultrasonographic appearance of the gallbladder has a high sensitivity to predict a positive bile culture (cats 96%, dogs 81%)
  - If concerned about biliary rupture due to abnormal appearance of gallbladder wall, blood culture recommended
- Definitive diagnosis of hepatic parenchymal infections in most cases requires laparoscopic or surgical liver biopsy, histopathologic evaluation, and bacterial culture and senstivity testing.
  - Fresh samples of the liver should be saved for atypical bacterial infections such as *Mycobacteria* and *Bartonella*.
  - Most special stains and fluorescence *in situ* hybridization (FISH) can be performed on formalin-fixed tissue.

TREATMENT

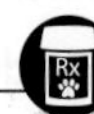

Treatment Overview

The treatment of bacterial hepatobiliary infection is a minimum of 4-6 weeks of continuous antimicrobial therapy based on the results of culture and sensitivity testing. Animals with extrahepatic biliary obstruction, hepatic abscessation, and bacterial cholecystitis may require surgery.

Acute General Treatment

- Withhold antimicrobials until samples for culture and sensitivity testing have been acquired unless signs of SIRS are observed.
- If recognized, address sepsis (p. 907) immediately.
- If prothrombin time (PT) and activated partial thromboplastin time (aPTT) are prolonged, administer vitamin K_1 (although many coagulopathies are not improved with vitamin K administration). Fresh or fresh frozen plasma transfusion may be required.
- Surgical resection is the preferred treatment for hepatic abscesses, and immediate surgical intervention is indicated in cases of a compromised gallbladder, severe extrahepatic biliary obstruction, or septic peritonitis (pp. 118 and 779).
- The ideal features of an antibiotic selected for empirical use include broad-spectrum bactericidal, therapeutic levels in bile, and no requirement for hepatic metabolism for activation or excretion. *E. coli* is the most commonly isolated organism, and susceptibility for this organism in empirical drug selection is recommended. Initial empirical choices may include:
  - Stable animal with cholangitis and mild to moderate signs of illness: amoxicillin-clavulanic acid 12.5-20 mg/kg PO q 12h (dog or cat) *or* pradofloxacin 7.5 mg/kg PO q 24h (cats)
  - Critically ill animal: ampicillin-sulbactam 22-30 mg/kg IV q 6-8h and enrofloxacin 10 mg/kg q 24h diluted slow IV (dog) *or* imipenem 10 mg/kg IV q 8h *or* cefoxitin 30 mg/kg IV q 8h and metronidazole 8-15 mg/kg IV q 8h
- Appropriate analgesia should be administered if indicated.

Chronic Treatment

- The choice of long-term antibiotic should be based on the results of culture of bile/liver and sensitivity tests. Prolonged therapy for a minimum of 4-6 weeks is required, and cessation of therapy should be based on negative culture and sensitivity testing if possible, along with normalization of laboratory abnormalities.
- Antioxidant therapy with *S*-adenosylmethionine (SAMe) or *N*-acetylcysteine are believed to restore glutathione levels that are reduced in liver disease (reduced glutathione can increase oxidative damage).
- The role of nutraceutical therapy is largely theoretical. Choleretics, such as ursodeoxycholic acid, are of value in promoting bile flow, and this is indicated unless extrahepatic biliary obstruction is present.

Nutrition/Diet

- Nutritional support is required, and the route is determined by clinical condition. An esophageal feeding tube may assist in caloric intake and drug administration (p. 1106).
- Protein restriction is indicated only if there are signs of hepatic encephalopathy.

Drug Interactions

Pharmacokinetics may be affected by altered liver function; avoid potentially hepatotoxic drugs.

Possible Complications

Sepsis, septic peritonitis, bile peritonitis, gallbladder rupture, recurrence with ineffective treatment, multidrug-resistant infection, hepatic lipidosis (cats) with prolonged anorexia or inadequate nutritional support

Recommended Monitoring

- Patients hospitalized for systemic involvement should be intensively monitored in a critical care setting, including frequent vital parameter assessment (heart and respiratory rate, temperature, blood pressure, body weight).
  - Serial serum biochemistry profile evaluation
  - Serial coagulation status assessment
  - Serial complete blood count evaluation
- Patients stable for outpatient therapy should be reassessed every 1-2 weeks with monitoring of serum liver enzymes and focused hepatobiliary ultrasonography as indicated until resolution.

PROGNOSIS & OUTCOME

- Bacterial cholangitis may be a single curable occurance, or become chronic in cases of ineffective antimicrobial therapy or in cases with surgically altered biliary anatomy. The prognosis is generally good with early diagnosis and appropriate treatment.
- Hepatic abscesses are life-threatening, with mortality rates > 50% in several studies.

PEARLS & CONSIDERATIONS

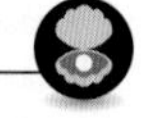

Comments

- Select cases (e.g., hepatic abscesses, bacterial cholecystitis/bactibilia) may require surgical management, and in the case of hepatic abscess, surgical management is preferred.
- Multidrug-resistant infections are common with ineffective or inappropriate antibiotic therapy, and treatment based on culture and sensitivity is recommended.

Technician Tips

Monitor patients closely for signs of SIRS (hypothermia, hyperthermia, tachycardia, bradycardia, tachypnea).

Client Education

Recurrence and persistent infection is possible even with appropriate antimicrobial therapy.

SUGGESTED READING

Webb CB: Canine inflammatory/infectious hepatic disease. In Ettinger SJ, et al, editors: Textbook of veterinary internal medicine, ed 8, St. Louis, 2017, Saunders.

AUTHOR: Yuri A. Lawrence, DVM, PhD, MS, MA, DACVIM
EDITOR: Keith P. Richter, DVM, MSEL, DACVIM

Hepatomegaly

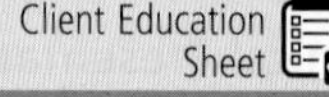

BASIC INFORMATION

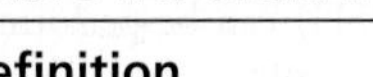

Definition

Liver enlargement

Epidemiology

SPECIES, AGE, SEX

Dogs > cats of any age but most often encountered in middle-aged to older patients; no sex predisposition

GENETICS, BREED PREDISPOSITION

Examples:

- Chronic hepatitis: Labrador retrievers, standard poodles, cocker spaniels
- Copper storage disease: Doberman pinschers, Labrador retrievers, Dalmations, West Highland white terriers, Skye terriers, Bedlington terriers
- Amyloidosis: Abyssinian cats, Chinese Shar-peis

RISK FACTORS

See Hepatomegaly (p. 1231).

ASSOCIATED DISORDERS

Hyperadrenocorticism (HAC), diabetes mellitus (DM), neoplasia, right-sided heart failure, hepatitis/cholangiohepatitis, and many other disorders that can cause hepatic enlargement

Clinical Presentation

HISTORY, CHIEF COMPLAINT

Hepatomegaly is a sign of an underlying disorder. Complete history, including vaccinations, medications and supplements, and changes in appetite, thirst, or behavior is required.

- Occasionally, abdominal distention due to hepatomegaly is the presenting complaint.
- Hepatomegaly may be an incidental finding on routine exam.
- Commonly, complaints are related to the underlying disease process causing hepatic enlargement. Complaints often include change in appetite or weight, polyuria/polydipsia, vomiting, or diarrhea.

PHYSICAL EXAM FINDINGS

- Other than cranial abdominal organomegaly, exam findings depend on underlying cause (e.g., hair loss, panting, and pendulous abdomen common with HAC; emaciation and icterus identified with some neoplastic disorders; right-sided heart murmur, jugular pulse, and ascites with right-sided heart failure).
- Hepatomegaly may not be appreciated on the exam of obese patients or those with tense ascites.

Etiology and Pathophysiology

Hepatomegaly can be caused by cellular infiltration (inflammatory, infectious, neoplastic), accumulation of metabolic by-products, hepatocyte swelling, hyperplasia, or congestion (p. 1231). Examples

- Exogenous glucocorticoid use or HAC lead to accumulation of glycogen in hepatocytes.
- Neoplastic lymphocytes infiltrate around hepatocytes in hepatic lymphoma.
- Right-sided heart failure leads to congestion of the portal veins.

Some causes of hepatomegaly are completely benign, but others indicate life- threatening disorders.

DIAGNOSIS

Diagnostic Overview

History, exam findings, minimum database, and radiographs guide additional diagnostic testing. For example, patients with polyuria/polydipsia, bilaterally symmetric alopecia, and hypercholesterolemia along with a high alkaline phosphatase level should be tested for HAC; whereas patients with weight loss, anorexia, vomiting, and hyperbilirubinemia should undergo early abdominal ultrasound.

Differential Diagnosis

Splenomegaly can be mistaken for hepatomegaly.

Initial Database

- CBC: may be normal
  - Anemia: inflammatory disease, hemorrhage due to ulcer, coagulopathy
  - Leukocytosis +/− left shift in inflammatory/infectious conditions
  - Stress leukogram: HAC, other illness
  - Thrombocytopenia: secondary to consumption
  - Thrombocytosis: HAC, gastrointestinal (GI) bleeding, neoplasia
- Serum biochemical profile
  - Some combination of increased alanine aminotransferase (ALT), alkaline phosphatase (ALP), aspartate aminotransferase (AST), gamma-glutamyltransferase (GGT) commonly identified
  - Hyperbilirubinemia may occur with intrahepatic bile stasis from cellular swelling/ infiltrates
  - Hypercholesterolemia seen with HAC, DM, or biliary obstruction
  - Hyperglycemia with DM
  - Low blood urea nitrogen (BUN) level, hypocholesterolemia, hypoglycemia, hypoalbuminemia, and hyperbilirubinemia may be apparent with hepatic dysfunction.
- Urinalysis
  - A low urine specific gravity often identified
  - Bilirubinuria may be present even in the absence of overt hyperbilirubinemia.
  - Ammonium biurate crystalluria may be seen with hepatic dysfunction.
- Abdominal radiographs: provides objective measure of liver size; difficult to interpret if marked ascites present
- Thoracic radiographs: warranted when right-sided congestive heart failure or neoplasia is suspected.

Advanced or Confirmatory Testing

- Abdominal ultrasound: evaluate hepatic parenchyma for mass lesions, changes in margination or echogenicity. Nonhepatic abnormalities (e.g., bilateral adrenomegaly, splenomegaly) may aid in diagnosis.
- Pursue diagnostic testing aimed at nonhepatic causes of hepatomegaly, as appropriate
  - Suspect HAC (p. 485)
  - Suspect right-sided heart disease: thoracic radiographs, echocardiogram
  - Suspect infectious disease: serologic titers or polymerase chain reaction (PCR) testing
- Abdominocentesis, if fluid present (pp. 1056 and 1343)
- Bile acids: assess hepatic function in animals with normal total bilirubin (p. 1312)
- Ammonia: often increased with hepatic encephalopathy (p. 440)
- Coagulation profile (p. 1325): prothrombin time, activated partial thromboplastin time may be prolonged. Always check before liver biopsy.
- Cholecystocentesis: if cholangiohepatitis suspected, bile samples submitted for cytology and aerobic/anaerobic culture
- Hepatic cytology: can establish diagnosis of hepatic neoplasia (e.g., lymphoma) or lipidosis
- Liver biopsy with histopathology: often required for definitive diagnosis of primary hepatic disease
  - Aerobic and anaerobic culture/sensitivity from tissue
  - Hepatic copper quantification
  - Special stains can be beneficial (e.g., Congo red stain for amyloidosis)

TREATMENT

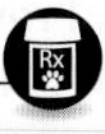

Treatment Overview

Treatment depends on the underlying cause and associated complications.

Acute General Treatment

- Supportive care is based on clinical signs, such as IV crystalloid fluids for rehydration and antiemetics (e.g., maropitant, ondansetron, dolasetron) for vomiting.
- Address hepatic encephalopathy (p. 440).
- Abdominocentesis for tense ascites (p. 1056)
- Transfusion, as appropriate (p. 1169)
- Address coagulopathy: vitamin K, transfusion (fresh or fresh-frozen plasma, whole blood)

Chronic Treatment

- Treatment is directed toward the underlying cause of hepatomegaly.
- Hepatoprotectants often considered
  - Denamarin
  - *S*-adenosylmethionine (SAMe)
  - Milk thistle
  - *N*-acetylcysteine (NAC)

Nutrition/Diet

Moderate- to low-protein diets indicated for hepatic encephalopathy; limited-copper diets used for copper storage disease (p. 458)

Drug Interactions

If hepatic dysfunction exists, avoid or consider dosage alteration for drugs with hepatic metabolism.

Possible Complications

Ascites, hepatic encephalopathy, coagulopathies

PROGNOSIS & OUTCOME

Prognosis depends on cause; good to guarded

PEARLS & CONSIDERATIONS

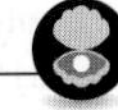

Comments

- Bile acids test is not indicated for icteric animals except to rule out hemolytic disease.
- Hepatic cytology often generates nonspecific results due to the inability to assess tissue architecture and hemodilution. Cytology should not be used to exclude diagnosis. For example, a finding of benign vacuolar change does not exclude the presence of other concurrent liver disease such as cholangiohepatitis or chronic hepatitis.
- Many causes of hepatomegaly (e.g., HAC, DM) are associated with relatively normal liver function.
- The absence of clinical signs does not exclude important liver disease/dysfunction, and hepatomegaly should not be ignored.

- Laparoscopic biopsies are preferred over needle biopsies due to the larger tissue sample obtained.

Prevention

Avoid prolonged use of glucocorticoids when possible.

Technician Tips

- Avoid jugular venipuncture until coagulation is assessed as normal.
- Blood for bile acids is collected after a 12-hour fast (preprandial) and 2 hours after feeding a fatty meal (postprandial).

SUGGESTED READING

Dirksen K, et al: Sensitivity and specificity of plasma ALT, ALP, and bile acids for hepatitis in Labrador Retrievers. J Vet Intern Med 31(4):1017-1027, 2017.

AUTHOR: Julie E. Trzil, DVM, MS, DACVIM
EDITOR: Leah A. Cohn, DVM, PhD, DACVIM

Hepatopathy, Copper-Associated

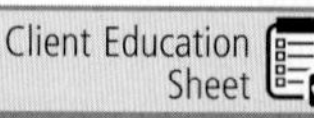

BASIC INFORMATION

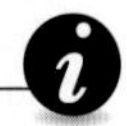

Definition

Accumulation of copper within hepatocytes, leading to hepatotoxicosis

Epidemiology

SPECIES, AGE, SEX

- Dogs: common; copper accumulates slowly, and clinical signs typically appear in middle age
- Cats: rare, younger (median age, 2 years)

GENETICS, BREED PREDISPOSITION

- Autosomal recessive in Bedlington terriers
- Predisposition in Dalmatians, West Highland white terriers, Labrador retrievers, Doberman pinschers and standard poodles
- Can happen sporadically in any breed of dog or cat

Clinical Presentation

DISEASE FORMS/SUBTYPES

- Subclinical
- Chronic hepatitis/cirrhosis
- Acute liver disease with hemolytic anemia (rare)

HISTORY, CHIEF COMPLAINT

- Patients usually present with features of chronic hepatic disease such as polyuria and polydipsia, lethargy, vomiting, abdominal distention, or encephalopathy (p. 440) or, less commonly, with acute liver failure (p. 442) and hemolytic anemia (p. 59).
- In early stages, patients may be asymptomatic with just increased serum liver enzyme activities, particularly serum alanine aminotransferase (ALT).

Etiology and Pathophysiology

- Copper is absorbed in the small intestine and extracted by hepatocytes. Copper is chaperoned around the hepatocyte before being released into the serum or excreted in bile. A small amount is stored in lysosomes.
- Copper homeostasis is maintained by biliary excretion of excess copper.
- Abnormal hepatic copper accumulation occurs because of a primary inborn error of metabolism or secondary to increased dietary consumption or acquired cholestatic liver disease.
  - In Bedlingtons, a defect in the *COMMD1* gene leads to decreased biliary excretion of copper.
  - Genetic basis for copper accumulation in other breeds is unknown, but some evidence for mutation in *ATP7B* (a copper transporter) in Labradors
- Secondary copper accumulation is due to cholestatic disease and impairment in biliary excretion. This is a rare cause of copper accumulation in the dog but occurs in cats.
- Emerging evidence suggests that many dogs accumulate excess copper in the liver associated with excess dietary copper content.
- Accumulating copper puts oxidant stress on the liver, predisposing it to damage.
- Excess copper damages hepatocytes by inducing the formation of free radicals.
- Rarely, copper storage hepatopathy is associated with renal Fanconi syndrome (p. 322).

DIAGNOSIS

Diagnostic Overview

The disorder may be suspected in two contexts: as part of any necroinflammatory or cholestatic liver disease (detected as part of evaluation of liver biopsy specimens) or in cases where copper accumulation is the dominant feature of hepatopathy in a dog (e.g., Bedlington terrier) with or without overt clinical signs. Definitive diagnosis requires quantification of hepatic copper content from a liver biopsy specimen.

Differential Diagnosis

Chronic:

- Infectious, immune, or toxic causes of inflammatory hepatic disease
- Hepatic neoplasia
- Congenital portosystemic shunts

Acute:

- Infectious, immune, drug, or toxin-induced (zinc) hemolytic anemia
- Exposure to hepatotoxic drugs or environmental toxins
- Infectious canine hepatitis, leptospirosis

Initial Database

Tests to rule out hemolytic anemia (p. 59), cirrhotic/fibrosing liver disease (p. 174), acute hepatic injury (p. 442), and chronic idiopathic hepatitis (p. 452)

Advanced or Confirmatory Testing

Determination of hepatic copper concentration: quantitative analysis on hepatic wedge or needle biopsies, digital image analysis of scanned rhodanine-stained histopathology slides; qualitative and semiquantitative assessment of rhodamine- or rubeanic acid–stained slides

- Normal hepatic copper levels: 200-400 mcg/g dry weight (DW) in dog and < 190 mcg/g DW in cats
- In Bedlingtons, genetic test, microsatellite marker (C04107) available, but may miss disease in some pedigrees (5%-10% false-negatives). No test for *COMMD1* mutation is available.
- In Bedlingtons, copper levels gradually increase with age and can reach very high levels (>10,000 mcg/g DW).
- Lower copper levels (500-2000 mcg/g DW) typically occur in Labradors and Dobermans.
- Cats > 700 mcg/g DW is consistent with primary copper hepatopathy.

Histopathologic findings:

- Inborn errors such as occur in Bedlingtons: initial finding is centrilobular copper accumulation with hepatocellular vacuolation, followed by degeneration/necrosis and then inflammation and fibrosis; progresses to become more panlobular with periportal orientation
- In secondary copper accumulation, copper staining is located primarily in areas of inflammation or degeneration (periportal), with more accumulation in macrophages.
- Cats with primary copper hepatopathy are predisposed to develop hepatocellular carcinoma.

TREATMENT

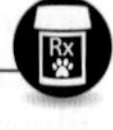

Treatment Overview

Decrease hepatic copper concentration, decrease copper absorption, and attenuate oxidant injury

Acute General Treatment

Manage the complications of acute or chronic hepatic disease (pp. 174 and 452).

Chronic Treatment

In dogs other than Bedlingtons and Dalmatians, the need to treat elevated hepatic copper concentrations is based on distribution of the copper in the biopsy, the presence of concurrent liver injury or inflammation, and evaluation of clinicopathologic markers of liver injury.

There is no hepatic copper concentration that is considered diagnostic of a primary copper hepatopathy in dogs. All dogs with inflammatory changes and high copper concentrations should be treated.

In cats with hepatic copper content of > 700 mcg/g DW in the presence of hepatic centrolobular necroinflammatory or vacuolar change, a primary copper storage hepatopathy should be considered.

- Copper chelators for initial de-coppering of liver and maintenance therapy
  - Penicillamine 10-15 mg/kg PO q 12h increases urinary copper excretion. Works slowly (removes ≈900 mcg/g per year), and copper levels take several months to decrease. The rate of de-coppering varies; dogs with higher initial values and those with inborn errors take longer. Side effects include vomiting and immune-mediated reactions (skin, kidney). The drug is also teratogenic.
  - Trientine 10-15 mg/kg PO q 12h increases urinary copper excretion and may block intestinal uptake. Fewer side effects than penicillamine but more expensive
  - Give medications on an empty stomach.
- Inhibit intestinal copper absorption.
  - Elemental zinc (dose poorly documented; 5-10 mg/kg PO q 8-12h)
  - Induces intestinal metallothionein, which binds copper, keeping it sequestered within the enterocyte, and decreases copper absorption. Side effects include vomiting (may give with small amount of food but decreases absorption) and hemolytic anemia. Keep serum zinc levels < 600 mcg/dL to avoid hemolysis. Effective zinc levels are > 200 mcg/dL.
  - Not recommended for initial de-coppering of the liver.
  - Do not use with penicillamine.
- Antioxidants
  - Induction of oxidant stress is central to copper-induced hepatic damage.
  - Vitamin E 10 IU/kg PO q 24h
  - *S*-adenosylmethionine (SAMe) 20 mg/kg PO q 24h

Nutrition/Diet

Reduce dietary intake of copper.

- Most dog foods are high in copper. Copper-restricted prescription diets are available. Avoid shellfish, nuts, and organ meats.
- Check copper in water supply if not public.

Possible Complications

- Chronic penicillamine therapy may be associated with vitamin B_6 deficiency. Supplement 25 mg/day PO
- Chronic zinc therapy can be associated with iron deficiency.

Recommended Monitoring

- Serum liver enzymes q 2-3 months
- Limited information on length of chelation necessary, must be individualized based on animal's response (normalization of serum liver enzymes and hepatic copper; repeat biopsy ideal)
- Maintenance therapy: poorly defined; dietary copper restriction for life +/− zinc or low-dose penicillamine

PROGNOSIS & OUTCOME

- Subclinical disease: excellent with therapy
- Chronic: depends on stage. Mild to moderate inflammatory disease: good. Severe inflammatory disease/cirrhosis: guarded.
- Acute: grave

PEARLS & CONSIDERATIONS

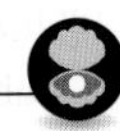

Comments

- All Bedlington terriers should be tested at 1 year of age by determination of hepatic copper concentration and/or genetic testing. Affected dogs should not be bred.
- All breeds predisposed to copper-associated chronic hepatitis (i.e., Labrador retrievers, West Highland white terriers, Doberman pinschers, and Dalmatians) should have hepatic copper analysis if hepatic biopsy is done.
- Rarely, reversible Fanconi syndrome (i.e., renal tubular dysfunction) has been documented along with copper hepatopathy.

Technician Tips

- Penicillamine-induced emesis can usually be avoided by slowly up-titrating to the required dose.
- Zinc-induced emesis is more difficult to manage. The dose can be reduced or given with food, although the latter practice decreases bioavailability.

SUGGESTED READING

Dirksen K, et al: Canine copper-associated hepatitis. Vet Clin North Am Small Anim Pract 47:631-644, 2017.

AUTHOR: Cynthia R. L. Webster, DVM, DACVIM
EDITOR: Keith P. Richter, DVM, MSEL, DACVIM

Hepatopathy, Copper-Associated, of Labrador Retrievers

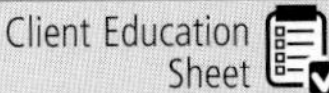

BASIC INFORMATION

Definition

Necroinflammatory hepatopathy affects Labrador retrievers as a response to a pathologic concentration of copper (Cu) in hepatocytes. This is a complex process involving dietary Cu, variable genetic mutations, and oxidative factors that concurrently stress hepatocytes. There can be acute, relapsing, and chronic syndromes. Copper-storage disease of other breeds is discussed on p. 458.

Synonyms

Copper-associated hepatitis (Cu-AH), copper storage hepatopathy

Epidemiology

SPECIES, AGE, SEX

More common in females

GENETICS, BREED PREDISPOSITION

- Breed: Labrador retrievers (Labrador cross-breeds, Labradoodles)
- Genetic testing is available and should be completed before breeding.
- Disease partially explained by recognized heritable factors
  - Missense mutation in Cu transporter *ATP7B* gene is inherited as an autosomal incomplete dominance pattern.
  - A protective mutation of the *ATP7A* gene is also recognized.
  - Other factors influence disease occurrence and severity.

RISK FACTORS

- Excess dietary Cu
- Other causes of inflammation and oxidative stress may precipitate a hepatocellular crisis.

ASSOCIATED DISORDERS

- Acute or chronic hepatitis
- Hepatic failure leading to hepatic encephalopathy

Clinical Presentation

DISEASE FORMS/SUBTYPES

- Subclinical: no clinical signs
- Acute: signs consistent with acute hepatocellular necroinflammatory disease where Cu-AH may be the primary disease or concurrent with another hepatic disorder (p. 442)
- Chronic: chronic ongoing or past elevations of alanine aminotransferase (ALT) and/or findings consistent with chronic liver disease (e.g., regenerative nodules, cirrhosis, acquired portosystemic shunts, ascites, fibrosis)

HISTORY, CHIEF COMPLAINT

- Subclinical Cu-AH
  - ALT elevation discovered inadvertently (e.g., preanesthesia lab testing or geriatric panel)
  - ALT may be normal in subclinically affected dogs; it is a poor biomarker (low sensitivity) for Cu accumulation.
- Acute Cu-AH: signs due to hepatocellular necrosis; chief complaints:
  - Can be mild to severe and develop over a few hours to days
  - Can include weakness, lethargy, vomiting, diarrhea, anorexia, variable jaundice, coagulopathies, hemolysis (rare), collapse
  - Hepatic encephalopathy (p. 440)
- Chronic Cu-AH: can include
  - History of past episodes of ALT elevations or unexplained illnesses
  - Slowly progressive or periods of lethargy, anorexia, vomiting, weight loss, diarrhea, polydipsia/polyuria
  - Ascites
  - Hepatic encephalopathy

PHYSICAL EXAM FINDINGS

- Subclinical Cu-AH: no abnormal findings
- Acute Cu-AH: weakness, variable jaundice, pallor, abdominal discomfort, ecchymoses
- Chronic Cu-AH: poor body condition, unkempt appearance, variable jaundice, abdominal effusion, bleeding

Etiology and Pathophysiology

- Risk increases with concentration of dietary Cu and the pattern of gene mutation. It is thought that elevated Cu concentration increases oxidative injury from other triggering events. These reactions induce hepatocellular death.
- Eventual lobular collapse occurs predominantly in zone 3. The ensuing necroinflammatory response stimulates fibrosis. Different lobules and regions of liver lobes may accumulate Cu at different rates and undergo varying degrees of necrosis so that severity of focal damage varies within the liver.
- This process allows for temporal ups and downs in serum ALT activities, clinical findings, as well as variable severity of biopsy findings.

DIAGNOSIS

Diagnostic Overview

Labrador retrievers with serum ALT elevations are logical suspects for Cu-AH. Confirmation depends on histopathology from liver biopsies showing zone 3–predominant hepatocellular necrosis, positive Cu staining, and abnormal quantitative Cu concentrations.

Differential Diagnosis

- Chronic hepatitis (inflammatory, immune mediated, infectious)
- Acute hepatic injury (hepatotoxic, infectious, other)
- Hepatic neoplasia
- Pancreatitis
- Bile duct obstruction or rupture

Initial Database

Laboratory and imaging findings are similar to those of any acute or chronic necroinflammatory hepatitis (pp. 174, 442, and 452).

Advanced or Confirmatory Testing

- Liver biopsy: laparoscopy (preferred [p. 1128]), laparotomy, or ultrasound guided
  - Ideally from ≥ 3 lobes (heterogenous disease), deeper and more surface oriented
  - Regenerative nodules may contain deceptively low Cu levels and should not be submitted for quantification.
- Histopathologic findings vary in severity of hepatocellular necrosis and often are worse in zone 3. Necroinflammatory response and lobular collapse are followed by bridging fibrosis.
- A panel of stains is superior for assessment.
  - Hematoxylin-eosin (H&E) for general assessment
  - Reticulin stain for lobular collapse
  - Masson's trichrome or Sirius red stain to highlight fibrosis
  - Rhodanine or rubeanic acid for Cu staining
- Quantitative Cu concentration often correlates with clinical severity.
  - Atomic absorption spectroscopy is most common test for quantitative Cu
  - Digital Cu quantification (DCQ) by computer processing of rhodanine-stained tissue correlates with the more common atomic absorption spectroscopy, providing an alternative method, and has the advantage of assessing multiple biopsies of different regions.
  - Affected dogs usually have values > 1000 mcg/g (mcg/g = ppm) dry weight liver (DWL), but normal is less than 400 mcg/g. Markedly affected dogs can exceed 2000-3000 mcg/g.

TREATMENT

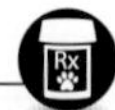

Treatment Overview

- Reduce Cu intake: food, supplements, potentially water sources
- Chelation therapy to help reduce hepatocellular Cu and increase elimination
- Antioxidants to reduce oxidative stress/ reactions within hepatocytes

Acute General Treatment

- Acute hepatic necrosis treatment (p. 442)
- Chelation therapy as soon as possible

Chronic Treatment

Chelation:

- D-penicillamine 10-15 mg/kg PO q 12h chelates Cu, promotes urinary Cu excretion, and provides other protective effects by binding of the Cu from oxidative reactions.
  - Initiate use if in affected patient hepatic Cu is > 500 mcg/g per DWL
  - Administer 1 hour before feeding to reduce nausea and vomiting, which is common.
  - Success results in histologic resolution of hepatitis; endpoint of therapy is sustained normalization of ALT.
  - Duration of chelation treatment varies; pre-treatment hepatic Cu concentration often correlates with the duration of therapy (higher concentration, longer treatment).
  - Repeated biopsy and Cu quantitation is helpful for clinical decision making.
  - Although it interferes with Cu uptake by enterocytes, zinc is not effective for de-coppering the liver.
- Transient dosing of prednisolone may aid in reducing hepatitis and improving patient well-being and appetite. However, negative concerns include potential of vacuolar hepatocellular swelling in a collapsed or regenerative nodule surrounded by fibrosis with increased cholestassis.
- Supplement pyridoxine (vitamin B_6) because D-penicillamine increases requirement for vitamin B_6.
- Chronic after Cu removal
  - Taper D-penicillamine by 50%, then every other day, and finally discontinue
  - Lifelong restriction of Cu intake
  - No benefit has been shown for providing zinc supplementation to Labradors eating only low-Cu diet.
- Trientine hydrochloride 5-7 mg/kg PO q 12h, an alternative Cu chelator, can be given if D-penicillamine is not tolerated (although it is very expensive).

Antioxidants:

- D-alpha-tocopherol (vitamin E 10 U/kg PO q 24h)
- *S*-adenosylmethionine (SAMe 20 mg/kg PO q 12-24h; give q 12h until the patient seems stable)

Hepatoprotectants:

- Ursodeoxycholic acid 15 mg/kg PO/day: in cases with significant necroinflammatory changes, notable suspected/proven fibrosis, and/or subsequent reduced hepatocellular function or cholestasis
- Silibinin (silybin): no proven benefit but safe; commercial preparation available in combination with SAMe (Denamarin)

Supportive care: see Chronic Hepatitis chapter (p. 452)

Nutrition/Diet

- Prescription diets for liver disease are low in Cu and should be fed during and after chelation therapy. These diets generally contain 3.5-7 ppm dry matter basis of Cu.
- In one study, hepatic Cu could be normalized in 50% of subclinically affected dogs with diet alone.

Drug Interactions

Oral zinc can impair chelation therapy.

Recommended Monitoring

- At 7-14 days after starting chelation and again in 3-4 weeks: include physical exam, CBC, serum chemistry profile, and urinalysis.

Monitoring q 1-3 months is adjusted based on response and tolerance of medications.
- Serum bile acid profile update at 3-4 months for nonicteric patients
- Long-term goal is serial trending of ALT toward the reference range.

PROGNOSIS & OUTCOME

- Affected by clinical severity, hepatic Cu concentration, and tolerance of medications
- Expect nodular regenerative response to be found on serial ultrasound scans that may not affect prognosis
- Pre-existing/acquired portosystemic shunts, cirrhosis, and ascites are negative factors.

PEARLS & CONSIDERATIONS

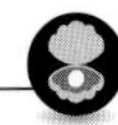

Comments

- Confirm that Cu staining findings correlate with quantitative assessment.
- Labrador retrievers with hepatitis can have a combination of chronic hepatitis (chronic active hepatitis, immune-mediated hepatitis) and Cu-AH. Disease may remain active after appropriate chelation therapy.
- Stain all liver biopsies for Cu.

Prevention

- Check for Cu-AH in pet's pedigree.
- Submit to genetic testing before breeding.
- Feed diets with reasonable Cu level.

Technician Tips

Control of nausea is critical because many of the desired treatments are PO.

Client Education

Low-Cu diet is needed lifelong.

SUGGESTED READING

Fieten H, et al: Long-term management of copper associated hepatitis in the Labrador retriever. J Vet Intern Med 28:721, 2014.

AUTHOR: Mark E. Hitt, DVM, MS, DACVIM
EDITOR: Keith P. Richter, DVM, MSEL, DACVIM

Hepatozoonosis

Bonus Material Online

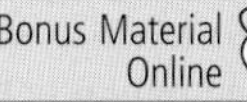

BASIC INFORMATION

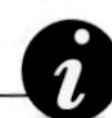

Definition

Emerging tick-borne protozoal disease of dogs has a gametocyte stage in white blood cells and a cystic stage in host tissues. *Hepatozoon americanum* is common in the Gulf Coast region of the southeastern United States, and *Hepatozoon canis* is found in the southeastern United States but is more commonly seen in many other parts of the world. Cats can be infected with *Hepatozoon* spp but rarely become ill.

Synonyms

Hepatozoon infection, New World hepatozoonosis *(H. americanum),* Old World hepatozoonosis *(H. canis)*

Epidemiology

SPECIES, AGE, SEX

Usually outdoor dogs

RISK FACTORS

Areas with large coyote populations and history of tick exposure or ingestion of wildlife carcass (typically 3-6 weeks before illness)

GEOGRAPHY AND SEASONALITY

- *H. americanum* is endemic in the Gulf Coast area of the United States and ranges from Oklahoma to Florida, with sporadic cases reported in California and the Pacific Northwest.
  - Most cases present in the summer and fall.
- *H. canis* is endemic in southern Europe, the Middle East, Africa, Southeast Asia, and South America and is uncommonly reported in dogs in the Gulf Coast area of the United States.
- Cats in Europe and the Middle East may be infected with *Hepatozoon felis, H. canis,* and *Hepatozoon silvestris* but are rarely ill.

ASSOCIATED DISORDERS

H. americanum: pyogranulomatous myositis, marked leukocytosis, fever of unknown origin, protein-losing nephropathy

Clinical Presentation

DISEASE FORMS/SUBTYPES

- *H. americanum*: chronic wasting disease characterized by waxing and waning muscle and bone pain and fever
- *H. canis*: subclinical most often but severe illness possible if there is comorbid disease or immunosuppression

HISTORY, CHIEF COMPLAINT

- *H. americanum*: fever, depression, reluctance to move, stiff gait, mucopurulent ocular discharge, weight loss despite normal appetite; transient bloody diarrhea can precede signs of muscle pain and fever. Signs wax and wane over time.
- *H. canis*: most often an incidental finding on blood smear; when illness occurs, signs are vague (lethargy, anorexia, depression)
- *H. felis*: usually subclinical but rarely depression, anorexia, weight loss, or hypersalivation

PHYSICAL EXAM FINDINGS

- *H. americanum*: fever, mucopurulent ocular discharge, hyperesthesia, neck guarding, ataxia, unwillingness to rise, muscle wasting, cachexia, paresis
- *H. canis*: normal, or pallor, tachycardia, fever
- *H. felis*: normal, or fever, lymphadenopathy, ulcerative glossitis

Etiology and Pathophysiology

- The protozoan parasites have a complex life cycle. Transmission is usually by ingestion of an infected tick (*H. americanum* in *Amblyomma maculatum* [Gulf Coast tick]; *H. canis* in *Rhipicephalus sanguineous* [brown dog tick]), but dogs can be infected *in utero* or by ingesting infected animal tissues.
- Sporozoites from ingested ticks penetrate the wall of the dog's gastrointestinal (GI) tract. They are phagocytized by macrophages and distributed throughout the body to form meronts, or cysts.
- The organisms replicate inside the cyst until it ruptures, releasing merozoites. *H. canis* cysts are primarily in the lymph nodes and spleen; *H. americanum* and *H. felis* cysts are primarily in skeletal muscle.
- When *H. americanum* merozoites are released, an intense inflammatory reaction occurs, resulting in painful myositis and fever. In cats, little inflammation is seen, and most infections are subclinical.
- Merozoites can enter leukocytes and become circulating gametocytes (gamonts) infectious to feeding ticks, or they enter a macrophage and undergo secondary merogony and continue the cycle of releasing merozoites causing repeated episodes of pyogranulomatous myositis.

DIAGNOSIS

Diagnostic Overview

H. americanum should be suspected in dogs with fever, pain, cachexia, ocular discharge, leukocytosis, and periosteal proliferation on long bones. Diagnosis is typically confirmed with polymerase chain reaction (PCR) testing or muscle biopsy because gametocytes are rarely seen on blood smear. In contrast, diagnosis of *H. canis* and *H. felis* is usually made by finding gametocytes on a blood smear.

Differential Diagnosis

H. americanum: meningitis, discospondylitis, polyarthritis, panosteitis, pyometra, amyloidosis, cancer, other vector-borne diseases (VBDs)

Initial Database

H. americanum:

- CBC: usually reveals extreme leukocytosis (20,000-200,000 cells/mcL; typically mature neutrophilia, left shift possible) and mild nonregenerative anemia. Platelet count is usually normal; thrombocytopenia may indicate co-infection with other VBD.
- Serum biochemistry profile: hypoalbuminemia, hyperglobulinemia, increased serum alkaline phosphatase activity, hypoglycemia (laboratory artifact associated with extreme leukocytosis), and low blood urea nitrogen. Creatinine kinase is usually normal despite myopathy.
- Urinalysis: proteinuria common due to glomerulonephritis or amyloidosis; increased urine protein/creatinine ratio.
- Long bone and spinal radiographs: periosteal proliferation secondary to adjacent muscle inflammation is common.
- Blood smear or buffy coat microscopy: rarely reveals gamonts (large, oblong inclusion in neutrophils) in circulating white blood cells. Gamonts of *H. canis* are almost identical but are more likely to be visualized than those of *H. americanum*.

Advanced or Confirmatory Testing

- PCR tests for *H. americanum, H. canis*, and *H. felis* are commercially available.
- If PCR is negative, definitive diagnosis of canine hepatozoonosis can usually be made by finding organisms in muscle biopsy. Any muscle can be sampled, but hindlimb muscles are most commonly used.

TREATMENT

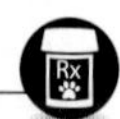

Treatment Overview

Acute antiprotozoal therapy eradicates circulating organisms, with rapid improvement in clinical signs. Chronic therapy is necessary for *H. americanum* to prevent relapses from intermittent release of merozoites from tissue cysts.

Acute General Treatment

- For *H. americanum*, combination therapy for 2 weeks: trimethoprim-sulfadiazine 15 mg/kg PO q 12h, clindamycin 10 mg/kg PO q 8h, and pyrimethamine 0.25 mg/kg PO q 24h. If clinical signs are still evident at 14 days, continue 2 more weeks.
  - Alternative: ponazuril 10 mg/kg PO q 12h × 14 days
  - Regardless of initial therapy, chronic treatment is necessary.
- For *H. canis*: imidocarb 5-6 mg/kg SQ repeated every 14 days until parasitemia has resolved. Pretreatment with atropine may minimize adverse effects.
- Nonsteroidal antiinflammatory drugs at standard doses for muscle pain
- Doxycycline 5-10 mg/kg PO q 12-24h if there is co-infection with other VBD
- IV fluids or transfusion (*H. canis*) may be needed for supportive care.

Chronic Treatment

For *H. americanum* only: decoquinate (Deccox 22.7 g/lb premix) 20 mg/kg (or 1 tsp/10 kg) mixed in food q 12h × 2 years or until PCR test result is negative; very safe for long-term use. Inhibits development of merozoites released from tissue cysts, preventing reinfection of the dog and cyclic bouts of illness.

Nutrition/Diet

Dogs with hepatozoonosis usually retain their appetite but often are too painful to move. They should be hand fed high-calorie diets and offered water until they become ambulatory.

Possible Complications

- If relapse occurs, acute therapy must be repeated. Subsequent relapse may be more difficult to control than initial disease.
- Protein-losing nephropathy may require therapy.

Recommended Monitoring

Repeat CBC and physical exam 2 weeks after initial treatment of *H. americanum*. If fever, muscle pain, or marked leukocytosis persists, continue combination therapy for 2 more weeks. PCR should be checked every 6 months because decoquinate can be discontinued when PCR is negative. Some dogs remain infected for > 5 years but remain free of clinical signs while receiving decoquinate.

PROGNOSIS & OUTCOME

- Without treatment, American hepatozoonosis can be fatal within several months.
- With acute antiprotozoal therapy alone, relapse will occur. Relapses become more frequent, more severe, and refractory to treatment. Without prolonged chronic therapy (i.e., decoquinate), death usually occurs within 1 year of diagnosis.
- Long-term cure (>5 years) can be achieved with acute antiprotozoal therapy followed by long-term decoquinate.

PEARLS & CONSIDERATIONS

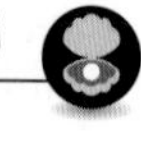

Comments

- Mucopurulent ocular discharge and fever are often the initial signs of relapse.
- Transmission is unusual for VBD because the dog ingests the tick rather than the tick inoculating pathogen during feeding.

Prevention

- Effective tick control
- Do not breed ill dogs.
- Prevent dogs from roaming to reduce the chance of predation or scavenging wildlife.

Technician Tips

- Making a buffy coat smear enhances the possibility of finding gametocytes (although still an insensitive means of diagnosis).
- Run blood glucose measurement immediately to avoid spurious hypoglycemia resulting from *in vitro* leukocyte glucose metabolism.

Client Education

- Clean matted eyes with a warm, moist towel as needed.
- Provide soft bedding.
- Bring food and water to dogs that are nonambulatory.
- Stopping decoquinate too early can result in relapse and death.

SUGGESTED READING

Allen KE, et al: Hepatozoon spp infections in the United States. Vet Clin North Am Small Anim Pract 41:1221-1238, 2011.

AUTHOR & EDITOR: Joseph Taboada, DVM, DACVIM

Herbal Drugs/Natural Supplements Toxicosis

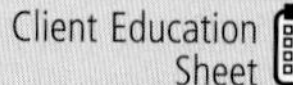

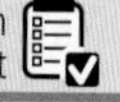

BASIC INFORMATION

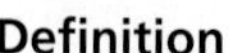

Definition

- Herbal preparations are obtained from plants. The use of herbal medications in humans is a multibillion-dollar industry around the world.
- Herbal medications are available in the form of nutritional or dietary supplements, extracts, teas, tablets, powders, creams, ointments, beverages, or tinctures as a single ingredient or multiple ingredients
- Toxicosis occurs when pets ingest large amounts of owners' medication (e.g., ma huang, guarana, 5-hydroxytryptophan [5HTP]) or when animal owners use concentrated herbal products (e.g., melaleuca oil) on the animal, assuming all natural products are safe. Adverse effects can also occur secondary to drug interactions with the herbal drugs (e.g., concurrent use of St. John's wort, antidepressants).

Toxicology of Commonly Used Herbal Ingredients

Common Names	Genus, Species	Toxin/Toxic Principle	Popular Uses	Toxicity Signs/Major Effect or Actions	Treatment Overview/ Comments
Chamomile	*Matricaria recutita, Chamaemelum nobile*	Hydroxycoumarin, bisabolol, chamazulene	Sedative, GI ulcers, wound healing, antibacterial, antiinflammatory	Vomiting, diarrhea, lethargy; rarely, anticoagulant effects; epistaxis, hematoma (cats)	Low toxicity; mild GI signs expected with acute ingestion; hematologic changes with chronic ingestion
ECGC (green tea), guarana, cocoa, cola, kola nut, chocolate	*Camellia sinensis, Paullinia cupana, Cola acuninata, Theobroma cacao*	Caffeine, theobromine (methylxanthines)	Weight loss, "herbal No-Doz"	Agitation, hyperactivity, polyuria, polydipsia, cardiac arrhythmias, seizures	Chocolate toxicosis (p. 159)
Evening primrose	*Oenothera biennis*	Oil contains 50%-70% *cis*-linoleic acid and other fatty acids	Supports cardiovascular function; used for rheumatoid arthritis, multiple sclerosis	Self-limited gastritis	Low toxicity; systemic effects not expected; mild vomiting or diarrhea possible
Ginkgo, ginkyo	*Ginkgo biloba*	Several flavonoids; terpenoids, alkaloid ginkgo toxin in the seed	Leaf extract used for antioxidant properties, dementia treatment, circulatory disorders, neuroprotection	From leaf extract: vomiting, diarrhea, lethargy From seeds: seizures, shaking, tremors possible	Mild effects from leaf extract; decontamination, diazepam, fluids if seeds involved (treat based on clinical signs)
Ginseng	*Panax quinquefolium; Panax ginseng*	Steroid-like compounds, ginsenosides, and panaxosides, saponins,	Roots, teas, cosmetics used for general well-being, aging, diabetes, neurosis, cancer	Vomiting, diarrhea, nervousness, excitation, lethargy, hypoglycemia possible	Good safety index in humans; decontamination of patient, fluids, and supportive care (treat based on clinical signs)
Grapefruit seed extract	*Citrus X paradise*	Quaternary ammonium compounds, cationic detergents	Disinfectant, antifungal, antimicrobial	Oral ulcers; hypersalivation, vomiting ± blood, weakness, anorexia, hyperthermia, dermal erythema, pain, ulceration	Cats more sensitive (p. 178) Dilution, bathing, GI protectants, pain control, supportive care
5-HTP	*Griffonia simplicifolia*	5-Hydroxytryptophan (5-HTP)	Depression, headaches, insomnia, obesity, over-the-counter antidepressant	Serotonin syndrome; sedation, vomiting, diarrhea, tremors, seizures, ataxia, hyperesthesia, hyperthermia	Antidepressant (SSRI/SNRI) (pp. 71 and 1281)
Kava, yangona, kawa	*Piper methysticum*	Kawain and several other lactones	Beverages prepared from roots used as a relaxant; euphoric effect; sedative	Expected clinical signs similar to benzodiazepines; sedation, ataxia, lethargy, visual disturbances	Benzodiazepine toxicosis (p. 116)
Khat, kat, gat, kus	*Catha edulis*	Alkaloid katin (amphetamine-like)	Used in East African countries; stimulant, mood elevator; leaves and stems chewed	Amphetamine-like effects; hyperactivity, agitation, seizures, tachycardia, hypertension	Amphetamine toxicosis (p. 50)
Kratom, mambog	*Mitragyna speciosa*	Mitragynine	Opium substitute, psychoactive substance	Low doses: sedation and ataxia Higher doses: hallucinations, agitation, and stimulation	Monitor cardiovascular system (heart rate and blood pressure), monitor for CNS signs, including ataxia, agitation, tremors, seizures Fluids, methocarbamol, diazepam, acepromazine
Ma huang, Indian common mallow, bitter orange	*Ephedra sinica, Sida cordifolia, Citrus aurantium*	Ephedrine, pseudoephedrine, synephrine	Weight loss, weight lifting, "herbal ecstasy," decongestants	Sympathomimetic effects; hyperthermia, hypertension, tachycardia, tremors, seizures, agitation	Decongestant toxicosis (p. 240)
Neem, nim, nimbi	*Azadirachta indica*	Azadirachtin as insecticide; neem oil	Insecticidal properties, birth control agent, hypoglycemic properties	Hypothermia, ataxia, lethargy, coma (cats)	Used for controlling fleas in dips/shampoos on cats; bathing, thermoregulation, supportive care
Purple coneflower, echinacea	*Echinacea purpurea*	Arabinogalactan	Cold and flu support, immune stimulant, wound healing	Signs due to allergenic effects; vomiting, diarrhea	Low toxicity; no systemic effects likely from acute exposure
St. John's wort	*Hypericum perforatum*	Hypericin	Antidepressant, insomnia, anxiety, wound healing, skin conditions	MAO inhibitor, depression, vomiting, diarrhea; rarely, tremors, seizures	Antidepressant (SSRI/SNRI) (pp. 71 and 1281)

Continued

Toxicology of Commonly Used Herbal Ingredients—cont'd

Common Names	Genus, Species	Toxin/Toxic Principle	Popular Uses	Toxicity Signs/Major Effect or Actions	Treatment Overview/ Comments
Tea tree oil, pennyroyal oil	*Melaleuca alternifolia, Mentha pulegium*	Melaleuca oil, pulegone, menthofuran	Germicidal, fungal infections, antiseptic, flea control, dermatitis	Terpenes; essential oils Oral: vomiting, diarrhea, CNS depression, hepatotoxicity, aspiration pneumonia Dermal: paresis, ataxia, weakness, hypothermia lasting 1-3 days	Cats more sensitive; bathing, fluids, thermoregulation; may need few days of supportive treatment
Thioctic acid, alpha-lipoic acid (ALA)	Alpha-lipoic acid (ALA)	Alpha-lipoic acid	Diabetic treatment, *Amanita* mushroom poisoning	Hypoglycemic effects; hypersalivation, vomiting, hypoglycemia, liver damage, kidney failure, death	Cats more sensitive; dextrose for hypoglycemia, hepatoprotectants, fluid support
Valerian	*Valeriana officinalis*	Valepotriates, monoterpenes, and sesquiterpenes	Sedative, sleep aid, antianxiety	Affects the GABA receptor; lethargy, sedation, muscle relaxation, ataxia	Decontamination, supportive care
Wintergreen extract /oil	*Gaultheria procumbens*	Oil contains 98% methyl salicylate; essential oils	Topical pain control; oral digestive	Vomiting, diarrhea, gastric ulceration, hyperthermia, sedation, coma, acute hepatic injury	Cats more sensitive; aspirin toxicosis
Yohimbine	*Pausinystalia yohimbine*	Alpha-2 adrenergic blocking agent	Stimulant; hypertension, angina, "herbal Viagra"	Signs due to alpha-2 adrenergic blocking activity; hyperactivity, agitation, tremors, seizures, vomiting, diarrhea, hypotension	Decontamination, diazepam, fluids, stabilize heart rate, blood pressure, thermoregulation

CNS, Central nervous system; *GABA*, gamma-aminobutyric acid; *GI*, gastrointestinal. *MAO*, monoamine oxidase; *SNRI*, serotonin, and norepinephrine reuptake inhibitor; *SSRI*, selective serotonin reuptake inhibitor.

Epidemiology

SPECIES, AGE, SEX

Acute toxicosis in dogs is reported commonly because of their indiscriminate eating habits. Dogs and cats of all breeds, ages, and both sexes are susceptible.

PEARLS & CONSIDERATIONS

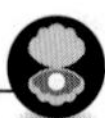

Comments

- Safety and efficacy of most herbal drugs in pets has not been evaluated.
- Concentration of active ingredients in the herbal supplement can vary between brands and from plant to plant because of environmental factors (e.g., growth stage, soil conditions, weather) or manufacturing processes.
- Many pet owners use herbal supplements as alternative/complementary/integrative therapy with or without discussing it with their veterinarian. Because there is usually no warning on the label, many pet owners do not consider herbal drugs/nutritional supplements hazardous and do not keep them out of reach of pets. Because pet owners do not consider herbal supplements medication, they may not include them in a medical history unless specifically asked.
- Most herbal supplements contain multiple ingredients, and if their mechanisms of action are similar, one supplement may cause additive or synergistic toxic effects (i.e., uncharacteristically severe signs). For example, presence of guarana and green tea or presence of ma huang and guarana together may lead to additive or synergistic toxic effects.
- The table above shows some of the most common ingredients, their actions, and treatments.

Technician Tips

Most herbal products/supplements contain multiple ingredients. Always ask the client to bring the container/label of the product involved.

SUGGESTED READING

DerMarderosian A, et al: The review of natural products, ed 8, St. Louis, 2014, Wolters Kluwer Health.

AUTHOR: Charlotte Means, DVM, MLIS, DABVT, DABT
EDITOR: Tina Wismer, DVM, MS, DABVT, DABT

Herpesviral Keratitis, Cats

Client Education Sheet

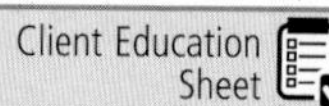

BASIC INFORMATION

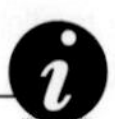

Definition

- Corneal inflammation associated with feline herpesvirus type 1 (FHV-1) infection
- Categorized clinically as nonulcerative (stromal) or ulcerative keratitis; categorized epidemiologically as primary or recrudescent herpesviral keratitis

Synonyms

- Herpetic keratitis
- Feline viral rhinotracheitis (FVR)

Epidemiology

SPECIES, AGE, SEX

- Highly species specific: domestic and wild cats of any age may be affected (p. 1006)
- Young kittens undergoing primary exposure usually display ulcerative disease; older cats undergoing viral reactivation may experience ulcerative or nonulcerative recrudescent disease along with conjunctivitis.

GENETICS, BREED PREDISPOSITION

- No proven breed predisposition (prevalence in breeding catteries may give false impression of breed susceptibility)

- Individual variation in susceptibility to recrudescent herpetic keratitis suggests immunologic predisposition.

RISK FACTORS

Stresses such as rehousing, concurrent disease, or pregnancy/parturition/lactation; glucocorticoid administration; multi-cat households or shelters; inadequate vaccination

CONTAGION AND ZOONOSIS

- Highly contagious to naive cats; carrier cats do not become reinfected (but virus may reactivate)
- Not zoonotic

GEOGRAPHY AND SEASONALITY

- Worldwide viral distribution without seasonality
- Because of higher susceptibility of kittens, trends in disease prevalence may be noted in association with feline breeding seasons.

ASSOCIATED DISORDERS

- FHV-1 also causes rhinitis, conjunctivitis, and dermatitis and may cause anterior uveitis secondary to corneal ulceration.
- FHV-1 is associated with corneal sequestra, symblepharon, and proliferative (eosinophilic) keratoconjunctivitis.

Clinical Presentation

DISEASE FORMS/SUBTYPES

- Ulcerative keratitis (seen most often on initial exposure but also in recurrent forms)
- Nonulcerative keratitis (seen most often in recurrent or chronic primary forms)

HISTORY, CHIEF COMPLAINT

- Ocular discharge (serous to mucopurulent)
- Blepharospasm
- Corneal opacification
- Upper respiratory signs may be seen, including nasal congestion, sneezing, and serous or mucopurulent nasal discharge.
- Ocular signs are typically bilateral in primary disease but often unilateral during recrudescence.

PHYSICAL EXAM FINDINGS

- Ocular discharge: epiphora, mucoid, purulent, sanguineous, or dry and crusty; sometimes dark red or black
- Blepharospasm
- Corneal ulceration: dendritic early; may become geographic; often chronic, nonhealing and sometimes with a lip of loose epithelium
- Deep or superficial corneal vascularization
- Corneal opacification due to white blood cell infiltration and/or edema and/or scarring
- Conjunctival or episcleral hyperemia
- Chemosis (conjunctival edema), blepharedema
- Reflex uveitis: miotic pupil; aqueous flare and/or inflammatory cells in the anterior chamber, low intraocular pressure (p. 1023)
- Proliferative (eosinophilic) keratoconjunctivitis: appears as raised, pink, sometimes chalky plaques extending from the limbus often with a leading zone of ulceration. Although this condition is seen in many polymerase chain reaction (PCR) FHV-1–positive cats, proof of a causal relationship has not been found.
- Corneal sequestration appears as a flat or raised, amber to black lesion on the axial to paraxial cornea, often surrounded by corneal vascularization and sometimes stromal inflammatory cell infiltration (p. 208). Sequestra most likely develop secondary to chronic corneal ulceration.
- Symblepharon (scarred fusion of conjunctival surfaces to each other or to the cornea)

Etiology and Pathophysiology

- FHV-1 is ubiquitous; the virus replicates in epithelial cells, especially those of the conjunctiva, and then ascends by axons to establish latency in the trigeminal ganglia.
- Primary disease is common and usually self-limited.
- At least 80% of affected cats become latently infected for life; periodic viral reactivation occurs in at least one-half of those latently infected.
- Periodic recrudescent disease occurs in a minority of cats undergoing viral reactivation.

DIAGNOSIS

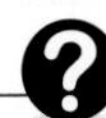

Diagnostic Overview

The frequency with which cats are vaccinated and the number of normal cats that shed virus at ocular sites make serologic testing (97% seroprevalence) and methods of viral detection (e.g., PCR) unhelpful. Inclusion bodies are rarely seen on cytologic specimens. Diagnosis is made based on visualization of dendritic ulcers or geographic ulcers, supportive signs, and/or response to therapy.

Differential Diagnosis

- There are no other recognized primary feline corneal pathogens.
- *Chlamydia felis* (formerly *Chlamydophila felis* or *Chlamydia psittaci*) causes conjunctivitis but is not known to cause keratitis.
- Feline calicivirus is not a primary corneoconjunctival pathogen but causes lesions of oral/pharyngeal mucosa.
- Noninfectious corneal disease (immune mediated, neoplastic, keratoconjunctivitis sicca, foreign body, traumatic) is uncommon in cats compared with dogs but should be considered.

Initial Database

- Thorough ophthalmic exam (p. 1137), including Schirmer tear testing, tonometry, and application of fluorescein and sometimes rose bengal or lissamine green stains
- Corneal or conjunctival cytologic evaluation important for diagnosing eosinophilic/proliferative keratoconjunctivitis; however, herpesviral inclusions are rarely seen.

TREATMENT

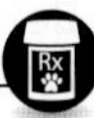

Treatment Overview

- Cats with primary and mild recrudescent herpetic keratitis may improve with supportive care only. Cats with severe or frequently recurrent keratitis require specific antiviral therapy.
- Many topical or systemic antiviral agents are limited by their toxicity and efficacy profiles.
- No antiviral drug has been developed to date for cats infected with FHV-1. Antiviral drugs developed for human herpesvirus infections are used. None has readily predictable safety in cats or efficacy against FHV-1.

Acute General Treatment

- Cats with concurrent respiratory signs may need supportive care (consider systemic antibiotics, fluid, and nutritional support).
- Cats with ulcerative keratitis require a topical broad-spectrum antibiotic because antiviral drugs are not antibacterial. Ophthalmic oxytetracycline (Terramycin) is a good choice because it is effective against *C. felis,* which is a common cause of conjunctivitis.
- Consider antiviral treatment for chronic, recurrent, or severe signs. Topical antiviral agents (e.g., idoxuridine, trifluridine, vidarabine) are virostatic and must be administered at least q 4h. The exception is cidofovir, which because of tissue accumulation may be administered q 12h. These medications should be administered for at least 1 week after ulcer resolution.
- Systemic acyclovir is not recommended due to toxicity. Valacyclovir is an acyclovir prodrug with fatal toxicity.
- Systemic famciclovir 90 mg/kg PO q 12h reduces clinical disease and viral shedding, produces effective plasma and tear drug concentrations, and appears to be well tolerated. Like other antimicrobials, it should be given beyond resolution of clinical signs and not tapered.
- Many cats benefit from mucinomimetic tear-replacement products, especially those containing hyaluronate.
- Avoid topical or systemic administration of corticosteroids, nonsteroidal antiinflammatory agents, cyclosporine, or tacrolimus.

Chronic Treatment

- Lysine 500 mg/CAT PO q 12h: lifelong treatment; may reduce viral replication in some cats with frequent recurrences. Give as q 12h bolus; do not add to food. Do not continue lifelong if a positive effect is not seen after a reasonable amount of time.
- Avoid prolonged topical antiviral administration due to corneal toxicity.
- Avoid topical or systemic administration of corticosteroids, nonsteroidal antiinflammatory agents, cyclosporine, or tacrolimus because they may lead to recrudescence.

Nutrition/Diet

High-lysine (≈5%) diets have proven counterproductive.

Behavior/Exercise

- Reduce known stresses.
- Reduce overcrowding in multi-cat situations.

Possible Complications

- Topical antiviral agents are epitheliotoxic.
- Acyclovir and its prodrug valacyclovir are toxic to cats.

Recommended Monitoring

- Frequent ophthalmic exams, especially for ulcerative keratitis
- Monitor CBC, urinalysis, and serum biochemistry panels if systemic antiviral agents are used.

PROGNOSIS & OUTCOME

- Primary disease is self-limited in most cats.
- A minority experience chronic and/or recrudescent disease.
- Treat recurrences early and aggressively.
- Secondary bacterial invasion of corneal ulcers can cause globe perforation.
- Chronic stromal herpetic keratitis is painful and can be blinding.

PEARLS & CONSIDERATIONS

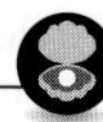

Comments

- FHV-1 is the most common cause of ulcerative and nonulcerative keratitis in cats.
- Diagnostic testing is not helpful due to viral shedding in apparently normal cats.
- Most topical antiviral agents must be administered frequently to be effective.
- Do not taper antiviral drug dose or frequency; use for at least 1 week after resolution of clinical signs.
- Cats with severe, chronic, or frequently recurrent corneal disease may benefit from referral to a veterinary ophthalmologist.

Prevention

Vaccination lessens signs but may not reduce recurrences or establishment of latency.

Technician Tips

- Minimize transfer of FHV-1 between cats by handwashing.
- Clean contaminated equipment with standard disinfectants.

Client Education

- Minimize known stresses.
- Early recognition of and therapy for recrudescent disease are important.

SUGGESTED READING

Thomasy SM, et al: A review of antiviral drugs and other compounds with activity against feline herpesvirus 1. Vet Ophthalmol 19(suppl 1):119-130, 2016.

AUTHOR: David J. Maggs, BVSc, DACVO
EDITOR: Diane V. H. Hendrix, DVM, DACVO

Herpesvirus, Dog

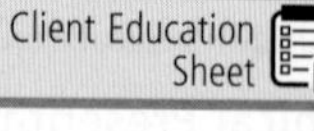

BASIC INFORMATION

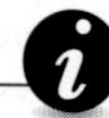

Definition

Viral infection of canids that can present one of five possible clinical scenarios:

- Upper respiratory infection
- Bilateral ocular disease
- Abortion (p. 2)
- Vaginitis/posthitis (p. 1030)
- Neonatal puppy mortality up to 8 weeks of age (p. 687)

Synonyms

Canine herpesvirus type 1 (CHV-1), fading puppy syndrome

Epidemiology

SPECIES, AGE, SEX

- Domestic dogs; wild canids (e.g., coyotes, wolves)
- Immunologically naive pregnant dams are most susceptible to the reproductive effects of CHV-1, and their offspring are most susceptible to systemic disease, with high puppy mortality.
- Immunologically suppressed adult dogs can experience systemic or ocular disease.

RISK FACTORS

There are 10 major risk factors: immunologic status of dog, pregnant dam (newborn pups), age, mating experience, reproductive cycle, breeding kennel, kennel size, breeding management (use of nonresident males), kennel cough, and kennel hygiene.

CONTAGION AND ZOONOSIS

- Highly contagious among canids only by saliva, ocular, and urogenital secretions
- Fomites may contribute to spread.
- Direct contact (saliva, ocular, urogenital secretions) is the most efficient mode of transmission, especially from dogs with clinical signs but possibly from latent carriers.
- The virus is readily inactivated outside the body by heat, drying, or disinfectants (diluted bleach, 1 part bleach to 30 parts tap water).
- Not zoonotic

GEOGRAPHY AND SEASONALITY

The virus persists in carrier dogs worldwide as a latent infection and may be exacerbated with stress-induced, pharmacologic, and/or physiologic/hormone-related immunosuppression (e.g., pregnancy) and radiation therapy in adult dogs.

ASSOCIATED DISORDERS

Surviving puppies may have deafness, ocular disease, neurologic dysfunction, or renal damage.

Clinical Presentation

DISEASE FORMS/SUBTYPES

- Dogs, usually < 2 years old: acute to chronic upper airway signs (e.g., cough)
- Adult dogs: mild to severe ocular disease (blepharitis, conjunctivitis, keratitis, and corneal ulceration)
- Dam aborts litter: usually with 100% puppy mortality if infection of dam occurs during last 3 weeks of gestation
- Dam infects her litter during whelping: usually 80%-100% puppy mortality if infection is a re-exacerbation of latent infection
- Naive dam gives birth to naive litter, and secondary contact with CHV-shedding dog carries virus back to litter. Mortality rate of 25%-80%, depending on virus challenge dose, age of puppies, and body temperature of puppies.
- Dam or sire presented for evaluation of papulovesicular lesions of the external genital organs

HISTORY, CHIEF COMPLAINT

As described above

PHYSICAL EXAM FINDINGS

Puppies appear painful with persistent crying and fail to nurse; decreased body weight; soft, yellow-green feces; no fever; rhinitis possible, with serous/mucopurulent/hemorrhagic nasal discharge; mucosal petechiae common. Puppies become lethargic and lose consciousness; may have opisthotonos and seizures before death. Adult dogs with ocular disease may present with unilateral, but usually bilateral, lesions. Adult dogs with upper airway infection as for canine infectious respiratory disease complex (CIRDC; p. 987)

Etiology and Pathophysiology

- CHV has a predisposition for lymphoid and neural cells, both of which may become latently infected (no mature viral production), but a dog remains a potential shedder if the virus is re-exacerbated due to stress (e.g., pregnancy, corticosteroids, irradiation).

- The optimal temperature for CHV replication is 33°C-35°C (i.e., temperature of the outer genital and upper respiratory tracts). This is the normal body temperature range for puppies < 3 weeks of age (poikilothermic), which increases the susceptibility to severe, systemic CHV disease in this age group.

DIAGNOSIS

Diagnostic Overview

Although a presumptive diagnosis of CHV-induced disease can be achieved by the observation of ill pups < 3 weeks of age, confirmation of CHV can be obtained histopathologically on fixed liver and kidney tissue of affected pups, virus isolation from fresh/frozen tissues, and/or polymerase chain reaction (PCR) assay of whole blood from pups. Carrier dogs can be identified by PCR testing of whole blood from adult dogs. Ocular swabs may be submitted for virus isolation or PCR testing.

Differential Diagnosis

- Acute-onset respiratory signs/respiratory distress of upper and lower airway passages: canine adenovirus type 2; canine parainfluenza; canine influenza (H3N8, H3N2); canine respiratory coronavirus; *Bordetella bronchiseptica*; upper-lower airway foreign body
- Reproductive disease: *Brucella canis*, *Streptococcus* spp; canine distemper virus; neosporosis; toxoplasmosis
- Ocular disease: primary bacterial infection, foreign body

Initial Database

CBC, serum biochemistry profile, urinalysis: values are usually nonspecific, but a marked thrombocytopenia may be observed. A marked increase in the alanine aminotransferase activity may be found in affected neonatal puppies. Be aware that many laboratory values differ in neonatal and adult dogs.

Advanced or Confirmatory Testing

Antemortem testing:

- Serologic titers from affected adult dogs (titers ≥ 1 : 2 indicate exposure/infection). Antibody titers do not correlate with active viral shedding but are good indicators of prior infection and latency status.
- Virus isolation from nasal/ocular/urogenital swabs indicates infection and active shedding.
- PCR of ocular swabs or whole blood indicates infection and active viremia or latency.

Postmortem testing (aborted/neonatal dead puppies):

- Virus isolation from lung, bronchiolar lymph nodes, liver, kidney, and spleen
- Histopathologic evaluation of lung, liver, kidney, spleen, small intestine, and brain. Depending on the stage of cellular infection and method of fixation, basophilic or acidophilic intranuclear inclusions may be noted. The intranuclear inclusion bodies are considered pathognomonic for CHV.
- No CHV immunohistochemical test is commercially available.
- PCR can also be done on the aforementioned selected tissues but is usually reserved for determining latency.

TREATMENT

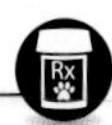

Treatment Overview

Treatment of CHV-induced neonatal disease requires rapid response on the part of owner and veterinarian. Usually by the time clinical signs occur, individually affected pups have a poor prognosis. Unaffected littermates may be treated with antiviral drugs and/or CHV-hyperimmune serum. The temperature of the puppy environment should be increased.

Acute General Treatment

- Treatment of neonatal puppies with CHV-induced disease is usually not recommended because of rapid progression, poor prognosis, and the potential for cerebellar and retinal dysplasias in surviving puppies.
- If only a portion of the litter demonstrates overt signs, the remaining littermates can be treated with immune serum (2 mL of serum from a dog with known anti-CHV titer, given intraperitoneally).
- Neonates should be maintained in an environment with high humidity (up to 55%) and elevated ambient temperatures of 36.6°C-37.7°C (98°F-100°F), given CHV's sensitivity to higher temperatures. Caution and constant rectal temperature monitoring are essential to avoid iatrogenic hyperthermia.
- Ocular disease: prevention of secondary bacterial infection (topical ocular antimicrobials), treatment for comfort (topical ocular atropine), antiviral therapy (0.1% idoxuridine, 1% trifluridine, or cidofovir 0.5% ophthalmic solution)
- Treatment of adult dogs with respiratory signs as for CIRDC

Chronic Treatment

Due to high incidence of life-threatening sequelae, treatment is not recommended if pup is presented already showing clinical signs.

Behavior/Exercise

Puppies will be in pain and crying. Keep as comfortable as possible.

Possible Complications

Treatment of clinically ill puppies may result in cerebellar and retinal dysplasias.

Recommended Monitoring

Puppies presented while showing clinical signs should be monitored every few hours because the prognosis is poor. Dam can be monitored by checking CHV antibody titers and by PCR testing of urogenital secretions (swabs).

PROGNOSIS & OUTCOME

- Prognosis for clinically ill neonates is poor; euthanasia should be considered.
- Unaffected neonatal puppies from an affected litter have a good prognosis with proper care.
- Dams that abort or have a naive litter that subsequently becomes infected by a secondary source of CHV commonly seroconvert and subsequently have normal litters. CHV passive immunity is passed to offspring through colostrum. Colostral immunity, which persists to 8 weeks, prevents clinical signs in the puppies but does not prevent primary infection and subsequent latency.
- Ocular disease can be self-limited or resolve after treatment with antivirals. Respiratory disease in adults has a good prognosis with supportive care.

PEARLS & CONSIDERATIONS

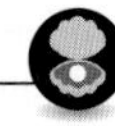

Comments

CHV is a manageable infection and a preventable disease (see Prevention and Client Education below).

Prevention

- Good hygiene: cleanliness of dam, rigorous handwashing or use of gloves by handlers
- Puppy environment with an ambient temperature that minimizes CHV replication (>35°C)
- No vaccine is available in the United States. A European product has been licensed, with good results reported when used before breeding.

Technician Tips

- Emphasize good prenatal and postnatal hygiene and biosecurity with clients.
- Incorporate kennel surveillance program for *B. canis* and CHV testing before breeding and arrival at kennel.
- Identify first-time pregnant dogs as high risk and quarantine from outside dogs/humans as much as possible.
- Advise clients that CHV disease (respiratory/ocular) can occur in older dogs of either sex.

Client Education

- Planned exposure of young (>6 months) puppies to older dogs to naturally immunize them before breeding and whelping. This induced infection rarely becomes clinically overt, but if it does as a respiratory disease, a 2-week quarantine is advised.
- Maintenance of a strict quarantine period to work within the 6-week danger period (3 weeks before and 3 weeks after whelping).
- Maintain temperature > 35°C because CHV replication is very heat sensitive.
- Be familiar with early signs of ocular disease, especially blepharitis and conjunctivitis, and seek immediate veterinary care.

SUGGESTED READING

Evermann JF, et al: Canine reproductive, respiratory, and ocular diseases due to canine herpesvirus. Vet Clin North Am Small Anim Pract 41:1097-1120, 2011.

AUTHOR: James F. Evermann, MS, PhD
EDITOR: Michelle A. Kutzler, DVM, PhD, DACT

Hiatal Hernia/Gastroesophageal Intussusception

Client Education Sheet 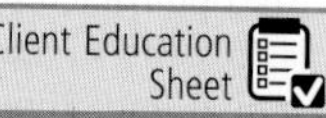

BASIC INFORMATION

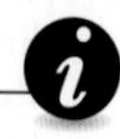

Definition

Hiatal hernia (HH) and gastroesophageal intussusception (GEI) are problems associated with the esophageal hiatus of the diaphragm. They represent very different clinical conditions in that HH is often subclinical and GEI is often an acute and potentially fatal problem. This difference emphasizes the need for accurate diagnosis of caudal esophageal mass lesions.

Epidemiology

SPECIES, AGE, SEX

- Congenital HH: primarily dogs < 1 year of age
- Acquired HH: dogs or cats of any age
- GEI: dogs usually < 3 months of age

GENETICS, BREED PREDISPOSITION

- Shar-peis and brachycephalic dog breeds may be predisposed to HH. Shar-peis may present at a young age (10-18 weeks).
- German shepherd dogs may be overrepresented for GEI.

RISK FACTORS

Trauma (HH and GEI)

ASSOCIATED DISORDERS

- Golden and Labrador retrievers: muscular dystrophy
- Esophageal hypomotility or megaesophagus
- Gastroesophageal reflux/esophagitis

Clinical Presentation

DISEASE FORMS/SUBTYPES

- Type I: sliding, or axial, HH
    - Longitudinal displacement of the abdominal esophagus, gastroesophageal junction, or stomach into the caudal mediastinum
- Type II: paraesophageal hernia
    - Gastroesophageal junction remains caudal to the hiatus, and the fundus of the stomach or other abdominal organ protrudes adjacent to and parallel to the gastroesophageal junction through the hiatus.
- Type III: axial (movement of the gastroesophageal junction into the thorax) with paraesophageal herniation (adjacent portion of the gastric fundus through the esophageal hiatus)
- GEI is a rare condition in which the cardia invaginates into the terminal esophagus and through the hiatus.
    - Associated with acute gastroesophageal obstruction and severe clinical signs in dogs

HISTORY, CHIEF COMPLAINT

- Absence of clinical signs: incidental finding on thoracic radiograph (50% of HH cases; small proportion of GEI cases)
- Intermittent signs with sliding HH: typically regurgitation, dysphagia, ptyalism, and weight loss or slow growth
- GEI
    - Acute vomiting or regurgitation, dyspnea, hematemesis, abdominal pain, and collapse
    - Chronic intermittent vomiting and regurgitation far less common

PHYSICAL EXAM FINDINGS

- May be unremarkable
- If signs are present, they may include:
    - Thin body condition
    - Dehydration
    - Ptyalism
    - Fever, harsh lung sounds, cough, dyspnea
- Possible aspiration pneumonia (p. 793)

Etiology and Pathophysiology

Cause:

- Congenital HH: abnormal diaphragmatic esophageal hiatus (abnormally large or abnormal laxity of the phrenicoesophageal ligament)
- Trauma: esophageal hiatal enlargement and/or stretching of the phrenicoesophageal ligament, esophageal hiatus, and the phrenicoesophageal ligament
- Severe respiratory disease: intense negative intrapleural pressure required for ventilation may be associated with HH in dogs and cats.

Mechanism:

- Loss of normal anatomic relationship adversely affects the normal high-pressure zone at the gastroesophageal junction, causing reflux esophagitis.
- Primary or secondary esophageal motility disorders and megaesophagus can exacerbate signs.
- Upper airway obstruction (e.g., brachycephalic syndrome, laryngeal paralysis) may result in increased negative intrapleural pressure required for inspiration, causing HH or gastroesophageal reflux.
- Diaphragmatic weakening may be associated with muscular dystrophy in predisposed breeds.
- Large hernias may allow other abdominal organs to enter the caudal mediastinum.

DIAGNOSIS

Diagnostic Overview

Diagnosis is suspected based on patient signalment, presenting history, physical exam findings, and above all, demonstration of a mass effect in the area of the terminal esophagus on thoracic radiographs. Elucidation of the diagnosis requires radiographic contrast studies and endoscopy.

Differential Diagnosis

- Megaesophagus
- Esophageal foreign body, stricture, or mass
- Vascular ring anomaly
- Mediastinal or pulmonary mass

Initial Database

- CBC: if neutrophilia with toxic changes and/or left shift associated with inflammation/infection, suspect aspiration pneumonia
- Serum biochemistry profile: hypoproteinemia possible (malnutrition)
- Thoracic radiographs
    - Increased density/mass lesion in the caudodorsal mediastinum on the lateral view
    - Disappearance/reappearance of mass on repeated radiographs is characteristic but not essential.
    - Radiographs can be normal if sliding hernia; compression of the abdomen while making the radiograph may aid in diagnosing a sliding hernia.

Advanced or Confirmatory Testing

- Fluoroscopy with positive contrast esophagram
    - Evaluate esophageal size and motility.
    - Confirm sliding HH when displacement is intermittent.
- Esophagoscopy
    - Assess presence and severity of esophagitis.
    - GEI: confirm diagnosis.

TREATMENT

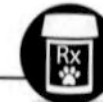

Treatment Overview

Treatment of HH is aimed at decreasing gastroesophageal reflux, providing nutritional support, and managing aspiration pneumonia if present. Surgery is performed on cases that do not respond to medical therapy. Treatment of paraesophageal hernia or GEI requires surgery to correct the malpositioning of organs through the esophageal hiatus.

Acute General Treatment

- Medical management
    - Correction of fluid and electrolyte deficits if present
    - Aggressive treatment of aspiration pneumonia
    - Treatment of gastroesophageal reflux/esophagitis
- Surgical management: patients showing clinical signs referable to HH or if GEI
    - Consider treatment of upper respiratory obstruction if present
    - Reduction of HH/GEI
    - Closure of esophageal hiatus to a smaller size
    - Left fundic gastropexy to prevent recurrence

Chronic Treatment

- Continuation of treatment of gastroesophageal reflux/esophagitis
- Surgical correction of HH in patients that do not respond to medical management within 30 days

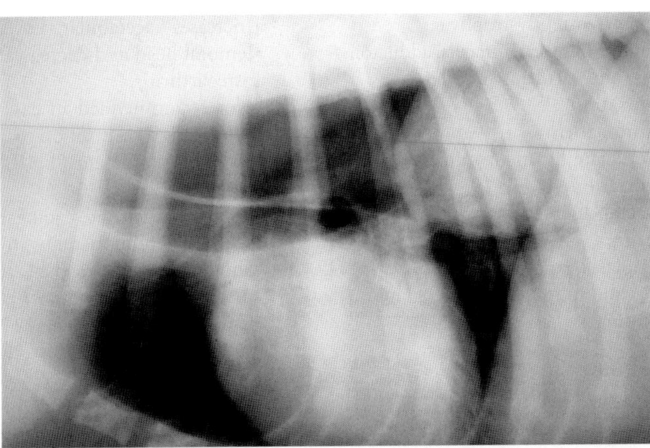

HIATAL HERNIA/GASTROESOPHAGEAL INTUSSUSCEPTION Lateral thoracic radiograph of a dog demonstrates a large, soft-tissue mass due to gastroesophageal intussusception, located characteristically in the caudodorsal thorax. The dog suffered strangulation injury when it became caught in a snare. Also visible is an air-filled esophagus, which demonstrates both sides of the dorsal tracheal membrane (tracheal stripe sign). A differential diagnosis for the radiographic appearance of the mass lesion is primary lung tumor. (Courtesy Dr. Richard Walshaw.)

Nutrition/Diet

Acute:

- Upright feeding of low-fat, small, frequent meals to promote normal function of the esophagus/gastroesophageal junction
- Feeding tube (percutaneous endogastric [p. 1109]) if oral intake inadequate

Chronic:

- Continuation of feeding regimen
- Upright feeding if megaesophagus associated with GEI

Possible Complications

- Failure of medical management to resolve clinical signs of esophagitis
- Overreduction of hiatal opening during surgery may worsen regurgitation.
- Recurrence of HH after surgical correction
- Development of esophageal stricture secondary to gastroesophageal reflux/esophagitis

Recommended Monitoring

Follow-up positive contrast esophagram (4-6 weeks):

- Demonstrate resolution of
  - HH/GEI
  - Gastroesophageal reflux
- Assess esophageal motility.
- Determine if continuation of feeding regimen and treatment of esophagitis still necessary

PROGNOSIS & OUTCOME

- Good prognosis
  - If the patient has no or mild clinical signs
  - With surgical intervention in the absence of aspiration pneumonia
- Guarded to poor prognosis associated with
  - Severe aspiration pneumonia
  - Severe esophagitis/stricture
  - Persistent megaesophagus

PEARLS & CONSIDERATIONS

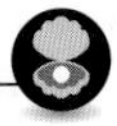

Comments

- Consider referral to a soft-tissue surgeon if surgical correction is indicated.
- Treatment for esophagitis should be continued postoperatively for any patient undergoing surgical correction of HH.
- Aspiration pneumonia requires intensive treatment before considering surgical intervention.

Technician Tips

- Pressure applied to the abdomen via a belly wrap or pressing a wooden spoon on the abdomen can improve the chance of observing HH on abdominal radiographs.
- Positioning on the surgery table with the abdomen lower than the head allows abdominal organs to fall caudally, thereby improving visibility and access to the diaphragm.

SUGGESTED READING

Cornell KL: Stomach. In Johnston SA, et al., editors: Veterinary surgery: small animal, ed 2, St. Louis, 2017, Elsevier pp 1700-1730.

AUTHOR: MaryAnn G. Radlinsky, DVM, MS, DACVS
EDITOR: Elizabeth A. Swanson, DVM, MS, DACVS

Hip Dysplasia

Client Education Sheet 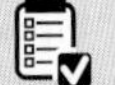  Video Available 

BASIC INFORMATION

Definition

A condition caused by abnormal development of the coxofemoral (i.e., hip) joint, characterized by joint laxity in young patients progressing to degenerative joint disease (DJD) of various degrees of severity

Epidemiology

SPECIES, AGE, SEX

- The condition is a developmental disease and occurs in young dogs. Clinical signs may become apparent at any age, or the condition may remain occult throughout life.
- No sex predisposition reported
- Less frequent in cats

GENETICS, BREED PREDISPOSITION

- Cause is not fully known, but the phenotypic expression of hip laxity that progresses to early DJD is due to the patient's genotype as well as environmental influences.
- Most common in large and giant breeds (Labrador retriever, golden retriever, German shepherd dog, rottweiler, Newfoundland)
- May be more common in Maine coon cats than other cat breeds

RISK FACTORS

- Being a large- or giant-breed dog
- Castration of young male dogs may promote expression of hip dysplasia.
- Excessive caloric intake causing rapid weight gain and growth
- Synovial inflammation of the hip joint

ASSOCIATED DISORDERS

Common concurrent genetic or developmental conditions include elbow dysplasia, osteochondrosis, stifle disease, panosteitis, and hypertrophic osteodystrophy. A causal relationship has not been identified, and it may simply be that these conditions are all common in large- and giant-breed dogs.

Clinical Presentation

DISEASE FORMS/SUBTYPES

Juvenile (up to 18 months):

- Hip laxity characterized by subluxation or luxation of the hip joint
  - Acetabular dysplasia
  - Femoral head/neck malformations

Mature:

- Degenerative joint disease secondary to hip instability and incongruity

HISTORY, CHIEF COMPLAINT

Juvenile patients typically have hindlimb lameness characterized by

- Bunny-hopping gait
- Unilateral or bilateral pelvic limb lameness
- Difficulty rising
- Exercise intolerance
- Description of an audible clicking when rising or walking
- Shifting of weight to the thoracic limbs and hyperextension of the hocks

Mature patients have progressively worsening hindlimb lameness characterized by
- Weight-bearing lameness
- Lameness after exercise
- Exercise intolerance
- Disuse atrophy of pelvic musculature
- Difficulty jumping

PHYSICAL EXAM FINDINGS

Juvenile patients:
- Pain during extension, external rotation, and abduction of the hip
- Hip joint laxity (positive Ortolani sign) characterized by dorsal subluxation of the femoral head with the limb adducted, followed by a palpable click with reduction of the femoral head when the limb is abducted
  - Angle of reduction is the measured point at which the femoral head slips back into the acetabulum as the limb is abducted.
  - Angle of subluxation is the measured point at which the femoral head slips out of the acetabulum as the limb is then adducted.
- Poor pelvic limb musculature
- Some dogs have tarsal hyperextension during weight bearing.
- Patient may appear to have an arched spine as weight is shifted cranially to the thoracic limbs.
- Narrow pelvic limb stance

Mature patient:
- Pain, sometimes crepitus during extension, external rotation, and abduction of the hip
- Decreased hip range of motion
- Ortolani sign is lost because periarticular fibrosis limits femoral head movement.
- Hindlimb muscle atrophy
- Exaggerated hip movement at a walk (see *Video*)

Etiology and Pathophysiology

- A combination of genetic and environmental factors causes hip joint laxity, resulting in joint instability and abnormal progression of endochondral ossification.
- Puppies with a genetic predisposition are born with hips that are grossly normal. Changes in the hip joint begin within the first few weeks after birth.
- Lameness and gait abnormalities appear between 3 and 8 months of age.
- In immature animals, lameness may improve/resolve over time as joint stability is gained through periarticular fibrosis. As degenerative changes accumulate, clinical signs of mature hip dysplasia develop.

DIAGNOSIS

Diagnostic Overview

Diagnosis is based on clinical signs of lameness, hip joint laxity or degeneration, and radiographs showing a malformed and/or arthritic joint.

Differential Diagnosis

Any cause of hindlimb lameness:
- In the immature patient
  - Panosteitis
  - Osteochondrosis
  - Physeal fractures of the femoral head
  - Hypertrophic osteodystrophy
  - Muscle injury (iliopsoas, gracilis, adductor, pectineus, and sartorius muscles)
  - Patellar luxation
- In the mature patient
  - Cranial cruciate ligament injury
  - Patellar luxation
  - Lumbosacral disease
  - Polyarthritis
  - Bone neoplasia
  - Rickettsial and fungal disease (geographic)
  - Muscle injury

Initial Database

- Orthopedic exam (p. 1143)
- In the young patient
  - Palpation of hip joints for Ortolani sign in addition to calculation of angles of subluxation and reduction (may require sedation/anesthesia)
  - Lateral and ventrodorsal pelvic radiographs

Advanced or Confirmatory Testing

- Orthopedic Foundation for Animals (OFA) radiographic protocol for subjective evaluation
- PennHIP or dorsolateral subluxation stress radiography protocols for objective evaluation of joint laxity to help predict likelihood of later osteoarthritis
- Hip arthroscopy to identify ligament and cartilage damage (clinical relevance is unknown)

TREATMENT

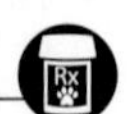

Treatment Overview

Goals are pain reduction, functional improvement, and restoration of hip congruity/stability if possible. In cases without complete hip luxation, medical therapy is typically the initial recommended treatment. In general, medical management and progression of DJD will not encumber future surgical intervention with hip replacement or excision arthroplasty.

Acute General Treatment

Medical management (p. 1425):
- Nonsteroidal antiinflammatory drugs (NSAIDs); dosages for dogs:
  - Carprofen 2.2 mg/kg PO q 12h, *or*
  - Deracoxib 1-2 mg/kg PO q 24h, *or*
  - Meloxicam 0.1 mg/kg PO q 24h, *or*
  - Grapiprant 2 mg/kg PO q24h for dogs > 3.6 kg, *or*
  - Firocoxib 5 mg/kg PO q 24h, *or*
  - Etodolac 10-15 mg/kg PO q 24h
- Analgesia (see Chronic Treatment)

Surgical management (p. 1425):
- Juvenile pubic symphysiodesis (JPS)
  - In immature patients with joint laxity and without DJD (14-20 weeks of age)
  - Minimally invasive; increases acetabular coverage of the femoral head
  - Not recommended in cases with severe subluxation or luxation
- Triple pelvic osteotomy (TPO) and double pelvic osteotomy (DPO)
  - In young dogs with joint laxity and without DJD
  - Increases acetabular coverage of the femoral head and decreases likelihood of osteoarthritis
  - Not recommended in cases with severe subluxation or luxation
- Total hip replacement (THR)
  - In mature dogs
  - Replaces degenerative joint structures with synthetic components
  - Should be performed by surgeons with specific training who do THR with some regularity
- Femoral head and neck ostectomy/excision (FHO or FHNE):
  - Young and mature dogs
  - Replaces the painful joint with a pseudoarthrosis
  - Associated with some mechanical gait deficit, fatigue with exercise in large dogs
  - Immediate postoperative physical rehabilitation needed for best outcome
  - After a hip has undergone this procedure, future THR becomes exceptionally difficult, with a high complication rate.
- Acetabular denervation
  - Neurotomy of nerve fibers in the periarticular region to partially desensitize the hip joint
  - Only a palliative procedure
  - Objective (force plate) evaluations question efficacy of the procedure.

Chronic Treatment

Medical management:
- Attaining lean body condition is the most important factor for long-term successful medical management (pp. 700 and 1077).
- Daily or prn NSAID administration (see above)
- Analgesia
  - Amantadine 2-4 mg/kg PO q 24h, *and/or*
  - Gabapentin 5-10 mg/kg PO q 12-24h, *and/or*
  - Tramadol 2-4 mg/kg PO q 8-12h, *or*
  - Codeine 0.5-2 mg/kg PO q 8-12h, *or*
  - Buprenorphine 0.01-0.03 mg/kg PO or via buccal mucosa q 6h (cats), *or*
- Adjunctive therapies
  - Acupuncture (p. 1056)
  - Rehabilitation with the goal of pain relief and improving/maintaining muscle mass
- Disease-modifying osteoarthritis agents may be beneficial.
  - Polysulfated glycosaminoglycan 5 mg/kg IM twice weekly × 4-6 weeks, *or*
  - Pentosan polysulfate 3 mg/kg SQ or IM once weekly, *or*
  - Oral formulations (glucosamine, chondroitin sulfate, hyaluronan): according to formulation/labeled instructions
- Nutrition (energy restricted diet, as appropriate)
  - High-omega-3 fatty acid diet

Surgical management:
- JPS or TPO is performed in some young animals with hip laxity and minimal degenerative change.
- FHO or THR is performed in mature animals with joint degeneration unresponsive

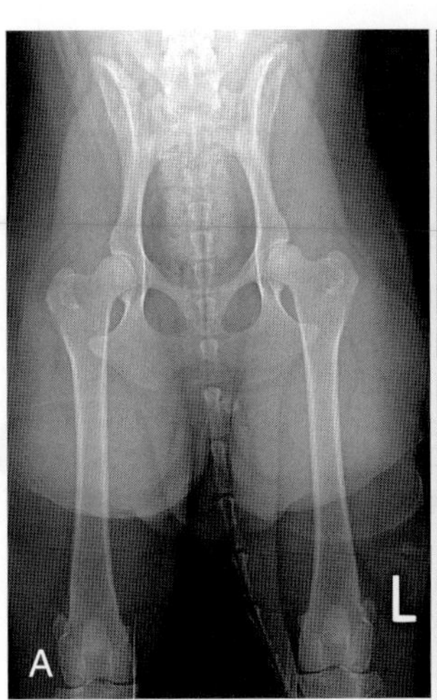

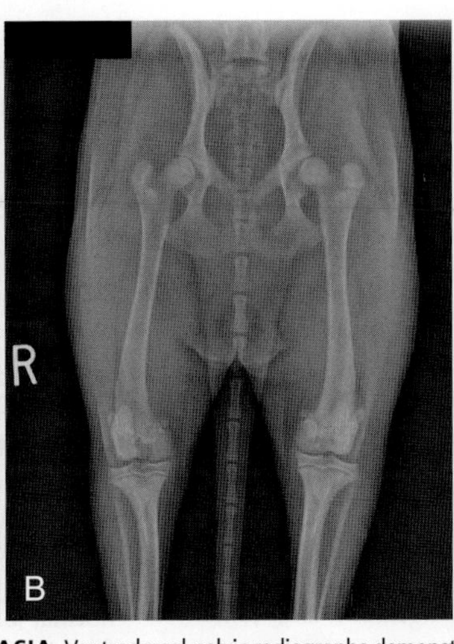

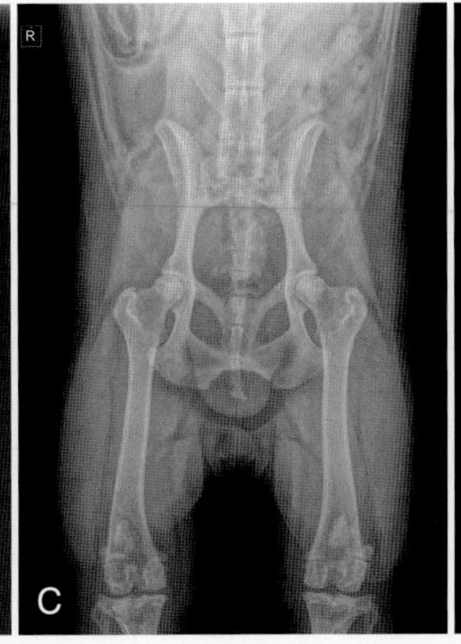

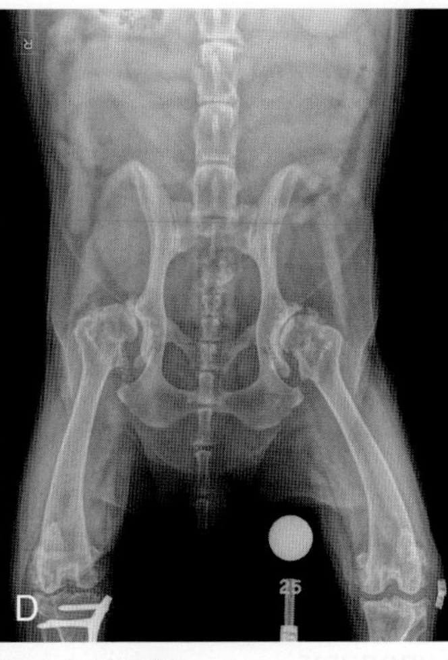

HIP DYSPLASIA Ventrodorsal pelvic radiographs demonstrate good hip conformation (**A**), dysplastic change (subluxation of the left femoral head) (**B**), mild degenerative changes in the hips (**C**), and severely dysplastic and osteoarthritic hips (**D**). Radiographic abnormalities (**D**) include severe subluxation of the femoral heads and remodeling of the shallow acetabula and femoral necks. This dog would be a candidate for total hip replacement or femoral head/neck ostectomies, based on clinical parameters described in the text.

to medical therapies or in situations that involve hip luxation.

Behavior/Exercise

- Exercise moderation; limit running, jumping, rough play
- Physical rehabilitation; increase low-impact activities to encourage muscular development: underwater treadmill, swimming, and walking

Possible Complications

Medical management:

- Adverse reaction to NSAID
- Failure of medical management to control pain, necessitating surgical intervention

Surgical management:

- DPO purportedly has reduced potential for complications (nerve injury, implant failure/loosening, pelvic canal narrowing) compared to TPO.
  - Nerve and/or urinary tract damage from TPO or JPS surgery
  - Implant failure/pelvic canal narrowing with TPO
- Surgical site infection +/− osteomyelitis
- Hip luxation, infection, implant subsidence/rotation, or femoral fracture with THR
- Poor limb use after FHO due to patient obesity, muscular atony, poor postoperative rehabilitation, or incomplete removal of femoral neck

Recommended Monitoring

- Laboratory monitoring of patients on NSAID therapy
- Weight, exercise level, clinical signs
- Radiographs if clinical signs progress

PROGNOSIS & OUTCOME

- The majority of patients improve with appropriate treatment.
- Postoperative rehabilitation is critical for good clinical recovery.

PEARLS & CONSIDERATIONS

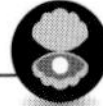

Comments

- Musculature asymmetry between pelvic and thoracic limbs suggests bilateral disease.
- Dysplastic animals acutely "down in the hind end" likely have concurrent bilateral cranial cruciate ligament rupture. Full orthopedic evaluation (p. 1143) should be performed before referral of these dogs for surgical management of hip dysplasia.
- Of medically managed juvenile patients that are lame due to hip joint laxity, 60%-75% return to acceptable clinical function with maturity.
- Radiographic signs do not always correlate with clinical signs.
- FHO significantly complicates further surgical procedures such as THR. If THR is an option, FHO should not be the first surgical intervention attempted.
- Routine radiographic monitoring of the clinically stable patient is generally not necessary.
- Practitioners should consider consultation and referral with an orthopedic surgeon for management of this condition.

Prevention

- Evaluation of at-risk breeds by a veterinarian able to perform JPS should be considered in animals by 14-16 weeks of age to ensure that the appropriate window for JPS is not lost; JPS is reportedly ineffective in puppies over 22 weeks.
- Screening and control of breeding animals for hip dysplasia
  - Avoid breeding animals that have not been evaluated for hip conformation or hip laxity using the OFA or the PennHIP method.
  - OFA evaluation has been the traditional and simpler method, but evaluation is subjective and performed on animals > 2 years old. Only dogs receiving excellent or good evaluations should be bred. The PennHIP method is an objective measure of hip laxity validated as early as 16 weeks of age. Breeding only dogs that are in the top 50% (dogs with less joint laxity) for the breed helps to decrease the incidence of hip dysplasia.
- Avoid high-energy diets for rapidly growing dogs.
- Activities such as walking, swimming, and underwater treadmill therapy under the guidance of a trained canine rehabilitation specialist may help increase muscle mass and improve hip congruity.

Technician Tips

- Sedation with analgesia is required for appropriately positioned radiographs to evaluate for hip dysplasia.
- When taking extended-leg VD views for OFA radiographs, patellas must be centered over the femoral condyles.
- In some animals chronic fibrotic changes in the hips may limit hip extension, in which case an angled radiographic beam may be required.

Client Education

- Knowledge about and careful screening of genetic history of the siblings and parents of potential pets
- Sterilization of affected dogs and dogs treated with TPO or JPS is a component of responsible pet ownership.
- Minimize clinical signs in affected dogs through diet, low-impact exercise (see Prevention above), and medical management.

SUGGESTED READING

Schulz KS: Hip dysplasia. In Fossum TW, editor: Small animal surgery, ed 4, St. Louis, 2013, Mosby, pp 1305-1316.

AUTHORS: Mathieu M. Glassman, VMD, DACVS; Spencer A. Johnston, VMD, DACVS
EDITOR: Kathleen Linn, DVM, MS, DACVS

Hip Luxation

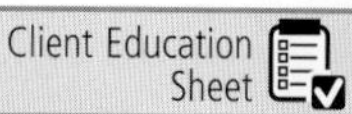

BASIC INFORMATION

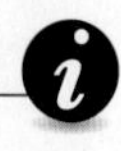

Definition

- Dislocation of the femoral head relative to the acetabulum, most frequently in a craniodorsal direction
- Luxation: complete displacement of the femoral head relative to the acetabulum
- Subluxation: partial or incomplete dislocation of the femoral head relative to the acetabulum (i.e., joint incongruity exists)

Synonyms

Coxofemoral luxation, dislocated hip

Epidemiology

SPECIES, AGE, SEX

Dogs and cats of either sex and any age

RISK FACTORS

Dogs with hip dysplasia are at risk for luxation with even minor trauma.

ASSOCIATED DISORDERS

Pelvic and proximal femoral fractures

Clinical Presentation

DISEASE FORMS/SUBTYPES

Craniodorsal luxation is most common; caudoventral is uncommon.

HISTORY, CHIEF COMPLAINT

- Trauma (falls, vehicular) causing acute non–weight-bearing lameness
- Intermittent lameness in chronic cases with unrecognized trauma

PHYSICAL EXAM FINDINGS

- Variable lameness
- With craniodorsal luxation, the limb appears shortened, with stifle rotated laterally and calcaneus medially.
- Palpation of hip reveals swelling, pain, crepitus, and abnormal position of greater trochanter.

Etiology and Pathophysiology

Coxofemoral luxations comprise 90% of all luxations in small animals.

- With craniodorsal luxation, femoral head is driven dorsally over the acetabular rim.
  - The femoral head ligament and joint capsule are torn.
  - Avulsion fracture associated with the ligament can occur.
  - Gluteal muscle contractions exacerbate craniodorsal displacement of proximal femur.
- With ventral luxation, transverse acetabular ligament is ruptured.

DIAGNOSIS

Diagnostic Overview

Orthogonal view radiography establishes the diagnosis and shows any concomitant fractures in the region.

Differential Diagnosis

Subluxation due to hip dysplasia, femoral capital physeal fracture, femoral neck fracture, acetabular fracture

Initial Database

- Physical exam (see Physical Exam Findings above)
- CBC, serum biochemistry panel, and urinalysis to assess anesthetic risk (American Society of Anesthesiologists classification system) (p. 1196)
- Limb and pelvic exams plus orthogonal view radiography to confirm the diagnosis and determine concomitant or inciting disorders

TREATMENT

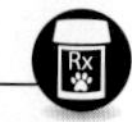

Treatment Overview

- With acute injury of a normal hip joint, the goal is closed or open anatomic joint reduction/stabilization.
- With an abnormal or chronically luxated normal joint, the goal is to return pain-free function with femoral head and neck excision (FHNE), also known as femoral head ostectomy (FHO), total hip replacement (THR), or pelvic osteotomy.

Acute General Treatment

- Closed reduction (p. 1158) and Ehmer sling application (p. 1161) if
  - Duration of injury is < 48 hours *and*
  - Hip is otherwise structurally normal *and*
  - Patient is sufficiently stable to undergo general anesthesia
- For craniodorsal luxation with patient in lateral recumbency (unaffected side down), the upper (affected) limb is externally rotated (toes out), abducted (lifted, as a male dog lifts the leg to urinate), and then internally rotated (toes in) while manual pressure on trochanter guides head into acetabulum.
- After reduction, extensive range-of-motion maneuvers are performed to force soft tissue out of acetabulum and test joint stability.
- Open (surgical) reduction is performed for failed or unstable closed reductions in patients with normal coxofemoral joints:
  - Extraarticular techniques: capsulorrhaphy, suture between origin of greater trochanter

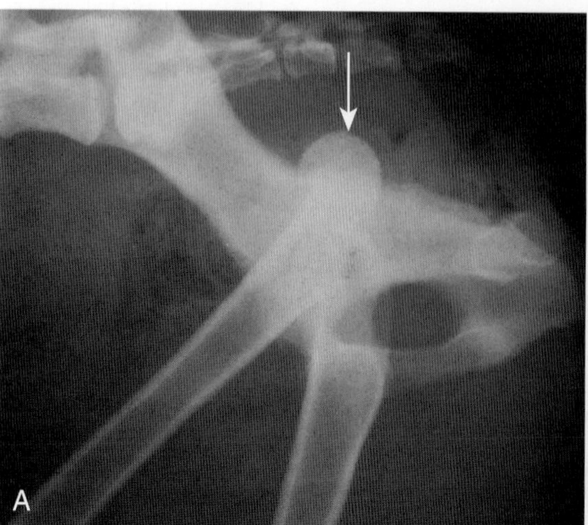

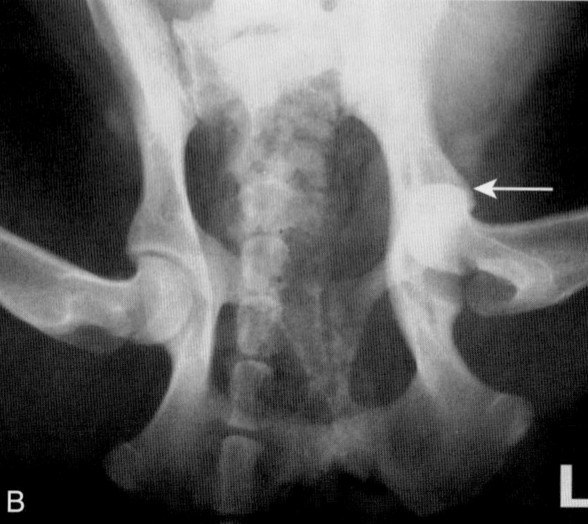

HIP LUXATION Lateral (**A**) and ventrodorsal (**B**) projections of a craniodorsal luxation of left hip joint. Note dorsal and cranial displacement of the femoral head relative to the acetabulum *(arrows)*.

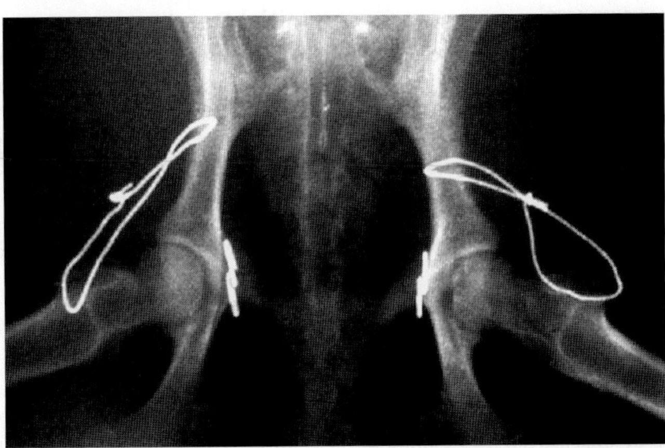

HIP LUXATION Postoperative ventrodorsal projection of hip joints of an obese 45-kg dog treated for traumatic bilateral hip luxation. Bilateral toggle pins and greater trochanter–to–ilium wires were used for stabilizing injuries.

and rectus femoris muscle, iliofemoral suture, synthetic sutures to replace capsule, gluteal muscle tenodesis
  - Intraarticular techniques: toggle pinning, fascia lata loop or sacrotuberous ligament transposition
- Triple or double pelvic osteotomy can be performed for mildly dysplastic, immature dogs with no degenerative joint changes.
- For chronic injuries, open reduction is difficult because of muscular contraction and tissue fibrosis; cartilage degeneration exists. FHNE or THR may be required in place of primary repairs.

Chronic Treatment

- Physical rehabilitation to maintain muscle tone, joint health, and overall limb functions
- Controlled activity to avoid reluxation, implant failures

- Nonsteroidal anti-inflammatory drugs (NSAIDs) as needed to reduce pain and inflammation
  - Carprofen 2 mg/kg PO q 12h (dogs), *or*
  - Deracoxib 1-2 mg/kg PO q 24h (dogs; may use 3-4 mg/kg PO q 24h for first 7 days only), *or*
  - Meloxicam 0.1 mg/kg (dogs), 0.05 mg/kg (cats) PO q 24h, *or*
  - Firocoxib 5 mg/kg PO q 24h (dogs)

Possible Complications

- Reluxation
- Implant failure
- Degenerative joint disease
- Infection

Recommended Monitoring

- For closed reduction
  - Frequent sling evaluations and removal 7-10 days after application
  - Limited activity for 1 month
  - Radiography after sling application and if lameness recurs
- For open repairs
  - Restricted ambulation for 1-2 months
  - Radiography if lameness recurs and based on fixation method

PROGNOSIS & OUTCOME

- Variable with closed reduction: 50% fail due to technical error or unrecognized joint disease
- Good to excellent with most operative procedures of acute injuries (i.e., previously normal joint)
- Guarded for dysplastic hips unless TPO, FHNE, THR performed

PEARLS & CONSIDERATIONS

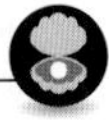

Comments

- With normal hips, reduction/stabilization is preferred over FHNE for all patient sizes.
- Extensive joint capsule and ligament damage impede successful closed reduction.
- Femoral head ligament avulsion fractures are often not recognized radiographically.

Technician Tips

Ehmer slings require frequent monitoring for pes ischemia or wounds beneath the tape.

SUGGESTED READING

Wardlaw JL, et al: Coxofemoral luxation. In Tobias KM, et al, editors: Veterinary surgery: small animal, ed 2, St. Louis, 2018, Elsevier, pp 956-964.

AUTHOR: Joseph Harari, DVM, MS, DACVS
EDITOR: Kathleen Linn, DVM, MS, DACVS

Histiocytic Diseases

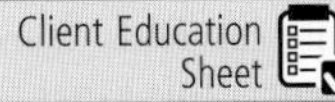

Client Education Sheet

BASIC INFORMATION

Definition

A complex group of syndromes resulting from an accumulation of histiocytes, which include cells of macrophage or dendritic origin and function as antigen-presenting cells. Clinical and histologic characteristics are needed to distinguish tumors and syndromes. Most arise from dendritic cells (DCs), specifically interstitial DCs, and less commonly from Langerhans DCs (in the epidermis). Histiocytic diseases occur in dogs and cats, although reports in cats are sparse and are limited to malignant neoplasia. Histiocytic disorders can be simplified into the following groups:

- Benign tumors
  - Histiocytoma: spontaneously regressing skin tumor of Langerhans cells common in young animals
  - Cutaneous Langerhans cell histiocytosis (LCH) includes multiple skin lesions that resemble histiocytomas and can involve lymph nodes.
- Reactive histiocytic disorders (from activated DCs, dogs only)
  - Cutaneous histiocytosis (CH): a benign accumulation of histiocytes in the skin with predisposition for the nasal planum, head, and neck
  - Systemic histiocytosis (SH): similar to cutaneous histiocytosis but characterized by lymph node and organ involvement
- Malignant histiocytic neoplasia (from interstitial DCs)
  - Histiocytic sarcoma (HS): focal or disseminated; the latter is commonly considered synonymous with malignant histiocytosis.
  - Hemophagocytic histiocytic sarcoma originates from macrophages.
  - Malignant fibrous histiocytoma: despite its name, this focal lesion is a unique soft-tissue sarcoma and is not discussed here. The histiocytic infiltrate is not neoplastic and is of questionable importance.

Synonyms

Histiocytic sarcoma (disseminated): malignant histiocytosis

Epidemiology

SPECIES, AGE, SEX

- Histiocytic diseases have predominantly been reported for dogs, but reports exist for cats (malignant histiocytosis).
- Cutaneous histiocytosis can occur in younger dogs, compared with systemic histiocytosis and disseminated HS in middle-aged dogs (median age, 6 years).
- Equal prevalence in males and females

GENETICS, BREED PREDISPOSITION

- Bernese mountain dogs (BMDs) are predisposed to many types of histiocytic disease. In BMDs, heritability is oligogenic and almost certainly *not* autosomal or sex-linked.
- Other breeds overrepresented in histiocytic diseases include golden retrievers, flat-coated retrievers (FCRs [44% of all tumors]), rottweilers (especially periarticular HS), and Doberman pinschers.
- Abnormalities in tumor suppressor genes (e.g., *RB1* [retinoblastoma], *PTEN*) have been implicated in HS in BMDs and FCRs.
- Shar-peis were overrepresented in LCH cases.
- Retrievers and Pembroke Welsh corgis may be overrepresented in central nervous system (CNS) HS.
- Irish wolfhounds may have a genetic predisposition for SH.
- No breed predisposition has been reported in cats.

RISK FACTORS

In a study of affected and unaffected BMDs, dogs with orthopedic disease were at greater risk for developing HS (OR = 2.5), and dogs treated with prescription anti-inflammatory medications had a lower risk (OR = 0.42).

GEOGRAPHY AND SEASONALITY

Initially, histiocytosis in BMD primarily affected dogs from Switzerland, where the breed originated. Many cases have now been reported in dogs born in the United States and the United Kingdom (especially FCRs).

Clinical Presentation

DISEASE FORMS/SUBTYPES

- As detailed above, histiocytic diseases are either local or diffuse, and are reactive, benign, or malignant. They can occur anywhere in the body, including the CNS or lungs as a primary site.
- A hemophagocytic variant that occurs in dogs and cats leads to anemia and thrombocytopenia. This variant is very aggressive.

HISTORY, CHIEF COMPLAINT

- Most dogs are presented for signs referable to the primary tumor (presence of a mass).
- Dogs with CH and SH are typically presented for evaluation of skin lesions.
- SH can have ocular involvement, and patients may be presented for evaluation of ocular signs.
- Dogs with periarticular HS are usually presented for evaluation of a soft-tissue mass or lameness.
- Disseminated HS is a much more insidious disease because masses are primarily visceral (spleen, liver, bone marrow, lymph nodes, lungs). Cutaneous and subcutaneous masses are uncommon.
- Affected dogs and cats are often presented for evaluation of nonspecific systemic signs such as lethargy and anorexia/weight loss.

PHYSICAL EXAM FINDINGS

- Histiocytomas occur most often as raised, hairless, erythematous masses and are commonly found on the extremities and head (especially the pinnae).
- Focal lesions typically involve a palpable mass, often on the extremities. If the mass is subarticular, lameness may be prominent, especially with bone involvement.
- Splenomegaly may be present with disseminated HS, is common with hemophagocytic HS, and can correlate with a worse prognosis.
- Dogs with disseminated HS often have significant pulmonary involvement and may be dyspneic with advanced disease. Cough is a common presenting complaint.
- With systemic histiocytosis, skin lesions may be seen on the nasal planum, muzzle, flank, scrotum, as well as the periocular tissues. Skin lesions in CH and SH are typically nodular to plaque-like.
- Generalized lymphadenopathy may be appreciated with systemic histiocytosis and disseminated HS.

Etiology and Pathophysiology

- Largely unknown in dogs, although oligogenic inheritance has been shown in BMDs, and 25% of BMDs are affected by clinical histiocytic sarcoma. Association with prior joint disease (e.g., arthritis) has been shown in this breed.
- Hemophagocytic histiocytic sarcoma is of macrophage origin and originates in the splenic red pulp or bone marrow.

DIAGNOSIS

Diagnostic Overview

Histiocytic diseases in dogs and cats can be distinguished from each other based on clinicopathologic findings, including site(s) of involvement. Diagnosis is based on cytology and histopathology, and the latter often requires immunohistochemistry to define ontogeny. After biopsy confirmation, staging should include general assessment to establish the health of the animal and a thorough evaluation of regional lymph nodes with cytology. Abdominal ultrasound is advised because visceral involvement is common with some forms. Thoracic radiographs are very important because pulmonary metastasis often occurs.

Differential Diagnosis

- Granulomatous disease
- Lymphoma
- Poorly differentiated mast cell tumor
- Anaplastic sarcoma or carcinoma
- Synovial sarcoma (joint tumors)
- Other soft-tissue or bone sarcomas (for local disease)
- Immune-mediated hemolytic anemia and immune thrombocytopenia (hemophagocytic form)

Initial Database

- CBC, serum chemistry profile, and urinalysis; no characteristic or specific findings with histiocytic diseases, except hemophagocytic syndrome results in Coombs-negative anemia and thrombocytopenia. Hypoalbuminemia may be present.
- Fine-needle aspiration of accessible masses and lymph nodes for cytologic exam (look for multinucleated giant cells and erythrophagocytosis by macrophages)
- Biopsy of affected tissue with immunohistochemistry (see Pearls & Considerations below)
- Radiography of affected area if bony involvement is suspected typically reveals a lesion that is permeative, punctate, or moth-eaten.
- Thoracic radiography to evaluate pulmonary parenchyma for nodules (often large) and lymphadenopathy (especially sternal or tracheobronchial)
- Abdominal ultrasound to screen for visceral involvement
- Bone marrow aspiration and cytology may be indicated if systemic disease is suspected and more than one cell line is abnormal (especially low) on CBC (p. 1068).

Advanced or Confirmatory Testing

- CT scan of affected area if focal and considering resection
- Immunohistochemistry on biopsy tissue (see Pearls & Considerations below)

TREATMENT

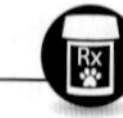

Treatment Overview

For benign/reactive disease, immunosuppression may suppress disease, but lesions are often resistant to treatment. These lesions can wax and wane, making it difficult to assess response to treatment. For malignant disease, if only local involvement is present, surgical removal should be followed by adjuvant CCNU-based chemotherapy. For disseminated disease, CCNU-based chemotherapy and palliative care may extend survival time, but long-term prognosis is poor. Dogs with anemia, thrombocytopenia, and hypoalbuminemia often survive less than 1 month, even with CCNU therapy. Histiocytomas often spontaneously regress through actions of $CD8^+$ T lymphocytes but can be bothersome enough to warrant surgical excision with an excellent prognosis.

Acute General Treatment

- Patients with malignant histiocytosis and significant erythrophagocytosis may require red blood cell transfusion (p. 1169), ideally in conjunction with initiation of therapy to abort red cell loss.
- Dyspneic patients with malignant histiocytosis may benefit temporarily from oxygen therapy, but the prognosis is grave when the disease has reached the point of producing respiratory compromise.

Chronic Treatment

- Reactive histiocytoses are typically treated with immunosuppressive therapy. Initially, prednisone 2 mg/kg PO q 24h is used until clinical response is noted; then a slow taper of 1 mg/kg PO q 24h for 1 month, 0.5 mg/kg PO q 24h for 1 month, 0.5 mg/kg PO q 48h for 3 months, and then stop or maintain at lowest effective dose.
- If no response is noted within 1 month of prednisone therapy or lesions relapse and no longer respond to prednisone, azathioprine 2 mg/kg PO q 24h, with the same taper schedule as prednisone or cyclosporine may be added.
- Evidence suggests efficacy of tetracycline and niacinamide (dogs < 10 kg: 250 mg of each drug PO q 8h, and dogs > 10 kg: 500 mg of each drug PO q 8h).
- All treatments can be used with or without antibiotics, depending on appearance of skin lesions and at the discretion of the treating clinician.
- Systemic malignant histiocytic diseases are poorly responsive to therapy, and remissions, if achieved, are typically short lived.
  - CCNU 60-90 mg/m^2 (p. 609); 29%-46% response with macroscopic disease. Dogs with metastasis limited to lymph nodes responded favorably (median survival time, 219 days; 38% 1-year survival). CCNU has been used in combination with other drugs with similar results.
  - Other chemotherapy drugs that have been used include doxorubicin 30 mg/m^2 IV (p. 609), epirubicin 30 mg/m^2 IV (p. 609), and dacarbazine 900-1000 mg/m^2 (p. 609) diluted in saline over 5 hours, although none provided durable responses.
  - Liposome-encapsulated clodronate, a novel formulation of a bisphosphonate capable of eliminating macrophage/dendritic cells, is not widely available but has been reported and may be useful in treatment.
  - TALL104 (cytotoxic T lymphocytes) therapy has been described but is not commercially available.
- Focal malignant histiocytic diseases respond well to surgical resection (amputation if joint or bone affected or complete resection with limb salvage impossible) ± irradiation.

Recommended Monitoring

- The involved site(s) should be monitored closely by regular observation and diagnostic imaging as appropriate.
- Three-view thoracic radiographs and physical exam, including lymph node palpation and exam of the site, should be performed every 3 months for the first year after diagnosis for localized HS and every 4-6 months thereafter.

PROGNOSIS & OUTCOME

- CH: good; may regress spontaneously or respond to immunosuppressive doses of prednisone
- SH and disseminated HS: poor. SH may wax and wane but is ultimately progressive, whereas disseminated HS is rapidly progressive, with both leading to death. Disseminated HS is considered uniformly fatal. Survival of dogs with SH ranges from months to years. Survival for dogs with disseminated HS averages 4 months, although chemotherapy in the adjuvant setting with CCNU may prolong survival to greater than 1 year for some dogs (see Treatment above). Prognosis to date for cats with malignant histiocytosis is similarly grave, and response to therapy has been poor.
- Focal histiocytic sarcoma: good if low grade and local control is achieved with surgery ± radiation therapy. Periarticular HS has a better prognosis than that at other sites, even with suspected metastasis at the time of diagnosis. CNS HS has a grave prognosis (3 days).
- More than 1 of 7 BMDs and FCRs die from HS.

PEARLS & CONSIDERATIONS

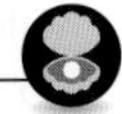

Comments

The following clinical and pathologic differences can help differentiate histiocytic syndromes:

- Clinical findings/behavior
  - Disseminated HS is a multiorgan disease typically arising from internal sites, including viscera, whereas SH involves skin and lymph nodes with occasional internal sites.
  - CH is limited to the skin and does not lead to HS.
  - Hemophagocytic HS may be confused with Evans syndrome (anemia and thrombocytopenia), but HS is Coombs negative.
- Histopathology and immunohistochemistry for dogs and cats
  - CD18$^+$ (leukocyte marker), CD3$^-$, and CD79a$^-$ are three stains and the immunohistochemical pattern most useful for diagnosing DC-origin disorders and ruling out lymphoma. Polymerase chain reaction (PCR) for antigen receptor rearrangement (PARR) may not adequately distinguish HS from lymphoma because of infiltrating clonal T cells in HS.
  - Newer markers include ionized calcium binding adaptor molecule 1 (IBA-1) with good sensitivity and specificity and CD204 with conflicting reports of utility.
  - Dendritic cells should be CD1a$^+$ or CD1c$^+$, CD11c$^+$, and MHC II$^+$ (Langerhans DCs are associated with E-cadherin positivity as in most histiocytomas, and interstitial DCs are CD90$^+$)
  - Macrophages (hemophagocytic HS) should be CD 1$^{low/-}$, CD11c$^-$, and CD11d$^+$ as well as lysozyme positive.
  - Malignant histiocytic diseases should be CD4$^-$, and reactive syndromes, CD4$^+$.

Prevention

Because histiocytic diseases are often inherited, careful documentation of pedigrees for affected animals may reduce disease through selective breeding. Inheritance of histiocytosis in BMDs has been calculated at a moderate 0.298, suggesting that careful breeding could be effective at eliminating this disease. This means that 29.8% of the risk of developing histiocytosis in the population of BMDs is attributable to genetic differences among individuals. The remainder of the risk is environmental, although specific factors have not been identified.

Technician Tips

Some tumor-bearing dogs have coagulopathies. Although peripheral veins may be preferred for routine blood draws, they may be needed to deliver intravenous chemotherapy.

Client Education

- Owners should contact the breeder or source of affected animals.
- An overtly (phenotypically) normal breeding pair of BMDs with one affected offspring will produce on average one in seven puppies that will ultimately succumb to histiocytosis.

SUGGESTED READING

Moore PF: A review of histiocytic diseases of dogs and cats. Vet Pathol 51(1):167-184, 2014.

AUTHOR: Kim A. Selting, DVM, MS, DACVIM, DACVR
EDITOR: Kenneth M. Rassnick, DVM, DACVIM

Histoplasmosis

Bonus Material Online Client Education Sheet 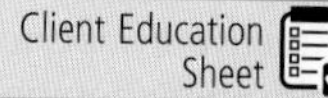

BASIC INFORMATION

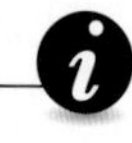

Definition

A systemic fungal disease caused by the soil-dwelling dimorphic fungus, *Histoplasma capsulatum*; affects companion animals and humans

Epidemiology

SPECIES, AGE, SEX

- Dogs and cats; cats slightly more susceptible than dogs
- Young adult, large-breed dogs; dogs 2-7 years of age are more likely affected than dogs < 2 years of age; females may be slightly more susceptible than males.
- Cats: mean age 4-9 years; females may be more susceptible

GENETICS, BREED PREDISPOSITION

Sporting (hunting) breeds, notably pointers, Weimaraners, and Brittany spaniels, may be overrepresented, likely due to greater environmental exposure.

RISK FACTORS

- Outdoor activities in endemic areas
- Contact with nitrogen-rich organic material such as moist soil containing bird or bat excrement
- Can occur in indoor-only cats and dogs

CONTAGION AND ZOONOSIS

Common-source exposure possible but true zoonosis does not occur (exception: accidental laboratory inoculation/inhalation)

GEOGRAPHY AND SEASONALITY

- *H. capsulatum* is endemic in many temperate and subtropical regions of the world.
- In the United States, histoplasmosis occurs most commonly in the Missouri, Mississippi, Tennessee, and Ohio River valleys.
- *H. capsulatum* may thrive in nonendemic regions if soil conditions favor fungal growth.
- Outside the typical geographic range, cats are more often affected than dogs.

Clinical Presentation

DISEASE FORMS/SUBTYPES

Disease may remain confined to the lungs or gastrointestinal (GI) tract or may become disseminated (commonly with GI involvement).

HISTORY, CHIEF COMPLAINT

- Clinical signs are determined by the major organ system(s) affected.
- History of time spent in an endemic area
- Nonspecific signs of disease are common, typically including depression, anorexia, and weight loss.
  - Clients may notice labored breathing in dogs and cats with pulmonary histoplasmosis (<50% of cats with histoplasmosis have respiratory signs).
  - Dogs with GI involvement may exhibit signs consistent with small- and/or large-bowel disease and recent weight loss. In cats, GI signs may be less specific (weight loss, anorexia).

PHYSICAL EXAM FINDINGS

- Dyspnea, tachypnea, coughing, abnormal lung sounds, pale mucous membranes
- Lymphadenopathy
- Poor body condition/emaciation
- Fever
- Hepatomegaly, splenomegaly (or both if disseminated disease)
- Cobblestone mucosa, hematochezia on rectal palpation
- Ocular lesions
- Dermal lesions (rare)
- Exam may be unremarkable

Etiology and Pathophysiology

- Eight clades of the organism have been identified by genetic analysis. Different clades tend to occur in different parts of the world and may have different pathogenicity.
- The primary reservoir appears to be bats, although high concentrations of the organism may also be found in bird guano.
- The mycelial stage (in soil; releases spores [microconidia and macroconidia]) of *H. capsulatum* is responsible for mammalian infections. Exposure most commonly occurs by inhaling microconidia, which are small enough to reach the lower airways. Oral exposure may result in disease, as evidenced by some animals developing only GI signs.
- After inhalation, microconidia convert to the yeast form in the lower respiratory tract, where they reproduce by budding.
- The organisms are phagocytosed by host alveolar macrophages, in which they undergo further replication. At this point, disease may remain limited to the respiratory system or become generalized by lymphatic and/or hematogenous dissemination.
- Dissemination to the GI tract, lymph nodes, spleen, liver, and bone marrow is common. The organism load in infected tissues is generally high, and affected tissues respond with pyogranulomatous inflammation.
- The incubation period may range from 2-3 weeks to years, depending on the extent of the immune response.
- Most exposed animals do not show clinical disease, and infection often remains subclinical.

DIAGNOSIS

Diagnostic Overview

Infection is suspected based on respiratory signs with a miliary or nodular pattern on thoracic radiographs in a dog or cat with exposure to an endemic region or with GI signs, lymphadenopathy, and hepatomegaly. Confirmation is ideally done by cytologic or histologic identification of yeast and pyogranulomatous inflammation. A urine antigen test for histoplasmosis is more sensitive than serologic testing.

Differential Diagnosis

- Other systemic mycoses (e.g., blastomycosis, cryptococcosis, coccidioidomycosis)
- Protein-losing enteropathy
- Severe infiltrative intestinal diseases (e.g., inflammatory bowel disease, GI lymphoma)

Initial Database

CBC, serum biochemistry profile:

- Normocytic, normochromic, nonregenerative anemia (most consistent, albeit nonspecific, finding with histoplasmosis); likely secondary to chronic disease, bone marrow infiltration, and/or GI blood loss
- Leukocyte parameters are variably affected. Thrombocytopenia and/or eosinophilia possible
- Intracellular organisms are rarely observed on blood smears.
- Hypoalbuminemia common; increased liver enzyme activities, hyperglobulinemia, hyperbilirubinemia, and/or hypercalcemia possible

Radiography:

- Cats with pulmonary histoplasmosis often exhibit a diffuse miliary interstitial or nodular pattern on thoracic radiographs consistent with mycotic pneumonia. Dogs may show alveolar, interstitial, and/or bronchial patterns; tracheobronchial lymphadenopathy is common. Mineralization of lesions is possible.
- Pleural effusion occasionally may be noted.
- Hepatomegaly and splenomegaly are possible.
- Osteolytic lesions occasionally occur in cats but rarely in dogs.

Abdominal ultrasound:

- Depends of organ(s) affected; may see abdominal lymphadenopathy, peritoneal effusion, enlarged and diffusely hypoechoic spleen and liver, as well as thickening of the intestinal walls

Advanced or Confirmatory Testing

- Cytologic evaluation:
  - Usually provides a definitive antemortem diagnosis
  - The organisms are usually observed in phagocytic cells and appear as single to multiple, round bodies with a basophilic center and clear, thin outer rim.
  - In dogs, tissues most rewarding for obtaining a diagnostic sample include rectal scrapings (p. 1157), colonic biopsy imprints, and aspirates of bone marrow (p. 1068), liver, spleen (p. 1064), lymph nodes, and lung (pp. 1073, 1074, and

1113), depending on the extent of disease. Organ enlargement and ease of access determine which organs are sampled.
  - In cats, tissues that may successfully be sampled include bone marrow, lung, and lymph nodes.
- Histology may be useful if cytology is inconclusive.
- Serologic testing for antibodies is not recommended because of poor diagnostic sensitivity.
- ELISA assay for *H. capsulatum* antigen (MiraVista Diagnostics, Indianapolis, IN) can be used on urine or serum and appears to have good sensitivity and specificity but cross-reacts with other fungal infections such as blastomycosis (p. 1365).
- False-negative antigen results can occur, especially in cases of focal disease (i.e., ocular). Therefore, a negative antigen test does not completely rule out infection.

TREATMENT

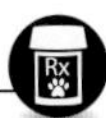

Treatment Overview

Oral azole antifungal agents are the mainstay of therapy for histoplasmosis, with itraconazole and fluconazole used most often. Newer-generation azoles (voriconazole and posaconazole) may be effective in cases that fail to respond well to itraconazole. Duration of treatment with oral antifungals typically is 4-6 months but depends on severity of disease and the patient's response to therapy.

Acute General Treatment

- Azole drugs
  - For mild to moderate disease (local involvement only, no overt or only mild respiratory signs, patient is eating and is not debilitated)
  - Itraconazole capsules 10 mg/kg PO q 24h (dogs), 10 mg/kg PO q 12h (cats), *or*
  - Itraconazole oral solution 5 mg/kg PO q 24h (cats, dogs)
  - Fluconazole tablets 5-10 mg/kg q 12h (dogs), 50 mg/CAT q 12h
- Itraconazole plus amphotericin B
  - In critically ill cases with disseminated disease or fulminant pulmonary, GI, or neurologic involvement, consider combination therapy of an oral azole with parenteral amphotericin B.
  - The drugs are started concomitantly, with the azole continued past cessation of amphotericin B therapy.
  - Sample protocol for amphotericin B: dog, 0.5 mg/kg IV q 48-72h up to 60 days or until signs of toxicosis; cat, 0.25 mg/kg IV q 48-72h or until signs of toxicosis. Cumulative dose of 9-12 mg/kg (dog) and 6-9 (cat) ideal
  - Sample protocol for lipid-complexed amphotericin B (lower risk of nephrotoxicosis) for dogs and cats: 1-2 mg/kg IV q 48-72h × 60 days or until signs of toxicosis. Cumulative dose of 24-30 mg/kg (dog) and 12-24 mg/kg (cat) ideal
  - Nephrotoxicity is the main side effect. Monitor blood urea nitrogen (BUN) and creatinine during treatment and stop if > 50% increase in either parameter.
- Prednisone 2 mg/kg PO q 24h hastens resolution of dyspnea in dogs with histoplasmosis-associated tracheobronchial lymphadenopathy (in the absence of systemic histoplasmosis). Taper after first week or two of antifungal therapy or as possible based on clinical signs.

Chronic Treatment

Itraconazole or fluconazole PO for at least 4-6 months. Fluconazole may require longer treatment and may not be as effective. Treatment should be continued for 1 month beyond resolution of clinical signs or when antigenuria is no longer present.

Possible Complications

- Acute kidney injury with amphotericin B
- Skin lesions from a drug-induced vasculitis may occur in dogs and cats treated with itraconazole (especially at higher doses). Itraconazole may also cause hepatopathy.

Recommended Monitoring

Response to treatment is monitored with periodic CBC and serum biochemistry profiles, weight checks, and monitoring for resolution of radiographic lesions. Urine antigen concentrations decrease with appropriate therapy and can be beneficial in deciding when to discontinue therapy as well as documenting relapse after treatment discontinuation. Therapuetic drug monitoring of itraconazole levels may be helpful in guiding dose adjustments.

PROGNOSIS & OUTCOME

- Prognosis varies from guarded to good, depending on the extent of disease; cats may have a better prognosis than dogs.
- Disease limited to the lungs typically carries a better prognosis compared with GI or disseminated histoplasmosis.
- Prognosis is guarded for return of vision with ocular involvement, depending on severity of retinal damage before treatment.

PEARLS & CONSIDERATIONS

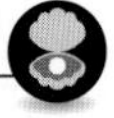

Comments

- Stable patients may be successfully treated with oral antifungals alone, and critically ill patients require more intense combination therapy and supportive care.
- Itraconazole capsules should be administered with food for increased bioavailability. Itraconazole liquid solution should be given on an empty stomach and has a greater bioavailability than capsules.

Prevention

Avoid contact with contaminated soil in endemic areas. Zoonotic transmission has not been reported, but common-source natural infection occurs. Dogs and cats with histoplasmosis may be sentinels for humans with the disease.

Technician Tips

Be cautious when collecting samples as transmission via needle stick injury is possible.

SUGGESTED READING

Dedeaux AM, et al: Blastomycosis and histoplasmosis. In Ettinger SJ, et al, editors: The textbook of veterinary internal medicine, ed 8, St. Louis, 2017, Saunders, pp 1027-1035.

AUTHORS: **Andrea Dedeaux, DVM, DACVIM; Joseph Taboada, DVM, DACVIM**
EDITOR: **Joseph Taboada, DVM, DACVIM**

Hit by Car

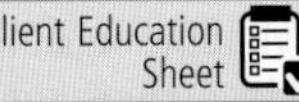

BASIC INFORMATION

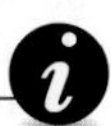

Definition

Trauma sustained after being struck by a motorized vehicle

Synonyms

HBC, vehicular trauma, motor vehicle accident (MVA)

Epidemiology

SPECIES, AGE, SEX

Young males are overrepresented for cats and dogs.

RISK FACTORS

The speculation is that male dogs roam more frequently, increasing risk of vehicular trauma.

GEOGRAPHY AND SEASONALITY

Anecdotally, more common during warmer months due to increased time outdoors

ASSOCIATED DISORDERS

Shock (hypovolemic, hypoxic), traumatic brain injury (TBI), microvascular thrombosis, systemic inflammatory response syndrome (SIRS), fractures, diaphragmatic rupture, proptosis, pneumothorax, pulmonary contusions, ventricular arrhythmias, uroabdomen, hemoabdomen

Clinical Presentation

HISTORY, CHIEF COMPLAINT

May be witnessed or inferred based on physical exam. Chief complaints can include difficulty breathing, bleeding, collapse, lameness, ocular or head injury, altered mentation, paresis, paralysis, abrasions, and degloving injuries.

PHYSICAL EXAM FINDINGS

Findings depend on injuries and may include the following:

- Cardiovascular: tachycardia, poor pulse quality, arrhythmia, cool extremities, pale mucous membranes, prolonged capillary refill time (CRT)
- Respiratory: quiet or absent breath sounds (auscultation), pulmonary crackles (auscultation), tachypnea, dyspnea, flail chest (p. 340), decreased chest wall/diaphragm excursions with neck injuries, paradoxical breathing (chest and abdominal walls move oppositely) with diaphragmatic hernia, or severe respiratory distress
- Neurologic: altered/abnormal mentation (dull, obtunded, stuporous, comatose, dysphoric), cranial nerve deficits, neck/back pain, paresis/paralysis, fecal/urinary incontinence
- Musculoskeletal: nonambulatory, pain or crepitus on bone palpation or joint manipulation, lameness, obvious fracture or dislocation
- Integument: abrasions/lacerations, degloving injuries, subcutaneous emphysema, bruising
- Ocular: proptosis, episcleral hemorrhage, detached retina, blindness, corneal ulcer, hyphema

Etiology and Pathophysiology

- The body's response to physical trauma is complex and individual. The acute inflammatory response is initally protective but can result in SIRS if excessive.
- Tissue factor exposed by endothelial damage activates coagulation. A hypercoagulable state may result and progress to disseminated intravascular coagulation (DIC [p. 269]).
- Coagulopathy was initially hypothesized to be a result of consumption, hemodilution, acidosis, and hypothermia; however, the acute hypocoagulable and hyperfibrinolytic state (acute traumatic coagulopathy) in trauma patients may occur solely due to hypoperfusion.
- Tissue hypoxia can result from hypovolemia and microvascular thrombosis.
- Multiple organ failure can ensue (p. 665).
- Head trauma can result in bleeding, cerebral edema, and brain herniation. Sympathetic stimulation can cause neurogenic pulmonary edema.

DIAGNOSIS

Diagnostic Overview

Diagnostics should complement exam findings and be used initially to rule out life-threatening derangements in major body systems. The use of a pulse oximeter, blood pressure, electrocardiogram (ECG), lactate, and focused assessment of sonography for trauma (FAST) scan (abdominal and thoracic) is advised. After major systems are adequately assessed and addressed, more comprehensive diagnostics may be pursued (e.g., investigation of possible fractures).

Differential Diagnosis

- Other forms of blunt trauma
  - Acceleration/deceleration (e.g., falls, being inside a car that was in an accident)
  - Crush/compression

Initial Database

- Neurologic exam (p. 1136)
  - Altered mentation or cranial nerve deficits increase suspicion for cerebral hemorrhage or edema. Skull fractures may be palpable.
  - Loss of proprioception, ataxia, paresis, or paralysis increase suspicion for spinal cord injury secondary to traumatic disc herniation, vertebral fracture, spinal luxation, hemorrhage causing cord compression, or spinal cord contusion.
- Orthopedic exam (p. 1143)
  - Careful palpation of all bones for crepitus, pain, and range of motion
  - Palpation of the pelvic floor per rectum may identify pelvic fractures.
- Blood pressure (p. 1065)
  - Hypotension often represents hypovolemia and requires immediate attention. It may also result from inappropriate vasodilation from SIRS.
  - Hypertension is commonly due to pain or increased intracranial pressure.
- Pulse oximetry (SpO_2)
  - Estimates arterial hemoglobin oxygen saturation (SaO_2). A value < 95% requires oxygen therapy and investigation of cause.
- ECG (p. 1096)
  - Ventricular arrhythmias (p. 1033) occur in 20%-25% of trauma patients. Treatment is recommended if there is hemodynamic compromise, sustained ventricular tachycardia with a rate > 180 beats/min, R-on-T phenomenon or polymorphic ventricular tachycardia. Arrhythmias may not occur until 12-24 hours after trauma.
  - Most trauma-associated ventricular arrhythmias resolve without specific therapy within 4 days (p. 1033).
- FAST scans (p. 1102)
  - Abbreviated ultrasound can identify free thoracic or peritoneal fluid, pneumothorax, or pulmonary contusions.
- Point-of-care blood tests
  - Packed cell volume (PCV) and total protein (TP) can identify the presence of hemorrhage. PCV may be low, normal, or high (due to splenic contraction in dogs) after hemorrhage; however, TP is always decreased and is a more sensitive early indicator of hemorrhage. Serial monitoring is recommended.
  - Elevated blood lactate concentrations can indicate poor perfusion (p. 1356)
  - Blood gas analysis can identify respiratory and metabolic disturbances.
- Thoracic radiographs
  - Common findings include pulmonary contusions, pneumothorax, diaphragmatic rupture, rib fractures, and pleural effusion.
- Abdominal radiographs
  - Common findings include peritoneal effusion, retroperitoneal effusion, and indistinct bladder. Free peritoneal gas may indicate a ruptured viscus or penetrating abdominal wound.
- CBC
  - Anemia secondary to hemorrhage
  - Leukocytosis due to inflammation, physiologic stress, or infection
  - Platelets may be decreased due to consumption
- Serum biochemistry
  - Hypoalbuminemia due to inflammation or hemorrhage
  - Increased liver enzyme activities due to hypoperfusion or liver trauma
  - Azotemia from hypovolemia, acute kidney injury, or uroabdomen
- Orthopedic radiographs: if abnormalities detected on physical exam
- Abdominocentesis (p. 1056)
  - Hemorrhage: confirm with PCV/TP
  - Urine: confirm by comparing effusion potassium and creatinine with serum values (p. 1343)
  - Bile: compare total bilirubin of the effusion to serum total bilirubin
  - Septic effusion (ruptured viscus): identify intracellular bacteria; compare blood glucose and lactate concentrations to those of effusion (p. 779)

Advanced or Confirmatory Testing

- Full-body CT scan is the gold standard imaging modality for trauma patients.
- Radiographic contrast studies to evaluate integrity of the urinary tract
- MRI (p. 1132) to assess extent of brain or spinal cord damage

TREATMENT

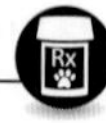

Treatment Overview

Treatment must be prioritized to address life-threatening problems first, with an initial goal of maximizing delivery of oxygen to tissues. Stabilization of cardiovascular, respiratory, and neurologic function should be performed immediately. In all cases, an intravenous catheter is useful, and blood can be obtained for point-of-care testing at the same time. If hypovolemia is suspected, a fluid bolus should be administered. Oxygen supplementation should be provided until it is proven that it is not needed. After initial triage assessment, pain medication should be administered.

Acute General Treatment

- Oxygen supplementation (oxygen cage, flow by/mask, nasal prongs or cannulas [p. 1146]); avoid nasal prongs with head trauma

- Fluid therapy for hypovolemia
  - Isotonic crystalloid bolus of 20 mL/kg IV over 15-20 minutes, then reassess perfusion parameters.
  - Repeat as necessary up to 60-90 mL/kg in a dog and 40-60 mL/kg in a cat.
  - If patient is hypovolemic but hydrated, a 7% hypertonic saline (HTS) bolus (3-5 mL/kg IV over 15 minutes) rapidly expands intravascular volume.
    - HTS also decreases intracranial pressure.
    - Caution in patients with cardiac disease.
    - Monitor serum sodium concentration
    - HTS should be followed with IV isotonic crystalloid.
- Treat hemorrhagic shock with transfusion of packed red blood cells (pRBCs) or fresh whole blood.
  - Approximately 1 mL/kg of pRBCs or 2 mL/kg of fresh whole blood will raise the PCV ≈1% (p. 1169).
- Oncotic support can be provided with colloids or albumin (canine or human).
- Analgesics are indicated in almost all cases; a pure mu opioid agonist is the drug of choice.
  - Methadone 0.1-0.3 mg/kg IM, IV q 4-6h
  - Hydromorphone
    - Dogs: 0.05-0.1 mg/kg IV, 0.05-0.2 mg/kg IM, SQ q 2-4h
    - Cats: 0.03-0.05 mg/kg IV, 0.05-0.1 mg/kg IM, SQ q 3-4h
  - Oxymorphone
    - Dogs: 0.03-0.1 mg/kg IM, IV q 2-4h
    - Cats: 0.01-0.05 mg/kg IM, IV q 2-4h
  - Fentanyl
    - Dogs: loading dose of 2-3 mcg/kg IV followed by infusion of 2-5 mcg/kg/h
    - Cats: loading dose of 1-3 mcg/kg IV followed by an infusion of 1-4 mcg/kg/h
- Thoracocentesis for pneumothorax or hemothorax (p. 1164)
- Sterile lubricant should be placed in wounds, the area clipped and cleaned and then flushed copiously, followed by sterile bandaging.
- Antimicrobials as needed if wounds or open fractures, after bacteriologic culture.
- Surgical procedures should occur after the patient has stabilized.

Chronic Treatment

- When neurologic or musculoskeletal injuries are sustained, physical therapy may be indicated for weeks to months.
- Limit exercise for a month if suspected or confirmed pulmonary or pleural space disease.

Nutrition/Diet

No special recommendations unless maxillofacial trauma necessitates tube feeding.

Behavior/Exercise

Exercise should be limited for 1 month; dogs that freely roam should be leash walked.

PROGNOSIS & OUTCOME

- Patients that survive the initial event have an excellent prognosis for survival. Mortality rates are 10%-12%.
- Factors that negatively affect survival include head trauma, fractures of the cranium, recumbency at admission, hematochezia, suspicion of acute respiratory distress syndrome, DIC, multiorgan dysfunction syndrome, development of pneumonia, requirement for positive-pressure ventilation, use of vasopressors, cardiopulmonary arrest, hyperlactatemia (≥ 4 mmol/L), modified Glasgow coma scale ≤ 17 (p. 404), and animal trauma triage score ≥ 5.

PEARLS & CONSIDERATIONS

Comments

- Frequent reassessment and close monitoring is essential.
- Radiographic evidence of pulmonary contusions may lag 12-24 hours behind clinical signs and may progress over 48 hours (p. 835).
- Autotransfusion can be considered if there is significant hemorrhage into a body cavity and blood products are not available. Blood must be filtered, and hemorrhage must be acute.
- Client education regarding at-home monitoring is vital because biliary tract rupture may take days to weeks to manifest.
- Tracheal rupture in cats may not manifest significant clinical signs until days after injury.

Prevention

The best way to prevent animals from vehicular trauma is to keep dogs on leash and cats indoors.

Technician Tips

- Large-gauge, short, intravenous catheters should be chosen.
- Signs of worsening condition include increased respiratory rate and effort, shallow breathing, persistent or worsening tachycardia, bradycardia, development of arrhythmias, rapid or prolonged CRT, pale or cyanotic mucous membranes, poor pulse quality, depressed mentation, vomiting, and progressive pain or paresis. Veterinary technicians are often the first to notice these signs due to close and frequent contact with the trauma patient.
- Recumbent patients should be propped in sternal recumbency or rotated every 4 hours to avoid atelectasis and pressure sores. Passive range-of-motion exercises may be indicated, and patients must be kept clean and dry.
- Observation of adequate urine production helps assess for possible urinary tract injury.

SUGGESTED READING

Simpson SA, et al: Severe blunt trauma in dogs: 235 cases (1997-2003). J Vet Emerg Crit Care 19(6):588-602, 2009.

AUTHORS: Sage M. De Rosa, DVM; Kenneth J. Drobatz, DVM, MSCE, DACVIM, DACVECC
EDITOR: Benjamin M. Brainard, VMD, DACVAA, DACVECC

Home-Prepared Diets

BASIC INFORMATION

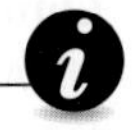

Definition

Home-prepared diets are an alternative to commercially available options.

Synonyms

Homemade diet, home-cooked diet

Epidemiology

SPECIES, AGE, SEX

Any dog or cat

RISK FACTORS

Animals with demanding requirements, such as those during growth or reproduction or those with underlying disease, are at higher risk for adverse effects of unbalanced or otherwise inadequate home-prepared diets. Most recipes found in books or on the Internet are unbalanced, imprecise, and lack appropriate strategies for supporting health or managing disease.

CONTAGION AND ZOONOSIS

Food-borne pathogens may affect pets or people in contact with the pet or the diet (particular concern for diets containing raw animal products).

ASSOCIATED DISORDERS

Some owners chose home-prepared diets to address poor pet acceptance of commercially available options. Poor acceptance of commercial diets may be due to behavioral issues (learned pickiness; fixed food preferences, especially in cats), but it also commonly occurs secondary to underlying illness that can predispose to food aversion (e.g., gastrointestinal disease, chronic kidney disease [CKD]).

Clinical Presentation

DISEASE FORMS/SUBTYPES

Always collect a thorough dietary history, which can reveal use of home-prepared diets.

HISTORY, CHIEF COMPLAINT

The feeding of a home-prepared diet may be discovered incidentally, or owners may seek veterinary help in initiating or continuing specific recipes out of preference or necessity. For some pets, a home-prepared diet is the only option to optimally manage their disease(s) if commercially available diets are not suitable.

PHYSICAL EXAM FINDINGS

Findings range from an apparently healthy pet (regardless of whether diet is balanced) to overt signs of nutritional deficiency or toxicity, such as dilated cardiomyopathy or blindness due to taurine deficiency in cats, poor skin and coat quality due to essential fatty acid deficiency, fractures due to calcium deficiency during growth, and poor body condition along with over or under ideal weight. Other abnormalities may be related to underlying disease that prompted consideration of diet change (e.g., small kidneys in pet with CKD).

DIAGNOSIS

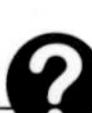

Diagnostic Overview

Dietary history should include specific types and amounts foods fed, including treats and supplements. If assessment of the diet does not meet the individual's needs (e.g., not addressing nutritionally-responsive disease, unbalanced home-prepared diet, inadequate calorie intake), adjustments should be implemented. When home-prepared diets are preferred or indicated for individual patients, the veterinarian is an important source of information to help ensure safe and effective use.

Differential Diagnosis

As home cooked diets are not a disease, there are no differential diagnoses. Other unconventional diets may or may not be balanced or otherwise appropriate (such as homemade-style commercial diets, commercial pre-mix products requiring the addition of meat, and refrigerated fresh commercial diets).

Initial Database

Nutritional assessment (including dietary history and physical exam with body weight, body condition score, and muscle condition score) as well as CBC, serum chemistry panel, and urinalysis are recommended before initiation of diet and then every 6 months. Home-prepared diet recipes can be qualitatively evaluated for provision of calories, protein source and amount, source of essential fatty acids, source of calcium, and source of trace minerals and vitamins.

Advanced or Confirmatory Testing

Comprehensive testing of nutritional status is not available. Few essential nutrients can be assessed by blood concentrations (e.g., cobalamin, amino acids), surrogate marker testing (e.g., transketolase enzyme activity for thiamin status), or liver biopsies (for copper status). Quantitative evaluation of recipes for a home-prepared diet requires specialized software, and a board-certified veterinary nutritionist should be consulted (www.acvn.org). The data can then be correlated with patient information to assess suitability and effectiveness of the diet.

TREATMENT

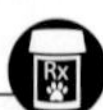

Treatment Overview

Obtaining a balanced and appropriate option or correcting an inadequate recipe for a home-prepared diet for individual pets is a service provided by some board-certified veterinary nutritionists (www.acvn.org).

Acute General Treatment

Urgency of diet correction depends on degree and chronicity of potential nutritional deficiency or toxicity, life stage of pet, and clinical presentation.

Possible Complications

Malnutrition

PROGNOSIS & OUTCOME

Excellent for pets on complete and balanced diets appropriate for their individual needs

PEARLS & CONSIDERATIONS

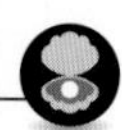

Comments

- Clinicians should discuss diet with every client and, for those invested in home-prepared options, understand their motivation as well as ability to provide an adequate and appropriate diet.
- Home-prepared diets typically require more financial, time, and space resources than commercially available options.

Technician Tips

- Provide valuable client education about the proper diet and feeding management of dogs and cats.
- Ensure that every patient is weighed, body condition scored, and has a dietary history recorded.
- Counsel clients regarding challenges as well as benefits of using home-prepared diets.

Client Education

Clients who want or need to provide home-prepared diets may require more logistical support. Board-certified veterinary nutritionists can help construct customized nutritional management plans that include home-prepared diets for healthy pets and those with disease. Reputable sources of recipes include Diplomates of the American College of Veterinary Nutrition (www.acvn.org) and www.balanceit.com.

SUGGESTED READING

Fascetti AJ, et al: Commercial and home-prepared diets. In Fascetti AJ, et al, editors: Applied veterinary clinical nutrition, Chichester, UK, 2012, Wiley-Blackwell, pp 95-107.

AUTHOR & EDITOR: Jennifer A. Larsen, DVM, PhD, DACVN

Hops Toxicosis

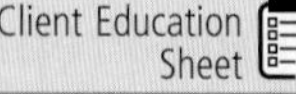

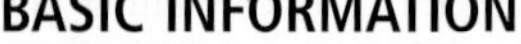

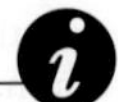

Definition

Humulus lupulus (hops) is a member of the Cannabaceae family. Hops may be cultivated in gardens as part of a landscape. It is used in herbal medications as a sleep aide. In most cases, intoxication results from exposure to hops (flowers, socks, plugs, or pellets) for use in the production of beer.

Synonyms

Common hops, beer hops, lupulin

Epidemiology

SPECIES, AGE, SEX

Dogs are the only known species to develop hyperthermia due to hops ingestion.

GENETICS, BREED PREDISPOSITION

Initially, greyhounds appeared to have a greater degree of susceptibility. However, as more cases are reported, toxicity has been reported in a wider variety of breeds.

RISK FACTORS

The presence of hops in the dog's environment (e.g., home brewers)

Clinical Presentation

DISEASE FORMS/SUBTYPES

Dogs develop a malignant hyperthermia–like syndrome.

HISTORY, CHIEF COMPLAINT

- History of ingesting new or spent hops, garden flowers
- Panting/tachypnea
- Agitation, anxiety, hyperactivity
- Vomiting

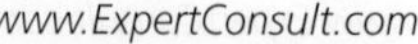

PHYSICAL EXAM FINDINGS

- Hyperthermia
- Tachycardia
- Tachypnea, panting
- Agitation, anxiety, hyperactivity, pacing
- Injected mucous membranes
- Death

Etiology and Pathophysiology

- Toxic principle is unknown.
- Although exact mechanism is unknown, theories include
  - Inhibition of electron transfer (oxidative uncoupling)
  - Alteration of mitochondrial activity
  - Serotonin syndrome

DIAGNOSIS

Diagnostic Overview

The medical history includes the presence of hops in the environment, as well as a potential ingestion. Clinical signs are expected as early as 30-60 minutes up to 12 hours after exposure. Most animals recover with therapy within 12-24 hours after ingestion. There are no rapid tests to confirm the ingestion of hops.

Differential Diagnosis

- Malignant hyperthermia
- Hyperthermia (heat stroke, exogenous heat source)
- Fever (infectious, immune-mediated, neoplasia, inflammatory)
- Amphetamines
- Selective serotonin reuptake inhibitors (SSRIs) (p. 1281)
- 5-Hydroxytryptophan
- Aspirin
- Metaldehyde

Initial Database

- Body temperature > 102.5°F
- Respiratory rate: tachypnea
- Heart rate: tachycardia
- CBC: mild elevations in white blood cells may be noted.
- Electrolytes: hyperkalemia, hypercalcemia, and hyperphosphatemia have been reported.
- Chemistry panel: creatine kinase (marked elevation), azotemia secondary to myoglobinuria
- Acid-base status
- Coagulation profile in cases of severe prolonged hyperthermia: possible disseminated intravascular coagulation (DIC)
- Urinalysis: myoglobinuria

TREATMENT

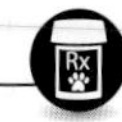

Treatment Overview

Soon after ingestion (<1 hour after ingestion), decontaminate asymptomatic patients. Symptomatic and supportive care is used to treat most clinical signs, although dantrolene is specific for the treatment of malignant hyperthermia.

Acute General Treatment

- Decontamination (p. 1087):
  - If ingestion occurred < 1 hour before presentation and dog is free of signs, induce emesis (p. 1188).
  - Enemas to stimulate fecal elimination of plant material (warm water, 10 mL/kg [p. 1099])
  - Activated charcoal 1-2 g/kg if asymptomatic
- Fluids, IV crystalloids to reduce risk of acute kidney injury (AKI) from myoglobinuria (p. 23)
  - Address electrolyte disorders, if present.
- External cooling (e.g., fans, cool water baths [p. 421])
- Methocarbamol 50-220 mg/kg slow IV to effect, no faster than 2 mL/min for tremors
- Diazepam 0.5-2 mg/kg IV *or* midazolam 0.5-1 mg/kg IV for significant stimulatory signs or tremors
- Specific antagonist:
  - To treat hyperthermia, dantrolene should be given at 2-3 mg/kg IV or 3.5 mg/kg PO, q 4-8h, depending on the recurrence of hyperthermia
  - If dantrolene is not available, cyproheptadine may be given at 1.1 mg/kg PO or per rectum q 4-6h. Reports of cyproheptadine efficacy in controlling malignant hyperthermia are mixed.
- Diazepam and acepromazine have NOT been effective for hyperthermia treatment.
- Address complications of hyperthermia, as necessary (p. 421).

Behavior/Exercise

Dogs should be kept caged and quiet until clinical signs resolve. Exercise should be restricted for 3-5 days after recovery to prevent additional myoglobinuria formation.

Possible Complications

Severe hyperthermia may cause DIC and/or myoglobinuria, resulting in AKI.

Recommended Monitoring

- Monitor temperature frequently, initially q 1-2h.
- Monitor heart rate and blood pressure.
- Monitor electrolytes and acid-base status.

PROGNOSIS & OUTCOME

Prognosis is good if addressed quickly but becomes guarded to poor in cases with severe hyperthermia.

PEARLS & CONSIDERATIONS

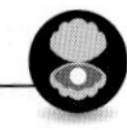

Comments

Many clients are not aware of the potential dangers of hops ingestions and assume hops are safe because they are used to make beer designed for human consumption. The client may not volunteer information about hops ingestion, believing the information is irrelevant. If clinical signs are consistent with hops ingestion, ask the client specifically about access to or ingestion of hops.

Prevention

- Prevent pets from hops exposure (dispose of spent hops immediately, choose different plants for landscaping).
- Do not put spent hops in compost piles.

Technician Tips

If dantrolene is not routinely part of the clinic's pharmacy, find out where dantrolene can be obtained quickly before an emergency, and keep the information in an easily accessible location.

Client Education

Educate clients about the dangers of hops to their dogs.

SUGGESTED READING

Duncan K, et al: Malignant hyperthermia-like reaction secondary to ingestion of hops in five dogs. J Am Vet Med Assoc 210:51, 1997.

AUTHOR: Charlotte Means, DVM, MLIS, DABVT, DABT
EDITOR: Tina Wismer, DVM, MS, DABVT, DABT

Hydrocephalus

Bonus Material Online 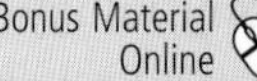 Client Education Sheet 

BASIC INFORMATION

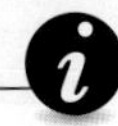

Definition

An increase in volume of cerebrospinal fluid (CSF) in the ventricular system of the brain that causes signs of encephalopathy

Epidemiology

SPECIES, AGE, SEX

- Congenital: dog, cat at birth or within several months of age
- Acquired: any

GENETICS, BREED PREDISPOSITION

- Toy breeds: Chihuahua, toy poodle, Pomeranian, Lhasa apso, pug, Pekingese, and Cairn, Yorkshire, Manchester, and Maltese terriers
- Brachycephalic breeds: Boston terrier, English bulldog

- Autosomal recessive inheritance in Siamese cats

RISK FACTORS

Vitamin A deficiency, toxicosis (cats: griseofulvin during pregnancy), infectious (cats: panleukopenia, feline infectious peritonitis; dogs: parainfluenza), ciliary dyskinesia

ASSOCIATED DISORDERS

Small birth size, short gestation periods, high stress at birth (dystocia)

Clinical Presentation

DISEASE FORMS/SUBTYPES

- Congenital: presumably associated with stenosis of mesencephalic aqueduct and malformation of the mesencephalon
- Acquired: caused by obstructive insults at any age (i.e., infection, trauma, neoplasia)
- Communicating: accumulation of CSF within the entire ventricular system resulting from obstruction of CSF outflow pathways (lateral aperture or arachnoid villi)
- Obstructive (noncommunicating): ventricular dilation resulting from lesion obstructing CSF flow within the ventricular system
- Subtypes based on location of CSF
  - Internal: accumulation of CSF within ventricular system
  - External: accumulation of CSF within the subarachnoid space
  - Compensatory: CSF accumulates in areas where there is loss of neural parenchyma; also called hydrocephalus ex vacuo

HISTORY, CHIEF COMPLAINT

- Changes in mentation: dullness, obtundation, disorientation, stupor
- Behavioral abnormalities: inability to learn (e.g., litter box use), loss of housebreaking, compulsive activities, aggression
- Visual deficits
- Progressive neurologic dysfunction (e.g., circling, pacing)
- Seizures
- Clinical signs may not be apparent.

PHYSICAL EXAM FINDINGS

- Domed-shaped head and persistent fontanelle are possible.
- Eye position typically will manifest ventral or ventrolateral strabismus.
- Neurologic exam (p. 1136): mentation changes, cognitive dysfunction; gait abnormalities can manifest as dysmetria, ataxia, circling, aimless wandering, central blindness, vestibular dysfunction; seizures

Etiology and Pathophysiology

- Pathologic changes include focal destruction of the ependymal lining, compromise of cerebral vasculature, damage to periventricular white matter, and injury to neurons.
- Secondary calvarial abnormalities depend on the stage of ossification at onset of fluid accumulation.
- Ventriculomegaly results from obstruction within the ventricular system, overproduction of CSF, or insufficient absorption of CSF at the arachnoid villi.
- Congenital
  - Fusion of the rostral colliculi and mesencephalic aqueductal stenosis. There is no other active disease process.
- Acquired
  - Exposure to teratogenic drugs, chemicals, and viral diseases during gestation
  - Obstruction of ventricular system by neoplastic mass, hemorrhage, or inflammation
  - Hydrocephalus also can be a component of other anomalous disorders (e.g., Chiari malformation, intracranial arachnoid cyst, Dandy-Walker syndrome, lissencephaly, cerebellar hypoplasia, ciliary dyskinesia).

DIAGNOSIS

Diagnostic Overview

Diagnosis is suspected based on the physical exam and signalment. Confirmation comes from diagnostic imaging (beginning with ultrasound and proceeding to CT/MRI if needed) and procedures assisting in determining underlying causes.

Differential Diagnosis

- Hydrocephalus usually produces signs of forebrain dysfunction.
- Encephalopathies
  - Degenerative disorders: storage diseases, leukodystrophies, multisystem atrophy
  - Anomalies (congenital): malformations (e.g., caudal occipital malformation syndrome, Dandy-Walker syndrome, hydranencephaly)
  - Metabolic: hepatic encephalopathy, organic acid disorders
  - Neoplasia: causes secondary obstructive hydrocephalus
  - Inflammatory: infectious (feline panleukopenia, feline infectious peritonitis, parainfluenza, canine distemper), noninfectious (breed specific, meningoencephalomyelitis of unknown cause)
  - Idiopathic: intracranial arachnoidal cysts
  - Trauma: hydrocephalus ex vacuo occurs with destruction of brain tissue (e.g., cerebrovascular accidents)
  - Toxin exposure: griseofulvin

Initial Database

- CBC, serum biochemistry profile, urinalysis: generally unremarkable for congenital causes
- Serologic titers: to rule out acquired infectious causes, if appropriate
- Skull radiography: decreased prominence of normal calvarial convolutions

Advanced or Confirmatory Testing

- Ultrasonography: through persistent bregmatic fontanelle to visualize enlarged ventricles as paired anechoic regions. Enlarged ventricles are a feature of hydrocephalus, but not all animals with ventriculomegaly have hydrocephalus.
- Cross-sectional imaging: to confirm hydrocephalus and rule out other contributing disorders and differentials that can mimic disease
  - CT: visualization of lateral ventricles
  - MRI (p. 1132): visualization of the ventricular system and the brain parenchyma (periventricular edema); periventricular hyperintensity indicates interstitial edema
- CSF analysis (pp. 1080 and 1323): to rule out inflammatory disorders, if appropriate
- Electroencephalography

TREATMENT

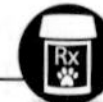

Treatment Overview

The treatment of hydrocephalus is guided by the underlying cause. Medical therapy offers temporary palliation of clinical signs. Surgical management using shunting procedures may offer a more permanent remedy.

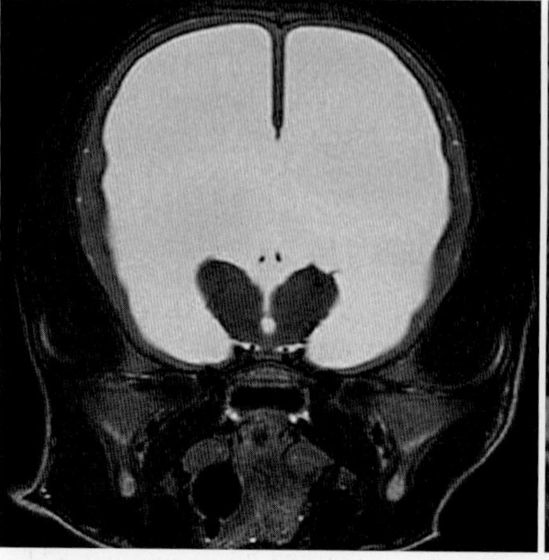

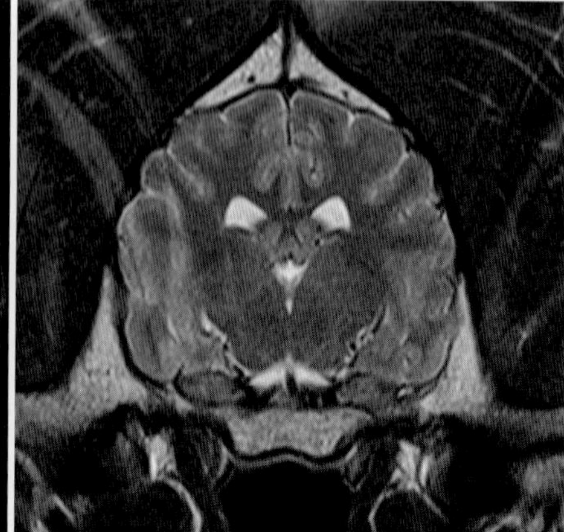

HYDROCEPHALUS Magnetic resonance imaging (transverse plane) of a dog with hydrocephalus *(left)* and a normal dog for comparison *(right)*. Cerebrospinal fluid appears white in these T2-weighted images. Note the marked dilation of both ventricles in the dog on the left and the normal ventricular volume in the dog on the right.

Acute and Chronic Treatment

Medical options:

- Prednisone (↓CSF production) 0.25-0.5 mg/kg PO q 12-24h, then tapered to lowest effective dose
- Furosemide (↓CSF production; Na-K cotransport inhibition) 0.5-2 mg/kg PO q 12-24h, taper to lowest effective dose
- Acetazolamide (↓CSF production; carbonic anhydrase inhibitor) 10 mg/kg PO q 8h
- Omeprazole (↓CSF production; proton pump inhibition) 0.7 mg/kg PO q 24h; 10 mg PO q 24h for dogs weighing < 20 kg or 20 mg q 24h PO for dogs weighing > 20 kg
- Mannitol (hyperosmolar therapy, decrease blood viscosity) 1 g/kg IV
- Antiepileptic drug therapy for seizure control

Surgical: indicated for worsening of clinical signs that do not respond to medical therapy:

- Ventriculoperitoneal shunt
- Ventriculoatrial shunt

Drug Interactions

Prolonged use of corticosteroids, furosemide, and acetazolamide can cause potassium depletion and other systemic disorders.

Possible Complications

- Generally, medical therapy results in only transient improvement of clinical signs.
- Complications of shunt placement include mechanical failure (breakage, migration, and disconnection), functional obstruction, infection, and overdrainage.

Recommended Monitoring

- Signs of acute decompensation: coma, seizures, behavior changes
- Seizure control

PROGNOSIS & OUTCOME

- Congenital: guarded; prognosis also is influenced by coexistence of other neural tissue abnormalities
- Acquired: prognosis depends on underlying cause

PEARLS & CONSIDERATIONS

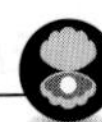

Comments

- Every attempt is made to determine the underlying cause.
- Early shunt placement is advocated to lessen residual neurologic deficits and behavior abnormalities.

Prevention

Limit prenatal exposure to toxins, viral infections, and vaccines.

Technician Tips

- Avoid excessive restraint and compression of the external jugular veins in these patients (can increase intracranial pressure).
- Counsel owners on monitoring for gastrointestinal ulceration if the animal is being treated with glucocorticoids.
- After surgery for shunt placement, monitor the skin over the shunt for signs of pressure necrosis, especially in small-breed dogs with tendency for thin skin.

Client Education

- Clinical signs of acute decompensation
- Guarded prognosis and likelihood of residual neurologic deficits with therapy
- Importance of maintaining the pet in a protective environment

SUGGESTED READING

Estey CM: Congenital hydrocephalus. Vet Clin North Am Small Anim Pract 46:217-229, 2016.

AUTHOR: Joan R. Coates, DVM, MS, DACVIM
EDITOR: Karen R. Muñana, DVM, MS, DACVIM

Hydronephrosis

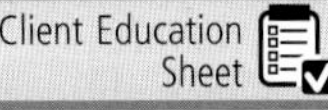

BASIC INFORMATION

Definition

Dilation of the renal pelvis and calices (pyelectasia) in one or both kidneys resulting in atrophy of the renal parenchyma, which typically results from ureteral (or rarely urethral) obstruction

Epidemiology

SPECIES, AGE, SEX

Dogs and cats of any age and either sex

RISK FACTORS

Any cause of ureteral (or urethral) obstruction, whether mechanical or functional:

- Bladder atonia/hypotonia
- Blood clots
- Celiotomy (inadvertent ligation/fibrotic entrapment of ureter)
- Congenital ureteral stenosis or stricture
- Ectopic ureter
- Prostatic carcinoma
- Reflex dyssynergia
- Retroperitoneal mass/fibrosis/infarction
- Trauma
- Ureteral fibroepithelial polyps
- Urinary tract neoplasia
- Urolithiasis (common cause)

ASSOCIATED DISORDERS

- Renal failure ± uremia
- Hypertension
- Urinary tract infection

Clinical Presentation

DISEASE FORMS/SUBTYPES

- Reversible or irreversible
- Unilateral or bilateral

HISTORY, CHIEF COMPLAINT

Often an incidental finding (patient is clinically normal); signs can include

- Vague abdominal pain (if renomegaly)
- Polydipsia/polyuria (with chronic kidney disease [CKD])
- Anorexia and vomiting (uremia)
- Pollakiuria, stranguria, dysuria, hematuria
- Urinary incontinence (if ectopic ureter)
- Oliguria or anuria (urethral obstruction or, rarely, bilateral ureteral obstruction)

PHYSICAL EXAM FINDINGS

Often normal; abnormalities can include

- Abdominal discomfort or back pain (severity related to rapidity of obstruction rather than degree of obstruction)
- Renomegaly
- Distended bladder (if urethral obstruction)
- Abdominal mass (kidney, bladder, prostate, granuloma)
- Urethral mass (by rectal palpation)
- Prostatomegaly
- Dehydration
- Halitosis (uremia)
- Oral ulcerations (uremia)

Etiology and Pathophysiology

- Illness varies depending on whether obstruction is unilateral or bilateral, degree and duration of obstruction, and pre-existing renal function.
- Clinical signs can be absent, chronic, or acute; acute signs are more likely when obstruction is complete.
- Obstruction results in increased hydrostatic pressure in renal pelvis, collecting ducts, and distal tubules, causing tubular dilation with flattening of the tubular cells.
- Concurrently, renal vasculature and blood supply are compromised. Renal blood flow progressively decreases, arterioles constrict, capillary pressure decreases, and many arterioles collapse, resulting in parenchymal atrophy.
- Changes may become irreversible after 14-45 days.

DIAGNOSIS

Diagnostic Overview

Hydronephrosis is usually diagnosed by renal imaging studies, including ultrasound or contrast studies, in conjunction with recognition of a functional or physical reason for urinary tract obstruction.

Differential Diagnosis

- Pyelectasia: pyelonephritis, iatrogenic fluid diuresis (mild)
- Renomegaly

Initial Database

- Digital rectal examination: lesions of the urethra and bladder trigone may cause hydronephrosis.
- Urethral catheterization: can rule out or confirm urethral obstruction from urolithiasis
- CBC: unremarkable; neutrophilia possible if concurrent pyelonephritis
- Serum biochemical profile: depending on degree of obstruction and/or nephron loss, azotemia, hyperphosphatemia, hyperkalemia, metabolic acidosis, increased anion gap, increased symmetric dimethylarginine (SDMA)
- Urinalysis: isosthenuria (e.g., if > 66% nephron loss), sometimes hematuria, pyuria
- Urine culture and sensitivity to rule out infection
- Blood pressure to rule out hypertension
- Abdominal radiographs: rarely renomegaly; additional findings may include
  - Urolithiasis
  - Urinary bladder distention
  - Prostatomegaly
  - Abdominal mass effect

Loss of contrast in retroperitoneal space or abdomen:

- Abdominal ultrasound
  - Pyelectasia
    - Dog renal pelvis diameter: normal = 1-3.8 mm (median 2 mm), fluid therapy = 1.3-3.6 mm (median, 2.5 mm), pyelonephritis = 1.9-12 mm (median, 3.6 mm)
    - Cat renal pelvis diameter: normal = 0.8-3.2 mm (median, 1.6 mm), fluid therapy = 1.1-3.4 mm (median, 2.3 mm), pyelonephritis = 1.7-12.4 mm (median, 4 mm)
  - ± Renomegaly, loss of medullary parenchyma, hydroureter, uroliths, masses in ureter/bladder/prostate/urethra

Advanced or Confirmatory Testing

- Additional testing is not usually required or beneficial.
- Excretory urography (EU)/intravenous pyelography (IVP): to assess perfusion of each kidney; percutaneous nephropyelography to assess structure of renal pelvis and ureter
  - Pyelectasia
  - Ureteral dilation or lack of filling (EU only)
  - May identify ectopic ureter
- CT scan with contrast
  - Findings of other imaging modalities may be confirmed on CT (e.g., ectopic ureter, uroliths)
- Renal scintigraphy or CT with contrast
  - Affected kidney contributes little to glomerular filtration rate.
- Other testing is aimed at characterizing underlying cause of hydronephrosis (e.g., quantitative analysis of uroliths, imaging studies to localize neurologic lesions contributing to reflex dyssynergia, cystoscopy for bladder abnormalities or ectopic ureter).

TREATMENT

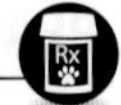

Treatment Overview

Hydronephrosis has no specific treatment. Instead, obstruction of urine flow should be corrected when possible, and complications of renal failure addressed. Treatment may not be necessary for incidentally discovered (chronic) hydronephrosis.

Acute General Treatment

- Relieve ureteral or urethral obstruction (pp. 1174, 1175, and 1176).
  - Subcutaneous ureteral bypass increasingly available (cats especially) for acute ureteral obstruction.
- Crystalloid fluid therapy for azotemia (pp. 23 and 169)
- Analgesia for abdominal pain (e.g., buprenorphine 0.01 mg/kg IM, IV, or SQ q 6-8h)
- Address electrolyte disorders and acidosis.
- Address uremia (pp. 23 and 169).

Chronic Treatment

- Antibiotics if indicated by results of urine culture and sensitivity
  - If infection cannot be cured medically and contralateral kidney function is adequate, nephrectomy may be indicated to remove infected, poorly functioning kidney.
- Address underlying cause of structural or functional urinary obstruction (e.g., therapeutic measures for urolithiasis, pharmacologic therapy of bladder atonia, reflex dyssynergia, ureteral stenting).

Nutrition/Diet

- If obstruction secondary to urolithiasis, diet appropriate for stone type
- Animals that remain azotemic should be fed a renal-appropriate diet (p. 167).

Possible Complications

- CKD/azotemia/uremia
- Urinary tract infection
- Urinary tract rupture and uroabdomen (septic peritonitis if urinary tract is infected)

Recommended Monitoring

- Ultrasound is repeated several weeks after urinary obstruction is relieved. If hydronephrosis persists after 6 weeks, changes are likely to be permanent.
- Animals with permanent hydronephrosis are monitored for CKD (pp. 167 and 169) with periodic urinalysis and culture, assessment of azotemia, electrolytes, and packed cell volume. Azotemic animals are monitored more intensively than nonazotemic animals.

PROGNOSIS & OUTCOME

- Depends on extent of renal damage, underlying cause and resolution of cause, duration, and concurrent infection. Hydronephrosis can be associated with severe renal failure or may be an incidental finding.
- Structural kidney changes may be irreversible.

PEARLS & CONSIDERATIONS

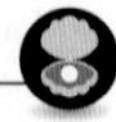

Comments

- Hydronephrosis is a consequence of obstructive urinary tract disease rather than a primary disease.
- Hydronephrosis can lead to CKD and uremia or may manifest only as subclinical pyelectasia.

Prevention

Strategies that limit the formation of uroliths are important for patients that have already demonstrated a predisposition to urolithiasis or those with known risk factors.

Technician Tips

- Monitor urine output via litterbox use or bladder size if no urinary catheter is in place. Alert clinician if there are any concerns.
- Abdomen may be painful; use caution when picking up patient.

Client Education

Urinary tract obstruction is life-threatening. Stranguria or oliguria should prompt immediate veterinary attention.

SUGGESTED READING

D'Anjou MA, et al: Clinical significance of renal pelvic dilatation on ultrasound in dogs and cats. Vet Radiol Ultrasound 52(1):88-94, 2011.

AUTHORS: Adam Mordecai, DVM, MS, DACVIM
EDITOR: Leah A. Cohn, DVM, PhD, DACVIM

Hyperadrenocorticism

Bonus Material Online Client Education Sheet 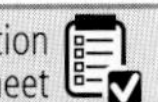

BASIC INFORMATION 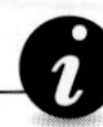

Definition

- Spontaneous hyperadrenocorticism (HAC) is a disorder caused by excessive adrenocortical cortisol production.
- Iatrogenic HAC results from exogenous glucocorticoid administration.

Synonyms

- Hypercortisolemia
- Cushing's syndrome: constellation of clinical signs due to excess glucocorticoid
- Cushing's disease: pituitary-dependent HAC

Epidemiology

SPECIES, AGE, SEX

- Common in dogs, rare in cats
- Dogs
  - Middle-aged to older; rare in dogs < 6 years
  - Possible predisposition toward females overall
- Cats: middle-aged to older; no known sex predisposition

GENETICS, BREED PREDISPOSITION

- Dogs
  - Can occur in any breed
  - Poodles, dachshunds, and boxers predisposed; German shepherds, Boston terriers, and beagles may be predisposed.
  - Dogs with adrenal tumors (ATs) more likely to be > 20 kg.
- Cats: no known breed predisposition

RISK FACTORS

Administration of any form of exogenous steroid by any route can cause iatrogenic HAC; the more potent the steroid and the more chronic the use, the more likely is iatrogenic HAC.

ASSOCIATED DISORDERS

- Urinary tract infections
- Pyoderma
- Calcium oxalate urolithiasis
- Systemic hypertension
- Diabetes mellitus (DM): more likely to occur in cats with HAC than in dogs
- Protein-losing nephropathy
- Neurologic signs with pituitary macroadenoma
- Pulmonary thromboembolism
- Ligament and tendon injury

Clinical Presentation

DISEASE FORMS/SUBTYPES

- Pituitary-dependent HAC (PDH)
- Adrenal tumor HAC (ATH)
- Iatrogenic HAC

HISTORY, CHIEF COMPLAINT

- Dogs
  - Classic complaints are polyuria/polydipsia (PU/PD), polyphagia, a potbellied appearance, and panting.
  - Alopecia and weakness are common.
  - Less common are lethargy, poor hair regrowth, issues related to infertility, bruising, and calcinosis cutis.
  - With a pituitary macroadenoma, anorexia, ataxia, disorientation, and uncommonly, seizures
- Cats
  - Approximately 80% of cats with HAC have DM with associated complaints (p. 251).
  - PU/PD uncommon in cats if DM not also present
  - Bilaterally symmetrical alopecia uncommon in cats with HAC, but thin skin can be severe, leading to spontaneous wounds

PHYSICAL EXAM FINDINGS

- Dogs
  - Common findings include pendulous abdomen, bilaterally symmetric alopecia, panting, hepatomegaly, and muscle weakness.
  - Less common findings include thin skin, comedones, hyperpigmentation, and pyoderma.
  - Uncommon findings are calcinosis cutis, bruising, testicular atrophy, facial nerve palsy, respiratory distress (due to pulmonary thromboembolism), ligament rupture, pseudomyotonia, neurologic signs such as ataxia and disorientation due to space-occupying effects of a pituitary macroadenoma, and space-occupying effects of an AT such as rear limb edema.
- Cats: pendulous abdomen, unkempt haircoat, alopecia, thin skin, and muscle wasting

Etiology and Pathophysiology

- Dogs
  - Approximately 85% of cases of spontaneous HAC (i.e., noniatrogenic) are due to PDH. A pituitary corticotroph tumor oversecretes ACTH, leading to bilateral adrenocortical hyperplasia and oversecretion of cortisol. Tumor almost always benign with nontumorous hyperplasia, and adenocarcinomas are rare.
  - Anterior pituitary involved in approximately 80%-85% of PDH cases, intermediate lobe of pituitary in the remaining cases
  - Pituitary macroadenomas (>1 cm in diameter) occur in 10%–25% of PDH cases.
  - In the remaining 15%-20% of spontaneous HAC cases, ATH is present; approximately one-half of ATs are malignant.
  - Food-induced HAC (p. 489) and ectopic ACTH secretion are rare causes of HAC.
- Cats: types appear similar to dogs; AT more likely to be malignant.
- Iatrogenic HAC can be due to exogenous glucocorticoid administration by any route.

DIAGNOSIS 

Diagnostic Overview

The suspicion that a patient has HAC is based on the history and physical exam. Endocrine tests should be performed only when clinical signs consistent with HAC are present. No test for the diagnosis of HAC is 100% accurate, and misdiagnosis and overdiagnosis may occur.

Differential Diagnosis

Depends on clinical and laboratory abnormalities:

- Hypothyroidism (p. 525)
- Alopecia X (p. 44)
- Sex hormone-secreting tumors (p. 35)
- DM (p. 251)
- Causes of PU/PD (p. 812)
- Causes of polyphagia (p. 809)
- Causes of alopecia (p. 47)
- Causes of panting (p. 1263)

Initial Database

- CBC: leukocytosis with mature neutrophilia, eosinopenia, and lymphopenia in most dogs; monocytosis, thrombocytosis, and mild erythrocytosis are less common. In cats, lymphopenia is most common finding.
- Serum chemistry
  - High cholesterol and liver enzymes (with elevation in alkaline phosphatase [ALP] greater than that of alanine aminotransferase [ALT]); ALP activity high in approximately 90% of dogs with HAC. Only about 33% of affected cats have elevated ALP values.
  - Hyperglycemia common; about 10% of dogs and 80% of cats with HAC have concurrent DM.
- Urinalysis: low specific gravity (usually < 1.020) and proteinuria common; pyuria may or may not be present with bacteriuria.
- Abdominal radiographs: hepatomegaly common; occasionally, cystic calculi, adrenal mass with or without mineralization
- Thoracic radiographs: bronchial mineralization possible; may see changes consistent with pulmonary thromboembolism (p. 842)
- Blood pressure: in dogs, hypertension common but usually mild

Advanced or Confirmatory Testing

Endocrine testing required to make a diagnosis of HAC.

- Cannot administer prednisone, prednisolone, hydrocortisone, or methylprednisolone within 12 hours before a test that measures cortisol (test interference)

To screen for HAC: ACTH stimulation test, low-dose dexamethasone suppression test

(LDDST) and/or urine cortisol/creatinine ratio (UC/CR)

- If clinical signs of HAC are present in a dog that has a nonadrenal illness, it is best to postpone testing for HAC until the nonadrenal illness has resolved, if possible.
- Sensitivity and specificity of the tests are unknown in cats.
- ACTH stimulation test
  - Only test that can diagnose iatrogenic HAC; diagnosis based on history of glucocorticoid exposure by any route, consistent clinical signs, and post-ACTH cortisol concentration below reference range.
  - Protocol (p. 1300): cosyntropin is the recommended form of ACTH to use; if using compounded ACTH, collect samples before and at 1 and 2 hours after ACTH administration so peak response not missed
  - A response greater than normal is consistent with a diagnosis of spontaneous HAC; cortisol concentrations below normal, often too low to be measured, are consistent with a diagnosis of iatrogenic HAC.
  - Overall sensitivity of the test is approximately 80%; for PDH, sensitivity is approximately 85%-90% and, for ATH, sensitivity is approximately 60%
  - Compared with LDDST, may have less chance of a false-positive result in a dog with nonadrenal illness
  - Can never differentiate between PDH and an ATH
- LDDST
  - Protocol (p. 1360): if using dexamethasone sodium phosphate, dose on concentration of parent compound, not the salt.
  - May be the preferred screening test for diagnosis of spontaneous HAC
  - Sensitivity is approximately 95% in dogs.
  - Relatively high chance of false-positive result exists, up to 50%, if nonadrenal illness present
  - If test positive for HAC, may also serve to differentiate PDH from ATH
    - If the 8-hour sample is > the cutoff value, result is consistent with HAC. If in addition, the 4-hour post-dexamethasone cortisol concentration is < the cutoff or the 4- and/or 8-hour post-dexamethasone concentrations are < 50% of baseline, results consistent with PDH
    - If criteria for PDH not met, chances approximately 50/50 for PDH versus ATH
  - If the baseline cortisol concentration is close to the cutoff value or suppression is just at 50%, PDH should be confirmed by other means.
  - If cortisol concentration 4 hours after dexamethasone is above the cutoff and the 8-hour sample is below, HAC is possible, and an ACTH stimulation test is recommended.
- UC/CR
  - Protocol (p. 1391): owner should collect sample at home when pet not stressed.
  - An elevated UC/CR may be a sensitive marker of HAC, found in 90%-100% of affected dogs in most studies. Some studies have found a sensitivity of only 75%.
  - False-positive results common; only 25%-30% of dogs with an elevated UC/CR have HAC.
  - Elevated ratio consistent with a diagnosis of HAC, but because the chance of a false-positive result is great, an ACTH stimulation test or LDDST must be done to confirm the diagnosis.
  - A protocol with reportedly high sensitivity and specificity exists in Europe; a minimum of two morning urine samples are collected, dexamethasone is then administered (3 doses PO over 24 hours) for differentiating purposes, and another urine sample is collected. Unfortunately, the cortisol assay used is proprietary and not commercially available. Because the accuracy of the protocol using cortisol assays commercially available in the United States has not been established, the method is not recommended for use in the United States and Canada.

After a diagnosis of HAC is made, a differentiation test should be performed (i.e., high-dose dexamethasone suppression test, endogenous ACTH concentration, or abdominal ultrasound) to determine if PDH or ATH present.

- Differentiation provides information crucial to therapeutic decisions and an accurate prognosis.
- High-dose dexamethasone suppression test (HDDST)
  - Protocol: same as for LDDST, but dexamethasone dose higher (p. 1353)
  - If the LDDST provided a diagnosis of HAC but did not differentiate between PDH and ATH, HDDST is unlikely to differentiate.
  - Two responses are consistent with PDH; if there is suppression to less than cutoff value at 4 and/or 8 hours after dexamethasone or the 4- and/or 8-hour post-dexamethasone samples are < 50% of baseline, PDH is present
  - If baseline values are close to cutoff value or suppression just at 50%, results are suspect, and PDH should be confirmed by other means.
  - HDDST can never confirm ATH; if criteria for PDH diagnosis are not met, there is a 50:50 chance the patient has PDH or ATH.
- Endogenous ACTH (eACTH) concentration
  - With PDH, eACTH concentration is inappropriately high. With ATH, eACTH is low or undetectable.
  - Protocol (p. 1299): proper sample handling is crucial.
  - Can confirm presence of ATH
  - Gray zone exists in results. If eACTH is in the gray zone (approximately 15% chance), results are not diagnostic. If eACTH measured again, almost 100% chance of obtaining differentiation. There is no way to predict when eACTH concentration will be in the gray zone.
- Abdominal ultrasound
  - Never use for screening. Bilateral adrenomegaly can be due to chronic nonadrenal illness, and ATs do not always cause HAC.
  - Maximal dorsoventral dimension of adrenal gland in a sagittal plane most informative parameter
  - Bilateral adrenomegaly present in > 90% of dogs with PDH
  - Defines location, size, and organ involvement of AT more precisely than radiography. Moderate asymmetry, contralateral adrenocortical atrophy, and destruction of normal tissue architecture are consistent with cortisol-secreting AT.
  - Indicators of malignancy are invasion of adjacent structures, presence of lesions suggestive of metastasis, and AT diameter > 2 cm.
- Pituitary imaging can be done if there is suspicion of macroadenoma.
- Abdominal CT: preoperatively if adrenalectomy is to be performed for ATH

TREATMENT

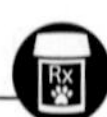

Treatment Overview

Treatment goal is resolution of clinical signs. For PDH, hypophysectomy ideal but of very limited availability. Medical therapy (trilostane or mitotane) is usually used in dogs with PDH, but response is inconsistent in cats (trilostane best for cats). If ATH, adrenalectomy is preferred in dogs and cats.

Acute General Treatment

Acute therapy unnecessary

Chronic Treatment

- Not all dogs with positive test results for HAC need to be treated. The decision should be made on a case-by-case basis. Consideration should be given to the dog's health, quality of life, owner needs and limitations, and severity of clinical signs.
- For medical therapy, mitotane and trilostane are preferred; L-deprenyl and ketoconazole are of low efficacy.
- For patients on medical therapy, owners should have prednisone 0.2 mg/kg available to administer at home if needed.
- Trilostane (Vetoryl)
  - Inhibits synthesis and secretion of adrenocortical steroids, particularly cortisol and, to a lesser extent, aldosterone.
  - Brand name product should be used due to variability in compounding.
  - Competitive inhibitor of the enzyme 3-beta-hydroxysteroid dehydrogenase
  - Goal is control of cortisol secretion.
  - Administer with food to enhance absorption.

- Twice-daily administration is recommended.
- See treatment algorithm on p. 1427.
- Mitotane (*o,p'*-DDD, Lysodren)
  - Causes selective destruction of adrenocortical glucocorticoid-secreting cells; zone that secretes aldosterone is relatively spared.
  - Goal is control of cortisol secretion by PDH and ATH.
  - For ATH, alternative goal is tumor destruction.
    - ATH treatment requires higher doses than PDH because AT is relatively resistant to mitotane.
  - Used in two treatment phases: 1) induction (or loading), which consists of daily administration, ideally q 12h; 2) maintenance, in which drug is dosed on a weekly basis, divided into 2-3 doses over the course of a week.
  - Should be given with food to increase drug absorption
  - See treatment algorithm on p. 1426.

Drug Interactions

- Mitotane: increases barbiturate and warfarin metabolism; decreases insulin requirements in diabetics.
- Trilostane: do not use in combination with other treatments for HAC.

Possible Complications

- For adrenalectomy (p. 35)
- For mitotane and trilostane
  - Gastrointestinal complications common
  - With mitotane, neurologic signs (e.g. ataxia) uncommon
  - Glucocorticoid deficiency common; if occurs by itself, adrenal glands recover function, usually within a few weeks but can take months
  - Glucocorticoid and mineralocorticoid deficiency uncommon; often permanent and treatment for hypoadrenocorticism needed (p. 512)
  - Mineralocorticoid insufficiency alone possible but less well understood
  - Hepatopathy with mitotane

Recommended Monitoring

- Frequent ACTH stimulation tests needed to assess efficacy of therapy and adjust dose; frequency depends on many factors (see treatment algorithms [pp. 1426, and 1427])
- Post-pill timing important with trilostane but controversial
  - Starting an ACTH stimulation test 2-6 hours after pill recommended
  - Post-pill interval should always be the same for a patient

PROGNOSIS & OUTCOME

- Untreated HAC: poor for quality of life; progression rate variable
- Treated PDH: good; median survival time approximately 2 years; dogs tend to die of causes unrelated to HAC
- Macroadenomas and neurologic signs: poor to grave; macroadenomas with no or mild neurologic signs: fair to good with radiation therapy and medical therapy
- Adrenal adenomas: good to excellent; small carcinomas (not metastasized): fair to good
- Large carcinomas and AT with widespread metastasis: poor to fair

PEARLS & CONSIDERATIONS

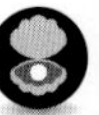

Comments

- The LDDST requires very small volumes of dexamethasone; it may need to be diluted for accurate dosing.
- Adrenal necrosis can occur with trilostane.
- If the patient cannot be adequately monitored (e.g., owner unwilling or unable to provide necessary follow-up for ACTH stimulation testing), mitotane and trilostane should not be used.

Technician Tips

For endocrine tests, it is best to consult with the laboratory concerning testing protocol and sample handling.

Client Education

Therapy is lifelong, and close monitoring is needed; the frequency of testing decreases with stabilization. Owners must be able to recognize hypoadrenocorticism and know how to intervene.

SUGGESTED READING

Behrend EN: Canine hyperadrenocorticism. In Feldman EC, et al, editors: Canine and feline endocrinology, St. Louis, 2015, Elsevier, pp 377-451.

AUTHOR & EDITOR: Ellen N. Behrend, VMD, PhD, DACVIM

Hyperadrenocorticism, Suspect/Conflicting Results

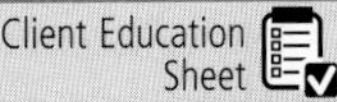

BASIC INFORMATION

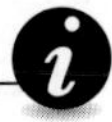

Definition

A scenario in which clinical features and results of general biochemical and/or endocrine testing conflict with regard to hyperadrenocorticism (HAC; Cushing's disease)

Epidemiology

SPECIES, AGE, SEX

Middle-aged to older dogs (i.e., those in which HAC occurs commonly)

Clinical Presentation

DISEASE FORMS/SUBTYPES

One clinical sign (e.g., polyuria/polydipsia, endocrine alopecia, systemic hypertension), one biochemical abnormality (e.g., increased alkaline phosphatase activity, proteinuria), or one other finding (e.g., vacuolar hepatopathy on biopsy) suggests HAC, but other results are normal or contradictory.

HISTORY, CHIEF COMPLAINT

- History sometimes includes clinical signs typical of HAC (p. 485): polyuria/polydipsia, polyphagia, panting, pot belly, and skin changes.
- The absence of polyuria/polydipsia makes a diagnosis of HAC unlikely.
- Ensure that the complaint is a new development (e.g., some dogs are always good eaters). If polyphagia is due to HAC, it should have developed recently.
- Finding suggesting HAC is sometimes discovered incidentally (e.g., increased alkaline phosphatase [ALP] value on predental blood tests).
- Inquire about the use of any type of glucocorticoid, including topical preparations.
- Clinical signs may be due to presence of a large pituitary tumor: inappetence, anorexia, stupor, pacing, behavior changes
- Clinical signs may be due to an adrenal tumor: ascites, hindlimb edema if it has invaded the vena cava

PHYSICAL EXAM FINDINGS

- Physical exam abnormalities present would be typical of HAC (p. 485): alopecia, thin skin, comedones, and others.
- Rarely, findings suggest abdominal mass or pituitary tumor.

Etiology and Pathophysiology

- HAC is a slowly progressive disease that can manifest in multiple ways.
- Clinical signs, for the most part, are the same whether the HAC is adrenal-dependent, pituitary-dependent, or iatrogenic.

- The possibility that a patient has HAC is based on history and physical exam findings. Endocrine tests should be performed only when clinical signs consistent with HAC are present.
- Not all animals with an adrenal or pituitary mass have HAC. Tumors can be nonsecretory or can secrete hormones unrelated to cortisol production (p. 34).

DIAGNOSIS

Diagnostic Overview

The primary indication for pursuing a diagnosis of HAC is the presence of one or more of the common clinical signs and physical exam findings. The more abnormalities identified, the stronger the indication to pursue testing. When only a single sign is present, it is usually polyuria/polydipsia or dermatologic abnormalities.

Differential Diagnosis

Differential diagnoses depend on the abnormalities present:

- Polyuria/polydipsia (pp. 812 and 1271)
- Polyphagia (pp. 809 and 1270)
- Panting (pp. 751 and 1263)
- Alopecia (pp. 47 and 1400)
- Proteinuria (p. 1272)
- Hypertension (pp. 501 and 1238)
- ALP elevation (p. 1304)

Initial Database

- Review the history and repeat exam to ensure no details that could support or refute HAC are missed. Of particular importance are questions regarding exposure to exogenous glucocorticoids by any route, even topical.
- CBC, biochemical profile, urinalysis, blood pressure measurement, and urine protein/creatinine ratio should be obtained. See p. 485 for findings typical of HAC.
  - No abnormality is pathognomonic for HAC.
  - Absence of abnormalities common in HAC (e.g., neutrophilic leukocytosis, thrombocytosis, increased ALP activity, dilute urine specific gravity, and proteinuria) should strongly decrease the suspicion of HAC.
- Abdominal ultrasound: if normal with respect to adrenal gland size and shape, HAC is unlikely. A large liver is an extremely nonspecific finding.

Advanced or Confirmatory Testing

- If mild suspicion of HAC still exists, a urine cortisol/creatinine ratio can be measured to help rule out the diagnosis (p. 1391).
  - Recently, sensitivity of this test has been reassessed and may be as low as 70%.
- If strong suspicion for HAC exists, consider low-dose dexamethasone suppression test or an ACTH stimulation test (pp. 1300 and 1360).
- Liver aspirates and cytology are not helpful for diagnosing HAC. Vacuolar hepatopathy is a nonspecific finding.
- When ACTH stimulation test and low-dose dexamethasone suppression test results are normal
  - If clinical signs are mild, wait and retest for HAC if progression occurs.
  - If clinical signs are moderate to severe and bilateral adrenomegaly is present on abdominal ultrasound
    - CT or MRI should be considered to identify a pituitary tumor causing early HAC.
    - Consider testing for occult hyperadrenocorticism (p. 490) or food-related HAC (p. 489).
  - If clinical signs are moderate to severe and the adrenal glands are normal on abdominal ultrasound, reconsider differential diagnoses.

TREATMENT

Treatment Overview

Treatment should be considered only if there are clinical signs consistent with HAC. Laboratory test abnormalities by themselves are insufficient grounds for treatment. No test for HAC is 100% sensitive or specific.

Acute General Treatment

Acute treatment of HAC is not warranted. Certain complications, such as pulmonary thromboembolism, may require immediate care.

Chronic Treatment

- Treatment for HAC is warranted only when there are clinical signs and positive tests for HAC.
- Trial therapy as a diagnostic test for HAC is not recommended because of the costs and potential side effects of treatment (p. 485).
- If mild signs of HAC are present, treatment need not be pursued immediately.
- Therapeutic recommendations vary among classic, occult, and food-related HAC.

Possible Complications

- Complications of treatment for HAC with mitotane or trilostane include gastrointestinal signs and hypoadrenocorticism.
- Hypoadrenocorticism, if not recognized and addressed promptly, can be fatal.

Recommended Monitoring

- If the diagnosis of HAC is not clear, continued monitoring is recommended. Owners should be on the lookout for the common clinical signs.
- A physical exam should be repeated every 3-4 months to identify new abnormalities.
- Testing can be repeated if clinical signs and physical changes progress.
- Potential complications of HAC that can be damaging to the body (i.e., proteinuria and hypertension) should be monitored q 2-3 months.
  - Treatment of either may be required if they worsen (p. 501).
  - Treatment for HAC is still not indicated if there are no clinical signs of it.

PROGNOSIS & OUTCOME

Depend on the disease present

PEARLS & CONSIDERATIONS

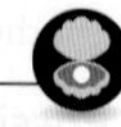

Comments

- Diagnosis of HAC can be challenging. Because it is typically a slowly progressive disease, a wait and watch approach is an option.
- No information exists that severe complications (e.g., pulmonary thromboembolism) occur before common clinical manifestations develop.
- If findings remain confusing, consultation with a specialist in veterinary internal medicine is indicated.

Technician Tips

Signs of worsening include increased drinking, urinating, appetite, and panting as well as reluctance to exercise (e.g., jump on furniture, get in and out of vehicles).

SUGGESTED READING

Behrend EN, et al: Diagnosis of spontaneous canine hyperadrenocorticism: 2012 ACVIM consensus statement (Small animal). J Vet Intern Med 27:1292-1304, 2013.

AUTHOR & EDITOR: Ellen N. Behrend, VMD, PhD, DACVIM

Hyperadrenocorticism, Food-Related

Client Education Sheet

BASIC INFORMATION

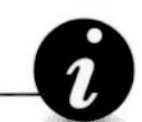

Definition

Food-dependent hyperadrenocorticism (FDH) is a syndrome caused by excess cortisol secretion as a result of aberrant expression of gastric inhibitory polypeptide (GIP) receptors in the adrenal cortex.

Synonym

Food-dependent hypercortisolism (FDH)

Epidemiology

SPECIES, AGE, SEX

- Middle-aged or elderly dogs
- No sex predisposition

ASSOCIATED DISORDERS

Adrenocortical tumor

Clinical Presentation

HISTORY, CHIEF COMPLAINT

Dogs present with the clinical signs of hypercortisolism: polyuria, polydipsia, polyphagia, pendulous abdomen, panting, alopecia, exercise intolerance, muscle atrophy, and obesity.

PHYSICAL EXAM FINDINGS

Thin skin, bilaterally symmetrical alopecia, hepatomegaly, abdominal enlargement, muscle wasting

Etiology and Pathophysiology

- GIP receptors in the adrenal cortex become functional and hyperactive.
- GIP is secreted from the intestines after a meal; binding of GIP to its receptors in the adrenal cortex results in cortisol secretion, identical to the response triggered by adrenocorticotropic hormone (ACTH) binding to its receptor.
- Secretion stimulated by GIP bypasses the normal negative feedback between the adrenal glands and the pituitary gland.
- Consequently, hypercortisolemia occurs despite low circulating ACTH concentrations.

DIAGNOSIS

Diagnostic Overview

FDH is characterized by clinical signs of hyperadrenocorticism with negative results on the standard screening tests for hyperadrenocorticism. The diagnosis is supported by testing of urinary cortisol concentrations before and after a meal and confirmed by an octreotide suppression test.

Differential Diagnosis

- Hyperadrenocorticism (p. 485)
- Atypical hyperadrenocorticism (p. 490)

Initial Database

- CBC: stress leukogram
- Serum biochemical profile: increased alkaline phosphatase (ALP), mild hyperglycemia
- Urinalysis: specific gravity < 1.020, +/− proteinuria
- Abdominal ultrasonography: hepatomegaly, bilateral adrenomegaly
- Endocrine tests for hyperadrenocorticism (i.e., ACTH stimulation and low-dose dexamethasone suppression): negative

Advanced or Confirmatory Testing

- Endogenous ACTH concentration is suppressed.
  - ACTH degrades quickly in plasma. Proper handling of sample is required (p. 1299).
- Urinary cortisol/creatinine ratio (UC/CR) before and after a meal
  - The samples should be collected by the owner at home.
  - Urine samples for UC/CR should be kept refrigerated until they are shipped to the laboratory.
  - The dog should be fasted for at least 8 hours, and then the first morning urine sample is collected.
  - The second urine sample is collected 3 hours after the dog has eaten its main meal.
  - The time of feeding does not need to be in the morning; the usual daily schedule should be followed.
  - An increase in the UC/CR after a meal of more than 50% compared with the morning (fasted) sample is suggestive of FDH.
- Octreotide test includes 2 days of testing.
  - Day 1
    - Two fasted, basal blood samples for cortisol measurement should be taken 30 minutes apart, and then the dog should be fed.
    - Four more blood samples for cortisol measurement are taken after the meal every 60 minutes.
    - In FDH, the cortisol concentration increases more than 50% after ingestion of a meal and remains elevated for at least 2 hours.
  - Day 2
    - 15 minutes after the first cortisol sample, octreotide (Sandostatin), which inhibits GIP secretion, should be administered 3 mcg/kg IM. The scheme of day 1 is followed thereafter.
  - In a patient with FDH, octreotide is expected to prevent hypercortisolemia after the meal.
  - The test is not well studied in veterinary medicine, and accuracy is unknown.
- CT or MRI
  - Pituitary gland: normal enhancement pattern and size
  - Adrenal glands: bilateral enlargement but normal structure; nodular changes are possible.

TREATMENT

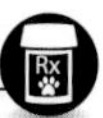

Treatment Overview

The main goal in treating FDH is resolution of clinical signs, which is achieved by suppressing hypercortisolemia.

Acute General Treatment

FDH is a mild and slowly progressive disease, and acute treatment is not indicated.

Chronic Treatment

Medical therapy with trilostane (Vetoryl):

- The timing of trilostane dosing is of utmost importance. The dog should be meal fed.
- Once-daily administration (2 mg/kg) at the time of the main meal is recommended. If the dog is fed twice daily, trilostane 1 mg/kg should be given with each meal.
- The same dosage protocol as for typical hyperadrenocorticism is used (p. 485).

Nutrition/Diet

FDH cannot be controlled by dietary manipulation.

Possible Complications

Gastrointestinal side effects are most common with trilostane; hypocortisolism and hypoaldosteronism can occur (p. 485).

Recommended Monitoring

- Monitoring of trilostane therapy is done as for typical hyperadrenocorticism (p. 485).
- Monitoring of the size of the adrenal glands by ultrasonography is recommended because aberrant GIP expression can lead to tumorigenesis.

PROGNOSIS & OUTCOME

- No data on survival for large groups of dogs with FDH are available.
- The dog described in the first case report (see reference) lived for 2 more years on medical therapy.

PEARLS & CONSIDERATIONS

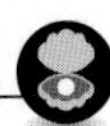

Comments

- FDH is a rare form of hyperadrenocorticism.
- Clinical signs might be mild and present years before a diagnosis is made.

Technician Tips

Ensure tubes for ACTH measurements are chilled before sampling and processed properly.

Client Education

Clients must be aware of the risks of trilostane therapy (p. 485).

SUGGESTED READING

Galac S, et al: ACTH-independent hyperadrenocorticism due to food-dependent hypercortisolemia in a dog: a case report. Vet J 177:141, 2008.

AUTHOR: Sara Galac, DVM, PhD
EDITOR: Ellen N. Behrend, VMD, PhD, DACVIM

Hyperadrenocorticism, Occult

BASIC INFORMATION

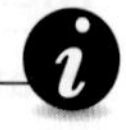

Definition

A syndrome in which a dog appears to have hyperadrenocorticism (HAC) based on history, physical exam, and clinicopathologic findings, but results of the low-dose dexamethasone suppression test (LDDST) and standard ACTH stimulation test fall into currently accepted reference ranges.

Synonym

Atypical hyperadrenocorticism

Epidemiology

SPECIES, AGE, SEX

Middle-aged to older dogs

Clinical Presentation

HISTORY, CHIEF COMPLAINT

History identical to that for classic HAC (i.e., HAC due to cortisol excess [p. 485])

PHYSICAL EXAM FINDINGS

Exam findings are identical to those for classic HAC.

Etiology and Pathophysiology

- The cause of occult HAC is unknown. Possibilities are:
  - Aberrant adrenocortical production and secretion of sex hormones
  - Cutoff values for the endocrine tests (LDDST, ACTH stimulation test) may be inappropriate.
  - Variable cortisol sensitivity may exist in dogs; those with high sensitivity may show clinical signs of HAC at cortisol concentrations considered normal.
  - Some dogs that appear to have occult HAC may have food-dependent HAC (p. 489).
- If occult HAC is related to sex hormone excess, progestins would be involved because they bind the glucocorticoid receptor.
- Although abnormalities such as sudden acquired retinal degeneration syndrome (SARDS [p. 883]) and hyperphosphatasemia in Scottish terriers have been linked to occult HAC, causative evidence is lacking.

DIAGNOSIS

Diagnostic Overview

Occult HAC should be suspected when history and clinical signs of HAC are present but both the LDDST and standard ACTH stimulation test are normal. If occult HAC is suspected, an ACTH stimulation test with measurement of sex hormones before and after ACTH should be considered.

Differential Diagnosis

- Classic HAC
- Adrenocortical neoplasia with secretion of a cortisol intermediate or progestin
- Food-induced HAC
- Any of the differential diagnoses for the clinical signs present

Initial Database

Perform initial database as for classic HAC; similar findings expected

Advanced or Confirmatory Testing

- Testing for classic HAC must be done before considering occult HAC (pp. 485, 1300, and 1360).
- If clinical signs are mild, wait and retest for classic HAC later if progression is noted.
- If clinical signs are moderate to severe, perform an abdominal ultrasound.
  - If an adrenal tumor is present, it may be the cause of the clinical signs (p. 35).
  - If the adrenal glands are normal, HAC is unlikely.
  - Bilateral adrenomegaly is supportive of, but is not specific for, HAC.
- If clinical signs are moderate to severe and abdominal ultrasound showed bilateral adrenomegaly, consider
  - Pituitary imaging to identify a tumor causing early HAC
  - Food-induced HAC (p. 489): urine cortisol/creatinine ratio before and after meal feeding, octreotide suppression
- If clinical signs are moderate to severe and all above are normal, perform an ACTH stimulation test (p. 1300) but instead of measuring only cortisol, sex hormone concentrations should be measured (https://vetmed.tennessee.edu/vmc/dls/Endocrinology/Pages/default.aspx)
  - Only the post-ACTH sex hormone concentrations should be used to make a diagnosis of occult HAC. Pre-ACTH concentrations of sex hormones are not helpful.
  - Test specificity is 70%; dogs with nonadrenal illness can have increased serum sex hormone concentrations.

TREATMENT

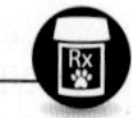

Treatment Overview

Treatment goal is resolution of clinical signs, and therapy should not be undertaken to resolve only laboratory abnormalities (e.g., elevated alkaline phosphatase [ALP]).

Acute General Treatment

Acute treatment is not needed.

Chronic Treatment

- Treatment of occult HAC with lignans (HMR lignan 10-40 mg/DOG q 24h) and melatonin 3-6 mg PO q 12h has been recommended, but efficacy is unknown.
- Treatment can be undertaken as for pituitary-dependent HAC (p. 485)
  - For occult HAC, whether dosages of mitotane or trilostane should be changed, as well as their efficacy, are unknown.
  - In theory, trilostane may be less effective than mitotane for treating occult HAC due to its mechanism of action. However, relative efficacy for occult HAC has never been evaluated, and either drug can be tried.

Possible Complications

- Complications of lignans and melatonin therapy are unknown but appear mild (e.g., lethargy).
- Hyperadrenocorticism (p. 485)

Recommended Monitoring

- If using lignans and melatonin, judge response subjectively based on clinical signs.
- If using trilostane or mitotane, monitor as for pituitary-dependent HAC. The best hormone to monitor is unknown.

PROGNOSIS & OUTCOME

Survival data unknown but likely similar to or better than for dogs with pituitary-dependent HAC

PEARLS & CONSIDERATIONS

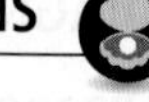

Comments

- Occult HAC should be considered only if clinical signs suggest HAC but results of an ACTH stimulation test with measurement of cortisol and an LDDST are normal.
- Abnormal laboratory results alone (e.g., elevated ALP) are not sufficient reason to treat.

Technician Tips

When performing an ACTH stimulation test with measurement of a sex hormone panel, 2 mL of serum is required in the pre- and post-ACTH samples.

Client Education

- Efficacy of treatment for occult HAC is unknown.
- If occult HAC warrants treatment and the patient responds, treatment is for life.
  - Hypoadrenocorticism is a potential complication if trilostane or mitotane are used.

SUGGESTED READING

Behrend EN, et al: Occult hyperadrenocorticism: is it real? In Bonagura J, et al, editors: Current veterinary therapy XV, St. Louis, 2014, Elsevier, pp 221-224.

AUTHOR & EDITOR: Ellen N. Behrend, VMD, PhD, DACVIM

Hypercalcemia

BASIC INFORMATION

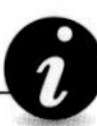

Definition

Increase in serum total and/or ionized calcium concentrations

Epidemiology

SPECIES, AGE, SEX

- Dogs or cats of either sex and any age, depending on the underlying cause
- Juvenile healthy dogs and cats: mild hypercalcemia is common.
- Hypercalcemia in adult dogs and cats is always worrisome.

GENETICS, BREED PREDISPOSITION

Depends on cause; inherited predisposition for primary hyperparathyroidism (PHPTH) in the keeshond

CONTAGION AND ZOONOSIS

Common-source infections possible with systemic mycoses

GEOGRAPHY AND SEASONALITY

Granulomatous diseases (systemic mycoses, schistosomiasis): specific geographic distributions

ASSOCIATED DISORDERS

Mineralization of nephrons due to hyperphosphatemia, despite serum calcium concentrations within reference ranges, may contribute to progression of chronic kidney disease (CKD). Hypercalcemia with low-normal to decreased serum phosphate concentrations (e.g., PHPTH) is not commonly associated with tissue mineralization or nephron damage.

Clinical Presentation

HISTORY, CHIEF COMPLAINT

- Polyuria/polydipsia (p. 812)
- Malaise: lethargy, weakness, inappetence, weight loss; mild with hypercalcemia alone.
- Lower urinary tract signs in 30%-50% of dogs with PHPTH due to cystic calculi and/or urinary tract infection (e.g., pollakiuria, stranguria, hematuria, and apparent incontinence)
- If the underlying cause is a condition other than PHPTH (e.g., neoplasia, toxin, Addison's disease), more worrisome signs may be present.

PHYSICAL EXAM FINDINGS

- No physical finding is pathognomonic for a specific cause of hypercalcemia.
- Various observations possible, depending on underlying cause
  - Lymphadenopathy possible with malignancy or granulomatous/fungal disease
  - Small kidneys in pets with CKD (p. 169).
  - Bone pain with some metastatic diseases
  - Slow heart rate and/or poor pulse quality may be noted with hypoadrenocorticism (p. 512).
  - Rectal palpation may reveal mass with anal sac apocrine gland adenocarcinoma (ASAGA [p. 29]). Because anal sac masses may be found incidentally, rectal palpation should be routine part of physical exam of dogs.

Etiology and Pathophysiology

- Approximate reference ranges for serum total and ionized calcium concentrations:
  - Dogs: total: 9.5-11.5 mg/dL (2.32-3.06 mmol/L); ionized: 1.2-1.4 mmol/L
  - Cats: total 9.0-11.5 mg/dL (2.20-3.04 mmol/L); ionized: 1.2-1.4 mmol/L
- Dystrophic, soft-tissue mineralization, specifically of nephrons, is more likely to occur if the product of calcium × phosphorus concentrations > 60-80 mg/dL.
- Approximately 50% of circulating calcium is ionized, 40% is protein bound (mostly to albumin), and 10% is bound to other molecules (e.g., lactate, citrate).

Dogs:

- The most common causes of hypercalcemia in dogs (% of affected dogs with hypercalcemia) include lymphoma (15%-30%), vitamin D toxicosis (expected), CKD (<5%), hypoadrenocorticism (≈25% in association with hyperkalemia), ASAGA (≈25%), PHPTH (expected), multiple myeloma (≈20%), histoplasmosis (uncommon), blastomycosis (uncommon), and various other malignancies (uncommon).
- In general, all these conditions in dogs are associated with worrisome clinical signs, *except* dogs with PHPTH.

Cats:

- Most commonly reported disease associations are malignancy (lymphoma, squamous cell carcinoma), kidney disease, idiopathic hypercalcemia, and urolithiasis.
- Less common disorders include PHPTH.

Mechanisms of causative disorders:

- PHPTH (p. 499)
  - Autonomous secretion of parathyroid hormone (PTH) activates osteoclastic resorption of calcium from bone, promotes renal conservation of calcium, and enhances intestinal absorption of calcium.
  - 50% of PHPTH dogs have serum PTH concentrations within reference limits, indicative of autonomous and excessive hormone secretion (e.g., adenoma)
- Hypercalcemia of malignancy: neoplastic cells elaborate parathyroid hormone–related protein (PTHrP; actions similar to parathyroid hormone).
- Granulomatous disease: elaboration of PTHrP-like substances
- Idiopathic hypercalcemia of cats (poorly understood) (p. 492)
  - Rule out underlying neoplasia.
  - Predisposed to urolith formation
- CKD: renal secondary hyperparathyroidism
- Vitamin D toxicosis (rodenticide or human prescription medications such as calcipotriene): heightened vitamin D–mediated intestinal calcium absorption, renal calcium conservation
- Juvenile: bone growth

DIAGNOSIS

Diagnostic Overview

History, absence or presence of worrisome clinical signs (e.g., anorexia, severe weight loss), physical exam, and serum phosphate concentrations should allow the differential diagnosis to be refined, directing additional testing (p. 1233).

Differential Diagnosis

See above and Hypercalcemia (p. 1232).

Initial Database

- CBC: depends on cause (e.g., nonregenerative anemia if CKD; monocytosis if systemic mycosis)
- Serum chemistry panel
  - Azotemia (i.e., increased blood urea nitrogen [BUN], creatinine, and phosphorus): severe dehydration, kidney disease, hypoadrenocorticism
  - Hyperkalemia: hypoadrenocorticism, acute kidney injury; NOTE: *in vitro* hemolysis can increase serum potassium in the Akita and Japanese Tosa breeds.
  - Hypophosphatemia: PHPTH, hypercalcemia of malignancy
  - Hyperphosphatemia: CKD, vitamin D toxicosis, hypoadrenocorticism

- Assess calcium × phosphorous (Ca • PO_4) product: if > 60, nephron damage is a concern. In PHPTH, typically < 45.
- Urinalysis
  - Uroliths and calcium-containing crystalluria are common.
  - All causes of hypercalcemia lead to poorly concentrated urine (by nephrogenic diabetes insipidus).
  - Persistent isosthenuria (1.008-1.012) with concurrent azotemia suggests kidney disease or hypoadrenocorticism.
  - Hyposthenuria, isosthenuria, or minimally concentrated urine associated with PHPTH (mean ≈1.011), with values as low as 1.002.
- Thoracic radiographs
  - Nodular lung patterns or lymphadenomegaly suggest neoplasia or fungal disease.
  - Cranial mediastinal mass common in dogs that have hypercalcemia secondary to lymphoma.
  - Lytic bone lesion suggests multiple myeloma or other metastatic cancer.
- Abdominal imaging (ultrasound ± radiographs)
  - Lesions suggesting malignancy (lymphadenopathy, hepatosplenomegaly, possible metastases, including lytic bone lesions)
  - Uroliths (calcium phosphate, calcium oxalate, or both) and bladder wall thickening: common in PHPTH
  - Assess renal structure. Renal dystrophic mineralization rarely is apparent radiographically or ultrasonographically.

Advanced or Confirmatory Testing

- Ionized calcium (i.e., biologically active component of the total serum calcium): normal or low with CKD, increased with most other causes of hypercalcemia (e.g., PHPTH, hypercalcemia of malignancy, vitamin D toxicosis)
- Serum PTH and PTHrP concentrations during hypercalcemia
  - PTH should be undetectable in response to hypercalcemia.
  - PTH values within or above reference range are consistent with PHPTH.
  - Undetectable PTH and detectable PTHrP concentrations are consistent with hypercalcemia of malignancy.
- Serum vitamin D concentrations: if suspect intoxication (p. 164)
- Cervical ultrasound
  - Parathyroid glands should be ≈1.3-3.3 mm in greatest width (dogs and cats).
  - In dogs with PHPTH, a mass is typically identified involving one or more parathyroid gland(s), usually 4-8 mm in greatest diameter.
  - Dogs with renal secondary hyperparathyroidism have enlargement of two, three, or all four parathyroid glands.
- Additional testing based on abnormalities identified (e.g., fine-needle aspiration of enlarged lymph nodes, fungal serology)

TREATMENT

Treatment Overview

Successful treatment of underlying cause lowers serum calcium. If (Ca • PO_4) is > 60, additional measures may be required. Rapid reduction in serum calcium, even with extremely increased values (15-23 mg/dL) is not necessary if (Ca • PO_4) is < 60, which is typical of PHPTH. Even when calcium is within reference range, if Ca • PO_4 is increased, nephron damage may ensue.

Acute General Treatment

Primary (most efficacious):

- IV fluid therapy (calcium free; avoid lactated Ringer's solution)
  - Dilution of serum calcium and phosphorus concentrations, improved glomerular filtration rate
  - Twice maintenance plus dehydration deficit should be administered over the first 24 hours, assuming no heart disease, oliguria, or other factor predisposing to intolerance of volume load; adjust according to clinical signs.
- Furosemide 2-3 mg/kg IV q 4-8h. Calciuric diuretic (unlike thiazide diuretics or spironolactone) is not recommended for pets with renal insufficiency.
- Glucocorticoids (prednisone or dexamethasone): decrease intestinal calcium absorption, increase renal calcium excretion. Diagnostic samples (e.g., lymph node aspirate, bone marrow aspirate, liver biopsy) should be obtained before treatment because steroids may mask lymphoma.

Secondary therapies (more expensive and not often required):

- Bisphosphonates
- Calcitonin
- Plicamycin
- Cinacalcet

Chronic Treatment

Treat inciting cause

Possible Complications

Overcorrection (hypocalcemia), urolithiasis, nephron damage (if Ca • PO_4 > 60)

Recommended Monitoring

- Serum total and ionized calcium concentrations
- Renal parameters
- Serum electrolytes

PROGNOSIS & OUTCOME

- Varies; depends on ability to achieve normocalcemia and correct underlying cause
- Excellent for PHPTH

PEARLS & CONSIDERATIONS

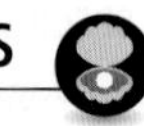

Comments

- Remember, renal failure is not caused by hypercalcemia alone.
- Correcting total calcium concentration for hypoalbuminemia or hyperalbuminemia is not reliable (instead, measure serum ionized calcium concentrations directly).
- Oral consumption of calcium alone does not cause hypercalcemia.
- Hypercalcemic dogs that are ill are not likely to have PHPTH.

Technician Tips

- Urolithiasis related to hypercalcemia can cause urinary obstruction. Straining to urinate is an emergent condition.
- Hypercalcemic dogs should always have drinking water available and should be given ample opportunity to urinate.

SUGGESTED READING

Skelly BJ: Primary hyperparathyroidism. In Ettinger SE, et al, editors: The textbook of veterinary internal medicine, ed 8, St. Louis, 2017, Elsevier, pp 1715-1727.

AUTHOR: Edward C. Feldman, DVM, DACVIM
EDITOR: Leah A. Cohn, DVM, PhD, DACVIM

Hypercalcemia, Idiopathic Feline

BASIC INFORMATION

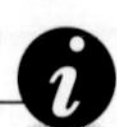

Definition

This poorly understood condition is the most common cause of increased ionized calcium (iCa) in cats.

Epidemiology

SPECIES, AGE, SEX

Cats of any age (often 5-10 years) and either sex

GENETICS, BREED PREDISPOSITION

Long-haired cats appear to be overrepresented.

RISK FACTORS

Genetics, diet, or the use of urinary acidifiers

ASSOCIATED DISORDERS

Calcium oxalate urolithiasis, chronic kidney disease (CKD)

Clinical Presentation

HISTORY, CHIEF COMPLAINT

- Usually an incidental finding (e.g., geriatric screening) or associated with vague clinical signs such as weight loss, diarrhea, constipation, vomiting, or anorexia
- The modest degree of hypercalcemia typical of the disorder is seldom associated with the most worrisome adverse effects of hypercalcemia (e.g., tissue mineralization).
- Sometimes, signs related to calcium oxalate urolithiasis (e.g., dysuria, periuria [p. 1014]) or concurrent CKD (e.g., polyuria/ polydipsia [pp. 167 and 169]) are noted.

PHYSICAL EXAM FINDINGS

No specific physical exam findings. Calcium oxalate urolithiasis can cause signs of urethral obstruction in some affected cats.

Etiology and Pathophysiology

- Extracellular total calcium fractions include biologically active iCa (≈52%), protein-bound calcium (≈40%), and calcium complexed to other molecules (≈8%). Calcium balance is closely controlled in health through intestinal absorption, renal excretion, and redistribution from bone.
- As the name implies, the cause of ionized hypercalcemia in affected cats remains unknown.

DIAGNOSIS

Diagnostic Overview

Typically, total calcium is measured first, and if above the upper end of the reference range, iCa is measured. If that too is above the reference range, attempts should be made to identify a cause of hypercalcemia. Idiopathic hypercalcemia is a diagnosis of exclusion.

Differential Diagnosis

Hypercalcemia (pp. 491 and 1232)

Initial Database

- Serum biochemistry profile: increased total calcium; phosphorus within reference range
    - Concurrent CKD associated with azotemia, hyperphosphatemia
- Ionized calcium: usually mild to moderate increase (80% between 1.5 and 1.75 mmol/L; 1.4 mmol/L is the upper end of the reference range)
    - If iCa cannot be measured quickly in house, sample should be collected anaerobically and transported on ice.
    - Exposure of sample to air can lead to loss of CO_2, resulting in decreased iCa.
    - Lactic acid accumulation alters the pH of stored samples, resulting in increased iCa.
- CBC: unremarkable
- Urinalysis: variable urine specific gravity, possible calcium oxalate crystalluria
- Total thyroxine (T_4): unremarkable
- Thoracic and abdominal imaging: rule out neoplasia

Advanced or Confirmatory Testing

Serum parathyroid hormone (PTH), parathyroid hormone–related protein (PTHrP), vitamin D profile:

- PTH: below or near the lower end of the reference range
- PTHrP: typically below limits of detection
- Vitamin D: 25(OH)D_3 and 1,25(OH)$_2$$D_3$ within reference range

TREATMENT

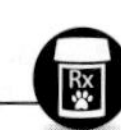

Treatment Overview

Because the degree of hypercalcemia is typically modest, emergent efforts to reduce calcium are not required. After other causes of hypercalcemia have been ruled out, dietary therapy is typically begun. If unsuccessful, medical management is attempted. Concurrent urolithiasis and/or CKD must be addressed, if present.

Acute General Treatment

Rarely, calcium oxalate urolithiasis results in urethral obstruction, requiring emergency intervention (p. 1009)

Chronic Treatment

- Many cats can be managed with dietary therapy alone.
- If ionized hypercalcemia persists after a 6-week diet trial, medical therapy with glucocorticoids or bisphosphonate drugs is recommended.
    - Prednisolone (not prednisone) 0.5-1 mg/kg PO q 12-24h. Avoid use until diagnostic testing is complete.
    - Alendronate 5-20 mg/CAT PO q 7 days. Begin with lower dose, and titrate up as needed. Administer after a 12-hour fast. Pills should not be cut because they can be highly irritating to the oral and esophageal surfaces. Follow pill with 5-10 mL of water to reduce risk of esophageal stricture. Liquid formulations are available but may not be palatable.
    - Occasionally, a combination of prednisolone and alendronate is required to control iCa.

Nutrition/Diet

- High-fiber diet and/or psyllium supplementation recommended
- Wet/canned foods preferred
- Oxalate prevention diets useful for cats with no evidence of CKD
- Renal diets are appropriate for cats with concurrent azotemia.

Possible Complications

- Uncontrolled hypercalcemia may result in calcium oxalate urolithiasis.
- Alendronate may cause esophageal stricture or irritation of mucous membranes.
- In humans, alendronate may cause osteonecrosis of the mandible and maxilla; if dental work is required, it should be completed before starting alendronate.

Recommended Monitoring

Recheck iCa 6 weeks after starting diet trial or 1-2 weeks after any change in medical therapy. Once controlled, iCa should be rechecked q 4-6 months. Serum chemistry profile (azotemia) and urinalysis (crystalluria) should be checked q 6-12 months.

PROGNOSIS & OUTCOME

With treatment, excellent. Without treatment, urolithiasis remains a concern.

PEARLS & CONSIDERATIONS

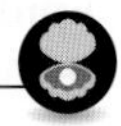

Comments

- Other causes of hypercalcemia may be associated with life-threatening disease and should be ruled out before instituting treatment for idiopathic hypercalcemia.
- Severe hypercalcemia is seldom caused by idiopathic hypercalcemia.
- Renal damage associated with hypercalcemia is related to the calcium × phosphorus product more than to the iCa. Because hypercalcemia is mild and phosphorus is within reference range, kidney damage is unlikely with idiopathic hypercalcemia alone.
- It is possible for a cat to have both CKD and idiopathic hypercalcemia, which can confuse the diagnosis (e.g., CKD can cause increased total calcium but normal iCa).
- Use of formulas to adjust calcium concentration based on albumin is not appropriate for cats with hypercalcemia. Instead, ionized calcium concentrations should be measured directly.

Technician Tips

Demonstrate for owners how to properly administer medications, including giving water afterward to minimize the risk of esophageal stricture with alendronate.

Client Education

Proper administration of medications

SUGGESTED READING

Finch NC: Hypercalcemia in cats: the complexities of calcium regulation and associated clinical challenges. J Feline Med Surg 18:387-399. 2016.

AUTHOR: Leah A. Cohn, DVM, PhD, DACVIM
EDITOR: Etienne Côté, DVM, DACVIM

Hyperemia

Bonus Material Online 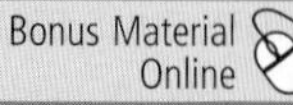

BASIC INFORMATION

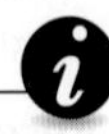

Definition

- Active hyperemia: increased volume of blood in an affected tissue or area due to arterial dilation
- Passive hyperemia: increased volume of blood in an affected tissue or area due to venous distention

Synonyms

- Active hyperemia: arterial hyperemia, reactive hyperemia, metabolic hyperemia
- Passive hyperemia: venous hyperemia

Epidemiology

SPECIES, AGE, SEX

Any dog or cat

RISK FACTORS

- Increased tissue metabolic demand (e.g., fever, physical exertion)
- Vascular occlusion: extravascular or intravascular

GEOGRAPHY AND SEASONALITY

Vasodilatory cooling related to high environmental temperature is a normal cause of hyperemia.

Clinical Presentation

DISEASE FORMS/SUBTYPES

- Primary complaint
  - Obvious extravascular occlusion such as limb constriction
  - Gross tissue changes
- Secondary finding
  - Abnormal finding during examination prompted by another problem
  - Incidental finding of no clinical significance (e.g., due to anxiety, physical activity, hot weather)
- Hyperemia may also be classified as regional or generalized.

HISTORY, CHIEF COMPLAINT

- Highly variable depending on underlying cause
- Examples of generalized hyperemia
  - Recent exposure to allergen (e.g., insect bite, vaccine, food allergen)
  - Exposure to toxic agent (e.g., smoke inhalation)
  - Exposure to high environmental temperature (e.g., thick haircoat, locked in car)
  - Systemic disease (e.g., pheochromocytoma, mast cell disease, shock)
  - Anxiety, restlessness (incidental finding during routine exam)

PHYSICAL EXAM FINDINGS

- Because hyperemia is a clinical sign and not a disease entity, physical findings depend on the underlying cause. Hyperemia usually manifests as erythema (redness of the skin and mucous membranes) due to vessel engorgement with oxygenated blood.
- Generalized hyperemia
  - Tachycardia, tachypnea, hyperthermia
  - Increased respiratory effort
  - Shortened capillary refill time
  - Episodic increased levels of activity
- Localized hyperemia
  - Regional dermal redness, swelling, and/or pain
  - Site may be warmer than normal and less functional

Etiology and Pathophysiology

- Arteriolar dilation usually is in response to tissue hypoxia, sympathetic neurogenic mechanisms, and/or exposure to vasodilatory metabolites released locally or systemically, such as adenosine, nitric oxide, lactate, potassium ion, and carbon dioxide.
- Venous distention, however, occurs in response to obstruction of blood outflow due to obstruction within the capillaries or veins due to thickening of the walls or thrombi or to external pressure such as from a tumor or tight bandaging.

DIAGNOSIS

Diagnostic Overview

Hyperemia is a clinical sign associated with a wide variety of conditions. Rule out obvious causes by a careful history and physical exam and determine whether the presence of hyperemia is clinically significant.

Differential Diagnosis

Hyperemia (p. 1234)

Initial Database

- Temperature, heart rate, respiration rate
  - Hyperthermia warrants consideration of true fever (e.g., infectious, inflammatory, drug reaction, neoplastic causes) versus environmental hyperthermia (e.g., hot weather, thick haircoat, anxiety, tremor).
- Diascopy: superficial lesions blanch with external pressure, such as with a glass slide.
  - This maneuver helps confirm whether hyperemia is present versus normal coloration or an area of subcutaneous hemorrhage.

Advanced or Confirmatory Testing

Use of these tests depends on determination of need. For example, in animals that are otherwise clinically normal (routine exam), behavioral agitation/anxiety, benign environmental hyperthermia, and exercise are common causes of hyperemia that do not warrant further evaluation.

- Blood pressure measurements (p. 1065)
  - Systemic
  - Localized (if embolic occlusion suspected)
- CBC (infectious, inflammatory, neoplastic, polycythemia)
- Serum biochemistry panel (hepatic, renal dysfunction)
- Radiographs (organomegaly, neoplasia)
- Neurologic evaluation (in cases of suspected intoxication or other systemic disorders with neurologic effects) (p. 1136)
- Abdominal ultrasound (neoplasm, infection/abscess, chronic passive congestion)
- Echocardiogram (endocarditis, embolic disorder, other [p. 1094])
- Aspirates and/or biopsies (masses, lesions)
- Tick-borne disease titers
- Blood gas analysis

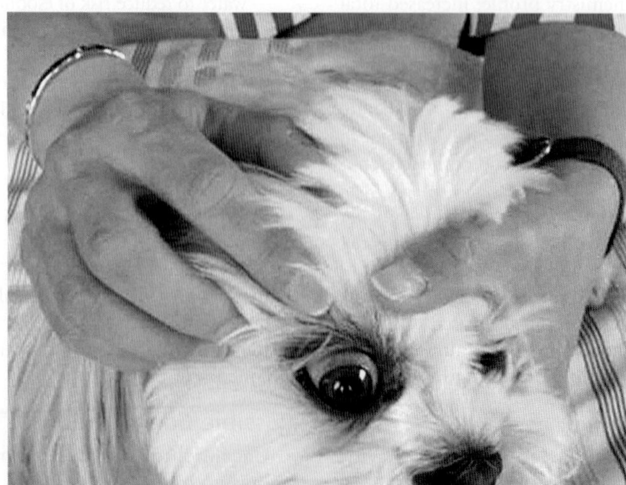

HYPEREMIA Conjunctival hyperemia in a 5-year-old shih tzu. The image was captured from a digital movie clip obtained by the owner at home. The chief complaint was episodic restlessness and generalized hyperemia, noted intermittently by the owner for a period of weeks. (Courtesy Dr. Etienne Côté.)

- Co-oximetry (carbon monoxide intoxication)
- CT or MRI (embolism evaluation)

TREATMENT

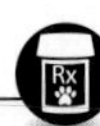

Treatment Overview

Goal of treatment is resolution of the underlying cause, with special attention paid to ensuring adequate tissue perfusion.

Acute General Treatment

- Supportive as needed: analgesia, oxygen supplementation (p. 1146), restoration of perfusion, cooling and/or elevation of the affected region
- Treat underlying disorder

Possible Complications

Reperfusion injury, tissue necrosis

PROGNOSIS & OUTCOME

Varies, depending on the underlying cause

PEARLS & CONSIDERATIONS

Comments

- Presenting signs (true chief complaint vs. routine visit for preventive/annual exam) are extremely valuable in determining the importance of a patient's hyperemia.
- Intermittent/episodic hyperemia associated with behavioral changes, cardiac arrhythmias, or other systemic signs should arouse the suspicion of mast cell tumor or pheochromocytoma.

Techician Tip

Good lighting is important in assessing if a perceived color change (e.g., reddening) is real.

SUGGESTED READING

Lima I, et al: The peripheral perfusion index in reactive hyperemia in critically ill patients. Crit Care 8(suppl 1):53, 2004.

AUTHOR: Adam J. Reiss, DVM, DACVECC
EDITOR: Leah A. Cohn, DVM, PhD, DACVIM

Hyperkalemia

BASIC INFORMATION

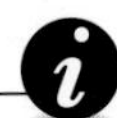

Definition

A serum potassium (K^+) concentration > 5.5 mEq/L; concentrations > 7.5 mEq/L are potentially harmful.

Synonym

Elevated serum potassium (K^+) concentration

Epidemiology

SPECIES, AGE, SEX

Any patient can be affected.

GENETICS, BREED PREDISPOSITION

- Hyperkalemia: hypoadrenocorticism (standard poodles)
- Pseudohyperkalemia: hemolysis or thrombocytosis in Japanese breeds (Akita, shiba); English springer spaniel with phosphofructokinase deficiency

RISK FACTORS

- Urinary obstruction
- Urinary bladder rupture
- Hypoadrenocorticism (i.e., Addison's disease)
- Oliguria and anuria
- Type 4 renal tubular acidosis
- Mineral acid metabolic acidosis (not organic acidosis such as lactic acidosis)
- Iatrogenic factors (drugs, oversupplementation)

ASSOCIATED DISORDERS

- Bradycardia
- Atrial standstill
- Abnormal electrocardiogram (ECG) complexes
- Skeletal muscle weakness

Clinical Presentation

DISEASE FORMS/SUBTYPES

Acute and chronic; subclinical or clinical

HISTORY, CHIEF COMPLAINT

- Acute: often dramatic and life-threatening; produces diffuse muscle weakness, mental depression, anorexia.
- Chronic: slower in onset and not as dramatic. Decreased appetite, weight loss, intermittent vomiting and diarrhea, and skeletal muscle weakness can occur.
- History often reflects cause of hyperkalemia (e.g., stranguria with lower urinary obstruction; vomiting with acute kidney injury (AKI) or hypoadrenocorticism).

PHYSICAL EXAM FINDINGS

- With severe hyperkalemia, may find:
  - Generalized muscle weakness
  - Weak pulse
  - Prolonged capillary refill time
  - Bradycardia, especially in setting of dehydration when heart rate should be increased
  - Irregular heart rate
  - Body temperature normal or hypothermia
- Other findings related to underlying cause (e.g., distended bladder from urethral obstruction)

Etiology and Pathophysiology

Cause of hyperkalemia: see Hyperkalemia (p. 1235)

- Decreased K^+ excretion, as in hypoaldosteronism, AKI, urinary bladder rupture or outflow obstruction, or type 4 renal distal tubular acidosis and with certain drugs (e.g., angiotensin-converting enzyme [ACE] inhibitors, potassium-sparing diuretics, beta-blockers)
- K^+ translocation from intracellular to extracellular fluid space (e.g., mineral acid–caused metabolic acidosis, hypertonicity, tumor lysis syndrome, hyperkalemic periodic paralysis, massive tissue destruction [rare])
- Miscellaneous conditions (cause poorly understood), such as whipworm enterocolitis, chylothorax, ascites, term pregnancy; these may be associated with hyponatremia (pseudo Addison's disease)
- Pseudohyperkalemia (e.g., thrombocytosis, extreme leukocytosis [>100,0000], hemolysis [especially Japanese breed dogs])
- Spurious

Mechanism of damage due to hyperkalemia:

- Affects primarily skeletal and cardiac muscle tissues
- Life-threatening effects on heart
  - Initially increased and subsequently depressed excitability and conduction velocity secondary to persistent depolarization and inactivation of the sodium channels in the cell membranes, causing cardiac conduction abnormalities
- Skeletal muscle weakness occurs.

DIAGNOSIS

Diagnostic Overview

Confirm accurate K^+ measurement. Cause is often readily identified by history, exam, and minimal laboratory testing and imaging studies. Unless mild, perform ECG.

Differential Diagnosis

- Pseudohyperkalemia
- Any cause of bradycardia (p. 1204)
- Primary myocardial disease
- Many of the causes of skeletal muscle weakness (p. 1295)

Initial Database

- Thorough history and physical exam
- CBC: eosinophilia, lymphocytosis, and anemia may occur with hypoadrenocorticism
- Serum biochemistry profile
  - Serum electrolytes: elevated K^+ with simultaneous decreased sodium concentrations can occur with hypoadrenocorticism,

enteritis, renal disease, pregnancy, pleural effusion, diabetes mellitus.
  - Blood urea nitrogen, creatinine: elevated with prerenal (e.g., hypoadrenocorticism), renal, or postrenal (e.g., urethral obstruction, urinary bladder rupture) azotemia.
  - Total CO_2/HCO_3^- decreased with metabolic acidosis
  - Glucose may be decreased in hypoadrenocorticism, sepsis or increased in diabetes mellitus.
- Urinalysis: isosthenuria concurrent with azotemia in renal failure or in hypoadrenocorticism.
- Blood gas: pH, HCO_3^- or total CO_2 typically decreased
- Abdominal imaging: small adrenal glands with ultrasonography (Addison's disease); abdominal effusion; small or large bladder (urinary rupture or obstruction)
- ECG: depending on severity, tented T waves, widened QRS complexes, accelerated idioventricular rhythm, bradycardia, atrial standstill, ventricular fibrillation

Advanced or Confirmatory Testing

- Measure plasma K^+ if pseudohyperkalemia is suspected.
- ACTH stimulation test for hypoadrenocorticism
- Assess effusions, if present.
- Urinary fractional excretion tests for renal tubular acidosis
- Other tests as necessitated by suspected cause

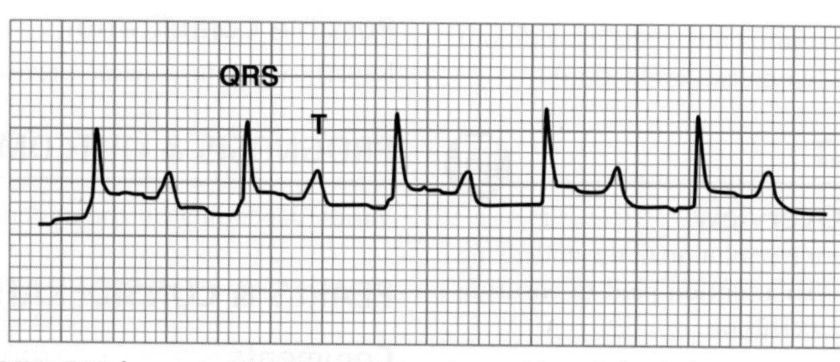

HYPERKALEMIA ECG for a cat with urethral obstruction and hyperkalemia (serum K^+ = 7.1 mEq/L) shows atrial standstill. No P waves are seen, but the R-R rhythm is regular, typical of atrial standstill. The heart rate is 210 beats/min, demonstrating that in cats, unlike dogs, a rapid heart rate is consistent with hyperkalemia. There is mild ST-segment elevation, suggesting myocardial hypoxia. Lead V_2, 25 mm/sec, 1 cm = 1 mV.

TREATMENT

Treatment Overview

- Antagonize myocardiotoxicity.
- Treat the underlying cause.
- Stop drugs known to increase serum K^+ concentration.

Acute General Treatment

- Calcium gluconate 10% solution 0.5-1.5 mL/kg IV immediately antagonizes myocardiotoxicity without actually lowering serum K^+ concentration.
- Emergent reduction of serum K^+
  - Sodium bicarbonate 1-2 mEq/kg IV bolus (minimally effective)
  - Regular insulin and glucose, give 0.25-0.5 units of insulin/kg IV, covering each unit of insulin administered with 2 g dextrose (2 g = 4 mL 50% dextrose)
  - Terbutaline or albuterol 0.01 mg/kg IV slowly over 3-5 minutes
  - Hemodialysis
  - Potassium-binding resins orally
- Treat the underlying cause (e.g., relieve urethral obstruction, DOCP for hypoadrenocorticism).

Chronic Treatment

Treat any underlying disease

Drug Interactions

Avoid ACE inhibitors and aldosterone antagonists as they can cause hyperkalemia.

Possible Complications

Cardiac arrest, death. Insulin administration can cause hypoglycemia.

Recommended Monitoring

- Monitor electrolytes until normalized or as dictated by underlying disease
- Monitor ECG until severe hyperkalemia is resolved.

PROGNOSIS & OUTCOME

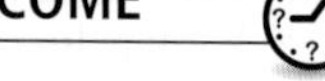

Prognosis depends on cause
- Guarded for AKI
- Good for hypoadrenocorticism, urethral obstruction

PEARLS & CONSIDERATIONS

Comments

- Do a lead II ECG on all patients suspected of having hyperkalemia.
- Bradycardia in a dehydrated patient is inappropriate; hyperkalemia should be considered as one of the causes.
- Calcium gluconate IV works within a few minutes, sodium bicarbonate IV works within 15 minutes, regular insulin and dextrose work within 30 minutes, and beta-agonists (albuterol and terbutaline) work within minutes.
- Blood samples put in ethylenediaminetetraacetic acid (EDTA) tubes cause pseudohyperkalemia because of the K^+ EDTA.
- In cats, hyperkalemia does not always cause bradycardia; hyperkalemic cats may be tachycardic even with severe hyperkalemia.
- On an ECG, peaked T waves are often normal; the transition from normal T wave to peaked T wave, however, is very suggestive of evolving hyperkalemia.
- When present, hyponatremia exaggerates the effects of hyperkalemia on cardiac myocytes.

Prevention

Monitor electrolytes when using parenteral fluids with large amounts of K^+.

Technician Tips

- Recognize ECG changes of hyperkalemia.
- Shut off outlet port of IV fluid line while adding K^+ to the bottle; mix well before administration.

Client Education

Straining to urinate or failure to urinate should prompt emergent visit.

SUGGESTED READING

Kogika MM, et al: A quick reference on hyperkalemia. Vet Clin Small Anim Pract 47:223-228, 2017. DOI: https://doi.org/10.1016/j.cvsm.2016.10.009.

AUTHOR: Michael Schaer, DVM, DACVIM, DACVECC
EDITOR: Leah A. Cohn, DVM, PhD, DACVIM

Hyperlipidemia

Client Education Sheet

BASIC INFORMATION

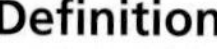

Definition

Increased fasting blood cholesterol and/or triglyceride (TG) concentrations; a common (dogs) to rare (cats) disorder in small animals

Synonyms

Hyperlipoproteinemia, lipemia

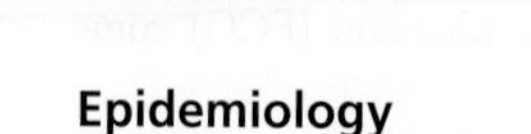

Epidemiology

SPECIES, AGE, SEX

- Postprandial: any animal for up to 12 hours after a meal

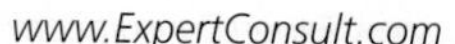

- Primary: middle-aged/older dogs; varies in cats
- Secondary: varies

GENETICS, BREED PREDISPOSITION

- Idiopathic hypertriglyceridemia: miniature schnauzers, Burmese cats
- Idiopathic hypercholesterolemia: Shetland sheepdogs, Briards, sporadic in other breeds
- Feline familial hyperlipidemia: autosomal recessive trait in domestic short-haired cats

RISK FACTORS

- Obesity (dogs)
- Drugs: glucocorticoids, phenobarbital (dogs), megestrol acetate (cats)
- High-fat diets or parenteral nutrition
- Negative energy balance (kittens)
- Hypothyroidism
- Hyperadrenocorticism
- Pancreatitis
- Diabetes mellitus
- Protein-losing nephropathy
- Cholestasis

ASSOCIATED DISORDERS

- Pancreatitis
- Vacuolar hepatopathy
- Gallbladder mucocele
- Insulin resistance
- Seizures
- Xanthomas
- Atherosclerosis
- Peripheral neuropathy
- Behavior changes

Clinical Presentation

DISEASE FORMS/SUBTYPES

Primary hyperlipidemias:

- Idiopathic hypertriglyceridemia (dogs)
  - Increased very low–density lipoprotein (VLDL) serum concentrations
  - ± Increased chylomicron (CM) serum concentrations
  - ± Hypercholesterolemia
- Idiopathic hypercholesterolemia (dogs)
  - Increased high-density lipoprotein (HDL) serum concentrations
  - ± Increased low-density lipoprotein (LDL) and VLDL serum concentrations
  - ± Hypertriglyceridemia
- Familial hyperlipidemia/hyperchylomicronemia (cats)
  - Increased CM and VLDL
  - Inactive lipoprotein lipase

Secondary hyperlipidemias: see Risk Factors above.

HISTORY, CHIEF COMPLAINT

- Clinical signs, when present, are usually the result of hypertriglyceridemia; hypercholesterolemia rarely causes clinical signs.
- Dogs: anorexia, lethargy, vomiting, diarrhea, abdominal discomfort, seizures
- Cats: inappetence, lethargy, cutaneous/subcutaneous masses, lameness

PHYSICAL EXAM FINDINGS

Physical exam may be unremarkable or may be compatible with underlying cause (e.g., alopecia due to hypothyroidism).

- Hypertriglyceridemia
  - Dogs: abdominal discomfort, hepatosplenomegaly, lipemia retinalis, lipemic aqueous humor, intraocular xanthogranuloma
  - Cats: xanthomas, decreased reflexes, pale mucous membranes, lipemia retinalis, lipid keratopathy, lipemic aqueous humor
- Hypercholesterolemia
  - Dogs: lipemia retinalis, lipid keratopathy, arcus lipoides corneae

Etiology and Pathophysiology

Lipoproteins

- Lipids (TG and cholesterol) do not circulate free; rather, they are complexed in varying proportions as circulating particles called *lipoproteins*.
- Four major types of lipoproteins exist: CM, VLDL, LDL, and HDL.

Mechanisms of hyperlipidemia

- Postprandial hyperlipidemia
  - CM in circulation 2-10 hours after fatty meal
- Primary hyperlipidemia
  - Inborn error in lipoprotein metabolism
    - Lack of lipoprotein lipase activity
    - Absence of surface apolipoproteins (i.e., CII)
- Secondary hyperlipidemia
  - Underlying disease (see Risk Factors) causing altered lipid metabolism
  - Secondary hyperlipidemias are more common than primary.

DIAGNOSIS

Diagnostic Overview

Lipemic serum suggests hypertriglyceridemia; hypercholesterolemia alone does not cause serum to appear lipemic. Persistent increases in serum TGs or cholesterol after a 12-hour fast should prompt investigation for causes of hyperlipidemia.

Differential Diagnosis

Postprandial hyperlipidemia

Initial Database

- CBC, serum biochemical profile (including serum cholesterol and TG concentrations), urinalysis
  - Perform after > 12-hour fast.
  - Point-of-care TG meters have been evaluated for screening (see Additional Suggested Readings); PTS CardioChek (Polymer Technology Systems Inc, Indianapolis, IN) is suitable as a screening device for hypertriglyceridemia in cats and dogs.
  - Identify abnormalities that suggest disease causing secondary hyperlipidemia.
- Subsequently, consider
  - Tests for hypothyroidism (p. 525)
  - Tests for hyperadrenocorticism (p. 485)
  - Urine protein/creatinine ratio (p. 1391)
  - Abdominal ultrasound
  - Serum canine and feline pancreatic lipase immunoreactivity (cPLI and fPLI, respectively) (p. 1370)

Advanced or Confirmatory Testing

If a cause of secondary hyperlipidemia is not found, additional tests may help define a primary hyperlipidemia.

- CM test: lipemic serum is left undisturbed for 12 hours at 4°C.
  - When CMs are present, they form a surface cream layer over a clear infranatant of serum. If CMs present, ensure patient was fasted before blood was drawn.
  - If the sample remains turbid, VLDL retention (and therefore a secondary hyperlipidemia) is likely.
  - Formation of a cream layer over turbid serum suggests a combined disorder.
- Lipoprotein electrophoresis, ultracentrifugation, and precipitation tests can be useful but are not routinely available.
- Lipoprotein lipase activity can be assessed by measuring TG (± lipoprotein) concentrations before and 15 minutes after heparin (dog: 90 IU/kg IV; cat: 40 IU/kg IV) administration. If no change, lipoprotein lipase inactivity is suspected.

TREATMENT

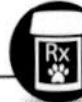

Treatment Overview

Treatment consists primarily of management of secondary causes and nutritional therapy. Medications are reserved for unresponsive severe cases of hyperlipidemia (TG > 500 mg/dL [5.65 mmol/L]; cholesterol > 800 mg/dL [20.7 mmol/L]). Goal of treatment is to reduce fasting TG or cholesterol concentrations to < 500 mg/dL (TG < 5.65 mmol/L; cholesterol < 12.95 mmol/L). Treatment is lifelong for primary hyperlipidemia.

Acute General Treatment

Treat any underlying diseases.

Chronic Treatment

- Hypertriglyceridemia (fasting, repeatable)
  - Dietary management should be the mainstay of treatment (see Nutrition/Diet below).
  - Menhaden fish oils 200-330 mg/kg PO q 24h (dogs)
  - Fibrates: gemfibrozil 10 mg/kg PO q 12h (dogs), 7.5-10 mg/kg PO q 12h (cats), *or* bezafibrate 4-10 mg/kg PO q 24h (dogs)
  - Niacin 50-200 mg/dose PO q 24h (dogs)
- Hypercholesterolemia (fasting, repeatable)
  - A cause is almost always present (e.g., hypothyroidism), and its control resolves the hypercholesterolemia. Otherwise, dietary management should be the mainstay of treatment (see Nutrition/Diet below).
  - Statins: atorvastatin 2-5 mg/kg PO q 24h (dogs) *or* lovastatin 10-20 mg/dose PO q 24h (dogs)

Nutrition/Diet

- Hypertriglyceridemia
  - Dietary fat restriction (dog: < 20% metabolizable energy [ME]; cat: < 25% ME)
  - If a low-fat diet is unsuccessful, a nutritionist can design an ultralow-fat (10%-12% ME) diet.
- Hypercholesterolemia
  - Low-fat diet with increased amounts of soluble fiber

Drug Interactions

- Statins should not be used concurrently with azole antifungals, cyclosporine, diltiazem, or gemfibrozil.
- Statins may increase the toxicity of digoxin.

Possible Complications

- Fibrates may cause myalgia and hepatopathy.
- Niacin may cause hyperglycemia, erythema, pruritus, myalgia, and hepatopathy.
- Statins may cause lethargy, diarrhea, myalgia, and hepatopathy.

Recommended Monitoring

- Monitor plasma TGs 4-8 weeks after initiation of low-fat diet, then every 6-12 months.
- Monitor hematologic/biochemical parameters with fibrates, niacin, or lovastatin.

PROGNOSIS & OUTCOME

- Successful management depends on adequate control of underlying disease(s) and reduction of plasma lipid concentrations.
- Cats with peripheral neuropathies generally have clinical signs resolve within 4-12 weeks of instituting diet change.

PEARLS & CONSIDERATIONS

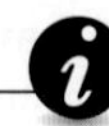

Comments

- Hyperlipidemia in patients fasted > 12 hours is abnormal.
- Lipemic plasma is an indication of hypertriglyceridemia, not hypercholesterolemia.
- Hypertriglyceridemia often signals underlying disease and may cause clinical disease.
- Hypercholesterolemia may indicate the presence of an underlying disorder but rarely causes clinical disease.

Prevention

- Treat predisposing disorders.
- Monitor TG concentrations in susceptible breeds.

Technician Tips

- Alert the attending veterinarian if the supernatant in a hematocrit tube or serum or plasma in a centrifuged tube is cloudy and the patient has not eaten in > 12 hours.
- Lipemia can increase total solids measured by refractometry and can interfere with multiple biochemical tests.

SUGGESTED READING

Xenoulis PG, et al: Canine hyperlipidaemia. J Small Anim Pract 56:595-605, 2015.

AUTHOR: Karen M. Tefft, DVM, MVSc, DACVIM
EDITOR: Ellen N. Behrend, VMD, PhD, DACVIM

Hypernatremia

BASIC INFORMATION

Definition

A serum sodium (Na^+) concentration above the reference range; caused by net water loss (most common) or Na^+ gain

Epidemiology

SPECIES, AGE, SEX

No species, age, or sex predisposition

GENETICS, BREED PREDISPOSITION

Essential adipsic hypernatremia rarely reported in schnauzers, other dog breeds, and cats; may have a genetic basis

RISK FACTORS

- Diuresis in the absence of adequate available water replacement
- Excessive water loss from nonrenal sources (e.g., vomiting, diarrhea, burns)
- Acute administration/consumption of large amounts of Na^+ (e.g., sea water consumption)

ASSOCIATED DISORDERS

Essential adipsic hypernatremia, diabetes insipidus, central nervous system (CNS) damage

Clinical Presentation

DISEASE FORMS/SUBTYPES

- Can be acute or chronic; accumulation of idiogenic osmols in chronic hypernatremia impact treatment
- Categorized by volume status as hypovolemic, normovolemic, or hypervolemic hypernatremia; volume status provides clues about the cause

HISTORY, CHIEF COMPLAINT

- Clinical signs (e.g., vomiting, diarrhea, polyuria/polydipsia [PU/PD]) often related to the underlying cause of hypernatremia
- Severity and rapidity of onset correlate with severity of signs attributed directly to hypernatremia, which can include
  - Mental dullness/ inappropriate mentation
  - Ataxia
  - Stupor/coma
  - Seizures
  - Muscle weakness

PHYSICAL EXAM FINDINGS

- Findings often relate to the underlying cause of hypernatremia.
- When Na^+ > 170 mEq/L, findings directly attributed to hypernatremia can become apparent (see Chief Complaint).
- Evidence of volume depletion or excess
  - Hydration usually adequate (from movement of water from intracellular space to extracellular space) until extreme water loss occurs
  - Volume depletion: loss of skin turgor, weak pulse, tachycardia, delayed capillary refill time
  - Volume excess: serous nasal discharge, tachypnea, harsh lung sounds

Etiology and Pathophysiology

- Na^+ and its anions account for ≈95% of osmotic activity in extracellular fluids; therefore, hypernatremia causes hyperosmolality.
- Acute hyperosmolality can cause brain cells to shrink because intracellular water is pulled into the extracellular fluid space, resulting in rupture of vessels and intracranial bleeding.
- If hypernatremia comes about more slowly, the brain can adapt through production of idiogenic osmoles, which hold water volume in the brain cells.
  - Overly rapid correction of long-standing hypernatremia causes water to be pulled into the brain cells by idiogenic osmoles, resulting in brain swelling and neurologic damage.
- Causes of hypernatremia (p. 1237)
  - Pure water deficit: normovolemic hypernatremia (e.g., water deprivation [especially with diabetes insipidus], adipsia)
  - Hypotonic fluid loss (most common): hypovolemic hypernatremia (e.g., diabetes mellitus, postobstructive diuresis, gastrointestinal (GI) fluid loss, burns, chronic kidney disease)
  - Increased Na^+ retention or intake: hypervolemic hypernatremia (e.g., hypertonic enema solutions, sea water consumption, excess hypertonic saline infusion)

DIAGNOSIS

Diagnostic Overview

Hypernatremia may be suspected in depressed animals with conditions known to predispose to hypernatremia, or it can be an incidental finding on serum biochemical profile. Signs of hypernatremia may not be apparent until Na^+ > 175-180 mEq/L.

Differential Diagnosis

- Encephalopathic signs: hypoglycemia, hyponatremia, hepatic encephalopathy, uremia, intoxications, hypoxia, CNS disorders
- Hypernatremia: pseudohypernatremia occurs occasionally in hyperproteinemic or hyperlipidemic animals. Confirm true hypernatremia with direct selective electrode measure.

Initial Database

- Review history for water consumption/thirst, urine production, possible salt ingestion/administration
- Serum biochemical profile
  - Na^+ above upper reference range (by definition; usually $Na^+ > 157$ mEq/L)
  - Hyperchloremia (common)
  - Azotemia (may accompany hypovolemia or kidney disease)
  - Hyperphosphatemia (may accompany kidney disease or sodium phosphate enema use)
  - Increased albumin in hemoconcentrated state
  - Serum osmolality (measured or calculated); always increased
- CBC: may show evidence of hemoconcentration
- Urinalysis, with urine osmolality (if available): hyposthenuria (e.g., diabetes insipidus), isosthenuria (e.g., kidney disease), or concentrated urine (e.g., salt intoxication, GI losses)

Advanced Diagnostic Testing

Additional testing is aimed at identification of the underlying cause of hypernatremia; choice of test depends on suspected cause. Common tests:

- Abdominal imaging: cause of vomiting or diarrhea, evaluation of kidneys and adrenal glands
- Brain imaging by MRI or CT: if hypothalamic lesion suspected
- Tests to confirm endocrinopathies, if indicated: diabetes insipidus (p. 250), hyperaldosteronism, diabetes mellitus (p. 251)

TREATMENT

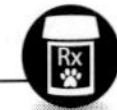

Treatment Overview

Acute hypernatremia (<24-hour duration) can be corrected rapidly, but longer-standing hypernatremia must be corrected slowly (often over 48-72 hours at < 8-12 mEq/L per 24 hours). Because frequent measures of serum Na^+ are required, animals with severe hypernatremia should be treated at 24-hour care facilities capable of monitoring electrolytes in real time.

Acute General Treatment

- See Hypernatremia Algorithm (p. 1428).
- For hypernatremia of short duration (<24 hours), rapid correction is appropriate (1.5-2 mEq/L/h) using no or low Na^+ fluids (e.g., 5% dextrose, 0.45% sodium chloride, one-half strength lactated Ringer's solution)
- For hypernatremia lasting for > 24 hours, correct no more quickly than 0.5 mEq/L/h (12 mEq/L/day). This rate may be difficult to achieve with very-low-sodium fluids; keep in mind that even fluids with a Na^+ concentration of 40 mEq/L (e.g., Normosol M, Plasma-Lyte 56) can provide necessary water with a lower Na^+ content than the patient's serum. Frequent (i.e., q 2-4h) rechecks of Na^+ are essential.
- For animals that are not vomiting and mentally appropriate, enteral water supplementation is useful.

Chronic Treatment

Address underlying cause of hypernatremia.

Possible Complications

Coma, seizures, and death

Recommended Monitoring

- During correction of chronic, severe hypernatremia, monitor serum Na^+ q 2-4h to be sure correction is not overly rapid.
- Repeat neurologic evaluations at least daily; signs of overly rapid correction may not be apparent for 48 hours or more after treatment.

PROGNOSIS & OUTCOME

- Prognosis depends on underlying cause as well as appropriate treatment. Often, hypernatremia is completely reversible if treated appropriately in a timely manner.
- Guarded to grave after coma occurs

PEARLS & CONSIDERATIONS

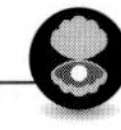

Comments

- Hypernatremia is more often the result of water loss rather than Na^+ gain.
- For slow-onset hypernatremia, correct slowly; for rapid onset of hypernatremia, correct rapidly.
- Hyperaldosteronism is rare and causes hypertension more often than hypernatremia (excess Na^+ pulls fluid into vascular space).

Prevention

- Provide ample access to water for any animal with polyuria or salt access.
- Do not allow dogs to drink sea water.
- Mix generous amounts of water in moist food for animals with adipsia.

Technician Tips

Any animal with polyuria should be provided access to water at all times (or IV fluids if GI/oral intake is not allowed) during any hospital stay, even if brief.

Client Education

Stress the importance of free-choice water for polydipsic pets.

SUGGESTED READING

Guillaumin J, et al. Disorders of sodium and water homeostasis. Vet Clin North Am Small Anim Pract 47:293-312, 2017.

AUTHOR: Michael Schaer, DVM, DACVIM, DACVECC
EDITOR: Leah A. Cohn, DVM, PhD, DACVIM

Hyperparathyroidism, Primary

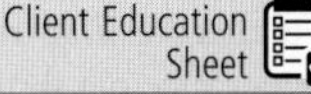

Client Education Sheet

BASIC INFORMATION

Definition

Primary hyperparathyroidism (PHPTH) is caused by increased synthesis and secretion of parathyroid hormone (PTH) by autonomously functioning parathyroid cells.

Epidemiology

SPECIES, AGE, SEX

- Dogs: uncommon; older dogs predominantly; no sex predisposition
- Cats: rare; older cats typically affected

GENETICS, BREED PREDISPOSITION

- Any breed
- Keeshond: inherited (autosomal dominant); a genetic test is available (http://ahdc.vet.cornell.edu/docs/PHPTInstructions.pdf).
- Hereditary neonatal PHPTH has been reported in two German shepherd dogs.

Clinical Presentation

HISTORY, CHIEF COMPLAINT

- Polyuria/polydipsia (≈50% dogs; ≈10% cats)
- Lower urinary tract signs (caused by infection or cystic calculi), including pollakiuria, stranguria, and hematuria (≈50% of dogs)
- Weakness, lethargy (≈40%-50% of dogs and cats)
- Inappetence (≈25%-30% of dogs; ≈40% of cats), vomiting (≈10% of dogs; ≈40% of cats)
- Some (≈30% dogs) have no clinical signs; hypercalcemia is an incidental finding.

PHYSICAL EXAM FINDINGS

- Physical exam: typically unremarkable

- A parathyroid mass is not usually palpable in dogs but may be palpable in the ventral neck in cats.

Etiology and Pathophysiology

- PHPTH is usually due to a solitary parathyroid adenoma (90%). Less common causes include hyperplasia of one or more glands or (rarely) carcinoma.
- Serum PTH concentration is normally controlled by blood ionized calcium concentrations by negative feedback. In PHPTH, the gland(s) function autonomously, and feedback inhibition is lost.
- Increased PTH causes hypercalcemia and hypophosphatemia.
- Clinical signs are due to hypercalcemia (p. 491).

DIAGNOSIS

Diagnostic Overview

- Concurrent hypercalcemia and low to low-normal serum phosphorus concentration are suggestive of PHPTH; however, these findings are also characteristic of humoral hypercalcemia of malignancy, a far more common disorder (p. 754). Presence of cystic calculi and/or the absence of clinical signs further increase suspicion for PHPTH.
- Parathyroid masses may be visible with ultrasonography; failure to visualize a parathyroid mass does not rule out the diagnosis.
- The diagnosis is established by measuring concurrent serum ionized calcium and PTH concentrations.

Differential Diagnosis

Hypercalcemia (pp. 491 and 1233)

Initial Database

- CBC, serum biochemical profile, urinalysis, urine culture (if lower urinary signs present): hypercalcemia, low or low-normal phosphorus concentration, and isosthenuria typical. Azotemia is uncommon. Urinary tract infection (UTI) is common (e.g., bacteriuria, pyuria).
- Confirm hypercalcemia by repeating the test on a new sample and/or, preferably, measuring serum ionized calcium concentration. Further testing to determine a cause of hypercalcemia should not be pursued unless ionized hypercalcemia is confirmed.
- Formulas to correct serum calcium to account for changes in serum albumin or protein values are not recommended.
- Abdominal radiographs: possible cystic calculi
- Other tests to rule out more common causes of hypercalcemia, particularly malignancy, include thoracic radiographs, abdominal ultrasound, aspiration of lymph nodes and/or bone marrow, and/or measurement of serum parathyroid hormone–related protein (PTHrP) concentration (p. 1371).

Advanced or Confirmatory Testing

- Concurrent serum ionized calcium and PTH concentrations: a serum PTH concentration within the upper half of the reference range is inappropriate with concurrent ionized hypercalcemia. Therefore, an ionized hypercalcemia with a serum PTH concentration that is high or within the upper half of the reference limits is consistent with a diagnosis of PHPTH.
- A serum PTH concentration within the lower half of the reference range in the face of hypercalcemia is suspicious for PHPTH.
  - Increased PTH: ≈25% of cases
  - PTH within reference range: ≈75% of cases; of these, more than one-half are in the lower half.
  - If PTH is in the lower half of the reference range, further diagnostics are needed to determine if PHPTH.
- Cervical ultrasonography requires an experienced ultrasonographer and sensitive equipment. Visualization of an enlarged parathyroid gland(s) in conjunction with compatible serum ionized calcium and PTH concentrations strongly support the diagnosis of PHPTH.

TREATMENT

Treatment Overview

Goals are to remove or ablate affected tissue and monitor/treat postoperative hypocalcemia. Referral is indicated if the clinician is unfamiliar with thyroid/parathyroid evaluation and surgery or if 24-hour care and in-house serum calcium monitoring cannot be provided during the immediate postprocedural period.

Acute General Treatment

- Nonspecific treatment of hypercalcemia while awaiting definitive diagnosis or surgery is not usually required. A decision to treat is made based on the presence of clinical signs and other factors (p. 491).
- Treatment of choice is removal/destruction of the affected gland(s). Surgical exploration of the neck with removal and histopathologic evaluation of the affected tissue is most common. Usually, a solitary parathyroid mass is easily identified and removed. Occasionally, identification of affected glands is difficult, and more than one gland may be removed.
- Percutaneous ultrasound-guided ethanol ablation and radiofrequency heat ablation are effective and less invasive options but technically challenging and still require general anesthesia. Both require an experienced ultrasonographer, and the latter requires specialized equipment.

Chronic Treatment

- Surgical or ablation therapy is curative in most patients, and chronic therapy is not required.
- If present, hypoparathyroidism and/or hypothyroidism require treatment (pp. 519 and 525).
- Medical therapy (cinalcet) is used in people but is cost-prohibitive in veterinary medicine.
- Address UTI (p. 232) and cystic calculi (p. 1014).

Possible Complications

- The most important complication with parathyroidectomy or ablation is postprocedural hypocalcemia.
- Unaffected parathyroid glands atrophy with prolonged hypercalcemia. After removal of affected gland(s), serum PTH and calcium concentrations may decline to below the reference range before remaining normal glands recover.
- Hospitalization recommended for 5 days after surgery to monitor for signs of hypocalcemia and serum calcium concentrations (q 12-24h).
- Treatment for hypocalcemia (vitamin D +/− calcium) must be individualized. Serum calcium concentration should be maintained in the slightly low/low-normal range (e.g. 8-9.5 mg/dL [2-2.4 mmol/L]) to prevent clinical signs of hypocalcemia while stimulating functional recovery of atrophied parathyroid glands.
  - If serum calcium concentration < 14 mg/dL (<3.5 mmol/L) before surgery, postoperative hypocalcemia is unlikely. Treatment is recommended only if total calcium falls below 8.5 mg/dL (2.1 mmol/L), if the rate of decline in calcium after surgery is rapid (e.g., > 25% in 1 day) or clinical signs of hypocalcemia occur (p. 515).
  - If clinical hypocalcemia occurs, administer 10% calcium gluconate (0.5-1.5 mL/kg IV, slowly over 15-30 minutes to effect).
  - If pre-treatment serum calcium concentration > 14 mg/dL (>3.5 mmol/L), begin prophylactic vitamin D treatment the morning of surgery.
  - If pre-treatment serum calcium concentration > 18 mg/dL (>4.5 mmol/L), begin prophylactic treatment 36 hours before surgery.
  - If a patient requires vitamin D, oral calcium supplementation (0.5-1.0 g/day divided, cats; 1.0-4.0 g/day divided, dogs) should be dispensed (p. 515). Calcium carbonate is preferred; it contains 40% calcium, so each gram contains 0.4 g of calcium.
  - If 1-3 parathyroid glands are removed, vitamin D and oral calcium treatment can be tapered over 3-6 months based on serum calcium levels.
  - Complications after parathyroid ablation occur uncommonly and include cough, voice change, and Horner's syndrome.

Recommended Monitoring

Recurrences may be observed > 12 months after successful treatment; evaluation of serum calcium is recommended q 3-6 months. Due to the genetic predisposition, recurrence is more likely in affected Keeshonden.

PROGNOSIS & OUTCOME

Prognosis is excellent after successful surgery or ablation.

PEARLS & CONSIDERATIONS 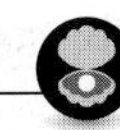

Comments

- Kidney injury, chronic kidney disease, and associated azotemia occur uncommonly with PHPTH.
- Serum PTH concentration within the reference range is suggestive of PHPTH when there is concurrent ionized hypercalcemia, because PTH should be low in response to high serum calcium levels.

Technician Tips

Signs of hypocalcemia (e.g., muscle fasciculations/twitching, facial pruritus, paw chewing, stiff gait, eventually seizures) postoperatively call for immediate measurement of serum calcium concentration.

SUGGESTED READING

Feldman EC, et al: Pretreatment clinical and laboratory findings in dogs with primary hyperparathyroidism: 210 cases (1987-2004). J Am Vet Med Assoc 227:756-761, 2005.

AUTHOR: Patty Lathan, VMD, MS, DACVIM
EDITOR: Ellen N. Behrend, VMD, PhD, DACVIM

Hypertension, Systemic

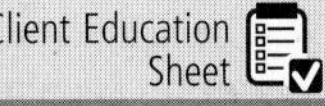

BASIC INFORMATION 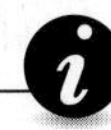

Definition

A sustained elevation in the arterial blood pressure (BP). In dogs and cats, systemic hypertension (SH) is suspected if sustained systolic BP > 160 mm Hg, diastolic BP > 95 mm Hg, or both.

Synonym

Arterial hypertension, high blood pressure

Epidemiology

SPECIES, AGE, SEX

SH occurs in dogs and cats, and there is no significant age or sex predisposition in either species. However, some systemic diseases commonly associated with SH (e.g., chronic kidney disease [CKD], hyperthyroidism, hyperadrenocorticism) are more common in older animals.

GENETICS, BREED PREDISPOSITION

There is no breed predisposition among cats. Sighthounds (e.g., deerhounds, Irish wolfhounds) have higher normal BP ranges than other breeds. Although essential hypertension has been diagnosed in one family of dogs, SH usually occurs secondary to other diseases and is not inherited.

RISK FACTORS

- Although *idiopathic hypertension* (i.e., cause unknown) may be diagnosed in veterinary patients, most cases of SH occur as a complication of another systemic disease. The most common diseases associated with SH in cats are CKD and hyperthyroidism. Many cats with hyperthyroidism have subclinical kidney disease; in these animals, it is unclear whether kidney disease, hyperthyroidism, or both are responsible for the hypertension. The prevalence of hypertension in cats with diabetes mellitus is still unclear.
- In dogs, the diseases most commonly associated with SH are CKD (especially proteinuric renal disease), hyperadrenocorticism, diabetes mellitus, and pheochromocytoma.
- Less typical causes of SH in either species include hyperaldosteronism, acromegaly, and use of hypertensive medications (e.g., phenylpropanolamine, excessive thyroxine supplementation).

ASSOCIATED DISORDERS

Target organ damage (TOD) may include retinal detachment, retinal hemorrhage, hyphema, intracranial hemorrhage, concentric left ventricular hypertrophy, and chronic aggravation of kidney injury.

Clinical Presentation

DISEASE FORMS/SUBTYPES

- SH can be diagnosed based on clinical signs (clinical SH) or as part of a diagnostic evaluation of a systemic disease, with the animal showing no overt clinical signs of SH (subclinical SH).
- SH can be divided into one of three categories: situational, secondary, or idiopathic. Idiopathic (i.e., primary) hypertension is rare in dogs and uncommon in cats.

HISTORY, CHIEF COMPLAINT

- Signs associated with the underlying disease
  - Lethargy, changes in activity or appetite, changes in mentation, excessive drowsiness; owners may interpret vague signs as signs of aging.
- Acute blindness, intraocular hemorrhage, photophobia
- Intracranial neurologic signs:
  - Generalized seizures
  - Focal facial seizures
  - Vestibular signs

PHYSICAL EXAM FINDINGS

- Signs of underlying systemic disease (e.g., small kidneys, thyroid nodule)
- Ocular TOD: vitreal or retinal hemorrhage, complete or partial retinal detachment, hyphema, vascular tortuosity, photophobia
- Nervous system TOD: signs of intracranial disease, changes in mentation (usually decreased but may include heightened anxiety), seizures (generalized or focal facial), vestibular signs
- Cardiovascular system TOD: new left-sided heart murmur, arrhythmia, gallop sound, concentric left ventricular hypertrophy on echocardiographic examination

Etiology and Pathophysiology

- Likely to be multifactorial; individual mechanisms may predominate in some diseases:
  - Abnormalities in renal sodium handling
  - Inappropriate activation of the renin-angiotensin-aldosterone system or sympathetic nervous system
  - Hypersensitivity to the effects of cortisol
  - Blood volume expansion secondary to underlying disease states

DIAGNOSIS 

Diagnostic Overview

The diagnosis is suspected in one of two clinical contexts: a patient is evaluated for clinical signs consistent with hypertensive decompensation (e.g., acute vision loss) or SH is identified in a compensated patient (e.g., as part of evaluation for CKD). BP measurement is a simple confirmatory test, but technical confounders, notably situational hypertension due to patient anxiety (i.e., white coat effect) and incorrect cuff size or placement must be avoided to achieve an accurate reading.

Differential Diagnosis

- Ocular signs: coagulopathies; uveitis; inflammatory, infectious, or neoplastic diseases, trauma
- Neurologic signs: intracranial lesions, idiopathic vestibular disease
- Cardiovascular signs: primary cardiac disease, other secondary cardiac diseases

Initial Database

- Initial diagnostic testing is guided by underlying disease if known.
- BP measurement (p. 1065)
- If SH is diagnosed in a patient without known predisposing disease
  - Dogs: CBC, serum chemistry profile, urinalysis with urine protein/creatinine ratio if proteinuria is present, complete funduscopic examination
  - Cats: CBC, serum chemistry profile, urinalysis, serum thyroxine if patient is ≥ 10 years old, complete funduscopic examination (p. 1137)
  - Both species: consider thoracic radiographs or abdominal ultrasound.

Advanced or Confirmatory Testing

Repeat BP measurement after several hours of acclimation is advisable if elevated BP is detected in an excited, anxious, or panting patient during the first measurement period.

TREATMENT 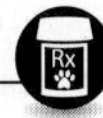

Treatment Overview

- SH with clinical signs referable to hypertensive TOD
  - First priority: prompt reduction of systolic BP to < 160-180 mm Hg

- If evidence of ocular or neurologic TOD is present, reduce systolic BP by 25% in the first 1-2 hours, with reduction to < 160 mm Hg recommended by 6 hours after beginning therapy.
  - Second priority: initiate clinical evaluation for causative disease
- SH found in conjunction with causative underlying disease but no clinical signs of hypertension are present
  - Institute optimal therapy of causative condition.
  - Confirm elevated BP values on more than one occasion to lessen the chance of false-positive due to anxiety- or excitement-related elevations of BP. Confirmatory BP measurements can be performed several hours to several days later.
  - If systolic BP > 180 mm Hg on more than one measurement occasion (preferably same day), begin antihypertensive therapy.
  - Systolic BP is 160-180 mm Hg on more than one measurement occasion
    - If underlying disease can be controlled or cured, monitor BP during therapy of underlying disease, and treat if systolic BP continues to exceed 160 mm Hg after optimal therapy of underlying disease.
    - If underlying disease is unknown or unlikely to be cured (e.g., CKD), begin antihypertensive therapy.

Acute General Treatment

- Discontinue any hypertensive medications.
- Emergency antihypertensive therapy for animals with acute ocular or neurologic signs
  - Dogs, oral or IV therapy (start at low end of dose and titrate to effect).
    - Nitroprusside 0.5-5 mcg/kg/min as continuous rate infusion IV, *or*
    - Hydralazine (oral) 0.5-2 mg/kg PO q 12h
  - Cats
    - Amlodipine 0.625 mg PO q 24h if cat ≤ 5 kg; 1.25 mg PO q 24h if cat > 5 kg, *or*
    - Hydralazine 0.5-2 mg/kg PO q 12h

Chronic Treatment

- Dogs
  - Transition from nitroprusside or hydralazine to amlodipine is recommended for chronic therapy.
    - Amlodipine 0.2-0.4 mg/kg PO q 24h
  - Angiotensin-converting enzyme inhibitors (ACEIs) can be added if proteinuria is present or if amlodipine alone is inadequate to control BP. ACEIs as monotherapy can be expected to lower systolic BP by approximately 10%.
    - Enalapril 0.5 mg/kg PO q 12-24h, *or*
    - Benazepril 0.25-0.5 mg/kg PO q 12-24h
- Cats
  - Calcium channel blockers (preferred first-line therapy)
    - Amlodipine 0.625 mg PO q 24h if cat ≤ 5 kg; 1.25 mg PO q 24h if cat > 5 kg
    - Cats with systolic BP > 200 mm Hg may benefit from beginning doses of 1.25 mg PO q 24h per cat, regardless of weight.
  - ACEIs are usually inadequate as monotherapy but may have additive effects when given with other medications or if proteinuria is present.
    - Enalapril 0.5 mg/kg PO q 12-24h
    - Benazepril 0.25-0.5 mg/kg PO q 24h
    - Beta-blockers are unlikely to be effective as monotherapy for SH.

Drug Interactions

- BP-lowering sedatives (e.g., acepromazine) should be used with caution in animals receiving any antihypertensive medication.
- Two medications from the same drug group should not be used together (e.g., benazepril and enalapril).

Possible Complications

- Hypotension
  - Resuscitate as needed; supportive fluid therapy may be necessary.
  - Reduce dose of BP medication.
  - Re-evaluate need for antihypertensive medication or reduce dose if weight loss has occurred.
- Uncontrolled hypertension despite drug therapy
  - Check compliance: review medications and administration information with caregiver.
  - Check BP measurement technique (i.e., cuff size, inadequate period of acclimation).
  - Add medications from other classes if needed.
  - Consult a specialist for further additions/modifications if hypertension is not controlled with two antihypertensive medications at upper end of dosing ranges.
- Previously controlled hypertension now out of desired target range
  - Dogs: hypertension may worsen over time, or underlying disease may be inadequately controlled:
    - Ensure optimal therapy of underlying disease.
    - Screen for hypertensive medications
    - Check post-pill serum thyroxine concentration in animals receiving thyroid supplementation.
    - Add additional antihypertensive medications or increase doses of current medications to high end of dosage range if tolerated.
  - Cats: hypertension control is usually stable once achieved. If BP continues to increase over time, treat as recommended above.

Recommended Monitoring

- After the underlying condition and SH are controlled, check BP in patients receiving antihypertensive therapy every 3 months.
- If doses/medications change, recheck BP in 3-5 days after change to ensure efficacy.
- Monitor weight at each visit to avoid accidental overdose if weight loss has occurred.

PROGNOSIS & OUTCOME

- If retinal detachment (p. 885) has occurred, the retina may reattach with good control of BP, but prognosis for return of vision varies.
- Prognosis for resolution of other clinical signs of hypertension (e.g., focal facial seizures, changes in mentation) is favorable if BP can be controlled with medication and with effective therapy of underlying diseases.
- Prognosis for SH may be affected by prognosis for causative disease.

PEARLS & CONSIDERATIONS

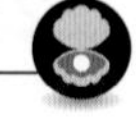

Comments

- SH is likely to be progressive over time in dogs even if initially well-controlled on medications. Monitoring BP during long-term therapy allows detection of progression of SH during therapy.
- SH usually remains controlled in treated cats and is seldom progressive, but monitoring over time is still required as changes in weight (especially decreases) might lead to hypotension if therapy is not adjusted.

Technician Tips

- Owners may interpret clinical signs of hypertension (e.g., lethargy, drowsiness) as signs of aging, and vigilance regarding monitoring of BP in animals at risk can detect subclinical cases.
- Any dog or cat with a systemic disease known to cause hypertension should have its BP monitored periodically regardless of clinical signs.
- High BP detected in young animals with no risk factors is often spurious.
- Pet owners may be taught to assess BP at home for chronic monitoring.

Client Education

- For optimal patient management, inform clients that
  - Hypertension is usually a complication of another disease rather than primary disease in itself.
  - Control of hypertension is necessary to avoid catastrophic ocular or neurologic damage and to minimize ongoing damage to susceptible organs (e.g., kidneys).
  - If the underlying disease is not curable, therapy for SH is likely to be lifelong.
  - Many patients require more than one medication to adequately control hypertension, and the need for medication may increase over time.

SUGGESTED READING

Acierno MJ, et al: ACVIM consensus statement: guidelines for the identification, evaluation, and management of systemic hypertension in dogs and cats. J Vet Intern Med 32(6):1803-1822, 2018.

AUTHOR: Rebecca L. Stepien, DVM, MS, DACVIM
EDITOR: Meg M. Sleeper, VMD, DACVIM

Hyperthyroidism

Client Education Sheet 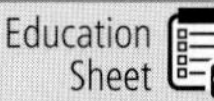

BASIC INFORMATION

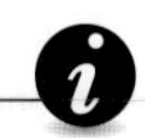

Definition

The clinical condition that results from continued excessive secretion of thyroid hormones

Epidemiology

SPECIES, AGE, SEX

- Cats
  - Older cats; range is 4-20+ years, but 95% of cats diagnosed with hyperthyroidism are > 8 years old.
  - No sex predisposition
- Canine hyperthyroidism is uncommon (p. 975).

GENETICS, BREED PREDISPOSITION

Purebred cats may be less likely to develop hyperthyroidism than domestic/mixed breeds (controversial).

RISK FACTORS

Likely multifactorial: genetic, nutritional, and environmental influences may play a role.

ASSOCIATED DISORDERS

- Concentric cardiac hypertrophy (ventricular thickening) can cause heart failure
- Systemic hypertension (p. 501)
- Hyperthyroidism may mask underlying chronic kidney disease (CKD).

Clinical Presentation

DISEASE FORMS/SUBTYPES

An unusual variant is apathetic hyperthyroidism (10% of cases): cat has decreased appetite and lethargy.

HISTORY, CHIEF COMPLAINT

- Weight loss despite normal to increased appetite (most common clinical sign)
- Polydipsia and polyuria
- Polyphagia
- Vomiting and/or diarrhea
- Hyperactivity, nervousness
- Tachypnea/panting
- Weakness, lethargy
- Decreased grooming activity
- Heat avoidance or seeking cool areas

PHYSICAL EXAM FINDINGS

- Poor body condition
- Unkempt haircoat
- Cardiac changes
  - Sinus tachycardia
  - Systolic heart murmur
  - Arrhythmia
- Abnormal retinal exam (tortuous retinal blood vessels, retinal tears, retinal detachment)
- Palpable thyroid gland(s)

Etiology and Pathophysiology

- In cats, benign thyroid neoplasia or adenomatous hyperplasia involving one or more often both (70%) thyroid lobes is most common.
- Thyroid carcinoma is found in < 2% of hyperthyroid cats.
- Canine hyperthyroidism is the result of a functional thyroid carcinoma (p. 975), excessive supplementation, or consumption of thyroid tissue.

DIAGNOSIS

Diagnostic Overview

The diagnosis should be suspected in a middle-aged to older cat with clinical signs of weight loss in the face of a normal to increased appetite; polyuria and polydipsia may be present. Confirmation is based on a high serum total thyroxine (T_4) concentration. When the serum T_4 level does not correlate with the clinical signs, further evaluation of the thyroid status is necessary.

Differential Diagnosis

- Polyphagia with weight loss in an adult/geriatric cat: diabetes mellitus, inflammatory bowel disease, gastrointestinal (GI) lymphoma. Rarely in cats: hyperadrenocorticism (pp. 809 and 1270)
- Polyuria/polydipsia (pp. 812, 1271, and 1442)
- Weight loss (pp. 1047 and 1295)
- Chronic vomiting (pp. 1042 and 1294)
- Chronic diarrhea (pp. 262 and 1213)
- Arrhythmias/tachycardia/murmur
  - Primary idiopathic hypertrophic cardiomyopathy (p. 505)
  - Restrictive/unclassified cardiomyopathy, feline (p. 881)

Initial Database

- CBC, serum biochemical profile, urinalysis: possible stress leukogram and mild erythrocytosis; increase in liver enzymes very common; urine specific gravity results vary.
- Serum T_4 measurement: usually increased, although values are sometimes in the upper half of the reference range, especially if concurrent disease is present.
- Thoracic radiographs: cardiomegaly common; rarely pulmonary edema and/or pleural effusion
- Systemic blood pressure measurement (p. 1065): hypertension (systolic blood pressure repeatedly > 180 mm Hg in calm environment) is possible, even after treatment of hyperthyroidism.
- Electrocardiogram (p. 1096), performed if an arrhythmia is present: sinus tachycardia is most common rhythm; atrial or ventricular arrhythmias are possible but uncommon.

Advanced or Confirmatory Testing

- Serum T_4 concentrations are usually increased and, if so, are diagnostic. If T_4 concentration is in the upper half of the reference range, but the thyroid gland is palpable and/or signs suggestive of hyperthyroidism are present, hyperthyroidism is still possible, and one of the following should be considered:
  - Re-evaluate T_4 in a few weeks (if clinical signs are mild).
  - Measure serum free T_4 using an equilibrium dialysis method (FT_4ED): an increased FT_4ED concentration in conjunction with a total T_4 concentration in the upper half of the reference range supports a diagnosis of hyperthyroidism.
- Serum thyroid-stimulating hormone (TSH) measured with a canine assay is highly sensitive (almost all hyperthyroid cats have suppressed TSH) but poorly specific for the diagnosis of feline hyperthyroidism. If used for diagnosis of hyperthyroidism, it should be measured in combination with T_4. The benefit of measuring TSH is more obvious for diagnosis of iatrogenic hypothyroidism (low T_4 and high TSH expected).
- Triiodothyronine (T_3) suppression test: generally replaced by FT_4ED measurement
- Radionuclide (technetium 99m) thyroid scan: besides confirming the diagnosis in challenging cases, can be used for determining whether one or both thyroid lobes are involved and whether ectopic functional thyroid tissue is present. Localization is of greatest interest if surgical thyroidectomy is contemplated.
- Echocardiography (p. 1094) can identify left ventricular hypertrophy. If it is symmetrical (whole left ventricle is thickened), hyperthyroidism, unrelated idiopathic hypertrophic cardiomyopathy (HCM), or other reasons for left ventricular hypertrophy may be the cause. If asymmetrical hypertrophy (e.g., interventricular septum thicker than left ventricular free wall) or hypertrophy is severe, idiopathic HCM (p. 505) or other causes are contributory, and hyperthyroidism alone is unlikely to be the only cause of the changes.

TREATMENT

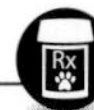

Treatment Overview

- Four therapeutic options are available: daily antithyroid medication, iodine-restricted diet, surgical thyroidectomy, and radioactive iodine therapy (^{131}I). Clinical status of the patient, owner motivation, and availability of modalities dictate which treatment option is best for an individual. Therapy of concurrent medical conditions such as CKD, cardiac hypertrophy, and systemic hypertension may be necessary.
- With reversible therapies (antithyroid medication and iodine-restricted diet), the cause (i.e., thyroid tumors) is not addressed, and the tumors continue to grow and may become malignant (occurs rarely, if at all).
- Ideally, therapy should restore serum T_4 to normal concentrations and eliminate clinical signs.

- Clinically, the therapeutic goal is to encourage weight gain, to improve body condition and haircoat, and to decrease polyuria, polydipsia, and polyphagia, with the overall goal of maximizing quality of life. In cats initially diagnosed with concomitant azotemia and hyperthyroidism, achieving T_4 concentrations within reference range may not be possible while avoiding signs of uremia.

Acute General Treatment

- Hyperthyroidism is a chronic disease, and urgent treatment usually is not needed.
- Concurrent congestive heart failure may require immediate intervention (p. 408).
- The existence of thyroid storm as described in humans, characterized by marked hyperthermia and decompensation of central nervous system signs, has not been documented in cats.
- However, hyperthyroid cats can get easily stressed, and some develop dyspnea/tachypnea or open-mouth breathing due to sympathetic simulation. Very gentle handling of hyperthyroid cats, ensuring as calm and quiet an environment as possible, is mandatory.

Chronic Treatment

See web algorithm Hyperthyroidism: Treatment.

- Antithyroid drugs and iodine-restricted diets are reversible options requiring lifelong therapy. Neither addresses the underlying disease.
- Renal function merits special attention. Two very different scenarios are recognized: cats having pre-existing azotemia at diagnosis of hyperthyroidism and cats developing a mild post-treatment azotemia. The second category of cats does not appear to have a shortened survival time if hypothyroidism is avoided or treated if it does develop.
- Thioureylene antithyroid drugs suppress thyroid hormone production.
  - Methimazole 2.5 mg/CAT PO q 12h or 5 mg/CAT PO q 24h, or carbimazole sustained-release tablets 10-15 mg/CAT PO q 24h (currently not available in North America).
  - Transdermal methimazole (from a compounding pharmacy) 2.5-5 mg/CAT applied inside the ear pinna q 12h has been used in cats that are not amenable to pill administration or that have sustained GI side effects with the oral form. Owners must wear gloves. Obtaining remission may take longer (4 weeks).
  - Regardless of the formulation used, dosage is adjusted such that serum T_4 concentrations are in the lower half of the reference range; hypothyroidism must be avoided.
  - Common but usually reversible side effects of methimazole and carbimazole include anorexia, vomiting, and lethargy.
  - Pruritus of the head and neck (and self-induced trauma), hepatotoxicosis, thrombocytopenia, agranulocytosis, and immune-mediated hemolytic anemia are uncommon and require cessation of drug administration. An alternative treatment must be used.
  - A beta-blocker (e.g., atenolol 6.25 mg/CAT PO q 12h) can be helpful in some cats to nonspecifically control tachypnea, severe tachycardia, hypertension, and hyperexcitability.
- Iodine-restricted diet (Hill's y/d)
  - Iodine restriction should lead to normalized T_4 concentrations within 4-8 weeks.
  - Patient must strictly eat the diet. Approximately 25% of patients will not eat this diet.
  - Clinicians should aim for resolution of clinical signs and T_4 concentrations within reference range.
- Thyroidectomy
  - Potentially curative
  - Eliminates grossly abnormal thyroid tissue, but ectopic tissue may remain if radionuclide imaging is bypassed.
  - Antithyroid medical treatment is essential for several weeks before surgery to improve the metabolic and cardiac status before anesthesia.
  - Unilateral thyroidectomy: contralateral thyroid gland can eventually become hyperplastic or adenomatous (recurrent hyperthyroidism).
  - Bilateral thyroidectomy: may involve loss of several or all parathyroid glands. Postoperative monitoring of serum calcium is required; if indicated, treat as for hypoparathyroidism (p. 519). Hypothyroidism is likely.
  - Other possible postoperative complications include Horner's syndrome and laryngeal paralysis (p. 574).
- ^{131}I therapy
  - This is considered the best treatment option for long-term control and cure of hyperthyroidism in many cats.
  - Treatment renders all hyperfunctional thyroid tissue, including ectopic tissue, nonfunctional.
  - Disadvantages: special handling facilities and post-therapy isolation for days to weeks are required. The length of isolation depends on the facility. Before therapy, the cat must be eating and able to tolerate the required time in isolation.
  - Consult the facility administering the radiotherapy to be informed about 1) discontinuing medical antithyroid drugs before treatment because duration is controversial and 2) owner requirements after discharge.

Possible Complications

- After therapy for hyperthyroidism, some cats develop renal azotemia (unmasking of CKD). These patients carry a prognosis similar to that of cats remaining nonazotemic as long as hypothyroidism does not develop or is treated if it does.
- If T_4 concentration is in the therapeutic range for a cat receiving antithyroid therapy, reducing the dose is not justified if only mild azotemia develops.
- If azotemia develops, therapy for CKD should be initiated (p. 169).
- Iatrogenic hypothyroidism must be avoided; diagnosis is based on clinical signs, a T_4 below the reference range, and an increased TSH concentration (measured with canine assay). Hypothyroid cats may have an increased TSH concentration but a T_4 level in the lower part of the reference range. If persistent hypothyroidism develops, therapy should be initiated (p. 525).

Recommended Monitoring

- General remarks
  - At each follow-up visit, besides history and physical exam, include systolic blood pressure, body weight, serum biochemistry profile (especially urea and creatinine), and T_4 and TSH measurement. Elevated TSH may be the best biochemical marker of hypothyroidism in cats.
  - Aim for T_4 well within reference range.
  - After euthyroidism is achieved, reassess q 6 months or earlier if adverse effects of treatment or signs of hyperthyroidism or hypothyroidism occur.
- Medical therapy: periodic CBC, serum biochemistry, and T_4.
- Thyroidectomy: besides the above, postoperative monitoring of serum calcium if bilateral thyroidectomy is important.
- ^{131}I: Effect of treatment on renal function can be assessed after 1 month. Hypothyroidism can occur transiently; unless the cat becomes azotemic, the cat should be monitored for a few months before treating for iatrogenic hypothyroidism. T_4 and TSH normalize in many cats.

PROGNOSIS & OUTCOME

- Prognosis is excellent for cats. With successful ^{131}I therapy or thyroidectomy, cure is obtained in most cases.
  - In geriatric patients, other conditions may be present or soon develop that affect survival; median survival time is approximately 2 years after diagnosis with medical therapy and 4 years with ^{131}I therapy.
  - Cats that are azotemic at the time of diagnosis of hyperthyroidism have shorter survival times.

PEARLS & CONSIDERATIONS

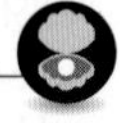

Comments

- Palpation of the ventral neck and measurement of serum T_4 concentrations should be routinely performed in geriatric cats to allow early detection of hyperthyroidism.
- Several effective therapeutic options are available. Clinicians should aim for resolution of clinical signs and serum T_4 well within the reference range.
- Monitoring T_4 and TSH concentrations is essential to avoid undertreatment or overtreatment.

- Renal function before and during treatment is important. Cats with an initial combination of azotemia and hyperthyroidism and cats developing post-treatment azotemia should be approached differently.

Prevention

Avoid foods containing soy isoflavones or cans with plastic linings or easy open lids (pop-tops).

Technician Tips

- Serum submitted for T_4 should be free of hemolysis.
- Serum submitted for FT_4ED should be free of hemolysis and lipemia; a fasted sample is recommended.

SUGGESTED READING

Carney HC, et al: AAFP guidelines for the management of feline hyperthyroidism. J Feline Med Surg 18:400-416, 2016.

AUTHOR: Sylvie Daminet, DVM, PhD, DACVIM, DECVIM
EDITOR: Ellen N. Behrend, VMD, PhD, DACVIM

Hypertrophic Cardiomyopathy

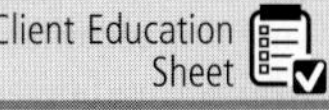

BASIC INFORMATION

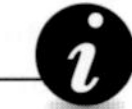

Definition

A common, primary myocardial disease characterized by increased left ventricular wall thickness (concentric left ventricular hypertrophy [LVH]) in the absence of secondary causes of hypertrophy such as systemic hypertension and hyperthyroidism

Synonyms

- Idiopathic hypertrophic cardiomyopathy (HCM)
- Hypertrophic obstructive cardiomyopathy (HOCM) if systolic anterior motion (SAM) of the mitral valve is present, which obstructs the left ventricular outflow tract

Epidemiology

SPECIES, AGE, SEX

- A common disease in cats, HCM is rarely recognized in dogs.
- Juvenile (6 months) to adult age routinely recognized; average age ≈6 years. Purebred cats often younger (average age at diagnosis: Ragdoll = 15 months, Maine coon = 2.5 years, Sphynx = 3.5 years, British shorthair = 2.3 years). The age is often older for Persian, domestic shorthair (DSH), and chartreux (8, 8, and 11 years, respectively).
- Males tend to be more severely affected, but there is no sex-linked heritability.

GENETICS, BREED PREDISPOSITION

- Autosomal dominant heritability with incomplete penetrance in Maine coon and Ragdoll cats. Two different missense mutations of the sarcomeric protein myosin-binding protein C cause HCM in these two breeds; there likely are additional causative mutations to be discovered in these and other breeds.
- Worldwide prevalence of genotypically affected Maine coon cats is 34% (91% of them are heterozygous).
- Autosomal dominant (one family of American shorthair cats); probable autosomal dominant heritability with incomplete penetrance (Sphynx)
- Other predisposed breeds: Siberian, British shorthair, Norwegian forest cat, Turkish van, Scottish fold, Bengal, Persian, Himalayan, Birman, and rex; DSH remains the most commonly diagnosed breed.

RISK FACTORS

- Precipitating events that can lead to congestive heart failure (CHF) in cats with previously compensated (asymptomatic) HCM include intravenous fluid administration, recent glucocorticoid administration (e.g., methylprednisolone acetate), and recent anesthesia/surgery.
- In Maine coon cats with the A31P myosin-binding protein C3 mutation, the risk ratio for developing LVH is 9.9 or 35.5 if heterozygous or homozygous, respectively.

ASSOCIATED DISORDERS

CHF (pp. 408 and 409), aortic thromboembolism (p. 74), sudden cardiac death

Clinical Presentation

HISTORY, CHIEF COMPLAINT

- Often, cats show no clinical signs, and HCM is discovered incidentally (e.g., murmur on physical exam).
- Respiratory abnormalities (CHF): tachypnea, dyspnea, orthopnea, uncommonly cough
- Nonspecific: lethargy, anorexia, vomiting
- Lameness, inability to move limb, signs of intense pain (aortic thromboembolism)
- Sudden death

PHYSICAL EXAM FINDINGS

- Systolic murmur (30%-80% of cases)
- Gallop (S_3 or S_4) heart sound: varies (≈30%), more likely with CHF
- Arrhythmia: premature beats, irregular rhythm (20%-70% of cases)
- Respiratory abnormalities common if CHF: tachypnea, dyspnea, increased breath sounds, paradoxic breathing, ventrally dampened lung sounds if pleural effusion
- Signs of arterial thromboembolism (ATE) (p. 74)

Etiology and Pathophysiology

- Initial defect is myocyte dysfunction due to primary sarcomeric defect; remaining sarcomeres develop compensatory concentric hypertrophy. Myocardial replacement fibrosis (dead myocardial cells and interstitial fibrosis) is likely mediated by angiotensin II and aldosterone levels +/− coronary artery abnormalities.
- Diastolic dysfunction from altered calcium handling, LVH, myofiber disarray, and myocardial fibrosis
- Elevated left ventricular filling pressure leads to elevated left atrial and pulmonary venous pressure and development of left-sided CHF (pulmonary edema +/− pleural effusion).
- Left atrial thrombus may form secondary to blood stasis in the dilated left atrium and can lead to ATE.

DIAGNOSIS

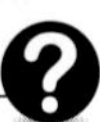

Diagnostic Overview

Diagnosis is made by echocardiographic demonstration of LVH with no identifiable cause. Thoracic radiographs are necessary to evaluate CHF, but radiographs alone cannot confirm or refute HCM and are often normal for cats with mild or moderate HCM without left atrial enlargement and/or CHF. Plasma N-terminal pro-brain-type natriuretic peptide (NT-pro-BNP) levels are elevated in a majority of symptomatic cats with clinically significant HCM.

Differential Diagnosis

Echocardiographically, HCM is a diagnosis of exclusion after other causes of LVH have been ruled out:

- Hyperthyroidism
- Systemic hypertension
- Subaortic stenosis
- Acromegaly

Initial Database

- Echocardiogram: interventricular septum and/or left ventricular free wall end diastolic thickness ≥ 6 mm. Papillary hypertrophy is often present (subjective or quantitative). SAM of the mitral valve with mitral regurgitation and left ventricular outflow tract obstruction may be variably present. Left atrial enlargement is variably present; a left atrial to aortic ratio greater than 1.5 or left

atrial diameter > 16 mm in the cat denotes left atrial enlargement, consistent with a more advanced disease state.
- Electrocardiogram (ECG): supraventricular or ventricular premature complexes are possible. Atrial fibrillation is possible but less common. Left axis deviation (mean electrical axis, 0° to −90°) or increased QRS amplitude > 1 mV may indicate LVH, but substantial overlap exists among normal cats.
- Clinicopathologic evaluation: CBC, serum biochemistry profile, urinalysis unremarkable unless ATE (p 74).
- Serum T_4 and systolic blood pressure: to rule out secondary LVH
- Thoracic radiographs: often normal if no left atrial enlargement. Moderate or severe cases may show evidence of left atrial enlargement and CHF (p. 408).
- NT-pro-BNP (Cardiocare, IDEXX Laboratories) often is markedly elevated in dyspneic cats with CHF (typically > 200 pmol/L; sensitivity 90%-95%, specificity 85%-88%) and may be elevated in some asymptomatic cats with moderate to severe HCM (>100 pmol/L). Use of NT-pro-BNP along with clinical information, including thoracic radiographs, may improve accuracy in diagnosing heart failure (accuracy increased from 69% to 87% with knowledge about NT-pro-BNP). The point-of-care NT-pro-BNP SNAP test may be useful to identify symptomatic cats with CHF and may be positive for cats with moderate to severe occult HCM (positive value is > 100 pmol/L).

Advanced or Confirmatory Testing

Tissue Doppler imaging (TDI) echocardiography (pulsed-wave Doppler or color TDI) to identify diastolic dysfunction may be abnormal before development of LVH as an early finding during screening for HCM in predisposed breeds.

TREATMENT

Treatment Overview

- Treatment of CHF: reduce the accumulation of pleural effusion or pulmonary edema.
- Antihypertrophic treatment in attempt to reduce the concentric hypertrophy of the left ventricle and decrease myocardial stiffness; unproven efficacy
- Reduce SAM if moderate or severe (pressure gradient > 50 mm Hg), which reduces the pressure overload of the left ventricle, reduces mitral regurgitation, and potentially reduces concentric hypertrophy in severe obstructions.
- Antiarrhythmic treatment for severe tachyarrhythmias such as ventricular tachycardia, supraventricular tachycardia, or atrial fibrillation
- Anticoagulant therapy in animals at high risk for ATE (spontaneous contrast, severe left atrial dilation, or a left atrial thrombus seen on echocardiogram) or in animals having previously suffered ATE

Acute General Treatment

Acute decompensated CHF (p. 408):
- Thoracocentesis if voluminous pleural effusion (p. 1164)
- Oxygen therapy in oxygen cage (p. 1146), minimize stress
- Furosemide 1-4 mg/kg IV
- +/− Nitroglycerin
- Concurrent fluid therapy is contraindicated.
- Avoid beta-blocker therapy during acute/critical CHF (unless severe tachyarrhythmia); controversial whether to start after CHF resolves

Chronic Treatment

Reduce SAM if moderate or severe: atenolol or diltiazem
- Atenolol 6.25-12.5 mg/CAT PO q 12-24h. Start at low dose (e.g., if asymptomatic, 6.25 mg/CAT PO q 12h), recheck in 1-2 weeks, and increase to 12.5 mg/CAT PO q 12h if heart rate (HR) remains > 170 beats/min and/or if SAM severity on echocardiogram is not improved. Do not increase atenolol if HR < 130 beats/min.
- Diltiazem: less effective than atenolol in reducing SAM and preventing tachycardia; fallen out of favor due to erratic drug levels of sustained release format and thrice-daily dosing of standard form. Dosage of diltiazem (regular) 7.5 mg/CAT PO q 8h; sustained-release diltiazem 30 mg/CAT PO q 12-24h (Dilacor-XR) or 10 mg/kg PO q 24h (Cardizem CD).

Benefit of antihypertrophic treatment for moderate to severe LVH (wall thickness > 7 mm) is unknown.
- Atenolol or diltiazem as above; may reduce LVH in some cases but controversial
- Angiotensin-converting enzyme (ACE) inhibitors or aldosterone antagonist (spironolactone) not likely to be of benefit in early compensated HCM

Pimobendan may be beneficial in cats with HCM and CHF, but it should be used with caution in cats with SAM because it can worsen dynamic obstruction.

Chronic CHF (p. 409): furosemide and an ACE inhibitor are standard therapy.
- Chronic refractory CHF
  - Addition of second diuretic: spironolactone 1-2 mg/kg PO q 24h; potential risk of cutaneous drug reaction in Maine coon cats. Hydrochlorothiazide occasionally used in refractory CHF in cats: consider conservative dose of 0.5-1 mg/kg PO q 24h, up-titrate to twice-daily dosage if necessary and azotemia is not prohibitive.
  - Consider switching from PO furosemide to torsemide (dosing not well defined in cats; consider $\frac{1}{10}$ of daily furosemide dose divided for twice-daily dosing)
  - Consider SQ administration (increased bioavailability compared with oral) of furosemide 1-2 times/week if persistent CHF despite furosemide 3-4 mg/kg PO q 8h.
  - ± Potassium supplement if serum K^+ ≤ 3 mEq/L (dosage 2-4 mEq/CAT PO q 8-12h)
- Anticoagulation for prevention of ATE
  - Clopidogrel is a potent platelet inhibitor (18.75 mg/CAT PO q 24h), *or*
  - One baby aspirin (81 mg ASA)/CAT or 5 mg/CAT PO q 3 days, *or*
  - Low-molecular-weight heparin (enoxaparin) 1.5 mg/kg SQ q 12h; pharmacokinetics and optimal dosing are still under investigation; if ATE has occurred or a thrombus or spontaneous contrast persists, q 12h dosing is changed to q 8h.
  - Combination anticoagulant therapy is controversial but has been done in cats with persistent spontaneous echo contrast or recurrent ATE.
- Antiarrhythmic therapy if persistently rapid supraventricular or ventricular tachycardia (pp. 96 and 1033)

Nutrition/Diet

Sodium restriction only if palatable and only with CHF; goal is to minimize diuretic requirement

Behavior/Exercise

Avoid encouraging intense physical activity (e.g., laser pointer toy), which increases HR and myocardial oxygen demand

Drug Interactions

- Diuretics and ACE inhibitors may exacerbate renal dysfunction.
- Concurrent use of beta-blockers and calcium channel blockers is generally contraindicated because they may cause bradycardia and hypotension.

Possible Complications

- The three main complications of severe HCM are ATE (12%-17%), CHF (46% in one study), and sudden death.
- Prerenal/renal azotemia and hypokalemia during treatment with diuretics
- Cats receiving high doses of diuretics may have mild to moderate azotemia but often maintain reasonable quality of life without requirement for concurrent fluid administration.
- ACE inhibitors occasionally may cause acute renal azotemia, which may reverse after discontinuation of the ACE inhibitor and supportive care.

Recommended Monitoring

- Baseline serum renal panel and urinalysis; repeat renal panel q 12-24h during acute in-hospital CHF treatment.
- Repeat renal panel 1-2 weeks after initiating ACE inhibitor, and decrease or discontinue ACE inhibitor (and reduce diuretic if possible) if moderate to severe azotemia is present.
- Thoracic radiographs to monitor CHF; recheck radiographs q 2-4 months once stabilized.

- Echocardiogram: q 3-12 months, depending on severity of HCM; monitor left atrial size as risk factor for development of CHF or ATE. Monitor LVH to assess possible progression of disease or assess potential antihypertrophic therapeutic effects.
- If systemic hypertension or hyperthyroidism is present, a recheck echocardiogram 3-4 months after cat is normotensive or euthyroid; should show regression of LVH. If hypertrophy is still present, the cat has concurrent HCM, or there is incomplete control of the systemic disorder.
- Systemic blood pressure and serum thyroxine q 6-12 months (adult HCM cats). Systemic hypertension and hyperthyroidism can worsen LVH but in a reversible way (see above).
- If arrhythmia: recheck ECG to assess emergence of new arrhythmia +/− response to antiarrhythmic therapy.

PROGNOSIS & OUTCOME

- Fair to good prognosis for cats with mild nonprogressive HCM. Cats with HCM and no clinical signs have a median survival time of 3 to > 5 years.
- Outcome for 647 occult HCM cats over 5 years: 17% (3.4%/yr) developed CHF; 8.5% (1.7%/yr) developed ATE; all-cause cardiac mortality was 22% (4.4%/yr).
- Young male cats and Ragdoll cats with significant LVH often progress more rapidly and die from their disease (often by 4 years of age).
- Severe HCM and CHF: poor long-term prognosis; median survival of 3 months, although survival times vary greatly, with over 2 years in some cats.
- Severe HCM and ATE: poor prognosis; median survival time of 2 months in early studies but varies greatly. Cats surviving the first month after ATE and then placed on clopidogrel had longer time to recurrent ATE (median, 443 days; recurrence rate, 43%) than cats treated with aspirin (median, 192 days; recurrence rate, 75%) in the FATCAT clinical trial.

PEARLS & CONSIDERATIONS

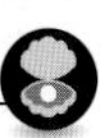

Comments

- Wide range of severity and progression of HCM in individual cats, which explains the large number of cats with this disease that live a normal life.
- In a multicenter, prospective, randomized, and blinded study, neither ACE inhibitors, atenolol, nor diltiazem were shown to improve survival over furosemide alone for cats with severe HCM and CHF or ATE.
- Pimobendan appears to benefit many cats with refractory CHF but can worsen left ventricular outflow tract obstruction (if SAM is present) and cause hypotension.
- Avoid long-acting glucocorticoid injections; avoid large volumes of SQ fluids (>100 mL) in cats with subclinical HCM.
- Anesthetic considerations: avoid high fluid rates (e.g., 5 mL/kg/h for low rate) and drugs that cause tachycardia. Consider induction with midazolam and propofol, Alfaxan, or etomidate; maintenance with isoflurane

Prevention

Genetic screening tests are available for Maine coon cats and Ragdolls. Breeding programs should be aimed at eliminating genetically affected cats. Echocardiograms are necessary to screen potential breeding candidates in all breeds, including Maine coon cats and Ragdoll cats because some of these cats may have HCM despite a normal genotype due to an unidentified mutation.

Technician Tips

- Cats with HCM and CHF tend to be very fragile and require careful handling to minimize stress. For thoracocentesis, cats may be maintained in a comfortable sternal position with minimal but effective restraint; mild sedation with butorphanol and midazolam may be considered.
- Blood pressure measurement should be performed before other diagnostic tests, with minimal but effective restraint/stress.
- Review with the owner techniques for administering oral medications because many cats with heart failure are on multidrug therapy. If clopidogrel is prescribed, discuss with owner that clopidogrel is bitter, and provide tips for administering it, such as placing in a gel cap or pill pocket, and avoiding crushing or putting in liquid.

Client Education

- In cats with CHF, teaching clients to monitor resting respiratory rate (RRR) and respiratory effort is helpful. Owner should contact the doctor when rates are consistently > 30-35 breaths/min. Technicians can review client-monitored RRR logs when calling back for updates or during recheck exams.
- Advise about risk of sudden death and ATE. It is difficult to prevent ATE when severe underlying cardiac disease is present.

SUGGESTED READING

Hogan DF, editor: The feline heart. J Vet Cardiol 17(suppl 1):1760-2734, 2015.

AUTHOR: Kristin A. MacDonald, DVM, PhD, DACVIM
EDITOR: Meg M. Sleeper, VMD, DACVIM

Hypertrophic Osteodystrophy

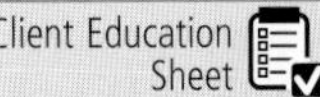

BASIC INFORMATION

Definition

A disease of the long bones of rapidly growing dogs, causing disruption of metaphyseal trabeculae, often accompanied by systemic inflammation

Synonyms

HOD, metaphyseal osteopathy, Barlow's disease, canine skeletal scurvy, idiopathic osteodystrophy, Moeller-Barlow disease, osteodystrophy types I and II

Epidemiology

SPECIES, AGE, SEX

- Dogs 2-8 months old; males > females
- Occasionally reported in kittens

GENETICS, BREED PREDISPOSITION

- Large and giant breeds
- Great Danes predisposed
- Reported in litters of Weimaraner puppies

RISK FACTORS

Rapid rate of growth; association with recent vaccination suggested in some

Clinical Presentation

DISEASE FORMS/SUBTYPES

- Lameness ± systemic disease
- Some Weimaraners: vaccine-associated onset
- Rarely, severe systemic disease with secondary sepsis

HISTORY, CHIEF COMPLAINT

- Acute onset of swelling of the distal antebrachial and/or distal tibial metaphyseal regions (generally bilateral)
- Peracute refusal to stand, anorexia, signs of pain, *or*
- Low-grade lameness of short duration

PHYSICAL EXAM FINDINGS

- Fever: temperature often ≥ 104°F (≥ 40°C)
- Metaphyses (most commonly of distal radius, ulna, and tibia) swollen, hot, painful on palpation
- Peracute cases can show lethargy, dehydration, and severe pain.

Etiology and Pathophysiology

- Unknown; *not* a deficiency of vitamin C or an excess of vitamin D, dietary minerals, or caloric intake
- Possible autoimmune inflammatory disease mediated by cytokines
- Links to canine distemper virus, bacterial infection proposed but unproven
- Associated with modified live vaccination in immunocompromised Weimaraners
- Disturbance of metaphyseal blood supply, causing delayed ossification of the physeal hypertrophic zone

DIAGNOSIS

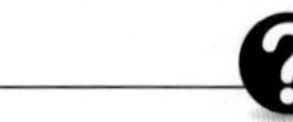

Diagnostic Overview

Acute presentation of swollen, warm metaphyses of the long bone(s) in a growing dog is highly suggestive. Radiographs (may need to be repeated) can support the diagnosis and rule out other disorders.

Differential Diagnosis

- Panosteitis
- Septic arthritis or osteomyelitis
- Rickets (failure to calcify the cartilaginous matrix of the growth plate)

Initial Database

- Radiographs: pathognomonic lucent line adjacent to the physis on the metaphyseal side (double physis or scorbutic line)
- CBC, urinalysis: results usually unremarkable, but leukocytosis or leukopenia may be present
- Serum biochemistry profile: rarely hypocalcemia of unknown significance

Advanced or Confirmatory Testing

Arthrocentesis (usually performed if inflammatory arthritis suspected [p. 1059]): increased volume of transparent, straw-colored fluid with normal viscosity and increased numbers of neutrophils; otherwise normal

TREATMENT

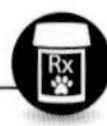

Treatment Overview

Pain relief and supportive care; usually self-resolves with time except in severe cases

Acute General Treatment

- Nonsteroidal antiinflammatory drugs (NSAIDs) such as carprofen, meloxicam, deracoxib, or firocoxib; see p. 721 for dosages, routes, and intervals.
- Glucocorticoids should be used instead of NSAIDs in Weimaraners.
- Rest, opioid analgesics, soft bedding, turning every 4-6 hours if nonambulatory
- Severe cases require more intensive management, including the use of intravenous glucocorticoids (rule out possibility of bacterial infection first), intravenous fluids, and nutritional support.

Chronic Treatment

- Monitor for development of angular deformities.
- Correct the use of inappropriate diet (see Technician Tips below).

Possible Complications

Relapses can occur until the patient reaches skeletal maturity.

PROGNOSIS & OUTCOME

- Most cases resolve, and significant relapses are uncommon.
- Rarely, severe systemic illness may lead to death or euthanasia
- Deformities of affected bones may persist.

PEARLS & CONSIDERATIONS

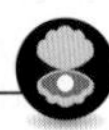

Comments

- Radiographic changes are pathognomonic.
- Ulnar ostectomy may prevent angular deformity if bridging of the distal ulnar physis is seen.

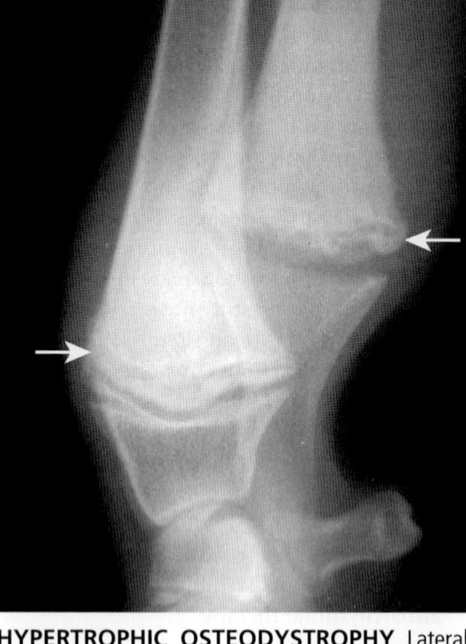

HYPERTROPHIC OSTEODYSTROPHY Lateral radiographic view of the distal radius and ulna of a 4-month-old Great Dane puppy with hypertrophic osteodystrophy (HOD). Note the radiolucent lines (scorbutic lines *[arrows]*) parallel to the epiphyseal growth plates and antebrachiocarpal joint, characteristic of HOD.

Technician Tips

- Use a lower-calorie puppy food; feed an amount that will achieve a lean body condition to minimize load on the developing skeleton.
- Do *not* supplement with minerals, vitamin D, or vitamin C.

SUGGESTED READING

Safra N, et al: Serum levels of innate immunity cytokines are elevated in dogs with metaphyseal osteopathy (hypertrophic osteodystrophy) during active disease and remission. Vet Immunol Immunopathol 179:32-35, 2016.

AUTHOR: Nicholas J. Trout, VetMB, MA, MRCVS, DACVS, DECVS
EDITOR: Kathleen Linn, DVM, MS, DACVS

Hypertrophic Osteopathy

Client Education Sheet

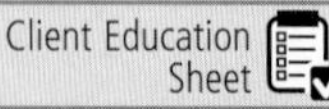

BASIC INFORMATION

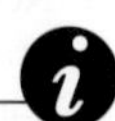

Definition

A periosteal reaction in the distal extremities of the limbs secondary to a mass or other disease in the thorax or abdomen

Synonyms

HO, hypertrophic pulmonary osteoarthropathy (HPOA), hypertrophic pulmonary osteopathy, Marie's disease, pulmonary osteoarthropathy

Epidemiology

SPECIES, AGE, SEX

- Mainly dogs; rare in cats
- Older animals because this disorder is often associated with neoplasia

GENETICS, BREED PREDISPOSITION

More common in large dog breeds

RISK FACTORS

- Thoracic mass (e.g., primary or metastatic pulmonary neoplasia, pulmonary abscess, esophageal carcinoma, *Spirocerca lupi* granuloma, granuloma of other causes)
- Heartworm disease
- Canine tuberculosis
- Megaesophagus
- Abdominal mass (e.g., urinary bladder rhabdomyosarcoma, liver adenocarcinoma, prostatic adenocarcinoma)

Clinical Presentation

HISTORY, CHIEF COMPLAINT

- Acute or gradual limb swelling, especially forelimbs
- Lethargy, low-grade lameness, or reluctance to move
- Incidental finding secondary to evaluation of a thoracic or abdominal mass

- Concerns may reflect underlying disorder (e.g., cough, weight loss, tachypnea)

PHYSICAL EXAM FINDINGS

- Swollen, hard extremities (e.g., distal long bones)
- Occasionally, pitting edema
- Decreased movement in joints secondary to soft-tissue swelling
- Other findings that suggest underlying disorder (e.g., palpable abdominal mass, abnormal lung sounds)

Etiology and Pathophysiology

Cause unknown:

- Autonomic neurovascular reflex increasing peripheral blood flow and causing periosteal congestion and new bone formation is speculated.
- Increased levels of platelet-derived growth factor (from megakaryocytes diverted from the pulmonary to the peripheral circulation) and vascular endothelial growth factor (often produced by tumors) may stimulate angiogenesis and new bone formation.

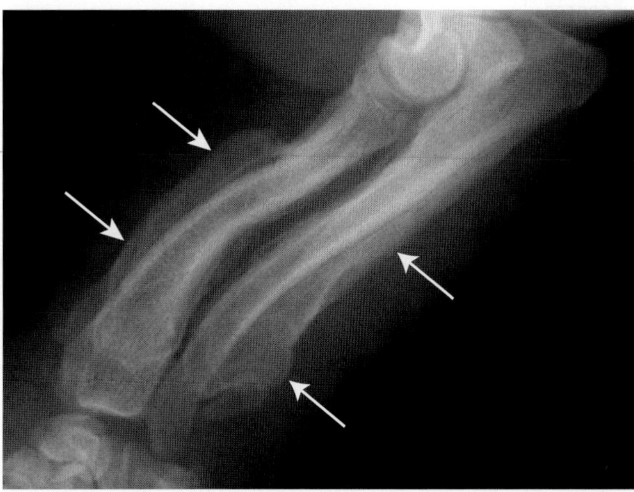

HYPERTROPHIC OSTEOPATHY Lateral radiograph of the radius and ulna of a 9-year-old, female, spayed dachshund dog with pulmonary carcinoma. Note the exuberant periosteal reaction *(arrows)* typical of hypertrophic osteopathy.

DIAGNOSIS

Diagnostic Overview

The combination of a characteristic limb lesion and a lung or abdominal mass defines HO.

Differential Diagnosis

Radiographic:

- Primary or secondary bone neoplasia
- Fungal bone disease
- Panosteitis
- Hepatazoon americanum

Initial Database

- CBC: neutrophilia, thrombocytosis, or thrombocytopenia possible
- Serum biochemistry profile and urinalysis: unremarkable or related to thoracic or abdominal disease; serum alkaline phosphatase elevation is common
- Radiographs of extremities: palisades of periosteal new bone on phalanges, metacarpi, metatarsi progressing to tibia/fibula, radius/ulna
- Thoracic and abdominal radiographs: mass usually identified in chest or abdomen; lung metastasis may be recognized

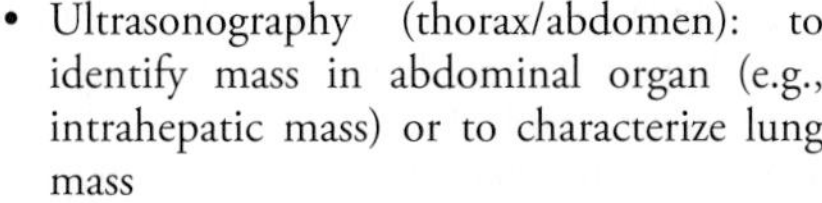

Advanced or Confirmatory Testing

- Ultrasonography (thorax/abdomen): to identify mass in abdominal organ (e.g., intrahepatic mass) or to characterize lung mass
- Biopsy or fine-needle aspiration of pulmonary/abdominal lesion for histologic diagnosis (pp. 1112 and 1113)

TREATMENT

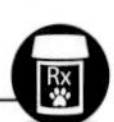

Treatment Overview

Treat the underlying thoracic or abdominal disease.

Acute and Chronic Treatment

- Surgical removal of mass lesion; removal of pulmonary metastases can also bring about resolution of HO.
- Medical treatment of mass when possible (e.g., infectious granuloma)
- Analgesic therapy if specific treatment is not feasible
- Bisphosphonate treatment is helpful in people; not yet reported for HO in dogs or cats

Recommended Monitoring

Follow-up radiographs of extremities to evaluate bone remodeling; monitoring as appropriate for primary disorder

PROGNOSIS & OUTCOME

- Depends on cause of underlying mass
- After treatment of the primary disease, bone lesions can take months to remodel and are not known to be fully reversible. Clinical lameness often improves.

PEARLS & CONSIDERATIONS

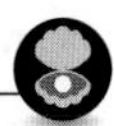

Comments

Swelling of the distal extremities of an older dog with radiographic evidence of characteristic palisading periosteal reaction calls for thoracic and abdominal imaging in search of an underlying primary lesion.

Technician Tips

New lameness or limb swelling in dogs treated for malignancy can signal the development of HO. Radiographs (including metacarpus or metatarsus) of at least one distal limb can confirm its presence.

SUGGESTED READING

Withers SS, et al: Paraneoplastic hypertrophic osteopathy in 30 dogs. Vet Comp Oncol 13(3):157-165, 2015.

AUTHOR: Nicholas J. Trout, VetMB, MA, MRCVS, DACVS, DECVS
EDITOR: Kathleen Linn, DVM, MS, DACVS

Hyperviscosity Syndrome

Client Education Sheet

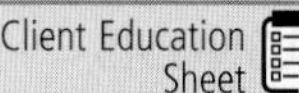

BASIC INFORMATION

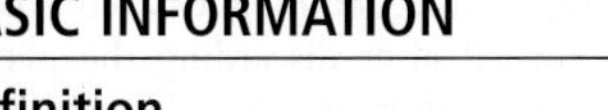

Definition

An uncommon sequela of diseases that may cause elevated blood viscosity; a constellation of secondary clinical signs may occur

Synonyms

Polycythemia indicates an increased number of all cell lines in the circulation; the term is often but mistakenly used interchangeably with *erythrocytosis,* an increase in circulating red blood cell mass.

Epidemiology

SPECIES, AGE, SEX

Dogs > cats; typically middle-aged to older animal

ASSOCIATED DISORDERS

- Neurologic signs from sludging of blood
- Bleeding disorders from platelet and coagulation factor inhibition
- Retinal lesions
- Volume overload and congestive heart failure
- Azotemia from decreased renal perfusion, infiltrative renal lesions, or associated hypercalcemia
- Immune suppression and secondary infection
- Pathologic fractures from infiltrative bone lesions (myeloma)

Clinical Presentation

HISTORY, CHIEF COMPLAINT

- Various combinations and severity of: lethargy, weakness, weight loss, polyuria/polydipsia, neurologic deficits, collapse, blindness, and overt bleeding
- Blood may be thick and difficult to collect by phlebotomy (especially from peripheral veins).

PHYSICAL EXAM FINDINGS

Ocular changes (retinal vessel engorgement/tortuosity, retinal hemorrhage or detachment, papilledema), neurologic deficits (blindness, altered mentation), epistaxis, mucosal hemorrhage or ecchymoses, or lymphadenopathy. If erythrocytosis present, red or cyanotic mucous membranes

Etiology and Pathophysiology

Viscosity is a function of the concentration and composition of blood components. A marked increase in plasma proteins or blood cells raises viscosity, leading to sludging in the microcirculation, causing clinical manifestations. Hyperviscosity may present insidiously with vague signs or acutely with neurologic and/or ophthalmic deficits.

Hyperviscosity syndrome can be caused by one of several hematologic conditions:

- Multiple myeloma (IgG or IgA)
- Waldenström's macroglobulinemia (IgM)
- Plasma cell leukemia
- Lymphoma
- Chronic lymphocytic leukemia (CLL)
- Amyloidosis
- Infectious disease: feline infectious peritonitis (FIP), ehrlichiosis, leishmaniasis
- Primary erythrocytosis (polycythemia vera)
- Secondary erythrocytosis
  - Hypoxemia (e.g., right-to-left patent ductus arteriosus, elevated altitude, chronic pulmonary disease)
  - Neoplasia (renal tumors, rarely sarcomas)

DIAGNOSIS

Diagnostic Overview

History and physical exam findings should raise suspicion; the clinical triad of neurologic, ophthalmic, and hemorrhagic findings suggests possible hyperviscosity. Diagnosis is further supported by routine CBC and serum biochemistry profile showing severe leukocytosis, erythrocytosis, or hyperglobulinemia. Any of these abnormalities warrants further evaluation to identify the underlying condition. Establishing a specific diagnosis (see list above) is essential for optimal treatment. Serum viscosity can be measured by a reference laboratory, but the clinical utility is low because treatment depends on the underlying cause.

Differential Diagnosis

- Lethargy, weakness, weight loss, polyuria/polydipsia are nonspecific signs, typically investigated with a CBC, serum biochemical profile, and urinalysis to identify abnormalities responsible for hyperviscosity.
- Acute visual deficits: retinal detachment, retinal hemorrhage, sudden acquired retinal degeneration
- Acute neurologic deficit: encephalitis, intracranial hemorrhage, hepatic encephalopathy
- Difficult phlebotomy: hypovolemia, technical difficulties

Initial Database

- CBC: markedly elevated hematocrit (i.e., > 60%) suggests erythrocytosis as cause of hyperviscosity; lymphocytosis may be apparent with leukemia.
- Serum biochemistry profile: hyperglobulinemia if hyperviscosity caused by Waldenström's macroglobulinemia, multiple myeloma, FIP, amyloidosis, or ehrlichiosis and possibly with CLL
- Urinalysis: no specific findings. Bence Jones proteins associated with multiple myeloma are not detected on routine urinalysis.
- Retinal exam: retinal arteries may be enlarged or tortuous; signs of uveitis or chorioretinitis may be present in FIP.

Advanced or Confirmatory Testing

- Serum or whole blood viscosity: measured by a reference laboratory to confirm hyperviscosity syndrome; rarely tested
- Blood pressure measurement (p. 1065): systemic hypertension may result from hyperglobulinemia.
- Thoracic radiographs: lytic bone lesions can be observed with multiple myeloma or rarely with lymphoma. Pulmonary changes if hypoxemia is the cause of secondary erythrocytosis
- Abdominal ultrasound
  - Diffuse hepatosplenomegaly or lymphadenopathy may be present with lymphoma, ehrlichiosis, or multiple myeloma (mainly splenomegaly).
  - Renal neoplasm (source of excess erythropoietin) as source of secondary erythrocytosis
- Serum protein electrophoresis (p. 1375): monoclonal protein spike with Waldenström's macroglobulinemia, multiple myeloma, or plasma cell leukemia or rarely with CLL. Polyclonal gammopathy usually with FIP, amyloidosis, or ehrlichiosis but occasionally monoclonal. Urine electrophoresis may reveal monoclonal spike for neoplastic disorders (less commonly used).
- Immunoelectrophoresis: further evaluation of a monoclonal gammopathy to assess concentrations of specific immunoglobulins
- Bence Jones proteinuria if hyperglobulinemia is cause of hyperviscosity
  - Excessive immunoglobulin light chains in urine
  - May be present with multiple myeloma, CLL, Waldenström's macroglobulinemia, or plasma cell leukemia
  - Alternatively, urine protein electrophoresis may be performed.
- Coagulation profile: bleeding disorders, especially platelet dysfunction (elevated buccal mucosal bleeding time; normal prothrombin time, activated partial thromboplastin time) may occur with hyperglobulinemia. Indicated if bleeding (epistaxis, petechia, hyphema, retinal hemorrhage) occurs.
- Bone marrow aspirate ± core biopsy: > 20% often abnormal plasma cells in multiple myeloma or plasma cell leukemia (p. 1068)
- Echocardiogram (p. 1094) with microbubble contrast: to identify right ventricular hypertrophy and right-to-left cardiac shunt
- *Ehrlichia canis* titer, *Leishmania* direct agglutination test; others: as indicated by geographic exposure and other clinical features

TREATMENT

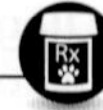

Treatment Overview

Hyperviscosity syndrome is a secondary condition. Patients may present with signs of hyperviscosity (e.g., epistaxis, blindness, retinal hemorrhage) and/or signs of the underlying condition. Identifying and treating the primary disease process is the cornerstone of care. Acutely, provide adequate hydration, supply tissue oxygenation, and ensure appropriate urine production. Phlebotomy or apheresis to reduce circulating blood components contributing to hyperviscosity syndrome may be used immediately if clinical signs are severe before definitive therapy for underlying condition.

Acute General Treatment

- To alleviate clinically significant neurologic or ophthalmic signs, phlebotomy is used to reduce the hematocrit to < 60%.
  - Remove up to 10-20 mL/kg whole blood (jugular vein preferred), with replacement of equivalent volume of isotonic crystalloids (peripheral IV catheter preferred).
  - If hypovolemia (tachycardia, weak pulses, hypotension, obtundation) develops, more conservative phlebotomy volumes and more aggressive crystalloid replacement are indicated during the initial treatments.
- When hyperglobulinemia is the cause of hyperviscosity, withdrawn blood can be centrifuged and autologous red blood cells returned after discarding the plasma component. Alternatively, plasmapheresis or therapeutic plasma exchange can be performed when patients have severe clinical signs.

Chronic Treatment

- Treatment of the underlying disorder (e.g., chemotherapy for leukemia, lymphoma, multiple myeloma; doxycycline for ehrlichiosis)
- Repeated plasmapheresis for Waldenström's macroglobulinemia
- Two options for polycythemia vera
  - Phlebotomy: a total of 10-20 mL/kg per treatment, repeated as needed based on clinical signs and hematocrit, *or*
  - Anti–RBC-precursor drugs: first decrease the hematocrit to < 60% using phlebotomy, then hydroxyurea 30-50 mg/kg PO q 24h initially for 7-10 days, followed by 30-50 mg/kg 2 or 3 times weekly as needed to maintain hematocrit < 60%. Monitor CBC for signs of myelotoxicosis.

Recommended Monitoring

- For erythrocytosis, monitor hematocrit.
- For hyperglobulinemia, monitor total protein, albumin, and globulin; repeated serum electrophoresis can be used for monitoring multiple myeloma.

PROGNOSIS & OUTCOME

Guarded; depends on underlying disease process

PEARLS & CONSIDERATIONS

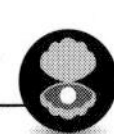

Comments

- Use glucocorticoids cautiously before establishing a diagnosis because biopsy or bone marrow results can be altered, making a diagnosis more difficult.
- Patients with hyperglobulinemia are predisposed to infection, and glucocorticoids further suppress the immune system.

Technician Tips

Blood collection is aided by using a larger-gauge needle.

SUGGESTED READING

Stein TJ: Paraneoplastic syndromes. In Ettinger SJ, et al, editors: Textbook of veterinary internal medicine, ed 8, St. Louis, 2017, Elsevier, pp 2126-2130.

AUTHOR: Jonathan F. Bach, DVM, DACVIM, DACVECC
EDITOR: Jonathan E. Fogle, DVM, PhD, DACVIM

Hyphema

Client Education Sheet

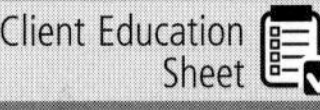

BASIC INFORMATION

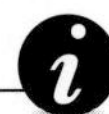

Definition

Blood in the anterior chamber of the eye

Epidemiology

SPECIES, AGE, SEX

Dogs and cats; any age, either sex

GENETICS, BREED PREDISPOSITION

Depends on the cause:

- Hereditary coagulopathies
- Inherited congenital ocular defects (e.g., collie eye anomaly [CEA] in rough and smooth collies, border collies, Australian shepherds, Lancashire heelers, and Shetland sheepdogs; persistent hyperplastic primary vitreous [PHPV] in Doberman pinschers, miniature schnauzers, and Staffordshire bull terriers; vitreoretinal dysplasias in shih tzus, Labrador retrievers, and Bedlington terriers) (p. 885)

RISK FACTORS

- Stimuli for preiridal fibrovascular membrane formation (PIFM, rubeosis iridis)
  - Retinal detachments
  - Intraocular neoplasia
  - Glaucoma
  - Uveitis
- Ocular trauma (e.g., blind animals, hunting dogs, exophthalmic animals, puppies exposed to cats)
- Any systemic disease causing vasculopathy and/or bleeding disorder
  - Systemic hypertension
  - Lymphoma
  - Immune-mediated diseases (thrombocytopenia, anemia)
  - Infectious diseases: feline leukemia virus, feline infectious peritonitis, rickettsial diseases (e.g., ehrlichiosis, Rocky Mountain spotted fever)
  - Hyperviscosity syndromes (multiple myeloma, polycythemia/erythrocytosis)
  - Severe liver disease
  - Rodenticide toxicity

Clinical Presentation

DISEASE FORMS/SUBTYPES

Acute:

- Various amounts of blood in anterior chamber
- Erythrocytes may settle in the ventral anterior chamber due to gravity or may be suspended throughout the anterior chamber.

Chronic:

- Various sizes of blood clots, ranging from dark red to dark brown
- Amount of blood varies with episodes of rebleeding.

HISTORY, CHIEF COMPLAINT

- Blood or redness in the eye
- Blindness or visual impairment
- Concerns related to systemic disease, if present

PHYSICAL EXAM FINDINGS

Ocular:

- Blood in the anterior chamber
- ± Fibrin clots with erythrocyte entrapment ± hypopyon
- Episcleral injection
- ± Corneal edema
- Miosis or mydriasis
- Variable intraocular pressure (IOP)
  - Normal (10-25 mm Hg): if uveitis is present with normal IOP, consider early onset of secondary glaucoma.
  - Reduced (<10 mm Hg): uveitis
  - Elevated (>25 mm Hg): glaucoma ± uveitis

General physical exam:

- Possible evidence of coagulopathy, trauma, or other systemic disease

Etiology and Pathophysiology

- Intraocular neovascularization (PIFM) is fragile, and disruption may cause spontaneous and recurring hyphema.
- Retinal detachment can cause recurring hyphema.
- Fibrinolysis, phagocytosis, and egress by the iridocorneal angle clear hyphema. Small bleeds resolve within 2-3 days; large bleeds may persist for weeks.
- Erythrocytes can clog the iridocorneal angle, increasing the risk of secondary glaucoma.

DIAGNOSIS

Diagnostic Overview

- Recognition of an underlying systemic disease is critical for overall health. Clinicians must determine if hyphema is due to ocular disease only (e.g., CEA, PHPV, primary intraocular neoplasia) or related to systemic disease (e.g., immune-mediated thrombocytopenia, metastatic neoplasia, infectious disease, intoxication).
- The fellow eye should also be examined for disease.
- Assessment of vision aids in prognostication.

Differential Diagnosis

- Intense corneal vascularization
- Rubeosis iridis (PIFM)
- Iridal hemorrhage can be secondary to many of the same causes as hyphema.

Initial Database

- Review history: trauma, travel, tick exposure, recent illness
- Ophthalmic exam (p. 1137)
  - Examine contralateral eye.
  - Examine periocular region (evidence of trauma).
  - Pupillary light and dazzle reflexes, menace response (vision prognosis)
  - Intraocular pressure (uveitis, glaucoma)
  - Fluorescein stain (corneal ulceration)
  - Examine cornea/sclera for evidence of perforating injury.
  - Aqueous flare and miosis support anterior uveitis.
  - Fundic exam (posterior hemorrhage, retinal detachment)
- General physical exam
  - Mucous membranes and skin exam (petechiae)
  - Abdominal and lymph node palpation (organomegaly and/or lymphadenopathy suggestive of systemic diseases)
  - Thoracic auscultation (pulmonary hemorrhage)
  - Neurologic exam (p. 1136) (head trauma, intracranial hemorrhage)
- Ocular ultrasound (p. 885) (posterior segment inflammation, retinal detachment, intraocular neoplasia, or intraocular foreign body)
- CBC, chemistry profile, and urinalysis (systemic disease)
- Blood pressure measurement (pp. 501 and 1065)
- Infectious disease testing

Advanced or Confirmatory Testing

- Coagulation profile
- Fine-needle aspirates/biopsy of organomegaly or enlarged lymph nodes
- Thoracic radiographs or CT (metastasis)
- Abdominal ultrasound or CT (metastasis)
- Skull radiographs (metallic foreign bodies)
- Ocular histopathology (after enucleation)

TREATMENT

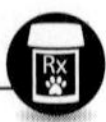

Treatment Overview

- Immediate treatment is necessary to limit bleeding and development of sequelae (secondary glaucoma, synechiae, cataract).
- Treatment of an underlying cause is the most important aspect of management.
- Management of inflammation and/or elevated intraocular pressures improves comfort and limits sequelae.
- Enucleation is the best treatment for patient comfort when the eye is permanently blind and painful.

Acute General Treatment

- Topical glucocorticoids (e.g., prednisolone acetate 1% or dexamethasone 0.1% q 6-8h)
  - Contraindicated in presence of corneal ulceration
  - Ophthalmic nonsteroidal antiinflammatory drugs (NSAIDs) such as flurbiprofen or diclofenac can be used in the setting of corneal ulceration.
- Topical atropine 1% solution q 24h if miosis present and IOP < 10-15 mm Hg (goal is to keep the pupil moving so that synechia does not develop)
- If IOP > 20-25 mm Hg (consistent with glaucoma), administer topical carbonic anhydrase inhibitors; other treatments are described on p. 387.
- Treat any identified systemic disease.
- Referral for surgical repair of corneal and/or scleral defects (p. 213)

Chronic Treatment

- Traumatic hyphema: refer for intracameral tissue plasminogen activator to dissolve clots.
  - Within 3-4 days of the hemorrhage
  - Slight risk of rebleeding
- Uncontrollable uveitis and/or secondary glaucoma (i.e., blind, painful eye)
  - Enucleation
- Surgical removal of hyphema rarely indicated

Behavior/Exercise

Restrict activity in acute cases of clotting disorders or trauma; cage rest with sedation if necessary

Drug Interactions

NSAIDs are often avoided to minimize secondary bleeding but may be necessary if glucocorticoids are contraindicated.

Possible Complications

Rebleeding, secondary glaucoma, synechiae, cataract, blindness, phthisis bulbi

Recommended Monitoring

Re-examine in 48-72 hours for resorption of blood or rebleeding and IOP changes. Close monitoring of IOP is necessary due to risk of secondary glaucoma.

PROGNOSIS & OUTCOME

- Varies; influenced by underlying cause
- Larger volume and blood in vitreous are associated with poorer outcome.
- Ocular sequelae (synechiae, cataract, glaucoma) can cause visual impairment, blindness, or loss of the eye.

PEARLS & CONSIDERATIONS

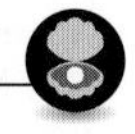

Comments

- Clinicians must rule out other causes of hyphema before presuming a traumatic cause, especially without confirmed history or visual evidence of trauma.
- Bilateral hyphema is rarely caused by trauma; a systemic disorder is more likely.

Prevention

- Avoid situations that predispose the animal to trauma (e.g., puppies interacting with feisty cats).
- Keep toxins (e.g., rodenticides) out of reach of animals.
- Tick control
- Avoid breeding dogs and cats with predisposing genetic diseases.
- Eye protection (goggles) for exophthalmic and blind dogs

Technician Tips

- Gentle restraint minimizes patient excitement and risk of further bleeding.
- Avoid jugular puncture for blood collection because coagulopathy may be present.

SUGGESTED READING

Telle MR, et al: Hyphema: considerations in the small animal patient. Top Companion Anim Med 30:97-106, 2015.

AUTHOR: Christine C. Lim, DVM, DACVO
EDITOR: Diane V. H. Hendrix, DVM, DACVO

Hypoadrenocorticism

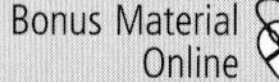

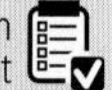

BASIC INFORMATION

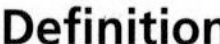

Definition

An endocrine disorder caused by adrenocortical insufficiency

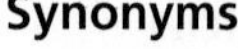

Synonyms

- Addison's disease
- Glucocorticoid-deficient hypoadrenocorticism (with normal serum electrolyte concentrations): atypical hypoadrenocorticism

Epidemiology

SPECIES, AGE, SEX

- Most common in young/middle-aged, female dogs, but any age, sex, or breed may be affected.

- Nova Scotia duck tolling retrievers (NSDTR) tend to be younger at time of diagnosis.
- Rare in cats; affected cats are typically young/middle-aged, although any age may be affected; no apparent sex predisposition

GENETICS, BREED PREDISPOSITION

- Increased risk: Great Danes, Portuguese water dogs, West Highland white terriers, bearded collies, poodles, rottweilers, soft-coated wheaten terriers, NSDTRs, and Leonbergers
  - Autosomal recessive inheritance in standard poodles, Portuguese water dogs, and NSDTRs
  - Highly heritable in bearded collies but precise mechanism unknown

Clinical Presentation

DISEASE FORMS/SUBTYPES

- Typical hypoadrenocorticism: signs of glucocorticoid and mineralocorticoid deficiency
- Atypical hypoadrenocorticism: signs only of glucocorticoid deficiency

HISTORY, CHIEF COMPLAINT

- Clinical signs are notoriously vague and often wax and wane over weeks or months (sometimes only apparent to owners in retrospect); worsening in stressful situations (e.g., travel, boarding) is possible. Severity of signs ranges from a mild, progressive, intermittent course to an acute, life-threatening crisis.
- Dogs
  - Most common: generalized weakness, lethargy, anorexia, vomiting
  - Less common: hindlimb weakness, diarrhea (possibly with melena or hematochezia), weight loss, trembling, polyuria/polydipsia (PU/PD), regurgitation (due to megaesophagus), and collapse. Rarely, seizures occur secondary to hypoglycemia.
- Cats: anorexia, weight loss, lethargy common; vomiting and PU/PD are uncommon.

PHYSICAL EXAM FINDINGS

- As described (see History, Chief Complaint above)
- Abdominal pain and muscle cramping may be detected.
- In crisis, signs may be severe. Mental depression, bradycardia (from hyperkalemia), and hypovolemic shock are possible.

Etiology and Pathophysiology

- Primary hypoadrenocorticism (typical and atypical): destruction of the adrenal cortices, usually due to idiopathic or immune-mediated processes. Other uncommon causes of adrenocortical destruction are granulomatous disease (e.g., histoplasmosis, blastomycosis, tuberculosis), infarction, neoplasia, and medications (e.g., mitotane, trilostane).
- Secondary hypoadrenocorticism (spontaneous): decreased secretion of ACTH from the pituitary, rarely due to destructive lesions or congenital defects.
- Secondary hypoadrenocorticism (iatrogenic): administration of exogenous glucocorticoids suppresses normal ACTH production, resulting in adrenocortical atrophy; sudden cessation of exogenous glucocorticoid administration then produces signs of cortisol deficiency.
- Clinical signs and laboratory findings are due to the absence of glucocorticoid and mineralocorticoid activity.
- Hypoadrenocorticism with clinical signs of glucocorticoid and mineralocorticoid deficiencies (typical hypoadrenocorticism; serum electrolyte concentrations are abnormal) is much more common than hypoadrenocorticism with signs of glucocorticoid deficiency only (atypical hypoadrenocorticism; electrolyte concentrations are normal).
- Consequences of glucocorticoid deficiency
  - Weakness, lethargy
  - Gastrointestinal (GI) signs (anorexia, vomiting, diarrhea, abdominal pain, melena, hematochezia, weight loss)
  - Hypoglycemia
  - Absence of a stress leukogram for an ill patient (failure of glucocorticoid-induced neutrophilia and lymphopenia), eosinophilia, mild anemia
- Consequences of mineralocorticoid (aldosterone) deficiency
  - Decreased renal sodium, chloride (and consequently water) reabsorption, resulting in hyponatremia (p. 518), hypochloremia, and volume depletion/dehydration
  - Loss of free water and sodium results in hypovolemia, hypotension, decreased cardiac output and poor tissue perfusion, solute diuresis and medullary solute washout. Consequences include prerenal azotemia, metabolic acidosis, weakness, depression, decreased urine concentrating ability, and PU/PD.
  - Decreased renal potassium excretion resulting in hyperkalemia (p. 495)
  - Metabolic acidosis due to decreased renal hydrogen ion excretion and poor tissue perfusion
- Additional reported findings for which a mechanism is not clearly defined include hypercalcemia (total and/or ionized calcium), hypoalbuminemia, hypocholesterolemia, and megaesophagus.

DIAGNOSIS

Diagnostic Overview

- Typical hypoadrenocorticism is suspected based on compatible historical/clinical findings in conjunction with hyponatremia and hyperkalemia. Bradycardia (or relative bradycardia) in the face of hypovolemia and/or absence of a stress leukogram in an ill patient increases the likelihood of the diagnosis.
- Atypical hypoadrenocorticism should be considered in dogs with historical/clinical signs of nonspecific illness (particularly GI signs) and any compatible laboratory finding, including absence of a stress leukogram, anemia, hypoalbuminemia, hypoglycemia, or hypocholesterolemia. Some dogs have only one clinicopathologic abnormality.
- The diagnosis (typical or atypical) is confirmed with an ACTH stimulation test. An algorithmic approach to diagnosis and management is outlined on p. 1429.

Differential Diagnosis

- Other causes of GI disease
- Hyperkalemia *and* hyponatremia: acute kidney injury/acute anuria, urinary tract obstruction, trichuriasis, severe GI disease, peritoneal or thoracic effusion, diabetes mellitus, pregnancy
  - Concurrent hyperkalemia, hyponatremia, prerenal azotemia, and isosthenuria can make it difficult to distinguish between hypoadrenocorticism and acute oliguric or anuric kidney failure. Differentiation is important because hypoadrenocorticism carries an excellent long-term prognosis. Initial treatment for both is similar, and the disorders can be distinguished using the ACTH stimulation test.
- Hyperkalemia (pp. 495 and 1235)
- Hyponatremia (pp. 518 and 1241)
- Hypercalcemia (pp. 491 and 1232)
- Hypoglycemia (p. 552)
- Hypoalbuminemia (p. 1239)

Initial Database

- CBC, serum biochemical profile, urinalysis
  - Typical hypoadrenocorticism: common findings include normocytic, normochromic nonregenerative anemia; absence of stress leukogram (p. 1283), hyponatremia, hypochloremia, hyperkalemia, metabolic acidosis, prerenal azotemia, and hypoalbuminemia. Hypoglycemia, hypercalcemia, and isosthenuria are also possible. A decreased Na/K ratio (<27) is suggestive of hypoadrenocorticism but is not pathognomonic and cannot be used to make a definitive diagnosis.
  - The most common reason for a missed diagnosis is failure to measure serum electrolyte concentrations because hyperkalemia and hyponatremia are usually the first clues pointing toward hypoadrenocorticism.
  - Atypical hypoadrenocorticism: similar to the typical form, with the exception that electrolyte concentrations are normal.
- Electrocardiogram (p. 1096): changes consistent with hyperkalemia possible, including increased T-wave amplitude, decreased P-wave amplitude, and bradycardia
- Thoracic radiographs: microcardia due to volume depletion common; signs of megaesophagus ± aspiration pneumonia possible
- Abdominal ultrasound: adrenal glands may be normal or slender; whereas slender adrenal glands are supportive of hypoadrenocorticism, normal adrenal gland size does not rule out the diagnosis.
- Basal serum cortisol level: if normal (>2 mcg/dL [>55 nmol/L]), hypoadrenocorticism is

highly unlikely. If low, ACTH stimulation test is required for confirmation.

Advanced or Confirmatory Testing

- ACTH stimulation test is the definitive diagnostic test for hypoadrenocorticism. Basal serum cortisol concentration will be low and cortisol fails to increase after ACTH administration (p. 1300).
- Dogs
  - 1) Collect blood sample for pre-ACTH cortisol level; 2) administer synthetic ACTH (cosyntropin/tetracosactide) 5 mcg/kg, up to 250 mcg/DOG IV; 3) collect blood sample 60 minutes later (post-ACTH cortisol level).
  - ACTH gel is not recommended due to variability in intramuscular absorption. If intramuscular gel is used, postcortisol samples should be obtained at 1 and 2 hours due to inconsistent results.
- Cats
  - 1) Collect blood sample for pre-ACTH cortisol level; 2) administer cosyntropin 125 mcg/CAT IV; 3) collect blood sample 60 minutes later (post-ACTH cortisol level).
- Endogenous ACTH can be measured to differentiate secondary (decreased ACTH) from primary hypoadrenocorticism (increased ACTH) if electrolyte values are normal. The difference can be important for prognosis and monitoring. Secondary hypoadrenocorticism never becomes typical with electrolyte abnormalities; patients with primary atypical hypoadrenocorticism can later develop electrolyte abnormalities.

TREATMENT

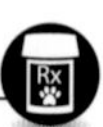

Treatment Overview

Initial therapy depends on severity of clinical signs. For animals in an Addisonian crisis, initial therapy is directed at correcting life-threatening conditions (hypotension, hypovolemia, hyperkalemia, acidosis, hypoglycemia). The cornerstone of treatment is IV fluid therapy. Patients with severe, typical clinical and laboratory abnormalities should be treated as if they have hypoadrenocorticism; delaying treatment until ACTH stimulation results are available may result in death of the patient. Chronic, lifelong therapy involves physiologic replacement of deficient hormones.

Acute General Treatment

- Isotonic replacement crystalloids
  - Traditionally, 0.9% NaCl has been recommended because of the high sodium content and lack of potassium. However, some clinicians prefer Plasma-Lyte A or lactated Ringer's solution because they correct the acidosis more quickly, and their low potassium content still allows for correction of hyperkalemia.
  - Hyponatremia should not be corrected too quickly or neurologic deficits can develop (p. 518).
  - If severely ill, dehydrated, and/or hypotensive, give one-third of the shock volume (that is, ≈20 mL/kg bolus repeated up to 90 mL/kg for dogs, 60 mL/kg for cats) IV bolus, then reassess and administer more if necessary. For maintenance and to correct dehydration, additional fluids should be given as needed over the next few days.
- Fluid therapy is the primary treatment for hyperkalemia and acidosis.
  - If hyperkalemia is life-threatening (>8.5 mEq/L and/or electrocardiographic abnormalities present), treat specifically (p. 495).
  - Bicarbonate is rarely needed to treat acidosis because fluids are almost always adequate.
- Glucocorticoid administration
  - Dexamethasone sodium phosphate (preferred by the author): rapid acting and is not detected by cortisol assay (ACTH stimulation test). Initially administer 0.25 mg/kg IV, then 0.1 mg/kg q 12h.
  - Alternatively, hydrocortisone (continuous-rate infusion) 0.5-0.625 mg/kg/h has both glucocorticoid and mineralocorticoid properties. However, it interferes with the cortisol assay and should not be administered until after completion of the ACTH stimulation test.
- Hypoglycemia: add dextrose to isotonic IV fluids to make a 2.5%-5% dextrose concentration. If hypoglycemia is severe or the patient has clinical signs of hypoglycemia, boluses of 25% dextrose solution, 1 mL/kg in 0.9% saline, may be given.
- After life-saving treatment has been initiated, perform ACTH stimulation test as above (p. 1300).
- Monitor urine production.
- Monitor electrolytes and glucose after initial fluid resuscitation and then q 8-12h until normal.
- Maintain fluid therapy until patient is eating.
- Use injectable glucocorticoids until oral prednisone can be instituted at 1 mg/kg PO q 24h until the patient goes home. Then taper the dose as below.
- Mineralocorticoid administration can be initiated after the diagnosis is confirmed.

Chronic Treatment

- Lifelong supplementation with glucocorticoids and mineralocorticoids (typical hypoadrenocorticism) or with glucocorticoids alone (atypical hypoadrenocorticism) is required.
- Glucocorticoid supplementation: prednisone 0.25-0.5 mg/kg PO q 12h initially, then taper to 0.1-0.25 mg/kg PO q 24h, depending on individual needs.
  - Increase dose if signs of hypoadrenocorticism persist, and decrease if signs of glucocorticoid excess are present.
  - Increased prednisone (2-3 times normal dose) is required during times of stress (e.g., travel, new pet or child, veterinary visit, other illness).
  - Prednisone doses < 0.1 mg/kg q 24h are often adequate and may be better tolerated, especially in larger dogs. Monitor for clinical signs of hypoadrenocorticism closely in these cases.
  - Patients receiving fludrocortisone acetate may not require additional daily glucocorticoid therapy long term, but those receiving deoxycorticosterone pivalate (DOCP) always do.
- Mineralocorticoid supplementation: DOCP injection or oral fludrocortisone
  - DOCP
    - Initial dose 2.2 mg/kg SQ or IM q ≈25 days
      - 1.5 mg/kg SQ or IM is effective in most dogs and is used by the author as an off-label starting dose.
    - Measure electrolytes on days 14 and 25 after treatment, and adjust dosing based on results.
    - If hyperkalemic or hyponatremic on day 14, increase the next dose by 5%-10%. If electrolytes are normal at 14 days but abnormal at 25 days, shorten the dosing interval by 48 hours. If electrolytes are normal at each recheck, dosing interval may be increased by several days. In one report, dose intervals of as long as 60 days were effective for some dogs.
    - If hypokalemic or hypernatremic on day 14, decrease the next dose by 10%.
    - After dosage and dosing interval are determined, clients can be taught to give DOCP at home.
  - Fludrocortisone acetate
    - Dogs: 0.01 mg/kg PO q 12h initially; dose often needs to be increased based on serum electrolyte concentrations over first 6-18 months to maintain normal electrolyte concentrations.
    - Cats: 0.05-0.1 mg/CAT PO q 12h initially; adjust based on serum electrolyte concentrations.
    - Prednisone should be given with fludrocortisone initially but may be tapered after normalization of electrolytes.

Possible Complications

- With Addisonian crises, death can occur if treatment is not prompt and intensive.
- Overly rapid correction of hyponatremia can result in demyelination (p. 518).
- Side effects of prolonged, excessive prednisone and/or fludrocortisone treatment include PU/PD and other signs of iatrogenic hyperadrenocorticism. In animals receiving fludrocortisone, if PU/PD cannot be resolved by tapering prednisone (to lowest dose needed to prevent signs of hypocortisolism), switching to DOCP is recommended.

Recommended Monitoring

- With fludrocortisone or prednisone, monitor serum biochemistry, including electrolytes,

every 7 days after diagnosis until stable. After electrolytes are stabilized, recheck monthly for 3-6 months, then q 3-6 months.
- With DOCP, see above.
- Subsequent ACTH stimulation testing is of no use in patients with spontaneous hypoadrenocorticism; adjustment of prednisone dose is based on clinical signs while adjustment of mineralocorticoid is based on measured electrolytes.

PROGNOSIS & OUTCOME

- With treatment and monitoring, prognosis is excellent, and a normal life span is expected.
- At the time of diagnosis of hypoadrenocorticism, azotemia with concurrent isosthenuria should not be taken to indicate renal failure and does not necessarily influence the prognosis (see Pearls & Considerations below). With treatment of hypoadrenocorticism, renal function usually returns to normal.

PEARLS & CONSIDERATIONS

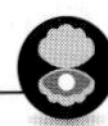

Comments

- This disease can mimic others that are more common (acute kidney injury/anuria, hepatic disease, GI disease), and the diagnosis of hypoadrenocorticism is commonly missed initially. The CBC can provide a valuable clue; absence of a stress leukogram in an ill animal suggests hypoadrenocorticism.
- DOCP is expensive. Reductions in the dose used or increases in the dosing interval can help control cost. However, initial monitoring to establish an effective dose/interval is essential to avoid potentially life-threatening complications.

Technician Tips

- Make sure that the ACTH is given IV for the diagnosis of hypoadrenocorticism.
- Owners can be taught to give SQ injections of DOCP at home.

Client Education

It is important to educate clients that this disease requires lifelong treatment and that failure to administer therapy (or delayed administration) may result in a life-threatening crisis. They must also understand the need for glucocorticoid dose adjustment in times of stress.

SUGGESTED READING

Lathan P: Hypoadrenocorticism in dogs. In Rand J, editor: Clinical endocrinology of companion animals, Ames, IA, 2013, Wiley-Blackwell, pp 1-21.

AUTHOR: Patty Lathan, VMD, MS, DACVIM
EDITOR: Ellen N. Behrend, VMD, PhD, DACVIM

Hypocalcemia

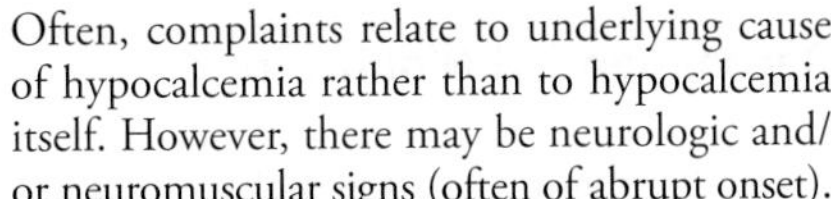

BASIC INFORMATION

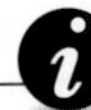

Definition

Serum total calcium < 9.0 mg/dL (<2.2 mmol/L) dogs; < 8.0 mg/dL (<2.0 mmol/L) cats; *or* serum ionized calcium < 5.0 mg/dL (<1.2 mmol/L) dogs; < 4.5 mg/dL (<1.1 mmol/L) cats

Epidemiology

SPECIES, AGE, SEX

- Dogs and cats of either sex and any age; predispositions depends on underlying cause
  - Eclampsia (p. 281)
  - Hypoparathyroidism (p. 519)
  - Protein-losing enteropathy (p. 600)

RISK FACTORS

- Homemade diets
- Lactation
- Massive transfusion
- Parathyroidectomy or bilateral thyroidectomy
- Phosphate enema
- Protein-losing enteropathy

Clinical Presentation

DISEASE FORMS/SUBTYPES

Asymptomatic hypocalcemia (common):
- Incidental finding on blood tests
- Hypocalcemia is mild or has been chronic.

Clinical hypocalcemia (less common):
- Patient presented for signs related to hypocalcemia.
- Hypocalcemia is moderate to severe or has developed acutely.

HISTORY, CHIEF COMPLAINT

Often, complaints relate to underlying cause of hypocalcemia rather than to hypocalcemia itself. However, there may be neurologic and/or neuromuscular signs (often of abrupt onset).
- Signs may be intermittent despite persistent hypocalcemia.
  - Facial rubbing, pawing at face
  - Ear twitching
  - Nervousness, excessive panting
  - Stiff, stilted, rigid gait
  - Muscle tremors
  - Seizures

PHYSICAL EXAM FINDINGS

Often, exam findings are related to underlying cause of hypocalcemia. However, signs may include
- Muscle rigidity, fasciculations
- Hyperthermia
- Tachyarrhythmias, soft heart sounds, weak pulses
- Raised nictitating membranes (cats)

Etiology and Pathophysiology

- Calcium homeostasis: 50% of total circulating calcium is ionized (biologically active form), 40% is bound to albumin (storage form), and 10% is complexed to anions (storage form).
- Clinical signs of hypocalcemia occur *only* when the ionized form is decreased.
- Serum calcium concentration is tightly regulated by parathyroid hormone (PTH), vitamin D, and calcitonin.
- PTH increases serum calcium by
  - Increasing osteoclastic bone resorption of calcium and phosphorus
  - Increasing calcium and decreasing phosphorus resorption from renal tubules
  - Stimulating conversion of vitamin D to its active form by the renal enzyme 1-alpha-hydroxylase
- Inactive vitamin D is absorbed in the intestine; transported to the liver, where it is hydroxylated to 25-dihydroxyvitamin D; it is then transported to the kidney, where it is hydroxylated by 1-alpha-hydroxylase to the active metabolite 1,25-dihydroxyvitamin D (calcitriol).
- Vitamin D increases serum calcium and phosphorus by
  - Increasing intestinal absorption of calcium, phosphorus, and magnesium
  - Facilitating PTH-induced bone resorption
  - Increasing renal tubular resorption of calcium and phosphorus
- Calcitonin decreases serum calcium and phosphorus by
  - Blocking bone resorption
  - Decreasing renal tubular resorption of calcium and phosphorus

DIAGNOSIS

Diagnostic Overview

The diagnosis is suspected based on the presence of facial pruritus, muscle fasciculations, stiff gait, and/or seizures, or more often, hypocalcemia is discovered on serum chemistry profile. Confirmation requires measurement of ionized calcium concentration (p. 1320).

Differential Diagnosis

See p. 1239 for detailed differential diagnoses.
- Decreased absorption
- Increased loss
- Laboratory error
- Sequestration

Initial Database

- CBC, serum biochemistry panel, urinalysis
- Serum ionized calcium concentration

Advanced or Confirmatory Testing

Specific testing depends on history, exam, and routine blood tests but may include
- Serum PTH concentration
- Serum magnesium concentration
- Ethylene glycol test
- Serum 25-hydroxyvitamin D and calcitriol concentrations

TREATMENT

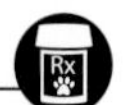

Treatment Overview

The goals of therapy are to increase serum calcium concentration to a level that alleviates clinical signs (but is not necessarily in the normal range), minimize the likelihood of hypercalcemia, and reduce the magnitude of hypercalciuria.

Acute General Treatment

Intravenous calcium infusion:
- Administer 10% calcium gluconate IV at a dose of 0.5-1.5 mL/kg or 5-15 mg/kg slowly to effect over 15-30 minutes.
- Electrographic monitoring is recommended during IV calcium administration. The infusion should be slowed/discontinued if bradycardia, ventricular premature complexes, or shortening of the QT interval is observed.

After clinical signs have improved, continue parenteral calcium administration. Calcium can be given as a continuous IV infusion at 60-90 mg/kg/day of elemental calcium (10% calcium gluconate contains 9.3 mg/mL of elemental calcium).

Chronic Treatment

- Vitamin D: calcitriol is the form recommended for maintenance therapy for its rapid onset of action and short half-life.
  - Loading dose is 10-15 ng/kg q 12h PO for 4 days.
  - Maintenance dose is 5-10 ng/kg q 12h PO. Adjust dose to maintain normocalcemia.
  - Maximal effect is seen in 1-4 days.
  - Recommend compounding as a liquid formulation to allow for small dosage adjustments.
- Calcium supplementation: calcium carbonate (1 g contains 400 mg of elemental calcium) is recommended at a dosage of 12.5-25 mg/kg elemental calcium q 12h PO.
- After normocalcemia is achieved, the dose of oral calcium can be slowly tapered and discontinued. Vitamin D must be continued until the underlying disorder is corrected.
- Therapy with synthetic PTH is not currently available.

Drug Interactions

Calcium salts should not be added to fluids that contain lactate, acetate, bicarbonate, or phosphates because calcium may precipitate.

Possible Complications

Subcutaneous administration of calcium should be avoided because cases of severe, extensive calcinosis cutis and epidermal necrosis resulting in euthanasia have been reported.

Recommended Monitoring

- Monitor total serum calcium. Target level is 8-9.5 mg/dL (2-2.4 mmol/L) (i.e., just below reference interval).
- Monitor for resolution of signs.

PROGNOSIS & OUTCOME

Depend on the underlying cause but are generally good.

PEARLS & CONSIDERATIONS

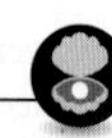

Comments

- Hypoalbuminemia is a common cause of incidental (total) hypocalcemia (ionized Ca^+ within reference range).
- The most common causes of clinical hypocalcemia are eclampsia, protein-losing enteropathy, and surgical removal of parathyroid glands (e.g., bilateral thyroidectomy).
- Do not measure calcium in EDTA-treated blood; EDTA chelates calcium, decreasing its concentration.
- Avoid the use of calcium chloride because it is caustic.
- Correction formulas used to compensate for hypoalbuminemia are not accurate; measure ionized calcium instead.

Prevention

- The modified intracapsular thyroidectomy technique reduces the occurrence of postoperative hypocalcemia.
- Maintain pregnant bitch on high-quality food throughout pregnancy.

Technician Tips

Facial pruritus is the earliest symptom of hypocalcemia patients may display.

Client Education

Patients receiving calcitriol should be monitored for signs of hypercalcemia: polydipsia, polyuria, anorexia, vomiting, and lethargy.

SUGGESTED READING

de Brito Galvão JF, et al: A quick reference on hypocalcemia. Vet Clin North Am Small Anim Pract 47:249-256, 2017.

AUTHOR: Karen M. Tefft, DVM, MVSc, DACVIM
EDITOR: Leah A. Cohn, DVM, PhD, DACVIM

Hypokalemia

BASIC INFORMATION

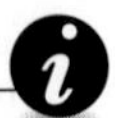

Definition

Serum potassium (K^+) concentration < 3.5 mEq/L

Epidemiology

SPECIES, AGE, SEX

Any animal is susceptible. Hypokalemia related to chronic kidney disease (CKD) is most likely in older cats. Hypokalemic periodic paralysis occurs in the first year of life.

GENETICS, BREED PREDISPOSITION

Hypokalemic periodic polymyopathy (Burmese, Bombay, Tonkinese cats, WNK3 mutation)

RISK FACTORS

Conditions that increase potassium loss (e.g., CKD, vomiting/diarrhea), or cause translocation of potassium between the fluid compartments

Clinical Presentation

DISEASE FORMS/SUBTYPES

Usually a complication of other disorders, hypokalemia can be severe and result in acute or chronic clinical manifestations or can be an incidental finding.

HISTORY, CHIEF COMPLAINT

History is often related to an underlying cause of K^+ loss (e.g., vomiting/diarrhea, postobstructive diuresis). However, signs attributable directly to hypokalemia include
- Muscle weakness or paralysis
- Limb discomfort
- Limp neck posture
- Mental dullness
- Bowel hypomotility (species susceptibility varies)
- Polyuria/polydipsia
- Episodic muscular weakness (periodic familial hypokalemia in cats)

PHYSICAL EXAM FINDINGS

Exam findings are often due to the underlying cause of K^+ loss (e.g., small, irregular kidneys).

However, findings attributable directly to hypokalemia (if present) may include

- Weakness
- Short, limited stride
- Flaccid ventral cervical flexion
- Shallow respiratory movements/apnea (K^+ < 2.4 mEq/L)
- Cardiac arrhythmias (K^+ < 2.4 mEq/L)

Etiology and Pathophysiology

See Hypokalemia on p. 516.
Pathophysiology:

- Two main causes: increased loss (most common/severe) and translocation between fluid compartments
- Hypokalemia increases cellular repolarization and adversely affects cell depolarization.
- Hypokalemia affects cardiac excitation and conduction, and renal function.

DIAGNOSIS

Diagnostic Overview

Potassium concentration should be measured in any animal with weakness or a disorder known to cause hypokalemia. Diagnostic efforts are typically geared toward the underlying disorder rather than the complication of hypokalemia.

Differential Diagnosis

Any cause of weakness (p. 1295)

Initial Database

CBC, serum chemistry profile, urinalyses, ± imaging studies performed to find cause of hypokalemia (by definition, serum/plasma K^+ < 3.5 mEq/L), with special attention to

- Creatinine and blood urea nitrogen (kidney failure)
- Urine specific gravity (isosthenuria in CKD, isosthenuria to hyposthenuria with diuresis)
- Serum sodium (increased if hyperaldosteronism)
- Serum chloride (hypochloremic metabolic alkalosis)
- Bicarbonate (increased with metabolic alkalosis, decreased with renal tubular acidosis)
- CK and AST (increase with rhabdomyolysis)

Advanced or Confirmatory Testing

As based on clinical suspicion; may include blood gas analysis, diagnostic imaging, measurement of aldosterone and renin, or genetic testing (periodic polymyopathy in cats)

TREATMENT

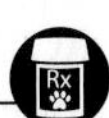

Treatment Overview

Must address the underlying disorder; K^+ supplementation (orally or parenterally, depending on presentation) is often indicated.

Recommended Amount Potassium Chloride and Rate of Infusion

Serum Potassium Concentration (mEq/L)	mEq KCl to Add to 250 mL Fluid	mEq KCl to Add to 1 L Fluid	Maximal Fluid Infusion Rate* (mL/kg/h)
<2.0	20	80	6
2.1-2.5	15	60	8
2.6-3.0	10	40	12
3.1-3.5	7	28	18
3.6-5.0	5	20	25

CAN DOSE ON BASIS OF mEq/L OVER 24 HOURS

Serum K^+ Concentration (mEq/L)	Dose of KCl in mEq/kg/24 Hours
3.0-3.5	2-3
2.5-3.0	3-5
<2.5	5-10

*So as not to exceed 0.5 mEq/kg/h. This rate can be exceeded in life-threatening hypokalemia by giving up to 1.5 mEq/kg/h with simultaneous electrocardiographic monitoring.

Modified from Greene RW, et al: Lower urinary tract disease. In Ettinger SJ, editor: Textbook of veterinary internal medicine, Philadelphia, 1975, Saunders, p 1572.

Acute General Treatment

- Potassium chloride typically favored for parenteral use as additive to intravenous fluids
- When there is coexisting hypophosphatemia (e.g., during treatment for diabetic ketoacidosis), potassium phosphate can be used to supply one-half of the K^+ supplementation.

Chronic Treatment

Oral potassium gluconate (commercial gel or powder): typical starting dose 1.0 mEq/kg/day divided two or three times per day; adjust based on recheck of [K^+]

Drug Interactions

Angiotensin-converting enzyme (ACE) inhibitors, beta-adrenergic blockers may lead to excess K^+ retention during supplementation.

Possible Complications

Post-supplementation hyperkalemia, cardiac arrhythmia/arrest from overly rapid supplementation

Recommended Monitoring

Appropriate K^+ supplementation is best gauged by repeat serum K^+ determinations. While on IV fluids, daily monitoring is ideal. For oral home supplementation, repeat measures once per week until stable; then recheck at routine appointments (p. 169).

PROGNOSIS & OUTCOME

Depends on ability to resolve/address underlying cause. Hypokalemic myopathy may cause chronic muscle functional impairment if fibrosis occurs.

PEARLS & CONSIDERATIONS

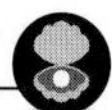

Comments

Recalcitrant hypokalemia sometimes improves when concurrent hypomagnesemia is addressed.

Prevention

- Supplement IV fluids with appropriate quantity of K^+, especially in anorexic animals or those with diuresis.
- Monitor K^+ regularly when there are conditions that predispose to hypokalemia.

Technician Tips

- Flaccid ventral neck flexion in a cat should prompt K^+ measurement.
- K^+-containing fluids should not be used for bolus administration as during cardiopulmonary resuscitation.

SUGGESTED READING

DiBartola SP: Disorders of sodium and water: hypernatremia and hyponatremia. In DiBartola SP, editor: Fluid, electrolyte and acid base disorders in small animal practice, ed 4, St. Louis, 2012, Saunders.

AUTHOR: Michael Schaer, DVM, DACVIM, DACVECC
EDITOR: Leah A. Cohn, DVM, PhD, DACVIM

Hyponatremia

Client Education Sheet 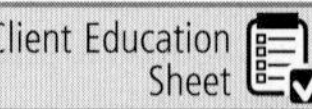

BASIC INFORMATION

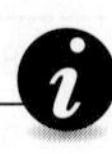

Definition

Serum sodium (Na^+) concentration below the lower end of the reference range. Clinical signs are most common with rapid rate of decline in Na^+ and are rarely seen until values fall below ≈132 mEq/L, with the most dramatic signs apparent at concentrations < 120 mEq/L.

Epidemiology

SPECIES, AGE, SEX

Hyponatremia can affect any animal. Young to middle-aged, female dogs may be predisposed to hypoadrenocorticism (p. 512), an important cause of hyponatremia.

GENETICS, BREED PREDISPOSITION

Dog breeds predisposed to hypoadrenocorticism: standard poodle, Portuguese water dog, Nova Scotia duck tolling retriever, bearded collie

RISK FACTORS

Parenteral administration of sodium-free fluids; disorders causing water gain or sodium loss

ASSOCIATED DISORDERS

Hypoadrenocorticism (Addison's disease); renal tubular dysfunction; conditions leading to appropriate or inappropriate secretion of antidiuretic hormone (ADH) with resultant water retention

Clinical Presentation

DISEASE FORMS/SUBTYPES

- Hyponatremia may be acute (<24 hours) or chronic and caused by water gain or Na^+ loss
- Patients with hyponatremia may be categorized by osmolality and volume status
  - Normosmolar
  - Hyperosmolar
  - Hypoosmolar (most common): hypovolemic, euvolemic, or hypervolemic

HISTORY, CHIEF COMPLAINT

- Most clinical signs are related directly to the underlying cause of hyponatremia (e.g., gastrointestinal [GI] signs, cough and respiratory distress due to congestive heart failure [CHF], icterus due to hepatic cirrhosis).
- Additional signs are related to chronicity and severity of hyponatremia.
  - Acute hyponatremia can cause nausea, vomiting, muscular weakness, mental dullness, disorientation, and seizures.
  - Signs of chronic hyponatremia are often subtle, but inappropriate medical management can cause devastating consequences. Overly rapid correction can cause more severe consequences than hyponatremia itself.
- Hyponatremia may not be suspected before electrolytes are measured.

PHYSICAL EXAM FINDINGS

- Examination is typically unremarkable, or abnormalities are related to the disorder responsible for hyponatremia. For example
  - Hypoadrenocorticism (p. 512): dehydration, bradycardia, weakness, prolonged capillary refill time
  - CHF (p. 408): murmur, tachycardia, tachypnea, audible pulmonary crackles (left-sided failure) or jugular pulses and diminished lung sounds (right-sided failure)
  - Hepatic cirrhosis (p. 174): icterus, abdominal effusion
  - Protein-losing nephropathy: peripheral edema, ascites, weight loss
- Gelatinous skin texture, transudative body cavity abdominal effusions, crackles on thoracic auscultation, and jugular distention can be signs of fluid retention.
- Mental dullness can occur with severe hyponatremia (especially if Na^+ < 120 mEq/L).

Etiology and Pathophysiology

- Na^+ accounts for the vast majority of serum osmolality. Rapid onset of hyponatremia allows water to enter cells in the brain, causing edema and neurologic signs or even death. If hyponatremia develops more slowly, brain cells can equilibrate (by loss of electrolytes, amino acids, and other osmolytes) so that clinical signs are less likely.
- Perhaps the most dangerous aspect of chronic (>24 hours) hyponatremia is overly rapid correction (>0.5-1 mEq/L/h). The adaptive changes that protect the brain against excessive swelling also render it susceptible to dehydration during the correction of hyponatremia.
  - Rapid correction can cause water to leave the brain cells, and brain shrinkage leads to vascular rupture and intracranial bleeding.
  - A delayed osmotic demyelination syndrome (i.e., central pontine myelinosis) can cause irreversible neurologic damage, producing ataxia, paresis, coma, and even death. This may not be evident for up to 2 weeks after the episode of hyponatremia.
- True hyponatremia results from sodium loss or water gain.
- Depending on the associated pathophysiology, it can be classified according to hydration state, plasma tonicity (hypotonic, isotonic, hypertonic), and plasma volume status (hypervolemic, euvolemic, hypovolemic).
- See causes of hyponatremia elsewhere (p. 1241).

DIAGNOSIS

Diagnostic Overview

Hyponatremia is confirmed by measurement of serum or plasma Na^+ after ruling out pseudohyponatremia or spurious hyponatremia. Additional diagnostic efforts are aimed at determining the underlying cause of hyponatremia.

Differential Diagnosis

- Pseudohyponatremia due to hyperlipidemia or hyperparaproteinemia
- Spurious hyponatremia occurs with rapid-onset hyperglycemia because of cellular water being dragged into the extracellular fluid space. Serum sodium decreases an average of 1.7 mEq/L for every 100 mg/dL increase in blood glucose concentration.

Initial Database

- Serum chemistry profile
  - By definition, Na^+ is below lower end of reference range.
  - Flame photometry or indirect potentiometry measurements can result in pseudohyponatremia if hyperproteinemia or hyperlipidemia is present.
  - Ion-selective electrode measurements can confirm true hyponatremia.
  - Hypochloremia is common.
  - Other abnormalities reflect cause for hyponatremia (e.g., hyperkalemia in hypoadrenocorticism, hypoalbuminemia due to protein-losing nephropathy, icterus due to cirrhosis, hyperglycemia due to diabetes mellitus)
- CBC: varies, depending on cause of hyponatremia
  - Normal eosinophil and lymphocyte numbers in a sick dog suggest hypoadrenocorticism.
- Urinalysis and, ideally, urine osmolality: variable
  - If concentrated urine suggests fluid retention, calculation of urine sodium fractional excretion can help differentiate between appropriate and inappropriate ADH secretion. Urine Na > 25 mEq/L and increased urine osmolality suggests syndrome of inappropriate ADH (SIADH).
- Thoracic and abdominal imaging studies for underlying disease

Advanced or Confirmatory Testing

As indicated by preliminary findings and necessary to confirm underlying disorder (e.g., ACTH stimulation test to confirm suspected hypoadrenocorticism; echocardiography to confirm cardiac disease; thyroid profile to confirm hypothyroidism)

TREATMENT

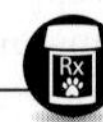

Treatment Overview

Goals of treatment are to correct hyponatremia at a safe rate (0.5 mEq/L/h for hyponatremia of > 24 hours' duration) while addressing the underlying disorder that originally caused hyponatremia. For animals with normal or excessive volume status, minimal parenteral fluids should be administered.

Acute Treatment

- Monitoring the rate of change in [Na^+] during correction is crucial.
- Direct treatment of the underlying disease is always in order. Sometimes, this may be the only treatment required for hyponatremia (e.g., furosemide to address CHF helps eliminate excess water and correct hyponatremia; dosoxycorticosterone [DOCP] to address hypoadrenocorticism increases [Na^+], although hypovolemia is likely to require crystalloid fluids).
- For animals that are not responsive to these treatments, calculate the Na^+ deficit.
  - Deficit = BW (kg) × 0.6 × (normal [Na^+] − patient [Na^+])
- If hyponatremia is of short duration (<24 hours), rapid correction with isotonic (0.9%) or hypertonic (3% or even 7.5%) saline is acceptable. Multiple formulas exist to determine infusion rate.
  - Administer the 3% saline at a rate of 0.5-2 mL/kg body weight (BW) per hour to increase the serum sodium level by 1-2 mEq/L/h.
  - For animals with hyponatremia-induced coma or seizures, can increase rate to 2-4 mL/kg/h until Na^+ is raised by 5-6 mEq/L (not to exceed 8-12 mEq/L/day).
  - Can give furosemide with saline to promote free-water excretion and prevent extracellular volume expansion, especially if the animal is not volume depleted (e.g., water intoxication).
- If hyponatremia has been present > 24 hours, gradual correction is essential. Rates should not exceed 0.5 mEq/L/h.
  - If the Na^+ is < 120 mEq/L, a maximum of only 10-12 mEq/L of sodium increase is recommended during the first 24-hour period and by no more than 18 mEq/L by 48 hours.
  - Rate (mL/h) = (0.6 × BW (kg) × (desired [Na^+] − measured [Na^+]) × 1000)/(fluid [Na^+] × hours) to target gradual correction.

Classification of Hyponatremia According to Plasma Tonicity and Volume Status

Plasma Tonicity		Example		Water and Na^+ Status
1	Isotonic		Pseudohyponatremia: hyperlipidemia, hyperproteinemia	Water normal, Na^+ normal
2	Hypertonic		Extreme hyperglycemia, mannitol infusion	Various effects; Na^+ can increase, or water can decrease
3	Hypotonic	a	Hypovolemic (overt volume contraction): GI loss, hemorrhage, Addison's disease, third spacing	Water and Na^+ depleted
		b	Hypervolemic (overtly edematous): CHF, cirrhosis, nephrotic syndrome	Water and Na^+ excess
		c	Euvolemic (volume status grossly clinically normal but mildly hypervolemic): SIADH, myxedema	Water excess, Na^+ normal

CHF, Congestive heart failure; *GI*, gastrointestinal; *Na^+*, sodium ion; *SIADH*, syndrome of inappropriate antidiuretic hormone. Isotonic = normosmolar; hypertonic = hyperosmolar; hypotonic = hypoosmolar.

Possible Complications

- Osmotic demyelination syndrome with too rapid correction
- Hypervolemia and cardiopulmonary overload when fluids are given to hypervolemic patient

Recommended Monitoring

During correction of hyponatremia of > 24 hours' duration, monitor serum sodium q 2-4h to avoid too rapid increase. Repeat neurologic evaluations several times each day.

PROGNOSIS & OUTCOME

Depend on underlying cause and ability to correctly restore serum Na^+ > 130 mEq/L in the absence of iatrogenic complications

PEARLS & CONSIDERATIONS

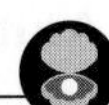

Comments

- If slow-onset hyponatremia, correct slowly. If rapid-onset hyponatremia, correct rapidly.
- Osmotic demyelination syndrome may not be evident for up to 2 weeks after overly rapid correction of hyponatremia.
- Water intoxication is uncommon but often is suggested by history (e.g., previously healthy dog on a recreational lake outing that develops sudden-onset ataxia and abnormal mentation).
- In humans, there are many reported causes of SIADH. Causes described in veterinary medicine include drugs, neoplasia, central nervous system disease, lung disease, and others.
- Hypoadrenocorticism is an important cause of low serum Na^+ with high potassium, but other causes include enterocolitis (e.g., whipworms), diabetes mellitus, renal disease, pregnancy, or effusive disease (e.g., chylothorax)

Prevention

Be alert to electrolyte abnormalities in any ill animal.

Technician Tips

Carefully monitor fluid rates during treatment of hyponatremia.

SUGGESTED READING

Guillaumin J, et al: Disorders of sodium and water homeostasis. Vet Clin Small Anim 47:293-312, 2017.

AUTHOR: Michael Schaer, DVM, DACVIM, DACVECC
EDITOR: Leah A. Cohn, DVM, PhD, DACVIM

Hypoparathyroidism, Primary

Client Education Sheet

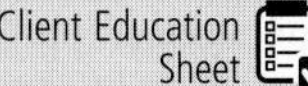

BASIC INFORMATION

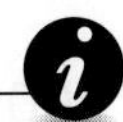

Definition

Absolute or relative deficiency of parathyroid hormone (PTH) due to parathyroid gland destruction or atrophy, causing hypocalcemia

Synonyms

Vitamin D_2: ergocalciferol; vitamin D_3: cholecalciferol; calcitriol: 1,25-dihydroxycholecalciferol, 1,25-dihydroxyvitamin D, activated vitamin D_3

Epidemiology

SPECIES, AGE, SEX

- Uncommon disorder of dogs; rare in cats
- Dogs: any age, either sex may be affected
- Cats: young to middle-aged, male predominance

GENETICS, BREED PREDISPOSITION

Toy poodles, miniature schnauzers, Saint Bernards (in Australia)

Clinical Presentation

HISTORY, CHIEF COMPLAINT

Sporadic or episodic signs related to hypocalcemia (p. 515)

- Most common
  - Focal or diffuse muscle tremors or twitching that may worsen with exercise or excitement
  - Seizures
  - Stiff gait, muscle pain/cramping

- Weakness, decreased activity (especially in cats)
- Less common
  - Facial rubbing
  - Biting/licking paws
  - Behavior changes (e.g., being restless, nervous, anxious, aggressive, reluctant to be touched)
  - Excessive panting
  - Vomiting, diarrhea, weight loss

PHYSICAL EXAM FINDINGS

- Neuromuscular signs; raised nictitans possible (cats)
- Additional findings may include hyperthermia (from muscle fasciculation), tense abdomen, thin body condition, or cataracts.
- Physical exam may be normal.

Etiology and Pathophysiology

- Naturally occurring disease is most commonly due to immune-mediated destruction or idiopathic atrophy of the parathyroid glands. Hypoparathyroidism can also result from parathyroid or thyroid surgery.
- In normal animals, hypocalcemia results in increased PTH secretion. However, with hypoparathyroidism, the parathyroid glands are unable to respond.
- Loss of PTH results in sustained, potentially severe hypocalcemia and hyperphosphatemia.
  - Hypocalcemia results from decreased calcium resorption from bone, decreased intestinal calcium absorption, and increased renal calcium excretion.
  - Hyperphosphatemia occurs due to decreased renal phosphate excretion.
- Loss of the membrane-stabilizing effect of ionized calcium on nerve cells causes increased central and peripheral nervous tissue excitability.

DIAGNOSIS

Diagnostic Overview

Concurrent hypocalcemia and hyperphosphatemia in a patient with normal renal function strongly suggests primary hypoparathyroidism. The diagnosis is confirmed by evaluating concurrent serum ionized calcium and PTH concentrations.

Differential Diagnosis

Hypocalcemia (pp. 515 and 1239)

Initial Database

- CBC and urinalysis: unremarkable
- Serum biochemical profile: hypocalcemia and hyperphosphatemia, normal renal parameters. Measure serum magnesium (Mg) as well.
- Confirm hypocalcemia.
  - Repeat calcium measurement on a separate blood sample. Use of EDTA plasma or EDTA contamination of sample causes a falsely low result.
  - Measure serum ionized calcium concentration.
  - Formulas to correct serum calcium to account for serum albumin or protein concentrations are NOT recommended.

Advanced or Confirmatory Testing

- Hypoparathyroidism is confirmed by evaluating concurrent serum ionized calcium and PTH concentrations; both usually are decreased.
- A low-normal serum PTH concentration is inappropriate if ionized calcium is low; in a patient with a low ionized calcium, a serum PTH concentration that is decreased or low-normal supports a diagnosis of hypoparathyroidism.

TREATMENT

Treatment Overview

- The goal of therapy is to increase serum total calcium above the threshold for clinical signs and maintain it just below or at the low end of the reference range (e.g., 8-9.5 mg/dL [2-2.4 mmol/L]). Lifelong therapy for primary hypoparathyroidism is required. Hypocalcemia caused by parathyroidectomy can be transient as long as ≥ 1 parathyroid gland remains.
- Therapy must be individualized, and frequent monitoring and adjustment of drug dosages are required. Overtreatment resulting in hypercalcemia must be avoided.
- The need for acute emergency therapy varies, depending on the severity of presenting signs.
- Referral is indicated if 24-hour care and in-house serum calcium monitoring cannot be provided during the stabilization period.

Acute General Treatment

For hypocalcemic tetany (p. 515)

Chronic Treatment

Subacute/early chronic treatment:

- Oral vitamin D
  - Calcitriol is the preparation of choice. It is faster- and shorter-acting than ergocalciferol and much less likely to cause hypercalcemia but more expensive. Initial dosage: 0.01-0.015 mcg/kg PO q 12h × 3-4 days. Maintenance dosage: 0.005-0.015 mcg/kg PO q 24h. Time to maximal effect is 1-4 days. Time required for relief of toxicosis is 1-14 days.
  - Ergocalciferol is rarely used due to its long half-life and potential for persistent hypercalcemia (up to 18 weeks).
  - Dihydrotachysterol is no longer available.
- Oral calcium
  - Dose: 25 mg/kg elemental calcium q 8-12h
  - The amount of elemental calcium per tablet varies with the preparation (p. 1205). Calcium carbonate is preferred; 750 mg of calcium carbonate contains 300 mg of elemental calcium.
  - After serum calcium concentration is stable and the patient is eating well, oral calcium can be tapered over 2-3 weeks and then discontinued because dietary calcium is usually adequate.
- Parenteral calcium administration is usually needed while awaiting oral vitamin D and oral calcium supplementation to take effect:
  - 10% calcium gluconate IV by constant-rate infusion (60-90 mg/kg q 24h; do not add to bicarbonate-containing fluids). SQ administration (p. 515) should not be used due to the potential for calcinosis cutis and skin necrosis. Calcium chloride is not recommended; perivascular administration can cause tissue necrosis and sloughing.
  - Monitor serum calcium concentrations q 12-24h and adjust dose to maintain serum calcium concentration between 8-9.5 mg/dL (2.0-2.4 mmol/L). When serum calcium concentrations have been consistently above 8 mg/dL (2 mmol/L) for 48 hours, parenteral calcium can be tapered and discontinued over 3-5 days by increasing the dosing interval.

Maintenance/long-term chronic treatment:

- Vitamin D should be slowly tapered to the lowest dose possible to maintain low-normal or slightly below normal calcium concentrations. Lifelong therapy is required for primary hypoparathyroidism.

Possible Complications

- Overzealous treatment with vitamin D may result in hypercalcemia and soft-tissue (renal) mineralization.
- Severe, extensive calcinosis cutis and epidermal necrosis after SQ administration of calcium gluconate for hypoparathyroidism have been described in dogs and a cat.
- Because lack of PTH results in hyperphosphatemia and calcitriol increases intestinal phosphorus absorption, hyperphosphatemia may occur. A low-phosphorus diet (e.g., formulated for chronic kidney disease) and a phosphate binder (e.g., aluminum hydroxide) may be indicated.

Recommended Monitoring

- During the stabilization phase, patients should be observed 24 hours/day for seizures and other signs of hypocalcemia.
- Initially, serum calcium and phosphorus concentrations should be measured at least q 12h, then with decreasing frequency as serum calcium concentration stabilizes. When patients are stable on maintenance oral vitamin D therapy, evaluation of serum calcium and phosphorus concentrations is recommended q 3-6 months.

PROGNOSIS & OUTCOME

With careful treatment and monitoring, prognosis is excellent.

PEARLS & CONSIDERATIONS

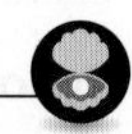

Comments

- Always measure serum Mg in a patient with apparent primary hypoparathyroidism. If

severe deficiency exists, correcting hypomagnesemia may resolve the hypoparathyroidism.
- Over-the-counter vitamin D supplements are not appropriate for treatment.
- Glucocorticoids may worsen/precipitate hypocalcemia associated with hypoparathyroidism.

Technician Tips

- Hyperthermia in hypocalcemic patients usually results from muscle fasciculations, not true fever. Cooling measures (e.g., moistening paw pads, fan/air circulation) may be appropriate, but antipyretic drugs (e.g., nonsteroidal antiinflammatories) are not.
- Compounded calcitriol formulations have variable stabilities. It is best to use an experienced compounding pharmacy and to heed the labeled expiration date.

Client Education

- Appropriate therapy requires repeated evaluation of serum calcium concentrations. Monitoring will become less intensive as serum calcium concentrations stabilize, but clients should be prepared for frequent rechecks.
- Treatment must be lifelong with naturally occurring hypoparathyroidism.

SUGGESTED READING

Henderson AK, et al: Hypoparathyroidism: pathophysiology and diagnosis. Compend Contin Educ Vet 27:270-279, 2005.

AUTHOR: Patty Lathan, VMD, MS, DACVIM
EDITOR: Ellen N. Behrend, VMD, PhD, DACVIM

Hypoplastic Trachea

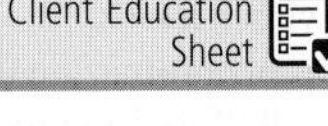

BASIC INFORMATION

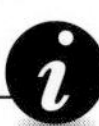

Definition

Congenital narrowing of the tracheal lumen

Epidemiology

SPECIES, AGE, SEX

Dogs < 1 year old but persists for life; 2:1 males:females; not reported in cats

GENETICS, BREED PREDISPOSITION

- Of reported dogs, 55% are bulldogs and 15% are Boston terriers.
- Reported as a recessive trait in Husky-mix puppies with blue eyes and partially white faces

ASSOCIATED DISORDERS

- Brachycephalic airway syndrome (BAS):
  - Hypoplastic trachea seen in 13% dogs with BAS
    - Elongated soft palate in 43% of dogs with hypoplastic trachea, stenotic nares in 22%
- Other congenital anomalies (pulmonic or aortic stenosis, megaesophagus) or respiratory abnormalities (bronchopneumonia, laryngeal paralysis, everted laryngeal saccules, laryngeal collapse) may be present.

Clinical Presentation

HISTORY, CHIEF COMPLAINT

- Incidental finding in ≈10% of affected dogs
- Recurrent respiratory infections poorly responsive to treatment
- Clinical signs associated with concurrent brachycephalic syndrome such as stertor, stridor, exercise intolerance, lethargy, coughing, gagging, regurgitation, syncope

PHYSICAL EXAM FINDINGS

- Physical exam can be unremarkable.
- Respiratory signs (e.g., dyspnea [predominantly inspiratory], cough, inspiratory stridor if laryngeal abnormalities, stertor if elongated soft palate), bronchopneumonia (e.g., increased lung sounds, fever, lethargy, tachypnea, increased respiratory effort)
- Hyperthermia

Etiology and Pathophysiology

- Trachea develops with rigid cartilaginous rings, ring ends apposed/overlapped, and dorsal membrane narrow/absent, narrowing the tracheal lumen.
- Narrowed tracheal lumen increases linear air velocity, tracheal resistance, and work of respiration.

DIAGNOSIS

Diagnostic Overview

Diagnosis is based on comparison of tracheal diameter to thoracic inlet diameter or by tracheoscopic evaluation. Normal tracheal diameter is smaller in bulldogs than in other breeds.

Differential Diagnosis

- Elongated soft palate
- Everted laryngeal saccules
- Stenotic nares
- Laryngeal paralysis or collapse
- Tracheal collapse
- Any cause of bronchopneumonia or tracheobronchitis
- Ciliary dyskinesia

Initial Database

- CBC: inflammatory leukogram ± left shift possible if bronchopneumonia present
- Serum biochemistry panel and urinalysis: usually normal
- Thoracic radiographs
  - Diffusely narrowed tracheal lumen
  - Bronchopneumonia in approximately 8% of cases at the time they present for care

Advanced or Confirmatory Testing

- Decreased tracheal diameter on lateral thoracic radiographs, CT, or tracheoscopy
  - On radiographs and CT, diffuse symmetrical (round) narrowing
  - TD/TI ratio is the ratio of tracheal diameter (TD) at the level of the thoracic inlet to the thoracic inlet diameter (TI). TI is the distance from the ventral aspect of the vertebral column at the midpoint of the first rib to the closest point on the inner surface of the manubrium. For dogs older than 6 months, radiographic TD/TI < 0.18 for breeds other than bulldogs and < 0.14-0.15 for bulldogs is diagnostic for tracheal hypoplasia.
  - CT measurements average 19% larger than tracheal measurements.
  - Persian cats have the same tracheal diameter as nonbrachycephalic cats.
  - Diameter measured with tracheoscopy does not correlate with CT or radiography.
- Tracheoscopy: luminal narrowing, mucosal swelling, overlapping tracheal cartilage rings, narrow dorsal membrane
- Airway lavage in dogs with bronchopneumonia for cytology plus bacterial culture and sensitivity (pp. 1073 and 1074)

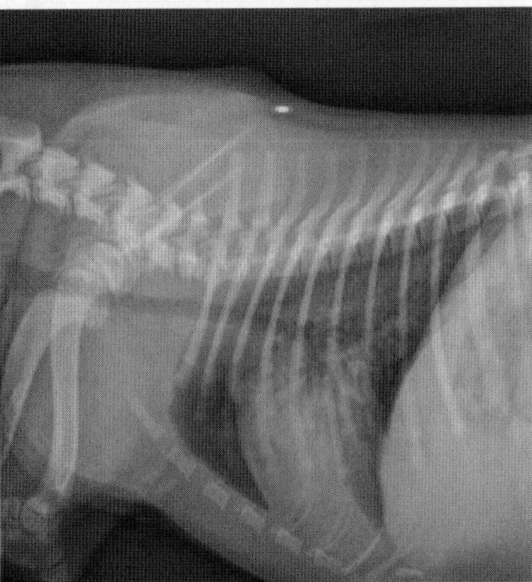

HYPOPLASTIC TRACHEA Hypoplastic trachea in a 4-month-old pug with seizures and stenotic nares. On necropsy, the puppy's trachea had complete (solid) cartilaginous rings and no dorsal longitudinal membrane.

TREATMENT

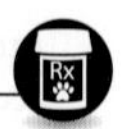

Treatment Overview

Animals with tracheal hypoplasia usually present with signs caused by other abnormalities (e.g., elongated soft palate, stenotic nares, pneumonia). Direct treatment toward correction of the abnormality that is the primary cause of clinical signs, and treat secondary infections when present. Delay surgery for stenotic nares and elongated soft palate in animals with pneumonia until lungs have improved radiographically, unless severe dyspnea is present.

Acute General Treatment

- Oxygen supplementation if needed (p. 1146)
- Sedation if dyspnea/ hyperpnea associated with stress
  - Acepromazine 0.03-0.05 mg/kg IV (e.g., 0.25-0.5 mg total dose for medium-sized dog) with butorphanol 0.2-0.4 mg/kg IV q 2-4h as needed
- For bronchopneumonia, broad-spectrum antibiotic treatment based ideally on results of culture and sensitivity (p. 795)

Chronic Treatment

- Reduce weight if obese
- Limit exercise, avoid heat (prone to hyperthermia)
- Reduce stress. Consider trazodone for home use (2-5 mg/kg PO; max dose 14 mg/kg).
- Correct associated structural respiratory defects (p. 128).

Possible Complications

Death from severe respiratory distress, bronchopneumonia, or hyperthermia

Recommended Monitoring

Repeat thoracic films for dogs with bronchopneumonia. Radiographic improvement can lag several days behind clinical improvement.

PROGNOSIS & OUTCOME

- In the absence of concurrent respiratory disease, hypoplastic trachea is well tolerated. Mortality rate (death or euthanasia) of 50% reflects associated respiratory disease or other defects (e.g., megaesophagus, cardiac disease).
- In bulldog puppies, TD/TI ratios can increase with growth to mature body size and resolution of bronchopneumonia.

PEARLS & CONSIDERATIONS

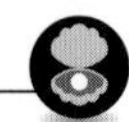

Comments

- Dyspnea is not related to the degree of tracheal lumen diameter narrowing but to presence of other diseases.
- Interobserver agreement on radiographic measuring techniques is poor, making them unreliable.
- Hypoplastic trachea does not affect outcome of surgery for elongated soft palate or stenotic nares.
- Some generalized increase in tracheal diameter, attributed to resolution of tracheal mucosal edema, may be seen after clinical improvement of respiratory event.
- Tracheal size may improve after bulldogs reach adulthood. Of young dogs with hypoplastic trachea, 60% are clinically normal > 6 months after diagnosis.

Prevention

Affected animals should not be bred.

Technician Tips

- Normal bulldogs have a smaller tracheal diameter than other breeds and therefore need smaller endotracheal tubes when undergoing general anesthesia.
- Trauma during intubation may cause mucosal swelling and edema, further narrowing the airway.

Client Education

- Consider thoracic radiographs of bulldogs and Boston terriers before breeding.
- Affected dogs have lifelong risk of respiratory infections and dyspnea.

SUGGESTED READING

Coyne BE, et al: Hypoplasia of the trachea in dogs: 103 cases (1974-1990). J Am Vet Med Assoc 2017:68-772, 1992.

AUTHOR: Karen M. Tobias, DVM, MS, DACVS
EDITOR: Megan Grobman, DVM, MS, DACVIM

Hypopyon

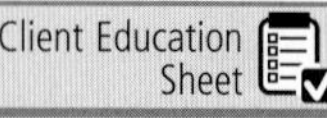

BASIC INFORMATION

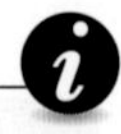

Definition

Presence of settled white blood cells in the anterior chamber

Synonyms

Purulent debris (pus) in the anterior chamber

Epidemiology

SPECIES, AGE, SEX

Dogs and cats, no age or sex predisposition

RISK FACTORS

- Keratomalacia (melting corneal ulcer) (p. 209)
- Any cause of anterior uveitis or endophthalmitis (bacterial, fungal, viral, parasitic or immune mediated) (p. 1023)
- Metastatic or primary ocular neoplasia (p. 559)
- Prior intraocular surgery (especially cataract surgery)

ASSOCIATED DISORDERS

Hypopyon is always secondary to anterior uveitis. Other concurrent diseases relate to causes of anterior uveitis.

Clinical Presentation

HISTORY, CHIEF COMPLAINT

Creamy white to light tan debris settled in the ventral aspect of the anterior chamber is often associated with a cloudy, red, painful eye. There may also be blepharospasm and an elevated nictitating membrane.

PHYSICAL EXAM FINDINGS

- Creamy white to light tan opacity settled in ventral anterior chamber. The cells may be subtle and obscured by the nictitating membrane or may fill much of the anterior chamber. Rarely is the entire anterior chamber involved.
- Aqueous flare
- ± Corneal edema
- Conjunctival/episcleral hyperemia
- ± Corneal neovascularization (p. 212)
- ± Keratitic precipitates
- Epiphora to mucopurulent discharge
- Intraocular pressure (IOP) may be low acutely, but with chronicity, secondary glaucoma may occur.
- ± Corneal ulceration
- ± Abnormal physical exam

Etiology and Pathophysiology

- Hypopyon is produced by a strong leukocyte stimulus such as local or systemic bacterial or fungal infections. Even in these cases, aqueous humor cultures are often negative, and therefore aqueocentesis is rarely indicated.
- Complicated corneal ulcers (infected or malacic) often lead to uveitis and hypopyon.
- Lymphoma and leukemia may increase anterior chamber cells to the point of producing hypopyon.
- The cells accumulate in ventral anterior chamber due to gravity and egress the eye by the iridocorneal angle.

DIAGNOSIS

Diagnostic Overview

The diagnosis is based on classic appearance with associated aqueous flare. Hypopyon can be difficult to appreciate if mild and hidden by an elevated nictitating membrane. Tilting the nose ventrally (causing the globe to rotate dorsally) can allow visualization of mild hypopyon.

Differential Diagnosis

- Lipid-laden aqueous humor: complete cloudiness of the anterior chamber with variably opaque, whitish aqueous humor with minimal hyperemia and blepharospasm. It is most commonly seen in dogs with diabetes mellitus or hyperlipidemia but also seen in dogs that eat a large amount of fat.
- Fibrin in the anterior chamber can occur with anterior uveitis. Fibrin is usually in strands and can be throughout anterior chamber. Conglomerations of fibrin may be noted but are less dense than hypopyon and more amorphous.

Initial Database

- Complete physical exam
- Complete ophthalmic exam (p. 1137)
- If no ocular cause (corneal ulceration, trauma) is found, advanced testing should be done.

Advanced or Confirmatory Testing

- CBC, serum biochemistries, urinalysis
- Thoracic radiographs
- Infectious disease diagnostics, depending on location or travel history
- Ocular ultrasound if posterior segment is not visible (to determine if a retinal detachment is present)
- Aqueocentesis for cytology and culture in selected cases (e.g., lymphoma suspects)

TREATMENT

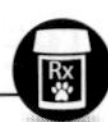

Treatment Overview

Treatment goal is to control the inciting cause if identified and treat underlying anterior uveitis.

Acute General Treatment

Topical antiinflammatory therapy:

- Corticosteroid (prednisolone or dexamethasone) q 6h initially. Do not use if corneal ulceration is present.
- Nonsteroidal antiinflammatory medications (e.g., diclofenac, ketorolac) q 6h initially; can be used in conjunction with topical steroids

Oral antiinflammatory therapy

- Corticosteroid (prednisone): do not use until systemic infectious disease has been ruled out and best to avoid with corneal ulceration.
- Nonsteroidal antiinflammatory medications (e.g., meloxicam, deracoxib) cannot be used in conjunction with oral steroids but can be used with either or both types of topical antiinflammatory drugs.

Cycloplegic:

- Atropine q 6-24h is used to stabilize the blood-aqueous barrier to lessen leukocyte influx into the anterior chamber. It minimizes posterior synechiae by causing mydriasis.
- Do not use if IOP are high-normal or elevated because atropine may increase risk of glaucoma.

Chronic Treatment

Treat underlying cause if present. The hypopyon usually resolves within several days of appropriate therapy.

Possible Complications

Ocular complications may include glaucoma, cataract, posterior synechiae, and endothelial cell degeneration (persistent corneal edema).

Recommended Monitoring

- Recheck daily to weekly initially until hypopyon and aqueous flare begin to resolve. Slowly wean down/off oral and then topical antiinflammatory medications over weeks to months after aqueous flare/hypopyon have resolved.
- Other monitoring is dictated by the underlying cause of the anterior uveitis/hypopyon.

PROGNOSIS & OUTCOME

Guarded, depending an inciting cause, degree of aqueous flare, degree of hypopyon, and presence of any secondary complications

PEARLS & CONSIDERATIONS

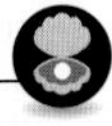

Comments

Differentiating lipid-laden aqueous humor from hypopyon is important. Lipid-laden aqueous humor is rarely painful and almost always fills the entire anterior chamber.

Technician Tips

Motion and shaking the head can rapidly change the appearance of the hypopyon.

Client Education

Trying to identify the underlying cause is important because it can dictate the prognosis.

SUGGESTED READING

Bergstrom BE, et al: Canine panuveitis: a retrospective evaluation of 55 cases (2000-2015). Vet Ophthalmol 20:390-397, 2017.

AUTHOR: Brian Skorobohach, DVM, DACVO
EDITOR: Diane V. H. Hendrix, DVM, DACVO

Hypothermia

BASIC INFORMATION

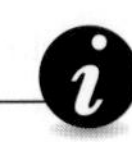

Definition

Core body temperature < 99.5°F (37.5°C) in dogs, < 100°F (37.8°C) in cats

Epidemiology

SPECIES, AGE, SEX

Any dog or cat

RISK FACTORS

- Neonates and geriatric patients
- General anesthesia
- Cold environment
- Cardiac disease (low rectal temperature, core temperature usually normal)
- Systemic inflammatory response/sepsis (cats)
- Hypothyroidism (dogs)
- Renal disease (generally mild hypothermia)
- Head trauma

Clinical Presentation

DISEASE FORMS/SUBTYPES

- Mild hypothermia: 90°F-99.5°F (32.2°C-37.5°C)
- Moderate hypothermia: 82°F-90°F (27.8°C-32.2°C)
- Severe hypothermia: <82°F (27.8°C)

HISTORY, CHIEF COMPLAINT

- Weak/collapsed patient
- Exposure to cold environmental temperatures
- Recovering from or undergoing general anesthesia

PHYSICAL EXAM FINDINGS

- Shivering
- Weakness, ataxia
- Cardiac arrhythmia (generally bradyarrhythmia)
- Hypotension
- Coma
- Other abnormalities may be related to underlying disease (e.g., dermatologic change related to hypothyroidism, heart murmur related to cardiac disease).

Etiology and Pathophysiology

- Initial compensation: peripheral vasoconstriction, shivering (not if patient anesthetized), piloerection
- Respiratory rate/effort

- Increased with mild hypothermia
- Decreased with moderate to severe hypothermia (central and reflex-mediated respiratory depression)
- Cardiovascular effects
  - Mild hypothermia initially induces mild tachycardia and increased cardiac output.
  - Moderate hypothermia may produce bradycardia, atrial fibrillation, and rarely Osborn or J waves (positive electrocardiographic [ECG] deflection after S wave).
  - Decreased vascular tone can result in hypotension.
  - Severe hypothermia can cause cardiac arrest from ventricular fibrillation.
- Central nervous system effects: shivering, stupor, unconsciousness, coma
- Gastrointestinal (GI) effects: GI tract ulceration, pancreatitis
- Renal effects
  - Cold-induced diuresis can lead to hypovolemia.
  - Impaired renal perfusion can lead to ischemic tubular necrosis.
- Clinicopathologic changes
  - Lactic acidosis secondary to hypoperfusion
  - Leukopenia
  - Hyperglycemia
  - Glucosuria
  - Hyperkalemia
  - Hemostatic dysfunction: thrombocytopenia (splenic sequestration), coagulopathy, slower rate of clot formation assessed by thromboelastography

DIAGNOSIS

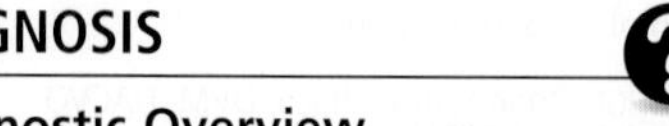

Diagnostic Overview

Diagnosis is made by measuring body temperature. Historical features increase the index of suspicion and are important for early recognition and treatment. Consideration of significant underlying disease predisposing to systemic hypoperfusion (and thus low rectal temperature) is especially important in cats (e.g., congestive heart failure, sepsis).

Differential Diagnosis

Artifactual low temperature with malfunction of thermometer or improper insertion

Initial Database

- Documentation of rectal or core body temperature < 99.5°F (37.5°C)
- Packed cell volume, total solids, glucose, serum electrolytes

Advanced or Confirmatory Testing

ECG:

- Sinus bradycardia: common, usually not treated beyond rewarming
- Ventricular arrhythmias are common (p. 1033).
- Mild changes (PR, QT, QRS prolongation). Osborn or J waves possible but less commonly observed.

Other diagnostics are aimed at discovering underlying cause of hypothermia (e.g., thyroid testing, echocardiogram) if cause is not obvious.

TREATMENT

Treatment Overview

- Restore body temperature to normal range.
- Treatment of hypothermia varies with
  - Degree of hypothermia
  - Underlying systemic diseases (cardiovascular, septic, neurologic, endocrine)

Acute General Treatment

- Place intravenous (IV) catheter. In the unconscious patient, endotracheal intubation and oxygen supplementation (reduce risk of aspiration pneumonia and arrhythmias) may be required.
- Rewarming: depending on severity of hypothermia, three methods are useful.
  - Passive external rewarming for mild to moderate hypothermia. Animal is wrapped in blankets, bubble wrap, or foil to prevent further loss of heat.
  - Active external rewarming for moderate to severe hypothermia. Apply heat (warm water bags, heating pads, warm incubator, Bair Hugger) to patient's torso. Be careful to limit direct contact with warming devices to prevent burns (i.e., always separate the warming device from the patient using a towel).
  - Active internal rewarming is reserved for refractory or severe hypothermia (<86°F [30°C]). Options include gastric, colonic, and/or urinary bladder lavage with 109°F (42.8°C) warm 0.9% NaCl; peritoneal dialysis with warm 0.9% NaCl at 10-20 mL/kg and an exchange rate of every 30 minutes; warmed IV fluids using dry heat fluid warmer; and/or increase inspired air temperature for animals on a ventilator.
- Continuous ECG
  - Bradyarrhythmia does not respond reliably to atropine (avoid); improvement in heart rate should occur with rewarming.
  - The hypothermic heart does not respond well to antiarrhythmic drugs until temperature is > 86°F (30°C). For ventricular arrhythmias, lidocaine is generally ineffective, and procainamide is associated with an increased incidence of ventricular fibrillation in humans.
  - The possibility for ventricular fibrillation exists, and defibrillation may be necessary. The cold heart is relatively resistant to defibrillation; if defibrillation is unsuccessful, rewarm patient, and again attempt defibrillation.
- Many hypothermic patients are dehydrated. Administer warm IV fluids (exception: cats with hypothermia caused by severe heart failure). Fluid rate needs to be monitored closely due to poor cardiac function and severe peripheral vasoconstriction. A conservative bolus (e.g., 10 mL/kg of isotonic crystalloid) can be given, with further boluses as needed.
- Once stable, assess for underlying predisposing factor.

Possible Complications

- During the rewarming process, the extremities reduce vasoconstriction, and sequestered cold blood mixes with the central circulation. Relatively warm core blood then perfuses the cold peripheral tissues. These two mechanisms cause afterdrop, a decrease in body temperature during the rewarming process.
- Burns may result from exuberant rewarming with high-temperature devices.

Recommended Monitoring

- Neurologic status during rewarming
- ECG
- Serum glucose, potassium, urea nitrogen, and creatinine levels
- Monitor fluid administration: heart rate, pulse quality, blood pressure urine output
  - Urine output target: 1-2 mL/kg/h

PROGNOSIS & OUTCOME

Depends on degree of hypothermia and cause

PEARLS & CONSIDERATIONS

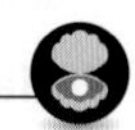

Comments

- Rewarming procedures should be tapered when the body temperature is still slightly below normal to avoid inadvertent hyperthermia.
- Because unconscious patients are unable to move away from a heat source, careful monitoring (e.g., body temperature q 15 minutes initially) is essential during rewarming. Burns and deaths associated with iatrogenic hyperthermia can result from inadequate monitoring.
- Intentional therapeutic hypothermia is uncommonly performed in animals compared with people. It may have neurologic advantages after successful cardiopulmonary resuscitation, but data for animals are unavailable.

Prevention

- Avoid exposure to low environmental temperature (especially in the very young or elderly).
- Avoid prolonged general anesthesia, and use measures to maintain normothermia during anesthesia.

Technician Tips

- Monitor rectal or esophageal temperature closely in pets at risk.
- Avoid more than mild hypothermia during anesthesia.

Client Education

Keep pets in a protected environment during cold weather. Do not allow dogs to play on ice-covered ponds or lakes.

SUGGESTED READING

Brodeur A, et al: Hypothermia and targeted temperature management in cats and dogs. J Vet Emerg Crit Care 27(2):151-163, 2017.

AUTHORS: Alex Lynch, BVSc, DACVECC, MRCVS
EDITOR: Benjamin M. Brainard, VMD, DACVAA, DACVECC

Hypothyroidism

Client Education Sheet

BASIC INFORMATION

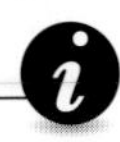

Definition

Clinical syndrome that occurs as a result of decreased circulating levels of serum thyroid hormones

Epidemiology

SPECIES, AGE, SEX

- Dogs: middle-aged at onset (2-9 years of age), no sex predisposition, rare in puppies (i.e., congenital form)
- Cats: spontaneous and congenital hypothyroidism rare; iatrogenic disease in middle-aged or older cats

GENETICS, BREED PREDISPOSITION

- Dogs: can occur in any breed, including mixed breeds
- Reported to be more prevalent in boxers, dachshunds, Doberman pinschers, golden retrievers, Great Danes, Irish setters, miniature schnauzers, poodles, and a number of other breeds
- Genetic risk loci have been identified in some breeds.

ASSOCIATED DISORDERS

Can rarely occur as part of an autoimmune polyglandular syndrome along with hypoadrenocorticism or diabetes mellitus

Clinical Presentation

DISEASE FORMS/SUBTYPES

- Primary hypothyroidism (most common): lymphocytic infiltration or atrophy of the thyroid gland
- Congenital hypothyroidism: rare
- Secondary hypothyroidism (rare): inadequate pituitary secretion of thyroid-stimulating hormone (TSH)
- Iatrogenic hypothyroidism resulting from treatment of hyperthyroidism (cats)

HISTORY, CHIEF COMPLAINT

- Acquired disease: signs are often nonspecific and gradual in onset.
  - Metabolic: weight gain, lethargy, mental dullness, exercise intolerance/inactivity, and cold intolerance are common.
  - Dermatologic: bilaterally symmetrical, truncal alopecia or thin hair, hyperkeratosis, seborrhea, hyperpigmentation, otitis, "rat tail," and pyoderma are often present, with alopecia or thin hair most common.
  - Reproductive: persistent anestrus, decreased libido, decreased survival of puppies born to hypothyroid dams
  - Neuromuscular: weakness/exercise intolerance sometimes seen; other signs (ataxia, seizures, facial drooping/paralysis, head tilt/circling [vestibular signs], and stridor/change in bark [laryngeal paralysis]) are uncommon.
  - Possible behavioral changes (e.g., aggression)
- Myxedema coma, characterized by profound mental dullness, stupor, hypothermia, hypoventilation, bradycardia, and hypotension, has been reported rarely.
- Congenital hypothyroidism: disproportionate dwarfism, short limbs, persistent puppy coat or alopecia/thin dull hair, broad head, thick protruding tongue, mental dullness/retardation, delayed dental eruption, constipation
- Iatrogenic hypothyroidism in cats: can follow treatment for hyperthyroidism. Signs may be absent or vague. If present, signs of lethargy, weight gain, inappetence, constipation, and dermatologic signs (especially seborrhea and ease of epilation) predominate.

PHYSICAL EXAM FINDINGS

- Exam findings are similar to signs described by the owners (see above).
- Additional findings (uncommon) include ocular changes (corneal lipid deposits most common), bradycardia, hypothermia, constipation, facial paresis, vestibular signs, and decreased spinal reflexes.

Etiology and Pathophysiology

- Primary hypothyroidism is usually due to lymphocytic thyroiditis or idiopathic thyroid gland atrophy (uncommonly due to infiltrative neoplasia).
- Secondary hypothyroidism (rare): decreased TSH secretion leads to atrophy of the follicular cells of the thyroid gland. Loss of TSH secretion can occur as a result of a congenital pituitary malformation or pituitary neoplasia.
- Tertiary hypothyroidism (decreased secretion of thyrotropin-releasing hormone [TRH]) has rarely been reported in dogs.
- Iatrogenic hypothyroidism can occur as a result of antithyroid medications (e.g., methimazole in cats), bilateral thyroidectomy, or radioiodine (I-131) therapy (p. 503).
- Clinical signs reflect the widespread metabolic effects of thyroid hormones.
- Surgery or anesthesia, a wide range of concurrent illnesses, and various nonthyroidal medications (e.g., glucocorticoids, phenobarbital, sulfonamides, carprofen, clomipramine) also decrease circulating thyroid hormone concentrations; clinical hypothyroidism does not result from any with the exception of sulfonamides.

DIAGNOSIS

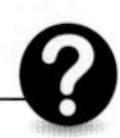

Diagnostic Overview

- The diagnosis should be suspected in a young to middle-aged dog presenting with one or more common clinical sign. Confirmation is not always straightforward, but the presence of typical clinical signs in conjunction with a decreased serum T_4 or free T_4 after equilibrium dialysis (FT_4ED) concentrations and an increased serum TSH concentration can be considered diagnostic.
- Diagnosis of iatrogenic hypothyroidism in cats is based on clinical signs combined with low serum T_4 and increased serum TSH concentrations (measured with a canine TSH assay).

Differential Diagnosis

- Alopecia (p. 47)
- Cutaneous cornification disorders (p. 214)
- Obesity/weight gain (p. 700)
- Hypercholesterolemia (p. 1234)

Initial Database

- CBC, serum biochemical profile, urinalysis: hypercholesterolemia is most common (must be differentiated from normal postprandial hypercholesterolemia [p. 1324]). A mild normocytic, normochromic, nonregenerative anemia; fasting hyperlipidemia/hypertriglyceridemia; mild increases in liver enzymes; and a mild increase in creatinine kinase may also be seen.
- Basal serum total thyroxine concentration [T_4]
  - Includes free (<1%) and protein-bound (>99%) T_4
  - Measurement of a concentration below the reference range in dogs has a sensitivity of 89%-100%, specificity of 75%-82%, and accuracy of 85%.
  - If T_4 is in the middle or upper end of the reference range, hypothyroidism is generally ruled out. An exception is the presence of antithyroid antibodies that interfere with some assays; if clinical signs strongly suggest hypothyroidism and T_4 or FT_4ED is normal, advanced thyroid testing is recommended.
  - T_4 that is low or at the low end of the reference range may be due to hypothyroidism, concurrent illness, or medications or may be normal (euthyroid). Be aware that certain breeds such as sighthounds, Alaskan sled dogs, and Chinese Shar-peis normally have significantly lower T_4 concentrations (approximately one-half of reference range of other breeds).
- Basal serum FT_4ED
  - Measures only free (i.e., metabolically available) T_4 fraction
  - An assay based on equilibrium dialysis should be used; it is more time intensive and expensive than radioimmunoassay but much more accurate.
  - Measurement of a concentration below the reference range in dogs has a sensitivity of 80%-98%, specificity of 93%-94%, accuracy of 95%.

  - Most accurate single-hormone test for diagnosis of hypothyroidism
- Basal serum TSH concentration: a validated canine TSH assay should be used. The test should not be evaluated alone but is best used in conjunction with T_4 and/or FT_4ED results.
  - High TSH with low T_4: sensitivity of 63%-67%, specificity of 98%-100%, accuracy of 82%-88%
  - High TSH with low FT_4ED: sensitivity of 74%, specificity of 98%, accuracy of 86%
  - Increased TSH with decreased T_4 or FT_4ED is strongly supportive of hypothyroidism.
  - A normal TSH in conjunction with decreased T_4 or FT_4ED does not rule out hypothyroidism, and if clinically relevant, advanced thyroid testing is recommended.
- See relevant laboratory tests (pp. 1385 and 1386).
- Measurement of serum T3 concentration is not helpful for the diagnosis of hypothyroidism.

Advanced or Confirmatory Testing

If basal thyroid hormone concentrations do not rule in/out hypothyroidism, additional options exist. TSH stimulation tests and thyroid scintigraphy are considered gold standards.

- TSH stimulation test
  - Several protocols exist; consult the laboratory performing the thyroid assays for the desired protocol and reference ranges for baseline and poststimulation T_4 concentrations.
  - Recombinant human TSH aliquoted and frozen in small syringes is used (50-150 mcg IV); evaluate serum T_4 concentrations in samples drawn before administration and 6-hour after administration. In patients with suspected or confirmed concurrent nonthyroidal systemic illness or receiving medication that may lower total T_4 concentrations, the higher dosage should be used.
- Thyroid scintigraphy can differentiate between hypothyroidism and nonthyroidal illness but is limited by availability.
- Serum thyroglobulin antibodies: increased levels suggest the presence of lymphocytic thyroiditis but occur in only ≈60% of hypothyroid dogs. Lymphocytic thyroiditis does not correlate with the presence of or always lead to hypothyroidism.
- Serum thyroid hormone antibodies: can interfere with testing and lead to spuriously high T_4 results, depending on the T_4 assay used
- Histopathologic evaluation of skin biopsies: epidermal and follicular infundibular hyperplasia is usually found. Vacuolated or hypertrophied erector pili muscles, increased dermal mucin, and a thickened dermis are consistent with hypothyroidism. If biopsy samples are taken from areas with alopecia, signs of hair growth cycle arrest are seen, and follicles are commonly in a hairless, telogen phase.
- Most patients, even those without hypothyroidism, temporarily show some response to therapy with thyroid hormones (e.g., increased activity). Therefore, response to therapy as a confirmatory test should be avoided whenever possible.

TREATMENT

Treatment Overview

The mainstay of treatment is oral thyroid hormone replacement. Therapy should be designed to raise serum T_4 values to the normal range and eliminate clinical signs. Therapy is lifelong.

Acute General Treatment

- Hypothyroidism usually is a chronic condition that seldom requires acute therapy.
- Myxedema coma (rare): levothyroxine for injection 5 mcg/kg IV q 12h until oral administration possible

Chronic Treatment

Oral thyroid supplementation: levothyroxine sodium (synthetic T_4):

- Initial dose (tablets)
  - In dogs, 0.01-0.02 mg/kg PO q 12h. Maximum dose 0.8 mg/DOG PO q 12h. If twice-daily administration is a problem, a once-daily dosage of 0.02 mg/kg is sufficient in many dogs.
  - In cats, initial dosage is 0.075 mg/CAT q 12h.
- A veterinary-licensed liquid formulation of L-thyroxine is available in many countries (not the United States); dose in dogs is 0.02 mg/kg PO q 24h.
- With concurrent heart failure, kidney disease, liver disease, hypoadrenocorticism, or diabetes mellitus, the initial dose should be decreased by 25%-50%, then slowly increased over the next 2-4 months.
- A brand-name veterinary preparation should be used because bioavailability of generic forms can vary.
- Adjust dose based on clinical response and serum T_4 concentrations (see Recommended Monitoring, below).
- Absorption kinetics vary between brands, and serum T_4 concentrations should be reassessed if the levothyroxine brand is changed.

Possible Complications

Iatrogenic hyperthyroidism

Recommended Monitoring

- A physical exam and serum thyroxine concentration (4-6 hours after pill) should be evaluated at 4-6 weeks, then q 6 months after euthyroidism is achieved.
  - Serum T_4 concentrations (4-6 hours after pill) should be in the upper one-half or just above the normal range. In most cases, monitoring serum TSH concentrations does not offer any additional advantage.
  - Standardize food administration (because it affects L-thyroxine absorption) and timing of blood sample between visits.
- Monitoring clinical signs: expected evolution of response
  - An increase in alertness and activity commonly is seen within 1-2 weeks.
  - Neurologic improvement may begin within the first month, but several months may be needed for full resolution; some neurologic manifestations do not resolve.
  - Dermatologic improvement often takes 1-4 months.
  - Resolution of reproductive manifestations may take several months.
- If major clinical improvement is not seen in 3 months despite normal serum T_4 concentrations, a concurrent but unidentified disease should be considered.

PROGNOSIS & OUTCOME

- Primary hypothyroidism: long-term prognosis is excellent with adequate lifelong therapy.
- Secondary hypothyroidism: long-term prognosis is usually guarded because pituitary neoplasia is the most common underlying cause.

PEARLS & CONSIDERATIONS

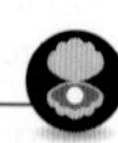

Comments

- The presence of nonthyroidal illness can make it difficult to obtain a definitive diagnosis of hypothyroidism. Sick euthyroid syndrome describes the condition that occurs when nonthyroidal illness results in decreased basal T_4 (and less commonly, FT_4ED) concentrations. Measurement of multiple thyroid hormones and advanced testing may be necessary.
- Subnormal T_4 concentrations are not an immediate indication for supplementation with levothyroxine, which may sometimes be deleterious. The history and physical exam findings must be critically evaluated for features supportive of hypothyroidism and signs of other illness that could be causing sick euthyroid syndrome. In the latter case, resolution/treatment of nonthyroidal illness returns T_4 concentrations to normal.
- Most obese dogs are not hypothyroid.
- Certain breeds (e.g., sighthounds, Shar-peis) have lower T_4 values than other breeds.
- Many drugs can decrease T_4 concentrations. Phenobarbital and especially sulfonamides can lead to increased TSH levels, making a reliable diagnosis very difficult. Sulfonamides should be stopped 2 months before thyroid evaluation. When a patient is receiving them, advanced thyroid testing is recommended (TSH stimulation or scintigraphy).

Prevention

Breeding of hypothyroid dogs risks perpetuating this disease; the presence of hypothyroidism should be considered together with the status of other heritable disorders in any particular dog before deciding on whether to breed it.

Technician Tips

- Serum submitted for FT_4ED should be free of hemolysis and lipemia; a fasted sample is recommended.
- T_4 is stable for 5 days if kept in plastic tubes. An artifactual increase in FT_4ED occurs if the sample is not kept cold.

SUGGESTED READING

Mooney CT: Canine hypothyroidism. In Ettinger SJ, et al, editors: Textbook of veterinary internal medicine, ed 8, St. Louis, 2017, Elsevier, pp 1731-1742.

AUTHOR: Sylvie Daminet, DVM, PhD, DACVIM, DECVIM
EDITOR: Ellen N. Behrend, VMD, PhD, DACVM

Hypoventilation

BASIC INFORMATION

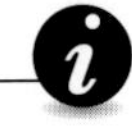

Definition

Pathologic increase in the partial pressure of carbon dioxide (PCO_2) in the blood secondary to factors that impair ventilation

Synonym

Ventilatory failure

Epidemiology

SPECIES, AGE, SEX

Dogs and cats of all ages, breeds, and sex may suffer from hypoventilation.

RISK FACTORS

- Use of narcotics, neuromuscular blockers (NMBs), sedatives, or general anesthesia
- Neuromuscular disease
- Trauma
- Tick exposure (e.g., *Dermacentor andersoni, Dermacentor variabilis, Amblyomma americanum*)
- Ingestion of raw, spoiled animal meat
- Small patients with weak ventilatory efforts under anesthesia
- Cisternal spinal tap

GEOGRAPHY AND SEASONALITY

- Dogs living in a warm, heavily wooded area where specific tick species are endemic
- Coral snakes can be found predominately in the southeastern United States.

Clinical Presentation

HISTORY, CHIEF COMPLAINT

History and clinical signs variable depending on the cause. Exposure to risk factors and clinical exam findings may raise index of suspicion for hypoventilation.

PHYSICAL EXAM FINDINGS

- Animals with abnormal respiratory mechanics: dyspnea (tachypnea, hyperpnea, orthopnea)
- Respiratory pattern localization: stridor = upper airway obstruction; decreased lung sounds with shallow inspiration = pleural space
- Animals with central nervous system (CNS) or lower motor neuron (LMN) disease: changes in mentation with deep, slow respirations; additional neurologic abnormalities (e.g., paralysis)
- Severe hypercapnia results in altered mentation (stupor or coma) and brainstem reflexes.

Etiology and Pathophysiology

- The partial pressure of arterial carbon dioxide ($PaCO_2$) is proportional to CO_2 production (VCO_2) and inversely proportional to alveolar ventilation.
- Decreases in alveolar ventilation and increases in VCO_2 therefore increase $PaCO_2$.
- Normal breathing requires flawless function and cooperation between the CNS, peripheral nervous system, neuromuscular junction (NMJ), respiratory muscles, and respiratory system. Disturbances in any of these areas can result in hypoventilation.

DIAGNOSIS

Diagnostic Overview

After hypercapnia ($PaCO_2$ > 36 mm Hg for cats and > 42 mm Hg for dogs) is confirmed, additional diagnostics can help determine if hypercapnia is due to hypoventilation, increased dead space ventilation (V_d), increased VCO_2, or rebreathing. Specific diagnostics aimed at identification of underlying condition depend on history and exam findings.

Differential Diagnosis

- CNS disease
  - Brain: drugs (e.g., narcotics, barbiturates, anesthesia), trauma, and space-occupying lesions (e.g., edema, granuloma, neoplasia, hemorrhage, inflammation)
  - Cervical spinal cord: trauma (e.g., fracture, hemorrhage), disc disease, infection, inflammation, or iatrogenic (after CSF tap or surgery)
- NMJ
  - Botulism, myasthenia gravis (MG), neuromuscular blockade, tick paralysis, polyradiculitis, coral snake envenomation, and organophosphates
- Respiratory dysfunction
  - Airways (e.g., laryngeal paralysis, tracheal collapse, asthma)
  - Parenchyma (e.g., edema, pneumonia, contusions, acute lung injury)
  - Pleural space (e.g., pneumothorax, hemothorax, diaphragmatic hernia)
  - Chest wall (e.g., flail chest, penetrating wound)

Initial Database

- Arterial or venous blood gas
- End-tidal CO_2 ($ETCO_2$) is a surrogate for $PaCO_2$ at end exhalation.
- Neurologic exam

Advanced or Confirmatory Testing

- CBC, chemistry analysis, urinalysis, ± thyroid panel
- Thoracic and cervical radiographs
- Functional laryngeal ± structural airway exam
- Titers/tests specific for neuromuscular disease
  - CT and/or MRI (± CSF)
  - Nerve or muscle biopsies (± electrodiagnostics) may be indicated for neuromuscular disease.

TREATMENT

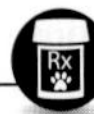

Treatment Overview

Treatment centers on resolution of the cause for hypoventilation and supportive care to maintain adequate $[CO_2]$ and $[O_2]$.

Acute General Treatment

- Establish and maintain a patent airway (tracheostomy, intubation if necessary).
- Low flow supplemental oxygen
- Sedation for mitigation of acute upper airway obstruction, if appropriate
- Treatment specific for cause:
  - Reverse narcotics
  - Status asthmaticus: bronchodilators (terbutaline, albuterol)
  - Tick paralysis: remove tick, apply ascridicides
  - Coral snake: antivenin
  - MG: anticholinesterase therapy
- Mechanical ventilation
- Sodium bicarbonate is not recommended for respiratory acidosis and will worsen hypercapnia.

Possible Complications

- Monitoring for aspiration pneumonia is essential in cases of CNS, spinal, or neuromuscular disease.

- Animals can require long-term mechanical ventilation for lung injury. Appropriate settings, analgesics, fluid therapy, and nursing care can minimize complications.

Recommended Monitoring

- Oxygenation: arterial blood gas or pulse oximetry
- Ventilation: blood gases or $ETCO_2$
- Blood pressure: invasive versus noninvasive
- Appropriate mechanical ventilator settings
- Monitor for clinical signs of volume overload (e.g., chemosis, serous discharge)

PROGNOSIS & OUTCOME

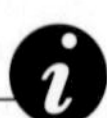

- Prognosis depends on the severity, presence of comorbidities, and reversibility of the underlying disease process.
- Client finances and access to 24-hour specialty care may alter prognosis for neuromuscular diseases requiring longer-term mechanical ventilation.
- Prognosis is good for animals if a reversible cause (e.g., drugs, tick paralysis, laryngeal paralysis) is rapidly identified and treated.

PEARLS & CONSIDERATIONS

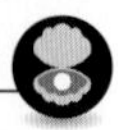

Comments

- Peripheral chemoreceptors initiate ventilation during periods of hypoxemia. Therefore, the use of high-inspired oxygen concentrations can worsen hypercapnia in chronically hypercapnic patients.
- Oxygen therapy can also decrease hypoxic pulmonary vasoconstriction, which prevents blood from entering alveoli with low ventilation. Decreasing this reflex increases ventilation-perfusion mismatch.

Technician Tips

- Venous $[CO_2]$ is less accurate if cardiac output or tissue perfusion is compromised because tissue CO_2 production increases with malperfusion.
- $ETCO_2$ is lower than $PaCO_2$ in conditions where CO_2 delivery is altered by severe parenchymal disease, low cardiac output, or thromboembolic disease.

SUGGESTED READING

Daly M: Hypoventilation. In Silverstein D, et al, editors: Small animal critical care medicine, ed 2, St. Louis, 2015, Saunders.

AUTHOR: Meghan Harmon, DVM, DACVECC
EDITOR: Leah A. Cohn, DVM, PhD, DACVIM

Icterus

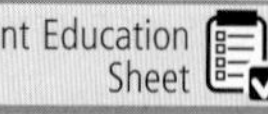

BASIC INFORMATION

Definition

Yellow discoloration of the tissues that results from bilirubin deposition when the serum bilirubin level exceeds 2.0 mg/dL. Causes can be categorized as pre-hepatic, hepatic, or post-hepatic.

Synonym

Jaundice

Epidemiology

SPECIES, AGE, SEX

- Dogs and cats of any age, either sex
- Pre-hepatic and post-hepatic causes of icterus are more common in dogs than cats.

GENETICS, BREED PREDISPOSITION

Based on underlying disorder

RISK FACTORS

- Pre-hepatic: risk of hemolytic anemia of any cause (pp. 59 and 60)
- Hepatic: risk of hepatic disease or injury of any cause (pp. 174, 442 and 444)
- Post-hepatic: risk of biliary obstruction (including pancreatitis) or rupture (pp. 160, 374, 740, and 742)

CONTAGION AND ZOONOSIS

There are many infectious but noncontagious causes of icterus; contagious causes (zoonosis*) include

- Dogs: canine infectious hepatitis, leptospirosis*, salmonellosis*
- Cats: feline infectious peritonitis, toxoplasmosis*, tularemia*

GEOGRAPHY, SEASONALITY

Some infectious causes of icterus are more common in a given region or season.

ASSOCIATED DISORDERS

- Pre-hepatic: hemolytic anemia, thromboembolic disease
- Hepatic: coagulopathy, hepatic encephalopathy
- Post-hepatic: pancreatitis, triaditis (cats), gallbladder mucocele, coagulopathy, peritonitis

Clinical Presentation

DISEASE FORMS/SUBTYPES

Categorized as pre-hepatic, hepatic, and post-hepatic based on the underlying mechanism for hyperbilirubinemia:

- Pre-hepatic: hemolytic anemia of any cause
- Hepatic: liver damage or disease (inflammatory, infectious, neoplastic, toxic), sepsis
- Post-hepatic: intrahepatic or extrahepatic cholestasis or biliary rupture

HISTORY, CHIEF COMPLAINT

Although rare, jaundice may be noticed by owners. Most patients present because of clinical signs associated with the underlying disease that has resulted in hyperbilirubinemia. Common signs:

- Pre-hepatic: clinical signs associated with anemia (e.g., lethargy, collapse)
- Hepatic: acute or chronic lethargy, anorexia, weight loss, gastrointestinal (GI) signs (e.g., vomiting, diarrhea)
- Post-hepatic: GI signs, anorexia, abdominal pain, lethargy

PHYSICAL EXAM FINDINGS

In addition to icterus (mucous membranes, sclera, skin), other common findings include

- Pre-hepatic: pale mucous membranes, tachycardia; tachypnea, bounding pulses, soft systolic heart murmur
- Hepatic: hepatomegaly or hepatic mass, abdominal distention with fluid wave
- Post-hepatic: abdominal pain, tachycardia, tachypnea, fever

Etiology and Pathophysiology

- Pre-hepatic: red blood cell (RBC) destruction releases heme, which is broken down to bilirubin. With accelerated hemolysis, bilirubin production overwhelms the ability of the liver to conjugate and secrete it into bile.
- Hepatic: abnormality in hepatic bilirubin uptake, conjugation, and/or excretion
- Post-hepatic: obstructive biliary disease (intrahepatic or extrahepatic) results in reduced bilirubin excretion in bile or rupture of biliary tree, allowing abnormal release of bile.

DIAGNOSIS

Diagnostic Overview

Icterus is a clinical feature that is always secondary to a primary disease/condition and always warrants thorough diagnostic investigation. The first step is a CBC to check for hemolytic anemia; if significant anemia is not present (packed cell volume [PCV] > 30% in dogs, > 25% cats), hepatic or post-hepatic icterus should be suspected. They are often differentiated with a chemistry profile and abdominal ultrasound.

Differential Diagnosis

Poor lighting or differences in visual perception can give a false impression of icterus; measurement of total bilirubin is confirmatory.

Initial Database

The myriad causes of icterus are reflected by variations in test results. Common findings:

- CBC
  - Pre-hepatic: anemia (often regenerative) ± autoagglutination ± spherocytes ± RBC parasites ± thrombocytopenia ± leukocytosis
  - Hepatic: ± mild anemia ± inflammatory or stress leukogram
  - Post-hepatic: ± mild anemia ± inflammatory or stress leukogram
- Chemistry panel (by definition, all demonstrate hyperbilirubinemia)
  - Pre-hepatic: mild increase in liver enzymes due to tissue hypoxia
  - Hepatic: increased liver enzymes (often proportional alanine aminotransferase [ALT] > alkaline phosphatase [ALP], gamma-glutamyltransferase [GGT]); potential for decreased in synthetic function (glucose, cholesterol, albumin, blood urea nitrogen [BUN]); azotemia with leptospirosis. Cats with hepatic lipidosis often have normal GGT.
  - Post-hepatic: increased liver enzymes (ALP, GGT > ALT), hypercholesterolemia, hypertriglyceridemia
- Urinalysis: bilirubinuria; hemoglobinuria with intravascular hemolysis; proteinuria with inflammatory or infectious disease
- Coagulation panel (prothrombin time/partial thromboplastin time [PT/aPTT]): normal to increased (disseminated intravascular coagulation secondary to immune-mediated hemolytic anemia [IMHA], severe hepatic dysfunction, or vitamin K deficiency)
- Blood ammonia concentration: may be increased with hepatic dysfunction
- Bile acids: seldom useful in icterus; increased with hepatic or post-hepatic causes
- Abdominal radiographs (may be normal)
  - Pre-hepatic: check for coin (zinc) in GI tract; hepatomegaly and/or splenomegaly may be present with hemolysis
  - Hepatic: microhepatica (chronic hepatopathy) or hepatomegaly (neoplasia, infectious hepatitis)
  - Post-hepatic: mass effect in cranial abdomen; loss of serosal detail (pancreatitis, bile peritonitis)
- Abdominal ultrasound (most useful in distinguishing between hepatic and post-hepatic cause)
  - Pre-hepatic: hepatomegaly and splenomegaly common with IMHA; evaluate for underlying cause of secondary IMHA
  - Hepatic: hypoechoic hepatic parenchyma (infectious hepatitis, neoplastic infiltrate), hyperechoic hepatic parenchyma (neoplasia), hepatic mass, large or small liver (size best assessed on radiographs), chronic hepatopathies may have mild echogenicity changes (hypoechoic, heterogenous) or may be normal in appearance
  - Post-hepatic: evaluate gallbladder, common bile duct, and extrahepatic structures/organs that may result in post-hepatic icterus (e.g., pancreatitis, extramural mass); peritonitis with free fluid if biliary rupture

Advanced or Confirmatory Testing

- Infectious disease testing, as appropriate
  - Pre-hepatic: vector-borne disease serology and polymerase chain reaction (PCR) (e.g., babesiosis, cytauxzoonosis)
  - Hepatic (dog*; cat†): leptospirosis* microscopic agglutination testing (MAT) and/or PCR (urine, blood), *Histoplasma capsulatum* urine antigen*†, adenovirus*, tularemia†, toxoplasmosis†, calicivirus†, bartonellosis*
- If effusion present, abdominocentesis and fluid analysis (pp. 1056 and 1343)
- Ultrasound-guided fine-needle aspiration (FNA) of liver or associated masses (p. 1112)
  - Often diagnostic for hepatic neoplasia (especially round cell neoplasia), hepatic lipidosis, and some infectious diseases
  - Less useful for chronic hepatopathy, hepatotoxicity
- Hepatic biopsy (ultrasound-guided needle biopsy, laparoscopic, laparotomy; coagulation profile first)
  - Histopathology, tissue copper quantification, and tissue/bile culture if suspect cirrhosis, chronic hepatitis, copper hepatopathy, or neoplasia (if FNA nondiagnostic)
- Exploratory laparotomy, if certain biliary disorders (e.g., bile peritonitis) are suspected

TREATMENT

Treatment Overview

Treatment depends on the underlying cause.

Acute General Treatment

- Pre-hepatic: RBC transfusion (packed RBCs or whole blood) may be necessary (p. 1169).
- Hepatic: discontinue hepatotoxic drugs, address fluid and electrolyte disorders, treat hepatic encephalopathy (p. 440), treat suspected infectious disease.
- Post-hepatic: bile peritonitis is considered a surgical emergency.

Chronic Treatment

Treatment depends entirely on underlying disease.

Nutrition/Diet

Nutritional support is a key aspect of treatment for some causes of icterus. Adequate nutrition is required for treatment of hepatic lipidosis, copper-restricted diets are necessary for copper-associated hepatopathy, and fat-restricted diets are appropriate for pancreatitis.

Drug Interactions

Hepatic metabolism and biliary excretion should be taken into account when prescribing medications to patients with hepatic and post-hepatic icterus, respectively.

Possible Complications

- There are multiple possible complications for the underlying disorders that cause icterus.
- In people, bilirubin accumulation in the brain leads to neurologic dysfunction (kernicterus); this does not seem to be a problem in dogs or cats.

Recommended Monitoring

- Pre-hepatic: vital parameters (as guide for transfusion need and indicator or thromboembolism), PCV, total solids
- Hepatic: signs of hepatic encephalopathy (dull mentation, hypersalivation in cats, nausea, seizures), appetite, serum biochemistry profile, abdominal effusion
- Post-hepatic: serum biochemistry profile, appetite, abdominal comfort

PROGNOSIS & OUTCOME

Prognosis depends on the underlying disease process and severity of disease, ranging from excellent (e.g., treatable cause of hemolysis) to grave (end-stage hepatic cirrhosis, metastatic neoplasia).

PEARLS & CONSIDERATIONS

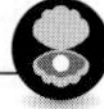

Comments

- Serum bilirubin concentration must be greater than 2 mg/dL before icterus can be visualized.
- Bile acids testing is generally not useful in animals with icterus because it does not help to differentiate between hepatic and post-hepatic causes of icterus.
- Imaging with abdominal ultrasound is important to differentiate between hepatic and post-hepatic icterus.
- Although theoretically unconjugated (indirect) bilirubin is increased more than conjugated (direct) bilirubin in animals with hemolysis, there is little practical benefit to testing for each type separately (as opposed to measuring total bilirubin and PCV).

Technician Tips

- An initial PCV is an important test for dogs and cats presenting with icterus because a normal PCV helps to rule out pre-hepatic icterus.

- Some causes of icterus are infectious or even zoonotic; practice biosecurity measures at least until the cause of icterus is determined.

SUGGESTED READING

Bradbury CA: Jaundice. In Ettinger SJ, et al, editors: Textbook of veterinary internal medicine, ed 8, St. Louis, 2017, Elsevier.

AUTHOR: Laura A. Nafe, DVM, MS, DACVIM
EDITOR: Leah A. Cohn, DVM, PhD, DACVIM

Idiopathic Tremor Syndrome

Client Education Sheet 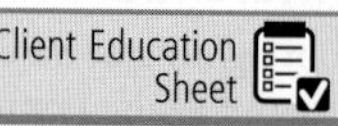

BASIC INFORMATION 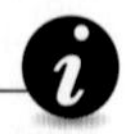

Definition

- A noninfectious meningoencephalitis primarily involving the cerebellum that manifests with whole-body tremors and is responsive to immunosuppressive glucocorticoids
- *Tremor* refers to an involuntary, rhythmic, oscillatory movement of a body part.

Synonyms

Corticosteroid-responsive tremor syndrome (CRTS), white dog shaker syndrome, shaker disease, idiopathic cerebellitis, sporadic acquired tremors of adult dogs, acquired action-related myoclonus

Epidemiology

SPECIES, AGE, SEX

- Most common in young (<5 years) and small-breed (<15 kg) dogs
- Rare in cats

GENETICS, BREED PREDISPOSITION

Although white dogs (West Highland white terrier and Maltese) are overrepresented, about 50% of cases reported are in dogs with nonwhite coats.

Clinical Presentation

HISTORY, CHIEF COMPLAINT

- Acute onset of whole-body tremors, worsening with stress or excitement
- Signs can progress over days to weeks and then typically remain static if left untreated.

PHYSICAL EXAM FINDINGS

- Characteristic finding is a high-frequency, low-amplitude, generalized tremor. Tremors are most evident in the head and limbs, often worsen with excitement and movement, and disappear during sleep.
- Additional cerebellovestibular neurologic abnormalities can be seen, including head tilt, menace response deficits, nystagmus, paresis, ataxia, and ocular tremors.
- Seizure activity has been reported in some affected dogs.
- Elevated temperature is possible.

Etiology and Pathophysiology

- Inflammatory disease of unknown cause, but an immune-mediated cause is strongly suspected
- Tremors are most likely due to a neurotransmitter imbalance.
- Similar characteristics to the human disease called stiff man syndrome, which is due to an autoimmune reaction against glutamic acid decarboxylase, an enzyme necessary for synthesis of GABA (an inhibitory neurotransmitter).

DIAGNOSIS 

Diagnostic Overview

Presumptive diagnosis can be based on signalment, history, and clinical signs. Advanced neurodiagnostic workup with MRI and cerebrospinal fluid (CSF) analysis can help rule out other causes of tremors.

Differential Diagnosis

Other types of tremors (p. 1288), toxicities, infectious encephalitis (cerebellitis, particularly *Neospora*), congenital abnormalities of myelin formation, or metabolic disorders

Initial Database

CBC, biochemistry profile, and urinalysis: normal

Advanced or Confirmatory Testing

- CSF analysis (pp. 1080 and 1323) is most useful diagnostic test; often shows a mild to moderate small mononuclear (e.g., lymphocytic) pleocytosis with an elevated protein. Occasionally, CSF results are normal or show albuminocytologic dissociation (normal nucleated cell count with elevated protein).
- MRI is most often normal. Changes consistent with mild meningoencephalitis may be seen.
- Histopathology can show a mild nonsuppurative meningoencephalitis with scattered lymphoperivascular cuffs within the CNS, especially the cerebellum.

TREATMENT 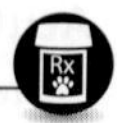

Treatment Overview

Medical management with immunosuppressive doses of glucocorticoids is typically effective at decreasing or eliminating the tremor. Diazepam can be used as adjunctive therapy. Glucocorticoid dose can be tapered after remission of clinical signs.

Acute General Treatment

- Immunosuppressive doses of glucocorticoids (e.g., prednisone 1-2 mg/kg PO q 12h); clinical signs often resolve within a few days
- Adjunctive diazepam therapy 0.2 mg/kg PO q 8h can be helpful in decreasing tremors.

Chronic Treatment

- After clinical signs are in remission, glucocorticoid dose can be slowly decreased over a 1-3 month period. Decreasing the dose by 25% or less at a time is recommended to avoid potential recrudescence of clinical signs.
- Most patients do not require therapy for longer than 3 months. However, some patients may require a long-term low dose, alternate-day glucocorticoid therapy to control signs.

Behavior/Exercise

Until clinical signs resolve, patient should avoid stairs, furniture, and other environments where a fall could result in injury.

Recommended Monitoring

Neurologic exam and clinical signs should be monitored as the glucocorticoid dose is tapered.

PROGNOSIS & OUTCOME 

Excellent

PEARLS & CONSIDERATIONS 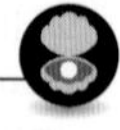

Comments

The term *white shaker dog syndrome* is a misnomer because about one-half of patients with idiopathic tremor syndrome do not have a white haircoat.

Technician Tips

- Hand feeding may be required if the tremors affect an animal's ability to properly reach the water and food bowls.
- Provide a well-padded, lower-level cage and nonslick surface to prevent falling or injury.
- Keep affected patients in environment with reduced stimuli (e.g., low/dark light and decreased noise) to help decrease tremor activity.

SUGGESTED READING

Lowrie M, et al: Classification of involuntary movements in dogs: tremors and twitches. Vet J 214:109-116, 2016.

AUTHOR: Devon Wallis Hague, DVM, DACVIM
EDITOR: Karen R. Muñana, DVM, MS, DACVIM

Immunodeficiency Syndromes, Dog

BASIC INFORMATION

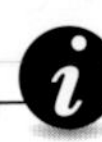

Definition

Primary immunodeficiency syndrome: an inherited defect involving the humoral (B-cell) or cell-mediated (T-cell) immune system, a combination of the two, or the phagocytic system

Epidemiology

SPECIES, AGE, SEX

- Signs often first manifest about 8-12 weeks of age, when the protective effects of maternal antibody are lost.
- No sex predisposition except for sex-linked severe combined immunodeficiency syndrome (X-SCID) in males
- More syndromes are described for dogs versus cats.

GENETICS, BREED PREDISPOSITION

- Humoral (B-cell) immunodeficiency disorders
  - Selective immunoglobulin A (IgA) deficiency: German shepherd dog, Shar-pei, and beagle
  - IgG deficiency: Cavalier King Charles spaniel
  - IgM-IgA-IgG deficiency: some lines of miniature dachshunds
- Complement deficiency: Brittany spaniel
- Cell-mediated (T-cell) immunodeficiency disorder
  - Thymic hypoplasia: dwarf Weimaraner
- Combined (B-cell and T-cell) immunodeficiency disorder
  - SCID: Jack Russell terrier, Frisian water dog
  - X-SCID: basset hound, Cardigan Welsh corgi
- Functional phagocytic immunodeficiency disorder
  - Canine leukocyte adhesion disorder (CLAD): Irish setter
  - Weimaraner immunodeficiency syndrome: Weimaraner
- Cyclical neutropenia: border collies, collie (gray)
- Trapped neutrophil syndrome (TNS): Border collies

CONTAGION AND ZOONOSIS

Most opportunistic infections that affect immunocompromised individuals are overgrowths or infections with organisms that otherwise are not pathogenic to immunocompetent hosts. However, immunocompromised animals are more susceptible than normal individuals to infection with organisms that are potentially zoonotic (e.g., dermatophytosis) or contagious to other dogs (e.g., respiratory tract pathogens).

Clinical Presentation

HISTORY, CHIEF COMPLAINT

- Recurrent infections seen at a young age that may or may not respond to appropriate therapy.
- Type of infection may vary with defect in the immune system.

PHYSICAL EXAM FINDINGS

- Humoral (B-cell) immunodeficiency disorder: physical exam findings are remarkable only for signs associated with chronic/recurring infections; increased incidence of chronic respiratory, skin, and intestinal infections
- Cell-mediated (T-cell) immunodeficiency disorder: absence of palpable lymph nodes; tonsils are not visible. Affected dogs typically have signs of growth retardation and unthriftiness compared with the other puppies in the litter.
- Combined (B-cell and T-cell) immunodeficiency disorder: similar findings as for humoral and cell-mediated immunodeficiency disorder
- Functional phagocytic immunodeficiency disorder: fever, generalized lymphadenopathy, dermatitis, pododermatitis, gingivitis, osteomyelitis; striking absence of exudate formation (CLAD), and poor wound healing

Etiology and Pathophysiology

- Humoral (B-cell) immunodeficiency: decreased concentrations or absence of certain immunoglobulins, with increased susceptibility to bacterial infections
  - IgA deficiency: mode of inheritance is unknown. Epidemiologic studies show that puppies born to dams with IgA deficiency are at increased risk for infections related to mucosal surfaces such as upper respiratory infections, recurrent bronchopneumonia, pyoderma, otitis, demodicosis, and enteritis.
- Cell-mediated (T-cell) immunodeficiency: affected animals have low numbers of or nonfunctional T cells. Findings include a small thymus and lack of lymph nodes, tonsils, and Peyer's patches on postmortem exam. Affected animals are at increased risk for infections with intracellular bacterial, fungal, protozoal, and viral organisms.
- Combined (B-cell and T-cell) immunodeficiency
  - SCID: autosomal recessive: affected individuals are unable to mount an appropriate antigen-specific immune response because of a lack of DNA protein kinase (DNA-PK) activity; DNA-PK is required for lymphocyte precursors to mature.
  - X-SCID: sex-linked mutation in the gamma chain of the interleukin 2 (IL-2) receptor required for normal B-cell and T-cell function. Affected male puppies are able to synthesize IgM, but IgG concentrations are significantly reduced, and IgA is not detectable.
- Complement deficiency: autosomal recessive mode of inheritance; dogs that are homozygous for the trait have no detectable C3, which is required for opsonization of bacteria. Affected individuals suffer recurrent sepsis, bronchopneumonia, pyometra, or wound infections.
- Functional phagocytic immunodeficiency: affected animals have an increased risk of systemic or superficial infections with pyogenic microorganisms.
  - Weimaraner immunodeficiency syndrome: inherited, exact mechanism unknown but there is neutrophil dysfunction at the site of lesions, and there appears to be a failure to produce IgA and IgG.
  - CLAD: deficiency of leukocyte surface glycoprotein (beta$_2$ integrin) associated with leukocyte adherence and egress into affected tissues; failure to express the beta$_2$ integrin CD18
  - TNS: retention of neutrophils in the bone marrow leads to neutropenia and secondary infections

DIAGNOSIS

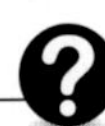

Diagnostic Overview

Affected puppies present with various, often nonspecific clinical signs and commonly with recurrent infections. It is the recurrence of the infections and the poor response to therapy that warrant further investigation of a primary immunodeficiency syndrome. Multiple animals in a litter may be affected.

Differential Diagnosis

- Humoral immunodeficiency: varies, based on presenting complaint
  - Upper respiratory infection: *Bordetella bronchiseptica*
  - Primary ciliary dyskinesia
  - Otitis
  - Stomatitis
  - Staphylococcal dermatitis
  - Atopic dermatitis
- Cell-mediated immunodeficiency
  - Fungal (cryptococcosis, aspergillosis, blastomycosis, dermatophytosis)
  - Protozoal (toxoplasmosis, giardiasis)
  - Viral infections can be seen after vaccination with modified live virus vaccine.
  - Intracellular bacteria (mycobacterial infections)
- Combined immunodeficiency: affected animals are susceptible to bacterial, viral, fungal, and protozoal agents.
- Functional phagocytic immunodeficiency
  - Sepsis
  - Bacteremia

- Chronic myelogenous leukemia
- Pelger-Huët anomaly: hyposegmentation of nuclei in granulocytes and monocytes; persistent degenerative left shift without toxic change or any signs of illness (incidental finding)
- Other infectious disease that can cause a neutrophilic leukocytosis with a left shift

Initial Database

Appropriate diagnostic testing based on clinical presentation:

- Minimal database: CBC, serum biochemistry profile, urinalysis with culture and sensitivity, fecal exam, thoracic radiographs can reflect concurrent infection (e.g., evidence of bacterial pneumonia)
- Other tests directed toward site of infection (e.g., airway lavage if pneumonia, biopsy of skin lesion)
- Humoral (B-cell) immunodeficiency disorder: no specific change
- Cell-mediated (T-cell) immunodeficiency disorder: normal/decreased lymphocyte count
- Combined (B-cell and T-cell) immunodeficiency disorder: normal/decreased lymphocyte count (average, 1000 cells/mcL); possibly low total protein due to low globulin levels; agammaglobulinemia (protein electrophoresis)
- Functional phagocytic immunodeficiency disorder: persistent leukocytosis with regenerative left shift; neutrophil count > 200,000 cells/mcL
- CLAD: marked leukocytosis; leukocytes cannot escape the vasculature
- Cyclic neutropenia: neutrophil count within or below reference range
- Trapped neutrophil syndrome: neutropenia

Advanced or Confirmatory Testing

If congenital immunodeficiency is suspected, consult with small animal internal medicine specialist or veterinary immunologist. Functional testing may require immediate assay.

- Specific tests are tailored to the suspected immunodeficiency.
- CLAD: biopsy of lesion shows bacteria ± necrosis but no neutrophil infiltration.
- Humoral immunodeficiency: serum protein electrophoresis to evaluate immunoglobulin concentrations, quantitation of serum immunoglobulin, and serum C3 for C3 deficiency
- Cell-mediated immunodeficiency: lymphocyte transformation (blastogenesis) evaluates the ability of the T cell to proliferate after stimulation; measurement of growth hormone or insulin-like growth factor 1 if dwarfism is suspected (available only in research laboratories)
- Cyclic neutropenia: bone marrow aspirate/biopsy
- Functional phagocytic immunodeficiency
  - Bactericidal assays: measure the ability of neutrophils to phagocytize or kill bacteria, or to generate reactive oxygen species
  - Polymerase chain reaction (PCR): to identify affected, normal, or carrier animals
- Genetic tests are available for some congenital immunodeficiency syndromes (e.g., TNS, CLAD).

TREATMENT

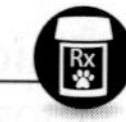

Treatment Overview

Substantial variation in severity may exist for a given immunodeficiency syndrome. Therefore, treatment intensity, treatment success, and prognosis are individually variable. Some individuals require minimal treatment (intermittent antimicrobial treatment during clinical exacerbation), whereas in others, euthanasia is the most humane option. Control opportunistic infections with antimicrobials and supportive care; hospitalize when necessary.

Acute General Treatment

Supportive care to treat opportunistic infections:

- Antibiotics are used for confirmed bacterial infections. Empirical antibiotics may be used initially, pending culture and sensitivity results. Antibiotic selection is based on suspected bacterial population of involved site.
  - Skin: gram-positive bacteria most common; consider cephalosporins (cephalexin 22 mg/kg PO q 8-12h) or penicillins (amoxicillin 22 mg/kg PO q 8h)
  - Oral cavity and respiratory tract
    - Gram-positive cocci: consider cephalosporins 22 mg/kg PO, IV q 8h *or* trimethoprim-sulfadiazine 15-30 mg/kg SQ, IM, IV q 12h (lower end of dosage range for larger dogs)
    - Gram-negative rods: trimethoprim-sulfadiazine 15-30 mg/kg SQ, IM, IV q 12h (lower end of dosage range for larger dogs) *or* enrofloxacin 5-10 mg/kg IV q 24h *or* gentamicin 8 mg/kg IV, IM, SQ q 24h
    - *Bordetella* infection: doxycycline 5 mg/kg IV, PO q 12h *or* chloramphenicol 50 mg/kg IV, SQ, PO q 8h; enrofloxacin 5-10 mg/kg slow IV, IM, PO q 24 h
    - Mixed populations: consider fluoroquinolones (enrofloxacin 5-10 mg/kg PO *or* slow IV q 24h) *or* beta-lactamase–resistant penicillins (amoxicillin-clavulanate 10-20 mg/kg PO q 12h) *or* macrolides (azithromycin 5-10 mg/kg PO q 24h × 1-5 days)
- Due to possibility of opportunistic fungal, viral, and protozoal infections, empirical antibiotic therapy may be inadequate or may select for resistant strains of bacteria; diagnostic samples for culture should be obtained before treatment, and judicious antibiotic use is warranted.
- Nebulization and coupage for bacterial pneumonia (p. 795)
- Disinfection of cutaneous wounds with diluted (0.05%) chlorhexidine solution
  - With standard 4% chlorhexidine solution, dilute 1 part chlorhexidine to 80 parts water to obtain a 0.05% concentration.
  - The same concentration may be used as an ear wash for otitis and as an oral antiseptic rinse for stomatitis.

Chronic Treatment

- Humoral immunodeficiency
  - Supportive therapy tailored to treating recurrent microbial infections
- Cell-mediated immunodeficiency
  - Supportive care with frequent monitoring for opportunistic infections; proceed with aggressive treatment when warranted
  - Dwarf Weimaraners respond to thymosin fraction 5 therapy (1 mg/kg SQ q 24h for 7 days).
- Combined (B-cell and T-cell) immunodeficiency
  - Bone marrow transplantation
- Phagocytic immunodeficiency
  - Bone marrow transplantation

Nutrition/Diet

- Caloric requirements of the critically ill patient may be less than those of a healthy animal.
  - Resting energy requirement (RER): RER = 70 × body weight (kg)$^{0.75}$
  - RER approximation: 30 × body weight (kg) + 70
- If anorexia persists after infection treated, feeding tubes may be required.

Drug Interactions

- When using chloramphenicol, consider human risks (myelosuppression, aplastic anemia; wear gloves).
- When using aminoglycosides, ensure that patient is well hydrated and has adequate renal function.
- Fluoroquinolones can affect cartilage in growing puppies.

Possible Complications

- Sepsis
- Recurring and resistant infections

Recommended Monitoring

Monitoring of appetite, activity, temperature, and CBCs can aid in the early detection of infection.

PROGNOSIS & OUTCOME

- Humoral immunodeficiency: fair to good
- Cell-mediated immunodeficiency: poor
- Combined (B-cell and T-cell) immunodeficiency: poor. Affected animals usually die between 2 and 4 months of age from systemic bacterial or viral infections.
- Phagocytic immunodeficiency: poor

PEARLS & CONSIDERATIONS

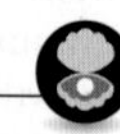

Comments

The diseases listed here are rare but are often severe, and several have a poor/guarded prognosis.

Prevention

- If molecular testing is possible, use genetic screening for predisposed animals.
- If congenital immunodeficiency is identified, avoid breeding related animals.

Technician Tips

- Wear gloves when handling immunocompromised patients.
- Protect yourself from opportunistic zoonotic infections by wearing protective shielding.
- Use sterile saline when performing nebulization.
- Encourage patient appetite by warming foods.

Client Education

Explain to the client that affected dogs will not be cured, the disease is heritable, and other puppies of the same litter may be affected. Affected puppies are at an extremely high risk for secondary infections and should avoid other ill animals.

SUGGESTED READING

Tizard JR: Primary immune deficiencies. In Tizard IR, editor: Veterinary immunology, ed 10, St. Louis, 2018, Elsevier.

AUTHOR: Jonathan F. Bach, DVM, DACVIM, DACVECC
EDITOR: Jonathan E. Fogle, DVM, PhD, DACVIM

Inappropriate Elimination, Cat

Client Education Sheet 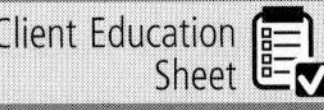

BASIC INFORMATION

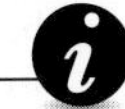

Definition

- Use of inappropriate areas (locations or surfaces) for elimination of urine or feces. As used here, this is a diagnosis associated with an anxiety disorder. Otherwise, inappropriate elimination is often elimination that is normal for the species but undesirable to clients.
- Urinary incontinence: passage of urine without awareness due to a medical problem; comparatively rare in cats.
- Marking: passage of urine or feces involving social interaction; very common in cats. Marking with urine may or may not involve spraying.

Synonyms

Toileting problems, litter box problems, undesirable litter box use, aversions/preferences to substrates/locations

Epidemiology

SPECIES, AGE, SEX

- Urine spraying: sexually intact animals > neutered animals; possibly males > females
- Marking behaviors (which need not involve spraying) may develop at sexual maturity (≈6 months) if about sexual advertisement or at social maturity (≈24-48 months) if about social stimuli, social anxiety, or stress or distress

GENETICS, BREED PREDISPOSITION

Long-haired cats possibly overrepresented with substrate (surface used for elimination) aversions

RISK FACTORS

Risk factors for elimination preferences and aversions:

- Dirty litter and/or litter boxes
- Litter boxes that are too high for cats to enter readily (e.g., arthritic cat)
- Litter boxes that are too small (<1.5 cat body length) and discourage active digging and exploration
- Styles (covered) and placement (in closets) that allow the cat using the litter box to be trapped by a child or another pet
- Placement of boxes in locations cats cannot reach because of pain (e.g., arthritis), access (e.g., doors closed), or social factors (e.g., being chased by the new puppy)
- Poor ventilation resulting in entrapped odors (covered boxes)
- Cystitis in offending cat (pain) or any household cat (e.g., odorant changes)

Risk factors for marking are based on social stress and distress; stressors:

- Addition or loss of another pet (including visits by outside cat)
- Change in the composition of the human household
- Change in the stress level of the household (e.g., illness, changes in jobs)
- Change of relationships between cats in the household (e.g., that are concomitant with social maturity)
- True intercat aggression

GEOGRAPHY AND SEASONALITY

Marking behaviors may intensify in spring, when more animals are let outside and visit indoor animals and when scents aerosolize. Marking increases in frequency (female and male, although males more readily noticed) when females enter estrus.

ASSOCIATED DISORDERS

- Comorbid intercat aggression is common; identifying relative victims and aggressors is essential to resolving the social conflict and fixing the toileting complaints.
- Medical issues may precipitate or worsen behavior issues due to pain and perceptual changes.

Clinical Presentation

DISEASE FORMS/SUBTYPES

Three classes of problems, all of which are normal behaviors in free-ranging cats:

- Substrate (texture/surface) preferences or aversions; sensory aspects of substrate is key
- Location preferences or aversions; location of area for elimination is key
- Marking
  - Nonspraying: elimination of small amounts of urine or feces in areas that have social, not tactile, significance
  - Marking: spraying is part of a normal signaling repertoire in cats. The cat treads on its front feet, raises its tail (quivering the tip), and sprays urine vertically. If the cat is not backed against a vertical surface, sprayed urine makes a linear pattern on horizontal surfaces. Only cats willing to be seen raise their tails.

HISTORY, CHIEF COMPLAINT

Clients find urine or feces in locations they consider unacceptable.

PHYSICAL EXAM FINDINGS

- Usually unremarkable
- Findings suggesting lower urinary tract disease, gastrointestinal problems, arthritis, or other nonbehavioral disorder warrant a diagnostic medical evaluation.

Etiology and Pathophysiology

- Behavior can be normal for the species but unacceptable to clients.
- Behavior can be an anxiety disorder and comorbid with intercat aggression or other behavioral conditions, such as comorbid inflammatory cystitis (p. 332).
- Association between crystalluria or anal sac disorders and periuria/perichezia (urinating/defecating outside the litter box) remains speculative.

DIAGNOSIS

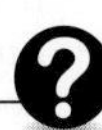

Diagnostic Overview

It is important to use history (video recordings in the home environment can be useful), physical exam, and routine lab tests to differentiate between behavioral and medical issues. For behavioral issues, you must determine whether marking or substrate/location preferences/aversions are involved because management and treatment plans are different. Cats with periuria/perichezia may progress to more anxious responses.

Differential Diagnosis

- Feline lower urinary tract signs/disease
- Bacterial cystitis
- Urethral obstruction
- Diabetes mellitus
- Cognitive dysfunction
- Hyperthyroidism
- Lower motor neuron disease
- Enteritis/colitis
- Parasitemia

Initial Database

- To rule out medical problems and before initiating medications: CBC, serum biochemistry profile, urinalysis, thyroid profile (if > 6 years old), urine culture (urination issue), fecal flotation and direct smear (defecation issue)
- Detailed history regarding toileting is essential: number, type, and placement of litter boxes; type of litter offered; surfaces/textures used for inappropriate elimination

Advanced or Confirmatory Testing

Client observations are essential. Videotaping, including interactions between cats in a multi-cat household, can be extremely informative. This is especially useful if the client is unable to determine which cat is eliminating inappropriately and/or is unable to understand social interactions and dynamics between the cats.

TREATMENT

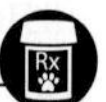

Treatment Overview

Treatment goals:

- Identify preferred locations/substrates (no litter, shredded paper towels, washable fabric, disposable vegetation)/box types/numbers/sizes/locations, and deploy. Appropriate and reliable use of intended substrates and locations for elimination when the problem is preference/aversion
- Identification and management of concurrent behavioral disorders (e.g., social factors involved in intercat aggression) that can contribute to elimination change when the above fail.

Acute and Chronic Treatment

- Identify previously preferred substrates (types of litter or atypical substrates [rags, shredded paper, no litter]) and locations, and replicate or use these.
- Ensure there is at least one more litter box than the number of cats.
- Ensure the litter boxes are at least 1.5 cat body lengths long (including tail). This is larger than virtually all commercially available litter boxes for cats, but research indicates this is the preferred size.
- Identify locations where the cat spends the most time, and place boxes accordingly.
- Litter box hygiene must be meticulous and lifelong. Ensure that clients are complying with an appropriate cleaning regimen:
  - Scoop litter multiple times daily.
  - Empty litter entirely, including recyclable multi-cat litters, two to three times per week (more often if more cats).
  - Wash, rinse, and dry the litter box at least weekly.
  - Avoid liners and scented litters.
  - If they must be used, ensure covered litter boxes have good ventilation.
- Use good odor elimination (e.g., Anti-Icky-Poo [AIP]) on all substrates where urine or feces has been inappropriately deposited.
- Pheromonal analog products have been suggested for use to calm animals, but they may make some animals more reactive. Studies of efficacy are poorly designed and involve medication; medication for underlying anxiety is likely more effective than pheromones.
- Identify and redress potential stressors or conflicts in the household. The most common of these may be relationships between cats in the household. Intercat aggression is a serious concern if
  - One cat is avoiding one or more other cats
  - One cat consistently leaves the room or a preferred resting spot when other cat(s) enter
  - One cat does not eat or drink in the presence of the others
  - One cat often hides
  - One cat is hyperreactive to noise or tactile stimuli
- If any of the previous conditions are identified, clients should separate cats when they are unsupervised. The more timid cat should have free range; the more aggressive cat should be confined in a space that is not highly contested/desirable (e.g., not the client's bedroom or the kitchen).
- If anxiety and aggression are involved, benzodiazepines (BZDs), gabapentinoids, tricyclic antidepressants (TCAs), or selective serotonin reuptake inhibitors (SSRIs) may be useful.
  - TCAs: amitriptyline or nortriptyline 0.5-1 mg/kg PO q 12-24h × 30 days minimum); clomipramine 0.5 mg/kg PO q 24h × 60 days minimum
  - SSRIs: fluoxetine or paroxetine 0.5 mg/kg PO q 24h × 60 days minimum
  - Gabapentinoids: gabapentin 3-5 mg/kg PO q 12-24h × 30 days minimum
  - BZDs: diazepam or oxazepam 0.2-0.4 mg/kg PO q 12-24h × 30 days minimum, alprazolam 0.01-0.025 mg/kg PO q 12-24h or as needed q 4-5h for panic
  - BZDs are helpful primarily in behavior modification programs involving food reward (e.g., teaching cats to tolerate each other).
  - TCAs and SSRIs can be extremely useful in helping overcome aversions and addressing anxiety involved in marking behaviors and intercat aggression.
- If the toileting issue is associated with intercat aggression and the victim needs to become more outgoing, the partial serotonin agonist buspirone 0.5-1 mg/kg PO q 24h × 60 days minimum can be used. However, clients should monitor carefully because the newly confident cat may engage in social interactions that result in a physical fight.
- If animals are added to the household, clients should expect social upheaval and be prepared to restart analysis of interaction and behavior.
- Attention should be paid to the victimized cat before the other cats.
- Outdoor or visitor cats should be kept to a minimum or excluded.
- If all else fails, consider allowing the cat to be an indoor/outdoor cat.

Possible Complications

- BZDs: hyperexcitability (less rare), severe hepatotoxicity (more rare), potential abuse by clients. Diazepam uses the *N*-desmethyldiazepam metabolic pathway; *N*-desmethyldiazepam has a long $T_{1/2}$ in cats and is highly sedative.
- Cats treated with monoamine oxidase inhibitors (some flea and tick collars) should not be treated with TCAs or SSRIs.

Recommended Monitoring

If on medications, exam and laboratory tests q 6-12 months

PROGNOSIS & OUTCOME

- Changes in hygiene and/or social management can resolve concerns for most cats.
- Without treatment, the prognosis is guarded. Inappropriate elimination is the single most common reason cats in North America are euthanized or relinquished. Many shelters consider cats that have litter box issues unadoptable and euthanize them.
- Prognosis is improved by early diagnosis, comprehensive treatment, attentive client monitoring, and open communication between clinician and client.

PEARLS & CONSIDERATIONS

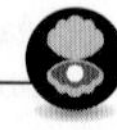

Comments

In the absence of meeting the cat's needs, attempts to constrain the cat to eliminate in places, on substrates, or in modes preferred by the client will likely result in a worsening of the problem and potentially create an anxiety disorder from an original hygiene/basic needs situation.

Prevention

- It is essential to ask clients about inappropriate elimination at every veterinary visit. Clients may not mention occasional inappropriate elimination, when correction is most easily accomplished. Allowed to go untreated, the problem is likely to worsen. On average, owners allow 2 years of occasional issues before the situation is considered untenable.

- Meeting the cat's needs by providing multiple, clean, large litter boxes (sweater boxes/canine litter boxes) and grouping cats by temperament is the best way to prevent elimination problems.

Client Education

- Clients should seek consultation after even one or two accidents.
- Treatment of behavioral conditions may be required for the life of the pet. Relapses may occur with treatment discontinuation or with added stressors.
- Physical illness is may promote a behavioral elimination problem where previously none existed.

SUGGESTED READING

Sung W, et al: Elimination behavior patterns of domestic cats *(Felis catus)* with and without elimination behavior problems. Am J Vet Res 67:1500–1504, 2006.

AUTHOR & EDITOR: **Karen L. Overall, VMD, MA, PhD, DACVB**

Inappropriate Elimination, Dog

BASIC INFORMATION

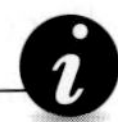

Definition

- Urination or defecation in a location other than areas acceptable to the client
- Marking: urination (or less commonly defecation) for communication purposes or as part of an anxiety disorder; usually involves small amounts of urine deposited in several places, often vertical surfaces
- Incontinence: inadvertent passage of urine or feces as a clinical manifestation of disease

Synonyms

Housesoiling, incomplete housebreaking, incomplete housetraining, soiling, toileting issues

Epidemiology

SPECIES, AGE, SEX

- Can affect dogs of any age and either sex
- Sexually intact dogs have increased rates of urine marking.
- Puppies first develop inhibition of elimination and associations with a preferred substrate (i.e., surface onto which they eliminate) at 8.5 weeks of age. It is therefore ideal to housetrain a dog between 7 and 9 weeks of age.
- Adult dogs (particularly neutered females) may experience urinary incontinence associated with urethral sphincter mechanism incompetence or other medical disorders. These are not behavioral abnormalities.

GENETICS, BREED PREDISPOSITION

Toy-breed dogs eliminate small volumes and may not be as strictly supervised or confined until fully housetrained as would be larger dogs; treatment may be more protracted or difficult, proportional to the length of time the dog has been eliminating in unwanted locations. Small bladder volume and greater metabolic rate also mean that smaller dogs need more frequent access to appropriate elimination areas.

RISK FACTORS

- Sexually intact status
- Presence of intact animals, especially if in estrus (provokes urinary marking by neutered and intact animals)
- Rehomed street and kennel-raised dogs may never have learned to inhibit elimination behaviors and need to learn inhibition and appropriate substrate and location preferences as adults
- Urinary and fecal marking and increased urgency can be nonspecific signs associated with anxiety disorders. Many dogs with chronic generalized anxiety disorder, for example, have episodic or chronic soft stools or diarrhea. Any dog given a diagnosis of inflammatory bowel disease should be fully screened for behavioral problems that may coexist.

CONTAGION AND ZOONOSIS

If the inappropriate elimination is due to incomplete housetraining, other dogs in the household also may mark.

GEOGRAPHY AND SEASONALITY

- Inclement weather may inhibit a dog's willingness to eliminate outside. Snow and ice should be cleared to allow access and good traction.
- Dogs should be exposed to a variety of surfaces/substrates (e.g., grass, cement, sand, stones, sawdust) that can meet with the seasonal and lifestyle requirements.

ASSOCIATED DISORDERS

Coprophagy (p. 204) may be exhibited by kennel-raised dogs. Dogs at risk may include puppy mill–sourced dogs or those adopted after an extended stay in shelters with limited space, labor, or other resources.

Clinical Presentation

DISEASE FORMS/SUBTYPES

Housesoiling may involve inappropriate urination, inappropriate defecation, marking with urine, marking with feces, or a combination. Not all urinary marking is vertical. Males and females can use a variety of positions to mark, and leg cocking is more often associated with unfamiliar social stimuli than with sex-based behaviors.

HISTORY, CHIEF COMPLAINT

- Client finds urine or feces inside the home
- Client may report that the dog was taken out and returned to eliminate in the house.
- Information on volume, frequency, appearance, and when the housesoiling occurs is critical in determining underlying cause.

PHYSICAL EXAM FINDINGS

- Findings, including rectal palpation, should be unremarkable in cases with a behavioral cause.
- Abnormal physical exam findings should raise the possibility of medical disorders causing urinary or fecal incontinence (pp. 537 and 538).

Etiology and Pathophysiology

- Inappropriate elimination is a nonspecific sign that may be normal (e.g., incomplete housetraining) or abnormal and associated with medical or behavioral disturbances, specifically with anxiety disorders.
- Any condition that triggers a fight-or-flight response can lead to involuntary voiding that may be misinterpreted by the client as purposeful, malicious, or vengeful.
- Olfactory stimulation for normal elimination and marking behaviors is extremely important to dogs and poorly understood by humans.
- Meeting the individual dog's age- and size-specific needs is essential to understanding the root of housesoiling and addressing it.

DIAGNOSIS

Diagnostic Overview

Inappropriate elimination is a complaint, not a diagnosis, and is not always a sign of abnormality because the pet's voiding location may just be incompatible with the client's wishes. Through careful behavioral history taking and after ruling out medical problems, diagnosis aims to determine whether the behavior is normal but requires some modification to better fit living in a human household or the elimination is a marker of an anxiety disorder.

Differential Diagnosis

Behavioral differential diagnoses:

- Incomplete housetraining: occurs regardless of client presence or absence. Large volume of urine is voided. Normal stool is deposited.

Certain areas of the house may be sought preferentially.
- Submissive or excitement urination: occurs on greeting a person or when the dog is excited. The dog often crouches down and starts to roll over when approached. Excited dogs may urinate while wagging or jumping.
- Marking behaviors: urine marking typically involves small quantities in several locations in the absence of another medical problem. Urine may be deposited on vertical (most common), horizontal, or a combination of surfaces. Fecal marking is less well understood, but small amounts of feces are deposited in response to the presence of unfamiliar animals. Texture and content of feces changes with frequency of marking.
- Separation anxiety (p. 905)
- Storm phobia (p. 787)
- Panic disorder
- Generalized anxiety disorder
- Canine cognitive dysfunction: loss of housetraining in a previously fully housetrained dog may be one of the many signs of the disorder (p. 188).

Medical differential diagnoses:
- Urinary and fecal incontinence (pp. 537 and 538) or polyuria/polydypsia (p. 812)

Initial Database

CBC, serum chemistry panel, urinalysis, and fecal flotation to assess possible causes of polyuria, pollakiuria, and abnormal stool consistency that may lead to inappropriate voiding

Advanced or Confirmatory Testing

- After any medical disorders are resolved, a behavioral diagnosis and treatment plan can be pursued if the inappropriate elimination persists because the inciting causes may be medical, but the maintenance causes may be behavioral.
- Behavioral diagnosis may be reached using detailed history; consultation with a veterinary behaviorist can help in devising a treatment plan.

TREATMENT

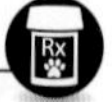

Treatment Overview

Treat any recognized underlying medical disorder(s). If inappropriate elimination persists, address behavioral sequelae to establish or restore housetraining.

Acute and Chronic Treatment

- Incomplete housetraining: fully confine or supervise when indoors, using a leash or crate. If the dog is caught eliminating, calmly take it outside to the chosen elimination area, allow the dog to finish, and praise lavishly. Take to eliminate after eating, after play, after any slowing in play, and after awakening. Any yelling or punishment is likely to hasten the voiding process and is entirely counterproductive.
- Submissive or excitement urination: client should maintain an emotionally calm approach, especially when greeting the dog. It may be necessary to ignore the dog until it is very calm or guide it outside to greet after elimination. Cornerstones of successful treatment are to keep the dog's bladder empty through frequent, well-timed walks outside to eliminate and to use positive reinforcement/rewards methods to teach the dog to sit without leaking or cringing. Use consistent rule structures that guide the pet to learn which behaviors are correct in the home and in social interactions. The clients should teach the dog that calm behaviors such as sitting and lying down get praise; attention lessens overall reactivity and encourages the dog to react calmly.
- Clients should be advised against punishing after the fact. This makes no sense to the dog, may force it to housesoil out of sight, and eliminates the opportunity to praise for correct behavior.
- For small dogs with higher metabolic rates or for less agile or ill dogs, canine litter boxes may be a good solution, especially in urban areas. Accustom the dog to the substrate to be used in the box at an early age. Commercially available boxes or homemade ones that accommodate the dog's size and mobility (low edges for arthritic dogs) can be filled with cat litter, specially made artificial turf, or lined with absorbent pads. Clients' objections tend to dissipate when it is pointed out that litter boxes, even large ones, are easier to clean than carpets and rugs.
- For marking behaviors in the house, it is important to address the social interactions between the animals. Screening for overt and covert aggression (p. 40) and other anxiety-related conditions in all of the household pets should be undertaken.
- For marking behaviors outside the house, decreasing exposure to outdoor stimuli is the only feasible management approach. If feral and roaming animals are triggers, clients can contact local animal control and shelter organizations to arrange for humane trapping.
- For intact male dogs that become distracted in the presence of female urine (a problem for many working dogs engaged in service, assistance, explosives detection), castration as early in the development of the marking behavior as possible largely resolves the situation in most cases.
- Veterinarians should screen all pets at each visit for elimination complaints; early intervention decreases the effect that learning has on the progression of any unwanted behavior.

Nutrition/Diet

When housesoiling involves defecation and the stool volume seems large, introducing a highly digestible, low-residue diet can assist in decreasing stool volume produced and frequency of elimination. Medical evaluation should rule out medical issues (e.g., exocrine pancreatic insufficiency, malabsorptive syndromes). Client compliance may improve because there is less stool to clean up and the interval between elimination bouts may lengthen, decreasing the number of times the dog needs to be taken outside.

Behavior/Exercise

Taking a dog out twice daily often is insufficient. Encourage clients to think of how often they eliminate every day and to understand the dog's metabolism is similar to theirs.

Possible Complications

Punishment is useless in resolving the problem or makes the problem worse, especially if anxiety is contributory.

Recommended Monitoring

Following up with the client by telephone or email can help keep clients on track with the treatment plan, particularly when the behavior is normal and the dog is being taught to eliminate in a location that the client favors. Weekly communication can address any problems or obstacles that the client may encounter before the client gets discouraged enough to give up on the dog.

PROGNOSIS & OUTCOME

- Prognosis is excellent in cases of incomplete housetraining or submissive or excitement elimination, as long as proper identification of underlying cause and thorough behavior modification are carried out.
- Prognosis for problematic marking behaviors is excellent if the associated behavioral concerns are competently addressed.
- Prognosis is guarded for an adult male dog that has urine marked for his entire life. Long-term learning is likely far more influential at this stage than any hormonal component.

PEARLS & CONSIDERATIONS

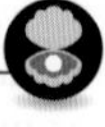

Comments

- Abuse of puppies (p. 9) and abuse of human children often starts with abusive behavior surrounding housetraining/toilet training.
- Lack of attention to the dog's need is the most common reason for poor housetraining or other nonmarking elimination problems in dogs.
- Fecal marking and increased urgency (e.g., sporadic diarrhea) can be nonspecific signs associated with anxiety disorders as much as with primary gastrointestinal disease. Dogs given a diagnosis of inflammatory bowel disease should be thoroughly screened for behavioral problems.

Prevention

- Ensure that dogs are not outside only for the purpose of elimination. If this is so, they may delay eliminating outside to have more opportunity to experience outdoor stimuli and may then eliminate indoors.

- Reward dogs for eliminating outside with play, freedom, exercise, praise, interaction with other dogs, and time to smell their canine world.

Technician Tips

Ask about housebreaking or litter box training at every puppy/kitten visit. When taking rectal temperatures, watch for perineal staining; it may point to abnormal stool consistency that the owners do not report.

Client Education

- Client education is key to preventing and resolving these problems. All veterinary practices should have handouts (see Additional Suggested Readings for other sources) that explain how to housetrain dogs. A designated staff member should be responsible for explaining and following up on training with clients.
- Quick screening at each veterinary visit for elimination complaints and other behavioral concerns saves lives. Clients are unlikely to talk about behavioral concerns and questions unless prompted to do so.

SUGGESTED READING

Houpt KA: Housesoiling by dogs. In Horwitz D, et al, editors: BSAVA manual of canine and feline behavioral medicine, Gloucester, UK, 2009, British Small Animal Veterinary Association.

AUTHOR: Soraya V. Juarbe-Diaz, DVM, DACVB
EDITOR: Karen L. Overall, VMD, MA, PhD, DACVB

Incontinence, Fecal

Client Education Sheet 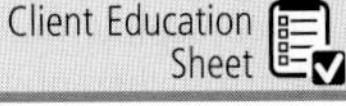

BASIC INFORMATION 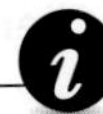

Definition

Involuntary loss of bowel control characterized by the inability to retain bowel contents, including flatus and fecal material

Epidemiology

SPECIES, AGE, SEX

Any species, age, breed, or sex

GENETICS, BREED PREDISPOSITION

- German shepherd dogs: lumbosacral stenosis
- Manx cats, English bulldogs, pugs: spinal malformations

RISK FACTORS

- Spinal cord/pelvic trauma
- Colorectal neoplasia
- Colorectal/perineal surgery
- Diffuse polymyoneuropathies/polyneuropathies

ASSOCIATED DISORDERS

May be associated with paraparesis, tetraparesis, or urinary incontinence in animals with neurologic causes of fecal incontinence (FI)

Clinical Presentation

DISEASE FORMS/SUBTYPES

Try to discern whether the animal senses and postures to defecate or defecation occurs without the animal's awareness. The former suggests a problem with fecal storage (storage or sphincter incontinence), and the latter suggests loss of neurogenic control (neurogenic incontinence).

HISTORY, CHIEF COMPLAINT

- Storage/sphincter incontinence: animal is aware of need to defecate but unable to control defecation as a result of colorectal or anal disease. Other signs may include
  - Tenesmus
  - Hematochezia
  - Small and/or frequent bowel movements
  - Malodorous stools or discharge
  - Excessive licking of perineal region
  - Tail chasing
  - Scooting
- Neurogenic incontinence: often unaware of the need to defecate. Often, there are other signs of neurologic disease (e.g., gait deficits, dysuria/urinary incontinence, spinal pain).

PHYSICAL EXAM FINDINGS

Depends on the cause:

- Visual inspection may reveal
  - Erythema, ulceration of perineum, anus
  - Anal mass/swelling
  - Aberrant tail movement/carriage
- Digital rectal exam
  - Absent anal sphincter tone
  - Thickened rectal mucosa
  - Abnormal stool consistency/composition
- Orthopedic exam
  - Pain when lifting tail
  - Evidence of pelvic or vertebral fracture
- Neurologic exam
  - Intracranial disease: altered mentation
  - T3-L3 myelopathy: paraparesis with intact pelvic limb reflexes (upper motor neuron)
  - L4-S3 myelopathy: paraparesis and decreased to absent pelvic limb reflexes and anal tone; large, flaccid bladder ± lack of tail movement (lower motor neuron)
  - Dysautonomia: lack of anal tone; large, flaccid bladder; fixed mid-range pupils; ocular/nasal discharge; weight loss; lack of heart rate increase with stress/exercise

Etiology and Pathophysiology

Fecal incontinence can be classified according to structural and neurogenic causes:

- Structural (storage/sphincter) FI results from inability to store feces because of colorectal disease or inability to form a seal around the feces because of disruption of the normal anal sphincter anatomy.
  - Includes anatomic and inflammatory conditions in the prostate, colon, rectum, or anus such as colorectal neoplasia, proctitis, colitis, anal fistulas, chronic constipation, and pelvic (e.g., whelping, vehicular) or iatrogenic (e.g., anal sacculectomy or rectal pull-through surgery) trauma
- Neurogenic FI results from impaired sensation or reduced neurologic control of defecation.
  - Includes peripheral neuropathies (e.g., diabetes mellitus), junctionopathies (e.g., myasthenia gravis), spinal cord disease or trauma (e.g., subarachnoid cysts, fibrocartilaginous embolism), intervertebral disc disease, constrictive myelopathy (e.g., articular process malformation, lumbosacral stenosis), dysautonomia, or age-related cognitive dysfunction

DIAGNOSIS 

Diagnostic Overview

History and physical exam findings should aid classification of structural versus neurogenic causes.

Differential Diagnosis

- Incontinence must be distinguished from behavioral issue resulting in inappropriate defecation.
- Severe diarrhea may result in some degree of fecal incontinence.

Initial Database

Depends on categorization as a structural or neurogenic cause

Advanced or Confirmatory Testing

Additional testing depends on suspicion of the cause (structural vs. neurogenic) of FI.

Structural:

- Abdominal imaging (abdominal radiographs and ultrasound)
  - Thickened colonic wall (inflammation, infection, neoplasia)
  - Generalized or focal dilation of colon
  - Lesions suggesting infection or neoplasia (lymphadenopathy, masses)
  - Ultrasound-guided transabdominal cytologic sampling of abnormalities identified on ultrasound (e.g., masses, lymphadenopathy)

- Thoracic imaging: if neoplastic or infectious causes suspected
- Centrifugation fecal flotation: helminths, *Giardia*, and *Tritrichomonas foetus* (cats only); sensitivity is moderate to low, especially for identification of cestodes with single fecal sample testing. Empirical anthelmintic therapy is recommended if clinical suspicion exists.
- Colonoscopy/proctoscopy with biopsies of affected areas may be indicated for inflammatory or neoplastic conditions.
- Rectal scrape if thickened mucosa (p. 1157)

Neurogenic:

- Advanced imaging (e.g., CT, MRI, myelography) to evaluate spinal cord lesion
- Cerebrospinal fluid analysis
- Electromyography and nerve conduction studies
- Specific infectious disease testing (e.g., distemper, *Neospora*, *Toxoplasma*), depending on history, exam findings, initial diagnostic tests, and the prevalence of infectious diseases in area
- Pilocarpine response test

TREATMENT

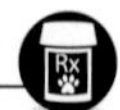

Treatment Overview

Successful treatment depends on the ability to identify and resolve cause.

Acute General Treatment

- Opioids may slow colonic transit time, but this rarely helps to resolve incontinence.
- Keep perineal area clean to prevent dermatitis.

Chronic Treatment

- For animals with incontinence as a result of external anal sphincter abnormalities, surgical options (e.g., silicone elastomer sling, muscle transfer flap) may be available.
- Some neurologic causes may be addressed surgically (e.g., intervertebral disease).

Nutrition/Diet

Highly digestible, low-fiber diets may decrease stool volume. If highly digestible diets worsen incontinence, addition of insoluble fiber to stimulate colonic contractions and improve fecal consistency may improve signs in animals with colitis-induced FI.

Possible Complications

- Perineal dermatitis
- Urinary tract infections, especially in female dogs

PROGNOSIS & OUTCOME

Depends on ability to resolve underlying cause

PEARLS & CONSIDERATIONS

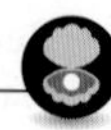

Comments

- A careful assessment of the history and physical exam is needed to differentiate true FI from a behavioral condition.
- Fecal incontinence may develop before other neurologic deficits in animals with neurogenic FI.

Prevention

Use a cautious approach to perineal and colorectal surgery.

Technician Tips

- Discuss risk of FI associated with perineal or colorectal surgery.
- Address perineal hygiene, and emphasize importance to owner.

Client Education

Take animal outside immediately after feeding.

SUGGESTED READING

Cave N: Fecal incontinence. In Washabau R, et al, editors: Canine & feline gastroenterology, St. Louis, 2013, Saunders, pp 118-123.

AUTHOR: M. Katherine Tolbert, DVM, PhD, DACVIM
EDITOR: Leah A. Cohn, DVM, PhD DACVIM

Incontinence, Urinary

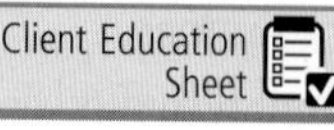

BASIC INFORMATION

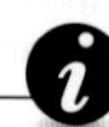

Definition

Lack of voluntary control over the passage of urine

Epidemiology

SPECIES, AGE, SEX

- Dogs more often than cats
- With young animals, congenital disorders are more likely.
- Older, spayed females are prone to incontinence due to urethral sphincter mechanism incompetence (USMI [p. 1011]).

GENETICS, BREED PREDISPOSITION

- Ectopic ureter: Siberian Husky, miniature and standard poodle, Labrador and golden retrievers, Newfoundlands, terriers
- Manx cats: spinal cord malformation

Clinical Presentation

HISTORY, CHIEF COMPLAINT

- Dribbling urine
- Trouble housebreaking: puppies
- Incontinence while sleeping: a hallmark of USMI in spayed female dogs and ectopic ureter(s) in puppies

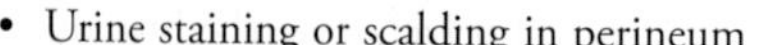

PHYSICAL EXAM FINDINGS

- Urine staining or scalding in perineum
- Urine dribbling from vulva or penis between urinations
- Neurologic deficits (if neurogenic cause)
- Bladder should be palpated before and after urination.
- Bladder expression
  - Easy: decreased outflow resistance
  - Difficult: normal or increased outflow resistance
- Rectal exam
  - Urethral thickening (inflammation or infiltration)
  - Prostatomegaly (p. 824)
  - Bladder trigone abnormalities

Etiology and Pathophysiology

Neurogenic:

- Lower motor neuron (LMN) (lesion at S1-S3 spinal cord segment or peripheral nerve disorder)
- Upper motor neuron (UMN) (lesion cranial to sacral spinal cord segment S1)

Non-neurogenic:

- Anatomic
- Functional

DIAGNOSIS

Diagnostic Overview

Any patient with a chief complaint of urinary incontinence should have a complete review of the medical history (notably to assess the possibility of behavioral causes and determine whether polyuria or pollakiuria is present); a physical exam, including abdominal palpation, rectal palpation when feasible, neurologic exam, and exam of the genitalia and reproductive tract; a urinalysis; and bacterial culture and susceptibility of urine.

Differential Diagnosis

Incontinence must be distinguished from behavioral issues (pp. 533 and 535), pollakiuria (p. 802), or polyuria (p. 812). Causes of incontinence (p. 538) can be divided as follows:

- Neurogenic
  - LMN disorders: S1-S3 segment or peripheral nerve disorders
  - UMN disorder: cranial to S1; usually characterized by urine retention; overflow incontinence can occur
- Non-neurogenic
  - USMI: most common cause in adult female dogs

- Urge incontinence/detrusor hyperspasticity: associated with lower urinary tract signs
- Anatomic abnormalities: ectopic ureter(s), vaginal stricture or diverticulum, patent urachus, others

Initial Database

Neurologic exam (p. 1136)

- UMN: firm, difficult to express bladder
- LMN: flaccid, easily expressed bladder; decreased/absent anal tone, bulbospongiosus reflex, perineal sensation
- Pain on tail lift: associated with lumbosacral disease
- Pain on spinal palpation; ataxia, proprioceptive deficits: associated with structural or inflammatory spinal cord disease or orthopedic spinal disease

Laboratory tests:

- Urinalysis
  - Cystocentesis preferred
  - Pyuria suggests inflammation (with or without infection), leading to increased urge
  - Hematuria suggests inflammation or neoplasia
- Urine culture and susceptibility: rule out bacterial infection (primary or secondary)
- CBC/serum biochemistry panel: no specific changes expected
- Retroviral testing: feline leukemia has been associated with urinary incontinence

Advanced or Confirmatory Testing

Diagnostic imaging:

- Abdominal radiographs/ultrasound: structural lesions
- Cystourethrography/vaginography: radiolucent defects
- Spinal radiography/myelogram/CT/MRI: spinal cord lesions

Endoscopy:

- Direct visualization of ectopic ureters and other anatomic defects
- Correction of anatomic defects
- If indicated, biopsy vaginal vault and mucosa of urethra and bladder
- Urethral pressure profile: rarely necessary

TREATMENT

Treatment Overview

Goals of treatment are to correct anatomic defects, treat secondary conditions, and palliate incontinence. Some dogs may respond better to one medication than another; if there is no response to a medication, review the diagnosis, and if unchanged, consider adding a second medication, changing to a medication in another class of action and/or pursuing further diagnostic testing.

Acute and Chronic Treatment

When an underlying disorder is present (e.g., urinary tract infection (UTI), prostatic disease, urethral neoplasia), treatment is directed at this primary cause.

- Surgical correction: ectopic ureter(s) (p. 282), penile/preputial/vulvar/vaginal conformational abnormalities, patent urachus, certain spinal disorders
- Medication: UTI (p. 232), USMI (p. 1011), urethral-detrusor dyssynergia, certain spinal disorders
- Multimodal treatment: neoplasia (e.g., transitional cell carcinoma [p. 991], leiomyoma or leiomyosarcoma of the vaginal vault)

PROGNOSIS & OUTCOME

- Outcome for dogs and cats with correctable structural abnormalities is good to excellent.
- Treatment is generally successful for USMI, although dosage adjustment is often required and UTI must be identified and treated.
- Although not an inherently life-threatening disorder, urinary incontinence may lead to euthanasia in refractory cases.

PEARLS & CONSIDERATIONS

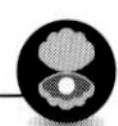

Comments

- Combination therapy of alpha-agonists and reproductive hormones is synergistic for treatment of USMI.
- Carefully question owner about thirst and urination. Polyuria may unmask USMI or a neurologic incontinence in an older patient.
- Carefully question owner that complains that a puppy is hard to housetrain. Incontinence may not be recognized in a juvenile patient.

Technician Tips

The signalment and an accurate history can narrow the differential list quickly. Congenital defects are present from a young age; USMI occurs in adult, spayed females; and neurologic patients often have a history of trauma or other neurologic signs.

SUGGESTED READING

Lane IF: Canine urinary incontinence (diagnostic tree). Clinician's Brief 11:18-19, 2013.

AUTHOR: Claire M. Weigand, DVM, DACVIM
EDITOR: Leah A. Cohn, DVM, PhD, DACVIM

Infertility, Female Dog

BASIC INFORMATION

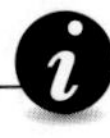

Definition

Includes failure to cycle, failure to ovulate, failure to accept the male, failure to become pregnant, failure to maintain pregnancy, and/or failure to deliver live puppies at term

Synonyms

Infecundity, sterility, persistent anestrus

Epidemiology

SPECIES, AGE, SEX

Canine, any time after puberty (≥6 months), female

GENETICS, BREED PREDISPOSITION

- More prevalent in inbred families of purebred dogs
- Anecdotal information indicates that some breeds of dogs have poor fertility (e.g., Norwich terriers, Bernese mountain dogs, and some sighthounds)
- Some conformation traits require assistance with breeding and parturition (e.g., bulldogs).

RISK FACTORS

- Advancing age can decrease fertility. Peak fertility is 2-4 years of age.
- Poor or incomplete breeding management is responsible for most apparent infertility in the bitch.
- Previous hormone therapy, abnormal hormone concentrations, and uterine disease also increase the risk of infertility.
- Anestrus, silent heat, persistent estrus, irregular estrus, abnormal sexual behavior, uterine disease, hypoluteoidism, structural abnormalities of the female reproductive tract, systemic illness, and inappropriate nutrition (excessive or inadequate caloric intake, raw diets contaminated with *Salmonella* spp and/or *Escherichia coli*) may predispose to infertility.

CONTAGION AND ZOONOSIS

Several bacterial and viral agents contributing to infertility are contagious. They can be spread by oral, inhalation, and venereal routes and include beta-hemolytic *Streptococcus*, *Mycoplasma*, and *Ureaplasma* spp, and canine herpesvirus (p. 466). The most significant canine venereal disease is *Brucella canis*.

GEOGRAPHY AND SEASONALITY

Female domestic dogs are nonseasonal, with the exception of the basenji, which enters pro-estrus only in the late summer/early fall.

ASSOCIATED DISORDERS

Pseudocyesis (p. 831) occurs in many bitches whether they are pregnant or not, and it has not been linked to infertility. Vaginal hyperplasia (p. 1028) may contribute to infertility by limiting or preventing natural service (does not interfere with artificial insemination).

Clinical Presentation

DISEASE FORMS/SUBTYPES

- Breeding management issues
- Abnormalities of the estrous cycle
- Uterine abnormalities
- Systemic or infectious disease

HISTORY, CHIEF COMPLAINT

Varies; medical history is the most important tool in the approach to infertility, including these important elements:

- General health history: vaccination status of the bitch; current and past medications (including heartworm preventative and topical medications, vitamins, and herbal supplements)
- Housing details: kennel, home, indoor, outdoor, and number of bitches in the household
- Bitch's age at first estrous cycle, which should occur by 24 months of age
- Length of each cycle from onset of vulvar swelling to diestrous cytology
- Interestrous interval; average is 7 months but shorter or longer could be normal or abnormal, depending on the individual
- Details of cycle: onset of vulvar swelling and vulvar discharge, onset of estrous behavior (flagging), dates of mating
- Method of mating: natural service or artificial insemination by bitch owner, stud owner, or veterinarian
- Artificial insemination, including type of semen (fresh, cooled/shipped, or frozen) and site of semen deposition (vagina or uterus)
    - Stud dog status: when did stud dog last sire puppies?
- Dates of last *B. canis* serologic testing for the bitch and the stud dog
- Method of pregnancy diagnosis: palpation, hormone assay, ultrasound, or radiographs
- Were hormone assays performed during the cycle? Was vaginal cytology and/or progesterone testing performed to determine optimal breeding time? If progesterone testing was done, was it quantitative or qualitative? Was ovulation confirmed after the luteinizing hormone (LH) peak?
- Was the bitch being campaigned or under any other stressful event such as a new home?
- Is there a history of infertility in the pedigree?

PHYSICAL EXAM FINDINGS

Physical exam is usually normal. Special attention should be paid to the external genitalia and mammary glands.

- Ambiguous genitalia may be an indicator of an intersex state (clitoral enlargement suggestive) and may be supportive of primary anestrus.
- Digital vaginal exam: to assess patency and accessibility of the vulva and caudal vagina
- Vaginal exams should be performed gently and atraumatically; may not be feasible in toy-breed bitches that are anestrous at the time of exam.
- Vaginal septa and circumferential strictures may interfere with natural service and with artificial insemination into the vagina.
- Visual inspection and palpation of the mammary glands

Etiology and Pathophysiology

- Mistimed breeding is by far the most common cause of infertility.
- Ovarian dysfunction: abnormalities in ovulation and maintenance of the corpus luteum, persistent estrus, and primary anestrus (can occur in XO bitches and XXY bitches)
- Silent heat must be differentiated from primary anestrus.
- Uterine dysfunction: lesions of the uterus (e.g.., cystic endometrial hyperplasia/pyometra, fibrosis with degeneration of endometrial glands), subclinical uterine infection, shortened interestrous interval resulting in implantation failure (i.e., canine uterus requires 130-150 days after the onset of proestrus to complete endometrial repair)

DIAGNOSIS

Diagnostic Overview

The diagnosis is based on a compilation of history (most important), physical exam, and results of laboratory evaluation. Historical information provided by the client is the cornerstone of the diagnostic process and must be elicited comprehensively. Without complete historical information, it is challenging to diagnose the cause of infertility and anestrus. A global approach to diagnosis and management is outlined on p. 1430.

Differential Diagnosis

- Pregnancy loss
- Ovulation failure
- Silent heat (endocrinologically normal estrous cycle with minimal to no external signs of proestrus or estrus)
- Stud dog infertility

Initial Database

- CBC, serum biochemistry profile, thyroid panel, *B. canis* serology, vaginal cytologic exam, vaginal culture if in estrus or if discharge is present
- Hypoproteinemia and/or renal dysfunction may contribute to infertility

Advanced or Confirmatory Testing

- Vaginoscopy
- Progesterone testing to document ovulation and assess luteal function. Progesterone testing is recommended monthly to assess cyclicity if the client has not observed cycles.
- Ultrasonography of the uterus and ovaries
- Canine herpesvirus titer
- Ovarian and/or uterine biopsy with histopathologic evaluation can be used in selected cases.
- In cases of primary anestrus, it is wise to determine the karyotype of the bitch to assess her chromosomal makeup; trisomy X or XO females and other abnormal chromosomal combinations have been reported. Many normal sighthound bitches do not cycle until nearly 24 months old.

TREATMENT

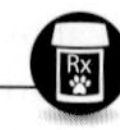

Treatment Overview

Targeted treatment is based on the underlying cause of the infertility. In most cases, correcting improper breeding management through client education can correct the problem.

Acute General Treatment

- Shortened interestrous interval: mibolerone 30-180 mcg/dose (small to large dog) PO q 24h (schedule IV controlled substance)
- Treatment for cystic endometrial hyperplasia/pyometra if present (p. 854)
- Treatment for persistent estrus if present (p. 822)
- There is no reliable therapy to induce fertile estrus in the bitch. There are many protocols in use with varying outcomes, but no controlled studies have been published. The most commonly attempted protocol includes the use of oral anti-prolactin medication cabergoline (5 mcg/kg PO q 24h until signs of proestrus develop).

Nutrition/Diet

- Diet with an Association of American Feed Control Officials statement that this diet is complete for all life stages, based on feeding trials
- If feeding a puppy food during the second half of gestation, it should be a small-breed puppy food.
- No controlled studies to support any claims of over-the-counter supplements that they can increase litter size, regulate estrous cycles, promote normal delivery, and so on; some may result in infertility
- Avoid calcium supplementation prepartum.

Behavior/Exercise

- A bitch that was removed from her littermates too early or that was herself a singleton puppy may never demonstrate normal breeding behavior because of her lack of appropriate interaction with littermates at an early age.
- A bitch that is the first canine in a household may not accept a male that is added to the

household at a later date (consider artificial insemination).
- Performance bitches may be allowed to continue training in the venue in which they compete but under optimal environmental and hygiene conditions to minimize risk to bitch and fetuses.

Drug Interactions

Use care in the selection of any medication used in a breeding bitch. For example, topical corticosteroids that are commonly found in otic preparations can be absorbed systemically and are not recommended.

Possible Complications

- Mibolerone causes clitoral hypertrophy, epiphora, and tear staining and may increase aggression toward other dogs. This drug can exacerbate existing liver enzyme elevation. Dogs with normal liver enzymes rarely have changes as a result of the drug.
- The progestational compounds may cause masculinization of female fetuses, mammary enlargement, and/or prolong gestation resulting in fetal death.

Recommended Monitoring

- Confirm pregnancy ultrasonographically 30 days after breeding.
- Serum progesterone concentrations at that time and weekly if there is any indication of variability in embryonic vesicle size or embryonic loss

PROGNOSIS & OUTCOME

- Good to excellent for clients who comply with breeding management recommendations
- Guarded for bitches with uterine disease and/or ovarian dysfunction
- Poor for bitches with primary anestrus due to chromosomal abnormalities

PEARLS & CONSIDERATIONS

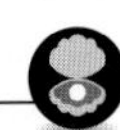

Comments

- Infertility of the stud dog is the second most common cause of female infertility after improper breeding management. The stud dog must also be evaluated and demonstrated to produce adequate numbers of motile and morphologically normal sperm, and the semen must be inseminated properly.
- Failure to cycle is often a failure to observe the bitch adequately for physical changes consistent with proestrus. The client should blot the vulva daily to detect vaginal discharge and change in vulvar size and shape ± monthly progesterone assays to detect ovulation with unobserved estrus.

Technician Tips

- Be prepared for many questions from clients whose dogs fail to produce puppies. Many clients think that all bitches should be bred on a particular pair of days from the onset of proestrus (e.g., 10th and 12th days) or every day while she is receptive, and these preconceived notions should be anticipated and addressed with medical facts.
- Ensure that serum samples for progesterone are collected in appropriate sample tubes.

Client Education

- Suggest a reproductive workup before the next anticipated estrous cycle.
- Educate about the value of vaginal cytologic evaluation, vaginal culture, and serum progesterone testing
- Importance of good semen and proper insemination technique

SUGGESTED READING

Wilborn RR, et al: Clinical approaches to infertility in the bitch. Vet Clin North Am Small Anim Pract 42(3):457-468, 2012

AUTHOR: Frances O. Smith, DVM, PhD, DACT
EDITOR: Michelle A. Kutzler, DVM, PhD, DACT

Infertility, Male

BASIC INFORMATION

Definition

- Spermiogram abnormalities may be categorized as follows:
  - Asthenozoospermia: decreased numbers of progressively motile spermatozoa per ejaculate (<30%-50%)
  - Teratozoospermia: increased numbers of morphologically abnormal spermatozoa per ejaculate (>40%-50%)
  - Oligozoospermia: abnormally low numbers of spermatozoa per ejaculate (<22 million spermatozoa/kg body weight in the dog or < 5 million total spermatozoa in the tom)
- Other causes of male infertility are listed on p. 1247.

Epidemiology

SPECIES, AGE, SEX

Dog or cat, intact males, any age

RISK FACTORS

Age, systemic disease (especially those resulting in increased body temperature), endocrinopathy, testicular disease or trauma, chemotherapy, hormone therapy

CONTAGION AND ZOONOSIS

Brucella canis

GEOGRAPHY AND SEASONALITY

Lower total number of spermatozoa and percentage of morphologically normal spermatozoa in summer months expected in North American dogs

ASSOCIATED DISORDERS

± Poor libido

Clinical Presentation

DISEASE FORMS/SUBTYPES

- Reversible versus irreversible
- Compensatory versus noncompensatory

HISTORY, CHIEF COMPLAINT

- Declining or consistently poor fertility
- Recent episode of malaise or fever
- Prior history of heavy physical training (possibility of performance-enhancing drugs)
- History of bloody penile or preputial discharge or pain with ejaculation
- History of chronic respiratory disease (asthenozoospermia)

PHYSICAL EXAM FINDINGS

- Libido may be normal or decreased.
- Testes may be small and soft or normal in size and consistency.
- Testes, epididymides, or spermatic cords may be enlarged (inflammation or neoplasia) and/or thickened.
- Scrotum may be enlarged or thickened (dermatitis, trauma, edema or fluid accumulation).
- Prostatomegaly possible (symmetrical or asymmetrical; painful or nonpainful)
- In dogs with asthenozoospermia due to primary ciliary dyskinesia/immotile cilia syndrome, additional signs may include recurrent nasal discharge and/or cough, hydrocephalus (open fontanelle, domed calvaria), or situs inversus (spleen is palpated on the right side of the abdomen; heartbeat is strongest on right hemithorax).
- ± Fever (infectious causes of infertility)

Etiology and Pathophysiology

Causes (all categories):

- Infectious or inflammatory (orchitis, epididymitis, prostatitis including infection with *B. canis*, mycoplasmas or other aerobic bacteria, or feline infectious peritonitis [FIP])

- Scrotal hyperthermia (due to fever, obesity with increased intrascrotal fat, hydrocele, hematocele, scrotal edema, or neoplasia)
- Toxin exposure or exogenous drug administration: glucocorticoids, anabolic steroids (human estrogen or testosterone patches or creams), other steroid hormones, chronic nonsteroidal antiinflammatory drug (NSAID) usage, gonadotropin-releasing hormone (GnRH) agonist/antagonists, chemotherapeutic agents
- Testicular degeneration (primary or secondary)
- Immune mediated (lymphocytic thyroiditis or spermatozoal autoantibodies)
- Unilateral or partial epididymal or tubular obstruction (granuloma, spermatocele)
- Congenital

Additional causes (specific to individual categories):

- Primary ciliary dyskinesia with abnormal spermatozoal midpiece formation (asthenozoospermia)
- Prostatic disease: benign prostatic hyperplasia, prostatitis, or squamous metaplasia (oligozoospermia, asthenozoospermia)
- Neoplasia (oligozoospermia, teratozoospermia)
- Hyperadrenocorticism (oligozoospermia)

DIAGNOSIS

Diagnostic Overview

Diagnosis is based on history (generally of suboptimal fertility), physical exam findings, semen evaluation, and cultures of semen or prostatic fluid in many cases. Remainder may require more advanced diagnostic testing.

Differential Diagnosis

Asthenozoospermia:

- Contaminated or improperly washed ejaculate collection equipment (e.g., disinfectant residues)
- Excessive use of lubricants
- Prolonged exposure of ejaculate to latex, heat, or cold
- Urine contamination of the ejaculate
- Infrequent ejaculate/collection, with accumulation of dead sperm in the epididymis and/or vas deferens

Teratozoospermia:

- Poor handling of semen after collection (especially if coiled tails or detached heads are present)
- Improper microscopic interpretation
- Prolonged sexual abstinence (increase in detached heads) or overuse, pubertal and geriatric patients (increases in cytoplasmic droplets)

Oligozoospermia:

- Retrograde ejaculation
- Fear or apprehension of mating (e.g., presence of dominant female, timid male, first time breeding)
- Overuse of males, resulting in depletion of epididymal sperm reserves

Initial Database

- Physical exam, including palpation of the scrotal contents, spermatic cords, and prostate
- Semen collection and libido evaluation
- Semen evaluation (including volume, motility, concentration, and morphology)
- Seminal and prostatic fluid cytologic analysis and culture (p. 1153)
- CBC, serum biochemistry panel, urinalysis
- Serologic titers, as appropriate: *B. canis*, feline coronavirus/FIP

Advanced or Confirmatory Testing

All categories:

- Scrotal and prostatic ultrasonography for structural lesions
- Endocrine testing: baseline testosterone, estradiol, follicle-stimulating hormone concentrations and/or prolactin
- Endocrine stimulation testing
  - Administer 2.2-3.3 mcg/kg GnRH IM or 44 IU/kg human chorionic gonadotropin (hCG) IM in dogs with baseline testosterone and luteinizing hormone (LH) and then sample for LH (10 minutes after injection) and testosterone (1 hour after injection)
  - 250-500 IU hCG IM or IV or 25 mcg GnRH IM in toms with baseline testosterone and post-stimulation samples taken 2 and 4 hours later for hCG or 1 hour after GnRH
  - Normal response: minimum of a twofold to fourfold increase in testosterone concentrations
  - Negligible or inappropriate response indicates a primary testicular lesion or a lesion of the hypothalamic-pituitary axis, resulting in failed feedback loop mechanisms.
- Testicular aspirate or biopsy
- Advanced semen diagnostics: sperm chromatin structure assay, electron microscopy, *in vitro* functional assays, flow cytometry

Asthenozoospermia:

- Radiography of the thorax, biopsy and electron microscopy of nasal or respiratory epithelium or spermatozoal midpieces for evaluation for primary ciliary dyskinesia
- Exam of ejaculate for pH and/or presence of urine crystals, indicating urine contamination
- Collection directly into semen extender at body temperature, with fractionation of ejaculate

Teratozoospermia:

- Detailed morphologic exam using special staining (i.e., Spermac, toluidine blue, Coomassie blue) and microscopic techniques (i.e., phase-contrast, differential interference contrast, or electron microscopy).

Oligozoospermia:

- Urinalysis after ejaculation to assess for retrograde ejaculation. Sample may be obtained by cystocentesis or catheterization.
- Seminal plasma alkaline phosphatase concentrations to confirm that ejaculation actually occurred with azoospermia.

TREATMENT

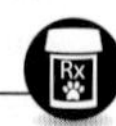

Treatment Overview

- Increase the number of total sperm, the number of total motile cells, and/or the number of normal cells per ejaculate.
- Manage use of the male to maximize fertility.

Acute General Treatment

All:

- Bacterial infections should be treated with appropriate antibiotics based on culture and sensitivity and on ability of drug to be effective in target tissue (e.g., blood-prostate barrier [p. 1443]). Individuals positively confirmed to be infected with brucellosis should be neutered or culled and all kennelmates tested.
- Hemicastration for unilateral inflammatory, obstructive, or neoplastic conditions

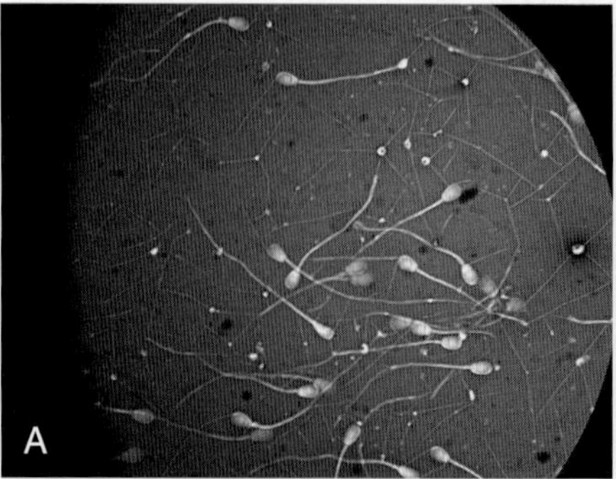

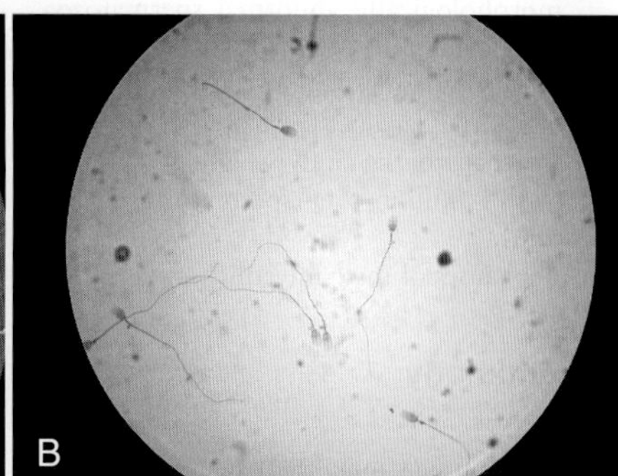

INFERTILITY, MALE Sperm morphology slides were made with an eosin-nigrosin (viability) stain (**A**) or Romanowsky (Diff-Quik) (**B**). With the viability stain, sperm that have damaged cell membranes (dead) stain red (pink), whereas sperm with normal cell membranes (live) do not take up the eosin and therefore appear white. With the Romanowsky stain, increased incubation time (at least 5 minutes for each stain instead of the typical 10 dips in the stain jar) is required for the sperm cells to take up adequate amounts of stain to determine morphology. Cytoplasmic droplets are not evident with Romanowsky stain.

- Cats that meet the clinical and laboratory criteria for FIP should be removed from catteries/multi-cat environments.

Asthenozoospermia:

- Careful cleaning, rinsing (at least twice with distilled water), and drying of artificial insemination equipment
- Sparing use of nonspermicidal lubricants
- Empty bladder immediately before collection to avoid urine contamination of ejaculate.
- In dogs, administer phenylpropanolamine at 1-2 mg/kg PO 1 hour before collection

Teratozoospermia:

- With scrotal overheating, waiting at least 65 days from insult should result in return to normal spermatozoal morphology.
- Weight reduction in obese males
- Centrifugation with sperm gradients to remove abnormal sperm

Oligozoospermia:

- With scrotal overheating, it requires at least 2-4 months from insult to have normal spermatozoal morphology return.
- For retrograde ejaculation: in dogs, phenylpropanolamine 1-2 mg/kg PO q 8-12h or 1-2 hours prior to collection; or, pseudoephedrine 1.5 mg/kg PO q 8h or up to 4-5 mg/kg PO 1-3 hours before breeding as a single dose (not to exceed 5 mg/kg/day); in toms, phenylpropanolamine 6.25-12.5 mg/CAT PO q 8-12h. Do not use either medication in dogs or cats with systemic hypertension.
- In dogs, administration of GnRH (Cystorelin 2.2 mcg/kg IM) to increase libido 20-30 minutes before collection or dinoprost tromethamine (Lutalyse 0.01-0.05 mg/kg SQ) 20 minutes before collection (results in sperm-rich ejaculate only ± full erection)
- Weight reduction in obese males
- Positive reinforcement for behavioral issues

Chronic Treatment

Asthenozoospermia:

- Immediate centrifugation of the ejaculate in cases of urine contamination, followed by re-extension with semen extender or centrifugation with sperm gradients
- Depo-testosterone enanthate (testosterone) plus pregnant mare serum gonadotropin (PMSG) every 2 weeks for 6 weeks has been advocated, but dosages, efficacy, and safety have not been established (50 mg/DOG testosterone enanthate with 250 IU/dog PMSG have been used successfully in 15-kg dogs).

Teratozoospermia, oligozoospermia ± asthenozoospermia:

- For testicular degeneration, long-term GnRH 3.3 mcg/kg IM q 1 week or hCG 500-1000 IU IM q 2 weeks in dogs or hCG 250-500 IU IM q 2 weeks in toms has shown some positive effects.
- In dogs, tamoxifen citrate 2.5-20 mg PO q 24h or anastrazole 0.25-1 mg PO q 24h can be used in individuals with high estrogen concentrations to alter negative hypothalamic/pituitary feedback, increasing local testosterone concentrations.
- In dogs and cats, long-acting GnRH analogs (e.g., buserelin 1 mcg/kg SQ q 1-2 weeks) can increase testosterone concentrations.

Nutrition/Diet

- Administration of daily glucosamine, omega-3 fatty acids, and DHA supplements may be of benefit for asthenozoospermia.
- Administration of daily zinc sulfate, carnitine, and vitamin E supplement may be of benefit for all conditions.

Behavior/Exercise

Excessive exercise and stress may result in infertility from chronic stress or overheating.

Recommended Monitoring

- Routine (monthly) microscopic re-evaluation of the spermiogram and reassessment of endocrine function as indicated, beginning 2 to 3 months after initiation of treatment
- Monitor pregnancy rates and litter size.

PROGNOSIS & OUTCOME

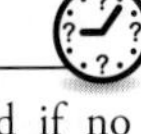

The prognosis for fertility is guarded if no response to treatment occurs within 3 months, poor if no response occurs within 6 months, and grave if no response occurs within a year. Some causes are never expected to improve (e.g., brucellosis, ciliary dyskinesia).

PEARLS & CONSIDERATIONS

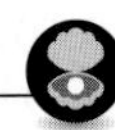

Comments

Optimize available sperm:

- Accurate breeding management and ovulation timing
- Reduce the number of matings per cycle.
- Use of transcervical or surgical insemination
- Breeding to young, fertile females

Avoid overuse:

- Do not collect more than every other day.
- Collection of males 7-10 days before anticipated matings in animals that have had prolonged abstinence to flush the ejaculatory tract of dead sperm
- Avoid strict raw-meat diets because they may result in amino acid or vitamin/mineral deficiencies.

Never diagnose sterility after a single exam.

Prevention

- Brucellosis screening biannually (dogs)
- Coronavirus/FIP screening of all new entries into catteries (p. 327)

Technician Tips

- When evaluating motility, dilute the sample enough to evaluate individual sperm movement.
- Encourage use of teaser bitch for all collections for infertility exams to prevent oligospermia due to lack of stimulation.

Client Education

- Monitor semen quality regularly for breeding males.
- Freeze semen when dogs are young and fertile.

SUGGESTED READING

Johnston SD, et al: Clinical approach to infertility in the male dog. In Johnston SD, et al, editors: Canine and feline theriogenology, Philadelphia, 2001, Saunders, pp 381-382.

AUTHOR: Cheryl Lopate, DVM, MS, DACT
EDITOR: Michelle A. Kutzler, DVM, PhD, DACT

Inflammatory Bowel Disease

Client Education Sheet

BASIC INFORMATION

Definition

Common intestinal disease characterized by chronic (>3 weeks) gastrointestinal (GI) signs of idiopathic origin, with inflammatory infiltration of small- and/or large-intestinal mucosa

Synonyms

IBD, chronic enteropathy (CE); depending on the infiltrating cell type: lymphocytic-plasmacytic, eosinophilic, suppurative, or granulomatous, and depending on location: enteritis, colitis, or enterocolitis

Epidemiology

SPECIES, AGE, SEX

Dogs and cats of all ages affected but moderate to severe forms more prevalent among middle-aged and old animals

GENETICS, BREED PREDISPOSITION

A U.K. study showed that German shepherds, Weimaraners, rottweilers, border collies, and boxers were at high risk of developing IBD in that country. Protein-losing enteropathy (PLE) occurs frequently in soft-coated wheaten terriers, Yorkshire terriers, and other small breeds; rottweilers; and lundehunds. Granulomatous colitis affects boxers and French bulldogs.

ASSOCIATED DISORDERS

- Dog: severe IBD may cause PLE and/or intestinal lymphangiectasia (p. 600)
- Cat: triaditis with concurrent IBD, cholangitis, and pancreatitis; prevalence unknown (pp. 160 and 740)

Clinical Presentation

DISEASE FORMS/SUBTYPES

- Clinical signs vary, depending on which segment of the intestine is involved.
- Subtypes are often described by the type of inflammation (i.e., lymphocytic-plasmacytic, eosinophilic, suppurative, or granulomatous [p. 395]).
- IBD or CE can be subtyped on the basis of clinical response, including food responsive (p. 347), antibiotic responsive (p. 260), or steroid responsive.

HISTORY, CHIEF COMPLAINT

- Mild IBD may cause intermittent clinical signs, whereas severe IBD is characterized by severe, progressive clinical signs.
- Dogs are presented for evaluation of chronic small- or large-bowel diarrhea (p. 1215).
  - Small-intestinal: decreased appetite, weight loss, vomiting, and lethargy
  - Large intestinal: characteristic diarrhea, occasionally vomiting
- Cats are usually presented for evaluation of chronic vomiting, which may or may not be associated with diarrhea. Hyporexia/anorexia, weight loss, and lethargy are common.

PHYSICAL EXAM FINDINGS

Small-intestinal disease:

- Poor body condition with poor haircoat is common with severe disease.
- Dehydration is possible.
- Thickened small-intestinal loops may occasionally be palpated (cats).
- Animals occasionally show pain or discomfort on abdominal palpation.
- Ascites, pleural effusion, and peripheral edema can occur in PLE.

Large-intestinal disease:

- Usually unremarkable; may be associated with abdominal discomfort in severe cases
- Mucoid and/or bloody stool during rectal exam; sometimes thickened or irregular rectal mucosa

Etiology and Pathophysiology

- Abnormal interactions between intestinal microbiota and innate/adaptive immune response
- Breakdown of the intestinal mucosal barrier and exposure of lamina propria to luminal antigens, with subsequent uncontrolled immune response
- Inflammation causes changes in mucosal architecture and ultracellular structure of enterocytes and ultimately results in abnormal function.
- Protein loss reflects poor absorptive function and/or inflammatory exudation or ulceration.
- In some instances, IBD is associated with mucosa-adhesive bacteria such as *Escherichia coli* (e.g., canine granulomatous colitis, feline IBD).
- IBD may predispose to GI lymphoma (p. 604)

DIAGNOSIS

Diagnostic Overview

The diagnosis of IBD requires exclusion of other causes for the clinical signs, and GI biopsies for confirmation of inflammation.

Differential Diagnosis

- For diarrhea (p. 1213)
- For chronic vomiting (p. 1294)
- For hypoalbuminemia (p. 1239), including lymphangiectasia (dog)

GI signs and histologic evidence of GI inflammation:

- Infiltrative intestinal neoplasia (e.g., alimentary lymphoma, especially in cats)
- Infectious diseases
  - Fungal enterocolitis (e.g., *Histoplasma*)
  - Bacterial enterocolitis (e.g., in dogs, *Campylobacter* spp, *Campylobacter perfringens, Campylobacter difficile*); rarely a primary disease
  - Granulomatous enteritis associated with pythiosis, protothecosis, or schistosomiasis

Initial Database

- Perform fecal parasitologic exams (flotation and direct) to rule out nematodes, protozoa, and *Giardia* (consider *Giardia* antigen test) in animals with diarrhea.
  - Alternatively, empirical treatment with broad-spectrum anthelminthic drug (e.g., fenbendazole 50 mg/kg PO q 24h for 3-5 days)
- If the animal seems well other than mild to moderate GI signs, a diet trial is a reasonable next step. Up to 70% of dogs with chronic diarrhea and 50% of cats with chronic GI signs respond within 2 weeks to empirical dietary trial using novel protein or hydrolyzed peptide diet (p. 347).
- Dogs that fail elimination trial may benefit from antibiotic treatment with tylosin 25 mg/kg PO q 12-24h or metronidazole 10-15 mg/kg PO q 12h (p. 260).
- If empirical treatment fails or animal demonstrates more than mild clinical signs, additional testing is required.
- CBC: useful to rule out other differential diagnoses
- Serum biochemistry: helps rule out or generate suspicion of other differential diagnoses (e.g., kidney or liver disease, hypoadrenocorticism)
  - Panhypoproteinemia associated with severe disease (dog)
  - Low total and ionized serum calcium reflect hypoalbuminemia (total calcium), malabsorption of vitamin D (ionized calcium)
  - Liver enzymes may point to concomitant liver or pancreatic disease (e.g., feline triaditis).
- Abdominal radiographs: rule out intestinal obstruction, especially if vomiting
- Abdominal ultrasound: fair sensitivity, good specificity. Focal or diffuse loss of intestinal wall layering, mucosal striations or spicules, wall thickening, enlarged and/or hypoechoic mesenteric lymph nodes may be detected. Localization of lesions may help decide best approach for biopsies (endoscopy or celiotomy).
- Serum cobalamin and folate concentrations (pp. 1325 and 1344)
- Consider baseline cortisol or ACTH stimulation test (dog) to rule out hypoadrenocorticism
- Serum thyroxine concentration (cat > 5 years) to rule out hyperthyroidism
- Rectal scrape (p. 1157): look for pathogens (e.g., *Histoplasma, Pythium*) if in endemic area

Advanced or Confirmatory Testing

- Upper and/or lower GI endoscopy (p. 1098): assess mucosa, sample at least eight deep biopsies per anatomic site.
- Celiotomy if endoscopy is not available, lesions are inaccessible by endoscopy, or full-thickness biopsies are desirable (avoid full-thickness biopsy of colon)
- Histopathologic analysis: objective is to confirm and evaluate severity of mucosal lesions (inflammation, architecture) and to rule out neoplastic or pathogen infiltration. Pathologists should use current reporting standards (i.e., World Small Animal Veterinary Association guidelines).
  - In cats, immunohistochemistry and polymerase chain reaction (PCR) for antigen receptor rearrangement (PARR) are recommended to differentiate IBD from alimentary small cell lymphoma.

TREATMENT

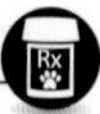

Treatment Overview

In cases with mild to moderate disease severity, a dietary elimination trial should be completed, and possibly followed by an antibiotic trial, before considering immunosuppressive therapy. Only if these fail and infectious causes of clinical signs have been reasonably excluded should immune suppression be considered. The goal of therapy is to control clinical signs because a cure may be unattainable.

Acute and Chronic Treatment

- Empirical deworming, as above
- Diet trial (hypoallergenic or novel antigen), as above
- Antibiotic trial (tylosin or metronidazole), as above
- Probiotics may have beneficial effects as adjunctive treatment.
- Supportive treatment (e.g., IV fluids, antiemetics) as necessary based on clinical findings

- Supplement hypocobalaminemic patients with PO or SQ vitamin B_{12} (p. 183).
- Address any infection (especially important for granulomatous colitis [p. 395])
- Noninfectious colitis may respond to sulfasalazine 10-30 mg/kg PO q 8h for 2 weeks, then taper to same dose q 12h for 2 weeks, then one-half dose q 12h for 2 weeks, and so on. Alternatively, olsalazine 10-20 mg/kg PO q 12h. Monitor tear production (risk of keratoconjunctivitis sicca with sulfa drugs).
- In severe IBD, in dogs with PLE, or in cases in which empirical approaches have failed, immune suppression with glucocorticoids is indicated.
  - Prednisone (dog) or prednisolone (cat) 2 mg/kg PO initially q 12h for a few days, then q 24h for 2-4 weeks. After remission of signs is achieved, decrease the dose by 25%-50% at 2-4 week intervals. Treatment and weaning period usually lasts for at least 8-12 weeks.
  - Budesonide (dog 3 mg/m^2 PO q 24h [p. 609] for body surface area conversion]; cat, 1 mg/CAT PO q 24h) can be substituted for prednisone. Budesonide undergoes some first-pass hepatic metabolism, and low systemic drug concentrations may cause fewer side effects.
  - Addition of metronidazole to glucocorticoid treatment does not appear beneficial.
- In glucocorticoid-refractory cases
  - Cyclosporine 5 mg/kg PO q 12-24h (dog, cat); *or*
  - Dogs only: azathioprine 2 mg/kg PO q 24h for 2 weeks, then q 48h (can be decreased to 1 mg/kg q 48h), *or*
  - Chlorambucil: may be used as supplemental immune-suppressive therapy in cats 2 mg/cat PO q 48h and in dogs with associated PLE 4-6 mg/m^2 PO q 24h for the first 7-21 days, then taper to q 48-72h, *or*
  - Mycophenolate mofetil 10 mg/kg PO q 12h may also be used in dogs, although the author does not recommend it for this indication. Up to 20% of dogs develop diarrhea and other GI signs.
- Dogs with PLE at increased risk for thromboembolism; clopidogrel 1-2 mg/kg PO q 24h after a loading dose of 10 mg/kg on first day, or low-dose aspirin 0.5 mg/kg PO q 12h for prophylaxis
- Ultimately, attempt to wean the patient off immunosuppressive therapy. If this is not feasible, find the lowest-dose/longest dosing interval regimen that achieves reasonable control of clinical signs.

Nutrition/Diet

- An elimination diet with novel proteins (requires detailed nutritional history) or hydrolyzed peptides is recommended in most dogs and cats with IBD and is often successful as a sole treatment in mild cases.
- Alternatively, an easily digestible diet with low fat content (<20% metabolizable energy as fat) may be preferable in cases of severe IBD and PLE.
- Consider adding soluble fiber (psyllium 1-2 teaspoons/10 kg body weight per meal) for colitis.

Possible Complications

- High doses of glucocorticoids may cause multiple systemic side effects (e.g., polyuria/polydipsia, panting).
- Side effects reported with cyclosporine use in dogs include decreased appetite and vomiting. Administering frozen capsules may help.
- Azathioprine has been associated with acute pancreatitis and hepatotoxicosis in dogs and may cause bone marrow suppression. Avoid use in patients with previous history of pancreatitis and liver disease. As with chlorambucil, regular monitoring of CBC is advised, and monitoring of serum liver enzyme levels is recommended at the beginning of treatment.
- Immunosuppressive medications predispose animals to secondary infections.

Recommended Monitoring

Regular evaluation of the body weight and overall clinical condition is essential to adapt treatment. Recheck abnormal laboratory parameters (e.g., serum albumin, cobalamin) to evaluate treatment success.

PROGNOSIS & OUTCOME

- Good for dogs and cats with mild forms that respond to an elimination diet
- Guarded for dogs with idiopathic intestinal dysbiosis because they may require repeated long periods of antibiotic treatment
- In dogs, negative prognostic factors include hypoalbuminemia, hypocobalaminemia, and severe mucosal lesions in the duodenum (endoscopy).
- Prognosis is guarded for dogs with moderate to severe IBD, and treatment failures are common. This may be due to incorrect diagnosis, severe disease, concurrent disease, or poor owner compliance.
- In cats, lack of response to treatment should motivate the clinician to reconsider the possibility of alimentary lymphoma. IBD in cats may progress to GI lymphoma.

PEARLS & CONSIDERATIONS

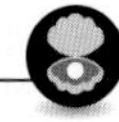

Comments

- IBD is a diagnosis of exclusion that requires a systematic approach. In mild cases, dietary elimination trial is frequently successful. Severe cases require a more intensive approach.
- Many cats may show only nonspecific signs. Differentiating IBD from small cell alimentary lymphoma in cats can be challenging.

Technician Tips

After intestinal parasites have been ruled out, many dogs with mild IBD respond within 2 weeks to an elimination diet. Obtain a very detailed diet history, and emphasize the importance of a very strict diet. Avoid anything other than the trial diet by mouth.

Client Education

- A realistic goal for treatment is to manage the intestinal disease. Because a definitive cure may not be attainable, the goal is to control clinical signs while limiting the side effects of treatment.
- Because diet is of central importance to treatment, every effort should be made to adhere closely to dietary recommendations.

SUGGESTED READING

Dandrieux JRS: Inflammatory bowel disease versus chronic enteropathy in dogs: are they one and the same? J Small Anim Pract 57:589, 2016.

AUTHOR: Frédéric Gaschen, Dr.med.vet., Dr.habil., DACVIM, DECVIM
EDITOR: Rance K. Sellon, DVM, PhD, DACVIM

Influenza, Canine

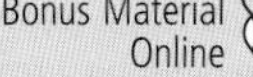

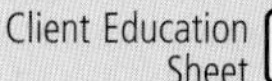

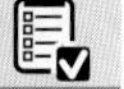

Bonus Material Online

Client Education Sheet

BASIC INFORMATION

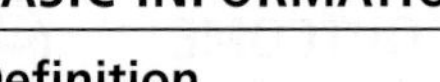

Definition

Canine influenza is an uncommon but highly contagious respiratory disease caused by type A influenza viruses that affect dogs. H3N8 evolved from an equine influenza and was first reported in Florida greyhounds in 2004. H3N2 came from an Asian avian influenza and was first reported in the Chicago area in 2015.

Synonyms

- Dog flu, canine influenza virus (CIV), H3N8 and/or H3N2
- Part of the canine infectious respiratory disease complex (CIRDC) (layman's term: kennel cough)

Epidemiology

SPECIES, AGE, SEX

- Dogs of any age; often, vaccinated for CIRDC pathogens other than CIV
- Cats have also been infected with H3N2.

GENETICS, BREED PREDISPOSITION

Any breed can be infected. Greyhounds have developed hemorrhagic pneumonia and sudden death from H3N8.

RISK FACTORS

- High-density canine populations (e.g., boarding kennels, shelters, grooming facilities, doggie day care, dog shows)
- Exposure to other dogs, especially during regional outbreaks
- Unvaccinated for CIV

CONTAGION AND ZOONOSIS

- Dog-to-dog transmission (spread through direct contact), fomites (e.g., humans, food bowls, leashes), and aerosol transmission
- H3N2: may be spread to cats
- H3N8 and H3N2: no reported zoonotic spread
- H1N1: undocumented reports of canine infection from contact with infected owners
- H7N2 (avian influenza): transmitted to cats in New York and subsequently infected the attending veterinarian. CDC considers the risk to humans to be low.
- Other type A influenza virus types (including seasonal influenza): rarely are transmitted from people to pets

GEOGRAPHY AND SEASONALITY

Confirmed CIV has occurred in numerous states with several hyperendemic foci that were identified in the Northeast, Midwest, western states, and Florida. There is no seasonality but may spread more rapidly during times of increased travel such as summer vacations or holidays.

ASSOCIATED DISORDERS

- Bacterial pneumonia
- Hemorrhagic pneumonia

Clinical Presentation

DISEASE FORMS/SUBTYPES

Three forms exist:

- Subclinical form: minimal/absent clinical signs (≈20% of exposed)
- Mild upper respiratory form: fever, cough, nasal discharge (most common)
- Severe form: as above, with signs of potentially life-threatening pneumonia (≈5%-20%)

HISTORY, CHIEF COMPLAINT

- Recent exposure to other dogs (especially high density), endemic geographic area with history of outbreaks
- Moist cough (productive or nonproductive), nasal discharge, lethargy, fever, anorexia, depression, and tachypnea/dyspnea

PHYSICAL EXAM FINDINGS

- Soft, moist paroxysmal cough (can be a dry cough, indistinguishable from mild tracheitis); most consistent finding
- Mucopurulent nasal discharge common
- Lethargy, fever, tachypnea and/or dyspnea, harsh lung sounds/crackles ± cyanosis: if pneumonia

Etiology and Pathophysiology

- Incubation time is 1-5 days after exposure.
- Clinical signs generally last 2-4 weeks.
- Peak shedding (2-4 days after infection) may occur before clinical signs begin.
- Although viral shedding may be shorter, dogs should be considered contagious for up to 4 weeks (H3N2 > H3N8).

DIAGNOSIS

Diagnostic Overview

Onset of clinical signs after recent exposure to high-density dog populations, especially in endemic areas, is suggestive. Confirmation requires a positive polymerase chain reaction (PCR) or positive CIV antibody titer. Because acute phase titer may be negative, paired samples should be taken at presentation and then 2-3 weeks later (convalescent phase). Combining paired serologic titers and PCR is optimal.

Differential Diagnosis

Other CIRDC pathogens:

- *Bordetella bronchiseptica*
- Canine parainfluenza virus
- Canine distemper virus
- Canine adenovirus 2
- Canine herpesvirus
- Canine pneumovirus
- Canine respiratory corona virus
- *Mycoplasma* spp
- Opportunistic bacterial pneumonia (*Pasteurella multocida, Klebsiella pneumoniae, Escherichia coli, Streptococcus* spp)

Initial Database

During confirmed outbreaks, complete diagnostic testing may be omitted when history and exam are highly suggestive of CIV, especially where cost is a concern.

- CBC, serum biochemistry profile, urinalysis: unremarkable, or neutrophilia ± immature neutrophils
- Thoracic radiographs: ± interstitial to alveolar pattern

Advanced or Confirmatory Testing

- Serologic testing: commonly used
  - First sample drawn as soon as possible after onset of clinical signs, second sample 2-3 weeks later
  - Fourfold increase in titer or seroconversion is confirmatory.
- PCR: nasal /pharyngeal swab samples to reference laboratory; specific but sensitivity depends on disease stage (best early)
- Influenza A ELISA: less sensitive than PCR but can be done as point-of-care test
- Virus isolation: most often used at necropsy (affected lung)
- Airway culture/susceptibility (p. 1073): typically done to characterize secondary bacterial infection or to rule out other cause of lung disease; neutrophilic infiltrate ± secondary bacteria

TREATMENT

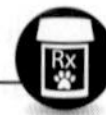

Treatment Overview

Treatment consists of supportive care and prevention/management of secondary bacterial infections. If CIRDC (including CIV) is suspected, isolation from other dogs is crucial. During outbreaks, coughing dogs may best undergo initial examination in the owner's vehicle. Outpatient treatment is preferred unless intensive treatment for pneumonia is required.

Acute General Treatment

- Maintain hydration (PO, SQ, or IV)
- Antibacterial drugs have no effect on CIV
  - If empirical treatment is deemed appropriate to address secondary bacterial infection, empirical choices include doxycycline 5 mg/kg PO q 12h for 7-10 days, azithromycin 5-10 mg/kg PO q 24h for 3-7 days, or cefovecin 8 mg/kg SC once.
  - Severe secondary bacterial pneumonia is best guided by airway culture and susceptibility using parenteral, bactericidal drugs (p. 795).
- Antiviral therapy (e.g., oseltamivir [Tamiflu]) is not approved for dogs, may promote emergence of resistant influenza strains, and is unlikely to be given to dogs quickly enough to provide benefit (must be given within 36 hours of exposure).
- Severe pneumonia may require additional treatment.
  - Nebulization and coupage q 6-8h (p. 1134)
  - Oxygen supplementation if necessary (p. 1146)

Chronic Treatment

See Bacterial Pneumonia (p. 795).

Possible Complications

Pneumonia, sepsis, pulmonary hemorrhage

Recommended Monitoring

- At home
  - Have owner monitor food and water intake, hydration, membrane color, temperature, and respiratory rate, and provide parameters to prompt re-evaluation.
- In hospital (pneumonia)
  - Repeat thoracic auscultation several times daily
  - Pulse oximetry or arterial blood gas (A:a gradient, PaO_2/FIO_2) if hypoxemia suspected
  - Thoracic radiographs if clinical deterioration

PROGNOSIS & OUTCOME

- Good with supportive care and antibacterial therapy
- Morbidity ≈80%
- Mortality 1%-5% (severe form: pneumonia)

PEARLS & CONSIDERATIONS

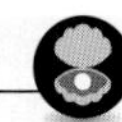

Comments

- Use proper isolation precautions (p. 987).
- Unless hospitalization required (e.g., oxygen therapy, IV fluids and medications), treat as outpatients.
  - Teach owners how to monitor hydration, temperature, respiratory rate/effort
  - Provide parameters for necessary return to hospital
- Progression to pneumonia may take 5-10 days.
- Coughing can continue for 10-30 days.

Prevention

- Conditional use of vaccines; CIV bivalent/univalent vaccines are inactivated vaccines given as initial series of two doses (2 weeks apart) with annual boosters.
  - Vaccine may not prevent infection but can reduce disease severity and viral shedding.
- Dogs presenting for veterinary care due to acute respiratory signs should be handled as if they have a contagious disease.
- Dogs with unexplained cough and/or nasal discharge should be kept isolated.
- Restrict access to high-density dog populations.

Technician Tips

- Wear gloves and wear protective gowns/clothing when handing dogs with CIRDC/CIV. Wash hands, and remove gown before handling other dogs.
- Strict isolation procedures: minimum 20-foot (6-meter) separation from other animals; when cleaning, use virucidal disinfectants with a minimum of 10 minutes contact time; dry surfaces well.
- Clear shower curtains hung in front of run/cage may reduce aerosol spread if separate isolation housing is unavailable.
- Clean nasal and ocular discharge with a warm moist disposable cloth.
- Warm food to enhance smell when offering food (nasal congestion) (p. 1199).
- Wash hands frequently and change clothes prior to handling non-exposed animals.

Client Education

- If treating at home, teach owner how to take temperature and monitor membrane color and breathing effort/respiratory rate.
- Keep separated from other pets, and vaccinate other dogs in the household.
- Do not take to public areas (e.g., dog parks, groomer) for a month after illness.

SUGGESTED READINGS

Crawford C, et al: Canine influenza. In Miller L, et al, editors: Infectious disease management in animal shelters, Ames, IA, 2009, Wiley-Blackwell, 173-180.

AUTHOR: Wendy Wolfson, DVM
EDITOR: Joseph Taboada, DVM, DACVIM

Infraspinatus Tendon Disorders

Client Education Sheet 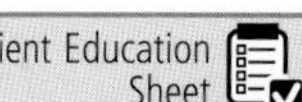 Video Available  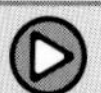

BASIC INFORMATION

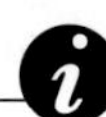

Definition

Disorders of the infraspinatus and teres minor muscles in the shoulder area of dogs, including myopathy and fibrotic contracture

Synonyms

- Infraspinatus contracture
- Fibrotic contracture of the infraspinatus muscle
- Infraspinatus myopathy

Epidemiology

SPECIES, AGE, SEX

Most commonly seen in medium-sized adult dogs

GENETICS, BREED PREDISPOSITION

Infraspinatus contracture is classically seen in hunting or working dogs.

RISK FACTORS

Overuse, trauma, or aging may play a role.

Clinical Presentation

DISEASE FORMS/SUBTYPES

- Acute, subtle to severe lameness
- Mechanical lameness resulting from fibrotic contracture

HISTORY, CHIEF COMPLAINT

Infraspinatus myopathy is associated with an acute lameness that resolves initially to be replaced by a chronic gait abnormality (external rotation of the manus in the swing phase) of gradual onset 4-8 weeks later.

PHYSICAL EXAM FINDINGS

- In the acute stage, there may be muscle swelling and pain on palpation caudal to the scapular spine.
- Chronic infraspinatus contracture has several distinguishing clinical signs.
  - Characteristic stance with adduction of the shoulder and elbow and external rotation of the distal limb.
  - Atrophy of the infraspinatus muscle, with supination of the distal limb (most evident when the dog is held up so the limb is not bearing weight)
  - During the swing phase, the distal limb circumducts in a lateral arc, producing a characteristic paddling gait (see *Video*).
  - Restriction to elbow flexion may disappear if the limb is held in normal alignment and externally rotated during manipulation.
  - Pain is usually not a feature of the chronic stage.

Etiology and Pathophysiology

- Infraspinatus contracture may be a result of trauma causing rupture of the muscle, which is then replaced with fibrotic tissue, leading to contracture over time.
- Compartment syndrome (muscle necrosis secondary to high pressure within a space constrained by a fascia) is suspected in at least some cases.

DIAGNOSIS

Diagnostic Overview

Infraspinatus contracture in the chronic stage is diagnosed on physical exam. In the acute phase, ultrasonography may reveal disruption of the normal architecture of the infraspinatus muscle.

Differential Diagnosis

- Bicipital tenosynovitis
- Shoulder osteoarthritis
- Shoulder instability/luxation
- Elbow dysplasia
- Osteosarcoma of the proximal humerus
- Nerve sheath tumor (especially before onset of neurologic dysfunction)

Initial Database

- Orthopedic (p. 1143) and neurologic (p. 1136) evaluations
- Radiography of the shoulder; lateral, craniocaudal, and cranioproximal-craniodistal views: findings usually normal
- CBC, serum biochemistry panel, urinalysis in older dogs

Advanced or Confirmatory Testing

- Localization of pain involves applying digital pressure to the insertion of the supraspinatus tendon (craniomedial greater tubercle of humerus), the bicipital tendon (intertubercular groove), and infraspinatus tendon of insertion (lateral and distal to greater tubercle).
- Ultrasonography of the infraspinatus muscle often reveals structural changes: hypoechogenicity during the acute phase and hyperechogenicity with development of fibrosis.
- The presence of mineralization alone is not diagnostic because it can be an incidental finding.

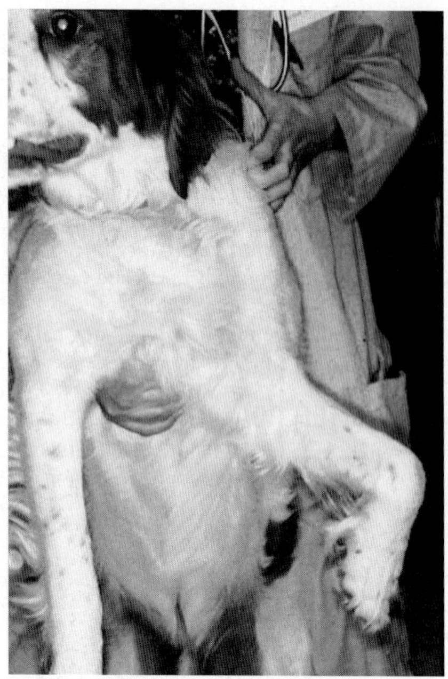

INFRASPINATUS TENDON DISORDERS Characteristic limb positioning of a dog with left infraspinatus contracture. (Courtesy Kathleen Linn.)

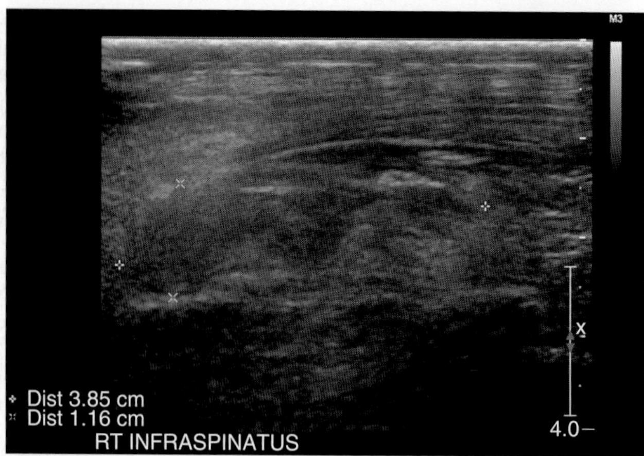

INFRASPINATUS TENDON DISORDERS Transverse ultrasonogram of an acute infraspinatus injury. Note the normal architecture in the top of the image, contrasting with the disrupted architecture outlined by the *white crossmarks.*

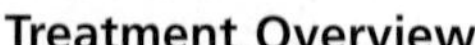

TREATMENT

Treatment Overview

Surgical treatment is usually indicated for infraspinatus contracture, with the goal of returning normal range of motion to the affected limb. Conservative therapy may be chosen because the contracture does not appear to be painful, but this strategy is unlikely to resolve the gait abnormality.

Acute General Treatment

- If acute infraspinatus trauma is suspected, early fasciotomy (with suturing of the muscle tear) may be indicated to decompress the muscle and avoid compartment syndrome. However, the acute phase often goes unrecognized.
- Injection of platelet-rich plasma (PRP) with ultrasound guidance into affected areas of the tendon and muscle shows promise if early acute injury can be detected. Controlled clinical studies are lacking at this point.
- Physical rehabilitation may be successful in maintaining range of motion and preventing fibrotic contracture in acute cases.

Chronic Treatment

Infraspinatus contracture treatment consists of infraspinatus (and sometimes teres minor) tenotomy and excision of the tendon insertion. Immediate ability to pronate the limb is achieved. Leash walks are performed immediately postoperatively, and normal activity is resumed 10-14 days after infraspinatus tenotomy.

Nutrition/Diet

Dietary management to prevent or treat obesity is likely beneficial for long-term management.

Behavior/Exercise

- Exercise is restricted for 2-4 weeks after surgery. Physical therapy with passive range-of-motion exercises and walking are recommended as soon as possible after surgery to aid the return of normal range of motion.
- Surgical treatment for infraspinatus contracture usually returns the dog to full function.

Possible Complications

- Seroma
- Infection
- Persistent lameness and restricted range of motion

PROGNOSIS & OUTCOME

Surgical treatment of infraspinatus contracture usually leads to an excellent outcome.

PEARLS & CONSIDERATIONS

Comments

- Contracture of the infraspinatus or teres minor muscles, or both, produces the characteristic gait abnormality.
- Lifting the dog's front end off of the ground or examining the dog in lateral recumbency with the affected limb on the nondependent side highlights the external rotation of the distal limb.

Technician Tips

- Early passive range of motion after transection of the infraspinatus tendon speeds recovery and prevents recurrence.
- It is essential to cycle the shoulder rather than the entire limb; have clients demonstrate the technique back to you after teaching them to ensure optimal compliance.

SUGGESTED READING

Devor G, et al: Fibrotic contracture of canine infraspinatus muscle: pathophysiology and prevention by acute surgical intervention. Vet Comp Orthop Traumatology 19:117-121, 2006.

AUTHOR: Peter Gilbert, BVSc, MVetSc, DACVS
EDITOR: Kathleen Linn, DVM, MS, DACVS

Inguinal Hernia

Client Education Sheet

BASIC INFORMATION

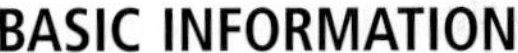
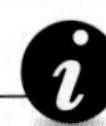

Definition

Defect in the inguinal ring, through which abdominal contents can protrude

Epidemiology

SPECIES, AGE, SEX

- Acquired: middle-aged to older, intact female dogs
- Congenital: young male small breeds; testicular descent likely delays inguinal ring narrowing
- Uncommon in cats

GENETICS, BREED PREDISPOSITION

- Acquired hernias
  - Toy breeds are overrepresented.
- Congenital hernias
  - Predisposed breeds include basenji, Pekingese, poodle, Cairn terrier, and West Highland white terriers
  - Polygenic inheritance suspected in cocker spaniels and dachshunds
- Traumatic inguinal hernia: no specific predispositions (rare)

RISK FACTORS

- Intact female, during or shortly after estrus or with pregnancy
- Obesity

ASSOCIATED DISORDERS

- Perineal hernia
- Obesity
- Cryptorchidism

Clinical Presentation

DISEASE FORMS/SUBTYPES

- Indirect inguinal hernia
  - Abdominal viscera herniate within the vaginal process.
  - Scrotal hernia in males (vaginal process is continuous with scrotum)
  - Narrowing of vaginal process at inguinal ring may cause organ entrapment/strangulation.
- Direct inguinal hernia
  - Less commonly seen
  - Organs pass through inguinal ring adjacent to evagination of the vaginal process.
  - Usually larger defect than indirect hernias

HISTORY, CHIEF COMPLAINT

- Swelling in the inguinal region
- No systemic signs if omentum/fat herniated or if no organ entrapment
- If organ entrapment/strangulation (devitalized tissue) within the hernia: abdominal pain, vomiting, diarrhea, dysuria/stranguria, vaginal discharge/hemorrhage, bruising, lethargy, depression

PHYSICAL EXAM FINDINGS

- Depends on size and contents of hernia
  - Hernia contents may include omentum/fat (most common), ovaries, uterine horns, intestine, bladder
- Uncomplicated inguinal hernia
  - Painless, unilateral or bilateral mass with a soft, doughy consistency
  - Mass is typically reducible (place in dorsal recumbency to palpate)
  - Enlarged inguinal ring is palpable just proximal and axial to the femoral triangle.
  - Hernia contents tracking along round ligament in females may appear perineal.
- Complicated inguinal hernia
  - Palpation less helpful due to swelling
  - Mass is often firm, nonreducible, and painful. Overlying skin is bruised/erythematous.
- Always palpate contralateral side; 35% are bilateral at time of diagnosis.

Etiology and Pathophysiology

- Pathogenesis is uncertain
- Anatomic: females seem predisposed due to a shorter, wider inguinal canal.
- Hormonal: sex hormones (estrogen) weaken the collagen in connective tissues.
- Nutritional/metabolic
  - Weakening of the abdominal wall secondary to glucocorticoid administration (autonomous or iatrogenic)
  - Weight of pregnant uterus or intra-abdominal fat stretches weakened inguinal ring.
- Traumatic: disruption/weakening of caudal abdominal muscles; rarely caused in isolation without other hernia (femoral or prepubic tendon)

DIAGNOSIS

Diagnostic Overview

Diagnosis is based largely on physical exam. Vomiting, abdominal pain, and depression suggest obstructed or devitalized intestine. Diagnosis is most often confirmed with manual reduction of hernia contents and palpation of an enlarged hernial ring(s). Imaging studies may be useful for complicated hernias.

Differential Diagnosis

- Abscess
- Inguinal lymphadenopathy
- Mammary tumor
- Lipoma
- Inguinal fat pad
- Mastitis: firm, enlarged, painful mammary glands

Initial Database

- CBC may show a leukocytosis with a left shift if intestinal strangulation is present.
- Chemistry panel may indicate mild electrolyte imbalances.
- Perform fine-needle aspiration if deemed appropriate but only under ultrasound guidance to avoid perforation of strangulated intestinal loop or gravid uterus.

Advanced or Confirmatory Testing

- Survey abdominal radiographs
  - Displaced uterus, intestines, urinary bladder
  - Loss of caudal abdominal and inguinal detail suggestive of herniation, although not definitive
- Contrast radiography
  - Retrograde contrast cystourethrogram to determine position of bladder
  - Upper gastrointestinal (GI) contrast studies are not recommended for evaluation of intestinal loops because of the risk of vomiting and subsequent aspiration.
- Abdominal ultrasound helps determine contents and timing of surgery for nonreducible hernias.
- Abdominal contrast CT useful for large, complicated hernias or in cases of blunt abdominal trauma.

TREATMENT

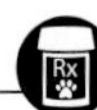

Treatment Overview

- Inguinal hernias are best repaired at time of diagnosis because delay can result in a more difficult procedure and greater risk of complications.
- Immediate surgical intervention is indicated for bladder, intestinal, or uterine incarceration; clinical signs of peritonitis; or intractable pain.

Acute General Treatment

- Goal: reduction or resection (if nonviable) of hernia contents, ligation of hernial sac, and tension-free closure of hernia ring
- Herniorrhaphy: must understand regional anatomy (e.g., exit point of genitofemoral nerve and external pudendal vessels)
  - An abdominal approach by a ventral midline incision is recommended for exploration because it allows simpler closure.
  - Alternative: external approach to inguinal ring by a ventral midline skin incision with subcutaneous dissection to hernia sac (avoids mammary tissue and allows bilateral access)
  - Complicated hernias may require combined approach for reduction of hernia contents and ligation of hernia sac.
  - Laparoscopic repair reported
  - Primary repair is preferably performed with patient's own tissues by partial closure of inguinal ring.

- Autologous muscle flaps or prosthetic materials may be necessary for large defects or recurrent herniation.

Possible Complications

- Preoperative
  - Incarceration or strangulation of involved organs and ensuing peritonitis
  - Intestinal strangulation occurs in < 5% of chronic inguinal hernias.
- Postoperative
  - Overall complication rate of 17%
  - Temporary stiffness when walking
  - Incisional infection/peritonitis
  - Intractable pain if genitofemoral nerve incorporated into repair

Recommended Monitoring

- Monitor surgical site pain, swelling, discharge, and dehiscence.
- Monitor for fever and signs of shock (peritonitis).
- Restrict exercise for 14-21 days.

PROGNOSIS & OUTCOME

- Congenital hernias may resolve spontaneously by ≈12 weeks of age. After this point, surgery is recommended.
- Excellent prognosis after repair of uncomplicated inguinal hernia

PEARLS & CONSIDERATIONS

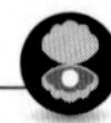

Comments

- Most commonly seen in middle-aged, intact bitches, especially if overweight, recently in heat, or pregnant
- Palpate both inguinal rings, and repair if enlarged.
- Easier to repair with fewer complications when hernias are small
- Animals with traumatic inguinal hernias should be carefully evaluated for other concurrent injuries.

Prevention

- Ovariohysterectomy decreases circulating estrogen.
- Preventing obesity may decrease risk.

Technician Tips

- Monitor and treat for signs of pain and discomfort; severe pain indicates entrapped nerve or tissue devitalization.
- Exercise restriction in postoperative period helps prevent recurrence.

Client Education

- Neuter nonbreeding animals.
- Do not breed male dogs with congenital inguinal hernias.

SUGGESTED READING

Smeak D: Abdominal wall reconstruction and hernias. In Tobias KM, et al, editors: Veterinary surgery: small animal, St. Louis, 2012, Saunders, pp 1353-1379.

AUTHOR: Jacob A. Rubin DVM, DACVS
EDITOR: Elizabeth A. Swanson DVM, MS, DACVS

Injection-Site Sarcoma

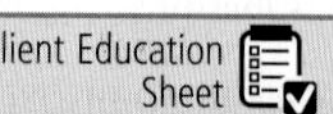

BASIC INFORMATION

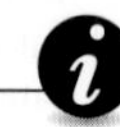

Definition

Commonly occurring tumors that arise from mesenchymal tissue secondary to vaccine administration or other injection

Synonyms

Vaccine-site sarcoma, vaccine-associated fibrosarcoma, vaccine-associated sarcoma

Epidemiology

SPECIES, AGE, SEX

- Almost exclusive to cats; rare reports involving dogs
- Younger age (7-9 years) compared with cats that develop sarcomas at nonvaccine sites

Clinical Presentation

DISEASE FORMS/SUBTYPES

Many tumor types have been identified at vaccination sites in cats, including fibrosarcoma, malignant fibrous histiocytoma, neurofibrosarcoma, nerve sheath tumor, hemangiopericytoma, schwannoma, leiomyosarcoma, rhabdomyosarcoma, undifferentiated sarcoma, osteosarcoma, chondrosarcoma, liposarcoma, and myofibroblastic sarcoma.

HISTORY, CHIEF COMPLAINT

- Cats are usually presented because their owners have noticed a progressively enlarging mass.
- A vaccination history should be obtained. Often, cats with vaccine-site sarcomas have a known prior history of having been vaccinated in a site near the tumor.

PHYSICAL EXAM FINDINGS

Cats usually present with a palpable, firm cutaneous mass. Typical locations include the interscapular area, dorsal lumbar area, flank, or lateral thorax and extremities. Often, the mass is hairless and/or ulcerated. The mass usually is not painful.

Etiology and Pathophysiology

- Injection-site sarcomas have been clearly linked to vaccination with certain inactive vaccines, particularly vaccines that contain aluminum hydroxide adjuvants. It is believed that inflammation at injection sites causes local cell proliferation, which may lead to tumor development.
- Small numbers of case reports and anecdotal reports suggest that these tumors may result from subcutaneous injection of medications, microchips, or fluids.

DIAGNOSIS

Diagnostic Overview

Definitive diagnosis can be confirmed only histopathologically, although adjunctive tests such as diagnostic imaging are often helpful in defining the extent of the tumor. Because an aggressive first surgery is more likely to result in tumor control, an incisional biopsy should be used first to confirm tumor type before planning definitive treatment (rather than an attempt at tumor removal, leaving incomplete margins histologically and requiring reoperation).

Differential Diagnosis

- Local inflammatory vaccine reaction
- Other subcutaneous tumor
- Abscess, granuloma

Initial Database

- Fine-needle aspiration and cytologic exam may help identify the tumor type before other tests.
- Thoracic radiographs to rule out pulmonary metastases

- Radiographs of the affected area may reveal involvement of underlying bone.
- Fine-needle aspiration of draining lymph nodes to help rule out metastasis

Advanced or Confirmatory Testing

- Histopathologic exam of an incisional biopsy specimen. Markers that may link the tumor with vaccine administration include peripheral lymphocytic infiltrate and macrophages in the tumor that contain aluminum adjuvant. In the absence of these markers, the location of the tumor, vaccination history, and diagnosis of a sarcoma can suggest that the tumor was caused by vaccination.
- Simple excisional biopsy is not recommended as a first step in obtaining a diagnosis for this tumor because the treatment is often inadequate. Reports suggest that aggressive surgical resection or multimodality therapy at the time of the first intervention is more likely to result in local disease control.
- Advanced imaging (i.e., CT or MRI) can delineate the local extent of the tumor. Many of these tumors have a peripheral region that is contrast enhancing, with a nonenhancing center. They also often have fingerlike projections that extend far into surrounding normal tissues, and identifying them helps with complete excision.

TREATMENT

Treatment Overview

Treatment goals are to eradicate the local tumor and, in some cats, to prevent or delay metastasis.

Acute and Chronic Treatment

- Radical surgical excision is the treatment of choice if physically possible.
  - Tumors on the distal limbs and tail may be successfully treated with amputation alone.
  - Tumors on the trunk are usually not amenable to radical excision. For these cases, a combination of radiation therapy and surgery (excision with as wide a margin as possible based on physical exam and advanced imaging) is usually indicated for successful treatment of the local tumor.
  - Rarely, surgery with complete excision may be possible and result in adequate local control of the tumor; however, in one report, 31% of cats with complete excision of the tumor based on histopathologically clean margins developed recurrence.
- Radiation therapy before surgery allows adequate treatment of the microscopic tumor extensions with smaller radiation fields; however, therapy interferes with the histopathologic evaluation of the primary tumor mass and the margins, and it may slightly increase risk of wound complications after surgery.
- Hypofractionated radiation therapy (small number of treatments) may be beneficial in controlling incompletely excised tumors for a significant period.
- The role of chemotherapy in the treatment of vaccine-site sarcoma is not well defined. Studies have not shown a definite advantage to using chemotherapy if local therapy (surgery, radiation therapy) is adequate. Nevertheless, many oncologists recommend chemotherapy (doxorubicin, cyclophosphamide, carboplatin, or ifosfamide).

Possible Complications

- Complications of surgery can include wound dehiscence and infection.
- Complications of radiation depend on the location of the tumor in relation to critical normal structures (e.g., spinal cord, kidneys) and the amount of radiation delivered to those structures.
- Chemotherapy complications (p. 152).

Recommended Monitoring

Due to the aggressive local nature of these tumors and the low risk of metastasis, long-term monitoring should include

- Routine exam by a veterinarian to monitor for local recurrence or side effects of treatment
- Routine thoracic radiographs to monitor for pulmonary metastases

PROGNOSIS & OUTCOME

- Prognosis depends on the stage and location of the tumor.
  - Cats with tumors that can be resected with a wide margin of normal tissue (tumors on the tail or distal limbs, small localized tumors) may have an excellent prognosis.
  - Cats with larger tumors that can still be removed with aggressive surgery and are treated with multimodality therapy (radiation, surgery, chemotherapy) may have an excellent prognosis for long-term tumor control; however, some of these cats will develop metastases or recurrence of the primary tumor.
  - Cats with large nonresectable tumors or metastases at the time of diagnosis have a poor prognosis regardless of treatment.
- Another factor that affects recurrence of injection-site sarcoma is the extent of surgery performed at the first intervention after identification of the tumor. Cats that had the first excision of their tumors at a referral institution had a longer time to recurrence than cats that had surgery performed by their regular veterinarian. This is likely due to the relatively aggressive nature of surgery performed at the referral institutions.

PEARLS & CONSIDERATIONS

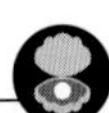

Comments

- Treatment of cats with injection-site sarcoma is usually best performed using a team approach. Specialists, including a surgeon, oncologist, and radiation oncologist, should be consulted early in the course of diagnostic testing to determine the best multimodality approach.
- Many different types of sarcoma have been identified at vaccine sites.

Prevention

- Early detection of tumors may lead to more successful treatment.
- Guidelines have been established by the American Veterinary Medical Association (AVMA) Vaccine-Associated Sarcoma Task Force for approaching a cat that has a mass in an injection site after vaccination. According to these guidelines, the following masses should be investigated with an incisional biopsy to determine whether further diagnostics or treatment are necessary:
  - A mass that is increasing in size 1 month after injection
  - A mass that is > 2 cm in diameter
  - A mass that persists > 3 months after injection
- Vaccination of cats in areas of the body that allow for aggressive surgical removal if a tumor develops (e.g., distal limb, tail) may prevent the tumors from requiring radiation or chemotherapy or from becoming life-threatening.
- Critical evaluation of vaccination protocols for animals that have a low risk of contracting infectious disease may help decrease the risk of vaccine-associated sarcomas.

Technician Tips

Record the location of administration (which site) for each vaccine given to allow long-term monitoring and follow-up of local adverse reactions.

Client Education

- Educate clients about the risks of tumor development after vaccination, as well as other risks of vaccination compared with the benefits of vaccination.
- Clients may also be educated on the importance of examining their cats regularly for new masses to allow early detection and treatment of tumors.

SUGGESTED READING

Lipták JM, et al: Soft tissue sarcomas. In Withrow SJ, et al, editors: Withrow and MacEwen's Small animal clinical oncology, St. Louis, 2013, Saunders, pp 356-380.

AUTHOR: John Farrelly, DVM, MS, DACVIM, DACVR
EDITOR: Kenneth M. Rassnick, DVM, DACVIM

Insulinoma

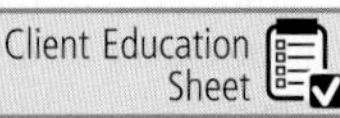

BASIC INFORMATION

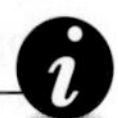

Definition

A malignant tumor of pancreatic beta cells that secretes insulin in an unregulated manner, often resulting in clinical signs of hypoglycemia

Synonyms

Beta-cell tumor, beta-cell carcinoma, insulin-secreting tumor

Epidemiology

SPECIES, AGE, SEX

- Dogs: older, with median age of 8.5-10 years; no sex predisposition
- Cats: rare; older, with median age of 14.7 years; no sex predisposition

GENETICS, BREED PREDISPOSITION

- Dogs: medium-large breeds with a median weight > 25 kg are overrepresented, although any dog can be affected.
- Cats: Siamese breed may be overrepresented.

ASSOCIATED DISORDERS

- Superficial necrolytic dermatitis (rare)
- Obesity

Clinical Presentation

DISEASE FORMS/SUBTYPES

Almost all insulinomas are malignant.

HISTORY, CHIEF COMPLAINT

- Signs resulting from hypoglycemia
  - Seizures, weakness, collapse most common
  - Ataxia
  - Muscle fasciculation
  - Depression, lethargy
  - Abnormal behavior
  - Polyphagia, weight gain
- Signs may be exacerbated by excitement, stress, or fasting.

PHYSICAL EXAM FINDINGS

- Often unremarkable
- Some dogs may show signs of peripheral neuropathy.
  - Paraparesis/tetraparesis
  - Facial nerve paralysis
  - Muscle atrophy
  - Reduced esophageal motility
  - Decreased anal tone
- Some dogs develop weight gain and obesity.

Etiology and Pathophysiology

- Tumors originate in pancreatic beta cells.
- Tumor cells secrete insulin without normal inhibition by hypoglycemia.
- These slowly growing tumors often metastasize to the liver and regional lymph nodes; lung metastasis is rare.
- Insulinoma cells can have an exaggerated response to hyperglycemic stimulus.
- Clinical signs result from hypoglycemia due to hyperinsulinemia.

DIAGNOSIS

Diagnostic Overview

Older animals with significant hypoglycemia should be suspected of having an insulinoma. Diagnosis requires demonstration of an inappropriately high level of serum insulin during hypoglycemia. The pancreas should be imaged to identify the tumor.

Differential Diagnosis

Hypoglycemia (p. 1240):

- Nonpancreatic tumors, most common
  - Adenocarcinoma
  - Leiomyosarcoma, leiomyoma
  - Hepatocellular carcinoma, hepatoma
- Hypoadrenocorticism
- Hepatobiliary disease
  - Portosystemic shunt
  - Liver failure (fibrosis, cirrhosis)
  - Hepatic necrosis
- Juvenile hypoglycemia
- Hunting dog hypoglycemia
- Sepsis
- Insulin overdose
- Toxins (xylitol, ethylene glycol)

Seizures (pp. 903 and 1279)
Collapse/weakness (pp. 192 and 1206)
Twitching/tremors (pp. 994 and 1288)

Initial Database

- CBC: often unremarkable
- Serum biochemical profile
  - Hypoglycemia; can be profound. Extremely low blood glucose in an animal with no or minimal clinical signs attests to chronicity of the condition.
  - Normal blood glucose concentration does not rule out an insulinoma.
  - Mild hypokalemia due to excess insulin driving potassium intracellularly
  - Liver enzymes may be elevated and may signal metastatic disease.
- Urinalysis: often unremarkable
- Thoracic radiographs are usually unremarkable with insulinoma but may identify metastasis associated with other tumors.
- Abdominal radiographs: usually unremarkable
- Abdominal ultrasound can identify up to 75% of pancreatic masses and may be used to identify potential metastatic lesions in the liver and lymph nodes.

Advanced or Confirmatory Testing

- Insulin and glucose should be measured on the same serum sample when the blood glucose is < 60 mg/dL. Serum insulin in the upper one-half of the reference range or above the reference range is consistent with insulinoma; in normal animals, insulin should be low to undetectable during hypoglycemic periods.
- An insulin level in the lower one-half of the reference range in the setting of hypoglycemia often means there is an insulinoma but not always.
- The animal may be fasted to achieve hypoglycemia, with blood glucose checked every 1-2 hours for detection of hypoglycemia.
- If serum insulin levels support the diagnosis of insulinoma and a mass cannot be identified on pancreatic ultrasound, consider contrast-enhanced CT imaging for localization and staging of disease. CT has almost 100% sensitivity for insulinoma detection.
- In some cases, a pancreatic mass cannot be identified with any imaging modality, and the insulinoma is found during surgical exploration.
- In rare cases, a definitive mass may not be found at surgery.
- Definitive diagnosis of insulinoma can be achieved by fine-needle aspiration of the pancreatic mass or histopathology of the tumor after surgical removal.

TREATMENT

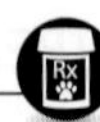

Treatment Overview

Surgical removal of the insulinoma is the treatment of choice, even if the entire tumor cannot be removed or there is metastatic disease. Insulinomas are slow growing; decreasing the amount of hormone-producing tissue makes a significant difference in control of clinical signs. Postoperative complications include hyperglycemia that may require insulin therapy until normal pancreatic beta cells become functional.

Acute General Treatment

- Acute treatment focuses on control of life-threatening hypoglycemia. Treat hypoglycemia only to relieve clinical signs.
- For acute, mild to moderate hypoglycemia, the treatment of choice is feeding small meals and avoiding simple sugars if possible.
- In cases of life-threatening hypoglycemia, administer a dextrose bolus of 1 mL/kg of 25% dextrose over 10 minutes, repeated as needed. Follow with IV fluids supplemented with 5% dextrose. Because insulinoma cells may be stimulated by the dextrose to secrete more insulin, this treatment should be used with caution and only if necessary.
- Dexamethasone 0.1 mg/kg IV to antagonize insulin effects
- Glucagon only when necessary for refractory hypoglycemia using a constant-rate infusion of 10-15 ng/kg/min; adjust as needed.

Surgery:

- Surgical removal of the tumor is the treatment of choice.

- Metastases should be removed if possible because they are usually functional (i.e., secrete insulin).

Chronic Treatment

- Because the tumor usually has metastasized by the time of surgery, hypoglycemia typically recurs eventually.
- Medical management should be instituted in addition to surgical removal if hypoglycemia is not controlled or when it recurs or in patients when surgery is not an option.
- Frequent feeding every 4-6 hours or free choice
- If frequent feeding fails to control hypoglycemia, institute prednisone/prednisolone at 0.5 mg/kg/day PO divided q 12h to antagonize insulin effects. The dose can be increased stepwise as needed up to 2 mg/kg/day.
- If the above therapies fail, diazoxide 5 mg/kg PO q 12h may be tried; often this is prohibitively expensive in medium-sized to large dogs.
- For refractory hypoglycemia, consider streptozotocin, a chemotherapeutic agent, at 500 mg/m^2 IV every 3 weeks; extensive diuresis is required during streptozotocin administration to prevent nephrotoxicity.

Nutrition/Diet

A diet high in protein and complex carbohydrates is desirable; avoid simple sugars such as those present in semimoist meals.

Behavior/Exercise

Moderate exercise, including short leash walks, is beneficial to promote insulin use and metabolism. Avoid strenuous exercise.

Possible Complications

- Pancreatitis is the most common complication after surgery; uncommonly, it can be fatal.
- Rarely, dogs may become permanently diabetic after surgical removal of the insulinoma; transient diabetes occurs in about 10%.

Recommended Monitoring

- Owners should watch for clinical signs of returning hypoglycemia.
- Dogs should have monthly blood glucose measurements.

PROGNOSIS & OUTCOME

- Median survival time is 12-24 months with surgical removal/debulking; postsurgical medical management can extend survival time significantly.
- Median survival time is 2-6.5 months with medical management alone.
- Dogs with stage III disease (tumor with distant metastasis) have significantly shorter survival times.
- Cats: median survival time is 6 months.

PEARLS & CONSIDERATIONS

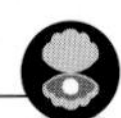

Comments

- Older dogs with no clinical signs in the face of significant hypoglycemia are likely to have an insulinoma.
- Treat hypoglycemia only to relieve clinical signs.
- In an acute setting, feeding is the best way to treat dogs with insulinoma and mild to moderate clinical signs of hypoglycemia.
- Consider referral to a specialty center for surgical removal of insulinoma; extensive postoperative monitoring and care are required.

Technician Tips

Avoid dextrose bolus/infusions unless absolutely necessary to control clinical signs of hypoglycemia.

Client Education

- Application of honey/molasses/Karo syrup on the gums may be used to treat clinical signs of hypoglycemia if pet will not eat; avoid simple sugars unless clinically necessary.
- Frequent feeding of good-quality food containing complex carbohydrates is important to maintain euglycemia.
- In dogs, insulinomas are almost always malignant, and they have metastasized by the time of diagnosis. Prognosis with surgery is still good, and surgery significantly prolongs survival even if surgery is not curative.

SUGGESTED READING

Nelson RW: Beta-cell neoplasia: insulinoma. In Feldman EC, et al, editors: Canine and feline endocrinology, ed 4, St. Louis, 2015, Elsevier.

AUTHOR: Cynthia R. Ward, VMD, PhD, DACVIM
EDITOR: Ellen N. Behrend, VMD, PhD, DACVIM

Interstitial Lung Diseases

Client Education Sheet

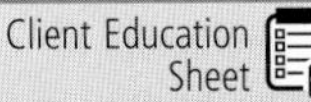

BASIC INFORMATION

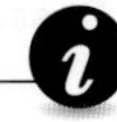

Definition

A heterogeneous group of pulmonary interstitial diseases that result from exaggerated inflammatory and/or reparative (fibrotic) processes, usually in response to inhaled or hematogenous insults

Synonyms

Interstitial lung diseases (ILDs):

- Bronchiolitis obliterans with organizing pneumonia (BOOP); the idiopathic form in people is cryptogenic organizing pneumonia (COP)
- Endogenous lipid pneumonia
- Eosinophilic pneumonia (i.e., eosinophilic bronchopneumopathy or pulmonary infiltrates with eosinophilia [PIE]) (p. 298)
- Pulmonary fibrosis (idiopathic, drug-induced)
- Lymphocytic interstitial pneumonia
- Pulmonary alveolar proteinosis
- Silicosis and asbestosis

Epidemiology

SPECIES, AGE, SEX

- Dogs or cats, usually middle-aged to older; eosinophilic pneumonia often occurs in younger animals
- No sex predisposition for most ILDs; females may be overrepresented among dogs with eosinophilic pneumonia

GENETICS, BREED PREDISPOSITION

Some specific syndromes have a breed predisposition:

- Pulmonary fibrosis: West Highland white terriers, Staffordshire bull terriers, schipperke
- Eosinophilic pneumonia: Siberian Huskies, Alaskan Malamutes, rottweilers

RISK FACTORS

Generally unknown; exceptions may include

- Pulmonary toxicant drugs (e.g., bleomycin, rabacfosadine [Tanovea-CA1])
- Inhaled chemical fumes (e.g., hydrocarbons)
- Mineral fibers
- Dusts
- Allergens

ASSOCIATED DISORDERS

- Eosinophilic pneumonia may occur alone or as part of the hypereosinophilic syndrome (e.g., rottweilers).
- Lymphocytic interstitial pneumonia (cats with feline immunodeficiency virus only)

Clinical Presentation

HISTORY, CHIEF COMPLAINT

Respiratory signs:

- Cough
- Tachypnea

- Respiratory distress
- Exercise intolerance
- Hemoptysis

Nonrespiratory signs:

- Fever
- Lethargy
- Anorexia
- Weight loss
- Syncope (associated with pulmonary hypertension [PH] or intermittent hypoxemia)

PHYSICAL EXAM FINDINGS

- Spontaneous or elicited cough (productive or nonproductive)
- Pulmonary crackles on auscultation (inspiratory, with pulmonary fibrosis)
- Increased respiratory rate and/or effort (inspiratory and expiratory)
- Right-sided systolic heart murmur may be ausculted if PH is present (with tricuspid regurgitation).
    - Unlike primary heart disease, tachycardia is absent, may have sinus arrhythmia
- Fever
- Poor body condition
- ± Cyanosis

Etiology and Pathophysiology

- ILDs result from injury to alveolar epithelial cells and a cycle of inflammation and reparative responses that proceed unchecked.
    - In humans, injury can be triggered by
        - Inhalation of toxins, irritants, or allergens
        - Vascular damage from drugs
        - Collagen-related vascular diseases
        - Systemic immune-mediated diseases
        - Infection
        - Neoplasia
    - Many veterinary cases are idiopathic.
- Alveolar epithelial cell injury leads to
    - Inflammatory cell influx
    - Release of proinflammatory and fibrogenic mediators
    - Deposition of extracellular matrix
    - Structural changes, including fibrosis
- Idiopathic pulmonary fibrosis appears to be a fibroproliferative disorder that originates independently of inflammation (i.e., inflammation is secondary).
    - Injured alveolar epithelial cells are still critical for triggering and sustaining fibrogenesis.

DIAGNOSIS

Diagnostic Overview

Diagnosis is suspected in patients with clinical signs and imaging features (radiographic, CT) consistent with ILD in which there is no evidence of infectious or neoplastic causes of respiratory disease. A definitive diagnosis requires lung biopsy for histopathologic exam.

Differential Diagnosis

Physical exam (cough/respiratory distress):

- Other airway diseases (e.g., chronic bronchitis, eosinophilic bronchitis, obstructive airway diseases)
- Pneumonia (infectious, aspiration, foreign body)
- Neoplasia
- Pulmonary thromboembolism
- Cardiogenic or non-cardiogenic pulmonary edema
- Pleural effusion or pneumothorax

Radiographic:

- Infectious pneumonia (bacterial, fungal, viral, protozoal, parasitic)
- Noncardiogenic pulmonary edema
- Neoplasia

Initial Database

- CBC
    - ± Inflammatory leukogram ± polycythemia if chronic hypoxemia
    - Eosinophilia present in 50%-60% of dogs with eosinophilic pneumonia
- Thoracic radiographs
    - Interstitial, alveolar (severe disease), or bronchointerstitial patterns
    - Interstitial nodules
    - Hypoinflation
    - ± Hilar lymphadenopathy
    - ± Right-sided cardiomegaly from cor pulmonale
- Arterial blood gas or pulse oximetry
    - ± Hypoxemia
    - ± Hypocarbia
- Six-minute walk test may provide an objective assessment of exercise tolerance.
- Fecal flotation or sedimentation (Baermann): respiratory parasites
- Infectious disease testing for agents endemic to patient's geographic region

Advanced or Confirmatory Testing

- CT provides more specific information on the extent, pattern, and location of disease. A ground-glass pattern is a common CT characteristic for dogs with pulmonary fibrosis.
- Bronchoscopy, bronchoalveolar lavage (p. 1074), and fine-needle aspiration (p. 1113) for cytologic evaluation and culture can provide evidence of underlying infection or neoplasia if microorganisms or neoplastic cells are identified:
    - Nonspecific inflammatory cells or poor cellularity is seen with ILDs.
    - Absence of microorganisms or neoplastic cells does not rule out these causes of respiratory disease.
- Lung biopsy is the only definitive means for diagnosis.
    - Can be performed by a keyhole technique, thoracoscopy, or thoracotomy
    - Special stains are indicated to rule out infectious agents.
- Echocardiogram (p. 1094) to evaluate for PH, if indicated.
- Various serum and bronchoalveolar lavage fluid biomarkers (e.g.; endothelin-1, CCLX, CXCL8) have shown promise in a research setting to aid in the diagnosis of idiopathic pulmonary fibrosis.

TREATMENT

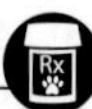

Treatment Overview

Treatment consists of removing or addressing the inciting cause if it can be identified. If no underlying cause can be identified, treatment is focused on decreasing inflammation. No treatments are known to directly halt the progression of fibrosis.

Acute General Treatment

Oxygen supplementation is indicated for hypoxemic patients in respiratory distress (p. 1146). Many affected patients are comfortable with mild to moderate chronic arterial hypoxemia.

Chronic Treatment

- Remove potential inciting causes.
    - Consider discontinuation of any drug not immediately critical for the patient's health.
- Eosinophilic pneumonias: treat underlying cause (e.g., heartworm, other parasites, fungi) if identified. If none found, treat with immunosuppressive doses of glucocorticoids.
    - Oral glucocorticoids are preferred for dogs > 10 kg. Inhaled glucocorticoid therapy (fluticasone) may be effective in small dogs and can reduce systemic side effects of long-term oral glucocorticoids (p. 298).
- If present, PH may be addressed with sildenafil 1-2 mg/kg PO q 12h.
- For most other ILDs, immunosuppression has been advocated (provided infection is definitively ruled out), starting with glucocorticoids (e.g., prednisone 2 mg/kg PO q 24h).
    - Empirically (i.e., without scientific evidence of their efficacy), other immunosuppressive drugs have been tried in refractory cases.

Behavior/Exercise

Minimize exposure to inhalant fumes, chemicals, dusts, or other known disease triggers.

Possible Complications

- Decompensation during and after bronchoscopy or lung biopsy, especially in patients with a significant degree of respiratory compromise at rest
- Immunosuppression can predispose to secondary infections.
    - After lung biopsy, allow the incision to heal before administering immunosuppressive medication.
- These patients may be predisposed to pneumonia due to compromise of normal respiratory defense mechanisms.

Recommended Monitoring

- Clinical signs
- Periodic physical exam, arterial blood gas (if significant respiratory compromise), thoracic radiographs, 6-minute walk test
- Echocardiogram (if indicated to monitor PH)

Diseases and Disorders

PROGNOSIS & OUTCOME 

- For eosinophilic pneumonia (without hypereosinophilic syndrome), with appropriate treatment, prognosis is fair to excellent.
- For BOOP, if the insult is removed and the animal responds well to glucocorticoids, the prognosis is good.
  - Relapse is common if glucocorticoids are tapered too quickly.
  - For animals with BOOP that do not respond well to therapy, prognosis is guarded to poor.
- For other ILDs, including idiopathic pulmonary fibrosis, prognosis depends on stage of the disease and rapidity of progression.
  - In general, long-term outcome is guarded to poor.

PEARLS & CONSIDERATIONS 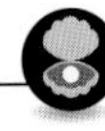

Comments

- Lung biopsy is critical for definitive diagnosis of ILDs.
- Pulmonary crackles on auscultation are common with interstitial fibrosis (crackles are not exclusive to pulmonary edema or pneumonia).
- High-resolution CT: useful in the diagnosis and staging of human ILDs, may become a useful noninvasive diagnostic technique as ILDs gain further recognition in veterinary medicine.

Technician Tips

Minimize stress and provide appropriate oxygen supplementation when handling distressed patients. Serial evaluation of arterial blood gases may help to assess oxygenation and oxygen needs of each patient.

Client Education

Over time, most ILDs are associated with permanent architectural changes, and treatment cannot reverse fibrosis. The likelihood that clinical signs will resolve depends on the balance of active inflammatory and reparative events versus fibrosis.

SUGGESTED READINGS

Reinero CR, et al: Interstitial lung diseases. Vet Clin North Am Small Anim Pract 37:937-947, 2007.

AUTHOR: Laura A. Nafe, DVM, MS, DACVIM
EDITOR: Megan Grobman, DVM, MS, DACVIM

Intervertebral Disc Disease

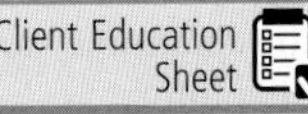

BASIC INFORMATION 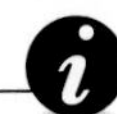

Definition

Intervertebral disc degeneration and displacement of disc material into the vertebral canal or intervertebral foramen, causing signs ranging from back pain to paresis or paralysis

Synonyms

IVDD, disc disease, disc protrusion or extrusion

Epidemiology

SPECIES, AGE, SEX

- Commonly occurs in dogs between 3 and 8 years of age; no sex predisposition
- Occasionally occurs in older cats.

GENETICS, BREED PREDISPOSITION

Dachshund, Pekingese, toy poodle, and beagles; some larger breeds (Labrador retriever, Doberman pinscher, Dalmatian) also are at increased risk.

RISK FACTORS

Disc degeneration (chondroid metaplasia) in chondrodystrophic breeds; rarely, direct external trauma

ASSOCIATED DISORDERS

Tetraparesis, paraparesis, paraplegia

Clinical Presentation

DISEASE FORMS/SUBTYPES

Cervical or thoracolumbar disc disease; disc extrusion; disc protrusion

HISTORY, CHIEF COMPLAINT

- Reluctance to jump, climb, or engage in other forms of activity
- With cervical disc disease: neck pain, carrying the head low, tetraparesis
- With thoracolumbar disc disease: arched back, reluctance to walk, pain when picked up, paraparesis
- Discomfort associated with thoracolumbar and lumbar disc disease may be misinterpreted as evidence of intraabdominal pain.
- Paresis (weakness): caused by disruption of normal nerve transmission between the brain and nerves to the limbs
- Ataxia (incoordination) and knuckling/tripping on digits (conscious proprioceptive deficits)
- Paralysis may occur acutely or progress over several days.

PHYSICAL EXAM FINDINGS

- Neurologic exam (p. 1136)
- Cervical disc disease: neck pain, forelimb lameness (root signature), tetraparesis or tetraplegia
- Thoracolumbar disc disease: focal pain on spinal palpation, upper motor neuron (UMN) reflexes in pelvic limbs, UMN bladder, loss of cutaneous trunci (panniculus) reflex two vertebral spaces caudal to the lesion, paraparesis/paraplegia
- Alterations in perception of and response to noxious stimuli (i.e., deep or superficial pain) are of localizing and prognostic significance.

Etiology and Pathophysiology

- Disc extrusion (Hansen type I disc disease): displacement of nucleus pulposus through a rent in the annulus fibrosis, causing spinal cord or nerve root compression. It is typically associated with chondroid disc metaplasia as seen in chondrodystrophic breeds. This is usually associated with acute/subacute onset of clinical signs.
- Disc protrusion (Hansen type II disc disease): bulging of the annulus fibrosis and herniation of nucleus pulposus within the annulus to produce a more diffuse mass effect within the vertebral canal; more common in nonchondrodystrophoid breeds. Clinical signs tend to develop more slowly and progressively.
- Hansen type III disc disease, or low-volume/high-velocity disc extrusion, causes concussive injury to the spinal cord.
- The neurologic dysfunction seen in dogs with intervertebral disc disease (IVDD) depends on the severity of the compressive or concussive injury and the type of nerve fibers affected. Conscious proprioception is initially lost due to injury to the superficial myelinated fibers, followed by loss of motor function from injury to the motor fibers and then loss of pain perception.

DIAGNOSIS 

Diagnostic Overview

Characteristic history and physical exam findings suggest disc disease, especially in overrepresented breeds of dogs. Compatible imaging results (myelography, CT, or MRI) support and refine the diagnosis, and the sum of this information is used for deciding whether to proceed medically or surgically.

Differential Diagnosis

Spinal fracture/luxation; spinal cord, nerve root, epidural or vertebral neoplasia; fibrocartilaginous embolism; spinal cord inflammation (myelitis); discospondylitis (intradiscal osteomyelitis); degenerative myelopathy; caudal occipital malformation syndrome with syringomyelia

Initial Database

- Orthopedic exam to rule out musculoskeletal disease (e.g., bilateral cruciate disease) (p. 1143)

- Neurologic exam (p. 1136)
  - Findings are consistent with a single focal spinal cord lesion (i.e., mentation and cranial nerve responses are normal)
  - Deficits and segmental reflexes help to localize the lesion.
- UMN signs in forelimbs and hindlimbs: C1-C5 lesion
- Lower motor neuron signs in forelimbs, UMN signs in hindlimbs: C6-T2 (cervical intumescence) lesion
- Forelimbs normal, UMN signs in hindlimbs: T3-L3 lesion
- Forelimbs normal, decreased patellar reflex: L4-6 lesion
- Forelimbs normal, decreased withdrawal in hindlimbs: L6-S2 lesion
- Cutaneous trunci reflex may help further localize in dogs with signs referable to a T3-L3 segment lesion, and might also help determine which side is preferentially affected.
- Palpation of epaxial muscles and vertebrae to determine presence and location of discomfort
- Determine a line of decreased or absent sensation, if possible.
  - Location of deficits helps determine the site of the lesion but does not confirm that intervertebral disc disease is the cause.
- CBC, serum biochemistry panel, and urinalysis to assess anesthetic risk; American Society of Anesthesiologists classification system (p. 1196). Urinary tract infection may accompany dysuria/urine retention.
- Survey radiography with orthogonal views of heavily sedated, properly positioned patient will rule out fractures/luxations and severe bone neoplasia. Calcified discs *in situ* are abnormal (degenerated) but may not be clinically significant.

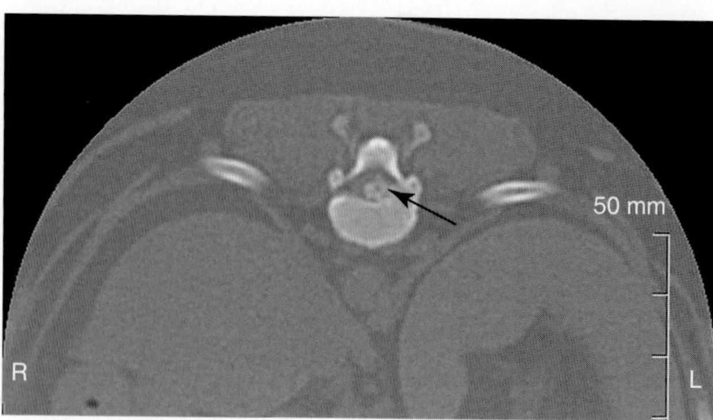

INTERVERTEBRAL DISC DISEASE Axial CT image shows intervertebral disc extrusion *(arrow)* at T12-13 on the left side.

Advanced or Confirmatory Testing

- Myelography, CT, CT combined with myelography, or MRI (p. 1132) may reveal location of spinal cord compression. MRI is the preferred method.
- Cerebrospinal fluid (CSF) analysis may be done in conjunction with myelography or after CT or MRI, especially if a disorder other than disc disease is suspected to be the cause of myelopathy (pp. 1080 and 1323).
- Advanced imaging is usually done when surgery is contemplated as a possible treatment. If a client has ruled out surgical intervention, the results of any imaging study are of academic value only and may have little influence on further treatment planning or prognostication.

TREATMENT

Treatment Overview

Goals of treatment are to alleviate discomfort and pain and reverse neurologic dysfunction by reducing swelling and compression of the spinal cord.

Acute General Treatment

- Choice of treatment is based on severity and progression of neurologic dysfunction and discomfort as well as on owner wishes. Discuss referral to a veterinary neurologist or surgeon for patients with paresis or paralysis.
- Patients with discomfort alone and no neurologic deficits or those with mild neurologic deficits that are not progressing rapidly: STRICT cage rest for 4-6 weeks (only activity is short walks to urinate/defecate) regardless of perceived improvement
- Treatment with muscle relaxants and analgesics (nonsteroidal antiinflammatory drugs [NSAIDs], opiates)
  - Muscle relaxant (e.g., methocarbamol [Robaxin] 15-20 mg/kg PO q 8h
  - NSAIDs: meloxicam 0.1 mg/kg IV, SQ, or PO q 24h, *or* carprofen 2.2 mg/kg PO q 12h or 4.4 mg/kg q 24h, *or* deracoxib 1-2 mg/kg PO q 24h. Do not use more than one NSAID at a time or an NSAID concurrently with glucocorticoids (risk of gastric ulceration).
- Glucocorticoids
  - Traditional but increasingly unpopular with neurosurgeons due to frequent adverse effects and lack of proven efficacy; higher success rates reported for NSAID therapy
  - Methylprednisolone sodium succinate (Solu-Medrol) 10-30 mg/kg IV once, within 12 hours of spinal cord injury; prednisone 0.5 mg/kg PO q 24h for 1-3 days; dexamethasone 0.1-0.2 mg/kg once
  - Dexamethasone has been associated with the highest incidence of adverse effects in treatment of IVDD.
- If acutely paraplegic/tetraplegic: IV fluids to maintain hydration for optimal spinal cord perfusion
- Patients with more severe neurologic signs (i.e., non-ambulatory paraparesis, loss of motor function, and loss of nociception) and evidence of cord compression on imaging should have decompressive surgery.
- Patients with recurrent signs of neurologic dysfunction, uncontrolled spinal pain despite strict medical management, and worsening neurologic signs are also candidates for surgery.

Chronic Treatment

- For animals that have lost motor function, the single most important aspect of treatment is bladder management to reduce the risk of urinary tract infection and bladder detrusor muscle damage from chronic overdistention. This may entail manual expression of the bladder every 4-6 hours or catheterization. In some cases, medication to help decrease urethral sphincter tone (e.g., phenoxybenzamine 0.25 mg/kg PO q 12h, avoid if hypotensive; prazosin 0.07 mg/kg PO q 8-12h) may be helpful.
- Reduce antiinflammatory medications and analgesics after the acute phase, based on patient comfort.
- Confined, padded rest areas; slings for assisted ambulation; hydrotherapy for cleanliness and to stimulate ambulation
- Physical rehabilitation including underwater treadmill use to strengthen axial and appendicular musculature and help retrain the nervous system
- Acupuncture may be helpful.
- Chiropractic maneuvers are controversial and may worsen neurologic status.

Nutrition/Diet

Control body weight to avoid obesity.

Behavior/Exercise

Avoid climbing and jumping activities that extend the spine during and after recovery to reduce risk of recurrence.

Drug Interactions

Concurrent use of glucocorticoids and NSAIDs can lead to severe gastrointestinal ulceration and is contraindicated.

Possible Complications

- Urinary tract infection from incontinence/urinary retention or improper catheter use/care
- Detrusor atony from chronic overdistention of the bladder

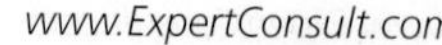

Diseases and Disorders

- Urine scalding of skin from overflow incontinence
- Worsened neurologic status due to iatrogenic spinal cord trauma or vascular changes during decompressive surgery
- Intraoperative hemorrhage or respiratory arrest requiring ventilator support during ventral slot for cervical decompression
- Ascending-descending myelomalacia: devastating complication that occurs in < 1% of acutely paraplegic dogs. Focal lesion, usually T3-L3 (perhaps more common with lower lumbar disc extrusions), rapidly deteriorates to expanding cord necrosis, causing signs of ascending and/or descending cord dysfunction over a period of hours. There is no known treatment for this complication, and the key is early recognition so humane euthanasia can be performed.

Recommended Monitoring

Discomfort level, bladder/bowel evacuations, evidence of pressure sores, and neurologic status, including evidence of myelomalacia, should be assessed frequently until the patient has recovered.

PROGNOSIS & OUTCOME

- The most important prognostic indicator for dogs without voluntary motor function is the presence or absence of nociception (deep pain sensation) because the unmyelinated pain fibers in the spinal cord are the least vulnerable to ischemic injury. This assessment is always subjective, but apparent loss of sensation caudal to the level of spinal cord injury suggests the possibility for permanent paralysis, regardless of treatment. Approximately 60% of dogs in this condition recover if treated with decompressive surgery.
- 90%-97% of dogs with intact nociception, even if they are paraplegic or tetraplegic, recover fully or almost fully with surgical decompression. However, the time frame for recovery is extremely variable (few days to many weeks or months).
- With nonsurgical treatment about 85% of ambulatory and 60% of non-ambulatory (but retaining pain perception) dogs ultimately recover.
- The recurrence rate (i.e., new disc extrusion at a different level) is low in nonchondrodystrophic breeds, although some of these dogs (especially German shepherds) may have signs attributable to Hansen type II disease at multiple levels simultaneously.
- For chondrodystrophic breeds treated with surgical decompression, recurrence rates vary between 5% and 25%.
- The recurrence rate for medically managed patients is about 40%.
- Dogs with signs attributable to ascending-descending myelomalacia have a grave prognosis.

PEARLS & CONSIDERATIONS

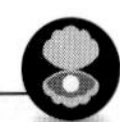

Comments

- Strict cage rest is critical for recovery in nonsurgical patients treated only with analgesics and antiinflammatory medications. Physical rehabilitation, weight control, and avoidance of jumping activities may reduce the risk of recurrence and future need for surgery.
- There is no direct correlation between severity of signs and amount of disc material displaced. Dogs with pain as their only sign or those with only mild deficits may have large amounts of displaced disc and marked spinal cord/nerve root compression. Conversely, some of the most severely affected dogs may have suffered a low-volume/high-velocity extrusion, which is not likely to be improved by surgery, even if done on an emergency basis.
- Dogs with thoracolumbar disc disease are often unable to urinate, but the resultant overflow from a distended bladder can give caretakers the mistaken impression that the dog is urinating frequently.
- Ongoing monitoring is essential to determine whether the current treatment course should be continued or if failure to improve, relapse of signs, or worsening of signs make a new strategy advisable.
- Referral to a veterinary neurology or surgical specialist should be offered if surgery is to be considered.

Prevention

- Avoidance of obesity and jumping activities for chondrodystrophic breeds may lessen the tendency for recurrence.
- Prophylactic disc fenestration or chemonucleolysis may reduce the risk of disc extrusion for treated disc spaces, but risks and the true benefit are unproven at this time.

Technician Tips

Close monitoring of bladder function and bladder expression or catheterization is important to prevent overdistention of bladder and detrusor atony. Check bladder size regularly, even in dogs that seem to be urinating, because overflow incontinence can be deceptive.

Client Education

- See Prevention above.
- For paralyzed patients, clients should be informed about bladder expression and nursing care to understand this component of management.

SUGGESTED READING

Dewey CW: Surgery of the cervical and thoracolumbar spine. In Fossum TW, editor: Small animal surgery, ed 4, St. Louis, 2013, Mosby, pp 1467-1507, 1508-1528.

AUTHOR: Suresh Sathya, BVSc, MVSc, MVetSc
EDITOR: Kathleen Linn, DVM, MS, DACVS

Intracranial Neoplasia

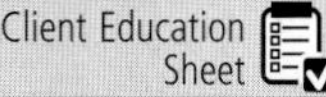

BASIC INFORMATION

Definition

- Primary brain tumors include meningioma, glioma (astrocytoma, oligodendroglioma), choroid plexus tumor, ependymoma, medulloblastoma, olfactory neuroblastoma, and primitive neuroectodermal tumor.
- Secondary brain tumors include pituitary tumors, tumors that invade by direct extension into the brain (e.g., nasal tumors, multilobular tumor of bone, osteosarcoma), and metastatic tumors to the brain (e.g., hemangiosarcoma, lymphoma).

Synonyms

Brain neoplasia; brain tumor

Epidemiology

SPECIES, AGE, SEX

- Dogs and cats of both sexes
- Incidence reported as high as 2.6% for dogs and 2.8% for cats
- Brain tumors typically occur in older dogs (most > 7 years old) and cats. Median age: 9 years (dogs), 11 years (cats)

GENETICS, BREED PREDISPOSITION

- Canine: dolichocephalic breeds (e.g., golden retriever, German shepherd dogs) tend to develop meningiomas. Brachycephalic breeds (e.g., boxer, Boston terrier) appear prone to developing gliomas.
- Feline: no breed predisposition. Meningioma is the most common brain tumor in cats (≈60%).

Clinical Presentation

DISEASE FORMS/SUBTYPES

- Meningioma: tumor of the arachnoid membrane
- Glioma: tumor of the cells that form the interstitial tissue of the central nervous system (CNS)
- Choroid plexus papilloma: tumor of the cells of the choroid plexus, the intracranial

vascular structure responsible for the formation of cerebrospinal fluid (CSF)
- Ependymoma: tumor of the ependymal cells that line the ventricular system
- Pituitary tumor: tumor of the pituitary gland, called macroadenoma when diameter > 1 cm
- Other neoplasms possible: primary CNS or generalized lymphoma, histiocytic sarcoma, nasal tumor, osteosarcoma and other primary bone tumors of the skull, metastatic tumors (e.g., hemangiosarcoma, melanoma, mammary tumor and others)

HISTORY, CHIEF COMPLAINT

- Intracranial neoplasia should be considered in any older patient with an insidious onset of slowly progressive neurologic signs and in any patient older than 5 years with a recent onset of seizures.
- Historic findings depend on lesion location. Clinical signs are often insidious and progressive; however, acute onset of clinical signs is possible.
- The most common chief complaints include seizures, circling, behavior change (aggression), altered consciousness, and nonspecific signs such as inappetence, lethargy, and inappropriate elimination.

PHYSICAL EXAM FINDINGS

- Neurologic exam findings vary, depending on lesion location (p. 1136).
- Findings generally reflect a focal lesion with asymmetric clinical signs. However, a large case series found that one-half of canine brain tumors occupy more than one anatomic region of the brain (e.g., forebrain and brainstem).
- Cerebral tumors: seizures, contralateral menace and postural reaction deficits, behavioral change, contralateral hemiparesis, altered mental status
- Brainstem tumors: ipsilateral cranial nerve deficits, hemiparesis or tetraparesis or tetraplegia, altered mental status, central vestibular dysfunction
- Cerebellar tumors: hypermetria, intention tremors, truncal sway, broad-based stance, paradoxical vestibular dysfunction

Etiology and Pathophysiology

- Cause is unknown.
- Usually occur as solitary masses, but multiple tumors can be seen with metastatic disease.
- Most commonly reported in the rostrotentorial compartment (rostral to the tentorium cerebelli, including the cerebrum and diencephalon)
- Biological behavior (benign vs. malignant) is generally irrelevant because neoplasia of the brain is detrimental due to space-occupying effects.

DIAGNOSIS

Diagnostic Overview

Neoplasia of the brain is suspected based on signalment, history, and neurologic exam results. Confirmation requires advanced intracranial imaging with CT or MRI.

Differential Diagnosis

- Infectious diseases (bacterial, viral, fungal, protozoal), depending on geographic location
- Inflammatory diseases (e.g., granulomatous meningoencephalomyelitis, necrotizing encephalitis)
- Cerebrovascular infarction if clinical signs are acute, nonprogressive, and asymmetrical
- Toxin and metabolic diseases if clinical signs are acute, nonprogressive, and symmetrical

Initial Database

- CBC, serum biochemistry profile, urinalysis: usually normal
- Thoracic and abdominal radiographs: often normal but performed to rule out extracranial neoplasia

Advanced or Confirmatory Testing

- CT or MRI (p. 1132)
  - MRI is markedly superior for soft-tissue detail (brain, spinal cord) and has higher resolution than CT. As a result, this is the current gold standard for brain imaging.
  - CT is an adequate imaging modality, is superior for bone lesions (e.g., skull tumors), is much faster, and is typically less expensive than MRI.
  - Focal mass identified for most brain tumors; however, diffuse neoplasia is possible (e.g., lymphoma) and multiple tumors may be identified with metastatic neoplasia.
  - CT and MRI features vary between tumor types.
- CSF analysis (p. 1080)
  - Used as an adjunct to advanced imaging, primarily to rule out encephalitis
  - With brain neoplasia, results are generally nonspecific and reveal normal to mildly elevated protein.
  - Albuminocytologic dissociation (elevated CSF protein with normal nucleated cell count) can occur but is not pathognomonic.
  - Neoplastic cells are rarely identified in the CSF; however, finding lymphoblasts in the CSF supports a diagnosis of CNS lymphoma.
- Histopathologic analysis of tissue is required for definitive diagnosis. Tissue samples can be obtained by surgical excision or stereotactic brain biopsy.

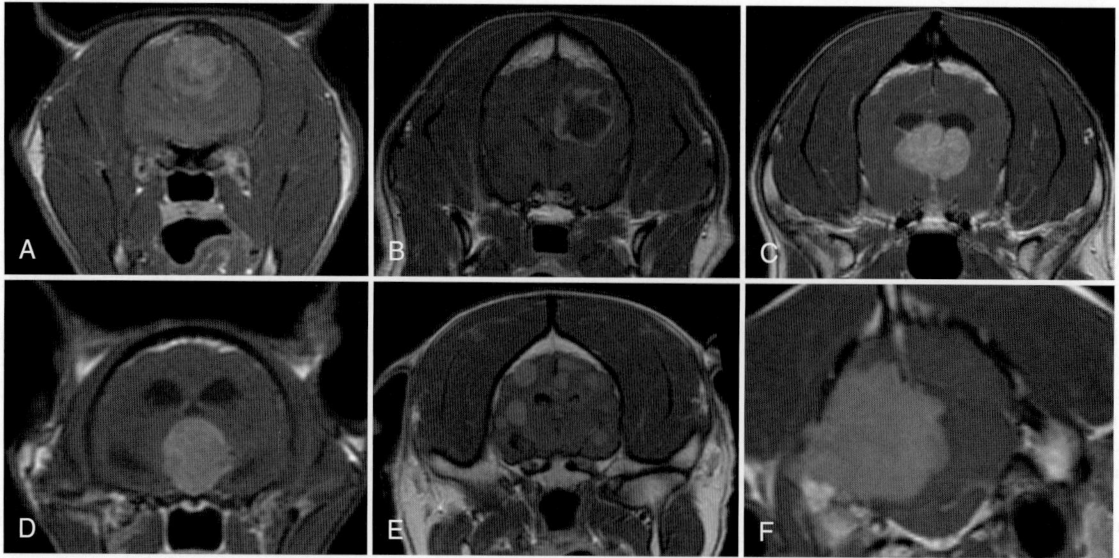

INTRACRANIAL NEOPLASIA Transverse, post-contrast, T1-weighted MR images of a variety of intracranial neoplasms. **A**, Meningioma in a cat. **B**, Oligodendroglioma in a dog. **C**, Choroid plexus tumor in a dog. **D**, Pituitary macroadenoma in a cat. **E**, Metastatic melanoma in a dog. **F**, Multilobular tumor of bone in a dog.

Diseases and Disorders

TREATMENT

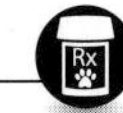

Treatment Overview

Definitive treatment involves surgical excision and/or radiation therapy and/or chemotherapy.

Acute General Treatment

- Surgical excision: used for removing or debulking the tumor if accessible and for providing a definitive histologic diagnosis
- Radiation therapy: used as adjunctive treatment to surgery or as a primary treatment modality (conventional radiation therapy or stereotactic radiosurgery); palliative radiation therapy may be pursued to improve quality of life if full-course radiation therapy cannot be performed
- Chemotherapy: most agents are not very effective because the blood-brain barrier (BBB) prevents chemotherapeutic agents from entering the brain. The exception is nitrosourea drugs.
  - Nitrosourea agents such as lomustine (CCNU 60-90 mg/m^2 PO q 4-6 weeks) or carmustine (BCNU 50 mg/m^2 IV q 6 weeks) (p. 609), which can cross the BBB, appear to have some effect in canine gliomas and canine CNS lymphoma.
  - The most serious potential adverse effects are myelosuppression (anemia, thrombocytopenia, leukopenia) and hepatotoxicosis.
  - Hydroxyurea 20 mg/kg PO q 24h can significantly increase survival times for dogs with meningiomas compared with use of prednisone alone. Side effects at this dose are typically mild. Monitor CBC weekly initially and then CBC/biochemical profile every 4 months.
- Cluster seizures or status epilepticus (p. 903)
- Cerebral edema/brain herniation: mannitol 0.5-1.0 g/kg IV slowly over 15-20 minutes or hypertonic saline (7%-7.5%) 2-4 mL/kg IV slowly over 15-20 minutes

Chronic Treatment

- Seizures: anticonvulsants should be used if there is more than one seizure every 2-3 months; see p. 903 for treatment options.
- Cerebral edema: prednisone 0.5 mg/kg PO q 12h initially, then taper to lowest dose that can control clinical signs

Drug Interactions

- Drug interactions or altered metabolism of medications have been reported between corticosteroids and amphotericin B, furosemide, thiazide diuretics, digitalis glycosides, cyclosporine, phenytoin, phenobarbital, and mitotane.
- Corticosteroids should not be given concurrently with nonsteroidal antiinflammatory drugs or other potentially gastric ulcerogenic medications.
- Phenobarbital may cause excessive sedation in dogs with intracranial mass lesions, even at low doses.

Possible Complications

Progression of clinical signs, including status epilepticus, brain herniation, and sudden death

Recommended Monitoring

- Serial neurologic exam every 4-6 weeks
- Serum phenobarbital level 2 weeks after starting medication, any change in dosage, or immediately after loading dose (p. 1372)
- Serum bromide (KBr) level 3-4 months after starting medication or after any change in dosage for dogs; 2 months after starting treatment in cats or immediately after loading dose (p. 1319)

PROGNOSIS & OUTCOME

- In general, the prognosis is fair to guarded for dogs and cats.
- For dogs, several small-scale reports have shown a median survival time of approximately 2-4 months with supportive care and nonspecific treatment only, 6-12 months with surgery alone, 7-24 months with radiation therapy alone, 6 months to 3 years with surgery and radiation, and 7-11 months with chemotherapy alone.
- There are no large-scale reports of survival times for cats, with the exception of meningiomas (average survival time is 2 years). However, the long-term prognosis for cats with other brain tumors is likely similar to that for dogs.

PEARLS & CONSIDERATIONS

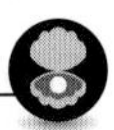

Comments

With neoplasia of the brain, asymmetrical neurologic deficits are much more common than symmetrical deficits. Symmetrical neurologic deficits make other diagnoses more likely.

Prevention

No known method to prevent disease

Technician Tips

Postoperative craniotomy patients are very vulnerable to brain trauma, and comprehensive care (e.g., padding of cage walls, prevention of self-trauma through gentle restraint and padding over the surgical site) can make the difference between an excellent outcome and a life-threatening complication.

Client Education

- Warn owner about corticosteroid side effects (e.g., polyuria, polydipsia, polyphagia, weight gain, gastrointestinal ulceration).
- Phenobarbital and KBr: short-term side effects include sedation/lethargy and pelvic limb weakness and ataxia. Long-term side effects include polyuria, polydipsia, polyphagia, and weight gain. Less common adverse effects include hepatotoxicosis and blood dyscrasias for phenobarbital and pancreatitis for KBr.

SUGGESTED READING

Dewey CW: Encephalopathies: disorders of the brain. In Dewey CW, et al, editors: Practical guide to canine and feline neurology, ed 3, Ames, IA, 2015, Wiley-Blackwell, pp 141-236.

AUTHOR: Mark T. Troxel, DVM, DACVIM
EDITOR: Karen R. Muñana, DVM, MS, DACVIM

Intraocular Neoplasia

Client Education Sheet 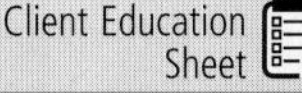

BASIC INFORMATION

Definition

- Primary intraocular neoplasms arise from the vascular intraocular tunic (uvea: iris, ciliary body, choroid) or limbal melanocytes. In cats, primary intraocular sarcoma arises from an undetermined cell population, most likely lens epithelium. Neoplasia of the fibrous tunic, adnexa (eyelids, conjunctiva, lacrimal glands), and orbit are covered in additional detail on pp. 644 and 716).
- Secondary intraocular neoplasia occurs through metastasis or (rarely) by extension from adjacent tissues.

Epidemiology

SPECIES, AGE, SEX

- Melanoma/melanocytoma affects dogs and cats, usually older adults (>7 years), although are also seen in young dogs < 4 years old.
- Medulloepithelioma usually affects animals 1-4 years of age.
- Primary intraocular sarcoma (feline ocular posttraumatic sarcoma) occurs in cats of any age.
- Lymphoma is the most common neoplasm to metastasize to the eye. Others include mastocytoma, chondrosarcoma, osteosarcoma, and carcinoma.

GENETICS, BREED PREDISPOSITION

Uveal melanoma and limbal melanoma have demonstrated genetic predisposition in Labrador retrievers, suspected in golden retrievers, German shepherds

ASSOCIATED DISORDERS

Uveitis, glaucoma, retinal detachment, and intraocular hemorrhage can occur secondary to intraocular neoplasia.

Clinical Presentation

HISTORY, CHIEF COMPLAINT

- Change in appearance of the eye: redness, cloudiness, swelling, darkening of iris, mass noted
- Pain, blepharospasm
- Loss of vision

PHYSICAL EXAM FINDINGS

Findings directly associated with tumor:

- Mass that may be pigmented (melanoma/melanocytoma) or pink in color (more likely ciliary body adenoma/adenocarcinoma or metastatic neoplasia) within the iris or pupil
- Not all melanomas are pigmented, nor are all pigmented masses melanomas (requires histologic diagnosis).
- Extension of mass through sclera (indicates more invasive tumor)
- Diffuse hyperpigmentation of iris (more often in cats)
- Dyscoria, anisocoria
- Shallow anterior chamber
- Hyphema
- Displacement of lens (p. 581)

Findings associated with secondary glaucoma/uveitis:

- Elevated intraocular pressure (glaucoma)
- Fixed, pupil
- Corneal edema
- Scleral injection
- Hyphema
- Aqueous flare
- Lens luxation
- If chronic glaucoma, retinal degeneration, optic nerve atrophy, and peripapillary (area around the optic disc) hyperpigmentation

Etiology and Pathophysiology

- Proliferation of uveal melanocytes or ciliary body epithelium, cause unknown
- Melanoma originates most commonly in the anterior uvea (iris and ciliary body), unlike in humans, in whom most are of choroidal origin.
- Primary intraocular sarcoma in cats occurs months to years after chronic uveitis or blunt or penetrating trauma to the eye. Damage to lens epithelium is implicated as initiating factor. Metastasis is common.
- Primary tumors in dogs are benign and, although locally invasive, rarely metastasize.
- Ciliary body tumors rarely metastasize.
- Uveal melanoma in cats may metastasize.
- Primary intraocular sarcoma in cats frequently metastasizes.

DIAGNOSIS

Diagnostic Overview

Goals of diagnosis are to confirm neoplasia versus other processes and differentiate primary from secondary and malignant from benign intraocular neoplasm.

Differential Diagnosis

- Iris cyst
- Diffuse iris melanocytosis, hyperpigmentation

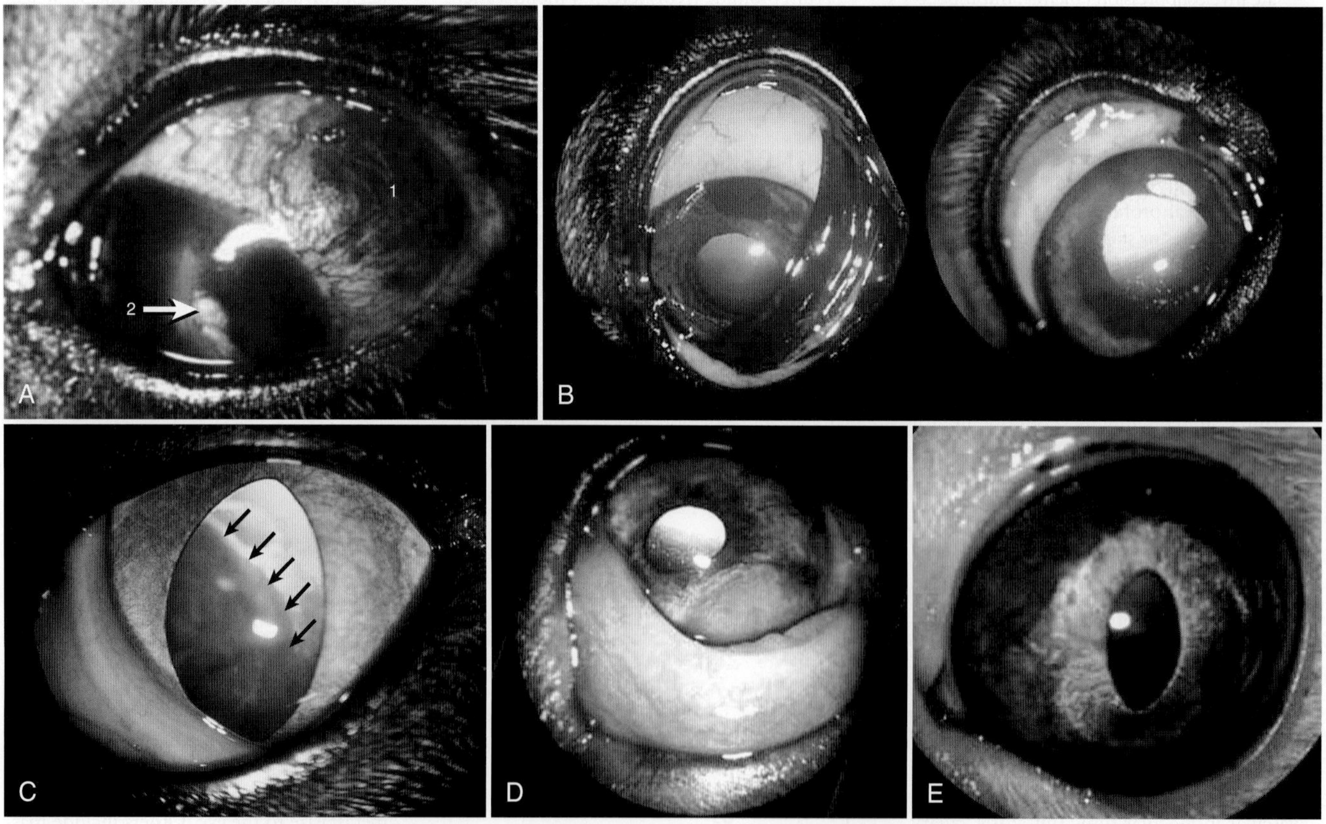

INTRAOCULAR NEOPLASIAS. A, Uveal melanoma in a dog with corneal and extrascleral extension (1). Note the white area of calcific corneal degeneration at leading edge of corneal extension (2). Enucleation is recommended. **B**, Localized, presumably benign, iris melanoma in a dog. Laser treatment was successfully performed as seen in the 6 months after the operative photo. **C**, Pink, vascular mass *(arrows)* is visible within the pupil in a cat. Appearance is typical of a ciliary body adenoma/adenocarcinoma, but metastatic neoplasia is also possible. **D**, Lymphoma metastatic to the iris and third eyelid in a dog. Diagnosis was made by biopsy of the third eyelid. **E**, Diffuse iris melanoma in a cat. Note the raised, velvety appearance distinguishing this from benign iris hyperpigmentation. Enucleation is recommended. (**D**, Courtesy Dr. Robert L. Peiffer, Jr.)

- Granulomatous uveitis with accumulation of inflammatory nodules within iris stroma
- Other causes of uveitis, glaucoma, intraocular hemorrhage

Initial Database

- Ophthalmic exam (p. 1137), including evaluation of vision and pupillary light reflexes, measurement of intraocular pressure; direct visualization of mass may allow conclusive diagnosis.
- Ocular ultrasonography may confirm and delineate mass that cannot be directly visualized because of location or lack of clarity of ocular media. Tumor appears as a hyperechoic mass within iris or ciliary body and may be difficult to differentiate from organized hemorrhage.
- Systemic evaluation to rule out metastatic disease (CBC, serum biochemistry panel, urinalysis, thoracic and abdominal radiographs and ultrasonography)

Advanced or Confirmatory Testing

- Aqueocentesis may not be diagnostic because tumors often do not exfoliate cells into the aqueous; most valuable for lymphoma
- Fine-needle aspiration of mass is often nondiagnostic due to inadequate size of sample.
- Biopsy of mass may be accompanied by hemorrhage.

TREATMENT

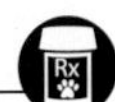

Treatment Overview

Treatment is based on assessment of presence of vision and potential to preserve comfortable globe. Goals are to prevent progressive growth of tumor (preserving vision and comfort) and alleviate discomfort caused by secondary glaucoma in blind eye.

Acute General Treatment

Primary intraocular tumors:

- Enucleation is indicated for irreversible blindness and pain due to secondary glaucoma
- Due to the metastatic potential, enucleation is indicated for iris melanoma and primary intraocular sarcoma in cats.
- Conservative monitoring alone may be justified in older dogs based on likely slow growth of primary tumor.
- Sector iridectomy may provide incomplete excision and is often accompanied by hemorrhage and secondary glaucoma; may be only surgical option other than enucleation for nonpigmented tumors
- Diode laser treatment, transcorneally or through a limbal incision, is often effective for pigmented uveal tumors.
- Diode laser treatment, possibly in combination with surgical debulking, is very effective for treatment of limbal melanomas.

Secondary intraocular tumors: treatment is directed at primary neoplasm if possible. If systemic prognosis warrants, enucleation may be indicated for comfort.

Possible Complications

- Laser treatment of large lesions may be accompanied by significant inflammation and may precipitate secondary glaucoma.
- Regrowth of tumor is possible after laser treatment.

Recommended Monitoring

Long-term monitoring to detect recurrent growth is indicated after laser treatment.

PROGNOSIS & OUTCOME

- Primary neoplasms of the iris, ciliary body, and limbus in dogs are almost always benign and rarely metastasize.
- Iris melanomas in cats are malignant tumors, and metastasis is possible.
- Primary intraocular sarcomas in cats are locally aggressive and often metastasize.

PEARLS & CONSIDERATIONS

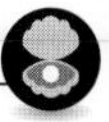

Comments

- Assessment of vision is the primary factor in determining treatment recommendation. If eye has functional vision, laser treatment should be considered for localized pigmented lesions; if eye is blind, enucleation is recommended.
- For malignant melanoma and sarcoma in cats, enucleation is advisable. Areas of progressive but localized iris hyperpigmentation, unconfirmed as neoplastic, can be treated by diode laser and monitored carefully.

Prevention

Iris melanoma in dogs: avoid breeding affected individuals or their close relatives.

Technician Tips

The appearance of intraocular neoplasia is extremely variable. It is important to monitor the intraocular pressure of these patients to check for secondary glaucoma.

SUGGESTED READING

Labelle AL, et al: Canine ocular neoplasia: a review. Vet Ophthalmol 16:3-14, 2013.

AUTHOR: Cynthia S. Cook, DVM, PhD, DACVO
EDITOR: Diane V. H. Hendrix, DVM, DACVO

Intussusception

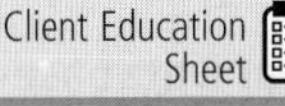

BASIC INFORMATION

Definition

- Invagination of one segment of the gastrointestinal (GI) tract into the lumen of an adjacent segment
- *Intussusceptum* is the invaginated segment, and the *intussuscipiens* is the outer or enveloping segment.

Epidemiology

SPECIES, AGE, SEX

- Intestinal intussusception usually occurs in animals < 1 year old unless associated with neoplasia.
- Gastroesophageal intussusception (GEI) is most common in dogs < 3 months old.

GENETICS, BREED PREDISPOSITION

Siamese and Burmese cats, German shepherds, and Shar-peis may be predisposed.

RISK FACTORS

- Infectious gastroenteritis (parasitic, bacterial, or viral), foreign body ingestion, intestinal mass/neoplasia, previous surgery peritonitis, organophosphate intoxication, parturition in queens
- Megaesophagus/abnormal esophageal motility for GEI.

Clinical Presentation

DISEASE FORMS/SUBTYPES

- Any of the following sites can be involved: gastroesophageal (p. 468), pylorogastric, duodenogastric, enteroenteric, enterocolic, cecocolic.
- Intussusception most commonly occurs in direction of normal peristalsis, with intussusceptum as proximal segment, but reverse can also occur (e.g., GEI).
- More than one site can be involved, or two invaginations may occur at the same site.

HISTORY, CHIEF COMPLAINT

- Diarrhea, hematochezia, vomiting, anorexia, lethargy, and weight loss
- Respiratory distress if GEI
- Signs can be acute or chronic.

PHYSICAL EXAM FINDINGS

- Palpable, sausage-shaped abdominal mass is characteristic but may not be present; palpation of mass may be precluded by abdominal guarding/pain.
- Signs of pain on abdominal palpation
- Dehydration, tachycardia (more severe signs associated with more proximal obstruction)
- Poor body condition can be seen in chronic cases.
- Intussusception may protrude from anus.

Etiology and Pathophysiology

- Proposed cause is structural or functional heterogeneity in the bowel wall, resulting in an alteration of intestinal pliability or motility.
- Intussusception produces partial or complete intestinal obstruction.
- Increased intraluminal pressure and kinking causes collapse of mesenteric blood vessels. Avulsion of vessels can also occur.
- Bowel wall becomes edematous and may become ischemic.
- Necrosis of the bowel wall, with leakage of contents contained by a fibrin seal between the layers of the intussusception, may occur. If leakage is not contained, peritonitis develops.

DIAGNOSIS

Diagnostic Overview

The diagnosis of enteroenteric (intestinal) intussusception is suspected based on history and typical physical exam findings. Confirmation is obtained with abdominal ultrasound exam or surgical exploration. GEI is confirmed with contrast imaging or endoscopy (p. 468).

Differential Diagnosis

- Gastroenteritis associated with infection or dietary indiscretion
- Intestinal obstruction associated with foreign body, neoplasia, abscess, or granuloma
- Physiologic ileus
- Rectal prolapse if intussusception protruding through anus (p. 866)

Initial Database

- CBC may show evidence of a stress leukogram or anemia. Increased red blood cell count may be seen with dehydration.
- Serum chemistry profile may show evidence of dehydration (increased total protein, azotemia), hypokalemia, hypochloremia, hyponatremia, or hypoproteinemia. Alkalosis may be seen with proximal obstructions.
- Abdominal radiographs may show fluid- or gas-distended intestinal loops. Tubular mass effect (sausage shape) of the intussusception may be seen in the small intestine or in a gas-filled colon.
- Thoracic radiographs: soft-tissue density within esophagus if GEI
- Fecal flotations are indicated to assess possible parasitic causes. Other tests (e.g., serologic assay for parvovirus) may be indicated in some cases.

Advanced or Confirmatory Testing

- Upper GI contrast radiographic study (p. 1098), barium enema, or pneumocologram for suspected ileocolic intussusception: filling defect caused by intussusceptum seen within intussuscipiens
- Ultrasonography: concentric rings in transverse plane (target sign) and hyperechoic or hypoechoic parallel lines in longitudinal views are characteristic. G-shaped or semilunar hyperechoic center (mesenteric fat) and visualization of the inner intussusceptum differentiate intussusception from other conditions. If mesenteric blood flow is identified with Doppler, the intussusception is more likely reducible at surgery.

TREATMENT

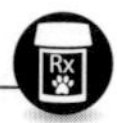

Treatment Overview

Immediate surgical intervention is indicated after hypovolemia is corrected. At surgery, an attempt is made to reduce the intussusception. If it is not reducible or there is bowel damage, resection and anastomosis are indicated. Enteroplication may be considered to prevent recurrence. Intestinal biopsy is indicated, particularly in older patients to evaluate for inflammatory bowel disease and neoplasia.

Acute General Treatment

- Intravenous crystalloids to correct dehydration or treat for shock. Colloids may be helpful with hypoproteinemia. If severe hypochloremia/hyponatremia, treat with 0.9% NaCl. Potassium supplementation if hypokalemic
- Administer perioperative antibiotics (e.g., cefazolin 22 mg/kg IV at induction and q 90 minutes during procedure +/− q 8h postoperatively)
- Enteroenteric or enterocolic intussusceptions; at the time of surgical exploration, reduce intussusception by applying pressure to intussuscipiens while *gently* pulling on intussusceptum.
    - Resection and anastomosis if unable to reduce intussusception, a mass is present, or there is nonviable bowel
- For enteroenteric intussusception, perform enteroplication if recurrence appears likely based on inability to correct underlying disease.
- For GEI, perform gastropexy of fundus and pylorus to prevent recurrence.

Chronic Treatment

- Opioid analgesia after surgery may decrease immediate risk of recurrence.
- Treat infectious enteritis that may have caused intussusception.
- Antibiotics should be continued after surgery if peritonitis is present.
- Enteroplication if not performed at first surgery and postoperative intussusception recurs

Possible Complications

- Recurrence of intussusception occurs in up to 20% of patients.
- Ileus
- Peritonitis associated with bowel rupture
- Leakage or dehiscence of intestinal suture line
- Entrapment and strangulation of bowel between enteroplication sutures
- Foreign body entrapment in bend of intestine created by enteroplication
- Persistent megaesophagus if GEI (p. 642)

Recommended Monitoring

- Monitor hydration status and serum electrolyte concentrations.
- Monitor for signs of intestinal suture line dehiscence and peritonitis (increased body temperature, abdominal pain, hypoglycemia).
- If clinical signs recur after surgery, repeat imaging to evaluate for possible recurrence of intussusception or complication associated with enteroplication.

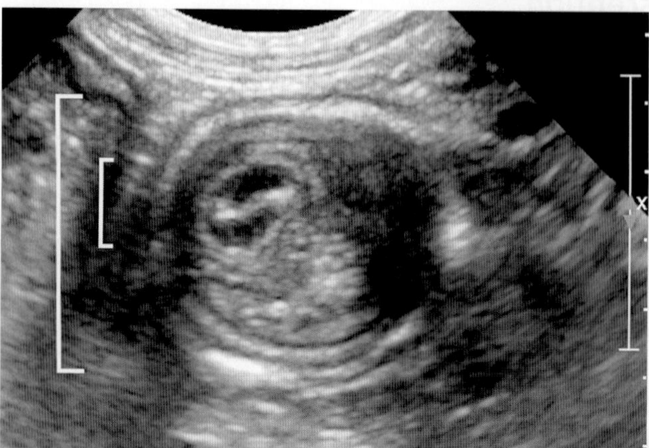

INTUSSUSCEPTION Ultrasound appearance (transverse view) of ileocolic intussusception in a dog. Note the typical target/bull's eye appearance created by the intussusceptum (*small bracket,* ileum) in the lumen of the intussuscipiens (*large bracket,* colon). The two structures are separated by ingesta/feces. (Courtesy Drs. Lesley Zwicker and Meghan Woodland, Atlantic Veterinary College, University of Prince Edward Island.)

PROGNOSIS & OUTCOME

- Depends on cause, location, and duration of intussusception
  - Good if fluid and electrolyte abnormalities are corrected and there is immediate surgical intervention
  - Patients with proximal GI tract intussusception, generalized peritonitis, or underlying malignant intestinal neoplasia have a worse prognosis.
- Severe complications have been associated with enteroplication, but recurrence may be seen if not plicated.

PEARLS & CONSIDERATIONS

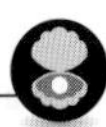

Comments

For each patient, the risk of recurrence must be weighed against the risk of complications associated with enteroplication:

- The decision to perform enteroplication is based largely on whether an underlying cause that can be corrected has been identified.
- If enteroplication is performed, create gentle loops along entire length of small intestine (from duodenocolic ligament to ileocolic junction); place sutures 5-10 cm apart.
- Spontaneous reduction of intussusception has been reported in dogs; however, recurrence that requires surgical intervention may occur.

Technician Tips

Young animals often have intussusception secondary to bacterial, viral, and/or parasitic causes. Therefore, the presence of intussusception is a signal to institute appropriate medical hygiene measures (e.g., gloving and gowning when handling patient, isolation when necessary).

SUGGESTED READING

Burkitt JM, et al: Signalment, history and outcome of cats with gastrointestinal tract intussusception: 20 cases (1986-2000). J Am Vet Med Assoc 234:771-776, 2009.

AUTHOR: Lori Ludwig, VMD, MS, DACVS
EDITOR: Elizabeth A. Swanson, DVM, MS, DACVS

Iris Abnormalities

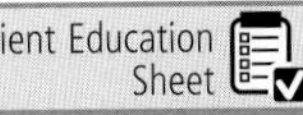

BASIC INFORMATION

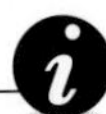

Definition

Iris abnormalities include any change in the color, character, or appearance of the iris, including acquired changes secondary to anterior uveitis, neoplasia, ocular melanosis or cyst formation, and developmental changes (e.g., persistent pupillary membranes [PPMs]). Other relevant definitions include those for rubeosis iridis (blood vessel formation on the surface of the iris) and synechia (adhesion of iris-to-cornea [anterior] or iris-to-lens [posterior]).

Synonyms

Uveal disease, ocular melanosis (once called pigmentary glaucoma)

Epidemiology

SPECIES, AGE, SEX

- Dogs and cats
- Anterior uveal neoplasia usually is seen in middle-aged to older animals.
- Ocular melanosis is seen in Cairn terriers and does not demonstrate age or sex predisposition.
- Uveal cysts are most frequently found in middle-aged to older animals (rare in cats).
- PPMs are congenital; pupillary membranes atrophy by 6 weeks of age in most puppies, but if not, PPMs may be detected in all age groups (rare in cats).

GENETICS, BREED PREDISPOSITION

- Uveal melanoma: suspected genetic predisposition in the Labrador retriever, golden retriever, and German shepherd.
- Ocular melanosis: inherited, probably autosomal dominant condition in Cairn terriers
- Uveal cysts: predisposed breeds include golden retrievers, Labrador retrievers, Boston terriers, Great Danes, rottweilers.
- PPMs: heritable cause suspected in basenjis, Pembroke Welsh corgis, chow chows, mastiffs, and others

Clinical Presentation

DISEASE FORMS/SUBTYPES

- Uveitis (p. 1023)
- Uveal neoplasia (p. 559)
- Uveal cysts
- PPMs

HISTORY, CHIEF COMPLAINT

Varies, depending on underlying cause; owner may report signs associated with any of the following:

- Anterior uveitis
- Uveal neoplasia
- Ocular melanosis
  - Darkening of the iris
  - ± Cloudy/hazy appearance to the eye in cases of secondary glaucoma
- Uveal cysts
- PPMs
  - Usually incidental finding
  - ± Cloudiness of eye if attached to cornea or lens

PHYSICAL EXAM FINDINGS

- See History, Chief Complaint above.
- Ocular melanosis: any or all of the following:
  - Dark brown thickening of the iris root/base
  - Episcleral/scleral pigment plaques
  - Release of pigment into aqueous humor, with pigment deposition in aqueous drainage pathways and on lens capsule
  - Pigmentation of the tapetal fundus ± on the surface of the optic disk
  - Secondary glaucoma in severe cases
- PPMs: any or all of the following:
  - Single or multiple fine strands of iris tissue originating from the iris collarette and inserting on:
    - Adjacent iris; typically benign, incidental finding
    - Anterior lens; often associated with anterior capsular cataracts
    - Corneal endothelium; associated with various degrees of corneal scarring and/or edema
    - Iris sheets; most severe form (sheet of tissue bridging pupil); associated with vision impairment (rare)
- Iris cysts
  - Variably pigmented spherical masses in anterior chamber
  - Cysts can be transilluminated or retroilluminated.

Etiology and Pathophysiology

Depend on underlying cause:

- The uveal tract (or vascular layer) of the eye is composed of the iris, ciliary body, and choroid. The iris is the most anterior of these and is a thin diaphragm containing blood vessels, connective tissue, melanocytes, and two muscles (iris sphincter and iris dilator). In the center of the iridal diaphragm is a circular aperture, the pupil.
- Anterior uveitis (p. 1023)
- Uveal neoplasia (p. 559)
- Ocular melanosis: inherited thickening and pigmentation of the iris caused by increased melanocytes and (to a lesser extent) melanophages, with release of pigmented material into the aqueous humor and pigment deposition in the episclera/sclera ± posterior segment. Secondary glaucoma can result from extensive pigment deposition in the aqueous drainage pathways.
- Uveal cysts
- PPMs: nonvascular remnants of the tunica vasculosa lentis, which appear as iris strands or sheets originating in the iris collarette (midway point between iris base and pupillary margin). PPMs extend across the iris

to insert on adjacent iris, lens, or cornea. When they insert on the lens or cornea, opacification of these structures may occur. PPMs are a developmental defect that may have a heritable component in some breeds.

DIAGNOSIS

Diagnostic Overview

The diagnosis is generally suspected because of the chief complaint or emerges as an incidental finding on ophthalmic exam. Characterization of an iris problem is based on a careful exam of the anterior chamber and iris surface with magnifying head loupes and diffuse and focal light sources.

Differential Diagnosis

Discoloration of iris:

- Increased pigmentation
  - Uveal melanoma: variable appearance in dogs (focal) vs. cats (mainly diffuse); solid tissue; may cause dyscoria (misshapen/distorted pupil) and/or anisocoria (unequal or asymmetrical pupils)
  - Ocular melanosis of cairn terriers
  - Uveal cyst: round to ovoid, single or multiple, often translucent
  - Chronic anterior uveitis
- Depigmentation
  - Chronic anterior uveitis
  - Uveal neoplasm
- Reddening
  - Rubeosis iridis; indicates chronic change
  - Iridal hemorrhage
  - Uveal neoplasm

Iris mass:

- Uveal neoplasm
- Uveal cyst

Iris strands:

- PPMs: arise from iris collarette; typically fine strands
- Synechiae: anterior forms typically arise from base of iris or pupillary margin; posterior: forms arise from pupillary margin or posterior aspect of iris; often result in dyscoria (abnormal pupil shape)

Initial Database

- Complete ophthalmic exam (p. 1137)
- Variable depending on underlying condition.

Advanced or Confirmatory Testing

- Varies, depending on underlying condition.
- Ocular ultrasound (differentiates uveal neoplasm from cyst)

TREATMENT

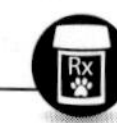

Treatment Overview

Treatment of iris abnormalities varies widely, but fortunately, diagnosis and subsequent treatment decisions are usually straightforward based on clinical signs.

Acute General Treatment

- Directed at underlying condition, when possible
- PPMs do not generally require treatment unless there is substantial corneal and/or lens opacification.
  - Iris-to-cornea PPMs may cause significant corneal edema, which may benefit from topical 5% hypertonic saline ophthalmic solution or ointment q 6-12h; continued long term if clinical improvement noted.
  - Iris-to-lens PPMs can lead to cataract formation; if cataract is causing vision impairment, cataract surgery may be warranted (p. 147).

Possible Complications

- Varies, depending on underlying condition
- Cataracts and corneal edema associated with PPMs are rarely progressive.

PROGNOSIS & OUTCOME

- Prognosis for anterior uveitis depends on severity at presentation, individual variation in severity and frequency of recurrences, underlying cause, and client compliance.
- Primary intraocular neoplasia usually carries a poor prognosis for saving the eye but good prognosis for systemic health.
- Ocular melanosis has a varied rate of progression and usually carries a poor prognosis for saving the eye if secondary glaucoma develops.
- Uveal cysts and PPMs rarely cause problems with vision or ocular comfort.

PEARLS & CONSIDERATIONS

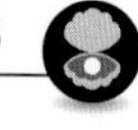

Comments

- Most iridal abnormalities can be readily diagnosed on the basis of clinical signs.
- Anterior uveitis requires immediate therapeutic intervention.

Prevention

Avoid breeding affected or closely related dogs predisposed to breed-related iris abnormalities.

Technician Tips

- Intraocular pressures should be checked in any cloudy eye.
- Pupillary light reflexes should be evaluated and documented before dilation with tropicamide.

SUGGESTED READING

Hendrix DVH: Diseases and surgery of the canine anterior uvea. In Gelatt KN, editor: Veterinary ophthalmology, ed 5, Ames, IA, 2013, Wiley-Blackwell, pp 1146-1198.

AUTHOR: Steven R. Hollingsworth, DVM, DACVO
EDITOR: Diane V. H. Hendrix, DVM, DACVO

Iron Toxicosis

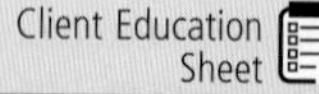

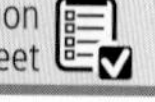

BASIC INFORMATION

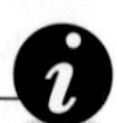

Definition

Iron toxicosis occurs when absorbable forms of iron are ingested, resulting in severe gastrointestinal (GI) effects and shock, followed by acidosis, central nervous system (CNS) depression, hepatic necrosis, and possibly kidney injury.

Epidemiology

SPECIES, AGE, SEX

Dogs are most commonly involved, but all species, ages, and both sexes can be affected.

RISK FACTORS

- Concurrent ascorbic acid (multivitamin) ingestion may increase iron absorption.
- Availability of multivitamins (notably prenatal vitamins), iron-based snail/slug baits, instant hand-warmers, heat patches or wraps, fertilizers, desiccants, and some birth control pills

Clinical Presentation

HISTORY, CHIEF COMPLAINT

- History or evidence of ingestion of iron-containing agent
- Mostly presented as an acute toxicosis
  - First stage (0-6 hours): vomiting, diarrhea (possibly severe/bloody), lethargy
  - Second stage (6-24 hours): latent period, apparent recovery, may be very short stage
  - Third stage (12-96 hours): lethargy, GI effects, acidosis, shock, hypotension, tachycardia, liver failure, coagulopathy, kidney injury
  - Fourth stage (2-6 weeks): possible scarring and stricture formation as GI ulcers heal

PHYSICAL EXAM FINDINGS

- Signs of hypovolemic shock (poor pulse quality, delayed capillary refill time, severe lethargy, tachycardia)
- Signs of dehydration
- Evidence of abdominal pain
- GI bleeding

Etiology and Pathophysiology

Mechanism of toxicosis:

- Direct corrosive damage to GI mucosa
- Causes free radical formation, which leads to lipid peroxidation and cell membrane injury.
  - All tissues are susceptible, but GI tract, liver, and heart have the most contact with free iron.

DIAGNOSIS

Diagnostic Overview

The combination of a history of exposure and consistent clinical signs is highly suggestive of iron toxicosis. Serum iron levels and serum iron-binding capacity are confirmatory. In patients already showing clinical signs, treatment of shock is instituted with only a presumptive diagnosis because aggravation of signs can occur while awaiting confirmation.

Differential Diagnosis

Depends on stage of intoxication

- Other intoxications that cause similar signs (GI and hepatotoxicosis): sago palm, caustics/corrosives, arsenic, copper, microcystin, xylitol, acetaminophen, mushrooms, phenols
- GI diseases that cause shock: infectious enteritis, hemorrhagic gastroenteritis, gastric dilation/volvulus, pancreatitis, GI obstruction, GI ulcer, peritonitis, and others
- Hepatopathies: neoplasia, leptospirosis, idiopathic chronic hepatitis

Initial Database

- CBC and serum biochemical profile to rule out other problems and assess liver function, coagulation, dehydration, acid/base status, and renal function
- Radiographs may show iron source in GI tract, but not all forms are radiopaque.

Advanced or Confirmatory Testing

- Serum iron
  - <300 mcg/dL usually does not justify chelation but may require treatment of GI signs
  - >400 mcg/dL along with clinical signs is significant and requires chelator treatment
- Some human hospital laboratories can measure serum iron and total serum iron-binding capacity (TIBC). Usually, serial samples are required at 2-4, 12, and 24 hours after exposure.
  - TIBC may indicate more free iron is available, which is toxic.
- Iron profile (p. 1355).

TREATMENT

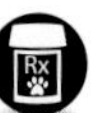

Treatment Overview

Initially, the goal is to decontaminate the patient if asymptomatic (first stage) or to stabilize the patient if hypovolemia is present (second-fourth stages). The next priority is diagnostic testing to determine if chelation is needed and to start chelation if indicated. If the animal is in the third stage (shock and acute liver injury), treatment is aimed at providing comprehensive supportive care and management of hepatic injury.

Acute General Treatment

Decontamination of the patient (p. 1087):

- Emesis induction (p. 1188), if exposure was within 2 hours and patient is not vomiting spontaneously. With large ingestions of multivitamins, emesis can be induced up to 6-8 hours after exposure because these tablets dissolve slowly.
- Gastric lavage (p. 1117) if a large number of tablets was ingested and not recovered in vomitus; however, tablets may form a pharmacobezoar or adhere to gastric mucosa.
- Activated charcoal is not indicated because it binds poorly to iron.
- Magnesium hydroxide 5-30 mL/DOG PO q 12h for 2-3 days may help reduce iron absorption; efficacy is questionable.

Stabilization:

- Intravenous fluids as needed
- Gastric protectants
  - Sucralfate 0.5-1 g PO q 8h, *and*
  - Famotidine 0.5-1 mg/kg PO, SQ, IM, or IV q 12-24h, *or*
  - Omeprazole 0.5-1 mg/kg PO q 24h
- Antiemetics if needed (e.g., maropitant 1 mg/kg SQ q 24h) or ondansetron 0.1-1 mg/kg PO q 12-24h or 0.2-0.5 mg/kg IV, IM, or SQ

Chelation:

- Deferoxamine (Desferal) is a specific iron chelator: 15 mg/kg/h continuous IV infusion (or 40 mg/kg IM q 4-8h for 24-72 hours) until serum iron levels fall below 300 mcg/dL. It can cause hypotension. Most effective within 24 hours of exposure and turns urine a pink-brown color (vin rose) while iron is being removed

Chronic Treatment

If needed: nonspecific support for liver dysfunction (e.g., *S*-adenosylmethionine 20 mg/kg PO q 24h for 1-3 months; give on empty stomach) (pp. 442 and 452).

Drug Interactions

Vitamin C can increase GI absorption of iron during toxicosis. Conversely, after iron is out of the GI tract, vitamin C can enhance chelation with deferoxamine and promote renal excretion.

Possible Complications

- Acute liver injury, liver failure
- Hypotension-induced kidney injury

Recommended Monitoring

- Hepatic function should be monitored for at least 96 hours after exposure in patients with overt clinical signs.
- If abdominal radiographs revealed evidence of the ingested iron source initially, follow-up radiographs after emesis or gastric lavage can help identify whether the iron-containing tablets have been removed.

PROGNOSIS & OUTCOME

- Varies, depending on how quickly treatment is started, severity of signs, amount ingested, and availability of chelator
- Excellent if only GI signs develop
- Guarded to poor if shock and liver damage occur

PEARLS & CONSIDERATIONS

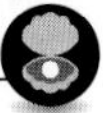

Comments

- Iron can vary in degree of solubility. Some forms, such as iron oxide (rust), present almost no risk because they are not absorbed.
- Iron can be present in many forms. It is necessary to convert to elemental iron to determine the dose ingested. Elemental iron content = iron form × percentage of elemental iron
  - Example: if a 20-kg dog ingests one 325-mg tablet of ferrous sulfate (20% elemental iron), elemental iron content = 325 mg × 0.2 = 65 mg elemental iron. For this dog, 65 mg/20 kg = 3.25 mg/kg elemental iron ingestion.
- In dogs, < 20 mg/kg elemental iron produces mild, self-limited GI signs, 20-60 mg/kg can cause mild to moderate GI signs that may require treatment, and > 60-80 mg/kg may cause severe signs and hepatic/renal injury.

Technician Tips

- Initial GI signs may worsen rapidly and can quickly lead to dehydration or shock; fluid status needs to be monitored closely.
- Deferoxamine can cause hypotension if given too rapidly or if used in a patient in shock; monitor blood pressure closely.
- Dogs ingesting iron-containing formulations can show black tarry stool color due to excreted iron oxides (not GI bleeding).

Percentage of Elemental Iron in Various Iron Salts

Compound	% Elemental Iron
Ferric ammonium citrate	15
Ferric chloride	34
Ferric EDTA	13
Ferric hydroxide	63
Ferric phosphate	37
Ferric pyrophosphate	30
Ferroglycine sulfate	16
Ferrous fumarate	33
Ferrous carbonate	48
Ferrous gluconate	12
Ferrous lactate	24
Ferrous sulfate (anhydrous)	37
Ferrous sulfate (hydrate)	20
Peptonized iron	17

Client Education

Vitamins may be palatable and need to be kept away from dogs.

SUGGESTED READING

Hall JO: Iron. In Peterson ME, et al, editors: Small animal toxicology, ed 3, St. Louis, 2013, Saunders, pp 595-600.

AUTHOR: Valentina Merola, DVM, MS, DABVT, DABT
EDITOR: Tina Wismer, DVM, MS, DABVT, DABT

Ivermectin Toxicosis

Client Education Sheet 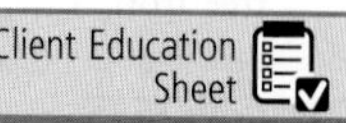

BASIC INFORMATION

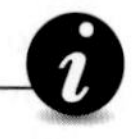

Definition

An acute or subacute intoxication resulting from accidental overdose, inappropriate owner administration, or ingestion of a common veterinary anthelmintic; characterized by neurologic signs

Synonyms

Agri-Mectin, Bimectin, DuraMectin, Eqvalan, EquiMax, Equimectrin, Heartgard, Iverhart, Ivomec, Tri-Heart, Vethical, Vetrimec, Zimectrin

Epidemiology

SPECIES, AGE, SEX

- Although any animal is susceptible, toxicity occurs far more often in dogs than cats.
- Young animals may be more susceptible due to a more penetrable blood-brain barrier.

GENETICS, BREED PREDISPOSITION

Breeds that have mutation in the *MDR1/ABCB1-Δ* gene (p. 638) that encodes for transmembrane pump P-glycoprotein responsible for keeping drugs out of the central nervous system (CNS) are more susceptible to intoxication:

- Collies
- Long-haired whippet
- Australian shepherd
- Miniature Australian shepherd
- McNab shepherd
- Silken windhound
- English shepherd
- Shetland sheepdog
- German shepherd
- Old English sheepdog
- Border collie
- Mixes of these breeds

RISK FACTORS

- Genetic susceptibility (i.e., *ABCB1* gene mutation)
- Pet owners' use of large-animal ivermectin products for pet animals or access of dogs to large-animal products (e.g., dog licking up flavored horse-product dropped on the ground)
- Dogs put on increasing doses of ivermectin for demodectic mange can develop clinical signs due to the long half-life of ivermectin in the dog.
- Veterinary miscalculation when giving an injection (decimal point error)

GEOGRAPHY AND SEASONALITY

Animals in rural areas or living on or near farms may have increased access to large-animal formulations of ivermectin.

Clinical Presentation

HISTORY, CHIEF COMPLAINT

- History of intentional administration or accidental ingestion
- Sudden onset of ataxia, visual difficulties, depression

PHYSICAL EXAM FINDINGS

- CNS
  - Depression
  - Coma
  - Ataxia
  - Tremors
  - Seizures
  - Disorientation
- Visual
  - Mydriasis
  - Blindness
- Cardiovascular
  - Bradycardia
- Gastrointestinal
  - Vomiting
  - Hypersalivation
- Respiratory
  - Hypoventilation
- Nonspecific
  - Dehydration
  - Hypothermia (with recumbency)
  - Hyperthermia (with tremors/seizures)

Etiology and Pathophysiology

- Ivermectin binds to glutamate-gated chloride ion channels in nerve and muscle cells, leading to hyperpolarization and ultimately paralysis and death of invertebrates.
- In mammals, gamma-aminobutyric acid (GABA)–mediated chloride channels that are sensitive to ivermectin are found in the CNS, which is normally protected by the blood-brain barrier and appropriately functioning P-glycoprotein. When normal protective mechanisms are overwhelmed or protective mechanisms do not function correctly, toxicosis occurs.

DIAGNOSIS

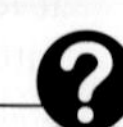

Diagnostic Overview

Diagnosis is typically based on presenting clinical signs and known exposure or potential access to ivermectin.

Differential Diagnosis

Toxic differentials:

- Alcohol
- 5-Hydroxytryptophan
- Amitraz
- Marijuana
- Smooth muscle relaxants
- Barbiturates
- Organophosphates or carbamate insecticides

Nontoxic differentials:

- Meningitis
- Intracranial neoplasia
- Portosystemic shunt

Initial Database

- CBC, serum chemistry profile, urinalysis: typically unremarkable
  - Monitor for hypernatremia with repeated doses of activated charcoal.
- Pulse oximetry and/or arterial blood gas if suspect hypoventilation
- Thoracic radiographs if suspect aspiration

Advanced or Confirmatory Testing

- Ivermectin can be detected in liver, adipose, tissue, or serum
- *ABCB1* gene testing for suspected breed sensitivity at Washington State University Veterinary Clinical Pharmacology Lab (vcpl.vetmed.wsu.edu)

TREATMENT

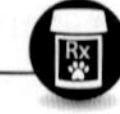

Treatment Overview

Decontamination and monitoring is key for animals presented with no clinical signs but known recent exposure. For patients already demonstrating signs of intoxication, care is largely symptomatic and supportive. Lipid emulsion therapy may be tried for more severely affected patients.

Acute General Treatment

- Decontamination in asymptomatic patient (p. 1087)
  - Induce emesis (p. 1188): apomorphine 0.03 mg/kg IV or 0.04 mg/kg IM (canine)
  - Gastric lavage in large exposures (p. 1117)
  - Activated charcoal 1-2 g/kg q 8h PO for 1-2 days
- Excision may be attempted for recent subcutaneous injections
- Control tremors/seizures
  - Methocarbamol 22-55 mg/kg IV, may need to go up to 150 mg/kg IV if signs are severe

  - Diazepam 0.5-1 mg/kg IV, *or*
  - Midazolam 0.1-0.3 mg/kg IV, IM
- Bradycardia: atropine 0.01-0.02 mg/kg IV, IM
- Lipid emulsion therapy 20% solution (p. 1127)
  - Initial bolus 1.5 mL/kg, then 0.25 mL/kg/min for 30-60 minutes; repeat every 4 hours provided no hyperlipemia is present and patient is responding to therapy. If no response after three doses, discontinue. If patient is hyperlipemic, discontinue until serum clears.
  - Adverse effects include potential binding of therapeutic lipophilic drugs, hyperlipemia, pancreatitis, hemolysis, liver enzyme elevation, and corneal lipid deposition.
- Nursing care for recumbent patients
  - Ocular lubricant
  - Appropriate bedding, frequent rotation to prevent decubital ulcers and urine scalding
  - Thermoregulation
- Fluid therapy for hydration and proper electrolyte balance
- Mechanical ventilation may be needed for more severely affected patients (p. 1185)
- Physostigmine 1-2 mg IV; nonspecific CNS stimulant; can wake dog up for 30-90 minutes so it can eat (repeated dosing to keep dog awake can cause seizures)

Nutrition/Diet

Feeding tube may be needed for recumbent/comatose patients as signs may last weeks (pp. 1106 and 1107)

Behavior/Exercise

Exercise restriction may be needed until signs fully resolve.

Drug Interactions

Avoid concurrent use of other drugs that can inhibit P-glycoprotein or may be G-glycoprotein substrates.

- Amiodarone
- Cyclosporine
- Diltiazem
- Erythromycin
- Fluoxetine, paroxetine
- Itraconazole, ketoconazole
- Spironolactone
- Spinosad
- Tacrolimus

Possible Complications

Watch for declining mental status, loss of gag reflex, or respiratory depression because they increase the risk of aspiration, particularly with administration of activated charcoal or vomiting.

Recommended Monitoring

Monitor mental status, cardiovascular, and respiratory systems closely.

PROGNOSIS & OUTCOME

Prognosis largely depends dose and severity of clinical signs. Animals that become symptomatic within the first 4 hours have a worse prognosis. In severe cases, significant care (ventilator, feeding tube, nursing care) may be needed for extended periods (days to weeks). No long-term sequelae are expected for patients that recover.

PEARLS & CONSIDERATIONS

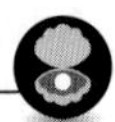

Comments

- When prescribing ivermectin for extra-label use, make sure strength and dose are clear on the label.
- Other drugs in this class (moxidectin, milbemycin, selamectin, doramectin, and abamectin) have similar toxic effects and treatment.
- Avoid use of extra-label doses of ivermectin with spinosad (spinosad affects P-glycoprotein and allows higher levels of ivermectin into the CNS).
- Activated charcoal is beneficial even with parenteral overdoses of ivermectin due to enterohepatic recirculation of ivermectin.

Prevention

- Double check strength and dose before sending home extra-label dosing.
- Do not use extra-label doses of ivermectin with spinosad-containing flea control products.
- Test at-risk breeds for *ABCB1* mutation before using ivermectin at doses higher than approved for prevention of heartworm.

Technician Tips

Check and double check math before giving any ivermectin by injection.

Client Education

- Educate owners to the dangers of using large-animal products in small animals because they can quickly lead to severe intoxication.
- Educate owner about potential adverse effects with extra-label dosing, and advise monitoring for ataxia and mydriasis with extended treatment.

SUGGESTED READING

Merola VM, et al: Toxicology of avermectins and milbemycins (macrocylic lactones) and the role of P-glycoprotein in dogs and cats. Vet Clin North Am Small Anim Pract 42(2):313-333, 2012.

AUTHOR: Kirsten Waratuke, DVM, DABT
EDITOR: Tina Wismer, DVM, MS, DABVT, DABT

Juvenile Cellulitis

BASIC INFORMATION

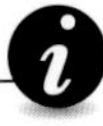

Definition

A sterile vesiculopustular to granulomatous skin disease of the face, pinnae, and submandibular lymph nodes primarily affecting dogs < 4 months old

Synonyms

Puppy strangles, juvenile sterile granulomatous dermatitis and lymphadenitis

Epidemiology

SPECIES, AGE, SEX

Puppies of either sex between 3 weeks and 4 months old are typically affected, although confirmed cases in young adults have been reported. One or more puppies in the same litter may be affected.

GENETICS, BREED PREDISPOSITION

Heritability is supported by an increased occurrence in certain breeds and breeding lines. Predisposed breeds include golden retrievers, Labrador retrievers, dachshunds, and Lhasa apsos, although mixed breeds can be affected.

Clinical Presentation

HISTORY, CHIEF COMPLAINT

Puppies are presented for an acutely swollen face (especially the eyelids, lips, and muzzle), edematous pinnae, and/or submandibular lymphadenopathy.

PHYSICAL EXAM FINDINGS

- Initially, acute swelling of face
- Within 24-48 hours, vesicles and pustules appear around mouth, eyes, and on muzzle. Lesions rapidly develop into a serous to purulent exudative dermatitis with or without fistulation.
- Serous to purulent bilateral otitis externa with edematous pinnae is common.
- Marked regional (submandibular and prescapular) to diffuse lymphadenopathy is common. Submandibular lymphadenopathy may occur as only clinical abnormality.

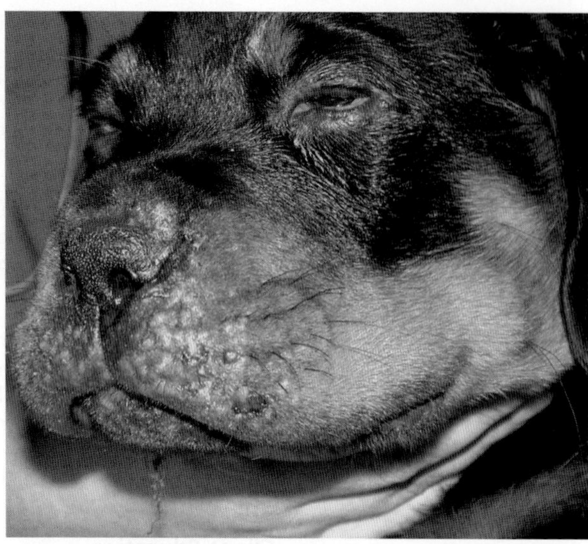

JUVENILE CELLULITIS Typical lesions in a 9-week-old rottweiler with edematous eyelids and papules, pustules, and swelling of the muzzle. (Courtesy Dr. Jocelyn Wellington.)

- Fistulation of affected lymph nodes is variable.
- Affected skin is frequently painful but rarely pruritic (p. 1091).
- Rarely, sterile subcutaneous nodules with or without fistulation develop on the trunk, preputial, or perineal regions.
- ≈50% of affected puppies are lethargic.
- Anorexia, fever, and lameness (sterile suppurative arthritis) are inconsistent findings.

Etiology and Pathophysiology

- The cause and pathogenesis of juvenile cellulitis are unknown. The presence of sterile lesions that respond to systemic glucocorticoids suggest immune dysfunction.
- Any evidence of infection usually reflects secondary pyoderma.

DIAGNOSIS

Diagnostic Overview

The diagnosis is suspected from the signalment, history, and physical exam.

Differential Diagnosis

- Angioedema: vaccine reaction or insect bite reaction
- Deep pyoderma/muzzle folliculitis
- Demodicosis
- Drug eruption (cutaneous drug reaction)

Initial Database

- Impression smears and cytologic evaluation of pustule (p. 1091): numerous neutrophils and macrophages (pyogranulomatous inflammation) without bacteria
- Skin scrapings: negative for *Demodex* mites

Advanced or Confirmatory Testing

Rarely required:

- Aerobic bacterial culture and susceptibility: usually sterile
- Skin biopsy of nontraumatized pustules or nodules: multiple discrete or confluent granulomas and pyogranulomas composed of nodular clusters of large epithelioid macrophages with variably sized neutrophilic centers
- Lymph node aspiration: pyogranulomatous lymphadenitis

TREATMENT

Treatment Overview

Early and aggressive immunosuppressive systemic therapy with predniso(lo)ne or dexamethasone is indicated to prevent secondary scarring. Concurrent systemic antibiotics are recommended if secondary pyoderma is found cytologically or marked fistulation is present.

Acute General Treatment

- Prednisone or prednisolone 2 mg/kg PO q 24h, or total dose can be divided q 12h until lesions resolve (≈1-4 weeks), then reduce to 2 mg/kg PO q 48h for 2 weeks, then taper prednisone over the next 2-3 weeks
- Some dogs respond better to dexamethasone 0.2 mg/kg PO q 24h. Gradually taper dosage (similar to prednisone).
- Oral cyclosporine can be combined with oral prednisone in recalcitrant cases.
- Bactericidal antibiotics for 3-4 weeks required with cytologic evidence of secondary pyoderma.
- Warm water soaks to remove crusts and exudates; topical astringents (e.g., 2% aluminum acetate [Burow's solution] q 12h) can be attempted.

PROGNOSIS & OUTCOME

Prognosis is good. Scarring may be extensive in severe cases.

PEARLS & CONSIDERATIONS

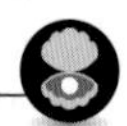

Comments

- Taper glucocorticoids gradually (over a few weeks) to reduce the risk of relapse.
- Adult dogs and dogs with panniculitis (subcutaneous nodules) require a longer treatment duration.
- If relapse occurs, restart immunosuppressive dosage of glucocorticoid immediately.
- Avoid routine vaccinations during therapy.

Technician Tips

Gentle wound care with an antimicrobial solution to remove crusts and exudate can reduce the need for systemic antibiotics.

SUGGESTED READING

Miller WH Jr, et al: Muller & Kirk's Small animal dermatology, ed 7, St. Louis, 2013, Saunders, pp 708-709.

AUTHOR: Jocelyn Wellington, DVM, DACVD
EDITOR: Manon Paradis, DMV, MVSc, DACVD

Keratoconjunctivitis Sicca

Client Education Sheet 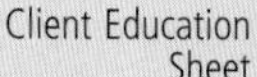 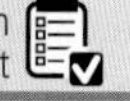

BASIC INFORMATION

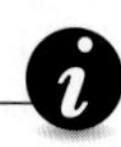

Definition

A common inflammatory condition of the cornea and conjunctiva secondary to a deficiency in the aqueous portion of the tear film

Synonyms

KCS, dry eye, quantitative tear film abnormality or deficiency, xerophthalmia

Epidemiology

SPECIES, AGE, SEX

- Common in dogs; rare in cats
- Age of onset varies, depending on underlying cause

- Increased predisposition reported for castrated male and spayed female dogs

GENETICS, BREED PREDISPOSITION

Predisposed breeds (dogs): English bulldog, West Highland white terrier, Lhasa apso, pug, American cocker spaniel, Pekingese, Yorkshire terrier, shih tzu, miniature schnauzer, Boston terrier, dachshund, Chihuahua, German shepherd, Doberman pinscher

RISK FACTORS

- Medications, metabolic disorders, dysautonomia, and infectious diseases (see Etiology and Pathophysiology below)
- Removal of gland of the third eyelid
- Systemic immune-mediated disease (e.g., systemic lupus erythematosus [p. 955])

CONTAGION AND ZOONOSIS

Infectious causes (e.g., canine distemper; feline herpesvirus type 1 [FHV-1]) are contagious.

ASSOCIATED DISORDERS

Conjunctivitis and ulcerative and nonulcerative keratitis

Clinical Presentation

HISTORY, CHIEF COMPLAINT

- Red eye (p. 870)
- Ocular pain
- Mucoid to mucopurulent ocular discharge

PHYSICAL EXAM FINDINGS

- Systemic: unremarkable unless associated with systemic disease
- Ophthalmic: any of the following
  - Mucoid to mucopurulent ocular discharge
  - Conjunctival hyperemia and chemosis
  - Blepharospasm
  - Protrusion of the third eyelid
  - Dry/lackluster corneal appearance
  - Corneal ulceration: range from superficial ulceration to corneal perforation
  - Signs of chronicity
    - Corneal vascularization
    - Corneal pigmentation
    - Corneal keratinization
  - Blepharitis
  - Periocular dermatitis secondary to exudates and/or self-trauma
  - Vision impairment secondary to chronic keratitis
- Cats often show fewer clinical signs than dogs.

Etiology and Pathophysiology

- Immune-mediated adenitis: most common (dogs)
- Congenital: lacrimal gland hypoplasia or aplasia (usually toy breeds)
- Drug-induced: general or topical anesthesia and atropine (transient keratoconjunctivitis sicca [KCS])
- Drug toxicity: some systemic medications (e.g., sulfonamides; phenazopyridine; 5-aminosalicylic acid; etodolac) may cause transient or permanent KCS.
- Iatrogenic: removal of the gland of the third eyelid increases risk of KCS, especially in predisposed breeds.
- Infectious disease (e.g., canine distemper, FHV-1)
- Metabolic disease (e.g., hypothyroidism, hyperadrenocorticism, diabetes mellitus)
- Neurogenic: may occur with facial nerve paralysis and denervation of parasympathetic fibers innervating the gland or after ocular proptosis.
- Chronic blepharoconjunctivitis due to obstruction of lacrimal ductules secondary to chemosis or ascending infection into lacrimal gland
- Chronic conjunctivitis may cause ductules to scar (e.g., FHV-1).
- Irradiation: when primary beam near or on periocular region

DIAGNOSIS

Diagnostic Overview

The diagnosis is suspected based on the presence of conjunctivitis or ulcerative and/or nonulcerative keratitis. The confirmatory test of choice is the Schirmer tear test (STT).

Differential Diagnosis

Dogs: other causes of keratoconjunctivitis:

- Conjunctivitis (p. 200)
- Corneal vascularization or pigmentation (e.g., pannus [pp. 212 and 748])
- Corneal exposure (e.g., lagophthalmos); common cause of misdiagnosis of KCS
- Corneal ulceration (p. 209)
- Blepharitis

Cats: other causes of keratoconjunctivitis:

- FHV-1 conjunctivitis/keratitis (p. 464)
- Proliferative keratoconjunctivitis: eosinophilic

Initial Database

Complete ophthalmic exam (p. 1137):

- STT
  - Normal: ≥ 15 mm/min in dogs; varies in cats
  - Early or subclinical KCS: 11-14 mm/min
  - Mild to moderate KCS: 6-10 mm/min
  - Severe KCS: ≤ 5 mm/min
- Fluorescein dye application: secondary corneal ulceration is common.
- Intraocular pressure (IOP): normal IOP values; normal IOP range is 15-25 mm Hg (dogs and cats)

Advanced or Confirmatory Testing

- Other quantitative test: phenol red-thread tear test
  - Dogs: normal 34.15 ± 4.45 mm/15 sec
  - Cats: normal 23.04 ± 2.23 mm/15 sec

TREATMENT

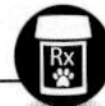

Treatment Overview

Treatment goals are to stimulate tear production, stabilize the tear film, and eliminate ocular pain by controlling ocular inflammation (conjunctivitis and nonulcerative keratitis), secondary bacterial infections, and corneal ulceration if present.

Acute General Treatment

- Lacrimostimulants
  - Cyclosporine 0.2% ointment or 0.5%-2% solution topically to affected eye(s) q 12h
- Lacrimomimetics (tear substitutes and stabilizers such as hyaluronic acid 0.4%, gels or ointments) applied topically to affected eye(s) q 4-6h
- Antimicrobials if secondary bacterial conjunctivitis and/or corneal ulceration
  - Topical broad-spectrum antibiotic (e.g., bacitracin-neomycin-polymyxin antibiotic solution) to affected eye(s) q 6-8h
- Antiinflammatories if severe conjunctivitis and/or corneal vascularization/pigmentation but only in the absence of corneal ulceration
  - Dexamethasone 0.1% solution topically to affected eye(s) q 6-8h
- Pilocarpine 1 drop 2% pilocarpine/10 kg body weight on food q 12h, gradually and cautiously increasing by 1-drop increments until increased tearing or systemic side effects (e.g., vomiting, diarrhea, anorexia, salivation, bradycardia; if systemic effects occur, decrease dose or discontinue immediately); effective only in some with neurogenic KCS

Chronic Treatment

Lacrimostimulants:

- Cyclosporine 0.2% ointment or 0.5%-2% solution topically to affected eye(s) q 8-24h (typically q 12h)
  - For STT values that remain 10 mm/min or less after 3-4 weeks of treatment, dosage may be increased to q 8h.
  - Dose frequency should not be decreased until STT values are ≥ 20 mm/min.
  - Dosage may be decreased to q 24h in rare cases if very favorable response occurs.
- Tacrolimus 0.02%-0.03% ointment or aqueous suspension q 12h
  - Used if no response to cyclosporine after 3-6 weeks of treatment
  - 51% of dogs that fail to respond to cyclosporine respond to tacrolimus.
  - Studies evaluating long-term safety have not been performed.
- Some ophthalmologists advocate increasing the concentration of the lacrimostimulant if there is no response (i.e., 0.2% cyclosporine ointment to 2% solution).
- Continue pilocarpine only if effective in neurogenic cases until the condition has resolved.
- Consider parotid duct transposition if no response to lacrimostimulants.

Possible Complications

- Corneal ulceration
- Vision impairment from progressive corneal vascularization/pigmentation (uncontrolled KCS)

Recommended Monitoring

- Varies, depending on underlying cause
- Complete ophthalmic examination with STT and corneal fluorescein staining performed every 3-4 weeks initially until KCS controlled, then every 3-4 months; more frequent rechecks if corneal ulceration is present

PROGNOSIS & OUTCOME

Varies, depending on underlying cause and severity at diagnosis

PEARLS & CONSIDERATIONS

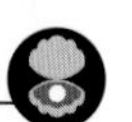

Comments

- Immune-mediated KCS usually requires lifelong treatment.
- Some forms of KCS may require transient treatment until tear production returns (e.g., topical atropine, topical or general anesthesia); lacrimomimetics may be sufficient.
- May take weeks to months of therapy before determining if favorable response to lacrimostimulants
- If frequency of administration of cyclosporine or tacrolimus is decreased to q 24h, STT should be monitored a few days and then a few weeks after reduction.
- Deep or infected ulcers should be stabilized with antibiotics and lacrimomimetics ± surgery before initiating treatment with cyclosporine or tacrolimus.

Prevention

For breeds predisposed to KCS, avoid breeding affected or closely related dogs.

Technician Tips

Owners should administer q 12h lacrimostimulants the morning of recheck appointments or the STT will not be reflective of the response to therapy.

Client Education

Immune-mediated KCS is a chronic disorder that is manageable but usually requires lifelong treatment.

SUGGESTED READING

Williams DL: Immunopathogenesis of keratoconjunctivitis sicca in the dog. Vet Clin North Am Small Anim Pract 38(2):251-268, 2008.

AUTHOR: **Phillip A. Moore, DVM, DACVO**
EDITOR: **Diane V. H. Hendrix, DVM, DACVO**

Lactation Disorders

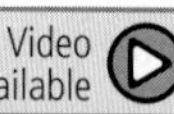

Video Available

BASIC INFORMATION

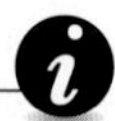

Definition

- Partial or complete failure to produce or secrete milk to meet puppies' demand
- Disorders include *agalactia* (complete failure to produce milk), *hypogalactia* (partial failure), and *galactostasis* (accumulation of milk in the mammary gland due to failure of ejection [letdown] from the gland).
- Primary agalactia is rare, and a delay in milk letdown is the most prevalent issue.

Synonyms

Agalactia or agalactosis, hypogalactia, hypolactation

Epidemiology

SPECIES, AGE, SEX

- Postpartum female dogs; young bitches seem more prone
- There is only one report of agalactia in queens.

GENETICS, BREED PREDISPOSITION

Any breed potentially can be affected. A genetic component may exist with agalactia.

RISK FACTORS

Inadequate nutrition, stress, anxiety, premature delivery or elective cesarean section, progesterone therapy, and systemic illness may trigger hypogalactia or poor milk letdown and galactostasis.

ASSOCIATED DISORDERS

Lactation disorders can coexist with other puerperal diseases, such as mastitis, metritis, and endotoxemia.

Clinical Presentation

DISEASE FORMS/SUBTYPES

Depending on the cause, agalactia can be classified as

- Primary, idiopathic, or true agalactia
- Secondary or poor milk letdown (galactostasis)

HISTORY, CHIEF COMPLAINT

History reveals the previous occurrence of (premature) parturition or elective cesarean section. Inadequate neonate weight gain and crying and restless puppies are frequent complaints due to insufficient lactation. Few puppies to nurse or abrupt weaning may precede galactostasis.

PHYSICAL EXAM FINDINGS

In cases of hypogalactia and agalactia, mammary development and milk appearance at nipple squeezing are scarce or absent. Galactostasis is characterized by engorged, firm, and painful mammary glands, which may be associated with nipple anatomic abnormalities.

Etiology and Pathophysiology

- Normal milk production is the consequence of an endocrine cascade of estrogens, progesterone, and prolactin, as well as other ancillary hormones. Idiopathic, primary agalactia may represent a disruption of the pituitary–ovarian–mammary gland axis of unknown origin.
- Failure of milk letdown (secondary agalactia) can be due to stress, anxiety, premature delivery, progesterone therapy, or systemic illness.

DIAGNOSIS

Diagnostic Overview

Crying puppies and a dam that is reluctant to nurse are suggestive of primary and secondary agalactia. Consideration of the environment where lactation is occurring and physical exam of the mammary glands help differentiate the two causes.

Differential Diagnosis

- Mastitis
- Mammary tumors
- Pseudocyesis
- Care should be taken because mastitis and mammary tumors can coexist with lactation disorders.

Initial Database

- History and physical findings (as previously described)
- CBC is normal if concurrent inflammatory illness is present.

Advanced or Confirmatory Testing

- Diagnosis is confirmed by exclusion of other diseases. Occult primary illness may require serum biochemistry profile, vaginal discharge exam, and ultrasound of the uterus.

- Cytologic evaluation of milk reveals cell counts > 3000 cells/mcL with macrophages and neutrophils when inflammation (p. 618) is present.

TREATMENT

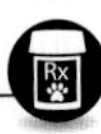

Treatment Overview

Agalactia treatment mainly consists of the administration of galactagogues (prolactin increasing drugs). Treatment should be continued for 3 days beyond when milk production appears. Failure of milk letdown requires treatment of primary cause (pp. 618 and 854). Conversely, galactostasis could be treated with prolactin-decreasing drugs (dopamine agonists or antiserotoninergics) if there are no puppies to nurse.

Acute General Treatment

- Because primary agalactia has no effective treatment, puppies should be hand reared.
- Hypogalactia or secondary agalactia can be treated with
  - Metoclopramide 0.1-0.2 mg/kg SQ q 6-8h
  - Domperidone 2.2 mg/kg PO q 12h for 4-6 days. Domperidone is a safer choice than metoclopramide because it does not cross the blood-brain barrier and therefore has no central side effects.
- Failure of milk letdown can be treated with nasal oxytocin spray 10 minutes before lactation q 8h.
- Anxious bitches may benefit from mild tranquilization with phenothiazine compounds (e.g., acepromazine 0.1-0.25 mg/kg PO or 0.05-0.1 mg/kg IM or SQ), which also increases prolactin release.
- In cases of galactostasis, reduction of milk production can be achieved by the administration of cabergoline 5 mcg/kg PO q 24h for 5-7 days. Diuretics and analgesics may also be beneficial when there are puppies to nurse and lactation cannot be interrupted.

Nutrition/Diet

Diminishing food intake (one-half) and water for 2 or 3 days may help resolve galactostasis.

Behavior/Exercise

- In hypogalactia or secondary agalactia, ensure puppies suckle vigorously so that natural stimulation of the glands occurs.
- Galactostasis may benefit from wrapping mammary area with an elastic bandage to protect from trauma. Any stimulation on the mammary glands (e.g., padding, touching, or milking) should be avoided if lactation is going to be terminated.

Drug Interactions

High metoclopramide doses (5 mg/kg) for more than 5 days usually cause behavioral side effects such as excitation and aggression. Domperidone provokes minimal (soft stools) or no side effects.

Possible Complications

When gross inflammatory changes of the mammary glands accompany the accumulation of milk, mastitis may be present.

PROGNOSIS & OUTCOME

Primary agalactia has a poor prognosis for lactation, and neonates should be hand reared. Failure in milk letdown and galactostasis typically respond to treatment or resolve spontaneously.

PEARLS & CONSIDERATIONS

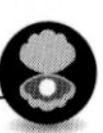

Comments

Lactation disorders do not pose a risk for the female's life, although they may cause considerable neonatal losses.

Prevention

- Provide a gradual increase of food intake during the second half of pregnancy, and 125%-150% maintenance requirements after whelping.
- Be sure mammary development is adequate before cesarean section.
- Gradual weaning prevents galactostasis.
- Considering the possible genetic component of primary agalactia, breeding affected bitches should be weighed against the potential of perpetuating the problem.

Technician Tips

- Slowly and calmly introduce puppies to dam after cesarean section. Anxious bitches may benefit from mild tranquilization with acepromazine. (See *Video*.)
- Galactostasis may benefit from wrapping mammary area with an elastic bandage to protect from trauma. Any stimulation of the mammary glands (e.g., padding, touching, or milking) should be avoided if lactation is going to be terminated.

Client Education

Teach clients to recognize lactation disorders early so puppies can be saved.

SUGGESTED READING

Romagnoli S, et al: Control of mammary gland function in the bitch and queen: a review. Clin Theriogenol 4:196-205, 2012.

AUTHOR: Christina Gobello, MV, DVM, DECAR
EDITOR: Michelle A. Kutzler, DVM, PhD, DACT

Lameness

BASIC INFORMATION

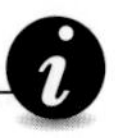

Definition

Alteration of gait caused by structural or functional abnormality in one or more limbs

Synonyms

Favoring leg, limping

Epidemiology

SPECIES, AGE, SEX

Dog or cat, any age, either sex

RISK FACTORS

Trauma, genetics, obesity, overnutrition during growth, tick bites, endocrinopathy

Clinical Presentation

HISTORY, CHIEF COMPLAINT

Thorough history is critical:

- Abnormal gait or limping observed by owner
- Determine which limb is affected.
- Difficulty rising
- Improves or worsens with exercise
- Holding limb up
- Dragging limb or inappropriate placement (knuckling)
- Shifting limb lameness
- Acute or gradual onset
- Progression over time

PHYSICAL EXAM FINDINGS

- Complete general physical looking for evidence of systemic abnormalities (e.g., fever)
- Complete orthopedic and neurologic exams (pp. 1143 and 1146). Orthopedic exam must include assessment of
  - Abnormal posture
  - Joint effusion, warmth
  - Bone, joint, or muscle pain
  - Muscle atrophy
  - Thickening or bony prominences at or near joints
  - Crepitus
  - Abnormal range of motion (ROM) in joints

- Observation at a walk and trot for gait abnormalities to help localize the limb that is affected
  - Failing to bear full weight on limb, leaning off affected limb when standing
  - Short stride on affected limb
  - Head bob (down on sound: head moves down when patient bears weight on normal limb and then up when bearing weight on affected limb to decrease weight on affected limb) with forelimb lameness
  - Toeing in or out
  - Dragging feet or scuffing nails
  - Bunny hopping (hindlimb weakness)
  - Stumbling
  - Ataxia
  - Hypermetria
  - Stiff, stilted gait: walking on egg shells
- When both hindlimbs are affected, weight may be shifted onto forelimbs, resulting in arched posture and abduction of the elbows.

Etiology and Pathophysiology

- Lameness secondary to pain from the musculoskeletal system: pain causes decreased weight bearing on the affected limb and shortness of stride. Severe, acute pain may cause non–weight bearing on affected limb.
- Mechanical lameness: may be caused by abnormal length or angulation of bones, joints, ligaments, or tendons
- Endocrine-related lameness: hyperadrenocorticism may cause myopathy, and diabetes mellitus may cause peripheral neuropathy.
- Neurologic disorders may cause ataxia, paresis, pain manifesting as lameness, or holding limb up as root signature
- Mono or polyarthropathy of any cause can result in lameness.

DIAGNOSIS

Diagnostic Overview

Accurate diagnosis of lameness combines a thorough history, clinical exam, and consideration of patient signalment. An orthopedic exam is indicated in every case, and additional tests such as radiographs are selected based on abnormalities identified in the exam and medical history.

Differential Diagnosis

See Lameness on p. 1249 for detailed differential diagnosis.

Initial Database

- Complete orthopedic and neurologic exams
- Radiographs of affected limb(s)

Advanced or Confirmatory Testing

- CBC, serum biochemistry panel, urinalysis: for abnormalities suggesting metabolic or systemic causes
- Serologic titers for infectious disease (e.g., Lyme disease, ehrlichiosis) as appropriate
- Arthrocentesis (p. 1059)
  - Can aid in differentiating degenerative joint disease from infectious, inflammatory, or immune-mediated joint disease
  - Culture and sensitivity: joint fluid should be cultured in blood culture medium for highest yield.
- Immunologic testing: rheumatoid factor (low yield), antinuclear antibody test if systemic lupus erythematosus suspected (p. 955)
- Ultrasound of tendons or muscles
- CT, MRI (p. 1132): CT is most useful for bones and joints, whereas MRI is most useful for soft tissue and spinal disease.
- Arthroscopy: can be used for diagnostic and therapeutic purposes.
- Arthrotomy
- Soft-tissue or bone biopsy of specific lesions
- Force plate and gait analysis
- Nuclear scintigraphy: used for localizing disease such as a difficult-to-diagnose lameness or metastatic tumors
- Electromyography (EMG): useful for evaluating neuromuscular conditions
- Muscle or nerve biopsy

TREATMENT

Treatment Overview

Treatment of lameness requires a multimodal approach to alleviate pain and treat the underlying disorder causing the lameness.

Acute General Treatment

Lameness is a clinical sign, not a specific disease. Treatment is based on determination of the underlying cause.

Chronic Treatment

- Depends on underlying cause
- Adjunctive/supportive treatment may include one or several of the following:
  - Weight loss, if indicated (p. 700)
  - Glycosaminoglycan administered intramuscularly or intraarticularly (p. 469)
  - Nonsteroidal antiinflammatory drugs (NSAIDs) (p. 469)
  - Analgesics (e.g., amantadine, tramadol, gabapentin) (p. 469)
  - Intraarticular hyaluronic acid or intraarticular corticosteroids can be administered for severe arthritis unresponsive to other therapies.
  - Platelet-rich plasma (PRP) therapy for osteoarthritis and soft-tissue injury
  - Stem cell therapy derived from autogenous adipose tissue has recently become available.
  - Acupuncture provides anecdotal relief for some dogs (p. 1056).
  - Physical/rehabilitative be useful.

Nutrition/Diet

Nutritional and dietary therapeutics include eicosapentaenoic acid (EPA)–rich diets and nutraceuticals such as chondroitin and glucosamine.

Behavior/Exercise

Behavioral and physical activity recommendations include moderation of physical activity, physical rehabilitation, stretching, and eliminating environmental risks such as slippery walking surfaces, stairs, and need for jumping. Toe grips, rough-surfaced booties, or painted-on pad products (e.g., PawFriction, Pawtology LLC) can be useful in some cases.

Drug Interactions

Glucocorticoids potentiate the gastrointestinal (GI) ulcerogenic effects of NSAIDs; this combination is contraindicated.

Possible Complications

NSAIDs may be associated with GI irritation for some patients. They should also be used cautiously in animals with pre-existing renal disease.

Recommended Monitoring

Response to therapy

PROGNOSIS & OUTCOME

Varies, depending on underlying cause of lameness. For example, most cases of panosteitis in growing dogs resolve spontaneously over time (prognosis excellent), whereas lameness due to osteosarcoma of a long bone has a poor long-term prognosis.

PEARLS & CONSIDERATIONS

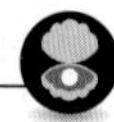

Comments

Attention to signalment, history, and thorough exam is essential for generating a short list of differential diagnoses. Common signalment profiles are provided on p. 1262.

Prevention

Weight management has been shown to reduce the incidence and severity of osteoarthritis and clinical signs in patients with orthopedic disease.

Technician Tips

Use a soft surface for patient and examiner comfort and to reduce patient stress.

SUGGESTED READING

Fossum TW: Orthopedic examination. In Fossum TW, editor: Small animal surgery, ed 4, St. Louis, 2013, Mosby, pp 931-941.

AUTHOR: David A. Puerto, DVM, DACVS
EDITOR: Leah A. Cohn, DVM, PhD, DACVIM

Laryngeal Masses

Client Education Sheet

BASIC INFORMATION

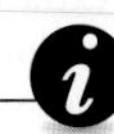

Definition

Benign or malignant proliferation of laryngeal tissues

Epidemiology

SPECIES, AGE, SEX

- Rare in dogs and cats; occurs most often in middle-aged or older animals
  - Benign lesions may be more common in younger animals.
- Higher incidence of laryngeal tumors in male dogs and cats

ASSOCIATED DISORDERS

- Signs associated with acute or chronic upper airway obstruction (p. 1004)
  - Stridor, dysphonia, collapse, cyanosis, dyspnea (increased inspiratory effort)
- Dysphagia (p. 277)
- Aspiration pneumonia (p. 1269)
- Extra-esophageal reflux

Clinical Presentation

DISEASE FORMS/SUBTYPES

Benign or malignant masses

HISTORY, CHIEF COMPLAINT

Any of the following are possible:

- Acute or progressive history of inspiratory stridor
- Dysphonia
- Exercise intolerance
- Dysphagia/gagging
- Dyspnea
- Cyanosis, collapse
- Cough
- Ptyalism
- Mass in the neck

PHYSICAL EXAM FINDINGS

- May be normal; mass can be an incidental finding at time of endotracheal intubation
- Inspiratory dyspnea, with gasping if severe
  - Dyspnea does not improve with open-mouth breathing.
- Stridor
- ± Palpable mass in the ventral laryngeal area
- Coughing and/or gagging due to laryngeal compression
- Weakness
- Ptyalism
- Halitosis

Etiology and Pathophysiology

- Laryngeal tumors cause obstruction by external compression or intraluminal obstruction.
- Primary
  - Benign: oncocytoma (do not metastasize but very locally aggressive), laryngeal cyst, laryngeal polyp, rhabdomyoma, granular cell tumor, lipoma
  - Malignant: squamous cell carcinoma and lymphoma (most common in cats); also chondrosarcoma, mast cell tumor, fibrosarcoma, rhabdomyosarcoma, osteosarcoma, melanoma, mixed cell tumor, adenocarcinoma, undifferentiated sarcoma
- Metastatic: lymphoma, plasma cell tumor, thyroid neoplasia

DIAGNOSIS

Diagnostic Overview

Diagnosis often hinges on direct observation of the larynx in an anesthetized or heavily sedated patient. Fine-needle aspiration (FNA) or biopsy is needed to identify type of mass.

Differential Diagnosis

- Laryngeal paralysis (dogs > cats)
- Laryngeal collapse
- Elongated soft palate (dogs, especially brachycephalic)
- Nasopharyngeal polyp (cats > dogs)
- Pharyngeal or laryngeal foreign body
- Granulomatous masses
- Laryngeal osseous metaplasia
- Retropharyngeal lymphadenopathy
- Cuterebra

Initial Database

- CBC, biochemistry panel, and urinalysis are usually unremarkable.
- Cervical radiographs may show a soft-tissue opacity in the area of the larynx, leading to laryngeal distortion or decreased laryngeal luminal space. The normal larynx of dogs, especially if mineralized, should not be confused with an abnormality (e.g., foreign body).
- Ultrasonography may allow identification of laryngeal masses because of the distortion of normal structural/anatomic relationships. It may also facilitate FNA of mass.
- Thoracic radiographs can demonstrate metastasis or aspiration pneumonia.
- Fluoroscopy can demonstrate soft-tissue opacity in the laryngeal area or dynamic obstruction. Free-standing protocols require minimal restraint.

Advanced or Confirmatory Testing

- Patients with laryngeal masses may be at the cusp of respiratory collapse despite showing only moderate (inspiratory) dyspnea and may be unable to recover from anesthesia without respiratory distress/suffocation. Therefore, *before* sedation/anesthesia for upper airway evaluation have the following ready:
  - An appropriate-sized endotracheal tube
  - A tracheostomy kit (p. 1166)
  - Clip hair from the ventral neck (preparation for tracheostomy if needed)
  - Discuss a contingency with the owner if the mass is nonresectable (e.g., recover with tracheostomy vs. euthanize).
- Functional laryngeal exam (sedation) to rule out laryngeal paralysis (pp. 574 and 1125) should precede laryngoscopy (general anesthesia) to directly visualize the mass.
- Cells should be obtained for diagnosis by FNA and/or endoscopic or surgical biopsy.
  - Cytologic analysis adequate for some tumor types (e.g., lymphoma, mast cell tumors)
  - A misleading cytologic or histologic diagnosis of lymphoid hyperplasia may be initially obtained by needle cytology or pinch biopsies in patients with primary laryngeal neoplasia.
- CT or MRI (p. 1132) can better show the extent of the mass and possible involvement of other regional structures.

TREATMENT

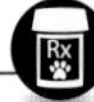

Treatment Overview

Immediate goal is to remove/reduce laryngeal luminal obstruction. Additional treatment depends on extent of lesion and type of mass.

Acute General Treatment

Patient stabilization as necessary:

- Oxygen by face mask, oxygen cage, or nasal cannula if needed (p. 1146)
- Sedation (e.g., acepromazine 0.005-0.01 mg/kg IV, with or without butorphanol 0.2 mg/kg IV)
- Endotracheal intubation
- Tracheostomy if in severe distress (p. 1166)

Chronic Treatment

- Small, benign lesions may be surgically excised by submucosal resection or partial laryngectomy.
- Laryngeal lymphoma is amenable to treatment with chemotherapy.
- Large, invasive lesions or malignant tumors are best removed surgically by total laryngectomy combined with a permanent tracheostomy.
  - Glucocorticoid administration (dexamethasone 0.05-0.1 mg/kg IV) at the time of surgery may help reduce laryngeal edema.
  - Permanent tracheostomy can palliate signs of respiratory distress in nonresectable cases or cases managed conservatively. Rarely successful in cats or small dogs because tracheal lumen becomes obstructed with secretions
- Certain tumors may be best treated with radiation therapy. Consultation with an oncologist is recommended.

Behavior/Exercise

Limit exercise and discourage barking for 2-4 weeks after surgery. Mild sedation may be helpful.

Possible Complications

- Postoperative swelling
- Dysphagia and/or gagging
- Pharyngeal dehiscence
- Laryngeal stenosis/webbing
- Hypoparathyroidism/hypothyroidism (if removed during laryngectomy)
- Tumor recurrence or metastasis
- Obstruction, self-trauma of tracheostoma
- Subcutaneous emphysema secondary to laryngeal/tracheal incision

Recommended Monitoring

- Monitor closely for upper airway obstruction secondary to postoperative pharyngeal swelling.
- Withhold water and food for at least 24-48 hours in the postoperative period.
- Routine laryngoscopic re-evaluation is recommended to identify tumor recurrence or laryngeal stenosis.
- Periodic physical and radiographic evaluation is recommended to check for recurrence or metastasis.

PROGNOSIS & OUTCOME

- The prognosis is good for benign lesions if complete resection is possible.
- Prognosis for malignant laryngeal tumors is guarded:
    - Advanced disease is often detected at the time of diagnosis.
    - May not be surgically resectable

PEARLS & CONSIDERATIONS

Comments

- Leaving the ventral part of the vocal cords intact may help prevent postoperative laryngeal webbing.
- A CO_2 laser works well for surgical dissection and results in minimal inflammation and hemorrhage.
    - When using a laser, ensure the endotracheal tube is protected from the laser beam.
- Some patients may benefit from a feeding tube for postoperative nutritional support (pp. 1106 and 1109).
- Rhabdomyoma, oncocytoma, and granular cell tumors share many cytologic and histologic features. These neoplasms should be differentiated using histochemical staining and immunohistochemical analysis.

Technician Tips

When preparing for exams of animals with laryngeal disease, have nearby a laryngoscope, tongue depressor (to move the soft palate), an extra endotracheal tube (if the first becomes occluded with blood and mucus), long cup biopsy forceps, formalin, 22- or 23-gauge needles of varying lengths (1-inch, 1/10 -inch, spinal needles), 6- or 12-mL syringes and microscope slides (for aspiration cytology), and cotton-tip swabs (or gauze sponges and forceps or suction) for clearing mucus or blood.

Client Education

Vocalization is lost after total laryngectomy.

SUGGESTED READING

Withrow SJ: Tumors of the respiratory system. In Withrow SJ, editor: Small animal clinical oncology, ed 5, Philadelphia, 2013, Saunders, pp 432-462.

AUTHOR: Michael B. Mison, DVM, DACVS
EDITOR: Megan Grobman, DVM, MS, DACVIM

Laryngeal Paralysis

Client Education Sheet 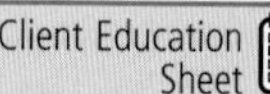

BASIC INFORMATION

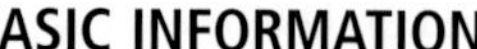

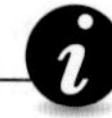

Definition

Lack of abduction of arytenoid cartilages and vocal folds secondary to cricoarytenoideus dorsalis muscle or recurrent laryngeal nerve dysfunction is common in old, large-breed dogs but rare in cats.

Epidemiology

SPECIES, AGE, SEX

- Dogs: males more common; no sex predisposition in cats
- Congenital form: animals < 1 year old
- Acquired form: middle-aged/older dogs and cats (mean, 9-11 years of age)

GENETICS, BREED PREDISPOSITION

- Acquired form commonly reported in Labrador retrievers, other large/giant breeds (Saint Bernards, Newfoundlands, Irish setters). No breed predisposition in cats.
- Congenital
    - Autosomal dominant: Bouviers des Flandres
    - Associated with laryngeal paralysis polyneuropathy complex: Leonberger dogs, rottweilers, Pyrenean mountain dogs, Dalmatians, and black Russian terriers
    - Other: bull terriers, Siberian Huskies, white-coated German shepherd dogs

RISK FACTORS

- Damage to the recurrent laryngeal nerve (blunt trauma, neoplasia, thoracic or cervical surgery)
- Any condition resulting in polyneuropathy or polymyopathy
    - Myasthenia gravis
    - Immune-mediated disorder
    - Diabetes mellitus
    - Hypothyroidism (cause/effect relationship not established)
    - Toxins (lead, organophosphates)
    - Progressive idiopathic polyneuropathy
- Extraesophageal reflux disease (EERD)
- Cervical/intrathoracic masses
- In cats, associations with tick paralysis, idiopathic polyneuropathy, bronchogenic carcinoma, trauma, and brainstem lesions have been reported.

GEOGRAPHY AND SEASONALITY

Hot weather/humidity and panting may increase severity of clinical signs.

ASSOCIATED DISORDERS

- Soft palate elongation occurs in 20% because of chronic increased inspiratory effort.
- Weakness and muscle wasting evident in up to 50% of chronically affected dogs.
- Dysphagia or megaesophagus is possible in dogs with polymyopathy, polyneuropathy, or reflux/esophagitis.
- Aspiration pneumonia/chronic aspiration-associated lung injury can develop secondary to dysphagia, EERD, esophageal or laryngeal dysfunction.
- Noncardiogenic pulmonary edema/acute respiratory distress syndrome with vigorous inspiration against upper airway obstruction

Clinical Presentation

DISEASE FORMS/SUBTYPES

- Unilateral: clinical signs mild or absent except in performance dogs or in cats
- Bilateral: clinical signs apparent in most animals

HISTORY, CHIEF COMPLAINT

- Varied progression over months to years
- Signs worsened by exercise and increased environmental temperature/humidity

Early:

- Inspiratory stridor; very common
- Voice change (i.e., dysphonia)
- Exercise intolerance with associated respiratory noise and/or breathlessness; very common
- Coughing, gagging when eating

With progression:
- Dyspnea
- Tachypnea
- Signs exacerbated with exercise, stress, hot weather, obesity
- ± Regurgitation if associated esophageal dysmotility

Severely affected animals:
- Dyspnea at rest
- Cyanosis
- Collapse
- Death

PHYSICAL EXAM FINDINGS
- Unremarkable in early stages
  - With panting, may recognize "hoarse" breathing noise
- With disease progression:
  - Increased inspiratory effort, inspiratory stridor
  - Increased upper airway sounds (referred on thoracic auscultation)
  - Coughing or gagging that may be induced by laryngeal compression
  - Paradoxical breathing (chest and abdomen move in opposition)
  - Weakness
  - Muscle atrophy, neurologic deficits if peripheral neuropathy/myopathy is present
  - ± Crackles from pneumonia or pulmonary edema
  - Severe hyperthermia ± signs of heat stroke (petechial hemorrhages, mucous membrane hyperemia, abnormal mentation) in severely dyspneic animals

Etiology and Pathophysiology

Causes:
- Nucleus ambiguus or axonal degeneration (congenital forms)
- Idiopathic: most common cause of acquired form; likely underlying generalized peripheral neuropathy
- Intrathoracic, peritracheal, or laryngeal masses or foreign bodies (rare)
- Other acquired causes include trauma to recurrent laryngeal nerve, polymyopathy, polyneuropathy, myasthenia gravis.

Whatever the cause, recurrent laryngeal nerve dysfunction results in loss of function of all intrinsic muscles of the larynx except the cricothyroideus, causing inability to abduct arytenoids during inspiration (loss of cricoarytenoideus dorsalis muscle function) or actively adduct arytenoids (close the rima glottidis) during swallowing.
- With increased inspiratory pressure, arytenoids are passively drawn inward, collapsing the airway during inhalation (paradoxical movement).
- Affected dogs also have decreased topical pharyngeal and laryngeal sensitivity and dysmotility of the cranial and caudal esophagus.

DIAGNOSIS

Diagnostic Overview

Definitive diagnosis is usually based on lack of active laryngeal movement ± presence of paradoxical movement on laryngeal exam under light anesthesia. Intravenous doxapram stimulates respiration in animals that have inhibition of respiration or reduced inspiratory motion because of sedative and anesthetic administration. Laboratory evaluations, thoracic radiographs, and complete neurologic exam (p. 1136) should be performed to assess the animal for signs of concurrent disease (e.g., polyneuropathy/myopathy, pneumonia, hypothyroidism). For dogs that present with dysphagia, evaluate for abnormal deglutition.

Differential Diagnosis

- Elongated soft palate
- Collapsing trachea
- Laryngeal collapse
- Reverse sneezing
- Laryngeal mass or other laryngeal/proximal tracheal obstruction
  - Laryngeal neoplasia: cats > dogs

Initial Database

- CBC, biochemistry panel, and urinalysis are usually unremarkable except in cases of systemic disease, dehydration, or heat stroke.
- Thoracic radiographs
  - Usually normal or age-related interstitial changes
  - ± Aspiration pneumonia
  - ± Megaesophagus in animals with polyneuropathy/polymyopathy
  - ± Diffuse alveolar pattern if noncardiogenic pulmonary edema
- Low total thyroxine (T_4) or free T_4 with normal/increased thyroid-stimulating hormone: hypothyroidism
- Pulse oximetry in dyspneic or cyanotic dogs; normal dogs have oxygen saturation ≥ 95%.

Advanced or Confirmatory Testing

- Definitive diagnosis with laryngoscopy (p. 1125)
  - May be performed without anesthesia during dyspneic crisis
  - Otherwise, light anesthetic plane (often propofol 2-6 mg/kg IV to effect, though can produce false-positives)
  - If no motion, administer doxapram HCl (1 mg/kg IV once):
    - In laryngeal paralysis, arytenoid and vocal fold motion are absent or paradoxical (inward collapse on inhalation, blown open on exhalation).
- May visualize lack of arytenoid movement on cervical ultrasound (cats especially)
- In patients with polymyopathy or polyneuropathy, electromyography or nerve conduction velocities may be abnormal.
- Esophageal dilation or lack of peristalsis on fluoroscopic contrast esophagram if there is concurrent esophageal motility disorder.
  - Progressive esophageal dysfunction in dogs with laryngeal paralysis reported
  - Esophagrams are not routinely performed because of risk of aspiration. Protocols employing free-feeding practices may mitigate these risks.
- Peripheral muscle and nerve biopsies are diagnostic for denervation polyneuropathy, even in dogs with no clinical signs of generalized neuromuscular disease.
- Coagulation panels may be abnormal for animals with hyperthermia or signs of heat stroke.

TREATMENT

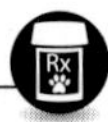

Treatment Overview

Mildly affected animals may respond to sedation and oxygen administration during acute exacerbations of clinical signs and remain stable with limited exercise or stress. Severely affected animals are most commonly treated with unilateral arytenoid lateralization, which improves survival rates but increases the risk of aspiration pneumonia.

Acute General Treatment

- Oxygen
  - Provide flow-by oxygen (mask or nasal catheter) if SpO_2 < 95% (p. 1146).
  - If SpO_2 cannot be maintained ≥ 95% on oxygen, perform tracheostomy (p. 1166), or intubate, and maintain under light anesthesia until swelling decreases, or immediate arytenoid lateralization.
- Reduce laryngeal edema (prednisolone 0.5-1 mg/kg IV q 24h; dexamethasone 0.1-0.2 mg/kg IV q 24h). Do not give steroids if on nonsteroidal antiinflammatory drugs (NSAIDs).
- Sedation (e.g., acepromazine 0.005-0.02 mg/kg or dexmedetomidine 2-5 mcg/kg with butorphanol 0.2-0.4 mg/kg IV q 2-4h as needed) for stressed animals
- Address hyperthermia, if present (p. 421)

Chronic Treatment

Nonsurgical (minimally affected/unilateral disease or comorbid disease likely to limit life expectancy):
- Weight loss
- Exercise restriction
- Stress reduction ± sedation (e.g., trazodone [dogs] starting at 2-5 mg/kg PO q 8-12h; maximal dose 14 mg/kg/day) when stress is expected
  - Trazodone has been used anecdotally in cats (25-50 mg/CAT PO q 24h)
- Treatment of underlying diseases (e.g., hypothyroid polyneuropathy)

Surgical:
- Unilateral arytenoid lateralization recommended because higher complication rates are seen with other surgical options (permanent tracheostomy, vocal fold excision, partial laryngectomy, castellated laryngofissure, muscle-nerve pedicle transposition)
  - Unilateral arytenoid lateralization is considered a referral procedure.
  - Lateralization should be accomplished with low-tension sutures to prevent excessive abduction of arytenoid.

- Unilateral arytenoid lateralization improves clinical signs in small-breed dogs with concurrent laryngeal paralysis and laryngeal collapse.
- Concurrent palate resection in dogs that also have elongated soft palate

Possible Complications

- Aspiration pneumonia reported in 8%-35% of dogs and 30% of cats after unilateral arytenoid lateralization
- Coughing/gagging in 10%-16% after unilateral arytenoid lateralization
- Respiratory distress requiring temporary tracheostomy; postoperative megaesophagus; concurrent respiratory tract, esophageal, neurologic, or neoplastic disease
- Bilateral arytenoid lateralization associated with increased risk of postoperative complications and death
- Complication rate higher (74% vs. 32%) in dogs with neurologic comorbidities

Recommended Monitoring

- Monitor for respiratory distress for 12-24 hours after surgery.
- Restrict exercise and reduce barking for 1-2 months after surgery.
- Re-evaluate laryngeal function and repeat chest films as needed if clinical signs recur.

PROGNOSIS & OUTCOME

- Reduction of respiratory signs and improved exercise tolerance in 90% of dogs after unilateral arytenoid lateralization
- Generalized neurologic signs commonly develop within 1 year of diagnosis of idiopathic laryngeal paralysis.
- Poor prognosis with progressive polyneuropathy (rottweiler, Dalmatian, others)
- Mortality rate of 14%; higher complication rates among older animals and those with concurrent respiratory, esophageal, or neurologic disease

PEARLS & CONSIDERATIONS

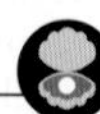

Comments

- Doxapram helps differentiate a deep anesthetic plane from laryngeal paralysis.
- Laryngeal function is inhibited in normal dogs with some anesthetic combinations (acepromazine/thiopental, acepromazine/propofol, ketamine/diazepam).
- Nonsurgical management is initially recommended for dogs with unilateral disease or clinical signs limited to coughing/dysphonia.
- Perioperative metoclopramide does not decrease the risk of aspiration pneumonia.
- Laryngeal paralysis is often an initial sign of generalized, progressive polyneuropathy.
- Surgical correction improves ability to breathe but does not reverse voice changes.

Prevention

Affected animals, especially members of predisposed breeds, should not be bred.

Technician Tips

- To assist during laryngeal exam, position the dog in sternal recumbency, and hold the upper jaw with a piece of rolled gauze.
- The examiner should pull the tongue down with a gauze sponge and use a videoendoscope or laryngoscope to visualize the larynx. Note each inhalation for the examiner so that normal opening of cartilages during inspiration can be differentiated from abnormal, paradoxical movement (abnormal: passive inward motion on inhalation, passive outward motion on exhalation).

Client Education

- Progressive polyneuropathy/polymyopathy, which may be identified in dogs with laryngeal paralysis, can increase the risk of surgical complications.
- Upper airway noise, change in/loss of bark, and coughing often persist after surgery.
- There is a lifelong risk of aspiration pneumonia after surgery, but survival improves with surgery.
- Some dogs do better when fed dry food from floor level. Try different food consistencies, bowl positions, and feeding strategies to reduce postoperative coughing and gagging and to slow down food intake.

SUGGESTED READING

Monet E: Surgical treatment of laryngeal paralysis. Vet Clin Small Anim 46:709-717, 2016.

AUTHOR: Karen M. Tobias, DVM, MS, DACVS
EDITOR: Megan Grobman, DVM, MS, DACVIM

Laryngeal Trauma

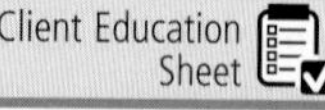

BASIC INFORMATION

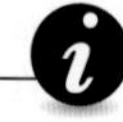

Definition

Trauma resulting in disruption of, or damage to, laryngeal structures (thyroid, cricoid, and arytenoid cartilages) and surrounding soft tissues

Epidemiology

SPECIES, AGE, SEX

- Dogs and cats; no age or sex predisposition
- Cats may be predisposed to iatrogenic laryngeal trauma from orotracheal intubation.

RISK FACTORS

- Animal fight/attack
- Access to outside while unsupervised poses general increased risk of trauma such as impalement, projectile missiles, foreign bodies, strangulation, and vehicular accidents.
- Use of choke collars
- Anesthesia with intubation
- Long-term intubation for positive pressure ventilation
- Bronchoscopy
- Surgery near the larynx (e.g., mass excision, tracheal stent)

ASSOCIATED DISORDERS

- Polytrauma: head/cervical trauma, respiratory compromise, cardiovascular shock
- Subcutaneous emphysema, pneumomediastinum, and potentially, pneumothorax and pneumoretroperitoneum

Clinical Presentation

HISTORY, CHIEF COMPLAINT

- ± History of witnessed trauma (e.g., bite wounds, penetrating missile, choking), recent prolonged or difficult intubation, surgery (cervical) or bronchoscopy
- Acute onset of dyspnea with stridor
- Exercise intolerance
- Dysphonia and/or dysphagia
- Cough/hemoptysis

PHYSICAL EXAM FINDINGS

- Tachypnea, dyspnea
- Stridor: usually more prominent on inspiration but can be both inspiratory and expiratory (fixed obstruction)
- Mucous membranes: ± pallor or cyanosis
- Thoracic auscultation: referred upper airway noise, ± harsh lung sounds, ± crackles (e.g., noncardiogenic pulmonary edema, pulmonary contusions, aspiration pneumonia)
- Subcutaneous emphysema in cervical region with penetrating wounds or laryngeal fracture and laceration
- ± Hyperthermia (dogs: inability to pant)
- Neurologic deficits associated with cervical spine injury

Etiology and Pathophysiology

- Rough or prolonged intubation can cause trauma to the mucosa, arytenoids, and vocal folds, resulting in hyperemia or edema, ulceration, and granulation tissue formation.

- Trauma (e.g., bite wounds, projectile missiles, strangulation) can cause penetrating or crush injury to the cartilages or recurrent laryngeal nerves.
- Airway lumen diameter can be drastically reduced if cartilages are crushed (e.g., choke chains) or with swelling/hemorrhage of surrounding soft tissues (e.g., stick foreign bodies).
- Decreased gas exchange from airway compromise: hypoxemia ± hypercarbia
- Worsened hypoxemia (ventilation/perfusion mismatch) if blood is aspirated into lungs or with noncardiogenic pulmonary edema from airway obstruction

DIAGNOSIS

Diagnostic Overview

Laryngeal injury is suspected based on respiratory distress with upper airway noise in a patient with a history of recent trauma to the cervical region or anesthesia with intubation. Confirmation relies on cervical radiographs, laryngoscopy, and/or tracheoscopy.

Differential Diagnosis

- Airway foreign body (p. 355)
- Insect sting/bite or other allergic reaction (pharyngeal swelling)
- Trauma to caudal pharynx or trachea (p. 486)
- Laryngeal paralysis/collapse (p. 574)
- Laryngeal/pharyngeal mass (neoplasm such as squamous cell carcinoma, abscess, granuloma, hematoma [p. 573])
- Pharyngeal/sublingual mucocele
- Epiglottic retroversion

Initial Database

- CBC, serum biochemistry profile, urinalysis: usually unremarkable
- Neurologic exam: deficits may support concurrent spinal trauma
- Pulse oximetry/arterial blood gas analysis
  - Hypoxemia (common)
  - Hypercarbia (severe airway obstruction)
- Cervical radiographs
  - Fractures, dislocations, or asymmetry in hyoid apparatus
  - Subcutaneous emphysema
  - Concurrent vertebral trauma
- Thoracic radiographs
  - Pneumomediastinum, pneumothorax, subcutaneous emphysema
  - Concurrent thoracic trauma (e.g., rib fractures, pulmonary contusions)
  - Noncardiogenic pulmonary edema secondary to airway obstruction
- Laryngoscopy under general anesthesia (p. 1125); exam can be performed after tracheostomy if patient does not have a patent airway, allowing for stabilization of patient first.
  - Evaluate symmetry and function of laryngeal structures.
  - Look for hematomas, exposed cartilage, foreign body, or flaps of laryngeal mucosa.
- ± Laryngeal function exam (rule out laryngeal paralysis)

Advanced or Confirmatory Testing

- Tracheoscopy/bronchoscopy (p. 1074); exam can be performed after tracheostomy if needed.
  - Evaluate larynx beyond the arytenoids.
  - Examine lower airways for evidence of trauma or foreign body.
- Esophagoscopy (p. 1098): rule out concurrent esophageal injury.
- CT may be useful in evaluating the hyoid apparatus for fractures or dislocations.
- Fluoroscopy: evaluate for dynamic obstruction (e.g., epiglottic retroversion)

TREATMENT

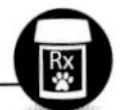

Treatment Overview

Treatment consists of stabilizing the patient (ensuring a patent airway, providing oxygen supplementation and additional supportive care), followed by surgical repair as needed. Initial stabilization may require an emergency tracheostomy if the patient cannot be intubated with an orotracheal tube.

Acute General Treatment

- Oxygen supplementation (p. 1146)
- Intubation if needed
- Emergency tracheostomy (p. 1166) if unable to pass endotracheal tube or if prolonged need anticipated
- Treat cardiovascular compromise (IV catheter, fluids) and other life-threatening injuries.
- Surgical exploration/repair or permanent tracheostomy, if indicated.
  - Approach: midline ventral thyrotomy or through thyroid cartilage fracture
    - Mucosal flaps: trim, appose edges
    - Reduce and immobilize cartilage fractures to prevent stenosis
    - Unilateral arytenoid lateralization (tieback) if traumatic laryngeal paralysis without fracture or arytenoid avulsion
    - Intraluminal stents may be used to prevent adhesions, collapse, and other complications
- Postoperative care
  - Antibiotics after obtaining cultures from contaminated wounds; continue 3-4 weeks postoperatively. Suggested empirical treatment while awaiting culture results:
    - Ampicillin 22 mg/kg IV q 8h and enrofloxacin 10-15 mg/kg diluted and given slowly IV or PO q 24h in dogs (5 mg/kg q 24h in cats) *or* pradofloxacin 7.5 mg PO q 24h (cats) *or*
    - Clindamycin 10 mg/kg IV or PO q 8h and either amoxicillin/clavulanic acid 15 mg/kg PO q 12h, *or* enrofloxacin as listed above
  - Glucocorticoids (dexamethasone sodium phosphate 0.1-0.2 mg/kg IV) at surgery to reduce inflammation; may repeat at 0.05-0.1 mg/kg IV q 12-24h for first 24-48 hours
  - Oxygen support as needed

Chronic Treatment

- Intraluminal stents require a second surgery 3-4 weeks later for removal.
- Permanent tracheostomy may be required if severe damage to larynx has occurred.

Behavior/Exercise

- Exercise restriction for 3-4 weeks after trauma or surgical repair
- No neck leads; harness only while leash-walking
- Sedation as needed
- Prevent hyperthermia

Possible Complications

- Respiratory arrest
- Stenosis or stricture over the ensuing 1-2 weeks, resulting in secondary airway compromise
- Obstruction of temporary or permanent tracheostomy site
- Laryngeal paralysis
- Infection

Recommended Monitoring

- Vital signs and frequent auscultation during initial admission and in the perioperative period
- Tracheostomy care
- Pulse oximetry and/or arterial blood gas analysis
- Respiratory rate and effort, respiratory noise, and exercise tolerance, during and after the recovery stage

PROGNOSIS & OUTCOME

- Depends on severity of trauma, concurrent injuries, and time to diagnosis and treatment
- If severe laryngeal trauma is present and veterinary care can be quickly obtained, permanent tracheostomy can allow for fair to good prognosis (with the exception of cats and very small dogs, in whom stoma obstruction with mucus may be recurrent and severe).

PEARLS & CONSIDERATIONS

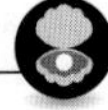

Comments

- Early temporary tracheostomy: stabilizes patient and allows imaging, including laryngoscopy, endoscopic exam, radiographs, and CT
- Surgical exploration/repair must occur early, optimally within 24 hours after injury.
- Surgical exploration is necessary if
  - Airway obstruction is severe enough to require temporary tracheostomy
  - There is emphysema in the cervical region and/or pneumomediastinum
  - There is exposed cartilage in the lumen of the larynx
  - The laryngeal cartilage is fractured

Prevention

- Selection of appropriate endotracheal tube and endoscope size along with lubrication may prevent iatrogenic trauma.

- Direct visualization of the larynx for intubation can reduce risk of iatrogenic trauma.
- Long-term intubation for positive-pressure ventilation can be maintained by temporary tracheostomy to prevent laryngeal damage.

Technician Tips

Careful monitoring is necessary because patients can develop acute airway obstruction. Any increased respiratory rate/effort or increase/change in respiratory sounds may indicate impending crisis. If possible, these patients are better monitored when not in an oxygen cage, allowing any airway noises caused by acute obstruction to be heard.

SUGGESTED READING

Basdani EE, et al: Upper airway injury in dogs secondary to trauma: 10 dogs (2000-2011). J Am Anim Hosp Assoc 52:291-296, 2016.

AUTHOR: Lori S. Waddell, DVM, DACVECC
EDITOR: Megan Grobman, DVM, MS, DACVIM

Lead Toxicosis

Client Education Sheet 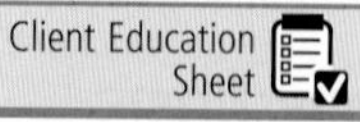

BASIC INFORMATION 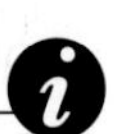

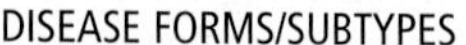

Definition

Lead toxicosis occurs most commonly when lead is ingested, resulting in neurologic, hematologic, and/or gastrointestinal (GI) effects.

Synonyms

Plumbism, lead poisoning

Epidemiology

SPECIES, AGE, SEX

Any dog or cat, although cats may be at higher risk due to grooming behaviors if there are lead particles available (e.g., flakes of lead-based paint). Younger dogs may be at higher risk due to an increased tendency to lick or chew objects. Immature animals absorb more lead from the GI tract than adults; immature animals are also at higher risk because lead can cross the blood-brain barrier more readily than in adults.

RISK FACTORS

- Living in a home that was built before 1977 may increase risk because this is when lead paint was banned. If a home painted with lead paint is remodeled or the paint is sanded or otherwise damaged, there is an increased risk of exposure to lead.
- Lead absorption can be increased in animals deficient in calcium, zinc, iron, or vitamin D.
- Availability of other lead sources: lead curtain or fishing weights, older painted toys, older gasoline or batteries, linoleum, lead solder, some foreign miniblinds, radiators, and hobbies such as stained-glass or pottery making.
- Feeding animals meat/scraps from hunting may also be a source of lead if shot is present in the carcass.

CONTAGION AND ZOONOSIS

Lead sources can be common to humans and animals living in the same environment. If an animal is diagnosed with lead intoxication, owners should be made aware of risks to themselves and to any infants and children living in the household.

Clinical Presentation

DISEASE FORMS/SUBTYPES

Can occur after a single acute exposure or after chronic exposure if lead accumulates in the body

HISTORY, CHIEF COMPLAINT

- Observed or suspected exposure to lead-containing agents
- Recent remodeling in older homes or agricultural buildings should increase suspicion of lead exposure.
- Acute toxicosis: vomiting, anorexia, ataxia, tremors, and seizures
- Chronic toxicosis: slow onset of vomiting, diarrhea, anorexia, abdominal pain, regurgitation (uncommon due to megaesophagus in cats, not dogs), lethargy, weight loss, weakness, behavior changes, ataxia, blindness, tremors and seizures

PHYSICAL EXAM FINDINGS

- Acute: vomiting, lethargy, ataxia, tremors, aberrant behavior, seizures
- Chronic: weight loss, vomiting, diarrhea, abdominal pain, lethargy, pale mucous membranes, aberrant behavior, tremors, ataxia, seizures
- Neurologic exam: mental dullness or lethargy is frequently seen. Ataxia, muscle tremors, and intermittent seizures may also be noted. Asymmetrical deficits are *not* consistent with lead poisoning.

Etiology and Pathophysiology

- Inhibition of enzymes associated with heme production results in microcytic, hypochromic, regenerative anemia with nucleated red blood cells (RBCs) and basophilic stippling.
- Competition with calcium ions results in storage of lead in bones, alteration of nerve and muscle transmission, and displacement of calcium from calcium-binding proteins.
- Inhibition of membrane-associated enzymes can result in increased RBC fragility and renal tubular epithelial injury.
- Lead may interfere with gamma-aminobutyric acid (GABA) production or activity in the central nervous system (CNS), leading to loss of inhibitory impulses and resulting in seizures.
- Lead can also interfere with vitamin D metabolism, resulting in derangements of calcium absorption and metabolism.

DIAGNOSIS 

Diagnostic Overview

Physical exam findings are nonspecific. Suspect lead intoxication if there are GI and neurologic signs or the history suggests lead in the animal's environment, with the characteristic RBC abnormalities or metallic foreign bodies in the GI tract on radiographs. Whole blood lead level is the confirmatory test of choice.

Differential Diagnosis

- Viral encephalitides (rabies, distemper)
- Sterile encephalitides (granulomatous)
- Toxoplasma
- Hepatic encephalopathy
- Idiopathic epilepsy
- Neoplasia
- Causes of vomiting (p. 1294)

Initial Database

- CBC (more common to see changes with chronic toxicosis)
  - Nucleated RBCs (nRBCs) found in 54% of dogs with lead intoxication
  - Between 5 and 40 nRBCs/100 white blood cells (WBCs) without severe anemia is highly suggestive of lead poisoning.
  - If > 40 nRBCs/100 WBCs, rule out myeloproliferative disease
  - Microcytic, hypochromic, regenerative anemia in approximately 8% of dogs with lead poisoning
  - Basophilic stippling can be seen in approximately 25% of dogs with lead toxicosis.
  - ± Anisocytosis, poikilocytosis, polychromasia, echinocytosis, target cells
  - ± Mature leukocytosis
- Serum chemistries and urinalysis are typically normal for lead intoxication; can help rule out other differentials (e.g., hepatic encephalopathy)
- Radiography
  - May show metal-density material in GI tract or joint spaces
  - Absence of metallic material does not rule out lead poisoning because source may be

Diseases and Disorders

too small to be seen (e.g., paint dust) or may have already passed through the GI tract.
  - Lead lines, dense radiograph opacities at the long bone metaphysis, are uncommonly identified in chronic lead poisoning.

Advanced or Confirmatory Testing

Blood lead level (BLL) done using whole blood in EDTA (purple-top) or heparin (green-top) tubes

- BLLs > 0.6 ppm are diagnostic of lead toxicosis.
- BLLs > 0.3-0.4 ppm suggest lead toxicosis and are considered diagnostic with appropriate clinical signs.
- BLLs of 0.1-0.3 ppm suggest significant exposure to lead.
- Normal background level is < 1 ppm.
- BLL is not always reflective of the total body burden of lead and may not correlate with clinical sign severity. In chronic exposures, BLL may be relatively low due to distribution of lead into bone.

TREATMENT

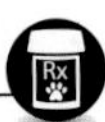

Treatment Overview

Treatment goals are to stabilize patient and manage any severe signs (seizures or anemia). Next priority is to remove lead objects from GI tract and start chelation therapy to bring BLL into normal range.

Acute General Treatment

- Manage seizures
  - Diazepam 0.5-2 mg/kg IV to effect or midazolam 0.1-0.5 mg/kg IV
  - If benzodiazepines are ineffective, phenobarbital 2-10 mg/kg IV to effect
  - Other options for intractable seizures: pentobarbital 3-15 mg/kg IV to effect, propofol 0.1-0.6 mg/kg/min, or gas anesthesia (p. 903)
- Correct any fluid and electrolyte abnormalities.
- Control vomiting (p. 1040).
- Remove lead from GI tract.
  - Remove lead before chelation; chelators (except for succimer) enhance absorption of lead from the GI tract.
  - Emesis (p. 1188), endoscopy, gastrostomy, cathartics, enemas, and whole-bowel irrigation may be useful.
  - Activated charcoal does not adsorb well to lead.
  - Magnesium sulfate 125-250 mg/kg PO may bind to lead in GI tract and cause catharsis.
- Chelation
  - Most lead chelators are nephrotoxic. Monitor renal parameters, and maintain adequate hydration.
  - Succimer (meso-2,3-dimercaptosuccinic acid [DMSA]): chelator of choice, least nephrotoxic, least likely to bind essential minerals; can be used if lead is still in GI tract; dogs: 10 mg/kg PO or PR q 8h for 10 days
  - Calcium disodium ethylenediaminetetraacetic acid (CaEDTA): nephrotoxic, useful if vomiting is severe; dogs: 25 mg/kg SQ q 6h diluted in 5% dextrose for 2-5 days; cats: 27.5 mg/kg in 15 mL 5% dextrose q 6h for 5 days; rest for 5 days, repeat if needed
  - Dimercaprol (British anti-Lewisite [BAL]): nephrotoxic, painful injections, contraindicated with hepatic disease; dogs 3-6 mg/kg IM q 6-8h for 2 days
  - Penicillamine: nephrotoxic, binds essential elements (zinc, iron, copper), vomiting is common adverse effect; dogs: 8-35 mg/kg PO q 6-8h for 1-2 weeks; cats: 125 mg/CAT PO q 12h for 5 days
  - Monitor chelation by monitoring BLL; decline in BLL should start at about 5 days after chelation. If signs persist and BLL not improving, need to make sure re-exposure is not occurring

Chronic Treatment

Prevent re-exposure in home environment. Manage CNS signs (e.g., seizures) if they persist.

Nutrition/Diet

A bland diet may be used after vomiting is controlled.

Behavior/Exercise

Aberrant behavior is possible with lead exposure.

Possible Complications

Neurologic injury can be permanent.

Recommended Monitoring

CBC, hematocrit, hydration, renal values, BLL

PROGNOSIS & OUTCOME

- Animals with mild to moderate signs have a good prognosis with treatment.
- BLL may rebound (increase) within 2 weeks of stopping chelation due to redistribution of tissue stores. If clinical signs are seen, re-dose with chelator; if no signs are seen, continue to monitor BLL q 14 days.

PEARLS & CONSIDERATIONS

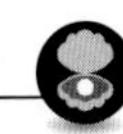

Comments

- Do not use sodium EDTA to chelate; it can result in hypocalcemia.
- The only chelator that should be used if lead still in GI tract is succimer.
- Lead embedded in soft tissue is not a significant source of lead toxicosis, but lead in joint spaces or areas of active inflammation can be absorbed.
- Although oral exposure is most important, inhalation of small particles/dust can also prove toxic.
- Lead is stored in bone and may be mobilized during time of increased bone resorption (lactation, fractures), resulting in delayed toxicosis.
- If chelation is not effective, ensure the patient is not having continued exposure to lead source.

Prevention

Remove lead objects and lead-based paint from environment.

Technician Tips

If patient is vomiting, note if foreign material is seen. All lead must be removed from GI tract before starting chelation (except for succimer). Make sure patient is well hydrated during chelation.

Client Education

Warn clients of risk in older homes if remodeling is to be done.

SUGGESTED READING

Wismer T: Lead. In Peterson ME, et al, editors: Small animal toxicology, ed 3, St. Louis, 2013, Saunders, pp 609-615.

AUTHOR: Valentina Merola, DVM, MS, DABVT, DABT
EDITOR: Tina Wismer, DVM, MS, DABVT, DABT

Leishmaniasis

BASIC INFORMATION

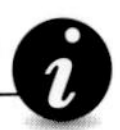

Definition

Leishmaniasis is a vector-borne, zoonotic, protozoal disease that is endemic in the Mediterranean region and South America (>80 countries worldwide). It has been reported in dogs in the United States.

Synonyms

Leishmaniosis, kala-azar

Epidemiology

SPECIES, AGE, SEX

Dogs, cats, foxes, jackals, humans

GENETICS, BREED PREDISPOSITION

Boxers; most dogs with leishmaniasis in the United States have been foxhounds.

RISK FACTORS

- Dogs that have traveled to endemic areas
- Outdoor dogs living in geographic areas where sandflies are endemic and without protection from specific topical insecticides
- In the United States, foxhounds are at increased risk.

CONTAGION AND ZOONOSIS

Dogs are an important reservoir for human disease. In people, the disease occurs most commonly in infants, children, and immunosuppressed or malnourished individuals.

GEOGRAPHY AND SEASONALITY

Disease is mostly limited to temperate or warm areas where vector sandflies are present. The sandfly vectors in the Old World (Middle East, southern Europe) are *Phlebotomus* spp and in the New World (Central and South America) are *Lutzomyia* spp.

Clinical Presentation

HISTORY, CHIEF COMPLAINT

One or more of the following: chronic weight loss, exercise intolerance, skin lesions, polyuria/polydipsia (due to renal injury), eye lesions/vision loss, lameness, epistaxis

PHYSICAL EXAM FINDINGS

- Lymphadenopathy
- Splenomegaly
- Skin lesions
  - Alopecia
  - Ulcerative skin lesions of pinnae, face, and limbs
  - Exfoliative dermatitis
  - Nodular dermatitis
  - Papular dermatitis
- Abnormal growth and elongation of nails (onychogryposis)
- Ocular discharge secondary to keratoconjunctivitis
- Miosis, photophobia secondary to uveitis

Etiology and Pathophysiology

- *Leishmania infantum* is the cause of human and canine visceral leishmaniasis in Europe, the Middle East, Africa, Asia, China, and the Americas. Other *Leishmania* species infect dogs, including *Leishmania braziliensis* in South America and *Leishmania tropica* and *Leishmania major* in Asia and North Africa.
- The parasite's life cycle is diphasic (vector and host phases). Female sandflies take a blood meal from an infected animal. Promastigotes develop in the gut of the sandfly and migrate to the proboscis. They are transmitted to the mammal host during a blood meal and are phagocytized by macrophages. Inside the macrophage, they become amastigotes and multiply by binary fission until the macrophage ruptures, and the amastigotes are then disseminated to other macrophages and throughout the body.
- Cats are infected by several species of *Leishmania,* and disease may manifest as primarily cutaneous or visceral and cutaneous in accordance with the infecting species. Feline leishmaniasis caused by *L. infantum* is similar to the canine disease caused by the same species.

DIAGNOSIS

Diagnostic Overview

- Highly sensitive and specific diagnostic serologic and molecular techniques to detect *Leishmania* infection are now widely available in commercial laboratories.
- Quantitative serologic and molecular (polymerase chain reaction [PCR]) techniques are the assays of choice. These should be used wisely and take into consideration that in endemic areas, a large part of the canine population may be infected subclinically and can present for veterinary care for unrelated reasons.
- Diagnostic testing is usually performed to confirm disease in dogs with suggestive clinical signs, monitor response to treatment, or evaluate possible infection in apparently healthy blood donors, imported dogs, or dogs that have traveled to endemic areas.
- Quantitative serology is the test of choice for confirmation of clinical disease in dogs with compatible clinical signs; quantitative PCR is the choice for confirmation of infection in dogs that do not necessarily have clinical signs. Bone marrow, lymph node, or spleen PCR are more sensitive than blood PCR.

Differential Diagnosis

- Tick-borne diseases: borreliosis, ehrlichiosis
- Leptospirosis
- Dirofilariasis
- Pyoderma
- Immune-mediated skin diseases, vasculitis, glomerulonephritis
- Demodicosis
- Lymphoma
- Malnutrition, poor husbandry

Initial Database

- CBC: may show leukopenia or leukocytosis, nonregenerative anemia, thrombocytopenia
- Serum chemistry profile: hyperglobulinemia, hypoalbuminemia ± azotemia
- Cytologic evaluation of lymph node, skin, splenic, and bone marrow aspirates may reveal amastigote forms of *Leishmania.*
- Urinalysis: may reveal isosthenuria and proteinuria secondary to immunoproliferative glomerulonephritis
  - Urine protein/creatinine ratio may be increased (>0.5).

Advanced or Confirmatory Testing

- Histopathologic evaluation and immunohistochemical staining of skin biopsies may reveal organisms.
- PCR test: most sensitive test; also can detect subclinically infected dogs
- Serologic tests: indirect immunofluorescent antibody test (IFAT) titers > 1:32 indicate suspected exposure; titers > 1:100 are consistent with active infection. Specific quantitative recombinant antigen rK39 ELISA, IFAT, or crude-antigen ELISA may also detect subclinical infection.

TREATMENT

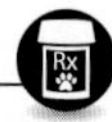

Treatment Overview

Current drugs used for treating canine leishmaniasis, including synergistic combinations of drugs, have limited efficacy and do not clear infection completely in most dogs. Long-term drug combination therapy decreases the parasite load in the dog's tissues and allows its immune system to recover and control the infection. Treatment of dogs is usually followed by clinical improvement, but treated dogs can remain latent carriers that may relapse.

Acute and Chronic Treatment

- Sodium stibogluconate (Pentostam; available from the Centers for Disease Control and Prevention in Atlanta, GA) 30 mg/kg q 24h IV or SQ for 3-4 weeks, *or*
- Meglumine antimonite (Glucantime) 50 mg/kg SQ q 12h or 100 mg/kg SQ q 24h for 4-6 weeks with allopurinol 10 mg/kg q 12h PO for 6-12 months
- Allopurinol 10 mg/kg q 12h PO for 6-12 months; can be administered in combination with meglumine antimoniate at the same doses and durations as above for both drugs
  - Consider stopping allopurinol treatment when the dog becomes seronegative and all clinical manifestations normalize.
- Miltefosine 2 mg/kg PO q 24h for 4 weeks with allopurinol 10 mg/kg q 12h PO for 6-12 months

Possible Complications

- Dogs may develop kidney disease during treatment.
- Xanthine urolithiasis with chronic allopurinol treatment
- Resistance to allopurinol may develop in dogs under treatment.

Recommended Monitoring

Repeat quantitative serology and PCR every 3-6 months during follow-up. Periodic monitoring of renal parameters every 3 months for dogs with no initial azotemia and more frequently in dogs with azotemia at admission.

PROGNOSIS & OUTCOME

- Prognosis is good for dogs with no renal disease and guarded for progressive stages.
  - Dogs with severe renal insufficiency and protein-losing nephropathy generally do not respond well to therapy.
- Infection may persist due to inability to completely eradicate the organism.
- Euthanasia should be considered for dogs with chronic, poorly responsive disease.

PEARLS & CONSIDERATIONS

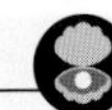

Comments

- *L. infantum* is transmitted in blood transfusions, and it is recommended to screen blood donors for infection in endemic regions or if the dogs originated from or have traveled to such an area. Foxhound donors in North America should be screened for infection by PCR.
- Evidence supports venereal and intrauterine transmission of leishmaniasis from dam to pup.

Prevention

- There is no vaccine available in the United States. Vaccines are marketed in Europe and Brazil. Vaccinated dogs may be seropositive to *L. infantum*.
- Specific insecticidal collars and topical insect repellent prevent vector transmission.
- If possible, keep pet dogs inside during dawn and dusk, the feeding times of sandflies.

Technician Tips

Response of dogs to treatment is slow, and it often takes a month or more before clinical improvement.

Client Education

- Leishmaniasis is a zoonotic disease that can be fatal in humans.
- Leishmaniasis is often a chronic infection in dogs that may not manifest for years after the initial exposure.

SUGGESTED READING

Solano-Gallego L, et al: LeishVet guidelines for the practical management of canine leishmaniosis. Parasit Vectors 4:86, 2011.

AUTHOR: Gad Baneth, DVM, PhD, DECVCP
EDITOR: Joseph Taboada, DVM, DACVIM

Lens Luxation

Bonus Material Online 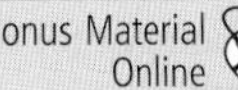 Client Education Sheet 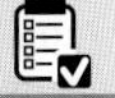

BASIC INFORMATION

Definition

Complete dislocation of the lens anteriorly (into the anterior chamber) or posteriorly (into the posterior segment/vitreous) from its normal position occurs as a result of abnormal development or degeneration (primary: usually a bilateral, inherited condition in dogs) or rupture or degeneration (secondary: acquired) of the lens zonules (fibers from the ciliary body that hold the lens in place).

Synonyms

Lens subluxation: partial dislocation of the lens

Epidemiology

SPECIES, AGE, SEX

- Primary: occurs most commonly in middle-aged dogs, especially terrier breeds
- Secondary: dogs and cats; any age

GENETICS, BREED PREDISPOSITION

- Primary: terrier breeds predisposed; typically 3-8 years old; due to a genetic mutation that is widespread in several dog breeds. DNA testing available (www.offa.org/dnatesting/pll.html).
- German shepherd, American Eskimo, Shar-pei, Lancaster heeler, border collie, and some spaniels may be predisposed.

ASSOCIATED DISORDERS

- Anterior uveitis
- Cataract
- Corneal endothelial-associated edema (anterior luxation)
- Glaucoma
- Vitreous degeneration
- Intraocular neoplasia
- Retinal detachment

Clinical Presentation

HISTORY, CHIEF COMPLAINT

- Signs of ocular pain in cases of anterior lens luxation, including tearing, redness, and squinting/blepharospasm
- The cornea may be focally or diffusely cloudy from edema secondary to corneal endothelial damage or increased intraocular pressure (IOP).
- Vision change noted by the owner, depending on the visual status of the contralateral eye

PHYSICAL EXAM FINDINGS

- Systemic: generally unremarkable
- Ophthalmic
  - Anterior chamber depth abnormal: shallow with anterior luxation; deep with posterior luxation
  - Iridodonesis (trembling of the iris)
  - Phacodonesis (trembling of the lens)
  - Aphakic crescent (visible edge of lens in the pupil creates a crescent-shaped area in the pupil where there is no lens)
  - Vitreous presentation in the anterior chamber (appears as fine white cotton strands)
  - Retina visualized without an ophthalmoscope (i.e., with penlight or transilluminator)
  - Focal or diffuse corneal edema from mechanical damage to corneal endothelium with anterior luxation
  - Glaucoma can result in secondary lens subluxation by buphthalmos; conversely, primary lens luxation can also result in secondary glaucoma.
  - Cataract with chronic lens luxation; a hypermature cataract may result in lens luxation or subluxation.
  - Blindness from cataract, glaucoma, retinal detachment

Etiology and Pathophysiology

- Primary lens luxation occurs because of an autosomal recessive inherited, progressive defect in the lens zonules and is usually bilateral.
- Secondary lens luxation occurs as a result of degeneration and/or stretching of the lens zonules; causes include
  - Chronic anterior uveitis (p. 1023)
  - Glaucoma with associated buphthalmos (p. 387)
  - Intraocular neoplasia (p. 559)
  - Hypermature cataract (p. 147)
  - Severe ocular trauma (results in other significant ocular damage)
  - Age-related (older dogs/cats)

DIAGNOSIS

Diagnostic Overview

Suspected on physical exam after owner presentation for reduced vision or observed ocular abnormality. A complete ophthalmic exam is indicated to confirm and characterize the luxation and identify predisposing causes that can be treated.

Differential Diagnosis

- Glaucoma
- Anterior uveitis

Initial Database

Ophthalmic exam (p. 1137):

- Menace response, dazzle and pupillary light reflexes
- Intraocular pressure (IOP); normal = 10-18 mm Hg with Tono-Pen or TonoVet
- Penlight or slit-beam exam to determine if lens luxation is primary or secondary, evaluate depth of anterior chamber, and assess cornea, lens, and vitreous for opacities
- Direct or indirect ophthalmoscopy to evaluate the posterior segment for retinal detachment and optic nerve and retinal degeneration
- Complete ophthalmic exam of the contralateral eye is indicated, especially in cases of primary lens luxation and in predisposed breeds.

Advanced or Confirmatory Testing

Ocular ultrasound if opacities of the lens or transmitting media prevent complete examination

TREATMENT

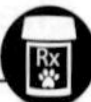

Treatment Overview

Therapeutic goals are to remove an anterior lens luxation or lens subluxation early to avoid secondary complications and to remove posterior lens luxation or prevent lens from entering anterior chamber by constriction of the pupil. Management of associated increased IOP and uveitis may also be indicated.

Acute and Chronic Treatment

Primary:

- Acute anterior lens luxation is considered an emergency.
- Determine IOP; treat if pressure elevated (p. 387).
- Prompt referral of acute anterior lens luxation to a veterinary ophthalmologist for surgical lens removal (lensectomy)
  - Intracapsular lens extraction (ICLE) (entire lens removed) or phacoemulsification ± intraocular lens sutured in place to restore emmetropia (normal vision, neither farsighted nor nearsighted; without an intraocular lens implant, animals are 14 diopters hyperopic [farsighted] with abnormal vision)
  - If lens only subluxated: phacoemulsification (ultrasonic fragmentation of the lens) with capsular tension ring and foldable acrylic intraocular lens (IOL)
  - To reduce risk of glaucoma, concurrent laser endocyclophotocoagulation (ECP) should be considered at the time of lens removal.
- If referral is not possible and the lens is luxated anteriorly, consider pupil dilation and intravenous mannitol to shrink the vitreous and shift the lens into the vitreous, then lifelong topical miotic treatment (e.g., prostaglandin analog [p. 387]) to trap the lens in the vitreous.
- Similarly, if lens luxation is posterior, topical miotic treatment can restrict lens movement. Consider referral for surgery because medical therapy alone does not prevent glaucoma or luxation-associated vision loss.
- Secondary: treat underlying cause.

Behavior/Exercise

Dogs with lens instability or lens luxation should avoid head shaking, and toys that elicit such behavior should be removed.

Possible Complications

- Lens luxation is associated with an increased risk for retinal detachment and glaucoma.
- Lenses that are luxated will become cataractous (p. 147).

Recommended Monitoring

- Monitor for cataract development (p. 147).
- Eyes with lens instability or lens luxation should be monitored q 2-4 months for increased IOP or progression of lens instability.
- Contralateral eye should be monitored for lens position in predisposed breeds; lens instability should prompt early referral for phacoemulsification.

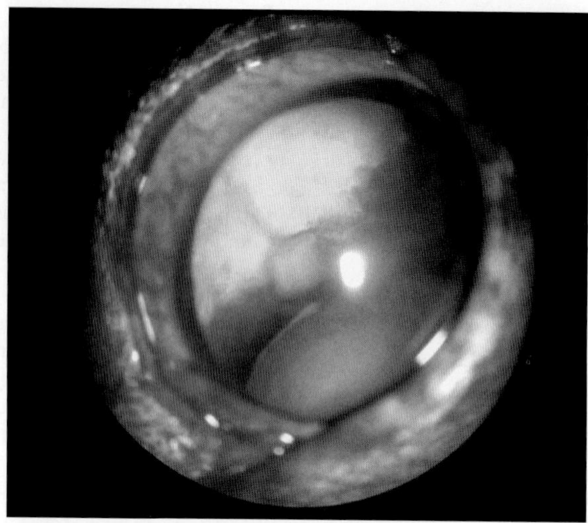

LENS LUXATION Canine eye with a posterior lens luxation (only the dorsal-most one-third of the lens is visible in the ventral margin of the pupil). The optic nerve and retinal vessels are visible without the aid of an ophthalmoscope.

PROGNOSIS & OUTCOME

- Varies, depending on underlying cause, duration, and extent of the lens displacement and anterior versus posterior luxations
- Most common complications are glaucoma and retinal detachment (≤50% of cases).
- Early surgical intervention by phacoemulsification while the lens is subluxated increases success.
- Lower risk of retinal detachment with phacoemulsification compared with ICLE
- Capsular tension ring and foldable acrylic IOL may restore normal vision, with reduced complications and risk of luxation.
- Lens phacoemulsification combined with ECP to manage secondary glaucoma results in the most favorable long-term prognosis.

PEARLS & CONSIDERATIONS

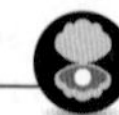

Comments

- Terriers affected with lens luxation, regardless of severity, should not be used for breeding.
- Dog breeders should be counseled and genetic testing considered for at-risk breeds (http://www.offa.org/dnatesting/pll.html).

Prevention

- Dilated ophthalmic exam of all individuals of predisposed breeds to detect early phacodonesis, aphakic crescent, and anterior vitreous presentation (vitreous rostral to the lens)
- Genetic testing of terriers to be used for breeding

Technician Tips

Ensure owners are aware of the early symptoms of glaucoma, uveitis, and the risk for involvement of the contralateral eye in terriers and the need for continued, long-term monitoring of both eyes.

Client Education

- Breed predisposition for bilateral involvement in terriers
- With or without surgical intervention, affected eyes are at increased risk for retinal detachment and glaucoma.
- Genetic testing is available to distinguish affected, carrier, and normal dogs. Homozygous affected dogs can luxate lenses between 4 and 8 years of age.
- Animals that undergo surgical removal of the lens and do not receive an IOL implant have vision that, in human equivalence, is worse than 20/400 and corresponds to being legally blind.

SUGGESTED READING

Davidson MG, et al: Diseases of the lens and cataract formation. In Gelatt KN, editor: Veterinary ophthalmology, ed 4, Ames, IA, 2007, Blackwell, pp 859-887.

AUTHOR: David A. Wilkie, DVM, MS, DACVO
EDITOR: Diane V. H. Hendrix, DVM, DACVO

Leptospirosis

Client Education Sheet

BASIC INFORMATION

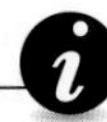

Definition

Leptospirosis is a zoonotic disease caused by thin, motile, gram-negative spirochetes of the genus *Leptospira*. *Leptospira* organisms are further classified by serogroups and serovars based on lipopolysaccharide antigens.

Synonyms

Weil disease, Fort Bragg fever, autumnal fever, canicola fever (England), swamp fever, mud fever, Nanukayami fever, hemorrhagic jaundice, 7-day fever (India), black jaundice, pretibial fever

Epidemiology

SPECIES, AGE, SEX

- Dogs: outdoor intact male working dogs may be at higher risk for infection.
- Cats: despite serologic evidence of exposure, clinical disease has not been clearly demonstrated.
- Dogs < 6 months of age are more likely to be severely affected and have signs of hepatic involvement.

RISK FACTORS

- Suburban or rural environments with exposure to wildlife or soil contaminated by their urine
- Contact with rodents or their urine
- Outdoor activities
- Exposure to livestock (potential carriers)
- Activities involving rivers, lakes, or streams; leptospires can live in water for months.
- Flooding

CONTAGION AND ZOONOSIS

- Leptospirosis is the most common zoonosis in the world and a common cause of acute kidney injury (AKI) in people. A reportable disease in people in the United States as of 2013, many states require reporting of canine cases.
- Those working with patients suspected to have leptospirosis should use personal protective equipment (PPE), and zoonosis warning labels should be placed on cages. The placement of a urinary catheter and sterile collection system can help avoid environmental contamination.
- Viable organisms may continue to be shed in urine for 2-3 days after starting antibiotic treatment. Urine must be inactivated before disposal; this can be performed by mixing urine 1:1 with an aqueous dilution of 10% bleach solution.
- The patient should be placed in a run or bottom cage to avoid contamination. Avoid using a spray hose to clean contaminated runs. Use disposable bedding for 3 days after starting appropriate antibiotic therapy, and treat bedding as biomedical waste.
- Those directly exposed to patient urine should seek medical attention. Those who are pregnant, planning to become pregnant, or immunocompromised should avoid all contact with the patient and its urine.

GEOGRAPHY AND SEASONALITY

- Worldwide distribution, including much of the United States
- Typically thought of as a disease of the tropics and subtropics (temperatures ≈80°F-90°F [30°C], rainfall), it is commonly found in the northeastern United States, and outbreaks in the Southwest have been confirmed.
- In general, leptospirosis can be found whenever there is sufficient rainfall, nonfreezing temperatures, and exposure to host animals or urine-contaminated water and soil.

Clinical Presentation

DISEASE FORMS/SUBTYPES

- Studies have failed to find a definitive association between specific serovars and clinical disease. Currently, no specific disease form/infecting serovars association can be made.
- Infection may be subclinical (carrier) or manifest as severe illness. Historically, renal, hepatic, and coagulation abnormalities have been most associated with leptospirosis, but pulmonary hemorrhage syndrome and vasculitis are also important.

HISTORY, CHIEF COMPLAINT

- Presentation is highly variable, from no obvious signs to severe systemic illness.
- Clinical signs in affected dogs often are nonspecific:
  - Lethargy
  - Anorexia
  - Vomiting
  - Polyuria
  - Increased respiratory effort

PHYSICAL EXAM FINDINGS

- Nonspecific signs predominate: lethargy, anorexia, vomiting, diarrhea, jaundice, signs of hypovolemia (e.g., weakness, mental dullness, weak pulse; may be severe), generalized muscle tenderness, reluctance to move, evidence of abdominal pain
- Kidney: signs consistent with AKI (p. 23). Quantify urine output because animals may be severely polyuric and at high risk for dehydration, and oliguric animals are at high risk for fluid overload and death.
- Liver: signs consistent with acute hepatic injury (e.g., icterus [p. 442])
- Ocular: conjunctivitis, uveitis
- Respiratory: increased lung sounds, tachypnea, dyspnea. Acute respiratory distress syndrome (p. 27) or leptospiral pulmonary hemorrhage syndrome possible; the latter may be more common than previously recognized.
- Coagulation abnormalities: petechiae, ecchymoses, hematemesis, hematochezia, hemoptysis, melena, epistaxis, and hematuria may be due to liver failure, vasculitis, and/or disseminated intravascular coagulation (DIC).
- Many experimentally infected dogs show no overt clinical signs. The percentage of naturally infected dogs that are subclinical or have only nonspecific signs is unknown.

Etiology and Pathophysiology

Leptospires are harbored in the renal tubules of reservoir hosts (deer, opossum, raccoon, rodents, skunk, and other wildlife or domestic animals) that become infected and then excrete *Leptospira* organisms in urine for long periods, contaminating the environment. Although leptospirosis is often transmitted directly between reservoir hosts through bite wounds, ingestion of infected tissues, and sexual secretions, most pets and people become infected though indirect contact with contaminated environment. Although leptospires do not appear to replicate outside the host, urine-contaminated soil can remain infective for months. Swimming in contaminated ponds, lakes, and streams is also a risk. Outbreaks of leptospirosis in dogs have been associated with periods of heavy rainfall and flooding.

- Leptospires enter the body by penetrating mucous membranes or damaged skin.
- Leptospiremia (7-10 days) causes dissemination to kidney, liver, spleen, central nervous system, eyes, and genital tract.
- Leptospires cause endothelial damage and vasculitis.
- Renal tubular epithelial cell colonization occurs in most infected dogs, causing shedding for months to years after infection if not appropriately treated.

DIAGNOSIS

Diagnostic Overview

Unexplained renal and/or hepatic insufficiency, especially with fever, should prompt consideration of leptospirosis. Diagnosis is multimodal; a serum titer alone is rarely sufficient, and a combination of history (exposure, clinical signs), physical exam, routine blood test results, serologic titers, and organism demonstration (by polymerase chain reaction [PCR]) contribute to confirming or refuting the clinical diagnosis.

Differential Diagnosis

- Other causes of AKI (e.g., toxin, pyelonephritis, heat stroke, shock [p. 23])
- Other causes of vasculitis (e.g., sepsis, rickettsial disease, pancreatitis)

- Other causes of hepatic injury (e.g., bacterial cholangiohepatitis, toxic hepatopathy, sepsis, idiopathic chronic hepatitis [p. 442])

Initial Database

- CBC
  - White blood cells (WBCs): neutrophilia; ± left shift, lymphopenia, monocytosis
  - Red blood cells (RBCs): mild to moderate nonregenerative anemia
  - Platelets: thrombocytopenia in > 50% of patients; may be severe
- Serum biochemistry profile
  - Azotemia and hyperphosphatemia are common.
  - Increased alanine aminotransferase (ALT), alkaline phosphatase (ALP), and bilirubin are common in azotemic patients; however, isolated hepatic injury is rare.
  - Electrolyte disturbances: hyponatremia, hypochloremia, and hypokalemia occur in some cases; however, dogs with oliguria or anuria develop hyperkalemia.
  - Metabolic acidosis (low pH on blood gas analysis, low bicarbonate concentration), often accompanied by increased anion gap
  - Hypoalbuminemia due to vasculitis or severe liver dysfunction
- Urinalysis
  - Isosthenuria/hyposthenuria
  - Signs of tubular damage: glucosuria, proteinuria, granular casts
  - Polyuria, oliguria, and anuria are all possible.
- Thoracic radiographs: interstitial to severe reticulonodular pattern, alveolar infiltrates with pulmonary involvement and effusion are possible.
- Abdominal radiography and ultrasonography: ± enlargement of liver, spleen, kidneys; renomegaly, pyelectasia, increased renal cortical echogenicity, perinephric effusion, and a medullary rim sign (medullary band of increased echogenicity)
- Coagulation profile (p. 1325): prolongations of prothrombin time and/or partial thromboplastin time with increased FDP are common.

Advanced or Confirmatory Testing

Microscopic agglutination test (MAT) and PCR are the most commonly used diagnostic tests. MAT titer should not be used to determine causative serovar:

- Initial titer with acute illness often negative
- Suggestive
  - Single titer ≥ 1:800 in unvaccinated animals
  - Titer ≥ 1:6400 in vaccinated animal, or titer > 800 to a nonvaccine serovar and a concurrent titer < 400 to a vaccine serovar
- Diagnostic
  - Paired titers 2-4 weeks apart with fourfold increase from first to second titer or seroconversion from negative to positive titer

PCR assays:

- Sensitive and specific; may be positive in early infection before rise in specific antibody detected by MAT is present.
- Identifies *Leptospira* but not serovars
- Leptospires appear in blood first and then persist in urine. Because the exact timing of appearance is not known, both urine and blood testing is recommended.
- False-negatives are possible and are especially likely after the start of antibiotic therapy.

Point-of-care assays:

- Point-of-care and laboratory ELISA tests are available.
- Formats that detect IgM (Witness Lepto, Zoetis) and IgG (SNAP Lepto, IDEXX) are available.
- Assays are subject to some of the same limitations as MAT testing, with the possibility of a false-negative early in disease and false-positive related to vaccination.
- As with other types of testing for leptospirosis, these point-of-care assays must be interpreted in light of history, signs, and often in combination with other types of tests.

Other (often unrewarding and not recommended)

- Dark-field microscopy: false-negatives common
- Organism identification in tissues section: invasive
- PCR of tissue section: invasive
- Urine or blood culture: fastidious organisms; false-negatives common

TREATMENT

Treatment Overview

Treatment goals are to eliminate leptospires, maintain renal perfusion and urine output, prevent disease progression, contain shedding in the environment, and treat associated conditions (kidney injury, hepatic insufficiency, DIC, uveitis).

Acute General Treatment

- Whenever possible, doxycycline should be used as the initial antimicrobial because it treats the leptospiremia and clears the carrier state that leads to environmental shedding. If urine is to be submitted for PCR testing, collect sample before or as soon as possible after antimicrobial treatment is begun.
  - Doxycycline 5 mg/kg PO or IV q 12h for 2 weeks
- Doxycycline concentrates in bile and is excreted in the feces, and supraphysiologic serum concentrations may occur in patients with liver disease. In these patients, beta-lactam antibiotics (e.g., penicillin, ampicillin) can be initially used to clear the leptospiremia. This must be followed with 2 weeks of doxycycline to clear the carrier state.
  - Ampicillin 20 mg/kg IV q 6h, with dose reduction for azotemic dogs, *or*
  - Penicillin sodium 25,000-40,000 U/kg IV q 12h, with dose reduction for azotemic dogs
- Intravenous fluid therapy as needed to replace initial deficits, guided by quantification of urine production. Polyuric patients may need large-volume fluid administration, whereas anuric/oliguric patients must not be fluid overloaded and may need dialysis.
- Management of kidney and liver injury and other consequences of infection (pp. 23, 269, and 442)

Recommended Monitoring

- Renal, hepatic, and electrolyte parameter monitoring to assess response to treatment and to adjust therapy
- Blood pressure because systemic hypertension may occur and require treatment (p. 1065)
- Urine output monitoring is essential in patients with AKI (p. 23).
- Monitor for development of complications (DIC, respiratory failure) (pp. 27 and 269).

PROGNOSIS & OUTCOME

- Survival rates for dogs with clinical leptospirosis: 70%-85%
- Patients with AKI may become oliguric or anuric. These patients benefit from dialysis or continuous renal replacement therapy (CRRT) and often do well after treatment.
- Patients may recover clinically but have persistent evidence of liver and kidney injury. Many continue to improve over the following months, whereas others have chronic disease (p. 167).

PEARLS & CONSIDERATIONS

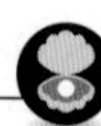

Comments

- Leptospirosis should be considered as a differential in any case of AKI, fever, vasculitis, and/or acute or chronic liver disease in a dog.
- Due to zoonotic potential, precautions should be taken when handling suspected leptospirosis patients.
- Early identification, isolation, and treatment (e.g., antibiotics) are important for the patient's recovery and to reduce the risk of transmission.
- Canine leptospirosis is a reportable disease in some U.S. states; contact regional authorities.
- Hemodialysis and CRRT are widely available and should be considered for AKI patients.

Prevention

- At-risk dogs should be vaccinated. Dogs at risk include pets living in urban areas if their environment could be contaminated by wildlife or rodents.
- Currently, bivalent vaccines containing *icterohaemorrhagiae* and *Canicola* serovars and vaccines containing *icterohaemorrhagiae, Canicola, grippotyphosa*, and *Pomona* serovars are available in North America. These vaccines produce serospecific immunity but may offer some immunity to antigenically similar

serovars. Generally, quadrivalent vaccines are preferred.
- Although there is a perception that adverse reactions have been reported with leptospirosis vaccines with a disproportionately high frequency, one large study demonstrated that they were no more likely to cause reactions than other canine vaccines.
- Rodent control, avoidance of contact with reservoir hosts, and proper sanitation/drainage are also important.

Technician Tips

- Leptospirosis can be transmitted from infected animals to humans. To prevent exposure of people and other animals, strict protective measures should be used in handling animals, their bedding, and all laboratory samples, especially urine. Spraying cages of infected animals with a hose should be avoided because aerosols can spread the organisms.
- Laundering patient bedding inactivates leptospires; however, those handling soiled laundry should wear PPE. Alternatively, disposable bedding may be used, and the bedding should be disposed of in biohazard bags.

Client Education

- Owners should be advised to contact a physician with expertise in infectious diseases for recommendations after exposure to an infected pet and should understand the greatest risk comes from contact with infected urine.
- The Centers for Disease Control and Prevention (CDC) maintains an informational page for pet owners: Leptospirosis and Your Pet (http://www.cdc.gov/leptospirosis/pets/).

SUGGESTED READING

Sykes JE, et al: 2010 ACVIM small animal consensus statement on leptospirosis: diagnosis, epidemiology, treatment, and prevention. J Vet Intern Med 25:1-13, 2011.

AUTHOR: Mark J. Acierno, MBA, DVM, DACVIM
EDITOR: Joseph Taboada, DVM, DACVIM

Lethargy

BASIC INFORMATION

Definition

An abnormal state that is characterized by a lower level of consciousness, listlessness, stupor, or inactivity. A common complaint during veterinary visits, alone or combined with other clinical signs, lethargy is nonspecific.

Synonyms

Fatigue, apathy, asthenia, weakness, malaise, depression

Epidemiology

SPECIES, AGE, SEX

- Puppies or kittens: infectious, metabolic (hypoglycemia), or congenital disease; toxin ingestion
- Older animals: endocrine, neoplastic, cardiovascular, orthopedic, or neurologic disease
- Males: hemophilia A and B, hypertrophic cardiomyopathy (cats), X-linked muscular dystrophy (dogs)
- Females: immune-mediated disease, patent ductus arteriosus

GENETICS, BREED PREDISPOSITION

Some conditions causing lethargy have a documented genetic basis, and others are congenital with a predisposition for specific dog or cat breeds. Some examples:

- Arrhythmogenic right ventricular cardiomyopathy in boxers, dilated cardiomyopathy in Dobermans, mitral valve endocardiosis in Cavalier King Charles spaniels
- Copper storage hepatopathy in Bedlington terriers
- Renal amyloidoisis in the Shar-pei dog and Bayesian cat
- Hypoadrenocorticism in the standard poodle

RISK FACTORS

- Conformation
  - Dolichocephalic: aspergillosis, meningioma
  - Brachycephalic: obstructive airway syndrome, chemodectoma
  - Toy breeds: hypoglycemia, patellar luxation, tracheal collapse
  - Large breeds: panosteitis, osteosarcoma, wobbler syndrome, hip dysplasia
- Geographic location: infectious disease (rickettsial, fungal, oomycotic, parasitic, or bacterial), snake envenomation, dysautonomia
- Obesity or malnutrition
- Electrolyte and/or acid-base disturbance
- Inflammatory or infectious disease
- Immune-mediated disease
- Organ dysfunction or disease (e.g., cardiovascular, respiratory, renal, hepatic)
- Drugs (e.g., tetrahydrocannabinol [THC], sedatives, beta-blockers)
- Physiologic stress or pain

Clinical Presentation

HISTORY, CHIEF COMPLAINT

A complete history must address the following questions:

- Duration of clinical signs
- Concurrent illness or clinical signs
- Current medications
- Vaccination status
- Timing of symptoms in relation to exercise, eating, or urination/defecation
- Environment (indoor, outdoor, roaming)

PHYSICAL EXAM FINDINGS

Findings depend on the underlying cause of lethargy; the exam is often key in narrowing the enormous list of potential causes of lethargy. When present, fever suggests infectious, inflammatory, or neoplastic disorders.

- Cardiovascular and thoracic auscultation: murmur, arrhythmia, mucous membrane color, pulse quality, stertor, stridor, crackles, wheezes, decreased heart/lung sounds
- Abdominal and lymph node palpation: mass effect, pain, fluid wave, organomegaly
- Rectal exam: masses, polyp, melena, hematochezia, lymph nodes
- Orthopedic exam: joint pain, crepitus, or effusion
- Neurologic exam: cranial nerves, reflexes, gait, postural reactions, hyperesthesia
- Ophthalmic exam: vision, glaucoma, uveitis, fundic lesions
- Dermatologic exam: petechiae, ecchymosis, wounds, masses

Etiology and Pathophysiology

Because the causes for lethargy are diverse, a systematic approach (see Differential Diagnosis below) is recommended.

DIAGNOSIS

Diagnostic Overview

Diagnostics should be tailored to the individual patient based on pertinent history and physical exam findings. In the absence of an identified higher yield problem, a minimal database (i.e., CBC, chemistry profile, urinalysis, and blood pressure) may provide diagnostic direction.

Differential Diagnosis

Organization of differentials can use any of the following methods:

- Organ system: cardiovascular, respiratory, gastrointestinal (GI), hepatic, renal, ocular, neuromuscular, hematologic
- Category: metabolic (electrolyte, acid-base disturbance), inflammatory, infectious, immune-mediated, hematologic (anemia), endocrine, nutritional disease or derangement
- DAMN-IT V scheme: degenerative or developmental, anomalous/allergic/autoimmune,

metabolic, nutritional/neoplastic, infectious/inflammatory/ischemic/immune-mediated, trauma/toxin, vascular disease
- VINDICATE'M scheme: vascular, infectious/inflammatory, neoplastic, degenerative/deficiency/drugs, idiopathic/intoxication/iatrogenic, congenital, autoimmune/allergic/anatomic, traumatic, endocrine or environmental, metabolic

Initial Database

- CBC, serum biochemistry profile, urinalysis with sediment exam
- Noninvasive blood pressure
- Retroviral testing (cats): feline leukemia virus/feline immunodeficiency virus (FeLV/FIV)

Advanced or Confirmatory Testing

Advanced testing depends on the results of initial diagnostic tests but may include:
- Diagnostic imaging: thoracic/abdominal radiographs, abdominal ultrasound
- Arterial or venous blood gas exam
- Endocrine testing: ACTH stimulation test, thyroxine/thyroid-stimulating hormone (T_4/TSH), low-dose dexamethasone suppression test (LDDST)
- Fluid analysis (abdominal, thoracic, joint, cerebrospinal fluid [CSF])
- Infectious disease testing/titers: consider regional prevalence, additional clues (e.g., puppy – parvovirus ELISA; Lyme serology in northeastern United States)
- Cytology or histopathology (fine-needle aspiration, bone marrow biopsy)
- Echocardiogram
- CT or MRI

TREATMENT

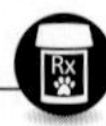

Treatment Overview

Treatment should be targeted to the definitive or suspected diagnosis and/or aid in the comfort of the patient. For most situations, antibiotics, glucocorticoids, and nonsteroidal antiinflammatory drugs (NSAIDs) should be withheld until a diagnosis is reached or when the potential benefits greatly outweigh patient risk (e.g., broad-spectrum antibiotics for fever of unknown origin).

Acute General Treatment

- Ideally, treatment should be specific to the underlying disease process.
- Symptomatic outpatient therapy (e.g., bland diet, gastroprotectants, ± antiemetic for animals with GI signs) may be appropriate for patients showing mild, nonspecific signs.
- Antibiotics should be administered only if infection is documented or highly suspected. Antibiotic choice should be based on the likely pathogen, confirmed by culture and sensitivity, and de-escalated when possible.

Possible Complications

Client follow-up is essential in cases of nonspecific lethargy because failure to respond to empirical therapy or time may warrant additional diagnostics, treatment, and/or referral.

PROGNOSIS & OUTCOME

Prognosis depends on the cause. The patient and diagnostic plan need to be re-evaluated if clinical signs persist or worsen despite initial treatment.

PEARLS & CONSIDERATIONS

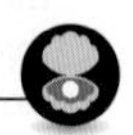

Comments

Glucocorticoids and NSAIDs inhibit the arachidonic acid cascade and therefore essential prostaglandins. Inhibition of prostaglandins may result in damage to the protective GI mucosal barrier and acute kidney injury. These treatments should be recommended on a case-by-case basis and should be avoided in situations of malperfusion or shock.

Technician Tips

Serial physical exams may aid in disease or problem localization. Frequent evaluation of mental status, respiratory rate/effort, pulse rate/strength, and comfort is essential.

SUGGESTED READING

Brewer FC: Weakness. In Ettinger SJ, et al, editors: Textbook of veterinary internal medicine, ed 8, St. Louis, Saunders, 2017, pp 91-94.

AUTHOR: Meghan Harmon, DVM, DACVECC
EDITOR: Leah A. Cohn, DVM, PhD, DACVIM

Leukemias, Acute

Client Education Sheet

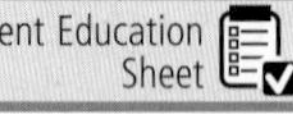

BASIC INFORMATION

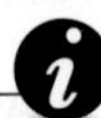

Definition

Acute leukemias (ALs) are clonal proliferations of malignant immature lymphoid or hematopoietic (myeloid) progenitor cells in the bone marrow/blood.

Epidemiology

SPECIES, AGE, SEX

- Young cats and dogs more commonly affected; acute lymphoblastic leukemias (ALLs) in dogs: median age of 7 years
- Purebred large-breed dogs predominate (e.g., German shepherd dogs and retrievers).

RISK FACTORS

- Feline leukemia virus (FeLV) infection: historically, > 60% of cats with ALL were FeLV positive and ≥ 90% of cats with acute myeloid leukemias (AMLs) were FeLV positive. Current infection rates are unknown but thought to be lower (p. 329).
- Myelodysplastic syndromes can progress to AML.

ASSOCIATED DISORDERS

- ALL in dogs: hypercalcemia
- AML in cats: myelofibrosis, hypercalcemia, glomerulonephritis

Clinical Presentation

DISEASE FORMS/SUBTYPES

Acute Lymphoid Leukemias:
- Contradictory reports of most common phenotype in dogs
- T-cell leukemia: most common immunophenotype in cats

Acute myeloid leukemias:
- Reports suggest more common than ALL
- Classified based on type of blasts (p. 1432)

HISTORY, CHIEF COMPLAINT

- Lethargy, weakness, inappetance, weight loss
- Vomiting, diarrhea
- Hemorrhage (e.g., epistaxis, petechiae)
- Lameness (bone pain)

PHYSICAL EXAM FINDINGS

- Lethargy, weakness, pallor, weight loss, dehydration
- Fever
- Tachypnea/dyspnea, tachycardia (anemia)
- Hepatomegaly, splenomegaly
- Lymphadenopathy (mild)
- Petechiae, ecchymoses, epistaxis, gastrointestinal (GI) bleeding
- Hyphema, uveitis, retinal hemorrhage
- Neurologic signs

Etiology and Pathophysiology

- ALs are diseases of the bone marrow. Leukemic cells crowd normal cells, change the marrow microenvironment, and secrete suppressor factors (myelophthisis). Normal hematopoiesis decreases, causing anemia, neutropenia, and thrombocytopenia. Cytopenias result in weakness, secondary infections, and hemorrhage.
- Hepatic and splenic infiltration results in organomegaly, abdominal distention, and loss of appetite. Other sites may be involved,

including lymph nodes, nervous system, kidneys, and GI tract.

DIAGNOSIS

Diagnostic Overview

Immature neoplastic cells on peripheral blood smears or increased numbers on bone marrow smears suggest a diagnosis of AL or stage V lymphoma. ALL, AML, and lymphoma are typically differentiated by immunophenotyping with flow cytometry. In the future, cytogenetic and molecular genetic/epigenetic analysis will allow more accurate classification and prognostication of AL. Mutations in genes associated with development of cancer have been identified in canine ALL and AML.

Differential Diagnosis

- ALL versus AML: it is extremely difficult to distinguish ALL from AML based on morphology (i.e., cytology).
- Available diagnostics do not allow typing of all ALs. ALs that do not express recognized markers are classified as acute undifferentiated leukemias (AUL). It is not always possible to distinguish ALL from stage V lymphoma.
- Stage V lymphoma
- Ehrlichiosis

Initial Database

- CBC/blood smear: leukocytosis with blasts and cytopenias. Nonregenerative anemia and thrombocytopenia common and may be severe. Neutropenia is more common, but neutrophilia is possible. Aleukemic or subleukemic patients have low-normal white blood cell (WBC) count with no or some circulating immature neoplastic cells, respectively.
- Flow cytometry is the primary diagnostic for confirming and classifying AL. Flow cytometry counts and immunophenotypes neoplastic cells. Blood in EDTA should be submitted for this test if blasts seen on CBC. Because cells must be alive, samples must arrive at lab within 24-48 hours.
- Polymerase chain reaction (PCR) for antigen receptor rearrangement (PARR) identifies clonal expression of genes for lymphoid receptors using blood or bone marrow smears. A recent study showed AML in dogs is frequently associated with clonal rearrangements of lymphoid receptors, so this test is not useful for differentiating ALLs from AMLs.
- Serum chemistry profile and urinalysis
- FeLV/feline immunodeficiency virus ELISA test (cats) ± FeLV PCR using bone marrow (p. 1342).
- *Ehrlichia* serology, if indicated (p. 285)
- Diagnostic imaging (for staging): thoracic radiography, abdominal ultrasonography
- ± Cytology of enlarged lymph nodes or organs: to detect infiltration

Advanced or Confirmatory Testing

Bone marrow aspiration or core biopsy is used for evaluation of cell morphology, percentage of neoplastic cells, and evaluation of cell lines. For aleukemic or subleukemic patients, evaluation of the bone marrow is necessary for diagnosis (p. 1068).
  - Neoplastic cell count ≥ 20% of nucleated cells in bone marrow is diagnostic for AL.
  - No studies are available to provide prognostic information or direct treatment based on bone marrow cytology results.
  - Phenotyping is performed on bone marrow aspirates with flow cytometry and on core biopsy samples with immunohistochemistry.

TREATMENT

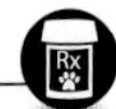

Treatment Overview

Goal is to eradicate leukemic cells with chemotherapy. Supporting the patient until normal hematopoiesis resumes is critical. ALL can respond to chemotherapy for short periods; AML is less responsive. Consultation with a veterinary oncologist is strongly suggested.

Acute General Treatment

- Intensive supportive care is important.
  - Broad-spectrum antibiotic therapy for treating/preventing secondary infections with severe neutropenia (prophylaxis not required in cats)
  - Intravenous fluid therapy
  - Peripheral veins for venipuncture/catheter placement if severe thrombocytopenia
  - Transfusions (p. 1169)
  - Nutritional support
- Chemotherapy: hospitalization for supportive care during induction period is indicated. Clinically significant myelosuppression is expected due to myelophthisis. Appropriate safety precautions must be taken when handling antineoplastic drugs.
  - Consultation with referral to an oncologist is recommended due to the need for intensive support, risk of severe adverse effects, and for AML, the requirement for intense chemotherapy protocols that are not routine.
  - ALL: L-CHOP (L- asparaginase, cyclophosphamide, hydroxydaunorubicin [doxorubicin], Oncovin [vincristine], and prednisone)–based chemotherapy protocols (p. 602). Radiation has been used for central nervous system (CNS) involvement; prednisone for palliative care
  - AML: protocols not well defined and results are disappointing. First-line therapy is cytosine arabinoside and doxorubicin; anecdotal responses to L-asparaginase plus corticosteroid
  - Bone marrow/stem cell transplantation limited by short remission times and difficulty identifying a suitable donor

Chronic Treatment

Patients responding to treatment receive chemotherapy for the remainder of their lives.

Possible Complications

- Myelosuppression: neutropenia, thrombocytopenia
- Anemia requiring transfusion
- GI toxicosis
- Tumor lysis syndrome

Recommended Monitoring

- Physical exam and CBC: q 1-2 weeks, more frequently during induction period; to monitor remission and myelosuppression
- Serum chemistry profile, urinalysis: 1 month after starting therapy, then at least q 3-4 months: more frequently if indicated

PROGNOSIS & OUTCOME

Prognosis is poor for AL. Most patients are ill at diagnosis, and survival times without treatment are 0-4 weeks. Because ALs are uncommon and many patients are euthanized at diagnosis, there is limited information describing treatment outcomes.

- CD34 (stem cell marker): in dogs, expression supports diagnosis of AL; possibly associated with poorer prognosis (median survival, 16 days; range, 3-128 days). CD34 is also expressed in some canine lymphomas.
- ALL: no available prognostic information for cats in post-FeLV era. Historically, 65% response rate for median of 7 months. Information about prognosis in dogs confounded by difficulty distinguishing ALL from stage V lymphoma and treatment with a variety of protocols; 30%-65% respond, with an average survival of days to 4 months. With CHOP-based protocols, 85% respond, with a remission duration 16-218 days (median, 41 days).
  - $CD8^+$ (cytotoxic T-cell) lymphocytosis (dog): abnormal cell counts > 30,000/mcL associated with shorter survival (131 vs. 1098 days).*
  - $CD21^+$ (B-cell) lymphocytosis with large cells (dog): median survival of 129 days*
  - This study(*) included dogs with stage V lymphoma, CLL, and ALL.
- AML: a few cases surviving 3-4 months have been reported. Treatments have minimal effect on the course of the disease, and prognosis is grave.

PEARLS & CONSIDERATIONS

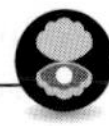

Comments

- Cytologic exam of a blood smear is imperative if leukocytosis or cytopenias on CBC.
- Patients with AL present with nonspecific signs. Cytologic evaluation of peripheral blood and bone marrow smears diagnoses AL, but flow cytometry is needed to differentiate ALL, AML, and stage V lymphoma. Because ALs progress rapidly, consultation with an oncologist should be pursued quickly and emergency referral considered.
- Owners should be advised of the poor prognosis and potential for adverse effects with treatment of AL. Supportive care is needed.
- Better characterization of AL and development of novel treatments targeting the

molecular abnormalities that cause them may improve the prognosis in the future.

Technician Tips

- Patients with AL are often sick and pancytopenic. With response to treatment, clinical signs may worsen before improving. Hospitalization for supportive care and monitoring is required.
- For severely neutropenic patients, wear gloves when handling, and avoid exposure to patients with infections.
- For severely thrombocytopenic patients, take precautions to avoid hemorrhage with venipuncture.
- Instruct owners to monitor for lethargy, loss of appetite, vomiting, diarrhea, bleeding, and signs of anemia and to call if noted.
- Instruct owners to avoid exposure to chemotherapy.

SUGGESTED READING

Young KM, et al: Hematopoietic tumors. In Withrow SJ, et al, editors: Small animal clinical oncology, ed 5, St. Louis, 2013, pp 608-678.

AUTHOR: Nicole C. Northrup, DVM, DACVIM
EDITOR: Kenneth M. Rassnick, DVM, DACVIM

Leukemias, Chronic

Client Education Sheet 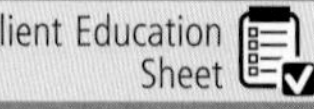

BASIC INFORMATION

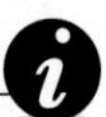

Definition

- Chronic leukemias (CLs) are clonal proliferations of malignant mature hematopoietic cells in the bone marrow.
- Chronic lymphocytic leukemia (CLL) is an indolent proliferation of mature lymphocytes, similar to low-grade lymphocytic lymphoma.
- Myeloproliferative neoplasms (MPNs), also called chronic myeloid leukemias (CMLs), are proliferations of mature granulocytes and/or monocytes, erythrocytes, platelets or of eosinophils, basophils, or mast cells.

Epidemiology

SPECIES, AGE, SEX

- CLL is uncommon in dogs and rare in cats; MPN is rare.
- Middle-aged to older dogs and cats

GENETICS, BREED PREDISPOSITION

- Primary erythrocytosis (i.e., polycythemia vera [PV]): *JAK2* mutations (dogs)
- Chronic myeloid leukemia (CML): *BCR-ABL* fusion gene (i.e., Raleigh chromosome)
- B-cell CLL: small breeds; Bichon frisé, Boston terrier, Cairn terrier, cocker spaniel, dachshund, English bulldog, Jack Russell terrier, Maltese, pit bull, Pomeranian, shih tzu, and Yorkshire terrier

RISK FACTORS

CLL is not associated with feline leukemia virus (FeLV) or feline immunodeficiency virus (FIV).

ASSOCIATED DISORDERS

- CLL: monoclonal gammopathy (English bulldogs predisposed), hyperviscosity syndrome, hypercalcemia, anemia
- PV: hyperviscosity syndrome
- CML: myelofibrosis
- Chronic basophilic leukemia (CBL) and MCL: hyperhistaminemia, urticaria, gastrointestinal (GI) signs/ulceration

Clinical Presentation

DISEASE FORMS/SUBTYPES

CLL (dogs):

- T-cell phenotype more common, large granular lymphocyte (LGL) common
- Atypical phenotypes: ≈15%

CLL (cats):

- T-cell phenotype more common

MPN:

- CML
- Chronic neutrophilic leukemia (CNL)
- Chronic monocytic leukemia (CMoL)
- Chronic myelomonocytic leukemia (CMML or CMMoL)
- Chronic eosinophilic leukemia (CEL)
- Chronic basophilic leukemia (CBL)
- Mast cell leukemia (MCL)
- Primary erythrocytosis (PV)
- Primary thrombocytosis (i.e., essential thrombocythemia [ET])

HISTORY, CHIEF COMPLAINT

- Incidental increased peripheral blood count of affected cell line
- Lethargy, loss of appetite, weight loss, and signs due to cytopenias (weakness, hemorrhage, infection)
- PV (rarely CLL): seizures, syncope, behavior changes, blindness, ataxia (due to hyperviscosity), polyuria/polydipsia
- CEL (cats): GI signs due to infiltration
- Some MPN signs are due to cytokines or other factors (e.g., CBL, MCL: GI signs due to histamine).

PHYSICAL EXAM FINDINGS

- Initially normal
- Hepatomegaly/splenomegaly as disease progresses
- CLL (dogs): lymphadenomegaly
- PV: brick red mucous membranes, neurologic signs, retinal hemorrhages, tortuous retinal vessels
- CEL (cats) and MCL: palpable GI thickening

Etiology and Pathophysiology

- CLs arise from uncontrolled proliferation of hematopoietic cells in bone marrow or spleen.
- Progression is insidious. Bone marrow infiltration results in myelophthisis (crowding of normal cells, changes in the marrow microenvironment, and secretion of suppressor factors) or myelofibrosis and consequent anemia, neutropenia, thrombocytopenia.
- Hepatic and splenic infiltration results in organomegaly, abdominal distention, and loss of appetite. Organ dysfunction is possible.
- Transformation may lead to blast crisis.

DIAGNOSIS

Diagnostic Overview

CL is diagnosed based on a high count of a cell line on CBC and/or bone marrow cytology or histopathology. CLL immunophenotype is determined with flow cytometry of blood or bone marrow. Distinction between CLL and low-grade lymphocytic lymphoma is not always possible.

Differential Diagnosis

- Based on type of cell(s) involved
- Lymphocytes: CLL, low-grade lymphocytic or LGL lymphoma, ehrlichiosis, viral infection (FeLV, feline herpesvirus type 1), chronic antigenic stimulation (e.g., inflammatory bowel disease, cholangiohepatitis), vaccination, stress/epinephrine (cats, typically < 20,000 cells/mcL), pure red cell aplasia, immune-mediated hemolytic anemia, hypoadrenocorticism, feline hyperthyroidism, thymoma
- Neutrophils: CML/CNL or extreme neutrophilia due to infection (e.g., pyometra, hepatozoonosis), tissue necrosis, autoimmune disease (e.g., immune-mediated hemolytic anemia), hemorrhage, drug reaction, congenital disorders (e.g., leukocyte adhesion deficiency), or paraneoplastic syndromes associated with nonhematologic or lymphoid cancers
- Monocytes: CMoL, CMML, chronic infection/inflammation, granulomatous disease
- Eosinophils: CEL, hypereosinophilic syndrome, parasites, eosinophilic granuloma complex, mast cell neoplasia, feline asthma,

eosinophilic enteritis, allergic diseases, paraneoplastic syndrome, hypoadrenocorticism
- Basophils: CBL, mast cell neoplasia, dirofilariasis
- Platelets: ET, hyperadrenocorticism, iron-deficiency anemia, hemolytic anemia, recovery from severe hemorrhage, splenectomy, chronic inflammatory disorders, acute infection
- Erythrocytes: relative erythrocytosis (dehydration, diuretics); breed variation (sighthounds); absolute erythrocytosis (PV, chronic hypoxemia [e.g., right-to-left cardiac shunts, chronic respiratory disease, high altitude], paraneoplastic erythropoietin); splenic contraction

Initial Database

- Laboratory tests
  - CBC: high leukemic cell count. Counts can be very high (hundreds of thousands or higher number of cells/mcL); for PV, packed cell volume (PCV) typically is 60% to ≥80%. Mature and immature forms of affected cell line may be present. Cytopenias are not generally observed until leukemic cell counts are very high. Mild anemia occurs with CLL and MPN.
  - Serum biochemistry profile and urinalysis: to evaluate overall health and identify paraneoplastic hyperglobulinemia or hypercalcemia
  - FeLV/FIV ELISA: typically negative
  - Erythropoietin level: normal or low with PV; may be high with autonomous erythropoietin source (e.g., renal neoplasm)
- Bone marrow cytology (p. 1068): indicated if CBC (with cytologic exam of blood smear) and flow cytometry insufficient to make the diagnosis
- Cytology of enlarged peripheral lymph nodes
- Imaging for staging and to identify concurrent abnormalities
  - Thoracic radiography
  - Abdominal ultrasonography

Advanced or Confirmatory Testing

Flow cytometry for CLL immunophenotyping

TREATMENT

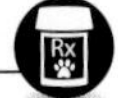

Treatment Overview

Goals are to eradicate leukemic cells and provide symptomatic care. Early in the disease, treatment may not be required.

Acute and Chronic Treatment

Supportive care (if indicated)
- Broad-spectrum antibiotic therapy for treating/preventing secondary infections if severe neutropenia (p. 152)
- Intravenous fluids: for infection, fever, inappetence/dehydration
- Avoid jugular venipuncture if severe thrombocytopenia or hyperviscosity syndrome
- Transfusions (p. 1169); uncommonly needed
- Phlebotomy for PV or plasmapheresis for hyperviscosity syndrome
- Nutritional support

Chemotherapy: special handling requirements needed, and severe adverse effects possible; consultation with or referral to a veterinary oncologist is recommended:
- CLL: treatment recommended for clinical signs, cytopenias, organ enlargement due to infiltration, significant lymphadenopathy, or lymphocyte counts > 60,000/mcL. Consider earlier treatment for dogs with atypical phenotype CLL and young dogs with B-cell CLL. If not treated, recheck q 1-2 months, and start treatment if indicated. Protocol includes prednisone (dogs) 1 mg/kg PO q 24h × 7 days, decrease to 0.5 mg/kg q 48h; prednisolone (cats) 1 mg/kg PO q 24h, and chlorambucil 20-30 mg/m^2 PO q 14 days (p. 609). Other drugs are used for lymphoma when it progresses (referral to/consultation with veterinary oncologist recommended).
- MPN: depends on diagnosis; referral to/consultation with veterinary oncologist is recommended.
  - PV, CML, and CEL: hydroxyurea (dogs) 30 mg/kg PO q 24h for 7-10 days, then 15 mg/kg PO q 24h; (cats) 125 mg PO q 3-4 days. Dosages are adjusted based on response and adverse events. It is important to know potential side effects of hydroxyurea before using this drug. Initially, PV may be managed with phlebotomy and fluid replacement.
  - Tyrosine kinase inhibitors (e.g., toceranib) may be an option for CML. Anecdotal responses have been observed by the author.

Possible Complications

- Myelosuppression: neutropenia, thrombocytopenia
  - Secondary infection
- Chronic bone marrow injury
- Hydroxyurea: methemoglobinemia (cats), anemia, skin/hair/nail changes
- GI toxicosis
- Rare hepatic, renal, pulmonary, or neurologic toxicoses

Recommended Monitoring

- Depends on diagnosis and severity
- Physical examinations: weekly during induction period; q 1-2 months after on maintenance therapy
- CBC: monitor myelosuppression and remission status, weekly during induction period and q 1-2 months on maintenance therapy to monitor for chronic bone marrow injury and relapse
- Serum biochemistry profile, urinalysis: 1 month after starting therapy and then q 3-4 months

PROGNOSIS & OUTCOME

CLs are indolent. Long-term survival is possible with CLL. There is less information for MPN.
- CLL: 80%-90% respond to chemotherapy; survival times of 1-3 years for dogs; median survival of 1.5 years for cats. Conflicting reports of survival with T-cell > B-cell CLL or no difference. Atypical phenotype has possibly shorter survival. For B-cell CLL, older dogs have longer survival. For T-cell CLL > 30,000 lymphocytes/mcL or anemia, shorter survival. Transformation into lymphoma/acute leukemia has a poor prognosis.
- MPN: prognosis depends on type. There is little or no information describing the prognosis for some of these conditions.
  - CML/CBL: dogs may live ≥ 1 year with treatment.
  - PV: survival times of 1 to > 6 years reported
  - CEL: in cats, limited response to treatment; survival times of a few months. Unclear if dogs develop CEL, but if they do, it is possibly prednisone responsive.
  - ET: typically nonresponsive to treatment but long-term control (>500 days) with busulfan in one dog

PEARLS & CONSIDERATIONS

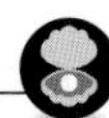

Comments

- CLs have a slow onset and progress slowly. Patients are initially normal and then show nonspecific signs.
- Diagnosis is based on identifying proliferating mature hematopoietic cells in blood and/or bone marrow with flow cytometry to immunophenotype if lymphocytic.
- There is diagnostic overlap between CLL and small cell lymphoma.
- Patients with CL can enjoy long survival times.
- Research is characterizing molecular abnormalities in CL as targets for therapy and prognostic indicators.

Technician Tips

- Patients with CL often undergo chronic chemotherapy.
- CBCs are monitored for chronic bone marrow injury and relapse.
- Owners should be educated on monitoring their pet and precautions to avoid chronic exposure to chemotherapy.

SUGGESTED READING

Vail EM, et al: Hematopoietic tumors. In Withrow SJ, et al, editors: Withrow and MacEwen's Small animal clinical oncology, ed 5, St. Louis, 2013, Saunders, pp 627-678.

AUTHOR: Nicole C. Northrup, DVM, DACVIM
EDITOR: Kenneth M. Rassnick, DVM, DACVIM

Lily Toxicosis

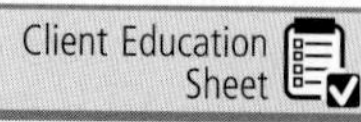

BASIC INFORMATION

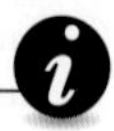

Definition

Lilies are a family of flowering ornamental plants that can cause acute kidney injury (AKI) when ingested by cats. Lily poisoning is a well-recognized and potentially fatal toxicosis in cats. In dogs, only mild gastrointestinal upset is expected with lily ingestion.

Synonyms

Lilies toxic to cats include daylilies (*Hemerocallis* spp), Easter lilies *(Lilium longiflorum)*, Rubrum or Japanese showy lilies *(Lilium speciosum, Lilium lancifolium)*, Stargazer lilies *(Lilium auratum)*, and tiger lilies *(Lilium tigrinum)*. Many new *Lilium* varieties are developed each year. All *Lilium* or *Hemerocallis* species should be considered toxic.

Epidemiology

SPECIES, AGE, SEX

Lily toxicosis has been reported only in cats and meerkats.

GENETICS, BREED PREDISPOSITION

All cats are susceptible.

RISK FACTORS

Younger cats may be more likely to eat plant material.

GEOGRAPHY AND SEASONALITY

- Easter lilies are most commonly sold in March and April. Other lilies are found year-round.
- Lilies grow naturally along the Pacific Coast of the United States. Lilies are frequently cultivated as garden plants or houseplants.
- Daylilies (*Hemerocallis* spp) are common landscape plants in the United States.

Clinical Presentation

HISTORY, CHIEF COMPLAINT

- History of plant ingestion and/or presence of lilies in owner's home
- Cats typically present vomiting (± plant material in vomitus), anorexic, and lethargic.
- Signs usually develop within 12 hours after exposure (range, 2 hours to 5 days).
- Polyuria, polydipsia, and AKI develop within 36-72 hours after ingestion.

PHYSICAL EXAM FINDINGS

- Unremarkable if ingestion was recent. Initial signs of vomiting, anorexia, and lethargy may appear to resolve without treatment.
- Signs progressing to oliguria and anuria, dehydration, lethargy, and vomiting
- Some cats also show vocalization, adipsia, drooling, tremors, ataxia, weakness, and seizures.

Etiology and Pathophysiology

Source:

- Lilies have large, showy, funnel-shaped flowers. The plants grow from bulbs and have erect stems 30-250 cm high. Lilies are frequently included in bouquets and floral arrangements. Daylilies are often grown in gardens.
- Peak incidence is during Christmas and Easter holidays because lilies are popular holiday ornamentals.

Mechanism of toxicosis:

- Intoxication occurs through ingestion. A single bite or even exposure only to pollen can cause the clinical syndrome.
- Mechanism of action is unknown. Toxin is believed to be a water-soluble fraction. All parts of the plant are considered toxic, including pollen. Flowers contain the highest amount of toxin.
- Affected cats develop AKI due to degeneration and necrosis of the proximal renal tubules. Sloughing of necrotic tubular epithelial cells results in tubular blockage and anuria.

DIAGNOSIS

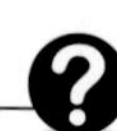

Diagnostic Overview

Diagnosis is based on history of vomiting in a cat with known exposure to lilies or unexplained/unexpected elevations in serum renal values, or both. In the absence of history of exposure, other potential causes for AKI must be ruled out, but empirical treatment should be initiated during diagnostic testing because of the potentially severe consequences of unchecked toxicosis. There is no specific confirmatory test for in-clinic use.

Differential Diagnosis

Toxicologic:

- Ethylene glycol
- Nonsteroidal antiinflammatory drugs
- Cholecalciferol or calcipotriene
- Oxalic acid
- Nephrotoxic antibiotics

Non-toxicologic, spontaneous (p. 23)

- Acute-on-chronic kidney disease (e.g., pyelonephritis, renal lymphoma, polycystic kidney disease)
- Acute glomerulonephritis (e.g., feline infectious peritonitis, autoimmune disease related)
- Renal thromboembolism

Initial Database

- Serum biochemistry panel: azotemia (blood urea nitrogen [BUN] > 34 mg/dL; creatinine is often disproportionately elevated), hyperkalemia, and hyperphosphatemia are common. Occasionally, hypercalcemia, elevated pancreatic enzymes
- Urinalysis: isosthenuria, epithelial granular casts, and glucosuria in the absence of hyperglycemia are typical.

Advanced or Confirmatory Testing

- There is no definitive confirmatory test for lily toxicosis.
- Ultrasound can aid in measuring renal size and cortical thickness and in ruling out other causes of AKI.
- Renal biopsy may help determine extent of renal damage and prognosis (rarely done because history and exclusion of other causes are usually sufficient).
- Histologically, the renal lesion includes acute necrosis of proximal convoluted tubules and mineralization. Pancreatic acinar cells also may show degeneration.

TREATMENT

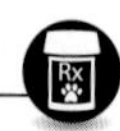

Treatment Overview

In asymptomatic cats, the aim of treatment is early decontamination (induction of emesis if within 2 hours and administration of activated charcoal) and to prevent the development of AKI. Such treatment, including therapy aimed at avoiding oliguria/anuria and uremic signs, is appropriate in all cases, including exposures that are suspected but unconfirmed because unchecked toxicosis may have devastating and irreversible results.

Acute General Treatment

- Decontamination of patient (no clinical signs) (p. 1087):
  - Emesis: for asymptomatic cats with recent ingestion (within a few hours), induce vomiting (p. 1087)
  - Give activated charcoal 1-4 g/kg PO. Protect airway with cuffed endotracheal tube if patient is unconscious.
- Prevent/slow development of kidney injury (if cat is suspected or known to have ingested lilies in the preceding 2 days). IMPORTANT: treatment is implemented regardless of whether signs are present:
  - Intravenous (IV) fluid diuresis for a minimum of 48-72 hours at 2-3 times maintenance rate plus volume deficit (adjust based on hydration, fluid volume tolerance, and response to treatment). Cats with normal serum renal values throughout diuresis may be weaned off fluids after 48 hours. In cats with azotemia, continue IV fluids until azotemia resolves. In some cases, this may mean days to weeks of treatment.
  - Monitor urine output in azotemic patients. For oliguria (urine production < 0.25 mL/kg/h), furosemide (begin with 1 mg/kg; increase as needed up to 4 mg/kg IV, IM, PO or SQ) may increase urine output (p. 1194).
  - Treat hyperkalemia (p. 495) if present.
- Supportive care
  - Persistent nausea: consider maropitant 1 mg/kg SQ q 24h, dolasetron mesylate

0.6 mg/kg IV q 24h, or metoclopramide 0.1-0.5 mg/kg SQ q 6-12h.
  - Abdominal pain can be managed with opiates such as buprenorphine 0.01-0.03 mg/kg IM, IV, buccal q 6-12h.
  - Peritoneal dialysis or hemodialysis if oliguria/anuria develops; renal transplantation can be considered if response is positive.
  - Control seizures with diazepam 0.5-2 mg/kg IV prn.

Recommended Monitoring

- Serum biochemistry profile baseline, 24, 48, and 72 hours (especially electrolytes and renal values). Recheck BUN and creatinine daily during clinical syndrome or for 72 hours if no abnormalities are seen.
- Urinalysis (baseline, 24, 48, 72 hours): ensure isosthenuria/hyposthenuria as sign of adequate fluid diuresis.
- If azotemia develops, monitor urine output.
- Monitor for fluid overload: respiratory rate and character, onset of gallop sound on cardiac auscultation, central venous pressure if possible.

PROGNOSIS & OUTCOME

- If treatment is initiated within 18 hours of ingestion, before onset of oliguria or uremic signs (from AKI), prognosis is good.
- Prognosis after onset of oliguria/anuria/uremic signs is guarded to poor.

PEARLS & CONSIDERATIONS

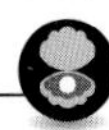

Comments

- Even when vomiting is mild and self-limited, the presence of plant material in vomitus makes it critical to initiate treatment, including IV fluids, to minimize AKI.
- Lily toxicosis should be high on the differential diagnosis list for any cat with AKI and an extremely high serum creatinine level.
- Neither lily-of-the-valley (*Convallaria majalis*) nor peace lily (*Spathiphyllum* spp) causes AKI in cats because they are not true lilies.

Prevention

Do not keep any *Lilium* or *Hemerocallis* species in environments with cats. In one study, 27% of cats actively sought out lilies that owners had attempted to keep out of reach.

Technician Tips

Some florists believe that plucking stamens out of lily flowers renders them nontoxic, which is incorrect. Therefore, any part of the lily plant in vomitus should be considered evidence of potentially toxic exposure.

Client Education

Clients should ensure plants are nontoxic before bringing them into environments with cats.

SUGGESTED READING

Hall JO: Lilies. In Peterson ME, et al, editors: Small animal toxicology, ed 3, St. Louis, 2013, Saunders, pp 617-620.

AUTHOR: Sharon M. Gwaltney-Brant, DVM, PhD, DABVT, DABT
EDITOR: Tina Wismer, DVM, MS, DABVT, DABT

Lipoma

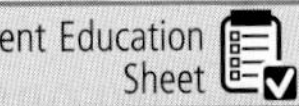

Client Education Sheet

BASIC INFORMATION

Definition

Benign tumor of mature fat cells/adipocytes; very common

Epidemiology

SPECIES, AGE, SEX

Occurs most commonly in older dogs, less frequently in older cats

Clinical Presentation

DISEASE FORMS/SUBTYPES

- Subcutaneous: most common
- Intermuscular
- Intrathoracic or intraabdominal
- Infiltrative: locally invasive into surrounding tissue
- Necrotic
- Myelolipoma: rare, benign tumor composed of well-differentiated adipocytes and hematopoietic cells; spleen, adrenal gland, and liver most common sites
- Liposarcoma: uncommon neoplasm arising from lipoblasts and mesenchymal tissue; cytologically characterized by spindle cells and immature adipocytes; low metastatic rate; malignant transformation from lipomas has not been reported

HISTORY, CHIEF COMPLAINT

- Generally incidental finding as reported by the owner or during the course of a routine physical exam
- Occasionally, a large lipoma (especially intrathoracic or intraabdominal) may cause clinical signs due to space-occupying effects.
- Rarely, systemic signs of illness are caused by torsion of a lipoma's vascular pedicle, creating a necrotic center and causing bacteremia/systemic inflammation.

PHYSICAL EXAM FINDINGS

- Solitary or multiple subcutaneous, nonpainful, movable masses of variable sizes and shapes; often soft but may be firm
- Intermuscular lipoma: palpable mass in caudal thigh (typically between semimembranous and semitendinosus fascial planes)
- Other locations (when accessible on exam): palpable, nonpainful mass

Etiology and Pathophysiology

- Benign tumor of adipocytes that grows by expansion rather than by invasion; nonmetastatic
- Medical significance, if any, generally arises from the physical presence of the mass, which can interfere with ambulation or internal organ function.

DIAGNOSIS

Diagnostic Overview

The diagnosis is suspected when aspiration of a soft subcutaneous mass is performed and cytologic evaluation yields only well-differentiated adipocytes.

Differential Diagnosis

- Subcutaneous mast cell tumors can appear identical on physical exam; cytologic evaluation readily distinguishes them from lipomas.
- Lipomas can appear firm on palpation if they develop deep to underlying muscle or fascia and may be confused with other subcutaneous tumors such as soft-tissue sarcomas.
- A lipoma may be mistaken for a more biologically harmful mass (especially intrathoracic or abdominal).

Initial Database

Fine-needle aspiration and cytologic evaluation reveal adipocytes.

Advanced or Confirmatory Testing

- Ultrasound echotexture consistent with fat: highly suggestive that an abdominal or intrathoracic mass may be a lipoma
- CT may be required for infiltrative or intermuscular lipomas to help determine full extent of tumor.
  - Fat-opacity mass that infiltrates surrounding tissue, sometimes with fine linear striations in infiltrated muscle; differentiation of infiltrative lipoma from adjacent normal subcutaneous fat is difficult.
  - No evidence of metastasis
- Definitive diagnosis of lipoma (and exclusion of other tumor types) requires histopathologic exam of tissue.

TREATMENT

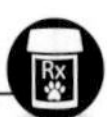

Treatment Overview

Surgical excision is recommended if masses interfere with function or mobility or are rapidly growing. The majority of tumors are asymptomatic and do not necessitate surgical removal.

Acute and Chronic Treatment

Infiltrative lipomas require aggressive initial surgery and may necessitate amputation; recurrence rate for incompletely excised tumors is > 50%. Radiation therapy should be considered for incompletely resected infiltrative lipomas to delay recurrence or for nonresectable tumors to delay progression.

PROGNOSIS & OUTCOME

- Subcutaneous, intermuscular, necrotic, intraabdominal, or intrathoracic lipomas can be cured with surgery.
- Infiltrative lipomas have high rate of local recurrence with incomplete excision and may necessitate multiple surgeries, aggressive surgery, and/or radiation therapy.

PEARLS & CONSIDERATIONS

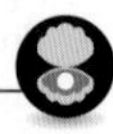

Comments

- Creation of a body map in the patient's medical record is recommended to monitor the size and appearance of subcutaneous lipomas.
- Occasionally, different tumor types can develop within a lipoma (e.g., mast cell tumors, soft-tissue sarcomas).
- Re-evaluation of lipomas should be done periodically, and re-aspiration or removal with histopathologic evaluation is suggested if the tumor's physical appearance is changing (e.g., rapidly growing or different feel on palpation).
- Lipoma should remain on the differential diagnosis for abdominal and intrathoracic masses because the prognosis for lipomas is generally better than the prognosis for other, more commonly encountered masses.

Technician Tips

Owners can mark skin masses with a marker or mascara or can shave the hair in the area at home, making locating the mass in question easier when having it evaluated by the veterinarian.

SUGGESTED READING

Spoldi E, et al: Comparisons among computed tomographic features of adipose masses in dogs and cats. Vet Radiol Ultrasound 58:29-37, 2017.

AUTHOR: Erin K. Malone, DVM, DACVIM
EDITOR: Kenneth M. Rassnick, DVM, DACVIM

Lumbosacral Stenosis, Degenerative

Client Education Sheet 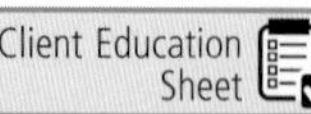

BASIC INFORMATION

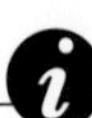

Definition

Progressive stenosis of the lumbosacral (LS) vertebral canal, leading to nerve root compression, dysfunction, and pain

Synonyms

Cauda equine syndrome, LS disease

Epidemiology

SPECIES, AGE, SEX

Mature, large breed, male dogs

GENETICS, BREED PREDISPOSITION

German shepherds overrepresented

RISK FACTORS

Transitional LS vertebrae

Clinical Presentation

HISTORY, CHIEF COMPLAINT

Owners may report one or more of the following:

- Pelvic limb lameness (unilateral or bilateral)
- Altered tail carriage/function
- Fecal/urinary incontinence
- Back pain
- Exercise intolerance and reluctance to stand, climb stairs, and jump
- Licking, chewing perineum or a limb

PHYSICAL EXAM FINDINGS

One or more may be noted:

- Pelvic limb lameness, paresis, proprioceptive deficits
- Pacing gait
- Plantigrade stance
- Tail paresis, low carriage, decreased sensation
- Atrophy of caudal thigh/leg muscles
- Reduced/absent pelvic limb reflexes
  - Patellar reflex may appear increased: pseudohyperreflexia
- Reduced/absent perineal reflex, anal tone
- Lower motor neuron bladder
- Pain on tail manipulation, LS palpation, hip extension
- Pain on palpation of vertebral bodies during rectal exam

Etiology and Pathophysiology

One or more of the following reduce the diameter of the vertebral canal:

- Intervertebral disc protrusion
- Articular remodeling
- Hypertrophy of interarcuate and dorsal longitudinal ligaments
- Vertebral malalignment/instability
- Osteophytes and foraminal stenosis

DIAGNOSIS

Diagnostic Overview

LS stenosis is suspected in dogs with signalment, clinical signs, and radiographic findings consistent with this disease, especially if lower motor neuron signs to the pelvic limbs are noted. However, advanced imaging (MRI, CT) is necessary to confirm diagnosis.

Differential Diagnosis

- Discospondylitis
- Intervertebral disc extrusion
- Neoplasia of nerve roots, nerves or vertebrae
- Hip osteoarthritis
- Cranial cruciate disease
- Fibrotic myopathy
- Iliopsoas injury
- Prostatic disease

Initial Database

- CBC, serum biochemistry and urinalysis often unremarkable
- Radiographic changes
  - LS disc space narrowing
  - LS endplate sclerosis and spondylosis
  - Misalignment of sacrum with L7
  - NOTE: these changes can also be seen in clinically unaffected dogs, and they may not be evident in affected dogs.

Advanced or Confirmatory Testing

- MRI and CT (p. 1132) provide the most detailed information of LS soft-tissue and osseous structures, respectively. It can be helpful to pursue both modalities in a single patient.
- Discography/epidurography can be helpful but are technically demanding and uncommonly used.
- Electromyography (EMG) and nerve conduction velocity (NCV) may suggest demyelination and/or an axonopathy.

TREATMENT

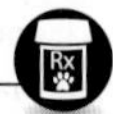

Treatment Overview

Surgical treatment is recommended if pain is refractory to medical management and/or neurologic signs are deteriorating. Goals of treatment are pain relief and return to function, although return to complete normalcy may not be possible.

Acute General Treatment

- Conservative management: strict cage rest (4-6 weeks), then gradually increasing activity over 6-8 weeks. Antiinflammatory/analgesic medication to control pain as needed. Consider tramadol 2-5 mg/kg PO q 8-12h and gabapentin 10 mg/kg PO q 8-12h in combination with a nonsteroidal antiinflammatory drug.
- Anxiolytics (trazodone 5-7 mg/kg PO q 12h; if combined with tramadol, reduce dose to 3.5 mg/kg) or sedatives (acepromazine 0.5-2 mg/kg PO q 8-12h) may be needed during cage rest, but avoid oversedation.
- Epidural injection of glucocorticoids (e.g., methylprednisolone acetate 1 mg/kg) was reported to confer improvement in up to 80% of dogs. Multiple injections may be required.
- Dogs with moderate to severe signs, fecal/urinary incontinence, or failure to improve despite conservative management are surgical candidates. Surgical treatment most frequently consists of decompression through dorsal laminectomy.
- Additional interventions can include foraminotomy, discectomy, and stabilization.

Chronic Treatment

- Strict confinement is necessary for 4-6 weeks after surgery, followed by gradual return to function over 2 months.
- Sling support may be necessary in the early postoperative period.
- Urinary bladder management is imperative until there is normal voluntary voiding. Consider placement of urinary catheter during early management.

Nutrition/Diet

Maintenance of ideal body condition is beneficial.

Behavior/Exercise

- Physical rehabilitation, including passive range of motion, acupuncture (p. 1056), and underwater treadmill, is often advantageous.
- High-impact activity such as jumping and climbing stairs should be avoided indefinitely.

Drug Interactions

Monitor for signs of serotonin syndrome if using both tramadol and trazodone (p. 1281)

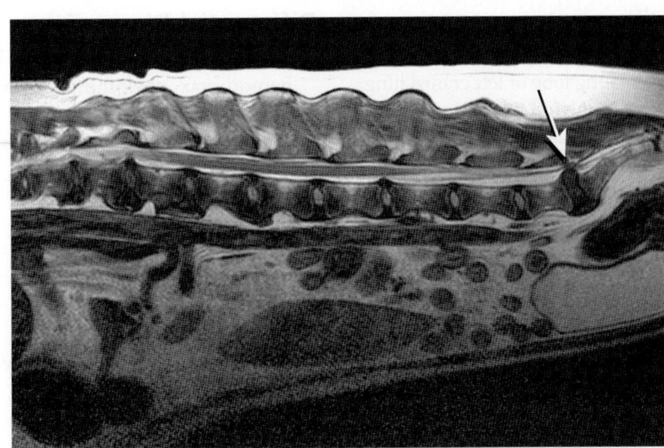

LUMBOSACRAL STENOSIS, DEGENERATIVE Sagittal T2-weighted MRI of the lumbar region of a mature dog with degenerative lumbosacral stenosis; cranial is to the left. The disc at the LS junction *(arrow)* is protruding into the spinal canal and shows low signal intensity that is consistent with degeneration.

Possible Complications

- Failure to improve
- Infection
- Increased LS instability
- Implant failure
- Laminectomy fibrosis

PROGNOSIS & OUTCOME

- 55% success rate with conservative management
- 70%-80% success rate with surgical management
- Surgical outcome is not typically negatively influenced by attempting medical management first.
- Recovery with fecal/urinary incontinence less favorable and may take weeks to months.
- Recurrence in 3%-18% of cases, with working dogs at increased risk

PEARLS & CONSIDERATIONS

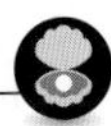

Comments

- When assessing pelvic limb reflexes, pay attention to reduced stifle and tarsal flexion during the withdrawal reflex. Hip flexion should be normal.
- LS discospondylitis can be difficult to distinguish from degenerative LS stenosis. In cases with osteolytic or severely proliferative changes, urine, blood, and if surgery is performed, the removed disc should be submitted for bacterial and fungal culture.
- The severity of stenosis/nerve root compression does not always correlate with severity of clinical signs.
- LS pain and lameness are the earliest and most consistent signs. Urinary and fecal incontinence are most likely to occur with progressive disease but may be the initial complaint.

Technician Tips

In patients with urinary incontinence, monitor closely for urine scald. Ensure patient is kept clean and dry at all times.

SUGGESTED READING

Dewey CW, et al: Disorders of the cauda equina. In Dewey CW, et al, editors: Practical guide to canine and feline neurology, ed 3, Ames, IA, 2016, Wiley-Blackwell.

RELATED CLIENT EDUCATION SHEETS

Consent to Perform Computerized Tomography (CT Scan)
How to Assist a Pet That Is Unable to Rise and Walk

Reproduced from the third edition in modified form. Third edition author: Boel A. Fransson, DVM, PhD, DACVS

AUTHOR: Danielle M. Zwueste, DVM, DACVIM
EDITOR: Kathleen Linn, DVM, MS, DACVS

Lung Lobe Torsion

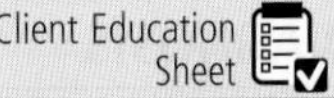

Client Education Sheet

BASIC INFORMATION

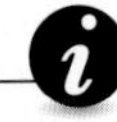

Definition

Rotation of a lung lobe along its long axis, with twisting of the bronchus and pulmonary vessels at the hilus

Epidemiology

SPECIES, AGE, SEX

- Dogs (and rarely, cats)
- Middle-aged dogs more commonly affected
- No sex predisposition.

GENETICS, BREED PREDISPOSITION

- Spontaneous lung lobe torsion (LLT): large breeds > small breeds
- Dogs with deep, narrow chests have a higher incidence.
- Afghan hounds are overrepresented.

- May be associated with chylothorax in this breed
- Right middle lung lobe or left cranial lung lobe are commonly affected.
- Also occurs in small-breed dogs (pugs, miniature poodles, miniature dachshund)
- Pugs are overrepresented.
    - Commonly affects the left cranial lobe

RISK FACTORS

Pre-existing conditions leading to atelectasis of lung lobes:

- Pleural effusion
- Pneumothorax
- Trauma
- Surgical manipulation

ASSOCIATED DISORDERS

Usually associated with marked pleural effusion (sometimes chylous)

Clinical Presentation

HISTORY, CHIEF COMPLAINT

Signs may be acute (more common) or insidious:

- Dyspnea (most common)
- History of pneumothorax, pneumonia, or trauma
- Cough
- Hemoptysis
- Anorexia ± weight loss
- Exercise intolerance
- Vomiting/hematemesis
- Depression

PHYSICAL EXAM FINDINGS

- Muffled heart and lung sounds (ventral with effusion or in area of affected lung lobe)
- Crackles
- Coughing, hemoptysis
- Dyspnea (inspiratory or paradoxical with pleural effusion)
- Pyrexia

Etiology and Pathophysiology

- Spontaneous LLT can occur.
- Any mechanism that increases the mobility of a lung lobe (e.g., pleural effusion, surgical manipulation) can lead to torsion.
- LLT leads to venous congestion from twisting/occlusion of pulmonary veins of the affected lobe and lung consolidation. Persistent venous congestion causes pleural effusion.
- Often associated with pleural effusion though the primary lesion is not always clear.

DIAGNOSIS

Diagnostic Overview

The diagnosis should be considered for any patient with pleural effusion. Suspicion is increased in an at-risk breed or by abnormalities (e.g., atelectasis) found on thoracic imaging (plain radiographs, ultrasonography, CT scans) or bronchoscopy.

Differential Diagnosis

- Other causes of pleural effusion: hydrothorax, hemothorax, chylothorax, pyothorax
- Pneumothorax
- Pneumonia
- Pulmonary thromboembolism
- Pulmonary contusion
- Pulmonary neoplasia
- Pulmonary atelectasis
- Diaphragmatic hernia

Initial Database

- Results of CBC, biochemistry panel, and urinalysis vary.
    - Stress or inflammatory leukogram common
- Pleural fluid may be a sterile, inflammatory serosanguineous effusion or chylous.
- Thoracic radiographs: findings vary with degree of effusion
    - Pleural effusion and lung consolidation (common)
        - Repeat radiographs after thoracocentesis (important)
    - Vesicular emphysema (pulmonary pattern with small, scattered gas bubbles) can occasionally be seen in the affected lobe on radiographs (CT is more sensitive)
- Thoracic ultrasound reveals hepatization of the torsed lung lobe (fluid-filled bronchi appear similar to hepatic vessels and fluid-filled pulmonary parenchyma resembling normal liver)

Advanced or Confirmatory Testing

Rarely needed or used

- Bronchoscopy (p. 1074) may demonstrate an obstructed orifice of the main bronchus supplying the affected lobe.
    - Bronchial mucosa may appear folded and edematous.
- Thoracic CT may demonstrate anatomic alterations of the affected bronchus, such as narrow, collapsed, or occluded bronchi with abrupt terminations.
    - Contrast-enhanced ultrasonography (CEUS) may improve the accuracy of conventional ultrasonography for detection of pulmonary blood flow compromise in dogs with LLT.
- For some patients, the diagnosis is confirmed at thoracotomy.

TREATMENT

Treatment Overview

Improve respiratory function, and stabilize patient before surgical removal of the affected lobe.

Acute General Treatment

- Thoracocentesis (p. 1164)
- Oxygen by face mask, nasal cannula, or oxygen cage (p. 1146)
- Fluid therapy as needed based on patient status, physical exam, and laboratory parameters

Chronic Treatment

Lobectomy of the affected lobe is the treatment of choice; spontaneous resolution is rare.

Behavior/Exercise

Restrict exercise for 2-4 weeks after thoracotomy.

Possible Complications

- Torsion of another lung lobe is possible.
- LLT may lead to chylothorax.

Recommended Monitoring

- Vital signs
- Respiratory pattern/rate
- Resolution of pleural effusion
    - Thoracic radiographs
    - Diminished fluid volume aspirated from chest tube in the postoperative period; 1 mL/kg/day of fluid production is expected from the presence of the chest tube alone.
- Postoperative pain

PROGNOSIS & OUTCOME

Good prognosis if lung lobectomy is performed

PEARLS & CONSIDERATIONS

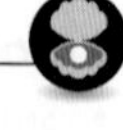

Comments

- Any lobe can torse, but the left cranial and right middle lung lobes are more frequently affected. LLT can occur in the mid-lobar region of the lung (partial lung lobectomy indicated).
- Air bronchograms can be seen for affected lobes early in the process, but bronchial air is absorbed and replaced by fluid within 2-3 days.
- During lobectomy, clamp the affected pedicle with noncrushing forceps before derotation to help prevent release of toxins into the bloodstream.
- Automated stapling devices (TA-30 V3) simplify surgery and decrease surgery time.
- Submit excised lung for culture and histologic exam.
- Thoracoscopy-assisted procedures have been described. This procedure, although more technically challenging, may decrease morbidities associated with a conventional thoracotomy approach.

Technician Tips

To stabilize the patient while prepping for surgery, evacuate pleural fluid just after anesthetic induction (p. 1164).

Client Education

Animals with concurrent chylothorax may have a poorer prognosis.

SUGGESTED READING

Monnet E: Lungs. In Johnston SA, et al, editors: Veterinary surgery: small animal, ed 2, St Louis, 2018, Elsevier.

AUTHOR: Michael B. Mison, DVM, DACVS
EDITOR: Megan Grobman, DVM, MS, DACVIM

Lung Parasites

BASIC INFORMATION

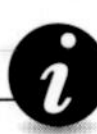

Definition

Infestation of major airways or pulmonary parenchyma with parasites, including *Oslerus osleri*, *Paragonimus kellicotti*, *Eucoleus aerophilus*, *Filaroides hirthi*, *Crenosoma vulpis*, and *Aelurostrongylus abstrusus*

Synonyms

Lungworms (LWs), *Oslerus osleri* (formerly *Filaroides osleri*), *Eucoleus aerophilus* (formerly *Capillaria aerophila*)

Epidemiology

SPECIES, AGE, SEX

- Dogs and cats
  - Dogs: *O. osleri, E. aerophilus, P. kellicotti, C. vulpis,* and *F. hirthi/milksi*
  - Cats: *P. kellicotti, E. aerophilus,* and *A. abstrusus*
- Clinical signs are most common in younger animals but can be seen in animals of any age.

RISK FACTORS

- Dogs clinically affected by *F. hirthi* often are immunocompromised.
- Free-roaming animals and those not receiving regular preventatives are at increased risk.
- Ingestion of paratenic or intermediate hosts

GEOGRAPHY AND SEASONALITY

Geographic distribution and seasonality are parasite specific. *P. kellicotti* is most often found in the Southeast, Midwest, and Great Lakes regions of the United States (snail and crayfish are intermediate hosts). *C. vulpis* is highly prevalent in Atlantic Canada (red fox reservoir).

ASSOCIATED DISORDERS

- Eosinophilic pneumonia
- Pneumothorax
- Cavitary lung disease
- Hemoptysis
- Bleeding diathesis
- Respiratory distress (p. 879)

Clinical Presentation

HISTORY, CHIEF COMPLAINT

- Can be an incidental finding
- Cough
- Wheeze
- Exercise intolerance
- Respiratory distress may be noted with pneumothorax or verminous pneumonia.

PHYSICAL EXAM FINDINGS

- Cough elicited on tracheal palpation (nonspecific finding): tracheal palpation may also elicit coughing in patients with other tracheal, bronchial, or pulmonary parenchymal diseases as well as in normal dogs.
- Thoracic auscultation is usually unremarkable.
  - Wheezes or crackles can be heard in severely affected animals.

Etiology and Pathophysiology

- Parasitic pulmonary disease may be caused by LW and other parasites.
- Parasites of the pulmonary vasculature (*Dirofilaria immitis* [pp. 415 and 481]) and *Angiostrongylus vasorum*) cause pulmonary pathology.
- Intestinal worms *Toxocara* sp and *Ancylostoma* sp undergo pulmonary migration and with a large worm burden may cause verminous pneumonia.
- For LWs, the final destination is the respiratory tract.

O. osleri:

- Transmission: direct transmission (ingestion) of larvae in regurgitated food, feces, or saliva
- Adults live in carina and mainstem bronchi and cause local nodular inflammation and fibrosis.

P. kellicotti:

- Transmission: ingestion of crayfish intermediate host or paratenic host such as rodents
- Adult flukes live in a subpleural cyst that communicates with a bronchus.
  - Rupture of cyst/bulla in patients with *P. kellicotti* can cause pneumothorax.

E. aerophilus:

- Transmission: direct transmission (ingestion) of eggs in respiratory secretions or feces or by ingestion of earthworm intermediate host
- Adults live in bronchial mucosa.

F. hirthi, F. milksi:

- Transmission: ingestion of larvae in feces
- Adult worms live in lung parenchyma (alveoli and terminal airways)
- Severe infection most likely in young, small-breed dogs, immunosuppressed dogs, or those with superinfections.

A. abstrusus:

- Transmission: ingestion of snail or slug intermediate host or paratenic host such as birds and rodents
- Adults live in terminal bronchioles, alveolar ducts, and alveoli.
- Important differential for asthma in endemic areas (p. 84)

C. vulpis:

- Transmission: ingestion of snail or slug intermediate host
- Adults live in bronchi.

DIAGNOSIS

Diagnostic Overview

Diagnosis is suspected based on age (typically young animals), signs of respiratory disease, exposure to paratenic or intermediate host, and compatible radiographic findings. Confirmation requires detecting the parasite and/or its egg in specialized fecal exam or in respiratory samples.

Differential Diagnosis

- Chronic bronchitis (p. 136)
- Infectious tracheobronchitis
- Asthma
- Pulmonary edema
- Bacterial or fungal pneumonia
- Pulmonary metastatic disease
- Pneumothorax
- Pulmonary granulomatosis
- Eosinophilic bronchopneumopathy (pulmonary infiltrates with eosinophils, eosinophilic bronchitis)

Initial Database

Thoracic radiographic abnormalities reflect the causative organism:

- *O. osleri:* tracheal and bronchial nodules
- *P. kellicotti*
  - Solid or cavitary mass lesion, most commonly in the right caudal lobe
  - ± Bulla
  - Pneumothorax
  - Bronchial or interstitial lung pattern on radiographs
- *E. aerophilus:* normal, or bronchial to bronchointerstitial pattern
- *A. abstrusus:* bronchial to diffuse miliary or nodular interstitial pattern most common early; generalized alveolar pattern in severely affected animals
- *F. hirthi:* nodular interstitial pattern or alveolar infiltrates
- *C. vulpis:* normal to mild-moderate bronchial or interstitial pattern

CBC/serum biochemistry panel/urinalysis: typically unremarkable

- Occasional eosinophilia, representing nonspecific parasitic infection or inflammation from other causes

Advanced or Confirmatory Testing

- Transtracheal/bronchial washes may demonstrate larvae or eggs (pp. 1073 and 1074).
- Bronchoscopy to identify nodules of *O. osleri*
- Fecal exam may show eggs or larvae (insensitive due to intermittent shedding)
  - Zinc sulfate flotation or Baermann technique is recommended for identification of ova or larvae, respectively, of *O. osleri, A. abstrusus, C. vulpis,* and *F. hirthi.*
  - Fecal flotations can identify *E. aerophilus* ova.
  - High-density fecal flotation or fecal sedimentation is preferred for identification of *P. kellicotti* ova.
- Use of nested polymerase chain reaction (PCR) has been studied and may prove helpful for diagnosis of *A. abstrusus* in cats (not routinely available).

TREATMENT

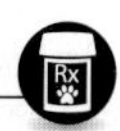

Treatment Overview

Administration of parasiticidal drugs to eliminate the parasite infestation, with other medications used as necessary to decrease clinical signs secondary to inflammation.

Acute General Treatment

- With severe respiratory signs (rare), oxygen administration may be necessary (p. 1146).
  - Although secondary inflammation is often seen with infection, glucocorticoid therapy (antiinflammatory doses) should be reserved for severe cases.
- Thoracocentesis (p. 1164) for pneumothorax
- Parasiticidal drugs
  - Fenbendazole 50 mg/kg PO q 24h for 10-14 days (14-21 days for *O. osleri*) can be used for all LW types.
  - Other approaches include
    - *A. abstrusus*: ivermectin 0.4 mg/kg SQ once and repeated in 2 weeks; selamectin 6 mg/kg topically once
    - *O. osleri*: ivermectin 0.4 mg/kg PO, SQ once every 2 weeks for 3 treatments
    - *P. kellicotti*: praziquantel 25 mg/kg PO q 8h for 3 days (dog), 10 mg/kg PO q 24h for 10 days (cat)
    - *C. vulpis*: milbemycin oxime 0.5 mg/kg PO once

Possible Complications

Certain breeds of dogs (e.g., collies) should not be treated with ivermectin without testing for *MDR1/ABCB1-Δ* gene mutations (p. 638). Ivermectin dosages used for treating lung parasites can cause ivermectin toxicosis in animals also taking flea and heartworm preventatives containing spinosad. Albendazole may be myelotoxic. Rare complications of fenbendazole (e.g., pancytopenia) have been reported.

Recommended Monitoring

Clinical signs, thoracic radiographs, fecal exams

PROGNOSIS & OUTCOME

Depends on severity of disease; generally good for recovery with appropriate treatment

PEARLS & CONSIDERATIONS

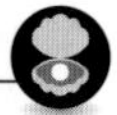

Comments

Lung parasites should be considered in any young animal presenting for coughing and with radiographic evidence of interstitial or bronchial lung disease.

Prevention

Limit exposure to intermediate or paratenic hosts.

Technician Tips

- False-negative results are common when examining stools for respiratory parasites.
- Fresh stool samples obtained per rectum are preferred for Baermann testing to limit contamination and confusion caused by soil nematodes.
- *ABCB1* testing is easily accomplished by submission of a cheek swab to the Veterinary Clinical Pharmacology Laboratory (www.vetmed.wsu.edu/depts-VCPL/).

Client Education

Reinfection is possible unless pets are limited in opportunities to ingest known paratenic hosts.

SUGGESTED READING

Cohn LA. Diseases of the pulmonary parenchyma. In Ettinger SJ, et al, editors: Textbook of veterinary internal medicine: diseases of the dog and the cat, ed 8, St. Louis, 2017, Elsevier, pp 1108-1130.

AUTHOR: Laura Ridge Cousins, DVM, MS, DACVIM
EDITOR: Megan Grobman, DVM, MS, DAVIM

Lyme and Other Borrelioses

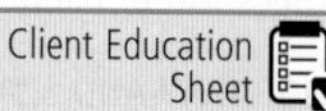

BASIC INFORMATION

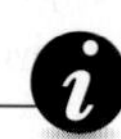

Definition

Lyme borreliosis is a disease caused by a bacterium that infects humans, other mammals, and birds. It is caused by a spiral-shaped, gram-negative spirochete that is transmitted primarily by *Ixodes* ticks. Other *Borrelia* bacteria can cause illness on occasion.

Synonyms

Lyme disease; non–Lyme borreliosis is tick-borne relapsing fever (TBRF)

Epidemiology

SPECIES, AGE, SEX

- Susceptibility: humans, dogs, cats (illness in cats is rare)
- Young and middle-aged dogs more commonly affected

GENETICS, BREED PREDISPOSITION

- Breeds associated with outdoor activities
- Labrador and golden retrievers appear predisposed to Lyme nephritis.

RISK FACTORS

Tick exposure in endemic areas

CONTAGION AND ZOONOSIS

- No direct transmission from pets to humans
- Seropositive dogs/cats are sentinels for potential human infection.

GEOGRAPHY AND SEASONALITY

- In 2015, 90% of human cases reported in the United States were from 14 northeastern, mid-Atlantic, and upper Midwest states (PA > NY > MA > NJ > CT > WI > MD > MN > VA > ME > RI > VT > NH > DE).
- Most human cases are reported between May and November.
- TBRF in dogs is seen in TX/FL (*Borrelia turicatae*) and northwestern states (*Borrelia hermsii*)

ASSOCIATED DISORDERS

Tick-borne coinfections are common, especially anaplasmosis (p. 393). Lyme nephritis can develop in predisposed animals.

Clinical Presentation

HISTORY, CHIEF COMPLAINT

- History of tick exposure in a Lyme-endemic area, although often tick bite is not recognized
- Incidentally seropositive dog (positive blood test result for antibodies to *Borrelia burgdorferi* in the absence of clinical signs of disease)
- Most seropositive dogs (95%) show no clinical signs. In highly endemic areas, 70%-90% of healthy dogs are seropositive.
- Less than 5% of seropositive dogs show the syndrome of Lyme arthritis (anorexia/fever/arthritis). This occurs 2-5 months after tick exposure in experimental beagle puppies (self-limited), whereas adults have shown no clinical signs.
- No experimental model exists for the less common syndrome of Lyme nephritis (protein-losing nephropathy [PLN] with glomerulotubular damage). Patients with this syndrome may present with signs of nephrotic syndrome, systemic hypertension, thromboembolic events, and/or signs of uremia (vomiting/anorexia).
- Cardiac, neurologic, or dermatologic manifestations as seen in people are not well documented in dogs.

PHYSICAL EXAM FINDINGS

- Most often, exam is unremarkable.
- Lyme arthritis: warm, swollen, painful joint(s), fever, local lymphadenopathy

- Lyme nephritis: dehydration (kidney failure), ascites/edema (nephrotic syndrome), saddle thromboembolism, dyspnea (pulmonary thromboembolism), retinal hemorrhage/detachment (hypertension)

Etiology and Pathophysiology

- *B. burgdorferi* is a small, microaerophilic spirochete.
- The agent in North America is *B. burgdorferi sensu stricto*, with at least 30 strains.
- The organism multiplies in the tick and enters the host at the end of the tick's blood meal (as OspA is down-regulated and OspC becomes expressed) after 36-48 hours of attachment.
- Replication in the skin at the tick bite site is followed by interstitial tissue migration.
- Clinical signs appear to be due to an immune-mediated pathogenesis (e.g., Lyme-specific antigen-antibody complexes are in glomeruli of dogs with Lyme nephritis).
- A persistent carrier state is likely in healthy-appearing carriers and clinically ill patients.
- Vectors are *Ixodes scapularis* (deer tick) in the eastern United States and *Ixodes pacificus* in the western United States. The white-footed deer mouse is the main reservoir and preferred host of larval and nymphal ticks. There is no transovarial transmission. Migratory birds are also carriers and disseminate infective ticks.
- There are 29 TBRF species with spirochetemia and transovarial transmission. *Ornithodoros* ticks, which feed for only 15-90 minutes, transmit *B. turicatae* and *B. hermsii,* causing illness in dogs (fever, lameness, uveitis, thrombocytopenia).
- It is unknown whether other *Borrelia* spp (e.g., *Borrelia miyamotoi*) that cause illness in people also do so in pets.

DIAGNOSIS

Diagnostic Overview

- A presumptive diagnosis of borreliosis includes 1) evidence of natural exposure antibodies, 2) clinical signs consistent with borreliosis, 3) consideration of other differentials, and 4) response to treatment, although Lyme nephritis may not respond well.
- Overdiagnosis should be avoided; in endemic areas, many dogs with no clinical signs are seropositive. Response to treatment does not confirm diagnosis and may occur by inadvertent treatment of co-infections (e.g., anaplasmosis, Rocky Mountain spotted fever [RMSF], ehrlichiosis, bartonellosis, leptospirosis) or the antiinflammatory/antiarthritic properties of doxycycline.
- All seropositive (clinical and nonclinical) dogs should be monitored for proteinuria. Treatment for nonclinical, nonproteinuric, seropositive carrier dogs is controversial. The dog's sentinel status is an opportunity to educate the owner about tick control and public health aspects of Lyme disease.

Differential Diagnosis

Lyme arthritis versus other causes for lameness:

- Tick-borne arthritides (anaplasmosis, ehrlichiosis, RMSF, bartonellosis), immune-mediated polyarthritis, systemic lupus erythematosus, rheumatoid arthritis, bacterial endocarditis, septic arthritis
- Degenerative joint disease, intervertebral disc disease, trauma
- Panosteitis, osteomyelitis, polymyositis, neoplasia
- Cardiopulmonary, metabolic, neurologic disease

Lyme nephritis:

- Proteinuria: leptospirosis, urinary tract infection, neoplasia, calculi
  - PLN: genetic, infectious, immune-mediated, amyloidosis, neoplasia
- Other causes for hypertension, hypercoagulopathy, edema/effusions, and/or kidney injury

Initial Database

To confirm exposure and rule out other causes of lameness/fever or PLN:

- CBC and serum biochemistry profile: thrombocytopenia possible; otherwise, no specific findings expected unless Lyme nephritis: hypoalbuminemia, hypercholesterolemia, ± azotemia, hyperphosphatemia, anemia
- SNAP 4Dx Plus test for heartworm antigen and antibodies to C6 peptide (specific for natural exposure to *B. burgdorferi*), *Ehrlichia canis/chaffeensis/ewingii*, and *Anaplasma phagocytophilum/platys*. This test replaces previous two-tier testing with Western blot for differentiating natural exposure from vaccine-induced antibodies because the C6 peptide of the VlsE antigen is not found in any Lyme vaccines.
  - AccuPlex4, Multiplex, and Abaxis Lyme test results may be confusing because OspA and OspC antibodies may occur in vaccinated and naturally exposed dogs.
  - Whole-cell IFA/ELISA/IgM/IgG titers are not helpful because of cross-reactions and because experimentally infected dogs do not show signs of Lyme disease until 2-5 months after exposure, well after seroconversion. Paired acute/convalescent titers are unnecessary.
- All Lyme-positive dogs should be screened for proteinuria by urinalysis, microalbuminuria, or urine protein/creatinine ratio testing. Lyme nephritis cases may also have glycosuria and/or active sediment due to tubular damage (rule out leptospirosis, pyelonephritis).
- If indicated, radiographs of limb(s) involved (nonerosive arthritis)
- If indicated, arthrocentesis (p. 1059): nonseptic suppurative inflammation
- Abdominal ultrasound and chest radiographs for dogs with PLN: rule out neoplasia

Advanced or Confirmatory Testing

- Specific quantitative serologic/antibody testing: C6 Quant. C6 antibody is detected 3-5 weeks post exposure, before clinical signs appear; paired titers are not necessary. C6 > 30 proves natural exposure (not cause) and is not an indication for treatment in nonclinical, nonproteinuric dogs. Magnitude of titer is not predictive of or correlated with illness.
- Polymerase chain reaction (PCR) assay or paired serologic titers for other infectious diseases: RMSF (if acute presentation), anaplasmosis/ehrlichiosis, babesiosis, bartonellosis, leptospirosis
- Renal biopsy: immune-complex glomerulonephritis, tubular necrosis/regeneration, interstitial lymphoplasmacytic inflammation
- Relapsing fever *Borrelia* spp cause spirochetemia (submit pre-treatment blood for PCR assay); antibodies may react on whole-cell IFA/ELISA Lyme tests.

TREATMENT

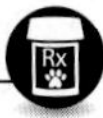

Treatment Overview

Goals of treatment:

- Avoid treating patients that have positive titers alone (exposure) in the absence of compatible clinical abnormalities.
- Resolution of lameness and fever if present
- Palliative/supportive care for complications of PLN

Acute General Treatment

- Doxycycline 10 mg/kg PO q 12-24h preferred (for coinfections, antiarthritic/antiinflammatory properties) or amoxicillin 20 mg/kg PO q 8h.
- Treatment for clinical cases is continued for 4 weeks to try to eliminate the carrier state.
- Treatment is not recommended for nonclinical, nonproteinuric carriers.

Chronic Treatment

- The length of time antibiotics are needed to clear the carrier state is unknown.
- Treatment for Lyme nephritis often includes long-term combination doxycycline, renin-angiotensin-aldosterone inhibitors (enalapril, benazepril, or telmisartan), antithrombotics (low-dose aspirin or clopidogrel), omega-3 fatty acids, possibly additional antihypertensives (amlodipine), colloids/crystalloids, and treatments for renal failure. Immunosuppressive therapy protocols (e.g., mycophenolate) may be indicated (p. 390).
- Supportive care of renal disease as appropriate (pp. 167 and 169)
- Avoid nonsteroidal antiinflammatories for pain relief (use opioids). Nonresponsive Lyme arthritis may be immune-mediated polyarthritis, for which glucocorticoids are added (e.g., prednisone 1 mg/kg PO q 12h, tapering to 0.5 mg/kg PO q 48h) (p. 803).

Recommended Monitoring

- Lyme nephritis is uncommon even in seropositive retrievers, but continue screening (duration/frequency unknown) all Lyme-positive dogs for proteinuria whether treated or not.

- In dogs that are treated, Quant C6 or OspF antibody testing is recommended at 0 and 3-6 months; the new baseline is for comparison if signs recur. High pre-treatment titers usually drop by at least 50%; lower titers may not. Qualitative C6 (SNAP 4Dx Plus) often remains positive after treatment.
- For Lyme nephritis: monitoring initially q 1-4 weeks for hematocrit, serum creatinine, blood urea nitrogen (BUN), albumin, urine protein/creatinine ratio, and blood pressure measurement, decreasing to q 3-6 months if clinically stable

PROGNOSIS & OUTCOME

- Prognosis is good for Lyme arthritis. Most dogs respond immediately without recurrence.
- Prognosis is guarded to poor for Lyme nephritis, especially in hypoalbuminemic, dehydrated, azotemic cases; life expectancy may be days to weeks.

PEARLS & CONSIDERATIONS

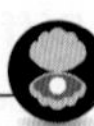

Comments

In humans, one day's dose of doxycycline taken within 72 hours of detaching an engorged *Ixodes* tick in Lyme-endemic areas helps prevent Lyme disease. The human *Borrelia* vaccine was removed from the market because of poor sales due to concern about possible immune-mediated sequelae in genetically predisposed individuals.

Prevention

- Tick prevention and control are paramount whether using vaccines or not. New tick control methods to prevent attachment or cause a fast kill of ticks include collars, topicals, and new oral isoxazolines.
- Available Lyme vaccines include bivalent bacterins (which induce OspA and OspC antibodies), recombinant subunit OspA, and a new chimeric recombinant OspA with 7 strains of OspC. Boosters may be needed q 6 months because of the short duration of immunity.
- Lyme disease vaccines are controversial because the most serious forms of Lyme disease in dogs have an immune-mediated pathogenesis; adequate tick control is paramount.

Technician Tips

All seropositive dogs need screening for proteinuria and better tick control.

Client Education

Proper tick removal, tick surveillance; prophylaxis for ectoparasites is lifesaving

SUGGESTED READING

Littman MP, et al: ACVIM consensus update on Lyme borreliosis in dogs and cats. J Vet Intern Med 32: 887-903, 2018.

AUTHOR: Meryl P. Littman, VMD, DACVIM
EDITOR: Joseph Taboada, DVM, DACVIM

Lymphadenopathy

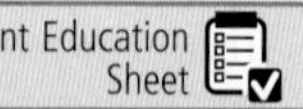

BASIC INFORMATION

Definition

Enlargement of a solitary, a regional group of, or all lymph nodes

Synonym

Lymphadenomegaly

Epidemiology

SPECIES, AGE, SEX

Dogs and cats, any age, either sex

GENETICS, BREED PREDISPOSITION

Lymphoma (p. 609)

RISK FACTORS

Infectious diseases: exposure to arthropod vectors

CONTAGION AND ZOONOSIS

- Few infectious causes of lymphadenopathy may be direct zoonosis (e.g., *Yersinia pestis*).
- Exercise caution when aspirating lymph nodes from animals with suspected infectious diseases (zoonosis by needlestick injury).

GEOGRAPHY AND SEASONALITY

Tick vectors are more prevalent in summer. Fleas and tick vectors are more prevalent in the tropics and subtropics. Many infectious agents (e.g., systemic mycosis) have specific geographic areas of prevalence.

Clinical Presentation

HISTORY, CHIEF COMPLAINT

Clinical signs generally reflect the underlying disorder and are not caused by the lymphadenopathy.

- Exception: mechanical obstruction due to marked lymph node enlargement may cause dysphagia, respiratory stridor, cough, regurgitation, cranial vena cava syndrome, swollen limb(s), or dyschezia.

PHYSICAL EXAM FINDINGS

- Evaluate all accessible lymph nodes during physical exam; the following nodes are palpable in dogs and cats:
  - Mandibular, prescapular (superficial cervical), and popliteal
  - Axillary and inguinal nodes are palpable if enlarged.
  - Enlarged sublumbar node may be palpable on rectal exam if enlarged.
  - Fat surrounding lymph nodes can be an imposter for lymphadenopathy; consider body condition.
- Node pain, erythema, heat, and adherence of node to underlying tissue suggest lymphadenitis.
- Patient may show vague signs of systemic illness from underlying disease (e.g., fever, anorexia, weight loss).
- Patients with chronic leukemias, post-vaccinal lymphadenopathies, and early lymphoma generally show subtle signs or no clinical signs other than node enlargement.
- Evaluate for apparent inciting cause in region of affected node.
  - Example: if a single popliteal node is enlarged, evaluate for lesions of the foot (dermatosis, foreign body, neoplasm).

Etiology and Pathophysiology

- Lymph nodes enlarge as a result of proliferation of normal cells within them or due to infiltration with normal or abnormal cells.
- Reactive hyperplasia
  - Proliferation of lymphocytes and plasma cells in response to antigens arriving through afferent lymphatics
  - Occurs mostly in response to inflammation in the tissues drained by the lymph node
  - After vaccination
  - Immune-mediated diseases
- Lymphadenitis
  - Migration of inflammatory cells into the node, usually caused by infection (bacterial, rickettsial, fungal, parasitic, viral)
- Neoplasia
  - Primary: lymphoma
  - Secondary: carcinomas, melanomas, sarcomas, mast cell tumors
- Extramedullary hematopoiesis (rare)
- Vascular changes: edema, congestion (rare)

DIAGNOSIS

Diagnostic Overview

Fine-needle aspiration of the lymph node for cytologic exam to classify the disease process is the first step. CBC, serum biochemistry profile,

Selected Lymph Nodes of the Dog and Associated Anatomic Regions of Lymphatic Drainage

Lymph Node (Alternative Name)	Location	Distribution of Lymphatics Contributing to the Node
Submandibular (mandibular)*	Ventral to the angle of the mandible; subcutaneous and mobile (vs. mandibular salivary glands, which are deeper, fixed structures)	Most structures of the head, except for the external ear and some parts of the skin of the dorsal muzzle
Prescapular (superficial cervical)*	Medial and dorsal to the point of the shoulder	Skin of the head, neck, and forelimb
Axillary	Dorsal to deep pectoral muscle and at the dorsal-most aspect of medial forelimb	Thoracic wall, deep structures of the forelimb
Inguinal (superficial inguinal)	Caudoventral abdomen, immediately caudal to the fifth mammary gland	Mammary glands, prepuce, scrotum, vulva, ventral abdominal wall up to the umbilicus
Popliteal*	Caudal surface of stifle (femorotibial joint)	All parts of the hindlimb distal to the node
Sublumbar (medial or external iliac)	Trifurcation of aorta (dorsal surface of pelvic canal/abdomen); may be palpable per rectum	Genital system, caudal part of the urinary and digestive systems, pelvis, hindlimbs, and dorsal half of the abdomen
Sternal (internal thoracic)	Medial to the second costal cartilage or intercostal space, cranioventral to the internal thoracic blood vessels	Peritoneal cavity, ribs, sternum, serous membranes, thymus, adjacent muscles, and mammary glands
Perihilar (tracheobronchial)	Immediately adjacent to the mainstem bronchi, distal trachea and hilar vessels, dorsal to proximal portions of the pulmonary veins and main pulmonary artery	Lungs, bronchi, heart, mediastinum; thoracic trachea, esophagus, and diaphragm

*Nodes that are normally palpable in the healthy dog and cat.

and urinalysis together with diagnostic imaging are often needed to determine the underlying cause. Lymph node biopsy may be necessary if no cause is found.

Differential Diagnosis

A detailed differential diagnosis is provided on p. 1251.

Initial Database

- Review history of travel to endemic infectious disease areas.
- Fine-needle aspiration of lymph nodes allows classification of the disease process and frequently yields infectious etiologic agents or neoplastic cells (e.g., lymphoma).
- CBC
  - Circulating blasts: lymphoma, acute leukemia
  - Neutrophilia: lymphadenitis, reactive lymph node hyperplasia, or neoplasia
  - Eosinophilia: allergic, parasitic
  - Thrombocytopenia: rickettsiosis, lymphoma
  - Monocytosis: granulomatous disease, mycosis, neoplasia, or immune-mediated disease
  - Anemia: ± depending on cause (e.g., anemia of inflammatory disease, anemia due to myelophthisis)
- Serum biochemistry profile
  - Hypercalcemia: lymphoma, multiple myeloma, anal sac adenocarcinoma
  - Hyperglobulinemia: neoplasia, rickettsiosis, chronic inflammatory diseases
- Test cats for feline leukemia virus and feline immunodeficiency virus infections.
- Imaging: radiographs, ultrasound, and/or CT to search for nidus of infection or neoplasia and determine the extent of lymph node involvement

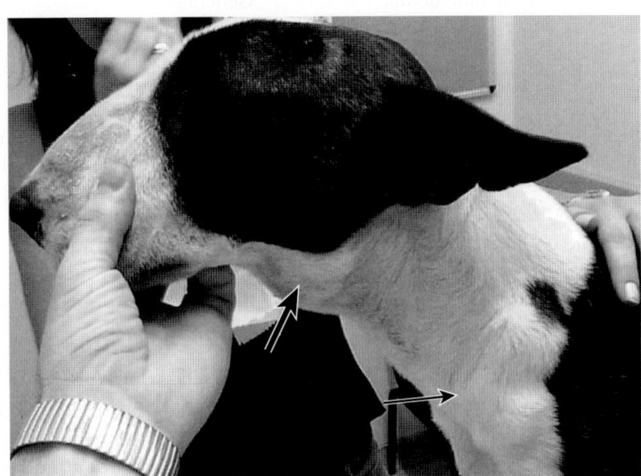

LYMPHADENOPATHY Lateral view of a bull terrier with evidence of severe submandibular (*thick arrow*) and prescapular (*thin arrow*) lymph node enlargement. (Courtesy Dr. A. Zambelli, Inanda Veterinary Hospital.)

Advanced or Confirmatory Testing

- Excisional lymph node biopsy (usually popliteal node) and histopathologic evaluation is ideal to confirm neoplasia and to perform immunophenotyping in lymphoma for prognostication.
  - Flow cytometry or PCR for antigen receptor rearrangement (PARR) testing may be useful when cytology is indeterminate for lymphoma before excisional biopsy.
- ± Aspiration and cytologic evaluation of spleen, liver, bone marrow
- ± Serologic tests for suspected infectious agents (e.g., *Blastomyces, Ehrlichia*)

TREATMENT

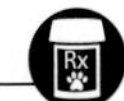

Treatment Overview

Treat the underlying cause of lymphadenopathy

Acute General Treatment

Prompt therapy (based on cause) is necessary if lymph nodes obstruct the airway or vessels.

PROGNOSIS & OUTCOME

Varies; determined by underlying cause

PEARLS & CONSIDERATIONS

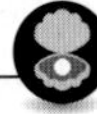

Comments

- Lymphadenopathy is most commonly associated with lymph nodes that are firm, irregular, painless, nonadherent to underlying tissue, and not warm to the touch.
- Nodes that are softer, warm, painful, and adherent to underlying tissue typically denote lymphadenitis.

- Metastatic lesions or lymphoma with extracapsular invasion of nodes are adherent to underlying tissue.
- Marked generalized lymphadenopathy (enlarged 5-10 times) occurs almost exclusively in dogs with lymphoma or in cats with lymphoma or lymph node hyperplasia.

Prevention

Tick and flea control

Technician Tips

- For generalized lymphadenopathy, the popliteal and prescapular lymph nodes are the most easily accessible for fine-needle aspiration and unaffected by oral disease (gingivitis).
- Ensure adequate platelets before lymph node aspiration.

SUGGESTED READING

Couto CG: Lymphadenopathy and splenomegaly. In Nelson RW, et al, editors: Small animal internal medicine, St. Louis, 2013, Mosby, pp 1264-1278.

AUTHOR: Paolo Pazzi, BVSc, MMedVet, DECVIM
EDITOR: Leah A. Cohn, DVM, PhD, DACVIM

Lymphangiectasia/Protein-Losing Enteropathy

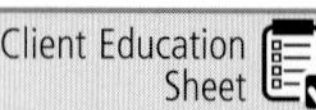

BASIC INFORMATION

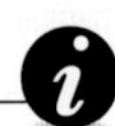

Definition

- Intestinal lymphangiectasia: intestinal lacteal (lymphatic) abnormalities commonly result in protein-losing enteropathy (PLE).
- PLE: gastrointestinal (GI) disease or dysfunction causing enteric protein loss; results in hypoalbuminemia ± hypoglobulinemia
  - Protein loss can occur with acute and chronic GI diseases.
  - The term *PLE* is usually reserved for chronic disorders.
  - May be associated with GI blood loss

Epidemiology

SPECIES, AGE, SEX

- Dogs affected more commonly than cats
- Any age; breed-associated disorders usually reported for young or middle-aged dogs

GENETICS, BREED PREDISPOSITION

- Basenji: immunoproliferative enteropathy
- Norwegian lundehund: intestinal lymphangiectasia
- Soft-coated wheaten terrier: PLE with protein-losing nephropathy (PLN)
- Yorkshire terrier: intestinal lymphangiectasia ± concurrent inflammatory bowel disease
- German shepherd, rottweiler, Chinese Shar-pei: all appear predisposed to PLE
- French bulldogs: appear predisposed to focal lipogranulomatous lymphangitis

CONTAGION AND ZOONOSIS

Chronic salmonellosis is possible in febrile or immunocompromised patients. Other infectious causes of chronic PLE are not directly contagious.

GEOGRAPHY AND SEASONALITY

Histoplasma capsulatum, *Heterobilharzia americana*, and *Pythium insidiosum* in endemic areas

ASSOCIATED DISORDERS

- Inflammatory bowel disease (IBD)
- Adverse food reactions (e.g., gluten-sensitive enteropathy)
- GI infection (e.g., histoplasmosis, salmonellosis, hookworms)
- Intestinal neoplasia (e.g., lymphoma, adenocarcinoma)
- Mechanical enteropathy (e.g., chronic foreign body, chronic intussusception)
- GI ulceration
- Lymphatic compromise/dysfunction
  - Confined to GI tract (i.e., intestinal lymphangiectasia)
  - Generalized
- Venous hypertension (portal hypertension, right-sided cardiac disease, pericardial disease)
- Low plasma oncotic pressure
  - Ascites, pleural effusion, pitting edema
- Anemia secondary to ulcerative or erosive GI disease
  - Microcytosis suggests iron deficiency.
- Thromboembolic complications from loss of antithrombin
  - May affect lungs, brain, and limbs

Clinical Presentation

HISTORY, CHIEF COMPLAINT

- May show no overt clinical signs; hypoalbuminemia may be an incidental finding.
- Weight loss is common and may be the only clinical sign.
- Chronic small-bowel diarrhea may or may not be present.
- Abdominal distention if ascites present
- Respiratory distress possible with pleural effusion, tense ascites, or pulmonary thromboembolism (PTE)
  - Thromboembolism may also cause central neurologic signs or limb dysfunction.

PHYSICAL EXAM FINDINGS

- Weight loss, emaciation
- Thickened intestinal loops or mass effects may be noted on abdominal palpation.
- Ascites and/or peripheral edema (generally when serum albumin < 1.5 g/dL)
- Dyspnea or tachypnea with pleural effusion, tense ascites, and/or PTE
- Soft stool or melena may be noted on rectal exam.

Etiology and Pathophysiology

- Hypoalbuminemia occurs when protein loss exceeds hepatic albumin synthesis.
- Several mechanisms (alone or in combination) contribute to intestinal protein loss (see Associated Disorders above).
  - Abnormalities of intestinal lymphatics cause leakage of lymph.
  - Increased intestinal permeability permits protein loss.
  - Intestinal mucosal erosion and ulceration results in protein loss.
  - Elevated venous pressures result in protein leakage.
- Hypoalbuminemia results in decreased oncotic pressure and leakage of fluid into interstitial spaces, causing peripheral edema, ascites, and/or pleural effusion.
- Loss of anticoagulant proteins, including antithrombin, results in a prothrombotic state.

DIAGNOSIS

Diagnostic Overview

Preliminary diagnostic tests confirm intestinal protein loss and rule out other causes of hypoalbuminemia. Not all patients have diarrhea, and the absence of GI signs does not exclude this diagnosis. More advanced testing defines the disorder and provides a targeted treatment plan.

Differential Diagnosis

Differential diagnosis for hypoalbuminemia:

- PLN, liver disease
- Glucocorticoid-deficient hypoadrenocorticism (i.e., atypical Addison's disease)
- Other causes of albumin loss from the vascular space
  - Peritonitis, pleuritis, vasculitis
  - Severe dermal burns or exudative dermatitis
  - GI bleeding or parasitism
- Protein malnutrition

Initial Database

- CBC
  - Anemia possible (GI hemorrhage, chronic inflammation); microcytosis, with/without hypochromasia, may reflect iron deficiency.
  - Lymphopenia common with lymphangiectasia; absence of lymphopenia may create suspicion for hypoadrenocorticism.

- Leukocytosis (usually neutrophilic) if underlying inflammatory or infectious disease
- Serum biochemistry profile
  - Hypoalbuminemia is the hallmark of severe or chronic PLE; serum albumin concentration may be at the low end of the reference range in the early stages or in patients with effective compensatory responses.
  - Globulins are often decreased, but this finding is variable.
  - Hypocholesterolemia is common.
  - Hypocalcemia (ionized and total) and hypomagnesemia are common in patients with lymphangiectasia and reflect reduced vitamin D absorption and compromised parathyroid hormone secretion.
  - Liver enzymes may be slightly elevated with GI disease; differentiate from primary liver disease with serum bile acid testing.
- Urinalysis
  - Rule out proteinuria as cause of hypoalbuminemia.
  - Hypoalbuminemia due to PLN is generally associated with a urine protein/creatinine ratio > 5.
  - PLN and PLE may occur concurrently (e.g., soft-coated wheaten terriers)
- Abdominal radiographs
  - May be unremarkable or demonstrate loss of serosal detail due to ascites
  - Underlying cause (e.g., mass, foreign body) may be apparent.
- Thoracic radiographs
  - May reveal pleural effusion due to hypoalbuminemia
  - Changes related to underlying cause (e.g., cardiac, fungal disease) or PTE possible
- Abdominal ultrasound
  - Ascites may be noted if serum albumin < 1.5 g/dL.
  - Intestinal walls may be thickened ± loss of normal layering.
  - Hyperechoic mucosal striations suggest lacteal dilation.
  - Focal intestinal lesions may be noted.
  - Lymphadenopathy suggests inflammatory, fungal, or neoplastic disease.
  - Extrahepatic shunt vessels may be noted in patients with portal hypertension.
- Fluid analysis of ascites or pleural effusion: consistent with pure transudate (pp. 1056 and 1343)
- Fecal evaluation for parasite and pathogen detection
  - Centrifuged flotation for helminth eggs and protozoal cysts
  - Saline preparation for trophozoites
- ± Serum cortisol > 2 mcg/dL (>55 nmol/L) excludes hypoadrenocorticism.

Advanced or Confirmatory Testing

- Canine fecal alpha-1 proteinase inhibitor can be assayed to confirm PLE.
  - This protein is similar in size to albumin and is resistant to digestion by intestinal proteinases.
  - Three voided fecal samples are collected into calibrated tubes (available from the GI Lab, Texas A&M University; http://www.vetmed.tamu.edu/gilab).
  - Primary use is confirming PLE in the presence of coexisting PLN or liver disease.
- Rectal scrapings can be examined cytologically for histoplasmosis or lymphoma (p. 1157).
- Serum folate and cobalamin concentrations should be measured.
  - Low folate level suggests duodenal disease.
  - Low cobalamin suggests ileal disease, exocrine pancreatic insufficiency, or changes in GI microflora.
- Enzyme-linked immunosorbent assay for *Histoplasma* antigen can identify histoplasmosis (p. 1365).
  - False-negative results have been reported for patients with GI infection.
  - Concurrent testing of serum and urine may improve sensitivity.
- Fecal polymerase chain reaction (PCR) assay can confirm infection with *H. americana.*
  - Test offered by GI Lab, Texas A&M University (http://vetmed.tamu.edu/gilab)
- GI endoscopy (p. 1098) allows evaluation of intestinal mucosa and collection of mucosal biopsy samples.
  - General anesthesia is required; this carries risk for severely hypoalbuminemic patients.
  - Samples may be collected from stomach, duodenum, ileum, and colon.
  - Lesions deeper in intestinal wall may be missed.
  - Feeding a small amount of corn oil or cream 2 hours before induction may increase visibility of dilated lacteals.
- Exploratory laparotomy allows visualization of the entire abdomen and serosal surface of intestine.
  - Full-thickness biopsies may be diagnostically superior.
  - Risk of infection or dehiscence, especially with hypoalbuminemic state

TREATMENT

Treatment Overview

- The long-term goal is to increase serum albumin concentrations.
- Ultralow-fat diet (<2 g fat/100 kcal) should be provided pending definitive diagnosis.
- Some patients need immediate intervention to
  - Mitigate third-space fluid accumulation
  - Provide nutritional support
  - Prevent or address thromboembolic complications
  - Address electrolyte imbalances (e.g., hypocalcemia and hypomagnesemia)

Acute General Treatment

- Colloidal support
  - Synthetic colloids (e.g., hetastarch, dextran) improve oncotic pressure and limit peripheral edema and ascites.
  - Starting dosages should be low (e.g., 5 mL/kg/day) because acute volume overload and pulmonary edema can occur due to shifts of interstitial fluid to the vascular compartment.
  - Plasma provides modest colloidal support and is unlikely to provide useful amounts of natural anticoagulants such as antithrombin.
  - Albumin administration provides only temporary improvement in colloidal status.
- Electrolyte disorders
  - Patients with severe hypocalcemia may not improve unless magnesium is also supplemented.
  - Crystalloids should be administered cautiously and used concurrently with colloids to minimize extravascular fluid accumulation.
- Abdominal drainage/thoracocentesis (p. 1164)
  - Fluid removal is required for patients with respiratory distress due to cavity effusion(s).
- Total or partial parenteral nutrition provides interim nutritional support in patients unable to absorb nutrients (p. 1148).

Chronic Treatment

- Effective treatment of PLE requires management of the underlying cause; this may not be possible in all patients, particularly those with intestinal lymphangiectasia.
- Immunosuppressive agents should be used in patients with idiopathic IBD.
  - Glucocorticoids are the mainstay of medical therapy (e.g., prednisone 1-2 mg/kg PO q 12h, tapering to lowest effective dose); may not be well tolerated by severely hypoalbuminemic dogs
  - Budesonide 0.5-3 mg/DOG q 24h may be substituted for prednisone to minimize iatrogenic hyperadrenocorticism.
  - Additional immunosuppressive agents (e.g., chlorambucil, cyclosporine, azathioprine) may be necessary in refractory patients or when chronic therapy is required.
- Glucocorticoids ± other immunosuppressive agents may be helpful in patients with lymphangiectasia.
  - Thought to decrease lipogranuloma formation and lymphangitis
  - Inflammation triggered by release of chylomicrons into adjacent tissue exacerbates lymphatic dilation, dysfunction, and leakage.
- Antibiotic therapy with tylosin (Tylan Soluble, Elanco 20 mg/kg PO q 12h × 4 weeks) may help control intestinal dysbiosis.
- Thromboembolism prophylaxis is warranted (e.g., clopidogrel 1-3 mg/kg PO q 24h) but should be discontinued before surgical procedures.
- Diuretics (spironolactone 1-2 mg/kg PO q 12h) do not mobilize cavitary effusions quickly but may delay return of fluid.

Nutrition/Diet

- Ultralow-fat, easily digestible diets should be fed to patients with intestinal lymphangiectasia to minimize fat malabsorption and lacteal flow.
  - Cottage cheese (1% fat), tilapia, and nonfat turkey breast mixed 1:2 with cooked white rice are excellent temporary options.
  - Prescription highly digestible diets containing < 2 g/100 kcal metabolizable energy from fat are also acceptable.
- Hydrolyzed protein or novel antigen diets should be considered for patients with concurrent IBD.
  - Most prescription diets in this category are not adequately fat restricted for patients with lymphangiectasia; consider a home-cooked diet or a hydrolyzed protein diet that is fat restricted.
- Gluten-free diets should be provided if gluten-sensitive enteropathy is suspected.
- Elemental enteral feeding products may be helpful for very compromised patients. These diets contain free amino acids to facilitate nutrient uptake by a compromised GI tract. Low-fat formulations (e.g., Vivonex T.E.N., Nestle) are appropriate for dogs with lymphangiectasia and can be administered through a small-gauge feeding tube.
- Cobalamin supplementation should be provided if serum concentrations are subnormal:
  - Cyanocobalamin 250-1000 mcg/PATIENT SQ q 7 days for 6 weeks, then q 3-4 weeks *or* 250-1000 mcg PO q 24h, depending on patient size (p. 1325)
- Folate supplementation if serum concentrations are subnormal (0.5 mg/PATIENT PO q 24h)
- Vitamin and mineral supplementation may be necessary in dogs with lymphangiectasia because uptake of fat-soluble vitamins (D, E, K) is substantially compromised.
  - Vitamin D supplementation requires careful monitoring to prevent overdose.
  - Supplementation with calcium 0.5-2 g of elemental calcium q 24h and magnesium 5-15 mL of magnesium hydroxide q 24h may be necessary.

Possible Complications

- Immunosuppressive therapy
  - May exacerbate infection if present
  - Glucocorticoids should be withheld until surgical sites have healed.
  - Iatrogenic hyperadrenocorticism with long-term glucocorticoid therapy
- Thromboembolic disease
  - Patients may present with respiratory distress, neurologic signs, or lameness.
  - Antithrombotic therapy should be considered for all patients with PLE unless specifically contraindicated (e.g., active bleeding, surgery).
  - Concurrent use of glucocorticoids may increase thromboembolic risk.
- Respiratory distress
  - From severe ascites or pleural effusion, necessitating abdominocentesis or thoracocentesis
  - PTE associated with PLE may also cause respiratory distress.

Recommended Monitoring

- Monitor serum albumin levels (assuming no other disease processes are contributing to hypoalbuminemia).
- Monitor calcium (preferably ionized) and magnesium concentrations.
- Monitor CBC if patients are receiving myelosuppressive agents.
- Monitor body weight regularly for third-space fluid accumulation.

PROGNOSIS & OUTCOME

Long-term prognosis depends on eventual diagnosis and response to therapy.

- Most patients with PLE secondary to IBD have a guarded to fair prognosis.
- Basenjis with immunoproliferative enteropathy have a guarded to poor prognosis.
- Yorkshire terriers with lymphangiectasia have a guarded long-term prognosis because secondary lipogranulomas may cause refractory dysfunction.
- Prognosis for patients with GI fungal infection or neoplasia (depending on type and extent) is guarded to grave.
- Hypovitaminosis D is associated with a poor outcome.

PEARLS & CONSIDERATIONS

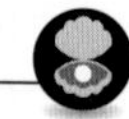

Comments

- Hypoalbuminemia or an unexplained decrease in serum albumin concentration should always be investigated, even if the patient appears otherwise healthy. Early recognition and treatment of PLE may improve outcome.
- Dietary modifications are an essential part of therapy in many cases.
- Always consider the risk of thromboembolism in patients with PLE.

Technician Tips

- Fluid therapy for dogs with PLE can be complicated; monitor respiratory rate hourly and check weight q 12h.
- Blood pressure must be carefully monitored during anesthesia in dogs with PLE.

Client Education

- Warn clients that intestinal lymphangiectasia and IBD are usually lifetime problems and that chronic therapy may be necessary.
- Dietary recommendations must be strictly followed to minimize the chances of relapse.

SUGGESTED READING

Simmerson SM, et al: Clinical features, intestinal histopathology, and outcome in protein-losing enteropathy in Yorkshire terrier dogs. J Vet Intern Med 8:331-337, 2014.

AUTHOR: Audrey K. Cook, BVM&S, DACVIM, DECVIM, DABVP
EDITOR: Rance K. Sellon, DVM, PhD, DACVIM

Lymphoma Chemotherapy Treatment Tables, Cat

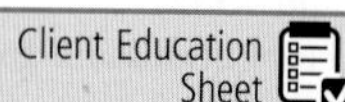

CBC Monitoring Guidelines for Cats

DOSAGE REDUCTION

- If neutrophils < 1000 cells/mcL on any CBC, decrease dosage of causative agent by 25% for future treatments, begin empirical prophylactic antibiotics (e.g., amoxicillin-clavulanate 11-22 mg/kg PO q 12h), and consider additional supportive care and diagnostic testing if cat is overtly ill.
- If platelets < 50,000 cells/mcL on any CBC, decrease dosage of causative agent by 25% for future treatments.

TREATMENT DELAY

- If neutrophils < 2000 cells/mcL on day treatment is due, postpone treatment, recheck CBC in 3-7 days, and resume treatment when neutrophil count is > 2000 cells/mcL.
- If platelets < 50,000 cells/mcL on day treatment is due, postpone treatment, recheck CBC in 3-7 days, and resume treatment when platelet count is > 50,000 cells/mcL.

AUTHOR: Laurel E. Williams, DVM, DACVIM
EDITOR: Kenneth M. Rassnick, DVM, DACVIM

COP Protocol (Cat)

Treatment and Monitoring	Week 1*	Week 2	Week 3	Week 4	Week 5	Week 6	Week 7	Week 8	Week 9	Week 10	Weeks 13, 16, 19, etc.[†]
CBC[‡]	•	•	•	•			•			•	•
Cyclophosphamide[§]	•			•			•			•	•
Vincristine[¶]	•	•	•	•			•			•	•
Prednisolone	•	•	•	•	•	•	•	•	•	•	•

*Day of first treatment.
[†]Continue 3-week cycle until relapse or until week 26 (Moore et al) or week 52 (Teske et al).
[‡]Complete blood count (CBC) once weekly for first 3-week treatment cycle, then every 3 weeks thereafter to screen for cytopenias, which could postpone or reduce treatment(s):
Cyclophosphamide 300 mg/m^2 PO q 3 weeks
Vincristine 0.75 mg/m^2 IV once weekly × 4 weeks, then q 3 weeks thereafter
Prednisolone 40-50 mg/m^2 PO q 24h
[§]The cyclophosphamide dosage in this protocol may be too high for some cats, and it may be preferable to start at a dosage of 200-250 mg/m^2 with subsequent consideration of escalation to 300 mg/m^2 if no toxicoses are noted.
[¶]The vincristine dosage in this protocol may be too high for some cats, resulting in gastrointestinal toxicoses (e.g., ileus); a dosage of 0.5 mg/m^2 may be preferable.
Data from Moore AS, et al: A comparison of doxorubicin and COP for maintenance of remission in cats with lymphoma. J Vet Intern Med 10(6):372-375, 1996; Teske E, et al: Chemotherapy with cyclophosphamide, vincristine, and prednisolone (COP) in cats with malignant lymphoma: new results with an old protocol. J Vet Intern Med 16(2):179-186, 2002.

CHOP Protocol (Cat)

Treatment and Monitoring	Week 1*	Week 2	Week 3	Week 4	Week 5	Week 6[†]	Week 7[†]	Week 8[†]	Week 9[†]	Week 10[†]
CBC	•	•	•	•		•	•	•	•	
L-Asparaginase	•									
Cyclophosphamide		•					•			
Doxorubicin				•					•	
Prednisolone	•	•	•	•	•	•			•	•
Vincristine	•		•			•		•		

*Day of first treatment.
[†]Continue/repeat 5-week treatment course (vincristine, cyclophosphamide, vincristine, doxorubicin, off) for two additional cycles to complete 20-week treatment protocol:
L-Asparaginase 400 U/kg SQ; if L-asparaginase is not available, the protocol can proceed without the inclusion of this drug.
Cyclophosphamide 200-250 mg/m^2 PO
Doxorubicin 25 mg/m^2 or 1 mg/kg IV as slow infusion (20 min)
Prednisolone 2 mg/kg PO q 24h for weeks 1 and 2; then 1 mg/kg PO q 24h for weeks 3 and 4; then 1 mg/kg PO q 48h for weeks 5 and 6; then taper and discontinue
Vincristine 0.5 mg/m^2 IV
CBC, Complete blood count.

Lymphoma Chemotherapy Treatment Tables, Dog

Client Education Sheet 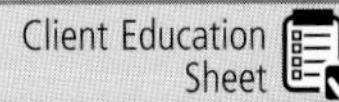

CBC Monitoring Guidelines for Dogs

DOSAGE REDUCTION

- If neutrophils < 1000 cells/mcL on any CBC, decrease dosage of causative agent by 25% for future treatments, begin empirical prophylactic antibiotics (e.g., amoxicillin-clavulanate 11-22 mg/kg PO q 12h for 7 days), and consider additional supportive care and diagnostic testing if animal is overtly ill.
- If platelets < 50,000 cells/mcL on any CBC, decrease dosage of causative agent by 25% for future treatments.

TREATMENT DELAY

- If neutrophils < 2000 cells/mcL on day treatment is due, postpone treatment, recheck CBC in 3-7 days, and resume treatment when neutrophil count is > 2000 cells/mcL.
- If platelets < 50,000 cells/mcL on day treatment is due, postpone treatment, recheck CBC in 3-7 days, and resume treatment when platelet count is > 50,000 cells/mcL.

AUTHOR: Laurel E. Williams, DVM, DACVIM
EDITOR: Kenneth M. Rassnick, DVM, DACVIM

COP Protocol (Dog)

Treatment and Monitoring	Week 1*	Week 2	Week 3	Week 4	Week 5	Week 6	Week 7	Week 8	Week 9	Week 10	Weeks 13, 16, 19, etc.†
CBC‡	•	•	•	•			•			•	•
Cyclophosphamide§	•			•			•			•	•
Predniso(lo)ne	•	•	•	•	•	•	•	•	•	•	•
Vincristine¶	•	•	•	•			•			•	•

*Day of first treatment.
†Continue 3-week cycle through week 52, then continue at 4-week cycle for an additional 6 months.
‡Complete blood count (CBC) once weekly for first 3-week treatment cycle, then every 3 weeks thereafter to screen for cytopenias, which could postpone or reduce treatment(s):
Cyclophosphamide 300 mg/m² PO q 3 weeks (administer furosemide 2 mg/kg single dose PO, immediately before to reduce risk of hemorrhagic cystitis; if cystitis develops, cyclophosphamide is terminated permanently and replaced with chlorambucil) or 300 mg/m² PO divided over 4 consecutive days q 3 weeks
Vincristine 0.75 mg/m² IV once weekly × 4 weeks, then q 3 weeks thereafter
Prednisolone 1 mg/kg PO q 24h for 3 weeks, then every other day
§The cyclophosphamide dosage in this protocol may be too high for some dogs, and it may be preferable to start at a dosage of 200-250 mg/m², with subsequent consideration of escalation to 300 mg/m² if no toxicoses are noted.
¶The vincristine dosage in this protocol may be too high for some dogs and result in toxicoses; a dosage of 0.5-0.7 mg/m² may be preferable as a starting point.
Data from Cotter SM: Treatment of lymphoma and leukemia with cyclophosphamide, vincristine, and prednisone: I. Treatment of dogs. J Am Anim Hosp Assoc 19:159-165, 1983.

CHOP Protocol (Dog)

Treatment and Monitoring	Week 1*	Week 2	Week 3	Week 4	Week 5	Week 6†	Week 7†	Week 8†	Week 9†	Week 10†
CBC‡	•	•	•	•	•	•	•	•	•	•
L-Asparaginase	•									
Cyclophosphamide§		•					•			
Doxorubicin				•					•	
Prednisone	•	•	•							
Vincristine	•		•			•		•		

*Day of first treatment.
†Continue/repeat 5-week treatment course (vincristine, cyclophosphamide, vincristine, doxorubicin, off) for two additional cycles to complete 20-week treatment protocol.
‡Complete blood count (CBC) to screen for cytopenias, which could delay, reduce, or cancel the week's treatment(s):
L-Asparaginase 10,000 IU/m² SQ (± pre-treatment with diphenhydramine 2 mg/kg IM 15-30 minutes before L-asparaginase dosing, at clinician's preference); patient monitored for hypersensitivity/anaphylaxis × 30 minutes, and if noted, L-asparaginase is terminated permanently. NOTE: If L-asparaginase is not available, the protocol can proceed without the inclusion of this drug.
Cyclophosphamide 200-250 mg/m² PO or IV (administer furosemide 2 mg/kg single dose PO or IV immediately before to reduce risk of hemorrhagic cystitis; if hemorrhagic cystitis develops, cyclophosphamide is terminated permanently and replaced with chlorambucil)
Doxorubicin for dogs > 10 kg, 30 mg/m² IV; for dogs ≤ 10 kg, 1 mg/kg IV
Prednisone 30 mg/m² PO q 24h for week 1, then 20 mg/m² PO q 24h for week 2, then 10 mg/m² PO q 24h for week 3, then stop
Vincristine 0.5-0.6 mg/m² IV for week 1, then 0.7 mg/m² IV for weeks 3, 6, 8, and thereafter
§In some citations, CHOP (cyclophosphamide + hydroxydaunorubicin [doxorubicin] + Oncovin [vincristine] + prednisone) is identical to COAP because hydroxydaunorubicin = doxorubicin = Adriamycin. However, in some, the A in COAP refers to ara-C, i.e., cytosine arabinoside, whereas in others, the A in COPA refers to asparaginase.
Additional lymphoma treatment/rescue protocols can be found at ExpertConsult.com.

Lymphoma, Gastrointestinal

Client Education Sheet 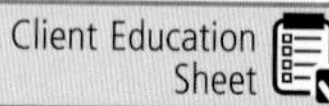

BASIC INFORMATION

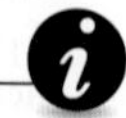

Definition

Gastrointestinal (GI) lymphomas/lymphosarcomas (LSAs) are malignant tumors of lymphoid cell origin that can arise at any location in the GI tract, including the stomach, small intestine, colon, and rectum. Lesions may be of B-cell, T-cell, or large granular lymphocyte subtypes and may be high or low grade, distinctions that are important prognostically.

Synonyms

Alimentary lymphoma, alimentary lymphosarcoma, gut-associated lymphoid tissue (GALT) lymphoma, enteropathy-associated T-cell lymphoma (EATCL), large granular lymphocyte lymphoma, mucosa-associated lymphoid tissue (MALT) lymphoma, neoplasm of globule leukocytes

Epidemiology

SPECIES, AGE, SEX

- GI LSA is the second most common form of lymphoid malignancy in dogs (after multicentric LSA), accounting for 5%-7% of all LSAs.
  - Dogs with GI LSA are middle-aged to older (mean 7.7 years).
- GI LSA is currently the most prevalent anatomic form of LSAs in cats now that feline leukemia virus (FeLV) infection, a cause of mediastinal and multicentric LSA in young cats, has been largely curtailed (p. 329).
  - Cats with GI LSA are typically 7-10 years old, although the disease can occur in much older and younger cats.
- No sex predisposition is noted for dogs or cats.

GENETICS, BREED PREDISPOSITION

Dog breeds predisposed include boxers, Shar-peis, golden retrievers, springer spaniels, Doberman pinschers, Labrador retrievers, and German shepherds.

RISK FACTORS

Cause of most cases of GI LSA is unknown.

- Chronic inflammatory bowel disease (IBD [p. 543]) is a predisposing factor.
- Epidemiologic studies implicate exposure to phenoxy herbicides (2,4-D) and environmental cigarette smoke in lymphomagenesis.
- *Helicobacter pylori* infection is implicated in human GI LSA, but that association has not been firmly established in veterinary medicine.
- Underlying immune disorders may predispose.

CONTAGION AND ZOONOSIS

No infectious or zoonotic cause is known in dogs. In cats, retroviral infection with FeLV and/or feline immunodeficiency virus (FIV) is rarely associated with GI lymphoma.

ASSOCIATED DISORDERS

- Anemia and panhypoproteinemia may occur secondary to chronic GI blood loss.
- Hypercalcemia may be associated with canine GI LSA, but it is rare in cats.
- LSA metastatic to the liver may be associated with biliary obstruction.

Clinical Presentation

DISEASE FORMS/SUBTYPES

- GI LSA may be of the B-cell, T-cell, or large granular lymphocyte (LGL) type. LGL LSA typically has a T-cell origin, although it can be a null cell phenotype of natural killer (NK) cells.
- Lesions may be focal masses or diffusely infiltrative throughout the gut.
- Lesions may be submucosal, epitheliotropic, or transmural.
- GI LSA may be a low-grade disease of cellular accumulation due to impaired apoptosis, as in human MALT lymphoma, or may be high-grade disease with rapid cell replication.

HISTORY, CHIEF COMPLAINT

- GI LSA is associated with GI signs:
  - Evidence of malassimilation such as weight loss
  - Anorexia
  - Vomiting and/or diarrhea, often chronic
  - Melena, hematemesis, hematochezia
- Polyuria/polydipsia if hypercalcemia present

PHYSICAL EXAM FINDINGS

- Poor body condition and ill-kempt appearance, especially cats
- Palpable abdominal mass(es) and intra-abdominal lymphadenomegaly
- With diffuse intestinal infiltration, turgid, thickened intestinal walls often palpable
- Signs of anemia (e.g., pallor, lethargy, tachycardia) or hypercalcemia (e.g., muscle weakness) may be evident.
- Hepatosplenomegaly may be present.
- Rectal exam may reveal melena, hematochezia, or abnormal rectal mucosa.
- Physical exam may be normal.

Etiology and Pathophysiology

Most lymphomas are thought to arise from abnormal somatic cell DNA recombination events, which may be random or induced by retroviral infection, environmental carcinogen exposure, or chronic infection/inflammation that increases lymphoid cell population expansion.

DIAGNOSIS

Diagnostic Overview

- The diagnosis is suspected in a patient with persistent vomiting, diarrhea, systemic signs such as weight loss, or some combination of these. Suspicion increases when abdominal ultrasound reveals gastric or intestinal wall thickening, GI masses or mesenteric lymphadenomegaly.
- Confirmation requires cytology or biopsy; endoscopic biopsies are less invasive but may be insufficient; full-thickness biopsies are the gold standard but require laparoscopy or laparotomy.
- Interpretation of histologic features in some cases is difficult and may require advanced staining or other techniques such as polymerase chain reaction for antigen receptor rearrangement (PARR), with some samples remaining permanently ambiguous.

Differential Diagnosis

Depends on the form and location of the LSA lesion(s):

- IBD
- Chronic endoparasitism
- GI foreign body or intussusception
- Chronic pancreatitis (especially cats)
- Other causes of liver disease such as hepatitis, cholangiohepatitis, toxic hepatopathy, or feline hepatic lipidosis
- Benign GI disease such as gastric ulcer, polyp, or adenoma
- Other GI tumors, including mast cell disease, adenocarcinoma, and mesenchymal tumors
- Granulomatous enteritis secondary to bacterial, fungal, algal, or oomycotic infection (p. 395)

Initial Database

- Minimum database: CBC, serum chemistry panel, urinalysis, fecal exam for parasites, *Giardia* antigen test, T_4 assay (cats), FeLV/FIV tests (cats)
  - Normal, or can find evidence of GI bleeding (e.g., anemia, hypoproteinemia, increased blood urea nitrogen [BUN]) or hepatopathy (e.g., increased liver enzymes, hyperbilirubinemia)
  - These tests are important to rule out alternative diagnoses, including parasitism, before undertaking more invasive tests (i.e., biopsy).
- Evaluation for chronic pancreatic or GI disease (trypsin-like immunoreactivity [TLI], cobalamin/folate, or pancreatic lipase immunoreactivity [PLI])
  - Hypocobalaminemia is associated with feline GI LSA
- Three-view thoracic radiographs to look for metastasis
- Abdominal ultrasonography with guided fine-needle aspiration cytology of thickened bowel and/or enlarged lymph nodes (p. 1112)
  - Normal bowel wall thickness (dog, cat) <5 mm
  - Any layer may be thickened; thickening may be focal or diffuse (diffuse more common), and mesenteric lymphadenomegaly is common but not specific to lymphoma. Intestinal mural layering is commonly preserved with diffuse disease.
  - Thickened small intestinal wall and muscularis propria layer is commonly observed in cats with small cell GI T-cell lymphoma; these changes are also common in cats with IBD.

Advanced or Confirmatory Testing

- Biopsy of gastric, duodenal, or colorectal lesions to make the diagnosis by histopathologic tissue exam
  - Endoscopy is less invasive and therefore generally preferred to surgical biopsy (p. 1098).
  - Surgical full-thickness biopsy may be necessary for LSA in the deeper layers of the GI tract or in portions of the intestine not reached by endoscopy (jejunum).
  - Avoid full-thickness biopsy of the colon.
- Tumor staging for extent of systemic involvement:
  - Bone marrow cytology for staging and/or as indicated by cytopenias (p. 1068)
  - Peripheral node aspiration or biopsy for staging and/or as indicated for lymphadenomegaly
- Immunohistochemical phenotyping for B-cell, T-cell, or LGL subtypes
  - CD3 for T-cell subset
  - CD79a or CD20 for B-cell disease
  - CD3 and CD57 for LGL subtype
  - PARR for monoclonality by B-cell (immunoglobulin gene rearrangement) or T-cell (T-cell receptor gene rearrangement) clonal expansion rather than polyclonal lesions seen in lymphoplasmacytic enteritis

TREATMENT

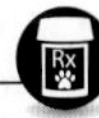

Treatment Overview

- It is extremely unlikely that dogs and cats with diffuse, nodal, or visceral organ involvement can be cured.
- For most cases, the goal is to prolong life with good quality while avoiding adverse effects of therapy.
- Focal GI LSA lesions can be surgically cured by excision with complete margins if neoplastic cells have not disseminated.

Acute General Treatment

General supportive care:

- Rehydration and restoring electrolyte homeostasis

- Managing anemia with transfusions and hematinics as needed (p. 1169)
- Antibiotics and emergency management for peritonitis (p. 779)
- Analgesics as indicated for pain
- Promotility agents are contraindicated in obstructive disease.
- Management of hypercalcemia of malignancy (pp. 491 and 754) by IV fluids and furosemide 1-2 mg/kg IV or PO q 12-24h after rehydration, bisphosphonates (e.g., pamidronate, zoledronate), or possibly calcitonin 4-8 IU/kg IV, IM, or SQ q 12h acutely. Management of hypercalcemia by treating the underlying malignancy should be started only *after* the cytologic or histopathologic diagnosis of GI LSA is established because treatment with glucocorticoids or other lympholytic agents can compromise detection of lymphoma.

Chronic Treatment

- Chemotherapy is generally the treatment of choice for GI LSA. A number of chemotherapy protocols (pp. 607 and 609) have been used to treat GI LSA.
- For high-grade disease, the University of Madison-Wisconsin or similar CHOP-based (cyclophosphamide, doxorubicin, vincristine, prednisone/prednisolone) protocols involve
    - Sequential treatment with CHOP drugs ± L-asparaginase over 19-25 weeks
    - Single-agent doxorubicin, mitoxantrone, ifosfamide, or lomustine and combination therapy with doxorubicin/dacarbazine have been used as rescue agents.
- For low-grade disease, treatment with milder chemotherapy protocols is helpful in prolonging life with good quality. Low-grade protocols include
    - Chlorambucil (commonly 20 mg/m^2 PO q 14 days [p. 609] or 2 mg PO q 48h) and prednisolone (various dosing schemes but often starting with 1-2 mg/kg PO q 24h for 7-14 days, then reducing to 0.5-1 mg/kg PO q 48h), or COP (cyclophosphamide, vincristine, and prednisolone)
- One study suggests lomustine as a rescue agent for cats with resistant small or intermediate cell GI LSA achieves a longer progression-free interval than for large cell GI LSA.
- Abdominal radiation therapy as a rescue protocol for feline GI LSA appears to be well tolerated and may increase median survival time.
    - Abdominal irradiation may be incorporated into the induction protocol. This is particularly helpful for cats that resist oral medication.
- Curative therapy for focal GI LSA lesions is through complete surgical excision.
    - Because of the high likelihood of systemic or local spread, these animals are followed with a course of chemotherapy.
- Cobalamin supplementation as needed (p. 183)

Nutrition/Diet

These animals are often thin; efforts should be made to provide adequate nutritional support. Appetite often improves if disease can be placed in remission.

Possible Complications

- Surgical wound dehiscence with secondary peritonitis, pneumoperitoneum
- Chemotherapy-induced neutropenia can predispose to infection, and thrombocytopenia can increase risk of hemorrhage.
- Chemotherapy can result in perforation of transmural lesions.

Recommended Monitoring

- CBC for chemotherapy-induced myelosuppression
- Ultrasonography is most practical for detecting intraabdominal metastasis or recurrence and may identify small amounts of peritoneal fluid as the first manifestation of peritonitis in cases of bowel rupture.
- Periodic restaging (physical exam monthly, laboratory evaluation, thoracic radiographs, abdominal ultrasound exam every other month) for patients in complete remission after surgical excision or completion of dose-intense therapy with CHOP-based protocols.

PROGNOSIS & OUTCOME

- GI LSA is a serious, life-threatening illness, but because of the widely different biological behaviors of various subtypes, predicting therapeutic response and duration of survival is difficult for individual animals.
- In general, low-grade disease is indolent and associated with longer survival than high-grade disease, depending on extent of disease at the time of diagnosis.
- T-cell phenotype is generally less responsive and associated with shorter survival duration than B-cell disease. Historically, median survival times for extranodal T-cell lymphomas were typically 6 months or less in dogs.
- Treatment efficacy remains variable, with reported median remission times of 3-12 months.
- Failure to achieve remission and diarrhea at presentation are negative prognostic indicators.
- Anatomic location may have prognostic significance for dogs. Colonic lymphoma is associated with a better prognosis than gastric or jejunal lymphoma.
- Cats with low-grade GI LSA require minimal therapy and may survive for years using treatment with chlorambucil, prednisolone, and cobalamin repletion.
- Antibiotic therapy (e.g., tylosin) for secondary dysbiosis may be helpful.

PEARLS & CONSIDERATIONS

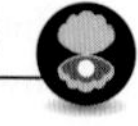

Comments

- Full-thickness surgical biopsies may be necessary to diagnose small-intestinal LSA because endoscopic access is limited to the duodenum or ileum.
- Fine-needle aspiration cytology of the intestinal wall is possible, but low-grade LSA is difficult to differentiate from reactive lymphocyte expansion.
- In general, the underlying cause of refractory diarrhea should be pursued aggressively because GI LSA is an important differential diagnosis.
- Treatment with glucocorticoids may impede the accurate diagnosis of LSA because lymphoblasts are rapidly lysed.

Prevention

- Aggressive management of lymphoplasmacytic enteritis is recommended. IBD may progress to GI LSA.
- Limiting exposure to lawn and agricultural chemicals and second-hand smoke is likely beneficial, but no specific preventive measures are known.

Technician Tips

These patients are very ill. Monitor for signs of hypotension and abdominal effusion that might indicate GI perforation.

Client Education

Response to initial therapy can be the best prognostic indicator.

SUGGESTED READING

WSAVA International Gastrointestinal Standardization Group: ACVIM consensus statement: endoscopic, biopsy, and histopathologic guidelines for the evaluation of gastrointestinal inflammation in companion animals. J Vet Intern Med 24:10, 2010.

AUTHOR: Barbara E. Kitchell, DVM, PhD, DACVIM
EDITOR: Rance K. Sellon DVM, PhD, DACVIM

Lymphoma, Multicentric (Cat)

Client Education Sheet

BASIC INFORMATION

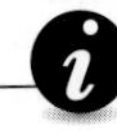

Definition

Systemic malignant neoplasm of lymphoid origin

Synonyms

Lymphosarcoma, malignant lymphoma, non-Hodgkin lymphoma (human)

Epidemiology

SPECIES, AGE, SEX

- Most common hematopoietic malignancy
- Disease forms/anatomic presentations have changed over the past decades, coincident with decreases in feline leukemia virus (FeLV) infection rates and FeLV-associated lymphoma.
- Can develop at any age
- Siamese cats may be at increased risk for certain forms of lymphoma.

RISK FACTORS

- FeLV and possibly feline immunodeficiency virus (FIV) infection status influences age and anatomic location at which lymphoma develops.
- Household exposure to environmental tobacco smoke (i.e., secondhand smoke). In one study, cats exposed to tobacco smoke had a 2.4-fold increased risk of lymphoma, which increased with duration of exposure and number of smokers in the house.

Clinical Presentation

DISEASE FORMS/SUBTYPES

- Histologic grade
  - High-grade or lymphoblastic lymphoma: most common; rapid onset and progression; affected cells are large lymphoblasts.
  - Low-grade or lymphocytic/small cell lymphoma: most often reported with gastrointestinal (GI) lymphoma; chronic insidious onset; affected cells are well differentiated and similar in appearance to small lymphocytes.
- Anatomic distribution
  - Multicentric: typically lymph node, spleen, and/or liver involvement; presenting signs and physical exam findings vary with organ(s) affected.
  - Alimentary (GI) (p. 604): older cats; majority are FeLV negative; presenting signs include anorexia, weight loss, vomiting, and diarrhea; physical exam may reveal palpable abdominal mass.
  - Mediastinal: young cats; most are FeLV infected; thymus, mediastinal, and sternal lymph nodes may be involved (rarely, superficial cervical nodes are affected); presenting signs include dyspnea, tachypnea; physical exam may reveal a noncompressible crainial thorax and suggest pleural effusion.
  - Renal: presenting sign is acute azotemia, which may largely or entirely resolve with chemotherapy; physical exam reveals marked bilateral renomegaly; central nervous system relapse is reported.
  - Spinal: often FeLV infected; presenting sign is hindlimb paraparesis; many have concurrent malignant lymphoblasts in bone marrow (p. 932).
  - Nasal: unique form of lymphoma, often localized and may be treated with radiation therapy
  - Cutaneous

HISTORY, CHIEF COMPLAINT

- Highly varied presentation (see Disease Forms/Subtypes above)
- Generalized peripheral lymphadenopathy is common in dogs but rare in cats with lymphoma.

PHYSICAL EXAM FINDINGS

Physical exam findings vary and reflect the organs involved (see Disease Forms/Subtypes above).

Etiology and Pathophysiology

- Rapid onset and disease progression over days to weeks (most types)
- Low-grade lymphoma (often GI) typically presents with chronic history.

DIAGNOSIS

Diagnostic Overview

Diagnosis is suspected based on detection of a mass lesion/infiltration in affected organ or site with associated clinical signs. Aspiration cytology of the mass or site is often diagnostic.

Differential Diagnosis

- Other neoplasms (e.g., leukemia, mast cell tumor)
- Multicentric: other neoplasms (e.g., mast cell tumor), cholangitis-cholangiohepatitis and other hepatopathies, pancreatitis
- Mediastinal: other neoplasms (e.g., thymoma, mesothelioma), heart disease, pyothorax, chylothorax, feline infectious peritonitis, diaphragmatic hernia
- Renal: acute kidney injury, polycystic kidney disease, pyelonephritis
- Nasal: other neoplasms (e.g., adenocarcinoma), rhinitis, inflammatory polyps, cryptococcosis
- Alimentary: inflammatory bowel disease, granulomatous bowel disease, parasitism, other neoplastic and non-neoplastic GI disorders

Initial Database

- CBC: to identify anemia, thrombocytopenia, and/or neutropenia (due to lymphoblast infiltration in marrow or secondary to immune-mediated destruction) or presence of circulating lymphoblasts (i.e., leukemia)
- Serum biochemistry panel: to identify liver or renal abnormalities that may develop secondary to organ involvement and may alter ability to metabolize or eliminate chemotherapeutic drugs
- Urinalysis ± urine culture and sensitivity: to further evaluate renal function and identify urinary tract infection secondary to immunocompromise
- FeLV serologic testing: FeLV antigenemia is associated with certain forms of lymphoma and may be prognostic (see Prognosis & Outcome below).
- Serum cobalamin level in cats with suspected low-grade alimentary lymphoma
- Aspiration and cytologic evaluation of affected organ(s) or site(s): to provide diagnosis

Advanced or Confirmatory Testing

- If lymphoma is identified cytologically, the following tests are indicated for staging before initiation of chemotherapy:
  - ± Biopsy of affected organ(s): for definitive diagnosis and histologic grading
  - Thoracic radiographs: to identify lymphadenopathy, cranial mediastinal mass, pleural effusion, pulmonary involvement
  - Abdominal ultrasound exam: to identify hepatic, splenic, renal, or GI involvement, lymphadenopathy, or other sites of lymphoma
  - Bone marrow aspiration for cytologic exam (p. 1068): to identify marrow involvement and/or develop better understanding of the cause of cytopenias
  - Phenotyping (flow cytometry, polymerase chain reaction [PCR] for antigen receptor rearrangement [PARR], immunocytochemistry, immunohistochemistry): to determine B-cell versus T-cell origin
- If financial restrictions prohibit these tests, one may elect to omit certain tests (e.g., if CBC results are unremarkable, okay to omit a bone marrow aspiration), provided client understands that sites of disease may be missed and staging and follow-up monitoring will be less certain.

TREATMENT

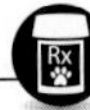

Treatment Overview

Treatment involves administration of chemotherapy to achieve complete remission while maintaining good quality of life for the patient. Special drug-handling requirements and potentially severe or life-threatening adverse patient effects exist with many chemotherapeutics; these concerns and rapid evolution of protocols warrant consultation with/referral to an oncologist.

Acute and Chronic Treatment

- Reports on single-agent chemotherapy, including prednisone, doxorubicin, mitoxantrone, and CCNU (lomustine) describe remission rates of 9%-40%, with remissions of 3-12 months. Prednisone may be used as a single agent. Although less clear in cats, its use before initiation of other chemotherapy should be avoided because it may decrease response to other agents.
  - Prednisolone 20-40 mg/m^2 PO q 24-48h as long as a clinical response is seen: mean survival of 1 month with spinal lymphoma
  - CCNU: 22% complete remission rate for median of 10 months in cats with intermediate-large cell GI lymphoma
  - Doxorubicin: 26% complete remission rate for median of 3 months
- Improved remission rates and durations are achieved with combination chemotherapy. Numerous protocols are reported with variations in scheduling, drug dosages, and dose intensity, with most using induction followed by maintenance chemotherapy. The most commonly used agents in these protocols include prednisone, L-asparaginase, vincristine, cyclophosphamide, and doxorubicin (p. 602). Complete response rates are between 50% and 70%, with remission of approximately 5-9 months. Options may include one of the following:
  - COP (p. 602): approximately 50% complete remission rate for median of 3-8 months, *or*
  - CHOP (p. 602): 40%-70% complete remission rate for median of 7-9 months (up to 18 months in one study); in cats with discrete high-grade GI lymphoma treated with surgical resection followed by CHOP, median 12-month disease-free interval reported, *or*
  - COP induction + doxorubicin maintenance: 47% complete remission rate for median of 9 months, *or*
  - Combination (cyclophosphamide, vincristine, prednisone, L-asparaginase, doxorubicin, methotrexate): 38%-74% complete remission rate for median of 9-22 months
- Studies have suggested that discontinuous chemotherapy protocols provide remission duration comparable to more traditional protocols relying on induction followed by maintenance chemotherapy.
  - 12-week CHOP: 46% complete remission for median of 13 months
- When a patient relapses and no longer responds to front-line chemotherapy, rescue chemotherapy can be considered with protocols such as MOPP (mechlorethamine, vincristine, procarbazine, prednisolone) or CCNU.
- Chemotherapy remains standard therapy. However, its use in combination with other treatment modalities, such as radiation therapy, may improve outcome. Whole-abdomen radiation therapy after abbreviated induction chemotherapy is well tolerated; efficacy studies are ongoing.
- Given the chronic indolent course of low-grade lymphoma, orally administered chemotherapy (chlorambucil and prednisolone) may be more appropriate than intensive, injectable chemotherapy for these cats.
  - Chlorambucil 6-8 mg/m^2 PO q 48h as long as clinical response is seen and prednisolone 20-40 mg/m^2 PO q 24-48h for 4-6 months or as long as clinical response is seen: 56%-69% complete remission rate for median of 21-30 months.
  - Cats with low-grade alimentary lymphoma often have hypocobalaminemia; testing or empiric cobalamin (vitamin B_{12}) supplementation is recommended (p. 183).
- Radiation therapy may be considered for nasal lymphoma.
  - Disease-free intervals of 6-69 months are reported after radiation therapy.
  - It has been suggested that radiation therapy, chemotherapy, or a combination of both modalities yields comparable survival times.

Possible Complications

- Systemic chemotherapy targets rapidly dividing cells. Due to their rapid and often abnormal division and defective repair mechanisms, tumor cells can be destroyed by chemotherapy.
- Some normal tissues have a high rate of cell turnover (GI mucosa, bone marrow, hair) and may be sensitive to chemotherapy, although unlike cancer cells, these normal tissues can repair chemotherapy-induced damage. Potential side effects of chemotherapy include GI upset 2-4 days after treatment, myelosuppression 7-10 days after treatment, and loss of whiskers (p. 152).
- All chemotherapeutic agents are potentially toxic, most are mutagenic or teratogenic, and at least some are proven carcinogens. Safe handling requires use of a vertical flow hood and closed-system drug transfer device.

Recommended Monitoring

- Regular monitoring of remission status
  - Complete remission: disappearance of all clinical evidence of cancer
  - Partial remission: decrease in volume of cancer by ≥ 50% without decrease to completely normal size
  - Stable disease: decrease in volume of cancer by < 50% or increase in volume of cancer by < 25%
  - Progressive disease: increase in cancer volume by ≥ 25% or appearance of new lesions
- CBC (including differential) monitoring after administration of chemotherapy

PROGNOSIS & OUTCOME

Several prognostic factors may help predict an individual's response to treatment:

- Stage of disease, including substage (asymptomatic vs. signs of systemic illness)
- Anatomic site of disease (mediastinal lymphoma may have a higher complete remission rate than other anatomic sites; nasal lymphoma has among the longest survival times)
- Histologic grade (low-grade lymphoma is often associated with longer remission and survival times with less intensive chemotherapy due to its chronic indolent nature)

BSA Correlations for Cats

Weight, kg (lb)	BSA, m^2
2 (4.5)	0.159
2.5 (5.5)	0.184
3 (6.5)	0.208
3.5 (7.75)	0.231
4 (8.75)	0.252
4.5 (10)	0.273
5 (11)	0.292
5.5 (12.25)	0.311
6 (13.25)	0.33
6.5 (14.25)	0.348
7 (15.5)	0.366
7.5 (16.5)	0.383
8 (17.5)	0.4
8.5 (18.75)	0.416
9 (19.75)	0.432
9.5 (21)	0.449
10 (22)	0.464

BSA, Body weight–to–body surface area correlation.

- FeLV status does not appear to influence rates of response to chemotherapy, but FeLV-positive cats have significantly shorter remission and survival times, possibly due in part to concurrent FeLV-related diseases.

PEARLS & CONSIDERATIONS

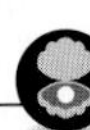

Comments

- Lymphoma is a common feline malignancy.
- The majority of cats can achieve complete or partial remission when treated with chemotherapy, and treatment can be rewarding for the pet owner and veterinarian.
- A variety of prognostic factors has been identified that may help predict an individual's response to treatment and guide the decision about whether to pursue treatment.
- An understanding of the relative efficacy and potential toxicoses of the various protocols aids in determining the best treatment protocol for an individual animal.

Technician Tips

Technicians handling chemotherapeutic drugs must have received appropriate training regarding drug handling, avoidance of unintended exposure, proper disposal, management of spills, and other complications.

SUGGESTED READING

Vail DM: Feline lymphoma and leukemia. In Withrow SJ, et al, editors: Withrow & MacEwen's Small animal clinical oncology, St. Louis, 2013, Saunders, pp 638-653.

AUTHOR: Laurel E. Williams, DVM, DACVIM
EDITOR: Kenneth M. Rassnick, DVM, DACVIM

Lymphoma, Multicentric (Dog)

Client Education Sheet 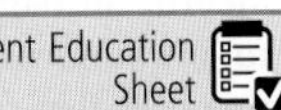

BASIC INFORMATION

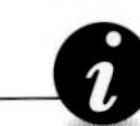

Definition

Well-recognized systemic malignant neoplasm of lymphoid origin

Synonyms

Lymphosarcoma, malignant lymphoma, non-Hodgkin lymphoma (human)

Epidemiology

SPECIES, AGE, SEX

- Most common canine hematopoietic malignancy: reported incidence of 24-114 cases per 100,000 dogs
- Typically middle-aged to older dogs, although may develop at any age
- No sex predisposition

GENETICS, BREED PREDISPOSITION

- Several breeds reported to be at increased risk, including golden retrievers, boxers, rottweilers, Scottish terriers, basset hounds, cocker spaniels, German shepherds, Airedales, bulldogs, and poodles; certain breeds (e.g., boxers) may be more likely to develop T-cell lymphoma.
- Genetic predisposition reported for a pedigree of bullmastiffs and a family of rottweilers and otter hounds

RISK FACTORS

- Reported association with 2,4-D herbicide use, but subsequent study nonconfirmatory
- Reported positive association with electromagnetic radiation exposure
- Residing in industrial areas and use of paints or solvents by owners reported to increase risk of lymphoma by 8.5- and 4.6-fold, respectively.
- Reported associations between hazardous waste emissions and lymphoma and for secondhand smoke and lymphoma in Italy

ASSOCIATED DISORDERS

Hypercalcemia secondary to elaboration of parathormone–related protein (PTH-rP) by tumor cells

Clinical Presentation

DISEASE FORMS/SUBTYPES

- Histologic grade
  - High-grade or lymphoblastic lymphoma: most common; rapid onset and progression; affected cells are large and blastic in appearance.
  - Low-grade or lymphocytic lymphoma: rare; chronic insidious onset; affected cells are well differentiated and similar in appearance to small lymphocytes.
- Stage: based on disease location/extent (e.g, lymph node, liver, spleen)

HISTORY, CHIEF COMPLAINT

- Generalized lymphadenopathy most common
- Owners usually report rapid increases in lymph node size over days to a few weeks.
- Lymph nodes generally are not painful, and dogs usually appear otherwise healthy in early stages of disease.
- Some patients present with nonspecific signs such as anorexia, weight loss, vomiting, diarrhea, dyspnea, fever, or polyuria.

PHYSICAL EXAM FINDINGS

- Marked generalized lymphadenopathy is most common physical exam finding, although occasionally, dogs present with only single or regional lymph node enlargement or single organ (e.g., spleen, gastrointestinal tract, thymus) involvement with or without regional lymph node enlargement.
- Hepatosplenomegaly may be noted in dogs with visceral involvement.
- Other findings, including dyspnea, fever, neurologic signs, may be reflective of other organ involvement or disease complications.

Etiology and Pathophysiology

- Rapid onset and disease progression due to malignant lymphocytes
- If untreated, most dogs succumb to disease in 1-2 months.

DIAGNOSIS

Diagnostic Overview

Diagnosis suspected based on marked generalized lymphadenopathy with minimal to no associated clinical signs in an otherwise healthy, middle-aged to older dog; confirmation begins with cytologic analysis of affected lymph node.

Lymphoma Staging

Stage	Characteristics
I	Single lymph node
II	Multiple regional lymph nodes
III	Generalized lymphadenopathy
IV	Hepatic and/or splenic involvement (± stages I-III)
V	Involvement of bone marrow, blood, and/or any nonlymphoid organ (± stages I-IV)
Substage a	No overt clinical signs of disease
Substage b	Overt clinical signs of disease

Differential Diagnosis

- Reactive lymphadenopathy
  - Infectious diseases (e.g., ehrlichiosis, bartonellosis, systemic mycotic infection)
  - Sepsis
  - Pyoderma causing lymphadenopathy
- Other neoplasms (e.g., leukemia, disseminated histiocytic sarcoma)

Initial Database

- CBC: to identify anemia, thrombocytopenia (due to lymphoblast infiltration in marrow or immune-mediated destruction), neutropenia, or circulating lymphoblasts (i.e., leukemia)
- Serum biochemistry panel: to identify paraneoplastic hypercalcemia or identify liver or renal value abnormalities that suggest organ involvement and may alter ability to metabolize chemotherapeutic agents
- Urinalysis ± urine culture and sensitivity: to identify urinary tract infections secondary to immunocompromise; to identify isosthenuria that, if associated with azotemia, suggests kidney disease (e.g., hypercalcemia-induced)
- Lymph node (or affected organ) aspiration and cytologic exam: may provide a definitive diagnosis of lymphoma

Advanced or Confirmatory Testing

- If lymphoma is identified cytologically, the following tests are indicated as routine staging before initiation of chemotherapy:
  - Lymph node biopsy: for definitive diagnosis, histologic grading, and possibly immunophenotyping
  - Thoracic radiographs: to identify lymphadenopathy, cranial mediastinal mass, pulmonary involvement
  - Abdominal ultrasound exam: to identify changes consistent with hepatic or splenic involvement, lymphadenopathy, or other sites of lymphoma
  - Bone marrow aspiration for cytologic evaluation (p. 1068): to identify marrow involvement and/or develop better understanding of etiology of cytopenias
- Phenotyping (flow cytometry, polymerase chain reaction [PCR] for antigen receptor rearrangement [PARR], immunohistochemistry): to determine B-cell versus T-cell origin
- If financial restrictions prohibit these tests, one may elect to omit certain tests (e.g., if CBC results are unremarkable, okay to omit bone marrow aspiration), provided the client understands that sites of disease may be missed and stage is uncertain.

TREATMENT

Treatment Overview

Treatment involves administration of chemotherapy to promote rapid complete remission (CR) of cancer while maintaining excellent quality of life for the patient. Special drug-handling requirements and potentially severe or life-threatening adverse patient effects exist with many chemotherapeutics; these concerns and rapid evolution of protocols warrant consultation with/referral to an oncologist.

Acute General Treatment

- Reports on single-agent chemotherapy, including prednisone, L-asparaginase, cyclophosphamide, doxorubicin, and rabacfosadine, describe response rates of 20%-80%, with remissions of 1-6 months. Although prednisone may be used as a single agent, its use before initiation of other chemotherapy should be avoided because this practice may decrease response to other agents.
  - Prednisone 30-40 mg/m^2 PO q 24h for 2-4 weeks, then continued at 20-40 mg/m^2 q 24-48h as long as clinical response is seen
  - Doxorubicin 50%-75% CR rate for 4-6 months
- Reports on dual-agent chemotherapy involving alternating rabacfosadine/doxorubicin report overall response rate of 85% with remission of 6 months.
- Improved remission rates and duration are achieved with combination chemotherapy. Numerous protocols are reported with variations in scheduling, drug dosages, and dose intensity, with most treatment protocols being of 6-12 months' duration. The most commonly used agents in these protocols include prednisone, L-asparaginase (some studies suggest that although very effective for inducing remission and associated with low risk of complications, inclusion of L-asparaginase may not significantly impact outcome for all patients), vincristine, cyclophosphamide, and doxorubicin. CR rates are 65%-90%, with remissions of approximately 6-11 months. Options may include
  - COP (p. 603): 70%-75% CR rate for median of 3-6 months, *or*
  - CHOP (p. 603): 80% CR rate for median of 9-10 months
- Several studies have suggested that discontinuous (i.e., 4-6 months) chemotherapy protocols provide remission duration comparable to more traditional protocols relying on induction followed by maintenance (i.e., up to 2-3 years) chemotherapy.
- Chemotherapy remains standard therapy; however, its use in combination with other treatment modalities, such as radiation therapy or bone marrow transplantation (BMT), may improve remission duration.
  - Half-body radiation therapy (HBRT) after shortened induction chemotherapy: results vary from superior (87% CR rate for median of 14 months) to not significantly different (66% CR rate for median of 8 months) from treatment without HBRT.
  - BMT in dogs achieving remission with chemotherapy may also improve outcome, with 90% successful engraftment reported and median disease-free intervals of 6 and 9 months, for T-cell and B-cell lymphoma, respectively, after BMT.
- Low-grade lymphoma: given the chronic indolent course of low-grade lymphoma, oral chemotherapy, consisting of chlorambucil 6-8 mg/m^2 PO q 48h as long as clinical response is seen and prednisone 20-40 mg/m^2 PO q 24-48h for 4-6 months or as long as clinical response is seen, may be more appropriate than intensive, injectable chemotherapy for this group of dogs.
- When a patient relapses and no longer responds to front-line chemotherapy, rescue chemotherapy can be considered. CR rates for relapsed lymphoma are generally lower, ranging from approximately 30%-50%, with remission durations of approximately 2-4 months (p. 612).

Nutrition/Diet

Dogs with lymphoma have alterations in carbohydrate, protein, and lipid metabolism and may benefit from a low-carbohydrate/moderate-quantity, high-quality protein diet. Supplementation with polyunsaturated fatty acids may also be of benefit.

Possible Complications

- Systemic chemotherapy targets rapidly dividing cells. Due to their rapid and often abnormal division and defective repair mechanisms, tumor cells can be destroyed by chemotherapy.
- Some normal tissues have a high rate of cell turnover (gastrointestinal mucosa, bone marrow, hair) and may be sensitive to chemotherapy, although unlike cancer cells, normal tissues can repair chemotherapy-induced damage. Potential side effects of chemotherapy include gastrointestinal upset 2-4 days after treatment, myelosuppression 7-10 days after treatment, and hair loss in breeds with continuously growing haircoats (e.g., poodle, Lhasa apso, Old English sheepdog, many terrier breeds [p. 152]).
- All chemotherapeutic agents are potentially toxic, most are mutagenic or teratogenic, and at least some are proven carcinogens. Safe handling requires the use of a vertical flow hood and closed-system drug transfer device.

Recommended Monitoring

- Regular monitoring of remission status (e.g., longest diameter of lymph node [LD])
  - CR: disappearance of all evidence of disease
  - Partial response (PR): ≥ 30% decrease in mean sum LD of target lesions compared with baseline
  - Stable disease (SD): insufficient decrease/increase to qualify for PR/PD
  - Progressive disease (PD): ≥ 20% increase in mean sum LD compared with smallest mean sum LD or progression of nontarget lesions
- CBC (including differential) monitoring after administration of chemotherapy

PROGNOSIS & OUTCOME

Several prognostic factors may help predict an individual's response to treatment:

BSA Correlations for Dogs

Weight, kg (lb)	BSA, m²	Weight, kg (lb)	BSA, m²
0.5 (1)	0.06	41 (90)	1.19
1 (2)	0.1	42 (92.5)	1.21
2 (4.5)	0.15	43 (94.5)	1.23
3 (6.5)	0.2	44 (97)	1.25
4 (9)	0.25	45 (99)	1.26
5 (11)	0.29	46 (101)	1.28
6 (13)	0.33	47 (103.5)	1.3
7 (15.5)	0.36	48 (105.5)	1.32
8 (17.5)	0.40	49 (108)	1.34
9 (20)	0.43	50 (110)	1.36
10 (22)	0.46	51 (112)	1.39
11 (24.5)	0.49	52 (114.5)	1.41
12 (26.5)	0.52	53 (116.5)	1.43
13 (28.5)	0.55	54 (119)	1.44
14 (31)	0.58	55 (121)	1.46
15 (33)	0.6	56 (123)	1.48
16 (35)	0.63	57 (125.5)	1.5
17 (37.5)	0.66	58 (127.5)	1.51
18 (39.5)	0.69	59 (130)	1.53
19 (42)	0.71	60 (132)	1.55
20 (44)	0.74	61 (134)	1.57
21 (46)	0.76	62 (136.5)	1.58
22 (48.5)	0.78	63 (138.5)	1.6
23 (50.5)	0.81	64 (141)	1.62
24 (53)	0.83	65 (143)	1.64
25 (55)	0.85	66 (145)	1.65
26 (57)	0.88	67 (147.5)	1.67
27 (59.5)	0.9	68 (149.5)	1.68
28 (61.5)	0.92	69 (152)	1.7
29 (64)	0.94	70 (154)	1.72
30 (66)	0.96	71 (156)	1.74
31 (68)	0.99	72 (158.5)	1.75
32 (70.5)	1.01	73 (160.5)	1.77
33 (72.5)	1.03	74 (163)	1.78
34 (75)	1.05	75 (165)	1.8
35 (77)	1.07	76 (167)	1.81
36 (79)	1.09	77 (169.5)	1.83
37 (81.5)	1.11	78 (171.5)	1.84
38 (83.5)	1.13	79 (174)	1.86
39 (86)	1.15	80 (176.5)	1.88
40 (88)	1.17		

BSA, Body weight–to–body surface area correlation.

- Sex (females better than males)
- Weight (small dogs better than large dogs, although possibly influenced by dosing regimen)
- Histologic grade (high-grade lymphoma has a higher CR rate than low-grade lymphoma, although low-grade lymphoma is often associated with comparable survival times with less intensive chemotherapy due to its chronic indolent nature)
- Stage and substage (I, II, or III better than IV or V; a better than b)
- Phenotype (B-cell better than T-cell lymphoma)
- Hypercalcemia (negative prognostic indicator, likely due to association with T-cell phenotype)
- Mediastinal mass (negative prognostic indicator, likely due to association with T-cell phenotype)
- Serum markers: thymidine kinase (sTK), lactate dehydrogenase (LDH), ferritin
- Administration of prior prednisone (negative prognostic indicator, possibly due to induction of multidrug resistance or masking of higher-stage disease)
- Other factors impacting prognosis: Ki67, AgNOR (argyrophilic nucleolar organizer region) staining, modified Glasgow prognostic score (mGPS), *CCND1* gene expression, chromosomal aberrations, older age, anorexia, anemia, fever, dyspnea, thrombocytopenia, hypoalbuminemia, and chronic inflammatory disease

PEARLS & CONSIDERATIONS

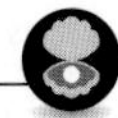

Comments

- Lymphoma is a common canine malignancy.
- The majority of dogs with lymphoma can achieve a CR when treated with chemotherapy, and treatment can be very rewarding for the pet owner and veterinarian.
- Identification of prognostic factors may help predict an individual's response to treatment and guide the decision on whether to pursue treatment.
- An understanding of the relative efficacy and potential toxicoses of the various protocols aids in determining the best treatment protocol for an individual animal.
- Differentiation of cell type (phenotype) is prognostic and may guide treatment decisions. B-cell lymphoma carries a more favorable prognosis than T-cell lymphoma ("B is better"), and B-cell lymphoma makes up the majority of cases of lymphoma in dogs.

Technician Tips

Technicians handling chemotherapeutic drugs must have received appropriate training regarding drug handling, avoidance of unintended exposure, proper disposal, management of spills, and other complications.

SUGGESTED READING

Vail DM: Canine lymphoma and lymphoid leukemias. In Withrow SJ, et al, editors: Withrow & MacEwen's Small animal clinical oncology, St. Louis, 2013, Saunders, pp 608-638.

AUTHOR: Laurel E. Williams, DVM, DACVIM
EDITOR: Kenneth M. Rassnick, DVM, DACVIM

Lymphoma Rescue Therapy

Client Education Sheets 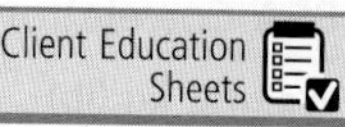

BASIC INFORMATION 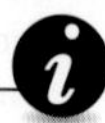

Definition

Rescue therapy attempts to induce remission in a patient with lymphoma that has failed first-line treatment or establish remission in a patient that has relapsed after previous treatment. *Relapse* is the return of signs of disease in a patient that previously attained and maintained clinical remission (CR) for at least 30 days after completion of treatment.

Synonyms

Reinduction therapy

Epidemiology

SPECIES, AGE, SEX

Dogs and cats, any age, either sex

RISK FACTORS

- Previous diagnosis of lymphoma (by definition)
- Immunophenotype (e.g., T cell)
- Anatomic location (e.g., gastrointestinal [GI], cutaneous)
- Poor treatment protocol compliance
- Pretreatment with corticosteroids (controversial)

Clinical Presentation

HISTORY, CHIEF COMPLAINT

- Relapse of lymphoma is usually determined by recognizing disease in the same organs(s) and/or tissue(s) where it was initially detected.
- Systemic signs (lethargy, inappetence, weakness, polyuria/polydipsia)
- Palpable mass (enlarged lymph node[s]; less commonly, primary neoplasm)

PHYSICAL EXAM FINDINGS

- Can include, but is not limited to, generalized lymphadenopathy, organomegaly, uveitis, pallor, and fever (pp. 607 and 609)
- Regular monitoring of disease status after treatment, including measuring and recording lymph node size, can allow early detection of relapse (NOTE: other tests performed at monitoring exams, such as bloodwork and possibly imaging studies, are often appropriate).

Etiology and Pathophysiology

- The main cause of lymphoma relapse is resistance to chemotherapy, which can be caused by pharmacokinetic factors (e.g., inability to achieve adequate drug concentrations in certain anatomic regions), inherent factors (e.g., measurable tumors are likely to contain 10-1000 inherently resistant cells), and acquired drug resistance (e.g., reduced drug uptake and/or accumulation).
- P-glycoprotein (P-gp/gp-170) is an example of an ATP-dependent efflux pump that extrudes cytotoxins and other harmful chemicals from cells. P-glycoprotein overexpression is a major contributor to the multidrug resistance (MDR) phenotype, causing simultaneous resistance to vinca alkaloids, doxorubicin, prednisone, and other drugs.
- Relapse of lymphoma can also result from controllable factors, including inadequate dosing (e.g., empirical dose reductions to reduce potential or actual side effects), inadequate treatment intervals (e.g., owners electing to postpone treatments), and pretreatment with corticosteroids (controversial).

DIAGNOSIS 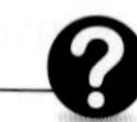

Diagnostic Overview

Relapse is suspected in a patient with lymphoma that has recurrence of node enlargement or organomegaly during a course of chemotherapy or after completion of a chemotherapy protocol. Patients typically have recurrent signs of illness similar to those at diagnosis of lymphoma. Relapse can be confirmed similar to diagnosis (e.g., using fine-needle aspirates of enlarged lymph nodes).

Differential Diagnosis

Nonspecific signs (lethargy, inappetence) may occur with disease relapse or with adverse effects of recently administered chemotherapy. Infectious disease, potentially related to therapeutic immunosuppression, can cause similar signs. Exam findings can help clarify the difference in some patients, whereas advanced testing (e.g., imaging) is needed in other patients to identify occult lymphoma.

Initial Database

- A minimal database, including CBC, serum biochemical panel, and urinalysis, can help rule out alternative diagnosis (e.g., infection), recognize changes related to lymphoma (e.g., hypercalcemia), and help select an optimal rescue protocol.
- Fine-needle aspiration and cytologic analysis of abnormal tissue (e.g., enlarged lymph nodes, spleen) can often provide a definitive diagnosis of relapse.
- Imaging studies, as guided by history (e.g., thoracic radiographs if respiratory signs present), physical exam (e.g., abdominal radiographs if splenomegaly present), or results of minimal database (e.g., abdominal ultrasound if liver enzymes increased)

Advanced or Confirmatory Testing

Diagnostic testing is guided by the specific clinical signs that are noted when relapse is confirmed.

- Serial exams (e.g., every few weeks), analysis of lymph nodes by flow cytometry, or polymerase chain reaction (PCR) for antigen receptor rearrangement (PARR) analysis may be needed for some patients.
- Bone marrow aspiration for cytologic analysis (p. 1068): to clarify cause of cytopenias

TREATMENT 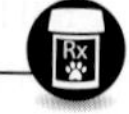

Treatment Overview

- The goal of rescue treatment for lymphoma is to reduce disease burden below that which causes clinical signs, while simultaneously avoiding adverse effects.
- Consultation with a veterinary oncologist is strongly recommended for treatment of relapsed disease.
- If the relapse interval is > 2 months after cessation of treatment, remission reinduction is attempted using the induction protocol that was initially successful.
- If the relapse interval is < 2 months after the cessation of treatment, reinduction using the initial protocol can be attempted, but rescue protocols may be more effective options in many cases.
- If reinduction chemotherapy does not achieve remission and the patient is resistant to first-line therapy: typically, single-drug or combination protocols that use drugs not employed in previous or standard protocols (e.g., CHOP: cyclophosphamide, hydroxydaunorubicin [doxorubicin], Oncovin [vincristine], and prednisone).
- Although achieving CR is ideal, in the rescue protocol setting, maintenance of a strong partial remission (PR) can also be a successful plan, as long as clinical signs resolve. Selecting a protocol that minimizes toxicosis while maximizing the chance of response is ideal.
- Many factors influence the choice and sequence of rescue protocols, including pet owner factors (e.g., cost, time commitment, concern about side effects), and clinician factors (e.g., limited access or experience with drugs, lack of experience with potential side effects, facilities).
- Rescue protocols may be inappropriate for animals with relapsed lymphoma that are ill from their disease (e.g., not eating and drinking on their own) because the chance of causing further adverse effects would likely exceed any potential benefit.

Acute General Treatment

Although the mainstay of treatment for relapsed lymphoma is chemotherapy, supportive care may be necessary for overtly ill patients before starting treatment (pp. 602 and 603).

Chronic Treatment

Consultation with or referral to a veterinary oncologist is recommended because of the complex nature of disease relapse. Special handling requirements and potentially life-threatening adverse effects exist with many of the following antineoplastic drugs.

Dogs:

- Alkylating agents are not affected by the MDR phenotype and rarely show cross-resistance to each other, making drugs in this class a good choice for rescue therapy:
  - Lomustine (CCNU) as single agent: 27% response rate for median of 86 days
  - LAP protocol (lomustine, L-asparaginase, and prednisone): 77% response rate (65% CR) for median of 70 days
  - Lomustine and dacarbazine (DTIC): 23% CR rate for median of 83 days, 12% PR rate for median of 25 days
  - MOPP protocol (mechlorethamine, vincristine [Oncovin], procarbazine, and prednisone): 31% CR for median of 63 days and 34% PR for median of 46 days
  - LOPP protocol (lomustine, vincristine, procarbazine, and prednisolone): 50%-61% overall response rate for median remission duration of 93-140 days
  - BOPP protocol (carmustine, vincristine, procarbazine, and prednisolone): 52% overall response rate (median CR duration, 112 days; PR duration, 85 days)
  - MOMP protocol (mechlorethamine, vincristine, melphalan, and prednisone): 12% CR rate for median of 81 days and 39% PR rate for median of 49 days
  - MPP protocol (mechlorethamine, melphalan, and prednisone): 17% CR rate for median of 238 days and 17% PR rate for median of 56 days
  - DMAC protocol (dexamethasone, melphalan, actinomycin D, and cytosine arabinoside): 44% CR rate for median of 112 days and 28% PR rate for median of 44 days
  - ADIC protocol (doxorubicin and dacarbazine) when resistant to single-agent doxorubicin: 33% CR rate for median < 42 days and PR in 20%
- Actinomycin D (single agent): 41% CR rate for median disease-free interval of 129 days
- Mitoxantrone (single agent): 47% CR rate for median of 84 days
- Vinblastine (single agent): 8% CR rate for median survival time of 46 days
- Combination carboplatin and cytarabine: overall response rate of 18%, with median survival time of 109 days

Cats:

- Extremely limited information (small-scale, heterogeneous studies)
- Doxorubicin ± lomustine: ≈10% CR rate, ≈10 PR rate, median progression-free interval of 39 days
- Radiation therapy (relapsed GI lymphoma): 90% response rate, 214 days median survival after radiation therapy, 355 days median overall survival time

Possible Complications

Doxorubicin cardiotoxicosis: a complete cardiac evaluation is recommended before the seventh (and before every treatment thereafter) cumulative lifetime dose in dogs, sooner if suspicion of cardiac disease (infiltration, cardiac arrhythmias) exists. Dexrazoxane can be coadministered with doxorubicin for cardioprotection.

Possible Complications

- Extensive list of potential adverse effects associated with chemotherapy agents (p. 152)
- Complications related to progression of lymphoma in any affected organ (e.g., kidney failure due to renal lymphoma, seizure due to central nervous system lymphoma, respiratory distress due to pulmonary lymphoma)

PROGNOSIS & OUTCOME

- Variety of protocols and heterogeneity of patient responses make prognoses highly varied.
- For dogs receiving rescue treatment with a CHOP protocol after having successfully completed an initial 6-month CHOP protocol, second remissions occur in 78% of cases for a median duration of 5 months. These second remissions are longer in dogs with first remissions that were > 9 months.
- Many protocols exist, and the order in which they are applied generates highly variable prognostic information. In general, 25%-50% of dogs respond to rescue therapy for a median of 2-6 months; longer and shorter times are possible.
- There is insufficient information in cats to generalize about the prognosis for rescue treatment.

PEARLS & CONSIDERATIONS

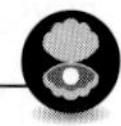

Comments

- Most cats and dogs with lymphoma experience a relapse regardless of initial therapy.
- Relapse occurs most often because neoplastic cells are resistant to treatment but may occur due to controllable (i.e., avoidable) factors.
- After resistance to first-line chemotherapy occurs, many different rescue protocols are available. Considerations for selection of rescue protocols include a combination of efficacy, side effects, cost, time commitment, and individual patient needs, including patient performance status.

Technician Tips

Technicians should be familiar with the chemotherapy drugs in rescue protocols, including proper handling, administration, disposal, anticipated reactions, and side effects.

Client Education

After relapse, treatment can often result in a second response with an excellent quality of life, but cure is not possible, and the disease will eventually relapse yet again.

SUGGESTED READING

Gustafson DL, et al: Cancer chemotherapy. In Withrow SJ, et al, editors Small animal clinical oncology, ed 5, St. Louis, 2013, Saunders, pp 157-179.

AUTHOR: Joanne L. Intile, DVM, MS, DACVIM
EDITOR: Kenneth M. Rassnick, DVM, DACVIM

Macadamia Nut Toxicosis

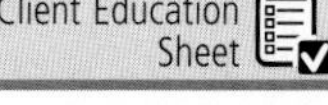

BASIC INFORMATION

Definition

- Acute and transient syndrome in dogs resulting from ingestion of macadamia nuts
- Common signs include lethargy, gastrointestinal (GI) upset, weakness, ataxia, trembling, and mild hyperthermia.

Epidemiology

SPECIES, AGE, SEX

Currently, macadamia nut toxicosis has been reported in dogs only. There does not appear to be a breed, age, or sex predisposition.

GEOGRAPHY AND SEASONALITY

Two tree species used for cultivating the edible nuts are *Macadamia integrifolia* and *Macadamia tetraphylla*. In the United States, macadamia nuts are cultivated mainly in Hawaii but are also found in Florida and California. Products containing the nuts are widely available year-round. Popularity increases during holiday seasons and risk of exposure for dogs is higher during these times.

Clinical Presentation

DISEASE FORMS/SUBTYPES

Other signs may be seen if macadamia nuts are part of a food item (e.g., chocolate toxicosis).

HISTORY, CHIEF COMPLAINT

- Evidence of exposure to macadamia nuts
- Macadamia nuts in stool or vomitus
- Presence of consistent clinical signs

PHYSICAL EXAM FINDINGS

- Lethargy, depression
- Vomiting, abdominal pain
- Ataxia, weakness (hindlimb > forelimb), tremors or trembling, muscle stiffness
- Hyperthermia

Etiology and Pathophysiology

- The mechanism of action for macadamia nut toxicosis in dogs is not known.
- 1 g/kg may warrant decontamination and monitoring (average weight is 2.6-5 g/nut).
    - Severity of signs correlates with dosage

DIAGNOSIS

Diagnostic Overview

The diagnosis is based on the history of known or suspected exposure to macadamia nuts and development of consistent clinical signs, usually within 12 hours of exposure. There are no diagnostic tests available.

Differential Diagnosis

- Toxins (e.g., ethanol, avermectins, barbiturates, benzodiazepines, DL-methionine, black walnut, organic fertilizer, bromethalin, ethylene glycol, marijuana, tremorgens)
- Orthopedic disorders
- Neuromuscular disorders
- Pancreatitis
- Infectious diseases
- Trauma
- Electrolyte disturbances
- Spinal disease

Initial Database

- Complete physical exam to rule out other causes for the signs
- Abdominal radiographs may reveal large amount of ingesta in stomach.
- Examine stomach contents (if vomiting) and feces for evidence of macadamia nuts.
- Serum biochemistry profile: mild elevations of serum triglycerides, lipase, and alkaline phosphatase have been reported; mild changes are expected to return to normal within 48 hours.

Advanced or Confirmatory Testing

Diagnostic lab tests as needed to rule out other causes for the signs

TREATMENT

Treatment Overview

Decontamination with emesis if exposure is recent and no signs are present. Activated charcoal is not typically indicated. Provide symptomatic and supportive care as needed. Many cases are self-limited and can be managed on an outpatient basis. Consider antiemetic, IV fluids, and thermoregulation for significant signs. Complications are rare, and signs are expected to resolve in 12-48 hours.

Acute General Treatment

- Decontamination of patient (p. 1087):
    - Emesis (within 4 hours of ingestion in asymptomatic dog) (p. 1188)
    - Apomorphine 0.03-0.04 mg/kg IV or IM, or crush tablet portion with water and instill into conjunctival sac, rinsing after emesis, *or*
    - Hydrogen peroxide 3% 2.2 mL/kg, max dose 45 mL PO, repeat in 10-15 minutes if no vomiting
    - Activated charcoal: not recommended. Macadamia nut toxicosis is not life-threatening, and there is some risk for potentially life-threatening complications associated with activated charcoal (e.g., aspiration pneumonia, hypernatremia).
    - Warm tap water enema 5-10 mL/kg may be considered for large ingestions to reduce transit time through the GI tract and potentially shorten the duration of signs.
- Symptomatic and supportive care
    - Antiemetic: maropitant 1 mg/kg SQ q 24h
    - IV fluids: if tremors, monitor urine color for myoglobinuria
    - Thermoregulation
    - Methocarbamol 55-220 mg/kg IV, repeat as needed; max dose (330 mg/kg/day) may be used to control tremors but is usually not needed

Possible Complications

Pancreatitis can be seen if macadamia nuts are part of baked goods or other food items.

Recommended Monitoring

In severe cases, monitor temperature, hydration status, and electrolytes.

PROGNOSIS & OUTCOME

Full recovery is expected within 12-48 hours.

PEARLS & CONSIDERATIONS

Comments

- Avoid overly aggressive decontamination and treatment. Activated charcoal may pose more serious risks than macadamia nut toxicosis and is not indicated in these cases.
- Ask owners about other potential concerns for toxicosis regarding the macadamia nut product, such as chocolate coating (p. 159), onion/garlic (p. 707), and spices.

Prevention

Keep all macadamia nuts away from dogs.

Technician Tips

If the dog is managed as an outpatient, advise owners to confine (away from furniture and stairs) at home to prevent injury if ataxia or weakness develops. Discuss nursing care, such as offering food and water by hand and assisting walking with a sling to facilitate elimination outside.

Client Education

Assure clients that the signs of macadamia nut toxicosis are transient and not life-threatening.

SUGGESTED READING

Gwaltney-Brant SM: Macadamia nuts. In Peterson ME, et al, editors: Small animal toxicology, ed 3, St. Louis, 2013, Elsevier, pp 625-627.

AUTHOR: Colette Wegenast, DVM
EDITOR: Tina Wismer, DVM, MS, DABVT, DABT

Malassezia Dermatitis

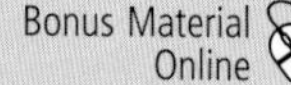
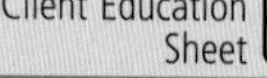
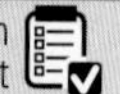

Bonus Material Online   Client Education Sheet

BASIC INFORMATION

Definition

This very common pruritic dermatosis is caused by the overgrowth of *Malassezia* spp yeast. Most infections are caused by the lipophilic unicellular organism *Malassezia pachydermatis.*

Epidemiology

SPECIES, AGE, SEX

Very common in dogs of all ages; uncommon in cats of any age; either sex

GENETICS, BREED PREDISPOSITION

- May occur in any breed of dog or cat
- Terriers, shih tzu, dachshund, Shar-pei, spaniel, basset hound, and German shepherd dogs seem to be predisposed, likely due to underlying conditions favorable to yeast overgrowth.
- Devon rex cats are more susceptible.

RISK FACTORS

- Excessive sebum production, poor sebum quality, cutaneous moisture accumulation (particularly in skin folds), a disrupted epidermal surface, and altered host immune defenses. These alterations are often the result of primary underlying diseases (e.g., allergy, endocrinopathy).
- Specific predisposing disorders include allergic skin disease (e.g., atopic dermatitis, food allergy, flea allergy, contact allergy), endocrinopathies (e.g., iatrogenic or spontaneous hyperadrenocorticism, hypothyroidism, hyperthyroidism, diabetes mellitus), primary or secondary cornification disorders, metabolic diseases (e.g., superficial necrolytic dermatitis, zinc-responsive dermatosis), nutritional deficiencies, cutaneous or internal neoplasia, and in cats, retroviral infections

CONTAGION AND ZOONOSIS

Malassezia yeasts have been transmitted from the contaminated hands of dog-owning health care workers to infants in an intensive care nursery, causing mycotic sepsis. *Malassezia* yeast should be considered a potential zoonotic agent, especially for immune-incompetent individuals.

GEOGRAPHY AND SEASONALITY

Malassezia dermatitis can occur more frequently in humid geographic regions and/or with underlying causes that worsen seasonally (e.g., atopic dermatitis).

Clinical Presentation

DISEASE FORMS/SUBTYPES

- Localized dermatitis: involving the face (perioral, muzzle, ears), ventral aspect of the trunk (neck, axillae, inguinal area), perineal region (ventral tail, perianal area), and paw (interdigital web and nail fold)
- Generalized dermatitis: involving several regions, as noted above

HISTORY, CHIEF COMPLAINT

- Intense pruritus: most common complaint
- Rancid offensive odor, an oily coat, alopecia, redness/erythroderma, lichenification, scaling, and/or relapsing and remitting dermatitis unresponsive to antibiotics or antipruritics are frequently observed.

PHYSICAL EXAM FINDINGS

- Skin lesions reflect existing pruritus and seborrhea and are not specific to *Malassezia* dermatitis.
- Lesional skin may be erythematous, hyperpigmented, hyperkeratotic, lichenified, scaly, greasy or dry, alopecic, saliva stained, and excoriated. Hyperpigmented lichenification implies chronicity.
- Intertriginous areas (skin folds) are typically affected. Occasionally, yellow/orange to slate gray seborrheic plaques are present in body folds.
- A brown, waxy discharge may be observed in the claw folds with extension onto the claws proper, signifying paronychia.
- Follicular casts (keratosebaceous material adhered to the proximal hair shaft) may suggest an underlying keratinization disorder.
- Cats, particularly Devon rexes, may present with alopecia, erythema, and greasy exudation of the axillae, groin, and paws. In some cats, the only manifestation is otitis externa with dark, waxy secretion.

Etiology and Pathophysiology

Malassezia spp. yeasts are part of the normal skin microbiota. They become opportunistic invaders when changes occur in the cutaneous microclimate (e.g., lipid composition, relative humidity) or defense mechanisms (e.g., epidermal barrier dysfunction, immunosuppression). After colonization takes place, yeasts release proteases and lipases that alter cutaneous homeostasis, allowing continued yeast overgrowth. In some atopic dogs, *Malassezia* may elicit a type 1 cutaneous hypersensitivity reaction.

DIAGNOSIS

Diagnostic Overview

Malassezia dermatitis should be considered for any pruritic dog or cat. Confirmation requires typical clinical signs, cytologic demonstration of yeast, and most importantly, response to antifungal therapy. Underlying primary conditions must be identified and corrected. Importantly, Devon rex cats may not have an identifiable predisposing disease.

Differential Diagnosis

Because *Malassezia* dermatitis is a secondary complication of an underlying disorder in most cases, identifying whether the underlying disorder (see Risk Factors above) exists in an uncomplicated state or secondary *Malassezia* dermatitis is also present is required.

Initial Database

- Skin cytologic exam is performed for every case with compatible historical/physical findings.
  - Specimens can be obtained by direct impressions, acetate tape preparations, or dry or wet swabs from representative lesions.
  - *Malassezia* are ovoid, monopolar budding yeasts that resemble the shape of footprints or peanuts. They are 3-8 microns in diameter (same size as or slightly smaller than a red blood cell).
  - Yeasts are best visualized using high-power (40×) or oil immersion (100×) microscopy.
- Multiple skin scrapings to exclude superficial and deep ectoparasites
- Especially with cats, dermatophyte culture to exclude ringworm

Advanced or Confirmatory Testing

- Biopsy and histopathologic analysis: rarely necessary
  - Suggestive but nonspecific findings include parakeratotic hyperkeratosis, epidermal hyperplasia, superficial perivascular dermatitis, and possibly eosinophilic microabscesses with or without the finding of yeast organisms.
  - Other histopathologic findings may represent changes associated with the underlying dermatosis.
- Elimination diet trial to exclude food allergy
- Intradermal and/or immunoglobulin E (IgE) serologic testing if history and clinical findings support atopic dermatitis

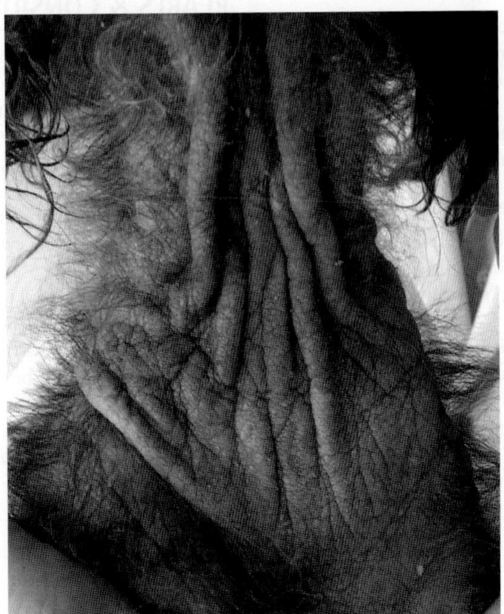

***MALASSEZIA* DERMATITIS** *Malassezia* dermatitis in a miniature poodle with alopecia, erythema, and lichenification on the ventral neck. (Copyright Dr. Manon Paradis.)

- CBC, serum chemistry panel, and urinalysis to screen for systemic internal diseases
- Hormonal testing (e.g., screening tests for endocrinopathies)
- Feline retroviral testing

TREATMENT

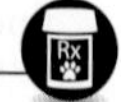

Treatment Overview

The main goal is to reduce pruritus and remove seborrhea. This is accomplished by killing yeast and controlling underlying primary diseases and risk factors.

Acute General Treatment

- Keratomodulating (antiseborrheic) and antiyeast topical therapies (e.g., sulfur/salicylic acid, phytosphingosine, ceramides, benzoyl peroxide, selenium sulfide, boric/acetic acid, miconazole, clotrimazole, climbazole, ketoconazole, terbinafine, enilconazole, lime sulfur, chlorhexidine) can be applied daily to weekly, depending on the formulation used (e.g., shampoo, solution, lotion, spray, wipe, mousse).
- Systemic antifungal therapy may be warranted for severe infections or those not responding to topical therapy alone. Duration of systemic therapy should persist beyond (e.g., 1-2 weeks) clinical and cytologic resolution (usually a minimum of 3-4 weeks). Griseofulvin has no effect against *Malassezia* species, and terbinafine may not be as effective as azoles.
    - Ketoconazole 5-10 mg/kg PO q 24h with food; other azoles better suited for cats, *or*
    - Itraconazole 5-10 mg/kg PO q 24h with (capsules) or without (suspension) food, *or*
    - Fluconazole 2.5-5 mg/kg PO q 24h, *or*
    - Terbinafine 30 mg/kg PO q 24h with food
- Because ≈40% of dogs with *Malassezia* dermatitis have concurrent superficial staphylococcal pyoderma, treating any associated bacterial infection with oral antibiotics at an appropriate dose and duration (minimum 3 weeks) can help improve cutaneous signs.

Chronic Treatment

- Therapy for underlying predisposing diseases
- Topical keratomodulating and/or antiyeast therapy at reduced frequencies of application if possible
- Pulse therapy with a systemic azole or terbinafine can be used for remitting and relapsing episodes of *Malassezia* dermatitis because these drugs concentrate in the skin. Typically, the same initial dosage is prescribed for 2 consecutive days per week or given daily for cycles of 1 week on/1 to 4 weeks off after the initial induction dose (see Acute General Treatment above).

Drug Interactions

Azole therapy may alter the metabolism or distribution of other prescribed medication by inhibiting cytochrome P450 metabolizing enzymes and P-glycoprotein transporting pumps. Terbinafine does not inhibit these enzymes. Specifically, azoles cannot be given with high-dose, extralabel macrocyclic lactones (e.g., avermectins); if needed, dosage reduction and close monitoring are required.

Possible Complications

- Idiosyncratic cutaneous adverse reactions to topical therapies
- Patient may have adverse reactions (e.g., vomiting, diarrhea, hepatotoxicosis, vasculitis, lightening of haircoat, pruritus) to systemic azoles.
- Ketoconazole may inhibit cortisol synthesis at dosages greater than 10 mg/kg/day.

Recommended Monitoring

- Clinical signs and cytologic evaluation every 3-4 weeks during therapy
- Other monitoring recommendations are at the discretion of the clinician and based on underlying predisposing diseases.

PROGNOSIS & OUTCOME

- Failure to detect and treat underlying disease(s) will result in partial treatment success, treatment failure, or relapse.
- For incurable diseases (e.g., primary cornification disorders), therapy for *Malassezia* dermatitis is often lifelong.

PEARLS & CONSIDERATIONS

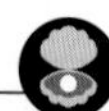

Comments

- *Malassezia* dermatitis is one of the most overlooked causes of pruritus in the dog.
- *Malassezia* dermatitis tends to occur in body areas rich in sebaceous glands and high in relative humidity, and it is commonly associated with allergic dermatitis.
- How many yeasts are cytologically significant? Finding any yeast from typical clinical lesions is significant. However, because false-negatives are possible with cytology, typical signs and pruritic distribution pattern (body folds) should not be taken lightly when making a diagnosis.
- Dogs with atopic dermatitis may be hypersensitive to *Malassezia*, resulting in yeast numbers disproportionate to the level of pruritus experienced by the animal.
- Skin culture for *Malassezia* yeast is not recommended in clinical practice because these organisms are residents on the skin.
- Biopsy with histopathologic evaluation is not considered superior to cytologic evaluation for the diagnosis of *Malassezia* dermatitis (most of the surface scale is lost during biopsy processing) but may be useful in the diagnosis of primary skin disorders in which *Malassezia* dermatitis is a secondary phenomenon.
- Do not use selenium sulfide on cats; it is too irritating to their skin.
- Enilconazole is not approved for small-animal use in some countries.
- When given in tablet or capsule form, the azole drugs ketoconazole and itraconazole are best absorbed systemically if administered with food; failure to do so may reduce bioavailability of these drugs by up to 40%.
- When not contraindicated, most allergic dogs benefit from a short course of antipruritic/antiinflammatory therapy (e.g., glucocorticoid, oclacitinib, lokivetmab) during the initiation of other antiyeast measures (p. 91).

Prevention

Correctly identifying and treating for all underlying predisposing factors favorable to yeast overgrowth

Technician Tips

Technicians managing patients with *Malassezia* dermatitis should be proficient in collection and exam of cytologic skin samples (p. 1091) and capable of instructing owners on appropriate use of topical therapy.

Client Education

- The identification of *Malassezia* dermatitis is only the beginning of the diagnostic process because yeast overgrowth is secondary to another condition.
- Show clients how to effectively use topical antiyeast treatments.

SUGGESTED READING

Negre A, et al: Evidence-based veterinary dermatology: a systematic review of interventions for *Malassezia* dermatitis in dogs. Vet Dermatol 20:1-12, 2008.

AUTHOR: Adam P. Patterson, DVM, DACVD
EDITOR: Manon Paradis, DMV, MVSc, DACVD

Malocclusion

Client Education Sheet

BASIC INFORMATION

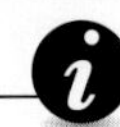

Definition

An abnormal position of one or more teeth. In dental malocclusion, one or more teeth are in an abnormal position, whereas in skeletal malocclusion, there is an upper/lower jaw size discrepancy.

Synonym

Malalignment of teeth

Epidemiology

SPECIES, AGE, SEX

Malocclusion can be seen in all species and age groups, and it is usually present from the time of eruption of the deciduous or permanent dentition.

GENETICS, BREED PREDISPOSITION

Occlusal development is determined by genetic and environmental factors. Most brachycephalic cats and dogs show malocclusion due to a shortened upper jaw.

RISK FACTORS

- Persistent deciduous teeth
- Orofacial trauma during tooth and jaw development
- Selective breeding for exaggerated head types

ASSOCIATED DISORDERS

- Discomfort and pain can result from maloccluding teeth.
- Linguoverted mandibular canines can traumatize the hard palate mucosa, leading to oronasal fistula formation.
- Maloccluding teeth may cause damage (attrition) to opposing teeth.
- Crowded teeth are at risk for development of early periodontitis from plaque retention.

Clinical Presentation

DISEASE FORMS/SUBTYPES

Dental malocclusion:

- Neutroclusion (class 1 malocclusion; normal rostrocaudal relationship of maxillary and mandibular dental arches, with malposition of one or more teeth)
  - Distoversion/mesioversion/linguoversion/palatoversion/labioversion/buccoversion: tooth in anatomically correct position in the dental arch is abnormally angled in a distal/mesial/lingual/palatal/labial/buccal direction, respectively.
  - Crossbite: malocclusion in which a mandibular tooth or teeth have a more labial or buccal position than the antagonist maxillary tooth
    - Rostral crossbite: one or more mandibular incisors are labial to opposing maxillary incisors when the mouth is closed.
    - Caudal crossbite: one or more mandibular cheek teeth are buccal to opposing maxillary cheek teeth when the mouth is closed.

Symmetrical skeletal malocclusion:

- Mandibular distoclusion (class 2 malocclusion; abnormal rostrocaudal relationship between the dental arches in which the mandibular arch occludes caudal to its normal position relative to the maxillary arch)
- Mandibular mesioclusion (class 3 malocclusion; abnormal rostrocaudal relationship between the dental arches in which the mandibular arch occludes rostral to its normal position relative to the maxillary arch)

Asymmetrical skeletal malocclusion:

- Maxillary-mandibular asymmetry in a rostrocaudal, side-to-side, or dorsoventral direction:
  - Rostrocaudal: mandibular mesioclusion or distoclusion is present on one side of the face, but the contralateral side retains normal dental alignment.
  - Side-to-side: there is loss of the midline alignment of the maxilla and mandible.
  - Dorsoventral: there is an *open bite* (abnormal vertical space between opposing dental arches when the mouth is closed).

HISTORY, CHIEF COMPLAINT

- Abnormal incisor occlusion (show and breeding dogs)
- Abnormal tooth position
- Obvious length difference between upper and lower jaws or between left and right

PHYSICAL EXAM FINDINGS

Normal occlusion:

- The maxillary incisors are positioned rostral to the mandibular incisors. The crown cusps of the mandibular incisors contact the cingula of the maxillary incisors.
- The mandibular canines are slightly inclined labially and bisecting the interdental spaces between the maxillary third incisors and canines.
- The maxillary premolars do not contact the mandibular premolars. The crown cusps of the mandibular premolars are positioned lingual to the maxillary premolars. The crown cusps of the mandibular premolars bisect the interdental spaces rostral to the corresponding maxillary premolars.
- The mesial crown cusp of the maxillary fourth premolar is positioned lateral to the space between the mandibular fourth premolar and first molar.

Dental malocclusion:

- Abnormal positioning of one or more teeth
- No jaw discrepancy
- Trauma to soft tissue or other teeth

Skeletal malocclusion:

- Abnormal maxillary-mandibular incisor relationship
- Loss of premolar interdigitation
- Incorrect mandibular canine occlusion
- Jaw length discrepancy (symmetrical or asymmetrical)
- Trauma to soft tissue or other teeth

Etiology and Pathophysiology

- Jaw length, tooth bud position, and tooth size are independently inherited. Unharmonious development of the upper and lower jaw and maxillary and mandibular teeth results in malocclusion.
- Persistent deciduous teeth are associated with malpositioned permanent teeth.
- Significant orofacial trauma at young age may lead to abnormal development and malocclusion.
- Significant facial trauma at any age may cause changes in jaw relationships.

DIAGNOSIS

Diagnostic Overview

The diagnosis is based entirely on physical exam to identify malpositioned teeth.

Differential Diagnosis

- Dental malocclusion versus skeletal malocclusion
- Functional (mal)occlusion versus clinically relevant malocclusion (causing discomfort or pain)

Initial Database

Physical exam:

- Look for persistent deciduous teeth.
- Differentiate between dental and skeletal malocclusion.

TREATMENT

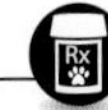

Treatment Overview

The goal of treatment is to have a pain-free, comfortable patient with a functional bite. Cosmetic considerations should not play a role.

Acute and Chronic Treatment

- Extract maloccluding deciduous teeth as early as possible (6-10 weeks of age) if they appear to cause discomfort or interfere with jaw growth.
- Treatment options for maloccluding permanent teeth causing trauma to soft tissue or other teeth
  - Extraction
  - Surgical crown reduction and vital pulp therapy
  - Orthodontic movement (passive or active)
- Linguoversion of mandibular canines: Verhaert's rubber ball technique is useful

for young dogs (<7 months of age) with normal jaw relationships and sufficiently wide diastema between maxillary third incisors and canines. The dog is stimulated to actively play with a smooth-surfaced hard rubber ball for at least 15 minutes three times daily.

Possible Complications

- Inappropriate extraction technique of deciduous teeth may cause trauma to developing permanent teeth.
- Surgical crown reduction may lead to pulpitis and pulp necrosis.
- Orthodontic treatment usually requires several corrective procedures under general anesthesia and may cause soft-tissue trauma from the appliance, root resorption, displacement of anchor tooth, overcorrection of target tooth, avulsion of anchor or target tooth, discomfort, and pain.

Recommended Monitoring

- Teeth treated by surgical crown reduction should be monitored radiographically after 4-6 months and then on a yearly basis.
- During orthodontic treatment, regular monitoring is necessary to assess tooth movement and to recognize possible complications at an early stage.

PROGNOSIS & OUTCOME

Prognosis is good after a functional bite has been accomplished.

PEARLS & CONSIDERATIONS

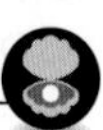

Comments

- Dental malocclusion is not considered inherited unless a familial predisposition exists (e.g., mesioverted maxillary canines in Shetland sheepdog).

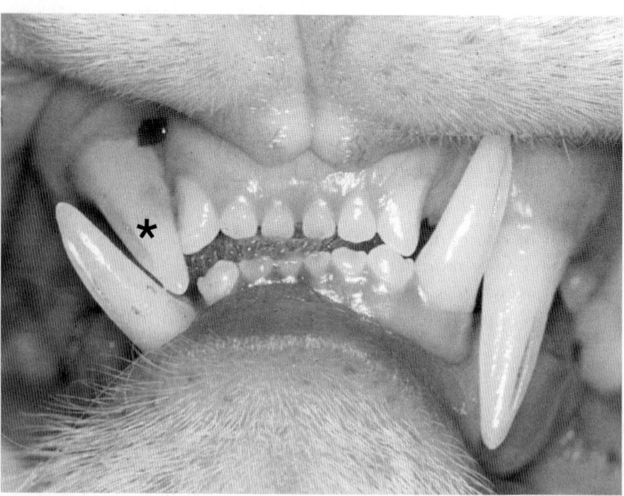

MALOCCLUSION Clinical photograph of a cat with mesioversion of the right maxillary canine tooth *(asterisk)*. There is no diastema between the right maxillary canine and third incisor, which the right mandibular canine tooth could occlude into when the mouth is closed (compare with normal left side). Mesioversion of the right maxillary canine tooth resulted in mild labioversion of the right mandibular canine tooth and an open bite (incomplete closure of the mouth). (Copyright Dr. Alexander M. Reiter, University of Pennsylvania.)

- Skeletal malocclusion is considered inherited unless a developmental cause (e.g., extensive orofacial trauma) can be identified.
- Inherited malocclusion should be corrected by orthodontic movement only if the animal is neutered.

Prevention

- Selective breeding
- Remove persistent deciduous teeth

Technician Tips

- Teach owners how to evaluate their pets' dentition twice weekly from the time of permanent tooth eruption (3 months of age) with special attention given to the timely shedding of deciduous canine teeth.
- Call patients in for occlusion control between 5.5 and 7 months of age.

Client Education

Neuter animals with skeletal malocclusion (if not normal for the breed).

SUGGESTED READING

American Veterinary Dental College: Recommendations adopted by the AVDC Board (website). https://www.avdc.org/Nomenclature/Nomen-Intro.html.

AUTHOR: Leen Verhaert, DVM, DEVDC
EDITOR: Alexander M. Reiter, DVM, Dr.med.vet, DAVDC, DEVDC

Mammary Disorders, Non-Neoplastic

BASIC INFORMATION

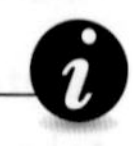

Definition

- Mastitis: inflammation of the mammary gland, usually septic; blood-milk barrier not intact
- Mammary hyperplasia: aseptic noninflammatory enlargement of mammary glands

Epidemiology

SPECIES, AGE, SEX

- Mastitis: most common in the postpartum bitch, less so in the bitch with overt pseudocyesis or the postpartum queen, uncommon in prepartum or spayed bitches; older bitches may be at greater risk.
- Mammary hyperplasia: usually young, intact female cats or pregnant queens but can occur in gonadectomized or intact cats of either sex

GENETICS, BREED PREDISPOSITION

Mastitis: short-legged dogs and dogs with pendulous mammary glands have greater risk of trauma.

RISK FACTORS

- Mastitis: poor hygiene, trauma (environmental or from nursing), infections from other sites in the body
- Mammary hyperplasia: cats of either sex with recent gonadectomy, cats of either sex receiving exogenous progestogens

CONTAGION AND ZOONOSIS

Common bacterial pathogens of the mammary gland are *Escherichia coli*, *Staphylococcus* spp, *Streptococcus* spp, *Pseudomonas* spp, *Klebsiella* spp, *Pasteurella* spp, and *Clostridium* spp. Secondary zoonotic potential exists with all of these pathogens.

GEOGRAPHY AND SEASONALITY

Mammary hyperplasia may be more prevalent during the spring, when queens begin to cycle;

incidence is 40%-50% after ovulation in cats with pseudocyesis.

ASSOCIATED DISORDERS

Mastitis:

- Galactostasis after weaning or overt pseudopregnancy
- Benign mammary hyperplasia in queens
- May be associated with mammary neoplasia

Mammary hyperplasia:

- Secondary mastitis and/or necrosis

Clinical Presentation

DISEASE FORMS/SUBTYPES

- Mastitis: acute, fulminant, or chronic/nearly subclinical
- Mammary hyperplasia: acute

HISTORY, CHIEF COMPLAINT

- Mastitis
  - Lactating bitch or queen: uncomfortable dam may or may not want to nurse offspring; neonates do not nurse (crying puppies or kittens)
  - Rarely occurs after an overt false pregnancy/pseudocyesis (bitch)
- Mammary hyperplasia: acute enlargement of mammary glands

PHYSICAL EXAM FINDINGS

Mastitis:

- Mammary signs: firm, warm, swollen, often painful mammary gland (one or more); it may be possible to express purulent or discolored milk from gland; gland may abscess, become ischemic, and rupture.
- Systemic signs: lethargy, dehydration, ± fever; may progress to septic shock
- Mammary hyperplasia: enlarged mammary glands (all glands usually involved; can be painful; can develop necrosis)

Etiology and Pathophysiology

Mastitis:

- Possible ascending bacterial infection (poor hygiene, traumatic nursing) or hematogenous spread of fungal infection (e.g., *Blastomyces dermatitidis*)
- Incidence highest for stimulated mammary glands; may be due to presence of abundant substrate (milk), open ducts, trauma from nursing, and increased trauma because glands are enlarged

Mammary hyperplasia:

- Hormonally-induced condition: hormones include progesterone (endogenous or exogenous), growth hormone, and prolactin.

DIAGNOSIS

Diagnostic Overview

History and physical exam are generally sufficient to formulate a diagnosis: enlarged, painful mammary glands (usually during lactation) in mastitis patients or rapidly enlarged, nonseptic mammary glands in cats with mammary hyperplasia.

Differential Diagnosis

- Mammary adenocarcinoma (inflamed or septic) usually in older females with no concurrent lactation (pp. 621 and 623)
- Galactostasis: dam not ill, nonseptic

Initial Database

- CBC: unremarkable or leukocytosis +/− left shift; leukopenia possible if acute sepsis (mastitis); within normal limits with mammary hyperplasia
- Cytologic exam of mammary secretions: in mastitis, many toxic neutrophils; in mammary hyperplasia, few to moderate epithelial cells
- Milk pH: normal milk pH = 6.3; with mastitis, pH of mammary secretions can influence an antibiotic's ability to penetrate the mammary gland. For example, when milk pH > 7.0, cephalosporins concentrate in the milk. The pH can be determined using a urine dipstick.

Advanced or Confirmatory Testing

- Bacterial culture and susceptibility of mammary secretions
- Serum and milk acute phase proteins (e.g., haptoglobin, C-reactive protein) can be used as an indicator of subclinical mastitis.
- Ultrasonography of mammary tissue (loss of distinct layering of the tissue is characteristic of mastitis and inflamed regions have reduced echogenicity)
- Biopsy of mammary tissue (to rule out neoplasia and benign mammary hyperplasia)

TREATMENT

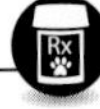

Treatment Overview

- Goals of treatment of mastitis are returning the patient to normal mammary function and preventing septicemia.
- Goals for treatment of mammary hyperplasia are to prevent mastitis.

Acute General Treatment

Mastitis:

- If mammary necrosis is present or milk is too contaminated for puppies and kittens (i.e., grossly purulent/malodorous milk or neonates are hungry, showing diarrhea/weight loss), offspring should be removed and the necrotic tissue surgically drained and debrided.

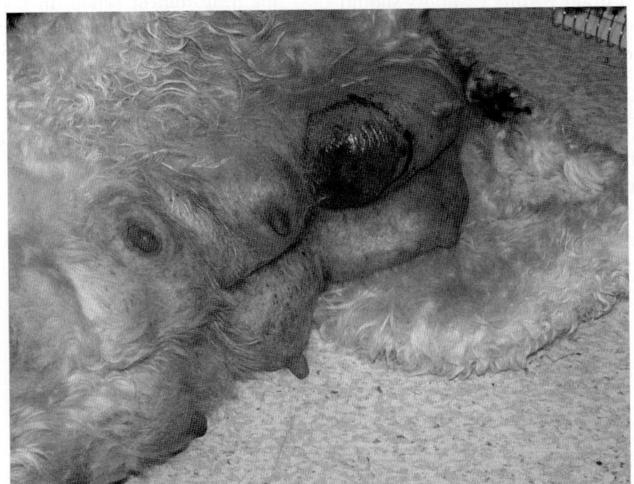

MAMMARY DISORDERS, NON-NEOPLASTIC Gangrenous mastitis in a Lagotto Romagnolo bitch. Affected area has been outlined with a black marker. (Used with permission from Cathy Gartley, DVM, DVSc, DACT.)

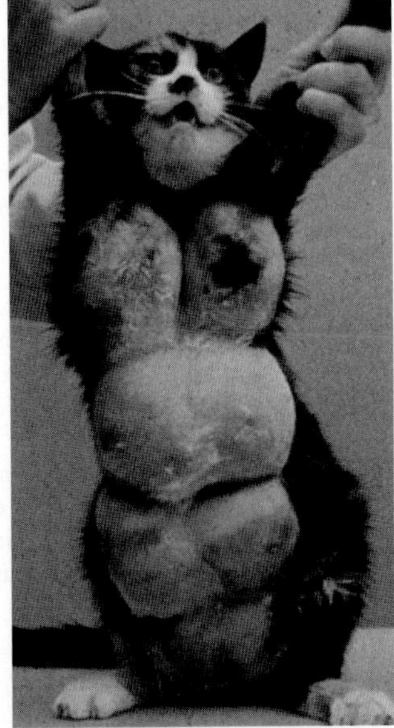

MAMMARY DISORDERS, NON-NEOPLASTIC Gross appearance of fibroepithelial hyperplasia in a young cat. (From Lana SE, et al: Tumors of the mammary gland. In Withrow & MacEwen's Small animal clinical oncology (4th ed) St. Louis, 2007, Saunders, pp 619-636.)

- Antiprolactin therapy may be administered to stop lactation (cabergoline 5 mcg/kg PO q 24h; response usually seen within 3-4 days; > 80% response by day 7).
- Systemic antibiotic treatment of the dam is required. General guidelines are initially based on Gram stain and milk pH and on whether neonates are still nursing. Subsequently, culture and susceptibility (C/S) results are used for definitive treatment. The therapeutic goal is to achieve significant antibiotic concentrations in the mammary tissue.
  - If neonates are still nursing, empirical options for gram-positive infections include amoxicillin-clavulanic acid 12.75 mg/kg PO q 12h or first-generation cephalosporins (e.g., cefadroxil 22 mg/kg PO q 8h); options for gram-negative infections include cefoxitin 30 mg/kg IV q 6h or chloramphenicol 40 mg/kg PO q 8h.
  - Antimicrobial choice can be adjusted as appropriate after C/S becomes available, while avoiding the use of aminoglycosides, sulfa drugs, tetracyclines, metronidazole, and floroquinolones (relative contraindication) if neonates are still nursing.
  - If the dam is no longer nursing neonates, empiric recommendations can include any of the drugs used for nursing mothers or quinolones (e.g., enrofloxacin 5 mg/kg PO q 12h for dogs or pradofloxacin 7.5 mg/kg PO q 24h for cats) for gram-negative aerobes; metronidazole 15 mg/kg PO q 12h or clindamycin 5-11 mg/kg PO q 12h for anaerobes; tetracyclines (e.g., doxycycline 5 mg/kg PO q 12h), erythromycin, or quinolones for *Mycoplasma.*
- Warm-packing and ongoing nursing: unless the gland is necrotic, continued nursing by the offspring and warm-packing the affected glands will prevent galactostasis and promote drainage.

Mammary hyperplasia: usually self-limited in 2-3 weeks:

- Progesterone withdrawal: if sexually intact, ovariectomy or ovariohysterectomy is recommended to prevent recurrence.
- Pain control
- Medical therapy
  - Progesterone receptor blocker: aglepristone 15 mg/kg SQ q 24h × 2 days. NOTE: not approved for use in cats in the United States; will abort pregnant cats; *or*
  - Prolactin inhibitor: bromocriptine mesylate 0.25 mg/CAT PO q 24h × 5-7 days. NOTE: not approved for use in cats in the United States; will abort pregnant cats; *or*
  - Androgens: testosterone enanthate or testosterone cypionate 2 mg/kg IM once. NOTE: not approved for use in cats in the United States.

Chronic Treatment

Mastectomy for intractable disease

Nutrition/Diet

To reduce galactostasis in dams if nursing offspring are removed, food intake should be reduced by 50%. Do not reduce food intake if neonates continue to nurse from lactating dams.

Behavior/Exercise

Limit activity that may induce mammary trauma (e.g., neonates biting or scratching mammary glands). This may include weaning puppies and kittens.

Drug Interactions

Antiprolactinics stop lactation. Some antibiotics are contraindicated for lactating bitches. Aglepristone is abortifacient in dogs and cats.

Possible Complications

Systemic antibiotic therapy in lactating dams may interfere with normal bacterial colonization of gastrointestinal flora in nursing neonates, resulting in diarrhea.

Recommended Monitoring

- Temperature, respiration, and heart rate
- Physical signs of septicemia
- Offspring that are nursing: weigh daily (neonates, twice daily) to determine adequate milk intake. Neonates should gain ≈10% of their body weight each day.

PROGNOSIS & OUTCOME

Prognosis is generally good unless sepsis occurs.

PEARLS & CONSIDERATIONS

Comments

- Abscessed mammary glands that do not rupture and drain within 12 hours should be surgically drained and debrided to prevent endotoxemia in the dam and toxic milk that puts the offspring at risk for infection.
- Ultrasound exam revealing decreased vascular flow to inflamed tissues indicates possible onset of gangrene.
- Pups/kittens 4½ to 5 weeks old should be allowed access to dam's food, and the bitch or queen should have an area where she can remove herself from the neonates (e.g., top of crate, raised platform).
  - Pups/kittens will start eating solid food for a portion of their caloric intake, decreasing the amount of time they are nursing on the dam. This also benefits the dam by greatly reducing her metabolic requirements.
- Older offspring with teeth nurse more aggressively and can cause bite and nail trauma to the mammary gland, greatly increasing the risk of inflammation and infection.
- Frequently, chronic subclinical mastitis has been suspected when neonates fail to thrive. However, subclinical mastitis has not been reported in dogs and cats.

Prevention

- Mastitis
  - Adequate husbandry, particularly clean bedding for mother and offspring
  - Keep mammary glands clean, monitor glands for trauma from offspring's nails or teeth.
  - Clipping offspring's toenails
- Mammary hyperplasia: limit the clinical use of exogenous progestogens.

Technician Tips

- Monitor neonates closely and record body weight twice daily. If neonates are hungry but spit the nipple out or they are not gaining weight, they should receive nutritional supplementation. If neonates are nursing, any ruptured gland should be covered. This protects the painful gland and prevents the neonates from exposure to bacteria.
- Cabbage leaf wraps on affected glands are reported to accelerate resolution.

Client Education

Primarily husbandry issues of proper hygiene and weaning instructions

SUGGESTED READING

Lopate C: Reproductive physiology of canine pregnancy and parturition and conditions of the periparturient period. In Lopate C, editor: Management of pregnant and neonatal dogs, cats, and exotic pets, Ames, IA, 2012, Wiley-Blackwell, pp 25-42.

AUTHOR: Michael Peterson, DVM, MS
EDITOR: Michelle A. Kutzler, DVM, PhD, DACT

Mammary Gland Neoplasia, Cat

Client Education Sheet

BASIC INFORMATION

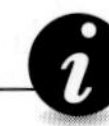

Definition

Mammary gland tumors are common tumors arising from mammary tissue. Mammary tumors can be benign or malignant.

Synonyms

- Mammary or breast cancer/tumor
- Specific mammary neoplasms: adenoma, fibroadenoma, carcinoma *in situ*, tubulopapillary carcinoma, solid carcinoma, cribriform carcinoma, inflammatory carcinoma

Epidemiology

SPECIES, AGE, SEX

- Mammary gland tumors represent up to 20% of all tumors in female cats.
- Third most common tumor in cats
- Mean age is 10-12 years.
- Most common: malignant epithelial carcinoma/adenocarcinoma
- Mixed mammary tumors (combination of epithelial and myoepithelial components) and sarcomas are rare.
- Siamese cats may develop mammary tumors at an earlier age than other breeds.
- Mammary tumors are rare in male cats (1%-2% of feline mammary carcinomas).

GENETICS, BREED PREDISPOSITION

- Siamese cats have a twofold risk of developing mammary gland tumors and have a higher incidence of malignant tumors with lymphatic invasion.
- Persian cats may have a higher incidence of benign mammary tumors.
- A genetic factor in the development of mammary tumors has not been identified. The following oncogenes/molecular markers have shown abnormal expression in selected feline mammary gland tumors:
  - *TP53*: gene encodes tumor protein 53, which regulates the cell cycle and functions as a tumor suppressor; mutation detected more frequently in carcinomas than benign tumors
  - *ERBB2 (HER2/NEU)*: gene involved in signal transduction and overexpression noted in more aggressive feline mammary tumors
  - *VEGF* (vascular endothelial growth factor): gene encodes an angiogenic factor that contributes to growth, invasion, and metastasis of tumor; overexpression seen in poorly differentiated tumors
  - *CCNA1/CCNA2* (cyclin A1/A2): gene regulates the cell cycle and may be associated with tumorigenesis in feline mammary carcinoma
  - *PTGS2* (prostaglandin-endoperoxide synthase 2/COX2): gene encodes an enzyme leading to conversion of arachidonic acid to prostaglandins; upregulated expression is associated with a poorer prognosis.

RISK FACTORS

- Ovariohysterectomy (OHE) reduces the risk of cats developing mammary tumors.
  - OHE < 6 months: 91% risk reduction compared with that of intact cats
  - OHE 7-12 months: 86% risk reduction compared with that of intact cats
  - OHE 13-24 months: 11% risk reduction compared with that of intact cats
  - OHE > 2 years: no benefit
- Treatment with progesterone and estrogen/progesterone combinations: threefold increased risk of development of benign and malignant mammary tumors in cats

Clinical Presentation

DISEASE FORMS/SUBTYPES

Clinical staging:

- Tumor: T1 < 2 cm; T2 2-3 cm; T3 > 3 cm
- Regional lymph node: N0, no metastasis; N1, metastasis detected
- Distant metastasis: M0, no metastasis; M1, metastasis detected

Stage Grouping	T	N	M
I	T1	N0	M0
II	T2	N0	M0
III	T1, T2	N1	M0
	T3	N0, N1	M0
IV	T1-3	N0, N1	M1

HISTORY, CHIEF COMPLAINT

- The owner may notice a swelling, lump, or ulcerated tissue in a cat's mammary chain.
- In cases of metastasis or inflammatory carcinoma, cats may be presented for general signs of illness or specific complaints attributable to a certain site of metastasis (e.g., dyspnea due to pulmonary metastases or pleural effusion).
- Duration of clinical signs varies, ranging from a few days to several months.

PHYSICAL EXAM FINDINGS

- >50% of cats have more than one mammary tumor, and both mammary chains may be affected simultaneously.
- Tumors may be firm on palpation and occasionally fixed to underlying structures.
- Discrete to infiltrative, soft to firm swelling in the mammary gland or overlying skin is most common.
- Ulceration is frequently present.
- Discharge from nipple is possible.
- Regional lymph nodes (inguinal and axillary) may be enlarged or normal on palpation.
- Lymph node enlargement can indicate metastasis or reactive change secondary to inflammation.
- Inflammatory carcinomas occur rarely in cats after mastectomy for mammary carcinoma and rarely as a primary entity. Cats with this form of mammary neoplasia present with local erythema, edema, pain, and involvement of the extremities.

Etiology and Pathophysiology

- The vast majority (>85%) of feline mammary tumors are malignant, with > 80% of feline mammary tumors classified as adenocarcinoma.
  - Metastasis is common (>80%). Common sites of metastasis include the lungs, pleura, and lymph nodes.
- Inflammatory carcinomas occur rarely in cats after mastectomy for mammary carcinoma.
  - These are aggressive anaplastic carcinomas with considerable inflammatory cell infiltrate, intradermal and dermal lymphatic invasion that leads to edema, pain, and rapid metastasis.
- Benign tumors, including adenomas, fibroadenomas, and duct papillomas, occur uncommonly in cats (<15%).

DIAGNOSIS

Diagnostic Overview

- The diagnosis is suspected based on the detection of a mass in the mammary chain. Histologic evaluation is required for definitive diagnosis and is usually obtained from an excisional biopsy.
- Incisional biopsy can be considered in cases where a benign tumor is suspected, but radical mastectomy with removal of all four glands and ipsilateral lymph node(s) is advised for firm, fixed, or ulcerated masses or when malignancy is confirmed. A diagnostic and treatment approach is presented on p. 1433.

Differential Diagnosis

- Fibroepithelial hyperplasia: involves one or multiple glands, most often in young intact females and spayed females given progesterone compounds.
- Mastitis
- Other cutaneous and subcutaneous tumors
- Inguinal/axillary lymphadenopathy (reactive, neoplastic)
- Inguinal hernia
- Enlarged inguinal fat pad

Initial Database

- Physical exam
  - Measure primary tumor (T).
  - Describe possible signs of invasiveness (ulceration, fixation).
  - Evaluate regional lymph nodes (N): palpation and cytologic analysis
- Thoracic radiographs (three views) for pulmonary metastasis
- Abdominal ultrasound in case of suspected metastasis to abdominal organs or lymph nodes
- Fine-needle aspiration and cytologic evaluation: limited utility but may be useful in differentiating neoplasia from fibroadenomatous hyperplasia
- CBC, serum biochemistry profile, urinalysis, coagulation profile in cases of suspected inflammatory carcinoma

Advanced or Confirmatory Testing

- Definitive diagnosis is by biopsy and histopathologic evaluation of mammary masses and associated lymph nodes
  - Histologic grading scheme is based primarily on mitotic activity, degree of tubule formation, and nuclear/cellular pleomorphism.
  - Because > 85% of feline mammary tumors are malignant, histopathologic exam most often is performed on tumor tissue obtained from a radical mastectomy.
  - When fibroepithelial hyperplasia (see Differential Diagnosis) or other nonmammary tumors are suspected, incisional (wedge) biopsies can be done.
- Lymph node evaluation
  - In general, the ipsilateral inguinal or axillary lymph node(s) should be removed during radical mastectomy and assessed histopathologically.
  - Axillary lymph nodes may be difficult to isolate, but fine-needle aspiration or biopsies can be done if they are enlarged. Ultrasound-guided aspiration cytology may be possible in some cases.
- Distant metastasis
  - Cytologic evaluation of pleural effusion can aid in the diagnosis of thoracic metastatic disease.
  - Advanced imaging (CT, MRI) may increase diagnostic accuracy of metastatic lesions in the thoracic and abdominal cavities.

TREATMENT

Treatment Overview

- Treatment consists of complete surgical removal of the mammary tumor(s). The recommended surgical approach for cats is radical mastectomy.
- Staged bilateral radical mastectomy is recommended for bilateral disease; bilateral radical mastectomy for cats with unilateral disease is of unproven benefit.
- Adjuvant chemotherapy is advised for cats with poor prognostic factors, although clinical studies to determine chemotherapy combinations/protocols that are most effective for increasing survival time need to be performed.

Acute General Treatment

Surgery:

- Radical mastectomy of the affected mammary chain(s) is recommended to reduce the risk of local recurrence.
- In contrast to individual mastectomies or lumpectomies, radical mastectomy significantly reduces the risk for local tumor recurrence.
- Affected lymph node(s) should be removed along with the mammary chain.
- Fixation of the tumor to underlying muscle or fascia necessitates en bloc removal of these structures.
- In cats with advanced metastatic disease, local mastectomy to remove ulcerated or infected mammary tumors may be palliative.
- Inflammatory carcinoma is nonresectable.

Chronic Treatment

Chemotherapy:

- Single-agent doxorubicin, doxorubicin in combination with cyclophosphamide, single-agent carboplatin, alternating doxorubicin and carboplatin or toceranib phosphate (Palladia) may lead to complete and partial responses in cats with metastatic disease or nonresectable mammary gland tumors.
- Adjuvant chemotherapy using the previously mentioned drugs as single agents or in combination is recommended in cats after radical mastectomy. However, a true survival benefit has yet to be proven.
- Special handling requirements and potentially severe, life-threatening adverse patient effects exist for these drugs. Consultation with a medical oncologist is recommended.

Radiation therapy:

- Used to palliate nonresectable disease may be an option in some cats

Immunotherapy:

- Treatment with levamisole, bacterial vaccines, and other immunomodulators has not led to improvement in local tumor control or survival.

Hormonal therapy:

- Because most malignant feline mammary gland tumors lack estrogen receptors, anti-estrogen therapy (tamoxifen) is not effective.

Analgesics:

- Should be used in cats that present with advanced disease

Possible Complications

Inflammatory carcinoma after mastectomy for mammary carcinoma is rare.

Recommended Monitoring

Regular examinations of the surgical site, local lymph nodes, and lung fields

PROGNOSIS & OUTCOME

- Local recurrence rate > 50% with incomplete excision
- Prognostic factors for cats with mammary gland carcinomas
  - Tumor size (survival times with surgery alone):
    - > 3 cm: median survival of 4-6 months (female), 1.6 months (male)
    - 2-3 cm: median survival of 1-2 years (female), 5.2 months (male)
    - < 2 cm: median survival of > 3 years after mastectomy (female), 14 months (male)
  - Type of surgery
    - Radical mastectomy significantly reduces the risk of local tumor recurrence compared with conservative surgery but does not appear to improve survival time.
  - Histologic grade: high grade is associated with a shorter survival time.
  - Clinical stage at presentation: median survival times for cats with stage I, II, III, and IV disease are 29, 12.5, 9, and 1 month(s), respectively.
  - Ulceration may be a poor prognostic indicator but likely is related to tumor size.
- Benign tumors and low-grade malignant tumors may be cured by wide excision.

PEARLS & CONSIDERATIONS

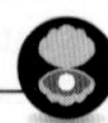

Comments

- Palpation of the mammary glands should routinely be performed as part of the physical exam.
- Mammary carcinoma in the cat is a highly malignant neoplastic disease that warrants early diagnosis and an aggressive treatment approach.
- Adjuvant chemotherapy should be considered in cats with resectable mammary carcinoma after radical mastectomy.
- In cats with advanced disease, palliative measures, including surgery, chemotherapy, radiation, and analgesics, may be considered.

Prevention

- OHE before age 6 months reduces the risk but does not prevent mammary carcinoma in female cats.
- Castration does not prevent mammary carcinoma in male cats.

Technician Tips

Because the timing of OHE is an important contributor to the risk of mammary tumor development, it is important to inquire about its timing when collecting a history on new patients.

Client Education

- Early OHE of queens not intended for breeding

- Regular examination of the mammary chain
- Prompt presentation for veterinary examination when abnormalities are found

SUGGESTED READING

De Campos CB, et al. Use of surgery and carboplatin in feline malignant mammary gland neoplasms with advanced clinical staging. In Vivo 28:863-866, 2014.

AUTHOR: Erin K. Malone, DVM, DACVIM
EDITOR: Kenneth M. Rassnick, DVM, DACVIM

Mammary Gland Neoplasia, Dog

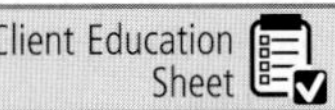

BASIC INFORMATION

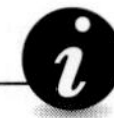

Definition

Mammary gland tumors are benign or malignant neoplasms arising from mammary tissue.

Synonyms

- Mammary or breast cancer/tumor
- Benign mammary tumors: adenoma/cystadenoma, benign mixed mammary tumor, duct papilloma, myoepithelioma, complex adenoma, fibroadenoma
- Malignant mammary tumors: carcinoma *in situ*, simple carcinoma (tubular/tubulopapillary, solid, cribriform, and anaplastic), complex carcinoma, inflammatory carcinoma (uncommon), carcinosarcoma (rare), sarcomas (fibrosarcoma, osteosarcoma, other; uncommon)
- Different pathologic classification schemes exist.

Epidemiology

SPECIES, AGE, SEX

- Mammary gland tumors are common tumors in female dogs, and the most common tumor in intact female dogs.
  - Incidence ≈2:1000
  - Due to the common practice of early-age ovariohysterectomy (OHE), the incidence has decreased in the United States. In European countries, mammary tumors represent 40%-70% of all tumors in female dogs.
- Mammary tumors affect middle-aged to older dogs; median age for malignant tumors is 10-11 years.
- Mammary gland tumors in male dogs are uncommon (≈1% of mammary tumors occur in males).

GENETICS, BREED PREDISPOSITION

- Breeds at increased risk
  - Spaniel breeds
  - Pointer breeds
  - Poodles
  - Dachshunds
  - German shepherds
  - Yorkshire terriers
- There seems to be a genetic factor in the development of mammary tumors, but a specific, common mutation has not been identified. The following genes have been found to be mutated in selected canine mammary gland tumors (p. 621):
  - *TP53*
  - *ERBB2 (HER2/NEU)*
  - *BCRA1, BCRA2*

RISK FACTORS

- Timing of OHE affects the relative risk of developing mammary gland tumors.
  - 0.5% of the risk of an intact bitch if OHE is performed before the first estrus
  - 8% of the risk of an intact bitch if OHE is performed between the first and second estrus
  - 26% of the risk of an intact bitch if OHE is performed between the second and third estrus
- Females spayed after 2 years of age have a sevenfold greater risk of mammary neoplasia than those spayed before age 6 months.
- Body condition/diet: reduced risk (odds ratio = 0.04) in dogs with lean body condition at age 9-12 months
- Hormone therapy: progesterone and/or estrogen administration may lead to a greater than twofold increase in the risk of benign and malignant mammary tumors.
- Pregnancy, lactation, pseudocyesis
  - Unlike in people, pregnancy does not afford a protective effect against the development of mammary tumors in dogs. Lactation and pseudocyesis also do not seem to have an influence.

ASSOCIATED DISORDERS

- Ovarian cysts, cystic endometrial hyperplasia
- Mammary tumors in male dogs may be associated with hormonal disturbances (e.g., estrogen-secreting testicular Sertoli cell tumor).
- Up to 21% of dogs with inflammatory carcinoma may have concurrent disseminated intravascular coagulation (DIC), and appropriate testing should be assessed accordingly (p. 269).
- Secondary inflammatory carcinoma may develop after (mean, 48 days) surgical removal of a mammary tumor; secondary inflammatory carcinoma typically behaves as aggressively as primary inflammatory carcinoma.

Clinical Presentation

DISEASE FORMS/SUBTYPES

- Clinical staging
  - Tumor: T1 < 3 cm; T2 3-5 cm; T3 > 5 cm
  - Regional lymph node: N0, no metastasis; N1, metastasis detected
  - Distant metastasis: M0, no metastasis; M1, metastasis detected

Stage Grouping	T	N	M
I	T1	N0	M0
II	T2	N0	M0
III	T3	N0	M0
IV	T1-3	N1	M0
V	T1-3	N0, N1	M1

- Histologic staging
  - 0: carcinoma *in situ*
  - 1: stromal invasion
  - 2: vascular/lymphatic invasion; lymph node metastasis
  - 3: distant metastases
- Histologic grading of carcinomas is based on tubule formation, nuclear pleomorphism, and mitotic index and offers prognostic significance. Low-, intermediate-, and high-grade tumors correspond to well, moderately, and poorly differentiated tumors.

HISTORY, CHIEF COMPLAINT

- Owners may notice a swelling, lump, or ulceration in their dog's mammary chain, or it may be an incidental finding on routine physical exam.
- Duration of clinical signs is highly variable, ranging from days to months.
- With metastasis or inflammatory carcinoma, dogs may be presented due to general signs of illness or specific complaints attributable to a certain site of metastasis (e.g., lameness in cases of bone metastasis, cough due to pulmonary metastasis).

PHYSICAL EXAM FINDINGS

- Varies, depending on extent and stage of the disease
- Single or multiple nodules may be present. Multiple tumors are common in dogs, and both mammary chains may be affected. The caudal glands are affected most frequently. Multiple tumor types among different glands are common.

- Signs of malignancy include fixation to skin or underlying structures, rapid increase in size, ill-defined borders, ulceration, pain, inflammation, and edema.
  - Absence of these signs does not exclude malignancy.
- Inflammatory carcinomas present with diffuse, firm, and painful swelling of the affected gland or chain. The adjacent extremity may be affected. Cutaneous involvement in the form of small, beadlike nodules may be found.
- Regional lymph nodes (inguinal and axillary) may be enlarged (due to metastasis or reactive hyperplasia) or normal on palpation. The internal iliac, popliteal, sternal, and prescapular nodes may also be affected.

Etiology and Pathophysiology

- Estimated malignancy rates: 30%-50%
- Tumors metastasize most commonly to the regional lymph nodes and lungs, although liver and bone metastases are frequently described.
- Tumors are classified according to their tissue of origin as epithelial, mesenchymal, and mixed tumors.
  - Inflammatory carcinoma is not a specific histologic subtype but an aggressive, high-grade carcinoma with invasion of the dermis and dermal lymphatics. The inflammatory cell infiltrate is moderate in most cases and consists of lymphocytes, plasma cells, and macrophages.
- Primary mesenchymal mammary tumors (e.g., fibrosarcoma, osteosarcoma) are uncommon. Malignant mesenchymal mammary tumors often behave aggressively, with frequent metastasis and a short survival time.
- Mixed mammary tumors consist of epithelial, myoepithelial, and mesenchymal tissue. Benign mixed mammary tumors (fibroepithelial) and malignant mixed mammary tumors (carcinosarcoma) have been described.
- Complex mammary tumors include epithelial and myoepithelial components.
- Cyclooxygenase 2 (COX2) is overexpressed in most mammary carcinomas. Prostaglandin E_2 (PGE_2), the product of COX2, may promote tumor development and angiogenesis/metastasis. COX-2 inhibitors may play a role in tumor control..

DIAGNOSIS

Diagnostic Overview

The diagnosis is suspected based on finding a mass in the mammary chain. Histologic evaluation is required for definitive diagnosis. A diagnostic and treatment approach is presented on p. 1434.

Differential Diagnosis

- Mastitis
- Dermatitis
- Fibroepithelial hyperplasia
- Other cutaneous and subcutaneous tumors, including benign lipoma
- Inguinal/axillary lymphadenopathy (reactive, neoplastic)
- Inguinal hernia

Initial Database

- Physical exam
  - Measure primary tumor (T).
  - Describe possible signs of invasiveness (ulceration, fixation).
  - Evaluation of regional lymph nodes (N): palpation and cytologic study
- CBC, serum biochemistry profile, urinalysis
- Thoracic radiographs (three views)
- Abdominal ultrasound in case of suspected metastasis to abdominal organs or lymph nodes
- Coagulation profile in cases of suspected inflammatory carcinoma (risk of DIC)

Advanced or Confirmatory Testing

- Biopsy of the tumor and thorough histologic exam are necessary to obtain a definitive diagnosis.
  - Fine-needle aspiration for cytologic exam of mammary masses may help distinguish nonmammary tumors (lipomas, mast cell tumors) from mammary tumors, although cytologic findings alone may not be helpful in distinguishing benign from malignant mammary tumors.
- Incisional biopsy may not represent the whole tumor but is recommended before excisional biopsy if malignancy is not initially suspected.
- Lymph node metastasis: fine-needle aspiration and cytologic evaluation of lymph nodes has been shown to increase diagnostic accuracy of mammary tumor metastasis. Metastases may be present in palpably normal nodes.
- Advanced imaging (CT, MRI [p. 1132]) may be more sensitive for detecting metastatic lesions in the thoracic and abdominal cavities and should be considered when metastasis is suspected but cannot be detected on radiographs or ultrasound.

TREATMENT

Treatment Overview

Treatment consists of complete surgical removal of the mammary tumor(s). The role of chemotherapeutics in delaying the onset of metastatic disease has not been well defined in dogs. For dogs with inoperable tumors or inflammatory carcinomas, palliation with antiinflammatory medications may improve quality of life.

Acute General Treatment

- Mainstay of treatment is surgical excision of sufficient width to completely remove the mammary tumor(s).
- Type of surgery (nodulectomy, regional or radical mastectomy) depends on the size, location, and number of tumors.
  - Type of surgery does not influence survival as long as the entire tumor is removed with histologically clean margins.
- Goal is to remove all tumor by simplest surgical procedure that ensures clean margins.
- Unilateral radical chain mastectomy decreases the chances of tumor development in the remaining mammary tissue. In one study, 58% of dogs that underwent a regional mastectomy for a solitary mammary tumor developed a new tumor in the ipsilateral mammary chain after the first surgery.
- Remove inguinal lymph nodes with caudal gland tumors; excise axillary nodes only if metastasis is suspected; always submit all excised tissue for histologic assessment.
- Inflammatory carcinoma is nonresectable; palliative surgery may be possible in select cases.

Chronic Treatment

- Chemotherapy: limited information available
  - Antitumor activity has been demonstrated *in vitro* in selected patients with gross metastatic disease and as adjuvant treatment in a small group of dogs with advanced-stage disease. Dogs with tumors at high risk for metastasis may benefit from adjuvant chemotherapy.
  - Chemotherapeutics studied for monotherapy include doxorubicin, 5-fluorouracil, cyclophosphamide, taxanes, and platinum compounds (i.e., cisplatin or carboplatin). Special handling requirements and potentially severe, life-threatening adverse patient effects exist for these drugs.
  - COX2 inhibition with nonsteroidal antiinflammatory drugs may have anticancer activity.
- OHE at time of mammary tumor surgery: benefit is controversial, with some studies reporting increased survival and others showing no difference.
- Radiation therapy: limited information is available; may be of use in the palliative setting or to improve local control in inoperable cases
- Anti-estrogen therapy (tamoxifen): not recommended. Most anaplastic mammary tumors lack estrogen receptors, and anti-estrogen therapy may not be beneficial for most cases in which systemic therapy is indicated. Estrogen-like side effects, including vulvar swelling, vaginal discharge, stump pyometra, signs of estrus, and urinary tract infection may occur.
- Pain medication: analgesics should be considered in the palliative treatment of advanced-stage disease or inflammatory carcinoma. Options include nonsteroidal antiinflammatories (including carprofen 2 mg/kg PO q 12h, deracoxib 1-2 mg/kg PO q 24h, meloxicam 0.1 mg/kg PO q 24h, firocoxib 5 mg/kg PO q 24h, or piroxicam 0.3 mg/kg q 24h).

Recommended Monitoring

Regular exam of surgical site and local lymph nodes: radiology or other imaging techniques if indicated (e.g., diagnosis of malignancy, respiratory signs, other signs suggesting internal metastasis)

PROGNOSIS & OUTCOME

- Dogs with benign mammary tumors are cured by complete surgical excision.
- Prognosis for dogs with malignant mammary gland tumors is extremely variable and ranges from a cure with surgery (especially low-grade malignancy) to rapid recurrence and metastasis within the first year after surgical excision. Prognostic factors include
  - Tumor size: tumors < 3 cm have a better prognosis than tumors > 3 cm.
  - Tumor histologic characteristics
    - Epithelial tumors (adenocarcinomas, cystadenocarcinomas, carcinomas) may have a better prognosis than sarcomas and carcinosarcomas. Median survival times are 6.5 months (solid carcinoma), 12 months (invasive tumor), 29 months (noninvasive tumor), 10 months (sarcoma), and 18 months (carcinosarcoma).
    - Inflammatory carcinomas have a grave prognosis.
    - Anaplastic and high-grade, invasive tumors with stromal or lymphatic or vascular infiltration carry a worse prognosis than well-differentiated, low-grade or noninvasive lesions.
  - Clinical stage: a worse prognosis is associated with
    - Large tumors (stages II-V)
    - Lymph node involvement (stages IV-V)
    - Distant metastasis (stage V)
- Disease-free interval of 24 months for malignant tumors in 27%-55% of cases

PEARLS & CONSIDERATIONS

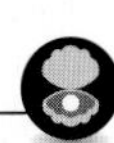

Comments

- Canine mammary tumors represent a heterogeneous group of tumors with different prognoses.
- Multicentric mammary tumors occur in > 50% of affected dogs; multiple tumor types occurring concurrently or sequentially are common.
- Highest-risk patients that can benefit most from postoperative adjuvant chemotherapy still need to be identified. They may include patients with advanced clinical stages (II-V), histologic evidence of vascular/lymphatic invasion, and/or high degree of anaplasia on histopathologic evaluation.
- The benefit of OHE at the time of mammary tumor surgery remains controversial, but a subset of dogs with differentiated estrogen receptor–positive tumors may benefit from concurrent OHE.

Prevention

OHE at age < 6 months can significantly reduce risk of mammary tumor development.

Technician Tips

Because the timing of OHE is an important contributor to the risk of mammary tumor development, it is important to inquire about its timing when collecting history on new patients.

Client Education

- Early-age OHE of bitches not intended for breeding
- Regular exam of the mammary chain
- Prompt presentation for veterinary exam when abnormalities are found

SUGGESTED READING

Kristiansen VM, et al: Effect of ovariohysterectomy at the time of tumor removal in dogs with mammary carcinomas: a randomized controlled trial. J Vet Intern Med 30:230-241, 2016.

AUTHOR: Erin K. Malone, DVM, DACVIM
EDITOR: Kenneth M. Rassnick, DVM, DACVIM

Marijuana Toxicosis

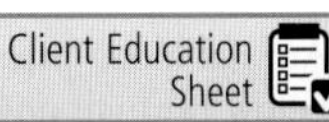

BASIC INFORMATION

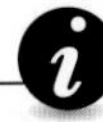

Definition

Common toxicosis resulting from ingestion of *Cannabis sativa* alkaloids and characterized by central nervous system (CNS) depression, ataxia, vomiting, hypothermia, urinary incontinence, bradycardia, hyperreflexia, possibly coma and seizures

Synonyms

Common names: marijuana, *Cannabis*, grass, hashish, hemp, Mary Jane, pot, reefer, Delta-9-tetrahydrocannabinol (THC)

Epidemiology

SPECIES, AGE, SEX

- Most commonly exposed animals: dogs (96%), cats (3%), other species (1%)
- Young dogs more commonly exposed

Clinical Presentation

HISTORY, CHIEF COMPLAINT

- History of exposure to marijuana or edibles/medibles (medicinal edibles) containing the active compound THC
- Ataxia, CNS depression, tremors, vomiting within 30 minutes of ingestion
- Specific history of exposure may be withheld by owner because of illicit nature of marijuana in some states.

PHYSICAL EXAM FINDINGS

- Common: bradycardia, hypothermia (body temperature: 98°F-99°F [36.7°C-37.2°C]), mydriasis, urinary incontinence/dribbling, weakness, ataxia
- Possible: hyperesthesia, ptyalism, recumbency, tachycardia, tremors, coma

Etiology and Pathophysiology

- *Marijuana* refers to a mixture of cut and dried flowers, leaves, and stems of the leafy green hemp plant, *Cannabis sativa*. It grows in warm, moist climates or is grown artificially indoors (greenhouses) and can be rolled into cigarettes or incorporated into food (e.g., brownies).
- Exposure by pet animals is mostly accidental, but occasionally, it is intentional or malicious. Sometimes, drug-detection dogs ingest marijuana accidentally.
- Marijuana is a Schedule I controlled substance commonly used as a recreational drug. Although considered illicit by U.S. federal regulations, it has been legalized for human use in many states.
- It is also used medicinally by humans (e.g., to treat nausea and improve appetite in cancer patients, reduce intraocular pressure in glaucoma patients) in the plant form or as synthetic THC (e.g., Marinol, Cesamet).

Mechanism of toxicosis:

- The predominant psychoactive portion of marijuana is THC, which is believed to act on a unique cannabinoid receptor in the brain that is primarily responsible for the CNS effects (ataxia and depression).
- Cannabinoids also enhance CNS formation of norepinephrine, dopamine, and serotonin; stimulate the release of dopamine; and enhance gamma-aminobutyric acid (GABA) turnover.
- When taken orally, THC goes through substantial initial hepatic metabolism (first-pass effect). It is highly lipophilic and distributes to the brain and other fatty tissues after absorption.
- Clinical signs in dogs may last 24-96 hours.
- Oral LD50 of THC in rats = 666 mg/kg, mice = 482 mg/kg. Clinical effects of marijuana are seen at much lower doses than this.
- THC content of marijuana (plant material) is 1%-8%, extract is 28%, and hash oil is up to 50%.

DIAGNOSIS

Diagnostic Overview

Intoxication is suspected based on typical clinical signs. Some clients may be reluctant to admit exposure or may not be aware that the agent is in their home. Exposure can be confirmed by testing the pet's urine with an over-the-counter illicit drug test kit. A low rate of life-threatening intoxications means a test kit can be obtained at some point during the first few hours of treatment/observation if definitive confirmation is needed (e.g., uncertain history).

Differential Diagnosis

Toxicologic:

- Ethylene glycol toxicosis
- Macadamia nut toxicosis
- Ivermectin toxicosis
- Other CNS depressants, such as benzodiazepines, barbiturates, and opioids

Spontaneous, non-toxicologic:

- The onset of clinical signs can mimic metabolic or toxic CNS disorders, but acute decompensation of primary CNS diseases (e.g., granulomatous meningoencephalitis, neoplasia, others) is possible, especially in an animal that is not closely observed by its owner.
- A sudden onset of signs with resolution and no recurrence within 24 hours makes intoxication much more likely than the non-toxicologic diagnoses.

Initial Database

- Arterial blood pressure (p. 1065): normal or below normal; normal (systolic) > 120 mm Hg in clinical setting
- CBC, serum biochemistry panel, urinalysis: unremarkable; used to assess for pre-existing conditions

Advanced or Confirmatory Testing

- Over-the-counter illicit drug test kits (urine) can help confirm exposure if used early in the course of exposure. CAUTION: the kits have not been validated in dogs; a negative result does not exclude exposure because false-negatives occur.
- Confirmatory testing can also be done at a diagnostic laboratory.

TREATMENT

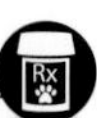

Treatment Overview

If presented soon after consumption, decontamination of the patient (induction of emesis, potential administration of activated charcoal) is indicated. In asymptomatic animals presenting > 1 hour after possible ingestion, treating with activated charcoal only and monitoring for onset of signs without further treatment is acceptable. After signs manifest, provide supportive care.

Acute General Treatment

Decontamination of the patient (p. 1087):

- Emesis (p. 1188) can be induced within 15-30 minutes of exposure in asymptomatic patients.
  - Dogs: use 3% hydrogen peroxide at 2.2 mL/kg PO, max 45 mL. Repeat once if emesis does not occur first time. Apomorphine may not work as an emetic because of the strong central antiemetic effect of marijuana.
- Activated charcoal: indicated for patients without clinical signs when emesis is absent. In patients with clinical signs or large ingestions, multiple doses may be used every 8 hours to reduce enterohepatic recirculation; 1-2 g/kg or labeled dosage of commercial products. CAUTION: risk of hypernatremia when using repeated doses of charcoal products.

Supportive care:

- IV fluids as needed for dehydration, hypovolemia
- Thermoregulation (heat source for hypothermia)
- Monitor cardiovascular function. Atropine 0.022-0.044 mg/kg IM or SQ for bradycardia in normotensive patients
- Control tremors with diazepam at a low dose of 0.25 mg/kg IV.
- Monitor for signs of aspiration pneumonia in recumbent animals. Pass cuffed endotracheal tube if needed, ensuring a mouth gag/speculum is also used to avoid the patient biting and transecting the tube when recovering.
- Control vomiting with metoclopramide 0.2-0.4 mg/kg q 6h PO, SQ, or IM or maropitant 1 mg/kg SQ or 2 mg/kg PO q 24h after ingested material has been expelled.

Drug Interactions

Other CNS depressants (barbiturates, benzodiazepines, opioids) may exacerbate signs.

Recommended Monitoring

Heart rate, blood pressure, body temperature

PROGNOSIS & OUTCOME

Excellent with treatment; fatalities are rare

PEARLS & CONSIDERATIONS

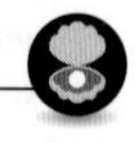

Comments

- Until proved otherwise, a dog presenting with acute-onset ataxia, CNS depression, and urinary incontinence that improves with stimulation and then gets worse again with decreased stimulation should be suspected of marijuana ingestion.
- Marijuana may be mixed with other substances for smoking (e.g., phencyclidine [PCP]), which may alter the patient's signs and prognosis.
- Legalization of marijuana use in some states may increase marijuana toxicosis incidence among dogs.
- Ingestion of synthetic marijuana, marketed as a legal high with street names such as K2 and spice, can cause much more severe CNS signs in dogs, sometimes lasting up to 3 days.

Technician Tips

With the increase in use of medical marijuana and legalization in some areas, the number of animal exposures is increasing. Some medical marijuana, including ones marketed to dogs, contain cannabinoids (CBDs), which are not expected to cause the neurologic signs associated with THC.

SUGGESTED READING

Meola SD, et al: Evaluation of trends in marijuana toxicosis in dogs living in a state with legalized medical marijuana: 125 dogs (2005-2010). J Vet Emerg Crit Care (San Antonio) 22:690-696, 2012.

AUTHOR: Eric Dunayer, VMD, MS, DABT, DABVT
EDITOR: Tina Wismer, DVM, MS, DABVT, DABT

Mass, Abdominal

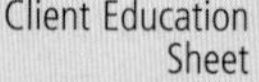

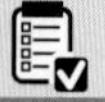

BASIC INFORMATION

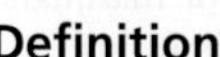

Definition

- An abnormal collection of cells and cellular components within the abdominal cavity that may cause abdominal distention
- Cystic structures or intestinal foreign body can cause a mass effect

Synonym

Abdominal tumor

Epidemiology

SPECIES, AGE, SEX

Any dog or cat; neoplastic masses tend to occur in older animals and intestinal foreign bodies in younger animals

Clinical Presentation

HISTORY, CHIEF COMPLAINT

- Highly variable, from an incidental exam finding to the cause of overt illness
- Common signs include gastrointestinal (GI) disturbance, weight loss, and lethargy.

PHYSICAL EXAM FINDINGS

Exam findings vary; may be normal if mass is small or may recognize

- Abdominal distention
- Palpable mass effect
- Abdominal pain
- Fluid wave (abdominal ballottement)
- Other findings depend on cause of mass (e.g., pallor and tachycardia due to bleeding abdominal hemangiosarcoma)
- Careful evaluation of peripheral lymph nodes and rectal palpation (dog) warranted

Etiology and Pathophysiology

Highly variable: malignant neoplasia, benign cellular organ infiltration, organ congestion, granuloma, cystic structures, abscess, abdominal lymphadenomegaly, intestinal intussusception, intestinal foreign body

DIAGNOSIS

Diagnostic Overview

Differential diagnosis often can be narrowed by location of the mass within the abdomen, as well as by signalment, history, and other exam findings. Diagnosis usually requires imaging studies coupled with cytology ± histopathology.

Differential Diagnosis

Common differential diagnoses for each organ system include the following:

- Cranial abdomen
  - Spleen: malignant neoplasia (hemangiosarcoma, fibrosarcoma, lymphoma, mastocytosis, chondrosarcoma), benign neoplasia (hemangioma, lipoma), splenic torsion, hematoma, congestion secondary to drug administration or other toxins, autoimmune disease, systemic infection/inflammation, normal folded spleen, abscess
  - Adrenal glands: malignant or benign neoplasia (adenocarcinoma/adenoma, pheochromocytoma, lymphoma), hyperplasia
  - GI tract: malignant neoplasia (leiomyosarcoma, GI stromal cell tumor [GIST], adenocarcinoma), benign neoplasia (leiomyoma), gastric dilation/volvulus (GDV), foreign body, trichobezoar, intussusception, mesenteric torsion, fecal material
  - Granuloma: secondary to retained foreign body (suture material, gauze [gossypiboma,], stick), infectious organisms such as protozoa or fungi, nodular fat necrosis (Bates body)
  - Pancreas: abscess, hemorrhagic pancreatitis, phlegmon (sequela of pancreatitis), rarely neoplasia (insulinoma)
- Mid-abdomen
  - Ovary: cyst, neoplasia (papillary adenoma/adenocarcinoma, granulosa cell tumor, teratoma)
  - Kidney: malignant neoplasia (renal cell carcinoma, nephroblastoma, lymphoma, hemangiosarcoma), benign neoplasia, renomegaly (hydronephrosis secondary to obstruction, pyelonephritis, toxin [ethylene glycol], portosystemic shunt), polycystic kidney, perirenal pseudocysts
  - Peritoneal cavity and mesentery: cyst, malignant neoplasia (carcinomatosis, hemangiosarcoma, mesothelioma), benign neoplasia (omental lipoma), sclerosing encapsulating peritonitis
- Caudal abdomen
  - Prostate: benign prostatic hypertrophy, prostatitis, prostatic abscess, prostatic cyst, paraprostatic cyst, neoplasia (prostatic or transitional cell carcinoma)
  - Testicles: typically benign neoplasm (Sertoli cell, seminoma, Leydig cell) or torsion of cryptorchid testicle
  - Urinary bladder: malignant neoplasia (transitional cell carcinoma, others), cystitis, urolithiasis, urethral obstruction, urinary retention from other causes (detrusor atony, neurologic)
  - Uterus: uterine torsion, pyometra, mucometra/hydrometra, pregnancy, neoplasia (adenocarcinoma, leiomyoma, leiomyosarcoma)

Initial Database

- CBC and serum biochemistry profile
- Urinalysis
  - Avoid cystocentesis if bleeding disorder or bladder tumor is suspected
- Urine culture and sensitivity for suspected urinary tract infection
- Survey abdominal radiographs
  - Evaluate location, size, mineralization of mass
  - Determine whether intestinal gas pattern suggests GI obstruction
  - Involvement or displacement of organs
  - Check for loss of serosal detail (suggests effusion) or free gas (viscus rupture)
- Abdominal ultrasound
  - Determine tissue of origin (may not be possible if mass is large and compresses other organs), consistency/echogenicity, vascularity, and invasiveness of mass
  - Evaluate distant organs for evidence of metastasis
  - Identify free fluid or gas
  - Ultrasound-guided sampling of free fluid for analysis ± culture
- Ultrasound-guided fine-needle aspiration of mass or enlarged organ for cytology (p. 1112) or needle biopsy for histopathology; avoid if thrombocytopenia/coagulopathy present or for bladder mass
- Three-view thoracic radiographs
  - Paraneoplastic syndromes (megaesophagus)
  - Aspiration pneumonia
  - Metastasis

Advanced or Confirmatory Testing

Choice of tests guided by initial findings but often includes

- CT is the imaging modality of choice for large masses.
- Diagnostic/exploratory celiotomy and mass removal or tissue sampling for histopathologic exam may be required for a diagnosis and treatment.

TREATMENT

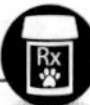

Treatment Overview

Often, removal of abdominal masses is indicated to minimize or prevent the following sequelae:

- Mechanical compression causing pain and/or organ dysfunction
- Localized or systemic infection
- Death from hemorrhage, metastasis, infection/sepsis, shock, or organ failure

Acute General Treatment

- Initial treatment includes stabilization as indicated by clinical condition.
  - Hypovolemic shock (p. 911)
  - Anemia (p. 57)
  - Peritonitis (p. 779)
  - Sepsis (p. 907)

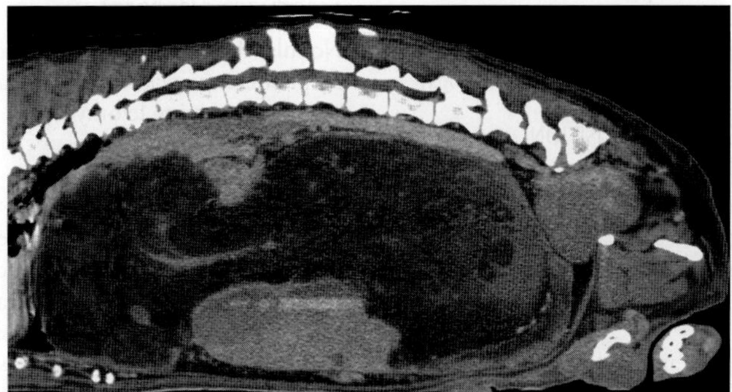

MASS, ABDOMINAL Large abdominal mass could not be identified on plain abdominal films or ultrasound. CT shows a very large, fat-attenuating splenic mass that was diagnosed as liposarcoma.

- Once stable, options include
  - Surgical intervention commonly indicated (e.g., bleeding splenic mass, intraabdominal abscess, uterine torsion, intestinal intussusception)
  - Medical treatment sometimes possible (e.g., chemotherapy for infiltrative lymphoma, medical treatment of fungal granuloma)
  - Palliative care: poor prognosis, costs, or owner's wishes
- In dogs at risk for GDV, consider gastropexy after removal of large masses

CHRONIC TREATMENT

Depends entirely on type/cause of mass

Nutrition/Diet

- Feeding tube placement during hospitalization (pp. 1106, 1107, and 1109) or surgery can help patients who have been or are expected to be anorexic.
- Supplemental nutrition is strongly advised in patients that are anorexic ≥ 5 days.

Possible Complications

Cross-sectional imaging for surgical planning of large/vascular masses and thorough knowledge of regional anatomy help minimize intraoperative complications.

Recommended Monitoring

General postoperative monitoring; specific parameters to monitor vary by disease/mass type

PROGNOSIS & OUTCOME

Varies, depending on diagnosis

PEARLS & CONSIDERATIONS

Comments

- Rule out normal processes (folded spleen, pregnancy) that cause an abdominal mass effect before proceeding to treatment.
- Some masses (including very large ones) are benign; presence of a mass does not by itself confer a particular prognosis.
- Prognosis is generally poorer for a patient with a nonresectable mass. Alternative therapies (e.g., chemoembolization for nonresectable liver mass) are available.
- Consider consultation with a veterinary specialist, especially for complicated or invasive abdominal masses (e.g., many adrenal tumors)

Technician Tips

Patients are often hypovolemic after removal of very large abdominal masses; monitor for tachycardia, low blood pressure, and tacky mucous membranes.

Client Education

Laboratory evaluation, imaging, and biopsy are usually necessary for definitive assessment of an abdominal mass.

SUGGESTED READING

Thamm DJ: Miscellaneous tumors. In Withrow SJ, et al, editors: Small animal clinical oncology, ed 5, St. Louis, 2013, Elsevier, p 679.

AUTHOR: Jacob A. Rubin DVM, DACVS
EDITOR: Elizabeth A. Swanson DVM, MS, DACVS

Mass: Cutaneous, Subcutaneous

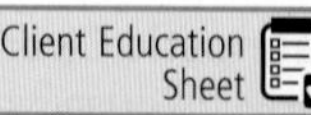

BASIC INFORMATION

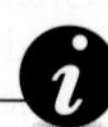

Definition

- A grossly detectable accumulation of cells in the skin (cutaneous) or soft tissue between the skin and underlying fascia, muscle, or bone (subcutaneous)
- Very common in dogs and common in cats

Epidemiology

SPECIES, AGE, SEX

- Older animals more commonly develop benign and malignant neoplasms.
- Eosinophilic lesions and plasma cell pododermatitis or stomatitis (cats)
- Canine juvenile cellulitis (puppies)
- Histiocytomas and viral papillomas (young dogs)
- Intact male cats are prone to abscesses because of fighting behavior.
- Mammary tumors (intact female dogs)
- Perianal gland tumors (intact male dogs)

GENETICS, BREED PREDISPOSITION

- Malignant tumors are more common in purebred versus crossbred dogs.
- Boxers are prone to a variety of benign and malignant neoplasms.
- Cutaneous histiocytoma (flat-coated retrievers)
- Keratinous cysts and nodular dermatofibrosis syndrome (German shepherds)
- Idiopathic focal mucinosis (Doberman pinschers)
- Dermatophyte pseudomycetoma (Persian cats)

RISK FACTORS

Long-term exposure to sunlight increases the risk of cutaneous hemangioma and hemangiosarcoma (dogs) and squamous cell carcinoma (dogs and cats).

CONTAGION AND ZOONOSIS

Transmissible venereal tumors and viral papillomas are contagious between dogs.

GEOGRAPHY AND SEASONALITY

- Transmissible venereal tumor is more prevalent in temperate climates.
- Fungal infections are more common in certain locales.

ASSOCIATED DISORDERS

Nodular dermatofibrosis syndrome in German shepherds is associated with renal adenocarcinoma and uterine leiomyoma.

Clinical Presentation

HISTORY, CHIEF COMPLAINT

- Most commonly, the pet owner sees or feels the mass, but it may be found incidentally by the veterinarian on physical exam.
- Historic information obtained should include
  - Evidence of systemic illness
  - Presence of similar lesions
  - Rapidity of onset/progression (malignant tumors tend to grow rapidly)
  - Evidence of pruritus or pain
  - Presence of other animals in the household
  - Possibility of exposure to anticoagulant rodenticides (hematomas)
  - Known trauma
  - In cats, indoor/outdoor status should be known (risk of bite or scratch wounds, foreign bodies, other trauma).

PHYSICAL EXAM FINDINGS

- Characterize the mass in terms of size, shape, location, consistency, depth, and ulceration and whether it is freely movable. Malignant tumors are more likely to be ulcerated, fixed to underlying structures, and have poorly defined margins.
- Examine local lymph nodes and possible sites of metastasis (e.g., lungs, abdomen). Local lymph nodes may be enlarged due to inflammation (i.e., reactive lymph node) or metastasis.
- A complete physical exam is essential to identify associated abnormalities.

Etiology and Pathophysiology

- A neoplasm is caused by progressive, uncontrolled growth of cells. Unlike benign neoplasms, malignant neoplasia shows a greater degree of anaplasia and exhibits invasive and metastatic properties. Most have an unknown cause, but some may be induced by irritation, trauma, viruses, vaccinations, ultraviolet radiation exposure, thermal injury, immunologic or genetic influences, or hormones.

- Cysts are accumulations of material (keratin, serum, glandular product) within a membrane that may have idiopathic, traumatic, congenital, follicular, or pilar causes.
- A granuloma is a focal accumulation of mononuclear inflammatory cells due to bacteria, mycoses, mycobacteria, dermatophytes, parasites, endogenous or exogenous foreign objects, allergic, or idiopathic causes. Pyogranulomas also include neutrophilic inflammation.
- Keratoses are solid, circumscribed lesions caused by overproduction of keratin.
- A hamartoma is a benign, disorganized overgrowth of normal cells within a tissue, whereas a nevus is a hamartoma arising from any skin component.
- A hematoma is local extravasation of blood due to trauma and/or bleeding disorder.
- Abscesses result from a local accumulation of neutrophils and necrotic tissue cells, usually secondary to a bacterial or fungal infectious agent.
- Urticaria is a group of wheals in the dermis caused by a hypersensitivity reaction to insect bites, food, irritants, drugs, allergens, or physical stimuli. Angioedema is a hypersensitivity reaction that occurs below the dermis.

DIAGNOSIS

Diagnostic Overview

Cytologic analysis of a fine-needle aspiration (FNA) sample, impression smear, scrape, or swab sample from a mass may provide a tentative or sometimes a definitive diagnosis. Histopathologic evaluation of an incisional or excisional biopsy may be necessary for final diagnosis.

Differential Diagnosis

- Neoplasm
  - Benign
  - Malignant: epithelial, glandular, mesenchymal, round cell
- Pseudoneoplasm
  - Cyst
  - (Pyo)granuloma
  - Keratoses
  - Hamartoma/nevus
  - Acral lick dermatitis
  - Feline plasma cell pododermatitis or stomatitis
  - Calcinosis cutis
  - Calcinosis circumscripta
  - Canine juvenile cellulitis
  - Nodular sterile panniculitis
  - Idiopathic lichenoid dermatitis (coalescent plaques)
  - Idiopathic focal mucinosis (Doberman pinschers)
  - Eosinophilic lesions: eosinophilic plaque, indolent ulcer, collagenolytic granuloma
- Hematoma
- Abscess
- Urticaria
- Angioedema
- Normal structures
  - Lymph node
  - Salivary gland
  - Bulbus glandis (transient preputial "mass" in male dogs)

Initial Database

- Confirm that the mass is not a normal structure (anatomic location).
- Cytologic exam of samples obtained from a mass by FNA, impression smear, scrape, or swab may provide a diagnosis.
- Cytologic evaluation of a local lymph node by FNA may help discern an inflammatory reaction from metastasis.
- Exam for evidence of distant metastasis by three-view thoracic radiographs and/or abdominal ultrasound
- Preoperative blood tests (e.g., CBC, serum biochemical profile, urinalysis, depending on the age of the patient) if a biopsy is planned

Advanced or Confirmatory Testing

Histopathologic evaluation ± bacterial and fungal culture of an incisional or excisional biopsy sample is sometimes necessary for a definitive diagnosis. Excisional biopsy may be diagnostic and therapeutic.

TREATMENT

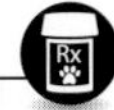

Treatment Overview

Benign neoplasms or pseudoneoplasms may not require treatment if they are not causing harm to the patient (e.g., lipoma, sebaceous cyst). Eliminating the mass by surgery and/or medical management may be ideal.

Acute and Chronic Treatment

- Often, masses are removed surgically for diagnosis and treatment.
- Drainage and antibacterial therapy (based on culture and sensitivity) recommended for most abscesses
- Medical therapy without surgical removal may be appropriate: eosinophilic lesions, urticaria and angioedema, dermatophytic pseudomycetoma, hematomas, and some round cell tumors

PROGNOSIS & OUTCOME

- Depends on the diagnosis
- Many benign masses can be cured with complete surgical removal or appropriate medical therapy (e.g., panniculitis, eosinophilic granuloma).
- Removal of malignant neoplasms can result in long remissions, or cure if metastasis is absent. For some tumor types, wide initial surgical margins are necessary (pp. 550, 634, and 927).

PEARLS & CONSIDERATIONS

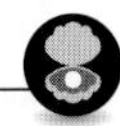

Comments

- Establishing a diagnosis by physical exam alone can lead to inappropriate patient outcomes.
- Cytologic exam of a sample obtained by FNA from a cutaneous or subcutaneous mass is a simple and inexpensive diagnostic aid that should be recommended in most cases (any mass > 1 cm diameter).
- Cytologic diagnosis before surgery may aid in surgical planning (i.e., are wide margins required?).

Technician Tips

Assisting in early recognition of new or changing masses can lead to rapid diagnosis and therapy and the best possible prognosis. Create body maps that allow any change in size of an existing mass to be recognized on future visits (p. 591).

SUGGESTED READING

Hauck ML: Tumors of the skin and subcutaneous tissues. In: Withrow SJ, et al, editors: Small animal clinical oncology, ed 5, St. Louis, 2013, Saunders, pp 305-320.

AUTHOR: Jeff D. Bay, DVM, DACVIM
EDITOR: Leah A. Cohn, DVM, PhD, DACVIM

Mass, Splenic

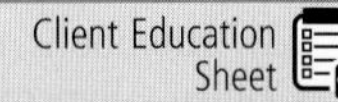

BASIC INFORMATION

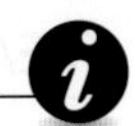

Definition

- Focal or diffuse enlargement of the spleen
- Causes include neoplastic and non-neoplastic infiltrative disorders, congestion, infection, inflammation, lymphoid hyperplasia, and extramedullary hematopoiesis.

Epidemiology

SPECIES, AGE, SEX

- Dogs: any dog, but often older, medium to large breed dogs of either sex
- Cats: diffuse splenomegaly is more common than nodular enlargement

GENETICS, BREED PREDISPOSITION

Labrador retrievers, German shepherds, and golden retrievers overrepresented

CONTAGION AND ZOONOSIS

Several vector-borne (e.g., cytauxzoonosis, babesiosis) and contagious (e.g., feline leukemia virus, brucellosis) infections can cause splenomegaly. Some are zoonotic (e.g., tularemia, leishmaniasis) (p. 1282).

GEOGRAPHY AND SEASONALITY

Some infectious diseases are associated with a geographic region or seasonality.

ASSOCIATED DISORDERS

Hemoabdomen, anemia, ventricular arrhythmias, disseminated intravascular coagulation (DIC), metastasis, vasculitis, thrombocytopenia

Clinical Presentation

DISEASE FORMS/SUBTYPES

Diffuse enlargement or focal mass-like lesion(s)

HISTORY, CHIEF COMPLAINT

Depends on cause but can include

- Minimal clinical signs; incidental finding on exam
- Inappetence, lethargy (may be intermittent), weight loss, vomiting, diarrhea
- Abdominal distention
- Weakness, collapse

PHYSICAL EXAM FINDINGS

Depends on size of mass and whether mass has ruptured but can include

- Palpable midabdominal mass
- Abdominal pain
- Abdominal distention
- Fluid (ballotable wave)
- Pale mucous membranes; weak, thready, or nonpalpable pulses; weakness; tachycardia
  - Hypovolemic shock caused by mass rupture and massive intra-abdominal hemorrhage
- Cardiac arrhythmias and pulse deficits; murmur due to anemia
- Other findings depend on cause of splenomegaly (e.g., peripheral lymphadenomegaly possible with lymphoma, fever due to infection or inflammation).

Etiology and Pathophysiology

- Splenomegaly is discussed on pp. 936 and 1282.
- Diffuse enlargement (generalized splenomegaly)
  - Infiltrative (e.g., lymphoma, mastocytosis [especially cats], histiocytic sarcoma, amyloidosis)
  - Congestion (e.g., splenic torsion, splenic vein thrombosis, right-sided heart failure)
  - Cellular hyperplasia (e.g., immune-mediated hemolytic anemia)
  - Inflammation/infection (e.g., erythrophagocytosis, infectious disease)
- Focal enlargement
  - Malignant neoplasia: cavitary tumors (e.g., hemangiosarcoma); solid tumors (e.g., leiomyosarcoma, liposarcoma)
  - Benign neoplasia: cavitary (e.g., hemangioma); solid (e.g., lipoma)
  - Trauma/hematoma
  - Nodular regeneration
  - Abscess

DIAGNOSIS

Diagnostic Overview

Splenic mass can be recognized by physical exam and diagnostic imaging. Although signalment, history, exam, and imaging findings often provide a strong suspicion about the cause, confirmation often requires additional testing, frequently including cytology and/or biopsy.

Differential Diagnosis

- Liver
  - Hepatic enlargement shifts gastric axis caudally
  - Diffuse hepatomegaly (lymphoma, hepatitis, cholangiohepatitis, hepatic lipidosis)
  - Benign neoplasia (cystadenoma, hepatoma)
  - Malignant neoplasia (massive hepatocellular carcinoma, hemangiosarcoma, biliary carcinoma)
- Kidney
  - Located retroperitoneally, displacing viscera ventrally
  - Neoplasia (renal cell carcinoma, lymphoma, hemangiosarcoma)
  - Severe hydronephrosis/pyelonephritis secondary to obstruction
  - Renal cyst
  - Perirenal pseudocyst
- Stomach: fluid-filled pylorus resembles a mass on right lateral radiographs.
- Abdominal cavity
  - Omental mass
  - Nodular fat necrosis: Bates body
  - Gossypiboma
- Lymph node
- Adrenal gland
  - Neoplasia (adenoma, adenocarcinoma, pheochromocytoma)

Initial Database

Varies broadly, with minimal changes possible

- CBC, serum biochemistry profile, urinalysis: depends on disorder, but can include
  - Evidence of hemorrhage
    - Acute: nonregenerative anemia, panhypoproteinemia
    - Chronic: regenerative anemia, hypoalbuminemia
    - A slightly low hematocrit with intermittent lethargy is highly suggestive of periodic minor hemorrhage.
  - Evidence of hemolysis (schistocytosis, spherocytes), red blood cell (RBC) parasites
  - Other organ system involvement (e.g., kidney, liver)
  - Hemoglobinuria/bilirubinuria
- Survey abdominal radiographs
  - To help identify splenic origin of mass
  - Poor serosal detail indicates free peritoneal fluid.
  - Size of spleen (larger size does *not* correspond to worse prognosis)
- Three-view thoracic radiographs
  - Pulmonary metastasis
  - Lymphadenopathy
  - Cardiomegaly suggestive of heart failure (congestion) or atrial tumor (hemangiosarcoma)
  - Sternal lymphadenopathy may indicate abdominal inflammation rather than metastasis

Advanced or Confirmatory Testing

- Abdominal ultrasound
  - Confirmation of origin and consistency of mass (e.g., cavitated lesions at greater risk for rupture)
  - Assess blood flow (splenic torsion)
  - Invasion of neighboring organs
  - Metastatic lesions
  - Localization of free abdominal fluid
- Abdominocentesis (blind or ultrasound guided [p. 1056])
  - Acute hemorrhage: abdominal packed cell volume (PCV) = peripheral PCV
  - Chronic hemorrhage: abdominal PCV > peripheral PCV
  - Previous hemorrhage: abdominal PCV < peripheral PCV
- Coagulation profile
  - Rule out rodenticide toxicity, bleeding disorders
  - Evaluation for DIC
- Electrocardiogram (ECG)
  - Accelerated idioventricular rhythms most common in patients with splenic masses and after splenectomy
  - Occasional ventricular premature contraction (VPC) usually associated with splenic capsule distention
  - Ventricular tachycardia
  - Other arrhythmias occasionally
- Fine-needle aspiration/cytology of spleen (ultrasound-guided)
  - Only for solitary masses or generalized splenomegaly; rarely able to differentiate tumor type or benign from malignant disease (exceptions: lymphoma, mastocytosis)
  - For cavitated masses, contraindicated due to low yield; risk of rupture or hemorrhage
- Echocardiography
  - Rule out right atrial hemangiosarcoma (8% of patients have splenic and cardiac masses); low-yield test
- Cross-sectional imaging
  - CT to identify the origin of large masses
    - Angiography may help identify early-onset metastatic lesions.
  - MRI may elucidate benign versus malignant lesions but is inherently flawed (long scan times and motion).

TREATMENT

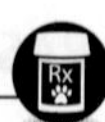

Treatment Overview

- In many cases, surgery should be performed to remove the spleen after the patient has been stabilized. Remove large, nonbleeding masses before they rupture. Treat hypovolemic

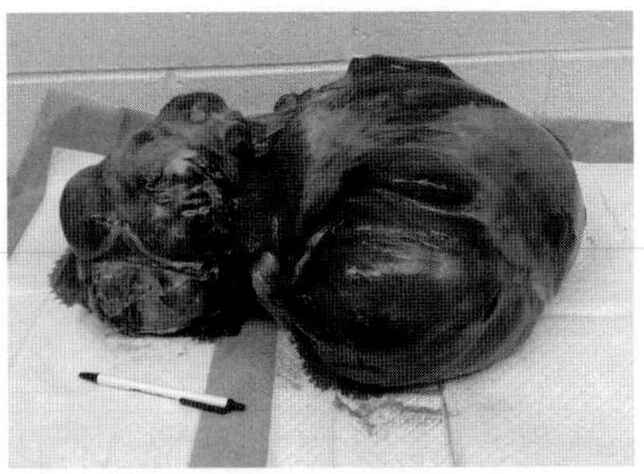

SPLENIC MASS The large splenic mass was removed and diagnosed as benign nodular hyperplasia. Size and shape of the mass are not a substitute for histopathologic diagnosis.

shock with IV fluids and blood products as needed. Immediate surgery is indicated for patients with active hemorrhage if pressures cannot be stabilized or if blood products are not available.
- Some causes of splenic mass are amenable to medical treatment (e.g., lymphoma, diffuse splenomegaly associated with congestion from right heart failure or from infectious [e.g., babesiosis, cytauxzoonosis] or inflammatory disease [e.g., immune-mediated hemolytic anemia]).

Acute General Treatment

- Initial stabilization for acute intraabdominal hemorrhage
  - IV fluid resuscitation (crystalloids ± colloids)
  - Blood product transfusion if needed (p. 1169)
  - Definitive surgical therapy is recommended after patient is stabilized.
  - Immediate surgery if patient cannot be stabilized (i.e., massive, ongoing internal hemorrhage)
- Treat coagulation disorders if prothrombin time/activated partial thromboplastin time (PT/aPTT) significantly prolonged (> 2 × normal) (p. 1325):
  - Fresh-frozen plasma, fresh whole blood
- Correct/control ventricular arrhythmias.
  - Correction of anemia/hypovolemia or electrolyte abnormalities often resolves ventricular arrhythmias without antiarrhythmic drugs.
  - Treat if arrhythmia persists and is pathologic (pp. 1033 and 1457).
- Complete splenectomy is necessary for control of hemorrhage and definitive diagnosis by histology.
  - Partial splenectomy is not recommended for splenic masses.
  - Consider liver biopsy ± lymph node biopsy for staging purposes.
- Nonsurgically treated splenic masses
  - Some neoplasms (e.g., lymphoma) treated with chemotherapy
  - Diffuse metastatic disease (e.g., hemangiosarcoma, histiocytic sarcoma): owner may elect palliative treatment only.
  - Diffuse splenomegaly associated with immune-mediated disorders, may/may not help underlying disease process
  - Splenectomy is contraindicated in cases of babesiosis and other hematologic infections.

Chronic Treatment

- Supportive care in the postoperative period
  - Analgesia
  - Fluid therapy must replace blood volume that was present in the mass.
  - Transfusion therapy (p. 1169)
  - Treatment of cardiac arrhythmias (pp. 1033 and 1457)
- Adjunct chemotherapy for malignant neoplasia

Drug Interactions

- Avoid acepromazine or other phenothiazine tranquilizers before surgery.
  - Causes splenic enlargement; may worsen bleeding and complicate removal
  - Can cause hypotension through central mechanisms and through alpha-adrenergic actions; may progress to cardiovascular collapse
- Avoid phenylephrine unless splenic mass is confirmed benign
  - Risk of seeding of tumor cells

Possible Complications

- Rupture of splenic mass
  - Hemoabdomen
  - Hypotension
  - Hemorrhagic/hypovolemic shock
  - Coagulation disorders
  - Cardiovascular collapse and death
- Intraoperative and postoperative complications
  - Hemorrhage
  - Ventricular arrhythmias
  - Damage to blood supply of pancreas
  - Pancreatitis from traumatic handling of pancreas
  - Chronic anemia from loss of red blood cell reservoir and decreased hematopoiesis
  - Diminished immune function (especially vector-borne and fungal disease)
  - Portal vein thrombosis (uncommon)
  - Gastric dilation/volvulus (uncommon); consider gastropexy in predisposed breeds

Recommended Monitoring

- Standard postoperative patient monitoring
- Serial PCV and total protein (TP) to monitor for hemorrhage
- Heart rate, blood pressure, and urine output to evaluate hydration status and restore euvolemia
- ECG monitoring for cardiac arrhythmias
  - Continuous ECG for first 24 hours postoperatively; spot checks thereafter if no arrhythmias noted and/or prior arrhythmias resolving
  - Ventricular arrhythmias may develop in first 3 days postoperatively (most within 24 hours) and typically resolve after 1-5 days.
- Long-term follow-up depends on diagnosis (e.g., thoracic radiographs q 3 months to monitor for pulmonary metastasis)

PROGNOSIS & OUTCOME

- Prognosis varies with cause for malignant and nonmalignant causes of splenic mass.
- Hemangiosarcoma (most common malignant splenic neoplasm in dogs); median survival time: 0-3 months with surgery alone, 4-8 months with surgery and chemotherapy
- Cats with systemic mastocytosis that undergo splenectomy often have extended survival times and may be cured.
- Prognostic indicators: NOTE: these findings are suspicious for but do not confirm a diagnosis. Only histopathologic evaluation of tissue can definitively differentiate malignant and benign disease.
  - Preoperatively, dogs with anemia, nucleated RBCs, abnormal RBC morphology, or splenic rupture are more likely to have malignant splenic neoplasia.
  - In one study, 50% of large incidentally discovered splenic masses in the absence of hemoabdomen were benign.

PEARLS & CONSIDERATIONS

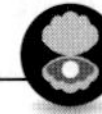

Comments

- In the dog, a splenic mass may be non-neoplastic (e.g., hematoma) or may be a benign (e.g., hemangioma) or malignant (e.g., hemangiosarcoma) neoplasm, and the *entire* mass and/or spleen should always be submitted for histopathologic exam.
- Be sure to section (bread-loaf) large masses into slices < 1-2 cm thick to allow appropriate penetration of formalin.
- It is impossible to differentiate splenic masses based on their gross appearance. Diagnosis is always based on histopathological exam.
- Accelerated idioventricular rhythms do not require treatment; however, monitor closely because they can convert to ventricular tachycardia.

Technician Tips

- The volume lost by removal of large masses frequently causes postoperative hypovolemia. Familiarity with the signs of hypovolemia is imperative for postoperative management.
- Be able to recognize accelerated idioventricular rhythm, R-on-T complexes and ventricular tachycardia to know when to alert the clinician for treatment of ventricular arrhythmias (pp. 1033 and 1457).

Client Education

- Bleeding splenic masses
  - Two-thirds are malignant, and two-thirds of those are hemangiosarcoma.
- Splenic masses may rupture and cause lethal intraabdominal hemorrhage.

- Splenectomy prevents exsanguination.
- Splenectomy improves the quality of life for the patient, but depending on diagnosis, it may not prolong life.

SUGGESTED READING

Thamm DG: Hemangiosarcoma. In Withrow SJ, et al, editors: Withrow and MacEwen's Small animal clinical oncology, St. Louis, 2013, Saunders, pp 679-684.

AUTHOR: Jacob A. Rubin DVM, DACVS
EDITOR: Elizabeth A. Swanson DVM, MS, DACVS

Mast Cell Tumors, Cat

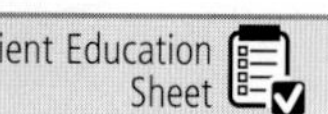

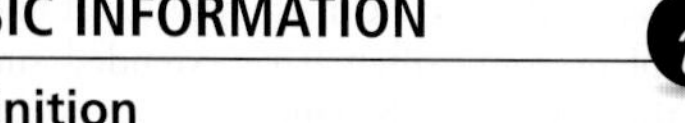

BASIC INFORMATION

Definition

Mast cell tumors (MCTs) are neoplastic accumulations of mast cells. MCTs produce deleterious effects when mast cells degranulate, resulting in release of bioactive substances that can produce cutaneous or systemic effects, depending on tumor location. Cutaneous MCTs are common. Visceral MCTs include splenic MCTs (uncommon) and gastrointestinal (GI) MCTs (rare).

Synonyms

Mastocytoma, splenic or visceral mastocytosis

Epidemiology

SPECIES, AGE, SEX

- Primarily a disease of older cats, although all ages can be affected
- Information on MCTs in dogs is provided on p. 634.

GENETICS, BREED PREDISPOSITION

Siamese (possibly)

RISK FACTORS

Mutations in the proto-oncogene *KIT* have occurred in feline MCT and may predispose cats to MCT development.

ASSOCIATED DISORDERS

Related to mast cell degranulation:
- GI ulceration
- Pruritus, cutaneous flushing, peritumoral edema, bruising
- Delayed wound healing

Related to visceral MCT (especially splenic):
- Pleural or abdominal cavity effusion (often containing mast cells)

Clinical Presentation

DISEASE FORMS/SUBTYPES

In cats, there are several distinct presentations:
- Cutaneous MCT (solitary or multiple)
- Splenic (i.e., visceral MCT; splenomegaly, occasionally concurrent with hepatic and/or bone marrow infiltration, and abdominal effusion)
- GI MCT (i.e., visceral MCT; commonly with hepatic and mesenteric lymph node [LN] infiltration)
- A unique form of feline visceral MCT is feline intestinal sclerosing MCT, a primary GI mass histologically characterized by GI mucosal ulceration, eosinophilic infiltrates, and poorly granulated MCTs.

HISTORY, CHIEF COMPLAINT

- Most cats with cutaneous MCTs are asymptomatic, although some lesions are pruritic and have peritumoral edema or bruising. MCTs often remain unchanged in appearance for years.
- Cats with visceral MCTs display nonspecific signs of illness (weakness, lethargy, anorexia) or GI ulceration–associated bruxism, vomiting, diarrhea, weight loss, and melena. Abdominal distention secondary to effusion and splenomegaly may also occur.

PHYSICAL EXAM FINDINGS

- Although most cutaneous MCTs are found on the head/neck, a thorough exam of the skin is indicated. Tumors are usually alopecic, small (<5 mm), round, and pink or white. Some MCTs are plaquelike. Regional

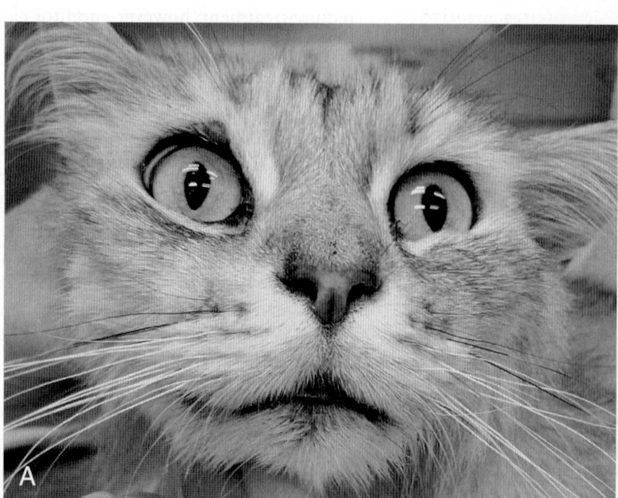

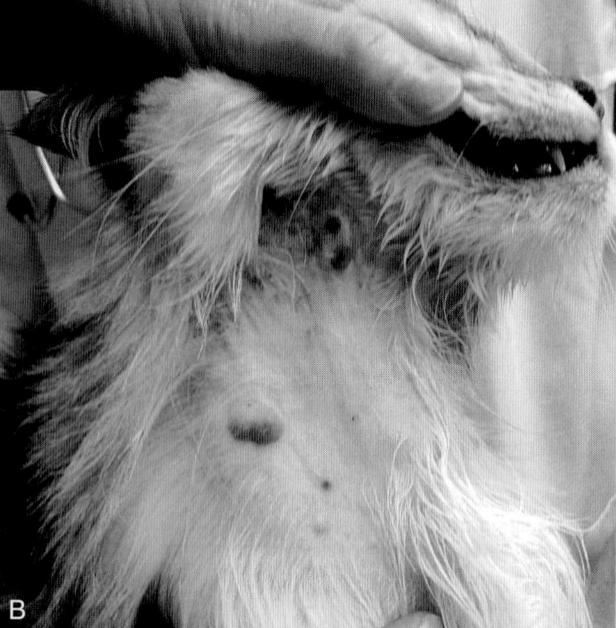

MAST CELL TUMORS, CAT A, Note the hairless, red MCT on the right dorsal eyelid. **B,** MCTs on the face and neck. On further exam, this cat had numerous cutaneous MCTs and splenic involvement.

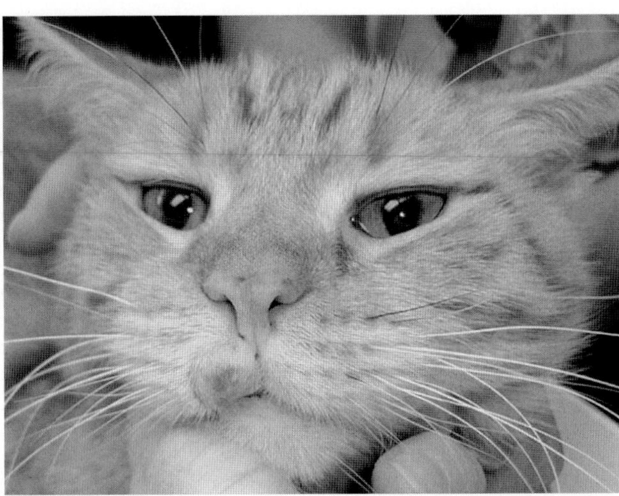

MAST CELL TUMORS, CAT This right lip MCT was present for several months before presentation and had not changed in size. The pink, hairless mass with mild, superficial ulceration is typical.

lymph nodes may be normal in size even with metastasis. About 15% of cats with cutaneous MCTs have concurrent splenic or visceral MCT.
- Visceral MCTs: splenomegaly, ascites, abdominal mass, bowel wall thickening, abdominal pain, and mucous membrane pallor secondary to anemia are possible.

Etiology and Pathophysiology
- Mast cells participate in allergic and inflammatory responses and are normally found in skin, visceral organs, bone marrow, and lungs.
- Mast cells harbor preformed granules that contain histamine, heparin, and other cytokines that are released on activation of the cells (degranulation). Cytokine release produces clinical signs. Degranulation may be spontaneous or secondary to manipulation of the tumor.
- MCTs may metastasize to regional LNs, spleen, liver, bone marrow, mesenteric LNs, and skin.
- Feline leukemia virus and feline immunodeficiency virus infections are not associated with the development of feline MCT.

DIAGNOSIS

Diagnostic Overview
- Cutaneous MCT should be suspected in cats with small, white or pink, hairless, pimplelike lesions of the head and neck; fine-needle aspiration (FNA) for cytologic exam is usually diagnostic. Cutaneous MCTs often temporarily bleed after aspiration.
- Any cat with splenomegaly should be suspected to have splenic MCT, and FNA of the spleen should be considered.
- GI MCT should be considered for any cat with an abdominal mass, although it is less common than other feline GI cancers. FNA of the mass is usually diagnostic.

Differential Diagnosis
- Cutaneous form: basal cell tumor, hair follicle or sweat gland tumor, squamous cell carcinoma, hemangioma/sarcoma, lymphoma, eosinophilic granuloma complex, and lipoma
- Splenic form: hemangiosarcoma, lymphoma, infectious splenitis, myeloproliferative disease
- GI masses or diffuse infiltration of the GI tract: lymphoma, intestinal adenocarcinoma, inflammatory bowel disease, leiomyosarcoma, histoplasmosis, or granulomas

Initial Database
Cutaneous form:
- FNA of the lesion for cytologic exam: cytologically, mast cells have a round nucleus and intracytoplasmic granules are almost always present.
- Before treatment: CBC, serum biochemistry panel, urinalysis, and a regional lymph node aspirate (if accessible) should be obtained.
  - CBC: mastocythemia (mast cells in peripheral circulation), eosinophilia, basophilia, and regenerative or nonregenerative anemia are possible. Serum chemistry may be normal or reflect protein loss or hepatic infiltration with mast cells.
  - LN aspirate and cytologic exams: normal; LN may contain scattered mast cells; increased numbers or clusters of mast cells in the LN draining an MCT suggest metastasis.
  - Buffy coat smear: more specific in cats than dogs. A positive test supports a diagnosis of mastocytosis in cats with MCTs.
- Staging for systemic mast cell disease is indicated before surgery in patients with lymph node metastasis, peritumoral edema or bruising, recurrent or multiple MCTs, or if there is suspicion of splenic or visceral MCTs.
  - Staging includes the tests listed above plus thoracic radiographs (rare pleural effusion), abdominal ultrasound (LN, splenic/hepatic enlargement/infiltration, GI mass or diffuse thickening), bone marrow aspiration (p. 1068); low yield in most cases with a normal CBC), splenic/liver aspiration (p. 1112), and fluid analysis (p. 1343).

Visceral forms (spleen, GI tract):
- Cats with visceral MCTs should have complete staging before definitive therapy.

Advanced or Confirmatory Testing
- The histologic grading system used for canine cutaneous MCTs is not applicable for cats.
- Histologic subtypes for feline cutaneous MCTs include mastocytic well-differentiated, mastocytic pleomorphic, and atypical/poorly granulated tumors. The mastocytic pleomorphic type has a higher mitotic index and a worse prognosis.
- Subtypes cannot be defined cytologically. *KIT* mutations occur in the majority of cutaneous or splenic MCTs but have not been shown to be prognostic for survival.

TREATMENT

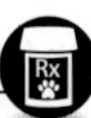

Treatment Overview
In most cases, the goal of therapy is to control the local disease with surgery or possibly radiation therapy (RT) to prevent recurrence and metastasis. In cases presenting with metastasis or nonresectable local disease, the goals are to minimize tumor volume and secondary GI signs and to maintain quality of life.

Acute and Chronic Treatment
Cutaneous form:
- Surgery is the primary treatment for cutaneous MCTs.
  - Preoperative diphenhydramine 1 mg/kg IM (not IV)
  - Wide surgical margins are not as important in cats as in dogs because recurrence after incomplete excision is uncommon in cats.
  - All tissue should be submitted for histologic evaluation; margins should be inked before placement in formalin.
  - Postoperative complications are uncommon; wound healing should be monitored after resection of large, infiltrative MCTs.
- MCTs in locations that may preclude complete excision (i.e., periocular, pinna) are common in cats. External beam RT (by linear accelerator) is uncommonly used; strontium-90 plesiotherapy (radiation source applied directly to small tumors) may be used instead of or after marginal excision.
- Chemotherapy and targeted therapy may play a role in cats with multiple, nonresectable, or metastatic cutaneous MCTs.

Visceral (splenic or GI) forms:
- Take care not to excessively manipulate tumor tissue because degranulation can result in anaphylaxis and hypotension. Perioperative diphenhydramine 1 mg/kg IM (not IV) and possibly dexamethasone sodium phosphate 1 mg/CAT IV (anecdotal) are recommended.

- Surgery is the primary treatment modality. Exploratory laparotomy/GI mass resection with liver and mesenteric lymph node biopsies, even if the tissue appears normal, are indicated.
- Splenectomy is the treatment of choice in cats with splenic MCTs, even if metastasis or cutaneous MCT is present. After splenectomy, disseminated disease may improve spontaneously and/or respond to chemotherapy or targeted therapy.

Chemotherapy and targeted therapy:
- Potential indications: multiple or recurrent cutaneous MCTs, metastasis at diagnosis, or before attempting surgical excision of large, infiltrative tumors.
- CCNU (lomustine) in cats with measurable MCT has a response rate of 50%, with a median duration of response of 168 days.
- Other drugs that may be effective include prednisone, chlorambucil, and vinblastine. Special handling requirements and potentially severe or life-threatening adverse patient effects exist with these chemotherapeutic drugs; these concerns and rapid evolution of protocols warrant consultation with/referral to an oncologist.
- Drugs that inhibit tyrosine kinase receptors (toceranib [Palladia]) may be used in conjunction with or instead of chemotherapy (3/14 cats that failed other treatments had partial or complete responses to Palladia), Consultation with an oncologist is advised before use.

Adjunctive therapies:
- Intralesional corticosteroids and de-ionized water are rarely useful and are not advised.
- Antihistamines are indicated for cats with MCTs before surgical excision or in cases of nonresectable or metastatic disease. Consider cyproheptadine 2 mg/CAT PO q 12-24h or diphenhydramine 1-2 mg/kg PO (most cats dislike the taste of the liquid suspension) or SQ (anecdotal) q 12h. Cyproheptadine is recommended for feline MCT due to its antiserotonin properties and ease of administration compared with diphenhydramine (side effects may include appetite stimulation). Proton pump inhibitors or H2 blockers should also be used in cats with measurable MCT.
- Supportive care, including nutritional and blood product support and analgesia, is indicated perioperatively as needed.

PROGNOSIS & OUTCOME

- The prognosis for cats with solitary cutaneous MCTs is good, and recurrence after excision or RT is uncommon. Cutaneous MCTs with > 5 mitoses/10 HPF have a worse prognosis. No factors are known to be predictive for development of multiple cutaneous MCTs, regional lymph node metastasis, or splenic or visceral MCTs.
- Cats with multiple cutaneous MCTs or cats with cutaneous tumors plus distant metastases have a median survival time of 582 days; longer median survival times are reached by cats with solitary dermal MCTs and by cats with cutaneous MCTs compared with cats that have splenic or visceral tumors.
- Prognosis for cats with solitary splenic MCTs: median survival time after splenectomy is ≈4-28 months. With involvement of additional sites (liver, skin), the prognosis varies, and chemotherapy or toceranib should be considered.
- Primary GI MCTs have the poorest prognosis (many cats die perioperatively or in 2-3 months postoperatively), which may improve if the lesions are surgically resectable. Chemotherapy or targeted therapy is recommended for these cats after surgery.

PEARLS & CONSIDERATIONS

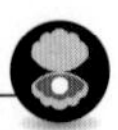

Comments

Many cats with mast cell disease develop additional MCTs, including cutaneous, splenic, and GI forms. Patients should be rechecked at least q 4-6 months by physical exams and possibly with restaging. The prognosis for feline MCTs varies widely, and individual cases should be discussed with an oncologist to devise an appropriate diagnostic/therapeutic plan and likely prognosis.

Technician Tips

In cats, MCTs are often located on the head and neck and have a white-to-pink pimplelike appearance. They may not change in appearance for years and are often overlooked. Aspiration cytology is diagnostic in most cases. In cats, clipping the fur (even the entire haircoat) may be indicated to identify all MCTs because they are often so small, but make sure to obtain owner permission.

Client Education

Client education about the pimplelike, small size of most feline MCTs is essential because early diagnosis and therapy are most likely to result in successful treatment. Any new skin mass or signs of illness should be evaluated as soon as possible.

SUGGESTED READING

Sabbatini S, et al: Prognostic value of histologic and immunohistochemical features in feline cutaneous mast cell tumors. Vet Pathol 47(4):643-653, 2010.

AUTHOR: Tracy Gieger, DVM, DACVIM, DACVR
EDITOR: Kenneth M. Rassnick, DVM, DACVIM

Mast Cell Tumors, Dog

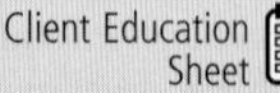

BASIC INFORMATION

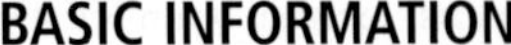

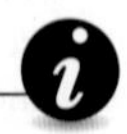

Definition

Canine mast cell tumors (MCTs) are neoplastic accumulations of mast cells. MCTs produce deleterious effects when the mast cells degranulate, releasing bioactive substances that can produce cutaneous or systemic effects, depending on location. In dogs, cutaneous and subcutaneous MCTs are common, and extracutaneous MCTs are uncommon.

Synonyms

Mastocytoma, systemic mastocytosis (metastatic MCT)

Epidemiology

SPECIES, AGE, SEX

Can occur in any age dog; the median age in dogs is 8 years.

GENETICS, BREED PREDISPOSITION

Breeds predisposed to MCT include boxer, Boston terrier, golden retriever, Labrador retriever, pug, Shar-pei, Staffordshire bull terrier, Jack Russell terrier

ASSOCIATED DISORDERS

Caused by mast cell degranulation: gastrointestinal ulceration, pruritus, hypotension, and delayed wound healing

Clinical Presentation

HISTORY, CHIEF COMPLAINT

- Most dogs show no clinical signs and are evaluated for an incidentally discovered cutaneous or subcutaneous mass. Lesions might be pruritic or have a history of shrinking and swelling. MCTs often remain unchanged in size for months before presentation or may be rapidly growing.
- Occasionally, dogs are evaluated because of signs related to gastric ulceration (vomiting, diarrhea, weight loss, melena) secondary to histamine-induced gastric acid secretion.

PHYSICAL EXAM FINDINGS

- MCTs have a highly variable appearance and may be mistaken for lipomas, skin tags, or insect bites. Skin and subcutaneous masses should always be aspirated and examined cytologically to obtain a diagnosis.
- Some dogs have multiple cutaneous MCTs, and a thorough exam of the entire skin surface is indicated.
- Because of the histamine in mast cell granules, MCTs might shrink and swell intermittently as degranulation (release of granules from the mast cell cytoplasm) occurs. Degranulation can result from manipulation of the tumor or can be spontaneous.
- Because of the presence of heparin in mast cell granules, MCTs may bleed excessively when aspirated, but this is rarely clinically significant.
- Peritumoral bruising and edema (i.e., Darier's sign) and hyperemia (p. 494) are uncommon but are associated with aggressive MCTs.
- Dogs with primary visceral or metastatic MCTs may have abdominal effusion containing mast cells, organomegaly (spleen/liver), a palpable abdominal mass, or abdominal pain on palpation.

Etiology and Pathophysiology

- Causes are further discussed on p. 632.
- The likelihood of MCT metastasis depends on tumor grade, mitotic index, location, and other factors, and it varies from 10%-50%. In dogs, MCTs most commonly metastasize to regional lymph nodes, followed by spleen, liver, mesenteric lymph nodes, other cutaneous sites, and bone marrow.
- Chronic dermatitis or mutations in a proto-oncogene *(KIT)* may predispose dogs to mast cell neoplasia. *KIT* encodes the tyrosine kinase receptor KIT, which promotes mast cell growth and differentiation. Mutations in *KIT* (≈20%-30% of canine MCTs) allow abnormal continuous activation of the receptor and predispose dogs to aggressive MCTs that are more likely to recur and metastasize. Inhibition of receptor tyrosine kinases through targeted therapies (see Treatment below) has a role in the treatment of advanced local or metastatic MCTs.

DIAGNOSIS

Diagnostic Overview

The diagnosis of MCT is generally straightforward. Microscopic exam of cytologic preparations or tissue samples reveals round cells with characteristic intracytoplasmic, metachromatic granules. Regional lymph nodes should be aspirated whenever possible before surgical removal of the primary tumor (most often the treatment of choice), and additional staging tests should be considered for lymph node metastasis or in patients with clinical signs of aggressive tumor behavior, including peritumoral edema, swelling, or bruising, and for recurrent tumors. A diagnostic and treatment approach is presented on p. 1436.

Differential Diagnosis

Gross appearance and palpation:

- Other tumor types: plasma cell tumor, histiocytoma, transmissible venereal tumor, lymphoma, amelanotic melanoma, squamous cell carcinoma, hemangiosarcoma or hemangioma, lipoma
- Phlebectasia
- Granuloma
- Abscess

Cytologically, other round cell tumors may have a similar appearance (p. 893).

Initial Database

- MCTs are readily diagnosed cytologically by their characteristic intracytoplasmic granules. In poorly differentiated MCTs, these granules may not be visible, especially with Diff-Quik stain (in-clinic stain). Wright stain (used in most university and commercial clinical pathology laboratories) is more sensitive for detecting granules.
- Before surgical excision, a CBC, serum chemistry panel, urinalysis, and regional lymph node aspiration (if accessible; regardless of size of the lymph node) should be obtained.
    - CBC abnormalities associated with MCTs can include eosinophilia, basophilia, and regenerative or nonregenerative anemia.
- Normal lymph nodes may contain scattered mast cells; increased numbers or clusters of mast cells in a lymph node draining an MCT suggest metastasis.
- Thoracic radiographs are of limited usefulness for dogs with MCT. Uncommonly, malignant pleural effusion containing mast cells occurs in cases with disseminated disease.
- Complete staging for systemic mast cell disease is indicated before surgery if lymph node metastasis, peritumoral edema, or bruising is present or tumors are recurrent. Consider staging for tumors located on the prepuce, scrotum, muzzle, digit, pinna or ear canal, or oral mucosa (locations potentially associated with a higher rate of metastasis).
- Complete systemic staging to examine patients for evidence of MCT metastasis includes the tests listed above and abdominal ultrasound possibly to include liver and spleen aspirates, bone marrow aspiration for cytologic evaluation (p. 1068), and biopsy of the primary tumor.
- Abdominal ultrasound
    - Affected lymph nodes may be enlarged, hypoechoic or hyperechoic, or irregular.
    - Splenic/hepatic infiltration: hypoechoic lesions throughout the parenchyma, rarely a solitary mass
- The liver, spleen, and bone marrow normally contain a few mast cells, but increased numbers or clusters of mast cells suggest MCT metastasis.
- The buffy coat smear to evaluate circulating mast cells has a high rate of false-positive results for dogs and is not recommended.

Advanced or Confirmatory Testing

- Historically, MCTs were categorized by grades based on their histologic appearance (Patnaik grading system): grade I = well-differentiated tumors, grade II = intermediately differentiated tumors, grade III = poorly differentiated tumors. Due to inconsistencies among pathologists (especially for classification of Patnaik grade II tumors), a two-tier histologic grading system (Kiupel, et al.) is also currently in use. This system evaluates cellular criteria such as mitotic figures and nuclear characteristics. Dogs with high-grade tumors have a higher metastatic rate and shorter survival time than dogs with low-grade tumors.
- Mitotic index (MI) is an important, independent predictor of prognosis. The MI (numbers of mitotic figures per 10 high-power fields) correlates with grade and prognosis. Dogs having cutaneous MCTs with an MI ≤ 5 had a median survival time of 70 months, compared with 5 months for an MI > 5.
- Mast cell granules may not be present or visible in highly anaplastic MCTs; CD117 (KIT) immunohistochemistry or toluidine blue staining can be used to confirm a diagnosis of MCT.
- A mast cell tumor prognostic panel is available at the Diagnostic Center for Population and Animal Health at Michigan State University (animalhealth.msu.edu); tumors

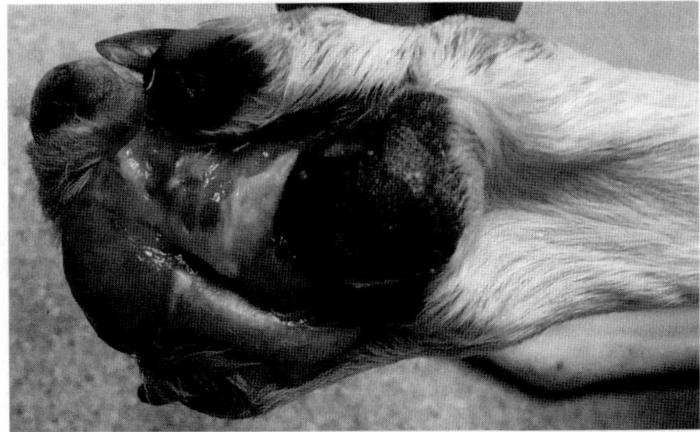

MAST CELL TUMORS, DOG Interdigital mast cell tumor in a dog. Note the ulceration, superficial infection, and displacement of the digits associated with this tumor.

are evaluated with both grading systems, immunohistochemistry for KIT and Ki-67, polymerase chain reaction (PCR) for KIT exon 8 and 11 mutations, and argyrophilic nucleolar organizer region (AgNOR) special staining. This panel may be useful to guide therapy for dogs with multiple or recurrent MCTs or tumors with aggressive biologic behavior or "borderline" histopathologic characteristics.

TREATMENT

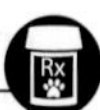

Treatment Overview

MCTs have a wide variety of biological behaviors and outcomes, and treatment can include surgery, radiation therapy (RT), chemotherapy, or a combination of these modalities. Targeted therapies (i.e., receptor tyrosine kinase inhibitors) are now widely available and may be indicated for patients with nonresectable or recurrent tumors. Consultation with an oncologist for current treatment options is warranted in these cases. A global overview of treatment is provided on p. 1436.

Acute General Treatment

- Surgery is the primary treatment modality for MCTs.
  - Preoperative H1 histamine blockers (such as diphenhydramine): begin therapy a few days before and premedicate immediately before surgery (and ongoing for nonresectable or metastatic disease)
  - Preoperative corticosteroids to attempt to shrink the tumor (measure and record at baseline first), making complete surgical resection more viable: prednisone 0.25-0.5 mg/kg PO q 24h × 5-7 days preoperatively, especially if MCT is difficult to access surgically
  - Proton pump inhibitors (omeprazole 0.5-1 mg/kg PO q 24h) and/or H2 histamine blockers are indicated for dogs with measureable MCT (preoperatively or in cases of nonresectable disease) to attempt to prevent or treat histamine-associated gastric ulceration.
  - For most MCTs, tumors should be surgically excised with 2 cm or greater lateral margins and 1 fascial plane deep to the tumor.
  - All tissue should be submitted for histologic evaluation of grade and margins. Margins should be inked before placement in formalin. Perioperative complications can include hypotension and hemorrhage. Postoperative complications can include poor wound healing after resection of large or infiltrative MCT.
- For tumors that are not surgically resectable because of size, invasiveness, or metastasis, chemotherapy, targeted therapy, or RT before or instead of surgery may be indicated.
- MCTs are responsive to RT.
  - Treating MCT in a microscopic disease setting (i.e., postsurgical resection) yields better results than when treatment is performed with macroscopic (measurable) disease.
  - Potential indications for RT for MCTs include incompletely excised, low-grade MCTs where wider surgical excision is not possible; as an adjunct to surgery and chemotherapy in dogs with high-grade MCT; and to attempt cytoreduction of nonresectable MCTs.
- The goal of chemotherapy is to delay or prevent metastasis and possibly local recurrence or attempt to cytoreduce or slow progression of nonresectable tumors or metastatic lesions. Potential indications for chemotherapy in dogs with MCT include
  - Dogs with high-grade MCT or tumors with MI > 5
  - Dogs with metastasis at diagnosis or with recurrent tumors
  - Dogs with tumors in locations associated with aggressive behavior (see above)
  - Before attempting surgical excision of large, fixed tumors or tumors with peritumoral edema or bruising
  - Chemotherapy drugs considered to be effective in the treatment of MCT include CCNU (lomustine), prednisone, vinblastine, vinorelbine, chlorambucil, cyclophosphamide, hydroxyurea, and others. Special handling requirements and potentially severe or life-threatening adverse patient effects exist with these chemotherapeutic drugs. These concerns and rapid evolution of protocols warrant consultation with/referral to an oncologist.
- Targeted therapies work by inhibiting cellular receptors. A receptor tyrosine kinase inhibitor (RTKI) currently in common use for MCT in dogs is toceranib phosphate (Palladia) for recurrent or metastatic grade II and III MCT. This drug has been used in combination with other therapies in many dogs with MCTs, and consultation with an oncologist is warranted for specific current treatment recommendations. This drug should be dispensed only by veterinarians familiar with its indications and side effects. Ongoing patient monitoring and veterinary follow-up for response to therapy and monitoring for adverse effects is warranted.

PROGNOSIS & OUTCOME

- The most significant prognostic indicator for MCT is tumor grade. For dogs with completely excised, low-grade MCTs, the prognosis is excellent: only ≈5% of these tumors recur locally or metastasize.
- For dogs with incompletely excised, low-grade MCTs where additional surgery (scar revision) is not possible, RT is the treatment of choice, with 80%-90% of dogs free of tumor 2-5 years after treatment. If RT is not an option, careful monitoring with routine exams is warranted. Benefit of treating dogs with incompletely excised, low-grade MCTs with corticosteroids, chemotherapy, or targeted therapies in an attempt to prevent recurrence remains unproved.
- For dogs with high-grade or high MI MCTs, survival times vary due to metastasis and tumor recurrence. Generally, additional therapy and monitoring are recommended (staging, chemotherapy, and/or targeted therapy). Case series of prolonged survival times in dogs with such tumors treated with aggressive local and systemic therapy exist, and owners should be made aware of all treatment options.
- Importantly, 10%-40% of affected dogs (especially pugs and boxers) develop additional cutaneous MCTs in their lifetime. Owners should be advised that any new skin mass should be addressed right away.
- Tumors located on mucous membranes may have a worse prognosis compared with MCTs of haired skin.

PEARLS & CONSIDERATIONS

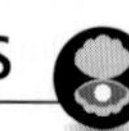

Comments

- Rechecks with physical exams at least q 4-6 months to detect and treat new MCTs as soon as possible
- Grossly, fine-needle aspirates of MCTs can look transparent and watery and are indistinguishable from fat. All fine-needle aspiration samples must be examined cytologically to differentiate fat from MCT.
- Because of the varied biologic behavior of MCT, factors such as tumor grade, MI, location and size of the tumor, regional and systemic metastasis, and completeness of surgical excision are essential for developing an appropriate treatment plan and prognosis.
- Intralesional therapies such as de-ionized water or corticosteroids may provide temporary shrinkage of MCTs but are rarely effective for long-term tumor control and are not recommended.

Technician Tips

Always aspirate skin and subcutaneous masses because some masses that feel like lipomas are MCTs.

Client Education

Any new masses on the skin should be evaluated as soon as possible.

SUGGESTED READING

Kiupel M, et al: Proposal of a 2-tier histologic grading system for canine cutaneous mast cell tumors to more accurately predict biologic behavior. Vet Pathol 48(1):147-155, 2011.

AUTHOR: Tracy Gieger, DVM, DACVIM, DACVR
EDITOR: Kenneth M. Rassnick, DVM, DACVIM

Masticatory Myositis

Client Education Sheet

BASIC INFORMATION

Definition

Masticatory myositis (MM) is a focal inflammatory myopathy of autoimmune origin that targets the unique muscle fibers (type 2M) of the muscles of mastication.

Synonyms

Masticatory muscle myositis (MMM), masticatory myopathy, historically: eosinophilic myositis (acute stage), atrophic myositis (chronic stage)

Epidemiology

SPECIES, AGE, SEX

- Canine, all ages, either sex
- Feline rarely reported

GENETICS, BREED PREDISPOSITION

- Large-breed, young adult (2-3 year old) to middle-aged (4-9 year old) dogs
- Overrepresented breeds: German shepherd, Labrador retriever, Doberman pinscher, and golden retriever
- Rottweilers are more prone to peripheral eosinophilia and eosinophilic muscle infiltrates due to their propensity for hypereosinophilic syndrome
- Cavalier King Charles spaniels: possible genetic predisposition; can develop signs of disease at a much younger age (12 weeks)

ASSOCIATED DISORDERS

MM has been documented to occur concurrently with myasthenia gravis, and masticatory muscle involvement can occur as an overlap syndrome with generalized polymyositis.

Clinical Presentation

DISEASE FORMS/SUBTYPES

Signs occur bilaterally in the muscles of mastication but are not always equal in severity or time of onset from one side to the other. Dogs can often be weeks into the acute stage of disease before owners present the dog for diagnosis. Signs can wax and wane during this time. Patients can present in the chronic stage without owner recognition of the acute phase.

Acute stage:

- Trismus: inability to open the jaw (even under anesthesia)
- Myalgia: pain on palpation of temporalis and masseter muscles
- Swelling of the muscles of mastication
- Ocular
  - Exophthalmos from swelling of the pterygoid muscles; can result in blindness from stretching of the optic nerve if severe, and also exposure conjunctivitis

Chronic stage:

- Atrophy of the muscles of mastication
- Enophthalmos (differs from acute stage)
- Permanent trismus

HISTORY, CHIEF COMPLAINT

- Dysphagia/jaw pain
- Ptyalism
- Abnormal facial appearance
- Weight loss
- Decreased activity/lethargy

PHYSICAL EXAM FINDINGS

Acute stage:

- Fever, lymphadenopathy (mandibular, prescapular)
- Trismus
- Pain on palpation and attempted forced opening of the jaw
- Swelling of the muscles of mastication
- Exophthalmos ± blindness ± decreased pupillary light responses (PLRs)

Chronic stage:

- Atrophy of the muscles of mastication
- Trismus
- Enophthalmos
- Rarely, inability to close the mouth

Etiology and Pathophysiology

- The muscles of mastication include the temporalis, masseter, pterygoid (medial and lateral), and rostral digastricus innervated by the mandibular branch of the trigeminal nerve that also innervates the tensor tympani and tensor veli palatine muscles.
- They have a unique embryologic origin (brachial arch vs. paraxial mesoderm), myofiber types (2M vs. 2A), and distinct myosin isoform compared with limb muscles.
- Autoantibodies are produced against masticatory myosin-binding protein-C; may involve molecular mimicry with bacterial antigens; results in necrosis and phagocytosis with fibrotic infiltrate of the muscles

DIAGNOSIS

Diagnostic Overview

Diagnosis is often based on clinical presentation and a positive serum 2M antibody titer. However, results of this test can vary according to the stage of disease (acute or chronic). It is important to consider a multimodal approach to the diagnosis of this disease, including serum testing and biopsy exam.

Differential Diagnosis

Acute disease: other causes of exophthalmos or pain on jaw opening:

- Extraocular myositis (EOM)
- Retrobulbar abscess
- Generalized polymyositis
  - Initially can present with only masticatory muscle involvement
- Infectious myopathy
  - *Toxoplasma gondii, Neospora caninum, Borrelia burgdorferi, Ehrlichia canis, Rickettsia rickettsii, Hepatozoon spp*
- Tetanus
- Disease of the temporomandibular joint or facial bones
  - Trauma, neoplasia, osteopathy, foreign body
- Idiopathic inflammatory polymyopathy in Hungarian Vizsla
- Phenobarbital-responsive hypersalivation

Chronic disease: other causes of masticatory muscle atrophy

- Loss of trigeminal nerve function
  - Peripheral nerve sheath tumor, inflammation, or other neoplasia

Initial Database

- Biochemistry profile: mild elevations in muscle enzymes creatine kinase (CK), alanine aminotransferase (ALT), aspartate aminotransferase (AST) in the acute phase (less than elevations associated with generalized polymyositis); hyperglobulinemia
- CBC: leukocytosis with neutrophilia or eosinophilia
- Urinalysis: ± proteinuria
- Muscle or lymph node aspirates can reveal lymphoplasmacytic or eosinophilic inflammation
- Thorough head and jaw evaluation (sedation may be required)
  - Measure the extent of jaw opening.
- Skull radiographs under sedation to rule out trauma, neoplasia, or foreign body

Advanced or Confirmatory Testing

- Serum 2M antibody: high specificity (100%) and sensitivity (85%-90%)
  - Negative < 1:100, borderline 1:100, positive > 1:100
  - Previous glucocorticoid therapy or the chronic form of the disease can result in false-negative
- Electromyography (EMG)
  - Fibrillation potentials; positive sharp waves; bizarre, high-frequency discharges in the acute phase
  - Decreased insertional activity in the chronic phase
  - Limb muscles should also be tested to differentiate generalized polymyositis
  - Muscle enzyme levels should be tested prior to EMG to prevent false enzyme elevations
- Muscle biopsy
  - Commonly biopsied muscles include the temporalis or masseter.
    - Care must be taken not to biopsy the thin frontalis muscle located superficial to the temporalis muscle.
    - Important not to biopsy areas where an EMG was performed
  - Necrosis and phagocytosis of muscle fibers
  - Perivascular infiltration of mononuclear cells
  - Perimysial and endomysial fibrosis

- Immunohistochemical staining for antibody deposits found in 85% of cases
- Advanced imaging (CT or MRI) (p. 1132)
  - CT is superior for imaging bones and joints.
  - MRI is more sensitive for identifying muscle inflammation than serum CK or CT.
  - Both show changes in the size of the muscle and in attenuation (CT) or intensity (MRI) associated with inflammation and provide ideal locations for biopsy.
  - It is proposed that MRI be used to assess response to therapy.

TREATMENT

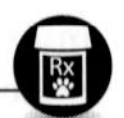

Treatment Overview

Successful treatment depends on prompt recognition of the disease and initiation of immunosuppressive glucocorticoid therapy. Delays in treatment can result in permanent disability secondary to fibrosis of the muscles of mastication and inability to open the jaw.

Acute General Treatment

- Prednisone/prednisolone: 1-2 mg/kg PO q 12h until resolution of clinical signs and return of serum 2M titers and CK to a normal range. In the acute stage, this can last for 2-4 weeks.
  - Expect muscle atrophy to occur during treatment and as a side effect of steroid therapy; do not assume this is a treatment failure.
- The chronic form of disease involves less inflammation and more fibrotic changes, and a lower dose of glucocorticoids 0.5-1mg/kg/day for a shorter duration (1 month) is recommended to determine if further steroid therapy will be effective.
- Do not attempt to force the jaw open. It does not affect the clinical outcome and can result in subluxation of the temporomandibular joint or mandibular fracture.

Chronic Treatment

- After the initial immunosuppressive treatment for the acute stage, a slow, tapering dose of glucocorticoid is administered until the lowest effective daily or every other day dosage is found.
- Tapering occurs over 4-6 months, with no more than a 50% reduction in dose each month. Some dogs can be withdrawn from therapy.
- Relapse occurs rapidly if treatment is tapered too quickly.

Nutrition/Diet

- A range of food consistencies should be offered to find one that is best for an individual dog.
- Feeding tubes may be needed temporarily in the acute phase or permanently in the chronic phase to maintain body condition and prevent starvation (pp. 1106 and 1109).

Behavior/Exercise

Physical therapy exercises for the jaw can be considered, such as offering rawhides or favorite toys to play with.

Possible Complications

Additional immunosuppressive medications such as azathioprine and cyclosporine have been used as adjuncts to glucocorticoids when side effects are unacceptable or clinical signs are resistant to monotherapy.

Recommended Monitoring

First month:

- Animals with difficulty eating should be weighed weekly to ensure proper nutritional intake.
- Hydration status should be monitored by the owner via urination habits, quantification of water consumption, and daily weighing.
- The owners can assess jaw mobility and comfort at home by watching the patient consume food, water, and treats. In the hospital, this can be quantified by physical exam and measurements.

Chronic monitoring:

- Serum 2M antibody titers can be monitored to assess response to therapy every 3-6 months initially and before glucocorticoid dose reductions or discontinuation.

PROGNOSIS & OUTCOME

- The acute phase offers a good prognosis when diagnosed and treated promptly with immunosuppressive doses of glucocorticoids, although treatment may be required lifelong.
  - Relapse occurs quickly with a premature reduction in dosage.
- Inadequate treatment of the acute phase or presentation in the chronic phase offers only a guarded to fair prognosis for return of normal jaw function. If left untreated, muscle necrosis leads to fibrosis of the muscles of mastication and inability to open the jaw. Muscle biopsy in the chronic phase can be used to assess the number of healthy versus fibrotic muscle fibers. If no viable muscle fibers remain, prognosis is worse.

PEARLS & CONSIDERATIONS

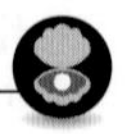

Comments

- Trismus can be severe enough to inhibit tracheal intubation. Care should be taken with anesthesia or sedation, and supplies should be in place to perform temporary emergency tracheostomy if needed.
- After initiation of treatment in the acute phase, muscle atrophy alone should not be considered evidence of treatment failure because steroid therapy causes muscle atrophy.

Technician Tips

- If feeding tubes are placed, knowledge of appropriate feeding protocols is required, with sufficient familiarity to teach owners.
- Monitor for tongue or pharyngeal swelling in patients under sedation or anesthesia because this can potentially occlude the airway during the procedure or recovery.

Client Education

- Because pets can have pain in the acute stages, owners with small children should be warned that painful dogs may be more prone to defensive biting if inappropriately handled by the children.
- If feeding tubes are required, owners should be provided instruction on appropriate feeding and maintenance of the tube.

SUGGESTED READING

Melmed C, et al: Masticatory muscle myositis: pathogenesis, diagnosis, and treatment. Compendium 26:590-604, 2004.

RELATED CLIENT EDUCATION SHEETS

Consent to Perform Computed Tomography (CT Scan)

How to Syringe-Feed, Tube-Feed, or Bottle-Feed a Pet

AUTHOR: Michaela J. Beasley, DVM, MS, DACVIM

EDITOR: Karen R. Muñana, DVM, MS, DACVIM

MDR1 Mutation

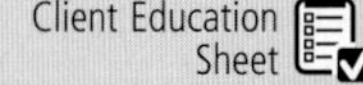

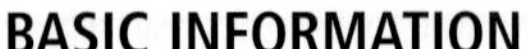

BASIC INFORMATION

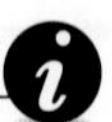

Definition

The *MDR1* (multidrug resistance 1) gene mutation is a common problem in many herding-breed dogs. It causes enhanced sensitivity to a number of drugs, and affected dogs are extremely susceptible to adverse drug reactions at doses of drugs well tolerated by normal dogs.

Synonyms

Ivermectin or avermectin sensitivity; *ABCB1* gene, *ABCB1-1Δ* gene mutation

Epidemiology

SPECIES, AGE, SEX

Dogs; similar mutation recently identified in cats

GENETICS, BREED PREDISPOSITION

Herding breeds (collie, Australian shepherd, Shetland sheepdog, Old English sheepdog,

English shepherd, border collie, German shepherd, McNab dog), sighthound breeds (long-haired whippet, silken windhound)

RISK FACTORS

Breed is a risk factor, based on the percentage of animals known to harbor the *MDR1* mutation:

- Australian shepherd: 50%
- Border collie: 5%
- Collie: 75%
- English shepherd: 15%
- German shepherd: 5%
- Long-haired whippet: 65%
- McNab: 30%
- Old English sheepdog: 35%
- Shetland sheepdog: 15%
- Silken windhound: 35%
- Mixed-breed dogs (presumed to be herding-breed crosses): 10%

ASSOCIATED DISORDERS

Relative adrenal insufficiency (*MDR1* mutant/mutant genotype)

Clinical Presentation

HISTORY, CHIEF COMPLAINT

- Depends on the particular drug to which the dog is exposed
  - Exposure to macrocyclic lactones (e.g., ivermectin, milbemycin, selamectin, moxidectin) may result in neurologic toxicosis. NOTE: use of these drugs as labeled for heartworm prevention is safe even for dogs with the *MDR1* mutation. Neurologic toxicosis occurs only with higher doses (e.g., treatment of mange, accidental overdose).
  - Exposure to loperamide may result in neurologic toxicosis.
  - Exposure to some chemotherapeutic drugs (vinca alkaloids, anthracyclines such as doxorubicin) can result in severe gastrointestinal signs and/or severe myelosuppression.
  - Exposure to vincristine has been documented to cause central neuropathy.
  - Exposure to some antiemetics (ondansetron, possibly maropitant) may result in neurologic toxicosis.
  - Exposure to some preanesthetic agents (acepromazine, butorphanol) may result in more profound and prolonged sedation than expected for the dose administered.
  - Exposure to emodepside has resulted in neurotoxicosis.
  - Exposure to apomorphine has resulted in central nervous system (CNS) depression.
- Onset of signs occurs in hours to days after drug exposure.
- Exposure to macrocyclic lactones can occur through ingestion of feces of animals, particularly livestock, recently treated with these agents. Several pesticides contain avermectins and have caused neurologic toxicosis in dogs that were inadvertently exposed.

PHYSICAL EXAM FINDINGS

Determined by drug to which the dog has been exposed (see above):

- Macrocyclic lactones: mydriasis, hypersalivation, ataxia, blindness, paresis, stupor, muscle tremors; may progress to coma
- Loperamide: paresis, ataxia, stupor
- Chemotherapeutic agents: anorexia; vomiting, diarrhea; signs of opportunistic infections or hemorrhage possible if neutropenia or thrombocytopenia, respectively
- Antiemetics: signs of mild to moderate CNS dysfunction (usually depression)
- Preanesthetic agents: prolonged and more profound CNS depression
- Emodepside: CNS depression
- Apomorphine: CNS depression

Etiology and Pathophysiology

- The *MDR1* gene mutation is inherited in a simple mendelian fashion.
- Heterozygotes and homozygotes experience enhanced drug sensitivity.
- The *MDR1* mutation is a 4–base pair deletion mutation that results in dysfunction of P-glycoprotein, the product of the *MDR1* gene.
- Normally functioning P-glycoprotein protects an individual from a number of drugs by restricting their access to the brain and enhancing their export from the body.

DIAGNOSIS

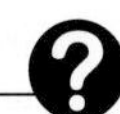

Diagnostic Overview

Screening for the *MDR1* mutation can be performed preemptively in a dog of a high-prevalence breed. Otherwise, the mutation is suspected when signs of drug toxicosis have occurred despite the use of normal drug dosages. In either situation, confirmation is done by genotyping.

Differential Diagnosis

- Idiopathic drug sensitivity
- Overdose

Initial Database

Initial diagnostic tests are those performed for any suspected case of toxicosis for the particular agent (e.g., CBC for chemotherapeutic drugs with myelosuppressive potential).

Advanced or Confirmatory Testing

Definitive diagnosis consists of genotyping the dog. A DNA sample (cheek swab, using purpose-made kit or EDTA blood) can be submitted to the Veterinary Clinical Pharmacology Laboratory at Washington State University. A DNA swab kit can be obtained at www.vetmed.wsu.edu/vcpl.

TREATMENT

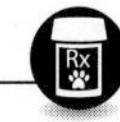

Treatment Overview

There is no treatment that can alter the dog's *MDR1* genotype, and treatment of clinical signs resulting from drug exposure should be aimed at the particular drug involved.

Acute and Chronic Treatment

- For macrocyclic lactones, supportive care is indicated (p. 152). Administration of CNS depressants such as diazepam should be avoided. Recently the use of IV lipid emulsion for reversal of macrocyclic lactone toxicity has been discussed, but there are no clinical studies in dogs at this time.
- The lipid rescue protocol (involving IV lipid emulsion administration) has not been effective for treating ivermectin toxicosis in *MDR1* mutant/mutant dogs.
- For loperamide, an opioid antagonist such as naloxone can reverse CNS depression.
- Chemotherapeutic agents, antiemetic agents, preanesthetic agents: supportive care (p. 152)

Drug Interactions

- Spinosad, ketoconazole, and cyclosporine can inhibit P-glycoprotein, causing an acquired P-glycoprotein deficiency in dogs that do not carry the *MDR1* mutation.
- Concurrent use of these P-glycoprotein–inhibiting drugs with macrocyclic lactones (high dose), vinca alkaloids, and doxorubicin should be avoided.

PROGNOSIS & OUTCOME

- Clinical signs tend to be milder, and clinical outcome better, in dogs heterozygous for the *MDR1* mutation (*MDR1* mutant/normal).
- For dogs homozygous for the *MDR1* mutation (*MDR1* mutant/mutant), the prognosis is guarded for those exposed to doses of ivermectin used for treating mange (300-600 mcg/kg or higher) and customary doses of vincristine 0.5-0.7 mg/m^2 and doxorubicin 30 mg/m^2 (p. 609).

PEARLS & CONSIDERATIONS

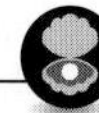

Comments

- The *MDR1* mutation and exposure to a macrocyclic lactone or loperamide should be considered in any herding-breed dog that develops unexplained signs of neurologic toxicosis.
- Before treatment with chemotherapeutic agents and/or off-label (i.e., anti-mange) doses of macrocyclic lactones, mixed-breed dogs or breeds listed above should be tested for the *MDR1* mutation.
- The *MDR1* mutation may explain the intolerance to stress and illness anecdotally observed in some breeds. In collies, the mutation is associated with lower plasma cortisol concentrations at baseline and after ACTH stimulation. Because P-glycoprotein limits glucocorticoid passage into the brain, *MDR1* mutation may favor such passage, increasing feedback inhibition and creating a state of relative adrenal insufficiency.
- A similar mutation has been identified in the feline *MDR1* gene and likely contributes to drug sensitivity in this species. Research is ongoing in the author's laboratory.

Prevention

Treatment planning for dogs identified as having the *MDR1* mutation (heterozygous or homozygous) depends on the drug involved.

Patients requiring treatment with the drugs listed above may need to receive a decreased drug dosage or an alternative drug. Studies to determine appropriate dosage adjustments have not yet been conducted.

Technician Tips

Attempts to save costs by off-label use of large animal ivermectin products in dogs is not appropriate and may be life-threatening in dogs with the *MDR1* mutation.

Client Education

Owners should be aware of drug sensitivities if the dog has the *MDR1* mutation. Breeders should consider the *MDR1* mutation as part of a comprehensive genetic assessment of their breeding program.

SUGGESTED READING

Mealey KL: Adverse drug reactions in herding-breed dogs: the role of P-glycoprotein. Compend Contin Educ Vet 28:23-33, 2006.

AUTHOR: Katrina L. Mealey, DVM, PhD, DACVCP, DACVIM
EDITOR: Leah A. Cohn, DVM, PhD, DACVIM

Mediastinal Disease

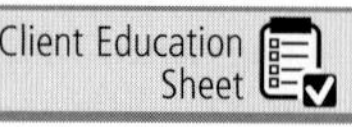

BASIC INFORMATION

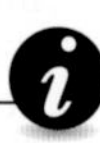

Definition

Disorders of the mediastinum (potential space between the right and left lungs)

Epidemiology

SPECIES, AGE, SEX

- Mediastinal lymphoma: young cats are overrepresented.
- Other mediastinal masses more commonly affect middle-aged or older animals.

GENETICS, BREED PREDISPOSITION

Mediastinal lymphoma: Asian-breed cats

RISK FACTORS

- Mediastinal lymphoma: feline leukemia virus infection (FeLV [p. 329])
- Pneumomediastinum: tracheal laceration/avulsion
- Mediastinitis: esophageal foreign body or rupture

CONTAGION AND ZOONOSIS

FeLV infection

ASSOCIATED DISORDERS

Mediastinal masses:

- Acquired myasthenia gravis (thymoma)
- Polyuria and polydipsia (lymphoma)

Clinical Presentation

DISEASE FORMS/SUBTYPES

- Pneumomediastinum
- Mediastinitis
- Mediastinal masses
- Mediastinal hemorrhage

HISTORY, CHIEF COMPLAINT

- Pneumomediastinum: recent trauma, anesthesia (overinflated endotracheal tube cuff or turning patient without disconnection of endotracheal tube), transtracheal wash or jugular venipuncture
  - ± Subcutaneous emphysema and/or dyspnea
- Mediastinitis (acute): obtundation, inappetence, dysphagia, regurgitation
- Mediastinal masses: inappetence, lethargy, polyuria/polydipsia, dysphagia or regurgitation, cough, dyspnea, facial/neck/forelimb swelling or edema, dysphonia if recurrent laryngeal nerve involvement
- Mediastinal hemorrhage: lethargy, weakness, tachypnea

PHYSICAL EXAM FINDINGS

Pneumomediastinum:

- Exam may be normal
- Subcutaneous emphysema
- Respiratory signs if severe: dyspnea, muffled breath sounds, hyperresonant thoracic percussion (pneumothorax)
- Jugular venous distention
- Shock

Mediastinitis:

- Fever
- Dyspnea, tachypnea, cough
- Edema (head, neck, forelimbs) secondary to cranial vena cava syndrome (p. 221)
- Dysphagia, regurgitation
- Thoracic pain
- Reduced thoracic compressibility (cats)
- Stridor

Mediastinal masses:

- Reduced thoracic compressibility (cats)
- Cranial vena cava syndrome
- Respiratory or gastrointestinal signs
- ± Paraneoplastic signs: weakness, regurgitation, stridor if secondary laryngeal paralysis, polyuria/polydipsia
- Horner's syndrome
- Stridor

Mediastinal hemorrhage:

- Pale mucous membranes
- Tachycardia
- Weakness

Etiology and Pathophysiology

Pneumomediastinum:

- Penetrating neck wounds
- Tracheal laceration/tear (traumatic; iatrogenic from endotracheal tubes)
- After esophageal surgery (uncommon)
- Positive-pressure ventilation
- Secondary to primary pulmonary pathology

Mediastinitis:

- Hematogenous infection
- Penetrating wounds (e.g., bites) and migrating foreign bodies
- Extension from surrounding tissues, commonly esophagus but also cervical tissues, trachea, pleural space
  - Esophageal foreign bodies
  - Rupture from esophagitis (after general anesthesia) or esophageal tear after stricture dilation
- Acute: *Staphylococcus* spp, *Streptococcus* spp, *Escherichia coli*, *Corynebacterium* spp
- Chronic: bacterial (*Nocardia*, *Actinomyces*, *Staphylococcus* spp) and fungal (histoplasmosis, blastomycosis, cryptococcosis) infection reported
- Spirocercosis (dogs)
- Clinical signs due to sepsis, pleural effusion, and compression of vascular or respiratory structures

Mediastinal masses:

- Lymphoma, thymoma, thyroid neoplasia, chemodectoma, thymic cysts, granulomas
- Clinical signs reflect compression of respiratory, cardiovascular, gastrointestinal structures, ± pleural effusion, ± neurologic abnormalities (Horner's syndrome, laryngeal paralysis)
- ± Paraneoplastic syndromes: hypercalcemia, myasthenia gravis

Mediastinal hemorrhage:

- Trauma
- Coagulopathy
- Spontaneous thymic hemorrhage
- Neoplasia
- Clinical signs related to acute blood loss.

DIAGNOSIS

Diagnostic Overview

Thoracic radiographs are typically the initial step in a diagnostic evaluation. If there is a mass lesion, advanced imaging such as CT is often indicated, but fine-needle aspiration and cytologic analysis or needle, thoracoscopic, or open surgical biopsy and histopathologic analysis of tissue typically is required to establish a definitive diagnosis.

Differential Diagnosis

- Pneumomediastinum: tracheal trauma, pneumothorax
- Mediastinitis: other causes of sepsis, mediastinal masses/fat/fluid, pleural effusions

- Mediastinal masses: mediastinitis, pleural space disease, pulmonary masses, thoracic wall masses, mediastinal fat or fluid, esophageal diverticulum, normal thymic enlargement (young animals)
- Mediastinal hemorrhage: mediastinitis, mediastinal fat or fluid, mediastinal mass, normal thymic enlargement (young animals), thymic hemorrhage (rare)

Initial Database

- Thoracic radiographs
  - Pneumomediastinum: visualization of mediastinal vascular structures not normally seen (e.g., branches of aorta) is pathognomonic; subcutaneous emphysema may also be present
  - Mediastinitis and mediastinal masses: mediastinal widening on dorsoventral or ventrodorsal views, dorsal displacement of trachea on lateral view possible, pleural fluid possible, gas in fascial planes of neck possible; may be unremarkable in acute mediastinitis
- Abdominal radiographs: pneumoretroperitoneum possible
- CBC: leukocytosis if inflammation, rarely cytopenias or leukemia; anemia if mediastinal hemorrhage
- Serum biochemistry panel: ± hypercalcemia (lymphoma)
- FeLV testing
- Thoracic ultrasonography may identify masses (e.g., branchial cysts), pleural effusion, lymphadenopathy, vascularity/vascular invasiveness of mass (impacts biopsy/excision possibilities), mediastinal fluid if hemorrhage
  - The presence of internal cysts or a heterogenous echogenicity in a mediastinal mass makes thymoma more likely than lymphoma.
- Fine-needle aspiration with cytologic evaluation
  - Risks include hemothorax, pneumothorax, or nondiagnostic sample.
  - Inflammatory: culture (aerobic, anaerobic, *Nocardia, Actinomyces,* ± fungal)
  - Good correlation between cytological and histological exam of mediastinal masses (single study)
- Thoracocentesis for cytologic evaluation and culture if fluid present (p. 1343)
- Acetylcholine-receptor antibody concentration if mediastinal mass and megaesophagus and/or generalized weakness (myasthenia gravis [p. 668])

Advanced or Confirmatory Testing

- Tracheoscopy/bronchoscopy if pneumomediastinum and patient stable (p. 1074)
- Contrast (water-soluble) esophagram for suspected rupture (p. 309)
- Esophagoscopy if suspect esophageal disease (p. 1098)
- Cytologic evaluation of respiratory wash samples if underlying pulmonary disease
- Echocardiography if heart base mass (p. 1094)
- Arterial blood gas to assess respiratory function
- Coagulation testing (prothrombin time [PT], partial thromboplastin time [aPTT]) if hemorrhage (p. 1325)
- CT or MRI (p. 1132) can better delineate the nature and extent of space-occupying disease and address possible metastatic disease (CT).
- Fungal serologic testing for possible fungal mediastinitis
- Scintigraphy (technetium or iodine 131) could confirm ectopic thyroid neoplasia.
- Thoracoscopic exam of the mediastinum
- Biopsy for histopathologic evaluation can be obtained transthoracically (Tru-cut) by thoracoscopy or thoracotomy.
- Flow cytometry analysis of aspirates can differentiate thymoma from thymic lymphoma.
- Polymerase chain reaction (PCR) for antigen receptor rearrangement (PARR) to demonstrate clonality for lymphoma

TREATMENT

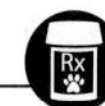

Treatment Overview

Nonlymphoid cranial mediastinal masses typically require surgical intervention, whereas lymphoid neoplasia is treated like other lymphoma (pp. 607 and 609). Pneumomediastinum usually resolves with time.

Acute General Treatment

Pneumomediastinum:

- Mild signs: cage rest; subcutaneous emphysema typically resolves in approximately 2 weeks.
- Marked signs: provide supplemental oxygen.
- Drain subcutaneous emphysema only if causing discomfort.
- If large tracheal tear/laceration, consider surgical repair (p. 986).
- Thoracocentesis if pneumothorax

Mediastinitis:

- Broad-spectrum empirical antimicrobial therapy pending culture/sensitivity
- Severe systemic signs may require IV fluids and/or additional supportive therapy.
- Esophageal laceration/rupture may require surgery.

Mediastinal masses:

- Surgery, chemotherapy, radiation therapy, or a combination based on type of mass
- Less invasive surgical techniques with video-assisted thoracic surgery/thoracoscopy have been described as alternatives to thoracotomy.
- Mediastinal cysts: drained transthoracically or excised.

Mediastinal hemorrhage:

- Volume support: crystalloid or colloids
- Blood transfusion if severe
- If coagulopathy due to vitamin K antagonism or deficiency, treat with vitamin K 2.5 mg/kg SQ in multiple sites initially and possibly a fresh-frozen plasma transfusion (p. 1169), followed by vitamin K 2.5 mg/kg PO q 12h.

Chronic Treatment

- Pneumomediastinum: cage rest
- Mediastinitis: long-term (minimum, 4-6 weeks) antimicrobial therapy based on culture and susceptibility results
  - Fungal mediastinitis may require months of therapy.
  - Large granulomas causing cranial vena cava syndrome may require surgical excision/debulking.
- Mediastinal masses
  - Chemotherapy or radiation therapy for lymphoma
  - Radiation therapy for incompletely resected or unresectable thymoma

Possible Complications

- Pneumothorax, pleural effusion, pyothorax from thoracostomy tubes
- Gastrointestinal and/or myelotoxicosis from chemotherapeutics
- Individual drug toxicoses
  - Renal: aminoglycosides, amphotericin B
  - Hepatic: azole antifungals
- Surgery entails risks of anesthesia, hemorrhage, and infection.

Recommended Monitoring

- Clinical signs
- Pulse oximetry, arterial blood gases
- Thoracic radiographs
- Pleural fluid volume and cytology if thoracostomy tube
- CBC (chemotherapy)
- Serum chemistries for renal and hepatic function, depending on drugs administered

PROGNOSIS & OUTCOME

- Pneumomediastinum: good if underlying disease resolves or can be corrected
- Mediastinitis: varies, depending on severity; chronic cases may be hard to resolve.
- Mediastinal masses
  - Lymphoma: chemotherapy usually palliative
  - Others: surgery for cure or palliation. The prognosis for dogs and cats with surgical excision of thymoma is generally good, even if invasive.
  - Cats: median 1-year survival rate: 89%
  - Dogs: median 1-year survival rate: 64%
- Mediastinal hemorrhage: prognosis varies with cause and severity.

PEARLS & CONSIDERATIONS

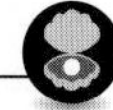

Comments

- Advanced imaging helps define internal structure and extent of mediastinal masses and detect pulmonary metastases.
- Patients at risk for foreign body inhalation (hunting or field trial dogs): consider *Nocardia, Actinomyces* as causes of mediastinitis.

Prevention

Avoid iatrogenic tracheal injury associated with

- Intubating using a stylet
- Overinflation of endotracheal tube cuffs

- Rotating a patient while attached to anesthetic circuit
- Traumatic jugular venipuncture

Technician Tips

- Complications of fine-needle aspiration of a mediastinal mass include pneumothorax and hemothorax. If a patient suddenly develops tachypnea and/or increased respiratory effort after the procedure, alert the attending clinician as soon as possible.
- Dogs that present with edema confined to the face, neck, and forelimbs may have mediastinal disease.
- Cats with mediastinal masses can be fragile (unstable respiratory/cardiovascular status). Minimize handling, and avoid ventrodorsal projection for thoracic radiographs.

SUGGESTED READING

Pintore L, et al: Cytological and histological correlation in diagnosing feline and canine mediastinal masses. J Small Anim Pract 55:28-32, 2014.

AUTHOR: **Graham Swinney, BVSc, DVCS, FACVSc**
EDITOR: **Megan Grobman, DVM, MS, DACVIM**

Megaesophagus

Client Education Sheet 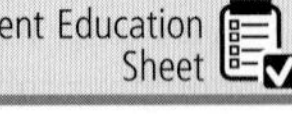

BASIC INFORMATION 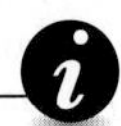

Definition

Esophageal dilation due to muscular weakness from any cause, which must be distinguished from esophageal dilation orad to an obstruction

Synonyms

Acquired esophageal weakness, congenital esophageal weakness

Epidemiology

SPECIES, AGE, SEX

- Dogs and cats (less commonly) of any age or sex
- Acquired megaesophagus usually occurs after 2-3 years of age.

GENETICS, BREED PREDISPOSITION

- Congenital megaesophagus
  - Cats: Siamese
  - Dogs: German shepherds, Great Danes, Labrador retrievers, miniature schnauzers, Irish setters, Shar-peis, fox terriers, Newfoundlands, but any dog can be affected
- Acquired megaesophagus in dogs: any dog can be affected

RISK FACTORS

Any cause of lower motor neuron weakness can produce acquired megaesophagus if the esophageal muscles are affected. Myasthenia gravis, hypoadrenocorticism, and dysautonomia are risk factors (feline dysautonomia, or Key-Gaskell syndrome, is now rare).

ASSOCIATED DISORDERS

- Coughing due to tracheobronchitis or aspiration pneumonia
- Death from aspiration pneumonia (most common cause)
- In some animals with acquired megaesophagus, generalized weakness due to myopathy, neuropathy, or junctionopathy

Clinical Presentation

DISEASE FORMS/SUBTYPES

- Congenital megaesophagus
- Acquired megaesophagus can be generalized or segmental (usually the cervical esophagus).

HISTORY, CHIEF COMPLAINT

- Regurgitation (distinguish from vomiting) is the most common complaint.
- Cough (due to aspiration): sometimes seen before regurgitation is reported
- Drooling (due to difficulty swallowing)

PHYSICAL EXAM FINDINGS

- Pulmonary crackles/easily elicited cough (due to aspiration pneumonia)
- Fever and signs of systemic illness (e.g., anorexia, lethargy) with severe aspiration pneumonia
- Bellows-like action at thoracic inlet, associated with breathing (due to filling and emptying of distended esophagus with air)
- Nasal discharge (with pneumonia or rhinitis secondary to regurgitation)
- Weight loss or failure to gain weight (if patient is losing excessive calories or has chronic pulmonary infection)

Etiology and Pathophysiology

Congenital or idiopathic megaesophagus:

- A defect in any part of the neuromuscular reflex that controls the pharyngeal and esophageal phases of swallowing, including sensory receptors, afferent nerves (glossopharyngeal and vagus), tractus solitarius (leading to the nucleus solitarius), swallowing center (near the lateral reticular formation), lower motor neurons of the nucleus ambiguus, efferent somatic and parasympathetic nerve fibers in the vagus, myoneural junction in the esophagus, esophageal striated muscle, and potentially esophageal smooth muscle in the cat
- Defect probably resides in the afferent limb of the reflex arc. This is supported by the fact that dogs with megaesophagus are prone to aspiration pneumonia, which is increased among dogs with loss of the afferent arc (abnormal respiratory reflexes also occur).

Secondary megaesophagus: muscular weakness due to some other lower motor neuron disease:

- Neurologic (e.g., polyradiculoneuritis, dysautonomia, demyelinating neuropathies, lead)
- Neuromuscular (botulism, tetanus, myasthenia gravis)
- Muscular (e.g., polymyositis, muscular dystrophy)

Other causes of megaesophagus include certain metabolic conditions (e.g., hypoadrenocorticism). Megaesophagus may also occur orad to esophageal obstruction (e.g., lower esophageal sphincter dysfunction/obstruction, persistent right aortic arch).

DIAGNOSIS 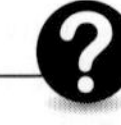

Diagnostic Overview

Megaesophagus is a differential for any regurgitating patient. It is important to differentiate vomiting from regurgitation; careful history taking helps but is not always accurate. Thoracic radiographs confirm megaesophagus in many cases, but some patients, especially those with segmental megaesophagus of the cervical region, require contrast esophagrams. Additional diagnostic tests are appropriate to look for underlying causes that present therapeutic opportunities.

Differential Diagnosis

Acquired megaesophagus in the dog:

- Myasthenia gravis (generalized or localized): most common identified cause
- Hypoadrenocorticism
- Dysautonomia (uncommon except in areas of the Midwest)
- Polymyopathies/polyneuropathies
- Lead intoxication (rare)
- Organophosphate intoxication (rare)
- Botulism or tetanus (rare)
- Esophagitis (rare cause of megaesophagus)
- Systemic lupus erythematosus (rare)
- Dermatomyositis (primarily collies and Shetland sheepdogs)
- Idiopathic (most common category)

Acquired megaesophagus in the cat:

- Dysautonomia (Key-Gaskell syndrome)
- Myasthenia gravis
- Idiopathic (most feline cases)

Initial Database

- CBC: look for evidence of inflammation consistent with aspiration pneumonia.
- Plain thoracic radiographs: look for megaesophagus (not always obvious) and for

pneumonia (especially but not limited to right middle lung lobe; need ventrodorsal, dorsoventral, or left lateral projection to reliably see).
- Contrast esophagram (radiographs)
  - Not needed if plain films show megaesophagus
  - Indicated if plain films are not diagnostic of esophageal disease or esophageal weakness cannot be distinguished from esophageal obstruction
- Contrast esophagram using fluoroscopy is most sensitive test for megaesophagus but is usually unnecessary. Segmental esophageal weakness (especially cervical esophagus) and partial loss of muscular tone can be especially difficult to diagnose (p. 1062).

Advanced or Confirmatory Testing

- Antibodies against acetylcholine receptors for diagnosis of myasthenia gravis (acquired megaesophagus) (p. 668)
- Resting serum cortisol concentration ± ACTH stimulation test to identify hypoadrenocorticism in dogs with acquired megaesophagus (pp. 512 and 1300)
- Serum creatine kinase determination: various myopathies
- Electromyography/motor nerve conduction velocity: polymyopathy/polyneuropathy
- Other tests as suggested by other findings (e.g., lead level, antinuclear antibody test)

TREATMENT

Treatment Overview

Treat acquired megaesophagus by resolving the underlying cause (possible in approximately 15%-20% of dogs); treat aspiration pneumonia if present. If an underlying cause cannot be found, treat as idiopathic megaesophagus by minimizing regurgitation with modified feeding practices and treating aspiration pneumonia when present.

Acute General Treatment

- Treat pneumonia if present (p. 793).
- Treat underlying cause if found.
- Feeding modification
  - Feed from an elevated platform so that the patient's esophagus is perpendicular to the floor and gravity aids in food/water passage from the esophagus into the stomach. Maintain this position for 5-10 minutes after eating to enhance food emptying into the stomach. The animal needs to be in a nearly perfectly upright position; a 50°-60° incline is often insufficient. Bailey chair can be used for feeding.
  - Feed different consistencies of food to find which is best tolerated: some animals fare better on canned or solid food or meatballs, whereas others do better with gruel.
  - Feed several small meals per day to minimize retention of large amounts in esophagus.
- Prokinetic drugs may be tried.
  - Only indicated when gastroesophageal reflux is suspected; increases normograde gastric emptying and reduces volume of acid reflux. Prokinetic drugs are often useful for treating gastric motility disorders, but they do not increase esophageal motility to any appreciable degree. Typical options:
    - Cisapride 0.1-0.5 mg/kg PO q 8-12h. Cisapride increases lower esophageal tone (most effective gastric prokinetic), which can worsen clinical signs if gastroesophageal reflux is not occurring.
    - Metoclopramide 0.2-0.4 mg/kg PO, IM, or SQ q 8-12h. The increase in lower esophageal sphincter tone described for metoclopramide is not thought to be clinically significant and does not contraindicate use in megaesophagus.
- Gastric acid–reducing therapy: recommended if gastroesophageal reflux is likely; omeprazole 1-2 mg/kg PO q 12h

Chronic Treatment

- Ongoing implementation of measures described in acute treatment
- Treat any identified specific conditions (e.g., hypoadrenocorticism, myasthenia gravis).
- Gastrostomy tube (p. 1109) is rarely required but can minimize regurgitation of food (especially if patient is having major problems with aspiration and is waiting for treatment of underlying cause to succeed)
  - Patient can still swallow, regurgitate, and aspirate saliva and other material despite gastrostomy tube
- Select dogs may improve after treatment with sildenafil, cisapride, or maropitant.

Possible Complications

- Aspiration pneumonia
- Infected stoma (gastrostomy tube)

PROGNOSIS & OUTCOME

- If the underlying cause can be found and cured, the outlook can be good. Esophageal function may normalize:
  - In some dogs with congenital megaesophagus
  - With resolution of myasthenia gravis, toxicity, botulism, or esophagitis
- As long as megaesophagus persists, aspiration poses a risk of pneumonia and death.
- If the underlying cause cannot be resolved, the outlook is guarded because these patients often die of aspiration pneumonia. Conservative management benefits many patients if the clients are determined and aggressive about making the patient eat in an almost perpendicular position.

PEARLS & CONSIDERATIONS

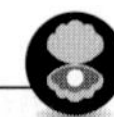

Comments

- Some drugs (especially sedatives like ketamine and alpha-2 adrenergic agonists xylazine and medetomidine) cause esophageal weakness, which can complicate the diagnosis.
- Megaesophagus spontaneously resolves in some dogs.
- Radiography/fluoroscopy is typically preferred to diagnose functional problems such as megaesophagus; endoscopy is preferred to diagnose anatomic esophageal problems such as strictures, foreign bodies, and esophagitis.
- The severity of radiographic esophageal dilation is not always proportional to the severity of clinical signs.
- Mild aspiration pneumonia is often missed on lateral radiographs; dorsoventral and opposite lateral projections increase sensitivity.
- Unexplained bacterial pneumonia in a dog could be caused by occult esophageal dysfunction; consider performing a contrast esophagram to look for esophageal weakness in dogs with unexplained pneumonia even if esophageal dilation is absent on plain radiographs.
- If a dog with megaesophagus vomits persistently, esophagitis typically occurs due to gastric acid entering and not exiting the esophageal lumen.
- Surgery (cardiomyotomy) has not been commonly used in dogs with megaesophagus; the role of true achalasia (which is helped by such surgery) is undetermined in dogs.

Prevention

Do not breed animals with known history of producing litters with megaesophagus.

Technician Tips

Watch closely for signs of aspiration (coughing, nasal discharge, tachypnea, dyspnea) in dogs with known esophageal dysfunction or neuromuscular diseases that may cause esophageal weakness.

Client Education

- Provide client with an education sheet: How to Provide Elevated Feedings.
- In cases with percutaneous endoscopic gastrostomy tube placement, provide client with an education sheet: How to Use and Care for an Indwelling Feeding Tube.
- Aspiration pneumonia can occur at any time, even in dogs with mild radiographic signs of megaesophagus.

SUGGESTED READING

McBrearty AR, et al: Clinical factors associated with death before discharge and overall survival time in dogs with generalized megaesophagus. J Am Vet Med Assoc 238:1622-1628, 2011.

AUTHOR: Michael D. Willard, DVM, MS, DACVIM
EDITOR: Rance K. Sellon, DVM, PhD, DACVIM

Melanoma

Bonus Material Online 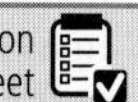 Client Education Sheet

BASIC INFORMATION

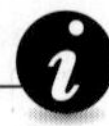

Definition

A common neoplasm that develops from melanocytes in dogs (rare in cats). Classification of melanomas by anatomic location generally has more clinical utility than by histologic subtype.

- Most oral melanomas are malignant, locally invasive, and highly metastatic (>60%) (p. 714).
- Subungual (nail bed) melanomas are locally invasive with a lower rate of metastasis (30%-60%).
- Cutaneous melanomas in dogs are generally (but not always) benign.
- Ocular melanoma (p. 559)

Synonyms

Malignant melanoma, melanocytic tumor (benign and malignant), melanocytoma (benign)

Epidemiology

SPECIES, AGE, SEX

Melanoma generally occurs in older patients (9-12 years).

GENETICS, BREED PREDISPOSITION

- Predisposed dog breeds include chow chow, Doberman pinscher, golden retriever, Gordon setter, Irish setter, giant schnauzer, miniature schnauzer, Scottish terrier (suggests an underlying genetic mechanism)
- Black dogs may be predisposed, but any color dog may be affected.

Clinical Presentation

HISTORY, CHIEF COMPLAINT

Oral melanoma:

- Detection of an oral mass by a veterinarian during routine exam or dental prophylaxis (common)
- Identification of an oral mass by the owner
- Recent-onset halitosis, ptyalism

Cutaneous or subungual melanoma:

- Identification of a mass by the owner or veterinarian

PHYSICAL EXAM FINDINGS

- Exam typically reveals a mass lesion.
- Oral exam should be thorough; some tumors are located at the base of the tongue or in the tonsils.
- Cutaneous and subungual tumors may become ulcerated.
- Melanomas may be pigmented (≈⅔) or amelanotic (≈⅓).
- Thorough exam of draining lymph nodes is always indicated; cytologic evaluation should be performed even if the nodes are of normal size.

Etiology and Pathophysiology

- Underlying genetic mutations and ultraviolet light exposure are known etiologic agents in humans.
- Melanomas do not have to arise in pigmented skin.

DIAGNOSIS

Diagnostic Overview

Biopsy of an identified mass is the test of choice to establish a diagnosis of melanoma. A diagnostic and treatment approach is presented on p. 1437.

Differential Diagnosis

- Oral: squamous cell carcinoma, fibrosarcoma, acanthomatous ameloblastoma
- Cutaneous: any mass lesion of skin (neoplastic or non-neoplastic)
- Subungual: squamous cell carcinoma, nail bed infection

Initial Database

CBC, serum biochemistry profile, urinalysis, lymph node aspiration, thoracic radiographs, and for patients with hindlimb or caudally located masses, abdominal ultrasound

Advanced or Confirmatory Testing

- Biopsy and histopathologic exam of tissue
- Immunohistochemical staining with S-100 or Melan-A may confirm the diagnosis of melanoma in undifferentiated and amelanotic tumors.
- Mitotic index may help distinguish benign from malignant canine cutaneous melanomas.
  - Determination of mitotic index requires histopathologic evaluation of tissue and cannot be reliably assessed on fine-needle aspiration/cytology.
  - Tumors with a mitotic index of < 3/10 high-power fields (HPF) are typically benign; those ≥ 3/10 HPF are generally malignant.

TREATMENT

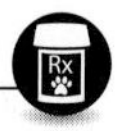

Treatment Overview

The treatment plan depends on the prognosis, and staging to identify local and metastatic disease is essential. Goals of treatment are long-term disease control in patients amenable to definitive therapy, and palliation of clinical signs in patients not treated definitively or those with metastatic disease (p. 1437).

Acute and Chronic Treatment

Oral melanoma:

- Radical excision of mass if
  - Wide surgical margins (>2 cm, including underlying bone) can be obtained, and
  - Patient has no regional lymph node or distant metastasis
- Removal of macroscopic (measurable) tumor plus definitive radiation therapy to primary tumor site and regional lymph nodes if
  - Radical excision is not possible or regional lymph node metastasis is identified, and
  - Patient has no distant metastatic disease
- Definitive radiation therapy alone to primary tumor and regional lymph nodes if
  - Removal of macroscopic tumor burden is not possible, and
  - Patient has no distant metastatic disease
- Palliative radiation therapy to tumor could be considered if
  - The patient has distant metastatic disease, and/or
  - Financial or other restrictions preclude definitive therapy

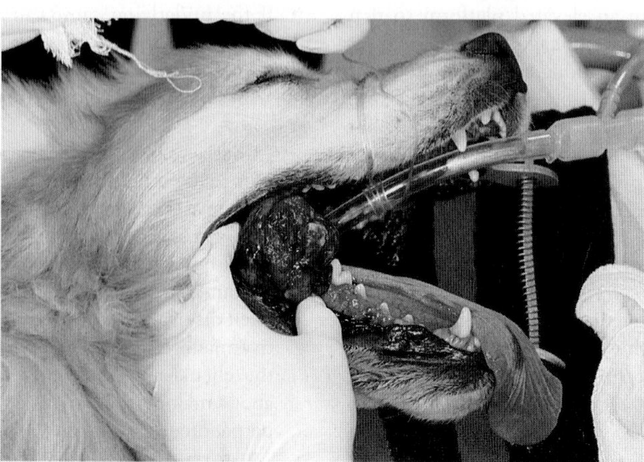

MELANOMA Oral malignant melanoma in the right mandibular gingiva of a 7-year-old golden retriever.

- Chemotherapy for all patients treated definitively with surgery and/or radiotherapy due to high rate of metastatic disease
  - Systemic therapy with carboplatin or cisplatin given reported activity of carboplatin in dogs with melanoma
  - Chemotherapy may benefit patients treated with palliative radiotherapy and those with evidence of distant metastasis.
- DNA-based melanoma vaccine (Oncept, Merial) is indicated for all patients for which local/regional control has been attained.

Subungual (nail bed) melanoma:
- Radical excision of mass if
  - Wide surgical margins (>2 cm, including underlying bone) are possible, and
  - Patient has no distant metastatic disease
- Limb amputation (plus excision of associated lymph nodes if metastasis) should be considered if wide surgical margins cannot be obtained with local resection (i.e., digital amputation).
- Removal of macroscopic tumor followed by definitive course of radiation therapy to primary tumor site and regional lymph nodes if
  - Digital amputation not possible, and
  - Regional lymph node metastasis is identified, and
  - Patient has no distant metastatic disease
- Palliative course of radiotherapy could be considered if
  - Patient has distant metastatic disease and clinical signs associated with local disease result in decreased quality of life
- DNA-based vaccine and possibly chemotherapy should be considered for all patients treated definitively with surgery and/or radiation therapy due to the high rate of metastatic disease in patients with subungual melanoma.

Cutaneous melanoma:
- Surgical resection is the treatment of choice for benign melanomas (<3 mitoses/10 HPF).
- Radical excision of malignant cutaneous melanoma (≥3 mitoses/10 HPF) if
  - Wide surgical margins (>2 cm) can be obtained, and
  - Patient has no regional lymph node or distant metastatic disease
- Removal of macroscopic tumor followed by definitive course of radiation therapy to primary tumor site and regional lymph nodes if
  - Radical excision is not possible or if regional lymph node metastasis is identified, and
  - Patient has no distant metastatic disease
- Palliative course of radiation therapy could be considered if
  - Patient has distant metastatic disease and clinical signs associated with local disease result in decreased quality of life
- DNA-based vaccine and possibly chemotherapy should be considered for all patients with malignant cutaneous melanomas treated definitively with surgery and/or radiation therapy.

Recommended Monitoring

Initially, patients should be monitored with physical exam (local disease status) and thoracic radiographs (to identify metastatic disease) every 2-3 months. Frequency is altered by individual factors.

PROGNOSIS & OUTCOME

Oral melanoma:
- Prognosis
  - Untreated: median survival of 65 days
  - Conservative surgery alone: median survival of 3-4 months; local recurrence rate > 70%
  - Radical surgery alone: median survival of 19 months for stage I (<2 cm), 4 months for stage II (2-4 cm without lymph node metastasis) and stage III (>4 cm or lymph node metastasis present); local recurrence rate of 22% after mandibulectomy and 48% after maxillectomy
  - Radical surgery with or without adjunctive treatment: median survival of 21-29 months for stage I, 8-27 months for stage II, and 6-7 months for stage III
  - Radiation therapy for microscopic tumors: median survival of 15 months; local recurrence rate of 26%
  - Radiation therapy for macroscopic tumors: response rate of 82%-94%; median survival of 5-12 months; local progression/recurrence rate of 45%
  - Chemotherapy for macroscopic tumors: response rate of 18%-37%.
  - Chemotherapy for microscopic tumors: progression-free interval of 9 months with adjuvant carboplatin after surgical resection or surgical resection combined with radiation therapy
  - Prognosis for definitively treated feline oral melanoma is not known.
- Prognostic factors
  - Stage
  - Mitotic index ≥ 4 mitoses/HPF has been associated with an increased risk of death within 1 year of diagnosis (90% sensitivity and 84% specificity).

Subungual melanoma:
- Prognosis
  - Surgical excision (local or limb amputation): median survival of 12 months; local recurrence rate of 30% (local resection only)
  - Role of radiation therapy and chemotherapy undetermined
  - Prognostic factors: none identified

Cutaneous melanoma:
- Prognosis
  - Surgical excision: median survival of 24 months (benign); 7-11 months (malignant)
  - Efficacy of radiation therapy and chemotherapy undetermined
  - Median survival for feline cutaneous melanoma treated with surgery alone is 12 months.
- Prognostic factors
  - Mitotic index is the most important prognostic factor: ≥ 3 mitoses/HPF indicates malignancy.
  - Breed: Doberman pinschers and miniature schnauzers more likely have benign melanoma (75%); miniature poodles more likely have malignant melanoma (85%).

PEARLS & CONSIDERATIONS

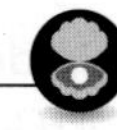

Comments

- Radiation treatment
  - Melanoma has a greater capacity for sublethal damage repair and therefore is best treated with a hypofractionated (larger doses per fraction) treatment protocol, such as 8-9 Gy/fraction 3-4 times instead of conventional protocols (e.g., 3-Gy/fraction 16-19 times).
  - For treatment of malignant melanoma, a hypofractionated protocol is used in most facilities, and a conventional radiation protocol is not used currently.
  - Four reported veterinary protocols for melanoma are 10 Gy × 3, 9 Gy × 4, 8 Gy × 3, and 4 Gy × 12.
  - Because late-responding normal tissues (bone, muscle, central nervous system) are more susceptible to toxicosis with larger doses of radiation, large doses (8-10 Gy) should be avoided in patients for which long-term survival (>12 months) is expected.
- Chemotherapy
  - In patients failing platinum-based chemotherapy, veterinary and human information may support the use of dacarbazine, melphalan, CCNU, piroxicam, and interferon.
- DNA-based vaccine
  - Studies indicate that patients with locally/regionally controlled disease may experience a longer survival when the tyrosinase DNA vaccine is administered.
  - The utility of tyrosinase DNA vaccination in patients with advanced disease is unclear.

Technician Tips

Do a complete oral exam during professional dental cleanings, and bring all identified oral masses, even very small masses, to the attention of the clinician for possible biopsy under the same episode of general anesthesia.

SUGGESTED READING

Bergman PJ, et al: Melanoma. In Withrow SJ, et al, editors: Small animal clinical oncology, ed 5, St. Louis, 2013, Elsevier, pp 321-334.

AUTHOR: Tetsuya Kobayashi, DVM, MSpVM, DACVIM, DAiCVIM
EDITOR: Kenneth M. Rassnick, DVM, DACVIM

Melena

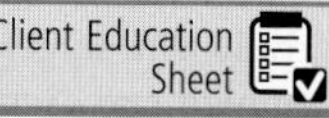

BASIC INFORMATION

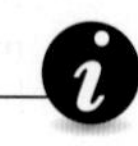

Definition

Black, tarry stool containing partially digested blood

Epidemiology

SPECIES, AGE, SEX

- More common in dogs than cats
- Neoplastic causes more common in older animals

RISK FACTORS

- Ulcerogenic drugs (e.g., nonsteroidal anti-inflammatory drugs [NSAIDs], high-dose corticosteroid, tyrosine kinase inhibitors)
- Anticoagulant exposure

ASSOCIATED DISORDERS

Anemia, panhypoproteinemia, increased blood urea nitrogen (BUN), and increased BUN/serum creatinine ratio

Clinical Presentation

DISEASE FORMS/SUBTYPES

- Commonly due to upper gastrointestinal (GI) disease that causes bleeding or hemostatic disorders or, less often, due to swallowed blood from respiratory tract disease
- Presentation may be chronic or acute, and the animal may be stable or critically ill.

HISTORY, CHIEF COMPLAINT

Pet owners may or may not recognize melena in their pet's stool. Other signs depend on severity and cause of bleeding.

- Lethargy, weakness may be caused by anemia or hypovolemia.
- GI disease: anorexia, regurgitation, vomiting, diarrhea, weight loss, hematemesis (raises suspicion for GI ulcers)
  - Include questions about ulcerogenic drugs
- Hemostatic disorder: other evidence of bleeding (e.g., ecchymosis, epistaxis, hematuria)
- Respiratory disease: epistaxis, stertor, coughing, exercise intolerance, dyspnea, hemoptysis

PHYSICAL EXAM FINDINGS

- Rectal exam: tarry stool
- If anemia and/or hypovolemia: pallor, tachypnea, tachycardia, thready pulses, dull mentation
- If GI disease, may find any of the following:
  - Loose stool in rectum
  - Pain on abdominal palpation
  - Abdominal mass effect
  - Thickened intestines
  - Oral cavity bleeding
  - Occasionally, hematochezia
- If hemostatic disorder, may see petechiae and ecchymoses; less often, epistaxis, hematuria, intracavitary hemorrhage
- If respiratory disease, may find tachypnea, dyspnea, epistaxis, stertor, adventitial lung sounds

Etiology and Pathophysiology

- Most commonly caused by bleeding originating from the oropharynx or upper GI tract due to local disease or hemostatic defects. Less often, swallowed blood from the respiratory tract or ingestion of blood causes melena.
- Further discussion of causes provided on p. 1252.

DIAGNOSIS

Diagnostic Overview

The history, physical exam, and initial database guide additional testing.

Differential Diagnosis

- Bismuth-containing products, iron, or charcoal can change fecal color and be confused with melena.
- Stool exposed to air may appear dark; the presence of melena should be judged on fresh stool.

Initial Database

- CBC
  - Acute bleeding: normal or regenerative anemia (i.e., reticulocytosis)
  - Nonregenerative anemia with microcytosis and hypochromasia, thrombocytosis, suggest chronic GI bleeding
  - Thrombocytopenia (<30,000 platelets/mcL) may explain cause of bleeding.
  - Neutrophil count > 50,000 neutrophils/mcL should raise suspicion for infectious disease or GI perforation.
  - Lack of stress leukogram compatible with hypoadrenocorticism
- Biochemical profile
  - BUN/creatinine ratio: often high end/above reference range (unless liver failure)
  - Total protein: often low end/below reference range due to loss of globulin and albumin, but if underlying disease (e.g., neoplasia, fungal infection) causes hyperglobulinemia, total protein may be within reference range
  - Electrolyte disturbances: may suggest primary GI or metabolic (e.g., hypoadrenocorticism)
  - Other abnormalities related to underlying disease (e.g., GI ulcers due to uremia or liver failure)
- Centrifugation fecal flotation: evaluate for helminths; sensitivity is low with single testing
- Abdominal radiographs/ultrasound
  - Thickened GI wall
  - Lesions suggesting infection or neoplasia (lymphadenopathy, hepatosplenomegaly, masses)
  - Abdominal effusion (severe hypoalbuminemia, portal hypertension)
  - GI foreign bodies
  - GI ulceration
- Coagulation profile for suspected hemostatic disorder (p. 1325)
- Primary hemostatic defects more likely to cause melena than secondary defects (i.e., thrombocytopenia/thrombocytopathy)

Advanced or Confirmatory Testing

- Thoracic imaging
  - Include in initial diagnostics if neoplastic or respiratory disease suspected
- Fecal sedimentation, wet mount, and Baermann fecal flotation test performed on fresh feces to evaluate for GI and respiratory parasites
- Esophagogastroduodenoscopy: to identify the source of GI bleeding ± biopsy. Capsule endoscopy can be used in dogs but cannot sample lesion.
- Imaging studies as appropriate for suspected respiratory bleeding (e.g., CT scan, pharyngoscopy/bronchoscopy)
- Specific disease testing may be recommended, depending on history, physical exam findings, results of initial tests, and the prevalence in the area.
  - Gastrinoma (p. 1346)
  - Hypoadrenocorticism (pp. 512 and 1300)
  - Heartworm disease (pp. 415, 418, and 1350)
  - Folate/cobalamin (pp. 1325 and 1344)

TREATMENT

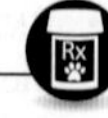

Treatment Overview

Successful treatment depends on the ability to resolve the cause, stabilize patient hemodynamics, and restore the GI mucosal barrier.

Acute General Treatment

- Severe anemia or shock: administer intravenous crystalloids, colloids, or blood products.
- Supportive therapy for proximal GI bleeding includes
  - Proton pump inhibitors (PPIs [e.g., omeprazole]) 1.0 mg/kg PO or IV q 12h. Do not use in combination with histamine-2 receptor antagonists (H2RAs) when treating ulcerative disease.
  - H2RAs (e.g., famotidine) are inferior to PPIs for GI bleeding.
  - Sucralfate 0.5-1.0 g (dogs) or 0.25 g (cats) q 6-8h PO administered as liquid or slurry is more effective for duodenal than gastric ulcers. Caution if concurrent kidney disease

- Misoprostol 3-5 mcg/kg PO q 8-12h (dogs) for NSAID toxicity
- Surgery may be necessary for patients with perforating GI ulcers, foreign bodies, or masses.
- If a definitive cause is not identified in a stable patient, administer fenbendazole 50 mg/kg q 24h PO for 5 days.

Chronic Treatment

- Iron dextran 5-10 mg/kg IM q 3-4 weeks for patients with iron-deficiency anemia (e.g., microcytosis, nonregenerative anemia). Pretreatment with diphenhydramine is advised.
- Other therapies depend on the cause of melena.

Nutrition/Diet

A canned, highly digestible, low-fat diet should be considered to promote gastric emptying and avoid further GI mucosal trauma.

Drug Interactions

- Sucralfate requires an acidic environment and interferes with the absorption of tetracyclines and ciprofloxacin. Delay administration of sucralfate by 2 hours when patient is receiving antibiotics, acid suppressants, or antacids.
- PPIs may have interactions with drugs metabolized by cytochrome P450 (e.g., itraconazole, cyclosporine) or those that depend on an acidic environment (e.g. sucralfate, antacids).

Possible Complications

- GI perforation and septic peritonitis if GI ulceration is present.
- Anemia may require transfusion ± iron supplementation.
- If injury to GI epithelium is severe, bacterial translocation may occur.

Recommended Monitoring

Activity, respiratory rate, and packed cell volume/total solids (PCV/TS) are used to assess for severity of bleeding.

PROGNOSIS & OUTCOME

Depends on ability to resolve cause, absence of GI perforation

PEARLS & CONSIDERATIONS

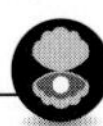

Comments

- In the absence of hemostatic disorders or ulcerogenic drugs, search for underlying neoplasia, especially in older animals with melena.
- The absence of abdominal ultrasound abnormalities does not rule out GI causes of melena.
- Capsule endoscopy may aid in identification of GI bleeding when GI endoscopy is not an option.

Prevention

- Avoid the use of ulcerogenic drugs in animals at risk for GI bleeding.
- Do not use corticosteroids and NSAIDS in combination. An exception to this rule is the coadministration of steroids and low-dose aspirin for patients at risk for thromboembolic disease.
- Misoprostol may decrease the risk of NSAID-induced GI ulceration.

Technician Tips

Advise clients to monitor for melena when administering ulcerogenic drugs, platelet inhibitors, or anticoagulants.

SUGGESTED READING

Willard M: Hemorrhage (gastrointestinal). In Washabau R, et al, editors: Canine & feline gastroenterology, St. Louis, 2013, Elsevier Saunders, 129-134.

AUTHOR: M. Katherine Tolbert, DVM, PhD, DACVIM
EDITOR: Leah A. Cohn, DVM, PhD DACVIM

Meningoencephalitis of Unknown Origin

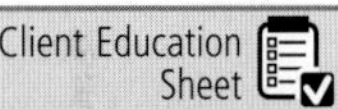

BASIC INFORMATION

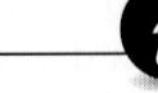

Definition

Meningoencephalitis of unknown origin (MUO) is the clinical diagnosis given to a group of noninfectious, inflammatory meningoencephal(omyel)itises of dogs. It can be further classified based on histopathology as granulomatous meningoencephalomyelitis (GME) or necrotizing encephalitis (NE).

Synonyms

Meningoencephalitis of unknown etiology (MUE; sometimes abbreviated MUA [atieology]), granulomatous meningoencephalomyelitis (GME), necrotizing encephalitis (NE), necrotizing leukoencephalitis (NLE), Yorkshire terrier encephalopathy, necrotizing meningoencephalitis (NME), pug (dog) encephalopathy, Maltese encephalopathy

Epidemiology

SPECIES, AGE, SEX

- Small to medium-sized breed (<10 kg), young adult (3-7 years old) dogs most commonly affected
- Dogs with GME are generally older (4-8 years) than those with NE (<4 years). Pugs with NE tend to be young (median age, 18 months)
- Slight female predisposition reported

GENETICS, BREED PREDISPOSITION

- GME: poodles and terriers are predisposed, but any breed and size can be affected.
- NE: pug, Maltese, Yorkshire terrier, Chihuahua, French bulldog, papillion, shih tzu, Pekinese, West Highland white terrier, Coton de Tuléar, Brussels griffon, miniature poodle
- Pugs with a mutation of the dog lymphocyte antigen (DLA) region of chromosome 12 have a 12.75 times greater likelihood of developing NE.

RISK FACTORS

MUO is thought to be autoimmune but recent vaccination has not been found to be a trigger.

GEOGRAPHY AND SEASONALITY

Possible higher incidence in spring and summer

Clinical Presentation

DISEASE FORMS/SUBTYPES

GME:
- Focal: often forebrain signs
- Disseminated: multifocal central nervous system (CNS) signs, including spinal cord
- Ocular: optic neuritis

NE:
- NME: forebrain signs, especially seizures
- NLE: forebrain and brainstem signs

HISTORY, CHIEF COMPLAINT

Subacute (days) to acute (weeks) focal or multifocal CNS signs; specific complaints vary based on region of nervous system involved

PHYSICAL EXAM FINDINGS

- Physical exam (other than neurologic exam): often unremarkable
- Any neurologic deficit referable to disease in the brain (or spinal cord) can be present.
- Common findings:
  - Forebrain signs: circling, seizures, blindness, ataxia

- Brainstem signs: central vestibular disease (head tilt, ataxia)
- Meningitis: cervical pain

Etiology and Pathophysiology

- Cause is unknown; presumed autoimmune or immune mediated
- Attempts to identify an inciting infectious cause have been unrewarding.
- Antibodies against neural elements (astrocytes, glial fibrillary acidic protein) have been identified in serum and cerebrospinal fluid (CSF) of affected dogs.
- Histopathology: nonsuppurative, mononuclear cell infiltration in the brain and/or meninges, especially $CD8^+$ T lymphocytes in GME

DIAGNOSIS

Diagnostic Overview

MUO should be considered based on signalment and presenting clinical signs. Initial diagnostics are performed to evaluate for other causes of neurologic disease. Diagnosis often requires referral for MRI and CSF analysis. MRI or CSF can occasionally be normal, highlighting the importance of a complete diagnostic workup.

Differential Diagnosis

- Infectious meningoencephalitis
  - Protozoal: *Toxoplasma gondii, Neospora caninum*
  - Bacterial
  - Viral: canine distemper, rabies
  - Tick-borne: *Ehrlichia canis, Anaplasma* spp, *Rickettsia rickettsii, Borrelia burgdorferi, Babesia canis, Bartonella henselae*
  - Fungal: *Cryptococcus neoformans, Blastomyces* spp, *Coccidioides immitis, Aspergillus* spp, *Histoplasma* spp
  - Other: *Prototheca* spp, *Cuterebra*
- Neoplasia
- Vascular: ischemic or hemorrhagic stroke
- Blindness (p. 123)

Initial Database

- Neurologic exam (p 1136): to localize lesion
- Testing to rule out other causes for clinical signs
  - CBC, serum chemistry, urinalysis
  - Bile acids, preprandial and postprandial
  - Infectious disease testing (tick-transmitted/protozoal/fungal infection)

Advanced or Confirmatory Testing

- MRI of brain (p. 1132): focal to multifocal T2- and FLAIR-weighted hyperintensities throughout cerebral cortex; occasional involvement of cerebellum and brainstem variable contrast enhancement
- CSF analysis (pp. 1080 and 1323): elevated nucleated cell count and total protein
- Cytology: > 50% mononuclear, varied lower percentages of nondegenerative neutrophils
- Paired distemper titers (serum ± CSF): normal
- Histopathology (surgical biopsy or necropsy): confirms GME or NE

TREATMENT

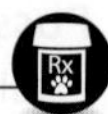

Treatment Overview

Glucocorticoids are the benchmark of treatment. The choice of add-on therapy varies based on clinician preference, owner finances, proximity to a hospital capable of administering chemotherapy, and owner health concerns (immune compromised/pregnant). Cytarabine, cyclosporine, procarbazine, azathioprine, mycophenolate mofetil, and radiation therapy have been used.

Acute General Treatment

- Prednisone/prednisolone is initiated at antiinflammatory dosages (e.g., 0.5-1 mg/kg PO q 24h) pending infectious disease titers. Some advocate for immediate immunosuppression (e.g., 2 mg/kg PO q 12h) after MRI and CSF, based on the low positive yields from infectious disease testing.
  - If severity of neurologic signs at the time of diagnosis precludes the administration of oral medications, consider drugs with IV formulations (dexamethasone, methylprednisolone sodium succinate, cytarabine, mycophenolate mofetil).
- Treat for common infectious diseases (doxycycline 5-10 mg/kg PO q 12h, clindamycin 15 mg/kg PO q 12h, fluconazole 5 mg/kg PO q 12h) while awaiting titer results.
- Seizure activity: IV benzodiazepines, then initiate maintenance antiepileptic therapy with parenteral formulation of phenobarbital or levetiracetam. Levetiracetam tends to be preferred and has less effect on dog's mental status than phenobarbital.
- Signs of elevated intracranial pressure (depressed mental attitude/poor pupillary light reflexes): mannitol 1 g/kg IV once or 3% hypertonic saline 4-6 mL/kg IV once.

Chronic Treatment

- Prednisone/prednisolone: immunosuppressive doses with a slow taper over the next year: 2 mg/kg PO q 12h for 3 days, then 1-1.5 mg/kg PO q 12h for 1-3 months, then decrease dose by 25% q 6-8 weeks until the lowest effective dose is achieved. Complete withdrawal is possible in some cases.
- Cytarabine 200 mg/m^2 IV constant-rate infusion (CRI) over 8 hours (25 $mg/m^2/h$ × 8 hours [p. 609]) *or* 50 mg/m^2 SQ q 12h for 4 doses. Repeat q 3 weeks for 4 cycles, increasing the treatment interval by 1 week q 4 cycles until q 8 week treatment schedule is reached. Recent studies suggest a longer survival time with CRI than SQ administration.
- Cyclosporine (Atopica) 5-10 mg/kg PO q 12h
  - To reduce cost, can be administered q 24h with ketoconazole 8 mg/kg PO q 24h
  - Targeted whole blood concentrations, measured 1 week after initiation of therapy or dosage change: 800-1400 ng/mL (peak), 400-600 ng/mL (trough)
  - Small size of many MUO patients may necessitate compounded formulations of cyclosporine; commercially available liquid formulation can be used (minimum dose of 10 mg/kg PO q 12h often required to achieve therapeutic concentrations). The microemulsified form (Neoral/cyclosporine modified) is recommended over Sandimmune.
  - Vaccines may be less effective in dogs on cyclosporine; avoid live attenuated vaccines.
- Procarbazine (Matulane, Alcami) 25-50 mg/m^2 PO q 24h decreasing to q 48h dosing after 1-3 months
- Azathioprine 2 mg/kg PO q 24h for 2-4 weeks, then 2 mg/kg PO q 48h
- Mycophenolate mofetil 20 mg/kg PO or IV q 12h, decrease to 10 mg/kg PO q 12h after 2-4 months, then 10 mg/kg PO q 24h for 2-4 months, for a final dosing schedule of 10 mg/kg PO q 48h. Capsules should not be opened, and the sodium enteric-coated tablets should be avoided.
- Tapering of medication dosages is contingent on the absence of recurrence of clinical signs.
- Lomustine 44-88 mg/m^2 PO q 6 weeks (p. 609). The use of live vaccines is discouraged.
- Radiation therapy 10 3-Gy treatments

Behavior/Exercise

While on immunosuppressive therapy, communal areas such as dog parks and boarding facilities should be avoided.

Drug Interactions

Cyclosporine, phenobarbital, and procarbazine are metabolized by the hepatic cytochrome P450 system; they alter the disposition of other drugs that depend on P450 enzymes for metabolism, necessitating a higher dose when used in combination.

Possible Complications

- Glucocorticoid side effects should be expected: polyuria, polydipsia, polyphagia, ± others (e.g., hepatopathy, iatrogenic hyperadrenocorticism)
- Gastrointestinal side effects are possible with all treatments: famotidine 1 mg/kg PO q 24h or omeprazole 1 mg/kg PO q 24h might help prevent gastric ulceration. Excessive vomiting, especially with blood, or anorexia necessitates a medication change.
  - Administer cyclosporine on an empty stomach; if excessive vomiting, freeze the capsule and/or administer metoclopramide or maropitant 30 minutes before dosing.
- Myelosuppression: perform complete blood counts to monitor
  - Cytarabine: 1 week after administration and before each treatment
  - Procarbazine: every week for the first month, then monthly

- Azathioprine: q 1-2 weeks, then q 1-3 months
- Mycophenolate: q 1-3 months
- Lomustine: 7-10 days after administration and before each treatment
- Monitor for secondary infections (respiratory, urinary, dermatologic).
- Gingival hyperplasia with chronic cyclosporine administration
- CNS depression and peripheral neuropathy with procarbazine
- Secondary infection due to immune suppression

Recommended Monitoring

- Serial neurologic exams
- Repeat CSF ± MRI at 3 months; relapse is more likely if CSF remains abnormal after 3 months of treatment or treatment is stopped before resolution of MRI abnormalities.
- Owners should monitor closely for recurrence of clinical signs. Any relapse should be treated aggressively because response to treatment can decline.

PROGNOSIS & OUTCOME

- Overall prognosis: fair to guarded (survival, 0-1834 days; median, 1-2 years). Breeds at higher risk for NE (pugs) have a worse prognosis.
- Dogs that respond to treatment in the first 24-72 hours and survive the first 3 months of treatment are likely to do well, reaching the median to higher range of survival. However, 15%-33% of dogs die in the immediate post-diagnostic period or first 2-3 months of treatment.
- Potential negative prognostic indicators: multifocal disease, seizures, altered mentation, MRI findings of herniation through the foramen magnum, decreased sulci depth of the cerebral cortex, or mass effect; partial instead of complete response to treatment

PEARLS & CONSIDERATIONS

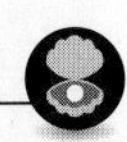

Comments

- If infectious disease titers are included in the initial minimal database, referral should not be delayed while awaiting results.
- Addition of a secondary immunomodulatory drug may allow more rapid taper of glucocorticoids and minimize associated side effects.
  - Procarbazine and radiation therapy are most expensive, followed by cyclosporine, mycophenolate, and lomustine.
  - Cytarabine and radiation therapy are limited by availability of a practice capable of administration.
- With resistant or recurrent disease, more aggressive treatment can be initiated with a tertiary immunomodulatory medication. Cytarabine can be administered with cyclosporine, procarbazine, azathioprine, or leflunomide. Avoid administration of procarbazine with cyclosporine due to potential cytochrome P450 interactions.

Technician Tips

- Cyclosporine concentrations are drawn in a purple-top tube; peak 2 hours after drug administration, and trough just before the next dosing.
- Blood should be collected from the jugular vein of dogs being administered cytarabine, saving the peripheral veins for catheter placement.

Client Education

Clients administering immunomodulatory/chemotherapeutic agents at home should be advised to wear gloves when handling the medication or bodily fluids from their pet.

SUGGESTED READING

Coates JR, et al: Perspectives on meningoencephalomyelitis of unknown origin. J Vet Clin North Am Small Anim Pract 44:1157-1185, 2014.

AUTHOR: Michaela J. Beasley, DVM, MS, DACVIM
EDITOR: Karen R. Muñana, DVM, MS, DACVIM

Mesenteric Volvulus

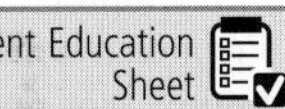

BASIC INFORMATION

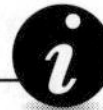

Definition

An uncommon disorder characterized by twisting of the intestine around the root of the mesentery; this process can be rapidly fatal.

Synonyms

Intestinal volvulus, mesenteric torsion

Epidemiology

SPECIES, AGE, SEX

Young adult male dogs are predisposed; also reported in cats

GENETICS, BREED PREDISPOSITION

Large-breed dogs, German shepherds, and English pointers

ASSOCIATED DISORDERS

Conditions that may be associated with mesenteric volvulus include exocrine pancreatic insufficiency, recent gastrointestinal (GI) surgery, GI foreign bodies, enteritis, intestinal neoplasia, blunt trauma, and gastric dilation/volvulus (GDV).

Clinical Presentation

HISTORY, CHIEF COMPLAINT

Acute-onset abdominal distention, pain, vomiting, and hematochezia

PHYSICAL EXAM FINDINGS

- Physical findings consistent with hypovolemic shock: tachycardia, weak pulses, pale mucous membranes, prolonged capillary refill time, weakness or collapse
- Abdominal distention, palpable gas-filled intestinal loops, abdominal pain
- ± Hematochezia on rectal palpation

Etiology and Pathophysiology

- Twisting of intestine occurs around mesenteric axis or root, causing vascular occlusion to the intestines.
- Thin-walled veins and lymphatics become obstructed, causing edema in the intestinal wall.
- Blood flow through cranial mesenteric artery and its branches is partially or completely occluded due to twisting.
- Ischemic necrosis of intestine occurs, and blood is lost into the intestinal lumen.
- Endotoxins and bacteria translocate into the abdomen through the damaged intestinal mucosa.
- Patients eventually die from circulatory shock and endotoxemia/sepsis.

DIAGNOSIS

Diagnostic Overview

The diagnosis is suggested by physical exam and appearance of abdominal radiographs. Differential diagnoses must be ruled out to the extent possible (e.g., ileus due to parvoviral enteritis: testing as appropriate). Confirmation of the diagnosis is made at the time of surgery.

Differential Diagnosis

Any condition associated with acute abdominal pain or hematochezia and vomiting (p. 21):

- GDV
- Cecocolic volvulus
- Intussusception
- Splenic torsion
- GI obstruction or rupture
- Peritonitis
- Pancreatitis

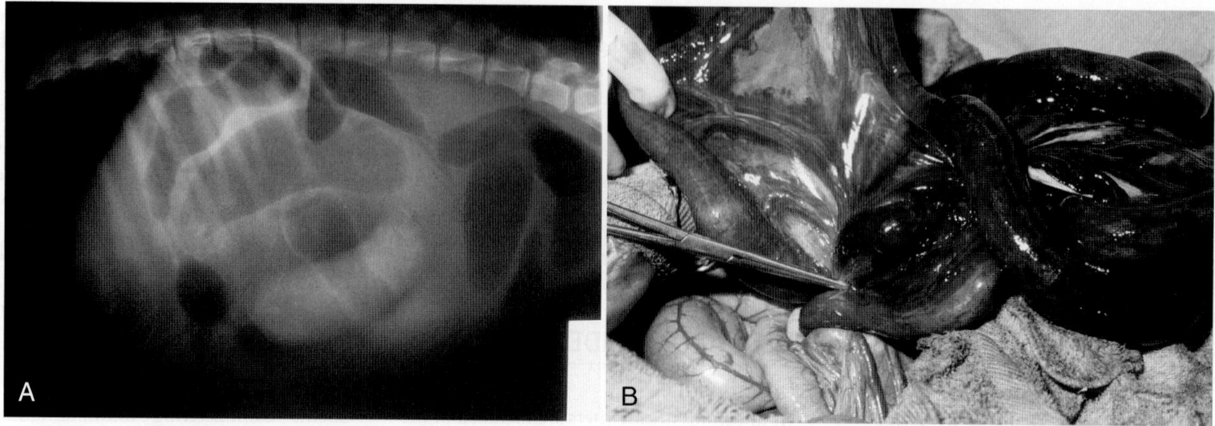

MESENTERIC VOLVULUS A, Lateral abdominal radiograph of a dog with mesenteric volvulus (cranial is to the left) and marked gas distention of bowel. **B**, In a different dog, gross appearance of bowel during exploratory laparotomy. Severe discoloration of much of small intestine and volvulus of the mesenteric root are diagnostic. (**B**, Courtesy Dr. Richard Walshaw.)

- Hemorrhagic gastroenteritis
- Parvoviral enteritis

Initial Database

- Abdominal radiography: multiple, severely distended, gas-filled intestinal loops; poor abdominal detail associated with peritoneal fluid; caudal displacement of the spleen; concurrent GDV
- CBC
  - Packed cell volume usually normal in dogs, low in cats
  - White blood cell count normal to elevated
- Serum biochemistry profile
  - Hypoproteinemia, hypokalemia
- Preoperative laboratory evaluation is often limited to on-site tests because of the potentially rapid deterioration of the patient's condition with mesenteric volvulus.
- Abdominocentesis (p. 1056) with fluid evaluation: modified transudate (early) or septic exudate (eventually, with bacterial translocation or peritonitis). With bowel necrosis, fluid may be dark and fetid.

Advanced or Confirmatory Testing

Surgical confirmation of diagnosis

TREATMENT

Treatment Overview

Patients with mesenteric volvulus should be treated for circulatory shock as appropriate and have rapid surgical intervention to correct the volvulus and resect diseased bowel.

Acute General Treatment

- Crystalloids should be administered for hypovolemic shock (p. 911): immediate bolus of 10-20 mL/kg, repeated as necessary based on reevaluation of clinical parameters, up to a maximum of 90 mL/kg in dogs and 45-60 mL/kg cats. Colloid boluses of 5 mL/kg can be administered simultaneously (up to 20 mL/kg dog, 5-10 mL/kg cat).
- Treat endotoxemia/sepsis with antibiotics.
  - Third-generation cephalosporin 22 mg/kg IV (e.g., cefotaxime 20-40 mg/kg IV q 6-8h or ceftriaxone 35 mg/kg IM or IV q 12h or ceftazidime 30 mg/kg IV q 6-8h; off-label use), *or*
  - Ampicillin 22 mg/kg IV q 6-8h combined with enrofloxacin 10 mg/kg IV q 24h for dogs
  - Ampicillin 22 mg/kg IV q 6h combined with cefoxitin 30 mg/kg IV q 6h (dogs and cats)
- Correct hypokalemia and acid-base abnormalities with fluid therapy.
- Resect only devitalized segment(s); do so without derotation to reduce reperfusion effects.
- If no normal bowel is seen, perform slow derotation of intestines and monitor for perfusion. Resect bowel that does not appear viable (i.e., dark color, no arterial pulsations).
- Perform thorough exploratory for associated conditions.
- Lavage abdomen, and consider postoperative drainage if peritonitis is present.

Possible Complications

- Septic peritonitis (p. 779) if diseased bowel not removed, contamination of abdomen not cleared, or resection and anastomosis site dehiscence
- Reperfusion injury
- Short-bowel syndrome may occur if > 50% of small intestine is resected.
- Persistent soft stool/diarrhea possible after ileocolic resection in dogs

Recommended Monitoring

- Postoperative monitoring of hydration and electrolyte concentrations
- Blood pressure monitoring for hypotension
- Body temperature and blood glucose monitoring for sepsis

PROGNOSIS & OUTCOME

- Grave prognosis unless volvulus is recognized and treated immediately
- Most reports of mesenteric volvulus cite a 100% mortality rate unless the volvulus is found incidentally during exploratory celiotomy.
- One study reported a 58% mortality rate for dogs with mesenteric volvulus presenting in shock; increased survival was attributed to rapid initiation of treatment.

PEARLS & CONSIDERATIONS

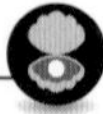

Comments

Surgery should not be delayed when an animal presents in shock with multiple, gas-filled intestinal loops on radiographs, but parvoviral enteritis should be ruled out before surgery.

Technician Tips

Any animal presenting with a distended, painful abdomen and vomiting should have treatment initiated immediately. Alert the clinician, and place an IV catheter promptly.

SUGGESTED READING

Junius G, et al: Mesenteric volvulus in the dog: a retrospective study of 12 cases. J Small Anim Pract 45:104-107, 2004.

AUTHOR: Lori Ludwig, VMD, MS, DACVS
EDITOR: Elizabeth A. Swanson, DVM, MS, DACVS

Mesothelioma

Client Education Sheet

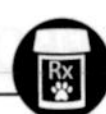

BASIC INFORMATION

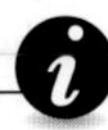

Definition

A neoplasm of mesodermal origin can arise from the pleural, pericardial, or peritoneal surfaces and has been reported arising from the scrotum or tunica vaginalis.

Epidemiology

SPECIES, AGE, SEX

Dogs > cats; males are overrepresented; generally older

GENETICS, BREED PREDISPOSITION

German shepherd dogs (particularly male) are overrepresented. Large-breed dogs are more commonly affected.

RISK FACTORS

- Possibly asbestos exposure, which causes mesothelioma in chronically exposed people
- Similar histopathologic findings (i.e., ferruginous bodies) have been noted in canine and human mesothelioma.

ASSOCIATED DISORDERS

Pleural, pericardial, and/or peritoneal effusion with dyspnea, acute cardiac tamponade and right-sided heart failure, or abdominal distention, respectively, are common.

Clinical Presentation

DISEASE FORMS/SUBTYPES

- Mesenchymal form: multiple focal nodules of solid or papillary neoplastic growth; historically, more common
- Sclerosing form: characterized by an intense fibroblastic reaction and thick fibrous adhesions involving all abdominal organs but most markedly affecting the stomach and prostate; uncommon in dogs

HISTORY, CHIEF COMPLAINT

Patients most commonly are presented for dyspnea or cough and possibly abdominal distention. This disease should be suspected in any adult patient with a cough that does not respond to standard treatment for nonspecific respiratory problems or with evidence of chronic disease and effusion in any body cavity. Depending on the anatomic location of the malignancy and the subsequent effusion, the patient may present with dyspnea, cough, weight loss, acute cardiac tamponade and right-sided heart failure, or abdominal distention.

PHYSICAL EXAM FINDINGS

- Dyspnea due to pleural effusion in dogs and cats is usually identified by shallow, inspiratory effort.
- Tachypnea, open-mouth breathing, cyanosis, muffled heart and lung sounds ventrally with increased bronchovesicular sounds dorsally, poor peripheral pulses, jugular distention, paradoxical breathing, and abdominal distention are possible.
- In cats, a noncompressible cranial thorax suggests other diagnoses: thymoma, mediastinal lymphoma
- In a standing patient, thoracic percussion may reveal a fluid line (zone of hyporesonance) ventrally.

Etiology and Pathophysiology

Mesothelioma involves a malignant transformation of mesothelial cells that line body cavities. Cavitary effusion from mesothelioma is most likely due to increased capillary permeability (parietal foci) secondary to vasculitis.

DIAGNOSIS

Diagnostic Overview

The diagnosis is suspected based on chronic, recurrent body-cavity effusions with no identified infectious, inflammatory, or other neoplastic cause. Often a diagnosis of exclusion, definitive diagnosis requires a biopsy.

Differential Diagnosis

- Pleural effusion (p. 791)
- Pericardial effusion (p. 773)
- Ascites (p. 79)

Initial Database

- Effusion should be sampled and evaluated with fluid analysis and cytologic assessment (p. 1343).
- CBC, serum biochemical analysis, and urinalysis: no specific changes
- These tests should be supplemented with fungal, viral, and parasitic (tick and heartworm) serologic evaluations and microbial (fungal and bacterial) culture as clinical suspicion and history warrant.
- Radiographs (especially after removal of as much fluid as possible)
- Ultrasonographic studies (abdomen, heart, and pleural space)

Advanced or Confirmatory Testing

- Contrast-enhanced ultrasonography (CEUS) may more precisely define lesion edges, define the presence of necrotic and devitalized areas, and the distribution of pulmonary vessels so that the diagnostic utility of cytology and percutaneous sampling may be enhanced.
- Cardiac MRI (if available) if pericardial effusion and echocardiographic findings are equivocal
- Definitive diagnosis requires tissue for histopathologic examination.
- A normal fibronectin level in the effusion could help rule out mesothelioma.

TREATMENT

Treatment Overview

The immediate goal of treatment is removal of body-cavity fluid that is causing clinical signs.

Acute General Treatment

- Stabilization of the patient by relieving the cardiovascular or respiratory embarrassment is paramount.
  - Remove large-volume effusions without delay if clinical signs are severe (pp. 1150 and 1164).
- Oxygen therapy (p. 1146) is often indicated before centesis or obtaining blood or urine samples if patients are extremely dyspneic or volatile in their behavior to prevent life-threatening cardiovascular or respiratory decompensation (especially cats).

Chronic Treatment

- For dogs with pericardial mesothelioma, surgical or thoracoscopic pericardectomy can palliate clinical signs and reduce tumor burden (disease cytoreduction).
- Periodic thoracocentesis (p. 1164) or pericardiocentesis (p. 1150) can be performed when fluid accumulation or symptoms are slow to return (weeks or more).
- Placement of a PleuralPort may aid in treatment. Some clients may be willing to learn proper care and use of such a device for home care.
- Administration of chemotherapy by intracavitary infusion on a q 3 weeks schedule can be attempted for long-term control. Chemotherapy options include cisplatin, carboplatin, mitoxantrone, bleomycin, and 5-fluorouracil.
- Potential benefits (unproven on a large scale) must be weighed against the real drawbacks of possible adverse reactions to these agents.
- At this time, only small numbers of patients have been evaluated, and efficacy remains unproven.
- IV chemotherapy with cisplatin, carboplatin, or doxorubicin may have a role in some patients.
- Consultation with an oncologist for the most current treatment recommendations is indicated, but because of the rarity of this disease, multicenter clinical trials are required to test and develop effective treatments.

Possible Complications

Pneumothorax, cardiac puncture, hemopericardium, hemothorax, infection

Recommended Monitoring

- Hourly for critical (ICU) patients: respiratory rates, degree of dyspnea, blood gases
- Daily to weekly for outpatients: respiratory rates, quality-of-life assessments, repeat thoracic radiographs as warranted or required

- As required per protocol for chemotherapy patients (e.g., CBC): quality-of-life assessments, repeat thoracic radiographs as warranted or required

PROGNOSIS & OUTCOME

- Poor to fair; survival depends on rate of accumulation of the fluid and degree of compensation, which are both variable from patient to patient.
- Many patients are euthanized at the time of diagnosis.
- For those that are treated, the reported survival time varies considerably (weeks to years).
- Some animals may have a dramatic improvement after centesis and a prolonged period (weeks to months) without clinical signs, whereas others have a recrudescence of fluid accumulation and return of tamponade or dyspnea in hours or days.
- A good quality of life for months to 1-2 years with pericardial or pleural mesothelioma is realistically possible if a good response to the first centesis occurs and owners are willing to follow-up regularly with centesis on an as-needed basis.
- In this author's experience, owners rarely agree to continue with repeat pericardiocentesis after more than two or three episodes of acute decompensation.

PEARLS & CONSIDERATIONS

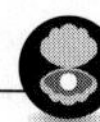

Comments

- Thoracocentesis should be considered before blood or urine sample acquisition or radiographic or ultrasonographic studies for patients that are unstable. The removal of even a small amount of fluid can dramatically relieve the respiratory embarrassment and stabilize the patient.
- Although it shares similarities with mesothelioma in terms of distribution (body cavity surfaces), *carcinomatosis* refers to seeding of pleural or peritoneal surfaces with malignant carcinoma cells.
  - Management of dogs and cats with carcinomatosis may include treatment with intracavitary chemotherapeutics as described for mesothelioma.

Technician Tips

- The pericardial effusion caused by mesothelioma is usually thick and hemorrhagic (indistinguishable from blood) but does not clot. If blood clots form in the discarded effusion during the pericardiocentesis procedure, this important observation should be brought to the attention of the clinician performing the procedure (catheter may be in the heart).
- When obtaining thoracic radiographs, the dorsoventral and ventrodorsal views are sometimes useful when identifying pleural effusion. Ask the clinician about her/his preferences.

Client Education

- Teaching the client to monitor respiratory rate can give the client and clinician an objective measure of progression and acuity of decompensation in the patient.
- PleuralPort management for dedicated clients

SUGGESTED READING

Rebhun RB, et al: Mesothelioma. In Withrow SJ, et al, editors: Withrow and MacEwen's Small animal clinical oncology, ed 5, St. Louis, 2013, Saunders, pp 696.

AUTHOR: Carlos O. Rodriguez, Jr., DVM, PhD, DACVIM
EDITOR: Kenneth M. Rassnick, DVM, DACVIM

Metaldehyde Toxicosis

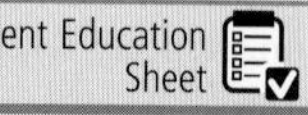

BASIC INFORMATION

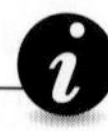

Definition

An acute intoxication from accidental ingestion of household molluscicide (snail bait), characterized by vomiting, tremors, and seizures

Synonyms

- Snail and slug bait or pellets
- Corry's Slug and Snail Death, Deadline Slug Bait, Eliminator Snail and Slug Bait, Ortho Bug-Geta, Vigoro Snail and Slug Killer, and many others

Epidemiology

SPECIES, AGE, SEX

- Dogs are more commonly exposed due to indiscriminate eating habits.
- All breeds, all ages, and both sexes are susceptible

RISK FACTORS

- Patients with pre-existing liver issues may be more sensitive to effects.
- Outdoor pets, use of snail bait in pet's environment

GEOGRAPHY AND SEASONALITY

Areas where slugs and snails are common pests: West Coast, particularly Northwest United States

ASSOCIATED DISORDERS

Hyperthermia and its complications (e.g., coagulopathy)

Clinical Presentation

HISTORY, CHIEF COMPLAINT

- History of exposure or access to product
- Signs consistent with exposure: ataxia, tremors, seizures

PHYSICAL EXAM FINDINGS

- Central nervous system (CNS)
  - Ataxia
  - Tremors
  - Seizures
  - Hyperesthesia
  - Nystagmus
- Gastrointestinal (GI)
  - Hypersalivation
  - Vomiting
  - Diarrhea
- Cardiovascular
  - Tachycardia
- Nonspecific
  - Dehydration
  - Hyperthermia (commonly severe, secondary to muscle activity)
  - Tachypnea, panting

Etiology and Pathophysiology

- In mollusks, the mechanism of action is fatal dehydration, seizures, and paralysis.
- The mechanism of action in mammals is not fully elucidated, but involvement of the CNS is evident. It is suspected that metaldehyde and its metabolite acetylaldehyde affect several neurotransmitters in the CNS, including 5-hydroxytryptamine, norepinephrine, gamma-aminobutyric acid (GABA), and monoamine oxidase (MAO).

DIAGNOSIS

Diagnostic Overview

Diagnosis is typically based on observed exposure, presence of toxin in environment, or clinical signs consistent with exposure. There are no clinically expedient tests available.

Differential Diagnosis

- Toxic
  - Bromethalin
  - Pyrethroid
  - Tremorgenic mycotoxin
  - Strychnine
  - Methylxanthines
  - Organophosphates, carbamates

- Nontoxic
  - Head trauma
  - Intracranial neoplasia
  - Meningitis
  - Encephalitis
  - Other causes of tremor or seizure (pp. 1279 and 1288)

Initial Database

- CBC: typically unremarkable; disseminated intravascular coagulopathy rarely reported
- Chemistry profile: may be normal on presentation, but liver injury is possible and is seen within 2-3 days of ingestion; prolonged tremors and seizures can increase creatine kinase level and cause azotemia due to rhabdomyolysis
- Blood gas analysis: ± acidosis
- Urinalysis: normal; if rhabdomyolysis present, may detect myoglobinuria

Advanced or Confirmatory Testing

Confirmatory testing can be performed on gastric content, urine, plasma, or liver tissues.

TREATMENT

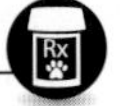

Treatment Overview

Because onset of signs (often severe) is rapid, prompt and aggressive control of tremors or seizures is paramount. If exposure is recent (<30 minutes) and patient is not showing clinical signs, decontamination recommended.

Acute General Treatment

- Decontamination (p. 1087)
  - Emesis (p. 1188): apomorphine 0.03 mg/kg IV, 0.04 mg/kg IM (canine)
  - Gastric lavage (p. 1117) for large exposures, particularly when emesis is not safe
  - Activated charcoal 1-2 g/kg with sorbitol
  - Enema 10 mL/kg water
- Tremors/seizures
  - Methocarbamol: start with initial bolus (50-150 mg/kg IV), followed by continuous-rate infusion (CRI) 10 mg/kg/h to start or repeat boluses 25-50 mg/kg IV as needed; maximum daily dose of 330 mg/kg/day may be exceeded, but monitoring for CNS depression is warranted.
  - Diazepam 0.5-1 mg/kg IV, 0.1-2 mg/kg/h as CRI, *or*
  - Midazolam 0.1-0.3 mg/kg IV or IM, 0.05-2 mg/kg/h CRI
  - If insufficient response to above therapies, general anesthesia may be warranted with gas anesthesia, propofol, or barbiturates.
- Nonspecific
  - Fluid therapy: treat or prevent dehydration, maintain electrolyte and acid base balance
  - Thermoregulation (e.g., cool IV crystalloid fluids, fans, alcohol spray)
  - If present, control acidosis.

Chronic Treatment

Manage liver injury, if present (p. 442).

Nutrition/Diet

Withhold food from patients that are vomiting, tremoring, or seizing.

Behavior/Exercise

Restrict activity, and minimize stimuli when signs are present.

Possible Complications

Aspiration is a concern due to rapid onset of severe neurologic signs. Use great care if inducing emesis or giving activated charcoal, and use these techniques only before signs are apparent. Control vomiting aggressively.

Recommended Monitoring

Monitor neurologic signs, hyperthermia, and acidosis. Rarely, rhabdomyolysis or disseminated intravascular coagulopathy may be a complication. Monitor for aspiration as complicating factor.

PROGNOSIS & OUTCOME

Due to rapid onset of severe neurologic signs and low margin of safety, prognosis is guarded. Difficulty controlling tremors or seizures, severe hyperthermia, large ingestion, liver injury, aspiration, or significant pre-existing disease worsen prognosis.

PEARLS & CONSIDERATIONS

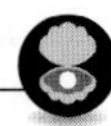

Comments

- Iron-based snail baits are becoming more popular; make sure to check active ingredients of product to which patient was exposed.
- Minimum lethal dose of metaldehyde in dogs is 100 mg/kg.
- Onset of signs can occur within 30 minutes to 4 hours of ingestion.

Prevention

Prevent access to areas where metaldehyde is used; use pet-friendly bait alternative.

Technician Tips

Monitor body temperature closely. Although hyperthermia is the usual concern, enemas or lavage can cause hypothermia.

Client Education

Educate owners to the dangers of common pesticide products, and explain that common bittering agents used as deterrents are frequently ineffective for canines.

SUGGESTED READING

Brutlag AG, et al: Metaldehyde. In Peterson ME, et al, editors: Small animal toxicology, ed 3, St. Louis, 2013, Saunders, pp 635-642.

AUTHOR: Kirsten Waratuke, DVM, DABT
EDITOR: Tina Wismer, DVM, MS, DABVT, DABT

Methicillin-Resistant Staphylococcal Infections

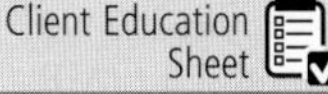

BASIC INFORMATION

Definition

Infections with methicillin-resistant staphylococci (MRS), which are staphylococci that have acquired the *mecA* gene. MRS are resistant to virtually all beta-lactam antimicrobials (penicillins, cephalosporins, carbapenems) and often acquire resistance to various other antimicrobials.

Synonyms

Methicillin and meticillin are synonymous.

Epidemiology

SPECIES, AGE, SEX

- Any animal, either sex, any age
- In dogs, methicillin-resistant *Staphylococcus pseudintermedius* (MRSP) predominates.

RISK FACTORS

- Influenced mainly by risk factors for whatever is predisposing to opportunistic infection (e.g., atopic dermatitis, wound)
- Prior antimicrobial exposure
- Veterinary hospital exposure increases the risk of MRSP infection. Direct or indirect human health care contact (e.g., hospital visitation, owned by recent hospital patient) increases the risk of methicillin-resistant *Staphylococcus aureus* (MRSA) infection.

CONTAGION AND ZOONOSIS

- MRSA can be transmitted between people and pets; transmission is most often from human to pet. MRSA can also be transmitted between pets.
- MRSA colonization rates are higher among veterinary personnel than in the general public. Colonized veterinary personnel can

also infect animal patients, with subsequent risk of exposure of other humans.
- MRSP is a potential zoonosis, but human infections are rare, and MRSP is no more likely to cause a zoonotic infection than methicillin-susceptible strains.
- Zoonotic risks of other MRS are inconsequential.
- In a household with at-risk (e.g., immunocompromised) humans, it is important to culture wounds or other potentially infected sites because of the increased likelihood of a multidrug-resistant infection and the potential human health implications.
  - The benefit is likely greater for the pet (i.e., pet is more likely to have an MRSA infection from the owner) than the owner (i.e., to indicate zoonotic disease risk).
- Routine screening of healthy animals for MRS carriage is not recommended.

Clinical Presentation

DISEASE FORMS/SUBTYPES

MRS cause a wide range of opportunistic infections, and clinical presentation of patients with MRS infections is not inherently different from that of other opportunistic infections. Pyoderma, otitis, soft-tissue infections, wound infections, and surgical site infections are most common, but infection of virtually any body system or site may occur.

HISTORY, CHIEF COMPLAINT

Historical factors are indistinguishable from those of routine, non-MRS infections (e.g., pyoderma [p. 851], urinary tract infection [p. 232], otitis externa [p. 728]). Although a history of previous antimicrobial therapy or hospitalization increases the risk, MRS infections can exist in any patient.

PHYSICAL EXAM FINDINGS

As expected with the primary disease process; see physical exam findings for pyoderma, bacterial cystitis, otitis externa, and other bacterial infections.

Etiology and Pathophysiology

- Any *Staphylococcus* species can be methicillin resistant. The most important are MRSP, MRSA, and *Staphylococcus schleiferi* (MRSS).
  - Coagulase-negative staphylococci are often resistant (MR-CoNS), but these tend to be of limited clinical consequence.
- Like their susceptible counterparts, MRS can be found as colonizers in healthy animals, particularly in the nose, mouth, intestinal tract, and skin.
- The biological behavior of MRS infections is indistinguishable from that of methicillin-susceptible staphylococcal infections, except for the limitation in treatment options (and accompanying risk of persistent/intractable infection).
- MRS infections develop no differently from those of any other opportunistic infection and typically require an inciting cause (e.g., atopic dermatitis, wound, surgical incision, immune compromise, abnormal lower urinary tract conformation) to cause disease.
- Transmission of MRS can occur in veterinary hospitals, and outbreaks can occur, but most MRS infections are sporadic and originate in the community.

DIAGNOSIS

Diagnostic Overview

- MRS are diagnosed by bacterial culture and susceptibility testing.
- The potential for contamination or isolation of an MRS that is merely colonizing the sampled site must be considered. This is particularly true for MR-CoNS organisms, which tend to be less virulent and are common contaminants.
- Cytology, imaging, and hematology may be necessary for some infection types and to help differentiate colonization or contamination from infection.
- Although polymerase chain reaction (PCR) screening tests are available for MRSA in humans, there are currently no validated rapid diagnostic assays for MRS in animals.

Differential Diagnosis

- MRS infections do not look any different than infections caused by susceptible staphylococci or other opportunistic pathogens.
- Some findings support MRS infection rather than nonpathogenic colonization by MRS:
  - Gross clinical findings consistent with infection versus sterile inflammation or other disease types
  - Evidence of staphylococcal infection on diagnostic tests (e.g., intracellular cocci on cytology, gram-positive cocci)
  - Sample unlikely to have been contaminated during collection

Initial Database

- As indicated by initial presentation (as clinically appropriate for pyoderma, suspected/confirmed cystitis, otitis externa)
- Routine bacterial culture and susceptibility testing can identify methicillin resistance, confirming the presence of MRS. This is usually performed by testing oxacillin or cefoxitin susceptibility as a marker of methicillin resistance (i.e., oxacillin- or cefoxitin-resistant staphylococci are MRS).
- Bacterial culture and susceptibility testing should be performed as clinically appropriate, and is considered particularly important in some cases:
  - There is initial treatment failure.
  - Clinical disease is severe.
  - The animal has had a previous MRS infection or has been in contact with an animal or person with a previous MRS infection.
  - Surgery is planned for some other issue (e.g., pyoderma patient is scheduled for orthopedic surgery).
  - There has been recent (past few months) antibiotic exposure.

Advanced or Confirmatory Testing

Erythromycin-resistant MRSA isolates should be tested by D-test (or equivalent) to confirm that inducible clindamycin resistance is not present. Confirmation of methicillin resistance can be performed by *mecA* PCR or PBP2a latex agglutination test. This should be performed for any isolate with equivocal results or multidrug-resistant staphylococci that appear to be methicillin susceptible because false-negative susceptibility results can occur.

TREATMENT

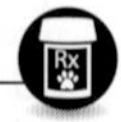

Treatment Overview

- In general, MRS infections are treated no differently than infections caused by susceptible staphylococci apart from the antimicrobial choice, which must exclude beta-lactam drugs.
- Alternatives to beta-lactams are almost always available, and selection depends on the type of infection, site of infection, patient factors, and other general principles of antimicrobial therapy.
- The goal of treatment is elimination of disease, not microbiologic cure, for infection of nonsterile (e.g., skin) sites.
- Re-culture after clinical cure is rarely indicated.
  - Persistence of MRS as colonizers in the nose, mouth, intestinal tract, or skin is common after resolution of clinical infection, particularly with MRSP, and some dogs may be prolonged (or even persistent) carriers.

Acute General Treatment

- Antimicrobial therapy is typically required and combined with supportive care as needed; measures to address inciting causes may be critical.
  - Beta-lactams (penicillins, cephalosporins, carbapenems) are not appropriate due to resistance.
- Surgery (e.g., removal of an infected surgical implant) if applicable
- With superficial bacterial folliculitis, topical application of biocides (e.g., 2%-4% chlorhexidine) may be effective (p. 851).
- Topical antimicrobials (e.g., mupirocin, fusidic acid) suitable for superficial infections
- Topical honey may be useful for wound infections.
- Nitrofurantoin is often an option for cystitis (p. 232).
- Regional therapy (e.g., antimicrobial-impregnated PMMA beads, collagen sponges) might be critical for deeper infections, particularly implant-associated infections.

Chronic Treatment

Uncommonly necessary, unless for an unaddressed nidus (e.g., foreign body, infected implant) or inability to control underlying disorder (e.g., atopic dermatitis) exists. In those situations, removal of the nidus (e.g., explantation) is the key.

PROGNOSIS & OUTCOME

Prognosis for MRS infections should be no different than for infections caused by susceptible microorganisms if there is a prompt diagnosis and institution of appropriate treatment.

PEARLS & CONSIDERATIONS

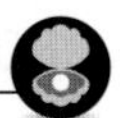

Comments

- Main clinical issues for MRS infections:
    - Difficulty in treating MRS infections because of limited drug options and options that may be undesirable
    - Potential for more severe disease if culture is not performed promptly because empirical treatment will likely fail
    - Zoonotic risk (mainly MRSA) and transmission of MRS to other high-risk animals, especially surgical patients, because MRSP surgical site infections can be a major concern
- MRS are not inherently more virulent than susceptible staphylococci, and the prognosis for MRS infections is usually good. The key is early recognition by culture to ensure that proper treatment is initiated and the risk of transmission is minimized.
- MRSA is a public health concern, and animal-human transmission can occur. Good general infection control practices should greatly minimize the risk. MRSP is of much less zoonotic risk, but rare human infections have been reported.
- Screening of veterinary personnel for MRS colonization is rarely, if ever, indicated.

Prevention

- Routine cleaning and disinfection kill MRS when performed properly.
- Quarantine of exam rooms for 24-48 hours after confirmation of MRS infection in a patient is *not* beneficial because if staphylococci were missed during cleaning and disinfection, they can be expected to persist for 1-2 weeks or until proper disinfection is completed.
- A focus on good routine infection control practices is recommended because MRS status is unknown initially for carriers and animals with active infections.
    - Routine cleaning and disinfection
    - Avoid contact between MRS cases and other animals. For example, any animal with known MRS infection or all animals with pyoderma should bypass the waiting room to avoid lying beside another patient being admitted for orthopedic surgery or receiving immunosuppressive treatment.
    - Good attention to hygiene, especially hand hygiene

Technician Tips

- Care must be taken to reduce the risk of transmission of MRS between patients and from patients to personnel.
- Because healthy animals may carry MRS, use of good general infection control practices (e.g., protective outerwear, handwashing) is important for any patient.
- Animals that are known to be infected or colonized should be handled with enhanced precautions. This can include protective outerwear (e.g., gown, gloves), restriction of movement in the clinic, and isolation if possible. Isolation is preferred during hospitalization when possible.
- MRS are killed by routine disinfectants if used properly.

Client Education

Client education helps ensure proper management and also can prevent an excessive response based on fear of MRSA. Providing reference materials from reputable sources (e.g., http://www.wormsandgermsblog.com, http://www.thebellamossfoundation.com) can help allay fears and improve patient care.

SUGGESTED READING

Morris DO, et al: Recommendations for approaches to methicillin-resistant staphylococcal infections of small animals: diagnosis, therapeutic considerations and preventative measures. Clinical Consensus Guidelines of the World Association for Veterinary Dermatology. Vet Dermatol 28:304-e69, 2017.

AUTHOR: J. Scott Weese, DVM, DVSc, DACVIM
EDITOR: Manon Paradis, DMV, MVSc, DACVD

Microvascular Dysplasia, Hepatic

Client Education Sheet

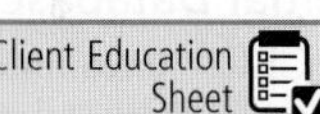

BASIC INFORMATION

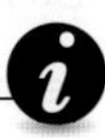

Definition

Hepatic microvascular dysplasia (HMD) involves a defect at the terminal branching of portal venules, with variable severity. This causes intrahepatic shunting of portal blood to the systemic venous return, causing intrahepatic portal venous hypoperfusion. Additional secondary microscopic alterations of the hepatic parenchyma compound the severity of shunting, with hepatic dysfunction proportional to the degree of portosystemic shunting. HMD can occur alone or be found in combination with macrovascular disorders such as primary portal vein hypoplasia or portal systemic vascular anomalies (PSVAs) such as portal systemic shunt (PSS).

Synonyms

HMVD, microvascular dysplasia (MVD), hepatoportal microvascular dysplasia, a form of portal venous hypoplasia (PVH) or portal vein hypoperfusion, microvascular portal dysplasia, portal venous atresia

Epidemiology

SPECIES, AGE, SEX

- More common in small, purebred dogs but may be seen in any breed or outcross
- Less common or rare in cats
- A congenital disease that may be diagnosed in older or younger patients based on severity of clinical signs or results of screening tests

GENETICS, BREED PREDISPOSITION

Predominantly toy breeds such as Yorkshire, Cairn, and Maltese terriers; also reported in other pure- and mixed-breed dogs, including pugs, dachsunds, miniature poodles, Lhasa apso, shih tzu, cocker spaniel, Havanese, and West Highland white terriers

Pattern of inheritance is thought to be tied to that of PSVA (p. 814) as an autosomal dominant mode, likely polygenic, and with simple to complex expression.

ASSOCIATED DISORDERS

- Concurrent PSVA and HMD offers an explanation for the frustrating persistence of symptoms and/or abnormal test values related to shunting despite apparent adequate surgical attenuation of PSVA.
- HMD can be concurrent with congenital PSVA, primary portal vein hypoplasia, portal vein atresia, hepatic arteriovenous fistula, and rare portal venous agenesis. Pursue advanced diagnostic imaging and liver biopsy during all PSVA surgeries.
- HMD has been reported concurrent with ductular plate malformations.

Clinical Presentation

DISEASE FORMS/SUBTYPES

- Most animals with HMD have minimal or no clinical signs.
- Rarely, signs suggesting PSVA or chronic hepatopathy occur, or there may be progression to noncirrhotic portal hypertension.
- Liver dysfunction may be discovered unexpectedly during assessment for other

disorders such as chronic enteropathies, ammonium biurate crystalluria, or seizures. It is difficult to determine the contribution of HMD to clinical signs (if any) when these disorders occur concurrently.

HISTORY, CHIEF COMPLAINT

Severity of signs associated with HMD is reflected as a spectrum of none to severe; most affected animals seem healthy. History can include signs found with congenital or acquired PSVA (e.g., behavioral abnormalities, lower urinary signs related to urate stones [p. 814]).

PHYSICAL EXAM FINDINGS

Unremarkable

Etiology and Pathophysiology

HMD involves shunting of portal blood to the hepatic venules and histologic changes consistent with hypoperfusion.

DIAGNOSIS

Diagnostic Overview

Diagnostics are initiated because of suspicion of PSVA or to follow-up on laboratory abnormalities discovered incidentally. Elevation of total serum bile acid (TSBA) concentrations without supportive findings of PSVA (acquired or congenital) or other causes of PVH or liver dysfunction suggest HMD. Abdominal imaging is useful to rule out PSVA.

Differential Diagnosis

- PSVA (congenital or aquired)
- Causes of hepatic encephalopathy (p. 440)

Initial Database

- CBC: uncommonly, microcytosis (low mean corpuscular volume [MCV]) without anemia
- Serum biochemical profile: often normal but can have mixed mild/modest patterns of elevations of alanine aminotransferase (ALT) and alkaline phosphatase (ALP), or rarely mild hypoalbuminemia
- Urinalysis: possibly hyposthenuria, rarely ammonium biurate crystalluria
- TSBA assay (with most emphasis on postprandial value): often range of 25-100 mmol/L. These concentrations can be higher and overlap with concentrations found in PSVA. Concentrations can vary day to day, and if results are discordant with clinical suspicion, repeat in 2 weeks.
- Coagulation profile: normal (assessed before liver biopsy)
- Abdominal radiographs: usually normal, sometimes microhepatica
- Abdominal sonography: ± microhepatica, lack of diminished intrahepatic portal vascular pattern (look at all lobes) versus PSVA; absence of PSVA and the PV/A ratio ≥ 0.8; normal renal volume/size. Percutaneous transsplenic injection of agitated saline has been used as contrast to highlight absence or presence of PSVA.
- Plasma protein C activity > 70% (normal) is supportive of diagnosis HMD in patients with elevated serum TSBA concentrations.

Advanced or Confirmatory Testing

- Abdominal computerized tomography (CT) scan with angiographic contrast to rule out PSVA
- Definitive diagnosis by histopathologic findings consistent with portal venous hypoplasia/hypoperfusion
  - Obtain 3-5 wedge or laparoscopic biopsies from different lobes. For needle biopsies, use 14-gauge needle with full throws of sampling notch/depth from different lobes.
  - Findings include arteriolization of central veins, arteriolar duplication, endothelial biliary hyperplasia, attenuation of lobular size, reduced sinusoidal flow, lipogranulomas, and diminished distance between terminal branches of portal and hepatic veins. Zone 3 degenerative hepatocelluar changes can be found in more severe cases.
  - There can be marked differences between liver lobes with caudate lobe often least affected. These histologic changes are seen with any cause of hypoperfusion and are not specific to HMD.
- Contrast portography shows diminished contrast filling of affected lobes without escape to vena cava or azygous vein.
- Transcolonic or transsplenic scintigraphy results are normal for HMD (shunt fraction < 15%). Largely replaced by contrast CT scan

TREATMENT

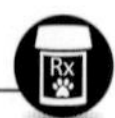

Treatment Overview

Most often requires no treatment, but if severe, the patients can be managed with medical management similar to that for PSVA

Acute General Treatment

If present, address hepatic encephalopathy (p. 440).

Chronic Treatment

If severe HMD is suspected, consider use of *S*-adenosylmethionine 15-30 mg/kg PO q 24h (or per product label), use of vitamin E 10 U/kg PO q 24h, and avoiding high-protein diets, with goal of providing an optimal microenvironment and reduction of oxidative stresses for hepatocytes over the long term.

Nutrition/Diet

Asymptomatic cases require no adjustments of diet. If symptomatic, consider a moderate, restricted-protein diet or as for hepatic encephalopathy.

Behavior/Exercise

Symptomatic cases of HMD may experience periodic atpyical behavior (aggression, passivity, hunger, confusion, inappropriate eliminations).

Drug Interactions

Caution is advised when choosing drugs that undergo hepatic metabolism.

Recommended Monitoring

Depends on clinical presentation, but repetition of CBC, serum biochemistry profile, and urinalsyis q 6-12 months is often appropriate for minimally affected pets.

PROGNOSIS & OUTCOME

- Prognosis is good to excellent for asymptomatic patients. Normal life expectancy is common.
- Prognosis is worse for the rare patients with significant hepatic dysfunction.

PEARLS & CONSIDERATIONS

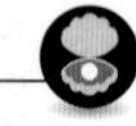

Comments

- HMD is often diagnosed in older patients during assessment for other diseases (e.g., protein losing enteropathies, hypoalbuminemia, chronic pancreatitis).
- CT angiogram is preferred over ultrasound to rule out PSVA.
- HMD is a diagnosis of exclusion of PSVA, then confirmation with biopsy. Biopsy alone cannot achieve a diagnosis as results are indistinguishable from histopathologic changes seen in PSVA.
- Animals with increased TSBA values < 100 mmol/L and normal serum biochemical profile are more likely to have HMD than PSVA.
- TSBA concentrations > 100 mmol/L or decreased serum albumin or blood urea nitrogen (BUN) concentrations should prompt continued diagnostic efforts to rule in or out PSVA or primary hepatic disease.

Prevention

Do not breed affected dogs.

Technician Tips

Ensure patients are fasted for 12 hours before bile acid panel testing or abdominal imaging intended to look for PSVA.

Client Education

Discuss patient-specific prognosis and breed-related concerns.

SUGGESTED READING

Christiansen JS, et al: Hepatic microvascular dysplasia in dogs: a retrospective study of 24 cases (1987–1995) J Am Anim Hosp Assoc 36:385-389, 2000.

AUTHOR: Mark E. Hitt, DVM, MS, DACVIM
EDITOR: Keith P. Richter, DVM, MSEL, DACVIM

Mitral Valve Dysplasia

Client Education Sheet

BASIC INFORMATION

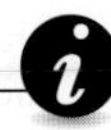

Definition

Congenital malformation of any component of the mitral valve apparatus (papillary muscles, chordae tendineae, leaflets, annulus) that results in valvular dysfunction

Epidemiology

SPECIES, AGE, SEX

Dogs and cats; usually identified early in life

GENETICS, BREED PREDISPOSITION

- Dogs: bull terrier, miniature bull terrier, English bulldog, Great Dane, German shepherd, Newfoundland, and Irish setter are predisposed.
- Cats: male Siamese cats are overrepresented (valvular and supravalvular stenosis).

RISK FACTORS

Predisposed breeds of dogs

ASSOCIATED DISORDERS

- Dogs (concurrent conditions)
  - Systolic anterior motion (SAM) of the mitral valve
  - Subaortic stenosis (SAS)
  - Patent ductus arteriosus (PDA)
  - Pulmonic stenosis
- Dogs and cats (associated conditions)
  - Congestive heart failure (CHF)
  - Pulmonary hypertension (PH)
- Cats (concurrent and associated condition): feline aortic thromboembolism

Clinical Presentation

DISEASE FORMS/SUBTYPES

- Mitral valve stenosis (MVS) involves the mitral valve leaflets (dog and cat).
- Supravalvular mitral stenosis

HISTORY, CHIEF COMPLAINT

- Exercise intolerance/episodic weakness
- Lethargy
- Cough
- Dyspnea (most common sign in cats)
- Syncope

PHYSICAL EXAM FINDINGS

- Left apical systolic murmur (if mitral regurgitation)
- Soft left apical diastolic murmur (MVS)
- With CHF
  - Tachycardia
  - Tachypnea
  - Pulmonary crackles and wheezes

Etiology and Pathophysiology

- Congenital (possibly heritable in predisposed breeds); presumed genetic, although specific mutations have not been identified.

Pathophysiology

- Mitral regurgitation
- Obstruction of the transmitral diastolic flow (increase in resistance to blood flow between the left atrium and ventricle) in MVS
- Obstruction of the left ventricular outflow tract with SAM
- Increase in left atrial, pulmonary venous, and pulmonary capillary pressures
- Pulmonary edema formation
- Exercise increases left atrial pressure; exercise-induced dyspnea/syncope may occur.
- PH can develop secondary to increased pulmonary capillary pressure.

DIAGNOSIS

Diagnostic Overview

The diagnosis is suspected in a young patient presenting with a left apical systolic heart murmur that may have cough, tachypnea, and dyspnea. Left heart enlargement is usually evident on thoracic radiographs, and an echocardiogram is required for confirmation.

Differential Diagnosis

- Radiographic/electrocardiographic
  - Left atrial enlargement: other types of cardiac disease (myxomatous mitral valve disease/endocardiosis, dilated cardiomyopathy, SAS, PDA, and [in cats] hypertrophic cardiomyopathy)
- Echocardiographic
  - Myxomatous mitral valve disease/endocardiosis
  - Bacterial endocarditis
  - Intracardiac neoplasia

Initial Database

- Thoracic radiographs: left atrial enlargement very common; signs of pulmonary edema if CHF
- Electrocardiogram (ECG): wide P waves in lead II, supraventricular premature complexes, atrial/supraventricular tachycardia, atrial fibrillation. Increased R-wave amplitude in lead II
- Echocardiogram
  - Two- (and three-) dimensional mode: abnormal mitral valve leaflets, abnormal valve motion, mitral regurgitation, left atrial dilation. Supravalvular membrane (cat), decreased mitral valve leaflet excursion, and diastolic doming of the leaflets (MVS)
  - M-mode: thickened mitral valve leaflets, increased left atrial/aortic (LA/Ao) ratio, incomplete leaflet separation in diastole and reduced mid-diastolic closure velocity (E-F slope) (MVS); SAM
  - Color-flow Doppler: systolic turbulent flow in the left atrium with mitral regurgitation and in the left ventricular outflow tract with SAM. Diastolic aliased or turbulent flow across the mitral valve (MVS)
  - Spectral Doppler: increased early diastolic filling (velocity of E wave > 1.1 m/s), prolonged pressure half-time (>50 ms), and reduced mitral valve area (MVS)

Advanced or Confirmatory Testing

- Cardiac catheterization: rarely necessary for confirming diagnosis but may yield quantitative information and help characterize unusual lesions
  - Angiogram: mitral regurgitation, thickened and/or restricted mitral valve leaflets, enlarged left atrium
  - Pressure measurements: increase in left atrial pressure and pulmonary artery pressure with PH or CHF
- Transesophageal echocardiography: better visualization of the mitral valve apparatus but requires general anesthesia

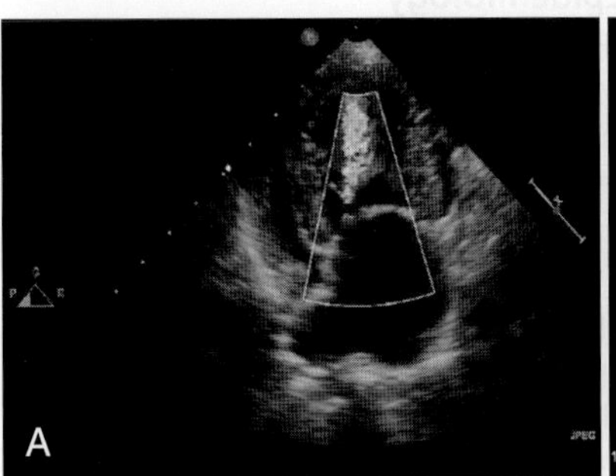

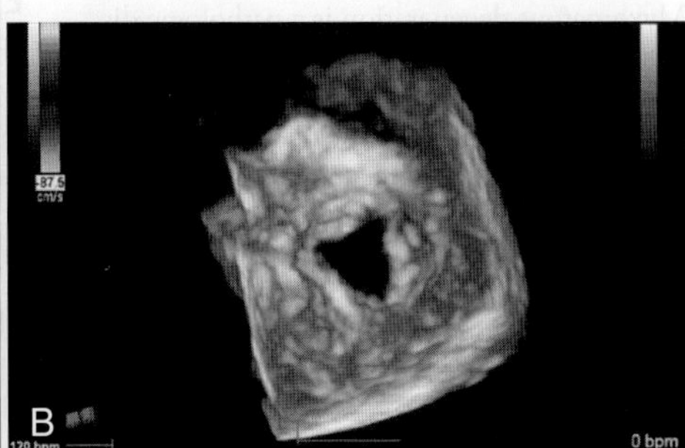

MITRAL VALVE STENOSIS A, Left parasternal four-chamber apical view of a dog with mitral valve stenosis demonstrates diastolic turbulent flow across the mitral valve. **B,** Mitral valve stenosis viewed from the apex of the left ventricle with real-time three-dimensional echocardiography. The commissural fusion is clearly visible, and the mitral valve orifice area is significantly reduced. (From Orvalho JS: Real-time three-dimensional echocardiography: from diagnosis to intervention. Vet Clin North Am Small Anim Pract 47:1005-1019, 2017.).

TREATMENT

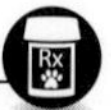

Treatment Overview

Treatment focuses on initial control of CHF signs, with therapy to reduce venous congestion (diuretics), improve function (inodilators), inhibit sodium/water retention, counteract vasoconstriction (angiotensin-converting enzyme [ACE] inhibitors, vasodilators), and control supraventricular arrhythmias (digoxin, calcium channel or beta-blockers). Consider referral to cardiologist for diagnosis and advice on treatment plan.

Acute General Treatment

- Management of CHF (p. 408)
- Digoxin, calcium channel blocker, or beta-blocker: management of supraventricular arrhythmias (pp. 94 and 96)
- For myocardial failure (advanced/end-stage state characterized by left ventricular hypocontractility): inodilators (pimobendan 0.2-0.3 mg/kg PO q 12h)

Chronic Treatment

- Medical therapy
  - Diuretics, ACE inhibitors, inodilators, and antiarrhythmics after acute treatment (p. 409)
  - In cats, antiplatelet and/or anticoagulant therapy for prevention of atrial thrombus formation (p. 74): clopidogrel, aspirin, warfarin, unfractionated heparin/low-molecular-weight heparins
  - Address PH, if present (p. 838).
- Surgical therapy
  - Mitral valve replacement or open mitral commissurotomy (MVS): requires cardiopulmonary bypass; postoperative management complications are common.
  - Balloon valvuloplasty (MVS): inconsistent results in canine patients; possible damage to the mitral valve apparatus with worsening of mitral regurgitation
  - Hybrid procedure (MVS): closed commissurotomy with balloon valvuloplasty

Behavior/Exercise

Restrict exercise and excitement in patients with collapsing or syncopal episodes.

Drug Interactions

- Excessive use of diuretics is contraindicated due to the decrease in preload, electrolyte disturbances, prerenal/renal azotemia, and increased risk of digitalis toxicity.
- ACE inhibitors may reduce glomerular filtration rate and cause azotemia; hypotension may occur when used with diuretics; risk of hyperkalemia when K^+ is supplemented or K^+-sparing diuretics are used concurrently.

Possible Complications

- Recurrence of signs due to progression of CHF
- Systemic thromboembolism (cats)
- Left atrial rupture (dogs)
- Postsurgical coagulation disturbances possible after mitral valve replacement, restenosis (MVS)

Recommended Monitoring

Recheck exams should include thoracic radiographs, serum renal panel (including electrolytes), systolic blood pressure measurement, digoxin levels (if applicable), and ECG.

PROGNOSIS & OUTCOME

- Long-term prognosis depends on the severity of the dysplasia: guarded in severe cases
- Surgical approach and new interventional procedures may offer a better outcome in the future.

PEARLS & CONSIDERATIONS

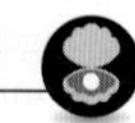

Comments

A disproportionate number of cases occurs in the bull terrier breed.

Prevention

Do not breed affected animals.

Technician Tips

These patients are at risk for pulmonary edema and CHF. Teaching the owner to keep a log of the patient's resting or sleeping breathing rate to monitor for changes can be an effective way to monitor progression of disease.

Client Education

- Monitor respiratory rate at rest, exercise tolerance, and appetite.
- Advise client not to breed affected animals.

SUGGESTED READING

Kittleson MD, et al: Congenital abnormalities of the atrioventricular valves. In Kittleson MD, et al, editors: Small animal cardiovascular medicine, New York, 1998, Mosby, pp 273-281.

AUTHOR: João S. Orvalho, DVM, DACVIM
EDITOR: Meg M. Sleeper, VMD, DACVIM

Mitral/Tricuspid Regurgitation Due to Myxomatous Valve Disease

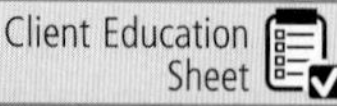

BASIC INFORMATION

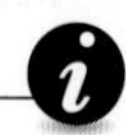

Definition

Myxomatous degeneration is a pathologic disturbance in the organization of the connective tissue of the atrioventricular (AV) heart valves. The disease most frequently includes the mitral valve, with or without changes of the tricuspid valve, and the disease is commonly referred to as myxomatous mitral valve disease (MMVD). Insufficient coaptation of the leaflets leads to AV valve regurgitation, particularly mitral regurgitation (MR), and subsequently, chronic volume overload with atrial and ventricular dilation. Eventually, the heart might become incapable of meeting the increased workload imposed on it, and congestive heart failure (CHF) develops.

Synonyms

Chronic valvular disease (CVD), chronic mitral valve disease, degenerative valvular disease, degenerative mitral valve disease (DMVD), mitral valve disease (MVD), endocardiosis

Epidemiology

SPECIES, AGE, SEX

MMVD is the most common cardiac disease in dogs. The prevalence increases with age. The disease is uncommon in young individuals but common in old dogs. Males develop the disease at a younger age than females.

GENETICS, BREED PREDISPOSITION

The age at which the disease develops is most likely inherited as a polygenetic threshold trait (i.e., multiple genes influence the trait, and a certain threshold has to be reached before the disease develops). Males have a lower threshold than females, leading to a higher disease prevalence at a given age. Although encountered in all breeds, the highest disease prevalence is seen among small to medium-sized breeds such as Cavalier King Charles spaniels, papillons, miniature poodles, Yorkshire terriers, Chihuahuas, and dachshunds.

ASSOCIATED DISORDERS

Myxomatous degeneration of the semilunar valves (very uncommon in dogs and, when present, seldom of clinical importance), pulmonary hypertension, CHF, and various cardiac arrhythmias

Clinical Presentation

DISEASE FORMS/SUBTYPES

American College of Veterinary Internal Medicine (ACVIM) Consensus Statement recommends staging into four classes (A to D):

- Class A: dogs at risk for developing heart disease but that have no identifiable structural disorder of the heart (e.g., Cavalier King Charles spaniels without heart murmurs)

- Class B: dogs without clinical signs but presenting with a systolic click (early stage) and/or systolic heart murmur. This class is divided into two subclasses:
  - Class B1: asymptomatic with heart murmur and (if an echocardiogram is performed) echocardiographic signs of AV valve lesions and regurgitation
  - Class B2: asymptomatic with AV valve lesions and hemodynamically significant regurgitation, as evidenced by radiographic or echocardiographic cardiomegaly ± electrocardiographic changes (electrocardiogram [ECG] is an insensitive method to detect cardiomegaly): P mitrale (increased P-wave duration) and/or P pulmonale (increased P-wave amplitude), increased R-wave amplitude, and increased QRS duration.
- Class C: dogs with AV valve lesions, hemodynamically significant regurgitation, and presenting with clinical signs of CHF (usually left-sided) or that have had episodes of CHF in the past that resolved with ongoing medical therapy
- Class D: dogs with end-stage disease; clinical signs of AV valve regurgitation–induced CHF that are refractory to standard CHF therapy

HISTORY, CHIEF COMPLAINT

- Often, incidental finding of murmur before CHF occurs
- Respiratory: tachypnea/dyspnea/orthopnea; cough (often worse at night)
- Systemic: lethargy, reduced exercise tolerance, syncope, anorexia, weight loss, ascites

PHYSICAL EXAM FINDINGS

Patients without overt clinical signs:
- Systolic click (early stage)
- Systolic heart murmur due to AV valve regurgitation; murmur increases in duration and intensity with progression of disease.

Patients showing overt clinical signs:
- Moderate to loud heart murmur, unless there is significant myocardial failure (e.g., with concurrent myocardial disease)
- Tachycardia and/or loss of respiratory sinus arrhythmia
- Arrhythmia and pulse deficit may be present, most commonly supraventricular premature beats, atrial fibrillation, or ventricular ectopies
- Weak femoral pulse
- Prolonged capillary refill time, pallor
- Tachypnea/dyspnea/orthopnea
- Respiratory crackles/rales
- Pink froth (i.e., pulmonary edema may be evident in the nostrils and oropharynx in cases with severe CHF)
- Ascites (tricuspid disease, pulmonary hypertension)

Etiology and Pathophysiology

- Primary inciting factor for the valvular degeneration is unknown. Current leading hypothesis is that a genetically determined dystrophic process initiates valve degeneration.
- Damage occurs to the endothelial cell lining covering the valve surface.
- The fibroblast-like valvular interstitial cells transform into a more active myofibroblast phenotype, and these cells can induce signaling pathways, resulting in an abnormal structural integrity of the valve, mediated through various proteolytic enzymes.
- Accumulation of glycosaminoglycans, proteoglycans, and collagen fibers lead to disorganization in the fibrosa layer and marked expansion of the spongiosa layer.
- The valve leaflets, which normally are thin, translucent, and soft, become thickened and elongated with disease progression.
- The chordae tendineae also are affected by myxomatous degeneration, resulting in elongation.
- Distortion of the valve architecture contributes to systolic atrial displacement of the valve leaflets.
- Insufficient coaptation of the leaflets leads to AV valve regurgitation and to chronic volume overload with atrial and ventricular dilation.
- Slight to moderate AV valve regurgitation is often completely compensated for years and is not expected to cause clinical signs of disease.
- Compensatory mechanisms include cardiac dilation and eccentric hypertrophy, increased force of contraction, increased heart rate, increased pulmonary lymphatic drainage (left-sided AV valve regurgitation), fluid retention, and neurohormonal modulation of cardiovascular function.
- With progression, valvular regurgitation can no longer be compensated, and CHF develops due to increased venous pressures and reduced cardiac output.
- Pulmonary edema develops with left-sided CHF, and ascites develops with right-sided CHF.

DIAGNOSIS

Diagnostic Overview

- The diagnosis is suspected based on the characteristic left apical location of a systolic heart murmur in an adult dog.
- Echocardiography is the diagnostic test of choice for demonstrating the valve lesion; a high index of suspicion usually exists before echocardiography is employed, and it functions as a confirmatory test, to identify severity of secondary changes, and for treatment decisions.
- Thoracic radiographs may alternatively be used for staging purposes (to assess for heart enlargement) and are indicated, particularly if cough and/or dyspnea is present, to differentiate pulmonary edema from unrelated comorbid conditions such as collapsing trachea or chronic bronchitis.

Differential Diagnosis

Physical:
- Other causes of systolic heart murmurs such as AV regurgitation caused by acquired (e.g., endocarditis) or congential heart disease, or functional flow murmurs
- Other causes of respiratory distress
  - Upper respiratory causes such as tracheal disease
  - Lower respiratory causes such as bronchial disease, pneumonia, pulmonary edema due to noncardiac or other cardiac diseases, pleural effusion, pneumothorax, hernias, or neoplasia
  - Nonrespiratory diseases such as neuromuscular disease, metabolic/endocrine disease, anemia, or abdominal disease
  - Other causes of respiratory effort, such as pain, fear, physical exertion, fever, heat, stress, obesity, or drug-related causes
- Other causes of reduced exercise capacity
  - Hypoxia of noncardiac causes such as anemia or respiratory disease, or other cardiac diseases.
  - Orthopedic- or neuromuscular-related disorders
  - Other systemic disease (e.g., renal or hepatic failure, and endocrinologic- or immune-related diseases)
- Other causes for syncope (p 953)
  - Arrhythmic syncope or sudden changes in heart rate
  - Cardiostructural syncope such as due to right-to-left shunting cardiac diseases or obstruction to blood flow
  - Neurologically mediated syncope, such as due to vasodepressor syncope (loss of sympathetic tone) or cardioinhibitory syncope (predominance of parasympathetic tone)
  - Conditions associated with reduced preload, such as dehydration, hemorrhage, hypotensive drugs, or cardiac tamponade
- Other causes of abdominal distention due to ascites
  - Liver disease, protein-losing enteropathy, glomerulopathy, right-sided heart failure caused by other cardiac/pericardial diseases, neoplasia, vasculitis, infectious diseases, pancreatitis, trauma, coagulopathies, or postoperative complications

Radiographic:
- Other causes of cardiac enlargement
  - Other heart diseases, hernia, pericardial effusion, or enlargement related to normal breed and/or individual variation
- Other causes of increased pulmonary interstitial or alveolar radiopacity due to
  - Pulmonary edema due to other cardiac and noncardiogenic processes
  - Primary respiratory or systemic disease processes
  - Artifacts or expiratory radiographs

Initial Database

Assessment of disease severity and complications; specific diagnostic tests chosen based on clinical progression
- Auscultation: a low-intensity murmur with or without a systolic click in an otherwise healthy dog usually indicates mild disease severity. Murmur intensity

generally increases with increasing disease severity.
- ECG: tachyarrhythmia (e.g., supraventricular premature beats, atrial fibrillation, ventricular ectopy) usually indicative of severe disease, presence of complication, or other cardiac diseases
- Radiography: vertebral heart score (VHS) index can be used when assessing cardiac size (p. 1187). Pulmonary congestion and edema indicate decompensated CHF. Other (noncardiac) causes for clinical signs of respiratory disease should be excluded.
- CBC, serum biochemistry panel, urinalysis: usually unremarkable in less severe cases; cases with CHF may have slightly increased levels of liver enzymes and evidence of prerenal azotemia.
- Echocardiography: atrial and ventricular size increases with increasing disease severity. Ventricular motion is usually exaggerated in advanced stages, whereas normal or reduced motion in the setting of severe regurgitation indicates myocardial failure. Detection of thickened/ballooning AV valve, identification of regurgitant jet (with Doppler echocardiography)
- Color Doppler echocardiography can semiquantify regurgitant volume, which generally increases with increasing disease severity. Spectral Doppler echocardiogram can assess regurgitant velocity (generally ≈5-6 m/s but may decrease in severe disease primarily due to high left atrial pressure).

Advanced or Confirmatory Testing

- Serum natriuretic peptides: brain natriuretic peptide (BNP) concentrations are often unremarkable in less severe cases. Moderate to severe disease is usually associated with increased concentrations, most markedly in cases with CHF. However, increased BNP concentration can also be seen in dogs with other heart diseases.
- Blood culture in case of suspicion of vegetative endocarditis

TREATMENT

Treatment Overview

- No treatment exists that slows or reverses the myxomatous valve lesions.
- Treatment is not indicated in mild disease (stage B1).
- Slow progression to clinical signs of CHF in dogs with cardiomegaly but no signs of CHF (stage B2).
- To alleviate clinical signs and improve quality of life and life expectancy in dogs with signs of CHF (stages C and D) by evacuating pulmonary edema/ascites and abolishing congestion, improving hemodynamic status, and protecting from detrimental exposure to neurohormones

Acute General Treatment

Acute CHF treatment is indicated when overt signs are caused by fluid retention (typically pulmonary edema and/or ascites) (p. 408).

Chronic Treatment

- Chronic treatment with pimobendan prolongs the preclinical period in dogs with cardiomegaly but no signs of CHF (stage B2)
- Long-term treatment consists of optimal medical management of chronic CHF (p. 409).
- Successful long-term management is based on titration and monitoring of medications that eliminate signs of CHF as completely as possible while causing as few adverse consequences as possible.
- Open-heart surgical repair of myxomatous mitral valve disease in dogs has been described but is rarely performed.

Drug Interactions

As described for CHF treatment (p. 409)

Possible Complications

- Syncopal events
- Arrhythmia, most commonly atrial fibrillation and ventricular ectopies
- Pulmonary hypertension
- Rupture of first-order tendinous chord(s), leading to a flail valve leaflet
- Atrial tear, leading to acquired atrial septal defect or pericardial effusion/cardiac tamponade

Recommended Monitoring

- Frequency of re-exams depends on severity of valvular regurgitation and severity of CHF (if present).
- Home monitoring of resting or sleeping respiratory rates and body weight is recommended for dogs with moderate to severe disease.
- Dogs without signs of CHF (stage B2)
  - Slight to moderate disease severity: q 6-12 months
  - Moderate to severe disease severity may require more frequent monitoring.
- Dogs with signs of CHF (stages C and D)
  - After acute CHF has been successfully treated, dogs can be treated at home.
  - Re-exam after 1-2 weeks of initiated therapy (check for signs of decompensated CHF, dehydration, electrolyte imbalance, renal dysfunction, and presence of any other complication). Thereafter, q 3-6 months; more severe cases may require more frequent monitoring.

PROGNOSIS & OUTCOME

Dogs without signs of CHF (stage B):
- Chronic disease progression: dogs with low-level disease severity may remain healthy for several years before signs of CHF develop.
- Pimobendan treatment prolongs the preclinical period in dogs with cardiomegaly but no signs of CHF (stage B2).
- Risk factors for progression: severity of valve lesions, age, and sex
- Risk factors for CHF: valvular regurgitant status, left atrial and ventricular sizes (especially an increase in size over time), high blood concentrations of natriuretic peptides

Dogs with CHF (acute or stabilized):
- Prognosis depends on age, left atrial and ventricular sizes, severity of CHF, development of complications, or presence of other diseases (e.g., chronic kidney disease).
- Clinical trials indicate a mean survival time from onset of CHF of 8-10 months, but this may vary from days to years for different dogs.
- Sudden death may occur but is uncommon, especially in the absence of preceding clinical signs of CHF.

PEARLS & CONSIDERATIONS

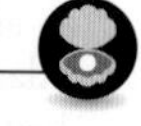

Comments

- If presence of valvular regurgitation is equivocal by auscultation, the murmur or regurgitant jet may become more obvious after stressing the dog slightly (e.g., exercise).
- CHF is unlikely in a dog diagnosed with MMVD with a respiratory sinus arrhythmia.
- Murmur severity usually increases with increasing disease severity.
- Loud musical murmurs can occur but are unusual. The intensity of this type of murmur is not usually related to disease severity.
- Mild pleural and/or pericardial effusion may develop from CHF. More pronounced accumulation of fluid in these locations raises the suspicion of other causes.

Prevention

- Because the liability for myxomatous AV valve disease in dogs is inherited, the disease prevalence among affected breeds should be reduced by breeding measures.
- Currently, no medication or management is known to prevent the disease or slow progression of valve changes, but onset of signs of CHF are delayed by pimobendan treatment in dogs with preclinical disease and cardiomegaly (stage B2).

Technician Tips

- Teach owners to maintain resting or sleeping respiratory rate logs to monitor for development of acute decompensated CHF.
- Teach owners how to administer medications and what signs should prompt a call or visit.

Client Education

- Mild disease severity is suggestive of a long period without clinical signs; moderate to severe disease indicates a shorter period.
- Pimobendan treatment delays the onset of clinical signs of CHF in dogs with cardiomegaly.
- If client is a breeder, inform about genetics of the disease and impact on future breeding.
- Discuss appropriate level of exercise (e.g., no restrictions for low disease severity, avoid strenuous exercise in moderate to severe cases).

- Monitor resting heart rate and sleeping respiratory rates at home (if indicated); describe when to contact veterinarian.
- Discuss diet (if indicated).

SUGGESTED READING

Ljungvall I, et al: Adult-onset valvular heart disease. In Ettinger SJ, et al, editors: Textbook of veterinary internal medicine: diseases of the dog and the cat, ed 8, 2015, Elsevier, pp 1249-1269.

AUTHORS: Ingrid Ljungvall, DVM, PhD, DECVIM; Jens Häggström, DVM, PhD, DECVIM
EDITOR: Meg M. Sleeper, VMD, DACVIM

Movement Disorders

Client Education Sheet 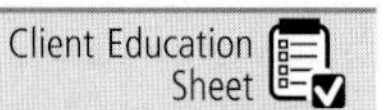

BASIC INFORMATION

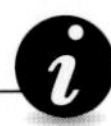

Definition

A diverse group of neurologic diseases, characterized by involuntary, sustained, or episodic movements of a body region (head, limb, trunk, or a combination) during activity or at rest, causing a paucity of movement (akinetic–rigid syndromes) or, more commonly, excessive involuntary movements (dyskinesia). Consciousness remains normal (p. 994).

- Classification of movement disorders
  - Tremor: involuntary, rhythmic, oscillatory movement of a body part
  - Myoclonus: sudden, brief, shock-like involuntary muscle contraction
  - Akinetic rigid syndrome: generalized muscular stiffness and paucity/slowness of movement
  - Paroxysmal dyskinesia: episodic excessive involuntary movement of variable duration (seconds to hours)

Synonyms

Tremors, tremor syndrome, myoclonus, paroxysmal dyskinesia, epileptoid cramping syndrome, episodic falling syndrome, Scottie cramp

Epidemiology

SPECIES, AGE, SEX

- Dogs > cats but both species affected
- Young dogs: anomalous (hypomyelination) or infectious disease (canine distemper virus) more likely
- Paroxysmal dyskinesia: varied age of onset; more common in young dogs
- Older dogs: idiopathic postural tremors and myoclonic epilepsy more likely
- Male predisposition (X-linked inheritance): suspected in Labradors with hypertonicity syndrome, confirmed in springer spaniels with hypomyelination

GENETICS, BREED PREDISPOSITION

Tremors:

- Hypomyelination: Bernese mountain dog, chow chow, Dalmatian, Samoyed, springer spaniel (*PLP* gene), Weimaraner, lurcher
- Idiopathic head tremor: Doberman pinscher, English bulldog
- Orthostatic tremor: Irish wolfhound, Scottish deerhound

Myoclonus:

- Hyperekplexia: Labrador retriever, Irish wolfhound (*SLC6A5* gene)
- Opsoclonus-myoclonus syndrome: springer spaniel
- Myoclonic epilepsy: basset hound, beagle (*EPM2B* gene), corgi, miniature wirehaired dachshund (*EPM2B* gene), pointer, poodle (miniature and standard)

Akinetic rigid syndromes:

- Hypertonicity syndrome: Labrador retriever
- Canine multiple system degeneration: Kerry blue terrier, Chinese crested

Dyskinesias:

- Paroxysmal dyskinesia: border terrier, Bichon frisé, boxer, Cavalier King Charles spaniel (*BCAN* gene), Chinook, Dalmatian, golden retriever, German short-haired pointer, Jack Russell terrier, Labrador retriever, Norwich terrier, Scottish terrier, soft-coated wheaten terrier (*PIGN* gene), springer spaniel, Weimaraner
- Autosomal recessive mode of inheritance suspected for most

Other movement disorders:

- Dancing Doberman disease: Doberman pinscher
- Idiopathic blepharospasm (focal dystonia): Great Dane
- Stiff dog syndrome: beagle, Labrador retriever

GEOGRAPHY AND SEASONALITY

Weather extremes can exacerbate paroxysmal dyskinesia in Jack Russell terriers and border terriers.

ASSOCIATED DISORDERS

Myoclonus secondary to canine distemper virus: can see ocular, dermatologic, gastrointestinal signs of infection (p. 271)

Clinical Presentation

DISEASE FORMS/SUBTYPES

Tremors:

- Hypomyelination
  - Generalized body tremors; subside at rest
  - Age of onset: 2-8 weeks
  - Ataxia, proprioceptive deficits can be present
  - Gradual improvement is possible (if due to delayed myelination)
- Idiopathic head tremor
  - Horizontal or vertical head bob
  - Distracting the animal (food, play) often causes the tremor to abate
- Idiopathic postural tremor
  - High-frequency pelvic limb postural tremor while standing
- Orthostatic tremor
  - Pelvic limb (± thoracic limb) tremors while standing; disappear when lying down or walking
  - Can involve head and trunk

Myoclonus:

- Myoclonus due to canine distemper virus
  - Continuous; can be generalized, segmental, or focal (>1 limb)
- Hyperekplexia
  - Excessive startle response with generalized muscle stiffness when handling
- Opsoclonus-myoclonus syndrome
  - Rapid, involuntary eye movements occurring in all directions (opsoclonus)
  - Myoclonus of the head
- Myoclonic epilepsy
  - Repetitive muscle contractions in response to sensory stimuli (visual, auditory)
  - Affected animals may also have seizures.

Akinetic rigid syndromes:

- Hypertonicity syndrome
  - Generalized muscular stiffness, forward flexed posture, and slow movements
- Canine multiple system degeneration
  - Cerebellar ataxia at 3-6 months of age
  - Akinesia
  - Postural instability, falling

Dyskinesias:

- Paroxysmal dyskinesia
  - Head, neck, and/or trunk rigidity (hunched back) in association with rigidity or uncontrolled flexion/extension of limb(s)
  - Restricts ambulation ± falls
  - Normal mentation

Other movement disorders:

- Dancing Doberman disease
  - Intermittent flexion of one or both pelvic limbs
  - Pelvic limb muscle atrophy, paresis, proprioceptive deficits
- Idiopathic blepharospasm (focal dystonia)
  - Bilateral blepharospasm, no ocular cause
- Stiff dog syndrome
  - Episodic muscular rigidity and lordosis, with gait impairment
  - Triggered by tactile stimulation

HISTORY, CHIEF COMPLAINT

- Observation of abnormal movements or posture

- Possible history of environmental factors that precipitate episodes

PHYSICAL EXAM FINDINGS

- Examination is typically normal.
  - Borborygmi can be observed in border terriers with paroxysmal dyskinesia.
- If tremors are observed, discern whether generalized or focal and whether they occur during movement (kinetic) or at a stance (postural).
  - With orthostatic tremor, tremor is abolished when the affected leg(s) is lifted from the ground, during walking, or when lying on the side. Tremor reappears when standing or when pressure is applied to the foot while lying down.

Etiology and Pathophysiology

- Pathophysiology is poorly understood for the majority of these disorders.
- An underlying genetic mutation has been identified in some instances.
  - Hypomyelination in springer spaniels: *PLP* encodes a major myelin protein.
  - Hyperekplexia in Irish wolfhound: *SLC6A5* dysfunction of presynaptic glycine transporter
  - Myoclonic epilepsy: *EPM2B*, glycogen metabolism disorder
  - Canine multiple system degeneration: *CFA1,* involved in protein degradation
  - Paroxysmal dyskinesia: *BCAN* in Cavalier King Charles spaniel (episodic falling syndrome) and *PIGN* in wheaten terrier; protein-encoding genes
- Myoclonus due to canine distemper virus: infection causes pathologic changes in the lower motor neurons of the spinal cord and cranial nerve nuclei, resulting in an autonomous pacemaker that gives rise to the rhythmic muscle contractions.
- Immune-mediated mechanism
  - Paroxysmal dyskinesia of border terrier: possible gluten sensitivity
  - Stiff dog syndrome in beagle: glutamic acid decarboxylase (anti-GAD) antibodies
  - Idiopathic tremor syndrome (suspected)
- Dancing Doberman disease: underlying myopathy and/or neuropathy

DIAGNOSIS

Diagnostic Overview

An accurate history and recognition of characteristic features is key. Episodic movement disorders must be differentiated from seizures, and determining the animal's state of consciousness is helpful in this regard. Observing video of an episode is particularly important for animals with episodic clinical signs and can often lead to a presumptive diagnosis of a movement disorder. More definitive diagnosis is made after exclusion of other potential causes. Brain imaging (MRI) and cerebrospinal fluid (CSF) analysis can rule out other central nervous system disease, whereas peripheral nervous system disorders are ruled out with electrophysiological studies.

Differential Diagnosis

Tremors (p. 1288)

- Generalized
  - Intoxication (mycotoxins, others)
  - Inflammatory (idiopathic tremor syndrome)
  - Cerebellar disease (inflammatory, neoplastic, vascular)
  - Pain
  - Weakness (metabolic, neuromuscular)
- Focal
  - Pain
  - Weakness

Myoclonus:

- Encephalitis (infectious, immune)

Dyskinesias:

- Seizures
- Drug induced (phenobarbital, propofol)

Other movement disorders:

- Dancing Doberman disease
  - Orthopedic disease: arthropathies
- Idiopathic blepharospasm (focal dystonia)
  - Ocular disease
- Stiff dog syndrome
  - Tetanus

Initial Database

CBC, chemistry profile, urinalysis: unremarkable

Advanced or Confirmatory Testing

- MRI of brain (p. 1132) and CSF analysis (pp. 1080 and 1323): rule out inflammatory, neoplastic, or vascular causes of brain disease
  - With canine multiple system degeneration, can see cerebellar atrophy, T2-weighted hyperintensity in substantia nigra and caudate nucleus
- Genetic testing, when available
- Electromyography
  - Orthostatic tremor: continuous discharges of 13-16 Hz muscle activity while standing
  - Hypertonicity syndrome: continuous motor unit activity in resting epaxial and proximal limb muscles (awake study)
  - Dancing Doberman disease: positive sharp waves, fibrillation potentials in gastrocnemius muscle; possible mild changes in appendicular muscles
  - Idiopathic blepharospasm: high-frequency discharges in orbicularis oculi muscle
  - Stiff dog syndrome: continuous motor unit activity in axial musculature
- Food trial (gluten-free diet): border terrier with paroxysmal dyskinesia
- Immunologic testing
  - Border terrier with paroxysmal dyskinesia: anti-transglutaminase 2 (TG2 IgA) and anti-gliadin (AGA IgG) antibodies
  - Stiff dog syndrome: glutamic acid decarboxylase (anti-GAD) antibodies

TREATMENT

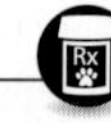

Treatment Overview

Because of the diversity of causes, there is no standard recommended therapy. Symptomatic therapy with muscle relaxants or antiepileptics is often attempted with various results.

Acute General Treatment

Benzodiazepines (diazepam 0.5-1.0 mg/kg PO q 8h) can be administered as a muscle relaxant.

Chronic Treatment

There is no effective treatment for many of the movement disorders. Treatment has been reported for the following:

- Orthostatic tremor
  - Transient improvement has been reported with phenobarbital 2.5-3.0 mg/kg PO q 12h and gabapentin 10 mg/kg PO q 8h.
- Myoclonus (canine distemper virus)
  - Mexiletine 8 mg/kg PO q 8h may lessen clinical signs.
- Myoclonic epilepsy
  - Antiepileptic medication (levetiracetam 20 mg/kg PO q 8h)
  - Dietary trial: antioxidant-rich diet
- Hypertonicity syndrome
  - Nonsteroidal antiinflammatory drugs
- Paroxysmal dyskinesia
  - Can respond unpredictably to different types of treatments such that symptomatic trial and error is often attempted.
  - Muscle relaxation with benzodiazepines and/or antiepileptic medications (clonazepam 0.5 mg/kg PO q 8h, phenobarbital 2.5-3.0 mg/kg PO q 8h) are often tried first, with various degrees of success.
  - Acetazolamide 4 mg/kg PO q 8h, baclofen 1.0 mg/kg PO q 8h, and fluoxetine 1.0 mg/kg PO q 12-24h have led to various degrees of response.
  - A gluten-free dietary trial has led to some improvement in border terriers.
- Idiopathic blepharospasm (focal dystonia)
  - Botulinum toxin injection
- Stiff dog syndrome
  - Symptomatic therapy: baclofen, gabapentin, phenobarbital
  - Immunotherapy: prednisone, intravenous immunoglobulin (IVIG)

Nutrition/Diet

Gluten-free diet is recommended for border terriers with paroxysmal dyskinesia.

Behavior/Exercise

Some paroxysmal dyskinesias are triggered by exercise.

Possible Complications

- Respiratory distress with severe disease (hyperekplexia)
- Hyperthermia (secondary to sustained muscle contractions)

Recommended Monitoring

Monitor respiration

PROGNOSIS & OUTCOME

Tremors:

- Prognosis depends on the nature and severity of the disorder.
- Improvement or spontaneous remission has been reported for some conditions.

- Hypomyelination: if clinical improvement is to occur, it typically is observed before 1 year.
- Idiopathic head tremor: 50%-66% remission rate
- Opsoclonus-myoclonus syndrome: spontaneous remission
- Paroxysmal dyskinesia: remission reported in Jack Russell terriers and Labrador retrievers

• Fair to good prognosis depending on severity of clinical signs
  - Idiopathic postural tremor (worsening with age possible)
  - Orthostatic tremor
  - Myoclonus due to canine distemper virus
  - Paroxysmal dyskinesia
  - Dancing Doberman disease
  - Idiopathic blepharospasm (focal dystonia)
  - Stiff dog syndrome
• Poor to guarded prognosis
  - Hyperekplexia
  - Myoclonic epilepsy
  - Hypertonicity syndrome: clinical signs worsen initially then stabilize; severity of signs can affect quality of life
  - Canine multiple system degeneration: affected animal often euthanized due to severity of clinical signs

PEARLS & CONSIDERATIONS

Comments

Obtaining video of a movement disorder is an important diagnostic tool because it often clarifies the state of consciousness of the patient and differentiates it from a seizure disorder. When in doubt, seek consultation with a veterinary neurologist.

Prevention

If a movement disorder occurs in a specific context (stress, noise, exercise, hot/cold weather), these potential triggers should be avoided.

Technician Tips

Movement disorders and seizures can look alike. Assessing the patient's mentation during the event is essential; if the patient responds to you, it is more likely a movement disorder. If possible, take a video of any observed episodes.

Client Education

Movement disorders are likely to cause imbalance and falls. Keep the pet away from stairs or sharp-edged furniture to avoid self-trauma. Maintain a diary of the events, noting context, event duration, and any mentation change.

SUGGESTED READING

Lowrie M, et al: Classification of involuntary movements in dogs: paroxysmal dyskinesias. Vet J 220:65-71, 2017.

AUTHOR: Julien Guevar, DVM, MVM, DECVN, MRCVS
EDITOR: Karen R. Muñana, DVM, MS, DACVIM

Multiple Myeloma and Plasma Cell Tumors

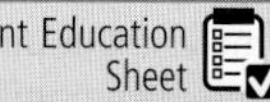

BASIC INFORMATION

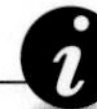

Definition

- Multiple myeloma (MM) is a disease of plasma cells derived from one clone in the bone marrow. It is a systemic disease, and multiple bone marrow sites are involved. Immunoglobulins (Igs) are produced by malignant plasma cells: IgM or IgG in the dog and IgA in the cat.
- Plasma cell tumors (PCTs) are solitary tumors composed of plasma cells originating in sites other than bone marrow (i.e., extramedullary tissue). PCTs can arise from skin, soft tissues, or bone. Serum Ig levels are often normal in this localized form of disease.

Synonyms

Plasmacytoma, myeloma-related disorder (MRD)

Epidemiology

SPECIES, AGE, SEX

- Uncommon disorder of older dogs and cats
- Male predominance in noncutaneous PCT; no sex predisposition in MM
- Extramedullary involvement (i.e., spleen, liver, and skin) at initial presentation is common in cats with MM.

GENETICS, BREED PREDISPOSITION

- MM: German shepherd
- PCT: Airedale terrier, cocker spaniel, Kerry blue terrier, Scottish terrier, standard poodle

ASSOCIATED DISORDERS

MM:

- Hyperviscosity syndrome
- Bence Jones proteinuria
- Pathologic fracture
- Bleeding diathesis
- Increased susceptibility to infection; immunosuppression
- Heart failure
- Renal disease
- Visual/ocular disturbances
- Amyloidosis
- Cryoglobulinemia (precipitation of Ig at colder temperatures vs. cold agglutinin disease [erythrocyte clumping at colder temperatures])

Clinical Presentation

DISEASE FORMS/SUBTYPES

- MM
- Waldenström's macroglobulinemia: IgM is the Ig type produced.
- Cutaneous PCT
- Extramedullary PCT (EMP)
- Solitary osseous PCT (SOP)

HISTORY, CHIEF COMPLAINT

- MM
  - Dogs usually present with lameness or skeletal pain. Bleeding (epistaxis, ecchymoses, mucosal hemorrhage), polyuria/polydipsia, central nervous system signs (seizures, dementia), and visual disturbances may also occur.
  - Cats tend to present with an insidious onset of nonspecific signs (anorexia, weight loss, lethargy). Other signs similar to those seen in dogs may rarely occur.
- Cutaneous PCT
  - Raised nodule on the trunk, limbs, head, or in the oral cavity
- EMP
  - Typically occur in the gastrointestinal (GI) tract and cause weight loss, anorexia, nausea, vomiting, and/or diarrhea
- SOP
  - Single lesion in bone; can cause bony swellings, lameness, neurologic deficits, and/or skeletal pain

PHYSICAL EXAM FINDINGS

- Skeletal pain, fractures
- Weight loss (MM, EMP)
- Lethargy (MM, EMP)
- Visual disturbances (MM)
- Depression, seizures, abnormal reflexes (MM)
- Epistaxis, gingival bleeding, ecchymoses
- Pallor, weak pulses, heart murmur, increased lung sounds (MM)
- Signs of congestive heart failure such as dyspnea (MM)
- Soft-tissue or bony masses
- Abdominal organomegaly

Etiology and Pathophysiology

- Malignant plasma cells produce large amounts of one type of Ig.
- The entire Ig can be produced or just a portion of it (e.g., light chain). The Ig or portion is referred to as the *M protein*; concentration is typically proportional to tumor burden in MM but not in PCT (low levels).

- Focal/diffuse bone lesions: due to proliferating malignant plasma cells (causing pathologic fractures in dogs but rarely in cats)
- M protein in blood increases serum viscosity, causing hyperviscosity syndrome (HVS [p. 509]).
- The light chain portion of the Ig, also called the *Bence Jones protein*, is small enough to be filtered by the normal glomerulus. They can be detected in the urine of patients with MM with the Bence Jones screening test or quantitative protein test (but not on a urine dipstick) (p. 1311).
- Kidney disease develops secondary to Bence Jones proteinuria, tumor infiltration into kidney, hypercalcemia, amyloidosis, and/or decreased renal perfusion.
- Hypercalcemia occurs from release of osteoclast-activating factor by neoplastic cells.
- Cytopenias develop from bone marrow infiltration and blood loss due to bleeding tendencies (from protein coating of platelets and inhibition of platelet and coagulation factor release).
- An increased susceptibility to infection is seen because of the suppression of normal Ig levels, leukopenias, and impaired cell-mediated immunity. Urinary tract infections and pneumonia are common manifestations.

DIAGNOSIS

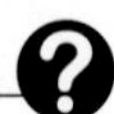

Diagnostic Overview

- MM typically is first considered when hyperglobulinemia is found on a serum biochemistry profile, osteolytic lesions are seen radiographically, or an unexplained bleeding disorder occurs. Diagnosis requires any two or more of these findings: monoclonal gammopathy on serum protein electrophoresis, lytic bone lesions on radiographs, Bence Jones proteinuria on specific urine assay, and/or plasma cell infiltration of bone marrow on bone marrow aspirate/biopsy.
- PCTs usually present as discrete masses (typically cutaneous); aspiration is often confirmatory because of the distinctive appearance of plasma cells.

Differential Diagnosis

Differentials for monoclonal gammopathy: ehrlichiosis, leishmaniasis, feline infectious peritonitis, pyoderma, lymphoma, leukemia, idiopathic (monoclonal gammopathy of unknown significance)

Initial Database

- Funduscopic exam: hemorrhage, retinal detachment, dilated/tortuous vessels may occur due to hyperviscosity
- CBC: cytopenias, thrombocytopenia, increased total protein
- Serum biochemistry panel: hypercalcemia, elevated total protein, hyperglobulinemia, azotemia possible
- Urinalysis: infection possible (immunosuppression), isosthenuria if in renal failure

Advanced or Confirmatory Testing

MM:

- In dogs, two of the following four criteria must be met: monoclonal gammopathy, lytic bone lesions, plasma cell infiltration of the bone marrow, and Bence Jones proteinuria.
  - Serum protein electrophoresis (p. 1375): monoclonal gammopathy
  - Survey radiographs: in dogs, multiple areas of bony lysis or diffuse osteopenias are common (vertebrae, scapulae, long bones) and/or pathologic fractures; not typically found in cats. A solitary area of lysis is typical of SOPs.
  - Bone marrow aspiration: > 10% plasma cells with atypia or > 20% plasmacytosis is required for the diagnosis of MM. Aspiration of multiple sites may be necessary. Marrow infiltration is uncommon in cats.
  - Heat precipitation or electrophoresis of urine (Bence Jones test): identifies Bence Jones proteins, which are not detected on urine dipstick.
- Abdominal ultrasound (especially in cats): to identify possible sites of organ involvement. In cats, abdominal organ infiltration (e.g., liver, spleen) by neoplastic plasma cells is more common, and ultrasound-guided fine-needle aspiration for cytology should be considered, especially if organomegaly is present and there are no contraindications (e.g., bleeding tendency).
  - If necessary, additional confirmatory diagnostics can be performed on cytology slides, including special stains to determine whether the cells noted are plasma cells and/or clonality testing to prove that a population of plasma cells is monoclonal (neoplastic) rather than polyclonal (inflammatory): immunocytochemistry for MUM-1, and polymerase chain reaction (PCR) for antigen receptor rearrangement (PARR), respectively.
- Serum or urine immunoelectrophoresis: identifies the Ig class (IgG, IgM, IgA)
- Serum viscosity may be measured in some labs to verify HVS.

PCT:

- Tissue biopsy confirmation of cutaneous PCT, EMP, and SOP
- Immunohistochemistry for the marker MUM-1 can help differentiate lymphoma from PCTs if needed.

TREATMENT

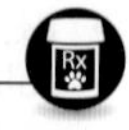

Treatment Overview

Goals of treatment are to reduce myeloma cell burden, relieve bone pain, allow skeletal healing, and decrease serum viscosity and Ig levels.

Acute General Treatment

- Stabilize fractures.
- Surgical excision of PCTs if possible; wide surgical margins generally are not necessary, but margins should be free of gross and microscopic evidence of neoplasia.
- IV fluids (if HVS) for hydration and diuresis to decrease serum viscosity, azotemia, and hypercalcemia
- Analgesia for bone pain
  - Bisphosphonate drugs (e.g., pamidronate 1-2 mg/kg diluted to 250 mL in sterile 0.9% NaCl and given as 2-hour IV infusion) are an option to reduce bone pain and may lower the risk of pathologic fracture in patients with lytic bone disease or osteopenia. Oral forms are not recommended (poor bioavailability in animals).

Radiation therapy can be palliative for SOP or a localized painful lytic bony lesion.

- Plasmapheresis to remove Bence Jones proteins (decrease serum viscosity) may be available at some institutions. Therapeutic phlebotomy (with donor red blood cell transfusion) can possibly achieve a similar effect.
- Prophylactic, broad-spectrum antibiotic therapy to treat infections (urinary, pneumonia), avoiding nephrotoxic or bacteriostatic antibiotics

Chronic Treatment

- Chemotherapy: melphalan and prednisone are the mainstay of treatment for MM in dogs and cats. Cyclophosphamide can alternatively be given initially in cases of widespread disease or severe hypercalcemia because this regimen is thought to have a more rapid clinical effect, but the benefit is unclear in dogs. Melphalan causes erratic myelosuppression in cats; substituting chlorambucil or cyclophosphamide has been advocated. Response rates and survival times with cyclophosphamide plus prednisolone are similar to melphalan plus prednisolone for cats. Chemotherapy can be attempted in cases of cutaneous PCT, EMP, or SOP that are nonresectable or if radiation therapy is not available. However, response information is limited. Other cytotoxic drugs (doxorubicin, vincristine, CCNU [lomustine], and Tanovea [rabacfosadine]) may have some activity in the rescue setting for some patients with MM. Consultation with an oncologist for the most current treatment options is recommended.
- Radiation therapy is the treatment of choice for SOP, some incompletely excised PCTs, and localized MM bony lesions.
- Surgical excision is curative for most cutaneous PCTs.

Recommended Monitoring

- Monitor CBCs frequently (myelosuppressive effects of melphalan), and alter dosage or schedule based on patient response.
- Monitor serum electrophoresis because size of monoclonal spike is proportional to tumor burden. Plasma globulin level can also be used for monitoring remission status.
- Monitor for evidence of infection, and treat with antibiotics as needed due to immunosuppression.

PROGNOSIS & OUTCOME

MM:

- Dogs: when treated with melphalan/prednisone, response rate is > 90%. A good response is defined as a 50% reduction of the initial M protein level. Long-term prognosis is guarded because recurrence is inevitable. Median survival time is 540 days with melphalan plus prednisone and 220 days for prednisone alone. Negative prognostic factors for dogs include hypercalcemia, Bence Jones proteinuria, and extensive bony lysis.
- Cats: reported response rates and survival times vary. Older reports suggest that prognosis is poor, most responses are partial, and median survival time is 137 days; however, newer information shows that 70%-80% of cats respond and median survival times are 252-394 days. Degree of differentiation of tumor predicts survival; cats with well-differentiated tumors have a median survival of 254 days, and cats with poorly differentiated tumors have a median survival of 14 days.

Cutaneous PCT:

- Benign biological behavior: surgical excision is generally curative.

EMP:

- EMPs at sites other than the oral cavity frequently metastasize, but long-term survival is possible with surgical excision and chemotherapy and/or radiation therapy. Oral plasmacytomas do not metastasize, and local control provides long-term control. Median survival of dogs with complete resection is 474 days.

SOP:

- Eventually progress to MM, but there may be a long disease-free interval
- Radiation therapy may provide control for 1 year or more.

PEARLS & CONSIDERATIONS

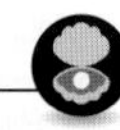

Comments

- Perform serum protein electrophoresis on any animal in which MM is suspected, even if globulin and serum viscosity are normal.
- Use size of monoclonal gammopathy to monitor response to treatment.
- Extensive infiltration of plasma cells in sites outside the bone marrow (e.g., abdominal organ involvement) is common for the initial presentation of cats.
- Cats experience more severe myelosuppression from melphalan than dogs.
- Multiple novel drug classes are used in the treatment of MM in people but have not been investigated in dogs or cats. Consultation with a veterinary oncologist is warranted for new developments in treatment.

Technician Tips

Patients with MM frequently have bony fragility and should be handled carefully to avoid causing pathologic bone fractures.

SUGGESTED READING

Vail MD: Myeloma-related disorders. In Withrow SJ, et al, editors: Withrow & MacEwen's Small animal clinical oncology, ed 5, St. Louis, 2013, Saunders Elsevier, pp 665-678.

AUTHOR: Andi B. Flory, DVM, DACVIM
EDITOR: Kenneth M. Rassnick, DVM, DACVIM

Multiple-Organ Dysfunction Syndrome (MODS)

BASIC INFORMATION

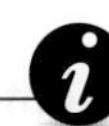

Definition

Multiple organ dysfunction syndrome (MODS) is a well-recognized complication of critical illness that is defined as the development of abnormal function in more than two organ systems in an acutely ill patient.

Synonym

Multiple-organ failure (MOF) is a similar term, specific to human trauma patients.

Epidemiology

SPECIES, AGE, SEX

Any animal can develop MODS.

RISK FACTORS

Sepsis, noninfectious systemic inflammatory response syndrome (SIRS) (e.g., pancreatitis, heat stroke), polytrauma (e.g., hit by car), neoplasia, abdominal compartment syndrome, any cause of hypovolemic shock (e.g., gastric dilation/volvulus)

ASSOCIATED DISORDERS

Sepsis, trauma, neoplasia, SIRS

Clinical Presentation

DISEASE FORMS/SUBTYPES

MODS is a sequela of systemic critical illness; its clinical appearance varies according to the organ systems affected.

HISTORY, CHIEF COMPLAINT

Any acute critical illness, with apparent progression to organ dysfunction in more than two organ systems

PHYSICAL EXAM FINDINGS

Exam findings reflect the organ systems affected and the primary disease process.

- Animals are almost invariably hemodynamically compromised (resulting in weakness or collapse, dull mentation, tachycardia or bradycardia, hypotension, tachypnea, mucous membrane pallor or injection).
- Hypovolemic shock may occur (p. 911).
- Cardiac arrhythmias may occur (pp. 96 and 1033).
- Urine production may be reduced with hypovolemia (physiologic/pre-renal) or with oliguric/anuric renal failure as a manifestation of MODS (p. 23).

Etiology and Pathophysiology

- MODS is characterized by new, often progressive dysfunction of the renal, cardiovascular, nervous, respiratory, gastrointestinal (GI), hepatobiliary, and/or hematologic systems. The major inciting cause is immune dysregulation leading to disordered and widespread systemic inflammation.
- Identification and treatment of underlying disease(s) is paramount.
- Mechanisms of organ injury leading to dysfunction include cytokine-mediated apoptosis, bacterial translocation, endotoxemia, ischemia/reperfusion injury, and endothelial cell activation.
- Three theories for MODS trigger
    - One-hit theory: primary event bad enough to promote massive inflammation and alter function of other organs (e.g., massive crush injury)
    - Two-hit theory: priming of the inflammatory, immunologic, and vascular systems after initial insult (e.g., shock). A second hit (e.g., infection, hypoxemia), even if minor, results in exaggerated host response and perpetuation of MODS.
    - Sustained-hit theory: continuous insult, such as ongoing inflammation in the GI tract, promotes systemic inflammation when endogenous antiinflammatory resources are expended.
- Dysfunction by organ system
    - Acute kidney injury (AKI [p. 23]): a common component of MODS and is likely due to acute tubular necrosis from ischemia, toxins (e.g., aminoglycosides), or sepsis. Pigment nephropathy (e.g., caused by hemolysis or rhabdomyolysis) may also promote renal injury.
    - Respiratory dysfunction: manifests as acute respiratory distress syndrome (ARDS [p. 27]). Damage to alveoli and pulmonary

endothelium are hallmarks of lung injury, which can be primary (e.g., pulmonary contusion) or secondary. Cytokine-mediated inflammation leads to pulmonary capillary leak and noncardiogenic pulmonary edema.
  - GI dysfunction: multifactorial, often presenting as ileus, GI bleeding, vomiting, or diarrhea. Hypoperfusion of splanchnic circulation and endotoxemia are risk factors. Secondary sepsis from bacterial translocation through the GI tract can occur due to increased GI permeability.
  - Neurologic dysfunction: likely due to hypotension, hypovolemia, and microthrombosis. Metabolic encephalopathy and hypoglycemia are also causes of neurologic deterioration.
  - Cardiovascular dysfunction: largely due to systemic inflammation and circulating cytokines, resulting in hypotension, myocardial dysfunction, and ectopy. Acid-base disturbances, hypoxemia, hypovolemia, and pain can contribute to cardiovascular dysfunction.
  - Hematologic dysfunction: due to widespread inflammation and activation of the coagulation cascade. Endothelial damage and tissue factor expression promote the development of consumptive coagulopathy (e.g., disseminated intravascular coagulation [DIC]) and microvascular thrombosis (p. 269).
  - Hepatic dysfunction: caused by ischemic injury, endotoxemia, and acute hepatocellular necrosis. Hepatic failure can lead to profound coagulopathy, hypoglycemia, and encephalopathy (pp. 440 and 442).

DIAGNOSIS

Diagnostic Overview

- The diagnosis is reached by identifying clinical and laboratory evidence of dysfunction of two or more organ systems in critically ill patient.
- Although anemia, leukopenia, and leukocytosis are not markers of organ dysfunction, they are common in critical illness.

Differential Diagnosis

SIRS and sepsis are the most important risk factors for MODS, but they can occur independent of organ dysfunction. Every effort should be made to rule out a septic focus in patients with systemic inflammation.

Initial Database

- Laboratory data: CBC/platelet count, serum biochemistry, blood gas analyses (arterial blood gas to assess for hypoxemia, arterial or venous to assess ventilation), urinalysis, coagulation profile (PT, aPTT, fibrinogen, and/or thromboelastography when available)

Organ System	Criteria for Dysfunction
Respiratory	Acute respiratory distress syndrome • Bilateral alveolar pulmonary infiltrates • Decreased pulmonary compliance • Absence of left-sided heart failure (pulmonary capillary wedge pressure < 18 mm Hg); normal echocardiogram • Hypoxemia (PaO_2/FIO_2 < 300)
Cardiovascular	Decreased cardiac output, decreased contractility, hypotension, arrhythmias
Renal	Creatinine ≥ 2-3 mg/dL (>176-264 mmol/L) (oliguria < 1-2 mL/kg/h) with normovolemia or rise in creatinine from baseline of ≥ 0.3-0.5 mg/dL (0.8-44 mmol/L) within 48 hours of hospitalization
Hematologic	Prolonged clotting times (PT or aPTT) > 125% of normal, thrombocytopenia < 80,000-100,000/mcL, evidence of DIC
Gastrointestinal	Ileus, intolerance of enteral feedings, GI ulceration, diarrhea
Hepatic	Progressive elevations in hepatocellular enzymes (ALT), increased bilirubin > 0.5 mg/dL (>8.55 mmol/L)
Neurologic	Decreased level of consciousness or intermittent loss of consciousness

ALT, Alanine aminotransferase; *aPTT*, activated partial thromboplastin time; *DIC*, disseminated intravascular coagulation; *GI*, gastrointestinal; *PT*, prothrombin time.

- Imaging: thoracic radiographs, abdominal radiographs or ultrasound, echocardiography
- Pulse oximetry: identify hypoxemia
- Blood pressure: identify hypotension, monitor trends
- Electrocardiogram: identify cardiac arrhythmias, monitor response to treatment.
- Aerobic (± anaerobic) cultures: urine, peritoneal, blood, wounds

TREATMENT

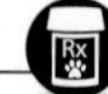

Treatment Overview

Treatment is targeted at the individual organ dysfunction and underlying disease.

Acute General Treatment

- Respiratory
  - Supplemental oxygen (p. 1146) and/or positive-pressure ventilation (p. 1185)
- Cardiovascular/hematologic
  - IV fluids are the mainstay of cardiovascular support in the absence of cardiac failure.
  - Positive inotropes and/or vasopressors are indicated in cases of refractory hypotension.
  - Replace coagulation factors and red blood cells (plasma/blood transfusions [p. 1169]).
  - Consider anticoagulant therapy in selected cases.
- Renal
  - Maintain renal perfusion.
  - Avoid hypervolemia and nephrotoxic medications (p. 1256).
  - Treat oliguria (fenoldopam, mannitol). Consider dialysis in anuric patients.
- GI
  - Gastroprotectants, antiemetics, and prokinetics (if no obstruction present)
  - Start enteral feedings as soon as possible or glutamate to support enterocyte health if full enteral feedings are not tolerated.

PROGNOSIS & OUTCOME

MODS conveys a poor prognosis: mortality rate for dogs with abdominal sepsis is 70% with MODS versus 50% without. In people, failure of more than four organs is almost 100% fatal.

PEARLS & CONSIDERATIONS

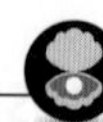

Comments

- The onset of MODS is a critical setback in therapy for any patient.
- Careful, serial monitoring and rapid treatment for new-onset abnormalities is vital.

Technician Tips

Careful monitoring is invaluable. Any change in a critically ill patient may be significant, with particular importance for changes in vital signs, laboratory values, and urine output.

Client Education

MODS is a severe complication of disease, with a guarded to poor outcome. Communication with owners regarding expectations is mandatory.

SUGGESTED READING

Osterbur K, et al: Multiple organ dysfunction syndrome in humans and animals. J Vet Intern Med 28(4):1141-1151, 2014.

AUTHORS: Melissa Bucknoff, DVM, DACVECC; Carsten Bandt, DVM, DACVECC
EDITOR: Benjamin M. Brainard, VMD, DACVAA, DACVECC

Mushroom Toxicosis

Client Education Sheet 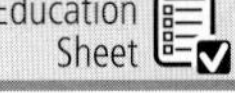

BASIC INFORMATION

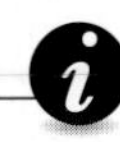

Definition

Condition resulting from ingestion of any of a variety of toxic mushrooms; toxic syndrome produced depends on mushroom type and amount ingested:

- Gastrointestinal (GI) irritant mushrooms: large variety of species
- Hallucinogenic mushrooms: *Psilocybe* spp, *Panaeolus* spp
- Hepatotoxic mushrooms: *Amanita* spp, *Galerina* spp, *Lepiota* spp
- Nephrotoxic mushrooms: *Cortinarius* spp
- Muscarinic mushrooms: *Inocybe* spp, *Clitocybe* spp
- Gyromitrin mushrooms: *Gyromitra* spp, *Helvella crispa, Helvella lacunosa*
- Isoxazole mushrooms: *Amanita gemmata, Amanita muscaria, Amanita smithiana, Amanita strobiliformis,* and *Tricholoma muscarium*

Epidemiology

SPECIES, AGE, SEX

All mammalian species are susceptible; dogs more likely to ingest than cats

GEOGRAPHY AND SEASONALITY

- Highest incidence of mushroom poisoning (all types) occurs from August to October.
- GI irritant mushrooms: wide distribution; long range of fruiting seasons
- Hallucinogenic mushrooms: wide distribution; Pacific Northwest and Gulf Coast; lawns, gardens, roadsides, open woods; cultivated in homes for recreational use
- Hepatotoxic mushrooms: wide distribution throughout United States; wide variation in habitats and fruiting seasons
- Nephrotoxic mushrooms: common in North America, especially Canada; grows in woods and forests; uncommon in urban areas
- Muscarinic mushrooms: wide distribution; forests or fields; fruits in fall, early winter in temperate areas, year-round in warm, moist climates
- Gyromitrin mushrooms: throughout North America, primarily in the spring
- Isoxazole mushrooms: eastern United States and Pacific Northwest; forests; fruits in spring/early summer and again in fall

Clinical Presentation

DISEASE FORMS/SUBTYPES

- GI: acute, self-limited GI distress
- Hallucinogenic: acute central nervous system (CNS) signs; generally self-limited
- Hepatotoxic: acute GI signs, then liver failure in 24-72 hours
- Nephrotoxic: renal tubular dysfunction
- Muscarinic: acute muscarinic signs
- Gyromitrin: GI signs followed by neurologic, hepatorenal, and/or hemolytic syndromes
- Isoxazole: acute inebriation followed by coma; generally self-limited

HISTORY, CHIEF COMPLAINT

- History of exposure; mushrooms in the vomitus
- GI: vomiting, diarrhea within 4 hours of ingestion
- Hallucinogenic: dysphoria, vocalization in 30 minutes to 4 hours of ingestion
- Hepatotoxic: acute, severe vomiting ± diarrhea in 8-24 hours; apparent recovery, then return of GI signs; evidence of acute liver failure in 24-72 hours; acute kidney injury possible in severe cases
- Nephrotoxic: acute kidney injury 12 hours to 8 days after exposure, polyuria, polydipsia
- Muscarinic: salivation, vomiting, diarrhea, lacrimation, bradycardia within 4 hours of ingestion
- Gyromitrin: GI signs in 6-8 hours, hepatorenal and hemolytic syndrome 36-48 hours after ingestion
- Isoxazole: vomiting, ataxia, disorientation, sleep/coma within 4 hours of ingestion

PHYSICAL EXAM FINDINGS

- GI: vomiting, diarrhea, dehydration possible, but generally unremarkable
- Hallucinogenic: vocalization, agitation
- Hepatotoxic: signs of abdominal pain, icterus, hypotension, hepatomegaly, coma
- Nephrotoxic: uremic signs (p. 23)
- Muscarinic: vomiting, hypersalivation, lacrimation, diarrhea, bradycardia, wet lung sounds
- Gyromitrin: vomiting, abdominal pain, icterus, hepatomegaly, hemoglobinuria, anemia
- Isoxazole: agitation, tremors, disorientation, GI signs

Etiology and Pathophysiology

- GI: several mechanisms; hypersensitivity, local irritation
- Hallucinogenic: stimulate serotonin and possibly norepinephrine receptors in central and peripheral nervous systems
- Hepatotoxic: cyclopeptides interfere with DNA synthesis, protein synthesis, resulting in cellular necrosis
- Nephrotoxic: orellanine causes energy depletion and tubulointerstitial nephritis; cortinarin causes oxidative membrane injury
- Muscarinic: bind muscarinic acetylcholine receptors in parasympathetic nervous system; prolonged duration due to lack of degradation; does not inhibit acetylcholinesterase
- Gyromitrin: metabolized to monomethylhydrazine, leading to metabolic alterations
- Isoxazole: muscimol mimics gamma-aminobutyric acid (GABA), causing sedation, mental dullness; ibotenic acid acts on glutamate receptors triggering CNS stimulation; combined effects result in hyperesthesia, sedation, intermittent agitation

DIAGNOSIS

Diagnostic Overview

Diagnosis is reached when nonspecific disorders (e.g., gastroenteritis, hepatotoxicity, neurologic disturbance) are combined with evidence of exposure, such as mushrooms in vomitus. There is no practical clinical confirmatory test.

Differential Diagnosis

- GI, muscarinic: parvoviral enteritis, foreign body, garbage toxicosis, organophosphate and carbamate pesticide toxicosis
- Hepatotoxic: other toxicoses (acetaminophen, iron, blue-green algae, *Cycas* spp), infectious hepatitis
- Nephrotoxic: ethylene glycol, grapes/raisins, nonsteroidal antiinflammatory drug (NSAID) toxicity, leptospirosis
- Isoxazole, hallucinogenic: encephalitis, portosystemic shunt, serotonergic drugs, cannabis, other illicit substances

Initial Database

- CBC, serum biochemistry profile, urinalysis, venous or arterial blood gas measurement: depends on type. Marked increase in liver enzymes ± bilirubin; azotemia; hypoglycemia; acidosis
- Coagulation profile: coagulopathy with severe liver injury; disseminated intravascular coagulation (hepatotoxic mushrooms)
- Rule out differential diagnosis depending on presentation (e.g., leptospirosis serology)

Advanced or Confirmatory Testing

- Abdominal imaging: hepatomegaly (hepatotoxic mushrooms)
- Liver biopsy (hepatotoxic): liver necrosis
- Urine: amatoxins can be detected in the urine as early as 90-120 minutes after ingestion of an amatoxin-containing mushroom.
- Urine: muscimol can be detected in urine; turnaround time is long and little value in acute cases

TREATMENT

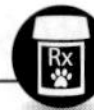

Treatment Overview

Initially, manage potentially life-threatening abnormalities (e.g., seizures, hypoglycemia, bleeding disorders). Further treatment consists of decontamination and supportive care: induction of vomiting and administration of activated charcoal to minimize absorption and treatment to minimize hepatic/renal injury, excessive muscarinic effects, and complications as they arise.

Acute General Treatment

Decontamination in asymptomatic animals (p. 1087):

- Emesis induction (effective within a few hours [p. 1188])
- Gastric lavage (p. 1117) can be attempted with a recent exposure to hepatotoxic or gyromitrin mushrooms.
- Activated charcoal
  - Use 1 g/kg with sorbitol or labeled dosage of commercial product given PO if safe to give. Repeat in 6-8 hours if hepatotoxic mushrooms ingested or suspected, one-half original dose

Manage clinical signs:

- Control CNS stimulation (for hallucinogenic, isoxazole, hepatotoxic mushrooms)
  - For agitation, disorientation, acepromazine 0.05-0.1 mg/kg prn
  - Diazepam 0.5-2 mg/kg IV or midazolam 0.5-1.0 mg/kg IV for seizures. Avoid benzodiazepine if isoxazole mushrooms could be involved. Respiratory depression and apnea due to potentiation of the muscimol-induced GABA effect may occur.
  - Barbiturates, other drugs if diazepam is ineffective (p. 903)
  - Pyridoxine 75-150 mg/kg slow IV for seizures (gyromitrin mushrooms)
- Atropine for excessive bronchial secretions and bradycardia (muscarinic) 0.04 mg/kg (give ¼ of dose IV, remainder IM), titrate up as needed. Contraindicated with isoxazole mushrooms
- Antiemetics
  - Maropitant 1 mg/kg SQ q 24h, *or* metoclopramide 0.2-0.4 mg/kg q 6h PO, SQ, or IM, or 1-2 mg/kg/day as constant-rate IV (CRI) infusion, *or* dolasetron 0.6-1 mg/kg IV q 12h
- Fluid diuresis for hepatotoxic/nephrotoxic mushrooms: fluid therapy for fluid/electrolyte/acid-base abnormalities for any mushroom exposure as needed based on signs (pp. 23 and 442).
- For hypoglycemia, dextrose 5% 1-2 mL/kg/h as needed (hepatotoxic mushrooms)
- Blood replacement/clotting factors, vitamin K_1 for coagulopathy (hepatotoxic mushrooms)
- Cyproheptadine (for dysphoria or serotonin syndrome–like signs associated with hallucinogenic mushrooms) 1.1 mg/kg PO or per rectum q 6-8h prn

Prevent/manage liver injury (hepatotoxic mushrooms):

- *N*-acetylcysteine 140 mg/kg IV or PO (5% solution), then 70 mg/kg PO q 6-8h for 7 doses
- Crystalline (sodium or potassium) penicillin G (interferes with enterohepatic recirculation of hepatotoxins) 0.5-1 million U/kg/day for 3 days as IV CRI
  - Do not use procaine penicillin G for IV administration (can be fatal).
- Silibinin and silymarin (extracts of milk thistle): veterinary formulation combines silybin and *S*-adenosylmethionine (SAMe; Denamarin): 20-40 mg/kg q 8-12h for 48 hours

Supportive care:

- Thermoregulation
- Pain management (fentanyl, buprenorphine, tramadol)

Chronic Treatment

SAMe 18 mg/kg PO q 24h for 2-3 months (hepatotoxic mushrooms)

Possible Complications

Hepatic insufficiency ± hepatic encephalopathy; chronic kidney disease

Recommended Monitoring

- Hydration, electrolytes for severe GI signs
- Hepatotoxic and gyromitrin mushrooms: CBC, liver enzymes, renal values, blood glucose, coagulation parameters
- Nephrotoxic mushrooms: renal values

PROGNOSIS & OUTCOME

- GI irritant, isoxazole, muscarinic, and hallucinogenic mushrooms: excellent with supportive care
- Hepatotoxic mushrooms: guarded to poor with evidence of liver injury
- Gyromitrin: guarded with hepatotoxicosis and hemolysis
- Nephrotoxic: guarded

PEARLS & CONSIDERATIONS

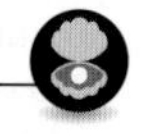

Comments

- Because of difficulty in differentiating toxic from nontoxic mushrooms, any ingestion of unidentified mushrooms by pets should prompt decontamination procedures (e.g., emesis, activated charcoal).
- Identification of mushrooms is best done by a mycologist; local college biology departments or museums are potentially useful sources of expertise. Internet can be used to help narrow and match pictures of the mushrooms involved.
- An excellent resource is the North American Mycological Association website (http://namyco.org/toxicology/poison_syndromes.html) for a case registry and a list of local area volunteers that can help identify the mushroom.

Technician Tips

Physical confinement and minimizing stimuli can be important to prevent injury for dysphoric, disoriented animals.

SUGGESTED READING

Puschner B: Mushrooms. In Peterson ME, et al, editors: Small animal toxicology, ed 3, St. Louis, 2013, Saunders, pp 659-676.

AUTHOR: Irina D. Meadows, DVM, DABT
EDITOR: Tina Wismer, DVM, MS, DABT, DABVT

Myasthenia Gravis and Myasthenic Syndromes

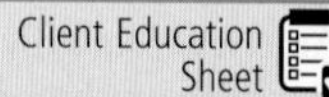

BASIC INFORMATION

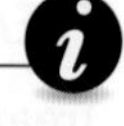

Definition

Myasthenia gravis is skeletal muscle weakness due to a decrease of acetylcholine receptors at neuromuscular junctions. Congenital myasthenic syndromes are hereditary disorders of neuromuscular transmission.

Epidemiology

SPECIES, AGE, SEX

- Congenital myasthenic syndromes are uncommon; signs occur by 8 weeks of age.
- Acquired myasthenia gravis is fairly common and occurs in adult dogs; bimodal age of onset (peaks at 3 and 10 years)
- Acquired myasthenia gravis is uncommon in adult cats.

GENETICS, BREED PREDISPOSITION

- Congenital myasthenic syndromes occur in Jack Russell terriers, smooth fox terriers, golden retrievers, Labrador retrievers, and sporadically in other breeds. They are rare in cats.
- Akitas, terriers, German short-haired pointers, and Chihuahuas have the highest relative risks for acquired myasthenia. German shepherds and golden retrievers are also commonly affected. A familial predisposition occurs in the Newfoundland and Great Dane.
- Abyssinians and Somalis are at increased risk for feline acquired myasthenia gravis.

RISK FACTORS

Methimazole increases the risk of acquired myasthenia gravis in cats.

ASSOCIATED DISORDERS

- In dogs, associated conditions include hypothyroidism, thymoma and other tumors, hypoadrenocorticism, and thrombocytopenia.
- Thymoma is common among cats with acquired myasthenia gravis.
- Megaesophagus and aspiration can occur with myasthenia.

Clinical Presentation

DISEASE FORMS/SUBTYPES

- Acquired: an autoimmune disorder characterized by circulating antibodies against acetylcholine receptors at the neuromuscular junction; can occur in generalized, focal, or acute fulminating forms
- Congenital: an inborn defect in the neuromuscular junction

HISTORY, CHIEF COMPLAINT

- Congenital: generalized weakness with or without regurgitation/dysphagia, evident by ≈8 weeks of age
- Generalized acquired: generalized limb weakness that can be precipitated by exercise, with or without regurgitation/dysphagia
- Focal acquired: dysphagia/regurgitation or facial weakness with no limb weakness
- Acute fulminating acquired: acute generalized weakness and dyspnea due to respiratory muscle weakness

PHYSICAL EXAM FINDINGS

- Generalized limb weakness is characterized by stiffness, tremor, and short-strided gait that may progress to inability to walk. Weakness may be more severe in the pelvic limbs, is often precipitated by 1-2 minutes of exercise, and improves with rest.
- No ataxia and proprioceptive positioning is usually normal when the patient's weight is supported. Muscle atrophy is absent, and tendon reflexes are usually preserved.
- Weak palpebral reflex, especially in cats; palpebral may become progressively weaker with rapid, repeated attempts to elicit the reflex (decremental palpebral)
- Cats often have neck ventroflexion.
- Abnormal lung sounds and fever possible if concurrent aspiration pneumonia

Etiology and Pathophysiology

- Congenital myasthenic syndromes are caused by mutations in genes coding for components of the neuromuscular junction.
- Acquired myasthenia gravis is caused by circulating autoantibodies against the acetylcholine receptor.

DIAGNOSIS

Diagnostic Overview

The diagnosis is suspected in one of four contexts (see History, Chief Complaint above), all characterized by weakness that often worsens with exercise and resolves with rest. Measurement of serum anti–acetylcholine receptor antibody levels is the diagnostic test of choice for acquired myasthenia gravis.

Differential Diagnosis

- Myopathies: polymyositis, degenerative myopathies
- Tick paralysis
- Acute idiopathic polyradiculoneuritis
- Botulism
- Polyneuropathy
- Metabolic disorders: hypokalemia, hypoglycemia, hypoadrenocorticism, hyperthyroidism in cats
- Orthopedic diseases: polyarthritis
- Focal acquired: megaesophagus (p. 642)

Initial Database

- CBC, serum biochemistry profile, urinalysis to rule out metabolic causes of weakness
- Thoracic radiographs to screen for megaesophagus, aspiration pneumonia
- Thyroid, adrenal function testing
- Edrophonium response test can help diagnose generalized myasthenia gravis. Administer edrophonium chloride 0.1-0.2 mg/kg IV during weakness. A positive response is obvious but short-lived improvement in strength within several minutes and suggests the diagnosis. False-negative results are common, and false-positive results are possible. Potential side effects include dyspnea due to bronchial constriction and secretions; treat with atropine.

Advanced or Confirmatory Testing

- Anti–acetylcholine receptor antibody test (p. 1298) for acquired myasthenia gravis
- Electrodiagnostic testing (single-fiber electromyography and repetitive nerve stimulation) is useful for the diagnosis and for excluding other causes of weakness.
- Definitive diagnosis of congenital myasthenic syndromes requires quantification of acetylcholine receptors from muscle biopsy or DNA testing.

TREATMENT

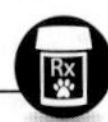

Treatment Overview

Treatment goals include improving neuromuscular transmission, administering supportive care, and immunosuppression (acquired form only).

Acute General Treatment

- Anticholinesterase drugs: pyridostigmine 0.5-3 mg/kg PO q 8-12h in dogs; 0.25 mg/kg PO q 8-12h in cats. Start at low end of dose range, and titrate dose based on response and side effects (hypersalivation, vomiting, diarrhea). If dysphagia/regurgitation precludes oral medication, neostigmine 0.04 mg/kg SQ q 6h is an alternative. Human intravenous immunoglobulin can be helpful for short-term management of acute fulminating myasthenia.
- Aspiration pneumonia (p. 793) is treated with antibiotics, nebulization and coupage, and oxygen if necessary.
- Endotracheal intubation and ventilatory support (p. 1185) may be necessary for the acute fulminating form or for patients with severe aspiration pneumonia.
- IV fluids as needed
- Nutritional support as needed: feedings with the head elevated or placement of a gastrostomy (preferred if megaesophagus present), nasogastric, or esophagostomy feeding tube (pp. 1109, 1107, and 1106)

Chronic Treatment

Immunosuppressive therapy (for acquired form only) is indicated when there is an inadequate response to anticholinesterase medication. Prednisone is the initial drug of choice (start at 0.5 mg/kg PO q 24h for 1-2 weeks, then increase to 2-4 mg/kg PO q 24h if needed; gradually taper if possible based on clinical response). Azathioprine, cyclosporine, or mycophenolate mofetil can be added if there is an inadequate response to prednisone or to allow decreased dose of prednisone in patients with severe glucocorticoid-related side effects.

Drug Interactions

- Avoid drugs that impair neuromuscular transmission, including ampicillin, aminoglycosides, fluoroquinolones, and phenothiazines.
- Organophosphates can increase toxicity of anticholinesterase drugs.
- In cats that develop myasthenia gravis while taking methimazole, the methimazole should be discontinued if possible.

Possible Complications

Aspiration pneumonia is the most common and serious complication in patients with pharyngeal/esophageal weakness.

Recommended Monitoring

- Client should monitor weakness and dysphagia/regurgitation at home daily.
- Monitor anti–acetylcholinesterase receptor antibody titer q 8-12 weeks in affected dogs. Normalization of titer indicates remission.

PROGNOSIS & OUTCOME

- Prognosis for the acquired form is good for patients without pharyngeal/esophageal weakness. Spontaneous remission occurs in almost 90% of affected dogs but is uncommon in cats.
- Prognosis is guarded for patients with dysphagia/regurgitation because aspiration pneumonia is common and carries an ≈50% 1-year mortality rate. If present, megaesophagus may or may not resolve.
- Relapse is rare but can be associated with stress (e.g., surgery) or vaccination.
- The prognosis for the acute fulminating form is poor; most affected dogs die from respiratory failure.

PEARLS & CONSIDERATIONS

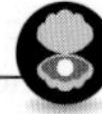

Comments

- Early diagnosis and treatment in an attempt to avoid aspiration pneumonia improves outcome.

- Serologic testing for antibodies to acetylcholine receptors should be evaluated in any adult dog with unexplained megaesophagus or dysphagia.

Technician Tips

Carefully assess respiratory strength in any patient with nonambulatory tetraparesis or tetraplegia. Intercostal paresis is evident as lack of chest movement with respiration (abdominal breathing) or paradoxical chest movement, in which the chest wall moves in rather than out on inspiration.

Client Education

For patients with megaesophagus, provide client education sheet: How to Provide Elevated Feedings.

SUGGESTED READING

Penderis J, et al: Junctionopathies: disorders of the neuromuscular junction. In Dewey CW, et al, editors: A practical guide to canine and feline neurology, ed 3, Ames, IA, 2016, Wiley-Blackwell, pp 521-558.

AUTHOR: William B. Thomas, DVM, MS, DACVIM
EDITOR: Karen R. Muñana, DVM, MS, DACVIM

Mycobacterial Diseases

BASIC INFORMATION

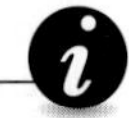

Definition

Infection by any species of *Mycobacterium*

Synonyms

Atypical mycobacteriosis, feline leprosy, leproid granuloma syndrome, rapidly growing mycobacterial (RGM) panniculitis, tuberculosis (TB)

Epidemiology

SPECIES, AGE, SEX

- Opportunistic mycobacterial infections are uncommon in cats, rare in dogs.
- Tuberculous and leproid forms are rare.

GENETICS, BREED PREDISPOSITION

Miniature schnauzers, basset hounds, and Siamese cats may be overrepresented with systemic forms of opportunistic infections.

RISK FACTORS

Traumatic injuries often precede opportunistic infection.

CONTAGION AND ZOONOSIS

- Zoonotic risk exists with all mycobacterial infections, especially among immunocompromised people.
- Tuberculosis (infection with *Mycobacterium tuberculosis*, and *Mycobacterium bovis* in some jurisdictions) is a reportable disease from the time of clinical suspicion or diagnosis.
- Tuberculous forms are a constant human health threat (especially exudates from cutaneous lesions). Gloves, mask, and eye protection are necessary during wound debridement and patient care.
- Anthroponosis (reverse zoonosis) is a common source of infection by tuberculous forms in companion animals.
- Common-source exposure is more likely than contagion in leproid and opportunistic forms; however, appropriate caution should be used in handling infected animals and their secretions, exudates, and tissues. The armadillo is an important source of zoonoses for leproid forms in the southern United States.
- Urine and feces do not pose a significant zoonotic risk to most immunocompetent people.

Clinical Presentation

DISEASE FORMS/SUBTYPES

Three clinical forms are commonly recognized:

- Opportunistic forms (most prevalent) are characterized by spreading, nonhealing subcutaneous lesions. Opportunistic species of the *Mycobacterium avium* complex and cutaneous *M. bovis* infections can progress to cause systemic disease.
- Tuberculous forms (rare) are characterized by skin and internal organ granulomas.
- Leproid forms (rare) consist of regionalized cutaneous nodules.

HISTORY, CHIEF COMPLAINT

- Opportunistic mycobacterial infections produce nonhealing exudative wound(s). Often, there is an associated history of partial response to prior antibiotic therapy with persistence of some portion of the lesion(s) or recurrence after therapy.
- Tuberculous forms often are subclinical or cause skin lesions, weight loss, lethargy, and coughing.
- Leproid forms are seen in young cats (rarely in dogs), with fleshy nodules on the face and forelimbs.

PHYSICAL EXAM FINDINGS

- Opportunistic: chronic intermittent serous/serosanguineous discharge from spreading skin lesions at sites of prior trauma, especially the inguinal fat pad in cats. If cutaneous lesions progress to generalized disease (*M. bovis*, *M. avium* complex), clinical signs mimic those seen with tuberculous forms.
- Tuberculous: systemic signs reflecting the location of visceral granulomas, with or without cutaneous lesions. Involvement of the lungs, spleen, and/or liver is common. In the tuberculous form (rare) in cats, the gastrointestinal tract may contain granulomas. Mediastinal or mesenteric lymphadenopathy may be noted on imaging.
- Leproid: multiple nonpainful, nonpruritic, fleshy cutaneous nodules, with or without ulceration. Usually, patients are otherwise well.

Etiology and Pathophysiology

- Mycobacteria are a large group of acid-fast, aerobic bacilli with widely varied pathogenicity.
- Opportunistic species (e.g., *M. avium* complex, *Mycobacterium smegmatis, Mycobacterium fortuitum*) are saprophytes, primarily acquired from water and wet soil across damaged or abraded skin.
- Tuberculous species (e.g., *M. tuberculosis, M. bovis*) are facultative intracellular parasites, and none has the dog or cat as the reservoir host.
- Leproid species *(Mycobacterium leprae, Mycobacterium. lepraemurium)* are obligate intracellular parasites transmitted to cats from rodents.
- Immune response is usually insufficient to clear infection but may confine bacteria in granulomas.

DIAGNOSIS

Diagnostic Overview

The most common form encountered is the opportunistic skin infection, which is suspected when a ventral abdominal, inguinal, or other wound fails to respond to appropriate cleaning, debridement, and antibiotic therapy. Cytologic exam of smears or biopsies obtained from a closed, intact portion of the involved skin are the most valuable diagnostic tools.

Differential Diagnosis

- Bacterial folliculitis
- Mycotic infections
- *Pythium* and *Lagenidium* infections
- Sterile nodular panniculitis
- Cutaneous or pulmonary neoplasia
- Foreign body reactions
- Drug eruptions

Initial Database

- CBC/serum biochemistry profile/urinalysis
  - Hypercalcemia of chronic granulomatous disease is possible and should not mislead the clinician into a diagnosis of neoplasia.

- Cytologic evaluation or biopsy of skin lesions reveals an acid-fast bacillus; cytology using routine stains can reveal apparent "holes" due to organisms that fail to take up stain.
- Thoracic and abdominal radiographs reveal granulomas in systemic forms.

Advanced or Confirmatory Testing

- Culture, including antibiotic susceptibility testing and speciation, is essential; identification of opportunistic forms by culture and takes ≈6 weeks.
- A specialized lab is required (e.g., National Jewish Center for Immunology and Respiratory Medicine in Denver, Colorado [www.nationaljewish.org/professionals/clinical-services/diagnostics/adx/about-us/lab-expertise/mycobacteriology]).
- Polymerase chain reaction (PCR) is increasingly available but technically challenging, prone to false-negatives; PCR has not replaced culture as the gold standard.
- Intradermal tuberculosis (skin) testing is not helpful in dogs and cats.

TREATMENT

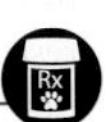

Treatment Overview

- Opportunistic forms can be curable with long-term treatment.
  - Treatment of opportunistic forms depends on aggressive resection and guided combination antibiotic therapy for a minimum of 3 months.
- Tuberculous forms pose a significant human health threat; treatment may not be recommended.
- Leproid forms are usually curable with aggressive surgical excision.
- Acute general treatment with wide surgical debulking of large opportunistic lesions is the first step in long-term management.
  - Submit surgical biopsies for species identification.
- Surgical excision of leproid granulomas is the treatment of choice.

Chronic Treatment

- Consultation with an internist specializing in infectious diseases is advised for drug recommendations; antibiotic resistance is prevalent, and protocols are evolving rapidly.
- Treatment of opportunistic forms, guided by species identification (and sensitivity testing when possible), requires a minimum of 3 months and typically longer.
  - Combination therapy with a fluoroquinolone plus clarithromycin, gentamicin, or doxycycline may be acceptable empirical therapy while definitive identification is pending.
- Treatment for tuberculous forms may not be recommended; if treatment is undertaken, combination antibiotic therapy must be administered for a minimum of 6-12 months.
- Medical therapy for leproid infections is indicated if complete surgical excision is not possible.

Possible Complications

- Surgical sites prone to dehiscence and recurrence of infection
- Risks of drug resistance, toxicosis, or intolerance with long-term antibiotic use

Recommended Monitoring

- Re-exam every 2-3 weeks for continued effectiveness of therapy
- Periodic lab tests for evidence of drug toxicosis

PROGNOSIS & OUTCOME

- Recurrence or incomplete clearance is likely.
- With appropriate intensive management, outcome of opportunistic infections can be good.
- Leproid forms have the best prognosis.

PEARLS & CONSIDERATIONS

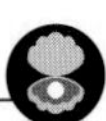

Comments

- Significant commitment of owner time and resources is required for positive outcome.
- Accurate species identification and current antimicrobial therapy recommendations are essential.
- Diagnosis of *M. tuberculosis* infection should result in a recommendation for in-contact people to be tested for TB. Infected in-contact people are likely the source of the infection for the pet.
- Euthanasia may be recommended over treatment of tuberculous forms (zoonotic risk).

Prevention

- Opportunistic forms are ubiquitous.
- Limiting rodent exposure reduces risk of leproid forms.
- Vaccination with human or large-animal products is not recommended.

Technician Tips

- Any chronic draining lesion in a dog or cat may contain mycobacteria or other agents transmissible to people.
- Always wear gloves and wash hands thoroughly.

SUGGESTED READING

Greene CE, et al: Mycobacterial infections. In Greene CE, editor: Infectious diseases of the dog and cat, ed 4, St. Louis, 2012, Saunders, pp 495-521.

AUTHOR: Kate E. Creevy, DVM, MS, DACVIM
EDITOR: Joseph Taboada, DVM, DACVIM

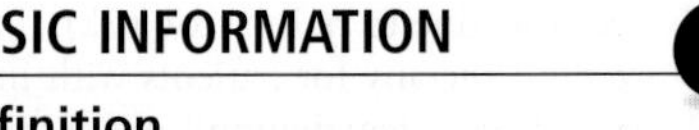

Myelodysplasia

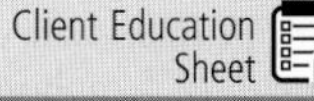

BASIC INFORMATION

Definition

- Myelodysplastic syndrome (MDS) describes a group of bone marrow disorders characterized by peripheral blood cytopenias and a hypercellular to hypocellular bone marrow containing < 20% blast cells. It is considered a precursor to acute leukemia, where the bone marrow blast population exceeds ≈25%.
- Morphologic signs of abnormal maturation (dysplasia) may be seen in the erythroid, myeloid, and/or megakaryocytic cells.

Synonyms

Ineffective hematopoiesis, refractory cytopenias, preleukemia, smoldering acute leukemia

Epidemiology

SPECIES, AGE, SEX

Dogs and cats; the prevalence of MDS in cats is decreasing as the prevalence of feline leukemia virus (FeLV) infection also decreases. MDS is occasionally associated with feline immunodeficiency virus (FIV) infections.

RISK FACTORS

- FeLV and FIV infections
- Some drugs: chloramphenicol, cephalosporins, melphalan, cyclophosphamide, estrogen, and vincristine
- Vitamin B_{12}/folate deficiency
- Lead toxicosis
- Exposure to radiation
- Immune-mediated diseases targeting the bone marrow
- Chronic exposure to alkylating chemotherapy drugs

CONTAGION AND ZOONOSIS

FeLV and FIV: contagious between cats

Clinical Presentation

DISEASE FORMS/SUBTYPES

Primary (no inciting cause known) or secondary (specific causative agent). MDS is classified as three subtypes based on cytologic exam of bone marrow. Although this classification offers quantification of blast populations, it does not provide specific prognostic information.

- MDS-ER (erythroid predominant): myeloid to erythroid (M:E) ratio < 1, blasts < 20% of nucleated bone marrow cells
- MDS-RC (refractory cytopenia): M:E ratio > 1, nonerythroid blasts < 5% of nucleated bone marrow cells
- MDS-EB (excess blasts): M:E ratio > 1, nonerythroid blasts 5%-19% of nucleated bone marrow cells

HISTORY, CHIEF COMPLAINT

- Nonspecific clinical signs related to anemia, including weakness, lethargy, tachypnea, and appetite changes (ranging from anorexia to pica)
- Recurrent/chronic infections if leukopenia or abnormal leukocyte function occurs
- Bruising/bleeding secondary to thrombocytopenia or platelet function disorders
- Drug history is important for identifying possible triggers.

PHYSICAL EXAM FINDINGS

- Weakness, tachycardia, syncope, heart murmurs, and pallor may indicate anemia.
- Fever due to secondary infections
- Epistaxis or petechiae due to thrombocytopenia or abnormal platelet/megakaryocyte maturation
- Hepatomegaly and splenomegaly are common in cats and may occur in dogs.
- Pleural effusion, possibly leading to muffled heart and lung sounds, has been reported in cats.

Etiology and Pathophysiology

- MDS may be primary (presumably due to mutations in hematopoietic progenitor cells) or secondary (associated with FeLV or FIV infections, drug therapy, or disorders such as lymphoma, multiple myeloma, myelofibrosis, or immune-mediated anemia/thrombocytopenia).
- In FIV-infected cats with peripheral cytopenias, FIV can be isolated from bone marrow mononuclear cells, megakaryocytes, and marrow stromal cells.
- A variety of chromosomal abnormalities and mutations in oncogenes and tumor suppressor genes have been identified in humans with MDS but have not been demonstrated in animals.
- MDS-associated clonal proliferation, apoptosis, and ineffective hematopoiesis can result in lethal cytopenias, or MDS may progress to acute leukemia.

DIAGNOSIS

Diagnostic Overview

History and physical findings are nonspecific, but CBC usually reveals at least one repeatable abnormality. The diagnosis is obtained on bone marrow exam performed because of persistent peripheral blood cell abnormalities without an identifiable cause. Additional tests for underlying causes (e.g., titers for rickettsial diseases) may be indicated.

Differential Diagnosis

- Acute leukemia
- Drug-induced bone marrow dyscrasia
- Hyperplasia of recovering bone marrow
- Nonregenerative anemia from chronic/inflammatory disease, renal disease, iron deficiency, drugs or toxins, or aplastic anemia
- Neutropenia: tissue demand, endotoxemia/sepsis, immune-mediated destruction, inherited/genetic leukocyte maturation/function abnormalities
- Thrombocytopenia: drug therapy, immune-mediated destruction
- Rickettsial (*Ehrlichia* and *Anaplasma* spp, Rocky Mountain spotted fever) organism-induced bone marrow dyscrasias
- Congenital conditions associated with dysplastic features
  - Miniature and toy poodles: familial nonanemic macrocytosis with dysplastic changes in erythroid precursors
  - English springer spaniels: congenital dyserythropoiesis, polymyopathy, and cardiac disease
  - Giant schnauzers: congenital malabsorption of vitamin B_{12} and myelodysplasia
  - Cavalier King Charles spaniels, Norfolk and Cairin terriers: idiopathic subclinical thrombocytopenia and dysplastic changes in megakaryocytes and platelets (macroplatelets)

Initial Database

- CBC: cytopenias and dysplastic blood cell morphology. Blood smear must be reviewed by a clinical pathologist for accurate assessment.
  - Nonregenerative anemia: often with many nucleated red blood cells; thrombocytopenia and/or leukopenia often present
  - Leukocyte abnormalities: ringed nuclei, micronuclei, nuclear fragments, abnormal cytoplasmic granulation, or maturation arrest
  - Giant platelets and dwarf megakaryocytes
- Bone marrow evaluation (biopsy is often superior to aspiration for establishing most accurate detail of bone marrow cellularity and marrow architecture) (p. 1068).
  - Exam of bone marrow is necessary to confirm MDS and identify the subtype.
  - By definition, < 20% of the marrow nucleated cells are blast cells (if > 25% blasts, the diagnosis is acute leukemia, and the prognosis is usually worse).
  - Asynchrony of nuclear and/or cytoplasmic maturation of affected cell lines
  - Bizarre nuclear morphologies resembling bowling pins, doughnuts, or abnormally small nuclei
- Serum biochemistry profile and urinalysis: no specific abnormalities
- All cats with MDS should be tested for FeLV and FIV.

Advanced or Confirmatory Testing

- Cytochemical stains, immunohistochemical stains, and/or flow cytometry may be useful to rule out myeloid and lymphoid malignancies.
- *Ehrlichia* and *Anaplasma* spp titers if indicated
- Serum iron, zinc, lead, and vitamin B_{12}/folate levels, as indicated
- Coombs' test to rule out antibodies directed against red blood cells

TREATMENT

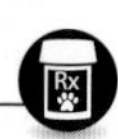

Treatment Overview

Therapy includes supportive care (if needed) until cytopenias resolve. Overall goals are to restore normal hematopoiesis, treat underlying cause (if appropriate), and eradicate dysplastic blast cells or neoplastic cells as possible.

Acute General Treatment

- Discontinue all drugs, especially agents associated with MDS.
- Intensive supportive care may be warranted for patients with severe cytopenias.
  - Transfusions (p. 1169)
  - Antibiotics for treating/preventing secondary infections
    - For prophylaxis, a common choice is trimethoprim-sulfadiazine 15 mg/kg PO q 12h (for dogs; cats do not usually need prophylactic antibiotics).
    - If fever or overt infection is present, IV broad-spectrum antibiotics, based preferably on culture and sensitivity or empirical use, are indicated. Example: a combination of a penicillin (e.g., ampicillin 22 mg/kg IV q 8h slow bolus) with an aminoglycoside (e.g., amikacin 20 mg/kg IV q 24h [only in hydrated patient without renal dysfunction]) or a fluoroquinolone (e.g., enrofloxacin 5 mg/kg diluted 1:1 in sterile water and given as a slow IV bolus q 12h [dogs]; 5 mg/kg q 24h in cats, but use judiciously in cats due to retinotoxic risk).
  - IV fluid therapy for patients with infection, fever, dehydration, or decreased appetite
  - Avoid jugular venipuncture or catheterization in cases of severe thrombocytopenia.
  - Nutritional support
- Recombinant granulocyte colony-stimulating factor (G-CSF) 5 mcg/kg SQ q 24h until neutrophil count normalizes, recombinant human erythropoietin (rh-Epo, Epogen) 100 IU/kg SQ q 48-72h until hematocrit rises, then q 7 days or as needed to maintain

low-normal hematocrit; anecdotally, darbepoetin (Aranesp) 0.45 mcg/kg SQ once weekly at first, then q 2-3 weeks adjusted for maintenance (may be less antigenic than recombinant erythropoietin), and/or thrombopoietin (currently experimental) may have a role in treating refractory cytopenias. Some recombinant human cytokines cause dogs and cats to form cross-reactive neutralizing antibodies to the recombinant products and their own cytokines, especially with chronic or repeated use.

- Immunosuppressive doses of prednisone/prednisolone 2 mg/kg PO q 24h have been effective for some dogs and cats with refractory cytopenias.
- Low-dose cytosine arabinoside (LD-AraC) 0.7-1.4 mg/kg (or 100 mg/m^2) SQ q 24h for 2-4 days has been attempted as a differentiation agent in the management of MDS in cats. A single complete response has been described. LD-AraC administered to a dog with MDS-Er at 10 mg/m^2 SQ q 12h for 3 weeks was ineffective (p. 609).

Chronic Treatment

- Patients responding to treatment will likely require lifelong therapy and chronic monitoring for progression to leukemia.
  - Supportive therapy as indicated (antibiotics, transfusions, hematopoietic cytokines)
  - Hematopoietic cytokines should be reduced/discontinued after cell counts are improved to reduce the risk of autoantibody formation.
- Patients with concurrent MDS secondary to drug administration should never receive that drug again.

Possible Complications

Chronic administration of rh-Epo and/or G-CSF can result in the production of antibodies that cross-react with feline or canine equivalent cytokines and have caused intractable cytopenias.

Recommended Monitoring

- Physical exams and CBC: q 1-2 weeks, more frequently during initial therapy. Blood smear review to monitor cytopenias, blasts and other abnormal cell morphology, and possible adverse effects of treatment. If lasting response to therapy is noted, interval may be extended to monthly.
- Serum biochemistry profile: at least q 2 months to monitor overall health

PROGNOSIS & OUTCOME

- In general, the prognosis for most animals with MDS is poor, with survival times ranging from a few days to a few months.
  - Primary MDS is considered to be a preneoplastic condition, progressing to acute leukemia in 40%-60% of cases. Animals may live a year or more but eventually succumb to acute leukemia or bone marrow failure.
  - The prognosis for animals with secondary MDS depends on successful elimination of the inciting disease or drug.
- Cats with refractory anemia can enjoy long survival times; however, cats with other types of MDS are typically euthanized due to cytopenias or may develop acute myeloid leukemia (AML) in weeks to months.
- The prognosis for cats with concurrent MDS and FeLV infection is especially grave; most do not survive 1 week after diagnosis. The prognosis is better for cats with FIV-associated MDS because progression is more chronic.
- Dogs with MDS-RC may have a better prognosis than those with MDS-EB. In one small study, dogs with refractory anemia lived longer (>6 months) than dogs with other MDS (mean, 2 weeks).
- In general, patients with high blast counts and/or poor clinical condition have a worse prognosis.
- Breed-related macrothorombocytopenia is inconsequential and does not require treatment.

PEARLS & CONSIDERATIONS

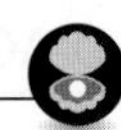

Comments

- MDSs are uncommon and can be challenging to accurately diagnose. When MDS is suspected based on clinical signs and evidence of hematologic abnormalities, bone marrow evaluation is indicated for definitive diagnosis.
- A thorough history is imperative to identify underlying causes of secondary MDS, especially in cases of environmental exposures and drug or medication reactions (including ingestion of medications not intended for veterinary use).
- Management of MDS is focused on identifying and treating underlying diseases (especially immune-mediated hemolytic anemia, immune-mediated thrombocytopenia, and lymphoma) and supportive care of secondary cytopenias.
- When considering these conditions, consultations with a veterinary clinical pathologist and a veterinary oncologist are highly recommended.
- Antineoplastic chemotherapy has not been shown to be beneficial for control of MDS or to prevent progression to leukemia.
- Although the overall prognosis for patients with MDS is poor, there is substantial interindividual variability; some patients respond well to therapy and enjoy longer survival times.

Prevention

All cats should be tested for feline retroviruses (FeLV; also FIV if > 6 months old) as kittens, and FeLV vaccination should be considered.

Technician Tips

- Because immunosuppression often accompanies MDS, nosocomial infection prevention protocols should be employed. This includes handling patients with gloves, using antibiotic scrub technique for blood collection and injections, and keeping patients away from other hospital patients.
- Blood collection should be performed using peripheral venipuncture, rather than jugular vein collection due to risk of thrombocytopenia. Apply bandages and monitor for swelling or bruising at collection sites.

Client Education

- Retrovirus-negative cats should be kept inside to prevent them from becoming exposed to cats harboring FeLV or FIV.
- There is a high risk of progression of primary MDS to acute leukemia.

SUGGESTED READING

Weiss DJ: Myelodysplastic syndromes. In Weiss DJ, et al, editors: Schalm's Veterinary hematology, ed 6, Ames, IA, 2010, Wiley-Blackwell, pp 467-474.

AUTHOR: Jennifer E. Locke, DVM, DACVIM
EDITOR: Jonathan E. Fogle, DVM, PhD, DACVIM

Myiasis

BASIC INFORMATION

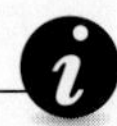

Definition

An infestation of living animals with the larvae (maggots) of dipteran (two-winged) flies, which may cause cutaneous, nasal, or other tissue lesions

Synonym

Maggot infestation

Epidemiology

SPECIES, AGE, SEX

- Dogs and cats may be affected; no age or sex predisposition
- Larvae are relatively species specific, but small animals may serve as aberrant hosts when housed near primary hosts.

RISK FACTORS

Wounded, soiled, debilitated, or weak animals living in temperate, wet regions known to harbor flies causing myiasis are predisposed. Some dipteran larvae can penetrate normal skin.

CONTAGION AND ZOONOSIS

- Emerging adult flies are a potential public health risk because they serve as fomites for bacteria found in animal waste.
- People with open wounds may be at risk for myiasis.
- Other implications: accidental reintroduction of screwworm *(Cochliomyia hominivorax),* which is mainly eradicated from the United States, is an ongoing threat because of the aggressiveness of infestations.
- Superficial wounds are a point of entry for screwworm larvae, which voraciously feed on living flesh and have fatally infected or "have completely eaten away the facial bones" of unconscious human victims (Bowman, 2013). Veterinarians play a key role in screwworm prevention through identification of larvae.

GEOGRAPHY AND SEASONALITY

Myiasis has a worldwide distribution, but larvae-specific infestations do occur in some countries. In the Northern Hemisphere, myiasis occurs during the summer months in temperate, moist areas.

Clinical Presentation

HISTORY, CHIEF COMPLAINT

A foul, putrid-smelling animal may be the only reason an owner seeks veterinary care, although occasionally, malodor may be absent or unnoticed. Other owners are aware that maggots are taking residence in their animal's skin. Occasionally, owners present an animal because of incontinence, debilitation, paresis, or skin fold dermatitis, and myiasis is an incidental finding.

PHYSICAL EXAM FINDINGS

- Maggot infestation typically occurs in moist locations: around the eyes, nose, mouth, genitalia, anus, or adjacent to wounded (traumatic or surgical) skin.
- Irregularly ulcerated to crateriform lesions are characteristic.
- Several lesions may coalesce to form large soft-tissue defects.
- Tracts dissecting through nearby soft-tissue structures may cause fistulation.
- Parasitized skin may present as a focal fistulated subcutaneous nodule.
- Aberrant larval migration can cause signs specific to other tissues.
- Findings associated with incontinence or debilitation (i.e., musculoskeletal, neurologic, or internal disease) might be identified in select cases. Severely infested animals may be in shock.

Etiology and Pathophysiology

- Eggs are laid on the moist skin of debilitated or wounded animals. Emerging larvae (maggots) secrete proteolytic enzymes that liquefy cutaneous tissue, creating full-thickness skin defects within hours. Occasionally, the initial larval infestation favors the strike of other myiasis-causing flies, resulting in disease propagation.
- Many dipteran flies (i.e., house, stable, horn, and black flies) can infest the skin of animals with risk factors (above). These flies cause the typical myiases seen in routine small animal practice.
- Blowflies (common in large animals), screwworm flies (reportable in many parts of the world), and flesh flies rarely infest the skin of small animals. However, their presence is alarming because of contagion implications.
- Although more common in rabbits and rodents, *Cuterebra* flies can cause myiasis in companion animals.

DIAGNOSIS

Diagnostic Overview

The diagnosis is confirmed based on the observation of maggots in the skin and surrounding soft tissue.

Differential Diagnosis

Direct visualization of maggots in representative cutaneous lesions confirms the diagnosis. Specific species identification is not usually required to treat most cases of myiasis.

Initial Database

- Direct visualization of maggots
- Cytologic evaluation of wounded and infested skin to identify secondary bacterial infection

Advanced or Confirmatory Testing

- Other diagnostic tests are done at the discretion of the clinician, but in most patients, a CBC, biochemistry profile, and urinalysis are beneficial to exclude concurrent and predisposing conditions.
- Bacterial culture and susceptibility testing for lesions that fail to heal rapidly or in septicemic animals
- Exam of the spiracle and stigmal plates on the maggot can aid in species identification.
- Larvae can be submitted to a regional veterinary office for precautionary identification and confirmation if a suspicion of screwworm myiasis exists.

TREATMENT

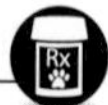

Treatment Overview

The goals are to remove and kill maggots, manage the wound(s), and identify and treat underlying predisposing conditions.

Acute General Treatment

- Stabilize the patient if needed (e.g., fluid resuscitation if hypotensive).
- Clip, clean, and surgically debride lesions (general anesthesia required).
- Mechanically remove larvae.
- Apply a non–alcohol-based pyrethrin or pyrethroid (dogs but not cats) spray on lesions to kill maggots.
- Systemically administered avermectins (ivermectin 0.2-0.4 mg/kg PO or SQ, may

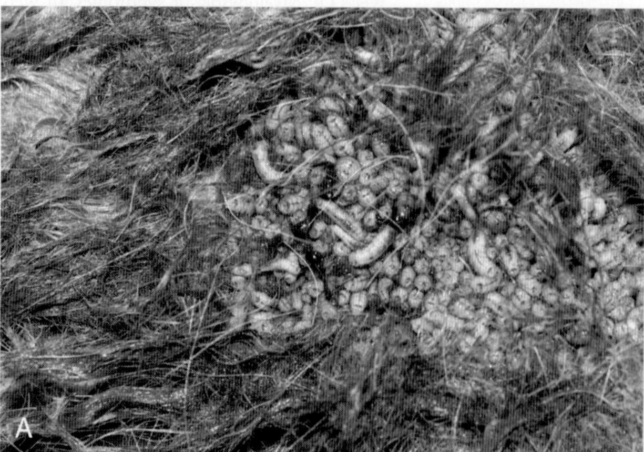

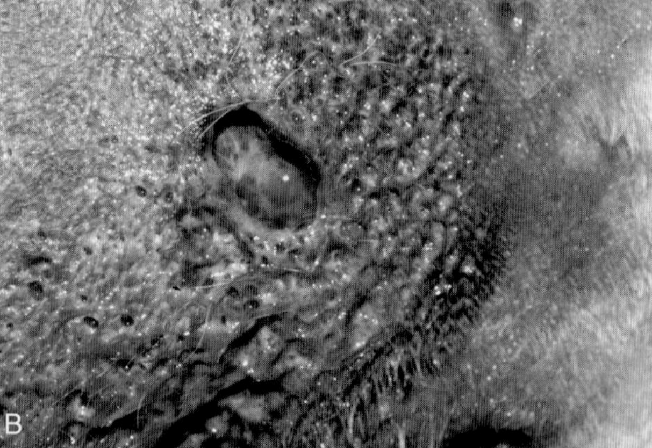

MYIASIS A, Numerous maggots packed into the open wound of a stray dog. **B,** The maggots have been removed, leaving a deep central ulcer with numerous satellite ulcers. (From Hnilica KA, et al: Small animal dermatology: a color atlas and therapeutic guide, ed 4, Philadelphia: 2017, Elsevier.)

repeat in 7-14 days) for dogs (negative for heartworms) can be used for killing maggots. CAUTION: avoid in susceptible individuals (p. 638).

- Although not approved for myiasis, topical or orally-administered isoxazolines (NexGard, Bravecto, Credelio, or Simparica), oral nitenpyram (Capstar), or spinosad/milbemycin (Triflexis) at routine dosages have shown a maggot-cidal effect. In the United States, these drugs are labeled by the U.S. Food and Drug Administration, not the Environmental Protection Agency.
- Wound care (p. 1189)
- House animal in fly-free area (e.g., indoors, screened-in patio).
- Empirical antibiotic therapy for secondary bacterial infection (e.g., cephalexin 22-30 mg/kg PO q 8-12h or clavulanic acid–potentiated amoxicillin 12.5-20 mg/kg PO q 12h for 21-30 days)

PROGNOSIS & OUTCOME

Guarded to good, depending on the severity of the infestation and underlying predisposing conditions

PEARLS & CONSIDERATIONS

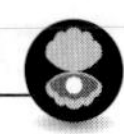

Comments

- Myiasis is a disease of neglect.
- Depending on the country, some types of myiases are reportable.
- Avoid crushing or cutting maggots *in vivo* because remaining body parts may cause allergic reactions.

Prevention

Animals with wounds (including perianal fistulas) should be housed indoors.

Technician Tips

In warm weather, myiasis is one of the reasons hygiene (avoidance of fecal staining or urinary scalding of the skin and haircoat) is so important, especially for recumbent patients.

Client Education

Basic hygiene care and early intervention when a pet is debilitated for any reason are essential for preventing myiasis.

SUGGESTED READING

Miller WH Jr, et al: Muller & Kirk's Small animal dermatology, ed 7, St. Louis, 2013, Saunders, pp 331-332.

AUTHOR: Adam P. Patterson, DVM, DACVD
EDITOR: Manon Paradis, DMV, MVSc, DACVD

Myocarditis

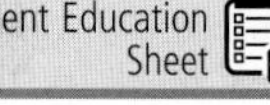

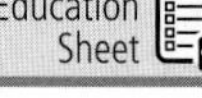

BASIC INFORMATION

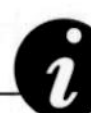

Definition

Myocarditis, which is inflammation of the heart muscle that is typically associated with myocytolysis, can result from infectious, chemical, or physical causes.

Epidemiology

SPECIES, AGE, SEX

Myocarditis occurs rarely and is recognized more often in dogs than in cats. No age predisposition (exception: parvoviral myocarditis in puppies 3-8 weeks of age).

RISK FACTORS

- Can result from an extension of infectious endocarditis (p. 294)
- Dogs and cats that roam are at risk for traumatic and vector-borne causes of myocarditis.

GEOGRAPHY AND SEASONALITY

- Chagas' myocarditis *(Trypanosoma cruzi):* southern United States, Latin America
- Lyme myocarditis *(Borrelia burgdorferi):* more common in the northeastern United States

ASSOCIATED DISORDERS

- Myocarditis is often associated with cardiac arrhythmias (especially ventricular tachyarrhythmias, but occasionally atrial tachyarrhythmias or atrioventricular [AV] block).
- Myocarditis, if chronic, may lead to dilated cardiomyopathy (DCM) and congestive heart failure (CHF).

Clinical Presentation

DISEASE FORMS/SUBTYPES

Myocarditis encompasses a range of etiologies resulting in many clinical and histologic manifestations. For viral myocarditis, three phases of disease are recognized:

- Phase 1: acute myocarditis associated with acute viremia, myocyte necrosis, and macrophage activation
- Phase 2: subacute myocarditis associated with viral clearing and overzealous immune response by cell-mediated and humoral immunity and cytokine activation
- Phase 3: chronic myocarditis, or DCM, associated with cardiac remodeling, fibrosis, cardiac dilation, and CHF

In veterinary medicine, myocarditis is most often recognized in the chronic phase in a young dog that is not of a breed commonly associated with DCM and that presents with acute CHF, DCM, and severe arrhythmias.

HISTORY, CHIEF COMPLAINT

Presenting complaint can be vague or specific to the cardiovascular system and may include

- Anorexia
- Lethargy/exercise intolerance
- Cough/dyspnea
- Syncope
- Sudden death
- With traumatic myocarditis, a history of having been hit by a car is common.

PHYSICAL EXAM FINDINGS

Possible findings include

- Signs of CHF (p. 408)
- Cardiac arrhythmias ± pulse deficits
- Possible fever or history of febrile illness
- Murmur
- Lymphadenopathy
- Skeletal muscle weakness
- With traumatic myocarditis, evidence of blunt chest trauma or generalized signs of trauma

Etiology and Pathophysiology

Mechanism:

- The heart's immune response to inflammation determines the structural and functional abnormalities in the cardiomyocyte; may result in subclinical disease that is often unnoticed, or substantial myocardial dysfunction and cardiac arrhythmias.

Etiology:

- Bacterial: *Bacillus piliformis, Citrobacter koseri*; streptococci, staphylococci, *Bartonella, Brucella, Leptospira, Salmonella* spp
- Spirochete: *Borrelia burgdorferi*
- Protozoan: *Trypanosoma cruzi, Toxoplasma gondii, Neospora caninum, Babesia* spp, *Leishmania infantum*
- Viral: parvovirus
- Other: doxorubicin chemotherapy, catecholamines, lead, arsenic, stinging insect and snake venom, hyperthermia, radiation therapy, blunt or penetrating trauma

DIAGNOSIS

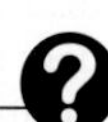

Diagnostic Overview

A clinical classification system for myocarditis in humans is based on the level of clinical certainty; it can be extrapolated to veterinary medicine:

- Possible subclinical myocarditis: subclinical patient with cardiac biomarkers,

electrocardiogram (ECG), and imaging abnormalities consistent with myocarditis
- Probable acute myocarditis: patient with acute CHF and cardiac biomarker, ECG, and imaging abnormalities (echocardiographic or MRI) consistent with myocarditis
- Definite myocarditis: histopathologic confirmation

Differential Diagnosis

- Infective endocarditis
- Idiopathic DCM
- Sepsis

Initial Database

- CBC, serum biochemistry profile, urinalysis: inflammatory leukogram possible
- Blood cultures for diagnosis of bacterial cause
- Cardiac troponin I (p. 1389) or other biomarker of cardiac necrosis: serum troponin levels usually are markedly elevated.
- Thoracic radiographs: may show signs of pulmonary edema and cardiomegaly
- Electrocardiogram (p. 1096): usually tachyarrhythmias (often ventricular arrhythmias [p. 1033]); occasionally bradyarrhythmias (AV block [p. 101])
- Echocardiogram (p. 1094): may show cardiac chamber dilation and global or regional myocardial dysfunction
- Infectious disease serologic tests for *Toxoplasma, Neospora, Bartonella*; based on geographic location, *Babesia*, Lyme, Chagas, and/or fungal titers may be indicated.

Advanced or Confirmatory Testing

- Endomyocardial biopsy and/or histopathologic evaluation (usually postmortem)
  - Considered the diagnostic gold standard
  - Rarely performed, due to invasive nature
  - Classic findings include lymphocyte infiltrates with myocyte necrosis (Dallas criteria); parvovirus inclusion bodies in cardiomyocytes are also possible.
- In acute viremia, parvovirus isolation may be attempted.
- MRI is an emerging modality, and early studies show high diagnostic accuracy for myocarditis.

TREATMENT

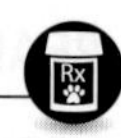

Treatment Overview

Treatment mainly consists of medications to control arrhythmias and CHF if present. If a bacterial or protozoal cause is suspected, antimicrobial treatment is recommended.

- Supportive care is the first line of therapy.
- Treatment of hemodynamically significant arrhythmias
- Pacemaker implantation for complete AV block
- Treatment of CHF with diuretics and vasodilators; support of cardiac output with positive inotropes may be necessary.
- Treatment with an antimicrobial agent if a bacterial or protozoan cause is suspected
- Immunosuppressive therapy has played an important role in some cases of myocarditis in humans; equivalent information for dogs and cats is lacking.

Acute and Chronic Treatment

- Severe ventricular arrhythmias (p. 1033)
- High-grade second-degree or third-degree AV block (p. 101)
- CHF (p. 408).
- Antimicrobial therapy: see specific infectious disease topics for recommendations.

Possible Complications

- Chronic CHF
- DCM
- Complete AV block
- Death

Recommended Monitoring

- Acute monitoring: continuous ECG, frequent blood pressure measurement (invasive or noninvasive), dyspnea watch and respiratory rate
- Chronic monitoring: periodic ECG or Holter monitor, echocardiogram, thoracic radiographs, renal and electrolyte parameters if receiving diuretics, convalescent serologic titers for suspected infectious diseases

PROGNOSIS & OUTCOME

Because myocarditis is an elusive diagnosis and uncommon disease, good information regarding prognosis and outcome is not known. The possibility of lethal arrhythmia and/or progression to DCM and CHF warrants an initial guarded prognosis.

PEARLS & CONSIDERATIONS

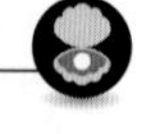

Comments

- In the author's clinical experience, myocarditis is strongly suspected when a dog presents with clinical signs attributable to a sudden onset of complex ventricular arrhythmias or complete AV block with no clear underlying cause.
- Myocarditis is likely an underdiagnosed cause of acute CHF in an atypical dog breed with DCM.

Technician Tips

Cardiac troponin I is the gold standard biomarker to assess myocardial cell damage.

SUGGESTED READINGS

Calforio ALP, et al: Myocarditis: a clinical overview. Curr Cardiol Rep 19:63, 2017.

Sagar S, et al: Myocarditis. Lancet 379:738-747, 2012.

AUTHOR: Teresa DeFrancesco, DVM, DACVIM, DACVECC

EDITOR: Meg M. Sleeper, VMD, DACVIM

Nasal Cutaneous Disorders

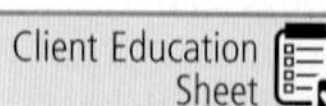

BASIC INFORMATION

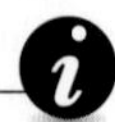

Definition

Dermatoses affecting the bridge of the nose (haired) or the nasal planum (hairless). This distribution of lesions is relatively common in dogs and cats, and lesions can be restricted to the nasal area or be part of a more generalized condition.

Epidemiology

SPECIES, AGE, SEX

- Affects dogs and cats
- Diseases more likely to appear in dogs < 1 year of age: demodicosis, dermatophytosis, dermatomyositis, hereditary nasal parakeratosis, juvenile cellulitis
- Epitheliotropic (cutaneous) lymphoma and nasodigital hyperkeratosis are more commonly seen in older dogs.

GENETICS, BREED PREDISPOSITION

- Nasal parakeratosis: Labrador retrievers
- Zinc-responsive dermatosis: Alaskan Malamutes, Siberian Huskies, bull terriers
- Dermatomyositis: collies, Shetland sheepdogs, Beauceron shepherds
- Uveodermatologic syndrome: Akitas, Alaskan Malamutes, Samoyeds, Siberian Huskies, chow chows, Australian shepherds, others
- Systemic lupus erythematosus (SLE) and cutaneous (discoid) lupus erythematosus (DLE): collies, Shetland sheepdogs, German shepherds
- Proliferative arteritis of the nasal philtrum: Saint Bernards
- Alopecia and melanoderma: Yorkshire terriers
- Familial vasculopathy: German shepherds, Scottish terriers
- Acrodermatitis: bull terriers
- Lentigo simplex: orange cats
- Vitiligo: Siamese cats, Belgian sheepdogs, rottweilers, Old English sheepdogs, Doberman pinschers
- Ulcerative nasal dermatitis: Bengal cat

RISK FACTORS

- Sun exposure can cause or aggravate canine and feline solar dermatitis, DLE, SLE, and pemphigus erythematosus.
  - Lack of skin pigmentation can predispose to sun damage.
- Susceptible dogs fed diets high in phytates (high-cereal content) or in minerals such as calcium can develop zinc-responsive dermatosis.

CONTAGION AND ZOONOSIS

Contagion (e.g., dermatophytosis) and/or zoonosis (e.g., feline sporotrichosis) possible, depending on the cause

GEOGRAPHY AND SEASONALITY

- Animals living in sunny climates more commonly develop photoaggravated dermatitis.
- Animals living in areas endemic for leishmaniasis are susceptible to the disease.

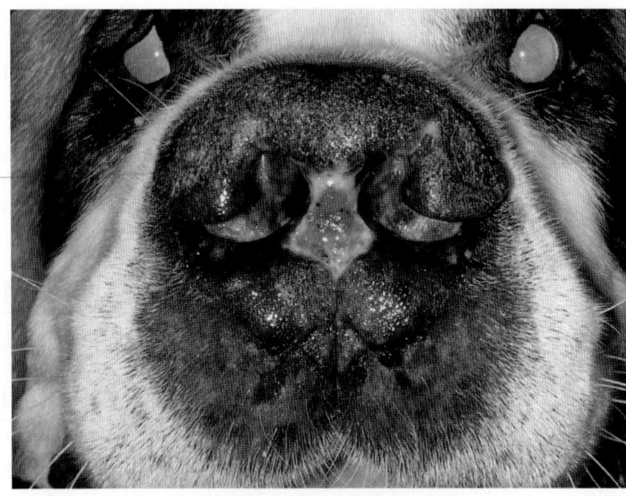

NASAL CUTANEOUS DISORDERS Proliferative nasal arteritis in an 8-year-old, male Saint Bernard. Note the ulcerative lesion on the nasal philtrum. (Courtesy Dr. Nadia Pagé.)

ASSOCIATED DISORDERS

- Granulomatous uveitis in uveodermatologic syndrome
- Systemic disease in SLE
- Hepatopathy or glucagon-producing pancreatic tumor in superficial necrolytic dermatitis

Clinical Presentation

HISTORY, CHIEF COMPLAINT

Presentation depends on the underlying disease:

- Nonpruritic hair loss confined to the bridge of the nose (e.g., localized demodicosis, localized dermatophytosis) or with a generalized dermatopathy (e.g., generalized demodicosis, dermatophytosis, endocrinopathies)
- Pruritus and facial rubbing, with secondary nasal alopecia in cases of allergic disease or intranasal foreign bodies (usually accompanied by sneezing and/or nasal discharge)
- Erosions and ulcers in cases of immune-mediated diseases or nodules and plaques (e.g., neoplastic, cutaneous histiocytosis, fungal diseases)
- Signs of systemic illness may be reported concurrently with generalized disorders (e.g., systemic mycoses, SLE, systemic histiocytosis).

PHYSICAL EXAM FINDINGS

Any of the following are possible, depending on the cause and severity:

- Nasal depigmentation or hyperpigmentation
- Alopecia
- Erythema
- Papules/pustules/vesicles
- Erosions/ulcers
- Crusts
- Hyperkeratosis
- Nodules/plaques

Etiology and Pathophysiology

Nasal lesions arise from various pathologic mechanisms:

- Infectious agents induce an immune response from the host, resulting in tissue inflammatory cell infiltrates (e.g., folliculitis, furunculosis, granulomatous lesions).
- Altered cornification process results in hyperkeratosis.
- Development of antibodies or activated lymphocytes against normal body constituents (autoimmune diseases) or against inciting antigens (drugs, bacteria, viruses) leads to tissue damage.
- Defective melanin production or destruction of melanocytes leads to pigment disorders; a disturbance at the dermoepidermal junction can cause hypopigmentation.
- Solar exposure of poorly pigmented nasal skin results in a phototoxic reaction (sunburn) and immune-mediated diseases, such as pemphigus erythematosus, SLE, and DLE; can also be photoaggravated.

DIAGNOSIS

Diagnostic Overview

The presenting complaint of nasal cutaneous abnormalities warrants a dermatologic exam. Selection of diagnostic tests is based on history and physical exam.

Differential Diagnosis

- Infectious
  - Bacterial: mucocutaneous pyoderma, nasal pyoderma, feline leprosy
  - Fungal: dermatophytosis, sporotrichosis, cryptococcosis, aspergillosis, blastomycosis, histoplasmosis
  - Parasitic: demodicosis
  - Protozoal: leishmaniasis
  - Rickettsial: canine Rocky Mountain spotted fever, canine ehrlichiosis
  - Viral: canine distemper; herpesvirus and calicivirus infections in cats
- Immune-mediated: pemphigus foliaceus and erythematosus, SLE, DLE, uveodermatologic syndrome, canine proliferative arteritis of the nasal philtrum, canine eosinophilic furunculosis, feline mosquito bite hypersensitivity
- Hereditary (see Genetics, Breed Predisposition above)
- Pigmentary: nasal depigmentation (Dudley nose), seasonal nasal hypopigmentation (snow nose), vitiligo, alopecia and melanoderma, lentigo simplex
- Metabolic/endocrine: superficial necrolytic dermatitis (hepatocutaneous syndrome), canine hypothyroidism
- Nutritional: zinc-responsive dermatosis
- Environmental/traumatic: phototoxicity (sunburn), contact dermatitis, local trauma
- Drug eruption: from topical or systemic administration
- Neoplastic: squamous cell carcinoma (SCC), basal cell carcinoma, epitheliotropic lymphoma, fibroma, feline sarcoid, others
- Miscellaneous: sterile granuloma/pyogranuloma syndrome, reactive cutaneous and systemic histiocytosis, nasodigital hyperkeratosis

Initial Database

- Wood's lamp (cats > dogs): dermatophytosis (fluorescent strains of *Microsporum canis* [p. 247])
- Skin cytologic exam (p. 1091): phagocytized bacteria, inflammatory cells, acantholytic keratinocytes (pemphigus), fungal organisms
- Skin scrapings (p. 1091): *Demodex* spp
- CBC, serum biochemistry profile, urinalysis (if concurrent systemic disease is suspected): results depend on underlying cause and are often normal or show nonspecific changes when cause is not systemic.
- Ocular exam (if vision loss or visible ocular lesions): uveitis (uveodermatologic syndrome) (p. 1137)
- Thoracic and abdominal imaging, if relevant, to confirm systemic disease or stage tumors

Advanced or Confirmatory Testing

- Skin biopsies for histopathologic evaluation: indicated when initial database is

inconclusive and nasal lesions persist. Using general anesthesia, nasal planum lesions can be biopsied with a 3- or 4-mm biopsy punch. The lesion should be centered in the specimen. If possible, multiple specimens should be taken of primary lesions (e.g., pustules, papules, bullae). Crusted lesions or depigmented lesions can also be useful.
- Culture: bacterial, fungal (evidence of bacterial/fungal infection and resistance to prior treatment)
- Antinuclear antibody (ANA) test: if SLE is suspected
- Endocrine or serologic testing if relevant

TREATMENT

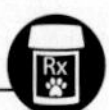

Treatment Overview

The goal of treatment is to achieve permanent cure or control of the disease. Topical treatment may be sufficient for localized and/or superficial skin disorders, whereas systemic therapy (ranging from simple to ongoing and intensive) may be needed when nasal cutaneous disorders are the first expression of a serious medical condition. For some benign conditions, treatment may not be warranted.

Acute General Treatment

Treatment depends on the cause of the lesions. Infectious diseases can be cured with appropriate treatment. Other diseases may need chronic maintenance treatment.

PROGNOSIS & OUTCOME

Varies, depending on the underlying disease

PEARLS & CONSIDERATIONS

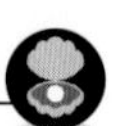

Comments

- Skin biopsies are often needed for diagnosis of nasal cutaneous disorders.
- Loss of pigment on the ventral nasal planum in areas of nasal discharge may suggest nasal aspergillosis.
- In addition to color change of the nasal planum, look for changes in the normal cobblestone texture. Inflammatory and infiltrative processes cause loss of this texture in addition to loss of pigment.

Prevention

- Prevent sun exposure, and use sunscreens on poorly pigmented animals and/or with photoaggravated diseases.
- Discourage breeding of animals with hereditary diseases.

Technician Tips

Some nasal cutaneous disorders worsen substantially with sunlight. Proper precautions (e.g., short walk, sunscreen) should be taken with patients with this type of problem.

SUGGESTED READING

Miller WH Jr, et al: Muller & Kirk's Small animal dermatology, ed 7, St. Louis, 2013, Elsevier.

AUTHOR: Nadia Pagé, DMV, MSc, DACVD
EDITOR: Manon Paradis, DMV, MVSc, DACVD

Nasal Discharge

BASIC INFORMATION

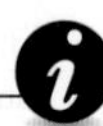

Definition

A common complaint in dogs and cats, nasal discharge may be the result of intranasal or extranasal (systemic) disease. Characterization of time course (acute or chronic), location (unilateral or bilateral), and character (serous, mucoid, purulent, hemorrhagic, or mixed) is necessary to determine the cause and treatment.

Synonyms

Hemorrhagic: epistaxis, nosebleed

Epidemiology

SPECIES, AGE, SEX

- Viral rhinitis is most common in young dogs (e.g., canine distemper virus) and cats (e.g., feline calicivirus).
- Foreign bodies (FBs) are most common in young dogs and cats. Usually accompanied by peracute sneezing
- Nasal tumors can occur at all ages but most often ≥ 5 years.

GENETICS, BREED PREDISPOSITION

- Primary ciliary dyskinesia can affect any breed, but Old English sheepdogs, English cocker spaniels, and Newfoundland dogs are overrepresented.
- Brachycephalic breeds have increased nasal mucosal contact points and aberrant caudal turbinates that may result in reduced antigenic clearance and intranasal stenosis.
- Mesocephalic and dolichocephalic dogs are at increased risk for sinonasal aspergillosis; brachycephalic cats are most commonly diagnosed with sinonasal/orbital aspergillosis.
- Doliocephalic dogs predisposed to nasal neoplasia

RISK FACTORS

- Lack of immunization and exposure to unvaccinated animals
- Severe periodontal disease

CONTAGION AND ZOONOSIS

Viral respiratory tract infections are highly contagious.

GEOGRAPHY AND SEASONALITY

- Dysautonomia occurs mostly in dogs in the Midwestern United States
- Grass awn FB more likely in some areas, seasons
- *Cryptococcus gattii* most often recognized in Australia, Pacific coastal areas of Canada and the United States

ASSOCIATED DISORDERS

Sneezing, stertor, cough, dysphonia, and pyrexia (if systemic infection)

Clinical Presentation

DISEASE FORMS/SUBTYPES

- Systemic disease (with nasal signs) or nasal disease
- Discharge character
  - Serous: clear (acellular)
  - Mucoid (M): clear and thick (acellular with high protein)
  - Purulent (P): yellow to brown and thick (neutrophilic with bacteria)
  - Hemorrhagic (epistaxis): frank blood
  - Combinations: mucopurulent (MP) most common
- Time course
  - Peracute/acute
  - Chronic
- Locations
  - Unilateral
  - Bilateral
  - Unilateral progressing to bilateral

HISTORY, CHIEF COMPLAINT

In addition to routine history questions (e.g., systemic signs, vaccinations, travel history, exposure to other animals), careful questioning about character and duration of discharge, laterality, progression, and response to prior treatment can provide key clues.

- Acute onset of epistaxis: suspect coagulopathy (p. 433) or less likely systemic disease (e.g., *Ehrlichia canis*, severe hypertension). Epistaxis can be the first sign of nasal neoplasia, fungal rhinitis, or FB.
- Acute onset of M or MP discharge: if pawing at face, suspect FB; if recent animal exposure or systemic illness, suspect viral infection
- Chronic, minimally progressive course: suspect structural nasal disease (e.g., stenosis, oronasal fistulae, chronic FB), inflammatory disease (e.g., lymphoplasmacytic rhinitis), or parasitic disease (i.e., mites)
- Chronic, progressive course (especially with unilateral to bilateral progression): suspect

nasal neoplasia, fungal rhinitis, or progressive severe dental disease
- Seizures raise concern about an infiltrative disease (e.g., neoplasia, mycoses) crossing the cribriform plate.

PHYSICAL EXAM FINDINGS

In addition to typical exam, note character and laterality of discharge (p. 1255), assess nasal airflow; condition of teeth, gums, and roof of mouth; facial symmetry; nasal planum pigmentation; eye position and ability to retropulse globes; and percussion of muzzle and frontal sinuses.

- Airflow can be assessed by 1) occlusion of each nostril one at a time, 2) holding a microscope slide in front of each nostril to visualize condensation, and 3) holding a wisp of cotton in front of each nostril to watch movement. Airflow may be reduced by neoplasia, granuloma, or mucus occlusion.
- Oral exam: look for tooth root abscess, oronasal fistulas, cleft palate, or other structural abnormalities
- Facial deformity suggests neoplastic or fungal disease. Feline cryptococcosis often causes a Roman nose.
- Nasal planum depigmentation is commonly identified in nasal aspergillosis (ventral depigmentation), immune-mediated disease (e.g., discoid lupus erythematosus)
- Inability to retropulse eye suggests a space-occupying lesion (e.g., abscess, neoplasia, granuloma).
- Ocular discharge suggests concurrent systemic disease (e.g., infection, dysautonomia, keratoconjunctivitis sicca with neurogenic rhinitis) or occlusion of nasolacrimal duct (tumor).
- Dysphonia, stertor, or Horner's syndrome suggests nasopharyngeal polyp.
- Pyrexia suggests systemic disease (e.g., canine distemper virus).
- Harsh lung sounds not referred from upper-airway or adventitial sounds suggest systemic disease.
- Submandibular lymphadenopathy suggests oral disease, metastatic neoplasia, or fungal infection

Etiology and Pathophysiology

- Nasal discharge may be a sign of systemic illness or may be due to local nasal pathology.
- Nasal pathology includes inflammatory, infectious, and neoplastic disorders, as well as structural issues.

DIAGNOSIS

Diagnostic Overview

Signalment, history, and exam influence the type and order of diagnostics. In some circumstances (e.g., young animals with acute-onset MP discharge thought to be from upper respiratory infection, chronic serous discharge believed to be from nasal mites), empirical therapy is appropriate without additional testing. Additional considerations include the owner's goals as well as diagnostic availability and costs.

Differential Diagnosis

Differential diagnoses are provided on p. 1255.

Initial Database

- CBC, serum chemistry profile, urinalysis, feline retroviral serology: assess health before anesthesia, rule out thrombocytopenia if hemorrhagic discharge
- If platelet count is normal with epistaxis, consider buccal mucosal bleeding time, coagulation profile, infectious disease serology (e.g., *E. canis*, *Bartonella* spp, *Anaplasma* spp), blood pressure
- Aspirate any enlarged submandibular lymph node for cytologic exam.
- Obvious mass or deformity may be amenable to fine-needle aspiration for cytology.
- Consider serologic tests for cryptococcosis (p. 223), sinonasal aspergillosis (p. 81), or systemic infection.
- Consider thoracic radiographs to rule out pneumonia, metastatic lung disease.
- Consider cytology of impression from nasal discharge; has extremely low sensitivity but occasionally recognizes fungal elements or neoplastic cells

Advanced or Confirmatory Testing

The choice of advanced diagnostic modalities depends on a patient-specific list of differentials, availability of diagnostics, and cost.

- Thorough oral exam requires anesthesia and may be combined with dental radiographs and cleaning.
  - In older animals or those with obvious dental disease, this is often the first step in evaluation of chronic MP nasal discharge.
- Imaging studies are often the next step in evaluation of chronic or progressive discharge.
  - Skull radiographs: multiple views (including open mouth) under general anesthesia; difficult to distinguish soft tissue from nasal discharge; generally inferior to other imaging modalities
  - Skull CT: modality of choice; ability to use contrast allows soft tissue to be distinguished from discharge, provides excellent bony detail (e.g., loss of turbinates) and better anatomic detail than radiographs, allows assessment of cribriform plate integrity, allows planning for radiation therapy
  - Skull MRI: excellent soft-tissue detail; sometimes used in place of CT
  - Findings on advanced imaging (CT/MRI) may be pathognomonic for some disease processes.
  - If owner is likely to consider radiation therapy should the diagnosis be nasal carcinoma, pet should be referred for advance imaging rather than starting with skull radiographs.
  - Imaging studies should precede rhinoscopy because bleeding will obscure images.
- Rhinoscopy allows direct visualization of the nasal passages and the choanae. Although tumors or fungal plaques are often recognized, FB may remain hidden (p. 1159).
- Nasal lavage, hydropulsion may be used to dislodge FB or tissue for exam.
- Nasal culture is rarely rewarding. Nasal discharge should never be cultured, but culture of nasal biopsy or deep nasal swabs is occasionally useful.
- Biopsies are required for histologic diagnosis of nasal neoplasia or inflammatory rhinitis. Ideally, biopsy collection is guided by imaging.

TREATMENT

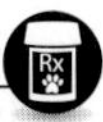

Treatment Overview

Treatment is aimed at addressing the cause for nasal discharge.

Acute General Treatment

- Nasal flush can be diagnostic and therapeutic.
- Dental disease or oronasal fistulas (pp. 7, 720, and 776)
- Nasopharyngeal polyp (p. 681)
- Nasal mites
- Nasal stenosis
- Sinonasal aspergillosis (p. 81)
- *Cryptococcus* spp (p. 223)
- Idiopathic lymphoplasmacytic rhinitis (p. 890)
- Nasal neoplasia (p. 680)
- Antibiotics are not routinely recommended. Many causes of nasal discharge result in secondary infection and improve temporarily with antibiotics, but discharge recurs unless the underlying issue is addressed.

Possible Complications

Nasal neoplasia may metastasize or invade into brain. Severe epistaxis can cause anemia/hypovolemia.

PROGNOSIS & OUTCOME

Depends on cause

PEARLS & CONSIDERATIONS

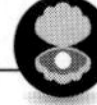

Comments

- Bacterial culture of nasal discharge is not useful.
- For devoted owners of pet with chronic nasal discharge, early referral for advanced diagnostics can save money and time.
- Rhinoscopy alone has limited diagnostic value and should be paired with advanced imaging.
- If advanced imaging is not possible, blind biopsies can be performed; it is important to educate the client that a diagnosis may be missed.
- For blind biopsy, premeasure the biopsy forceps to the medial canthus of the eye, and do not biopsy beyond that.
- Identifying the cause of chronic nasal discharge is often more rewarding in dogs than in cats.
- Without specific identification of an underlying cause, treatment of chronic nasal

discharge is often extremely frustrating for the veterinarian and pet owner.

Prevention

Nasal mites are prevented by routine use of heartworm and ectoparasites prophylactics.

Technician Tips

Physical manipulation of cats with reduced nasal airflow can prompt respiratory distress. Abort handling, and notify a veterinarian if a cat begins to open-mouth breathe.

SUGGESTED READING

Cohn LA: Canine nasal disease. Vet Clin North Am Small Anim Pract 44:75-89, 2014.

AUTHOR: Jared Jaffey, DVM, MS, DACVIM
EDITOR: Leah A. Cohn, DVM, PhD, DACVIM

Nasal Neoplasia

Client Education Sheet 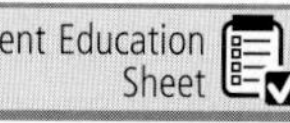

BASIC INFORMATION

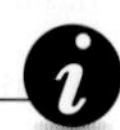

Definition

Neoplastic growth originating in the nasal passageways or sinuses

Synonyms

Nasosinal tumor, nasal tumor

Epidemiology

SPECIES, AGE, SEX

- Nasosinal tumors are ≈2% of canine neoplasia and are common in older dogs (mean, 9-10 years, youngest reported is 1 year).
- Nasosinal tumors are ≈1% of feline neoplasia and are common in older cats (mean, 8-10 years, youngest reported is 2 years).

GENETICS, BREED PREDISPOSITION

More common in dolichocephalic dogs

RISK FACTORS

Possible association with urban environments and smoke exposure

CONTAGION AND ZOONOSIS

Transmissible venereal tumor is contagious among dogs.

ASSOCIATED DISORDERS

- If the tumor extends into the brain, neurologic signs such as seizures can occur.
- Nasal lymphomas can progress to a systemic lymphoma with clinical signs reflecting the organ systems infiltrated.

Clinical Presentation

DISEASE FORMS/SUBTYPES

Malignant:

- Epithelial
  - Two-thirds of canine nasal tumors; adenocarcinoma and, less frequently, squamous cell carcinoma and anaplastic carcinoma
  - Uncommon in cats; adenocarcinoma and squamous cell carcinoma
- Mesenchymal
  - One-third of canine nasal tumors; chondrosarcoma and, less frequently, osteosarcoma and fibrosarcoma. Olfactory neuroblastoma is rare.
  - Rare in cats
- Round cell
  - Rare in dogs; transmissible venereal tumor in dogs living in endemic locations
  - Solitary nasal lymphoma is the most common nasal tumor in cats. Some cats eventually develop systemic lymphoma.

Benign:

- Inflammatory polyps (p. 681)
- Oral tumors may also extend into the nasal cavity.

HISTORY, CHIEF COMPLAINT

Most patients have had signs for 2-4 months before presentation.

- Unilateral or bilateral epistaxis or nasal discharge
- Sneezing/reverse sneezing
- Stertor
- Facial deformity or pain
- Dysphagia with invasion of the oral cavity
- Seizures with invasion into the brain

PHYSICAL EXAM FINDINGS

Signs may be unilateral or bilateral, depending on the stage.

- Decreased nasal airflow
- Stertor
- Epistaxis or nasal discharge
- Reduced or painful ocular retropulsion
- Mass effect above the soft palate
- Facial deformity or pain
- Enlarged mandibular lymph nodes ipsilateral to tumor

Etiology and Pathophysiology

Exposure to poor air quality (environmental contaminants) may increase the risk of neoplastic transformation.

DIAGNOSIS

Diagnostic Overview

Further evaluation is indicated if nasal discharge persists for more than 2-3 weeks or recurs after treatment, or for any pet with epistaxis.

Differential Diagnosis

- Epistaxis
  - Systemic disorders: coagulopathy (e.g., thrombocytopathy, thrombocytopenia, anticoagulant rodenticide intoxication), hypertension, hyperviscosity syndrome, vasculitis, ehrlichiosis
  - Nasal disease (p. 678)
- Nasal discharge/sneezing (pp. 678 and 1255)
- Facial deformity
  - Tooth root abscess
  - *Cryptococcus* (cats)

Initial Database

- CBC, biochemical profile, and urinalysis are typically unremarkable but can indicate chronic inflammation/hemorrhage.
- Mandibular lymph node aspirates (bilateral) to screen for local metastasis
- Thoracic radiographs to screen for pulmonary metastasis (uncommon at diagnosis)

Advanced or Confirmatory Testing

- Skull radiographs: not sensitive or specific; can show evidence of soft-tissue/fluid opacity in the nasal passages, displacement of midline, or bone destruction. High-quality images require general anesthesia.
- CT: preferred over nasal radiographs; allows tumor staging and treatment planning and extremely useful to distinguish fungal rhinitis from neoplasia. Perform scan before rhinoscopy or biopsy to prevent artifacts.
- MRI (p. 1132): provides excellent soft-tissue detail but not useful for radiation planning
- Biopsy (blind, transnasal, guided): if possible, use the location determined by CT to direct sampling. Be careful not to advance biopsy instrument past the medial canthus of the eye.
- Rhinoscopy (p. 1159): may not visualize tumor. Rhinoscopic biopsy specimens are frequently nondiagnostic.
- Abdominal ultrasound: for cats with nasal lymphoma to rule out systemic involvement

TREATMENT

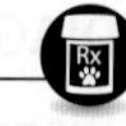

Treatment Overview

Malignant nasal tumors are rarely cured but are often well managed. The primary goal is controlling discomfort and morbidity.

Acute General Treatment

Urgent or acute treatment is seldom required. If epistaxis is profuse or sustained, consider:

- Sedation
- Intranasal epinephrine

- Icing the muzzle
- Packing the nasal cavity with gauze
- Ligation of the ipsilateral carotid artery for life-threatening hemorrhage
- Transfusion (p. 1169) for anemia due to blood loss is rarely required.

Chronic Treatment

External beam radiation therapy:
- Definitive-intent radiation is the most effective treatment option for dogs and cats with nasosinal tumors.
- Palliative-intent radiation provides less durable tumor control, but the acute side effects are reduced.

Chemotherapy:
- For dogs, chemotherapy can palliate clinical signs. Most protocols combine nonsteroidal antiinflammatory drugs (NSAIDs) with carboplatin, doxorubicin, or Palladia.
- For cats with nasal lymphoma, combining irradiation with chemotherapy does not improve survival compared with radiation therapy alone. With systemic involvement, a CHOP-based chemotherapy protocol is the primary treatment modality (p. 607).

Surgery:
- Surgery alone is not effective for controlling nasal tumors.
- Exenteration of the nasal cavity after radiation can improve survival but also increases side effects significantly.

Palliative medical management:
- Pain management, antiinflammatory agents (prednisolone in cats, NSAIDs in dogs), and antibiotics (e.g., clindamycin, amoxicillin plus clavulanic acid)

Possible Complications

- Acute radiation side effects develop 2-3 weeks into radiation and resolve after 2-3 weeks. They include mucositis, conjunctivitis, and moist desquamation. Typically, well controlled with pain medications, antibiotics, and comfort care
- Chronic radiation side effects are rare but can develop after 6-12 months. They can include bone necrosis, oronasal fistulas, keratoconjunctivitis sicca (KCS), and secondary tumor formation.
- Chemotherapy side effects are uncommon (20%-25% of patients) and vary depending on the medication. They typically resolve in 1-2 days with supportive care. The most common include gastrointestinal upset 2-3 days after treatment and neutropenia or thrombocytopenia 5-7 days after treatment. Serious complications, including septic neutropenia, are possible.

Recommended Monitoring

Recheck every 3 months. Monitor clinical signs, and do routine imaging (chest radiographs in dogs, abdominal ultrasound in cats) to monitor for systemic spread.

PROGNOSIS & OUTCOME

A range of median survival times (MST) are provided below to reflect the results of multiple studies.

Dogs:
- The overall median survival time (MST) with definitive radiation is ≈12 months. MST is ≈24 months for tumors limited to the nasal cavity, ≈10 months with SQ/oropharyngeal/orbital involvement, and ≈6 months with brain involvement.
- MST with palliative radiation therapy is ≈6-7 months.
- MST with chemotherapy is ≈5-7 months.
- MST with palliative medical management is ≈4 months.

Cats:
- MST for nasal lymphoma treated with definitive radiation is ≈18 months. With complete remission (CR), MST is ≈3 years; partial remission (PR) MST is ≈4 months.
- MST for nasal lymphoma treated with chemotherapy alone is 4-5 months. With CR, MST is ≈2 years, and PR MST is ≈2 months.
- MST for nonlymphoma nasal tumors treated with definitive radiation is ≈12 months.
- MST for all nasal tumors with palliative medical management is ≈2-4 months.

PEARLS & CONSIDERATIONS

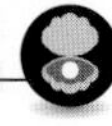

Comments

- If an animal owner is considering radiation therapy for treatment of a pet with possible nasal neoplasia, early referral for advanced imaging (e.g., CT scan) is suggested rather than pursuing nasal radiographs (can save time and money).
- Nasal tumors are rarely cured but are often well managed. The primary goal is controlling discomfort and morbidity from local disease.
- In dogs, distant metastasis develops late in the course of disease, and most dogs are euthanized due to failure of local disease control rather than for signs related to metastatic disease.
- In cats with nasal lymphoma, local control can result in prolonged survival. However, systemic involvement develops in 15% of cases. Cats can come out of remission even if there is no evidence of systemic involvement at the time of diagnosis. Cats with systemic involvement should be treated with a CHOP-based chemotherapy. Radiation can be used concurrently for palliation of nasal signs. Survival time depends on the organ systems involved and the response to chemotherapy.

Technician Tips

- Oronasal fistulas may be present and cause an increased risk of aspiration.
- Draw blood only from the jugular vein during the 72 hours before IV chemotherapy to spare peripheral veins for catheter placement.

Client Education

- Persistent or recurrent nasal discharge often requires advanced imaging and a biopsy to obtain a diagnosis.
- Nasal tumors are treatable but not curable. The side effects of treatment options are usually temporary and can be well controlled with oral medications at home.

SUGGESTED READING

Vail DM, Page RL: Nasosinal Tumors. In Withrow & MacEwen's Small animal clinical oncology, St. Louis, 2013, Saunders.

AUTHORS: Sarah B. Rippy, DVM; Melanie Moore, BVM&S, DVM
EDITOR: Megan Grobman, DVM, MS, DACVIM

Nasopharyngeal Polyps

Client Education Sheet 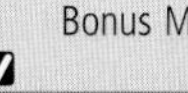 Bonus Material Online 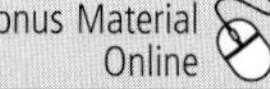

BASIC INFORMATION

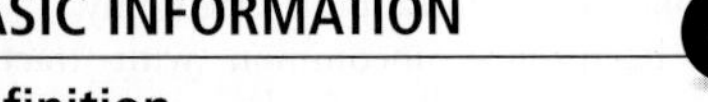

Definition

Non-neoplastic pedunculated mass originating from the middle ear or auditory tube epithelium

Synonym

Inflammatory polyp

Epidemiology

SPECIES, AGE, SEX

Well-recognized disorder in young adult cats but can occur at any age; rare in dogs

RISK FACTORS

Chronic inflammation of the upper respiratory tract or any process that obstructs middle ear drainage are proposed; may have a congenital origin.

ASSOCIATED DISORDERS

- Otitis media, interna, or externa
- Horner's syndrome

Clinical Presentation

DISEASE FORMS/SUBTYPES

- Nasopharyngeal polyp
- Ear (aural) polyp if mass grows into external ear canal instead of nasopharynx

HISTORY, CHIEF COMPLAINT

- Stertor
- Nasal discharge
- Sneezing
- Dyspnea
- Dysphagia
- Gagging
- Voice change
- ± Head shaking or pawing at ears in cases of concurrent otitis externa; concurrent nasopharyngeal and aural polyps reported in 18% of cats
- ± Vestibular signs or Horner's syndrome if concurrent otitis externa progresses to otitis media/interna

PHYSICAL EXAM FINDINGS

- Increased inspiratory noise (often stertor)
- Mucoid to mucopurulent nasal discharge (unilateral or bilateral)
- Gagging
- Unilateral deafness in 35% of cats because of concurrent middle ear disease (hard to recognize)
- Uncommon signs include otitis externa, submandibular swelling, regurgitation, head tilt, ataxia, nystagmus, or facial nerve palsy.
- ± Horner's syndrome: miosis, ptosis, enophthalmos, and third eyelid prolapse on affected side
- ± Rarely, severe inspiratory dyspnea

Etiology and Pathophysiology

- Exact cause is unknown, but proposed causes include inflammatory conditions and congenital persistence of branchial arches.
  - The significance of herpesvirus, calicivirus, bacteria, or fungi recovered from polyps is questionable.
- Proliferation of the auditory (eustachian) tube or tympanic bulla mucosal epithelium likely obstructs drainage from the middle ear. The resulting fluid accumulation and inflammation (otitis media) can extend into the inner ear (otitis interna) or drain through the tympanic membrane (otitis externa) and provokes formation of a fibrous polyp.
- Enlarged mass fills the nasopharyngeal region, obstructing caudal nasal drainage and airflow, and eventually impedes inspiration and swallowing causing nasal discharge.
- Alternatively, the tympanic membrane ruptures, and the mass extends into the horizontal ear canal.

DIAGNOSIS

Diagnostic Overview

The primary method of diagnosis is visualizing a firm, pink mass dorsal to the soft palate on oral exam under anesthesia. Confirmation is based on histologic analysis.

Differential Diagnosis

- Neoplasia (e.g., lymphoma, squamous cell carcinoma)
- Infectious rhinitis
- Nasal/nasopharyngeal foreign body
- Nasopharyngeal stenosis
- Laryngeal paralysis
- Granuloma (cryptococcosis)
- Hamartoma

Initial Database

- CBC, biochemistry panel, and urinalysis are usually normal.
- Otoscopic exam (p. 1144):
  - Bulging of tympanic membrane from fluid or mass if otitis media present
  - Aural polyp can extend through tympanic membrane into external ear canal.
  - Otitis externa if tympanic membrane ruptured

Advanced or Confirmatory Testing

- Oral exam under anesthesia (p. 1125):
  - Palpable mass dorsal to soft palate or mass protruding into oropharynx
  - Retraction of the soft palate may increase visualization
  - Often, this is the only confirmatory test required.
  - Removal may be performed immediately (see Acute Treatment).
- Skull radiographs (seldom necessary)
  - Increased soft-tissue density in pharynx (lateral or oblique lateral view)
  - Evidence of otitis media: enlarged or thickened bulla containing increased soft-tissue density (rostrocaudal view)
  - May be normal
- CT
  - Focal, contrast-enhancing, soft-tissue nasopharyngeal mass with stalk
  - Rim enhancement on CT differentiates from fluid and other neoplasia
  - Increased fluid and soft-tissue density in bulla. Bulla wall is thickened and pathologically expanded. Bilateral bulla disease in 31%
  - Enlarged ipsilateral medial retropharyngeal lymph node in 62%
- Endoscopy: both ear canals and nasopharynx
  - Aural polyps: pink-red, multilobulated masses in the ear canal/tympanic cavity. Waxy cerumen is common, If intact, thickening/bulging of the tympanum due to impaired auditory tube drainage is often seen. Myringotomy may be performed after exam.
  - Nasopharyngeal polyps: direct visualization of mass in the nasopharynx
- Histologic exam
  - Well-vascularized fibrous tissue covered by stratified squamous or columnar epithelium
  - Inflammatory cells, primarily lymphocytes, plasma cells, and macrophages, present in the stroma

TREATMENT

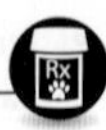

Treatment Overview

Nasopharyngeal polyp removal by gentle, steady traction and avulsion can cure many cats. Recurrence rates are lower if combined with oral prednisolone therapy or bulla osteotomy. Surgical removal may be required for aural polyps in dogs.

Acute General Treatment

- Oxygen supplementation (p. 1146) if in respiratory distress
- General anesthesia, intubation, and removal of the polyp: retract soft palate rostrally (spay hook, stay sutures, or Babcock forceps), and grasp the polyp gently at the base with Allis tissue forceps. Apply slow, steady traction to avulse stalk of polyp from auditory tube/middle ear. Minor to moderate hemorrhage may occur, requiring a short period of digital pressure or local packing.
- To reduce recurrence rate, oral prednisolone 1-2 mg/kg PO q 24h for 2 weeks, then 0.5-1 mg/kg PO q 24h for 1 week, then 0.5-1 mg/kg PO q 48h for 7-10 days or ventral bulla osteotomy with removal of the epithelial lining; culture from the bulla is also indicated at the time of surgery.
- Perendoscopic transtympanic traction (PTT) and laser ablation have been described for aural poly removal and may be associated with lower recurrence rates.

Chronic Treatment

Antibiotics if bacterial otitis media is suspected (e.g., amoxicillin-clavulanate 62.5 mg/CAT PO q 12h until culture results return)

Possible Complications

- Horner's syndrome: ≈80% of cases after bulla osteotomy; can also occur with polyp traction avulsion alone. Usually resolves within 1 month
- Otitis interna: ≈40% of cases after ventral bulla osteotomy; ataxia and head tilt can affect quality of life.

Recommended Monitoring

- Re-evaluate nasopharynx, bulla, and external ear canal if clinical signs recur.
- Repeat otoscopic exam and otic cytologic exam if otitis externa is present.

PROGNOSIS & OUTCOME

- Polyp regrowth occurs in 11%-50% of cats treated with traction avulsion without concurrent ventral bulla osteotomy.
  - Recurrence uncommon with traction removal followed by postoperative prednisolone
  - Ventral bulla osteotomy prevents recurrence in most cats after traction removal.
- Deafness in affected ear often persists after polyp removal.

PEARLS & CONSIDERATIONS

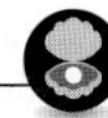

Comments

- Cats can have concurrent nasopharyngeal and aural polyps; both areas should be examined under anesthesia.
- CT is more sensitive than survey skull radiographs for detecting otitis media.
- For a broad-based mass, fine-needle aspiration and cytologic evaluation are indicated to rule out lymphoma.
- The feline tympanic bulla has two chambers; the epithelial lining of both chambers should be removed during bulla osteotomy, but dorsal curettage should be avoided.
- Sympathetic fibers are superficial in the feline bulla; development of Horner's syndrome is likely after bulla osteotomy and may occur with traction alone.

Technician Tips

- Cats with large nasopharyngeal polyps can be difficult to intubate. An IV catheter placed before induction permits administration of IV anesthetics, and a stylette may be needed for intubation.
- A laryngoscope and several sizes of cuffed endotracheal tubes should be available before induction. Mucus and saliva may collect in the caudal pharynx; suction or swabs may be needed during intubation.
- The endotracheal tube may need to be tied to the lower jaw to allow soft palate retraction.
- The cuff of the endotracheal tube should be inflated because hemorrhage is possible after polyp extraction.

Client Education

Complications with bulla osteotomy are common but usually temporary.

SUGGESTED READING

Anderson DM, et al: Management of inflammatory polyps in 37 cats. Vet Rec 147:684-687, 2000.

AUTHOR: Karen M. Tobias, DVM, MS, DACVS
EDITOR: Megan Grobman, DVM, MS, DACVIM

Neck Pain

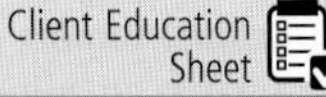

BASIC INFORMATION

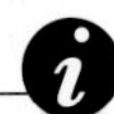

Definition

Sensation of discomfort or distress associated with the cervical spine or surrounding tissues

Synonyms

Cervical hyperesthesia or hyperpathia

Epidemiology

SPECIES, AGE, SEX

Dogs and cats of any age and either sex

GENETICS, BREED PREDISPOSITION

- Atlantoaxial instability: toy breeds: Chihuahua, toy poodle, Pomeranian, Pekingese
- Intervertebral disc disease (IVDD): chondrodystrophoid breeds: dachshund, beagle, basset hound, Pekingese, shih tzu, other breeds
- Cervical spondylomyelopathy (CSM) (e.g., wobbler syndrome): Great Dane, Doberman pinscher, many other large breeds
- Corticosteroid-responsive meningitis/arteritis: beagles, Bernese mountain dog, boxer, Nova Scotia duck tolling retriever

CONTAGION AND ZOONOSIS

- Canine distemper viral (CDV) myelitis: dog to dog
- *Brucella canis*–associated discospondylitis: dog to dog

ASSOCIATED DISORDERS

- Horner's syndrome possible with caudal cervical spinal lesions
- Nerve root signature may be sign of nerve root pain.

Clinical Presentation

DISEASE FORMS/SUBTYPES

- Spinal disease
  - Congenital: CSM in young Great Danes, atlantoaxial instability
  - Acquired/degenerative: IVDD, CSM in Doberman pinschers
  - Traumatic
- Infectious disease: canine distemper myelitis, systemic fungal myelitis, discospondylitis
- Inflammatory: cranial cervical pain sometimes found with meningitis
- Traumatic: cervical fractures, instability, penetrating pharyngeal or neck wounds
- Neoplastic: spinal tumors, axial skeletal osteosarcoma, nerve sheath tumor, and other such growths

HISTORY, CHIEF COMPLAINT

- Reluctance to rise
- Reluctance to walk on stairs
- Reluctance to jump
- Crying out when changing positions or moving head
- Shaking

PHYSICAL EXAM FINDINGS

- Abnormal head posture: holding head down, reluctant to turn head
- Arched neck or back
- Pain on manipulation of the neck or palpation ventral process of C6
- Pain on palpation of the cervical musculature
- Reluctance to walk
- Abnormal gait if animal is neurologically impaired
- Heat and swelling in cervical tissues
- Hypersalivation possible with pharyngeal injuries
- Fever associated with infections or meningitis
- Root signature

Etiology and Pathophysiology

Epaxial musculature:
- Traumatic muscle injury
- Myositis from penetrating injury or foreign body (stick or grass awn migration)
- Inflammatory myositis: immune mediated, parasitic, bacterial, or protozoal

Spinal column:
- IVDD: progressive degeneration of intervertebral disc, resulting in protrusion or herniation of disc material into the spinal canal. The annulus fibrosus is the portion of the disc that contains pain receptors. Typically affects dogs 3-8 years of age but can also occur in cats
- Discospondylitis: bacterial infection of vertebral body endplates; the caudal cervical region is one of the predisposition sites.
- Malformation: CSM in Great Danes, hemivertebrae, spinal canal stenosis
- Instability: atlantoaxial malformation, CSM, vertebral subluxation, traumatic fracture or luxation
- Neoplasia: osteosarcoma, hemangiosarcoma, fibrosarcoma, chondrosarcoma, or metastatic tumors involving the vertebrae

Meninges:
- Inflammatory, parasitic, protozoal, bacterial, and neoplastic processes

Spinal nerves:
- Nerve root compression, ischemia
- Inflammation: immune mediated, infectious (protozoal, viral, parasitic)
- Neoplasia

DIAGNOSIS

Diagnostic Overview

The diagnosis of neck pain is made by observation of the patient and physical exam. Determining the underlying cause of neck pain begins with orthopedic and neurologic exams and a review of the history to identify duration and severity of signs and response to treatment.

Differential Diagnosis

A detailed differential diagnosis is provided on p. 1256.
- IVDD
- Meningitis
- Cervical spondylomyelopathy

- Foreign body/abscess
- Trauma/fracture
- Neoplasia

Initial Database

- Neurologic and orthopedic exams (p. 1136 and 1143)
- CBC, serum biochemistry panel, urinalysis
- Neck radiographs

Advanced or Confirmatory Testing

- Myelography, CT, or MRI (p. 1132): very useful for spinal imaging
  - Myelograms with dynamic views (under careful patient manipulation) may be useful for diagnosis of CSM and for IVDD and some spinal tumors.
  - MRI is best for spinal cord and nerve lesions and increasingly used for IVDD.
  - CT is best for evaluating bony lesions (spinal tumors or fractures) and can be used as an adjunct to myelography.
- Cerebrospinal fluid (CSF) tap if meningitis or neoplasia is suspected (pp. 1080 and 1323)
- Serologic titers or polymerase chain reaction (PCR) testing of blood or CSF as appropriate (e.g., CDV, *Brucella* card test)
- Aspiration or biopsy of abnormal tissues
- Ultrasound of soft tissues to locate an abscess, foreign body, neoplasm, or other such abnormalities
- Surgical exploration: histopathologic evaluation of tissue samples, bacterial culture and susceptibility (C&S)
- Urine culture ± blood culture (p. 1333) if there is a concern about discospondylitis

TREATMENT

Treatment Overview

In most cases, therapeutic tenets are relief of pain, immobilization if movement is detrimental or painful, and treatment of underlying disease process.

Acute General Treatment

- Animals with acute severe neck pain are often initially treated with cage rest and medications such as analgesics (hydromorphone 0.1-0.2 mg/kg SQ, IM, or IV q 4-6h, buprenorphine 10-30 mcg/kg IV q 6-8h, or butorphanol 0.1-0.2 mg/kg IV as needed up to q 4h) and/or muscle relaxants (methocarbamol 20-50 mg/kg PO q 8h). Empirical glucocorticoids given before ruling out infectious causes can exacerbate infectious diseases.
- If spinal instability is suspected, a neck brace for immobilizing the neck can provide pain relief and prevent further tissue damage. Cage rest and exercise restriction are important for the same purpose.

Chronic Treatment

Specific treatment of the underlying cause is paramount. Nonspecific treatment should not interfere with diagnosis or treatment of the underlying cause:

- Nonsteroidal antiinflammatory drugs (NSAIDs (e.g., carprofen 2 mg/kg PO q 12h, etodolac 10-15 mg/kg PO q 24h, deracoxib 1-2 mg/kg PO q 24h, firocoxib 4-5 mg/kg PO q 24h, grapiprant 2 mg/kg PO q 24h, or meloxicam 0.1 mg/kg PO q 24h)
- Low-dose glucocorticoids: never combine with NSAIDs. Glucocorticoids should be tapered after improvement. Typical recommended course: prednisone 0.25-0.5 mg/kg PO q 12h × 4-5 days, then q 24h for 4-5 days, then q 48h for 4-5 doses
- Amantidine 3-5 mg/kg PO q 24h, tramadol 1-4 mg/kg PO q 8-12h, or gabapentin 10 mg/kg PO q 8h for adjunctive pain control
- Acupuncture (p. 1056)
- Surgery if indicated by imaging, emergent disorder, and/or lack of response to conservative therapy
- Treatment of specific infectious disease if identified

Behavior/Exercise

- Exercise restriction
- Use of a harness instead of a collar for walks
- Elevation of food and water bowls

Drug Interactions

Do not coadminister NSAIDs with glucocorticoids due to risk of serious or life-threatening gastroenteritis and gastrointestinal (GI) ulceration.

Possible Complications

- Adverse reactions to the medication, especially GI ulceration caused by taking glucocorticoids and NSAIDs simultaneously
- Pneumonia is a common complication in dogs that have tetraparesis and are recumbent.
- Respiratory obstruction is possible with a neck brace; it is important to adjust the brace so it fits properly, and the owner and clinician should monitor the animal.
- Paralysis or death is possible with acute spinal injury.

Recommended Monitoring

Any dog with signs of neck pain should be closely monitored for the development of neurologic conditions such as ataxia, paresis, paralysis, and respiratory impairment. These conditions often warrant further intervention and intensive care.

PROGNOSIS & OUTCOME

Varies, depending on underlying disease process

PEARLS & CONSIDERATIONS

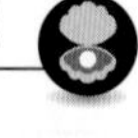

Comments

- Neck pain in certain dog breeds is a common problem in clinical practice.
- All dogs being considered for nonspecific supportive treatment should first have cervical spinal radiographs.
- Cage rest, typically for at least 4 weeks, is a critical component of conservative treatment for dogs with IVDD.
- If a dog does not respond appropriately to nonspecific supportive therapy, the clinician should perform further diagnostic testing.

Technician Tips

- Observe for any signs of developing weakness or neurologic deficits.
- Progressive swelling/pain and heat may alert to need for additional diagnostics and treatment.

Client Education

- Owners should be informed to use a harness for walks.
- Cage rest is critical in conservative management of IVDD.
- The clinician should inform the owner about exercise restrictions.

SUGGESTED READING

Platt SR, et al: Cervical spine. In Tobias KM, et al, editors: Veterinary surgery: small animal, St. Louis, 2012, Saunders, pp 410-448.

AUTHOR: David A. Puerto, DVM, DACVS
EDITOR: Leah A. Cohn, DVM, PhD, DACVIM

Necrotizing Fasciitis

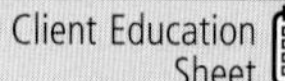

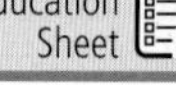

Client Education Sheet

BASIC INFORMATION

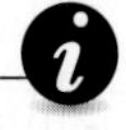

Definition

Fulminant, rapidly progressing infection of the skin, subcutis, and fascia that can lead to tissue necrosis, severe pain, and septic shock

Synonyms

Flesh-eating disease, flesh-eating bacteria

Epidemiology

SPECIES, AGE, SEX

Dogs and cats of any age or sex

RISK FACTORS

Injury, such as a bite wound or motor vehicle accident

CONTAGION AND ZOONOSIS

The risk of zoonosis is low, but humans can have the same clinical disease caused by the same/similar organisms. Considering the potential severity of disease, good hygiene practices should be employed, especially in cases of broken skin or mucous membrane contact. Risk may be increased for immunocompromised individuals.

ASSOCIATED DISORDERS

Toxic shock syndrome

Clinical Presentation

DISEASE FORMS/SUBTYPES

Type II (single-organism) infections of beta-hemolytic group G *Streptococcus* predominate in dogs, but other causative agents have been identified.

HISTORY, CHIEF COMPLAINT

Many patients have a history of penetrating trauma, but cases have also been reported after vaccination and nonpenetrating wounds. Swelling and lameness may be noted by owner.

- Concurrent sepsis results in typical clinical signs: anorexia, depression, lethargy, and weakness, leading to hypotension, shock, and multiorgan failure (p. 907)
- Clinical disease is acute and rapidly progressive

PHYSICAL EXAM FINDINGS

- Signs include localized heat, swelling, erythema, and pain (severe).
  - Muscle bellies may be hard and severely painful on palpation.
- Skin is variously affected, ranging from normal to soft and exudative to an erythematous/blackened eschar
- Limb involvement is commonly reported in dogs.
- Systemic signs include fever, tachycardia, and dehydration.

Etiology and Pathophysiology

- Causative organism: Lancefield group G, beta-hemolytic *Streptococcus* consistent; *Streptococcus canis* is most commonly cultured. *Staphylococcus pseudintermedius, Clostridium* spp, *Pasteurella multocida, Pseudomonas aeruginosa,* and other bacteria have been reported to cause necrotizing fasciitis.
- Bacterial exotoxins and proteases cause tissue destruction/necrosis and clinical signs.
- An extremely rapid course of progression (line of tissue inflammation/edema visibly advances over minutes to hours) is a hallmark of necrotizing fasciitis, ultimately leading to sepsis and/or the systemic inflammatory response syndrome (SIRS).

DIAGNOSIS

Diagnostic Overview

A presumptive diagnosis is made when soft-tissue pain is disproportionate to evident trauma and subcutaneous tissues can be easily dissected. On palpation and probing of the affected area, a lack of resistance of affected fascial planes is characteristic. Fractures as a source of pain are ruled out with radiographs. Confirmation requires bacterial culture and histopathology, but treatment must be instituted before results of these tests are available.

Differential Diagnosis

- Cellulitis
- Subcutaneous abscess, seroma, or hematoma
- Soft-tissue or orthopedic trauma
  - Fractures
  - Blunt trauma
  - Bites
  - Penetrating projectiles (e.g., gunshot)
- Envenomation, especially snake bite

Initial Database

- CBC, serum biochemistry profile, urinalysis
  - Nonspecific abnormalities consistent with severe inflammation (e.g., neutrophilic leukocytosis with left shift)
- Radiographs of affected areas to rule out fractures and other lesions as causes of pain
- Advanced or septic cases have abnormalities consistent with sepsis and/or disseminated intravascular coagulation (DIC [p. 269]).

Advanced or Confirmatory Testing

Cytology of fluids or affected tissues may reveal exudate with cocci in pairs or chains in cases with *Streptococcus,* increasing clinical suspicion for the disease. Diagnostic confirmation is made by histopathology and culture of the causative organism, but treatment must be instituted before these results are available.

TREATMENT

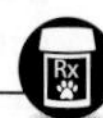

Treatment Overview

Immediate, aggressive treatment consists of wide surgical excision of affected tissue, appropriate antimicrobial therapy, intensive pain management, and medical therapy for shock and sepsis if present.

Acute General Treatment

- Immediate aggressive treatment for SIRS and septic shock, if present (p. 907)
- Early, aggressive surgical debridement
  - Immediate owner consent for amputation for limb infections; guarded prognosis and risk of reoperation should be discussed
  - Debridement of all necrotic and questionable tissue and drainage (often by fasciotomy) are indicated; copious surgical lavage with warm isotonic fluids ± chlorhexidine 0.05%
  - Wet-to-dry bandaging until infection is controlled; the bandage should contain a thick absorptive layer.
  - Negative-pressure wound therapy has been used successfully as an additional management tool.
- IV antibiotics: beta-lactamase–resistant antibiotics are generally effective against *S. canis*; initially broad-spectrum antimicrobial therapy may be superior due to the risk of polymicrobial infections.
  - Clindamycin 11 mg/kg IV q 12h; clindamycin is considered a drug of choice for human necrotizing fasciitis, *or*
  - Cefoxitin 30 mg/kg IV q 6h, *or*
  - Cefazolin or ampicillin/sulbactam 22 mg/kg IV q 6h plus enrofloxacin 20 mg/kg IV q 24h (dogs) or 5 mg/kg q 24h (cats); alternatively, cefazolin or ampicillin/sulbactam as above plus amikacin 20 mg/kg IV q 24h (dogs and cats)
  - Enrofloxacin may be associated with increased risk of streptococcal toxic shock syndrome and should be used with caution when *Streptococcus* species are suspected in necrotizing fasciitis.
- Hyperbaric oxygen therapy and pentoxofylline (15-30 mg/kg PO q8-12h) may improve outcome and assist with wound management.
- Aggressive analgesia, titrated to need
  - Opioids (e.g., morphine sulfate 0.05-0.15 mg/kg/h IV constant rate infusion or buprenorphine 0.02 mg/kg IV q 6h) combined with a nonsteroidal antiinflammatory drug (NSAID) such as carprofen 2.2 mg/kg SQ or PO q 12h unless contraindicated
  - Previous concerns that NSAIDs caused poorer outcomes in humans was not substantiated in prospective and retrospective studies.

Chronic Treatment

Chronic wound management may be needed.

Nutrition/Diet

Enteral feeding is preferred over parenteral unless contraindicated. Feed twice the basal requirements.

Drug Interactions

NSAIDs: avoid in septic shock or dehydrated animals

Possible Complications

Delaying treatment waiting for diagnostic results or not treating aggressively enough increases risk of sepsis, SIRS, and death.

Recommended Monitoring

- Monitor patients for septic shock, DIC, and infection progression that would warrant further debridement.
- Monitor bandages for amount and character of exudate.

PROGNOSIS & OUTCOME

Surgical delay, incomplete debridement, and concurrent sepsis are negative prognostic factors.

Prognosis appears to be much better for dogs (>80% survival) than humans. Prognosis appears to be worse for cats.

PEARLS & CONSIDERATIONS

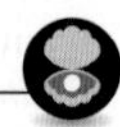

Comments

Early recognition and aggressive surgical and medical management are important for a favorable outcome. Referral to a 24-hour care facility (in a timely manner) is ideal.

Technician Tips

Close monitoring of vital signs and affected tissues and wounds can be helpful for identifying whether the infection is progressing and further surgery is warranted. A Sharpie-type pen can be used to mark skin along edge of affected area to help monitor disease progression.

Client Education

Owners should be aware that treatment is frequently drastic, is costly, and should be pursued quickly.

SUGGESTED READING

Naidoo SL, et al: Necrotizing fasciitis: a review. J Am Anim Hosp Assoc 41:104-109, 2005.

AUTHOR: Michelle Woodward, DVM, MS, DACVD
EDITOR: Joseph Taboada, DVM, DACVIM

Neonatal Isoerythrolysis

BASIC INFORMATION

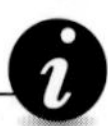

Definition

Neonatal isoerythrolysis (NI) is a hemolytic disease occurring in newborn kittens (and rarely in puppies). It is a type II hypersensitivity reaction in which antibodies from the mother's colostrum are directed against the red blood cells (RBCs) of the newborn.

Epidemiology

SPECIES, AGE, SEX

Far more common in neonatal cats than dogs

GENETICS, BREED PREDISPOSITION

Feline breeds with a high prevalence of B blood type, such as British shorthair, Birman, Devon rex, Scottish fold, Somali, Turkish van, Persian, or Abyssinian, are at higher risk for NI (p. 1203).

RISK FACTORS

- Kittens with blood type A that are born to queens of blood type B
- Puppies born to dams that have previously received blood transfusions

GEOGRAPHY AND SEASONALITY

Cats with type B blood are found more often in some locations (e.g., Australia, Greece, California)

Clinical Presentation

HISTORY, CHIEF COMPLAINT

The kittens/puppies are typically normal at birth and nurse vigorously. They begin to fade 48-72 hours after birth, exhibiting lethargy and weakness.

PHYSICAL EXAM FINDINGS

- Weak, lethargic kitten(s)
- Reduced vocalization
- Hypothermia
- Pale/white mucous membranes, sometimes icterus
- Urine that is dark red/brown (hemoglobinuria)
- Tail tip necrosis (common in survivors)

Etiology and Pathophysiology

- Colostrum is the antibody-rich fluid found in the mammary gland at parturition. After about 48-72 hours, the mammary gland switches from colostrum to milk, which is rich in immunoglobulins G (IgG) and A (IgA).
- The mammalian gut absorbs colostrum for ≈24 hours after birth (highest in the first 16 hours). After gut closure occurs, antibody is no longer absorbed into circulation but acts locally in the gut.
- Cats with blood type B have naturally occurring anti-A antibodies without prior exposure (sometimes referred to as "isoantibodies"). If the queen is type B, these antibodies will be found in the colostrum.
- If the tom has type A blood (dominant to type B), any type A offspring will ingest maternal antibody (naturally occurring anti-A antibodies from the type B queen) when suckling colostrum.
- Colostrum-derived antibodies (especially IgG) targeting the kitten's RBCs induces hemolysis similar to immune mediated-hemolytic anemia (p. 60).
- Cats with type A blood can develop anti-B antibodies. However, the anti-B reaction is much less vigorous and the clinical signs much less severe.
- In dogs, maternal antibodies may develop to a specific foreign blood group from previous transfusions but not from prior pregnancies.

DIAGNOSIS

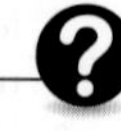

Diagnostic Overview

Blood type A kittens born to type B queens are at high risk for NI. The diagnosis is usually suspected based on history and clinical signs.

Differential Diagnosis

Heritable RBC disorders, hemolytic toxins, severe parasitism

Initial Database

- Packed cell volume
- Blood smear for cytologic evaluation of RBCs: evidence of agglutination and/or spherocytosis is consistent with NI
- Pigmenturia in fading kittens strongly suggests NI.

Advanced or Confirmatory Testing

- Blood typing of both parents (NI occurs when queen is type B, tom type A)
- Cord blood can be used to type kittens if a risky mating is known or suspected and the tom is not available for typing.
- The diagnosis is confirmed by screening maternal serum, plasma, or colostrum against the neonatal RBCs or paternal RBCs; in essence a cross-match (p. 1084).

TREATMENT

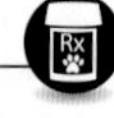

Treatment Overview

Treatment for NI is supportive; early identification and intervention is key.

Acute General Treatment

- Remove nursing animals from the queen until blood types are established for all kittens in the litter. Type B kittens can be returned to a type B queen immediately.
- Remove blood type A kittens from queens for about 24 hours after birth.
    - Bottle-feed using a high-quality kitten milk replacer until returned to queen.
    - Kittens deprived of colostrum are at increased risk for infection.
    - Adult serum (type A donor) can provide antibody to colostrum-deprived kittens.
- Anemic kittens may require transfusion (p. 1169). If IV catheterization is impossible, the intraosseous route may be used.

PROGNOSIS & OUTCOME

The prognosis is guarded if NI is not recognized early.

PEARLS & CONSIDERATIONS

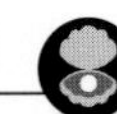

Prevention

- Blood type the queen and tom before mating; avoid mating type B queen with type A tom.
- If a risky mating has occurred, the kittens should not be allowed to nurse from the queen until they have been confirmed as blood type B or after the first 24 hours.
- Be alert for this complication in a bitch that has received transfusion before pregnancy.

Technician Tips

- A body stocking on the queen is a good method to prevent kittens from nursing, if needed. This allows the queen to continue care for the kittens (e.g., warmth, stimulation of elimination).
- Cord blood is useful for blood typing kittens in at-risk breeds.

Client Education

Counsel feline breeders on the breeds at risk and the need to have the queen and tom blood typed before mating.

SUGGESTED READING

Silvestre-Ferreira A, et al: Feline neonatal isoerythrolysis and the importance of feline blood types. Vet Med Int 2010:753726, 2010.

AUTHOR: Jonathan E. Fogle, DVM, PhD, DACVIM
EDITOR: Leah A. Cohn, DVM, PhD, DACVIM

Neonatal Losses

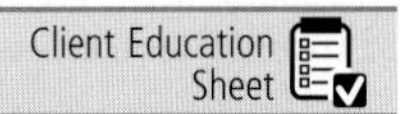

BASIC INFORMATION

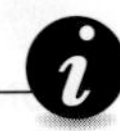

Definition

Life-threatening illness occurring between birth and 4 weeks of age

Synonyms

Fading kittens, fading puppies, stillbirth

Epidemiology

SPECIES, AGE, SEX

- Canine or feline; both sexes
- Neonatal mortality rates: 5%-30%
  - Greatest incidence occurs within the first week of birth.
  - Kittens have second peak in mortality at 3-4 weeks, usually of viral origin

GENETICS, BREED PREDISPOSITION

- Purebred puppies and kittens are more prone to congenital and hereditable defects.
- Dogs: breeds prone to anasarca and cleft palate
- Cats: British shorthair, Scottish fold, Devon rex, Abyssinian, Birman, Himalayan, Persian, Somali

RISK FACTORS

- Dam condition
- Premature labor
- Dystocia, causing fetal distress
- Prolonged labor (6-12 hours)
- Low birth weight or failure to grow
- Lack of colostrum ingestion, immunodeficiency
- Endometritis in the dam
- Congenital anomalies
- Malnutrition or nutritional diseases
- Assisted feeding (potential aspiration pneumonia)
- Unhygienic environment, maternal stress, low ambient temperature
- Parasitism
- Infectious diseases
- Inbreeding
- Cats: tom with blood type A having mated with queen with blood type B (p. 686)

CONTAGION AND ZOONOSIS

- *Brucella canis* infection
- Herpesvirus infection
- *Bartonella* infection
- Toxoplasmosis
- Parvovirus
- Feline leukemia virus (FeLV) or feline immunodeficiency virus (FIV) infections

GEOGRAPHY AND SEASONALITY

Colder climates may negatively affect neonatal survival.

ASSOCIATED DISORDERS

Failure to thrive (weight loss), vomiting, diarrhea, respiratory distress

Clinical Presentation

HISTORY, CHIEF COMPLAINT

- Low birth weight, low weight gain, and/or failure to gain weight
- Separation from the dam or other littermates
- Sudden onset of illness is characterized by depression, anorexia, bradycardia, hypothermia, persistent crying, abdominal distention/pain, and failure to suckle. Death can occur in 18-24 hours or less.
- Primarily respiratory and gastrointestinal (GI) signs in puppies and hemolytic or respiratory signs in kittens. With infectious causes, clinical signs vary according to the route and time of infection.
- Severity of presenting signs influences survival.

PHYSICAL EXAM FINDINGS

- General: weakness, diarrhea, gasping/panting/labored breathing/respiratory distress
- Red-tinged abdominal skin and nail bed tips
- Decreased activity, decreased muscle tone, pale mucous membranes, decreased GI sounds, dehydration, hypothermia
- Neonatal isoerythrolysis (cats): pallor, icterus, tail tip necrosis, tachypnea, discolored urine (hemoglobinuria)

Etiology and Pathophysiology

- Mechanisms
  - Hypoglycemia, dehydration, hypoxemia, and hypothermia are the main mechanisms for neonatal losses in dogs and cats.
  - Hypothermia causes failure to suckle and intestinal ileus, which causes bacterial translocation. This process occurs at body temperatures < 96°F (<35.6°C). The most common route of entry for bacterial organisms is through the umbilicus, but oronasal exposure and contact with infectious vaginal fluids are also important.
  - Meconium aspiration may cause pneumonia and systemic bacterial infection.
  - Neonatal isoerythrolysis (p. 686)

DIAGNOSIS

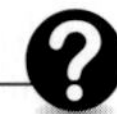

Diagnostic Overview

The syndrome is defined by the death of pups or kittens or by persistent crying, anorexia, weakness, lack of weight gain, hypothermia, abdominal pain, or a combination of these in puppies and kittens younger than 2-3 weeks of age. Specific cause of illness can sometimes be determined by careful history, exam of dam and offspring, and performing additional diagnostic tests.

Differential Diagnosis

See Etiology and Pathophysiology above.

Initial Database

- CBC, serum chemistry profile, urinalysis
  - Volume of blood withdrawn should be conservative due to small body size (maximum: of 1 mL/100 g body weight/wk). In very small patients, minimal database should consist of hematocrit, total protein, glucose, blood urea nitrogen, and urinalysis.
  - Neonates normally have mild serum alkaline phosphatase and phosphorus elevations, and mild blood urea nitrogen, albumin, globulin, cholesterol, and

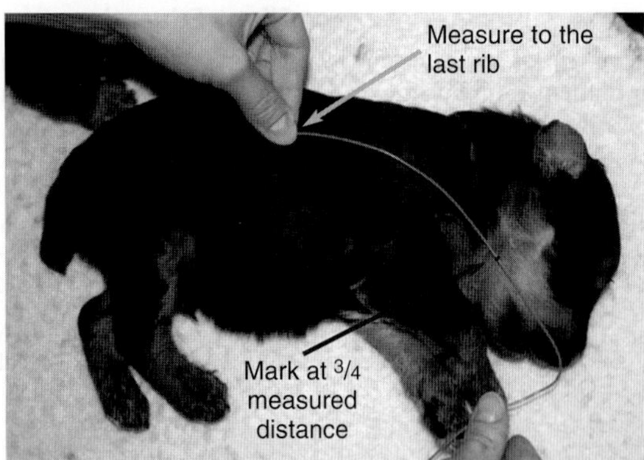

NEONATAL LOSSES Preparing for tube feeding. The distance from the tip of the nose to the last rib should be measured first. Then, with a permanent marker, 75% of that distance should be measured and marked on the catheter. (From Rickard V: Birth and the first 24 hours. In Peterson ME, et al, editors: Small animal pediatrics, St. Louis, 2010, Saunders.)

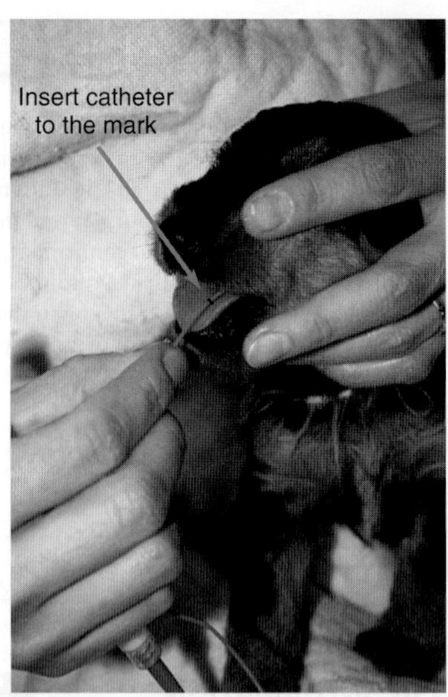

NEONATAL LOSSES Passing the orogastric tube. While holding the neonate upright with its neck flexed (not extended), insert the tip of the tube along the roof of the mouth, following the path of least resistance. (From Rickard V: Birth and the first 24 hours. In Peterson ME, et al, editors: Small animal pediatrics, St. Louis, 2010, Saunders.)

hematocrit reductions compared with adult normal ranges.
- Compare serum gamma-glutamyl transferase (GGT) and alkaline phosphatase (ALP) levels to assess transfer of colostrum.
  - Adequate colostral transfer: neonate's serum levels should be 30 (GGT) to 100 (ALP) times higher than adult values during days 1-3 of life.
- FeLV/FIV test
  - Positive FIV test can be due to maternal antibody rather than infection of kitten.
- Fecal flotation
- Thoracic and abdominal radiographs
  - Lack of fat causes poor serosal detail on abdominal images.

Advanced or Confirmatory Testing

- Urine culture
- Infectious disease tests, as appropriate
  - Serologic titers: *Brucella canis,* canine herpesvirus, *Toxoplasma, Neospora,* parvovirus antigen test
  - Polymerase chain reaction (PCR) test is confirmatory for herpesvirus.
  - Virus isolation
- Blood typing (purebred cats)
- Pleural/abdominal fluid analysis
- Ultrasound of the skull for patients presenting with hydrocephalus
- Necropsy of any/all animals that die

TREATMENT

Treatment Overview

Treatment is generally supportive, based on the test results and affected body systems. Not all treatments need to be instituted at once because it is very easy to overstress puppies and kittens of such young age. Assess organ involvement and institute/revise treatments as clinical signs dictate.

Acute General Treatment

- Management of specific disorders if present (e.g., isoerythrolysis in kittens [p. 686], canine herpesvirus [p. 466])
- Hypothermia: gradual correction over 30 minutes to 2 hours at a maximal rate of 1°F (0.5°C) per 30 minutes to avoid delayed organ failure
- If immune compromise due to insufficient colostrum ingestion, frozen colostrum, or fresh-frozen plasma (FFP) administration: FFP can be given PO (<24-hour-old neonate), IP, SQ, or IV: 3-5 mL/lb (6-10 mL/kg); maximum of 10 mL/dose. FFP should not be mixed with any solution, including milk replacer, IV fluids, or water. The first 3 doses should be given at birth, 12 hours, and 24 hours.
- Start administering broad-spectrum bactericidal antibiotics (e.g., ceftiofur [Naxcel] 2.5 mg/kg SQ q 12h for 5 days, which is considered very safe and has minimal effects on intestinal flora).
- Correct dehydration with warmed, balanced crystalloid fluids (lactated Ringer's solution or Normosol-R and 5% dextrose 1 mL/30 g body weight IP or intraosseous [IO] initially, then as needed based on response).
- Correct hypoxemia by administration of oxygen at 30%-40%.
- Vitamin K_1 0.01-0.1 mg SQ once because puppies < 2 days old have reduced thrombin levels
- Correct hypoglycemia if present (p. 552).
- Correct hypokalemia if present (p. 516).
- After the patient is stable, provide supportive nursing. In weaker patients with an inadequate suckle reflex, tube feeding is better than bottle feeding because it is a more reliable method to minimize possibility of aspiration (p. 1117). During the first week of life, feeding guidelines for kittens are 100-175 kcal/lb (220-380 kcal/kg); for puppies, requirements are 105-120 kcal/lb (230-260 kcal/kg) divided equally into 6-8 feedings daily.
- Viral replication can be inhibited by maintaining body temperature above 101°F-102°F (38.3°-38.8°C). Clinicians should monitor neonates closely to avoid overheating (not more than 103.5°F [39.7°C]). Incubator should be at a temperature of 85°F-95°F (29.4°-35°C) with a relative humidity of 55%-65%.

Chronic Treatment

- Supportive care
- Use commercial milk replacement if mother's milk is not available. Caloric requirements are 155 kcal/kg/d for week 2, 175-198 kcal/kg/d for week 3, and 220 kcal/kg/d for week 4.

Drug Interactions

- Avoid drugs contraindicated for neonates (e.g., glucocorticoids, immunosuppressive agents, nonsteroidal antiinflammatory drugs [NSAIDs], fluoroquinolones, tetracyclines, aminoglycosides, trimethoprim-sulfadiazine, and chloramphenicol).
- Drug absorption, metabolism, and excretion in dog or cat neonates differ from those of adults and vary according to the drug; detailed drug information should be obtained before use in neonates.

Possible Complications

- Transient organ injury (e.g., GI, respiratory) from the disease process
- Fluid volume overload
- Aspiration pneumonia
- Death of additional members of litter

Recommended Monitoring

- Body weight q 12h is very important to identify early changes and the need for heightened nutrition/diagnostic testing/treatment. Puppies and kittens should gain

2-7 g/day for each kilogram of anticipated adult weight and should double their birth weight by 10 days of age.
- Monitor color and amount of urine to assess for dehydration (sample can be obtained by manual stimulation with a warm, wet cotton ball).

PROGNOSIS & OUTCOME

Supportive care is the cornerstone of successful treatment.

PEARLS & CONSIDERATIONS

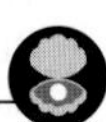

Comments

- Instituting intensive early treatment is the key because neonates can deteriorate rapidly.
- FFP is salty. If given PO, it should be followed with a little drop of sugar, honey, or STAT solution (concentrated nutritional supplement; PRN Pharmacal, FL) on the tongue.

Prevention

Incidence of neonatal problems is reduced when clinicians
- Avoid administering modified live vaccines during pregnancy.
- Avoid administering teratogenic drugs and chemicals to a pregnant dam or queen.
- Avoid incompatible matings for cats, and check blood type before breeding.
- Ensure that neonates have ingested colostrum within the first 24 hours to acquire passive immunity. Administer FFP if immunity status is questionable.
- Administer broad-spectrum anthelmintic therapy to the dam/queen 2 weeks before birthing and then to neonates every 2-3 weeks starting at 3 weeks of age and continuing until 12 weeks old.
- Administer appropriate vaccination protocols.
- Maintain excellent hygiene in whelping and nesting areas.

Technician Tips

- Urine collection: touch the vulva/prepuce with a warm, wet cotton ball.
- Fecal sample collection: gentle insertion and removal of a soft thermometer with manual stimulation over the anus with a warm, wet cotton ball
- Tube feeding guidelines
  - Use a 5-Fr or 8-Fr red rubber catheter.
  - Measure from the nose to last rib, and mark 75% of that distance.
  - Preload 6-mL syringe with milk replacer, empty all air out of the catheter by squeezing the syringe until milk starts to drip from the edge of the catheter.
  - Squeeze toe to make neonate cry just before advancing catheter along the roof of the mouth along the path of least resistance until it reaches the mark.
  - Pull back on the syringe to make sure there is negative pressure (no air in the syringe, which would indicate intratracheal location [contraindicated]).
  - Feed appropriate amount of milk replacer over 5-10 seconds, kink the catheter, and pull it out.
  - This technique can also be used for FFP administration if colostral ingestion is questionable.
  - If sepsis is suspected, look at the color of the abdomen and tips of nail beds, which will be red.

SUGGESTED READING

Peterson ME: Neonatal mortality. In Peterson ME, et al, editors: Small animal pediatrics, St. Louis, 2011, Saunders, pp 82-87.

AUTHOR: Valeria Rickard, DVM
EDITOR: Michelle A. Kutzler, DVM, PhD, DACT

Nephrolithiasis

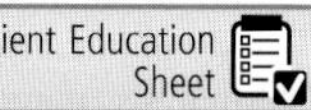

BASIC INFORMATION

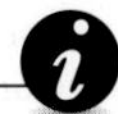

Definition

Deposition of crystallized minerals in the kidney occurs less commonly than in the lower urinary tract, but the incidence (or recognition) is increasing.

Synonyms

Kidney stones, renal urolithiasis, renolithiasis

Epidemiology

SPECIES, AGE, SEX

- Feline: prevalence increases with age; up to 47% of cats with chronic kidney disease (CKD) may be affected.
- Canine: middle-aged to older dogs

GENETICS, BREED PREDISPOSITION

Dogs (data extrapolated from general uroliths):
- Oxalate: miniature schnauzer, Lhasa apso, Yorkshire terrier, Bichon frisé, Pomeranian, shih tzu, miniature poodle (p. 1014)
- Struvite: miniature schnauzer, shih tzu, Bichon frisé, miniature poodle, cocker spaniel, and Lhasa apso (p. 1016)
- Urate: Dalmatian, English bulldog, miniature schnauzer, shih tzu, Yorkshire terrier (urate/biurate [p. 1019])

RISK FACTORS

- Struvite: pyelonephritis
- Calcium oxalate: hyperadrenocorticism, hypercalcemia (any cause), diet
- Urate: portosystemic shunt, breed

ASSOCIATED DISORDERS

- Hydronephrosis/hydroureter
- Ureteral obstruction
- Pyelonephritis
- Renal failure/CKD
- Acute kidney injury

Clinical Presentation

DISEASE FORMS/SUBTYPES

- Unilateral or bilateral
- Unobstructed or obstructed (partial or complete)
- Urolith type: calcium oxalate, struvite, urate and other purines, xanthine, silica, cystine, compound/mixed

HISTORY, CHIEF COMPLAINT

Clinical signs may be absent or may include
- Abdominal pain
- Anorexia
- Depression
- Hematuria
- Pollakiuria
- Polyuria and polydipsia (PU/PD)
- Stranguria
- Vomiting
- Weight loss

PHYSICAL EXAM FINDINGS

Physical exam may be unremarkable or may reveal
- Signs of abdominal pain
- Dehydration
- Renomegaly or small kidneys
- Halitosis/oral ulcers (uremia; rare)

Etiology and Pathophysiology

- Nephroliths (1%-4% of analyzed uroliths) are less common than cystoliths. The actual prevalence is likely higher because nephroliths are less frequently removed for analysis.
- The most common nephrolith types in dogs are calcium oxalate (≈40%), struvite (≈33%), and urate (≈12%). The most common nephroliths in cats are calcium oxalate.

DIAGNOSIS

Diagnostic Overview

Nephrolithiasis may be an incidental finding or may be associated with urinary tract obstruction, renal failure (acute or chronic), or recurrent urinary tract infections.

Differential Diagnosis

- Radiopaque renal opacities
  - Nephrocalcinosis
  - Radiopaque intestinal content
  - Mineralized lymph nodes
  - Mineralized adrenal glands
  - Neoplastic mineralization
  - Other ectopic mineralization
- Clinical signs
  - Urolithiasis (ureters, bladder, urethra)
  - Feline lower urinary tract signs/disease (FLUTS/D)
  - Pyelonephritis or cystitis
  - Acute kidney injury
  - Overt CKD
  - Urinary tract neoplasia
  - Prostatic disease
  - Causes of hematuria (p. 1229)

Initial Database

- CBC: often unremarkable
  - Normocytic, normochromic, nonregenerative anemia (if overt CKD)
  - Leukocytosis ± left shift (if pyelonephritis)
- Serum biochemical profile: often unremarkable, but depending on degree of renal dysfunction and/or urinary obstruction, may reveal
  - Azotemia
  - Hyperphosphatemia
  - Hypokalemia/hyperkalemia
  - Metabolic acidosis
- Urinalysis: may be unremarkable or reveal hematuria, proteinuria, pyuria, bacteriuria, crystalluria, and/or isosthenuric urine
- Urine culture and sensitivity (C/S) to rule out infection
- Blood pressure to rule out hypertension associated with CKD
- Abdominal radiography: depending on urolith composition, radiopaque density apparent in one or both renal pelvises
  - Radiopaque: calcium phosphate, calcium oxalate, struvite; small uroliths are difficult to detect radiographically.
  - Radiolucent: urate, cystine
  - Concurrent ureteral, cystic, or urethral calculi are sometimes present.
  - Enlarged or atrophied kidneys
- Ultrasound is a sensitive means of detection but may overestimate nephrolith size (acoustic shadowing in renal pelvis, concurrent pyelectasia or hydronephrosis)

Advanced or Confirmatory Testing

- If nephroliths are recovered, quantitative urolith analysis and culture
- If definitive therapy is anticipated
  - Nuclear scintigraphic or CT assessment of glomerular filtration rate (GFR) to determine contribution of each kidney to global GFR
  - Excretory urogram (p. 1101) or CT to confirm urolith location in kidney

TREATMENT

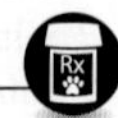

Treatment Overview

Incidentally discovered nephroliths often do not require therapeutic intervention. Nephroliths may remain stationary, pass into the bladder, or become lodged in the ureter and result in renal dysfunction. Urinary tract obstruction should be relieved and uremia addressed directly. Whenever possible, measures to dissolve or prevent urolith growth are undertaken.

Acute General Treatment

- Complete urinary tract obstruction is rare, but when present, it requires interventional (radiological, surgical, endoscopic) treatment.
- Address renal failure, including electrolyte and acid-base disorders (pp. 23, 167, and 169).
- Address pyelonephritis (p. 849).

Chronic Treatment

- Medical dissolution is possible for some types of nephrolithiasis (pp. 1014, 1016, and 1019).
- Invasive intervention is not routinely required, and benefit must be carefully weighed against risk.
- Indications for surgery (nephrotomy, pyelolithotomy, or nephrectomy)
  - Complete obstruction to urine flow
  - Recurrent infection (nephrolith may be nidus)
  - Marked, persistent renal hematuria
  - Progressive nephrolith enlargement (despite medical management) accompanied by reduction in renal function or in a solitary functional kidney
- Lithotripsy (extracorporeal shock wave, laser, or electrohydraulic)
  - Results in fragmentation or crushing of calculi; may require multiple treatments, depending on calculi shape, size, location, and type
  - Indications similar to those for surgical intervention
  - Shock wave availability limited (e.g., in United States: Universities of Tennessee and Pennsylvania, Purdue, Tufts, Animal Medical Center in New York City); can cause renal damage
  - Laser lithotripsy more readily available (several large referral centers) but technique best suited to larger animals

Nutrition/Diet

- Diets to support dissolution or prevention of nephroliths, depending on stone type (pp. 1014, 1016, and 1019)
- Patients with CKD should be fed a suitable diet (p. 167).

Possible Complications

- Nephrolith may lodge in ureter, causing obstructive nephropathy, which is particularly likely when calculi shrink (e.g., medical dissolution, lithotripsy).
- Surgical trauma may further damage renal parenchyma.
- Some medical conditions may be worsened by calculolytic diets (pp. 1014, 1016, and 1019).
- Recurrence rates are high, especially for calcium oxalate nephroliths.

Recommended Monitoring

- Routine monitoring (pp. 1014, 1016, and 1019).
- Repeated abdominal ultrasound or excretory urography (contrast is potentially nephrotoxic) should be considered in patients with radiolucent stones.

PROGNOSIS & OUTCOME

- Depends on urolith composition, degree of obstruction, remaining renal function, concurrent infection, and ability to identify and treat underlying cause
- Surgical intervention does not address causation; recurrence rates are high.

PEARLS & CONSIDERATIONS

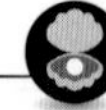

Comments

- Small nephroliths can be incidental findings requiring no therapy.
- Medical management of nephroliths mirrors medical management of cystoliths of identical composition.

Prevention

- Promote water consumption.
- Identify and address risk factors.

Technician Tips

Nephroliths can cause kidney pain; avoid abdominal pressure when picking up animals with renal pain.

Client Education

Strict adherence to dietary recommendations is crucial.

SUGGESTED READING

Ross SJ, et al: A case-control study of the effects of nephrolithiasis in cats with chronic kidney disease. J Am Vet Med Assoc 230:1854, 2007.

AUTHOR: Adam Mordecai, DVM, MS, DACVIM
EDITOR: Leah A. Cohn, DVM, PhD, DACVIM

Nephrotic Syndrome

Client Education Sheet

BASIC INFORMATION

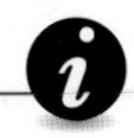

Definition

The presence of pathologic proteinuria, hypoalbuminemia, hypercholesterolemia, and edema is an uncommon but important complication of protein-losing nephropathy.

Epidemiology

SPECIES, AGE, SEX

- More common in dogs than in cats
- More common in middle-aged to older dogs (average, 6.2 years of age)
- For most causes, no sex predisposition

GENETICS, BREED PREDISPOSITION

- Labrador and golden retrievers may be overrepresented.
- Hereditary nephritis: bull terrier, Dalmatian, English cocker spaniel, Samoyed, American Eskimo, beagle, mixed-breed dog (p. 875)
- Amyloidosis: Chinese Shar-pei

RISK FACTORS

Any glomerular disease associated with substantial protein loss can be the underlying cause of nephrotic syndrome. However, immune complex–mediated glomerulonephritis and amyloidosis are often associated with the highest protein losses. Neoplasia and infectious and noninfectious inflammatory diseases predispose to these glomerular diseases (p. 390).

CONTAGION AND ZOONOSIS

Some causes of glomerular disease are zoonotic (p. 390).

ASSOCIATED DISORDERS

- Thromboembolic disease
- Chronic kidney disease
- Systemic hypertension
- Dyspnea from pulmonary thromboembolism or, less commonly, pleural effusion
- Ascites
- Reduced renal perfusion and possibly acute kidney injury from decreased plasma oncotic pressure

Clinical Presentation

DISEASE FORMS/SUBTYPES

Incomplete nephrotic syndrome (edema absent): the most common form

HISTORY, CHIEF COMPLAINT

Patients may not show overt clinical signs. When present, signs may be nonspecific (e.g., weight loss, lethargy) or caused by

- Fluid retention (e.g., edema, abdominal distention)
- Renal failure/uremia (e.g., polyuria and polydipsia [PU/PD], vomiting, halitosis)
- Thromboembolism (e.g., dyspnea, collapse)
- Systemic hypertension (e.g., blindness)
- Related to predisposing disease

PHYSICAL EXAM FINDINGS

May be unremarkable; abnormalities may include

- Subcutaneous edema, ascites, pleural effusion
- Evidence of thromboembolism (e.g., dyspnea, decreased peripheral pulse)
- Evidence of hypertension (e.g., choroidopathy, central nervous system signs, new cardiac murmur)
- Evidence of predisposing disease
- Variably sized kidneys

Etiology and Pathophysiology

- Proteinuria results from altered glomerular capillary wall permselectivity and abnormal (inadequate) filtration of plasma proteins, primarily albumin.
- Hypoalbuminemia develops when the renal loss of plasma proteins exceeds hepatic regenerative capacity.
- The pathogenesis of hypercholesterolemia is complex and incompletely understood. Hypoalbuminemia or decreased oncotic pressure stimulates hepatic protein synthesis, including lipoprotein synthesis, leading to hypercholesterolemia. Altered lipid catabolism may contribute to the condition.
- Sodium retention and decreased plasma oncotic pressure contribute to edema formation.

DIAGNOSIS

Diagnostic Overview

The diagnosis of partial nephrotic syndrome is based on the combination of proteinuria, hypoalbuminuria, and hypercholesterolemia; complete nephrotic syndrome includes the presence of fluid retention. Further investigation is required for either.

Differential Diagnosis

- The combination of proteinuria, hypoalbuminemia, hypercholesterolemia, and edema/effusion is pathognomonic for nephrotic syndrome.
- Glomerular diseases that cause severe proteinuria: immune complex–mediated glomerulonephritis (i.e., membranous nephropathy/glomerulonephritis, membranoproliferative glomerulonephritis, and mixed glomerulonephritis), amyloidosis, hereditary nephritis, minimal change disease, focal segmental glomerulosclerosis

Initial Database

- CBC, biochemical profile, urinalysis: assess glomerular filtration (creatinine, blood urea nitrogen [BUN], symmetrical dimethylarginine [SDMA]), renal tubular function (urine specific gravity). Identify evidence of predisposing disease, and rule out other causes of proteinuria (p. 1272).
- Urine protein/creatinine (UPC) ratio: confirm nephrotic range proteinuria (UPC > 2), and establish pretreatment baseline. UPC is accurate only when urine sediment is inactive and urine has not been discolored by hematuria.
- Urine culture and susceptibility testing (C&S) to rule out infection
- Blood pressure measurement (p. 1065): hypertension is common. High risk of end-organ damage if systolic blood pressure > 180 mm Hg

Advanced or Confirmatory Testing

- Identify predisposing diseases with abdominal ultrasound, thoracic radiographs, infectious disease testing (e.g., heartworm, ehrlichiosis), and antinuclear antibody (ANA) serologic analysis.
- Renal biopsy allows definitive diagnosis of glomerular lesion and should include light, electron, and immunofluorescent microscopic evaluation. It may provide prognostic information. Contact the International Veterinary Renal Pathology Service, Ohio State University (Dr. Rachel Cianciolo's lab).

TREATMENT

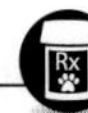

Treatment Overview

The goals of treatment are to reduce the magnitude of proteinuria, manage uremia, control systemic hypertension, and reduce patient discomfort (e.g., relief from edema, effusion).

Acute General Treatment

- Initiate angiotensin antagonism.
  - Angiotensin-converting enzyme (ACE) inhibitor therapy: starting dosage of enalapril or benazepril 0.5 mg/kg PO q 24h; can increase up 1 mg/kg PO q 12h, *or*
  - Angiotensin receptor blocker: starting dose of telmisartan 1 mg/kg PO q 24h; can increase up 3 mg/kg PO q 24h.
  - Start at lower doses and gradually increase in patients that are considered to be unstable. Correct volume depletion before starting.
- Address edema and effusion.
  - Abdominocentesis (p. 1056) if ascites impinging on ventilation; thoracocentesis rarely required
  - Appropriate diuretic use:
    - If plasma volume is reduced (e.g., dehydration), diuretics may be ineffective and dangerous, increasing risk of uremia or thromboembolism.

- If plasma volume is normal, spironolactone 1-2 mg/kg PO q 12h may help delay return of third-space fluid and provide benefit of inhibiting aldosterone.
  - Low-level exercise may help mobilize edema.
- Address components of uremia if present (p. 169).
- Initiate aspirin 2 mg/kg PO q 12h or clopidogrel 1.1 mg/kg PO q 24h therapy as anticoagulant to reduce risk of thromboembolism.
- Add additional medications as needed to control systemic hypertension (p. 501).
- Address concurrent/underlying disease when possible.
- Uremic crisis may require colloid support for appropriate diuresis.

Chronic Treatment

- Disease-specific treatment is indicated on basis of renal biopsy and other test results.
- If proteinuria is not reduced by > 50% with an ACE inhibitor or telmisartan, another inhibitor of the renin-angiotensin-aldosterone system (RAAS) should be added.
- Consider immunosuppressive therapy.

Nutrition/Diet

Diet formulated for renal disease

Behavior/Exercise

Moderate, comfortable physical activity is encouraged; inactivity may worsen peripheral edema.

Drug Interactions

- Hypoalbuminemia increases the unbound (often active) fraction of highly protein-bound drugs; dosages may need to be adjusted.
- Warfarin is avoided in the face of hypoalbuminemia.
- Heparin is an ineffective anticoagulant when antithrombin is depleted.

Possible Complications

- Hypotension from ACE inhibitor and calcium channel blocker or severe reduction in plasma oncotic pressure
- Hyperkalemia from ACE inhibitor
- Bleeding tendency from aspirin or clopidogrel (rare at recommended dose)
- Worsening azotemia as a result of ACE inhibition or calcium channel blockade (rare)
- Worsening of ascites/edema after parenteral fluid administration

Recommended Monitoring

The UPC, urinalysis, blood pressure, serum albumin and creatinine, body weight, and body condition score should be monitored regularly, weekly to monthly initially and after therapeutic adjustments. Once stable, re-evaluate every 3 months unless changes in therapy are initiated or changes are noted in clinical condition. Urine culture indicated at least twice per year. Ideally, UPC should be evaluated in several samples collected over a few days. Alternatively, equal aliquots from several samples can be pooled for UPC evaluation.

PROGNOSIS & OUTCOME

- Varies but usually guarded
- Prognosis improves if underlying disease causing proteinuria can be identified and corrected.
- Azotemia, systemic hypertension, and marked tubulointerstitial lesions on biopsy may be negative prognostic indicators.
- Nephrotic syndrome due to Lyme nephritis has a poor prognosis.

PEARLS & CONSIDERATIONS

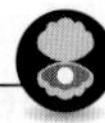

Comments

- Nephrotic syndrome is pathognomonic for glomerular disease.
  - The clinical condition can deteriorate rapidly, and prompt intervention is warranted.
- Nephrotic syndrome is a predisposing factor for thromboembolic disease.

Prevention

- Urinalysis screening during routine health evaluations may allow early detection of protein-losing nephropathy.
- Early intervention when proteinuria is first detected might prevent the development of nephrotic syndrome.

Technician Tips

Affected dogs need frequent evaluation because they can destabilize rapidly.

Client Education

Rapid deterioration is possible; frequent rechecks are necessary.

SUGGESTED READING

Klosternam ES, et al: Comparison of signalment, clinicopathologic findings, histologic diagnosis, and prognosis in dogs with glomerular disease with or without nephrotic syndrome. J Vet Intern Med 25:206, 2011.

AUTHOR: Shelly Vaden, DVM, PhD, DACVIM
EDITOR: Leah A. Cohn, DVM, PhD, DACVIM

Nerve Sheath Tumors

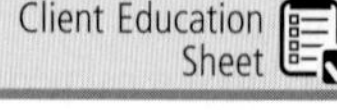

BASIC INFORMATION

Definition

Benign or malignant tumors arising from cells of the peripheral nerve sheath, nerve sheath tumors can affect peripheral nerves, spinal nerve roots, or cranial nerves. About 80% of nerve sheath tumors occur in the brachial plexus region. The remaining ≈20% involve cranial nerves (most commonly, the trigeminal nerve) or other spinal nerve roots.

Synonyms

Peripheral nerve sheath tumor (PNST), malignant nerve sheath tumor (MNST)

Epidemiology

SPECIES, AGE, SEX

- Common in medium-sized to large-breed dogs, less common in cats
- Reported age range is 3-13 years (dogs) and 8-19 years (cats).

Clinical Presentation

DISEASE FORMS/SUBTYPES

Nerve sheath tumors include

- Ganglioneuroma
- Peripheral neuroblastoma
- Paraganglioma
- Peripheral nerve sheath tumors
  - Benign peripheral nerve sheath tumors (schwannoma, neurofibroma, perineuroma)
  - Malignant peripheral nerve sheath tumors (malignant schwannoma, neurofibrosarcoma)

HISTORY, CHIEF COMPLAINT

- Chronic, progressive lameness
- Pain or paresthesia
- Muscle atrophy
- Weakness
- Ataxia

PHYSICAL EXAM FINDINGS

Varies with respect to tumor location and nerve root(s) affected; abnormalities can include

- Localized muscle atrophy (often severe): involving thoracic limb with tumor of brachial plexus and involving masticatory muscles with tumor of trigeminal nerve
- Progressive lameness and/or weakness
- Proprioceptive deficits
- Hyporeflexia
- Sensory deficits
- Pain on palpation of tumor site (e.g., axilla)
- Ipsilateral loss of cutaneous trunci reflex (can occur with involvement of C8-T1 spinal segments)
- Ipsilateral Horner's syndrome (can occur with cervical or brachial plexus nerve sheath tumors)

Etiology and Pathophysiology

Undetermined; a point mutation in the *neu* oncogene has been suggested.

DIAGNOSIS

Diagnostic Overview

A presumptive diagnosis can be made with history, clinical signs, and diagnostic imaging; cytologic or histopathologic evaluation is required for definitive diagnosis.

Differential Diagnosis

- Other soft-tissue tumors (e.g., fibrosarcoma, chondrosarcoma, lymphoma) can invade or compress nerves and result in similar neurologic deficits and imaging appearance.
- Abscess, granuloma
- Orthopedic abnormalities (e.g., osteoarthritis, osteochondrosis desiccans [OCD], biceps tenosynovitis)
- Other cranial neuropathies (e.g., tumors of the brainstem or cavernous sinus)
- Other neuropathies (e.g., lateralized disk herniation)
- Traumatic brachial plexus injury

Initial Database

- Neurologic exam (p. 1136)
- Radiographs of the affected limb to rule out orthopedic conditions
    - It is important to avoid overinterpreting the presence of osteoarthritis, which can be a concurrent condition and not the primary cause of presentation.
- Spinal radiographs may show subtle osteolysis at the vertebral foramen.

Advanced or Confirmatory Testing

- Electrophysiologic studies (electromyography and motor nerve conduction velocity)
    - Differentiate neurologic from orthopedic conditions.
    - Determine specific nerve roots involved to aid in surgical planning.
- Cerebrospinal fluid (CSF) evaluation (pp. 1080 and 1323): occasionally, albuminocytologic dissociation (disproportionate elevation in CSF protein concentration compared with nucleated cell count)
- Myelography
    - May indicate local invasion into spinal canal
    - Can rule out lateralized disk herniation
- Advanced imaging
    - MRI (p. 1132) is the preferred modality for identifying soft-tissue and intracranial lesions. However, a normal MRI scan does not completely rule out a small or diffuse nerve sheath tumor.
    - CT can be particularly useful in evaluating compressive spinal lesions when performed in conjunction with a myelogram.
- Fine-needle aspiration for cytologic exam
- Biopsy (percutaneous or surgical excision)
- Tumor staging
    - Thoracic radiographs
    - Abdominal ultrasound
    - Lymph node aspirates

TREATMENT

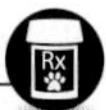

Treatment Overview

Complete tumor excision if possible and pain relief are the desired goals; radiation therapy can be used for palliation.

Acute General Treatment

- Surgical exploratory/excision
    - Radical excision (i.e., limb amputation ± hemilaminectomy) provides the optimal chance of complete excision and is recommended in most cases.
- Radiation therapy
    - Adjunctive to surgical excision
    - Can be used as monotherapy in nonresectable cases
- Adjunctive chemotherapy
    - Rarely used as monotherapy
    - Doxorubicin, metronomic therapy

Chronic Treatment

- Analgesics
- Glucocorticoids may help alleviate some discomfort and reduce peritumoral inflammation; however, there is insufficient research to support or refute their use for treating this condition.

Drug Interactions

- Concurrent administration of nonsteroidal antiinflammatory drugs (NSAIDs) and glucocorticoids is NOT recommended.
- Other potential drug interactions depend on the specific therapeutic modalities chosen; clinicians should consult appropriate references.

Possible Complications

- Local invasion into adjacent tissues (e.g., brainstem, spinal cord)
- Metastatic rates for nerve sheath tumors have not been established, although they appear to be low.

Recommended Monitoring

Monitor for progressive/recurrent neurologic deficits and/or pain.

PROGNOSIS & OUTCOME

- Varies; histopathologic grade, tumor location (surgical accessibility), and stage are prognostic.
- Although complete excision can be curative, local invasion into the spinal cord or brainstem often has already occurred by the time of diagnosis, making cure unlikely.
    - For tumors close to the spinal cord, the median postoperative survival time is 5-6 months, with a disease-free interval of about 1 month.
    - Survival times of untreated trigeminal nerve sheath tumors were 5-21 months.

PEARLS & CONSIDERATIONS

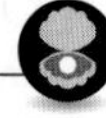

Comments

- Early diagnosis increases the potential for complete excision.
- Orthopedic conditions typically do not produce neurologic deficits; if proprioceptive deficit or localized muscle atrophy is present, a nerve sheath tumor may be the cause.
- Even advanced imaging may fail to identify the tumor if it is small or diffuse.

Technician Tips

- Chronic lameness with significant muscle atrophy should raise suspicion for a nerve sheath tumor.
- Patient can have paresthesia in the lame limb or in the axillary/inguinal regions.

Client Education

- Clients should understand the potential for progression/recurrence.
- Clients should be counseled regarding quality-of-life issues that pertain to their pets.

SUGGESTED READING

Brehm DM, et al: A retrospective evaluation of 51 cases of peripheral nerve sheath tumors in the dog. J Am Anim Hosp Assoc 31:349-359, 1995.

AUTHOR: David M. Brewer, DVM, DACVIM
EDITOR: Karen R. Muñana, DVM, MS, DACVIM

Nodular Skin Disorders

BASIC INFORMATION

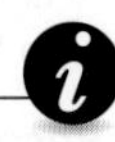

Definition

Nodules are > 1 cm in diameter, and they can occur in or below the skin. They are common and have three causes: neoplasia (benign or malignant), infections, and granulomas.

Epidemiology

SPECIES, AGE, SEX

Dogs and cats; no age or sex predisposition

GENETICS, BREED PREDISPOSITION

- Nodular dermatofibrosis: German shepherd dogs
- Histiocytic diseases (p. 473): Bernese mountain dog, rottweiler, golden retriever
- Sterile nodular panniculitis (p. 747): dachshunds
- Mucinosis: Shar-pei
- Pseudomycetoma: Persian cats

RISK FACTORS

- Any disease or medication that causes immune compromise predisposes animals to infections, which may cause nodular dermatoses.
- Phaeohyphomycoses are emerging opportunistic infections, especially in dogs or cats receiving high doses of cyclosporine.
- Foreign body penetration, bite wound: increased risk of infectious nodular dermatitis
- Mineralizing fat necrosis/panniculitis in dogs with pancreatitis or pancreatic carcinomas
- Working/hunting dogs are predisposed to kerion reactions.

CONTAGION AND ZOONOSIS

Dermatophytic granuloma (p. 247), sporotrichosis (p. 938), and systemic mycoses may be contagious between animals and/or transmissible to humans under various conditions.

GEOGRAPHY AND SEASONALITY

- Straelensiosis reported in France, Spain, and Portugal
- *Cuterebra* in summer and fall
- Many others, depending on organism's endemic region (pp. 121, 184, 476, 860, and 938)

ASSOCIATED DISORDERS

Renal cystadenocarcinoma is typically a concurrent finding with nodular dermatofibrosis.

Clinical Presentation

HISTORY, CHIEF COMPLAINT

Animals present with acute to chronic onset of single or multiple cutaneous or subcutaneous nodules, with or without draining tracts and potentially with accompanying systemic signs such as fever, cough, rhinitis, anorexia, or lethargy.

PHYSICAL EXAM FINDINGS

Lesions are elevations above the epidermal surface of 1 cm or greater in diameter. They can be solitary or multiple, localized or generalized, firm or fluctuant, draining or intact, and pruritic or nonpruritic, depending on the underlying cause.

Etiology and Pathophysiology

Nodules, which are larger than papules (<1 cm in diameter), are usually the result of a massive infiltration of inflammatory and/or neoplastic cells into the dermis or subcutis. The inflammatory cells are in response to an infectious, antigenic, or neoplastic cause.

DIAGNOSIS

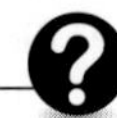

Diagnostic Overview

There are a variety of causes for nodular skin disorders. Fine-needle aspirates for cytologic exam may allow a diagnosis. Biopsies for histopathologic exam and/or bacterial and fungal cultures are often required to obtain a definitive diagnosis.

Differential Diagnosis

- Noninfectious granuloma/pyogranuloma: idiopathic sterile pyogranuloma/granuloma (sterile nodular panniculitis), juvenile cellulitis (p. 567), foreign-body reaction, acral lick dermatitis (p. 16), sarcoidosis, histiocytic diseases (histiocytoma, cutaneous or systemic histiocytosis [p. 473]), cutaneous xanthomatosis
- Infectious granuloma/pyogranuloma: fungal (blastomycosis, histoplasmosis, cryptococcosis, coccidioidomycosis, sporotrichosis, phaeohyphomycosis, eumycotic mycetoma, zygomycosis, dermatophyte kerion, true mycetoma), oomycotic (pythiosis, lagenidiosis), bacterial (mycobacterial infection, actinomycosis, nocardiosis, botryomycosis, methicillin-resistant bacteria, bacterial furunculosis, abscess, feline leprosy, canine leproid granuloma), *Rhodococcus equi* infection, viral papillomatosis, opportunistic mycobacteriosis, plague, tuberculosis, feline cowpox.
- Parasitic: tick-bite granuloma, cuterebriasis, toxoplasmosis (p. 984), leishmaniasis, demodicosis, dirofilariasis, dracunculiasis
- Lymphocytic/plasmacytic: lupus profundus (panniculitis associated with systemic lupus erythematosus [SLE] [p. 955]), vaccine reaction, drug eruption (p. 227), erythema nodosum, plasma cell pododermatitis (p. 799), lymphomatoid granulomatosis, pseudolymphoma, epitheliotropic lymphoma, plasmacytoma (p. 663)
- Neutrophilic: deep pyoderma (e.g., *Pseudomonas, Staphylococcus*), familial vasculopathy of German shepherd dogs, abscess
- Eosinophilic: eosinophilic granuloma, eosinophilic furunculosis, insect-bite granuloma, straelensiosis, dracunculiasis, dirofilariasis, pythiosis, ruptured hair follicle
- Anatomic: hygroma, callus, tail gland hyperplasia, ceruminous cystomatosis
- Other fibrosing, dysplastic, or neoplastic cells: follicular cysts/intraepidermal inclusion cyst, dermoid cyst/pilonidal cyst, acral pruritic nodule/fibropruritic nodule, calcinosis circumscripta, nodular dermatofibrosis, mucinosis, hemangioma, sebaceous gland hyperplasia/adenoma, collagenous nevus, follicular cyst, mast cell tumors (pp. 632 and 634), cutaneous lymphoma, melanoma (p. 644), transmissible venereal tumor (p. 993)

Initial Database

- Dermatologic exam (p. 1091) to rule out *Cuterebra* infestation, protruding foreign bodies, and any other grossly visible causes
- Skin scrapings and hair trichogram to identify possible *Demodex* mites, *Dirofilaria,* or *Pelodera*
- Impression smears from draining material for cytologic exam; numerous impression smears (≥4) should be taken and unfixed unstained specimens sent to the laboratory for special testing.
- Fine-needle aspiration to acquire cells for cytologic exam or parasites
- Cytologic exam of an impression smear or fine-needle aspirate to help identify evidence of infectious organisms
  - Cocci (*Staphylococcus* spp) or rod-shaped (*Pseudomonas* spp) bacteria
  - Gram-positive, branching, filamentous organisms: *Actinomyces* spp (non–acid-fast); *Nocardia* (partially acid-fast)
  - Diff-Quik: yeast or fungal elements of systemic mycoses sometimes detectable
  - Acid-fast bacilli: atypical mycobacteria, feline *Mycobacterium lepraemurium* infection
  - Spindle- to crescent-shaped protozoal organisms *(Toxoplasma gondii* or *Neospora caninum)*
  - Amastigotes in Giemsa-stained smears (leishmaniasis)
  - Nematodes (dracunculiasis) or microfilaria (dirofilariasis)
  - Organisms in foamy macrophages (may be seen)
- Cytologic exam may also reveal important noninfectious findings.
  - Foamy macrophages without evidence of infectious agents often detected with sterile nodular panniculitis
  - Eosinophils noted with eosinophilic granulomas, eosinophilic furunculosis, foreign body, or insect bite reactions
  - Neoplastic cells: round cell tumors (e.g., histiocytes, mast cells, plasmacytoma)

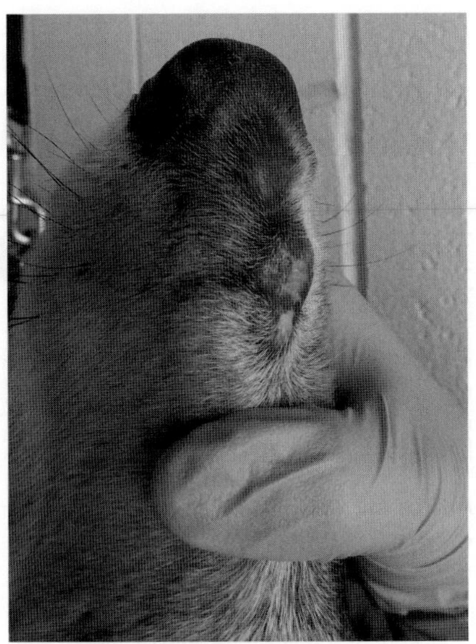

NODULAR SKIN DISORDERS Sterile nodular lesion on nose of dog

- Surgical biopsies to obtain a sufficiently deep sample to incorporate the panniculus. Optimal samples are obtained by deep wedge biopsy; otherwise, infectious agents may be missed. If using a punch biopsy, be certain to double punch to obtain the subcutaneous fatty tissue. Use an 8-mm skin biopsy punch.
- Dermatohistopathologic evaluation required to
  - Differentiate the cellular infiltrate (neutrophils, histiocytes, plasma cells, lymphocytes, eosinophils, multi-nucleated giant cells, neoplastic cells)
  - Identify the presence of infectious organisms with the aid of special stains (Gomori-Grocott methenamine silver [GMS], periodic acid–Schiff [PAS], and Fite acid-fast stains)
  - Help direct advanced diagnostics

Advanced or Confirmatory Testing

- A biopsy specimen should be submitted aseptically for tissue maceration and culture; this often needs to be an explicit request to the laboratory.
- Be certain to notify the laboratory of suspected organisms (adjustments to culture media selection and incubation times; precautions).
  - Bacterial culture and susceptibility testing: aerobic *(Staphylococcus* spp, *Rhodococcus equi, Nocardia)* and anaerobic *(Actinomyces)*
  - Rapidly growing atypical mycobacterial culture
  - Fungal culture for deep mycosis (many are biohazards; never culture these in house). Negative cultures support a diagnosis of sterile nodular panniculitis, lupus profundus, sterile pyogranuloma/granuloma syndrome, immune-mediated conditions, or neoplasia.
- For the detection of antibody deposition (lupus) and identification of infectious agents that are sometimes difficult to culture or typically found low in numbers (canine sporotrichosis with direct immunofluorescence [DIF], leishmaniasis with polymerase chain reaction [PCR]): DIF, fluorescent antibody testing, immunoperoxidase staining, immunohistochemistry, immunostaining with polyclonal bacillus Calmette-Guérin (BCG) antibody (promising method), PCR
- Serologic testing
  - *Coccidioides, Blastomyces, Cryptococcus, Histoplasma, Leishmania*
  - Urine antigen test for *Blastomyces*
- Additional laboratory tests
  - Feline leukemia virus/feline immunodeficiency virus (FeLV/FIV)
  - Antinuclear antibody (lupus profundus, SLE) testing
  - CBC/serum biochemistry/urinalysis
    - Rule out metabolic disturbances causing immunosuppression.
    - Evidence of concurrent immune-mediated process (e.g., autoimmune hemolytic anemia)
    - Baseline before commencing any long-term medications
- Diagnostic imaging
  - Radiographs: metastasis or infection dissemination
  - Abdominal ultrasound: clinicians should evaluate concurrent factors (pancreatitis, hyperadrenocorticism) and invasion of neoplasms (mast cell tumor, histiocytic sarcoma) into abdominal organs.

TREATMENT

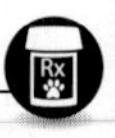

Treatment Overview

Because the group of nodular skin disorders encompasses a wide variety of causes, treatment depends on identification of the specific cause.

PROGNOSIS & OUTCOME

Varies: good to poor depending on the ability to identify and specifically treat the underlying cause.

PEARLS & CONSIDERATIONS

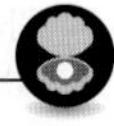

Comments

A thorough and methodical diagnostic protocol is often necessary to confirm a specific cause. Most common mistake is inadequate submission of tissue. Take multiple deep wedge biopsy specimens and/or use 8-mm skin biopsy punch.

Technician Tips

- Always wear gloves.
- Prepare for excisional biopsy or use 8-mm skin biopsy punch.
- Make at least four extra unstained slides from fine-needle aspirates for special staining by referral laboratory.

Client Education

A thorough diagnostic evaluation is cost-effective and allows targeted therapy. Many diseases presenting as nodules have a limited window of treatment success before the disease disseminates, making cure or durable remission impossible.

SUGGESTED READING

Miller WH Jr, et al: Muller & Kirk's Small animal dermatology, ed 7, St. Louis, 2013, Saunders.

AUTHOR: Karen Moriello, DVM, DACVD
EDITOR: Manon Paradis, DMV, MVSc, DACVD

Nonsteroidal Antiinflammatory Drug Toxicosis

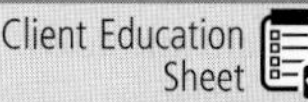

BASIC INFORMATION

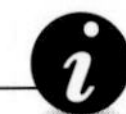

Definition

The common toxicosis is due to acute overdose or chronic administration of a nonsteroidal antiinflammatory drug (NSAID), most commonly affecting the gastrointestinal (GI) tract or kidneys. Although uncommon, hepatopathy, central nervous system (CNS), and hematologic effects are also possible.

Epidemiology

SPECIES, AGE, SEX

- Most cases are reported in dogs.
- Cats are generally more sensitive than dogs because of a deficiency in enzymes that metabolize these drugs.
- Elderly and very young animals are at higher risk.

GENETICS, BREED PREDISPOSITION

Labrador retrievers are not considered at greater risk for hepatopathies from carprofen, despite the fact that one-third of the initially reported cases of hepatic syndrome were in Labradors (likely reflecting popularity of the breed).

RISK FACTORS

- Pre-existing GI, renal, cardiovascular, or hepatic disease may increase severity of signs.
- Dehydration, hypotension, and concurrent use of other potentially nephrotoxic drugs can potentiate signs.
- Concurrent use of NSAIDs with other NSAIDs or glucocorticoids can lead to life-threatening complications.
- Hypoproteinemia or concurrent use of other highly protein-bound drugs can result in higher active drug levels.

Clinical Presentation

DISEASE FORMS/SUBTYPES

- Acute toxicosis: single, large ingestion (usually 5-10 times the recommended dose)
- Chronic toxicosis: in sensitive animals after NSAID use for days, weeks, or months at recommended doses

HISTORY, CHIEF COMPLAINT

- History of exposure (acute or chronic) to an NSAID
- Clinical signs can begin within hours after acute exposure, or days to weeks later with repeated/chronic therapeutic use or when hepatopathy develops.
- Vomiting (± hematemesis), anorexia, lethargy, diarrhea (melena) due to GI irritation/ulcer
- Polyuria, polydipsia due to kidney disease/kidney injury
- CNS signs are possible.

PHYSICAL EXAM FINDINGS

Varies from minor GI signs to signs caused by life-threatening GI perforation or kidney injury

- Minor to moderate toxicosis: signs of abdominal pain, vomiting, diarrhea, lethargy
- Severe toxicosis: dehydration, pallor, tachycardia, icterus, bruising (aspirin), hyperthermia (aspirin), sudden death
- CNS signs (lethargy, ataxia, coma, seizures) can be seen with large doses of some NSAIDs (ibuprofen, phenylbutazone).
- Neither hematemesis or melena is reliably linked to GI perforation. Absence of hematemesis does not indicate absence of perforation.

Etiology and Pathophysiology

- Examples of commonly implicated NSAIDs:
  - Acetic acid derivatives: diclofenac, etodolac (EtoGesic),* indomethacin, nabumetone, ketorolac
  - Fenamic acids: meclofenamic acid
  - Oxicams: meloxicam (Metacam),*† piroxicam
  - Propionic acids: carprofen (Rimadyl),* flurbiprofen, ibuprofen, ketoprofen, naproxen
  - Azole derivatives: phenylbutazone, tepoxalin
  - Salicylic acid derivatives: aspirin, flunixin meglumine
  - Cyclooxygenase 2 (COX2) inhibitors: celecoxib, firocoxib (Previcox),* deracoxib (Deramaxx),* robenacoxib (Onisor)*†
  - Prostaglandin E_2 EP4 receptor blocker: grapiprant (Galliprant)*
- NSAIDs inhibit COX enzymes, blocking prostaglandin (PG) production. PGs formed by COX1 are important for normal physiologic function (GI protection, renal medullary blood flow). PGs formed by COX2 mediate inflammation. Adverse effects are generally fewer when COX2 is selectively inhibited; however, in overdose situations, selectivity is lost.
- Platelet aggregation can be affected by NSAIDs because they inhibit the formation of platelet thromboxane through COX inhibition.
- NSAID hepatopathy is thought to result from formation of antigenic proteins that trigger an immune-mediated attack against the liver.

*Approved for use in dogs in the United States.
†Approved for use in cats in the United States

DIAGNOSIS

Diagnostic Overview

In most cases, exposure is known (whether acute overdose or ongoing therapeutic administration). In acute overdoses, history and clinical signs may be sufficient to make the diagnosis. In chronic treatment-associated toxicosis, detailed diagnostic testing and/or drug discontinuation for regression of signs is needed to distinguish NSAID toxicosis from other naturally occurring disorders mimicking NSAID toxicosis.

Differential Diagnosis

Any disease process that can cause GI, renal, hepatic, CNS, or hematologic adverse effects

Initial Database

- CBC: anemia from GI hemorrhage (usually regenerative), leukocytosis (stress or peritonitis) is possible.
- Serum chemistry profile: azotemia (prerenal or primary renal insult [usually within 24-48 hours after exposure in acute toxicosis]) or elevated liver enzymes and bilirubin (hepatopathy)
- Urinalysis: hematuria, glycosuria, pyuria, proteinuria, casts, and isosthenuria possible with renal injury
- Abdominal radiographs: free air in peritoneal cavity strongly suggests GI tract perforation.

Advanced or Confirmatory Testing

- Usually, serum/plasma drug levels are not useful clinically.
- Endoscopy (with persistent nonspecific GI signs to rule out GI ulceration/irritation/perforation)
- Histopathologic evaluation of tissues
  - Stomach (endoscopic or surgical): irritation/duodenal ulceration/hemorrhage; peritonitis if gastric perforation
  - Kidneys (postmortem): renal tubular or papillary necrosis or interstitial nephritis
  - Liver (if persistent enzyme elevation; rarely performed): multifocal to bridging hepatocellular degeneration and necrosis (apoptosis), with mild to moderate periportal inflammation (neutrophils and lymphocytes)

TREATMENT

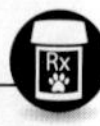

Treatment Overview

Treatment goals are decontamination (acute ingestion; induce vomiting and potentially repeated doses of activated charcoal); preventing/managing/monitoring GI, renal, hepatic and hematologic effects; and supportive care

Acute General Treatment

- Decontamination (p. 1087):
  - Induction of emesis (p. 1188): indicated in the first 1-2 hours in acute overdose patient not showing clinical signs
  - Activated charcoal 1-2 g/kg PO (or as labeled) with a cathartic if over a potential renal toxic dose, repeated (one-half dose) q 6-8h to reduce enterohepatic recirculation of NSAID if indicated
- Prevent and/or manage GI effects with combination therapy (sucralfate + proton pump inhibitor [PPI] + misoprostol):
  - For dogs, misoprostol 2-5 mcg/kg PO q 8-12h; prostaglandin analog helps replace NSAID-induced PG depletion.
  - PPI: omeprazole 0.5-1 mg/kg PO q 12-24h (dogs, cats), or esomeprazole 0.5-1 mg/kg PO q 12-24h, or pantoprazole 0.7-1 mg/kg IV over 15 minutes q 24h
  - Sucralfate 0.25-1 g PO q 6-12h (dogs, cats), given in addition to PPI
- Prevent and/or manage renal effects.
  - Fluid diuresis (2-3 times maintenance rate, barring cardiovascular disease; monitor renal output) to enhance NSAID excretion and maintain renal perfusion for 48 hours if potential renal toxic dose has been ingested (72 hours for naproxen due to long half-life)
- Manage hepatic effects.
  - Discontinue use of NSAID.
  - IV fluids
  - Administer vitamin K_1 1-5 mg/kg PO if evidence of coagulation disruption.
  - *S*-adenosyl-l-methionine (SAMe) 18 mg/kg PO q 24h for 1-3 months
- Supportive care
  - Control vomiting with maropitant 1 mg/kg SQ q 24h or metoclopramide 0.2-0.5 mg/kg q 6-8 h PO, SQ, or IM or 0.01-0.09 mg/kg/hr IV as constant-rate infusion
  - Correct fluid losses and electrolyte changes.
  - Control seizures with diazepam 0.5-1 mg/kg IV.
  - Blood transfusion if needed (p. 1169)
  - Treat GI tract perforation or enteropathy (laparotomy, antibiotics) if suspected.

Nutrition/Diet

Use appropriate prescription diets for patients with kidney or liver dysfunction.

Drug Interactions

- Concurrent use of glucocorticoids and NSAIDs increases the risk of adverse effects.
- Increased serum drug levels: phenytoin, valproic acid, oral anticoagulants, sulfonamides, sulfonylurea hypoglycemic agents, ketoconazole, methotrexate, and fluconazole
- Increased risk of nephrotoxicosis: aminoglycosides, angiotensin-converting enzyme (ACE) inhibitors, and diuretics

Possible Complications

- Chronic kidney disease
- Hepatopathy
- GI perforation and peritonitis

Recommended Monitoring

- Blood urea nitrogen, serum creatinine, electrolytes, urinalysis (baseline, 24, 48, and 72 hours in acute cases)
- Serum liver enzymes and bilirubin (for hepatopathy)

PROGNOSIS & OUTCOME

- Excellent with mild to moderate GI irritation/ulceration
- Guarded to poor with GI tract perforation
- Renal effects of NSAIDs are usually reversible if discovered early and treated intensively.
- Recovery from idiosyncratic hepatic toxicity is good when NSAID is discontinued and with supportive care.

PEARLS & CONSIDERATIONS

Comments

- For most NSAIDs, the minimal toxic/lethal dose is unknown. Generally, an acute overdose of 5-10 times more than the recommended dose could cause potentially severe GI irritation/ulceration in dogs.
- Some NSAIDs (naproxen and meclofenamic acid) have a much longer half-life in dogs due to extensive enterohepatic recirculation (naproxen: 74 hours).
- Check baseline CBC and serum biochemistry profile in all patients before long-term use of NSAIDs.
- Before starting long-term therapy, discuss common adverse effects associated with NSAIDs with clients.

Prevention

Keep all NSAIDs, especially chewables, out of the reach of pets.

Technician Tips

Misoprostol is an abortifacient. Do not handle if pregnant.

Client Education

Owners should not give any medications to their pets at home without first consulting a veterinarian.

SUGGESTED READING

Khan SA, et al: Toxicology of frequently encountered nonsteroidal anti-inflammatory drugs in dogs and cats. Vet Clin North Am Small Anim Pract 42:289-306, 2012.

AUTHOR: Camille DeClementi, VMD, DABT, DABVT
EDITOR: Tina Wismer, DVM, MS, DABVT, DABT

Nutritional Secondary Hyperparathyroidism

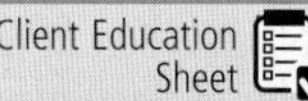

Client Education Sheet

BASIC INFORMATION

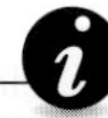

Definition

Chronic elevation of circulating parathyroid hormone (PTH) resulting from low serum ionized calcium (iCa) concentrations due to deficiency of absorbed calcium or vitamin D or a calcium/phosphorus (Ca:P) imbalance

Synonyms

- Nutritional secondary hyperparathyroidism (NSHP), nutritional osteodystrophy
- The term *rickets* describes bony changes consistent with vitamin D deficiency.

Epidemiology

SPECIES, AGE, SEX

Young, rapidly growing animals of any sex or species that have been fed an improperly formulated diet; occasionally affects older animals, especially those with malabsorptive disorders

RISK FACTORS

- Animals fed improperly formulated homemade (especially all-meat) diets, particularly during growth. Such diets typically contain deficient calcium and/or excessive phosphorus, with a calcium-to-phosphorus ratio (Ca:P) ≤ 1 : 16 (1 : 1 to 2 : 1 for dogs and 1 : 1 to 1.5 : 1 for cats is recommended) and inadequate vitamin D.
- Exotic pets because dietary requirements for calcium, phosphorus, and vitamin D are not always known and diets fed are often inappropriate
- Animals with severe gastrointestinal disease that limits calcium or vitamin D absorption

GEOGRAPHY AND SEASONALITY

The condition may be more common in winter months in some indoor-housed exotic pets because of decreased exposure to sunlight. This does not apply to cats and dogs because they cannot make vitamin D in skin.

ASSOCIATED DISORDERS

Animals may have decreased bone density or fractures related to increased circulating PTH.

Clinical Presentation

DISEASE FORMS/SUBTYPES

- Inadequate dietary calcium or vitamin D concentration or altered dietary Ca:P ratio
- Inadequate absorption of dietary calcium and vitamin D due to intestinal disease

HISTORY, CHIEF COMPLAINT

- History of a poorly formulated homemade diet or exclusive use of a commercial diet intended for supplemental feeding only
- Excessive use of supplements such as meats, vitamins, and minerals
- History of malabsorption due to intestinal disease
- Reluctance to walk, stiff gait, bone pain, lameness, or limb deformities (pathologic bone fractures); difficulty with prehension; tooth loss, ± neurologic signs if the axial skeleton is involved
- Signs of hypocalcemia: twitching, tremors, stiffness, or seizures (rare)

PHYSICAL EXAM FINDINGS

- Bone palpation may elicit pain; fractures may be noted.
- Swelling of costochondral junctions or metaphyses may be evident.

Etiology and Pathophysiology

- Inadequate calcium absorption decreases iCa, increasing PTH production.
- Inadequate absorbed vitamin D decreases calcitriol production, decreasing iCa and increasing PTH production.
- PTH stimulates renal 1,25-dihydroxyvitamin D (calcitriol, the active metabolite of vitamin D) synthesis and bone resorption and increases renal calcium resorption and phosphorus excretion.
- Calcitriol also stimulates bone resorption to raise iCa into the normal range and decreases PTH production.
- Excessive PTH production reduces bone density, and pathologic fractures may occur.

- Excess circulating phosphorus also inhibits calcitriol synthesis and can lower iCa by the mass law effect.

DIAGNOSIS

Diagnostic Overview

The diagnosis is strongly suspected in young animals with a history of an inadequate diet, radiographic evidence of diffuse bone loss, and pathologic fractures.

Differential Diagnosis

- Other causes of lameness, bone pain, loss of bone density, or fractures, including congenital problems in young animals
- Renal secondary hyperparathyroidism (p. 878) (ruled out based on serum biochemistry profile and urinalysis)
- Hyperadrenocorticism-associated secondary hyperparathyroidism in older dogs (ruled out based on adrenal function testing and clinical signs)
- Genetic defects in calcitriol production or use (vitamin D–dependent rickets type 1 or 2); clinical signs are the same in the absence of compatible diet history or malabsorptive disorder.

Initial Database

- CBC and serum biochemical profile: serum total calcium concentration normal to low. NOTE: Serum phosphorus and alkaline phosphatase may be elevated in normal animals relative to the laboratory reference range, especially in those that are young and growing.
- Radiography of the skull, axial skeleton, and limbs: diffusely decreased cortical bone density; fractures possible
- Diet history

Advanced or Confirmatory Testing

- Measure serum PTH (increased), iCa (low to normal), and 25-hydroxyvitamin D (25-OH-D; typically low) concentrations to confirm the diagnosis.
- Serum calcitriol determination (usually increased)
- Vitamin/mineral analysis of homemade diets may be useful, but diet history is usually sufficient to help confirm suspected diagnosis.

TREATMENT

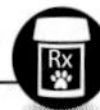

Treatment Overview

Goals of treatment are to increase intestinal absorption of calcium and vitamin D and decrease PTH production.

Acute General Treatment

- Feed a properly formulated, complete, and balanced diet.
- Stop use of all supplements.
- Supportive therapy for pain or fractures (cage rest or limited activity as indicated)
- Treatment of malabsorption when present
- Dietary supplementation with oral calcium 25-50 mg/kg elemental Ca (e.g., 62.5-125 mg/kg calcium carbonate) daily if clinical signs of hypocalcemia (p. 515) are present, discontinuing when signs resolve

Chronic Treatment

- Ensure that a properly formulated diet is fed.
- If a homemade diet is fed, ensure use of an appropriate and balanced recipe for long-term use.
- Supplemental oral calcium may be indicated in cases of chronic malabsorption but are not necessary if the diet is inadequate and subsequently corrected.

Nutrition/Diet

Feed a properly formulated commercial or homemade diet appropriate for the life stage.

Possible Complications

- Clinicians should repeat tests of PTH, iCa, and 25-OH-D concentrations 3-4 weeks after initiating treatment. PTH should be decreased and 25-OH-D increased compared with pretreatment values. Clinicians should monitor the animals monthly until levels are normal.
- Clinicians should measure PTH, iCa, and 25-OH-D concentrations every 3-4 months, even if secondary hyperparathyroidism has resolved, especially when intestinal malabsorption is present.
- Clinicians should order repeat radiography tests to assess bone density and fracture healing.

PROGNOSIS & OUTCOME

- Depends on presence and location of pathologic fractures, which worsen the prognosis because of pain and a potentially long convalescent period
- Incidentally discovered NSHP that is due to inappropriate diet typically carries a good prognosis.
- For animals with malabsorption, the prognosis depends on the underlying cause and effectiveness of therapy.

PEARLS & CONSIDERATIONS

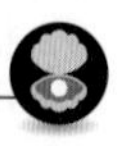

Comments

- Animals fed homemade diets should be monitored as part of a routine nutritional assessment.
- Review balanced homemade diet recipes with owners at every visit to ensure that substitutions or omissions have not occurred.

Prevention

Clinicians should inform owners to

- Feed their pets nutritionally complete and balanced pet foods rather than improperly formulated homemade diets.
- Avoid supplementing balanced diets with meats, vitamins, or minerals.

Technician Tips

Be careful when handling or walking affected animals because fractures can easily occur. Cage rest during healing is critical for recovery.

Client Education

- Clinicians should explain the risks of serious skeletal problems associated with nutrient imbalance to clients feeding homemade diets, especially to young, growing animals.
- Clinicians should have the adequacy of homemade diets verified by a veterinary nutritionist.

SUGGESTED READING

Cook SD, et al: A quantitative histologic study of osteoporosis produced by nutritional secondary hyperparathyroidism in dogs. Clin Orthop 175:105-120, 1983.

AUTHOR: Patricia A. Schenck, DVM, PhD
EDITOR: Jennifer Larsen, DVM, PhD, DACVN

Nystagmus

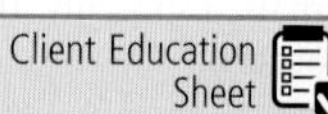

BASIC INFORMATION

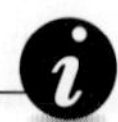

Definition

- Involuntary rhythmic movement of the globe of the eye; nystagmus occurs in a horizontal, rotary, or vertical direction.
- *Jerk nystagmus* with a fast and slow phase is most common.
- Nystagmus direction is named after the direction of the fast phase.
- *Pendular nystagmus* is characterized by eye movements of equal speed without a fast or slow phase.

Epidemiology

SPECIES, AGE, SEX

Any age, breed, or sex

GENETICS, BREED PREDISPOSITION

- Cats: pendular nystagmus occurs in otherwise normal Siamese and Himalayan

cats. Pathologic nystagmus is a congenital abnormality in Siamese, Tonkinese, and Burmese breeds.
- Dogs: pathologic nystagmus is a congenital abnormality in Doberman pinscher, cocker spaniel, German shepherd, and other breeds

ASSOCIATED DISORDERS

Vestibular disease

Clinical Presentation

DISEASE FORMS/SUBTYPES

Types of nystagmus:
- Physiologic nystagmus: occurs in normal animals (vestibulo-ocular reflex) with head rotation and consists of a slow phase in the opposite direction of head movement and a fast phase occurring in same direction of head rotation.
- Pathologic nystagmus: spontaneous
  - Present when the head is stationary and in a normal position
  - Often resolves within several days of onset of vestibular signs
- Pathologic nystagmus: positional
  - Nystagmus occurs in changing or unusual head positions (head extension, dorsal or lateral recumbency).
  - Possible at onset of vestibular dysfunction or after spontaneous nystagmus has resolved
  - Occurs with peripheral or central vestibular lesions
  - Nystagmus that changes direction with different head positions usually suggests a central lesion.
- Pendular nystagmus
  - Typically nonpathologic
- Disconjugate nystagmus
  - Direction of oscillation is different for each eye (e.g., horizontal for the left eye [OS] and vertical for the right eye [OD]).
  - Indicates central lesion

HISTORY, CHIEF COMPLAINT
- Pathologic nystagmus usually has acute onset.
  - Most commonly with vestibular disease
  - Nystagmus may be unnoticed if animal moves quickly or with vestibular compensation (positional nystagmus possibly induced).
- Pendular nystagmus or congenital nystagmus is present from birth/adolescence and is not associated with deteriorating vestibular function.

PHYSICAL EXAM FINDINGS

Nystagmus from peripheral vestibular disease (not all signs may be present):
- Jerk nystagmus
  - Horizontal or rotary most common
  - Fast phase: away from side of vestibular lesion and contralateral to head tilt
  - Direction unchanged with head position
  - Vertical rare with peripheral vestibular disease
  - Convergence–retraction nystagmus is an irregular jerk nystagmus with simultaneous rhythmic convergence and eyeball retraction of both eyes (OU)
- Positional nystagmus possible after spontaneous nystagmus resolves
  - Important to evaluate different head positions
- Head tilt (ipsilateral)
- Ataxia
- Circling (ipsilateral)
- Falling can occur (ipsilateral)
- Ventral strabismus (ipsilateral)

Nystagmus from central vestibular disease (not all signs may be present):
- Jerk nystagmus
  - Horizontal, rotary, or vertical
  - Vertical suggests central disease
  - Disconjugate indicates central disease
- Convergence-retraction indicates central lesion, often in dorsal midbrain
  - Fast phase can occur in either direction relative to the vestibular lesion
  - Direction can change with head position
- Positional nystagmus possible after spontaneous nystagmus resolves
  - Important to evaluate different head positions
- Head tilt (ipsilateral, unless paradoxical)
- Circling (ipsilateral, unless paradoxical)
- Ataxia
- Proprioceptive deficits (ipsilateral)
- Ventral strabismus (ipsilateral)
- Cranial nerve deficits (ipsilateral)
- Obtundation

Etiology and Pathophysiology
- Physiologic nystagmus occurs in normal animals with head rotation. Jerk nystagmus results in the plane of rotation. Fast phase occurs in same direction as movement, and slow phase occurs in opposite direction of movement. The fast phase is induced by visual stimuli. This vestibulo-ocular reflex preserves image stability on the retina.
  - Afferent initiating stimuli from semicircular canals travel to vestibular nuclei.
  - Vestibular nuclei interconnect with motor nuclei that control extraocular muscle movement in brainstem (cranial nerves III, IV, and VI through the medial longitudinal fasciculus).
  - Head movement causes reciprocating afferent stimuli from semicircular canals in the plane of movement through vestibular nuclei, allowing coordinated and conjugate eye movements.
- Pathologic nystagmus occurs with a unilateral lesion (e.g., single semicircular canal). Asymmetrical neural activity is perceived as head rotation, despite the head being at rest/motionless, inducing nystagmus.
- Vestibulocochlear nerve provides input from semicircular canals to central vestibular system (vestibular nuclei and rostral cerebellum).
- Damage to the peripheral or central vestibular system produces nystagmus.

DIAGNOSIS

Diagnostic Overview

Pathologic nystagmus indicates vestibular dysfunction. Diagnostic testing focused on central and peripheral vestibular centers and diseases affecting these regions.

Differential Diagnosis

Peripheral causes:
- Infection (otitis media/interna)
- Idiopathic
- Otopharyngeal polyps
- Neoplasia
- Hypothyroidism (rare)
- Trauma
- After middle ear surgery or ear cleaning (if tympanum not intact)
- Intoxication (e.g., aminoglycosides, cleaning solutions)
- Congenital/hereditary

Central causes:
- Neoplasia
- Idiopathic
- Vascular
- Inflammation (granulomatous meningoencephalitis, necrotizing leukoencephalitis)
- Infection (bacterial, viral, fungal, protozoal or central extension of otitis media/interna)
- Toxic (metronidazole, marijuana, anesthesia induction/recovery)
- Nutritional (thiamine deficiency)
- Trauma
- Congenital/developmental

Pendular nystagmus: congenital abnormality affecting visual pathway

Initial Database
- Neurologic exam (p. 1136)
  - Attempt to induce positional nystagmus.
  - Absent vestibulo-ocular reflex may indicate bilateral vestibular disease.
- Otoscopic exam (p. 1144)
- CBC, chemistry, T_4, and urinalysis: usually normal
- Tympanic bulla radiographs (limited benefit)
- Thoracic radiographs and abdominal ultrasound evaluates for metastatic/systemic disease

Advanced or Confirmatory Testing
- MRI (p. 1132): preferred, due to superior soft-tissue resolution
- CT: high resolution of inner ear, less for brain
- Cerebrospinal fluid (CSF) (p. 1323) analysis if intracranial disease suspected or to further evaluate for central extension of otitis media/interna
- Myringotomy (cytology and culture) indicated for otitis media/interna
- Infectious serology considered based on MRI/CSF results and environmental risk factors
- Brainstem auditory evoked response testing can help localize vestibular disease.

TREATMENT

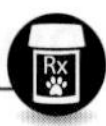

Treatment Overview

- Supportive care
- Alleviate nausea if present.
- Treat underlying cause.

Acute and Chronic Treatment

- Vestibular: supportive care (pp. 403 and 1037) and treatment of the inciting disorder
  - Prolonged use of antinausea drugs can delay vestibular compensation/recovery.
  - Discontinue metronidazole.

Possible Complications

Use caution when cleaning external ear canals. If tympanic membrane is ruptured, most cleaning solutions and antibiotics can cause damage.

PROGNOSIS & OUTCOME

- Spontaneous nystagmus often resolves within the first several days of a vestibular event.
- Vestibular: varies, based on underlying cause
  - Metronidazole toxicosis: typically good prognosis with discontinuation of metronidazole and supportive care. Diazepam therapy may speed improvement.

PEARLS & CONSIDERATIONS

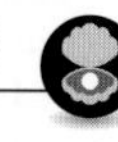

Comments

- Nystagmus is usually absent with bilateral vestibular disease.
- Physiologic nystagmus can persist for a few seconds after head rotation has stopped.
- Idiopathic peripheral vestibular disease usually causes nystagmus; nystagmus should resolve spontaneously in 1-2 weeks.
  - Compensation can also occur initially with other disease processes.
  - When compensation occurs with causes other than idiopathic vestibular disease or vascular causes, then decompensation/relapse typically occurs.
- Many (but not all) patients with nystagmus caused by central vestibular disease have other CNS signs (mentation changes, cranial nerve deficits, proprioceptive deficits).

Technician Tips

- Use caution when cleaning external ear canals.
- Patients often do better with self-induced movement. Quick movements can exacerbate vestibular disease.

Client Education

- Signs often improve within several days.
- Diagnostics evaluate possible causes, need for specific treatment, and help determine prognosis.
- Harness and sling helps patient handling.
- Nightlights can help. Loss of balance (vestibular disease) together with low visibility can make it difficult for animals to stay oriented and upright.

SUGGESTED READING

Rossmeisl JH: Vestibular disease in dogs and cats. Vet Clin North Am Small Anim Pract 40:81-100, 2010.

AUTHOR: James Lavely, DVM, DACVIM
EDITOR: Leah A. Cohn, DVM, PhD, DACVIM

Obesity

Bonus Material Online 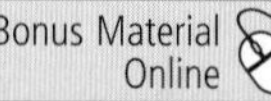 Client Education Sheet 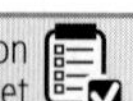

BASIC INFORMATION

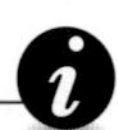

Definition

In companion animals, obesity is defined as 25% above ideal body weight, which corresponds to a body condition score (BCS) of 7 on a 9-point scale.

Epidemiology

SPECIES, AGE, SEX

Prevalence ranges up to 63% in some canine populations and 59% among cats. Incidence increases with age in both species. Female dogs and male cats appear to be predisposed.

GENETICS, BREED PREDISPOSITION

- Predisposed dog breeds include Labrador and golden retrievers, Cairn and Scottish terriers, collies, basset hounds, Cavalier King Charles and cocker spaniels, dachshunds, rottweilers, Saint Bernards, and Newfoundlands. A mutation in the proopiomelanocortin gene *(POMC)* is associated with body weight, adiposity, and greater food motivation in Labrador retrievers.
- Crossbreed, mixed-breed, and Manx cats are at higher risk for obesity.

RISK FACTORS

- Neutering (dogs and cats)
- Age (dogs and cats)
- Female sex (dogs)
- Male sex (cats)
- Strict indoor housing (cats)
- Apartment living (dogs and cats)
- Orthopedic or neuromuscular disease impeding mobility
- Medications such as phenobarbital and glucocorticoids (dogs > cats)
- Endocrine disease (e.g., hypothyroidism, hyperadrenocorticism, acromegaly)

ASSOCIATED DISORDERS

- Hyperlipidemia/dyslipidemia (dogs and cats)
- Insulin resistance and glucose intolerance (pre-diabetes; dogs and cats)
- Diabetes mellitus (dogs and cats)
- Hepatic lipidosis (cats)
- Orthopedic disease (dogs and cats)
- Dermatological disease (dogs and cats)
- Oral cavity disease (cats)
- Hypertension (dogs)
- Pancreatitis (dogs)
- Feline lower urinary tract disease (cats)
- Urolithiasis (cats and possibly dogs)
- Respiratory compromise (dogs and cats)
- Dystocia (dogs and cats)
- Exercise intolerance (dogs and cats)
- Heat intolerance (dogs and cats)
- Decreased immune function (dogs and cats)
- Increased anesthetic risk (dogs and cats)
- Decreased life span (dogs and cats)

Clinical Presentation

Noted on routine wellness consultation or with associated concurrent disease

HISTORY, CHIEF COMPLAINT

Associated concurrent issue, such as exercise intolerance or impaired mobility. Many owners do not recognize or acknowledge that their pet is obese.

PHYSICAL EXAM FINDINGS

Excessive adipose tissue is generally readily recognized, but ascites or organomegaly may be confounding factors. Abnormalities related to cause of obesity, such as haircoat changes in a dog with hypothyroidism or hyperadrenocorticism, may be noted.

Etiology and Pathophysiology

Obesity results when energy intake exceeds expenditure, but it has a heterogeneous pathophysiology that can involve genetics, diet, feeding habits, environment, and microbiota.

DIAGNOSIS

Diagnostic Overview

Identify any concurrent, predisposing, or resulting disorder.

Differential Diagnosis

- Ascites
- Abdominal mass or organomegaly
- Hyperadrenocorticism
- Pregnancy

Initial Database

- A nutritional assessment should be performed for every animal at every visit (includes body weight, BCS, and diet history). Compare with historical data.
  - BCS assesses body fat with visualization and palpation. Each score above ideal represents 5% increase in body fat corresponding to 10%-15% body weight (see Body Condition Score Charts for Dogs and Cats).
- CBC, biochemistry panel, urinalysis, and thyroid panel to look for clues as to contributing or associated conditions

TREATMENT

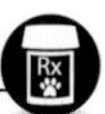

Treatment Overview

Weight loss plans involve calorie restriction. Monitoring is critical to assess for potential complications and evaluate rate of loss to make adjustments as needed (p. 1077).

Nutrition/Diet

- A veterinary therapeutic weight loss diet is recommended.
  - Reduced-energy density; increased nutrient-to-calorie ratio, including higher protein; strategies for satiety such as higher-fiber and moisture content
- Calculate initial target of daily calories.
  - Ideally, determine total current intake, and reduce this amount by 20%.
  - Alternatively, calculate starting amount as

Dog = resting energy requirement ($70 \times$ BW [current body weight in kg]$^{0.75}$)

Cat = $0.8 \times$ resting energy requirement ($70 \times$ BW [current body weight in kg]$^{0.75}$)

- For accuracy and ease of adjustments, provide daily target amount in grams rather than cup or can amounts.
- Provide treat options if needed to make up no more than 10% of daily calories. Fruits and vegetables are recommended due to their low energy density. Be sure pet owner is aware of foods that are dangerous for pets (e.g., grapes, avocado).

Behavior/Exercise

- Increasing activity and exercise is encouraged for mental and physical stimulation. Consider food toys, training, walks and play, and creating opportunities to chase or seek all or part of food allowance.
- Restricting access to other food sources is important, especially in multipet households. All family members and visitors should be aware of the weight loss plan.

Drug Interactions

Side effects of some medications, such as glucocorticoids or phenobarbital, may result in increased appetite or decreased energy expenditure.

Possible Complications

- Excessive loss of lean body mass if > 2% of body weight is lost per week
- Weight regain
- Hepatic lipidosis in cats
- Poor satiety leading to begging, stealing, or scavenging

Recommended Monitoring

- Assess body weight at least once weekly initially and then every 2-3 weeks using the same scale. Review diet history at every recheck to ensure and reinforce compliance.
- Target loss rate is 1%-2% body weight per week.
- Adjust the daily caloric intake by 5%-10% to maintain target rate of loss.
- Counsel owners that depending on the animal's BCS, it could take up to 1 year until ideal body condition is reached, although improvement in well-being and comorbidities is expected before an ideal BCS is achieved.

PROGNOSIS & OUTCOME

Outcome depends on compliance and severity of concurrent disease. Regaining excessive body weight is likely if feeding of controlled amounts is not practiced because fewer calories may be needed for rebound and to maintain an obese condition than before initial weight loss.

PEARLS & CONSIDERATIONS

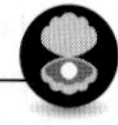

Comments

- Regular monitoring and owner diligence is crucial to reverse obesity as well as to prevent it in pets, especially those that are neutered. Owner education is paramount for success.
- Troubleshooting to improve satiety may involve switching to another weight loss diet with lower caloric density, dividing the daily food amount over more daily feedings, increasing food moisture content, or using food toys.

Prevention

- Communicate benefits of obesity prevention, and provide guidance on appropriate diet types and amounts to feed.
- Promote activity and regular exercise, especially in strictly indoor cats.
- Discuss the importance of regular assessment to enable food adjustment to maintain ideal BCS, especially after neutering.

Technician Tips

- Encourage use of gram scales to weigh foods for accuracy and ease of adjustments to maintain target rate of loss.
- Encourage and provide positive reinforcement to the owner when the animal meets its weekly target goals for weight loss. Focus on the process rather than the end goal.
- Technicians play a key role in continued support of weight loss efforts through frequent client communication and feedback regarding progress toward goals.

SUGGESTED READING

Farcas AK, et al: Small animal obesity. Vet Clin North Am Small Anim Pract 46:761-940, 2016.

AUTHOR: Aarti Kathrani, BVetMed, PhD, DACVIM, DACVN
EDITOR: Jennifer Larsen, DVM, PhD, DACVN

Obsessive-Compulsive Disorder

BASIC INFORMATION

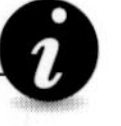

Definition

Mood/behavioral disorders characterized by repetitive, invariant, patterned behaviors that are exaggerated in intensity, frequency, and duration given the inciting stimuli (i.e., expressed out of context). The behavior interferes with health and well-being.

Synonyms

Compulsive disorders, stereotypies, stargazing, air or fly snapping, spinning/tail chasing, self-mutilation, OCD

Epidemiology

SPECIES, AGE, SEX

Dogs and cats of any age

GENETICS, BREED PREDISPOSITION

Dogs: genetic predisposition is suspected. Anecdotally, certain syndromes are more commonly associated with some breeds:

- Acral lick dermatitis: large and giant dog breeds
- Air/fly snapping, checking (hindquarter area), star gazing: miniature schnauzer
- Flank sucking: Doberman pinscher
- Spinning/tail chasing: German shepherd dog, bull terrier, Parson Russell and Jack Russell terriers

Cats: fabric chewing or ingestion is anecdotally associated with Asian breeds (e.g., Siamese, Tonkinese, Burmese).

RISK FACTORS

- Stressful or traumatic event, especially for cats
- Lack of a daily routine or change in a well-established routine

CONTAGION AND ZOONOSIS

Characteristically, OCD is not induced in conspecifics (e.g., housemates) by affected individuals.

ASSOCIATED DISORDERS

The patient may have multiple diagnoses of other impulsive or anxiety-based disorders.

Clinical Presentation

HISTORY, CHIEF COMPLAINT

- Repetitive behavior that is out of context (might have been exacerbated over time or begun suddenly)
- Inciting triggers may be identifiable, or the behavior may occur spontaneously.
- Earlier in the course, the owners might have been able to stop the behavior, but that may not be the case at the time of presentation, and the pet may not stop until exhausted.
- The pet may hide (to perform the behavior), become aggressive when the owners try to stop the behavior, or may begin avoiding the owners.
- Distress vocalizations (whining, crying, yowling, or growling) may occur before, during, or after performance of the compulsive behavior.
- When owners do not identify the behavior as abnormal, the chief complaint may be damage to self (alopecia, granuloma, weight loss, change in voice, recurring gastrointestinal obstruction due to pica), damage to the home, or altered social interactions.
- The chief complaint may suggest partial seizures or dysphoria.
- With chronicity, some owners may not consider the behavior problematic or abnormal.

PHYSICAL EXAM FINDINGS

- Often unremarkable
- Skin lesions possible with overgrooming/self-mutilation
- Weight loss if near-constant

Etiology and Pathophysiology

- A genetic contribution is suspected.
- In humans, the current hypothesis for OCD involves dysfunction in a neuronal circuit traversing from the orbital frontal cortex to the cingulate gyrus, caudate nucleus, putamen (i.e., striatum), globus pallidus, thalamus, and back to the frontal cortex.
- Dysfunction involving glutamate and/or gamma-aminobutyric acid (GABA) is an additional focus of research.
- Acral lick dermatitis appears to involve interplay between behavioral, neurologic, and dermatologic conditions in many cases (p. 16).

DIAGNOSIS

Diagnostic Overview

Performance of repetitive, invariant behaviors that are spontaneous or triggered, are difficult or impossible to interrupt, and interfere with normal maintenance and social behaviors are characteristic of OCD.

Differential Diagnosis

- Attention-seeking (behavior occurs only when the owner is present)
- Separation anxiety (behavior occurs only when the owners are absent)
- Cognitive dysfunction (middle-aged/geriatric animals that pace or stare)
- Hyperthyroidism (primarily cats)
- Neuropathic pain disorders (e.g., feline hyperesthesia, neck and shoulder hyperesthesia in syringomyelia in the Cavalier King Charles spaniel)
- Degenerative joint disease, anal sac disease, cystitis, and less commonly, endoparasitism (excessive licking or hindquarter checking)
- Circling, spinning, and air-snapping patients should be evaluated for peripheral or central vestibular disease, psychomotor seizures, or other central nervous system lesions.

Initial Database

- CBC, urinalysis, and serum chemistry profile: usually within reference limits (assess for systemic disorders before initiation of medications). Fecal exam warranted for hindquarter checking.
- Neurologic examination (p. 1136)
- Dermatologic diagnostic tests (p. 1091) if skin lesions are a feature

TREATMENT

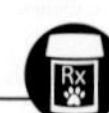

Treatment Overview

- All cases of OCD warrant intervention, which is individualized and based on frequency and severity of clinical signs.
- Treatment is a combination of behavioral and environmental modification and psychotropic medication.
- The goal is to minimize and, if possible, eliminate bouts of compulsive behavior and the concomitant focused, anxious states that accompany them.

Acute and Chronic Treatment

- Owner should identify and eliminate trigger events/situations whenever possible.
- No punishment should ever be used because it can heighten anxiety and worsen, not improve, the problem.
- If possible, the pet can be redirected to an alternative and incompatible behavior, such as licking food from a toy instead of licking the skin, as long as the redirection does not make the pet more anxious.
- The pet should be calmly rewarded for any spontaneous calm behavior.
- Keeping a structured daily routine helps decrease anxiety.
- The most successful medications used in the treatment of OCD in people include selective serotonin reuptake inhibitors (SSRIs) and clomipramine, a tricyclic antidepressant (TCA). In dogs and cats, the most commonly used are
  - Clomipramine (Clomicalm): dogs, 2-3 mg/kg PO q 12h; cats, 0.5 mg/kg PO q 24h
  - SSRI drugs (fluoxetine [Prozac]): dogs, 1 mg/kg PO q 24h; cats, 0.5 mg/kg PO q 24h, paroxetine (Paxil): dogs, 1 mg/kg PO q 24h; cats, 0.25-0.5 mg/kg PO
  - Treat for a minimum of 16 weeks; many OCD patients require lifelong medication.
- Very distressed pets may need concomitant use of benzodiazepines (BDZs); anxiolytics have faster onset of action
  - Diazepam or oxazepam (oxazepam for cats, obese patients, liver disease) 0.2-0.4 mg/kg PO q 12-24h, alprazolam 0.01-0.025 mg/kg PO q 8-24h, or clonazepam (dogs) 0.01-0.05 mg/kg PO q 12-24h for the first 2-3 weeks of treatment. Adjust to ideal dose based on response and lack of adverse (e.g., hepatic) effects. May also be used preemptively when stress or change in routine is anticipated
- Gabapentin, a GABA analog, is another useful adjunct medication; dogs, 3-5 mg/kg PO q 12h; cats 5-10 mg/kg PO q 12h starting low and titrating to effect
- *N*-methyl-D-aspartate (NMDA) antagonists hold promise as a potential treatment of OCD as single pharmacologic agents or as an adjunct to SSRIs.
- Skin lesions secondary to overgrooming may require treatment with antibiotics, analgesics, and/or antiinflammatories. Cold laser therapy can be used to decrease pain and inflammation and to speed healing of acral lick granuloma lesions. The underlying mood disorder that led to excessive grooming needs to be managed (p. 16).
- Typically, TCA or SSRI therapy is necessary for longer periods than other anxiety-based disorders (months to years, depending on

severity and duration of the disorder). Lifelong medication use is not unusual in severe cases.

Behavior/Exercise

Some patients benefit from activities that serve as a controlled outlet for the compulsive behavior (e.g., retrieving, herding, agility, flyball), although they can be too arousing for others; tailor treatment to the individual.

Drug Interactions

- TCAs and SSRIs should not be given with monoamine oxidase inhibitors (MAOIs), which are found in many flea and tick collars and dips and in some medications to treat cognitive dysfunction.
- TCAs: use with caution in cases with cardiac arrhythmias or liver or thyroid disorders.
- Use of SSRIs with tramadol, which has a weak serotonin reuptake inhibiting effect, may increase the risk of serotonin syndrome (p. 1281). Coadministration of fluoxetine, paroxetine, and possibly sertraline may result in decreased plasma concentrations of tramadol's active demethylated metabolite by inhibition of hepatic cytochrome P450 enzymes. If their use together is necessary, starting both at reduced doses, titrating each to effect, and keeping watch for signs of serotonin syndrome reduces but does not eliminate the risk. The client should be informed and should learn to monitor heart rate for profound increases as one way of assaying an early sign of serotonin syndrome.

Possible Complications

- Paroxetine: avoid in kidney disease; anecdotal reports of constipation in cats
- Gabapentin dose reduction is warranted in patients with renal disease.

Recommended Monitoring

- Cats receiving paroxetine: monitor stool consistency (reports of diarrhea).
- Animals taking BDZs require a physical exam every 6 months in most U.S. states. The potential for human diversion warrants vigilance regarding refill requests.
- Performing a yearly physical exam, CBC, serum chemistry profile, urinalysis, and thyroid screen (twice yearly in senior pets) should be a minimum for animals taking other psychotropic medications.

PROGNOSIS & OUTCOME

- Prognosis is highly variable from guarded to very good for management of the clinical signs of OCD and is contingent on a number of variables:
    - Time at which treatment is first instituted (the earlier, the better the prognosis)
    - Owner compliance with all (and not just portions) of the treatment recommendations
    - Frequent communication and follow-up is necessary between the owner and the clinician because the treatment plan will need adjustment based on the pet's response and changing life circumstances
    - Untreated OCD seldom improves and very commonly worsens over time.

PEARLS & CONSIDERATIONS

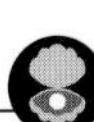

Comments

- Because repetitive behaviors are commonly thought of by clients as entertaining or as quirks in their pet's personality and seldom understood to be potential early markers of this disease, many pets suffer greatly throughout life while their owners are ignorant of the distress associated with OCDs.
- Early intervention is a significant factor in the successful treatment of OCDs, but owners seldom talk about behavior during a veterinary visit unless prompted. It is extremely important to incorporate specific questions about behavior in all wellness and sick exams. "Any behavior that is new, different, or peculiar since the last veterinary exam?" is sufficient to open the door and encourage owners to talk about their pet's behavior.
- Boredom is an insufficient explanation for OCD, and simply "blaming" boredom precludes essential early intervention.

Prevention

- Consider temperament when selecting breeding stock.
- At the onset of any repetitive behaviors, the owners should be instructed to watch for a worsening of signs or specific triggers that may initiate the behavior. Keeping a diary, written or preferably on video media, is helpful to track onset and progression.

Technician Tips

OCD may create a home situation that is disrupted compared with an owner's expectations. Support from the entire veterinary staff in identifying and treating this disorder correctly is rewarding for all and lifesaving for the pet.

Client Education

Treatment of OCD is never static, often lifelong, and subject to adjustment based on changing conditions. Relapses may occur with treatment discontinuation or profound life changes/stressors. Planning in advance of added stressors can help minimize their effect on an OCD patient.

SUGGESTED READING

Overall KL, et al: Clinical features and outcome in dogs and cats with obsessive-compulsive disorder: 126 cases (1989-2000). J Am Vet Med Assoc 221:1445-1452, 2002.

AUTHOR: Soraya V. Juarbe-Diaz, DVM, DACVB
EDITOR: Karen L. Overall, MA, VMD, PhD, DACVB

Ocular Discharge

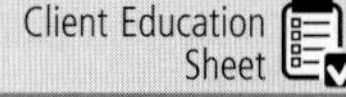

BASIC INFORMATION

Definition

- Abnormal secretions on or around the eye(s)
- Secretions can be watery (serous), contain mucus (mucoid), or contain white blood cells, mucus, and bacteria/fungi (mucopurulent).
- An abnormal overflow of tears down the face is *epiphora*.

Epidemiology

SPECIES, AGE, SEX

Dogs and cats; age of onset varies, depending on cause

GENETICS, BREED PREDISPOSITION

Depends on cause:

- Breeds predisposed to distichia, ectopic cilia, and trichiasis
- Breeds predisposed to congenital atresia, ectopia, and/or imperforate lacrimal puncta
- Breeds predisposed to entropion and/or ectropion
- Breeds predisposed to keratoconjunctivitis sicca (KCS)
- Dolichocephalic breeds of dogs with narrow skull conformation and deep medial canthal areas (i.e., medial canthal pocket syndrome)

RISK FACTORS

Outdoor animals prone to infectious causes of conjunctivitis and ocular trauma

CONTAGION AND ZOONOSIS

Certain infectious causes of conjunctivitis are contagious (e.g., feline herpesvirus type 1 [FHV-1]) and/or zoonotic (e.g., *Chlamydia* spp).

Clinical Presentation

HISTORY, CHIEF COMPLAINT

- Clear, watery, white to gray, mucoid or green-yellow, thick secretions on the eye(s) or eyelids
- Sudden, progressive, or persistent in nature

PHYSICAL EXAM FINDINGS

Unilateral or bilateral, serous, mucoid, or mucopurulent ocular secretions with one or more of the following:

- Blepharitis: inflammation of the eyelids
- Conjunctivitis (pp. 199 and 200)
- Corneal ulceration (p. 209)
- KCS (p. 568)
- Qualitative tear film abnormality (e.g., mucin and/or lipid deficiency)
- Entropion and/or ectropion (p. 296)
- Distichiasis/ectopic cilia/trichiasis (p. 273)
- Anterior uveitis (p. 1023)
- Glaucoma (p. 387)
- Globe size abnormalities (p. 705)
- Orbital disease (p. 716)
- Congenital anomalies or infection of nasolacrimal system (e.g., dacryocystitis)

Etiology and Pathophysiology

Serous discharge:

- Corneal mechanical irritation
  - Distichiasis/ectopic cilia/trichiasis
  - Entropion
  - Eyelid agenesis (partial absence of palpebral margin): more common in cats
  - Eyelid neoplasia
- Obstruction of nasolacrimal system, congenital
  - Imperforate lacrimal punctum (commonly ventral lacrimal punctum not open)
  - Micropunctum (small ventral lacrimal punctum; common)
  - Nasolacrimal aplasia (lack of opening into nasal cavity; rare)
  - Obstruction of nasolacrimal duct in dogs by dacryops (cysts originating from lacrimal tissue) or nasal cyst (rare)
- Blockage of nasolacrimal system, acquired
  - Dacryocystitis (inflammation of the nasolacrimal system)
  - Neoplasia: primary (rare); secondary (more common) (e.g., nasal; maxillary sinus)
  - Foreign body
  - Trauma to medial canthus/eyelid, involving lacrimal punctum/puncta and/or canaliculus/canaliculi
- Ocular pain
  - Conjunctivitis
  - Simple or indolent/recurrent corneal ulceration
  - Qualitative tear film abnormality (e.g., mucin and/or lipid deficiency)
  - Anterior uveitis
  - Glaucoma

Mucoid to mucopurulent discharge:

- Blepharitis
- Conjunctivitis
- KCS
- Melting/infected corneal ulceration
- Orbital abscess/cellulitis
- Dacryocystitis
- Nasolacrimal foreign body (e.g., grass awn, parasite)

DIAGNOSIS

Diagnostic Overview

Ocular discharge is apparent on physical exam. The underlying cause should be initially investigated with a review of the history, physical exam, and complete ophthalmic exam. If the cause is not elucidated, specific ocular tests (some requiring referral) may be warranted.

Differential Diagnosis

- Ocular discharge with red eye(s) is often associated with overproduction of tears (i.e., linked with causes of corneal mechanical irritation, infection, or ocular pain).
- Ocular discharge with quiet eye(s) (i.e., no evidence of ocular pain or eyelid conditions) is often associated with impaired drainage of tears (e.g., congenital or acquired blockage of nasolacrimal system).

Initial Database

- Complete ophthalmic exam (p. 1137):
  - Careful examination with magnification of the eyelids
  - Schirmer tear test (normal 15-25 mm/min; excessive lacrimation > 25 mm/min with corneal irritation)
  - Fluorescein dye application (corneal dye retention with corneal ulceration; dye exiting nares helps confirm patent nasolacrimal system)
  - Intraocular pressure (IOP) (pressures > 25 mm Hg with glaucoma; may be low at < 15 mm Hg with uveitis; both are painful conditions)
- Conjunctival and/or corneal (if infected corneal ulcer) swabs
  - Cytologic exam to determine cell type and possible cause
  - Culture and susceptibility (C&S): aerobic; anaerobic and fungal pathogens are rare

Advanced or Confirmatory Testing

- Varies depending on underlying cause
- Polymerase chain reaction (PCR): FHV-I, *Chlamydia* spp, and *Mycoplasma* spp
- Blockage of nasolacrimal system can be investigated with nasolacrimal flush; if no fluorescein dye exits nares, blockage is suspected. If results are unclear, confirmation is possible with nasal radiographs with a contrast study of the nasolacrimal system. Contrast CT is best to assess the integrity of the nasolacrimal system.

TREATMENT

Treatment Overview

Treatment is directed at the underlying cause. If discharge persists or progresses, referral to a veterinary ophthalmologist should be considered.

Acute General Treatment

- Treat the underlying cause (see Etiology and Pathophysiology above).
- Blockage of nasolacrimal system: treat the primary lesion causing the obstruction (may be difficult to diagnose; if so, consult a veterinary ophthalmologist).

Chronic Treatment

May be required with certain diseases (e.g., KCS)

Possible Complications

- Conjunctivitis due to FHV-1 may lead to symblepharon (i.e., adhesions of conjunctiva to surrounding tissues), KCS, ulcerative keratitis, and stromal keratitis (p. 464).
- Chronic epiphora can lead to focal facial dermatitis at the medial canthus.

Recommended Monitoring

Varies, depending on the underlying cause

PROGNOSIS & OUTCOME

Prognosis is guarded to excellent, depending on the underlying cause.

PEARLS & CONSIDERATIONS

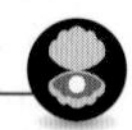

Comments

- Routine aerobic bacterial C&S tests should be done in cases of mucopurulent discharge, especially those nonresponsive to therapy, to identify the implicated bacteria or fungus.
- Fungal infections rarely cause ocular discharge in cats and dogs.
- Serous ocular discharge in cats is common with FHV-1 infection.
- A thorough examination of the *entire* conjunctival sac, including dorsally throughout the dorsal surface of the globe and ventrally on both sides of the third eyelid, may be necessary to identify any retained foreign material.

Technician Tips

The type of ocular discharge can be important in the diagnosis of the inciting cause. It is best if all the discharge is not removed before the veterinarian evaluates the patient.

Client Education

At the first sign of abnormal ocular discharge in their pets, owners should consult their veterinarian.

SUGGESTED READING

Pena MT, et al: Canine conjunctivitis and blepharitis. Vet Clin North Am Small Anim Pract 38:233-249, 2008.

AUTHOR: Chantale L. Pinard, DVM, MSc, DACVO
EDITOR: Diane V. H. Hendrix, DVM, DACVO

Ocular Size Abnormalities

Client Education Sheet

BASIC INFORMATION

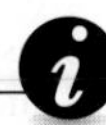

Definition

- Buphthalmos: a larger than normal globe; an acquired condition resulting from glaucoma
- Microphthalmia: a smaller than normal globe; a congenital and potentially inherited condition sometimes associated with other ocular anomalies
- Phthisis bulbi: a shrunken globe; an acquired condition due to severe ocular trauma or chronic intraocular inflammation (e.g., uveitis)

Synonyms

Buphthalmia (buphthalmos), microphthalmos (microphthalmia)

Epidemiology

SPECIES, AGE, SEX

- Buphthalmos may occur and microphthalmia does occur congenitally.
- Phthisis bulbi: no age predisposition

GENETICS, BREED PREDISPOSITION

- Glaucoma resulting in buphthalmos is inherited in several breeds (p. 387).
- Microphthalmia is inherited in several breeds and is commonly associated with multiple ocular defects (recommend consultation with a veterinary ophthalmologist).

ASSOCIATED DISORDERS

Buphthalmos associations:

- Lagophthalmos (incomplete closure of the eyelids) with or without secondary corneal ulceration and chronic keratitis
- Lens subluxation/luxation
- Intraocular neoplasia (p. 559)

Microphthalmia associations:

- Other congenital ocular anomalies, including cataracts, anterior segment dysgenesis, and retinal dysplasia/folds
- Collie eye anomaly, including choroidal hypoplasia with or without optic nerve coloboma, staphyloma, retinal detachment, and intraocular hemorrhage

Phthisis bulbi associations:

- Untreated or poorly responsive intraocular inflammation (e.g., uveitis [p. 1023] or severe ocular trauma [p. 213])

Clinical Presentation

HISTORY, CHIEF COMPLAINT

Condition is most likely unilateral but can be bilateral.

- Buphthalmos: enlargement of globe due to congenital, primary, or secondary glaucoma
- Microphthalmia: small eye from birth
- Phthisis bulbi: progressive shrinkage of globe associated with severe uveitis or trauma

PHYSICAL EXAM FINDINGS

Buphthalmos: larger globe and signs of glaucoma:

- Red eye (congested conjunctival and episcleral blood vessels)
- Diffuse corneal edema with possible stria (white streaks in the cornea from breaks in Descemet's membrane)
- Corneal vascularization secondary to chronic exposure (e.g., lagophthalmos)
- Fixed and dilated pupil if secondary to primary glaucoma or miotic pupil if glaucoma is secondary to uveitis
- Lens subluxation/luxation
- Blindness

Microphthalmia: smaller globe and the following:

- Appearance of enophthalmos (caudal displacement of the eye)
- Prolapsed third eyelid (p. 970)
- Other intraocular abnormalities (cataracts, retinal folds/dysplasia)
- ± Small palpebral fissure (e.g., small eyelid opening) or entropion and/or conjunctivitis if eyelids are normal length despite small eye
- Vision may be normal, reduced, or absent.

Phthisis bulbi: shrunken globe and the following:

- Appearance of enophthalmos
- Prolapsed third eyelid
- ± Corneal edema; deep corneal vascularization
- ± Entropion, conjunctivitis, posterior synechiae, cataract, iris atrophy
- Vision typically reduced or absent

Etiology and Pathophysiology

- Buphthalmos: result of untreated, poorly managed, or progressive glaucoma
- Microphthalmia: congenital deficiency of optic vesicle or failure of normal growth and expansion of optic cup; inherited condition
- Phthisis bulbi: acquired condition that usually follows chronic intraocular inflammation or severe trauma

DIAGNOSIS

Diagnostic Overview

The definitive diagnosis depends on the general appearance of the ocular globe and signalment of the patient.

Differential Diagnosis

- Buphthalmos: exophthalmos (forward displacement of the globe)
- Microphthalmos, phthisis bulbi: ruptured globe, enophthalmos

Initial Database

- Complete ophthalmic exam (p. 1137):
  - Measurement of intraocular pressure (IOP): may be elevated (>25 mm Hg, indicating active glaucoma) or normal (chronic glaucoma) with buphthalmos; typically low (<10 mm Hg) with phthisis bulbi
  - Fluorescein dye application with buphthalmos to rule out corneal ulcer secondary to exposure keratitis
  - Neuro-ophthalmic exam (p. 1136) to assess vision (e.g., menace response)
- Additional tests vary, depending on underlying cause (e.g., uveitis).

Advanced or Confirmatory Testing

- Buphthalmos: ocular ultrasound if corneal or ocular media opacities preclude evaluation of intraocular structures (e.g., assess for cataract or intraocular mass)
- Ocular histopathologic exam if eye is enucleated due to blindness and ocular pain (common with buphthalmos)

TREATMENT

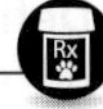

Treatment Overview

The management of ocular pain is paramount, independent of the appearance of the globe. Pain control may require enucleation. No treatment may be required if the ocular size abnormality is not accompanied by evidence of discomfort, inflammation, or elevated IOP.

Acute and Chronic Treatment

- For buphthalmos: if the animal's globe is blind and if glaucoma remains medically uncontrolled, options include
  - Enucleation, evisceration with intraocular prosthesis, or chemical ablation of blind eyes with chronic primary glaucoma; chemical ablation is not recommended in cats
  - Enucleation of eyes with intraocular neoplasia
  - Enucleation of eyes with congenital glaucoma
- For microphthalmos: enucleation is warranted if eye is blind and entropion or chronic conjunctivitis occurs.
- For phthisis bulbi: treatment of underlying uveitis; recommend enucleation if eye is blind and entropion or chronic conjunctivitis occurs; if phthisis bulbi occurs in a cat, enucleation is warranted to prevent trauma-induced ocular sarcoma (p. 559)

PROGNOSIS & OUTCOME

- Prognosis for vision is grave in cases of buphthalmos and phthisis bulbi.
- Prognosis for vision varies for microphthalmia because it depends on the degree of severity and the presence of other ocular anomalies.

PEARLS & CONSIDERATIONS

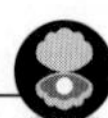

Comments

- Measure the corneal horizontal diameter of each eye (limbus to limbus) to document ocular size abnormality.
- Recommend against breeding animals affected with microphthalmia if the condition is deemed to be breed related or inherited in nature.
- Abnormal ocular size requires prompt evaluation and may or may not indicate an immediate need to treat; a proper and complete clinical ophthalmic exam determines the need for intervention.

Technician Tips

Acquiring accurate intraocular pressures in eyes with severe exposure keratitis (uneven corneal surface) or phthisis bulbi (very low pressures) can be difficult.

Client Education

Clinicians should advise clients to seek veterinary care for their pets as soon as the eye becomes red and/or the eye changes in appearance.

SUGGESTED READING

Moore PA: Examination techniques and interpretation of ophthalmic findings. Clin Tech Small Anim Pract 16:1, 2001.

RELATED CLIENT EDUCATION SHEETS

Consent to Perform Computed Tomography (CT Scan)
Consent to Perform Enucleation
Glaucoma

AUTHOR: Chantale L. Pinard, DVM, MSc, DACVO
EDITOR: Diane V. H. Hendrix, DVM, DACVO

Oleander Toxicosis

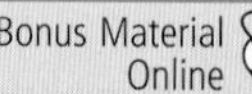
Bonus Material Online

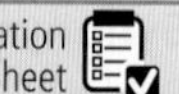
Client Education Sheet

BASIC INFORMATION

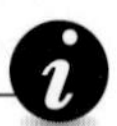

Definition

Acute poisoning occurs after ingestion of dried or fresh parts of an oleander plant (genus *Nerium* or *Thevetia*). Clinical manifestations are similar to those of clinical digoxin toxicosis: gastrointestinal (GI) signs initially, with possible subsequent cardiac arrhythmias

Synonyms

- Nerium oleander: oleander
- Thevetia neriifolia: yellow oleander

Epidemiology

SPECIES, AGE, SEX

Animals of all ages, all breeds, and both sexes are susceptible; dogs are more commonly affected.

RISK FACTORS

Availability of oleander plant in pet's environment

GEOGRAPHY AND SEASONALITY

Oleander is an ornamental evergreen shrub widely cultivated all over the world and most of the southern United States, notably California, Texas, and Florida. It can also be purchased as a patio plant in colder climates.

Clinical Presentation

HISTORY, CHIEF COMPLAINT

- Observed or suspected exposure to plant
- Vomiting, with plant material in the vomitus
- Owners may note lethargy, salivation, signs of abdominal pain, diarrhea, weakness, and tremors within 6 hours of ingestion.

PHYSICAL EXAM FINDINGS

- See History, Chief Complaint above.
- Cardiac arrhythmias: tachycardias (premature beats or runs of tachycardia) or bradycardias. A pattern of bradycardia, initially present for 24 hours, followed by tachycardia and ventricular arrhythmia has been described.
- Central (seizures) and peripheral (tremors, weakness) nervous system effects leading to coma and death

Etiology and Pathophysiology

- Oleander contains cardiac glycosides (e.g., oleandrin, neriine) that inhibit the sodium/potassium–adenosine triphosphatase (Na^+/K^+-ATPase) pump, which is essential for normal cellular function in multiple body systems, notably the cardiovascular and nervous systems.
- Inhibition of the Na^+/K^+-ATPase pump leads to an abnormal accumulation of potassium outside the cell and sodium inside the cell, producing a cascade of calcium release that results in cardiac arrhythmia and myocardial ischemia or necrosis (in severe cases).
- The toxic effects are indistinguishable from those of digoxin toxicosis.

DIAGNOSIS

Diagnostic Overview

A functional diagnosis is made when a pet has appropriate clinical signs (GI and cardiac arrhythmias) and there is the possibility of exposure in areas where oleanders are accessible. Diagnosis can be confirmed (generally retrospectively) by showing presence of oleandrin in body fluids by thin-layer chromatography (TLC) or high-performance liquid chromatography (HPLC).

Differential Diagnosis

- Advanced primary heart disease (e.g., cardiomyopathy, valvular heart disease, traumatic myocarditis)
- Primary bradycardias (third-degree atrioventricular block, sick sinus syndrome, atrial standstill/hyperkalemia)
- Systemic causes of ventricular arrhythmias (p. 1033)
- Exposure to other cardiac glycoside-containing plants (p. 143)

Initial Database

- CBC, serum chemistry profile: hypokalemia or hyperkalemia possible. Hypokalemia may be particularly detrimental; it fosters ventricular arrhythmia and makes animal refractory to antiarrhythmics (e.g., lidocaine, quinidine, mexiletine).
- Electrocardiogram (ECG [p. 1096]) to determine type of cardiac arrhythmia

Advanced or Confirmatory Testing

- Confirmation of oleandrin in body fluids, stomach, and intestinal contents by using TLC and HPLC techniques (available in some veterinary diagnostic laboratories)
- Postmortem exam may reveal oleander plant material in the GI tract, pericardial effusion, possibly pulmonary edema, and varying degrees of thrombi and hemorrhages in epicardial surfaces.
- Histologic examination of the heart tissue may reveal evidence of myocardial inflammation, degeneration, and necrosis.

TREATMENT

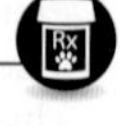

Treatment Overview

When exposure is known or suspected in an asymptomatic patient, induction of vomiting is indicated, followed by administration of activated charcoal. If overt signs are present (or emerge), treatment is directed at decontamination and palliation of consequences (e.g., antiarrhythmic therapy) while also addressing potentially complicating factors (e.g., hypokalemia, retention of plant material). Anti-digitalis antibodies are indicated in critical cases with severe signs when not cost-prohibitive.

Acute General Treatment

Decontamination of patient (p. 1087):

- Induction of emesis if appropriate within 1-2 hours after ingestion (p. 1188)

- Activated charcoal: administration of activated charcoal after inducing emesis or if few hours have elapsed after exposure 1-2 g/kg with a cathartic such as 70% sorbitol 3 mL/kg PO

Treating cardiac arrhythmias:
- Sinus bradycardia that occurs within 24 hours of exposure: treat if severe (heart rate < 60-80 beats/min in an awake and standing, large- to small-breed dog, respectively) or if the condition is associated with overt signs (e.g., lethargy): atropine 0.02 mg/kg IV
- Ventricular arrhythmias (p. 1457)
- Supraventricular arrhythmias (p. 96): extremely rapid, persistent supraventricular tachycardias may need to be controlled (propranolol 0.1-0.5 mg IV total dose per bolus; no more frequently than 1 bolus q 1-3 min to 5 mg maximum for large dogs). The goal is to lower heart rate to acceptable level (e.g., by 20%) and not cause an overly rapid suppression.

Use of specific antibodies (FAB, Digibind) in severe cases:
- IV anti-digitalis antibodies: inactivate significant proportion of circulating cardiac glycoside
- Extremely expensive and reserved for cases in which animals are profoundly ill or manifesting severe arrhythmias and in which cost of treatment is unimportant to the owner

Supportive care:
- IV fluids as needed; avoid fluids that contain calcium (e.g., lactated Ringer's solution).
- Treatment of diarrhea, severe vomiting, and abdominal pain as needed
- Correction of electrolyte imbalances (potassium) if needed

Recommended Monitoring
- ECG
- Serum chemistry profile, especially electrolytes

PROGNOSIS & OUTCOME

- Poor prognosis with severe cardiac arrhythmias; animals are often found dead.
- Clinical signs of toxicosis may persist for 24 hours or longer in animals that ultimately survive; hospitalization for > 24 hours is appropriate, and outcome can be successful.

PEARLS & CONSIDERATIONS

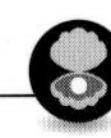

Comments
- Animals that survive may or may not have permanent cardiac sequelae (myocardial infarct with severe intoxications).
- Oleander leaves can be identified by a characteristic venation pattern and stromata; they have a prominent middle rib with parallel veins extending to the periphery.
- All parts of oleander are toxic; ingestion of dry leaves/clippings is the most common cause of poisoning in animals.
  - The dry leaves/clippings taste sweet compared with green leaves, which are bitter.
- A 0.005% of an animal's body weight in oleander leaves (e.g., 10-12 leaves) may be lethal.
- Intoxication can occur by drinking water in which oleander was soaked.

Prevention
Avoid growing oleander close to animal housing or on premises.

Technician Tips
If unsure about the type of plant/flower, consult with a plant nursery or floral shop.

Client Education
Do not grow oleander in pet's environment.

SUGGESTED READING

Pao-Franco A, et al: Successful use of digoxin-specific immune Fab in the treatment of severe *Nerium oleander* toxicosis in a dog. J Vet Emerg Crit Care 5:596-604, 2017.

AUTHOR: Eric Dunayer, VMD, MS, DABT, DABVT
EDITOR: Tina Wismer, DVM, MS, DABVT, DABT

Onion or Garlic Toxicosis

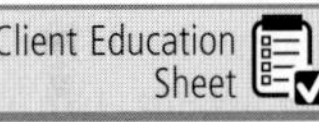

Client Education Sheet

BASIC INFORMATION

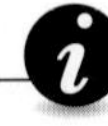

Definition
Intoxication results from consumption of a plant in the genus *Allium,* which includes garlic, onions, leeks, scallions, shallots, and chives. Most of these plants are perennial, rhizomatous, or bulbous herbs. Most have a distinctive odor.

Epidemiology
SPECIES, AGE, SEX

Cats are more susceptible than dogs.

GENETICS, BREED PREDISPOSITION

Japanese dog breeds such as the Akita, shiba inu, and Tosa inu are more susceptible to oxidative damage of red blood cells (RBCs).

RISK FACTORS
- Dogs' indiscriminate feeding behavior and the likelihood of being fed table scraps increase the risk of ingestion.
- Cats are more likely to be exposed from eating baby food with onion or garlic powder as a flavoring (chronically) or chewing on potted chives.

Clinical Presentation
HISTORY, CHIEF COMPLAINT
- History of exposure to raw, cooked, dried, or powdered chives, onions, garlic, leeks, shallots, or scallions
- Common physical signs: weakness, lethargy, pale mucous membranes, discolored urine
- Less common: halitosis, hypersalivation, vomiting, and/or diarrhea
- The owner of any dog with hemolytic anemia should be asked about exposure to onions/garlic.

PHYSICAL EXAM FINDINGS
- Lethargy, weakness, and/or ataxia
- Mild hypersalivation, vomiting, and/or diarrhea
- Pale mucous membranes (anemia), tachypnea, tachycardia
- Discolored (red to brown) urine (hemoglobinuria)

Etiology and Pathophysiology
Source:
- These plants grow wild and are widely cultivated.

Mechanism of toxicosis:
- *Allium* spp contain sulfoxides (provide the characteristic odor) that are hydrolyzed to thiosulfinates, which decompose to dipropyl sulfide. Dipropyl sulfides oxidize RBC membranes, resulting in hemolysis, Heinz bodies, anemia, and less commonly methemoglobinemia.
- Poisoning can result from ingesting raw, dried, powdered, or cooked onions and garlic; cooking or drying does not inactivate the toxic principle.
- Dogs fed onion soup equivalent to 30 g of raw onion/kg q 24h for 3 days develop marked Heinz body anemia. Similarly, a significant increase in Heinz bodies is seen 12 hours after feeding dogs 200 g ($\frac{1}{2}$ lb) of boiled onions (approximate dose of 17 g onions/kg).
- Dogs given an extract equivalent to 5 g of whole garlic/kg PO q 24h for 7 days develop anemia 9-11 days after dosing.
- Generally, most dogs need to eat at least 10-15 g/kg body weight to develop onion toxicosis, unless the dog is of a sensitive breed (see Genetics, Breed Predisposition above).

As cats are much more sensitive, as little as 5 g/kg body weight poses a risk.

DIAGNOSIS

Diagnostic Overview

Diagnosis is based on historical evidence of *Allium* species ingestion and the delayed onset (usually 2-5 days) of compatible signs (anemia, pale mucous membrane color, hemoglobinuria, hemolysis).

Differential Diagnosis

Toxicologic:

- Oxidative damage, hemolysis, anemia, or methemoglobinemia: acetaminophen, brown recluse spider, chlorates, hydroxyurea, local anesthetics, methylene blue, naphthalene mothballs, phenazopyridine, phenols, propylene glycol, zinc

Spontaneous, nontoxicologic:

- Anemia, hemolytic
- Anemia, immune-mediated hemolytic (p. 1197)
- Anemia, blood loss (p. 57)

Initial Database

- CBC: hematologic changes (e.g., hemolysis, Heinz body anemia, methemoglobinemia) may occur as early as 12 hours after ingestion but generally take 2-5 days to develop
  - Decreased hematocrit, elevated white blood cell count
  - Smears should be examined for Heinz bodies, evidence of regeneration
  - With methemoglobinemia (p. 1365), blood may appear brown and fail to turn red when exposed to air.
- Serum biochemical profile depends on degree of anemia, but increase in liver enzymes is possible.
- Urinalysis
  - Reddish brown color suggests hemoglobinuria (rule out hematuria, myoglobinuria).
  - Urine dipstick is positive for blood with hemoglobinuria or hematuria.
  - Centrifuged urine remains reddish brown with hemoglobinuria, whereas the supernatant of centrifuged urine clears with hematuria.
- If exposure history is unconfirmed, other tests may be indicated to explore alternative causes for anemia/hemolysis

Advanced or Confirmatory Testing

Co-oximetry (measures percentage of methemoglobin) and methemoglobin assays exist but are not typically available in the limited time frame of an intoxication.

TREATMENT

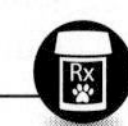

Treatment Overview

If no clinical signs are present and recent ingestion (less than 4 hours) of significant amounts (>5 g/kg in cats, > 10 g/kg in dogs) of onion is confirmed, treatment can include induction of vomiting and administration of activated charcoal (if emesis unsuccessful). If the patient is showing overt signs compatible with toxicosis, care is supportive.

Acute General Treatment

No clinical signs apparent:

- Minimal exposure requires no treatment.
- For substantial, recent consumption (>5 g/kg for cats or > 10 g/kg for dogs), decontamination is beneficial.
  - Induction of vomiting (p. 1188)
  - Activated charcoal 1-2 g/kg PO (dose according to packaging label of product; p. 1087); especially useful if emesis unsuccessful

Patient showing clinical signs:

- Packed RBCs or whole blood transfusion if necessary. NOTE: new RBCs remain at risk for hemolytic damage if toxicant is still in the blood (p. 1169).
- Oxygen supplementation is of limited benefit because oxygen saturation of intact hemoglobin remains high and methemoglobin binds oxygen poorly even with supplementation.
- If necessary, manage hypotension, vomiting, or diarrhea.

Behavior/Exercise

Limit exercise pending resolution of anemia.

Drug Interactions

Garlic has an antithrombotic effect, and concomitant use of garlic and drugs that alter platelet function (e.g., aspirin, clopidogrel) may produce additive antithrombotic effects.

Possible Complications

- Hemoglobinuria-associated renal tubular damage possible in severe cases
- Abortions can occur secondary to severe hypoxemia if pronounced anemia is present.

Recommended Monitoring

CBC/hematocrit/blood smear; renal function; urinalysis

PROGNOSIS & OUTCOME

- Generally good with prompt veterinary care of patients showing overt clinical signs
- Guarded with severe anemia or secondary renal damage

PEARLS & CONSIDERATIONS

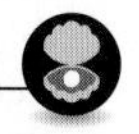

Comments

- Many commercial garlic or onion powder products list the conversion for a clove of garlic (e.g., $\frac{1}{4}$ tsp of garlic powder equals one clove of garlic, or 1 Tbsp onion powder equals $\frac{1}{2}$ cup chopped onion).
- One pearl onion weighs about 14 g, a small onion (2 inches [5 cm] in diameter) weighs 56-85 g, a medium onion (3 inches [7.5 cm] in diameter) weighs 226-255 g, and a large onion (4 inches [10 cm] in diameter) weighs 425-450 g.
- A medium onion yields about 1 cup of coarsely chopped onion.

Prevention

Owners should keep foods containing onion or garlic out of their pets' reach. Garlic and onion should not be used to flavor foods or treats for pets.

Technician Tips

When recommending baby food to stimulate appetite, it is important to remind clients to avoid products with garlic or onion powder, especially for cats.

Client Education

Garlic supplementation for the prevention of fleas or heartworm disease is unsubstantiated and contraindicated.

SUGGESTED READING

Tang X, et al: An experimental study of hemolysis induced by onion *(Allium cepa)* poisoning in dogs. J Vet Pharmacol Ther 31:143-149, 2008.

AUTHOR: Brandy R. Sobczak, DVM
EDITOR: Tina Wismer, DVM, MS, DABVT, DABT

Open-Mouth Jaw Locking

Client Education Sheet

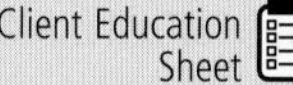

BASIC INFORMATION

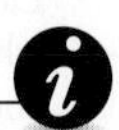

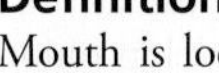

Definition

Mouth is locked wide open due to displacement of the coronoid process of the mandible ventrolateral to the zygomatic arch.

Synonyms

Often confused with classic rostrodorsal luxation of the temporomandibular joint (TMJ) but showing different clinical/radiographic signs and requiring entirely different treatment approaches

Epidemiology

SPECIES, AGE, SEX

Cats and dogs of either sex; usually adult animals

GENETICS, BREED PREDISPOSITION

- Cats: primarily Persian
- Dogs: primarily basset hound; occasionally other breeds

RISK FACTORS

- Head shape (e.g., brachycephalic cats)
- Specific anatomic configuration of the TMJ (relating to capsule, articular disk, condylar process, mandibular fossa, retroarticular process) and adjacent tissues (coronoid process of mandible, zygomatic arch, masticatory muscles)
- Dysplasia, subluxation/luxation of the TMJ, and laxity of the mandibular symphysis

ASSOCIATED DISORDERS

- TMJ luxation
- TMJ dysplasia (bony and/or soft tissue)
- Abnormal extrusion of maxillary and/or mandibular canine teeth
- Trauma to TMJ, mandible (condylar process, coronoid process), and mandibular symphysis

Clinical Presentation

DISEASE FORMS/SUBTYPES

- TMJ dysplasia without mandibular displacement
- TMJ dysplasia with subluxation/luxation of the TMJ but no open-mouth jaw locking
- Open-mouth jaw locking with the mouth locked wide open due to displacement of the coronoid process of the mandible ventrolateral to the zygomatic arch

HISTORY, CHIEF COMPLAINT

- Episodes of open-mouth jaw locking after yawning, grooming, or vocalizing
- Frequency: once per month to several times per day
- Duration: a few seconds/minutes to many hours/days
- Spontaneous correction possible, sometimes associated with an audible click
- Drooling of saliva and dropping of food due to inability to close mouth and swallow
- Pawing at face, rubbing muzzle on ground, shaking head, and vocalizing during locking episodes
- Dehydration and weight loss due to inability to swallow water and food (if untreated)

PHYSICAL EXAM FINDINGS

Usual presentation (compare with TMJ luxation):

- Mouth locked wide open (lower jaw cannot be closed when pushed against the upper jaw)
- No contact between upper and lower teeth
- Slight rostral protrusion of ipsilateral mandible
- More ventrally positioned dental arch at ipsilateral mandible
- Facial protuberance from displaced coronoid process sometimes palpable (and occasionally even visible under skin) ventrolateral to ipsilateral zygomatic arch
- Drooling of saliva (due to inability to close the mouth and difficulty to swallow) and moist fur at chin and neck region
- Hair accumulation at dorsocaudal tongue surface (in cats that continue grooming but cannot swallow)
- Bilateral exophthalmos and reduced retropulsion of globes

Etiology and Pathophysiology

Dysplasia of TMJ or adjacent tissues:

- Resulting in progressive TMJ laxity and subluxation/luxation of the condylar process
- Medial pulling of the mandibular body on contraction of pterygoid muscles at maximal mouth opening (e.g., immediately after yawning) and lateral flaring of the coronoid process of the mandibular ramus eventually causing displacement of the tip of the coronoid process ventrolateral to the zygomatic arch

Trauma of TMJ or adjacent tissues:

- Flattening of the zygomatic arch
- Displacement of the coronoid process
- Thickening (callus formation) of the zygomatic arch and/or coronoid process
- Laxity of the mandibular symphysis
- Laxity of the TMJ

Iatrogenic:

- After unilateral total mandibulectomy

Other:

- Abnormal extrusion of maxillary and/or mandibular canine teeth, causing them to contact the opposing canine teeth on closure of the mouth; subsequent levering forces resulting in increased mandibular symphyseal laxity, TMJ laxity, and rotational movement of the mandibular body

DIAGNOSIS

Diagnostic Overview

- History, clinical signs, and radiography (often sufficient to make a diagnosis)
- CT is of academic interest but not required for diagnosis.

Differential Diagnosis

- Traumatic TMJ luxation with rostrodorsal displacement of the mandibular condyle (lower jaw shifting to opposite side, inability to fully close mouth due to contact between upper and lower teeth, dorsoventral radiographic view showing no contact between mandibular coronoid process and zygomatic arch)
- Mandibular neurapraxia (trigeminal neuritis)
- Bilateral mandibular fracture (similar to mandibular neurapraxia, lower jaw can usually be moved against the upper jaw)
- Periorbital/caudal mandibular/caudal maxillary neoplasia
- Mandibular ramus/zygomatic arch fracture

Initial Database

Routine preanesthetic blood tests

Advanced or Confirmatory Testing

- Dorsoventral/ventrodorsal radiographic view of the head (most useful)
- Lateral oblique radiographic view (showing TMJ dysplasia when present)
    - Wide joint space
    - Shallow, flat, or irregular mandibular fossa
    - Hypoplastic articular eminence
    - Flattened or enlarged condylar process
    - Hypoplastic or thickened retroarticular process

TREATMENT

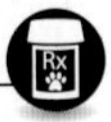

Treatment Overview

Immediate relief by manual unlocking in the sedated or anesthetized patient and temporary maxillomandibular fixation to avoid recurrence of locking, followed by definitive surgery the same or next day

Acute General Treatment

- Manual unlocking by opening the mouth a little further, carefully pressing the affected mandible medially, and gently closing the mouth
- Maxillomandibular fixation (e.g., placement of a tape muzzle to restrict full range of mouth opening until definitive surgery)

Chronic Treatment

Recommended:

- Partial resection of the zygomatic arch
- Partial reduction of the coronoid process
- Combination of zygomatic arch resection and coronoid process reduction (preferred by the author)
- Symphysiotomy, symphysiectomy, and intermandibular fixation (if laxity of the mandibular symphysis was the leading cause of open-mouth jaw locking)
- Skin suture removal 10-14 days postoperatively

Not recommended:

- Imbrication/plication of the lateral TMJ capsule
- Mandibular condylectomy

Nutrition/Diet

Soft food for 2 weeks postoperatively

Possible Complications

Recurrence of open-mouth jaw locking

- Unlikely if resective surgery was properly performed
- Possible with partial zygomectomy only or partial coronoidectomy only (particularly when insufficient bony tissue was removed)

Open-mouth jaw locking occurring on opposite side:

- If possibility of bilateral locking had not been evaluated before surgery of one side only

Recommended Monitoring

Observing animal closely when yawning, particularly when having had history of open-mouth jaw locking

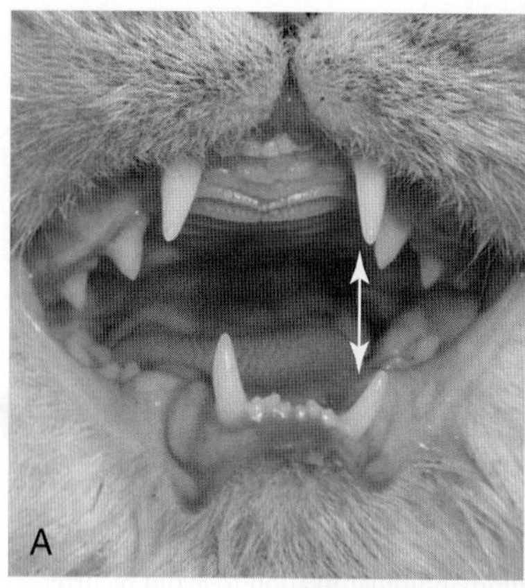

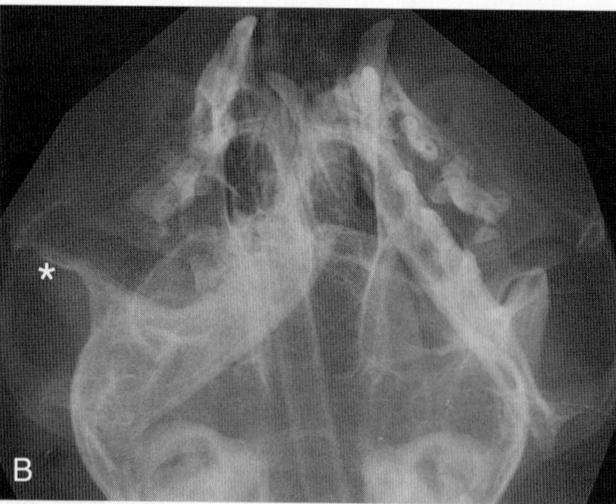

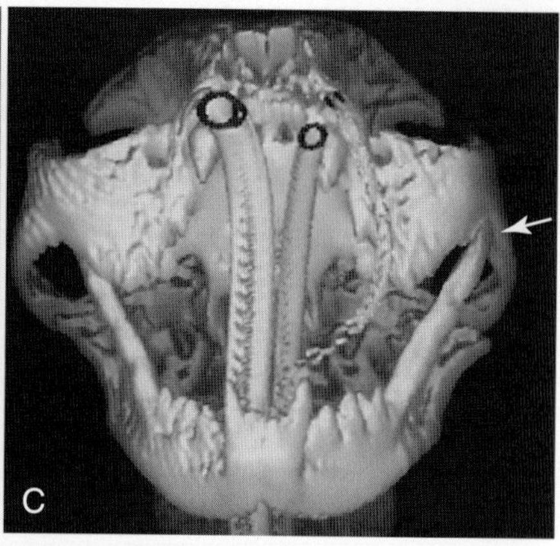

OPEN-MOUTH JAW LOCKING A, Clinical photograph of a cat with the mouth in a fixed, wide-open position *(double-headed arrow)*; note the more ventrally positioned left mandibular dental arch and no contact between upper and lower teeth. **B**, Dorsoventral radiographic view of the same cat shows the left mandibular coronoid process *(asterisk)* contacting the zygomatic arch. **C**, Three-dimensional CT reconstruction of the same cat demonstrates displacement of the left mandibular coronoid process *(arrow)* ventrolateral to the zygomatic arch. (Copyright Dr. Alexander M. Reiter, University of Pennsylvania.)

PROGNOSIS & OUTCOME

- Poor with conservative therapy (manual unlocking and tape muzzling) due to high rate of recurrence
- Excellent with resective surgery

PEARLS & CONSIDERATIONS

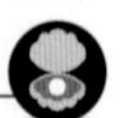

Comments

- Size 4 dental films or phosphor plates are very useful for taking dorsoventral/ventrodorsal, lateral oblique, and rostrocaudal radiographic projections of the temporomandibular joints in the cat.
- Manual locking of an apparently unaffected side should be attempted before surgery of the affected side because both sides can be affected (requiring resective surgery on both sides).

Technician Tips

- Practice how to fabricate a tape muzzle.
- Know the difference between rostrodorsal TMJ luxation and open-mouth jaw locking.
- Be able to use size 4 dental films or phosphor plates for imaging the TMJ and associated tissues.

Client Education

Selective breeding

SUGGESTED READING

Reiter AM: Symphysiotomy, symphysiectomy and intermandibular arthrodesis in a cat with open-mouth jaw locking—case report and literature review. J Vet Dent 21:147, 2004.

AUTHOR & EDITOR: Alexander M. Reiter, DVM, Dr.med. vet., DAVDC, DEVDC

Opiate/Opioid Toxicosis

Client Education Sheet

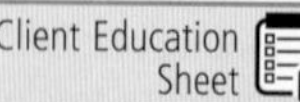

BASIC INFORMATION

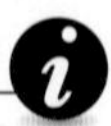

Definition

Opioids are naturally occurring, semisynthetic, and synthetic substances that act at opioid receptors to inhibit presynaptic release and postsynaptic response to excitatory neurotransmitters, thereby impeding pain transmission. Opioids are used in human and veterinary medicine to treat pain (severe, moderate, or chronic), diarrhea, and cough and are a drug of abuse in humans. Originally opiates referred to the natural alkaloids, and opioids were the synthetics; now *opioid* is used for the entire family.

Epidemiology

SPECIES, AGE, SEX

Accidental exposures more often reported in dogs than cats.

GENETICS, BREED PREDISPOSITION

Dogs with the *MDR1/ABCB1-Δ* (p. 638) gene mutation and all cats are more sensitive to opioids.

RISK FACTORS

- Young animals with incomplete blood-brain barriers may show more severe signs.
- Neonates with underdeveloped livers may be unable to adequately metabolize opioids.
- Geriatric animals with underlying hepatic or renal disease may have inadequate metabolism or delayed excretion.
- Narcotic dogs in all fields of service are at risk for accidental exposure.

Clinical Presentation

HISTORY, CHIEF COMPLAINT

- Recognized accidental exposure: owner gave his/her own medication to the pet in error, bottle of medication chewed open, pills dropped on the floor, and so on
- Clinical signs indicating possible exposure: lethargy, weakness, vocalization, ataxia

PHYSICAL EXAM FINDINGS

- Lethargy or depression
- Ataxia
- Gastrointestinal (GI) signs: diarrhea (dogs), vomiting (cats)
- Bradycardia or tachycardia
- Tachypnea (cats)
- Body temperature normal or low in dogs, may be increased in cats
- Respiratory rate may be depressed
- Mydriasis
- Hypersalivation

Etiology and Pathophysiology

- Opioids have various uses in veterinary medicine, including analgesia, emetic, antidiarrheal, cough suppression, and sedation.
- Opioids are classified as agonist, agonist/antagonist, partial agonist, or antagonist. They target specific opioid receptors, which include mu, kappa, and delta that are found in various organs throughout the body. The receptor targeted by the specific drug determines the clinical response.
- Mu receptors are responsible for analgesic effects as well as for respiratory depression.
- Kappa receptors are potently analgesic but are also responsible for dysphoria, dissociation, and sedation.
- Delta receptors are involved in spinal analgesia but also have antidepressant and neuroprotective effects.

DIAGNOSIS

Diagnostic Overview

Diagnosis is based on the presenting clinical signs and history of ingestion. Due to the illicit nature of some opioids, many owners are not forthcoming with complete or accurate histories. Over-the-counter illicit drug test kits can be used to confirm suspicion of exposure, but they have not been validated in animals.

Differential Diagnosis

- Other drugs causing central nervous system (CNS) depression, including barbiturates, benzodiazepines, phenothiazines, ivermectin, marijuana, ethylene glycol, and alcohol
- In the absence of known drug exposure, it is important to rule out nontoxic causes of signs (e.g., hypoglycemia, meningoencephalitis, neoplasia, hepatic encephalopathy).

Initial Database

- Blood pressure: decreased or sometimes increased
- Blood gas: may see respiratory acidosis
- O_2 saturation: may be low.
- CBC, chemistry, and urinalysis are expected to be normal.

Advanced or Confirmatory Testing

Urine or blood can be sent to a veterinary diagnostic lab for an illicit drug screen or tested in house with point-of-care kit (not validated in pets).

TREATMENT

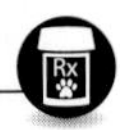

Treatment Overview

With known very recent ingestion and no clinical signs, decontamination can be attempted by inducing emesis (monitor respiratory status closely if using apomorphine). If symptoms are present, stabilize respiration, and use naloxone (specific agonist for opioids).

Acute General Treatment

- Decontamination is rarely performed due to quick time frame of clinical signs and existence of reversal agent (p. 1087).
- Provide ventilatory support, including intubation and positive-pressure ventilation in severe cases (p. 1185).
- Naloxone 0.02-0.04 mg/kg IV, IM, or SQ for dogs and cats. Doses up to 0.1 mg/kg may be required to reverse buprenorphine, fentanyl, and tramadol; may need to repeat dosing
- IV fluids for cardiovascular support; avoid overhydration and monitor for noncardiogenic pulmonary edema
- Diazepam 0.25-1.0 mg/kg slow IV for seizures and dysphoric reactions. Monitor respiratory rate and effort closely (respiratory depression).
- Cyproheptadine 1.1 mg/kg PO or per rectum for serotonin syndrome–like effects

Drug Interactions

- CNS depressants (e.g., barbiturates, phenothiazines, centrally acting muscle relaxants, tranquilizers, alcohol) increase respiratory and CNS depression.
- Diuretics may have decreased efficacy in some congestive heart failure patients.
- Monoamine oxidase (MAO) inhibitors (amitraz, selegiline) may have additive effects or increase CNS depression.
- *S*-adenosylmethionine (SAMe) may increase serotonergic effects.
- Erythromycin, itraconazole, fluconazole, cimetidine, rifampin, and digoxin decrease clearance and increase toxicity due to prolonged half-life and decreased metabolism.
- Some opioids may potentiate anticoagulant activity of warfarin.

Possible Complications

- Constipation due to decreased peristalsis
- Aspiration pneumonia

Recommended Monitoring

Heart rate, blood pressure, respiratory rate and effort, body temperature, oxygen saturation, CNS depression

PROGNOSIS & OUTCOME

- Prognosis is generally good when naloxone has been used to reverse opioid effects and respiratory and cardiovascular status is properly maintained.
- Prognosis is guarded when seizures occur or if prompt veterinary care (and antidote) is not available.

PEARLS & CONSIDERATIONS

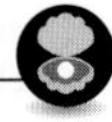

Comments

- Used fentanyl patches or the sticks from the fentanyl lollipops still contain enough drug to cause toxicosis.
- Naloxone may be administered intranasally if IV access is not available.

Prevention

- Keep all medications out of reach of pets.
- Handlers of narcotics detection dogs should carry naloxone at all times.

Technician Tips

- Confirm with the owner that the opioid ingested is not combined with acetaminophen.
- Make all efforts to obtain an accurate, honest history, especially when exposure to illicit drugs is suspected.

Client Education

Keep all medications away from pets.

SUGGESTED READING

Bischoff K: Toxicity of drugs of abuse. In Gupta RC, editor: Veterinary toxicology, ed 2, Waltham, MA, 2012, Elsevier, pp 475-477.

AUTHOR: Jodi Carlson, VMD, MS
EDITOR: Tina Wismer, DVM, MS, DABVT, DABT

Oral Tumors, Benign

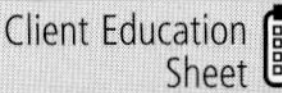

BASIC INFORMATION

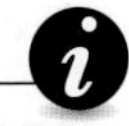

Definition

Benign and malignant masses are common in the mouths of dogs. In cats, oral masses tend to be malignant more often than benign. Although benign tumors do not metastasize to distant sites, some (e.g., acanthomatous ameloblastoma) may be locally invasive.

Synonyms

- Benign oral neoplasia
- Epulis (plural, epulides) is a nonspecific clinical descriptive term referring to a local exophytic growth on the gingiva (e.g., focal fibrous hyperplasia, peripheral odontogenic fibroma [fibromatous epulis and ossifying epulis], acanthomatous ameloblastoma [acanthomatous epulis]) (p. 306).

Epidemiology

SPECIES, AGE, SEX

- Dogs: usually gingival hyperplasia, peripheral odontogenic fibroma, acanthomatous ameloblastoma; occasionally pyogenic granuloma, dentigerous cyst, odontoma, papilloma, osteoma, plasmacytoma; rarely giant cell epulis, amyloid-producing odontogenic tumor (APOT)
- Cats: usually proliferative inflammatory tissue; occasionally giant cell epulis, osteoma, plasmacytoma; rarely peripheral odontogenic fibroma, acanthomatous ameloblastoma, inductive ameloblastoma (feline inductive odontogenic tumor), APOT, odontoma, gingival hyperplasia
- Benign oral tumors can occur at any age.
- Oral papillomas (p. 752) usually occur in dogs < 2 years old or older dogs with concurrent immunopathy.
- Feline inductive odontogenic tumor usually occurs in cats < 2 years old.
- Odontogenic tumors (arising from tooth-forming tissue) can occur at any age, but tumors in young pets are more likely to be of odontogenic origin.

GENETICS, BREED PREDISPOSITION

- Peripheral odontogenic fibroma (previously called fibromatous epulis and ossifying epulis): more common in brachycephalic dog breeds
- Oral tumors in cats are rarely benign.

CONTAGION AND ZOONOSIS

Oral papillomas in young dogs are caused by species-specific canine papillomavirus.

ASSOCIATED DISORDERS

- Gingival hyperplasia
- Malignant oral tumors

Clinical Presentation

DISEASE FORMS/SUBTYPES

- Gingival hyperplasia: abnormal increase in the number of normal cells in a normal arrangement, resulting in clinical enlargement or thickening of gingiva
- Pyogenic granuloma: usually developing on gingiva/alveolar mucosa caudobuccal to the mandibular first molar in cats; consisting of markedly vascular granulation tissue with endothelial proliferation, generally ulcerated and inflamed, commonly with hemosiderin deposits
- Dentigerous (tooth-containing) cyst (follicular cyst): develops around the crown of an unerupted tooth
- Odontoma: not a true tumor but considered to be a hamartoma (accumulation of normal epithelial and mesenchymal odontogenic cells arranged in an abnormal manner but allowing for induction of dental hard tissues)
    - Compound odontoma: hard tissues produced in a relatively organized manner, resulting in tooth-like structures
    - Complex odontoma: dental hard tissue bearing no resemblance to a tooth
- Peripheral odontogenic fibroma (also called fibromatous and ossifying epulides): ossifying epulides may contain bone-, dentin-, or cementum-like tissue within the soft-tissue swelling; minimally invasive
- Giant cell granuloma (giant cell tumor, giant cell epulis): rare; rapid growth with inflammatory and ulcerative changes, osteoid and woven bone formation; multinucleated giant cell is main component in mass; rapid recurrence after incomplete excision; thought to be a variant of the peripheral odontogenic fibroma
- Ameloblastoma: central (intraosseous) or peripheral (extraosseous); both locally invasive, but central ameloblastoma often exhibiting cystic bony changes; acanthomatous ameloblastoma in dogs historically classified as acanthomatous epulis but probably similar to peripheral ameloblastoma
- Feline inductive odontogenic tumor: rare; occurs most commonly in the rostral maxilla of cats < 2 years of age; may be locally invasive but does not metastasize
- APOT: rare; previously called calcifying epithelial odontogenic tumor; may be locally invasive in dogs and cats but does not metastasize
- Plasmacytoma (plasma cell tumor): extramedullary variant at nasal, pharyngeal, and oral mucosa that has no apparent primary bone involvement; sessile or polypoid sessile and usually solitary oral masses appear to remain localized
- Osteoma: slow growing; composed of well-differentiated, densely sclerotic, compact bone
- Cementoma: odontogenic neoplasm of mesenchymal origin, consisting of cementum-like tissue deposited by cells resembling cementoblasts
- Granular cell tumor (myoblastoma): uncertain histogenesis, most commonly occurring on the tongue

HISTORY, CHIEF COMPLAINT

- Focal swelling of gingiva and/or alveolar mucosa commonly noted as an incidental finding
- Benign oral tumors rarely present with oral bleeding or halitosis unless they are large enough to be traumatized by opposing teeth on closure of the mouth. Bleeding at the lesion site is a common complaint in dogs with a large acanthomatous ameloblastoma.

PHYSICAL EXAM FINDINGS

- Focal swelling of gingiva/alveolar mucosa is often circumscribed and rarely ulcerated.
- Benign tumors that are locally invasive (e.g., canine acanthomatous ameloblastoma) may cause disfigurement secondary to invasion of the maxilla or mandible.
- Displaced teeth (but uncommonly mobile)
- Mandibular lymph nodes are often normal.
- Appetite and activity level are usually unaffected.

Etiology and Pathophysiology

- Cause is unknown, but genetic predisposition may play a role.
- Some benign masses are suspected to undergo malignant transformation, although this seems to be rare.

DIAGNOSIS

Diagnostic Overview

Diagnosis of benign oral masses usually requires histopathologic exam of an incisional or excisional biopsy specimen because many oral masses do not exfoliate well on cytologic sampling.

Differential Diagnosis

- Normal anatomy (e.g., incisive papilla caudal to maxillary incisors in dogs and cats; lingual molar gland caudolingual to mandibular first molar teeth in cats): if the mass is located directly on the midline or is bilateral, consult an anatomy textbook to rule out normal structures before performing a biopsy.
- Scar tissue (chewing lesions from traumatizing buccal or sublingual mucosa)
- Eosinophilic granuloma (p. 300): on tongue, lips, and palate
- Inflammatory swelling due to foreign body
- Apical abscess (p. 7)
- Osteomyelitis/bone sequestrum: usually seen in the incisive bone or bilaterally in the caudal mandible or maxilla; often appears as bony swelling with gingival recession, erosion, and ulceration; exposed bone; and fetid odor. Cocker spaniels and dachshunds may be overrepresented.
- Gingival hyperplasia
- Dentigerous cyst: arising around tooth that has not erupted
- Craniomandibular osteopathy (CMO): most commonly seen in West Highland white, Scottish, and Cairn terriers; mandibular swellings associated with CMO are often bilateral.
- Malignant oral tumors (p. 714)

Initial Database

- CBC, serum biochemistry profile, and urinalysis: generally unremarkable
- Thoracic radiographs: benign tumors do not cause metastasis

Advanced or Confirmatory Testing

- Anesthetized oral exam (p. 1140)
- Dental radiography: various bony changes
- CT: particularly helpful for maxillary masses
- Cytologic exam of aspirated oral masses and lymph nodes
- Histopathologic evaluation of incisional or excisional biopsy

TREATMENT

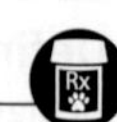

Treatment Overview

- Marginal resection (removal of the mass and a small amount of unaffected surrounding

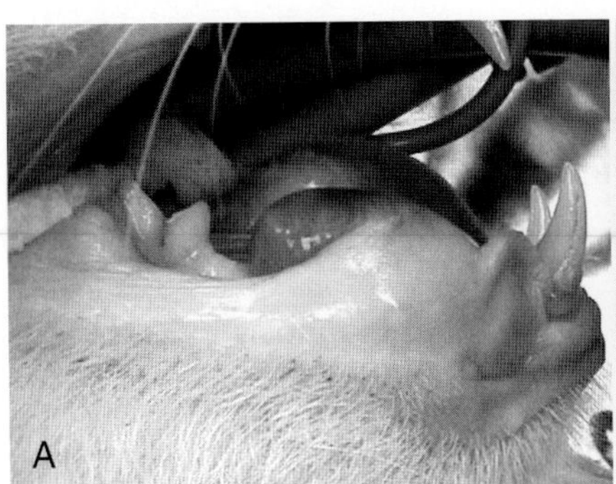

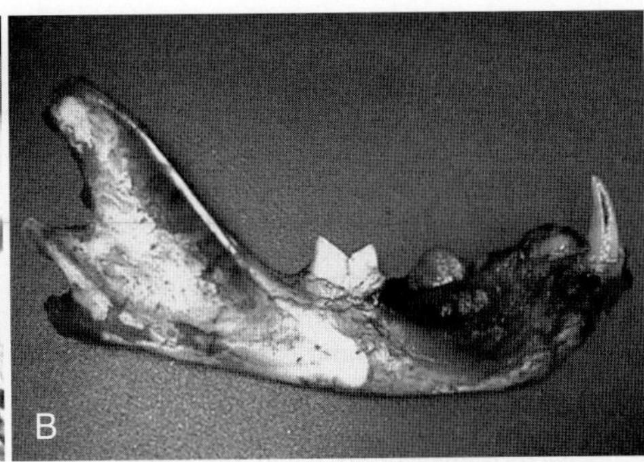

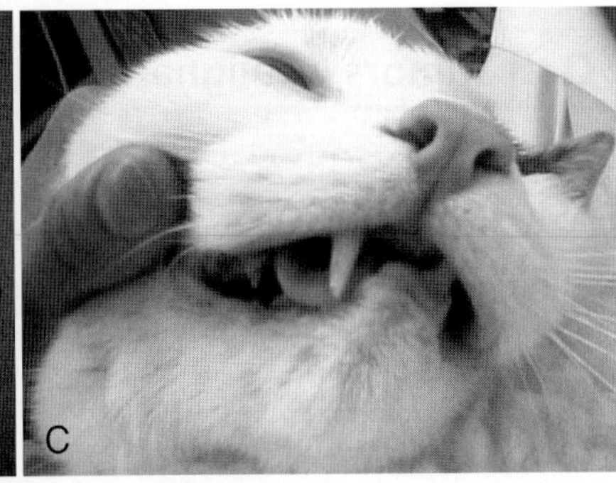

ORAL TUMORS, BENIGN A, Total mandibulectomy: preoperative image of a cat with a right mandibular amyloid-producing odontogenic tumor (APOT), which is a benign but locally aggressive neoplasm. **B,** Total mandibulectomy: intraoperative image shows resected right mandible from same cat. **C,** Total mandibulectomy: postoperative image of the same cat presenting several months later for a recheck shows excellent healing of the surgical site and no tumor recurrence. (Copyright Dr. Alexander M. Reiter, University of Pennsylvania.)

tissue) usually prevents local recurrence of benign lesions. For tumors such as acanthomatous ameloblastoma, wide resection (removal of the mass and 1-2 cm of surrounding tissue) is indicated.
- When surgical excision is not an option, efforts should be made to decrease the rate of growth (e.g., radiation therapy) and provide relief from discomfort (extraction of teeth impinging on the tumor, administration of pain medications).

Acute General Treatment

- Removal of a circumscribed mass to the normal level of the surrounding gingiva often serves as an adequate biopsy but may not prevent local recurrence. Peripheral odontogenic fibromas may recur if the associated tooth/teeth and the inciting gingival connective tissue/periodontal ligament have not been removed.
- Incisional biopsies of large masses are warranted to provide information before considering radical surgery.

Chronic Treatment

- Depending on biopsy result and tumor extent, surgery or radiation therapy may be good long-term options.
- Intralesional chemotherapy has been reported to be successful for treatment of some benign tumors (e.g., acanthomatous ameloblastoma). Systemic chemotherapy may be used as an adjunctive therapy but is rarely effective by itself against most oral tumors.
- Radiation therapy offers excellent long-term control for treatment of acanthomatous ameloblastoma, but malignant tumors may develop in the irradiated area in 3.5%-12.5% of dogs.

Possible Complications

- Recurrence of primary tumor
- Intraoperative or postoperative bleeding
- Dehiscence of the surgical site: use of electrocautery may obscure histologic exam of margins of excised tissue and increase the likelihood of wound dehiscence in oral surgery.

Recommended Monitoring

Repeat oral exam, including head/neck lymph node palpation, to monitor for recurrence at 6-month intervals.

PROGNOSIS & OUTCOME

- Prognosis is excellent with benign tumors if they are amenable to complete surgical resection or respond to radiation therapy.
- When clients are reluctant to pursue surgery, radiation therapy has been documented to provide a good long-term clinical outcome for treatment of canine acanthomatous ameloblastoma.

PEARLS & CONSIDERATIONS

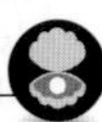

Comments

- For larger oral masses, start with an incisional biopsy to obtain more information before definitive resection. Biopsy results help determine the required extent of definitive surgical resection and other treatment options. When submitting excisional biopsies, clinicians should request that the pathologist evaluate margins for presence of neoplastic cells. Clean margins according to histologic exam do not rule out the possibility of recurrence, but animals with clean margins do have a better long-term prognosis.
- Dental radiography is invaluable for providing diagnostic and treatment planning information for oral tumors. Benign tumors tend to displace teeth that often remain firmly seated, whereas aggressive tumors cause root and alveolar bone resorption, which may manifest as very mobile (floating) teeth. Benign tumors may have a smooth layer of reactive bone surrounding the neoplastic tissue, whereas a malignant tumor often exhibits destruction of cortical bone with formation of a classic sunburst appearance.
- Right or left total mandibulectomy (previously called hemimandibulectomy) and maxillectomy surgeries carry with them the potential for profuse bleeding. Blood type and cross-matching may be warranted preoperatively.

Technician Tips

- Technicians are on the frontline of identifying oral tumors during professional dental cleanings. Do a complete oral exam on each anesthetized patient, including the sublingual area and tonsils. Bring all identified oral masses to the attention of the clinician for possible biopsy during the same anesthetic episode.
- Provide as much information as possible on histopathologic evaluation forms. Include size (in three dimensions), surface characteristics (ulcerated, smooth, verrucous), complete history, and specific location of tumors.

Client Education

- Complete surgical removal of oral tumors provides the best long-term prognosis. Clinicians should advise new pet owners to acclimate puppies and kittens to periodic exam of the oral cavity (as well as routine at-home dental care).
- Animals adapt remarkably well after radical resection of oral tumors, and altered cosmesis is usually well accepted by owners if enough function can be restored to allow for independent eating and drinking. Clients should be shown before and after pictures of similar surgical cases to ensure their understanding of cosmetic changes.

SUGGESTED READING

Goldschmidt SL, et al: Clinical characterization of canine acanthomatous ameloblastoma (CAA) in 263 dogs and the influence of postsurgical histopathological margin on local recurrence. J Vet Dent 34(4):241-247, 2017.

AUTHOR: John R. Lewis, VMD, FAVD, DAVDC
EDITOR: Alexander M. Reiter, DVM, Dr.med.vet., DAVDC, DEVDC

Oral Tumors, Malignant

Bonus Material Online Client Education Sheet

BASIC INFORMATION

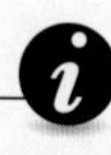

Definition

Neoplastic oral disease is locally invasive and can metastasize to distant sites. Oral tumors comprise approximately 6% of all tumors in dogs and 10% of all tumors in cats.

Synonyms

Malignant oral neoplasia, oral cancer

Epidemiology

SPECIES, AGE, SEX

- Malignant oral tumors can occur at any age, but middle-aged and geriatric pets are overrepresented.
- Canine papillary squamous cell carcinoma (SCC) occurs most commonly in adolescent and young adult dogs.
- The most common canine malignant oral tumor is malignant melanoma (melanosarcoma [p. 644]), seen most often in dogs > 10 years of age.
- The most common feline malignant oral tumor is SCC (p. 939), representing 70% of oral tumors in cats. Average age of onset is 10 years, but cats as young as 5 months have been affected.

GENETICS, BREED PREDISPOSITION

Breeds with pigmented oral mucosa may be predisposed to malignant melanoma.

RISK FACTORS

Factors that increase the risk of feline SCC threefold to fivefold:

- Exposure to flea collars
- High intake of canned cat food
- Regular ingestion of canned tuna

CONTAGION AND ZOONOSIS

Canine transmissible venereal tumor (p. 993) can manifest as a primary or metastatic tumor on the lips, buccal mucosa, and palatine tonsils.

Clinical Presentation

DISEASE FORMS/SUBTYPES

- Dogs: malignant melanoma, SCC, fibrosarcoma, osteosarcoma, multilobular tumor of bone (multilobular osteochondrosarcoma), mast cell tumor, hemangiosarcoma, peripheral nerve sheath tumor, lymphoma (epitheliotropic lymphoma), adenocarcinoma
- Cats: SCC, fibrosarcoma, osteosarcoma, hemangiosarcoma, malignant melanoma (rare)

HISTORY, CHIEF COMPLAINT

- Swelling of mandible or maxilla
- Oral bleeding, halitosis
- Dysphagia if the mass is large enough to affect masticatory function and deglutition
- Appetite and activity level often unaffected

PHYSICAL EXAM FINDINGS

Halitosis, oral bleeding, facial/oral swelling, enlarged mandibular lymph nodes; additional specific findings may vary with tumor type:

- Malignant melanoma is pigmented (melanotic) or nonpigmented (amelanotic) and often lobulated, ulcerative, and friable; necrosis may occur when the tumor outgrows its blood supply. A benign variant of melanoma may occur in the oral cavity (melanocytoma), which is usually less than 1 cm in diameter and well circumscribed.
- Fibrosarcoma is often smooth and firm and may cause generalized disfigurement but rarely bleeds spontaneously.
- Peripheral nerve sheath tumor tends to grow along larger nerves (e.g., infraorbital nerve into infraorbital canal and inferior alveolar nerve into mandibular canal).
- SCC is pink, friable, often verrucous (cauliflower-like), and may be proliferative or ulcerative. Desmoplasia (formation of fibrous tissue) secondary to SCC development may result in a firm tumor on palpation.
- Osteosarcoma can manifest as a diffuse swelling of the maxilla or mandible but often also exhibits a fleshy, pink or red proliferative component that bleeds readily.
- Multilobular tumor of bone is locally invasive but slow to metastasize and usually located at the mandibular ramus, caudal maxilla, zygomatic arch, or calvarium.
- Adenocarcinoma is an invasive, malignant epithelial neoplasm derived from glandular tissue of the oral cavity, nasal cavity, or salivary tissue (major or accessory).
- Hemangiosarcoma is a malignant neoplasm of vascular endothelial origin characterized by extensive metastasis. It has been reported in the gingiva, tongue, and hard palate.
- Maxillary, retro-orbital, and caudal pharyngeal masses: decreased ability to retropulse the eye globes and decreased range of mouth opening if tumor involves the caudal maxilla, zygomatic arch, mandibular coronoid process, or temporomandibular joint.

Etiology and Pathophysiology

Cause is unknown, but a genetic predisposition may play a role.

DIAGNOSIS

Diagnostic Overview

Diagnosis of malignant oral masses usually requires histopathologic analysis of a biopsy, because many oral masses do not exfoliate well on fine-needle aspiration, or vascularity results in hemodilution. Incisional (rather than excisional) biopsy is the preferred initial step for suspected malignancies to provide the clinician and client with further information before deciding on radical surgery and/or radiation therapy.

Differential Diagnosis

As for benign oral tumors (p. 711)

Initial Database

CBC, serum biochemistry profile, urinalysis, and thoracic radiographs: to assess for concurrent illnesses, metastasis

Advanced or Confirmatory Testing

- Anesthetized oral exam (p. 1140)
- Dental radiography
- CT: particularly helpful for maxillary and caudal mandibular masses
- Cytologic exam of oral masses (fine-needle aspiration, woodpecker technique, or scraping from tumor cut surface)
- Cytologic exam of aspirated lymph nodes or histopathologic exam of resected lymph nodes
- Histopathologic evaluation of incisional or excisional biopsy

TREATMENT

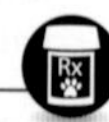

Treatment Overview

- Debulking of aggressive oral tumors is rarely helpful. After a diagnosis is obtained, the mass and a margin of normal surrounding tissue should be removed comprehensively to prevent local recurrence.
- If complete removal is not an option, radiation therapy or chemotherapy may decrease the rate of growth, depending on tumor type.

Acute General Treatment

- Removal of a circumscribed mass to the normal level of the surrounding gingiva often serves as an adequate biopsy but may not prevent local recurrence. Incisional biopsies of large masses are warranted to provide information before performing a radical maxillectomy or mandibulectomy.
- Aspiration and/or removal of head and neck lymph nodes is warranted for staging of animals with malignant oral tumors.

Chronic Treatment

- Depending on biopsy results and tumor extent, radical surgery and/or radiation therapy may be treatment options. Even when surgery is an option, consult with a medical oncologist and/or radiation oncologist regarding the need for adjuvant or postoperative treatment. Chemotherapy may be used as an adjunctive therapy but is rarely effective by itself against most oral tumors. Immunotherapy of certain tumors shows promise, and a commercial melanoma vaccine is available (p. 644).

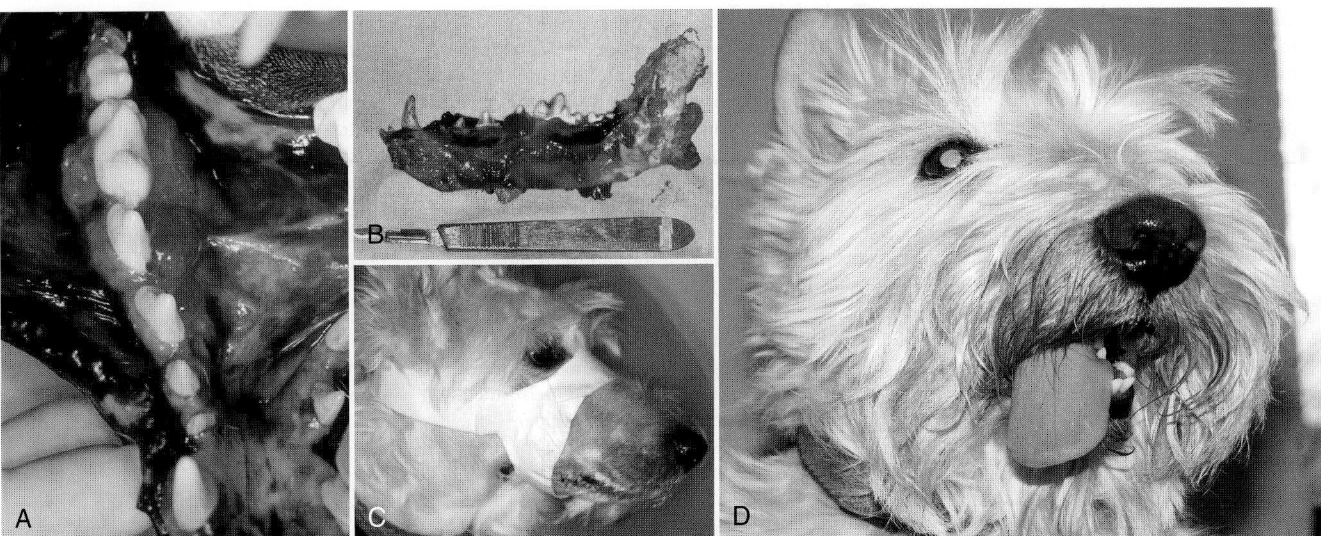

ORAL TUMORS, MALIGNANT Clinical photographs of a 9-year-old dog with malignant spindle cell sarcoma at the right mandibular body. **A,** Rostrodorsal view at right mandible, with tumor located in the area of the third and fourth premolars (P3 and P4) and first molar (M1). **B,** Right total mandibulectomy (resected specimen is shown); right commissuroplasty and crown reduction with vital pulp therapy of left mandibular canine tooth were performed. **C,** Same dog presenting for its 2-week re-exam; note sutures at lip skin still in place and an adhesive tape muzzle in position that limits range of mouth opening postoperatively. **D,** Dog presenting for its 1-year re-exam. This dog had an excellent quality of life for 4.5 years postoperatively and died of unrelated causes. (Copyright Dr. Alexander M. Reiter, University of Pennsylvania.)

- Radiation therapy offers good long-term control for treatment of microscopic disease, but bulky tumors rarely respond well.
- Piroxicam 0.3 mg/kg PO q 24h in dogs may slow the progression of some carcinomas. Short-term (10 days) use of piroxicam in cats appears to be safe at 0.3 mg/kg PO q 24h. Further studies are necessary to determine long-term gastrointestinal safety in cats. If prescribed long-term for cancer palliation, the author prescribes 0.3 mg/kg q 48h.

Nutrition/Diet

Soft food/esophagostomy tube (p. 1106) if necessary because of inability to prehend or chew food

Drug Interactions

Piroxicam and other nonsteroidal antiinflammatories may cause extensive gastric ulceration; avoid concurrent use of corticosteroids, and consider gastric protectants such as misoprostol.

Possible Complications

- Recurrence of primary tumor; at least 1 cm of clinically and radiographically healthy tissue surrounding malignant tumors should be removed; many locally aggressive tumors (fibrosarcoma, peripheral nerve sheath tumor, malignant melanoma) require even wider margins.
- Intraoperative or postoperative bleeding: having blood products available is important for mandibulectomy and maxillectomy procedures (p. 1169).
- Dehiscence of the surgical site: avoid using electrocautery on mucosal edges because it can obscure histologic exam of margins of excised tissue and may increase the likelihood of wound dehiscence, which can result in the need for further surgical intervention (e.g., repair of an oronasal fistula).
- Sublingual or cervical sialoceles may occur if transection of salivary ducts is necessary; these ducts should be ligated if transected.

Recommended Monitoring

- Oral exam to monitor for local recurrence 1 month after surgery and at a maximum of 6-month intervals thereafter.
- Thoracic radiographs and lymph node palpation should be performed every 6 months.

PROGNOSIS & OUTCOME

- Median survival time for most malignant oral tumors after surgical excision has been 7-12 months. However, when surgeons obtain clean surgical margins in the absence of microscopic metastasis, patients can be cured.
- Prognosis for SCC is good if found while still surgically resectable.
- Malignant melanomas > 8 cm^3 (2 × 2 × 2 cm) have a high incidence of microscopic metastasis at the time of diagnosis.
- Mandibular osteosarcoma has been reported to have a lower metastatic rate and better prognosis than appendicular osteosarcoma.
- Tonsillar SCC in dogs commonly metastasizes to regional lymph nodes, with 85% having regional metastasis at necropsy.

PEARLS & CONSIDERATIONS

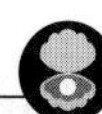

Comments

- Incisional biopsy should be performed for larger oral masses. Excisional biopsy may be curative but carries the risk of inadequate tumor removal. When submitting excisional biopsies, request that the pathologist evaluate margins for neoplastic cells. Clean margins according to histologic exam do not rule out the possibility of recurrence, but animals with clean margins have a better long-term prognosis.
- Dental radiography is invaluable for providing diagnostic and treatment planning information for oral tumors. Benign tumors tend to displace teeth that often remain firmly seated, whereas more aggressive tumors cause root and alveolar bone resorption, which can manifest as very mobile (floating) teeth. Benign tumors may have a smooth layer of reactive bone surrounding the neoplastic tissue, whereas a malignant tumor often exhibits destruction of cortical bone, with formation of a classic radiographic sunburst appearance.
- Right or left total mandibulectomy (incorrectly called hemimandibulectomy) and maxillectomy surgeries carry with them the potential for profuse bleeding. Blood type and cross-matching may be warranted preoperatively.
- Sublingual edema seen within 48 hours after mandibulectomy should not be confused with a sublingual sialocele (ranula). Edema usually resolves without treatment.
- Pigmentation is not a reliable indicator of tumor type. About 40% of oral malignant

melanomas may be amelanotic (unpigmented). Malignant tumors other than melanoma may be partially pigmented if the patient's oral mucosa is normally pigmented.
- Removal of regional lymph nodes may be beneficial at the time of oral surgery. A single surgical approach to parotid, mandibular, and medial retropharyngeal lymph nodes has been described.
- If the biological behavior of a tumor does not match histopathologic results, the biopsy should be reread or retaken. A type of fibrosarcoma exists that appears histologically benign but is biologically (clinically) very aggressive.
- Nonhealing dental extraction sites, particularly in cats, may be a clinical manifestation of SCC; biopsy any suspicious tissues at the time of extraction.
- Dehiscence and inappropriate healing often occur when oral surgery is performed on irradiated sites.
- Oral tumors in cats are more often malignant than benign.

Technician Tips
- Technicians are on the front line of identifying oral tumors during professional dental cleanings. Do a complete oral exam on each anesthetized patient, including the sublingual area, palate, and tonsils. Bring all identified oral masses to the attention of the clinician for possible biopsy under the same anesthetic episode.
- Provide as much information as possible on histopathologic forms. Include size (in three dimensions), surface characteristics (ulcerated, smooth, verrucous), complete history, and specific location of tumors. When an excisional biopsy is performed, ask the pathologist to evaluate the specimen for evidence of clean or dirty margins.

Client Education
- Complete surgical removal of oral tumors provides the best long-term prognosis. Tumors that are detected early are likely to be operable. Advise new pet owners to acclimate puppies and kittens to feel comfortable with periodic exam of the oral cavity as well as routine dental care.
- Animals adapt remarkably well after radical resection of oral tumors (mandibulectomy or maxillectomy), although one study noted that 12% of cats did not regain the ability to eat on their own.
- Altered cosmesis is usually well accepted by owners if masticatory function can be restored. Clients should be shown before and after pictures of similar surgical cases to ensure their understanding of cosmetic changes.
- Lymph node aspirates and thoracic radiographs are important for preoperative staging, but microscopic metastasis cannot be totally ruled out by these tests.

SUGGESTED READING

Bertone ER, et al: Environmental and lifestyle risk factors for oral squamous cell carcinoma in domestic cats. J Vet Intern Med 17:557, 2003.

AUTHOR: John R. Lewis, VMD, FAVD, DAVDC
EDITOR: Alexander M. Reiter, DVM, Dr.med.vet., DAVDC, DEVDC

Orbital Diseases

Client Education Sheet 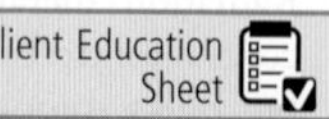

BASIC INFORMATION 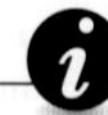

Definition
Orbital diseases encompass several conditions that frequently lead to an abnormal position of the eye in the orbit. These abnormal positions include exophthalmos (rostral displacement of the eye), enophthalmos (caudal displacement of the eye), and strabismus (deviation of the axis of the resting eye position). Orbital diseases can be congenital or acquired and have vascular, inflammatory, traumatic or neoplastic causes.

Synonyms
Exophthalmia, enophthalmia, retrobulbar disease, orbital or retrobulbar abscess and/or cellulitis, orbital neoplasia, retrobulbar neoplasia

Epidemiology
SPECIES, AGE, SEX
- Orbital abscess and cellulitis are more common in younger animals.
- Orbital neoplasia is more common in older animals.

GENETICS, BREED PREDISPOSITION
- Ocular proptosis is more common in brachycephalic breeds.
- Myositis is more common in German shepherds, Weimaraners, golden retrievers, and Labrador retrievers (masticatory myositis); extraocular polymyositis is more common in golden retrievers.
- Craniomandibular osteopathy is more common in West Highland white terriers.
- Congenital strabismus may be seen in Akita and Shar-pei dogs, as well as in Siamese and some shorthair cats.

ASSOCIATED DISORDERS
Masticatory myositis (exophthalmos or enophthalmos)
Exophthalmos:
- Head trauma (proptosis)
- Nasal or metastatic neoplasms (and/or strabismus)
- Dental disease
- Pharyngeal abscess (p. 6)
- Systemic mycoses

Enophthalmos:
- Facial fractures
- Primary ocular diseases (i.e., corneal ulceration, uveitis)
- Horner's syndrome
- Emaciation
- Dehydration (severe)
- Tetanus

Clinical Presentation
HISTORY, CHIEF COMPLAINT
Sudden or progressive change in position of the eye; abnormal eye position from birth

PHYSICAL EXAM FINDINGS
Bilateral or unilateral:
- Exophthalmos with any of the following:
  - Reduced ability or inability to retropulse the globe in the orbit
  - Lagophthalmos with or without corneal ulceration
  - Third eyelid protrusion
  - Conjunctival hyperemia, chemosis
  - Exposure keratitis (corneal neovascularization, corneal edema, corneal ulceration)
  - Periocular swelling
  - Pain on opening the mouth (orbital abscess/cellulitis; myositis)
  - Blindness (especially with proptosis)
- Enophthalmos with any of the following:
  - Third eyelid protrusion
  - Ptosis (drooping upper eyelid)
  - Miosis
  - Corneal ulceration
  - Corneal edema, aqueous flare, hypopyon, fibrin clot, hyphema (uveitis)
  - Extraocular and/or masticatory muscle atrophy
  - Entropion
  - Emaciation (loss of orbital fat results in enophthalmos)
- Strabismus
  - Deviation of the eye(s): dorsal, ventral, medial, lateral, or a combination of these eye positions
  - ± Exophthalmos or enophthalmos

- Variable systemic signs, depending on underlying cause
- Inflamed oral mucosa or draining fistula behind the last upper molar with orbital abscess

Etiology and Pathophysiology

Exophthalmos caused by space-occupying orbital lesion caudal to the eye:

- Congenital
  - Orbital varix, arterial to venous shunts (rare)
  - Orbital cysts and dermoids (rare)
- Acquired
  - Ocular proptosis: usually unilateral, peracute, trauma associated
  - Orbital abscess/cellulitis: usually unilateral, peracute to acute, painful resistance to ocular retropulsion and mouth manipulation
  - Orbital hemorrhage: secondary to coagulopathy or head trauma
  - Orbital neoplasia: usually unilateral, progressive, typically not painful, primary or secondary, predominantly malignant
  - Feline restrictive orbital myofibroblastic sarcoma (FROMS; previously orbital pseudotumor [cats]): rare, progressive debilitating neoplastic orbital disease; restricts mobility of the eyelids and globe; may become bilateral condition
  - Mucocele: unilateral, progressive, arising from zygomatic salivary gland
  - Myositis: bilateral, enophthalmia occurring in late stages

Enophthalmos: caused by loss of orbital volume or space-occupying lesion rostral to the eye:

- Acquired
  - Facial fractures with associated displacement of orbital tissues
  - Loss of orbital fat or muscle (e.g., weight loss, orbital fractures, cachexia)
  - Ocular pain
  - Dehydration
  - Horner's syndrome
  - Secondary to atrophy of the masticatory muscles from myositis episode or age
  - Neoplasia anterior to the eye (e.g., rostral orbit)
  - Tetanus (rare)

Strabismus; typically caused by lesions restricting extraocular muscle mobility or affecting their innervation:

- Congenital
  - Unilateral or bilateral, progressive juvenile fibrosis of the medial rectus muscle seen in Shar-pei dogs
  - Bilateral medial strabismus (esotropia) in Siamese cats
- Acquired
  - Trauma-induced extraocular muscle avulsion or scarring
  - Extraocular muscle scarring from previous inflammation
  - Abnormal innervation of extraocular muscle(s) (e.g., cranial nerve [CN] III, IV, and/or VI lesions)

DIAGNOSIS

Diagnostic Overview

The diagnosis is suspected based on the time frame of clinical signs, signalment, and clinical appearance of the affected eye. Orbital imaging may be necessary for a definitive diagnosis if the globe is normal.

Differential Diagnosis

Exophthalmos:

- Buphthalmos
- Episcleritis/scleritis

Enophthalmos:

- Microphthalmia
- Phthisis bulbi
- Ruptured globe

Initial Database

- Complete ophthalmic exam (p. 1137)
- Complete neurologic exam, especially cranial nerves (p. 1136)
- Oral exam if orbital abscess suspected (e.g., buccal pain and/or purulent drainage)
- Nasal airflow if nasal neoplasm with secondary orbital invasion suspected
- CBC, serum biochemistry profile, urinalysis, skull radiographs, thoracic radiographs, fine-needle aspiration of submandibular lymph nodes if enlarged, abdominal ultrasound if orbital neoplasm suspected
  - CBC may reveal evidence of inflammation (bands, toxic changes in neutrophils) with orbital abscess
- Pharmacologic testing (topical 1% or 10% phenylephrine) for Horner's syndrome

Advanced or Confirmatory Testing

- Ocular/orbital ultrasound if exophthalmos (differentiates orbital abscess, cellulitis, and mass)
- CT or MRI if exophthalmos (fully assess orbital mass or foreign body)
- Ultrasound-guided fine-needle aspiration or biopsy of orbital mass, abscess, or mucocele under general anesthesia (referable procedure)
- Masticatory or extraocular muscle biopsies under general anesthesia (e.g., myositis; referable procedure)

TREATMENT

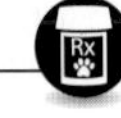

Treatment Overview

Although treatment of orbital abscesses and myositis may not always require referral, treatment options for orbital neoplasms are likely to require referral to a veterinary ophthalmologist, surgeon, and oncologist.

- If possible, return the eye to its normal position.
- Alleviate pain.
- Preserve vision (optic neuropathy and/or retinal detachment may occur with space-occupying orbital lesions).

Acute General Treatment

Treat underlying cause:

- Ocular proptosis (p. 823)
- Orbital abscess/cellulitis:
  - Abscess is suspected if the oral mucosa caudal to last upper molar is abnormal and conjunctiva and eyelids are inflamed. In such cases, medical stabilization (e.g., rehydration) is warranted if necessary, followed by surgical drainage by blunt dissection under general anesthesia with small hemostats. Samples should be obtained for aerobic and anaerobic culture and susceptibility (C&S). Often, oral lesion is not visible, and in those cases, empirical treatment with broad-spectrum oral antibiotics is advised.
  - Systemic nonsteroidal antiinflammatory drugs (NSAIDs) for 7 days; may require longer depending on resolution of pain and inflammation.
    - Dogs: carprofen 2.2 mg/kg PO q 12h, meloxicam 0.1 mg/kg PO q 24h, *or* deracoxib 1-2 mg/kg PO q 24h
    - Cats: tolfenamic acid 4 mg/kg SQ, IM, or PO q 24h for 3-5 days, robenacoxib 1 mg/kg q 24h PO for 3 days, *or* meloxicam 0.3mg/kg once SQ
  - Broad-spectrum oral antibiotics for 14-28 days (amoxicillin-clavulanic acid 13.5 mg/kg PO q 12h [dogs] or 62.5 mg PO q 12h [cats]). Amoxicillin-clavulanic acid is the first-choice antibiotic for this condition.
  - Hospitalization with supportive treatment for first postoperative 24-48 hours (if necessary)
- Orbital neoplasia
  - Surgical excision (exenteration, orbitotomy, or orbitectomy) may require referral to a veterinary ophthalmologist or surgeon.
  - Adjunctive radiation therapy or chemotherapy, depending on type of neoplasm (consult veterinary oncologist)
- Feline restrictive orbital myofibroblastic sarcoma: Exenteration with adjunctive radiotherapy and/or chemotherapy (referral to a veterinary oncologist) has been suggested as a treatment, but most patients are euthanized due to the grave prognosis.
- Mucocele: surgical excision (typically curative); may require referral to a veterinary ophthalmologist or surgeon (p. 894)
- Myositis: prednisone 1-2 mg/kg PO q 12h, tapered gradually after response to treatment is noted (p. 637). This is long-term therapy that should be tapered every 2-4 weeks pending response to treatment. Additional immunosuppressive drugs may be required if response to treatment is not seen within 1-2 weeks.

Possible Complications

- Permanent strabismus or third eyelid protrusion
- Blindness
- Loss of the eye
- Systemic complications possible (potentially death), depending on extent of disease process

Recommended Monitoring

Weekly or bimonthly re-examination for inflammatory diseases

PROGNOSIS & OUTCOME

- Favorable with orbital abscess if treated adequately
- Guarded with myositis
- Poor with orbital neoplasia

PEARLS & CONSIDERATIONS

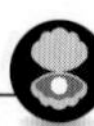

Comments

Orbital disease should be investigated in a timely fashion to alleviate discomfort and potentially preserve vision.

Technician Tips

Check the intraocular pressure on all dogs with orbital disease as glaucoma can have a similar appearance.

Client Education

- Consult a veterinarian as soon as an alteration in position of the eye(s) is noted.
- Relapses can occur with myositis or when an orbital foreign body persists.

SUGGESTED READING

Betbeze C: Management of orbital diseases. Top Companion Anim Med 30:107, 2015.

AUTHOR: Chantale L. Pinard, DVM, MSc, DACVO
EDITOR: Diane V. H. Hendrix, DVM, DACVO

Organophosphate and Carbamate Insecticide Toxicosis

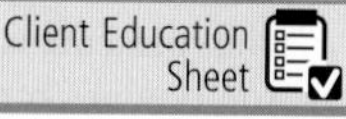

BASIC INFORMATION

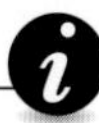

Definition

Organophosphate (OP) and carbamate insecticides are used for controlling insects in agriculture, around the home, and on or around animals (e.g., controlling fleas and ticks). Toxicosis results from dermal or oral exposure and is characterized by any combination of increased salivation, lacrimation, urinary incontinence, diarrhea, dyspnea, and emesis (SLUDDE), bradycardia, tremors, shaking, ataxia, seizures, and/or sudden death.

Synonyms

Acetylcholinesterase (AChE) inhibitors, cholinesterase inhibitors

Epidemiology

SPECIES, AGE, SEX

- All breeds and both sexes
- Very young, elderly, or debilitated animals are more susceptible.
- Cats are particularly sensitive to chlorpyrifos; the onset of clinical signs is usually delayed (1-5 days) after exposure, and signs can last 2-4 weeks.

RISK FACTORS

Exposure to other AChE inhibitors

GEOGRAPHY AND SEASONALITY

Toxicosis is more common in summer months (insecticide use).

Clinical Presentation

HISTORY, CHIEF COMPLAINT

- Known dermal or oral exposure to an OP or carbamate
- Recent history (usually within 24 hours before onset of clinical signs) of using an OP or carbamate insecticide in the yard/house
- Rapid onset of clinical signs (typically minutes to hours after exposure)
- Salivation, vomiting, diarrhea, lacrimation, dyspnea
- Tremors, muscle weakness, ataxia, seizures; acute death possible
- Cats may not show typical OP toxicosis signs from chlorpyrifos intoxication. Clinical signs, which begin 1-5 days after exposure, can consist of anorexia, depression, vomiting, tremors, salivation, ataxia, seizures, and ventroflexion of the neck.

PHYSICAL EXAM FINDINGS

- Muscarinic signs: SLUDDE, miosis, and bradycardia
- Nicotinic signs: muscle tremors, weakness, and paresis progressing to paralysis
- Central nervous system (CNS) signs: hyperactivity, depressed respiration, and seizures
- Muscarinic signs may be overridden by sympathetic stimulation, resulting in opposite effects (e.g., mydriasis, tachycardia).

Etiology and Pathophysiology

Source:

- Organophosphates (OPs) are aliphatic carbon, cyclic, or heterocyclic phosphate esters.
    - Commonly used OPs are disulfoton, acephate, terbufos, phorate, parathion, chlorpyrifos (Dursban), fenthion, diazinon, and malathion.
- Carbamates are cyclic or aliphatic derivatives of carbamic acid.
    - Commonly used carbamates are aldicarb, carbofuran, methomyl, propoxur, and carbaryl (Sevin).

Mechanism of toxicosis:

- OPs and carbamates competitively inhibit AChE by binding to its esteric site. Acetylcholine (ACh) then accumulates in the synapse and causes excessive synaptic neurotransmitter activity, leading to muscarinic, nicotinic, or CNS effects. Competitive inhibition of AChE explains the result of confirmatory testing with OP or carbamate toxicosis (low blood AChE level).
- Some OPs undergo aging, rendering the phosphorylated (inactivated) cholinesterase enzyme very stable so that recovery of AChE activity occurs only through the synthesis of new enzyme. Inhibition of AChE by the OPs tends to be irreversible, whereas inhibition by the carbamates is reversible, which allows a spontaneous regeneration of the enzyme. Both carbamates and OPs respond initially to atropine, but only carbamates continue to do so. OPs become refractory to atropine treatment.
- Atropine blocks the effects of the excess ACh at the neuromuscular junction. Atropine can control only the muscarinic signs, not the nicotinic signs.
- Death occurs secondary to respiratory failure from excessive bronchial secretions, bronchiolar constriction, paralysis of intercostal muscles or diaphragm, or respiratory paralysis (CNS effects).

DIAGNOSIS

Diagnostic Overview

A tentative diagnosis is based on history of exposure (recent use of pesticide on the animal or in the environment) and presence of one or several SLUDDE signs. Serum AChE levels are the clinical confirmatory test of choice, but treatment generally needs to be initiated before availability of results.

Differential Diagnosis

- Some *Solanaceae* family plants; anatoxin-a(s) found in some blue-green algae
- Muscarinic signs: muscarinic mushrooms, tremorgenic mycotoxins
- Nicotinic signs: nicotine, pyrethrins/pyrethroids, organochlorine-type pesticides, caffeine, strychnine, sodium fluoroacetate (compound 1080), 4-aminopyridine, metaldehyde, zinc phosphide, lead
- CNS signs: any disorder that can cause seizures (p. 903)

Initial Database

- CBC, urinalysis (usually normal)
- Serum biochemistry profile: possible mild increase in liver and pancreatic enzymes with some OPs (disulfoton)

Advanced or Confirmatory Testing

- AChE levels (p. 1299): serum, plasma, whole blood (preferred), brain, or retina:
  - An AChE result that is < 50% of normal indicates significant exposure is likely, and AChE activity < 25% of normal indicates toxicosis (activity can remain depressed for 6-8 weeks).
  - Because carbamates are reversible inhibitors of AChE, the results may be normal even in the face of carbamate toxicosis.
- AChE insecticide screen: liver, kidney, gastrointestinal tract contents, and source material to look for specific insecticide

TREATMENT

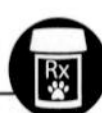

Treatment Overview

Triage identifies cases with life-threatening clinical effects on presentation, which are treated with atropine, pralidoxime (for OPs), ventilator support if hypoventilation, seizure control if needed, and supportive care. Decontamination and other treatment measures are carried out after the animal has been stabilized. The treatment process is summarized in an algorithm found on p. 1438.

Acute General Treatment

- Treat life-threatening signs first if present.
  - Atropine sulfate (dogs/cats) 0.1-0.5 mg/kg; one-fourth dose IV and rest of dose IM or SQ to reduce muscarinic signs; repeat as needed to control bradycardia and bronchial secretions.
  - Pralidoxime chloride (2-PAM; Protopam) (dogs/cats) 20 mg/kg IM, SQ, or very slow IV q 12h for controlling the nicotinic signs, although some benefit may be seen by controlling CNS signs. 2-PAM should not be used with carbamates because it would not be beneficial. Oximes reverse binding of toxin to AChE, but carbamate binding to AChE is inherently reversible. If the OP-intoxicated animal shows no response after 3 doses, discontinue treatment with 2-PAM. Oximes such as pralidoxime are ineffective once OP aging has occurred, but because the time of aging varies with the compound, pralidoxime may be effective even days after exposure.
- Seizure control
  - Diazepam 1-2 mg/kg IV, repeat as needed, *or*
  - Phenobarbital 2-5 mg/kg IV bolus, repeated in 20 minutes up to two times
  - Pentobarbital to reach desired effect; repeat as needed
  - Controlling tremors: methocarbamol 50-100 mg/kg IV; repeat as needed without exceeding 330 mg/kg/day
- Oxygen and ventilatory support as needed for animals in respiratory distress (pp. 1146 and 1185)
- Decontamination of the animal: indicated after any potentially life-threatening hemodynamic, neurologic, and respiratory abnormalities have been addressed (p. 1087).
  - Dermal exposure: bathe the animal with a mild dishwashing liquid, then rinse thoroughly, dry and keep patient warm. Wear gloves.
  - Emesis induction: only in asymptomatic patients; effective only within a few hours of ingestion (p. 1188)
  - Gastric lavage: when a large amount of poison has been ingested or emesis is contraindicated (comatose); use a short-acting anesthetic and cuffed endotracheal tube to protect airway (p. 1117).
  - Activated charcoal 1-2 g/kg PO or labeled dosage of commercial product. In animals showing overt clinical signs, repeat in 8 hours (one-half the original dose).
- Supportive care: IV fluids as needed

Nutrition/Diet

Tube feeding (p. 1106) or other nutritional support may be necessary for cats that may be anorectic for days to weeks after being exposed to chlorpyrifos.

Drug Interactions

Avoid:

- Enhancing toxicity: phenothiazine tranquilizers (e.g., acepromazine), opiates, aminoglycoside antibiotics, theophylline
- Administering neuromuscular blocking agents (levamisole, succinylcholine, nicotine, and curare) can enhance the nicotinic effects of OPs.

Possible Complications

- Pancreatitis, hemorrhagic enteritis, and increased liver enzymes can occur in some animals after OP toxicosis (disulfoton).
- Certain OPs can cause a delayed neuropathy 2-3 weeks after acute poisoning. This complication is characterized by hindlimb ataxia, hypermetria, and proprioceptive deficits. Chlorpyrifos (experimentally at high doses) is possibly associated with this neuropathy in cats.
- There are usually no long-term effects in animals that recover from acute OP or carbamate toxicosis unless there have been prolonged seizures.

Recommended Monitoring

- Heart rate
- Respiratory rate and effort, and lung sounds
- CNS signs

PROGNOSIS & OUTCOME

- Prognosis good unless the animal suffers from respiratory distress (excessive bronchial secretions, aspiration pneumonia) or seizures
- Duration of signs depends on treatment, dose, compound, and species of animal.

PEARLS & CONSIDERATIONS

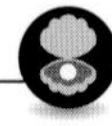

Comments

- The main difference of clinical importance between carbamates and OPs is that AChE inhibition is generally irreversible in cases of OP toxicosis but reversible in cases of carbamate toxicosis.
  - Pralidoxime (2-PAM, Protopam) is indicated for treatment of OP toxicosis but not carbamate toxicosis (ineffective).
  - Carbamates are generally short-acting chemicals.
- SLUDDE signs can have several causes. If history of exposure to an anticholinesterase insecticide is not known, a test dose of atropine can be given to determine whether the signs are caused by an anticholinesterase (OP or carbamate) insecticide.
  - Record baseline heart rate.
  - Administer preanesthetic dose of atropine (i.e., 0.02 mg/kg IV for dogs and cats), and monitor the animal's response for 15-30 minutes.
  - If the heart rate increases and mydriasis occurs, the muscarinic signs are NOT due to OP or carbamate toxicosis (it takes ≈10 times the preanesthetic dose of atropine to resolve signs caused by cholinesterase inhibitor insecticides).
- For dead animals, submit one-half the brain (sagittal section, frozen) to the lab (put the other half in formalin for histopathologic exam) but only if rabies is definitively ruled out (otherwise, the material could be hazardous to personnel opening the skull and handling tissue).
- With the availability of safer insecticides for controlling insects, the incidence of OP and carbamate toxicoses in animals has decreased.
- The table shows toxicity ratings.

Technician Tips

Exposure to aldicarb- and methomyl-containing carbamates by dogs can cause rapid seizures and death (within minutes). Ask the client to bring the patient to the clinic immediately if such an exposure is encountered.

Toxicity Ratings

Toxicity Rating	LD50	Substances
Highly toxic	<50 mg/kg	Disulfoton, coumaphos, famphur, phorate, terbufos, methomyl, aldicarb
Moderately toxic	50-1000 mg/kg	Acephate, chlorpyrifos, diazinon, carbaryl, phosmet, propoxur
Lower toxicity	>1000 mg/kg	Malathion, tetrachlorvinphos

LD50: Dose that is lethal for 50% of exposed individuals.

Client Education

- Pet owners should use insecticides according to label directions and keep all insecticides away from pets.
- Safer flea and tick treatments are now available for use on pets.

SUGGESTED READING

Means C: Organophosphate and carbamate insecticides. In Peterson ME, et al, editors: Small animal toxicology, ed 3, St. Louis, 2013, Saunders, pp 715-724.

AUTHOR: Camille DeClementi, VMD, DABT, DABVT
EDITOR: Tina Wismer, DVM, MS, DABVT, DABT

Oronasal Fistula

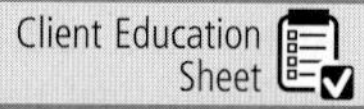
Client Education Sheet

BASIC INFORMATION

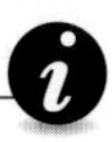

Definition

An abnormal connection forms between oral and nasal cavities, usually due to severe periodontal disease or after tooth extraction. It typically results from oral disease extending dorsally and is virtually never caused by nasal disease extending ventrally.

Synonym

Oronasal communication

Epidemiology

SPECIES, AGE, SEX

- Older dogs, typically small breeds/mixes with narrow muzzles (dolichocephalic)
- Older cats concurrently affected by tooth resorption, alveolar bone expansion, and abnormal tooth extrusion

GENETICS, BREED PREDISPOSITION

- Conformation of skull and predisposition to development of periodontal disease
- Miniature poodles, Chihuahuas, Yorkshire terriers, miniature schnauzers, dachshunds

RISK FACTORS

Periodontal disease (p. 776)

ASSOCIATED DISORDERS

Halitosis, nasal discharge

Clinical Presentation

DISEASE FORMS/SUBTYPES

- Area of the maxillary canine tooth is most often affected
- Occasionally seen in the premolar tooth area; may be present although the tooth is still in place (e.g., palatal aspect of a maxillary canine tooth)

HISTORY, CHIEF COMPLAINT

- Acute: epistaxis after tooth extraction
- Chronic: history of tooth loss or extraction, nasal discharge, sneezing, halitosis

PHYSICAL EXAM FINDINGS

- Mucopurulent nasal discharge
- Round or oval defect at junction of palatal and gingival/alveolar mucosa if tooth is missing (oral epithelium in continuity with nasal epithelium)
- Severe plaque and calculus accumulation, tooth mobility, and deep periodontal pocketing if tooth is still present

Etiology and Pathophysiology

Periodontitis results in alveolar bone loss and loss of the oral and nasal epithelium that normally separates the oral and nasal cavities.

DIAGNOSIS

Diagnostic Overview

The diagnosis is purely visual and made on physical exam. If uncertainty exists, oronasal communication can be demonstrated by irrigation (see below).

Differential Diagnosis

- Oronasal communications not related to periodontitis
- Other causes of chronic nasal discharge (p. 678). Clinicians should always thoroughly examine the mouth and teeth of animals with nasal discharge.

Initial Database

- CBC, serum chemistry profile, urinalysis (before anesthesia): results generally unremarkable
- Thoracic radiographs if the chief complaint, history, and physical exam findings raise the possibility of metastatic disease or pneumonia

Advanced or Confirmatory Testing

- Periodontal probing and dental radiographs under general anesthesia can reveal the extent of alveolar bone loss.
- Injection of water into the oral defect (and while the head is positioned lower than the neck) shows water flowing from the ipsilateral nostril.
- Other areas of the mouth should be evaluated because periodontal disease is likely generalized and severe in patients with oronasal fistula.

TREATMENT

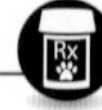

Treatment Overview

Surgical repair prevents continued entry of food or fluid into the nasal cavity.

Acute General Treatment

- After tooth extraction in the area of the oronasal fistula (if the tooth is still present), the first step is careful tissue debridement and irrigation to remove the epithelial lining and debris.
- Single-flap technique: two divergent releasing incisions are made, extending from the gingiva over the mucogingival junction.

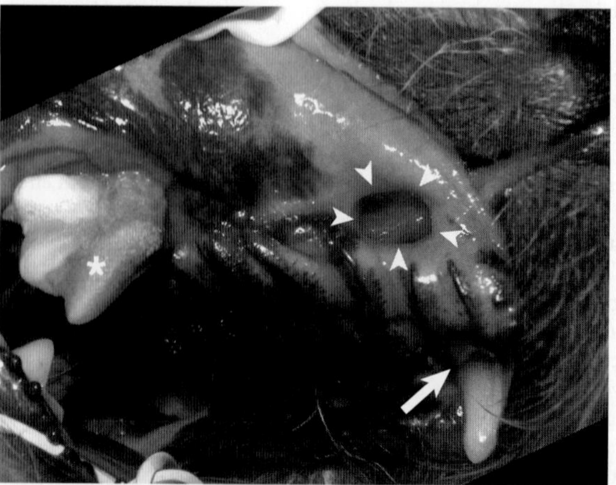

ORONASAL FISTULA Chronic oronasal fistula *(arrowheads)* in the area of a missing right maxillary canine tooth in a dog. The incisors and most cheek teeth also are missing. The left canine *(arrow)* and right fourth premolar *(asterisk)* are affected by severe periodontal disease. (Copyright Dr. Lenin A. Villamizar.)

into alveolar mucosa. The labial mucosa (epithelium and supporting connective tissue) is dissected free from its maxillary attachments. The epithelium lining the oronasal fistula on the palatal side is resected. Necrotic or injured tissue is trimmed from the flap edges. Sharp bony surfaces are smoothed. The periosteum at the base of the flap is incised to make it tension free. The wound is rinsed again. The edges of the flap are gently apposed and sutured to freshly incised edges of epithelium. A barrier material (auricular cartilage, flexible bone membrane) may be placed under the flap.
- Double-flap technique: initially, a full-thickness mucoperiosteal palatal flap is raised but remains hinged at the medial margin of the defect. The flap should be transposed to cover the defect (palatal epithelium becomes nasal epithelium). A labial-based flap is then raised, advanced, and sutured over the connective tissue side of the first flap.
- Treatment of periodontal disease in other areas of the mouth is important. This often requires extraction of other maxillary teeth on the same side; closure of these extraction sites after thorough debridement and irrigation of the wound can be combined with closure of the flap covering the oronasal fistula.

Nutrition/Diet

Soft food for 2 weeks

Behavior/Exercise

No hard treats and toys for 4 weeks

Possible Complications

Dehiscence: avoid tension as previously described. If the flap tissue tends to pull back when placed across the defect before sutures are placed, it is too tight, and additional dissection is required.

PROGNOSIS & OUTCOME

Excellent

PEARLS & CONSIDERATIONS

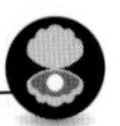

Comments

Gentle tissue handling and avoidance of tension at the suture line improves healing.

Prevention

Preventative care and prophylactic treatment information is provided on pp. 776 and 1090.

Technician Tips

The teeth of animals with nasal discharge should always be examined by means of periodontal probing.

Client Education

Teach owners about good home oral hygiene and provide related client education sheets.

SUGGESTED READING

Reiter AM, et al: Applied feline oral anatomy and tooth extraction techniques—an illustrated guide. J Feline Med Surg 16:900, 2014

AUTHOR: Lenin A. Villamizar-Martinez, DVM, MS, PhD
EDITOR: Alexander M. Reiter, DVM, Dr.med.vet., DAVDC, DEVDC

Osteoarthritis

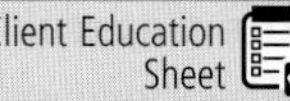

BASIC INFORMATION

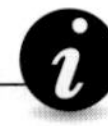

Definition

Progressive, noninflammatory, irreversible deterioration of articular cartilage

Synonyms

Degenerative joint disease, osteoarthrosis, OA

Epidemiology

SPECIES, AGE, SEX

Dogs and cats; increasing prevalence with age

GENETICS, BREED PREDISPOSITION

- Elbow dysplasia: rottweilers, Labrador retrievers, Bernese mountain dogs
- Hip dysplasia: many breeds
- Cranial cruciate ligament rupture, patellar luxation: many breeds
- Arthropathy: Scottish fold cats

RISK FACTORS

- Joint instability (hip dysplasia, cranial cruciate ligament rupture, trauma)
- Joint incongruity (elbow dysplasia, trauma)
- Obesity
- Work duty or athletics

Clinical Presentation

DISEASE FORMS/SUBTYPES

- Primary (idiopathic) osteoarthritis: unknown cause; more common in cats
- Secondary osteoarthritis: commonly results from trauma or joint instability, incongruity, immobilization, or osteochondrosis

HISTORY, CHIEF COMPLAINT

- Reluctance to ambulate or jump
- Lameness and stiffness after exercise or prolonged rest
  - Pet owners are more likely to recognize lameness due to OA in pet dogs than in cats.
- Irritable behavior when approached or touched
- Decreased grooming, elimination outside of litter box in cats may be seen without recognized lameness

PHYSICAL EXAM FINDINGS

Orthopedic exam (p. 1143):
- Lameness
- Stiff or altered gait (e.g., bunny hopping)
- Joint pain, crepitus, instability, and/or decreased range of motion
- Joint effusion, thickening
- Muscle atrophy

Etiology and Pathophysiology

- Disruption in joint homeostasis begins with abnormalities in cartilage or joint biomechanics, which induces extracellular matrix degradation by cytokines and other inflammatory mediators.
- Chondrocytes attempt to repair the damaged collagen network, but eventually, repair activity cannot keep up, resulting in progressive and irreversible loss of articular cartilage structure and function.
- Periarticular fibrosis develops as a secondary process directed toward stabilizing the joint.

DIAGNOSIS

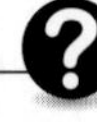

Diagnostic Overview

Osteoarthritis is suspected based on signalment, history, and especially physical findings (lameness; thickened, painful joint). Confirmation requires imaging (primarily radiographs).

Differential Diagnosis

- Infectious arthritis
- Immune-mediated arthritis (erosive or nonerosive)
- Neoplasia (synovial sarcoma, osteosarcoma)

Initial Database

- Clinical exam localizing joint pain
- Radiography: subchondral sclerosis, joint space narrowing, osteophytosis, enthesophytosis, joint capsule thickening, subchondral sclerosis, intraarticular calcified bodies, soft-tissue calcification or subchondral cysts, bone remodeling, joint effusion

Advanced or Confirmatory Testing

- Arthrocentesis (p. 1059) and synovial fluid analysis (p. 1384): rarely necessary but can rule out other forms of arthritis (e.g., septic, immune-mediated)
  - Total cell count < 5,000 nucleated cells/mcL; mononuclear cells/macrophages predominate; < 10% polymorphonuclear cells. Fluid is clear, hazy, or pale yellow with normal to decreased viscosity.
- Other tests used on rare occasions
  - Arthroscopy: view articular cartilage
  - CT: confirm joint incongruity
  - MRI (p. 1132): morphologic change of articular cartilage
  - Nuclear scintigraphy: localize osteoarthritis or inflammation to specific joint

TREATMENT

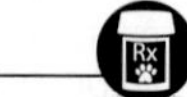

Treatment Overview

The goal of treatment is to alleviate pain, improve function, limit disease progression, and facilitate joint reparative processes. Treatment may include surgical correction of the primary cause of osteoarthritis (correction of malalignment or instability), joint replacement or excision, or arthrodesis if other treatments are not possible. Nonsurgical management includes analgesics/antiinflammatories, exercise modification, and weight management.

Acute General Treatment

- Surgical treatment for cause of joint degeneration: repair of an articular fracture, removal of osteochondral lesion, stabilization of an unstable joint, as necessary
- Nonsteroidal antiinflammatory drugs (NSAIDs) to reduce inflammatory mediators and pain; give one of the following (dosages are for dogs unless stated otherwise):
  - Carprofen 2.2 mg/kg PO q 12h
  - Deracoxib 1-2 mg/kg PO q 24h (may use 3-4 mg/kg PO q 24h for first 7 days only)
  - Etodolac 10-15 mg/kg PO q 24h
  - Firocoxib 5 mg/kg PO q 24h
  - Meloxicam 0.1 mg/kg PO q 24h; for cats, 0.1 mg/kg PO on day 1, then 0.05 mg/kg PO q 24h for 4 days, then 0.05 mg/kg every other day thereafter
  - Robenacoxib 1-2 mg/kg PO q 24h; for cats, 1 mg/kg q 24h for 3 days
- Non–cyclooxygenase (COX)-inhibiting prostaglandin receptor antagonist: grapiprant 2 mg/kg PO q 24h
- Disease-modifying agents
  - Polysulfated glycosaminoglycan 5 mg/kg IM once weekly for 4-6 weeks (dogs)
  - Pentosan polysulfate 3 mg/kg SQ or IM once weekly (dogs or cats)
  - Oral formulations (omega-3 fatty acids, glucosamine, chondroitin, avocado-soy unsaponifiables): according to formulation/labeled instructions
- Opioids (e.g., fentanyl patch 2-4 mcg/kg/h for 3-5 days) or synthetic opiate agonists (e.g., tramadol 2-5 mg/kg PO q 8-12h) if necessary to decrease pain
- *N*-methyl-D-aspartate (NMDA) receptor antagonist: amantadine 3-5 mg/kg PO q 24h (dog or cat) given along with an NSAID

Chronic Treatment

- NSAIDs
- Oral omega-3 fatty acids
- Disease-modifying agents
- Intraarticular injection of platelet rich plasma or mesenchymal stem cell products
- Arthroplasty of severely affected hip, stifle, and elbow joints
- Arthrodesis of severely affected joints
- Excision arthroplasty (hip, shoulder, metacarpo-/metatarsophalangeal joints)
- Acupuncture (p. 1056)

Nutrition/Diet

- Weight control to maintain a lean body condition score (p. 1077)
- Diets high in omega-3 fatty acids (e.g., Hill's j/d, Purina JM)

Behavior/Exercise

- Encourage low-impact activity such as leash walks and swimming rather than high-impact activity such as unrestricted off-leash activity and jumping.
- Physical activity/therapy can help strengthen muscle mass and improve function.
- Nonslip surfaces or products to increase traction (e.g., PawFriction) can be helpful for some dogs.

Drug Interactions

- Gastrointestinal irritation, hemorrhage, gastric ulceration, and perforation with NSAIDs
- NSAID-induced nephrotoxicity possible with hypovolemia or pre-existing renal disease
- Hepatotoxicity with carprofen (idiosyncratic)
- Decreased platelet aggregation with NSAID therapy (especially aspirin)
- Do not give NSAID drugs to animals receiving glucocorticoids for any cause.

Possible Complications

Polysulfated glycosaminoglycan is a heparin analog; caution if given with NSAIDs to an animal with a bleeding disorder.

Recommended Monitoring

- Palpate for joint effusion and/or periarticular fibrosis.
- Quantify muscle mass with palpation and tape measure.
- Measure range of motion with a goniometer during exam.
- Monitor joint pain and gait during exam or with force plate analysis.
- Assess serial radiographs.
- Assess animal's attitude, appetite, body condition score, body weight, and activity level.
- Scoring systems have been developed for repeated owner assessment of severity of signs.

PROGNOSIS & OUTCOME

- Osteoarthritis is typically an irreversible, slowly progressive disease.
- Medical and/or surgical treatment often permits a good quality of life.

PEARLS & CONSIDERATIONS

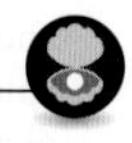

Comments

- Radiographic signs of osteoarthritis may not correlate with clinical signs. Treatment decisions cannot be made on the basis of radiographic findings alone.
- Efficacy of cartilage modifiers is not as well documented as efficacy of NSAIDs.
- Comparative efficacy of various NSAIDs is debatable.
- Use of glucocorticoids in place of NSAIDs is controversial; using both together is contraindicated because of severe, potentially life-threatening gastrointestinal ulceration.
- In cats, low-dose regimens of ketoprofen, meloxicam, robenacoxib, or butorphanol and treatment with tramadol and omega-3 fatty acids have been described (see Additional Suggested Readings, Lascelles).

Prevention

Prompt recognition and early intervention may delay progression of disease.

Technician Tips

Nonslick floors and slow leash walks with slings to support body weight (especially during rising) may improve dogs' comfort.

Client Education

- Treatment is palliative (no magic bullet), and disease will likely progress.
- Client participation is necessary for long-term management.
- Animals in pain are more likely to bite; use caution in handling.
- Be sure that cats with OA can comfortably access food, water, and litter box.
- Educate clients regarding potential adverse effects of NSAID use (e.g., monitor appetite, watch for signs of melena in stools).

SUGGESTED READING

Sanderson RO, et al: Systematic review of the management of canine osteoarthritis. Vet Rec 164(14):418-424, 2009.

AUTHORS: Desiree D. Rosselli, DVM, DACVS; Spencer A. Johnston, VMD, DACVS
EDITOR: Kathleen Linn, DVM, MS, DACVS

Osteochondrosis

Client Education Sheet

BASIC INFORMATION

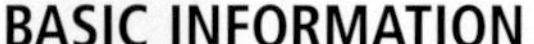

Definition

- Osteochondrosis is an abnormality of endochondral ossification that disturbs the ordered transition of epiphyseal or physeal cartilage to bone. The resultant cartilage thickening inhibits the ability of nutrients to diffuse to the articular surface, and chondrocyte death ensues. This can lead to loosening of the articular cartilage from the underlying subchondral bone, causing painful and clinically overt osteochondritis dissecans (OCD).
- OCD may lead to osteoarthritis (p. 721), also called degenerative joint disease (DJD), which is a deterioration of articular cartilage and joint capsule tissues causing decreased joint function.
- It is a common heritable/developmental disorder in dogs.

Synonyms

Osteochondritis, osteochondritis dissecans (OCD), osteochondrosis dissecans

Epidemiology

SPECIES, AGE, SEX

- Large- and giant-breed dogs
- More common in males
- First signs may appear at maximal growth rate (4-8 months of age)

GENETICS, BREED PREDISPOSITION

Predisposition among these breeds is seen in certain bloodlines, but the mode of inheritance is unknown:

- Border collie, German shepherd, golden retriever, Great Dane, Irish wolfhound, Labrador retriever, Newfoundland, rottweiler, Saint Bernard, Bernese mountain dog, others

RISK FACTORS

- Genetic predisposition
- Rapid growth rate
- Excessive dietary calcium (Ca) and calorie intake proposed
- Hormonal effects (i.e., male dogs, calcitonin)
- Increased joint loading and trauma from intense exercise

ASSOCIATED DISORDERS

- Hip dysplasia
- Disturbances in endochondral ossification also are seen with nontraumatic premature distal ulnar physis closure and ununited anconeal processes, supraglenoid tubercles, and medial humeral epicondyles
- Medial coronoid disease

Clinical Presentation

HISTORY, CHIEF COMPLAINT

- Young dogs in good general health (typically)
- Chief complaint is usually lameness of various degrees and durations
  - Unilateral or bilateral
  - May become clinically overt after skeletal maturity due to secondary osteoarthritis
- History may include use of homemade diet or supplemented commercial dog food during growth

PHYSICAL EXAM FINDINGS

- Lameness may manifest as a short-stepping gait if bilateral.
- Joint pain, swelling, crepitus, instability, decreased range of motion
- Occasionally, only joint swelling and fibrosis are noted
- Muscle atrophy of the affected limb(s)

Etiology and Pathophysiology

- Nutritional excess implicated but not proven as a causal factor
  - Excessive caloric (but not protein) intake
  - Increased calcium (or increased vitamin D with normal calcium/phosphorus [Ca/P]) intake disturbs endochondral ossification in Great Danes, potentially other large dogs
- At least in horses and pigs, osteochondrosis begins with failure of the blood supply in growth cartilage, leading to chondrocyte death
- Disturbed endochondral ossification leads to cartilage thickening, resulting in cartilage malnutrition and further chondrocyte necrosis
- Clefts develop at the junction of viable and nonviable layers. During normal joint motion, vertical fissures develop in the articular cartilage, resulting in the formation of a cartilage flap.
- The flap may remain attached to the remaining cartilage tissue or may completely detach (joint mouse).
- Inflammatory mediators are released, and osteoarthritis results.
- Joints most commonly affected:
  - Shoulder: caudal humeral head
  - Elbow: medial humeral condyle
  - Hock (tarsocrural joint): medial or lateral trochlear ridges of the talus
  - Stifle: lateral or medial femoral condyle
  - Also identified in the vertebral articular processes and caudal border of glenoid

DIAGNOSIS

Diagnostic Overview

OCD is suspected based on age (juvenile), breed (large/giant), history, diet, unilateral or bilateral lameness, and radiographic signs of a subchondral bone defect in typical locations.

Differential Diagnosis

- Shoulder: humeral or scapular fracture; biceps tenosynovitis, insertional myopathy, scapulohumeral luxation
- Elbow: medial coronoid disease, ununited anconeal process, ununited medial epicondyle, incongruity, collateral ligament injury, fracture
- Stifle: cranial cruciate ligament rupture or avulsion, meniscal injury, collateral ligament injury, extensor tendon avulsion, patella luxation, femoral or tibial fracture
- Tarsus: collateral ligament rupture, fracture
- Radius curvus syndrome: shortening of antebrachium as in chondrodystrophy, curvature due to physeal injury

Initial Database

- Radiographs of the affected and contralateral joints:
  - Indentation, flattening, or saucer shape of the subchondral bone
  - Mineralized density may be seen in the joint
  - Varying degrees of osteoarthrosis
  - Subchondral sclerosis in advanced cases
  - Multiple views may be required for lesion identification in some joints (e.g., tarsus)
- Review dietary history, including food intake and body condition score
- Not diagnostic: blood Ca, P, and vitamin D concentrations

Advanced or Confirmatory Testing

- Contrast radiography or CT imaging may be necessary. Scintigraphy and MRI are uncommonly used.
- Arthrocentesis for synovial fluid analysis when joint effusion is present. Mild increase in mononuclear cell counts with OCD and DJD
- Arthroscopy can be used for diagnosis if radiography and CT are inconclusive.

TREATMENT

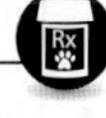

Treatment Overview

- Surgery (arthrotomy or arthroscopy) is used to remove the devitalized cartilage and help stimulate new cartilage formation. Joint congruity cannot usually be completely restored. Surgery is superior to medical management for shoulder OCD; controversy remains about whether medical or surgical management is better for other joints.
- Medical management (alone or with surgery) aims to reduce inflammation, pain, lameness, and improve joint health.
- Nutrition should be adjusted if necessary.
- Modify excessive activity in juvenile large-breed dogs.

Acute General Treatment

Conservative management:

- Exercise restriction for 6 weeks
- Nonsteroidal antiinflammatory drugs (NSAIDs): never administer more than one at a time nor with concurrent corticosteroids: carprofen 2.2 mg/kg PO q 12h, etodolac 10-15 mg/kg PO q 24h, deracoxib 1-2 mg/kg PO q 24h, firocoxib 5 mg/kg PO q 24h, ketoprofen 0.25-1 mg/kg PO q 24h, meloxicam 0.1 mg/kg PO q 24h, or grapiprant 2 mg/kg PO q 24h
- Targeted analgesics can be used in addition for multimodal pain management: tramadol 2-5 mg/kg PO q 8-12h, amantadine 3-5 mg/kg PO q 24h, or gabapentin 5-10 (can increase up to 20 mg/kg if needed) mg/kg PO q 8-12h

Surgical management:

- Arthrotomy or arthroscopy to debride loose or devitalized cartilage, cartilage flaps, and intraarticular osteochondral fragments
- Curettage and forage (drilling) of the subchondral bone lesion to stimulate fibrocartilage formation
- The talus is NOT curetted to avoid creating additional joint instability
- Autogenous osteoarticular grafting and prosthetic resurfacing of defects has been reported.

Chronic Treatment

DJD may occur at a later age:

- Prevent joint overload (activity moderation and weight management) and administer NSAIDs and analgesics as listed above for osteoarthritis pain

Disease-modifying agents help relieve discomfort, reduce degradative and inflammatory enzyme levels, and stimulate production of synovial fluid, proteoglycan, and collagen:

- Glucosamine hydrochloride, chondroitin sulfate, manganese ascorbate, and avocado/soybean unsaponifiables combination product (Dasuquin)
- Polysulfated glycosaminoglycans (PSGAG) 4.4 mg/kg IM q 3-4 days for up to 4 weeks (maximum of 8 injections)
- Pentosan polysulfate: intraarticular 5-10 mg/joint weekly, IM or SQ 3 mg/kg once weekly for 4 weeks, or PO 10 mg/kg weekly for 4 weeks, repeated every 3 months
- Hyaluronan 3-5 mg intraarticular
- Acupuncture, cold laser therapy, physical rehabilitation
- Platelet-rich plasma (PRP) and adipose tissue–derived stem cells

Nutrition/Diet

- Avoid feeding excessive calories, calcium (bones, bone meal, milk, tablets, powder), or vitamin D (drops, tablets, fish diets).
- The lowest risk of diet-induced disease is found in animals whose body condition score is maintained at 2/5 during the period of growth.
- Dogs should not be fed ad libitum; volume of food should be based on the animal's body condition score. Calculated energy requirements and manufacturers' recommendations should only be used as starting points (p. 1077).
- During growth, owners should feed their pets a commercially available dog food with a calcium content not exceeding 3.5 g/1000 kcal and energy density < 4 kcal/g (<17% fat). Optimal calcium levels are found in many purpose-made large/giant-breed puppy foods; owners should not feed adult dog food to puppies.
  - Owners should not add supplements.
  - These feeding guidelines are especially important in the preweaning and postweaning periods.

Behavior/Exercise

- Limit/control activity to low impact.
- For joint instability, consider commercially available, custom-fitted support wrap.

Drug Interactions

Intraarticular glucocorticoid injections increase lesion severity and are contraindicated.

Possible Complications

- Untreated cartilage flaps irritate the joint and cause more DJD. In OCD of the shoulder joint, the flap can loosen and migrate into the biceps tendon sheath or attach to the joint capsule and grow (ossicle).
- Perioperative and postoperative complications:
  - Seroma formation due to excessive postoperative physical activity occurs commonly after arthrotomy.
  - Swelling from irrigating fluid leaking into the periarticular soft tissue may occur after arthroscopy.
  - Infection (uncommon)
  - Failure to remove all the osteochondral fragments
  - Tarsocrural joint instability

Recommended Monitoring

- The contralateral joint is often affected and should be evaluated clinically and radiographically.
- If lameness persists, synovial fluid analysis and culture, radiographs, arthroscopy, CT, or MRI may be indicated.

PROGNOSIS & OUTCOME

- Shoulder: good after treatment, even in cases with DJD. Most dogs become sound 4-8 weeks after surgery.
- Elbow: fair to good when cartilage damage is small in young animals and DJD is minimal; fair to poor when combined with medial coronoid disease and/or severe cartilage damage
- Stifle: varies; a large lesion in a young animal may carry a poor prognosis.

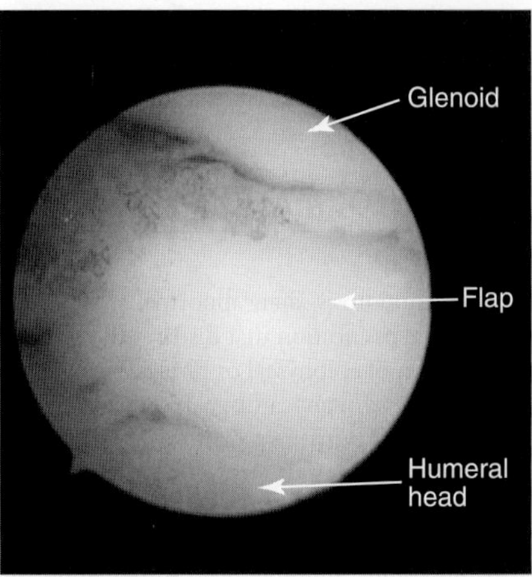

OSTEOCHONDROSIS Arthroscopic view of OCD of the humeral head.

- Hock: fair; joint capsule thickening helps stabilize the joint, although residual instability remains, and DJD is likely.

PEARLS & CONSIDERATIONS

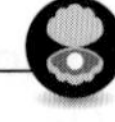

Comments

Although lameness may be unilateral, radiographs of the contralateral joint are indicated.

Prevention

- Only breed animals screened for OCD (and other hereditary diseases); affected dogs and their relatives (parents and siblings) should not be bred.
- Diet management (see above)

Technician Tips

- Application of cold compress immediately after surgery and continued at intervals for the first 2-3 days can minimize swelling and inflammation.
- Application of heat compress is recommended after swelling and inflammation have subsided.

Client Education

- Pre-purchase knowledge of lineage/parental history of heritable orthopedic disorders
- Dietary management
- Owners should give the puppy time to grow and should not train the dog too heavily or too early.

SUGGESTED READING

Fitzpatrick N, et al: Early clinical experience with osteochondral autograft transfer for treatment of osteochondritis dissecans of the medial humeral condyle in dogs. Vet Surg 38:246, 2009.

AUTHOR: Joseph C. Glennon, VMD, DACVS
EDITOR: Kathleen Linn, DVM, MS, DACVS

Osteomyelitis

Bonus Material Online 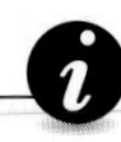 Client Education Sheet 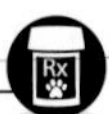

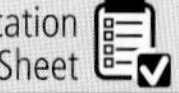

BASIC INFORMATION

Definition

An acute or chronic inflammatory process of bone secondary to hematogenous or traumatic infection with pyogenic organisms.

Epidemiology

SPECIES, AGE, SEX

- Any dog or cat
- Young, male dogs: traumatic osteomyelitis

GENETICS, BREED PREDISPOSITION

German shepherds: *Aspergillus* infection

RISK FACTORS

- Open fractures secondary to trauma, bite wounds
- Fracture repair, orthopedic procedures with direct or hematogenous contamination
- Extension of soft-tissue infections
- Compromised immunity, allowing hematogenous dissemination
- Young animals are prone to deposition of blood-borne bacteria near physes.

GEOGRAPHY AND SEASONALITY

- Blastomycosis and histoplasmosis: states south of the Ohio River and east of the Mississippi; Canadian prairies
- Coccidioidomycosis in the southwestern United States and Central and South Americas
- Actinomycosis associated with grass awns (p. 398) in summer in California and Florida

ASSOCIATED DISORDERS

Periodontitis, bulla osteitis, discospondylitis or paronychia, depending on location of infected bone

Clinical Presentation

HISTORY, CHIEF COMPLAINT

- Orthopedic surgery, trauma, or travel (systemic fungal infection) may be in the recent history.
- Owner may have noted lethargy, anorexia, lameness, swelling, signs of pain, or cutaneous draining tracts.

PHYSICAL EXAM FINDINGS

- Acute osteomyelitis: fever, lethargy, anorexia, limb or joint swelling/pain, lameness
- Chronic osteomyelitis: draining tracts, normothermia, disuse muscle atrophy, lameness, limb deformity

Etiology and Pathophysiology

- Neonatal osteomyelitis may originate from an umbilical infection.
- Acute postoperative osteomyelitis causes clinical signs 2-7 days after surgery.
- Radiographic changes are evident 2 weeks after trauma or surgery.
- Glycocalyx (biofilm) is deposited on surgical implants with bacteria present, forming a barrier that protects bacteria from antibodies and drugs.
- 50%-60% of cases are monomicrobial, with *Staphylococcus* spp most common (50%).
- 40%-50% of cases are polymicrobial, with a mixture of aerobes and anaerobes.
- Anaerobes, including *Actinomyces, Clostridium, Bacteroides, Fusobacterium,* and *Peptostreptococcus* spp, are reported in up to 70% of infections in some studies.
- Other common isolates are *Streptococcus, Escherichia coli, Pasteurella, Pseudomonas, Proteus,* and *Klebsiella* spp.

DIAGNOSIS

Diagnostic Overview

Osteomyelitis is suspected based on history, clinical, and radiographic findings and is confirmed with direct bacterial or fungal cultures.

Differential Diagnosis

- Bone infarct, neoplasia, or cellulitis
- Callus of healing bone can be mistaken for osteomyelitis but it typically has a smoother radiographic appearance.

Initial Database

- CBC, serum biochemistry panel: results can be normal or there can be an inflammatory leukogram. Monocytosis is sometimes seen with systemic fungal disease.
- Craniocaudal and mediolateral radiographs of affected bone: usually an area of mixed lysis and new bone formation is evident. Sequestra, if present, are sclerotic, have sharp edges, and may be surrounded by an area of lucency.
- Thoracic and abdominal radiographs if fungal cause suspected
- Arthrocentesis (p. 1059) with cytologic exam, culture and susceptibility (C&S) for joint involvement
- Aerobic and anaerobic C&S of deep fine-needle aspirates of tissues (not of draining tracts)
- Fungal titers/antigen testing: as appropriate for geographic exposures

Advanced or Confirmatory Testing

- Ultrasonography may reveal soft-tissue abscess or periosteal elevation.
- Contrast fistulogram to localize source or sequestrum
- Radionuclide bone scan with technetium-99m: detects inflammatory lesions; more specific if performed with leukocytes labeled with gallium-67 or indium-111 and best if animal has a confirmed leukocytosis
- Bone biopsy for culture and histopathology
- Blood and/or urine cultures if systemic infection suspected (p. 1333)

TREATMENT

Treatment Overview

Treatment is based on identification and elimination of the source of infection. Infected fractures must be stabilized for healing to occur, and removal of infected bone may be necessary.

Acute General Treatment

- Acute osteomyelitis requires 4-6 weeks of antimicrobials based on C&S results.
- Initial antibiotics may be given IV.
- Because *Staphylococcus* spp are most common, initial therapy can involve
  - Clavulanic acid/amoxicillin 10-25 mg/kg PO q 8-12h, *or*
  - Cephalexin 22-30 mg/kg PO q 8h, *or*
  - Marbofloxacin 2.75-5.5 mg/kg PO, SQ q 24h (avoid in growing dogs), or
  - Clindamycin 11-33 mg/kg PO q 12h (dogs), q 24h (cats), *or*
  - Chloramphenicol 40-50 mg/kg PO, IV, IM q 8h (dogs), 15-50 mg/kg q 12h (cats) for otherwise resistant infections
- Definitive (medium- and long-term) antibiotic selection depends on results of bacterial C&S.
- Request extended-spectrum agent if initial sensitivity results do not support oral medications.
- Choices for fungal osteomyelitis include itraconazole, fluconazole (not for aspergillosis), or amphotericin B.

Chronic Treatment

- May require surgical exploration and removal of sequestrum (dead bone) with curettage of surrounding bone
- Remove loose implants, retain stable implants until union is achieved, and consider adding external fixation if further support is needed.
  - Fracture-associated infection will not clear unless fracture is stable.
  - Exchange of implants may be possible.
  - Because of glycocalyx, implants may need to be removed after bone healing for infection to fully resolve.
- A cancellous bone graft may be indicated after infection has subsided.
- Open drainage with lavage or closed drainage with ingress/egress
- Antibiotic-impregnated beads or gels may be implanted around the bone.
- Continue antibiotics for a minimum of 6-8 weeks.

Drug Interactions

- Use cautions for human exposure to chloramphenicol.
- Avoid administering quinolones to skeletally immature dogs (risk of cartilage defects).
- Monitor renal values if on amphotericin B.

- Monitor hepatic values if on itraconazole or fluconazole.

Possible Complications

- Bone abscess
- Bacteremia
- Fracture/limb deformity
- Implant failure
- Cellulitis
- Draining tracts
- Delayed/nonunion
- Sequestrum formation

Recommended Monitoring

- Radiographs at 4-6 week intervals to evaluate healing
- Aspirate and reculture if animal shows signs of recurrence.

PROGNOSIS & OUTCOME

- Acute osteomyelitis can be eradicated with early, aggressive treatment.
- Chronic osteomyelitis can recur weeks to years after the initial treatment.
- Fungal osteomyelitis may require several months of treatment, and outcome is guarded to poor.
- Involvement of joints may result in osteoarthrosis and limb disuse.

PEARLS & CONSIDERATIONS

Comments

- Obtaining a culture only from the drainage tract can be misleading because contaminants (skin organisms and gram-negative bacteria) are common.
- Leukocytosis is common with acute disease; typically it is absent with chronic infection.
- Antibiotic-coated implants are being used for prevention and treatment.
- Radiographic appearance of fungal osteomyelitis and primary bone tumors is similar.

Prevention

- Aseptic surgical technique
- Appropriate antimicrobial prophylaxis and therapy

Technician Tips

- Animals with active draining infections should be isolated to reduce the possibility of cross-contamination of other surgical patients.
- Disposable gowns, mask, and gloves should be worn for wound care/bandage changes.

Client Education

Treatment of chronic osteomyelitis can be costly and lengthy.

SUGGESTED READING

Robinson R: Osteomyelitis and implant-associated infections. In Johnston SA, et al, editors: Veterinary surgery: small animal, ed 2, St. Louis, 2018, Elsevier, pp 775-783.

AUTHOR: Mary E. Somerville, DVM, DACVS
EDITOR: Kathleen Linn, DVM, MS, DACVS

Osteosarcoma

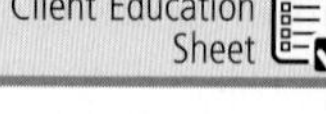

BASIC INFORMATION

Definition

Osteosarcoma (OSA) is a primary malignant tumor of mesenchymal tissue that always includes the production of bone (osteoid) by malignant osteoblasts.

Epidemiology

SPECIES, AGE, SEX

- In dogs, OSA accounts for up to 85% of all primary bone tumors.
    - Median age is 7-9 years, with a smaller peak incidence at 1.5-2 years of age.
    - No obvious sex predisposition
- In cats, primary bone tumors are uncommon, but OSA accounts for 70%-80% of those seen.
    - Extraskeletal OSA can occur at sites of previous vaccinations (p. 550).

GENETICS, BREED PREDISPOSITION

- Body size (height and weight) is a more important predictor than breed.
- Compared with small-breed dogs (weighing < 10 kg [22 lb]), the risk of OSA is 60 times higher in dogs weighing > 30 kg (66 lb) and 8 times higher in dogs weighing 20-30 kg (44-66 lb).
- Appendicular OSA accounts for 95% of all cases in dogs weighing > 40 kg but only 40%-50% of all cases in dogs weighing < 15 kg.

Clinical Presentation

DISEASE FORMS/SUBTYPES

- 75% of OSA arises from the appendicular skeleton. In the forelimb, the distal radius and proximal humerus are affected most commonly. In the hindlimb, lesions are evenly distributed among the distal femur, proximal tibia, and distal tibia.
- 25% of OSA arises from the axial skeleton. The mandible, maxilla, vertebra, ribs, and pelvis are most commonly affected.
- Extraskeletal OSA is rare. Mammary gland is one of the more frequently reported sites.

HISTORY, CHIEF COMPLAINT

- Appendicular OSA usually is associated with progressive lameness. Occasionally, lameness is acute and severe due to a pathologic fracture. A palpable swelling might or might not be present.
- Axial OSA can present with a variety of signs. Localized swelling with or without pain is common. Tumors arising from the mandible or maxilla can be associated with halitosis, dysphagia, pain on opening the mouth, or nasal discharge. Vertebral tumors may induce neurologic deficits. Rarely, rib tumors are associated with respiratory signs.
- The first clinical signs of pulmonary metastasis usually are vague, including lethargy and anorexia. The animal may cough, but overt respiratory distress is uncommon. Rarely, lameness develops in one or more limbs secondary to hypertrophic osteopathy.

PHYSICAL EXAM FINDINGS

- Dogs with appendicular OSA exhibit lameness ranging from minimal to non–weight-bearing. A palpable swelling might or might not be present.
- Dogs with axial OSA can have variable physical exam findings (see History, Chief Complaint). Signs of pain or discomfort are not as consistent as with appendicular tumors. Depending on the size and location of the tumor, a mass might or might not be visible or palpable.

Etiology and Pathophysiology

Cause is largely unknown, but OSA has been associated with fracture sites, metallic orthopedic implants, chronic osteomyelitis, bone infarction, osteochondromatosis, and ionizing radiation.

DIAGNOSIS

Diagnostic Overview

The diagnosis is strongly suspected based on patient signalment, history, physical exam findings, and radiographic evidence of an aggressive bone lesion. Cytology can further support the diagnosis, but histopathology is required for a definitive diagnosis.

Differential Diagnosis

- Other primary bone tumors: chondrosarcoma, fibrosarcoma, hemangiosarcoma
- Metastatic bone tumors: transitional cell, prostatic, mammary, thyroid, anal sac carcinomas, pulmonary carcinoma (cat only)
- Tumors that locally invade adjacent bone: synovial cell sarcoma, histiocytic sarcoma, oral tumors (squamous cell carcinoma [SCC], melanoma, fibrosarcoma, ameloblastoma), digital tumors (SCC, melanoma)
- Hematopoietic tumors: myeloma, lymphoma. Radiographic lesions typically are purely lytic.
- Bacterial or fungal (e.g., blastomycosis, coccidioidomycosis) osteomyelitis

Initial Database

Radiographic imaging of OSA:

- Aggressive bone lesions are associated with neoplasia and infection, and they are characterized by one or more of the following radiographic signs:
  - Presence of bone disruption, particularly involving the cortex
  - Bone lysis; permeative and moth-eaten patterns always are aggressive; geographic lysis can be aggressive or benign.
  - Nonhomogeneous, interrupted periosteal bone formation, or amorphous new bone deposited haphazardly in the soft tissues surrounding the bone
  - Ill-defined or indistinct transition zone between normal and abnormal bone
- Appendicular OSA is usually located in the metaphyseal region of long bones. Extension across joints is uncommon.

After a radiographic or histologic diagnosis, animals should be completely staged:

- CBC, serum biochemistry panel, urinalysis
- Three-view thoracic radiographs
  - <10% of animals have visible pulmonary metastatic lesions at initial diagnosis.
  - Most dogs with OSA ultimately develop visible metastatic disease, even if the primary tumor is surgically removed, indicating metastasis occurred before initial presentation.
- <5% of dogs have lymph node metastasis, but any enlarged regional lymph nodes should be evaluated with cytology and/or histopathology.

Advanced or Confirmatory Testing

- Fine-needle aspiration (FNA) with cytologic analysis is minimally invasive and can help support a diagnosis of OSA.
  - FNA can be considered for lesions with associated cortical destruction. Ultrasound guidance can be used for sample collection.
  - Cytologic analysis can distinguish between malignant and nonmalignant lesions with an accuracy of 70%-85%. In samples diagnostic for cancer, alkaline phosphatase cytochemistry is a highly sensitive and fairly specific marker for OSA and can help distinguish OSA from other bone tumors.
- Histopathologic evaluation is required to definitively diagnose OSA.
  - An incisional biopsy can be performed using a Jamshidi bone biopsy needle. Tumors are distinguished from benign lesions with an accuracy of 90%; the specific tumor type is diagnosed with an overall accuracy of 80%.
    - Biopsy core(s) should be taken from the lesion's center. Samples taken from the periphery are likely to be nondiagnostic, containing only reactive bone.
  - If signalment, history, and initial database all support a diagnosis of OSA, and the owners are willing to treat aggressively, it is reasonable to surgically remove local disease (amputation or limb-sparing procedure), with biopsy submission after surgery.
- CT imaging is recommended for axial tumors to more accurately stage local disease and help with planning surgery and/or radiation therapy (RT). If CT is performed, lungs should be included in imaging to screen for pulmonary metastasis.
- Whole-body bone survey radiography and nuclear scintigraphy (i.e., bone scan) are not routinely recommended; however, any suspicious lesions or painful areas should be imaged.

TREATMENT

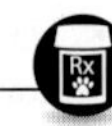

Treatment Overview

Definitive treatment includes surgery or stereotactic radiosurgery (SRS) for the primary tumor, followed by adjuvant chemotherapy to help delay the onset of visible metastasis. Palliative therapy focuses primarily on pain control and is indicated when patients present with gross metastatic disease or owners decline definitive therapy.

Acute and Chronic Treatment

- Surgical removal of the primary tumor
  - Amputation is the standard treatment for appendicular OSA. Most animals function well after surgery; osteoarthritis is rarely a contraindication.
  - In limb-sparing techniques, only the neoplastic portion of the affected bone is excised, and the weight-bearing axis is re-established using a variety of strategies. Candidates should have tumors arising from the distal radius, distal ulna, or proximal femur, and the tumor should involve < 50% of the bone, with minimal extension into the surrounding soft tissues.
    - Compared with amputation, survival times are similar, but complication rates are higher (infection, implant failure, local tumor recurrence).
  - For animals with axial OSA, wide surgical excision is recommended whenever possible. Complete excision is often more difficult because of the tumor's proximity to vital structures. When complete excision is not possible, surgery can be combined with conventional RT, or SRS can be considered in place of surgery (see below).
- SRS is a specialized form of RT in which a large dose of radiation is precisely delivered to the primary tumor, usually in 1-3 daily treatments. Candidates should have minimal cortical lysis to minimize risk of subsequent pathologic fracture.
  - Compared with amputation, survival times with SRS are similar. In contrast, conventional RT is inferior to amputation.
  - SRS also can be used for axial tumors that are not amenable to surgery. However, because OSA contains bone mineral, the extent of tumor shrinkage and return to function varies for vertebral tumors and other tumors compressing adjacent normal structures.
- The most commonly used adjuvant chemotherapy drug is carboplatin. Cisplatin and doxorubicin also have efficacy. Protocols typically include one or more of these drugs for a total of 4-6 treatments.
- Toceranib phosphate (Palladia) can help slow disease progression in some dogs with visible pulmonary metastasis.
- A genetically engineered *Listeria*-based vaccine has been developed that targets *ERBB2 (HER2/NEU)*, an oncogene expressed on some canine OSAs. This vaccine has been used in combination with amputation and carboplatin. The vaccine is not commercially available at the time of publication.
- A variety of palliative treatments can be used to help control the pain associated with the primary tumor. Multimodal therapy is more effective, and pain is easier to prevent than reverse.
  - Nonsteroidal antiinflammatory (NSAID) choices (use only one at a time) include aspirin 10-25 mg/kg PO q 8-24h, carprofen 2 mg/kg PO q 12h, deracoxib 1-2 mg/kg PO q 24h; may use 3-4 mg/kg PO q 24h for first 7 days only, meloxicam 0.1 mg/kg PO q 24h, and firocoxib 5 mg/kg PO q 24h.
  - Other oral analgesic drugs include acetaminophen with codeine (Tylenol #4 [300 mg acetaminophen, 60 mg codeine]) 0.5-2 mg/kg PO q 6-8h with dosing based on codeine (acetaminophen is contraindicated in cats), tramadol 2-5 mg/kg PO q 6-12h, gabapentin 10-15 mg/kg PO q 8-12h, amantadine 3-5 mg/kg PO q 24h.
  - Bisphosphonates decrease bone resorption and increase bone mineral density.
    - Pamidronate 1-2 mg/kg IV q 3-4 weeks decreases lameness in 30% of dogs.
    - Zoledronate 0.1 mg/kg IV q 4 weeks decreases lameness in 75% of dogs.
  - Palliative RT reduces pain in 75%-90% of dogs with OSA. Analgesia persists for a median of 2-3 months.
  - Animals with pulmonary metastasis often benefit from oral glucocorticoids at antiinflammatory doses, such as prednisone 0.5-1 mg/kg PO q 24h (do not combine with NSAIDs).

Recommended Monitoring

Clinicians should evaluate patients every 2-3 months for evidence of local recurrence and metastatic disease. Ideally, this includes a thorough physical exam and three-view thoracic radiographs. Imaging of the site of the primary tumor may be indicated, depending on location, completeness of excision, and clinical signs.

PROGNOSIS & OUTCOME

- Most animals with OSA ultimately succumb to the effects of the primary tumor and/or metastatic disease.
  - The lungs are the most common site for metastasis, followed by other bones and then various soft tissues.

- For animals with appendicular OSA
  - With amputation alone, median survival is 4-5 months; the 1-year survival rate is 10%, and the 2-year survival rate is 2%.
  - When amputation, limb salvage, or SRS is combined with adjuvant platinum-based chemotherapy, median survival improves to 10-12 months, and 2-year survival rate improves to 15%-25%.
  - When local therapy is combined with single-agent doxorubicin, median survival is 8 months, the 1-year survival rate is 35%, and the 2-year survival rate is 17%.
  - Prognosis using combinations of carboplatin/doxorubicin or cisplatin/doxorubicin is comparable to that seen with single-agent platinum therapy.
  - Proximal humerus location, elevated serum alkaline phosphatase level, monocytosis, and lymphocytosis are negative prognostic factors.
  - With palliative care alone, survival times are up to 4-5 months, depending on how well the pain associated with the primary tumor can be controlled.
  - After metastatic disease is visible, survival times typically are < 2-3 months, regardless of therapy (palliative or aggressive).
- For most animals with axial OSA, prognosis is similar or more guarded, depending on completeness of excision with surgery or return to function with SRS.
- Mandibular OSA carries a better prognosis. With mandibulectomy alone, metastatic rate is ≈60%, and median survival is ≈17 months. The benefit of adjuvant chemotherapy is uncertain.
- Nasal and digital OSA might also have a lower metastatic rate, but information is limited.

PEARLS & CONSIDERATIONS

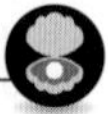

Comments

Animals that are non–weight-bearing lame on a limb affected by OSA have already demonstrated the degree to which they will be able to ambulate after amputation.

Technician Tips

When OSA is suspected, use caution when positioning the patient for radiographs to minimize pain and risk of pathologic fracture.

SUGGESTED READING

Selmic LE, et al: Comparison of carboplatin and doxorubicin-based chemotherapy protocols in 470 dogs after amputation for treatment of appendicular osteosarcoma. J Vet Intern Med 28:554, 2014.

AUTHOR: Dennis B. Bailey, DVM, DACVIM
EDITOR: Kenneth M. Rassnick, DVM, DACVIM

Otitis Externa

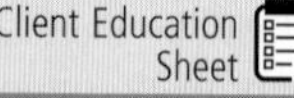

BASIC INFORMATION

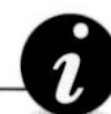

Definition

Acute or chronic inflammation of the external ear canal that may also involve the pinnae

Epidemiology

SPECIES, AGE, SEX

Dogs, less commonly cats

GENETICS, BREED PREDISPOSITION

- Canine: cocker spaniel, Brittany spaniel, and many others
- Feline: Himalayan and Persian cats

RISK FACTORS

- Swimming, moisture in the ear canal
- Plucking hair from external ear canal

CONTAGION AND ZOONOSIS

- Contagion: ear mites (*Otodectes cynotis)* are contagious among animals (p. 731).
- Zoonosis: zoonotic transmission of bacterial infections from the ears of dogs to humans is very uncommon. It is prudent to advise owners to wash their hands frequently or wear gloves while handing their pet with known or suspected drug-resistant infectious otitis externa.

ASSOCIATED DISORDERS

Allergic diseases (e.g., cutaneous adverse food reaction, atopic dermatitis), aural hematoma, pyotraumatic dermatitis on face/neck, infectious otitis media

Clinical Presentation

HISTORY, CHIEF COMPLAINT

- Otic pruritus manifests as head shaking, scratching, or rubbing ears on the floor.
- Otic erythema, otic exudate and odor, otic pain
- Vestibular signs, hearing loss, Horner's syndrome, nystagmus, and facial paresis/paralysis may occur with middle and inner ear involvement.
- Additional clinical signs (e.g., pedal pruritus, indicating primary underlying allergic disease) may be present and help with determination of the primary cause of the otitis externa.

PHYSICAL EXAM FINDINGS

- Alopecia and excoriations of the pinnae
- Thickening and/or calcification of the ear canals is indicative of chronic to end-stage otitis.
- Erythema, exudation, hyperplasia, stenosis, and ulcerations of the ear canals
- Sometimes, pain when opening the mouth, hearing loss, facial paralysis or paresis, head tilting, circling, Horner's syndrome, and nystagmus

Etiology and Pathophysiology

- Predisposing factors facilitate inflammation by permitting alteration of the normal microenvironment.
  - Conformation: stenotic canals, excessive hair in the ear canals, pendulous pinnae
  - Moisture
  - Treatment errors: use of cotton-tipped applications to clean ears, plucking hair from the ear canals
- Primary causes: conditions or disorders that initiate the inflammatory process
  - Allergic disease: atopic dermatitis, cutaneous adverse food reaction
  - Parasites: *O. cynotis, Demodex canis, Demodex cati, Otobius megnini*
  - Foreign bodies
  - Juvenile cellulitis
  - Cornification disorders
  - Endocrine disorders
  - Autoimmune diseases
  - Masses: neoplasia, nasopharyngeal polyps
- Perpetuating factors sustain and aggravate the inflammatory process, prevent resolution, or worsens an already present otitis externa.
  - Bacteria
  - Yeast
  - Progressive pathologic changes of the ear canal (e.g., stenosis, hyperplasia)
  - Otitis media
- Successful treatment of otitis externa depends on identification and on controlling or eliminating these factors and causes. Treating the complicating infection without addressing the primary cause or eliminating the primary cause without control of the secondary infection likely will result in treatment failure.

DIAGNOSIS

Diagnostic Overview

The diagnosis of otitis externa is based on obtaining a complete history and assessment of the results of the clinical and cytologic exam.

Initial Database

- Physical exam: to identify the underlying dermatologic disease that triggered the otitis. In the dog, the most common causes are allergic diseases (e.g., cutaneous adverse food reaction, atopic dermatitis), and in the cat, *O. cynotis* and nasopharyngeal polyps are more common primary causes of otitis than allergies.
- Otic exam: to evaluate the vertical and horizontal ear canal for evidence of hyperplasia, stenosis, and ulceration, as well as to evaluate the amount, consistency, and color of the otic exudate. If possible, the tympanic membrane is examined.
- Otic cytology: CRITICAL diagnostic test is used for identification of bacterial (rods, cocci) and yeast organisms and for leukocytes. Any rod bacteria detected cytologically should be considered abnormal.
- Ear swab: mite identification. A second sample should be obtained from each ear and mixed with mineral oil to assess for *Otodectes* and *Demodex* mites.
- Otic culture: bacterial culture and susceptibility testing is done to identify the organism(s) in the ear and to guide the use of systemic (oral) antimicrobial therapy because the results indicate the attainable levels in the plasma. Susceptibility testing is generally not clinically useful for determining the appropriate topical otic antimicrobial agent.

Advanced or Confirmatory Testing

- Video otoscopy (p. 1144) allows greater visualization and detail resolution of the ear canal and tympanic membrane.
- Radiographic imaging: plain radiology, CT, and MRI are used to image the external, middle, and internal parts of the ear. Abnormal findings indicate otitis media, but normal radiographic findings do not rule out otitis media.
- Ear flush under anesthesia: to completely clean the external ear canal when further exam is needed
- Audiologic testing: brainstem auditory evoked response (BAER) testing is an objective test used to measure the animal's auditory response to sound stimulation.
- Allergy workup: elimination diet trial; intradermal allergy testing, and serum allergy testing (pp. 91 and 345)
- Neurologic exam (p. 1136)
- Mass removal/biopsy

TREATMENT

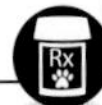

Treatment Overview

Goals of management of otitis externa:

- Reduce inflammation of the ear canal with glucocorticoids.
- Clean the ear by having the owner use an otic cleaning and drying agent at home or by an in-hospital ear flush under anesthesia.
- Resolve infection with topical otic antimicrobial agents, and monitor response to therapy.
- Prevent recurrence by diagnosing and managing the primary cause, perpetuating causes, and predisposing factors.

Mainstay of therapy for otitis externa is topical otic therapy, with the choice of topical otic medication based on

- Results of otic cytology are used to choose the active ingredient in the topical otic medication.
  - Options for bacterial otitis externa include aminoglycosides, polymyxin B, florfenicol, silver sulfadiazine, tris-EDTA, and fluoroquinolones.
  - Options for yeast otitis externa include nystatin, thiabendazole, clotrimazole, miconazole, ketoconazole, posaconazole, and terbinafine.
- Results of the otic exam are used for selection of the vehicle of the topical otic medication.
  - Solution, lotion, emulsion, flush, or gel if the ear canals range from no stenosis and hyperplasia to moderate to severe stenosis and/or hyperplasia
  - Suspension or ointment if there is minimal or no stenosis or hyperplasia
- Chronicity of the otitis is used to select the specific topical otic medication.
  - Acute or occasional otitis externa: first-line topical otic medication
  - Chronic otitis externa: second-line topical otic medication

Topical Otic Treatments for Otitis Externa

	PRODUCT OPTIONS FOR ORGANISMS CYTOLOGICALLY DETECTED		
Otic Exam	**Rods, Cocci, and Yeast *or* Rods and Yeast *or* Rods**	**Cocci and Yeast *or* Cocci Only**	**Yeast**
Treatment of Acute Otitis Externa			
Minimal or no stenosis or hyperplasia; *first-line topical otic medication, active ingredients based on cytologic evaluation of otic exudate containing any vehicle*	• EasOtic suspension • Mometamax suspension • Otomax ointment • Surolan suspension • Tresaderm solution*	• Claro otic solution • EasOtic suspension • Mometamax suspension • Osurnia otic gel • Otomax ointment • Surolan suspension • Tresaderm solution*	• Claro otic solution • EasOtic suspension • MalAcetic Ultra otic flush* • Mal-A-Ket plus TrizEDTA flush* • Miconazole 1% lotion† • Miconazole 1% lotion/dexamethasone (2 mg/mL injectable)† (1 : 1 vol. conc.), extralabel • Mometamax suspension • Osurnia otic gel • Otomax ointment • Surolan suspension • Tresaderm solution* • TrizUltra + Keto flush* • T8 Keto flush*
Moderate to severe stenosis or hyperplasia; *first-line topical otic medication, active ingredients based on cytologic evaluation of otic exudate containing solution, lotion, emulsion, flush, or gel vehicle*	• Tresaderm solution*	• Claro otic solution • Osurnia otic gel • Tresaderm solution*	• Claro otic solution • Mal-A-Ket plus TrizEDTA flush* • Miconazole 1% lotion† • Miconazole 1% lotion/dexamethasone (2 mg/mL injectable)† (1 : 1 vol. conc.), extralabel • Osurnia otic gel • Tresaderm solution* • TrizUltra + Keto flush* • T8 Keto flush*

Continued

Topical Otic Treatments for Otitis Externa—cont'd

	PRODUCT OPTIONS FOR ORGANISMS CYTOLOGICALLY DETECTED		
Otic Exam	**Rods, Cocci, and Yeast *or* Rods and Yeast *or* Rods**	**Cocci and Yeast *or* Cocci Only**	**Yeast**
Treatment of Chronic Otitis Externa			
Minimal or no stenosis or hyperplasia; *second-line topical otic medication, active ingredients based on cytologic evaluation of otic exudate containing any vehicle*	• Baytril (2.27% injectable)/ miconazole 1% lotion/ dexamethasone (2 mg/mL injectable) solution† (1 : 1 : 1 vol. conc.), extralabel • Posatex suspension	• Baytril (2.27% injectable)/Cort/Astrin solution† (1 : 4 vol. conc.), extralabel • Baytril (2.27% injectable)/ dexamethasone (2 mg/mL injectable)/ saline solution† (1 : 1 : 1 vol. conc.), extralabel • Baytril otic emulsion • Posatex suspension	• Claro otic solution • EasOtic suspension • MalAcetic Ultra otic flush* • TrizEDTA flush* • Miconazole 1% lotion† • Miconazole 1% lotion/dexamethasone (2 mg/mL injectable)† (1 : 1 vol. conc.), extralabel • Mometamax suspension • Osurnia otic gel • Otomax ointment • Tresaderm solution* • TrizUltra + Keto flush* • T8 Keto flush*
Moderate to severe stenosis or hyperplasia; *second-line topical otic medication, active ingredients based on cytologic evaluation of otic exudate containing solution, lotion, emulsion, flush, or gel vehicle*	• Baytril (2.27% injectable)/ miconazole 1% lotion/ dexamethasone (2 mg/mL injectable) solution† (1 : 1 : 1 vol. conc.), extralabel	• Baytril (2.27% injectable): Cort/Astrin solution† (1 : 4 vol. conc.), extralabel • Baytril (2.27% injectable)/ dexamethasone (2 mg/mL injectable)/ saline solution† (1 : 1 : 1 vol. conc.), extralabel • Baytril otic emulsion	• Claro otic solution • MalAcetic Ultra otic flush* • TrizEDTA flush* • Miconazole 1% lotion† • Miconazole 1% lotion/dexamethasone (2 mg/mL injectable)† (1 : 1 vol. conc.), extralabel • Osurnia otic gel

*Products for use in cats.
†Products not specifically for use in the ear.
-Active ingredients of otic products:
Baytril (2.27% injectable)/dexamethasone (2 mg/mL injectable)/saline solution† (1 : 1 : 1 vol. conc.), extralabel
Baytril (2.27% injectable)/miconazole 1% lotion/dexamethasone (2 mg/mL injectable) solution† (1 : 1 : 1 vol. conc.), extralabel
Baytril (2.27% injectable): Cort/Astrin solution†: (1 : 4 vol. conc.), extralabel
Baytril otic emulsion: enrofloxacin, silver sulfadiazine
Claro otic solution: florfenicol, terbinafine, mometasone furoate
EasOtic suspension: gentamicin sulfate, miconazole, hydrocortisone aceponate
MalAcetic Ultra otic flush*: ketoconazole, acetic acid, boric acid, hydrocortisone
Mal-A-Ket plus TrizEDTA flush*: chlorhexidine gluconate, ketoconazole, tris-EDTA
Miconazole 1% lotion†
Miconazole 1% lotion/dexamethasone (2 mg/mL injectable)†(1 : 1 vol. conc.), extralabel
Mometamax suspension: gentamicin sulfate, clotrimazole, mometasone furoate
Osurnia otic gel: florfenicol, terbinafine, betamethasone acetate
Otomax ointment: gentamicin sulfate, clotrimazole, betamethasone valerate
Posatex suspension: orbifloxacin, posaconazole, mometasone furoate
Surolan suspension: miconazole, polymyxin B, prednisolone
T8 Keto flush*: tris-EDTA, ketoconazole
Tresaderm solution*: neomycin sulfate thiabendazole, dexamethasone
TrizUltra + Keto flush*: ketoconazole, tris-EDTA

Additional Topical Medications for Acute or Chronic Otitis Externa

- Ear cleaning and drying agents
  - Recommended for at-home cleaning
  - May be used daily or as needed
- Ceruminolytic agent
  - Used for in-clinic anesthetic flush or at-home cleaning
  - Ceruminolytic agents are considered ototoxic until proved otherwise
  - Non-ototoxic product option
    - Cerumene* (25% squalene)
- Glucocorticoids
  - Used if specific otic medication for infection does not contain a glucocorticoid
  - Used for management of allergic otitis externa
  - Product options
    - Cort/Astrin* (Burow's solution, 1% hydrocortisone)
    - Synotic (0.01% fluocinolone acetonide, 60% dimethyl sulfoxide)
- Tris-EDTA
  - Recommend using a tris-EDTA–containing product any time the otic infection is due to rod (gram-negative) bacteria
  - Pre-treat before using a specific otic medication for the bacterial infection
  - Product options
    - Mal-A-Ket plus TrizEDTA flush*: chlorhexidine gluconate, ketoconazole, tris-EDTA
    - TrizUltra + Keto flush*: ketoconazole, tris-EDTA
    - T8 Keto flush*: tris-EDTA, ketoconazole
    - TrizChlor flush*: chlorhexidine, tris-EDTA

*Products for use in cats.
†Products not specifically for use in the ear.

Chronic Treatment

In end-stage otitis, the ear canal is completely or nearly completely occluded, often accompanied by palpable fibrosis/mineralization, and is nonresponsive to treatment with glucocorticoids. Treatment at that point is surgical total ear canal ablation and bulla osteotomy.

Possible Complications

Para-aural abscesses, draining tracts, infectious otitis media, and otitis interna

Recommended Monitoring

An otoscopic exam along with otic cytology should be performed by the veterinarian every 2 to 4 weeks to monitor improvement in the clinical signs of the otitis and resolution of the infection.

PROGNOSIS & OUTCOME

If the primary cause of the otitis externa is identified and managed, the prognosis is good. Causative primary factors for otitis externa must be evaluated or the condition is likely to become

chronic, resulting in an irritable patient and an unhappy owner.

PEARLS & CONSIDERATIONS

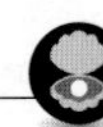

Comments

Dogs with atopic dermatitis or cutaneous adverse food reaction may present with signs of otitis externa only. Complete resolution of ear problems is unlikely unless predisposing, primary, and perpetuating factors are identified.

Technician Tips

Otic cytology should be performed for both ears at the first visit as well as at each recheck to monitor response to therapy.

SUGGESTED READING

Diseases of the eyelids, claws, anal sacs, and ears. In Miller WH, et al, editors: Muller & Kirks Small animal dermatology, ed 7, St. Louis, Mosby, 2013.

AUTHOR: Lynette K. Cole, DVM, MS, DACVD
EDITOR: Manon Paradis, DMV, MVSc, DACVD

Otodectic Mange

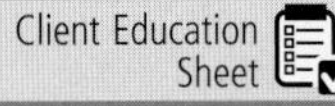

BASIC INFORMATION

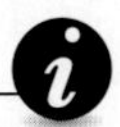

Definition

Contagious, primarily aural mite infestation caused by *Otodectes cynotis*

Synonyms

Otodectic acariasis, otoacariasis, ear mite infestation

Epidemiology

SPECIES, AGE, SEX

- Very common in cats; common in dogs
- More common in puppies and kittens but may occur at any age

RISK FACTORS

Contact with stray animals; shelter, boarding, or grooming facility

CONTAGION AND ZOONOSIS

- Very contagious
- Transmission by direct contact and fomites
- Very low zoonotic risk

GEOGRAPHY AND SEASONALITY

Worldwide, not seasonal

Clinical Presentation

HISTORY, CHIEF COMPLAINT

- Aural/periaural pruritus evidenced by head shaking and ear scratching
- Asymptomatic carriage occurs.

PHYSICAL EXAM FINDINGS

- Otitis externa characterized by erythema and dark brown, ceruminous otic exudate ("coffee grounds")
- Erosions, ulcers, crusts found on inner pinna and entrance of the ear canal
- Occasional ectopic infestations evidenced by alopecia, erythema, papules, and crusts of periaural region, head, neck, feet, and tail when mites escape from ears
- Cats may occasionally present with one or a combination of cutaneous patterns: erosive and crusting dermatosis of the head and neck, miliary dermatitis, symmetric alopecia, or eosinophilic granuloma complex.
- Positive ear-pedal reflex is possible, particularly in cats: animal scratches with ipsilateral hindlimb when ear canal is swabbed.
- Ear mites can be visualized by otoscopic exam (p. 1144), appearing as moving white specks.

Etiology and Pathophysiology

These psoroptic, non–host-specific, nonburrowing mites cause a hypersensitivity reaction by feeding on epidermal debris and tissue fluids of ear canal lining.

DIAGNOSIS

Diagnostic Overview

Diagnosis established through historical and physical exam findings and visualization of mites and/or eggs on direct otoscopic or microscopic exam. If mites/eggs cannot be found, a positive response to treatment can be used for presumptive diagnosis.

Differential Diagnosis

- Hypersensitivities (atopic dermatitis, flea-bite allergy, food allergy, contact allergic dermatitis, adverse drug reaction)
- Ectoparasites (*Sarcoptes*, cheyletiellosis, fleas, lice)
- Otodemodicosis
- Bacterial and fungal otitis externa
- Neoplasia, polyps

Initial Database

Microscopic exam of ear swab samples placed in mineral oil is the most effective method for identifying ear mites and eggs. If the skin is involved, collect a minimum of three broad, superficial skin scrapings (p. 1091). Crusts and papules are the best areas to scrape, but mites may be hard to find.

TREATMENT

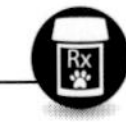

Treatment Overview

Clean ear canal with a ceruminolytic ear cleaner, and then apply topical (inside ear canal) or systemic acaricidal products. Animals that do not tolerate or resent topical therapy can be treated systemically. Treatment with an acaricidal-only spot-on agent does not resolve the secondary bacterial and fungal infections, nor does it directly resolve inflammation. Using a treatment that combines acaricidal, antibiotic, antifungal, and antiinflammatory agents results in faster relief of symptoms.

Acute General Treatment

Spot-on acaricidal products with systemic effects:

- Selamectin (Revolution/Stronghold; apply in interscapular region) in dogs as young as 6 weeks of age and cats as young as 8 weeks of age. Two doses are administered 30 days apart for optimal control. Kills ear mites as early as 10-12 hours after administration with increasing effect over time.
- Moxidectin (Advantage Multi/Advocate; apply in scapular region) in cats as young as 8 weeks of age. Two doses are administered 28 days apart for optimal control; also labeled for dogs for this use in some countries

Topical (otic) acaricidal product:

- Thiabendazole (Tresaderm) applied in affected ears q 12h for up to 7 days. Off-label use: 10 days minimum

Topical (otic) products labeled for use in cats

- Ivermectin (Acarexx) applied in affected ears in cats as young as 4 weeks of age; kills ear mites as early as 10-12 hours after administration with increasing effect over time
- Milbemycin oxime (MilbeMite) applied in affected ears in cats as young as 4 weeks of age
- Permethrin (Oridermyl) applied once daily for 10 consecutive days in affected ears in cats as young as 8 weeks of age; also contains neomycin, nystatin, and triamcinolone for the treatment of associated inflammation, secondary bacterial/yeast infections
- Any of the above topical otic treatments should be used in conjunction with an appropriate whole-body (or systemic) acaricide to eliminate ectopic mites.

Off-label acaricidal treatments:

- Ivermectin (Ivomec, 200-400 mcg/kg PO or SQ) q 1-2 weeks for up to 4 treatments or diluted 1:9 in propylene glycol and apply a few drops in each ear once daily for 21 days or apply 0.05 mL (500 mcg)/EAR once each week for 5 weeks
- Moxidectin (Cydectin, 200 mcg/kg PO or SQ) for 2 treatments 10 days apart
- Fipronil (Frontline Spot-on) 2 drops applied in affected ears once or twice (1 month apart)

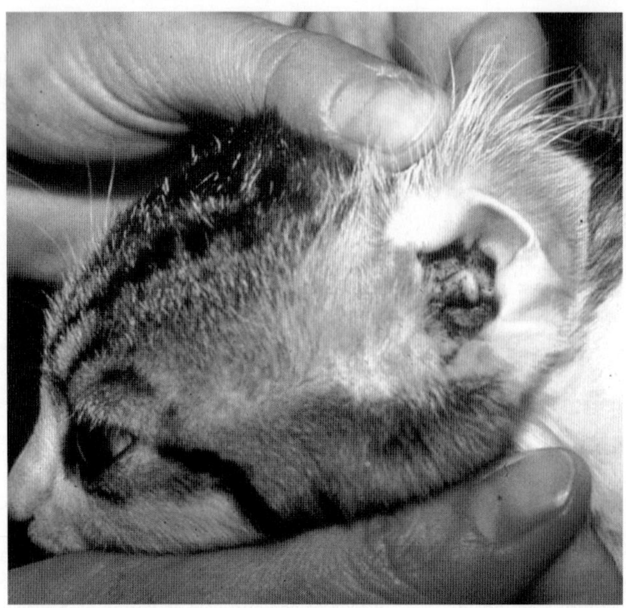

OTODECTIC MANGE Gross appearance of a young cat with otodectic mange. The pinna appears normal, but copious specks of characteristic exudate ("coffee grounds") are visible in the ear canal. (Copyright Dr. Manon Paradis, University of Montreal.)

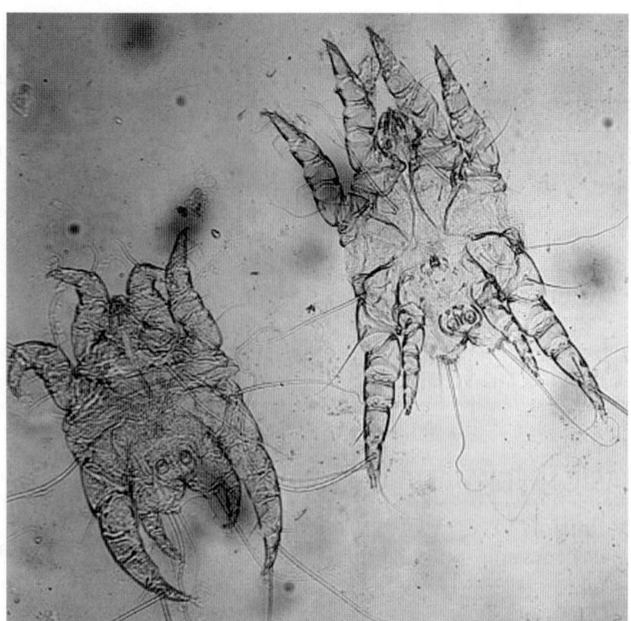

OTODECTIC MANGE Microscopic appearance of ear mites *(Otodectes cynotis)*. (Copyright Dr. Manon Paradis, University of Montreal.)

Isoxazolines:

- Dogs
  - Fluralaner (Bravecto 25 mg/kg PO) as a single oral dose
  - Sarolaner (Simparica 2 mg/kg PO) as a single oral dose or 2 treatments 30 days apart
- Cats
  - Fluralaner (Bravecto spot-on solution, 40 mg/kg) applied topically once
  - A combination of selamectin plus sarolaner spot-on formulation (Revolution Plus, Stronghold Plus) applied topically once

Drug Interactions

Off-label doses of ivermectin or moxidectin should not be used in sensitive canine breeds unless the *MDR1/ABCB1-Δ* gene mutation is confirmed to be absent (p. 638).

Possible Complications

Otitis media

Recommended Monitoring

Repeat ear swab and physical exam 1 month after first treatment if clinical signs persist.

PROGNOSIS & OUTCOME

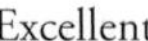

Excellent

PEARLS & CONSIDERATIONS

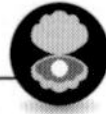

Comments

- Other household pets such as ferrets can become infested.
- Ear mites can be eradicated only if all animals in contact are treated simultaneously, even if signs of disease are absent.

Prevention

- Ear mites have a 3-week life cycle and a 2-month life span. They can live off the host for weeks. Environment may require thorough cleaning and treatment in cattery or kennel situations.
- When Revolution/Stronghold or Advantage Multi/Advocate is used as flea control, it has the added benefit of ongoing ear mite prevention.

Technician Tips

Diagnosis may be falsely based on typical appearance of otic exudate alone, without visualization of parasites on microscopy. This is often misleading.

Client Education

Many pet owners seeing inflamed ears with discharge assume it is an ear mite infestation, often leading to weeks of inappropriate treatment with over-the-counter treatments.

SUGGESTED READING

Taenzler J, et al: Efficacy of fluralaner against *Otodectes cynotis* infestations in dogs and cats. Parasit Vectors 10(1):30, 2017.

AUTHOR: Vincent E. Defalque, DVM, DACVD
EDITOR: Manon Paradis, DMV, MVSc, DACVD

Ovarian Remnant Syndrome

BASIC INFORMATION

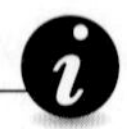

Definition

Presence of functional ovarian tissue in a previously ovariectomized bitch or queen

Epidemiology

SPECIES, AGE, SEX

Female dog or cat; months to years after ovariectomy (OVE) or ovariohysterectomy (OHE)

GENETICS, BREED PREDISPOSITION

Large-breed dogs may have increased incidence.

RISK FACTORS

OVE during estrus or at time of cesarean section may increase risk.

GEOGRAPHY AND SEASONALITY

Seasonality (spring) of estrous signs possible in cats, and recurrence at typical cycle interval (4-12 months) in dogs

ASSOCIATED DISORDERS

- As with intact females, ovarian tumors can occur.
- Stump pyometra and mammary neoplasia may occur secondary to progesterone exposure during the estrous cycle.

Clinical Presentation

HISTORY, CHIEF COMPLAINT

Behavioral estrus, attracting males, licking vulva excessively

PHYSICAL EXAM FINDINGS

Swollen vulva, bloody or serosanguineous vulvar discharge

Etiology and Pathophysiology

- Ovarian tissue remaining after OVE/OHE becomes revascularized and hormonally active.
- Ovarian tissue may remain in the abdomen due to improper placement of clamps, poor visualization of surgical field, tissue dropped during surgery, or ectopic/accessory tissue in the broad ligament (latter more common in cats).
- It may take months to years after OVE/OHE for ovarian remnant to become active (cause unknown).

DIAGNOSIS

Diagnostic Overview

The diagnosis is suspected based on overt clinical evidence of estrogen and/or progesterone influence in a spayed female. Confirmation requires histopathologic evaluation of remnant ovarian tissue.

Differential Diagnosis

- Exogenous estrogen and/or progesterone source (e.g., owner's hormone replacement cream)
- Other endogenous estrogen source (e.g., adrenal disease)

Initial Database

- Vaginal cytology demonstrating cornified epithelial cells (p. 1183)
- Negative serum luteinizing hormone (LH) test: females with ovarian remnants, like intact females, have low/undetectable serum LH barring the preovulatory LH surge, whereas LH concentrations should remain persistently elevated in OVE/OHE females (absence of inhibition from estrogen) (p. 1361).
- Serum progesterone > 5 ng/mL (p. 1375)

Advanced or Confirmatory Testing

- Positive anti-mullerian hormone (AMH) test: AMH is produced by the ovaries. A positive result indicates the presence of ovarian tissue (p. 1308).
- Vaginoscopy: to rule out other causes of vulvar discharge (e.g., mass, foreign body)
- Ultrasound: occasionally useful, but ovarian tissue is usually small and difficult to identify.
- Histopathologic exam of tissue: to confirm ovarian tissue removed surgically

TREATMENT

Treatment Overview

Complete removal of ovarian tissue by exploratory laparotomy

Acute and Chronic Treatment

Surgery is best performed during estrus to facilitate identification of ovarian tissue.

Possible Complications

Remnant ovarian tissue may be difficult to find surgically. Careful exam of the ovarian pedicles and broad ligament is required with removal of any suspicious tissue. If no obvious tissue is found, both ovarian pedicles should be further resected and submitted for histopathologic evaluation.

Recommended Monitoring

Monitor for recurrence of clinical signs.

PROGNOSIS & OUTCOME

Prognosis is good if remnant ovarian tissue is found and removed.

PEARLS & CONSIDERATIONS

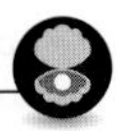

Comments

Positive LH test result indicates a spayed female or an intact female during the preovulatory LH surge. Confirm all positive results 1-2 weeks later because the normal LH surge has a short duration. Alternatively, use AMH test.

Prevention

Complete removal of ovarian tissue at initial OVE/OHE surgery prevents this condition. Consider laparoscopy for improved access to ovaries in large or deep-chested breeds.

Technician Tips

- Some females may allow breeding to occur and should be kept isolated from males.
- When obtaining a vaginal cytology sample, use a large otoscope cone as a speculum to avoid contamination from the vestibule.

SUGGESTED READING

Ball RL, et al: Ovarian remnant syndrome in dogs and cats: 21 cases (2000-2007). J Am Vet Med Assoc 236(5):548-553, 2010.

AUTHOR: Kara A. Kolster, DVM, DACT
EDITOR: Michelle A. Kutzler, DVM, PhD, DACT

Ovarian Tumors

Bonus Material Online 
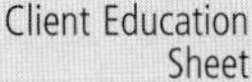
Client Education Sheet 

BASIC INFORMATION

Definition

Ovarian tumors are uncommon and are classified by cell type origin as sex cord (granulosa cell tumor, Sertoli-Leydig), epithelial (adenocarcinoma, adenoma, cyst adenocarcinoma), or germ cell (dysgerminoma, teratoma).

Synonyms

Ovarian neoplasia, ovarian cancer

Epidemiology

SPECIES, AGE, SEX

Canine, intact females:

- Epithelial tumors (40%-50% of all ovarian tumors): median age of 9.6 years (adenomas, 10.5 years; adenocarcinomas, 9.3 years). Metastasis rate ≥ 60%.
- Sex cord tumors: median age of 8 years (granulosa cell tumor, 7 years; Sertoli, 5 years; Sertoli-Leydig, 12 years).
- Germ cell tumors: median age of 6.4 years (dysgerminoma, 9 years; teratoma, 5 years; teratocarcinoma, 5 years)

Feline, intact females:

- Sex cord tumors (most common): median age of 9 years (granulosa cell tumor, 10 years). More than 50% are malignant.
- Epithelial tumors: median age of 10 years (cystadenoma, 10 years)
- Germ cell tumors: median age of 6 years (dysgerminoma, 6 years; teratoma, 8 years)

ASSOCIATED DISORDERS

Persistent estrus, hyperestrogenism (anemia and thrombocytopenia), pyometra, and/or cystic endometrial hyperplasia are sometimes associated with sex cord tumors.

Clinical Presentation

DISEASE FORMS/SUBTYPES

- Epithelial tumors (adenoma, adenocarcinoma, carcinoma, cystadenoma, cystadenocarcinoma): 5% of all pathologic exam reports, no case reports
- Sex cord tumors (granulosa cell tumor, Sertoli, Sertoli-Leydig): 31% of all pathologic exam reports, 50% of case reports
- Germ cell tumors (dysgerminoma, teratoma, teratocarcinoma): 15% of all pathologic exam reports, 50% of case reports

HISTORY, CHIEF COMPLAINT

Dog:

- Abdominal enlargement and ascites (adenomas, adenocarcinoma, granulosa cell tumor, dysgerminoma, teratoma, teratocarcinoma)
- Depression (dysgerminoma, teratocarcinoma)
- Estrous cycle abnormalities such as prolonged estrus (granulosa cell tumor)
- Vulvar enlargement and discharge (adenocarcinoma, granulosa cell tumor)
- Incidental finding during ovariohysterectomy or necropsy (adenomas, teratoma)
- No common findings (Sertoli and Sertoli-Leydig cell tumors)

Cat:

- Estrous cycle abnormalities such as persistent estrus (granulosa cell tumor)
- Depression (granulosa cell tumor)
- Incidental finding during ovariohysterectomy or necropsy (cystadenoma, dysgerminoma, teratoma)

PHYSICAL EXAM FINDINGS

- Estrus (vaginal smear for cytologic exam)
- Vulvar discharge
- Abdominal enlargement/effusion
- Palpable abdominal mass (cats)
- Fever, pallor, weakness, and heart murmur possible if pancytopenia secondary to estrogen myelosuppression

Etiology and Pathophysiology

Clinical signs can be related to hormone production by sex cord tumors; the signs can also be related to organ impingement by space-occupying masses or metastasis for other types. Abdominal distention can occur secondary to carcinomatosis (abdominal effusion).

DIAGNOSIS

Diagnostic Overview

The diagnosis is expected if an older intact animal has persistent estrus, vulvar discharge, or abdominal enlargement. The diagnosis is aided by abdominal imaging and is confirmed by surgery and histopathologic exam of tissues.

Differential Diagnosis

- Estrus
- Pyometra
- Gastrointestinal or other intraabdominal disease

Initial Database

- Routine lab tests (CBC including platelet count, urinalysis, and serum chemistry panel): generally unremarkable unless estrogen myelosuppression is present
- Vaginal cytologic exam
    - Confirmation of estrus
    - Assessment for pyometra or other infection

Advanced or Confirmatory Testing

- Abdominal radiographs
- Abdominal ultrasound
- Abdominocentesis (p. 1056) and fluid analysis (cytologic evaluation for ovarian carcinoma)
- Thoracic radiography for metastasis
- Exploratory surgery
- Histopathologic exam of tissue

TREATMENT

Treatment Overview

Surgical excision is the most common treatment; chemotherapy has been used in some patients.

Acute General Treatment

Ovariohysterectomy or unilateral ovariectomy if owner desires to preserve fertility. A small litter has been reported after unilateral ovariectomy of an ovarian tumor.

Chronic Treatment

- Chemotherapy should be considered if there is histologic evidence of vascular or lymphatic invasion or evidence of metastasis in the peritoneal cavity during surgery (carcinomatosis).
    - Cisplatin (not in cats) or cyclophosphamide and chlorambucil and nitrosourea have been used for treating metastatic carcinomas in a few dogs, resulting in a median 9-month survival.
    - Additional chemotherapeutics that can be considered include doxorubicin, carboplatin, and 5-fluorouracil. Intracavitary chemotherapy may be indicated for effusions.
    - Consultation with an oncologist is recommended.

Possible Complications

Metastasis:

- Canine
    - Epithelial tumors: adenomas and adenocarcinoma in 50% of cases according to pathologic exam reports
    - Germ cell tumors: dysgerminoma is rare; teratoma reported at a rate of 50% in one study; teratocarcinoma is common.
    - Sex cord tumors: granulosa cell tumors in up to 20% of cases
- Feline sex cord: granulosa cell tumor with metastasis to the lung, liver, and spleen has been reported.

Recommended Monitoring

- In dogs, abdominal enlargement and estrous cycle abnormalities (e.g., prolonged estrus, vaginal discharge, vulvar enlargement) should be monitored.
- In cats, estrous cycle abnormalities (e.g., persistent estrus) should be monitored.
- In either species, evidence of anemia, hemorrhage, or opportunistic infection warrants consideration of estrogen-induced myelosuppression.

PROGNOSIS & OUTCOME

- Excellent if benign and no metastasis has occurred
- Poor if distant metastasis or carcinomatosis is present at the time of diagnosis

PEARLS & CONSIDERATIONS

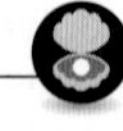

Comments

- May be unilateral or bilateral
- Ovarian tumors are possible in animals after ovariohysterectomy if an ovarian remnant remains.

Prevention

Ovariectomy or ovariohysterectomy

Technician Tip

Avoid cystocentesis in pets with abdominal effusion.

Client Education

Ovariohysterectomy eliminates the risks of ovarian and uterine tumors.

SUGGESTED READING

Arlt SP, et al: Cystic ovaries and ovarian neoplasia in the female dog—a systematic review. Reprod Domest Anim 51:3-11, 2016.

AUTHORS: Jose A. Len, DVM, MS, PhD, DACT; Bruce E. Eilts, DVM, MS, DACT

EDITOR: Michelle A. Kutzler, DVM, PhD, DACT

Pain

Client Education Sheet

BASIC INFORMATION

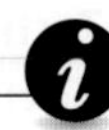

Definition

An unpleasant sensory or emotional experience associated with actual or potential tissue damage

Epidemiology

SPECIES, AGE, SEX

Animals of any species, age, or sex may experience pain, although pain thresholds and response characteristics vary between individual animals. The experience of pain depends on physiologic, psychological, and contextual factors.

GENETICS, BREED PREDISPOSITION

Although there are likely genetic differences in susceptibility to pain, the clinical significance is unknown at this time.

RISK FACTORS

Trauma, surgery, degenerative disease processes, inflammation, viscus organ distention (e.g., ileus), and neoplasia can be associated with pain. Intensity does not always correlate with degree of tissue damage. An animal may experience pain without apparent tissue damage.

ASSOCIATED DISORDERS

See Risk Factors.

Clinical Presentation

DISEASE FORMS/SUBTYPES

- Acute pain is short-term pain (days to weeks) usually caused by tissue damage. Acute pain is considered physiologic and self-limited.
- Chronic pain persists for a long duration (weeks to months), or longer than normal healing time. Chronic pain is considered pathologic and without biological purpose.
- Pain may also be classified as nociceptive, inflammatory, or neuropathic.

HISTORY, CHIEF COMPLAINT

Owners may observe changes in behavior that can be attributed to pain (e.g., decreased activity, altered mentation, decreased appetite, lameness).

PHYSICAL EXAM FINDINGS

Although a variety of physiologic parameters (i.e., heart rate, blood pressure, and respiratory rate) may be altered by pain, changes are not specific to pain. Unfortunately, signs of pain are often subtle, nonspecific, and variable between animals.

Etiology and Pathophysiology

See Suggested Readings.

DIAGNOSIS

Diagnostic Overview

- Veterinarians should follow a routine evaluation for pain in their patients (see Initial Database below). Pain should be treated as a fourth vital sign, in addition to temperature, pulse, and respiration.
- No individual physical exam finding or laboratory value is specific for pain, and an integrated approach using history, physical exam, and laboratory evaluation findings is the best way to estimate the degree of discomfort.
    - In some scenarios, even when easily identified evidence of pain is absent, it is reasonable to assume that there is some degree of occult pain (for instance, in the postoperative period).
- After pain has been identified and characterized, the veterinarian should investigate the underlying cause and develop a suitable treatment plan.

Differential Diagnosis

- Distress (e.g., restraint, restrictive bandaging, confinement, separation from owners)
- Opioid-induced dysphoria (exacerbated by additional administration of opioids)

Initial Database

A routine evaluation for pain often includes

- Signalment, history, and physical exam findings
- Use of a scoring system is important for pain assessment. Most pain scales involve
    - An observation of behavior when undisturbed (preferably with the animal unaware that it is being observed). Appetite, posture, facial expression, voluntary movement, social interaction, and interaction with the environment are assessed.
    - Observation of behavior during interaction
        - Palpation
        - Directed movement (e.g., trotting)
    - Repeated assessment over time

Advanced or Confirmatory Testing

- Although there is no single test that can be used to diagnose pain, patient-appropriate tests may be useful. For example, radiography may be used to confirm the cause of lameness and suspected hindlimb pain in a dog with a fractured femur.
- Increased plasma or salivary cortisol concentration or decreased heart rate variability may indicate pain. Unfortunately, these changes are not specific for pain and may be caused by a number of nonpainful stressors.

TREATMENT

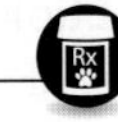

Treatment Overview

The goal of treatment is to improve the animal's quality of life and address the underlying cause of pain. Effective pain control often requires a multimodal approach in which two or more agents or techniques are used concurrently. Effective management may also be improved when pre-emptive analgesia is used. If pain is unresponsive to treatment and quality of life is significantly affected by pain, euthanasia should be considered.

Acute General Treatment

- Approach to management depends on species, pain intensity, and underlying cause.
- Pharmacologic treatment of acute pain commonly includes one or more of the following:
    - Alpha-2 receptor agonists
    - Opioids
    - Nonsteroidal antiinflammatory drugs (NSAIDs)
    - Local anesthetics
        - Local anesthetic agents may be used systemically, regionally, or locally to alleviate pain.
    - *N*-methyl-D-aspartate receptor antagonists (i.e., ketamine)
- Other pharmacologic adjuncts or analgesics may also be considered (but are probably more useful in chronic pain management)
    - Gabapentin
    - Glucocorticoids
- Nonpharmacologic modification may be useful in managing pain.
    - Icing/temperature modulation
    - Neuromodulation/trigger point therapy

Chronic Treatment

- Pharmacologic management
    - NSAIDs
        - Prostaglandin receptor antagonists (i.e., grapiprant)
    - Opioids
    - Other pharmacologic adjuncts or analgesics
        - Tramadol
        - Gabapentin
        - Amantadine
- Nonpharmacologic management
    - Icing/temperature modulation
    - Neuromodulation/trigger point therapy/acupuncture
    - Physical therapy
    - Laser therapy
    - It should be noted that the effectiveness of some nonpharmacologic approaches is questionable, limited, or has not been adequately evaluated.

Nutrition/Diet

Decreasing body weight may be important in modifying pain in musculoskeletal disease. Manipulation of diet to decrease inflammation is also an active area of research.

Behavior/Exercise

Physical therapy and regular exercise help to manage pain caused by osteoarthritis.

Drug Interactions

- Opioids reduce the requirement for anesthetic drugs and sedative agents.

- Certain opioids (e.g., meperidine) may interact with monoamine oxidase-B inhibitors (e.g., selegiline [L-deprenyl], amitraz) and produce serotonin syndrome (p. 1281).
- Coadministration of NSAIDs and glucocorticoids is contraindicated due to risk of gastrointestinal (GI) ulceration.

Possible Complications

Each class of pharmacologic agents is associated with its own set of potential complications:.

- NSAIDs may be associated with GI and renal toxicity. Consider other options in patients with hypovolemia, receiving nephrotoxic drugs, or at risk for GI ulceration.
- Opioids may be associated with
  - Respiratory depression
  - Altered GI motility/emesis
  - Dysphoria/excitement
  - Bradycardia
  - Histamine release

Recommended Monitoring

Serial evaluation of pain is important.

PROGNOSIS & OUTCOME

- Acute pain is expected to resolve within the period of normal tissue healing.
- When pain persists beyond the period of normal tissue healing, persistent disease, recurrent injury, or chronic (pathologic) pain should be considered.

PEARLS & CONSIDERATIONS

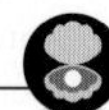

Comments

- Multimodal and pre-emptive approaches should be considered.
- Consider consulting with a veterinarian who has advanced training in pain management for difficult cases.
- Veterinarians should be aware of the abuse potential of drugs used in pain management. In addition to being vigilant for pet owners who may use a pet as an excuse to obtain opioid drugs, veterinarians must take appropriate steps to prevent drug diversion by hospital employees, including associates or practice owners.

Prevention

Pre-emptive approaches should be considered whenever possible (e.g., administration of analgesic drugs before surgery).

Technician Tips

Careful patient monitoring and behavioral assessment enable early recognition of pain in animal patients.

SUGGESTED READING

McKune CM, et al: Nociception and pain. In Grimm KA, et al, editors: Veterinary anesthesia and analgesia, ed 5, Ames, Iowa, 2015, John Wiley & Sons.

RELATED CLIENT EDUCATION SHEET

How to Provide General Postoperative Care at Home, Especially Lifting or Picking Up a Pet, and Pain Control

AUTHORS: John R. Dodam, DVM, MS, PhD, DACVAA; Leigh A. Lamont, DVM, MS, DACVAA
EDITOR: Leah A. Cohn, DVM, PhD DACVIM

Pallor

BASIC INFORMATION

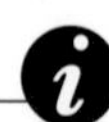

Definition

Pale tissues, especially mucous membranes and/or nonpigmented paw pads

Epidemiology

SPECIES, AGE, SEX

Any dog or cat

GENETICS, BREED PREDISPOSITION

Hereditary causes of anemia exist (p. 59)

CONTAGION AND ZOONOSIS

Infectious causes of anemia (e.g., feline leukemia virus–associated anemia, babesiosis, hemotropic mycoplasmosis) exist

Clinical Presentation

DISEASE FORMS/SUBTYPES

- Generalized (more common) or regional (less common) pallor
- Generalized pallor: anemia (most common) or inadequate perfusion
  - Anemia: perfusion is adequate, but circulating red blood cell (RBC) mass is low.
  - Inadequate perfusion: circulating RBC mass is normal, but perfusion poor (e.g., shock).
- Regional pallor: always due to inadequate regional perfusion (e.g., aortic thromboembolism → pale rear paw pads).

HISTORY, CHIEF COMPLAINT

Owners rarely report pallor but instead notice signs related to anemia (e.g., weakness, tachypnea, collapse) or poor perfusion (e.g., dyspnea with cardiogenic shock).

PHYSICAL EXAM FINDINGS

- Pale mucous membranes (gingiva, tongue, conjunctiva, anus, penis, vulva) and/or nonpigmented nose or paw pads
- Tachypnea, tachycardia, weakness, and collapse may be seen with either anemia or shock.
  - Extremities (paws, pinnae) often cool with poor perfusion but not with anemia.
- Capillary refill time (CRT): should be normal (<2 seconds) in an anemic animal but is prolonged by poor perfusion.
  - May be impossible to gauge CRT in severely anemic animals
- Other findings vary with cause:
  - Aortic thromboembolism: absent femoral pulse, rear limb paralysis
  - Cardiogenic shock: poor pulse, arrhythmia, heart murmur
  - Blood loss anemia: evidence of bleeding (e.g., melena, petechial or ecchymotic hemorrhage)

Etiology and Pathophysiology

- Anemia causes pallor due to decreased RBCs traversing through easily seen capillary beds, creating a pale rather than pink color in the mucous membranes.
- Shock leads to poor perfusion of blood through capillary vessels, causing pallor. Shock is a peracute condition, but the underlying cause may be chronic in nature.
- Severe anemia can lead to shock, and both conditions may exist in the same animal.
- Regional obstruction to blood flow can lead to localized pallor of extremities.

DIAGNOSIS

Diagnostic Overview

Physical exam is often adequate to distinguish between anemia and poor generalized or regional perfusion. Blood pressure (BP) and packed cell volume (PCV) measurements confirm the suspicion, and additional testing can provide a specific diagnosis.

Differential Diagnosis

Ambient lighting and visual perception may lead to a mistaken impression of pallor, and dark pigmentation can impede recognition of pallor.

Initial Database

- Anemic animals, by definition, have a diminished PCV. Severity of pallor correlates with severity of anemia.
- BP (p. 1065) is usually diminished in cases of shock. Unless the anemia is severe or acute, BP is typically normal in anemic animals.
- CBC, biochemical profile, and urinalysis are warranted in most cases of pallor to assist in determining the underlying cause.
  - Reticulocyte count and RBC indices are used to characterize type of anemia.
- Feline leukemia virus (FeLV) infection status for cats

Advanced or Confirmatory Testing

Next diagnostic steps depend on initial findings

- Anemia (pp. 56, 57, 59, 60, and 63)
- Shock (pp. 907 and 911)

- Heart failure (pp. 263 and 408)
- Aortic thromboembolism (p. 74)

TREATMENT

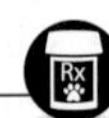

Treatment Overview

Stabilization of the animal (e.g., blood transfusion for severely anemic patients, intravenous fluids for noncardiogenic shock) followed by treatment of specific cause.

Acute and Chronic General Treatment

- Patients with severe anemia or acute blood loss may require transfusion of packed RBCs or whole blood if packed RBCs are not available (pp. 57 and 1169).
- Hypovolemic, traumatic, and septic shock cases are usually treated with intravenous crystalloids ± colloids (pp. 907 and 911).
- Cardiogenic shock requires supplemental oxygen (p. 1146) and attempts to improve perfusion, such as with pericardiocentesis (if cardiac tamponade) and medications (e.g., positive inotropes, antidysrhythmics) (pp. 263, 408, and 1033).
- Regional perfusion impairment is addressed according to cause (p. 74).

Recommended Monitoring

Frequent initial assessment of vital parameters and PCV in patients with anemia, BP in shock

PROGNOSIS & OUTCOME

Determined by the underlying cause; ranges from excellent (e.g., hemotropic mycoplasma, hookworm infestation) to grave (e.g., cardiogenic shock with dilated cardiomyopathy)

PEARLS & CONSIDERATIONS

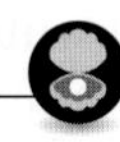

Comments

Most causes of pallor are serious, requiring timely evaluation and therapy.

Technician Tips

Be cognizant of membrane color because pallor is often a sign of serious disease.

SUGGESTED READING

Ohad DG: Pallor. In Ettinger SJ, et al, editors: Textbook of veterinary internal medicine, ed 8, St. Louis, 2017, Elsevier, pp 206-207.

AUTHOR: Jeff D. Bay, DVM, DACVIM
EDITOR: Leah A. Cohn, DVM, PhD, DACVIM

Palm (Cycad/Sago) Toxicosis

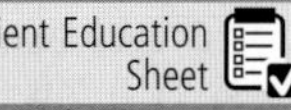

BASIC INFORMATION

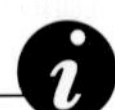

Definition

Acute, potentially fatal toxicosis occurring from ingesting cycad palm leaves, seeds, bark, or roots and characterized by vomiting and diarrhea, anorexia, lethargy, acute liver failure (2-3 days later), coagulopathies, and neurologic signs.

Synonyms

Cycad palm/plant, sago palm (includes *Zamia* and *Cycas* spp)

Epidemiology

SPECIES, AGE, SEX

All animals are susceptible; most poisoning cases are reported in dogs.

RISK FACTORS

Presence of palm in the pet's environment

GEOGRAPHY AND SEASONALITY

- Indoor ornamental plants; landscaping in the southern part of the United States and Hawaii
- Intoxication occurs mostly in summer months; availability of indoor potted sago palms makes intoxication possible throughout the year.

Clinical Presentation

HISTORY, CHIEF COMPLAINT

- Exposure to sago palm (any part of the plant)
- Within 24 hours, onset of vomiting, diarrhea, lethargy, and anorexia; chewed leaves, seeds, plant material may be in vomitus.
- Ataxia, weakness, or seizures
- Occurrence/recurrence of lethargy, anorexia, vomiting 2-3 days after ingestion, due to acute hepatic injury/failure (p. 442)

PHYSICAL EXAM FINDINGS

- As above (see History, Chief Complaint)
- Abdominal pain, dehydration
- Hypovolemic shock (depressed mentation, weakness/collapse, poor perfusion, weak pulse)
- Petechiae, ecchymoses
- Central nervous system (CNS) signs: ataxia, seizures

Etiology and Pathophysiology

- Sago palms (cycad plants) are palmlike plants in the family Cycadaceae. They are woody, coarse plants with leaves originating from a thickened stem and are found in dry, sandy soils of tropical and subtropical regions throughout the world.
- *Cycas revoluta* is the species most commonly involved in poisoning cases.
- Toxins: cycasin and methylazoxymethanol, a neurotoxic amino acid, and an unidentified high-molecular-weight compound
- The glucose molecule on cycasin is hydrolyzed by the gut bacterial enzyme alpha-glycosidase, yielding sugars and methylazoxymethanol, which then alkylates DNA and RNA. This process causes hepatotoxic, teratogenic, carcinogenic, and gastrointestinal (GI) effects.
- Azotemia secondary to decreased renal perfusion resulting from systemic hypotension/hypoperfusion is possible.

DIAGNOSIS

Diagnostic Overview

Diagnosis is based on history/evidence of exposure to plant and presence of vomiting, anorexia, lethargy, and diarrhea within 24 hours. High liver enzymes 1-3 days after exposure offer further support. There is no definitive diagnostic test.

Differential Diagnosis

- Toxic: mushroom *(Amanita)* poisoning, acetaminophen, blue-green algae toxicosis (microcystin), iron, xylitol (dogs)
- Nontoxic: chronic hepatitis, viral hepatitis, leptospirosis, other causes of acute hepatic injury

Initial Database

- CBC: leukocytosis, thrombocytopenia (mild, due to blood loss)
- Serum biochemistry panel: increased alanine aminotransferase (ALT) and alkaline phosphatase (ALP) levels, hyperbilirubinemia, hypoalbuminemia/hypoproteinemia, azotemia (prerenal and/or renal)
- Coagulation profile: increased prothrombin time (PT), activated partial thromboplastin time (aPTT) (liver damage–related coagulopathy)
- Urinalysis: glucosuria, bilirubinuria, hematuria possible

Advanced or Confirmatory Testing

Histopathologic lesions of liver include marked focal centrolobular and midzonal coagulation necrosis.

TREATMENT

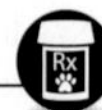

Treatment Overview

Asymptomatic animals thought to have ingested sago palm should undergo prompt decontamination (emesis, activated charcoal). In patients showing clinical signs (GI, CNS), treatment is aimed at stabilization. Signs of hepatic dysfunction should prompt treatment/prophylaxis for hepatic encephalopathy and coagulopathy.

Acute General Treatment

Decontaminating the animal (p. 1087):

- Emesis (p. 1188): in asymptomatic animals; within a couple of hours of ingestion
- Gastric lavage (p. 1117) only if a large dose has been ingested and emesis cannot be induced (e.g., comatose animal)
- Activated charcoal 1-2 g/kg PO; weigh risk of aspiration and hypernatremia (p. 1087)
- Cholestyramine, which binds bile acids, 300 mg/kg PO, sprinkled on canned food q 8-12h for 3-5 days, may reduce toxin uptake by the liver

Controlling CNS and GI signs:

- Seizures: diazepam 0.5-2 mg/kg IV or midazolam 0.5-1 mg/kg IV as needed; other anticonvulsants if refractory (p. 903)
- Vomiting, gastric ulceration
    - Ondansetron 0.11 mg/kg slow IV q 6-12h; *or* maropitant 1 mg/kg SQ q 24h or 2 mg/kg PO q 24h; *or* metoclopramide 0.1-0.4 mg/kg PO, SQ, or IM q 6h; combination of antiemetic agents may be needed
    - GI protectants: omeprazole 0.5-1 mg/kg PO q 12-24h *or* pantoprazole 0.5-1 mg/kg IV q 24h ± sucralfate 0.5-1 g for a dog or 125-250 mg for a cat PO q 8-12h if evidence of gastric ulceration

Treating signs of liver damage (p. 442):

- Monitor and treat secondary effects of acute hepatic failure, such as hepatic encephalopathy (p. 440), coagulopathy (p. 433), and hypoproteinemia.
- *S*-adenosylmethionine (SAMe) 20-40 mg/kg PO q 24h
- Vitamin K_1 3 mg/kg PO or SQ if prolonged coagulation factors noted ± blood transfusions (p. 1169) if hemorrhage
- Consider using *N*-acetylcysteine (Mucomyst) 140 mg/kg PO or IV (use a 5-micron filter for IV) followed by 70 mg/kg PO q 6h for 5-7 treatments; efficacy for treating sago palm toxicosis has not been determined.

Supportive care:

- IV fluids (recommend adding dextrose to 5% even if no evidence of hypoglycemia)

Chronic Treatment

SAMe 20 mg/kg PO q 24h × 1-3 months if evidence of persistent liver insult (e.g., serum ALT and/or bilirubin elevation)

Possible Complications

Chronic liver disease (cirrhosis/fibrosis)

Recommended Monitoring

- CBC: PCV, platelets
- Serum biochemistry profile: liver enzymes (baseline, 24, 48, and 72 hours), albumin, and total protein
- Coagulation profile

PROGNOSIS & OUTCOME

- Poor prognosis if evidence of severe liver injury
- Fair to good prognosis with early and intensive decontamination and supportive care

PEARLS & CONSIDERATIONS

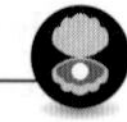

Comments

- All exposures should be taken seriously because the mortality rate for dogs can be as high as 67%.
- All plant parts are considered toxic, and seeds concentrate more toxin; one or two ingested seeds can be lethal for a medium-sized dog.
- Clinical signs of toxicosis can last from a few days to weeks, depending on the severity of liver injury.

Prevention

Keep pets out of areas where sago palm plants are growing.

Technician Tips

- Be aware of the biphasic nature of this intoxication. Initial clinical signs occur within hours of ingestion of the plant, and after initial recovery, a second clinical syndrome (due to liver failure) should be anticipated, monitored, and treated. Onset may be delayed for 2-3 days after the initial signs are noted.
- Educate pet owners about common toxins, including toxic plants.

SUGGESTED READING

Clarke C, et al: Cycad palm toxicosis in 14 dogs from Texas. J Am Anim Hosp Assoc 53(3):159-166, 2017.

AUTHOR: Mary Schell, DVM, DABT, DABVT
EDITOR: Tina Wismer, DVM, MS, DABVT, DABT

Pancreatic Adenocarcinoma

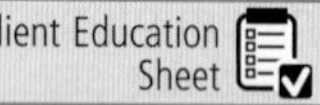

BASIC INFORMATION

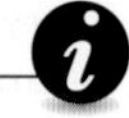

Definition

Malignant epithelial tumor of the pancreas of ductular or acinar origin

Epidemiology

SPECIES, AGE, SEX

- Uncommon tumor of dogs and cats (<0.5% of all cancers)
- Older dogs and cats (dogs: median age of 9.2 years; cats: 8-18 years)
- More common in female dogs; no sex predisposition in cats

GENETICS, BREED PREDISPOSITION

Spaniel dog breeds may be at higher risk.

ASSOCIATED DISORDERS

- Paraneoplastic alopecia in cats (p. 754)
- Bile duct obstruction
- Secondary pancreatitis
- Carcinomatosis with or without ascites and metastasis to distant sites
- Diabetes mellitus (rare)
- Exocrine pancreatic insufficiency secondary to pancreatic duct obstruction (rare)
- Superficial necrolytic dermatitis (hepatocutaneous syndrome, metabolic epidermal necrosis, necrolytic migratory erythema): more common in dogs

Clinical Presentation

HISTORY, CHIEF COMPLAINT

- Typically vague and nonspecific: anorexia, weight loss, lethargy, vomiting, constipation, diarrhea, abdominal distention (mass, ascites), and paraneoplastic alopecia (cats)
- Owners may note icterus if the neoplasm is occluding the common bile duct.
- Signs related to metastasis: ascites, dyspnea, cough, lameness/bone pain
- Signs related to effects of superficial necrolytic dermatitis on paws (dogs): reluctance to walk or signs of paw pain when walking

PHYSICAL EXAM FINDINGS

- Abdominal mass and/or ascites
- Icterus if common bile duct obstruction
- Dyspnea or cough due to pleural effusion or pulmonary metastasis
- Pododermatitis due to superficial necrolytic dermatitis (dogs)
- Paraneoplastic alopecia; alopecia of ventral abdomen/caudal thighs can reveal "shiny" appearing skin (cats)

Etiology and Pathophysiology

- Clinical signs are related to local disease (mass), metastatic disease (carcinomatosis and systemic), and metabolic effects.
- Metastasis to regional or distant sites is commonly noted at diagnosis.

DIAGNOSIS

Diagnostic Overview

Clinical signs are vague and nonspecific. In some cases, there is a palpable abdominal mass, ascites (associated with carcinomatosis), and/or icterus (associated with extrahepatic biliary obstruction). Confirmation is based on detection of a pancreatic mass (usually with ultrasound or at exploratory laparotomy) in an older patient and cytologic or histopathologic exam of tissue specimens from the mass or metastatic sites or cytologic evidence of malignant epithelial cells from abdominal effusion.

Differential Diagnosis

- Pancreatitis: primary pancreatitis or pancreatitis secondary to the tumor
- Pancreatic acute fluid collections or pseudocyst
- Pancreatic abscess
- Pancreatic nodular hyperplasia
- Other pancreatic tumors (islet cell tumor, adenoma, sarcoma, and lymphoma)

Initial Database

- CBC, serum biochemical profile, and urinalysis
  - Can be unremarkable
  - Variable neutrophilia, anemia, hyperbilirubinemia, hyperglycemia, and elevations in hepatic enzymes
  - Serum lipase activities: marked hyperlipasemia may be a noninvasive indicator and biochemical marker for neoplasia of the pancreas; activity > 25 times normal is probably diagnostic for exocrine pancreatic carcinoma, particularly if the serum amylase activity is minimally increased.
- Abdominal radiographs: nonspecific; may reveal cranial abdominal mass effect, compression of the duodenum, and/or loss of abdominal organ detail due to ascites.
- Thoracic radiographs (three views): to evaluate for pulmonary metastasis and/or pleural effusion
- Abdominal ultrasound (high yield)
  - In most cases, a soft-tissue mass can be identified in the region of the pancreas. It may not be possible to conclusively identify the mass as pancreatic in origin on ultrasound exam. Contrast-enhanced ultrasonography has been reported for the diagnosis of pancreatic neoplasia and has shown different enhancement patterns for adenocarcinoma and insulinoma.
  - Benign pancreatic nodular hyperplasia, a common incidental finding in cats, must be considered when pancreatic nodules are identified. There is a tendency for neoplastic lesions to manifest as a single, larger lesion and for nodular hyperplasia to manifest as multiple smaller lesions, although there can be overlap of the imaging findings for these entities. A mass > 2 cm in cats is suggestive of pancreatic neoplasia rather than nodular hyperplasia.
  - Allows identification of metastatic lesions (liver target lesions, peritoneal masses, lymphadenopathy) and ascites, but these are not specific for pancreatic adenocarcinoma.
  - Benign lesions such as hepatic nodular regeneration/hyperplasia, accessory splenic tissue, and others can be identified on ultrasound and should not be misidentified as metastases.

Advanced or Confirmatory Testing

- Cytologic or histologic diagnosis is essential due to the inability to grossly differentiate pancreatic adenocarcinoma, chronic pancreatitis, and pancreatic nodular hyperplasia.
- Evaluation of ascites (pp. 1056 and 1343) may reveal neoplastic cells. Flow cytometry can help distinguish between malignant and nonmalignant effusions.
- Ultrasound-guided percutaneous fine-needle aspirate for cytologic exam (varied yields; neoplastic cells may not exfoliate and differentiation between neoplastic lesions and nodular hyperplasia may be difficult)
- Ultrasound-guided percutaneous core biopsy, laparoscopic biopsy (p. 1128) or surgical biopsy to obtain tissue for histopathologic evaluation
- Pancreatic lipase immunoreactivity (PLI): has not been evaluated for pancreatic neoplasia; increased levels would be expected if there is secondary pancreatitis.
- Abdominal CT or MRI (surgical planning and staging [p. 1132])

TREATMENT

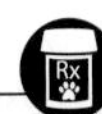

Treatment Overview

- Surgical excision of the tumor may be palliative but is not indicated if metastasis is present (majority of cases).
- Aggressive surgical procedures (complete pancreatectomy or pancreaticoduodenectomy) have been described, but they carry high operative morbidity and mortality without meaningful cure rates.

Acute General Treatment

- Supportive therapy if there is secondary pancreatitis (pp. 740 and 742)
- Surgery is indicated for solitary masses without evidence of metastasis, although a high early metastatic rate makes this situation uncommon.
- Palliative surgery if there is intestinal or biliary obstruction

Chronic Treatment

- No effective chemotherapy or radiation therapy protocols have been described.
- Gemcitabine (Gemzar) is approved for the treatment of pancreatic adenocarcinoma in human patients, and although cures are rare, gemcitabine has improved survival times for these patients; other chemotherapeutic agents used in humans have not been evaluated in veterinary patients.
- A single cat with carcinomatosis of pancreatic origin was treated with toceranib phosphate; achieved 792-day survival.
- Successful treatment of superficial necrolytic dermatitis in a dog has been reported after treatment with octreotide.
- Palliation of pain with analgesics (opioids, tramadol, gabapentin)
- Palliation of gastrointestinal signs (maropitant and ondansetron for nausea and emesis; mirtazapine, capromorelin, or cyproheptadine for appetite stimulation)

Nutrition/Diet

Nutritional support utilizing an esophagostomy tube (p. 1106) may be considered.

Possible Complications

Postoperative pancreatitis; preoperative and perioperative octreotide (Sandostatin) 5-10 mcg/kg SQ q 8h may be protective.

PROGNOSIS & OUTCOME

- Very poor to grave
- Survival time of greater than 1 year is rare.
- In one study, cats with pancreatic adenocarcinoma that underwent surgery and/or chemotherapy had a median survival time of 97 days (overall) to 165 days (with chemotherapy or their masses removed surgically), with a range of 1 day to 17 months. Those with abdominal effusions at the time of diagnosis had a median survival of 30 days.
- A recent report described survival times of > 300 days in several cats that underwent surgical removal of localized exocrine pancreatic carcinoma.

PEARLS & CONSIDERATIONS

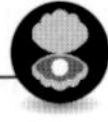

Comments

- Pancreatic adenocarcinoma is an aggressive malignancy with high potential for metastasis and generally no effective treatment, although cases with solitary masses without evidence of metastasis are candidates for surgery.
- Must be differentiated from non-neoplastic pancreatic lesions. It is important to have a cytologic or histologic diagnosis because chronic pancreatitis may closely resemble pancreatic adenocarcinoma grossly.
- Suspected metastatic lesions in the liver may be benign nodules (p. 449).

Technician Tips

Technicians can help pet owners as they consider difficult decisions related to the very poor to grave prognosis for this disease.

SUGGESTED READING

Withrow SJ: Cancer of the gastrointestinal tract: exocrine pancreatic cancer. In Withrow SJ, et al, editors: Small animal clinical oncology, ed 5, St. Louis, 2013, Saunders, pp 401-402.

AUTHORS: Steve Hill, DVM, MS, DACVIM; Brenda Phillips, DVM, DACVIM
EDITOR: Keith P. Richter, DVM, MSEL, DACVIM

Pancreatitis, Cat

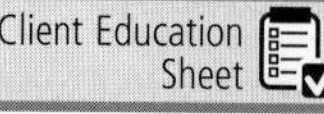

BASIC INFORMATION

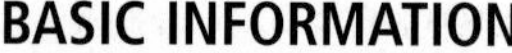
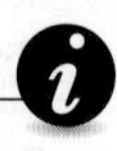

Definition

A common inflammatory condition of the pancreas that can be acute or chronic. Chronic pancreatitis, which can be differentiated from acute pancreatitis only based on histopathologic findings, is more common than acute pancreatitis in cats and is associated with permanent changes (i.e., pancreatic fibrosis and/or atrophy).

Epidemiology

SPECIES, AGE, SEX

No known age or sex predispositions

RISK FACTORS

In most cats, pancreatitis remains idiopathic, but some risk factors have been identified:

- Blunt abdominal trauma
- Hypercalcemia
- Pancreatic hypoperfusion
- High-fat diets (e.g., low-carbohydrate diets, diets for patients with chronic kidney disease)
- Pharmaceuticals: organophosphates and others
  - There is no evidence that corticosteroids cause pancreatitis in cats.
- Infections: *Toxoplasma gondii,* hepatic fluke infestation *(Amphimerus pseudofelineus),* possibly feline infectious peritonitis (FIP), and others

ASSOCIATED DISORDERS

- Feline pancreatitis can occur concurrently with cholangitis and/or inflammatory bowel disease (called *triaditis* when inflammation occurs in all three sites at the same time), but a cause-and-effect relationship has not been demonstrated.
- Pancreatitis can cause extrahepatic bile duct obstruction (EHBO [p. 118]).

Clinical Presentation

DISEASE FORMS/SUBTYPES

- Acute or chronic
- Subclinical (no clinical signs), mild (not associated with systemic or pancreatic complications), or severe (associated with systemic and/or pancreatic complications)

HISTORY, CHIEF COMPLAINT

Vague clinical signs (e.g., lethargy, inappetence) are typical. About one-third of cases experience vomiting.

PHYSICAL EXAM FINDINGS

There are no specific findings. Lethargy is common. In severe cases, dehydration and/or hypothermia may be recognized. Abdominal pain is reported in about one-fourth of cases. Icterus can occur with EHBO or concurrent hepatopathy (e.g., cholangitis, lipidosis), triaditis (p. 160), or secondary hepatic lipidosis (p. 444).

Etiology and Pathophysiology

- In most cats with pancreatitis, the underlying cause remains unknown, but several risk factors have been identified (see Risk Factors section, above).
- In general, premature activation of pancreatic digestive enzymes leads to initiation of pancreatitis, and the inflammatory response leads to progression of the disease and systemic complications.

DIAGNOSIS

Diagnostic Overview

Serum feline pancreatic lipase immunoreactivity (fPLI) concentration, as measured by Spec fPL, is the most sensitive and specific laboratory test currently available for feline pancreatitis. However, integration of all clinical data available affords the most accurate diagnosis. A point-of-care rapid assay (i.e., SNAP fPL) is available. A negative test result makes pancreatitis highly unlikely and should prompt the clinician to look for other disorders. A positive test result should be followed by quantitative laboratory Spec fPL measurement.

Differential Diagnosis

- Primary acute or chronic gastrointestinal (GI) disorders
- Acute or chronic metabolic or systemic disorders: hepatobiliary, renal, thyroid, systemic, or (less likely) central nervous system (CNS) or heartworm disease

Initial Database

- A CBC and chemistry profile should be evaluated for all patients suspected of having pancreatitis. Although findings are variable and nonspecific for pancreatitis, results from both are critical for assessing disease severity, identifying complications, and ruling out other disorders.
  - Serum calcium and fasting triglyceride concentrations should be assessed in cats with pancreatitis, and conditions (e.g., hyperlipidemia of other causes, hypocalcemia of other causes) causing abnormalities in these parameters should be managed before the changes are attributed to pancreatitis.
- Retroviral testing is appropriate for all sick cats.
- Abdominal radiographs are not useful for diagnosing pancreatitis but are useful for ruling out other differential diagnoses of pancreatitis.

Advanced or Confirmatory Testing

- Abdominal ultrasound can be useful in the diagnosis of feline pancreatitis.
  - Diagnostic criteria: pancreatic enlargement or mass effect, fluid accumulation around the pancreas, hypoechoic (necrosis) or, less common, hyperechoic (fibrosis) pancreas, hyperechoic peripancreatic fat (peripancreatic fat necrosis), or dilated pancreatic duct
  - False-negative and false-positive results are possible for ultrasonographic recognition of feline pancreatitis and are somewhat machine and operator dependent.
- Measurement of serum amylase activity is neither sensitive nor specific for feline pancreatitis.
- Serum total lipase activity can be measured using various substrates and assays, but none (including 1,2-diglyceride, triolein, 1,2-*O*-dilauryl-rac-glycero-3-glutaric acid (6′-methyl resorufin) ester [DGGR]) specifically measures pancreatic lipase. Sensitivities vary largely and cannot be compared even when using the same substrate.
- Serum feline trypsin-like immunoreactivity (fTLI) concentration has a limited diagnostic value for feline pancreatitis.
- Point-of-care fPLI assay can help rule out pancreatitis or provide support for the diagnosis.
- Serum fPL immunoreactivity (Spec fPL) concentration
  - Measures concentration of pancreatic lipase in serum (many other lipases contribute to total serum lipase activity)
  - Reference interval: 0.1-3.5 mcg/L; cutoff value for pancreatitis: 5.4 mcg/L
  - Highly specific for exocrine pancreatic function, although positive tests do not always reflect primary pancreatic disease (specificity is approximately 80%)
  - Highly sensitive for acute and chronic pancreatitis, but false-negative results are possible (sensitivity is 85%-90%)
  - Serial measurements allow for monitoring of disease progression in a specific animal.
- Because of the potential relationship between pancreatitis and intestinal disease (as occurs in cases of triaditis), measurement of serum folate and cobalamin may be useful (p. 543).
- Specific infectious disease testing may be appropriate in some cases (e.g., *Toxoplasma* serology [p. 984]).

TREATMENT

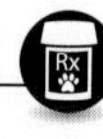

Treatment Overview

The mainstay of pancreatitis therapy is supportive care to treat clinical signs that cause morbidity (e.g., abdominal pain, vomiting), identify and treat systemic and pancreatic complications, and provide nutritional support.

Acute General Treatment

- If possible, remove potential risk factors (e.g., medications or infections implicated in pancreatitis).

- Aggressive but judicious crystalloid fluid therapy
- Analgesia is very important. Abdominal pain should be assumed to be present in any cat with pancreatitis, whether clinically apparent or not. Analgesia can be achieved with intermittent dosing or continuous-rate infusion. Acceptable options include one of the following:
  - Meperidine 2-4 mg/kg IM, as needed; short half-life or adverse effects can be limiting
  - Butorphanol 0.1-0.4 mg/kg SQ, IM, or IV q 8h
  - Buprenorphine 0.005-0.015 mg/kg IM or IV q 8h
  - Morphine 0.05-0.2 mg/kg q 2-6h SQ or IM, may cause dysphoria or nausea
  - Fentanyl 0.002-0.003 mg/kg IV once; then if needed, as a constant-rate infusion: 0.001-0.004 mg/kg/h IV
- Antiemetic therapy for vomiting
  - Maropitant has peripheral and central antiemetic properties (1 mg/kg IV, SQ, or PO q 24h).
  - Dolasetron and ondansetron are 5-HT_3 receptor antagonists with strong antiemetic properties. Dolasetron 0.3-0.6 mg/kg IV, SQ, or PO q 12-24h and ondansetron 0.1-0.2 mg/kg slowly IV q 12h can be used safely in cats.
  - Simultaneous use of maropitant and 5-HT_3 antagonists can provide additive effects.
  - Metoclopramide is a dopamine antagonist and a weak antiemetic but may also have a negative impact on pancreatic perfusion and therefore is not the first drug of choice.
- Monitor for complications as early intervention can be lifesaving.
- Antibiotic therapy should be implemented only when there is a specific suspicion for an infectious complication of pancreatitis.
- Glucocorticoid therapy may be helpful, especially if there is concurrent histologically confirmed (or suspected) inflammatory bowel disease and/or cholangitis.
- Although nothing *per os* was recommended in years past, nutritional support is crucial. If anorexia is prolonged, nasoesophageal or esophagostomy tube feeding may be warranted (see below).

Chronic Treatment

- Cats with concurrent inflammatory bowel disease (IBD) and/or cholangitis (triaditis when inflammation exists in all three sites) benefit from appropriate management of comorbid conditions.
- Avoid diets that are high in fat content, such as low-carbohydrate diets and diets intended for patients with chronic kidney disease.
- Many cats with chronic pancreatitis have a lymphocytic infiltration of the pancreas, similar to humans with autoimmune pancreatitis. If no risk factors are identified and the patient does not improve spontaneously, a therapeutic trial with an immunosuppressive agent can be undertaken. A baseline serum fPLI concentration is measured, and prednisolone 1-2 mg/kg PO q 12h is given for 10 days or cyclosporine 5 mg/kg PO q 24h for 3 weeks. A second serum fPLI concentration measured at this point indicates whether to stop treatment (fPLI the same or higher and/or clinical signs unaltered or worsened) or continue on a tapering schedule based on positive response (i.e., fPLI decreased and/or clinical signs improved).

Nutrition/Diet

- Nutritional support, preferably enteral nutrition, has numerous beneficial effects, including reduction of risk for anorexia-associated hepatic lipidosis.
- In cats that are eating and not vomiting, a low-fat diet should be offered in small amounts and given multiple times per day.
- Tube feeding (nasogastric, esophagostomy, percutaneous endoscopic gastrostomy, or jejunostomy tube [pp. 1106, 1107, and 1109]) should be considered for cats that refuse food for more than 3 to 4 days.
- If vomiting despite the use of antiemetics precludes enteral nutrition, total or partial parenteral nutrition (TPN or PPN [p. 1148]) should be considered.

Drug Interactions

Avoid any drugs implicated in causing pancreatitis.

Possible Complications

- Pancreatic abscessation has been reported for only two cats.
- Pancreatitis can lead to EHBO; most such obstructions resolve with supportive care.
- Systemic complications are rare in cats but may include disseminated intravascular coagulation (DIC), thrombocytopenia, acute kidney injury and uremia, pleural effusion, and peritonitis.
- Chronic recurrent pancreatitis may be a risk factor for endocrine (i.e., diabetes mellitus) or exocrine (i.e., exocrine pancreatic insufficiency) pancreatic dysfunction.

Recommended Monitoring

- Short-term monitoring: CBC, serum biochemistry profile, coagulation panel, fPLI (every 2-3 days for cats with acute disease and every 2-3 weeks for patients with chronic disease)
- Ultrasound is of little value in monitoring short-term progress.
- Long-term monitoring: fPLI (initially every 2-3 weeks; less frequently as patient normalizes)

PROGNOSIS & OUTCOME

The prognosis for cats with pancreatitis is directly related to the severity of the disease. Mild disease without pancreatic and systemic complications carries a good prognosis. Severe disease with pancreatic (e.g., pancreatic necrosis, pancreatic or peripancreatic fluid accumulations; other) or systemic complications carries a poor to grave prognosis.

PEARLS & CONSIDERATIONS

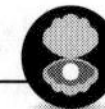

Comments

Pancreatitis is diagnosed with increasing frequency in cats. It is intriguing to speculate that at least some cats with chronic pancreatitis have a condition that is similar to autoimmune pancreatitis in humans and, like humans with this disease, may benefit from immunosuppressive therapy (see above).

Technician Tips

Cats with pancreatitis should be frequently and carefully reassessed for evidence of abdominal discomfort.

SUGGESTED READING

Steiner JM: Exocrine pancreas. In Steiner JM, editor: Small animal gastroenterology, Hannover, 2008, Schlütersche-Verlagsgesellschaft, pp 283-306.

AUTHOR: Jörg M. Steiner, Dr.med.vet., PhD, DACVIM, DECVIM, AGAF
EDITOR: Keith P. Richter, DVM, MSEL, DACVIM

Pancreatitis, Dog

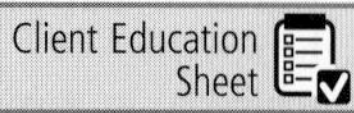

BASIC INFORMATION

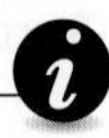

Definition

Pancreatitis is an inflammatory condition of the pancreas. It can be acute or chronic, which can be differentiated only histopathologically.

Epidemiology

SPECIES, AGE, SEX

No known age or sex predispositions

GENETICS, BREED PREDISPOSITION

Miniature schnauzers appear to be more commonly affected. As in some humans with hereditary pancreatitis, a mutation of the *SPINK* gene may be responsible. In the United Kingdom, English cocker spaniels are considered to be more commonly affected by chronic pancreatitis.

RISK FACTORS

- Dietary indiscretion
- Blunt abdominal trauma
- Hypercalcemia
- Pancreatic hypoperfusion
- Pharmaceuticals: potassium bromide, phenobarbital, L-asparaginase, azathioprine, trimethoprim-sulfadiazine, and others
  - There is little evidence that corticosteroids cause pancreatitis in dogs, and pancreatitis or a history of pancreatitis are not considered contraindications for corticosteroid use.
- Severe hypertriglyceridemia and disorders of lipid metabolism

ASSOCIATED DISORDERS

- In patients with severe disease, acute kidney injury, respiratory failure, myocarditis, disseminated intravascular coagulation (DIC), peritonitis, and multiorgan failure
- Pancreatitis can cause extrahepatic bile duct obstruction (EHBO).

Clinical Presentation

DISEASE FORMS/SUBTYPES

- Acute or chronic
- Subclinical (no clinical signs), mild (not associated with systemic or pancreatic complications), or severe (associated with systemic and/or pancreatic complications)

HISTORY, CHIEF COMPLAINT

- Often, a history of dietary indiscretion (especially high-fat foods)
- Anorexia and vomiting are common (91% and 90%, respectively, of dogs with severe pancreatitis).
- Weakness
- Abdominal pain is reported for about one-half of dogs with severe pancreatitis.
- Diarrhea is reported for about one-third of dogs with severe pancreatitis.

PHYSICAL EXAM FINDINGS

- Abdominal pain
- Dehydration
- Fever
- Possible icterus

Etiology and Pathophysiology

- The cause of pancreatitis in many dogs remains unknown.
- In general, premature activation of pancreatic digestive enzymes leads to initiation of pancreatitis, and the inflammatory response leads to progression of the disease and systemic complications.

DIAGNOSIS

Diagnostic Overview

Serum levels of canine pancreatic lipase immunoreactivity (cPLI) are measured with the Spec cPL test, which is the most sensitive and specific laboratory test currently available for pancreatitis, but the diagnosis rests on a combination of all available clinical findings.

Differential Diagnosis

- Primary acute or chronic gastrointestinal disorders
- Acute or chronic metabolic or systemic disorders: hepatic, renal, adrenal, thyroid (less likely), reproductive, or central nervous system (CNS) disease

Initial Database

- CBC findings are variable and nonspecific.
- Findings on a serum chemistry profile vary and are nonspecific; they are most useful in assessing the patient for systemic complications and ruling out other disorders with overlapping clinical signs.
- Abdominal radiographs are not useful in diagnosing pancreatitis but are useful in ruling out other differential diagnoses of pancreatitis.

Advanced or Confirmatory Testing

- Abdominal ultrasound is useful for the diagnosis of canine pancreatitis.
  - Diagnostic criteria: enlargement of the pancreas, fluid accumulation around the pancreas, pancreatic mass effect, hypoechoic pancreas (necrosis), hyperechoic peripancreatic fat (peripancreatic fat necrosis), and/or a dilated pancreatic duct
  - Resolution of equipment and operator expertise have increased significantly over the past 2 decades.
  - Clinicians must exercise caution not to overdiagnose pancreatitis based on ultrasonographic findings.
  - Useful to detect secondary extrahepatic EHBO
- Measurement of serum amylase activity is neither sensitive nor specific for canine pancreatitis.
- Serum total lipase activity can be measured using various substrates and assays, but none (including 1,2-diglyceride, triolein, 1,2-di-*O*-lauryl-rac-glycero-3-(glutaric acid 6-methyl resorufin ester [DGGR]) specifically measures pancreatic lipase. Sensitivities vary widely and cannot be compared, even when using the same substrate.
- A semiquantitative point-of-care test (i.e., SNAP) is available for immediate rule-out of canine pancreatitis. A negative test result should prompt the clinician to evaluate the patient for other differential diagnoses. A positive test result should be confirmed by measurement of a quantitative Spec cPL test.
- New point-of-care tests have become available (e.g., VetScan cPL, Vcheck cPL) but have not yet been shown to be repeatable or reproducible.
- Serum cPLI concentration (now measured by the Spec cPL assay)
  - Measures the concentration of pancreatic lipase in serum (many other lipases contribute to serum lipase activity measurement).
  - Reference interval: < 200 mcg/L; cutoff value for pancreatitis: 400 mcg/L
  - Highly specific for exocrine pancreatic function, but positive tests can occur due to diseases other than primary pancreatitis. This is especially likely when results fall in the gray zone between 200 and 400 mcg/L.
  - Highly sensitive for acute and chronic pancreatitis
  - One-time measurement does not allow assessment of disease severity, but serial measurements do allow monitoring of disease progression in a specific patient.
  - Measurement of cPLI in abdominal fluid (if present) is highly reliable for the diagnosis of pancreatitis. Cutoff value for pancreatitis: 500 mcg/L

TREATMENT

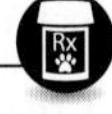

Treatment Overview

- Address any identified risk factors.
- Treat clinical signs that cause morbidity (e.g., pain, vomiting, anorexia).
- Identify and treat complications
- Nutritional support

Acute General Treatment

- If the clinician can identify a known risk factor, it should be addressed appropriately. For example, discontinue any medication that has been implicated in causing pancreatitis. Medications the patient requires for a concurrent condition should be switched to a different class of drug with the same or similar effect.

- The mainstay of pancreatitis therapy is supportive care. This includes aggressive fluid therapy and careful monitoring for signs of ensuing complications. After a complication has become established in a patient, treatment of it may become increasingly difficult.
- Abdominal pain is a key clinical sign in people with pancreatitis and should be assumed to be present in any dog with pancreatitis, whether or not this is clinically apparent. Analgesia is of paramount importance and can be achieved with intermittent dosing or continuous-rate infusion. Acceptable options include one of the following:
  - Meperidine 5-10 mg/kg IM or slowly IV as needed (q 1-4h); short half-life can be limiting.
  - Butorphanol 0.2-0.7 mg/kg SQ, IM, or IV q 3-6h
  - Buprenorphine 0.01-0.02 mg/kg IM or IV q 4-8h
  - Fentanyl 0.002-0.01 mg/kg SQ, IM, or IV once, then as a constant-rate infusion at 0.003-0.006 mg/kg/h; alternatively, may be administered as transdermal patch, which takes > 12 hours to take effect
- Antiemetic therapy can be important.
  - Maropitant 1 mg/kg IV or SQ q 24h or 2 mg/kg PO q 24h is an NK_1 receptor antagonist, which has peripheral and central antiemetic properties.
  - Dolasetron and ondansetron are $5\text{-}HT_3$ receptor antagonists that have strong antiemetic properties. Dolasetron 0.3-0.6 mg/kg IV, SQ, or PO q 12-24h and ondansetron 0.1-0.2 mg/kg slowly IV, or 0.4-1 mg/kg SQ, or PO q 6-12h can be safely used in dogs.
  - Patients can be treated with a $5\text{-}HT_3$ and an NK_1 inhibitor simultaneously. Because both classes of drugs act through different mechanisms, effects are additive.
  - Metoclopramide is a dopamine antagonist and may have a negative impact on pancreatic perfusion and therefore is not the drug of first choice.
- Dogs with severe pancreatitis associated with dehydration, electrolyte and acid-base abnormalities, DIC, and/or other systemic complications may benefit from plasma transfusions on a daily basis (e.g., 10 mL/kg IV for 1-2 hours [p. 1169]), although there is little scientific evidence that plasma administration is clinically useful in humans or dogs with pancreatitis. However, many veterinary gastroenterologists think there appears to be a clinical benefit.
- Antibiotics have failed to show benefit in human patients with pancreatitis. Dogs with pancreatitis rarely develop infectious complications of pancreatitis, and antibiotic therapy should be implemented only when there is suspicion of a concurrent infectious complication (e.g., aspiration pneumonia).
- There is no evidence that any other therapeutic strategy is clinically efficacious in dogs with pancreatitis. Exploratory laparotomy is rarely indicated but may be necessary for the rare patient with suspected pancreatic necrosis.

Chronic Treatment

- Dogs with chronic pancreatitis should be evaluated for potential risk factors for pancreatitis. An 18-hour fasting serum triglyceride concentration should be measured, and treatment measures should be employed for hyperlipidemic animals to keep the serum triglyceride concentration below 500 mg/dL (p. 496).
- The serum calcium concentration should be measured and a detailed drug history taken.
- Dietary measures are important in the successful treatment of dogs with chronic pancreatitis (see below). Antioxidants may be of benefit.
- Measurement of serum Spec cPL concentration can be used to objectively monitor dogs with chronic pancreatitis.

Nutrition/Diet

- Although once standard therapy for acute pancreatitis, withholding food and water is no longer recommended. Nutritional support, preferably enteral nutritional support unless uncontrollable vomiting prevents it, can have beneficial effects in dogs with pancreatitis, especially in those with severe disease.
- If uncontrollable vomiting persists for several days, total or partial parenteral nutrition (TPN or PPN [p. 1148]) should be considered for nutritional support. Alternatively, a jejunostomy tube placed surgically or by endoscopy can be used for nutritional support.
- Dogs with pancreatitis should be fed an ultralow-fat diet. Care should be taken to avoid treats that may be high in fat. Owners should be encouraged to switch treats to vegetables, fruits, or commercial ultralow-fat treats.

Drug Interactions

Avoid drugs implicated in causing pancreatitis (see Risk Factors above).

Possible Complications

- Pancreatic fluid collections or pseudocyst (an encapsulated fluid collection in the region of the pancreas) rarely develop in dogs with pancreatitis. Little is known about appropriate management in dogs. In humans, pancreatic pseudocysts are carefully monitored and are drained only if they increase in size.
- Pancreatic abscesses have been reported in only a few dogs. Most were not infected. Surgical drainage may be the best option. Intensive antibiotic therapy should be instituted after draining the abscess, at least until culture results show an absence of infectious organisms.
- Pancreatitis can lead to EHBO. In most cases, the obstruction resolves with supportive care. However, rare patients need surgery to reroute the bile duct (p. 118).
- Systemic complications may include DIC, thrombocytopenia, acute kidney injury, pulmonary emboli, myocarditis, peritonitis, and/or aspiration pneumonia.

Recommended Monitoring

- Short-term monitoring: CBC, serum biochemistry profile, coagulation panel, Spec cPL
- Ultrasound is of little value in monitoring short-term progress.
- Long-term monitoring: serum Spec cPL concentration

PROGNOSIS & OUTCOME

The prognosis for dogs with pancreatitis directly correlates with the severity of disease and level of supportive care. Mild disease without pancreatic and systemic complications carries an excellent prognosis. Severe disease with pancreatic (e.g., pancreatic necrosis, pancreatic fluid accumulations, other) or systemic (e.g., kidney injury, respiratory failure, DIC, other) complications carries a poor to grave prognosis.

PEARLS & CONSIDERATIONS

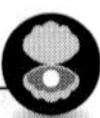

Comments

Pancreatitis is being diagnosed with increasing frequency in dogs. Most dogs that die for any reason have histopathologic changes of the exocrine pancreas, suggesting that subclinical exocrine pancreatic disease and inflammation are common in dogs.

Prevention

Eliminating risk factors aids in the prevention of pancreatitis.

Technician Tips

The vital parameters for dogs with severe forms of acute pancreatitis can change rapidly. Frequent re-evaluation is essential for recognizing changes early, before complications manifest.

SUGGESTED READING

Steiner JM. Canine pancreatitis: diagnosis and treatment. In Ettinger SJ, et al, editors: Textbook of veterinary internal medicine, ed 8, St. Louis, 2017, Elsevier, pp 1683-1688.

AUTHOR: Jörg M. Steiner, Dr.med.vet., PhD, DACVIM, DECVIM, AGAF
EDITOR: Keith P. Richter, DVM, MSEL, DACVIM

Panic Disorders and Canine Post-Traumatic Stress Disorder

BASIC INFORMATION

Definition

- Extreme responses (e.g., avoidance, escape, anxiety) driven by the sympathetic nervous system in response to an innate perception (panic disorder [PD]) or exposure to an identifiable stimulus/situation from which escape is impossible (canine post-traumatic stress disorder [C-PTSD])
    - C-PTSD signs develop only after the terrifying incident that triggered the disorder.
- May include mania or catatonia concomitant with decreased sensitivity/responsiveness to pain or social stimuli
- Repeated exposure to any aspect of the circumstance that triggered the original response (or its memory) results in the characteristic response.

Epidemiology

SPECIES, AGE, SEX

- PD: any dog; little is understood about PD in cats, although it likely occurs
- C-PTSD: any dog

GENETICS, BREED PREDISPOSITION

There may be a genetic influence (as in humans).

RISK FACTORS

- PD: prior episodes of panic; likely genetic/neurochemical liability
- C-PTSD: exposure to inescapable traumatic event(s) from which the patient was helpless to escape

ASSOCIATED DISORDERS

Separation anxiety, chronic or sporadic diarrhea

Clinical Presentation

- PD: acute anxiety in odd contextual circumstances that are repeatable and consistent
- C-PTSD: working dogs lose focus, appear distracted, are reluctant to emerge from their kennels or try to return quickly, show increased hesitance in work until refusing or being unable to do so
- Pet dogs actively resist being left in any social/physical circumstance associated with the provocative event(s). They pant, salivate, shake, tremble; have an oblique, darting gaze; and experience muscle fasciculations, lowered body postures, cringing, and tail tucks. Dogs may have nightmares that manifest these signs, and signs appear on exposure to a triggering stimulus (e.g., fire alarm, someone who resembles an abusive trainer).

DISEASE FORMS/SUBTYPES

Unlike panic, which can be idiopathic, all forms of C-PTSD are induced by trauma.

HISTORY, CHIEF COMPLAINT

- PD: change in behavior associated with some circumstances or pattern of behaviors
- C-PTSD: change occurs with acute trauma and associated sensory triggers in an environment where the dog cannot escape or gain control.

PHYSICAL EXAM FINDINGS

Dogs may be acutely fearful and avoidant or hyperreactive and explosive. Weight loss is common. Coat condition may be poor, and teeth/claws may have been broken attempting escape.

Etiology and Pathophysiology

- C-PTSD is reported in U.S. military working dogs proportionately to soldiers. It also can occur in pet dogs subjected to inescapable abuse or trapped in terrifying situations (e.g., dogs in crates during fires/burglaries, bait dogs for dog fights, prolonged or repeated threat by another dog, injury and entrapment in car accidents).
- Hyperresponsivity to environmental events and hypervigilance, behaviors aimed at escaping or avoiding previously positive or neutral environments or tasks, changes in social interaction with human handlers (for working dogs) or owners/friendly humans (for pet dogs), and failure to perform previously mastered tasks.
- Removal from the situational environment does not alleviate PD or C-PTSD. Signs persist continuously or sporadically.
- Human/rodent models suggest a key role for the amygdala in hyperresponsivity and hypervigilance. Caudate nuclei volume differs in matched affected and unaffected twin humans.

DIAGNOSIS

Diagnostic Overview

Diagnosis is based on behavioral evaluation and in ruling out other differential diagnoses.

Differential Diagnosis

Lack of early social exposure, lack of early exposure to novel environments; traumatic brain injury (TBI), organic brain disease (e.g., neoplasia)

Initial Database

- CBC, serum biochemistry profile, urinalysis: to rule out medical disorders and in anticipation of medical treatment. Stress leukogram is common (p. 1283).
- Other tests for common illnesses that owner/handler may mistake for signs of PD or C-PTSD (e.g., thyroid profile, vector-borne disease titers)

Advanced or Confirmatory Testing

None. In humans, fMRI confirms association between stimuli and regional brain response.

TREATMENT

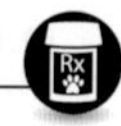

Treatment Overview

Treatment decreases hyperreactivity and hyperarousal associated with stimuli (or remembrance of stimuli) and ultimately gives the dog control over how he responds to such stimuli by allowing him to engage in a set of learned, calming behaviors that minimize arousal and fear (i.e., cognitive behavioral modification).

Acute General Treatment

- If the dog is sleeping fitfully, medication to encourage restorative sleep is essential: benzodiazepines (alprazolam 0.02-0.04 mg/kg to start; clonazepam 0.125-1.0 mg/kg); gabapentinoids (gabapentin 10-20 mg/kg PO q 8-12h or prn before sleep).
- Panicolytic: alprazolam; Sileo (i.e., dexmedetomidine, 125 mcg/m^2) and fast-acting anti-anxiety medications (benzodiazepines) daily while giving tricyclic antidepressants and/or selective serotonin inhibitors (clomipramine 2-3 mg/kg PO q 12h; fluoxetine 1 mg PO q 24h; sertraline 1-2 mg/kg PO q 24h).
- Agents that affect peripheral responses: beta-blockers (propranolol 0.5-1 mg/kg) or alpha-agonists (clonidine 0.01-0.05 mg/kg; Sileo 125 mcg/m^2 [p. 609]) can be given multiple times daily.
- Medications can be combined (e.g., fluoxetine q 24h; gabapentin q 12h; clonazepam q 24h before sleep; Sileo q 4-6h prn).
- Any situation that renders the dog calmer (darkened rooms, eye shades, white noise, certain toys, clothes/bedding that smells like the client) should be provided.

Chronic Treatment

Treatment is lifelong. Cognitive behavior modification teaches the dog to use practiced calming behaviors to alter his physiologic state. Daily medication helps facilitate and maintain these responses.

Behavior/Exercise

Cognitive games (e.g., find it, the shell game, nosework) or exercise may help. Any task engendering engagement should be rewarded, even if it is just sitting and looking happy for a treat.

Possible Complications

If the client is unable to protect the dog from the provocative stimuli (e.g., police/ambulance sirens), recovery will be more difficult.

Recommended Monitoring

Close contact with the client is necessary until issues have improved. For dogs receiving medications, repeat serum biochemistry 1-2 times per year.

PROGNOSIS & OUTCOME

- Guarded, depending on client needs
- One-half of military working dogs with C-PTSD return to service; one-half retire.

PEARLS & CONSIDERATIONS

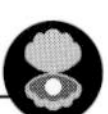

Comments

C-PTSD is usually recognized only when fully developed. Treatment must be aggressive and involve avoidance of triggers.

Prevention

Dogs should be provided an environment in which no human or animal can entrap and torment them. Humane dog training that uses only techniques designed to provide information about how the dog can get rewards should replace punitive training. Inescapable tragedies and disasters are, by definition, unpreventable, and putting dogs (or humans) in war zones has known, serious risks.

Technician Tips

Clients have difficulty understanding that PD is driven by the dog's perception.

Client Education

Educate clients about protection, the role of arousal, and behavior modification as a script for calming dogs.

SUGGESTED READING

Burghardt WF: Preliminary evaluation of case series of military working dogs affected with canine post-traumatic stress disorder (N = 14). In Proceedings ACVB/AVSAB veterinary behavior symposium, Chicago, 2013, American College of Veterinary Behaviorists/American Veterinary Society of Animal Behavior, pp 5-9.

AUTHOR & EDITOR: **Karen L. Overall, VMD, MA, PhD, DACVB**

Panleukopenia, Feline

BASIC INFORMATION

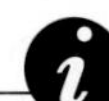

Definition

Highly contagious parvovirus infection of cats typically causes severe, sometimes acute gastroenteritis with degeneration of intestinal villi and leukopenia. Although uncommon in pet cats due to effective vaccination protocols, it is a re-emerging problem in shelters.

Synonyms

Feline parvovirus (FPV) infection, panleuk

Epidemiology

SPECIES, AGE, SEX

- All Felidae susceptible: domestic cats, tigers, lions, cheetahs
  - Also affects raccoons, mink, foxes, and monkeys
  - Can replicate in ferrets without causing disease
- Clinical disease most recognized in (unvaccinated) kittens > 6 weeks old but < 1 year old
  - Vaccinated kittens 8-20 weeks old, when maternal antibodies wane but may still neutralize vaccine-induced antibodies
- Kittens born to pregnant queens receiving modified live virus vaccine or infected during pregnancy are at risk for cerebellar hypoplasia. Because hypoplasia is permanent, cats of any age can be recognized as having persistent static cerebellar signs.

RISK FACTORS

Dense feral or shelter populations; inappropriate vaccination; immunosuppression (e.g., glucocorticoids, neoplasia, chronic kidney disease) that suppresses antibody response

CONTAGION AND ZOONOSIS

- Highly contagious to other cats; isolation of infected cats required
- Virus is shed in all body secretions (high loads in feces) for several days. For some cats, shedding may persist up to 6 weeks.
- Virus is extremely stable in environment (up to 1 year). Susceptible cats are infected by exposure to infected feces, secretions, or fomites. Virus can be transmitted *in utero*.

GEOGRAPHY AND SEASONALITY

Worldwide

Clinical Presentation

DISEASE FORMS/SUBTYPES

- Subclinical infection without illness (estimated > 75% of infections)
- Classic feline enteritis: kittens and susceptible adults
- Silent abortion/fetal death: queens (first trimester)
- Central nervous system (CNS) form: kittens infected *in utero* in second or third trimester or up to 9 days postpartum
  - Virus infects replicating neurons, especially those in external granule cell layer of developing cerebellum and postmitotic Purkinje cells.
  - Neurologic signs are primarily cerebellar and nonprogressive after birth; affected kittens can still make good pets.

HISTORY, CHIEF COMPLAINT

- Classic enteritis, acute onset: vomiting, diarrhea, anorexia
- Fading kitten syndrome: weakness/lethargy, failure to thrive, or sudden death
- Cerebellar hypoplasia in young kittens (infection *in utero* or shortly after birth): intention tremors, cerebellar ataxia, and wide-base stance noted after kittens start to walk (10-14 days old).
  - Less commonly, altered mentation and dullness (usually not noted until several weeks old) or seizures

PHYSICAL EXAM FINDINGS

- Classic enteritis: kittens infected with FPV
  - Fever or hypothermia in severe cases
  - Marked dehydration or hypovolemia
  - Vomiting, diarrhea
  - Thickened bowel loops, abdominal discomfort
- Cerebellar form: mother was infected or vaccinated when pregnant
  - Cerebellar ataxia, hypermetria, intention tremors, wide-base stance
  - Optic nerve hypoplasia, dark foci/retinal folding, streaking of retina
  - Mental dullness, behavioral abnormalities

Etiology and Pathophysiology

- Single: standard non-enveloped DNA virus affecting cats; isolates of canine parvovirus (CPV2a and CPV2b) can also affect cats.
- Replicates in rapidly dividing cells; clinical signs reflect destruction of these cells
  - Lymphoid tissue: lymphopenia, lymph node necrosis
  - Bone marrow: panleukopenia; occasionally, other short-lived cell lines (thrombocytes)
  - Intestinal mucosal crypt cells: damage results in malabsorption diarrhea, increased permeability, increased risk of bacterial translocation.
  - Nervous system: cerebellar hypoplasia, hydrocephalus, retinal dysplasia from destruction of neural tissue

- Unlike canine parvovirus type 2 (CPV2), feline parvovirus has no role in endomyocarditis (EMC) and left ventricular endomyocardial fibrosis (LVEF), clinically known as endomyocardial restrictive cardiomyopathy in cats.

DIAGNOSIS

Diagnostic Overview

Diagnosis is typically based on history, signalment, clinical signs, and initial laboratory findings. Severe gastroenteritis with neutropenia in a young kitten strongly suggests the diagnosis. Diagnosis of the cerebellar form is largely clinical.

Differential Diagnosis

- Gastroenteritis
  - Foreign body
  - Other bacterial or viral infection (coronavirus, *Salmonella* spp, *Clostridium* spp)
  - Toxin ingestion
  - Other causes of vomiting (p. 1293) and diarrhea (p. 1213)
- Leukopenia
  - Feline leukemia virus (FeLV) infection
  - Salmonellosis
  - Sepsis

Initial Database

- CBC: mild anemia unless severe gastrointestinal (GI) bleeding; leukopenia and especially neutropenia are typical but normal leukogram does not rule out FPV infection; thrombocytopenia due to bone marrow suppression or disseminated intravascular coagulation (DIC)
- Serum biochemistry: often unremarkable; prerenal azotemia and increases in alanine aminotransferase/bilirubin possible
- Retroviral testing: FeLV and feline immunodeficiency virus (FIV)
- Fecal exam: rule out parasites
- Coagulation panel: occasionally, evidence of DIC
- Abdominal radiographs: rule out foreign body obstruction

Advanced or Confirmatory Testing

- Canine parvovirus fecal ELISA test kits can reliably detect FPV antigen. False-positive results can occur up to 3 weeks after (modified live) vaccination.
- Confirmatory tests for FPV enteritis include serologic titer (paired samples), immunofluorescence antibody testing, polymerase chain reaction (PCR) assay, and virus isolation.
- For the cerebellar form, history and neurologic exam revealing stable cerebellar signs in a young cat can be assumed to be due to *in utero* or perinatal FPV infection.
- Although unnecessary, advanced brain imaging (e.g., MRI) can confirm cerebellar hypoplasia.

TREATMENT

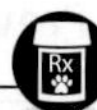

Treatment Overview

Comprehensive supportive care is required for acute enteritis. There is no treatment for the neurologic form, but clinical signs are not progressive.

Acute General Treatment

- IV crystalloid fluids to correct dehydration/hypovolemia, provide maintenance needs, and address ongoing losses
  - Address electrolyte abnormalities (e.g., hypokalemia).
- Broad-spectrum antibiotics (e.g., ampicillin ± sulbactam 20-30 mg/kg IV q 8h) to combat secondary bacterial infections.
- Antiemetic (e.g., ondansetron 0.5 mg/kg IV q 12-24h, maropitant 1 mg/kg SQ q 24h, or metoclopramide 0.2-0.4 mg/kg SQ q 8h (or 0.01-0.09 mg/kg/hr as an IV constant-rate infusion)

Nutrition/Diet

- If vomiting is controlled, consider tube feeding (p. 1107). Trickle feeding of a liquid diet through a nasogastric tube may improve gut healing and hasten return to appetite.
- Appetite stimulant (for adult-sized cats, cyproheptadine 2 mg/kg/CAT PO q 12h or mirtazapine 3.75 mg PO q 72h; dosing for small kitten may be difficult). Appetite stimulants are not often successful if the animal is still nauseous/ill.
- See tips for coax feeding (p. 1199).
- Vitamin B_{12} 0.25 mg/CAT IM or SQ once

Recommended Monitoring

- Vital parameters (heart and respiratory rate, temperature, body weight, capillary refill time) monitored closely during severe illness
- Rebound leukocytosis (24-48 hours) is expected; if leukopenia persists, rule out other causes (e.g., bacterial sepsis, retrovirus).

PROGNOSIS & OUTCOME

- Guarded (short term) for acute gastroenteritis, but complete recovery common
- Guarded to good for kittens with cerebellar hypoplasia, depending on ability to compensate for deficits; neurologic signs are not treatable but are nonprogressive.
- Grave to poor for kittens with forebrain signs (rare)

PEARLS & CONSIDERATIONS

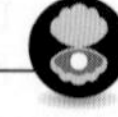

Comments

- Kittens cannot simultaneously have both neurologic signs and signs of enteritis from panleukopenia because neurologic signs occur from *in utero* infection of the queen.
- Routine vaccination has profoundly decreased the incidence of disease. Disease is maintained due to persistence of FPV in the environment and birth of susceptible animals in unvaccinated populations.

Prevention

- Modified live vaccines (MLVs) are preferred because they provide rapid and effective immunity.
  - Vaccinate after 8 weeks of age to avoid inactivation by maternal antibodies (maternal antibodies can persist up to 12 weeks in some kittens) and then approximately 3 and 6 weeks after first vaccination.
  - Kittens from high-exposure environments (e.g., shelters, feral colonies) may benefit from an additional booster between 16 and 20 weeks.
  - Initial vaccination may provide lifelong immunity, but triennial revaccination is recommended.
- MLV is contraindicated in pregnant queens or kittens < 4 weeks old.
- A negative titer in adult cats does not indicate lack of protection against the disease.
- Distal tail is considered an acceptable site for vaccination. It is well tolerated and produces similar serologic responses to vaccination in the distal limb 1-2 months after vaccination.

Technician Tips

- Because the virus is easily spread by fomites (e.g., towels, bowls, shoes) and persists up to 1 year, strict isolation and disinfection protocols are essential (e.g., disposable gowns, booties, gloves). Monitoring equipment such as stethoscope and thermometers cannot leave the isolation area.
- Disinfection of the environment or fomites requires 1 : 32 diluted sodium hypochlorite (bleach), formaldehyde gas, and glutaraldehyde, as for parvovirus in puppies.

Client Education

Breeders should vaccinate any new cat before introduction to cattery.

SUGGESTED READING

Greene CR: Feline parvovirus intentions. In Greene CE, editor: Infectious disease of the dog and cat, ed 4, St. Louis, 2012, Elsevier. pp 80-90.

AUTHOR: Harmeet Aulakh, BVSc & AH, MVSc, DACVIM
EDITOR: Joseph Taboada, DVM, DACVIM

Panniculitis

BASIC INFORMATION

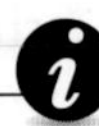

Definition

Inflammation of the subcutaneous adipose tissue (i.e., panniculitis) is different from cellulitis, which is an acute, diffuse, and suppurative inflammation of loose connective tissue, particularly the deep subcutaneous tissues, and sometimes muscle, most commonly resulting from infection of a wound, ulcer, or other skin lesion. Panniculitis is not a definitive diagnosis but rather an inflammatory condition with numerous causes.

Epidemiology

SPECIES, AGE, SEX

Uncommon in dogs and cats

GENETICS, BREED PREDISPOSITION

Sterile nodular panniculitis: dachshunds, collies, and miniature poodles

RISK FACTORS

- Outdoor pets (penetrating foreign body, bite wound): infectious panniculitis
- Obesity: mycobacteriosis
- Immunocompromised cat (e.g., feline leukemia virus [FeLV], feline immunodeficiency virus [FIV]) or dog (e.g., iatrogenic hyperadrenocorticism): greater risk of dissemination of infectious organisms
- Unbalanced diets low in antioxidants (e.g., low levels of vitamin E)
- Recurrent pancreatitis: panniculitis and steatitis (inflammation of body fat)
- Pancreatitis or pancreatic carcinomas: mineralizing fat necrosis/panniculitis

CONTAGION AND ZOONOSIS

- Dermatophytic granulomatous panniculitis: *Microsporum canis* and *Trichophyton mentagrophytes* are potentially contagious to other animals and are zoonotic.
- Sporotrichosis: risk of cat-to-human transmission is extremely high; dog-to-human transmission has not been reported.
- Blastomycosis, coccidioidomycosis, histoplasmosis: risk of zoonosis by aerosol from culture plates; in-house culture is always contraindicated.

GEOGRAPHY AND SEASONALITY

Sporotrichosis has a worldwide distribution but may occur in regional outbreaks (e.g., Brazil).

ASSOCIATED DISORDERS

Interscapular panniculitis may be a precursor of injection-site sarcoma in cats.

Clinical Presentation

HISTORY, CHIEF COMPLAINT

Acute to chronic onset of single or multiple subcutaneous nodules or draining tracts, potentially with accompanying constitutional signs such as lethargy, anorexia, and pyrexia

PHYSICAL EXAM FINDINGS

- Lesions typically involve the trunk and may be single or multifocal.
- Subcutaneous nodules/swellings may become cystic-like and painful, especially before rupturing or developing draining tracts.
- Skin superficial to nodules may be atrophic.
- Panniculitis and subsequent fat necrosis are characterized by an oily yellow-brown to blood-tinged discharge.
- Lesions often heal with crusting, pigmentation, and scarring.

Etiology and Pathophysiology

- Panniculitis is caused by inflammation and/or infection of the panniculus (subcutaneous fat) with subsequent oxidative damage to the lipocytes.
- Result: release of free lipids into subcutis, resulting in fat saponification with further worsening of inflammation and granulomatous reactions.

DIAGNOSIS

Diagnostic Overview

Panniculitis has several causes but is initially suspected based on physical finding of subcutaneous swellings/nodules (pseudotumor) that may or may not be painful or have developed draining tracts. Biopsies for histopathologic evaluation and culture (bacterial and fungal) are required for diagnosis. Idiopathic sterile nodular panniculitis is diagnosed with 1) supportive histopathologic findings, 2) exclusion of an infectious cause, and 3) failure to identify other known causes of panniculitis.

Differential Diagnosis

Inflammatory:

- Infectious: abscess, bacterial/botryomycosis, actinomycosis, nocardiosis, atypical mycobacteriosis, feline leprosy, *Bartonella* spp (bacillary angiomatosis), dermatophytic pseudomycetoma, subcutaneous and systemic mycoses, oomycoses, leishmaniasis
- Noninfectious: trauma (including surgical sites), foreign body (e.g., suture), ruptured follicular cyst, insect bite, vitamin E deficiency, pancreatitis/pancreatic carcinoma, injection-site reaction (e.g., repository glucocorticoids, rabies vaccination), sterile vasculitis, lupus erythematosus, drug reaction, feline cutaneous lymphocytosis, calcinosis cutis, idiopathy (sterile nodular panniculitis)

Neoplastic:

- Benign: follicular tumors, lipoma
- Malignant: mast cell tumor, cutaneous lymphoma, malignant histiocytosis, liposarcoma

Initial Database

- Cytologic examination; to identify infectious organisms, if present
  - Gram-positive, branching, filamentous organisms: *Actinomyces* sp (nonacid-fast); *Nocardia* sp (partially acid-fast)
  - Diff-Quik: fungi possible (systemic mycoses)
  - Acid-fast bacilli: atypical mycobacteria, feline *Mycobacterium lepraemurium*
  - Organisms may be seen within foamy macrophages.
- Full-thickness skin (epidermis plus subcutaneous fat) biopsy; panniculus must be included; consider double-punch technique. Histopathologic analysis:
  - Qualify cellular infiltrate (neutrophilic, eosinophilic, granulomatous, pyogranulomatous).
  - Identify infectious organisms (special stains).
  - Severity of lesions (necrosis, fibrosis, vasculitis)

Advanced or Confirmatory Testing

- Clinicians should aseptically submit part of a biopsy specimen for tissue maceration and culture and possibly polymerase chain reaction (PCR) (tissue or swabs).
  - Consult laboratory for suspected organism(s), preference of culture media, incubation times, and necessary precautions for lab personnel.
  - Bacterial culture and sensitivity testing
  - Rapid-growing, atypical mycobacterial culture
  - Fungal culture (not usually for systemic mycoses; other tests are safer to personnel)
  - PCR for mycoses and leishmania
- Serologic evaluation: systemic mycoses
- Direct fluorescent antibody testing for *Sporothrix* antigen
- Abdominal ultrasound: pancreatic diseases may be a contributing factor (rare).

TREATMENT

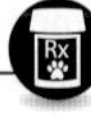

Treatment Overview

Because panniculitis has a variety of causes, selection and duration of treatment depend on identification of the specific cause.

Acute General Treatment

- Surgical excision of solitary lesions for diagnosis and possibly cure
- Appropriate antifungal, antibacterial, antimycobacterial, or antiprotozoal treatment if indicated

Chronic Treatment

Sterile panniculitis (e.g., rabies vaccine–induced, systemic lupus erythematosus, vasculitis, sterile nodular):

- Vitamin E 10-20 IU/kg PO q 8-12h may control mild cases.
- Tetracycline and niacinamide 500 mg of each for dogs > 10 kg or 250 mg of each for dogs < 10 kg, PO q 8h until improvement (about 2-3 months), then taper gradually; doxycycline 5-10 mg/kg PO q 12h or minocycline 10-25 mg/kg PO q 12h may be used in place of tetracycline.
- Pentoxifylline 20-30 mg/kg PO q 12h until resolved, then taper gradually
- Topical or intralesional glucocorticoid (e.g., dexamethasone, triamcinolone) administration when systemic/oral glucocorticoids are not tolerated
- Systemic glucocorticoid: prednisone 2 mg/kg PO q 24h (dogs), prednisolone 3-4 mg/kg PO q 24h (cats) until resolution (about 2-6 weeks), then gradually taper
- Azathioprine 1.5-2 mg/kg PO q 24h (dogs), chlorambucil 0.1-0.2 mg/kg PO q 24h (cats and small dogs), mycophenolate 10-15 mg/kg PO q 12h or cyclosporine 5-10 mg/kg PO q 24h or divided q 12h are glucocorticoid-sparing alternatives for long-term treatment. After a 2- to 6-week lag phase, q 48h (or longer) administration can be staggered with q 48h glucocorticoids (if still required).

Nutrition/Diet

Dietary elimination trial: adverse food reaction may be a trigger in immune-mediated panniculitis (rare).

Possible Complications

Adverse effects of treatments (e.g., glucocorticoids)

Recommended Monitoring

CBC, platelet count, serum chemistry profile, and urinalysis typically after 2-4 weeks (initially) to q 3-6 months (when stable) if using immunosuppressive agents

PROGNOSIS & OUTCOME

- Variable, from guarded to good; healed lesions may leave scars.
- Most cases of panniculitis involve lengthy treatment (months).

PEARLS & CONSIDERATIONS

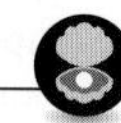

Comments

- A complete diagnostic workup to identify the underlying cause leads to the most appropriate and successful treatment plan and outcome.
- Clinicians should review the complexity of the differential diagnoses with clients and ensure they are willing to pursue prolonged treatment before starting extensive diagnostic testing beyond histologic confirmation. Consider referral to dermatology or internal medicine specialist.
- A biopsy punch may not reach the hypodermis (subcutaneous fat), impeding proper diagnosis. Wedge biopsy may be preferred.
- Nonsteroidal immunosuppressive drugs are sometimes prescribed for long-term control to minimize glucocorticoid side effects.

Prevention

- Weight loss for obese animals reduces amount of fat to which the body can react.
- Owners should minimize pets' access to high-risk areas (swamps, riverbeds) and should rinse/bathe the pet after high-risk area exposure

Technician Tips

- Wear gloves when patients with draining nodules present in the exam room.
- In some cases, a biopsy punch may not reach the hypodermis (subcutaneous fat), impeding proper diagnosis. Therefore wedge biopsy may be preferred if panniculitis is suspected.

Client Education

- Extensive diagnostic testing can be involved; need to determine infectious versus noninfectious cause
- Treatment is generally lengthy, especially when addressing atypical mycobacteria, *Actinomyces, Nocardia,* and intermediate/systemic fungal infections; but with appropriate therapy, the prognosis in most cases is positive. Healed lesions may leave scars, however.

SUGGESTED READING

Hnilica KA, et al: Small animal dermatology—a color atlas and therapeutic guide, ed 4, St. Louis, 2017, Elsevier, pp 279-280.

AUTHOR: Adam P. Patterson, DVM, DACVD
EDITOR: Manon Paradis, DMV, MVSc, DACVD

Pannus (Chronic Superficial Keratitis)

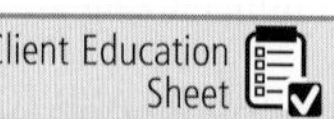

BASIC INFORMATION

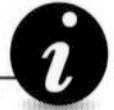

Definition

The typically bilateral, progressive, immune-mediated, inflammatory disease of the cornea is characterized by infiltration of vessels and granulation tissue and/or pigmentation.

Synonyms

Chronic superficial keratitis (CSK), pannus, degenerative pannus, German shepherd pannus, Uberreiter's syndrome

Epidemiology

SPECIES, AGE, SEX

- Dogs only
- Age of onset: 2-5 years of age; depends on breed and altitude

GENETICS, BREED PREDISPOSITION

- Primarily affects large-breed dogs but may occur in any breed
- Breed predisposition: German shepherd, greyhound, Belgian Tervuren, Belgian sheepdog, dachshund, border collie, Shetland sheepdog, Siberian husky, Scotch collie, Australian shepherd, miniature pinscher, pointer, Dalmatian, English springer spaniel, Airedale terrier

RISK FACTORS

Ultraviolet radiation exposure

GEOGRAPHY AND SEASONALITY

Increased incidence and severity of disease in geographic regions with high altitude (≥4500 feet [1500 m]) and intense sunlight. Dogs that live at lower altitudes respond better to therapy.

ASSOCIATED DISORDERS

Lymphocytic/plasmacytic conjunctivitis (atypical pannus, plasmoma) (p. 970)

Clinical Presentation

DISEASE FORMS/SUBTYPES

- Early pannus: lesions occur in the lateral to lateroventral cornea
- Chronic pannus: lesions may extend across the entire cornea
- Pannus may present as a
    - Vascular form
    - Pigmentary form
    - Combination of vascular and pigmentary forms in same eye or between eyes

HISTORY, CHIEF COMPLAINT

- Corneal discoloration: rapidly or slowly progressive; reddish and/or brown film covering surface of the eyes
- Progressive loss of vision

PHYSICAL EXAM FINDINGS

- Typically bilateral; often symmetrical
- Generally nonulcerative, pinkish red, vascularized, cloudy, and/or pigmentary superficial

corneal lesions commencing in the lateral to ventrolateral cornea and progressively involving the medial, ventral, and dorsal aspects of the cornea, including the central cornea
- Conjunctivitis present in most cases
- Multifocal white, crystalline lipid deposits often present at the leading edge of the corneal lesions
- ± Third eyelid involvement as evidenced by pink proliferative lesions and depigmentation along leading edge of third eyelid (atypical pannus)
- Early pannus
  - Vascularization and/or pigmentation at lateral to ventrolateral cornea adjacent to limbus
  - Progresses centrally
- Chronic pannus
  - Fleshy lesion (i.e., granulation tissue) with corneal vascularization and/or pigmentation
  - Entire cornea may be affected, predisposing the animal to blindness.

Etiology and Pathophysiology

- Increased expression of major histocompatibility complex (MHC) class II genes (particularly dog leukocyte antigen [DLA] class II genes) indicates pannus is an immune-mediated disease.
- Tissue-specific antigens in the cornea are altered by ultraviolet radiation exposure.
- Dogs with pannus develop a hypersensitivity response to corneal proteins, predisposing them to chronic inflammation.
- Pannus is more rapidly progressive and severe in young dogs (<3 years of age).

DIAGNOSIS

Diagnostic Overview

Diagnosis is based on the clinical presentation of typically bilateral corneal vascularization and pigmentation in large-breed dogs.

Differential Diagnosis

- Keratoconjunctivitis sicca
- Other causes of corneal vascularization (p. 212)
- Other causes of corneal pigmentation (p. 206)

Initial Database

Complete ophthalmic exam (p. 1137):
- Schirmer tear test (typically normal with pannus)
- Fluorescein dye application (typically no corneal dye retention with pannus but the dye may settle in rough areas in the cornea)
- Intraocular pressures normal (15-25 mm Hg)
- Careful exam of the conjunctiva and cornea

Advanced or Confirmatory Testing

- Usually not required; diagnosed by clinical findings, dog's signalment, and ruling out other causes of corneal vascularization and pigmentation
- Cytologic exam of corneal and conjunctival swabs/scrapings reveals lymphocytes and plasma cells.
- If a keratectomy is performed, histopathologic findings consist of lymphocyte, plasma cell, macrophage, and melanocytic cell infiltrations with corneal vascularization and fibroplasia.

TREATMENT

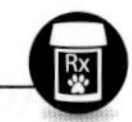

Treatment Overview

The treatment goal is to suppress the disease process with intensive initial treatment and to maintain the disease remission with continued therapy. Generally, treatment with topical corticosteroids is initiated and then tapered as treatment with cyclosporine or tacrolimus is initiated when the pannus is in remission.

Acute General Treatment

- Topical corticosteroids (dexamethasone 0.1% solution or ointment or prednisolone acetate 1% suspension) q 6-8h for 3 weeks, followed by slow reduction to a maintenance dose
- Cyclosporine 0.2% ointment or 0.5%-2% solution topically q 12h or tacrolimus 0.02%-0.03% ophthalmic ointment or aqueous suspension q 12h

Chronic Treatment

- Requires lifelong therapy
- Maintenance therapy consists of topical ophthalmic corticosteroids and/or cyclosporine or tacrolimus q 12-24h or lowest effective dose. Best to discontinue corticosteroids if possible to decrease risk of lipid corneal degeneration.
- Maintenance of remission is possible in some dogs with once daily application of cyclosporine.
- For nonresponsive and severe cases, clinicians can consider
  - Adjunctive subconjunctival injections of corticosteroids (e.g., methylprednisolone acetate, 4-8 mg; triamcinolone acetonide 4-12 mg [dose depends on size of dog]) q 2-3 weeks
  - Referral to veterinary ophthalmologist for beta-irradiation (i.e., strontium-90) or superficial keratectomy

Possible Complications

- Corneal ulceration (p. 209); if it occurs, clinicians should discontinue corticosteroid for the animal and commence/continue cyclosporine or tacrolimus until corneal ulcer has healed.
- Granuloma at site of subconjunctival corticosteroid injection

Recommended Monitoring

- Response to therapy is monitored every 3-4 weeks initially, then every 4-6 weeks. Pannus is in remission when the active vessels have receded. The pigment takes months to thin and never completely resolves if severe.
- Once stable, the patient is reevaluated every 3-6 months.

PROGNOSIS & OUTCOME

- Pannus is a chronic disorder that typically responds to intensive medical therapy.
- Maintenance therapy is needed to keep the disease in remission.

PEARLS & CONSIDERATIONS

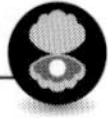

Comments

- A common error in treatment is failure to provide intensive therapy in the early stages of disease.
- The disease should be treated proactively with topical corticosteroids ± cyclosporine or tacrolimus, and the frequency should be slowly reduced over weeks to reach a maintenance therapy.
- Pannus is a chronic disease that requires lifelong treatment.

Prevention

- Owners should limit exposure of pets to ultraviolet light.
- They should also avoid breeding affected or closely related dogs.

Technician Tips

Most dogs with severe or blinding pannus gain functional vision with intense and prolonged treatment. Continued owner compliance is very important.

Client Education

- Pannus is an immune-mediated disease that is manageable but not curable.
- Lifelong treatment is required.

SUGGESTED READING

Ledbetter EC, et al: Diseases and surgery of the canine cornea and sclera. In Gelatt KN, editor: Veterinary ophthalmology, ed 5, Ames, IA, 2013, Wiley-Blackwell.

AUTHOR: Phillip A. Moore, DVM, DACVO
EDITOR: Diane V. H. Hendrix, DVM, DACVO

Panosteitis

Bonus Material Online 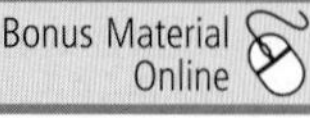

BASIC INFORMATION

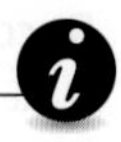

Definition

A spontaneous, self-limiting, painful condition of diaphyseal and metaphyseal portions of long bones that is common in young dogs

Synonyms

Enostosis, eosinophilic panosteitis; common lay terms include pan-O, eopan, and growing pains

Epidemiology

SPECIES, AGE, SEX

- Medium to giant-breed dogs; not reported in cats
- Young (5-18 months, occasionally up to 5 years of age in German shepherds)
- Males > females

GENETICS, BREED PREDISPOSITION

Very common in German shepherds but occurs in a variety of medium to large breeds; occasionally occurs in small-breed dogs

Clinical Presentation

HISTORY, CHIEF COMPLAINT

- The hallmark complaint is acute lameness of varied severity in a single limb or as a recurrent shifting leg lameness.
- Clinical signs typically last 1-3 weeks (per affected bone), waxing and waning in severity.
- Systemic signs (fever, anorexia, lethargy, reluctance to rise) can occasionally be sufficiently severe to warrant supportive care.

PHYSICAL EXAM FINDINGS

- Pain on deep (firm) palpation of the diaphyseal and distal metaphyseal portions of affected bones is characteristic, although pressure on nearby muscles or nerves can elicit a false-positive response.
- Most frequently affected bones: ulna (42%), radius (25%), humerus (14%), femur (11%), and tibia (8%)
- Fever, lethargy may be present

Etiology and Pathophysiology

- Cause is unknown.
- Infectious agents (bacteria, canine distemper virus, modified live viral vaccines) suggested but never proved to cause panosteitis
- Other suggested causes: localized vascular congestion, metabolic diseases, genetic disorder, parasitism, hyperestrinism, and hemophilia
- Panosteitis is associated with bone remodeling after the death of intramedullary adipocytes and hematopoietic cells. Cell death is attributed to vascular congestion and increased intramedullary pressure, but the underlying cause remains unknown.
- The necrotic marrow cells are replaced with fibrous tissue and then with woven bone. Endosteal bone formation is a prominent histologic finding.
- Periosteal new bone formation is present in some cases.
- Eventually, endosteal bone resorption occurs, and normal vascularity and marrow adipose tissue are re-established.

DIAGNOSIS

Diagnostic Overview

Panosteitis is typically a mild, self-limited condition. Persistence of lameness suggests another cause. Typical signalment, history, and physical exam findings should prompt radiographic exam, which is the clinical diagnostic test of choice.

Differential Diagnosis

Septic arthritis, osteomyelitis, polyostotic lymphoma, bone infarcts, immune-mediated arthropathies, and other developmental diseases (e.g., hypertrophic osteodystrophy, elbow dysplasia, osteochondrosis, hip dysplasia)

Initial Database

- High-quality radiographs of affected bones show characteristic lesions:
  - Patchy areas of increased intramedullary opacity
  - Increased radiographic lucency near the nutrient foramen of the bone
  - Increased periosteal bone formation
  - Characteristic lesions may not be present during the acute phase of the disease, and the typical radiographic appearance of panosteitis may be seen in bones that are no longer painful.
- CBC: eosinophilia present during the acute phase in ≤ 50% of dogs
- Serum biochemical panel/urinalysis, if indicated by clinical signs

Advanced or Confirmatory Testing

Nuclear scintigraphy if radiographs inconclusive

TREATMENT

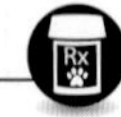

Treatment Overview

There is no specific therapy; analgesics are used during acute phase to reduce lameness and provide comfort.

Acute and Chronic Treatment

- For severely affected dogs, supportive care can require parenteral fluids, intravenous analgesics, and nutritional support (as needed; hospitalization is rarely required)
- Nonsteroidal antiinflammatory drugs (NSAIDs) generally provide adequate analgesia for dogs with panosteitis.
  - Carprofen 2 mg/kg PO q 12h, *or*
  - Deracoxib 1-2 mg/kg PO q 24h, *or*
  - Meloxicam 0.1 mg/kg PO q 24h, *or*
  - Firocoxib 5 mg/kg PO q 24h
  - Misoprostol (synthetic prostaglandin E_1 analog 2-5 mcg/kg PO q 8-12h can be given to decrease the risk of gastrointestinal ulceration but is seldom required.
- There is no indication for the use of glucocorticoids in panosteitis.
- Other analgesics can be added to or substituted for NSAIDs:
  - Gabapentin at 10-20 mg/kg PO q 8-12h, *or*
  - Tramadol 2-4 mg/kg (can be titrated up to a maximum of 10 mg/kg if needed) PO q 6-8h

Nutrition/Diet

- Excessive (3 times recommended intake) dietary calcium *increases* risk of panosteitis in young puppies. Diets containing 1%-2% calcium have not been implicated in this disease, nor have calcium/phosphorus imbalances.
- Use of vitamin, mineral, or nutraceutical supplements has not been shown to alter the course of panosteitis and could exacerbate development of other orthopedic conditions.
- A well-balanced, maintenance-type diet for the appropriate age should be used.

Behavior/Exercise

Restricted activity is recommended to improve patient comfort.

Drug Interactions

- Gastric ulceration and other side effects occasionally occur with use of NSAIDs.
- Glucocorticoids should not be used in patients receiving NSAIDs due to increased risk of gastric ulceration.

Possible Complications

- Most complications arise from treatment rather than disease. NSAIDs use can be associated with
  - Gastrointestinal hemorrhage, ulceration, and perforation
  - Renal dysfunction or hepatotoxicosis
  - Excessive bleeding (rare)

Recommended Monitoring

- Radiographic exam if other limbs become affected
- Repeated evaluation of dogs with protracted lameness to rule out other developmental diseases
- CBC (blood-loss anemia), biochemical profile (changes in liver or renal parameters), and urinalysis (urine specific gravity, sediment for evidence of renal casts) are recommended with long-term NSAID use.

PROGNOSIS & OUTCOME

- Lameness usually resolves within a month.
- The condition may shift among limbs.
- Long-term prognosis is very good.

PEARLS & CONSIDERATIONS

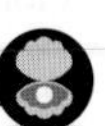

Comments

- Panosteitis may have a waxing and waning clinical course with repeated exacerbations over several months as the condition moves to different long bones, but it is rare for panosteitis to return to a previously affected bone.
- If lameness within a single limb does not resolve within a month, it is most likely due to another orthopedic disease (e.g., elbow dysplasia), even if panosteitis is evident radiographically.

Technician Tips

Dogs with panosteitis are in pain; use caution when handling (e.g., radiographic positioning) to avoid bite injury.

Client Education

- Clients should be reminded that panosteitis is a self-limited condition that will resolve with minimal treatment in the majority of dogs.
- Because panosteitis can mask other developmental orthopedic conditions, the dog should be re-evaluated if lameness persists.

SUGGESTED READING

Towle Millard HA, et al: Miscellaneous orthopedic conditions. In Johnston SA, et al, editors: Veterinary surgery small animal, ed 2, St. Louis, 2018, Elsevier, p 1307.

Reproduced from the third edition in modified form. Third edition author: D. Michael Tillson, DVM, MS, DACVS

AUTHOR AND EDITOR: Kathleen Linn, DVM, MS, DACVS

Panting

BASIC INFORMATION

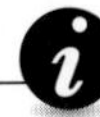

Definition

- Rapid, shallow breathing with a small tidal volume, usually with the mouth open
- Although it is a normal thermoregulatory mechanism in dogs, cats rarely pant.
- Dogs pant in response to warm ambient temperature, exercise, or anxiety (e.g., visit to the veterinarian's office).
- Excessive panting can be related to disease.

Synonyms

Hyperventilation, hyperpnea, polypnea, and tachypnea are distinct phenomenon

Epidemiology

SPECIES, AGE, SEX

- Depends on cause
- All dogs pant as a normal physiologic function, but cats rarely pant other than during stressful situations (e.g., car ride).
- There are age predispositions for some disease states associated with excessive panting. For example, middle-aged to older dogs more often develop hyperadrenocorticism or pheochromocytoma, and older cats develop hyperthyroidism.

GENETICS, BREED PREDISPOSITION

Brachiocephalic dogs

RISK FACTORS

Warm ambient temperature, emotional stress

GEOGRAPHY AND SEASONALITY

Summer (normal thermoregulation in dogs)

Clinical Presentation

DISEASE FORMS/SUBTYPES

Normal panting must be distinguished from inappropriate panting due to underlying disease. Diseases associated with panting include respiratory, cardiac, endocrine, central nervous system (CNS), and neoplastic disorders and pain from any source.

HISTORY, CHIEF COMPLAINT

Pet owners rarely complain about normal, physiologic panting. If increased amount of panting or panting at inappropriate time prompts a veterinary visit, an underlying disorder is likely. Specific additional complaints depend on the cause of pathologic panting. Questions should consider

- Perceived evidence of pain
- Glucocorticoid or narcotic drug administration
- Changes in water consumption or urination (hyperadrenocorticism, pheochromocytoma)
- Changes in food consumption or weight (e.g., hyperthyroidism, hyperadrenocorticism)
- Seizures, abnormal mentation (brain disease)
- Exercise intolerance, lethargy, coughing, dyspnea (e.g., cardiac, respiratory disease)

PHYSICAL EXAM FINDINGS

Findings other than intermittent panting (i.e., extremely rapid, shallow breathing without evidence of respiratory distress) depend on reason for panting. Many healthy dogs, and occasional cats, pant due to excitement and stress when presented for veterinary care. Additional findings:

- Elevated body temperature (panting due to hyperthermia is appropriate for dogs)
- Signs of pain (anywhere)
- Truncal hair loss, pot-bellied appearance, hepatomegaly (canine hyperadrenocorticism)
- Enlarged thyroid, tachycardia, heart murmur, or gallop heart sound (feline hyperthyroidism)
- Neurologic deficits (CNS disease)
- Heart murmur, tachyarrhythmia (cardiac disease)
- Harsh or adventitial lung sounds (lung or airway disease)
- Pallor (anemia)
- Obesity

Etiology and Pathophysiology

Panting is the primary means of thermoregulation in dogs by evaporative cooling; upper airway ventilation is increased with a decrease in tidal volume. Muscular work of breathing is minimally increased during panting. If severe or prolonged, respiratory alkalosis is possible. Pathologic causes of excessive panting:

- Phobias or anxiety
- Obesity
- Anemia
- Any respiratory (lung, airway) disease
- Cardiac disease and tachyarrhythmias
- Endocrine diseases
  - Hyperadrenocorticism
  - Pheochromocytoma
  - Hyperthyroidism
- Drug administration (e.g., glucocorticoids, narcotics)
- Hypocalcemia/eclampsia
- CNS disorders

DIAGNOSIS

Diagnostic Overview

Complete history and physical exam findings can help determine whether panting is normal (e.g., thermoregulation, anxiety) or a sign of disease. They also aid in ranking the importance of additional tests, which can be varied and extensive.

Differential Diagnosis

Tachypnea, respiratory distress, hyperpnea, hyperventilation

Initial Database

- CBC, biochemistry profile, and urinalysis can provide clues to underlying disease (e.g., hyperadrenocorticism → stress leukogram, thrombocytosis, increased alkaline phosphatase (ALP) and cholesterol, and minimally concentrated urine).

- Blood pressure (p. 1065): moderate to severe hypertension possible with hyperthyroidism or pheochromocytoma; mild hypertension possible with severe anxiety
- Thoracic radiographs: evidence of heart, lung, or airway disease
- Pulse oximetry: SpO_2 < 95 mm Hg suggests respiratory disease with hypoxemia; arterial blood gas can be used instead (PaO_2 of < 85 mm Hg)
- Serum T_4 (cats) to rule out hyperthyroidism

Advanced or Confirmatory Testing

Specific testing depends on history, exam, and initial database. Chapters on specific disorders provide diagnostic recommendations.

TREATMENT

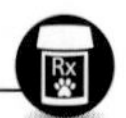

Treatment Overview

The goal is to treat the underlying condition.

Acute General Treatment

- If hypoxemia is suspected or confirmed, give oxygen supplementation (p. 1146).
- If hyperthermia is identified, institute cooling measures (p. 421) as well as other necessary treatments (e.g., ensuring adequate hydration).
- Provide analgesia for perceived pain.
- Reduce anxiety, and for short-term relief (e.g., panting during storms), consider use of sedative or anxiolytic drugs (e.g., trazodone 2-7 mg/kg PO q 8-24h [dog]) if animal is severely stressed.
- Manage recognized underlying disorders as appropriate (e.g., antiarrhythmic therapy for ventricular tachyarrhythmias, bronchodilator for feline asthma, calcium supplementation for eclampsia, transfusion for anemia).

Chronic Treatment

Address underlying disorder.

Nutrition/Diet

Initiate program for weight loss if the animal is obese.

PROGNOSIS & OUTCOME

Highly variable, due to broad range of underlying causes.

PEARLS & CONSIDERATIONS

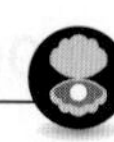

Comments

With the exception of cats that pant only under predictable conditions of stress, all panting cats should be evaluated for underlying disease.

Technician Tips

- Until proved otherwise, assume panting cats require immediate care, including oxygen supplementation.
- Ask owners of dogs that are panting on arrival for care whether panting is also an issue at home or it reflects the stress/excitement of the veterinary visit.

SUGGESTED READING

Hackner SG: Panting. In King LG, editor: Textbook of respiratory disease in dogs and cats, St. Louis, 2004, Saunders, pp 46-48.

AUTHOR: Jeff D. Bay, DVM, DACVIM
EDITOR: Leah A. Cohn, DVM, PhD, DACVIM

Papillomas, Oral and Cutaneous

BASIC INFORMATION

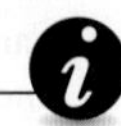

Definition

Benign tumors of the skin and oral cavity caused by infection with one of the numerous strains of canine or feline papillomaviruses

Synonyms

Warts, verrucae, cutaneous horns

Epidemiology

SPECIES, AGE, SEX

- Lesions occur in young, adult, or older dogs, depending on the clinical syndrome.
- Immunocompromised dogs or cats may be predisposed.

GENETICS, BREED PREDISPOSITION

- Cutaneous papillomas: cocker spaniels, Kerry blue terriers
- Multiple pigmented plaques: miniature schnauzers and pugs

RISK FACTORS

- Young and immunologically naive individuals with damaged skin or mucous membranes
- Immunosuppressed or immunocompromised individuals (e.g., glucocorticoids, oclacitinib, and/or oral cyclosporine; severe combined immunodeficiency [dogs])

CONTAGION AND ZOONOSIS

- Canine papilloma virus (CPV) is highly contagious, resistant to many common disinfectants, and persists in the environment.
- Generally species specific (nonzoonotic), although bovine papilloma virus (BPV) specifically has been implicated as the causative agent of equine and feline sarcoids.

ASSOCIATED DISORDERS

- Association with malignant transformation to squamous cell carcinoma (SCC) in the dog is controversial.
- Increasing evidence that viral plaques may progress to SCC *in situ* or invasive SCC in cats

Clinical Presentation

DISEASE FORMS/SUBTYPES

Disease in dogs can be classified as a variety of clinical subtypes. Clinical presentation depends on viral strain, individual immunocompetence, virulence, and other comorbidities.

- Canine oral papillomatosis
- Cutaneous exophytic papilloma
- Cutaneous endophytic papilloma
- Pigmented plaques
- *In situ* and invasive SCC (NOTE: majority of SCCs in dogs and cats are not associated with papillomaviruses)

Cats have at least three clinical presentations:

- Feline plaques
- Feline sarcoids (BPV1 and BPV2 associated)
- Bowenoid *in situ* carcinoma, invasive SCC

HISTORY, CHIEF COMPLAINT

- Intraoral nodule(s); oral discomfort, dysphagia, halitosis, and ptyalism (dog or cat)
- Cutaneous nodule or plaque (dog or cat)

PHYSICAL EXAM FINDINGS

- Canine oral papilloma virus (COPV or CPV1) infection presents with multiple growths in the oral cavity (few millimeters to 1 cm in diameter). They initially develop as smooth, white nodules before progressing to gray, pedunculated masses with fronds.
- Cutaneous lesions in dogs are normally solitary and can manifest as
  - Pedunculated exophytic growth with multiple fronds; found anywhere on the body (head, eyelids, and feet most commonly affected); rarely > 1 cm in diameter
  - Inverted endophytic papilloma with a small central keratin pore (ventral trunk and abdomen most common); typically 1-2 cm in diameter
  - Pigmented, sessile plaques/nevi/lentigines dispersed in numbers from 3 or 4 up to 80, involving the ventral neck, trunk, and

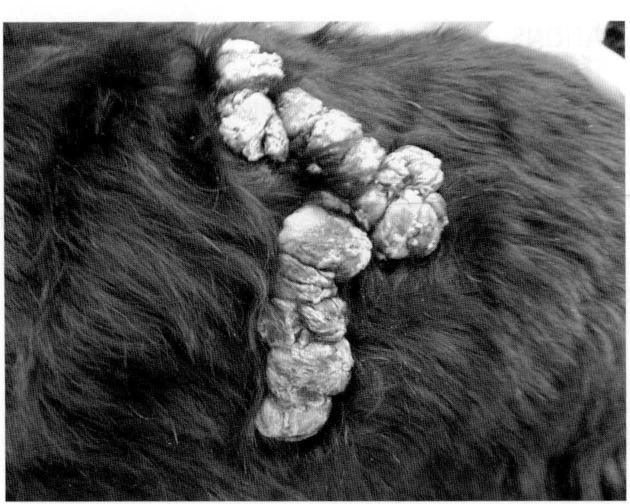

PAPILLOMAS, ORAL AND CUTANEOUS Cutaneous papillomatosis in an adult cocker spaniel dog. (Copyright Dr. Karen Moriello.)

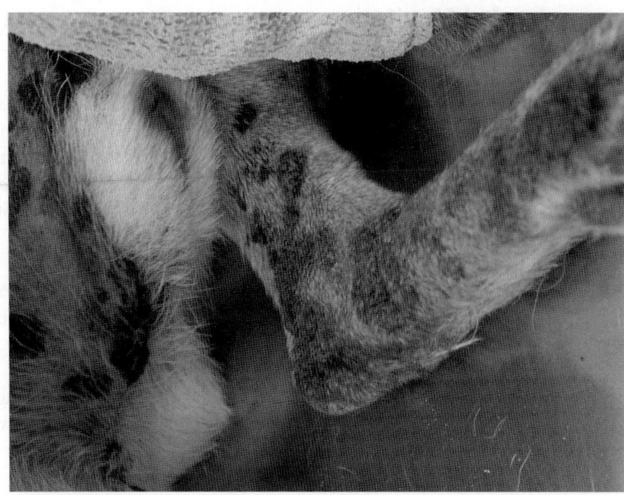

PAPILLOMAS, ORAL AND CUTANEOUS Pigmented viral plaques in an adult pug dog. (Copyright Dr. Karen Moriello.)

medial surfaces of limbs, usually in pugs and miniature schnauzers
- Papillomas affecting the footpads of dogs. Firm, hyperkeratotic, hornlike growths that occur on multiple footpads, sometimes resulting in lameness

- Cats
  - Multiple oral, raised, oval, flat-topped, 4-8 mm masses, especially on ventral tongue
  - Variably sized 3-mm to 3-cm masses on haired skin and progress from pigmented macules to hyperkeratotic plaques, which can transform into the ulcerated lesions of SCC.
  - Small, pedunculated masses

Etiology and Pathophysiology

- Papillomaviruses are host specific and relatively site specific, non-enveloped, double-stranded DNA viruses that can induce proliferative cutaneous and mucosal tumors.
- Infection requires inoculation through breaks in the epidermal or mucosal barrier by means of direct contact with an animal or transmission by fomite. Immunosuppression or immunodeficiency may be necessary for development of some forms (e.g., feline and canine plaques, disseminated papillomatosis).
- Incubation period is 1-8 weeks; regression typically occurs in 1-5 months, and lesions occasionally persist for 24 months or more.

DIAGNOSIS

Diagnostic Overview

For young dogs, diagnosis of canine oral papillomatosis is often visual. All other clinical presentations require definitive diagnosis by skin biopsy and histologic exam of tissue; polymerase chain reaction (PCR) testing may be required for confirmation of diagnosis.

Differential Diagnosis

- Canine oral papillomas
  - Fibromatous epulis
  - Transmissible venereal tumor
  - SCC (especially if ulcerated)
- Cutaneous papilloma
  - Pedunculated with fronds: sebaceous adenoma/hyperplasia
  - Pigmented: melanoma
  - Inverted: intracutaneous cornifying epitheliomas

Initial Database

Skin biopsy and histologic exam: Classic findings for exophytic papillomas include epidermal hyperplasia, orthokeratotic hyperkeratosis, ballooning degeneration of epidermal cells, koilocytosis, variably present intranuclear inclusion bodies and prominent keratohyaline granules in the stratum spinosum. Exam may reveal SCC *in situ* or invasive SCC (p. 939).

Advanced or Confirmatory Testing

- Most diagnostic laboratories can make a definitive diagnosis based on histologic findings. PCR, immunohistochemistry, and *in situ* hybridization can often help support or confirm a diagnosis.
- Electron microscopy is the gold standard for diagnosis but is primarily used for research purposes.

TREATMENT

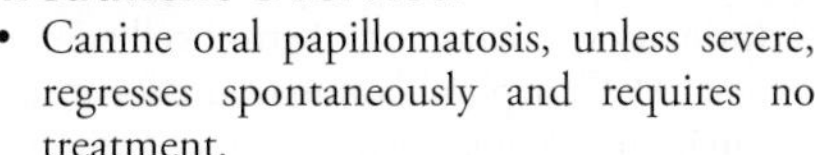

Treatment Overview

- Canine oral papillomatosis, unless severe, regresses spontaneously and requires no treatment.
- Consideration of an underlying immunosuppressive disease is warranted for adult animals.

Acute General Treatment

- Lesions often regress spontaneously in 2-3 months.
- Anecdotal reports exist that crushing lesions spurs resolution, but this has never been proved in controlled studies.
- Single-case series demonstrated varied response of canine oral papillomatosis to azithromycin 5-10 mg/kg PO q 12-48h.
- Surgical removal: CO_2 laser ablation, excision, cryosurgery, or electrosurgery. This often needs to be repeated. Most important in cases when normal physiologic functions are compromised by disease (e.g., airway obstruction, dysphagia)
- Discontinue use of systemic glucocorticoids, oclacitinib or cyclosporine, particularly if oral or cutaneous disease reoccurs or persists.

Chronic Treatment

- Interferon (IFN) at immunostimulatory low dosages (0.1 mL of 30,000 IU/mL solution, = 3000 IU/dose) PO q 24h or high dosages (1-1.5 million IU/m^2 SQ q 48-72h [p. 609]) for 4-8 weeks pending response
- Imiquimod 5% (Aldara) is applied topically to affected areas q 24-72h. Human-approved immunomodulator that activates toll-like receptors upregulates interleukin-6 (IL-6), IL-12, tumor necrosis factor-alpha (TNF-alpha), IFN-alpha, and IFN-gamma; activates Langerhans cells; and provides antiproliferative and antiviral effects. Local irritation is anticipated as part of the upregulated immune response against the virus-infected keratinocytes and can sometimes be difficult to differentiate from resolving lesions.
- Autogenous vaccines are not recommended because they have been associated with injection-site neoplasms several years later.
  - Modified papillomavirus vaccines containing codon-optimized E1, E2, E4, and E7 are protective against experimental and natural infection without inducing injection-site neoplasia.

Recommended Monitoring

- If benign neglect is chosen, clinicians should monitor lesions for ulceration, purulent exudation, and proliferation of growths; if noted, additional intervention is appropriate.
- Clinicians should monitor for abnormal persistence (e.g., development into a large or ulcerated mass), which could warrant biopsy because of the potential for malignant transformation of affected cells to SCC.

PROGNOSIS & OUTCOME

- Prognosis usually good
- Spontaneous regression is likely, with subsequent lifelong immunity.

PEARLS & CONSIDERATIONS

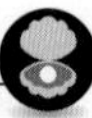

Comments

Once thought to be a nuisance and often treated by benign neglect with spontaneous regression, persistent lesions should be addressed sooner to minimize the potential risk of malignant transformation to SCC.

Prevention

Owners should separate dogs with oral papillomatosis from other susceptible individuals.

Technician Tips

- Thorough cleaning of exam tables and instruments used to treat dogs with papillomas; use dilute bleach 1 : 10
- Oral lesions in cats should be noted at the time of exam, especially under the tongue.

Client Education

Not a zoonotic disease

SUGGESTED READING

Hnilica KA: Small animal dermatology—a color atlas and therapeutic guide, ed 4, Philadelphia, 2017, Elsevier, pp 175-177.

AUTHORS: Karen Moriello, DVM, DACVD; Britt Levy, VMD

EDITOR: Manon Paradis, DMV, MVSc, DACVD

Paraneoplastic Syndromes

BASIC INFORMATION

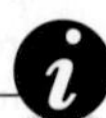

Definition

Pathologic changes in structure or function that develop secondary to and distant from a primary neoplasm. Certain paraneoplastic syndromes (PNSs) occur frequently, whereas others are rare. PNSs most commonly arise secondary to hormonal or cytokine factors produced by the tumor. In some instances, PNSs are more harmful than the physical tumor.

Epidemiology

SPECIES, AGE, SEX

Dogs and cats; generally no sex predisposition, with few exceptions (e.g., feline acromegaly associated with pituitary adenomas occurs more commonly in males)

GENETICS, BREED PREDISPOSITION

- PNSs are rarely directly induced by genetic factors, with occasional exceptions. One exception is nodular dermatofibrosis associated with an autosomal dominant heritable mutation of the Birt-Hogg-Dubé syndrome gene *(FLCN)* in German shepherds. Affected dogs commonly develop bilateral renal cysts or cystadenocarcinomas. Female dogs may develop uterine leiomyoma.
- Certain purebreds are predisposed to individual cancers, resulting in relatively higher incidence of PNS (e.g., boxers have higher incidence of T-cell lymphoma; boxers, pugs, and Labrador retrievers have higher incidence of mast cell tumors [MCTs]).

RISK FACTORS

Individual PNSs associated with specific tumors:

- Hypercalcemia: T-cell lymphoma, anal sac apocrine gland adenocarcinoma, parathyroid adenoma most common; also reported sporadically with malignant melanoma, squamous cell carcinoma, mammary adenocarcinoma, thyroid carcinoma, bronchoalveolar carcinoma, multiple myeloma, and others.
- Cachexia: multiple tumor types
- Hypoglycemia: beta-cell tumor (insulinoma), gastrointestinal leiomyosarcoma, hepatocellular carcinoma most common; others sporadically
- Gastroduodenal ulceration: MCT, pancreatic gastrinoma (Zollinger-Ellison syndrome)
- Erythrocytosis: renal tumors, nasal fibrosarcoma, lymphoma, others
- Disseminated intravascular coagulopathy: hemangiosarcoma (HSA), acute leukemia, lymphoma
- Hyperviscosity syndrome: multiple myeloma, lymphoma, leukemia, primary polycythemia
- Hyperadrenocorticism: pituitary adenoma, adrenocortical adenoma/carcinoma
- Cardiac arrhythmias/altered blood pressure: pheochromocytoma, HSA
- Anemia: HSA, lymphoma, leukemia, multiple myeloma, estrogen-producing tumors (Sertoli cell), other chronic neoplasia
- Thrombocytopenia: lymphoma, leukemia, multiple myeloma, HSA
- Leukocytosis: lung tumor, renal transitional cell carcinoma (TCC), lymphoma, thymoma
- Peripheral neuropathy: many tumors
- Alopecia: pancreatic carcinoma, hepatocellular carcinoma, lymphoma
- Hypertrophic osteopathy: lung tumor (primary or metastatic), Sertoli cell tumor, renal TCC, nephroblastoma, adrenocortical carcinoma, *Spirocerca lupi*–induced esophageal sarcoma
- Myasthenia gravis: thymoma, osteosarcoma
- Acromegaly: pituitary adenoma (cats), mammary adenocarcinoma (dogs)
- Superficial necrolytic dermatitis (hepatocutaneous syndrome): glucagonoma

ASSOCIATED DISORDERS

- Chronic hypercalcemia can cause renal injury by tubular mineralization and ischemic damage.
- Hyperglobulinemia/hyperviscosity syndrome can cause coagulopathy and hypertension, resulting in retinal detachment, seizures, renal infarction, cerebral/pulmonary thromboembolism, and congestive heart failure.
- Hypoglycemia usually causes depression, ataxia, and seizures.
- Gastroduodenal ulceration from excessive histamine-induced gastric hydrochloric acid (HCl) production results in melena, hematemesis, and anemia.
- Pancytopenia predisposes to opportunistic infections and spontaneous hemorrhage.
- Myasthenia gravis–induced megaesophagus predisposes to aspiration pneumonia.
- Hypertrophic osteopathy causes fever, lameness.
- Hyperadrenocorticism predisposes to thromboembolism, hypertension, glomerulosclerosis.
- Acromegaly commonly causes insulin resistance, upper airway obstruction, hypertrophic cardiomyopathy, and renal failure.

Clinical Presentation

HISTORY, CHIEF COMPLAINT

- Hypercalcemia: most common clinical signs include polyuria and polydipsia (PU/PD). Others are lethargy, inappetence, vomiting from uremia (p. 491).
- Cachexia: loss of lean body mass, often despite normal appetite
- Hyperviscosity syndrome: signs depend on organ system(s) affected: seizures, blindness, syncope, dyspnea (p. 509)
- Hypoglycemia: depression, ataxia, seizures
- Gastroduodenal ulceration: anorexia, melena, hematemesis (p. 380)

- Myasthenia gravis: regurgitation, dyspnea (secondary to aspiration pneumonia), weakness/collapse (p. 668)
- Hypertrophic osteopathy: lameness, lethargy (p. 508)
- Hyperadrenocorticism: PU/PD, polyphagia, bilaterally symmetric alopecia, muscle wasting, pendulous abdomen, comedones, calcinosis cutis (p. 485)
- Acromegaly: PU/PD, weight gain, enlarged head/limbs, exercise intolerance (p. 17)
- Peripheral neuropathy: cranial nerve deficits, altered proprioception, urinary/fecal incontinence
- Superficial necrolytic dermatitis: ulcerated cutaneous lesions, cracked/painful paw pads (p. 952)

PHYSICAL EXAM FINDINGS

Depends on tumor type (see History, Chief Complaint)

Etiology and Pathophysiology

- Hypercalcemia: due to excessive parathyroid hormone (PTH) production by parathyroid adenomas or humoral production of PTH-related peptide (PTHrP) and other cytokines (interleukin-1 [IL-1], transforming growth factor-beta [TGF-beta]), prostaglandins, receptor activator of nuclear factor kappa B ligand (RANKL)
- Cachexia: complex metabolic derangement due to altered cytokine milieu (especially increased IL-1beta, IL-6, tumor necrosis factor-alpha [TNF-alpha]), increased anaerobic glycolysis, misappropriation of nutrients
- Hypoglycemia: excessive insulin or insulin-like growth factor 2 (IGF-2) production
- Gastroduodenal ulceration: usually result of hyperhistaminemia leading to excessive gastric acid in mast cell tumors; rarely hypergastrinemia in pancreatic gastrinoma
- Erythrocytosis: excessive production of erythropoietin
- Bleeding disorder: antibody coating of platelets, platelet loss/sequestration/consumption, or inappropriate activation of secondary coagulation cascade
- Hyperviscosity syndrome: excessive immunoglobulin production and subsequent antibody coating of red blood cells, leading to aggregation
- Hyperadrenocorticism: excessive cortisol production in adrenal glands; usually due to excessive ACTH release from pituitary tumors but may be primarily produced by adrenal tumors or rarely ectopically
- Cardiac arrhythmias/altered blood pressure: excessive catecholamine production, hypoxia, sepsis
- Cytopenias: hemorrhage, chronic inflammation, immune-mediated hemolysis, hormone-induced suppression, myelophthisis
- Leukocytosis: excessive production of granulocyte-macrophage colony-stimulating factor (GM-CSF) or G-CSF
- Myasthenia gravis: antibody production targeted against acetylcholine receptors at neuromuscular junctions
- Acromegaly: excessive growth hormone (GH) and/or IGF-1 production

DIAGNOSIS

Diagnostic Overview

When animals present with signs related to a PNS, discovery of the underlying malignancy is essential.

Differential Diagnosis

- Hypercalcemia: granulomatous disease, hypoadrenocorticism, renal secondary hyperparathyroidism, hypervitaminosis-D, young/growing, spurious, osteogenic disease
- Cachexia: intestinal parasites, poor-quality diet, inadequate feeding, malabsorptive/maldigestive disorder, heart disease, infectious disease, renal disease
- Hypoglycemia: sepsis, iatrogenic (insulin overdose), spurious/old sample (p. 1240)
- Gastroduodenal ulceration: nonsteroidal antiinflammatory drugs (NSAIDs), corticosteroids, foreign body, toxins, uremia, liver failure, other
- Erythrocytosis: hemoconcentration, breed-related variation (greyhounds, sled dogs), dehydration, hypoxemia, other
- Bleeding disorder: anticoagulant rodenticide ingestion, sepsis, idiopathic immune-mediated thrombocytopenia, others (p. 433)
- Hyperadrenocorticism: iatrogenic (corticosteroid administration)
- Cardiac arrhythmias/altered blood pressure: primary cardiac disease, renal failure, others
- Cytopenias: infectious disease (especially *Rickettsiae*)
- Myasthenia gravis: hypothyroidism, hypoadrenocorticism, lead intoxication, esophagitis, idiopathic megaesophagus, others

Initial Database

CBC, chemistry panel, urinalysis, coagulation profile, thoracic radiographs, abdominal ultrasound, tumor aspiration/biopsy to confirm neoplasia

Advanced or Confirmatory Testing

- Hypercalcemia: measure PTH/PTHrP, ionized calcium to identify inappropriate function of hormone axis; parathyroid gland ultrasound to identify tumor; bone marrow aspiration to identify sequestered neoplasia
- Hypoglycemia: measure serum insulin; concentration should be below reference range; if level is high or within reference range with concurrent hypoglycemia, this suggests inappropriate function of hormonal feedback axis.
- Pancytopenia: bone marrow aspiration to evaluate for infiltrative disease, maturation arrest of cell lines
- Hyperviscosity syndrome: serum/urine protein electrophoresis to document monoclonal gammopathy
- Hyperadrenocorticism: urine cortisol/creatinine ratio, ACTH stimulation test, dexamethasone suppression test, endogenous ACTH to identify inappropriate pituitary-adrenal axis
- Myasthenia gravis: measure serum acetylcholine receptor antibody titer to prove autoimmunity.
- Acromegaly: measure serum GH, IGF-1 to confirm inappropriate hormone secretion.

TREATMENT

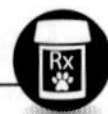

Treatment Overview

The severity of a PNS often parallels the status of the neoplasm. Direct treatment of the primary tumor (surgical excision, chemotherapy, or radiation therapy) should be the ultimate goal and can resolve the PNS. Some patients may be debilitated by the PNS and initially unable to undergo definitive therapy. Supportive measures include

- Hypercalcemia: saline diuresis, loop diuretics, corticosteroids, bisphosphonates, calcitonin to reduce serum calcium
- Hyperviscosity syndrome: phlebotomy, plasmapheresis to reduce serum globulins
- Gastroduodenal ulceration: gastroprotectants (histamine receptor antagonists, proton-pump inhibitors, coating agents, prostaglandin analogs) to reduce/protect against excess gastric HCl production; antiemetics, antidiarrheals as needed
- Myasthenia gravis: cholinesterase inhibitors and/or immunosuppressive therapy to improve esophageal muscular tone; upright feedings or gastrostomy tube to reduce risk of aspiration
- Cytopenias: blood product transfusion as needed; prophylactic antibiotics to prevent opportunistic infection if neutropenic
- Hypoglycemia: dextrose, corticosteroids, and diazoxide to increase serum glucose concentration; frequent small meals with complex carbohydrates to prevent spikes in serum glucose
- Seizures: anticonvulsant medications, corticosteroids, mannitol (as needed for increased intracranial pressure)
- Hypertrophic osteopathy: nonsteroidal antiinflammatories, opioids, bisphosphonates as needed for analgesia

PROGNOSIS & OUTCOME

Depends on individual tumor type, although some PNSs influence long-term prognosis:

- Hypercalcemia shortens survival for lymphoma ± anal sac apocrine gland adenocarcinoma.
- Myasthenia gravis: megaesophagus shortens survival for thymoma patients.
- Gastroduodenal ulceration: patients with MCT and clinical signs have shorter survival times.

PEARLS & CONSIDERATIONS

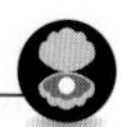

Comments

- Recrudescence of a PNS can indicate cancer relapse.
- If cause for hypercalcemia cannot be determined based on history and baseline diagnostic testing, consider bone marrow aspiration to investigate occult neoplasia.

Technician Tips

- PNS can cause clinical signs not typically associated with individual cancer types.
- Understanding the dynamic behavior of PNS can be helpful in distinguishing recurrence of cancer from treatment-related complications.

SUGGESTED READING

Withrow SJ, et al: Paraneoplastic syndromes. In Withrow SJ, et al, editors: Withrow & MacEwen's Small animal clinical oncology, ed 5, St. Louis, 2013, Saunders, pp 83-97.

AUTHOR: Michael A. Kiselow, DVM, DACVIM
EDITOR: Kenneth M. Rassnick, DVM, DACVIM

Paresis, Forelimb

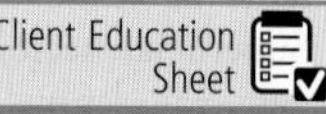

BASIC INFORMATION

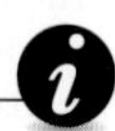

Definition

- Monoparesis: partial loss of motor function in one limb; voluntary movement exists but patient cannot initiate gait and is unable to support weight.
- Monoplegia/paralysis: complete loss of motor function in one limb
- Mononeuropathy: disease or injury of a peripheral nerve or its nerve roots

Epidemiology

SPECIES, AGE, SEX

Any dog or cat can be affected.

ASSOCIATED DISORDERS

- Horner's syndrome
- Loss of cutaneous trunci (panniculus) reflex
- Self-mutilation/trauma to affected limb

Clinical Presentation

HISTORY, CHIEF COMPLAINT

Weakness, lameness, or inability to use a forelimb

PHYSICAL EXAM FINDINGS

- Lower motor neuron (LMN) signs for the affected limb: weakness and decreased muscle tone
- Various: mild forelimb lameness to complete loss of sensory and motor function
- Denervation atrophy of forelimb musculature, usually within 7-10 days of nerve injury; differentiate from disuse atrophy, which is slower to develop and generally less severe
- Nerve root signature: lameness and pain of affected forelimb caused by entrapment of a nerve root within the brachial plexus
- Suspicion of neoplasia if chronic progressive monoparesis, nerve root signature and denervation atrophy
- Variable exam findings
    - Horner's syndrome (ipsilateral); common with traumatic injuries to the brachial plexus
    - Loss of cutaneous trunci (panniculus) reflex (ipsilateral) may be seen with brachial plexus injuries.
    - Palpable mass in axilla (uncommon)
    - Dysesthesia/paresthesia of limb and secondary self-trauma
    - Traumatic injury/fracture

Etiology and Pathophysiology

- Central nervous system (CNS)
    - Lesions affecting spinal cord segments C6-T2 can cause LMN forelimb signs.
    - Flaccid forelimb monoparesis
    - Basis: injury to LMN cell bodies that innervate forelimb musculature
    - Usually associated with upper motor neuron signs for ipsilateral pelvic limb
- Peripheral nervous system
    - Spinal/peripheral nerve disorders cause sensory and motor dysfunction distal to the lesion (permanent nerve damage or temporary, self-resolving trauma called *neurapraxia*).
        - Trauma: brachial plexus avulsion and radial nerve injury are examples.
        - Neoplasia: commonly affected are brachial plexus and dorsal nerve roots.
- Cervicothoracic spinal cord, nerve roots, sympathetic trunk: Horner's syndrome (ipsilateral)
- Lateral thoracic nerve (C8, T1) disruption: loss of panniculus reflex (ipsilateral)

DIAGNOSIS

Diagnostic Overview

A complete orthopedic and neurologic exam (including distribution of sensory loss) is the best means of differentiating musculoskeletal disease from neural involvement. Although uncommonly performed, electromyography and nerve conduction may aid in confirming the diagnosis of a nerve injury, determining the distribution, estimating the prognosis, and monitoring recovery. Advanced imaging and/or surgical exploration and biopsy may be necessary for definitive diagnosis.

Differential Diagnosis

- Degenerative (e.g., intervertebral disc disease [p. 555])
- Neoplasia (e.g., peripheral nerve sheath tumor [p. 692])
- Infectious (e.g., discospondylitis [p. 266])
- Inflammatory (e.g., granulomatous meningoencephalomyelitis [p. 647])
- Trauma (e.g., brachial plexus abnormalities)
- Vascular (e.g., fibrocartilaginous embolism [p. 336])

Initial Database

- CBC, serum biochemistry panel, urinalysis: generally unremarkable
- Orthopedic (p. 1143) and cardiovascular evaluation: rule out concurrent diseases
- Neurologic exam (gait, posture, spinal reflexes; p. 1136)
    - Distribution and severity of sensory loss aids in localizing the injury to a particular nerve or spinal cord segment; most important test for establishing prognosis for peripheral nerve injuries
- Forelimb and spinal radiographs (bone fractures, luxations, neoplasia, or infection)

Advanced or Confirmatory Testing

- Myelography, computed tomography scan (CT), or magnetic resonance imaging (MRI [p. 1132]) to localize unilateral spinal cord compression (intervertebral disc disease [IVDD] or neoplasia)
- MRI or CT to evaluate nerve/nerve sheath tumors
- Electrodiagnostics (electromyography [EMG], motor nerve conduction) to localize the dysfunctional spinal cord segment, nerve root, or peripheral nerve
    - EMG used for determining whether LMN, myelin, or muscle fibers may be the site of the lesion. Fibrillation potentials, positive sharp waves, and fasciculations can be seen beginning 5 days after denervation.
    - Nerve conduction is polyphasic and prolonged with LMN disease and absent with avulsion injury.
- Cerebrospinal fluid analysis (CSF [p. 1323]) to evaluate for infection, inflammation, or exfoliating neoplasia
- Surgical exploration (based on imaging results)
    - Biopsy, histopathologic exam for suspected neoplasia
    - Evaluation of type, extent, and severity of nerve injury

TREATMENT

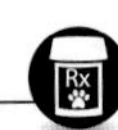

Treatment Overview

Short-term treatment is dictated by the cause, anatomic localization, and severity of the lesion/injury. Long-term treatment may involve medical therapy, physical rehabilitation, protection of affected limb from trauma, and an adequate duration of supportive care to allow for recovery/reinnervation.

Acute General Treatment

As indicated by underlying cause and its effects

Possible Complications

- Failure to regain adequate function of affected limb
- Local recurrence of nerve root tumors
- Persistent trauma, self-mutilation, or contracture of paretic limb, necessitating amputation

Recommended Monitoring

- Monitoring of limb daily for signs of trauma or self-mutilation
- Serial neurologic exams for up to 6 months to evaluate limb for reinnervation
- Serial electrodiagnostics to monitor recovery
- Monitoring for evidence of recurrence of nerve root tumor by physical exam and MRI or CT if indicated

PROGNOSIS & OUTCOME

- Largely depends on the neurologic exam at presentation and response to treatment
- Central
  - Intervertebral disc herniation
    - Fair to excellent with intact deep pain perception
    - Guarded to poor with absent deep pain sensation if addressed in 24-48 hours
    - Poor to grave if absent deep pain sensation and addressed after 24-48 hours
  - Fibrocartilaginous embolism
    - Poor to excellent based on magnitude/distribution of spinal cord lesion and nociception status
  - Neoplasia
    - Guarded to poor based on surgical accessibility and follow-up care
- Peripheral
  - Brachial plexus avulsion
    - Generally poor; often requires amputation
    - Guarded to fair if there is deep pain sensation
  - Brachial plexus neuritis
    - Guarded but recovery is possible
  - Peripheral nerve injuries
    - Fair to good for mild neurologic deficits, sharp lacerations with prompt surgical repair and short distance from site of injury to end organ
    - Guarded to poor for severe neurologic deficits; stretching, crushing, and avulsion injuries; contaminated wounds with delayed surgical repair; and large distance from site of injury to end organ (>30 cm)
  - Ischemic thromboembolic neuromyopathy
    - Prognosis more favorable for forelimb emboli
  - Nerve sheath tumors
    - Guarded to poor because local recurrence is common

PEARLS & CONSIDERATIONS

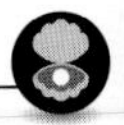

Comments

Brachial plexus avulsions with severe traction on the nerve roots may cause damage to the spinal pathways, resulting in pelvic limb deficits that are usually ipsilateral but can be bilateral.

Technician Tips

- Use caution when manipulating patients with suspected fractures or luxations to avoid secondary injuries to peripheral or spinal nerves.
- Use sling support and/or a protective boot to prevent trauma to the foot when walking a patient with a paretic limb(s).

Client Education

- Inform clients about prognosis, expected duration of forelimb paresis, and potential for failure to regain adequate function of limb, which necessitates amputation.
- Perform or recommend physical rehabilitation techniques.

SUGGESTED READING

de Lahunta A, et al: Lower motor neuron: spinal nerve, general somatic efferent system. In de Lahunta A, et al, editors: Veterinary neuroanatomy and clinical neurology, ed 4, St. Louis, 2015, Elsevier, pp 102-161.

AUTHOR: Dan Polidoro, DVM, DACVS
EDITOR: Leah A. Cohn, DVM, PhD, DACVIM

Paresis, Hindlimb

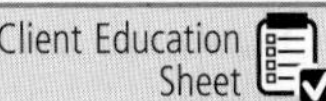

BASIC INFORMATION

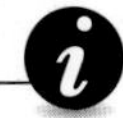

Definition

Paraparesis is defined as partial loss of motor function in the pelvic limbs. Paraparalysis or paraplegia is a complete loss of motor function in the pelvic limbs.

Epidemiology

SPECIES, AGE, SEX

Any dog or cat can be affected.

GENETICS, BREED PREDISPOSITION

- Young to middle-aged chondrodystrophoid dogs (e.g., dachshunds) are predisposed to intervertebral disc disease (IVDD), especially Hansen type I.
- Middle-aged to older nonchondrodystrophoid dogs (e.g., German shepherds) are predisposed to IVDD, especially Hansen type II.
- German shepherds are overrepresented in cases of degenerative myelopathy.

Clinical Presentation

DISEASE FORMS/SUBTYPES

Hindlimb paresis or paralysis is the difficulty or inability to use the hindlimbs due to weakness, ataxia (incoordination), or spasticity (limb stiffness) caused by a neurologic lesion. Weakness suggests a lower motor neuron or neuromuscular lesion. Spasticity and ataxia suggest an upper motor neuron lesion.

HISTORY, CHIEF COMPLAINT

Weakness, lameness, or inability to use hindlimb(s)

PHYSICAL EXAM FINDINGS

- Assessment of the femoral pulse; if absent, consider aortic thromboembolism
- Orthopedic examination (p. 1143) to rule out orthopedic causes of weakness
- Palpation of the bones of limbs, pelvis (including rectal exam in dogs), and vertebral column for fractures/luxations
- Fundic exam: evidence of multifocal/diffuse central nervous system (CNS) inflammation
- Neurologic exam (p. 1136) findings depend on location and severity of lesion.
  - Gait varies from mild pelvic limb lameness to complete loss of sensory and motor function.
  - Spinal reflexes (e.g., patellar)
    - Hyporeflexia: lesion in L4-S2 spinal cord segments
    - Hyperreflexia: lesion in T3-L3 spinal cord segments
  - Spinal hyperpathia (back pain on palpation)
    - Presence: may indicate IVDD, neoplasia, trauma, infectious or inflammatory myelopathy

- Absence: may indicate embolism or degenerative myelopathy
  - Muscle tone
    - Increased (spasticity): lesion in T3-L3 spinal cord segments
    - Decreased: lesion in L4-S2 spinal cord segments

Etiology and Pathophysiology

- IVDD (p. 555)
  - Degenerative disc changes lead to disc herniation into the spinal canal: Hansen types I, II, III
- Fibrocartilaginous embolization (p. 336)
  - Herniation of disc material into vertebral body and entrance into the venous plexus
- Degenerative myelopathy (p. 241)
  - Progressive, diffuse degeneration of spinal cord myelin and axons
- Spinal/peripheral nerve disorders
  - Cause sensory and motor dysfunction distal to the lesion (e.g., trauma, neoplasia)

DIAGNOSIS

Diagnostic Overview

A complete orthopedic and neurologic exam (including distribution of sensory loss) is the best means of differentiating musculoskeletal disease from neural involvement. Advanced imaging (myelography, CT, or MRI) is often required when a neurologic disease is suspected.

Differential Diagnosis

- Degenerative (e.g., IVDD [p. 555])
- Neoplasia (e.g., vertebral osteosarcoma)
- Infectious (e.g., discospondylitis [p. 266])
- Inflammatory (e.g., granulomatous meningoencephalomyelitis [p. 647])
- Trauma (e.g., spinal fracture/luxation [p. 369])
- Vascular (e.g., fibrocartilaginous embolism [p. 336])
- Orthopedic disease can cause hindlimb weakness.

Initial Database

- CBC, serum biochemistry panel, urinalysis: may reflect stress or underlying infectious cause (less common)
- Complete orthopedic (p. 1143), neurologic (p. 1136), and cardiovascular evaluations to rule out concurrent disease
- Spinal and pelvic limb radiographs to evaluate for bony lesions such as fracture, neoplasm, or infection

Advanced or Confirmatory Testing

- Myelography, CT, or MRI (p. 1132): spinal cord compression secondary to IVDD, neoplasia, and infectious or inflammatory disease process
- Cerebrospinal fluid (CSF) analysis (p. 1323): evidence of infection, inflammation, exfoliating neoplasia
- Titers and polymerase chain reaction (PCR) assay of serum and CSF: to assess for infectious causes, especially if CSF analysis suggests active inflammation
- Blood, urine, and CSF culture if infectious cause is suspected
- Electrodiagnostics: electromyography, motor nerve conduction

TREATMENT

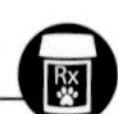

Treatment Overview

Treatment should address the underlying cause: surgical decompression if a compressive lesion is found (e.g., IVDD) or medical management (antibiotics, antiinflammatories, antifungals) as indicated. The goal of treatment is pain relief and resolution of the neurologic dysfunction.

Acute General Treatment

As dictated by the underlying cause

Possible Complications

Ascending myelomalacia from severe cord injury is somewhat unpredictable and has a grave prognosis.

Recommended Monitoring

- Reevaluate neurologic function at 4-week intervals until satisfactory pelvic limb function is achieved.
- A canine cart is an option for dogs that fail to regain adequate pelvic limb function.

PROGNOSIS & OUTCOME

- Based on preoperative neurologic exam and underlying disease
- Type I disc herniation with intact deep pain perception: 80%-95% have functional recovery with surgery.
- Type I disc herniation with absent deep pain perception: guarded to poor prognosis (50% functional recovery) if surgery performed within the first 24-48 hours and poor to grave after 48 hours
- Type II disc herniation (chronic) with intact deep pain perception: fair to good prognosis with surgical decompression, depending on number of lesions and duration of clinical signs, with the prospect of a longer recovery period
- Nonsurgical spinal cord disease has a variable prognosis depending on the underlying cause.

PEARLS & CONSIDERATIONS

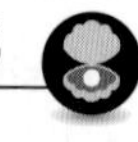

Comments

- Immediate referral to a surgeon or neurosurgeon is warranted for an animal that is decompensating neurologically.
- IV glucocorticoid administration (methylprednisolone sodium succinate, dexamethasone) has no proven benefit for spinal cord injuries in dogs and cats and may cause adverse effects: gastrointestinal disorders, infection, and immunosuppression.

Technician Tips

Use care and rigid support when moving patients with acute hindlimb paresis and an unknown trauma history.

Client Education

- Approximately 40% of dogs treated medically for presumptive intervertebral disc herniation have a relapse of clinical signs or fail to respond.
- It is essential to comply with a recommended period of cage rest/confinement.

SUGGESTED READING

Aikawa T, et al: Long-term neurologic outcome of hemilaminectomy and disk fenestration for treatment of dogs with thoracolumbar intervertebral disk herniation: 831 cases (200-2007). J Am Vet Med Assoc 241:1617-1626, 2012.

AUTHOR: Dan Polidoro, DVM, DACVS
EDITOR: Leah A. Cohn, DVM, PhD, DACVIM

Parturition, Normal

Client Education Sheet 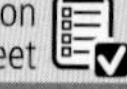  Video Available 

BASIC INFORMATION

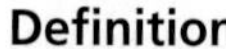

Definition

The act or process of giving birth to puppies or kittens

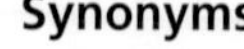

Synonyms

- Queening: parturition in the queen (female cat)
- Whelping: parturition in the bitch

Epidemiology

SPECIES, AGE, SEX

Dogs and cats: postpubertal, female

CONTAGION AND ZOONOSIS

Brucella canis, canine herpesvirus (p. 466), and *Coxiella burnetti* can be shed in lochia (parturient uterine fluids) during term parturition, preterm parturition, and/or abortion.

GEOGRAPHY AND SEASONALITY

- With the exception of the basenji, bitches are nonseasonal, meaning that parturition occurs year-round. In the basenji, ovulation occurs only in October, and parturition associated with a resulting pregnancy occurs only in December.
- In contrast, queens are seasonal, long-day breeders; estrous cycles cease during October to December (Northern hemisphere) unless they are exposed to 14 hours of light (natural and artificial). Parturition associated with any resulting pregnancy can be expected about 65 days from breeding (February to December).

ASSOCIATED DISORDERS

- Dystocia
- Premature parturition
- Abortion

Clinical Presentation

DISEASE FORMS/SUBTYPES

- Spontaneous
- Induced

HISTORY, CHIEF COMPLAINT

Bitch or queen is uncomfortable about 60 days after breeding and may have a vaginal discharge.

PHYSICAL EXAM FINDINGS

- In the bitch, rectal temperature is normal to low normal (98°F-100°F; 36°C-37°C) in the hours before parturition and increases to normal or slightly higher than normal during parturition. In the queen, rectal temperature is normal to low normal (100.5°F-102.5°F; 37.8°C-39.3°C), with additional variation based on environment, body condition, and other factors.
- Respiration and heart rates are slightly increased to normal.
- Uterine contractions may be visible through the abdominal wall.
- Examiner may be able to palpate fetuses transabdominally.

Etiology and Pathophysiology

- Three stages of labor
  - Stage 1: cervical dilation, 3-6 hours
  - Stage 2: fetal expulsion, 3-6 hours (depends on litter size) (see *Video*)
  - Stage 3: placental expulsion occurs at the same time or within minutes of each fetal expulsion; however, two fetuses and then two placentas may be delivered.
- Dystocia may occur for a variety of reasons (p. 278).

DIAGNOSIS

Diagnostic Overview

Parturition is identified when a gravid dam is at term gestation and is showing clinical signs of labor and/or has begun delivering fetuses.

Differential Diagnosis

- Abortion
- Dystocia
- Pseudopregnancy
- Premature birth
- Pyometra

Initial Database

- Pups or kittens are detected on abdominal palpation.
- Confirmation of fetal skeletons in the normal position and not too large for dam's bony pelvis: abdominal radiography after 42 days' gestation
- Abdominal ultrasound: fetal heart rates should be > 180 beats/min. Sustained fetal heart rates < 180 beats/min are associated with fetal distress.

Advanced or Confirmatory Testing

Tocodynamometry can be used externally to monitor uterine contractility.

TREATMENT

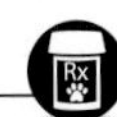

Treatment Overview

- Goal: delivery of healthy puppies or kittens without compromising mother's health
- Bitches and queens with normal parturition do not require any treatment or intervention.

Acute General Treatment

- In normal, spontaneous parturition, treatment is not needed.
- For the induction of canine parturition at days 59-61 after estimated ovulation day, aglepristone 15 mg/kg SQ once, followed 24 hours later by oxytocin 0.15 IU/kg SQ q 2h until onset of parturition, is a safe and effective protocol.
- If parturition is not normal (dystocia [p. 278])

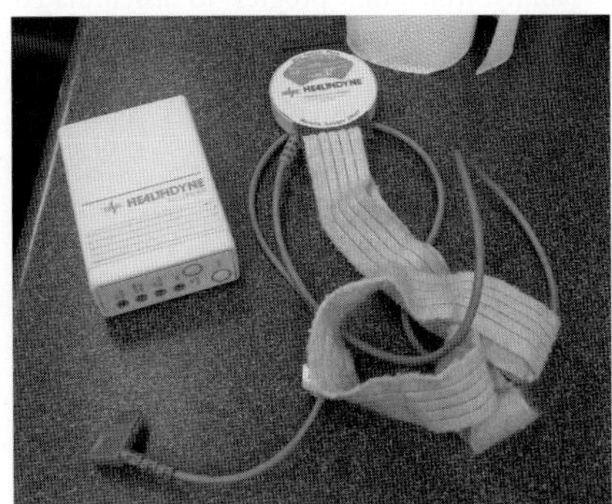

NORMAL PARTURITION Tocodynamometer for external measurement of uterine contractility in dogs and cats.

Nutrition/Diet

Administration of a calcium carbonate tablet (e.g., Tums 1 tablet/30 lb of body weight PO) at the onset of parturition may increase the strength of uterine contractions and prevent dystocia secondary to uterine inertia. However, administration of any calcium supplementation before parturition is contraindicated.

Behavior/Exercise

Dams can have unrestricted exercise before and during parturition.

Drug Interactions

- Aglepristone (Alizine) is not manufactured in the United States but is approved for the termination of pregnancy in cats and dogs in most other countries.
- Oxytocin should not be used at dosages in excess of those cited previously (0.15 IU/kg SQ q 2h). Higher dosages of oxytocin (>10 IU) cause placental vasculature constriction and fetal hypoxia.

Possible Complications

If the bitch or queen has prolonged abdominal contractions without delivery of a fetus or appears to be in constant intense pain, she should be evaluated by a clinician (p. 278).

Recommended Monitoring

- Clinicians can monitor the puppy or kitten delivery and be available to assist if needed (e.g., dystocia occurs, fetuses experience distress).
- Clinicians should make sure a placenta is delivered after each fetus.

PROGNOSIS & OUTCOME

- Good if parturition is normal
- Fair to guarded in cases of dystocia

PEARLS & CONSIDERATIONS

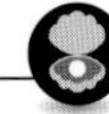

Comments

- Because parturition is a normal process, it is appropriate for most females to deliver pups or kittens at home in familiar surroundings. However, for high-risk pregnancies or in breeds prone to dystocia, scheduling an elective cesarean section may provide the lowest maternal and fetal morbidity and mortality rates.
- Oxytocin treatment should be used only if the cervix is open, which can be assessed only by vaginoscopy (p. 1184).
- Dark green vaginal discharge before the delivery of any pups in the bitch is an indication of premature placental separation. The bitch should be evaluated for fetal viability by abdominal ultrasonography and may require a caesarean section to remove viable fetuses.
- Keeping a placenta in the freezer after delivery can be useful if the dam rejects a newborn; it can be thawed out (microwave), allowed to cool, applied to the puppy, and then given to the dam to eat (which she will). Then

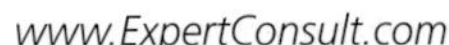

the dam is likely to lick the placenta liquid off the puppy. The placenta cannot be from another litter, however (risks problems such as cannibalism), and this approach works in dogs but not cats.

Prevention

Prevention of pregnancy can be accomplished by medical contraception or surgical sterilization.

Technician Tips

Technicians involved in whelping/queening should be familiar with

- Basic asepsis and hygiene of neonates
- Normal neonatal responses that indicate viability (e.g., rooting and suckling) versus signs of distress (e.g., vocalization)
- Normal maternal behavior
- Neonatal resuscitation

Client Education

For prepartum bitches, the client should monitor the rectal temperature two to three times daily beginning at 56 days after breeding. Rectal temperature decreases by 1°F-2°F (0.5°C-1°C) about 8-12 hours before whelping.

SUGGESTED READING

Beccaglia M, et al: Determination of gestational time and prediction of parturition in dogs and cats: an update. Reprod Domest Anim 51(suppl 1):12-17, 2016.

AUTHOR & EDITOR: Michelle A. Kutzler, DVM, PhD, DACT

Parvoviral Enteritis

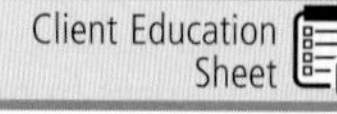

BASIC INFORMATION

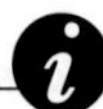

Definition

Viral infection targets small intestinal germinal epithelial cells and bone marrow hematopoietic progenitor cells, resulting in hemorrhagic enteritis, leukopenia, sepsis, and cardiovascular compromise.

Epidemiology

SPECIES, AGE, SEX

- Dogs: greatest risk to unvaccinated puppies between 7 weeks and 12 months of age
- Cats: discussed elsewhere (p. 745).

GENETICS, BREED PREDISPOSITION

Breed-related risks were identified in Doberman pinschers, German shepherds, rottweilers, and American pit bull terriers. Genetic predisposition may be related to variations in cytokine production.

RISK FACTORS

- Inappropriate or absence of vaccination
- Intestinal parasitism, immunosuppressive conditions, poor husbandry, and recent stress contribute to overall disease severity. Dogs receiving anthelmintic therapy are at lower risk of contracting canine parvovirus (CPV).
- Exposure to other dogs, especially in dense housing situation (e.g., shelter environment)

CONTAGION AND ZOONOSIS

- Highly contagious due to viral shedding in feces and persistence of CPV in the environment.
- Feces are infectious as early as 3-4 days after CPV exposure; significant viral shedding continues for approximately 10-14 days.
    - Viral shedding may continue up to 4 weeks after infection; infectivity for other dogs during this extended time is not known.
- Fomites facilitate CPV transmission; avoid contact with contaminated fur or inanimate objects.
- CPV survives in the soil for up to 7 months. Sunlight or drying conditions shorten infectivity, whereas cold weather may prolong it.
- About 23% of healthy dogs shed CPV DNA after routine modified live vaccination; DNA may be detectable in feces using polymerase chain reaction (PCR) for up to 28 days. It is unlikely these dogs pose an infectious threat to other dogs.
- No zoonotic risk

GEOGRAPHY AND SEASONALITY

CPV is distributed worldwide; infections are more common during the warmer months.

ASSOCIATED DISORDERS

- Concurrent intestinal diseases include parasitism (e.g., coccidiosis, helminthiasis, giardiasis), other viral enteritis (e.g., coronavirus, circovirus), and intestinal intussusception, which may occur subsequent to gastrointestinal (GI) hypermotility.
- CPV-induced neutropenia and bacterial translocation predispose to bacterial sepsis.
- Systemic inflammation induces hypercoagulability, which may progress to disseminated intravascular coagulation.
- Myocarditis has been observed in neonatal infection, often preceding GI signs and resulting in peracute death.

Clinical Presentation

DISEASE FORMS/SUBTYPES

- The more virulent strain of CPV (type 2) involves three antigenic variants (2a, 2b, and 2c). Vaccination with CPV2b provides protection against all type 2 variants.
- CPV2b and CPV2c predominate in naturally occurring disease in North America; research has not identified a difference in disease severity or clinical outcome when comparing types 2b and 2c.
- Variation in disease severity among dogs is likely related to age, breed, presence or absence of maternal antibodies, vaccination status, comorbidities, and regional differences in CPV genetic strain.

HISTORY, CHIEF COMPLAINT

Clinical disease occurs 7-14 days after oronasal exposure to CPV-contaminated feces. Nonspecific signs of illness (e.g., lethargy, hyporexia) occur during the peracute phase of disease. Vomiting, diarrhea, generalized weakness and depression occur shortly thereafter. Diarrhea ranges from mucoid to hemorrhagic and is large in volume, frequent, and liquefied.

PHYSICAL EXAM FINDINGS

- Vomiting and diarrhea result in dehydration. Vital signs are consistent with systemic inflammation and include fever, tachycardia, and tachypnea. Severely decompensated dogs may present with bradycardia and hypothermia. Mucous membranes can be injected due to sepsis-induced vasodilation or pale due to hypovolemic shock and/or anemia.
- Ongoing fluid losses lead to depletion of intravascular volume and hypovolemia, detected by abnormal perfusion parameters (e.g., tachycardia, prolonged capillary refill time, weak or absent peripheral pulses, obtundation, low arterial blood pressure, and elevated blood lactate concentration).
- Due to severe enteritis, most dogs display moderate to severe abdominal pain. Abdominal palpation elicits nausea, regurgitation, and discomfort. Intestinal loops palpate distended and fluid filled. Sometimes, intussuscepted bowel segment is palpable. Rectal exam produces (often hemorrhagic) liquid feces.

Etiology and Pathophysiology

- After oronasal exposure and during the incubation period, viral replication occurs

in the lymphoid tissues of the oropharynx, thymus, and regional lymph nodes.
- Marked plasma viremia occurs 1-5 days after infection, allowing viral movement into the small intestinal crypt cells. Necrosis and collapse of these cells impair intestinal function. GI signs cause progressive dehydration, hypovolemia, and blood electrolyte disturbances. The compromised blood-gut barrier results in translocation of gram-negative and anaerobic bacteria from the intestinal lumen into systemic circulation.
- Destruction of other rapidly dividing cells (i.e., hematopoietic progenitor cells in the bone marrow) leads to leukopenia. Profound neutropenia combined with bacteremia leads to sepsis, coagulation disorders, and possible death.

DIAGNOSIS

Diagnostic Overview

- Diagnosis is typically confirmed by point-of-care enzyme-lined immunosorbent assay (ELISA) from feces or rectal swabs, but false-negative results are common (up to 50%). In such cases, PCR has a higher sensitivity for detecting CPV antigen in feces.
- Maintain biosecurity precautions for any young dog displaying clinical signs consistent with CPV. Use serial ELISA testing, PCR testing, and/or exam of clinicopathologic data to verify diagnosis.
- Minimum diagnostics at presentation should include a CPV ELISA point-of-care test, CBC with packed cell volume (PCV) and total solids (TS), and venous blood gas with lactate and electrolyte panel.

Differential Diagnosis

- Other GI infections (viral, bacterial, or parasitic)
- Gastroenteritis
- Mechanical obstruction
- Intussusception
- Intoxication

Initial Database

- CBC: neutropenia due to destruction of myeloblasts and peripheral neutrophil consumption; lymphopenia due to depletion of lymphoid tissue (may be a negative prognostic indicator); anemia related to age, GI hemorrhage, and hemodilution after fluid therapy; thrombocytopenia associated with platelet consumption and coagulation disorders; hypoproteinemia
- Venous blood gas and electrolyte panel: mixed acid-base disturbances are common. Metabolic acidosis may be secondary to hyperlactatemia, pre-renal azotemia, or sodium/bicarbonate loss in diarrhea. Metabolic alkalosis occurs with vomiting of upper GI contents and loss of chloride and/or hypoalbuminemia. Hypokalemia secondary to decreased intake and GI loss can be profound and require aggressive supplementation. Hypomagnesemia can contribute to refractory hypokalemia. Hypoglycemia occurs with a combination of anorexia, sepsis, and/or decreased liver function.
- Blood lactate concentration can be used to guide IV fluid resuscitation and should be used in conjunction with other perfusion parameters, including arterial blood pressure.
- Biochemical profile can be useful to assess kidney and liver function and plasma albumin concentration.
- Urinalysis or urine specific gravity is needed to confirm azotemia as prerenal in origin.
- Abdominal imaging helps exclude other causes of GI signs (e.g., foreign body, intussusception).
- Fecal wet mount and flotation can identify co-infection with intestinal parasites.
- If initial ELISA is negative and parvovirus still suspected, consider PCR of rectal swab or feces or repeat ELISA the next day.
- Puppies that die peracutely should be necropsied.

TREATMENT

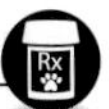

Treatment Overview

Immediate cardiovascular stabilization with IV fluid resuscitation, correction of glucose and electrolyte derangements, initiation of antimicrobials, control of vomiting, and analgesia are paramount.

Acute General Treatment

- IV fluid resuscitation: administer one-fourth to one-half of the calculated blood volume (90 mL/kg) over 15 minutes using an isotonic crystalloid (i.e., Plasma-Lyte A, Normosol-R, lactated Ringer's solution, or 0.9% NaCl) without additives. Smaller aliquots (10-20 mL/kg) of volume can be titrated until cardiovascular parameters normalize.
  - If response is poor, administer hypertonic saline (7.2% NaCl) at a bolus dose of 4 mL/kg IV over 10 minutes. Avoid hypertonic saline in cases of severe dehydration.
  - Alternatively, a colloid (6% hetastarch or VetStarch) can be administered at a bolus dose of 2-5 mL/kg IV over 10 minutes.
- After the patient is normovolemic, transition to maintenance fluid therapy using a balanced isotonic crystalloid. Daily fluid requirements in juvenile dogs depend on age; an adult rate of 60 mL/kg/day is appropriate for pups > 16 weeks, and rates of 80-120 ml/kg/day are more appropriate for younger pups. In addition to the baseline fluid rate, calculate the following:
  - Correct for dehydration (mL to replace = % dehydration × BW_{kg} × 10); provide this volume over the first 24 hours of hospitalization.
  - Estimate ongoing losses (e.g., vomiting, diarrhea), and replace the volume lost (mL) every 6-12 hours. Continue replacing losses throughout hospitalization.
- If hypoglycemic (≤60 mg/dL), administer 50% dextrose (0.5-1 mL/kg) diluted 1 : 2 (central line) or 1 : 4 (peripheral line) with sterile water, and give IV over 3-5 minutes.
  - After the patient is normoglycemic, initiate dextrose by continuous-rate infusion (CRI) by adding 50% dextrose (50 mL of 50% dextrose per 1 L bag = 2.5% solution; 100 mL of 50% dextrose per 1 L bag = 5% solution) to a 1 L bag of isotonic crystalloids, provided at a maintenance fluid rate.
- If severely hypokalemic (≤2.0 mEq/L), begin an IV CRI of potassium chloride (KCl) up to a maximum rate of 0.5 mEq/kg/h. Recheck serum potassium q 2h and continue CRI until serum potassium is ≥ 2.5 mEq/L.
  - Mild to moderate hypokalemia may then be corrected by providing KCl in the maintenance fluids at a dose of 0.1-0.2 mEq/kg/h, as indicated by blood potassium concentrations.
- Administer parenteral, broad-spectrum antimicrobials. Recommended drugs include extended-spectrum penicillins, second-generation cephalosporins, or a penicillin paired with a fluoroquinolone. Examples:
  - Ampicillin-sulbactam 50 mg/kg IV q 8h
  - Cefoxitin 30 mg/kg IV q 6-8h
  - Ampicillin 22 mg/kg IV q 6-8h plus enrofloxacin 10 mg/kg IV q 24h (dilute and infuse slowly; concern for cartilage damage in growing puppies)
- Add metronidazole 7-15 mg/kg IV q 12h to the above for extended anaerobic coverage or profusely hemorrhagic diarrhea.
- Treat nausea and vomiting using at least one of the following antiemetics:
  - Maropitant citrate 1 mg/kg IV q 24h
  - Ondansetron 0.3-0.5 mg/kg IV q 8h or dolasetron 0.5-1 mg/kg IV q 24h
  - Metoclopramide 1-2 mg/kg/24 hours IV CRI
  - Chlorpromazine 0.1-0.5 mg IM q 8h
- Provide analgesia using an opioid as a CRI (i.e., fentanyl 2-5 mcg/kg/h, hydromorphone 0.01-0.05 mg/kg/h, or butorphanol 0.03-0.4 mg/kg/h). For mild cases, buprenorphine 0.01-0.02 IV q 6h is an acceptable alternative.
  - Refractory abdominal pain should prompt further investigation for CPV-related complications (e.g., intussusception).
  - Multimodal analgesia is helpful for enteritis-related discomfort. Add ketamine 2-4 mcg/kg/h or lidocaine 10-30 mcg/kg/min to opioid CRI.
  - Avoid nonsteroidal antiinflammatories due to adverse GI and renal effects.
- Ancillary treatments provided on an individual basis
  - Magnesium supplement as an IV CRI using MgCl or $MgSO_4$ in the maintenance fluids: 0.75 mEq/kg q 24h for hypokalemia that does not respond to KCl supplementation.
  - Prokinetics: metoclopramide 1-2 mg/kg/day IV CRI for persistent regurgitation; anecdotal concern for intestinal

hypermotility and intussusception; determine need for prokinetics based on degree of regurgitation and/or absence of borborygmi.
  - Gastric acid suppressants: pantoprazole 1 mg/kg IV q 12h or famotidine 0.5-1 mg/kg IV q 12h for hematemesis or melena.
  - Parasite control: fenbendazole 50 mg/kg PO q 24h for 3-5 days or sulfadimethoxine 50 mg/kg PO q 24h for 5-20 days as indicated (after vomiting resolved).
  - Colloidal support: synthetic colloids 10-20 mL/kg q 24h or fresh-frozen plasma 10 mL/kg over 4-6 hours in cases of severe hypoalbuminemia with persistent cardiovascular instability. Canine albumin may also be used (0.5-1 g/kg, IV), if available.
  - *N*-acetylcysteine 70 mg/kg IV q 24h consecutively for 5 days has been shown to ameliorate oxidative stress and minimize duration of hospitalization.
  - Recently, fecal microbiota transplantation (p. 1105) was associated with faster resolution of diarrhea.

Chronic Treatment

Limited finances may dictate treating CPV on an outpatient basis. Outpatient success (80% survival) is best achieved with highly compliant owners and when the puppy is briefly stabilized in hospital (e.g., IV fluid resuscitation, supplementation of dextrose and KCl). Recommended outpatient protocol:

- Cefovecin 8 mg/kg SQ once
- Isotonic crystalloid fluids 30 mL/kg SQ q 6h
- Maropitant 1 mg/kg SQ q 24h
- Syringe feed q 6h (see below)
- 60% of outpatient dogs develop hypokalemia; 50% develop hypoglycemia. If electrolytes cannot be monitored on an outpatient basis, provide oral supplementation using potassium gluconate (2 mEq/4.5 kg body weight PO q 6-12h) and high-fructose corn syrup (1-5 mL buccally q 6h).
- Buprenorphine 0.02 mg/kg SQ prn up to q 6h
- External warming to maintain rectal temperature > 37.2°C (99°F)

Nutrition/Diet

- Early enteral nutrition is associated with more rapid clinical improvement in CPV dogs compared with withholding food. Begin nutrition within the first 12-24 hours of hospitalization, ideally through a nasogastric or nasoesophageal tube and with control of vomiting (p. 1107).
- Syringe feeding is an acceptable alternative but may predispose to food aversion and aspiration pneumonia.
- Choose a calorically dense food; options include Hill's Science Diet a/d (1.1 kcal/mL), Royal Canin Recovery Support (1.0 kcal/mL), or Purina ProPlan Critical Nutrition (1.3 kcal/mL).
- Calculate resting energy requirement (RER) based on hydrated body weight (daily kilocalorie requirement = $[BW_{kg} \times 30] + 70$).
  - Begin with one-fourth of the calculated RER on day 1, dividing the daily volume over 4-6 feedings.
  - If tolerated, increase feedings by 25% per day until full RER is attained.
- Supplements aimed at improving GI recovery (e.g., prebiotics, omega 6/3 fatty acids, essential amino acids) may enhance voluntary appetite and caloric intake. The author's institution has used Viyo Recuperation with success (10 mL q 12h if body weight 0-10 kg, 15 mL q 12h if body weight 10-25 kg).
- After voluntary appetite returns, many dogs prefer dry food. Offer dry food staggered with the prescribed diet during hospitalization. Free-choice water should be available at all times.

Possible Complications

- Intestinal intussusception
- Bacterial sepsis, consumptive coagulopathy
- Pneumonia (e.g., aspiration, hematogenous, or opportunistic viral)
- Phlebitis or thrombosis at IV catheter site

Recommended Monitoring

- Every 24 hours: PCV/TS, venous blood gas and electrolyte panel, more frequently for critically ill patients
- Every 12 hours: body weight, arterial blood pressure, more frequently for critically ill patients
- Every 6 hours: vital signs, pain assessment, more frequently for critically ill patients
- CBC and biochemical profile as needed during hospitalization; repeated blood sampling can lead to anemia and hypovolemia in small dogs

PROGNOSIS & OUTCOME

- Prompt diagnosis, hospitalization, and aggressive supportive care result in a high survival rate (≥90%).
- Persistent lymphopenia and elevated C-reactive protein have been associated with mortality in select studies.

PEARLS & CONSIDERATIONS

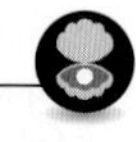

Comments

- False-positive ELISA is unlikely after vaccination.
- Immunotherapies have not been found to significantly influence clinical recovery or survival; the aforementioned cornerstones of therapy remain integral to overall success.

Prevention

Puppies should be vaccinated q 3-4 weeks between the ages of 6 and 16 weeks. Limit susceptible puppy's potential exposure to CPV until fully protected.

Technician Tips

- Central venous catheter placement is helpful for serial blood sampling.
- Evaluate the IV catheter site daily because neutropenia predisposes to secondary infection and phlebitis/cellulitis is commonly observed.

Client Education

- Husbandry considerations include prevention, disinfection, and reducing the risk of transmission.
- Properly disinfect nonporous surfaces using dilute bleach (1 part sodium hypochlorite to 30 parts water) or quaternary ammonium disinfectants; allow ≥ 10 minutes of exposure time. Porous objects should be discarded.
- Although puppies that survive infection have a high level of immunity against CPV, they still require wellness exams and vaccination for other preventable diseases.

SUGGESTED READING

Venn E, et al: Evaluation of an outpatient protocol in the treatment of canine parvoviral enteritis. J Vet Emerg Crit Care 21(7):52-65, 2017.

AUTHOR: Lauren Sullivan, DVM, MS, DACVECC
EDITOR: Benjamin M. Brainard, VMD, DACVAA, DACVECC

Patellar Luxation

Video Available

BASIC INFORMATION

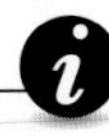

Definition

Medial or lateral displacement of the patella from the femoral trochlear groove is usually a developmental disease. Medial patellar luxation (MPL) is the most common form.

Epidemiology

SPECIES, AGE, SEX

Occurs in dogs and cats of both sexes; onset usually during growth but condition persists throughout life

GENETICS, BREED PREDISPOSITION

- Most common in Newfoundlands and toy and miniature dogs, but occurs in most breeds
- Heritability has been established for many dog breeds.
- Some reports of increased incidence among Maine coon, Persian, Devon rex, and Abyssinian cats

RISK FACTORS

- Varus/valgus deformities of the distal femur or proximal tibia
- Trauma to the bone or soft tissues of the hindlimb or neurogenic muscle contracture
- Previous stifle surgery that included lateral arthrotomy with patellar luxation

ASSOCIATED DISORDERS

- Cranial cruciate ligament instability (present in 15%-42% of stifles with chronic patellar luxation)
- Hip dysplasia (weak association in dogs and cats)

Clinical Presentation

DISEASE FORMS/SUBTYPES

- MPL: the most common form of patellar luxation in cats and dogs of all sizes
- Lateral patellar luxation (LPL): uncommon but seen in dogs of all sizes as well as cats
- Traumatic luxation: uncommon; usually the patella displaces medially after retinacular injury.
- Grading system for degree of luxation
  - Grade 1: patella is in place most of the time and spontaneously reduces if it does luxate.
  - Grade 2: patella moves in and out of the trochlear groove, often with every stride. This is the grade most commonly associated with consistent, painful lameness.
  - Grade 3: patella is luxated all of the time but can be moved back into the trochlear groove by an examiner. This and grade 4 luxation produce a mechanical lameness due to deformity from abnormal joint positioning, but it is not evidently painful.
  - Grade 4: patella is luxated all the time and cannot be manually reduced. Resultant limb malpositioning is severe.

HISTORY, CHIEF COMPLAINT

- Low-grade luxation: transient skipping gait (holding hindlimb flexed and non–weight bearing for a few steps at a time) when walking or running; grade 2 luxation may be associated with a consistent limp.
- High-grade luxation: sustained lameness due to secondary limb deformity
- Weakness in jumping or reluctance to jump
- Acute lameness or increase in lameness in a limb with chronic patellar luxation suggests recent cranial cruciate ligament rupture.

PHYSICAL EXAM FINDINGS

- Patella can be manually displaced into and out of the trochlear groove during flexion and extension with grades 1 and 2 luxations; crepitus may be palpable with grade 2.
- With higher grades, patella may sometimes be palpated medial or lateral to femoral condyle; trochlear groove may be palpable.
- Stifle may flex excessively when bearing weight.
- Animals with MPL may demonstrate genu varum and metatarsal varus (bow-legged and pigeon-toed, respectively) when patella is luxated (see first *Video*)
- Animals with LPL demonstrate genu valgum (walking knock-kneed), with external rotation of the distal limb when the patella is luxated (see second *Video*)

Etiology and Pathophysiology

Skeletal changes are associated with asymmetrical pull of the quadriceps mechanism. Which comes first is unknown because many of the changes in high-grade patellar luxation *result* from the abnormal directional pull of the quadriceps.

- Medial patellar luxation
  - Distal femoral varus/genu varum, external rotation
  - Tibial internal rotation/metatarsal varus
  - Shallow femoral trochlear sulcus
  - Tight, thick medial retinaculum; loose, thin lateral retinaculum
- Lateral patellar luxation
  - Distal femoral valgus/genu valgum, internal rotation
  - External tibial rotation
  - Tight, thick lateral retinaculum; loose, thin medial retinaculum

DIAGNOSIS

Diagnostic Overview

- Diagnosis of patellar luxation is based on physical exam.
- Radiographs may be normal if taken when the patellae are in place, but they are useful for planning surgical intervention and identifying changes with concurrent cranial cruciate ligament rupture. However, interpretation of apparent angular and torsional deformities must be done with caution because natural curvatures of the femur and tibia can give the impression of abnormal conformation, especially if radiographs include a degree of rotational malpositioning.

Differential Diagnosis

- Aseptic necrosis of the femoral head (Legg-Calvé-Perthes disease): young, small dogs only
- Coxofemoral luxation
- Cranial cruciate ligament rupture (often concurrent)
- Osteochondrosis of the lateral femoral condyle
- Immune-mediated polyarthritis
- Lumbosacral compressive disease

Initial Database

- Palpation of the stifle joints (in flexion and extension) for patellar instability and cranial cruciate ligament rupture
- Radiographs
  - Include the hip and/or tarsus to better assess angular and torsional deformities of femur and tibia.
  - Take views with patellae in normal position if possible.
  - Craniocaudal views should be taken with the x-ray beam perpendicular to the thigh because slight variations from the ideal can cause the femurs to appear falsely angled.

Advanced or Confirmatory Testing

- Measurement of varus/valgus angles of femur and tibia
- CT scan with three-dimensional reconstruction

TREATMENT

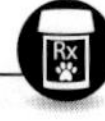

Treatment Overview

- Only animals showing overt clinical signs should have surgery. Patellar luxation produces surprisingly little osteoarthritis, which is typically slow to progress.
- In all but very young puppies and kittens, correction of bone deformities as well as soft-tissue repairs are necessary if surgery is performed. Without bone correction, a soft-tissue repair alone, even if it feels stable on the operating table, usually allows patellar reluxation by 3 weeks after surgery.
- Concurrent cranial cruciate rupture (p. 218) must be addressed during the patellar luxation operation because cruciate ligament

rupture is frequently the chief source of the lameness being treated.

Acute General Treatment

Medical management:

- Nonsteroidal antiinflammatory drugs (NSAIDs) in dogs
  - Carprofen 2 mg/kg PO q 12h, *or*
  - Deracoxib 1-2 mg/kg PO q 24h, *or*
  - Meloxicam 0.1 mg/kg PO q 24h, *or*
  - Grapiprant 2 mg/kg PO q 24h

Physical rehabilitation for mild patellar luxations (grade 1 ± grade 2):

- Exercises to strengthen quadriceps muscle function

Surgical management:

- Soft-tissue reconstruction
  - Imbrication of loose and release of tight pericapsular tissues based on direction of luxation; release of the rectus femoris or sartorius muscle for MPL
  - Derotational suture from fabella to patella or tibial tuberosity
- Trochleoplasty to deepen the femoral trochlear groove
  - Trochlear chondroplasty in immature dogs
  - Abrasion trochleoplasty
  - Block or wedge recession trochleoplasty
- Tibial tuberosity transposition opposite to direction of luxation (very common in dogs, sometimes omitted in cats because it is associated with a higher complication rate)
- Femoral or tibial corrective osteotomies: usually performed when angular deformity is severe (>15° varus for the distal femur in MPL)
- Stifle arthrodesis may be performed as a salvage procedure for severe luxations not amenable to other treatments (more functional in small dogs than large ones).
- Concurrent cranial cruciate ligament rupture should be treated along with the MPL; osteotomy techniques such as tibial plateau leveling osteotomy (TPLO) or tibial tuberosity advancement (TTA) can be modified so that the tibial osteotomy also transposes the tibial tuberosity.

Chronic Treatment

- Same as in acute cases but may require long-term medical management for the treatment of osteoarthritis
- Disease-modifying agents
  - Polysulfated glycosaminoglycan 4-5 mg/kg IM once to twice weekly for 4-6 weeks
  - Pentosan polysulfate 3 mg/kg SQ once weekly; 10 mg/kg PO or SQ weekly up to 4 weeks
  - Oral formulations (glucosamine, chondroitin sulfate, avocado soy unsaponifiables): according to labeled instructions

Nutrition/Diet

Weight control (p. 1077)

Possible Complications

Medical management:

- Gastrointestinal, hepatic, renal, or other systemic reactions to NSAIDs
- Continued progression of degenerative joint disease
- Failure of medical management to control pain

Surgical management:

- Patellar reluxation (occurs in 10%-30% of cases, especially in dogs when tibial tuberosity transposition has not been done)
- Implant failure/tibial tuberosity avulsion

Recommended Monitoring

- Laboratory monitoring of animals on NSAID therapy
- Weight, exercise levels, and clinical signs as dictated by the patient's condition
- Postoperative rehabilitation enhances clinical recovery.

PROGNOSIS & OUTCOME

- Generally good to excellent for return to normal limb function if appropriate techniques are used
- Degenerative joint disease progresses (radiographically, not necessarily symptomatically) despite treatment.

PEARLS & CONSIDERATIONS

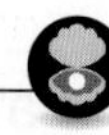

Comments

- Severity of lameness may not correlate with grade of patellar luxation. Animals with grade 2 luxation are often the most painful because their patellae are repeatedly grinding across the trochlear ridges. Animals with higher-grade luxations are not painful but are instead impeded by joint misalignment.
- Patellar luxation is usually a developmental condition, and the grade of luxation may increase as the animal matures.
- In bilateral luxations, the grade of patellar instability may differ between stifles.
- Soft-tissue stabilization techniques alone are not sufficient to stabilize moderate or severe luxations.
- Block or wedge trochleoplasty is the preferred method to deepen the femoral trochlear groove because it preserves the articular cartilage.
- In older animals with chronic patellar instability and acutely worsening lameness, concomitant cranial cruciate ligament rupture is likely.

Prevention

Screening and control of breeding animals for prevention of patellar luxation

Technician Tips

To take straight craniocaudal views of the femur, image only one limb at a time. Hold the dog in a sitting position, or angle the beam so that it is perpendicular to the femur. Do not allow the stifle to splay laterally.

SUGGESTED READING

Kowaleski MP, et al: Stifle joint. In Johnston SA, et al, editors: Veterinary surgery small animal, St. Louis, 2018, Elsevier, pp 1141-1159.

AUTHOR & EDITOR: **Kathleen Linn, DVM, MS, DACVS**

Patent Ductus Arteriosus

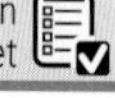

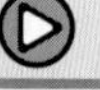

BASIC INFORMATION

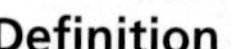

Definition

An arterial shunt between the aorta and pulmonary artery is normally present in fetuses but should constrict and close within 24 hours after birth. Patency (incomplete closure) results in a channel, the diameter of which determines the amount and direction of blood flow through the shunt and the impact on the patient. It is the most common congenital heart defect in dogs, occurring in 1 of 1000.

Synonym

PDA

Epidemiology

SPECIES, AGE, SEX

- All species, but much less common in cats
- Recognized most frequently in young animals
- Moderate predominance in females

GENETICS, BREED PREDISPOSITION

Sporadic or hereditable defect occurring most frequently in small, relatively nonmuscular dog breeds such as Maltese, Pomeranians, Yorkshire terriers, Shetland sheepdogs, and toy and miniature poodles

RISK FACTORS

In-breeding

GEOGRAPHY AND SEASONALITY

Breed predispositions may vary due to regional differences in the gene pool.

ASSOCIATED DISORDERS

- Arrhythmias
- Congestive heart failure (CHF)
- Pulmonary hypertension
- Erythrocytosis (right-to-left shunting PDA)

Clinical Presentation

DISEASE FORMS/SUBTYPES

- Clinical/gross classification: type 1 = small PDA, type 2 = medium PDA, type 3A = large PDA, type 3B = large PDA with CHF, type 4 = large PDA with pulmonary hypertension and right-to-left or bidirectional shunt
- Angiographic classification of PDA morphology: type 1 (5%) = gradual tapering from aorta to pulmonary artery, type IIa (most common, 54%) = gradual tapering from aorta to pulmonary artery plus abrupt taper at pulmonary artery insertion, type IIb (32.5%) = parallel walls of PDA plus abrupt tapering at pulmonary arterial insertion, type III (8%) = walls of PDA are parallel for the length of the PDA (tubular)

HISTORY, CHIEF COMPLAINT

- Varies with PDA diameter and age
- Most often recognized as an incidental heart murmur in a young animal presented for vaccination and not showing overt clinical signs
- When clinical signs are present, they include exercise intolerance, failure to thrive, and signs of CHF (p. 408).

PHYSICAL EXAM FINDINGS

Varies with PDA diameter (see classification systems above)

- Type 1, small: characteristic focal continuous murmur at left heart base
- Type 2, medium: type 1 signs plus continuous murmur audible at apex and precordial thrill at left heart base
- Type 3A, large: types 1 and 2 signs plus bounding pulses, prominent cardiac impulse at left apex, and systolic murmur of mitral regurgitation at left apex
- Type 3B, large with CHF: types 1, 2, and 3A signs and signs of CHF (e.g., dyspnea, pulmonary crackles, ascites [occasionally]); arrhythmias, especially atrial fibrillation, possible
- Type 4, large PDA with pulmonary hypertension: no heart murmur; prominent right apical impulse, split second heart sound, caudal cyanosis (differential cyanosis), hindlimb collapse with exercise

Etiology and Pathophysiology

- The principal cause of PDA in dogs is site-specific hypoplasia of ductus smooth muscle, coupled with reciprocal excess elastic tissue in the wall of the ductus. To varying degrees, the hypoplastic smooth muscle does not encircle the lumen, and muscle contraction does not completely constrict the lumen postpartum.
- Typically, pulmonary vascular resistance decreases after birth and postnatal blood flow through the PDA is from the aorta to the pulmonary artery (left-to-right type), causing increased flow through the pulmonary circulation, left atrium, left ventricle, and ascending aorta, resulting in enlargement of these chambers and left ventricular hypertrophy (eccentric). Established left-to-right types rarely develop enough pulmonary hypertension to cause reversed PDA flow (right-to-left type).
- In animals with a large PDA and pulmonary hypertension (type 4, persistent fetal circulation), there is right ventricular hypertrophy, and blood flows through the ductus predominantly from the pulmonary artery to the aorta (as in the fetus), resulting in caudal cyanosis and secondary erythrocytosis.

DIAGNOSIS

Diagnostic Overview

The diagnosis is made easily by auscultating a continuous murmur over the left heart base (types 1-3) and palpating a precordial thrill (types 2 and 3). Chest radiographs reveal the degree of cardiomegaly and the urgency of PDA closure.

Differential Diagnosis

- Combined abnormalities producing systolic and diastolic heart murmurs such as a ventricular septal defect and aortic insufficiency due to an unsupported aortic valve leaflet
- Aorticopulmonary window
- Arteriovenous fistula

Initial Database

- Thoracic radiographs to assess heart and lung vessel size and lung parenchyma
- Electrocardiogram (p. 1096) to identify cardiac arrhythmias and findings supportive of ventricular hypertrophy
- Packed cell volume (PCV) to determine presence of anemia or erythrocytosis

Advanced or Confirmatory Testing

- Two-dimensional echocardiography (p. 1094) to determine chamber sizes, wall thickness, systolic ventricular function, presence of any concurrent cardiac defects, and an approximate measurement of ductal diameter in anticipation of device-based surgical closure
- Color Doppler echocardiography to verify turbulent blood flow in the pulmonary artery
- Spectral Doppler echocardiography to determine flow velocity in the PDA and estimate the aorta/pulmonary artery pressure gradient. If tricuspid or pulmonic insufficiencies are present, respective estimates of right ventricular systolic and pulmonary artery diastolic pressures can be made.

TREATMENT

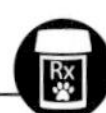

Treatment Overview

PDA closure is recommended for all left-to-right cases (types 1-3) but contraindicated in right-to-left cases (type 4). In type 4 cases, phlebotomy and/or chemotherapy is used to reduce and maintain hematocrit at 60%-65%, which improves blood flow characteristics.

Acute General Treatment

- Type 3B: for large PDA, preoperative diuretic and cage rest to alleviate CHF and then closure of PDA are indicated.
- Types 1-3: surgery or transarterial coil or Amplatz duct occluder to occlude PDA (see *Video*)
- Type 4: phlebotomy to reduce erythrocytosis. Goal is PCV of 60%-65%; volume removed varies, but 10 to 15 mL/kg (with or without crystalloid volume replacement) is reasonable initially.

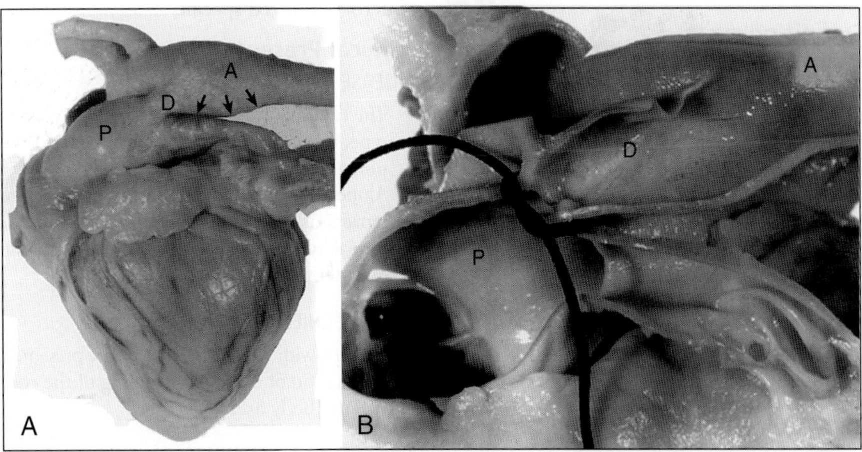

PATENT DUCTUS ARTERIOSUS A, Postmortem photograph of the heart, aorta *(A)*, and pulmonary artery *(P)* of a 4-month-old dog with a PDA *(D)* and ductal-aortic aneurysm *(arrows)*. **B**, Sagittal section photograph of the great vessels and a ligature demonstrates PDA ligation at surgery (thoracotomy). Most of the PDA lies within the wall of the aorta in dogs and constitutes a ductal-aortic aneurysm commonly referred to as a *ductus diverticulum*. The typical ridge at the pulmonary artery opening (at the level of the ligature in this image) limits PDA diameter and determines blood flow through the PDA.

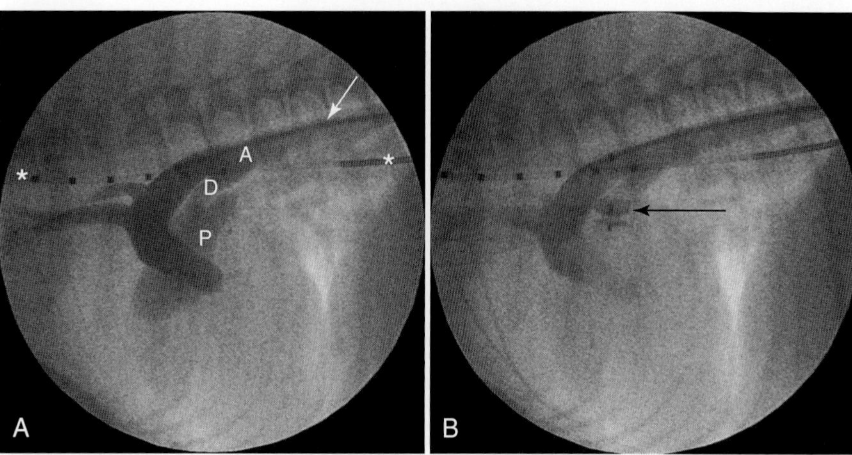

PATENT DUCTUS ARTERIOSUS Aortic injection angiograms in a dog with PDA before (**A**) and after (**B**) PDA occlusion with a canine ductal occluder by a catheter-based (minimally invasive) approach. **A,** An injection of contrast through a catheter in the aorta *(arrow)* opacifies the aorta *(A)*, PDA *(D)*, and pulmonary arteries *(P)*, demonstrating patency of the ductus. A measuring catheter *(asterisks)* is placed in the esophagus for scale (1-cm markers). **B,** The ductal occluder *(arrow)* has been deployed, and an aortic injection demonstrates absence of flow through the PDA. (Image courtesy Dr. Etienne Côté, copyright 2013.)

Chronic Treatment

Type 4:

- Sildenafil 1-2 mg/kg q 8h may reduce severity of pulmonary hypertension and therefore right-to-left shunting (pp. 838 and 1274).
- Hydroxyurea to suppress erythrocytosis at the bone marrow level 25-30 mg/kg PO every other day; titrated downward as needed based on resulting hematocrit

Possible Complications

- Uncontrolled (type 1-3): refractory CHF, refractory arrhythmias
- Uncontrolled (type 4): complications caused by hyperviscosity (p. 509)
- Pulmonary artery dissection may be a rare complication of uncorrected PDA in dogs. Closure of the duct appears to improve outcome.
- Iatrogenic: surgical hemorrhage, occlusion device embolization into the aorta or a pulmonary artery branch, hematoma at arteriotomy site

PROGNOSIS & OUTCOME

- Types 1-3A: 90%-98% successful correction with experienced interventionalist/surgeon. After correction, most will live a normal life span.
- Type 3B: 98% initially successful if heart failure and arrhythmia are controlled preoperatively and can live for years but life span is usually shortened
- Type 4: may live for years if erythrocytosis is controlled

PEARLS & CONSIDERATIONS

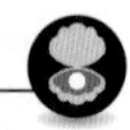

Prevention

Avoid breeding affected animals.

Technician Tips

PDA closure confers an important survival benefit for affected animals, with similar results whether the procedure is performed with a thoracotomy or minimally invasive approach.

SUGGESTED READING

Buchanan JW: Patent ductus arteriosus: morphology, pathogenesis, types and treatment. J Vet Cardiol 3:7-16, 2001.

AUTHOR: James W. Buchanan, DVM, M Med Sci, DACVIM
EDITOR: Meg M. Sleeper, VMD, DACVIM

Pattern Alopecia, Canine

BASIC INFORMATION

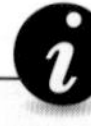

Definition

Canine pattern alopecia (CPA) is a relatively common, likely heritable, noninflammatory alopecic disorder of specific breeds. It encompasses several distinct syndromes.

Synonyms

CPA, canine pattern baldness

Epidemiology

SPECIES, AGE, SEX

- Dogs of either sex and of any reproductive status
- Early onset (usually < 1 year of age)

GENETICS, BREED PREDISPOSITION

- CPA, ventral type, is seen in dogs with fine, short coats such as dachshunds, Chihuahuas, miniature pinschers, whippets, greyhounds, Boston terriers, and boxers.
- CPA, pinnal type, is seen mainly in dachshunds.
- Alopecia and melanoderma of Yorkshire terriers is breed specific.

Clinical Presentation

DISEASE FORMS/SUBTYPES

- The two main forms of CPA are the ventral type, the most common syndrome, and the pinnal type.
- Alopecia and melanoderma of Yorkshire terriers is clinically very similar to CPA, pinnal type, and it is most likely the same disorder.

HISTORY, CHIEF COMPLAINT

Dogs born with a normal hair coat are presented for evaluation of a gradual thinning of the coat in specific body areas.

PHYSICAL EXAM FINDINGS

- CPA, ventral type: progressive alopecia developing along the ventral neck, thorax, abdomen, caudomedial aspect of thighs, perineum, and postauricular regions (base of the ear pinnae)
- CPA, pinnal type: progressive alopecia of the convex aspect of the ear pinnae, starting around 6 months of age. Alopecia of the bridge of the nose also can occur.
- Alopecia and melanoderma of Yorkshire terriers: alopecia and hyperpigmentation of the convex aspect of the ear pinnae and the bridge of the nose

Etiology and Pathophysiology

CPA may be an overshoot reaction to artificial selection pressure favoring the fine, delicate coat sought by breeders. Over past decades, smooth-hair dachshund breeders have been able to markedly decrease the incidence of CPA, ventral type, by selective breeding, but as a result, dogs generally have a coarser haircoat.

DIAGNOSIS

Diagnostic Overview

The diagnosis is based on history, dermatologic exam, and exclusion of endocrinopathies and inflammatory diseases such as alopecia areata.

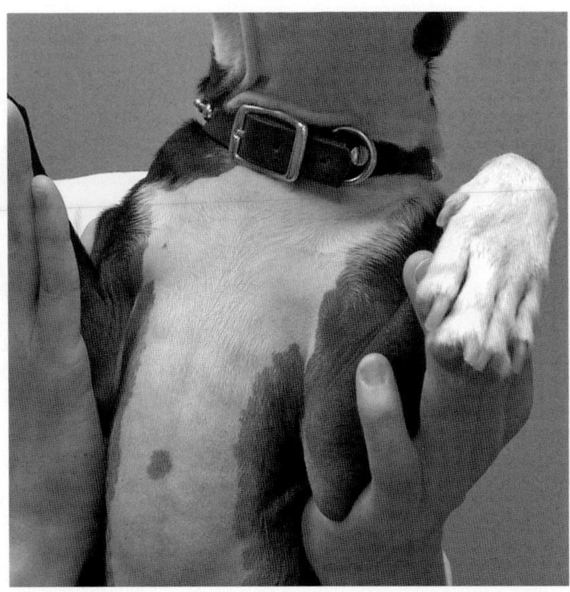

PATTERN ALOPECIA, CANINE Pattern alopecia (ventral type) in a 2-year-old neutered male Boston terrier. Note loss of hair and lack of signs of inflammation on the ventral neck and thorax. (Copyright Dr. Manon Paradis.)

The early onset, breed predisposition, and absence of inflammation and pruritus are distinctive.

Differential Diagnosis

- Endocrinopathies (hypothyroidism, hyperadrenocorticism, hyperestrogenism)
- Follicular dysplasias
- Alopecia areata
- Infectious process (pyoderma, demodicosis, dermatophytosis) in some clinical presentations

Initial Database

- History and physical exam findings are generally sufficient.
- Ruling out other differentials may involve thyroid testing, adrenal function testing, and dermatologic diagnostic tests such as skin scraping based on lesion distribution and appearance.

Advanced or Confirmatory Testing

Skin biopsies: changes are characterized by miniaturization of anagen hair follicles. Biopsies are rarely performed because biopsy at affected sites often requires general anesthesia, biopsy healing may lead to permanent visible scarring, and histopathologic changes can be subtle and wrongly suggest endocrinopathies.

TREATMENT

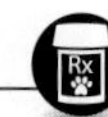

Treatment Overview

The goal is to try to promote hair regrowth if this is the desire of the owner; it may protect the dog from cold climate.

Acute and Chronic Treatment

Anecdotal evidence exists for the efficacy of melatonin (3-6 mg/DOG PO q 8-12h for 2 months) to stimulate hair growth. Improvement, if any, should occur within 2 to 3 months.

PROGNOSIS & OUTCOME

- Dogs affected by this genetically based dermatosis are healthy otherwise.
- It is not known whether dogs initially responding to melatonin will eventually become refractory to this form of treatment.

PEARLS & CONSIDERATIONS

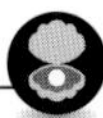

Comments

The early-onset, pattern-linked alopecia and breed predisposition make the diagnosis straightforward in many cases.

Technician Tips

The main impact of this disorder is cosmetic rather than medical.

SUGGESTED READING

Paradis M: Canine pattern alopecia. In Mecklenburg L, et al, editors: Hair loss disorders in domestic animals, Ames, IA, 2009, Wiley-Blackwell, p 164.

AUTHOR & EDITOR: Manon Paradis, DMV, MVSc, DACVD

Pediculosis

BASIC INFORMATION

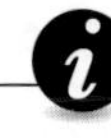

Definition

Louse infestation

Epidemiology

SPECIES, AGE, SEX

Affects dogs and cats of any age, with young patients predisposed

RISK FACTORS

Dogs: frequent contact with other dogs (grooming, day care), neglect, overcrowding

CONTAGION AND ZOONOSIS

- Contagious to same species only; not zoonotic
- Transmitted by direct contact, grooming instruments, premises

GEOGRAPHY AND SEASONALITY

- Possibly more common in winter
- Rare in many parts of the world (especially areas where flea control is routinely practiced) but common in other regions (e.g., canine sucking lice in Western Canada)

ASSOCIATED DISORDERS

- Anemia, debilitation (puppies)
- See Physical Exam Findings

Clinical Presentation

DISEASE FORMS/SUBTYPES

Chewing versus sucking lice: differentiate by microscopy; broad head on chewing lice; slender, tapered head on sucking lice

HISTORY, CHIEF COMPLAINT

- Pruritus may be severe and affect several animals. Often, no history of skin disease
- Lice or nits (small, white ova) are often noticed by owners or groomers.
- Weakness (puppies with sucking lice)

PHYSICAL EXAM FINDINGS

- Unless parasites are seen, exam findings are nonspecific. Lice are smaller than fleas but visible to the naked eye. They accumulate around ears and body openings. Detection is difficult if numbers are low. Nits are often seen attached to hair. In some cases, excoriations, scaling, matted hair, alopecia, and other findings:

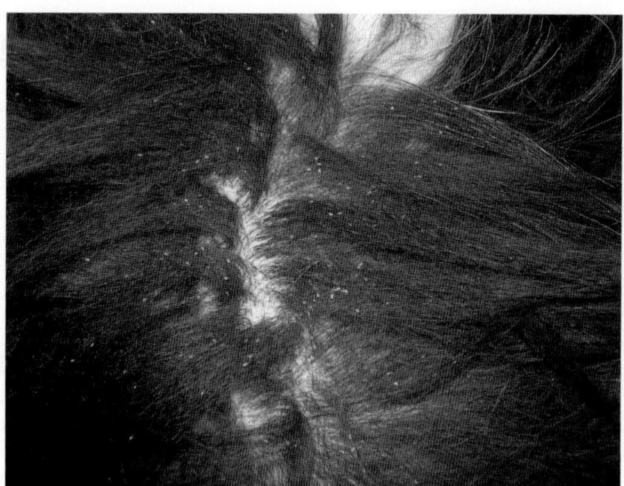

PEDICULOSIS Louse nits attached to hairs on a black dog. (Courtesy Dr. Kinga Gortel)

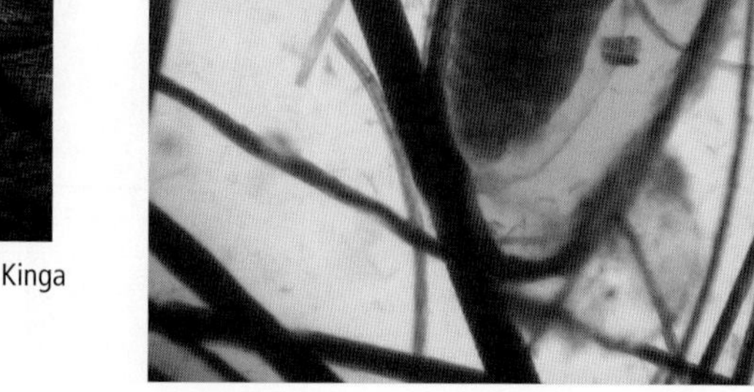

PEDICULOSIS Microscopic exam of dog hair with attached louse nit. (Courtesy Dr. Kinga Gortel.)

    - In dogs, secondary pyoderma and pyotraumatic dermatitis (hot spots)
    - In cats, miliary dermatitis
- Occasionally, weakness, pale mucous membranes in puppies (sucking lice)

Etiology and Pathophysiology

- Infestation by insects of the suborder Anoplura (sucking lice, which feed on blood) or Mallophaga (chewing or biting lice, which feed on skin debris and hair)
- Dogs: sucking louse *Linognathus setosus* and chewing louse *Trichodectes canis*
- Cats: chewing louse *Felicola subrostratus*
- Rarely, other louse species
- Lice have a 2- to 3-week life cycle spent entirely on the host and survive only a short period off host.
- Lice may be capable of transmission of *Bartonella* and *Rickettsia* spp in some animals, but their importance as vectors for dogs and cats is not known.
- *T. canis* can act as the intermediate host of the tapeworm, *Dipylidium caninum*.

DIAGNOSIS

Diagnostic Overview

The diagnosis is confirmed by finding lice or nits on physical and microscopic examination.

Differential Diagnosis

- Other ectoparasite infestations, particularly fleas, *Sarcoptes*, *Cheyletiella*
- Various hypersensitivity disorders

Initial Database

Attempt to find and identify ectoparasites, including lice, in pruritic cats and dogs (p. 1091).

- Thorough direct examination of skin and hair can reveal lice and nits. This is aided by adequate lighting and magnification (if available). Suspect material is transferred to microscope slide with a drop of mineral oil and examined at low magnification:
    - Clear tape can be used to pick up parasites and nits
    - Hair can be plucked or clipped from suspected areas because nits are firmly adhered to hairs.
- Hair and surface samples can be collected using a flea comb and similarly examined.

Advanced or Confirmatory Testing

Response to therapy can be used but is not specific for pediculosis.

TREATMENT

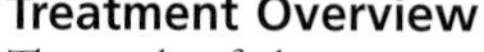

Treatment Overview

The goals of therapy are eradication of lice from the patient and in-contact animals and amelioration of associated clinical signs.

Acute General Treatment

- Treat the affected pet and same-species, in-contact animals.
- Wash the premises, bedding, collars, and grooming equipment at least once.
- Clip matted hair.
- Bathe the pet, unless debilitated, to remove lice.
- Treat secondary pyoderma (p. 851).
- Pruritus is reduced in 2-4 weeks. If severe, consider extralabel coadministration of antipruritic therapy such as oclacitinib (adult dogs) or antiinflammatory doses of corticosteroids (dogs or cats).
- Lice succumb to many insecticidal agents. Nits are more resistant, and repeated treatment after 2-4 weeks is needed for products without residual efficacy.
- In many countries, imidacloprid-containing products are labeled for canine pediculosis. Most other commonly used treatments are used extralabel.
- Treatments considered effective for lice include
    - Imidacloprid and imidacloprid + permethrin spot-ons; labeled in some countries
    - Selamectin and fipronil spot-ons
    - Various pyrethrin, carbamate, lime sulfur, and (for dogs only) permethrin preparations
    - Isoxazoline drugs: reports of success, anecdotal at this time
    - Ivermectin is not recommended due to safety concerns.
- Follow-up is recommended to ensure complete eradication of lice. Treatment failures are sometimes seen.
- In weak, anemic puppies, additional supportive care (including blood transfusion) as needed

Recommended Monitoring

Recheck patients after 4-6 weeks.

PROGNOSIS & OUTCOME

The prognosis, with the exception of severely anemic or debilitated animals, is excellent.

PEARLS & CONSIDERATIONS

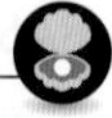

Comments

- Nits attached to hairs may be mistaken for skin scales but are of uniform size and almost impossible to remove from hair shafts. They are harder to see on light-colored hair.
- Close examination with a good light source is key.
- Consider treatment trial if history is suggestive.

Prevention

Because pets regularly receiving flea control products are less likely to contract lice, protection should be considered in lice-endemic areas.

Technician Tips

- Clients become understandably concerned about a diagnosis of lice in their pet. They may inquire whether a household pet could be the source of a human infestation (no). Counsel clients about the highly host-specific nature of this parasite.
- Stress the importance of follow-up to assess efficacy because treatment failures are possible.

SUGGESTED READING

Miller WH Jr, et al, editors: Muller & Kirk's Small animal dermatology, St. Louis, 2013, Mosby, pp 320-322.

AUTHOR: Kinga Gortel, DVM, MS, DACVD
EDITOR: Manon Paradis, DMV, MVSc, DACVD

Pemphigus Complex

Bonus Material Online 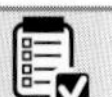 Client Education Sheet

BASIC INFORMATION 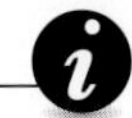

Definition

The pemphigus complex is a group of autoimmune skin diseases characterized by acantholysis. The two major subsets are pemphigus foliaceus (PF) (most common) and pemphigus vulgaris (PV). Rare variants are pemphigus vegetans (PVeg), paraneoplastic pemphigus (PNP), and pemphigus erythematosus (PE). Spontaneous, drug-induced, and paraneoplastic forms are reported.

Epidemiology

SPECIES, AGE, SEX

Dogs and cats; PF is the most common autoimmune skin disease, typically affecting middle-aged animals (range, 0.5-16 years)

GENETICS, BREED PREDISPOSITION

- PF: Akita, chow chow, and many other breeds (drug-induced PF in Doberman pinscher and Labrador retriever)
- PE: collie and German shepherd

RISK FACTORS

PF and PE may be aggravated by sunlight. Some cases of pemphigus are triggered by drug reactions. PF cases in dogs after various topical ectoparasiticides have been well documented. Chronic skin disease may be a risk factor. PNP in dogs has been associated with underlying lymphoma, thymoma, and Sertoli cell tumor.

GEOGRAPHY AND SEASONALITY

Prevalence of PF appears higher in warmer regions. Seasonal exacerbation of lesions may occur during months of increased sunlight exposure.

Clinical Presentation

DISEASE FORMS/SUBTYPES

Subsets of pemphigus, in decreasing order of frequency:

- Superficial pemphigus complex: PF, PE (possible local and milder variant of PF), panepidermal pustular pemphigus (PPP; possibly a more extensive subtype of PF)
- Deep variants: PV, PVeg, and PNP

HISTORY, CHIEF COMPLAINT

- PF: progressive multifocal or generalized skin disease, often with facial and footpad involvement. Degree of pain is variable. Pruritus occurs in 30%-50% of the cases. The initial complaint can be lameness due to footpad disease.
- PV, PNP: intraoral lesions are common, and presenting signs include hypersalivation, halitosis, anorexia, and weight loss.
- Fever, anorexia, lethargy, and limb edema are reported in severe cases of pemphigus.

PHYSICAL EXAM FINDINGS

- PF: a pustular and crusting dermatitis, with crusts on the trunk and/or the facial area being the most common lesion. Concave pinnae and dorsal muzzle are often the first areas affected, and the disease can stay restricted to the head and face. Other commonly involved areas are the footpads and nail beds (nail beds often affected in cats; sometimes the only physical exam abnormality). The disease progresses and becomes multifocal or generalized in most cases. Range of lesions noted includes erythema; pustules; dry, honey-colored crusts; scales; alopecia; and erosions bordered by collarettes. Secondary bacterial pyoderma (≈one-third of PF cases) and peripheral lymphadenopathy are common.
- PE: a milder form of PF with crusts, erosions, alopecia, and scales restricted to the face

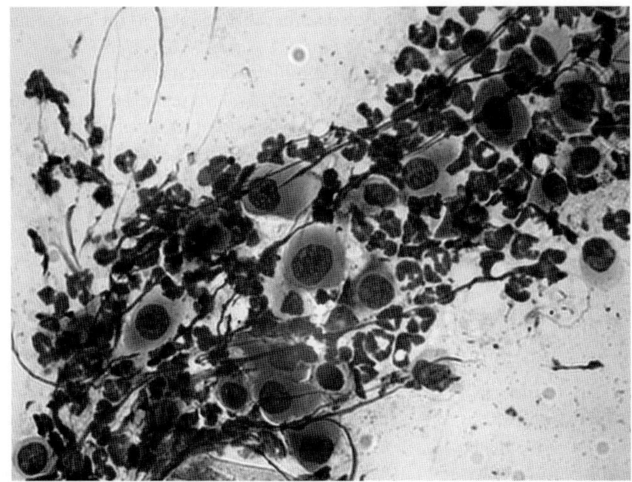

PEMPHIGUS COMPLEX Impression smear of a pustule from a dog with pemphigus foliaceus shows numerous acantholytic keratinocytes and neutrophils. (Courtesy Dr. Manon Paradis.)

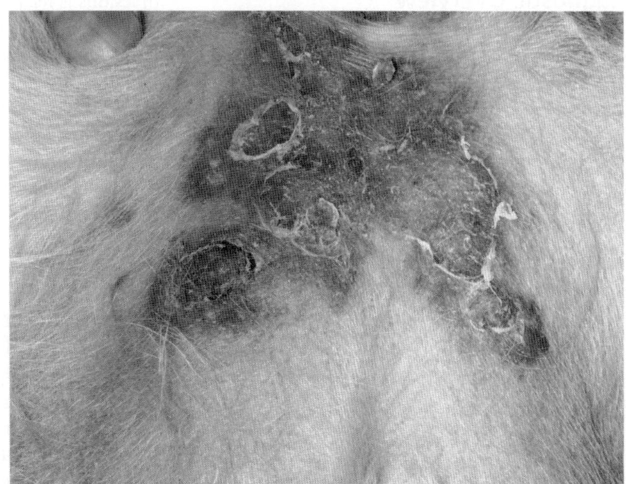

PEMPHIGUS COMPLEX Pemphigus foliaceus in 4-year-old Bichon frisé: close-up view of typical lesions on the abdomen. Note pustules, epidermal collarettes, and honey-colored crusts. (Courtesy Dr. Caroline de Jaham.)

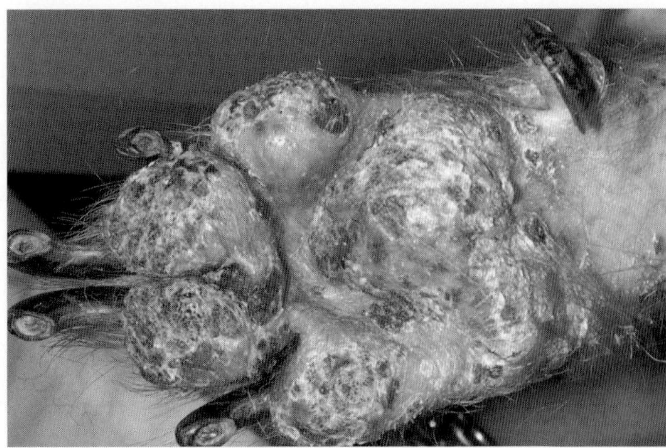

PEMPHIGUS COMPLEX Pemphigus foliaceus in 7-year-old terrier cross: close-up view of lesions affecting the feet (pododermatitis). Note almost complete loss of normal footpad architecture. (Courtesy Dr. Caroline de Jaham.)

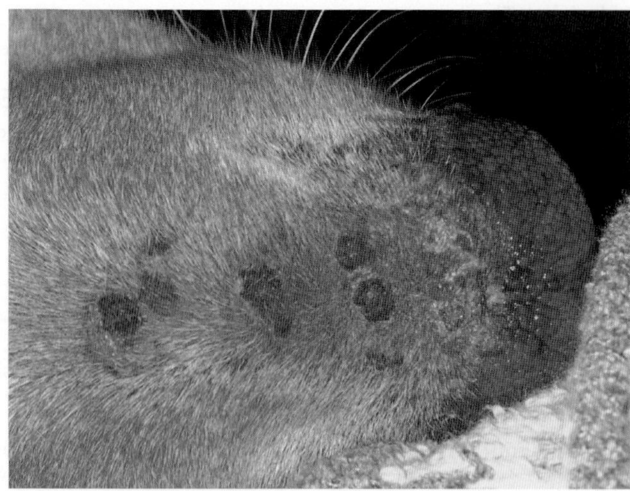

PEMPHIGUS COMPLEX Pemphigus erythematosus in 3-year-old collie. Note superficial erosions and crusts on bridge of nose. Depigmentation of the nasal planum is also observed. (Courtesy Dr. Caroline de Jaham.)

- PV: a deep and severe form of pemphigus presenting with transient, flaccid vesiculopustules that are rapidly replaced by large erosions and ulcers of the mucosal surfaces and mucocutaneous junctions. Affected areas include oral cavity (>70% of cases), concave pinnae, nasal planum, lip margins, genitalia, and anus. Erosions of the nail beds are reported in 14% of cases. A milder form of PV is reported where lesions are restricted to one body area (e.g., nail beds, nasal planum, oral cavity).
- PVeg and PPP: severe erosions and ulcerations of the oral cavity, nose, vulva, and haired skin

Etiology and Pathophysiology

Intraepithelial acantholysis (loss of intercellular cohesion between keratinocytes) leads to vesicles/pustules formation due to autoantibodies (IgG) binding to components of desmosome complex.

DIAGNOSIS

Diagnostic Overview

The diagnosis of PF, the most common form of pemphigus, is suspected in a dog or cat presented for evaluation of a bilaterally symmetrical, progressive, crusting, and pustular dermatitis that does not typically respond to appropriate systemic antibiotic therapy. The definitive diagnosis requires skin biopsies showing histopathologic changes of acantholysis.

Differential Diagnosis

- PF, PE, and PNP: bacterial folliculitis, demodicosis, dermatophytosis, eosinophilic folliculitis and furunculosis, cornification disorders, cutaneous (discoid) and systemic lupus erythematosus, leishmaniosis, drug eruptions
- PV and PPP: bullous pemphigoid, epidermolysis bullosa acquisita, erythema multiforme, toxic epidermal necrolysis, Stevens-Johnson syndrome, epitheliotropic lymphoma, ulcerative stomatitis, vesicular cutaneous lupus erythematosus, mucocutaneous lupus erythematosus, systemic lupus erythematosus

Initial Database

- Cytologic exam of content of intact pustules or exudate under a crust may strongly suggest pemphigus. Intact neutrophils, various numbers of eosinophils, and clusters of acantholytic keratinocytes can be seen in most cases, but skin biopsies are still required because other disorders may have similar findings.
- CBC, serum biochemistry profile: nonspecific changes, mild to moderate leukocytosis with neutrophilia, mild nonregenerative anemia, and hypoalbuminemia

Advanced or Confirmatory Testing

- Skin biopsies: confirmatory test. Histopathologic findings of acantholysis with pustule formation are diagnostic. Epidermal location of lesions is related to depth of autoantibody deposition: subcorneal and intragranular layers in PF and PE, suprabasilar level in PV and PPP, and panepithelial in PNP.
- Immunohistochemical and immunofluorescent analysis of skin biopsies or serum may be helpful but depends on the sensitivity of the methods being used; not routinely performed.

TREATMENT

Treatment Overview

The treatment goal is to implement immunosuppressive therapy after a firm diagnosis of pemphigus is made that can induce and maintain remission of skin lesions without significant or life quality–altering side effects. This is best achieved by using combination drug therapy. The therapeutic modalities and response to treatment vary with the type of pemphigus and the species treated. Cases refractory to initial systemic glucocorticoids should be referred to a dermatologist.

Acute General Treatment

Systemic glucocorticoids alone induce remission in most cases of PE and in one-third of cases of PF in dogs and most cats. Other forms of pemphigus are more refractory. Response should be seen within 10-14 days.

- Dogs (initially): prednisone/prednisolone 2-4 mg/kg PO q 24h; these drugs can also be used as high-dose pulse therapy (e.g., 10 mg/kg PO q 24h for 3 consecutive days followed by reduced daily dosage [<2 mg/kg]).
- Cats (initially)
  - Prednisolone 2-4 mg/kg PO q 24h, *or*
  - Dexamethasone 0.2-0.4 mg/kg PO q 24h, *or*
  - Triamcinolone 1-2 mg/kg PO q 24h

Chronic Treatment

- Maintenance dosages of drugs are the lowest doses that result in a stable degree of disease that is acceptable to the owner and clinician.
- When combinations of medications are used, the first ones to be tapered are those with the greater likelihood of adverse effects.
- The glucocorticoid dosage is slowly reduced on a daily basis over 30-40 days after remission of active skin lesions is attained (2-4 weeks). Lowering to an alternate-day regimen with an ideal maintenance dose of 1 mg/kg q 48h of prednisone/prednisolone or less is the ultimate goal.
- Concurrent immunosuppressive drugs are used in conjunction with glucocorticoids (initially or added later) to achieve and maintain remission with fewest/no glucocorticoid adverse effects.
  - Azathioprine 2.2 mg/kg PO q 24-48h in conjunction with prednisone/prednisolone; first choice in dogs, contraindicated in cats, *or*

- Cyclosporine 5-10 mg/kg PO q 24h with glucocorticoids for PF; first choice in cats, *or*
- Chlorambucil 0.1-0.2 mg/kg PO q 24-48h in conjunction with prednisolone (cats), *or*
- Mycophenolate mofetil 15 mg/kg PO q 12h with prednisone/prednisolone; more recent promising option, potentially less myelotoxicity/hepatotoxicity than azathioprine
- Alternative immunosuppressive drugs
  - Tetracycline and niacinamide: milder or localized cases of PF and PE (250 mg of each PO q 8h for dogs < 10 kg; 500 mg of each PO q 8h for dogs > 10 kg) for 2-3 months to achieve remission, then gradually decrease to q 12-24h or alternate days if remission is maintained
- Topical therapy is indicated as a sole treatment for some localized forms of PF and PE and in conjunction with systemic therapy for persistent focal lesions that remain active despite satisfactory control of the overall disease. Person applying treatment must wear gloves.
  - Potent topical glucocorticoid initially: fluocinolone acetonide, triamcinolone, betamethasone valerate; when adequate response, treatment is changed to 1%-2% hydrocortisone for maintenance
  - Tacrolimus 0.1%: has shown efficacy for treating both PE and PF.

Drug Interactions

- Ketoconazole potentiates cyclosporine activity; adjust dosage accordingly and monitor serum cyclosporine levels (p. 1333).
- Azathioprine is contraindicated in cats because of a profound myelosuppressive effect in this species.

Possible Complications

- Side effects are common with long-term oral glucocorticoid therapy (signs of iatrogenic hyperadrenocorticism, urinary tract infections, pyoderma).
- Persistent use (daily for > 14 days) of potent topical glucocorticoids can create skin atrophy, alopecia, and comedone formation.

Recommended Monitoring

- Semiannual CBC, serum biochemistry profiles, urinalysis, and urine cultures for all patients receiving long-term oral glucocorticoids
- Azathioprine, chlorambucil: CBC monitoring for cytopenias q 2-3 weeks for the first 3 months, then q 3-6 months. For azathioprine, also monitor liver and pancreatic enzyme activity.

PROGNOSIS & OUTCOME

- PF: fair to good prognosis, with the majority achieving partial or complete remission with oral glucocorticoid ± other immunosuppressive drugs. Time to improvement with therapy is 2-6 weeks; time to complete remission is 3-9 months. Mortality (euthanasia) rate for dogs with PF is 20%-30% within the first year due to lack of response or adverse effects of treatment, notably glucocorticoids (implying a need to use combination therapy before triggering adverse effects that are unacceptable to the owner, deleterious to the patient, or both). Mortality rate for cats with PF is < 10% in first 6 months of therapy. Persistence of long-term remission of PF after discontinuation of therapy has been reported for 7%-22% of cases.
- PV: 39% mortality rate (death or euthanasia); milder variants have better prognosis.
- PNP: poor prognosis

PEARLS & CONSIDERATIONS

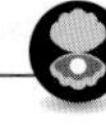

Comments

- Because response to treatment and prognosis vary with the forms of pemphigus, it is essential to make a specific diagnosis.
- A significant percentage of cases can be cured.
- Side effects of drug therapy are a major cause for euthanasia, and this can be avoided.
- Combination drug therapy is generally more effective and acceptable than monotherapy.
- Although acantholytic keratinocytes and neutrophils on skin cytology exams suggest pemphigus, clinicians may also see these cells in cases of pustular dermatophytosis (*Trichophyton* spp) and in some cases of canine pyoderma. Biopsies (including special stains such as periodic acid–Schiff) are needed for confirmation.
- Clinicians should consider prophylactic antibiotic treatment during initial immunosuppression or (in milder cases) before starting immunosuppressive therapy (p. 851).
- If new cutaneous lesions occur during treatment, first rule out pyoderma, demodicosis, or dermatophytosis before increasing immunosuppression.

Technician Tips

Acanthocytes, which are acantholytic keratinocytes, are uncommonly seen on microscopic cytologic exams. They appear as large, rounded, dark blue cells with a violet nucleus. When seen, especially in clusters, they should alert the clinician that biopsies may be required.

Client Education

Owners must be well informed about the chronic nature of the disease, as well as the potential side effects of immunosuppressive drug therapy. Gloves must be worn when applying topical immunosuppressive medications.

SUGGESTED READING

Miller WH Jr, et al: Muller & Kirk's Small animal dermatology, ed 7, St. Louis, 2013, Saunders, pp 438-448.

AUTHOR: Caroline de Jaham, DMV, MScV, DACVD
EDITOR: Manon Paradis, DMV, MVSc, DACVD

Perianal Fistula

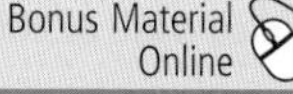

BASIC INFORMATION

Definition

Potentially severe inflammation of the perianal tissue leading to draining tracts/fistulas in the tissue adjacent to and/or surrounding the anus.

Synonyms

Anal furunculosis

Epidemiology

SPECIES, AGE, SEX

Dogs, often middle-aged (4-7 years); no sex predisposition

GENETICS, BREED PREDISPOSITION

German shepherds are the most commonly affected breed, but others can be affected.

RISK FACTORS

German shepherds that express the dog leukocyte antigen allele DLA-DRB1*00101 are at greater risk for developing perianal fistulas than those that do not express the allele.

ASSOCIATED DISORDERS

Colitis has been described in approximately 50% of dogs with perianal fistulas. Anal sacculitis occurs in some.

Clinical Presentation

HISTORY, CHIEF COMPLAINT

Historical complaints:

- Low tail carriage/reluctance to lift tail
- Pain on lifting tail

- Perianal licking/chewing
- Scooting
- Painful defecation
- Constipation/obstipation
- Foul odor and exudate
- Large-bowel diarrhea (if colitis)
- Tenesmus
- Hematochezia
- Increased frequency of defecation
- Ribbon-like stool

PHYSICAL EXAM FINDINGS

- Pain when tail is lifted
- Epithelial ulcerations adjacent to or surrounding the anal opening, potentially with fistulous tracts extending into the deeper underlying tissue
- Purulent perianal discharge
- Foul odor
- Thickened or ruptured anal sacs or rectal stricture possible

Etiology and Pathophysiology

The underlying pathophysiology has not been determined. Improvement with immunosuppressive therapy and/or diet modifications incriminates a pathologic immune response to bacterial and/or dietary antigens.

DIAGNOSIS

Diagnostic Overview

Diagnosis is usually made by observing characteristic perianal lesions during physical examination of a dog with compatible history and clinical signs.

Differential Diagnosis

- Anal sac neoplasia (primarily adenocarcinoma)
- Anal sacculitis or anal sac abscess
- Chronic colitis of many causes (e.g., antibiotic responsive, diet responsive, infectious)
- Colonic neoplasia

Initial Database

Results of CBC, biochemical profile, and urinalysis are usually normal/unremarkable.

Advanced or Confirmatory Testing

Colonoscopic biopsies, if obtained, can show lymphocytic/plasmacytic mucosal infiltrates characteristic of colitis of many causes.

TREATMENT

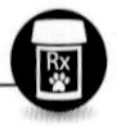

Treatment Overview

A best treatment for this disease is not established. Resolution of inflammation and associated clinical signs has been accomplished with medical therapy (immunosuppressive drugs, diet modification), surgery, or combinations of the two. The role of surgery in the early management has diminished given the responses typically expected with medical therapy, but surgery may play a role for some dogs (see Chronic Treatment below). Some have argued that surgery can reduce the long-term expense of medical treatment.

Acute General Treatment

- Cyclosporine 2-5 mg/kg PO q 12h until no evidence of lesions
  - Preferred drug given reported high response rates
  - Ketoconazole 10 mg/kg PO q 24h administration can reduce cyclosporine dosage to as low as 1 mg/kg PO q 12h and thereby reduce treatment cost.
  - Microemulsified forms offer more consistent and predictable gastrointestinal absorption.
- Tacrolimus 0.1% ointment applied topically to affected tissues q 12-24h is also associated with high response rates.
  - May be given in conjunction with prednisone
  - For dogs initially too painful for topical application, may implement after improvement is achieved with cyclosporine
- Prednisone 2 mg/kg PO q 24h until no evidence of lesions, then tapered to lowest effective dose
- Azathioprine 1-2 mg/kg PO q 24h until lesions improve, then q 48h; often given in conjunction with prednisone
- The benefits of the immunosuppressive drugs mycophenolate mofetil or leflunomide have not been explored.
- Cleaning of perineum (under sedation or anesthesia) may be needed for some dogs.
- Analgesics
- Antibiotics (e.g., cephalexin 22 mg/kg PO q 8h, metronidazole 10 mg/kg PO q 12h for 14 days) are commonly given before or in conjunction with immunosuppressive therapy, but their role in disease management has not been critically evaluated. Because antibiotics alone rarely resolved, or minimally improved, lesions in the cases described in the literature, their value has to be questioned.

Chronic Treatment

- Some dogs require maintenance immunosuppressive therapy to maintain remission.
- Anal sacculectomy may benefit a population of dogs that respond incompletely to medical therapy, those that have anal sac involvement, or those with recurrence in the face of diminishing doses of immunosuppressive drugs.
- Some dogs may need surgical resection of residual inflamed tissue.
- Some of the literature supports a period of initial medical therapy to improve lesions before surgery with the goal of reducing the amount of tissue to surgically remove.

Nutrition/Diet

Feeding a novel protein/novel carbohydrate or hydrolyzed protein is often advocated with the potential of allowing immunosuppressive drugs to be given at low dosages, long dosing intervals, intermittently (tacrolimus), or not at all. These diets can benefit dogs with concurrent colitis.

Drug Interactions

Interaction of cyclosporine with many drugs can increase or decrease blood cyclosporine concentrations; consult a formulary before giving with other drugs.

Possible Complications

- If lesions recur with drug dose reductions, resume high-dose treatment.
- Surgical complications (recurrence, stricture, incontinence)
- Constipation, obstipation, or anorectal strictures may be managed with stool softeners.
- Azathioprine can cause hepatopathy, or bone marrow suppression that usually manifests as thrombocytopenia or neutropenia in dogs.

Recommended Monitoring

Physical exam at intervals to document resolution or persistence of lesions is typically sufficient. Improvement in many dogs is appreciated within 2-4 weeks of starting cyclosporine.

- Therapeutic monitoring of cyclosporine can be considered, especially for dogs not improving in response to treatment.
  - Trough drug concentrations are often suggested, but the analyzing laboratory should be consulted for the timing of sample collection and target drug concentration because results and recommendations can vary with assays and drug formulations.
  - Pharmacodynamic monitoring based on suppression of T-lymphocyte function has been available through the Mississippi State University College of Veterinary Medicine (http://www.cvm.msstate.edu/animal-health-center/pharmacodynamic-laboratory).
- For dogs administered azathioprine
  - Liver enzymes: weekly for the first month (hepatopathy uncommon after 4 weeks)
  - CBC: weekly for the first 6-8 weeks, then monthly

PROGNOSIS & OUTCOME

Prognosis for most dogs is fair to good. Anal sac involvement may decrease the likelihood of durable control with medical therapy alone.

PEARLS & CONSIDERATIONS

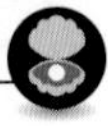

Comments

Tapering immunosuppressive drugs to the lowest effective dose or longest dosing interval to control lesions is encouraged. Transition to topical tacrolimus often reduces treatment costs, especially for dogs needing long-term treatment.

Prevention

There is no means of preventing this disease. Given the genetic predisposition of German shepherds, affected dogs should not be bred. This may be true of affected dogs of other breeds.

Technician Tips

Because of marked pain and discomfort in the perianal area, some dogs require sedation to accomplish a good exam, including rectal exam, of the perianal region.

Client Education

- Prolonged, potentially lifelong, medical and dietary therapy to control lesions and clinical signs is necessary for some dogs.
- Contact of tacrolimus ointment with human skin must be avoided; wear gloves when handling.

SUGGESTED READING

Patricelli AJ, et al: Cyclosporine and ketoconazole for the treatment of perianal fistulas in dogs. J Am Vet Med Assoc 220:1009, 2002.

AUTHOR & EDITOR: Rance K. Sellon, DVM, PhD, DACVIM

Pericardial Effusion

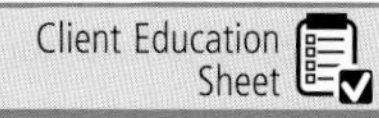

BASIC INFORMATION

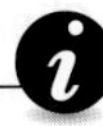

Definition

Fluid accumulation within the pericardial sac (composed of blood, plasma, pus, chyle, or mixed)

Epidemiology

SPECIES, AGE, SEX

Depends on underlying cause; dogs: middle age or older (neoplastic, idiopathic)

GENETICS, BREED PREDISPOSITION

- Dogs: golden retrievers, Labrador retrievers, German shepherds, boxers, bulldogs
- Cats: possibly purebreds with predisposition to hypertrophic cardiomyopathy (Maine coons, Ragdolls, Sphinx)

RISK FACTORS

- Dogs: mesothelioma associated with asbestosis; speculative link between lymphoma and exposure to volatile chemicals
- Cats: multi-cat household, feline infectious peritonitis (FIP), congestive heart failure (CHF)

CONTAGION AND ZOONOSIS

Cats: FIP (cat-to-cat only)

Clinical Presentation

DISEASE FORMS/SUBTYPES

- Cardiac tamponade produces clinical signs of right-sided CHF and/or low cardiac output.
- May occur as an incidental finding
  - During echocardiography
  - Cardiomegaly on radiographs
  - Electrocardiographic (ECG) changes

HISTORY, CHIEF COMPLAINT

- Acute collapse or weakness
- Lethargy or exercise intolerance
- Abdominal distention
- Dyspnea, orthopnea, coughing
- Pale mucous membranes
- Inappetence

PHYSICAL EXAM FINDINGS

- Tachycardia
- Soft or muffled heart sounds
- Weak pulses or pulsus paradoxus (decreased femoral pulse strength with inspiration)
- Abdominal distention, palpable fluid wave
- Jugular distention and pulsation
- Dyspnea/attenuated lung sounds if pleural effusion

Etiology and Pathophysiology

Cause:

- Neoplasia: hemangiosarcoma, heart base tumors (chemodectoma, ectopic thyroid adenocarcinoma), mesothelioma in dogs; lymphoma, rhabdomyosarcoma, fibrosarcoma in dogs and cats
- Idiopathic pericarditis in dogs
- Structural heart disease: CHF (rarely in cardiac tamponade), left atrial rupture
- Infectious: FIP (cats), bacterial, systemic fungal (endemic)
- Traumatic (migrating foreign bodies, e.g., grass awn, porcupine quill)
- Metabolic or toxic: uremia, coagulopathy (rodenticide toxicosis, disseminated intravascular coagulopathy)

Mechanism:

- Cause, rate and volume of pericardial effusion (PE) accumulation, and pericardial distensibility determine onset of clinical signs (cardiac tamponade).
- Cardiac tamponade is the result of intrapericardial pressure exceeding filling pressure of the cardiac chambers (right atrium and ventricle). Diastolic filling is impeded, resulting in elevated caval pressures and decreased stroke volume.

DIAGNOSIS

Diagnostic Overview

PE is suspected in patients with a history of clinical signs and/or physical exam findings consistent with cardiac tamponade. Confirmation requires echocardiography. Further investigation of primary cause (by echocardiography, thoracic radiographs, abdominal sonography, and routine complete blood and urine testing) is warranted. Less commonly, PE is diagnosed incidentally in patients without clinical signs of cardiac tamponade.

Differential Diagnosis

- Physical
  - Hypovolemia
  - Hypotension
  - Causes of ascites (p. 79) and pleural effusion (p. 791)
- Radiographic
  - Cardiac enlargement from heart disease
  - Expiratory radiograph
  - Normal variation/breed conformation
- Echocardiographic
  - Pleural effusion
  - Marked left auricular enlargement (may mimic PE in some views)
  - Oblique views (may mimic mass)

Initial Database

- Radiographs
  - Thoracic: enlarged or globoid cardiac silhouette (only ≈80% sensitive and less specific), widened caudal vena cava, pleural effusion; thoracic mass, pulmonary metastasis possible but uncommon
  - Abdominal: hepatomegaly, poor serosal detail (ascites)
- Echocardiogram: anechoic fluid in the pericardial space; possible cardiac mass (right atrial/auricular or heart base most common); diastolic right atrial (± right ventricular) collapse when cardiac tamponade is present
- CBC, serum biochemistry panel, and urinalysis: varies based on cause
- ECG: electrical alternans (≈30% of canine cases), low-amplitude QRS complexes, sinus tachycardia, possible ventricular arrhythmias
- Plasma cardiac troponin I levels: higher in dogs with PE compared with normal dogs; may be significantly higher when PE is caused by hemangiosarcoma
- If clinical suspicion warrants: coagulation profiles and/or infectious disease titers

Advanced or Confirmatory Testing

- Echocardiography is confirmative. CT is superior to echocardiography in detection of pulmonary metastasis but not cardiac tumors. MRI appears superior for detection of cardiac tumors.

- Effusion cytology: generally low yield; higher with infectious cause, lymphoma, and effusates with hematocrit < 10%
- Histopathology of pericardium ± mass tissue after pericardiectomy and sample collection

TREATMENT

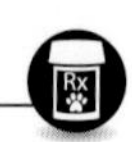

Treatment Overview

- Short-term: pericardiocentesis to relieve cardiac tamponade but not indicated if no evidence of cardiac tamponade, as usually occurs when PE is secondary to CHF
- Long-term: treatment of primary cause; pericardiectomy can reduce/prevent recurrence of tamponade in many cases.

Acute General Treatment

- Pericardiocentesis (p. 1150): necessary to resolve cardiac tamponade; relatively contraindicated in coagulopathy, left atrial rupture, and acute hemorrhage
  - Ascites resorbs over 24-48 hours after relief of tamponade and does not require drainage unless it is causing respiratory compromise or overt discomfort.
- Treatment of primary cause
- Diuretics contract intravascular volume and are contraindicated for treating cardiac tamponade acutely.

Chronic Treatment

- Management/resolution of systemic disorder if present
- Recurrent pericardiocentesis as needed
- Pericardiectomy may prevent recurrent cardiac tamponade caused by idiopathic pericarditis or heart base mass.
- Diuretics are indicated for animals with CHF (secondary PE) due to myocardial or valvular heart disease; otherwise, chronic diuretic treatment for delaying recurrence of primary PE is controversial.
- Antiinflammatory doses of glucocorticoids are controversial but can be used in dogs with presumed idiopathic effusion when pericardiectomy is not pursued.

Possible Complications

- Recurrent effusion
- Constrictive pericarditis can develop with recurrent effusions regardless of cause.
- Cardiac arrhythmias and/or sudden cardiac death (depends on cause)
- Dyspnea from severe pleural effusion or ascites
- Pericardiocentesis related (p. 1150)

Recommended Monitoring

Follow-up exam and echocardiography 2-4 weeks after pericardiocentesis or depending on return of clinical signs

PROGNOSIS & OUTCOME

- Guarded (average: days to months) with hemangiosarcoma
- Guarded to fair with heart base tumors and idiopathic effusion; survival time increased with surgical pericardiectomy
- Hemorrhagic effusion that recurs hours to days after pericardiocentesis is rarely benign; prognosis is worse.

PEARLS & CONSIDERATIONS

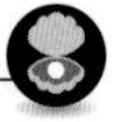

Comments

- Malignant PE and benign PE can appear equally hemorrhagic; cytology is rarely helpful for differentiation.
- Normal cardiac silhouette on radiographs does not rule out PE.
- PE is rapidly depleted of clotting factors and should not clot during/after pericardiocentesis; if clotting is observed, suspect acute hemorrhage or intravascular stick and sample.
- Reactive mesothelial cells on pericardial cytology reports may be present with either mesothelioma and benign pericarditis.

Technician Tips

- Dogs undergoing pericardiocentesis often feel much better partway through the procedure; adequate restraint is critical.
- If the procedure must be terminated prematurely, PE usually resolves anyway because the PE continues to leak through the pericardiocentesis site.

Client Education

- Monitor for recurrence of presenting signs as a sign of recurrent PE.
- Rapid deterioration (including sudden death) is possible.
- Surgical pericardiectomy may prevent recurrence and improve survival time (depends on cause).

SUGGESTED READING

Cagle LA, et al: Diagnostic yield of cytologic analysis of pericardial effusion in dogs. J Vet Intern Med 28(1):66-71, 2014.

AUTHOR: Erin Anderson, VMD, DACVIM
EDITOR: Meg M. Sleeper, VMD, DACVIM

Perineal Hernia

Client Education Sheet

BASIC INFORMATION

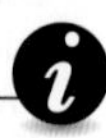

Definition

Atrophy and breakdown of the muscles of the pelvic diaphragm with prolapse of tissue/organs

Epidemiology

SPECIES, AGE, SEX

- Primarily canine: highest incidence (83%-93% of cases) among middle-aged to older, intact male dogs or dogs castrated later in life
- Rare in cats and female dogs (often secondary to trauma)

RISK FACTORS

- Older intact males or males castrated late in life
- Any cause of tenesmus
  - Prostatitis/prostatomegaly
  - Constipation
  - Anal sacculitis
  - Diarrhea: inflammatory bowel disease, lymphoma, parasites, other
- History of anal sacculectomy
- Cats: history of tenesmus, megacolon, previous perineal surgery (perineal urethrostomy), trauma

ASSOCIATED DISORDERS

- Constipation

Clinical Presentation

HISTORY, CHIEF COMPLAINT

- Tenesmus
- Ribbon-like stools
- Dysuria (bladder or prostate entrapment)
- Unilateral or bilateral perineal swelling lateral to the anus that may change in size
- Vomiting, abdominal pain (intestinal entrapment)

PHYSICAL EXAM FINDINGS

- Unilateral or bilateral swelling in the perianal region
- External digital exam: may reduce hernia contents
- Rectal palpation: may need to manually evacuate feces
  - Weakened and/or disrupted pelvic diaphragmatic muscles with possible rectal sacculation to the side of the hernia
  - Large rectal ampulla if bilaterally affected

Etiology and Pathophysiology

- Likely multifactorial in nature
- Congenital or acquired weakness of the pelvic diaphragm
  - Potentially androgen mediated
  - Relaxin produced by prostate may inhibit collagen synthesis

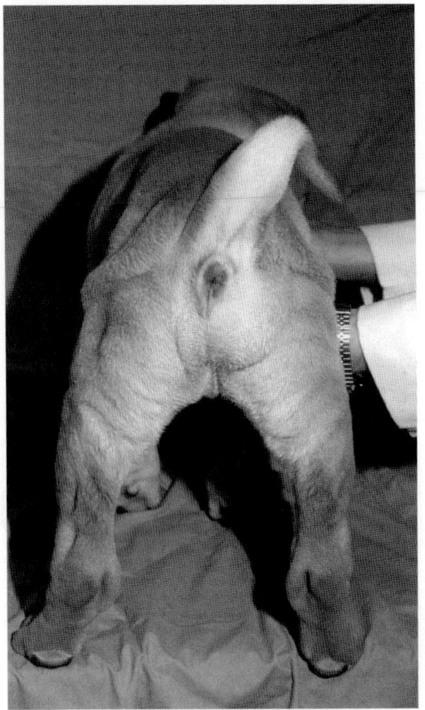

PERINEAL HERNIA Large, right-sided perineal hernia with omental herniation. Note the deviation of the rectum to the left. (Courtesy Dr. Bryden Stanley.)

- Tenesmus causes excessive strain on pelvic diaphragm.
- Neurogenic atrophy of pelvic diaphragm muscles
- Trauma in cats and female dogs

DIAGNOSIS

Diagnostic Overview

Perineal hernia is suspected in cases of unilateral or bilateral perineal swelling. It may be identified during workup of tenesmus. Rectal exam is necessary for confirmation. Bilateral pelvic diaphragmatic muscle weakness is often identified, even when perineal swelling is unilateral.

Differential Diagnosis

- Perianal adenoma
- Anal sac adenocarcinoma
- Anal sac abscess
- Colorectal mass

Initial Database

- CBC, serum biochemistry profile, urinalysis
  - Presurgical screening
  - Bladder entrapment (renal and/or postrenal azotemia)
  - Elevated white blood cell count, toxic changes (entrapped/incarcerated bowel or tissue)
- External perineal and rectal exam
  - Unilateral versus bilateral
  - Rule out rectal/colonic neoplasia and prostatic disease.
- Survey abdominal and pelvic radiographs.
  - Position of bladder/prostate
  - Evaluation of contents of hernia

Advanced or Confirmatory Testing

- Ultrasound exam
  - Prostatic evaluation
  - Identify bladder herniation
  - If history of castration status of male dog is unknown, search for testicle(s)
- Gonadotropin-releasing hormone (GnRH) stimulation testing if castration status unknown

TREATMENT

Treatment Overview

Perineal hernias require surgical repair for successful resolution. Goals of surgical intervention are to replace the herniated contents into the abdomen and reconstruct the pelvic diaphragm. Complicated hernias may require an additional abdominal approach to surgically fix herniated organs in place. Concurrent castration decreases risk of recurrence. Medical management consisting of stool softeners and a high-fiber diet may be instituted if other medical conditions make the patient a poor surgical candidate.

Acute General Treatment

- Emergency treatment to relieve urinary obstruction caused by a retroflexed bladder
  - Passage of a red rubber catheter can alleviate the obstruction.
  - Percutaneous cystocentesis
  - Indwelling urinary catheter
- Constipation/impaction relief
  - Manual evacuation under sedation
  - Stool softeners/dietary management
- Surgical repair (herniorrhaphy)
  - Ensure organ viability, and replace herniated contents into abdomen.
  - Use tension-free closure with reconstruction of the pelvic diaphragm. The internal obturator flap technique is the surgical procedure of choice (<25% recurrence rate)
  - Uncomplicated hernias can be repaired using a perineal approach.
  - Complicated hernias may require additional abdominal approach for cystopexy ± vas deferens–pexy for bladder entrapment or colopexy for severe rectal sacculation (consider staged procedures).
- Prevent recurrence
  - Castration: to remove androgen effect on pelvic diaphragm muscles
  - Treatment of underlying cause of tenesmus (e.g., castration for prostatomegaly, enrofloxacin 10 mg/kg PO q 24h for prostatitis)
- Bilateral herniorrhaphy often is necessary, but more affected side should be performed first.

Chronic Treatment

- Prevention of tenesmus in the postoperative period
  - Dietary management
  - Stool softeners
- Identification of causes of prostatomegaly
- Cystopexy ± vas deferens–pexy may be necessary for bladder herniation.
- Colopexy may be necessary for severe sacculation

Nutrition/Diet

- Postoperatively
  - Prevention of tenesmus
  - Easily digestible fiber diets produce soft but formed stool.
  - Stool softeners (e.g., lactulose, psyllium) if pain or tenesmus is noted during defecation

Possible Complications

- Complications associated with perineal hernia
  - Urinary obstruction
  - Urinary incontinence secondary to pelvic or pudendal nerve entrapment and dysfunction
  - Constipation
  - Compromised intestinal segments
- Complications associated with herniorrhaphy
  - Up to 27% recurrence rate when an internal obturator flap is used
  - Tenesmus postoperatively led to higher rate of recurrence and contralateral side herniation.
  - A 2.7 times greater risk of recurrence when left sexually intact (male dogs)
  - Incisional dehiscence and infection
  - Fecal incontinence (<15%)
  - Sciatic nerve entrapment (<5%)

Recommended Monitoring

Routine rectal exam to evaluate integrity of pelvic diaphragm repair

PROGNOSIS & OUTCOME

- Good to excellent outcome with successful herniorrhaphy and no other concurrent diseases
- Fair to poor prognosis if the patient cannot undergo surgical correction, there is recurrence after appropriate surgical correction, and/or cannot resolve cause of tenesmus/dysuria
- Highest complication rate seen with continued tenesmus after surgery and if not concurrently castrated

PEARLS & CONSIDERATIONS

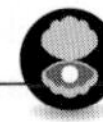

Comments

- Perineal hernia may be a hormonally related disease in the male dog.
- Herniorrhaphy plus castration is the treatment of choice; consider referral to a soft-tissue surgeon.
- Diagnosis and elimination of underlying causes of tenesmus are important for a successful outcome.
- Revision perineal herniorrhaphy is challenging and should not be undertaken by inexperienced surgeons.

Prevention

- Prevention of tenesmus plays a role in slowing the development or progression of perineal hernia.

- Castration reduces or eliminates the risk of benign prostatomegaly and secondary perineal hernia.

Technician Tips

- Important points regarding postoperative care
  - Maintain appropriate level of analgesia.
  - Prevent tenesmus to avoid undue stress on surgical repair.
- Consider epidural anesthesia.
- Ice pack on the area to decrease swelling and ease discomfort

Client Education

- Prevention and control of risk factors such as constipation, prostatomegaly, and colitis
- Surgery is the definitive treatment for perineal hernia.

SUGGESTED READING

Shaughnessy M, et al: Internal obturator muscle transposition for treatment of perineal hernia in dogs: 34 cases (1998–2012). J Am Vet Med Assoc 246:321-326, 2015.

AUTHOR: Jacob A. Rubin DVM, DACVS
EDITOR: Elizabeth A. Swanson DVM, MS, DACVS

Periodontal Disease

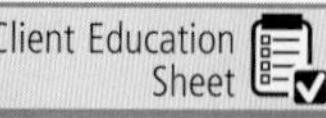

BASIC INFORMATION

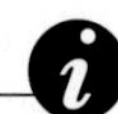

Definition

Plaque-induced inflammation of the gingiva, periodontal ligament, and alveolar bone

Synonyms

Gingivitis (inflammation of gingiva), periodontitis (inflammation of deeper periodontal tissues)

Epidemiology

SPECIES, AGE, SEX

- Most common disease in companion animals; affects dogs and cats of any breed
- More common and severe in small-breed dogs
- More severe with increasing age

GENETICS, BREED PREDISPOSITION

Small-breed dogs have relatively large teeth compared with small size of jaws, causing crowding of teeth.

RISK FACTORS

- Soft-food diet; lack of dietary abrasion permits accumulation of plaque and calculus
- Malocclusion (dental crowding)

CONTAGION AND ZOONOSIS

All clinically normal animals carry the putative causative organisms in their mouths. There is a potential risk of bacterial transmission between dogs or cats and people.

GEOGRAPHY AND SEASONALITY

Dogs and cats in less developed parts of the world are less prone to develop severe periodontal disease because they have a more varied diet that encourages natural chewing activity.

ASSOCIATED DISORDERS

Coexists with many other oral conditions (gingival hyperplasia, tooth resorption, endodontic disease and osteomyelitis) and may mask the appearance of diseases with a worse prognosis (oral neoplasms); found in almost every animal with stomatitis (p. 943)

Clinical Presentation

DISEASE FORMS/SUBTYPES

- Severity of inflammation varies relative to extent of plaque and calculus accumulation and local/general immunologic health.
- Juvenile periodontitis, rapidly progressive periodontitis, acute periodontitis, and chronic periodontitis

HISTORY, CHIEF COMPLAINT

- Halitosis (p. 402)
- Teeth covered by calculus (tartar)
- Gingiva: swollen, bleeding, or ulcerated
- If oronasal fistulas, nasal discharge

PHYSICAL EXAM FINDINGS

Wide variation in the severity of the disease may become apparent when comparing one part of the mouth with another in the same animal. Exam of molars is crucial.

- Halitosis, plaque, and calculus (although their absence does not rule out a diagnosis of periodontal disease)
- Gingivitis, gingival bleeding (on probing or spontaneously), gingival recession (root exposure)
- Furcation exposure (space between roots of multirooted teeth), periodontal pocket formation
- Mobile, displaced, and missing teeth
- Pathologic jaw fracture
- Oronasal fistula (p. 720), often with chronic rhinitis

Etiology and Pathophysiology

- Caused by bacteria in dental plaque adjacent to gingival margin and in gingival sulcus/periodontal pocket (primarily gram-negative anaerobic rods and spirochetes)
- Gingival inflammation leads to destruction of periodontal ligament, causing resorption of alveolar bone and gradual loss of attachment of the tooth to the jaw (increased mobility)
- Gingiva may recede with worsening bone loss or remain in place with a deepening pocket between the gingiva and root as the bone loss worsens.
- Inflammation resolves after the tooth (and its root) is out, and gingiva grows over the edentulous area.

DIAGNOSIS

Diagnostic Overview

Initial diagnosis is based on oral exam in the conscious patient. Anesthetized oral exam and dental radiographs determine full extent of the disease, treatment plan, and prognosis.

Differential Diagnosis

- Periodontal disease is almost always present when other oral diseases are present.
- Oral tumors (pp. 711 and 714) may appear as ulcerated gingival lesions, but unlike tumors, periodontal disease is typically symmetrical, and teeth with greater amounts of plaque and calculus deposition are more severely affected.
- Gingival enlargement due to hyperplasia: firm and symmetrical gingiva, irregular surface contour, partly or completely covering the tooth crown; usually not inflamed or ulcerated; juvenile hyperplastic gingivitis seen in young adult cats
- Abnormalities in periodontal disease are limited to gingiva, periodontal ligament, and alveolar bone. Abnormalities in other oral tissues/locations may be secondary to periodontal disease (inflammatory tooth resorption, draining tracts, osteomyelitis) or manifest as a different condition (stomatitis, tumors).

Initial Database

- General physical exam, CBC, and serum chemistry profile; urinalysis in selected cases to identify extraoral disease (e.g., renal, hepatic) that could contribute to halitosis, and for anesthesia planning
- Conscious oral exam: lower jaw manipulation should be done carefully in small-breed dogs because bone resorption around mandibular teeth can risk pathologic fracture.

Advanced or Confirmatory Testing

Oral exam under general anesthesia:

- Visual exam of color and swelling of gingiva
- Insertion of periodontal probe between gingiva and crown or exposed root to assess periodontal pocket depth (distance between gingival margin and bottom of pocket,

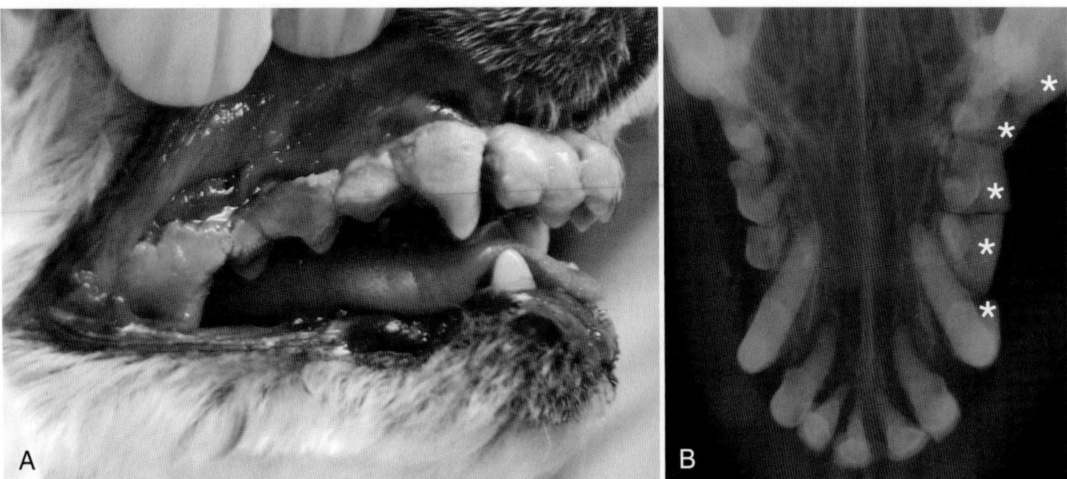

PERIODONTAL DISEASE A, Clinical photograph of a dog with severe periodontal disease; note generalized extensive plaque and calculus accumulation. **B**, Radiograph of upper jaw in same patient (labial mounting; rostral is at bottom of image, patient's left is on right of image). Note extensive calculus accumulation *(asterisks)* at the left maxillary teeth (calculus had already been grossly removed on the contralateral side) and generalized alveolar bone loss (particularly visible in the incisor region). (Copyright Dr. Alexander M. Reiter, University of Pennsylvania.)

normally ≤ 3 mm in dogs and ≤ 0.5 mm in cats) and attachment loss (distance between cementoenamel junction and bottom of pocket, normally 0 mm)
- Because gingival recession occurs as part of periodontal tissue loss, the measured pocket depth may underestimate the quantity of attachment loss.
- Pressure against the side of the tooth determines mobility (assessed on 0-3 [least to most] mobility index).
- Dental radiography to establish a treatment plan for each tooth
- Horizontal or vertical alveolar bone loss on radiographs
- Secondary endodontic disease on radiographs (extension of periodontal disease to the apical periodontium and pulp involvement)

TREATMENT

Treatment Overview
- Each tooth is a "patient."
- The goal is to decrease inflammation and prevent further attachment loss by removal of plaque and calculus and inflamed/infected tissue.
- If the owner is willing to provide long-term home oral hygiene after initial treatment, moderately affected teeth may be candidates for periodontal surgery.

Acute General Treatment
- Professional dental cleaning (scaling and polishing of all teeth by a trained veterinary health care provider)
- For moderately affected but retainable teeth (periodontal pockets > 5-6 mm and mobility of 1-2), many procedures are available. Which procedure is selected depends on whether the gingival cuff around the tooth is intact, the furcation is exposed, extent of bone surrounding the root, and experience of and equipment/materials available to the veterinarian. Options include closed and open periodontal debridement, periodontal flaps or gingival grafts to enhance gingiva around the tooth, and bone augmentation techniques.
- When mobility is rated as 2 or > 50% of the root length has lost attachment, involved therapy or extraction is indicated.
- When tooth mobility is rated as 3, extraction is performed.

Chronic Treatment
- Annual (or q 6 months for small-breed dogs) professional dental cleaning is necessary to control the disease.
- Home oral hygiene (toothbrushing, oral rinses/gels, appropriate chew toys and treats, dental diet food) to prevent progression of periodontal disease

Nutrition/Diet
The dental diets available are a useful means of retarding plaque and calculus accumulation.

Drug Interactions
Gingival hyperplasia can result from long-term phenytoin, cyclosporine, or amlodipine therapy.

Possible Complications
- Distant organ disease from periodontitis-related bacteremia or systemic release of inflammatory or bacterial degradation products; associations between periodontal disease and microscopic changes in the kidney, liver, and cardiac muscle; systemic acute-phase proteins decreasing after periodontal treatment
- Pathologic mandibular fracture due to extensive bone loss around teeth in small-breed dogs
- Secondary endodontic disease (perio-endo lesions)
- Damage to adjacent soft tissues (jaw, eye, tongue) during tooth extraction
- Oronasal fistula and rhinitis

Recommended Monitoring
Periodic re-exams:
- At 1 month and 2-3 months after involved periodontal surgical procedures to ensure that tissues are responding as expected and that home oral hygiene performed by owner is effective (if not, rescaling/repolishing of teeth and adjustments in home oral hygiene should be considered)
- Maximum of 6 months between re-exams after less involved periodontal surgery and maximum of 1 year between re-exams after professional dental cleaning

PROGNOSIS & OUTCOME

- Prevention of periodontal disease by plaque and calculus control is very effective.
- Periodontal surgery has a better prognosis if owner and patient cooperate with home oral hygiene instructions.
- Treatment of severe lesions is more problematic, and very mobile teeth should always be extracted.
- If teeth have been lost or are extracted, the tooth that would normally occlude against the missing tooth is more at risk of plaque and calculus accumulation.

PEARLS & CONSIDERATIONS

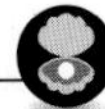

Comments
- The impact of periodontal disease on the rest of the body is a topic of research.
- A conscious oral exam should be performed whenever an animal is seen by a veterinarian

for any reason. It does not take much time.
- The Veterinary Oral Health Council (www.vohc.org) provides a standard for efficacy of products marketed to control plaque and calculus accumulation and awards its Seal of Acceptance to those that have been shown to meet its standards.

Prevention

- Home oral hygiene: owner education about the combination of brushing or rubbing the tooth surfaces (once daily or every other day), the use of oral health care products, and offering pets nutritionally complete diets formulated to reduce plaque and calculus accumulation (i.e., dental diets).
- An effective prevention strategy should be built into every animal's wellness program from a young age.

Technician Tips

- Proper toothbrushing can easily be demonstrated to owners and is a vital part of long-term maintenance of oral health.
- The technician can help the owner to select oral health care products (dental diets, treats, toys, gels, and rinses) based on scientific information.

Client Education

- Dogs and cats manage very well without teeth.
- Clinicians should teach owners about methods of prevention.

SUGGESTED READING

McFadden T, et al: Consequences of untreated periodontal disease in dogs and cats. J Vet Dent 30:266, 2013.

AUTHOR: Ana C. Castejon-Gonzalez, DVM, PhD, DAVDC, DEVDC
EDITOR: Alexander M. Reiter, DVM, Dr. med. vet., DAVDC, DEVDC

Peritoneopericardial Diaphragmatic Hernia

Bonus Material Online 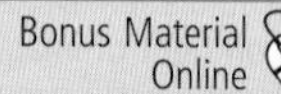 Client Education Sheet 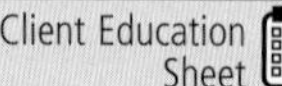 Video Available 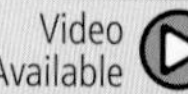

BASIC INFORMATION

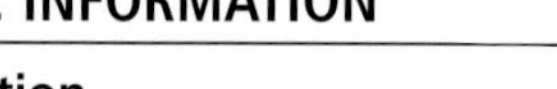

Definition

- Embryologic malformation of the diaphragm results in communication between peritoneal and pericardial cavities and allows herniation of cranial abdominal organs and omentum into the pericardial space (from most to least common: liver, gallbladder, small intestine, spleen, stomach).
- Can result in vascular compromise or obstruction of herniated organs and cardiac tamponade

Synonyms

Pericardioperitoneal diaphragmatic hernia, pericardial diaphragmatic hernia, PPDH

Epidemiology

SPECIES, AGE, SEX

- Uncommon defect; prevalence in cats > dogs
- Age at diagnosis variable (30% diagnosed at > 4 years of age)
- No sex predisposition

GENETICS, BREED PREDISPOSITION

- Not known to be hereditary
- Predisposed breeds: domestic long-haired cat, Maine coon, Persian, Himalayan, Weimaraner

RISK FACTORS

Prenatal injury, systemic illness, or toxin exposure affecting pregnant dam

ASSOCIATED DISORDERS

- Cranioventral abdominal hernia
- Caudal sternal abnormalities (pectus excavatum, malformed/absent sternebrae)
- Ventricular or atrial septal defect, pulmonic stenosis, pericardial cyst
- Portosystemic shunt
- Chylothorax

Clinical Presentation

HISTORY, CHIEF COMPLAINT

- Incidental finding in up to 50% of cases
- Nonspecific signs (lethargy, anorexia, pyrexia, weight loss)
- Respiratory signs most common (dyspnea, tachypnea, coughing)
- Gastrointestinal (GI) signs (vomiting, diarrhea)
- Uncommonly, signs of cardiac tamponade and right-heart failure (weakness, collapse, ascites)

PHYSICAL EXAM FINDINGS

- May be normal
- Muffled heart sounds (most common abnormality)
- Displaced heart sounds
- Cardiac murmur (physiologic or concurrent structural heart disease)
- Decreased lung sounds
- Palpable sternal or cranial abdominal defects
- Inability to palpate cranial abdominal organs
- Borborygmi (GI sounds) over heart

Etiology and Pathophysiology

- Abnormal development of septum transversum (forms ventral portion of the diaphragm) ± pleuroperitoneal folds (form dorsolateral diaphragm), resulting in joined peritoneal and pericardial cavities
- A congenital abnormality, not acquired

DIAGNOSIS

Diagnostic Overview

Definitive diagnosis can be made based on history, physical exam, and thoracic radiographs.

Differential Diagnosis

- Other causes of generalized cardiomegaly
  - Pericardial effusion
  - Congenital or acquired cardiac diseases
- Pleuroperitoneal diaphragmatic hernias do not involve the presence of abdominal viscera in the pericardial space.

Initial Database

- CBC and serum biochemistry panel: Often unremarkable. Elevated alanine aminotransferase (ALT) concentration most common finding in dogs; elevated calcium level in cats
- Thoracic radiographs
  - Cardiomegaly
  - Silhouetting of caudal cardiac border with diaphragm
  - Discontinuity of diaphragm
  - Irregular and heterogeneous radiopacities (soft tissue, fat, gas) within cardiac silhouette
  - Dorsal mesothelial remnant on lateral view in cats: curvilinear soft-tissue opacity ventral to caudal vena cava, representing dorsal aspect of hernia
  - Pleural effusion (uncommon)
  - Sternal deformities possible
- Abdominal radiographs
  - Small or absent liver
  - Cranial displacement or absence of stomach or spleen
  - GI gas pattern extending from abdomen into pericardial space

Advanced or Confirmatory Testing

- Ultrasound: fat or abdominal organs within pericardial sac ± small amount of pericardial effusion and discontinuity of diaphragm (see first *Video*). Consolidation of the accessory lung lobe can be a misleading impostor for peritoneopericardial diaphragmatic hernia (PPDH) ultrasonographically (see second *Video*). If uncertainty exists, a radiologist's evaluation is strongly recommended.
- Echocardiography: indicated in the presence of a heart murmur to investigate concurrent structural heart disease or for signs of cardiac tamponade.

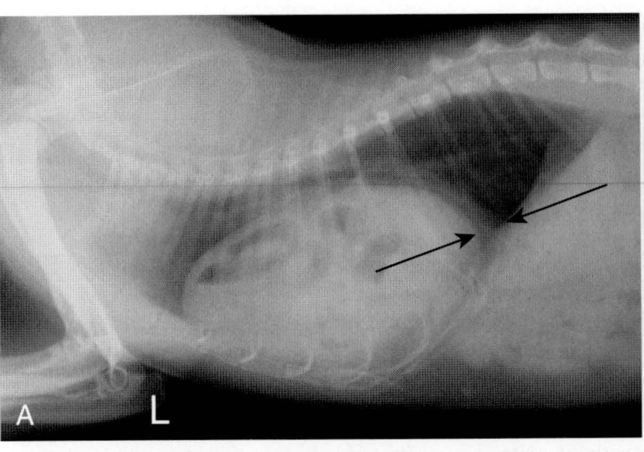

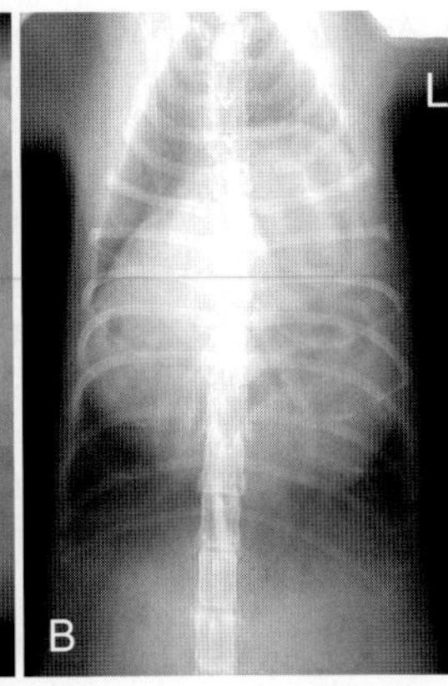

PERITONEOPERICARDIAL DIAPHRAGMATIC HERNIA Lateral (**A**) and dorsoventral (**B**) thoracic radiographs of a 1-year-old cat with PPDH. Note cardiomegaly, irregular soft tissue, fat, and gas opacities over the heart, indistinct diaphragm, and dorsal mesothelial remnant *(arrows)*. (Courtesy Dr. Stephanie Nykamp.)

- Additional testing is rarely needed. Upper GI barium series or contrast peritoneography (1-2 mL/kg of water-soluble, nonionic, iodinated radiopaque contrast agent injected aseptically into peritoneal cavity, followed by elevation of the caudal end and thoracic radiography) may confirm PPDH if other tests are inconclusive, but false-negatives are common.

TREATMENT

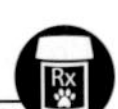

Treatment Overview

Surgical correction is indicated to eliminate clinical signs and prevent vascular compromise or obstruction of organs. It may be appropriate not to pursue surgical repair in some cases (e.g., animal without clinical signs, small incidentally discovered PPDH).

Acute General Treatment

- Oxygen supplementation
- Surgical correction by laparotomy: return of all abdominal organs to correct locations and closure of diaphragmatic defect. Caudal sternotomy may be required for adhesions or reconstruction of a large defect.
- Assessment of liver function before general anesthesia

Possible Complications

- Left uncorrected, the risk of hepatic or splenic incarceration, bowel obstruction, or cardiac tamponade and right-heart failure persists.
- Surgical complication rate is low but may include difficulty ventilating, hypotension, re-expansion pulmonary edema, and pleural effusion. Postoperative pericardial cyst and constrictive pericarditis have each been reported in one cat.

PROGNOSIS & OUTCOME

- Excellent prognosis with effective surgical correction; resolution of clinical signs in 85% of cases
- Postoperative mortality rates of 5%-14%
- Left uncorrected, the patient may remain free of clinical signs, but the risk of complications persists.

PEARLS & CONSIDERATIONS

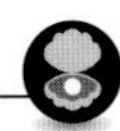

Comments

- PPDH is the most common congenital pericardial disorder in dogs and cats.
- PPDH is a congenital defect, in contrast to a pleuroperitoneal diaphragmatic hernia, which may be congenital or the result of trauma.
- PPDH is important to rule out for cardiomegaly, particularly in young animals with cranial abdominal or sternal defects.

Technician Tips

- Ventilation techniques allowing slow and controlled re-expansion of the lungs postoperatively may diminish the risk of re-expansion pulmonary edema.
- For the uncorrected PPDH patient, it is critical to educate clients about monitoring for signs of respiratory, GI, or circulatory compromise as listed above.

SUGGESTED READING

Burns CG, et al: Surgical and non-surgical treatment of peritoneopericardial diaphragmatic hernia in dogs and cats: 58 cases (1999-2008). J Am Vet Med Assoc 242:643-650, 2013.

AUTHOR: M. Lynne O'Sullivan, DVM, DVSc, DACVIM
EDITOR: Meg M. Sleeper, VMD, DACVIM

Peritonitis, Septic

Client Education Sheet
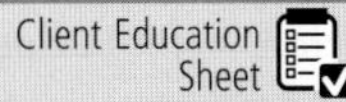

BASIC INFORMATION

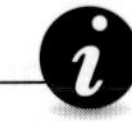

Definition

Peritonitis is local or generalized inflammation of the peritoneum. A diagnosis of bacterial septic peritonitis is based on identification of intracellular bacteria or other infectious agents (e.g., *Candida*) in abdominal effusion.

Epidemiology

SPECIES, AGE, SEX

Younger animals prone to ingesting foreign material, older animals with gastrointestinal (GI) neoplasia or biliary disease, and intact animals are predisposed.

RISK FACTORS

GI surgery, GI ulcer/necrosis, liver lobe torsion or neoplasia, closed pyometra, septic prostatitis, urinary tract obstruction with urinary tract infection, severe colitis, trauma (blunt or penetrating)

Clinical Presentation

DISEASE FORMS/SUBTYPES

- GI tract perforation or dehiscence
- Leakage or translocation of bacteria from other abdominal organ (e.g., pyometra, prostatic or hepatic abscesses, cholecystitis, urinary tract)
- Penetrating abdominal trauma

HISTORY, CHIEF COMPLAINT

- History suggestive of precipitating cause:
  - Medications predisposing to GI ulceration (e.g., nonsteroidal antiinflammatory drugs, glucocorticoids)
  - Penetrating wounds, foreign object ingestion, or prior GI surgery
- Lethargy, anorexia, collapse
- Vomiting, regurgitation
- Owners may notice abdominal distention or pain.

PHYSICAL EXAM FINDINGS

- Tachycardia (bradycardia possible in cats) and signs of hypovolemic or septic shock (p. 907)
- Abdominal pain indicated by tension, guarding, or prayer position (may be disproportionately subtle for the degree of inflammation or be mimicked by apprehension or back pain)
- Abdominal effusion
- Fever or hypothermia
- Altered mentation
- Other findings related to cause (e.g., distended uterus ± purulent vaginal discharge if

pyometra; wounds if penetrating abdominal trauma)

Etiology and Pathophysiology

- Bacteria gain access to the abdominal cavity most frequently by GI tract perforation, although leakage or translocation from other internal sources (genitourinary tract, liver) and external sources (penetrating trauma) are possible.
- Infection in the abdominal cavity causes inflammation, cellular infiltration (primarily macrophages and neutrophils), and fibrin production.
- The peritoneum responds with increased vascular permeability, and systemic manifestations of inflammation (e.g., fever, vasodilation, hyperdynamic shock) develop.
- Electrolytes, plasma proteins, and erythrocytes extravasate and are lost through third spacing into the abdominal cavity. These losses may cause hypovolemia, hemoconcentration, and metabolic derangements.

DIAGNOSIS

Diagnostic Overview

The diagnosis of septic peritonitis, regardless of the underlying cause, is based on demonstration—typically by cytologic evaluation of fluid obtained by abdominocentesis—of intraperitoneal toxic, degenerative neutrophils containing intracellular organisms. A diagnostic and treatment algorithm is presented on p. 1439.

Differential Diagnosis

- For abdominal pain or distention (i.e., acute abdomen): acute pancreatitis, gastric dilation/volvulus, intestinal or mesenteric torsion, pyometra, splenic, hepatic, renal, or GI neoplasia, biliary tract obstruction, ureteral obstruction (pp. 21 and 1192)
- For suppurative abdominal effusion: feline infectious peritonitis, acute necrotizing pancreatitis, ischemia or thrombosis of GI tract, sterile bile peritonitis

Initial Database

- CBC, serum chemistry panel, urinalysis with culture
  - Common findings on CBC include neutrophilia or neutropenia with a left shift, thrombocytopenia, and/or anemia. Neutrophilic toxic changes are often noted.
  - Metabolic derangements common (e.g., acidosis, electrolyte disorders, hyperglycemia/hypoglycemia)
  - Urine sample should be obtained by catheterization if possible; cystocentesis may inadvertently retrieve septic fluid or puncture a pyometra.
- Abdominal radiographs may document GI foreign body obstruction, intraabdominal neoplasia, or free intraabdominal air or fluid.
  - Free air highly suggestive/specific for septic peritonitis unless air is result of prior abdominal surgery in the preceding weeks
- Abdominal ultrasound: identify free abdominal fluid, mucocele, pyometra, GI foreign body, neoplasia, granuloma/abscess
- Coagulation profile (p. 1325): disseminated intravascular coagulation complication of septic peritonitis (p. 269)

Advanced or Confirmatory Testing

- Abdominocentesis (p. 1056) and diagnostic peritoneal lavage (DPL) are safe and reliable for evaluating a patient suspected of having septic peritonitis; however, with the emergence of rapid abdominal ultrasonography (FAST [p. 1102]), DPL is rarely performed.
  - For patients with physical exam consistent with abdominal sepsis but without ascites, recheck of FAST scan after IV fluid resuscitation may reveal fluid that has extravasated during resuscitation.
- Diagnosis of septic peritonitis is based on the finding of degenerate neutrophils with intracellular bacteria or fungal organisms in the abdominal fluid (p. 1343).
  - An effusion glucose level of at least 20 mg/dL (1.1 mmol/L) less than that of peripheral blood is very specific and moderately sensitive for septic effusion.
  - In dogs, abdominal fluid lactate > 2 mmol/L greater than the blood lactate level predicts abdominal sepsis.
  - Fluid should be submitted for bacterial culture and susceptibility.

TREATMENT

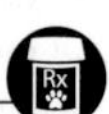

Treatment Overview

Stabilize patient; identify and control source of infection if possible (i.e., surgical correction)

Acute General Treatment

- Initial treatment directed toward stabilization of the metabolic consequences of peritonitis.
- IV crystalloid fluids (up to 60-90 mL/kg), fresh-frozen plasma (10-15 mL/kg), packed red blood cells, or whole blood may be necessary to maintain cardiac output (see p. 907).
  - Maintain hematocrit above a target of 21%.
- IV antibiotic therapy should be started as soon as sepsis is suspected. Broad-spectrum options:
  - Ampicillin or ampicillin/sulbactam + enrofloxacin 10 mg/kg IV q 24h in dogs, 5 mg/kg IV q 24h in cats
    - Enrofloxacin should be diluted 1:9 in saline and given over at least 10 minutes; IV use is off-label in dogs and cats
  - Ampicillin 30 mg/kg IV q 6h or ampicillin/sulbactam 30 mg/kg IV q 8h plus gentamicin 6 mg/kg IV q 24h or amikacin 15 mg/kg IV q 24h
    - Aminoglycoside therapy only after the animal is hydrated and producing urine.
  - Cefoxitin 30 mg/kg IV q 6-8h
- Upgrade antibiotic selection for hospital-acquired infections pending culture results.
  - De-escalate antibiotics based on culture and sensitivity.
- Exploratory laparotomy is warranted promptly after adequate stabilization.
  - Repair of the lesion
  - Biopsy/removal of affected tissues and intraoperative cultures
  - Lavage
  - Closed-suction drainage (warranted in almost all cases)
  - Open abdominal drainage if extensive contamination is present

Possible Complications

- Disseminated intravascular coagulopathy (p. 269)
- Multiple organ dysfunction syndrome (p. 665)
- Dehiscence of prior repair (usually occurs 3-5 days after initial surgery)
- Hypoalbuminemia

Recommended Monitoring

- Hydration and vascular volume status
- Serum total protein, albumin, electrolyte, and glucose levels
- Vital parameters, body weight, and blood pressure
- Renal function/urine output
- Pain management

PROGNOSIS & OUTCOME

Prognosis variable, and worsens with organ failure. The reported mortality rate for dogs and cats with all-cause septic peritonitis is 27%-70%.

PEARLS & CONSIDERATIONS

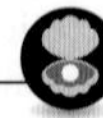

Comments

- Gastric perforations may result in a large volume of free intraabdominal air without fluid or fluid with low numbers of bacteria.
- Linear foreign bodies are particularly prone to causing GI perforation.
- Severely dehydrated animals may not develop significant volumes of abdominal effusion until after fluid resuscitation.
- Consider nasogastric tube placement at the time of surgery to facilitate early enteral nutrition (p. 1107).

Technician Tips

- Monitor closed-suction drain fluid for changes in character or volume.
- A return of sepsis (e.g., from intestinal dehiscence) may be recognized by unexplained tachycardia, hypotension, increased drain volume/ascites, or decline in patient awareness.

SUGGESTED READING

Bentley AM, et al: Comparison of dogs with septic peritonitis: 1988-1993 versus 1999-2003. J Vet Emerg Crit Care 17(4):391-398, 2017.

AUTHORS: Mary Aslanian, DVM, DACVECC; Danna M. Torre, DVM, DACVECC
EDITOR: Benjamin M. Brainard, VMD, DACVAA, DACVECC

Petechiae and Ecchymoses

BASIC INFORMATION

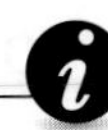

Definition

Petechiae and ecchymosis are clinical signs rather than a specific disease.

- Petechiae are pinpoint (1-3 mm) hemorrhages that occur due to capillary bleeding and are specific for defects in primary hemostasis (i.e., platelet number/function) or vasculitis.
- Ecchymoses are larger (>1 cm) subcutaneous hemorrhages occurring due to arteriole or venule bleeding caused by defects in primary or secondary (i.e., coagulation cascade) hemostasis.

Synonym

Purpura

Epidemiology

SPECIES, AGE, SEX

- Dogs more than cats
- Age varies with cause (e.g., congenital platelet disorders in young animals, immune-mediated thrombocytopenia during middle age, coagulopathy secondary to malignancy in older animals)

GENETICS, BREED PREDISPOSITION

Certain breeds are predisposed to conditions that may result in petechiae or ecchymoses (pp. 972 and 1043).

CONTAGION AND ZOONOSIS

Several infectious diseases can cause thrombocytopenia or vasculitis, resulting in petechiae or ecchymosis. Many are vector transmitted rather than directly contagious, and many are indirect zoonoses (e.g., Rocky Mountain spotted fever, anaplasmosis).

RISK FACTORS

Any cause of thrombocytopenia, thrombocytopathy, or vasculitis can result in petechiae; these or any secondary hemostatic defect can cause ecchymosis.

ASSOCIATED DISORDERS

Anemia and evidence of bleeding from the gastrointestinal (GI) tract, urinary tract, or respiratory tract are often identified.

Clinical Presentation

DISEASE FORMS/SUBTYPES

Petechiae and ecchymosis can occur as a sign of an underlying coagulation disorder or as a complication of systemic disease.

HISTORY, CHIEF COMPLAINT

Rarely are patients presented due to owner observation of petechiae and/or ecchymoses. More commonly, they are presented for signs related to bleeding (e.g., epistaxis, hyphema, hematuria), signs related to anemia (e.g., weakness, collapse), or signs related to an underlying disease process (e.g., signs of acute kidney injury with leptospirosis, signs of heat stroke). The clinician should obtain a thorough history to include current medications, recent vaccinations, access to toxins/drugs, travel, ectoparasites prophylaxis or exposure, and any history of prolonged or spontaneous hemorrhage.

PHYSICAL EXAM FINDINGS

Exam should focus on identifying areas of petechiae (e.g., mucous membranes, inner pinnae, nonhaired regions) and ecchymoses (e.g., ventral abdomen, inguinal region, sites of recent venipuncture) and should confirm that they are truly regions of hemorrhage as opposed to surface/cutaneous lesions (i.e., skin disease). Petechiae and ecchymoses should NOT blanch with pressure. Careful exam should look for other evidence of hemorrhage (e.g., rectal exam for melena and/or hematochezia). Pallor, tachycardia, and a soft systolic heart murmur are often recognized with severe anemia. Other findings reflect underlying disease.

Etiology and Pathophysiology

- Thrombocytopenia (<30,000 platelets/mcL) is the most common cause of petechiae and/or ecchymoses.
  - Decreased production (e.g., bone marrow disorders, drugs or toxins, immunologic attack on platelet precursors); often part of pancytopenia
  - Platelet destruction (e.g., primary or secondary immune-mediated thrombocytopenia [IMT], *Anaplasma platys* infection)
  - Platelet consumption (e.g., disseminated intravascular coagulation [DIC], vasculitis)
- Thrombocytopathy (must be severe to result in spontaneous hemorrhage)
  - Congenital/inherited platelet disorders (e.g., Glanzmann's thrombasthenia)
  - Drugs/toxins (e.g., aspirin, clopidogrel, nonsteroidal antiinflammatory drugs [NSAIDs], colloids)
  - Concurrent diseases (e.g., hepatic disease, uremia, rickettsial infections)
  - von Willebrand factor deficiency
- Vasculitis: rickettsial disease, drug reaction, immune-mediated vasculitis
- Secondary hemostatic defects (e.g., vitamin K rodenticide toxicosis) can cause ecchymosis but not petechiae
- Often, multiple mechanisms contribute to signs simultaneously.

DIAGNOSIS

Diagnostic Overview

History and exam guide diagnostic evaluation, but the most important initial test is a CBC with slide review (use peripheral veins in animals with suspected coagulopathy). If this cannot be done quickly, a blood smear evaluation with platelet estimate and packed cell volume/total protein (PCV/TP) should be performed. Routine chemistry and (free-catch) urinalysis can assess for concurrent disease. Coagulation profile or specific tests of coagulation may also be helpful. In general, dogs with coagulation disorders and no other systemic disease (e.g., primary IMT, congenital coagulation disorder) are less ill than dogs with other causes of hemorrhage.

Differential Diagnosis

- Erythema: blanches with pressure (diascopy) as opposed to petechiae/ecchymosis
- Cutaneous hemangiomas or hemangiosarcoma
- Burns (chemical, thermal)
- Cutaneous drug reaction
- Traumatic dermatitis

Initial Database

- CBC
  - Rule out thrombocytopenia (manual count if automated is decreased). Microscopic slide review is important because platelet clumping (best seen on the feathered edge) can result in artifactual decrease in count. Spontaneous hemorrhage occurs only if platelet count is < 30,000/mcL unless complicated by thrombocytopathy or vasculitis. Large platelets suggest platelet regeneration, as is common in IMT.
  - Anemia and low TP may reflect severe hemorrhage.
  - Pancytopenia suggests bone marrow disease.
  - Neutrophilia suggests infection or inflammatory disease.
- Platelet estimate (if CBC cannot be performed rapidly)
  - Each platelet observed in a high-power field (hpf, 1000×) suggests ≈15,000 platelets (i.e., average number of platelets/hpf × 15,0000 = platelet estimate per mcL)
  - Normal dogs and cats should have > 10 platelets/hpf, but spontaneous hemorrhage is unlikely due to thrombocytopenia alone if > 2 platelets/hpf
- Chemistry panel: ± increased blood urea nitrogen (BUN) if GI bleeding, ± hypoproteinemia from blood loss, ± hyperglobulinemia from infection/inflammation
- Urinalysis (free-catch sample): ± hematuria, ± proteinuria
- Coagulation panel (prothrombin time/ activated partial thromboplastin time [PT/aPTT] [p. 1325]): not required if thrombocytopenia confirmed unless DIC suspected; useful to assess secondary hemostasis for ecchymotic hemorrhage

Advanced or Confirmatory Testing

- Radiographs or ultrasound (thorax, abdomen) as appropriate to assess the cause or effects of hemorrhage (e.g., neoplastic abdominal mass → DIC; pulmonary hemorrhage)
- Infectious disease serology and/or polymerase chain reaction (PCR): relevant infection → vasculitis and/or thrombocytopenia/thrombocytopathia (e.g., *Rickettsia rickettsia,* leptospira titers)
- Flow cytometry for platelet-bound antibodies if IMT suspected (rarely performed)
- Bone marrow aspirate ± core biopsy (p. 1068) to evaluate for causes of thrombocytopenia
- Buccal mucosal bleeding time (p. 1076): suspect von Willebrand or thrombocytopathy
- von Willebrand factor deficiency testing (p. 1393)
- DNA screening for inherited thrombocytopathia (Auburn University, https://www.vetmed.auburn.edu/academic-departments/dept-of-pathobiology/diagnostic-services/)
- Platelet function evaluation (platelet function analyzer PFA-100, Sonoclot, thromboelastography)

TREATMENT

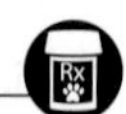

Treatment Overview

Treat for cause of clinical sign. Transfusion of red blood cells may be required for anemic animals, but platelet product transfusions are short lived and rarely indicated.

Acute General Treatment

Treatment is aimed at the underlying cause (i.e., disorder of platelet number or function, vasculitis, or other hemostatic defect) as well as at providing supportive care.

- Animals with clinical signs of anemia require transfusion of packed red blood cells or whole blood (pp. 57 and 1169)
- Platelet transfusion in the form of platelet concentrate, fresh whole blood, or platelet-rich plasma is reserved for animals with life-threatening hemorrhage, such as bleeding into the central nervous system or lungs.
    - A dose of 1 mL/kg whole blood increases platelet count by only ≈10,000/mcL.
    - Platelet-rich plasma is typically dosed at 1 unit/3 kg body weight.
    - Frozen platelet concentrate has the advantages of a longer shelf life and lower volume; typical dose is 1 unit/10 kg of body weight.
    - Recently, freeze-dried, shelf-stable platelet product has become available (StablePlate RX); 1 vial per 5 kg body weight.
- Severe thrombocytopenia without evidence of DIC is often treated presumptively as for IMT (p. 972) with glucocorticoids ± doxycycline for potential rickettsial disease trigger.
- Hemorrhage may warrant other supportive measures (p. 433).

Chronic Treatment

See chapters on the specific disorder or disease identified.

Behavior/Exercise

Activity should be limited to reduce the risk of trauma that may result in hemorrhage. Animals should be kept in low cages for the same reason.

Drug Interactions

Drugs that result in platelet dysfunction (e.g., aspirin, clopidogrel) should be avoided.

Recommended Monitoring

Monitor closely for worsening of petechiae and/or ecchymoses or other signs of hemorrhage (feces, urine). It can be helpful to use permanent marker to draw the edges of ecchymosis to determine whether they are expanding or contracting or new lesions develop. Monitor vital parameters and PCV/TP to assess need for transfusion.

PROGNOSIS & OUTCOME

Depends on the existing disease/condition

PEARLS & CONSIDERATIONS

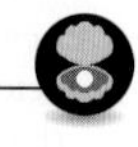

Comments

- Perform platelet count/estimate quickly; if thrombocytopenia is only mild to moderate, consider conditions that result in vasculitis and/or thrombocytopathia.
- Patients with secondary hemostatic disorders may develop ecchymosis but should not develop spontaneous petechiae.

Prevention

Ectoparasite prevention; prepare for planned surgery for animals with known congenital coagulation disorders

Technician Tips

- For patients with petechiae and/or ecchymoses, venipuncture should be performed using a peripheral vein, and a pressure wrap should be applied for 5-10 minutes after venipuncture.
- Cystocentesis should NOT be performed in patients with petechiae and/or ecchymoses.

SUGGESTED READING

Blois S: Petechiae and ecchymoses. In Ettinger SJ, et al, editors: Textbook of veterinary internal medicine, ed 8, St. Louis, 2017, Elsevier.

AUTHOR: Laura A. Nafe, DVM, MS, DACVIM
EDITOR: Leah A. Cohn, DVM, PhD, DACVIM

Petroleum Distillates/Turpentine Toxicosis

BASIC INFORMATION

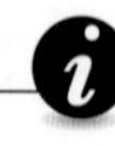

Definition

Toxicosis can result from petroleum distillates, which are hydrogen- and carbon-containing chemicals (i.e., hydrocarbons [HCs]) originating from the distillation of crude oil or petroleum. Some compounds originate from the steam distillation of plants. Toxicosis is usually due to accidental dermal or oral exposure to HC-containing products. Signs can range from dermal irritation, to vomiting and aspiration, to severe central nervous system (CNS) effects.

Synonyms

- HC-containing products include naphtha, gasoline, kerosene, paint thinners/strippers, engine cleaners/degreasers, diesel fuel, heating fuels, lamp and furniture oils, waxes, lubricating oils, grease, paraffin wax, tar, asphalt
- Plant distillate examples include turpentine and linseed oil.

Epidemiology

SPECIES, AGE, SEX

- Dogs are more commonly exposed than cats.
- Due to the grooming behavior of cats, topical exposures quickly become oral exposures.

RISK FACTORS

Free-roaming animals are at a higher risk for accidental exposures (automobiles, garages, workshops, sheds, construction).

GEOGRAPHY AND SEASONALITY

Warmer months involve an increased use of HC-containing products outdoors (lighter fluid use for BBQ), with increased opportunities for exposure.

Clinical Presentation

HISTORY, CHIEF COMPLAINT

- Evidence or suspicion of exposure to HC-containing product (smell of product on breath or fur)
- Onset of clinical signs is generally 1-3 hours after exposure.
- Owner may notice hypersalivation, vomiting, retching, excessive licking motions, and coughing.

PHYSICAL EXAM FINDINGS

- Presence of the product on the feet, muzzle, or fur
- HC/distillate smell on the coat or breath
- Dermal discomfort (tender and inflamed interdigital skin or other exposed areas)
- Anxious, agitation, pacing, crying/whimpering
- Oral exposure: hypersalivation, vomiting, excessive licking motions, hacking, retching, panting, wheezing, coughing, crackles on auscultation
- Ocular: blepharospasm, blepharitis

Etiology and Pathophysiology

- The physical and chemical properties of a particular HC determine its toxicity. Hydrocarbons with lower boiling points (more flammable), lower viscosities (thinner), and lower surface tension are more dangerous due to a greater ability to penetrate lipid membranes (increased systemic absorption) and increased volatility, increasing risk of aspiration.
- Volatile HC can damage nerve endings and solubilize subdermal/submucosal fat, resulting in acute, generalized pain and discomfort. Systemic absorption can result in dissolution of cellular lipids and cell necrosis with generalized systemic inflammation and congestion. Some HCs can cause more direct organ damage (e.g., benzene causes myelotoxicosis).

DIAGNOSIS

Diagnostic Overview

History of known or suspected exposure, clinical signs, and the presence of a volatile scent of petroleum distillates are the major components of diagnosis. If the patient vomits, a spot test can help confirm ingestion of petroleum distillates (see Advanced or Confirmatory Testing below).

Differential Diagnosis

- Vomiting (p. 1293)
- Respiratory distress (p. 879)
- Allergic or other dermal toxins (topical toxicity)
- Organophosphate or carbamate insecticides, zinc phosphide

Initial Database

- CBC: leukocytosis, neutrophilia; possible septic changes if pneumonia is a complication; possible hemoconcentration
- Serum biochemistry profile: hypoglycemia possible
- Urinalysis: unremarkable
- Thoracic radiographs if aspiration suspected
- Pulse oximetry or arterial blood gas measurement if aspiration suspected

Advanced or Confirmatory Testing

- Spot test: mix warm water and vomitus; distillates rise to the surface, and the characteristic odor of volatile distillates (e.g., gasoline, charcoal lighter fluid) becomes apparent.
- Confirmatory analysis of the distillate is possible but is usually not useful in terms of clinical management due to turnaround time; collect samples in airtight containers and refrigerate.
- In animals with aspiration, airway lavage with Gram stain and/or culture can assist with antibiotic selection (p. 1073).

TREATMENT

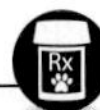

Treatment Overview

Due to the risk of aspiration, induction of vomiting and activated charcoal are NOT recommended. Bathe the animal with liquid dishwashing liquid to decrease continued dermal exposure. Treat pain due to skin lesions and aspiration as needed.

Acute General Treatment

- Emesis, gastric lavage, and administration of activated charcoal are CONTRAINDICATED because there is an increased risk of aspiration with ingestion of petroleum distillates.
- Oxygen supplementation (p. 1146) if required due to aspiration
  - Mechanical ventilation may be necessary, depending on oxygen concentration (p. 1185)
- Use IV fluids to maintain hydration and perfusion; forced diuresis is not effective at increasing the elimination of HCs.
- Pain control if needed (opioids such as buprenorphine 0.005-0.04 mg/kg IV, IM, or SQ); dermal exposures can be painful
- Prophylactic antibiotics with aspiration pneumonia is controversial; HC pneumonitis has a low risk of bacterial pneumonia complications
- Dermal decontamination: bathe well with a mild liquid hand dishwashing detergent solution, rinse thoroughly, do not allow pet to get chilled
- Ocular exposure: flush eyes with saline, fluorescein stain to assess for corneal ulcer

Chronic Treatment

For aspiration pneumonitis: oxygen supplementation, mechanical ventilation as necessary

Possible Complications

- Aspiration and chemical pneumonitis
- Volatile HC can cause CNS depression and ataxia.

Recommended Monitoring

- Clinical parameters, including respiratory rate and effort
- Arterial blood gas or pulse oximetry for animals with respiratory signs

PROGNOSIS & OUTCOME

Prognosis is good unless aspiration pneumonia occurs.

PEARLS & CONSIDERATIONS

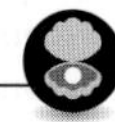

Comments

- Most commercial or industrial products containing petroleum distillates are labeled: "May be harmful or fatal if swallowed." This warning is not specific to the individual product and does not automatically imply a poor prognosis. It is more useful to consider the volatility of the product when determining the relative clinical risk to the animal, with greater volatility carrying a higher risk.
- Petroleum distillates are listed in terms of their volatility: tar (least volatile); paraffin wax, lubricating oil, fuel oil, kerosene (intermediate); mineral spirits, gasoline, petroleum naphtha, petroleum ether (most volatile).
- Risk of aspiration pneumonia/pneumonitis from viscous or solid petroleum distillates, including motor oil, transmission oil, waxes, other lubricating oils, grease, paraffin wax, and asphalt, is low. Most of these exposures result in mild, self-limited vomiting, lethargy, and diarrhea.
- Delayed (12-24 hours after exposure) gastrointestinal and respiratory effects can be seen when waterproofing sprays (used on leather products) containing volatile HCs such as heptane, butane, benzene, or trichloroethylene are used around pets.

Prevention

Keep animals away from all HC-containing products.

Technician Tips

Make sure to wear gloves when bathing animal to reduce dermal exposure to yourself.

Client Education

Keep all HC products locked away in a safe location; childproof does not mean animal-proof.

SUGGESTED READING

Raisbeck MF: Petroleum hydrocarbons. In Peterson ME, et al, editors: Small animal toxicology, ed 3, St. Louis, 2013, Saunders, pp 755-761.

AUTHOR: Elizabeth Cripe, DVM
EDITOR: Tina Wismer, DVM, MS, DABVT, DABT

Phenylpropanolamine Toxicosis

Client Education Sheet 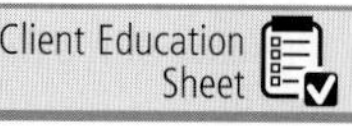

BASIC INFORMATION 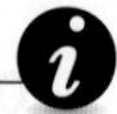

Definition

Adverse effects are caused by exposure to phenylpropanolamine (PPA), a synthetic sympathomimetic amine used to control urinary incontinence in dogs due to urinary sphincter incompetence (p. 1011).

Synonyms

PPA, Proin toxicosis

Epidemiology

SPECIES, AGE, SEX

Exposure occurs more commonly in dogs than cats.

GENETICS, BREED PREDISPOSITION

Large-breed dogs and potentially greyhounds may have a higher risk of developing significant cardiac effects, including ventricular arrhythmias and myocardial necrosis.

RISK FACTORS

Animals with pre-existing renal compromise (renal excretion) or pre-existing cardiac disease may be at a higher risk.

Clinical Presentation

HISTORY, CHIEF COMPLAINT

- History of exposure to PPA; onset of signs most commonly occurs within 3 hours of exposure.
- Most common clinical signs on presentation: agitation or lethargy, vomiting, mydriasis, piloerection, and dermal erythema

PHYSICAL EXAM FINDINGS

Bradycardia (occasionally tachycardia), piloerection, erythema, occasionally ventricular arrhythmias, rarely hyphema and retinal detachment due to hypertension

Etiology and Pathophysiology

- PPA is a sympathomimetic that acts mainly by causing release of norepinephrine, but it also has direct agonist activity at some adrenergic receptors. Release of norepinephrine indirectly stimulates alpha and beta receptors. Most effects are on the alpha receptors, with weak effects on beta receptors.
- Excessive amounts of norepinephrine can have multisystemic effects: cardiovascular (hypertension, tachycardia or bradycardia, arrhythmias, myocardial necrosis), musculoskeletal (rhabdomyolysis), renal (myoglobinuria), ocular (hyphema and retinal detachment), and endocrine (hypoglycemia has been seen)
- Animals are initially agitated and tachycardic; then as their blood pressure rises, they become lethargic, and a reflex bradycardia occurs.
- Excessive catecholamines and sympathetic amines can cause myocardial necrosis in humans and animals.
- Disseminated intravascular coagulation (DIC) has developed in critically ill patients.

DIAGNOSIS 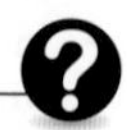

Diagnostic Overview

Diagnosis is based on a history of exposure to PPA and supporting clinical signs. Diagnostics are performed to evaluate the physiologic effects of PPA. There is no clinically relevant testing available to determine exposure. Troponin 1 assays can be performed if myocardial necrosis is suspected.

Differential Diagnosis

- Amphetamine and cocaine toxicosis: most commonly with these agents, tachycardia is seen, and agitation or hyperactivity is more pronounced.
- Phenylephrine toxicosis
- Sumatriptan and other selective serotonin subtype 1 agonist toxicosis

Initial Database

- CBC, clinical chemistry: often unremarkable, but thrombocytopenia possible with DIC, azotemia possible with renal injury or dehydration, and hypoglycemia reported
- Urinalysis: ± myoglobinuria
- Electrocardiogram (p. 1096): bradyarrhythmia or tachyarrhythmia
- Blood pressure (p. 1065): hypertension

Advanced or Confirmatory Testing

- Troponin 1 assay
- Echocardiogram to evaluate cardiac function

TREATMENT 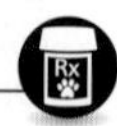

Treatment Overview

Treatment is focused on controlling the clinical signs and physiologic effects of PPA.

Acute General Treatment

- Decontamination includes emesis (p. 1188) and activated charcoal (p. 1087) if overdose is suspected before onset of clinical signs.
- Treatment of hypertension
  - Acepromazine 0.02 mg/kg IV, can repeat 2-3 times, but if hypertension is not controlled use other pharmacologic intervention.
  - Nitroprusside continuous-rate infusion (CRI) 1-2 mcg/kg/min initially, increasing by 1 mcg/kg every 3-5 minutes until improvement is noted, *or*
  - Phentolamine 0.02-1 mg/kg IV bolus followed by a CRI, *or*
  - Hydralazine 0.5-3 mg/kg IV q 12h or a 0.1 mg/kg IV loading dose followed by a CRI of 1.5-5 mcg/kg/min
- Treatment of cardiac arrhythmias
  - Do NOT use atropine to increase the heart rate (bradycardia is a reflex from hypertension and should resolve after the blood pressure is normalized)
  - A specific beta-1 blocker may be given for significant supraventricular tachyarrhythmias: esmolol 5-100 mcg/kg/min CRI
  - Ventricular premature contractions (VPCs) or ventricular tachycardia: lidocaine 2-4 mg/kg IV over 1-2 minutes, followed by 0.5-2 mg/kg q 20-60 minutes or 0.4-0.8 mg/kg/min CRI, if required (p. 1033)
- Central nervous system (CNS) stimulatory signs: acepromazine (see above)
- IV crystalloid fluids are used to maintain hydration, meet maintenance needs, and protect renal function. Avoid fluid loading until hypertension is controlled.

Chronic Treatment

If myocardial necrosis occurs, ongoing treatment of heart disease may be necessary (p. 409).

Behavior/Exercise

Exercise restriction may be indicated when myocardial necrosis is suspected or confirmed.

Drug Interactions

- Caffeine seems a very important co-ingestant, potentially triggering significant hypertensive episodes.
- Any agent that can cause an increase in blood pressure can worsen clinical signs.

Possible Complications

- DIC
- Myocardial necrosis
- Retinal detachment
- Renal damage

Recommended Monitoring

Heart rate, blood pressure, renal parameters, and ocular function

PROGNOSIS & OUTCOME 

With prompt and appropriate treatment, a full recovery is expected for most patients.

PEARLS & CONSIDERATIONS 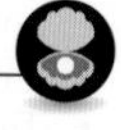

Comments

- Significant hypertension can be present even in patients that look relatively normal.
- Severe signs can be seen in dogs at doses as low as 3.5 mg/kg (therapeutic dose 1-2 mg/kg).

Prevention

Prevent access to medication.

Technician Tips

Monitor blood pressure and for ventricular arrhythmias.

Client Education

Chewable formulations increase the likelihood that pets will ingest a large number of tablets.

Never leave bottles of medications on counters or other areas that pets may be able to reach.

SUGGESTED READING

Holding J: Phenylpropanolamine toxicosis in dogs and cats. Vet M 107:18-19, 2012.

AUTHOR: Judy K. Holding, DVM, RN
EDITOR: Tina Wismer, DVM, MS, DABVT, DABT

Pheochromocytoma

Video Available Client Education Sheet

BASIC INFORMATION

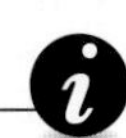

Definition

Catecholamine-producing tumor derived from adrenal medulla chromaffin cells (most common) or extraadrenal sympathetic ganglia (paragangliomas). Most involve a single adrenal gland (90%), but 10% are bilateral. Tumor hormone secretion is episodic and sporadic.

Epidemiology

SPECIES, AGE, SEX

- Dogs: uncommon; middle-aged/older (mean, 11 years; range, 1-18 years)
- Cats: rare; older (mean, 14.5 years)

ASSOCIATED DISORDERS

- May occur as part of multiple endocrine neoplasia syndrome
- Concurrent tumors can include cortisol-secreting adrenocortical tumors, adrenocorticotrophic hormone-secreting tumors or hyperplasia, thyroid tumors and insulinomas
- Non-endocrine tumors may occur concurrently.

Clinical Presentation

HISTORY, CHIEF COMPLAINT

- Antemortem diagnosis is challenging because clinical signs are varied, intermittent, and often nonspecific.

Dogs:

- Intermittent weakness, lethargy, and collapse most common; panting/tachypnea, agitation, anorexia, weight loss, polyuria and polydipsia (PU/PD), tachycardia, vomiting, diarrhea, seizures, or sudden death possible
- Signs often episodic and complicated by a high incidence of concurrent disease
- Many show no clinical signs, and the diagnosis is made incidentally during abdominal ultrasonography or necropsy.

Cats:

- Vague signs, with PU/PD, lethargy, and anorexia most common

PHYSICAL EXAM FINDINGS

- Physical exam commonly unremarkable
- Potential abnormalities include tachypnea, generalized weakness (often episodic), tachycardia or other cardiac arrhythmias, pale mucous membranes, epistaxis, muscle tremors, blindness, retinal hemorrhage/detachment, and signs of abdominal pain.
- An abdominal mass is not usually palpable.

Etiology and Pathophysiology

- Tumors usually are solitary, slow growing, and highly vascular. Rarely, bilateral pheochromocytomas or adrenal pheochromocytomas with a contralateral adrenocortical tumor have been reported.
- Clinically detected pheochromocytomas are considered to be malignant in at least 50% of cases, with local invasion (e.g., caudal vena cava) and metastasis to liver and regional lymph nodes most common.
- Clinical signs related to excessive catecholamine secretion (most common) and/or from space-occupying or invasive behavior of the tumor or from distant metastasis (less common).
- Excess catecholamines cause arteriolar vasoconstriction and systemic hypertension, cardiac arrhythmias, mydriasis, increased smooth muscle sphincter tone, and increased hepatic gluconeogenesis and glycogenolysis.

DIAGNOSIS

Diagnostic Overview

A presumptive diagnosis rests on identification of an adrenal mass and concurrent, often episodic cardiovascular abnormalities (e.g., sinus tachycardia; premature ventricular complexes; systemic hypertension; syncope; pulmonary thromboembolism) ± testing to document elevations in urine or plasma catecholamines (epinephrine and norepinephrine) and catecholamine metabolites (metanephrine and normetanephrine). Measurement of catecholamines and catecholamine metabolites is recommended; catecholamines are secreted episodically, and metabolites (metanephrines) are secreted continuously from the tumor. No consensus exists on preference for plasma or urine testing. If urine used, normetanephrine to creatinine ratio has higher sensitivity and specificity than metanephrine, epinephrine, or norepinephrine to creatinine ratios for the diagnosis. Similarly, measurement of plasma free normetanephrine is superior to measurement of free epinephrine, norepinephrine, or metanephrine. To help differentiate from a cortisol-secreting adrenocortical tumor, serum inhibin can be measured, if available; if inhibin is detectable in serum, an adrenal gland tumor is most likely cortical, and an undetectable level is highly supportive of a pheochromocytoma. Definitive diagnosis requires histopathologic exam of the excised adrenal gland.

Differential Diagnosis

- Adrenal mass
  - Nonfunctional adrenal mass
  - Functional adrenocortical mass
- Systemic hypertension; other causes such as renal disease or hyperadrenocorticism may need to be investigated.
- Collapse/weakness; other causes such as hypoglycemia, cardiac or respiratory disease may need to be investigated.
- Sinus tachycardia; other causes such as systemic disease or anxiety/excitement/pain should be considered.

Initial Database

- CBC, serum biochemical profile, and urinalysis: normal or may show nonspecific changes (e.g., mild nonregenerative anemia, mature neutrophilia, increased liver enzymes, proteinuria)
- Multiple arterial blood pressure (BP) measurements (p. 1065): hypertension (sustained systolic pressure > 160 mm Hg and/or diastolic pressure > 100 mm Hg) is well recognized (40% of cases), but normotension does not rule out a pheochromocytoma because tumor catecholamine secretion is intermittent.
- Abdominal radiographs: low sensitivity for detecting pheochromocytomas but may reveal a perirenal mass ± mineralization.
- Thoracic radiographs: pulmonary metastasis in 10% of affected dogs; cardiomegaly, or pulmonary edema or congestion (rare). Pulmonary thromboembolism (p. 842) is recognized with pheochromocytoma and may cause tachypnea and, rarely, acute cor pulmonale and/or right-sided congestive heart failure.
- Electrocardiography (ECG [p. 1096]): intermittent or sustained tachycardia (sinus tachycardia, ventricular arrhythmias) is common. A 24-hour Holter monitor (p. 1120) may be needed to document intermittent arrhythmias.

- Abdominal ultrasonography: usually unilateral adrenal tumor with normal-size contralateral adrenal gland; may also identify intraabdominal metastasis or tumor invasion of adjacent structures (see *Video*). Careful evaluation of the regional vena cava using Doppler ultrasound is important to identify tumor thrombi (basis for anticoagulation; prognosis more guarded); large thrombi are possible.
- Tests for hyperadrenocorticism (p. 485) should be normal.

Advanced or Confirmatory Testing

- Contrast radiography (nonselective venography or excretory urography) for evaluating tumor invasion of the caudal vena cava or kidney, respectively
- Abdominal CT or MRI (p. 1132) with or without contrast: strongly recommended when surgical intervention is planned; usually shows an adrenal mass and helps identify any local invasion or distant metastasis within the abdomen and to the lungs.
- Increased serum and urine catecholamines and urinary catecholamine metabolites (e.g., normetanephrine): high-performance liquid chromatography superior technique but not available in North America at this time. A nonvalidated species-specific assay is available.
  - Urine normetanephrine concentration (≥4 times normal) in dogs and high plasma normetanephrine concentration in cats strongly suggest pheochromocytoma.
  - Stress associated with hospitalization, critical illness, hyperadrenocorticism, and some medications (e.g., opioids, high-dose dexamethasone) can increase urine catecholamine excretion (i.e., false-positive result); urine collection should occur at home after a few days of adaptation to the sampling procedure. Urine must be acidified, chilled, and protected from light. It is recommended to call the laboratory ahead of time for instructions on collection and shipping of samples.
- Although experimental, functional imaging using ^{123}I-labeled metaiodobenzylguanidine (MIBG), octreotide-DTPA scintigraphy, or positron emission tomography scan with ^{18}F-MIBG may be useful for detecting a pheochromocytoma not found on CT or MRI.
- Histopathologic exam and positive immunohistochemical staining for chromogranin A and synaptophysin of the excised tumor are required for a definitive diagnosis. Biochemical testing for catecholamines can provide additional proof of diagnosis. No histologic features (e.g., invasion of blood vessels or surrounding tissue) are predictive of metastatic behavior.

TREATMENT

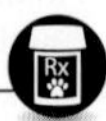

Treatment Overview

Adrenalectomy is the preferred treatment if there is no evidence of (nonresectable) metastasis. Surgical removal should always be preceded by initial medical stabilization to control patient's BP and cardiac arrhythmias. Medical therapy for 1-3 weeks before surgery with an orally administered alpha-antagonist (phenoxybenzamine) is indicated to limit intraoperative complications associated with sudden catecholamine release (hypertensive crisis, cardiac arrhythmias, pulmonary edema, and cardiac ischemia). Mortality rates after adrenalectomy are significantly lower after pretreatment with phenoxybenzamine. Concurrent vena caval venotomy is required when caudal vena caval invasion is present.

Acute General Treatment

- Alpha-antagonist: phenoxybenzamine 0.25 mg/kg PO q 12h initially, then increased to every few days until hypertension controlled, without lethargy/weakness/signs of hypotension, for the 1-3 weeks preceding surgery. Maximal dosage 1.5 mg/kg PO q 12h in dogs (cats, maximum of 0.5 mg/kg PO q 12h) can be reached. Prazosin or amlodipine are alternatives.
- Beta-blocker drugs (e.g., atenolol beginning at 0.5 mg/kg PO q 12h and titrating up to 1 mg/kg PO q 12h if needed) may be used for controlling sinus tachycardia but only after alpha-adrenergic blockade has been initiated.

Chronic Treatment

- Careful anesthetic selection is needed to minimize intraoperative complications; isoflurane or sevoflurane are typically used for maintenance. Direct arterial BP and ECG should be monitored during surgery and for at least 24 hours postoperatively.
- If surgical resection is incomplete or not possible, long-term treatment with an alpha-antagonist ± beta-blockade is indicated.
- Other treatments used in people for nonresectable pheochromocytoma include the radioisotope ^{131}I-MIBG and metyrosine. Metyrosine inhibits tyrosine hydroxylase, the rate-limiting step in catecholamine synthesis, and is used in patients with signs refractory to phenoxybenzamine.

Drug Interactions

Avoid administering monoamine oxidase inhibitors and metoclopramide because either may exacerbate hypertension.

Possible Complications

- Sudden blindness, seizures, or death from a hypertensive crisis
- Perioperative complications include hypertension, hypotension, arrhythmias, respiratory distress, and hemorrhage. Most animals become normotensive 24-48 hours after surgery.

Recommended Monitoring

- In hospital: monitor BP and central venous pressure perioperatively.
- After discharge: assess BP and ECG monthly. Given tendency for pheochromocytomas to be malignant, routine follow-up with ultrasound is recommended q 3 months.

PROGNOSIS & OUTCOME

- Prognosis depends on tumor size, metastasis or local tumor invasion, perioperative complications, and concurrent diseases, which are common (older animals).
- Animals with a surgically excisable tumor have a guarded to good prognosis. If animals survive the immediate postoperative period, a survival time of 18-24 months is possible.

PEARLS & CONSIDERATIONS

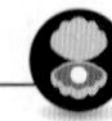

Comments

Pheochromocytomas are difficult to diagnose antemortem, and perioperative management is complex. Referral to an experienced surgeon and anesthesiologist team is recommended.

Technician Tips

Preoperatively and immediately postoperatively, patients may have marked fluctuations in BP and arrhythmias. Close monitoring and preparation for treatment when necessary (monitoring parameters/guidelines should be made clear) are essential.

SUGGESTED READING

Gostelow R, et al: Plasma-free metanephrine and free normetanephrine measurement for the diagnosis of pheochromocytoma in dogs. J Vet Intern Med 27:83-90, 2013.

AUTHOR: Elisabeth Snead, DVM, MSc, DACVIM
EDITOR: Ellen N. Behrend, VMD, PhD, DACVIM

Phobias

BASIC INFORMATION

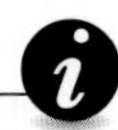

Definition

Behaviors are characterized by persistent and extreme anxiety and avoidance that occur only in response to specific triggers. The fear response is out of proportion given the objective threat, is beyond voluntary control, and may be preceded by anticipatory anxiety.

Epidemiology

SPECIES, AGE, SEX

- Dogs and cats of any age
- As with most behavioral conditions, phobias most commonly develop during social maturity (12-36 months in dogs, 24-48 months in cats).

GENETICS, BREED PREDISPOSITION

Predispositions are suspected, but modes of inheritance, population, and breed variability are mostly unproven. Candidate gene regions are associated with noise-reactive phenotypes in Australian shepherds, border collies, and German shepherds.

RISK FACTORS

Mild signs may exacerbate quickly after exposure to a trigger of large magnitude.

CONTAGION AND ZOONOSIS

A young dog that seems well adjusted and joins a home with a phobic dog may learn (and/or may react to) some of the behaviors associated with the phobia (e.g., reactive barking), especially if these behaviors engender attention.

GEOGRAPHY AND SEASONALITY

Holidays that are celebrated with fireworks, gunfire, or cannon blasts; seasonal thunderstorms

ASSOCIATED DISORDERS

Comorbidity of thunderstorm phobia and separation anxiety (p. 905) is high.

Clinical Presentation

DISEASE FORMS/SUBTYPES

- Thunderstorm/storm phobia
- Noise phobia (single or combination noise types such as booming, metallic, electronic, other noises)
- Neophobia (fear of new objects or circumstances)
- Panic
- Other phobias (e.g., reflective surfaces or floors, nighttime, other animals)

HISTORY, CHIEF COMPLAINT

- Exposure to or anticipation of exposure to discrete triggering events elicits observable signs of sympathetic arousal (e.g., tremor, pacing, hypervigilance, scanning of the environment, restlessness, vocalization, mydriasis, piloerection, ptyalism, elimination, anal sac expression, immobility, repeated startle responses, and behaviors associated with avoidance).
- The onset may be acute, with or without an identifiable trigger, or may worsen over time. If escape attempts are interrupted, growling, snarling, lunging, or biting may be elicited.
- The aroused state may persist for minutes/hours.
- Clients' chief complaints may be only destructive behavior, excessive vocalization, or house soiling, without awareness of their meaning as markers of anxiety. Because many clients crate their dogs to resolve such behaviors, it is important to query clients regarding the reason they do so; otherwise, signs may be missed until the dog escapes the crate, frequently injuring himself/herself in the process.
- Cats may show signs that the clients may misinterpret as normal, such as frequent and extended hiding out of context with the situations that trigger the behaviors (i.e., scaredy cats).

PHYSICAL EXAM FINDINGS

- Generally unremarkable exam findings; damage to teeth, nails, or feet in extreme cases
- Self-inflicted injuries as dogs attempt to break out of crates in which they are confined as "treatment" for anxiety-associated behaviors

Etiology and Pathophysiology

Dogs, like humans, may have susceptibility genes for development of pathologic anxieties. Dysfunction or dysregulation of caudate nuclei in the brain has been implicated in some phobic states. Inadequate *in utero* nutrition has also been associated with heightened reactivity. Cats may remain aroused for 24-48 hours after an event of profound hypothalamic stimulation. The worse the panic, the more insensitive the animal is to routine physical or social stimuli.

DIAGNOSIS

Diagnostic Overview

From the behavioral history, a diagnosis is made when extreme fear or anxiety (anticipatory fear) is provoked by specific triggers and the severity of the fearful response is out of context with the risk the trigger represents.

Differential Diagnosis

- Generalized anxiety disorder
- Separation anxiety
- Learned fear after a traumatic event
- Attention-seeking behavior

Initial Database

- CBC, serum chemistry profile, urinalysis: generally unremarkable; used to assess systemic illness triggering or contributing to phobic states or before initiating medication (if indicated)
- Perform additional tests based on history and physical exam findings (e.g., feline leukemia virus, feline immunodeficiency virus, serum T_4 assays in most adult cats).

Advanced or Confirmatory Testing

If signs of neurologic dysfunction are present or develop, a primary behavioral abnormality is virtually never the sole diagnosis. Extracranial and intracranial medical disorders should be investigated as appropriate.

TREATMENT

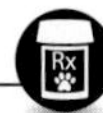

Treatment Overview

The goal is to produce a decreased or ablated response to the inciting trigger as evidenced by a reduction in or elimination of overt signs of sympathetic arousal.

Acute and Chronic Treatment

- The client should help the pet avoid exposure to the panic-inciting stimulus if it has been identified.
- The client should reward any spontaneous decrease in reactivity to phobic triggers.
- Benzodiazepines (BZDs) for their quick onset of action and specific panicolytic effects should be prescribed in combination with other psychotropic medications such as tricyclic antidepressants (TCAs) or selective serotonin reuptake inhibitors (SSRIs). Clonidine and gabapentin are also options as adjuncts to TCAs or SSRIs.
- Trazodone, a serotonin antagonist and reuptake inhibitor (SARI) may be a useful adjunct in combination with an SSRI or TCA when other combinations do not reduce symptoms. A dexmedetomidine oromucosal gel (Sileo) is FDA approved to treat noise aversion and provides almost immediate relief of sympathetic signs.
  - TCA medications
    - Amitriptyline 1-2 mg/kg PO q 12h (dogs); 0.5-1 mg/kg PO q 12-24h (cats). Treat for a minimum of 30 days. First drug of choice in mild cases without contraindications to their use; inexpensive
    - Clomipramine 2-3 mg/kg PO q 12h (dogs); 0.5 mg/kg PO q 24h (cats). Treat for a minimum of 8 weeks. Most successful when the behaviors have a ritualistic or elimination component
  - SSRI medications
    - Fluoxetine (Prozac) 1 mg/kg PO q 24h (dogs); 0.5 mg/kg PO q 24h (cats). Treat for a minimum of 8 weeks.

    - Paroxetine (Paxil) 1 mg/kg PO q 24h (dogs); 0.25-0.5 mg/kg PO q 24h (cats). Treat for a minimum of 8 weeks.
    - Sertraline (Zoloft) 1 mg/kg PO q 24h (dogs); 0.5 mg/kg PO q 24h (cats). Treat for a minimum of 8 weeks. Can be successful for situations in which other medications have been less helpful
  - BZD medications
    - Diazepam or oxazepam 0.2-0.4 mg/kg PO q 12-24h. Treat for a minimum 30 days.
    - Alprazolam 0.01-0.025 mg/kg PO q 8-24h or q 4-6h for panic (dose should be increased to a maximum of 2 mg/dose for a medium-sized dog until effect or sedation before deciding the medication is not effective)
    - Clonazepam 0.01-0.05 mg/kg PO q 12-24h or q 4-6h for panic as needed (dogs)
    - Response to benzodiazepines is very individualized, and constant communication between practitioner and client is necessary to achieve adequate titration of the patient's dose.
  - SARI medications
    - Trazodone 3-7 mg/kg PO, used prn or q 8-24h (dogs); 3-8 mg/kg or 25 mg/CAT (cats). If given daily, using one-half of the target dose for 3 days may diminish the likelihood of side effects. Trazodone is well tolerated by dogs, but starting at the lower end of the range and carefully titrating upward is advised while monitoring for signs of serotonin syndrome. Alone, prn treatment is usually not sufficient to abort a phobic response.
  - Gabapentin (GABA analog) 3-5 mg/kg PO q 12h (dogs); 5-10 mg/kg PO q 12h (cats), starting low and titrating to effect
  - Adrenergic agonists
    - Clonidine 0.01-0.05 mg/kg PO q 8-12h (dogs)
    - Dexmedetomidine 125 mcg/m^2 (p. 609), delivered as an oromucosal gel (Sileo) (dogs)
- Using positive reinforcement, clients should teach dogs to relax while making eye contact with them so that this new behavior can be used when the dog encounters a situation about which it is anxious or unsure. Clients should learn to monitor facial cues, body postures, pupil size and shape, and respiration associated with relaxation versus anxiety.
  - Avoidance of exposure to the panic-inciting stimulus
  - Desensitization to the triggers can be accomplished if triggers can be identified and reproduced faithfully and in a systematic and incremental fashion.
  - Clients should offer positive reinforcement to their animals for all relaxed and calm behaviors, particularly when facing phobic triggers.

Drug Interactions

- BZDs, TCAs, SSRIs, and SARIs can be combined at lower than normal dosages if needed, but there is potential for sedation, and patient response must be evaluated on a case-by-case basis.
- TCAs, SARIs, and SSRIs should not be given with monoamine oxidase inhibitors (MAOIs), found in some flea and tick collars and dips and in some cognitive dysfunction medications.
- Use of SSRIs and SARIs with tramadol may increase the risk of serotonin syndrome and should be avoided if possible. If they must be combined, start both at reduced doses, titrate each to effect, and watch for signs of serotonin syndrome; risk is reduced but not eliminated, and the client should be informed.
- TCAs should be used with caution in patients with cardiac arrhythmias, existing hepatic or thyroid disease.
- Paroxetine should be avoided in animals with renal disease, and gabapentin should be used with caution. Anecdotal reports of constipation are more common in cats, and their owners should be cautioned to monitor stool consistency.

Possible Complications

- Generalization to triggers that are similar to the original stimulus (e.g., a thunder-phobic dog begins to respond to firework displays and then reacts to all loud noises in general)
- Phobias are almost always comorbid conditions; screen for comorbidities (most common are separation anxiety, panic disorder, and generalized anxiety disorder).
- BZDs have the potential for drug diversion and abuse by clients.

Recommended Monitoring

- Animals that take BZDs require a physical exam every 6 months in most U.S. states. The potential for human diversion warrants vigilance regarding refills.
- Yearly CBC, serum chemistry profile, urinalysis, and thyroid screen (q 6 months for geriatric pets) if taking psychotropic medications. Cardiac monitoring is recommended if syncope or other suspected cardiac signs are involved in panic.

PROGNOSIS & OUTCOME

Prognosis varies and depends on
- Timeliness of diagnosis (prognosis more favorable for early diagnosis)
- Frequent and thorough communication between clinician and client allows treatment to be adjusted according to the animal's response and needs: prognosis is more favorable.
- Client factors
  - Diligence of treatment (comprehensive, persistent treatment plan, and follow-up: prognosis more favorable)
  - Client compliance (good compliance: prognosis more favorable)
- If the best outcome is to be obtained, early intervention is essential.
- If the problem is chronic before treatment is sought, treatment may well be lifelong, especially with other comorbid anxiety-related conditions.

PEARLS & CONSIDERATIONS

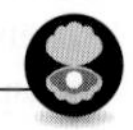

Comments

- Client observations and reports are critical in data collection; it is important to spend time understanding the client's use of language. Asking clients to describe what they see their pet do, rather than their interpretation of the behavior, is key in obtaining behavioral data.
- The single best tool for evaluating behavior is observing the behavior itself. Video recording with smart phones and webcams make this possible. Consider having a video camera clinicians can use in the practice and lend to clients.

Prevention

- When selecting breeding stock, temperament, conformation, and medical phenotypes should be assessed because genetic predisposition is suspected to be a strong contributor to mood disorder development.
- At the first sign of any fearful behavior, clients should watch for worsening of the behavior and possible triggers that might indicate the development of a phobia.
- Veterinarians should screen for fear and phobias as a routine part of every appointment.

Technician Tips

Noise-phobic dogs may startle repeatedly in response to any small sound.

Client Education

- Most behavioral conditions are due to chemical and functional brain abnormalities (areas of the limbic system and prefrontal cortex) and therefore are not willful acts of disobedience by a pet.
- Treatment of behavioral conditions is an ongoing process, often for the duration of the pet's life. Relapses may occur with treatment discontinuation or with added stressors.

SUGGESTED READING

Overall KL, et al: Phenotypic determination of noise reactivity in 3 breeds of working dogs: A cautionary tale of age, breed, behavioral assessment, and genetics. J Vet Behav Clin Appl Res 16:113-125, 2016.

AUTHOR: Soraya V. Juarbe-Diaz, DVM, DACVB
EDITOR: Karen L. Overall, MA, VMD, PhD, DACVB

Pinnal Diseases

Bonus Material Online 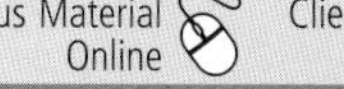 Client Education Sheet 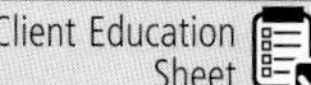

BASIC INFORMATION

Definition

Diseases affecting the skin, cartilage, or other tissues of the pinna (externally visible part of the ear) are often part of a more widespread dermatologic disease but can involve the pinna exclusively.

Epidemiology

SPECIES, AGE, SEX

Depends on cause

GENETICS, BREED PREDISPOSITION

Breed predispositions exist for some pinnal diseases:

- Acquired pattern alopecia (p. 766): dachshund, Boston terrier
- Ear margin seborrhea: dachshund
- Sebaceous adenitis: standard poodle, others
- Canine familial dermatomyositis: Shetland sheepdog, collie
- Primary seborrhea (p. 214): cocker spaniel
- Actinic keratoses, squamous cell carcinoma, hemangioma: light-colored cats
- Canine leproid granuloma syndrome: boxers, other short-coated dogs
- Pigmented viral plaques: pug, miniature schnauzer
- See Differential Diagnosis for other breed predispositions

CONTAGION AND ZOONOSIS

Contagious and zoonotic causes include dermatophytes, *Sarcoptes, Notoedres,* and *Otodectes. Demodex gatoi* and lice are contagious but not zoonotic. Leishmaniasis is a vector-transmitted zoonosis.

GEOGRAPHY AND SEASONALITY

A distinct geographic distribution exists for leishmaniasis, notoedric mange, *D. gatoi* infestation, and leproid granuloma syndrome.

Clinical Presentation

HISTORY, CHIEF COMPLAINT

- Some conditions are pruritic or painful; others only alter pinnal appearance.
- Clients may note folding of an erect pinna.
- Pinnal lesions often accompany more generalized dermatologic disease.
- Conditions can have a predilection for the concave or convex aspect of the pinna, its distal tip, or its margins.

PHYSICAL EXAM FINDINGS

- Various presentations: excoriations, crusts, scales, ulcers, alopecia, nodules, plaques, edema, lichenification, pigmentary changes, erythema, hemorrhage, tissue loss, diffuse thickening or deformation of the normal shape of the pinna
- Other physical exam findings, such as tail tip or footpad lesions with vasculitis, can be suggestive of the cause.

Etiology and Pathophysiology

- The pinna consists of skin and cartilage, and a disease process affecting either tissue can result in pinnal lesions.
- Certain diseases are more likely to affect the pinna than other cutaneous sites.
  - Ear margin seborrhea, proliferative and necrotizing feline otitis externa, proliferative thrombovascular necrosis of the pinna, and aural hematomas are limited to this location.
  - Vasculitis and other ischemic conditions affect the pinna because of its limited collateral blood supply.
  - The feline pinna is prone to UV-induced damage and frostbite.
  - Canine leproid granuloma syndrome and fly bites have a predilection for this site.
- Conversely, the pinna is rarely affected by pyoderma, otherwise the most common cause of cutaneous crusting in dogs.

DIAGNOSIS

Diagnostic Overview

- Localization of lesions to the pinnae should prompt complete dermatologic and physical exam. Palpate the ear canals, and perform otoscopic exam of both ears.
- Pruritic animals should be assessed for a pinnal-pedal reflex: rub the edge of one pinna and observe for a scratching motion in the ipsilateral hind leg.
- Unless the diagnosis is apparent from physical exam alone, skin scrapings for ectoparasites and cytologic analysis of pinnal lesions are often performed. Further testing is based on the differential diagnoses (see below).

Differential Diagnosis

Parasitic causes:

- Sarcoptic mange (dogs): positive pinnal pedal reflex, but it may be difficult to find mites on skin scrapings
- Notoedric mange (cats): usually easy to find mites on skin scrapings
- Demodicosis (dogs): may cause erythema in concave pinna and/or alopecia on convex pinna
- Pediculosis (louse infestation): convex pinna common site
- Other: trombiculiasis, insect bites (often *Stomoxys calcitrans,* affecting ear tips or folds),

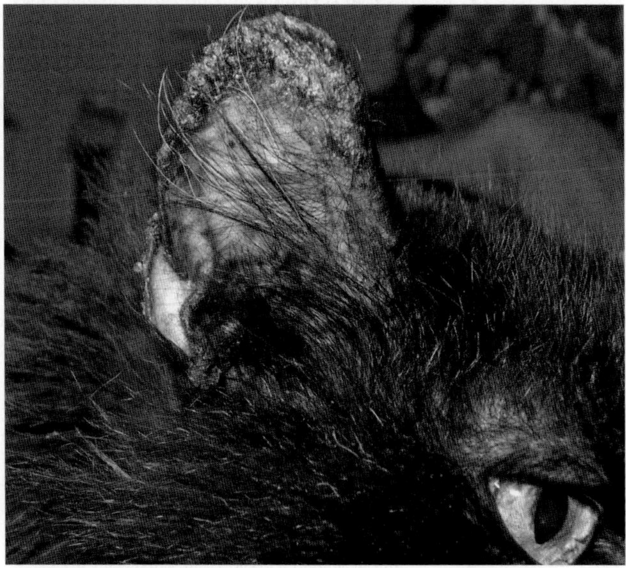

PINNAL DISEASES Pinnal crusting in a cat with pemphigus foliaceus.

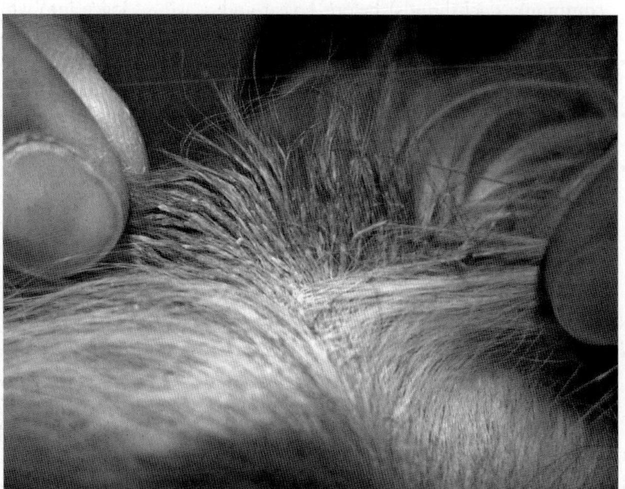

PINNAL DISEASES Pinnal margin follicular casts in a dog with sebaceous adenitis.

Otodectes (primarily affects the ear canal), *D. gatoi* (cats)

Infectious causes:
- Dermatophytosis (feline > canine)
- Canine leproid granuloma syndrome: nodules on convex pinna caused by a novel species of mycobacteria with a distinct geographic distribution
- Leishmaniasis (dogs > cats): pinnal scaling and alopecia; infected animals are systemically ill
- Pigmented viral plaques: darkly pigmented macules or slightly raised papules

Hypersensitivity disorders:
- Atopic dermatitis and food allergy: commonly cause pinnal erythema and pruritus
- Contact hypersensitivity: most often due to topically applied ear medications (e.g., neomycin, propylene glycol); suspect when ear worsens rather than improving with treatment despite resolution of infection on cytology
- Mosquito bite hypersensitivity (cats): seasonal; convex pinna is a common site

Immune-mediated disorders:
- Pemphigus foliaceus: may resemble pyoderma, which is rare on the pinna. Common site of lesions in cats
- Vasculitis and ischemic dermatopathy: fairly common cause of pinnal lesions in dogs; this diverse group of diseases can be idiopathic, hereditary (e.g., Jack Russell terriers), or iatrogenic (e.g., rabies vaccine induced). Ulcerative and crusted lesion, often on the distal concave pinna; distal extremities and tail tip can be affected
- Less common, also affecting other sites: pemphigus erythematosus, discoid lupus erythematosus, bullous pemphigoid, cold agglutinin disease, alopecia areata, familial cutaneous vasculopathy of German shepherd dogs
- Less common, limited to the pinna: proliferative thrombovascular necrosis (dogs), auricular chondrosis (swollen, misshapen, painful pinnae)

Hereditary causes:
- Acquired pattern alopecia: affects dogs (most commonly dachshunds) before 1 year and progresses to complete pinnal alopecia
- Canine familial dermatomyositis: lesions usually manifest by 6 months of age.
- Color dilution alopecia: progressive hair loss in blue- or fawn-colored dogs
- Other: primary seborrhea, psoriasiform-lichenoid dermatosis of English springer spaniels, exfoliative cutaneous lupus erythematosus of German short-haired pointers, congenital hypotrichosis, black hair follicular dysplasia

Neoplastic diseases:
- Squamous cell carcinoma: most common in light-colored cats; often preceded by premalignant actinic keratoses (small areas of crusting and hyperkeratosis). Pinnal lesions on light-colored cats warrant investigation.
- Histiocytoma and sebaceous gland tumor: commonly occur on the canine pinna
- Basal cell tumor: commonly occurs on the feline pinna

Miscellaneous conditions:
- Aural hematoma (p. 104): hemorrhage within or along the cartilage of the pinna. Assess for causes of head shaking (e.g., otitis externa, sometimes in the contralateral ear)
- Ear margin seborrhea: pendulous-eared dogs, particularly dachshunds. Keratinous deposits occur on concave and convex margins; fissures may form in chronic cases.
- Sebaceous adenitis: scaling and follicular casts
- Acquired folding of feline ear pinnae: associated with iatrogenic hyperadrenocorticism (topical or systemic steroid use)
- Proliferative and necrotizing otitis externa of cats: highly characteristic: adherent, dark, keratinous debris on the concave aspect of the pinna, usually in young cats
- Canine sterile eosinophilic pinnal furunculosis
- Melanoderma and alopecia of Yorkshire terriers: also affects bridge of nose

Initial Database

Varies, depending on differential diagnoses but may include
- None; diagnosis may be presumptive (e.g., aural hematoma, acquired pattern alopecia)
- Skin scrapings (p. 1091)
- Pinnal-pedal reflex: ≈82% sensitivity and ≈94% specificity for *Sarcoptes* (p. 900); sensitivity higher than skin scrapings for this parasite
- Cutaneous cytology (p. 1091)
- Wood's lamp exam, fungal culture
- Trichography (demodicosis, color dilution alopecia, pediculosis, sebaceous adenitis)
- Fine-needle aspiration of nodular lesions
  - Acid-fast stain of aspirates if mycobacteria suspected
- Skin biopsies
  - Advise clients that pinnal biopsies can result in permanent cosmetic changes. It is not usually necessary to provide cartilage, and so full-thickness biopsies are not often required.
  - Procedure often requires general anesthesia because there is very little subcutaneous space into which to inject lidocaine. The proximal convex pinna can be an exception.
  - The pinna can be clipped to help visualize blood vessels. Close surgical clipping is not recommended because it can remove diagnostically important material.
  - Pinnal margin lesions
    - For a good cosmetic outcome, sample using a thin shave biopsy of the pinnal margin; using a #15 scalpel blade, shave the skin down to the level of the cartilage.
    - Larger wedges can be removed, leaving skin distal to the cartilage for closure.
    - With extensive pinnal necrosis, affected tissue can be excised to create a more proximal margin.
  - Nonmarginal lesions
    - Use a biopsy punch (usually 6 mm unless pinna is small). Take care NOT to cut through underlying cartilage; otherwise, a permanent hole will result. A small (<0.25 mL) volume of normal saline or lidocaine injected under the biopsy site on the convex pinna elevates the skin to protect the cartilage but may result in some distortion of the dermis.
  - If direct pressure does not stop bleeding, epinephrine can be applied to the surgical wound with a cotton-tipped applicator.
  - Suture or allow skin to heal by second intention. The latter causes less puckering of the ear.
  - Always include crusts in the biopsy. Because pinnal biopsies are very thin, place them on a piece of heavy paper, dermis side down, before placing in formalin.
- CBC, serum chemistry profile, thyroid hormone levels, urinalysis, antinuclear antibody titers, and other tests as appropriate
- Response to empirical therapy (e.g., *Sarcoptes*)

TREATMENT

Treatment Overview

Varies, depending on cause. For aural hematomas, various surgical and medical techniques are described (p. 104).

PROGNOSIS & OUTCOME

Varies, depending on cause

PEARLS & CONSIDERATIONS

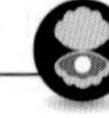

Comments

- Due to the difficulty of collecting diagnostic skin biopsies from the pinna, seek out and sample other similarly affected areas of skin.
- Although both diseases are most common in dachshunds, ear margin seborrhea is characterized by scaling and skin lesions, whereas pattern alopecia is not.
- Consider empirical treatment for *Sarcoptes* in dogs with pinnal pruritus, even with negative skin scrapings and no pinnal-pedal reflex.

Technician Tips

Head shaking greatly exacerbates hemorrhage after pinnal biopsies or injury. A gentle technique to protect the pinnae from this self-trauma uses a surgical stockinette tube placed over the head and secured to the forehead by surgical tape. The stockinette may be used in a single layer or doubled over with loose holes cut out for the ears in the bottom layer. The stockinette is placed over the head such that the ears rest in an anatomically normal position. The stockinette must not be tight. The aim is to keep the ears from flapping when the head is shaken.

SUGGESTED READING

Marignac G: Diseases that affect the pinna. In Gotthelf LN, editor: Small animal ear diseases, ed 2, St. Louis, 2005, Saunders, pp 235-263.

AUTHOR: Kinga Gortel, DVM, MS, DACVD
EDITOR: Manon Paradis, DMV, MVSc, DACVD

Pleural Effusion

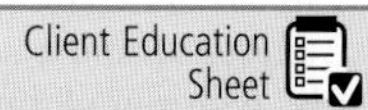

BASIC INFORMATION

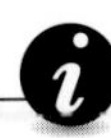

Definition

Accumulation of fluid within the pleural space is relatively common.

Synonyms

- General: pleural fluid, thoracic effusion
- Specific: hydrothorax (pure or modified transudate), hemothorax, chylothorax, pyothorax, neoplastic exudate
- Chylothorax, hemothorax, and pyothorax are discussed elsewhere on pp. 172, 436, and 857, respectively.

Epidemiology

SPECIES, AGE, SEX

Dogs and cats of either sex; age at presentation varies with underlying cause

GENETICS, BREED PREDISPOSITION

Breed predispositions depend on underlying cause (e.g., lung lobe torsion [LLT] in pugs and Afghan hounds; heart failure Maine coon cat)

RISK FACTORS

- Heart disease (cats > dogs)
  - Pleural effusion may be seen with right- and left-sided congestive heart failure (CHF) in cats, but only right-sided failure is likely to cause effusion in dogs
- Hypoalbuminemia
- Neoplasia
- LLT
- Vasculitis

CONTAGION AND ZOONOSIS

Based on specific underlying cause (e.g., feline infectious peritonitis [FIP])

Clinical Presentation

DISEASE FORMS/SUBTYPES

Classified by fluid type (p. 1343):
- Hydrothorax (i.e., transudate)
- Hemothorax (p. 436)
- Chylothorax (p. 172)
- Pyothorax (p. 857)

HISTORY, CHIEF COMPLAINT

- Severity of clinical signs varies with underlying cause, volume of effusion, and rate of fluid accumulation.
  - If rate is slow, large volumes may be present before clinical signs are apparent (especially cats).
- Dyspnea, tachypnea, orthopnea
- Lethargy, exercise intolerance
- Chronic cough (uncommon)
- Signs related to underlying disease (e.g., pallor, weight loss, abdominal effusion, diarrhea, signs of trauma)

PHYSICAL EXAM FINDINGS

General:
- Dyspnea: wide chest excursions, abducted elbows when standing, extension of the neck, orthopnea, anxiousness, flared nostrils
  - Affected animals may have a prolonged inspiratory and short expiratory phase (inspiratory effort) or dyssynchrony between the thoracic cage and abdomen (paradoxical breathing; very common in cats)
- Muffled heart and lung sounds ventrally
- Normal to increased bronchovesicular lung sounds dorsally
- Ventral hyporesonance with thoracic percussion; fluid line may be detected
- Other signs associated with specific underlying cause (e.g., pallor, fever, abdominal fluid wave, jugular pulse, heart murmur)

Etiology and Pathophysiology

Respiratory dysfunction reflects hypoventilation and ventilation/perfusion mismatch. Pathophysiologic mechanisms determine fluid classification:
- Reduced plasma colloid oncotic pressure (hydrothorax: pure transudate)
  - Hypoalbuminemia: protein-losing nephropathy (e.g., glomerulonephritis, amyloidosis); protein-losing enteropathy (e.g., inflammatory bowel disease, lymphangiectasia, neoplasia); protein-losing dermatopathy (e.g., burns, exudative skin disease (uncommon); vasculitis (infectious or noninfectious, modified transudate more common); synthetic failure (e.g., chronic hepatopathy, portal vascular anomalies) (p. 1239)
- Increased capillary hydrostatic pressure (hydrothorax: modified transudate)
  - CHF; Budd-Chiari–like syndromes; thoracic or mediastinal neoplasia (also exudate); LLT (cause vs. effect of LLT and pleural effusions is unclear; torsion may cause effusion, but effusion can also predispose to torsion); caval syndrome; heartworm disease (HWD)
- Reduced lymphatic drainage/lymphatic obstruction: hydrothorax (modified transudate), chylothorax
- Pyothorax: modified transudate to exudate
- Thoracic or pulmonary neoplasia: chylothorax, pyothorax, neoplastic exudate
- Increased vascular permeability (exudate)
  - Pyothorax, FIP, systemic disease (e.g., pancreatitis, vasculitis)
- Disruption of vascular integrity/hemostatic abnormalities (hemothorax)
  - Rupture of neoplastic mass, coagulopathy, trauma, LLT, and infection (abscess, granuloma)

DIAGNOSIS

Diagnostic Overview

Pleural effusion can be suggested by physical exam and confirmed with thoracic radiographs, thoracic ultrasound, or thoracocentesis. Thoracocentesis and fluid analysis provide precise information on the nature of the fluid and perhaps the underlying cause.

Differential Diagnosis

- Other pleural space disease
  - Masses
  - Pneumothorax
  - Constrictive/fibrosing pleuritis: can occur concurrently with pleural effusion (chylothorax or pyothorax) and causes rounded lung lobe contours that may be difficult to distinguish radiographically from pleural effusion
- Pulmonary parenchymal/airway disease
- Thoracic wall defects
- Diaphragmatic hernia, including peritoneal/pericardial hernia
- Neuromuscular disease

Initial Database

Thoracocentesis (p. 1164)
- Diagnostic/therapeutic
  - With severe dyspnea, consider thoracocentesis before thoracic radiographs.
  - Thoracic ultrasonography can also demonstrate effusion.
- Thoracocentesis first
  - Therapeutic value: removal of effusion, improved oxygenation for patient
  - Diagnostic value: fluid analysis, improved radiographic visualization of parenchymal structures: mediastinal masses, consolidated lung lobes, pulmonary masses, and abdominal organs in the thoracic cavity (hernia)
  - Use caution if other clinical signs of coagulopathy found on physical exam.
- Radiographs first
  - Diagnostic value: confirms effusion; identify displacement of cardiac silhouette (avoid during thoracocentesis).
  - Care with positioning not to cause excess stress
- Ultrasound first
  - Diagnostic value: confirm effusion, guide thoracocentesis, estimate volume of effusion (see above)

Diagnostics: fluid in EDTA (lavender-top) and plain (red-top) tubes for analysis: total nucleated and red cell counts, total protein, and cytology; prepare fresh smears (p. 1343)
- Send fresh smears with fluid for outside analysis; prevents cellular degradation during shipping
- Pyothorax culture and susceptibility (C&S): aerobic and anaerobic in all cases

- Chylothorax: compare effusion and serum triglyceride and cholesterol concentrations
- FIP: albumin/globulin ratio of > 0.8 makes FIP unlikely (exception: if protein clot forms *in vitro,* false-negative), positive Rivalta test suggests FIP (p. 327)
- Hemothorax: compare packed cell volumes (PCVs) (peripheral and effusion)

Thoracic radiographs: signs of pleural effusion vary with fluid volume; at a minimum, two-view thoracic radiography is recommended in all cases, but three-view radiographs are preferred:

- Radiographic changes: first apparent with approximately 10 mL/kg of fluid
- General: retraction (scalloping) of lungs from thoracic wall with interposed fluid opacity, obscured diaphragm, widened mediastinum; with trauma, fractured ribs, diaphragmatic hernia, and orthopedic injuries may be present
- Specific views: dorsoventral (DV) view: obscured cardiac silhouette; lateral view: increased opacity dorsal to the sternum and scalloping of lung margins (lateral view prone to misinterpretation); ventrodorsal (VD) view: visualization of small volumes, blunting of lung margins and costophrenic angles; horizontal beam: may reduce patient stress
- Pyothorax/chylothorax: may cause fibrosing pleuritis; prevents full expansion of lungs after thoracocentesis with rounded lung lobe contours. Difficult to distinguish from effusion
- Radiographs after thoracocentesis recommended to evaluate for underlying disease (improved visualization)

Clinicopathologic abnormalities (depend on cause):

- CBC: inflammatory leukogram, thrombocytopenia, anemia with some causes
- Serum biochemical panel: depending on cause, may find hypoalbuminemia, hypoglobulinemia/hyperglobulinemia, hypoglycemia, hypocholesterolemia, azotemia, electrolyte abnormalities, or increased liver enzyme concentrations
- Urinalysis: proteinuria if protein-losing nephropathy

Thoracic ultrasonography (p. 1102)

- Before thoracocentesis to improve the acoustic window, unless the animal is uncomfortable/ dyspneic during restraint for the exam

Advanced or Confirmatory Testing

Testing is based on nature of effusion and prior diagnostic test results:

- Hydrothorax: for pure transudate (effusion total protein < 2.5 g/dL, total nucleated cell count < 1000), consider
  - Protein-losing nephropathy: urine protein/ creatinine ratio
  - Hepatic failure/portal systemic shunt: bile acids/ammonia, abdominal imaging
  - Protein-losing enteropathy: serum folate/ cobalamin, intestinal biopsies (surgical or endoscopic)
- Hydrothorax: for modified transudate (effusion total protein = 2.5-5 g/dL; no cytologic evidence of infection or hemorrhage), consider
  - Heart disease: echocardiography (p. 1094), NT-pro-BNP (p. 1369)
  - Thoracic mass: thoracic ultrasound exam, CT (useful for identifying and characterizing pleural space lesions; post-contrast images can help delineate pleural lesions from effusion), fine-needle aspiration and cytologic exam of lung or mass if lesion is identified (p. 1113), thoracoscopy or thoracotomy for pleural or lung biopsy
- FIP (p. 327)
- Chylothorax (p. 172)
- Hemothorax (p. 436)
- Pyothorax (p. 857)

TREATMENT

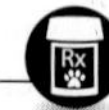

Treatment Overview

Thoracocentesis is commonly needed acutely to improve respiratory function. Ultimately, correction of the underlying disease provides the best chance for resolution of effusion.

Acute General Treatment

- Oxygen supplementation (p. 1146) if dyspneic
- Minimize stress
- Thoracocentesis
- Specific acute treatment as indicated by type/ cause of pleural effusion
- Support of circulatory and respiratory function

Chronic Treatment

Correction of the underlying disorder may resolve effusion with or without repeated thoracocentesis. See specific disease condition for treatment information.

- Chronic effusions refractory to therapy: consider placement of a PleuralPort device, which allows owners to drain the effusion at home using a Huber needle placed into a subcutaneous drainage hub.

Possible Complications

- Iatrogenic pneumothorax and hemothorax from thoracostomy tube
- Constrictive/fibrosing pleuritis (pyothorax or chylothorax)
- Disseminated intravascular coagulation (DIC) or systemic inflammatory response syndrome (SIRS) from pyothorax
- Recurrence of pyothorax if migrating foreign body remains or inappropriate antibiotics are used or used for an insufficient duration
- Complications of thoracocentesis (and corresponding precautions) include:
  - Lung laceration and pneumothorax: less likely if needle is introduced and withdrawn in linear fashion, without side-to-side or rotatory motions after the needle tip is in the pleural space
  - Re-expansion pulmonary edema: less likely if large-volume effusions are withdrawn periodically over several hours rather than all at once and more likely with chronic effusions
  - Pleural shock: sudden bradycardia of vagal origin caused by needle contact with the pleura (no prevention; responds to immediate administration of atropine 0.04 mg/kg IV)
  - Bronchopleural fistula: constrictive/ fibrosing pleuritis prevents further lung expansion during thoracocentesis, and ongoing fluid withdrawal creates excessive negative pressure in the pleural space; rupture of the bronchial wall into the pleural cavity may occur (possibly less likely to occur if large-volume effusions are withdrawn periodically over several hours rather than all at once), especially if lung lobes are very round on radiographs

Recommended Monitoring

- Clinical signs, including respiratory rate
- Thoracic radiographs to assess resolution or progression
- Daily cytologic exam/Gram stain of chest tube fluid withdrawn from pyothorax cases to assess antimicrobial response

PROGNOSIS & OUTCOME

- Varies with cause and severity of underlying disease (e.g., grave prognosis for FIP, good prognosis for hemothorax due to coagulopathy after initial stabilization)
- Pleural effusion may worsen the short-term prognosis for the underlying disease by causing acute respiratory compromise.

PEARLS & CONSIDERATIONS

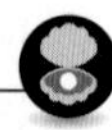

Comments

- If pleural effusion is suspected, consider thoracocentesis, which can be diagnostic and therapeutic, before thoracic radiographs.
- Thoracic percussion may increase suspicion of pleural effusion and supports pre-radiograph thoracocentesis.
- Even partial drainage of the effusion can improve respiratory function.
- Obtain dorsoventral view first, which is often sufficient to confirm effusion.
  - Alternatively, a brief ultrasound exam may confirm pleural effusion, justifying thoracocentesis. Radiographs may then be taken more safely after thoracocentesis.
  - Ultrasonography with patient in sternal recumbence or standing can visualize effusion with minimal restraint and stress.
- Because cats with pleural effusion can be easily stressed by radiographs, consider thoracocentesis early (especially if paradoxical breathing occurs without expiratory wheezing).
- Hemothorax usually develops from trauma, coagulopathies, or neoplasia.
- Grass awns can be located in multiple sites, including the pericardial sac, in dogs with pyothorax.

- Retrosternal fat and interindividual variation may give the false impression of pleural effusion on lateral radiographic projections of animals without pleural effusion. For this reason and to determine whether effusion is unilateral or bilateral, a minimum of two-view thoracic radiographs is indicated.

Prevention

Avoid trauma and exposure to anticoagulant rodenticides.

Technician Tips

- Animals with large-volume pleural effusions are fragile and susceptible to stress with handling. Minimal handling is important.
- Supplemental oxygen should be provided to all dyspneic patients.
- Avoid dorsal recumbence (ventrodorsal view) for radiographs in animals with pleural effusions.
- Supplies for emergency thoracocentesis: clippers, skin preparation materials, butterfly needle or needle with an extension set, 3-way stopcock, and syringes
- Complications of thoracocentesis (e.g., pneumothorax, hemothorax): if patient suddenly develops a tachypnea or increased effort after pleural drainage, alert the attending clinician as soon as possible.

SUGGESTED READING

Dempsey SM, et al. A review of the pathophysiology, classification, and analysis of canine and feline cavitary effusions. J Am Anim Hosp Assoc 47:1-11, 2011.

AUTHOR: Graham Swinney, BVSc, DVCS, FANZCVS
EDITOR: Megan Grobman, DVM, MS, DACVIM

Pneumonia, Aspiration

Client Education Sheet

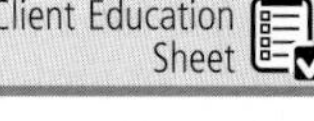

BASIC INFORMATION

Definition

- Infection associated with inhalation of oropharyngeal secretions, foodstuffs, other foreign material, or gastric contents
- In veterinary medicine, the term is often used in reference to aspiration pneumonitis, which is chemical injury caused by inhalation of gastric contents (most commonly) or other materials (e.g., barium, mineral oil).

Synonym

Aspiration pneumonitis

Epidemiology

SPECIES, AGE, SEX

Most often male dogs, but dogs (and less often, cats) of either sex and any age

GENETICS, BREED PREDISPOSITION

Large breeds of dogs are overrepresented. Irish wolfhound may be predisposed.

RISK FACTORS

- Diseases of
  - Pharynx or larynx (e.g., laryngeal paralysis, before and after arytenoid lateralization; extraesophageal reflux)
  - Esophagus (e.g., megaesophagus, severe esophagitis)
  - Stomach or intestine (e.g., pyloric or upper intestinal obstruction)
- Forced enteral administration of drugs or foods
- Impaired protective reflexes (e.g., anesthesia, seizure)

ASSOCIATED DISORDERS

- Acute respiratory distress syndrome
- Bacterial pneumonia
- Hypoxemia
- Lung lobe abscessation
- Pneumothorax
- Shock
- Airway obstruction

Clinical Presentation

DISEASE FORMS/SUBTYPES

- Acute or chronic
- Fulminant or insidious

HISTORY, CHIEF COMPLAINT

Clinical signs may be absent or severe; when present, they may include
- Anorexia
- Collapse
- Cough
- Lethargy
- Respiratory distress
- Others that reflect predisposing cause (e.g., regurgitation, anesthetic episode)

PHYSICAL EXAM FINDINGS

Findings may be absent or severe; when present, they may include:
- Tachypnea
- Cough
- Inspiratory and expiratory distress
- Auscultatory abnormalities (may be localized if present)
  - Increased or harsh bronchovesicular sounds (≈50%)
  - Decreased bronchovesicular sounds (≈6%)
  - Crackles (≈10%)
  - Wheezes (≈2%)
- Cyanosis (rare)
- Fever (<50% are febrile)
- Shock (rare)
- Others that reflect predisposing cause (e.g., exercise intolerance with myasthenia gravis–related megaesophagus)

Etiology and Pathophysiology

Inhalation of particulates or fluid into the larynx and lower respiratory tract triggers injury.
- Gastric contents are typically sterile, but acid and particulate matter can cause potentially severe damage.
  - Acid causes direct, caustic epithelial injury that is followed by inflammation.
  - Particulate material may obstruct airways.
- Infection may follow aspiration of contaminated oropharyngeal secretions or as a secondary (opportunistic) complication of respiratory damage.

Severity of injury depends on volume, toxicity, pH, particulates, and pathogen content of aspirated material. Sequelae may include
- Airway obstruction
- Bronchoconstriction
- Pulmonary hemorrhage
- Epithelial necrosis
- Pulmonary inflammation or edema

DIAGNOSIS

Diagnostic Overview

Differentiation of aspiration pneumonia from bacterial pneumonia or pulmonary edema often depends on circumstantial evidence such as history of vomiting or regurgitation or involvement of the typical dependant lung lobes.

Differential Diagnosis

- Infectious pneumonia
- Cardiogenic or noncardiogenic pulmonary edema
- Neoplastic infiltrates

Initial Database

- Neurologic exam (p. 1136) reflects underlying neurologic disease, if present.
- CBC: neutrophilic leukocytosis ± left shift common
- Serum biochemical profile and urinalysis: no specific changes
- Thoracic radiographs: abnormalities may lag aspiration event by up to 24 hours

- Both right and left lateral views should be acquired.
- Alveolar or interstitial pattern, or consolidation in affected lung lobes. Changes found in the lobes that were dependent at the time of aspiration; if the patient was conscious during aspiration, abnormalities are often seen in the right middle, right cranial, or caudal portion of the left cranial lung lobe.

Advanced or Confirmatory Testing

- Pulse oximetry and/or arterial blood gas (ABG) analyses to assess oxygenation
- Respiratory (tracheal or bronchoalveolar [p. 1073]) lavage (submit samples for cytological exam and culture and susceptibility [C&S])
  - Neutrophilic inflammation ± bacteria
  - Hemorrhage
  - Particulates/debris
  - Lipid-laden macrophages
- Search for predisposing cause of aspiration (e.g., acetylcholine receptor antibody titer for myasthenia gravis–related megaesophagus)

TREATMENT

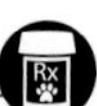

Treatment Overview

Severity of aspiration pneumonia varies, and therefore intensity of therapeutic intervention varies as well. Adequate oxygenation must be ensured and further aspiration prevented when possible. Antimicrobial drugs may be needed to treat secondary bacterial infection. A step-by-step approach to treatment is shown on p. 1440.

Acute General Treatment

- If aspiration is witnessed, immediately suction material from pharynx/airways, and ensure airway patency.
- If respiratory distress or evidence of hypoxemia exists, administer supplemental oxygen using the lowest effective oxygen concentration (typically, FIO_2 ≈40%) (p. 1146).
  - If PaO_2 < 60 mm Hg or if PCO_2 > 60 mm Hg despite oxygen supplementation, intubate for positive-pressure ventilation.
- Bronchodilators may relieve bronchospasm (cats especially): terbutaline 0.01 mg/kg SQ, inhaled albuterol (nebulized or by metered dose inhaler), or aminophylline (dosage depends on preparation)
- IV crystalloid fluids
  - Maintenance rate of 60 mL/kg/day after correction of dehydration; more if there are ongoing losses. CAUTION: excessive parenteral fluids may precipitate edema in the damaged lung.
- Antimicrobials are often suggested because secondary infection is common.
  - Choice ideally based on C&S (respiratory lavage)
  - Often more than one type of bacteria present (*Escherichia coli, Mycoplasma, Pasturella,* and *Staphylococcus* spp most common)
  - Initial choice pending culture often parenteral broad-spectrum antibiotics (e.g., combination of ampicillin 22 mg/kg IV q 8h and enrofloxacin 5 mg/kg IM or IV q 12h [dogs] or 5 mg/kg q 24h [cats])
- Physiotherapy: coupage, movement
- Saline nebulization
- If aspiration is suspected but respiratory distress is absent, careful observation without additional treatment may be sufficient.

Chronic Treatment

- Prevent further aspiration or reduce severity of injury from aspiration (see Prevention below).
- Discontinue oxygen when PaO_2 remains above 65 mm Hg and the animal can breathe comfortably without it.
- Traditionally, antibiotics continued for 3-4 weeks; a shorter duration of therapy may be adequate.

Nutrition/Diet

Animals with severe ongoing vomiting/regurgitation should not be fed by mouth.

Behavior/Exercise

- Recumbent animals with severe pneumonia should NOT be allowed to lie with the most functional lobes on the down side.
- Movement may facilitate beneficial cough and airway clearance.

Possible Complications

- Administration of high concentrations of oxygen for prolonged periods can contribute to respiratory epithelial injury.
- Parenteral fluids/colloids may worsen noncardiogenic pulmonary edema.

Recommended Monitoring

- Oxygenation (ABG or pulse oximetry), depending on severity of disease, q 4-24h until normalized
- Thoracic radiographs: frequency determined by severity or progression of clinical signs; ideally repeated 1-2 weeks after discontinuation of antibiotics
- CBC: rechecked at least weekly until leukocytosis resolved

PROGNOSIS & OUTCOME

- Depends on volume and character of aspirated material but generally good
- Prognosis worsens when > 1 lobe involved

PEARLS & CONSIDERATIONS

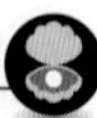

Comments

- Because aspiration pneumonia rarely occurs in the absence of an underlying cause, animals should be evaluated for risk factors.
- Absence of known regurgitation or vomiting does not rule out aspiration pneumonia because these events can be silent.
- Cough suppression is contraindicated.

Prevention

- Address underlying diseases that predispose to aspiration.
- Fast animals at least 6 hours before general anesthesia, and use properly inflated, cuffed endotracheal tubes during anesthesia.
- For animals at high risk, consider administration of antacids (proton pump inhibitors) to increase gastric pH or administration of prokinetic agents (e.g., metoclopramide) to enhance gastric emptying and increase lower esophageal sphincter tone. Unfortunately, these measures have not been shown to improve outcomes in humans at high risk for aspiration, and perioperative metoclopramide administered to dogs undergoing unilateral arytenoid lateralization did not reduce risk of aspiration pneumonia.
- Use caution with forced administration of drugs or foodstuffs.
- Feeding tubes should not cross the lower esophageal sphincter unless gastric evacuation is required.

Technician Tips

- Sudden respiratory signs in hospitalized animals should be brought to the attending veterinarian's attention immediately.
- For animals with regurgitation, maintain an upright position with the head and chest elevated above the stomach for at least 30 minutes after oral feeding.
- Use appropriately sized endotracheal tube with cuff inflated during general anesthesia.

Client Education

When a predisposing cause is not reversible (e.g., idiopathic megaesophagus), repeated aspiration events are likely.

SUGGESTED READING

Tart KM, et al: Potential risks, prognostic indicators, and diagnostic and treatment modalities affecting survival in dogs with presumptive aspiration pneumonia: 125 cases (2005-2008). J Vet Emerg Crit Care 20:319, 2010.

AUTHOR: Leah A. Cohn, DVM, PhD, DACVIM
EDITOR: Megan Grobman, DVM, MS, DACVIM

Pneumonia, Bacterial

Client Education Sheet 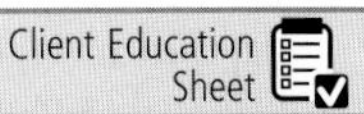

BASIC INFORMATION

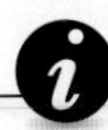

Definition

Inflammation of the pulmonary parenchyma (small airways, interstitium, and alveoli) from bacterial infection

Epidemiology

SPECIES, AGE, SEX

Dogs are diagnosed more often than cats. Puppies acquired from community situations (shelters, pet stores) are more likely to have pneumonia from *Bordetella bronchiseptica* than from other pathogens. Bacterial pneumonia secondary to congenital defects (e.g., primary ciliary dyskinesia) is more common in young animals, but bacterial pneumonia occurs at any age and in either sex.

GENETICS, BREED PREDISPOSITION

Breed or genetic predispositions associated with underlying primary diseases or associated conditions. Irish wolfhounds are reported to be at increased risk.

RISK FACTORS

Any disease that increases the potential for aspiration:

- Laryngeal disease: laryngeal paralysis post tieback surgery, laryngeal neoplasia, etc.
- Dysphagia
- Gastroesophageal reflux
- Esophageal disease (p. 873): esophagitis, megaesophagus, stricture, foreign body
- Altered consciousness
- Chronic vomiting

Any disorder that compromises respiratory defenses:

- Bronchial masses or foreign bodies
- Bronchiectasis
- Viral respiratory infection (e.g., distemper)
- Congenital immune deficiencies
- Immune suppression
- Primary ciliary dyskinesia

Exposure, especially in dense housing conditions, to other animals with respiratory signs may be a risk factor for *B. bronchiseptica*, *Mycoplasma* spp, or streptococcal pneumonia.

ASSOCIATED DISORDERS

- Sepsis
- Systemic inflammatory response syndrome
- Multiple organ dysfunction syndrome
- Respiratory foreign body (recurrent pneumonia)
- Bronchial obstruction (foreign body, mass)
- Hemothorax (uncommon)

Clinical Presentation

DISEASE FORMS/SUBTYPES

Bronchopneumonia involves inflammation of airways and alveolar/interstitial compartments.

HISTORY, CHIEF COMPLAINT

Chief complaint may be related to pneumonia or the predisposing disease:

- Pneumonia
  - Cough (absence of cough does not rule out pneumonia)
  - Nasal discharge ± sneezing
  - Exercise intolerance
  - Anorexia, lethargy
  - Hemoptysis (uncommon)
  - Acute death (uncommon)
- Predisposing disease
  - Regurgitation
  - Vomiting
  - Recurrent/persistent infections (usually respiratory but occasionally other)
- Mild, vague signs (e.g., delayed postoperative recovery) may be the earliest manifestations of the onset of bacterial pneumonia as a complication of another disorder (e.g., sepsis, systemic inflammatory response syndrome, multiple organ dysfunction syndrome).
- Absence of clinical signs of respiratory disease does not exclude the diagnosis; some animals with pneumonia demonstrate no clinical signs.

PHYSICAL EXAM FINDINGS

Physical exam may be unremarkable or may reflect only signs related to an underlying predisposing disorder. Lack of physical exam abnormalities referable to the respiratory system cannot exclude the diagnosis. Findings are variable but often include

- Cough (hemoptysis possible)
- Nasal discharge
- Pulmonary auscultation
  - Loud or harsh bronchovesicular sounds
  - Crackles or wheezes, sometimes focal
  - Focal absence of breath sounds
- Fever (≈50%)
- Tachypnea
- Increased respiratory effort or overt respiratory distress (p. 879)

Etiology and Pathophysiology

- Bacterial pneumonia is most often a complication of another disease that disrupts or overwhelms mechanical or immunologic pulmonary clearance and defense mechanisms:
  - Aspiration of gastric or oropharyngeal contents
  - Impaired mucociliary clearance
  - Impaired reflex closure of the glottis
  - Absent or impaired cough reflex
  - Abnormal immune function: innate or acquired
- *B. bronchiseptica* can cause disease as a primary pathogen in dogs or cats without other underlying risk factors or concurrent disease.
- Bacteria most often enter lungs through airways but can enter hematogenously. With impaired or overwhelmed clearance and defense mechanisms, bacteria can proliferate and initiate local inflammatory responses:
  - Common isolates in dogs and cats include *Escherichia coli, Klebsiella, Bordetella, Pasteurella, Mycoplasma* spp, and *Staphylococcus* spp. Polymicrobial infection is common.
  - Acutely fatal pneumonia caused by *Streptococcus equi* subsp *zooepidemicus* and associated with fever, hemothorax, and bleeding into airways can occur in dogs from dense housing situations.
  - Regionally endemic bacterial diseases, such as plague and tularemia, can cause pneumonia.
- Local inflammatory responses cause pulmonary lesions, impair lung function, and contribute to respiratory and systemic disease manifestations.

DIAGNOSIS

Diagnostic Overview

Definitive diagnosis of bacterial pneumonia hinges on demonstration of bacteria by culture and sensitivity testing (C&S, most sensitive) or cytologic exam of respiratory wash samples. Pursuit of an underlying or concurrent disease that increases risk of bacterial pneumonia is strongly encouraged.

Differential Diagnosis

Many diseases share clinical and diagnostic similarities:

- Noninfectious inflammatory respiratory diseases
- Pulmonary neoplasia
- Respiratory parasites
- Pulmonary edema
- Fungal pneumonia, particularly blastomycosis and coccidioidomycosis in dogs

Initial Database

- CBC: inflammatory leukogram (with or without left shift) expected, although not seen in all cases
  - Neutropenia is possible, especially with sepsis. Conversely, bacterial pneumonia can develop secondary to primary neutropenic disorders (e.g., myelosuppression from chemotherapy).
- Serum biochemical profile/urinalysis: often normal unless sepsis/systemic inflammation present
- Thoracic radiographs
  - Obtaining right and left lateral and ventrodorsal (VD) or dorsoventral (DV) views is recommended because infiltrates may be apparent only in nondependent lung.
  - Minimally, two views (at least one lateral and either VD or DV) is necessary in all cases. Three views (right and left lateral and either VD or DV) are strongly encouraged.

- Alveolar pattern, often most severe in dependent regions of lung lobes, is expected in most cases.
    - Right middle lung lobe is commonly affected and may be obscured by the heart on right lateral projections.
    - Distribution may be variable in patients that are non-ambulatory or aspirate after surgery.
- Interstitial patterns, with or without alveolar patterns, are possible.
- In some cases, lobar consolidation is the prominent radiographic abnormality.
- Other abnormalities that reflect underlying primary disease (e.g., megaesophagus, bronchiectasis, pulmonary mass)

Advanced or Confirmatory Testing

Confirmatory tests help rule out other diseases or predisposing diseases/risk factors:

- Respiratory washes and bronchoalveolar lavage (pp. 1073 and 1074)
    - Primarily septic, suppurative inflammation
    - Bacteria are not always evident in cytologic exams, and samples should be submitted for C&S testing irrespective of cytologic findings.
    - Specific requests are often required for *Mycoplasma* culture. Because *Mycoplasma* spp can be difficult to culture, polymerase chain reaction (PCR) may be preferred.
- Bronchoscopy (p. 1074):
    - Endobronchial masses or foreign bodies may be evident in some cases.
    - Mucopurulent exudate in airways of affected regions may be seen.
    - Dilated/sacculated airways (bronchiectasis)
    - Can guide sampling to a specific affected lung lobe
- CT: superior delineation of the extent of pneumonia but seldom needed if good-quality thoracic radiographs are consistent with the diagnosis
- Fine-needle aspiration for cytologic analysis: may diagnose fungal pneumonia or neoplasms (p. 1113)
- Barium esophagram is occasionally useful if esophageal disease suspected, but there is a risk of barium aspiration in patients with esophageal disease. Free-feeding swallow study protocols may increase utility while decreasing risk of aspiration.
- Arterial blood gas (ABG) analysis (p. 1058)
    - Hypoxemia and hypocapnia are the most common abnormalities; when present, generally indicate severe pneumonia or presence of a complicating factor (e.g., acute respiratory distress syndrome [ARDS] [p. 27]) and therefore a more guarded prognosis.
- Tests specific for underlying diseases (e.g., serum acetylcholine receptor antibody titers for myasthenia gravis–induced megaesophagus)

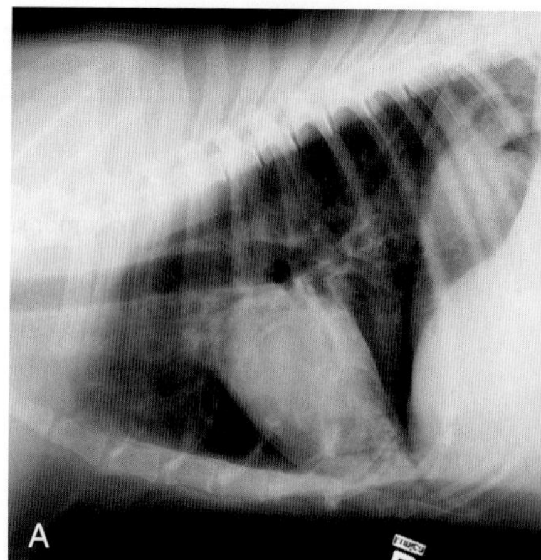

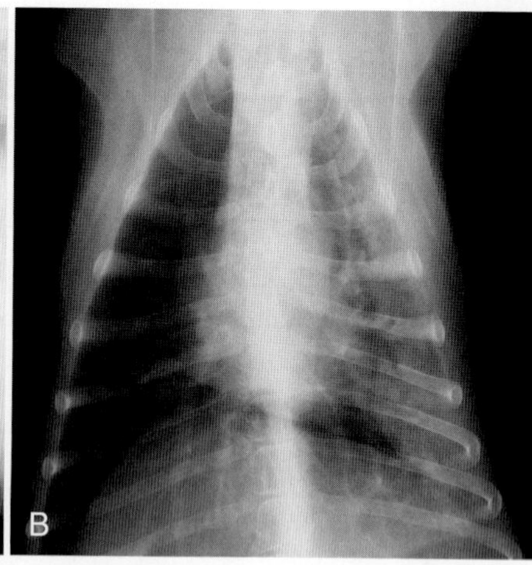

PNEUMONIA, BACTERIAL A, Left lateral thoracic radiograph of a 14-year-old, mixed-breed dog with pneumonia. Alveolar infiltrates are visible over the cardiac silhouette (especially the apex) but are not striking. Microcardia suggests hypovolemia. **B**, Dorsoventral thoracic radiograph of same dog. Left-sided alveolar infiltrates are more obvious than in **A**, where they were obscured by being on the dependent side and overlying the cardiac silhouette.

TREATMENT

Treatment Overview

Administration of antimicrobials; supportive care, including oxygenation support if needed; and addressing predisposing factors to the extent possible are key.

Acute General Treatment

Broad-spectrum antibiotics:

- Frequent *in vitro* resistance to empirically chosen antimicrobials underscores the benefit of C&S testing.
- Clinically unstable animals should be treated with broad-spectrum (ideally, parenteral) antibiotics.
    - Ampicillin 22-30 mg/kg IV, SQ q 8h, cefazolin 22 mg/kg IV, IM q 6h, or clindamycin 10 mg/kg SQ q 12h (dogs), 10-15 mg/kg SQ q 12h (cats) AND enrofloxacin 5-20 mg/kg IM, IV q 24h (dogs), 5 mg/kg IM, IV (cats) or pradofloxacin 5 mg/kg PO q 24h (dog; extra-label use in the United States), 7.5 mg/kg PO q 24h (cats)
    - Severe clinical disease may warrant therapy before obtaining respiratory samples for culture; blood culture can be an alternative for such patients.
- Mildly affected stable animals may be treated with oral antibiotics, ideally based on C&S testing. Empirical choices while awaiting results:
    - Ampicillin or amoxicillin/clavulanate 22 mg/kg q 8h, or
    - Doxycycline 5 mg/kg PO q 12h, particularly for animals that show no response to other antibiotics or *Bordetella* is suspected.
- Oxygen (nasal cannula, oxygen cage, face mask) for hypoxemic animals or those in respiratory distress (p. 1146)
- IV fluids are typically needed for moderately or severely affected animals.
- Saline nebulization and coupage, several times daily. Change in position and encouraging movement are also beneficial.
- Bronchodilator use is controversial. They may be beneficial for some animals, especially before nebulization.
    - Theophylline: dosage varies with formulation.
    - Terbutaline 1.25-5 mg/DOG PO q 8h; 0.625-1.25 mg/CAT PO q 12h or 0.01-0.02 mg/kg SQ or IM once (cat)

Chronic Treatment

- Manage underlying causes when identified.
- Antibiotic therapy continued at least 1 week beyond clinical and radiographic resolution of infection has been typical, but recently, the need for such prolonged treatment has come into question. Shorter courses based on clinical resolution of signs are likely appropriate.
- Lung lobectomy is occasionally needed to resolve infection when extensive single-lobe involvement has failed medical therapy or is associated with recurrent infection.
    - Foreign-body pneumonia or underlying neoplasia may be discovered.

Possible Complications

- Lung lobe abscess
- Bronchiectasis
- Pyothorax
- Recurrence if underlying cause not identified and treated
- Joint cartilage and dental abnormalities secondary to fluoroquinolone or tetracycline (respectively) administration to growing puppies or kittens

Recommended Monitoring

- Clinical signs (e.g., respiratory rate, effort; attitude, appetite)
    - Carefully re-evaluate animals that are not clinically better within 48-72 hours of starting treatment or that deteriorate substantially at any time; consider pursuing more diagnostic tests and/or changing therapy.
- Assessment of oxygenation, if needed (e.g., arterial blood gas analysis, pulse oximetry)

- Thoracic radiographs: changes can lag as much as 48 hours behind clinical changes.
- Evaluate (physiologic, hematologic, radiographic exam) patient by 10-14 days after starting treatment and base decisions to extend treatment on results of evaluation.
  - Repeating thoracic radiographs approximately 1 week after cessation of antibiotics may demonstrate focal primary diseases (e.g., neoplasia) not evident on initial radiographs.

PROGNOSIS & OUTCOME

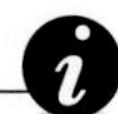

Varies with severity of disease and nature of predisposing factors:

- Prognosis for uncomplicated pneumonia is generally good.
- Prognosis for animals with risk factors depends on ability to treat/resolve the risk factor.
  - Recurrent infections are common in animals with unresolved primary diseases.

PEARLS & CONSIDERATIONS

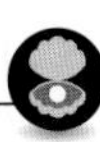

Comments

Bacterial pneumonia should be viewed as a complication of another underlying disease; *B. bronchiseptica* infections are an exception. Patients should be rigorously evaluated for risk factors if they are not immediately apparent.

Technician Tips

- Puppies with bacterial pneumonia, particularly those that came from pet stores or shelters, should ideally be isolated from other animals in the hospital, including cats, because *B. bronchiseptica* is common in those animals.
- For respiratory washes, make sure the wash solution does not contain bacteriostatic agents.

Client Education

- Home treatment may include
  - Respiratory humidification by inhalation of cold steam is best accomplished by having a pet in a closed, unventilated bathroom (but not in the bath/shower) for 10-15 minutes once to three times per day while a warm shower runs.
  - This is often followed by coupage, which is a series of brusque pats to both sides of the chest, performed for 10-30 seconds after each humidification session, with the intention of loosening pulmonary secretions and pus to facilitate expectoration.
  - Pet owners should perform these treatments only on the recommendation of a veterinarian; they can make a condition worse if used inappropriately.

SUGGESTED READING

Lappin MR, et al: Antimicrobial use guidelines for treatment of respiratory tract disease in dogs and cats: Antimicrobial Guidelines Working Group of the International Society for Companion Animal Infectious Diseases. J Vet Intern Med 31:279, 2017.

AUTHOR: Rance K. Sellon, DVM, PhD, DACVIM
EDITOR: Megan Grobman, DVM, MS, DACVIM

Pneumothorax

Client Education Sheet 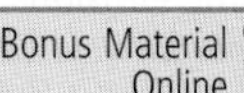 Bonus Material Online 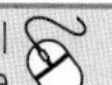

BASIC INFORMATION

Definition

Accumulation of air within the pleural space

Synonym

Collapsed lung

Epidemiology

SPECIES, AGE, SEX

Young, large-breed male dogs are predisposed to trauma and subsequent pneumothorax.

GENETICS, BREED PREDISPOSITION

Northern breeds (Siberian Husky or Alaskan Malamute) are predisposed to spontaneous pneumothorax, as are golden retrievers and possibly Gordon setters and sighthounds.

RISK FACTORS

- Trauma (e.g., hit by car, bite wounds, falls from elevated heights)
- Surgical intervention (e.g., cranial abdominal, intervertebral disc, pulmonary surgery)
- Pleural effusion (e.g., iatrogenic after thoracocentesis)
- Airway or pulmonary disease (e.g., neoplasia, parasites)

GEOGRAPHY AND SEASONALITY

Trauma is more common in warmer months.

ASSOCIATED DISORDERS

- Pulmonary contusions
- Diaphragmatic hernia
- Flail chest
- Fracture
- Asthma in cats
- Pleural effusion

Clinical Presentation

DISEASE FORMS/SUBTYPES

- Traumatic: due to damage to the pulmonary parenchyma or chest wall
- Spontaneous: due to abnormal pulmonary parenchyma without trauma
- Iatrogenic: due to damage to the lung parenchyma after thoracocentesis for removal of pleural effusion, aspiration of a pulmonary mass, or thoracic surgery

HISTORY, CHIEF COMPLAINT

- Trauma
- Acute-onset, tachypnea, respiratory distress, coughing, or restlessness
- Worsening tachypnea after a medical intervention

PHYSICAL EXAM FINDINGS

- Dyspnea/increased respiratory effort is the hallmark finding.
  - Restrictive respiratory pattern: shallow inspiration. Paradoxical breathing (chest and abdomen move in opposition) sometimes identified. Inspiratory distress with stridor suggests upper airway disease rather than pneumothorax.
  - May be absent in mild cases
- Other evidence of trauma, blunt (e.g., hit by car) or penetrating (e.g., bite, gunshot, stabbing)
- Dull or muffled lung sounds (auscultation) ± hyperresonance (percussion)

Etiology and Pathophysiology

- Air may enter the pleural space from damage to the pulmonary parenchyma (e.g., rupture of a pulmonary bleb or bullae, laceration of a lung lobe) or damage to the chest wall.
- When the lung parenchyma is normal, small injuries (e.g., needlestick during centesis) heal rapidly.
  - Intrapleural volumes of air of up to 45 mL/kg cause no clinical signs and take about 2 weeks to resorb spontaneously in healthy dogs.
  - Iatrogenic pneumothorax occurring during thoracocentesis is almost invariably associated with chronic effusions (especially chylothorax), diseased lung tissue, an uncooperative patient, or an inexperienced operator.
  - Iatrogenic pneumothorax may also result from unexpandable lung; in this case, the pleura has constricted around the lung, and when pleural effusion is removed, the resulting negative pressure results in a tear of the scarred pleura and subsequent air leakage.
- Diseased lung or distal airways (e.g., neoplasia, parasites) can rupture spontaneously, causing pneumothorax.
- Tension pneumothorax is a severe pneumothorax from any cause that results in cardiovascular collapse due to inadequate cardiac filling.

- Rarely, foreign bodies (e.g., grass awns [p. 398], wooden toothpicks, porcupine quills) may migrate intrathoracically and cause pneumothorax.

DIAGNOSIS

Diagnostic Overview

The diagnosis is suspected based on a history of thoracic trauma (field or surgical), dyspnea, or both. The confirmatory test of choice is thoracic radiography, although thoracic ultrasound (p. 1102) is also useful for detecting pneumothorax (absence of the glide sign) and may be performed without moving the animal.

Differential Diagnosis

Dyspnea after trauma:

- Pleural effusion/diaphragmatic hernia
- Pulmonary contusions
- Primary lung or airway disease
- Pain
- Hypovolemia

Dyspnea in absence of trauma:

- Pneumonia
- Congestive heart failure
- Neoplasia
- Pulmonary thromboembolism
- Pleural effusion
- Upper airway disease
- Others

Initial Database

- Thoracic radiographs are the test of choice for patients who can tolerate the procedure; left lateral recumbency is the most sensitive view for detecting small volumes of air in the pleural space. Thoracic ultrasound can detect pneumothorax as well and is less stressful.
- In animals with suspected pneumothorax when respiratory distress makes the animal unstable for radiographs and ultrasound is unavailable, thoracocentesis may be diagnostic as well as therapeutic.
- Arterial blood gas (ABG [p. 1058]) or pulse oximetry may help elucidate whether dyspnea in a traumatized animal with pneumothorax is due to the pneumothorax itself (e.g., PaO_2 < 85 mm Hg on room air and/or SpO_2 < 95%) or to pain, hypovolemia, or other conditions associated with trauma. Pulmonary contusions may also cause hypoxemia and desaturation.
- Routine laboratory testing (CBC, serum chemistry profile, urinalysis): generally unremarkable

Advanced or Confirmatory Testing

- CT often is useful for identification of pulmonary bullae or abscesses.
- Analysis of pleural effusion obtained by thoracocentesis (pp. 1164 and 1343)

TREATMENT

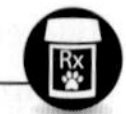

Treatment Overview

The course and severity of the patient's clinical signs and suspected inciting cause help determine whether to pursue conservative management or thoracotomy. Treatment goals for conservative management include removal of air from the pleural space and measures that encourage formation of a seal to prevent further leakage; surgical treatment aims to eliminate the source of the leak.

Acute General Treatment

- Supplemental oxygen (p. 1146) produces more rapid resolution of a closed (not ongoing) pneumothorax because the trapped air is higher in nitrogen, and if inhaled oxygen is administered, the trapped air moves more quickly down its concentration gradient.
- Traumatic pneumothorax
  - No clinical signs and identified incidentally on radiographs: no treatment; monitoring is important
  - Clinical signs: thoracocentesis warranted (p. 1164). If large volumes (>200 mL/kg), no endpoint, or recurrent pneumothorax, place thoracostomy tubes (p. 1082). Apply the three-strikes rule: if three or more thoracocenteses are required within 24 hours after trauma, a thoracostomy tube should be placed.
- Spontaneous pneumothorax (no trauma)
  - If a bulla or bleb is suspected (no masses on radiographs), a thoracotomy is often warranted (p. 834).
  - If a necrotic neoplasm or pulmonary abscess is suspected, thoracic CT followed by thoracotomy is warranted.
  - If underlying feline asthma or chronic bronchitis is suspected, conservative therapy may be adequate.
- Iatrogenic
  - If there are no clinical signs (radiographic diagnosis only or a small volume of air was aspirated during thoracocentesis), monitoring (e.g., regular respiratory rate, effort, SpO_2) is adequate.
  - If the patient is showing clinical signs, repeating the thoracocentesis and monitoring the animal closely are recommended. The animal may require a thoracostomy tube or exploratory thoracotomy if not responsive. Underlying disease may require specific treatment.

Chronic Treatment

- Correction of the underlying cause if applicable
- If surgery is not an option, intrathoracic installation of autologous fresh whole blood (i.e., "blood patch") may help seal ongoing pulmonary air leaks (p. 834).

Possible Complications

Ongoing pneumothorax or effusion

Recommended Monitoring

- Respiratory rate and effort
- Pulse oximetry
- Keep track of volume of air removed

PROGNOSIS & OUTCOME

- Fair to good; often with trauma, the associated injuries are more likely to predict outcome.
- Dyspnea and duration of intensive care are negative prognostic factors for dogs and cats with pneumothorax.

PEARLS & CONSIDERATIONS

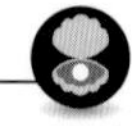

Comments

- Traumatic pneumothorax rarely requires surgical correction; most cases rapidly resolve (within 72 hours).
- Spontaneous pneumothorax in dogs commonly requires surgical treatment because many cases do not resolve without surgery. Cats with spontaneous pneumothorax are more likely to resolve without surgery.

Prevention

Prevent free roaming of pets, and use caution when performing thoracocentesis.

Technician Tips

Technicians involved in caring for patients with pneumothorax should be familiar with management of chest tubes.

SUGGESTED READING

Mooney ET, et al: Spontaneous pneumothorax in 35 cats (2001-2010). J Feline Med Surg 14(6):384-391, 2012.

AUTHOR: Elizabeth Rozanski, DVM, DACVIM, DACVECC
EDITOR: Benjamin M. Brainard, VMD, DACVAA, DACVECC

Pododermatitis

Client Education Sheet

BASIC INFORMATION

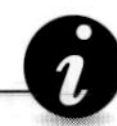

Definition

- An inflammatory skin disease affecting the paw
- Footpad disorders are discussed on p. 350.

Synonyms

Interdigital dermatitis, interdigital pyoderma, pedal dermatitis

Epidemiology

SPECIES, AGE, SEX

- Dogs and cats of any age and either sex
- Pododermatitis is more common in dogs than cats. Paw lesions in cats more commonly involve the footpads, claws, and periungual areas, whereas dogs often present with interdigital lesions.

RISK FACTORS

- In cats, immunosuppression caused by feline leukemia virus (FeLV), feline immunodeficiency virus (FIV), or diabetes mellitus can predispose to infectious pododermatitis.
- Lack of routine prophylactic parasiticide use

CONTAGION AND ZOONOSIS

Dermatophytosis is contagious and zoonotic. Sporotrichosis (especially feline, which is a zoonotic hazard) and systemic mycoses (common-point source of infection or accidental inoculation) also may affect humans.

GEOGRAPHY AND SEASONALITY

Atopic dermatitis and allergic or irritant contact dermatitis can be seasonal. Systemic fungal infection may have regional distribution (e.g., blastomycosis seen most often surrounding Ohio and Mississippi River valleys and the Great Lakes).

Clinical Presentation

HISTORY, CHIEF COMPLAINT

Owners can observe lesions on a single paw or multiple paws. Licking or chewing of the affected areas and lameness may also be apparent. Pododermatitis also may be part of a more generalized skin condition.

PHYSICAL EXAM FINDINGS

Lesions can occur on the dorsal and/or the ventral aspects of the paw. One or several interdigital spaces can be affected. Possible lesions:

- Erythema
- Nodules
- Swelling of the paw
- Interdigital serosanguineous or seropurulent exudates, bullae, or draining tracts
- Ulcers and erosions
- Scales and crusts
- Alopecia
- Paronychia (inflammation/infection of the claw folds)
- Eosinophilic plaques (cat)
- Salivary staining
- Occasional pitting edema of associated metatarsus or metacarpus
- Regional lymphadenopathy may be present.

Etiology and Pathophysiology

Pododermatitis can arise through various pathologic mechanisms:

- Contact with irritant substances or physical trauma that can induce skin injury and inflammation
- Infectious agents that can induce an immune response from the host, resulting in tissue inflammatory cell infiltrates
- Hormonal imbalances (hypothyroidism, hyperadrenocorticism, diabetes mellitus) that can predispose to infectious pododermatitis
- Allergic disease: self-trauma can result in skin lesions, alopecia, and salivary staining
- Immune-mediated disorders: development of antibodies or activated lymphocytes against normal body constituents or inciting antigens (drugs, bacteria, viruses) can cause tissue damage.
- Neoplastic cell infiltrates can disturb the normal structure of the skin.

DIAGNOSIS

Diagnostic Overview

Pododermatitis is apparent on physical exam; the cause is determined based on number of paws affected, appearance of lesions, possible environmental triggers, and results of tests selected based on lesion distribution and extradermatologic physical exam findings.

Differential Diagnosis

Lesions restricted to one paw:

- Foreign bodies, trauma
- Neoplasia
- Localized bacterial or fungal infection
- Osteomyelitis

Multiple paws involved:

- Environmental/traumatic: contact chemical dermatitis, clipper burn
- Infectious: bacterial, fungal (dermatophytosis, *Malassezia* dermatitis, sporotrichosis, mycetoma, blastomycosis, cryptococcosis), parasitic (demodicosis, hookworm and *Pelodera* dermatitis, trombiculiasis), rickettsial (Rocky Mountain spotted fever), viral (papillomatosis)
- Allergic: food hypersensitivity, atopic dermatitis, contact allergic dermatitis
- Immune-mediated: pemphigus (foliaceus, erythematosus, vulgaris), bullous pemphigoid, systemic lupus erythematosus (SLE), and immunomodulatory-responsive lymphocytic plasmacytic pododermatitis (dog) and plasma cell pododermatitis (cat)
- Metabolic/endocrine: superficial necrolytic dermatitis (hepatocutaneous syndrome, metabolic epidermal necrosis); hypothyroidism and hyperadrenocorticism can predispose an animal to bacterial or dermatophyte-induced pododermatitis and to adult-onset demodicosis
- Miscellaneous: behavioral (self-induced lesions), zinc-responsive dermatosis, foreign-

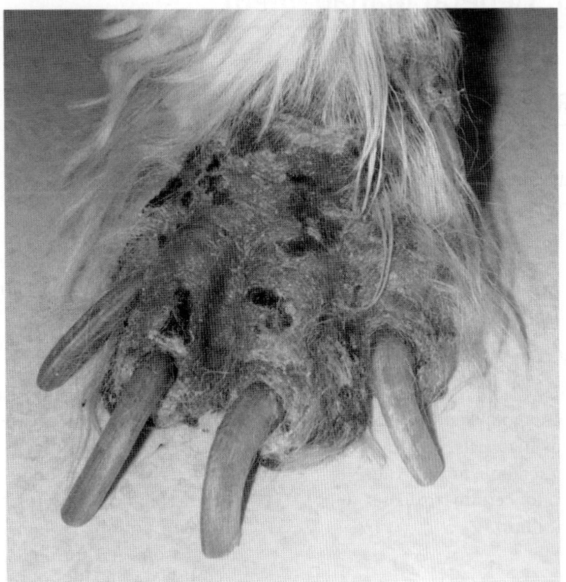

PODODERMATITIS Alopecia, erythema, and crusting of the skin of the paw of a 12-year-old dog with adult-onset generalized demodicosis and bacterial pyoderma. (Courtesy Dr. Nadia Pagé.)

body reaction (occasionally affects multiple feet), sterile pyogranulomas, nodular dermatofibrosis (German shepherd dogs)

Initial Database

Selection of diagnostic tests (p. 1091) is based on evidence provided by the history and physical exam:

- Skin scrapings: *Demodex* spp
- Wood's lamp exam: dermatophytosis (fluorescent strains of *Microsporum canis*)
- Cytologic exam: fungal organisms, bacteria and inflammatory cells (bacterial pododermatitis), acantholytic keratinocytes (pemphigus), neoplastic cells
- Elimination diet: food allergy
- Intradermal skin testing and/or serologic allergy testing: atopic dermatitis
- Fecal flotation: hookworm ova
- Radiographs: osteomyelitis, radiopaque foreign bodies
- CBC, biochemistry panel, urinalysis: results depend on the underlying cause; often normal or nonspecific unless systemic disease

Advanced or Confirmatory Testing

- Culture: bacterial, fungal
- Skin biopsy: foreign bodies, demodicosis or other parasites, bacterial or fungal infections, neoplasia, immune-mediated diseases, superficial necrolytic dermatitis, zinc-responsive dermatosis
- Antinuclear antibody (ANA): positive in most animals with SLE; typically done if there is other evidence of immune mediated disease (e.g., glomerulonephritis. polyarthritis)
- Endocrine tests and serologic titers, if relevant

TREATMENT

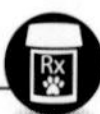

Treatment Overview

The goal of treatment is to achieve cure or control of the disease. Sometimes, palliative treatment is the only option (e.g., nonresectable tumors).

Acute and Chronic Treatment

Specifics depend on the underlying cause:

- Minimizing paw trauma (e.g., owner education; use of booties)
- Draining lesions can benefit from soaks in a magnesium sulfate solution (Epsom salts) 30 mL/L of warm water q 12-24h until drainage stops (5-7 days).
- Surgery: neoplastic lesions, surgical exploration (foreign bodies), or debridement laser surgery can be useful for removing cystic lesions and sinuses (dogs).
- Bacterial pododermatitis, most often caused by *Staphylococcus pseudintermedius,* can necessitate 8-12 weeks of appropriate systemic antibiotics (e.g., cephalexin 22-30 mg/kg PO q 12h, amoxicillin-clavulanate 13.75-25 mg/kg PO q 12h).
- If other bacteria are involved or the empirical choice of antibiotic is not effective, antibiotic selection should be based on culture and susceptibility (C&S) results.
- Manage parasitic or fungal infections with appropriate medications.
- Atopic dermatitis often requires management with combination therapy: antipruritic agents, allergen-specific immunotherapy, various topicals (e.g., moisturizers, antipruritics, antiseptics), and antimicrobial drugs to control secondary bacterial or yeast infections (p. 91).
- Immunosuppressive treatments are usually required for treating immune-mediated diseases.

PROGNOSIS & OUTCOME

Varies, depending on the cause of pododermatitis

PEARLS & CONSIDERATIONS

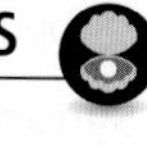

Comments

- Interdigital pyoderma is often frustrating to treat. Even after resolution of infection, the remaining fibrosis and scarring may predispose the animal to relapse.
- In severe, refractory cases, clinicians may have to consider drastic surgical measures (fusion podoplasty).
- Cases of canine pododermatitis with substantial footpad involvement are more commonly seen with autoimmune diseases, drug reactions, zinc-responsive dermatosis, superficial necrolytic dermatitis, and distemper.

Technician Tips

Patients with pododermatitis may have painful paws. Their reluctance to walk should not be misinterpreted as stubbornness, and they may need support to walk comfortably.

SUGGESTED READING

Miller WH Jr, et al: Muller & Kirk's Small animal dermatology, ed 7, St. Louis, 2013, Elsevier.

AUTHOR: Nadia Pagé, DMV, MSc, DACVD
EDITOR: Manon Paradis, DMV, MVSc, DACVD

Poisoning, General Management

Client Education Sheet

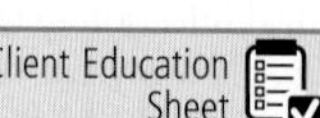

BASIC INFORMATION

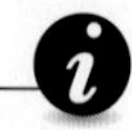

Definition

A poison is a substance that causes death or injury when introduced into or absorbed by a living organism.

Synonyms

Intoxication, toxicosis

Epidemiology

SPECIES, AGE, SEX

- Young animals are more likely to accidentally ingest poisonous materials.
- A cat's unique metabolism may cause it to be predisposed to certain toxicoses (e.g., acetaminophen, lilies).

RISK FACTORS

- Lack of supervision
- Access to poisonous materials
- Individual behavior (some animals routinely ingest materials but others seldom do)
- Poisoning of companion animals is rarely malicious.

CONTAGION AND ZOONOSIS

Several animals may be affected simultaneously by exposure to the same source.

Clinical Presentation

HISTORY, CHIEF COMPLAINT

- Key components of the history may include witnessed exposure, evidence of exposure (e.g., chewed medication container), and characteristic behavior or clinical signs. It is common for owners to believe their animal has been poisoned when it becomes ill for any reason. A thorough history can help establish the likelihood of poisoning.
- Additional important information may include the exact nature of the poison (if known), maximum possible dose ingested, time elapsed since ingestion, and time elapsed since clinical signs were first observed.

PHYSICAL EXAM FINDINGS

Depends on the poison involved; common categories of signs:

- Central nervous system (CNS) alterations and seizures (e.g., lead, metaldehyde, organophosphates, carbamates, tremorgenic mycotoxins, alcohol, blue-green algae, marijuana, chocolate, ivermectin)
- Muscle weakness, paresis, and paralysis (e.g., coral snakes, black widow spiders, phenoxy herbicides [including 2,4-D], macadamia nuts, marijuana)
- Acute blindness (e.g., avermectins, salt)
- Oral mucosal lesions (e.g., corrosive acids, alkalis, cationic detergents, liquid potpourri, formaldehyde)

- Acute kidney injury (e.g., ethylene glycol, lily plants [cats], raisins)
- Acute hepatic damage (e.g., mushrooms, blue-green algae, iron, sago, cycad palm plants/trees)
- Severe anemia (e.g., onions, garlic, naphthalene mothballs, zinc, anticoagulant rodenticides, acetaminophen [cats])
- Cardiac arrhythmias (e.g., foxglove, lily of the valley, oleander, azalea/rhododendron, yew, *Bufo* toads)
- Gastrointestinal (GI) signs (e.g., several already listed; arsenic, castor beans, nitrogen-phosphate-potassium fertilizers, zinc oxide, oxalate-containing plants)

Etiology and Pathophysiology

The possibility of poisoning should be considered when a previously healthy animal exhibits an acute onset of neurologic signs, organ failure, or other systemic signs and after all other common diseases have been ruled out or with confirmed exposure to a poison.

DIAGNOSIS

Diagnostic Overview

When an inciting cause is unknown, owners may express concern that their pet has been poisoned. The clinician should remember that unless clinical signs are consistent with poisoning and there is a reasonable chance of exposure to the poison based on the history, the illness is likely caused by something other than malicious poisoning.

Differential Diagnosis

Other systemic or metabolic diseases

Initial Database

- Careful history review for known/potential exposures
- Packed cell volume/serum total protein
- Blood glucose
- Urine specific gravity and dipstick
- Serum biochemical profile
- Samples of urine, blood, and gastric contents should be saved for possible toxicologic analysis.

Advanced or Confirmatory Testing

Serum levels or tissue analysis for specific toxin

TREATMENT

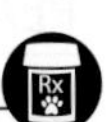

Treatment Overview

Treatment of poisoning should focus on maintaining cardiovascular, respiratory, and neurologic stability and preventing further absorption of toxin. ASPCA Animal Poison Control (888-426-4435) or the Pet Poison Helpline (800-213-6680) are useful resources to determine specific treatments for particular toxins. Goals of treatment:

- Achieve cardiovascular stability.
- Prevent further absorption of the toxin.
- Administer antidote if available.

Acute General Treatment

- Triage principle: any life-threatening complications must be addressed first. Start with the animal, not the toxin.
  - Airway support or intubation if respiratory arrest
  - IV catheter placement if animal is showing systemic signs
  - Electrocardiogram (ECG [p. 1096]), blood pressure (BP [p. 1065]), and pulse oximetry monitoring as dictated by physical exam findings
  - IV fluid and oxygen support (p. 1146) as indicated by cardiovascular and respiratory status
- Decontamination of the patient (p. 1087)
  - Emesis (p. 1188): consider if ingestion has occurred within 2 hours of visit. Contraindicated in animals that ingested potentially caustic substances (acids, alkalis, petroleum distillates) or are unable to protect the airway because of depression, seizures, or other neurologic dysfunction.
  - Gastric lavage (p. 1117): used when emesis is contraindicated because of the animal's inability to protect its airway; requires induction of general anesthesia and endotracheal intubation. A large-bore stomach tube is introduced into the stomach and 5-10 mL/kg of tepid water are infused. The water is then withdrawn through the tube with gravity flow. Lavage is repeated until gastric contents are clear. If indicated, activated charcoal can be administered by this tube before removal.
  - Activated charcoal: the most commonly used general treatment for intoxications; dose is 1-4 g/kg PO (suspension: 5-10 mL/kg PO). It is ineffective in removing heavy metals or alcohols (e.g., ethylene glycol). Some animals eat the activated charcoal willingly (alone or mixed with a small amount of dog food), but some require oral syringe or orogastric administration. Clinicians must be careful to prevent aspiration pneumonia. Elimination of toxins that undergo enterohepatic circulation may be hastened by additional doses of activated charcoal q 4-6h for up to 24 hours. Owners must be made aware that the animal will have black stool for several days.
  - Cathartics: accelerate fecal elimination of toxin. Sorbitol is most commonly used combined with activated charcoal, and only a single dose should be administered. Other available cathartics include sodium sulfate, magnesium sulfate, or citrate. Contraindications include GI obstruction, recent bowel surgery, volume depletion, electrolyte imbalance, and ingestion of a corrosive substance.
  - Fluid diuresis may accelerate elimination of renally excreted toxins (e.g., methylxanthines).
  - Skin: dermal exposure (i.e., topical pyrethrin exposure) warrants bathing with warm water and a mild dishwashing detergent (e.g., Dawn). Care should be taken to prevent hypothermia.
  - Lipid emulsion for intoxication (p. 1127) is a useful method to address intoxications with lipophilic drugs and toxicants (e.g., ivermectin, baclofen).

PROGNOSIS & OUTCOME

Prognosis depends on the toxin, total dose of exposure, and severity of clinical signs.

PEARLS & CONSIDERATIONS

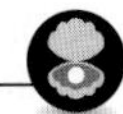

Comments

- Most specific intoxications seen in small animal practice are discussed individually and in detail elsewhere in this book.
- Many poisons cause signs similar to those caused by other common diseases. The diagnosis of toxicity should not be reached without strong historical or physical evidence of exposure.

Prevention

Owners should prevent their pets from accessing toxins.

Technician Tips

- Verify that animals have normal mentation and swallow reflex before administering activated charcoal.
- If performing phone triage, encourage client to bring in any packaging for the ingested toxin to facilitate identification.

Client Education

Information on common poisonings should be made available to clients.

SUGGESTED READING

Koenigshof AM, et al: Effect of sorbitol, single, and multidose activated charcoal administration on carprofen absorption following experimental overdose in dogs. J Vet Emerg Crit Care 25(5):606-610, 2015.

AUTHOR: Scott P. Shaw, DVM, DACVECC
EDITOR: Benjamin M. Brainard, VMD DACVAA, DACVECC

Pollakiuria and Stranguria

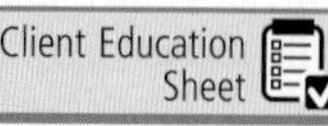

BASIC INFORMATION

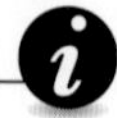

Definition

- Pollakiuria: increased frequency of attempts to urinate
- Stranguria: straining to urinate
- Both are common clinical signs of lower urinary tract inflammation, infection, and/or obstruction.

Epidemiology

SPECIES, AGE, SEX

Any species or age; either sex

Clinical Presentation

HISTORY, CHIEF COMPLAINT

- Owners may confuse these clinical signs with inappropriate elimination, polyuria, tenesmus, or incontinence.
- Other clinical signs can include discolored and malodorous urine.
- Often, pollakiuria/stranguria is the only presenting clinical sign.

PHYSICAL EXAM FINDINGS

Important to determine whether pollakiuria/stranguria is caused by urethral obstruction:

- Obstruction: bladder enlarged/firm, nonexpressible, often painful
- No obstruction: bladder is small (often empty), soft, expressible; bladder wall may be thickened and often painful

Observe voiding attempts and assess urine stream. Bladder should be palpated before and after the patient voids:

- Uroliths, masses, and bladder wall thickness/irregularities may be assessed more easily in the flaccid bladder.

Rectal exam may reveal urethral, prostatic, or bladder trigone abnormalities.

Etiology and Pathophysiology

- Any disease that causes lower urinary tract inflammation or obstruction can cause pollakiuria or stranguria.
- Localizes the lesion to the lower urinary tract (bladder, prostate, urethra)

DIAGNOSIS

Diagnostic Overview

Beyond a complete history and physical exam, a sterile urine sample for urinalysis and bacterial culture and susceptibility (C&S) should be the first diagnostic tests. Diagnostic imaging should be considered before performing cystocentesis if bladder cancer seems likely (e.g., older dog, Scottish terrier breed). Imaging is also indicated for a patient with pollakiuria/stranguria with a negative culture, poor response to therapy, or recurrence.

Differential Diagnosis

Distinguish from inappropriate elimination, polyuria, or tenesmus. Potential causes of pollakiuria/stranguria (p. 1270):

- Feline
  - Feline lower urinary tract signs (FLUTS [p. 332]), also called *feline idiopathic cystitis* (FIC), *feline urologic syndrome* (FUS), and *feline lower urinary tract disorder* (FLUTD), is the most common cause.
  - Primary bacterial infection: rare in young cats (<2% of cats < 10 years of age with lower urinary tract signs), more common in cats ≥ 10 years of age
  - Urolithiasis
  - Neoplasia
- Canine
  - Bacterial cystitis: most common
  - Nonbacterial causes of cystitis: fungal, drug induced
  - Other bladder diseases: cystic calculi/uroliths, neoplasia
  - Prostatic diseases: infection, benign hyperplasia, neoplasia
  - Urethral disease: infection, granulomatous inflammation, neoplasia

Initial Database

CBC and serum biochemistry panel:

- Sometimes identifies diseases that predispose to infection or calculi (e.g., diabetes mellitus, hypercalcemia)

Urinalysis:

- Cystocentesis preferred unless bladder cancer suspected (alternative, catheterized sample)
- Comparison with free-catch sample may assist in anatomic localization of lesion.
- Presence of white blood cells and red blood cells does not confirm infection. Sterile lesions can cause inflammation.

Urine C&S:

- Cystocentesis preferred
- Confirms or rule out bacterial infection

Abdominal radiographs:

- Mass effect
- Prostatomegaly
- Radiopaque calculi

Abdominal ultrasound:

- Thickened bladder wall
- Bladder mass (inflammatory, neoplastic, or blood clot)
- Calculi
- Abnormal prostate
- Thickened, irregular urethra

Advanced or Confirmatory Testing

- Advanced imaging (double-contrast cystogram, excretory urethrogram)
- Cystoscopy (biopsy of mass or bladder wall, culture of bladder wall, removal of small calculi)
- Voiding urohydropulsion (p. 1175): appropriate if small calculi are present
- Cystotomy (biopsy, removal of calculi, culture of bladder wall)
- If calculi are present, chemical analysis is needed to determine appropriate, preventative diet and medications.

TREATMENT

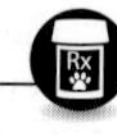

Treatment Overview

Goals of treatment are to relieve discomfort and treat underlying cause.

Acute General Treatment

Of greatest immediate concern is urethral obstruction (p. 1009). No matter the cause, urine flow must be established to prevent life-threatening hyperkalemia (p. 495) if complete obstruction is present (urinary bladder moderately to markedly enlarged) (pp. 1175 and 1176).

- Assess azotemia and potassium level.
- Gently try to pass a urinary catheter using retrograde hydropulsion if obstruction is met.
- If catheterization is unsuccessful, options include
  - Cystocentesis
  - Urethrotomy (males)
  - Cystostomy tube
- Provide fluid and electrolyte support while diagnostic tests are pursued.
  - Consider IV fluid (e.g., 0.9% NaCl) without potassium as first choice until serum potassium level is known.

Chronic Treatment

Depends on accurate diagnosis of underlying cause

Possible Complications

- Hyperkalemia associated with obstruction may cause life-threatening cardiac arrhythmia.
- Bladder rupture and uroperitoneum are possible with obstruction due to devitalization of the bladder wall.

PROGNOSIS & OUTCOME

Depends on cause and response to therapy

PEARLS & CONSIDERATIONS

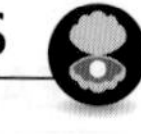

Comments

- Pollakiuria and stranguria localize the problem to the lower urinary tract.
- With any episode of pollakiuria or stranguria, urinary obstruction must be ruled out as soon as possible.
- Although bacterial infection is the most common cause in dogs, it is rare in cats < 10 years of age.
- FLUTS (FLUTD/FUS/FIC) is the most common cause of pollakiuria and stranguria in young cats.
- At a diagnostic minimum, urinalysis is warranted for all animals with pollakiuria/stranguria.

Technician Tips

- Any client who calls with concerns about pollakiuria/stranguria should be advised about the risk of urethral obstruction and urged to bring the pet in for exam without delay. Owners often misidentify stranguria as constipation (both involve straining), and a telephone question regarding constipation likewise warrants an immediate evaluation to rule out urethral obstruction.
- Immediate, careful palpation of the bladder to rule out obstruction should be done as soon as possible on presentation.

SUGGESTED READING

Cooper ES: Controversies in the management of feline urethral obstruction. J Vet Emerg Crit Care 25:130-137, 2015.

AUTHOR: Claire M. Weigand, DVM, DACVIM
EDITOR: Leah A. Cohn, DVM, PhD, DACVIM

Polyarthritis

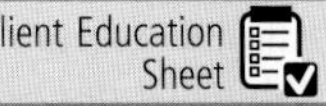

BASIC INFORMATION

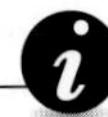

Definition

Inflammation of multiple joints

Epidemiology

SPECIES, AGE, SEX

- Dogs and cats of any age and either sex
- Rheumatoid arthritis: usually middle-aged dogs
- Polyarthritis of Akita dogs < 8 months old
- Infectious polyarthritis in dogs: male > female
- Feline chronic progressive polyarthritis: male > female

GENETICS, BREED PREDISPOSITION

- Certain histocompatibility alleles are associated with rheumatoid arthritis, usually in small-breed dogs.
- Juvenile-onset polyarthritis is seen in the Akita.
- Familial amyloidosis is a cause of polyarthritis in the Shar-pei.
- Sulfonamide-induced polyarthritis has been seen mostly in Doberman pinschers.
- Systemic lupus erythematosus (SLE) is overrepresented in certain breeds (p. 955).

RISK FACTORS

- Dogs: recent vaccination, treatment with sulfonamides or other drugs, exposure to ticks (e.g., tick-transmitted Lyme, ehrlichiosis, anaplasmosis), infection (e.g., bacterial endocarditis, pyometra, discospondylitis, urinary tract infection, neoplasia), and intestinal disease such as inflammatory bowel disease
- Cats: calicivirus vaccination (especially kittens)

ASSOCIATED DISORDERS

Immune-mediated polyarthritis (IMPA) may occur in association with meningitis (steroid-responsive meningitis arteritis), SLE, and other systemic disease.

Clinical Presentation

DISEASE FORMS/SUBTYPES

- Noninfectious, nonerosive IMPA
  - Breed-associated (e.g., Akita, Weimaraner, Shar-pei)
  - Triggered by an immune response to antigens outside the joint (reactive polyarthritis) (see Risk Factors)
  - Associated with SLE
  - Idiopathic
- Infectious, erosive and nonerosive arthritis
- Noninfectious erosive arthritis (rare)
  - Feline progressive polyarthritis: periosteal new bone formation and bony erosions; acute (more common, young cats) or chronic (less common, slower onset, older cats)
  - Canine rheumatoid arthritis (p. 888)
  - Polyarthritis of greyhounds

HISTORY, CHIEF COMPLAINT

- Difficulty walking; weakness, inability to rise, stiffness, lameness
  - Owners may not recognize lameness when multiple limbs involved
- Inappetence
- Lethargy, weight loss, vomiting, diarrhea
- Idiopathic IMPA typically is sudden onset with multiple symmetric joint involvement.

PHYSICAL EXAM FINDINGS

- Joint pain, swelling
  - May be difficult to localize source of stiffness; sometimes articular pain may be absent initially.
  - Firm, complete flexion of carpi should be performed and may reveal signs of pain that otherwise would escape notice.
  - Distal, symmetrical joint involvement (commonly carpi and tarsi) in IMPA
  - Usually one (monoarthritis) but occasionally two or more proximal joints involved with septic bacterial polyarthritis
- Fever; in some cases of IMPA, fever may be the only sign.
- Lymphadenopathy
- Other signs of underlying disease (e.g., heart murmur, arrhythmia, neck pain)

Etiology and Pathophysiology

- Noninfectious, nonerosive IMPA is common.
  - Most IMPA cases are idiopathic.
  - Breed-associated polyarthritides may have a genetic basis.
  - Possible mechanisms for reactive polyarthritis include immune complex deposition in joints in response to infection or inflammation remote from the joint (i.e., type III hypersensitivity reaction), and molecular mimicry, in which antibodies to bacteria, viruses, tumors, drugs, vaccines, or diets cross-react with joint antigens.
  - After joint inflammation has occurred, autoantigens (e.g., altered collagen) are produced that perpetuate the inflammation.
  - With SLE, autoantibodies to nuclear material, immune complex formation, and subsequent deposition in tissues cause multisystemic disease that commonly manifests with nonerosive polyarthritis, dermatitis, and/or glomerulonephritis (GN).
- Recognized causes of infectious polyarthritis
  - Vector transmitted: Lyme disease *(Borrelia burgdorferi)*, ehrlichiosis *(Ehrlichia ewingii)*, *Anaplasma phagocytophilum*, Rocky Mountain spotted fever, *Hepatozoon, Leishmania, Bartonella*
  - Other: calicivirus, *Streptococcus, Staphylococcus, Corynebacterium, Escherichia coli*, L-form bacteria, *Mycoplasma*, and systemic fungal infections
  - Nonvector-transmitted bacterial infection occurs after joint penetration (surgery, trauma, bite wound, arthrocentesis) or from hematogenous spread. Bite wounds are common in cats, whereas hematogenous spread from an unidentified source of infection can occur in dogs. Pre-existing damage to a joint may predispose to infection. Single joint involvement is more common, but infection may spread to other joints.
  - Multiple joint involvement can occur with systemic bacterial infections (e.g., bacterial endocarditis), which may also cause IMPA.
- Noninfectious erosive IMPAs include rheumatoid arthritis (rare in cats) and periosteal proliferative polyarthritis (common in cats). Least common causes of polyarthritis:
  - Rheumatoid arthritis is usually associated with autoantibodies to immunoglobulin G (rheumatoid factor).
  - Periosteal proliferative polyarthritis is characterized by periosteal new bone formation and bony erosions. It affects young adult cats, often castrated males, and is usually acute in onset. Chronic progressive polyarthritis is a milder form, is insidious in onset and affects older cats.

DIAGNOSIS

Diagnostic Overview

Polyarthritis can be suspected from the history and physical exam alone. Fever, lethargy, lameness, and painful or swollen joints (especially distal) should arouse suspicion. Confirmation rests on arthrocentesis with fluid analysis of multiple joints and radiography to evaluate erosive changes. Further testing (tick titers, cultures, screening for cancer) is required to identify an underlying cause and guide management. Successful management requires that any underlying cause be identified and treated. A diagnostic and treatment approach is presented on p. 1441.

Differential Diagnosis

- Neurologic disease (e.g., spinal cord or brain disorders, neuromuscular diseases)
- Muscular disease (e.g., polymyositis)
- Orthopedic disease (e.g., bilateral cranial cruciate ligament rupture, degenerative joint disease)
- Cardiac disease (e.g., pericardial effusion)
- Metabolic disease (e.g., hypoglycemia, hypocalcemia)
- Hematologic disease (e.g., acute blood loss)

Initial Database

- Orthopedic (p. 1143) and neurologic (p. 1136) exams to rule out other disorders
- CBC, serum biochemistry profile, urinalysis
  - Anemia and leukocytosis are common in idiopathic polyarthritis but are nonspecific. Thrombocytopenia may suggest vector-borne infection.
  - Serum chemistry profile to assess organ function
  - Proteinuria may be indicative of GN (immune mediated) or amyloidosis
- Radiographs to distinguish erosive from nonerosive polyarthritis
  - Erosive polyarthritis is characterized by subchondral bone destruction, seen as an irregular joint surface or punched-out erosion of bone at the joint space (p. 888). In advanced cases of joint deformity, loss of mineralization of the epiphysis and calcification of soft tissues of the joint may be seen. Often affects distal joints most severely.
  - Nonerosive polyarthritis has no bony abnormalities; signs of joint effusion and soft-tissue swelling may be apparent.

Advanced or Confirmatory Testing

- Arthrocentesis (p. 1059); two or more joints should be sampled.
  - The tarsi and carpi are especially useful because of frequency of involvement and ease of access.
  - Gross appearance: normal synovial fluid is viscous (tenacious), scant in volume, and clear, whereas synovial fluid of animals with polyarthritis is generally thin/watery and may be copious (several milliliters) and potentially turbid (more so with infectious/septic polyarthritis).
  - Synovial fluid analysis: neutrophils predominate in inflammatory polyarthritis (distinguishing them from the more common degenerative arthropathies), and total cell counts are always > 3000/mcL, often ≥ 40,000/mcL. Cytologic exam is seldom helpful in distinguishing septic from nonseptic arthritis (only occasionally are organisms seen), although the presence of degenerate or toxic neutrophils suggests septic arthritis.
  - Culture: synovial fluid cultures are often negative (false-negative rates of 20%-70%). When septic arthritis is suspected, consider additional cultures of synovial membrane, blood, and/or urine. Special media may be required to culture L-form bacteria and *Mycoplasma*.
- Titers and/or polymerase chain reaction (PCR): *B. burgdorferi*, *E. ewingii*, *A. phagocytophilum*, *Bartonella* spp, *Leishmania*
- Echocardiogram: suspected bacterial endocarditis (e.g., heart murmur, especially if recent onset and/or diastolic [p. 294])
- Serum antinuclear antibody and rheumatoid factor: suspected SLE or rheumatoid arthritis, respectively; the tests have limited accuracy.
- Cerebrospinal fluid tap (pp. 1080 and 1323) if meningitis is suspected
- Thoracic radiographs and abdominal ultrasound exam to evaluate remote infection, GI disease, or neoplasia

TREATMENT

Treatment Overview

Treatment depends on cause. Sometimes, despite treating the underlying cause, a course of prednisone is required to resolve the polyarthritis. For cases of IMPA, immunosuppressive doses of predniso(lo)ne are the treatment of choice, and after resolution of clinical signs, usually within 2 weeks, glucocorticoids should be slowly tapered over 4-6 months. Insufficient dosages and/or administration for insufficient periods are important causes of treatment failure.

Acute General Treatment

- Doxycycline 10 mg/kg PO q 24h for 28 days for tick-borne infections, *Mycoplasma*, and L-form bacteria
  - Instruct clients to administer a bolus of water or morsel of food after each dose to enhance esophageal transit.
- Prednisone/prednisolone 1.1 mg/kg PO q 12h initially for nonerosive and erosive noninfectious IMPA
- Cyclosporine or leflunomide are effective alternative treatments for IMPA.
- Broad-spectrum antibiotics (e.g., amoxicillin-clavulanate 22 mg/kg PO q 12h) or cephalosporins (e.g., cephalexin 22 mg/kg PO q 8h [dogs], 20 mg/kg PO q 12h [cats] or cefadroxil 22 mg/kg PO q 12-24h [dogs and cats]) pending cultures in suspected or confirmed cases of septic arthritis
- Surgical joint lavage and drainage sometimes are required for septic arthritis.
- Analgesia may be required, but avoid combination of nonsteroidal antiinflammatory drugs (NSAIDs) and glucocorticoids. Pain often resolves quickly with appropriate treatment of IMPA or vector-transmitted disease. Shar-pei fever or other arthropathies not treated with glucocorticoids may be treated with NSAIDs (e.g., meloxicam 0.1 mg/kg PO q 24h).

Chronic Treatment

- IMPA: prednisone/prednisolone 1.1 mg/kg PO q 12h (20 mg/m^2 PO q 12h for dogs > 25 kg; [p. 609] for body surface area conversion) until resolution of signs (usually 2-4 weeks), then slowly reduce the dose and administer q 48h. Average of 3-6 months but rarely lifelong treatment is required.
- If glucocorticoid's adverse effects are marked or high doses are necessary to suppress signs, consider other immunosuppressive drugs such as azathioprine, leflunomide, cyclosporine, cyclophosphamide, with lower dosages of glucocorticoids.
- Shar-pei fever requires intermittent long-term treatment.
- Septic arthritis: antibiotics required until 2 weeks after infection has resolved; often a minimum of 6 weeks.

Nutrition/Diet

Caloric control is necessary to avoid weight gain by patients receiving glucocorticoids.

Drug Interactions

Consult a formulary for possible interactions.

Possible Complications

- Secondary infections from immunosuppressive drugs
- Prednisone has many potential adverse effects.
- Azathioprine: myelosuppression, hepatotoxicity, acute pancreatitis; avoid in cats
- Leflunomide: hepatotoxicity, gastrointestinal upset, cytopenias

Recommended Monitoring

- Primarily resolution of clinical signs; ideally, repeat arthrocentesis to see if cell counts have returned to normal.
- Monthly CBC, liver enzymes for animals receiving immunosuppressive drugs.

PROGNOSIS & OUTCOME

- Nonerosive IMPA: good to guarded, ≈30% of cases relapse and may be difficult to control or may require lifelong treatment
- Juvenile hereditary arthritis of Akitas: very poor; does not respond to immunosuppressive therapy
- Calicivirus infection of cats: excellent; generally resolves in 3 days with supportive care
- Noninfectious erosive arthritis: guarded; arthrodesis or splints may improve quality of life
- Infectious arthritis: provided the arthritis is nonerosive and the infection can be treated, the prognosis is good.

PEARLS & CONSIDERATIONS

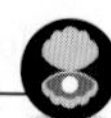

Comments

- Polyarthritis should be suspected in any animal that is reluctant to walk or in any case of fever of unknown origin. Even in the absence of joint pain or swelling, arthrocentesis of multiple joints is indicated to confirm or refute a diagnosis of IMPA.

- Cats with polyarthritis may be described only as lethargic by owners; polyarthritis can be missed unless cats are observed walking in the exam room.
- A thorough workup is required to rule out underlying causes, especially infectious disease.
- In any animal with polyarthritis, fever, and a newly recognized murmur, promptly rule in/rule out endocarditis.
- More than 50% of cases of IMPA are idiopathic.

Prevention

Tick prevention

Technician Tips

- Pain associated with polyarthritis should not be mistaken for reluctance or other behavioral traits; these patients may be too painful to walk, may be more prone to aggression if handled, or both.
- Joints should be clipped and aseptically prepared for arthrocentesis to avoid inadvertent introduction of infection.

Client Education

- Close monitoring is required for patients receiving immunosuppressive therapy.
- Relapses are possible.
- Genetic counseling for hereditary forms

SUGGESTED READING

Stull JW, et al: Canine immune-mediated polyarthritis: clinical and laboratory findings in 83 cases in western Canada (1991-2001). Can Vet J 49: 1195-1203, 2008.

AUTHOR: Orla Mahony, MVB, DACVIM, DECVIM
EDITOR: Jonathan E. Fogle, DVM, PhD, DACVIM

Polycystic Kidney Disease

Bonus Material Online 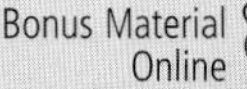 Client Education Sheet 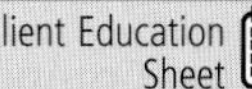 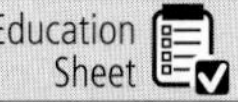

BASIC INFORMATION 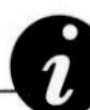

Definition

Inherited form of chronic kidney disease (CKD) characterized by development of multiple cysts in the kidney and occasionally in the liver, pancreas, or uterus. The condition is common in Persian and Persian-related cats.

Synonyms

PKD, autosomal dominant polycystic kidney disease (ADPKD), autosomal recessive polycystic kidney disease (ARPKD)

Epidemiology

SPECIES, AGE, SEX

- Cats and dogs, both sexes
- Although the diagnosis can be made in kittens, clinical signs usually appear at 3-10 years of age (average, 7 years).
- Infrequently reported in dogs. Bull terriers manifest signs as adults, and other breeds manifest signs as puppies.

GENETICS, BREED PREDISPOSITION

- Persians and related breeds (e.g., Himalayans), long-haired cats, and exotic shorthair cats are commonly affected; increasingly documented in domestic shorthair cats
- Autosomal dominant trait in cats and bull terriers (*PKD1* gene in Persians, bull terriers)
- In cats, PKD is not strictly associated with a long haircoat or brachycephalic facial conformation.
- About 40% of all Persians and Persian-related cats are affected; prevalence in bull terriers is unknown.
- Autosomal recessive polycystic kidney and liver disease has been reported in Cairn terriers and West Highland white terriers; onset of clinical signs occurs at an early age (≤2 months).
- Most reported bull terriers are from Australia.

ASSOCIATED DISORDERS

- CKD
- Polycystic liver disease
- In bull terriers, glomerulopathy (hereditary nephritis) may occur simultaneously; affected bull terriers have a higher incidence of cardiac disease.

Clinical Presentation

HISTORY, CHIEF COMPLAINT

- Animals with overt manifestations of illness present with signs of CKD such as polyuria, polydipsia, anorexia, lethargy, nausea, vomiting, weight loss, or poor body condition.
- Young animals presented for screening appear healthy.

PHYSICAL EXAM FINDINGS

- Early disease: normal
- Moderate disease: enlarged kidneys but contour may be smooth
- Advanced disease: bilaterally enlarged, irregular kidneys; may not be symmetrical
- Other findings of overt CKD (p. 169)

Etiology and Pathophysiology

- Abnormalities in integral membrane proteins polycystin 1 and polycystin 2 are the result of mutations in the polycystic kidney genes *PKD1* and *PKD2*, respectively, although alternative genetic and structural abnormalities may result in cyst formation.
- Cysts are abnormal dilations of renal tubules. Any section of the renal tubule may be affected by cyst formation.
- Cysts (usually multiple) that are present at birth slowly enlarge, compressing adjacent renal and other affected tissue. When sufficient renal parenchymal damage exists, CKD results. Rate of progression varies.

DIAGNOSIS 

Diagnostic Overview

Genetic testing (cats) or renal ultrasound can be used to diagnose PKD.

Differential Diagnosis

For enlarged kidneys: acute intrinsic kidney injury (e.g., pyelonephritis, nephrotoxicant), fungal nephritis, perinephric pseudocysts, renal lymphoma and other neoplastic diseases, ureteral obstruction with hydronephrosis, feline infectious peritonitis, amyloidosis, hematoma, perinephric abscess, and compensatory hypertrophy (unilateral)

Initial Database

- Healthy-appearing young cats presented for screening: renal ultrasound or genetic testing
- Clinically ill cats with enlarged kidneys: CBC, biochemistry profile, urinalysis and urine culture to assess renal function and identify uremia-associated complications (p. 169), abdominal ultrasound, and blood pressure (especially in azotemic animals)

Advanced or Confirmatory Testing

- Abdominal ultrasound can establish the diagnosis (75% sensitivity for diagnosis in cats < 16 weeks of age, 90% sensitivity in cats by 36 weeks). Cysts are anechoic, spherical structures with smooth, sharply marginated walls and far field enhancement. Cysts are easier to identify in the cortex than medulla.
- Genetic testing *(PKD1)* is available for cats > 8 weeks old (Veterinary Genetics Laboratory, University of California, Davis: www.vgl.ucdavis.edu). Buccal swab samples can be collected by owner.

- Cats may have ultrasonic evidence of PKD with a negative *PKD1* genetic test. Consider a different mutation in the *PKD1* or candidate genes or other causes of renal cysts (e.g., neoplasia, age-related cysts).

TREATMENT

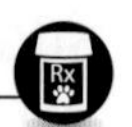

Treatment Overview

Affected animals should not be used for breeding. Animals with clinical signs related to PKD should be managed as other animals with CKD.

Acute General Treatment

No treatment is specific for PKD; treat for CKD and associated complications. Draining the cysts does not provide any advantage and introduces the risk of bacterial contamination.

Chronic Treatment

Same as for CKD (pp. 167 and 169)

Possible Complications

Cysts can become infected. Alkaline and lipid-soluble antibiotics, including fluoroquinolones, clindamycin, chloramphenicol, and trimethoprim-sulfonamide, penetrate cysts well.

Recommended Monitoring

- Routine recheck, including physical exam, weight, CBC (or packed cell volume), and serum biochemistry panel; frequency depends on disease severity
  - Stage I-II CKD: recheck every 3-6 months.
  - Stage III CKD: recheck every 2-3 months.
  - Stage IV CKD: recheck monthly.
- Urinalysis (with consideration for urine protein/creatinine ratio) ± urine culture should be performed at least annually.
- Blood pressure measurement should be performed at least q 3 months or 1 week after antihypertensive drug dose adjustments.
- Changes in clinical signs also warrant recheck.

PROGNOSIS & OUTCOME

- Not all cats with PKD develop azotemia.
- PKD tends to progress more slowly than many other types of CKD. After azotemia develops, long-term prognosis is poor.

PEARLS & CONSIDERATIONS

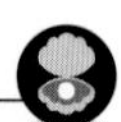

Comments

Although hypertension is common in people with PKD, it occurs infrequently in healthy cats with PKD.

Prevention

Eliminate affected animals from breeding population.

Technician Tips

Owners and breeders can collect and submit samples for genetic testing at home. Technicians can help instruct clients on obtaining cheek swab samples.

Client Education

- Because most PKD is due to an autosomal dominant trait, 50% of offspring from an affected animal will have the mutant *PKD1* gene. Screening (genetic or ultrasound) and subsequent removal of positive animals is suggested in commonly affected breeds.
- Kittens can be screened by ultrasound at < 16 weeks, but if negative, screening should be repeated when the cat is at least > 10 months of age, or genetic testing should be performed.
- Genetic screening can be completed in cats > 8 weeks old.
- If an individual cat with PKD is important to a breeding program, breed only to PKD-negative cats, and screen offspring. Assuming the affected parent is heterozygous for the mutant *PKD1* gene, one-half of the offspring will be affected and should be neutered; the unaffected individuals can be bred.

SUGGESTED READING

Domanjko-Petric A, et al: Polycystic kidney disease: a review and occurrence in Slovenia with comparison between ultrasound and genetic testing. J Feline Med Surg 10:115-119, 2008.

AUTHORS: Catherine E. Langston, DVM, DACVIM; Adam Eatroff, DVM, DACVIM
EDITOR: Leah A. Cohn, DVM, PhD, DACVIM

Polycythemia Vera

BASIC INFORMATION

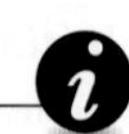

Definition

An inappropriate, absolute increase in red blood cell (RBC) mass as measured by RBC count, hematocrit (HCT), and hemoglobin (Hb) concentration

Synonyms

- Polycythemia rubra vera
- Strictly speaking, primary erythrocytosis is the more accurate term for this disorder; however, even though polycythemia implies increases in all circulating blood cell lines, the term polycythemia vera is used more commonly.

Epidemiology

SPECIES, AGE, SEX

Usually middle-aged to older dogs or cats

ASSOCIATED DISORDERS

Hyperviscosity syndrome (p. 509)

Clinical Presentation

HISTORY, CHIEF COMPLAINT

Mainly caused by or associated with hyperviscosity

- Neurologic changes (e.g., behavior, motor, or sensory), mental dullness, seizures
- Lethargy, exercise intolerance, collapse
- Hemorrhage (e.g., epistaxis, hyphema)

PHYSICAL EXAM FINDINGS

None, one, or many may be present:

- Hyperemic or cyanotic mucous membranes
- Erythema of the skin
- Polyuria and polydipsia (PU/PD)
- Splenomegaly

Etiology and Pathophysiology

- Absolute primary erythrocytosis
- Autonomous production of RBCs (erythropoietin independent)
- Myeloproliferative clonal disease
- Arises from a multipotent hematopoietic progenitor cell in the bone marrow, resulting in the accumulation of morphologically and functionally normal RBCs
  - *JAK2* gene mutation occurs in 90% of human polycythemia vera patients and has been identified in a dog with polycythemia vera.
- Erythrocytosis may lead to the hyperviscosity syndrome and resultant clinical signs.

DIAGNOSIS

Diagnostic Overview

The goals are to determine whether a true increase in red cell mass is present and then rule out erythrocytosis secondary to increased erythropoietin. Because polycythemia vera is an autonomous increase in red cells, repeatable elevations in HCT, RBC count, and Hb are expected. Polycythemia vera is a diagnosis of exclusion, and a complete diagnostic workup is indicated to rule out all other possibilities in the differential diagnosis.

Differential Diagnosis

- Relative erythrocytosis (pseudoerythrocytosis): elevated HCT, with normal or decreased RBC mass
  - Decrease in plasma volume is associated with severe dehydration and increased serum total protein (TP) concentration.
- Absolute secondary erythrocytosis: erythropoietin dependent; appropriate or inappropriate response
  - Appropriate (secondary to decreased tissue oxygenation)
    - High altitude
    - Chronic pulmonary disease
    - Right-to-left cardiovascular shunts (ventricular septal defect, reversed patent ductus arteriosus [PDA], tetralogy of Fallot, atrial septal defect)
    - Hemoglobinopathies (abnormal hemoglobin, methemoglobin reductase deficiency)
  - Inappropriate (normal tissue oxygenation)
    - Renal neoplasia (e.g., lymphoma, nephroblastoma, carcinoma, fibrosarcoma)
    - Other renal disease (e.g., polycystic kidney disease, rarely amyloidosis or glomerulonephritis)
    - Other neoplasms (e.g., cecal leiomyosarcoma, hepatic tumors)

Initial Database

- CBC: persistently increased HCT, RBC count, and Hb concentrations with normal total protein concentration; RBC morphology is normal.
- Serum biochemistry profile, urinalysis: generally unremarkable
- Arterial blood gas (ABG) analysis: to rule out hypoxemia as a cause of secondary erythrocytosis; normal oxygenation in polycythemia vera
- Abdominal ultrasound
  - To identify renal masses or other potential erythropoietin-producing tumors
  - Nonspecific findings (hyperechoic kidneys or splenomegaly noted in 25% of cats and 10% of dogs with polycythemia vera)
- Thoracic radiographs: bronchial or interstitial changes are nonspecific. If pulmonary disease is suspected as the cause of hypoxemia (and erythrocytosis secondarily), ABG measurement is indicated for confirmation.
- Echocardiography: to identify myocardial hypertrophy (secondary to hyperviscosity [left ventricle, mild] or right ventricular outflow obstruction/pulmonary hypertension [right ventricle, marked]), right-to-left shunts, or other abnormalities that could cause secondary erythrocytosis

Advanced or Confirmatory Testing

- Measurement of plasma erythropoietin concentration (rarely performed)
  - Generally normal to low in polycythemia vera
  - Test has low diagnostic specificity; substantial overlap with the normal range; other types of erythrocytosis (e.g., relative erythrocytosis) are associated with similar results.
  - Measurement can help rule out secondary erythrocytosis (high plasma erythropoietin concentration).
  - Bone marrow aspiration and cytologic exam or bone marrow core biopsy: not useful because it cannot distinguish primary from secondary erythrocytosis

TREATMENT

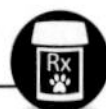

Treatment Overview

Decrease blood viscosity and RBC mass to reduce or resolve clinical signs (palliation).

Acute General Treatment

Initial treatment is phlebotomy:

- Collect 20 mL/kg of blood from external jugular or other central vein.
- Avoid hypotension due to volume depletion (rarely a problem) by replacement with equivalent volume of IV crystalloid fluid.
- Target HCT is < 55% in dogs, < 50% in cats
- Replacement of coagulation factors and albumin if multiple phlebotomies in short period (rare). Autologous plasma (centrifuge phlebotomized blood, discard RBCs, and administer patient's own plasma) and allogenic fresh-frozen plasma are suitable options.

Chronic Treatment

- Periodic phlebotomies if needed
- Alternatively, hydroxyurea (Hydrea) 30 mg/kg PO q 24h for 7-10 days, then decrease to 15 mg/kg PO q 24h, and titrate dose to maintain normal HCT; reduces RBC production. Monitor CBC for myelosuppression.
- Other chemotherapy agents such as chlorambucil have been used less often.
- Radioactive phosphorus (^{32}P) for myelosuppression: rarely used in animals; available only in specialized centers

Possible Complications

Hydroxyurea can cause myelosuppression. With chronic use, adverse effects, including onychomadesis (sloughing of the claws), macrocytosis (increased mean corpuscular volume [MCV]), methemoglobinemia (cats), and induction of secondary neoplasia (including leukemia), have been reported.

Recommended Monitoring

- CBC weekly at first until HCT stabilizes, then q 4-6 weeks
- Physical exam and diagnostic testing as needed; opportunistic infections, myelosuppression, and other complications of various degrees of concern can occur during treatment with chemotherapeutic agents.

PROGNOSIS & OUTCOME

Polycythemia vera can be successfully managed for years.

PEARLS & CONSIDERATIONS

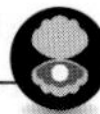

Comments

- The diagnosis is made by excluding other causes of polycythemia.
- Most pets tolerate treatment well.

Technician Tips

As a result high blood viscosity in patients with erythrocytosis, it may be difficult to obtain a blood sample through a relatively small (e.g., 19-gauge) catheter.

Client Education

Infections can occur secondary to myelosuppression. Routine follow-up evaluations are necessary during treatment, even when clinical signs are well controlled.

SUGGESTED READING

Couto G: Erythrocytosis. In Nelson RW, et al, editors: Small animal internal medicine, ed 5, St. Louis, 2013, Mosby, pp 1227-1229.

AUTHOR: Pascale Salah, Dr.vet.med., DACVIM
EDITOR: Jonathan E. Fogle, DVM, PhD, DACVIM

Polyneuropathy

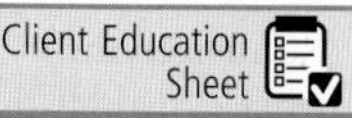

BASIC INFORMATION

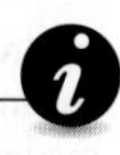

Definition

The diverse group of disorders affects the peripheral nerves. Although motor and sensory nerves can be affected, animals most often present with generalized lower motor neuron deficits reflecting involvement of motor nerves. Sensory deficits can be seen in conjunction with motor deficits in some disorders and are the only clinical signs in sensory polyneuropathies.

Synonyms

Peripheral neuropathy

EPIDEMIOLOGY

SPECIES, AGE, SEX

- Dogs, less common in cats; either sex
- Age of onset varies, depending on underlying cause.
- Inherited polyneuropathies can have a juvenile, adult, or geriatric onset, depending on the specific condition.

GENETICS, BREED PREDISPOSITION

- Mixed (motor and sensory) polyneuropathies without laryngeal paralysis: German shepherd dog, Great Dane, Bouvier des Flandres, Siberian Husky, rottweiler, golden retriever, Tibetan mastiff, boxer
- Laryngeal paralysis–polyneuropathy complex: Labrador retriever, Leonberger, rottweiler, Black Russian terrier, Dalmatian, Alaskan Malamute, Italian spinone, Great Pyrenees
- Sensory polyneuropathies: border collie, German short-haired pointer, English pointer, long-haired dachshund, golden retriever

Clinical Presentation

DISEASE FORMS/SUBTYPES

- Motor or mixed polyneuropathies: generalized limb involvement ± megaesophagus
  - Laryngeal paralysis is a presenting sign of certain disorders (laryngeal paralysis–polyneuropathy complex)
- Sensory neuropathies: sensory deficits only

HISTORY, CHIEF COMPLAINT

- Motor or mixed polyneuropathies
  - Weakness, usually affecting all four limbs; pelvic limbs can be more severely affected
  - Dysphagia, regurgitation
  - Signs of respiratory distress and stridor with laryngeal involvement
- Sensory polyneuropathies
  - Self-mutilation, ataxia

PHYSICAL EXAM FINDINGS

- Motor or mixed polyneuropathies
  - Ambulatory or non-ambulatory tetraparesis, sometimes paraparesis; in severe cases, tetraplegia or paraplegia
  - Decreased or absent segmental spinal reflexes
  - Muscle atrophy
  - With pure motor polyneuropathies, proprioception is usually normal unless patient is too weak to move limb.
  - Plantigrade stance (common in feline diabetic polyneuropathy)
  - Signs of cranial nerve involvement: laryngeal paralysis, megaesophagus, dysphonia
  - With laryngeal paralysis, stridor and inspiratory effort (p. 574)
- Sensory polyneuropathies
  - Self-mutilation, proprioceptive deficits, proprioceptive ataxia

Etiology and Pathophysiology

Motor and mixed polyneuropathies:

- Inflammatory, noninfectious
  - Idiopathic polyradiculoneuritis (coonhound paralysis) (p. 810)
  - Other immune-mediated conditions (brachial plexus neuritis, chronic inflammatory neuropathy): uncommon
- Infectious: protozoal (*Neospora caninum*)
- Inherited: multiple breeds; whether disease affects axons, myelin sheath, or both varies
- Paraneoplastic: insulinoma, others (carcinomas, multiple myeloma)
- Metabolic/endocrine
  - Diabetic polyneuropathy in cats
  - Hypothyroidism

Sensory polyneuropathies:

- Inherited
- Toxic

DIAGNOSIS

Diagnostic Overview

Polyneuropathy should be considered in an animal with generalized lower motor neuron signs and/or diffuse sensory deficits. Initial diagnostic testing is used to screen for inflammatory or metabolic disease. Thoracic radiographs are indicated to evaluate for aspiration pneumonia, megaesophagus, or metastatic neoplasia. Electrodiagnostics and nerve biopsy are required to reach a definitive diagnosis.

Differential Diagnosis

Motor polyneuropathies:

- Disorders of the neuromuscular junction
  - Botulism
  - Tick paralysis
  - Coral snake envenomation
  - Myasthenia gravis (fulminant form)
  - Polymyositis
  - Myopathies (hereditary, metabolic/endocrine)
  - Rabies

Mixed polyneuropathies:

- Severe, acute cervical spinal cord lesion
- If only one limb is affected
  - Peripheral nerve sheath tumor
  - Trauma to the nerve or partial avulsion of the nerve plexus

Sensory polyneuropathies:

- Mild cervical spinal cord lesion: if ataxia and proprioceptive deficits are only signs

Initial Database

- Neurologic exam (p. 1136): evidence of lower motor neuron disease
- Serum biochemistry profile, including creatine kinase (to rule out myopathy) and glucose (to screen for diabetes mellitus)
- Thoracic radiographs: evaluate for megaesophagus, aspiration pneumonia, metastatic neoplasia
- Thyroid testing
- *Neospora caninum* titers

Advanced or Confirmatory Testing

Motor and mixed polyneuropathies:

- Electrodiagnostic testing
  - Electromyography (EMG): changes seen 5-7 days after onset of clinical signs
  - Nerve conduction velocity (NCV): abnormalities in velocity and/or amplitude, depending on whether underlying disease results in demyelination or axonopathy
- Laryngeal exam to assess for laryngeal paralysis (p. 1125)
- Cerebrospinal fluid (CSF) analysis (pp. 1080 and 1323): increased protein levels possible in polyradiculoneuritis
- Muscle biopsy: changes compatible with denervation
- Nerve biopsy: axonal and/or myelin abnormalities; pattern dependent on cause
- Abdominal ultrasound to rule out or confirm neoplasia
- DNA testing for hereditary disease

Sensory polyneuropathies:

- Electrodiagnostics: sensory nerve conduction velocity
- DNA testing for hereditary disease

TREATMENT

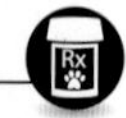

Treatment Overview

- Motor and mixed polyneuropathies: treat any identified underlying cause, and provide supportive care, including ventilatory support, if needed. Glucocorticoids not shown to be of benefit (with possible exception of paraneoplastic or autoimmune neuropathies)
- Sensory polyneuropathy: no specific treatment available; prevent self-mutilation

Acute General Treatment

Motor and mixed polyneuropathies:

- Supportive care: fluid therapy, hand feeding or feeding tube, soft bedding, rotating sides, and ventilatory support, if needed
  - Positive-pressure ventilation is indicated only for reversible causes of polyneuropathy (e.g., botulism, tick paralysis [p. 1185]).

- Diabetic or hypothyroid polyneuropathy: treat underlying disease
- Laryngeal paralysis–polyneuropathy complex: if respiratory distress, consider laryngoplasty surgery to manage laryngeal paralysis symptomatically; underlying polyneuropathy cannot be treated.
- Protozoal polyneuropathy: clindamycin 11 mg/kg PO q 12h for 6 weeks

Sensory polyneuropathies:

- Cleaning and debridement of wounds: e-collar to prevent further self-mutilation; no specific treatment available. Most dogs are euthanized soon after diagnosis. Avoid breeding carrier or affected dogs.

Nutrition/Diet

If patient is unable to eat due to respiratory effort or dependence on ventilatory support, feeding tube placement or parenteral nutrition should be considered. Elevated feeding is indicated in cases of megaesophagus.

Behavior/Exercise

Physical rehabilitation consists of passive range-of-motion and standing exercises.

Possible Complications

- Aspiration pneumonia, pressure sores, muscle atrophy
- Muscle atrophy cannot be avoided in chronic cases, but physical rehabilitation can help to minimize it.

Recommended Monitoring

Regular monitoring of body temperature and auscultation of the lungs to check for signs of aspiration pneumonia

PROGNOSIS & OUTCOME

Varies, based on underlying cause and severity:

- Idiopathic polyradiculoneuritis: favorable, if no severe complications occur
- Paraneoplastic polyneuropathy: depends on type of underlying neoplasia
- Protozoal polyneuropathy: depends on severity of clinical signs
- Inherited polyneuropathies: depends on age of onset and rate of progression
  - In some breeds (e.g., Labrador retrievers), manifests as slowly progressive disease in older dogs. Dogs can have a good quality of life but some need surgical correction of laryngeal paralysis to improve respiration.

PEARLS & CONSIDERATIONS

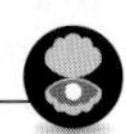

Comments

Motor and mixed polyneuropathies are more common than sensory polyneuropathies. Polyradiculoneuritis is the most commonly seen polyneuropathy. Creatine kinase levels are important to rule out polymyositis, a potentially treatable condition.

Technician Tips

Severely affected patients need to be turned frequently and have clean and dry bedding to prevent pressure sores. They benefit from passive range-of-motion exercises to minimize muscle atrophy.

Client Education

- Prognosis varies, depending on the underlying cause.
- Despite the best care, some dogs develop pressure sores or aspiration pneumonia.
- Clients need to be aware that some dogs will require ventilatory support, which is associated with high costs and potential complications.

SUGGESTED READING

Anor D: Lower motor neuron tetraparesis. Vet Clin Small Anim 44:1201-1222, 2014.

RELATED CLIENT EDUCATION SHEETS

Consent to Perform Cerebrospinal Fluid Tap
Diabetes Mellitus (Cats)
How to Assist a Pet That Is Unable to Rise and Walk
How to Perform Range-of-Motion Exercises
How to Use and Care for an Indwelling Feeding Tube
Hypothyroidism
Laryngeal Paralysis
Megaesophagus

AUTHOR: Daniela A. Mauler, DVM, DECVN
EDITOR: Karen R. Muñana, DVM, MS, DACVIM

Polyphagia

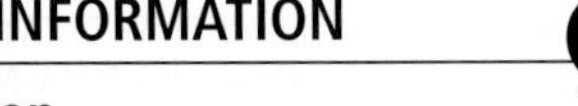

Client Education Sheet

BASIC INFORMATION

Definition

Excessive hunger or food intake

Epidemiology

SPECIES, AGE, SEX

- Any species or age, either sex
- Neutering may lead to weight gain ± increased appetite

GENETICS, BREED PREDISPOSITION

Certain breeds are more likely to eat excessively (e.g., Labrador retriever, Shetland sheepdog, dachshund, cocker spaniel, others)

RISK FACTORS

Neuter status, cold weather, increased exercise, drug (e.g., glucocorticoids, phenobarbital, antihistamines, progestins, benzodiazepines, cyproheptadine, mirtazapine), growth, pregnancy, lactation, various disease states (see Associated Disorders)

ASSOCIATED DISORDERS

- Result of polyphagia: obesity
- Cause of polyphagia: endocrinopathy such as diabetes mellitus (DM), hyperadrenocorticism (HAC), hyperthyroidism, insulinoma, or acromegaly; pancreatic enzyme insufficiency; gastrointestinal (GI) disease (e.g., inflammatory bowel disease, lymphangiectasia, lymphocytic lymphoma-cats); GI parasites (especially in young); sudden acquired retinal degeneration (mimics HAC [p. 883]); hepatic encephalopathy; neoplasia (early); destruction of satiety center (e.g., trauma, mass, infection/inflammation)

Clinical Presentation

DISEASE FORMS/SUBTYPES

Polyphagia with weight gain (more common) or weight loss

HISTORY, CHIEF COMPLAINT

- Increased appetite (e.g., begging for food, stealing food)
- Weight gain or loss
- Other findings related to cause (e.g., polyuria, polydipsia with DM or HAC)

PHYSICAL EXAM FINDINGS

Excess or inadequate body condition is possible. Other findings are related to cause of polyphagia.

- Excess weight: more common with behavioral causes, drugs (e.g., phenobarbital, glucocorticoids), and some endocrinopathies (e.g., HAC)
- Underweight: more common with pancreatic enzyme insufficiency, GI disease, some endocrinopathies (e.g., DM, hyperthyroidism)

Etiology and Pathophysiology

Polyphagia may be behavioral, compensation for inadequate caloric intake, increased caloric use, increased metabolic demands, related to issues affecting satiety, or due to other (often poorly understood) causes.

DIAGNOSIS

Diagnostic Overview

Actual caloric intake should be calculated because owners may underestimate needs (leaving the pet hungry). In addition to routine medical history, a thorough diet history is paramount; ask open-ended questions about the patient's feeding and eating habits to help rule out behavioral issues. A CBC, serum chemistry profile, urinalysis, and thyroid level often provide clues to metabolic and endocrine causes. If a cause is still not identified (especially if polyphagia accompanied by weight loss), GI investigation is in order.

Differential Diagnosis

Appropriate hunger may be misinterpreted as excessive.

Initial Database

- Calculate caloric intake compared with caloric needs (p. 1077).
- CBC
  - Anemia (chronic disease, GI blood loss)
  - Leukocytosis (HAC)
  - Eosinophilia (parasitism)
- Chemistry panel
  - Hypoalbuminemia (GI loss)
  - Elevated liver enzymes (endogenous or exogenous steroids)
  - Hyperglycemia (diabetes mellitus)
  - Hypoglycemia (insulinoma)
- Urinalysis
  - Glucose, ketones (diabetes mellitus)
  - Protein: rule out renal loss if patient hypoalbuminemic
- Thyroid level
  - Hyperthyroidism (cats with weight loss)
  - Hypothyroidism (dogs with weight gain, polyphagia is uncommon)
- Fecal (ova and parasite)

Advanced or Confirmatory Testing

Guided by previous results.

- Suspect HAC (p. 485)
- Suspect DM (p. 251)
- Suspect hyperthyroidism (p. 503)

GI panel (especially with weight loss, vomiting, or diarrhea):

- Cobalamin and folate levels: intestinal function (pp. 1325 and 1344)
- Trypsin-like immunoreactivity (TLI): test of choice for exocrine pancreatic insufficiency (p. 317)

Abdominal ultrasound:

- Adrenal size and shape
- GI tract layering, thickness, and appearance
- Pancreatic size, echogenicity
- Rule out pregnancy in intact female patient

Chest radiographs

- Help rule out metastatic neoplasia

Endoscopy (especially with weight loss, vomiting, diarrhea, or GI imaging abnormalities):

- Obtain mucosal stomach and intestinal biopsies
- Minimally invasive, safe in face of severe hypoalbuminemia

Exploratory laparotomy (if less invasive tests have failed and especially with weight loss):

- Full-thickness stomach and intestinal biopsies
- Invasive: not recommended with severe hypoalbuminemia (albumin < 2.0 g/dL)

CT/MRI (if central nervous system disease suspected)

TREATMENT

Treatment Overview

Address any identified underlying disease. Pet owner should be counseled on the appropriate diet (type and quantity) for the animal's needs. If polyphagia seems to be behavioral or related to a necessary medication, a switch to a lower-caloric-density food and increased exercise may help avoid weight gain.

Chronic Treatment

Depends on accurate diagnosis of underlying cause

Nutrition/Diet

Calculate daily caloric need for ideal weight, and have owner measure food. Obesity is discussed on p. 700.

Behavior/Exercise

For healthy dogs with a large appetite, increased exercise may help avoid excess weight gain.

Possible Complications

Obesity can worsen orthopedic, neuromuscular, and respiratory disorders.

Recommended Monitoring

Weight, body condition, and muscle condition scores

PROGNOSIS & OUTCOME

Depends on cause

PEARLS & CONSIDERATIONS

Comments

- Young dogs with polyphagia and weight loss must be tested for pancreatic enzyme insufficiency.
- Older cats with polyphagia and weight loss must be tested for hyperthyroidism.
- Although both HAC and DM cause polyphagia, polyuria, and polydipsia, HAC generally causes weight gain rather than weight loss.
- Exogenous glucocorticoids given by any route (including topical therapy) can lead to increased appetite.
- Protein-losing enteropathy includes poor absorption of nutrients with loss of nutrients, and weight loss can be extreme, even in the face of polyphagia.

Technician Tips

A complete history is vital to diagnosis.

- Discuss all medications, including topicals and supplements.
- Dietary history, including changes in diet, is crucial.

Client Education

It is best to give clients calories per day and measurements for dry and canned food. For example, "to feed 350 calories per day, the patient should receive ½ cup dry and ¼ canned of food twice each day."

SUGGESTED READING

Daminet S: Polyphagia. In Ettinger SJ, et al, editors: Textbook of veterinary internal medicine, ed 8, St. Louis, 2017, Elsevier, pp 100-103.

AUTHOR: Claire M. Weigand, DVM, DACVIM
EDITOR: Leah A. Cohn, DVM, PhD, DACVIM

Polyradiculoneuritis

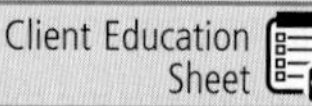

BASIC INFORMATION

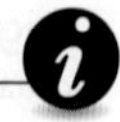

Definition

The idiopathic inflammatory disorder primarily involving axons and myelin of ventral nerve roots is probably the most common polyneuropathy in dogs. An analogous polyneuropathy has been described in cats (much less common).

Synonym

Coonhound paralysis. Similar to Guillain-Barré syndrome in humans.

Epidemiology

SPECIES, AGE, SEX

Dogs, usually adults, of any breed and either sex

GENETICS, BREED PREDISPOSITION

Hunting dogs, specifically coonhounds of certain lineages, may be predisposed.

RISK FACTORS

Raccoon bites or scratches in a genetically susceptible animal. Raw chicken consumption and *Campylobacter* infection may also be risk factors.

ASSOCIATED DISORDERS

- Aspiration pneumonia
- Urinary tract infections
- Muscle atrophy/contracture
- Pressure-induced skin ulcerations
- Hypoventilation/respiratory paresis or paralysis

Clinical Presentation

DISEASE FORMS/SUBTYPES

Two subcategories appear identical in terms of onset, clinical signs, disease course, diagnostics, and pathology and are likely representative of the same disease syndrome:

- Coonhound paralysis (CHP)
  - History of being bitten or scratched by a raccoon 7-10 days before onset of signs
- Acute idiopathic polyradiculoneuritis (PRN)
  - Identical disorder with no exposure to raccoons

HISTORY, CHIEF COMPLAINT

- Acute-onset lower motor neuron (LMN) paresis/plegia, usually beginning in pelvic limbs and progressing to thoracic limbs. Some dogs can initially develop a short, choppy gait.
- Progression to nonambulatory tetraparesis/tetraplegia, typically within 10 days of onset (as quickly as 72 hours)
- Clinical signs occasionally begin in the thoracic limbs and progress to pelvic limbs or present as acute-onset tetraparesis/tetraplegia.
- Duration of paralysis varies from several weeks to 2-5 months, depending on degree of axonal versus myelin damage (more prolonged recovery with axonal involvement).

PHYSICAL EXAM FINDINGS

- Nonambulatory LMN paraparesis/plegia or tetraparesis/plegia
- Normal mentation
- Afebrile patient
- Decreased to absent spinal reflexes (with exception of perineal reflex)
- Hypotonia/atonia
- Generalized, severe (neurogenic) muscle atrophy commonly develops within 7-10 days.
- Sensory function is normal to heightened; some dogs are hyperesthetic.
- Hypoventilation and/or development of a life-threatening respiratory paralysis can occur, especially in acute-onset, rapidly progressive cases.
- Loss of voice (dysphonia, aphonia) is common.
- Cranial nerves are usually normal; occasionally slight facial weakness
- Proprioceptive placing is normal in animals that retain some motor function.
- Patients retain the ability to urinate and defecate and readily eat and drink if the head is supported.

Etiology and Pathophysiology

Presumptive cause:

- The antigenic stimulus in dogs is currently unknown, although raccoon saliva is thought to be one source. Findings from a seroprevalence study suggest that *Toxoplasma gondii* infection may serve as a potential trigger for PRN in some dogs.
- There may also be a genetic predisposition for this disease in coonhound breeds.

Pathophysiology:

- After exposure to the specific antigen (e.g., raccoon saliva, vaccine, infectious agent), alteration of the patient's immune system occurs. An autoimmune reaction against axons and myelin of the ventral nerve roots is theorized. Antibodies directed against gangliosides, a major component of neuronal membranes, have been identified in affected humans and dogs.
- In humans with PRN (Landry-Guillain-Barré syndrome), molecular mimicry and concurrent infection with *Campylobacter jejuni* (gastroenteritis) are thought to be involved in the pathogenesis. The bacterium's capsular antigens mimic the components found on peripheral nerves. After the immune system is exposed to *C. jejuni,* the antibody response destroys the bacterium and the peripheral nerve.
- Numerous exogenous antigens have components that mimic molecules found in canine axons; molecular mimicry may be involved in the pathogenesis.

DIAGNOSIS

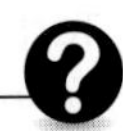

Diagnostic Overview

PRN is a diagnosis of exclusion. A working clinical diagnosis is based on the typical clinical presentation of an acute-onset LMN paraparesis/plegia that rapidly progresses to tetraparesis/plegia. Although not confirmatory, ancillary testing is helpful in ruling out other differential diagnoses.

Differential Diagnosis

Botulism, tick paralysis (United States and Australia), myasthenia gravis, protozoan polyneuritis/polymyositis, paraneoplastic neuropathy

Initial Database

- Three-view thoracic radiographs: unremarkable unless secondary aspiration pneumonia or metastasis; useful in ruling out paraneoplastic neuropathies and megaesophagus
- CBC, serum biochemistry profile, urinalysis: unremarkable unless secondary urinary tract or respiratory infection present
- Antiacetylcholine receptor antibody test: negative; useful in ruling out myasthenia gravis
- Lumbar cerebrospinal fluid (CSF) tap: an increase in protein with a normal nucleated cell count (albuminocytologic dissociation) supports the diagnosis (p. 1323)
- Serum muscle enzyme levels: normal or only mildly elevated due to recumbency (compared with marked elevations in polymyositis)
- Carefully examine entire dog for ticks. Consider rapid-acting ectoparasite treatment even if tick is not seen to help rule out tick paralysis.

Advanced or Confirmatory Testing

- Electrodiagnostic testing (electromyography and motor nerve conduction studies): affected dogs exhibit abnormal electromyographic activity (fibrillation potentials and positive sharp waves consistent with denervation) with normal or slightly reduced motor nerve conduction velocities (NCVs).
- Nerve biopsy: demyelination, leukocytic infiltration, axonal degeneration, and segmental demyelination are consistent with PRN but nonspecific because the inflammatory process occurs primarily at the ventral nerve roots.
- Arterial blood gas analysis: helps determine whether mechanical ventilation is warranted

TREATMENT

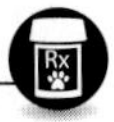

Treatment Overview

Therapy is nonspecific, supportive, and often very protracted (major determinant of prognosis). Cornerstones are persistent supportive care and rehabilitation to prevent secondary complications. Most patients show signs of improvement within 3 weeks and complete recovery by 3-5 months. Rarely, severe, rapidly progressive cases require mechanical ventilation.

Acute General Treatment

Monitor pulmonary function and ventilatory status with arterial blood gas analysis in recumbent patients. If hypoventilation is evident, provide mechanical ventilatory support (p. 1185).

Chronic Treatment

- Supportive care, physical rehabilitation, and proper nutrition are essential for recovery.
  - Animals should be turned at least 6-8 times daily to prevent complications secondary to prolonged recumbency (e.g., hypostatic lung congestion, decubital ulcers).
  - Passive range-of-motion exercises and massage of limbs should be performed at least four to five times daily to keep joints flexible and muscles supple.
  - Hydrotherapy provides exercise and helps preclude muscle atrophy.
  - Proper bedding is essential to prevent pressure-induced skin ulcerations; waterbeds are useful.
  - Assisted feedings help prevent aspiration pneumonia.
  - Ensure the patient's environment is clean and dry.
  - Monitor for bladder overdistention, and intervene as necessary.
- Glucocorticoid treatment has been suggested, but there is no evidence of efficacy.
- The role of plasmapheresis and intravenous immunoglobulin (IVIG) administration, an established treatment for humans with signs of PRN, has not been proved in dogs. A pilot clinical study demonstrated a trend toward faster recovery in dogs treated with IVIG compared with controls.

Possible Complications

- Aspiration pneumonia, pressure-induced skin ulcerations, and urinary tract infections occur secondary to prolonged recumbency.
- Severe muscle atrophy and contracture
- Respiratory paresis/paralysis can occur in severe cases.

Recommended Monitoring

If patient is not hospitalized, weekly recheck exams to assess recovery progress

PROGNOSIS & OUTCOME

- Prognosis for full recovery is usually favorable. Due to the transient nature of the inflammatory phase, damaged axons remyelinate and to some degree regrow over 3-6 weeks. If respiration is unaffected, with adequate supportive care, most animals show signs of improvement in 3 weeks and full recovery in 3-5 months.
- Large/heavy dogs, dogs living in dense urban environments, and dogs whose owners or families are unable to provide supportive care may have a worse prognosis because of the difficulties these factors impose on home care.
- If mechanical ventilation is needed or severe disease complications such as aspiration pneumonia and significant muscle contracture are present, recovery may be significantly prolonged or incomplete.
- Animals with significant axonal degeneration may not show clinical improvement.

PEARLS & CONSIDERATIONS

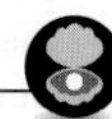

Comments

- After an animal has been affected with PRN, recurrence of clinical signs is possible if the patient is subsequently re-exposed to the inciting antigen.
- Chronic forms of this disease exist and are characterized by waxing and waning clinical signs. Tetraplegia is generally not seen with these forms of disease.

Prevention

Avoid exposure to raccoons, especially by dogs having recovered from CHP, because it may trigger a relapse.

Technician Tips

Treatment success greatly relies on intensive daily nursing care and physical rehabilitation. Patience and persistence over extended periods tend to be rewarded with recovery. Sometimes, it can take months for patients to recover.

Client Education

- For recumbent patients being cared for at home, provide client with a client education sheet: How to Perform Range-of-Motion Exercises.
- Clients need to be aware of and persistent about at-home nursing care and physical rehabilitation. They must also be aware of secondary complications. Frequent rechecks are necessary.
- Veterinary physical rehabilitation centers are available to aid with physical therapy.

SUGGESTED READING

Añor S. Acute lower motor neuron tetraparesis. Vet Clin North Am Small Anim Pract 44:1201-1222, 2014.

SECOND EDITION AUTHOR: **Lauren R. Talarico, DVM, DACVIM**
EDITOR: **Karen R. Muñana, DVM, MS, DACVIM**

Polyuria/Polydipsia

Client Education Sheet

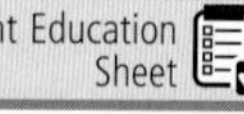

BASIC INFORMATION

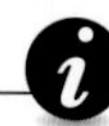

Definition

- Polydipsia (PD): excessive consumption of water (definitions vary)
  - >60-100 mL/kg/day for dogs
  - >40-60 mL/kg/day for cats
- Polyuria (PU): production of excessive urine volumes (dogs and cats, >30-50 mL/kg/day)

Epidemiology

SPECIES, AGE, SEX

Any dog or cat of any age

Clinical Presentation

PU and PD are clinical signs that vary dramatically from none to subtle to obvious. Underlying conditions and their clinical signs may overshadow PU/PD.

DISEASE FORMS/SUBTYPES

- PU with secondary PD (common)
- PD with secondary PU (uncommon)

HISTORY, CHIEF COMPLAINT

- Drinking more frequently, unusually large volumes and/or for prolonged periods
- Water-starved behavior (seeking water from unusual or poorly accessible locations)
- Urinating more frequently
- Prolonged duration of urination
- Urinating in inappropriate locations
- Need to change litter with increased frequency (cats)
- May be described as incontinence rather than excessive urination by owner

Often impossible to determine whether PU is primary with secondary PD or vice versa by history alone; questions to ask:

- Features suggestive of pollakiuria rather than PU (e.g., stranguria, hematuria), incontinence (e.g., seeming unaware of urination), or behavioral issues (e.g., spraying)
- Water consumption and urine output compared with 1, 4, or 8 weeks (or even 3, 6, or 12 months) earlier; AVOID leading the owner; do not ask whether water consumption has increased.
- Basic questions: diet, duration between walks (most healthy dogs urinate about every 8-12 hours), new pets or family members, new environment (behavior/marking or exposure to toxins), and change in litter type, location, or hygiene (cats).
- Medication history: glucocorticoids (dogs), phenobarbital, diuretics, and thyroid supplementation can cause PU/PD.
- Intoxication history: nephrotoxicants (e.g., ethylene glycol, grapes, raisins, lilies [cats], and nephrotoxic medications [p. 23]).

PHYSICAL EXAM FINDINGS

Hyperadrenocorticism, hyperthyroidism, pyometra, liver disease, and many other conditions that cause PU/PD may have exam findings that allow rapid refinement of differential diagnoses.

- Dehydration: consistent with any cause of PU/PD other than psychogenic PD
  - Pets with primary (psychogenic) PD, by definition, should be overhydrated.
  - Pets with a primary polyuric condition should be underhydrated.
- Thin body condition
  - Diabetes insipidus (DI): some drink excessively and choose water over food.
  - Large pituitary tumors may cause poor or no appetite and weight loss.
  - Serious illness (e.g., chronic kidney disease, lymphoma) can cause weight loss.
- Panting (excessive) may be noted with hyperadrenocorticism or hyperthyroidism.
- Bilaterally symmetrical truncal alopecia: hyperadrenocorticism
- Cervical palpation: thyroid mass or slip causing hyperthyroidism
- Thoracic auscultation: murmur, gallop with hyperthyroidism
- Rectal exam: apocrine carcinoma of the anal sac causing PU/PD through hypercalcemia or any cause of incontinence other than PU (urethral, trigone, prostatic abnormalities).
- Vaginal exam: purulent exudate if pyometra (pp. 1183 and 1184)
- Abdominal palpation
  - Kidneys: small (e.g., chronic kidney disease [CKD]), large (e.g., polycystic kidney disease, renal lymphoma, other renal neoplasia), painful (rarely) in pyelonephritis
  - Hepatomegaly: primary hepatopathies, hyperadrenocorticism, diabetes mellitus, iatrogenic (glucocorticoids, barbiturates), lymphoma
  - Splenomegaly: lymphoma (malignancy-associated hypercalcemia), hemangiosarcoma has been associated with PU in some dogs.
  - Uterine enlargement: pyometra

Etiology and Pathophysiology

Mechanisms of PU/PD in selected conditions:

- CKD: excessive urea and sodium presented to distal tubules causes osmotic diuresis
- Pyelonephritis: countercurrent concentrating mechanisms disrupted
- Hyperadrenocorticism: antidiuretic hormone (ADH) deficiency/inefficacy
- Liver failure: impaired urea synthesis (primary PU, secondary PD)
- Hypokalemia: interferes with renal tubular action of ADH
- Hypoadrenocorticism: hyponatremia depletes the renal medullary concentration gradient
- Diabetes mellitus: glucosuria creates an osmotic diuresis (primary PU, secondary PD)
- Diabetes insipidus (DI): ADH deficiency (central DI) or ineffective ADH action (nephrogenic DI); both cause primary PU with secondary PD
- Intoxication (ethylene glycol): osmotic diuresis initially then renal failure
- Psychogenic PD: secondary renal medullary washout: primary PD and secondary PU
- Hyperthyroidism: secondary decreased renal medullary concentration gradient (primary PU, secondary PD)
- Pyometra: *Escherichia coli* endotoxin interferes with ADH action on renal tubules (primary PU, secondary PD).
- Hypercalcemia: calcium in excess interferes with the action of ADH at renal tubular level (reversible acquired nephrogenic DI; primary PU, secondary PD).

DIAGNOSIS

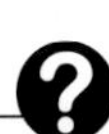

Diagnostic Overview

PU and/or PD typically are reported by owners; request that the owner of any pet with concerns regarding inappropriate urination bring a free-catch urine sample to the appointment. The sample (a teaspoon [5 mL] is more than adequate) should be placed in a clean, dry container. History, physical exam, and basic laboratory tests are usually sufficient to identify the cause of PU/PD (diagnostic approach outlined on p. 1442).

Differential Diagnosis

Benign causes of increased water intake (usually without associated PU):

- Diet (e.g., formulation [dry kibble versus moist/canned], salt content)
- High environmental temperatures
- Exercise, panting
- Diarrhea

Causes of apparent or false PU:

- Pollakiuria
- Stranguria
- Inappropriate elimination/incontinence
  - Hormone-responsive incontinence (p. 1011)
  - Other anatomic, neuromuscular, or physical concerns (p. 538)
  - Behavior issues (pp. 533 and 535)
- Urinary marking/spraying
- Dogs fed extremely low-protein diets

Initial Database

- Urinalysis: (first and most important)
  - Free-catch sample brought from home is ideal.
  - Concentrated urine (urine specific gravity [USG] > 1.025) without glucosuria *not* consistent with PU/PD
  - True PU: usually associated with USG < 1.012 (sometimes USG > 1.012 but < 1.022) or glucosuria
  - Isosthenuria (USG = 1.008-1.012) can be associated with almost any cause of PU/PD but is expected for CKD.
  - Marked PU (repeatable USG < 1.008) often associated with hyperadrenocorticism (dogs), hypercalcemia (dogs), hyperthyroidism (cats or dogs), DI (cats or dogs), or atypical leptospirosis (dogs). USG < 1.008 is not consistent with CKD.
  - Diabetes mellitus causes PU but relatively concentrated urine (USG often 1.025 or higher).
  - Calcium oxalate dihydrate crystals suggest post-acute ethylene glycol ingestion.
  - Ammonium biurate crystals are consistent with liver failure (e.g., shunt, cirrhosis).
- CBC
  - Anemia of chronic disease is associated with a few causes of PU/PD
  - Stress leukogram: nonspecific (e.g., hyperadrenocorticism, pyelonephritis)
  - Neutrophilia with evidence of inflammation (band forms, toxic changes in neutrophils): rule out pyometra; may not be present with pyelonephritis (counterintuitive)
  - Normal lymphocyte and eosinophil counts despite severe illness: rule out hypoadrenocorticism.
- Serum chemistry profile
  - Hyperglycemia: rule out diabetes mellitus (clinical signs, glucosuria, fructosamine).
  - Increased blood urea nitrogen (BUN), creatinine, and phosphorus with isosthenuria (USG = 1.008-1.012): most consistent with CKD; less commonly with prerenal azotemia due to hypoadrenocorticism or DI
  - Hypoalbuminemia, low BUN, hypocholesterolemia, hypoglycemia, hyperbilirubinemia (all or any combination): consider liver failure (many causes of PU, such as DI or hyperadrenocorticism, lead to decreases in BUN)
  - Hypercalcemia: rule out malignancy, primary hyperparathyroidism (both usually have concurrent low-normal to hypophosphatemia), vitamin D toxicosis, CKD (phosphorus usually normal or elevated), and other conditions. Idiopathic hypercalcemia (cats) is not usually associated with PU/PD.
  - Hyperkalemia with hyponatremia suggests hypoadrenocorticism.
- Urine culture and sensitivity (C&S) should be considered for any animal with PU/PD. Urinary tract infection may complicate any cause of PU/PD, may not be associated with additional overt clinical signs, often escapes diagnosis on urinalysis alone due to dilute urine, and is treatable. Urine for C&S should be obtained by cystocentesis.
- Serum thyroxine (cats > 6 years of age): rule in or out hyperthyroidism
- Blood pressure
  - Normal to decreased blood pressure: consistent with primary PU conditions
  - Normal to increased blood pressure: consistent with primary PD conditions
- Serum osmolality (Osm)
  - Normal to decreased serum osm: consistent with primary PD conditions
  - Normal to increased serum osm: consistent with primary PU conditions

Advanced or Confirmatory Testing

- Abdominal imaging (ultrasound especially useful): evaluate kidneys (CKD, pyelonephritis, neoplasia); urinary bladder (signs of cystitis, urolithiasis, or mass/neoplasm producing pollakiuria or stranguria rather than PU); GI tract (evidence of neoplastic infiltration); liver (chronic hepatopathy, portosystemic shunt, nonspecific enlargement, and hyperechogenicity [diabetes mellitus, hyperadrenocorticism, others]); adrenal glands (mass; subtle changes related to pituitary-dependent hyperadrenocorticism, although 40%-60% of dogs with pituitary-dependent hyperadrenocorticism have structurally normal shaped and sized adrenal glands on ultrasound exam); and uterus (pyometra)
- Other tests as dictated by suspected diagnosis (e.g., urine cortisol/creatinine ratio, leptospira serology, low-dose dexamethasone suppression test, ACTH stimulation test)
- Water deprivation test (never recommended; consult with internal medicine specialist before considering)
  - Rarely used to differentiate central DI, nephrogenic DI, and primary PD
  - Essential to first exclude other causes of PU or PD
  - Test is time consuming and labor intensive; can result in severe and potentially fatal dehydration, and results may not be reliable

TREATMENT

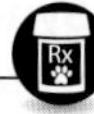

Treatment Overview

Successful treatment requires identification of cause. PU and PD are not diseases but clinical manifestations of primary underlying disorders, and nonspecific treatment such as withholding water may be dangerous and is never recommended.

Acute General Treatment

Withholding water can be dangerous or life-threatening in all cases of PU/PD for which the underlying disease produces primary PU with secondary PD (see Etiology and Pathophysiology above).

Possible Complications

- Dehydration, electrolyte disturbances
- Progression of the primary problem if not identified and addressed

Recommended Monitoring

Physical exam, including body weight; recheck USG and assess for glucosuria; further testing as indicated by underlying disease process and evolution of case

PROGNOSIS & OUTCOME

Depends on underlying cause and response to treatment

PEARLS & CONSIDERATIONS

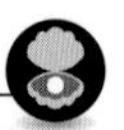

Comments

- Anytime an owner is concerned about any problem with urination, they should be instructed to collect about a teaspoon (5 mL) of urine to bring in at the time of exam. This allows easy separation of a pet with lower urinary tract disease (e.g., bladder stones, bacterial cystitis) from one with diabetes mellitus (glycosuria) or one with nondiabetic PU/PD.
- Isosthenuria (USG = 1.008-1.012) implies that the USG is the same as the specific gravity of plasma. Because dehydrated animals can have hyperosmolar plasma, USG up to 1.020 may still be consistent with isosthenuria in some cases.
- Dogs may drink excessively (or inadequate amounts) during hospitalization. Do not overinterpret in-hospital PD if the owner does not complain of PU.
- Dogs with weak but previously adequate urethral sphincter tone (usually spayed females) may develop urinary incontinence along with PU.

Technician Tips

- Urine brought in by owner should have specific gravity and dipstick evaluation before veterinarian sees pet.
- Do not underestimate how much water is consumed or how frequently polyuric dogs and cats need to urinate.
- Frequent walks are far better than forcing house-trained dogs to retain their urine or to urinate in their cage or run.

SUGGESTED READING

Shiel RE: Polydipsia and polyuria. In Ettinger SE, et al, editors: The textbook of veterinary internal medicine, ed 8, St. Louis, 2017, Elsevier, pp 181-184.

AUTHOR: Edward C. Feldman, DVM, DACVIM
EDITOR: Leah A. Cohn, DVM, PhD, DACVIM

Portosystemic Shunt

Client Education Sheet 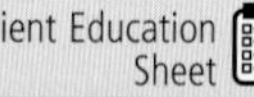

BASIC INFORMATION

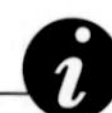

Definition

- Congenital portosystemic shunts (PSSs) are macroscopic malformations of portal venous anatomy that create communications of the portal venous return directly with the systemic venous blood flow, bypassing the liver. These malformations connect the portal vein or its branches to the caudal vena cava or, less commonly, the azygous vein or other systemic veins, allowing portal blood to bypass the liver. Congenital PSSs may be intrahepatic or extrahepatic; they are usually single (≈75%), but multiple (2-3) shunts can occur.
- Acquired PSSs (APSSs) are typically multiple, extrahepatic shunts that develop in response to portal hypertension (p. 174).

Synonyms

- Portosystemic vascular anomoly (PSVA), liver shunt
- APSS refers to a specific type of PSS.

Epidemiology

SPECIES, AGE, SEX

- Extrahepatic shunts (dogs and cats); intrahepatic shunts (mostly dogs)
- Congenital PSS
  - Large shunt fraction often results in clinical signs in animals < 3 years.
  - Less severe shunts can be identifed in older patients.
- APSS: often recognized in middle-aged to older animals

GENETICS, BREED PREDISPOSITION

- Extrahepatic PSS: any dog or cat
  - More common in small, purebred dogs: Yorkshire terrier, Maltese, Cairn terrier, Norfolk terrier, dachsund, pug, Havanese, miniature poodle, Dandie Dinmont terrier, Skye terrier, miniature schnauzer, Chihuahua, Scottish deerhound
  - Cat breeds: domestic shorthair, Persian, Siamese, Himalayan, and Burmese
  - Heritability partially defined in some dog breeds; often a complex trait with nonsimple inheritance
- Intrahepatic shunts: more common in larger-breed dogs
  - Irish wolfhound, Labrador retriever, golden retriver, Australian cattledog, Australian shepherd
  - Autosomal dominant mode with incomplete penetrance (Irish wolfhound)

ASSOCIATED DISORDERS

- Hepatic microvascular dysplasia (HMD) concurrent with PSS (p. 655)
- Hepatic encephalopathy (HE [p. 440])
- APSS: cirrhotic/fibrosing liver disease (p. 174)

Clinical Presentation

DISEASE FORMS, SUBTYPES

- Congenital versus acquired
- Extrahepatic versus intrahepatic

HISTORY, CHIEF COMPLAINT

Clinical signs are related to the degree of shunting present and hepatic insufficiency.

- Reduced body stature (i.e., runt dogs with congenital PSS); often slightly underweight (dogs or cats)
- Signs of HE, sometimes precipitated by feeding/protein rich meal
  - Behavioral changes
  - Blindness
  - Ataxia
  - Disorientation
  - Seizures
  - Dull/obtunded
- Lower urinary signs (e.g., stranguria, hematuria) related to urate uroliths; usually in older dogs
- Ptyalism (especially cats)
- Vague complaints of "not doing well," poor appetite, or occasional gastrointestinal signs
- APSS: signs of hepatic failure/portal hypertension (e.g., icterus, abdominal distention, vomiting/diarrhea)

PHYSICAL EXAM FINDINGS

Congenital PSS may be normal or

- Small stature (dog), underweight
- ± Abnormal mentation, vision, or neurologic findings (i.e., HE)
- Copper-colored irises common in cats
- Hepatic AV malformations can create an auscultable abdominal bruit.
- Cryptorchidism in male dogs and cats (one report of higher incidence)
- Findings may relate to urolithiasis (p. 1019)

APSS: findings typical of liver failure/cirrhosis (e.g., icterus, ascities, small or large liver, petechial or echymotic hemorrhage [p. 174]) or signs of HE

Etiology and Pathophysiology

- Congenital PSS is caused by developmental failure of the embryonic circulatory system of the liver and splanchnic veins.
    - *In utero*, the oxygen-rich blood from the placenta should bypass the liver and flow into circulation through the ductus venosus. A failure of the ductus venosus to close causes an intrahepatic shunt.
    - Extrahepatic shunts are usually a developmental abnormality of the vitelline veins. They should become the portal vein and its branches that deliver blood to the sinusoids. Failure of one or more to develop results in a persistent connection to the caudal vena cava or, less commonly, the azygous vein or another systemic vein.
    - Rarely, primary portal vein hypoplasia or atresia or hepatic arterioportal fistula occur.
- APSSs form as a result of portal hypertension due to cirrhotic liver disease (most common), noncirrhotic portal hypertension, congenital portal vein atresia, hepatic AV malformations, ductal plate malformations, portal vein thrombosis or stricture, or outflow obstruction through hepatic veins (Budd-Chiari syndrome, veno-occlusive syndrome).
- With PSS, venous blood from splanchnic organs bypasses the hepatic sinusoids and mixes with the systemic venous circulation before detoxification (ammonia, others); hepatocytes are also denied necessary substances.

DIAGNOSIS

Diagnostic Overview

- In a young animal with findings suggesting HE or a mature (non-Dalmation, non-bulldog) animal with urate cystoliths, the most useful initial test is measurment of total serum bile acids (TSBAs). The combination of (12-hour) fasted and (2-hour) postprandial serum samples represents a bile acid panel, which is preferred to a single TSBA measurement. Values of bile acids in younger patients that are > 200 mmol/L commonly represent congenital PSS (sensitivity ≈99% but false-positives occur).
- Most animals with APSS are older, and clinical signs of hepatic failure (p. 174) occur in addition to signs of HE.
- Imaging studies and/or surgical explorations are necessary to confirm the diagnosis of PSS, but such studies are often not important for APSS.

Differential Diagnosis

- HMD (for congenital PSS)
- Any hepatopathy resulting in hepatic failure (for APSS)
- HE must be differentiated from other neurologic disorders.

Initial Database

Congenital PSS:

- CBC: microcytosis, often with absent or minimal anemia, poikilocytosis in cats
- Serum biochemistry profile: liver enzymes (alanine aminotransferase [ALT], alkaline phosphatase [ALP], gamma-glutamyltransferase [GGT]) normal or increased (ALP normally higher in dogs < 6 months of age); low blood urea nitrogen (BUN), hypocholesterolemia, and hypoalbuminemia common; hypoglycemia sometimes recognized
- Urinalysis: specific gravity varies but often < 1.025 ± ammonium urate (biurate) crystals ± hematuria
- Bile acids: increase often in fasting and postprandial samples, but often a marked increase in postprandial sample compared with fasted sample. Sensitive but not specific for congenital PSS (p. 1312)
- Urine bile acid to creatinine (UBA/UCre) ratio: less sensitive for detecting PSS than total serum bile acids (p. 1312)
- Blood ammonia (fasting or ammonia tolerance testing): rarely performed due to difficulties of proper sample handling (p. 1305) but often increased with HE
- Coagulation profile: usually normal
- Fecal exam: all young dogs and cats to rule out parasites
- Abdominal radiographs: microhepatica and plump kidneys common; although urate calculi are radiolucent, can be radiopaque if complexed with magnesium and phosphate

APSS: results overlap with PSS except

- Hyperbilirubinemia suggests APSS.
- Coagulation times may be prolonged.
- Radiographs may show peritoneal effusion.

Advanced or Confirmatory Testing

Imaging: selection of techniques is often a balanced decision involving availability of the method, skills, and experience of operator, probability of obtaining actionable information, and potential costs.

- Abdominal ultrasound confirmation of a PSS relies on excellent equipment, fortuitous patient echogenic features, and advanced skills/experience of sonographer (estimated accuracy of 85% for congenital PSS).
    - Subjectively small liver; often nodular with APSS (regenerative nodules)
    - Intrahepatic PSS is generally easier to identify than extrahepatic PSS.
    - Turbulence of flow within the caudal vena cava has good correlation with an intrahepatic or extrahepatic PSS.
    - ± Increased portal blood flow velocity as a calculated value (technically difficult)
    - Measurements of vascular diameters are used to obtain ratios of the major vessels. Portal vein/aorta (PV/Ao) ratio that is < 0.65 is supportive for presence of extrahepatic PSS or noncirrhotic portal hypertension. If the PV/Ao and portal vein/caudal vena cava (PV/CVC) are > 0.75 and > 0.80, respectively, an extraphepatic shunt is much less likely.
    - Hepatofugal (reverse) portal blood flow has a high correlation with APSS but can be hard to confirm.
    - Ultrasound contrast bubble study uses agitated saline or saline diluted autologous anticoagulated blood that is shaken to produce microbubbles. This is then injected into the splenic parenchyma. If microbubbles are detected in right ventricle, a shunt is present because normal hepatic sinusoidal blood flow would trap microbubbles.
    - ± Uroliths
    - ± Ascites (APSS)
- CT with contrast angiography has become the imaging study of choice for noninvasive confirmation of PSS. It provides location and number of shunts and can demonstrate calculi or concurrent abnormalities.
- Contrast mesenteric venous portography or splenic portography was a standard method of demonstrating presence and location of PSS in past decades. Positive iodinated contrast is injected into a catheterized mesenteric or splenic vein or splenic pulp by surgery or as an ultrasound-guided injection. If the most caudal point of shunt is cranial to T13, it is likely intrahepatic.
- MRI with contrast angiography creates diagnostic images but requires more time under anesthesia and is more expensive; CT is preferred in most cases.
- Nuclear medicine/portal scintigraphy: technetium pertechnetate isotope delivery to the liver compared with delivery to the heart imaged after adminstration per rectum (less detail but even very caudal abdominal shunts are found) or ultrasound-guided splenic injection (better detail). Answers broad question of whether a shunt is present but does not give anatomic detail.

Laboratory testing:

- Protein C levels are commonly < 70% of normal for PSS, whereas dogs with HMD usually have levels > 70%. Protein C does not distinguish between PSS and other hepatobiliary diseases and liver failure. When PSS is corrected, protein C levels return to normal.

Liver biopsy:

- Biopsy is recommended to determine specific hepatic disease in APSS and during surgical correction of congenital PSS. For congenital PSS, biopsy can assess the degree of hypoperfusion or presence of other hepatopathies. Findings that reflect portal venous hypoperfusion are nonspecific.

TREATMENT

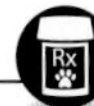

Treatment Overview

Address HE with medical management. For congenital PSS, surgical correction of the shunt(s) is the treatment of choice. Treatment of APSS includes treatment of the underlying hepatopathy, and continued medical management of HE and complications of liver disease (e.g., gastric ulcers, vomiting).

Acute General Treatment

- If present, address HE immediately (p. 440): lactulose PO or by enema, antibiotics, other treatment

- Address severe hypoglycemia, if present (p. 552).
- If seizures continue despite previously described medical treatment, use anticonvulsant therapy (p. 903).
- If present, address urinary obstruction (p. 1009) or infection (p. 232) secondary to urolithiasis.
- If suspected, address gastrointestinal ulcers (p. 380).

Chronic Treatment

Congenital PSS:

- Best option is usually surgical correction to reduce shunting blood flow; surgery is more difficult for intrahepatic than extrahepatic shunts. Referral to a veterinary surgeon is strongly reccomended.
  - Goal is to achieve normal life expectancy and wellness without need for dietary or medical interventions.
  - Medical stabalization usually is indicated for a period of weeks to months before surgery.
  - Ameroid occluder: slow occlusion over several days to weeks; may not always completely close or may close too quickly
  - Cellophane banding: partial immediate ligation followed by slow occlusive perivenular fibrosis with thrombosis occurring over period of weeks
  - Direct ligation (silk ligature): attenuated shunted flow; best to measure portal venous pressure before and after attenuation (largely replaced by other techniques)
  - Intrahepatic PSS: coil placements by interventional radiology (IR) technique (percutaneous transvenous coil embolization) is used to create occlusive clot; multiple attempts may be needed.
- If surgery is not an option (e.g., costs, referral distance), medical treatment can be sustained. Some animals do well for many years with medical management alone.

APSS:

- Surgery is contraindicated for APSS (exception: resectable arterioportal malformation)
- Medical management of HE and complications: as for congenital PSS
- Address underlying hepatopathy or cirrhosis (pp. 174, 452, and 458).

Drug Interactions

Caution when using drugs that require hepatic metabolism and for sedative or analgesic medications

Possible Complications

Varies (life-threatening to minor): postoperative complications can occur hours to weeks after surgery and include seizures, failure to adequately occlude shunt, portal venous hypertension, failure of liver portal vasculature to handle redirected blood flow, hypothermia, hypoglycemia, ascites, and infection.

Recommended Monitoring

- Monitor closely for seizures or evidence of portal hypertension in the postoperative period. Over the next weeks to months after shunt ligation, watch for resolution of clinical signs, recheck serum biochemical profiles, reassess TSBA (may not normalize if HMD present or shunt ligation incomplete), reassess protein C (reversion to normal), resolution of ammonium urate crystalluria. Often, dietary restrictions and medications can be withdrawn.
- Monitoring patients with APSS as for cirrhosis and HE or for specific cause of hepatopathy.

PROGNOSIS & OUTCOME

Congenital PSS:

- Although serious complications are possible around the time of surgical correction (more so for intrahepatic shunt), surgery can offer an excellent long-term prognosis.
- Partial PSS ligation can have good results based on degree of attenuation of shunted blood flow. Patients with incomplete shunt correction (or concurrent HMD) often benefit from chronic dietary and medical management.
- Progressive occlusion of shunt flow can occur over many months after surgery (depending on techinique used).
- Extent of closure for ameroid occluders and cellophane banding is not specifically known but can be reflected in bile acid test results and protein C level. May also require repeat advanced imaging
- Dogs diagnosed late in life (>5 years) and without signs of HE can have excellent surgical outcomes, but survival may be similar with surgical versus medical management.

APSS due to underlying hepatopathy:

- Depends on specific diagnosis, severity, and potential for medical intervention, but often poor if associated with cirrhosis

PEARLS & CONSIDERATIONS

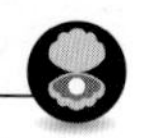

Comments

- Consider PSS as a differential diagnosis for young dogs and cats having intermittent central neurologic problems; periods of suspected blindness; unexplained ptyalism; poor growth; prolonged effects of anesthesia, sedatives, or drugs metabolized by the liver; vague gastrointestinal upsets or poor appetite; failure to train or behavior swings (including aggression); and in any non-Dalmation, non-bulldog patient with ammonium urate crystalluria or urolithiasis.
- Perioperative mortality rate with surgery for intrahepatic shunts is higher than that with extrahepatic PSS. IR-assisted placement of intravascular coils shows promise for intrahepatic and extrahepatic shunt correction, but it requires specific expertise and is not foolproof.

Prevention

Do not breed affected dogs.

Technician Tips

- Patients should be fasted for 12 hours before bile acid testing or abdominal imaging studies.

SUGGESTED READING

Greenhalgh SN, et al: Long-term survival and quality of life in dogs with clinical signs associated with a congenital portosystemic shunt after surgical or medical treatment. J Am Vet Med Assoc 245:527-533, 2014.

AUTHOR: Mark E. Hitt, DVM, MS, DACVIM
EDITOR: Keith P. Richter, DVM, MSEL, DACVIM

Pregnancy

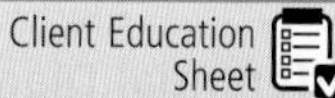

BASIC INFORMATION

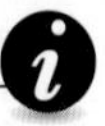

Definition

- The period of gestational development in the uterus, beginning at conception and continuing through parturition
- Bitch: gestational length is 65 days from the luteinizing hormone (LH) surge or 63 days from ovulation (54-60 days from the first day of diestrus and 57-72 days from breeding).
- Queen: gestational length is 64 days from the LH surge. Cats are induced ovulators, and the LH surge corresponds to 24 hours after the first breeding date.

Epidemiology

SPECIES, AGE, SEX

Canine and feline: postpubertal intact female (usually > 6 months old)

GENETICS, BREED PREDISPOSITION

Fertility (pregnancy rate) and fecundity (litter size) are heritable traits. Mixed breeds and outcross matings generally result in higher pregnancy rates and larger litter sizes. Litter size also depends on maternal size; smaller breeds have fewer offspring/litter.

RISK FACTORS

Intact females exposed to intact males

GEOGRAPHY AND SEASONALITY

- Canine: most domestic breeds cycle twice yearly irrespective of season, with the potential to become pregnant during each estrous cycle. Wolf hybrids cycle annually during the spring (long-day breeders), and basenjis and Tibetan mastiffs cycle annually during autumn (short-day breeders).
- Feline: cats are polyestrous, long-day breeders (queening during spring and summer) with seasonal anestrus during the winter months. It is possible for a queen to have multiple litters each year. Indoor housing with extended hours of artificial lighting may eliminate the anestrus period.

ASSOCIATED DISORDERS

- Insulin resistance (pregnancy-associated diabetes)
- Pregnancy anemia
- Pyometra (p. 854)
- Hydrops (amnion, allantois, or fetal anasarca)
- Overt false pregnancy/pseudocyesis (p. 831)
- Abortion (p. 2) or early embryonic loss
- Mammary hyperplasia (cats)

Clinical Presentation

HISTORY, CHIEF COMPLAINT

- Intentional breeding
- Unintentional breeding
- Unexplained weight gain
- Unexplained mammary development and lactation
- Nesting behavior

PHYSICAL EXAM FINDINGS

- Embryonic vesicles or fetuses palpable abdominally
  - Embryonic vesicles are palpable approximately 25-35 days after the LH surge.
  - Fetuses are palpable approximately 45 days after the LH surge.
- Mammary development and lactation usually emerge in the last 2 weeks of pregnancy.

Etiology and Pathophysiology

- Ovulation occurs 48 hours post LH surge in dogs and 48 hours after breeding in cats.
  - Bitches are most fertile 2-4 days after ovulation (4-6 days post LH surge); however, pregnancy can result from breedings preceding ovulation by as much as 7 days if the sperm survive in the uterine tubes until the ova mature.
- Fertilization occurs in the uterine tube (ampulla-isthmus junction), and the embryos enter the uterus approximately 10-11 days post LH surge in the bitch (5-6 days post LH surge in the queen).
- Embryos migrate within the uterus and may implant in the horn ipsilateral or contralateral to ovulation.
- Implantation occurs 15-17 days post LH surge in the bitch (14-15 days post LH surge in the queen).
- Pregnancy is progesterone dependent throughout gestation. Corpora luteal production of progesterone is required for pregnancy maintenance. Prolactin is luteotropic and maintains the corpus luteum during the second half of pregnancy in dogs and cats.

DIAGNOSIS

Diagnostic Overview

Transabdominal ultrasound (>20 days post LH surge) is the most informative method to confirm pregnancy, but it also requires the greatest experience. All methods of diagnosis may result in misdiagnosis if performed too early in gestation and warrant repeat evaluation 1-2 weeks later if a definitive diagnosis cannot be made.

Differential Diagnosis

- Pyometra
- Mucometra
- Overt false pregnancy/pseudocyesis
- Ectopic pregnancy

Initial Database

- Transabdominal ultrasound: embryonic vesicles can be detected as early as 20 days post LH surge (16 days post LH surge in cats). The embryo can be detected after 25 days post LH surge.
  - False-positives (diagnosis of pregnancy in a nonpregnant animal) may result from misinterpretation of early pyometra or mucometra or misidentifying fluid-filled loops of bowel.
  - False-negatives (diagnosis of no pregnancy in a pregnant animal) may occur in early pregnancy if the ultrasonographer is inexperienced or the embryonic vesicle is too small to visualize or obscured by viscera.
  - Fetal viability can be readily assessed by evaluating fetal heart rates after 25 days post LH surge.
  - Gestational age can be estimated by fetal measurements and presence of fetal structures.
  - Litter size can only be approximated. Accurate counts are especially difficult in late gestation or with large litters.
- Serum relaxin: relaxin is a hormone produced by the placenta and is a confirmatory test of pregnancy 30 days post LH surge. A commercially available test is labeled for dogs and has been validated for use in cats.
  - False-positives may result when relaxin levels remain elevated after fetal death (up to 2 days) or in cases of large ovarian cysts (queens).
  - False-negatives can occur in early pregnancy or in singleton litters that do not generate sufficiently elevated relaxin for detection.
  - Litter size and fetal viability do not correlate with relaxin concentrations.
- Abdominal radiographs: pregnancy can be diagnosed by visualization of ossified fetal skeletons after 45 days post LH surge.
  - False-negatives may occur with small litters if a full colon obscures fetuses.
  - False-negatives may occur before 45 days post LH surge.
  - Fetal loss of viability can be evaluated by fetal posture (appearance of disarticulation), bone juxtaposition (especially skull), and presence of intrafetal gas.
  - Estimation of whelping date based on fetal structures (tooth buds and digits) is unreliable.
  - Litter size is most reliably estimated by late-term radiographs during the last week of gestation.

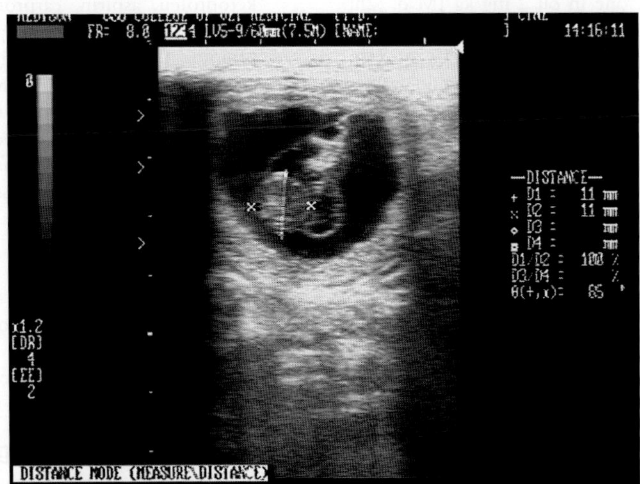

PREGNANCY Transabdominal ultrasonogram from a pregnant bitch demonstrates a gestational sac containing a fetus. The body diameter measurement made between the cursors indicates that gestational age of this fetus is 34 days past the luteinizing hormone surge (31 days before whelping). (Courtesy Dr. Michelle A. Kutzler.)

Advanced or Confirmatory Testing

- Serum progesterone levels can be monitored to ascertain if endogenous levels are high enough to maintain pregnancy (>2 ng/mL).
  - May be assessed for bitches diagnosed nonpregnant to rule out luteal insufficiency as the cause (pp. 539 and 1375)
  - May be run for bitches with high-risk pregnancy to monitor progesterone supplementation therapy
- Uterine monitoring (www.WhelpWise.com) may be required for high-risk pregnancies.

TREATMENT

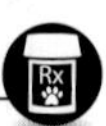

Treatment Overview

- Intentional, normal pregnancies require no treatment.
- Unintentional, unwanted pregnancies may be terminated (p. 819).
- High-risk, threatened pregnancies require advanced and continuous monitoring. Many therapeutic options are inferred from human medicine, have no proven efficacy, and may be detrimental to the welfare of the dam or the fetuses.

Acute General Treatment

- To halt premature uterine contractions: terbutaline 0.01-0.03 mg/kg PO or SQ q 8h, titrated to effect based on uterine monitoring
  - If ongoing terbutaline treatment is required, it should be discontinued 24 hours before the due date.
  - Safety and efficacy in dogs have not been properly researched. Efficacy of oral treatment is disputed in human literature.
  - Tachycardia is a common and potentially life-threatening side effect of terbutaline. The effect on fetuses is uncertain.

Chronic Treatment

- For maintenance of pregnancy when endogenous progesterone levels prematurely fall below 2 ng/mL
  - Progesterone in oil 2 mg/kg IM q 72h; discontinue 3 days before due date.
  - Altrenogest 0.088 mg/kg PO q 24h; discontinue 24 hours before due date.
- Serum progesterone levels can be used for monitoring endogenous progesterone if altrenogest is used but not if progesterone in oil is used. Altrenogest is a synthetic progestogen that is not reliably measured with standard progesterone assays.

Nutrition/Diet

- No supplemental nutrition is required during pregnancy if the bitch or queen is receiving high-quality feed. Supplementing calcium during pregnancy may be detrimental to whelping or result in postpartum complications (p. 281).
- Caloric intake should be increased 1.5- to 3-fold after whelping/queening to sustain the dam's energy requirements during lactation.

Behavior/Exercise

No alteration of normal physical activity is required during pregnancy. Active and athletic dogs may continue normal activity throughout gestation. Obese dogs may be encouraged to increase exercise during pregnancy to improve muscle tone and reduce fat stores (decreasing feed is not recommended for weight loss during pregnancy).

Drug Interactions

- Certain drugs may be detrimental to the developing fetuses and should be avoided unless benefit to the health of the dam outweighs the risk to the fetus. Consult package inserts for all drugs before use. Selected examples:
  - Antifungals (e.g., ketoconazole, griseofulvin) are teratogenic.
  - Antibiotics: penicillins and cephalosporins are the antibiotics of choice in pregnant animals.
    - Fluoroquinolones (e.g., enrofloxacin) inhibit cartilage formation.
    - Tetracyclines inhibit dental enamel production.
    - Chloramphenicol suppresses bone marrow.
    - Aminoglycosides may be neurotoxic (gentamicin appears to be safe but should be used with caution and owner consent).
  - Chemotherapeutics are teratogenic or abortifacient.
  - Cimetidine may decrease androgen production, resulting in increased risk of cryptorchidism.
  - Glucocorticoids may cause anasarca or induce abortion (prednisone is recommended if treatment it unavoidable as it is less likely to cross the placenta).
  - Hormone supplementation (e.g., altrenogest, diethylstilbestrol, estradiol benzoate, testosterone) may affect sexual development.
  - Nonsteroidal antiinflammatories (e.g., ketoprofen, aspirin, carprofen): teratogenesis
  - Opioids (e.g., buprenorphine) are the analgesics of choice during pregnancy and lactation. However, chronic use has been associated with adverse fetal effects; overdosage may result in the dam's inattention to neonates and accidental smothering.

Possible Complications

- Dystocia (p. 278)
- Abortion (p. 2)
- Early embryonic loss (fetal resorption)
- Mastitis
- Insulin resistance (pregnancy-associated diabetes)

Recommended Monitoring

- In high-risk, threatened pregnancies, serum progesterone levels should be monitored every other day or as needed to confirm that levels are > 2 ng/mL.
- Uterine monitoring (www.WhelpWise.com) may be required for high-risk pregnancies in bitches with a history of premature labor or uterine inertia.

PROGNOSIS & OUTCOME

Parturition usually occurs without complications.

PEARLS & CONSIDERATIONS

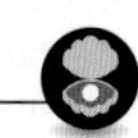

Comments

- Superfecundation: a bitch bred to multiple males can have pups in the same litter that are from different sires. Paternity can be determined for registration by DNA testing.
- Elevated serum progesterone levels do not indicate pregnancy. Progesterone concentrations remain elevated throughout diestrus whether pregnancy is established or not. Progesterone concentrations remain elevated for ≥ 65 days post LH surge in the nonpregnant bitch and for 40 days post LH surge in the nonpregnant queen.

Prevention

Preventing unwanted pregnancies: surgical neuter of nonbreeding animals and proper supervision of intact animals

Technician Tips

Pregnant dogs and cats brought to the veterinary clinic for pregnancy diagnosis are generally healthy. Because other patients visiting the veterinary clinic may have contagious diseases detrimental to pregnancy (e.g., herpesvirus, parvovirus, *Leptospira* spp infections), it is recommended that bitches or queens presenting for pregnancy diagnosis be escorted out of the public waiting room as soon as possible to await evaluation in a clean and disinfected exam room.

Client Education

- More than 4 million unwanted dogs and cats are euthanized annually in humane societies.
- Breeding is recommended to improve the breed standard and is not encouraged to witness the miracle of birth.
- Designer breeds that are early-generation crosses of purebred dogs (e.g., the product of a mating between a poodle and a golden retriever) do not breed true to their own phenotype and should not be purchased as breeding animals.

SUGGESTED READING

Concannon PW, et al: Recent advances in small animal reproduction. International Veterinary Information Service (IVIS) (website), 2001. http://www.ivis.org/advances/Concannon/wanke/chapter_frm.asp/.

AUTHOR: Richard Wheeler, DVM, DACT
EDITOR: Michelle A. Kutzler, DVM, PhD, DACT

Diseases and Disorders

Pregnancy Termination

Bonus Material Online 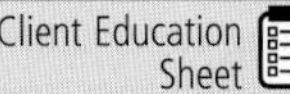 Client Education Sheet 

BASIC INFORMATION

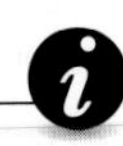

Definition

Elective nonsurgical abortion of a litter before 55 days' gestation, with gestation based on days from the luteinizing hormone (LH) surge (term = 65 ± 1 days)

Synonyms

Abortion (elective), mismating/misalliance options

Epidemiology

SPECIES, AGE, SEX

Postpubertal intact bitches and queens

RISK FACTORS

Intact cycling females

ASSOCIATED DISORDERS

Depending on the method of pregnancy termination and on timing, pyometra, pseudocyesis, or delivery of premature viable offspring may occur.

Clinical Presentation

DISEASE FORMS/SUBTYPES

Stages when pregnancy termination may be performed:

- Before pregnancy diagnosis (<20 days past the onset of the LH surge)
- Before fetal ossification (20-44 days past the onset of the LH surge)
- After fetal ossification (>44 days past the onset of the LH surge)

HISTORY, CHIEF COMPLAINT

Female bred to an unintended male and/or at an unintended time

PHYSICAL EXAM FINDINGS

- Typically healthy female
- Abdominal palpation of focal, discrete uterine enlargements during the fourth week of gestation. Accuracy depends on the expertise of the examiner and the stage of pregnancy.

Etiology and Pathophysiology

- Ovarian progesterone production from the corpora lutea (CLs) is required for the entire duration of a canine or feline pregnancy.
- Pregnancy in the bitch and queen can be terminated by administration of drugs that prematurely lyse CLs.

DIAGNOSIS

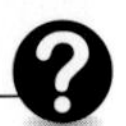

Diagnostic Overview

Pregnancy diagnosis (p. 816)

Differential Diagnosis

For pregnancy:

- Pseudopregnancy
- Pyometra
- Mucometra/hydrometra

Initial Database

The diagnosis of pregnancy can be made with abdominal ultrasound, serum relaxin assay, or abdominal radiographs. Advantages, drawbacks, and expected results of each are discussed on p. 816.

TREATMENT

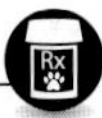

Treatment Overview

- Reduce serum progesterone concentrations to < 2 ng/mL by lysis of the CLs (luteolysis) for a period of >48 hours.
- Perform a complete evacuation of the uterus.
- The owner and clinician should discuss the advantages and drawbacks of medical versus surgical (ovariohysterectomy) pregnancy termination to develop an appropriate treatment plan.

Acute General Treatment

Depending on the protocol, luteolysis can be induced before or after a pregnancy diagnosis has been made.

- Prostaglandin F_{2alpha} (PGF_{2a}) therapy can be initiated as soon as day 5 of diestrus, as determined by vaginal cytologic exam, and as late as day 45.
  - Canine: dinoprost 0.1-0.25 mg/kg SQ q 8-12h to effect, usually 3-9 days of therapy is needed, or cloprostenol 1-2.5 mcg/kg q 24-48h for 4-5 injections is needed.
  - Feline: dinoprost 0.25-0.5 mg/kg SQ q 8-12h to effect; usually 3-9 days of therapy is needed.
- Combination (preferred method) of PGF_{2a} with a prolactin inhibitor (may cause severe vomiting in cats)
  - PGF_{2a} SQ q 8h (dosage as listed above); PGF_{2a} may be needed for an additional 1-2 days after the last treatment with a prolactin inhibitor for complete uterine evacuation.
  - Prolactin inhibitor: bromocriptine 10 mcg/kg (0.01 mg/kg) or cabergoline 5 mcg/kg (0.005 mg/kg) PO q 8h. Usually, 3-4 days of therapy are needed. Protocols using prolactin inhibitors are initiated during the middle third of pregnancy (20-44 days from the onset of the LH surge), when the clinician is able to verify the diagnosis of pregnancy by palpation or ultrasonography.
- Prolactin inhibitor in queens: cabergoline 25-50 mcg/CAT PO q 24h for 3-5 days
- Dexamethasone (in bitches) 0.1-0.2 mg/kg PO q 8-12h at decreasing dose for 5-10 days or 5 mg IM q 12h for 10 days (large dog). Fetal death occurs 5-13 days after treatment, and fetal expulsion starts at 7-15 days. Treatment efficacy is highest when treated up to 10 days after day 35 of gestation. Treatment failure has been reported in bitches treated between 30 and 35 days' gestation. Concurrent treatment with PGF_{2a} does not improve efficacy.
- Aglepristone (in bitches and queens) 10 mg/kg SQ, two doses 24 hours apart. Aglepristone is a progesterone receptor antagonist and has few side effects. It is not manufactured in the United States. It may be administered during mid-pregnancy and has been successful in terminating pregnancies between 23-42 days after breeding. Side effects include localized swelling at the injection site.

Chronic Treatment

If pregnancy termination does not occur after an initial treatment, and pregnancy termination is still desired, the protocol should be continued or a different treatment regimen should be used.

Behavior/Exercise

Depending on the pregnancy termination method used, pseudocyesis (inappropriate lactation) may develop. If this occurs, dams should not be allowed to lick the mammary glands because it may stimulate further lactation.

Possible Complications

- Side effects secondary to pregnancy termination include anorexia, vaginal discharge, discomfort, depression, and shortened interestrous interval at the first estrus after treatment.
- Side effects of PGF_{2a} (occur 30-40 minutes after injection; decrease with subsequent injections) include salivation, panting, vomiting, defecation/diarrhea, and vocalization in queens.

Recommended Monitoring

Ultrasonography and serum progesterone concentrations to verify completion of abortion and uterine evacuation

PROGNOSIS & OUTCOME

Good prognosis for future fertility

PEARLS & CONSIDERATIONS

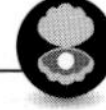

Comments

- Because >50% of bitches are not pregnant after a misalliance situation, waiting until the pregnancy is positively diagnosed to begin a protocol to terminate a pregnancy is recommended.
- Administration of estrogen during estrus has been reported to be effective, but it is not considered standard of care for pregnancy termination.
- The combination protocols using PGF_{2a} and prolactin inhibitors achieve success more

quickly and with fewer side effects than using either individually.
- If pregnancy termination protocols are initiated after 50 days' gestation, birth of viable puppies or kittens may occur and is not recommended.
- Gonadotropin-releasing hormone (GnRH) agonists, GnRH antagonists, GnRH vaccines, as well as progesterone antagonists are effective treatments for misalliance in dogs. Currently these products are not available in the United States.

Prevention

- Effective physical control of cycling bitch or queen during estrus
- Ovariectomy or ovariohysterectomy prevents the problem of unwanted pregnancy permanently.

Technician Tips

- Side effects of pregnancy termination include anorexia, vaginal discharge, discomfort, depression, and lactation.
- Side effects of PGF_{2a} (occur 30-40 minutes after injection; decrease with subsequent injections) include salivation, panting, vomiting, defecation/diarrhea, and vocalization in queens.

Client Education

- In the bitch or queen not intended for breeding, ovariectomy or ovariohysterectomy should be performed as early in gestation as possible.
- Shortening the luteal phase shortens the interestrous interval. Clients should be advised to expect the next cycle to occur sooner than normally expected.

SUGGESTED READING

Eilts BE: Pregnancy termination in the bitch and queen. Clin Tech Small Anim Pract 17:116-123, 2002.

AUTHOR: Julie T. Cecere, DVM, MS, DACT
EDITOR: Michelle A. Kutzler, DVM, PhD, DACT

Preputial Discharge

BASIC INFORMATION

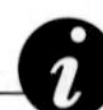

Definition

Characterized by the presence of normal or abnormal secretions from the penile sheath (prepuce).

Synonym

Penile discharge

Epidemiology

SPECIES, AGE, SEX

- Canine, male
- Juvenile or adult

GENETICS, BREED PREDISPOSITION

Intact males and brachycephalic breeds tend to have more normal preputial discharge than other dogs.

RISK FACTORS

- Anatomic abnormalities (acquired or congenital)
- Hormonal imbalances (acquired or iatrogenic)
- Poor hygiene/kennel management
- Canine herpesvirus type 1 or *Brucella canis* infection
- Prostatic disease
- Hemostatic disorder (acquired vs. genetic)
- Foreign body (e.g., grass awn)

CONTAGION AND ZOONOSIS

Preputial discharge may be contagious if caused by canine herpesvirus type 1 or *B. canis* (zoonotic).

GEOGRAPHY AND SEASONALITY

No geographic or seasonal trends have been established.

ASSOCIATED DISORDERS

- Balanitis (inflammation of the penis)
- Balanoposthitis (inflammation of the penis and prepuce)
- Urinary tract infection (UTI)
- Prostatic disease

Clinical Presentation

DISEASE FORMS/SUBTYPES

Juvenile onset versus adult onset

HISTORY, CHIEF COMPLAINT

- Preputial or penile discharge
- Excessive licking of prepuce
- ± Preputial discomfort/pain
- ± Visible lesions or abnormalities of the penis/prepuce
- ± Urinary incontinence/distress (e.g., stranguria, hematuria, pollakiuria)
- ± Constipation, ribbon-like stool, tenesmus

PHYSICAL EXAM FINDINGS

Depends on cause
- Discharge (smegma, mucoid, purulent, or hemorrhagic)
- Preputial anatomic abnormalities
- Preputial or penile lesions
- Pain during manipulation
- Atrophy of preputial opening
- Preputial mucosal vesicles (canine herpesvirus)
- Enlarged preputial/inguinal lymph nodes
- Prostatomegaly
- Masses (transmissible venereal tumor [TVT])
- Systemic signs (e.g., lethargy, fever)
- Petechiation or bruising (hemostatic defect)

Etiology and Pathophysiology

- Normal preputial discharge
  - Small amount of yellow-white smegma
- Abnormal preputial discharge
  - Clear/mucoid (can be copious): hormone imbalance in prepubertal dogs
  - Hemorrhagic: coagulopathy, trauma, neoplasia, prostatic or testicular disease
  - Purulent: infection, foreign body

DIAGNOSIS

Diagnostic Overview

The age of the animal helps differentiate juvenile-onset from adult-onset forms of preputial discharge. In younger dogs, the forms are generally benign and involve hormonal imbalances rather than infectious processes. Adult-onset forms are generally chronic and require a thorough diagnostic workup.

Differential Diagnosis

- Clear/mucoid discharge
  - Persistent penile frenulum
  - Hypospadias
  - Traumatic penile adhesions
  - Phimosis
  - Infectious (canine herpesvirus, calicivirus, abnormal microbiologic flora)
  - Neoplasia
  - Hormonal imbalance (e.g., puberty, exogenous steroids)

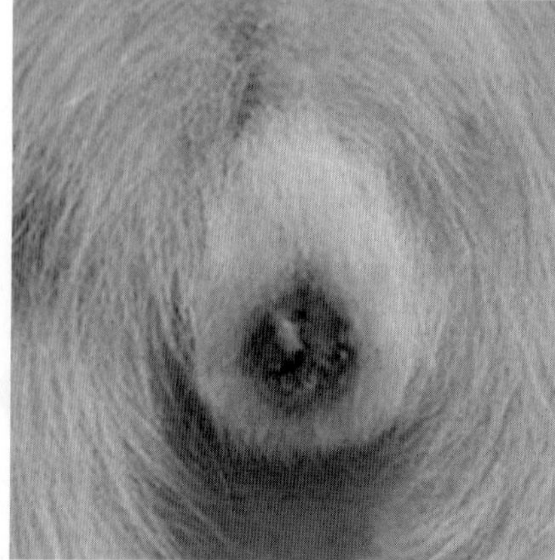

PREPUTIAL DISCHARGE Normal preputial discharge in a prepubertal male dog.

- UTI or incontinence
- Poor hygiene
- Hemorrhagic discharge
  - Trauma (penile or preputial)
  - Foreign body
  - Infectious (canine herpesvirus, *B. canis*, abnormal microbiologic flora)
  - Balanoposthitis or prostatitis (p. 827)
  - Benign prostatic hyperplasia (BPH [p. 824])
  - Neoplasia
  - Hormonal imbalance (exogenous steroids, endogenous estrogens)
  - UTI or urolith
  - Coagulopathy
  - Poor hygiene
- Purulent discharge
  - Persistent penile frenulum
  - Hypospadias
  - Trauma
  - Foreign body
  - Phimosis
  - Infectious *(B. canis)*
  - Balanoposthitis, prostatitis (p. 827), orchitis, epididymitis
  - Neoplasia
  - UTI or urolith
  - Poor hygiene

Initial Database

- General health exam
  - CBC, serum chemistry panel
  - Urinalysis and urine culture (p. 232)
  - *B. canis* screening
  - If hemorrhagic discharge, coagulation profile and platelet count
- Complete reproductive exam
  - Retraction of the prepuce caudal to the bulbus glandis (sedation or general anesthesia may be required)
  - Rectal exam to evaluate prostate
- Preputial/penile culture and cytology (p. 1071)
  - Culture (preputial swab, prostatic wash)
    - Heavy growth of a single bacterium in combination with clinical signs suggests infection.
    - Antibiotics are not indicated if a mixed flora is cultured.
    - Normal flora may include *Escherichia coli, Pseudomonas* spp, *Streptococcus* spp, *Pasturella* spp, *Staphylococcus* spp, *Klebsiella* spp, *Mycoplasma* spp, *Ureaplasma* spp.
  - Cytology (preputial swab, prostatic wash)
    - Cornification may indicate hyperestrogenism

Advanced or Confirmatory Testing

- Advanced imaging
  - Ultrasound of the prostate, bladder, urethra
  - Radiographs (e.g., os penis, bladder)
- Endoscopic exam of prepuce (foreign body, mass, etc.)
- Biopsy and/or cytologic exam of preputial masses

TREATMENT

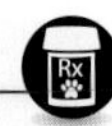

Treatment Overview

Treatment depends on the cause and can vary from improving hygiene to surgery or systemic antibiotics.

Acute General Treatment

- Varies, depending on origin or causative agent
- Excessive discharge should be flushed with warm saline (98°F/38°C), dilute (weak tea-colored) povidone-iodine solution, or a 0.05% chlorhexidine diacetate.
- Surgical correction may be necessary for anatomic defects or removal of masses.
- Benign neglect is reasonable for hormonal imbalances
- Removal of foreign body
- Discourage licking
- Antibiotics based on culture and sensitivity (e.g., prostatitis, cystitis)

Chronic Treatment

- Probiotics are recommended if patient is treated with long-term antibiotics.
- Treat benign prostatic hyperplasia (neuter, antiandrogens or gonadotropin agonists).
- For recurrent infection, investigate primary source of infection (e.g., prostatic, urinary tract).
- Chronic cases refractory to basic treatment may be referred to a theriogenologist, especially if the future reproductive potential is a concern.

Behavior/Exercise

Owners should prevent the dog from excessive licking of the prepuce and/or penis.

Possible Complications

- Recurrent and/or chronic infections (e.g., UTI, prostatitis)
- Canine herpesvirus and *B. canis* are associated with infertility and are transmissible to other dogs.

Recommended Monitoring

Varies with cause; if discharge worsens, additional diagnostic testing may be warranted.

PROGNOSIS & OUTCOME

- Good for juvenile animals
- Fair to guarded for adults; depends on cause of secretions

PEARLS & CONSIDERATIONS

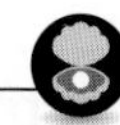

Comments

- A small amount of yellow-white discharge is normal in male dogs of any age and/or neuter status.
- Juvenile cases may be more of an annoyance than a real disease, except in cases of anatomic defects or with systemic illness (e.g., infection, coagulopathy)
  - Generally resolve spontaneously without treatment.
- In older animals, preputial discharge is often secondary to an underlying disease.

Prevention

- In prepubertal (juvenile) dogs, hormonal imbalances are impossible to prevent.
- Avoid exposure to dogs infected or potentially infected with canine herpesvirus and *B. canis*.

Technician Tips

- Preputial discharge can be normal and of no clinical significance in most dogs, *except* if abundant or associated with other clinical signs.
- Analgesia should be considered at the time of exam and during treatment if the dog appears to be painful.
- Dogs used for breeding may need to be cleaned with physiologic saline before semen sample collection to minimize discharge contamination of the ejaculate.

Client Education

- The benign nature of most discharge should be discussed with the client. Do not begin antimicrobial therapy without culture of bacterial pathogens.
- Clients should call their veterinarian if the discharge seems excessive or is associated with extensive licking or apparent pain.

SUGGESTED READING

Foster RA: Common lesions in the male reproductive tract of cats and dogs. Vet Clin North Am Small Anim Pract 42(3):527-545, 2012.

AUTHOR: Eleas M. Wu, DVM, DACT
EDITOR: Michelle A. Kutzler, DVM, PhD, DACT

Prolonged Estrus

Bonus Material Online   Client Education Sheet

BASIC INFORMATION

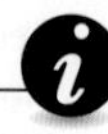

Definition

- In the dog, combined proestrus and estrus of > 6 weeks or a cytologic estrus that lasts for > 21 days
- In the queen, estrus lasting longer than 10 days is considered prolonged.
- Ovarian remnant syndrome (ORS) refers to clinical signs indicating functional ovarian tissue in a previously ovariohysterectomized bitch or queen and is discussed in detail on p. 732.

Synonyms

Persistent estrus (heat), nymphomania

Epidemiology

SPECIES, AGE, SEX

Female dogs and cats > 4 months of age

GENETICS, BREED PREDISPOSITION

Asian cat breeds (e.g., Siamese) are predisposed to overlapping follicular waves that can present as prolonged or persistent estrus.

RISK FACTORS

Young and very old bitches; previous history of follicular cysts; abnormal karyotype

ASSOCIATED DISORDERS

Secondary to chronic estrogen exposure, bone marrow suppression, uterine disease, and mammary disease may occur.

Clinical Presentation

HISTORY, CHIEF COMPLAINT

- More than 21 days (dog) or 10 days (cat) of behavioral estrus
    - Estrous behaviors in the bitch include receptivity to males, vulvar edema, and serosanguineous vulvar discharge. In the queen, lordosis and vocalization occur.
- History of use of estrogens to treat urinary incontinence or deslorelin (gonadotropin-releasing hormone [GnRH] agonist) for contraception
    - Recent use of estradiol cypionate as an abortifacient for unintended breedings is sometimes reported, although not recommended.

PHYSICAL EXAM FINDINGS

- Bitch or queen may be in good health.
- Chronic exposure to estrogen can result in disease states manifesting as cystic endometrial hyperplasia-pyometra complex, bone marrow suppression (anemia, agranulocytosis, thrombocytopenia), mammary and uterine neoplasia, and endocrinologic alopecia.
- Palpable unilateral abdominal mass (ovarian tumor)

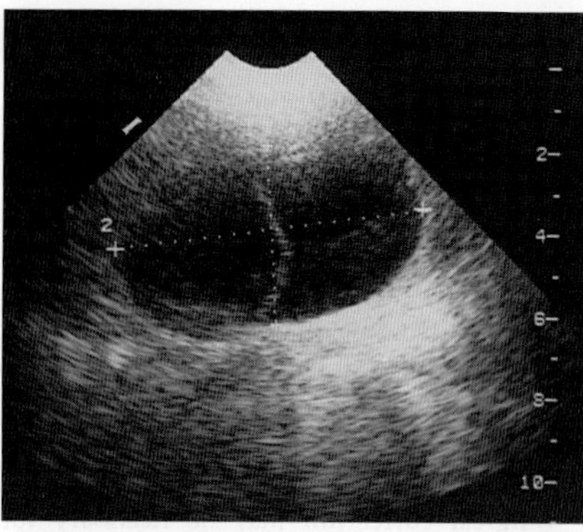

PROLONGED ESTRUS Abdominal ultrasonography of a bitch with ovarian cysts that caused prolonged proestrus. (From Feldman EC, et al: Canine and feline endocrinology and reproduction, ed 3, St. Louis, 2004, Saunders.)

Etiology and Pathophysiology

Prolonged estrus:

- Cause depends on source of persistently circulating estradiol (exogenous or endogenous).
- Estrogen-secreting follicular cysts or granulosa cell tumors can result in persistent estrus.
    - Follicular cysts have been reported to occur in 3%-62% of dogs with ovarian cystic disorders. These cysts occur as single or multiple, thin-walled structures that contain a clear, serous fluid.
- In the queen, persistent estrus may result from the overlapping waves of maturing ovarian follicles, resulting in prolonged high concentrations of estradiol.

DIAGNOSIS

Diagnostic Overview

The diagnosis is suspected based on the presence of estrous behaviors in an ovariohysterectomized animal or prolonged in an intact bitch or queen. Confirmation requires identification of the source of estradiol (exogenous or endogenous) and functional ovarian tissue.

Differential Diagnosis

- Persistent proestrus
- Split estrus (proestrus without subsequent estrus followed by a normal cycle in about 4 weeks)
- Recurrent estrus (low progesterone level or premature luteal failure)
- Pyometra
- Vaginitis
- Coagulopathy
- ORS

Initial Database

- CBC (anemia, thrombocytopenia), serum biochemistry profile, urinalysis
- Exfoliative vaginal cytologic exam indicative of estrus: > 90% cornification of epithelial cells (p. 1183)
- Abdominal ultrasonography to look for endogenous sources of estradiol
    - Identification of abnormal ovarian structures: anechoic spherical regions in the ovary (follicles) or mixed echogenicity of a tumor
    - Identification of ovarian remnant in an ovariohysterectomized animal

Advanced or Confirmatory Testing

- Vaginoscopy (p. 1184) to rule out foreign body and vaginitis
- Exclusion of abnormal karyotype
- Coagulation panel to rule out coagulopathy

TREATMENT

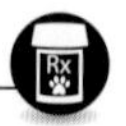

Treatment Overview

Treatment of abnormal estrus consists of removing the source of estradiol. For persistent estrus, induction of follicular luteinization with subsequent monitoring of progesterone concentrations and vaginal cytology for signs of diestrus or alternatively performing an ovariohysterectomy

Acute and Chronic Treatment

Medical:

- Follicular cysts in dogs and cats can be treated with GnRH 25 mcg/dose IM; use 2.2 mcg/kg if > 11 kg or with human chorionic gonadotropin (hCG) 500-1000 IU/dose IM, which results in luteinization of the follicles.
- Monitor serum progesterone, and perform a vaginal cytologic exam (p. 1183) weekly after GnRH or hCG administration; monitor for signs of diestrus or anestrus.

Surgical:

- When genetic qualities of the dam are not superior, ovariohysterectomy is the treatment of choice after reduction of current hyperestrogenic state.

Possible Complications

Pyometra sequelae (p. 854):

- Progesterone promotes endometrial growth and glandular secretion while decreasing myometrial activity. Cystic endometrial hyperplasia and accumulation of uterine secretions result, providing an excellent environment for bacterial growth.
- Chronic estradiol production by the cystic follicles upregulates progesterone receptors in the uterus. This enhances the effect of the progestins produced after treatment to luteinize the cystic follicles.

Myelotoxicosis sequelae:

- Chronic endogenous or exogenous estradiol may induce production of myelopoiesis-inhibitory factor with subsequent myelosuppression (causing anemia, thrombocytopenia, leukopenia) and a poor prognosis if untreated.

Recommended Monitoring

Monitor signs of estrus, which should subside within 5-7 days of treatment.

PROGNOSIS & OUTCOME

- Recurrence is possible, but prognosis is good if signs of diestrus follow treatment.
- If estrus persists, increased suspicion of neoplasia or abnormal karyotype yields a poorer prognosis for subsequent fertility, and an ovariohysterectomy is indicated.

PEARLS & CONSIDERATIONS

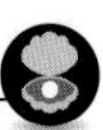

Comments

Although ovarian cancer is rare in the bitch or queen, failure of medical treatment to end signs of behavioral estrus or decrease circulating estradiol concentrations greatly increases the possibility of this diagnosis.

Prevention

In animals of nonbreeding stock, complete ovariohysterectomy prevents reproductive abnormalities and their sequelae.

Technician Tips

- Vaginal cytology swabs should be gently rolled, not smeared.
- Pyometra can be as pronounced as vaginal discharge or as subtle as depression or lethargy with a fever.
- Tumors should be staged with histopathology.

Client Education

- Train owners to recognize signs of estrus or discuss outward signs of behavioral estrus for the bitch and queen.
- Clinicians and owners should discuss multiple benefits of spaying nonbreeding stock while young.
- Recurrence is more likely in animals with previous follicular cysts.

SUGGESTED READING

England GCW: Infertility in the bitch and queen. In Noakes DE, et al, editors: Arthur's veterinary reproduction and obstetrics, Philadelphia, 2001, Saunders, pp 639-670.

RELATED CLIENT EDUCATION SHEETS

Consent to Perform Abdominal Ultrasound
Consent to Perform Ovariohysterectomy (Spay), Canine
Consent to Perform Ovariohysterectomy (Spay), Feline

AUTHOR: Timothy Hazzard, DVM, PhD
EDITOR: Michelle A. Kutzler, DVM, PhD, DACT

Proptosis of the Globe

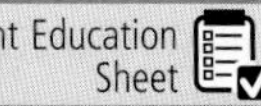

BASIC INFORMATION

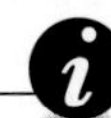

Definition

Acute rostral displacement of the globe (exophthalmos), with caudal entrapment of eyelids

Epidemiology

GENETICS, BREED PREDISPOSITION

Brachycephalic breeds of dogs and cats are at higher risk; however, if traumatic forces are sufficient, proptosis can occur in any breed of either species.

RISK FACTORS

Traumatic forces to the head: mild for brachycephalic; moderate to severe for mesocephalic and dolichocephalic breeds

ASSOCIATED DISORDERS

Retrobulbar mass or severe orbital abscess or cellulitis (p. 716) may predispose the eye to proptosis.

Clinical Presentation

HISTORY, CHIEF COMPLAINT

Caused by peracute event, usually blunt head trauma (e.g., hit by car, fighting) or restraint around neck (in severely brachycephalic dogs)

PHYSICAL EXAM FINDINGS

Exophthalmos with eyelids trapped caudal to globe, along with any or all of the following:

- Ocular: conjunctival hyperemia or hemorrhage, corneal desiccation and/or ulceration, abnormal pupil size (constricted or dilated), intraocular inflammation and/or hemorrhage, ruptured globe, avulsion of extraocular muscle(s) (mainly medial and/or ventral oblique recti), optic nerve rupture/transection, orbital fractures
- Extraocular: other fractures (facial, axial, or appendicular skeleton), neurologic deficits from brain trauma, hypovolemic shock, intrathoracic abnormalities (diaphragmatic hernia, pulmonary contusions, hemothorax, pneumothorax)

Etiology and Pathophysiology

- Force(s) applied to the head (e.g., trauma), leading to rostral displacement of the globe and caudal entrapment of eyelids
- In brachycephalic animals, the orbit encircles a lesser proportion of the globe (i.e., is shallower), allowing proptosis to occur despite a comparatively mild trauma.
- The medial rectus is the first extraocular muscle to avulse during trauma, leading to lateral strabismus. Multiple extraocular muscle avulsions produce a greater degree of proptosis, resulting in a grave prognosis for vision.

DIAGNOSIS

Diagnostic Overview

History and physical exam provide the diagnosis. Additional evaluation is directed at assessing vision and identification of trauma to the rest of the body.

Differential Diagnosis

- Exophthalmos secondary to orbital abscess (opening mouth may cause pain), benign or malignant orbital mass (opening mouth is rarely painful), and congenital vascular anomalies (opening mouth is rarely painful; forward displacement of globe that may be positional, but eyelids are in a normal position; rarely peracute) (p. 716)
- Buphthalmos secondary to congenital, primary, or secondary glaucoma (enlarged globe; eyelids in normal position; rarely acute) (p. 387)

Initial Database

- Ophthalmic exam (p. 1137)
  - Pupillary light reflexes; a midrange, unresponsive pupil (direct and consensual) carries a grave prognosis for vision because optic nerve stretching, avulsion or transection is likely.
  - Fluorescein dye application
  - Intraocular pressure (IOP > 30 mm Hg with glaucoma; low [<10-15 mm Hg] with uveitis). IOP measurement should be performed only after the globe has been replaced in the orbit, releasing the eyelids' pressure on the globe.
- Chest radiographs if hit by car, signs of trauma beyond the face, and/or dyspneic
- Skull radiographs if suspect orbital and/or skull fractures (e.g., extensive facial/cranial trauma, bony crepitus, and neurologic compromise such as obtundation)

TREATMENT

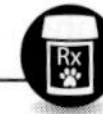

Treatment Overview

Although the primary goal is to return the globe to its proper anatomic location, enucleation may be preferable if there are grave prognostic indicators for vision.

Acute General Treatment

- Hemodynamic, respiratory, and neurologic stabilization if trauma is severe
- Keep cornea lubricated. If surgical correction is not immediately possible (e.g., grave

anesthetic risk), hourly topical ointment application (alternating between bacitracin-neomycin-polymyxin antibiotic q 2h and sterile lubricant q 2h) is recommended.
- Place an Elizabethan collar to prevent self-inflicted trauma.
- Reposition the globe, with patient under general anesthesia
  - Lateral canthotomy: 1-2 cm skin incision at the lateral canthus to relieve pressure on the eyelids
  - Unroll eyelids and replace over globe
  - Simple interrupted skin sutures to close lateral canthotomy
  - Two to three horizontal mattress sutures exiting meibomian gland openings (4-0 to 6-0 suture material) with stents made of Penrose drain or IV tubing to distribute tension evenly on upper and lower eyelids
  - Removal of medial-most suture in 1-2 weeks and lateral sutures in 2-3 weeks, depending on resolution of exophthalmos
  - Vision, tear production, cornea, and intraocular structures (e.g., lens, retina) assessment within 2-3 weeks after surgery
- Enucleation if globe is ruptured, optic nerve is transected, and/or three or more extraocular muscles are avulsed

Chronic Treatment

- Topical atropine in medial canthus q 12h for 3 days
- Topical antibiotic solution q 6h for 2 weeks (e.g., bacitracin-neomycin-gramicidin or tobramycin)
- Nonsteroidal antiinflammatory drugs (NSAIDs) systemically for 5-7 days. Dogs: carprofen 2.2 mg/kg PO q 12h; or meloxicam 0.1 mg/kg PO q 24h. Cats: tolfenamic acid 4 mg/kg SQ, IM, or PO q 24h for 3-5 days; robenacoxib 1 mg/kg PO q 24 h for 3 days.
- Broad-spectrum systemic antibiotics for 5-7 days (e.g., cephalexin 20 mg/kg PO q 8h)
- Elizabethan collar until suture removal
- After repositioning and healing of the globe (days/weeks later), enucleation is still necessary if
  - Affected eye is blind and painful (e.g., chronic uveitis, glaucoma, complex corneal ulcer); critical in cats due to the risk of development of posttraumatic ocular sarcoma (p. 559)

Possible Complications

- Corneal ulceration
- Keratoconjunctivitis sicca (KCS)
- Blindness
- Repeat proptosis in brachycephalic breeds (soon after suture removal)
- Strabismus (frequently lateral or dorsolateral due to avulsion of medial rectus or medial and ventral oblique recti muscles, respectively)
- Glaucoma
- Uveitis
- Lagophthalmos (incomplete closure of eyelids due to CN V or VII damage)
- Neurotrophic keratitis (damage to ophthalmic branch of trigeminal nerve supplying cornea, such as in corneal denervation) with chronic corneal ulceration

Recommended Monitoring

Recheck suture placement 24-48 hours postoperatively because eyelid swelling may have dramatically improved, causing loosening of sutures and risking corneal-suture contact.

PROGNOSIS & OUTCOME

- Varies, depending on the extent of trauma (e.g., hyphema is a poor prognostic sign)
- Most affected eyes with mild trauma can be salvaged.
- Overall prognosis for vision varies
  - Poor to grave (dolichocephalic breeds and cats; midrange unresponsive pupil; marked proptosis [globe displaced several centimeters rostral to the orbit])
  - Guarded (brachycephalic breeds)

PEARLS & CONSIDERATIONS

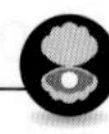

Comments

- True ocular emergency
- Avoid using topical corticosteroids (corneal ulceration is common).
- A blind comfortable eye can have an excellent cosmetic appearance.

Prevention

Permanent partial tarsorrhaphy (surgery to shorten length of eyelid opening) in brachycephalic breeds of dogs

Technician Tips

In the postoperative stage, avoid excessive pressure around the neck to avoid recurrence (e.g., use harness instead of collar).

Client Education

- If globe is replaced but remains blind and painful in the postoperative stage, enucleation, or evisceration with intraocular prosthesis if cornea and STT are normal, is warranted.
- Early enucleation of blind and painful eyes in cats is done to prevent posttraumatic ocular sarcoma.

SUGGESTED READING

Mandell DC, et al: Ophthalmic emergencies Vet Clin North Am Small Anim Pract 35:455, 2005.

RELATED CLIENT EDUCATION SHEETS

Consent to Perform Enucleation
Consent to Perform General Anesthesia
How to Administer Eye Medications
How to Assemble and Use an Elizabethan Collar

AUTHOR: Chantale L. Pinard, DVM, MSc, DACVO
EDITOR: Diane V. H. Hendrix, DVM, DACVO

Prostatic Enlargement (Noninfectious, Non-Neoplastic)

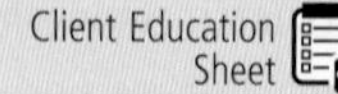

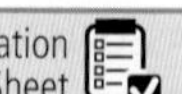

BASIC INFORMATION

Definition

Prostatic cell hypertrophy and hyperplasia are ongoing processes with progressive expansion over time. Noninfectious/non-neoplastic prostate enlargement should be considered a normal physiologic process without pathologic consequences for most intact dogs. Loss of androgen influence after castration or by pharmacologic blockade causes regression of the prostate to an immature, rudimentary state.

Synonyms

Prostatomegaly, benign prostatic hyperplasia (BPH), cystic BPH

Epidemiology

SPECIES, AGE, SEX

- BPH is observed only in dogs (and men). BPH is a normal age-related change in intact male dogs (80% of intact dogs > 5 years and 95% > 9 years of age). Histologic evidence of BPH can be encountered at a young age, with a reported 16% prevalence among 2-year-old, intact male beagles. However, the true prevalence of BPH is difficult to determine. A study focusing on dogs that died of diseases unrelated to the prostate found a 45% prevalence of subclinical BPH.
- Diseases of the prostate gland are rare in cats and prostatomegaly in cats has been described only in association with neoplastic lesions, bacterial prostatitis, and prostatic abscess.

GENETICS, BREED PREDISPOSITION

Prostatic size correlates with body weight and breed. Scottish terriers are reported to have prostates that are four times larger than those from other breeds of similar weights. German shepherds and Doberman pinschers have a higher reported incidence of all prostatic diseases.

RISK FACTORS

Prolonged androgen exposure (endogenous or exogenous)

CONTAGION AND ZOONOSIS

Environmental shedding of *Brucella canis* organisms may be increased from intact male dogs with BPH due to increased prostatic secretions eliminated in urine and preputial discharge.

GEOGRAPHY AND SEASONALITY

The prevalence of BPH is higher in countries where dogs are rarely castrated and lower in countries where castration is common.

ASSOCIATED DISORDERS

BPH can progress to prostatic cyst formation and predispose dogs to acute or chronic bacterial prostatitis or prostatic abscesses. Chronic prostatitis can progress to cystitis, epididymitis, and orchitis.

Clinical Presentation

DISEASE FORMS/SUBTYPES

BPH should be differentiated from cystic BPH because the latter can predispose dogs to acute or chronic bacterial prostatitis or prostatic abscesses.

HISTORY, CHIEF COMPLAINT

- Most dogs with BPH are asymptomatic.
- Clinical signs associated with BPH occur mostly in advanced stages. Symptoms include lower urinary tract signs (e.g., hematuria, dysuria), gastrointestinal signs (e.g., tenesmus, obstipation), and reproductive signs (e.g., sanguineous preputial discharge, hematospermia, infertility).
- In advanced stages or with complications, caudal abdominal pain, stiff gait, reluctance to move, and severe systemic manifestations consistent with sepsis may occur.

PHYSICAL EXAM FINDINGS

Physical exam findings can include a middle to caudal abdominal mass in an otherwise healthy male dog. The normal prostate is bilobed, symmetrical, smooth, movable, and nonpainful. When symmetrical, nonpainful, prostatomegaly is an incidental physical exam finding in an otherwise normal, healthy, older, intact male dog, a tentative diagnosis of BPH is justified.

Etiology and Pathophysiology

- Although normal prostatic growth is achieved by about 2 years of age, prostatic cells undergo ongoing hypertrophy and hyperplasia under the influence of androgens.
- Age-related changes in the androgen-estrogen ratio appear to be important in the pathophysiology of BPH.
  - Dihydrotestosterone (DHT) is the main mediator of prostatic hyperplasia by promoting growth of stromal and glandular elements, whereas estradiol induces cellular metaplasia of prostatic epithelial cells, with glandular obstruction, retention of prostatic fluid and blood, and formation of parenchymal cysts of various sizes that may or may not communicate with the urethra.
  - Testosterone has only minor direct biological activity in the prostate because of lower receptor affinity.
  - Intraprostatic conversion of testosterone to DHT by the enzyme 5-alpha-reductase and subsequent activation of the androgen-binding receptor (ABR) and translocation of the DHT-ABR complex to the nucleus leads to prostatic cell hypertrophy and hyperplasia.
  - 17-beta-estradiol increases the number of ABRs and decreases the degradation of DHT, promoting androgen-associated prostatic growth.

DIAGNOSIS

Diagnostic Overview

A presumptive diagnosis of BPH can be made on signalment, history, physical exam (including transrectal digital prostate palpation), prostatic fluid exam, and transabdominal ultrasonography of the prostate. A definitive diagnosis of BPH requires prostatic biopsy, which is difficult to justify when less invasive methods strongly support BPH.

Differential Diagnosis

- Prostatitis (acute or chronic)
- Prostatic abscess
- Prostatic adenocarcinoma

Initial Database

- Dogs with BPH have a symmetrically enlarged prostate that is moderately firm and not painful on palpation. Prostate asymmetry can be palpated in dogs with large prostatic cysts (p. 1272)
- Serum canine prostate–specific arginine esterase (CPSE) is a biomarker for BPH but is not clinically useful because it does not distinguish between BPH, bacterial prostatitis and prostatic carcinoma.
- Seminal fluid of dogs with BPH contains blood with or without minimal mononuclear inflammation. Quantitative bacterial culture should yield fewer than 100 bacteria per milliliter.
- Transabdominal ultrasound reveals prostatomegaly with a diffuse hypoechogenic to hyperechogenic echotexture. The size of the normal canine prostate varies considerably by body weight and age. The size of the prostate can be measured in three dimensions using ultrasonography and compared with the prostate volume of dogs unaffected by BPH using the following formula: volume (cm^3) = ($0.867 \times$ BW [kg]) + ($1.885 \times$ age [year]) + 15.88.
- Ultrasonography is especially important to evaluate possible parenchymal cysts and to rule out other differentials such as abscesses or neoplasia. The sublumbar lymph nodes should not be enlarged in uncomplicated BPH.
- When complicated forms of BPH (e.g., cystic BPH) and focal lesions (e.g., prostatic abscess) can be ruled out by ultrasonography, the presumptive diagnosis of BPH can be confirmed by therapeutic androgen suppression.

Advanced or Confirmatory Testing

- Fine-needle aspiration (FNA) and cytology reveal the typical characteristics of hypertrophic prostatic cells.
- Biopsy is very seldom indicated for BPH.

TREATMENT

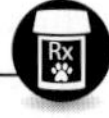

Treatment Overview

Dogs with no clinical signs of BPH do not require treatment. The goal of treatment is to reduce prostatic size and thereby alleviate clinical signs and decrease the risk of complications (e.g., prostatitis, prostatic abscess).

Acute General Treatment

Surgical treatment: castration:

- Castration is the first-choice treatment for most dogs. It causes rapid reduction in prostatic volume by more than 50% in 3 weeks and 75% in 3 months.
- Approximately 3 weeks after castration, involution of the prostate should be verified by rectal palpation or by ultrasound to rule out concurrent neoplasia or abscess previously masked by BPH.

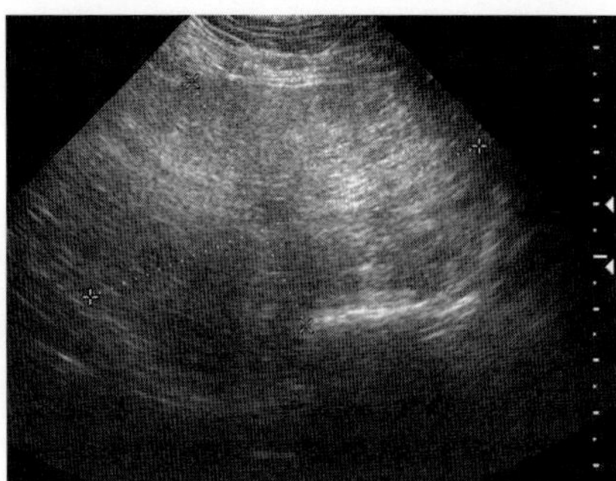

PROSTATIC ENLARGEMENT Transabdominal ultrasound image of the prostate from a 10-year-old, intact, male German shepherd with benign prostatic hyperplasia reveals prostatomegaly with a diffuse hypoechogenic to hyperechogenic echotexture.

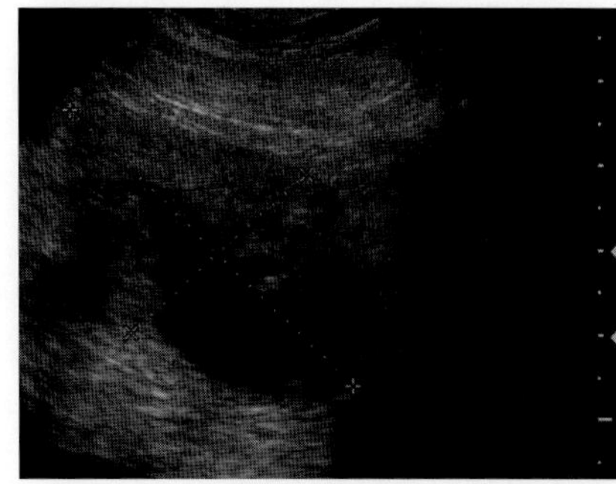

PROSTATIC ENLARGEMENT Transabdominal ultrasound image shows a prostate from a 5-year-old, intact, male Doberman pinscher with benign prostatic hyperplasia and single large intraprostatic cyst. The cystic fluid is hypoechoic and flocculent.

Medical treatment can act within weeks (see Chronic Treatment).

Chronic Treatment

Reversible medical therapy should be considered for breeding dogs or older dogs with significant anesthesia risks. These forms of therapy are safe and practical, even for long-term treatment and for breeding dogs. Therapeutic response should be evaluated, even with complete resolution of clinical signs, because of the risk of concurrent infection or neoplasia. Between 3 and 4 weeks after initiation of therapy, BPH should have sufficiently regressed, and coexisting diseases are more likely to be detected.

- Finasteride 0.1-0.5 mg/kg (maximum 5 mg/DOG) PO q 24h is a synthetic steroid that inhibits prostatic type II 5-alpha-reductase, which blocks conversion of testosterone to DHT.
  - This results in selective blockade of prostatic androgen effects, prostatic atrophy, and decrease in prostatic volume of 50%-70% in 2-4 weeks. Clinical signs associated with BPH begin to resolve after 1 week of therapy, and most dogs are asymptomatic within 4 weeks.
  - Prostatic DHT concentrations decrease, but serum testosterone concentrations remain unchanged. Dogs therefore maintain libido and fertility, and they can be bred successfully. Semen volume decreases without negative effect on semen quality.
  - Treatment should be continued for 1-4 months or longer. However, the prostate will return to its original size in 4-8 weeks after discontinuing therapy.
- Osaterone acetate (Epostane, Virbac 0.25 to 0.5 mg/kg PO q 24h) is a synthetic testosterone analog with antiandrogen and progestogen effects. It blocks the absorption of testosterone in the prostate and competitively inhibits prostatic DHT receptors.
  - Osaterone decreases prostatic volume by approximately 27% after 1 week and 40% after 2 weeks. One-half of treated dogs exhibit resolution of BPH clinical signs in 2 weeks and 83% in months.
  - Because osaterone does not suppress testosterone production itself but only its effect on the prostate, it should have no effect on sperm quality and fertility. However, osaterone can decrease serum cortisol concentrations and may interfere with ACTH response in hormonal testing and induce adrenocortical insufficiency.
- Synthetic progesterone analogs (medroxyprogesterone acetate 3-4 mg/kg SQ as necessary, megestrol acetate 0.5 mg/kg PO q 24h) exert antiandrogen activity by decreasing testosterone concentrations through negative feedback at the level of the hypothalamus and by inhibiting prostatic 5-alpha-reductase.
  - The clinical effects of synthetic progesterone analogs combine good efficacy for prostatic hyperplasia with only mild to moderate systemic antiandrogenic effects, including decreased libido and fertility.
  - One injection of medroxyprogesterone acetate resulted in complete resolution of clinical signs in 84% of dogs in 4-6 weeks, and 68% remained asymptomatic for at least 10 months.
- Deslorelin (Suprelorin, Virbac) is a gonadotropin-releasing hormone (GnRH) agonist available in an SQ sustained-release implant. Administration induces down-regulation of pituitary GnRH receptors and subsequent complete suppression of gonadotropins (luteinizing hormone [LH], follicle-stimulating hormone [FSH]) and gonadal hormones (testosterone, estradiol).
  - This product causes reversible but complete nonselective chemical castration with infertility and suppressed semen quality. Testicular and prostatic size reduction is achieved reliably for at least 6-12 months.

Nutrition/Diet

An herbal supplement derived from the berry of the saw palmetto plant reportedly improves urinary flow rates in men with BPH. However, use of this supplement for 3 months in dogs with BPH did not reduce prostate size.

Behavior/Exercise

Exposure to estrous females may increase prostatic fluid secretions and exacerbate clinical signs associated with BPH.

Drug Interactions

All progestogens can increase appetite, suppress the adrenal axis, and increase susceptibility to insulin resistance and diabetes mellitus.

Possible Complications

Complications associated with FNA of the prostate include periprostatic hemorrhage, hematuria, dissemination of a concurrent prostate infection, laceration of major blood vessels, urethral fistulation, orchitis, or inadvertent puncture of adjacent organs. Avoid FNA before examining prostatic fluid obtained by ejaculation or prostatic massage. Risk may be increased in febrile animals or those with leukocytosis.

Recommended Monitoring

- Record prostate size for all male dogs (intact and neutered) with each physical exam.
- If asymmetrically enlarged or enlargement is associated with clinical signs in an intact dog, perform transabdominal ultrasound to rule out coexisting conditions.

PROGNOSIS & OUTCOME

For BPH with or without cysts, the prognosis is excellent. Dogs not showing clinical signs may remain symptom free for months to years. Castration is curative of clinical signs of BPH, and intraparenchymal prostatic cysts will decrease in size.

PEARLS & CONSIDERATIONS

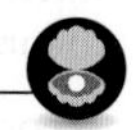

Comments

- Young, valuable breeding dogs with prostatic disease are more likely to be asymptomatic and should be regularly screened for prostatic disease by prostatic ultrasound and a semen evaluation.
- CPSE is a biomarker for BPH but is not clinically useful because it does not distinguish BPH, bacterial prostatitis, or prostatic carcinoma.
- Semen evaluation and freezing may be performed during finasteride treatment and does not interfere with fertility.

Prevention

Surgical castration

Technician Tips

- Counsel owners of young healthy breeding dogs regarding the high incidence of BPH, and discuss semen cryopreservation for valuable breeding stock.
- Recommend annual prostate exams with breeding evaluations and *B. canis* screening.

Client Education

- BPH should be considered a normal age-related change in intact male dogs, and most dogs are asymptomatic. Symptoms associated with BPH occur mostly in advanced stages and include lower urinary tract signs (e.g., hematuria, dysuria), gastrointestinal signs (e.g., tenesmus, obstipation), or reproductive signs (e.g., sanguineous preputial discharge, hematospermia, infertility).
- The goal of BPH treatment is to reduce prostatic size and thereby alleviate clinical signs and decrease the risk of complications (e.g., prostatitis, prostatic abscess). Treatment options involve surgical castration (permanent) or medical management (reversible).

SUGGESTED READING

Kutzler M: Prostatic diseases. In Ettinger SJ, et al, editors: Textbook of veterinary internal medicine, ed 8, St. Louis, 2017, Elsevier, pp 2031-2036.

AUTHOR & EDITOR: Michelle A. Kutzler, DVM, PhD, DACT

Prostatic Infections (Prostatitis, Prostatic Abscessation)

Client Education Sheet

BASIC INFORMATION

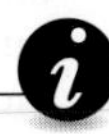

Definition

- Prostatitis usually occurs secondary to bacteria ascending the urethra in conjunction with a compromised prostatic defense mechanisms. Prostatitis may be acute or chronic.
- Animals with acute infection are systemically ill; signs may be absent or vague in chronic infections.
- Prostatic abscesses usually form as a sequela to chronic prostatitis. Clinical signs vary depending on the extent of the infection and systemic involvement.

Epidemiology

SPECIES, AGE, SEX

- Dogs: predominantly intact males > 6 years of age
- Cats: rare

GENETICS, BREED PREDISPOSITION

Large-breed dogs

RISK FACTORS

Older, intact male dogs with benign prostatic hyperplasia (BPH), prostatic cysts, or squamous metaplasia of the prostate

CONTAGION AND ZOONOSIS

Brucella canis

ASSOCIATED DISORDERS

- BPH (p. 824)
- Prostatic cysts (p. 824)
- Sertoli cell tumor (p. 962)
- Urinary tract infection (p. 232)

Clinical Presentation

DISEASE FORMS/SUBTYPES

- Acute prostatitis presents as an acute illness with fever, stranguria, tenesmus, stiff-legged gait, and signs of sepsis if prostatic abscessation or septicemia are present. Treatment consists of antimicrobial therapy and supportive care. Surgery may be warranted for prostatic abscessation. Uncomplicated cases often respond quickly and have a good short-term prognosis, but patients with sepsis have a poorer prognosis.
- Chronic prostatitis may have no clinical signs or manifest with infertility or chronic urinary tract infection. Treatment consists of antimicrobial therapy and castration.

HISTORY, CHIEF COMPLAINT

- Urinary symptoms such as hematuria, pollakiuria, stranguria, dysuria, pyuria, and incontinence frequently occur with prostatitis or abscessation.
- Systemic symptoms such as depression, hyporexia, fever, or hypothermia are most likely to occur with acute prostatitis and prostatic abscessation.
- Lumbar pain and reluctance to breed may be noted with acute prostatitis.
- Gastrointestinal signs such as tenesmus, diarrhea, and abdominal pain may be noted with prostatic abscessation or acute prostatitis.
- Chronic prostatitis may be asymptomatic or associated with chronic urinary tract infection.
- Dogs < 6 years of age are more likely to present for infertility.

PHYSICAL EXAM FINDINGS

- Signs of acute prostatitis/abscessation are related to bacterial inflammation and include fever and pain on prostate palpation. A stiff gait may be noted.
- Asymmetry of the prostate, an abdominal mass, and severe systemic signs (e.g., depression, shock, marked pain) more frequently occur with prostatic abscessation.
- Exam is often normal for chronic prostatitis, although prostatomegaly is possible.

Etiology and Pathophysiology

- Normal prostatic defense mechanisms include urine flow, urethral tone, bactericidal prostatic fluid, and local immunoglobulin A (IgA) production.
- Prostatitis and abscessation are associated with disruption of the normal prostatic defense mechanisms.
- The usual route of bacterial infection is urethra ascension, but hematogenous spread is possible.
- *Escherichia coli* is isolated most often. Other pathogens include *Mycoplasma* spp, *Staphylococcus* spp, *Streptococcus* spp, *Klebsiella* spp, *Proteus mirabilis*, *Pseudomonas* spp, and *B. canis*.
- There are case reports of infection with *Blastomyces* spp, *Cryptococcus* spp, *Pythium* spp, *Leishmania* spp, and *Bartonella henselae*.

DIAGNOSIS

Diagnostic Overview

Diseases of the prostate present with overlapping clinical signs. Correct diagnosis requires consideration of signs in conjunction with diagnostic tests. Although transrectal prostate palpation is a useful physical exam tool, it is neither sensitive nor specific enough to make a definitive diagnosis. A minimal database and semen evaluation are appropriate initial diagnostics. Further evaluation with transabdominal ultrasound and, if indicated, contrast-enhanced CT are advised. Culture, serology, cytology, and histopathology may facilitate the diagnostic process.

Differential Diagnosis

- Prostatic disease: cysts, BPH, neoplasia, squamous metaplasia
- Urinary disease: urolithiasis, transitional cell carcinoma of the prostatic urethra, cystitis
- Gastrointestinal disease: colitis, colonic neoplasia

Initial Database

- CBC: inflammatory leukogram ± left shift (acute prostatitis/abscess)
- Serum biochemical analysis: low albumin (negative acute-phase protein response in sepsis)
- Urinalysis: active sediment (white blood cells, pyuria, high pH, bacteria)
- Urine culture and susceptibility: cultures are typically positive with bacterial prostatitis; antimicrobial minimal inhibitory concentration (MIC) aids treatment choice
- *Brucella* serology: breeding males should have regular *Brucella* screening.
- Transrectal digital prostate palpation (p. 1272): The prostate may be palpated transrectally while transabdominally pushing the neck of the bladder and the prostate into the pelvic canal. Sensitivity for prostatic disease using this method alone is low at 53%.
- Abdominal radiographs: the normal canine prostate should not exceed 50% of the width of the pelvic inlet on ventrodorsal views. Prostatic dimensions > 90% of the pubic-sacral promontory distance are more consistent with neoplasia, abscessation, or paraprostatic cysts.
- Transabdominal ultrasound: the normal prostate is homogenous and ≈ walnut sized. Cystic lesions with flocculent content support prostatic abscessation. Focal or diffuse heterogenous increase in echogenicity supports prostatitis and/or BPH.
- Prostatic mineralization: is highly associated with prostatic neoplasia in castrated dogs, but this is not true for intact dogs.

Advanced or Confirmatory Testing

- Semen evaluation (pp. 1061 and 1381): the third fraction is composed of prostatic fluid. Red blood cells may be present due to concurrent BPH. Leukocytes (with or without phagocytized bacteria) in prostatic fluid are highly predictive of prostatitis.
- Prostatic fluid culture: single organism with a colony count greater than 10,000/mL or ≥ 2 log higher colony count compared with urethral swab cultures for paired prostatic and urethral samples supports a diagnosis of bacterial prostatitis. Prostatic fluid may be obtained by ejaculation or prostatic massage (p. 1153).
- Prostatic fine-needle aspiration: used to obtain fluid or tissue for cytology or culture.

Aspiration is best performed with ultrasound guidance.

- Prostatic biopsy: minimal improvement in definitive diagnosis compared with fine-needle aspiration (66% vs. 50%); may be obtained with a perirectal approach or exploratory. Complications include seeding of neoplasia or infection and urethral damage.
- CT imaging with contrast: more sensitive tool for evaluation of prostate size, density, and other alterations compared with trans-abdominal ultrasound.

TREATMENT

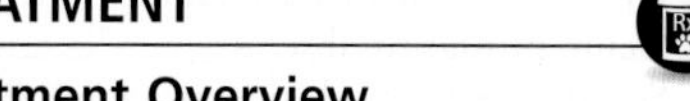

Treatment Overview

Primary focus for treatment is control of the infectious agent, with supportive care as needed for cases with systemic involvement. The secondary focus is correction of underlying risk factors if possible and prevention of recurrence, which may require medical treatment, surgical procedures such as abscess drainage or omentalization, or castration.

Acute General Treatment

- Antimicrobial treatment is ideally based on culture and sensitivity and the ability to penetrate the blood-prostate barrier.
  - Antimicrobials of choice include enrofloxacin 5-20 mg/kg PO q 24h (bactericidal; often first choice), trimethoprim-sulfadiazine 15 mg/kg PO q 12h, (bactericidal), chloramphenicol 30-50 mg/kg PO q 8h (bacteriostatic), and doxycycline 5 mg/kg PO q 12h (bacteriostatic)
  - Clindamycin and macrolides can be used but only after culture identifies a susceptible gram-positive pathogen.
  - Antimicrobial penetration is greater in cases of acute prostatitis because the blood-prostate barrier is disrupted.
- Isolation, serologic testing of other exposed animals and humans, and notification of public health authorities should be initiated for cases of confirmed *B. canis*.
- Supportive care (e.g., intravenous fluids, analgesia, coagulation support) should be instituted where required (pp. 907 and 1448).
- Castration or antiandrogen therapy (finasteride 0.1-0.5 mg/kg [maximum of 5 mg] PO q 24h) may be required to decrease prostate size and facilitate treatment.
- Large prostatic abscesses or cases with septic peritonitis may benefit from surgical intervention.

Chronic Treatment

- Antimicrobial administration typically continues for 4-6 weeks.
- If castration is refused, finasteride may be continued long term as needed to manipulate prostate size.

Possible Complications

Patients receiving antimicrobial treatment for 4-6 weeks should be monitored per drug formulary recommendations (e.g., trimethoprim-sulfadiazine can cause keratoconjunctivitis sicca).

Recommended Monitoring

- Repeat physical exam and transabdominal ultrasound should be performed every 2 weeks during treatment.
- Urine or prostatic fluid cytology and culture should be evaluated 3-5 days after discontinuing antimicrobials, and a complete exam and culture should be repeated 3-4 weeks later.

PROGNOSIS & OUTCOME

- Any systemic involvement carries a poorer prognosis based on the severity of illness.
- The prognosis for resolution of acute prostatic infection without neutering is good.
- Chronic prostatitis generally carries a poor prognosis for complete resolution without castration.
- The prognosis for prostatic abscessation varies depending on the extent of the infection, systemic involvement, and surgical intervention required.
- Any disease associated with fever may interfere with spermatogenesis and alter short- and long-term reproductive potential.

PEARLS & CONSIDERATIONS

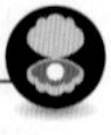

Comments

- Young breeding dogs are more likely to be asymptomatic and should be regularly screened for prostatic disease by prostatic ultrasound and a semen evaluation.
- Serum canine prostate–specific arginine esterase (CPSE) is a biomarker for BPH, but it is not clinically useful because it cannot distinguish between BPH, bacterial prostatitis, or prostatic carcinoma.
- Semen evaluation and freezing may be performed during finasteride treatment and will not interfere with fertility.
- Prostatitis is rare in castrated males (unless recently castrated).

Prevention

Surgical castration

Technician Tips

- Counsel owners of young, healthy breeding dogs regarding the high incidence of prostatic disease among animals > 6 years old, and discuss semen cryopreservation for valuable breeding stock.
- Recommend regular breeding evaluations and *Brucella* screening for all breeding animals.

Client Education

- Chronic prostatitis is frequently asymptomatic or associated with chronic urinary tract infection.
- Dogs < 6 years of age with prostatic disease are more likely to present for infertility than illness.
- Systemic illness associated with prostatic disease may result in damage to the blood-testis barrier and a subsequent loss of normal spermatogenesis.

SUGGESTED READING

Smith J: Canine prostatic disease: a review of anatomy, pathology, diagnosis, and treatment. Theriogenology 70:375-383, 2008.

AUTHOR: Sophie A Grundy, BVSc, MACVS, DACVIM
EDITOR: Michelle A. Kutzler, DVM, PhD, DACT

Prostatic Neoplasia

Video Available Bonus Material Online Client Education Sheet

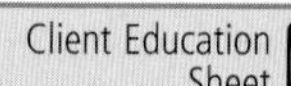

BASIC INFORMATION

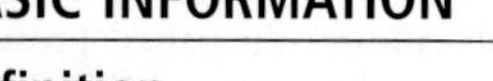

Definition

The most common tumor types of the prostate gland include adenocarcinoma, urothelial carcinoma, and undifferentiated carcinoma. Prostate tumors are locally invasive and highly metastatic.

Epidemiology

SPECIES, AGE, SEX

Prostate tumors occur almost exclusively in dogs (castrated or intact); sporadic cases are reported in cats. Median age at diagnosis in dogs is 10 years.

GENETICS, BREED PREDISPOSITION

The Bouvier des Flandres, Doberman pinscher, Shetland sheepdog, Scottish terrier, beagle, miniature poodle, German short-haired pointer, Airedale terrier, and Norwegian elkhound may be at increased risk for prostatic carcinoma.

RISK FACTORS

The effects of reproductive status on the development of prostate tumors are not fully understood. Exposure to endogenous androgens has been associated with development of prostatic adenocarcinoma in dogs. Castration at a young age appears to increase the risk of other types of prostate tumors.

ASSOCIATED DISORDERS

Secondary bacterial cystitis (p. 232)

Clinical Presentation

DISEASE FORMS/SUBTYPES

Histologic types include adenocarcinoma, urothelial carcinoma (i.e., prostatic extension of urethral transitional cell carcinoma), and undifferentiated carcinoma. The natural behavior of and diagnostic approach to each subtype are identical.

HISTORY, CHIEF COMPLAINT

Clinical signs are often chronic, linked to the urinary tract, and most commonly include hematuria, incontinence, and stranguria. Rarely, patients may present with complete urethral obstruction. Animals with large masses may present with tenesmus and/or altered stool shape (flattened stools) caused by compression of the colon by the tumor. Local invasion into the lumbar vertebrae or bone metastasis may cause signs of pain and/or lameness.

PHYSICAL EXAM FINDINGS

External physical exam is often unremarkable. A large, irregular mass that may be firmly adhered to surrounding pelvic structures is typically found on rectal palpation. Animals with bone metastases may display evidence of pain during orthopedic exam of the spine, pelvis, and/or hindlimbs (p. 1143). The sublumbar lymph node may be enlarged.

Etiology and Pathophysiology

Intact and castrated dogs develop prostatic carcinoma. Tumor location often precludes early diagnosis; most tumors are consequently locally advanced and have metastasized (70%-80%) at the time of diagnosis:

- The ultimate metastatic rate for prostate tumors is 85%-100%.
- The most common sites for metastasis include lungs (50%), lymph node (>30%), and bone (15%-45%). The pelvis and lumbosacral spine are the most common sites of bony metastasis.

Cyclooxygenase 2 (COX2) expression may play a role in tumor development and progression because 75% of prostatic carcinomas have been shown to express COX2 protein, whereas such expression is not evident in normal prostatic tissue.

DIAGNOSIS

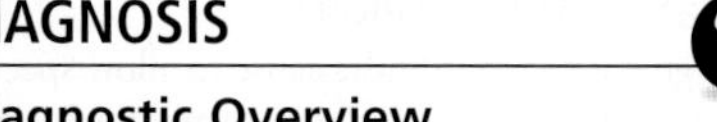

Diagnostic Overview

The diagnosis is suspected based on the presence of lower urinary tract signs in a patient with a large, irregular prostate on rectal exam. Castrated dogs with radiographic and/or ultrasonographic prostatic mineralization are very likely to have prostatic neoplasia. Intact dogs are unlikely to have prostatic neoplasia if no mineralization is found. Confirmation of prostatic neoplasia requires cytologic or histopathologic evaluation.

Differential Diagnosis

- Other prostatic disorders (largely limited to intact dogs)
  - Benign prostatic hyperplasia (BPH)
  - Paraprostatic cyst
  - Prostatic abscess
  - Prostatitis
- Locally invasive transitional cell tumor of the urinary bladder

Initial Database

- CBC, serum biochemistry profile, urinalysis, ± urine culture. Midstream catch or catheterized (culture) samples preferred; avoid cystocentesis
- Thoracic and abdominal radiographs (including evaluation of bony structures for metastasis; sublumbar lymph node)
- Abdominal ultrasound (see *Videos*)
- Aspirates of regional lymph nodes if indicated to identify the presence of metastatic disease

Advanced or Confirmatory Testing

- Cytologic evaluation of a prostatic aspirate or wash may aid in establishing a diagnosis (p. 1153). Transdermal aspiration or biopsy of the prostate may be associated with a risk of tumor seeding. However, the need to establish a definitive diagnosis usually supersedes the risk.
- Histopathologic confirmation should be obtained before a patient undergoes definitive therapy. Traumatic catheterization under ultrasound guidance or digital palpation from the rectum is useful to obtain sample for cytologic and histopathologic evaluation with minimal risk of urethral obstruction or tumor seeding.
- CT for surgical or radiation treatment planning.
- Detection of *BRAF* mutation in urine DNA may be helpful for making a diagnosis of canine urothelial and prostatic carcinoma (https://www.sentinelbiomedical.com/braf-vets/).

TREATMENT

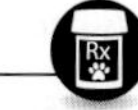

Treatment Overview

Long-term disease control is the ultimate goal but is often not possible due to extensive local or metastatic disease. For patients with lesions not amenable to definitive therapy, palliation of clinical signs is the primary goal.

Acute General Treatment

Definitive therapy:

- Curative therapy should be considered only for dogs with no evidence of metastases.
- Reports describing definitive therapy for dogs with localized prostate tumors are limited. The following treatments can be considered:
  - External beam radiotherapy to prostate ± regional lymph nodes
  - Partial prostatectomy with preservation of the urethra (animals with focal prostatic lesions)
  - Complete prostatectomy with urethral resection/permanent cystostomy tube placement
  - Given the high metastatic rate, chemotherapy (e.g., doxorubicin, mitoxantrone, carboplatin, cisplatin) is indicated in definitively treated animals. The efficacy of chemotherapy has not been established conclusively.
  - COX2 inhibition with piroxicam 0.3 mg/kg PO q 24-48h (or possibly other selective COX2 inhibitors) can be beneficial in animals with prostatic adenocarcinoma or prostatic carcinoma of urothelial origin.

Chronic Treatment

Palliative therapy:

- Palliative care should be considered in animals with metastatic disease and those with advanced localized disease not amenable to definitive therapy. The efficacy of palliative treatments has not been established conclusively.
- Palliative radiotherapy may provide short-term relief from urinary obstruction or other clinical signs resulting from local disease.
- Placement of a urethral stent may provide similar short-term relief from obstruction.
- Permanent cystostomy tube placement/urinary bladder marsupialization may provide relief from urinary obstruction.
- Electrosurgical transurethral resection may result in significant palliation of clinical signs.
- Castration may provide alleviation of signs in intact dogs with concurrent prostatic hyperplasia.
- Systemic treatment with chemotherapy and/or piroxicam
- Use of stool softeners may be helpful in dogs with tenesmus.

Drug Interactions

Patients receiving piroxicam therapy should not be given corticosteroids or other nonsteroidal antiinflammatory medications.

Possible Complications

Potential complications of chemotherapy (e.g., gastrointestinal toxicity, bone marrow suppression) and radiation treatment (e.g., tissue irritation) are similar to those observed for other tumors. Piroxicam therapy may be associated with gastrointestinal ulceration and kidney injury.

Recommended Monitoring

After treatment, recommended monitoring includes routine physical exam, abdominal ultrasound, and thoracic radiographs. For chemotherapy, routine monitoring should be undertaken based on protocol.

PROGNOSIS & OUTCOME

- Due to the severity of clinical disease (advanced local and distant metastasis), most dogs with clinical signs caused by prostate tumors are euthanized within 1 month of diagnosis.
- The prognosis for definitive therapy is largely unknown, with the exception of radiotherapy. Animals treated with a single 30-Gy dose of intraoperative radiation have had a median survival time of 4 months; animals treated with conventional external beam radiotherapy (57 Gy) have had a median survival time of 7 months.
- Dogs receiving COX2 inhibition therapy have a median survival time of 7 months, compared with a median survival of < 1 month for those not receiving such therapy.

PEARLS & CONSIDERATIONS

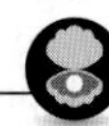

Comments

- With rare exception, the prognosis for animals with prostatic tumors is poor; advanced disease at the time of diagnosis is the major causative factor for a poor prognosis.
- Advances in the treatment of dogs with prostate tumors will more likely come from earlier detection rather than improved treatment.

Technician Tips

Cystocentesis should not be performed on animals with hematuria until the clinician is reasonably certain that the animal 1) does not have a coagulopathy and 2) does not have a bladder or prostatic tumor.

SUGGESTED READING

Lawrence JA, et al: Tumors of the male reproductive system. In Withrow SJ, et al, editors: Small animal clinical oncology, ed 5, St. Louis, 2013, Elsevier, pp 561-565.

AUTHOR: Tetsuya Kobayashi, DVM, MSpVM, DACVIM, DAiCVIM
EDITOR: Kenneth M. Rassnick, DVM, DACVIM

Pruritus

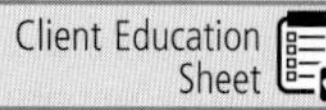

BASIC INFORMATION

Definition

Unpleasant sensation that triggers the desire to scratch, chew, rub, lick, or bite at the skin

Synonym

Itch

Epidemiology

SPECIES, AGE, SEX

- Most common symptom in veterinary dermatology
- Sex and age of onset depend on the underlying cause.
- Contagious acarioses (mite infestations) are more common in young animals.
- Canine atopic dermatitis is first seen in young adults (6 months to 3 years of age).
- Food allergy, although seen most commonly in young adults, may develop at any age.

Clinical Presentation

HISTORY, CHIEF COMPLAINT

Animals scratch, chew, rub, lick, or bite at the skin. Cats can be secretive lickers and may present only for extensive self-induced alopecia.

PHYSICAL EXAM FINDINGS

- Skin lesions vary according to cause.
- Self-induced alopecia, excoriation, and erythema are common findings.
- Typically, no primary skin lesions are noted in canine atopic dermatitis.
- Papules and/or pustules are noted in infectious or parasitic conditions.
- In cats: miliary dermatitis, eosinophilic granuloma complex, self-induced symmetrical alopecia, or self-induced ulcerative facial dermatitis

Etiology and Pathophysiology

- Neurophysiology of pruritus is remarkably complex. A variety of exogenous (e.g., chemicals, parasites, microbial agents, proteases) and endogenous mediators (e.g., histamine, tryptase, kallikreins, interleukins [IL-2, IL-31], leukotriene B_4, prostaglandin E_2, substance P) are involved in pruritus.
- Causes of pruritus are numerous (p. 1445). For most parasitic infestations, a hypersensitivity reaction develops and is responsible for most if not all of the pruritus (often disproportionate to the number of parasites found).
- Pyoderma and yeast dermatitis are frequent causes of pruritus in dogs but are uncommon in cats.

DIAGNOSIS

Diagnostic Overview

Causes of pruritus are numerous, and the signalment, history (notably environment), and dermatologic exam (e.g., lesion distribution) help focus the differential diagnosis. Diagnostic procedures aimed at identifying infections or infestations should be selected first because these disorders are common, and treatment is generally straightforward. A precise diagnosis is necessary to administer a specific treatment.

Differential Diagnosis

- Parasitic: fleas, contagious acarioses (*Sarcoptes*, *Notoedres*, *Cheyletiella*, *Otodectes* spp), lice, *Trombicula* (chiggers), and *Pelodera* spp
- Bacterial: staphylococcal pyoderma
- Fungal: *Malassezia* spp dermatitis and otitis
- Allergic: flea bite hypersensitivity, atopic dermatitis, food hypersensitivity, contact hypersensitivity, drug reaction
- Miscellaneous: calcinosis cutis, cutaneous lymphoma

Initial Database

- Complete history and dermatologic examination (p. 1091)
  - Skin scrapings
  - Skin cytology
  - Wood's lamp and dermatophyte culture (in cats)

Advanced or Confirmatory Testing

- Therapeutic trial with broad-spectrum antiparasitic agents (an integral part of the case workup) is always indicated whenever there is any possibility of a parasitic problem despite of negative skin scrapings.
- Therapeutic trials with antimicrobial agents are often used in dogs to document the contribution of bacteria and yeast in the degree of pruritus seen.
- A hypoallergenic dietary trial should be initiated only after infections and infestations have been excluded/controlled (p. 345).
- Intradermal skin test and/or serologic allergy test for identifying allergen involved in atopic dermatitis (p. 91)
- Skin biopsies are useful in unusual cases (e.g., calcinosis cutis, cutaneous lymphoma) and may be considered if the diagnosis remains elusive despite approaches described above or the clinician suspects these unusual disorders from other aspects of the case. Biopsies may corroborate the diagnosis of allergic skin disease but rarely confirms a specific cause and are therefore less useful for suspected allergic conditions.

TREATMENT

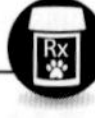

Treatment Overview

The goal is to identify the cause to allow specific treatment. When possible, treatment is limited to one medication at a time to facilitate interpretation of response. When doing therapeutic trials, the most effective treatment regimen that is available and safe should be used to eradicate parasites or infections so interpretation of response is clear.

Acute General Treatment

An acute, intense pruritic episode can be treated with IM or IV short-acting glucocorticoids (dexamethasone sodium phosphate 0.1-0.2 mg/kg), followed by a few days of prednisone or prednisolone 1 mg/kg PO q 24h. Short-term use of glucocorticoids seldom causes serious problems. Oclacitinb (Apoquel) can be an alternative in such cases.

Chronic Treatment

- In long-term management of pruritus, as in cases of canine atopic dermatitis (p. 91), clinicians rely on immunotherapy (hyposensitization), glucocorticoids, oral cyclosporine (Atopica), oclacitinib, interleukin-31caninized monoclonal antibodies (Cytopoint), antihistamines, and/or essential fatty acid supplementation.
- Long-term administration of glucocorticoids should be avoided, unless the maintenance dose is low (e.g., < 0.25 mg/kg of prednisone q 48-72h in dogs) and/or if the treatment is intermittent. In dogs, induction and maintenance doses of prednisolone are typically ≈30% lower than prednisone doses, at least when administered concomitantly with trimeprazine (Temaril-P, Vanectyl-P [Canada]). A long-term treatment goal with these combination products is to administer the minimal effective dose q 48h.
- In cats, prednisone is generally not effective. Oral prednisolone, methylprednisolone, dexamethasone, or triamcinolone is preferred.
- For food hypersensitivity, clinicians must find a commercial hypoallergenic diet that maintains the animal free of clinical signs (p. 345).
- In flea bite hypersensitivity, maintain an effective flea elimination treatment (p. 342).

Recommended Monitoring

Animals receiving chronic glucocorticoid therapy should be monitored every 6 months for signs of iatrogenic hyperadrenocorticism or other complications (e.g., urinary tract infection, pyoderma, weight gain).

PROGNOSIS & OUTCOME

- Varies according to the cause
- Excellent for most parasitic and infectious skin problems and food hypersensitivity
- Atopic dermatitis is an incurable disease that requires long-term management of pruritus.

PEARLS & CONSIDERATIONS

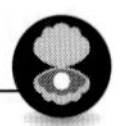

Comments

- Treatment of pruritic dermatoses does not always imply use of antipruritic drugs specifically. Antiparasitic drugs, antibiotics, and antifungal drugs (for yeast dermatitis), which are not inherently antipruritic, are among the most useful antipruritic drugs. They have a key role in pruritus management because they control or eliminate the underlying cause. Superficial pyoderma is a frequent cause of pruritus in dogs.
- Always rule out parasitic and infectious causes of pruritus before administering long-term antipruritic drugs or before initiating an elimination diet (food trial).
- If pruritus is refractory to a usual maintenance dose of glucocorticoid (i.e., > 0.5 mg/kg q 48h of prednisone in dogs), consider the following diagnoses: sarcoptic mange, *Malassezia* dermatitis, pyoderma, food hypersensitivity, calcinosis cutis, contact allergic dermatitis, and epitheliotropic lymphoma.
- More than one disease may be contributing to pruritus; for example, dogs with atopic dermatitis often have secondary bacterial and/or yeast infections.

Technician Tips

Explain to the owner how to quantify the pruritus level using a validated pruritus severity scale (http://www.cavd.ca/images/CAVD_ITCH_SCALE.pdf).

Client Education

- Owners of dogs with canine atopic dermatitis must be well informed about the chronic and multifaceted nature of the disease.
- A pruritus score (http://www.cavd.ca/images/CAVD_ITCH_SCALE.pdf) is very useful for evaluating response to treatment or disease progression. It adds a measure of objectivity and may reduce the owner's perception that treatment is ineffective or may support the severity of pruritus perceived by the owner.

SUGGESTED READING

Tater KC: An approach to pruritus. In Jackson H, et al, editors: BSAVA manual of canine and feline dermatology, ed 3, Gloucester, 2012, British Small Animal Veterinary Association, pp 37-45.

AUTHOR & EDITOR: Manon Paradis, DMV, MVSc, DACVD

Pseudocyesis

BASIC INFORMATION

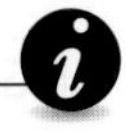

Definition

The common syndrome observed in nonpregnant diestrous or early anestrous bitches is characterized by different degrees of maternal behavior, mammary gland enlargement, and lactation.

Synonyms

Nervous anorexia, pseudopregnancy, overt false pregnancy

Epidemiology

SPECIES, AGE, SEX

Postpubertal female dogs of any age; has not been described in cats

GENETICS, BREED PREDISPOSITION

- Any breed; incidence is higher among Dalmatians, basset hounds, and pointer-breed dogs.
- German shepherds and beagles are rarely affected.

RISK FACTORS

Exogenous administration of progestins, diestrous ovariectomy, and/or hypothyroidism may trigger its occurrence.

ASSOCIATED DISORDERS

May predispose to mastitis

Clinical Presentation

DISEASE FORMS/SUBTYPES

Depends on intensity of clinical signs:

- Covert: physiologic, although recognizable from the rest of the estrous cycle
- Overt: physical and behavioral manifestations become a clinical problem (clinical pseudocyesis)

HISTORY, CHIEF COMPLAINT

- Estrus 6-12 weeks before, without ensuing pregnancy
- Chief complaints: mammary problems (engorgement, lactation, licking of the glands) and abnormalities associated with aberrant maternal behavior (nesting, digging, adoption of animals or objects)
- Depression or anxiety, anorexia, and excessive vocalization (whining) are possible.

PHYSICAL EXAM FINDINGS

- Mammary enlargement, ranging from turgid nipples to painful engorgement and galactostasis, is most evident in the caudal pair of glands.
- Mammary dermatitis occasionally occurs if excessive licking occurs.

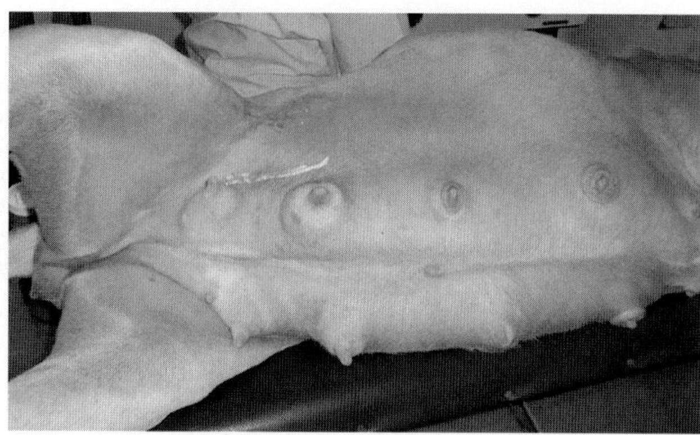

PSEUDOCYESIS Enlargement of mammary glands in a 3-year-old bitch suffering from clinical pseudocyesis.

Etiology and Pathophysiology

- Associated with a high plasma concentration of prolactin at the end of the luteal phase, when progesterone concentrations decrease abruptly
  - Pseudocyesis is maintained when owners relieve galactostasis by milking or when the bitch excessively licks the mammary glands and elicits milk letdown (self-milking).
- Individual and breed sensitivity to these hormonal changes and environmental factors may influence its occurrence.

DIAGNOSIS

Diagnostic Overview

The diagnosis is suspected in any diestrous, nonpregnant bitch with mammary enlargement (and milk secretion) in which other mammary disease has been ruled out. Diagnostic imaging confirms absence of pregnancy if necessary.

Differential Diagnosis

- Pregnancy
- Pyometra
- Mastitis
- Mammary tumors
- Any other cause of anorexia, depression, or anxiety should be ruled out.
- Pseudocyesis can coexist with pyometra, mastitis, and mammary tumors.

Initial Database

CBC results are unremarkable.

Advanced or Confirmatory Testing

Ultrasonographic or radiographic confirmation of the absence of pregnancy or pyometra

TREATMENT

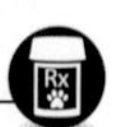

Treatment Overview

Treatment is not necessary in mildly affected bitch. When appropriate, treatment mainly consists of the administration of antiprolactinic drugs (dopamine agonists or anti-serotonergic compounds).

Acute General Treatment

- Administer dopamine agonists with food to reduce digestive side effects. Cabergoline 5 mcg/kg PO q 24h for 5-7 days is a safer choice compared with other antiprolactinic drugs.
- Avoid steroid hormones (progestins/androgens) because they usually postpone the problem.
- Treat local dermatitis (p. 851).

Chronic Treatment

Clinical chronic, unresponsive, or recurring pseudocyesis cases should be treated surgically (ovariectomy) after the acute phase of the syndrome has been controlled and during anestrus.

Nutrition/Diet

One study reported that short-term (7 days) partial food restriction (30%-50% of maintenance) did not cure pseudocyesis, but it did hasten resolution of clinical signs.

Behavior/Exercise

- Discourage maternal behavior using aversion methods.
- Avoid stimulation of the mammary glands (e.g., hot or cold packing, touching, or milking).
- If necessary, Elizabethan collars can be used for preventing licking and self-milking.

Drug Interactions

- Avoid administering phenothiazine drugs and metoclopramide during pseudocyesis because they increase plasma prolactin concentrations.
- Do not administer antiserotonergic drugs (e.g., metergoline) for anxious and restless bitches because they can potentiate pseudocyesis behavior.

Possible Complications

- Mammary dermatitis is the most frequent complication and may have an influence in perpetuating the problem.
- Repeated episodes of pseudocyesis have been hypothetically associated with the future development of mammary tumors.

Recommended Monitoring

Follow cases until complete resolution. If pseudocyesis does not resolve spontaneously, look for predisposing causes (see Risk Factors above).

PROGNOSIS & OUTCOME

Pseudocyesis typically resolves spontaneously within 2 or 3 weeks from its onset but can occasionally persist until the next estrous cycle.

PEARLS & CONSIDERATIONS

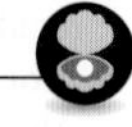

Comments

- Pseudocyesis is a good indicator of ovulatory estrous cycles.
- Predisposed bitches usually suffer the syndrome after each estrous cycle, and the disorder becomes more severe throughout life.

Prevention

- Ovariectomy in predisposed bitches
- Pregnancy does not prevent future episodes.

Technician Tips

- Avoid stimulation of the mammary glands (e.g., hot or cold packing, touching, or milking).
- If necessary, Elizabethan collars can be used for preventing licking and self-milking.

Client Education

Teach clients to recognize pseudocyesis and ask for treatment if it becomes clinically relevant.

SUGGESTED READING

Gobello C, et al: A review of canine pseudocyesis. Reprod Domest Anim 36(6):283-288, 2001.

AUTHOR: Cristina Gobello, MV, DMV, DECAR
EDITOR: Michelle A. Kutzler, DVM, PhD, DACT

Ptyalism

BASIC INFORMATION

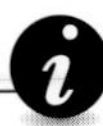

Definition

Production of excessive amounts of saliva, commonly manifested as drooling

Synonyms

Hypersalivation, polysialia, sialorrhea

Epidemiology

SPECIES, AGE, SEX

- Any dog or cat
- Young animals: oral foreign body, portosystemic shunts (PSSs; especially in cats)
- Older animals: oral neoplasia, dental abscess, megaesophagus

GENETICS, BREED PREDISPOSITION

Depends on underlying cause

RISK FACTORS

- Trauma of oral/pharyngeal region or nerves
- Exposure to toxins (e.g., organophosphates, mushrooms, frogs/toads)
- Esophageal disorders (esophagitis, esophageal obstruction, megaesophagus)
- Oral foreign bodies
- Severe dental disease, including abscesses
- Metabolic or physical disorders causing nausea or abdominal pain
- Neurologic disorders
- Nausea
- Infectious disease

CONTAGION AND ZOONOSIS

Contagion: viral infections causing oral lesions (e.g., calicivirus in cats) or nausea (e.g., parvovirus)

Clinical Presentation

HISTORY, CHIEF COMPLAINT

Inquire about potential toxicant exposures, especially if acute onset. All or some may be recognized:

- Salivary gland enlargement
- Dysphagia
- Pawing at mouth
- Halitosis
- Oral discomfort with oral or pharyngeal causes
- Anorexia or weight loss
- Coughing and/or dyspnea (from aspiration pneumonia)
- Gagging, retching, or vomiting
- Seizures, facial twitching, behavioral changes (intoxications or PSS)

PHYSICAL EXAM FINDINGS

Depending on cause, may identify:

- Saliva around mouth, salivary staining of fur
- Oral lesions (e.g., masses, foreign bodies, abscesses, stomatitis, gingivitis, dental diseases)
- Swelling of salivary glands, facial paralysis, atrophy of temporal or facial muscles
- Loss of gag reflex, inability to use tongue, dysphagia
- Mentation changes, seizures, tremors, or anxiety
- Nausea, lip licking, painful abdomen

Etiology and Pathophysiology

- Cause is discussed on p. 1274.
- Pathophysiology: oral secretions are produced by submandibular, parotid, and sublingual salivary glands. Innervation of salivary glands is controlled by the autonomic nervous system, with primary control by the parasympathetic nervous system. Many environmental, physical, or metabolic events can stimulate increased saliva production.

DIAGNOSIS

Diagnostic Overview

A complete medical history and thorough oral exam, possibly under sedation, often leads the clinician in the right direction for diagnosis. For instance, an outdoor cat with acute onset of drooling may have oral ulcers, evidence of intoxication, or a foreign body.

Differential Diagnosis

Certain conformations of the lips cause drooling with normal saliva production. History (conformation-associated drooling is chronic) and physical exam of the lips are generally sufficient for correct identification. Drooling can also be caused by disorders that prevent swallowing normal volumes of saliva.

Initial Database

- CBC: possible evidence of infectious/inflammatory disease
- Serum biochemistry profile and urinalysis: possible evidence of metabolic disorders
- Neurologic exam (p. 1136)
- Thoracic, abdominal, and neck/head radiographs, if indicated

Advanced or Confirmatory Testing

- Oral exam with sedation or anesthesia (pp. 1125 and 1140)
- If PSS suspected, serum bile acids
- Abdominal ultrasound
- Electroencephalogram, CT, and/or MRI to evaluate central nervous system lesions
- Endoscopy to evaluate esophageal or gastric lesions
- Specific tests, such as toxin screen, acetylcholine (ACh) receptor antibody testing for myasthenia gravis, or infectious disease testing, as indicated

TREATMENT

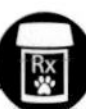

Treatment Overview

Ptyalism is a clinical sign, and treatment is aimed at the underlying cause.

Acute and Chronic Treatment

- Supportive and nonspecific; possible use of anticholinergics, antinausea, or antianxiety medications
- Address underlying cause.

Behavior/Exercise

Behavioral modification and antianxiety medication for stress-related hypersalivation

Possible Complications

- Aspiration, potentially leading to pneumonia
- Anticholinergics often cause tachycardia, constipation, and behavioral changes; they require frequent dosing. Antiemetics such as chlorpromazine may cause sedation.
- Antisialagogues may reduce salivary output but do not correct the underlying problem.
- Antianxiety medications may cause sedation, anorexia, gastrointestinal upset.

Recommended Monitoring

Monitor for coughing, breathing difficulty, and fever, which may suggest aspiration.

PROGNOSIS & OUTCOME

- Depends on response to treatment of underlying cause of ptyalism
- Removal of foreign bodies, resolution of dental disease, repair of traumatic injury, and response to decontamination of toxins have very favorable outcomes.
- Prognosis is guarded with more serious disease processes such as neoplasia.

PEARLS & CONSIDERATIONS

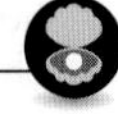

Comments

- Ptyalism is often a sign of a more serious disorder and deserves attention aimed at identifying the underlying cause.
- Owners may find that their pet's ptyalism is unacceptable even if caused by minor problems, prompting consideration of euthanasia if unresolved.
- Bilaterally symmetrical salivary gland enlargement accompanied by ptyalism, gagging, weight loss, hyporexia, ± vomiting suggests phenobarbital-responsive sialadenosis.

Technician Tips

- Monitor patients for coughing, dyspnea, or retching, which could indicate aspiration pneumonia or choking. Monitor ability to prehend, chew, and swallow food or water.

- Although rare, remember rabies as a potential cause of difficulty swallowing and salivation. Wear gloves and use caution (p. 861).

SUGGESTED READING

Heinze C, et al: Ptyalism and halitosis. In Ettinger SJ, et al, editors: Textbook of veterinary internal medicine, ed 8, St. Louis, 2017, Elsevier, pp 146-152.

AUTHOR: Diana M. Schropp, DVM, DACVECC
EDITOR: Leah A. Cohn, DVM, PhD, DACVIM

Pulmonary Bullae and Blebs

Client Education Sheet 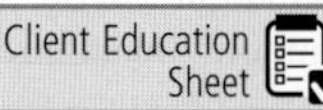

BASIC INFORMATION

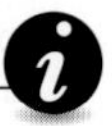

Definition

The focus of this chapter is idiopathic bullae and blebs rather than the bullae created by recognized parenchymal disease (e.g., neoplasia, parasites).

- Bulla: an air-filled space within the pulmonary parenchyma that arises from alveolar distention or destruction of alveolar walls
- Bleb: an accumulation of air within the mesothelial covering and layers of elastic fibers/connective tissue cells that comprise the visceral pleura

Synonym

Bullous emphysema

Epidemiology

SPECIES, AGE, SEX

Idiopathic bullae are reported most commonly in middle-aged dogs, although dogs of any age can be affected. Cats are rarely affected.

GENETICS, BREED PREDISPOSITION

- A familial or genetic predisposition has not been demonstrated.
- Large, deep-chested dog breeds are considered at greater risk for pulmonary blebs and bullae.

RISK FACTORS

- Congenital bronchial hypoplasia (uncommon) reported in dogs and cats
- Chronic obstructive small airway diseases are a risk factor for people and may be for dogs and cats.

ASSOCIATED DISORDERS

- Congenital bronchial hypoplasia
- Congenital bronchial cartilage hypoplasia/dysplasia
- Inflammatory airway disease
- Spontaneous pneumothorax
- Pneumomediastinum (uncommon)
- Subcutaneous emphysema (uncommon)
- Pneumopericardium (uncommon)

Clinical Presentation

DISEASE FORMS/SUBTYPES

- Usually an acquired disease
- Congenital forms of bullous/emphysematous lung disease, usually secondary to bronchial hypoplasia or bronchial cartilage defects, have been described.

HISTORY, CHIEF COMPLAINT

Animals may be clinically normal:

- A pulmonary bleb or bulla may be found incidentally during thoracic imaging, thoracotomy, or thoracoscopy.

Clinical signs, when present, can be acute, intermittent, or slowly progressive:

- Anorexia
- Lethargy
- Respiratory distress
  - Rupture of a bleb or bulla, causing spontaneous pneumothorax, is typically associated with acute respiratory distress.
- Cough
- Exercise intolerance

PHYSICAL EXAM FINDINGS

- Respiratory distress
- Increased inspiratory effort (pneumothorax)
- Increased expiratory effort (pulmonary emphysema without pneumothorax)
- Tachypnea
- Tachycardia
- Diminished heart and lung sounds on one or both sides if pneumothorax (p. 797)
- Subcutaneous emphysema (occasional)

Etiology and Pathophysiology

- Histopathologic assessment of resected tissues classifies lesions as blebs or bullae.
- Mechanisms leading to idiopathic bulla or bleb formation are not defined.
  - Suspected to reflect the effects of distensile or traction forces on the lung surface or effects of inflammation or degradative enzymes in the alveoli that break down alveolar walls
  - Increased alveolar pressure relative to transpleural pressure may also contribute.
  - Obstructive small airway disease potentially could contribute to air trapping and increased alveolar pressure.

DIAGNOSIS

Diagnostic Overview

In patients with spontaneous pneumothorax, definitive diagnosis usually depends on exclusion of other causes of pneumothorax after evaluation of patient history, physical exam, radiographic imaging, and then surgical observation of typical lesions.

Differential Diagnosis

- Other causes of pneumothorax: blunt or penetrating trauma to the thoracic wall, trachea, esophagus, or pulmonary parenchyma
- Inflammatory lung disease
- Neoplastic lung disease
- Parasitic lung disease, especially *Paragonimus kellicotti* and *Dirofilaria immitis*
- Obstructive airway disease
- Migrating foreign bodies

Initial Database

- Thoracic radiographs
  - May demonstrate pneumothorax (p. 797)
  - Lung parenchyma often unremarkable; observation of a bleb or bulla is uncommon.
  - Animals with paragonimiasis may have thick-walled bullae that are evident, even with pneumothorax.
  - Thoracic radiographs may show air-filled dilations within the parenchyma.
  - Occasionally, animals may have pneumomediastinum, pneumopericardium, or subcutaneous emphysema.
- Thoracic ultrasound can be used to quickly and safely detect pneumothorax (p. 1102)
- Results of a CBC, biochemical profile, and urinalysis are typically normal.
- Hypoxemia is the most common abnormality on arterial blood gas analysis.
- Fecal exams (flotation and sedimentation techniques) to rule out respiratory parasites

Advanced or Confirmatory Testing

- Definitive diagnosis is usually made by detection of bullae, blebs, or air leaking from the lung surface during thoracotomy or thoracoscopy and confirmed with histopathologic exam of resected tissue.
  - Median sternotomy is the preferred approach in patients with spontaneous pneumothorax.
  - Cranial lung lobes are most commonly affected, although other lung lobes can have lesions.
- Tracheoscopy, bronchoscopy, and esophagoscopy results are usually normal for patients with bullous lung disease unless airway hypoplasia is present.
- Thoracic CT is more sensitive than plain thoracic radiographs for the detection of bullae in dogs with spontaneous pneumothorax but cannot detect all lesions.

TREATMENT

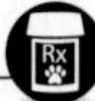

Treatment Overview

- Improve respiratory function and oxygenation, typically by thoracocentesis, in

patients with respiratory distress induced by pneumothorax.
- Remove bullae or blebs, if possible.
- Treat any underlying obstructive disease.

Acute General Treatment

- Thoracocentesis if pneumothorax is present (p. 1164)
  - Thoracostomy tubes with continuous suction may be needed in some patients for management of persistent air accumulation.
- Oxygen provided by mask, nasal catheter, or oxygen cage (p. 1146)
- Cage rest
- Instillation of whole blood into the thoracic cavity (i.e., blood patch) has been used to address pneumothorax (see Suggested Readings).

Chronic Treatment

- Long-term resolution of spontaneous pneumothorax from ruptured blebs or bullae, if not from parasitic diseases, is most reliably achieved by surgical resection of diseased lung (partial or complete lobectomy) by thoracotomy or thoracoscopy.
  - Persistence or recurrence of clinical signs is more likely if patient is managed nonsurgically.
  - If bullae are found in multiple lung lobes, surgery may not be an option.
  - The use of pleural ports to successfully manage persistent/recurrent pneumothorax has been described; this may be an option for patients that cannot have surgery.
- Treat underlying obstructive disease.

Possible Complications

- Pneumothorax from leakage at lobectomy site
- Postoperative complications of infection, wound dehiscence
- Recurrence of pneumothorax

Recommended Monitoring

Clinical signs; thoracic radiographs for recurrence of pneumothorax

PROGNOSIS & OUTCOME

Prognosis is generally good with surgical resection of bullous lung lesions.

PEARLS & CONSIDERATIONS

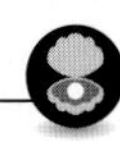

Comments

- In dogs with spontaneous pneumothorax of uncertain origin and no history of trauma, bleb or bulla rupture ultimately is often found to be the underlying cause.
- Unlike dogs, cats with spontaneous pneumothorax almost always have an identifiable underlying respiratory disease.
- Some animals can be successfully managed with nonsurgical methods (thoracocentesis, thoracostomy tubes), but the literature supports early lung lobectomy for the best long-term outcomes.
- Affected animals can have multiple lesions scattered over different lung lobes, and lung lobes on both sides of the thoracic cavity can be affected. It is imperative to examine the entirety of both lungs during thoracotomy or thoracoscopy.

Prevention

Animals with congenital bronchial hypoplasia should probably not be bred.

Technician Tips

- Thoracocentesis is most often done at about the seventh or eighth intercostal space, and these areas should be clipped in preparation for the procedure.
- Thoracocentesis to remove air can be performed in whichever position the patient is most comfortable, including sternal recumbency.

Client Education

Nonsurgical treatment approaches are more likely to be associated with persistence or recurrence of clinical signs. Postsurgical outcomes are usually excellent.

SUGGESTED READING

Puerto DA, et al: Surgical and nonsurgical management of and selected risk factors for spontaneous pneumothorax in dogs: 64 cases (1986-1999). J Am Vet Med Assoc 220:1670, 2002.

AUTHOR: Rance K. Sellon, DVM, PhD, DACVIM
EDITOR: Megan Grobman, DVM, MS, DACVIM

Pulmonary Contusions

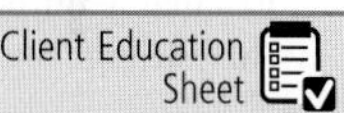

BASIC INFORMATION

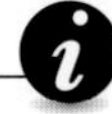

Definition

A lesion consisting of intrapulmonary hemorrhage and inflammation secondary to blunt trauma

Epidemiology

SPECIES, AGE, SEX

Young male dogs are at increased risk for trauma; small-breed dogs are more likely to have penetrating thoracic wounds.

RISK FACTORS

Free-roaming behavior; exposure to larger dogs

GEOGRAPHY AND SEASONALITY

More common in warmer months

ASSOCIATED DISORDERS

- Pneumothorax
- Diaphragmatic hernia
- Flail chest, rib fractures
- Hit by car (HBC) injury
- Fractures

Clinical Presentation

HISTORY, CHIEF COMPLAINT

Traumatic event; increased respiratory rate and effort, occasionally hemoptysis

PHYSICAL EXAM FINDINGS

- External evidence of trauma: cutaneous abrasions or lacerations, fractures
- Increased respiratory rate and effort
- Increased bronchovesicular sounds
- Pale mucous membranes associated with shock
- Tachycardia

Etiology and Pathophysiology

- Trauma results in intraparenchymal pulmonary hemorrhage. Extracapillary hemorrhage results in recruitment of inflammatory cells and protein into the alveolar and interstitial spaces.
- Pulmonary hemorrhage results in ventilation/perfusion mismatch and the potential for hypoxemia.
- Sequelae of pulmonary contusion may vary from very mild to rapidly fatal.

DIAGNOSIS

Diagnostic Overview

Suspected clinically because of association with blunt trauma; clinical confirmation is generally radiographic. Thoracic ultrasound may confirm the presence of B lines, which are associated with intrapulmonary fluid (p. 1102).

Differential Diagnosis

- Nontraumatic pulmonary hemorrhage (anticoagulant rodenticide, neoplasia, thrombocytopenia)
- Congestive heart failure (pulmonary edema)
- Pneumonia
- Pain (tachypnea)

Initial Database

- Thoracic radiographs: patchy to diffuse interstitial to alveolar pattern
  - Radiographic changes may lag behind clinical signs.
  - May be indistinguishable from other patchy interstitial infiltrates, especially pulmonary edema in cats

- CBC, serum biochemistry profile: generally unremarkable but may indicate hemorrhage or other associated injuries

Advanced or Confirmatory Testing

- Arterial blood gas (ABG) analysis or pulse oximetry: characterize the degree of hypoxemia. These tests are especially useful for determining whether tachypnea is due to pain (results are normal) or pulmonary lesions (hypoxemia commonly observed).
- Central venous pressure monitoring (CVP), pulmonary wedge pressure measurement: assess right- and left-sided vascular pressures, respectively (helps rule out cardiogenic causes). Pulmonary wedge pressure measurement is rarely performed clinically, and CVP may not provide significant extra information.

TREATMENT

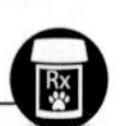

Treatment Overview

Treatment goals are to maintain adequate intravascular volume but avoid overhydration/hypervolemia, which may worsen pulmonary contusions, and to provide supplemental oxygen and rest.

Acute General Treatment

- Administration of supplemental oxygen (p. 1146), as appropriate
- Judicious administration of IV fluids as needed to maintain perfusion
  - Administration of boluses of 5-10 mL/kg of crystalloid fluids (e.g., lactated Ringer's solution) until adequate blood pressure (BP) and pulse quality are obtained
  - Colloids may also be considered for vascular volume support, depending on the patient.
- Address other associated injuries (e.g., head trauma, limb fractures).
- Glucocorticoids, antibiotics, and diuretics are NOT indicated for treatment of pulmonary contusions.
- If contusions are associated with penetrating thoracic wounds, exploratory thoracotomy may be warranted.

Behavior/Exercise

Cage/house rest until respiratory rate and effort are normal

Possible Complications

- Infection (rare)
- Respiratory failure
- Severe pulmonary contusion may require positive-pressure ventilation (p. 1185) with positive end-expiratory pressure (PEEP) and may progress to acute respiratory distress syndrome (p. 27).

Recommended Monitoring

Hourly respiratory rate and effort; pulse oximetry/ABG if concerned about respiratory failure

PROGNOSIS & OUTCOME

- Guarded to good prognosis
- Most animals that survive the trip to the hospital also survive pulmonary contusions with appropriate supportive care.
- Concurrent injuries (e.g., vertebral body fractures) are more likely to compromise the prognosis.
- Other than very severe cases, pulmonary contusions generally resolve with supportive care.

PEARLS & CONSIDERATIONS

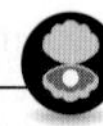

Comments

- Avoid excessive volume resuscitation; administer IV fluids judiciously, and adjust the rate frequently based on the animal's response and evolution of the case.
- Avoid diuretic therapy (e.g., furosemide) because intravascular volume contraction may be detrimental.

Prevention

Animals should be on leash or otherwise protected from trauma (e.g., indoor cats).

Technician Tips

Animals with pulmonary contusions can have a very dynamic clinical course and must be monitored closely for changes in respiratory effort.

Client Education

Pulmonary contusions are lung bruises. The injured animal often gets worse over the first 24 hours, and the lesions then regress in the next 48 hours.

SUGGESTED READING

Powell LL, et al: A retrospective analysis of pulmonary contusion secondary to motor vehicle accidents in 143 dogs: 1994-1997. J Vet Emerg Crit Care 9:127-136, 1999.

AUTHOR: Elizabeth Rozanski, DVM, DACVIM, DACVECC
EDITOR: Benjamin M. Brainard, VMD, DACVAA, DACVECC

Pulmonary Edema, Noncardiogenic

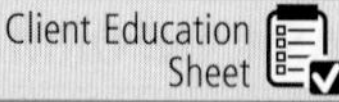

BASIC INFORMATION

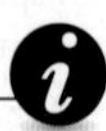

Definition

Extravascular fluid accumulation in the pulmonary interstitium and/or alveolar space secondary to a noncardiac cause

Synonyms

Selected forms of noncardiogenic pulmonary edema (NPE) are referred to as increased permeability edema, neurogenic pulmonary edema, negative-pressure pulmonary edema, and acute respiratory distress syndrome (ARDS [p. 27]).

Epidemiology

SPECIES, AGE, SEX

- More common in dogs than cats
- Although any animal can develop NPE, predispositions are recognized for some causes (e.g., young animals are more likely than older animals to chew electric cords).

GENETICS, BREED PREDISPOSITION

Obstructive airway disease is more likely in brachycephalic dogs (p. 128) and retrievers (laryngeal paralysis [p. 574]).

RISK FACTORS

- Seizures
- Electrocution
- Specific toxin or drug ingestion (see Differential Diagnosis)
- Aggressive thoracocentesis or mechanical ventilation
- Smoke inhalation/inhaled irritants
- Acute upper airway obstruction (e.g., laryngeal paralysis, tracheal foreign body)
- Vasculitis
- Anaphylaxis
- Near drowning
- Sepsis or systemic inflammatory response syndrome
- Severe lung injury of any cause
- Severe trauma resulting in pulmonary contusions, head trauma, or coagulopathy
- Multiple blood transfusions
- Hypercoagulable state secondary to inflammatory, infectious, endocrine, or protein-losing diseases

ASSOCIATED DISORDERS

See Risk Factors above.

Clinical Presentation

DISEASE FORMS/SUBTYPES

- Increased permeability edema
- Mixed pulmonary edema (PE) due to permeability and hydrostatic pressure change

  - Neurogenic
  - Reexpansion
  - Negative pressure

HISTORY, CHIEF COMPLAINT

- History might identify known risk factors (e.g., smoke inhalation, near drowning, choking episode)
- Varying degrees of respiratory distress (p. 879)

PHYSICAL EXAM FINDINGS

- Acute respiratory distress and tachypnea
  - Often mixed inspiratory and expiratory effort
  - Cyanosis, serous nasal discharge, and cough possible
- Thoracic auscultation
  - Often harsh or loud bronchovesicular sounds ± fine crackles, especially in the dorsocaudal lung fields
  - Murmur, arrhythmia, or gallop increases suspicion for cardiogenic pulmonary edema but do not rule out NPE.
- Other findings can reflect cause of NPE:
  - Lingual ulceration due to electric cord electrocution
  - Stridor with laryngeal paralysis or obstruction
  - Uremic breath and/or small kidneys with uremia

Etiology and Pathophysiology

- Increased permeability edema secondary to direct endothelial and/or alveolar epithelial injury, resulting in proteinaceous fluid accumulation in the alveoli
  - Any cause of ARDS (p. 27)
  - Pulmonary thromboembolism (p. 842)
  - Toxins/drugs: petroleum distillates, paraquat, zinc phosphate, arsenic, smoke inhalation, organophosphate/carbamate, calcium channel blockers, cisplatin (cats), cytarabine, oxygen toxicity (prolonged, high FIO_2), others
- Mixed PE: a combination of increased permeability and increased hydrostatic pressure from increased sympathetic nervous system (SNS) discharge, resulting in increased systemic and pulmonary capillary pressure
  - Re-expansion PE: acute re-expansion of chronically atelectic lung lobes
  - Neurogenic PE: head trauma, seizures, electrocution, near drowning
  - Negative pressure PE: strangulation, choking, upper airway obstruction
- Arterial hypoxemia and respiratory distress secondary to ventilation perfusion mismatching and, to a lesser extent, diffusion impairment
- Edema fluid from noncardiogenic cause has protein content equal to plasma, and cardiogenic edema fluid has a low protein content.
- Reduced oncotic pressure alone is unlikely to cause PE because of generous pulmonary lymphatics, but low colloid oncotic pressure can worsen edema severity.

DIAGNOSIS

Diagnostic Overview

Provide oxygen and minimize stress during diagnostic investigation. History often provides clues that NPE is likely, as does physical exam. Imaging studies confirm pulmonary infiltrates. If the cause of NPE is not clear based on history or exam, testing to determine a cause can begin after the patient is stabilized.

Differential Diagnosis

- Cardiogenic PE (pp. 408 and 409)
- Primary respiratory disease
  - Infectious pneumonia: bacterial (p. 795), viral (pp. 987 and 545), verminous (p. 595)
  - Aspiration pneumonia (p. 793)
  - Foreign body (p. 355)
  - Neoplasia (p. 134)
  - Pulmonary contusions (p. 835)
  - Interstitial lung disease (p. 553)
  - Lung lobe torsion (p. 593)
- Heartworm disease (pp. 415 and 418)
- Pleural space disease (p. 791)

Initial Database

- Thoracic radiographs: varies
  - Mixed interstitial and alveolar (≈77%) > interstitial (≈26%) pattern
  - Peripheral (≈90%) > central distribution
  - Focal or multifocal (≈77%) > diffuse
  - Bilateral (≈77%) > unilateral
  - Dorsal (≈58%) > ventral
- CBC/serum biochemistry profile/urinalysis: may be unremarkable or reflect systemic disease (e.g., uremia, pancreatitis, sepsis)
- Pulse oximetry: depends on severity of NPE; < 95% on room air suggests respiratory impairment

Advanced or Confirmatory Testing

- Point-of-care test for N-terminal pro-brain-type natriuretic peptide (NT-pro-BNP) to rule out a cardiac cause for respiratory distress in cats; a positive test warrants an echocardiogram
- Echocardiogram to rule out cardiogenic PE (especially if cardiac exam abnormal)
- Cage-side lung ultrasound exam (veterinary bedside lung ultrasound exam [Vet BLUE]) can detect changes suggestive of pulmonary edema (i.e., B lines in the dorsocaudal lung field) or alternative causes of distress (e.g., pleural effusion, left atrial enlargement).
- Arterial blood gas is nonspecific for NPE but can reveal hypoxemia.
- Heartworm antigen (dog) or antigen and antibody (cat) testing
- If pneumonia or other lung disease is suspected, bronchoscopy with bronchoalveolar lavage (pp. 1073 and 1074) for infectious/inflammatory disease; with NPE, proteinaceous alveolar fluid expected

TREATMENT

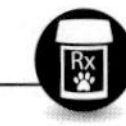

Treatment Overview

Minimize stress and handling of patients in respiratory distress, and focus on alleviation of hypoxemia. Identify and treat underlying disease whenever possible. Additional therapies, such as IV fluid therapy, should be tailored to the patient's needs.

Acute General Treatment

- Oxygen supplementation (flow-by, face mask, or oxygen cage [p. 1146]); if head trauma recognized, avoid nasal cannulas to minimize increases in intracranial pressure (ICP).
- A trial dose of furosemide 2 mg/kg IV or IM may be used to assess response to therapy before additional doses are prescribed. Diuretics are seldom useful in NPE because increased hydrostatic pressure is absent or transient.
- IV fluids should be administered judiciously as gauged by the animal's hydration and volume status and to avoid dramatic increase in capillary hydrostatic pressure.
- Whenever possible, address the underlying cause of NPE.
  - Upper airway obstruction (pp. 1004 and 1166)
  - Control seizures that can precipitate NPE (p. 903)
  - Treat sepsis (p. 907), uremia (pp. 23 and 169), or other systemic disease
  - Unfortunately, many causes of NPE cannot be readily resolved (e.g., near drowning, smoke inhalation, severe pancreatitis). Supportive care allows time for the injury/illness to resolve.
- Mechanical ventilation (p. 1185) if patient has a sustained increase in work of breathing, SpO_2 < 90%, PaO_2 < 60 mm Hg, or $PaCO_2$ > 55 mm Hg despite oxygen therapy.
- Unless needed to treat the underlying cause of NPE, there is no indication for antibiotics, glucocorticoids, or nonsteroidal antiinflammatory drugs.

Chronic Treatment

Depends on the underlying disease process

Possible Complications

- Mechanical ventilation: acute lung injury, hypotension, pneumothorax, and pneumonia.
- Appropriate ventilator settings, analgesia, fluid therapy, and nursing care can minimize complications.

Recommended Monitoring

- Frequent assessment of vital parameters with focus on respiratory rate and effort
- Blood pressure (invasive, Doppler, oscillometric)
- Oxygenation: arterial blood gas (p. 1058) or pulse oximetry
- Ventilation: blood gas analysis or $ETCO_2$
- Serial thoracic radiographs or CT if improvement lacking or to assess resolution

PROGNOSIS & OUTCOME

Prognosis depends on the cause, severity, and duration of NPE and on comorbidities.

Although conditions that result in increased permeability edema often carry a guarded prognosis, animals with neurogenic or negative-pressure PE often recover with hospitalization, time (24-48 hours), and supportive care.

PEARLS & CONSIDERATIONS

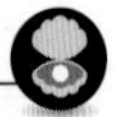

Comments

- Focus on fluid strategies that minimize increases in pulmonary capillary pressure because minor increases can exacerbate increased permeability edema.
- Hypertonic saline (7.5%) at doses of 2-4 mL/kg (dog) and 1-2 mL/kg (cat) provides low-volume resuscitation in cases of head trauma and increased ICP.

Technician Tips

- Monitor for clinical signs of volume overload, including weight gain, serous nasal discharge, chemosis, worsening respiratory rate or effort, gelatinous skin, and peripheral edema.
- Monitor respiratory rate for all hospitalized animals, and notify the clinician if the rate or effort change markedly.

SUGGESTED READING

Adamantos S, et al: Pulmonary edema. In Silverstein D, et al, editors: Small animal critical care medicine, ed 2, St. Louis, 2013, Saunders.

AUTHOR: **Meghan Harmon, DVM, DACVECC**
EDITOR: **Megan Grobman, DVM, MS, DACVIM**

Pulmonary Hypertension (Arterial)

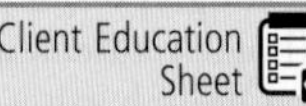

BASIC INFORMATION

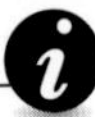

Definition

Pulmonary hypertension (PH) is increased pulmonary arterial pressure (PAP): systolic > 30 mm Hg and/or diastolic > 19 mm Hg. World Health Organization (WHO) classification of chronic PH adapted for dogs is based on similarities in pathophysiologic mechanisms:

- Group 1: pulmonary arterial hypertension (PAH): progressive vasoproliferative conditions
  - Idiopathic (formerly primary PH [PPH]): no underlying cause is found, characteristic histologic abnormalities in small pulmonary arteries
  - Associated with congenital systemic-to-pulmonic shunts, drugs, toxins, inflammatory conditions
- Group 2: left heart disease
  - Left ventricular or atrial disease
  - Left-sided valvular disease (i.e., myxomatous mitral valve disease [MMVD])
- Group 3: respiratory disease and/or hypoxemia
  - Airway/interstitial disease
  - Chronic upper airway obstruction
  - High altitude (chronic)
- Group 4: thrombotic/embolic disease
  - Primary pulmonary arterial lesion (e.g., *Dirofilaria immitis, Angiostrongylus vasorum*)
  - Diseases predisposing to pulmonary thromboembolism (PTE)
  - Tumor embolism
- Group 5: miscellaneous (e.g., neoplasm compressing pulmonary arteries)

Epidemiology

SPECIES, AGE, SEX

- Dogs > cats
- Group 1: PAH
  - Idiopathic: any age (rare)
  - Young animals (cats > dogs) with congenital cardiac shunt
  - Dogs of any age after elimination of *A. vasorum*
- Group 2: left heart disease
  - Middle-aged to older small-breed dogs with MMVD; most common cause for PH (dogs)
  - Cats are resistant to PH from chronic left-sided heart disease.
- Group 3: respiratory disease and hypoxemia
  - Signalment varies with cause of hypoxemia
  - Older dogs (rarely cats) with chronic interstitial lung disease
  - Middle-aged to older dogs (rarely cats) with chronic upper airway, laryngeal or tracheal, and chronic bronchial disease
- Group 4: thrombotic/embolic disease
  - Chronic PTE is a rare cause of PH in dogs and even less common in cats.
  - PTE secondary to *A. vasorum* (dogs) or *D. immitis* (dogs or cats) at any age
- Group 5: miscellaneous, pulmonary arterial compression
  - Older dogs: chemodectoma compressing pulmonary artery (older dogs, rare)

GENETICS, BREED PREDISPOSITION

Depends on underlying cause:

- MMVD: poodles, dachshunds, terriers, Cavalier King Charles spaniels, and other small breeds
- Chronic obstructive upper airway disease: brachycephalic dogs
- Pulmonary fibrosis: terrier breeds; West Highland white, Staffordshire, or other terriers

RISK FACTORS

- PTE (p. 842)
- Potential genetic risk for some causes of PH
- Lack of heartworm prophylaxis (*D. immitis*), snail ingestion (*A. vasorum* [French heartworm])
- Acute respiratory distress syndrome (ARDS [p. 27])

GEOGRAPHY AND SEASONALITY

- *D. immitis*: worldwide distribution (temperate climates)
- *A. vasorum*: in Europe and Newfoundland, Canada; probably most important cause of acute PH in endemic areas due to interstitial lung disease (group 3) and thrombosis (group 4)
- High altitude (hypobaric hypoxia): contributes to PH, but dogs at 3500 m altitude (11,500 feet) and mean arterial PO_2 of 52 mm Hg had a mean systolic PAP of only about 40 mm Hg as determined by Doppler evaluation of tricuspid regurgitation (TR).
- Atypical *Ehrlichia canis* infection (interstitial pneumopathy) may be a cause of PH in endemic areas.

Clinical Presentation

DISEASE FORMS/SUBTYPES

- Acute (e.g., ARDS, PTE, pulmonary veno-occlusive disease [PVOD])
- Chronic (e.g. MMVD, PAH)
- Acute-on-chronic (e.g., pulmonary edema in left-sided congestive heart failure, hypoxic pulmonary artery vasoconstriction)

HISTORY, CHIEF COMPLAINT

- May be an incidental finding (e.g., right ventricular hypertrophy on radiographs obtained for unrelated reason)
- Signs associated with acute moderate or severe chronic PH
  - Exercise intolerance
  - Collapse/syncope
  - Respiratory distress
  - Coughing
  - Abdominal distention
- Signs related to underlying cause of PH (e.g., rear limb weakness from reverse patent ductus arteriosus [PDA], coagulopathy from *A. vasorum* infection); often, signs due to the cause of PH are identical to the signs of PH (e.g., cough associated with MMVD, congestive heart failure, or heartworm infection)

PHYSICAL EXAM FINDINGS

Group 1: PAH; may be unremarkable or may demonstrate

- Pale mucous membranes or cyanosis
- Respiratory distress (p. 879)
  - May be precipitated/exacerbated by exercise
- Cough
- Tachycardia

- Weak pulse
- Right-sided congestive heart failure (CHF) (e.g., jugular distention or jugular pulse, ascites)
- Split-second heart sound (pulmonic valve closing after aortic valve)
- TR murmur (systolic, right-sided)
- Pulmonic regurgitation murmur (rare; diastolic, left heart base)
- Hyperemic mucous membranes due to erythrocytosis (response to hypoxemia)
- Differential cyanosis in reverse PDA (often only after exercise)

Group 2: PH with left-sided heart disease; same as PAH plus

- Loud mitral regurgitation murmur, increased lung sounds/crackles with CHF
- Intensity of mitral murmur may decrease with progression of PH; intensity of TR murmur may increase.

Group 3: PH with respiratory disease/hypoxia; same as PAH plus

- Stertor or stridor with upper respiratory obstruction
- Abnormal lung sounds (e.g., harsh, loud, wheezes, crackles)
- Altered pattern of respiration, if present, can aid in disease localization (p. 879).

Group 4: PH due to thrombotic/embolic disease; same as PAH plus

- Hemoptysis
- Increased lung sounds
- Sometimes palpable tumor (e.g., neoplastic embolism)
- Exam findings suggestive of cause for PTE (e.g., signs of hyperadrenocorticism or protein-losing nephropathy)

Etiology and Pathophysiology

- Regardless of cause, PH can lead to cor pulmonale (right ventricular hypertrophy secondary to PH) and eventually to right-sided heart failure.
- In PAH, genetically mediated susceptibility to vascular injury is thought to be a final common response to inciting factors such as mechanical lesions (overperfusion), drugs, toxins, and infections.
- PH is a common complication of cardiac and extracardiac diseases causing increased left atrial pressure and increased pulmonary vascular resistance.
- Important causes:
  - Cardiac: pulmonary venous hypertension due to increased left atrial pressure in left myocardial failure, most common in advanced MMVD and occasionally in dilated cardiomyopathy, cor triatriatum sinister, and mitral stenosis
  - Congenital left-to-right cardiac shunt: causes pulmonary overcirculation and, in some individuals, pulmonary arterial remodeling and constriction leading to PAH. This results in right-to-left shunt in the minority of patients (i.e., Eisenmenger physiology)
  - Hypoxic vasoconstriction: chronic obstructive lower airway disease (bronchitis, emphysema); chronic obstructive upper airway disease; high-altitude hypoxia
  - Pulmonary vascular bed occlusion: PTE; parasites (*D. immitis, A. vasorum*); embolism (e.g., tumor)
  - Pulmonary parenchymal disease: interstitial pneumonia (*A. vasorum, E. canis*); interstitial lung disease (p. 553); ARDS (p. 27)
  - Multiple mechanisms can occur simultaneously (e.g., heartworm infection causing obstruction by intravascular parasites, vasculitis, thrombosis, hypoxic vasoconstriction, and vascular remodeling)

DIAGNOSIS

Diagnostic Overview

A clinical diagnosis of PH is made when high-velocity valvular regurgitation (tricuspid, pulmonic, or both) is documented by Doppler echocardiography in the absence of pulmonic stenosis.

Differential Diagnosis

- Right-sided heart failure
  - Congenital cardiac disease: pulmonic stenosis, tricuspid dysplasia, tricuspid stenosis, cor triatriatum dexter
  - Acquired cardiovascular disease: severe myxomatous/degenerative tricuspid valve disease, right ventricular cardiomyopathy, pericardial effusion, heartworm
- Right ventricular hypertrophy
  - Pulmonic stenosis, tetralogy of Fallot

Initial Database

- Thoracic radiographs; dorsoventral view is particularly important.
  - Right ventricular and main pulmonary artery enlargement; nonspecific, reversed D, and increased sternal contact on the lateral view are often overinterpreted in normal dogs and cats (expiratory films, rotation of patient, thoracic conformation).
  - Tortuous/enlarged peripheral pulmonary vasculature
  - Peripheral pulmonary arterial markings may abruptly stop with PTE.
  - Enlarged left atrium and congested pulmonary veins with underlying left atrial, ventricular, or mitral valve disease; left-sided cardiac enlargement may decrease in chronic MMVD and associated chronic PH.
  - Underlying bronchial, interstitial, or alveolar pulmonary disease may be evident (e.g., classic peripheral interstitial to alveolar opacities in *A. vasorum*) but importantly may also be unremarkable in severe interstitial and thromboembolic lung disease.
  - Noncardiogenic pulmonary edema, responsive to sildenafil, may occur in dogs with chronic pulmonary disease.
- Echocardiogram
  - Identify causes of PH, including (acquired) left ventricular heart disease (MMVD), *D. immitis* (worms in pulmonary arteries, right ventricle, or right atrium), and congenital cardiovascular shunt.
  - Qualitative confirmation of PH: characteristic two-dimensional (2D) and M-mode findings in moderate to severe PH are dilation of right ventricle and atrium, thickening of right ventricular wall and papillary muscles, septal flattening, prominent pulmonary artery, and decreased left ventricular chamber size. CAVEAT: 2D abnormalities are usually prominent only if PH is severe or acute.
  - Quantitative confirmation of PH: Doppler exam is the most useful noninvasive clinical tool to confirm and quantitate severity of PH. Velocity of TR correlates with right ventricular systolic pressure and therefore, barring pulmonic stenosis, with pulmonary arterial systolic pressure. Vmax > 3-3.5 m/s reflects mild, 3.5-4.5 indicates moderate, and > 4.5 indicates severe PH. In chronic PH, Vmax < 4.0 m/s does not usually cause clinical signs due to PH. CAVEAT: loading conditions, right ventricular systolic function and sedation may significantly affect peak velocities. For Doppler quantification of pulmonary valve insufficiency (PI), peak velocity correlates with mean PAP and end-diastolic velocity with diastolic PAP.
- Electrocardiogram (ECG): document right ventricular hypertrophy (deep S waves in leads I, II, III, aVF), right axis deviation, and possible arrhythmias; in acute PH, ECG abnormalities may not be present; in chronic PH, PH must be marked to cause abnormalities, and ECG therefore is not a sensitive tool.
- Serology or other parasite testing (e.g., *D. immitis* or *A. vasorum* serology; Baermann fecal exam)
- Platelet count, coagulation profile, and parameters associated with hypercoagulability (e.g., antithrombin and D-dimer) may be abnormal with vasculitis and acute thrombosis but mostly normal in chronic PTE.
- Arterial blood gas analysis (p. 1058): hypoxemia in primary respiratory disease or right-to-left cardiovascular shunt
- CBC/biochemistry panel/urinalysis: abnormalities may suggest parasitic disease (eosinophilia, basophilia; not commonly found with *A. vasorum*), chronic inflammation (thrombocytosis, hyperglobulinemia), and systemic disease predisposing to PTE (e.g., proteinuria, hypoalbuminemia, increased liver enzyme activities consistent with steroid hepatopathy)
- Natriuretic peptides may be increased in PH; the combination of respiratory distress and increased natriuretic peptides is not proof for respiratory distress being caused by heart failure.

Advanced or Confirmatory Testing

- Contrast (microbubbles) ultrasound of the heart and descending aorta can exclude right-to-left shunt. Shunt is also possible due to pulmonary arteriovenous anastomoses secondary to PH; in this case, bubbles take ≥ 3 cardiac cycles from appearance in the right atrium until appearance in the left atrium.

- Pulmonary angiography: tortuous pulmonary arteries indicate PH; perfusion deficits occur in PTE.
- Pulmonary CT much more sensitive to identify/rule out parenchymal disease
  - CT-angiography for PTE: less sensitive and specific than expected
- Pulmonary ventilation/perfusion scintigraphy to rule out PTE (rarely performed)
- Pulmonary wedge pressure: estimate of left atrial pressure, systolic and diastolic pulmonary artery pressure; evaluate therapeutic response
- Pulmonary histopathology: not recommended to diagnose PH but may be necessary to identify the underlying disease process

TREATMENT

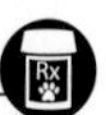

Treatment Overview

Lower PAP in patients with signs of right ventricular failure, improve oxygenation in patients with hypoxemia, and correct/improve underlying disease.

Acute General Treatment

- Oxygen therapy (cage or nasal), as necessary (p. 1146)
- Sildenafil 2-3 mg/kg q 8-12h PO to lower PAP if clinical signs plausibly due to PH.
- Pimobendan 0.2-0.3 mg/kg PO q 12h to increase systolic function in CHF due to MMVD
- Careful fluid balance in cases with suspected increased pulmonary vascular permeability: balance of close to zero or negative fluid balance to avoid additional pulmonary edema
- Clopidogrel 1-3 mg/kg PO q 24h for potential thrombotic pulmonary vascular disease

Specific treatments:

- PH secondary to congenital cardiovascular shunt may be reversible. Patients with newly developing PH and known PDA and patients with PDA and moderate to severe PH but still with left-to-right shunting should be sent for correction as soon as possible.
- Cardiogenic pulmonary edema: reduce preload with diuretics and left- and right-sided afterload with amlodipine (p. 408)
- ARDS and acute severe interstitial lung disease: consider ventilator if underlying disease and its prognosis justify; extracorporal membrane oxygenation if available.
- Right-heart failure due to parasitic pulmonary vascular disease–induced PTE: *D. immitis* (pp. 415 and 418); *A. vasorum*: recommend slow worm kill (i.e., fenbendazole 50 mg/kg PO q 24h for 21 days)
- Suspected pulmonary artery vasculitis *(D. immitis, A. vasorum, E. canis)*: prednisolone 1 mg/kg q 12h for 1 week, with slow taper over 1 month; similar protocol recommended for *A. vasorum* as for *D. immitis* (p. 418)

Chronic Treatment

Because optimal medical treatment for naturally occurring PH in pets is unknown, the following are merely treatment considerations:

- Amlodipine (mild to moderate PH; author's first choice for PH due to MMVD): 0.05 mg/kg PO q 24h, dose titrated based on response while avoiding systemic hypotension
  - If PH is associated with MMVD, add an angiotensin-converting enzyme (ACE) inhibitor (e.g., enalapril, benazepril).
  - If systemic hypotension occurs before reduction in PH, change to sildenafil.
- Sildenafil 1-3 mg/kg PO q 8-12h (titrated to effect) is considered by many to be the treatment of choice and is the author's first choice for causes other than MMVD. Can improve clinical condition despite only mild reduction in PAP.
  - In pulmonary venous hypertension (e.g., MMVD, PVOD), decreasing PAP but not systemic arterial pressure can increase pulmonary capillary blood volume and increase risk of pulmonary edema.
- Specific treatment of underlying mechanism or disease in secondary PH

Possible Complications

- PH: right ventricular failure and systemic arterial hypotension
- Treatment: systemic arterial hypotension with syncope, prerenal azotemia; potential risk of pulmonary edema with sildenafil in dogs with MMVD

Recommended Monitoring

- Clinical parameters: general attitude, exercise tolerance, respiration, severity of ascites
- Systemic blood pressure
- Velocity of TR and pulmonic regurgitation

PROGNOSIS & OUTCOME

Varies with disease/stage:

- Good: parasitic pulmonary vasculature disease with acute PH if patient survives acute episode and no progressive vascular remodeling occurs
- Fair: right-to-left cardiovascular shunts, MMVD, PH secondary to chronic parasitic pulmonary vasculature disease
- Poor: advanced PAH (idiopathic or secondary), advanced pulmonary fibrosis, ARDS, nonparasitic PTE, right-sided heart failure

PEARLS & CONSIDERATIONS

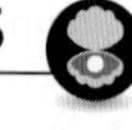

Comments

- PH is rarely a primary process but occurs secondary to another disease.
- PTE and right-to-left PDA may be missed if not considered.
- Radiographs lack sensitivity to detect even severe interstitial or vascular pathology.
- Diagnosis of idiopathic PAH is one of exclusion and histologic confirmation.

Technician Tips

Oxygen should be administered to patients with respiratory distress (p. 1146). Owners should be advised about the importance of parasite prevention in endemic areas.

Client Education

In dogs with cardiac disease, travel to a higher altitude (>7000 feet [2200 m]) may aggravate PH to a clinically relevant degree.

SUGGESTED READING

Goldberg AB, et al: Pulmonary hypertension: diagnosis, imaging techniques, and novel therapies. Cardiovasc Diagn Ther 7:405-417, 2017.

AUTHOR: Tony M. Glaus, Dr.med.vet.habil., DACVIM, DECVIM
EDITOR: Megan Grobman, DVM, MS, DACVIM

Pulmonary Nodules

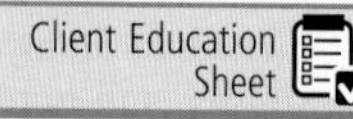

BASIC INFORMATION

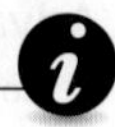

Definition

Single or multiple masses of varying sizes occurring in the lung parenchyma; usually detected radiographically

Epidemiology

SPECIES, AGE, SEX

- Dogs: 9-11 years
- Cats: 11-12 years
- Females may be at increased risk.
- The prevalence of pulmonary nodules in dogs and cats is not known. Pulmonary neoplasms have an average reported incidence of 5.6/100,000 (dogs) and 2.2/100,000 (cats).

RISK FACTORS

Exposure to secondhand smoke may be a risk factor.

ASSOCIATED DISORDERS

Paraneoplastic syndromes are reported to occur secondary to primary or metastatic lung neoplasms (hypertrophic osteopathy; hypercalcemia; fever; feline lung-digit syndrome; elevated ACTH with associated signs of hyperadrenocorticism).

Clinical Presentation

DISEASE FORMS/SUBTYPES

- Benign or malignant
- Malignant nodules may be metastatic or primary.

Most primary lung neoplasms are adenocarcinomas (75%) or carcinomas (20%).

HISTORY, CHIEF COMPLAINT

- Pulmonary nodules or masses may be found incidentally in patients undergoing radiography for other reasons.
- When lung neoplasms cause clinical signs, the most frequent complaints from the owner are cough and dyspnea.
- Sputum with or without blood or hemoptysis is possible.
- Other possible signs are weight loss, fever, dysphagia, vomiting, regurgitation, and wheezing.
- Cats often manifest signs related to metastatic disease to their digits rather than respiratory signs.

PHYSICAL EXAM FINDINGS

- Physical exam: often normal
- If due to metastatic disease: physical abnormalities from the primary tumor may be found in other parts of the body.
- If due to fungal or other disorder: abnormalities related to the lungs (e.g., tachypnea, crackles) or systemic illness (e.g., fever, lymphadenopathy due to systemic mycosis)
- Careful evaluation of the common sites of origin for tumors that metastasize to the lungs is indicated (e.g., oral cavity, area of the thyroid, mammary glands).
- In cats, careful evaluation of each claw (paying particular attention to the quick) and of the fundus is important; both of these sites are predisposed to primary and secondary metastasis of angioinvasive pulmonary tumors.
- A rectal exam is essential in every dog with pulmonary nodules (assess prostate, anal sacs, bladder/urethra, sublumbar lymph nodes).
- A fundic exam (p. 1137) and careful dermatologic evaluation may be helpful in identifying disseminated fungal disease.

Etiology and Pathophysiology

- The main concern for patients with pulmonary nodules is malignancy; neoplasms from virtually any part of the body, including primary lung tumors, may metastasize to the lungs.
- Metastatic neoplasia may reach the lungs through lymphatics or the bloodstream; both can produce a nodular pulmonary pattern.
- Development of metastasis is a complex, multistep process, and failure to complete any of the steps prevents development of a metastatic focus. It is estimated that < 1 in 100 neoplastic cells that leave the primary tumor survive the metastatic cascade.
- The multistep process includes induction of neovascularization, detachment of the tumor cell from the primary tumor, dissolution of the basement membrane and invasion into the bloodstream, evasion of the host immunity and survival in the bloodstream, margination in a new capillary and attachment to the endothelium, dissolution of the basement membrane and extravasation into the extracellular matrix, survival in the new tissue by evading the host immunity, and induction of neovascularization to support continued growth of the new metastatic focus. Neovascularization begins the process again.

DIAGNOSIS

Diagnostic Overview

Recognition of pulmonary nodules is usually made with a radiographic evaluation. A systematic approach is paramount to rule out infectious or granulomatous causes (as warranted by geography) or other foci of neoplasia (i.e., primary lesions elsewhere that have resulted in the identified pulmonary nodules).

Differential Diagnosis

- Solitary lung mass: primary neoplasia, metastatic neoplasia, granuloma, cyst, infarct, localized hemorrhage, focal pneumonia, abscess
- Multiple pulmonary masses: primary or metastatic neoplasia, fungal disease (e.g., blastomycosis, histoplasmosis), pulmonary osteomas (rarely > 3-4 mm in diameter and more radiopaque than soft-tissue nodules because of mineral composition), eosinophilic bronchopneumopathy. Bacterial abscesses and granulomas uncommonly cause multiple pulmonary masses.
- One or more cutaneous or subcutaneous nodules, one or more nipples, and intrahepatic mineralizations can be mistaken for focal pulmonary lesions, especially if only one radiographic projection is made.

Initial Database

- Thoracic radiographs
  - Most often source of initial identification of pulmonary nodules (less commonly found at surgery or necropsy)
  - Three views should be obtained.
- Repeated meticulous physical exam (with particular attention to the mammary chains, anal sacs, oral cavity, skin, fundus and digits)
- CBC, serum biochemistry profile, and urinalysis: typically unremarkable in patients with incidentally discovered pulmonary nodules. Hypercalcemia may occur with neoplasia, fungal, and other granulomatous diseases. Eosinophilia may accompany parasites or eosinophilic bronchopneumopathy.
- Pleural effusion, if present, should be sampled and evaluated with fluid and cytologic analysis (pp. 1164 and 1343).

Advanced or Confirmatory Testing

- Ultrasonographic studies
  - Abdomen and heart to screen for primary sites of disease
  - Nodule itself, with aspiration for diagnosis if possible (p. 1113)
- CT to assess for lesions too small to be identified with plain film radiography and/or to be used for CT-guided aspiration or biopsies
- Fungal and microbial testing based on clinical suspicion and history
- Airway lavage sometimes beneficial (pp. 1073 and 1074)
- Thoracotomy with histopathologic evaluation of biopsy specimens. The hilar lymph nodes and lung lobes should be carefully evaluated and sampled as necessary.

TREATMENT

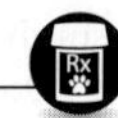

Treatment Overview

Goals are resolution of clinical signs and control or elimination of primary disease process (exception: clinically unimportant pulmonary nodules such as pulmonary osteomas)

- Single pulmonary masses are commonly addressed surgically (focal process).
- Multiple pulmonary masses typically are part of a generalized process (e.g., neoplastic, fungal). Identification of cause and systemic (medical) treatment are most important.

Acute General Treatment

- Supportive care (p. 1146) may or may not be required.
- After a lesion has been identified, surgical excision should be considered.
  - Treatment of choice for primary pulmonary neoplasia (single pulmonary nodule in which the diagnosis was established with aspiration or biopsy)
- Surgical excision may be considered for solitary pulmonary nodules/masses of unknown tissue type. The slow-growing nature of some single pulmonary nodules means that other concerns (e.g., concurrent illnesses, patient age) may supersede the need for thoracotomy.
- In specific cases, metastasectomy (excision of metastases) can be performed. Consultation with an oncologist is recommended beforehand.

Chronic Treatment

- Chemotherapy may be attempted for primary pulmonary neoplasia deemed unresectable or with evidence of lymphatic metastasis at the time of diagnosis. Options may include doxorubicin, platinum compounds (cisplatin, carboplatin), gemcitabine, vinorelbine, or tyrosine kinase inhibitors.
- Chemotherapy is largely unproven in the management of pulmonary tumors in veterinary medicine.

- Address infection, parasitism, granuloma or other cause as needed (e.g., blastomycosis [p. 121], eosinophilic bronchopneumopathy [p. 298])

Possible Complications

- Hypertrophic osteopathy typically resolves with removal of pulmonary disease.
- Digital or ocular metastasis (cats), particularly with angioinvasive neoplasms
- Pneumothorax: ruptured cyst or tumor

Recommended Monitoring

- Monthly to quarterly radiographs to assess for recurrence, progression, or changes (cavitation is not uncommon but is often misinterpreted as abscess/infection)
- As required per protocol for chemotherapy patients (e.g., CBC), quality-of-life assessments

PROGNOSIS & OUTCOME

Guarded and extremely variable (median survival times in parentheses):

- Dogs with primary lung tumors
  - 50% of dogs without clinical signs and having peripheral, solitary, small (<5 cm), well-differentiated, low-grade pulmonary adenocarcinomas without lymph node metastasis or pleural effusion have median survival time > 1 year (12-20 months).
  - In contrast, median survival time is shorter (8 months) for patients with clinical signs referable to the pulmonary nodule/mass or with a large solitary (>5 cm or 100 cm^3) neoplasm, one that involves an entire lobe, squamous cell carcinoma histologically, or nodal metastasis (1-2 months).
- Cats with primary lung tumors: median survival time of 4 months after lobectomy. Cats with poorly differentiated tumors or enlarged tracheobronchial lymph nodes: median of 2 months
- The use of chemotherapy has not been well studied in the management of pulmonary carcinoma, but carboplatin, cisplatin (dogs only), doxorubicin, and vinorelbine may have efficacy in its treatment, particularly when surgery is not possible or lymphatic metastasis are identified.

PEARLS & CONSIDERATIONS

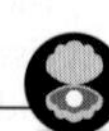

Comments

- Metastatic neoplasia is much more common than primary pulmonary neoplasia.
- One-half of patients with newly diagnosed pulmonary neoplasia are deemed inoperable because regional or systemic extension is identified at presentation.
- Pulmonary osteomas are benign mineralizations often identified incidentally on the radiographs of older dogs. The diagnosis of osteoma versus metastasis can be made empirically based on size and relative opacity. The limit of detection for soft-tissue lesions in the pulmonary parenchyma is considered to be 5-10 mm. Because osteomas have mineral or bone density, they can be identified in the 2-5 mm range.
- Eosinophilic bronchopneumopathy can closely mimic metastatic lung cancer and should be considered in young dogs, especially in predisposed breeds.
- In this author's experience, cats with pulmonary metastases tend to show overt signs, have more advanced disease at the time of presentation, and have markedly shorter survival times compared with dogs.

Technician Tips

- If pleural effusion is present, both dorsoventral and ventrodorsal thoracic radiographic views can be useful. Ask the clinician about her/his preferences.
- Vinorelbine is a vinca alkaloid drug that is used in the management of pulmonary tumors. It is imperative that with absolute certainty vinorelbine (not vincristine or vinblastine) is drawn up for administration because the dosage for vinorelbine is 5 to 10 times higher than for the other two drugs. Inadvertent substitution of the latter two drugs for the former would likely prove fatal.

SUGGESTED READING

Rebhun RB, et al: Tumors of the respiratory system and pulmonary neoplasia. In Withrow SJ, et al, editors: Withrow and MacEwen's Small animal clinical oncology, ed 5, St. Louis, 2013, Saunders, pp 453-459.

AUTHOR: Carlos O. Rodriguez, Jr., DVM, PhD, DACVIM
EDITOR: Kenneth M. Rassnick, DVM, DACVIM

Pulmonary Thromboembolism

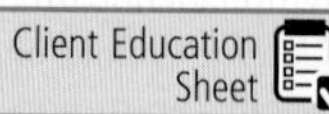

BASIC INFORMATION

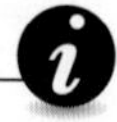

Definition

Pulmonary thromboembolism (PTE) is the occlusion of a pulmonary artery or arteriole by a thrombus that forms in the systemic venous system/right heart (embolism) or in the pulmonary arterial system (*in situ* thrombus).

Epidemiology

SPECIES, AGE, SEX

- Dogs: any age; median of 11 years
- Cats: any age; median of 7 years

RISK FACTORS

Many predisposing conditions for PTE have been identified, and treatment of the underlying cause is the cornerstone of management.

- Neoplasia
- Heartworm disease
- Sepsis
- Hyperadrenocorticism
- Disseminated intravascular coagulation
- Immune-mediated hemolytic anemia
- Protein-losing nephropathy/enteropathy
- Central catheters
- Vasculitis
- Pancreatitis
- Cardiac disease
- Surgical procedures, especially total hip replacement
- Trauma
- Glucocorticoid administration

ASSOCIATED DISORDERS

Hypoxemia, right-sided congestive heart failure, pulmonary hypertension (PH)

Clinical Presentation

HISTORY, CHIEF COMPLAINT

- Acute-onset dyspnea/tachypnea; may be mild or progressive when PTE is small or gradual, respectively
- Signs of the underlying disorder may predominate.
- Occasionally, signs of right-sided heart failure (abdominal distention, exercise intolerance)
- Uncommonly, cough or hemoptysis
- Nonspecific signs (lethargy, anorexia/inappetence, weight loss, collapse)

PHYSICAL EXAM FINDINGS

Depends on degree of vascular occlusion and hypoxemia.

- Tachypnea/dyspnea
- Pulmonary auscultation is often normal, but increased bronchovesicular sounds/crackles might be heard.
- Cyanosis (if severe hypoxemia)
- Tachycardia and weak pulses
- Findings reflecting the predisposing condition (e.g., pallor if hemolytic anemia)
- Occasionally, findings are consistent with right-sided congestive heart failure (jugular venous distention/pulsation, ascites).
- Right apical murmur or split-second heart sound is possible with PH (p. 838).

Etiology and Pathophysiology

- PTE is secondary to an underlying condition that causes venous stasis, endothelial damage, and/or hypercoagulability (Virchow's triad).
- PTE leads to obstruction of a pulmonary artery or arteriole and reactive pulmonary vasoconstriction, reducing blood flow to the affected region of lung. Other forms of emboli, including parasites, neoplastic cells, fat, or gas, may also cause pulmonary vascular obstruction.
- Although small PTEs are often clinically silent and resolve rapidly, large or numerous PTEs cause hypoxemia due to ventilation-perfusion mismatch, sometimes complicated by pulmonary edema and atelectasis.
- Because the lung has a dual blood supply with bronchial arteries from the aorta perfusing the lung parenchyma with oxygenated blood, PTE generally does not cause lung infarction.
- Increased pulmonary vascular resistance due to pulmonary vascular obstruction and pulmonary vasoconstriction may cause PH, which can lead to right-sided heart failure when severe.

DIAGNOSIS

Diagnostic Overview

Clinical diagnosis is challenging, and definitive diagnosis requires advanced imaging. Often, a presumptive diagnosis is based on strong clinical suspicion from identifying a known risk factor and diagnostic test results consistent with PTE.

Differential Diagnosis

- Pulmonary parenchymal disease (e.g., aspiration pneumonia, bronchopneumonia, pulmonary edema, neoplasia, contusion)
- Upper or lower airway disease (e.g., bronchitis/asthma, neoplasia, obstruction)
- Pleural space disease (e.g., pleural effusion, pneumothorax)
- Other causes of PH (p. 838)

Initial Database

- Thoracic radiographs: initial test of choice, although minimally specific and sensitive: main pulmonary artery dilation, abrupt distal pulmonary artery attenuation, regional oligemia (hypovolemia), interstitial or alveolar pulmonary pattern (often with lobar distribution), right heart enlargement, pleural effusion. Radiographs can be normal.
- CBC, serum biochemistry panel, and urinalysis: not specific for diagnosis of PTE but important for recognition of predisposing diseases.
  - Mild to moderate thrombocytopenia may be recognized or decrease in platelet count from (recent) prior value.
- Arterial blood gas analysis: hypoxemia; hypocapnia or normocapnia; metabolic acidosis; increased alveolar-arterial (A-a) gradient (>15 mm Hg) is sensitive but not specific.
  - A-a gradient = FiO_2 (P_b-P_{H2O}) − ($PaCO_2$/R) − PaO_2, in which FiO_2 = fraction of inspired oxygen (e.g., 0.21 for room air; 0.4 for 40% oxygen), P_b = barometric pressure (627-643 mm Hg; www.weather.com), P_{H2O} = 47 mm Hg, R = 0.8, and PaO_2 and $PaCO_2$ are obtained from the arterial blood gas results.
- Coagulation profile: not useful because coagulation time below reference interval does not indicate a hypercoagulable state

Advanced or Confirmatory Testing

- Plasma D-dimer concentration (p. 1334): poor specificity, but high concentrations are consistent with thromboembolic disease in the dog (>250 ng/mL is 80% sensitive, > 103 mg/mL is 100% sensitive).
- Thromboelastography: can detect a hypercoagulable state but does not confirm PTE
- Echocardiography: evidence of PH, right atrial and ventricular enlargement, and occasionally, visible thrombus
- Nuclear ventilation/perfusion scanning: safe and noninvasive but very limited availability
- Pulmonary angiography: previous gold standard for definitive diagnosis. Invasive; unstable patient condition may preclude sedation/anesthesia.
- CT angiography: confirmatory test of choice. Noninvasive and can be performed under sedation without breath holding using newer multidetector CT scanners.

TREATMENT

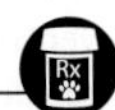

Treatment Overview

PTE can be a life-threatening emergency, and initial treatment focuses on respiratory support. If clinical suspicion is strong or a definitive diagnosis can be made, specific therapy should be provided.

Acute General Treatment

- Oxygen therapy (p. 1146)
- Ventilation with positive end-expiratory pressure if warranted (PaO_2 < 60 mm Hg despite oxygen supplementation) (p. 1185)
- Judicious parenteral fluid therapy to maintain tissue perfusion without exacerbating right heart failure
- Anticoagulant therapy to prevent additional thrombus formation
  - Unfractionated heparin 100-150 U/kg IV followed by 18-37.5 U/kg/h IV continuous-rate infusion (CRI) to prolong activated partial thromboplastin time (aPTT) to 1.5-2.5 times baseline, *or*
  - Low-molecular-weight heparin (LMWH): effective doses not established; dalteparin 150 U/kg SQ q 6-12h or enoxaparin 1 mg/kg SQ q 6-12h
- Antiplatelet therapy
  - Aspirin 1-2 mg/kg PO q 12-24h (dogs); 5-20 mg PO q 3 days (cats), *or*
  - Clopidogrel loading dose of 10 mg/kg PO followed by 2-3 mg/kg PO q 24h (dogs); 18.75 mg/CAT PO q 24h (cats)
- Thrombolytic therapy may be useful in acute stage, but experience is very limited in veterinary medicine, and adverse effects appear to be common.
  - Tissue plasminogen activator (Alteplase) 0.25-1 mg/kg/h IV CRI up to 1-2 days
- Catheter-directed thrombectomy/thrombolysis is possible but requires anesthesia and specialized equipment.

Chronic Treatment

- Treatment of underlying condition
- Anticoagulant therapy
  - LMWH: dalteparin or enoxaparin as above, *or*
  - Warfarin 0.05-0.2 mg/kg PO q 24h titrated to attain an international normalized ratio (INR) of 2-3. Not generally recommended due to narrow therapeutic index and frequent bleeding complications
  - Rivaroxaban and other direct factor Xa or thrombin-inhibiting oral anticoagulants have recently been used in veterinary medicine, but experience is limited.
- Antiplatelet therapy: aspirin or clopidogrel as above

Possible Complications

- PH and right-sided heart failure
- Potentially severe hemorrhage is possible with any anticoagulant or thrombolytic therapy. This limits the use of warfarin and thrombolytics, but risk appears low with heparin or platelet antagonists.

Recommended Monitoring

- Respiratory rate, arterial blood gas analysis or pulse oximetry, and thoracic radiography provide relative indications of response to therapy or deterioration of patient condition.
- Careful monitoring of coagulation times with unfractionated heparin or warfarin therapy; consider monitoring anti-factor Xa activity, if testing available, with LMWH

PROGNOSIS & OUTCOME

Varies, depending on thrombus size and degree of pulmonary vascular occlusion. Thrombi resulting in occlusion of large portions of the pulmonary vascular bed are associated with a poor prognosis.

PEARLS & CONSIDERATIONS

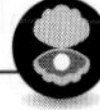

Comments

- PTE should be considered in any patient with dyspnea and/or hypoxemia and normal thoracic radiographs.
- PTE should be suspected in patients with a predisposing cause, lower respiratory signs, increased D-dimer concentrations, and an abnormal A-a gradient.
- Even with management of an underlying disease, recurrence is possible, and long-term anticoagulant therapy may be necessary.

Prevention

Elimination of predisposing conditions is imperative. Prophylactic anticoagulant therapy may be considered when this is not possible.

Technician Tips

IV catheters, especially central catheters, should be removed or replaced in patients suspected of having PTE because they may be a nidus for thrombus formation.

SUGGESTED READING

Goggs R, et al: Pulmonary thromboembolism. J Vet Emerg Crit Care 19:30-52, 2009.

AUTHOR: Herbert W. Maisenbacher, III, VMD, DACVIM
EDITOR: Meg M. Sleeper, VMD, DACVIM

Pulmonic Stenosis

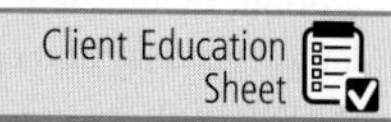

BASIC INFORMATION

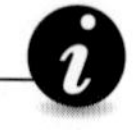

Definition

A fixed or dynamic obstruction of flow from the right ventricle to the pulmonary artery. The obstruction may be infundibular (within the outflow tract), subvalvular, valvular, or supravalvular (at the level of the main pulmonary artery).

Synonyms

Pulmonary stenosis, pulmonary valve dysplasia

Epidemiology

SPECIES, AGE, SEX

Pulmonic stenosis is among the three most common congenital heart defects in dogs. It is uncommon in cats. Some studies suggest that male dogs may be overrepresented.

GENETICS, BREED PREDISPOSITION

- Inherited as a polygenic trait in beagles, although specific mutations have not been identified
- Small terrier breeds, English bulldogs, boxers, mastiffs, miniature schnauzers, Chihuahuas, miniature pinschers, Labrador retrievers, and Samoyeds are also overrepresented.

ASSOCIATED DISORDERS

Pulmonic stenosis most commonly occurs as an isolated congenital defect, although it may occur in conjunction with other congenital cardiac defects, including patent ductus arteriosus, aortic stenosis, ventricular septal defects, and defects of the conotruncal septum (e.g., tetralogy of Fallot). Significant tricuspid valve dysplasia is present in 10%-20% of cases. A patent foramen ovale is present in 8%-40% of cases.

Clinical Presentation

DISEASE FORMS/SUBTYPES

- The pathophysiologic consequences of stenosis are similar, regardless of the level of the obstruction (infundibular, subvalvular, valvular or supravalvular). Nevertheless, accurate anatomic characterization is important in determining an appropriate surgical or interventional approach.
- Two categories of valvular stenosis are recognized in dogs: type 1 (valve cusps are mildly thickened and fused) and type 2 (valve cusps are moderately to severely thickened and the valve annulus may be hypoplastic).
- Annular hypoplasia may be present without valve cusp abnormalities.

HISTORY, CHIEF COMPLAINT

Pulmonic stenosis may be detected as an incidental finding on auscultation, or animals may present with a history of exercise intolerance and/or syncope. In severely affected animals, possible sequelae include right-sided congestive heart failure (CHF) and sudden death.

PHYSICAL EXAM FINDINGS

A systolic, left basilar heart murmur, which may radiate cranioventrally, is typically detected. Arterial pulse quality is usually normal. Signs of right-sided CHF include ascites, jugular distention and pulsation, and positive hepatojugular reflux. In cases with concomitant intracardiac shunts (e.g., patent foramen ovale, atrial or ventricular septal defects), right-to-left shunting of blood may cause cyanosis.

Etiology and Pathophysiology

- The right ventricle must generate sufficient pressure in systole to overcome the outflow tract obstruction, resulting in concentric right ventricular hypertrophy (increased wall thickness) that is proportional to the severity of the obstruction.
- Infundibular hypertrophy may create a dynamic right ventricular outflow tract obstruction, exacerbating the stenosis. The dynamic obstruction may worsen after an acute decrease in pressure gradient across the primary stenosis (e.g., after balloon valvuloplasty), resulting in a sudden, severe decrease in right ventricular stroke volume (i.e., suicide right ventricle).
- Diastolic compliance decreases with increasing wall thickness, resulting in impaired ventricular filling and increased right atrial pressures, which are exacerbated by any concurrent tricuspid valve regurgitation (due to dysplasia or damage during balloon valvuloplasty).

DIAGNOSIS

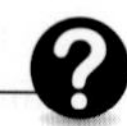

Diagnostic Overview

The diagnosis is suspected in a patient with a typical murmur. The most common differential for a left basilar systolic murmur is subaortic stenosis; the index of suspicion for pulmonic stenosis is increased on the basis of breed predispositions, direction of murmur radiation, pulse quality, and radiographic findings. Echocardiography is required for confirmation.

Differential Diagnosis

Other conditions, such as subaortic stenosis or tetralogy of Fallot, can cause a left basilar systolic murmur. Soft basilar murmurs can also be physiologic, with no underlying structural heart disease.

Initial Database

- Thoracic radiography: evidence of right ventricular hypertrophy and post-stenotic dilation of the main pulmonary artery are frequently appreciated, especially on dorsoventral projections. The pulmonary vasculature usually appears normal, although a right-to-left shunting intracardiac defect may result in pulmonary undercirculation and decreased vessel width.
- Electrocardiography (p. 1096): changes consistent with right ventricular hypertrophy are frequently observed (right-axis deviation with deep S waves in leads I, II, III, aVF, CV6LL and CV6LU and slightly increased QRS duration). Arrhythmias may be detected (e.g., ventricular premature complexes, atrial fibrillation).
- Echocardiography (p. 1094): two-dimensional echocardiography allows identification of the level of stenosis, annulus measurement, and assessment of the anatomic features of the lesion and any post-stenotic dilatation. The region of the pulmonic valve is best visualized on the right parasternal short-axis view, the left cranial view, or by transesophageal echocardiography. The severity of stenosis is assessed by estimation of the pressure gradient across the narrowing using Doppler echocardiography flow velocity measurements with the modified Bernoulli equation (pressure gradient = 4 × velocity^2). Severity of stenosis is categorized as mild (10-49 mm Hg), moderate (50-80 mm Hg), or severe (>80 mm Hg).

Advanced or Confirmatory Testing

Direct angiography is performed before balloon valvuloplasty using a right ventricular contrast injection, allowing further assessment of valve morphology (cusp fusion and/ or thickening, annular hypoplasia), right ventricular hypertrophy, post-stenotic dilatation, tricuspid regurgitation, and identification of intracardiac shunting lesions (e.g., patent foramen ovale). If a single coronary ostium with anomalous prepulmonic coronary artery is suspected, a left-sided injection should be performed to assess coronary anatomy due to the risk of coronary artery rupture during balloon valvuloplasty. These abnormalities are most commonly reported in boxers and bulldog breeds.

TREATMENT

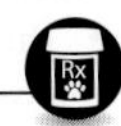

Treatment Overview

The goal of treatment is to reduce clinical signs and myocardial workload to decrease the risk of CHF and sudden death.

Acute General Treatment

- Treatment is not necessary in animals with mild or moderate stenosis that is not associated with clinical signs.
- Animals with severe, fixed obstruction and/or clinical signs referable to pulmonic stenosis (e.g., exercise intolerance, syncope or signs of right-sided CHF) should be referred for interventional or surgical reduction in pressure gradient. The precise approach chosen (e.g., balloon valvuloplasty, pulmonary patch graft) depends on the anatomic location and characteristics of the lesion and presence or absence of concurrent congenital defects.
- Type 1 valvular lesions are most amenable to balloon valvuloplasty. Surgery may be necessary in cases of annular hypoplasia or significant subvalvular obstruction.
- Dynamic obstructions that are exacerbated by increased sympathetic tone may respond to adrenergic beta-receptor blockade (e.g., atenolol 0.5-1.5 mg/kg PO q 12h). These dynamic obstructions may persist after interventional or surgical treatment for fixed stenosis, requiring ongoing treatment.
- In cases of severe obstruction in which interventional or surgical treatment is not feasible, exercise restriction and beta-blocker therapy are frequently recommended to control clinical signs and reduce the risk of sudden death, although the latter benefit remains unproven.

Possible Complications

In severe obstruction, progressive right ventricular hypertrophy, tricuspid regurgitation, and increased right atrial pressure may result in worsening exercise tolerance, recurrent syncope, arrhythmias, CHF, and sudden death.

Recommended Monitoring

For dogs not undergoing interventional or surgical treatment, serial echocardiography is recommended to monitor progressive right ventricular hypertrophy or right atrial enlargement. The pressure gradient sometimes increases as puppies grow toward maturity. After interventional or surgical treatment, short- and long-term success is assessed by longitudinal echocardiographic monitoring of the pressure gradient. Detected arrhythmias should be assessed and monitored electrocardiographically.

PROGNOSIS & OUTCOME

- Animals with mild pulmonic stenosis often have a good quality of life and relatively normal life expectancy.
- Prognosis is guarded for dogs with severe obstructions due to the risk of right-sided CHF or sudden death. Prognosis is also negatively affected by significant right ventricular hypertrophy or tricuspid regurgitation.
- Balloon valvuloplasty improves outcome, especially in those patients in which severity is reduced into the mild to moderate range.
- Restenosis occurs infrequently after balloon valvuloplasty.

PEARLS & CONSIDERATIONS

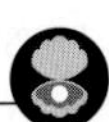

Comments

Careful auscultation over the left heart base is key to detection, especially in animals with no clinical signs.

Prevention

Dogs with confirmed pulmonic stenosis should not be used for breeding.

Technician Tips

Common signs of disease progression include the development or worsening of exercise intolerance or arrhythmias, increasing frequency of syncope, and development of clinical signs of right-sided CHF, such as ascites. Situations likely to result in increased sympathetic tone (e.g., stress, excitement, exertion) should be avoided in cases of severe pulmonic stenosis because they are likely to exacerbate clinical signs. Calm, gentle handling is paramount, especially for cats.

Client Education

Puppies with persistent heart murmurs often benefit from referral to a veterinary cardiologist for echocardiography. Balloon valvuloplasty or surgical correction should be offered in cases of severe stenosis. Owners should be warned of the risk of right-sided CHF or sudden death in these cases.

SUGGESTED READING

Stafford JM, et al: Pulmonic stenosis in dogs: balloon valvuloplasty improves outcome. J Vet Intern Med 18:656-662, 2004.

AUTHOR: Melanie Hezzell, VetMB, MA, PhD, DACVIM
EDITOR: Meg M. Sleeper, VMD, DACVIM

Pulse Abnormalities

Client Education Sheet 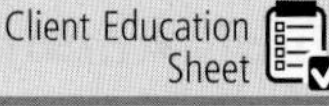

BASIC INFORMATION

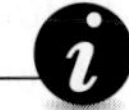

Definition

The arterial pulse is produced by the fluctuation between diastolic and systolic arterial pressure and can be palpated as an impulse in superficial arteries, such as the femoral artery. *Pulse deficit* refers to a heartbeat that is heard on auscultation or felt on the chest wall but does not generate a palpable arterial pulse.

Synonyms

- Hyperkinetic pulse: strong, bounding, or water-hammer pulse
- Hypokinetic pulse: weak or thready pulse

Epidemiology

SPECIES, AGE, SEX

Dogs and cats of either sex and any age

ASSOCIATED DISORDERS

A detailed differential diagnosis is discussed on p. 1275.

- Reduced pulse amplitude (hypokinetic pulse): decreased cardiac output or left ventricular outflow tract obstruction. With aortic or subaortic stenosis, the pulse may be decreased and delayed *(pulsus parvus et tardus).*
- Increased pulse amplitude (hyperkinetic pulse): increased stroke volume or decreased diastolic arterial pressure. Example: diastolic runoff through a patent ductus arteriosus causes a greater difference between systolic and diastolic pressures (greater pulse pressure) and a correspondingly stronger pulse.
- Pulse deficits (missing pulses compared with cardiac auscultation): tachyarrhythmias, severe myocardial failure (pulsus alternans; pulse amplitude alternates between a strong pulse and a weak or absent pulse)
- Variation in pulse rhythm: tachyarrhythmias (atrial fibrillation, premature beats) or bradyarrhythmias (second-degree atrioventricular block)
- Regular variation in pulse amplitude: exaggerated effect of respiration: pulsus paradoxus (pericardial effusion with cardiac tamponade). The pulse is stronger during expiration and weaker during inspiration.
- Regional variation in pulse amplitude: arterial thromboembolism (feline myocardial disease, infective endocarditis, hypercoagulable states)

Clinical Presentation

HISTORY, CHIEF COMPLAINT

Varies widely, depending on underlying cause

PHYSICAL EXAM FINDINGS

- Systemic or primary cardiac problems may alter the pulse, and a complete physical exam is necessary.
- Femoral pulses are easiest to palpate in cats and dogs.
- The dorsal metatarsal pulse is also readily palpable.
- Auscultate heart sounds simultaneously (by definition, a pulse deficit exists when a heart sound does not have a corresponding palpable peripheral pulse).
- Pulse quality relates mainly to pulse amplitude (also affected by rate of rise of arterial pressure in systole and affected by pulse duration).

Etiology and Pathophysiology

- Pulse pressure: difference between systolic and diastolic blood pressure (BP)
  - Pulse pressure can be widened by an increase in stroke volume or decreased diastolic BP (e.g., aortic insufficiency, patent ductus arteriosus), increasing pulse amplitude.
- With premature beats, the weak ventricular contraction may not generate sufficient systolic pressure to open the aortic valve, and no S_2 or pulse is produced (S_1 is still normally heard).
- Variations in stroke volume also occur with the phase of respiration with cardiac tamponade, in which increased filling of the right heart during inspiration leads to decreased filling of the left heart and a reduced pulse pressure.
- Pulsus alternans is an uncommon finding characterized by alternate pulses that are very weak or absent despite consistent electrical activation (due to abnormal intracellular calcium cycling in myocardial failure). It should not be confused with electrical alternans, an electrocardiographic finding consisting of alternating tall-short QRS complexes, that suggests pericardial effusion and is unrelated to pulsus alternans.

DIAGNOSIS

Diagnostic Overview

A pulse abnormality is a physical exam finding, and its significance may vary from harmless (e.g., seemingly weak pulse in an obese patient) to indicative of cardiac or systemic disturbances. An intermittent pulse deficit should be investigated initially with an electrocardiogram; a weak pulse should be assessed with evaluation of the patient's intravascular volume status (hydration) and cardiac function (auscultation, thoracic radiographs, echocardiogram).

Differential Diagnosis

- Hypokinetic pulse: obesity, arterial disease/disorder. The combination of hypokinetic pulse and a palpably strong or hyperdynamic heartbeat (apex beat) strongly suggests outflow obstruction (e.g., moderate to marked aortic stenosis; less commonly, pulmonic stenosis).
- Hyperkinetic pulse: thin body condition
- Variation in pulse amplitude: normal variation as occurs with respiratory sinus arrhythmia (pulse is stronger after pause)

Initial Database

- Pulse deficits should prompt the recording of an electrocardiogram (p. 1096).
- Alternate pulse deficits with normal sinus rhythm (pulsus alternans): thoracic radiographs and an echocardiogram

TREATMENT

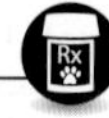

Treatment Overview

Manage the underlying cause.

PROGNOSIS & OUTCOME

Varies widely, depending on underlying cause

PEARLS & CONSIDERATIONS

Comments

- Palpation of the peripheral arterial pulse can give useful information about stroke volume and cardiac output.
- Palpation of the arterial pulse is not useful for detecting systemic hypertension.
- Presence of a hyperkinetic pulse may be more obvious than a diastolic murmur with severe aortic insufficiency (as with infective endocarditis of the aortic valve).
- Pulsus paradoxus is a very helpful finding when cardiac tamponade is suspected, but it may be difficult to detect if the dog is panting.

Technician Tip

Absent metatarsal pulses can be an indication of hypotension.

SUGGESTED READING

Perloff JK: The arterial pulse. In Perloff JK: Physical examination of the heart and circulation, ed 4, Shelton, CT, 2009, People's Medical Publishing House, pp 55-91.

RELATED CLIENT EDUCATION SHEET

Consent to Perform Echocardiography

AUTHOR: Virginia Luis Fuentes, VetMB, MA, PhD, DVC, DACVIM, DECVIM
EDITOR: Leah A. Cohn, DVM, PhD, DACVIM

Pupil Abnormalities

BASIC INFORMATION

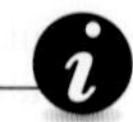

Definition

Abnormalities include pupils that are inappropriately dilated or constricted and those with a distorted shape.

- Anisocoria: unequal or asymmetrical pupils
- Dyscoria: misshapen/distorted pupil
- Miosis: constricted pupil
- Mydriasis: dilated pupil

Epidemiology

SPECIES, AGE, SEX

- Dogs and cats
- Iris atrophy is an aging change and is therefore seen in older animals.
- Iris coloboma (absence of or defect in the iris) is a developmental/heritable condition that is usually first noticed in young animals, most frequently dogs.

GENETICS, BREED PREDISPOSITION

- Distorted pupil: a distorted pupil, such as iris coloboma, may be breed related in dogs. Australian shepherds and Dalmatians are overrepresented.
- Dilated pupil
  - Glaucoma, primary (predisposed breeds)
  - Toy and miniature poodles are predisposed to optic nerve hypoplasia.
  - Heritable retinal degeneration in many breeds of dogs

Clinical Presentation

DISEASE FORMS/SUBTYPES

Conditions that lead to pupil abnormalities can be divided into those that cause

- Pupillary dilation (mydriasis)
- Pupillary constriction (miosis)
- Abnormal pupil shape (dyscoria)

HISTORY, CHIEF COMPLAINT

Abnormalities in pupil size and shape may be noted by the owner. Veterinarians may notice the pupil abnormalities during routine exams or in animals presenting for painful, red, or blind eyes.

PHYSICAL EXAM FINDINGS

Dilated pupil and the following:

- Scalloping at pupillary margin
  - Iris coloboma: focal; young animal
  - Iris atrophy: typically multifocal and/or moth-eaten effect in iris stroma and/or at pupillary margin; typically age-related change (i.e., older animals)
- Blindness (negative menace response)
  - See chapters on blindness, retinal degeneration, and retinal detachment (pp. 123, 883, and 885).

- Optic nerve lesion (e.g., optic nerve hypoplasia, congenital, glaucoma [p. 387], optic neuritis)
- Optic chiasmal lesion
- Quiet (i.e., nonred) sighted (visual) eye
  - Internal ophthalmoplegia (paralysis of the iris and ciliary muscles) caused by pharmacologic pupillary dilation (e.g., parasympatholytics such as atropine and topical tropicamide), iris atrophy, or lesions involving the parasympathetic fibers of the oculomotor nerve (cranial nerve [CN] III, rare)
  - Fearful animal (i.e., sympathetic stimulation): transient mydriasis; resolves after animal becomes calm
  - Horner's syndrome: other signs include ptosis (drooping of upper eyelid), enophthalmos (caudal displacement of the eye), and third eyelid protrusion.

Constricted pupil and the following:
- Red eye with or without vision impairment
  - Anterior uveitis (p. 1023)
  - Corneal ulceration and axon reflex miosis through trigeminal and oculomotor nerves (CN V and III)
  - Pharmacologic pupillary constriction (e.g., parasympathomimetic, such as topical pilocarpine, demecarium, or synthetic prostaglandins; analogs include latanoprost, bimatoprost, and travoprost; may cause conjunctival hyperemia)

Distorted pupil and the following:
- Scalloping at pupillary margin
  - Iris coloboma: focal; young animal
  - Iris atrophy: typically multifocal and/or moth-eaten effect in iris stroma; typically age-related change (i.e., older animals)
- Red eye with or without vision impairment
  - Adhesions of iris to lens and/or iris to cornea (posterior and anterior synechiae, respectively) from current or past anterior uveitis
  - Iris prolapse through full-thickness corneal lesion
  - Iridodonesis (tremulousness of the iris on eye movement) noted, with loss of iris support subsequent to lens subluxation/luxation (p. 581)

Anisocoria:
- Primary iridal disease (age-related atrophy); heritable or developmental coloboma, active inflammatory process causing miosis; chronic inflammation leading to degeneration and/or posterior synechia
- Primary neurologic cause (CN III abnormality, Horner's syndrome)
- Pharmacologic agents (miotics such as pilocarpine, mydriatics such as atropine and tropicamide)

Unresponsive pupils:
- Retinal disease
- Optic nerve disease
- Iridal disease
- Pharmacologic agents
- Posterior synechia secondary to anterior uveitis

Etiology/Pathophysiology
- Anisocoria: Horner's syndrome, breed related (Siamese cats), iris atrophy, ophthalmoplegia
- Dyscoria: iris atrophy, iris neoplasia, congenital disorder of iris, iris coloboma
- Miosis: bright light, uveitis, synechia, Horner's syndrome, drugs (e.g., latanoprost, pilocarpine, dexmedetomidine)
- Mydriasis: dim light, sympathetic stimulation, iris atrophy, blindness from retinal or optic nerve disease, glaucoma, drugs (e.g., diazepam, diphenhydramine)

DIAGNOSIS

Differential Diagnosis
Abnormalities of pupillary size or shape are recognized on visual examination of the eye. Although there are a variety of different causes for these abnormalities (see Etiology/Pathophysiology), the only thing that might be mistaken for a pupillary abnormality would be the use of poor lighting for the assessment of pupil size/response.

Diagnostic Overview
Diagnosis of pupil abnormalities requires consideration of the entire eye, as well as the orbit and brain. Pupil abnormalities frequently indicate serious but nonocular problems.

Initial Database
Complete ophthalmic exam (p. 1137):
- Neuro-ophthalmic exam (p. 1136) (i.e., menace response; dazzle, palpebral, pupillary light, and vestibulo-ocular reflexes)
- Fluorescein stain application (miosis commonly occurs in animals with corneal ulceration)
- Intraocular pressures (>30 mm Hg with glaucoma; often low [<10-15 mm Hg] with uveitis)

Advanced or Confirmatory Testing
Varies, depending on underlying condition:
- Pharmacologic testing (e.g., 2.5% phenylephrine) for Horner's syndrome
- Advanced imaging (p. 1132); cerebrospinal fluid tap (pp. 1080 and 1323) for diseases of the neurologic system (e.g., optic neuritis; optic chiasmal lesions) or orbital disorders
- Electroretinogram to assess retinal function

TREATMENT

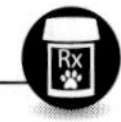

Treatment Overview
If a specific systemic cause of oculomotor neuropathy, optic neuropathy, anterior uveitis, or Horner's syndrome can be identified, treatment should address the cause. Treatment is not indicated or not available for iris atrophy, iris coloboma, optic nerve hypoplasia, retinal degeneration, and optic nerve atrophy/degeneration.

Acute and Chronic Treatment
Directed at underlying cause

PROGNOSIS & OUTCOME

- Prognosis varies widely, depending on underlying condition and cause.
- Many causes of pupil abnormalities are completely innocuous, whereas others may be life-threatening.

PEARLS & CONSIDERATIONS

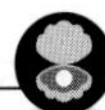

Comments
Many pupil abnormalities can be diagnosed with careful consideration of the signalment and presence or absence of other ophthalmic signs.

Technician Tips
Pupillary light reflexes should be evaluated and documented before dilation with tropicamide.

Client Education
- Pupil abnormalities can be an early sign of serious disease.
- Early detection may improve prognosis.

SUGGESTED READING
Grahn BH, et al: Neuro-ophthalmology. In Veterinary ophthalmology essentials, Philadelphia, 2004, Butterworth Heinemann, pp 200-224.

AUTHOR: Steven R. Hollingsworth, DVM, DACVO
EDITOR: Diane V. H. Hendrix, DVM, DACVO

Pustular and Crusting Skin Disorders

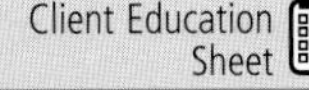

BASIC INFORMATION

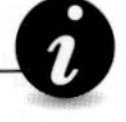

Definition
Pustules and crusts are common skin lesions. Pustules are small, circumscribed elevations of the skin filled with pus. Healing or ruptured pustules may form crusts, the dried accumulation of exudate (blood, pus, serum) over a lost or damaged epidermis.

Epidemiology
SPECIES, AGE, SEX
- In dogs, impetigo, demodicosis, juvenile cellulitis, and dermatophytosis are typically seen in young animals.

Pemphigus is more common in middle-aged adults.
- Hereditary mechanobullous disease: epidermolysis bullosa develops shortly after birth.
- Drug eruptions can occur at any age.

GENETICS, BREED PREDISPOSITION
- Juvenile cellulitis (p. 567): dachshund, golden and Labrador retrievers, Gordon setters, pointers. More than one puppy can be affected in a litter.
- Superficial suppurative necrolytic dermatitis: miniature schnauzer
- Pemphigus foliaceus: Akita, chow chow
- Drug eruption (especially sulfonamides): Doberman pinscher

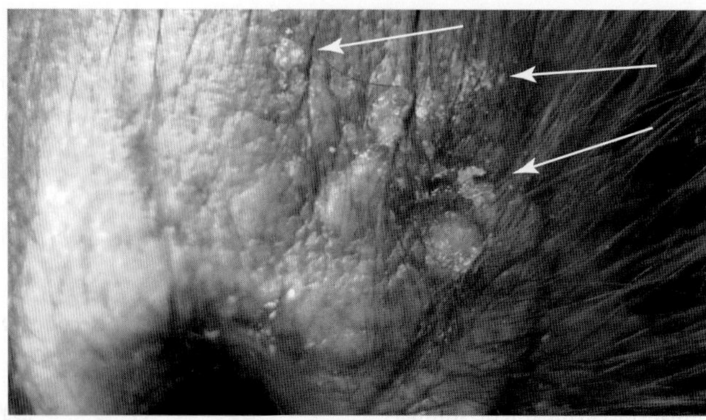

PUSTULAR AND CRUSTING SKIN DISORDERS Honey-colored crusts *(arrows)* on the pinna of a dog with pemphigus foliaceus. (Courtesy Dr. Caroline de Jaham.)

RISK FACTORS
- Pyoderma, the most common cause of pustular and crusting dermatitis in dogs, is often secondary to a predisposing skin disease (e.g., atopic dermatitis, food allergy, demodicosis, endocrinopathies).
- With the exception of abscesses, pyoderma is relatively uncommon in cats.
- Cats affected with feline immunodeficiency virus (FIV) are more susceptible to dermatophytosis.

CONTAGION AND ZOONOSIS

Dermatophytosis is contagious to other animals and is zoonotic.

GEOGRAPHY AND SEASONALITY
- Pemphigus foliaceus and pemphigus erythematosus can be aggravated by exposure to sunlight.
- Pyodermas associated with underlying atopic dermatitis may have a seasonal occurrence.

ASSOCIATED DISORDERS

Bullous impetigo in adult dogs is often associated with immunosuppression (e.g., hyperadrenocorticism, diabetes mellitus, hypothyroidism).

Clinical Presentation

HISTORY, CHIEF COMPLAINT
- Pustules are usually short-lived and may go unnoticed. Scaling and crusting are often the dominant presentation.
- Pruritus varies with the skin disorder. It can be a major presenting complaint in pyodermas, with or without underlying allergies or ectoparasitism.
- Some degree of hair loss may accompany follicular damage.
- Lethargy and anorexia can be part of the presenting picture with juvenile cellulitis, pemphigus foliaceus, cutaneous drug eruptions, or superficial suppurative necrolytic dermatitis of the miniature schnauzer.

PHYSICAL EXAM FINDINGS
- Pustules are most commonly yellow. Green pustules may indicate the presence of gram-negative bacteria or toxic change. Larger, flaccid pustules are more common with the pemphigus complex and bullous impetigo.
- Scales, epidermal collarettes, crusts of various colors (brown, honey colored) and texture (adherent, flaky), alopecia, erythema, and focal areas of hyperpigmentation or hyperkeratosis may be noted. The extent and location of lesions may vary, depending on the condition and severity.

Etiology and Pathophysiology

Pustules result from a loss of epidermal intercellular cohesion (e.g., edema, degeneration, inflammation, autoantibody formation), causing epidermal or subepidermal cavities that eventually fill with inflammatory cells.

DIAGNOSIS

Diagnostic Overview

The combination of crusts and pustules narrows the differential diagnosis, but pustules can be short-lived, and the clinician should perform a careful exam before confirming their absence. Cytologic exam of the content of an intact pustule or from the exudates under a crust is an important step to orient the diagnosis. When pustules or crusts are seen on dogs, skin scrapings should always be performed to rule out demodicosis. Skin biopsies are recommended in most cases presenting with pustules and crusts after pyoderma, demodicosis, and dermatophytosis have been ruled out. A diagnostic approach is outlined on p. 1446.

Differential Diagnosis

An asterisk indicates that intact pustules often occur with the disease.
- Infectious: pustules most often have a follicular orientation with the exception of impetigo.
  - Bacterial: pyoderma (bacterial folliculitis,* impetigo,* furunculosis), dermatophilosis
  - Fungal: dermatophytosis
  - Parasitic: demodicosis,* *Pelodera* dermatitis
  - Protozoal: leishmaniasis
- Immune-mediated: juvenile cellulitis, pemphigus complex (especially pemphigus foliaceus*), canine eosinophilic folliculitis* and furunculosis, canine sterile eosinophilic pustulosis,* subcorneal pustular dermatosis,* and canine linear IgA pustular dermatosis*
- Drug eruption: superficial suppurative necrolytic dermatitis of schnauzers (associated with shampoo therapy), drug-induced pemphigus foliaceus, and eosinophilic pustulosis (subcorneal to follicular neutrophilic pustulosis)

Initial Database
- The medical history of the animal is important in determining cause: age of onset, breed, presence or absence of pruritus, previous medications, other animals affected, progression, chronicity, and seasonality
- Lesion distribution is important to orient the diagnosis.
  - Face (lips, muzzle, eyelids, ear pinnae): juvenile cellulitis, pemphigus erythematosus, demodicosis, eosinophilic folliculitis and furunculosis, nasal pyoderma, mucocutaneous pyoderma, drug eruption
  - Feet: pyoderma, dermatophytosis, demodicosis, pemphigus foliaceus
  - Trunk: superficial pyoderma, demodicosis, subcorneal pustular dermatosis, pemphigus foliaceus, drug eruption, impetigo (abdomen)
- Cytologic exam of pustular contents
  - Bacteria: phagocytized bacteria (often cocci because staphylococcal organisms are the primary isolates from dogs and cats with pyoderma)
  - Neutrophils: pyoderma, pemphigus complex, subcorneal pustular dermatosis, and canine linear IgA pustular dermatosis
  - Eosinophils: abundant eosinophils with eosinophilic folliculitis/furunculosis and sterile eosinophilic pustulosis; eosinophils are also associated with superficial pyodermas with parasitic or allergic disorders, deep pyodermas (furunculosis), drug eruptions, and pemphigus foliaceus.
  - Acantholytic keratinocytes: seen in pemphigus complex in conjunction with numerous neutrophils
- Skin scrapings: *Demodex* spp
- Fungal culture: dermatophytosis
- CBC, serum biochemistry profile, and urinalysis if systemic disease is suspected; results often unremarkable besides mild/moderate neutrophilic or eosinophilic leukocytosis

Advanced or Confirmatory Testing

- Skin biopsies for histopathologic evaluation
- Bacterial culture and sensitivity (C&S) indicated when
  - Bacilliform bacteria are noted on cytologic exam
  - Poor response to previous appropriate antibiotic therapy
  - Antibiotic treatment in the past 6 months or another known risk factor for antimicrobial resistance (p. 653)
- Endocrine tests if history and physical exam suggest underlying endocrinopathy
- Serologic testing for FIV, feline leukemia virus (FeLV), and leishmaniasis based on history and environment

TREATMENT

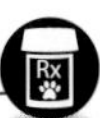

Treatment Overview

Pyoderma is the most common cause of pustules and crust formation in dogs. Most pyodermas are successfully addressed with antibiotic therapy. Because causes of crusting and pustular skin diseases are often infectious or parasitic, glucocorticoids should not be used until a final diagnosis has been reached.

Acute General Treatment

Depends on the cause of the disorder:

- Antibiotic therapy: common empirical choices include cephalexin 25-30 mg/kg PO q 12h or amoxicillin-clavulanate 15-20 mg/kg PO q 12h, usually for 1-2 weeks beyond resolution of lesions. A more specific selection can be made based on results of culture and sensitivity testing, which is strongly recommended.
- Antifungal therapy: itraconazole 5 mg/kg PO q 24h for 3-6 weeks (pulse or continuous) is a good first-choice therapy for cats with dermatophytosis.
- Antiparasitics: choice depends on the parasite identified
- Glucocorticoids for immune-mediated disorders such as juvenile cellulitis, pemphigus complex, eosinophilic folliculitis/furunculosis, eosinophilic pustulosis
  - Prednisone/prednisolone is a common first choice for dogs, usually for 10-14 days at high induction dosage (2-4 mg/kg PO q 24h), then gradually tapered according to clinical response. Prednisolone is preferred for cats.

PROGNOSIS & OUTCOME

- Varies according to the disease
- Excellent for most parasitic and infectious skin diseases
- Excellent for some immune-mediated skin diseases such as juvenile cellulitis, eosinophilic folliculitis, and furunculosis

PEARLS & CONSIDERATIONS

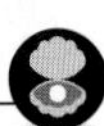

Comments

- Crusts alone are noted in certain diseases, such as in cornification disorders or zinc-responsive dermatosis.
- Crusts secondary to excoriations are frequently seen in atopic dermatitis, food intolerance, and flea bite dermatitis.
- Treat for and rule out pyoderma before taking biopsies.

Technician Tips

- Cytologic exam of pustular content is best performed by rupturing the top of the pustule with a needle or the sharp corner of the glass microscopic slide. Smears are then done by direct impression on the open pustule.
- Bacterial culture samples should be made from pustular content whenever possible or by vigorously rubbing the swab under a freshly lifted crust.

Client Education

In lay terms, pustules are pimples, and crusts are scabs.

SUGGESTED READING

Miller WH, et al: Diagnostic methods. In Miller WH, et al, editors: Muller and Kirk's Small animal dermatology, ed 7, St. Louis, 2013, Saunders, pp 57-107.

AUTHOR: Caroline de Jaham, DMV, MScV, DACVD
EDITOR: Manon Paradis, DMV, MVSc, DACVD

Pyelonephritis

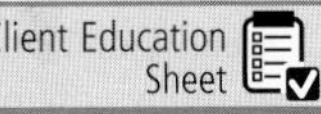

BASIC INFORMATION

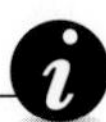

Definition

Inflammation of the renal pelvis and interstitium is typically associated with bacterial infection. Acute pyelonephritis is uncommon; chronic pyelonephritis is more common but often clinically inapparent.

Synonym

Pyelitis

Epidemiology

SPECIES, AGE, SEX

- Dogs and cats are susceptible, with females predisposed.
- Most common in older animals or in younger animals with predisposing cause (e.g., congenital urinary malformations, uroliths).

RISK FACTORS

Anatomic abnormalities:

- Ectopic ureter(s)
- Urethral/ureteral obstruction
- Hydroureter/hydronephrosis
- Perineal urethrostomy
- Urolithiasis
- Vulvar conformational abnormalities

Functional abnormalities:

- Urine retention (>0.25 mL/kg after complete voiding)
- Urine reflux due to increased intravesicular pressure
- Urinary incontinence
- Isosthenuria, hyposthenuria (any cause)
- Immunocompromise
- Indwelling urinary catheter or repeated catheterization

Lower genitourinary tract infection:

- Dogs and cats: various bacteria; *Escherichia coli* most common isolate in urinary tract infections (UTIs)
- Fungal and yeast pyelonephritis possible, especially in immunocompromised animals
- Bacterial prostatitis: intact male dogs

CONTAGION AND ZOONOSIS

Rarely, shared clones of bacteria involved in UTIs have been found in people and their dogs.

ASSOCIATED DISORDERS

- Acute kidney injury
- Chronic kidney disease (CKD)
- Hypokalemia (cats)
- Bacterial cystitis
- Urolithiasis
- Hydronephrosis

Clinical Presentation

DISEASE FORMS/SUBTYPES

- Ascending pyelonephritis: most common
- Hematogenous pyelonephritis: rare; may be sequela of septicemia
- Acute pyelonephritis: less common, often causes systemic illness
- Chronic pyelonephritis: more common, often insidious

HISTORY, CHIEF COMPLAINT

Clinical signs may be absent; chronic pyelonephritis can be a complicating factor in CKD. When present, clinical signs may include

- Polyuria and polydipsia (PU/PD; acute or chronic pyelonephritis)
- Malaise (usually acute pyelonephritis)

- Hematuria
- Pollakiuria, stranguria (if concurrent lower UTI)
- Abdominal, lumbar, or general discomfort (usually acute pyelonephritis)
- Recurrent lower UTIs (chronic pyelonephritis)
- Possible history of predisposing cause may be present (e.g., urinary catheterization, uroliths)

PHYSICAL EXAM FINDINGS

Exam may be normal, especially in the more common chronic form of infection. Abnormalities, when present, may include

- Fever (acute pyelonephritis)
- Dehydration
- Renomegaly (acute pyelonephritis)
- Renal asymmetry (chronic pyelonephritis)
- Abdominal/renal/lumbar pain (more often acute pyelonephritis)
- Oral ulcerations/halitosis (if uremia)
- Debris or secretions (vomitus, saliva) in the oral cavity (if uremia or sepsis)
- Bladder discomfort (if concurrent lower UTI)

Etiology and Pathophysiology

- Infectious agents (bacteria, fungi) usually ascend to renal pelvis from lower urinary tract. Rarely, agents infect the kidneys hematogenously.
- Onset may be acute or insidious.
- Renal response to injury causes clinical signs.
  - Acute infection results in nephritis (renal inflammation), causing renomegaly, renal pain, and often systemic signs of sepsis.
  - Acute or chronic infection causes nephrogenic diabetes insipidus through bacterial toxin actions on antidiuretic hormone receptors.
  - Chronic infection results in renal scarring, smaller than normal kidneys, and loss of renal function.
  - Emphysematous pyelonephritis is rare.
- Infection may result in acute or chronic renal failure or exacerbation of pre-existing CKD.

DIAGNOSIS

Diagnostic Overview

The diagnosis of pyelonephritis should be considered for any animal with pyuria and/or bacteriuria (especially in the absence of lower urinary tract signs such as dysuria), polyuria/polydipsia, azotemia, CKD, chronic cystitis, and/or immunocompromise. Although acute pyelonephritis may cause dramatic illness, chronic pyelonephritis with obscure clinical signs occurs more commonly.

Differential Diagnosis

- PU/PD (pp. 812, 1271, and 1442)
- Bacteruria (p. 232)
- Pyelectasia (p. 483)

Initial Database

- Careful evaluation of vulvar/preputial/penile conformation, especially in obese (female) dogs, to identify anatomic abnormalities
- CBC: may be normal (chronic pyelonephritis) or show leukocytosis with left shift (acute pyelonephritis); normocytic, normochromic nonregenerative anemia is possible with concurrent CKD.
- Serum biochemical profile: often normal but may demonstrate azotemia (elevated blood urea nitrogen [BUN], creatinine), hyperphosphatemia, hypokalemia or hyperkalemia, and/or metabolic acidosis
- Urinalysis: isosthenuria is common; bacteruria may be absent despite bacterial urinary infection (emphasizing the value of urine bacterial culture and antimicrobial susceptibility [C&S]) testing; occasionally, leukocyte casts (acute pyelonephritis), pyuria, hematuria, and/or crystalluria are noted.
- Blood pressure: CKD associated with chronic pyelonephritis may cause hypertension, and sepsis associated with acute pyelonephritis may cause hypotension.
- Abdominal radiographs: varied renal shadow (normal, large, or small and irregular). Radiopaque urinary (upper or lower) calculi (suspect struvite) are sometimes present.
- Abdominal ultrasound: renal pelvic dilation can occur (normal dog renal pelvis diameter = 1-3.8 mm [median, 2 mm], on fluid therapy = 1.3-3.6 mm [median, 2.5 mm], pyelonephritis = 1.9-12 mm [median, 3.6 mm]; normal cat renal pelvis diameter = 0.8-3.2 mm [median, 1.6 mm], on fluid therapy = 1.1-3.4 mm [median, 2.3 mm], pyelonephritis = 1.7-12.4 mm [median, 4 mm]) and may mimic hydroureter due to ureteral obstruction; renomegaly, or small and irregular kidneys. Alterations in renal parenchymal echogenicity and other changes may be present.
- Urine C&S: before treatment when suspicion of pyelonephritis exists, even if urine sediment inactive
  - In occult pyelonephritis, urine C&S can be negative, and repeated C&S is justified if other features (e.g., renal ultrasound findings, intermittent pyuria) suggest pyelonephritis.

Advanced or Confirmatory Testing

- Confirmatory tests are used rarely. Presumptive diagnosis is based on compatible history, physical, laboratory (including C&S), and ultrasonographic findings.
- Ultrasound-guided pyelocentesis to obtain urine directly from the renal pelvis for C&S; begin with routine cystocentesis instead, and choose pyelocentesis if trying to pinpoint source of infection to one kidney (rarely necessary).
- Blood cultures can be helpful, especially with acute pyelonephritis.
- Excretory urogram and/or cystourethrogram to rule out anatomic abnormalities for recurrent UTIs (abdominal ultrasound is used first)
- Rule out other causes of recurrent UTI as appropriate (e.g., hyperadrenocorticism).
- Renal cortex biopsy: typically not helpful due to localization of disease (renal pelvis and interstitium)

TREATMENT

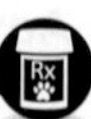

Treatment Overview

The mainstay of treatment is therapy with appropriate antimicrobial drugs. It is often a challenge to obtain a positive urine C&S result, despite renal infection. Because pyelonephritis often occurs secondary to another disease process, recurrence is common unless the predisposing condition can be addressed. Renal failure is addressed as needed (pp. 23, 167, and 169).

Acute General Treatment

- Antimicrobial therapy
  - Antibiotic selection is based on C&S results whenever possible. Interpret susceptibility data using serum rather than urine antimicrobial breakpoints.
  - Oral route is often adequate, but vomiting or septicemia warrants parenteral therapy.
  - Pending results or if C&S is negative despite clinical suspicion of pyelonephritis, therapy is indicated using a renally excreted bactericidal antibiotic with gram-negative spectrum. Examples:
    - Fluoroquinolone (e.g., enrofloxacin 5-20 mg/kg q 24h IV, IM, or PO [dogs] or 5 mg/kg q 24h [cats], pradofloxacin 5 mg/kg PO q 24h [cats], marbofloxacin, or orbifloxacin)
    - Augmented penicillin: amoxicillin-clavulanate 22 mg/kg PO q 8-12h or ampicillin-sulbactam. Beta-lactams may be less efficacious in pyelonephritis than cystitis.
    - Trimethoprim-sulfadiazine: only the trimethoprim portion is likely to achieve high renal concentrations.
  - For intact male dogs: antimicrobial that penetrates blood-prostate barrier (e.g., fluoroquinolone, trimethoprim-sulfadiazine)
  - Although evidence regarding optimal duration of antimicrobial treatment is lacking, due to issues of renal medullary blood flow, duration should be greater than for bacterial cystitis. Traditionally, 3-6 weeks of treatment has been recommended, but much shorter courses are used in humans (7-14 days) and might be adequate in dogs and cats.
  - If initial urine sediment was active, a repeat urinalysis ≈1 week after starting antibiotic therapy is recommended (ensure resolution of bacteruria, pyuria).
  - If predisposing cause cannot be resolved, urine C&S should be repeated regularly to identify future infections.
  - Fungal pyelonephritis may be more difficult to eradicate than bacterial pyelonephritis.
- Hospitalization is not indicated if the patient is drinking and eating enough to maintain hydration. For animals with sepsis (uncommon), fluid therapy and blood pressure maintenance are key management factors (p. 907).
- Treatment of uremic renal failure starts with isotonic crystalloid fluid therapy (pp. 23 and 169).

- Uremic signs are managed as for acute kidney injury and CKD (pp. 23 and 169).
- Medical therapy for hypokalemia (p. 516)

Chronic Treatment

- Identification, treatment, or cure of predisposing cause if possible (e.g., vulvar/preputial conformational abnormality, hyperadrenocorticism, ectopic ureter, urolithiasis)
- Other treatments for CKD as necessary (pp. 167 and 169).

Nutrition/Diet

A diet restricted/optimized in protein and phosphorus is ideal for animals with CKD. Regardless, ensure the availability of fresh drinking water at all times.

Drug Interactions

Treatment with a fluoroquinolone that is FDA approved for use in cats is recommended. Avoid trimethoprim-sulfa antibiotics in Doberman pinschers or dogs with keratoconjunctivitis sicca.

Possible Complications

- Failure to resolve infection: bacterial resistance is common if there is infection secondary to an underlying disease process or a structural lesion, or if antimicrobials have been used in the recent past for any infection (e.g., pyoderma, cystitis).
- Urolithiasis (nephrolithiasis), ureteral obstruction due to urolithiasis
- Renal damage after pyelonephritis may be permanent; CKD

Recommended Monitoring

- Repeat urine C&S 1-2 weeks after completion of antibiotics and ≈1 and 2 months later to ensure negative C&S.
- If predisposing cause cannot be resolved, monitoring should include urinalysis and urine C&S q 3-6 months to identify recurrence.
- When initial urine C&S is negative despite clinical suspicion of pyelonephritis, monitoring should include water consumption before and after initiation of antibiotics to assess efficacy of therapy. If water consumption decreases within 2 weeks of antimicrobial therapy, treatment should be continued for a total of 3-6 weeks.

PROGNOSIS & OUTCOME

- Guarded to good, depending on ability to correct predisposing cause and antimicrobial susceptibility of pathogen
- Prognosis for recurrent pyelonephritis is guarded because infections can cause renal failure and recurrent infections tend to develop resistance to multiple antimicrobials.

PEARLS & CONSIDERATIONS

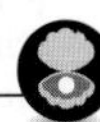

Comments

- Pyelonephritis is often difficult to confirm, especially after initiation of antimicrobial therapy.
- Evidence of renal pelvic dilation (pyelectasia) on ultrasound without other supportive clinical findings may indicate a past infection with permanent renal injury or be due to fluid therapy.
- Chronic pyelonephritis can occur without producing any overt clinical signs and without changes on CBC, serum biochemical profile, or urine sediment exam.
- A urine C&S is warranted in the management of any chronic renal disorder. Because pyelonephritis may be clinically silent and difficult to detect (e.g., diluted urine may give the mistaken appearance of an inactive sediment), urine C&S is warranted periodically in the management of any chronic kidney disorder.
- Pyelonephritis is treatable, and early intervention allows reversal of renal tubular damage.

Prevention

- Address conditions that predispose to UTI directly (e.g., correct anatomic urinary abnormalities).
- If predisposing causes cannot be avoided, use periodic urine C&S to identify recurrent infections as early as possible.

Technician Tips

- Because urethral catheterization can introduce bacteria, use strict aseptic technique.
- Animals that are hospitalized should be allowed to empty their bladder on a regular basis. Dogs that are particularly well housetrained can retain urine when kenneled, which can predispose to ascending pyelonephritis. Cats may have preferences for the type of cat litter used. Monitoring frequency and volume of urine output in hospitalized animals is vitally important.

Client Education

- In animals with recurrent UTI or complicating factors (p. 232), urine C&S is essential, rather than empirical antimicrobial therapy.
- Treatment of resistant strains of bacteria causing pyelonephritis may be costly and require prolonged therapy; consider consultation with veterinary internist, pharmacologist, or microbiologist.
- CKD may predispose animals (especially cats) to recurrent renal infections.

SUGGESTED READING

Olin SJ, et al: Urinary tract infections: treatment/comparative therapeutics. Vet Clin North Am Small Anim Pract 45:721-746, 2015.

AUTHOR: Marie E. Kerl, DVM, MPH, DACVIM, DACVECC
EDITOR: Leah A. Cohn, DVM, PhD, DACVIM

Pyoderma

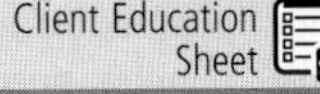

BASIC INFORMATION

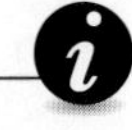

Definition

A bacterial infection of the skin and one of the most common diseases of dogs

Synonym

Bacterial dermatitis

Epidemiology

SPECIES, AGE, SEX

- Common in dogs, rare in cats
- Impetigo (superficial form of pyoderma, typically in puppies): sometimes in conjunction with immunosuppression, poor nutrition, endoparasitism, or poor hygiene
- Acne is a type of pyoderma that occurs more commonly in young dogs.
- Feline: deep bacterial infections (cellulitis, abscess) are more common in outdoor animals.

GENETICS, BREED PREDISPOSITION

- Intertrigo (skinfold pyoderma): English bulldogs and other brachycephalic breeds
- Mucocutaneous pyoderma: German shepherd, Bichon frisé, poodle
- Familial idiopathic deep pyoderma: German shepherd
- Acne: short-coated breeds such as boxers, Doberman pinschers, bulldogs, Great Danes, and others

RISK FACTORS

- Some forms of pyoderma, particularly superficial bacterial folliculitis (SBF) and bacterial overgrowth syndrome (BOGS), are often secondary to underlying disorders such as hypersensitivity skin disease (atopic dermatitis, food allergy, flea bite hypersensitivity), endocrinopathies (hypothyroidism, hyperadrenocorticism), parasitic skin disease (*Sarcoptes, Demodex* spp), immune-mediated diseases, or cornification disorders.
- Deep pyoderma may be associated with underlying immunoincompetence.

CONTAGION AND ZOONOSIS

Staphylococcus pseudintermedius, the most common cause of canine pyoderma, is considered to be rarely pathogenic to humans.

GEOGRAPHY AND SEASONALITY

Warm and humid environments predispose animals to pyoderma.

Clinical Presentation

DISEASE FORMS/SUBTYPES

Surface pyoderma: infection restricted to the surface layer of the epidermis:
- Dog: intertrigo (skinfold pyoderma), acute moist dermatitis (pyotraumatic dermatitis, hot spots), BOGS

Superficial pyoderma: infection involving the epidermis and the infundibular portion of the hair follicle:
- Dog: impetigo, SBF, exfoliative superficial pyoderma (ESP, superficial spreading pyoderma), mucocutaneous pyoderma

Deep pyoderma: bacterial infection extending beyond the hair follicle to involve the dermis and subcutis, which may lead to cellulitis:
- Dog: acne, pyotraumatic furunculosis, nasal folliculitis (inflammation of the hair follicle) and furunculosis (simultaneous occurrence of many furuncles, which are inflamed hair follicles that have ruptured, triggering pyogranulomatous dermal inflammation), interdigital furunculosis/pododermatitis, infected acral lick dermatitis (lick granuloma), callus pyoderma, and postgrooming furunculosis; German shepherd: deep pyoderma
- Cat: bite wounds, cellulitis, abscess, feline acne

HISTORY, CHIEF COMPLAINT

Animals typically are presented for evaluation of skin changes: pustules, crusts, epidermal collarettes, hair loss, and/or pruritus. Animals with deep pyoderma may show signs of pain.

PHYSICAL EXAM FINDINGS

- Impetigo: small nonfollicular pustules and crusts on the ventral abdomen
- BOGS: pruritus, greasy coat, offensive odor, erythema, lichenification, hyperpigmentation, excoriations, and alopecia
- SBF: papules, pustules, and epidermal collarettes with patchy alopecia, producing a moth-eaten appearance of the haircoat over the trunk. Resolving lesions may show central hyperpigmentation (bull's-eye lesion).
- ESP: large epidermal collarettes with an erythematous leading edge noted over the trunk; associated exudate may form crusts.
- Canine acne: deep folliculitis and furunculosis, with crusting and possible scarring on the lips and chin of young dogs
- Mucocutaneous pyoderma: crusts and erosions affecting the lip margin, nasal planum, eyelid margin, vulva, prepuce, and perianal area
- Pyotraumatic folliculitis and furunculosis: may occur anywhere on the body, depending on underlying cause; atypical acute moist dermatitis with superficial ulceration but also a component of deep folliculitis and occasional furunculosis. Clinically, this lesion may be thickened and plaquelike and have satellite papules and pustules.
- Nasal folliculitis and furunculosis: initially a papular/pustular eruption on the bridge of the nose that progresses to ulceration, crusting, and hemorrhage
- Pedal furunculosis (bacterial pododermatitis): interdigital papulonodules, hemorrhagic bullae, and ulceration with draining tracts and fibrosis; alopecia secondary to licking
- Callus pyoderma: develops over pressure points. Skin is thickened, fibrotic, and hyperpigmented with foci of papules, pustules, and ulceration.
- Postgrooming folliculitis/furunculosis: papular/pustular rash, crust formation, self-induced alopecia
- German shepherd deep pyoderma: lesions include ulcerations and draining tracts on the lateral thighs, trunk, and groin ± lips.
- Infected feline acne: comedones, papules, pustules, and alopecia confined to the mandibular and perilabial areas
- Feline bite wounds/abscess/cellulitis: swelling, pain, and alopecia in the affected area; possible dermal and cutaneous necrosis with ulceration, purulent exudate, and hemorrhage

Etiology and Pathophysiology

- Canine skin is characterized by a relatively thin stratum corneum, a paucity of intercellular lipids, lack of a follicular plug, and a higher pH than that of humans and other domestic species. This predisposes the dog to overgrowth of commensal flora and colonization by potentially pathogenic bacteria.
- Superficial infection may occur if the integrity of the skin is weakened by trauma or there are changes in surface immunity.
- Deep bacterial infections are generally an extension of a superficial pyoderma. As infection progresses deeper into the hair follicle, rupture of the follicle (furuncles) occurs. This leads to a pyogranulomatous endogenous foreign-body reaction on the part of the host. This reaction occurs initially in the dermis and is an inflammatory response to keratin, bacterial organisms, and cellular debris.
- More than 90% of cases in dogs are caused by coagulase-positive *S. pseudintermedius,* a normal component of canine skin flora. A small number of cases are caused by *Staphylococcus aureus,* the most common human pathogen. Other staphylococcal bacteria (e.g., the coagulase-positive *Staphylococcus schleiferi* subsp *coagulans* and the coagulase-negative *Staphylococcus schleiferi* subsp *schleiferi*) are less commonly associated with bacterial pyoderma.
  - *Staphylococcus intermedius* was reclassified as *S. pseudintermedius* in 2007.
- The gram-negative organisms, *Proteus* spp, *Escherichia coli,* and *Pseudomonas* spp, may act as secondary invaders. Deep pyoderma is occasionally associated with *Actinomyces, Nocardia,* mycobacteria, and *Actinobacillus* spp.
- In cats, *Pasteurella multocida* and beta-hemolytic *Streptococcus* are routinely involved.

DIAGNOSIS

Diagnostic Overview

The dermatologic exam alone may provide a strong suspicion of pyoderma (see signs listed above). With clinical signs of deep pyoderma, systemic signs, or recurrence despite therapy, additional tests beyond basic dermatologic testing are often indicated to rule out predisposing causes.

Differential Diagnosis

- Demodicosis
- Dermatophytosis
- *Pemphigus foliaceus*
- Cutaneous epitheliotropic lymphoma

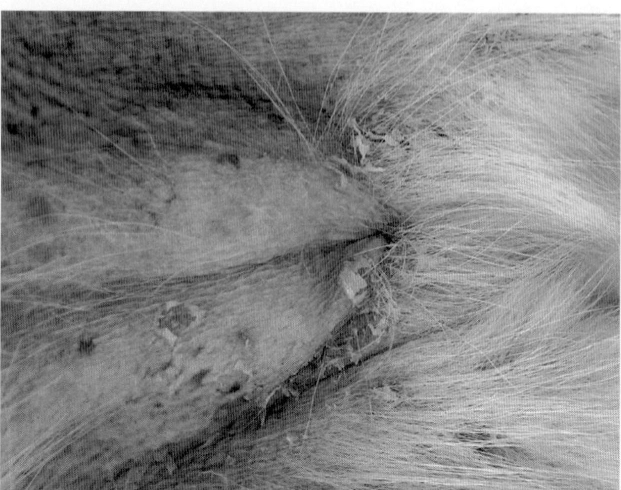

PYODERMA Epidermal collarettes on the ventral abdomen of a dog with superficial bacterial folliculitis. (Copyright Dr. Manon Paradis.)

- Subcutaneous mycoses (deep pyoderma)
- Atypical mycobacterial infections (deep pyoderma)
- Hookworm (deep pedal pyoderma)
- Foreign-body granulomas (deep pyoderma)

Initial Database

- Skin scrapings to confirm or rule out *Demodex* and *Sarcoptes*
- Skin cytologic exam (p. 1091): direct smear from pustule reveals bacteria, neutrophils in varying stages of degeneration, and active bacterial phagocytosis.
- Fungal culture (for dermatophytes and possibly for deep mycosis if draining tracts are present)

Advanced or Confirmatory Testing

- Culture and susceptibility (C&S) testing: when there has been a failure to respond to rational antibiotic therapy or bacilli are noted on skin cytologic exam
- Skin biopsy and histopathologic exam: not performed unless cases are not responding to appropriate antibiotic therapy. Findings include intraepidermal neutrophilic pustules, folliculitis, or furunculosis ± underlying cause (e.g., *Demodex*, pemphigus foliaceus, epitheliotrophic lymphoma, calcinosis cutis).
- Endocrine status: thyroid function and adrenal function tests may be warranted
- Allergy testing: intradermal or serum allergy testing for environmental allergies, and elimination diet trial for food allergy may be warranted.

TREATMENT

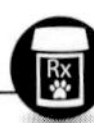

Treatment Overview

The main goals are to treat the infection and determine the underlying cause(s).

Acute General Treatment

Topical therapy:

- Topical therapy alone is a desirable approach for most cases of surface pyoderma and many cases of superficial pyoderma (e.g., impetigo, mild or localized SBF) and to help prevent recurrence of SBF while pursuing diagnostic procedures for primary underlying skin disease.
- Chlorhexidine shampoos 2%-4% (typically twice weekly) and/or daily chlorhexidine 2%-4% spray or wipes are most commonly used.
- Shampoos containing benzoyl peroxide, ethyl lactate, and povidone-iodine may also be used.
- Topical antibiotics: mupirocin, fusidic acid (Fucidin) most commonly used. Silver sulfadiazine and benzoyl peroxide 5% gels are also available, as are nisin wipes.
- Topical barrier membrane enhancing products; ceramides
- Clip affected areas.
- Deep pyoderma: bathe animal or soak lesion with Epsom salts solution (magnesium sulfate, 2 tablespoons/L of lukewarm water) or Burrow's solution (aluminum acetate solution) daily.

Systemic antibiotic therapy:

- Systemic antibiotic therapy is required to treat widespread superficial pyodermas and deep pyodermas.
- Bactericidal antibiotics are generally recommended for skin infections; however, bacteriostatic drugs may be effective in an immunocompetent animal. The chosen drug should have a narrow spectrum to limit the effects on the normal flora of the skin and gastrointestinal (GI) tract.
- Cases should be treated for a minimum of 3-4 weeks or 7-14 days beyond clinical cure. Deep pyoderma may take as long as 12 weeks to resolve. Regular re-exam is recommended to minimize overly prolonged use of antibiotics.
- The most commonly used antibiotics (generally monotherapy) include
    - Cephalexin 22-30 mg/kg PO q 8-12h (most common choice for dogs)
    - Clavulanic acid–potentiated amoxicillin 12.5-25 mg/kg PO q 12h
    - Clindamycin 5.5-11 mg/kg PO q 12h
    - Cefovecin injectable 8 mg/kg SQ q 14 days
- Other suggested drugs/dosages include (generally monotherapy, all PO) cefpodoxime 5-10 mg/kg q 24h, oxacillin 22 mg/kg q 8h, erythromycin 10-20/kg q 8h (vomiting and diarrhea common), lincomycin 15-25 mg/kg q 12h, azithromycin 5 mg/kg q 24h, tylosin 10-20 mg/kg q 12h, trimethoprim-sulfadiazine 15-30 mg/kg q 12h, enrofloxacin 5-20 mg/kg q 24h (not in immature animals), marbofloxacin 2.75-5.5 mg/kg q 24h (not in immature animals), pradofloxacin 3-4.4 mg/kg q 24h (labeled for cats only in the United States), or doxycycline 5 mg/kg (day 1), then 2.5 mg/kg q 12h
- Appropriate pain management

Chronic Treatment

- In face of an idiopathic recurrent pyoderma (typically SBF) that recurs fewer than three or four times per year, it is economical and reasonable to treat each event with an appropriate course of antibiotics. Repeated use of antibiotics increases the importance for culture and susceptibility testing. p. 653.
- In cases of idiopathic recurrent pyoderma in which several episodes occur annually and/or total annual antibiotic administration is > 12 weeks, adjunctive immunomodulatory therapy or extended antibiotic regimens (both controversial in veterinary dermatology) may be needed to maintain clinical remission.
    - Immunomodulatory therapy: Staphage Lysate (SPL, Delmont Laboratories) may decrease recurrences of pyoderma in up to 35% of dogs. The dog should initially receive a 4- to 6-week course of oral antibiotic in conjunction with a 20- to 30-week course of SPL (0.5 mL twice weekly SQ). If the pyoderma does not recur during that period, the frequency of injections is gradually reduced to once weekly and then to every other week.
    - Extended regimens of antibiotic therapy (or pulse therapy): in light of emerging multidrug-resistant *Staphylococcus* spp, pulse therapy should be considered a last resort and should be used only with regular C&S monitoring (p. 653).
- Antimicrobial shampoo or lotions used on a regular basis may assist in the prevention of relapses by limiting the bacterial surface flora.

Possible Complications

- Many antibiotics occasionally cause vomiting and diarrhea.
- Fluoroquinolones can cause cartilage damage in growing puppies.
- Potentiated sulfonamides: keratoconjunctivitis sicca, polyarthritis, uveitis, immune-mediated dermatitis, hepatobiliary disease, drug interaction, decreased thyroid function (possible hypothyroidism at high dose), blood dyscrasias
- Benzoyl peroxide gel has to be used with care because it may be irritating with repeated use and causes fabric and hair discoloration.
- Drug-induced pemphigus foliaceus (beta-lactams)

Recommended Monitoring

It is important to assess response to therapy before the antibiotic course is completed to determine the appropriate duration of antibiotic administration and also to determine if there is residual pruritus, which would suggest underlying allergy, ectoparasite, or concurrent *Malassezia* dermatitis.

PROGNOSIS & OUTCOME

- Superficial pyoderma: good prognosis as long as underlying factors are addressed adequately
- Deep pyoderma: some cases of deep pyoderma result in scarring.
- Affected animals are often immunosuppressed or have other concurrent diseases.

PEARLS & CONSIDERATIONS

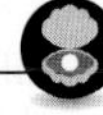

Comments

- Epidermal collarettes are extremely useful secondary skin lesions to look for (clip some hair if needed); they are strongly suggestive of a superficial pyoderma.
- Any therapeutic plan for controlling pyoderma without considering underlying predisposing factors is destined to fail.
- Most dermatologists use cephalexin as their first drug choice because it has been shown to be an effective drug against *S. pseudintermedius*. However, there are increasing concerns about emerging resistance. C&S testing should be considered more frequently (p. 653).
- Pemphigus foliaceus, calcinosis cutis, and epitheliotrophic lymphoma may manifest as

pyodermas that fail to respond to appropriate antibiotic therapy. Skin biopsy is indicated.
- The use of immunomodulating therapy and an extended antibiotic regimen should be limited to veterinary dermatologists.

Technician Tips

- When medicated shampoos are used, it is important to respect the contact time, typically 5-10 minutes. Using a timer aids in providing sufficient contact time.
- Clipping the haircoat may facilitate topical treatment and accelerate healing. However, one needs the client's permission first.

Client Education

Counsel clients concerning the potential chronicity of the disease because of underlying predisposing factors. The need of long-term antibiotic therapy regimens, importance of treating for 1-2 weeks beyond cure, and need for recheck must be explained thoroughly.

SUGGESTED READING

Miller WH Jr, et al: Muller & Kirk's Small animal dermatology, ed 7, St. Louis, 2013, Saunders, pp 184-222.

AUTHOR: Michael Hannigan, BVMS
EDITOR: Manon Paradis, DMV, MVSc, DACVD

Pyometra

Bonus Material Online 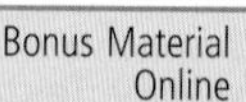 Client Education Sheet 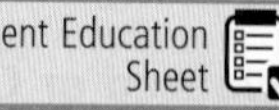

BASIC INFORMATION

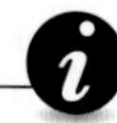

Definition

Pyometra (Greek *pyon* = pus and *metra* = womb) is an acute or chronic, suppurative metritis in bitches and queens with at least one partial (remnant) or intact ovary and a partial or intact uterus.

Synonyms

Cystic endometrial hyperplasia, suppurative metritis

Epidemiology

SPECIES, AGE, SEX

Female dogs and cats, any age (most common in middle to old age)

GENETICS, BREED PREDISPOSITION

Anecdotal familial predisposition in certain lines:
- Dogs: spaniels, golden retrievers, rottweilers, rough-coated collies. Lower risk for German shepherds, dachshunds, drevers, and Swedish hounds.
- Cats: purebred, oriental breeds (e.g., Sphinx, Siberian, ocicat, Korat, Siamese), Ragdoll, Maine coon, Bengal, Burmese

RISK FACTORS

- Affected females commonly middle-aged to older (mean age, 7.25 years)
- Nulliparous bitches more commonly affected
- Higher risk for females that have a history of exogenous steroid hormone treatment (e.g., mismating shot, use of progestogens for estrus prevention)
- Bitches usually presented within 12 weeks after estrus
- Cats usually present within 4 weeks after estrus

ASSOCIATED DISORDERS

Cystic endometrial hyperplasia (CEH) is an underlying disease entity that enables development of pyometra, but pyometra can also arise *de novo* (without CEH), and in some cases, CEH occurs secondary to pyometra as a result of the uterine reaction to bacterial infection.

Clinical Presentation

DISEASE FORMS/SUBTYPES

- Open-cervix pyometra: mucopurulent blood–tinged vaginal discharge is often the only sign.
- Closed-cervix pyometra: animals often systemically ill due to bacteremia/endotoxemia

HISTORY, CHIEF COMPLAINT

Because of the possibility of an ovarian remnant, pyometra should be ruled out in any intact or spayed bitch or queen that presents with any of the following signs: vaginal discharge, depression, abdominal discomfort, vomiting, anorexia, polyuria/polydipsia, and/or pyrexia.

PHYSICAL EXAM FINDINGS

- Vaginal discharge and systemic signs depend on patency of cervix.
  - Open: mucopurulent vaginal discharge (± hemorrhagic) may be only physical abnormality.
  - Closed: pyrexia, depression, abdominal distention, abdominal discomfort, dehydration, tachycardia, ± pallor, ± petechia (if secondary coagulopathy due to sepsis)
- Abdominal palpation usually reveals tubular enlarged uterus in case of closed-cervix pyometra. Great care should be taken to avoid uterine rupture.

Etiology and Pathophysiology

- Bacteria suspected to ascend through an open cervix during proestrus/estrus
  - *Escherichia coli* is the most common isolate from pyometra.
  - Bacterial binding through fimbriae on uterine epithelium is the first step.
- Progesterone (exogenous or endogenous) is essential for the occurrence of pyometra (ovariectomized females with an intact or partial uterus are at risk if they are treated with exogenous progesterone).
  - Progesterone influence during diestrus suppresses the immune response, reduces myometrial contractions, closes the cervix, and promotes uterine gland proliferation and secretions, which aids in bacterial proliferation.
- CEH is a common uterine pathology in older bitches in response to empty estrous cycles.
  - Cystic/hyperplastic effects are cumulative and enhanced by estrogen exposure during the preceding estrous period.
  - Older dogs that were never pregnant are at highest risk.
- In cats, pyometra is believed to be associated with spontaneous ovulation, which occurs in certain cat breeds quite commonly. The prolonged progesterone influence is thought to have similar predisposing effects in queens as in bitches.

DIAGNOSIS

Diagnostic Overview

Diagnostic process should always include a transabdominal ultrasonographic exam and CBC.

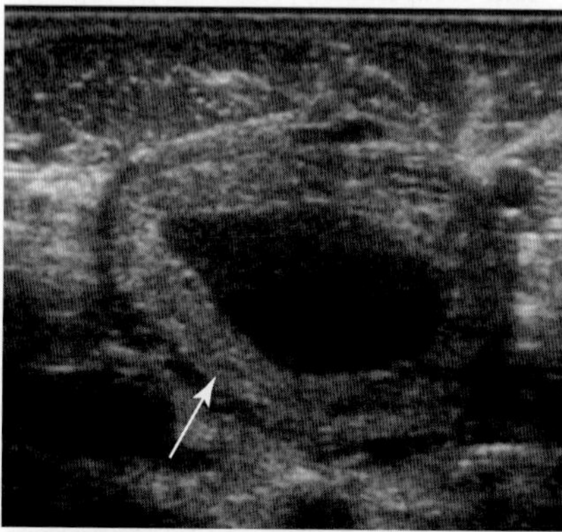

PYOMETRA Ultrasonographic image of the caudal abdomen of a bitch with pyometra. Note the fluid-filled uterus and thickened uterine wall with evidence of cystic changes *(arrow)*. (Used with permission from Krekeler N, et al: Pyometra. In Monnet E, editor: Small animal soft tissue surgery, Ames, IA, 2013, Wiley-Blackwell, pp 625-634.)

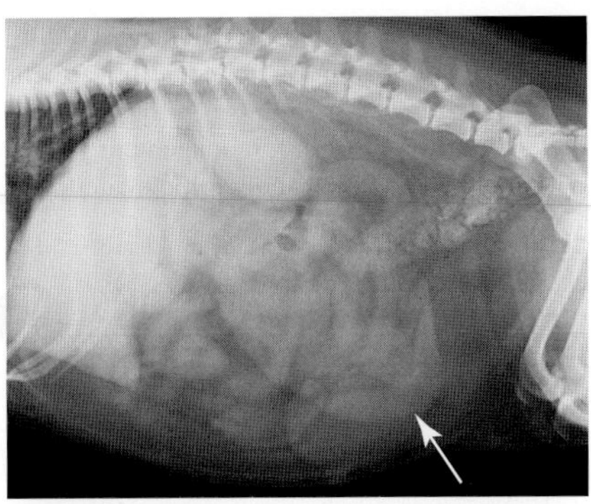

PYOMETRA Lateral abdominal radiographic image. Note the fluid-filled uterus *(arrow)*. (Used with permission from Krekeler N, et al: Pyometra. In Monnet E, editor: Small animal soft tissue surgery, Ames, IA, 2013, Wiley-Blackwell, pp 625-634.)

Differential Diagnosis

- Uterine enlargement
  - Pregnancy: ruled out by ultrasonography performed > 25 days after the luteinizing hormone (LH) peak
  - Mucometra or hematometra: not associated with systemic clinical signs and neutrophilia
- Systemic clinical signs
  - Polyuria/polydipsia (pp. 812 and 1271)
  - Abdominal discomfort or distention (p. 21)
- Vulvar discharge (p. 1045)

Initial Database

- Diagnostic imaging
  - Ultrasonography is strongly recommended. The uterine horns are convoluted and filled with anechoic to hypoechoic fluid (± flocculation); uterine wall can be thickened, and cystic endometrial hyperplastic changes may be visible
  - If abdominal radiography is performed, fetal ossification is visible only after day 42, and distinction of uterine enlargement between pregnancy and pyometra is not possible earlier.
- CBC
  - Leukocytosis (>35 × 10^9/L) common; neutrophilia with left shift (± toxic change)
  - Decreased white blood cell count may be observed due to pooling of neutrophils inside uterine lumen.
- Biochemistry
  - Hyperproteinemia, hypergammaglobulinemia, hypoalbuminemia, hypercholesterolemia, and elevation of C-reactive protein level
  - Increase in serum liver enzymes, azotemia (response to sepsis and dehydration)
  - Electrolyte imbalances (if vomiting and diarrhea)
- Urinalysis
  - Bacteriuria, glucosuria, isosthenuria and proteinuria
  - Cystocentesis under ultrasound guidance to minimize risk of uterine puncture
  - Midstream urine sample is likely to be contaminated by vaginal discharge.

Advanced or Confirmatory Testing

- Culture and cytology of vaginal discharge
  - Cytology findings (degenerate polymorphonuclear cells and phagocytized bacteria) often indistinguishable from other causes of vaginal discharge (e.g., foreign object, vaginitis)
  - Bacterial culture: usually detects normal vaginal flora (often *E. coli*), and bacterial culture is therefore important only for appropriate antibiotic choice and not diagnosis. Sample for culture should be collected from the cranial vagina with a guarded swab or from the uterus with the use of endoscope.
- Additional blood tests
  - Serum progesterone usually > 2 ng/mL
  - Prostaglandin F_{2a} (PGF_{2a}) metabolites useful to rule out hydrometra and mucometra (elevated only in cases of pyometra)

TREATMENT

Treatment Overview

- Complete ovariohysterectomy (OHE) is the treatment of choice for any animal that is not intended for breeding.
- Medical management is recommended only for young (<4 years), valuable breeding animals without significant systemic illness.

Acute General Treatment

Medical management:

- Medical treatment can be used on closed-cervix pyometra cases using appropriate pharmacologic agents and protocols.
- The rationale of medical treatment is to remove progesterone and to eliminate bacteria from the uterus.
- To evacuate the uterus, the cervix needs to be open. If bitch has a closed-cervix pyometra, it is paramount to immediately initiate a treatment protocol that removes the influence of progesterone and opens the cervix. Aglepristone (Alizin) is drug of choice because it does not cause uterine contractions so the risk of uterine rupture is low.
  - Aglepristone is a progesterone antagonist that competitively prevents progesterone binding to its receptor, which results in luteolysis without uterine contractions.
  - Works well in combination with PGF_{2a} in open- and closed-cervix pyometra cases
    - In closed-cervix pyometra, aglepristone should be given first to induce luteolysis and cervical opening; cervical opening occurs 26 hours (± 13 hours) after first aglepristone injection.
    - Aglepristone 10 mg/kg SQ given twice 24 hours apart; can follow with injection 8 days later
    - PGF_{2a} treatment can be started 24 hours after the last injection of aglepristone to accelerate uterine evacuation.
- If only PGF_{2a} is used, it is critical to start with low doses to minimize ecbolic effect of the drug until the cervix opens (risk of uterine rupture). After the cervix opens, the dose can be incrementally increased depending on patient tolerance, and evacuation of uterus is the desired effect of treatment.
  - Natural PGF_{2a}: dinoprost tromethamine (Lutalyse)
    - Dose of 10-15 mcg/kg q 8h for 1 day SQ; 25 mcg/kg q 8h for 2 days SQ; 50-100 mcg/kg q 8h for 3 days SQ
    - Dose can be adjusted; some animals are more sensitive and react with more side effects, but it is rare to see side effects at these low, incrementally increased doses. Others may need doses up to 100 mcg/kg for 2-3 days to evacuate uterus effectively.
  - Synthetic PGF_{2a} analog cloprostenol
    - At higher dosages, it can have side effects; stimulates less uterine contractions, prolonging resolution of pyometra compared with natural form of PGF_{2a}
    - Convenience of q 24h administration, reported to be effective if given at a dose of 1-2.5 mcg/kg q 24h for 10 days (started with 1 mcg/kg)
  - Side effects of PGF_{2a} are dose dependent and diminish after several injections.
    - Side effects (i.e., tachypnea, vomiting, diarrhea, urination, and anxiety) start about 20 minutes after treatment and last for about an hour.
    - Walking the bitch for 15 minutes after administration seems to alleviate side effects; should be hospitalized for at least 1 hour after treatment for observation
    - Animals should not be fed before PGF_{2a} treatment but rather an hour after side effects have disappeared.
- Misoprostol (synthetic PGE1 analog)
  - PGE1 causes uterine contractions and cervical relaxation, thereby assisting in evacuation of pus from the uterus. However, misoprostol does not have a luteolytic action, so it must be combined with aglepristone and/or a PGF-2a.
  - Oral dose 10 mcg/kg PO once. Vomiting can occur after oral administration. Or,
  - Dissolve tablets in saline (200 mcg for bitches < 20 kg and 400 mcg for bitches > 20 kg) and deliver intravaginally using a long soft pipette to deposit the PGE1 as close to the cervix as possible.
- Dopamine agonists: cabergoline; prolactin antagonist
  - Cabergoline 5 mcg/kg PO q 24h for 7-14 days; can be used 25 days after ovulation to treat pyometra
  - Cabergoline is most effective when used with PGF_{2a} because it potentiates the luteolytic effect and results in rapid decline in progesterone (<24-48 hours).
  - Cabergoline has minimal or no side effects.

- Antimicrobial therapy
  - Initiate antimicrobial therapy immediately with broad-spectrum antibiotic (presumption of *E. coli* infection).
  - Continued antimicrobials are based on culture and susceptibility, ideally from sample of uterine contents obtained transcervically (alternative is cranial vaginal culture) until at least 14 days after resolution of vaginal discharge.
  - Initial empirical therapy: amoxicillin/clavulanic acid 12.5-25 mg/kg PO q 12h, cephalosporins (e.g., cephazolin 22 mg/kg IV q 8h), and potentiated sulphonamides (care with renal function).

Surgical management:

- Complete removal of ovaries, uterus, and entire cervix recommended in any animal not intended for breeding, > 4 years old, presents systemically ill, or has evidence of prior CEH changes in uterine wall.
- Prior medical stabilization often indicated (p. 907)
  - If animal's health is in critical condition, medical stabilization may be possible only for a few hours before surgery is required.
  - If patient is in a more stable condition, surgery can be delayed 12-24 hours while medical treatment with aglepristone is given to aid in dilation of cervix and subsequent drainage of pus from uterus.
  - Presurgical treatment with aglepristone facilitates patient stabilization before surgery and reduces risk of uterine rupture and leakage of pus during surgery.
- It is important to monitor animal's cardiac (arrhythmia common), metabolic (acidosis common), and hydration status before, during, and after surgical procedure.
- Great care must be taken when removing uterus in a case of closed-cervix pyometra because it can be very friable. Saline-soaked laparotomy sponges can help prevent leakage of purulent discharge into abdominal cavity.
- Postoperatively, the animal should be intensively monitored for signs of acid-base/electrolyte imbalances, dehydration, hypoglycemia, hypoproteinemia, and anemia. IV fluids should be administered for a minimum of 24 hours after surgery or until bitch is eating or drinking
- Pain management can include opioids: buprenorphine 0.01 mg/kg SQ q 8h or morphine 0.1-0.2 mg/kg IV q 4-6h

Other therapy:

- Transcervical endoscopic catheterization and flushing with warm saline and subsequent intrauterine instillation of 10-15 mcg/kg of dinoprost and 10 mg/kg of cefazolin has been described.
- Care should be taken to ensure the cervix is open (e.g., flush on day 2 or 3 after initiation of antiluteolytic treatment in cases of closed pyometra).
- Uterine rupture and leakage resulting in peritonitis has not been reported but should be considered a risk.

Possible Complications

Retention of fluid in the uterus after 5 days of treatment is a poor prognostic sign for future fertility. Complete OHE should be performed in these cases.

Recommended Monitoring

- Ultrasonography is the most important tool in assessing response to medical treatment. Significant reduction in uterine wall thickness and absence of intraluminal fluid should be seen 5-7 days after initiation of treatment.
- Hematologic parameters should return to normal in about 7-15 days after treatment.
- Vaginal discharge should change from purulent to serous and significantly reduce in volume over 5 days.
- Clinical improvement in demeanor and appetite should be seen 48 hours after onset of treatment in most cases.
- Serum progesterone levels are difficult to interpret if aglepristone is used. If only PGF_{2a} is used, reduction in serum progesterone is seen within 48 hours, and serum levels are < 2 ng/mL in 5-7 days. If treatment is stopped before progesterone levels are < 2 ng/mL, pyometra can recur.
- Medical treatment can result in shortened interestrous interval, which can adversely affect a bitch's fertility in the next estrus. The subsequent estrus can be postponed with mibolerone treatment for 2-3 months starting 1 month after end of pyometra treatment, which ensures a minimal interestrous interval of 6 months.

PROGNOSIS & OUTCOME

- At 1 month after the end of therapy, reduction in ultrasonographic evidence of CEH is a good indicator of future fertility.
  - Bitches that respond to treatment within 5-7 days have a better prognosis in regards to future fertility than bitches that are slow to respond.
- Case selection is critical to success and future prognosis. Bitches < 4 years of age have a much better prognosis in regards to future fertility than bitches > 5 years of age.
- The likelihood of the bitch becoming pregnant after appropriate medical treatment during the subsequent estrus is high (>80%) with optimal breeding management and in cases with no ultrasonographic evidence of CEH.

PEARLS & CONSIDERATIONS

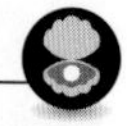

Comments

- Any animal not intended for breeding should be spayed.
- Animals that have been medically treated for pyometra should be bred the following cycle; early ultrasonographic examination for pregnancy (>21 days post LH surge) can detect the recurrence of pyometra as early as possible and before systemic clinical signs develop.

Prevention

- Do not treat females with a partial or complete uterus with exogenous progestins long-term and at high doses.
- Complete OHE if not intended for breeding
- Because of potential familial predisposition, do not breed female offspring from dams treated for pyometra.

Technician Tips

It is important to remember that the uterus can be extremely friable, and great care should be taken during abdominal palpation.

Client Education

- Animals should be bred at a young age because the incidence of pyometra increases at > 4 years.
- Breeding females should be spayed as soon as desired number of litters has been achieved.
- Animals should be bred when young (<4 years).
- Early ultrasonographic pregnancy exams should be encouraged to detect recurrence of pyometra.

SUGGESTED READING

Krekeler N, et al: Pyometra. In Monnet E, editor: Small animal soft tissue surgery, Ames, Iowa, 2013, Wiley Blackwell, pp 625-634.

AUTHORS: Natali Krekeler, Dr. med. vet., PhD, DACT; Fiona K. Hollinshead, BVSc, PhD, DACT
EDITOR: Michelle A. Kutzler, DVM, PhD, DACT

Pyothorax

Bonus Material Online Client Education Sheet 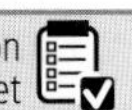

BASIC INFORMATION

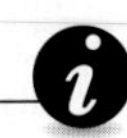

Definition

Accumulation of purulent exudate in the pleural space is associated with significant pleural inflammation.

Synonyms

Pleural empyema, thoracic empyema

Epidemiology

SPECIES, AGE, SEX

Dogs and cats:

- Medium and large dog breeds overrepresented
- Males of both species overrepresented
- Median age of occurrence: 4 years

GENETICS, BREED PREDISPOSITION

Dogs: hunting breeds subject to increased risk of inhaled foreign (plant) material

RISK FACTORS

Cats: higher risk if from multi-cat household and young. Cat fight wounds and upper respiratory infection are risk factors. Role of feline retrovirus infection not proved. No difference in risk for indoor versus outdoor

Clinical Presentation

HISTORY, CHIEF COMPLAINT

- Slowly progressive onset of dyspnea, inappetence, and weight loss, *or*
- Acute decompensation with dyspnea/tachypnea/collapse from pleural effusion

PHYSICAL EXAM FINDINGS

- Respiratory: dyspnea (p. 879), tachypnea; muffled heart and lung sounds on auscultation (unilateral/bilateral), ventral hyporesonance on thoracic percussion
- Systemic: depression, weight loss, ± pyrexia (or hypothermia, especially in cats), ± pale mucous membranes
- Cats: possibly decreased compressibility of cranial thorax on palpation
- Sometimes, findings suggest septic shock (e.g., prolonged capillary refill time [p. 907])

Etiology and Pathophysiology

- Septic pyothorax (most common): potential causes of pleural space infection:
  - Penetrating/migrating plant material (p. 398)
  - Inhaled plant material
  - Penetrating injury
    - Bite, stab, gunshot wounds
  - Esophageal perforation
    - Foreign body
    - *Spirocerca lupi* infection
  - Hematogenous spread
  - Extension from discospondylitis
  - Pneumonia or lung abscess
  - Pulmonary or intrathoracic neoplasia
  - Gastric foreign body migration
- Pleuritis (and nonseptic pyothorax) can be associated with canine hepatitis, leptospirosis, canine distemper, feline infectious peritonitis, toxoplasmosis, or feline upper respiratory tract infection.

DIAGNOSIS

Diagnostic Overview

The diagnosis is suspected based on presenting history and physical exam findings. Confirmation requires appropriate analysis of pleural fluid; cytologic exam provides a working clinical diagnosis, and culture can confirm bacterial contribution.

Differential Diagnosis

- Pulmonary parenchymal disease (e.g., pneumonia, edema)
- Pleural effusion
  - Chylothorax
  - Heart failure
  - Hemothorax
  - Feline infectious peritonitis
  - Neoplastic effusion
- Diaphragmatic hernia
- Intrathoracic neoplasia

Initial Database

- CBC
  - Usual: neutrophilic leukocytosis with or without a left shift
  - Possible: leukopenia, thrombocytopenia if sepsis
- Serum biochemistry profile
  - Multiple abnormalities (e.g., hepatic and renal parameters, electrolytes, hypoalbuminemia) can occur secondary to sepsis (p. 907).
- Survey thoracic radiographs
  - Identify pleural effusion; hold off if animal in severe respiratory distress until after thoracocentesis
  - After thoracocentesis: to evaluate pleural space, mediastinum, and pulmonary parenchyma for potential primary cause of pyothorax
- Thoracic ultrasound exam
  - Thoracic focused assessment of sonography for trauma (TFAST) can confirm pleural fluid for animals in distress (p. 1102).
  - Identify masses, and evaluate their internal structure.
  - Identify site of greatest pleural effusion for centesis (if overall small volume of effusion).
  - Identify foreign material in the pleural space if possible (may be challenging).
- Pleural fluid evaluation (pp. 1164 and 1343)
  - Fluid typically blood tinged; may be opaque; often foul odor (anaerobes). Macroscopic yellow clumps (sulfur granules) strongly suggest *Actinomyces* (p. 20).
  - Exudate: protein > 3 g/dL, nucleated cell count > 7×10^9/L, often > 30×10^9/L
  - Degenerate neutrophils predominate, with macrophages and activated mesothelial cells also present; intraleukocytic bacteria are diagnostic (septic pyothorax).
- Gram stain of fluid: guides initial empirical antimicrobial therapy
  - Oropharyngeal bacteria (e.g., *Pasteurella* spp, *Bacteroides* spp, *Fusobacterium* spp) common in cats; *Escherichia coli* in dogs (all gram-negative rods)
  - *Actinomyces* (anaerobe) and *Nocardia* (aerobe): important potential pathogens in dogs from regions where grass awns are endemic (p. 398); both gram-positive short rods and filaments
- Anaerobic and aerobic bacterial culture and susceptibility (C&S):
  - For planning long-term antimicrobial therapy
  - Dogs: most commonly mixed anaerobes and aerobes
  - Cats: oropharyngeal anaerobes and *Pasteurella* spp, *Streptococcus* spp, and *Mycoplasma* spp; include specific request for *Mycoplasma* culture

Advanced or Confirmatory Testing

CT

- Potentially identify cause of pyothorax.
- Evaluate mass(es) in thoracic cavity, and determine if resectable

TREATMENT

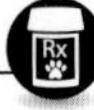

Treatment Overview

Patient stabilization, pleural drainage (thoracostomy tubes for pleural lavage), ± surgical exploration and debridement of the thoracic cavity, and long-term antimicrobial therapy based on results of microbiologic C&S testing are the standard of care.

Acute General Treatment

- Stabilize respiratory compromise
  - Therapeutic (and diagnostic) thoracocentesis (p. 1164)
  - Oxygen administration (p. 1146)
- Correct fluid and electrolyte deficits and address shock if present (p. 907).
- Antimicrobial therapy: empirical therapy active against aerobic and anaerobic bacteria (combination therapy typical)
  - Gram stain results (as previously described)
  - Amoxicillin/ampicillin 22 mg/kg IV or PO q 8h if *Actinomyces* suspected
  - Trimethoprim-sulfadiazine 15 mg/kg PO q 12h if *Nocardia*, *E. coli*, or *Pasteurella* suspected

- Enrofloxacin 10 mg/kg IV q 24h for dogs, 5 mg/kg IV q 24h for cats (use with caution); does not treat anaerobes
- Cefoxitin 22 mg/kg IV q 8h for dogs/cats
- Medical management
  - Bilateral thoracostomy tube placement (p. 1082)
  - Consider thoracic lavage q 6-8h with body-temperature sterile saline.
  - Serial cytologic evaluation of pleural fluid to assess success of lavage therapy. Improvement includes change from degenerate neutrophils with intracellular or extracellular bacteria to nondegenerate neutrophils without bacteria.
- Surgical management (more commonly indicated for dogs): thoracotomy indicated if
  - Definitive cause identified and retained in thoracic cavity (foreign body, lung lobe abscess)
  - Fluid loculated in the pleural space (lavage cannot access portions of fluid accumulation)
  - Patient fails to respond to intensive medical therapy (4-5 days of pleural lavage and antibiotics)
  - *Actinomyces* (in dogs, notoriously poor response to medical management alone)
- Surgical management: aggressive debridement of the pleural space, removal of underlying cause if identified, thorough intraoperative lavage, and postoperative intermittent pleural aspiration, lavage, and antimicrobial therapy
  - Video-assisted thoracic surgery has been described for debridement in dogs. Significant adhesions or inability to visualize critical structures should prompt conversion to median sternotomy.

Chronic Treatment

- Thoracostomy tube removal based on overt clinical and cytologic resolution of infection. The incidence of infection related to thoracostomy tube placement in healthy dogs suggests avoidance of long-term indwelling thoracostomy tubes.
- Long-term antibiotic therapy in all cases (4-6 weeks minimum)
  - Based on accurate identification of organism(s) involved
  - Up to 3 months of therapy may be required.

Possible Complications

Failure to resolve/recurrence of pyothorax:
- Cause not removed
- Failure of medical management:
  - Ineffective pleural lavage
  - Ineffective/inappropriate antibiotic therapy

Recommended Monitoring

Thoracic radiographs at completion of antibiotic therapy and q 3 months for first year after recovery

PROGNOSIS & OUTCOME

- Surgical management, which may include thoracoscopic debridement, is associated with a better prognosis than medical management in dogs with pyothorax in some studies; disease-free at 1 year: 78% (surgical) versus 25% (medical)
- Development of fibrosing pleuritis is associated with poor outcome.
- Lower heart rate and hypersalivation are associated with poorer outcomes for cats.
- Overall, 66% of cats and 80% of dogs can survive if treated appropriately.

PEARLS & CONSIDERATIONS

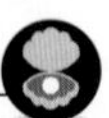

Comments

- Intensive therapy should start immediately on diagnosis. Undertreatment is thought to be a major contributor to morbidity/mortality.
- Surgical treatment has been associated with a better outcome than medical treatment alone for dogs. However, this varies by study and may not apply in regions where grass awns are rarely identified.
- Cats are more often successfully treated with bilateral thoracostomy tubes and appropriate antimicrobial therapy.
- Benefit of saline lavage as opposed to drainage alone is uncertain. Animals with thicker, more flocculent fluid are more likely to benefit.
- Addition of antimicrobials or other drugs to lavage fluid is not indicated.
- Bilateral thoracostomy tubes are helpful in aspiration and lavage of the pleural space.
- Antimicrobial therapy should be guided by culture and susceptibility, with attention paid to *Actinomyces* and *Nocardia* and to *Mycoplasma* in cats.
- Obligate anaerobes are common in pyothorax and are found in combination with aerobes; antimicrobial treatment should be aimed at both types of bacteria until culture results are available.

Technician Tips

Knowledge of and experience in working with thoracostomy tubes is important in the management of patients with pyothorax:
- Used as the primary treatment modality for nonsurgical thoracic drainage and lavage
- Used in the postoperative period for continued thoracic drainage ± lavage

SUGGESTED READING

Stillion JR, et al: A clinical review of the pathophysiology, diagnosis, and treatment of pyothorax in dogs and cats. J Vet Emerg Crit Care 25:113-129, 2015.

AUTHOR: MaryAnn G. Radlinsky, DVM, MS, DACVS
EDITOR: Elizabeth A. Swanson, DVM, MS, DACVS

Pyrethrins/Pyrethroids Toxicosis

BASIC INFORMATION

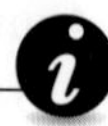

Definition

- Pyrethrins are derived from *Chrysanthemum* flowers, and pyrethroids are synthetic pyrethrins.
- Pyrethroids are further divided into type I (lack a cyano group) and type II (with an alpha-cyano group). Type I pyrethroids include allethrin, bifenthrin, etofenprox, permethrin, phenothrin, resmethrin, and tetramethrin. Type II pyrethroids include cyfluthrin, cyhalothrin, cypermethrin, cyphenothrin, deltamethrin, esfenvalerate, fenvalerate, flumethrin, lambda-cyhalothrin, and tralomethrin.
- Pyrethrins and pyrethroids can be found in a number of household and garden products as well as topical flea and tick products.
- Concentration is important in determining toxicosis. Low-concentration products are relatively safe for dogs and cats, but concentrated products can be toxic, especially to cats.
- Except for bifenthrin, most small exposures to pyrethroids in dogs do not result in significant clinical signs, but any concentrated exposure in cats can lead to severe signs.

Epidemiology

SPECIES, AGE, SEX

Cats are more sensitive to pyrethroids than dogs.

RISK FACTORS

Use of pyrethrins/pyrethroids in the environment or on the animal

GEOGRAPHY AND SEASONALITY

More exposures during flea and tick season and summer (home and lawn use)

Clinical Presentation

DISEASE FORMS/SUBTYPES

- Ingestion can cause oral paresthesia, which can manifest as hypersalivation, retching, gagging, and vomiting. Signs can be quite dramatic, but systemic toxicosis is not expected.
- Dermal exposure to pyrethrins/pyrethroids can result in dermal paresthesia in dogs (e.g.,

pruritus, twitching, behavior changes). Signs can last hours to days and typically resolve after the product is removed.
- Dermal or oral exposure to concentrated pyrethroids in cats can cause significant clinical signs, including seizures and severe tremors. Bifenthrin exposures in dogs can also result in these signs.

HISTORY, CHIEF COMPLAINT

- Cats may present with severe tremors or seizures. Often, it is reported that a flea and tick product was applied to the cat. Further investigation can reveal the active ingredient of the product as well as whether the product was intended for cats or dogs. Occasionally, cats can become clinically ill after dermal exposure to a dog that had a flea and tick product applied.
- Dogs may present with hypersalivation, retching, vomiting, rubbing on furniture, or walking a few steps, sitting down, and looking at their back. Usually, this is seen within hours of application of a flea and tick product containing a pyrethroid.

PHYSICAL EXAM FINDINGS

- Hypersalivation, licking, gagging, vomiting
- Mild to severe muscle tremors, seizures, agitation, hyperthermia
- Local dermal irritation (erythema to excoriation) near the site of application of a flea and tick product

Etiology and Pathophysiology

Pyrethrins/pyrethroids bind to the membrane lipids of nerve cells near the sodium channels, which slows normal opening and closing of the channel. Pyrethrins and type I pyrethroids cause repetitive discharges, leading to tremors and seizures. Type II pyrethroids cause conduction blocks and lead to weakness and paralysis.

DIAGNOSIS

Diagnostic Overview

Diagnosis typically revolves around whether an insecticide was used in the environment or a flea and tick medication was applied to the pet recently and on the clinical signs.

Differential Diagnosis

- Toxic: tremorgenic mycotoxins, organophosphates/carbamates, metaldehyde, methylxanthines, nicotine; prescription drugs (amphetamines, phenylpropanolamine, pseudoephedrine, isoniazid, serotonergics, dopaminergics, antidepressants, albuterol); sodium (table salt, paintballs, charcoal), ethylene glycol, hops, mushrooms, bromethalin, strychnine, organochlorines, zinc phosphide, marijuana, 5-hydroxytryptophan (5-HTP)
- Nontoxic: intracranial disorders (neoplasia, encephalitis, trauma, idiopathic epilepsy); metabolic disorders (e.g., hypocalcemia, portosystemic shunt)

Initial Database

- CBC, serum biochemistry with electrolytes: extended tremors can cause increased creatine kinase (CK) levels and azotemia secondary to rhabdomyolysis.
- Urinalysis: myoglobinuria secondary to rhabdomyolysis
- Coagulation panel: if hyperthermia is severe, disseminated intravascular coagulation (DIC) is possible.

Advanced or Confirmatory Testing

Pyrethrins/pyrethroids can be detected in hair, stomach contents, fat, liver, brain, serum, and urine, but testing is not necessary in most cases.

TREATMENT

Treatment Overview

- First, stabilize the patient neurologically and hemodynamically. Dermal decontamination then can take place by bathing with a liquid dish soap.
- Symptomatic and supportive care, including fluid therapy, close monitoring of central nervous system (CNS) status, and temperature as well as urine color until recovery (typically 24-72 hours)

Acute General Treatment

- Bathing
  - May be the only treatment needed for mildly affected animals
  - Bathe entire body with liquid dishwashing detergent
  - Bathing should be delayed if CNS signs are present until animal is stable
  - Avoid hypothermia after bath because it can potentiate tremors.
  - Vitamin E and cool compresses can be applied to the product application site to reduce irritation.
- Oral signs: dilute with milk, water, or a tasty treat to address hypersalivation and gagging/retching
- Neurologic signs
  - Methocarbamol (50-150 mg/kg slow IV to effect as needed) is the drug of choice for tremor control; if giving > 330 mg/kg/day, monitor for respiratory depression. Oral or rectal administration can be used when the injectable is not available (delayed onset).
  - Diazepam 0.5-1 mg/kg IV can be used for seizure control.
  - Intralipid therapy (p. 1127) has been suggested, but efficacy and safety have not been proved.
- Supportive care
  - IV fluids
  - Thermoregulation (p. 421)

Possible Complications

- Tremors cause breakdown of muscle (rhabdomyolysis); myoglobinuria can lead to acute renal tubular injury.
- DIC due to prolonged hyperthermia and seizure (rare)

Recommended Monitoring

CNS status, temperature, urine color

PROGNOSIS & OUTCOME

- With medical attention, prognosis is good, and recovery typically occurs in 1-3 days.
- Guarded if seizures are prolonged or refractory to treatment

PEARLS & CONSIDERATIONS

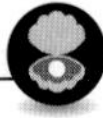

Comments

- Concentration is most important in determining toxicosis. Most household products have very low concentrations and are not expected to cause more than mild gastrointestinal signs.
- Pyrethroids are often combined with an insect growth regulator (methoprene, pyriproxyfen) and one or more synergists (piperonyl butoxide, MGK-264).

Prevention

- Never apply flea and tick products marketed for dogs to cats.
- Pyrethroid-treated dogs should be kept separate from cats until the product has dried completely (≈24 hours).
- If insecticides are applied in the environment, allow to dry completely before allowing pets in the area.

Technician Tips

Stabilize the patient before bathing. Bathing before stabilization can lead to further stress on the pet and worsen the clinical signs.

Client Education

Use only feline-approved flea and tick products on cats, and keep cats away from pyrethroid-treated dogs until the product has dried.

SUGGESTED READING

Sobczak B: Managing exposure to permethrin. Clinician's Brief May:87-89, 2012.

AUTHOR: Michelle Carlino, DVM
EDITOR: Tina Wismer, DVM, MS, DABVT, DABT

Pythiosis and Lagenidiosis

Bonus Material Online Client Education Sheet

BASIC INFORMATION

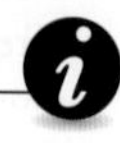

Definition

Oomycotic infections of the gastrointestinal (GI) tract *(Pythium)* or skin (*Pythium, Lagenidium*, and *Paralagenidium*) of dogs and cats caused by *Pythium insidiosum, Lagenidium* spp, and *Paralagenidium karlingii*, respectively

Synonyms

Oomycosis, phycomycosis, swamp cancer

Epidemiology

SPECIES, AGE, SEX

Dogs (young to middle-aged) affected more often than cats (any age but often < 1 year)

GENETICS, BREED PREDISPOSITION

Dogs: any breed, especially large, outdoor working breeds

RISK FACTORS

Recurrent exposure to warm freshwater lakes, swamps, and ponds that may contain *Pythium, Paralagenidium*, or *Lagenidium* zoospores, but disease in house pets without such exposure has been reported.

CONTAGION AND ZOONOSIS

Motile zoospores cause infections in mammalian species, including humans; no direct contagion or zoonotic potential

GEOGRAPHY AND SEASONALITY

- Endemic in warm, humid regions such as the southern United States, especially along the Gulf coast, and in California, Southeast Asia, Central and South America, and eastern coastal Australia
- Sporadic cases in temperate climates and areas using soil from endemic regions for landscaping
- Infections most often diagnosed in fall, winter, and early spring.

Clinical Presentation

DISEASE FORMS/SUBTYPES

- Pythiosis: GI disease, cutaneous disease
- Lagenidiosis/paralagenidiosis: cutaneous disease initially, usually progressing to systemic involvement when diagnosis is established; large vessels often affected

HISTORY, CHIEF COMPLAINT

- GI infection: weight loss with chronic vomiting and/or diarrhea; large-bowel diarrhea is common; dogs usually continue to feel well and have a good appetite despite marked weight loss.
  - Regurgitation if esophagus affected
- Cutaneous infection: nonhealing wounds and invasive skin masses containing ulcerated nodules and draining tracts

PHYSICAL EXAM FINDINGS

Dog:

- GI infection: severe weight loss in an otherwise active, alert dog; abdominal mass often palpable. Colonic mucosa may feel thickened/cobblestone on rectal exam.
- Cutaneous infection: nonhealing wounds and invasive masses that contain ulcerated nodules and draining tracts, most often involving extremities, tailhead, ventral neck, or perineum

Cat:

- Nasopharyngeal infection: nasal discharge and upper respiratory signs; ulcerated caudal oral masses
- Cutaneous infection: invasive subcutaneous masses (especially in inguinal, tailhead, and periorbital regions) or ulcerated plaquelike lesions on extremities
- GI infection: occasionally seen

Etiology and Pathophysiology

- Infection follows exposure of the immunocompetent host to motile zoospores in warm, freshwater environments.
- Hyphal growth in affected tissues causes massive inflammation resulting in masses, draining lesions, and regional lymphadenopathy. Transmural GI thickening may cause obstruction.
- Dogs with *Pythium* infection may have any portion of the GI tract affected; pylorus, proximal duodenum, and ileocolic junction are affected most often. Mesenteric lymphadenopathy is common. Invasion of mesenteric vessels may result in infarction. Esophagus is affected less often.
- Dogs with *Lagenidium* spp infection have progressive dermal or subcutaneous nodular lesions (often multifocal) involving extremities, mammary region, perineum, or trunk.
- In contrast to *Pythium* infection, dogs with paralagenidiosis have lesions in distant sites, including great vessels, sublumbar and inguinal lymph nodes, lung, pulmonary hilus, and cranial mediastinum.

DIAGNOSIS

Diagnostic Overview

The diagnosis of pythiosis is suspected in one of two contexts: chronic weight loss with vomiting and/or diarrhea (marked intestinal thickening/mass raises the differential diagnosis of neoplasia) or chronic, invasive, often ulcerated subcutaneous masses. Confirmation is by serology or histologic demonstration of the organism on biopsy. If cutaneous oomycotic infection is noted, systemic disease should be suspected in *Lagenidium* or *Paralagenidium* infections.

Differential Diagnosis

Gastrointestinal presentations:

- GI neoplasia
- Other causes of esophageal disease
- Pyloric outflow obstruction due to hypertrophy, intussusception
- Zygomycosis and other hyphal fungal infections

Cutaneous presentations:

- Mycobacterial, nocardial, and actinomycotic infections of skin
- Other cutaneous fungal infections (sporotrichosis, blastomycosis, cryptococcosis, hyalohyphomycosis)

Initial Database

- CBC: eosinophilia and nonregenerative anemia possible
- Serum biochemistry panel: hyperglobulinemia is common. Hypercalcemia has been reported.
- Abdominal radiographs: abdominal mass effect; evidence of intestinal obstruction
- Abdominal ultrasound
  - Pythiosis: severe segmental thickening of the GI tract, mesenteric lymphadenopathy

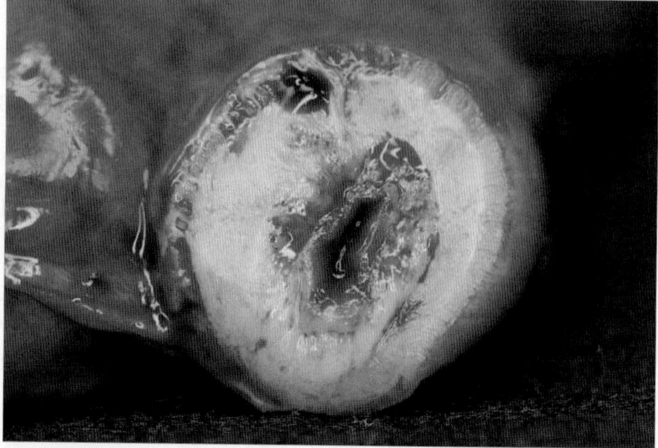

PYTHIOSIS AND LAGENIDIOSIS Cross-section of distal small intestinal *Pythium insidiosum*–induced lesion. Note characteristic mural thickening and loss of normal intestinal architecture that will eventually result in bowel obstruction.

- ◦ Paralagenidiosis: great vessel aneurysmal dilations

Advanced or Confirmatory Testing

- Cytologic preparation from fine-needle aspirate (e.g., ultrasound-guided aspirate of intestinal mass) sometimes demonstrates oomycotic hyphae.
- Rectal scrape cytology may be diagnostic with distal GI involvement (p. 1157).
- Histopathologic exam of tissue: eosinophilic pyogranulomatous inflammation; *Pythium* hyphae are difficult to visualize on hematoxylin-eosin–stained sections, whereas *Lagenidium/Paralagenidium* hyphae are easier to see.
  - ◦ Broad, rarely septate, occasionally branching hyphae are seen on silver stains. *Lagenidium/Paralagenidium* hyphae are much wider than *Pythium* hyphae.
- Culture using fungal media
- Serologic testing: ELISA, immunodiffusion, hemagglutination, and immunochromatographic tests have been developed. Cross-reactivity exists between *Lagenidium/Paralagenidium* and *Pythium*.
- Molecular phylogeny using ribosomal DNA sequencing allows speciation.

TREATMENT

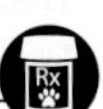

Treatment Overview

Complete surgical resection if possible.

Acute General Treatment

Complete surgical resection is the treatment of choice; segmental GI lesions are occasionally completely resectable. Amputation is recommended for cutaneous lesions limited to a single extremity. Local postoperative recurrence is common. Resection of *Lagenidium* lesions is less likely to be curative.

Chronic Treatment

- Medical therapy with itraconazole 10 mg/kg PO q 24h and terbinafine 5-10 mg/kg PO q 24h is recommended for at least 2-3 months after surgery. Some animals (<20%) respond to long-term medical therapy alone. Positive response may take months. Medical therapy for lagenidiosis/paralagenidiosis is typically ineffective.
- Adding prednisone 1 mg/kg PO q 24h may improve response rates of patients with GI pythiosis, reduce lesion size, and resolve clinical signs.
- Susceptibility of cutaneous lesions may be enhanced by topical use of essential oils.
- Treatment with a *Pythium* vaccine has been recommended but has not been well evaluated, and inconsistent results have been reported.

Possible Complications

Sudden death is associated with *Pythium* infarction or invasion of mesenteric vessels; rupture of a *Paralagenidium*-induced aneurysm of the aorta or vena cava can occur.

Recommended Monitoring

ELISA serologic titers should be used for monitoring response to medical therapy or recurrence after surgical resection.

PROGNOSIS & OUTCOME

- Pythiosis: fair to guarded if lesions appear surgically resectable; fair to guarded if medical therapy for GI disease includes prednisone
- Lagenidiosis: guarded
- Paralagenidiosis: grave

PEARLS & CONSIDERATIONS

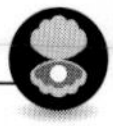

Comments

- GI pythiosis is often mistaken for diffuse intestinal neoplasia at surgery.
- Aggressive surgery with wide surgical margins is critical to cure.
- ELISA testing offers a noninvasive diagnosis and can be used for monitoring treatment.

Technician Tips

- Oomycotic hyphae are difficult to see when cytologic sample is stained with Diff-Quik; special stains may be needed.
- Affected dogs can look emaciated but maintain a good attitude and appetite. Dogs should initially be managed like a partial GI obstruction.
- Gloves should be worn while working with samples, but zoonotic disease has not been reported.

Client Education

Chronic weight loss and vomiting in a dog that spends time in the water in endemic areas should prompt early evaluation for *Pythium* infection.

SUGGESTED READING

Grooters AM: Pythiosis, lagenidiosis, and zygomycosis. In Sykes J, editor: Canine and feline infectious diseases, St. Louis, 2014, Elsevier, pp 668-678.

AUTHOR: Joseph Taboada, DVM, DACVIM
EDITOR: Rance K. Sellon, DVM, PhD, DACVIM

Rabies

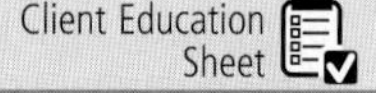

BASIC INFORMATION

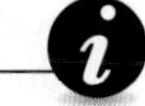

Definition

Fatal polioencephalitis of warm-blooded animals and humans caused by a virus of the genus *Lyssavirus* and generally transmitted by the bite of an infected mammal

Epidemiology

SPECIES, AGE, SEX

Warm-blooded animals of all ages are susceptible:

- Bats, foxes, coyotes, wolves, and some rodents are highly susceptible.
- Moderately susceptible species include dogs, cats, horses, sheep, goats, and humans.
- Worldwide, the dog is the most likely domestic animal to be infected, but in the United States, cats are the domestic species most frequently reported to be rabid, with 200-300 cases/year.
- Rabies has been reported in ferrets, rabbits, and one guinea pig.
- Often endemic in wild animals, with periodic outbreaks (epizootics)
- In the United States, the most important species-adapted strains are in the fox, raccoon, skunk, and bat.
- Salivary gland infections occur in vampire bats without producing clinical signs in the bats, resulting in prolonged viremia. Insectivorous bats may also be infected.

RISK FACTORS

- Contact with wildlife, especially bats, raccoons, skunks, foxes, and mongoose
- Lack of vaccination against rabies
- Exposure to aerosols in bat caves
- Vaccines for dogs and cats in the United States are inactivated and therefore pose no risk of infection, but modified live vaccines left out for wildlife (i.e., bait vaccines) or used in other parts of the world might pose a minor risk of infection for pets.

CONTAGION AND ZOONOSIS

- Highly zoonotic disease
- Transmission is most commonly by bite.
  - ◦ The risk of human infection is far greater through a rabid animal's bite (5%-80%) than a scratch (0.1%-1%).

GEOGRAPHY AND SEASONALITY

- Worldwide
  - ◦ Rabies-free regions include New Zealand, some Caribbean islands, the British Isles, parts of Scandinavia, Japan, and Hawaii.
- Rabies is primarily a disease of wildlife in the United States.
  - ◦ Raccoons: mainly eastern part of the United States

- Skunks: mainly in California and the north central and south central states
- Bats: 48 contiguous United States and responsible for most human cases in the past 20 years
- Foxes: Arctic fox in Alaska, red and gray fox in southeast United States
- Mongoose: Puerto Rico

- The dog is the primary species involved in transmission of rabies in Central America and the Southern Hemisphere.

Clinical Presentation

DISEASE FORMS/SUBTYPES

Clinical signs are variable but predominantly arise from central nervous system (CNS) dysfunction.

- Prodromal form
  - Change in behavior, which may include anxiety, solitude, and apprehension
  - Fever may occur.
  - Pruritus may occur at the site of exposure.
  - Lasts 2-3 days
- Paralytic (dumb) form (majority of canine cases, minority of feline cases)
  - Lethargy, difficulty swallowing, ptyalism, voice or bark change, dropped jaw, and lower motor neuron paralysis, often first in the wounded limb
  - Lasts 1-7 days, from onset of overt signs to death
- Furious form (majority of feline cases, minority of canine cases)
  - Aggression, biting, altered voice, paralysis, seizures, and ataxia
  - Hyperesthesia and hyperresponsiveness to auditory and visual stimuli are possible.
  - Lasts 2-4 days, from onset of overt signs to death

HISTORY, CHIEF COMPLAINT

- History of wound may or may not exist. Given the pathophysiology of rabies, neurologic clinical signs beginning within 1 week of the occurrence of a wound are extremely unlikely to be related to rabies infection by the wound.
- Behavioral changes are very common and can vary.
  - Aggression, viciousness, irritability, excitability, nervousness, apprehension, and anxiety
  - Abnormal or erratic behaviors, such as licking, biting, wandering, disorientation, ataxia, seizures, or paralysis
- Ptyalism and change in bark
- No clinical signs; exposure is suspected but not confirmed.

PHYSICAL EXAM FINDINGS

Timing of the onset of clinical signs varies: signs begin 2 weeks to several months after exposure. Signs include fever, dropped jaw, ptyalism, inability to swallow, and mandibular and laryngeal paralysis. Lower motor neuron limb signs, ataxia, and cranial nerve deficits may be present.

Etiology and Pathophysiology

- Single-stranded RNA virus of the genus *Lyssavirus,* family Rhabdoviridae
- Transmission
  - Virus in saliva is transmitted through a wound or mucous membranes.
  - Inhalation of aerosolized virus may occur with exposure to bats/bat caves.
  - Ingestion of infected tissues is also possible as a route of infection but is rare.
  - By organ transplantation (humans)
- Virus replicates in local tissues, where it enters neuromuscular junctions and neurotendinous spindles.
  - Virus is vulnerable to immune-mediated destruction (e.g., vaccine induced) in local tissues but becomes protected after it reaches peripheral nerves or the CNS.
- Spreads by intraaxonal flow through peripheral nerves to the spinal cord and brain, replicates in the CNS, and then moves outward through peripheral, sensory, motor, and cranial nerves.
- Large amount of virus is present in salivary glands, where it is shed. Salivary virus excretion begins up to 2 weeks before the onset of neurologic signs.
- The incubation period varies and depends on innervation at the bite site, distance of the bite site to the CNS, virus variant, and amount of virus in the exposure; can range from 2 weeks to > 6 months
- After clinical signs are apparent, death ensues within 10 days.

DIAGNOSIS

Diagnostic Overview

Diagnosis is suspected in any animal with an unknown or incomplete rabies vaccination history that develops acute neurologic signs. Confirmation requires direct immunofluorescence assays of brain/nervous tissue.

Differential Diagnosis

- Encephalitis: viral (canine distemper, feline leukemia virus, feline immunodeficiency virus, feline infectious peritonitis); immune mediated (e.g., granulomatous meningoencephalitis); rarely, protozoal, rickettsial, bacterial, or fungal
- Pseudorabies
- Intoxication (e.g., lead)
- Cerebral cysticercosis caused by larval *Taenia solium* mimics rabies in dogs.
- Portosystemic shunt
- Hypoglycemia
- Neoplasia
- Trauma
- Trigeminal neuropathy
- Causes of ptyalism (p. 833)

Initial Database

- The clinical suspicion of rabies is based on history and physical exam in unvaccinated or poorly vaccinated animals.
- CBC, serum chemistry panel, and urinalysis are unhelpful.

Advanced or Confirmatory Testing

- Cerebrospinal fluid (CSF) analysis may show nonspecific increases in protein and leukocytes.
- Direct IFA testing of nervous tissue is the confirmatory test of choice.
  - Chill—do not freeze—the body or brain of any dead/euthanized rabies suspect.
  - Immediately submit the brain to a state-approved laboratory for rabies IFA testing.
  - Use extreme caution in obtaining samples and shipping specimens; zoonosis can occur if rabies virus is aerosolized (e.g., when an electric saw is used for opening the skull and proper protection is not used) or is inadvertently inoculated.
- A new reverse transcription polymerase chain reaction (RT-PCR) method is useful with small samples such as saliva and spinal fluid and has been shown to be as rapid as the IFA test.
- Direct IFA testing of dermis: skin biopsy of sensory vibrissae of the maxillary area should not be used (false-negative results).

TREATMENT

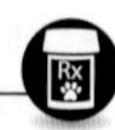

Treatment Overview

- Fatal; recovery is extraordinarily rare. There have been 15 reports of human survival after confirmed rabies infection to date, and the best outcome appears to be after bat virus transmission.
- The first reported survival of a human who did not receive rabies pre-exposure or post-exposure prophylaxis was recently described, with a treatment called the Milwaukee protocol: rifampin, amantadine, and the induction of a ketamine/midazolam coma.
- Dogs or cats that have bitten a person or are believed to have had contact with a wild animal must be confined and quarantined.

Recommended Monitoring

- Management of rabies suspects varies with immunization status and local laws. The attending veterinarian should contact the local state/regional veterinarian.
- Most public health laws require a 10-day confined observation period for dogs/cats that bite a human.
  - Virus shedding in saliva begins 1-5 (possibly up to 13) days before the onset of neurologic signs in infected animals.
- A healthy dog or cat that bites or scratches an individual should be securely confined and monitored for behavioral changes and/or neurologic signs suggesting rabies for 10 days.
  - If clinical signs do not develop in the dog/cat within 10 days of bite/scratch, there has been no human exposure to rabies virus.
  - If clinical signs consistent with rabies develop in the dog/cat during the 10-day quarantine period, or if there were neurologic signs consistent with rabies at the

time of the bite, the dog or cat must be euthanized and its brain submitted immediately for exam. If infection is confirmed within 24-48 hours, there is adequate time to begin human postexposure prophylaxis.
- Unvaccinated dogs or cats that are exposed to a known rabid animal or to any bat or wild, carnivorous mammal
  - Unowned animals are often euthanized at presentation for immediate rabies testing.
  - If the animal is wanted, the dog/cat is placed in quarantine for up to 6 months.
  - The dog/cat must be monitored for the onset of clinical signs and euthanized immediately if signs consistent with rabies occur. It the animal remains healthy, it should be vaccinated for rabies 1 month before release.
- Vaccinated dogs or cats that are exposed to a known rabid animal or to any bat or wild, carnivorous mammal
  - Immediate revaccination for rabies is indicated.
  - A period of monitoring must follow, typically for 45 days.
- When a dog or cat with an expired rabies vaccination status is exposed to a rabid animal, individual factors determine the recommended course. Clinicians should contact the state/regional veterinarian.

PROGNOSIS & OUTCOME

- Cats and dogs typically succumb within 7-10 days after onset of clinical signs.
- The human Milwaukee protocol is no longer recommended due to 26 reports of failure.
- Experimental treatment with nanoviricides has shown a 30% survival rate compared with standard treatment (0% survival); currently being investigated by the Centers for Disease Control and Prevention for use in humans with rabies.

PEARLS & CONSIDERATIONS

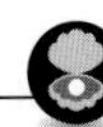

Comments

- If clients are concerned regarding possible or known human exposure to rabies, they must see their physician immediately.
- Veterinarians should notify the local public health officials about potential human exposure.
- Signs take weeks to months to develop after exposure, but after signs occur, death ensues quickly (<2 weeks).
- The 10-day quarantine of pets after a bite does not guarantee that the animal is not harboring rabies virus but ensures that the pet was not shedding virus in saliva at the time of the bite.
- Travel to rabies-free areas has been facilitated by a vaccinate-microchip-and-blood test protocol that shows adequate neutralizing antibody levels (e.g., > 0.5 IU/mL) and no clinical signs of rabies typically over a 6-month period before departure. This reduces the burden of travel on the pet (previously a 6-month quarantine in the destination country/state). The specific jurisdiction can provide detailed requirements (e.g., for the United Kingdom, www.gov.uk/take-pet-abroad).
- A new Rabies Rapid Screen Saliva test (Dyne Immune) has not yet undergone sensitivity and specificity testing and cannot be recommended at this time.
- Worldwide, > 50,000 people per year die of rabies; more than one-half of these are children.

Prevention

- A new initiative by the CDC aims to eliminate dog-transmitted human rabies deaths by 2030 by mass vaccination campaigns.
- All dogs and cats should be vaccinated for rabies after 12 weeks of age, again at 12 months of age, and then every 3 years or yearly, depending on state regulations.
- An immediate booster vaccination in immunized dogs and cats potentially exposed to rabies is advised.
- Avoid modified live vaccine (MLV) for pet animals.
- Disinfect contaminated cages, food dishes, and instruments with a diluted solution of 1 part bleach to 32 parts tap water.

Technician Tips

- Gloves should be worn during exam of all unknown or unvaccinated animals and during exam of bite wounds of unknown origin as protection against rabies.
- The classic vicious, foaming at the mouth image is true for only ≈10% of rabid dogs. A majority of dogs with rabies are lethargic and poorly responsive but highly infectious. Strict precautions to avoid being bitten are warranted around animals with these signs.
- Document rabies vaccination date for every patient so that the information is available in case a bite occurs during veterinary care.

Client Education

- Emphasize the importance of rabies vaccination for all dogs and cats.
- Keep pets from roaming (leash laws).
- Inform clients about state and local policies.
- Advise the client to bring the animal to a veterinarian immediately if exposure is suspected. With human exposure, individuals should immediately contact a physician.
- Additional travel/quarantine information is available at www.aphis.usda.gov/animal_welfare/pet_travel/pet_travel.shtml

SUGGESTED READING

Wallace RM, et al: Elimination of dog-mediated human rabies deaths by 2030: needs assessment and alternatives for progress based dog vaccination. Front Vet Sci 4:9, 2017.

AUTHOR: **Maureen A. McMichael, DVM, DACVECC**
EDITOR: **Joseph Taboada, DVM, DACVIM**

Raw Diets

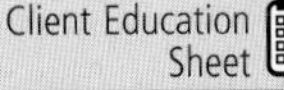

BASIC INFORMATION

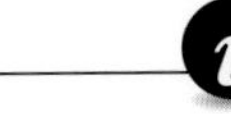

Definition

Raw diets are based on uncooked ingredients of animal origin and can include skeletal muscle, offal, bones, and eggs or dairy. Plant ingredients can also be included. Raw diets may be home prepared or commercial products (fresh, frozen, or freeze dried).

Synonyms

Biologically appropriate raw food (BARF; a trademarked term by a raw diet company for its associated products)

Epidemiology

A 2008 survey found that 16.2% of dogs and 9.6% of cats in the United States and Australia were fed raw meat or bones daily, and an additional 7.4% of dogs and 0.9% of cats were fed these items at least weekly.

SPECIES, AGE, SEX

Dogs and cats of any age and sex

CONTAGION AND ZOONOSIS

- The U.S. Food and Drug Administration (FDA) does not recommend feeding raw diets to pets due to the public health risk posed by the handling of contaminated meat and potential for zoonotic transmission of pathogens from the dog or cat to humans, even when the pet does not show any signs of disease. Although dry commercial foods (kibble) can also be contaminated, it is much less common than for raw animal products due to the thermic processes applied to kibble for microbiological safety.
- The FDA analyzed hundreds of pet foods for *Salmonella* and *Listeria monocytogenes* and found that 31.6% of the raw samples were positive for either microorganism, but only 0.4% of the kibble samples were positive

for *Salmonella*. Several studies have reported fecal shedding of pathogenic bacteria by dogs fed contaminated raw food, and illnesses in people owning raw-fed pets have been documented and linked to the diet.

Clinical Presentation

DISEASE FORMS/SUBTYPES

- Raw feeding is a risk factor for several problems.
- Bones are common foreign bodies associated with gastrointestinal obstruction (including esophageal) and have also been associated with tooth fractures and constipation.
- Nutritional imbalances (e.g., nutritional secondary hyperparathyroidism) have been reported in dogs and cats fed raw diets, particularly home prepared.
- Infectious disease caused by microorganisms (manifested clinically as vomiting and/or diarrhea or other disease) has also been associated with raw food feeding.
- Many raw food diets are very high in fat and may risk obesity or acute canine pancreatitis.

HISTORY, CHIEF COMPLAINT

Diet history includes feeding of raw animal products. Animals may be well, but complaints can include vomiting, diarrhea, regurgitation, constipation, ataxia, limb pain, or difficulty prehending food.

PHYSICAL EXAM FINDINGS

Physical exam of pets fed raw diets can be completely normal. Potential findings include dehydration secondary to vomiting and diarrhea and pain on limb palpation.

Etiology and Pathophysiology

- Unbalanced raw diets can result in nutritional deficiency or excess. One of the most common is calcium and/or vitamin D deficiency, resulting in nutritional secondary hyperparathyroidism (rickets during growth, osteomalacia in adults).
- Some raw diets have resulted in hyperthyroidism in dogs after the consumption of necks or gullets including thyroid tissue.
- Bones can cause oral and gastrointestinal problems (e.g., foreign bodies).
- Consumption of pathogenic bacteria or endotoxins from contaminated raw meat can result in gastroenteritis and septicemia.

DIAGNOSIS

Diagnostic Overview

Feeding of raw animal products is identified by a thorough and complete diet history as part of the nutritional assessment. Raw treats (rawhide, bully sticks, pig ears) should also be noted because they are associated with *Salmonella* contamination. Note whether the diet is commercial or home prepared (the latter is more likely to cause nutrient imbalances). An extended nutritional evaluation is indicated for these patients.

Differential Diagnosis

- Foreign bodies (other than bones)
- Gastroenteritis
- Hereditary vitamin D disorders
- Primary or renal secondary hyperparathyroidism

Initial Database

Physical exam; depending on presenting complaint and exam findings, CBC, serum chemistry, urinalysis, radiographs, or ultrasound may be indicated.

Advanced or Confirmatory Testing

If indicated, vitamin D panel (calcium, vitamin D, parathyroid hormone, parathyroid hormone–related protein), thyroid panel, or canine pancreatic lipase immunoreactivity (Spec cPL) may confirm suspected complications of raw diets.

TREATMENT

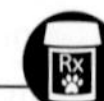

Treatment Overview

Not all dogs and cats will get sick from eating raw food. However, switching to a cooked balanced diet is strongly recommended to prevent problems and to reduce risk to humans in contact with the food and the pet. If illness does occur, treatment varies, depending on the specific problem caused by the raw diet, but the patient should be switched to a complete and balanced home-cooked or commercial diet if raw food has caused illness.

Acute and Chronic Treatment

Diet change, supportive care, and specific treatment that varies with the problem caused by raw feeding.

Nutrition/Diet

Pet owners should be encouraged to change to a complete and balanced home-cooked or commercial diet as indicated by health concerns (consult with a board certified veterinary nutritionist for balanced home-cooked diets [www.acvn.org]). For owners who decline these recommendations, feeding a balanced commercial raw diet and following FDA hygiene guidelines (https://www.fda.gov/animalveterinary/resourcesforyou/animalhealthliteracy/ucm373757.htm#tips) is indicated but does not eliminate risk of infectious disease for the pet or humans interacting with it.

PROGNOSIS & OUTCOME

Prognosis varies depending on the specific disease. For nutritional secondary hyperparathyroidism, acute pancreatitis, and foreign-body obstruction, the prognosis is guarded.

PEARLS & CONSIDERATIONS

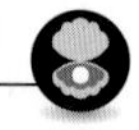

Comments

- Raw foods do not always cause illness, but they increase the risk of certain illnesses.
- Provide owners with objective resources such as the FDA (https://www.fda.gov/animalveterinary/resourcesforyou/animalhealthliteracy/ucm373757.htm) science-based information regarding raw diets for pets. Propose that owners contact manufacturers to ask how nutritional adequacy and microbiological safety are determined.
- Develop a hospital policy for handling raw pet foods as well as handling pets eating these diets to have a plan for those that require hospitalization or boarding.

Prevention

Pets that consume raw diets and demonstrate diarrhea can pose a risk of contagion or zoonosis. These animals and their waste products should be handled appropriately, and the dogs should not be allowed to use a common pet relief area at the clinic, nor should they be taken to dog parks.

Technician Tips

A complete and thorough diet history for each patient at each visit is critical to identify patients at risk for disease due to raw feeding practices.

SUGGESTED READING

Freeman LM, et al: Current knowledge about the risks and benefits of raw meat-based diets for dogs and cats. J Am Vet Med Assoc 243:1549, 2013.

AUTHOR: Cecilia Villaverde, BVSc, PhD, DACVN, DECVCN
EDITOR: Jennifer A. Larsen, DVM, PhD, DACVN

Rectal Masses

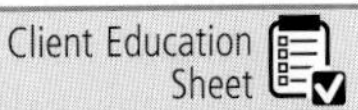

BASIC INFORMATION

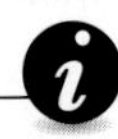

Definition

Tumors of the distal gastrointestinal (GI) tract can be benign or malignant. The most common benign tumors are adenomatous polyps; others include leiomyoma, fibroma, plasmacytoma, ganglioneuroma, inflammatory pseudopolyposis, and idiopathic eosinophilic masses. The most common malignant rectal tumor is adenocarcinoma; others include lymphoma, leiomyosarcoma, hemangiosarcoma, extramedullary plasmacytoma, mast cell tumor, melanoma, and fibrosarcoma.

Epidemiology

SPECIES, AGE, SEX

Benign masses:
- Adenomatous polyps: more frequent in males
- Benign GI masses are rare in cats.

Malignant masses:
- More common in older dogs
- Adenocarcinoma: higher incidence in males
- Adenocarcinoma in cats: median age of 12.5 years

GENETICS, BREED PREDISPOSITION

Benign masses:
- Collies and West Highland white terriers are predisposed to adenomatous polyp formation.
- Rottweilers and purebred, large-breed dogs are predisposed to eosinophilic masses.
- Medium- to large-breed dogs appear predisposed to leiomyomas.

Malignant masses:
- Medium- to large-breed dogs are overrepresented.
- German shepherds and poodles are predisposed.

Clinical Presentation

HISTORY, CHIEF COMPLAINT

Clinical signs include dyschezia, hematochezia, hemorrhage, tenesmus, abnormal feces, emaciation, anal biting/licking or scooting, and diarrhea. Leiomyomas and adenocarcinomas may cause signs secondary to extraluminal obstruction, such as vomiting, diarrhea, and weight loss.

PHYSICAL EXAM FINDINGS

Benign masses:
- Principal physical abnormalities are found on rectal palpation.
- Adenomatous polyps can be single (80%) or multiple (20%) and raised, sessile, or pedunculated.
- Most commonly found at the distal rectum and anorectal junction
- Leiomyomas are intramural and well-circumscribed.

Malignant masses:
- Cachexia
- ± Dehydration, signs of abdominal pain
- Sublumbar lymphadenopathy (may be palpable per rectum) suggests neoplasia.
- Rectal adenocarcinomas can spread circumferentially or radially through bowel wall as pedunculated (mid-to-distal rectum), ulcerative, cobblestone, or infiltrative masses.
  - Sedated rectal exam may be required to palpate deeper infiltrative masses.
  - Circumferential or stenotic lesions (colon to midrectum) suggest adenocarcinoma.
- Lymphoma can be discrete or diffusely infiltrative.

Etiology and Pathophysiology

- Malignant transformation of benign masses occurs in 20%-50% of dogs, more commonly in masses that have been present for longer durations.
  - *Carcinoma in situ* refers to polyps that undergo carcinomatous change, invading the intestinal lamina propria and submucosa but not the basement membrane, and have a metastatic potential.
- Hematochezia is usually not seen with leiomyomas and leiomyosarcomas because they do not involve the mucosa.
- Chronic bleeding may result in anemia, thrombocytopenia, and hypoproteinemia.
- Smooth muscle tumors may cause hypoglycemia.
- Plasmacytomas may cause hyperproteinemia and monoclonal gammopathy.

DIAGNOSIS

Diagnostic Overview

Type of tumor is suspected based on appearance and location. Definitive diagnosis requires biopsy and histopathologic analysis. Endoscopic exam can localize the primary lesion and help determine if other lesions are present.

Differential Diagnosis

- Perineal hernia
- Perianal neoplasia
- Colonic adenocarcinoma (p. 30)
- Perianal gland hyperplasia
- Anal sacculitis
- Anal sac neoplasia
- Rectal pythiosis
- Benign rectal stricture

Initial Database

- CBC, serum biochemistry profile, urinalysis: paraneoplastic leukocytosis can occur with adenomatous rectal polyps; eosinophilia, neutrophilia, hypocholesterolemia, and hypoalbuminemia may be seen with idiopathic eosinophilic masses.
- Abdominal and thoracic radiographs: for metastasis, additional mass lesions

Advanced or Confirmatory Testing

- Abdominal ultrasound: pelvis can interfere with imaging distal colon
- CT: optimal structural evaluation
- Endoscopy/proctoscopy/colonoscopy
  - Evaluate primary lesion location and determine whether other lesions exist.
  - Biopsy samples obtained by this method are usually small and superficial, which can result in an incorrect diagnosis.
- Incisional/excisional biopsy: recommended
  - Depending on mass location, full-thickness biopsy by laparotomy or partial-thickness biopsy by rectal eversion technique may be necessary.
  - Adenomatous polyps are composed of branching lamina propria covered by abnormal epithelial tissue that is continuous with normal rectal mucosa.
  - Leiomyomas arise from the outer smooth muscle and lack mucosal involvement.
- Misdiagnosis common with cytology

TREATMENT

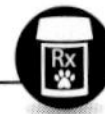

Treatment Overview

Surgical excision is the treatment of choice for most rectal tumors except lymphoma. The surgical approach is determined by tumor type and location. Strict aseptic technique is required because of the risk of infection associated with rectal flora; systemic perioperative antibiotics include gentamicin or amikacin plus second- or third-generation cephalosporin or metronidazole. Postoperative antibiotic administration is controversial, but antibiotics should be continued if contamination has occurred. Enemas should not be administered preoperatively because liquid feces may increase the risk of surgical site contamination.

Acute General Treatment

- Surgical excision
  - Rectal eversion and submucosal resection may be used for noninvasive masses such as polyps or carcinoma *in situ*.
  - Benign polyps can be excised down to the level of the muscularis, ligated, or removed by electrocautery.
  - Cryosurgery can be considered for treatment of polyps and has been used for local excision of adenocarcinomas; evidence for this method is limited.
- Resection and anastomosis of larger lesions
  - Anal, ventral, dorsal, or lateral approach, depending on mass location
  - Rectal pull-through technique
  - Caudal midline celiotomy with pubic symphysiotomy or ischial pubic flap

osteotomy to access colorectal junction or cranial third of rectum
 - EEA stapling device transrectally
- Postoperatively, analgesia, stool softeners, and cool compresses for the first 2 days, followed by warm compresses, should be used.
- Antiinflammatory drugs therapeutically or palliatively (e.g., piroxicam)
- Chemotherapy or radiation therapy
- Colostomy

Possible Complications

- Postoperatively
 - Bleeding, mild tenesmus, stricture formation, stenosis, rectal prolapse, perineal hernia formation secondary to tenesmus, perirectal abscesses, and recurrence
 - Septic peritonitis with colonic dehiscence
 - Fecal incontinence if pelvic plexus is damaged, distal 1.5 cm of rectum is removed, or long rectal resection (>4 cm) has been performed
 - Colostomy may result in skin excoriation.

PROGNOSIS & OUTCOME

- Good after resection of rectal polyps, carcinoma *in situ,* and leiomyomas
 - Adenomatous polyps: median survival time = 2 years; 0%-41% recurrence rate
 - Carcinoma *in situ:* median survival time = 5-24 months; 55% recurrence rate
- Guarded for malignant masses (p. 30)
 - Metastatic rate varies.
 - Adenocarcinoma: mean survival time of 24 months with cryosurgery, 18-29 months with electrocautery
 - Radical surgery (e.g., rectal resections of more than 4 cm, colonic resection cranial to the peritoneal reflection) can have a high complication rate and poor survival (<1 week).
 - Annular masses are poor prognostic indicators, with a median survival time of 1.6 months.
 - Nodular or cobblestone masses have a median survival time of 12 months.
 - Single pedunculated masses that are completely excised can have a median survival time of 32 months.

PEARLS & CONSIDERATIONS

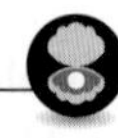

Comments

- Histopathology is required to determine tumor type because cytology alone can result in misdiagnosis.
- Endoscopy helps with assessment, but biopsies obtained by this method may lead to an incorrect diagnosis.
- Careful surgical technique and strict asepsis can decrease the risk of complications.

Technician Tips

Monitor for depression, high fever, abdominal pain, vomiting, ileus, and perineal inflammation, which may indicate infection or septic peritonitis.

SUGGESTED READING

Baines SJ, et al: Rectum, anus, and perineum. In: Johnston SA, et al, editors: Veterinary surgery—small animal. ed 2, St. Louis, 2018, Elsevier, pp 1783-1827.

AUTHORS: Dena L. Lodato, DVM, MS, DACVS, CCRP; Jennifer L. Wardlaw, DVM, MS, DACVS
EDITOR: Elizabeth A. Swanson, DVM, MS, DACVS

Rectal Prolapse

Client Education Sheet

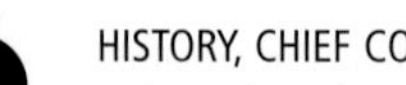

BASIC INFORMATION

Definition

Eversion of the anal mucosa or full-thickness rectal wall through the anal opening

Epidemiology

SPECIES, AGE, SEX

Can occur at any age, but young dogs and cats are most frequently affected.

GENETICS, BREED PREDISPOSITION

Manx cats may be predisposed.

RISK FACTORS

Recent perineal surgery, tenesmus

ASSOCIATED DISORDERS

Any condition that causes tenesmus may be associated with rectal prolapse: gastrointestinal (GI) parasitism; neoplasia of the colon, rectum, or anus; rectal foreign bodies; colitis; perineal hernia; prostatic disease; urinary disease; dystocia

Clinical Presentation

DISEASE FORMS/SUBTYPES

- Partial prolapse (mucosa only)
- Complete prolapse (all layers of the rectal wall)

HISTORY, CHIEF COMPLAINT

- Visualization of red tissue protruding from anus
- Straining to defecate (tenesmus) or urinate
- Diarrhea

PHYSICAL EXAM FINDINGS

- Partial prolapse: a few millimeters of red, swollen mucosa protruding through anus
- Complete prolapse: cylindrical mass protruding from anus; tissue may be red, ulcerated, or necrotic.
- Other findings consistent with underlying cause for straining (e.g., enlarged prostate, palpable neoplastic mass)

Etiology and Pathophysiology

- Animal affected by underlying disease that causes straining
 - In young/immature animals, intestinal parasites common
- Repetitively increased intraabdominal pressure from straining causes weakness of perirectal and perianal connective tissue or muscles, resulting in prolapse.
- Inflammation or edema of mucosa may result in more straining and can exacerbate prolapse.
- Prolapsed tissue may become traumatized or desiccate, resulting in ulceration and necrosis.

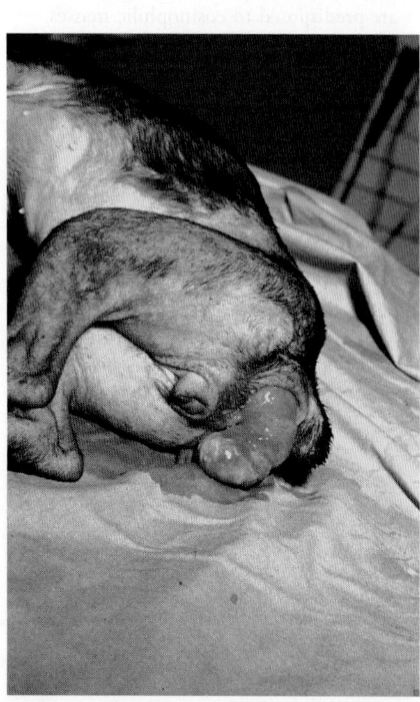

RECTAL PROLAPSE Clinical image of rectal prolapse in a dog. (Courtesy Dr. Richard Walshaw.)

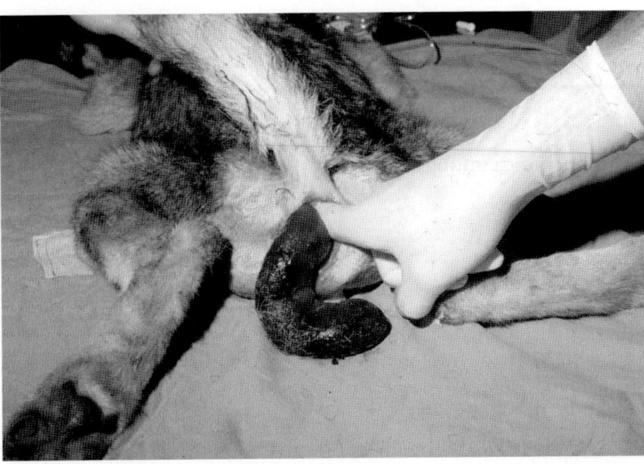

RECTAL PROLAPSE Clinical image of colonic intussusception, an important differential diagnosis for rectal prolapse. In this condition, a digit may be passed into the rectum, as shown in this anesthetized animal. With rectal prolapse, bowel is everted at the anus, not within the colon, and rectal palpation is not possible. (Courtesy Dr. Richard Walshaw.)

DIAGNOSIS

Diagnostic Overview

The diagnosis is made by visual inspection and rectal palpation.

Differential Diagnosis

- Prolapsed intussusception: must be differentiated from rectal prolapse because intussusception requires laparotomy, whereas rectal prolapse does not.
- Neoplastic mass protruding from anus

Initial Database

- Rectal exam: carefully insert a blunt probe between prolapsed tissue and rectal wall. The probe cannot be passed cranially with rectal prolapse but does pass at least a few centimeters into a fornix created by everted colon in cases of prolapsed intussusception.
- CBC, serum chemistry profile, urinalysis, and urine culture may identify the underlying cause of straining and indicate an animal's metabolic status.
- Abdominal radiographs may demonstrate conditions associated with rectal prolapse (e.g., neoplastic masses, prostatomegaly, urinary calculi).
- Fecal analysis (direct and flotation) for intestinal parasitism

Advanced or Confirmatory Testing

- Abdominal ultrasonography to identify associated conditions
- Proctoscopy and biopsy to rule out potential underlying causes (colitis, neoplasia); indicated in older animals but rarely for young animals

TREATMENT

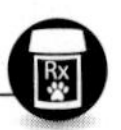

Treatment Overview

Treatment consists of correction of the prolapse by manual reduction (if viable) or surgical resection (if necrotic) and prevention of recurrence by treating the underlying cause of straining.

Acute General Treatment

- Acute treatment with patient under general anesthesia to prevent tenesmus during prolapse reduction
- Lavage prolapsed tissue with saline, and inspect viability.
- Apply lubricant, and manually reduce (gentle digital pressure) if tissue is viable.
  - Apply dextrose (50%), cold water, or copious amounts of sugar to tissue and wait several minutes to decrease edema and aid in reduction.
- Place purse-string suture around rectum at mucocutaneous junction to maintain reduction. The purse-string suture should be tight enough to prevent prolapse but should still allow for passage of soft stools. Tightening the suture over a syringe case (3 mL in most small animals is adequate) may prevent overtightening.
- Resection and anastomosis of diseased tissue if tissue is not viable
  - If tenesmus expected postoperatively, place a purse-string suture for 1-2 days.
- Consider performing epidural to prevent tenesmus during recovery from procedure.
- Initiate treatment for underlying cause (e.g., deworming for intestinal parasites).

Chronic Treatment

- Maintain purse-string suture for 3-5 days, and begin treatment of underlying cause of straining.
- If the patient undergoes resection and anastomosis, he/she should receive a low-residue diet and stool softeners to reduce postoperative straining.
- Perform a colopexy if prolapse repeatedly recurs after appropriate acute treatment.
- Laparoscopic colopexy has been described in a cat with recurrent prolapse.

Possible Complications

- Continued tenesmus
- Dyschezia, hematochezia
- Recurrent prolapse
- Leakage, dehiscence, and stricture if resection performed

PROGNOSIS & OUTCOME

Good prognosis if surgically treated and underlying cause reversible

PEARLS & CONSIDERATIONS

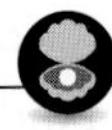

Comments

- Place a lubricated finger or small syringe case in rectum while tightening purse-string suture to prevent overtightening.
- Apply a local anesthetic to the rectal tissue after removal of the purse-string suture, which may help prevent recurrence.
- Empirically treat all young animals with rectal prolapse for intestinal parasitism, even if fecal flotation result is negative.

Technician Tips

Important points regarding postreduction/postoperative care:

- Maintain appropriate level of analgesia/sedation
  - Pain control
  - Prevention of tenesmus (to prevent recurrence)
- Perianal/perineal hygiene
  - Especially after defecation
  - Warm-pack the area to decrease swelling and ease discomfort.
- Diet
  - Prevent tenesmus, constipation, and diarrhea.
  - GI diet (e.g., Iams Low Residue) to promote formed but soft stool
  - Stool softener (e.g., Metamucil, Miralax) to promote pain-free defecation and no tenesmus

SUGGESTED READING

Baines SJ, et al: Rectum, anus, and perineum. In Johnston SA, et al, editors: Veterinary surgery—small animal, ed 2, St. Louis, 2018, Elsevier, pp 1783-1827.

AUTHOR: Janet Kovak McClaran, DVM, DACVS, DECVS, MRCVS
EDITOR: Elizabeth A. Swanson, DVM, MS, DACVS

Rectoanal Stricture

Bonus Material Online 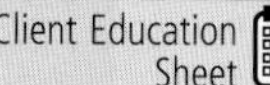 Client Education Sheet 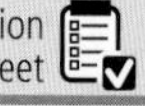

BASIC INFORMATION

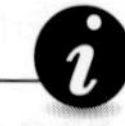

Definition

Uncommon disorder involving circumferential narrowing of anal or rectal lumen diameter

Synonym

Anorectal stricture

Epidemiology

SPECIES, AGE, SEX

Although atresia ani is a congenital failure to form a normal anal opening and is seen in young puppies and kittens, stricture formation is generally a sequela of disease processes that occur in middle-aged to older animals.

RISK FACTORS

Anal trauma or surgery

Clinical Presentation

HISTORY, CHIEF COMPLAINT

- Tenesmus, diarrhea, hematochezia, and ribbon-like stools
- Animals with advanced or metastatic malignancy may present with weight loss, anorexia, and lethargy.

PHYSICAL EXAM FINDINGS

Stricture is usually palpable on digital rectal exam.

Etiology and Pathophysiology

Primary causes of rectoanal stricture:

- Neoplasia
  - The most common malignant tumor of the rectum is adenocarcinoma (p. 30).
  - Other tumor types include lymphoma, leiomyosarcoma, and hemangiosarcoma.
  - Benign neoplasia may include adenoma, fibroma, or leiomyoma.
- Inflammatory disease such as colitis
- Infectious disease: histoplasmosis has been reported to cause rectal stricture in one dog.

Secondary causes of rectoanal stricture:

- Trauma: direct or from bone ingestion
- Scar formation secondary to surgery (e.g., anal sacculectomy, perianal fistula repair, mass excision), enema, or radiation therapy

DIAGNOSIS

Diagnostic Overview

Diagnosis is suspected based on presenting history and physical/rectal exam findings. Confirmation of the cause of the stricture may require endoscopy and biopsy.

Differential Diagnosis

- Rectal masses
- External compression from intrapelvic mass(es)
- Malunion pelvic fracture resulting in narrowed pelvic canal
- Enlarged prostate

Initial Database

- Gentle digital rectal palpation
- Assessment of location (identifying possible organ of origin), symmetry (circumferential versus focal), pain, and evidence of metastasis (palpation of sublumbar lymph nodes)
- CBC, serum chemistry analysis, and urinalysis: usually unremarkable
- Abdominal radiographs
  - Potential for visualizing area of stenosis, as well as megacolon cranial to stricture
  - Evidence of underlying cause of stricture, metastatic disease (± thoracic radiographs)

Advanced or Confirmatory Testing

- Negative (air) or positive contrast radiography may help localize stricture.
- Abdominal ultrasound can help assess diffuse metastatic disease.
- Colonoscopy should be used for visualizing extent of stricture formation and to acquire biopsy samples.
- CT of caudal abdomen and pelvis can assess intrapelvic disease and determine extent of stricture

TREATMENT

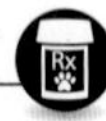

Treatment Overview

Treatment is aimed at increasing luminal size through the strictured area and preventing recurrence by treating the underlying cause.

Acute General Treatment

- With the animal under general anesthesia, mild strictures can be dilated using gentle digital or balloon bougienage.
  - Subsequent use of stool softener or psyllium supplementation is beneficial.
  - Local triamcinolone injections after dilation are reported to improve signs with non-neoplastic stricture.
- Surgical intervention, if possible, may be indicated to resect stricture or cause of stricture and to obtain a definitive biopsy sample:
  - Use a rectal pull-through or dorsal rectal approach.
  - Colostomy has been reported as an option for rectal obstruction or perforation in dogs but is poorly tolerated.

Possible Complications

Surgical complications include temporary or permanent incontinence, dehiscence, infection, and recurrence of stricture or neoplasia.

PROGNOSIS & OUTCOME

- Prognosis is related to histopathologic findings. Approximately 50% of rectal neoplasms are malignant. Reported outcome for adenocarcinoma is poor.
- Regardless of the underlying cause, there is a high likelihood for stricture reformation. Multiple balloon or surgical procedures may be required to correct the problem, and this should be discussed with the owner before initiating treatment.

PEARLS & CONSIDERATIONS

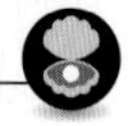

Comments

- It is common to cause iatrogenic tears of the rectum or anus during stricture treatment, and care is warranted when performing digital or balloon bougienage.
- If resection of stricture is performed, avoid enema administration for 24 hours before surgery to reduce intraoperative fecal contamination (fecal spillage from the anus during surgery).

Technician Tips

- Close observation of the patient's ability to defecate is required in postoperative or post-treatment period. Adjustments in diet (type and consistency) plus the addition of stool softeners (e.g., psyllium mucilloid) may be necessary.
- Temporary postoperative or post-treatment fecal incontinence necessitates good perineal hygiene.
- Pain control and patient comfort is vital.

SUGGESTED READING

Webb C, et al: Rectal strictures in 19 dogs: 1997-2005. J Am Anim Hosp Assoc 43:332-336, 2007.

RELATED CLIENT EDUCATION SHEETS

Consent to Perform Abdominal Ultrasound
Consent to Perform Endoscopy, Lower GI (Colonoscopy)
Consent to Perform Radiography

AUTHOR: Janet Kovak McClaran, DVM, DACVS, DECVS, MRCVS
EDITOR: Elizabeth A. Swanson, DVM, MS, DACVS

Recurrent Flank Alopecia, Dog

BASIC INFORMATION

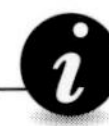

Definition

Skin disorder of unknown origin is characterized by episodes of truncal hair loss with spontaneous regrowth that often occurs on a recurrent basis.

Synonyms

Canine recurrent flank alopecia (CRFA), canine idiopathic cyclic flank alopecia, cyclic follicular dysplasia, seasonal flank alopecia

Epidemiology

SPECIES, AGE, SEX

- Dogs of both sexes, intact or neutered
- Age at onset of first episode: 8 months to 11 years (mean, 4 years)

GENETICS, BREED PREDISPOSITION

Boxers may account for about one-half of all cases, but other breeds at high risk include English bulldog, Airedale terrier, and all sizes of schnauzers. Although CRFA seems to affect numerous breeds, the condition appears to be rare to absent in the plush-coated Nordic breeds, German shepherds, and cocker spaniels.

GEOGRAPHY AND SEASONALITY

Characteristically, most dogs have an onset of alopecia between November and March (Northern Hemisphere).

Clinical Presentation

HISTORY, CHIEF COMPLAINT

Fairly abrupt onset of bilateral alopecia affecting the thoracolumbar region

PHYSICAL EXAM FINDINGS

- Nonscarring alopecia, usually bilaterally symmetrical, with well-demarcated borders
- Marked hyperpigmentation of the alopecic skin is common.
- The alopecia is usually confined to the dorsolateral thoracolumbar region, but on rare occasions, the condition is seen in association with alopecia on the dorsum of the nose, base of the ears, base of tail, and perineum.
- Spontaneous regrowth of a normal coat occurs in 3-8 months (range, 1-14 months) in most dogs.
- Most dogs develop recurrent alopecic episodes every year, but some dogs have an occasional year when the alopecia does not recur.
- The degree of alopecia is variable, with some dogs developing a virtually identical hair loss (size and duration) year after year, and other dogs developing larger areas and/or longer episodes of hair loss as years go by.
- In a few cases, hair regrowth may become less complete after several episodes; it may even progress to an end-stage permanent flank alopecia and marked hyperpigmentation.
- Occasionally, a dog may have only one isolated episode of alopecia during its lifetime.

Etiology and Pathophysiology

- The high incidence in some breeds and the familial character of CRFA suggest a genetic influence.
- The seasonal nature and annual recurrence suggest that photoperiod may be involved. The higher incidence of CRFA at higher latitudes (around or north of the 45th parallel in the Northern Hemisphere) supports the implication of light exposure in this disorder.

DIAGNOSIS

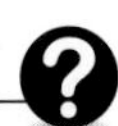

Diagnostic Overview

Diagnosis is based on history, clinical findings, and ruling out other differentials (e.g., exclusion of concomitant hypothyroidism in dogs > 2 years of age). The rapid onset of well-demarcated truncal alopecia with spontaneous hair regrowth in predisposed breeds and the absence of inflammation and pruritus make it quite distinctive.

Differential Diagnosis

- Endocrinopathies (hypothyroidism, hyperadrenocorticism, hyperestrogenism)
- Other follicular dysplasias
- Telogen defluxion

Initial Database

- Thyroid testing for adult dogs
- Other endocrine testing if indicated by history and physical exam findings

Advanced or Confirmatory Testing

Skin biopsies for dermatohistopathologic exam:

- Nonspecific changes suggestive of endocrinopathies may be observed. Truncated, keratin-filled atrophic primary and secondary hair follicles (witches feet) are suggestive of, but not pathognomonic for CRFA.
- Biopsies may further support the diagnosis but are not always performed if signalment and characteristic lesions are seen.

TREATMENT

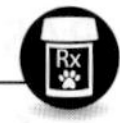

Treatment Overview

The goal is to reduce or prevent hair loss.

Acute General Treatment

- Melatonin 3-6 mg/DOG PO q 8-12h for 1-2 months may be beneficial in up to 50%-75% of cases (whether initiated before or shortly after the onset of alopecia).
  - To prevent hair loss, administer melatonin 1-2 months before the expected episode of alopecia.
  - To shorten the duration of an existing alopecic episode, start melatonin administration as soon as possible after the onset of alopecia.

PROGNOSIS & OUTCOME

Dogs affected with CRFA are healthy otherwise, and benign neglect is a valuable therapeutic approach.

PEARLS & CONSIDERATIONS

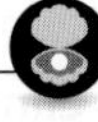

Comments

The unpredictable course of CRFA and the spontaneous regrowth of hair render the

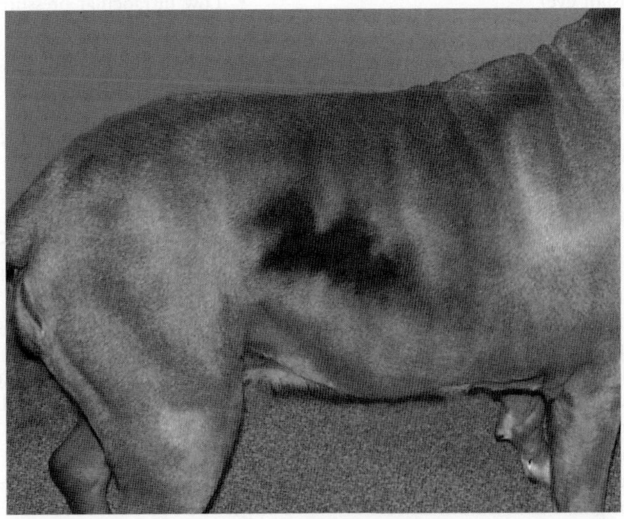

RECURRENT FLANK ALOPECIA, DOG Recurrent flank alopecia in a boxer. Note characteristic distribution of alopecia and hyperpigmentation. (Copyright Dr. Manon Paradis.)

evaluation of any therapeutic agent difficult, whether used for preventing the condition or to shorten an existing episode of alopecia.

Technician Tips

Discuss sun protection with owners, particularly if alopecic skin is lightly pigmented.

SUGGESTED READING

Paradis M: Canine recurrent flank alopecia. In Mecklenburg L, et al, editors: Hair loss disorders in domestic animals, Ames, IA, 2009, Wiley-Blackwell, pp 155-161.

AUTHOR & EDITOR: Manon Paradis, DMV, MVSc, DACVD

Red Eye

Client Education Sheet 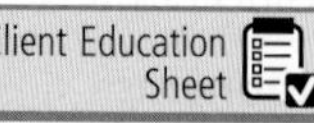

BASIC INFORMATION

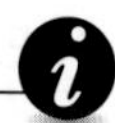

Definition

- Conjunctival, episcleral/scleral, or palpebral hyperemia
- The term *red eye* does not traditionally apply to redness in the anterior chamber (i.e., hyphema).

Synonyms

Conjunctival hyperemia, conjunctival injection, episcleral/scleral hyperemia or injection

Epidemiology

SPECIES, AGE, SEX

Dogs and cats, no age or sex predisposition

RISK FACTORS

- Trauma
- Systemic infectious or inflammatory diseases
- Coagulopathy
- Current therapy with potentially irritating topical ophthalmic medications (e.g., pilocarpine, neomycin, prostaglandin analogs, aminoglycosides)

Clinical Presentation

HISTORY, CHIEF COMPLAINT

Varies but may include any or all of the following:

- Red eye, by definition (layperson's description: bloodshot eye)
- Blepharospasm
- Ocular discharge
- Cloudiness of eye
- Loss of vision

PHYSICAL EXAM FINDINGS

- Conjunctival vessel hyperemia: diffuse conjunctival redness
  - Usually indicates ocular surface (i.e., superficial) disease, including
    - Conjunctivitis
    - Superficial keratitis
  - Vessels appear to originate in conjunctival fornix and branch as they approach limbus.
- Episcleral/scleral hyperemia: discrete engorgement and tortuosity of episcleral vessels
  - Usually indicates intraocular disease, deep corneal disease, or episcleritis/scleritis
  - Vessels originate near limbus and follow a deep, straight course toward the conjunctival fornix.
- Conjunctival and episcleral/scleral vessel injection can occur in the same eye. Ocular discharge and blepharospasm are nonspecific signs; other signs depend on the underlying cause of red eye:
  - Blepharitis; hyperemic, swollen eyelids
    - ± Mucopurulent ocular discharge
    - Normal intraocular exam
  - Conjunctivitis; hyperemic conjunctiva
    - Chemosis (conjunctival swelling)
    - Ocular discharge
    - Normal intraocular exam
  - Keratitis
    - Corneal opacities
    - Corneal vascularization
    - Corneal vessels that cross the limbus and branch suggest superficial corneal disease.
    - Vessels that start at the limbus and form a dense, straight pattern on cornea suggest deep corneal disease and/or intraocular disease.
    - ± Fluorescein dye retention
  - Uveitis; any or all of the following
    - Aqueous cells or flare
    - Constricted pupil
    - Abnormal appearance to iris
    - Hyphema
    - Fibrin clot in anterior chamber
    - Hypopyon
    - Low intraocular pressure
  - Glaucoma
    - Dilated pupil
    - Diffuse corneal edema
    - ± Buphthalmos
    - Fundic exam: optic disk cupping
    - Lens luxation: consistent with primary or secondary glaucoma

Etiology and Pathophysiology

Dilation of conjunctival and/or episcleral/scleral vessels:

- Typically inflammatory response to superficial and/or deep ocular disease
- May be caused by passive congestion (e.g., large, space-occupying orbital lesion)

DIAGNOSIS

Diagnostic Overview

Initial suspicion comes from history and/or physical exam. Diagnosis of the cause of red eye is achieved with a comprehensive ophthalmic exam. A diagnostic approach is outlined on p. 1447.

Differential Diagnosis

- See Etiology and Pathophysiology above.
- A red eye may also involve more than one ocular disease (e.g., corneal ulceration with secondary uveitis).

Initial Database

Complete ophthalmic exam (p. 1137):

- Schirmer tear test; a low result (<5-10 mm/min) indicates keratoconjunctivitis sicca (KCS).
- Fluorescein stain application; a positive result (stain retention) indicates corneal ulceration.
- Intraocular pressure measurement; elevated level (>30 mm Hg) is diagnostic of glaucoma; level is typically low (<10 mm Hg) with uveitis.

Advanced or Confirmatory Testing

- Variable depending on results of initial exam and testing (i.e., suspected cause)
- Corneal or conjunctival swabs for cytologic exam ± culture and susceptibility (C&S) for conjunctivitis, corneal ulcers, keratitis, or blepharitis
- CBC, serum chemistry panel, titers for infectious disease; radiography, ultrasonography for certain causes of uveitis
- Biopsy of lesion and histopathologic exam for refractory or complex blepharitis or episcleritis/scleritis

TREATMENT

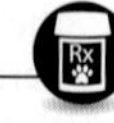

Treatment Overview

Treatment goals are to control/resolve underlying cause, decrease inflammation, eliminate infection if present, normalize intraocular pressure, eliminate ocular pain, and maintain vision.

Acute General Treatment

- Loss of vision is an emergency that requires immediate determination and treatment of underlying cause (p. 123). Glaucoma, severe uveitis, and severe keratitis should be considered in acute or progressive vision loss concurrent with red eye(s).

- Blepharitis
  - Determine underlying cause.
  - Patient often needs systemic antibiotic and/or antiinflammatory therapy.
  - Juvenile cellulitis and pemphigus complex are discussed on pp. 567.
- More information is available in chapters on keratoconjunctivitis sicca (p. 568), conjunctivitis in cats (p. 199), conjunctivitis in dogs (p. 200), corneal ulceration (p. 209), uveitis (p. 1023), glaucoma (p. 387), episcleritis/scleritis (p. 304), and orbital disease (p. 716).

Chronic Treatment

Varies, depending on underlying condition and cause; may include treatments to delay or avoid

- Loss of eye
- Loss of vision
- Worsening of systemic disease

PROGNOSIS & OUTCOME

- Varies, depending on underlying cause
- Lack of vision at presentation is often a poor prognostic indicator (return of vision uncommon).

PEARLS & CONSIDERATIONS

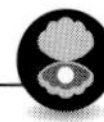

Comments

Avoid the following:

- Topical corticosteroids in any eye with positive fluorescein dye retention or unknown fluorescein status
- Systemic corticosteroids until preliminary diagnostic tests are performed or a diagnosis is reached because these drugs are generally contraindicated for treating infectious systemic disease

Technician Tips

- Avoid pressure on eye when handling affected animal.
- Increased ocular redness or pain indicates worsening of ocular disease.

Client Education

Seek veterinary attention promptly at first sign of red eye because many causes of red eye are globe and/or vision threatening.

SUGGESTED READING

Miller PE: Ocular emergencies. In Maggs DJ, et al, editors: Slatter's Fundamentals of veterinary ophthalmology, ed 4, Philadelphia, 2008, Saunders, p 419.

AUTHOR: Ellison Bentley, DVM, DACVO
EDITOR: Diane V. H. Hendrix, DVM, DACVO

Reflex Dyssynergia

BASIC INFORMATION

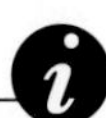

Definition

Upper motor neuron (UMN) dysfunction prevents coordinated urinary bladder contraction and urethral sphincter relaxation during micturition. Sacral spinal cord lesions, diseases associated with the urethra, or an idiopathic condition can mimic reflex dyssynergia.

Synonyms

Detrusor-sphincter dyssynergia or incoordination, functional urethral obstruction, UMN bladder

Epidemiology

SPECIES, AGE, SEX

- Affects dogs and cats of any age, depending on causation
- More often observed in male dogs; an idiopathic dyssynergia-like condition affects predominantly large-breed male dogs

RISK FACTORS

- Thoracolumbar spinal cord injury/disease
- Dyssynergia-like condition
  - After relief of urethral obstruction
  - Sacral spinal cord injury/disease

ASSOCIATED DISORDERS

- Bladder atony/hypotonia
- Urinary tract infection
- Urinary incontinence

Clinical Presentation

DISEASE FORMS/SUBTYPES

- True reflex dyssynergia: neurogenic suprasacral lesions
- Dyssynergia-like conditions: neurogenic and non-neurogenic disorders

HISTORY, CHIEF COMPLAINT

- Frequent attempts at voiding with inability to empty bladder completely are characteristic.
- Normal initiation of voiding with interruption of urine stream; short spurts of urine followed by cessation of urine flow
- Animal may strain with no urine produced.

PHYSICAL EXAM FINDINGS

- Manual bladder expression difficult
- Clinicians should palpate the bladder before and after voiding: turgid, incomplete emptying of bladder and increased residual urine volume are expected.
- Perineal reflex is present or exaggerated.
- Neurologic dysfunction unrelated to urination may be present.
- Rectal and vaginal exams are indicated to assess structural causes (e.g., sacral vertebral lesion) versus other causes of dysuria (e.g., urethral lith or mass). Anal tone is normal/good.
- Observation of urination: thin, interrupted urine stream

Etiology and Pathophysiology

- Disorders of urinary retention caused by central nervous system (CNS) lesions located between the pontine micturition center and the sacral spinal cord (suprasacral spinal cord: L7 to brainstem)
- UMN lesion causes a loss of inhibitory pathways.
  - To sympathetic innervation of the internal urethral sphincter (smooth muscle)
  - To somatic innervation (pudendal nerve) of the external urethral sphincter (striated muscle)
- Additional factors include increased sensory input (sacral nerves), increased sympathetic output, and bladder neck hypertrophy.
- Neurogenic dyssynergia-like conditions occur when pelvic nerve damage results in weakened detrusor contraction that cannot override urethral sphincter tone.
- In animals with non-neurogenic dyssynergia-like conditions, there is a similar failure of simultaneous relaxation of the internal or external urethral sphincter with detrusor contraction. This may be idiopathic or may follow irritation/disease of the urethra.

DIAGNOSIS

Diagnostic Overview

A diagnosis of primary reflex dyssynergia is made by exclusion of other conditions that mimic signs. The diagnostic plan should include eliminating conditions that cause mechanical (anatomic) obstruction of the urethra. The physical and neurologic exams can define an anatomic or neurologic differential.

Differential Diagnosis

Anatomic urethral obstruction:

- Intraluminal (e.g., urethral plug/lith, transitional cell carcinoma, urethritis)
- Extraluminal (e.g., prostatomegaly, pelvic granuloma)

Functional urethral obstruction (dyssynergia-like conditions):

- Neurogenic
  - Suprasacral and sacral spinal cord disease

- Pelvic plexus injury
- Cauda equina disease
- Non-neurogenic
  - Idiopathic
  - After relief of urethral obstruction
  - Secondary urinary tract infection
  - Bladder neck obstruction
  - Prostate disease
  - Alpha-adrenergic agonist administration (e.g., phenylpropanolamine, pseudoephedrine)
  - Myopathic disease
  - Detrusor muscle atony

Initial Database

- Urethral catheterization: unobstructed but residual urine volume increased (normal, 0.2-0.4 mL/kg in dogs or < 10 mL in dogs and < 2 mL in cats)
- Rectal exam: good anal tone, no pelvic/urethral mass
- Neurologic exam (p. 1136), including perineal and bulbocavernosus reflexes
  - Neuroanatomic lesion localization: spinal cord, usually T3-L3
- Clinical pathologic exam
  - CBC and serum biochemistry: unremarkable
  - Urinalysis and urine culture: secondary urinary tract infection common
- Caudal abdominal and pelvic radiographs, abdominal ultrasound: no urethral obstruction or mass, possible vertebral injury/disease

Advanced or Confirmatory Testing

- Contrast urethrography (p. 1181): rule out urethral obstruction if necessary.
- Cystoscopy and urethroscopy (p. 1085): identify masses, obtain biopsies, and remove small calculi.
- Neurodiagnostic procedures: confirm lesion localization, extent of lesion, and suspected cause.
  - Myelography to evaluate for intramedullary or extramedullary compressive disease
  - Electromyography of the anal sphincter muscle to assess pudendal nerve
  - Somatosensory-evoked response testing to evaluate ascending sensory pathways
  - Cross-sectional imaging: CT, MRI (p. 1132)
- Urodynamic procedures
  - Cystometry to assess bladder function
  - Urethral pressure profile to assess urethral tone, which is the only means to confirm idiopathic dyssynergia-like condition
  - Leak point pressure measurement to assess urethral resistance

TREATMENT

Treatment Overview

It is important to treat the underlying cause. Supportive therapies include bladder emptying and pharmacologic management. Bladder emptying prevents secondary bladder atony (p. 89) and urine retention that predispose to urinary tract infection. Pharmacologic therapy is often empirical; starting at lower end of the dosage range, response to therapy is noted and dose adjusted.

Acute General Treatment

- Urinary bladder catheterization
  - Indwelling urinary catheter (closed-collection system) (p. 1182)
  - Intermittent catheterization has a lower risk of inducing urinary tract infection.
- Urethral sphincter relaxation
  - Smooth muscle relaxation (alpha-antagonists)
    - Phenoxybenzamine 0.25 mg/kg PO q 12-24h (dogs); 1.25-5 mg/CAT PO q 12h (cats). Onset of action is delayed up to 4 days. Possible side effects include hypotension, tachycardia, and increased intraocular pressure. Contraindications are cardiovascular disease, glaucoma, and renal insufficiency. (Commercially prepared product, Dibenzyline 10-mg capsules, has become cost-prohibitive; USP-grade powder for compounding is more cost-effective.)
    - Prazosin 1 mg/15 kg PO q 8-12h (dogs); 0.25-0.5 mg/CAT PO q 12-24h (cats). Possible side effects are hypotension and mild sedation; contraindications are same as those for phenoxybenzamine.
    - Tamsulosin 0.01-0.03 mg/kg, or 0.4 mg/DOG, PO q 12-24h (dogs). Possible side effect: hypotension
  - Striated muscle relaxation (skeletal muscle relaxants)
    - Diazepam 2-10 mg/DOG PO q 8h; 2-5 mg/CAT PO q 8h or 0.2-0.5 mg/kg IV as needed. Possible side effects of the centrally acting muscle relaxant: sedation, excitation, and idiosyncratic acute hepatocellular necrosis in cats
    - Methocarbamol 15-20 mg/kg PO q 8h (dogs); initial dose 33 mg/kg PO q 8h, then 20 mg/kg PO q 8h (cats). Possible side effects of the centrally acting muscle relaxant: weakness, sedation, lethargy, and vomiting
- May add drugs to stimulate detrusor muscle contraction
  - Bethanechol (parasympathomimetic) 5-25 mg/DOG PO q 8h; 1.25-5 mg/CAT PO q 8h. Start with low dose and titrate to effect. Possible side effects are ptyalism, vomiting, diarrhea, and bronchoconstriction; contraindications are urinary or gastrointestinal (GI) tract obstruction.
  - Cisapride (prokinetic; enhances acetylcholine release) 0.5 mg/kg PO q 8h (dogs); 1.25-5 mg/CAT PO q 8-12h (cats). Possible side effects are diarrhea and abdominal pain.

Chronic Treatment

- Resolution of underlying disorder
- Intermittent bladder catheterization or manual bladder expression
  - Complete emptying with manual expression may take several attempts; allow the animal to relax between attempts.
- Long-term drug therapy
- Address secondary urinary tract infection (p. 232).
- Sacral nerve stimulation and newer alpha-antagonists (e.g., silodosin, tamsulosin) may be other treatment options and are new to veterinary medicine at this time.

Drug Interactions

Start treatment with an alpha-antagonist (e.g., prazosin) before bethanechol. Bethanechol may enhance urethral sphincter tone (has nonspecific cholinergic effects on the caudal mesenteric ganglia, causing further stimulation to the hypogastric nerve).

Recommended Monitoring

- Observe voiding activity daily.
- Monitor residual urine volume.
- Perform a periodic urine culture/urinalysis after removal of indwelling catheter and at least every 3 months until condition has resolved.

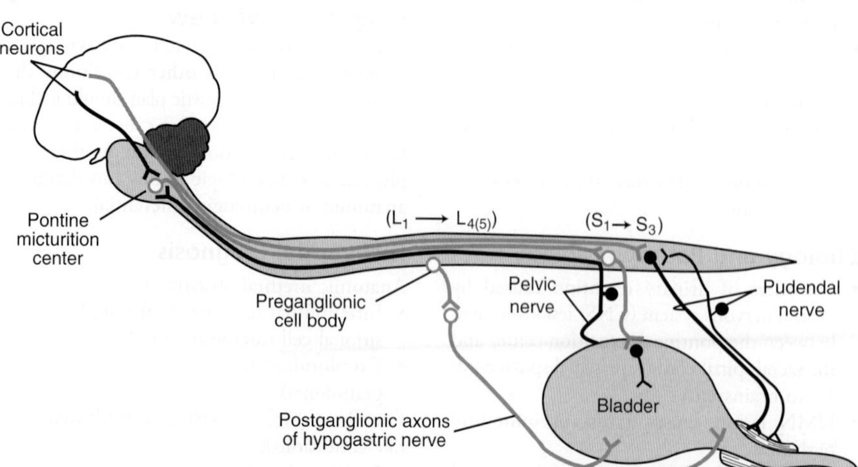

REFLEX DYSSYNERGIA Neuronal pathways to and from the urinary bladder.

PROGNOSIS & OUTCOME

- Good prognosis with resolution of underlying disease but may require weeks to resolve
- Good prognosis for resolution of dyssynergia-like conditions when underlying cause eliminated (e.g., urethral inflammation)
- Fair prognosis for medical control of idiopathic dyssynergia-like condition

PEARLS & CONSIDERATIONS

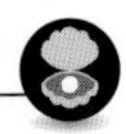

Comments

- Reflex dyssynergia is a common sequela of severe suprasacral spinal cord injury.
- If prolonged recovery from the spinal cord injury is expected, initiate an alpha-antagonist early (3-5 days to onset of action), barring hypotension.

Prevention

Successful management depends on identification and treatment of underlying disorder.

Technician Tips

- Aseptic protocols (cleanse external catheter and genital areas; change collection bag) to reduce risks for urinary tract infection should be instituted in patients requiring urinary catheterization.
- Secondary urine overflow increases risks of urine scald and decubitus ulceration. The patient should be kept clean and dry on a padded surface with frequent (q 4h) rotation if recumbent.

Client Education

- Manual bladder expression or intermittent catheterization may be required.
- Watch for signs of urinary tract infection (e.g., change in color or odor).

SUGGESTED READING

Byron JK. Micturition disorders. Vet Clin Small Anim 45:769-782, 2015.

AUTHOR: Joan R. Coates, DVM, MS, DACVIM
EDITOR: Leah A. Cohn, DVM, PhD, DACVIM

Regurgitation

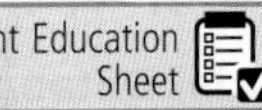

Client Education Sheet

BASIC INFORMATION

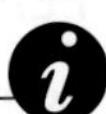

Definition

Passive retrograde expulsion of food and/or liquids from the esophagus secondary to functional (dysmotility) or mechanical obstruction

Synonym

Esophageal dysphagia

Epidemiology

SPECIES, AGE, SEX

More commonly recognized in dogs than cats; age of onset depends on underlying cause:
- Congenital: clinical signs from birth or weaning. In dogs, esophageal maturation may continue up to 1 year.
- Acquired: usually adults

GENETICS, BREED PREDISPOSITION

Megaesophagus (ME) is the most common esophageal disorder (dogs >> cats). Idiopathic esophageal dysmotility (IED) and functional/mechanical obstruction may precede focal or generalized ME.
- IED: Chinese Shar-pei, Bouvier des Flandres, terrier breeds
- Vascular ring anomalies: German shepherd dogs, Irish setter
- Gastroesophageal intussusception: German shepherds
- Hiatal hernia: brachycephalic breeds, Chinese Shar-pei
- Hereditary ME: wire-haired fox terriers, miniature schnauzer
- Congenital ME: Labrador retrievers, Newfoundlands, Chinese Shar-peis, Great Danes, German shepherds, Irish setters
- Familial ME: Great Danes, German shepherds, Irish setters, Newfoundlands, Siamese cats

RISK FACTORS

- Recent anesthesia
- Gastric reflux/esophagitis (p. 312)
- Mechanical esophageal obstruction
- Stricture: (e.g., oral drugs: doxycycline or clindamycin) (cats > dogs) (p. 310)
- Vascular ring anomaly (e.g., persistent right aortic arch)
- Foreign body (p. 351)
- Mass (neoplasia, granuloma, abscess): intraluminal or extraluminal/compressive
  - Lower esophageal sphincter (LES) pseudo-achalasia: circumferential LES mass
- Gastroesophageal intussusception
- Hiatal hernia (p. 468)
- Pyloric outflow obstruction (less common)
- Hairballs (cats)
- Diverticula

Functional esophageal obstruction:
- IED
- ME: Primary or secondary (p. 642)
- LES achalasia-like syndrome

Neurologic disorders:
- Peripheral neuropathy (e.g., polyradiculoneuritis, polyneuritis) (p. 808)
- CNS lesions: brainstem
- Dysautonomia
- Myasthenia gravis (p. 668)

Toxicity: lead, thallium, organophosphates, botulism, tetanus (see individual intoxications)

CONTAGION AND ZOONOSIS

- *Spirocerca lupi* (p. 933)
- *Pythium insidiosum* (p. 860)
- *Neospora caninum* (p. 984)
- Canine distemper (p. 271)

GEOGRAPHY AND SEASONALITY

Dysautonomia: midwestern United States and United Kingdom; winter

ASSOCIATED DISORDERS

- Aspiration pneumonia (can be life-threatening)
- Chronic aspiration lung injury
- Rhinitis
- Weight loss/poor body condition
- See Risk Factors

Clinical Presentation

HISTORY, CHIEF COMPLAINT

- Regurgitation/vomiting: regurgitation is often confused with vomiting
- Weight loss
- Coughing ± nasal discharge
- Respiratory distress
- Weakness
- Polyphagia

PHYSICAL EXAM FINDINGS

Specific findings vary:
- General: poor body condition/weight loss, halitosis, weakness, neurologic abnormalities, nasal discharge
  - Respiratory disease: tachypnea, harsh lung sounds, ± respiratory distress, ± fever
  - Esophageal dilation: fluid-filled esophagus bulging at neck

Etiology and Pathophysiology

- Pathophysiology varies (p. 1277)
- Regurgitation: nonspecific feature of esophageal dysfunction with or without ME

DIAGNOSIS

Diagnostic Overview

- The first step is to differentiate between regurgitation (passive) and vomiting (active), although both can occur in the same patient. Careful questioning, filming, or feeding and observation of episodes in hospital may provide clarification.
- The list of potential causes of regurgitation is different for pets with ME and those without, and for otherwise healthy pets with ME (e.g., idiopathic or structural cause) and those with ME and evidence of systemic illness (e.g., endocrinopathy, toxicity, infection, metabolic diseases). Recognition of systemic illness or its absence often guides next diagnostic steps.
- Idiopathic ME/IED is a diagnosis of exclusion.

Differential Diagnosis

- Vomiting
- Expectoration
- Oral/pharyngeal dysphagia

Initial Database

- CBC: often unremarkable; inflammatory leukogram (aspiration pneumonia), erythrocyte basophilic stippling (lead)
- Chemistry: often unremarkable; electrolyte changes with systemic metabolic disturbances (e.g., hypoadrenocortisolism)
- Urinalysis: often unremarkable
- Radiographs (cervical and thoracic): identify esophageal abnormalities (e.g., ME, esophageal foreign body, mass, diverticulum), and screen for lung injury/pneumonia.

Advanced or Confirmatory Testing

- Acetylcholine receptor antibody titers: rule out myasthenia gravis as cause of ME, which is indicated for all adult animals with ME unless another cause is known.
- Fluoroscopy: capable of identifying most functional and mechanical obstructions
  - Simultaneous evaluation of swallow and LES relaxation (or manometry) needed to diagnose LES achalasia-like syndrome
  - Freely fed videofluoroscopic swallow study may reduce the risk of aspiration.
- Esophagoscopy: strictures, esophagitis, and diverticula; less reliable than radiography for identifying ME
  - Unless esophageal mass identified, biopsy seldom indicated
- Reflux scintigraphy: reflux disease/aspiration (not widely available)
- ACTH stimulation test: rule out hypoadrenocortisolism
- Thyroid testing: thyroid-stimulating hormone and free T_4 by equilibrium dialysis to rule out hypothyroidism
- Dilute pilocarpine test: rule out dysautonomia
- Toxin screen: rule out lead, thallium, other toxins
- Fecal floatation (sugar or sodium nitrate [$NaNO_3$]): rule out *S. lupi*
- Bioassay: tetanus and botulism (pp. 127 and 964)
- Thoracic CT ± angiogram: esophageal or thoracic mass, vascular ring anomaly

TREATMENT

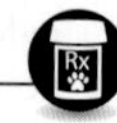

Treatment Overview

Identify and treat underlying disease. In idiopathic ME and IED, treatment is limited to symptomatic and supportive care.

Acute General Treatment

- If present, address respiratory distress due to aspiration (pp. 793 and 879)
- Correction of underlying disease process
  - Immediate intervention for esophageal foreign body (e.g., endoscopy)
  - Address emergent manifestations of metabolic disorders (e.g., hypoadrenocortisolism, hypothyroidism)

Chronic Treatment

Varies with the underlying disease process:
- Metabolic disorders (see specific disorder)
- ME (p. 642)
  - Upright feeding of various food consistencies often useful
  - Sildenafil 1 mg/kg PO q 8-12h: improved clinical signs reported in some dogs with ME
- LES achalasia-like syndromes
  - Pneumatic dilation ± botulinum toxin A: improved clinical signs, weight gain, and improved esophageal motility anecdotally described
  - Heller myotomy and Dorr fundoplication may be beneficial in a subset of patients with LES achalasia-like syndrome
- Promotility drugs: metoclopramide 0.2-0.5 mg/kg PO q 8-12h: increased LES tone and increased gastric emptying
  - Controversial in dogs with ME, helpful in cases of reflux
  - Drugs increasing LES tone: contraindicated for LES achalasia-like syndromes
  - Impendence to bolus flow may occur in cases of IED.
- Reflux esophagitis: acid reducers (omeprazole 1 mg/kg PO q 12h 30 minutes before meals)

Nutrition/Diet

- Small, frequent meals
- Upright feeding (maintained upright 5-10 minutes after feeding) may improve esophageal transit (p. 642)
- Gastrostomy/percutaneous endoscopic gastrostomy (PEG) tubes in dogs not responsive to upright feeding
- Reflux: low-fat meals may facilitate gastric emptying.
- No ideal food texture: consider controlled diet trials with different consistencies

Possible Complications

Weight loss and aspiration pneumonia/aspiration lung injury are the most common complications. Pharyngitis, rhinitis, and laryngeal paralysis are also reported. Other complications vary with the underlying disease process.

Recommended Monitoring

- Frequent evaluations of weight and body condition
- Quantify episodes of regurgitation to gauge response to therapy.
- Thoracic radiographs of patients with increased respiratory rate/effort or to monitor for resolution of pre-existing pathology. Serial radiographs of asymptomatic patients are not recommended.

PROGNOSIS & OUTCOME

Depends on the underlying disease process. Idiopathic ME carries a guarded to poor long-term prognosis, although dogs may do well for months to years. In juvenile dogs with IED, the esophagus may continue to mature and motility may improve up to 1 year of age.

PEARLS & CONSIDERATIONS

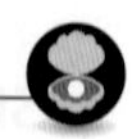

Comments

- Discrimination between regurgitation and vomiting is critical.
  - Unlike vomiting, with regurgitation there is no active abdominal effort, no apparent nausea beforehand, and expectorated material does not contain bile.
- Aspiration pneumonia may exist in the absence of an inflammatory leukogram and fever.
- Antibiotics are not required for all cases of aspiration pneumonia, particularly when pets are asymptomatic.

Prevention

- Fast pets before general anesthesia to reduce risk of esophagitis/stricture.
- Administer water after pilling pets.
- Monthly moxidectin/imidacloprid to prevent *S. lupi*

Technician Tips

When clients report vomiting, ask questions necessary to distinguish vomiting (active) from regurgitation (passive).

Client Education

Monitor respiratory rate and effort at home.

SUGGESTED READING

Pollard R: Imaging evaluation of dogs and cats with dysphagia. ISRN Vet Sci 2012, 2012:238505.

AUTHOR: Megan Grobman, DVM, MS, DACVIM
EDITOR: Leah A. Cohn, DVM, PhD, DACVIM

Renal Dysplasia

Client Education Sheet 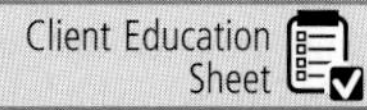

BASIC INFORMATION

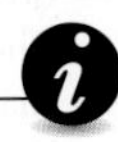

Definition

Disorganized renal development resulting from arrested or anomalous cellular processes; uncommon in dogs and rare in cats

Synonyms

Familial renal disease, progressive juvenile nephropathy

Epidemiology

SPECIES, AGE, SEX

Dogs (rarely cats) of either sex; onset of signs ranges from weeks to years of age, with most animals developing signs before 2 years

GENETICS, BREED PREDISPOSITION

Familial; reported in some common breeds (e.g., golden retriever, boxer, cocker spaniel, Lhasa apso, shih tzu, beagle, miniature schnauzer) and less common breeds (e.g., Dutch kooiker, Finnish harrier, soft-coated wheaten terrier, standard poodle)

RISK FACTORS

In utero viral infection (e.g., canine herpesvirus, feline panleukopenia)

ASSOCIATED DISORDERS

- Chronic kidney disease (CKD), stages I to IV (pp. 167 and 169)
- Stunted growth
- Renal (fibrous) osteodystrophy
- Systemic hypertension

Clinical Presentation

DISEASE FORMS/SUBTYPES

- Familial
- Nonfamilial

HISTORY, CHIEF COMPLAINT

Clinical signs may be absent. When present, abnormalities may include

- Polyuria and polydipsia (PU/PD): common
- Anorexia/wasting (stage III or IV CKD)
- Vomiting/diarrhea (stage III or IV CKD)
- Depression/lethargy (stage III or IV CKD)
- Poor wound healing (stage III or IV CKD)
- Bone pain (if osteodystrophy)
- ± Anestrus
- ± Stunted growth

PHYSICAL EXAM FINDINGS

Physical exam may be unremarkable, or abnormalities can include

- Calcinosis circumscripta: uncommon
- Dehydration (stage III or IV CKD)
- Enlarged and pliable mandible/maxillae (rubber jaw), pathologic fractures (if osteodystrophy)
- Muscular twitching (if osteodystrophy)
- Oral ulceration/halitosis (uremia)
- Pallor (stage III or IV CKD) ± poor haircoat
- Small or irregular kidneys on abdominal palpation common but inconsistent finding
- Small stature/poor body condition common but inconsistent finding

Etiology and Pathophysiology

- The microscopic appearance of kidneys should be mature by 70 days of age (some development and histologic change normally continues during the first 2 months of life). Disorganized parenchymal development with immature or anomalous structures characterizes renal dysplasia with histologic features inappropriate for the animal's age.
- Poorly developed kidneys result in renal failure and eventual death.
- Diminished renal conversion of vitamin D to the active form, calcitriol, contributes to secondary hyperparathyroidism and subsequent renal osteodystrophy. This complication is more pronounced in juvenile renal disease.

DIAGNOSIS

Diagnostic Overview

Renal dysplasia should be suspected in juvenile animals with clinical features consistent with CKD. Definitive diagnosis is established from exam of kidney biopsies.

Differential Diagnosis

Azotemia:

- Prerenal (e.g., dehydration, gastrointestinal [GI] bleeding)
- Renal (e.g., acute kidney injury, CKD of any cause)
- Postrenal (e.g., urinary obstruction, urinary tract rupture)

Initial Database

- Blood pressure (pp. 501 and 1065)
- CBC: nonregenerative anemia common in later stages of CKD
- Serum biochemical profile: abnormalities become more likely and more severe as stage of CKD progresses. Common findings include azotemia, hyperphosphatemia, hypokalemia, hypercalcemia/hypocalcemia, metabolic acidosis, hypercholesterolemia, hypoalbuminemia
- Serum symmetric dimethylarginine (SDMA) test: can detect renal dysfunction sooner than routine biochemical profile
- Urinalysis: isosthenuric or minimally concentrated urine expected, proteinuria, glucosuria, occasionally hematuria
- Urine culture and sensitivity to rule out secondary infection
- Abdominal radiography
  - Small kidneys
  - Poor abdominal detail (young age, poor body condition)
  - Soft-tissue mineralization
- Abdominal ultrasonography
  - Small, irregularly shaped kidneys
  - Thin renal cortex
  - Hyperechoic renal parenchyma
  - Poor corticomedullary distinction
  - Soft-tissue mineralization

Advanced or Confirmatory Testing

- Serum parathyroid hormone (PTH) concentration is initially normal, then rises. Calcitriol therapy may delay PTH increase.
- Serum ionized calcium to confirm biologically significant hypercalcemia: may be normal initially and then may increase as PTH concentration rises.
- Assessment of glomerular filtration rate: occasionally used in nonazotemic animals with suspected renal dysplasia
- Renal histopathologic exam confirms the diagnosis.
  - Asynchronous nephron development
  - Immature glomeruli and/or tubules
  - Persistent fetal mesenchyme
  - Persistent metanephric ducts
  - Atypical tubular epithelium
  - Dysontogenic metaplasia

TREATMENT

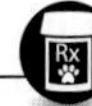

Treatment Overview

Renal dysplasia cannot be reversed or cured; the goal of therapy is to delay progression of kidney disease, maintain hydration, address signs of uremia, and address complications of overt CKD such as anemia and electrolyte disorders.

Acute General Treatment

Acute treatment addresses uremia, dehydration, electrolyte, and acid-base disorders.

Chronic Treatment

- More information is provided on pp. 167, 169, and 887. Besides those described below, other treatments to consider address hyperphosphatemia, systemic hypertension, GI ulceration, anorexia, anemia, hypokalemia, and acidosis.
- Vomiting: address promptly because dehydration may lead to rapid deterioration of renal function. Commonly used antiemetics include maropitant 2 mg/kg PO q 24h for 5 days (dogs), metoclopramide 0.2-0.5 mg/kg SQ or IM q 8h, and ondansetron 0.1-0.2 mg/kg IV q 12h (consider dose reduction for advanced stage CKD). Provide crystalloid fluid therapy as needed.
- Bone pain (renal osteodystrophy): opioids (e.g., full mu agonists such as oxymorphone 0.03-0.2 mg/kg SQ, IM, or IV; fentanyl patch; or buprenorphine 0.01-0.02 mg/kg

SQ, IM, or IV q 6-8h). Avoid administering nonsteroidal antiinflammatory drugs (NSAIDs), which have potentially negative renal effects.

- Early calcitriol therapy may delay or prevent bone changes and should be considered before hyperphosphatemia occurs.
  - Initial dosage 1.65-3.63 ng/kg (= 0.00165-0.00363 mcg/kg) PO q 24h (dogs and cats); dosage is adjusted based primarily on serum calcium and phosphorus concentrations (± PTH concentrations).
  - Maintain total serum Ca (mg/dL) × P (mg/dL) product of < 70; avoid hypercalcemia; if total calcium elevated, confirm with ionized calcium.
  - Ideally, PTH level should be within reference range during treatment. If low, dose is decreased; if high, dose is increased.
  - Calcitriol loses efficacy when phosphorus > 8 mg/dL (>2.6 mmol/L). Typically, calcitriol is used in conjunction with a phosphorus-reducing diet and non–calcium-containing phosphate binders.

Nutrition/Diet

Renal diets are indicated (p. 167).

Drug Interactions

- Vascular calcium channel blockers (amlodipine) and angiotensin-converting enzyme (ACE) inhibitors used concurrently may produce hypotension.
- Phosphate binders can interfere with absorption of orally administered medications.
- Concurrent use of calcitriol and calcium-containing phosphate binders, thiazide diuretics, corticosteroids, and barbiturates should be avoided.
- Nephrotoxic drugs (e.g., aminoglycosides) or drug combinations (e.g., NSAIDs plus ACE inhibitors) should be avoided.
- Drugs that undergo renal elimination may need adjustment in dosage or frequency of administration in animals with CKD.

Possible Complications

- Hypotension may result from use of a calcium channel blocker and/or ACE inhibitors.
- Calcitriol may lead to hypercalcemia, cystic uroliths and/or ectopic mineralization of tissues.
- Complications of CKD include uremia, systemic hypertension, GI ulceration, anemia, electrolyte disorders, acidosis, and renal osteodystrophy.

Recommended Monitoring

- Monitor calcium and phosphorus levels 2 weeks after beginning calcitriol therapy and at least monthly thereafter for dosage adjustment. Ideally, measure PTH levels before and 1-2 months after therapy is started.
- The clinician is advised to monitor the animal as he/she would for other animals with CKD (p. 169); monitoring includes complete physical exam; blood pressure measurement; serum biochemistry profiles and blood gas determinations to assess azotemia, electrolyte, and acid-base status; and urinalysis ± urine culture.

PROGNOSIS & OUTCOME

- Depends on degree of dysplasia, age at onset of signs, severity of dysfunction at diagnosis, and subsequent treatment
- Renal dysplasia is an irreversible condition; long-term prognosis is generally poor.

PEARLS & CONSIDERATIONS

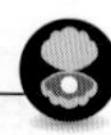

Comments

- Renal dysplasia can occur in any breed of dog or cat.
- There is no specific therapy, but animals are managed as for CKD and its complications.

Prevention

- Do not breed affected animals.
- Inform owners of appropriate vaccination of cats against panleukopenia.

Technician Tips

End-stage patients may have oral ulcers or facial bone pain. One should take extra care when restraining difficult patients, especially with a muzzle. An Elizabethan collar may be less stressful and painful.

Client Education

- Owners should research breed-associated diseases before considering adoption or purchase.
- Breeders should be informed of the diagnosis. Owners of littermates should consider screening their apparently healthy pets.

SUGGESTED READING

Greco DS: Congenital and inherited renal disease of small animals. Vet Clin North Am Small Anim Pract 31:393, 2001.

AUTHOR: Adam Mordecai, DVM, MS, DACVIM
EDITOR: Leah A. Cohn, DVM, PhD, DACVIM

Renal Neoplasia

Client Education Sheet

BASIC INFORMATION

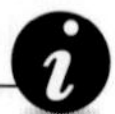

Definition

Neoplasms arising in the kidney parenchyma of epithelial (carcinoma), mesenchymal (sarcoma), or mixed embryonal (nephroblastoma) origin, and lymphoma

Synonyms

Wilms' tumor (nephroblastoma), kidney tumors

Epidemiology

SPECIES, AGE, SEX

- Dogs: older adults; nephroblastomas reported in young dogs
- Cats: older adults, but young cats may develop feline leukemia virus (FeLV)–related lymphoma

GENETICS, BREED PREDISPOSITION

Nodular dermatofibrosis genetically associated with multiple, bilateral renal cystadenocarcinomas in German shepherds through mutation of the *BHD* gene

RISK FACTORS

- Dogs: no sex predominance, except possibly sarcomas in females
- Cats: FeLV infection associated with renal lymphoma

CONTAGION AND ZOONOSIS

Cats: FeLV-related lymphoma (cat to cat)

ASSOCIATED DISORDERS

Paraneoplastic erythrocytosis; nodular dermatofibrosis with renal cystadenocarcinoma

Clinical Presentation

DISEASE FORMS/SUBTYPES

- Primary renal tumors are associated with minimal clinical signs until advanced stage.
- Renal lymphoma in cats may disseminate to the central nervous system (CNS).

HISTORY, CHIEF COMPLAINT

- Hematuria
- Lethargy
- Inappetence
- Abdominal mass
- Weight loss
- Vomiting
- Polyuria/polydipsia (PU/PD)
- Flank pain
- Behavior changes
- Acute collapse

PHYSICAL EXAM FINDINGS

- Renomegaly
- Abdominal mass
- Pale mucous membranes, or dark red membranes if erythrocytosis present
- Abdominal distention ± fluid wave
- Shock (if actively bleeding)

Etiology and Pathophysiology

- Lymphoma may occur spontaneously (dogs and cats) or be associated with FeLV (cats).
- Carcinoma: renal cell carcinoma, transitional cell carcinoma, or adenocarcinoma with tubular or papillary differentiation
  - Mass in renal parenchyma leads to hematuria and proteinuria.
  - Pyuria (common); may be secondary to inflammation from tumor or bacterial infection
  - Anemia secondary to blood loss (with hypoalbuminemia) or diminished renal erythropoietin production
  - Erythrocytosis (rare) due to erythropoietin or erythropoietin-like secretion
  - Metastasis common (16%-48% at diagnosis, 61% at death)
  - Unilateral or (rarely) bilateral
- Sarcoma: hemangiosarcoma, renal sarcoma, leiomyosarcoma, fibrosarcoma, malignant fibrous histiocytoma, and spindle cell sarcomas reported
  - May be metastatic from other site
  - Hematuria common
  - Hypoalbuminemia less common
  - Erythrocytosis (rare)
  - Flank pain more common than in carcinomas
  - Metastasis common
- Nephroblastoma
  - Anemia
  - Associated with young dogs but reported in older dogs
  - Metastasis common
- Benign tumors
  - Hemangioma most common in dogs
  - Renal adenomas and leiomyomas most common in cats

DIAGNOSIS

Diagnostic Overview

A renal tumor should be suspected in cases of persistent hematuria, evidence of abdominal/flank pain, erythrocytosis, or retroperitoneal mass. Confirmation requires imaging, including radiography, ultrasonography, or advanced planar imaging.

Differential Diagnosis

Physical exam:

- Abdominal mass ± pain ± ascites
  - Urinary tract infection, urolithiasis, bladder tumor
  - Mass in spleen, mesenteric lymph node, or retroperitoneal space
  - Ruptured splenic or hepatic mass with hemoperitoneum
  - Abdominal trauma or coagulopathy with peritoneal or retroperitoneal bleeding
  - Renal cysts
  - Hydronephrosis
- Renal pain without mass
  - Pyelonephritis
  - Ethylene glycol ingestion

Radiography:

- Mass in spleen, mesenteric lymph node, or retroperitoneal space
- Ruptured splenic or hepatic mass with hemoperitoneum
- Retroperitoneal fluid: blood or urine
- Renal cyst or hydronephrosis

Ultrasonography:

- Renal abscess or granuloma
- Metastatic neoplasia

Urinalysis:

- Urinary tract infection
- Urolithiasis
- Ureter or bladder tumor
- Idiopathic renal hematuria

Initial Database

- CBC, serum biochemistry profile, urinalysis: anemia or erythrocytosis possible, thrombocytopenia occasionally, azotemia (prerenal and renal), hypoalbuminemia, proteinuria, and hematuria possible
- Abdominal radiographs: mass, possibly peritoneal or retroperitoneal fluid
- Thoracic radiographs: metastasis (16%-48% at diagnosis)
- Abdominal ultrasound: renal mass and possibly metastasis to any abdominal organ, including adrenal gland and caudal vena cava
- Prothrombin time and partial thromboplastin time if disseminated intravascular coagulation suspected

Advanced or Confirmatory Testing

- Cytology or biopsy necessary for diagnosis
- Renal scintigraphy or excretory urogram to assess functional renal mass before nephrectomy
- Anecdotally, the veterinary bladder tumor antigen (V-BTA) test may detect renal pelvic transitional cell carcinoma.
- Echocardiogram if hemangiosarcoma to rule out cardiac mass
- Cerebrospinal fluid (CSF) tap and bone marrow aspiration and cytologic analysis if lymphoma (to stage disease)

TREATMENT

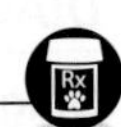

Treatment Overview

The goal of treatment is to remove the source of bleeding, pain, or erythrocytosis. Surgery is the primary treatment modality, with demonstrated benefit for tumors other than lymphoma. Complete resection is ideal and therapeutic goal.

Acute General Treatment

- Stabilize with crystalloids, colloids, and oxygen-carrying capacity.
- Address renal insufficiency with fluid diuresis.
- Surgically remove bleeding mass.
- Begin chemotherapy for lymphoma with caution.
  - L-Asparaginase 10,000 U/m^2 IM once on day 1 (pp. 607 and 609)
  - Cytosine arabinoside 50 mg/m^2 SQ q 12h × 3 days for first week starting day 1
  - Vincristine 0.5 mg/m^2 IV q 7 days starting day 1
  - Cyclophosphamide 50 mg/m^2 PO once daily for 4 days each week starting day 1 if no evidence of cystitis
- Alleviate pain with opioids.

Chronic Treatment

- Lymphoma: if remission is achieved with the COAP (cyclophosphamide, vincristine, cytosine arabinoside, prednisone) protocol (pp. 602 and 603), after 6 weeks, administer doxorubicin IV at 30 mg/m^2 for dogs > 30 kg or 1 mg/kg for dogs < 30 kg and cats, q 3 weeks (pp. 607 and 609).
- Others
  - No prospective clinical trials exist.
  - Most literature reports based on doxorubicin or actinomycin D
  - Anecdotal reports of response to carboplatin for carcinomas
  - Carcinomas may express cyclooxygenase 2 (COX2), and 0.3 mg/kg piroxicam PO q 24h is recommended if azotemia absent
  - Carcinomas may express KIT protein, suggesting a possible role for toceranib (2.5-3 mg/kg) for management with anecdotal reports of response in metastatic disease (pp. 632 and 634).

Drug Interactions

Avoid combining drugs with similar toxicity profiles, such as cisplatin and piroxicam.

Possible Complications

Neutropenia, thrombocytopenia, sepsis, and renal injury secondary to chemotherapy

Recommended Monitoring

- Monitor CBC before every chemotherapy treatment and 7-10 days later.
- Monitor blood urea nitrogen (BUN), creatinine, and urine specific gravity for renal function.
- Monitor CBC, serum biochemistry profile, urine protein/creatinine ratio for toceranib.

PROGNOSIS & OUTCOME

- Benign: good
- Lymphoma: guarded to poor (60% remission rate; median duration of 4 months [cats])
- For solid tumors, survival depends on therapy: median of 16 months with surgery, median < 1 month without surgery; chemotherapy not demonstrated to make a difference
  - Carcinomas: guarded to poor, rare survivals > 1 year
  - Sarcomas: guarded to poor, reportedly more aggressive than carcinomas
  - Nephroblastomas: guarded to poor, rare reports of long survival

- Metastatic potential of all tumors is high.
  - Lymphoma metastasis to CNS is lower with cytosine arabinoside in chemotherapy protocol.
  - Chemotherapy effect on metastasis of carcinomas, sarcomas, nephroblastomas unevaluated

PEARLS & CONSIDERATIONS

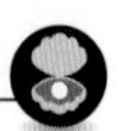

Comments

- Hematuria in the absence of other clinical signs may suggest renal neoplasia.
- Early detection is critical for successful treatment.
- Definitive diagnosis is necessary for prognosis and therapeutic decisions.
- Complete resection offers best chance for long survival.
- Erythrocytosis usually resolves with nephrectomy.

Technician Tips

- Erythrocytosis (packed cell volume > 55%-65%, depending on breed) may be a sign of renal tumor.
- Careful handling of all excreta from dogs receiving chemotherapy is important to prevent exposure to active metabolites.

Client Education

Because signs are subtle and nonspecific, advanced diagnostic tests and imaging are most useful early. Nephrectomy may be palliative and maximize quality of remaining life.

SUGGESTED READING

Bryan JN, et al: Primary renal neoplasia of dogs. J Vet Intern Med 20:1155-1160, 2006.

AUTHOR: Jeffrey N. Bryan, DVM, MS, PhD, DACVIM
EDITOR: Leah A. Cohn, DVM, PhD, DACVIM

Renal Secondary Hyperparathyroidism

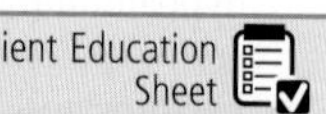

BASIC INFORMATION

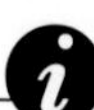

Definition

Renal secondary hyperparathyroidism (RSHP) results from the effects of excessive production of parathyroid hormone (PTH, parathormone) in animals with azotemic and nonazotemic chronic kidney disease (CKD). RSHP occurs as an important component of CKD–metabolic bone disease (CKD-MBD) complex.

Epidemiology

SPECIES, AGE, SEX

Any animal with CKD (pp. 167 and 169)

RISK FACTORS

CKD: International Renal Interest Society (IRIS) stages 3 and 4 very frequently; stage 2 commonly; stage 1 up to 30%

ASSOCIATED DISORDERS

Hyperphosphatemia, hypocalcemia, CKD (azotemic and nonazotemic)

Clinical Presentation

HISTORY, CHIEF COMPLAINT

History of CKD; obvious clinical signs or inapparent to owner (i.e., occult CKD)

PHYSICAL EXAM FINDINGS

- Variable combinations of signs of CKD (pp. 167 and 169)
- Skull and jaw lesions (rubber jaw) occasionally occur with advanced stages of RSHP.

Etiology and Pathophysiology

- Declining kidney function increases phosphorus retention, which leads to increased secretion of PTH and fibroblast growth factor 23 (FGF23).
  - Increased circulating phosphorus inhibits renal synthesis of calcitriol, the active form of vitamin D, effectively increasing PTH concentration by lessening calcitriol-mediated genomic inhibition of PTH synthesis.
  - FGF-23, a phosphatonin secreted by osteocytes, promotes phosphaturia, decreases calcitriol synthesis, and decreases PTH synthesis early in CKD.
  - Low concentrations of circulating 1,25-dihydroxyvitamin D and 25-hydroxyvitamin D increase PTH synthesis (failed inhibition of synthesis).
- Increased secretion of PTH stimulates calcitriol synthesis until advanced CKD; normal calcitriol concentrations are maintained in early stages of CKD from this mechanism.
- Decline in renal calcitriol synthetic capacity and resultant lower circulating concentrations decrease calcium (Ca) entry into the circulation from bone and intestine, decreasing serum ionized calcium (iCa) concentrations. Excessive PTH rarely results in hypercalcemia (tertiary hyperparathyroidism).

DIAGNOSIS

Diagnostic Overview

Should be suspected in all patients with CKD

Differential Diagnosis

- Primary hyperparathyroidism (p. 499)
- Tertiary hyperparathyroidism
- Hypovitaminosis D; nutritional secondary hyperparathyroidism (NSHP [p. 697])

Initial Database

- Laboratory assessment of CKD (pp. 167 and 169)
- Serum phosphorus is important: concentration is often increased in later IRIS CKD stages. Serum phosphorus of 4.5-5.5 mg/dL (upper end of reference range) predicts RSHP for many dogs.
- Total serum Ca: usually normal to low
- Serum iCa, which may not parallel serum total Ca, is more reliable than total Ca (especially with azotemia).

Advanced or Confirmatory Testing

- Serum PTH concentration (p. 1370): increased serum PTH can occur within reference range (usually upper half) in early stages of CKD.
- Measure iCa at the same time to determine appropriateness of the response.
- Serum FGF23 concentration (if commercially available): biomarker is elevated earlier than PTH in CKD and RSHP.
- Serum 25-hydroxyvitamin D concentration: low concentrations are common even in early stages of CKD.
  - Decreased proximal renal tubular reabsorption of this form of vitamin D bound to vitamin D–binding protein contributes to reduced concentrations.
  - Some increase in PTH may be due to low circulating 25-hydroxyvitamin D secondary to reduced hepatic conversion of vitamin D to 25-hydroxyvitamin D in CKD and/or from inadequate vitamin D intake.
- Radiography may reveal diffuse bone demineralization. Pathologic fractures are rare. Earliest lesions are detected in facial bones by loss of the lamina dura dentes, seen using high-definition dental technique.
- High-frequency ultrasonography of the neck reveals multiple parathyroid gland enlargement.

TREATMENT

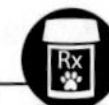

Treatment Overview

The initial goals of treatment are to decrease circulating PTH and slow CKD progression through reduction of phosphorus intake. Doing so increases endogenous renal synthesis of calcitriol, and additional benefit can be gained from exogenous calcitriol supplementation. The target serum phosphorus concentration in dogs or cats with CKD is ≈4 mg/dL (≈1.3 mmol/L; middle to lower half of reference range) versus the upper limit of many reference ranges for adults (<6 mg/dL [<1.94 mmol/L]).

Acute and Chronic Treatment

- Reduce phosphorus intake by providing a phosphorus-restricted (veterinary therapeutic) diet (target: 0.4-1.4 mg P/kcal).
  - If phosphorus restriction fails to reduce serum phosphorus to targeted concentrations or phosphorus-restricted diets are refused, intestinal phosphorus binders should be prescribed.
- Calcitriol 9 ng/kg PO twice weekly after serum phosphorus < 6 mg/dL can prevent parathyroid gland hyperplasia and increased PTH. Increased PTH can be restored to lower concentrations.
  - Calcitriol should be prescribed when serum phosphorus and iCa concentrations are below the upper limit of the reference range. Otherwise, soft-tissue mineralization may occur.
- Additional therapy for animals with CKD as appropriate (pp. 167 and 169)

Possible Complications

- Ionized hypercalcemia (> 6 mg/dL [1.5 mmol/L] in dogs; 5.5 mg/dL [1.37 mmol/L] in cats)
- Increased total serum Ca occurs in 10%-20% of dogs and cats with CKD before treatment, but iCa may be high, normal, or low.
- Hypercalcemia is dangerous only when iCa is increased; when it is,
  - Decrease the daily dose of calcitriol by 50%.
  - Give calcitriol at night on an empty stomach to help minimize intestinal calcium absorption.
- If serum phosphorus is low (lower 25% of the reference range or less), increase dietary phosphorus or reduce phosphorus binder.
- Change to non–calcium-containing phosphate binder if relevant, or decrease the daily dose by 50%. In general, administering calcium-containing phosphate binders is NOT recommended when calcitriol will be used to treat CKD.

Recommended Monitoring

- Measure serum PTH and iCa (from the same sample) after 1, 3, and 6 months of therapy and q 6 months thereafter for stable animals. Goal is to have both within reference range. Calcitriol dosage should be adjusted based on PTH and iCa results: increase if serum PTH is too high, and decrease if serum iCa is too high.
- Measure serum phosphorus to ensure control of hyperphosphatemia; adjust dietary phosphorus and phosphorus binders accordingly.
- Refer animals with persistently increased iCa for evaluation of primary or tertiary hyperparathyroidism or idiopathic hypercalcemia in cats (p. 492).
- Monitor CKD as dictated for the individual patient.

PROGNOSIS & OUTCOME

- Survival of months to years is possible, depending disease severity at diagnosis and initiation of treatment for CKD. Prognosis is guarded to poor (weeks) for animals with advanced CKD and uncontrolled RSHP.
- Long-term survival in cats with treatment of CKD is far more common than for dogs.
- Worse for animals with uncontrollable hyperphosphatemia
- Survival increases with appropriate PTH-lowering therapy.

PEARLS & CONSIDERATIONS

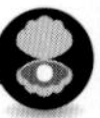

Comments

- Almost impossible to lower PTH or FGF23 if serum phosphorus remains > 6 mg/dL
- Reference ranges for serum phosphorus levels often include results from growing animals, which are much higher than for adult animals. Normal mature animals typically have serum phosphorus levels < 5.0 mg/dL.
- Conversion to metric for calcium (total or ionized): 1 mg/dL = 0.25 mmol/L. Conversion to metric for phosphorus: 1 mg/dL = 0.323 mmol/L

Prevention

Appropriate phosphorus restriction can control/prevent development of RSHP in early CKD but does not prevent development of CKD in the first place.

Technician Tips

Technicians are instrumental in providing client education about proper diet and feeding management. There are many options for phosphorus-restricted diets in different forms and flavors that can be tried to accomplish adequate intake of an appropriate diet.

Client Education

Evaluation is recommended q 3-4 months for stable CKD and more often if poorly controlled.

SUGGESTED READING

Harjes LM, et al: Fibroblast growth factor-23 concentration in dogs with chronic kidney disease. J Vet Intern Med 31:784-790, 2017.

AUTHORS: Joao Felipe de Brito Galvao, MV, MS, DACVIM; Dennis J. Chew, DVM, DACVIM
EDITOR: Jennifer Larsen, DVM, PhD, DACVN

Respiratory Distress

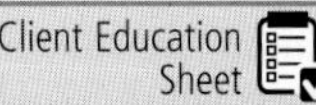

Client Education Sheet

BASIC INFORMATION

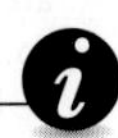

Definition

Respiratory distress refers to difficult or labored respiration. Although often used synonymously, the term *dyspnea* refers to a conscious sensation of air hunger and is therefore anthropomorphic.

Synonyms

Dyspnea, increased respiratory effort, shortness of breath, belly breathing

Epidemiology

SPECIES, AGE, SEX

Any dog or cat but a particular cause of distress may be more likely in certain animals (e.g., laryngeal paralysis in older dogs; asthma in young to middle-aged cats)

GENETICS, BREED PREDISPOSITION

Breed predispositions exist for some specific causes of respiratory distress.

RISK FACTORS

May be precipitated by factors related to the underlying disease process:

- Laryngeal paralysis, collapsing trachea: heat and humidity
- Feline asthma: aeroallergen exposure, dust
- Aspiration pneumonia: anesthesia, vomiting, regurgitation
- Infectious pneumonia: group housing, inappropriate or absent vaccination

CONTAGION AND ZOONOSIS

Pathogens of tracheobronchitis (pp. 271 and 987) are contagious; rarely, *Bordetella bronchiseptica* infects immunosuppressed people. Other systemic contagions occasionally cause respiratory distress (e.g., leptospirosis [p. 583], feline infectious peritonitis [p. 327]), and some are also zoonotic (e.g., plague).

ASSOCIATED DISORDERS

Stridor, syncope, cyanosis, orthopnea, regurgitation, exercise intolerance, dysphonia, or others, depending on cause of distress

Clinical Presentation

DISEASE FORMS/SUBTYPES

- Inspiratory distress: upper airway obstruction (above the thoracic inlet), severe abdominal distention, or pleural space disease. Upper airway obstruction may also be associated with an externally audible noise (e.g., stridor/stertor). A history of dysphonia localizes disease to the upper airway (larynx).
- Expiratory distress: lower airway disease (below the thoracic inlet); may be associated with expiratory wheeze, expiratory effort is associated with abdominal contraction during exhalation
- Inspiratory-expiratory distress: mixed inspiratory and expiratory effort is typically associated with pulmonary parenchymal or mixed disorders.
- Paradoxical breathing: pleural space disease, airway obstruction, and diaphragmatic paralysis; dyssynchronous movement of the chest and abdomen. A focal paradoxical pattern of chest movement is seen with flail chest.
- Respiratory effort in vascular disorders (e.g., pulmonary thromboembolic disease [PTE], pulmonary capillary hemangiomatosis [PCH]) varies.
- Look-a-like diseases, including anemia, stress, pain, or metabolic disorders, may be mistaken for respiratory distress.

HISTORY, CHIEF COMPLAINT

Labored, rapid, or noisy breathing, open-mouth breathing (cats), and collapse are common presenting complaints. Anorexia, restlessness, exercise intolerance, and hiding behavior (cats) may be reported. Cough, hemoptysis, and cyanosis are sometimes reported. Many cat owners fail to recognize cough, and cats with paroxysms of cough may present for vomiting or hairballs.

PHYSICAL EXAM FINDINGS

Special attention should be paid early in the exam (before excessive handing) to phase of respiratory effort, rate, and depth of excursions.

- Features of respiratory distress may include an anxious facial expression, abducted elbows, neck extension, flaring nostrils, and restlessness, orthopnea, or open-mouth breathing (cats).
- Ocular/nasal discharge (suggestive of an infectious process; may warrant containment to prevent contagion)
- Consider pattern of distress: inspiratory, expiratory, mixed, paradoxical (see Disease Forms/Subtypes above)
- Muddy or cyanotic mucous membranes with severe hypoxemia (p. 231)
- Audible noises (p. 945)
  - Stertor: seldom associated with cause of distress because it reflects obstruction above the larynx
  - Stridor: laryngeal or upper tracheal obstruction; inspiratory
- Thoracic palpation
  - Evidence of trauma (e.g., rib fracture, fail segment)
  - Lack of compressibility (cats) suggests cranial mediastinal masses or pleural effusion.
  - Palpable thrill from high-grade heart murmur
- Thoracic percussion
  - Hyporesonance suggests effusion, consolidation, or mass effect.
  - Hyperresonance suggests pneumothorax.
- Thoracic auscultation
  - Murmurs/arrhythmias due to heart disease
  - Crackles suggest edema, pneumonia, contusions, or fibrosis; often inspiratory
    - Cough may enhance ability to auscultate crackles (post-tussive crackle).
  - Wheezes suggestive of airway narrowing (e.g., bronchoconstriction, exudate); often expiratory
  - Increased bronchovesicular sounds suggest increased airflow, early edema, or pneumonia.
  - Dull or absent bronchovesicular sounds ventrally or dorsally may suggest pleural fluid or pneumothorax, respectively.
  - Tracheal auscultation to assess referred upper airway sounds
- Hyperthermia may be identified with upper airway obstruction or infectious disease.
- Profound abdominal distention (e.g., ascites, gastric distention) can cause shallow, inspiratory distress.
- Poor body condition may be seen in cases of chronic disease (e.g., neoplasia, fungal pneumonia).
- Other findings may reflect underlying disease (e.g., skin lesions due to blastomycosis, abdominal mass associated with metastatic pulmonary neoplasia).

Etiology and Pathophysiology

- Respiration depends on coordination of central and peripheral O_2 and CO_2 sensors, the respiratory control center (medulla oblongata and pons), and external effector muscles (diaphragm, intercostal muscles).
- Respiratory distress may be triggered by hypoxemia or hypercarbia ($PaO_2 < 60$ mm Hg; $PaCO_2 > 50$ mm Hg)
- Causes of hypoxemia
  - Decreased fraction of inspired oxygen (FIO_2)
  - Ventilation-perfusion (VQ) mismatching (e.g., PTE, asthma, pulmonary veno-occlusive disease [PVOD], PCH)
  - Hypoventilation (e.g., central nervous system disease, sedation)
  - Diffusion impairment across the alveolocapillary membrane (e.g., pulmonary fibrosis); rarely causes hypercarbia due to differences in solubility of gasses.
  - Shunt (blood from the right heart enters the left side without taking part in gas exchange) (e.g., acute respiratory distress syndrome [ARDS], alveolar collapse)
- Causes of hypercarbia
  - Hypoventilation
  - VQ mismatching

DIAGNOSIS

Diagnostic Overview

Disease localization is critical to prompt treatment in an emergency setting. Upper airway obstruction (inspiratory effort with stridor), lower airway obstruction (expiratory effort, wheeze), pleural space disease (inspiratory/paradoxical effort, decreased ventral/dorsal lung sounds), flail chest, and abdominal distention are identifiable during initial physical exam, allowing specific intervention before extensive diagnostics.

Differential Diagnosis

- Panting
- Reverse sneezing
- Look-a-like diseases: abnormal respiratory rate/pattern without respiratory pathology (e.g., anemia, acidemia, stress, pain, methemoglobinemia)
  - Differentiated from respiratory disease by normal arterial blood gas or pulse oximetry (pulse oximetry reads low with methemoglobin) on room air

Initial Database

Provide supplemental oxygen immediately, including during all diagnostic testing.

- CBC/serum biochemical profile/urinalysis: changes depend on underlying disorder, often nonspecific
- Thoracic/cervical radiographs: minimum of three-view thoracic radiographs recommended; inspiratory and expiratory views that include the thoracic and cervical trachea are needed in cases of collapsing trachea (p. 1155)
  - Radiographic positioning may not be tolerated until respiratory distress is improved.
- Pulse oximetry: ensure a good waveform corresponding to auscultated heart rate; anemia should not cause interference when packed cell volume > 15%-18%
- Thoracic focused assessment of sonography for trauma (TFAST) scan if pneumothorax or pleural effusion is suspected (p. 1102)

Advanced or Confirmatory Testing

Choice of tests depends on prior results but often includes

- Oral/pharyngeal exam: may require sedation; evaluate above the soft palate (e.g., nasopharyngeal polyps) and below the tongue
- Laryngeal function exam (p. 574)
- Plasma N-terminal pro-brain-type natriuretic peptide (NT-pro-BNP) may be increased in disease of cardiac origin such as congestive heart failure (CHF) (pp. 408 and 1369).
- Echocardiography (pp. 408 and 838): CHF and pulmonary hypertension
- Arterial blood gas (p. 1058); if can be obtained without additional distress, allows accurate assessment of O_2, CO_2
- Respiratory fluoroscopy: dynamic airway collapse/obstruction (e.g., tracheal collapse, mainstem bronchial collapse, epiglottic retroversion)
- Thoracic CT can be performed quickly and provides more detail than thoracic radiographs.
- Bronchoscopy with bronchoalveolar lavage for culture and cytology (p. 1073)
- Bronchoalveolar lavage (blind) or transtracheal wash (p. 1073)
- Diagnosis of interstitial lung diseases (p. 553) might require lung biopsy.
- Infectious disease testing, as appropriate

TREATMENT

Treatment Overview

Provide oxygen supplementation immediately. Specific intervention may be necessary before diagnostic testing to control respiratory crisis (e.g., thoracocentesis to remove fluid or air, endotracheal intubation or tracheostomy to bypass laryngeal obstruction). The eventual goal is to address the underlying cause.

Acute General Treatment

- Oxygen supplementation (p. 1146)
- Specific treatments depend on underlying cause.
  - Upper airway obstruction: ensure patency of the airway (e.g., endotracheal tube; tracheostomy [p. 1166]), sedation (p. 574), external cooling as needed
  - Lower airway obstruction: sedation, bronchodilators (p. 84)
  - CHF: diuretics (p. 408)
  - Pleural effusion, pneumothorax: thoracocentesis (p. 1164)
  - Address abdominal distention (e.g., ascites, bloat).
  - Positive-pressure ventilation may become necessary, typically when $PaO_2 < 60$ mm Hg or $PaCO_2 > 60$ mm Hg despite oxygen supplementation (p. 1185).

Possible Complications

Uncontrolled respiratory distress may lead to progressive hypoxemia, cyanosis, respiratory fatigue, and death.

Recommended Monitoring

During period of respiratory distress, frequent monitoring of respiratory effort and rate is essential. Pulse oximetry and/or arterial blood gas analysis allow assessment of oxygenation. Thoracic imaging may need to be repeated.

PROGNOSIS & OUTCOME

Depends on underlying disease process and severity

PEARLS & CONSIDERATIONS

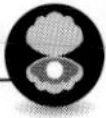

Comments

Patients in respiratory distress are fragile and prone to decompensation. Avoid excessive handling and restraint.

Technician Tips

Provide supplemental oxygen to any animal with respiratory distress. Minimize handling and stress. Animals in respiratory distress may bite when handled.

Client Education

- Sustained open-mouth breathing is never normal in a cat and should prompt veterinary assessment.
- At home resting respiratory rates can help monitor for disease progression.

SUGGESTED READING

Sumner C, et al: Management of respiratory emergencies in small animals. Vet Clin North Am Small Anim Pract 43:4, 2013.

AUTHOR: Megan Grobman, DVM, MS, DACVIM
EDITOR: Leah A. Cohn, DVM, PhD, DACVIM

Restrictive Cardiomyopathy, Feline

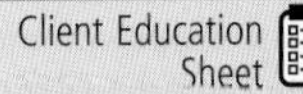

BASIC INFORMATION

Definition

Restrictive cardiomyopathy (RCM) is a primary myocardial disease that occurs more commonly in cats than dogs. It is characterized by impaired ventricular filling, severe biatrial enlargement, normal (nonhypertrophied) ventricular wall thickness, normal (nondilated) ventricular chamber size, and normal to mildly reduced systolic function in the absence of valvular lesions. Some classification schemes also consider RCM to be characterized by normal to mildly thickened ventricular myocardium. In unclassified cardiomyopathy, the echocardiographic anatomic changes are similar, but ventricular filling cannot be assessed (i.e., due to heart rate).

Synonyms

End-stage hypertrophic cardiomyopathy (HCM) and unclassified cardiomyopathy (UCM) are difficult to differentiate from each other and from RCM. UCM and end-stage HCM are characterized by severe left atrial or biatrial enlargement; mixed changes to the ventricles, including areas of thickening and areas of thinning (scarring); ventricular dilatation; and depressed systolic function.

Epidemiology

SPECIES, AGE, SEX

- RCM is reported to be the second most common cardiomyopathy in cats, although true prevalence is difficult to determine given the inconsistent diagnostic characterizations used previously.
- Middle- to older-aged cats are most often affected, although RCM has been reported in cats as young as 4 months of age to as old as 19 years. Varied sex predisposition has been reported with no apparent consensus.

GENETICS, BREED PREDISPOSITION

RCM has been described in many cat breeds, with possible predominance in domestic shorthair, Siamese, Persian, and Burmese.

ASSOCIATED DISORDERS

- Acute and chronic left or biventricular congestive heart failure (CHF)
- Arterial thromboembolism (ATE): may be more common with RCM than HCM
- Syncope/sudden cardiac death: typically arrhythmogenic

Clinical Presentation

DISEASE FORMS/SUBTYPES

It is important to differentiate RCM from restrictive physiology. Restrictive physiology (resulting from a stiff, noncompliant left ventricle and high left atrial pressure) can be seen in many forms of primary cardiomyopathies (RCM, UCM, HCM, dilated cardiomyopathy), valvular diseases, in secondary cardiomyopathies (hypertensive and thyrotoxic cardiomyopathy). Restrictive physiology is typically seen with RCM but is not pathognomonic of RCM.

HISTORY, CHIEF COMPLAINT

- Tachypnea and/or dyspnea: murmurs are often absent, making early detection difficult; many cats present with signs of CHF in the form of pulmonary edema and/or pleural effusion and rarely ascites
- Paresis/pain and other clinical signs consistent with arterial thromboembolic disease (p. 74) with or without CHF; transient weakness/lameness may be a historical complaint
- Syncope: significant arrhythmias can result in syncope and/or transient weakness and altered consciousness

PHYSICAL EXAM FINDINGS

Exam findings are variable but include:

- Gallop heart sound: common
- Jugular venous distention: common
- Heart murmurs: uncommonly, a soft systolic ejection murmur may be present
- Acute dyspnea/tachypnea
- Muffled lung and heart sounds (pleural effusion ± pericardial effusion)
- Pulmonary crackles (pulmonary edema)
- Palpable abdominal fluid wave: ascites, uncommon
- Signs of ATE: absent femoral pulses, pale and cold footpads, cyanotic nail beds, painful and firm limb(s)
- Irregular heart rhythm with pulse deficits

Etiology and Pathophysiology

- Cause unknown: thought to be multifactorial with hypotheses including viral or immune-mediated endomyocarditis with reparative fibrosis. Some hypothesize that within the spectrum of HCM, RCM represents an end-stage form of HCM.
- RCM secondary to infiltrative disorders (amyloidosis, sarcoidosis, neoplasia) and storage disease are common in people but rarely or not reported in cats.
- Typical pathologic features include endomyocardial scarring and myocardial fibrosis, predominately of the left ventricle.
    - Ventricular changes result in impaired ventricular filling and high atrial pressure (diastolic heart failure).
    - Atrial enlargement results in blood stasis that can lead to thrombus formation and subsequent thromboembolism to systemic and coronary arteries.
    - Ventricular scarring can serve as nidus for arrhythmias.

DIAGNOSIS

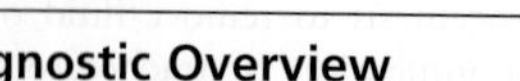

Diagnostic Overview

Diagnosis of RCM is ultimately made with echocardiography. Other diagnostic tests (e.g., thoracic radiographs, abdominal aortic ultrasound) can be helpful when determining presence/severity of the consequences of RCM (CHF, ATE, arrhythmias).

Differential Diagnosis

The findings listed below for RCM can also occur with other cardiomyopathies. Consider the following differentials:

- Pulmonary edema: noncardiogenic pulmonary edema, pulmonary hemorrhage, neoplasia
- Pleural effusion: neoplasia, idiopathic chylothorax, pyothorax, hemothorax
- Jugular distension: fluid overload, cranial vena cava obstruction
- Atrial and ventricular arrhythmias: myocarditis, electrolyte disturbances, hyperthyroidism, systemic diseases, drugs and toxins, autonomic imbalance
- Arterial thromboembolism: endocarditis, pulmonary neoplasia/abscess, trauma

Initial Database

- CBC: in the presence of CHF and/or ATE, will often see changes consistent with stress leukogram
- Chemistry: with ATE, may see elevations in creatine kinase (CK), aspartate aminotransferase (AST), and alanine aminotransferase (ALT)
- N-terminal pro-brain-type natriuretic peptide (NT-pro-BNP): test rarely done because murmurs are uncommon and many RCM cases are diagnosed late in disease (when NT-pro-BNP is typically significantly elevated). NT-pro-BNP is most often used as a screening test to differentiate functional from pathologic murmurs in cats.
- Thoracic radiographs: left atrial or biatrial enlargement, changes consistent with CHF when present (venous ± arterial distention, pulmonary edema, pleural effusion), generalized cardiomegaly may be present with pericardial effusion
- Electrocardiogram (ECG): atrial and ventricular ectopy common (p. 1096)
- Two-dimensional (2D) echocardiogram (p. 1094):
    - Biatrial enlargement, often severe
    - Nondilated, nonhypertrophied left ventricular chamber/walls
    - Normal to mildly reduced ventricular systolic function
    - ± Areas of hyperechoic endocardium/myocardium
    - ± Left atrial/auricular spontaneous echogenic contrast ("smoke")
    - ± Left atrial/auricular thrombus
    - ± Pleural and/or pericardial effusion

Advanced or Confirmatory Testing

- Spectral Doppler echocardiogram
    - Restrictive left ventricular filling pattern (increased E-wave amplitude with shortened deceleration time; reduced A-wave amplitude; E:A wave ratio > 2)
    - Reduced isovolumic relaxation time (IVRT)
    - Diastolic-dominant pulmonary venous flow
    - Depressed left auricular emptying velocity
- Tissue Doppler echocardiogram
    - Severely reduced E′ velocity
    - E:E′ ratio ≫ 12

TREATMENT

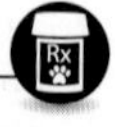

Treatment Overview

There are no proven treatments for reversing or preventing the progression of RCM. Treatment is aimed at the consequences of the disease: CHF, ATE, and arrhythmias. Treatment involves stabilizing the patient (acute therapy) and preventing further clinical signs (typically lifelong chronic therapy).

Acute General Treatment

Acute treatment is directed at complications secondary to RCM:

- Congestive heart failure (p. 408)
- Thromboembolic disease (p. 74)
- Cardiac arrhythmias (pp. 94 and 1033)

Chronic Treatment

- Standard chronic therapy for CHF includes furosemide and an angiotensin-converting enzyme (ACE) inhibitor
    - Furosemide 1-4 mg/kg PO q 8-12h (start and maintain at lowest dose possible and increase as necessary for persistent/recurrent congestion)
    - ACE inhibitors: enalapril or benazepril 0.25-0.5 mg/kg PO q 12-24h
    - Other therapies to consider in refractory cases
        - Torsemide: typically dosed at one-tenth the dose of furosemide being used in cases of refractory CHF; torsemide replaces furosemide; monitor for azotemia and hypokalemia
        - Pimobendan 0.25-0.3 mg/kg PO q 12h; used when depressed systolic function present
- Antithrombotic therapy for cats at risk for ATE
    - Clopidogrel 18.75 mg/CAT PO q 24h for ATE prevention
    - Aspirin 20-81 mg/CAT PO q 72h for ATE prevention; clopidogrel is superior but the two sometimes used in combination
    - Enoxaparin 1 mg/kg SQ q 12-24h for ATE prevention; sometimes used in combination with clopidogrel or aspirin
    - Dalteparin 100 IU/kg SQ q 24h for ATE prevention; sometimes used in combination with clopidogrel or aspirin

- Antiarrhythmic therapy for cats with clinically significant ventricular arrhythmias
  - Sotalol 1-2 mg/kg PO q 12h; used to treat ventricular arrhythmias
  - Atenolol 6.25-12.5 mg/CAT q 12-24h; used to treat ventricular arrhythmias (CHF should be controlled before starting)

Nutrition/Diet

Moderately salt-restricted diets with normal protein and taurine levels are recommended.

Behavior/Exercise

- Cats with heart disease can typically set their own pace.
- Although it is rare for cats on antithrombotics to experience spontaneous bleeding, it is usually recommended that cats be kept indoors.

Drug Interactions

- Azotemia can result from diuretic and ACE inhibitor administration. A renal panel is recommended 5-7 days after starting these medications.
- Bleeding can be seen with antithrombotic therapy, especially with combination therapy.
- For cats with CHF and comorbidities requiring steroids: short-term antiinflammatory doses of oral prednisolone can typically be tolerated well; methylprednisolone acetate (Depo-Medrol) should be avoided. Topical glucocorticoids (e.g., fluticasone inhaler for asthma) are preferred when possible.

Possible Complications

Recurrent episodes of CHF are common. Other common complications include ATE, syncope, and sudden cardiac death.

Recommended Monitoring

- Monitor for signs of CHF, including tachypnea and dyspnea.
- Monitor for signs of ATE, including unexplained lameness, pain, and/or behavioral changes.
- Monitor renal values and for signs of azotemia (lethargy, anorexia, vomiting, hiding, altered mentation).
- Intermittent monitoring of thoracic radiographs and echocardiogram recommended, depending on clinical signs.
- Some anticoagulant therapies (except platelet inhibition) require periodic monitoring.

PROGNOSIS & OUTCOME

- Poor to guarded prognosis for long-term survival of cats with RCM (typically months, not years)
- Guarded to good prognosis for acute CHF
- Guarded to poor prognosis for acute cardiogenic shock
- Guarded prognosis for ATE

PEARLS & CONSIDERATIONS

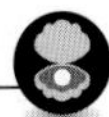

Comments

- Cats with ATE should be offered treatment. Once stabilized, median time from first to second ATE event is 1.2 years (443 days) for cats treated with clopidogrel.
- Although cats with RCM and CHF can typically be stabilized, it is common to have recurrent episodes of CHF.
- Clopidogrel is very bitter; consider the use of gel capsules to combine medication dosages and avoid ptyalism.

Technician Tips

- Care should be taken with venipuncture in cats receiving antithrombotics. Although jugular venipuncture can safely be performed, this approach should be avoided if possible.
- Cats with CHF are especially fragile; avoid stressful handling/restraint. Sedation (typically with butorphanol 0.1-0.3 mg/kg IM) should be used to reduce stress when performing diagnostics.
- Cats with this form of heart disease often lack an audible murmur.

Client Education

- Owners should monitor resting respiratory rate at home (should be < 30-35 breaths/min), allowing early intervention for CHF relapses to be initiated.
- Owners should be educated on the signs associated with ATE.

SUGGESTED READING

Fox PR, et al: Spontaneously occurring restrictive nonhypertrophied cardiomyopathy in domestic cats: a new animal model of human disease. Cardiovasc Pathol 23:28-34, 2014.

AUTHOR: Jaylyn Rhinehart, DVM, MS, DACVIM
EDITOR: Meg M. Sleeper, VMD, DACVIM

Retinal Degeneration

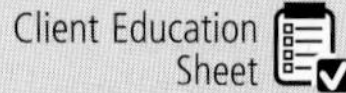

BASIC INFORMATION

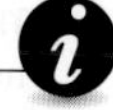

Definition

Deterioration of the retina due to primary inherited retinal disorders or secondary to other intraocular or systemic disease (acquired) may be focal, multifocal, or generalized. Extent of retinal involvement determines degree of vision impairment.

Synonym

Retinal atrophy

Epidemiology

SPECIES, AGE, SEX

Affects dogs and cats; age of onset and sex predisposition vary with underlying cause:

- Inherited
  - Progressive retinal atrophy (PRA): early onset (i.e., dysplasia at 12 weeks of age) and late onset (i.e., degeneration; typically detected by 2 to 8 years of age) in dogs and cats
  - Retinal pigment epithelial dystrophy (RPED); young dogs; uncommon
- Acquired
  - Sudden acquired retinal degeneration syndrome (SARDS) typically affects middle-aged to older dogs; females are predisposed.

GENETICS, BREED PREDISPOSITION

- Dogs
  - PRA: autosomal recessive in most predisposed breeds, including poodles, cocker spaniels, Irish setters, collies, whippets (novel form), and other breeds
  - RPED: Briards, English cocker spaniels in association with familial vitamin E deficiency
  - Multifocal retinopathy: Great Pyrenees, coton de Tuléar, Australian shepherd, dachshunds, boerboel
  - Multifocal chorioretinopathy: borzoi
- Cats: PRA is seen in Abyssinians as autosomal dominant (dysplasia) and autosomal recessive (degeneration) disorders; also seen in Bengals as early-onset autosomal recessive disorder and in Persians

RISK FACTORS

Primary retinal degeneration: genetics
Secondary retinal degeneration:

- Glaucoma (pp. 387)
- Retinal detachment (p. 885)
- Posterior uveitis/chorioretinitis (p. 1023)
- Nutritional deficiency (e.g., taurine in cats; vitamin A or E in dogs and cats)
- Toxicosis

  - Fluoroquinolone-induced retinal degeneration in cats (e.g., enrofloxacin, typically at high dosages [>5 mg/kg/day]) due to feline-specific amino acid changes in ABCG2 causing its dysfunction at the blood-retinal barrier
  - Griseofulvin in cats
  - Ivermectin in dogs and cats
- Metabolic (e.g., mucopolysaccharidosis, dogs and cats)

ASSOCIATED DISORDERS

- Cataracts
- Retinal detachment
- Systemic diseases causing uveitis
- Hyperadrenocorticism-like signs (p. 485), regarding SARDS
- Taurine deficiency in cats (p. 960)

Clinical Presentation

DISEASE FORMS/SUBTYPES

- Bilateral or unilateral
- Inherited versus acquired
- Acute onset versus progressive
- Focal, multifocal (chorioretinal scars), generalized

HISTORY, CHIEF COMPLAINT

Varies, depending on underlying cause; owner may report any or all of the following:

- Acute or progressive vision impairment or blindness
- Red eye and/or other signs of glaucoma or uveitis
- Greenish reflection to eye (tapetal reflection in dilated pupil)
- Enlarged eye (illusion due to dilated pupil or caused by buphthalmos)
- Polyuria/polydipsia (SARDS)

PHYSICAL EXAM FINDINGS

- Absence of clinical signs possible if focal degeneration
- Generalized
  - Often bilateral
  - Dilated pupils and sluggish to absent pupillary light reflexes (PLRs)
  - Vision disturbances: ranging from impaired night vision (nyctalopia) and/or impaired day vision (hemeralopia; rare) (e.g., PRA) to complete blindness (e.g., SARDS; end-stage PRA)
  - Diffuse tapetal hyperreflectivity
  - Depigmentation of nontapetum
  - Retinal vascular attenuation
  - With/without signs of
    - Active or inactive uveitis
    - Glaucoma
    - Cataracts
    - Systemic disease (acquired)
- Focal, multifocal
  - Areas of tapetal hyperreflectivity ± associated pigmentation
  - ± Retinal vascular attenuation in affected areas
  - ± Signs of active or inactive uveitis

Etiology and Pathophysiology

- Inherited: breed-specific genetic abnormality in photoreceptor metabolism (*PRA* gene)
  - PRA: always bilateral; variable rate of progression; leads to blindness when both rods and cones affected
    - Early onset: photoreceptors fail to develop normally (i.e., dysplasia)
    - Late onset: photoreceptors develop normally but degenerate
- Typically, rods affected first, causing nyctalopia
- Eventually, cones also affected, resulting in hemeralopia and blindness
  - RPED is a genetic abnormality affecting the retinal pigment epithelium, with secondary effects on the neural retina (nine inner retinal layers); rare.
  - Multifocal retinopathy manifests in affected puppies at 3-4 months of age as multifocal serous retinal detachments.
- Acquired
  - SARDS is idiopathic, always bilateral, dogs only
    - Sudden blindness within days or 1-2 weeks
    - Normal fundic exam acutely; when disease is chronic, generalized retinal degeneration is indistinguishable from PRA
- Secondary
  - Occurring after resolution of posterior uveitis: distemper, systemic mycoses, toxoplasmosis, hypertension, hemorrhage, others
  - Occurring after retinal reattachment
  - Chronic glaucoma

DIAGNOSIS

Diagnostic Overview

Exam of the posterior segment of the eye (i.e., fundic exam) is the cornerstone of diagnosis but can be difficult, and making a diagnosis of retinal degeneration can be challenging. Prompt referral to a veterinary ophthalmologist is advisable for all cases of vision impairment or blindness of undetermined cause.

Differential Diagnosis

Acute, nonred, quiet-eye blindness (e.g., SARDS):

- Optic neuritis
- Optic chiasmal lesion
- Postchiasmal/cortical blindness (pupil size and PLRs usually normal)

Progressive blindness (e.g., PRA):

- Slowly progressive cataracts
- Progressive corneal opacification

Red eye blindness:

- Glaucoma
- Uveitis/chorioretinitis (may have resolved)
- Lens luxation
- Complex corneal ulceration

Initial Database

Ophthalmic exam (p. 1137)

Advanced or Confirmatory Testing

- Electroretinogram
- Other diagnostics commensurate with clinical signs and suspected causes

TREATMENT

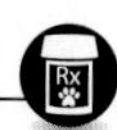

Treatment Overview

No treatment exists to regenerate the retina, and the presentation of these patients for vision loss often means the disease process has affected the retina extensively. Treatment of retinal degeneration consists of controlling or reversing an underlying cause when one can be identified.

Acute General Treatment

- Treat underlying cause (e.g., glaucoma, uveitis) when possible to prevent progression of acquired retinal degeneration.
- Investigational treatments include gene therapy and retinal allograft transplantation.

Possible Complications

- Cataracts
- Corneal/scleral trauma due to vision impairment

Recommended Monitoring

- Varies, depending on underlying cause
- Monitor for secondary cataracts and lens-induced uveitis.
- If SARDS is suspected but cannot be confirmed with an electroretinogram, repeated fundic exams at 3, 6, and 12 months are indicated to assess clinical signs of progressive retinal degeneration.

PROGNOSIS & OUTCOME

- Permanent blindness with SARDS and PRA
- Prognosis is typically good with focal retinal degeneration caused by scarring from previous posterior uveitis and/or retinal detachment, assuming disease process does not recur.

PEARLS & CONSIDERATIONS

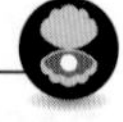

Comments

- There is no available treatment to regenerate the retina.
- Avoid enrofloxacin doses greater than 5 mg/kg/day in cats.
- Maze testing can help confirm early PRA. Create a maze with chairs or other objects in a small room and observe the dog's navigation in semi-dark and light conditions. Dogs with early PRA act differently in dark conditions.

Prevention

- Ophthalmic screening by a veterinary ophthalmologist of animals used for breeding and registration through the Orthopedic Foundation for Animals (www.offa.org/eye_evaluation.html) can help remove PRA- and RPED-affected animals from the breeding population.

- Genetic testing of blood samples or buccal swabs for breed-specific inherited ocular diseases helps detect carrier and affected animals.

Technician Tips

Place blind patients in lower cages to prevent falls.

Client Education

- Retinal degeneration alone does not cause ocular pain.
- Animals often adjust to blindness.

SUGGESTED READING

Narfström K, et al: Diseases of the canine ocular fundus. In Gelatt KN, editor: Veterinary ophthalmology, ed 5, Ames, IA, 2013, John Wiley & Sons, pp 1303-1392.

AUTHOR: Cheryl L. Cullen, DVM, MVetSc, DACVO
EDITOR: Diane V. H. Hendrix, DVM, DACVO

Retinal Detachment

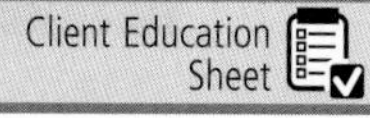

Client Education Sheet

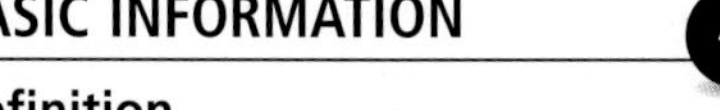

BASIC INFORMATION

Definition

Separation of the neural retina (inner nine layers) from the underlying retinal pigment epithelium (RPE) because of primary inherited retinal disease or secondary to other intraocular or systemic disease (acquired) may be focal, multifocal, or complete. Extent of retinal involvement determines degree of vision impairment.

Epidemiology

SPECIES, AGE, SEX

Affects dogs and cats; age of onset and sex predisposition vary with underlying cause.

- Inherited (dogs)
  - Severe retinal dysplasia: congenital
  - Multifocal retinopathy: nonprogressive, multifocal, serous retinal detachments that manifest between 3 and 4 months of age
  - Collie eye anomaly (CEA): retinal detachments occur in up to 10% of CEA-affected dogs; commonly young pups; may also develop later in life
- Acquired
  - Secondary to liquefaction/degeneration of the vitreous; usually older dogs
  - Systemic hypertension; typically older dogs or cats
  - Posterior uveitis (chorioretinitis); typically associated with systemic disease

GENETICS, BREED PREDISPOSITION

Dogs:

- Retinal dysplasia: presumed autosomal recessive in many predisposed breeds, including English springer spaniels, Bedlington terriers, American cocker spaniels, and miniature schnauzers; an incomplete dominant inheritance in breeds with associated skeletal deformities, including Labrador retrievers and Samoyeds; presumed autosomal dominant inheritance pattern in American pit bull terriers
- Multifocal retinopathy: autosomal recessive condition in coton de Tuléar, Great Pyrenees, Australian shepherds, dachshunds, boerboels
- CEA: predisposed breeds include collies, Shetland sheepdogs, border collies, and Australian shepherds.
- Shih tzus are predisposed to vitreous degeneration and rhegmatogenous (retina is torn) retinal detachments.

RISK FACTORS

Acquired:

- Systemic hypertension (p. 501)
- Uveitis (p. 1023)
- Cataracts (p. 147)
- Surgical lens removal (lensectomy)
- Intraocular or systemic neoplasia (p. 559)
- Lens luxation (p. 581)
- Bleeding disorder (e.g., coagulopathy due to anticoagulant rodenticide intoxication)
- Ocular trauma

ASSOCIATED DISORDERS

- Cataracts
- Hyphema (p. 511)
- Retinal degeneration (p. 883) if chronic or patient has had previous bouts
- Systemic diseases causing uveitis
- Diseases causing systemic hypertension
- Neoplasia (e.g., multiple myeloma, lymphoma)

Clinical Presentation

DISEASE FORMS/SUBTYPES

- Bilateral or unilateral
- Inherited versus acquired
- Rhegmatogenous (retinal tear) versus nonrhegmatogenous
- Nonrhegmatogenous: bullous with subretinal transudate (serous), exudate, or blood
- Focal, multifocal, complete
- Tractional

HISTORY, CHIEF COMPLAINT

Various visual deficits, depending on whether the retinal detachment is unilateral or bilateral, partial or complete, ± bleeding inside eye

PHYSICAL EXAM FINDINGS

May produce no clinical signs if detachment is focal or multifocal, but typical findings in complete detachment are

- Pupil(s) dilated
- Pupillary light reflex (PLR) decreased (i.e., sluggish and incomplete) or absent
- ± Anisocoria (asymmetrical pupil size, especially if unilateral lesion; only pupil of affected eye is dilated)
- Blindness (variable vision impairment if incomplete)
- Gray to white membrane (retina) with blood vessels and/or hemorrhage often visible with a penlight or transilluminator through pupil behind lens
- With or without signs of uveitis, hyphema, glaucoma, cataracts, or systemic disease (acquired)

Etiology and Pathophysiology

- A potential space exists between the neural retina and the RPE (subretinal space).
- Bullous: exudative/nonexudative
  - Breakdown of the blood-retinal barrier, allowing the following into the subretinal space:
    - Serous fluid ± hemorrhage (e.g., hypertension; hyperviscosity; vasculitis; idiopathic or steroid-responsive retinal detachment)
    - Exudative fluid (e.g., posterior uveitis due to systemic bacterial or mycotic infection or feline infectious peritonitis)
- Rhegmatogenous
  - Tear in retina allows vitreous to enter the subretinal space (e.g., hypermature cataracts, after lensectomy, CEA, old age, breed predisposition to vitreous degeneration/liquefaction, retinal degeneration) or severe head trauma (seen most commonly in herding dogs).
- Tractional
  - Fibrous or fibrocellular tissue pulling on the retina, with separation of the neural retina from RPE (e.g., ocular trauma resulting in vitreous hemorrhage, posterior

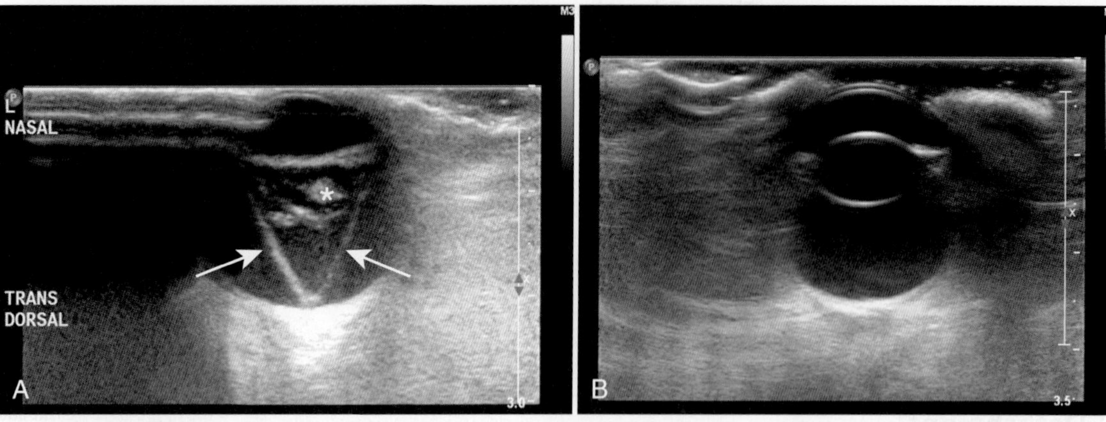

RETINAL DETACHMENT A, Ultrasound image of an eye (anterior/rostral is at the top) shows retinal detachment *(arrows)*. Note the globoid hyperechogenicity consistent with vitreous hemorrhage and/or degeneration *(asterisk)* posterior to the misshapen hyperechoic lens, which is compatible with a hypermature cataract. **B,** Ultrasound image of a normal eye for comparison. The separated, linear echogenicity (retina) seen in **A** is not apparent in a normal eye. (Images Courtesy Dr. Lee Ann Pack, Atlantic Veterinary College, University of Prince Edward Island, Canada.)

uveitis, and hyalitis [inflammation of the vitreous])

- Causes: see Risk Factors above.

DIAGNOSIS

Diagnostic Overview

The diagnosis rests on exam of the fundus, typically through a complete ophthalmic exam (ocular ultrasound if the ocular medium is opaque [hyphema or cataract]). Exam of the posterior segment of the eye can be difficult, and making a diagnosis of retinal detachment can be challenging. Prompt referral to a veterinary ophthalmologist is advisable for all cases of vision impairment or blindness of undetermined cause.

Differential Diagnosis

Other causes of blindness (p. 123)

Initial Database

Complete physical exam and ophthalmic exam (p. 1137):

- Direct or indirect ophthalmoscopy to assess the posterior segment of the eye
  - Optic nerve: optic disk hidden by torn retina with complete rhegmatogenous detachment
  - Tapetum: hyporeflective/grayish, dull discoloration ± hemorrhage with most forms of bullous retinal detachment; hyperreflective/brighter with complete rhegmatogenous form because retina remains attached at/hangs off optic disk and no longer covers underlying tapetum
  - Nontapetal fundus: whitish/gray discoloration ± hemorrhage with retinal detachment
  - Retinal vasculature: normally, well-focused, small arteries and larger veins come from the optic disk and course peripherally. With retinal detachment, blood vessels change their course and become out of focus. With some cases of retinal detachment, blood vessels may be visualized in the pupil behind the lens.

Advanced or Confirmatory Testing

- Ocular ultrasound if ocular media opaque
- Histopathologic evaluation of enucleated eye if eye is blind and painful
- Systemic workup such as CBC, chemistry panel, electrolytes, blood pressure, urine antigen testing, thoracic radiographs as indicated
- Referral for additional workup is advisable for all cases of blindness of undetermined cause.

TREATMENT

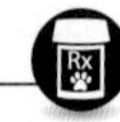

Treatment Overview

Treat underlying cause and restore vision or preserve remaining vision when possible.

Acute General Treatment

- Varies, depending on underlying cause, duration, extent, and type of retinal detachment
- Treat underlying cause when possible to prevent progressive retinal detachment.
- Promptly refer animals with acute blindness of undetermined cause to a veterinary ophthalmologist for early diagnosis and treatment (medical and/or surgical).

Possible Complications

- Permanent blindness
- Cataracts
- Retinal degeneration
- Hyphema
- Corneal/scleral trauma due to vision impairment

Recommended Monitoring

- Varies, depending on underlying cause
- Monitor for secondary cataracts and uveitis ± glaucoma.

PROGNOSIS & OUTCOME

- Varies, depending on underlying cause, duration, extent, and type of retinal detachment
- Prognosis for vision with focal or multifocal forms is typically good, especially if underlying cause is addressed and does not recur.
- Prognosis for vision with complete retinal detachment is typically guarded.

PEARLS & CONSIDERATIONS

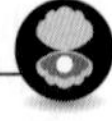

Comments

Irreversible retinal degeneration occurs quickly after retinal detachment. Prompt diagnosis and treatment of underlying cause (when possible) are crucial.

Prevention

Ophthalmic screening of animals used for breeding by a board-certified veterinary ophthalmologist and registration through the Orthopedic Foundation for Animals (https://www.ofa.org/diseases/eye-certification) helps remove animals with inherited forms of retinal detachment from the breeding population.

Technician Tips

Ideally, place blind patients in a floor-level cage to avoid falls from an open cage door.

Client Education

- Retinal detachment may indicate systemic disease and may or may not be reversible, depending on cause. Diagnostic testing is advised.
- Animals often adjust to blindness.

SUGGESTED READING

Leblanc NL, et al: Ocular lesions associated with systemic hypertension in dogs: 65 cases (2005-2007). J Am Vet Med Assoc 238:915-921, 2011.

AUTHOR: Cheryl L. Cullen, DVM, MVetSc, DACVO
EDITOR: Diane V. H. Hendrix, DVM, DACVO

Diseases and Disorders

Reverse Sneezing

Video Available

BASIC INFORMATION

Definition

Repeated paroxysmal, snoring-like inspiratory efforts secondary to nasopharyngeal irritation, during which the owner often thinks the animal is suffocating; common in dogs but rare in cats.

Synonym

Mechanosensitive aspiration reflex

Epidemiology

SPECIES, AGE, SEX

- Dogs of any sex or age, depending on the underlying cause
- Reverse sneezing can be induced in cats.

ASSOCIATED DISORDERS

Reverse sneezing can be a physiologic occurrence in many dogs but can also be associated with any nasal or nasopharyngeal disease. Sudden increase in body weight can exacerbate or induce reverse sneezing.

Clinical Presentation

DISEASE FORMS/SUBTYPES

- Incidental episodes: no clinical significance
- Frequent episodes secondary to an underlying nasal or nasopharyngeal disease

HISTORY, CHIEF COMPLAINT

- Incidental episodes of reverse sneezing are typically short in duration (few seconds to 1 minute) and self-limited. Between episodes, the animal is normal.
- Frequent episodes of reverse sneezing may be a reflection of underlying disease and associated with signs of nasal/nasopharyngeal disease such as sneezing, nasal discharge, epistaxis, stertor, or retching.

PHYSICAL EXAM FINDINGS

Incidental episodes of reverse sneezing: normal physical exam. Reverse sneezing secondary to an underlying disease:

- Nasal/nasopharyngeal inflammation, foreign body; unilateral or bilateral serous, mucopurulent, or bloody nasal discharge; sneezing; stertor; decreased or sometimes increased nasal air passage; systemic signs are rare.
- Nasopharyngeal stenosis
- Nasopharyngeal reflux (anecdotal)
- Nasal/nasopharyngeal tumor: unilateral or bilateral serous, mucopurulent, or bloody nasal discharge; sneezing; stertor; decreased nasal air passage (unilateral or bilateral); epiphora (secondary to nasolacrimal duct obstruction); decreased ability to retropulse eye if periorbital invasion; facial or hard/soft palate deformity if malignant tumor (occasionally)
- Sinonasal aspergillosis: unilateral or bilateral serous, mucopurulent, or bloody nasal discharge; sneezing; depigmentation of nasal planum; pain during palpation of facial bones possible; increased nasal air passage; decreased appetite and poor body condition are possible.
- Nasal parasite (*Pneumonyssoides caninum* or *Eucoleus boehmi*): sneezing; reverse sneezing, which may be the only abnormality in some dogs; serous nasal discharge; facial pruritus; hyposmia

Etiology and Pathophysiology

- Incidental reverse sneezing can be a normal occurrence.
- Receptors and myelinated trigeminal nerve endings in the lateral aspects of the nasopharynx respond to local stimulation, implying a reflex pathway. Any local stimulation can activate the reflex, which causes a strong inspiration of material from the nasopharynx to the oropharynx through a decreased nasopharyngeal opening.

DIAGNOSIS

Diagnostic Overview

The diagnosis is based on recognition of the characteristically loud, stertorous inspiratory episode that is sudden in onset and termination. It most often occurs in an animal that is usually otherwise healthy. When other nasal signs are present, it requires further investigation.

Differential Diagnosis

- Reverse sneezing might be confused with stertor, which is typically less abrupt in onset and offset and more commonly associated with activity or excitement; snoring, which only occurs during sleep; retching/gagging, which often involves expectoration and an open mouth or cough, when owners do not know how to describe the sign.
- When reverse sneezing occurs frequently (daily or several times per day) and/or is accompanied by other clinical signs, a nasal or nasopharyngeal disease should be suspected.
    - Foreign body
    - Neoplasia (nasopharyngeal)
    - Abscess
    - Mycotic infection
    - Chronic lymphoplasmacytic rhinitis, sinusitis
    - Nasopharyngitis
    - Nasal parasites
    - Reflux

Initial Database

- Results of CBC, biochemistry panel, and urinalysis are usually unremarkable.
    - Eosinophilia may be present in some cases of nasal mites.
- If the episodes occur only at home (not in the veterinary hospital), and it is unclear whether they are consistent with reverse sneezing, clinicians can make the diagnosis by instructing the owner to record videos of the episodes.
- It can also be helpful to play videos for pet owners of reverse sneezing in other dogs; they frequently corroborate that this is what they are seeing in their own pet (see *Video*).
- Radiographs are rarely useful for the diagnosis of underlying diseases.

Advanced or Confirmatory Testing

For animals with a recent onset of reverse sneezing or recent increase in frequency of events, consider

- Direct rhinoscopy and results of culture and cytologic and histopathologic evaluation of nasal samples (primary nasal diseases), retrograde rhinoscopy for nasopharyngeal diseases
- CT and/or MRI for neoplasia, aspergillosis
- Fluoroscopy may detect dynamic pharyngeal collapse. Swallow studies may detect reflux.

TREATMENT

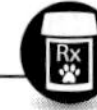

Treatment Overview

Sporadic reverse sneezing requires no therapy. Reduce nasopharyngeal irritation by treating the underlying disorder when possible.

Acute General Treatment

Acute episodes of reverse sneezing associated with perceived severe discomfort of the animal can be shortened by calming the dog or giving the animal something to lick or drink.

Chronic Treatment

- Incidental episodes need no treatment.
- Increased frequency of episodes without any other sign of nasal or nasopharyngeal disease
    - A short period of glucocorticoid therapy (e.g., prednisolone 0.5 mg/kg PO q 12h for 1 week) may limit repeated episodes induced by local inflammation.
    - Treatment for nasal mites if suspected: ivermectin 0.1-0.4 mg/kg (100-400 mcg/kg; use caution in herding breeds [p. 638]) PO or SQ once every 3 weeks for 3 treatments or milbemycin oxime 0.5-1 mg/kg PO once weekly for 3 consecutive weeks
    - Diet when sign follows weight gain
    - Empirical treatment for gastric reflux (e.g., omeprazole)
- Related to nasal or nasopharyngeal disorders: treatment dictated by the underlying condition

PROGNOSIS & OUTCOME

- Excellent for incidental episodes or with antiparasitic treatment when the underlying cause is nasal mite infestation
- The episodes themselves pose no danger to pet.

PEARLS & CONSIDERATIONS

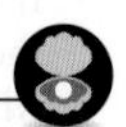

Comments

The presence of clinical signs that suggest nasal or nasopharyngeal disease in conjunction with reverse sneezing should prompt diagnostic testing to detect underlying diseases.

Technician Tips

Nasal lavage by direct or retrograde methods in conjunction with exam of nasal lavage fluid can be helpful to both clean the nasal cavity when occluded and provide material for culture, cytologic, and histopathologic exams.

Client Education

Clients should be told not to worry during acute episodes of reverse sneezing because there is in fact no real danger of suffocation.

SUGGESTED READING

Doust R, et al: Nasal discharge, sneezing, and reverse sneezing. In King LG, editor: Textbook of respiratory diseases in dogs and cats, St. Louis, 2004, Saunders, pp 19-20.

AUTHOR: Cécile Clercx, DVM, PhD, DECVIM
EDITOR: Megan Grobman, DVM, MS, DACVIM

Rheumatoid Arthritis

Client Education Sheet 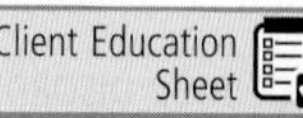

BASIC INFORMATION

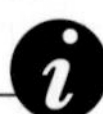

Definition

A progressive, noninfectious, immune-mediated, inflammatory polyarthropathy characterized by erosion of articular cartilage and bone

Synonyms

Rheumatoid arthritis (RA), erosive immune-mediated polyarthritis (IMPA), idiopathic erosive polyarthritis

Epidemiology

SPECIES, AGE, SEX

- Uncommon in dogs, rare in cats (see Associated Disorders)
    - Estimated 15% of dogs with IMPA have the erosive type
- Young to middle-aged animals
- No sex predisposition

GENETICS, BREED PREDISPOSITION

- Small-breed dogs most commonly affected but can occur in larger dog breeds
- No inheritance patterns known

ASSOCIATED DISORDERS

- Cranial cruciate ligament (CCL) rupture: 10 of 13 dogs with RA in one report
- Semi-erosive polyarthritis of greyhounds 3-30 months of age
- Feline chronic progressive polyarthritis (FCPP)
    - Any age, especially young (1-5 years old) adult male cats
    - Some association with feline syncytium-forming virus
- Leishmania infection causing reactive IMPA
- Felty's syndrome: RA, splenomegaly, and neutropenia (humans)
- Some association of RA with reactive amyloidosis (humans)

Clinical Presentation

HISTORY, CHIEF COMPLAINT

- Acute or chronic, single or multiple leg weight-bearing lameness and arthralgia; severity may wax/wane over time
- Systemic signs may occur (one-third of cases): unexplained fatigue, anorexia, fever
- Late stages: chronic distal limb joint laxity and deformity

PHYSICAL EXAM FINDINGS

- Joint effusion and pain in multiple limbs, distal limbs (carpus especially) most common and severely affected
- Possibly fever and mild lymphadenopathy if systemic involvement
- Associated joint laxity (CCL rupture)

Etiology and Pathophysiology

- Cause unknown, some genetic variation likely due to breed/dog size predisposition
- Type III (immune complex) hypersensitivity reaction is similar in all types of IMPA.
- Immune dysregulation (failure of self-tolerance) or production of immunogenic immunoglobulin G (IgG) antigen results in formation of pathogenic autoantibodies (rheumatoid factors [RFs], IgM, and IgA) by synovial lymphocytes and plasma cells.
- Immune complexes deposit in joints and activate complement, causing synovial proliferation and attracting neutrophils.
- Activated synoviocytes, macrophages, and neutrophils release inflammatory mediators and enzymes (interleukin-1 [IL-1], collagenases, prostaglandin E_2 [PGE_2], matrix metalloproteases), causing joint damage.
- Osteoclasts are activated and resorb subchondral bone (cysts).
- Inflamed synovium forms a pannus (intraarticular granulation tissue composed of inflammatory leukocytes) and results in fibrosis of joint capsule.
- Chronic bone loss and joint inflammation damages supporting ligaments, leading to joint instability and/or limb deformity.

DIAGNOSIS

Diagnostic Overview

CBC, serum biochemistry profile, urinalysis, radiographs, and arthrocentesis of multiple joints (cytologic analysis/culture) are indicated to distinguish RA from other causes of polyarthritis. Table outlines diagnostic criteria for RA.

Differential Diagnosis

- Nonerosive IMPA
- Septic arthritis (bacterial, fungal)
- Systemic lupus erythematosus (SLE)
- Reactive polyarthritis
- Joint neoplasia

Initial Database

- CBC, serum biochemistry profile, urinalysis: often unremarkable
    - Leukocytosis, neutrophilia, hyperglobulinemia, hyperfibrinogenemia, and proteinuria possible with systemic disease
- Radiographs of multiple joints: findings vary with duration of illness
    - Early: periarticular soft-tissue swelling; minimal or no bony changes
    - Middle: irregular joint margins, discrete subchondral lucencies, diffuse generalized osteopenia (epiphyses especially)
    - Late: extensive bone destruction, joint space collapse, joint malformation with associated subluxations/luxations
    - FCPP: marked periosteal new bone; focal erosions, especially hocks and carpi
- Arthrocentesis of multiple joints (p. 1059)
    - Synovial fluid analysis: poor viscosity (watery), increased total nucleated cell

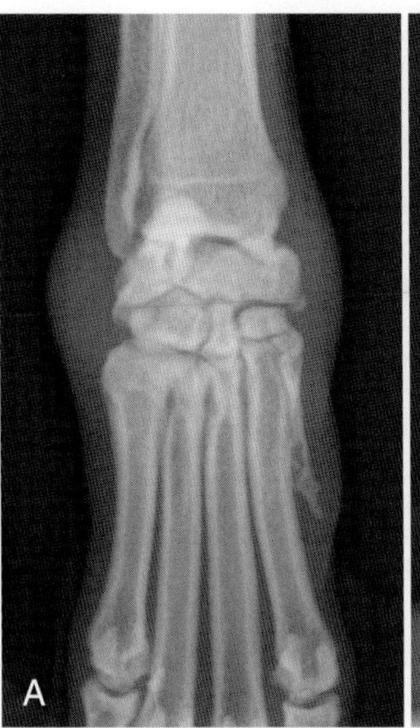

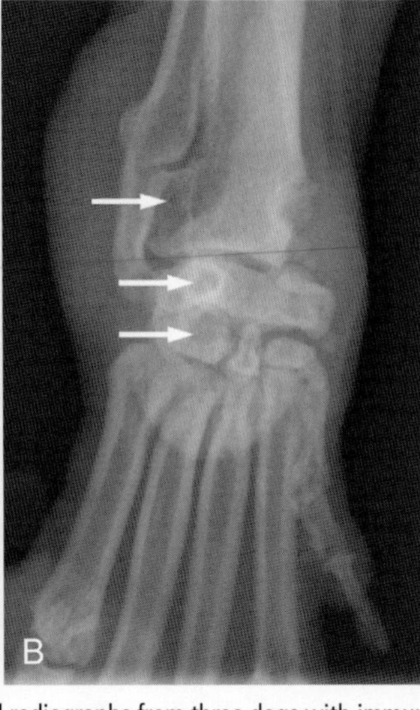

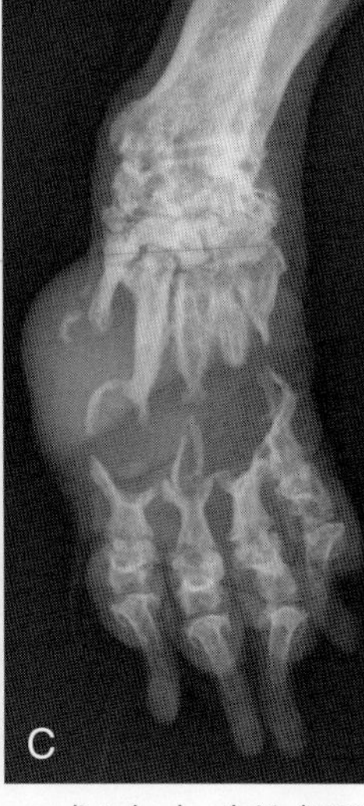

RHEUMATOID ARTHRITIS Carpal radiographs from three dogs with immune-mediated polyarthritis (IMPA). **A,** Nonerosive IMPA: soft-tissue swelling focused on the carpus, normal osseous structures. **B,** Erosive IMPA, early-middle stage: focal subchondral lucencies *(arrows)* in the bones of the radius/ulna, carpus, and metacarpus associated soft-tissue swelling. **C,** Erosive IMPA, late stage: extensive bone destruction of the distal limb, including loss of joint space, irregular joint margins, numerous coalescing subchondral lucencies, complete destruction of metacarpal bones, and limb malformation.

Criteria for Diagnosis of Rheumatoid Arthritis*

1	Stiffness after rest
2	Pain or tenderness in at least one joint
3	Swelling (not bony overgrowth alone) in at least one joint
4	Swelling of at least one other joint within 3 months
5	Symmetrical joint swelling
6	Subcutaneous nodules over bony prominences or extensor surfaces or in juxtaarticular regions
7	Destructive radiographic changes typical of rheumatoid arthritis
8	Positive agglutination test for serum rheumatoid factor
9	Poor mucin precipitate from synovial fluid
10	Characteristic histopathologic changes in the synovial membrane with three or more of the following: marked villous hypertrophy, proliferation of superficial synovial cells, marked infiltration of chronic inflammatory cells (lymphocytes and plasma cells predominating) with tendency to form lymphoid nodules, deposition of fibrin, foci of cell necrosis
11	Characteristic histopathologic changes in nodules showing granulomatous foci with central zones of cell necrosis, surrounded by proliferated fixed cells and peripheral fibrosis and chronic inflammatory cell infiltration, predominantly perivascular

*Criteria 1-5 should be present for > 6 weeks. Classic RA: ≥ 7 criteria; definite RA ≥ 5 criteria. Additionally, two of criteria 7, 8, and 10 should be satisfied as most specific for canine RA.

Adapted from criteria for RA in humans. Aletaha D, et al: Rheumatoid arthritis classification criteria: an American College of Rheumatology/European League Against Rheumatism collaborative initiative. Arthritis Rheum 62:2569-2581, 2010.

count (TNCC) of 5,000-80,000, elevated neutrophils (>12% of TNCC)
  - Culture negative
  - Mucin clot test negative

Advanced or Confirmatory Testing

- RF: lacks sensitivity/specificity; positive in ≈25% of dogs with RA
- C-reactive protein (CRP): lack specificity, may be useful in monitoring response to therapy
- Antinuclear antibody (ANA): useful only if SLE is suspected
- Synovial biopsy: proliferative synovitis with lymphocytes, plasma cells, and macrophages (rarely needed to confirm)

TREATMENT

Treatment Overview

There are no curative treatments; clinical remission is the goal. Lifelong immunosuppressive drugs are the mainstay of treatment to slow progression of disease. Owners should be counseled on chronic lifestyle changes and realistic outcomes.

Acute General Treatment

Immunosuppressive therapy with single or multiple agents:

- Prednisone 1-2 mg/kg PO q 12h for 4 weeks, then taper based on monitoring
- Leflunomide 3-4 mg/kg PO q 24h for 6 weeks, then dose reduction
  - Consider initiation with prednisone in combination for 4 weeks until therapeutic levels of leflunomide are achieved.
- Cyclosporine initially 5 mg/kg PO q 12h, then taper dosage based on serum levels
- Azathioprine 2 mg/kg PO q 48h (dogs)
- Cyclophosphamide 2 mg/kg PO q 24h, 4 consecutive days weekly

Analgesics for symptomatic pain control:

- Acetaminophen with codeine: 1-2 mg/kg PO q 8-12h (based on the codeine component, do not exceed 15 mg/kg acetaminophen, do not use in cats)
- Gabapentin: 5-10 mg/kg PO q12h
- Tramadol: 4-6 mg/kg PO q 8-12h
- Nonsteroidal antiinflammatory drugs (NSAIDs): AVOID when using glucocorticoids

Chronic Treatment

Taper immunosuppression to lowest dosage that maintains clinical remission. More likely to require combination therapy and lifelong treatment compared with nonerosive IMPA.

Ancillary treatment options:

- Chrysotherapy (gold salts): limited outcome data but thought to work by modulation of T lymphocytes; requires concurrent oral immunosuppression (glucocorticoids)
- Splints fitted to pet may provide joint stability, improving comfort and mobility; especially useful for carpi

Nutrition/Diet

- Maintain lean body condition score
- Impact of joint nutraceuticals (omega-3 fatty acids, glucosamine/chondroitin) is unclear

Behavior/Exercise

- Activity restriction and lifelong modification with focus on low-impact activities that do not exacerbate lameness
- Physiotherapy and tissue massage to maintain joint mobility (active/passive range-of-motion exercise) and muscle mass

Possible Complications

- All immunosuppressive agents: bone marrow suppression and opportunistic infections
- Long-term glucocorticoids: hyperadrenocorticism and associated side effects
- Cyclophosphamide (cystitis), azathioprine (hepatotoxicity, pancreatitis), and gold salts (dermatitis, glomerulonephritis, stomatitis)

Recommended Monitoring

- Clinical assessment: physical exam and activity monitoring
- Evaluate arthrocentesis/synovial fluid cytology initially monthly, then based on clinical assessment; may not directly correlate
- Consider CRP as less invasive option for systemic inflammatory status (efficacy as monitoring tool questionable)
- Other routine bloodwork (CBC/biochemistry) based on treatment regime to detect myelosuppression or organ damage
- Pharmacokinetic or pharmacodynamic monitoring for cyclosporin or some other adjunct immunosuppressive agents

PROGNOSIS & OUTCOME

- Even with appropriate therapy, the condition of most patients deteriorates over time.
- Surgical salvage (arthrodesis) may be considered for poor clinical function associated with joint breakdown (laxity, subluxation, chronic pain); most amenable in carpus and hock joints to improve ambulatory function
- Arthroscopic synovectomy, arthroplasty, and total joint replacement have unclear benefit
- Prognosis for semi-erosive polyarthritis of greyhounds and FCPP is poor

PEARLS & CONSIDERATIONS

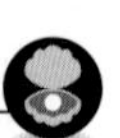

Comments

- An accurate diagnosis of RA is multifactorial, involving physical exam, radiographs, and arthrocentesis/joint fluid analysis using established criteria.
- The name of this condition implies that RF blood testing is important; however, the test is positive in only ≈25% of affected dogs.
- RA may initially resemble non-erosive IMPA, but eventually joint destruction becomes apparent radiographically.

Technician Tips

- Use caution when handling affected animals because they may be too painful to walk and become aggressive.
- Adequate sedation is required for arthrocentesis; consider hydromorphone 0.05 mg/kg and dexmedetomidine 3-5 mcg/kg IV; use lowest dosage possible (and with caution) in dogs with cardiovascular disease.
- Submit synovial fluid samples in blood culture media to improve detection of bacterial organisms (distinguish RA from septic arthritis)

Client Education

- Poor prognosis for cure
- Progressive disabling disease requires lifelong medical therapy, activity modification, and frequent rechecks.

SUGGESTED READING

Shaughnessy ML, et al: Clinical features and pathologic joint changes in dogs with erosive immune-mediated polyarthritis: 13 cases (2004-2012). J Am Vet Med Assoc 249:1156-1164, 2016.

AUTHOR: Jason Bleedorn, DVM, MS, DACVS-SA
EDITOR: Jonathan E. Fogle, DVM, PhD, DACVIM

Rhinitis, Lymphoplasmacytic

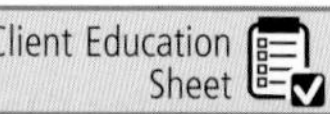

BASIC INFORMATION

Definition

Chronic, progressive inflammatory nasal disease characterized by infiltration of the nasal mucosa with lymphocytes and plasma cells frequently (≈33%) affects dogs and cats with chronic nasal disease. Causes of secondary inflammation must be ruled out to diagnose idiopathic lymphoplasmacytic rhinitis (LPR).

Synonyms

LPR (dogs), chronic rhinitis/rhinosinusitis (CRS) (cats), chronic inflammatory rhinitis, immune-mediated rhinitis, allergic rhinitis

Epidemiology

SPECIES, AGE, SEX

- Dogs: any age, either sex
- Cats: young adult to middle-aged cats, either sex

GENETICS, BREED PREDISPOSITION

Often seen in large-breed dogs, although the dachshund and Yorkshire terrier may be overrepresented.

RISK FACTORS

- Lymphoplasmacytic inflammation reflects a nonspecific response to disease.
- Diseases predisposing to chronic inflammation, epithelial erosion, turbinate lysis/remodeling, recurrent infections (e.g., feline infectious upper respiratory tract disease, fungal infection), foreign bodies, extra-esophageal reflux, and anatomic abnormalities can provoke lymphoplasmacytic nasal infiltrates.

Clinical Presentation

HISTORY, CHIEF COMPLAINT

- Nasal discharge (most common)
- Sneezing
- Snoring, stertor
- Reverse sneezing
- Ocular discharge and rubbing at the nose (occasionally)
- In cats, dysorexia may occur because of inability to smell food.

PHYSICAL EXAM FINDINGS

- Bilateral or unilateral (≈35%) nasal discharge; often mucopurulent, but serous, mucoid, or blood-tinged discharge may occur.
- ± Decreased air passage through one or both nares
- ± Submandibular lymph node enlargement
- General condition is normal

Etiology and Pathophysiology

- Hypothesized to be a chronic inflammatory response to an inhaled irritant, pollutant, or allergen, or an immune-mediated process
- In dogs, the local tissue immune response mounted is distinct from that of sinonasal aspergillosis, and the disease is not due to undiagnosed sinonasal aspergillosis.
- Chronic inflammation causes loss of epithelium and squamous metaplasia, reduced population of ciliated cells, hyperplasia of subepithelial glands, increased amount of viscid mucus, and impaired ciliary clearance.
- Retention of mucus plugs, inhaled bacteria, and irritating particles maintain and aggravate inflammation.
- Role for *Bartonella* spp or saprophytic fungi has not been documented.

DIAGNOSIS

Diagnostic Overview

Lymphoplasmacytic infiltration of nasal mucosa can be a sequela of many chronic nasal diseases. Diagnosis of the idiopathic condition is made by exclusion of other causes of rhinitis and histopathologic confirmation of infiltrate.

Differential Diagnosis

Other causes of nasal discharge (pp. 678 and 1255)

Initial Database

- CBC, biochemistry panel, and urinalysis are usually normal.
- Thorough oral exam under anesthesia or heavy sedation helps rule out oronasal fistulae or dental disease.
- Plain radiographs (with anesthesia) of the nasal cavities, sinuses, nasopharynx, and dental roots may help eliminate some causes of chronic nasal discharge, but radiographs lack sensitivity and specificity.
- Culture of nasal secretions is discouraged. Bacterial cultures from nasal swabs or biopsies can be positive or negative; positive cultures rarely reflect a primary role of bacteria in pathogenesis.

Advanced or Confirmatory Testing

- CT and/or MRI (p. 1132) of the nasal cavities and sinuses can identify differentials with more accuracy than plain radiographs but cannot confirm LPR. For animals with chronic nasal discharge, referral for advanced imaging is often warranted.

- Rhinoscopy (p. 1159) findings are variable and can include
  - Copious, thick mucus or mucopurulent discharge
  - Mucosal hyperemia
  - Proliferative or thickened nasal mucosa
  - Turbinate lysis or remodeling
  - Pseudopolypoid appearance of mucosa
  - Absence of other causes of nasal discharge (e.g., neoplasia, aspergillosis, foreign bodies)
- Histopathologic exam of nasal mucosal biopsies is necessary for diagnosis of LPR and demonstrates mild to severe lymphoplasmacytic infiltration sometimes mixed with mild neutrophilic or eosinophilic infiltration.

TREATMENT

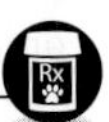

Treatment Overview

Treatment can be challenging. There is no therapy that has been proven consistently effective for all patients.

Acute General Treatment

- Generally, antibiotics are of little benefit.
  - Anecdotally, azithromycin or doxycycline has been helpful in some cases.
  - Some cats respond to repeated courses of amoxicillin, likely as treatment for secondary bacterial rhinitis.
- Glucocorticoids are useful in some, but not all, dogs and cats.
  - Prednisone 1-2 mg/kg PO q 12-24h for 7-10 days, tapered to lowest dose that controls clinical signs (or until switched to topical corticosteroids)
  - If systemic glucocorticoids improve condition, may switch to topical (nasal spray, drops, or aerosols) treatments (e.g., fluticasone propionate 125-250 mcg q 12h nasal spray or metered-dose inhaler; prednisolone ophthalmic drops 2 drops per nostril q 12h)
- Anecdotal reports of benefit for other anti-inflammatory agents; piroxicam 0.3 mg/kg PO q 24h
- Anecdotal reports of benefit for other immunosuppressive or immunomodulatory agents
  - Oclacitinib 0.4-0.6 mg/kg PO q 12h for 2 weeks, then q 24h (dogs)
  - Azathioprine 1-2 mg/kg PO q 24h for 10-14 days, then q 48h (dogs only), *or*
  - Cyclosporine 3-5 mg/kg PO q 12-24h for 2-4 weeks and then q 48h; monitor serum concentrations
- Antihistamines are rarely effective but may reduce discharge in some pets.
- Mucolytic drugs
  - *N*-acetylcysteine 5-10 mg PO q 12h, up to 100 mg/kg PO q 12h has been reported. Intranasal or aerosol delivery of 5%-20% solution q 8-12h has been described. *N*-acetylcysteine aerosol therapy is contraindicated in cats because it can induce bronchospasm.
  - Bromhexine hydrochloride 0.5-2 mg/kg PO q 12-24h or through aerosol delivery
  - Flushing and aspiration of all nasal secretions during rhinoscopy can help before initiating therapy.

Chronic Treatment

- Humidification of nasal cavities with saline (drops or aerosol delivery) to moisten and help clear nasal secretions.
- Mucolytic drugs (as above)
- Long-term glucocorticoids (oral or topical), potentially in combination with cyclosporine or azathioprine; use lowest therapeutic dose
- Desensitization therapy according to allergy testing has been anecdotally helpful in a few dogs.

Possible Complications

- Secondary bacterial rhinitis
- Chronic sinusitis

Recommended Monitoring

Identify and treat episodes of secondary bacterial rhinitis.

PROGNOSIS & OUTCOME

- Cure is uncommon, and mild to moderate clinical signs often persist despite treatment.
- Maintenance therapy is generally successful in minimizing clinical signs, although relapses are common if treatment is discontinued.
- Some cases remain refractory to any treatment, although the disease is rarely life-threatening.
- Owners should prevent their pets' exposure to exacerbating factors (e.g., cigarette smoke, perfumes).

PEARLS & CONSIDERATIONS

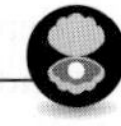

Comments

- Diagnosis of LPR is established by elimination of other causes of chronic lymphoplasmacytic nasal infiltrates. Referral for advanced imaging can be extremely useful in ruling out other conditions.
- The disease is chronic and progressive, and cure is rarely achieved.
- There is no therapeutic gold standard. Treatment trials should be used to determine what works best for each case.

Technician Tips

Nebulization of nasal cavities with saline q 8-12h can help moisten and clear nasal secretions.

Client Education

- Owner should be warned that this is a frustrating condition to treat. Cure is rare, but trial and error often allows identification of a regimen that can minimize clinical signs.
- Treatment must be sustained because relapses are common.
- Potentially exacerbating factors should be avoided.

SUGGESTED READING

Lobetti R: Idiopathic lymphoplasmacytic rhinitis in 33 dogs. J S Afr Vet Assoc 85(1):1151, 2014.

AUTHOR: Frédéric Billen, DVM, MS, PhD, DECVIM
EDITOR: Megan Grobman, DVM, MS, DACVIM

Rocky Mountain Spotted Fever

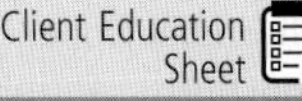

BASIC INFORMATION

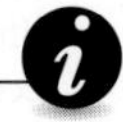

Definition

An acute, potentially life-threatening, tick-borne rickettsial disease affecting dogs and people

Epidemiology

SPECIES, AGE, SEX

- Species: dogs and people are primarily affected. Seropositive cats are not clinically ill.
- Young dogs (<2 years) are at greater risk.

GENETICS, BREED PREDISPOSITION

Purebred dogs, especially German shepherds, may be predisposed.

RISK FACTORS

Tick exposure, failure to use tick preventatives

CONTAGION AND ZOONOSIS

Direct transmission does not occur from dogs to people. Dogs are short-term reservoirs and sentinels.

GEOGRAPHY AND SEASONALITY

Rocky Mountain spotted fever (RMSF) is found in North, Central, and South America. The majority of cases in the United States occur in the southeast, south central, and mid-Atlantic states; disease occurrence is highest from March to October.

ASSOCIATED DISORDERS

Co-infection with other tick-borne diseases such as ehrlichiosis can occur.

Clinical Presentation

DISEASE FORMS/SUBTYPES

- Clinical and subclinical illnesses have been reported.
- Systemic disease is common, but localized signs (dermatologic, neurologic, ocular) may predominate.

HISTORY, CHIEF COMPLAINT

- Acute onset of illness with nonspecific signs; depression, anorexia, musculoskeletal pain, and sometimes vomiting are noted.
- Varied presentations: epistaxis, head tilt, limb/scrotal edema, stiff gait

PHYSICAL EXAM FINDINGS

- Fever: commonly seen within 2-3 days of exposure
- Evidence of pain or stiff, stilted gait common (arthralgia/myalgia, abdominal pain)
- Cutaneous lesions: petechial/ecchymotic hemorrhages (especially on mucous membranes), edema, hyperemia, vesicles, and macules are all possible.
- Ocular (uveitis/chorioretinitis) and/or neurologic abnormalities (e.g., head tilt)
- Splenomegaly, lymphadenopathy
- Dyspnea/cough occasionally recognized (interstitial pneumonitis)

Etiology and Pathophysiology

- *Rickettsia rickettsii* is an obligate intracellular parasite. Ticks become infected by horizontal transmission, transstadially, or by transovarial passage.
- Vectors: *Dermacentor variabilis* (American dog tick, eastern United States), *D. andersoni* (wood tick, western United States), *Rhipicephalus sanguineus* (brown dog tick, Arizona/California), and *Amblyomma americanum* (lone star tick)
- Transmission to the host requires at least 5-20 hours of tick attachment.
- Incubation is 2-14 days after tick exposure. There is no carrier state.
- Pathogen invades vascular endothelial cells, leading to vasculitis, local necrosis, thrombosis, and plasma loss.
- Thrombocytopenia is due to consumption (vasculitis), antiplatelet antibodies, and/or whole blood loss. Disseminated intravascular coagulation is rare.

DIAGNOSIS

Diagnostic Overview

Seasonal occurrence, clinicopathologic changes, and response to therapy suggest the diagnosis. Clinical suspicion justifies treatment while confirmation is pending because a fulminant course may occur in some individuals. Convalescent serologic titers 1-3 weeks later are confirmatory.

Differential Diagnosis

- Acute ehrlichiosis/anaplasmosis/rickettsiosis (CBC, oculoneural signs, lameness, proteinuria)
- Bacterial sepsis (CBC, shock)
- Babesiosis (CBC, neurologic signs, proteinuria)
- Borreliosis (lameness, proteinuria)
- Leptospirosis (CBC; gastrointestinal, renal, ocular, hepatic changes)
- Immune-mediated diseases (e.g., immune-mediated thrombocytopenia, polyarthropathy, glomerulonephritis)
- Canine distemper (ocular, neurologic, respiratory, gastrointestinal signs)
- Bacterial discospondylitis, intervertebral disc disease (stiff, painful gait)
- Vestibular disease, acute meningoencephalitis (neurologic signs)

Initial Database

- CBC: thrombocytopenia most common; leukopenia or leukocytosis (left shift possible); mild to moderate anemia
- Serum biochemistry profile: hypoalbuminemia, azotemia, low Na/Cl/K/Ca levels, increased liver enzyme activities
- Fluid analysis (joint [p. 1059] or cerebrospinal fluid [pp. 1080 and 1323] if affected): mild increase in protein and cells, initially neutrophils, then monocytes
- Proteinuria due to vasculitis/glomerulonephritis

Advanced or Confirmatory Testing

- IFA documentation of seroconversion or fourfold or greater increase between acute/convalescent titers or an acute titer ≥ 1:1024 with compatible clinical signs is confirmatory.
- Cross-reactivity with nonpathogenic rickettsial organisms may occur. Some nonpathogenic rickettsiae are proving to be pathogenic, but not all cross-react with RMSF.
  - A positive titer, even a high positive, cannot confirm infection if the history and signs do not suggest RMSF.
- Direct FA testing for antigen (skin/tissue samples) before antibiotics are started can confirm infection
- Polymerase chain reaction (PCR) testing (blood/tissue) for RMSF and other rickettsiae is insensitive because the pathogen does not live inside blood cells.

TREATMENT

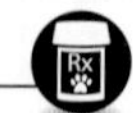

Treatment Overview

Early recognition and prompt treatment with appropriate antimicrobial therapy is associated with a good response and excellent prognosis. Delayed therapy carries a more guarded prognosis.

Acute General Treatment

- Doxycycline 5-10 mg/kg PO or IV q 12h for 7-14 days is the treatment of choice; minocycline 5-12.5 mg/kg PO q 12h for 7-14 days may be effective if doxycycline unavailable, *or*
- Enrofloxacin 5 mg/kg PO slow IV or IM q 12h for 7-14 days, *or*
- Chloramphenicol 25-30 mg/kg PO, SQ, IV, or IM q 8h for 7-14 days
- Prednisolone 1-2 mg/kg PO q 24h does not potentiate severity in experimental infections and may minimize immune-mediated complications.
- Fluid and supportive therapies (e.g., analgesia) to improve perfusion; caution to avoid exacerbating tissue edema

Recommended Monitoring

Cases are often seronegative acutely; repeated serologic testing 1-3 weeks after initial onset confirms seroconversion (negative to positive) or fourfold rise (e.g., 80 to 320) in acute/convalescent titers. Early antibiotics may blunt rise.

PROGNOSIS & OUTCOME

- With early diagnosis and treatment, prognosis is usually excellent.
- Delayed diagnosis, fulminant disease, and/or the use of ineffective antibiotics (e.g., penicillins, cephalosporins) increase mortality.
- Long-term sequelae may include scarring from thrombosis and acral gangrenous necrosis of digits, nasal planum, and other sites, or kidney damage.
- In intact dogs, scrotal edema and dermatitis are common and may be severe.

PEARLS & CONSIDERATIONS

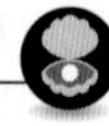

Comments

- Despite the name, the disease is not found primarily in the Rocky Mountains, and a spotted rash may not be apparent.
- Owners are often unaware of a specific tick bite before illness.
- RMSF causes an acute vasculitis, from which the dog will recover or die within a few weeks. Chronic illness is not reported in cases of RMSF, and a positive titer (even a high titer) in an animal with chronic illness does not support RMSF as a cause for clinical signs.

Prevention

- Adequate tick control is ideal, especially for dogs that roam outdoors in wooded areas.
- Lifelong immunity may follow disease recovery.

Technician Tips

- Do not remove ticks with your bare hands; transmission of RMSF may occur if cracked cuticles are exposed to infected tick contents.
- Cystocentesis and jugular venipuncture are contraindicated in severely thrombocytopenic dogs.

Client Education

- RMSF in dogs is a warning to owners that ticks in their area carry RMSF (other dogs and people may be exposed).
- Ticks removed from pets must not be removed by unprotected fingers, lest owners' cuticles be exposed to infective tick hemolymph/feces.

SUGGESTED READING

Greene CE, et al: Rocky Mountain and Mediterranean spotted fevers, cat-flea typhuslike illness, rickettsialpox, and typhus. In Greene CE, editor: Infectious diseases of the dog and cat, ed 4, St. Louis, 2012, Saunders, pp 259-270.

AUTHOR: Meryl P. Littman, VMD, DACVIM
EDITOR: Joseph Taboada, DVM, DACVIM

Round Cell Tumors

Bonus Material Online 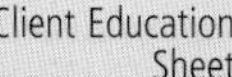 Client Education Sheet 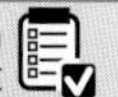

BASIC INFORMATION 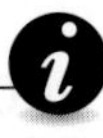

Definition

- Cells can be classified based on certain common cytologic features: epithelial, mesenchymal, and round cells. After cell types are identified, additional cytologic criteria are used to help determine whether cells are normal or part of an inflammatory or neoplastic process.
- Round cells are often called *discrete cells* because they exist individually in tissues rather than adhere to other cells or a matrix. Round cell tumors are typically composed of a homogeneous population of cells that have well-defined cytoplasmic margins, are round, and have a round nucleus. Exceptions to this include histiocytic sarcomas (multinucleate giant cells with irregular nuclear shapes are common) and melanoma (cells have variable appearances and can be round, epithelial, or mesenchymal cells). Distinct cytologic characteristics of each type of round cell aid in definitive diagnosis.
- Round cell tumor types include lymphoproliferative diseases (e.g., lymphoma, plasma cell tumor, multiple myeloma), mast cell tumor (MCT), transmissible venereal tumor, histiocytic tumors (i.e., histiocytomas, cutaneous and systemic histiocytosis, and histiocytic sarcoma), and melanocytic tumors. Each of these is discussed in greater detail in individual chapters.

Synonym

Discrete cell tumors

Epidemiology

SPECIES, AGE, SEX

Depends on tumor type

Clinical Presentation

DISEASE FORMS/SUBTYPES

- Lymphoproliferative diseases
  - Lymphoma (malignant lymphoma, lymphosarcoma) is seen in dogs and cats of all ages and can affect any organ system. Lymphocytic (small cell) and lymphoblastic (large cell) forms have varied presentations, clinical signs, and treatment options. In dogs, the most common form is lymphoblastic lymphoma, affecting the lymph nodes and lymphoid organs. In cats, solitary-site lymphocytic and lymphoblastic lymphoma can occur, affecting tissues that include gastrointestinal (GI), nasal/pharyngeal, mediastinal, central nervous system (CNS), and kidneys; multicentric lymphoma can also occur, especially in cats with feline leukemia virus (FeLV).
  - Solitary plasma cell tumors most commonly occur in dogs as skin and subcutaneous masses (plasmacytomas) but have also been reported in bones and the GI/respiratory tracts. Multiple myeloma is the systemic form of plasma cell cancer and can affect organ systems such as the bone marrow and lymphoid organs.
- MCTs (mastocytomas, mast cell sarcomas)
  - In dogs, the most common form is skin/subcutaneous masses. The prognosis varies and depends on tumor grade, clinical presentation, breed, and stage of disease.
  - In cats, skin, splenic, and visceral forms may occur.
- Transmissible venereal tumors (TVT) are transplanted from dog to dog by direct contact (sniffing/licking/sexual contact). TVT is most commonly seen in intact dogs in the genital regions and oral and nasal cavities and might regress in dogs with a competent immune system.

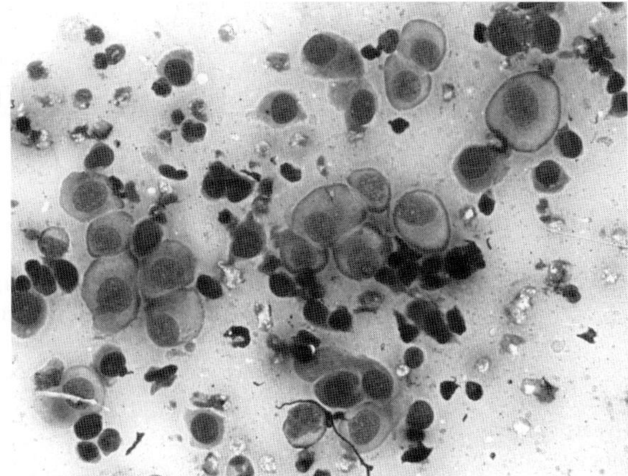

ROUND CELL TUMORS Histiocytoma (cutaneous mass, aqueous Romanowsky stain [Diff-Quik]). Round cells with a fried egg appearance contain moderate to large amounts of cytoplasm and fairly uniform paracentral to eccentric oval nuclei. Small lymphocytes are seen, and lymphocytic or mixed inflammation may be prominent in aspirates, particularly as tumors regress. (Courtesy Dr. Mary Leissinger, University of Florida.)

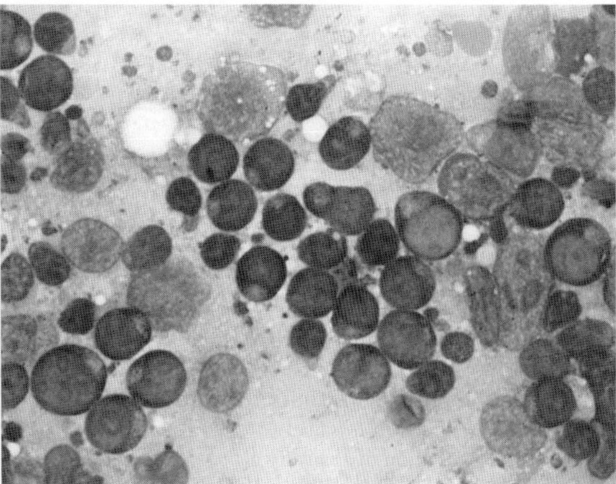

ROUND CELL TUMORS Lymphoma (lymph node aspirate, Wright-Giemsa stain). Intermediate to large lymphoblasts predominate, admixed with few small lymphocytes, many large pale-staining free nuclei, and small basophilic cytoplasmic fragments. The cells have open chromatin with prominent nucleoli and a small amount of deeply basophilic cytoplasm. The cells contain a prominent perinuclear clearing (Golgi zone), as can be seen in plasma cell tumors, but the high nuclear-cytoplasmic ratio and chromatin pattern are typical of neoplastic lymphocytes. (Courtesy Dr. Mary Leissinger, University of Florida.)

- Histiocytic cancers
    - Histiocytomas occur more commonly in young dogs (<3 years of age). They are usually small (<2 cm diameter), red, raised, round, and alopecic. They usually spontaneously regress and may become ulcerated/inflamed as they regress.
    - Cutaneous and systemic histiocytosis are rare, reactive, immune-mediated diseases.
    - Histiocytic sarcomas may be solitary (e.g., around joints, retroperitoneal, primary lung) or disseminated. The disseminated form often results in rapid onset of illness, with disease progression through lymph nodes and viscera.
- Melanomas are most commonly seen in the skin, oral cavity, and digits of dogs. The prognosis is highly variable and depends on the site and tumor grade.

HISTORY, CHIEF COMPLAINT

Depends on tumor type

PHYSICAL EXAM FINDINGS

Depends on tumor type

Etiology and Pathophysiology

Depends on tumor type

DIAGNOSIS

Diagnostic Overview

The diagnosis of round cell tumors is generally straightforward, with cytologic exam of aspirates or smears. Recommended staging tests/treatment and prognosis depend on tumor type.

Differential Diagnosis

Depends on tumor type (see chapters on specific tumors)

Initial Database

- Cytologic evaluation can confirm the cell type (diagnosis) for many round cell tumors.
- The following cytologic characteristics are commonly seen in these specific cell types:
    - Lymphoma (lymphoblastic): high nuclear-cytoplasmic ratio, multiple nucleoli, numerous mitotic figures
    - Plasma cell tumor: perinuclear clear zone adjacent to nucleus, eccentrically positioned nucleus, large amount of dark blue cytoplasm, binucleation and trinucleation can be seen, but does not correlate with the degree of malignancy.
    - MCT: nuclear details obscured by pink to purple intracytoplasmic granules that occur in most MCTs (in some poorly differentiated MCTs, granules are absent); eosinophils are often present
    - TVT: cytoplasmic vacuolation is common and distinctive; inflammatory cells such as lymphocytes and plasma cells may be seen when tumors are regressing.
    - Histiocytoma: anisocytosis and anisokaryosis are common; the cytoplasm is pale and may contain fine granules; mitotic figures are occasionally seen; inflammatory cells are present when tumors are regressing.
    - Histiocytic sarcoma: multinucleate giant cells with marked cellular atypia are common.
    - Melanoma: varied appearance; green, brown, or black intracytoplasmic granules often seen

Advanced or Confirmatory Testing

- Occasionally, the tumor type is not readily distinguished cytologically; a biopsy and histopathology of the lesion or immunocytochemistry (available through some commercial or university clinical pathology labs) may further delineate the cell type.
    - Special stains such as toluidine blue or Giemsa can identify granules in MCTs.
    - Immunohistochemical staining involves the use of antibodies directed against specific cell antigens that are markers of individual cell types (i.e., CD3/CD4/CD8 for T lymphocytes)
    - In some cases, flow cytometry of fluid samples (blood, bone marrow, liver or spleen aspirates) may be used to determine the cell lineage.

TREATMENT

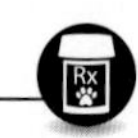

Treatment Overview

Depends on tumor type

Acute and Chronic Treatment

Depends on tumor type

PROGNOSIS & OUTCOME

Depends on tumor type

PEARLS & CONSIDERATIONS

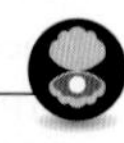

Comments

All new or growing masses should be evaluated by fine-needle aspiration as cytology from aspiration is a noninvasive method of obtaining a diagnosis for inflammatory and neoplastic diseases.

Technician Tips

Most round cell tumors exfoliate easily, and resulting cytology smears are highly cellular. Well-made slide preparations that result in a thin layer of cells is critical for accurate interpretation. One slide from each site should be stained and examined before submission to the lab to ensure diagnostic quality.

SUGGESTED READING

DeNicola DB: Round cells. In Valenciano AC, et al, editors: Diagnostic cytology and hematology, ed 4, St. Louis, 2014, Elsevier, pp 70-79.

AUTHOR: Tracy Gieger, DVM, DACVIM, DACVR
EDITOR: Kenneth M. Rassnick, DVM, DACVIM

Salivary Gland Disorders

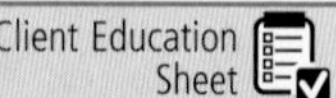

BASIC INFORMATION

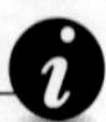

Definition

- Sialocele: accumulation of saliva that has leaked from a salivary gland or its duct into subcutaneous or submucosal tissue and consequent tissue reaction to saliva
- Sialadenitis: inflammation of a salivary gland
- Sialadenosis: noninflammatory, non-neoplastic enlargement of a salivary gland
- Necrotizing sialometaplasia: squamous metaplasia of the salivary gland ducts and lobules, with ischemic necrosis of the salivary gland lobules
- Salivary neoplasia: benign or malignant lesion arising from salivary glandular or ductal tissue

Synonyms

- Sialocele, salivary mucocele, ranula (sublingual sialocele)
- Necrotizing sialometaplasia, salivary gland necrosis or infarction

Epidemiology

SPECIES, AGE, SEX

- Sialocele: typically dogs 2-4 years old
- Sialadenitis: typically older dogs
- Sialadenosis and necrotizing sialometaplasia: dogs of all ages, most often 3-8 years old
- Salivary neoplasia: older dogs (mean, 10 years old); prevalence in cats almost twice that among dogs

GENETICS, BREED PREDISPOSITION

- Sialocele: German shepherds, miniature poodles overrepresented
- Sialadenosis and necrotizing sialometaplasia: small dog breeds (especially terriers) predisposed
- Salivary neoplasia: spaniel breeds and poodles predisposed

RISK FACTORS

Sialocele: oral trauma and activity of young dogs; however, experimental duct ligation, duct laceration, rupture of the mandibular salivary gland capsule with damage to glandular tissue, and subcutaneous injection of mucocele fluid have not caused salivary mucoceles in healthy dogs, suggesting a developmental predisposition in some dogs.

CONTAGION AND ZOONOSIS

Necrotizing sialometaplasia: *Spirocerca lupi* infestation (esophageal granulomas), megaesophagus, esophagitis, esophageal diverticulum, giardiasis, autoimmune sialadenitis

Clinical Presentation

DISEASE FORMS/SUBTYPES

Sialocele:
- Sublingual sialocele (ranula): in sublingual tissue
- Cervical sialocele: in intermandibular or cervical area; most common
- Pharyngeal sialocele: in pharyngeal wall
- Zygomatic sialocele: in orbit

Salivary neoplasia: carcinoma or adenocarcinoma most common

HISTORY, CHIEF COMPLAINT

Sialocele:
- Acute, painful intermandibular swelling: initial stage of cervical salivary mucocele resulting from an inflammatory response; uncommon presentation
- Swelling in the cranioventral neck region: cervical salivary mucocele at later stages, when inflammation has subsided (more common presentation); typically found incidentally by owner; slowly enlarging or intermittently large, fluid-filled, and usually nonpainful
- Ptyalism, blood-tinged saliva secondary to masticatory trauma, poor prehension of food, and reluctance to eat: sublingual salivary mucocele
- Dyspnea/dysphagia secondary to pharyngeal obstruction: pharyngeal salivary mucocele
- Periorbital mass and either enophthalmos or exophthalmos: zygomatic salivary mucocele (infrequently reported in dogs)

Sialadenitis:
- Painful swelling (depends on location) along the vertical ear canal, caudal to the mandible, or orbital/retrobulbar area with exophthalmos
- Lymphadenopathy, fever
- Pain associated with palpation of the affected gland
- Pain associated with mouth opening
- Dysphagia secondary to pain or enlarged inflamed gland that physically inhibits mouth opening

Sialadenosis:
- Regional swelling (depends on location), exophthalmos, but no apparent pain
- Retching and gulping elicited by mild excitement and occurring several times per day
- Weight loss, reluctance to exercise, snorting, lip smacking, nasal discharge, hypersalivation, inappetence, depression

Necrotizing sialometaplasia:
- Depression, nausea, anorexia
- Hypersalivation, persistent swallowing, lip smacking
- Retching, gagging, regurgitation, chronic vomiting, weight loss
- Cough, tachypnea, dyspnea, abdominal respiration
- Painful swelling caudal to the mandible, pain associated with mouth opening

Salivary neoplasia:
- Sometimes painful swelling (depends on location) around the vertical ear canal or caudal to the mandible
- Exophthalmus from orbital or retrobulbar swelling
- Pain on palpation of the involved gland
- Pain associated with mouth opening
- Dysphagia secondary to pain or neoplastic gland that physically inhibits mouth opening

PHYSICAL EXAM FINDINGS

All: see History/Chief Complaint above.

Sialocele:
- Fluid-filled, generally painless swelling in the cervical, sublingual, pharyngeal, or periorbital region
- Patient otherwise normal with no signs of systemic disease
- Sublingual gland most commonly affected

Sialadenitis:
- Pain on palpation of the gland
- Pain on gentle retropulsion of the eye through closed eyelids
- Systemic signs of inflammation: fever, malaise, inappetence
- Mucopurulent discharge may be noted at the duct opening in the oral cavity.
- Soft palate asymmetry from an enlarged, inflamed zygomatic salivary gland
- Zygomatic and mandibular glands most commonly affected

Sialadenosis:
- Usually bilateral salivary gland enlargement
- Mandibular gland most commonly affected
- Exophthalmos if zygomatic gland affected
- Hypersalivation, retching, and gulping but no signs of pain

Necrotizing sialometaplasia:
- Enlarged, painful, hard salivary gland
- Mandibular gland most commonly affected
- Very sensitive on palpation of pharyngeal area
- Dyspnea, cough, reverse sneezing
- Hypersalivation, lip smacking, persistent swallowing, retching, vomiting
- Weight loss

Salivary neoplasia:
- Painful swelling in the cervical, periauricular, or periorbital region; distinct mass; rarely any fluid accumulation
- Pain on gentle retropulsion of the eye through closed eyelids
- Occasionally, cancer cachexia or signs of other paraneoplastic disorders
- Parotid and mandibular glands most commonly affected

Etiology and Pathophysiology

Sialocele:
- Contrary to a true cyst, which is lined by epithelium, a sialocele represents a tissue reaction to extravasation of saliva from a gland/duct complex and has a nonepithelial, nonsecretory lining consisting primarily of fibroblasts and capillaries.
- Damage to salivary gland or duct associated with orofacial trauma may cause leakage of saliva into adjacent tissues. Generally, this leakage is self-limited and does not lead to mucocele.
- The defect is most often associated with the portion of the sublingual gland/duct complex caudal to the lingual nerve.

Sialadenitis:
- Salivary gland inflammation with enlargement
- Sialoliths may be a contributing factor because they can occur in dogs and are reported commonly in humans with sialadenitis. The associated ductal obstruction can lead to inflammation of the glandular tissue.

Sialadenosis:
- Salivary gland enlargement without cytologic or histologic abnormalities; excessive saliva production may be associated with increased parasympathetic activity or changes in sympathetic innervation.
- No evidence of cytologic or histologic abnormalities in affected salivary glands; usually no abnormalities noted on esophageal endoscopy

Necrotizing sialometaplasia:
- Squamous metaplasia of salivary gland ducts and lobules, with ischemic necrosis of the salivary gland lobules
- Neurogenic pathogenesis suspected to be associated with abnormalities of the vagal nerve
- Associations with *S. lupi* infestation, megaesophagus, esophagitis, esophageal diverticulum, giardiasis, autoimmune sialadenitis

Salivary neoplasia:
- No cyst or mucocele formation unless there is saliva accumulation secondary to ductal obstruction or leakage

DIAGNOSIS

Diagnostic Overview

Among other signs, the presence of any swelling in the periorbital, sublingual, intermandibular, subhyoid, parotid, pharyngeal, and cranioventral neck regions; exophthalmos; or being unable or reluctant to open the mouth should prompt suspicion of disease of the salivary gland/duct complex. Fine-needle aspiration for cytologic evaluation is valuable (particularly for sialoceles: saliva-like fluid). Definitive diagnosis for all others requires biopsy and histologic evaluation.

Differential Diagnosis

- Edema, pharyngeal remnant cyst, cyst, seroma, hematoma, abscess
- Trauma, foreign body, sialolith
- Lymphadenitis, neoplasia affecting lymph nodes
- Aural or ocular neoplasia

Initial Database

Sialocele:
- Fine-needle aspiration and cytologic evaluation: clear or nontransparent, stringy,

sometimes blood-tinged, often brownish fluid with a very low cellular content
- Mucin and amylase analyses of the fluid are not reliable diagnostic procedures.
- If cervical sialocele appears on ventral midline, place patient in exact dorsal recumbency (awake, sedated, or anesthetized):
  - Sialocele usually shifts to the originating side and is more easily mobile on the originating side.
  - Essential for correct identification of the affected side if surgical intervention is contemplated

Sialadenitis, sialadenosis, necrotizing sialometaplasia, salivary neoplasia:
- Fine-needle aspiration of gland and cytologic evaluation (zygomatic salivary gland may require per os aspiration)
- Fine-needle aspiration of regional lymph nodes
- Bacterial culture and sensitivity
- Three-view thoracic radiographs to rule out conditions associated with necrotizing sialometaplasia and thoracic metastasis

Advanced or Confirmatory Testing
- Regional radiographs or ultrasonography if sialolith is suspected or palpated
- Sialography: radiographic contrast study of a salivary gland/duct complex; most common indication for a sialogram is to determine the location of a salivary gland/duct defect in patients with sialocele
- CT, MRI (p. 1132)
- Incisional biopsy for histopathologic evaluation

TREATMENT

Treatment Overview
Combination of immediate relief through aspiration or incision for some disorders is followed by surgical excision, radiation therapy, or others, depending on diagnosis.

Acute General Treatment
Sialocele:
- Needle drainage of mucocele; not recommended as a repeat treatment option due to rapid recurrence and risk of iatrogenic infection
- Complete removal of involved salivary gland/duct complex with ligation of remaining duct and drainage of sialocele and surgical site
- Marsupialization of a sublingual or pharyngeal sialocele (creation of a large window in the mucosa overlying the swelling to allow for intraoral drainage of saliva) is not as effective as removal of the involved gland/duct complex because granulation tissue may result in closure of the window.

Sialadenitis, sialadenosis, and necrotizing sialometaplasia:
- Surgical removal of the affected salivary gland produces minimal if any improvement.
- If needle aspirate yielded mucopurulent fluid, per os or percutaneous drainage to alleviate mucopurulent fluid accumulation and associated pressure causing discomfort
  - Percutaneous drainage using a closed suction system rarely required
  - Per os drainage after stab incision using a #15 scalpel blade through the soft palate into the affected zygomatic salivary gland (hemostatic forceps can be used to enlarge the stab wound and facilitate drainage)

Salivary neoplasia:
- Complete excision of a salivary neoplasm: only if entirely intracapsular, otherwise not recommended
- Surgical debulking procedure recommended if part of a multimodality treatment plan that involves cytoreduction of the neoplasm
- Pain management

Chronic Treatment
Sialadenitis, sialadenosis, and necrotizing sialometaplasia:
- Pain management, antibiotics (based on culture and sensitivity of the fluid/tissue aspirate), nonsteroidal antiinflammatory drugs (NSAIDs), antiinflammatory doses of glucocorticosteroids (do not combine with NSAIDs), and control of internal parasites have resulted in favorable responses in some cases.
- Phenobarbital 1-2 mg/kg PO q 12h administration has resulted in dramatic improvement in some cases, providing more support for a neurogenic pathogenesis.

Salivary neoplasia:
- Radiotherapy
- Surgical debulking

Possible Complications
- Injury to the lingual nerve during removal of mandibular/sublingual gland/duct complex (lingual nerve is located dorsal and rostral to the gland/duct complex)
- Recurrence of mucocele due to failure of having completely excised all affected gland(s)
- Seroma/hematoma formation due to failure of having appropriately drained the sialocele and surgical site
- Injury to major neurovascular structures during incisional biopsy procedures
- Ocular trauma associated with the zygomatic salivary gland during drainage of mucopurulent fluid
- Failure to completely excise all affected tissue (any salivary neoplasm)
- Ocular complications of radiotherapy if ipsilateral eye is in the treatment field

Recommended Monitoring
Surgical site for evidence of seroma/hematoma formation

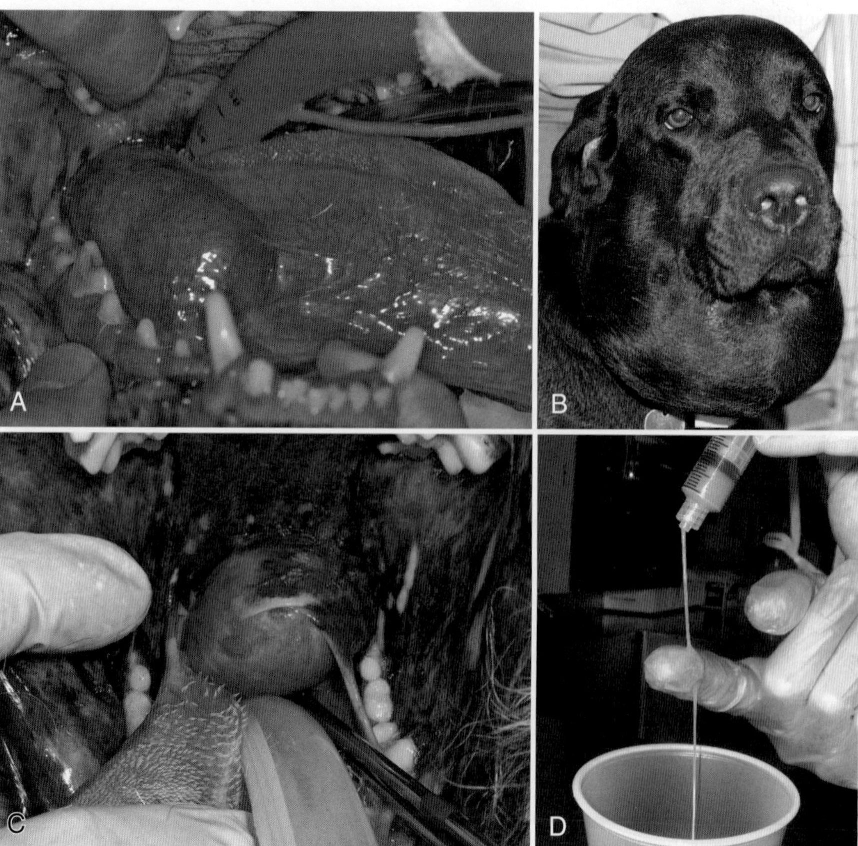

SALIVARY GLAND DISORDERS Sialoceles in dogs. **A,** Sublingual (right-sided). **B,** Cervical (originating from the right side). **C,** Pharyngeal (left-sided). **D,** Nontransparent, stringy, brownish fluid aspirated from a sialocele. (Copyright Dr. Alexander M. Reiter, University of Pennsylvania.)

PROGNOSIS & OUTCOME

- Sialocele: excellent with complete removal of the gland/duct complex, with appropriate drainage of the sialocele and surgical site
- Sialadenitis: excellent/good, depending on identification of initiating cause and response to treatment
- Sialadenosis: excellent/good with phenobarbital treatment
- Necrotizing sialometaplasia: good/guarded, depending on response to medical treatment (such as phenobarbital)
- Salivary neoplasia: guarded/poor; treatment generally considered palliative

PEARLS & CONSIDERATIONS

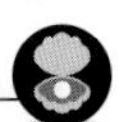

Comments

Sialocele:

- Placement of the patient in exact dorsal recumbency can lateralize cervical sialoceles that otherwise seem to be on the ventral midline, which is essential for knowing which side to approach surgically.
- Sialoliths are concretions of calcium phosphate or calcium carbonate and may occur with chronic sialocele.
- The intimate anatomic association of the sublingual and mandibular salivary glands and their ducts requires removal of both structures when a sialocele affects one of them.
- If left untreated, a sialocele may result in
  - Physical problems associated with a large cranioventral cervical mass
  - Trauma, ulceration, secondary infection
  - Dysphagia (sublingual sialocele), dyspnea/dysphagia (pharyngeal sialocele), exophthalmos, strabismus, and other ocular complications (zygomatic sialocele)
- Injury to the parotid duct (e.g., after animal bites, caudal maxillectomy, masseter muscle biopsy, open extraction of caudal cheek teeth) or foreign-body entrapment at the parotid papilla may occasionally cause progressive duct enlargement. A finger-sized, tubular, soft, movable and fluid-filled structure can then be felt underneath the skin overlying the masseter muscle.
  - This pathology more likely represents a salivary cyst than a sialocele because the enlarged duct is lined by epithelium.
  - Treatment requires ligation of the parotid duct at its caudal aspect close to where it emerges from the parotid gland and resection of the enlarged portion rostrally.
  - Repeat drainage of saliva from the enlarged duct may only temporarily reduce the size of the duct and bears the risk of iatrogenic infection.

Sialadenitis, sialadenosis, and necrotizing sialometaplasia:

- Be careful to differentiate these conditions from salivary neoplasia because they can have similar clinical signs.
- Complete surgical excision of affected salivary gland/duct complexes is virtually impossible, often unhelpful, and usually not necessary.
- Be mindful of the many neurovascular structures in anatomic areas where drainage of salivary glands is required.
- It is speculative whether sialadenosis can progress to necrotizing sialometaplasia.

Salivary neoplasia:

- Be careful to differentiate this from sialadenitis, sialadenosis, and necrotizing sialometaplasia because they can produce similar clinical signs.
- Complete excision of a salivary neoplasm is unlikely and may increase morbidity; generally, lesions are large and invasive at the time of diagnosis.
- Be mindful of the many neurovascular structures in anatomic areas where salivary gland neoplasms are likely to occur.
- Salivary neoplasia should be staged according to the tumor-node-metastasis (TNM) system (p. 623) to enable appropriate prognostication and a treatment plan.

Phenobarbital-responsive sialadenosis:

- An uncommon disorder associated with nonpainful salivary gland enlargement and systemic signs such as nausea, retching, gagging, weight loss, and vomiting
- There is no diagnostic test other than response to therapy for this idiopathic condition.
- As the name implies, the disorder responds rapidly to phenobarbital administration.

Technician Tips

Technicians should be able to distinguish mandibular lymph nodes from salivary glands on neck palpation (lymph node in front).

SUGGESTED READING

Reiter AM, et al: Oral and salivary gland disorders. In Ettinger SJ, et al, editors: Textbook of veterinary internal medicine, ed 8, Philadelphia, 2017, Saunders, pp 1469-1476.

AUTHOR & EDITOR: Alexander M. Reiter, DVM, Dr. med. vet., DAVDC, DEVDC

Salmon Poisoning

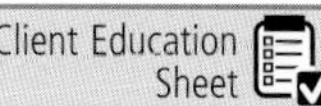

BASIC INFORMATION

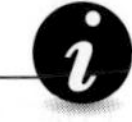

Definition

A febrile rickettsial infection of dogs in the Pacific northwestern United States and British Columbia, associated with ingestion of raw fish

Synonym

Neorickettsia helminthoeca infection

Epidemiology

SPECIES, AGE, SEX

Intact males and Labradors overrepresented

RISK FACTORS

Exposure to a stream, beach, or sites where fish are cleaned or fish fertilizer is common.

GEOGRAPHY AND SEASONALITY

Infections are limited to the habitat range of the intermediate snail host *(Oxytrema silicula)* in western British Columbia, Washington, Oregon, northern California, and more sporadically in areas where fish carrying the causative organism, *N. helminthoeca,* are transported. Dogs have the greatest access to dead fish during spawning seasons (late summer to early winter), but cases can be seen year-round.

Clinical Presentation

DISEASE FORMS/SUBTYPES

- Acute, severe febrile illness usually 5-7 days after fish ingestion; often fatal
- A more moderate illness may be seen as late as 14-33 days after exposure, particularly with the Elokomin fluke fever disease variant.

HISTORY, CHIEF COMPLAINT

- Acute onset of anorexia, lethargy, and fever
- Vomiting and bloody diarrhea common
- Oculonasal discharge and tremor occasionally reported

PHYSICAL EXAM FINDINGS

- Fever
- Lymphadenomegaly
- Signs of hypovolemic shock or dehydration

Etiology and Pathophysiology

- Dogs acquire the causative organism *(N. helminthoeca)* from a fluke parasite *(Nanophyetus salmincola)* carried in salmon and rarely from other fish or salamanders.

- Rickettsial infection is transmitted when flukes mature in the canine gastrointestinal (GI) tract.
  - Fluke maturation in the GI tract involves release of the rickettsiae, which are taken up by macrophages and disseminate to lymph nodes (especially mesenteric).
  - Replication of the organism occurs in the lymph nodes, where the lesions are most profound (other than the inflammation in the GI mucosa when flukes and rickettsiae elicit an immune response).
- Systemic rickettsial replication results in clinical disease in dogs.

DIAGNOSIS

Diagnostic Overview

Diagnosis is based on compatible clinical signs (fever, hemorrhagic gastroenteritis, lymphadenomegaly) in a dog with a history of raw fish ingestion, finding flukes on a fecal exam, or response to tetracycline therapy.

Differential Diagnosis

- Parvoviral enteritis
- Acute hemorrhagic diarrhea syndrome (AHDS; formerly hemorrhagic gastroenteritis [p. 259])
- Sepsis (e.g., due to foreign body perforation, cholangiohepatitis)
- Pancreatitis
- Neoplasia, especially GI lymphoma

Initial Database

- CBC and serum biochemical findings may include thrombocytopenia, lymphopenia, eosinophilia, hypoalbuminemia, and elevated alkaline phosphatase.
- Operculated fluke eggs are most easily seen on zinc sulfate fecal flotation or sediment exam but may be seen on direct smear.
  - Combining fecal flotation and sedimentation exams yields sensitivity of > 90% for fluke eggs.

Advanced or Confirmatory Testing

- Giemsa-stained lymph node aspirates may reveal intracytoplasmic rickettsial bodies. Polymerase chain reaction (PCR) amplification of rickettsial DNA is also possible.
- Abdominal ultrasound often reveals moderate mesenteric lymph node enlargement.

TREATMENT

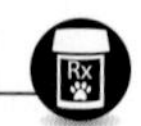

Treatment Overview

Hospitalization for treatment with fluids, supportive care, and tetracyclines is indicated. Ideally, the fluke vector should be eliminated by treatment with praziquantel, although spontaneous resolution can occur.

Acute General Treatment

- IV fluid support and alleviation of vomiting (p. 1040) and diarrhea (p. 257)
- Mild cases: rickettsial infection can be treated with oral doxycycline 10 mg/kg q 12h, minocycline 10 mg/kg q 12h, or tetracycline 22 mg/kg q 8h for 7-14 days.
- Severe cases: parenteral doxycycline 5-10 mg/kg IV q 12h until oral form is tolerated; oxytetracycline 7 mg/kg IV q 8h × 3 days has also been effective
- Praziquantel 10-30 mg/kg PO or SQ once for elimination of flukes

Possible Complications

Parenteral oxytetracycline rarely has been associated with acute kidney injury. Doxycycline can cause elevated liver enzymes.

PROGNOSIS & OUTCOME

- Prognosis is fair to good for aggressively managed cases; improvement is usually noted in 2-3 days after treatment initiation.
- Death is likely in 5-10 days if the disease remains untreated.

PEARLS & CONSIDERATIONS

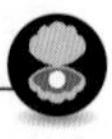

Comments

- Salmon poisoning is an important cause of fever, lymphadenomegaly, and severe GI signs in dogs in the Pacific northwestern United States and Pacific coastal Canada.
- Clinical signs are similar to AHDS, but affected dogs are typically febrile.
- Fecal exams and treatment with tetracycline antibiotics are recommended for febrile dogs when possible ingestion of raw fish is noted in disease-endemic regions.

Prevention

Restrict access to raw fish in the Pacific Northwest.

Technician Tips

- Ask owners about potential fish ingestion when a febrile dog presents with vomiting or diarrhea.
- Always follow oral doxycycline administration with water or food because esophagitis can develop.

Client Education

- Early aggressive treatment is required for salmon poisoning, or death is likely.
- Do not allow dogs to consume raw fish.

SUGGESTED READING

Sykes JE, et al: Salmon poisoning disease in dogs: 29 cases. J Vet Intern Med 24:504-513, 2010.

AUTHOR: Polly B. Peterson, DVM, DACVIM
EDITOR: Rance K. Sellon, DVM, PhD, DACVIM

Salmonellosis

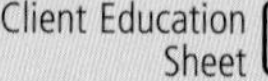

BASIC INFORMATION

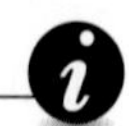

Definition

Infection of susceptible patients with pathogenic *Salmonella* spp

Synonyms

- Songbird fever (cats)
- Fading puppy/kitten syndrome (one of many causes)

Epidemiology

SPECIES, AGE, SEX

- Many species can be infected, including cats, dogs, and people.
- Cats appear to be more resistant to *Salmonella* infection than dogs.
- Younger animals are more commonly affected.

RISK FACTORS

- Young, stressed, or immunocompromised patients
- Feeding raw or undercooked meat products, eggs, or diets, especially containing chicken (p. 863)
- Overcrowded, unsanitary, or stressful conditions
- Concurrent gastrointestinal (GI) infections
- Antibiotic therapy

CONTAGION AND ZOONOSIS

- Infected dogs and cats are a major risk to people, especially immunocompromised persons.
- Risk to people increases if pets are eating raw meat diets due to increased fecal shedding.
- Undercooked meat is also a risk for people if ingested or when contamination of human food preparation areas/utensils occurs.
- Outbreaks from contaminated pet foods have occurred.

GEOGRAPHY AND SEASONALITY

Salmonellosis occurs worldwide, but songbird fever is primarily reported in the northeastern

United States and Sweden and occurs primarily in cats feeding on songbirds during seasonal migrations.

ASSOCIATED DISORDERS

Focal organ infections can be found anywhere but especially likely are:

- Abscesses, pneumonia, pyothorax
- Meningitis
- Osteomyelitis
- *In utero* infection resulting in abortion, stillbirth, weak puppies or kittens
- Acute hepatic necrosis and associated hepatic failure

Clinical Presentation

DISEASE FORMS/SUBTYPES

- Up to 30% of dogs and 18% of cats are subclinical carriers.
- Primarily acute enterocolitis
- Chronic diarrhea rare
- Septicemia/endotoxemia
- Localized infections (see Associated Disorders)
- Cats may develop chronic, febrile illness (songbird fever)

HISTORY, CHIEF COMPLAINT

Animals can appear healthy or have signs of illness related to localized infection or sepsis. The most common historical findings of illness due to salmonellosis are GI-related: watery to mucoid diarrhea with or without blood, straining or increased urgency to defecate, vomiting, anorexia, lethargy/depression, and weight loss

PHYSICAL EXAM FINDINGS

Exam can be normal, or findings can reflect GI, localized, or systemic infection:

- Fever
- Abdominal pain
- Dehydration, possibly severe
- Pale mucous membranes, tachycardia, tachypnea, weakness, weak pulses if septicemic
- Conjunctivitis in cats

Etiology and Pathophysiology

- *Salmonella* spp: gram-negative, facultative anaerobic, motile, non–spore-forming rods from the family Enterobacteriaceae
- Ubiquitous, most commonly transmitted through contact with contaminated food, water, or fomites
- Bacterium survives for up to 6 weeks in environment.
- Clinical signs occur secondary to mucosal invasion and epithelial injury.
  - *Salmonella* spp also produce an enterotoxin, resulting in secretory diarrhea.
- Organism persists in phagocytic cells of intestinal mucosa and mesenteric lymph nodes, liver, and spleen:
  - Results in persistent shedding for 3-6 weeks after infection
- Bacteremia and endotoxemia may occur secondary to mucosal invasion, resulting in systemic infection, disseminated intravascular coagulation (DIC), and/or systemic inflammatory response syndrome (SIRS).
- Persistence and severity of infection depend on the patient's immune status.

DIAGNOSIS

Diagnostic Overview

Diagnosis is suspected in animals with acute or chronic GI illness, especially if young, immunocompromised, or eating raw meat diets. Diagnosis is based on isolation of *Salmonella* from feces, blood, or infected tissues. Because prevalence of organism is similar in stool from healthy and diarrheic animals, diagnosis must be made in conjunction with appropriate clinical signs.

Differential Diagnosis

- Diarrhea due to other causes (p. 1213)
- Septicemia due to other causes (p. 907)

Initial Database

- CBC, biochemistry profile, and coagulation changes are generally nonspecific or represent signs of endotoxemia/sepsis.
  - Neutropenia with left shift and toxic neutrophils in acute phase or systemic disease
  - Neutrophilia if chronic illness
  - Nonregenerative, possibly hypochromic anemia may be noted.
  - Thrombocytopenia in severe cases, with septicemia leading to DIC
  - Prolonged coagulation times in severe cases with DIC
  - Hypoproteinemia due to GI loss
  - Sometimes hyponatremia and hyperkalemia (similar to hypoadrenocorticism)
  - Hypoglycemia, azotemia, or hyperbilirubinemia suggests endotoxemia/sepsis.
- Fecal flotation, culture, and ELISA testing as needed to rule out other causes of diarrhea.

Advanced or Confirmatory Testing

- Fecal bacterial culture
  - Best results using enrichment broth or selective culture media
  - Positive fecal culture establishes infection but does not necessarily confirm that signs are due to salmonellosis because subclinical carriers are common.
  - False-negative results are possible because the organism grows fastidiously.
- Fecal polymerase chain reaction (PCR) may improve sensitivity of detection.
- Blood culture or culture from other infected sites; positive culture from blood, bile, or other normally sterile samples strongly indicative of salmonellosis.

TREATMENT

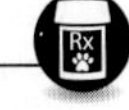

Treatment Overview

For uncomplicated gastroenteritis, treatment consists of supportive care without antibiotics. For systemic disease or immunocompromised patients, aggressive therapy with antibiotic use is warranted. No therapy is recommended for subclinical carriers.

Acute General Treatment

- Mild cases are often self-limited and require only supportive therapy and good hygiene to prevent contagion or zoonotic infection.
- IV fluid support, including plasma or colloids if necessary, is recommended for dehydration or septicemia (p. 907).
- Antibiotic therapy is controversial.
  - May induce a carrier state and prolong fecal shedding of organisms
  - May induce drug-resistant strains while suppressing endogenous (beneficial) flora
  - Antibiotics are indicated if the patient is febrile, evidence of sepsis or SIRS exists, the patient is immunocompromised and shows GI signs, or blood cultures are positive.
  - Combination of enrofloxacin 5-10 mg/kg PO or slow IV q 24h in dogs or 5 mg/kg PO or slow IV q 24h in cats and amoxicillin or ampicillin 10-20 mg/kg PO or IV q 8h is advocated as empirical therapy but ideally should be based on susceptibility testing.
  - Others reported to be effective include trimethoprim-sulfadiazine 15 mg/kg PO q 12h or chloramphenicol.
  - Antibiotic therapy should initially be administered for 10 days, but some cases may require longer-term administration.

Recommended Monitoring

Monitor carefully for signs of sepsis (p. 907) or SIRS.

PROGNOSIS & OUTCOME

- Prognosis for mild cases is good; infections usually resolve spontaneously or with supportive care only.
- Prognosis for septicemic patients is guarded; potential disease complications include electrolyte imbalances, septic shock, SIRS, and DIC.

PEARLS & CONSIDERATIONS

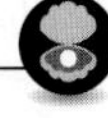

Comments

Patients fed raw food diets are at increased risk for salmonellosis.

- *Salmonella* isolated from 66%-80% of samples of raw food (e.g., bones, raw food [BARF] diet)
- *Salmonella* isolated from 30%-93% of stool samples from dogs fed BARF diets; there is an increased risk for human exposure and infection.

Prevention

- Avoid feeding raw or undercooked meat diets.
- Isolate infected animals, and practice good hygiene.

Technician Tips

- Contact precautions should be taken to avoid spread between infected patients and other hospitalized patients or personnel.

- Food/water containers and grooming utensils should not be shared with other patients.
- Use caution when handling fecal samples from patients fed raw food diets.

Client Education

- Owners should be informed that this is a zoonotic disease and that humans are very susceptible.
- Avoid raw diets, or use caution when handling raw foods or feces from pets fed raw food diets (human infection possible).

SUGGESTED READING

Marks SL, et al: Enteropathogenic bacteria in dogs and cats: diagnosis, epidemiology, treatment, and control. J Vet Intern Med 25:1195-1208, 2011.

AUTHOR: Katherine D. Scott, DVM, DACVIM
EDITOR: Rance K. Sellon, DVM, PhD, DACVIM

Sarcoptic Mange

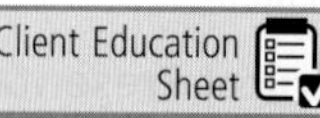

BASIC INFORMATION

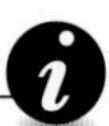

Definition

A nonseasonal, highly contagious, intensely pruritic cutaneous infestation caused by a small, obligate, burrowing mite, *Sarcoptes scabiei* var. *canis*

Synonyms

Canine scabies, sarcoptic acariasis

Epidemiology

SPECIES, AGE, SEX

Dogs (all breeds, both sexes, all ages) are commonly affected.

RISK FACTORS

Animal shelters, pet shops, dog shows, grooming/boarding facilities, stray dogs, and rural dogs in direct or indirect contact with infested foxes or coyotes: increased risk

CONTAGION AND ZOONOSIS

- Transmission occurs most commonly from direct contact with an infested dog or wild Canidae but can also occur from a contaminated environment and fomites.
- Humans exposed to an infested dog can develop a pruritic papular eruption, which resolves after mites are eradicated from the animal. Rarely, a dog may acquire the parasite from a human infested with *S. scabiei* var. *humanis.*

Clinical Presentation

HISTORY, CHIEF COMPLAINT

The primary complaint is pruritus. In chronic cases, the condition can present as nonseasonal intense pruritus that has responded poorly to various dermatologic therapies, including corticosteroid therapy.

PHYSICAL EXAM FINDINGS

- Typically, the ear margins, elbows and hocks, ventral abdomen, chest, and eventually legs (the dorsum is usually spared) show intense pruritus, papules, erythema, crusting, excoriations, and alopecia.
- A positive pinnal-pedal reflex (scratching action with the dog's hindlimb when the examiner rubs or scratches the margin of the dog's pinna) is seen in ≈80% of dogs with sarcoptic mange and in ≈7% of dogs with pruritus caused by other diseases.

Etiology and Pathophysiology

- The life cycle lasts ≈3 weeks, and adult mites usually survive off the host for up to 6 days at room temperature.
- *S. scabiei* var. *canis* is not totally host specific, given that it has been isolated from foxes, coyotes, and rarely from immunosuppressed cats.
- Infestation with *Sarcoptes* mites (as for many other parasitic infestations) leads to a hypersensitivity reaction, the latter being responsible for the intense pruritus in sensitized dogs. The precise incubation period is not known, but in first-time infestations, the first clinical signs are usually expected 3-4 weeks after exposure.

DIAGNOSIS

Diagnostic Overview

The diagnosis is suspected from the history and clinical signs; a positive pinnal-pedal reflex is strongly suggestive of the disease. Consider *S. scabiei* infestation when presented with any dog with an apparent sudden onset of intense itching.

Differential Diagnosis

- Ectoparasites (*Cheyletiella, Otodectes,* fleas, lice, chiggers, *Pelodera* dermatitis)
- Hypersensitivities (atopic dermatitis, food, flea bite and other ectoparasites, contact)
- Pyoderma
- *Malassezia* dermatitis

Initial Database

- Confirmation of the diagnosis relies on a positive skin scraping (mites, mite eggs, or mite fecal pellets) or occasionally on histopathologic analysis of skin biopsies or fecal flotation. The ear margins, elbows or hocks, and unexcoriated papules are the preferred sites for scrapings. However, the mites are notoriously difficult to find (p. 1091).
- Test for the pinnal-pedal reflex.

Advanced or Confirmatory Testing

- A serodiagnostic (ELISA) test is available in some countries for the diagnosis of canine scabies, with a sensitivity of 82%-92% and specificity of 92%-96%.
- Therapeutic trials with reliable scabicides are essential to confirm or rule out scabies in pruritic dogs with negative skin scrapings.

TREATMENT

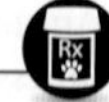

Treatment Overview

- The goal of treatment is to thoroughly eradicate the mites. Affected and all in-contact dogs should be treated with a scabicide regardless of presence or absence of clinical signs.
- All clinically suspected *S. scabiei* cases should be treated even if multiple skin scrapings are negative.
- Traditional topical scabicides (lime sulfur, amitraz, organophosphates) have been largely replaced by labeled and off-label use of macrocyclic lactones and, more recently by isoxazolines.

Acute and Chronic Treatment

- Selamectin (Revolution, Stronghold) and moxidectin/imidacloprid (Advantage Multi, Advocate) are approved as topical scabicides given once q 30 days for two treatments, although many veterinary dermatologists recommend a minimum of three treatments q 2 weeks.
- Isoxazoline (afoxolaner [NexGard], fluralaner [Bravecto], sarolaner [Simparica]) appear highly effective and safe at labeled doses.
- The off-label use of ivermectin remains a therapeutic alternative but should never be used in collies or other breeds with a high prevalence of the *MDR1/ABCB1-Δ* mutation (p. 638). The injectable product (Ivomec 1% injection for cattle and swine) is usually given at a dosage of 0.3 mg/kg PO or SQ q 7-14 days for a 4-6 week course of treatment. The 0.5% alcohol-based, pour-on ivermectin formulation (Ivomec Pour-on for cattle) is also effective and practical when applied to the interscapular skin q 14 days at 0.5 mg/kg for two to three treatments.

- Concomitant antimicrobial therapy (chlorhexidine shampoos, oral antibiotics) may be required if secondary pyoderma is present.
- Short-term corticosteroid or oclacitinib administration may be considered for severely pruritic dogs. The use of an environmental acaricidal is generally not required, although grooming equipment and bedding can be treated with an appropriate acaricidal spray.

Possible Complications

In collies, Australian shepherds, and many other canine breeds carrying the *MDR1/ABCB1-Δ* mutation, intoxication can occur with dosages of ivermectin or other off-label macrocyclic lactones that are tolerated by normal dogs. Pretreatment testing for the gene mutation (and/or selection of alternate treatment) is recommended in at-risk breeds.

Recommended Monitoring

Follow-up exam, including skin scrapings and cytologic analysis, is recommended if clinical signs persist or worsen 1-2 months after initiating scabicidal treatment.

PROGNOSIS & OUTCOME

- Prognosis with appropriate treatment is excellent.
- It can take 2 to several weeks for complete resolution of pruritus. In some dogs, an increase in pruritus (probably associated with an immunogenic response to the dying mites) may occur in the first few days after treatment.
- In humans, the zoonotic infestation is transient, with the pruritic papular eruption resolving when the mites are eradicated from the dog.

PEARLS & CONSIDERATIONS

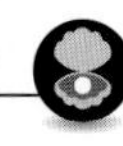

Comments

- Crusting of the elbows, hocks, and pinnal ear margins accompanied by intense pruritus are strongly suggestive of *S. scabiei.*
- Look for a pinnal-pedal reflex, and treat for scabies if this reflex is noted.
- Feline scabies is caused by a different parasite, *Notoedres cati;* however, cats in close contact with dogs affected with *S. scabiei* var. *canis* may be temporary reservoirs for the mite and occasionally develop transient pruritus. Rarely, immunosuppressed cats may develop persistent pruritic lesions when infested with *S. scabiei* var. *canis.*
- Due to cross-sensitization, a positive intradermal skin test response to house dust mite antigen is seen in ≈75% of dogs with a confirmed diagnosis of scabies. All clinical signs resolve after acaricidal therapy, and all intradermal reaction to dust mites are generally negative within 6 months of eradication of the mites. This illustrates the importance of ruling out scabies before testing for atopic dermatitis.

Technician Tips

- Sarcoptic mange has zoonotic potential. Try to limit direct contact with the affected dog. Hospital environment should be decontaminated.
- An acaricide (e.g., pyrethrin) is indicated for disinfecting surfaces such as exam tables and floors, but for patients that have low mite burdens, these surfaces may be adequately treated using routine disinfectants.
- Home environment is rarely treated, except for the dog's bedding.

Client Education

Humans transiently affected with *S. scabiei* mites may develop a pruritic papular eruption, especially on the arms and trunk. This should spontaneously resolve within 3 weeks when the mites are eradicated from the dog. Persistent symptoms should prompt the person to consult with a physician.

SUGGESTED READING

Miller WH Jr, et al: Muller & Kirk's Small animal dermatology, ed 7, St. Louis, 2013, Saunders, pp 315-319.

AUTHOR & EDITOR: **Manon Paradis, DMV, MVSc, DACVD**

Sebaceous Adenitis

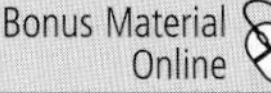
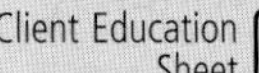
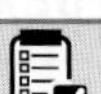

Bonus Material Online   Client Education Sheet

BASIC INFORMATION

Definition

Sebaceous adenitis (SA) is a destructive inflammatory disease of the sebaceous glands.

Epidemiology

SPECIES, AGE, SEX

Uncommon in dogs, rare in cats; signs tend to appear in young-adult to middle-aged dogs (1.5-7 years)

GENETICS, BREED PREDISPOSITION

Any breed can be affected, but the condition appears to be inherited in the Akita, Samoyed, and standard poodle (autosomal recessive). Other breeds frequently reported are the English springer spaniel, Havanese, vizsla, German shepherd, Lhasa apso, Hovawart, and Bernese mountain dog.

ASSOCIATED DISORDERS

Pyoderma (p. 851), *Malassezia* dermatitis (p. 614), and otitis externa (p. 728)

Clinical Presentation

DISEASE FORMS/SUBTYPES

- Marked variability of clinical presentation depending on individual breeds and severity. May be divided into:
  - Generalized SA: in long-coated breeds, such as Akita and standard poodle
  - Multifocal SA: in short-coated breeds, such as vizsla and in cats
- SA can also be subclinical and identifiable only by histologic exam of predisposed breeds (e.g., standard poodles)

HISTORY, CHIEF COMPLAINT

Progressive areas of hair loss, change in hair color or quality, poor haircoat, excessive scaling, and musty odor. Pruritus is variable but may be marked, especially with secondary bacterial or yeast infection.

PHYSICAL EXAM FINDINGS

- Generalized SA: presents with dramatic amounts of scaling. Typically, scales are adherent to hairs (follicular casts) and skin, and haircoat is often dry to the touch. Hypotrichosis on the top of the head, back of the neck, and dorsum is observed as the disease progresses. The dorsal midline and ears are often the first and most affected areas. In the Akita, in which the disease can be more severe, fever, anorexia, and lethargy have been reported.
- Multifocal SA: clinical presentation seen in vizslas presents with coalescing patches of scaly alopecia and annular plaques, with adherent scales developing mainly on the face, head, and trunk.

Etiology and Pathophysiology

- A genetically inherited, cell-mediated immune reaction directed against a component of the sebaceous glands is suspected.
- Another theory is that the initial defect may be an abnormality in cutaneous lipid metabolism.

DIAGNOSIS

Diagnostic Overview

The diagnosis is suspected based on clinical presentation in a predisposed breed, and skin biopsy is confirmatory.

Differential Diagnosis

- Generalized form: cornification disorders (primary seborrhea, ichthyosis), pyoderma, *Malassezia* dermatitis, demodicosis, dermatophytosis, endocrinopathies, leishmaniosis
- Multifocal form: pyoderma, demodicosis, dermatophytosis, zinc-responsive dermatosis, pemphigus foliaceus

Initial Database

- Cytologic exam (p. 1091) to assess for presence of secondary bacterial or *Malassezia* infection
- Skin scrapings to rule out ectoparasites
- Wood's lamp and dermatophyte culture to rule out dermatophytosis
- Trichography shows casts of keratosebaceous material adherent to hair shafts.
- CBC, serum biochemistry profile, urinalysis, and thyroid function tests: no abnormalities expected

Advanced or Confirmatory Testing

Skin biopsies of early lesions, preferably in areas with active scaling and little alopecia, show dermatohistopathologic findings that are diagnostic, including a pyogranulomatous inflammation around the sebaceous glands with sebaceous glands in various stages of destruction. In the late stage, the inflammation resolves, leaving an absence of sebaceous glands. Marked orthokeratotic hyperkeratosis is also seen.

TREATMENT

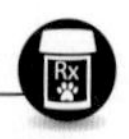

Treatment Overview

SA is incurable, but acceptable control of clinical signs (for patient comfort, reduction of risk of secondary infections, and esthetics) can be reached with lifelong topical and/or systemic therapy. The mainstay of topical treatment involves the use of keratolytic product. Nutritional supplements may be beneficial but are unproved.

Acute General Treatment

- Treat bacterial infections with appropriate systemic antibiotic therapy. An acceptable empirical choice initially is cephalexin 25-30 mg/kg PO q 12h for 3 weeks (p. 851).
- There is no gold standard for treatment of SA in dogs; the protocols have been published, all with variable efficacy.
- Mild cases: intensive topical therapy may lead to effective control of scaling and some hair regrowth. Mild keratolytic shampoos and emollient rinses; weekly baby oil soaks 30 minutes to 2 hours before shampoo are highly effective in dissolving the keratin. Weekly soaks and baths are needed at first (6-8 weeks), but the frequency usually can be decreased to q 2-3 weeks when signs improve.
- For more stubborn cases, topical application of 50%-75% propylene glycol as a rinse daily, then decrease frequency as needed
- Options for more severe or refractory cases:
  - For effectively reducing sebaceous gland inflammation, alopecia, and follicular casts, cyclosporine 5 mg/kg PO q 24h for 4 months, then gradual dosage reduction that maintains clinical control (typically q 48h). A combination of systemic cyclosporine and topical treatments further improves the skin and coat condition.
  - Synthetic retinoids (isotretinoin, acitretin) 1-3 mg/kg PO q 12-24h until remission (approximately 6 weeks); then the lowest, most infrequent dose (reported effective in vizsla, variable results in other breeds). Hepatotoxicity, hypertriglyceridemia, and keratoconjunctivitis sicca are common, and monitoring is indicated. CAUTION: severe human and animal teratogen
  - Tetracycline and niacinamide each 250-500 mg/DOG PO q 8h, with or without concurrent vitamin A, have been tried with varied benefits.

Nutrition/Diet

- Omega-3 fatty acids PO q 24h (eicosapentaenoic acid 180 mg/5 kg body weight)
- Vitamin A 1000 IU/kg PO q 24h (only weak clinical evidence of benefit)

Drug Interactions

Combining cyclosporine (2.5-3 mg/kg PO q 24h) and ketoconazole (2.5-3 mg/kg PO q 24h) reduces dosage and associated cost of cyclosporine required to control the disease; monitor serum cyclosporine levels (p. 1333).

Recommended Monitoring

Animals receiving synthetic retinoids should have liver enzyme activity and triglyceride levels monitored q 1-2 months and tear production monitored q 3 weeks for first 2 months, then q 1-2 months. Animals receiving cyclosporine should be examined for gingival hyperplasia and have urinalysis performed q 6 months to screen for bacterial cystitis.

PROGNOSIS & OUTCOME

- Early diagnosis and treatment improve the prognosis for long-term control.
- Infection control with appropriate systemic and topical antimicrobial therapy is key in management of body odor and pruritus.
- Even though the disease is not lethal, dogs with SA are sometimes euthanized because the treatment is lifelong and labor intensive. A clinically and cosmetically acceptable result is sought but not always obtained.

PEARLS & CONSIDERATIONS

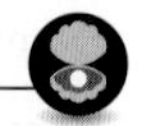

Comments

- Subclinical states of SA may progress with time. Early diagnosis can be made with skin biopsies.
- Hair regrowth can be straight rather than curled and of a different color in affected standard poodles.

Prevention

- Discourage the breeding of affected animals.
- Screening is performed by histologic analysis of at least two 6-mm biopsies taken from skin with scaling and hair loss or, if there are no lesions, on the dorsal midline between the neck and lumbosacral region (https://www.ofa.org/pdf/saapp_bw.pdf).

Technician Tips

Do not shave, scrub, or wipe with alcohol or antiseptic the biopsy site before performing skin punch biopsies because this can hamper diagnosis.

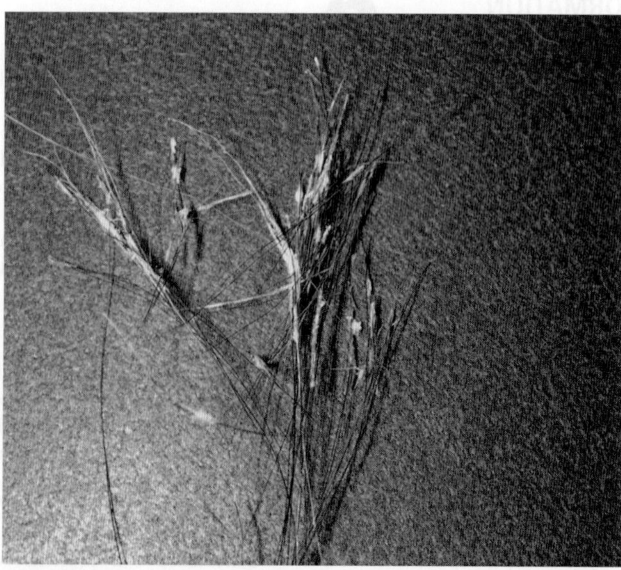

SEBACEOUS ADENITIS When hairs of patients with sebaceous adenitis are epilated, follicular casts adhere to hair shafts. (Courtesy Dr. Caroline de Jaham.)

Client Education

- Owner education about the chronic nature of the disease, varied response to therapies, and importance of infection control is essential to minimize client frustration.
- The Orthopedic Foundation for Animals (OFA) provides a database and guidelines on canine sebaceous adenitis (www.offa.org).

SUGGESTED READING

Miller WH Jr, et al: Muller & Kirk's Small animal dermatology, ed 7, St. Louis, 2013, Saunders, pp 695-699.

AUTHOR: Caroline de Jaham, DMV, MVSc, DACVD
EDITOR: Manon Paradis, DMV, MVSc, DACVD

Seizures

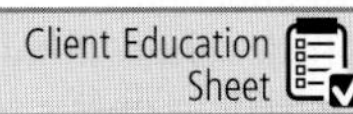

Client Education Sheet

BASIC INFORMATION

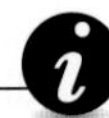

Definition

An epileptic seizure is a transient, paroxysmal disturbance in brain function characterized by increased neuronal excitability and synchronization. Clinical manifestations depend on the specific area(s) of the brain involved and can include alterations in consciousness, behavioral changes, involuntary motor activity, and autonomic signs.

Synonyms

Convulsion, ictus, fit

Epidemiology

SPECIES, AGE, SEX

- Dogs and cats, any age or sex
- In dogs, certain conditions are more likely based on age of seizure onset.
  - Congenital or anomalous conditions (e.g., hydrocephalus, portosystemic shunt): juvenile dogs
  - Idiopathic epilepsy: 6 months to 6 years
  - Intracranial neoplasia: older (median age in dogs, 9 years)

GENETICS, BREED PREDISPOSITION

- Idiopathic epilepsy: heritable in Australian shepherd, beagle, Belgian shepherd, Belgian Tervuren, Bernese mountain dog, border collie, Dalmatian, English springer spaniel, Finnish spitz, golden retriever, greater Swiss mountain dog, Irish wolfhound, keeshond, Labrador retriever, Lagotto Romagnolo, petit basset griffon Vendéen, standard poodle, Vizsla
- Other breeds are predisposed, but inheritance not yet discerned.

Clinical Presentation

DISEASE FORMS/SUBTYPES

- Generalized seizure: characterized by abnormal neuronal activity that originates from or rapidly involves networks in both cerebral hemispheres. It typically manifests as symmetrical tonic-clonic contractions of somatic muscles, altered consciousness, and autonomic discharge. Other generalized seizure types (atonic, myoclonic, absence) are less common in veterinary medicine.
- Focal seizure: originates in neuronal cortical or subcortical networks in an isolated area or single side of the brain. Typical clinical manifestations include involuntary movement of a region of the body or behavioral signs and can secondarily become generalized.

HISTORY, CHIEF COMPLAINT

- One or more episodes of transient (<5 minutes) neurologic impairment, which can include involuntary motor activity (single limb, face, jaw, or entire body), alteration in consciousness, and autonomic signs (salivation, urination, defecation, mydriasis, piloerection); signs occur most commonly at rest.
- Usually followed by a postictal period of ataxia, disorientation, fatigue, agitation, hunger, or blindness that can persist for minutes to hours.

PHYSICAL EXAM FINDINGS

- Usually normal
- Occasionally: findings are related to underlying cause of seizures (e.g., metabolic or cardiovascular disease).
- A complete neurologic exam (p. 1136) should be performed. Interictal neurologic abnormalities suggest an increased likelihood of underlying intracranial disease (neoplasia, inflammatory, vascular). However, a normal neurologic exam does not rule out structural disease because seizures are frequently the sole presenting sign.

Etiology and Pathophysiology

- Reactive seizures arise from extracranial causes, and metabolic (endogenous) or toxic (exogenous) disturbances secondarily impair normal brain function.
  - Metabolic disease: hypoglycemia, hypoxia, hepatic disease, renal disease, electrolyte disturbances, hyperlipidemia
  - Environmental toxins: heavy metals, ethylene glycol, pesticides, caffeine/methylxanthines, mycotoxins, others
- Epilepsy: recurrent seizures due to a primary intracranial abnormality
  - Idiopathic epilepsy: no underlying cause aside from a presumed genetic predisposition; likely due to defect at the molecular level
  - Structural epilepsy: associated with an identifiable congenital or acquired structural brain abnormality (neoplasia, inflammatory disease, congenital malformation, cerebrovascular disease)
  - Epilepsy of unknown cause: structural cause not identified, but age of seizure onset makes idiopathic epilepsy less likely

DIAGNOSIS

Diagnostic Overview

Seizures, being episodic, are usually not witnessed by the veterinarian. A thorough history should be obtained to help differentiate seizures from other episodic events and to aid in ranking possible causes. Blood tests are performed to evaluate for metabolic causes. Idiopathic epilepsy (p. 301) is the most common cause of seizures in dogs and is presumptively diagnosed based on signalment, normal physical and interictal neurologic exam, and unremarkable serum chemistry profile and CBC. Animals with suspected structural epilepsy based on interictal neurologic deficits should undergo brain MRI and cerebrospinal fluid (CSF) analysis.

Differential Diagnosis

- Syncope often occurs with exercise, is characterized by brief (seconds) loss of consciousness and muscle tone that are normal afterward; possible evidence of cardiovascular disease on exam
- Narcolepsy/cataplexy: often precipitated by excitement (play, feeding); abrupt onset of sleep and collapse, lasting seconds to minutes; normal after event
- Transient vestibular attacks: ataxia, disequilibrium, head tilt, nystagmus lasting seconds to hours; no loss of consciousness; can see disorientation after episode
- Behavioral (compulsive) disorders: possible triggers (fear, separation); characterized by vocalization, anxiety, chasing objects, chewing; duration minutes to hours
- Movement disorders: precipitated by activity, exercise, or stress; manifest as abnormal movement or muscle tone; no loss of consciousness; last seconds to hours

Initial Database

- Neurologic exam: often abnormal postictal; persistent interictal deficits raises suspicion for structural brain disease
- Fundic exam: examine for inflammatory disease, evidence of hypertension
- Blood pressure measurement: systolic blood pressure > 180 mm Hg, consider hypertensive encephalopathy
- CBC, chemistry profile, urinalysis: evaluate for metabolic disease
- Bile acid tolerance: screen for hepatic dysfunction
- Toxic screen: if indicated by history
- Infectious disease testing: recommended in cats (feline immunodeficiency virus [FIV], feline leukemia virus [FeLV], toxoplasmosis, cryptococcosis); performed in dogs as supported by history (canine distemper if unvaccinated, tick-borne disease, toxoplasmosis, neosporosis, systemic fungal disease)

Advanced or Confirmatory Testing

- Electrocardiogram (ECG): evaluate for arrhythmias to rule out syncope
- Ultrasound of brain: through open fontanelle to evaluate for ventriculomegaly, characteristic of hydrocephalus
- Electroencephalogram (EEG): necessary to confirm electrical activity in brain is characteristic of seizure; infrequently performed in veterinary medicine
- MRI of brain (p. 1132): evaluate for structural brain disease
- CSF analysis (pp. 1080 and 1323): evaluate for inflammatory disease

TREATMENT

Treatment Overview

Any identified underlying cause should be treated. Antiepileptic drugs are the mainstay of long-term seizure management, with seizure freedom being the primary goal. However, this is not achievable in most animals, and treatment is tailored to maximize seizure control with minimal medication-related adverse effects. An isolated seizure every 4-6 weeks is often considered acceptable. In most cases, therapy is lifelong.

Acute General Treatment

For cluster seizures or status epilepticus:

- Address emergent issues (ventilation, oxygenation, heart rate/rhythm, blood pressure, body temperature)
- Check blood glucose and electrolytes
  - If glucose < 60 mg/dL, administer 50% dextrose 0.5 g/kg diluted 1:3 in 0.9% NaCl as slow IV bolus
  - If total serum calcium < 7.0 mg/dL or ionized calcium < 0.8 mmol/L, administer 10% calcium gluconate 0.5-1.5 mL/kg IV over 20-30 minutes
- Administer a benzodiazepine; repeat up to 3 times as needed
  - Diazepam 0.5-2.0 mg/kg IV, per rectum, intranasal (IN)
  - Midazolam 0.1-0.3 mg/kg IV, 0.2-0.5 mg/kg IM
  - Lorazepam 0.2 mg/kg IV, IN
  - Can use benzodiazepine as constant-rate infusion (CRI) if seizure activity recurs after initial response
- Follow with a longer-acting (second tier) antiepileptic.
  - Phenobarbital 4-6 mg/kg IV; repeat q 30-120 minutes to achieve loading dose of 16-24 mg/kg, *or*
  - Levetiracetam 30-60 mg/kg IV
- If seizures persist, administer an anesthetic agent.
  - Propofol 1-4 mg/kg IV, then 0.1-0.6 mg/kg/min
  - Pentobarbital 3-15 mg/kg IV; then 0.5-4.0 mg/kg/h
  - Isoflurane 1%-2% minimal alveolar concentration (MAC)
  - Ketamine 5 mg/kg IV, then 5 mg/kg/h
- Animals with structural epilepsy: mannitol 0.5-1.0 g/kg or hypertonic saline 7.5%, 4 mL/kg; 3%, 5.3 mL/kg administered IV over 15-20 minutes if concerned about increased intracranial pressure

Chronic Treatment

- Treat any identified underlying cause.
- Guidelines for initiating maintenance antiepileptic drug therapy: seizure frequency > q 4-6 weeks, history of cluster seizures or status epilepticus, seizure severity
  - Phenobarbital 2.5-3.0 mg/kg PO q 12h (dog); 1.5-2.5 mg/kg PO q 12h (cat)
  - Bromide 30 mg/kg PO q 24h (dog); not recommended for cats due to potential adverse effect of bronchial constriction
  - Zonisamide 5-10 mg/kg PO q 12h (dog); 5 mg/kg PO q 12h (cat)
  - Levetiracetam (dogs, cats) 20 mg/kg PO q 8h

Drug Interactions

- Phenobarbital alters the disposition of other drugs metabolized by the hepatic cytochrome P450 system, including antiepileptic drugs (zonisamide, diazepam); a dosage adjustment may be necessary.
- Phenobarbital coadministration increases the clearance of levetiracetam in dogs.

Possible Complications

- With status epilepticus: hyperthermia, hypoxia, acidosis, hypotension, renal failure, disseminated intravascular coagulation, cardiopulmonary failure, brain edema, death
- With anticonvulsant drugs: see formulary for specific drugs

Recommended Monitoring

- Measure serum antiepileptic drug concentrations.
  - Phenobarbital: 2-3 weeks after dosage adjustment; q 6-12 months
  - Bromide: 1 and 3 months after dosage adjustment; q 6-12 months
  - Zonisamide, levetiracetam: not routine; performed as needed to optimize treatment
- Physical, neurologic exam, CBC, serum chemistry profile: annually
- Ask owner to keep log of seizure activity and notify if becoming more frequent or severe

PROGNOSIS & OUTCOME

- Reactive seizures: good to excellent; most conditions are reversible with toxin removal or correction of metabolic derangement, with exception of those due to neoplasia or end-stage organ dysfunction
- Idiopathic epilepsy: good; many dogs have normal life span, although at increased risk for premature death compared with general dog population
- Structural epilepsy: depends on cause and availability of definitive treatment; reported median survival of 4.5 years

PEARLS & CONSIDERATIONS

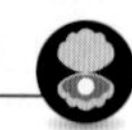

Comments

- Obtaining videotape of an episode can help discriminate seizures from other events, particularly those with unusual clinical manifestations.
- Seizures arising from a metabolic disturbance tend to respond poorly to acute treatment until the primary derangement (e.g., hypoglycemia, hypocalcemia) is corrected.
- For dogs prone to cluster seizures, a rescue protocol can be prescribed for home use; most commonly, a benzodiazepine (IN, rectal) in conjunction with additional oral doses of maintenance antiepileptic medication

Technician Tips

- Meticulous nursing care is important for animals hospitalized for recurrent seizures to avoid complications associated with recumbency (e.g., urine scald, aspiration pneumonia).
- Animals can paddle their limbs when recovering from the effects of recurrent seizures and antiepileptic medication, and this can look like a seizure. Observe for other subtle signs of seizure activity (e.g., salivation, orofacial muscle twitching) to help differentiate.

SUGGESTED READING

Moore SA: A clinical and diagnostic approach to the patient with seizures. Top Companion Anim Med 28:46-50, 2013.

AUTHOR & EDITOR: Karen R. Muñana, DVM, MS, DACVIM

Separation Anxiety

Client Education Sheet

BASIC INFORMATION

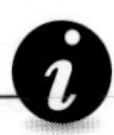

Definition

Physical or behavioral signs of distress are exhibited only in the absence of or lack of access to the client and can manifest as destruction, elimination, vocalization, withdrawal, salivation, pacing, freezing, or other forms. The term *separation distress* includes normal behaviors as well as the behavioral pathology of separation anxiety.

Epidemiology

SPECIES, AGE, SEX

- Prevalence estimated at 14% of dogs seen in the average U.S. private practice. In the absence of uniform screening, this may be an underestimate.
- Dogs reported > cats; age of onset usually overlaps with social maturity (dogs: 12-36 months; cats: 24-48 months).

RISK FACTORS

- Long absences (>4 hours) that leave the pet without human contact may increase risk of separation anxiety.
- Trauma during a client's absence (e.g., fire, burglary) can precipitate a sudden onset of separation anxiety.
- Rehomed dogs may be at increased risk. Repeated rehoming without treatment worsens fears of abandonment, and dogs with separation anxiety are frequently relinquished and rehomed.
- The popular beliefs that dogs with separation anxiety are spoiled, are only dogs, or have never learned to be left alone are incorrect.

ASSOCIATED DISORDERS

Phobias (p. 787) are commonly coexistent. Probabilities of separation anxiety given a diagnosis of storm or noise phobia are 87% and 88%, respectively.

Clinical Presentation

HISTORY, CHIEF COMPLAINT

- Complaints range from subtle to extreme
  - Destruction of property (e.g., chewed slipper, destroyed walls)
  - Inappropriate elimination (urine and/or feces)
  - Primary (e.g., chewing paw) or secondary (e.g., injury during escape attempt) mutilation
  - Vocalization (unless reported by neighbors, may go unrecognized)
  - Otherwise unexplained diarrhea (often assumed to have inflammatory bowel disease)
  - Signs often occur within 30 minutes of being left.
- Observant clients may notice manifestations of anxiety with signs of impending absence (e.g., putting on a coat).
- Some dogs become withdrawn; these patients are underdiagnosed but suffering.

PHYSICAL EXAM FINDINGS

- Self-induced injury: broken teeth; lingual, nasal, buccal, or cutaneous lacerations; torn or broken claws
- Abdominal palpation: evidence of ingestion of drywall, plastic, and other such items
- Often thin body condition: anxiety may increase activity (e.g., pacing)

Etiology and Pathophysiology

- Multiple mechanisms are likely given the wide variety of anxiety manifestations.
- Longer duration of the disorder may lead to additional or more intense manifestations and worse response to treatment.
- Dogs, like humans, may have susceptibility genes for the development of problematic anxieties.

DIAGNOSIS

Diagnostic Overview

The diagnosis is based entirely on history and, ideally, a video of behaviors after separation. Physical exam findings may be supportive.

Differential Diagnosis

- Generalized anxiety disorder (GAD), panic disorder: signs are similar to separation anxiety, but in patients with separation anxiety, signs occur only around owner's absence.
- Attention-seeking behavior (as a pathology): signs occur only in the owner's presence and generally improve with proper management (redirecting needy behaviors such as pawing can be redirected to retrieving a plush toy or to lying down for a massage; rewarding any offered good behavior by praise or interaction) and medication for profound anxiety.
- Incomplete housetraining: signs are confined to elimination and occur continually (daily for months or more), regardless of owner's presence.
- Age-associated destruction and elimination problems (puppy behavior or old age [cognitive dysfunction; physical compromise])
- Pseudocyesis-like reaction: destructive behavior is typically confined to bedding and responds to hormonal supplementation.
- Systemic medical conditions can produce changes in behavior, including hyperthyroidism (cats), hypothyroidism (dogs), neurologic disease (e.g., some seizure disorders, rare brain tumors, rabies), and urinary tract disorders.

Initial Database

- A complete and detailed history is the cornerstone of diagnosis.
- The most powerful diagnostic tool for separation anxiety is a video camera. Client should video the animal when left alone routinely.
  - Identification of distressed but nondestructive patients
  - Identification/ruling out provocative stimuli for destructive behavior
  - Assess improvement by comparison with a later video.
- Neurologic exam (p. 1136): no abnormalities expected
- CBC, serum biochemistry panel, urinalysis ± thyroid profile: typically unremarkable but may reflect chronic stress

Advanced or Confirmatory Testing

If neurologic signs are identified or develop, a full neurologic evaluation, including spinal fluid analysis and imaging (CT or MRI) may be indicated (pp. 1132 and 1136).

TREATMENT

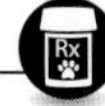

Treatment Overview

The ultimate goal is to allow the pet to be calm when left alone. Separation anxiety can be a veterinary emergency that harms the patient.

Acute General Treatment

- Until medications can take effect or if clients are unwilling to use medication, patients must not be left alone. Options include dog and cat sitters, day care, boarding, or bringing the patient to work.
- Ensure clients recognize signs of anxiety and associated reactivity and have them reward any spontaneous decrease in reactivity, even if they are staying home. Reward calm or happy behaviors.
- Implement behavior modification designed to teach the pet to relax. Substitute a new and calming rule structure for the pet that panics. Teach clients to avoid rewarding or punishing signs of anxiety. Accidental reinforcement of anxiety-related behaviors occurs frequently (e.g., think their frantic dog is just glad to see them and do not work to calm the greeting response).
- Clients should redirect signs of anxiety to a calmer behavior while actively engaging with the patient only if it is sitting calmly and quietly. Talking calmly, softly, and reassuringly can help induce calmer behaviors and ensure that the patient is not ignored. Clients can add to the behavior modification to teach the dog to sit and self-calm in a variety of increasingly complex contexts. After patients discover that they have a choice about reacting with distress, they can learn to exhibit contrasting behaviors. Patients should be rewarded with praise and food treats when calm.

- The pace of the behavior modification must proceed at an appropriate rate that allows improvement. If the patient is distressed, the owner is trying to progress too quickly or is not recognizing/rewarding the correct behaviors. Video the dog/client team.
- If panic, noise phobia, or storm phobia coexist (p. 787), consider
  - Alprazolam (dogs) 0.01-0.1 mg/kg (likely most effective range: 0.02-0.04 mg/kg) PO q 4-6h prn; (cats) 0.0125-0.025 mg/kg PO q 12-24h prn. NOTE: some published sources recommend a 10-fold higher dose, which is an error.
  - Diazepam (dogs) 0.5-2 mg/kg PO q 4-6h prn; (cats) 0.2-0.4 mg/kg PO q 12-24h prn, which is more sedative. Give one-half to a full dose 2 hours before the expected provocative event and repeat 30 minutes beforehand. Can give one-half to a full dose the night before and/or on awakening in the morning and then give the same dose 30 minutes before departure.
  - Clonidine 0.01-0.05 mg/kg PO q 12h (total daily amount typically 0.9 mg for most dogs) may help very reactive dogs.
  - Gabapentin 10-20 mg/kg (starting dose) PO q 8-12h can help many dogs in combination with other medications.
  - Dexmedetomidine (Sileo, Zoetis) can be used in dogs off-label for arousal associated with departure (125 mcg/m^2) (p. 609) given at least 30 minutes before leaving.

Chronic Treatment

- Dogs should be taught to relax while making eye contact with people as a new default behavior when the dogs encounter a situation about which they are anxious/unsure. Clients should learn to monitor facial cues, body postures, pupil size and shape, and respiratory behavior associated with relaxation. Periodic videotaping, reviewed by the clients with their veterinarian, is priceless.
- Avoid exposing dogs to circumstances likely to distress them (e.g., boarding dogs in a kennel).
- Desensitization to the triggers can be accomplished if two criteria can be met: triggers can be identified and are limited, and they can be reproduced faithfully in a systematic and incremental fashion. Many dogs learn to react earlier only if gradual departure desensitization programs are inappropriately conducted. Trainers may not appreciate this.
- Crates may represent entrapment to some patients and can make the patients worse. Use crates as part of treatment only if the pet enjoys the crate.
- After the patient has improved, it is important that the owners consistently continue the behavior modification. A decreased response to an inciting trigger is the desired goal.
- Humane treatment of separation anxiety likely requires long-term treatment with antianxiety medications.
  - Amitriptyline (minimum of 30 days) 1-2 mg/kg PO q 12h (dogs); 0.5-1 mg/kg PO q 12-24h (cats); tricyclic antidepressant (TCA) is drug of choice in mild cases.
  - Clomipramine (Clomicalm, Novartis, minimum of 8 weeks) 2-3 mg/kg PO q 12h (dogs); 0.5 mg/kg PO q 24h (cats); TCA licensed for use in separation anxiety and most successful when the behaviors have a ritualistic or elimination component
  - Selective serotonin reuptake inhibitors (SSRIs) (minimum of 8 weeks): fluoxetine (Prozac/Reconcile) 1 mg/kg PO q 24h (dogs); 0.5 mg/kg PO q 24h (cats) or sertraline (Zoloft) 1 mg/kg PO q 24h (dogs); 0.5 mg/kg PO q 24h (cats)
  - Polypharmacy (adding benzodiazepines, alpha-agonists, gabapentinoids) may help by combining prn and daily treatment.
  - Long-term treatment is the rule. When using medication with behavior modification, medications are typically continued at least 4-6 months.

Nutrition/Diet

Polyunsaturated fatty acids may help protect neurons from oxidative stress.

Behavior/Exercise

Regular aerobic exercise may help but is not a substitute for treatment.

Drug Interactions

- Benzodiazepines, TCAs, and SSRIs can be combined at lower-than-normal dosages if needed, but the potential for sedation and interaction must be evaluated.
- TCAs and SSRIs should not be given with monoamine oxidase inhibitors (MAOIs) that are found in many ectoparasite control products and in some cognitive dysfunction medications.

Possible Complications

- Abrupt cessation of medications with short half-lives is not recommended for TCAs and SSRIs; wean over 10-14 days.
- TCAs should be used cautiously or not at all in patients with heart disease.
- Cats and dogs receiving serotonergic medications rarely manifest serotonin-like syndromes with hyperactivity, unpredictability, and ultimately, seizures.

Recommended Monitoring

- Frequent and thorough communication between clinician and client is essential to allow treatment plan adjustment according to the patient's response.
- Physical exam and routine laboratory testing (CBC, chemistry profile, urinalysis) are repeated q 6 to 12 months for pets taking medications.
- To reduce risk of owner abuse of benzodiazepines, do not allow automatic refills, and schedule frequent follow-up appointments.
- Clients can monitor heart rate at home to detect tachycardia associated with anxiety or drug therapy.

PROGNOSIS & OUTCOME

- Prognosis is improved by early diagnosis, aggressive treatment, and dedicated clients.
- With chronic separation anxiety, treatment may be lifelong, especially if there are comorbid anxiety-related conditions.

PEARLS & CONSIDERATIONS

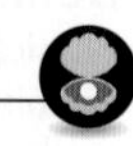

Comments

- If a veterinarian is not comfortable treating separation anxiety, the patient should be referred to a specialist immediately (www.dacvb.org for a listing in the United States). Screen for and treat any comorbid anxieties, especially those associated with noise.
- Dog trainers may have mistaken beliefs regarding separation anxiety that could do real harm.

Prevention

- Dogs obtained by rescue or from puppy mills should be screened aggressively for separation anxiety to facilitate early intervention.
- Veterinarians should inquire about behavioral problems as a routine part of every appointment. Left undiagnosed and untreated, separation anxiety worsens.
- Breeders should consider medical and behavioral issue when selecting breeding stock. Propensity for anxiety disorders is likely heritable.

Technician Tips

Technicians should review all signs of anxiety with clients, review patient video, and note improvement or worsening of signs. Resources include the Pet Professional Guild (www.petprofessionalguild.com) and the Society of Veterinary Behavioral Technicians (www.SVBT.org).

Client Education

- Pets with separation anxiety are distressed; they are not vindictive, jealous, spoiled, or disobedient.
- Under no circumstances should patients be punished or physically disciplined because it will increase anxiety.
- Treatment should be long term and often is lifelong.
- Relapses may occur with treatment discontinuation or added stressors. If stressors are anticipated, premedication may be helpful.
- Clients must understand and screen for comorbid anxieties so that they can be addressed.

SUGGESTED READING

King JN, et al: Results of a follow-up investigation to a clinical trial testing the efficacy of clomipramine in the treatment of separation anxiety in dogs. Appl Anim Behav Sci 89:233-242, 2004.

AUTHOR & EDITOR: Karen L. Overall, VMD, MA, PhD, DACVB

Sepsis and Septic Shock

Client Education Sheet

BASIC INFORMATION

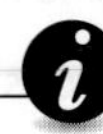

Definition

- *Sepsis* was classically defined as the systemic inflammatory response to infection. In 2016, the definition of sepsis in humans was revised to "life-threatening organ dysfunction caused by a dysregulated host response to infection," which was previously called *severe sepsis*. There is no consensus definition of sepsis in veterinary medicine.
- Sepsis is clinically identified in an animal that fulfills criteria for the systemic inflammatory response syndrome (SIRS) and has evidence of infection. In human medicine, the revised clinical definition of sepsis requires identification of an acute increase of ≥ 2 sequential organ failure assessment (SOFA) points as an indicator of organ dysfunction in addition to confirmed or suspected infection.
- *Septic shock* is sepsis with hypotension that is refractory to fluid therapy, requiring vasopressor therapy. The current clinical criteria for septic shock in human medicine is sepsis with hypotension requiring vasopressors to maintain mean arterial pressure (MAP) ≥ of 65 mm Hg and having blood lactate concentration > 2 mmol/L despite adequate volume resuscitation.

Epidemiology

SPECIES, AGE, SEX

Dogs and cats of any age and either sex; predispositions vary by cause:
- Sexually intact female dogs: pyometra
- Sexually intact male dogs: infectious prostatitis, orchitis
- Immunologic immaturity: increased risk of infection and subsequent sepsis in very young animals after maternal immunity wanes and before complete vaccination
- Immunoaging: increases risk of sepsis in geriatric patients.

RISK FACTORS

- Established infections
- Congenital or acquired immunodeficiency
- Treatment with immunosuppressive drugs
- Compromise of normal protective barrier functions by iatrogenic interventions or tissue damage (e.g., IV or urinary catheters, prolonged endotracheal intubation, burns)

CONTAGION AND ZOONOSIS

Particular pathogens causing sepsis in some animals may be contagious (e.g., canine parvovirus) or zoonotic (e.g., leptospirosis).

GEOGRAPHY AND SEASONALITY

Particular pathogens causing sepsis may have geographic (e.g., systemic mycoses) or seasonal (e.g., tick-borne pathogens) distribution.

ASSOCIATED DISORDERS

Multiple organ dysfunction syndrome (MODS [p. 665]), disseminated intravascular coagulopathy (DIC [p. 269])

Clinical Presentation

DISEASE FORMS/SUBTYPES

The manifestation of sepsis differs among patients in the location of the original infection and the organ dysfunctions that result. Clinical manifestation is also determined by a variety of host and pathogen factors, including the immunologic status of the host, genetics, and pathogen virulence.

HISTORY, CHIEF COMPLAINT

Complaints vary, depending on the source.
- Abdominal sources: vomiting, diarrhea, anorexia, signs of abdominal pain are possible.
- Thoracic sepsis: cough, respiratory distress
- Occult source: localizing signs may be absent; vague signs (e.g., anorexia, lethargy)

PHYSICAL EXAM FINDINGS

General:
- By definition (i.e., SIRS criteria), animals with sepsis have derangements in one or more of the following:
  - Fever (>39.4°C [>103°F]) or hypothermia (e.g., <37.8°C [<100°F])
  - Tachycardia (>120-140 beats/min in dogs; >220 beats/min in cats) or bradycardia (<80 beats/min in dogs, <160 beats/min in cats)
  - Tachypnea
- Abnormal perfusion parameters
  - Altered level of consciousness, heart rate, pulse quality, mucous membrane (mm) color, capillary refill time (CRT), and extremity temperature
  - Vasoconstrictive shock, when compensatory mechanisms (vasoconstriction in response to decreased cardiac output) are intact, is characterized by decreased level of consciousness (obtundation to stupor), progressive tachycardia, weak/absent peripheral pulses, pale mm, delayed CRT, and cold extremities
  - Vasodilation, occurring in distributive shock with loss of vasomotor tone, manifests as injected mm, warm extremities, and bounding pulses
- Collapse

Specific signs may indicate the source of infection:
- Signs of abdominal pain or distention (abdominal sepsis)
- Swollen limb or infected cutaneous wound or incision
- Lameness and joint effusion (e.g., infected joint)
- Dyspnea suggests pneumonia or pyothorax.
- Hematuria, stranguria, pollakiuria, or dysuria suggests a lower urinary tract source.
- Mucopurulent vulvar discharge suggests pyometra.
- Mucopurulent nasal discharge suggests respiratory tract infection.

Etiology and Pathophysiology

- Bacteria, viruses, fungi, and protozoa can cause sepsis.
- Localized immune and inflammatory responses are vital for successful pathogen elimination; a dysregulated host response results in the systemic derangements of sepsis.
- The immunologic response to infection involves recognition of pathogen-associated molecular patterns (PAMPs) by the innate immune response.
- Activated innate immune response produces inflammatory mediators such as cytokines (e.g., tumor necrosis factor-alpha, interleukin-1, interleukin-6), chemokines, and products of the complement cascade.
- Early proinflammatory cytokines recruit leukocytes to the site of infection to perform their phagocytic function. Cytokines also act on the hypothalamus to induce fever, activate downstream processes (e.g., coagulation, arachidonic acid cascade, production of acute phase proteins [e.g., globulins, C-reactive protein]), and induce nitric oxide synthase to produce nitric oxide. Nitric oxide–induced vasodilation contributes to distributive shock.
- Sepsis is also associated with increased microvascular permeability, resulting in leakage of fluid from the vascular space and reduced effective circulating volume.
- Shock (p. 911) can result from hypovolemic, cardiogenic, distributive, and/or obstructive causes.
- Decreased oxygen delivery to tissues contributes to cellular injury and MODS.

DIAGNOSIS

Diagnostic Overview

Sepsis should be suspected in a patient with an infection that fulfills the SIRS criteria. Septic shock should be considered in a septic animal that remains hypotensive despite adequate fluid resuscitation.

Differential Diagnosis

Causes of
- Fever (p. 334)
- Abdominal pain without infection (e.g., pancreatitis, nephro-/ureterolithiasis, neoplasia)
- Abdominal distention

Initial Database

- CBC: typically neutrophilia (± bands, toxic change) or neutropenia. Thrombocytopenia suggests DIC or vasculitis.

- Serum biochemistry panel
  - Azotemia may be prerenal, renal, or postrenal.
  - Elevated hepatocellular enzyme activities from primary hepatopathy, hepatic hypoperfusion, or bacterial showering from a compromised gastrointestinal (GI) tract
  - Hyperbilirubinemia
  - Hypoalbuminemia
  - Hypoglycemia (from consumption, changes in hepatic gluconeogenesis, and/or insulin-like growth factor production)
- Blood lactate concentration > 2 mmol/L is an important marker of shock in dogs with sepsis.
  - Hyperlactatemia often resolves quickly after initiation of IV fluid therapy.
  - Hyperlactatemia despite fluid resuscitation is a negative prognostic indicator.
- Urinalysis with culture and susceptibility (C&S) helps rule out urosepsis. Urine is obtained by cystocentesis for culture unless contraindicated (e.g., pyometra, coagulopathy).
- Coagulation testing (p. 1325) helps identify coagulopathy.
- Point-of-care testing for infectious diseases may include a vector-borne disease or parvovirus test in dogs, feline immunodeficiency virus/feline leukemia virus (FIV/FeLV) testing in cats
- Diagnostic imaging, including chest and abdominal radiographs, computerized tomography, and/or ultrasound, is often necessary to elucidate the source of sepsis.

Advanced or Confirmatory Testing

- Abdominocentesis (p. 1056) for abdominal effusion and SIRS. Neutrophilic inflammation with intracellular bacteria is diagnostic of septic effusion. Ascitic fluid glucose 20 mg/dL (1.1 mmol/L) or more below the blood glucose level can support a diagnosis of abdominal sepsis.
- Thoracocentesis (p. 1164) and cytologic evaluation; bacterial culture to identify pyothorax in animals with pleural effusion
- Consider transtracheal wash or bronchoalveolar lavage (pp. 1073 and 1074) for cytologic analysis and culture if radiographic evidence of pneumonia
- Echocardiography (p. 1094) if source of sepsis is difficult to identify, especially with a new-onset heart murmur. Valvular vegetative lesions suggest endocarditis. Echocardiography also is used for the diagnosis of secondary myocardial dysfunction.
- Blood cultures are indicated in any critically ill animal whose source of sepsis remains elusive despite routine testing.

TREATMENT

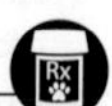

Treatment Overview

Treatment involves early IV antibiotics, identifying and treating shock, early aggressive source control, and supportive care (particularly for organ dysfunctions). A step-by-step approach to treatment is shown on p. 1448.

Acute General Treatment

Antibiotic treatment:

- Give appropriate antibiotics IV as early as possible. Empirically, consider broad-spectrum coverage, including drugs effective against gram-positive aerobes (e.g., ampicillin, amoxicillin + sulbactam, cefazolin), gram-negative aerobes (e.g., enrofloxacin, cefotaxime, amikacin), and anaerobes (e.g., metronidazole).
- Single-agent, broad-spectrum antibiotic therapy can also be considered with drugs such as ampicillin ± sulbactam, meropenem, or piperacillin + tazobactam.
- Antimicrobial treatment is adjusted per C&S results.

Hemodynamic stabilization:

- Treat shock: intravascular volume expansion with isotonic crystalloids (e.g., lactated Ringer's solution) is the mainstay of therapy; colloids may be indicated for animals with hypoalbuminemia. Fluid resuscitation should continue to effect to normalize perfusion parameters, heart rate, lactate, blood pressure, and mentation.
- Vasopressor therapy for septic shock is indicated if hypoperfusion persists despite appropriate fluid therapy; consider dopamine 6-15 mcg/kg/min IV, norepinephrine 0.05-2 mcg/kg/min IV, or vasopressin 0.5-5.0 mU/kg/min IV. The Surviving Sepsis Guidelines in human medicine recommend norepinephrine as first-line vasopressor. Vasopressors should ideally be given through a central venous catheter (can be commenced through a peripheral catheter until a central line can be placed) and titrated based on direct arterial blood pressure monitoring to achieve a MAP ≥ 65 mm Hg.
- If decreased myocardial contractility is present by echocardiography, dobutamine 5-15 mcg/kg/min (dogs) or 1-5 mcg/kg/min (cats) may be required; may cause seizures in awake cats.

Source control:

- As soon as possible after hemodynamic stabilization; may include drainage of abscesses or thorax, surgical thoracotomy, celiotomy, arthrotomy, or an exploratory procedure

Support of organ function:

- Supplemental oxygen (p. 1146) if hypoxemia; mechanical ventilation (p. 1185) if PaO_2 < 60 mm Hg despite oxygen supplementation
- GI dysfunction: injectable antacids (e.g., famotidine, pantoprazole), antiemetics (e.g., maropitant, dolasetron/ondansetron, metoclopramide), and/or oral gastroprotectants (e.g., sucralfate)
- Oligoanuric acute kidney injury (p. 23) may require pharmacologic therapy (e.g., furosemide, fenoldopam, or mannitol to encourage urine output) or renal replacement therapy.
- Hemorrhage associated with DIC or the need for surgery in a patient with prolonged clotting times is an indication for fresh-frozen plasma transfusion (p. 1169). It is not recommended to give plasma for prolonged clotting times in the absence of clinical bleeding. Conversely, a hypercoagulable state, especially with evidence of thromboembolism, may be an indication for anticoagulation.

Nutrition/Diet

After stabilization, enteral nutrition (pp. 1106 and 1107) is considered superior to parenteral nutrition (p. 1148) to preserve gut function and integrity.

Possible Complications

Organ dysfunction, thromboembolism, and intractable hypotension leading to cardiac arrest

Recommended Monitoring

- Heart rate/rhythm, pulse quality, blood pressure, mentation, respiratory rate/effort, and body temperature: continuously, hourly, or as indicated by case evolution
- Direct arterial blood pressure monitoring is recommended for patients receiving vasopressors
- Continuous electrocardiogram (ECG [p. 1096]): all animals with arrhythmias
- Hematocrit, total protein, blood glucose, lactate, and electrolyte concentrations: at least daily
- Urine output: at least q 4h
- Body weight as a guide to fluid balance: at least daily
- Fluid cytology from indwelling closed suction drains: daily (a fresh sample of effusion should be acquired for cytology, versus collection directly from the drain balloon)

PROGNOSIS & OUTCOME

- Mortality rates for sepsis in animals is 30%-70% and increases with increasing number of dysfunctioning organs
- Severity of underlying disease and provision of early, intensive, and appropriate therapy are important factors influencing mortality.

PEARLS & CONSIDERATIONS

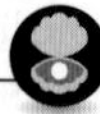

Comments

Delayed recognition of sepsis (and specifically delayed administration of antibiotics) can result in increased morbidity and mortality.

Prevention

- Treat infections aggressively before they progress to sepsis.
- Take precautions to prevent nosocomial infection (e.g., good hand hygiene, use of aseptic technique for procedures, removing indwelling devices as soon as possible).

Technician Tips

Close patient monitoring, ideally with continuous monitoring devices, is essential; any deterioration in patient status should be communicated to the veterinarian immediately.

SUGGESTED READING

Lewis DH, et al: The immunopathology of sepsis: pattern recognition, systemic inflammation, the compensatory anti-inflammatory response, and regulatory T cells. J Vet Intern Med 26(3):457-482, 2012.

AUTHOR: Claire R. Sharp, BVMS, MS, DACVECC
EDITOR: Benjamin M. Brainard, VMD, DACVAA, DACVECC

Diseases and Disorders

Shearing/Degloving Wounds

Bonus Material Online Client Education Sheet 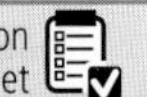

BASIC INFORMATION 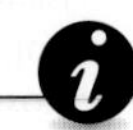

Definition

Traumatic soft-tissue injury commonly associated with the limbs and tail

Epidemiology

SPECIES, AGE, SEX

Dogs and cats, any age, either sex

RISK FACTORS

Roaming; areas with high automobile traffic (vehicular trauma is the primary cause)

Clinical Presentation

DISEASE FORMS/SUBTYPES

Any of the following is possible: laceration, contusion, crushing, shearing, penetration, perforation, avulsion, thermal injury, bite wound

HISTORY, CHIEF COMPLAINT

- An open wound, bleeding, or swelling of the injured area
- Necrotic tissue
- Absence or avulsion of tissue and underlying tissues: exposure of bone
- Purulent discharge
- Lameness in association with limb injury
- The patient may display pain by vocalization, guarding the injured area, or defensive posturing.

PHYSICAL EXAM FINDINGS

- Open wounds
  - Skin laceration
  - Partial or complete loss of skin and underlying tissues
  - Avulsion or partial detachment of skin segments
  - Necrotic tissue
  - Exposure of tendons, ligaments, bones, and joints
  - Varied development of granulation tissue in older wounds
- Evidence of hemorrhage
- Intact skin with the presence of contusion (ecchymosis/bruising)
- Local swelling due to edema, hematoma formation
- Condition and viability of the digital and metacarpal/metatarsal pads; severity of tissue trauma
- Evidence of underlying orthopedic injury
  - Fracture
  - Joint instability associated with soft-tissue trauma and bone loss
  - Partial, tangential loss of bone and cartilage
- Pain with manipulation of the affected limb(s)
- The overall health status of the animal depends on a variety of factors, including body region(s) involved, extent of trauma, degree of circulatory compromise, blood loss, and presence of necrotic tissue/infection.

Etiology and Pathophysiology

- Wounds are the result of the transfer and absorption of energy by the body; severity depends on the type of trauma and surface area(s) absorbing it.
- Lacerations are the result of contact with a sharp, bladelike object (e.g., glass, metal) or impact against a hard-edged surface such as a curb. Bite wounds may create an irregular laceration as a result of the cutting and tearing of tissues.
- Crushing wounds are the result of compression, either from impact with a heavy object or contact with a mechanical device or from a powerful bite.
- Cutaneous surfaces may be stripped or avulsed from the extremity, damaging the circulation to the traumatized skin segment (typically from vehicular or bite trauma).
- Shearing wounds are the result of tangential impact with a hard surface, dragging of a body region on a hard road surface, or entrapment of an extremity beneath the tire of a moving vehicle.
- Accurate assessment of tissue circulation at the time of injury can be incomplete. Progressive loss of circulation can result in vascular stasis and necrosis that may not be evident for 4 or more days after the initial injury.

DIAGNOSIS 

Diagnostic Overview

The diagnosis is made from the history and physical exam findings, although the full extent of bony lesions and other internal injuries may be appreciated only with radiographs and/or ultrasound.

Differential Diagnosis

- Vehicular trauma
- Bite wounds
- Penetrating/perforating objects (gunshot, impalement)
- Sharp objects
- Thermal injuries, including contact burns (muffler/engine contact)

Initial Database

- CBC, serum biochemistry profile, urinalysis: provides baseline; various abnormalities; can suggest concomitant injury (e.g., azotemia due to urinary rupture from vehicular trauma)
- Radiographs (two orthogonal views) of the injured area to rule out orthopedic trauma
- Thoracic radiographs to rule out diaphragmatic hernia, lung contusions, pneumothorax, and fractured ribs from vehicular trauma
- Bacterial culture and susceptibility of infected wounds to select the most appropriate antibiotic

Advanced or Confirmatory Testing

As indicated by the severity and type of trauma

TREATMENT 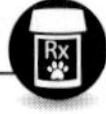

Treatment Overview

Treatment goals:

- Provide hemodynamic stability before anesthesia; other injuries (e.g., pneumothorax, diaphragmatic hernia) may exist.
- Assess severity of soft-tissue and orthopedic injury.
- Assess wound for tissue viability.
- Provide definitive wound care and closure if indicated.
- Prevent or manage infection.
- Stabilize local fractures or joint instability.

Acute General Treatment

- Consider sedation, pain medication, muzzling, or placing an Elizabethan collar to reduce the risk of being bitten.
- Cover open wounds with a sterile dressing.
- Initiate systemic antibiotic therapy: empirical therapy for broad aerobic coverage (e.g., cefazolin 22 mg/kg IV q 90 minutes perioperatively), then based on bacterial culture and sensitivity
- General anesthesia is preferable for definitive wound care because manipulation of the affected area can be painful.
  - Regional nerve blocks can be used for patient comfort.
- Liberally remove fur from around the circumference of a shearing wound.
- Povidone iodine or chlorhexidine surgical scrub is used for preparing the skin, alternated with swabbing the area with sterile-saline–impregnated sponges.
- Aseptically drape the wound.
- Explore the wound and remove nonviable tissue and foreign debris; perform copious lavage of the wound with sterile saline to remove contaminants.
  - Chlorhexidine solution (1:40 dilution) or povidone iodine solution (1:9 dilution) may be added to the sterile saline.
- Gentle pressure lavage is useful to remove contaminants, using a fluid bag and pressure cuff or a 35-mL syringe and 18-gauge needle (moderate pressure only).
- In the absence of infection and necrotic tissue (creating a surgically clean wound)
  - Skin borders can be approximated with sutures.
  - Partial closure or delayed primary closure if substantial incisional tension and/or unresolved edema

  - Wound drainage (drains, or leaving a portion of the wound open for drainage)
- Joint injury associated with shearing wounds
  - Repair collateral ligament damage (screws/anchor + suture material/surgical steel wire); persistent instability may warrant arthrodesis.
  - Perform copious lavage for open joints; in the absence of infection, the joint capsule can be closed if sufficient tissue is available.
- With extensive bruising and swelling, open wound management should be considered until circulation improves, evidenced by resolution of these two conditions.
- Open wound management varies with severity of trauma and extent of the wound. Common options include
  - Judicious surgical debridement with resection of nonessential tissues of questionable viability
  - Especially with extremity wounds, it is advisable to delay debridement of skin of questionable viability (daily reassessment) due to the limited availability of loose elastic skin to facilitate wound closure.
  - Important tissue structures of questionable viability should be managed conservatively until their status becomes apparent. If necrotic, debridement is instituted.
  - Wet-to-dry dressings are a form of mechanical debridement that may be used in the setting of extensive contamination/local infection. Cotton sponges are moistened with saline (or dilute povidone iodine or chlorhexidine [see above]) and are placed onto the wound. Residual necrotic tissue adheres to the cotton fibers along with partial retention of the exudate. Stripping the partially dry dressing off the wound helps remove this debris. Consider using for 3-4 consecutive days to achieve mechanical debridement. Use sedation and analgesics, including topical lidocaine, as needed to reduce the pain of dressing removal and replacement.
  - Negative-pressure wound therapy is an alternative method of managing problematic open wounds after surgical debridement and lavage to remove necrotic tissue and contaminants.
  - Other suitable dressing and topical agents include
    - Hydrogel and hydrocolloid products (topical application or as an occlusive dressing)
    - Occlusive dressings (most effective when a healthy granulation bed is forming and infection/tissue necrosis is absent)
    - Absorptive dressings, including the alginates (to promote healing and provide a matrix to absorb exudate, especially in the early days of open wound care)
    - A thick layer of honey (especially manuka honey; sterile honey dressings are available) or sugar; these substances are antibacterial and hydrophilic
    - Nonadherent/low-adherent dressings with a topical antimicrobial ointment or gel to create a (partially) occlusive environment
  - A protective bandage is required to maintain a topical dressing, with thicker absorptive bandages initially for better retention of discharge from highly exudative wounds.
    - Typically, bandage changes are needed daily (1-2 times) over the first week of open wound management, then less frequently over the subsequent weeks as discharge decreases.
    - Occlusive dressings are normally changed according to the manufacturer's guidelines and the judgment of the clinician (usually q 3-5 days) when applied to a healthy wound bed. Any protective bandage is changed accordingly.
  - Large open wounds may require closure with skin grafts or skin flaps if wound closure by contraction/epithelization is unlikely.
    - Remember that edema and the elastic retraction of the skin exaggerate wound size, especially during the first week of wound care. With resolution of swelling, the wound is often appreciably smaller.
    - In general, wounds affecting less than 90 degrees of the extremity's circumference may heal by second intention in 6-8 weeks after injury.
  - Extensive extremity trauma with severe circulatory compromise and tissue necrosis usually necessitates amputation. The total cost of limb salvage (treatment without amputation) plays a role in the decision-making process with many pet owners.

Chronic Treatment

- Bandage and dressing changes
- Progressive loss of circulation secondary to trauma requires serial wound debridement that may include digit amputation. Severe loss of blood supply over time may necessitate limb amputation.
- Extensive skin loss, especially involving the lower extremities, may require closure with skin grafts or skin flaps. Loss of the metacarpal or metatarsal pads may require reconstruction with digital pad transplantation.
- Osteostixis can be used to facilitate granulation tissue coverage over viable exposed bone surfaces. This may be useful in preparing the wound for skin graft application.
- Arthrodesis may be necessary to correct chronic instability of the carpal and tarsal joints involved in extensive shearing wounds.
- Wound contracture secondary to excessive scarring may warrant surgical intervention (skin graft/flap application) and physical rehabilitation to reestablish regional range of motion.
- Formation of a fragile scar may result in repeated injury to the thin epithelial surface; skin grafting or skin flaps may be required.
- Failure to completely heal usually necessitates wound closure with a skin graft or flap.
- Platelet-rich plasma (PRP) has been used to improve the processes of second intention closure in open wounds that have failed to close in a timely fashion.

Possible Complications

- Infection of the soft tissues, underlying bone, or exposed joint
- Failure to heal
- Persistent instability of a shearing wound involving a joint
- Associated fracture nonunion
- Formation of a fragile scar surface that is subject to reinjury

Recommended Monitoring

- Bandage care and periodic wound assessment
- Serial radiographs to assess bone healing as needed

PROGNOSIS & OUTCOME

- Prognosis is generally good for return to function for mild to moderate shearing injuries with appropriate wound care.
  - Many shearing wounds heal by second intention.
- Prognosis is guarded to good for extensive shearing injuries, depending on degree and severity of the injury.
  - Massive trauma to the extremities may necessitate limb amputation.
  - The need for amputation may not be immediately apparent, as in cases with extensive loss of tissue viability over time or development of severe osteomyelitis.

PEARLS & CONSIDERATIONS

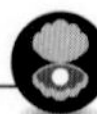

Comments

- Most cases of soft-tissue trauma that are presented to veterinarians are relatively simple to manage.
- Early tissue edema and the elastic retraction of the traumatized skin margins exaggerate the size of the wound.
- Initial partial wound closure, when possible, reduces the magnitude of the granulation bed and helps promote faster closure by second intention healing.
- In the face of infection, open wound management provides optimal drainage and facilitates daily inspection of the entire wound.
- Combined closure techniques can be used effectively together. In some cases, wounds can be supported while second intention healing progresses. If the wound does not close within 8 weeks, the wound likely will be smaller; closure may be accomplished with a smaller local flap or skin graft.
- In general, the goal of wound care is to promote formation of a healthy wound bed. In open wound management, the formation

of granulation tissue is a key indicator of underlying tissue viability. Moreover, the wound may be a suitable candidate for surgical closure.

- With the formation of a healthy granulation bed, systemic antibiotics are usually discontinued unless infection is present.
- Surgical closure of problematic wounds may be more cost-effective than prolonged open wound management.

Prevention

Confining a pet to the house or yard or pet restraint by leash dramatically reduces risks associated with vehicular trauma, bites, and malicious injury.

Technician Tips

- Understand bandage care to optimize patient management; monitor for strike-through, wet, or slipped bandages, swollen digits, odor, and patient discomfort.
- Always wear gloves when handling a bandage/wound.

Client Education

- Treating open wounds can take several weeks. A frank discussion on time and cost commitments is necessary.
- In open wound management, many willing owners can be trained to perform simple bandage changes and manage wound drains to reduce costs.

SUGGESTED READING

Pavletic MM: Atlas of small animal wound management and reconstructive surgery, ed 4, Ames, IA, 2018, Wiley-Blackwell.

AUTHOR: Michael M. Pavletic, DVM, DACVS
EDITOR: Elizabeth A. Swanson, DVM, MS, DACVS

Shock, Hypovolemic

BASIC INFORMATION

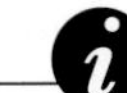

Definition

Decreased circulating blood volume resulting in insufficient tissue oxygen delivery

Synonyms

- Hemorrhagic shock
- Relative hypovolemic or distributive shock is caused by normal blood volume that is inappropriately distributed in the vasculature.

Epidemiology

SPECIES, AGE, SEX

All species, ages, and both sexes

RISK FACTORS

- Behaviors that increase risk of trauma
- Concurrent disease that can increase fluid loss or decrease fluid intake

ASSOCIATED DISORDERS

- Blood loss: trauma, neoplasia (e.g., hemangiosarcoma), coagulopathy, ulcer
- Increased fluid loss: kidney disease, diabetes mellitus/insipidus, hypoadrenocorticism or hyperadrenocorticism, vomiting/diarrhea
- Decreased fluid intake: intracranial disease, starvation

Clinical Presentation

DISEASE FORMS/SUBTYPES

Whole blood volume loss (i.e., hemorrhage) or plasma fluid volume loss (i.e., secondary to renal or gastrointestinal [GI] loss)

HISTORY, CHIEF COMPLAINT

Acute collapse is common. Other complaints can include trauma (internal/external hemorrhage), abdominal distention, or vomiting/diarrhea.

PHYSICAL EXAM FINDINGS

- Quiet or dull mentation
- Pale mucous membranes with prolonged capillary refill time (CRT > 2 seconds)
- Tachypnea
- Tachycardia (bradycardia in cats); dogs with decompensatory shock may display bradycardia.
- Weak or thready pulses, which may be bounding in some cases of compensatory shock
- Distended abdomen (e.g., hemoperitoneum)
- Signs of severe dehydration: tacky mucous membranes, enophthalmos, decreased skin turgor

Etiology and Pathophysiology

Hypovolemic shock is always secondary and can be caused by whole blood loss (external or internal hemorrhage) or plasma fluid loss (commonly of GI or renal origin)

Pathophysiology of hypovolemic shock:

- Blood or fluid loss leads to decreased circulating volume, which at significant levels (>20% loss) causes decreased tissue perfusion resulting in inadequate delivery of oxygen and nutrients to tissues.
- Without enough oxygen, cells convert from aerobic to anaerobic metabolism, resulting in decreased adenosine triphosphate (ATP) produced for each molecule of glucose and increased lactate production.
- Decreased cellular energy (ATP) leads to cellular enzyme failure and cell injury/death that can lead to organ dysfunction.

DIAGNOSIS

Diagnostic Overview

History and physical exam:

- Possible sources of blood or fluid loss
- Shock
    - Tachycardia, tachypnea, and potentially normal pulse pressure and blood pressure (BP): compensatory shock
    - Bradycardia, hypothermia, weak/thready pulses, low BP, variable respiratory rate, hypothermia: decompensatory shock
- Other exam parameters: dull mentation, pale mucous membranes, prolonged CRT, and abdominal distention with a fluid wave

Differential Diagnosis

- Distributive shock (e.g., obstructive, neurogenic, and septic)
- Cardiogenic shock
- Hypoxemia from primary respiratory disease
- Metabolic shock (e.g., hypoglycemia and carbon monoxide or other toxins)
- Dehydration without shock that requires rehydration over time, not immediate fluid boluses

Initial Database

- BP: systemic hypotension (p. 1065) (systolic arterial pressure < 90 mm Hg) is consistent with decompensated hypovolemic shock.
- Packed cell volume/total protein (PCV/TP): decreased PCV/TP may indicate blood loss; increased PCV/TP likely indicates dehydration. Peracute blood loss may show a normal PCV and low TP due to splenic contraction.
- Blood glucose: exclude hypoglycemia as cause of shock.
- CBC and serum biochemistry profile: electrolyte disturbances may be present with vomiting or upper GI obstruction (e.g., hypochloremia). Thrombocytopenia may indicate immune-mediated destruction (p. 972) or a consumptive coagulopathy (p. 269).
- Urinalysis: evaluate for infection or decreased concentrating ability (associated with urinary fluid loss and subsequent hypovolemia)

- Coagulation profile: severely prolonged coagulation times may raise concerns about anticoagulant rodenticide ingestion, and mildly prolonged times are consistent with a consumptive coagulopathy
- Abdominal and thoracic ultrasound: focused assessment of sonography for trauma (FAST) (p. 1102) is used to quickly identify intracavitary bleeding, evaluate intravascular volume status, and exclude other causes of shock (e.g., heart failure). Full abdominal ultrasonography may be indicated to evaluate extent of intraabdominal neoplasia, assess cause of vomiting or diarrhea, and plan surgical treatment.
- Abdominal and thoracic radiographs: evaluate for effusions or GI disease/obstruction, as well as heart and blood vessel size
- If fluid present, abdominocentesis (p. 1056)/ thoracocentesis (p. 1164) with fluid analysis (p. 1343): avoid if risk of anticoagulant rodenticide exposure; otherwise, a hemorrhagic effusion suggests intracavitary hemorrhage as the cause of hypovolemia.
- Echocardiography: complete evaluation of heart disease and intracardiac volume status

Advanced or Confirmatory Testing

Blood lactate level (p. 1356): hyperlactatemia (>2.5 mmol/L) is an easy and reliable measure of the degree of hypovolemic shock. Must be differentiated from elevated lactate due to hypoxia, trembling, seizures, or struggling during restraint for venipuncture, and type B hyperlactatemia, as with diabetes mellitus, neoplasia, sepsis, toxins, or hypoglycemia.

TREATMENT

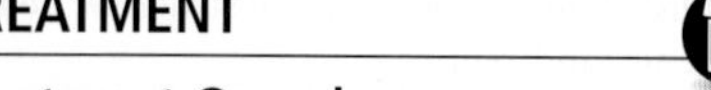

Treatment Overview

- Primary goal is to restore circulating volume and tissue perfusion. This usually means rapid and continued IV fluid or blood product administration with frequent re-evaluation of patient status.
- Early determination of the need for surgical intervention is essential. Otherwise, chasing severe, ongoing, intraabdominal hemorrhage with crystalloids and blood, rather than surgical intervention perpetuates shock in the face of ongoing hemorrhage.
- Specific treatment of underlying disease (e.g., plasma and vitamin K_1 for anticoagulant rodenticide toxicity) is critical.
- A step-by-step approach to treatment is described on p. 1449.

Acute General Treatment

- Restoration of intravascular volume
    - Crystalloids: isotonic replacement fluids (e.g., lactated Ringer's solution, Normosol-R) 20-30 mL/kg IV boluses (typically over 15-20 minutes) and repeated as necessary to stabilize physical exam parameters
    - Synthetic colloids (e.g., VetStarch, hetastarch) 5-10 mL/kg IV boluses to reach desired effect (up to 50 mL/kg/day for VetStarch and 20 mL/kg/day for hetastarch)
    - Blood transfusions (p. 1169): initiated early if blood loss is cause of hypovolemia; packed red blood cells 10 mL/kg or 20 mL/kg of fresh whole blood. Calculations can estimate the expected increase in PCV from transfusion, assuming that further blood loss is absent.
    - Plasma transfusions: if coagulopathy is cause of bleeding or to prevent dilutional coagulopathy if large quantities of crystalloid fluids (e.g. > 80 mL/kg) are given. Typically, 10 mL/kg but repeated doses may be required until normalization of coagulation times if treating coagulopathy.
- Often, fluid type is not as important as expedient return of adequate circulating volume, but the cause of hypovolemia and results of laboratory testing (e.g., PCV/TS and electrolytes) may inform fluid selection.
- Fluid therapy is goal-directed to correct abnormal exam parameters and hypotension, if present. Central venous pressure (CVP) may be useful to monitor intravascular volume status. Serial blood lactate measurements can be made during resuscitation to monitor for resolution of shock.

Chronic Treatment

- Medical and/or surgical control of inciting cause
- Fluid replacement must continue past initial stabilization to meet ongoing loss and maintenance fluid needs and should be adjusted for the individual patient.

Possible Complications

Prolonged shock can cause acute kidney injury, loss of GI integrity with bacterial translocation, myocardial dysfunction, cerebral hypoxia, loss of vascular tone, systemic inflammatory response syndrome, disseminated intravascular coagulation, acute respiratory distress syndrome, and sepsis.

Recommended Monitoring

- Serial physical exams focused on previously abnormal findings after each resuscitative treatment is crucial.
    - Return of normal mucous membrane color and CRT and improvement in mentation is a fast and reliable indicator of return to adequate perfusion.
    - If tachycardia does not resolve, but other parameters do, evaluate for other causes, such as anxiety or pain.
- Serial BP monitoring: target is systolic arterial pressure (SAP) > 90 mm Hg for initial resuscitation.
    - In acute hemorrhage, when surgical intervention is planned, a lower endpoint (SAP > 60-70 mm Hg) can be used to avoid rebleeding that can occur with a large increase in vascular pressure (i.e., low-volume/hypotensive resuscitation).
- Serial CVP monitoring is best used for individual patient trends during fluid resuscitation, but vascular volume is generally adequate if CVP > 8 cm H_2O.
- Monitor PCV/TP for evidence of ongoing hemorrhage and need for transfusions.
- Serial blood lactate measurements can be made during resuscitation to monitor resolution of shock.

PROGNOSIS & OUTCOME

- Depends on cause of hypovolemia and the rapidity with which the volume deficit has been corrected
- Prolonged shock may cause multiple organ dysfunction (p. 665), which carries a poor prognosis.

PEARLS & CONSIDERATIONS

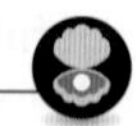

Comments

- Hypovolemic shock requires early identification and treatment to avoid life-threatening secondary organ damage.
- Dull mentation, pale mucous membranes, tachycardia (bradycardia in some cats and dogs with decompensatory shock), hypotension, and a known cause of blood or fluid loss are hallmarks of the clinical diagnosis of hypovolemic shock.
- Elevated blood lactate level concentration can indicate inadequate tissue oxygen delivery, and normalization can provide an endpoint for resuscitation.

Technician Tips

Repeated reassessment is of utmost importance to ensure adequate resuscitation (and not over-resuscitation). Physical parameters (mentation, heart rate, BP, pulse quality, mucous membrane color, and CRT) should be rechecked serially, and clinicians should be alerted when parameters are persistently abnormal.

SUGGESTED READING

Pachtinger GE, et al: Assessment and treatment of hypovolemic states. Vet Clin North Am Small Anim Pract 38(3):629-643, 2008.

AUTHOR: Gary Puglia, DVM, DACVECC
EDITOR: Benjamin M. Brainard, VMD, DACVAA, DACVECC

Shoulder Luxation

Bonus Material Online Client Education Sheet 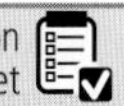

BASIC INFORMATION 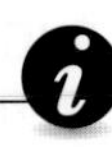

Definition

Traumatic or congenital separation of the scapulohumeral joint

Epidemiology

SPECIES, AGE, SEX

- Traumatic luxation
  - Any dog or cat
- Congenital luxation
  - Toy/small-breed dogs
  - Puppies or young adults

RISK FACTORS

Congenital: laxity of the soft-tissue supporting structures and/or deformity of the glenoid and humeral head

Clinical Presentation

DISEASE FORMS/SUBTYPES

- Congenital
  - Medial luxation
- Traumatic
  - Medial or lateral luxation
  - Rarely cranial or caudal luxation

HISTORY, CHIEF COMPLAINT

- Congenital
  - Intermittent or continuous lameness without trauma
- Traumatic
  - Acute lameness after trauma

PHYSICAL EXAM FINDINGS

- Congenital
  - Intermittent or continuous lameness
  - Flexion, abduction, and external rotation of the distal forelimb
  - Variable shoulder pain
- Traumatic
  - Continuous non–weight-bearing lameness
  - Shoulder pain and crepitus
  - Medial luxation: flexion, abduction, and external rotation of the limb
  - Lateral luxation: flexion, adduction, and internal rotation of the limb
  - Other findings related to the traumatic event are often identified.

Etiology and Pathophysiology

- Congenital
  - Laxity in the medial supporting structures (joint capsule, collateral ligament, and subscapularis tendon)
  - Dysplasia of the glenoid cavity (shallowing, erosion of medial rim) and humeral head (flattening)
  - Often bilateral
- Traumatic
  - Caused by a jump/fall or blunt trauma while bearing weight
  - Rupture of the supporting soft tissues (joint capsule, collateral ligament, cuff tendons) results in luxation.

DIAGNOSIS 

Diagnostic Overview

Diagnosis relies on shoulder palpation and radiographic confirmation.

Differential Diagnosis

- Periarticular fracture
- Shoulder instability/subluxation
- Bicipital tenosynovitis
- Supraspinatus tendinosis
- Infraspinatus contracture
- Neoplasia
- Nerve root or brachial plexus injury

Initial Database

- Orthopedic exam (p. 1143)
  - Displacement of the greater tubercle relative to the acromion process
  - Laxity on shoulder drawer test
  - Increased abduction angle (>45 degrees)
- Neurologic exam (p. 1136)
  - Rule out deficits in trauma patients
- Radiographs
  - Document luxation and direction, rule out concurrent fractures, and allow assessment of dysplasia.
  - Stress radiographs document dynamic instability.
  - Thoracic radiographs rule out concurrent injury in trauma patients.
- Clinical pathology: CBC, chemistry, urinalysis
  - Possibly elevated alanine aminotransferase (ALT), aspartate aminotransferase (AST), or anemia in trauma patients

Advanced or Confirmatory Testing

CT, MRI, and/or musculoskeletal ultrasound: sometimes indicated to rule out other differentials and assess degree of periarticular soft tissue damage

TREATMENT 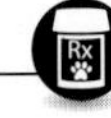

Treatment Overview

Treatment is focused on restoring joint congruity and stability to resolve lameness and pain.

Acute General Treatment

Traumatic luxation:

- Closed reduction: extend the limb and apply pressure on the humeral head toward the glenoid cavity while maintaining counterpressure on the scapular neck.
- Open reduction and stabilization
  - Performed when closed reduction is not possible or luxation recurs
  - Joint is stabilized through prosthetic ligament reconstruction with nonabsorbable sutures passed through bone anchors or tunnels at the origin/insertion of the damaged glenohumeral ligament; can be performed arthroscopically or arthroscopically assisted
  - Transposition of the biceps tendon in the direction of the damaged glenohumeral ligament has also been used to provide stability.
- After closed or open reduction
  - Lateral luxation: support joint with a spica splint.
  - Medial luxation: apply a Velpeau sling or use a shoulder support brace with hobbles (Shoulder Stabilization System, DogLeggs).
  - Maintain external support for 2-12 weeks, depending on type of support and patient energy level and tolerance.
  - Crate confinement with gradual increase in leash walks over 12 weeks, followed by a gradual return to normal activity
  - Physical rehabilitation: initially gentle flexion/extension exercises if permitted by external coaptation, followed by muscle strengthening exercises later in recovery period. Abduction/adduction should be avoided.

Congenital luxation:

- Closed reduction
  - Typically unsuccessful due to dysplasia
  - If luxation is intermittent and closed reduction is possible, application of a shoulder support brace (Shoulder Stabilization System, DogLeggs) may provide sufficient stability.
- Open reduction may be unsuccessful due to dysplasia.

Alternative procedures for congenital luxation or failed repair of a traumatic luxation:

- Shoulder arthrodesis: spica splint and crate confinement until complete fusion is documented
- Glenoid excision arthroplasty: activity is gradually increased with exercises to strengthen the periarticular musculature.

Chronic Treatment

Long-term management of osteoarthritis:

- Ideal body condition
- Regular, low-impact exercise
- Chondroprotectant therapy (omega-3 fatty acids, glucosamine/chondroitin sulfate supplements, glycosaminoglycan therapy)
- Rehabilitation therapy to strengthen shoulder cuff tendons and maintain joint mobility
- Nonsteroidal antiinflammatory therapy as needed for pain relief
- Ancillary modalities: platelet-rich plasma (PRP), stem cell therapy, laser therapy, therapeutic ultrasound, extracorporeal shock wave therapy, acupuncture

Behavior/Exercise

Muscle strengthening exercises in the later recovery period, avoiding abduction/adduction with increased movement of the scapula and limb circumduction.

Possible Complications

- Reluxation with closed reduction or implant failure
- Infection
- Traumatic or iatrogenic nerve injury
- Mid-substance biceps tearing after transposition

PROGNOSIS & OUTCOME

Closed and open treatment of traumatic cases generally results in a good outcome, with resolution or only occasional lameness for the majority of patients. Some degree of osteoarthritis is anticipated. Excision arthroplasty and shoulder arthrodesis can result in acceptable function with increased movement of the scapula and limb circumduction.

PEARLS & CONSIDERATIONS

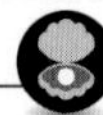

Comments

- Amputation is contraindicated with bilateral shoulder instability or dysplasia.
- Shoulder support brace (Shoulder Stabilization System, DogLeggs) is ideal for external support of closed and open reductions.
  - Minimal morbidity allows for longer use
  - Temporary removal permits passive range-of-motion therapy.

Technician Tips

A Velpeau sling must be applied with great care to avoid neurovascular damage to the distal limb.

Client Education

Any attempts of self-mutilation or malodor associated with bandages should prompt early return for a bandage change.

SUGGESTED READING

Kunkel K, et al: A review of lameness attributable to the shoulder in the dog: part one. J Am Anim Hosp Assoc 44:156, 2008.

AUTHOR: Courtney Fitzpatrick, DVM, DACVS
EDITOR: Kathleen Linn, DVM, MS, DACVS

Shoulder Soft-Tissue Injuries

Video Available 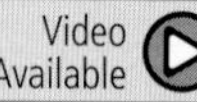 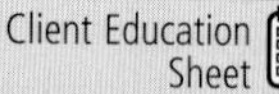 Client Education Sheet 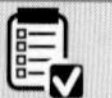

BASIC INFORMATION

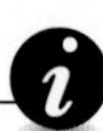

DEFINITION

Injuries to the ligaments, joint capsule, and tendons of the shoulder. These injuries are fairly common in dogs but tend to be underdiagnosed.

Synonyms

Biceps tenosynovitis, supraspinatus calcifying tendinopathy, supraspinatus tendinopathy, collateral ligament tears, rotator cuff injuries

Epidemiology

SPECIES, AGE, SEX

Adult dogs of both sexes

GENETICS, BREED PREDISPOSITION

Most common in medium to large working and sporting dogs; toy- and small-breed dogs are prone to shoulder instability and luxation secondary to glenoid dysplasia.

ASSOCIATED DISORDERS

Lameness (pp. 571 and 1249)

Clinical Presentation

DISEASE FORMS/SUBTYPES

- Supraspinatus tendinopathy
- Biceps tendinopathy
- Medial and lateral glenohumeral ligament disruptions
- Subscapularis tendon tears
- Infraspinatus myopathy, contracture

HISTORY, CHIEF COMPLAINT

Forelimb lameness is the primary complaint; may range from mild to non–weight-bearing status

PHYSICAL EXAM FINDINGS

The key to diagnosing soft-tissue shoulder lameness is a systematic forelimb lameness exam. Compare the affected forelimb with the unaffected one. Perform these tests with the dog awake and again under sedation; persistence of pain under sedation makes findings more compelling.

- Palpate shoulder for swelling.
- Check position of the greater tubercle of the humerus and the acromion process of the scapula relative to each other.
  - Lateral shoulder luxation: greater tubercle is lateral to acromion.
  - Medial luxation: greater tubercle is medial to acromion.
  - If the shoulder joint is lax, the anatomic landmarks may or may not be out of position, depending on whether the shoulder is in a reduced or luxated position.
- Extend and flex the shoulder (if it is grossly stable), being careful to minimize manipulation of the elbow. Check for a pain response, and see if the shoulder can flex and extend in a straight line.
  - Infraspinatus contracture causes the humerus to be externally rotated.
  - Pain is a feature of many shoulder injuries, but a pain response may be absent even with an injury.
- Isolated full flexion of the shoulder: fully flex the shoulder with minimal manipulation of the distal limb. Many patients with shoulder discomfort show a response to this test and not to other tests.
- Flex the shoulder while slowly extending the elbow: pain response suggests biceps tendinopathy (see first *Video*).
- Apply direct pressure over the insertion of the supraspinatus tendon on the proximal medial humerus: pain response suggests supraspinatus tendinopathy.
- Palpate for medial to lateral and cranial to caudal laxity, comparing shoulders.
- Abduction test: with the dog in lateral recumbency and with the shoulder extended, abduct the humerus. Excessive abduction compared with the normal side suggests medial glenohumeral ligament injury (see second *Video*).
  - Some toy breeds have bilateral medial instability, and there is not a normal contralateral side.

Etiology and Pathophysiology

- Biceps and supraspinatus tendinopathies can result from acute injury or chronic repetitive strain.
- Infraspinatus contracture is thought to start after an acute injury to the muscle, which may create a compartment syndrome.
- Glenohumeral ligament tearing can be purely traumatic or associated with conformational tendency for instability/luxation (toy breeds).

DIAGNOSIS

Diagnostic Overview

- Physical exam: key to diagnosis of all shoulder problems; often makes the diagnosis of infraspinatus contracture, gross instabilities, and luxations
- Ultrasonography: useful for diagnosis of myopathies, supraspinatus and biceps tendinopathies
- MRI (p. 1132): useful for diagnosis of tendinopathies and glenohumeral ligament tears

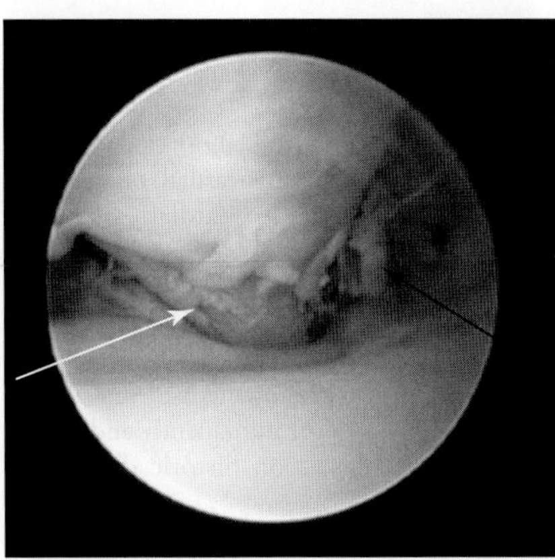

SHOULDER SOFT-TISSUE INJURIES Arthroscopic image of chronic canine biceps tendinitis. Note disruption of tendon fibers *(white arrow)* and hypertrophied synovial fronds *(black arrow).*

- Arthroscopy: used for confirming diagnosis of biceps tendonitis, glenohumeral ligament tears, and subscapularis tearing

Differential Diagnosis

- Immune-mediated and septic arthropathies
- Elbow lameness
- Cervical nerve compression
- Neoplasia involving scapula, humerus, or brachial plexus

Initial Database

- Systematic orthopedic exam (p. 1143)
- Shoulder radiographs: useful for ruling out problems such as proximal humeral osteosarcoma and fractures. Changes tend to be nonspecific (mild degenerative changes) for many soft-tissue shoulder injuries. Some findings suggest a specific diagnosis:
  - Calcification cranial to the greater tubercle on lateral projections: supraspinatus tendinopathy. However, this is also a common incidental finding unassociated with lameness.
  - Blunting, enthesopathy, or small avulsions from the supraglenoid tubercle suggest injury to the biceps origin.
  - Calcification in the intertubercular groove on a skyline view suggests biceps tendinopathy.
- Elbow radiographs: taken to rule out elbow disease, which can be difficult to distinguish from shoulder disease on physical exam

Advanced or Confirmatory Testing

- Ultrasound, MRI, and arthroscopy
- Arthrocentesis if inflammatory arthropathy is a differential diagnosis

TREATMENT

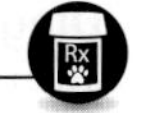

Treatment Overview

Many soft tissue shoulder injuries resolve with time. Surgical treatment should be considered when lameness persists for more than 2 months despite rest and and conservative treatment.

Acute General Treatment

- Biceps tendinopathy
  - Mild: antiinflammatory and analgesic medication (p. 218)
  - Controlled exercise (6 weeks) and rehabilitation
  - Intraarticular injection of sodium hyaluronate, repositol corticosteroid, and/or platelet-rich plasma
  - Stem cell therapy may be helpful; efficacy not yet established
- Supraspinatus tendinopathy
  - Antiinflammatory and analgesic medication (p. 218)
  - Physical rehabilitation
  - Shock wave therapy
  - Stem cell therapy, platelet-rich plasma injections may be considered
- Glenohumeral ligament instability, subscapularis tears
  - Mild or acute injury: medical treatment as for biceps tendinopathy
  - Bracing to limit abduction for medial instability reported but untested for efficacy (p. 913)
  - Degenerative joint disease may progress, depending on patient size and degree of instability.

Chronic Treatment

- Biceps tendinopathy: for severe cases or cases that do not respond to conservative therapy, biceps tendon release (can be done arthroscopically or by small arthrotomy); biceps tenodesis
- Supraspinatus tendinopathy: removal of mineralized material in the supraspinatus insertion by longitudinal tendinotomies; resection of diseased portion of insertion
- Glenohumeral ligament instability: prosthetic ligament stabilization, with or without arthroscopy

PROGNOSIS & OUTCOME

Prognosis and outcome depend on the specific injury, its extent, and the treatment involved. In most reports, success rates are 60%-80% for surgical treatment of biceps and supraspinatus tendinopathies, subscapularis tears, and glenohumeral ligament instabilities.

PEARLS & CONSIDERATIONS

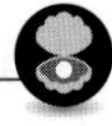

Comments

- Soft-tissue injuries of the shoulder are treatable and relatively easy to diagnose. The most important factor is a careful physical exam followed by the appropriate diagnostic imaging technique.
- Supraspinatus calcification is a common incidental finding on radiographs of asymptomatic dogs; this radiographic finding does not prove that lameness is due to supraspinatus tendinopathy. Other diseases should be ruled out by further diagnostic testing.
- Most soft-tissue shoulder injuries come with nonspecific radiographic findings at best; it is prudent to rule out elbow disease (with radiographs and possibly with CT and arthroscopy) in cases where diagnosis is challenging.

Technician Tips

When clipping the patient for arthroscopic biceps tendon release, make sure that the cranial extent of the prep goes up to the caudal aspect of the mandible. This prep allows easy maintenance of the sterile field while the release is performed.

SUGGESTED READING

Rochat MC: The shoulder. In Tobias KM, et al, editors: Veterinary surgery: small animal, St. Louis, 2012, Elsevier, pp 692-708.

AUTHOR: Andrew E. Sams, DVM, MS, DACVS
EDITOR: Kathleen Linn, DVM, MS, DACVS

Sick Sinus Syndrome

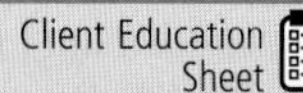

BASIC INFORMATION

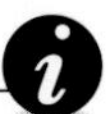

Definition

Sick sinus syndrome (SSS) produces a spectrum of cardiac arrhythmias that represent diffuse cardiac conduction system disease and disorders of impulse generation. Variable degrees of sinoatrial (SA) nodal dysfunction (sinus bradycardia, sinoatrial block, or sinus arrest) and/or atrioventricular (AV) nodal dysfunction are common. Because subsidiary pacemakers often display depressed automaticity, prolonged episodes of sinus arrest are accompanied by periods of asystole and syncope. Some dogs have episodes of supraventricular tachycardia alternating with bradyarrhythmias, producing the so-called bradycardia-tachycardia syndrome. Increased autonomic tone plays a role in some cases. It is one of the two most common indications for cardiac pacemaker implantation in dogs. The disease can be divided into symptomatic (SSS) or asymptomatic (sinus node dysfunction).

Synonyms

Sinus node dysfunction (SSS), bradycardia-tachycardia (brady-tachy) syndrome, chronotropic incompetence, sinoatrial syncope, sinoatrial node disease

Epidemiology

SPECIES, AGE, SEX

Small-breed, older dogs

GENETICS, BREED PREDISPOSITION

Middle-aged to older, female miniature schnauzers are most commonly afflicted. West Highland white terriers and cocker spaniels and their crosses are also overrepresented.

ASSOCIATED DISORDERS

Because of their similar breed and age predispositions, SSS and chronic degenerative valvular disease often occur at the same time. However, there is no known causative link between the two.

Clinical Presentation

HISTORY, CHIEF COMPLAINT

Sinus node dysfunction may be recognized because of sinus bradycardia on routine exam or during general anesthesia. Clinical signs associated with SSS include syncopal/seizure-like episodes or, less commonly, episodic weakness. Some animals with severe, long-standing sinus bradycardia may develop congestive heart failure (CHF) and are presented with respiratory distress.

PHYSICAL EXAM FINDINGS

- Bradyarrhythmia with prolonged episodes of asystole (due to sinus arrest without activation of subsidiary AV or intraventricular pacemakers) is classic.
- Paroxysms of tachycardia followed by pauses (brady-tachy syndrome) may be detected.
- Varied-intensity, left apical systolic murmurs of mitral insufficiency are common but unrelated (small breed, older dogs).
- Exam may be normal if high sympathetic tone associated with veterinary visit overcomes bradycardia; this may obscure the diagnosis.

Etiology and Pathophysiology

- The etiologic basis for SSS in dogs has not been determined.
- Fibrosis and/or fatty infiltration with atrophy of the SA node have been identified in humans and dogs with SSS.
- The absence of morphologic abnormalities in some humans with sinus node dysfunction suggests that alterations of neural innervation or neural regulation may contribute to the bradyarrhythmias.
- Autoantibodies to proteins isolated from sinus node cells have been identified in humans, suggesting an immune-mediated process in some cases.
- Changes in ion channels, often sodium, or gap junctions within the sinus node may account for the development of SSS in humans.
- Occlusion or sclerodegenerative changes of the sinus node artery rarely play a role in the development of this disease.

DIAGNOSIS

Diagnostic Overview

The two most common clinical contexts that would raise the suspicion of this disorder are a history of syncope in a dog of a susceptible breed and incidental discovery of contextually inappropriate bradycardia. The diagnosis is confirmed electrocardiographically. In some patients, an in-hospital resting electrocardiogram (ECG [p. 1096]) is sufficient; in others, the intermittent nature of the arrhythmia mandates the use of telemetry or ambulatory ECG (p. 1120).

Differential Diagnosis

Other bradyarrhythmias:

- High-grade second-degree AV block
- Third-degree AV block
- Persistent atrial standstill
- Vagally mediated bradyarrhythmias
- Metabolic disorders that slow SA nodal activity
  - Hyperkalemia (p. 495)
  - Hypothermia (p. 523)
  - Hypothyroidism (p. 525)
  - Dysautonomia
- Seizures of any cause (p. 903)

Initial Database

- ECG: essential to characterize the bradyarrhythmia and diagnose SSS
  - Although exact criteria have not been established for the diagnosis of SSS, sinus arrest with or without various degrees of AV block or supraventricular tachycardia raises suspicion.
- Atropine response test can determine whether the bradyarrhythmia is vagally (entirely or partially) mediated. If vagally mediated (i.e., physiologic), the test reveals increased heart rate. If pathologic, there is no change in the ECG.
  - Obtain initial ECG.
  - Administer atropine 0.04 mg/kg IV, IM, or SQ. Obtain follow-up ECG approximately 10 minutes later (if administered IV) or 20-30 minutes later (if IM or SQ).
  - An increase of at least 50% in the heart rate is expected when the bradycardia is vagally mediated (i.e., physiologic). A positive atropine response test predicts the success of medical treatment.
  - The absence of any response to atropine in a dog with appropriate signalment and clinical signs is strongly suggestive of SSS.
- CBC, serum chemistry profile, and urinalysis to detect underlying electrolyte imbalances or metabolic disorders that may contribute to bradyarrhythmias or seizures.
- Thoracic radiographs: cardiomegaly or CHF may develop in the face of long-standing bradyarrhythmias, especially when complicated by degenerative valvular disease in older small-breed dogs.
- Echocardiography (p. 1094) can assess the severity of valvular, myocardial, or structural (including neoplastic) cardiac disease, if present.

Advanced or Confirmatory Testing

- Video recording of episodes by the owner may help differentiate syncope from seizures if the episodes occur infrequently and cannot be classified based on historic description alone.
- A 24-hour Holter monitor or cardiac event monitor may be indicated in cases when the history, clinical signs, ECG, and atropine response test are inconclusive. A Reveal/Linq device (ECG loop recorder) can be implanted when episodes are very infrequent.

TREATMENT

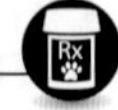

Treatment Overview

- Dogs showing no overt clinical signs (incidentally discovered arrhythmia): periodic monitoring and client education to detect progression of disease
- Dogs showing overt clinical signs such as syncope
  - Bradycardia: increase the heart rate to alleviate the syncopal episodes using medical therapy or pacemaker implantation.
  - Brady-tachy syndrome: bradyarrhythmia should be addressed before starting therapy aimed at reducing the supraventricular tachycardia (p. 96).

Acute General Treatment

- In the absence of syncope, significant cardiomegaly, or CHF, periodic ECGs and client education are indicated. General anesthesia should be avoided, or if unavoidable, temporary cardiac pacing should be available.
- Dogs showing overt clinical signs
  - Vagolytic drugs display variable and often temporary efficacy in animals with SSS, although a positive atropine response helps predict the likelihood of success for medical therapy. One option is to begin with a sympathomimetic agent (e.g., theophylline, terbutaline), and if clinical signs persist, add a parasympatholytic (anticholinergic such as propantheline).
    - Theophylline 10 mg/kg PO q 8h
    - Terbutaline (instead of theophylline) 1.25-5 mg/kg PO q 8-12h
    - Propantheline bromide 0.25-0.5 mg/kg PO q 8h
  - Pacemaker implantation: dogs with overt clinical signs caused by SSS that fail to respond or become refractory to positive chronotropic drugs require permanent cardiac pacing.

Chronic Treatment

- Positive chronotropic drugs: if animals are responsive, therapy is maintained lifelong;

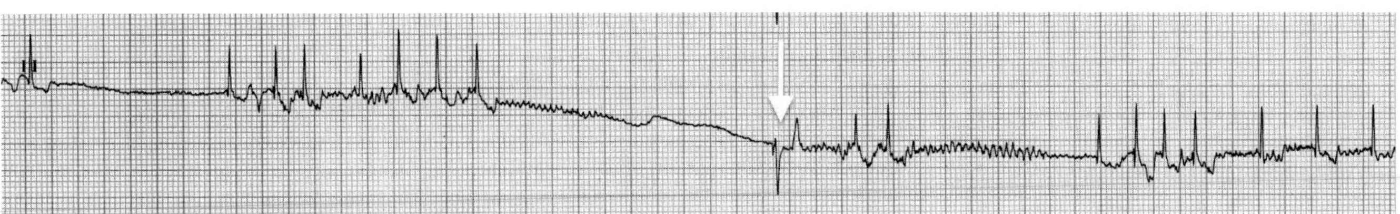

SICK SINUS SYNDROME Electrocardiogram for an 8-year-old miniature schnauzer with sick sinus syndrome. Note the long pauses and ventricular escape complex *(arrow)* followed by periods of supraventricular tachycardia. Lead II, 25 mm/s and 1 cm/mV.

some dogs become refractory over time and may require a pacemaker.
- Pacemaker therapy: biannual re-evaluations with annual pacemaker interrogation are indicated. Because this population tends to be older, battery life is not usually an issue.

Drug Interactions

Theophylline:
- Arrhythmias may develop when used with additional sympathomimetic agents.
- Cimetidine, erythromycin, allopurinol, thiabendazole, clindamycin, and lincomycin may increase its effects.
- Phenobarbital or phenytoin may decrease its effects.
- Enrofloxacin or ciprofloxacin inhibit the metabolism of theophylline and may promote toxicosis.

Possible Complications

- Administration of sympathomimetic agents: nervousness/anxiety, hyperactivity, vomiting, diarrhea, polyuria and polydipsia (PU/PD), and anorexia. Administration of anticholinergic drugs (e.g., propantheline): dry mouth, dry eyes, urinary hesitancy, constipation, and vomiting
- Pacemakers: lead dislodgement, infection, seroma formation, failure to sense or oversensing, ventriculoatrial conduction, caval obstruction, or skeletal muscle stimulation (if a unipolar pacemaker is implanted)

Recommended Monitoring

- ECG: periodic monitoring or as dictated by recurrence of syncopal episodes
  - Incidentally discovered: q 3-4 months to evaluate for progression of bradyarrhythmia-tachyarrhythmia; atropine response test may have to be repeated.
  - Overt clinical signs: whether medical therapy or pacemaker implantation has been performed, ECGs should be repeated q 6 months to assess the long-term response to vagolytic agents or appropriate functionality of the pacemaker.
  - If clinical signs recur, re-examination including ECG is indicated immediately.
- Thoracic radiographs: q 6 months, especially in the face of valvular disease; assessment for progressive cardiomegaly and CHF; assessment of the integrity of the pacemaker
- Pacemaker interrogation: at 1 and 6 months, followed by annual interrogations; evaluation of the pacing and sensing threshold, lead impedance, and battery life

PROGNOSIS & OUTCOME 

- The risk of sudden death with SSS appears low, and some affected animals never develop clinical signs.
- If syncope occurs, the episodes tend to increase in frequency over time, and the risk of sudden death may increase.
- Medical therapy is usually well tolerated, although the response is variable and in some cases is short-lived.
- The prognosis and response to therapy after successful pacemaker implantation are good for animals with SSS. Episodes of syncope often resolve, animals become more suitable anesthetic candidates, and episodes of supraventricular tachycardia can be managed with medications if necessary.

PEARLS & CONSIDERATIONS 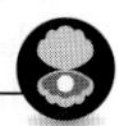

Comments

- SSS should always be on the differential list for older miniature schnauzers, West Highland white terriers, and cocker spaniels that display syncope or seizure-like activity.
- A normal heart rate at the time of exam does not exclude SSS.
- Even in the absence of syncope during Holter monitoring, many animals with SSS display significant and prolonged episodes of sinus arrest. Analysis of the Holter recording is still warranted when no episodes have occurred during the monitoring period.
- Although ventricular-based pacemakers readily alleviate the clinical signs, atrial-based pacing may be the most appropriate if AV nodal function is normal.

Technician Tips

Seizures and syncope can be very similar in appearance, and the underlying cause is difficult to confirm. Seizures often have a preictal and/or postictal period of altered behavior, whereas syncope does not.

Client Education

- Response to medical therapy may be short-lived.
- Artificial pacemaker implantation is most commonly performed by a transvenous approach, markedly reducing the pain and recovery time for older dogs.

SUGGESTED READING

Ward JL, et al: Outcome and survival in canine sick sinus syndrome and sinus node dysfunction: 93 cases (2002-2014). J Vet Cardiol 18:199-212, 2016.

AUTHOR: Simon Swift, VetMB, MA, DECVIM
EDITOR: Meg M. Sleeper, VMD, DACVIM

Sinusitis and Other Sinus Disorders

Bonus Material Online 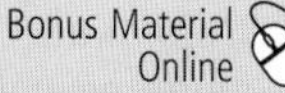

BASIC INFORMATION 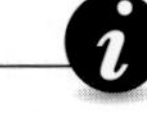

Definition

Mucosal inflammation, or other disease, associated with one or more of the sinuses: the frontal or maxillary sinuses in dogs and the frontal or (less commonly) sphenoidal sinuses in cats

Epidemiology

SPECIES, AGE, SEX

Cats:
- No sex predisposition
- Chronic idiopathic rhinosinusitis: young to middle age
- No age or sex predisposition for upper respiratory tract aspergillosis (both sinonasal and sino-orbital forms)
- Sinus tumors: older animals
- Trauma: any age

Dogs:
- No sex predisposition

- Tumors associated with frontal sinusitis: older dogs
- Aspergillosis: young adults
- Chronic idiopathic sinusitis: young to middle-aged dogs
- Cilary dyskinesia: young dogs
- Trauma: any age

GENETICS, BREED PREDISPOSITION

- Cats: brachycephalic breeds, especially Persian and Himalayan for upper respiratory tract aspergillosis (both sinonasal and sino-orbital forms), any breed for other diseases
- Dogs: primarily dolichocephalic breeds for frontal sinusitis associated with tumors, aspergillosis, or chronic idiopathic sinusitis

ASSOCIATED DISORDERS

- Nasal tumors
- Nasal aspergillosis
- Chronic idiopathic or lymphoplasmacytic rhinosinusitis
- Nasal or frontal sinus trauma
- Abscessation of roots of the upper fourth premolar (apical dental abscess), causing maxillary sinus empyema
- Feline herpesvirus (rhinotracheitis)

Clinical Presentation

DISEASE FORMS/SUBTYPES

See Associated Disorders above.

HISTORY, CHIEF COMPLAINT

- Nasal discharge
- Intermittent sneezing
- Focal facial swelling or deformity (tumor, trauma)
- Signs related to local pain
  - Dullness or lethargy
  - Decreased movements of the head
  - Anorexia

PHYSICAL EXAM FINDINGS

- Unilateral nasal discharge of variable nature: mucoid, mucopurulent, or blood tinged; often bloody with nasal neoplasia
- Diminished airflow through nasal passages/nares if nasal cavity affected, except aspergillosis (increased airflow)
- Focal swelling, firm enlargement, facial deformity, and/or pain with atrophy or lysis of the frontal or nasal bones:
  - Depressions or defects in frontal/nasal bone integrity from osteolysis may be noted during palpation.
  - Dogs with maxillary sinusitis from fourth premolar tooth root abscessation may have a swelling or fistulous tract and drainage ventral to the eye on affected side.
- Enlargement of submandibular lymph nodes is possible. Both lymph nodes may be affected due to overlapping drainage territories (lymphosomes).
- Percussion of the sinus may induce pain or be associated with reduced resonance.

Etiology and Pathophysiology

- Sinusitis is usually secondary to another primary nasal or frontal sinus disease (see Associated Disorders) that disrupts normal nasal/sinus anatomy and impairs mucociliary clearance or obstructs mucus drainage.
- Due to physical continuity between the chambers, frontal sinus tumors can extend into the nasal cavity, and nasal tumors can extend in the frontal sinus.
- Mycotic sinusitis and rhinitis can affect the nasal cavity and sinus individually or in combination. Periorbital involvement is seen in cats.
- Chronic lymphoplasmacytic inflammation in dogs can be a sequela to many other sinonasal diseases (p. 890).
- Chronic lymphoplasmacytic rhinosinusitis in cats can be a sequela to bacterial, viral (feline upper respiratory tract infection complex), as well as mycotic infections.
  - As in dogs, the condition can be idiopathic in cats, possibly related to an allergic cause.
- Primary bacterial rhinitis is rare, with most bacterial infections occurring secondary to an underlying disease process. The exception is bacterial rhinitis associated with ciliary dyskinesia, which results in recurrent bouts of sinusitis, rhinitis, and pneumonia due to defective mucociliary clearance.

DIAGNOSIS

Diagnostic Overview

Sinus diseases are generally associated with nasal diseases and probably secondary to nasal disease in most cases.

Differential Diagnosis

Nasal diseases of various origins:

- Fungal rhinitis
- Nasal neoplasia
- Dental disease/dental root infection (maxillary sinus)
- Foreign bodies
- Lymphoplasmacytic rhinitis
- Nasal mites
- Chronic viral upper respiratory tract infection in cats

Initial Database

- For some cases, plain radiographs of the nasal cavities, sinuses, and dental roots can be helpful in the diagnosis of trauma or structural lesions secondary to neoplasia, fungal rhinitis/sinusitis, and dental disease but cannot discriminate among the various causes of nasal/sinus disease not involving structural changes. Generally considered both poorly sensitive and poorly specific.
- CBC, serum biochemical profile, and urinalysis are often unremarkable.
- For cases in which there is swelling or lysis (which can be palpable) of nasal/facial bones or the frontal sinus area, fine-needle aspiration (FNA) cytology can show neoplasia or inflammation.
- Submandibular lymph node aspirates (bilateral) may help detect metastatic neoplasia.

Advanced or Confirmatory Testing

- CT and/or MRI of the nasal cavities and sinuses can differentiate neoplasia, fungal rhinitis, and dental disease with more accuracy than plain radiographs but cannot confirm the diagnosis in all cases. Biopsy with histopathology is frequently necessary.
- The frontal sinus can be examined by direct rhinoscopy in some dogs, but access to and visualization of the frontal sinus is often possible only in animals with severe turbinate destruction.
- Trephination of the frontal sinus for exam and biopsy may be necessary to confirm the presence of neoplasia, fungal rhinitis, or inflammation, especially if disease is confined to the frontal sinus. Trephination may also have therapeutic value for cases of fungal rhinitis in dogs (p. 81).

TREATMENT

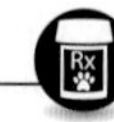

Treatment Overview

When possible, the best opportunity for resolution of sinusitis is treatment of the underlying primary nasal disease.

Acute General Treatment

- Treatment of the underlying disease.
  - Fungal sinusitis/rhinitis: antimycotic therapy (p. 81)
  - Frontal sinus tumors: radiation therapy, and occasionally, surgical resection
  - Traumatic injuries causing fractures of the frontal bone: removal of bone fragments in the frontal sinus and possibly reconstruction; check patency of the nasofrontal ostium (nasofrontal opening); broad-spectrum antibiotics
  - Apical dental (tooth root) abscess: surgical extraction of the tooth, including roots, or endodontic treatment; broad-spectrum antibiotics
- For acute infection, as well as in chronic idiopathic inflammation with episodes of secondary bacterial infections, oral or injectable antibiotics (amoxicillin 20 mg/kg PO q 8h, cefadroxil 20 mg/kg PO q 8h, or amoxicillin-clavulanate 15 mg/kg PO q 12h) and possibly mucolytics may be needed.
  - The frontal sinus is a combination of several large cavities surrounded by bone; systemically administered drugs often do not achieve high concentrations in the sinus. Even very high doses of highly soluble drugs, preferred for systemic therapy, may not reach adequate concentrations throughout the entire sinus cavity.
  - Effect of drug nebulization is unproved; the amount of drug delivered into the frontal sinus is unknown.

Chronic Treatment

In cases of concomitant nasal disease with loss of the protective filter provided by normal

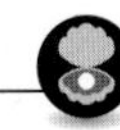

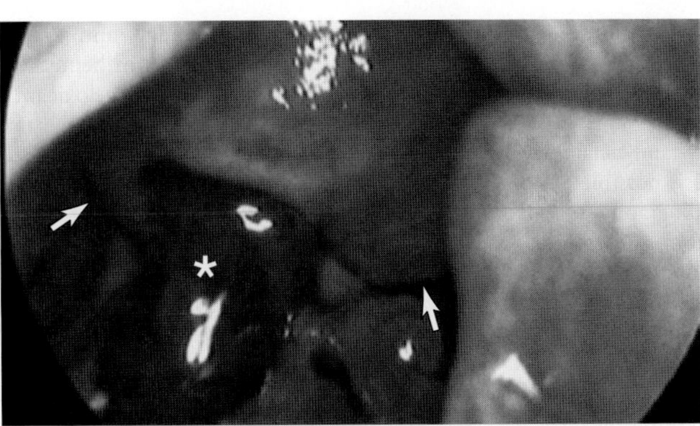

SINUSITIS AND OTHER SINUS DISORDERS Endoscopic view of the frontal sinus of a dog. A large, smooth convex mass occupies the center of the image *(arrows)*, and its appearance strongly suggests neoplasia. An adjacent blood vessel is seen *(asterisk)*.

turbinates and decreased mucociliary clearance along the distal nasal cavity, recurrent secondary bacterial infections are common and are treated each time with antibiotics and mucolytics, preferably using intranasal administration.

Possible Complications

In animals with chronic sinusitis, repeated episodes of bacterial infection can be expected.

Recommended Monitoring

Monitoring depends on the cause of the condition and persistence of clinical signs. For example, in lymphoplasmacytic inflammation of the frontal sinus after treatment of aspergillosis, diagnostic workup is warranted in cases with recurrence of severe clinical signs to differentiate secondary bacterial infection from recurrence of aspergillosis because the latter must be treated with antifungal agents.

PROGNOSIS & OUTCOME

- Prognosis and outcome depend on the cause, whether the cause can be eliminated or treated, and whether there is chronic, irreversible damage to the turbinates and sinus mucosa.
- Poor for most patients with frontal sinus tumors, which are usually malignant
- Favorable prognosis for the sinonasal form of feline aspergillosis (SNA) and poorer prognosis for the more invasive sino-orbital form, the most common form (65% of cases)
- Cure of chronic sinusitis is rarely achieved, but response to ongoing therapy is generally good.

PEARLS & CONSIDERATIONS

Comments

- In acute cases, quickly find the cause using appropriate diagnostic tests, and promptly treat to avoid chronic irreversible sequelae.
- When sinusitis is related to extension of nasal disease, it is often a chronic condition with consequent remodeling, and cure is rare; secondary bacterial infections can always occur.

Technician Tips

Although of low diagnostic yield, cytologic exam of nasal exudate can occasionally identify another underlying cause (e.g., cryptococcosis, rarely nasal neoplasia) of nasal cavity disease. Culture of nasal exudate is not recommended.

Client Education

Treatment must be repeated for relapses, which are common in chronic idiopathic sinusitis. The disease rarely totally resolves, and often, mild clinical signs persist despite treatment. If severe signs persist, repeating a complete diagnostic evaluation is indicated, with the intent of identifying an underlying cause.

SUGGESTED READING

Venker-van Haagen AJ, et al: Disease of the nose and nasal sinuses. In Ettinger SJ, et al, editors. Textbook of internal veterinary medicine, St. Louis, 2010, Elsevier, pp 1030-1040.

AUTHORS: Cécile Clercx, DVM, PhD, DECVIM; Frédéric Billen, DVM, MS, PhD, DECVIM
EDITOR: Megan Grobman, DVM, MS, DACVIM

Smoke Inhalation

Client Education Sheet

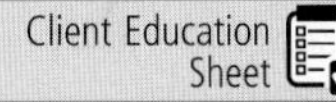

BASIC INFORMATION

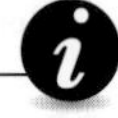

Definition

Injury to the respiratory system results from breathing harmful gases, vapors, and particulate matter contained in smoke. Neurologic dysfunction and burns may occur concurrently.

Synonyms

Smoke exposure, smoke intoxication

Epidemiology

SPECIES, AGE, SEX

Any animal can suffer smoke inhalation.

RISK FACTORS

Exposure to closed-space fires

GEOGRAPHY AND SEASONALITY

More residential fires in winter

ASSOCIATED DISORDERS

Carbon monoxide (CO) intoxication, acute respiratory distress syndrome (ARDS), burns, secondary bacterial pneumonia, systemic inflammatory response syndrome (SIRS)

Clinical Presentation

DISEASE FORMS/SUBTYPES

Inhalation injury generally manifests in three clinical stages:

- Hypoxic injury
- Neurologic compromise
- Secondary lung injury

HISTORY, CHIEF COMPLAINT

- Complaint of respiratory difficulties after smoke inhalation
- Weakness, stupor, or coma after rescue

PHYSICAL EXAM FINDINGS

- Respiratory distress, coughing, tachypnea, short or shallow respirations, harsh or moist airway sounds, crackles, wheezes, and loud laryngeal or tracheal sounds; in milder cases, signs may be limited to the nasal cavity (inflammation-induced nasal congestion, obstruction to nasal airflow).
- Mentation and motor dysfunction may include ataxia, weakness, depression, stupor, or coma.
- Mucous membranes may be hyperemic (due to carboxyhemoglobin [COHb], cyanide [CN], or vasodilation), pale, or cyanotic.
- Dermatologic findings include smoky smell, singed or burnt hair and skin, soot, or skin lacerations.
- Altered mental status, abnormal respiratory effort, and hypothermia may be associated with a higher blood level of CO.

Etiology and Pathophysiology

Causes of respiratory injury:

- Thermal damage is usually limited to the upper-airway mucosa, owing to rapid heat dissipation. Steam, soot (particles < 2.5 mm), and volatile and explosive gases, however, may also cause thermal injury to lower airways.
- Asphyxiation
  - Atmospheric oxygen deficit due to combustion
  - CO toxicosis: tissue hypoxia from COHb formation and subsequent decrease in the

oxygen-carrying capacity of blood. A left shift of the hemoglobin-oxygen dissociation curve also reduces peripheral oxygen delivery.
  - Combustion of plastics, polyurethane, fiber, rubber, and paper produces cyanide gas, which arrests cellular respiration by binding to cytochrome a_3.
  - Methemoglobinemia occurs secondary to heat denaturation of hemoglobin and release of oxides and nitrites.
- Pulmonary irritants cause direct tissue injury (depends on particle size, water solubility, and acidity), bronchospasm, and inflammation. Leukocyte activation with cytokine release and nitric oxide upregulation lead to pulmonary vascular hyperpermeability and edema. Pulmonary hypertension and atelectasis due to acute surfactant inactivation contribute to hypoxemia.
  - Impaired macrophage function and decreased mucociliary clearance may predispose the animal to bacterial pneumonia.
- Neurologic dysfunction: central nervous system (CNS) hypoxia

DIAGNOSIS

Diagnostic Overview

Diagnosis of smoke inhalation is almost always straightforward based on history of known exposure to fire and smoke and compatible clinical signs. Diagnostic testing is used for monitoring progress.

Differential Diagnosis

- Anaphylaxis
- ARDS
- Asthma (cats)
- Congestive heart failure (CHF)
- Pneumonia
- Pneumothorax
- Pulmonary thromboembolism
- Primary CNS disorders

Initial Database

- Arterial blood gas (ABG) and pulse oximetry (p. 1058)
  - ABG may confirm hypoxemia or hypercarbia.
  - Pulse oximetry is less useful for determining tissue oxygenation in the face of CO exposure and methemoglobinemia, and co-oximetry must be used to quantify the different hemoglobin species.
  - With smoke inhalation, standard pulse oximetry cannot evaluate the severity of hypoxemia because it does not differentiate between oxygenated Hb and COHb.
- CBC
  - Increased packed cell volume (PCV) (hypovolemia, splenic contraction): dogs with a more severe inhalation injury tend to have a higher PCV (mean, 58%) than milder cases (mean, 50%).
  - Neutropenia: pulmonary neutrophil sequestration
- Serum chemistry profile
  - May reflect hypoxic organ damage (e.g., increased hepatic enzyme levels, azotemia)
  - Electrolyte (and lactate) levels: high anion gap acidosis possible
- Thoracic radiography
  - May be normal after initial smoke inhalation but useful to establish a baseline
  - Findings may include atelectasis, aspiration pneumonia, and pulmonary edema.
- Fluorescein stain corneas for evidence of ulceration.

Advanced or Confirmatory Testing

- Bronchoscopy (p. 1074): may demonstrate the severity of airway damage and indicate impending airway obstruction. A bronchoalveolar lavage (cytologic exam, culture) can be helpful in stable animals to assess for secondary processes such as bacterial pneumonia.
- Transtracheal wash or endotracheal wash (p. 1073): if secondary infection is suspected

TREATMENT

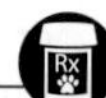

Treatment Overview

Early oxygen supplementation is a cornerstone of treatment to optimize these patients' chances for survival. Close attention should be paid to maintaining normal tissue perfusion and general nursing care. Additional goals are to maintain airway patency, restore normal gas exchange, and assess for and treat secondary complications such as bacterial pneumonia or ARDS. A step-by-step approach to treatment is provided on p. 1450.

Acute General Treatment

- High-flow humidified oxygen therapy (p. 1146) is crucial to reverse hypoxia and accelerate CO elimination:
  - COHb half-life: 4 hours (room air) versus 1.5 hours (100% oxygen)
  - Hyperbaric oxygen treatment at 2 atm (3 absolute atm) can reduce CO half-life to 45 minutes.
- Severe cases: mechanical ventilation with positive end-expiratory pressure (PEEP) (p. 1185)
- Administration of IV fluids as needed to maintain normal cardiac output and tissue perfusion
- Nebulization of saline and coupage may facilitate clearance of respiratory secretions (p. 1134)
- Drug therapy
  - Secondary pneumonia: prophylactic use of antimicrobials is not indicated because it increases the risk of developing fungal or resistant bacterial pneumonias. Monitor for development of bacterial pneumonia (worsening respiratory character or rate, purulent nasal discharge or sputum; radiographic changes, ± results of airway lavage).
  - Glucocorticoids: probably contraindicated
  - Nonsteroidal antiinflammatory drugs for analgesia in hemodynamically stable patients only: meloxicam 0.1-0.2 mg/kg SQ or PO q 24h or carprofen 2.2 mg/kg PO or SQ q 12h
  - Opioids: hydromorphone 0.05-0.1 mg/kg IV or IM q 4-6h, methadone 0.1-0.3 mg/kg IV q 4-6h, buprenorphine 0.01-0.02 mg/kg IV or IM q 6-8h, or fentanyl 1-5 mcg/kg/h IV as a continuous-rate infusion. All provide effective and relatively safe analgesia without greatly affecting respiratory drive.
  - Bronchodilators: albuterol 90-mg inhaler 1-2 puffs per large-breed dog q 8h as needed or aminophylline 6-10 mg/kg IM or diluted IV q 8h, may alleviate reflex bronchospasm
  - Diuretics: not indicated (decrease intravascular volume without major benefits on pulmonary function and edema)
  - Specific (rarely used) antidotes include
    - 20% sodium thiosulfate 30-50 mg/kg IV q 8-12h for treatment of cyanide intoxication
    - Sodium nitrite no longer recommended (can cause methemoglobinemia)

Nutrition/Diet

Nutritional support to preserve body condition and immune status (pp. 1106 and 1107)

Possible Complications

- ARDS and respiratory failure (p. 27)
- Superimposed bacterial infections: common cause of deterioration (p. 795)
- Immediate or delayed neurologic complications

Recommended Monitoring

- Careful monitoring of airway patency, gas exchange, hydration, and cardiovascular function
- Repeat thoracic radiographs

PROGNOSIS & OUTCOME

- The duration of smoke exposure, type of burn material, and availability of immediate oxygen supplementation impact recovery.
- Severe skin burns, other internal organ injury, and deteriorating respiratory function within 24 hours carry a poor prognosis.
- Animals with signs of neurologic dysfunction who are stable or improving at 24 hours have a good prognosis; worsening neurologic function at 24 hours is a poor prognostic indicator.
- Delayed neurologic sequelae of CO intoxication may manifest 4-6 days after exposure.

PEARLS & CONSIDERATIONS

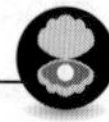

Comments

- Substantial pulmonary damage may not manifest until several hours after admission.

- Early treatment with high-flow oxygen or hyperbaric oxygen therapy (in stable patients) is critically important.

Technician Tips

- Early oxygen supplementation is essential; it should be administered from the time of triage. Standard monitoring for animals with respiratory distress (e.g., pulse oximetry) may not be helpful for animals with smoke inhalation; monitoring respiratory rate and character and serial radiography are superior.
- Good nursing care is vital, especially for patients with skin wounds (keeping clean and uncontaminated, changing dressings, pain management) or who have neurologic deficits (protection from self-injury).

Client Education

Alert firefighters to pets in household.

SUGGESTED READING

Drobatz KJ, et al: Smoke exposure in dogs: 27 cases (1988-1997). J Am Vet Med Assoc 215(9):1306-1311, 1999.

AUTHOR: Gareth J. Buckley, VetMB, MA, DACVECC
EDITOR: Benjamin M. Brainard, VMD, DACVAA, DACVECC

Snake Envenomation (Coral)

BASIC INFORMATION

Definition

Injury resulting from the envenoming bite of a coral snake

Synonym

Snake envenomation

Epidemiology

SPECIES, AGE, SEX

Any age or species; either sex

RISK FACTORS

- Environment: exposure to outdoors in warm climates where coral snakes dwell
- Behavior: curiosity

CONTAGION AND ZOONOSIS

Coral snakes are also extremely poisonous to humans, although fatalities are very unusual if the required antivenom is available.

GEOGRAPHY AND SEASONALITY

- Coral snakes belong to the Elapidae family.
- Three major species are found in the United States.
  - *Micrurus fulvius*: eastern coral snake found from North Carolina to Louisiana, most prevalent in Florida
  - *Micrurus tener*: Texas coral snake found in the southwestern United States, west of the Mississippi
  - *Micrurus eurxanthus*: Sonoran or Arizona coral snake, found in the Sonora desert, Arizona
- Most bites occur during warmer months, although bites of the eastern coral snake have been reported year-round.

ASSOCIATED DISORDERS

- Neurologic dysfunction
  - Progressive lower motor neuron (LMN) paralysis
  - Respiratory failure
- Hemolysis (reported in dogs only)
  - Anemia
  - Acute kidney injury (AKI)
  - Multiorgan failure

Clinical Presentation

DISEASE FORMS/SUBTYPES

- Animals can appear normal or demonstrate neurologic abnormalities.
- Onset of neurologic signs can be delayed up to 36 hours after envenomation.
- About 25% of human bites are reportedly *dry*, with no envenomation.

HISTORY, CHIEF COMPLAINT

- Most common presentation is a clinically normal animal found in the vicinity of a dead or injured snake
- Some animals are presented due to onset of neurologic signs with no witnessed snake encounter (more common for cats)
- Many animals have an episode of vomiting shortly after the bite.
- Can show hiding or behavioral changes in the early stages of envenomation

PHYSICAL EXAM FINDINGS

- It is rare to find bite marks; if found, they are tiny red puncture or scratch wounds ranging from 2-4 mm in size, small hematomas, or small contusions with minimal tissue reaction, typically on the lips of dogs or the paws of cats.
- Cats
  - Tetraparesis with LMN hyporeflexia
  - Mental depression
  - Proprioceptive deficits
  - Hypothermia
  - Vocalization associated with anxiety
  - Vomiting
  - Changes in respiratory pattern: short, shallow respiratory movements indicate imminent danger of respiratory paralysis
- Dogs
  - Generalized progressive LMN paralysis
  - Ptyalism associated with bulbar paralysis
  - Changes in respiratory pattern: short, shallow respiratory movements indicate imminent respiratory paralysis
  - Muscle tremors/fasciculation
  - Loss of gag reflex (part of bulbar paralysis that can involve other cranial nerves, especially CN 7, 9, and 10)
  - Proprioceptive deficits
  - Poor muscle tone
  - Vomiting or retching
  - Red or port wine discolored urine if hemolysis present

Etiology and Pathophysiology

Elapid venom is neurotoxic and hemolytic in dogs and rodents and only neurotoxic in cats and humans:

- Initial signs can occur up to 36 hours after envenomation.
- Mental depression and LMN signs predominate due to postsynaptic blockade of nicotinic acetylcholine (ACh) receptors by alpha-neurotoxins (different than elapids in other parts of the world, where ACh activity predominates).
- Produces a nondepolarizing (curare-like) effect on the muscle fiber membrane
- Phospholipases specific to coral snake venom can cause hemolysis (dogs and rodents only), as well as being toxic to skeletal and smooth muscle (including cardiac tissue).
- Unlike the vipers, protease activity is low, with little local tissue reaction or swelling, and effects on coagulation are not clinically significant.

DIAGNOSIS

Diagnostic Overview

Diagnosis is typically by history of known exposure to a coral snake with or without consistent clinical signs. For animals with no known history of coral snake exposure, it depends on compatible clinical signs and supportive laboratory testing, although clinical course of the disease is often the most helpful indicator (NOTE: combination of hemolysis and LMN disease in coral snake–endemic areas is virtually pathognomonic of envenomation in dogs).

Differential Diagnosis

- Hemolysis
  - Immune-mediated hemolytic anemia
  - Zinc toxicity
  - Other causes of hemolysis (e.g., *Babesia*, drugs, other toxins)
- Generalized LMN signs
  - Tick paralysis
  - Polyradiculoneuritis

- Botulism
- Myasthenia gravis
- Toxicity (e.g., baclofen)

Initial Database

- Urinalysis: in dogs, hemoglobinuria, proteinuria (from heme protein) is a common finding.
- Serum biochemistry profile: in dogs, aspartate aminotransferase (AST) and alanine aminotransferase (ALT) activity may be moderately elevated.
- CBC: hemolysis occurs in 50%-60% of dogs; mild to moderate anemia can rarely occur in severely affected dogs. Echinocytes and spherocytes are rare after coral snake envenomation.
- Pulse oximetry or arterial blood gas to assess for hypoxia (SpO_2 < 95% or PaO_2 < 80 mm Hg warrants oxygen supplementation and close patient monitoring), SpO_2 < 92% or PaO_2 < 65 mm Hg with normal lung function may indicate hypoventilation from neuromuscular dysfunction.
  - PCO_2 > 60 mm Hg on arterial blood gas indicates hypoventilation

Advanced or Confirmatory Testing

No confirmatory test is available; however, known exposure to a coral snake warrants treatment. If hemolysis or compatible clinical signs are present, treatment must not be delayed.

TREATMENT

Treatment Overview

- Neutralize the toxin if antivenom is available.
- Victims can survive without antivenom if patient support is optimal.
- Nursing and supportive care of animals with LMN paralysis
- Avoid development of aspiration pneumonia by not feeding dysphagic animals.
- Ventilator support is necessary for animals with respiratory failure.
- Manage complications of hemolysis.

Acute General Treatment

- Antivenom is not widely available for use in animals in the United States.
  - Only limited amounts of expired Pfizer/Wyeth anticoral snake antivenom are available under strict U.S. Food and Drug Administration allocation.
  - Coralmyn antivenom is produced by Instituto Bioclon in Mexico and has been shown to be effective in neutralizing the venom of eastern and Texan coral snakes. Suero Antiofidico Anticoral, manufactured in Costa Rica, is also effective against eastern and Texas coral snakes. Both products are available to veterinarians but require a U.S. Department of Agriculture import permit.
  - If available, it is recommended to treat animals that have a convincing history of exposure with 1-2 vials of antivenom before clinical signs develop.
  - The antivenom dose is empirical and is influenced by the high cost of the drug.
  - If clinical signs develop, higher doses of antivenom may be needed, but progression to respiratory failure may still occur.
- Turning regularly to prevent sores in recumbent patients and physical therapy such as passive range-of-motion exercises are important parts of the treatment protocol.
- Mechanical ventilation (p. 1185) is required for patients who progress to respiratory failure. Due to the rapid progression of signs, transfer of coral snake victims to a facility that can provide 24-hour intensive care, including ventilation, is recommended. Duration of mechanical ventilation is typically less than 3 days.
- Hemolysis does not occur in every case and can be mild and self-limited. In severe cases, treatment of the complications of hemolysis is required.
  - If present, AKI requires management (p. 23). If pigmenturia is severe, urinary alkalization can be considered to reduce the nephrotoxic effects.
  - Anemia is usually mild, but in severe cases, blood transfusion using packed red cells may be required, although this is rarely required (p. 1169).

Chronic Treatment

Continue physical rehabilitation until ambulating normally

Nutrition/Diet

- Oral nutrition or nasoesophageal feeding should be withheld from animals with severe neurologic compromise due to the risk of aspiration pneumonia.
- For dogs that recover quickly (2-3 days), no intervention is required.
- Rarely, animals requiring longer-term care (e.g., those on mechanical ventilation) may require tube feeding (pp. 1107 and 1109).

Behavior/Exercise

Physical rehabilitation is important, but excessive exercise early in the course of disease can worsen clinical signs.

Drug Interactions

- Antivenin may cause an anaphylactic reaction (p. 54).
- Monitor vital signs during infusion; if signs of anaphylaxis develop (sudden collapse, vomiting, diarrhea, restlessness, urticaria), temporarily stop the infusion, administer diphenhydramine and/or epinephrine, and then restart the infusion at a slower rate when signs have subsided.
  - Epinephrine 0.01-0.02 mg/kg IM or IV (if very unstable) should be used in cases of severe anaphylaxis. The dose should be ready to administer when antivenom is used.
- Drugs causing respiratory depression (e.g., opioids, sedatives) are contraindicated unless the patient is mechanically ventilated.
- Drugs potentially affecting synaptic transmission (e.g., aminoglycosides) should be avoided.

Possible Complications

AKI or anemia can occur in patients with severe hemolysis.

Recommended Monitoring

- Mildly affected or exposed but normal animals: monitor for worsening clinical signs for minimum of 36 hours after snake exposure.
- Severely affected animals: cardiovascular monitoring, serial neurologic exams, arterial or venous blood gases to assess for hypoxia or hypoventilation, packed cell volume/total solids (PCV/TS), serum color, urine output and clarity

Prognosis and Outcome

- Prognosis for clinically normal animals and animals without ventilatory compromise given antivenom is excellent.

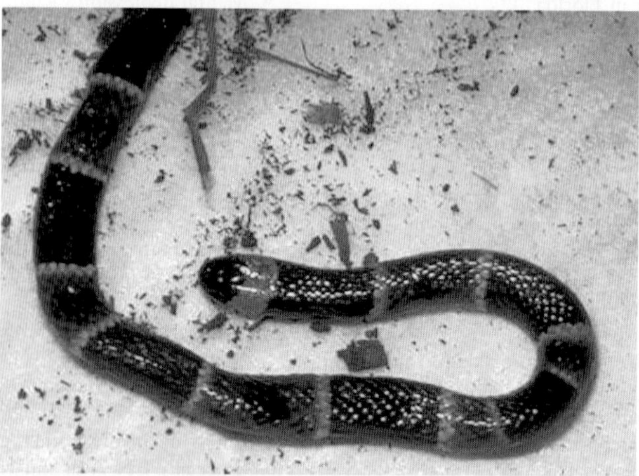

SNAKE ENVENOMATION (CORAL) Red on yellow kills a fellow: rhyme used to identify the poisonous eastern coral snake, *Micrurus fulvius*. (Photograph courtesy Dr. Michael Schaer.)

- Animals showing neurologic signs demonstrate a > 75% survival to discharge (most common cause of death is euthanasia due to cost of care). Those aggressively treated have a good to excellent survival rate.
- Even animals becoming ventilator dependent have a fair to good prognosis, with more than 66% surviving. Most animals requiring mechanical ventilation are weaned from the ventilator within 3 days.
- Recovery is complete without any neurologic sequelae.

PEARLS & CONSIDERATIONS

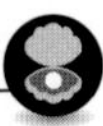

Comments

- Clinical signs are often delayed (up to 36 hours), and normal animals can become ventilator dependent very quickly.
- The eastern coral snake is identified by its black head and red and yellow adjacent rings along the snake's body. This color pattern changes in different geographic locations among Western Hemisphere elapids. King snakes have adjacent black and red stripes and are not poisonous.

Prevention

- The best way to prevent snake bites is to avoid snakes.
- Prevent unsupervised roaming of pets if possible.

Technician Tips

- Observe exposed animals frequently and closely in an easily visible area of the clinic due to potential for rapid decline.
- Ptyalism and difficulty rising can be a first signs of LMN paralysis.

Client Education

- Most clients who live in areas where the snake is endemic are well educated about the dangers of snake bite. Pets in areas of high coral snake activity should not be allowed to roam.
- Due to the potential for delayed signs, the importance of seeking veterinary attention in the event of suspected coral snake exposure (even if the animal is clinically normal) cannot be stressed enough.

SUGGESTED READING

Perez-Gonzalez M, et al: A retrospective evaluation of coral snake envenomation in dogs and cats: 20 cases (1996-2011). J Vet Emerg Crit Care 22(6):682-689, 2012.

AUTHORS: Gareth J. Buckley, VetMB, MA, DACVECC, DECVECC; Michael Schaer DVM, DAVIM, DACVECC; Mayrim L. Perez-Gonzalez, DVM, DACVIM
EDITOR: Benjamin M. Brainard, VMD, DACVAA, DACVECC

Snake Envenomation (Pit Viper)

BASIC INFORMATION

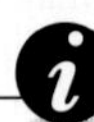

Definition

Injury and associated syndrome resulting from envenomation by a pit viper

Synonyms

Crotalid envenomation, snake bite

Epidemiology

SPECIES, AGE, SEX

Dogs or cats of any age and either sex

RISK FACTORS

Dogs and cats that spend time outdoors in snake-endemic areas

GEOGRAPHY AND SEASONALITY

- There are two main groups of pit vipers:
  - Rattlesnakes (*Crotalus* and *Sistrus* spp)
  - Cottonmouths and copperheads (*Agkistrodon* spp)
- Although found throughout the United States, bites are more common in the southern United States.
- Increased incidence of bites in the late spring and summer months

ASSOCIATED DISORDERS

Local tissue necrosis, severe coagulopathy, and multisystemic disease (cardiovascular collapse, multiorgan failure)

Clinical Presentation

DISEASE FORMS/SUBTYPES

Disease severity varies from mild (i.e., small amount of venom is inoculated or envenomation occurs by a snake with low-potency venom) to severe (i.e., large amount of highly potent venom is inoculated).

HISTORY, CHIEF COMPLAINT

- Observed bite
- Unobserved bite: facial, neck, or limb swelling and pain or collapse after being outdoors

PHYSICAL EXAM FINDINGS

- Pair of fang marks with swelling and bruising around the area (may require careful inspection and/or clipping hair) typically is detected within 15 minutes after envenomation. The animal may show signs of mild discomfort to profound hemorrhagic, cardiovascular, and neurologic alterations.
- Hemorrhagic lymphedema (hallmark finding)
- Swelling, pain, erythema, ecchymoses
- Cyanosis and tissue sloughing (later stage)
- Tachycardia and ventricular arrhythmias are common.
- In severe cases, poor pulse quality and pale mucous membranes indicate severe hypovolemic shock (p. 911).
- Dull mentation or neurologic signs such as paresis (more common in cats or after bites by certain snakes; see below)

Etiology and Pathophysiology

Crotalid venom is vasculotoxic and necrogenic.

- Bites are most often inflicted on the face and head and occasionally on the limbs (cats especially).
- Swelling typically worsens over the first 24 hours after the bite, and the swollen tissue may appear like a hematoma.
- The venom also has systemic effects, causing potentially severe coagulopathy that can be clotting factor mediated, with hyperfibrinolysis and with or without thrombocytopenia; cardiac arrhythmias; systemic hypotension; and neurologic signs (e.g., obtundation, loss of motor function)
- The Mojave rattlesnake primarily causes neurologic signs with less swelling and tissue necrosis than that of the other rattlesnakes. Neurologic signs include dull mentation, difficulty swallowing, and severe lower motor neuron muscle weakness, which can lead to collapse or respiratory muscle paralysis.
- Eastern diamondback rattlesnake venom has historically been associated with cardiovascular, coagulopathic and hematologic changes and tissue necrosis, but neurotoxin may cause obtundation and profound weakness.

DIAGNOSIS

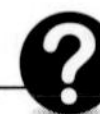

Diagnostic Overview

Suspected when a patient develops acute swelling with bruising, often around the face or forelimbs, in a geographic region known to harbor venomous snakes. Identification of puncture marks in the skin from the bite is confirmatory.

Differential Diagnosis

Other animal attacks or wounds

Initial Database

- CBC with platelet count: hemoconcentration, leukocytosis, echinocytosis, or thrombocytopenia
- Serum biochemistry profile is typically initially unremarkable, except for hypokalemia;

in severe cases, azotemia and hepatic enzyme elevations can occur as injury progresses. Creatine kinase level may be increased secondary to tissue damage.
- Urinalysis: hematuria, hemoglobinuria, or myoglobinuria is possible (avoid cystocentesis).
- Baseline arterial blood pressure measurement (p. 1065): normal or low
- Coagulation profile (p. 1325): prolonged activated clotting time (ACT), prothrombin time (PT), partial thromboplastin time (aPTT); thromboelastography (TEG) evidence of hypocoagulability and/or hyperfibrinolysis

Advanced or Confirmatory Testing

Echinocytes on a blood smear are a common finding in envenomated animals. Echinocytes are burred red blood cells that appear soon after envenomation and last in circulation 24-48 hours.

TREATMENT

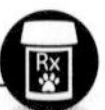

Treatment Overview

Goals are management/prevention of hypotension, neutralization of venom (minimizing local and systemic effects), pain management, and avoidance of iatrogenic complications (particularly during administration of antivenom).

Acute General Treatment

- All animals that are bitten by a snake, regardless of their apparent hemodynamic stability, should be hospitalized for a minimum of 8 hours to assess for delayed clinical signs that manifest during this period.
- IV fluid therapy
  - First line of therapy is to treat hypotension or hypovolemic shock (p. 911).
  - Crystalloids (e.g., lactated Ringer's solution) to replace deficit and provide replacement of ongoing losses and normal maintenance. For hypovolemic patients, initial bolus doses of 20-30 mL/kg over 10-15 minutes followed by reassessment and repeat as required.
- Antivenin (Crotalidae) polyvalent
  - Administered immediately for viper bites that cause moderate to severe systemic signs (e.g., hypotension, hemorrhage, neurologic abnormalities). It increases survival when given closer to time of bite, but beneficial effects noted for at least 60 hours after envenomation. Most victims of pygmy rattlesnake and copperhead bites do not require antivenom.
  - A dosage of up to 6-25 vials of polyvalent immune Fab-ovine is recommended in humans after crotalid envenomation; however, patients with less severe clinical signs may not require this amount of antivenom. For dogs, a mild case (mild localized swelling only, no other clinical signs) usually does not require antivenom treatment. For moderate cases (more severe swelling, mild systemic signs), typically 1-2 vials of antivenom are given over 30-60 minutes, and the patient is reassessed. For severe cases (very severe swelling or severe cardiovascular signs), 2-4 vials can be administered at initiation of treatment. These severely affected patients may require further treatment with antivenom even if their signs initially stabilize; watch for recurrence of clinical signs. Dosing of antivenom is controversial because venom concentration assays are not rapidly available; the key is to use enough antivenom to control and reverse the clinical signs. In general, the more severely affected the patient, the more antivenom is required. Provide adequate antivenom promptly and continually reassess the patient's need for ongoing treatment.
  - Several antivenoms are now available in the United States.
    - Lyophilized products requiring reconstitution: Antivenin Crotalidae Polyvalent (ACP; Boehringer Ingelheim, St Joseph, MO); CroFab (polyvalent immune Fab-ovine; BTG International, West Conshohocken, PA); the Fab1 product is less antigenic, dissolves more rapidly and is more potent but is extremely expensive.
    - New equine-origin products that do not require reconstitution: VenomVet (Instituto Biologica Argentino, Buenos Aires, Argentina) and Rattler Antivenin (Mg Biologics, Ames, IA)
- Antibiotics (controversial): not usually required. If wound infection occurs (usually after day 3), choose a broad-spectrum antibiotic with adequate gram-negative coverage while cultures are pending. Routine culture of bite wounds is probably not helpful.
- Analgesics: opioids should be used judiciously. Avoid sedation initially because mental status is an excellent clinical indicator of response to treatment. Options include buprenorphine 0.01-0.02 mg/kg IV q 6-8h, hydromorphone 0.05-0.1 mg/kg IV q 4-6h, fentanyl continuous-rate infusion (CRI) 2-5 mcg/kg/h after loading dose of 1-3 mcg/kg IV.
- Nonsteroidal antiinflammatory drugs should be avoided due to potential for nephrotoxicosis in hypovolemic patients and their effects on platelet function.
- Glucocorticoids and antihistamines: not recommended (unless anaphylaxis)
- Urgent airway management: rarely needed in dogs; dogs with bites inside the mouth (e.g., on the tongue) are the exception (p. 1166).
- Transfusion (p. 1169) is indicated in patients with clinically significant anemia secondary to hemorrhage or hemolysis. Fresh-frozen plasma is sometimes used when a coagulopathy is not improving, but the best treatment for venom-induced coagulopathy is adequate treatment with antivenom.

Chronic Treatment

Surgical debridement of necrotic tissue is sometimes necessary; most cases of necrosis become apparent by day 3-5. Occasionally, wounds with severe necrosis become infected; antibiotic therapy is indicated in these cases. Rarely, a recurrence of envenomation occurs after improvement with antivenom administration; it is thought that this is due to a depot of venom that was mobilized anew. This is associated with a worsening of clinical signs and may merit another treatment with antivenom.

Nutrition/Diet

Almost all snake bite victims surviving the initial intoxication begin to eat in 1-3 days. In patients with severe wounds around the mouth, nasoesophageal or esophagostomy feeding tubes may be indicated until they can comfortably eat (pp. 1106-1107).

Behavior/Exercise

Rest until recovered

Possible Complications

Monitor during infusion because antivenom may cause an anaphylactic reaction (p. 54).
- Signs of mild to moderate anaphylaxis include salivation, vomiting, abdominal pain, hives, and fever.
- Signs of severe anaphylaxis also include collapse, pale or white mucous membranes, severe hypotension, cardiac arrhythmias, or sudden death.
- Anaphylaxis can usually be treated if recognized at an early stage. Life-threatening reactions can occur with infusion of even tiny amounts of antivenom.
- Treatment includes
  - Epinephrine 0.01 mg/kg IV in severe cases or IM in milder cases; in very severe cases, repeated doses q 3-5 minutes or CRI may be necessary.
  - Glucocorticoids (e.g., dexamethasone 0.25 mg/kg IV or IM)
  - H1-blockers (e.g., diphenhydramine 2 mg/kg IM)
  - H2-blockers (e.g., famotidine 1 mg/kg IV or IM)
- Acute kidney injury can occur due to pigmenturia from hemolysis and/or rhabdomyolysis. Risk is reduced by use of antivenom to prevent further hemolysis, adequate crystalloid fluid therapy, and avoidance of artificial colloids.

Recommended Monitoring

- Respiratory rate and effort, blood pressure, electrocardiogram, urine color/output, and mentation
- Reassess fully if deteriorating mentation is recognized. Recheck packed cell volume (PCV), total protein, blood lactate concentration, ± coagulation status q 6-12 hours for

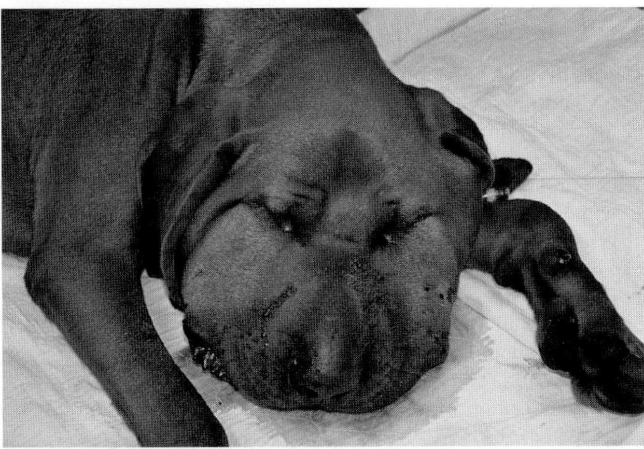

SNAKE ENVENOMATION (PIT VIPER) Dog with recent envenomation by an eastern diamondback rattlesnake. Note the severe local swelling, visible fang marks, hemorrhagic lymphedema, and active bleeding from the bite site. (Photograph courtesy Dr. Michael Schaer.)

the first 1-2 days, depending on the severity of the envenomation.

PROGNOSIS & OUTCOME

- Most dog or cat snake bite victims survive without permanent sequelae if treated early. The prognosis is worse for animals with high-venom burdens or cardiovascular collapse at the time of presentation.
- Although death may occur despite the timely use of crotalid-specific antivenom, a higher survival rate has been found in dogs that received antivenin than in dogs that did not.

PEARLS & CONSIDERATIONS

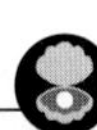

Comments

- Tissue swelling often becomes dramatically worse in the 24-48 hours after a viper bite. Warn owners in advance to prevent the perception that treatment is unsuccessful.
- Ineffective first-aid techniques include tourniquet application, incision and suction of the bite, electroshock of the bite, and hot or cold pack application.
- Effective first aid involves minimizing exertion and immediate transport to a hospital for treatment as outlined previously.
- Early intensive treatment with antivenom, although costly, may ultimately save clients' money by shortening recovery time.
- Rattlesnakes can bite for up to 30 minutes after they are killed, including after they have been decapitated. The body or head of a snake that has bitten and is then killed and transported for identification should be kept in a rigid, closed container, and the head should not be handled directly.

Prevention

The best way to prevent snake bites is to avoid snakes.

- Vipers bite in self-defense, when they are surprised, or to immobilize and consume prey, such as small rodents.
- Vipers strike with unavoidable speed (8 ft [2.5 m]/s) but typically for a distance corresponding only to one-half the snake's length (e.g., one-half of 3-5 ft [1-1.6 m]).
- Keeping dogs in enclosed areas with concrete walls or on leashes while outside may help prevent contact with snakes.
- Keeping cats indoors helps to prevent contact with snakes.
- Vaccination may offer some protection against ill effects of bite from Western diamondback rattlesnake for dogs at high risk of exposure.

Technician Tips

- Monitor constantly during and 1-2 hours after administration of antivenom for signs of anaphylaxis.
- Deteriorating mentation can be the first sign of a crisis.
- Do not bandage any bite wound to avoid compromising blood supply to the tissues. Blood oozing from the bite site for the first several hours is of no consequence.

Client Education

- There is almost always severe or extreme swelling around the location of the bite, even if treatment is working.
- Most snakes bite when surprised or threatened; vigilance and avoidance of snakes during warm months are the best approach to preventing bites. In the event that a dog or cat is bitten, rapid transport to a veterinary hospital capable of providing antivenom treatment along with 24-hour intensive care is recommended.
- Animals recovered from a bite do not learn to avoid snakes.

SUGGESTED READING

Armentano RA, et al: Overview and controversies in the medical management of pit viper envenomation in the dog. J Vet Emerg Crit Care 21(5):461-470, 2011.

AUTHOR: Gareth J. Buckley, MA, VetMB, DACVECC, DECVECC
EDITOR: Benjamin M. Brainard, VMD, DACVAA, DACVECC

Sneezing

BASIC INFORMATION

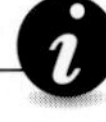

Definition

- The explosive release of air from the lungs through the nasal cavity and mouth with the purpose of rapidly removing irritants from the nasal epithelial surface
- Commonly associated with nasal discharge
- Reverse sneezing: loud, paroxysmal, inspiratory noise typically initiated by nasopharyngeal irritation (p. 887)

Epidemiology

SPECIES, AGE, SEX

- Viral rhinitis is most common in young dogs (e.g., canine distemper virus [CDV]) and cats (e.g., feline calicivirus [FCV]).
- Foreign bodies (FBs) (e.g., plant material) are most common in young animals.
- Nasal tumors can occur at all ages, but most often at > 5 years of age.

RISK FACTORS

- Lack of appropriate immunization and exposure to unvaccinated animals
- Severe periodontal disease
- Possible precipitating factors for idiopathic lymphoplasmacytic rhinitis in dogs include aeroallergens, infections, and inhaled irritants (e.g., cleaning products, cigarette smoke).

CONTAGION AND ZOONOSIS

Viral respiratory tract infections are highly contagious.

GEOGRAPHY AND SEASONALITY

Geographic locations where grass awns are common

ASSOCIATED DISORDERS

Nasal discharge

Clinical Presentation

DISEASE FORMS/SUBTYPES

- Sneezing versus reverse sneezing
- Time course
  - Peracute/acute
  - Chronic

HISTORY, CHIEF COMPLAINT

The time course and presence or absence of additional signs (e.g., nasal discharge, coughing) vary with the cause of sneezing.

- Peracute onset with pawing at the face should increase suspicion for a nasal FB (p. 355).
- Acute sneezing by animals recently exposed to other animals (e.g., shelter, boarding, parks, groomer) suggests viral infection, especially if accompanied by other signs (e.g., cough, ocular discharge, hyporexia).
- Chronic sneezing with mild serous nasal discharge or absent any other signs suggests nasal mites.
- Sneezing associated with chronic nasal discharge may reflect any number of disorders (p. 678).

PHYSICAL EXAM FINDINGS

Findings reflect the underlying cause. In addition to typical exam, evaluation of the head should be similar to that described for nasal discharge (p. 678).

- Exam may be entirely normal.
- Nasal discharge is commonly identified; characterize type and laterality.
- Nasal airflow may be reduced from one or both nostrils due to space-occupying mass or copious mucus accumulation.
- Stertor may be associated with nasopharyngeal disease.
- Depigmentation of nasal planum suggests infection (e.g., sinonasal aspergillosis) or immune-mediated disease (e.g., discoid lupus erythematosus).
- Facial deformity may be associated with nasal neoplasia, tooth root abscess, or infection (e.g., *Cryptococcus* spp).
- Oral exam may demonstrate tooth-root abscess, oronasal fistula, mucosal ulceration (FCV), or cleft palate.
- Inability to retropulse eyes suggests space-occupying lesion (e.g., abscess, neoplasia).
- Ophthalmic exam may demonstrate ocular discharge or other findings suggestive of viral infection (e.g., feline herpesvirus) or systemic disease (e.g., keratoconjunctivitis sicca associated with neurogenic rhinitis).
- Fever suggests systemic or respiratory infection (e.g., FCV, CDV).

Etiology and Pathophysiology

Sneezing is a protective reflex that removes nasal irritants or particulates. All causes of nasal discharge are potential causes of sneezing (p. 1255).

DIAGNOSIS

Diagnostic Overview

Signalment, history, and physical exam often allow reasonable prioritization of differential diagnoses and appropriate diagnostic testing. For some animals, empirical treatment may be appropriate without additional testing. For example, trial treatment for nasal mites is appropriate for an otherwise healthy dog with sneezing ± serous nasal discharge, and empirical therapy may be appropriate for a young dog or cat with history and exam findings suggestive of acute respiratory infection (p. 141). There is much overlap in investigation of sneezing and nasal discharge (p. 1255).

Differential Diagnosis

Reverse sneeze can be mistaken for sneeze by pet owners.

Initial Database

- CBC, serum chemistry profile, urinalysis, feline retroviral serology: assess health before anesthesia, rule out thrombocytopenia if sneezing is associated with hemorrhagic discharge
- Aspirate any enlarged submandibular lymph node for cytologic exam.
- Obvious mass or deformity may be amenable to fine-needle aspiration for cytology.
- Consider serologic tests for cryptococcosis (p. 223), sinonasal aspergillosis (p. 81), or systemic infection.
- Consider thoracic radiographs to rule out pneumonia and metastatic lung disease.
- Consider cytology of impression from nasal discharge; very low sensitivity but occasionally recognizes fungal elements or neoplastic cells.

Advanced or Confirmatory Testing

The choice of advanced diagnostic modalities depends on a patient-specific list of differentials, availability of diagnostics, and cost.

- If nasal FB is suspected, nasal lavage ± choanal exam and rhinoscopy (p. 1159) may be undertaken before imaging studies.
  - Nasal FBs tend to be located in the nasal passages of dogs and at the choanae of cats; retroflexed visualization of the choanae is a crucial portion of the exam.
  - Rhinoscopy may identify fungal plaques, turbinate destruction, or mass effects and facilitate direct sampling of identified lesions.
  - Nasal FB may remain hidden on rhinoscopic exam (FB cannot be ruled out by negative rhinoscopy)
  - Nasal lavage may be performed in antegrade and retrograde fashion.
- Thorough oral exam requires anesthesia and may be combined with dental radiographs and cleaning.
  - In older animals or those with obvious dental disease, this is often the first step in evaluation of chronic mucopurulent nasal discharge.
- Imaging studies are often necessary for evaluation of sneezing or chronic, progressive nasal discharge. Skull CT or MRI offers significant advantage over radiographs.
- Biopsies are required for histologic diagnosis of nasal neoplasia or inflammatory rhinitis (p. 890). Ideally, biopsy collection is guided by imaging studies.

TREATMENT

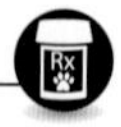

Treatment Overview

Treatment depends on cause of sneezing.

Acute General Treatment

- If sneezing is accompanied by respiratory distress, oxygen supplementation (p. 1146) may be required.
- Nasal FB should be removed promptly. Sedation or placement of an Elizabethan collar may be necessary to prevent self-trauma if sneezing is accompanied by aggressive pawing/rubbing of the face.
- See chapters on specific disease conditions for treatment options.

PROGNOSIS & OUTCOME

Depends on cause

PEARLS & CONSIDERATIONS

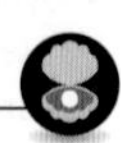

Comments

- It can be difficult to identify nasal FBs, even with advanced imaging (CT/MRI) and rhinoscopy.
- Animals with an acute onset of sneezing and a history of exposure to other animals should be handled as if they have a contagious infectious disease (i.e., limit exposure to other animals).

Prevention

Many heartworm preventatives and isoxazoline compounds can prevent nasal mite infestation.

Technician Tips

- Animals with a recent onset of sneezing should be directed into an exam room immediately to limit exposure of other animals to a potential infectious agent. The exam room should be cleaned immediately afterward.
- Physical manipulation of cats with reduced nasal airflow can prompt respiratory distress. Abort handling, and notify a veterinarian if a cat begins to open-mouth breathe.

SUGGESTED READING

Cohn LA: Canine nasal disease. Vet Clin North Am Small Anim Pract 44:75-89, 2014.

AUTHOR: Jared Jaffey, DVM, MS, DACVIM
EDITOR: Leah A. Cohn, DVM, PhD, DACVIM

Soft-Tissue Sarcoma

Client Education Sheet

BASIC INFORMATION

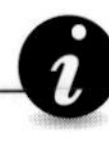

Definition

A group of common tumors arising from various mesenchymal tissues, they are classified together because of similar biological behavior and treatment. They include fibrosarcoma, hemangiopericytoma, malignant fibrous histiocytoma, nerve sheath tumor, neurofibrosarcoma, malignant schwannoma, leiomyosarcoma, rhabdomyosarcoma, liposarcoma, myxosarcoma, lymphangiosarcoma, and synovial cell sarcoma. Although it is also a mesenchymal tumor arising from soft tissue, hemangiosarcoma is often excluded from this group because of its aggressive biological behavior.

Synonym

Soft-part sarcomas

Epidemiology

SPECIES, AGE, SEX

- Common in middle-aged to older dogs
- Soft-tissue sarcomas at sites other than injection sites are less common in cats.

GENETICS, BREED PREDISPOSITION

They tend to occur more commonly in larger breeds, but direct inheritance of these tumors has not been reported.

RISK FACTORS

- Certain sarcomas have been associated with metal implants, previous exposure to ionizing radiation, implanted microchips, and parasites *(Spirocerca lupi).*
- Sarcomas at injection sites are well described in cats (p. 550) but rare in dogs.

ASSOCIATED DISORDERS

Hypoglycemia and diabetes insipidus have been reported as uncommon paraneoplastic syndromes in dogs with intestinal leiomyosarcoma.

Clinical Presentation

HISTORY, CHIEF COMPLAINT

- Most animals present for a progressively enlarging mass noticed by the owner.
- Animals with sarcoma in certain locations are presented because of clinical signs related to the location of the tumor. Dogs with oral tumors often present due to halitosis, difficulty eating or prehending food, oral bleeding, or a visible oral mass. Dogs with intestinal sarcomas often are presented because of signs related to an intestinal mass, including vomiting and diarrhea.

PHYSICAL EXAM FINDINGS

- Visible or palpable mass. Regional lymphadenopathy may be present secondary to inflammation caused by the tumor or (rarely) lymph node metastasis.
- Sarcomas in specific sites may present with physical exam findings related to the location of the tumor (e.g., abdominal pain, weight loss, dehydration).

Etiology and Pathophysiology

- Soft-tissue sarcomas arise spontaneously in dogs and cats. Genetic and environmental factors may be involved in tumor development, but these factors are poorly understood.
- Specific lesions and overt clinical manifestations caused by soft-tissue sarcomas depend on location of the primary tumor and invasion into and destruction of surrounding normal structures.

DIAGNOSIS

Diagnostic Overview

Definitive diagnosis can be confirmed only by histopathologic exam, although additional tests such as diagnostic imaging are useful for defining the extent of the tumor. An aggressive first surgery is more likely to result in tumor control. An incisional biopsy should be performed first to establish the diagnosis. After the tumor type is confirmed, definitive treatment can be planned and performed correctly. A global approach to diagnosis and management is outlined on p. 1451.

Differential Diagnosis

- Mast cell tumors
- Other skin and subcutaneous tumors: lipoma, histiocytoma, others
- Other masses: abscess, granuloma

Initial Database

- Fine-needle aspiration and cytologic exam may help identify the type of soft-tissue sarcoma or differentiate it from other tumor types.
- Thoracic radiographs to rule out pulmonary metastases
- Radiographs of the affected area may (rarely) reveal involvement of underlying bone.
- Fine-needle aspiration of draining lymph nodes to help rule out metastasis

Advanced or Confirmatory Testing

- CT or MRI may be necessary to delineate the local extent of the tumor and plan for surgery or radiation therapy.
- Diagnosis is based on histopathologic evaluation of tissue. Occasionally, special stains are necessary to differentiate various types of soft-tissue sarcomas, especially poorly differentiated tumors.
- Histopathologic grade of the tumor is necessary for determining prognosis and treatment of most soft-tissue sarcomas.

TREATMENT

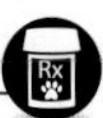

Treatment Overview

- The goal of treatment for soft-tissue sarcomas in dogs or cats is complete eradication of the primary tumor.
- In cases where the tumor cannot be eliminated entirely, the goal of treatment is prevention or delayed development of metastases.
- Palliative treatment options, such as palliative irradiation, may help control pain or discomfort in patients with advanced tumors or when definitive treatment is not an option.
- Consultation with an oncologist is recommended.

Acute General Treatment

Surgery:

- Commonly, these tumors appear encapsulated at surgery. This can be misleading because the capsule is usually a pseudocapsule made of compressed tumor cells, and viable tumor cells are often present beyond the pseudocapsule.
- Surgery should be aimed at an aggressive resection of the mass with as wide a margin of normal tissue as possible from around the tumor. When this is not possible because of the size and/or location of the tumor, radiation therapy may be indicated in addition to surgery.

Radiation therapy:

- May be used before surgery when the tumor is not easily resectable due to location or size. In cases where surgery is attempted first but resection is incomplete based on histologic evaluation, patients should be treated with radiation therapy after surgery.
- Hypofractionated radiation (fewer treatments with larger doses per treatment) may be beneficial in controlling soft-tissue sarcomas with or without surgery.

Chemotherapy:

- May be indicated for patients with high-grade tumors, tumors in certain locations, certain tumor types, and in patients that develop metastatic disease
- Chemotherapy drugs that have been used for soft-tissue sarcoma include doxorubicin, mitoxantrone, platinum drugs, ifosfamide, and combinations.
- Metronomic chemotherapy, using daily low doses of chemotherapy, has been shown to slow the time to recurrence for incompletely excised canine soft-tissue sarcomas. It may be considered as an alternative to irradiation for some cases.
- Marginal tumor excision with intralesional chemotherapy beads can result in long-term control and may be considered as an alternative to radiation therapy for some cases.

Hyperthermia:

- Hyperthermia has been shown to increase response rates for macroscopic tumors treated with radiation. However, hyperthermia has limited availability, and recurrence of tumors often occurs rapidly after treatment.

Possible Complications

Complications of treatments for sarcomas depend on types of treatments and location of the primary tumor:

- Surgery may result in wound complications, including infection, dehiscence, or loss of function of a limb.
- Radiation therapy can cause short-term complications (dermatitis, mucositis) in skin and mucosa involved in the radiation field. Long-term complications, including bone necrosis, are uncommon but are permanent when they do occur.
- Chemotherapy complications may include bone marrow suppression, gastrointestinal effects, and haircoat changes along with other side effects caused by specific chemotherapy drugs (p. 152).

Recommended Monitoring

After appropriate local treatment of the primary tumor, follow-up exams should be done on a routine basis to monitor for local recurrence and metastasis. High-grade tumors may require more frequent monitoring for metastasis during and after chemotherapy administration.

PROGNOSIS & OUTCOME

Prognosis is variable depending on type, location, clinical stage, and histologic grade of tumor:

- Certain tumor types may have higher metastatic rates (e.g., leiomyosarcoma) or more aggressive local behavior (e.g., histologically low-grade, biologically high-grade sarcomas of the oral cavity).
- Soft-tissue sarcomas located in the abdomen (spleen, intestines) are typically more likely to lead to metastasis.
- Soft-tissue sarcomas in certain locations (e.g., oral tumors) may be more difficult to treat with local therapy (surgery or irradiation), resulting in lower rates of local disease control.
- Soft-tissue sarcomas that are large or have metastasized at the time of diagnosis usually have a poor prognosis.
- Histologic grading of canine soft-tissue sarcomas is based on: (1) degree of differentiation, (2) mitotic index, and (3) percent necrosis. Metastasis is more likely for high-grade (grade 3) tumors. Typical metastatic rates are $\approx$40% for grade 3 tumors, up to 20% for grade 2 tumors, and 10% or less for grade 1 tumors. It is unclear whether this grading scheme is applicable to feline soft-tissue sarcomas.

PEARLS & CONSIDERATIONS

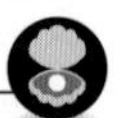

Comments

Many patients with soft-tissue sarcomas can be successfully treated with wide surgical excision alone. Patients with soft-tissue sarcomas that may be more difficult to treat (e.g., oral sarcomas, grade 3 sarcomas, nonresectable tumors) should be referred for consultation with specialists, including a surgeon, oncologist, or radiation oncologist, to develop a multimodality treatment approach.

Prevention

Prevention of soft-tissue sarcomas is not possible. Early detection and treatment may result in easier treatment and better prognosis. Administration of vaccines to cats on the distal limb or tail can facilitate surgical treatment if sarcoma occurs at injection site.

Technician Tips

Measuring and documenting the location (on a body map) of all palpable masses aids in future monitoring.

Client Education

Owners should be educated to monitor for emergence of palpable masses and have them evaluated quickly. Early detection may allow easier treatment by surgery and help avoid the need for radiation therapy.

SUGGESTED READING

Liptak JM, et al: Soft tissue sarcomas. In Withrow SJ, et al, editors: Small animal clinical oncology, Philadelphia, 2013, Saunders, pp 356-380.

AUTHOR: John Farrelly, DVM, MS, DACVIM, DACVR
EDITOR: Kenneth M. Rassnick, DVM, DACVIM

Spider Envenomation

BASIC INFORMATION

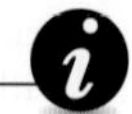

Definition

Of the approximately 40,000 species of spiders in the world, there are few whose bite can cause severe clinical signs. Members of the genus *Latrodectus* (widow spiders) can cause systemic signs, including generalized muscle pain, weakness, paralysis, and (rarely) death. The *Loxosceles* (recluse spiders) can cause nonhealing, necrotizing wounds and occasionally systemic signs.

Synonyms

- Lactrodectism
- Loxoscelism, necrotic arachnidism

Epidemiology

SPECIES, AGE, SEX

Cats are thought to be more sensitive to widow envenomation.

RISK FACTORS

Widow spiders: underlying respiratory or cardiac disease

GEOGRAPHY AND SEASONALITY

See Etiology and Pathophysiology.

Clinical Presentation

HISTORY, CHIEF COMPLAINT

- Rarely, witnessed or suspected spider near pet
- Widow spider: mild local swelling or erythema; reluctance to move (30-120 minutes after envenomation), muscle pain, stiffness
- Recluse spider: pain, pruritus, erythema within 10-30 minutes; expanding (nonhealing), necrotizing wound

PHYSICAL EXAM FINDINGS

- Widow spider: see History, Chief Complaint plus vomiting, hypersalivation, muscle cramping or fasciculations, tachypnea, tachycardia, rigidity, tremors, vocalization, hypertension (cats)
- Recluse spider: see History, Chief Complaint plus expanding bull's-eye lesion, tissue sloughing (may be gravity dependent), and healing that can take months; systemic signs (hemolysis, pyrexia, myalgia, vomiting) are rare and develop 24-72 hours after envenomation

Etiology and Pathophysiology

Widow spiders:

- The name comes from the female's practice of killing the male after insemination, although this may occur only if the female has not eaten recently. Female *Latrodectus* spp have red or orange marks on the abdomen. Males are $\frac{1}{20}$ the size of females and do not have large enough fangs to envenomate humans.

- Prefer dark, undisturbed places (homes, garage, wood pile); bite only if disturbed
- Venom contains proteolytic enzymes and latrotoxins. Alpha-latrotoxin is a neurotoxin. It causes release and depletion of acetylcholine and norepinephrine at motor nerve ending and postganglionic sympathetic synapses, resulting in blocked neurotransmission. The muscle cramping is thought to be secondary to acetylcholine release and the tachycardia/hypertension secondary to norepinephrine release.
- *Latrodectus mactans* (black widow spider, southern black widow) has an orange to red hourglass pattern on ventral abdomen but occasionally has a row of red spots (unconnected hourglass) instead; found throughout North America
- *Latrodectus hesperus* (western black widow spider) has a white to yellow to orange to red hourglass, occasionally broken into two separate spots; found in western North America
- *Latrodectus. various* (northern widow spider) has two separate, elongated spots; found in middle Atlantic United States, southern Ontario
- *Latrodectus bishopi* (red widow spider, red-legged widow) has red legs and cephalothorax with the red hourglass reduced to a single red elongated marking; found in central Florida
- *Latrodectus geometricus* (brown widow spider) has a yellow to red hourglass on a brown body; found in southern North America

Recluse spiders:

- Females possess twice the venom of males, and larger spiders have more venom; site of bite effects toxicity
- Nocturnal, not aggressive
- Venom contains several necrotizing enzymes, including hyluronidase, esterase, and phospholipase D. Sphingomyelinase D, a phospholipase, appears to be responsible for most of the clinical signs. It binds to cell membranes and attracts and activates neutrophils (contributing to the local lesions) and inactivates serum hemolytic complement, leading to rapid coagulation and occlusion of small capillaries, which increases the tissue necrosis. Depletion of clotting factors, hemolysis, platelet activation, and thromboembolic disease can also occur.
- *Loxosceles reclusa* (brown recluse spider, fiddleback spider) has a fiddle-shaped mark on its back, three pairs of eyes; found in south central United States
- *Loxosceles rufescens* (Mediterranean recluse spider), *Loxosceles deserta* (desert recluse), *Loxosceles arizonica* (Arizona brown spider, Arizona recluse): less severe lesions than *L. reclusa*; found in western United States

DIAGNOSIS

Diagnostic Overview

Envenomation by spiders is usually not witnessed. Diagnosis is based on clinical signs and geographic area. There are no diagnostic tests to confirm envenomation.

Differential Diagnosis

- Widow spiders: tetanus, bromethalin, macadamia nuts (dogs), marijuana; meningoencephalitis, intervertebral disc disease, neoplasia
- Recluse spiders: *Allium* spp toxicosis, zinc toxicosis; immune-mediated hemolytic anemia, necrotizing bacterial infection, cellulitis

Initial Database

Widow spider:

- Vital signs (respiratory and heart rate, blood pressure, temperature): all increased
- CBC: potential leukocytosis
- Serum chemistry panel: increased creatine phosphokinase level, hyperglycemia

Recluse spider:

- CBC: hemolysis, anemia (rare), thrombocytopenia; leukocytosis if secondary infection
- Coagulation profile: evidence of disorder (rare)
- Urinalysis: hemoglobinuria (rare)

TREATMENT

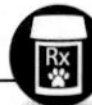

Treatment Overview

- Widow spider: hospitalize and control systemic signs (muscle relaxants, antihypertensives); pain control is important; antivenin if available
- Recluse spider: dermal lesions should be kept clean and managed until healed; systemic signs may require fluids and blood transfusions.

Acute General Treatment

Widow spider:

- Control pain (opioids are most effective): buprenorphine 0.005-0.04 mg/kg IM, IV, SQ, buccal q 6-12h *or* hydromorphone 0.1-0.2 mg/kg SQ, IM, IV q 2-4h or prn
- Hypertension usually resolves with pain control.
- Clean wound (if found) with antiseptics (p. 909).
- Fluid therapy IV (protect kidneys from myoglobinuria, regulate body temperature) (p. 1367)
- Muscle relaxants (methocarbamol 50-150 mg/kg IV, PO, titrate up as needed)
- Antivenom is rarely available but is indicated in severe cases.

Recluse spider:

- Local wound care: monitor size and migration of lesion; clean and debride as needed, sugar/honey bandages (p. 909), antibiotics if secondary infection (amoxicillin-clavulanate 10-20 mg/kg PO q 12h)
- Dapsone 1 mg/kg/day for 10 days (dogs) may limit severity of lesion because it inhibits neutrophil migration
- Diphenhydramine 2.2 mg/kg IV, PO q 8h if pruritic
- Control pain (opioids or nonsteroidal antiinflammatory drugs [NSAIDs]): buprenorphine 0.005-0.04 mg/kg IM, IV, SQ, buccal q 6-12h *or* carprofen 2.2 mg/kg (dogs) PO q 12h
- IV fluids for systemic signs (protect kidneys from hemoglobinuria) (p. 1352)
- Whole blood transfusion or packed red blood cells if hemolysis and anemia occur (p. 1169)
- Monitor and treat disseminated intravascular coagulation (DIC) if present (p. 269).

Chronic Treatment

Recluse spider: manage open wound

Possible Complications

Scarring from recluse spider bite wounds

Recommended Monitoring

Recluse spider: periodic recheck CBC, platelets, coagulation profile until normalized

PROGNOSIS & OUTCOME

- Clinical effects and prognosis are based on both spider and victim.
  - The size of the spider, amount of venom injected, and time of year may affect the outcome.
  - The species envenomated, size of animal, location of the bite, underlying health problems, and age can affect the outcome.
- Widow spiders: prognosis is generally good, and fatalities are rare.
- Recluse spiders: prognosis is generally good because most animals have only mild local signs; prognosis decreases with systemic signs (rare).

PEARLS & CONSIDERATIONS

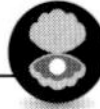

Comments

- Tarantulas produce venom that can cause local pain but is not likely to cause systemic signs. Ingestion of the still hairs by dogs can cause oral irritation, salivation, and vomiting.
- A single widow bite can be life-threatening, but dry bites are also possible. Spiders can control the amount of venom released.

Prevention

Keep pets away from spiders if possible.

Technician Tips

Although rare, systemic signs can occur with recluse bites; monitor vital signs and hematologic changes.

Client Education

Most spider bites in pets are mild, but a few types can cause severe signs.

SUGGESTED READING

Gwaltney-Brant SM, et al: Terrestrial zootoxins. In Gupta RC, editor: Veterinary toxicology basic and clinical principles, ed 2, London, 2012, Academic Press, pp 969-992.

AUTHOR & EDITOR: Tina Wismer, DVM, MS, DABVT, DABT

Spinal Cord Injury

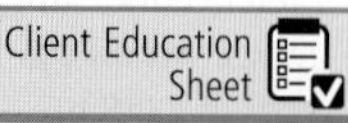

BASIC INFORMATION

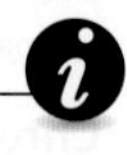

Definition

Any insult to the spinal cord resulting in neurologic impairment. Most common causes of acute spinal cord injury (SCI):

- Intervertebral disc herniation (IVDH)
  - Hansen's type I
  - Hansen's type II
  - Acute noncompressive nucleus pulposus extrusion (ANNPE)
- Vertebral column trauma (including fractures, subluxations, and luxations)
- Fibrocartilaginous embolism (FCE)

Synonyms

- SCI, spinal cord trauma
- For ANNPE: missile disc; traumatic disc; high-velocity, low-volume disc herniation

Epidemiology

SPECIES, AGE, SEX

- Any species, age, or sex, depending on the underlying cause
- IVDH: type I tends to affect middle-aged (3-7 years) chondrodystrophic dog breeds; type II predominantly affects slightly older (6-8 years), nonchondrodystrophic dog breeds. IVDH tends to occur in older cats.
- ANNPE or FCE typically affects middle-aged, medium- to large-breed dogs; uncommon but reported in cats
- Vertebral column trauma can occur at any age but is more common in younger animals.

GENETICS, BREED PREDISPOSITION

IVDH: chondrodystrophic dog breeds (e.g., dachshund, basset hound, French and English bulldog, shih tzu, miniature schnauzer, Pekingese, beagle, Lhasa apso, Bichon frisé, Tibetan spaniel, Cavalier King Charles spaniel, Welsh corgi)

RISK FACTORS

- Breed for IVDH
- ANNPE and FCE have been associated with physical activity.
- Free-roaming animals at greater risk of trauma

ASSOCIATED DISORDERS

Urinary and fecal incontinence: depend on injury severity

Clinical Presentation

HISTORY, CHIEF COMPLAINT

- Acute SCI is characterized by peracute to acute onset of neurologic deficits affecting 1 to 4 limbs, ranging from pain (back or neck), mild paresis and ataxia to paralysis and loss of pain perception.
- Signs can be progressive (e.g., IVDH, unstable fracture) or nonprogressive (ANNPE, FCE).
- Discomfort is common with IVDH and vertebral column trauma.
- Possible history of prior episodes of pain or neurologic deficits with IVDH.
- ANNPE and FCE: progression up to 24 hours after onset is possible; pain is described but atypical; neurologic deficits frequently asymmetrical; history of physical activity common; blunt force trauma noted with traumatic disc herniation
- Traumatic event (e.g., being hit by car, falling from a height) may be witnessed or suspected

PHYSICAL EXAM FINDINGS

- Neurologic deficits: paraspinal pain, paresis (weakness), ataxia (incoordination), paralysis with loss of pain perception
- Specific deficits depend on the neuroanatomic localization.
- With acute, severe thoracolumbar injury, spinal shock and a Schiff-Sherrington posture may be present characterized by flaccid hindlimbs with reduced spinal reflexes and increased forelimb extensor tone.
- With severe thoracolumbar injury (typically paraplegia with loss of pain perception secondary to IVDH), there may be signs of progressive ascending/descending myelomalacia. They include decreased trunk and abdominal tone, rapidly changing neurologic exam findings such as cranial progression or loss of the cutaneous trunci reflex, loss of hindlimb spinal reflexes, flaccid bladder, absent anal tone, progression to forelimb abnormalities and breathing difficulty.
- With tetraplegia, hypoventilation is possible.
- With trauma, there may be signs of external trauma (abrasions, lacerations or other wounds). Concurrent injuries are common with signs referable to the body system affected. Excessive patient manipulation should be avoided.

Etiology and Pathophysiology

Cause:

- ANNPE: herniation of relatively normal nucleus pulposus material causing a contusive injury to the spinal cord with little or no residual extradural compression; associated with exercise and can occur secondary to blunt force trauma
- See chapters on intervertebral disc disease (IVDD [p. 555]), FCE (p. 336), and vertebral fractures (p. 369).

Pathogenesis:

- Primary injury: mechanical insult to the spinal cord causing contusion, shearing, laceration, compression, hemorrhage, and ischemia; spinal stabilization and/or decompression prevent further primary injury, if indicated.
- Secondary injury: cascade of pathologic events that perpetuate and exacerbate the primary injury, including hemorrhage, inflammation, excitotoxicity, free radical production, and apoptosis resulting in progressive tissue destruction; therapies are being investigated to address secondary injury.

DIAGNOSIS

Diagnostic Overview

Thorough neurologic exam is key to accurate neuroanatomic localization, diagnosis, and initiation of appropriate therapy. If trauma is suspected, complete physical exam is essential to evaluate for concurrent injury. The initial diagnostic plan consists of spinal radiographs and testing to establish general health status and suitability for general anesthesia. Further testing includes advanced imaging and possibly cerebrospinal fluid (CSF) analysis. For more severely affected animals (nonambulatory or worse), prompt referral to a neurologist or surgeon is recommended.

Differential Diagnosis

- Vertebral neoplasia causing pathologic fracture
- Meningomyelitis (infectious or immune-mediated causes)
- Neuromuscular weakness (e.g., neuropathy, junctionopathy, myopathy)
- Orthopedic: bilateral cranial cruciate ligament rupture (dogs), hip fractures
- Non–nervous system: hemoabdomen, aortic thromboembolism (especially cats), severe systemic illness or end-stage disease (e.g., cancer), abdominal pain

Initial Database

- Neurologic exam (p. 1136): neuroanatomic localization depends on location of SCI
- CBC and serum biochemical profile: typically unremarkable; preanesthesia screening test
- Urinalysis: can be unremarkable or show hematuria, pyuria, or bacteruria
- Thoracic radiographs, abdominal radiographs, or ultrasound: screening tests considered for older animals and trauma cases
- Spinal radiographs: often unremarkable, especially for ANNPE or FCE; lack of visible abnormalities does not rule out IVDH or trauma. May reveal: mineralized discs *in situ*, narrowed disc space, mineralized material in the spinal canal, spondylosis, fractures, subluxation or luxation

Advanced or Confirmatory Testing

- MRI (p. 1132): excellent soft-tissue detail allows visualization of the spinal cord; gold standard for definitive diagnosis of cause of the SCI

- CT: excellent bony detail, useful for identification of mineralized disc herniation and bony abnormalities secondary to trauma
- Myelography: less commonly used given widespread availability and superior diagnostic capability of MRI; useful to evaluate compressive SCI
- Cerebrospinal fluid analysis (pp. 1080 and 1323): recommended when advanced imaging is inconclusive; nucleated cell count and protein level can be normal or elevated.

TREATMENT

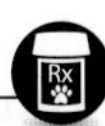

Treatment Overview

Treatment depends on the nature and severity of signs. For nonambulatory or paralyzed animals with compressive or unstable injuries (i.e., IVDH or trauma), prompt surgical decompression ± stabilization is usually recommended. Pain management, excellent nursing care, and bladder evacuation are essential.

Acute General Treatment

- Stabilization for cases of trauma includes immobilization of the spine (backboard or external coaptation) and ensuring respiratory and circulatory function.
  - Evaluate SpO_2 (ideal > 97%), blood gas ($PaCO_2$ < 60 mm Hg), blood pressure (MAP > 60 mm Hg)
  - Address concurrent injuries as indicated.
- Referral to a neurologist or surgeon with access to 24-hour, comprehensive care is recommended for more severe or extensive injuries.
- Surgical treatment
  - Surgical decompression ± stabilization typically recommended for nonambulatory or paralyzed animals with compressive or unstable injuries
  - Paralysis with or without pain perception considered a surgical emergency
- Medical treatment
  - Pain management
    - Opioids: hydromorphone 0.1 mg/kg IV q 4-6h or methadone 0.1 mg/kg IV q 4-6h or fentanyl 2-5 mcg/kg/h IV
    - Nonsteroidal antiinflammatory drugs (NSAIDs): carprofen 2.2 mg/kg PO q 12h or meloxicam 0.1 mg/kg IV, SQ, PO q 24h
  - Glucocorticoids are not recommended as routine therapy for acute SCI.
  - Manual bladder evacuation or urinary catheterization (paralyzed animals)

Chronic Treatment

- For IVDH or trauma managed medically or postoperatively
  - Confinement/activity restriction (4-6 weeks)
  - Rehabilitation with a rehabilitation-certified veterinarian/technician or at-home exercises by owner
  - Pain management: gabapentin 5-15 mg/kg PO q 8-12h × 2-4 weeks), NSAIDs as above × 1-2 weeks, or fentanyl transdermal patch 2-4 mcg/kg
  - Bladder management: manual expression 2-3 times per day until return of voluntary urination; pharmacologic assistance with diazepam 0.25-0.5 mg/kg PO q 8h given 30 minutes before bladder expression and phenoxybenzamine 0.25 mg/kg PO q 12h or prazosin 1 mg/DOG < 15 kg, 2 mg/DOG >15 kg; 1 mg/CAT
  - Nursing care: padded, dry bedding; turning/moving nonambulatory animals; regular bathing and change of bedding
- For ANNPE or FCE: cage rest to prevent further injury of neurologically impaired animals. Rehabilitation is recommended; bladder management and nursing care as above
- See chapters on IVDD (p. 555), vertebral fractures (p. 369), and FCE (p. 336) for more information.
- Future therapies for acute and chronic SCI may include neuroprotective strategies, stem cell transplantation, or other multimodal approaches to treatment.

Possible Complications

- For nonambulatory animals: decubital ulcers, urine scald, aspiration pneumonia, disuse atrophy; meticulous nursing care can help to prevent
- Neurologic worsening: implant failure or infection, recurrent IVDH, or ascending/descending myelomalacia
- Urinary tract infection (UTI): bladder dysfunction is common in animals with SCI, increasing risk of UTIs; regular bladder expression is important (p. 232).

Recommended Monitoring

- Re-evaluation after 7-10 days or at any time if neurologic status worsens for animals with IVDH or trauma managed medically
- Recheck exam 4 weeks after injury.

PROGNOSIS & OUTCOME

- Prognosis for recovery from acute SCI depends on the underlying cause and severity of neurologic injury. The prognosis for a successful outcome (defined as independent ambulation and continence) is fair to excellent regardless of cause as long as pain perception is maintained below the injury. After pain perception is lost, prognosis is fair (secondary to IVDH managed surgically) to guarded (all other causes).
- Prognostic indicators associated with a worse outcome
  - Presence and dimensions of intramedullary hyperintensity on T2-weighted MRI for IVDH, ANNPE, and FCE
  - CSF elevations of nucleated cell count, percentage of macrophages, and macrophage to monocyte ratio in severe IVDH
- For IVDH, conflicting reports regarding onset and duration of signs and outcome; there is no definitive relationship between breed, age, body weight, prior surgery, or administration of glucocorticoids and outcome.

PEARLS & CONSIDERATIONS

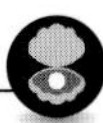

Comments

- Surgery is generally recommended for nonambulatory dogs (due to IVDH or trauma), but medical management remains a viable option with a reasonable chance of recovery as long as pain perception is maintained.
- Interpret leaking urine in a paralyzed animal with caution; it frequently represents overflow rather than voluntary urination.

Technician Tips

- Avoid extensive manipulation of the patient in cases of suspected or confirmed vertebral column trauma.
- Technicians caring for paralyzed animals should be skilled at manual bladder expression.

Client Education

- Manual bladder expression should be performed 3 times/day for paralyzed animals; failure to evacuate any urine over a 24-hour period should prompt a veterinarian visit for assistance.
- Padded bedding that is changed frequently, more frequent bathing, and regular turning are important for nonambulatory/recumbent patients.
- Rest and rehabilitation exercises are important for return of function.

SUGGESTED READING

Granger N, et al: Acute spinal cord injury: tetraplegia and paraplegia in small animals. Vet Clin Small Anim 44:1131-1156, 2014.

AUTHOR: Melissa J. Lewis, VMD, PhD, DACVIM
EDITOR: Karen R. Muñana, DVM, MS, DACVIM

Spinal Cord Neoplasia

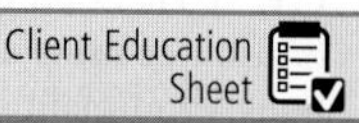

BASIC INFORMATION

Definition

- Spinal neoplasms encompass a wide range of cancers. Vertebral neoplasms are often included in discussions of spinal neoplasms because they secondarily impact the spinal cord and thereby result in clinical signs of neurologic dysfunction.
- Spinal neoplasms are divided into primary and secondary (metastatic or extension from extravertebral tissues) tumors.
- Primary neoplasms can arise from vertebrae, meninges, or neuroparenchyma.
  - Vertebral neoplasia: osteosarcoma, fibrosarcoma, hemangiosarcoma, plasma cell tumor/multiple myeloma, lymphoma, cartilaginous exostosis/osteochondroma
  - Meningeal: meningioma
  - Neuroparenchyma: nerve sheath tumors (NSTs), glial tumors (oligodendroglioma, astrocytoma, oligoastrocytoma, gliomatosis cerebri), ependymoma, metastatic choroid plexus carcinoma, cordoma
  - Mesenchymal tumors: myxoma/myxosarcoma, histiocytic sarcoma, nephroblastoma
  - Secondary neoplasia: metastatic cancers such as prostatic, mammary adenocarcinoma, osteosarcoma, transitional cell carcinoma, melanoma, thyroid carcinoma, pheochromocytoma, and those that secondarily invade the vertebral column ± spinal cord (i.e., infiltrative lipoma/liposarcoma)

Epidemiology

SPECIES, AGE, SEX

- Canine: middle-aged to older, large-breed dogs
  - Possible male predisposition for meningioma (p. 557)
  - Boxer and golden retriever predisposition for meningioma
- Feline: lymphoma; any age but in young (median, 2-3 years) cats often have concurrent feline leukemia (FeLV) infection

Clinical Presentation

HISTORY, CHIEF COMPLAINT

- Clinical signs are related to the anatomic location of the lesion. Lesions affecting the cervical spinal cord to the level of the cranial thoracic spinal cord (spinal cord segments T1 and T2) present with tetraparesis, whereas lesions affecting the thoracolumbar spinal cord caudal to the T2 spinal cord segment present with paraparesis. Lesions affecting the sacral spinal cord may cause urinary and fecal incontinence.
- Canine: chronic progressive paresis and/or general proprioceptive (GP) ataxia (scuffing digits, knuckling, crossing limbs)
  - Mean duration of signs ≈6 weeks, range is 1 day to 1 year. In one study, duration of clinical signs before diagnosis was longest for intradural/extramedullary tumors, followed by extradural tumors. Shortest duration was for intramedullary tumors. Acute presentation also observed, notably with lymphoma
  - Intramedullary neoplasms: dogs with secondary neoplasms (metastasis) tend to be older and have a shorter duration of clinical signs before presentation compared with dogs with primary intramedullary neoplasms.
- Feline lymphoma: acute onset (often ≤ 7 days)

PHYSICAL EXAM FINDINGS

- Neurologic exam (p. 1136). Deficits depend on location and are often asymmetrical. Pain may be noted on palpation of the vertebral column.
- Neurologic signs can often be localized to a region of the spinal cord:
  - C1-C5 spinal cord segments: upper motor neuron (UMN) tetraparesis/plegia and GP ataxia, postural reaction deficits, normal to exaggerated myotatic reflexes, normal withdrawal reflexes, normal to increased muscular tone
  - C6-T2 spinal cord segments: tetraparesis/plegia, postural reaction deficits all four limbs; thoracic limbs: short, choppy gait, decreased withdrawal reflexes, decreased muscular tone, muscle atrophy: pelvic limbs: GP ataxia/UMN paresis, normal to exaggerated myotatic reflexes, normal withdrawal reflexes, normal to increased muscular tone
  - T3-L3 spinal cord segments: GP ataxia/UMN paraparesis/plegia; pelvic limbs: normal to exaggerated myotatic reflexes, normal withdrawal reflexes, normal to increased muscular tone; normal thoracic limbs
  - L4-S3 segments, roots or spinal nerves: paraparesis/plegia; short-strided and crouched pelvic limb posture and gait, postural reaction deficits, decreased myotatic and withdrawal reflexes, decreased muscular tone, muscle atrophy in pelvic limbs; decreased perineal reflex, urinary incontinence, and/or fecal incontinence; decreased tail function

Etiology and Pathophysiology

- Cause is unknown.
- Canine
  - Meningioma commonly affects first three cervical spinal cord segments.
  - Osteosarcoma may occur in prior radiation therapy fields.
  - Nephroblastoma (rare): dogs < 2 years old, intradural/extramedullary, between T10 and L2 vertebrae
  - Multiple cartilaginous exostosis/osteochondroma can undergo malignant transformation to osteosarcoma or chondrosarcoma.
- Feline lymphoma: FeLV infection

DIAGNOSIS

Diagnostic Overview

Presumptive diagnosis is based on cross-sectional imaging. MRI is the gold standard. Lesion location (extravertebral, vertebral, extradural, intradural/extramedullary, or intramedullary), lesion intensity, lesion topography (borders, shape), and degree of contrast enhancement may suggest a specific histologic type. In dogs with an intramedullary lesion, MRI is sensitive imaging modality for discrimination of intramedullary neoplasms from other causes. Despite this, definitive diagnosis requires histologic evaluation.

Differential Diagnosis

- Canine: intervertebral disc herniation, discospondylitis, infectious meningomyelitis (canine distemper virus [CDV], rabies, fungal, *Neospora caninum/Toxoplasma gondii*, bacterial), granulomatous meningoencephalomyelitis, trauma, cervical spondylomyelopathy, fibrocartilaginous embolic myelopathy, orthopedic disease
- Feline: infectious meningomyelitis (feline infectious peritonitis virus, feline immunodeficiency virus [FIV], *Toxoplasma gondii*, rabies, fungal, bacterial), trauma, aortic thromboembolism, intervertebral disc herniation

Initial Database

- CBC, serum biochemical profile, urinalysis, and radiographs of thorax, abdomen, and vertebral column
- Depending on clinical suspicion: serologic testing
  - Feline: serologic testing for FeLV, FIV, *Cryptococcus neoformans, T. gondii*
  - Canine: serologic testing for *C. neoformans, N. caninum, T. gondii,* paired titers (cerebrospinal fluid [CSF]/serum) for CDV

Advanced or Confirmatory Testing

- Cross-sectional imaging: MRI (p. 1132) is the gold standard; CT, combined CT/myelography, myelography may be helpful for vertebral neoplasms
  - MRI characterization
    - Meningioma is often a broad-based, intradural/extramedullary lesion demonstrating uniformly strong contrast enhancement and dural tail.

- NSTs often result in enlargement and abnormal contrast enhancement of the spinal nerves and roots and may extend into the spinal cord.
  - CT may allow appreciation of bony lysis or proliferation.
- CSF analysis (pp. 1080 and 1323)
- Fluoroscopic-guided needle aspiration/biopsy of vertebral lesion
- Spinal lymphoma: further staging is required. FeLV/FIV testing, cytologic evaluation of bone marrow, ± kidney, lymph node, liver, or spleen
- Presumptive diagnosis based on lesion location and imaging characteristics
  - Vertebral: osteosarcoma, fibrosarcoma, hemangiosarcoma, plasma cell neoplasia, lymphoma, metastatic neoplasia
  - Extradural: lymphoma, NST
  - Intradural/extramedullary: NST, meningioma, nephroblastoma (young dog)
  - Intramedullary: neuroparenchymal tumors (e.g., glial tumors), metastatic neoplasia, hematopoietic neoplasms)
- Definitive diagnosis: histopathologic exam

TREATMENT

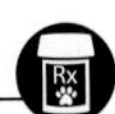

Treatment Overview

In general, surgery is the basis for treatment of most neoplasms. Complete resection is often impossible, but cytoreduction enables decompression of the spinal cord and allows return of function. Adjunctive therapy may include radiation therapy and/or chemotherapy. For hematopoietic neoplasms, chemotherapy alone or in conjunction with radiation therapy may be used, depending on degree of compression and neurologic function of the animal. Surgery should be performed by a board-certified neurologist or surgeon.

Acute General Treatment

- Hemilaminectomy/dorsal laminectomy for decompression and cytoreduction
- Palliation with glucocorticoids and analgesics
- Vertebral tumors: palliation with radiation, bisphosphonate, glucocorticoids
- Spinal lymphoma: systemic chemotherapy, radiation therapy
- Plasma cell tumor/multiple myeloma: systemic chemotherapy, radiation therapy

Chronic Treatment

- Same as for acute general treatment
- For incompletely excised neoplasms, postoperative radiation therapy should be considered.

Behavior/Exercise

- Postoperative exercise restriction; 3-4 weeks' duration
- Controlled physical rehabilitation under the guidance of trained personnel may be beneficial.

Possible Complications

Radiation myelopathy

Recommended Monitoring

- Periodic neurologic exam
- Repeat imaging studies
- Chemotherapy necessitates hematologic and serum biochemical profile monitoring.

PROGNOSIS & OUTCOME

- Variable based on tumor type, completeness of resection, and severity of neurologic deficits
  - Patients lacking motor function and nociception (sensation) have a grave prognosis.
- Canine
  - Surgical resection alone: in a study of dogs with various neoplasms, the overall median survival was 240 days.
  - Meningioma with surgical resection alone: median survival of 19 months; ranges from < 30 days to 1440 days; postoperative radiation may prolong survival time
  - Vertebral tumors (osteosarcoma and fibrosarcoma): median survival of 135 days (range, 15-600 days)
  - NST: varies, depending on the proximity to the spinal cord
    - With surgery alone: median survival of 203 days (range, 120-300 days); proximal neoplasms have shorter survival times
    - In one study of 10 dogs treated with radiation alone, the mean progression-free survival was 240 days, whereas the overall mean survival was time 371 days.
  - In dogs with intramedullary neoplasms: median survival time is 20 days (range, 1-202 days).
  - Surgical resection and postoperative radiation: in one report of 9 dogs (6 with meningiomas), overall median survival was 510 days.
- Feline: lymphoma (p. 607)

PEARLS & CONSIDERATIONS

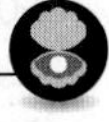

Comments

- MRI may help exclude other differential diagnoses and may provide insight into histologic type of neoplasm.
- Definitive diagnosis requires histopathologic evaluation.
- Long-term remission is possible regardless of completeness of excision.

Technician Tips

- Severely affected animals require intensive nursing care.
  - Animals may not be able to urinate and therefore require manual bladder expression or maintenance of a urethral catheter and indwelling closed urinary collection system. Development of urinary tract infection is common.
  - Affected animals require soft, padded bedding and frequent changes in their recumbency to prevent decubital ulcers. Passive range of motion of paralyzed limbs and other physical therapy exercises may be performed to assist in recovery.
- Affected animals are often painful preoperatively and in the early postoperative period, necessitating analgesic therapy.

SUGGESTED READING

Levy MS, et al: Spinal tumors in 37 dogs: clinical outcome and long-term survival (1987-1994). J Am Anim Hosp Assoc 33:307-312, 1997.

AUTHOR: Marc Kent, DVM, DACVIM
EDITOR: Kenneth M. Rassnick, DVM, DACVIM

Spirocercosis

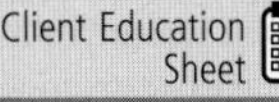

BASIC INFORMATION

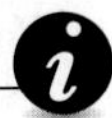

Definition

A disease of dogs caused by the nematode *Spirocerca lupi* and characterized by lesions that can affect the esophagus (with potential for transformation to esophageal malignancy), aorta, and vertebrae

Epidemiology

SPECIES, AGE, SEX

- Primarily affects dogs
- Young to middle-aged dogs overrepresented; dogs < 1 year old unlikely to develop disease

GENETICS, BREED PREDISPOSITION

Medium- and large-breed dogs predisposed, but genetic and breed predisposition unknown.

CONTAGION AND ZOONOSIS

Not zoonotic

GEOGRAPHY AND SEASONALITY

This parasite is found in the southern United States and many tropical and subtropical regions. In some endemic areas, there is a disproportionately high prevalence among urban dogs compared with rural dogs, but this varies with geographic region.

ASSOCIATED DISORDERS

- Esophageal neoplasia (osteosarcoma, fibrosarcoma, undifferentiated sarcoma) may occur secondary to esophageal granuloma formation from the encysted worms.
- Hypertrophic osteopathy
- Thoracic aortic aneurysm and/or thrombosis may occur secondary to migration of *S. lupi* from the gastrointestinal (GI) tract into the aortic wall.
- Thoracic vertebral spondylitis has been reported secondary to migration and granuloma formation.
- Salivary gland necrosis, esophageal perforation with associated mediastinitis and pyothorax have also been reported.

Clinical Presentation

HISTORY, CHIEF COMPLAINT

May be subclinical or clinical signs reflecting location of lesion: vomiting or regurgitation, odynophagia, ptyalism, weakness, respiratory difficulty, coughing, anorexia, melena, paraparesis

PHYSICAL EXAM FINDINGS

In addition to the chief complaints listed above, the most common abnormalities are weight loss and fever.

Etiology and Pathophysiology

- Spirocercosis is caused by migration of the nematode *S. lupi*. Carnivores are infected by ingestion of an intermediate host (coprophagous beetles) or other paratenic hosts (e.g., birds, hedgehogs, lizards, mice, rabbits) in which the parasite does not undergo further development during its passage.
- Adult *S. lupi* generally live in esophageal and gastric nodules. *Spirocerca* eggs pass with feces, and they are ingested by coprophagous beetles. The definitive host may acquire the infection by ingesting the beetle intermediate host or other paratenic host.
- L3-stage larvae penetrate the stomach wall of the definitive host, migrate in the walls of the gastric arteries to the thoracic aorta, and then migrate to the esophagus. The prepatent period, the time from infection of the host to the first ability to detect the infection with diagnostic evaluation, is approximately 5-6 months.
- Clinically significant lesions reflect the migration route and final destination of the parasite. The most common scenario is esophageal granuloma formation.

DIAGNOSIS

Diagnostic Overview

Spirocercosis typically is suspected in a patient living in an endemic area presented for evaluation of regurgitation. Thoracic radiographic findings often support the diagnosis, but direct visualization through endoscopy is required for confirmation before treatment.

Differential Diagnosis

- Regurgitation: other esophageal disorders such as megaesophagus, esophagitis, foreign bodies, esophageal stricture, gastroesophageal reflux disease
- Esophageal mass: esophageal neoplasia, granuloma of other origin
- Vomiting: gastrointestinal (GI) (inflammatory, infectious, parasitic, neoplastic, dietary) and extra-GI (metabolic, endocrine, pancreatitis) causes

Initial Database

- CBC, serum biochemical profile, urinalysis; no characteristic abnormalities
  - Anemia (53% of cases) typically normocytic, normochromic, and nonregenerative
  - Leukocytosis (primarily neutrophilia)
  - Elevation in serum creatine kinase level: most common biochemical abnormality (54% of cases)
  - Hyperproteinemia due to hyperglobulinemia
- Fecal flotation $NaNO_3$ (specific gravity [SG] 1.22), $MgSO_4$ (SG 1.29), $ZnSO_4$ (SG 1.30), or sugar (SG 1.27)
  - May reveal characteristic small, elongated eggs; positive result in 42%-67% of endoscopically confirmed cases ($NaNO_3$ best)
- Thoracic and abdominal radiographs are indicated (dorsoventral and right lateral projections most accurate for thoracic films) and may reveal
  - Esophageal and stomach lesions (soft-tissue masses with/without calcification): a mass is noted in the caudal esophagus in 53%-86% of cases of spirocercosis. Most affected dogs have more than one granuloma, but not all are visible radiographically.
  - Insufflation of the esophagus with air (sedated/anesthetized patient) significantly improves diagnostic yield.
  - Bony changes in the thoracic vertebrae
  - Evidence of metastasis possible when esophageal neoplasia is present
- Limb radiographs of patients with lameness or hard swelling of distal limbs to assess for hypertrophic osteopathy

Advanced or Confirmatory Testing

- Esophagoscopy and gastroscopy (p. 1098) may allow visualization of granulomas and biopsy. In most cases of spirocercosis, endoscopy is the confirmatory diagnostic procedure of choice.
- Thoracic CT identifies significantly more esophageal masses, aortic aneurysms, aortic mineralization, and aortic thrombi.
- Postmortem exam of patients with sudden death or that have been euthanized can provide a definitive diagnosis.

TREATMENT

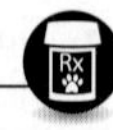

Treatment Overview

Treatment goals:

- Resolution of regurgitation or vomiting
- Prevent development of esophageal neoplasia or hypertrophic osteopathy.
- Prevent sudden death due to rupture of aneurysm.

Acute General Treatment

- Doramectin is treatment of choice. Permanent resolution/cure is expected for many or most dogs in 6 weeks or less. Two protocols are recognized:
  - Intermittent SQ protocol: 200 mcg/kg SQ q 14 days for 3 treatments; if necessary (incomplete resolution of lesions), retreatment with 500 mcg/kg PO q 24h × 6 weeks has been successful and safe.
  - Daily PO protocol: 500 mcg/kg PO q 24h × 42 days (65% cured); if lesions persist, can retreat × 42 days once (further 25% cured) or twice (remaining 10% cured) more
- Fenbendazole 50 mg/kg PO q 24h × 5-7 days or ivermectin 200-400 mcg/kg SQ q 14-28 days has been used for treating spirocercosis.

Possible Complications

Do not use ivermectins (like doramectin) in collies, Shetland sheepdogs, Australian shepherds, or other susceptible breeds or individuals unless *MDR1/ABCB1-Δ* mutation negative (p. 638).

PROGNOSIS & OUTCOME

Prognosis is variable:

- With appropriate treatment, cure is expected for many or most dogs in 6 weeks or less.
  - Daily protocol: > 97% of dogs have resolution of clinical signs after 7-10 days of treatment.
- Esophageal neoplasia, aortic aneurysm, or large masses obstructing flow of ingesta worsens the prognosis.
- Hypertrophic osteopathy signifies a worse prognosis (39% of cases with esophageal malignancy, 0% of cases without esophageal malignancy)
- Radiographic evidence of spondylitis (68% vs. 38%) and bronchial displacement (52% vs. 17%) is significantly more likely in those with malignancy.
- Sixty-three percent of dogs with spirocercosis may die or be euthanized within 1 month of admission.

PEARLS & CONSIDERATIONS

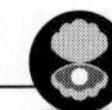

Comments

- In North America and Europe, spirocercosis is a rare disease and is considered only when there is a high index of clinical suspicion.
- The characteristic lesion is a soft-tissue mass in the caudal esophagus; radiographically and clinically, foreign-body ingestion is an important differential diagnosis.
- A minority of dogs develops neoplastic transformation of esophageal granulomas (e.g., 13 of 14 dogs with spirocercosis had esophageal masses, but only 1 of 13 had esophageal neoplasia).
- Significantly lower serum vitamin D concentrations in dogs with *Spirocerca* granulomas (and even lower levels in those with esophageal neoplasia) may offer new insights in the mechanism and/or treatment of spirocercosis.

Prevention

Prevent dogs from eating beetles or paratenic hosts.

Technician Tips

Testing for the *MDR1/ABCB1-Δ* mutation is easily accomplished by submitting an EDTA blood sample or cheek swab to the Washington State University Veterinary Clinical Pharmacology Lab (https://vcpl.vetmed.wsu.edu/).

SUGGESTED READING

Lobetti R: Successful resolution of oesophageal spirocercosis in 20 dogs following daily treatment with oral doramectin. Vet J 193(1):277-278, 2012.

AUTHOR: **Steven L. Marks, BVSc, MS, DACVIM**
EDITOR: **Rance K. Sellon, DVM, PhD, DACVIM**

Splenic Torsion

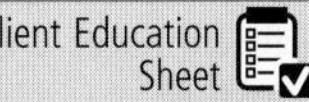

BASIC INFORMATION

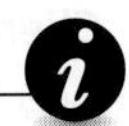

Definition

Twisting and rotation of the spleen around its vascular pedicle, resulting in occlusion and thrombosis of vasculature and splenic congestion and ischemia

Epidemiology

SPECIES, AGE, SEX

Dogs:
- Deep-chested large and giant breeds (Great Dane, Saint Bernard, German shepherd, Irish setter)
- No age predisposition
- Males more commonly affected

RISK FACTORS

Spontaneously resolving gastric dilation and volvulus (GDV) can occur in conjunction with splenic torsion

ASSOCIATED DISORDERS

- GDV (can occur following splenectomy for splenic torsion)
- Splenic infarction

Clinical Presentation

DISEASE FORMS/SUBTYPES

- Acute
- Chronic

HISTORY, CHIEF COMPLAINT

Acute:
- Collapse
- ± GDV and associated signs
- Signs of hypovolemic or toxic shock

Chronic:
- Vague, nonspecific history: difficult to distinguish from other disorders that cause signs of abdominal pain
- Signs may be present for up to 3 weeks.
- Lethargy, anorexia, vomiting, diarrhea, polyuria/polydipsia, discolored urine, weight loss

PHYSICAL EXAM FINDINGS

- Abdominal distention
- Mid-abdominal mass/splenomegaly
- Signs of hypotensive shock if acute form (tachycardia, pallor, prolonged capillary refill time, weak peripheral pulse)

Etiology and Pathophysiology

- Twisting of vasculature results in venous occlusion first. The arterial system remains patent, resulting in a large and painful spleen.
- Proposed mechanism
  - Gastric distention repeatedly stretches gastrosplenic and splenocolic ligaments, allowing splenic hypermotility.
  - Spontaneous resolution of GDV may leave the spleen in a rotated position.
- Intravascular microangiopathic hemolysis is a common complication.

DIAGNOSIS

Diagnostic Overview

Diagnosis is suspected based on patient signalment, history, and physical exam findings. Abdominal diagnostic imaging (radiography, ultrasound) demonstrates the uniformly enlarged, malpositioned spleen.

Differential Diagnosis

- Splenic mass
- Neoplasia of other abdominal organs
- GDV
- Mesenteric volvulus

Initial Database

- CBC: anemia, leukocytosis (stress leukogram common)
- Serum biochemistry profile: increased alkaline phosphatase, alanine aminotransferase, bilirubin concentrations. Hemolysis of sample often noted
- Coagulation profile
- Urinalysis: hemoglobinuria common
- Abdominal radiographs: splenomegaly
  - Spleen may have a reversed C shape.
  - Gas opacities in spleen in chronic torsions
  - Loss of abdominal detail consistent with effusion
  - Displacement of small intestine
- Abdominal ultrasound
  - Generalized splenomegaly
  - Lacy, diffusely hypoechoic splenic parenchyma
  - Thrombi located within splenic vasculature
  - Color-flow Doppler: decreased blood flow to the hilar vessels
- Electrocardiogram (ECG): ventricular arrhythmias are common.

Advanced or Confirmatory Testing

CT: corkscrew-like soft-tissue mass in the location of the splenic artery and vein

TREATMENT

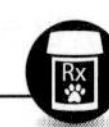

Treatment Overview

Splenectomy is the required treatment and should be performed as soon as the patient is stable. Intensive postoperative care is necessary.

Acute General Treatment

Preoperative patient stabilization
- Correct fluid and electrolyte imbalances.
- Blood transfusion: if hematocrit < 20% (p. 1169)
- Treat cardiac arrhythmias (pp. 1033 and 1457)
- Preoperative and perioperative broad-spectrum antibiotics

Surgical treatment: as soon as the patient is stable:
- Do not reposition/untwist the spleen, which releases microthrombi or thrombi, vasoactive amines, and cellular breakdown products (e.g., free radicals, tumor necrosis factors, toxins).
- Splenectomy: submit for histopathologic analysis
- Gastropexy: performed unless the patient is unstable

Postoperative supportive care:
- Intravenous fluid therapy: must replace volume lost in spleen
- Electrolyte and acid-base correction
- Additional blood products based on hematocrit
- ECG monitoring for arrhythmias

Possible Complications

- Undiagnosed or delay in treatment: splenic necrosis, septic peritonitis, hemolytic anemia, disseminated intravascular coagulation possible
- Pancreatitis (compromised vascular supply of the left limb of the pancreas)

PROGNOSIS & OUTCOME

Prognosis is good to guarded.
- Chronic torsion has a better prognosis than acute torsion.
- In acute form, early treatment improves prognosis.

PEARLS & CONSIDERATIONS

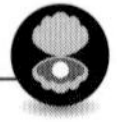

Comments

- Splenic torsions can be acute or chronic and can occur in association with a GDV or as an isolated event.

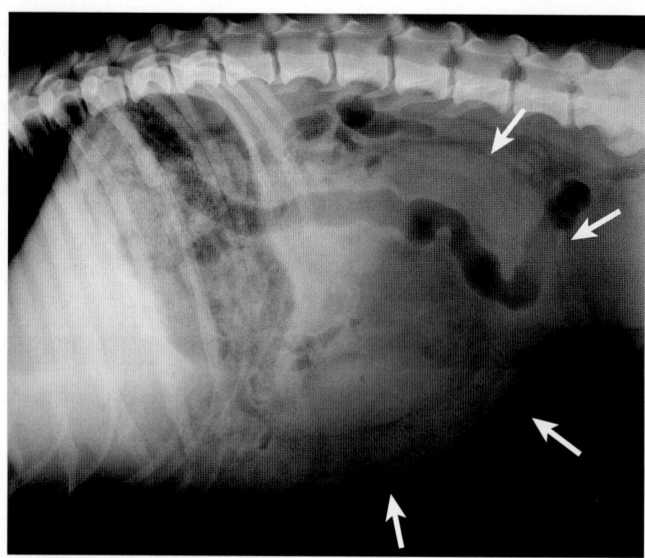

SPLENIC TORSION Lateral abdominal radiograph of a dog with splenic torsion shows the characteristic reversed C shape of the torsed spleen *(arrows)*. (Courtesy Dr. Richard Walshaw.)

- Breeds associated with a high incidence of GDV are also at risk for splenic torsion.
- Gastropexy should be performed after splenectomy to prevent GDV.

Technician Tips

- Be familiar with the signs of hypovolemia to help guide postoperative fluid management.
- Be able to recognize accelerated idioventricular rhythm, R-on-T complexes, and ventricular tachycardia to know when to alert a clinician for treatment of ventricular arrhythmias (pp. 1033 and 1457).

Client Education

Large/giant-breed dogs are at risk for developing a splenic torsion, and chronic splenic torsion can produce vague, nonspecific abdominal signs.

SUGGESTED READING

DeGroot W, et al: Primary splenic torsion in dogs: 102 cases (1992-2014). J Am Vet Assoc 248:661-668, 2016.

AUTHOR: Otto I. Lanz, DVM, DACVS
EDITOR: Elizabeth A. Swanson, DVM, MS, DACVS

Splenomegaly

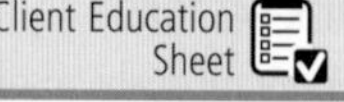

BASIC INFORMATION

Definition

Focal or diffuse splenic enlargement

Epidemiology

SPECIES, AGE, SEX

Dogs or cats of any age and either sex

GENETICS, BREED PREDISPOSITION

- German shepherd dogs have a large spleen normally.
- Certain breeds are predisposed to conditions that commonly result in splenomegaly (e.g., Staffordshire bull terriers and *Babesia gibsoni*; poodles and immune-mediated hemolytic anemia [IMHA]; golden retriever and hemangiosarcoma [HSA]).

CONTAGION AND ZOONOSIS

Several infectious diseases can cause splenomegaly (p. 1282).

ASSOCIATED DISORDERS

Thrombocytopenia, arrhythmia

Clinical Presentation

DISEASE FORMS/SUBTYPES

Diffuse or focal enlargement

HISTORY, CHIEF COMPLAINT

Depends on cause, but nonspecific signs (e.g., lethargy, anorexia) are common.

PHYSICAL EXAM FINDINGS

- Palpable cranial to mid-abdominal mass; usually left-sided but may extend to the right side
- Other exam findings depend on the cause of splenomegaly:
  - Lymphoma may result in generalized lymphadenopathy.
  - Immune-mediated thrombocytopenia (ITP) may result in petechiae.
  - Splenic torsion may result in hypovolemic shock.
  - Ruptured splenic HSA may result in pallor and arrhythmia.

Etiology and Pathophysiology

- There are myriad causes of diffuse or focal splenomegaly (p. 1282).
- Extramedullary hematopoiesis is a common cause of splenomegaly, usually in response to bone marrow disorders.
- Neoplasia is another common cause of splenomegaly. The most common splenic cancers in dogs are lymphoma (diffuse) and HSA (focal), and mast cell tumor is common in cats.
- Many infectious diseases cause splenomegaly (p. 1282).
- Splenic congestion may be drug induced or related to disease (e.g., portal hypertension, right-sided heart failure, splenic torsion).

DIAGNOSIS

Diagnostic Overview

Diagnostic plan depends on other historical and exam findings but often includes abdominal imaging. Radiographs are preferred for assessing size of the spleen, whereas ultrasound is preferred for differentiating focal and diffuse enlargement and assessing splenic parenchyma. Minimal laboratory data may guide prioritization of differential diagnoses and aid in determining whether the platelet count is adequate to perform a fine-needle aspiration (FNA) of the spleen (if appropriate). Diseases commonly diagnosed by cytology with an ultrasound-guided FNA sample include extramedullary hematopoiesis (EMH), lymphoma, mast cell neoplasia, and some infectious diseases (e.g., histoplasmosis, cytauxzoonosis).

Differential Diagnosis

Enlargement of other abdominal organs can be mistaken for splenomegaly.

Initial Database

CBC:

- Nonregenerative anemia: bone marrow infiltrative disease with secondary EMH
- Regenerative anemia: IMHA, splenic mass hemorrhage/rupture, erythrocyte organisms (e.g., *Babesia* spp)
- Thrombocytopenia: vector-borne disease, ITP, platelet consumption, splenic sequestration
- Blood smear evaluation for RBC organisms, spherocytosis (IMHA), schistocytosis (HSA)

Chemistry panel:

- Hypercalcemia: lymphoma, other neoplastic disease, fungal/granulomatous disease
- Hyperglobulinemia: neoplasia (multiple myeloma, lymphoma), feline infectious peritonitis (FIP), nonspecific inflammatory disease

Urinalysis:

- Bilirubinuria, hemoglobinuria: hemolysis

Imaging:

- Abdominal radiographs: confirm splenomegaly and identify additional issues (e.g., effusion, concurrent hepatomegaly)
- Abdominal ultrasound: diffuse or focal (i.e., mass) enlargement, echogenicity of spleen, metastatic disease or involvement of other abdominal organs (e.g., liver), vascular occlusion (splenic torsion, thrombosis)
- Thoracic radiographs: metastatic disease, right-sided cardiac enlargement
- Advanced imaging of the abdomen (CT or MRI): provides more detailed information but costly and requires anesthesia/sedation

Advanced or Confirmatory Testing

Choice of tests determined by initial data:

- Specific infectious disease testing, when appropriate
  - *Babesia* spp polymerase chain reaction (PCR) and serology
  - *Cytauxzoon felis* PCR
  - *Ehrlichia* spp serology and/or PCR
  - *Histoplasma capsulatum* urine antigen
  - Retroviral testing feline leukemia virus/feline immunodeficiency virus (FeLV/FIV)
  - Bartonella serology and PCR
  - Others as suggested by other findings
- Advanced diagnostics for disease suspected to cause splenomegaly:
  - Immune-mediated disease (e.g., Coombs' test, flow cytometry)
  - Lymphoid neoplasia (e.g., PCR for antigen receptor rearrangement [PARR], flow cytometry)
  - Right heart failure (e.g., echocardiogram, heartworm test)
  - Extramedullary hematopoiesis (e.g., bone marrow aspirate ± core biopsy)
- FNA (ultrasound guided): allows for identification of infiltrative neoplasia (lymphoma, mast cell tumor) and some infectious diseases (e.g., histoplasmosis).
  - Not usually indicated for cavitated splenic mass due to risk of hemorrhage/splenic rupture and low diagnostic yield
- Splenic biopsy (splenectomy or, less commonly, incisional biopsy): histopathologic evaluation ± culture.

TREATMENT

Treatment Overview

Treatment is aimed at the underlying disease. Diffuse enlargement of the spleen is rarely an indication for splenectomy because it could worsen the clinical condition (e.g., *Babesia* spp, EMH). Most causes of diffuse splenomegaly are treated medically. However, splenic torsion or focal enlargement (i.e., splenic mass) often calls for complete (or sometimes partial) splenectomy.

Acute General Treatment

- Red blood cell (RBC) transfusion (packed RBC or whole blood): sometimes indicated for hemoabdomen due to splenic mass hemorrhage/rupture or severe anemia secondary to IMHA or ITP
- Splenectomy: patients with a bleeding splenic mass benefit therapeutically and diagnostically from prompt splenectomy. Patients can stabilize on their own if the bleeding stops and they reabsorb peritoneal hemorrhage.
- Antiarrhythmic agents (e.g., lidocaine 2 mg/kg IV bolus): treatment of ventricular arrhythmias is indicated in patients with ventricular tachycardia or frequent ventricular ectopy (especially if resulting in hemodynamic instability).

Chronic Treatment

Chronic management is specific for the disease process resulting in splenomegaly.

Behavior/Exercise

Animals with a splenic mass should be handled with caution to reduce the risk of rupture.

Possible Complications

- The spleen has an important role in controlling some infectious diseases, and these infectious diseases (e.g., *Babesia* spp, hemotrophic *Mycoplasma* spp) are harder to clear after splenectomy.
  - Splenectomy can predispose to certain infections (e.g., *Mycoplasma haemocanis*).
- Splenectomy can predispose to GDV. Although controversial, gastropexy should be considered at the time of splenectomy in selected patients (e.g., deep-chested dog breeds).

Recommended Monitoring

Monitor for coagulopathy, ventricular arrhythmias, and anemia requiring blood transfusion in patients with HSA. Monitor severity of anemia in patients with IMHA, ITP, and erythrocytic infections.

PROGNOSIS & OUTCOME

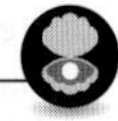

- Prognosis depends on the underlying disease process resulting in splenomegaly.
- Benign masses of the spleen generally carry a good prognosis with removal (64% alive at 1 year).

PEARLS & CONSIDERATIONS

Comments

- Degree of splenomegaly cannot be used to predict malignancy or likelihood of disease recovery. Splenic hematoma can cause profound splenomegaly but is a benign condition.
- If a systemic disease or drug is recognized as a likely cause of splenomegaly, specific splenic sampling may not be indicated.
- Diffuse splenomegaly is rarely an indication for splenectomy (splenic torsion is an exception).
- Ultrasound-guided FNA samples can provide important cytologic evaluation of the spleen but is not advised if cavitation is recognized.
- If the whole spleen is removed, the entire spleen should be submitted for histopathologic evaluation. Use adequate volume of formalin for diagnostic submission, and slice excised spleen to allow proper fixation.

Prevention

Tick prevention reduces the chance of vector-borne disease.

Technician Tips

Patients with splenic mass or undergoing splenectomy should be monitored by continuous electrocardiogram (p. 1096) for arrhythmia.

SUGGESTED READING

Argyle DJ, et al: Nonneoplastic diseases of the spleen. In Ettinger SJ, et al, editors: Textbook of veterinary internal medicine, ed 8, St. Louis, 2017, Elsevier.

AUTHOR: Laura A. Nafe, DVM, MS, DACVIM
EDITOR: Leah A. Cohn, DVM, PhD, DACVIM

Sporotrichosis

BASIC INFORMATION

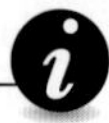

Definition

The mycotic disease is caused by the dimorphic fungus *Sporothrix schenckii,* which clinically manifests with chronic granulomatous skin lesions. *Sporothrix brasiliensis* is emerging as a more pathogenic form in Brazil and neighboring South American countries.

Epidemiology

SPECIES, AGE, SEX

- Cats, dogs, humans, horses, pigs, and cattle; young to middle-aged cats and dogs predominate.
- Rose-grower's disease in humans

RISK FACTORS

- The disease is often acquired by inoculation from puncture wounds, and outdoor-roaming dogs are overrepresented. For cats, prevalence is higher among fighting, intact males.
- A higher concentration of organisms exists in soils rich in decaying organic matter, barberry and rose bush thorns, sphagnum moss, and tree bark.
- Immunosuppression allows for dissemination.

CONTAGION AND ZOONOSIS

- Cat-to-cat or cat-to-human transmission is considered possible, especially to immunosuppressed people (by wounds or contaminated claws).
- Dog-to-dog or dog-to-human transmission is unlikely/rare due to low numbers of organisms found in lesions.

GEOGRAPHY AND SEASONALITY

- Worldwide distribution; temperate to tropical climates
- Found in Mississippi and Missouri River valleys; infrequent in California and southwestern United States

Clinical Presentation

DISEASE FORMS/SUBTYPES

- Three clinical forms: cutaneous, lymphocutaneous, and multifocal disseminated
- Dogs: predominantly cutaneous, lymphocutaneous
- Cats: all three forms

HISTORY, CHIEF COMPLAINT

- Cutaneous lesions (nodular to ulcerated), possibly with draining tracts
- Lethargy
- Anorexia

PHYSICAL EXAM FINDINGS

- Fever: suggests possible disseminated disease and immunocompromised state
- Depression
- Cats: ≈97% of affected cats have one or multiple skin lesions, commonly on the distal limbs, tail base, or head (face or nasal plenum), often with mucosal involvement.
  - Draining puncture wounds, abscesses, or cellulitis
  - Ulcerations, purulent exudate, and large crusted lesions
  - ≈44% of affected cats have respiratory tract signs
- Dogs: multinodular truncal or head lesions; dermal or subcutaneous
  - Ulcerations with purulent exudate and crust formation are possible.
  - Lymphocutaneous form: nodules on distal limb, ascending through lymphatics, and associated lymphadenopathy

Etiology and Pathophysiology

- Inoculation of mycelial form of *S. schenckii* into tissues leads to production of the yeast form.
- Incubation period of ≈1 month
- Pyogranulomatous inflammation occurs, with organisms seen in macrophages and neutrophils.
- Lymphatic dissemination to spleen, liver, lung, eyes, bones, central nervous system, muscles, mammary gland, testis, and epididymis
  - Lung and liver are predominant sites for dissemination in cats.
- Dissemination is rare in dogs but may occur in up to 50% of cats, especially with immune-suppressive dosages of corticosteroids.

DIAGNOSIS

Diagnostic Overview

Diagnosis is based on geography, history, and physical exam findings, with positive cytologic results. Suspicion is also warranted with skin wounds that are not responding to standard antibiotic therapy.

Differential Diagnosis

- Deep cutaneous bacterial infection
- L-form bacterial infection
- Systemic mycosis
- Squamous cell carcinoma
- Immune-mediated disease, systemic lupus erythematosus, pemphigus, vulgaris, allergy, drug eruption
- Leishmaniasis (dogs)

Initial Database

- CBC, serum biochemistry profile, urinalysis: anemia, leukocytosis with neutrophilia, hypoalbuminemia, and hyperglobulinemia commonly observed
- Feline leukemia virus (FeLV) and feline immunodeficiency virus (FIV) serologic testing: positive in < 1% and 8% of affected cats, respectively
- Cytologic exam from aspirates, exudates, or skin preps: diagnostic
  - Organism is small (3-5 mcm in diameter and 5-9 mcm long [slightly smaller than erythrocytes]) and round, oval, or cigar shaped. Large numbers of organisms are found in exudate in cats; small numbers are found in dogs.
- Positive bacterial cultures from secondary infection, often *Staphylococcus pseudintermedius*

Advanced or Confirmatory Testing

- Histopathologic exam of nodules: diagnostic
- Fungal culture: notify laboratory of the possibility of *Sporothrix* organisms because of the infectious nature of sample to humans (zoonosis risk). For the same reason, never culture suspected sporotrichosis lesions in house.
- The Centers for Disease Control and Prevention, Atlanta, can perform fluorescent antibody testing on exudates or tissue.

TREATMENT

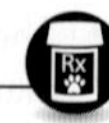

Treatment Overview

- Antifungal treatment of organisms, with treatment continuing for 30 days beyond apparent cure
- Corticosteroids or other immunosuppressives are contraindicated.

Acute and Chronic Treatment

Dogs: options include one of the following:

- Itraconazole or fluconazole 5-10 mg/kg PO with food q 12-24h for 30 days beyond apparent cure, *or*
- Supersaturated solution of potassium iodide (SSKI) 40 mg/kg PO with food q 8-12h for 30 days beyond apparent cure, *or*
- Ketoconazole 5-15 mg/kg PO with food q 12h for 30 days beyond apparent cure
- Terbinafine 25-30 mg/kg/day for 30 days beyond apparent cure

Cats:

- Itraconazole is the treatment of choice for cats; better absorption with suspension formula; or 5-10 mg/kg (capsules) PO q 12-24h for 30 days beyond apparent cure
- Itraconazole 5-10 mg/kg q 12-24h with SSKI (2.5-20 mg/kg/day) may be a better combination for resistant infections in cats.

Possible Complications

- SSKI can cause systemic iodination (ocular and nasal discharge, dry haircoat with scaling, vomiting, depression, collapse). If signs are mild, discontinue the medication for 1 week and reinitiate; if signs are severe, change to different therapy.

- Ketoconazole can be hepatotoxic, especially in cats.
- Itraconazole is hepatotoxic in 10% of dogs treated with a dosage of 5 mg/kg q 12h; better tolerated, fewer side effects in cats, although hepatotoxicity can occur.

Recommended Monitoring

With itraconazole or ketoconazole administration, monitor liver enzymes q 2-4 weeks for duration of therapy.

PROGNOSIS & OUTCOME

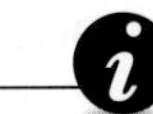

- Response of cutaneous or lymphocutaneous forms is fair to good. Of 266 cats treated in one study, 68 (26%) were cured, irrespective of extracutaneous signs or FIV status.
- Disseminated disease carries a guarded prognosis.

PEARLS & CONSIDERATIONS

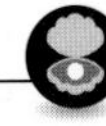

Comments

- Even after treatment is completed, use of immunosuppressive dosages of corticosteroids is contraindicated due to reports of recurrence.
- Duration of therapy is often ≥ 3 months.
- Cats have been given iodide and ketoconazole, but because of high sensitivity, these are not recommended.

Prevention

- Limit outdoor roaming, especially in wooded areas.
- Castrate male cats to diminish fighting.

Technician Tips

- Wear gloves when handling infected animals.
- Wash hands and forearms with chlorhexidine or povidone-iodine scrub after wearing gloves.

Client Education

- Sporotrichosis is a zoonotic disease, especially in cats.
- Separation of infected animals from immunosuppressed people is necessary.

SUGGESTED READING

Viana PG, et al: Successful treatment of canine sporotrichosis with terbinafine: case reports and literature review. Mycopathologia 183:471-478, 2018.

AUTHOR: Mauria A. O'Brien, DVM, DACVECC
EDITOR: Joseph Taboada, DVM, DACVIM

Squamous Cell Carcinoma

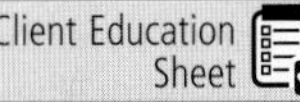

BASIC INFORMATION

Definition

A malignant tumor arising from squamous epithelium

Epidemiology

SPECIES, AGE, SEX

Nasal planum (nonhaired, rostral, external part of nose):

- Dog: rare site
- Cat: squamous cell carcinoma (SCC) is the most common tumor in this site; older cats

Aural: occurs in older animals:

- Dog: SCC is the second most common ear canal tumor (after ceruminous gland adenocarcinoma).
- Cat: SCC may affect the pinna, often in cats with planum and periocular SCC; may also affect the ear canal, where it is the most common tumor type, equal in frequency to ceruminous gland adenocarcinoma.

Digital:

- Dog: SCC is the most common digital tumor, 35%-55% of such tumors; age 7-11 years
- Cat: primary SCC of the digit is rare (<10%). Digital carcinomas usually occur as metastasis from a bronchogenic carcinoma in older (mean, 13 years) cats.

Oral:

- Dog: SCC is one of the three most common malignant oral tumors, with nontonsillar SCC having a prevalence rate of approximately 7 per 100,000 dogs. Gingival area is most frequently affected, followed by lips, tongue, palate, and pharynx. Middle-aged to older dogs affected for most oral SCCs; no sex predisposition. Gingival papillary SCC reported in young (<1-year-old) dogs; also may be seen in adult dogs. Papillary SCC in adults can have a bone invasive or noninvasive pattern.
- Cat: SCC is the most common oral tumor. SCC makes up 75% of feline oral tumors and occurs in the gingival and sublingual area in equal frequency. Older cats affected; no sex predisposition

GENETICS, BREED PREDISPOSITION

Planum:

- Cat: lightly pigmented animals; Siamese breed underrepresented

Aural:

- Cat: on pinna; lightly pigmented animals; Siamese underrepresented

Digital:

- Dog: ≈75% large-breed dogs, ≥ 70% having dark coats. Breeds at increased risk include giant, standard, and miniature schnauzers, Gordon setter, standard and miniature poodles, Scottish terrier, Labrador retriever, rottweiler, and dachshund.

Oral:

- Dog: large dogs may be more likely to develop nontonsillar SCC; poodles, Labrador retrievers, and Samoyeds may be predisposed to lingual SCC.

RISK FACTORS

- Solar exposure in white-coated cats associated with increased risk of nasal planum, pinnal, and periocular SCC.
- Exposure to air pollution may be associated with development of tonsillar SCC in dogs.
- Gingival SCC reported to develop after oral radiation therapy in dogs.
- Oral SCC in cats may be associated with flea collar use, canned cat food or tuna consumption, and (possibly) environmental tobacco smoke.
    - In one study, cats with SCC exposed to environmental smoke were more likely to overexpress mutant TP53 than cats with SCC from smoke-free environments.

GEOGRAPHY AND SEASONALITY

- High altitude may increase the risk of solar exposure–induced SCC, as does living in countries with lower ozone coverage (e.g., New Zealand).
- Tonsillar SCC is 10 times more likely to occur in dogs from urban areas versus those in rural areas.

Clinical Presentation

HISTORY, CHIEF COMPLAINT

- Planum and pinna: crusted or ulcerated lesions or an actual mass ± bleeding or sneezing.
- Aural, external ear canal: visible mass, ear discharge, odor, pruritus, pain, facial nerve paralysis, head tilt, or circling. Cats are more likely to present with neurologic signs versus dogs.
- Digital
    - Dog: lameness, digit swelling, abnormal nail growth, fractured nail, licking/chewing at digit; often animals have a history of chronic nail bed infection with no improvement with antibiotics.
    - Cat: lameness; despite the fact that digital carcinoma in cats is usually metastatic from a primary lung tumor, cats rarely have respiratory signs.

- Oral
  - Difficulty eating, reluctance to eat, drooling, halitosis, bloody oral discharge, pawing at mouth, facial mass, oral mass, loose teeth, or weight loss. Tonsillar SCC: presenting complaint may be "lumps under jaw" from metastasis to the mandibular lymph nodes, with no other clinical signs.

PHYSICAL EXAM FINDINGS

- Planum and pinna: lesion may be proliferative or erosive; mass, crusting, and/or ulcerative lesion may be present. Regional lymph node may be enlarged.
- Aural, external ear canal: otic exam shows raised irregular mass, often ulcerated. Palpation of vertical ear canal may reveal large mass invading the area in late-stage cases.
- Digital
  - Dog: painful swollen digit with an abnormal or absent claw ± ulceration. Regional lymph node may be enlarged.
  - Cat: swollen digit, ulcerated skin with purulent discharge; constant exsheathment, deviation, or loss of nail; 80% of cats with digital carcinoma metastasis from a primary lung tumor present with multiple digits involved. The less common primary SCC of the digit usually involves only one digit with possible local extension into an adjacent digit.
- Oral
  - Gingival SCC: swelling or raised mass along gingival margin may be irregular, ulcerated. Cats can have normal gingiva, with the tumor affecting the mandible/maxilla leading to bone mass.
  - Tonsillar SCC: enlarged mandibular lymph nodes and enlarged irregular tonsils may be seen. Tonsillar enlargement is usually unilateral.
  - Sublingual SCC: irregular mass under tongue; in dogs, lingual SCC often involves the ventral aspect of the tongue with limited dorsal involvement noted on physical exam.
- Multicentric SCC *in situ* (MSCCIS, Bowen's disease, bowenoid *in situ* carcinoma [BISC]) is an uncommon disease reported mainly in cats. Lesions are multifocal; occur most commonly over the head, neck, dorsal thorax, abdomen, and proximal limbs. Lesions found in haired and darkly pigmented skin; not solar induced.

Etiology and Pathophysiology

- Planum and pinna: may begin as actinic keratosis and become locally invasive; low metastatic rate, possible association in some cases with papillomavirus
- Aural, external ear canal: locally invasive, more aggressive in cats than dogs; low metastatic rate (about 5%-15% local lymph nodes)
- Digital
  - Dog: locally invasive with digital (P3) bony destruction, low metastatic rate (5%-20% lymph node or pulmonary)
  - Cat: locally invasive with digital (P3) destruction; usually, metastatic lesions from a pulmonary tumor. Lymph node involvement not documented.
- Oral
  - Gingival and sublingual SCC: locally invasive with a low metastatic rate (5%-10% regional lymph nodes, 3% lung)
  - Tonsillar SCC: invasive and highly metastatic (98% regional lymph nodes, 63% lung)

DIAGNOSIS

Diagnostic Overview

The diagnosis of SCC is suspected based on signalment, physical exam, at times cytologic analysis, but is confirmed by histopathologic evaluation from incisional/excisional biopsy sample.

Differential Diagnosis

Planum:

- Fungal lesion (particularly *Cryptococcus* in cats)
- Other neoplasms: cutaneous lymphoma, mast cell tumor, fibrosarcoma, melanoma, eosinophilic granuloma
- Immune-mediated dermatopathy

Aural:

- Canal: severe hyperplasia in dogs with chronic otitis, ceruminous gland adenocarcinoma, adenoma, papilloma, polyp, plasmacytoma, basal cell tumor, melanoma, granuloma
- Pinna: consider trauma, frostbite, insect bites (see Planum above).

Digital:

- Dog: melanoma, mast cell tumor, soft-tissue sarcoma, osteomyelitis, paronychia
- Cat: usually metastatic lung tumor; bacterial paronychia; other primary tumors much less likely

Oral:

- Gingival mass in a dog: melanoma, fibrosarcoma, acanthomatous ameloblastoma (acanthomatous epulis). Less likely are osteosarcoma, plasma cell tumor, tooth root abscess, fungal disease, and other primary tumors.
- Gingival mass in a cat: fibrosarcoma, dental disease. Less likely are melanoma and other primary tumors.
- Tonsillar mass in a dog: lymphoma. Less likely is bacterial or fungal infection.
- Sublingual mass in a cat: foreign body, fungal infection, other neoplasia
- Lingual mass in a dog: melanoma, hemangiosarcoma, fibrosarcoma, granular cell tumor, plasma cell tumor, papilloma

Initial Database

Dog, all sites:

- CBC, serum biochemistry profile, urinalysis; usually unremarkable
- Aspirate and cytologic exam from regional lymph nodes (mandibular, also superficial cervical nodes [prescapular] for aural masses) to assess for metastasis in all cases; unlikely to be positive (except tonsillar SCC) but an easy test with prognostic value
- Three-view thoracic radiographs to assess for metastasis; usually negative
- Fine-needle aspiration (FNA) and cytologic exam of the primary mass; it may be possible to obtain the samples on animal that is awake, but if sedation is needed, plan to biopsy as well.
  - Cytologic exam can provide a definitive diagnosis, but severe inflammation can hamper interpretation of malignancy, necessitating a biopsy.

Cats:

- Planum and aural (see Dog above): hypercalcemia rarely seen as paraneoplastic syndrome in ear canal SCC
- Digital: three-view thoracic radiographs almost always reveal lung neoplasia; usually solitary mass but may be multiple. FNA and cytologic exam of the digital mass can provide a definitive diagnosis, but at times extreme inflammation of the tumor can make interpretation of the epithelial cells difficult. These cells, although usually pulmonary adenocarcinoma in origin, may have some squamous differentiation. FNA of the lung mass can confirm a lung tumor if the digit lesion is nondiagnostic.
- Oral: mandibular lymph node FNA and cytologic exam to assess for metastasis in all cases. Hypercalcemia may be seen as a paraneoplastic syndrome in some cats with oral SCC. Three-view thoracic radiographs to assess for metastasis

Advanced or Confirmatory Testing

- Incisional or excisional biopsy of the primary mass for histopathologic diagnosis
- Radiographs, CT scan of lesion to assess tumor extent and bone involvement and to plan surgery or radiation therapy

TREATMENT

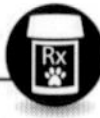

Treatment Overview

Excision of primary tumor with wide margins is often curative, as indicated by low metastatic rates for most primary locations except the tonsil. Due to location and extent of lesion in many cases, however, wide excision may be difficult or impossible.

Acute General Treatment

Wide surgical resection; if margins are not complete on histologic evaluation, irradiation is effective for microscopic disease.

- Planum
  - Dog: excising the premaxilla along with the planum in cases with very large masses may provide better cosmesis.
  - Cat: excision is an excellent option if the tumor is not too extensive along the bridge of the nose or does not involve the lip or surrounding skin. Irradiation, photodynamic therapy, cryotherapy, intralesional chemotherapy (intralesional carboplatin: complete remission for > 9 months in 6/6

cats), and curettage with thermocautery can be effective for small superficial lesions, with decreasing effectiveness for larger lesions.
- Aural: total ear canal ablation with bulla osteotomy provides best survival times. In cats, the tumors can invade aggressively into the skull bones, precluding surgical excision.
- Digital
  - Dog: digital amputation; adjuvant therapy usually unnecessary; can discuss chemotherapy as below
  - Cats: therapy unrewarding if metastatic lesion; if thoracic films are normal and only one digit is involved, amputation of the digit is recommended.
- Bowen's disease
  - Daily topical imiquimod has shown some efficacy in cats: median survival time > 3 years in series of 12 cats. This imidazoquinoline works by binding to surface toll-like receptors 7 and 8 on macrophages, which leads to innate and cell-mediated immune responses resulting in tissue-specific apoptosis. Systemic therapy was not shown to be of benefit.
- Oral
  - Gingival: aggressive resection, including partial mandibulectomy or maxillectomy. Definitive radiation for residual microscopic disease if surgery does not provide tumor-free margins
  - Tongue, dog: if rostral to midlingual, surgical resection (40%-60% of the tongue can be removed with good function remaining, possibly more). Dogs with tumors < 2 cm live significantly longer.
  - Tonsillar: usually poor treatment options due to invasiveness and metastatic behavior; multimodality therapy includes surgical debulking, if possible, of primary mass and involved lymph nodes, followed by chemotherapy and radiation therapy; may extend survival times
  - Sublingual and gingival, cat: very poor treatment options. Surgical excision is usually not feasible. Radiation therapy and photodynamic therapy have been tried with limited success. Gemcitabine as a radiation sensitizer with palliative radiation has significant hematologic and normal tissue toxicosis and therefore cannot be recommended.

Chemotherapy:
- Piroxicam 0.3 mg/kg PO q 24h (caution regarding gastric ulcerative effects); has some effect against gross SCC in dogs (18% complete and partial remission, 29% stable disease).
- Cisplatin + piroxicam: ≈40% renal toxicoses, so the combination is not recommended
- Carboplatin ± piroxicam has been reported in several small case series to have effect against canine SCC in a variety of primary sites.
- Docetaxel with cyclosporine gavage in dogs with oral SCC: 50% (6/12) response rate
- In 31 cats with SCC in a variety of oral locations, carboplatin combined with an accelerated radiation therapy protocol provided a median survival of 163 days, with long-term survivors (>2 years) noted with tonsil or cheek locations.

Chronic Treatment
- Cyclooxygenase 2 (COX2) expression was shown in 40 of 40 canine SCC cases, and therapy with piroxicam or other nonsteroidal antiinflammatory drugs (NSAIDs) may be of benefit.
- COX2 expression also has been detected in 27/27 cats with cutaneous SCC and 4/9 cats with actinic keratosis.

PROGNOSIS & OUTCOME

- Planum: excellent prognosis for cure if complete surgical resection. Median survival of cats with planum and/or pinna SCC: 673 days with surgery alone
- Aural, canal: excellent prognosis for cure if treated early; unfortunately, tumors in cats have often progressed massively before identification, leading to a median survival time of only 3.8 months.
- Digital
  - Dog: good prognosis, with 95% 1-year and 75% 2-year survival rates. Median survival not reached in recent study (>1700 days)
  - Cat: for metastatic lesion, digital amputation median survival is only 1-2 months; for primary digital SCC, reported survival time with surgery varies (3 weeks to 2 years).
- Oral
  - Dogs with rostral SCC: wide surgical resection can be curative.
  - Dogs with mandibular or maxillary nonresectable SCC: radiation therapy. Median survival time is 450 days. Control time for dogs with tumors greater than 4 cm in diameter is generally shorter.
  - Histologic grade may be predictive for survival, with significantly worse survival for dogs with grade 3 tumors.
  - Dogs with tonsillar SCC: surgery and radiation therapy. Median survival is 100 days. With surgery, irradiation, and chemotherapy (doxorubicin and cisplatin), median survival is 270 days. If only one tonsil is affected and no metastasis, surgery and chemotherapy may provide prolonged survival (median, 637 days in one small study).
  - Dogs with lingual SCC: rostral to midlingual masses can be cured with wide resection if < 2 cm. Dogs with nonresectable lingual SCC can be treated with radiation therapy, but survival is generally short (median, 4 months), with dogs euthanized due to local proliferation.
  - Cats with mandibular SCC: radiation therapy and mitoxantrone or carboplatin; without surgery, generally poor response; median survival of 180 days. Mandibulectomy and irradiation: median survival of 14 months; euthanasia usually due to local recurrence.
  - Cats sublingual: poor response to therapy; survival time < 3 months

PEARLS & CONSIDERATIONS

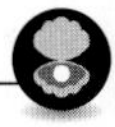

Comments
- Planum: cosmesis and quality of life after a nosectomy are generally good to excellent, with high owner satisfaction. Early treatment when the lesion is small enough for a surgical cure is strongly recommended when possible.
- Aural
  - Canal: complete ear ablation is needed; simple debulking is inadequate because the tumor will continue to invade inward, making a surgical cure impossible later.
  - Pinna: preneoplastic changes can extend along the entire edge of the pinna; complete pinnectomy may be required for cure. If lesion is very small, simple removal of the affected tip of the ear can be considered, with a later decision made according to need for further excision based on histopathologic exam results.
- Digital
  - Dog: tumors often go undiagnosed for extensive amounts of time due to treatment for a nail bed infection. Any questionable, non–antibiotic-responsive digital swelling must be biopsied.
  - Cat: primary digit tumors are rare; three-view thoracic radiographs are essential before surgery because digital tumors are usually secondary.
- Oral
  - Mandibular, maxillary, and lingual SCC in rostral locations in dogs can be cured with aggressive resection.
  - SCC in cats and in other locations in the mouth in dogs is difficult to address due to invasiveness and/or metastasis.
  - Multimodality therapy may extend survival times, but quality of life can be an issue with the treatments.
    - Dogs with tonsillar SCC can have pronounced dysphagia and discomfort; surgical debulking may not alleviate clinical signs, and radiation therapy can contribute to local discomfort for several weeks.
    - Cats with mandibular or maxillary SCC can have temporary responses to chemotherapy and radiation therapy, but side effects may necessitate placement of a feeding tube. The occasional cat with a small lesion may have a greatly extended survival time with surgery.
    - Case selection for multimodality treatment is important for dogs and cats, and owners need to have realistic expectations for the success of the therapy.

Prevention
Planum and pinna: limit sun exposure in light-coated cats.

Technician Tips

Superficial aspects of SCC have inflammation. Cytology samples must be obtained from deeper areas. Do not attempt impression smears.

SUGGESTED READING

Supsavhad W, et al: Animal models of head and neck squamous cell carcinoma. Vet J 210:7-16, 2016.

AUTHOR: Laura D. Garrett, DVM, DACVIM
EDITOR: Kenneth M. Rassnick, DVM, DACVIM

Steroid-Responsive Meningitis-Arteritis

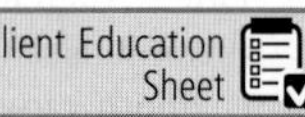

BASIC INFORMATION

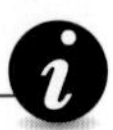

Definition

Steroid-responsive meningitis-arteritis (SRMA) is a suspected autoimmune disorder characterized by meningitis and leptomeningeal arteritis, occurring most commonly in the cervical spinal cord.

Synonyms

Corticosteroid-responsive meningomyelitis, aseptic meningitis, beagle pain syndrome, canine juvenile polyarteritis syndrome, sterile suppurative meningitis, juvenile polyarthritis

Epidemiology

SPECIES, AGE, SEX

Young adult dogs (6-18 months old) but any age is possible

GENETICS, BREED PREDISPOSITION

- Genetic factors are possible but have not been proved.
- Any breed can be affected, but beagles, boxers, Bernese mountain dogs, Weimaraners, and Nova Scotia duck tolling retrievers are overrepresented.

RISK FACTORS

Immune response can occur secondary to environmental or infectious causes. No association between SRMA and time of year, vaccination, geographic location, sex, or neuter status

CONTAGION AND ZOONOSIS

Infectious cause has not been demonstrated.

ASSOCIATED DISORDERS

Can occur concurrently with immune-mediated polyarthritis

Clinical Presentation

DISEASE FORMS/SUBTYPES

- Classical (acute)
- Chronic

HISTORY, CHIEF COMPLAINT

- Acute (classical): cervical hyperesthesia and rigidity, fever, stiff gait, lethargy
- Chronic: as with acute disease but with additional complaints suggestive of spinal cord dysfunction (proprioceptive deficits, paresis, ataxia)

PHYSICAL EXAM FINDINGS

- Typical of meningitis: cervical pain and rigidity; stiff, stilted gait; fever; lethargy
- In more protracted cases: gait abnormalities, proprioceptive deficits, back pain. Other neurologic signs are less commonly reported.

Etiology and Pathophysiology

- Idiopathic: possibly an autoimmune condition
- Acute (classical): histologic analysis demonstrates moderate to marked meningitis characterized by infiltration of neutrophils, macrophages, lymphocytes, and plasma cells, as well as degenerative changes and perivascular inflammation of the leptomeningeal arteries. Lesions are most commonly found in the cervical spinal cord.
- Chronic: histologic analysis demonstrates moderate to marked fibrosis and patchy mineralization of the meninges.

DIAGNOSIS

Diagnostic Overview

The diagnosis is suspected when a (typically young) dog has signs of cervical pain. Advanced imaging helps rule out other differential diagnoses, and cerebrospinal fluid (CSF) analysis provides the most characteristic abnormalities.

Differential Diagnosis

- Infectious meningitis (bacterial, viral, protozoal, fungal)
- Discospondylitis
- Inflammatory, noninfectious meningitis (e.g., granulomatous meningoencephalomyelitis [GME])
- Intervertebral disc disease
- Neoplasia (e.g., spinal meningioma, lymphoma, malignant histiocytosis)

Initial Database

- CBC: leukocytosis, neutrophilia ± left shift; can be normal in chronic cases
- Serum biochemistry profile: usually normal
- Urinalysis: usually normal
- Survey spinal radiographs: should be normal

Advanced or Confirmatory Testing

- Paired serum and CSF immunoglobulin A (IgA) is often elevated and supports the diagnosis. A study demonstrated 91% sensitivity and 78% specificity.
- C-reactive protein (CRP) is often elevated in serum and CSF but not pathognomonic. CRP level can be used to monitor remission status.
- CSF analysis (p. 1080) often reveals an elevated protein level and nucleated cell count with sterile neutrophilic pleocytosis in the acute stage of disease. Chronic cases can have normal CSF or mononuclear pleocytosis.
- CSF culture: negative.
- Infectious disease titers and/or advanced imaging (MRI [p. 1132], CT, myelography) may be required to rule out other diseases.
- Arthrocentesis if concurrent joint pain or swelling: sterile neutrophilic inflammation

TREATMENT

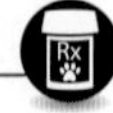

Treatment Overview

The cornerstone of treatment is judicious immunosuppression adjusted to optimal response with fewest/no adverse effects.

Acute General Treatment

- Prednisone initially 2 mg/kg PO q 12h for 3-5 days if severe clinical signs, then reduce to 1 mg/kg PO q 12h for 1-2 months, then 1 mg/kg PO q 24h for 1-2 months, and then taper to lowest effective dose. Every-other-day dosing in the later stages of dose reduction may reduce adverse effects.
- Consider gastrointestinal (GI) protective agents (e.g., famotidine 0.5 mg/kg PO q 12-24h, sucralfate 0.25-1 g PO q 8h) while giving glucocorticoids (controversial).
- Analgesics (e.g., gabapentin 10 mg/kg PO q 8-12h; amantadine 2-3 mg/kg PO q 12h for 4-6 weeks).

Chronic Treatment

Additional immunosuppressive medications may be required to control disease while minimizing adverse drug effects (p. 60). Consider azathioprine (Imuran 2 mg/kg PO q 24h × 5 days, then q 48h), cyclosporine 2-10 mg/kg PO q 24h or divided q 12h, or mycophenolate 10 mg/kg PO q 12h.

Drug Interactions

- All immunosuppressive drugs carry the risk of excessive immune suppression, and some can have other effects (e.g., bone marrow suppressant).

- Glucocorticoids should not be given concurrently with nonsteroidal antiinflammatory drugs (NSAIDs) or other potentially ulcerogenic medications.

Possible Complications

Glucocorticoid side effects: polyuria, polydipsia, polyphagia, weight gain, GI ulceration, iatrogenic hyperadrenocorticism, and others

Recommended Monitoring

- Neurologic exam every 4-6 weeks. Repeat CBC, biochemistry profile, and urinalysis as needed to monitor for adverse drug effects (e.g., hepatopathy due to azathioprine).
- Ideally, CSF analysis should be repeated every 4-6 weeks before planned reduction in medication dosage.
- In lieu of repeat CSF analyses, serial CRP levels have been used to monitor for remission.

PROGNOSIS & OUTCOME

- Acute (classical): generally good to excellent prognosis if treated early and aggressively
- Chronic: prognosis is fair to guarded due to frequent relapses.
- A recent retrospective analysis of 74 dogs with SRMA (Biedermann et al., 2016) found more than one-half of dogs had no evidence of relapse after initial treatment. Approximately one-third of dogs had at least one relapse, with up to four relapses reported.

PEARLS & CONSIDERATIONS

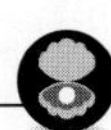

Comments

- SRMA has a good to excellent prognosis when treated early.
- CSF analysis should be performed early in the course of disease.

Technician Tips

Neck pain is the hallmark sign of this disorder. Avoid neck leads. Be aware of the possibility of pain-associated aggression.

Client Education

Warn owners of glucocorticoid side effects; they should know that if effects are intolerable, alternative immunosuppressive treatments are available but that treatment should never be discontinued abruptly.

SUGGESTED READING

Tipold A, et al: Inflammatory diseases of the spine in small animals. Vet Clin Small Anim 40:871-879, 2010.

AUTHOR: Mark T. Troxel, DVM, DACVIM
EDITOR: Karen R. Muñana, DVM, MS, DACVIM

Stomatitis

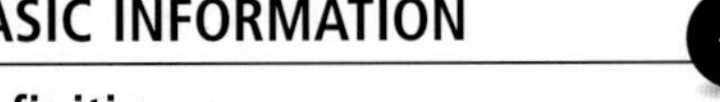

Bonus Material Online 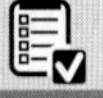 Client Education Sheet

BASIC INFORMATION

Definition

In clinical use, *stomatitis* is inflammation of the mucous lining of any of the structures in the mouth. The term should be reserved to describe widespread oral inflammation (beyond gingivitis and periodontitis) that may also extend into submucosal tissues.

Synonyms

Lymphocytic-plasmacytic stomatitis, gingivostomatitis (cats); ulcerative stomatitis (dogs); alveolar, labial/buccal, sublingual, and caudal stomatitis

Epidemiology

SPECIES, AGE, SEX

Adult cats and dogs

GENETICS, BREED PREDISPOSITION

- Cats: no known predispositions
- Dogs: ulcerative stomatitis considered a familial disorder in Maltese dogs; terrier breeds more frequently affected

RISK FACTORS

Cats: sometimes seen in group-housed families; may be pathogen-associated; exposure to viral diseases such as feline calicivirus (FCV), feline herpesvirus (FHV), or feline immunodeficiency virus (FIV)

CONTAGION AND ZOONOSIS

Cats: FCV, FHV, and FIV

ASSOCIATED DISORDERS

- Juvenile hyperplastic gingivitis: cats <1 year old, presenting with severe gingival inflammation and enlargement; unknown whether progresses to adult stomatitis
- Cats with stomatitis often show periodontal disease (p. 776) and resorption of multiple teeth (p. 982).

Clinical Presentation

DISEASE FORMS/SUBTYPES

Ulcers and inflammation on gingiva, alveolar mucosa, and mucosa of lip, cheek, and tongue

HISTORY, CHIEF COMPLAINT

Pain when eating, yawning, palpation of mouth; decreased grooming; drooling; weight loss

PHYSICAL EXAM FINDINGS

Cats:

- Poor body condition and haircoat if condition is chronic
- Symmetrical, bright red, ulcerated lesions of gingiva, alveolar, sublingual, labial and buccal mucosa (rostral stomatitis), and/or the area of and lateral to the palatoglossal folds (caudal stomatitis)
- Sometimes affecting the lateral margins of the tongue and rostromedial aspects of the pharyngeal walls (but usually no hard palate involvement)

Dogs:

- Halitosis, drooling, and reluctance to chew on hard food
- Ulcers most commonly on labial and buccal mucosa facing plaque-laden tooth surfaces, lateral margins of tongue, and palatal mucosa adjacent to teeth
- Ulcers occasionally on areas that do not contact teeth
- Necrosis and osteomyelitis in severe cases

Etiology and Pathophysiology

- Immune-mediated disease related to degree of plaque accumulation; plaque bacteria play a role in disease progression, and control of oral bacteria can be a critical contributor to successful management.
- The most reliable treatment in both species is extraction of teeth in affected areas ± extraction of all teeth, eliminating bacteria-laden plaque deposits.
- FCV and FHV infection may play a role in the immune system's aberrant response to plaque; 88% of stomatitis cats shed both viruses (versus 21% of cats without stomatitis). FCV polymerase chain reaction (PCR) assay is positive for 97% of cats with caudal stomatitis.

DIAGNOSIS

Diagnostic Overview

The diagnosis is based on clinical presentation (bilaterally symmetrical inflammation that extends beyond the gingiva and mucogingival junction into other mucosal linings). Anesthesia at the time of initial presentation allows for biopsy, dental radiography, professional dental cleaning, and extraction of teeth.

Differential Diagnosis

- Periodontal disease (p. 776)
- Squamous cell carcinoma or other less common neoplasia: usually unilateral (pp. 711 and 714)
- Eosinophilic granuloma (p. 300)
- Erythema multiforme
- Epitheliotropic lymphoma (mycosis fungoides)
- In dogs, stomatitis may occasionally be a manifestation of autoimmune disease (pemphigus vulgaris, bullous pemphigoid, discoid/systemic lupus erythematosus); look for other signs of autoimmune disease.

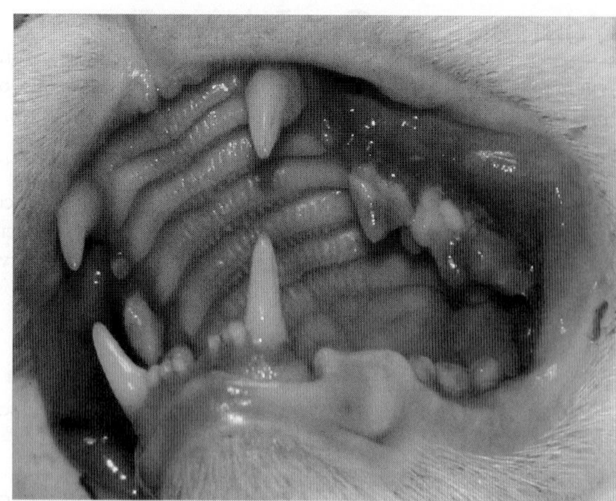

STOMATITIS In a cat with inflammation of gingiva, alveolar mucosa, and labial and buccal mucosa, the palatal mucosa immediately adjacent to the cheek teeth also is inflamed. There is severe plaque and calculus accumulation and loss of attachment on cheek teeth (gingival recession, periodontitis). (Copyright Dr. Alexander M. Reiter, University of Pennsylvania.)

Initial Database

- CBC, serum chemistry profile, urinalysis to rule out distant organ disease or systemic disease; hypergammaglobulinemia due to polyclonal gammopathy is most common.
- FIV and FeLV tests for cats

Advanced or Confirmatory Testing

Biopsy of representative lesions; mixture of acute and chronic inflammatory cells (particularly lymphocytes and plasma cells); rule out autoimmune disease or neoplasia

TREATMENT

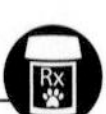

Treatment Overview

Extraction of selected (partial-mouth extraction) or all teeth (full-mouth extraction) to remove the plaque-retentive surfaces; up to 80% of cases improve after tooth extraction. If extraction is not an option or is ineffective, treat with strict plaque control, immunomodulators, ± antimicrobials.

Acute General Treatment

- Initial approach with anesthetized oral exam, dental radiographs, biopsy (if not already performed), extraction of diseased teeth (e.g., those with periodontal disease, tooth resorption), and scaling/polishing of remaining teeth
- Pain management with opioids (e.g., transmucosal buprenorphine 0.01 mg/kg q 6-8h [cats], 0.02 mg/kg q 6-8h [dogs]; codeine 2 mg/kg PO q 8h), gabapentin 5-20 mg/kg PO q 8-12h
- Glucocorticoids (prednisolone 0.5-1 mg/kg PO q 12-24h; taper dose slowly over months to determine the lowest dose that controls clinical signs). Alternative is nonsteroidal antiinflammatory drugs (NSAIDs) (e.g., meloxicam 0.1 mg/kg SQ or PO on first day, followed by 0.05 mg/kg PO q 24h), but NSAIDs should not be combined with steroids. Either may temporarily provide comfort together with pain medications; if possible, avoid depot formulations (methylprednisolone 1-2 mg/kg SQ) due to long-term side effects (e.g., diabetes mellitus, congestive heart failure).
- Daily home oral hygiene with topical antiseptics (chlorhexidine gel or zinc ascorbate gel PO q 12h) and/or antimicrobials (e.g., amoxicillin-clavulanate 13.75 mg/kg PO q 12h); nursing care (nutritional support, grooming)
- Re-exam 1- 2 weeks after initial treatment; if significant improvement, continue home oral hygiene regimen (including toothbrushing if tolerated) and re-examine the patient in 3, 6, and 12 months.

Chronic Treatment

Cats:

- Extraction of otherwise healthy teeth (partial-mouth or full-mouth extraction)
- CO_2 laser: effective in selected cases of severely proliferative disease but requires multiple anesthesia sessions ± placement of an esophagostomy tube (p. 1106)
- Recombinant feline interferon (Virbagen Omega, Virbac): vial of 10 MU is injected in a 100-mL bag of sodium chloride and frozen in ten 10-mL aliquots; client gives 1 mL orally every 24 hours for 100 days; the 10-mL fraction in use is refrigerated, and the other aliquots are kept frozen until needed
- Cyclosporine (Neoral 2.5 mg/kg PO q 12h as a starting dose) resulted in improvement in 85% of cats with refractory stomatitis.
- Bovine lactoferrin spray 6 mg/CAT PO q 12h and piroxicam 0.3 mg/kg PO q 48h in combination resulted in improvement in 77% of cats.

Dogs:

- Some dogs may start to develop lesions (and oral pain) soon after initial treatment; in such cases, metronidazole 20 mg/kg PO q 24h for 1-2 weeks may help, then gradually reducing the dose. Continuous treatment at 10 mg/kg PO q 48h provides good control in animals that relapse.
- If there is no improvement with initial treatment, extract all remaining teeth, and start prednisone treatment 0.5-1 mg/kg PO q 12-24h, tapering down to the lowest dose/frequency that controls clinical signs.

Nutrition/Diet

- Soft food during healing
- Esophagostomy tube placement if severe oral discomfort precludes prehension and chewing of food

Drug Interactions

Do not combine glucocorticoids and NSAIDs.

Possible Complications

- Outcome is unpredictable. Some patients have poor quality of life regardless of treatments.
- Exacerbation of pre-existing infections (toxoplasmosis, FIV) due to immunosuppressive drug use; other adverse effects of glucocorticoids

Recommended Monitoring

- Glucocorticoids: monitor for adverse drug effects.
- Cyclosporine: assess blood levels after 4-6 weeks and every 6-12 months thereafter (target levels at 12 hours post blood sample are > 300 ng/mL)

PROGNOSIS & OUTCOME

Variable; response to full-mouth or almost full-mouth extraction: 28%-60% fully cured, 20%-38% clinically cured (some inflammation, no need for further medical therapy, but continued home oral hygiene), 13%-26% slightly improved (but needing further medical therapy), and 7% unimproved (nonresponsive)

PEARLS & CONSIDERATIONS

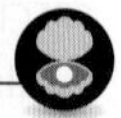

Comments

- Tooth extraction provides the most reliable results without long-term side effects; partial-mouth or full-mouth extraction should be considered as an early option.
- Affected dogs and cats usually show decreased appetite or abnormal oral behavior but usually do not stop eating; rule out other causes of anorexia/hyporexia (e.g., chronic kidney disease, neoplasia) before surgery.

Prevention

- Good home oral hygiene program may decrease the inflammatory response in at-risk animals.
- Exercise caution when introducing new cats into the household with unknown oral health or FeLV/FIV status.

Technician Tips

- Home oral hygiene is challenging for cats and dogs with painful, inflamed mouths.

When teaching clients how to brush teeth, wait until after professional dental cleaning has been performed and inflammation and pain has been decreased by medical therapy.
- Full-mouth extraction requires a long duration of general anesthesia. To minimize anesthesia time, practice four-handed dentistry. Be ready and anticipate the surgeon's needs.
- Cats and dogs with severe inflammation and oral pain need assisted nutrition by changing the consistency of the food (slurry to slightly soft) or by using feeding tubes. Knowledge of routine care of the tubes and administration of food through the tube are recommended.

Client Education

Clients should understand that stomatitis is often controlled rather than cured. Some owners may decline surgery because it seems too aggressive or they believe that the patient cannot eat without teeth. Sharing "happy ending stories" of other patients (pictures, owner's comments) with them may decrease owner anxiety.

SUGGESTED READING

Jennings MW, et al: Effect of tooth extraction on stomatitis in cats: 95 cases (2000-2013). J Am Vet Med Assoc 246:654, 2015.

AUTHOR: Ana C. Castejon-Gonzalez, DVM, PhD, DAVDC, DEVDC
EDITOR: Alexander M. Reiter, DVM, Dr. med. vet., DAVDC, DEVDC

Stridor and Stertor

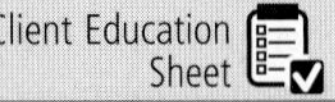

BASIC INFORMATION

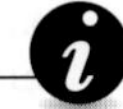

Definition

- Stridor: a harsh, high-pitched sound usually occurring during inspiration that results from partial upper airway obstruction at or below the larynx
- Stertor: a sonorous breathing sound similar to a snore that results from partial upper airway obstruction above the larynx (i.e., nasal passages, choanae, or nasopharynx)

Epidemiology

SPECIES, AGE, SEX

More common in dogs than cats but occurs in both species

GENETICS, BREED PREDISPOSITION

- Brachycephalic dog breeds are predisposed to stertor.
- Breed predispositions exist for laryngeal paralysis (p. 574).

RISK FACTORS

- Nasal/nasopharyngeal disorders through primary obstruction (mass, foreign body [FB], mucosal edema) or obstruction by discharge
- Pharyngeal, laryngeal, and tracheal disorders

ASSOCIATED DISORDERS

- Laryngeal paralysis, nasal and nasopharyngeal tumors, nasopharyngeal polyps, brachiocephalic airway syndrome, airway FBs
- Powerful, sustained inspirations against an obstructed upper airway are associated with the development of noncardiogenic pulmonary edema.

Clinical Presentation

HISTORY, CHIEF COMPLAINT

- Owners may report these respiratory sounds as a chief complaint or concurrently with other signs of respiratory disease (coughing, nasal discharge, sneezing, dyspnea, epistaxis), pharyngeal disease (gagging, dysphagia), decreased exercise tolerance, or syncope.
- Clinical signs are often exacerbated by excitement, high environmental temperature, or increased activity; animals may show no signs at rest.
- Owner may report voice change with laryngeal involvement. Owners may consider stertor a normal sound, especially in brachiocephalic dogs.

PHYSICAL EXAM FINDINGS

Abnormal sounds may be intermittent; other findings can include:
- Stertor: nasal discharge, occlusion of airflow from one or both nostrils, stenotic nares in brachycephalic breeds, periodontal disease with evidence of tooth root abscessation or tooth loss; sound may disappear with open-mouth breathing
- Stridor: coughing, gagging, dyspnea, hyperthermia, open-mouth gasping (inspiratory effort exaggerated), panting, paradoxical breathing, unilateral discharge from the ear (sometimes seen in cats with nasopharyngeal polyps)

Etiology and Pathophysiology

- During inspiration, air pressure in the upper airway is low, allowing air to flow in through the nares or mouth and fill the lungs.
- Obstruction narrows airway diameter, causing audible turbulence proximal to the obstruction during inspiration.
- Dynamic obstruction occurs when the airway narrows on inspiration due to pressure effects; fixed obstruction exists regardless of phase of respiration.
- Noise may be absent on expiration if the pressure of exhaled air opens the airway (e.g., laryngeal paralysis, other dynamic obstructions).

DIAGNOSIS

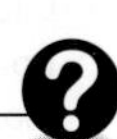

Diagnostic Overview

Physical exam and upper/lower airway radiographs help localize the lesion causing respiratory stridor. Rhinoscopy, laryngoscopy, tracheoscopy, and/or CT are often necessary to determine the exact cause of the airway obstruction.

Differential Diagnosis

These noises are clinical signs, not disorders. A list of stridor causes is provided on p. 1283.

Initial Database

- CBC, serum biochemistry profile, and urinalysis: rule out systemic diseases
- Stertor
  - Thorough examination of head, including oral and otic exams. Note nares/muzzle confirmation, symmetry, and color. Retropulse eyes, percuss sinus and muzzle, and evaluate submandibular lymph nodes.
  - Assessing airflow through both nostrils, using a wisp of cotton ball or a cold glass slide (warm, moist, expired air fogging the glass if the nasal passage is patent)
- Stridor
  - If severe open-mouth inspiratory dyspnea: may be possible to visualize caudal pharynx and larynx with patient awake (e.g., pharyngeal FB, laryngeal/pharyngeal mass), using only a bright light source
  - Cervical radiographs to rule out laryngeal and tracheal masses and FBs. The normal larynx (especially if mineralized and/or radiographed obliquely) should not be misinterpreted as an FB
  - Thoracic radiographs: intrathoracic trachea, lungs (rule out secondary noncardiogenic pulmonary edema)

Advanced or Confirmatory Testing

- Stertor
  - Thorough and complete oral/pharyngeal exam under sedation/anesthesia
  - Dental radiographs (apical dental/tooth root abscesses)
  - CT of nasal cavity and pharynx
  - Rhinoscopy (p. 1159), including choanal exam with biopsies and cytologic exam if discharge is present

- Stridor
  - Laryngoscopy (p. 1125) under light general anesthesia to evaluate laryngeal and oral anatomy and rule out laryngeal paralysis
  - Pharyngoscopy and tracheoscopy with biopsies, cytologic exam, ± bronchoalveolar lavage (p. 1074)
  - If available, flouroscopy may be useful.
- Coagulation profile: rule out coagulopathies, if appropriate

TREATMENT

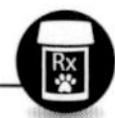

Treatment Overview

Reduce/remove obstruction of the upper airway when possible. If respiratory effort is increased, oxygen supplementation and sedation may be required. In severe cases, tracheotomy may be necessary to restore airflow to the lungs (p. 1004).

Acute General Treatment

- Stertor: rarely associated with crisis as open-mouth breathing can circumvent obstruction.
- Stridor: if associated with severe obstruction, may cause (in increasing order of severity) severe upper airway dyspnea, cyanosis, collapse, and respiratory arrest
- Patients with marked stridor associated with exaggerated, severe inspiratory efforts require immediate attention.
  - Calm environment
  - Oxygen supplementation (p. 1146)
  - Sedation, especially if the degree of inspiratory dyspnea is severe and the patient is known to be otherwise healthy (e.g., butorphanol 0.1-0.3 mg/kg IV)
- With deterioration or failure to improve despite the measures described above
  - If the obstruction is cranial to the mid-cervical trachea and stridor and dyspnea are severe, consider anesthesia and endotracheal intubation or a tracheostomy if intubation is not possible (p. 1166).
  - If the obstruction is caudal to the midcervical trachea and stridor and dyspnea are severe despite the treatments mentioned above, immediate preparations should be made for tracheoscopy and/or surgical intervention.
  - If the site of obstruction is unknown, the patient must undergo radiography or direct visualization of the pharynx and larynx to determine the best intervention.

Chronic Treatment

Correction of underlying causes, as applicable. For example:

- Brachycephalic airway surgery (p. 128)
- Laryngeal paralysis: arytenoid lateralization (p. 574)
- Surgical excision of masses, removal of polyps
- Endoscopic or surgical retrieval of FBs (pp. 1074 and 1159)

Recommended Monitoring

Respiratory effort, mucous membrane color (pallor/cyanosis), pulse oximetry, and arterial blood gas analysis if severely affected

PROGNOSIS & OUTCOME

Depends on the underlying disease

PEARLS & CONSIDERATIONS

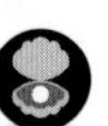

Comments

- Stridor can be a sign of a serious or life-threatening airway obstruction. Conversely, dogs with stertor can often breathe simply by opening the mouth.
- Cats are much more reluctant than dogs to breathe with their mouths open. As a result, significant nasal cavity obstruction can cause marked respiratory distress in a cat, whereas a dog would mouth breathe to bypass the obstruction.
- Stridor is often exacerbated by excitement and exercise.
- Tracheal collapse above the thoracic inlet is most apparent on inspiratory radiographs and below the thoracic inlet on expiratory films.

Technician Tips

- Keep the environment around an acutely dyspneic animal as calm as possible. Do not force an oxygen mask on the animal if it is resisting, but consider flow-by oxygen or an oxygen cage. Sedation may help calm the animal and reduce dyspnea.
- Animals with stridor on a hot day often become hyperthermic; be sure to check body temperature and actively cool animals if necessary.

SUGGESTED READING

O'Sullivan ML: Tachypnea, dyspnea, and respiratory distress. In Ettinger SJ, et al. editors: Textbook of veterinary internal medicine, ed 8, St. Louis. 2017, Elsevier.

AUTHOR: Peter M. Foley, MSc, DVM, DACVIM
EDITOR: Leah A. Cohn, DVM, PhD, DACVIM

Stunted Growth

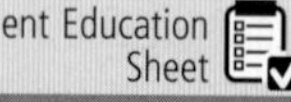

BASIC INFORMATION

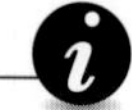

Definition

Slower growth rate or failure to attain expected body size/stature

Synonyms

Failure to thrive, delayed growth, poor-doer

Epidemiology

SPECIES, AGE, SEX

- Dogs and cats
- Male and female; sex predispositions vary with cause.
- Stunted growth is usually observed in the first year of life, although pet owners may recognize the problem later.

GENETICS, BREED PREDISPOSITION

- Pituitary dwarfism: German shepherd, Saarloos wolfhound, Karelian bear dog
- Congenital hypothyroidism: toy fox terrier, rat terrier, boxer, giant schnauzer, Abyssinian
- Osteochondrodysplasia: Alaskan Malamute, beagle, bull terrier, English pointer, Great Pyrenees, Irish setter, Labrador retriever, miniature poodle, Newfoundland, Norwegian elkhound, Samoyed, Scottish deerhound
- Cleft palate: shih tzu, English bulldog, pointers, Swiss sheepdog, Brittany spaniel
- Congenital megaesophagus: Irish setter, German shepherd, Labrador retriever, miniature schnauzer
- Vascular ring anomaly: German shepherd, Irish setter
- Pancreatic acinar atrophy: German shepherd
- Portosystemic shunt (PSS [p. 814])
- Polycystic kidney disease (p. 805)
- Familial renal diseases (pp. 51, 390, 875)
- Juvenile hyperparathyroidism: German shepherd (rare)

RISK FACTORS

- Malnutrition: poor-quality feed/parasitic infestation
- Group housing/lack of hygiene: infectious diseases

CONTAGION AND ZOONOSIS

Some gastrointestinal (GI) parasites (e.g., *Toxocara, Giardia*) present a zoonotic risk.

GEOGRAPHY AND SEASONALITY

Certain infectious organisms are endemic to a specific geographic area, whereas they are rarely encountered in other regions (e.g., *Histoplasma, Pythium*).

ASSOCIATED DISORDERS

- Juvenile diabetes mellitus: pancreatic acinar atrophy and exocrine pancreatic insufficiency
- Pituitary dwarfism: hypoadrenocorticism
- PSS: urate urolithiasis, microvascular dysplasia
- Megaesophagus: myasthenia gravis, vascular ring anomaly, congenital cardiac disease (e.g., persistent ductus arteriosus [PDA])
- Cleft palate: middle ear abnormalities

Clinical Presentation

DISEASE FORMS/SUBTYPES

Subdivision according to body condition score (BCS; good or poor thrift) and according to body stature (proportionate or disproportionate) is particularly helpful in the approach to patients with stunted growth.

HISTORY, CHIEF COMPLAINT

- Pet lags behind littermates in growth/does not have the expected body stature.
- Quantity and palatability of the diet, deworming history, and onset and progression of signs are important.
- ± Signs of mental dullness
- ± Regurgitation (since weaning), diarrhea or voluminous stools
- ± Polyuria/polydipsia
- ± Medication exposure (e.g., glucocorticoids, androgens, estrogens)
- May be unnoticed by owner or noticed at a late stage

PHYSICAL EXAM FINDINGS

- Determine BCS to distinguish between good and poor body condition.
- Determine whether the patient has proportionate or disproportionate body stature.
  - Congenitally hypothyroid patients and chondrodysplastic patients are disproportionate dwarfs (limbs are exceptionally short). By contrast, with proportional dwarfism (e.g., due to growth hormone deficiency), the limbs, trunk, and head are of appropriate relative sizes.
- Examine patient for
  - Mental dullness or disorientation
  - Cleft palate
  - Cough, respiratory distress
  - Heart murmur, arrhythmia
  - Bloated abdomen
  - Signs of diarrhea staining coat

Etiology and Pathophysiology

Common underlying disease types:

- Nutritional
- Gastrointestinal (GI)
- Esophageal
- Endocrine
- Cardiac
- Systemic disease (infectious/metabolic)

See Small Stature and Body Condition table.

DIAGNOSIS

Diagnostic Overview

History (nutrition, parasite control, accompanying clinical signs) and a thorough physical exam (distinction between good/poor BCS, proportionate or disproportionate dwarfism, cardiac auscultation) are the cornerstone in the diagnosis of disorders causing stunted growth. Laboratory tests and diagnostic imaging modalities are then selected as needed based on most likely differentials.

Differential Diagnosis

Small stature and poor body condition:

- Nutritional: poor-quality diet, underfeeding
- GI: parasites, inflammatory bowel disease, food intolerance/allergy, exocrine pancreatic insufficiency, obstruction
- Esophageal disease: megaesophagus, congenital myasthenia gravis, vascular ring anomaly
- Cardiac: congenital malformations
- Systemic disease
  - Metabolic: PSS (or other hepatic disease), kidney disease, glycogen storage disease
  - Infectious: respiratory infections (e.g., bacterial pneumonia), GI infections, other
- Endocrine: diabetes mellitus, hypoadrenocorticism, diabetes insipidus, juvenile hyperparathyroidism (rare)

Small stature and good body condition or overweight:

- Disproportionate stature: chondrodystrophy, endocrine (congenital hypothyroidism)
- Proportionate stature: hyposomatotropism (growth hormone deficiency), hyperadrenocorticism (rare)

A detailed differential diagnosis is provided in Section 3.

Initial Database

- First rule-outs: nutritional causes and GI parasites
  - Diet history: good-quality diet, appropriate daily quantity (p. 1077)
  - Fecal flotation, deworming
- CBC/serum biochemistry panel/urinalysis for systemic disease
- If no significant abnormalities are found with these tests and physical exam is otherwise unremarkable, proceed to advanced testing.

Advanced or Confirmatory Testing

- Disproportionate dwarfism: congenital hypothyroidism → joint radiographs (epiphyseal dysgenesis and delayed skeletal formation); thyroxine (T_4), thyroid-stimulating hormone (TSH), and advanced thyroid function testing may be necessary.
- Proportionate dwarfism: hyposomatotropism → serum level of insulin-like growth factor
- Trypsin-like immunoreactivity: exocrine pancreatic insufficiency
- Thoracic/abdominal radiographs: look for megaesophagus, cardiac shape change, microhepatica, other
- Abdominal ultrasound: kidney disease, PSS
- ACTH-stimulation test: hypoadrenocorticism
- Echocardiography: congenital heart defects
- Scintigraphy: PSS, ciliary dyskinesia

TREATMENT

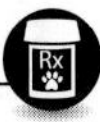

Treatment Overview

Correct diseases that are reversible as soon as possible.

Chronic Treatment

- Nutritional: provide a good-quality, balanced diet in appropriate quantity.
- Parasitic: deworming
- GI: supplementation of pancreatic enzymes (exocrine pancreatic insufficiency), hypoallergenic diet (food intolerance/allergy), supportive treatment (megaesophagus) ± surgical correction (vascular ring anomaly)
- Congenital hypothyroidism: supplementation with levothyroxine
- Hyposomatotropism: porcine growth hormone or progestins (the latter only after ovariohysterectomy, side effects: pyoderma, mammary gland tumors, acromegaly, skeletal maldevelopment, diabetes mellitus, cystic endometrial hyperplasia), often in combination with levothyroxine when there is also TSH deficiency
- Cardiac: interventional or surgical correction if amenable
- Systemic disease: as indicated for specific condition

Possible Complications

Early diagnosis and intervention are crucial to prevent major complications for certain conditions such as PSS, cardiac disease, vascular ring anomalies.

Recommended Monitoring

Body weight, BCS

PROGNOSIS & OUTCOME

- Many underlying diseases are reversible, but for some disorders, prognosis depends greatly on early diagnosis and intervention.
- Osteochondrodysplastic dogs can fare well, but the disorder is irreversible.

PEARLS & CONSIDERATIONS

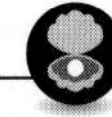

Comments

- Key to correct diagnosis is distinction between good and poor BCS and proportionate and disproportionate dwarfism.
- A thorough physical exam including careful cardiac auscultation is essential for diagnosis.
- Adequate nutrition and effective deworming should be assured before performing expensive diagnostic tests.

Technician Tips

Patient monitoring and handling greatly depends on the underlying condition (e.g., megaesophagus: upright position during and after feeding, monitoring for respiratory signs, which could be indicative of aspiration pneumonia).

SUGGESTED READING

Kooistra HS: Failure to grow. In Ettinger SJ, et al, editors: Textbook of veterinary internal medicine, ed 8, St. Louis, 2017, Elsevier, pp 88-91.

AUTHORS: Pascale M. Y. Smets, DVM, PhD, DECVIM; Sylvie Daminet, DVM, PhD, DACVIM, DECVIM
EDITOR: Leah A. Cohn, DVM, PhD, DACVIM

Subaortic Stenosis

Client Education Sheet 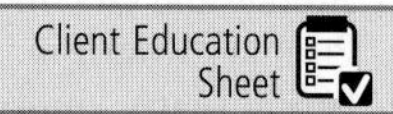

BASIC INFORMATION 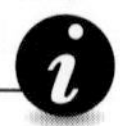

Definition

- Most common cardiac congenital malformation of large-breed dogs
- Hallmark is a narrowing of the left ventricular outflow tract (LVOT) just below the aortic valve.
- May be fixed (fibrous nodule, band, annulus, fibromuscular tunnel) or dynamic (systolic anterior motion of the mitral valve [SAM])

Synonyms

Subvalvular aortic stenosis (SAS)

Epidemiology

SPECIES, AGE, SEX

- First noted in puppies < 12 months old (usually after 4-8 weeks of age)
- The severity of narrowing is progressive (or rarely regressive) during a puppy's growth, and the true severity of SAS cannot be determined until the dog is fully grown (12-18 months, depending on breed).
- Depending on the study, SAS is the most common congenital heart defect of dogs or is second to patent ductus arteriosus (PDA).
- Uncommon in cats, but dynamic LVOT obstruction occurs commonly with hypertrophic obstructive cardiomyopathy (p. 505).

GENETICS, BREED PREDISPOSITION

- Large-breed dogs (especially Newfoundlands, golden retrievers, rottweilers, boxers, German shepherds, Bouvier des Flandres, Bernese mountain dogs, bullmastiffs, and dogues de Bordeaux)
- Bull terriers are predisposed to valvular aortic stenosis (thickened leaflets and hypoplastic valvular annulus), a different disease but with the same result of obstruction between left ventricle (LV) and aorta.
- Hereditary transmission has been demonstrated in Newfoundland dogs (autosomal dominant abnormality in the *PICALM* gene), golden retriever, bullmastiffs, and dogue de Bordeaux (autosomal recessive in these breeds).
- No apparent sex linkage
- Mildly affected dogs can produce more severely affected offspring.

RISK FACTORS

A decreased (steeper) aortoseptal angle is often seen with SAS and represents a predisposing anatomic factor for SAS development in the boxer, dogue de Bordeaux, golden retriever, and possibly other breeds.

ASSOCIATED DISORDERS

- Mild/moderate aortic regurgitation/insufficiency: very commonly observed echocardiographically in dogs with SAS; generally inaudible on auscultation
- Mitral valve dysplasia, PDA, and a variety of aortic arch abnormalities have been associated with some SAS cases.
- Jet lesions associated with SAS can damage the aortic valvular endothelium and predispose to bacterial endocarditis.

Clinical Presentation

DISEASE FORMS/SUBTYPES

Many distinct malformations are grouped under the heading of SAS.

Fixed obstruction:

- Grade I: small, raised nodules of thickened endocardium
- Grade II: narrow ridge of thickened endocardium that partially encircles the LVOT
- Grade III: fibrous band, ridge, or collar completely encircles the LVOT
- This grading system is used for gross pathologic findings. It is unrelated to murmur intensity or clinical signs.

Dynamic obstruction:

- Systolic anterior motion of the mitral valve
  - Narrowing of the LVOT and papillary muscle distortion caused by left ventricular hypertrophy allows slight displacement of the mitral valve such that a small amount of mitral regurgitation occurs.
- Septal hypertrophy or malalignment
  - The left ventricular hypertrophy induced by SAS may further contribute to left ventricular outflow obstruction because of hypertrophy of the interventricular septum.
  - The aortic arch may be congenitally malaligned with the long axis of the interventricular septum, resulting in SAS due to protrusion of the interventricular septum into the subvalvular area.

HISTORY, CHIEF COMPLAINT

In most cases, the condition causes a heart murmur in an apparently healthy/asymptomatic puppy. However, severe cases may exhibit

- Exertional fatigue or syncope
- Congestive heart failure (CHF) (rare)
- Sudden death; sometimes the first clinical sign in severe cases
- Moderate cases often show exaggerated or long-lasting panting after exercise as their only clinical sign.

PHYSICAL EXAM FINDINGS

They are often unremarkable except for a systolic, ejection-type (crescendo-decrescendo) heart murmur, heard loudest at the left heart base (between the third and fifth intercostal spaces) or at the thoracic inlet (immediately lateral to the trachea). This murmur results from the turbulent blood flow in the LVOT and ascending aorta.

- Intensity of the heart murmur grossly correlates with severity of disease:
  - Grades I-III/VI: mildly to moderately affected dogs
  - Grades IV-VI/VI: severely affected dogs
- Murmur may radiate cranially up the carotid arteries to the neck and head or to the right hemithorax.
- A weak and late-rising femoral pulse *(pulsus parvus et tardus)* is typical in severe cases as a consequence of the obstructive lesion and delayed rate of left ventricular ejection.
- A diastolic heart murmur is rarely heard with aortic valve insufficiency.
- Premature beats and pulse deficits (due to ventricular arrhythmias) may be detected in severe cases.

Etiology and Pathophysiology

- Predisposing anatomic characteristics of the LVOT such as increased mitral-aortic separation, decreased (steep) aortoseptal angle, malaligned interventricular septum, and a small aortic annulus (which increases the shear stress and stimulates cellular proliferation in the LVOT) are strongly suspected.
  - The persistence of embryonal endocardial tissue that retains potential capacity for chondrocyte proliferation was historically suspected, but evidence is lacking.
  - Some of these predisposing factors are suspected to be heritable, especially in the golden retriever, boxer, and dogue de Bordeaux.
  - Other dogs with SAS have LVOT obstruction without evidence of the anatomic abnormalities listed above.
- An important consequence of SAS, regardless of subtype or causative mechanism, is left ventricular pressure overload that results in
  - An increase in left ventricular systolic pressure and a pressure gradient across the stenotic lesion

- Increased blood flow velocity through the LVOT
- Compensatory left ventricular concentric hypertrophy in moderate and severe cases
- This process may rarely lead to left-sided CHF in some severe cases.
- With worsening SAS over time, left ventricular thickening may exceed intramyocardial (coronary) blood supply, which does not grow along with the hypertrophied myocardial cells. Together with coronary arterial changes, the result is inadequate perfusion of left ventricular tissue and ventricular arrhythmias or, less commonly, myocardial infarction. These adverse consequences are especially likely during high myocardial oxygen demand, which explains the value of exercise restriction in severely affected dogs.
- Either process may be responsible for sudden death (common in severe SAS).

DIAGNOSIS

Diagnostic Overview

The diagnosis is first suspected on auscultation of a systolic heart murmur loudest at the left heart base or cranial sternal region. Electrocardiography and thoracic radiographs may help raise or lower the likelihood of SAS, but Doppler echocardiography is the most accurate diagnostic test.

Differential Diagnosis

Other systolic heart murmurs heard at the left heart base:

- Pulmonic stenosis
- Tetralogy of Fallot
- Atrial septal defect
- Incompletely ausculted PDA

High-output states:

- Hyperthyroidism
- Anemia
- Fever
- Exercise: physical activity increases the heart rate, which may reveal a murmur of SAS that was not audible at rest. The distinction between this phenomenon and a benign, exercise-induced heart murmur requires echocardiography.

Juvenile innocent heart murmur:

- Puppies and kittens < 4 months old
- Soft heart murmur, grade I-II/VI, short (early to midsystolic)
- Sometimes disappears with a change in body position or exercise/increase in heart rate
- Electrocardiogram (ECG), thoracic radiographs, and echocardiogram are normal

Initial Database

ECG (p. 1096):

- Often normal in mild to moderate cases
- Left ventricular hypertrophy pattern often present (R wave > 3 mV in lead II) in severe cases; unreliable as a screening tool
- ST segment may be slurred, depressed, or elevated in severe cases (consistent with myocardial hypoxia) especially while exercising.
- Ventricular arrhythmias are seen in severe cases. Ambulatory ECG recording is more sensitive than a brief ECG, especially if arrhythmias are precipitated by exercise.

Thoracic radiographs:

- Often normal; unreliable as a screening tool because hypertrophy of the LV is concentric.
- Variable left-sided cardiomegaly (left ventricular and atrial enlargement), usually only with moderate to severe cases
- Helpful mostly to rule out congestive heart failure (rare), Post-stenotic dilation of the aortic root may be visible in some dogs, often greater in severe cases. It appears as a loss of the cranial waist on the lateral views and widening of the mediastinum on the dorsoventral view.

Echocardiogram (p. 1094) for definitive diagnosis:

- Two-dimensional (2D)
    - Often normal in mildly affected dogs
    - Subvalvular obstructive lesion or narrowed left ventricular outflow tract
    - A decreased/steeper aortoseptal angle can be seen in severe cases.
    - Various degrees of left ventricular concentric hypertrophy
    - Papillary muscles and the endocardial surface of the LV may appear hyperechoic.
    - Various degrees of dilation of the left atrium
    - Dilated ascending aorta (poststenotic dilation) in some cases
- M-mode study
    - Normal to increased left ventricular fractional shortening
    - Normal to increased left ventricular wall thickness
    - SAM sometimes observed
- Doppler study
    - Turbulent, high-velocity systolic signal in the LVOT and aortic root. Normal range (controversial) = up to 2 m/s; gray zone = 2-2.3 m/s; > 2.3 m/s = suggestive of SAS when corresponding murmur and breed are also present; exception in the boxer breed and possibly others, where such elevated velocities may be normal (requiring 2D aortic measurements for further evaluation)
    - Determination of the peak pressure gradient in combination with the indexed effective orifice area (IEOA) estimates the severity of disease; peak pressure gradient = 4 × (Doppler-derived LVOT peak velocity in m/s^2). This classification remains arbitrary.
    - 16-40 mm Hg = mild SAS; 40-99 mm Hg = moderate SAS
    - >100 mm Hg = severe SAS. IEOA < 0.6 cm^2/m^2 = severe SAS
    - >125-130 mm Hg usually associated with clinical signs and worse prognosis
    - Diastolic signal of aortic regurgitation is present in most cases of SAS.

TREATMENT

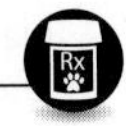

Treatment Overview

- Only severe cases benefit from therapy. Moderate and mild cases are usually asymptomatic and do not need therapy.
- No definitive treatment exists for curing SAS.
- Excision of the stenotic tissue by open-heart surgery or dilation of the stenosis by noninvasive balloon valvuloplasty has not yet been shown to provide an outcome that is superior to conservative, medical management.
- Recurrence of the stenotic lesion is often observed after balloon dilation or surgery, possibly as a result of anatomic characteristics of the LVOT that were left unaltered after surgery (e.g., abnormal aortoseptal angle).
- A dilation technique using cutting and high-pressure balloons has been described and can be beneficial in symptomatic dogs. Long-term and survival benefits of this procedure remains controversial.

Acute General Treatment

- Syncopal dogs should be kept at complete rest until a complete cardivascular evaluation is performed (ECG, echocardiogram, ± chest radiographs and Holter monitoring or "in-house" telemetry).

Chronic Treatment

Mild SAS:

- No treatment

Moderate SAS:

- Treatment not universally implemented
- Mild exercise restriction (avoid vigorous activity) may be advised for dogs at the higher velocities of the moderate SAS range (80-100 mm Hg).
- Beta-blockade may be instituted in individual cases.

Severe SAS:

- Open resection of the obstructing lesion is possible, but long-term survival is unchanged compared with medical management.
- Balloon dilation of the stenosis: survival not longer than with medical management
- Cutting balloon and high-pressure balloon dilation may be beneficial short-term (12 months) when aortoseptal angle > 160 degrees. Promising but still unknown whether survival is superior to medical management alone
- Exercise restriction: limit to walks on a leash and light exercising, and avoid vigorous exercise.
- Beta-blockers to prevent or control ventricular arrhythmias, decrease myocardial oxygen consumption, and improve coronary artery flow
    - Atenolol 0.5-1.5 mg/kg PO q 12h; begin at low dose and increase titration over 2-4 weeks until upper end of dose range or signs of intolerance (lethargy, inappetence, hypotension) warranting dosage reduction, *or*
    - Sotalol 1-3 mg/kg PO q 12h, up-titration as per atenolol. Sotalol might be more effective in certain breeds (e.g., boxers).

SAS with CHF (pp. 408 and 409)

Behavior/Exercise

Severe SAS cases: exercise restriction is recommended, especially avoidance of vigorous activity. Sudden death typically occurs during or shortly after strenuous exercise. However, this recommendation must be weighed against quality of life.

Drug Interactions

- Concurrent use of antacids can alter the bioavailability of atenolol.
- Calcium channel blockers may cause hypotension and bradycardia when administered together with atenolol.
- Effects of theophylline can be blocked by beta-blocking agents such as propranolol.

Possible Complications

- Ventricular arrhythmias/ventricular tachycardia
- Exertional syncope or sudden death
- Left-sided heart failure
- Aortic valve endocarditis: antibiotics may be indicated during periods of anticipated bacteremia (dental procedures, surgery, wounds, other concurrent bacterial disease).

Recommended Monitoring

- Control ventricular arrhythmias when present (p. 1033). Ambulatory ECG is recommended if syncope is noted and for monitoring efficacy of antiarrhythmic treatment (p. 1120).
- SAS can progress during puppyhood, and a cardiac evaluation should be done at full maturity to stage the severity of disease.

PROGNOSIS & OUTCOME

- Mild to moderate SAS: good
  - Normal quality of life and longevity, especially for dogs with peak pressure gradient < 50 mm Hg and when follow-up visit shows no progression of SAS
- Severe SAS: guarded
  - Depending on studies, median survival time is 19-61 months when untreated.
  - Medical management is associated with a median survival of 4.5 years.
  - Most dogs with pressure gradients > 125-130 mm Hg develop serious complications or die suddenly in the first 3 years of life.

PEARLS & CONSIDERATIONS

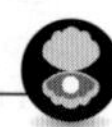

Comments

- SAS is a problematic disease; it is difficult to diagnose mildly affected dogs, and there is no definitive cure for severely affected dogs, which remain at risk of sudden death even after surgical intervention.
- The combination of a ≥ grade IV/VI ejection left-sided heart murmur that radiates cranially to the thoracic inlet and over the carotid arteries along with a weak femoral pulse in a large-breed puppy is highly suggestive of severe SAS.
- The severity of ventricular arrhythmias detected by extended (24-hour) ambulatory ECG recordings correlates with the severity of disease.
- Because of the progressive nature of SAS during growth, the lesion/heart murmur may be clinically silent in very young puppies but becomes increasingly prominent at 2-3 months of age.
- Breeding dogs affected by mild SAS may generate severely affected offspring.
- Overtly healthy boxer dogs may have systolic murmurs without obvious SAS. This phenomenon is potentially caused by a relatively smaller outflow tract/aorta in that breed, predisposing them to increased ejection velocity and development of murmurs.
- Differentiation between SAS and the normal state in the most mildly affected dogs is challenging and requires a combination of physical exam, echocardiography (left ventricular thickening, left atrial enlargement, steep aortoseptal angle, and aortic insufficiency suggest SAS) and regular follow-up exams (progression of these abnormalities and of Doppler-derived pressure gradient suggest SAS).

Prevention

- Screening of breeding dogs for SAS
- Genetic testing may become available in the near future.

Technician Tips

Avoid stress and intense activity in dogs with severe SAS dogs because of risk of syncope or sudden death.

Client Education

- In cases of severe SAS, avoid prolonged or vigorous exercise.
- Contact breeders to notify them of SAS cases; do not breed SAS dogs.

SUGGESTED READING

Beijerink NJ, et al: Aortic stenosis. In Ettinger SJ, et al, editors: Textbook of veterinary internal medicine, ed 8, St. Louis, 2017, Elsevier, pp 1234-1240.

AUTHOR: Marie-Claude Bélanger, DVM, MSc, DACVIM
EDITOR: Meg M. Sleeper, VMD, DACVIM

Subinvolution of Placental Sites

Bonus Material Online Client Education Sheet 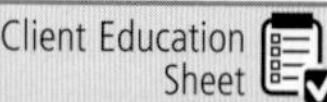

BASIC INFORMATION

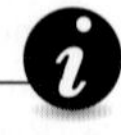

Definition

Persistent bright red, bloody vulvar discharge is usually observed in young primiparous bitches with failure of or delayed uterine involution beyond 12 weeks after whelping. These dogs are not systemically ill unless the retained placental remnants become infected or there is severe uterine bleeding (metrorrhagia).

Synonyms

Postpartum metrorrhagia, postpartum placentitis, SIPS

Epidemiology

SPECIES, AGE, SEX

- Incidence in dogs (histopathologic evaluation of postpartum uteruses): 8%-21%
  - Does not occur in cats
- Any age but more prevalent after the first parturition, especially in bitches < 3 years old
- Litter size has no effect.

GENETICS, BREED PREDISPOSITION

No breed predisposition

RISK FACTORS

Low parity (especially after the first pregnancy)

ASSOCIATED DISORDERS

- Anemia (rarely hemorrhage is so severe that it requires a hysterectomy)
- Postpartum metritis (secondary to infected placental remnants)
- Uterine rupture can occur as a result of SIPS (rare).

Clinical Presentation

HISTORY, CHIEF COMPLAINT

- History of recent whelping or abortion
- Hemorrhagic vulvar discharge is persistent even after pups are weaned.
- Bitch is otherwise in good health.

PHYSICAL EXAM FINDINGS

- Bright red discharge rather than normal brown lochia
- Slight pallor of mucous membranes if discharge is copious
- Abdominal palpation may reveal discrete uterine swellings of various sizes.
- Physical exam generally reveals an otherwise healthy animal.

Etiology and Pathophysiology

- Normally, expulsion of the fetal membranes and lochia occurs immediately postpartum,

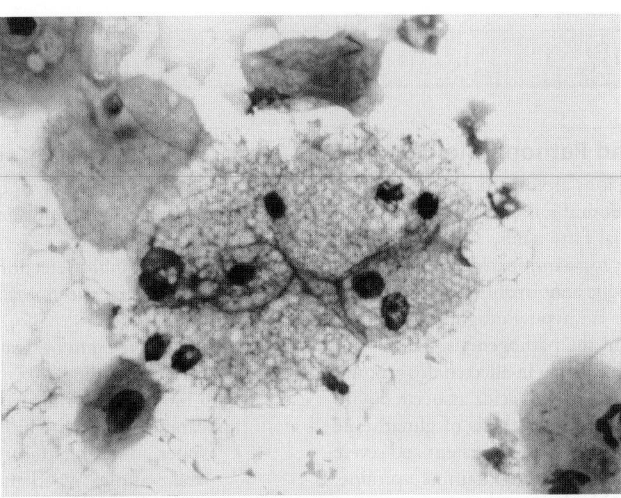

SUBINVOLUTION OF PLACENTAL SITES A vestibular smear from a dog with subinvolution of placental sites (SIPS). A trophoblast cell is visible as a polynucleated, vacuolated giant cell. (Courtesy Auke C. Schaefers-Okkens.)

and a mild serosanguineous discharge may last 3-5 weeks postpartum.
- With SIPS, placental cells (trophoblasts) continue to invade the endometrium and myometrium after the placentas have been delivered.
- Failure of these cells to regress prevents normal uterine involution, resulting in chronic hemorrhagic vulvar discharge.

DIAGNOSIS

Diagnostic Overview

- The diagnosis is based on hemorrhagic vulvar discharge that ranges in severity from self-limited and not producing overt signs to life-threatening metrorrhagia requiring transfusion.
- The diagnosis is often presumptive, unless accompanied by uterine histopathology.

Differential Diagnosis

- Exogenous estrogens
- Metritis
- Vaginitis
- Vulvar, vaginal, or uterine tumor
- Urinary tract hemorrhage (e.g., bacterial cystitis, calculi)
- Coagulopathies
- Brucellosis
- Trauma

Initial Database

- CBC, serum biochemistry profile, urinalysis: unremarkable. NOTE: mild normocytic, normochromic anemia is normal in postpartum bitches.
- Vaginal cytologic exam: a typical finding is trophoblasts.

Advanced or Confirmatory Testing

- Definitive diagnosis: histologic exam based on biopsy specimen of placental sites (rarely done)
- Vaginoscopy (p. 1184): to distinguish vaginal bleeding from blood derived from the uterus
- Abdominal ultrasonography: focal thickenings of the uterine wall and a fluid-distended lumen; color Doppler velocity measurements of blood flow differentiates SIPS from normally involuting uteruses.
- Abdominal radiographs: focal areas of uterine irregularity

TREATMENT

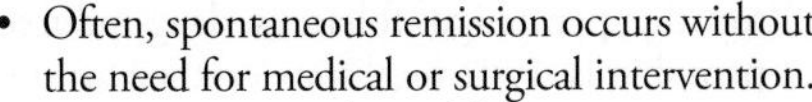

Treatment Overview

- Often, spontaneous remission occurs without the need for medical or surgical intervention.
- Hysterectomy and possibly curettage is necessary in acute cases with severe metrorrhagia.

Acute General Treatment

- Observation (benign neglect)
  - Erosion through the uterine wall resulting in peritonitis is possible but rare.
  - In most cases, SIPS resolves spontaneously.
- Curettage may be attempted if bitch is intended for future breeding and/or hemorrhage is severe.
- Hysterectomy is indicated if the bitch is not intended for future breeding and hemorrhage is severe.
- Acute life-threatening uterine bleeding may require blood transfusion (p. 1169).
- Systemic and intrauterine antibiotics may be indicated when metritis or peritonitis is present.

Recommended Monitoring

Serial weekly/biweekly clinical, hematologic, and ultrasonographic exams. Recheck animals showing any signs of systemic illness, and look for complications (e.g., anemia, rarely uterine perforation and peritonitis).

PROGNOSIS & OUTCOME

- Good: many females recover without treatment.
  - With spontaneous remission, future reproductive success is not compromised.
  - Affected bitches are not predisposed to SIPS in subsequent pregnancies.
  - Rarely, trophoblastic cells cause uterine perforation and subsequent peritonitis.
- Poor: if acute exsanguination (rare); uterine perforation and peritonitis (rare)

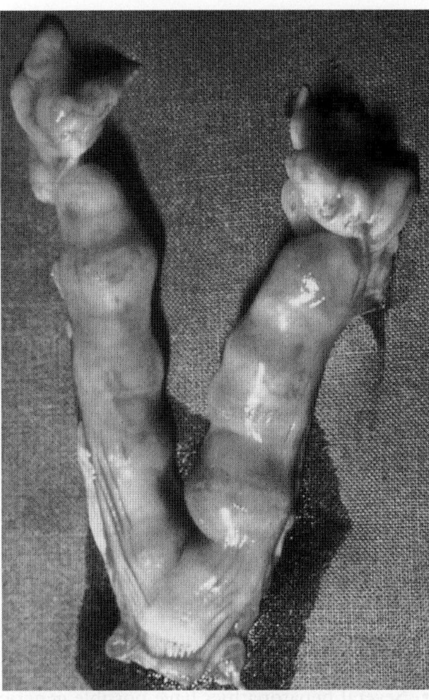

SUBINVOLUTION OF PLACENTAL SITES Enlarged uterine segments were visible at the time of ovariohysterectomy in a bitch with severe metrorrhagia. They may be palpable per abdomen. (Courtesy Auke C. Schaefers-Okkens.)

PEARLS & CONSIDERATIONS

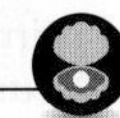

Comments

SIPS is the most common cause for persistent postparturient serosanguineous vulvar discharge in an otherwise healthy bitch.

Prevention

Hysterectomy or not breeding an intact female dog prevents this problem from occurring.

Technician Tips

Advise client to monitor the color of mucous membranes for signs of anemia.

Client Education

Careful monitoring for complications such as systemic illness and metritis (foul-smelling discharge)

SUGGESTED READING

Dickie MB, et al: Diagnosis and therapy of the subinvolution of placental sites in the bitch. J Reprod Fertil Suppl 47:471, 1993.

AUTHOR: Carlos M. Gradil, DVM, MS, PhD, DACT
EDITOR: Michelle A. Kutzler, DVM, PhD, DACT

Superficial Necrolytic Dermatitis

Client Education Sheet 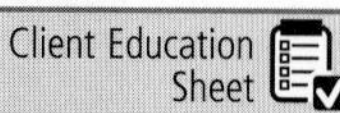

BASIC INFORMATION

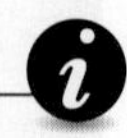

Definition

Progressively debilitating skin disease associated with severe internal disease process

Synonyms

Hepatocutaneous syndrome, glucagonoma syndrome, metabolic epidermal necrosis, necrolytic migratory erythema

Epidemiology

SPECIES, AGE, SEX

- Uncommon in dogs, rare in cats
- Middle-aged to geriatric patients

GENETICS, BREED PREDISPOSITION

- Possible heritable component in shih tzus
- Several hepatopathies have possible genetic component (p. 450)

RISK FACTORS

- Administration of phenobarbital
- Ingestion of mycotoxin

ASSOCIATED DISORDERS

- Most cases are associated with hepatopathy.
- Few cases are associated with functional pancreatic alpha-cell (glucagon-secreting) tumor.
- Diabetes mellitus reported to occur in 25%-40% of dogs with hepatic form
- Other associated conditions in dogs: hepatic cirrhosis, idiopathic vacuolar hepatopathy, extrapancreatic glucagonoma (liver, spleen, adrenal glands, and mesenteric lymph nodes), copper storage disease, hyperglucagonemia, and intestinal disease
- Associated diseases in cats: pancreatic carcinoma, hepatopathies, and thymic amyloidosis

Clinical Presentation

HISTORY, CHIEF COMPLAINT

Owners usually observe footpad lesions first because dermatologic changes may precede onset of clinical signs of internal disease. Lethargy, anorexia, weight loss, lameness, reluctance to walk/signs of pedal pain, and pruritus are frequently reported. Other chief complaints may include polyuria and polydipsia.

PHYSICAL EXAM FINDINGS

Dermatologic lesions are characterized by thickening, fissuring, and crusting of footpads and interdigital erythema. Crusts, erosions, and ulcers can affect pinnae, mucocutaneous junctions (oral cavity, eyes, anus, and genitalia), elbows and other pressure points, and ventral abdominal and inguinal regions. Regional lymphadenopathy and hyperthermia are possible.

Etiology and Pathophysiology

- The skin lesions are due to degeneration of keratinocytes, and it is thought that deficiencies (essential fatty acids, zinc, biotin, and particularly hypoaminoacidemia) resulting from metabolic abnormalities caused by liver dysfunction or hyperglucagonemia play a major role in the pathogenesis.
- Hypoaminoacidemia in affected dogs prominently involves amino acids associated with the urea cycle and synthesis of glutathione and collagen. The most consistent and severe abnormalities involve glutamine, proline, cysteine, and hydroxyproline.
- Dysfunction of specific amino acid transporters and wasting of amino acids essential for collagen synthesis are evidenced by marked lysinuria and prolinuria in affected dogs.

DIAGNOSIS

Diagnostic Overview

Diagnosis is usually based on clinicopathologic, ultrasonographic, and histopathologic findings.

Differential Diagnosis

- Autoimmune/immune-mediated dermatopathy: pemphigus foliaceus, drug-induced pemphigus, systemic lupus erythematosus, paraneoplastic pemphigus, cutaneous vasculitis, erythema multiforme, toxic epidermal necrolysis
- Infectious dermatopathy: bacterial (pyoderma), fungal (dermatophytosis, *Malassezia* dermatitis), protozoal (leishmaniasis)
- Parasitic dermatopathy: demodicosis
- Nutritional dermatopathy: zinc-responsive dermatosis
- Neoplastic dermatopathy: epitheliotropic lymphoma
- Idiopathic: nasodigital hyperkeratosis

Initial Database

- Deep skin scrapings (typically negative, although secondary demodicosis may occur), cytologic evaluation of the skin (patients often have a bacterial or *Malassezia* overgrowth) ± dermatophyte culture (typically negative) (p. 1091)
- CBC (nonregenerative anemia and leukocytosis are possible), serum biochemistry profile (elevated alkaline phosphatase, alanine aminotransferase, serum glucose and fructosamine levels; hypoalbuminemia; decreased blood urea nitrogen), and urinalysis (glucosuria if diabetic)

Advanced or Confirmatory Testing

- Abdominal ultrasonography
  - Changes in hepatic parenchyma are highly characteristic: hypoechoic nodules with a hyperechoic trabecular network throughout the liver, resulting in a honeycomb or Swiss cheese pattern. Occasionally, hepatic metastases are detected.
  - Ultrasonographic detection of pancreatic and extrapancreatic glucagonomas can be difficult.
- Histopathologic exam of tissue (± immunohistochemical staining)
  - Skin biopsy: epidermis has a French flag appearance (i.e., red-white-blue layers):
    - Upper layer (stratum corneum): parakeratotic hyperkeratosis staining red (eosinophilic)
    - Middle layer (stratum spinosum): intracellular edema, vacuolation, and necrosis of the keratinocytes staining white (pallor)
    - Deep layer (stratum basale): hyperplasia staining blue (basophilic)
- Ultrasound-guided hepatic biopsy: first perform platelet count, arterial blood pressure, and coagulation panel to assess bleeding risk; hepatic neoplasia or idiopathic vacuolar hepatopathy
- Other assays
  - Fasting and postprandial bile acid values are frequently elevated (nonspecific).
  - Complete plasma amino acids (hypoaminoacidemia supportive of diagnosis of superficial necrolytic dermatitis [SND]) testing is available at Amino Acid Analysis Laboratory Service, University of California, Davis. Generalized hypoaminoacidemia, with numerous amino acid concentrations < 50% of mean reference values. Contact laboratory for sample handling and cost (https://www.vetmed.ucdavis.edu/labs/amino-acid-laboratory).
  - Urinalysis: marked lysinuria and prolinuria
  - Pancreatic tumors may not be readily visible with abdominal ultrasonography; therefore, measurement of plasma glucagon is also recommended.

TREATMENT

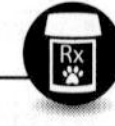

Treatment Overview

Treatment consists of a three-pronged approach: supportive therapy for dermatologic manifestations, management of internal disease process (which may require hospitalization), and surgical removal of neoplasm when possible.

Acute General Treatment

- Pain management
- Treat secondary bacterial and fungal infections with appropriate therapy (avoid systemic azole antifungal therapy because of potential hepatotoxicosis).
- Gentle shampoo therapy

Chronic Treatment

- Amino acid infusions: 25 mL/kg slow IV over 6-8 hours. Several crystalline amino acid solutions are available with varying compositions; no data suggest that one product is more efficacious than another. Solutions without additional electrolytes are preferred.
    - 10% crystalline amino acid solution (Aminosyn); high-osmolality solution and a jugular venous catheter is recommended to avoid thrombophlebitis (p. 1123)
    - 3% amino acid and electrolyte solution (Procalamine, B. Braun) is an alternative product. Lower cost; less hypertonicity (can therefore be injected in peripheral veins).
    - No defined protocols for frequency of administration (i.e., may be performed bimonthly, monthly, or when clinical signs return)
    - Most patients demonstrate clinical improvement in 5-10 days. Some dogs show dramatic improvement in demeanor with resolution of skin lesions after receiving infusion.
- Insulin therapy if indicated (p. 251)
- Octreotide (somatostatin analog inhibits glucagon release) 2-3 mcg/kg SQ q 12h in nonresectable or recurrent glucagonoma-associated disease: can improve skin lesions and systemic clinical signs. Anorexia is likely side effect.

Nutrition/Diet

- High-quality protein diet. Adding 3-6 entire hard-boiled eggs per day may be beneficial.
- Oral amino acid supplementation: Promod 1 scoop/10 kg PO q 24h
- Oral vitamin E supplementation: 400 IU/DOG PO q 12h
- Oral essential fatty acids
- Oral zinc methionine supplementation: Zinpro 1.5 mg/kg PO q 24h
- Oral *S*-adenosylmethionine may attenuate liver damage.
- Consultation with a veterinary nutritionist may be helpful.

Drug Interactions

Using antiinflammatory doses of oral glucocorticosteroids is controversial. It may give temporary relief, but diabetes and deterioration of the liver are possible complications.

Possible Complications

- Discomfort while walking may become sufficiently severe to constitute a reason for euthanasia.
- Monitor for signs of encephalopathy (slow down infusion rate if indicated) when using IV amino acid infusions.
- Postsurgical pancreatitis and biliary obstruction may occur.

PROGNOSIS & OUTCOME

- Prognosis is generally poor: most dogs die or are euthanized within 5 months of developing skin lesions. However, 20% of dogs in one study were maintained for 12 months or more with oral protein hyperalimentation and periodic IV amino acid infusions. In one study of affected dogs with a history of phenobarbital administration, patients were often euthanized within 12 weeks of diagnosis despite drug discontinuation.
- Surgical excision of pancreatic tumor may result in remission.
- Superficial necrolytic dermatitis in cats: poor

PEARLS & CONSIDERATIONS

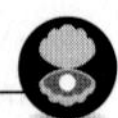

Comments

- The visually distinctive skin lesions of superficial necrolytic dermatitis are recognizable markers of an underlying systemic disease.
- Dermatologic signs often precede onset of clinical signs of internal disease.
- Hyperkeratotic, fissured footpads in an older dog are highly suggestive of superficial necrolytic dermatitis.

Technician Tips

Pododermatitis may be extremely painful. Use care and a gentle approach when walking dogs suspected or confirmed of having SND (may be reluctant to walk due to intense footpad pain).

SUGGESTED READING

Hall-Fonte DL, et al: Hepatocutaneous syndrome in shih tzus: 31 cases (1996-2014). J Am Vet Med Assoc 248(7):802, 2016.

AUTHOR: Vincent E. Defalque, DVM, DACVD
EDITOR: Manon Paradis, DMV, MVSc, DACVD

Syncope

Client Education Sheet

BASIC INFORMATION

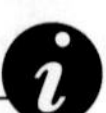

Definition

A sudden, temporary loss of consciousness resulting in collapse, followed by spontaneous recovery and caused by a transient cerebral deficiency of oxygen.

Synonyms

- Faint, collapse
- Neurocardiogenic syncope: vasovagal syncope
- Tussive syncope: cough-drop phenomenon

Epidemiology

SPECIES, AGE, SEX

- Depends on underlying cause: cardiac versus noncardiac causes
- Acquired heart disease: middle-aged to older animals
- Congenital heart disease: young animals

GENETICS, BREED PREDISPOSITION

- Tussive syncope: older, small-breed dogs with pulmonary or airway disease
- Neurocardiogenic syncope: boxer, golden retrievers, brachycephalic breeds
- According to underlying heart disease: many breed predispositions

RISK FACTORS

- Cardiac disease/arrhythmia
- Pulmonary hypertension
- Autonomic dysfunction (neurocardiogenic syncope)
- Drugs: beta-blockers, diuretics, vasodilators (hypotensive syncope)
- Anemia, hypoglycemia

Clinical Presentation

HISTORY, CHIEF COMPLAINT

- Acute collapse, with altered or loss of consciousness
- No clinical signs or brief staggering or ataxia before the event
- Exercise, excitement, or coughing may precipitate the event.
- ± Clonic movements (usually absent)
- ± Involuntary urination or defecation (usually absent)
- No postictal phase (i.e., mentation normal after event)
- Duration: seconds (and virtually always < 1 minute; otherwise, likely to be fatal)
- Recovery: complete and rapid

PHYSICAL EXAM FINDINGS

Depends on underlying disorder(s):

- Cardiac: murmur, arrhythmia, altered arterial pulse quality, pulse deficits, cyanotic mucous membranes, and pulmonary rales or crackles are possible.
- Neurologic exam (p. 1136): cranial nerve abnormalities, altered reflexes, proprioceptive deficits, and altered mentation are possible.
- Upper airway exam: stenotic nares, hypoplastic trachea, everted laryngeal saccules, elongated soft palate (i.e., brachiocephalic airway syndrome)

Etiology and Pathophysiology

A detailed list of causes are provided on p. 1284.

Cardiac:

- Bradyarrhythmias: syncope can result when there is a 6-8 second pause in electrical activity (i.e., failure of subsidiary pacemaker in third-degree atrioventricular [AV] block, sinus arrest associated with sick sinus syndrome [SSS]) or physical exertion that is not matched by an increase in cardiac output in a patient with inappropriate bradycardia (e.g., third-degree AV block).

- Tachyarrhythmias: rates > 300 beats/min for > 6 seconds (i.e., supraventricular tachycardia [SVT] or ventricular tachycardia) in dogs; cats uncommonly experience syncope with tachyarrhythmias but more so with bradycardias. Heart rate and time necessary for syncope can vary, depending on underlying cardiac structure (i.e., a slower heart rate for a shorter duration may cause syncope in an animal with underlying myocardial or valvular heart disease). Various outcomes: nonsustained tachyarrhythmia results in a return to sinus rhythm; overdrive suppression leads to sinus arrest or possibly ventricular fibrillation.
- Outflow obstruction (i.e., pulmonic stenosis, subaortic stenosis, cor pulmonale due to heartworm disease with secondary pulmonary hypertension)
  - Classic theory: exercise results in vasodilation of systemic arterioles. Fixed obstruction to flow results in inadequate increase in cardiac output, leading to hypotension and syncope.
  - Alternate theory: systolic function, cardiac output, and flow increase through stenosis during exercise. Increased left ventricular systolic pressure causes overstimulation of left ventricular mechanoreceptors. Reflex activation of cardiac afferent vagal fibers results in increased parasympathetic tone to heart and systemic blood vessels, resulting in bradycardia, vasodilation, and subsequent syncope.
- Cyanotic heart disease (e.g., right-to-left patent ductus arteriosus, tetralogy of Fallot): syncope is due to hypoxemia and/or hyperviscosity of blood from erythrocytosis, or else is caused by arrhythmias.
- Masses obstructing inflow or outflow of blood (rare): intracardiac mass lesions reduce cardiac output by restricting blood flow through atrioventricular valves or obstructing a ventricular outflow tract.
- Pericardial disease: compromises cardiac output by interfering with systemic venous return (i.e., cardiac tamponade)
- Congestive heart failure: syncope mechanism presumed to be similar to autonomic dysfunction (see below)

Noncardiac:

- Neurologic syncope: increased intracranial pressure with resultant decrease in cerebral perfusion (e.g., cerebral edema, brain tumors, meningitis, encephalitis, cerebral vascular obstructions, acute bleed). Seizures are far more likely than syncope with these diseases.
- Metabolic syncope: abrupt decrease in oxygen or nutrient delivery (i.e., glucose) to the brain. Oxygen concentration is affected by blood flow, hemoglobin concentration, and oxygen tension; seizures > syncope
- Tussive syncope: proposed mechanisms
  - Increased intrathoracic pressure transiently increases intracranial pressure and diminishes cardiac venous return and resultant cardiac output; cerebral blood flow is decreased during paroxysms of coughing.
  - Coughing stimulates vagal afferent transmission to the vasomotor center in the medulla, with subsequent stimulation of vagal efferents to the heart and blood vessels (bradycardia, hypotension).
- Autonomic dysfunction: excessive baroreflex resulting in cardiac inhibition and/or peripheral vasodilation (i.e., neurocardiogenic syncope, carotid sinus sensitivity, carotid body tumor)
- Peripheral vasomotor dysfunction: abnormality of peripheral vasoconstriction, muscle tone, heart rate, and/or respiration, resulting in syncope (postural hypotension)
- Undetermined: ≈40% of human syncope cases despite extensive testing; likely similar percentage in veterinary medicine

DIAGNOSIS

Diagnostic Overview

Diagnosis is largely based on patient signalment; historical events before, during, and after the episode; and complete cardiovascular and neurologic exams (p. 1136). Because the episode often is not witnessed directly by the veterinarian (to confirm or refute syncope), request video recording by the owner when an event occurs at home. Confirmatory testing may involve ambulatory electrocardiogram (ECG) monitoring and/or central nervous system (CNS) imaging, depending on the suspected cause. Consider consultation with and/or referral to a veterinary cardiologist ± veterinary neurologist.

Differential Diagnosis

- Seizures (p. 1280)
- Narcolepsy/cataplexy
- Weakness/collapse (e.g., metabolic, neuromuscular)

Initial Database

- CBC: often unremarkable; ± anemia, thrombocytopenia
- Serum biochemistry panel: often unremarkable; ± electrolyte abnormalities, metabolic derangements
- Urinalysis: often unremarkable; ± proteinuria (antithrombin loss and subsequent hypercoagulable state leading to thromboembolism)
- Blood pressure (p. 1065): normal result does not rule out transient hypotension.
- Heartworm testing: antigen test, microfilaria test
- Thoracic radiographs: to identify structural heart disease, pulmonary parenchymal abnormalities (e.g., pulmonary artery abnormalities with heartworm disease, cardiogenic pulmonary edema)
- Echocardiogram (p. 1094): ± congenital or acquired heart disease, estimation of pulmonary arterial pressure (p. 838)
- Resting ECG (p. 1096): ± rhythm abnormalities

Advanced or Confirmatory Testing

- Holter monitor (p. 1120): 24-hour ECG; helpful in establishing a diagnosis in 42% of patients
- Cardiac event recorder (p. 1120): digital loop recorder that is patient or owner activated, programmed to capture the heart rate and rhythm before and after the syncopal episode(s); diagnostic yield is 85%
- Cardiac troponin I level is increased in dogs with cardiac syncope as compared with seizure, but overlap in values occurs so that troponin cannot be used to distinguish between the disorders.
- Assessment of oxygenation: pulse oximetry, arterial blood gas analysis (p. 1058)
- CT/MRI/cerebrospinal fluid tap: neurologic disease (pp. 1080 and 1132)
- Other tests may be useful, as indicated by prior findings (e.g., abdominal ultrasound, bronchoalveolar lavage, fine needle aspirate or lung biopsy)

TREATMENT

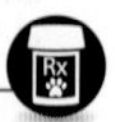

Treatment Overview

Treatment involves addressing the primary cause to alleviate syncopal episodes and prevent sudden death.

Acute General Treatment

Acute treatment is aimed at the underlying cause or stabilization procedures:

- Blood loss: fluids, blood products, others
- Pericardial effusion with cardiac tamponade: pericardiocentesis
- Bradyarrhythmias
  - SSS, third-degree AV block: medical management may be effective if arrhythmia is due to excessive vagal tone and atropine responsive (i.e., anticholinergics [propantheline] and beta-agonists [terbutaline]; see individual diseases for specific treatment recommendations). Temporary pacemaker if bradyarrhythmia is refractory to medical management and animal is showing persistent clinical signs.
- Tachyarrhythmias (p. 1457)
  - Ventricular tachycardia: oral or intravenous medical management, depending on severity of the arrhythmia (i.e., oral options: mexiletine, sotalol, amiodarone, atenolol; intravenous options: lidocaine, procainamide, amiodarone, esmolol. Cautious use or avoidance of beta-blockers in cases with systolic dysfunction/dilated cardiomyopathy

Chronic Treatment

- Treatment of underlying systemic disorder, if identified

- Bradyarrhythmias: medically refractory SSS, high-grade second-degree AV block, third-degree AV block: permanent pacemaker
- Tachyarrhythmias (p. 1033)
- Severe outflow obstructions: limit exertion in all cases.
  - Subaortic stenosis (SAS [p. 948]): beta-blockers if severe ± cutting balloon valvuloplasty
  - Pulmonic stenosis (p. 844): ± balloon valvuloplasty and beta-blockers if severe
  - Hypertrophic obstructive cardiomyopathy (p. 505): beta-blocker or calcium channel blocker
  - Heartworm disease with secondary pulmonary hypertension (pp. 415 and 418)
- Pulmonary hypertension: sildenafil (p. 838)
- Cyanotic heart disease–induced erythrocytosis: phlebotomy or hydroxyurea 50 mg/kg PO q 48-72h, adjusted based on response
- Congestive heart failure (p. 409)
- Neurologic syncope: treat underlying cause
- Metabolic syncope: treat underlying cause
- Tussive syncope: cough suppressant (e.g., butorphanol 0.1-0.5 mg/kg PO q 8-12h), bronchodilator (aminophylline 10 mg/kg PO q 8h), treatment with diuretics (e.g., furosemide 2 mg/kg IV, SQ) for pulmonary edema
- Autonomic dysfunction: anticholinergics (e.g., propantheline bromide 0.5-1 mg/kg PO q 8h if bradycardia related), beta-blocker (e.g., atenolol 0.25-1 mg/kg PO q 12h if tachycardia related). Treatment modalities are aimed at maintaining heart rate and/or preventing sympathetic surge. Medical management fails to address hypotensive component of reflex arc, and animals may continue to faint, potentially requiring a pacemaker.

Behavior/Exercise

Limit exertion/excitement in cases of outflow obstructions, cyanotic heart disease, impending/decompensated left-sided congestive heart failure, ventricular arrhythmias, and neurocardiogenic syncope.

Drug Interactions

Beta-blockers, diuretics, and vasodilators can exacerbate hypotension.

Possible Complications

Sudden death

Recommended Monitoring

Depends on cause

PROGNOSIS & OUTCOME

Highly dependent on underlying cause:

- Excellent for bradyarrhythmias treated with pacemaker implantation
- Fair to good with supraventricular tachycardia responsive to medical therapy
- Guarded with ventricular tachycardia treated medically; poor if systolic dysfunction/dilated cardiomyopathy present
- Varied prognosis for outflow obstructions (i.e., severe SAS has a poor long-term prognosis)
- Good with tussive syncope if cough responds well to medical therapy
- Prognosis is good for autonomic dysfunction. Treatment is usually unrewarding. Fortunately, sudden death is not common.

PEARLS & CONSIDERATIONS

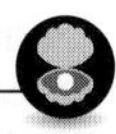

Comments

- Syncopal episodes may be difficult to differentiate from seizures. Videorecording and ECG event monitoring are simple, noninvasive tests that greatly help differentiate the two.
- Syncope, although uncommon in cats, occasionally occurs with hypertrophic obstructive cardiomyopathy and with bradyarrhythmias (e.g., third-degree AV block).
- In SSS, bradyarrhythmias (e.g., sinus arrest) typically cause syncopal episodes but seldom result in death (p. 915).
- In 40% of human cases, a cause is never identified; similar percentages are suspected in veterinary medicine.

Prevention

- Tussive syncope: cough suppressant, bronchodilator, treatment with diuretics if pulmonary edema is present
- Autonomic dysfunction: anticholinergics, beta-blocker

Technician Tips

- In-house ECG telemetry is useful for identifying bradyarrhythmias and tachyarrhythmias.
- Seizure bells can be placed on hospitalized patients presenting for syncope to help alert the staff when an animal has an episode.

Client Education

Distinguishing between seizures and syncope is crucial but not always obvious. Discuss unique features of each, and encourage videorecording of events.

SUGGESTED READING

Davidow EB, et al: Syncope: pathophysiology and differential diagnosis. Compend Contin Educ Pract Vet 23(7):609-618, 2001.

AUTHOR: Sarah J. Miller, DVM, DACVIM
EDITOR: Leah A. Cohn, DVM, PhD, DACVIM

Systemic Lupus Erythematosus

Client Education Sheet

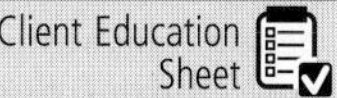

BASIC INFORMATION

Definition

A multisystemic autoimmune disease affecting at least two different organ systems

Epidemiology

SPECIES, AGE, SEX

More commonly reported in dogs than cats; young to middle-aged animals are predisposed.

GENETICS, BREED PREDISPOSITION

- Systemic lupus erythematosus (SLE) is heritable in dogs; experimental SLE colonies have been established.
- German shepherds may be overrepresented.

GEOGRAPHY AND SEASONALITY

Exposure to UV light may trigger cutaneous lesions.

ASSOCIATED DISORDERS

See Disease Forms/Subtypes below. New clinical signs may be due to additional manifestations of SLE or complications of treatment.

Clinical Presentation

DISEASE FORMS/SUBTYPES

The diagnosis of SLE is made when any three of the following occur concurrently or over any period:

- Cutaneous lesions, especially skin exposed to sunlight and/or at mucocutaneous junctions
- Oral mucosal ulcers
- Nonseptic, nonerosive polyarthritis
- Glomerulonephritis
- Hemolytic anemia and/or thrombocytopenia
- Leukopenia
- Polymyositis or myocarditis
- Serositis (nonseptic inflammatory effusion in the abdominal, pleural, or pericardial cavity)
- Neurologic disorder (seizures, psychosis, or polyneuritis)
- Significant serum antinuclear antibody (ANA) titer

HISTORY, CHIEF COMPLAINT

- Lameness is the most common primary complaint in dogs.
- Nonspecific lethargy and poor appetite
- Skin lesions

- Signs may wax and wane, confusing response to treatment.
- Other complaints relate to specific manifestation (e.g., abdominal distention due to nephrotic syndrome)

PHYSICAL EXAM FINDINGS

Depends on manifestations, which may include
- Lameness with swollen, painful joints; the carpi, tarsi, elbows, and stifles are most frequently involved.
- Intermittent fever
- Lymphadenopathy and/or splenomegaly
- Cutaneous lesions: erythema, scaling, crusting, depigmentation, and alopecia. Lesions may develop on the skin, mucocutaneous junctions, and oral cavity.

Etiology and Pathophysiology
- SLE occurs when a stimulus triggers the appropriate susceptibility genes in a patient.
- Triggering factors can include vaccination, drug administration, stress, infection, or exposure to UV radiation.
- Antibodies are directed against a broad range of nuclear, cytoplasmic, and cell membrane molecules. Antibodies against the patient's own DNA are detected with the ANA test.

DIAGNOSIS

Diagnostic Overview
The diagnosis of SLE is not based on a single test but on the constellation of clinical signs (see Disease Forms/Subtypes above) and exclusion of other possible causes.

Differential Diagnosis
- Tick-borne disease
- Neoplasia and paraneoplastic syndromes
- Bacterial, fungal, or viral infection
- Other immune-mediated diseases

Initial Database
- CBC, including manual differential: may show anemia, leukocytosis, or leukopenia; platelet count may be normal or low
- Serum biochemical profile: abnormalities reflect the site of inflammation (e.g., azotemia and hypoalbuminemia with glomerular involvement)
- Urinalysis: ± proteinuria; if present, perform urine protein/creatinine ratio, urine culture and susceptibility (C&S) testing
- Skin biopsies may reveal inflammatory infiltrates at the dermoepidermal junction and vacuolar change in the basal columnar cells.
- Radiographs of affected joints may reveal nonerosive joint swelling.
- Arthrocentesis of multiple joints (p. 1059) may reveal sterile neutrophilic inflammation.
- Serum ANA titer (p. 1308)
  - Serum ANA commonly stated as a requirement for the diagnosis of SLE, but sensitivity and specificity of this test are not known for the dog and cat.
  - Normal ranges are determined by individual laboratories.
  - False-positive results can occur with various medications (nonsteroidal antiinflammatory drugs [NSAIDs], antibiotics, others) or infections (e.g., heartworm, ehrlichiosis).
  - False-positive or false-negative results can occur as a result of different laboratory standardization, varied quality control protocols, and other factors.
- Lupus erythematosus (LE) cell test is rarely useful (p. 1361)
- Thoracic radiographs may reveal pleural or pericardial effusion (usually subtle).
- Abdominal ultrasonography: usually normal
- Tick-borne disease titers to rule out diseases that can mimic SLE (e.g., glomerulonephritis, polyarthritis, hematologic changes)
- Cats: feline leukemia virus (FeLV) and feline immunodeficiency virus (FIV) serologic tests

Advanced or Confirmatory Testing
- See Disease Forms/Subtypes above
- Coombs' test: indicated if anemia present but often negative
- Platelet autoantibodies: rarely useful
- Rheumatoid factor: usually negative
- Immunohistologic evaluation of skin biopsies (immunoperoxidase and immunofluorescent staining) may demonstrate immunoglobulin and complement deposits at the epidermal basement membrane, which are specific for immune-mediated dermatopathies.

TREATMENT

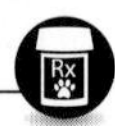

Treatment Overview
At least three aspects of treatment should be considered:
- Resolve clinical signs
- Prevent kidney injury
- Because of the natural waxing and waning of the disease, aggressive therapy may not be indicated for all cases.

Acute General Treatment
- Prednisone/prednisolone 1 mg/kg PO q 12-24h initially
- With severe disease, the addition of adjunctive immunosuppressants (e.g., mycophenolate mofetil 10 mg/kg PO q 12h) should be considered (p. 60).
- Proteinuria may be lessened with enalapril 0.5 mg/kg PO q 12h along with dietary protein optimization/restriction; may add omega-3 fatty acid supplementation (p. 390)

Chronic Treatment
- After all clinical and laboratory abnormalities have resolved, attempt to taper drugs. In general, decrease doses by one-half every 2-4 weeks while monitoring clinical and laboratory abnormalities.
- The minimal duration of immunosuppressive therapy should be 4-6 months.
- If signs recur during drug taper, increase level to the previous dose, and attempt to taper more slowly.

Behavior/Exercise
Avoid outdoor activity and/or use topical sunscreen for patients showing cutaneous or mucocutaneous lesions.

Drug Interactions
- Concurrent NSAID and glucocorticoid administration should be avoided because of the potential for GI ulceration.
- Mycophenolate mofetil may cause diarrhea.

Possible Complications
- Progressive kidney disease
- Infections (e.g., urinary tract infection) from long-term immunosuppression

Recommended Monitoring
- If prednisone is administered, monitor body weight and avoid obesity.
- If immunosuppressive medications are needed chronically, a urine culture is indicated q 3 months even in the absence of clinical signs of infection.
- Monitor CBC, serum biochemistry profile, and urinalysis q 3 months after in remission
- Serum ANA may be useful to detect relapse.

PROGNOSIS & OUTCOME

- Not well-known; many cases wax and wane
- Good for most cases
- Progressive renal disease indicates guarded prognosis.

PEARLS & CONSIDERATIONS

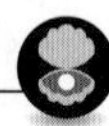

Comments
- The diagnosis of SLE is not based on a single test but on the constellation of clinical signs and exclusion of other possible causes.
- Treatment with doxycycline is useful to exclude infectious causes of polyarthropathy.
- Perform arthrocentesis on at least three joints, even if not swollen or painful.
- Biopsy of skin lesions must include intact epithelium. Ulcerated lesions are inherently nondiagnostic. Erythematous areas adjacent to ulcers yield the most conclusive results.
- Many animals are euthanized not because of progressive disease but due to adverse effects of glucocorticoids. Avoid obesity, and routinely monitor for infection of the skin and urinary tract.
- Combination immunosuppressive therapy with mycophenolate mofetil is often more effective and has fewer adverse effects than prednisone/prednisolone alone.

Prevention
Although a link has not been proved, vaccinations should be limited to those considered essential after the diagnosis of SLE.

Technician Tips
Many of the effects of SLE, notably polyarthritis, may be painful. Patients showing clinical signs that are known or suspected to be caused by SLE should be handled and walked as gently

as possible, with an awareness that pain may cause them to be uncooperative or aggressive even with normal handling.

Client Education

- Routine monitoring should be scheduled to detect relapse of disease and adverse effects of immunosuppressive medications.
- Many dogs live normal lives after the diagnosis.

SUGGESTED READING

Stone MS. Systemic lupus erythematosus. In Ettinger SJ, et al, editors: Textbook of veterinary internal medicine, ed 8, St. Louis; 2017, Elsevier, pp 861-866.

AUTHOR: Michael Stone, DVM, DACVIM
EDITOR: Jonathan E. Fogle, DVM, PhD, DACVIM

Tail Paralysis

BASIC INFORMATION

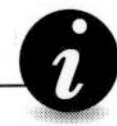

Definition

Severe impairment or loss of tail motor function

Epidemiology

SPECIES, AGE, SEX

Depends on underlying cause

GENETICS, BREED PREDISPOSITION

- Pugs, bulldogs (spina bifida, sacrocaudal dysgenesis)
- Chondrodystrophic breeds (disc herniation)
- Working dogs (limber tail, cold tail syndrome, or acute caudal myopathy)

RISK FACTORS

- Outdoor cats (trauma)
- Free-roaming dogs
- Cardiomyopathies in cats (aortic thromboembolism [p. 74])
- Type I disc herniation with severe paraparesis
- Degenerative lumbosacral stenosis (cauda equina syndrome)

ASSOCIATED DISORDERS

- Cutaneous wounds of the tail
  - Self-inflicted if sensation altered by neurologic disease
  - Secondary to external trauma (e.g., hit by car, falls)
- Tail fracture
- Feline cardiomyopathy

Clinical Presentation

HISTORY, CHIEF COMPLAINT

- Trauma involving the hindquarters (e.g., hit by car, falls, stepped on)
- Trauma involving traction injury on the tail (e.g., malicious, caught in door)
- Unwillingness to jump up (e.g., lumbosacral diseases)
- Acute-onset vocalization and hindlimb paresis/paralysis (aortic thromboembolism)
- Painful partially limp tail, generally after intense activity (limber tail syndrome)

PHYSICAL EXAM FINDINGS

- Impaired tail motility with or without hindlimb paresis
- Skin wounds (limbs, trunk, abdomen, and/or tail)
- Concurrent fractures of the axial skeleton, pelvis, pelvic limbs, and/or thoracic limbs
- Urinary and/or fecal incontinence, urine- or feces-soiled tail and/or perineum
- Pain originating from the pelvic area or the base of the tail
- Shock if massive trauma
- Tachycardia, heart murmur, gallop, weak or absent pulses, cyanosis/cold extremities of the pelvic limbs, possibly with signs of congestive heart failure (if feline cardiomyopathy-associated thromboembolism)
- Transverse myelopathy (T3-L3 or L4-S3 or Cd1-Cd5 only)
  - Large, distended bladder
  - Easy to empty if spinal lesion involves lumbar intumescence (lower motor neuron bladder)
  - Difficult to empty if spinal lesion is cranial to lumbar intumescence (upper motor neuron bladder)
- Rectal exam: painful and might induce sacrocaudal instability if associated with trauma

Etiology and Pathophysiology

Musculoskeletal:

- Spinal/coccygeal fracture
- Degenerative lumbosacral stenosis
- Coccygeal muscle injury (suspected in limber tail syndrome)

Neurologic:

- Spinal malformations
- Spinal fracture
- Nerve root avulsion (lumbar intumescence/coccygeal)
- Disc herniation (with or without paraparesis)
- Tumor of the spine/spinal canal/cord

Cardiac/vascular:

- Feline thromboembolic disease
- Vascular compromise secondary to trauma (arterial avulsion or thrombosis)
- Fibrocartilaginous embolism

DIAGNOSIS

Diagnostic Overview

Tail paralysis is apparent on physical exam. A complete neurologic exam helps identify the extent of the causative lesion, which contributes to determining the prognosis and whether or not treatment is likely to require tail amputation.

Differential Diagnosis

- Anomalous (spina bifida, hemivertebra, sacrocaudal dysgenesis, dermoid sinus)
- Degenerative lumbosacral stenosis (stenosis of vertebral canal, type II disc at L7-S1 space, sacral osteochondrosis, instability and misalignment of L7-S1, articular facet arthritis)
- Intervertebral disc disease (type I or type II)
- Spinal trauma/fracture/avulsion
- Vascular (feline thromboembolism, fibrocartilaginous embolism)
- Neoplasia
- Discospondylitis
- Limber tail/cold tail syndrome or acute caudal myopathy

Initial Database

- Rectal exam to document pain, swelling, instability, mass effect
- Complete neurologic exam to localize the lesion (p. 1136)
- Radiographs of the spine, including sacrocaudal region (malformations, fracture/trauma/avulsion, discospondylitis, osteolytic/osteoproliferative tumor, intervertebral disc disease)
- CBC, serum biochemistry panel, urinalysis depending systemic involvement
- Thoracic radiographs
  - To assess for lesions secondary to trauma
  - To assess for metastases if neoplasia is suspected
- Ultrasound
  - Thoracic (for feline cardiomyopathy)
  - Abdominal (suspected pelvic canal tumor or aortic thromboembolus)

Advanced or Confirmatory Testing

- Advanced imaging modalities: myelography, CT, MRI (p. 1132) may be indicated for assessing underlying spinal abnormalities
- Electromyography (rare instances of neuromuscular disease, also reported in limber tail syndrome)
- Fine-needle aspiration if possible for cytologic evaluation (masses, discospondylitis)
- Ultrasound-guided biopsy (masses)

TREATMENT

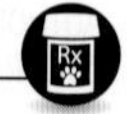

Treatment Overview

Musculoskeletal or neurologic:

- Treatment to address underlying cause
- Medical management of fractures, using pain management, bandages for immobilization
- For limber tail syndrome, the use of antiinflammatories might improve the symptoms.
- Amputate tail if vascular compromise
  - Leave 3-4 coccygeal vertebrae if well vascularized
  - Amputate to the level of healthy skin margins if tail is devascularized

Cardiovascular/thromboembolic disease:

- Tail amputation if tail is soiled by urine and/or feces or if tail has not revascularized well
- Address underlying cardiac disease.

Neoplasia:

- Wide surgical excision if possible
- Radiation therapy or chemotherapy if indicated and if possible

Skin wound of the tail (p. 909):

- With vascular compromise, amputate tail at appropriate level.
- Without vascular compromise, treat by local debridement (wet-to-dry bandaging or surgical debridement).
- Use second-intention healing (bandages with hydrogel).
- If wound closure impossible by second-intention healing, use secondary closure (local skin flaps, free skin grafts).

Acute General Treatment

- If identified, treat shock, concurrent trauma, or cardiac disease
- Consider corticosteroids if tail paralysis is secondary to spinal cord/nerve compression (controversial [p. 555]).
- After patient is stable, treatment depends on underlying cause.

Chronic Treatment

- Hygiene
- Bladder catheterization if necessary
- Physical therapy for paraparetic patients

Possible Complications

- Depends on therapeutic options
- Beware of corticosteroid administration: associated with gastrointestinal ulceration, colonic perforation

Recommended Monitoring

Depends on primary cause and therapeutic options

PROGNOSIS & OUTCOME

- Trauma
  - Intact deep pain perception and normal vascularization: guarded. Generally, these patients regain enough motor activity to maintain hygiene.
  - Absence of deep pain for more than 48 hours: poor prognosis for return of motor activity but good if tail amputated and normal voluntary hindlimb activity and bladder control
- Limber tail syndrome: condition is self-limited and resolves in 7-21 days (anecdotal). Recurrence is possible.
- Guarded to poor if feline thromboembolic disease (recurrence risk, heart failure)

PEARLS & CONSIDERATIONS

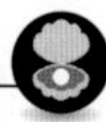

Comments

- The most common causes of tail paralysis are trauma and degenerative lumbosacral stenosis; prognosis depends on deep pain perception and vascular supply.
- In dogs and cats, the tail is not essential to life; tail amputation in patients with normal limb function and bladder control provides excellent quality of life.
- Beware: pain originating from the pelvic canal (e.g., prostatic abscess, degenerative lumbosacral stenosis) can mimic tail paralysis.

Technician Tip

Hygiene and topical care to prevent urine/fecal contact dermatitis is a key to chronic care: bathing, keeping area dry and clean, clipping perianal/perineal region, and protective ointment if necessary.

SUGGESTED READING

de Lahunta A, et al: Veterinary neuroanatomy and clinical neurology, ed 3, St. Louis, 2009, Saunders.

AUTHOR: Bertrand Lussier, DMV, MSc, DACVS
EDITOR: Leah A. Cohn, DVM, PhD, DACVIM

Tarsal Trauma

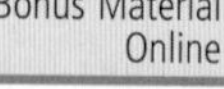
Bonus Material Online
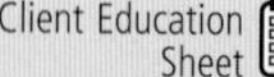
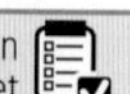
Client Education Sheet

BASIC INFORMATION

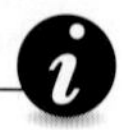

Definition

Tarsal trauma includes ligament damage, luxation/subluxation of individual tarsal bones, fractures, shearing injuries

Synonym

Tarsal breakdown

Epidemiology

GENETICS, BREED PREDISPOSITION

- Racing greyhounds: central tarsal bone fractures
- Border collies: central tarsal bone fracture/luxation
- Shelties and collies: superficial digital flexor tendon luxation
- Cats: tibiotarsal luxation with lateral malleolar fracture

RISK FACTORS

Racing/agility activities; hindlimb trauma

Clinical Presentation

DISEASE FORMS/SUBTYPES

Sprains, fractures, shearing/degloving wounds, coaptation-related injuries

HISTORY, CHIEF COMPLAINT

Hindlimb trauma; lameness after competition/exercise

PHYSICAL EXAM FINDINGS

- Lameness
- Swelling
- Open wounds
- Pain/crepitation
- Instability with plantigrade stance
- Mediolateral/rotational instability
- Tarsal deformity

Etiology and Pathophysiology

- Racing on counterclockwise tracks predisposes to right-sided injuries.
- In racing greyhounds, there is a classic triad of fractures involving the central tarsal bone, calcaneus, and the fifth proximal metatarsal bone.
- In border collies, cause of central tarsal bone subluxation/fracture is unknown.

DIAGNOSIS

Diagnostic Overview

Most injuries are diagnosed by physical/radiographic examinations.

Differential Diagnosis

- Autoimmune polyarthropathy (systemic lupus erythematosus, rheumatoid arthritis)

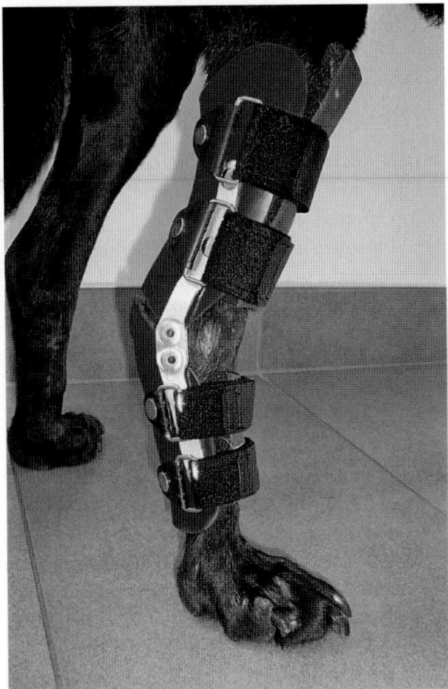

TARSAL TRAUMA A hinged orthosis is used by this 6-year-old Labrador retriever only when running/playing with other dogs because of mild persistent instability after short and long collateral ligaments prosthetic reconstruction.

- Infectious (e.g., Lyme borreliosis, rickettsial disease) polyarthropathy
- Achilles mechanism disruption

Initial Database

- Careful palpation/evaluation of mediolateral instability with tarsus in extension (long collaterals) and tarsocrural internal/external rotation instability with tarsus in flexion (short collaterals) (p. 1143)
- Orthogonal radiographs
- CBC, serum biochemistry panel, and urinalysis to assess anesthetic risk; the American Society of Anesthesiologists Classification is provided on p. 1196.

Advanced or Confirmatory Testing

- Oblique radiography and/or CT (nondisplaced fractures)
- Stress radiography (mediolateral radiograph with tarsus manually forced into dorsal and plantar extension and a dorsoplantar radiograph with mediolateral stress) to identify location of instability

TREATMENT

Treatment Overview

The goal of therapy is anatomic/functional restoration of tarsal functions:

- Fractures: anatomic reduction/stabilization
- Ligamentous injuries: reestablishment of joint support by repairing collateral ligaments or arthrodesis/ankylosis
- Shearing injuries: wound management, surgical stabilization if needed

Acute General Treatment

- Minimally displaced, nonarticular fractures and ligament sprains with no or minimal instability can be stabilized for 4-8 weeks with an external splint.
- Luxated joints, intraarticular fractures, and high-grade sprains are supported in a modified Robert Jones bandage or splint until surgery (p. 1161).
    - Short/long collateral ligament disruption requires stabilization with tension band principle (malleolar fractures) or replacement with prosthetic suture.
    - Individual tarsal bone fractures require lag screw fixation, except for lesions of the calcaneus, which require bone plate or tension band repair.
    - Plantar and mediolateral intertarsal and tarsometatarsal subluxations are unstable and require partial tarsal arthrodesis.
    - Dorsal intertarsal and tarsometatarsal subluxations are stable (compressed) when bearing weight. Surgical repair is needed only if lameness persists.
- Superficial digital flexor tendon luxation is treated by suturing torn retinacular tissues.
- Shearing injuries require wound management.
    - Lavage open wounds using warm saline, lactated Ringer's, or dilute chlorhexidine solutions.
    - Tissue coverage with moistened gauze sponges is useful in debridement (wet-to-dry bandages); change daily.
    - Alternatively, direct application of sugar or honey has been used for reducing infection and promoting healing, although the role of such treatment in the joint is unclear.
    - Final surgical debridement/lavage can be performed during orthopedic stabilization surgery.
    - Wounds with healthy granulation tissue and early epithelialization can be sutured or covered with nonadherent dressings and allowed to heal by second intention.
- Pantarsal arthrodesis should be considered for shearing injuries with severe/critical loss of bone/cartilage and for some comminuted fractures.

Chronic Treatment

Surgical repairs require 4-12 weeks of external coaptation and exercise restriction.

Possible Complications

- Reduction/implant failure
- Delayed/failed arthrodesis
- Vascular injury
- Wound infection
- Coaptation-related morbidity
- Degenerative joint disease

Recommended Monitoring

- Lameness evaluation 1-3 months after injury/treatment
- Serial radiographs to evaluate fracture healing/arthrodesis progression

PROGNOSIS & OUTCOME

- Good to excellent for noncompeting dogs; variable for return to preinjury status for competing dogs
- Residual/recurrent instability at some point throughout range of motion is not uncommon in collateral ligament reconstruction; synthetic ligaments are anchored from point A to point B, which differs from the multiple attachment sites of a normal ligament.
- In noncompeting animals, solitary intertarsal joint fusion/ankylosis (i.e., calcaneotarsal, calcaneoquartal, quartalmetatarsal) can lead to near-normal function.
- Despite extensive damage in shearing injuries, acceptable function is possible with various reconstructive efforts. Cases with neurovascular compromise may necessitate amputation.

PEARLS & CONSIDERATIONS

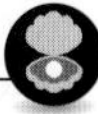

Comments

- When conservatively managed, intraarticular fractures rarely heal with osseous bridging, leading to degenerative joint disease. Surgical treatment is recommended to reduce the risk of such adverse consequences.
- Patients with mild, persistent instability after collateral ligament reconstruction can be normal while walking but lame during more intense activities; a custom-made, hinged thermoplastic orthosis can be very useful to stabilize the tarsus when needed.

Technician Tips

- When tarsal trauma confirmed, prepare for modified Robert-Jones bandaging with or without splinting.
- Prepare for wound irrigation and management, if applicable.

SUGGESTED READING

DeCamp CE, et al: Fractures and other orthopedic injuries of the tarsus, metatarsus, and phalanges. In Permattei DL, et al, editors: Brinker, Piermattei, and Flo's Handbook of small animal orthopedics and fracture repair, ed 5, St. Louis, 2016, Elsevier, pp 707-752.

AUTHOR: Louis Huneault, DMV, MSc, DACVS
EDITOR: Kathleen Linn, DVM, MS, DACVS

Taurine Deficiency

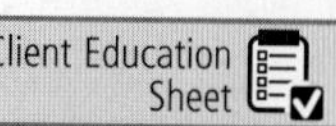

BASIC INFORMATION

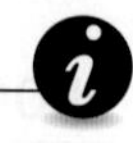

Definition

Deficient blood taurine concentrations result from inadequate intake, synthesis, or availability of dietary taurine and can cause clinical disease.

Epidemiology

SPECIES, AGE, SEX

- Cats: taurine is an essential amino acid in the diet of cats because they lack the ability to synthesize adequate amounts from the precursor amino acids cysteine and methionine.
- Dogs: taurine is not an essential amino acid in dogs as they can normally synthesize taurine from precursor amino acids. However, taurine can become a conditionally essential amino acid in some dogs and under some conditions.

GENETICS, BREED PREDISPOSITION

In dogs, taurine-deficient dilated cardiomyopathy (DCM) has been identified in a variety of breeds, including American cocker spaniels, golden retrievers, Newfoundlands, and dogs with cystine and urate urolithiasis consuming protein-restricted diets.

RISK FACTORS

- Cats: inadequately supplemented commercial or home-prepared diets
- Dogs: low-protein diets; vegetarian diets (plant protein sources are devoid of taurine); lamb meal and rice diets; grain-free diets with legumes such as chickpeas, peas, and lentils; and diets supplemented with beet pulp, presumably due to inadequate or unavailable dietary sulfur amino acids. Large breeds and dogs with lower than predicted energy requirements may be at higher risk.

Clinical Presentation

DISEASE FORMS/SUBTYPES

- Cats: central retinal degeneration (CRD), reproductive failure, growth retardation, and DCM
- Dogs: DCM in susceptible breeds or individuals

HISTORY, CHIEF COMPLAINT

- Cats: blindness, signs of congestive heart failure (CHF) such as dyspnea, respiratory distress, lethargy, and anorexia (pp. 408 and 409), or reproductive failure. Compatible diet history (poorly formulated commercial or home-prepared diet) is suggestive.
- Dogs: signs of CHF; possible history of restricted diet (very-low-protein diets; vegetarian diets; dry dog food with lamb meal, rice, or both as the primary ingredient; grain-free and boutique diets)

PHYSICAL EXAM FINDINGS

- Cats and dogs: if in CHF, variable combinations of tachypnea, dyspnea, tachycardia, systolic murmur, gallop sound, lethargy, dehydration, and hypothermia
- Cats only: initially, increased granularity in the area centralis, which progresses to hyperreflectivity that can eventually extend across to the nasal retina and finally result in diffuse retinal atrophy

Etiology and Pathophysiology

- Taurine is a sulfur-containing amino acid. Unlike most other amino acids, it is not incorporated into proteins but rather remains one of the most abundant free amino acids in the body.
- Taurine, synthesized from methionine and cysteine, is required for a variety of cellular homeostatic functions. In cats, synthesis is very limited and cannot maintain taurine balance in the absence of adequate intake. Dogs have a greater ability to synthesize taurine than do cats, but occasionally, they develop taurine deficiency. Obligatory loss occurs in both species because only taurine can be used for conjugation of bile acids; most other species can substitute glycine for taurine.
- In cats and likely in dogs, excessive taurine-conjugated bile salt loss in feces may occur secondary to type of diet processing, protein source, fiber type and concentration, changes in location and/or numbers of intestinal microflora, and/or increased secretion of bile salts due to changes in the release of cholecystokinin.

DIAGNOSIS

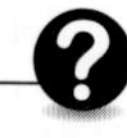

Diagnostic Overview

Taurine deficiency should be considered with a compatible diet history and signs of cardiac dysfunction (DCM in dogs, cats) or blindness or reproductive failure (cats).

Differential Diagnosis

- Idiopathic DCM
- Other causes of myocardial failure
- Retinal detachment or degeneration (cats)

Initial Database

- Thoracic radiography to determine presence of CHF
- Fundic exam (cats [p. 1137])

Advanced or Confirmatory Testing

- Echocardiography for diagnosis of DCM: dyskinesis (reduced systolic motion) of the left ventricular walls, increased end-diastolic diameter, and reduced shortening fraction.
- Assessment of both plasma and whole blood taurine concentrations (lithium heparin [green top] tubes [p. 1384]) provides the most accurate estimate of taurine status provided samples are collected and processed properly. Since plasma taurine concentrations may decrease with prolonged fasting (2-3+ days), low values in such patients should be interpreted with caution.
  - Plasma: immediately centrifuge blood, separate plasma from cells, and immediately freeze plasma. Avoid contaminating plasma with cells from buffy coat. If sample is hemolyzed, draw new sample.
  - Whole blood: freeze whole blood sample immediately in appropriate plastic tube (to lyse red blood cells).
  - Plasma and whole blood taurine reference ranges (reference intervals may vary, depending on the laboratory)
- Dogs: plasma: normal = 60-120 nmol/mL; deficient: < 40 nmol/mL; whole blood: normal = 200-350 nmol/mL; deficient: < 150 nmol/mL
- Cats: plasma: normal = 60-120 nmol/mL; deficient: < 40 nmol/mL; whole blood: normal = 300-600 nmol/mL; deficient: < 200 nmol/mL

TREATMENT

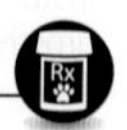

Treatment Overview

The goals of treatment are to restore taurine homeostasis and improve cardiac function. DCM due to taurine deficiency may be reversible in some patients.

Acute General Treatment

- Supportive care for CHF and DCM (pp. 263 and 409)
- Taurine supplementation while waiting confirmation of blood analysis

Chronic Treatment

- Ongoing treatment as needed for CHF
- Cats: taurine supplementation with 250-500 mg/CAT PO q 12h
- Dogs: taurine supplementation with 500-1000 mg/DOG PO q 8-12h for dogs < 25 kg or 1-2 g/DOG PO q 8-12h for dogs > 25 kg
  - Concurrent carnitine supplementation 50-100 mg/kg PO q 8h is recommended for American cocker spaniels and dogs consuming protein-restricted diets.
- Echocardiogenic improvement in cardiac function can take 3-4 months. Do not stop supplementation prematurely.

Nutrition/Diet

Ensure a nutritionally balanced diet with adequate sulfur amino acid content.

Possible Complications

Taurine is an extremely safe substance, even when given at pharmacologic doses.

Recommended Monitoring

- Clinical condition, including daily resting respiratory rate to predict CHF (until resolution of DCM)

- Plasma and whole blood taurine levels should be re-evaluated in 1-2 months.
- Radiography, echocardiography as needed to monitor resolution of heart disease

PROGNOSIS & OUTCOME

- Clinical improvement (improved energy, appetite) is often noted after a few weeks of supplementation before echocardiographic improvement.
- Early treatment can be curative, but chronic disease may allow for extensive, permanent change in the myocardium.
- Blindness is irreversible.

PEARLS & CONSIDERATIONS

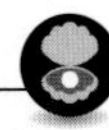

Comments

- Echocardiographic improvement may require 3-4 months of supplementation.
- A recently identified association between grain-free diets and dilated cardiomyopathy has not been confirmed to be entirely due to taurine deficiency.

Prevention

Feeding a properly formulated diet

Technician Tips

A diet history should be collected for every patient at every visit. Risk factors for many potential problems may be identified and corrected before clinically significant disease develops.

Client Education

Explain the importance of feeding pets a properly formulated diet.

SUGGESTED READING

Sanderson SL: Taurine and carnitine in canine cardiomyopathy. Vet Clin North Am Small Anim Pract 36:1325-1343, 2006.

AUTHOR: Sherry Lynn Sanderson, DVM, PhD, DACVIM, DACVN
EDITOR: Jennifer Larsen, DVM, PhD, DACVN

Tenesmus

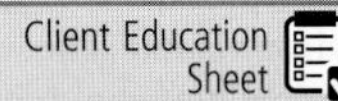

BASIC INFORMATION

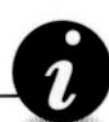

Definition

Ineffectual or painful straining to eliminate wastes; generally applies to straining to defecate, most often due to obstruction or inflammatory lesions of distal colon, rectum, or anus

Epidemiology

SPECIES, AGE, SEX

Dogs and cats, any age, either sex

ASSOCIATED DISORDERS

- Rectal prolapse (greater incidence in puppies, kittens)
- Megacolon (if chronic constipation/obstipation)

Clinical Presentation

HISTORY, CHIEF COMPLAINT

- Frequent posturing to defecate/urinate without producing feces/urine
- Excessive licking/chewing of perineal region
- Vocalizing when posturing (cats > dogs)
- Inappropriate defecation or refusal to defecate (severe pain/constipation)
- Common error in cats is overassumption of constipation, whereas careful history/observation might reveal lower urinary tract signs (i.e., stranguria [p. 802]).

PHYSICAL EXAM FINDINGS

- Examine anus/perianal area: erythema of anal/perineal region, porphyrin-stained fur, altered skin pigmentation (suggesting excessive licking/chewing), perineal fistulas/masses, pseudocoprostasis (anal obstruction due to severe matting of fur with feces)
- Abdominal palpation: mass, signs of discomfort, organomegaly, stool in colon
- Rectal palpation (with sedation/general anesthesia if painful)
    - Rule out perineal hernia, mass, prostatomegaly, pelvic fractures, stricture, foreign body
    - Assess fecal consistency
    - Palpate urethra ventrally: assess size/shape/texture/presence of mass, urethrolith, or stricture
    - Palpate anal sacs (mass/impaction/infection/abscess/rupture). Express anal sacs if full and re-palpate for presence of a mass.
- Examine bladder size and vulva/vagina or prepuce/penis to identify genitourinary causes of straining (misinterpreted as straining to defecate).

Etiology and Pathophysiology

- Colonic, rectal, or anal inflammation triggers an afferent impulse in parasympathetic pathways through the pelvic nerve, sacral spinal cord, and cerebral cortex.
- The resultant efferent signal is carried by parasympathetic efferent nerve fibers in the pudendal nerve, leading to stimulation of the colon, rectum, anus, and pelvic muscles.
- Intraabdominal pressure is increased by posturing, contraction of the diaphragm and abdominal muscles, and closing of the glottis.

DIAGNOSIS

Diagnostic Overview

- Tenesmus is a clinical sign, not a disease; successful management requires identification of the underlying cause.
- Diagnostic test selection is highly dependent on obtaining a clear history, observing the animal urinating and defecating, and performing a thorough exam (rectum, perineal, and perianal areas). Some diagnoses (e.g., perianal fistulas) may not require additional testing.

Differential Diagnosis

- Genitourinary tract disorders, especially in cats, may mimic straining to defecate.
- Causes of tenesmus are detailed on p. 1285.
    - Rectal disease (e.g., colitis, constipation, other obstruction)
    - Anal, perianal, perineal disorders (e.g., proctitis, perianal fistula, anal stricture, anal sac disorders)
    - Pelvic disorders (e.g., mass, misaligned healed fracture)
    - Lumbosacral disease
    - Prostatomegaly

Initial Database

- Observe the animal defecating/urinating
    - Position of tail: low carriage/resentment of tail elevation suggests sacrocaudal discomfort.
    - Posture: arched back suggests abdominal, back, or joint pain.
    - Presence/absence of gross fecal abnormalities (e.g., diarrhea, hematochezia)
- Neurologic exam (p. 1136): perineal reflex, anal/perineal tone, lumbosacral/back pain
- CBC, serum biochemical profile, urinalysis, fecal flotation: elucidate possible urinary or systemic abnormalities, or parasites
- Radiographs (abdominal/pelvic): distended colon, pelvic narrowing, sublumbar lymphadenomegaly, mass effect, enlarged prostate

Advanced or Confirmatory Testing

- Abdominal ultrasonography: gastrointestinal (GI)/pelvic mass ± lymphadenopathy, urogenital tract, GI motility, distention/wall thickening
- Colonoscopy: rigid and/or flexible to identify and biopsy polyps, masses, strictures, or infiltrative lesions; facilitate biopsy
- Intrarectal ultrasonography: specific probes required

TREATMENT

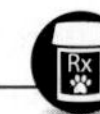

Treatment Overview

The goals of treatment are to address the underlying cause and relieve patient discomfort.

Acute and Chronic Treatment

Depends on cause of tenesmus:

- Systemic medications (e.g., colitis, perianal fistulas)
- Topical treatment (e.g., proctitis, pseudocoprostasis)
- Fluid resuscitation and enemas (e.g., constipation/obstipation)
- Surgical treatment (e.g., certain anal sac disorders; pelvic, rectal, or anal mass lesions)
- Stool softener may be appropriate (e.g., MiraLax, lactulose)

Nutrition/Diet

- ± High-soluble fiber diet
- ± Hypoallergenic diet if inflammatory bowel disease/food sensitivity suspected

Behavior/Exercise

Modification to address stressors (e.g., environmental/schedule change, renovations, multipet household) if contributing to inability or unwillingness to defecate

Possible Complications

- Recurrent tenesmus, colonic/rectal obstruction causing obstipation, perineal hernia, or rectal prolapse (uncommon; usually patients < 6 months old)
- Megacolon due to chronic obstipation
- Surgery: risk of postoperative fecal incontinence

PROGNOSIS & OUTCOME

- Colonic/rectal inflammatory lesions: medical therapy often successful
- Anal sac disease/perineal hernias/wounds in and surrounding anorectal area: better prognosis than strictures/malignant neoplasia
- Perianal fistulas: improved prognosis with cyclosporine but costly. Topical tacrolimus is less expensive but may be less effective (p. 771).

PEARLS & CONSIDERATIONS

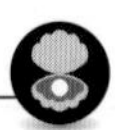

Comments

- Stranguria is a common impostor for tenesmus, especially in cats.
- Tenesmus is a clinical sign, not a disease; an underlying cause must be sought.

Technician Tips

- Technicians should be able to differentiate tenesmus from stranguria when communicating with the owner; may be lifesaving.
- Triage of patient: assess urinary bladder size (ensure urethra is not obstructed).

SUGGESTED READING

Jergens AE: Dyschezia and tenesmus. In Washabau RJ, et al, editors: Canine and feline gastroenterology, St. Louis, 2013, Saunders, pp 109-113.

AUTHOR: Lisa Carioto, DVM, DVSc, DACVIM
EDITOR: Leah A. Cohn, DVM, PhD, DACVIM

Testicular Tumors

Bonus Material Online 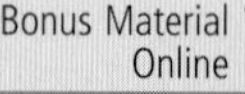 Client Education Sheet 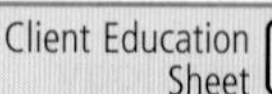

BASIC INFORMATION

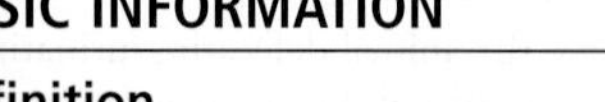

Definition

Neoplasia arising from testicular germ cells or sex cord–stromal cells; common in dogs, uncommon in cats

Synonyms

- Germ cell tumor: seminoma
- Mixed tumors: germ cell/stromal tumors
- Sex cord–stromal tumor: Leydig (interstitial) cell tumor, Sertoli (sustentacular) cell tumor

Epidemiology

SPECIES, AGE, SEX

Dogs:

- Incidence: common (75% of all tumors affecting the male urogenital tract)
- Age: aged patients, most > 7 years
- Equal incidence of seminoma, Leydig cell tumor; Sertoli cell tumor much less common

Cats: all tumor types are rare.

GENETICS, BREED PREDISPOSITION

- All tumors: Shetland sheepdogs and collie (fivefold higher prevalence), Maltese dogs overrepresented
- Seminoma: boxer and Norwegian elkhound are predisposed.
- Sertoli cell: miniature schnauzers with persistent müllerian duct syndrome, Shetland sheepdogs, and collies are predisposed.

RISK FACTORS

Dogs, cryptorchidism:

- Overall risk of testicular tumor development increased 13-14 times
- Risk of Sertoli cell tumor increased 20 times
- Approximately one-half of Sertoli cell tumors occur in cryptorchid testes.
- Approximately one-third of seminomas occur in cryptorchid testes.

Cats: none identified

ASSOCIATED DISORDERS

Sertoli cell tumor: hyperestrogenism occurs in approximately 20%-30% of affected dogs. Pancytopenia also can occur.

Clinical Presentation

DISEASE FORMS/SUBTYPES

- Primary: unilateral or bilateral, focal or multifocal
- Metastatic (rare)

HISTORY, CHIEF COMPLAINT

- Testicular enlargement ± atrophy of unaffected testis (most severe associated with Sertoli cell tumor but can occur with other neoplasms, especially larger tumors)
- Sertoli cell tumor: symmetrical hair loss, feminization (gynecomastia, attractiveness to other male dogs, pendulous penile sheath, lethargy, loss of libido, redistribution of body fat). Occasionally, complaints related to anemia, thrombocytopenia, or leukopenia

PHYSICAL EXAM FINDINGS

Testicular enlargement ± atrophy of contralateral testis; if cryptorchid, intraabdominal mass may be palpable

- Seminoma: soft to slightly firm texture
- Sertoli cell tumor: very firm texture, discrete mass
- Leydig cell tumor: soft texture, discrete mass
- Mixed germ cell/stromal tumors: various textures, generally discrete and focal
- Sertoli cell with hyperestrogenism: endocrine dermatopathy, gynecomastia, pendulous penile sheath, redistribution of body fat, marked contralateral testicular atrophy

Etiology and Pathophysiology

Cryptorchidism: altered testicular environment due to increased testicular temperature favors neoplastic transformation of Sertoli cells and (less commonly) germ cells.

DIAGNOSIS

Diagnostic Overview

Diagnosis relies on palpation of an enlarged testis or an abnormal firm area in a normal-sized testis. Ultrasound and cytologic evaluation may aid in diagnosis, but in most cases, excision of the affected testis and submission for histopathologic evaluation confirms neoplasia and allows classification of the tumor.

Differential Diagnosis

- Testicular torsion
- Abscess
- Cyst

Initial Database

- CBC: rule out bone marrow suppression due to Sertoli cell tumor–associated hyperestrogenism.
- Semen evaluation and/or testicular biopsy with histologic exam of unaffected testis can aid in decision for unilateral or bilateral castration in breeding dogs.

Advanced or Confirmatory Testing

- Ultrasound, all tumor types: hypoechoic or mixed echotexture
- Cytologic evaluation of abnormal testis
- Gross pathologic exam of excised testis
  - Seminoma signs include soft to slightly firm testis; homogeneous, gray/white, glistening appearance; possible areas of discoloration due to hemorrhage or necrosis; focal to multifocal
  - Sertoli cell tumor signs include very firm testis that are discrete, white or gray, with possible tan or yellow hemorrhagic areas; usually focal
  - Leydig cell tumor signs include soft testis that are discrete and yellow/brown, bulges on section, areas of hemorrhage or cystic change common, focal to multifocal
  - Mixed germ cell/stromal tumor signs include various textures and pale white or gray appearance; generally discrete and focal
- Bilateral tumors are common, and multiple tumor types often occur in the same testis.
- Histopathologic exam: include spermatic cord to evaluate for local invasion; multiple tumor types can occur in the same testis.

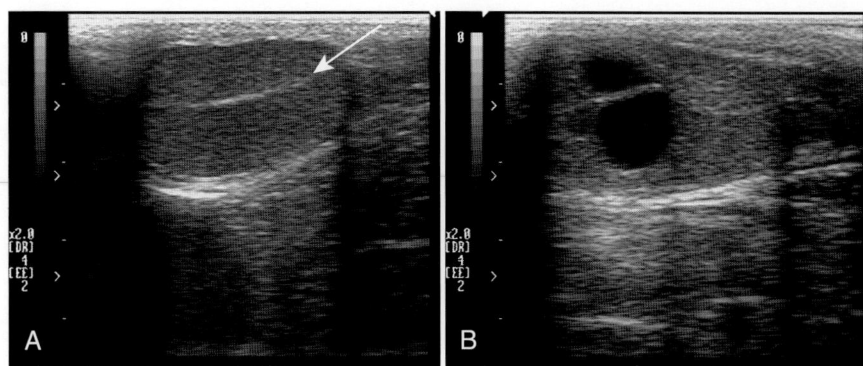

TESTICULAR TUMORS A, Transscrotal ultrasonogram of left testis of a normal fertile male dog. Echotexture of the parenchyma is homogeneous, with the exception of the hyperechoic mediastinum (rete testis; *arrow*). **B,** Transscrotal ultrasonogram of left testis of an infertile male dog. Two anechoic cystic structures are seen within the parenchyma on either side of the mediastinum. Differential diagnoses include cystic neoplasia or testicular cyst. (Courtesy Dr. Michelle A. Kutzler.)

TREATMENT

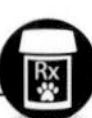

Treatment Overview

Therapy consists of surgical removal of the affected testis.

Acute General Treatment

- Testicular removal: castration; unilateral castration if contralateral testis is normal to small and future breeding with the dog is desired
- Supportive care for dogs with Sertoli cell tumor–associated bone marrow suppression

Chronic Treatment

For metastatic seminoma, both chemotherapy and radiation therapy have been described. Methotrexate, vincristine, and cyclophosphamide; cisplatin; bleomycin; and radiation therapy have been reported to have some degree of efficacy.

Behavior/Exercise

Avoid estrous females, and restrict physical activity for approximately 1 week after surgery.

Possible Complications

- Bone marrow suppression (hyperestrogenism) from Sertoli cell tumors
- Behavioral changes (hyperandrogenism) from Leydig cell tumors

Recommended Monitoring

- Seminoma, Leydig cell tumor, nonactive Sertoli cell tumor, mixed sex cord–stromal tumor: yearly physical exam
- Sertoli cell tumor with bone marrow suppression: close follow-up resolution of anemia, thrombocytopenia, and leukopenia; yearly physical exam after marrow recovery

PROGNOSIS & OUTCOME

- Seminoma: excellent after testicular removal; metastasis is rare.
- Sertoli cell tumor: excellent after testicular removal; metastasis is rare, but risk of metastasis is increased for tumors > 2 cm diameter.
- Leydig cell tumor: excellent after testicular removal; metastasis is not expected.
- Mixed sex cord–stromal tumor: excellent after testicular removal; metastasis is not expected.

PEARLS & CONSIDERATIONS

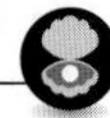

Comments

- Histopathologic exam is needed for determination of tumor type.
- Unilateral castration may result in up to 50% compensatory hypertrophy of the remaining testis. Return to fertility after unilateral castration depends on the severity of testicular atrophy secondary to hormonal downregulation and presence of underlying disease (testicular degeneration with loss of spermatogonia).

Prevention

Testicular removal, especially of cryptorchid testes

Technician Tips

- Make a longitudinal incision into testes greater than 2.5 cm in diameter to aid in fixation for histopathology submission.
- When fixing, use an adequate amount of formalin (1 part tissue to 9 parts formalin).

Client Education

- Regular exam of testes and evaluation of the semen in breeding animals
- Prompt presentation for veterinary exam if an abnormality is detected

SUGGESTED READING

Agnew DW, et al: Tumors of the genital systems. In Meuten DJ, editor: Tumors in domestic animals, ed 5, Ames, IA, 2017, Wiley Blackwell, pp 706-714.

AUTHOR: Beth A. Valentine, DVM, PhD, DACVP
EDITOR: Michelle A. Kutzler, DVM, PhD, DACT

Tetanus

Bonus Material Online  Client Education Sheet 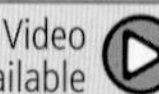 Video Available

BASIC INFORMATION 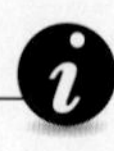

Definition

Tetanus is an infectious disease caused by a potent neurotoxin produced by the bacterium *Clostridium tetani,* resulting in a sustained tonic contraction of the muscles.

Synonym

Lockjaw

Epidemiology

SPECIES, AGE, SEX

All domestic animals are susceptible; cats are more resistant than dogs.

RISK FACTORS

Open wounds; exposure to organism in feces or in the environment

GEOGRAPHY AND SEASONALITY

Ubiquitous in the environment; no seasonality

Clinical Presentation

DISEASE FORMS/SUBTYPES

Focal versus generalized depends on inoculation site; the generalized form is more common.

HISTORY, CHIEF COMPLAINT

- Cutaneous/soft-tissue wound: cut, puncture, surgical (e.g., ovariohysterectomy)
- Progressively worsening gait stiffness

PHYSICAL EXAM FINDINGS

- Extreme sensitivity to tactile and auditory stimulation: mildly to extremely exaggerated reaction to sound or touch
- Characteristic facial expression due to facial muscle spasm: ears held erect, forehead wrinkled, lips drawn back (risus sardonicus)
- Trismus (teeth clenching)
- Protrusion of third eyelids, enophthalmos, strabismus, hypersalivation, laryngeal spasm, dysphagia
- Mild hyperthermia due to excessive muscular activity
- Dyspnea, coughing possible from aspiration pneumonia
- Progression to periodic generalized tonic muscle contraction possible
- Autonomic storms: cardiac arrhythmias, hypotension or hypertension
- Death can result from respiratory compromise.

Etiology and Pathophysiology

- *C. tetani* typically enters the body through wounds.
- A potent neurotoxin (tetanospasmin) is formed in the patient's body during vegetative growth of *C. tetani.*
- Tetanospasmin enters the neuromuscular endplate of motor nerves and migrates to the neuronal cell body in the spinal cord or brainstem.
- Tetanospasmin blocks inhibitory neurotransmitter release (glycine, gamma-aminobutyric acid [GABA]), facilitating muscle contraction.
- Tetanospasmin's binding to presynaptic sites of inhibitory neurons is irreversible; recovery depends on sprouting of new axon terminals.
- Signs occur within 5-10 days of injury but can be delayed up to 3 weeks.
- Wounds close to the head are associated with a more rapid onset of signs than those in the extremities.

DIAGNOSIS

Diagnostic Overview

Tetanus is diagnosed based on clinical signs and history of a recent wound; there is no practical clinical confirmatory test. The source of infection or wounds is not always immediately apparent.

Differential Diagnosis

Hypocalcemic tetany

Initial Database

The following test results can be seen, but none is required for a diagnosis of tetanus:

- CBC: leukocytosis (neutrophilia with left shift)
- Serum biochemistry profile: elevated serum creatine phosphokinase (CPK)
- Cerebrospinal fluid (CSF) analysis: unremarkable
- Electrocardiogram (ECG): tachyarrhythmias or bradyarrhythmias (atrioventricular [AV] block, sinus arrest) possible
- Thoracic and abdominal imaging: megaesophagus with or without aspiration pneumonia possible; abdominal effusion possible if source of *C. tetani* is septic peritonitis (metritis, enteritis, ruptured abscess)
- Muscle biopsy: usually unremarkable
- Serum antibody titers to tetanus toxin may support the diagnosis (compared with control animals).
- Attempts at isolation of *C. tetani* from wounds are unrewarding.

Advanced or Confirmatory Testing

No specific confirmatory test

TREATMENT 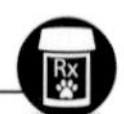

Treatment Overview

Treatment is mostly supportive and can be protracted: resolution of clinical signs can take days to weeks, depending on form (generalized or localized) and individual response (see *Video*).

Acute General Treatment

- As much as possible, keep the animal in a quiet, soundproof area with minimal stimulation.
- Wound debridement and resection of necrotic tissue; wounds are left open (avoid anaerobic conditions).
- Antitoxin: equine antitetanus serum (ATS) is given IM or IV or human tetanus immunoglobulin (TIG) given IM. Equine ATS:
  - Give the initial test dose 0.1-0.2 mL SQ or ID 15-30 minutes before IV administration; monitor for anaphylaxis.
  - If no anaphylaxis, therapeutic dose is 2.5-25 IU/kg IV; continue to monitor

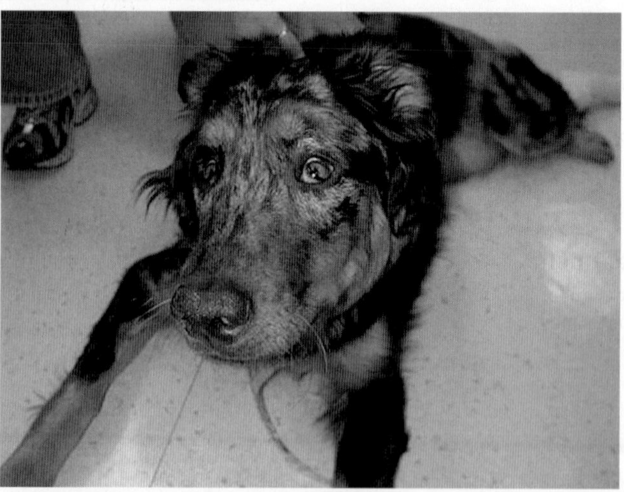

TETANUS Dog with tetanus secondary to ovariohysterectomy. Note the highly characteristic facial expression with pinnae drawn far toward the dorsal midline, upper eyelids drawn dorsomedially giving an anxious appearance, and canthi of lips drawn caudally, producing the sardonic grin.

for anaphylaxis during and immediately after administration.
  - Intralesional injection appears promising (experimental studies).
  - Antitoxin prevents further toxin binding to axons but does not eliminate currently bound toxin.
- Sedation with one of the following is recommended: diazepam (helps enhance GABA inhibition), acepromazine, phenobarbital, or chlorpromazine
- Muscle relaxation: methocarbamol, diazepam, or midazolam
- Pain control: cautious use of opioids (see Drug Interactions)
- Antibacterial treatment *(C. tetani):* sodium or potassium penicillin 20,000-50,000 IU/kg slow IV q 6h for 10 days and metronidazole 10 mg/kg PO or IV q 8h for 10 days

Chronic Treatment

- Physical rehabilitation
- Intensive nursing care to include IV fluids and nasogastric, esophageal, or percutaneous endoscopic gastrostomy (PEG) tube feedings (pp. 1106, 1107, and 1109)
- Prevention of decubital ulcers
- Indwelling urinary catheter (p. 1182)

Nutrition/Diet

Nutrition can be provided by indwelling feeding tube with a high-quality, blendable diet.

Behavior/Exercise

Passive range-of-motion exercises can be challenging given the nature of the limb contracture.

Drug Interactions

- Narcotic analgesics (e.g., opiate drugs) can depress the respiratory center and stimulate other areas of the central nervous system.
- Parasympatholytic drugs such as atropine should be avoided in routine cases.

Possible Complications

- Aspiration pneumonia (p. 793)
- Decubital ulcers
- Respiratory paralysis: some animals may require intubation (or tracheostomy) and ventilation (p. 1185)

Recommended Monitoring

- Heart and respiratory rates
- Temperature monitoring
- Seizure watch
- Urine output

PROGNOSIS & OUTCOME

- Guarded; better with mild clinical signs and localized disease
- In mildly affected animals, normal function usually returns within 3 weeks of the initial treatment.
- Reported survival rate in dogs is 50%-92%.

PEARLS & CONSIDERATIONS

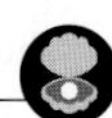

Comments

- Acepromazine is indicated due to its sedative and antianxiety effects.
- Patient should be in a quiet and nonobtrusive environment.

Prevention

- Avoid exposure to potential sources of infection.
- Routine immunoprophylaxis (tetanus toxoid) is not recommended for dogs and cats.
- Appropriate (open) care of infected wounds and rational antibiotic therapy

Technician Tips

Patients can be exquisitely sensitive to light and sound; any efforts to prevent stimulating them (e.g., signs to alert clinic staff, selection of an appropriate location in the hospital for housing and recovery) are important during convalescence. Monitor for dyspnea and regurgitation.

Client Education

- Treatment of the disease can take weeks, but a cure is possible.
- Seek veterinary attention in cases of open wounds.

SUGGESTED READING

Burkitt JM, et al: Risk factors associated with outcome in dogs with tetanus: 38 cases (1987-2005). J Am Vet Med Assoc 230:76-83, 2007.

AUTHOR: Karen L. Kline, DVM, MS, DACVIM
EDITOR: Karen R. Muñana, DVM, MS, DACVIM

Tetralogy of Fallot

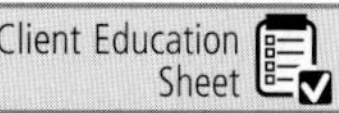

BASIC INFORMATION

Definition

The complex congenital heart defect consists of a ventricular septal defect (VSD), overriding of the interventricular septum by the aortic root, obstruction of the right ventricular (RV) outflow tract, and secondary hypertrophy of the right ventricle.

Synonyms

Fallot's tetralogy, Fallot's syndrome

Epidemiology

SPECIES, AGE, SEX

Dogs and cats; present at birth; possible male predisposition in cats

GENETICS, BREED PREDISPOSITION

- Keeshond, terrier breeds, retriever breeds, Siberian Huskies, toy poodles, English bulldog, and French bulldog
- Conotruncal malformations in keeshond, including tetralogy of Fallot (TOF), have been found to be oligogenic.

ASSOCIATED DISORDERS

- Patent ductus arteriosus (PDA) and atrial septal defect (ASD) may be seen concurrently.
- Systolic anterior motion (SAM) of the mitral valve may be seen secondary to the RV hypertrophy and altered left ventricular geometry.
- Secondary polycythemia is commonly seen due to systemic hypoxemia.

Clinical Presentation

DISEASE FORMS/SUBTYPES

Patients often present with cyanosis, but some may be acyanotic (pink tet). The severity of the RV obstruction often determines the degree or lack of cyanosis. Signs of hyperviscosity syndrome, most commonly neurologic, may occur due to erythrocytosis. Right-sided congestive heart failure is rare with TOF.

HISTORY, CHIEF COMPLAINT

- Cardiac murmur in puppy or kitten
- Cyanosis
- Exercise intolerance
- Syncope
- Stunted growth

PHYSICAL EXAM FINDINGS

- Systolic murmur is most commonly heard at the left basilar area. The murmur grade varies, depending on the severity of the defect and blood viscosity.
- Cyanosis may be aggravated by exercise or other systemic illness (especially respiratory).

Etiology and Pathophysiology

- The combination of RV obstruction and VSD allows central admixing of venous and arterial blood.

- The overriding aorta acts as a conduit that further contributes to the right-to-left shunting of blood.
- Severity of the RV obstruction often determines direction and volume of shunting.
- Flow direction and volume can additionally be altered by systemic blood pressure.
- Exercise and systemic hypotension are likely to increase the right-to-left shunting.
- Increased blood flow through bronchial artery collateral vessels increases venous admixture and further lowers the arterial PO_2.
- Chronic hypoxemia caused by the right-to-left shunting can lead to erythrocytosis and signs of hyperviscosity.

DIAGNOSIS

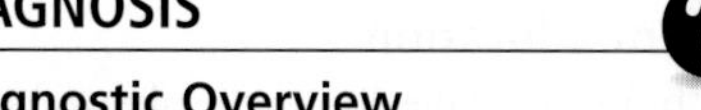

Diagnostic Overview

TOF should be suspected based on young age of animal, left basilar systolic murmur, and cyanosis. CBC, electrocardiography, and thoracic radiographs may help raise or lower the likelihood of TOF, but the most useful diagnostic test is a complete echocardiogram.

Differential Diagnosis

- Pulmonic stenosis with VSD or ASD
- ASD, VSD, or PDA with pulmonary hypertension (Eisenmenger's physiology)
- Double-chamber right ventricle with a VSD
- Double-outlet right ventricle
- Truncus and pseudotruncus arteriosus
- Extracardiac causes of erythrocytosis (pulmonary, renal, and bone marrow)

Initial Database

- CBC: erythrocytosis
- Thoracic radiography: thoracic radiographs commonly have minor abnormalities despite the significant cardiovascular changes present. RV, right atrial, and pulmonary artery (best seen on the ventrodorsal or dorsoventral views) enlargement may be seen. Thoracic radiographs are most helpful in ruling out primary respiratory disease.
- Electrocardiography (ECG): RV hypertrophy pattern is typically present.
- Systemic blood pressure: clinical assessment of systemic vascular resistance should be assessed before treatment with beta-blockers.

Advanced or Confirmatory Testing

- Echocardiography with color Doppler: should allow confirmation of all four components of TOF. Contrast echocardiography (bubble study) may be beneficial if there is equivocal right-to-left shunting or bidirectional shunting.
- Cardiac catheterization and angiography are typically not needed but may be considered if definitive surgical correction is planned.
- CT/MRI are typically not needed but may be beneficial if definitive surgical correction is planned.

TREATMENT

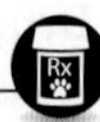

Treatment Overview

There are surgical and palliative medical management strategies. Definitive surgical repair may need to be delayed if patient size is not amenable. Palliative surgical options may be considered to allow patient to grow to a larger size for definitive repair. Alternatively, palliative surgical and medical options may provide relief of symptoms for a period of time.

Acute General Treatment

- The asymptomatic patient may not need acute treatment.
- Sedation with butorphanol 0.2-0.3 mg/kg may be beneficial if the patient is anxious and dyspneic. Avoid sedatives and anxiolytics that can decrease systemic blood pressure.
- Supplemental oxygen, although of little benefit with right-to-left shunts, should be provided when clinical signs are apparent. In addition to oxygen therapy, the quieter environment of oxygen cages may provide a buffer from hospital noise. Monitor temperature in cage and avoid hyperthermia.
- If necessary, increase systemic vascular resistance with an alpha-adrenergic agonist (phenylephrine) to reduce right-to-left shunting.
- If packed cell volume (PCV) or hematocrit is > 70%, perform a phlebotomy with a target of 10%-12% drop in PCV. Replace the removed volume with a balanced crystalloid (100%-200%).

Chronic Treatment

- Definitive surgical repair is available but requires cardiac bypass and open-heart surgery. Veterinary facilities that can provide cardiac bypass are limited at this time.
- Palliative surgical options to create a systemic to pulmonary shunt (e.g., modified Blalock-Taussig shunt) can improve pulmonary blood flow and increase systemic arterial oxygen concentrations. This surgical option does not require bypass and can be performed by an experienced thoracic surgeon.
- Another palliative surgical option is balloon valvuloplasty if the pulmonic stenosis is valvular. Caution is warranted because overdilation with the balloon catheter can lead to severe left-to-right shunting and acute pulmonary edema.
- Control of erythrocytosis (PCV > 70%) with periodic phlebotomy may be necessary.
- If frequent phlebotomies are needed to control PCV, consider hydroxyurea at 30-50 mg/kg PO q 24-48h; titrate based on PCV.
- Propranolol, a nonselective beta-adrenergic blocker, should be considered. The beta-2-blocking effects may reduce systemic vasodilation, minimizing right-to-left shunting. It may also reduce dynamic RV obstruction from RV hypertrophy. The dose range for propranolol is 0.5-1.0 mg/kg q 8h starting at the lower dosage and titrating upward based on symptoms and resting heart rate.
- Aspirin or clopidogrel should be used if a surgical shunt is performed to reduce the risk of thrombosis.

Behavior/Exercise

Vigorous or extended exercise restrictions should be implemented.

Drug Interactions

Hydroxyurea may be difficult to dose with the commercially available product, especially in patients with low body weights. Compounding is frequently needed, and caution is warranted when chronically administering a chemotherapeutic drug. Periodic monitoring of the CBC is warranted.

Recommended Monitoring

- Monitor PCV or hematocrit; CBC if patient receiving hydroxyurea
- If surgical shunt is created, serial echocardiograms are warranted to monitor for patency.
- Resting heart rate, especially when using beta-blockers; resting respiratory rate

PROGNOSIS & OUTCOME

Median survival time reported in one recent publication was approximately 2 years for dogs and cats being treated medically. Palliative surgery can significantly improve clinical outcome. A low-grade murmur appears to have poorer prognosis than a higher-grade murmur with TOF. Sudden cardiac death is common.

PEARLS & CONSIDERATIONS

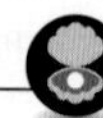

Comments

Erythrocytosis is commonly seen with TOF secondary to hypoxemia, but hydration status is commonly overlooked.

Prevention

Breeding of affected dogs and their immediate relatives is not recommended.

Technician Tips

If routine phlebotomy is indicated, care should be taken to preserve vessels during venipuncture.

Client Education

If animals acquire heartworm infection, it could be a fatal combination with TOF. Heartworm preventives should be given regularly, especially in endemic areas.

SUGGESTED READING

Chetboul V, et al: Epidemiological, clinical, and echocardiographic features and survival times of dogs and cats with tetralogy of Fallot: 31 cases (2003-2014). J Am Vet Med Assoc 249:909-917, 2016.

AUTHOR: Ryan Baumwart, DVM, DACVIM
EDITOR: Meg M. Sleeper, VMD, DACVIM

Tetraplegia/Tetraparesis

Client Education Sheet 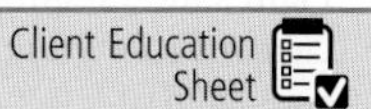

BASIC INFORMATION 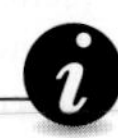

Definition

The suffix *-plegia* signifies complete paralysis; *-paresis* signifies muscle weakness. Either may manifest with upper motor neuron (UMN) or lower motor neuron (LMN) signs. *Tetraplegia* is complete paralysis of all limbs; *tetraparesis* is weakness of all limbs.

Synonyms

- Tetraplegia: quadriplegia
- Tetraparesis: quadriparesis

Epidemiology

SPECIES, AGE, SEX

Dogs and cats of any age and either sex

GENETICS, BREED PREDISPOSITION

- Toy-breed dogs: atlantoaxial instability
- Older Doberman pinschers, young Great Danes, and other large-breed dogs: cervical spondylomyelopathy
- Chondrodystrophic dog breeds: cervical intervertebral disc protrusion
- Burmese cats: hypokalemia
- Labrador retrievers: exercise-induced collapse
- Various cat/dog breeds: breed-associated motor neuron diseases
- Various cat/dog breeds: breed-associated muscular dystrophies and myopathies

RISK FACTORS

- Exposure to carrion: botulism (dogs)
- Exposure to toxins (e.g., 2,4-D herbicide; organophosphates/carbamates)
- Penetrating wounds (tetanus)
- Areas endemic for coral snakes; black widow spiders (*Latrodectus* spp); *Dermacentor* spp, *Amblyomma* spp, and *Ixodes* spp of ticks (tick paralysis)

Clinical Presentation

HISTORY, CHIEF COMPLAINT

Tetraplegia:

- Inability to bear weight, voluntarily move limbs, or ambulate

Tetraparesis:

- Impaired locomotion, ranging from mild weakness or spasticity (usually with ataxia) to recumbency
- Ability to voluntarily move limbs even if recumbent
- Tetraparetic/tetraplegic animals with diseases involving the cerebral cortex and/or brainstem show other abnormal neurologic signs.
    - Abnormal mentation and/or seizures (cerebral cortex or diencephalon)
    - Dullness, stupor, or coma (brainstem) (i.e., midbrain, pons, medulla oblongata)
    - Cranial nerve disturbances (brainstem)
    - Abnormal respiratory character (brain, cervical spinal cord)

PHYSICAL EXAM FINDINGS

- Varies (see specific diseases)
- It is important to neuroanatomically localize the lesion (p. 1136).
- Tetraplegia or tetraparesis can be seen with UMN and/or LMN signs.
- Symmetry or asymmetry of paresis should be noted because this finding may help narrow the differential diagnosis.
- Animals may have UMN or LMN bladder, depending on the neuroanatomic location of the lesion(s).
- Animals with tetraplegia or tetraparesis have a disease involving one of the following regions:
    - Tetraplegia or tetraparesis to all four limbs
        - Bilateral cerebral cortex
        - Bilateral brainstem
        - Bilateral cervical spinal cord
    - Tetraplegia or tetraparesis with hindlimb UMN (as above) and forelimb LMN signs (decreased muscle tone, hyporeflexia)
        - Bilateral C6-T2 spinal cord involvement
    - Tetraplegia or tetraparesis with LMN signs to all four limbs
        - Disease affecting motor neurons of C6-T2 and L4-S2
        - Disease affecting peripheral nerves (motor component) of all four limbs
        - Disease affecting the neuromuscular junction
        - Disease affecting the skeletal muscle
- If one particular region cannot be logically identified, disease process is likely multifocal.

Etiology and Pathophysiology

- UMNs are found in the brain and control LMNs.
- LMNs transmit information from the central nervous system (CNS) to an effector organ-like skeletal muscle.
- Conditions affecting UMNs and/or their axons result in UMN signs.
    - Paralysis or paresis
    - Normal to increased spinal reflexes
    - Later-onset muscle atrophy (disuse atrophy)
    - Normal to increased muscle tone
- Conditions that affect LMNs, their axons, and the neuromuscular junction result in LMN signs.
    - Paralysis or paresis
    - Decreased or absent spinal reflexes
    - Rapid, severe muscle atrophy (neurogenic atrophy)
    - Decreased muscle tone
- Primary or systemic diseases affecting skeletal muscle cause impaired muscular function and can manifest as tetraplegia or tetraparesis.

DIAGNOSIS 

Diagnostic Overview

Tetraparesis/tetraplegia implies a neurologic syndrome; severe systemic disturbances must be ruled out with physical exam and minimal laboratory testing (CBC, chemistry profile). A neurologic exam is pivotal in establishing an anatomic diagnosis, which narrows the differential diagnosis and allows the clinician to choose specific diagnostic tests.

Differential Diagnosis

Intracranial:

- Neoplasia
- Vascular (e.g., cerebrovascular accident)
- Trauma
- Encephalitis (various causes, including infectious and immune-mediated meningoencephalitis of unknown origin [MUE] diseases)
- Hydrocephalus
- Postictal state

Cervical spinal cord:

- Intervertebral disc disease
- Trauma
- Cervical spondylopathy
- Atlantoaxial instability
- Myelitis (various causes, including infectious and immune-mediated [MUE] diseases)
- Osteochondromatosis
- Synovial or arachnoid cysts

Peripheral nerves or neuromuscular junction:

- Tick paralysis
- Idiopathic polyradiculoneuritis
- Snake or spider envenomation
- Myasthenia gravis
- Botulism
- Hypothyroidism
- Various toxins

Muscle:

- Immune-mediated polymyositis (primary or secondary to another disease, such as neoplasia)
- Hypokalemia
- Endocrine disease (hyperthyroidism [cats], hypothyroidism, hyperadrenocorticism)
- Various breed-related muscular dystrophies and myopathies

Initial Database

- Assess patient stability (some may present with impaired respiratory function and/or cardiac arrhythmias)
- Complete physical and neurologic exams
- CBC, serum chemistry profile, and urinalysis for assessment of systemic causes and preanesthetic evaluation

Advanced or Confirmatory Testing

Choice of test depends on neurolocalization and most likely diagnosis.

- Plain skull or spinal radiographs
- Cerebral spinal fluid (CSF) analysis (pp. 1080 and 1323)
- Myelography
- MRI (p. 1132) or CT
- Electrodiagnostic and histopathologic evaluation of affected muscle and nerves
- Detection of antibodies to acetylcholine receptors in cases of fulminant myasthenia gravis

TREATMENT

Treatment Overview

Treatment goals are to eliminate the inciting cause and provide adequate supportive nursing care.

Acute General Treatment

- Treat underlying condition if possible.
- Intensity of nursing care depends on the individual needs of the animal.
- Some supportive therapies to be considered
  - Assisted pulmonary ventilation (p. 1185): if inadequate spontaneous ventilation
  - Caloric intake: hand-feeding (p. 1199), feeding by esophagostomy/gastrostomy tube (p. 1106)
  - Hydration: appropriate fluid therapy
  - Muscle contracture: passive range-of-motion exercises
  - Pressure sores: turn animals frequently, and treat the lesions early and intensively if they occur.
  - Urinary bladder (e.g., catheterization) and bowel management (e.g., stool softener)
  - Hygiene: regular cleaning of perineum; ensure animals are kept on clean, dry bedding.

Chronic Treatment

Long-term supportive therapy may be necessary.

Possible Complications

Complications associated with tetraplegia or severe tetraparesis:

- Decubital ulcers/pressure sores
- Urinary tract infections (with chronic urinary bladder catheterization)
- Fecal impaction
- Pneumonia

Recommended Monitoring

- Complete physical exams two times per day to identify complications from recumbency
- Regularly scheduled and frequent neurologic assessments to monitor disease progression
- Severe or progressive CNS or neuromuscular disease: regular assessment of respiratory function

PROGNOSIS & OUTCOME

Varies, depending on underlying cause

PEARLS & CONSIDERATIONS

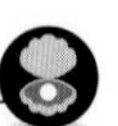

Comments

- Referral to an appropriate treatment center is often necessary.
- Nursing care is often intensive, extensive, and expensive.

Technician Tips

Technicians caring for these patients should be able to turn the patients regularly to minimize the risk for pressure sores, be familiar with precautions to be taken when moving patients that have spinal cord disease, be familiar with urinary catheter management, and be able to perform range-of-motion exercises.

Client Education

- Diseases resulting in tetraplegia or tetraparesis can be costly to diagnose and treat.
- When applicable, provide a Client Education Sheet: How to Perform Range-of-Motion Exercises.

SUGGESTED READING

Comparative Neuromuscular Laboratory, University of California, San Diego, Department of Pathology, School of Medicine (website). http://vetneuromuscular.ucsd.edu.

AUTHOR: Aubrey A. Webb, DVM, PhD
EDITOR: Leah A. Cohn, DVM, PhD, DACVIM

Thiamine Deficiency

BASIC INFORMATION

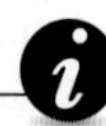

Definition

Deficiency of thiamine (i.e., vitamin B_1), a water-soluble vitamin, may result from inadequate intake or alterations of thiamine absorption, retention, and metabolism.

Epidemiology

SPECIES, AGE, SEX

- All dogs and cats, irrespective of signalment
- Cats are more susceptible due to higher dietary thiamine requirement and frequent consumption of fish-based diets.
- Growth and reproduction also increase thiamine requirement.

RISK FACTORS

- Low dietary thiamine intake
  - Consumption of unbalanced homemade diets; can occur when the diet is not formulated by a specialist in nutrition or when pet owner deviates from a balanced recipe
  - Excessive losses during conventional pet food production; processing conditions are destructive to thiamine, especially canning. Typically, manufacturers overcome predicted losses by adding synthetic thiamine before processing.
  - Consumption of antagonists that inactivate thiamine; thiaminases that degrade thiamine are found in raw seafood, certain ferns, and some bacterial species. Cooking destroys these enzymes. Natural polyhydroxyphenols (caffeic acid, phenols, flavonoids, and tannins), which are heat-stable compounds found in plants, can transform thiamine to nonabsorbable thiamine disulfide. Sulfur dioxide and sodium disulfide are antithiamine factors used to preserve meats and have been implicated in cases of thiamine deficiency in dogs and cats; these are prohibited by the U.S. Department of Agriculture.
  - Hyporexia or anorexia
- Alterations of thiamine absorption and metabolism
  - May occur despite adequate intake due to chronic gastrointestinal (GI) diseases and subsequent malabsorption or maldigestion.
  - Feline leukemia virus (FeLV) subgroup A attaches to the thiamine transporter 1 (THTR1), which subsequently prevents thiamine uptake. Because THTR2 is not affected, the risk of thiamine deficiency as a result of FeLV may be low.
  - Alaskan Husky encephalopathy, a fatal juvenile neurologic disease, is thought to be caused by a mutation of the *SLC19A3* gene encoding THTR2 in nervous tissue.
- Excessive renal excretion of thiamine
  - Increased urinary thiamine excretion occurs with polyuria/polydipsia or administration of diuretics (furosemide, chlorothiazide). Surprisingly, dogs with chronic kidney disease (CKD) have higher blood thiamine diphosphate concentrations compared with healthy controls.

Clinical Presentation

DISEASE FORMS/SUBTYPES

Primarily affects nervous system, although multiple organ systems may be involved.

- Induction stage: within 1 week of severe deficiency
- Critical stage: if not identified and reversed during the induction stage
- Terminal stage: after approximately 1 month of severe deficiency; death occurs. Most cases are diagnosed in terminal stage.

HISTORY, CHIEF COMPLAINT

- Diet and medical history compatible with risk factors
- Clinical signs are variable and nonspecific.
  - GI signs initially: hyporexia or anorexia, lethargy, depression, weight loss, hypersalivation (cats), vomiting, and diarrhea or constipation.
  - Progression to neurologic signs: blindness, ataxia, paresis, weakness, cervical ventroflexion (cats), tremors, seizures, and coma
  - In terminal stage, rapid worsening of signs until death occurs.

PHYSICAL EXAM FINDINGS

- Dogs: tachypnea, tachycardia, weak femoral pulses; cats: sinus arrhythmia, bradycardia
- Neurologic exam (p. 1136): altered mentation, poor proprioception, abnormal postural reaction, absence of deep and superficial pain in all limbs, and hyperesthesia
- Cats: spastic ventroflexion of head and neck that worsens and persists despite being held upside down
- Ocular exam (p. 1137): nystagmus, anisocoria, mydriasis, unresponsive dilated pupils, and lack of menace response. Fundic exam may reveal retinal venous dilatation and hemorrhage.
- Electrocardiographic changes (p. 1096): flattening or inversion of the T wave, QRS prolongation, or prolongation of the ST segment

Etiology and Pathophysiology

- Thiamine can be obtained only from the diet and is not stored in the body. Excess thiamine is excreted in the urine.
- Thiamine exists in the blood as free form or phosphorylated (thiamine monophosphate, diphosphate, and triphosphate).
- Critical role in carbohydrate metabolism and energy production; clinical signs of deficiency may relate to dependence of neuronal and cardiac tissue on energy
- Role in neural function (synaptic transmission and cell membrane conductance and stimulates activity in the spinal cord and cerebellum).

DIAGNOSIS

Diagnostic Overview

Thiamine deficiency is suspected based on clinical signs and presence of risk factors on nutritional assessment. These findings justify prompt initiation of treatment. Response to treatment strongly supports the diagnosis.

Differential Diagnosis

- Intoxication
- Inflammatory or infectious central nervous disease
- Multifocal intracranial neoplasia
- Other nutritional disease
- Metabolic disease

Initial Database

- Nutritional assessment, including body weight, body condition score, muscle condition score, food intake and diet history, followed by assessment of nutritional risk factors.
- Question owners about possibility of toxin ingestion.
- CBC, serum biochemical profile, urinalysis, and CSF analysis are generally unremarkable.

Advanced or Confirmatory Testing

- Treatment with thiamine results in rapid response in 12-48 hours; response is considered confirmatory for suspected diagnosis.
- Erythrocyte transketolase activity: indicator of thiamine status; limited availability; requires specific blood sample preparation.
- High-performance liquid chromatography for whole blood and serum thiamine analyses: limited availability; lack of reference ranges
- Elevated plasma pyruvate and urinary lactate concentrations in dogs
- MRI of the brain: symmetrical bilateral lessons in the brainstem; primarily affects gray matter
- Histopathology: lesions may be spongy or may involve cell degeneration and hypertrophy; especially occur in the nuclei of the caudal colliculi
- Laboratory analyses of diet for thiamine (± sulfur dioxide)

TREATMENT

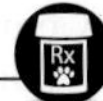

Treatment Overview

Parenteral thiamine supplementation is recommended; acute treatment with oral supplementation is considered for longer-term use. Dietary correction is indicated if nutritional thiamine deficiency is suspected.

Acute General Treatment

- Crystalloid fluids IV
- Anticonvulsant medications, if required (p. 903)
- Thiamine hydrochloride 100-250 mg IM or SQ q 12-24h until neurologic signs subside (3-5 days). The ideal dose is currently unknown. Dosages described after improvement of neurologic signs are 25-150 mg in cats, 100-600 mg in dogs PO q 12h.

Chronic Treatment

- Continue with oral thiamine supplementation for an additional 2-4 weeks.
- Correct dietary or medical issues.

Nutrition/Diet

Dietary correction:

- Eliminate any raw food, especially raw fish.
- Discontinue suspected deficient diet.
- Feed an appropriate, balanced commercial or home-cooked diet.

Assisted feeding if diminished food intake:

- Veterinary therapeutic critical care diet offered orally or administered through feeding tube
- Introduce food gradually; begin at one-fourth to one-third of the patient's resting energy requirement (RER), increase to one-half to two-thirds after 24 hours, and so forth to full RER.

Possible Complications

- Animals can experience discomfort during or after SC or IM thiamine injection. Rarely, allergic reactions to SQ thiamine have occurred.
- Thiamine supplementation IV should be avoided because severe hemodynamic effects (hypotension, cardiac arrhythmias, neuromuscular and ganglionic blockage, apnea, and death) have been reported.

PROGNOSIS & OUTCOME

Clinical signs begin to resolve within hours after supplementation, although some signs may persist for days to months. Full recovery may not be possible if severe neurologic damage has occurred. Exercise intolerance and some degree of ataxia can persist for years after treatment.

PEARLS & CONSIDERATIONS

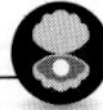

Prevention

- Feed a balanced commercial diet in accordance with the patient's life stage, or feed a balanced homemade diet formulated by board-certified veterinary or PhD nutritionist
- Do not feed raw food, especially raw fish.
- Note the "best before" date on pet food packaging and ensure proper pet food storage (original packaging, avoid exposure to heat and light).

Technician Tips

Nutritional assessment and diet history are most important tools to diagnose thiamine deficiency.

Client Education

Explain the dietary risk factors associated with thiamine deficiency and the importance of feeding a balanced diet in accordance with the pet's life stage.

SUGGESTED READING

Kritikos G, et al: The role of thiamine and effects of deficiency in dogs and cats. Vet Sci 4(4):59, 2017.

AUTHOR: Adronie Verbrugghe, DVM, PhD, DECVCN
EDITOR: Jennifer Larsen, DVM, PhD, DACVN

Third Eyelid Abnormalities/Protrusion

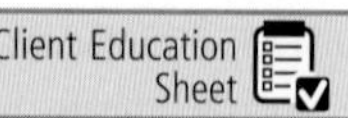

BASIC INFORMATION

Definitions

- Prolapsed gland of the third eyelid: dorsal displacement and prolapse of the gland from its normal position at the base of the third eyelid
- Everted cartilage of the third eyelid: a malformed leading edge of the third eyelid that rolls outward
- Protrusion of the third eyelid: a third eyelid that is resting in an elevated or more dorsal position, covering the ocular surface
- Atypical pannus: localized proliferative inflammation of the third eyelid found in German shepherds and greyhounds (p. 748)
- Third eyelid neoplasia: any neoplastic growth originating from the gland or conjunctiva of the third eyelid

Synonyms

- Third eyelid: membrana nictitans, nictitating membrane
- Bilateral third eyelid protrusion: Haw's syndrome
- Prolapsed gland of the third eyelid: cherry eye
- Everted cartilage: scrolled cartilage, bent cartilage, protruding third eyelid cartilage tips
- Atypical pannus: plasmoma

Epidemiology

SPECIES, AGE, SEX

- Prolapsed gland of the third eyelid: young dogs and cats, most often less than 2 years of age
- Everted cartilage of the third eyelid: congenital or early developmental malformation
- Third eyelid protrusion secondary to ocular pain, enophthalmos, and exophthalmos: dogs and cats of any age (pp. 705 and 716)
- Third eyelid gland neoplasia: most common in older dogs and cats
- Follicular conjunctivitis: dogs and cats typically < 18 months of age (pp. 199 and 200)

GENETICS, BREED PREDISPOSITION

- Prolapsed gland of the third eyelid: most common in beagles, American cocker spaniels and brachycephalic breeds, especially the English bulldog; Burmese cats are predisposed
- Everted cartilage of the third eyelid: inherited in German shorthair pointers. giant-breed dogs are predisposed, including Great Danes, Newfoundlands, mastiff breeds, and St. Bernard dogs; reported in Burmese and British blue cats
- Atypical pannus: German shepherds, greyhounds, and others
- Follicular conjunctivitis: primarily large-breed dogs (especially retrievers)

RISK FACTORS

- Prolapsed gland of the third eyelid: concurrent follicular conjunctivitis may induce prolapse
- Bilateral third eyelid protrusion: cats living in multi-cat households; association with gastrointestinal disease, diarrhea, feline leukemia virus (FeLV), and a toravirus-like agent
- Third eyelid protrusion secondary to ocular pain and enophthalmos: consider keratoconjunctivitis, corneal ulceration, uveitis, and glaucoma
- Third eyelid protrusion secondary to exophthalmos or enophthalmos
- Follicular conjunctivitis: high exposure to allergens (e.g., field trial dogs)

ASSOCIATED DISORDERS

Prolapsed gland of the third eyelid:
- Conjunctivitis (pp. 199 and 200)

Third eyelid protrusion:
- Secondary to ocular pain and resultant enophthalmos
- Exophthalmos or enophthalmos (p. 716)
- Otitis and nasopharyngeal polyps
- Horner's syndrome
- Rabies
- Tetanus
- Cannabis intoxication
- Dysautonomia
- Other systemic illness (e.g., cytauxzoonosis)

Third eyelid inflammation:
- Atypical pannus
- Follicular conjunctivitis
- Keratoconjunctivitis: eosinophilic, cats

Clinical Presentation

HISTORY, CHIEF COMPLAINT

Common layperson descriptions:
- Droopy eyelids (describing ptosis and third eyelid protrusion seen in Horner's syndrome)
- Membrane covering the eye (describing third eyelid protrusion)

PHYSICAL EXAM FINDINGS

- Prolapsed gland of the third eyelid
  - A smooth, round, pink or red protrusion over the leading edge of the third eyelid. Size varies significantly based on breed and chronicity.
  - Evidence of conjunctivitis, including mucoid discharge, epiphora, lymphoid follicles, and hyperemia
  - ± Low Schirmer tear test values
- Everted cartilage of the third eyelid
  - The entire leading edge of the third eyelid scrolls anteriorly (rostrally) away from the ocular surface due to a bend in the shaft of the cartilage.
  - Anterior (rostral) protrusion of the cartilaginous tips of the leading edge of the third eyelid (less common)
  - Inversion of the cartilage toward the ocular surface, causing keratitis (rare)
  - Evidence of conjunctivitis, including mucoid ocular discharge, epiphora, lymphoid follicles and hyperemia
  - May have concurrent prolapsed gland of the third eyelid
- Protrusion of the third eyelid
  - One or both third eyelids extend more dorsally and temporally than normal.
  - ± Evidence of ocular pain: blepharospasm
  - ± Other signs of Horner's syndrome
  - ± Exophthalmos or enophthalmos
- Atypical pannus
  - Various surface irregularities and pigment loss on leading edge of third eyelid
- Third eyelid gland neoplasia
  - Various findings, depending on tumor type and location
    - Adenomas and adenocarcinomas arise from the gland on the posterior aspect of the third eyelid.
    - Hemangiomas, hemangiosarcomas (red masses), and squamous cell carcinoma (pinkish/white masses) most often arise from the anterior surface or leading margin of the third eyelid.
  - Mandibular lymph node enlargement may be present.

Etiology and Pathophysiology

- Prolapsed gland of the third eyelid: possible polygenic inheritance; may occur secondary to loosening of retinacular attachments of the gland to the shaft of the third eyelid cartilage
- Everted cartilage of the third eyelid: disparate growth rate of posterior aspect of third eyelid cartilage relative to the anterior aspect
- Protrusion of the third eyelid (four pathophysiologic causes)
  - Active retraction of the globe (enophthalmos) by retractor bulbi contraction from ocular pain, leading to passive protrusion of the third eyelid
  - Disruption of smooth muscle tone on the orbital cone from Horner's syndrome, infection (rabies, tetanus), dysautonomia or toxin (cannabis intoxication), leading to enophthalmos resulting in passive protrusion of the third eyelid
  - Imbalance of orbital volume secondary to enophthalmos (pain or loss of orbital contents), exophthalmos (e.g., retrobulbar neoplasia, orbital cellulitis), microphthalmos, or phthisis bulbi leading to passive protrusion of the third eyelid
  - Voluntary control of third eyelid protrusion (only seen in cats) leading to active protrusion of the third eyelid
- Atypical pannus: immune-mediated
- Neoplasia of the third eyelid

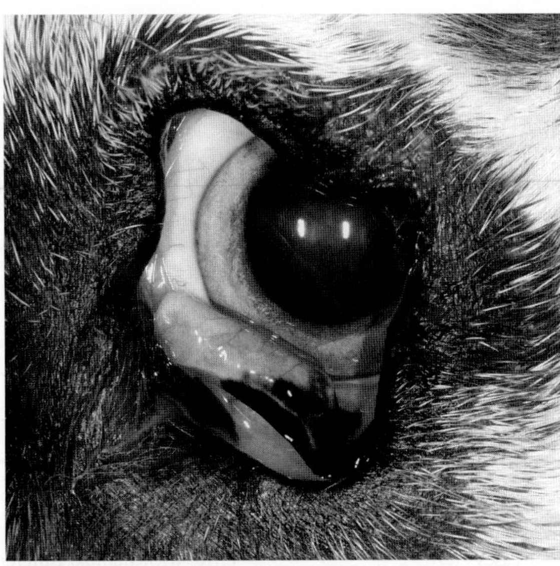

THIRD EYELID ABNORMALITIES/PROTRUSION Scrolled cartilage of the third eyelid in a dog. Note the anterior scrolling of the leading edge of the third eyelid.

   - Various causes and pathophysiology, depending on tumor type
   - Hemangiomas/hemangiosarcomas and squamous cell carcinomas have been associated with UV light exposure.

DIAGNOSIS

Diagnostic Overview

Most conditions associated with the third eyelid are diagnosed based on clinical appearance, but a complete ophthalmic exam should be done.

Differential Diagnosis

Differentials for a mass or swelling of third eyelid:
- Prolapsed gland of the third eyelid, everted cartilage of the third eyelid, atypical pannus, and some third eyelid neoplasms
- Chemosis
- Onchocerca granuloma

Differentials for protrusion of the third eyelid:
- Pain
- Orbital disease
- Variation in degree of pigmentation of third eyelids. Often, one that is not pigmented appears more obvious than a pigmented third eyelid.

Initial Database

- Prolapsed gland of the third eyelid and everted cartilage of the third eyelid: diagnosis is typically straightforward based on appearance and expected signalment
- Protrusion of the third eyelid secondary to Horner's syndrome: most cases also have miosis, ptosis and enophthalmos
- Atypical pannus: diagnosis is typically straightforward based on appearance and expected signalment.
- Complete ophthalmic exam (p. 1137)
   - Pupillary light reflexes: miosis is often present with Horner's syndrome
   - Schirmer ear test: low values (<15 mm wetting/minute) may occur with chronic prolapsed gland of the third eyelid.
   - Fluorescein stain: ensure there is a lack of corneal stain uptake to rule out ulceration as a cause of pain because topical steroids are occasionally indicated to reduce inflammation before surgical repair

Advanced or Confirmatory Testing

- Neoplasia of the third eyelid
   - Obtain a biopsy, taking care to avoid exposing the cartilage of the third eyelid, which can cause irritation to the ocular surface.
   - Palpate the ipsilateral mandibular lymph node, and obtain a fine-needle aspirate for cytology if enlarged.
   - Tumor staging and complete third eyelid excision are indicated for malignant tumors.
- Advanced diagnostic imaging modalities may be indicated if third eyelid protrusion is suspected to be secondary to orbital disease.

TREATMENT

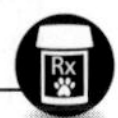

Treatment Overview

Medical or surgical therapies are specific to each third eyelid disorder.

Acute General Treatment

Prolapsed gland of the third eyelid:
- Expedient surgical repair reduces the likelihood of progressive inflammation and loss of tear production.
- Multiple options for surgical repair exist, and selection depends on surgeon preference:
   - Imbrication of bulbar conjunctiva over the gland (pocket technique)
   - And/or suture anchoring to ventral orbital periosteum
   - And/or suture anchoring to the cartilage of the third eyelid
- NOTE: use caution when passing suture blindly through the ventral orbital periosteum because inadvertent globe penetration can cause blinding ocular injury.
- CONTRAINDICATION: excision of a prolapsed gland of the third eyelid. Removal of this gland may permanently reduce tear function and often leads to keratoconjunctivitis sicca months or years after the procedure.

Everted cartilage of the third eyelid:
- Everted cartilaginous tips of the leading edge of the third eyelid may not require therapy.
- Surgical options for scrolled third eyelid cartilage:
   - Surgical excision of the bent aspect of the shaft third eyelid cartilage with the conjunctiva left to heal by second intention
   - And/or application of low temperature cautery can be applied to the convex side of the bent cartilage; causes cartilage contraction, straightening affected areas
   - NOTE: excessive application of cautery can cause overcorrection.

Neoplasia of the third eyelid gland:
- Local excision, with or without adjunctive therapies (e.g., cryotherapy, radiation therapy, chemotherapy) is dictated by size and predicted biologic behavior.
- Complete excision of the third eyelid is indicated for diffuse or malignant neoplasms of the third eyelid gland.
- NOTE: all excised samples should be submitted for histopathology.
- NOTE: an empirical trial of topical corticosteroids (dexamethasone 0.1% solution or ointment q 6-8h for 10-14 days) can be used to differentiate inflammatory disorders from neoplastic lesions.

PROGNOSIS & OUTCOME

- Prolapsed gland of the third eyelid: good after surgical repair. Repeated prolapse occurs commonly (up 20%), and attempts at repair should be repeated. Bulldogs may have a lower success rate than other breeds. Consider referral to an ophthalmologist with repeated prolapses.
- Everted cartilage of the third eyelid: good after surgical repair. Surgical correction can restore normal anatomic appearance and function in most cases.
- Protrusion of the third eyelid secondary to orbital disease: depends on underlying process
- Atypical pannus: good prognosis for control with topical therapy

PEARLS & CONSIDERATIONS

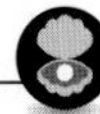

Comments

- The gland of the third eyelid should be excised only when neoplasia is present.
- The bulbar surface of the third eyelid can be examined by retropulsing the globe and using thumb forceps to gently grasp the leading edge of the third eyelid and extending

it rostrally. This should be done when attempting to look for a cause of corneal ulceration.
- Third eyelid flaps are not indicated in cases of infected ulcers, melting ulcers, descemetoceles, or corneal perforations.

Technician Tips

Technicians skilled at performing the Schirmer tear test, fluorescein stain, and tonometry are invaluable in aiding veterinarians in establishing an underlying diagnosis for third eyelid abnormalities.

SUGGESTED READING

Multari D, et al: Pocket technique or pocket technique combined with modified orbital rim anchorage for the replacement of a prolapsed gland of the third eyelid in dogs: 353 dogs. Vet Ophthalmol 19:214-219, 2016.

AUTHOR: Lucien V. Vallone, DVM, DACVO
EDITOR: Diane V. H. Hendrix, DVM, DACVO

Thrombocytopenia, Immune-Mediated

Client Education Sheet 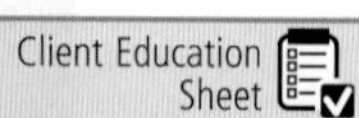

BASIC INFORMATION 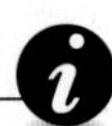

Definition

Thrombocytopenia resulting from immune-mediated platelet destruction in the absence of an identifiable cause

Synonym

Idiopathic thrombocytopenic purpura (ITP)

Epidemiology

SPECIES, AGE, SEX

Dogs > cats; either sex, 8 months to 15 years of age, with middle-aged females predisposed

GENETICS, BREED PREDISPOSITION

Cocker spaniels, Old English sheepdogs, German shepherds, and poodles are overrepresented.

ASSOCIATED DISORDERS

Immune-mediated diseases may affect multiple body systems; immune-mediated thrombocytopenia (IMT) may be associated with polyarthritis or proteinuria. Anemia may be due to blood loss (especially gastrointestinal [GI]) or concurrent immune-mediated hemolytic anemia (Evans syndrome).

Clinical Presentation

DISEASE FORMS/SUBTYPES

Primary IMT is idiopathic. Secondary IMT occurs in association with infection, drug therapy, or neoplasia.

HISTORY, CHIEF COMPLAINT

Owners commonly notice bleeding in the skin, from the nose or mouth, or associated with minor trauma. Hematochezia, melena, or hematuria may be observed. The patient may continue to act normally, although some present with lethargy and weakness. Signs caused by bleeding into vital organs (brain, spinal cord) are uncommon.

PHYSICAL EXAM FINDINGS

- Petechiae, ecchymoses
- Ocular hemorrhage/hyphema
- GI bleeding manifesting as melena or hematochezia
- Pale mucous membranes
- Fever in < 20% of cases

Etiology and Pathophysiology

- Occurs when a stimulus triggers a patient with the appropriate susceptibility genes
- Identification and inheritance of predisposing genes are unknown.
- Triggering factors may include vaccination, drug administration, stress, or infection.
- Bleeding does not occur until the platelet count is < 25,000/mcL, although bleeding may occur in the face of higher platelet counts if there is platelet dysfunction (thrombocytopathia).

DIAGNOSIS 

Diagnostic Overview

The diagnosis is suspected in patients showing overt signs of bleeding in the history, physical exam, or both, and it is confirmed by demonstrating repeatable, severe thrombocytopenia (<25,000/mcL) in the absence of an identifiable cause.

Differential Diagnosis

- Breed-associated physiologic thrombocytopenia (greyhounds, Cavalier King Charles spaniels, Norfolk terriers)
- Tick-borne disease (e.g., ehrlichiosis, anaplasmosis, Rocky Mountain spotted fever)
- Splenic disease (neoplasia, torsion, infarction)
- Drug administration (antineoplastic chemotherapy, antibiotics, estrogen, nonsteroidal anti-inflammatory drugs [NSAIDs], albendazole, griseofulvin, propylthiouracil, ketoconazole)
- Bacterial sepsis, vasculitis, disseminated intravascular coagulation
- Bone marrow disease (e.g., myelofibrosis, myelodysplasia, necrosis, myelophthisis)
- Thrombocytopathia (e.g., drug-related, inherited such as von Willebrand disease)
- Severe hemorrhage (e.g., anticoagulant rodenticide, trauma)
- Cats: feline leukemia virus (FeLV), feline immunodeficiency virus (FIV) infections

Initial Database

- CBC with manual differential:
  - Bleeding may cause anemia (regenerative after 3-5 days)
  - By definition, severe thrombocytopenia: platelet count usually < 25,000/mcL; may be few to no visible platelets (p. 1373)
- Serum biochemical profile: usually normal
- Urinalysis (voided)
  - Usually normal or may show hematuria
  - Avoid cystocentesis in severely thrombocytopenic patients.
- Coagulation profile: usually normal, but activated clotting time (ACT) may be prolonged.
- Thoracic radiographs: usually normal
- Abdominal ultrasonography: usually normal or may show mild splenomegaly
- Serum titers for tick-borne diseases in endemic areas

Advanced or Confirmatory Testing

- Bone marrow cytologic exam is rarely necessary (e.g., if there is concurrent leukopenia or nonregenerative anemia): may show increased (peripheral platelet destruction; more common) or decreased (marrow-based destruction) megakaryocyte numbers
- Testing for platelet-bound antibody is usually unnecessary.
- Antinuclear antibody testing only if there are multiple systems involved to suggest systemic lupus erythematosus.

TREATMENT 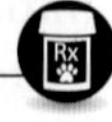

Treatment Overview

Stable patients can be treated as outpatients, with therapy aimed at raising the platelet count into the normal range. If signs of anemia or severe bleeding are apparent, hospitalization and transfusion are required.

Acute General Treatment

- Prednisone/prednisolone 2.2 mg/kg PO q 24h or divided q 12h; for large-breed dogs 40 mg/m^2/day (alternative: dexamethasone 0.3 mg/kg IV q 24h or divided q 12h)

- Vincristine 0.02 mg/kg (or 0.5 mg/m^2 [pp. 607 and 609]) IV once weekly (author preference)
- Mycophenolate mofetil 10 mg/kg PO q 12h (author preference)
- Red blood cell (RBC) transfusions (fresh whole blood, packed cells) as needed (p. 1169)
- Platelet transfusions are usually impractical because platelets are rapidly destroyed.
  - Life-threatening, uncontrolled hemorrhage may require platelet-rich plasma (6-12 mL/kg IV; >5 × 10^9 platelets/kg IV), frozen platelet concentrate, or lyophilized platelets (StablePlate RX).

Chronic Treatment

- Discontinue vincristine after platelet count is > 50,000/mcL or if no response.
- Taper prednisone/prednisolone and mycophenolate after platelet count has normalized.
  - Decrease doses by 25%-50% every month (in general) while monitoring platelet count.
  - The minimum duration of therapy is typically 4-6 months.
  - If the platelet count falls during the drug tapering, increase to the previous dose, and attempt to taper more slowly.
  - Attempt to taper completely off prednisone; treatment with mycophenolate alone is used in patients requiring long-term immunosuppression.
  - It may be preferable to allow mild thrombocytopenia to persist to decrease medications to tolerable levels.

Behavior/Exercise

Activity and excitement should be minimized to avoid self-trauma until a safe platelet count (>25,000/mcL) is achieved.

Drug Interactions

- Extravasation of vincristine causes severe skin necrosis; use an indwelling IV catheter.
- Avoid drugs that inhibit platelet function (e.g., NSAIDs).

Possible Complications

- Avoid cyclophosphamide in these patients; hemorrhagic cystitis may be fatal.
- Glucocorticoid-induced side effects are common with long-term administration (polyuria, polydipsia, polyphagia; weight gain, panting, behavioral change, coat thinning, calcinosis cutis, and/or muscle weakness).
- Mycophenolate mofetil may cause diarrhea.

Recommended Monitoring

Platelet counts every other day until > 50,000/mcL, then weekly until normal

PROGNOSIS & OUTCOME

- Prognosis is initially guarded, with fatal bleeding into the brain or spinal cord possible.
- Response often takes 3-10 days.
- After the platelet count normalizes, the prognosis is fair to good; survival rate is 84% for dogs treated at referral hospitals.
- Many pets are tapered completely from immunosuppressive medications, although relapse remains possible (10%-40% recurrence rate for dogs).

PEARLS & CONSIDERATIONS

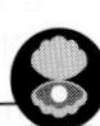

Comments

- The presence of severe thrombocytopenia (<25,000/mcL) in an otherwise healthy-appearing animal is most likely due to IMT.
- If bleeding is present when the platelet count is > 25,000/mcL, an additional problem such as clotting factor deficiency, thrombocytopathia, or vasculitis must be present.
- Combination immunosuppressive therapy with mycophenolate mofetil is often more effective and has fewer adverse effects than prednisone/prednisolone alone.
- Anecdotal reports suggest melatonin 3 mg (<10 kg) or 6 mg (>10 kg) PO q 12h as adjunct therapy.
- Additional immunosuppressants (azathioprine, cyclosporine, leflunomide) and/or splenectomy may be beneficial in refractory cases. Consultation with an internal medicine specialist is recommended.
- Many animals are euthanized due to adverse effects of glucocorticoids. Strategies to decrease glucocorticoid-induced adverse effects include avoidance of obesity, use of an additional immunosuppressive agent to lower glucocorticoid dosage, and routine monitoring for infections of the skin and urinary tract.

Prevention

- Future vaccinations should be limited to those considered essential.
- Stressful circumstances should be avoided during severe thrombocytopenia to reduce the risk of self-trauma.

Technician Tips

Venipuncture should be performed with the least possible trauma and pressure maintained over the vein for a full 60 seconds. Venipuncture from the jugular veins should be avoided.

Client Education

- Frequent monitoring is necessary to prevent side effects of immunosuppressive medications.
- Obesity must be prevented; body weight should be carefully monitored.

SUGGESTED READING

O'Marra SK, et al: Treatment and predictors of outcome in dogs with immune-mediated thrombocytopenia. J Am Vet Med Assoc 238:346-352, 2011.

AUTHOR: Michael Stone, DVM, DACVIM
EDITOR: Jonathan E. Fogle DVM, PhD, DACVIM

Thymoma

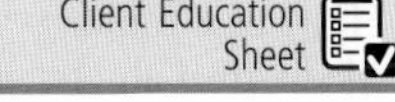

BASIC INFORMATION

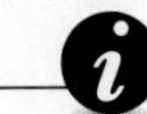

Definition

A benign or malignant primary tumor in the cranial mediastinum that originates from the thymic epithelium. The presenting complaints for animals with thymoma are signs caused by the space-occupying nature of the mediastinal mass or paraneoplastic syndromes such as myasthenia gravis, megaesophagus, or hypercalcemia.

Epidemiology

SPECIES, AGE, SEX

- Dog: average age is 8-10 years.
- Cat: average age is 9-12 years.

GENETICS, BREED PREDISPOSITION

Dog: large-breed dogs (Labrador retriever, German shepherd) may be more commonly affected.

ASSOCIATED DISORDERS

- Paraneoplastic syndromes associated with thymoma
  - Myasthenia gravis (11%-50% of dogs with thymoma [p. 668])
  - Hypercalcemia (p. 491)
- Immune-mediated syndromes (less common)
  - Polymyositis, dermatitis (e.g., feline thymoma-associated exfoliative dermatitis), and myocarditis
- Megaesophagus (p. 642)
- Cardiac arrhythmias: rare
- Cranial vena cava syndrome (p. 221): rare

Clinical Presentation

DISEASE FORMS/SUBTYPES

Epithelial cell–dominant, lymphocyte-dominant, and mixed forms exist and can make diagnosis by fine-needle aspiration difficult.

HISTORY, CHIEF COMPLAINT

- Respiratory signs: very common chief complaints (tachypnea, dyspnea, coughing); signs may be surprisingly mild given size of thymoma.

- Anorexia and weight loss also common
- Weakness: associated with myasthenia or hypercalcemia
- Regurgitation: if megaesophagus is present
- Polyuria/polydipsia if hypercalcemic
- Dermatitis in cats (12%)

PHYSICAL EXAM FINDINGS

- Respiratory system: muffled or absent lung and heart sounds due to pleural effusion and/or space-occupying nature of mass
  - Increased, harsh lung sounds: aspiration pneumonia
- Weakness: episodic or sustained; associated with loss of muscle tone, decreased spinal reflexes. Can be focal, associated with the pharyngeal, laryngeal, or facial muscles
- Decreased chest wall compliance is noted with manual compression of the cranial thorax.
  - Important physical finding in cats with medium to large thymomas

Etiology and Pathophysiology

- Neoplastic transformation of thymic epithelial cells
- Cranial mediastinal mass ± pleural effusion: clinical signs of respiratory compromise
- Paraneoplastic syndrome of myasthenia gravis result of aberrant immune stimulation

DIAGNOSIS

Diagnostic Overview

The diagnosis of thymoma is suspected based on presenting history, physical exam findings, and demonstration of a well-defined cranial mediastinal mass on thoracic radiographs. Ultrasound-guided fine-needle aspirates or needle biopsies are required to confirm the diagnosis and rule out other causes such as mediastinal lymphoma. Computerized tomography (CT) helps determine whether the mass is surgically resectable.

Differential Diagnosis

- Thymic lymphoma, hyperplasia, or hemorrhage
- Branchial cyst
- Ectopic thyroid or parathyroid neoplasia
- Neurogenic tumor
- Heart base tumor
- Mediastinal abscess or granuloma

Initial Database

- CBC, serum biochemical profile, and urinalysis: evaluate for hypercalcemia (5%-35% of dogs hypercalcemic), which does not change survival time; poorly concentrated urine if hypercalcemia present; inflammatory leukogram if aspiration pneumonia due to megaesophagus
- Feline leukemia virus (FeLV) and feline immunodeficiency (FIV) serologic testing in cats: thymic lymphoma often associated with FeLV-positive status
- Survey thoracic radiographs (three views): extent of primary neoplasm, evidence of metastasis, evidence of megaesophagus and/or aspiration pneumonia (secondary to myasthenia gravis), pleural effusion
- Thoracic ultrasound: morphologic exam of mass, including association with/invasion of vascular structures, presence or absence of cysts; fine-needle aspiration or needle biopsy of mass (rule out lymphoma); collection of pleural fluid (cytologic exam [pp. 1164 and 1343])
- Survey abdominal radiographs, ultrasound: rule out abdominal organ involvement (lymphoma)

Advanced or Confirmatory Testing

- MRI (p. 1132) or CT: determine whether surgical excision is a viable treatment option. Evaluate compression, displacement, invasion, or incorporation of adjacent structures (e.g., vessels, esophagus, trachea, thoracic wall) and metastasis. Evaluation of invasion of major vessels, including the cranial vena cava, is difficult. Contrast administration does not assist in determining cell type of mediastinal masses. Extent of mediastinal masses is often unknown until surgery.
- Acetylcholine (ACh) receptor antibody titers: positive with thymoma-associated myasthenia gravis
- Flow cytometry of samples collected by fine-needle aspiration and stored in fetal bovine serum may be useful in differentiating thymoma from lymphoma. The test uses T-cell marker expression of CD4 and CD8 on T cells; > 20% expression of CD4 and CD8 is consistent with thymoma, and lack of CD4 and CD8 expression rules out thymoma.

TREATMENT

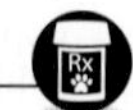

Treatment Overview

Complete surgical resection is the recommended treatment.

Acute and Chronic Treatment

- Complete surgical excision is often feasible with thymoma. May be carried out thoracoscopically for noninvasive thymoma
- Incomplete surgical excision is more likely when thoracic ultrasonography reveals invasion into or attachment to local vessels. The size of thymoma is not necessarily predictive of complete or incomplete resection.
  - Chemotherapy: lymphoma protocol (pp. 607 and 609)
  - Radiation therapy
- Nonresectable masses: radiation therapy ± chemotherapy
- Myasthenia gravis (p. 668)
  - Resolution after complete resection of neoplasm
  - Prednisone 2 mg/kg PO q 24h for 4 weeks, then tapered
- Hypercalcemia (p. 491)
- Aspiration pneumonia (p. 793): antibiotic therapy based on culture and susceptibility (C&S) testing
- Megaesophagus (p. 642): consider tube gastrostomy for medical and nutritional support (p. 1109)
- Therapeutic thoracocentesis (p. 1164)
  - If respiratory compromise due to pleural effusion
  - Preanesthetic patient stabilization

Possible Complications

Inability to resolve the associated myasthenia gravis:

- Persistent regurgitation/megaesophagus
- Recurring aspiration pneumonia
- Intraoperative hemorrhage
- Disseminated intravascular coagulation
- Perioperative mortality of 20% in dogs and 22% in cats due to nonresectable disease, hemorrhage, or cardiopulmonary arrest

Regrowth of thymoma: occurs in some cases after complete surgical resection, as well as in cases with incomplete surgical resection. Monitoring with exam and imaging studies is essential regardless of completeness of resection.

Recommended Monitoring

- After surgical resection (complete or incomplete): q 3 months (exam, thoracic radiographs) for 1 year, then q 6 months
- If patient is receiving chemotherapy: as determined by protocol

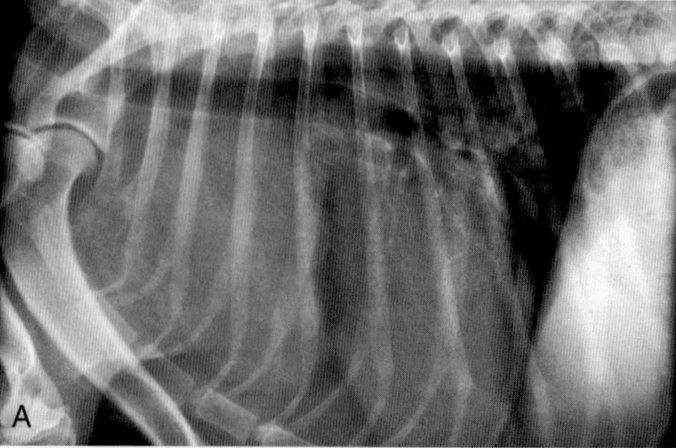

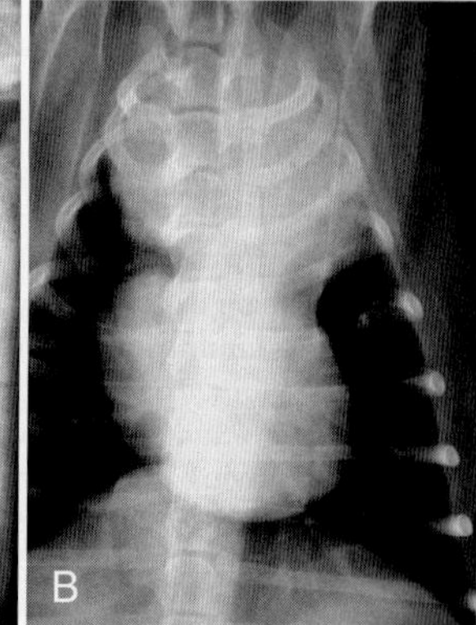

THYMOMA A, Lateral thoracic radiograph shows a large soft-tissue/fluid opacity mass occupying the entire cranial thorax of this dog and elevating the trachea. **B,** Dorsoventral radiographic view of the same animal. The midline location suggests a mediastinal mass. Surgical excision and histopathologic analysis confirmed a thymoma. (Courtesy Dr. Richard Walshaw.)

PROGNOSIS & OUTCOME 

Dog:
- Resectable thymoma without megaesophagus
  - 70%-80% 1-year survival rate, 50% 3-year survival in one study; 55% 1-year, 44% 2-year, 44% 3-year, and 44% 4-year survival in another study. Median survival time is 616-635 days.
- Nonresectable thymoma: poor
- Presence of myasthenia gravis or megaesophagus: guarded to poor; may resolve over a period of months

Cat:
- Resectable thymoma
  - 70% 1-year, 63% 2-year, 63% 3-year, and 47% 4-year survival rates. Median survival is 1354 days.

PEARLS & CONSIDERATIONS 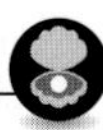

Comments
- It is critical to differentiate thymoma from mediastinal lymphoma, especially in cats, because the former is surgically treated and the latter is treated medically.
- Adjuvant radiation therapy ± chemotherapy may benefit animals with nonresectable thymoma.
- Closely monitor animals for development of aspiration pneumonia and myasthenia gravis.

Technician Tips
- Knowledge of and experience in working with thoracostomy tubes is important in the postoperative management of patients who have undergone a thoracotomy.
- Patients with megaesophagus will require nutritional support (p. 1109).

Client Education
For dogs with megaesophagus, provide client education sheet: How to Provide Elevated Feedings.

SUGGESTED READING

Zitz JC, et al: Results of excision of thymoma in cats and dogs: 20 cases (1984-2005). J Am Vet Med Assoc 232:1186, 2008.

AUTHORS: MaryAnn G. Radlinsky, DVM, MS, DACVS; Don R. Waldron, DVM, DACVS
EDITOR: Elizabeth A. Swanson, DVM, MS, DACVS

Thyroid Neoplasia

Client Education Sheet 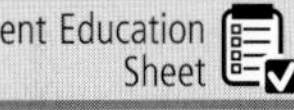

BASIC INFORMATION 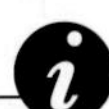

Definition
Cancer of the thyroid gland in dogs is most often carcinoma or adenocarcinoma and may (10%) or may not (90%) be functional, causing hyperthyroidism. This chapter deals specifically with thyroid tumors in dogs.

Epidemiology
SPECIES, AGE, SEX
- Most often occurs in older dogs
- Thyroid neoplasia in cats is rarely (2% of cases) malignant, as discussed on p. 503.

GENETICS, BREED PREDISPOSITION
- Increased expression of genes encoding proteins involved in a major cell survival pathway (PI3K/AKT) occurs in some dogs.
- Predisposed breeds include beagles, golden retrievers, boxers, and Siberian Huskies.

RISK FACTORS
- Radiation exposure
- Untreated hypothyroidism

ASSOCIATED DISORDERS
- Hyperthyroidism (p. 503)
- Hypothyroidism (p. 525)
- Uncommonly, part of multiple endocrine neoplasia syndrome
- Laryngeal paralysis (p. 574)
- Horner's syndrome

Clinical Presentation
DISEASE FORMS/SUBTYPES
- Benign adenoma in dogs very uncommon (<10%); usually silent and are found incidentally
- Histologic subtypes
  - Follicular cell origin: includes compact (solid), follicular, anaplastic, and papillary; first two constitute majority in dogs
  - Parafollicular (i.e., C-cell or medullary thyroid) carcinomas; have a lower metastatic rate
- Can be classified as functional (secretes thyroid hormones) or nonfunctional

HISTORY, CHIEF COMPLAINT

Common clinical signs:
- Visible or palpable mass in ventral neck
- Dysphonia
- Dyspnea
- Dysphagia
- Unexplained weight loss, if functional

PHYSICAL EXAM FINDINGS
- Palpable mass in mid-cervical region, unilateral or bilateral
- Masses can occur between base of the tongue and the base of the heart but usually in cranial to middle, ventral neck; occasionally intimately associated with larynx or sublingual region
- Nodal enlargement of mandibular and superficial cervical lymph nodes if metastases present
- Referred upper airway noise on thoracic auscultation

Etiology and Pathophysiology
- Increased circulating thyroid-stimulating hormone (TSH) is associated with an increased risk of thyroid cancer (untreated hypothyroid beagles) and tumor relapse (humans). In dogs, thyroid supplementation to suppress TSH is typically combined with surgery or radiation therapy (RT) for local disease.
- Metastasis present in 30%-40% at time of presentation, 80% at time of death
- Increased metastasis risk with tumors > 23 cm^3; metastasis almost 100% if tumor > 100 cm^3 and with bilateral tumors

DIAGNOSIS 

Diagnostic Overview
Malignant thyroid neoplasia is diagnosed using exam findings (e.g., mass location), cytology, and imaging. Due to high vascularity, significant bleeding can occur during aspiration or biopsy. Test sequence is very important because some tests can interfere with evaluation and treatment.

Differential Diagnosis
- For a cervical mass
  - Other primary tumors: lipoma (p. 591), soft-tissue sarcoma, mast cell tumor (pp. 632 and 634), or lymphoma (p. 609); carotid body tumor if tumor located high (cranial) on neck
  - Metastatic oral tumor
  - Abscess
  - Salivary mucocele

Initial Database
- CBC, chemistry, urinalysis for general health assessment; fasting hypercholesterolemia can occur with hypothyroidism.
- Thyroid panel (total T_4, free T_4 by equilibrium dialysis method, and TSH) (p. 525)
- Cytology of mass
  - Significant bleeding can occur.
  - Sample can be hemodiluted.

  - Use passive aspiration. Do not attach syringe, or if a syringe is used to maneuver the needle, do not actively aspirate. Redirect needle only.
- Cytology of regional lymph nodes (superficial cervical and mandibular): possible metastasis
- Three-view thoracic radiographs: possible metastasis
- Ultrasound
  - Evaluate carotid artery and jugular vein for invasion.
  - Use to guide a needle for aspiration or biopsy to avoid vascular structures.

Advanced or Confirmatory Testing

- CT or MRI: do NOT perform a contrast-enhanced CT until radioiodine has been determined to not be a treatment option (see below).
- Scintigraphy
  - ^{99m}Tc-pertechnetate commonly available and less expensive, with better resolution compared with ^{123}I
  - ^{123}I or tracer dose of ^{131}I can distinguish thyroid from salivary gland; pertechnetate cannot.
- Immunohistochemistry of biopsy to differentiate follicular and parafollicular tumors.

TREATMENT

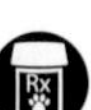

Treatment Overview

Optimal treatment depends on location and resectability, owner's goals, and availability of RT. Most freely moveable tumors are resected. Invasive or attached tumors are surgically cytoreduced to microscopic disease and then treated with RT or treated with RT alone.

Acute Treatment

- In cases of severe respiratory compromise, consider tracheostomy (p. 1166).
- Occasionally, dogs with functional tumors can experience a thyroid storm (i.e., sudden release of excessive amounts of or exaggerated response to thyroid hormone) that causes acute tachycardia and hypertension. Treat symptomatically with supportive care (beta-blockers).
- For dogs with hyperthyroidism, methimazole is sometimes used. Suggested starting dose is 5 mg q 8-12h, then adjusted to effect. Because it is unknown whether this affects radioiodine uptake in dogs, avoid if possible before radioiodine therapy. If used, consider a minimum 3-day withdrawal before radioiodine therapy (based on Society of Nuclear Medicine recommendation for humans).
- Treat hypothyroidism if present (see below), but NOT before radioiodine therapy because it decreases iodine uptake.

Chronic Treatment

- Surgical excision alone if freely moveable
- Surgery plus RT: external beam, or if preoperative scintigraphy showed uptake, postoperative ^{131}I can be considered
- Surgery plus chemotherapy
- RT: external beam or ^{131}I
  - Treatment of malignant tumors with ^{131}I requires large doses and is limited to < 10 facilities in North America.
  - Dose should not exceed 5 mCi/kg to avoid unacceptable myelosuppression.
  - Radioiodine spares normal tissues compared to external beam radiation.
- Chemotherapy
  - ≈50% response seen to doxorubicin, cisplatin, mitoxantrone, actinomycin D, and metronomic chlorambucil.
  - 80% of dogs responded to toceranib phosphate in an early study (25% had tumor size reduction; remainder had stable disease).
- Thyroid hormone supplementation is typically provided after RT or bilateral thyroidectomy (p. 525). Keep serum T_4 concentration in high-normal range to suppress TSH.

Nutrition/Diet

- Restricted-iodine diets may be recommended before radioiodine to cause increased iodine uptake.
- An iodine-restricted diet and methimazole were used in one dog to palliate clinical signs of hyperthyroidism resulting from a thyroid mass.

Possible Complications

- Thyroid tumors or their treatment (surgery or RT) can cause laryngeal paralysis and Horner's syndrome.
- Surgical removal of bilateral thyroid tumors can result in hypoparathyroidism and hypocalcemia; if this is anticipated, consider perioperative calcitriol and calcium (p. 519).
- Hypothyroidism is expected with bilateral thyroidectomy and is possible with definitive RT (p. 525).
- Myelosuppression with high-dose ^{131}I

Recommended Monitoring

- Assessment of the neck (exam and possibly ultrasound or CT) and lungs (thoracic radiographs) q 3 months.
- Monitor thyroid function (total T_4 and TSH) 1 month after definitive treatment and q 3-6 months thereafter.
- Monitor CBC weekly for 4-6 weeks (until neutrophils have reached a nadir and then recovered) after radioiodine therapy.

PROGNOSIS & OUTCOME

- With no treatment, median survival time (MST) is 3 months; dogs with sublingual tumors can have long MST.
- Surgery
  - Tumors contained within the thyroid gland capsule and freely moveable, MST is 3 years.
  - With extracapsular invasion, MST is 6-12 months.
- No clear benefit for chemotherapy after surgery but should be considered; dogs with tumoral vascular invasion or other negative prognostic factors might benefit.
- Radioiodine therapy: MST of 1 year with metastasis present, > 2 years without metastasis
- External beam RT: 80% survival at 1 year; MST 2 years.
  - Dogs can survive a long time (MST ≈2 years) even with pulmonary metastasis if primary tumor is addressed with RT.
  - After RT, takes at least 8 months to achieve full effect.
- Negative prognostic factors with regard to local invasion and resectability or metastatic behavior, or both, include increased size, location (ectopic or bilateral), attachment to underlying structures, high Ki-67 activity, and vascular invasion (macroscopic and microscopic).

PEARLS & CONSIDERATIONS

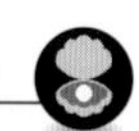

Comments

- First, decide whether radioiodine will be considered for treatment. If radioiodine is a possibility, it is CRITICAL to NOT perform a contrast-enhanced CT because doing so decreases treatment efficacy for at least 4 weeks.
- If considering surgery, the most important consideration is whether the tumor is attached to underlying structures.

Technician Tips

- The jugular vein may be displaced. Shaving hair over the venipuncture site may be helpful.
- Jugular venipuncture should not be performed before CT or scintigraphy because it can create artifact.

Client Education

- Owners must be prepared to manage endocrine complications of therapy for thyroid neoplasia, including accurate, timely, and lifelong administration of calcitriol and/or levothyroxine.
- Pulmonary metastasis tends to progress slowly, and dogs can still benefit from treatment.

SUGGESTED READING

Nadeau ME, et al: Evaluation of the use of chemotherapy and other prognostic variables for surgically excised canine thyroid carcinoma with and without metastasis. Can Vet J 2011;52:994-998.

AUTHOR: Kim A. Selting, DVM, MS, DACVIM, DACVR
EDITOR: Ellen N. Behrend, VMD, PhD, DACVIM

Tick Paralysis

Client Education Sheet

BASIC INFORMATION

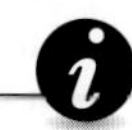

Definition

An acute, rapidly progressive, generalized lower motor neuron (LMN) paralysis that results from neuromuscular blockade due to a salivary neurotoxin produced by certain gravid, female tick species

Epidemiology

SPECIES, AGE, SEX

- Any age or breed; both sexes
- North American tick paralysis (*Dermacentor* ticks) affects dogs but not cats; Australian tick paralysis (*Ixodes* ticks) affects dogs and cats.

RISK FACTORS

Tick exposure, lack of tick prevention

CONTAGION AND ZOONOSIS

Some ticks can cause tick paralysis in humans; animal-to-animal or zoonotic transmission does not occur.

GEOGRAPHY AND SEASONALITY

- Worldwide, notably United States and Australia
- Most frequent in summer months

Clinical Presentation

DISEASE FORMS/SUBTYPES

Based on the geographic location of the tick (see below)

HISTORY, CHIEF COMPLAINT

- History of hindlimb and then forelimb stiff gait, progressing to flaccid paralysis
- Mentation, behavior, and ability to urinate and defecate remain normal.

PHYSICAL EXAM FINDINGS

North America (*Dermacentor* spp ticks most often but also *Amblyomma* spp):

- Hindlimb weakness rapidly progressing to generalized weakness, then complete flaccid paralysis. Tail wag often is preserved.
- Pain sensation is preserved, but hyperpathia is rare.
- Cranial nerve involvement is rare; nystagmus, mild facial palsy possible
- Voice change and intercostal muscle paresis can be observed, potentially leading to respiratory paralysis.

Australia (*Ixodes* spp ticks):

- Hindlimb weakness, pain sensation: as for North America
- Signs of facial paralysis, dysphagia, and megaesophagus are common and may be profound.
- Autonomic signs (mydriasis, arterial and pulmonary hypertension) can be observed and, if untreated, may lead to respiratory paralysis and death.

Etiology and Pathophysiology

- Gravid female tick of the species *Dermacentor variabilis* (Eastern wood or dog tick), *Dermacentor andersoni* (Rocky Mountain wood tick) in the United States, and *Ixodes holocyclus* in Australia
- Adult *D. variabilis* and *D. andersoni* female ticks elaborate the neurotoxin; adult female, nymphs, and larvae of *Ixodes* ticks are incriminated.
- The neurotoxin is secreted by the engorged feeding female tick; the toxin inhibits depolarization in the terminal portions of motor nerves or blocks the release of acetylcholine (ACh) from the motor nerve terminals at the neuromuscular junction.
- In most cases, hindlimb weakness begins 5-9 days after tick attachment, rapidly followed by generalized weakness and complete flaccid paralysis and areflexia in 24-72 hours.

DIAGNOSIS

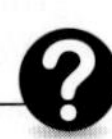

Diagnostic Overview

The diagnosis rests entirely on finding one or more ticks on an animal with compatible clinical signs. Delay in finding and removing tick(s) can affect prognosis markedly.

Differential Diagnosis

- Polyradiculoneuritis
- Early stages of botulism
- Fulminant myasthenia gravis
- Rabies

Initial Database

- Response to tick removal is confirmatory: patient's rapid clinical improvement after tick removal (within 24 hours for *Dermacentor* spp and return to normalcy in 48-72 hours; clinical signs may initially progress for 24-48 hours after tick removal for *Ixodes* spp)
- Exclusion of other causes of rapidly progressive LMN diseases (see Differential Diagnosis above)
- CBC and serum biochemical profile are usually unremarkable.

Advanced or Confirmatory Testing

- Chest and abdominal radiographs are usually unremarkable (exception: megaesophagus [*Ixodes* spp]).
- Electromyography
  - Shows no evidence of denervation
  - Amplitude of evoked motor potentials is markedly reduced.
  - Repetitive stimulation does not cause further decrement in amplitude.
- Nerve conduction velocity (motor and sensory) may be slightly slower; terminal conduction times may be prolonged.

TREATMENT

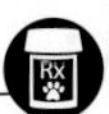

Treatment Overview

Because tick removal is diagnostic and therapeutic, additional treatment consists of supportive care until clinical signs resolve.

Acute General Treatment

- Tick removal can be curative; remember to remove the tick's head because the toxin resides in the salivary glands.
- Insecticide if ticks are not found (e.g., isoxazolines)
- Whole-body shaving of long-haired patient (tick search)
- Hyperimmune serum 0.5-1 mL/kg IV recommended for dogs with respiratory compromise as it binds circulating neurotoxin and prevents further progression; caution regarding anaphylaxis risk
- Autonomic dysfunction can be treated with a combination of phenoxybenzamine hydrochloride 1 mg/kg as a 0.1% solution given IV over 15 minutes q 12-24h and acepromazine 0.05-0.1 mg/kg IV q 6-12h.
- Oxygen supplementation (p. 1146) and ventilatory support (p. 1185) as necessary for animals with respiratory compromise

Chronic Treatment

- Supportive care
- Physical rehabilitation
- Sanitation
- Provision of food and water

Nutrition/Diet

High-quality diet in the recuperation period

Behavior/Exercise

- Physical rehabilitation is essential in the recovery period.
- Passive range-of-motion exercises and sanitation are of utmost importance.

Drug Interactions

Avoid aminoglycosides (associated with neuromuscular blockade).

Possible Complications

- Respiratory paralysis (especially with recurrent exposure)
- Decubital ulcers
- Aspiration pneumonia

Recommended Monitoring

- Respiratory rate and character
- Urination/defecation
- Progression of signs

PROGNOSIS & OUTCOME

- Highly dependent on timely identification and removal of tick(s)

- Excellent if rapid removal of *Dermacentor* tick (in United States); fatal if undiagnosed/untreated
- Guarded with *Ixodes* ticks (Australia); fatal if undiagnosed/untreated
- Recurrence is possible with re-exposure.

PEARLS & CONSIDERATIONS

Comments

- Consider time of the year in the differential diagnosis.
- Note rapid (24-72 hours) progression to areflexic flaccid paralysis, which should raise the suspicion of tick paralysis and prompt a meticulous exam of the skin and coat.
- Make sure whole tick is removed because the toxin lies in the tick's head (salivary glands).
- Application or administration of rapidly acting ascridicides may be warranted for dogs with LMN paralysis even if no tick is found.

Prevention

- Avoid tick exposure.
- Use ascridicides regularly at appropriate doses.

Technician Tips

- Identifying and removing a tick (including mouth parts) from the skin of a patient with a presumptive diagnosis of neuromuscular disease can be lifesaving.
- Shaving of a patient with a thick coat may expose ticks that are otherwise hidden.

Client Education

- The recovery period can vary, and return to function will be gradual.
- In most cases, a full recovery is attainable.

SUGGESTED READING

Holland CT: Asymmetrical focal neurological deficits in dogs and cats with naturally occurring tick paralysis *(Ixodes holocyclus)*: 27 cases (1999-2006). Aust Vet J 86:377-384, 2008.

AUTHOR: Karen L. Kline, DVM, MS, DACVIM
EDITOR: Karen R. Muñana, DVM, MS, DACVIM

Toad Intoxication

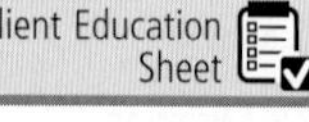

BASIC INFORMATION

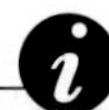

Definition

Toxicosis associated with exposure to *Bufo*, *Anaxyrus*, *Rhinella*, or *Incilius* spp of toads, characterized by gastrointestinal (GI), neurologic, or cardiovascular effects

Synonym

Bufo poisoning

Epidemiology

SPECIES, AGE, SEX

Dogs are more likely to kill and ingest toads than cats.

RISK FACTORS

Underlying cardiac disease may increase risk of severe signs.

GEOGRAPHY AND SEASONALITY

- Toads of concern (*Rhinella marina* [formerly *Bufo marinus*] or cane toad, *Incilius alvarius* [formerly *Bufo* alvarius], Colorado river toad, or Sonoran desert toad) are located in Florida, California, Hawaii, New Mexico, and Arizona. Toads in other places in the United States may cause drooling and vomiting if ingested, but no serious cardiac problems are expected.
- Peak months are June to September.

Clinical Presentation

DISEASE FORMS/SUBTYPES

- Taste reactions (drooling, gagging, and vomiting) can occur with the less toxic toads.
- Severe cardiovascular and neurologic reactions can occur with exposure to *R. marina* or *I. alvarius*

HISTORY, CHIEF COMPLAINT

Witnessed or suspected exposure to toads due to location and clinical signs of hypersalivation, gagging, and potentially collapse

PHYSICAL EXAM FINDINGS

- Hypersalivation, vomiting, gagging, face rubbing
- Weakness, lethargy, vocalization
- Tachypnea
- Ataxia
- Arrhythmia (tachyarrhythmia or bradyarrhythmia)
- Pale mucous membranes, poor capillary refill time
- Muscle rigidity
- Seizures

Etiology and Pathophysiology

- Modified toad parotid glands excrete cardiac toxins (bufogenins, bufagins, bufadienolides, bufotoxins) that mimic digoxin. Toxins inhibit Na^+/K^+-ATPase pumps in myocardial cells, leading to increased intracellular calcium and extracellular potassium. Increased intracellular calcium causes delayed afterpolarization, leading to cardiac arrhythmias.
- Bufogenins may also have sodium channel blocking effects.
- Bufotenines are indolealkylamines with oxytocic and pressor actions. They are oral irritants and potentially hallucinogenic.
- Other toxins include catecholamines (epinephrine, norepinephrine) and serotonin.

DIAGNOSIS

Diagnostic Overview

Diagnosis is based on witnessed/suspected exposure and clinical signs. There are no clinically expedient tests available.

Differential Diagnosis

- Cardiac glycosides: digoxin, *Digitalis* spp (foxglove), *Convallaria majalis* (lily of the valley), *Nerium oleander* (oleander), *Thevetia peruviana* (yellow oleander), *Apocynum cannabinum* (dogbane), *Asclepias* spp (milkweed)
- Organophosphates, pyrethrins, metaldehyde, methylxanthines, pseudoephedrine, amphetamines
- Other cardiac pharmaceuticals (e.g., calcium channel blockers, beta-blockers)
- Grayanotoxins: *Rhododendron* spp (rhododendron, azalea), *Kalmia* spp (mountain laurel), *Aconitum* spp (monkshood)
- *Taxus* spp (yew)

Initial Database

- Blood pressure (BP): hypotension (p. 1065)
- Electrocardiogram (ECG): arrhythmias (tachycardia or bradycardia) (p. 1096)
- Electrolytes: hyperkalemia or hypokalemia; baseline, repeat in 2-4 hours

Advanced or Confirmatory Testing

- Serum digoxin assay can confirm exposure, but levels do not correlate well with clinical signs.
- Chromatography can be used to detect bufogenins in tissues.

TREATMENT

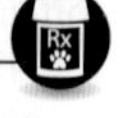

Treatment Overview

After exposure to minimally toxic species or if a more toxic toad was involved but not consumed, rinse the dog's mouth, and monitor for clinical signs. If a more toxic toad was ingested or systemic signs manifest, more aggressive therapy is needed. Cardiovascular signs can change, and treatment is tailored to the arrhythmia present.

Acute General Treatment

- Rinse mouth with water for at least 5 minutes (toward rostrum).
- If toad was swallowed and animal is asymptomatic, consider emesis (p. 1188).
- Activated charcoal may bind toxins; weigh risks (p. 1087). Most effective within the first hour

- Cholestyramine 300 mg/kg PO q 6h enhances elimination of digitoxin in humans and may be tried.
- Non–calcium-containing IV fluids correct potassium disorders, if present.
- Maropitant 1 mg/kg SQ
- Seizures: diazepam 0.5-1 mg/kg IV
- Arrhythmias: treat as appropriate (pp. 1033 and 1457)
    - Atropine 0.02-0.04 mg/kg IV for bradycardia
    - Propranolol 0.02-0.06 mg/kg IV for supraventricular arrhythmias, *or*
    - Esmolol (dogs) 0.25-0.5 mg/kg IV over 1-2 minutes, then 25-200 mcg/kg/min constant-rate infusion (CRI)
    - Phenytoin 2 mg/kg up to 10 mg/kg IV (dogs) for ventricular arrhythmias (disrupts reentrant pathways and improves conduction through AV node), *or*
    - Lidocaine 2 mg/kg IV up to 8 mg/kg, 25-80 mcg/kg/min CRI (dogs); 0.25-0.5 mg/kg IV (cats)
- Oxygen (p. 1146)
- Antidote: digoxin Fab fragments (Digibind) can be given in severe cases. Start with 1-2 vials administered slowly over 30 minutes; response occurs within 20-90 minutes (very expensive: $2000+).
    - Fragments bind directly to digoxin, rendering them unavailable to interact at the binding sites.

Drug Interactions

- Amiodarone increases serum glycoside concentration.
- Calcium channel blockers, beta-blockers: use only when needed, can have additive effects on the AV node
- Calcium increases arrhythmias.

Possible Complications

- Concern for renal injury with prolonged hypotension
- Potential for permanent myocardial damage

Recommended Monitoring

- ECG, BP, oxygen saturation
- Neurologic status
- Potassium

PROGNOSIS & OUTCOME

- Good if signs are just limited to mild GI; guarded if cardiac signs develop
- Signs last 1-2 hours if toad is licked/mouthed and up to 36 hours if ingested.

PEARLS & CONSIDERATIONS

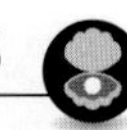

Comments

- Eggs may be more toxic than adult toads.
- Tadpoles are similar in toxicity to adults.
- Do not use atropine to treat hypersalivation because it can worsen tachyarrhythmias.

Prevention

Try to limit pet access in areas with toads during peak toad activity.

Technician Tips

Closely monitor arrhythmias because they can change frequently.

Client Education

Secretions from the skin can contaminate water bowls. Do not leave full water bowls out overnight in areas where the most toxic toads live.

SUGGESTED READING

Peterson ME, et al: Toads. In Peterson ME, et al, editors: Small animal toxicology, ed 3, St. Louis, 2013, Saunders, pp 833-839.

AUTHOR & EDITOR: Tina Wismer, DVM, MS, DABVT, DABT

Tonsillar Disorders

BASIC INFORMATION

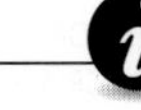

Definition

Abnormal structure or function of the palatine tonsils usually manifests as increased size, often with protrusion from the tonsillar fossa.

Synonym

Palatine tonsillar disorder

Epidemiology

SPECIES, AGE, SEX

- Occasionally seen in dogs; less frequent in cats of either sex
- Acute tonsillitis appears to be more frequent in animals < 1 year of age.

CONTAGION AND ZOONOSIS

- Group A *Streptococcus pyogenes* ("strep throat" in humans) does not cause signs of tonsillitis in dogs or cats.
- Rates of infection in dogs or cats from contact with infected humans appear low; in rare circumstances, infected dogs or cats not showing clinical signs may serve as a source of reinfection for humans in the household.

Clinical Presentation

HISTORY, CHIEF COMPLAINT

Tonsillar enlargement often is an incidental finding; signs may include dysphagia/retching, coughing, ptyalism, stridor, and inappetence. The clinical signs of the underlying disease may often be more clinically significant than the signs attributable to tonsillar enlargement.

PHYSICAL EXAM FINDINGS

- Bilaterally or unilaterally enlarged palatine tonsils; with tonsillitis, the tonsils are often bright red and protrude from the tonsillar crypts. There may be petechiae or a purulent exudate on the tonsils or in the tonsillar crypts.
- Fever is common with infectious disease.
- Inspect for evidence of infection or inflammation that could cause secondary tonsillar reactivity by licking behavior (e.g., anus, external genitalia) and the teeth/gums.

Etiology and Pathophysiology

- The palatine tonsils are sentinels for exposure to antigens that enter through the mouth and nose. Unlike lymph nodes, they have no afferent drainage region, and reactive tonsillar enlargement arises from exposure through the oral cavity.
- Primary tonsillitis: bacterial or viral colonization of the lymphatic tissue of the tonsils. The tonsils are a common portal of entry for enteric bacteria and viruses.
- Secondary tonsillitis results from chronic pharyngeal irritation, such as recurrent vomiting, regurgitation, or coughing; it may also result from chronic pharyngitis secondary to elongated soft palate, immunosuppression from feline immunodeficiency virus (FIV), chronic contamination of the oropharynx with pathogenic bacteria in cases of chronic periodontal disease, or licking of distant infected sites such as skin or anal sacs.
- Swallowed foreign bodies such as grass awns or wood splinters may become lodged in the tonsillar crypt.
- Tonsillar cyst: embryonic remnant
- Neoplasia: squamous cell carcinoma (SCC) or lymphoma may develop from the epithelial or lymphoid components of the tonsils, respectively.

DIAGNOSIS

Diagnostic Overview

Most cases of bilateral tonsillar enlargement are benign and secondary to processes such as licking infected material. The diagnostic goal is to rule out neoplasia. If a single tonsil is irregular and enlarged, suspect SCC or foreign body. If both tonsils are enlarged along with other lymphoid tissues such as peripheral lymph nodes, suspect lymphoma. Suspected neoplastic cases can be confirmed with fine-needle aspiration (FNA) or biopsy.

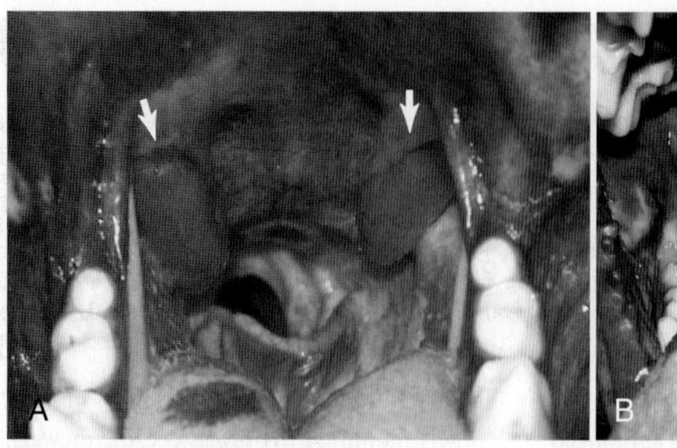
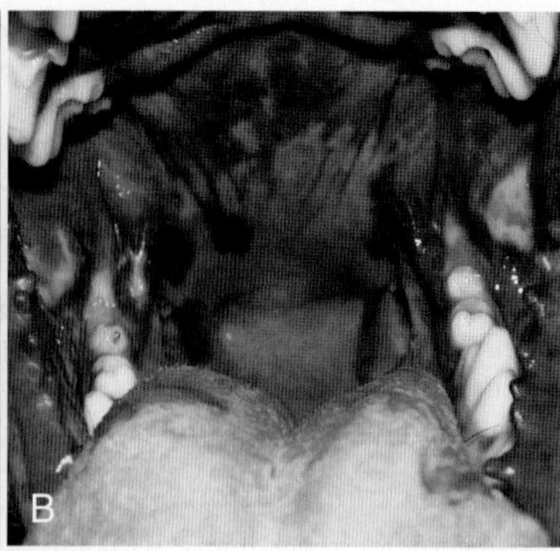

TONSILLAR DISORDERS A, Intraoral view of a dog with marked bilateral enlargement of the tonsils *(arrows)*. **B,** Intraoral view of tonsils in a normal dog for comparison.

Differential Diagnosis

A detailed list of potential causes is provided on p. 1287.

Initial Database

- CBC, serum biochemistry profile, and urinalysis to identify underlying systemic disease
- Feline leukemia virus (FeLV) and feline immunodeficiency virus (FIV) testing of cats

Advanced or Confirmatory Testing

- Bacterial culture and susceptibility (C&S) or virus isolation in cases of primary tonsillitis that fail to respond to routine antibiotics
- If peripheral lymph nodes are enlarged, FNA of representative nodes for cytologic exam can identify lymphoma.
- General anesthesia and tonsillar FNA cytologic exam or biopsy
  - Specific indications: unilateral tonsillar enlargement or tonsillar enlargement that does not resolve (or worsens) despite identification and treatment of underlying disease

TREATMENT

Treatment Overview

- Treat the underlying disease.
- Tonsillectomy is indicated only for the following:
  - Chronic recurrent tonsillitis unresponsive to antibiotic therapy and elimination of source of antigen (e.g., licking infected area)
  - Marked tonsillar enlargement interfering with swallowing or breathing
  - Neoplasia: SCC

Acute and Chronic Treatment

- Incidentally discovered bilateral/symmetrical tonsillar enlargement is often most appropriately only monitored (watchful waiting) while the underlying cause is sought and treated.
  - Remove any recognized foreign body.
  - Address dental and periodontal disease.
  - Address distant infection/inflammation and minimize licking.
- Primary tonsillitis with clinical signs and no identifiable cause
  - Acute: broad-spectrum antibiotics (e.g., amoxicillin 20 mg/kg PO q 8h for 10-14 days)
  - Chronic: based on C&S results
- Tonsillar lymphoma (pp. 607 and 609)
- SCC: surgical excision followed by chemotherapy and radiation therapy (p. 939)

PROGNOSIS & OUTCOME

- Tonsillitis: good prognosis, usually resolves with underlying disease
- Neoplasia: poor long-term prognosis

PEARLS & CONSIDERATIONS

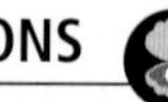

Comments

- Therapeutic intervention for enlarged tonsils is rarely required.
- The most common cause of symmetrical/bilateral tonsillar enlargement is a reactive change in response to oral exposure to antigen, such as the pet licking his/her anal sacs or genitalia. Diagnostic investigation and treatment should focus on these processes first and then on the tonsils only if necessary.

Technician Tips

If tonsillar enlargement is observed during endotracheal intubation for any anesthetic procedure, notify the veterinarian so that investigation can be made into cause.

SUGGESTED READING

Radlinsky MG: Surgery of the oral cavity and oropharynx. In Fossum TW, editor: Small animal surgery, ed 4, St. Louis, 2013, Elsevier, pp 394-396.

AUTHOR: Peter M. Foley, MSc, DVM, DACVIM
EDITOR: Leah A. Cohn, DVM, PhD, DACVIM

Tooth Fractures

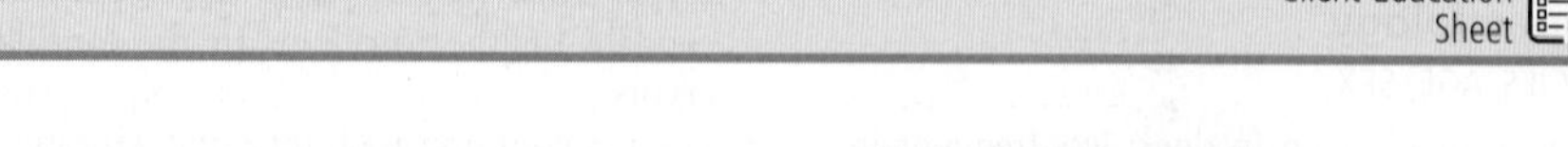

BASIC INFORMATION

Definition

Breaking of enamel, dentin, and/or cementum of the crown or root (or both) of a tooth; common in dogs and cats

Synonyms

- Dental fracture
- Slab fracture: fracture of the labial/buccal (or lingual/palatal) surface of a tooth

Epidemiology

SPECIES, AGE, SEX

Any age (including deciduous teeth)

- Dogs: canine and maxillary fourth premolar teeth commonly affected (due to aggressive chewing or other trauma)
- Cats: more common in canine teeth (due to trauma) or any teeth weakened by tooth resorption (p. 982)

RISK FACTORS

- Dogs: chewing on bones, ice cubes, nylon toys, cow hooves, rocks, deer antlers, and cages
- Cats: high-rise syndrome, vehicular trauma, tooth resorption

ASSOCIATED DISORDERS

Attrition (wear from tooth-to-tooth contact), abrasion (wear from contact of teeth with nondental materials), pulpitis (pulpal inflammation), displacement injuries (tooth luxation or avulsion), tooth resorption (p. 982), and caries (bacterial infection causing tooth demineralization)

Clinical Presentation

DISEASE FORMS/SUBTYPES

American Veterinary Dental College (AVDC) Tooth Fracture Classification (www.avdc.org):

- Enamel infraction: incomplete fracture (crack) of the enamel without loss of tooth substance
- Enamel fracture: fracture with loss of crown substance confined to the enamel
- Uncomplicated crown fracture: fracture of the crown that does not expose the pulp
- Complicated crown fracture: fracture of the crown that exposes the pulp
- Uncomplicated crown-root fracture: fracture of the crown and root that does not expose the pulp
- Complicated crown-root fracture: fracture of the crown and root that exposes the pulp

- Root fracture: fracture involving the root

HISTORY, CHIEF COMPLAINT

- Tooth fractures commonly noted as incidental findings on routine physical exam
- History of falling from a height, vehicular trauma, fights with other animals, aggressive chewing tendencies, or other trauma

PHYSICAL EXAM FINDINGS

- Commonly no overt clinical signs, especially if fracture is uncomplicated
- Oral bleeding with complicated fractures
- Hypersalivation with acute complicated fractures
- Appetite rarely affected; chewing on opposite side resulting in greater calculus accumulation on affected side
- Calculus may obscure a slab fracture of the maxillary fourth premolar; compare with crown height and shape of the contralateral tooth.
- Acute pulp exposure: red spot in tooth defect ± bleeding from exposed pulp, painful on probing
- Chronic pulp exposure: dark brown/black spot in tooth defect, asymmetrical calculus accumulation (greater on affected side), regional facial swelling ± draining tracts at mucogingival junction or through skin

Etiology and Pathophysiology

- Uncomplicated fracture: exposure of dentinal tubules causes sensitivity and may allow bacterial access to the pulp. Odontoblasts may respond by forming tertiary dentin, sealing off exposed tubules.
- Complicated fracture: pulp exposure results in pulpitis and bacterial infection; most develop pulp necrosis and periapical disease (p. 7).

DIAGNOSIS

Diagnostic Overview

A sedated/anesthetized oral exam and dental radiography are needed to determine whether the fracture is complicated or involves the root.

Differential Diagnosis

- Abrasion/attrition
- Tooth resorption
- Caries
- Displacement injury (luxation/avulsion)

Initial Database

CBC, serum chemistry panel, urinalysis: generally unremarkable (preanesthetic)

Advanced or Confirmatory Testing

- Anesthetized oral exam using a dental explorer (#11/12, 17, or 23) to determine pulp exposure (p. 1140)
- Dental radiographs are indicated to identify extent of lesion and state of adjoining teeth; possible findings include structural crown and/or root defect, arrested root development (open root apex, wide root canal compared with healthy, contralateral tooth), diffuse root canal mineralization, apical root resorption, and/or periapical lucency.

TREATMENT

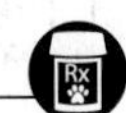

Treatment Overview

Endodontic therapy or extraction is indicated for fractured teeth with pulp exposure. Fractured teeth with no pulp exposure require radiographic evaluation and monitoring because they may also develop endodontic disease. A wait-and-see approach for fractured teeth with pulp exposure is below the standard of care because tooth fractures cause discomfort and invite infection of endodontic and periapical tissues.

Acute General Treatment

- Uncomplicated crown fractures may not require treatment or benefit from smoothing the rough tooth surface and sealing dentinal tubules of exposed dentin with a bonding agent.
- Acute complicated crown fracture: vital pulp therapy (partial pulpectomy, direct pulp capping, and restoration) within 48 hours of pulp exposure. Administer antibiotics (e.g., intraoperative ampicillin 22 mg/kg IV q 6h, followed by amoxicillin/clavulanic acid, 14 mg/kg PO q 12h × 7 days, or clindamycin 11 mg/kg PO q 12h × 7 days).
- Extraction of fractured deciduous or permanent teeth

Chronic Treatment

- Chronic, complicated crown fractures (adult animals): root canal therapy or extraction
- Fractures extending below the gingival attachment (crown-root fractures) may require periodontal surgery to prevent focal periodontal pocketing.
- Prosthodontic crowns are indicated after root canal therapy to protect the remainder of the crowns in dogs.

Possible Complications

- Failure of endodontic therapy: repeat root canal therapy, perform apicoectomy and retrograde filling, or extract the tooth.
- Uncontrolled force during tooth extraction
  - Fracture and incomplete removal of the tooth/root, resulting in periapical abscess (p. 7)
  - Trauma to soft tissues (eye, brain, tongue, salivary gland ducts, and neurovascular structures)

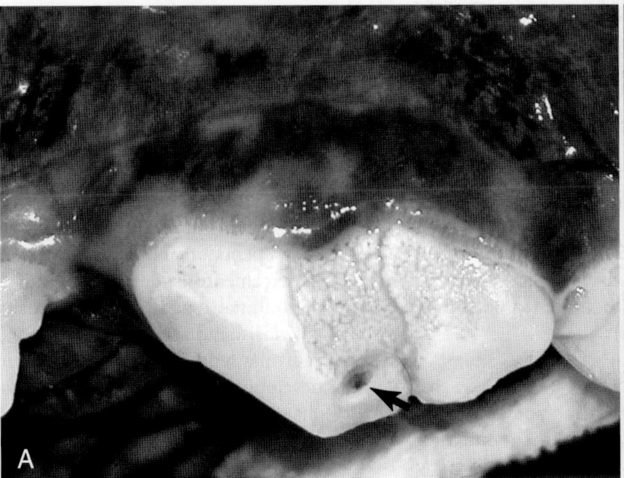

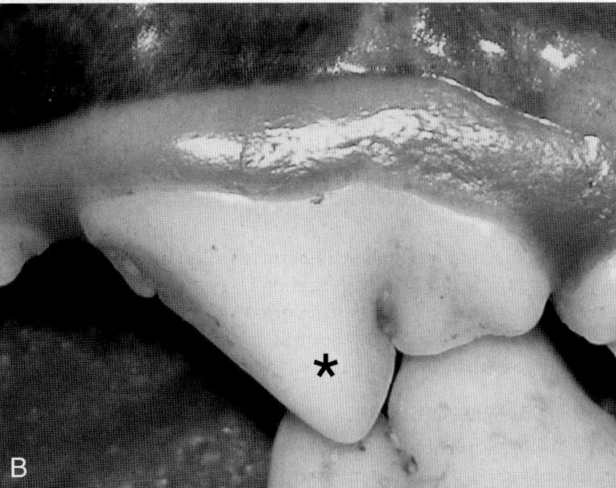

TOOTH FRACTURES **A**, Slab fracture of the left maxillary fourth premolar in a dog. The main cusp is fractured off; there is pulp exposure *(arrow)* and moderate calculus accumulation. Amount of calculus indicates fracture occurred more than 1-2 months before the visit, but bleeding pulp tissue indicates fracture may not be older than 6-12 months. **B**, Normal left maxillary fourth premolar for comparison. The tooth (notably the main cusp *[asterisk]*) is structurally intact; mild calculus accumulation is seen in developmental groove. (Copyright Dr. Alexander M. Reiter, University of Pennsylvania.)

- ◦ Transposition of tooth/root into mandibular/infraorbital canal and nasal passages
- ◦ Iatrogenic jaw fracture

Recommended Monitoring

Endodontic procedures require follow-up radiography under sedation/anesthesia at 6 months postoperatively and yearly thereafter.

PROGNOSIS & OUTCOME

- Excellent with extraction if entire tooth has been removed
- Root canal therapy fails in only 6% of treated roots (depends on skill of the operator).
- Animals that continue abusive chewing habits may benefit from placement of prosthodontic crowns.

PEARLS & CONSIDERATIONS

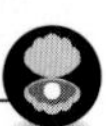

Comments

- Functionally important teeth (i.e., those for chewing, prehending, cosmesis) should be preserved with endodontic therapy rather than being extracted.
- Although root canal therapy can be performed for almost any dog tooth, endodontic therapy in cats is often not feasible because of size, except for the canine teeth.

Prevention

- Control aggressive chewing behavior.
- Avoid chewing on hard objects.

Technician Tips

- Discuss with owners appropriate chewing habits, treats, and toys during wellness visits.
- Technicians may be the first to notice subtle tooth fractures during professional dental cleanings. Bring these fractures to the veterinarian's attention and become accustomed to taking dental radiographs of fractured teeth.

Client Education

- Complicated crown fracture in immature permanent teeth is considered a true emergency if the objective is to save the tooth. Vital pulp therapy must be performed as soon as possible.
- Root canal therapy causes less postoperative discomfort than tooth extraction.

SUGGESTED READING

Soukup JW, et al: Classification and epidemiology of traumatic dentoalveolar injuries in dogs and cats: 959 injuries in 660 patient visits (2004-2012). J Vet Dent 32:6, 2015.

AUTHOR: Lenin A. Villamizar-Martinez, DVM, MS, PhD
EDITOR: Alexander M. Reiter, DVM, Dr. med. vet., DAVDC, DEVDC

Tooth Resorption

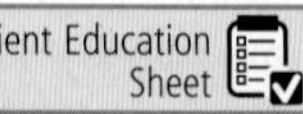

BASIC INFORMATION

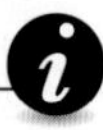

Definition

Loss of tooth substance due to resorption by odontoclasts

Synonyms

- Feline odontoclastic resorptive lesion (FORL), odontoclastic resorptive/resorption lesion, external root resorption, cervical line erosion/lesion, feline caries, neck lesion
- The term *neck lesion* is a topographic distinction only. The terms *erosion* and *caries* are inappropriate because the dental defect is resorptive in nature and not caused by acidic or bacterial insult, respectively.

Epidemiology

SPECIES, AGE, SEX

The condition affecting multiple or all permanent teeth is seen predominantly in domestic cats 4 years of age or older, with a reported prevalence of 25%-75%. It is now seen more frequently in dogs than in years past.

GENETICS, BREED PREDISPOSITION

No obvious breed predisposition; purebred cats have been reported to be affected at a younger age

RISK FACTORS

- Periodontal disease
- Trauma from occlusion
- Dietary composition
- Increased vitamin D levels in commercial diets

ASSOCIATED DISORDERS

- Thickening of bone at the alveolar margin (alveolar bone expansion)
- Abnormal tooth extrusion (particularly canine teeth)

Clinical Presentation

DISEASE FORMS/SUBTYPES

Tooth resorption is classified based on severity (stages 1-5) and radiographic appearance (types 1-3) (https://www.avdc.org/Nomenclature/Nomen-Intro.html):

- Dentoalveolar ankylosis (ankylotic fusion between root and bone) and replacement resorption (resorption followed by bone replacement)
- Inflammatory resorption (vascular and inflamed granulation tissue filling a resorptive defect) and alveolar bone resorption (near the resorptive defect)

HISTORY, CHIEF COMPLAINT

Patients may present with red spots on their teeth (crown defect filled with granulation tissue), repetitive lower jaw motions (jaw opening reflex; teeth chattering), fractured crowns, root remnants, and missing teeth. These animals may also have difficulty eating hard food and may refuse to drink cold water. The majority of cats are diagnosed with tooth resorption from dental radiography.

PHYSICAL EXAM FINDINGS

Oral exam (p. 1140) can reveal crown defects filled with inflamed granulation tissue, fractured crowns, root remnants, bulging gingiva in areas of missing teeth, thickening of bone at the alveolar margin of canine teeth, and abnormal extrusion of canine teeth.

Etiology and Pathophysiology

- Suggested causes include periodontal disease, anatomic peculiarities, mechanical trauma, increased vitamin A and vitamin D intake, abnormal calcium homeostasis, and viruses causing immunosuppression.
- Association of multiple tooth resorption in cats with excessive dietary intake of vitamin D (not proved):
  - ◦ Histologic exam of healthy teeth from cats with tooth resorption of other teeth shows periodontal ligament degeneration, hypercementosis, decreased width of the periodontal space, and dentoalveolar ankylosis, indicating that inflammatory cells may not play a primary role in the development of tooth resorption. Similar changes can be found after administration of high doses of vitamin D or vitamin D metabolites in experimental animals.
  - ◦ Cats with tooth resorption have significantly higher serum levels of 25-hydroxyvitamin D compared with cats without tooth resorption, indicating that those with tooth resorption must have had a higher intake of dietary vitamin D.

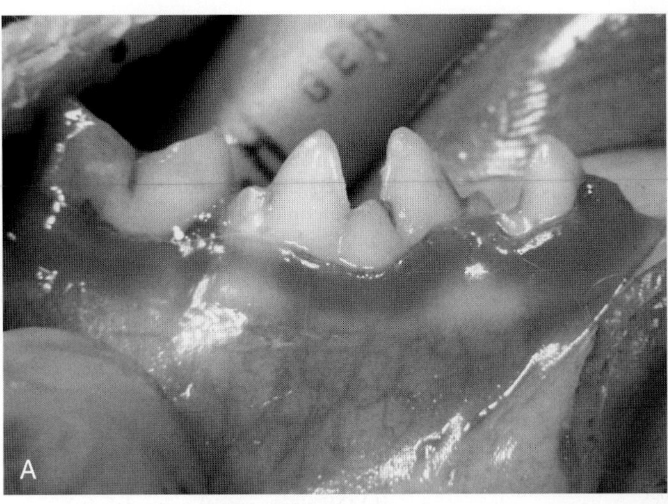

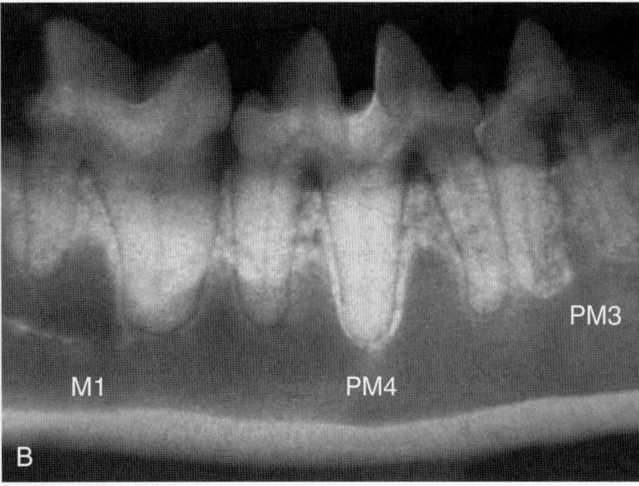

TOOTH RESORPTION A, Clinical picture of right mandibular third and fourth premolars and first molar in a cat (rostral is to the right) shows generalized moderate gingivitis with focalized gingival hyperplasia and possible tooth resorption on the third premolar and first molar. Fourth premolar shows gemination (division of a tooth bud, resulting in the formation of partially or completely separated crowns). **B**, Radiograph of the same area shows generalized mild to moderate horizontal alveolar bone loss, tooth resorption on the third premolar (PM3, with inflammatory resorption near cervical region and furcation and dentoalveolar ankylosis and replacement resorption at distal root) and first molar (M1, with inflammatory resorption near cervical region on mesial tooth surface). Geminated fourth premolar (PM4) does not show obvious radiographic signs of tooth resorption. (Copyright Dr. Alexander M. Reiter, University of Pennsylvania.)

DIAGNOSIS

Diagnostic Overview

Full-mouth dental radiography is of utmost importance in identifying and assessing tooth resorption in cats.

Differential Diagnosis

- Periodontal disease
- Fractured teeth
- Root remnants
- Tooth resorption due to local causes (e.g., periapical abscess, orthodontic tooth movement, trauma, neoplasia)
- Caries (dogs)

Initial Database

Preanesthesia CBC, serum biochemistry profile, urinalysis

Advanced or Confirmatory Testing

Full-mouth (intraoral) dental radiographs show dentoalveolar ankylosis (fusion between alveolar bone and tooth), replacement resorption (root resorption followed by alveolar bone replacement, giving the tooth its moth-eaten appearance on radiographs), and inflammatory resorption closer to the crown (when the resorptive defect becomes exposed to the oral cavity, and an inflammatory component joins the initially noninflammatory lesion).

TREATMENT

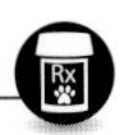

Treatment Overview

Goals of treatment are to make the mouth free of pain, preserve masticatory function, and prevent abscess formation and local osteomyelitis.

Acute General Treatment

- Closed or open extraction of root remnants and teeth affected by resorption
- Flaps should be closed with synthetic absorbable suture material.
- Administration of antibiotics is not usually necessary after tooth extraction unless there is another medical condition or extensive tissue trauma at the extraction site.
- Pain management: regional nerve block(s) intraoperatively (0.2-0.4 mL of 0.5% bupivacaine per block) followed by opioid medications on extubation (methadone 0.1-0.2 mg/kg IV or buprenorphine 0.01-0.02 mg/kg IV) and opioid medications postoperatively for 3-4 days (butorphanol 0.2-0.4 mg/kg PO q 8h or buprenorphine 0.01-0.02 mg/kg buccal transmucosal q 8h); transdermal fentanyl patch (25 mcg) if multiple extractions were performed

Possible Complications

- Fractured teeth and roots
- Root remnants
- Regional trauma due to improper extraction technique
- Infection
- Future development of resorption on other teeth

Recommended Monitoring

- Exam in 2 weeks to evaluate extraction sites
- Clinical exam and full-mouth dental radiography once per year

PROGNOSIS & OUTCOME

- Excellent for extraction site healing
- Fair when preventing the development of resorption on other teeth

PEARLS & CONSIDERATIONS

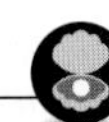

Comments

- Usually more than one tooth is affected.
- Dental radiography is an invaluable tool for diagnosing tooth resorption that is missed on clinical exam.

Prevention

There is no reliable prevention strategy available at this time.

Technician Tips

- Learn how to detect subtle resorptive defects by means of careful assessment of the tooth surface with a dental explorer.
- Become an expert in obtaining full-mouth dental radiographs in cats and dogs.

Client Education

Inform clients about the likelihood of development of resorption on other teeth and the need for continued clinical and radiographic monitoring.

SUGGESTED READING

Reiter AM, et al: Update on the etiology of tooth resorption in domestic cats. Vet Clin North Am Small Anim Pract 35:913, 2005.

AUTHOR & EDITOR: Alexander M. Reiter, DVM, Dr. med. vet., DAVDC, DEVDC

Toxoplasmosis/Neosporosis

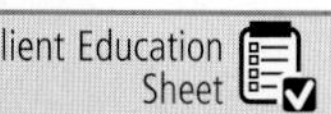

BASIC INFORMATION

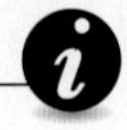

Definition

Infections with *Toxoplasma gondii* or *Neospora caninum,* which are obligate intracellular coccidian parasites that infect mammals, including humans

Epidemiology

SPECIES, AGE, SEX

Felids are definitive and intermediate hosts for *T. gondii.*

- All mammals, including dogs, serve as intermediate hosts.
- Clinical disease can be severe in transplacentally or lactationally infected kittens.
- Cats of any age can be affected.

Dogs are intermediate and definitive hosts for *N. caninum.*

- *N. caninum* infections are known to occur in dogs, cattle, sheep, goats, horses, and deer.
- Puppies are more severely affected, but dogs of any age can be infected.
- Most canine infections are subclinical.
- *N. caninum* antibodies have been detected in cats and people, but neither species is known to develop clinical neosporosis, and exposed cats do not shed *N. caninum* oocysts.

GENETICS, BREED PREDISPOSITION

It is unclear whether any dog or cat breeds are more susceptible to clinical illness from *N. caninum* or *T. gondii,* and so these agents should be on the differential list for all appropriate clinical problems.

RISK FACTORS

- Ingestion of tissue cysts in prey species is the greatest risk factor for feline toxoplasmosis.
- Ingestion of bovine placental tissues or sporulated oocysts in canine feces is the greatest risk factor for canine neosporosis.
- Concurrent immunosuppression (from glucocorticoids or antineoplastic drugs) or concomitant illnesses, such as ehrlichiosis, canine distemper, feline leukemia virus (FeLV), feline immunodeficiency virus (FIV), feline infectious peritonitis (FIP), or *Mycoplasma haemofelis* infection, may potentiate clinical illness. However, both parasites can be primary pathogens.

CONTAGION AND ZOONOSIS

T. gondii is zoonotic:

- Many people are infected by ingesting sporulated oocysts that contaminate the environment or by ingesting undercooked meat.
- A healthy cat positive for *T. gondii*–specific antibodies is of little risk to its owner because it is unlikely to shed oocysts again if exposed.

N. caninum antibodies have been detected in people, suggesting zoonotic transmission, but the agent has not been associated with disease in people.

GEOGRAPHY AND SEASONALITY

- Worldwide; nonseasonal
- Approximately 30% of cats and 15% of dogs in the United States have antibodies against *T. gondii.*
- There is a higher prevalence of antibodies against *N. caninum* among rural or farm dogs than urban dogs.

Clinical Presentation

DISEASE FORMS/SUBTYPES

- Subclinical infection is most common result of infection with *T. gondii* and *N. caninum.*
- Clinical findings of canine toxoplasmosis and neosporosis are similar.

HISTORY, CHIEF COMPLAINT

Toxoplasmosis:

- Approximately 10% of cats have small bowel diarrhea for several days after the first exposure to *T. gondii.*
- If appropriate immune responses occur, most cats and dogs do not develop noticeable clinical signs of *T. gondii* or *N. caninum* infections.
- Transplacental infection with *T. gondii* can lead to abortion or stillbirth in dogs or cats.
- Kittens infected by the transplacental or lactational routes but survive present as fading kittens with nonspecific findings such as anorexia, lethargy, respiratory distress, ocular, and central nervous system (CNS) signs.
- Dogs and cats with *T. gondii* infections in the postpartum period commonly present with nonspecific findings of lethargy and anorexia and occasionally fever.
- Older dogs and cats with *T. gondii* infections can present with anorexia, vomiting, diarrhea, weight loss, lethargy, dyspnea, ocular signs, lameness, possible muscle pain, and signs of CNS dysfunction (ataxia, paresis, seizures, cranial nerve deficits).

Neosporosis:

- In young dogs (<6 months), particularly those with transplacental infections, acute ascending paralysis is typical. Dysphagia, incontinence, and muscle atrophy are also seen.
- Older dogs may present with dermatitis, respiratory signs (cough, dyspnea), gastrointestinal (GI) signs, or neurologic signs (lameness, seizures).

PHYSICAL EXAM FINDINGS

Toxoplasmosis:

- Most infections with *T. gondii* result in no physical exam abnormalities.
- Prenatally infected kittens: hepatomegaly, ascites, dyspnea, and fever
- Clinical infection in cats (as opposed to neonatal kittens) is characterized by uveitis, chorioretinitis, dyspnea, abdominal distension, icterus, fever, stiff gait, hyperesthesia, and neurologic deficits (spinal cord or brain).
- Young dogs (≤1 year old) have generalized infections resulting in fever, icterus, dyspnea, and tonsillitis.
- Older dogs more commonly have neuromuscular signs, including muscle atrophy, stiffness, abnormal gait, and multifocal neurologic deficits involving the spinal cord or brain (seizures, ataxia, lower motor neuron [LMN] signs, cranial nerve deficits).
- Arrhythmias or, rarely, heart failure may be present in some older dogs.

Neosporosis:

- Puppies are more severely affected and show ascending rigid paralysis, with hindlimbs worse than forelimbs.
  - Muscle atrophy and stiffness, muscle contractures leading to arthrogryposis and hyperesthesia. Cervical weakness, dysphagia, and variable CNS signs may also be seen.
- Older dogs may have LMN flaccid paralysis or show multifocal CNS signs (cranial nerve deficits, seizures, blindness).
- Systemic signs include fever, dyspnea, cough, skin lesions, vomiting, icterus, cardiac arrhythmias, megaesophagus, and regurgitation.

Etiology and Pathophysiology

- *T. gondii* exists in three infectious stages: sporozoites, tachyzoites, and bradyzoites.
  - Sporozoites occur in oocysts, which are excreted in feces, whereas tachyzoites infect all cells with formation of bradyzoites in tissue cysts as immune responses develop.
- Transmission can occur through ingestion of infected tissues or ingestion of oocysts in contaminated food or water; transmission can also occur transplacentally or lactationally (proved only for *T. gondii* in kittens, not puppies).
- The enteroepithelial life cycle (and fecal shedding) occurs in cats only after ingestion of intermediate hosts infected with tissue cysts or ingestion of sporulated oocysts. Infection ultimately results in oocyst formation, with millions passed into the environment. Sporulation occurs in 1-3 days, and then the oocysts are infectious.
- The extraintestinal life cycle occurs in all hosts, including cats:
  - After ingestion of oocysts or tissue cysts, the organism invades the small intestine and spreads to many extraintestinal tissues through blood and lymph, where it causes focal necrosis. The CNS, muscles, liver, lungs, and eyes are commonly affected.
  - The organism localizes in tissues as cysts, resulting in chronic infection. The cysts

may rupture, resulting in clinical relapses during immunosuppression.

- The life cycle of *N. caninum* involves three infectious stages: tachyzoites, tissue cysts found primarily in the CNS, and oocysts.
  - Tissue cysts and tachyzoites are found in intermediate hosts.
  - Transmission is suspected to occur through ingestion of sporulated oocysts, ingestion of infected tissues, or transplacentally.
  - Transplacental transmission may be the predominant route in dogs.
  - The organism may be found in macrophages, polymorphonuclear cells, spinal fluid, and neural cells (brain, spinal cord, peripheral nerves, retina), as well as other cells, causing focal necrosis.

DIAGNOSIS

Diagnostic Overview

The diagnosis of toxoplasmosis or neosporosis is based on the combination of clinical findings and results of specific diagnostic tests.

Differential Diagnosis

- Uveitis: infectious (FeLV, FIV, FIP [coronavirus]), immune-mediated, trauma
- Respiratory signs: feline asthma, pneumonia (bacterial, *Mycoplasma,* parasitic, fungal), pulmonary edema, neoplasia, heartworm disease, trauma
- Hepatic: hepatic lipidosis (cats), cholangitis/cholangiohepatitis (cats), infectious hepatitis, neoplasia, toxic hepatopathy
- GI: infectious (bacterial, viral, parasitic), dietary, endocrine (hypoadrenocorticism), obstructive, pancreatitis
- Neurologic signs: meningoencephalitis (FeLV, FIV, FIP, canine distemper, ehrlichiosis, Rocky Mountain spotted fever, rabies, fungal disease, parasitic disease, thiamine deficiency [cats], immune-mediated disease)
- Neuromuscular: hepatozoonosis, Lyme borreliosis, immune-mediated disease (polyradiculoneuritis, polymyositis)

Initial Database

- CBC, serum biochemistry profile, urinalysis
  - Nonregenerative anemia, neutrophilic leukocytosis, lymphocytosis, monocytosis, and eosinophilia are possible with either infection.
  - Leukopenia (lymphopenia, neutropenia, degenerative left shift) is possible in cats severely affected with toxoplasmosis.
- Serum biochemistry profile may show elevated activities of alanine aminotransferase (ALT), aspartate aminotransferase (AST), alkaline phosphatase (ALP), amylase, lipase, and creatine kinase (CK) in dogs or cats with either infection. Hyperbilirubinemia, hyperglobulinemia, hypoalbuminemia, hypoproteinemia, proteinuria, and bilirubinuria may also occur.
- Radiographs
  - Thoracic radiographs may show a diffuse interstitial to alveolar pattern and mild pleural effusion.
  - Abdominal radiographs may show hepatomegaly, ascites, intestinal masses, or mesenteric lymphadenopathy.
- Other tests
  - Oocysts may be detected in the feces of cats with clinical toxoplasmosis or dogs with clinical neosporosis, but shedding has often already stopped by the time clinical illness is noted, leading to false-negative results.
  - Cytologic exam of ascitic fluid, tracheal washes, and pleural fluid may reveal tachyzoites of either organism.

Advanced or Confirmatory Testing

Toxoplasmosis:

- A presumptive diagnosis is usually based on the combination of appropriate clinical signs, positive results of serologic tests, exclusion of other causes for clinical signs, and positive response to treatment.
  - Serologic testing: ELISA tests designed specifically for dogs or cats should be used. A fourfold rise in immunoglobulin (Ig) G over a 2-3 week period or a high IgM titer suggests active infection.
  - Positive IgM titers can have a short duration, but 80% of cats with clinical disease associated with toxoplasmosis have positive IgM titers.
  - IgG reflects only past exposure, but a positive titer along with appropriate clinical signs may suggest toxoplasmosis.
- Cytologic detection of tachyzoites in body fluids or histologic detection of bradyzoites associated with inflammation in tissues suggests toxoplasmosis, and the agent can be confirmed by polymerase chain reaction (PCR) assays.
- *T. gondii* DNA can be amplified from blood, aqueous humor, CSF, and tissues and is positive in clinically ill cats.

Neosporosis:

- A presumptive diagnosis is usually based on the combination of appropriate clinical signs, positive results in serologic tests, exclusion of other causes for clinical signs, and positive response to treatment.
  - Serologic testing with IFA, ELISA, and direct agglutination tests.
- Cytologic detection of tachyzoites in body fluids or histologic detection of bradyzoites associated with inflammation in tissues suggests neosporosis, and the agent can be confirmed by PCR assays.

Both organisms:

- Can be grown in cell culture and in mice
- CSF analysis and aqueous humor may have elevated protein levels and leukocytes in toxoplasmosis and neosporosis.

TREATMENT

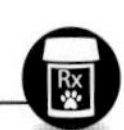

Treatment Overview

Treatment is predominantly supportive, with antimicrobials used as appropriate for the organism. Drugs suppress replication of *T. gondii* and are not completely effective at killing the organism. There is limited information on effectiveness of treatment of neosporosis.

Acute and Chronic Treatment

- Toxoplasmosis: clindamycin is the treatment of choice in dogs and cats.
- Neosporosis should be treated early in the disease with the same drugs used for treating toxoplasmosis. Treatment should continue at least 2 weeks after resolution of clinical signs.
- Clindamycin (dogs) 10-20 mg/kg PO q 12h for at least 2 weeks
- Clindamycin (cats) 12-25 mg/kg PO q 12h for a minimum of 2-4 weeks
- Azithromycin (cats) 10 mg/kg PO q 24h for 4 weeks is also a good choice.
- Alternatively, trimethoprim-sulfonamide 15-30 mg/kg PO q 12h for 2-4 weeks may be used if the patient cannot tolerate clindamycin.
- Ponazuril 20 mg/kg PO q 24h for 28 days was used successfully in one dog with toxoplasmosis and has been used to lessen tissue cysts in rodent models. This drug can be considered in dogs or cats with toxoplasmosis that are intolerant to other drugs.
- Barring corneal ulceration or conjunctivitis, uveitis should be treated with 1% prednisolone acetate ophthalmic drops.

Possible Complications

- Clindamycin may cause anorexia, vomiting, and diarrhea with higher doses.
- Trimethoprim-sulfonamides are associated with bone marrow suppression (anemia, leukopenia, thrombocytopenia), keratoconjunctivitis sicca (KCS), depression, immune-mediated disease, cutaneous drug eruptions, kidney injury, GI signs, and hepatotoxicosis (especially in Doberman pinschers). Reduce dose of trimethoprim-sulfadiazine in kidney disease, and avoid use in hepatic disease, anemia, leukopenia, and congenital bleeding disorders. Cats dislike the taste of sulfa drugs (hypersalivation).
- In cases of fulminant infection, some patients worsen after antimicrobials are started.

Recommended Monitoring

Clinical findings and routine laboratory abnormalities can be rechecked at appropriate intervals for the individual patient. There is no evidence indicating that *T. gondii–* or *N. caninum–*specific tests are of clinical utility, and treatment decisions should be based on clinical responses.

PROGNOSIS & OUTCOME

- Most affected kittens or puppies or immune-suppressed animals with fulminant disease will die or require euthanasia.
- Animals may survive acute disease if treated intensively and rapidly.
  - Guarded for complete resolution of neuromuscular signs

- Clinical improvement is not likely in severe cases of neosporosis with muscle contracture.
- In milder systemic cases, clinical signs of systemic illness usually begin to resolve in 1-2 days after institution of therapy.
- Uveitis should resolve in 1 week with therapy.
- Neuromuscular deficits should partially resolve within 2 weeks of initiation of therapy; however, in most puppies with neosporosis, some signs may be permanent.
- Older puppies (>16 weeks) and adult dogs generally respond better to treatment for *N. caninum*.

PEARLS & CONSIDERATIONS

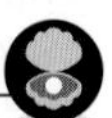

Comments

- Patients with suspected neosporosis or toxoplasmosis should respond to appropriate therapy within several days. If the patient is not responding or progressing, there may be concurrent disorders.
- No drug clears either organism from the tissues of dogs or cats, and relapses may occur.

Prevention

- Do not allow dogs or cats to hunt or eat uncooked meats.
- Clean litter boxes daily (oocysts need 1-5 days to sporulate and become infective).
- Disinfect litter boxes with boiling water at least once weekly.
- Cover outdoor sandboxes to keep feral cats out.
- Immune-suppressed or pregnant cat owners should have someone else clean the feline litter box or clean it daily while wearing gloves.
- Do not allow dogs to defecate in food animal or dairy operations.

Technician Tips

Risk of infection to veterinary staff is minimal to nonexistent with appropriate handling, such as keeping feline feces refrigerated until handled, wearing gloves, and hand washing.

Client Education

- Wash hands and surfaces after handling raw meat or cleaning litter boxes.
- Wear gloves when gardening, and wash vegetables and hands thoroughly to prevent contamination from soil.
- Do not eat undercooked meat or unpasteurized dairy products.
- Boil or filter drinking water from unreliable sources.
- Pregnant women must avoid contact with soil, cat litter, raw meat, and cats excreting oocysts.
- Produce should always be washed thoroughly or cooked because it is now known that people are commonly exposed to *T. gondii* sporulated oocysts in this way.
- Although *T. gondii* has been potentially linked to a number of human behavioral abnormalities, the associations are weak, and owners usually do not acquire toxoplasmosis from their cats.

SUGGESTED READING

Dubey JP, et al: Toxoplasmosis and neosporosis. In Greene CE, editor: Infectious diseases of the dog and cat, St. Louis, 2012, Elsevier, pp 806-827.

AUTHOR: Michael R. Lappin, DVM, PhD, DACVIM
EDITOR: Joseph Taboada, DVM, DACVIM

Tracheal Avulsion

Client Education Sheet

BASIC INFORMATION

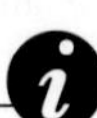

Definition

Disruption in the continuity of or a tear in the trachea

Synonyms

Tracheal laceration, tracheal rupture, tracheal transection

Epidemiology

SPECIES, AGE, SEX

Reported primarily in small dogs and cats; no age or sex predisposition

RISK FACTORS

- Choke chains
- Overinflation of endotracheal tube cuff
- Traumatic intubation
- Cervical trauma
- Thoracic trauma

ASSOCIATED DISORDERS

- Pneumomediastinum
- Pneumothorax
- Subcutaneous emphysema
- Musculoskeletal injury consistent with trauma (cervical/thoracic)

Clinical Presentation

HISTORY, CHIEF COMPLAINT

- History of blunt or penetrating trauma or recent general anesthesia and subsequent dyspnea
- Intermittent, continuous, or progressive respiratory distress
- Chronic onset of dyspnea and exercise intolerance days to weeks after traumatic event
- Initial dyspnea may persist, worsen, or resolve until subsequent stenosis or displacement causes return of clinical signs.

PHYSICAL EXAM FINDINGS

- Increased respiratory effort: decreased heart and breath sounds if pneumothorax
- Subcutaneous emphysema (inflated, crepitant subcutaneous space)
- Precipitation of severe dyspnea with neck flexion
- Severity of signs depends on severity of tear

Etiology and Pathophysiology

- Direct injury to the trachea due to blunt or penetrating trauma to the cervical or thoracic area (e.g., bite wounds, hit-by-car)
- Violent hyperextension of the head and neck can stretch the trachea and cause tracheal transection.
  - The carina and lungs are a fixed point that is stronger than the tracheal wall.
  - As the trachea is stretched, the intrathoracic trachea ruptures cranial (1-4 cm) to the carina.
- The dorsal tracheal membrane is the most common site of tear from overinflation of an endotracheal tube cuff (cats > dogs).
- Peritracheal tissues (adventitia or mediastinum) can maintain tracheal continuity (psuedotrachea).

DIAGNOSIS

Diagnostic Overview

Tracheal avulsion is suggested by a history of cervical trauma or recent anesthesia, especially in the presence of subcutaneous emphysema, pneumomediastinum, or obvious radiographic disruption of the trachea. These patients typically present 2-3 weeks after the initial injury with signs of airway obstruction.

Differential Diagnosis

- Tracheal foreign body
- Collapsing trachea
- Tracheal stenosis
- Tracheal neoplasia or mass
- Laryngeal paralysis
- Laryngeal collapse
- Tracheobronchitis
- Pneumothorax/pneumomediastinum from other causes
- Pulmonary disease

Initial Database

- Results of CBC, serum biochemistry panel, and urinalysis are usually unremarkable.
- Cervical radiographs (lateral view) may show discontinuity of the tracheal wall. Site of rupture may be obscured by the humeri or

scapulae, requiring retaking radiographs with the forelimbs repositioned.
- Cervical and/or thoracic radiographs may show peritracheal air accumulation, subcutaneous emphysema, and/or pneumomediastinum.
  - Pneumothorax is rare.
  - Tracheal stenosis can occur with chronicity.

Advanced or Confirmatory Testing

- Tracheoscopy (p. 1074) can confirm tracheal rupture, especially of the dorsal tracheal membrane, if a radiographic diagnosis is not definitive.
- Thoracic CT may be more sensitive for detecting tracheal injury than thoracic radiographs based on studies in human patients.

TREATMENT

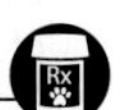

Treatment Overview

- The goals of treatment are to stabilize the patient and if necessary, repair or resect damaged trachea or stenosis to resolve respiratory distress.
- Surgery is not always needed; see guidelines below (Chronic Treatment)

Acute General Treatment

- Oxygen supplementation if dyspneic (p. 1146)
- For animals in respiratory distress, induction of anesthesia or heavy sedation with intubation per os or through a cervical tracheal laceration (if present) is indicated to quickly gain control of the airway:
  - Intubation through a cervical laceration/avulsion is accomplished in similar fashion to tracheostomy (p. 1166).
  - Distal cervical tracheal lacerations may require retrieval of the distal trachea from the thoracic inlet by traction sutures.
- Thoracocentesis may be indicated if pneumothorax is present (p. 1164).
- Prepare the animal for exploration of all structures in the injured area to determine extent of injury and provide the opportunity for primary repair.
- Treat any additional wounds.
- Antibiotics are indicated, especially if traumatic injuries are present.
- Coverage against skin organisms (*Staphylococcus* or *Streptococcus* spp) is considered most important.
  - Ampicillin 22 mg/kg PO or IV q 8-12h, cefazolin 22 mg/kg PO or IV q 12h, or clavulanic acid/amoxicillin 12.5-25 mg/kg PO q 8-12h (dogs), 62.5 mg PO q 8-12h (cats)
  - Enrofloxacin 5-20 mg/kg PO or IV q 24h if concerned about gram-negative organisms (maximum 5 mg/kg PO q 24h in cats)
  - Pradofloxacin 7.5 mg/kg PO q 24h in cats

Chronic Treatment

Closure and debridement of tracheal laceration:
- Surgery is indicated for repair of tracheal defects if
  - The cause is from injury associated with contamination (e.g., bite wounds or other penetrating injury).
  - The animal is not improving or getting worse with conservative (nonsurgical) treatment (see Acute General Treatment above).
  - There is stenosis or stricture causing respiratory difficulty.

Resection of damaged or stenotic trachea and anastomosis of normal ends:
- Minimize tension.
- May need to use tracheal tubes/stents
- Use a tape neck splint to hold the neck in a flexed position to reduce tension on the trachea postoperatively. Try to keep the splint in place for 2 weeks if it is needed.

Behavior/Exercise

Restrict exercise for 2-4 weeks.

Possible Complications

- Dehiscence if excessive tracheal suture tension is present
- Narrowing of the tracheal lumen (stricture) due to scar tissue secondary to tracheal anastomosis
- Infection

Recommended Monitoring

- Monitor for respiratory distress.
- Drainage of peritracheal area may be indicated if area is contaminated.
- Small areas of tracheal granulation tissue may be removed through a bronchoscope at periodic exams during the healing period.
- Removal of tubes/stents is indicated when the mucosal surface is healed.

PROGNOSIS & OUTCOME

- Good for long-term resolution of clinical signs
- Tracheal stricture may be a complication postoperatively.
- Nerve damage postoperatively has been reported in rare cases.

PEARLS & CONSIDERATIONS

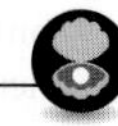

Comments

- Trauma is the most common cause of tracheal tear in small dogs.
- Overinflation of the endotracheal tube is the most common cause of tracheal tear in cats.
  - Tears can occur from overinflation of low-volume/high-pressure cuffs or high-volume/low-pressure cuffs.

Technician Tips

- When managing a patient with a suspected tracheal tear intraoperatively, have a sterile endotracheal tube readily available in case the trachea within the sterile field needs to be intubated. Have an extra-long endotracheal tube handy in case the avulsed trachea needs to be temporarily bridged.
- Be very careful not to overinflate endotracheal cuffs during general anesthesia.

Client Education

Recurrence of clinical signs is possible secondary to tracheal stenosis.

SUGGESTED READING

White RN, et al: Surgical management of intrathoracic tracheal avulsion in cats: long-term results in nine consecutive cases. Vet Surg 29:430, 2000.

AUTHOR: Michael B. Mison, DVM, DACVS
EDITOR: Megan Grobman, DVM, MS, DACVIM

Tracheobronchitis, Infectious (Dog)

Bonus Material Online 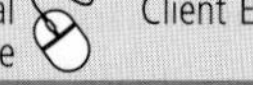 Client Education Sheet 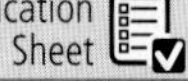

BASIC INFORMATION

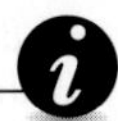

Definition

The common, acute, highly contagious respiratory disease complex of dogs is caused by a number of potential pathogens alone or in combination. The common manifestations include cough, sneezing, oculonasal discharge, lethargy, decreased appetite, and occasionally bronchopneumonia. More information on this disease in cats is provided on p. 1006.

Synonyms

Canine infectious respiratory disease complex (CIRDC); infectious tracheobronchitis; kennel cough

Epidemiology

SPECIES, AGE, SEX

- Common in dogs of all ages, with puppies prone to more severe disease
- Brachycephalic breeds may be more susceptible.

RISK FACTORS

- Unvaccinated status: higher incidence and infections are more severe
- Exposure to infected dogs
- Higher prevalence in group housing or multi-dog settings
- Stress and crowded conditions increase risk of disease.

CONTAGION AND ZOONOSIS

- Highly contagious among dogs; some pathogens (e.g., *Bordetella bronchiseptica*) may also be contagious to cats.
- Immunocompromised people or those with respiratory disease are at a small risk from some but not all involved pathogens.
- Incubation periods are variable, depending on which pathogens are involved (2 days for influenza, up to 6 weeks for distemper virus).
- All CIRDC pathogens can be shed before clinical signs are apparent (i.e., dogs may be contagious before they become ill). Shedding typically lasts 7 days but is variable with each infective agent, and some may be shed for months (e.g., *Bordetella*, distemper).

ASSOCIATED DISORDERS

Secondary bacterial pneumonia

Clinical Presentation

DISEASE FORMS/SUBTYPES

- Most illnesses are characterized by coughing, sneezing, and mild oculonasal discharge. Lethargy and decreased appetite may be noted.
- Unvaccinated dogs (especially puppies) or immunodeficient dogs may develop severe systemic disease with pneumonia.

HISTORY, CHIEF COMPLAINT

- Usually, history of recent exposure to groups of unfamiliar dogs (e.g., animal shelter, boarding, groomer, dog show)
- Cough ranges from soft and moist to deep and hacking, often followed by terminal retch (may be misinterpreted by client as vomiting).
- Owners often think the dog has "something stuck in its throat."
- Signs of pneumonia (p. 795)

PHYSICAL EXAM FINDINGS

- Common: serous to mucoid nasal discharge; ocular discharge with possible conjunctivitis; easily elicited or spontaneous cough (productive or dry, often harsh and hacking)
- Pneumonia: depression; harsh lung sounds with or without crackles and wheeze; tachypnea ± fever, dyspnea, and/or cyanosis

Etiology and Pathophysiology

- Usually, the multi-etiologic disease involves one or more agents: *B. bronchiseptica* (p. 125), canine parainfluenza virus (CPIV), canine adenovirus 2 (CAV-2), canine influenza virus (CIV, H3N2, H3N8 [p. 545]), canine herpesvirus (CHV), canine pneumovirus, canine respiratory coronavirus (CRCV), *Mycoplasma* spp, *Streptococcus equi* subsp *zooepidemicus,* pneumovirus, and canine distemper virus (CDV [p. 271]). Recently identified canine hepacivirus and canine bocavirus may also contribute to CIRDC.
    - The most frequently identified pathogens differ with locality and vaccination status; *B. bronchiseptica** and *Mycoplasma* spp are the most commonly identified bacterial culprits; CRCV, CPIV*, pneumovirus, and CAV-2* are common viral pathogens (*vaccine-preventable).
    - Depending on infectious agent, transmission occurs through direct contact, aerosol, fomite, or oral/fecal route.

DIAGNOSIS

Diagnostic Overview

Presumptive diagnosis is made on history (exposure, vaccination status) and clinical signs. Similar illness in multiple exposed dogs greatly strengthens clinical suspicion of CIRDC. For an individual pet, diagnostic tests may be performed to exclude other, more serious disorders, leaving infectious tracheobronchitis as a diagnosis of exclusion. In complicated cases or during outbreaks (e.g., boarding facilities, animal shelters), tests may be indicated to identify specific pathogens.

Differential Diagnosis

Acute cough: aspiration pneumonia, airway foreign body, heartworm disease, congestive heart failure, noncardiogenic pulmonary edema, pulmonary thromboembolism, exacerbation of chronic condition such as collapsing trachea

Initial Database

- For dogs with a simple cough, presumptive diagnosis based on history and exam is sufficient.
- For dogs with suspected pneumonia
    - CBC: normal, or neutrophilic leukocytosis ± left shift, lymphopenia
    - Serum chemistry panel and urinalysis: assess systemic health; often normal
    - Thoracic radiographs: normal or diffuse, unstructured interstitial pattern (viral pneumonia), or focal or diffuse alveolar pattern (bacterial pneumonia), hyperinflation or atelectasis, or complete lobar consolidation
    - Airway lavage (p. 1073; fluid analysis; culture and susceptibility): neutrophilic inflammation ± bacteria
    - Oxygenation assessment

Advanced or Confirmatory Testing

Identification of specific pathogens during an outbreak can be useful to guide preventive measures. Polymerase chain reaction (PCR) testing with a CIRDC panel from nasal or pharyngeal swabs may be the most cost-effective and least invasive testing method.

- Multiple animals should be tested as early in the course of illness as possible. Testing 3-5 dogs, or 10%-30% of affected animals, is ideal. Because secondary pathogens are common and false-negatives occur, testing multiple dogs allows detection of the common denominator of infected dogs.
- Timing of collection of samples is crucial. For example, CIV is shed early in the course of the disease before clinical signs, and even a few days' delay in testing can give false-negative results.
- False-positive PCR results can occur if modified live vaccines have been given recently. Some laboratories can help differentiate vaccination from infection.
- *Mycoplasma* spp are difficult to grow in culture; PCR offers a more sensitive means of detection.
- Contact the laboratory before sample collection for methodologic details. PCR tests are susceptible to contamination and error; use only laboratories with stringent quality control.

TREATMENT

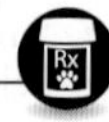

Treatment Overview

- For uncomplicated disease, the goal of treatment is cough suppression and prevention of secondary infection; the cough resolves spontaneously (7-14 days).
- For dogs with pneumonia, the goals are to identify and eradicate any causative bacteria, maintain oxygenation and respiratory epithelial health, and provide supportive care.

Acute General Treatment

For dogs with uncomplicated disease, at home care is preferred.

- Antitussives (contraindicated in pneumonia)
    - Hydrocodone 0.2-0.5 mg/kg PO q 6-12h prn
    - Butorphanol 0.5-1 mg/kg PO, SQ, or IM q 6-12h prn
    - Dextromethorphan (available in over-the-counter human cough suppressants) 1-2 mg/kg PO q 6-8h. Warn owners to avoid products that contain other ingredients such as antihistamines and decongestants.
- Antimicrobial therapy is usually *not* required. If it is to be given due to concern regarding secondary infection or early/mild pneumonia, make reasonable empirical choices:
    - Doxycycline or minocycline 5-10 mg/kg PO q 12h
    - Amoxicillin/clavulanic acid 12-25 mg/kg PO q 8-12h
    - Azithromycin 5-10 mg/kg PO q 12-24h

For dogs with pneumonia, hospitalization in isolation from other dogs may be required depending on disease severity. Infection is highly contagious, and strict biosecurity is essential.

- Antibiotic selection should be based on culture and sensitivity (C&S) results (p. 795).
- Further therapy, including oxygen supplementation (p. 1146), bronchodilators, aerosol

therapy (p. 1122), judicious IV crystalloid fluids, and supportive care, may be required, depending on disease severity.

Behavior/Exercise

- Keep away from communal dog areas such as dog parks.
- Limit exercise during recovery to avoid eliciting cough.
- Avoid neck collars to decrease tracheal stimulation.

PROGNOSIS & OUTCOME

Prognosis for dogs with uncomplicated disease is excellent. Prognosis for those with pneumonia is guarded to good, depending on age of animal and severity of disease.

PEARLS & CONSIDERATIONS

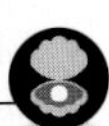

Prevention

Vaccines are available for some but not all agents of CIRDC. CDV and CAV-2 are considered core vaccines, whereas vaccines for CPIV, *B. bronchiseptica*, and CIV are conditional-use vaccines.

- Single-component and multivalent vaccines are available for most listed agents.
- Depending on the agent, vaccines may be available as intranasal, oral, or injectable formulations.
- Vaccination protocols and duration of immunity vary by product.

Considerations for vaccine use:

- Likelihood of exposure (e.g., boarding, dog sports)
- Geographic considerations (e.g., endemic foci of CIV)
- Underlying health issues: animals with chronic cardiorespiratory disease may be less able to withstand CIRDC and benefit from vaccination; animals with a history of immune-mediated disease may be more likely to develop complications.
- Breed: hemorrhagic pneumonia is reported in greyhounds with CIV; brachiocephalic breeds may develop pneumonia due to CIRDC more often than mesocephalic breeds.
- The owner's perception of risks and rewards of vaccination

Technician Tips

- Wear gloves, wash hands, and strictly isolate patients to prevent spread to other hospitalized dogs. If ill animals cannot be moved to an isolation building, isolation distances of 25 feet should be maintained between ill and healthy dogs.
- Clean nasal and ocular discharge with a warm, moist cloth.
- Warm food to enhance smell when offering it (p. 1199).
- Damp environments increase spread of disease; do not allow damp kennels.
- To prevent cross-species transmission, house cats separately.

Client Education

- Limit exposure to other dogs, especially in high-density populations such as boarding kennels, shelters, and dog parks.
- If exposure is unavoidable, recommend complete vaccination 5-14 days before potential risk.
- Educate clients that antimicrobials do not cure or shorten the course of viral infections and that most causes of CIRDC are viral.

SUGGESTED READING

Ellis JA, et al: A review of canine parainfluenza virus infection in dogs. J Am Vet Med Assoc 240:273-284, 2012.

AUTHOR: Wendy Wolfson, DVM

EDITOR: Joseph Taboada, DVM, DACVIM

Transfusion Reactions

BASIC INFORMATION

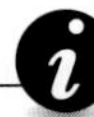

Definition

Adverse effects develop due to the infusion of blood products (p. 1169). Reactions can be classified as acute (minutes to 48 hours later) or delayed (days to weeks after transfusion) and as immunologic or nonimmunologic.

Epidemiology

SPECIES, AGE, SEX

Dogs and cats of any age and either sex

GENETICS, BREED PREDISPOSITION

Certain cat breeds have a higher prevalence of type B blood and are at greater risk of receiving noncompatible blood (p. 686).

RISK FACTORS

Previous blood transfusions

CONTAGION AND ZOONOSIS

Infection can be a type of nonimmunologic delayed adverse transfusion reaction, and some of these infections are transmissible (e.g., feline leukemia virus).

Clinical Presentation

DISEASE FORMS/SUBTYPES

Acute immunologic:

- Acute hemolytic transfusion reaction (AHTR): pre-existing antibodies in the recipient's plasma target antigens on donor red blood cells (RBCs) (incompatible blood type). Reaction severity is proportional to the volume of blood transfused.
- Febrile nonhemolytic transfusion reaction (FNHTR): pre-existing antibodies in the recipient interact with antigens on the donor's leukocytes, platelets, or proteins. Characterized as a 1°C or greater increase in body temperature during or shortly after a transfusion that cannot be attributable to an underlying cause
- Allergic reaction: recipient with pre-existing antibodies that bind to an allergen (antigen, protein) in the donor plasma, causing a hypersensitivity reaction

Acute nonimmunologic:

- Transfusion-related sepsis: infusion of bacterially contaminated blood products, usually due to a lack of aseptic collection, storage, or administration; subclinical infection in the donor; and long infusion times (>4 hours)
- Citrate toxicity (hypocalcemia): during large-volume, rapid transfusions or in patients with significant hepatic dysfunction, the normal metabolism of the anticoagulant citrate is overwhelmed, allowing binding of the recipient's calcium (by citrate), causing hypocalcemia and preventing thrombus formation.
- Volume overload: in normovolemic patients, especially with compromised cardiac or renal function, rapid or large-volume transfusions can cause hypervolemia, particularly in cats and small dogs.
- Hypothermia: infusion of large volumes of refrigerated or frozen blood products, especially in small patients
- Dilutional coagulopathy: dilution or loss of platelets and clotting factors during massive transfusions (>1 blood volume in 24 hours [rare])
- *In vitro* hemolysis: improper handling of blood products (freezing, overheating, inappropriate infusion devices) can cause hemolysis.
- Hyperammonemia: older units of stored blood accumulate ammonia. Infusion in recipients with poor hepatic function can cause hyperammonemia.

Delayed immunologic:

- Delayed hemolytic transfusion reaction (DHTR): recipient develops antibodies to donor antigens 3-14 days after transfusion and shortens the life span of transfused RBCs.

Delayed nonimmunologic:

- Infectious disease transmission

Transfusion-related acute lung injury (TRALI):

- Can be classified as acute or delayed and immunologic or nonimmunologic
- Pulmonary endothelial damage results in vascular leakage and neutrophil activation (humans). Anecdotal reports in dogs and cats.

HISTORY, CHIEF COMPLAINT

Current (acute reaction) or recent (delayed reaction) transfusion of whole blood, packed RBCs (pRBCs), platelets, or plasma

PHYSICAL EXAM FINDINGS

Initial signs of a transfusion reaction may be subtle, but if unnoticed, the recipient's condition can rapidly decline.

Clinical signs associated with acute immunologic reactions:

- Whole blood/pRBCs: vomiting, fever, hemolysis (pallor, tachycardia, weakness), pigmenturia, jaundice, anaphylaxis, tachypnea/dyspnea, urticaria, pruritus, hypotension (weak pulse), ventricular arrhythmias, apnea
- Platelets: fever, vomiting
- Plasma: urticaria, edema, pruritus, erythema

Clinical signs associated with acute nonimmunologic reactions:

- Transfusion-related sepsis: signs of sepsis (fever, weak pulse, tachycardia), hemoglobinuria, vomiting
- Citrate toxicity: vomiting, tremors, tetany, excessive hemorrhage
- Volume overload: dyspnea, tachypnea, tachycardia, cough (dry, soft initially), vomiting
- Dilutional coagulopathy: excessive hemorrhage
- Improper collection, *in vitro* hemolysis: vomiting
- Hyperammonemia: neurologic signs

Clinical signs associated with delayed immunologic reactions:

- Whole blood/pRBCs: fever, jaundice, premature recurrence of anemia
- Platelets: thrombocytopenia (post-transfusion purpura [rare]), spontaneous hemorrhage

Clinical signs associated with delayed nonimmunologic reactions: disease transmission; signs vary with pathogen

Clinical signs associated with TRALI: dyspnea (noncardiogenic pulmonary edema), tachypnea

Etiology and Pathophysiology

Immunologic: a sensitized recipient mounts an immune response to a specific antigen (cellular or protein) in transfused blood.

- Acute: patients receiving incompatible blood.
  - Dogs: usually dog erythrocyte antigen (DEA) 1.1 incompatibility
  - Cats: usually incompatibility with A/B blood types; reactions severe in type B cats receiving type A blood. In the United States, purebred cats are more likely than domestic shorthair cats to have type B blood.
- Delayed: immune response with antibodies to minor RBC antigens

Nonimmunologic: bacterial contamination, improper unit selection, handling, or administration

DIAGNOSIS

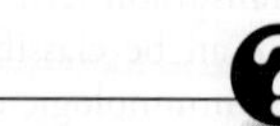

Diagnostic Overview

For acute transfusion reactions, clinical signs usually develop during or immediately after completion of the transfusion. For delayed reactions, clinical signs typically occur several days or longer after a transfusion and may present similar to a recurrence of the primary disorder (e.g., hemolysis). Additional diagnostic testing may be required based on the type and severity of the reaction.

Differential Diagnosis

- Hemolysis: underlying hemolytic disorder (p. 59)
- Fever: acute hemolytic transfusion reaction, sepsis, underlying inflammatory or infectious disease
- TRALI: volume overload (difficult to distinguish from each other)

Initial Database

- CBC, serum biochemistry
  - Hemoglobinemia (red/pink serum; repeat blood sampling to rule out hemolysis due to collection technique or sample handling)
  - Bilirubinemia
  - Leukocytosis
- Urinalysis: hemoglobinuria, bilirubinuria
- Hypocalcemia (ionized): citrate toxicity
- Blood pressure: hypotension (p. 1065)
- Thoracic radiographs
  - Suspected volume overload or TRALI (rule out pulmonary edema)
  - Enlarged pulmonary vasculature supports fluid volume overload.
- Prothrombin time (PT)/activated partial thromboplastin time (aPTT)/platelet count: before and during massive transfusions

Advanced or Confirmatory Testing

- AHTR: confirm hemolysis in recipient (centrifuge); perform major cross match, ideally with pretransfused recipient blood (p. 1084); Coombs' test on recipient
- Inspect transfused unit for contamination.
  - Dark discoloration, clots, air bubbles
  - *In vitro* hemolysis (unit and administration set)
  - Gram stain and culture (aerobic/anaerobic)
- Echocardiography (p. 1094) and central venous pressure may help distinguish volume overload from TRALI.
- Specific testing if infectious disease transmission suspected (e.g., blood culture, serology, polymerase chain reaction [PCR])

TREATMENT

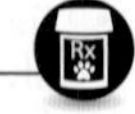

Treatment Overview

Treatment depends on the type and severity of reaction. In mild reactions, slowing or stopping the transfusion might be sufficient, but in severe reactions, aggressive fluid and pharmacologic therapy may be required. Supportive care is necessary while the cause of the reaction is identified and corrected.

Acute General Treatment

- The initial action should be to stop the transfusion; it can often be restarted at a slower rate when the patient is stable.
- AHTR: treat for hypotensive shock (IV fluids, vasopressor agents for persistent hypotension). Glucocorticoids are not likely beneficial.
- FNHTR: temporarily stop or slow the infusion rate. If the fever is significant, antihistamines or nonsteroidal antiinflammatory drugs (NSAIDs) might reduce the fever. Discontinue the transfusion if the fever persists or worsens.
- Volume overload: diuretics (furosemide 2 mg/kg IV) and oxygen (p. 1146)
- Sepsis: obtain samples for culture, IV antibiotics, and IV fluids
- Dilutional coagulopathy: transfuse fresh-frozen plasma if prolonged PT or aPTT (p. 1169).
- TRALI: oxygen supplementation, maintain blood pressure (IV fluids ± vasopressors). Glucocorticoids are controversial; avoid diuretics. May require ventilatory support (p. 1185)

Chronic Treatment

Recognition of infectious disease may be delayed; treatment varies with pathogen type.

Possible Complications

- AHTR and reactions to contaminated blood may be severe and require an aggressive therapeutic response. Most other reactions, when detected early, respond to conservative management.
- AHTR from contaminated blood: hypotension, shock, renal failure, disseminated intravascular coagulation
- Volume overload, TRALI: hypoxemia
- TRALI: hypotension, hypoxemia

Recommended Monitoring

Monitor mentation, temperature, vital parameters, hematocrit before, during, and after transfusion, with very close monitoring of mentation and vital parameters (q 15 minutes) through at least the first 60 minutes.

PROGNOSIS & OUTCOME

- Stable patients: good with early recognition and intervention
- Critical patients: guarded

PEARLS & CONSIDERATIONS

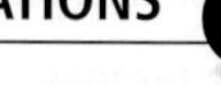

Comments

- Pretreatment with antihistamines or glucocorticoids *may not* prevent immunologic reactions.
- Severe reactions usually occur during or shortly after transfusion.
- Most AHTRs can be prevented by using DEA 1.1–negative canine blood donors (for nontyped recipients) and using typed and matched feline blood donors.
- With the discovery of new RBC antigens (e.g., Mik in cats; Dal in dogs), pretransfusion cross-matching should be performed for all cats and all previously transfused dogs.

- Major cross-matches detect antibodies against donor RBCs. Nonimmune reactions or reactions from antibodies targeting leukocytes, platelets, or proteins are not detected.

Prevention

- All donors should be blood typed and screened regularly for infectious diseases, use flea and tick prevention, and have blood collected using a sterile technique.
- Recipients should be blood typed (all cats) and cross-matched if possible, especially if they have received previous transfusions.
- Never use outdated or hemolyzed products.
- Consider the recipient's underlying disorders when choosing blood product and administration rate.
- Follow strict guidelines for storage, handling, and administration (p. 1169).
- Monitor (mentation, temperature, vital parameters) transfusions carefully.

Technician Tips

- Inspect all units before infusion and discard if discolored, hemolyzed, or expired.
- Monitor patients closely during the transfusion using a checklist to ensure early recognition of potential reactions.
- All staff should be familiar with signs of transfusion reactions.

SUGGESTED READING

Tocci LJ: Transfusion medicine in small animal practice. Vet Clin North Am Small Anim Pract 40:485-494, 2010.

AUTHOR: John M. Thomason, DVM, MS, DACVIM
EDITOR: Jonathan E. Fogle, DVM, PhD, DACVIM

Transitional Cell Carcinoma

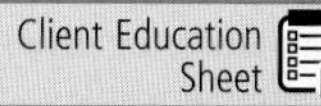

BASIC INFORMATION

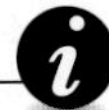

Definition

Neoplasms of epithelial origin that arise in the bladder parenchyma are relatively common in dogs but rare in cats.

Epidemiology

SPECIES, AGE, SEX

- Dogs: typically, older adults (median age, 11 years). Females are at higher risk than males.
- Cats: affects older adults rarely; males at increased risk

GENETICS, BREED PREDISPOSITION

Scottish terriers (up to 20-fold increased risk), Shetland sheepdogs, West Highland white terriers, wirehaired fox terriers, Airedales, beagles, and collies have higher incidences.

RISK FACTORS

- Dogs: female predominance. Exposure to herbicides and insecticides is associated with an increased risk that is worsened in the presence of obesity, possibly due to accumulation of inert ingredients. Spot-on flea products do not appear to increase risk. Cyclophosphamide administration and chronic urinary tract infection (UTI) appear to increase risk.
- Cats: possibly associated with chronic UTI; older cats at greatest risk

ASSOCIATED DISORDERS

- Bacterial cystitis
- Hypertrophic osteopathy
- Urethral obstruction
- Bladder atonia/hypotonia

Clinical Presentation

DISEASE FORMS/SUBTYPES

- Most common form is invasive cancer into muscularis, most often in trigone region.
- Early form of superficial cancer may be identified that may be more responsive to therapy.

HISTORY, CHIEF COMPLAINT

- Pollakiuria (common)
- Hematuria (common)
- Stranguria (common)
- Tenesmus (occasional)
- Abdominal pain (occasional)
- Abdominal distention (occasional)
- Lameness and joint thickening (rare; associated with hypertrophic osteopathy)

PHYSICAL EXAM FINDINGS

- Abdominal tenderness +/−
- Caudal abdominal mass +/−
- Urethral mass on rectal exam +/−
- Distended urinary bladder +/−
- Abdominal distention with fluid wave if bladder ruptured (rare)

Etiology and Pathophysiology

- Bladder mass most commonly in trigone region (dogs).
- Urethral or prostate involvement is common, often leading to obstruction.
- Lymph node metastasis present in ≈15% of cases at the time of diagnosis
- Distant metastasis common (49% at death)
- Metastatic sites include lymph node, lung, liver, kidney, spleen, uterus, gastrointestinal (GI) tract, bone, muscle, cystocentesis needle tracts.
- Secondary bacterial cystitis is common.

DIAGNOSIS

Diagnostic Overview

Middle-aged to older animals with signs of recurrent UTI should be screened for bladder masses, and dogs of at-risk breeds (particularly Scottish terriers) should be screened early. Early diagnosis allows the best outcome.

Differential Diagnosis

Pollakiuria, stranguria, hematuria:

- UTI
- Urolithiasis
- Feline lower urinary tract disease/interstitial cystitis
- Other bladder tumor such as botryoid rhabdomyosarcoma (in young, large-breed dogs) or leiomyosarcoma

Abdominal distention/tenderness or abdominal mass:

- Mass in spleen, mesenteric lymph node, or retroperitoneal space
- Ruptured splenic or hepatic mass with hemoperitoneum
- Abdominal trauma or coagulopathy with peritoneal or retroperitoneal bleeding
- Rectal mass
- Prostatic abscess, cyst, or neoplasia
- Pyelonephritis
- Hydronephrosis or hydroureter

Radiographic:

- Other bladder neoplasm or radiolucent urolithiasis
- Ruptured splenic, renal, or hepatic mass with hemoperitoneum
- Traumatic bladder rupture

Ultrasonographic:

- Papillary cystitis
- Leiomyosarcoma
- Botryoid rhabdomyosarcoma
- Lymphoma (rare)
- Other rare carcinomas or sarcomas

Urinalysis:

- UTI
- Urolithiasis
- Other bladder tumor
- Idiopathic renal hematuria

Initial Database

- CBC, serum biochemistry profile: no specific findings. Azotemia and hyperkalemia if obstruction present
- Urinalysis: proteinuria and hematuria are common and may be complicated by secondary bacterial UTI with pyuria, bacteruria. Cystocentesis has been associated with needle-tract neoplastic cell implantation and should be avoided if transitional cell carcinoma (TCC) is suspected or confirmed; recommend catheterization or free-catch method.
- Veterinary bladder tumor antigen test (VBTA): ≈85% sensitive for TCC but only

45% specific in the presence of other urinary tract disease. It can be used as a screening test (negative result is 85% reliable), but a positive result does not confirm TCC.
- Test for *BRAF* V595E mutation (CADET): polymerase chain reaction (PCR) assay of urine for a common mutant gene in bladder cancer is 85% sensitive and 100% specific for bladder cancer.
- Abdominal radiographs: visualization of bladder mass is uncommon. Bladder distention may be seen, and with rupture, peritoneal or retroperitoneal fluid may be present.
- Thoracic radiographs: metastases may be present. Pulmonary lesions may be nodular interstitial, unstructured interstitial, cavitated, or alveolar in appearance; bone lesions possible
- Abdominal ultrasound: bladder mass or wall thickening with possible metastasis to abdominal organs or nodes; prostate or urethra is commonly involved. Study is insensitive for monitoring tumor size.
- CT: useful for monitoring total tumor volume and staging for metastasis to lymph nodes and lungs

Advanced or Confirmatory Testing

- Cytologic analysis from guided diagnostic catheterization or biopsy from cystoscopy necessary for diagnosis (p. 1085)
- Positive *BRAF* mutation may substitute if tissue is not diagnostic.
- Contrast cystography/ureterography or CT scan may be used for delineating ureteral involvement and impending urethral obstruction.

TREATMENT

Treatment Overview

The therapeutic goals are to alleviate clinical signs, control the primary tumor, and prevent or delay metastasis.

Acute General Treatment

- Surgically manage urinary bladder rupture if present (p. 1012).
- Surgically remove lesions at bladder apex if operable. Surgery may be of greater benefit in cats. Surgery reduces clinical signs but has not been shown to extend survival.
- Address complicating bacterial UTI with culture and minimum inhibitory concentrations (MIC)–guided antimicrobials (p. 232).
- Begin chemotherapy to palliate clinical signs and address metastatic disease.
  - Piroxicam 0.3 mg/kg PO q 24h if renal function is normal or firocoxib 5 mg/kg PO q 24h. For cats, meloxicam 0.02-0.05 mg/kg PO q 24h has been evaluated and can be used alone or in combination with chemotherapeutic drugs.
  - Mitoxantrone 5 mg/m^2 IV q 21 days for 4 cycles, *or*
  - Doxorubicin 30 mg/m^2 IV q 21 days for 4 cycles (dogs) or 1 mg/kg IV q 21 days (cats and small dogs); body surface area conversion charts are provided on pp. 607 and 609.
  - Vinblastine 2.0 mg/m^2 IV q 14 days for 4 cycles (dogs); can be escalated incrementally (2.0 mg/m^2, then 2.33 mg/m^2, then 2.67 mg/m^2, then 3.0 mg/m^2) but should not exceed 3.0 mg/m^2.
  - Chlorambucil 4.0 mg/m^2 PO once daily if other therapies have failed or oral therapy is the only option.
  - CBC and blood urea nitrogen (BUN)/creatinine/urine specific gravity should be checked before each dose, and CBC should be checked 1 week later.
  - Cisplatin cannot be recommended in combination with piroxicam due to nephrotoxicosis.
  - Intravesicular therapy of bacillus Calmette-Guérin (BCG) or thiotepa used in humans has been poorly effective in veterinary patients.
- If bladder distended initially, maintain urinary drainage to avoid detrusor hypotonia (p. 89).
- Address metabolic imbalances occurring secondary to obstruction (pp. 495 and 1009).

Chronic Treatment

- Continue piroxicam indefinitely barring adverse GI or renal effects.
- May repeat mitoxantrone or vinblastine after first four doses if clinical signs recur
- Cumulative doxorubicin dosages greater than 180-240 mg/m^2 are associated with risk of cardiotoxicosis.
- Late bone marrow suppression is not uncommon in dogs treated chronically with chlorambucil.
- Urinary diversion surgery or intraluminal stenting (p. 1179) may prolong life if obstruction is imminent.

Nutrition/Diet

Feeding vegetables may reduce risk.

Drug Interactions

- Avoid combining drugs with similar toxicity profiles (e.g., cisplatin and piroxicam).
- Piroxicam should not be given in combination with other nonsteroidal antiinflammatory drugs or glucocorticoids.

Possible Complications

- Neutropenia, thrombocytopenia, sepsis, and renal injury secondary to chemotherapy
- GI ulceration or nephrotoxicosis secondary to piroxicam
- Urethral or ureteral obstruction secondary to tumor growth

Recommended Monitoring

- Monitor CBC before every chemotherapy treatment and 7-10 days later.
- Monitor BUN, creatinine, and urine specific gravity for renal function every 3-12 weeks.
- Monitor frequently for UTI (avoid cystocentesis).

PROGNOSIS & OUTCOME

This disease is locally aggressive with significant metastatic potential.

Dogs:
- Median reported survival treated with piroxicam alone is 6-7 months.
- Median reported survival treated with piroxicam and mitoxantrone is ≈12 months, with or without surgery.
- Median reported survival treated with surgery alone is ≈3.5 months.

Cats:
- Median reported survival is ≈8.5 months.
- Surgical resection may improve prognosis significantly for cats.

PEARLS & CONSIDERATIONS

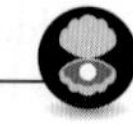

Comments

- Repeated urinary tract signs, especially in older animals, warrant screening for TCC.
- Early detection is critical for best response to treatment.
- VBTA or *BRAF* mutation test may allow early detection in geriatric at-risk breeds of dogs with lower urinary signs.
- Definitive diagnosis necessary for prognosis and therapeutic decisions requires cytologic exam or biopsy.
- Bacterial UTI is a frequent complication.

Technician Tips

Because cystocentesis can allow peritoneal seeding and accelerate metastasis, it should be avoided in older dogs (especially in predisposed breeds) with signs of dysuria before screening for TCC by imaging, VBTA, or *BRAF* mutation test and in dogs with known TCC.

Client Education

- Because signs are subtle and nonspecific, advanced diagnostics are most useful early.
- Urethral obstruction is often the life-limiting complication, and urinary diversion may be beneficial.

SUGGESTED READING

Knapp DW, et al: Randomized trial of cisplatin versus firocoxib versus cisplatin/firocoxib in dogs with transitional cell carcinoma of the urinary bladder. J Vet Intern Med 27:126-133, 2013.

AUTHOR: Jeffrey N. Bryan, DVM, MS, PhD, DACVIM
EDITOR: Leah A. Cohn, DVM, PhD, DACVIM

Diseases and Disorders

Transmissible Venereal Tumor

Bonus Material Online 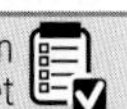 Client Education Sheet

BASIC INFORMATION

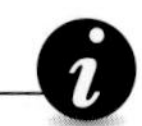

Definition

A contagious, neoplastic disease transmitted by transplantation of viable tumor cells during coitus

Synonyms

Canine condyloma, contagious lymphoma, contagious venereal tumor, infectious sarcoma, Sticker's sarcoma, transmissible venereal sarcoma, venereal granuloma, TVT

Epidemiology

SPECIES, AGE, SEX

- Species: canids (dogs, foxes, coyotes, jackals)
- Age: mostly young, sexually active animals; average age of 4-5 years
- Sex: both sexes; females > males

GENETICS, BREED PREDISPOSITION

Higher prevalence in mixed-breed dogs

RISK FACTORS

- More commonly occurs in free-roaming, sexually active dogs
- Grows more rapidly in neonatal or immunosuppressed dogs

CONTAGION AND ZOONOSIS

By definition, transmissible venereal tumor (TVT) is contagious among members of the family *Canidae*. It has not been identified as a zoonotic disease, although personal protection apparel (e.g., exam gloves) is recommended when examining and treating TVT lesions.

GEOGRAPHY AND SEASONALITY

- Worldwide distribution
- Greatest prevalence in tropical and subtropical urban environments

ASSOCIATED DISORDERS

- Urinary tract infections (UTIs) due to TVT masses in the vestibulovaginal junction (females) and phimosis (males), with inability to extrude the penis from the prepuce. Both conditions interfere with urination.
- Tumors are easily traumatized and ulcerated; secondary bacterial infection is common.

Clinical Presentation

DISEASE FORMS/SUBTYPES

Genital and extragenital forms

HISTORY, CHIEF COMPLAINT

- Initial persistent or intermittent bloody genital discharge (often foul smelling), constant licking, genital malformation, or swelling
- Eventually, masses can be seen protruding from the vulva or penis.
- Clinical signs of TVT typically last 40-100 days but may last longer, depending on the tumor size and location, immune status of the animal, and occurrence of secondary bacterial infections.

PHYSICAL EXAM FINDINGS

- Nodular lesions in the external genitalia
- Solitary or multiple masses progressing to cauliflower-like, papillary, multilobulated, or pedunculated masses
- Appearance is typically gray or pinkish gray.
- Texture is firm but friable; masses bleed easily when manipulated, resulting in genital bleeding in both sexes.
- In the oronasal presentation, epistaxis and frequent sneezing with epistaxis, halitosis, ptyalism, dyspnea, loss of teeth, and ulcerative lesions in gingivae and palate
- In the skin, nodular masses may be ulcerated, and regional lymph nodes may be enlarged.

Etiology and Pathophysiology

- Transmitted by coitus; affecting mainly external genital organs, and spreading to internal genitalia
- Transmitted more easily if there are abrasions or breaks in the integrity of the mucosal surface
- Social behavior (e.g., licking/sniffing affected areas) can produce extragenital TVT in the skin and eyes and in oral and nasal cavities.
- Metastasis is rare, but when it occurs, it affects regional lymph nodes, subcutaneous tissues, abdominal and thoracic viscera, brain, pituitary, spleen, and kidneys. Metastatic disease can also occur without the presence of a primary genital tumor.
- Cell origin of TVT is unknown but is presumed to be an undifferentiated round cell neoplasm of histiocytic origin.
- Chromosome number of tumor cells is 59 ± 5, whereas the normal canine complement is 78.
- *Leishmania* spp amastigotes have been isolated from TVT tissue, which could represent an alternative route of venereal transmission of leishmaniasis.

DIAGNOSIS

Diagnostic Overview

The diagnosis is suspected based on history/presence of a hemorrhagic mass on the genital mucosa. Confirmation is achieved with cytologic assessment of impression smears and a biopsy (which may serve to debulk the mass).

Differential Diagnosis

- Tumor type is suspected by the history, location, and appearance of the mass.
- Especially when there is no evidence of a primary genital tumor, TVT can be confused with other round cell tumors such as mast cell tumor, histiocytoma, and lymphoma. Also to be considered are malignant melanoma, squamous cell carcinoma (SCC), and fibrosarcoma.
- Clinical signs may be similar to those found with prostatitis, estrus, urethritis, and cystitis.

Initial Database

Cytologic exam of impression smears stained with Wright's or new methylene blue reveal homogeneous sheets of round to oval cells with prominent nucleoli and a small amount of cytoplasm with multiple mitotic figures.

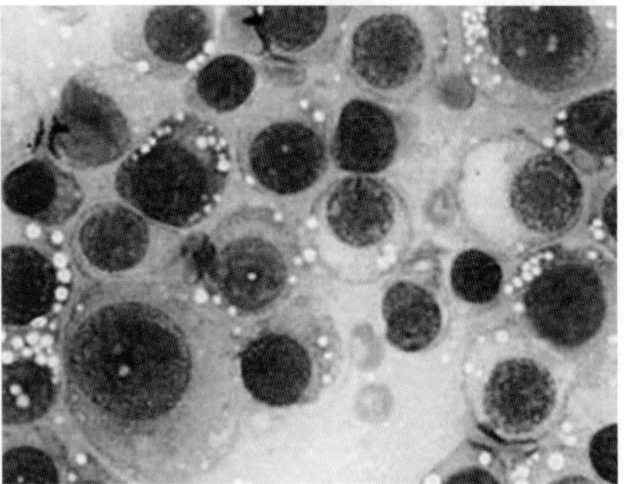

TRANSMISSIBLE VENEREAL TUMOR Cytologic exam of a TVT on impression smears stained with Wright's reveal homogeneous sheets of round to oval cells with prominent nucleoli and a small amount of cytoplasm with multiple mitotic figures.

Advanced or Confirmatory Testing

Definitive diagnosis is made by polymerase chain reaction assay or histologic classification of a biopsy specimen (after formalin fixation and staining with hematoxylin and eosin) and by immunochemistry testing to determine degree of malignancy.

TREATMENT

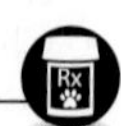

Treatment Overview

The goal of treatment is elimination of the tumor. Spontaneous regression occurs in experimental and clinical cases.

Acute General Treatment

- Surgical excision: physically removes the mass and induces an immune response. Effective for small masses; excision of large tumors (>2 cm in diameter) is often followed by tumor regrowth.
- Intratumoral injection (1-4 treatments) with vincristine 0.5-0.7 mg/m^2 and interleukin-2 (IL-2) 2 × 10^6 units has impressive therapeutic effects. However, IL-2 alone did not cause tumor regression in all cases.
- Chemotherapy with vincristine 0.7 mg/m^2 IV (highly corrosive if extravascular [pp. 152 and 609] for precautions) once weekly for 6 weeks until complete tumor regression is the treatment of choice for metastatic or multifocal TVT.
- Orthovoltage radiotherapy is effective (100% cure with a single radiation dose of 10 Gy); it requires an appropriate facility.

Chronic Treatment

Electrochemotherapy with bleomycin has been tried for vincristine-resistant TVT.

Behavior/Exercise

- Breeding should be avoided when TVT is present (contagion risk).
- Erection from excitement with preputial extrusion of the penis with a TVT tumor may result in paraphimosis.

Drug Interactions

Severe bronchospasm has been reported in humans when vinca alkaloids are used in combination with mitomycin C.

Possible Complications

- Extravasation injuries associated with perivascular injection of vincristine can range from irritation to necrosis and tissue sloughing.
- Combined chemotherapy with vincristine causes more side effects (vomiting, diarrhea, and neutropenia) than vincristine alone.

Recommended Monitoring

- Monitor for efficacy (tumor reduction).
- Monitor for toxicosis, using peripheral neuropathic clinical signs, CBCs with platelets, and liver tests before, during, and after treatment.

PROGNOSIS & OUTCOME

Despite the location or pattern of metastasis, the prognosis for TVT is excellent with recommended therapy.

PEARLS & CONSIDERATIONS

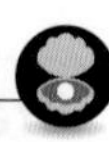

Comments

With any kind of vaginal or preputial bleeding

- Cytologic exam for TVT cells
- Visual exam of clitoral fossa and preputial fornix for gross TVT lesions

Prevention

Pet dogs should avoid contact with stray dogs.

Technician Tips

There has been an increased incidence of TVT lesions in pet (nonbreeding) dogs coincident with the increased movement of dogs within and between countries, especially the movement of dogs into U.S. shelters for adoption from Mexico, the Caribbean, and South America. TVT should be considered as a rule-out for any dog presenting with a friable, hemorrhagic mass.

Client Education

In areas where TVT is endemic, pet dogs should be confined and spayed or neutered to reduce the risk of disease transmission.

SUGGESTED READING

Ganguly B, et al: Canine transmissible venereal tumour: a review. Vet Comp Oncol 14(1):1-12, 2016.

AUTHOR: Rosa María Páramo-Ramírez, MVZ, PhD
EDITOR: Michelle A. Kutzler, DVM, PhD, DACT

Tremors and Myoclonus

BASIC INFORMATION

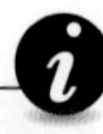

Definition

- Tremor: involuntary rhythmic oscillatory contraction of a muscle group
- Myoclonus: sudden, brief, sporadic, or repetitive contraction of a group of muscle cells followed by immediate relaxation (p. 661)

Synonyms

- Tremor: trembling, twitching
- Myoclonus: jerk, spasm

Epidemiology

SPECIES, AGE, SEX

Any dog or cat; age may vary with underlying cause

- Dogs: puppies (hypomyelination/dysmyelination, familial myoclonus); older adults (senile tremors)
- Cats: kittens (hypomyelination)

GENETICS, BREED PREDISPOSITION

Dogs:

- Idiopathic/glucocorticoid-responsive tremor syndrome: Maltese, West Highland white terriers, other small-breed white or nonwhite dogs (p. 530)
- Idiopathic head tremors: English bulldog, Doberman pinscher, Shetland sheepdog, others
- Idiopathic head tremor, familial myoclonus: Labrador retriever
- Orthostatic tremor: Great Dane, Scottish deerhound
- Hypomyelination/dysmyelination: springer spaniel, Samoyed, chow chow, Weimaraner, lurcher, Bernese mountain dog, Dalmatian, Siamese cats
- Central axonopathy: Scottish terriers

RISK FACTORS

Exposure to tremorgenic drugs or toxins, lack of vaccination

CONTAGION AND ZOONOSIS

Canine distemper virus (myoclonus); *in utero* panleukopenia virus in cats (intention tremor)

Clinical Presentation

DISEASE FORMS/SUBTYPES

- Action-related generalized tremor: diffuse, high-frequency skeletal muscle tremor that worsens with activity and resolves with sleep
  - Congenital: hypomyelination or dysmyelination; present at birth
  - Acquired: idiopathic glucocorticoid-responsive tremor syndrome, toxicosis
- Postural tremor
  - Episodic (several-minute duration) head tremor that is a high-frequency "yes or no" movement of the head and is often confused with focal seizures
  - Pelvic limb tremor in older dogs (benign) or young Great Danes (orthostatic), which occurs while standing but resolves when moving or recumbent

- Intention tremor: tremor of the head and neck that occurs when focusing on something such as a food bowl; associated with cerebellar disorders. Other localizing signs (e.g., hypermetria, disequilibrium) are present.
- Constant repetitive myoclonus: constant rhythmic jerking, usually of one limb every 1 to several seconds. Persists during activity, rest, and sleep, and may involve several limbs or muscles such as the diaphragm or masticatory muscles.
- Sporadic myoclonus: sudden contraction of a muscle group such as a facial twitch or limb jerk that may be benign or may represent focal seizure activity.

HISTORY, CHIEF COMPLAINT

- Must differentiate tremor or myoclonus from seizure (p. 903)
- Tremor may worsen with exercise/excitement and abate with rest or sleep.
- Littermates may be affected: tremor associated with hypomyelination/dysmyelination typically begins between 12 days and 3 weeks of age. Signs worsen with exercise but often resolve with rest.
- Idiopathic head tremors are episodic and may be confused for focal seizures. They are often precipitated by excitement or particular head positions, and owners may describe a characteristic "yes or no" movement of the head and normal consciousness. Mentation and gait remain normal during episodes.
- Orthostatic tremor is a fine tremor of the postural muscles that occurs only while standing, squatting to urinate/defecate, or attempting to lie down and subsides when walking, running, or in recumbency.
- Scottish terriers with central axonopathy develop tremors and ataxia at 10-12 weeks of age.
- Exposure to tremorgenic toxins and vomiting support intoxication.
- Recent (preceding weeks/months) history of respiratory disease, ill thrift, or adoption from a shelter suggests canine distemper-associated myoclonus.
- Recent whelping suggests hypocalcemic tetany (p. 281).

PHYSICAL EXAM FINDINGS

- The presence of tremors or myoclonus may be the only abnormality found on the physical or neurologic exam (p. 1136).
- Exam is normal between episodes of idiopathic head tremor.
- Seizures, stupor, and coma may be seen concurrently with intoxication or metabolic derangement.
- Ocular tremors and menace deficits often accompany idiopathic tremor syndrome. Head tilt and vestibulocerebellar ataxia occur occasionally.
- Intention tremor (i.e., tremor precipitated by the onset of voluntary movement, such as responding to a command), if associated with a fine head tremor, dysmetria, and nystagmus, is characteristic of cerebellar disease.
- Pelvic limb tremors in older dogs (senile tremors)

Etiology and Pathophysiology

Tremors and myoclonus may be a primary disorder or a manifestation of systemic disease. The most common and important cause of myoclonus in dogs is canine distemper virus. Common causes of tremor are provided on p. 1288.

DIAGNOSIS

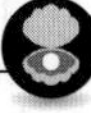

Diagnostic Overview

A presumptive diagnosis is often made based on the signalment, history, and clinical findings.

Differential Diagnosis

- Shivering
- Tetany
- Weakness
- Seizure

Initial Database

- Complete physical and neurologic exam (p. 1136)
- CBC, serum biochemistry, and urinalysis to assess for metabolic causes (e.g., hypocalcemia)

Advanced or Confirmatory Testing

- Cerebrospinal fluid (CSF) analysis (pp. 1080 and 1323) may be normal or reveal increased numbers of leukocytes (usually lymphocytes) with increased levels of protein, reflecting a nonsuppurative meningoencephalitis.
- Infectious disease serology (blood or CSF)
- Advanced imaging techniques (CT or MRI)

TREATMENT

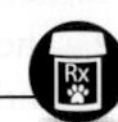

Treatment Overview

Treatment depends on underlying cause. It is not required for idiopathic head tremor or postural pelvic limb myoclonus in older dogs. Treatment not possible for several congenital disorders (e.g., myelination disorders, congenital cerebellar hypoplasia).

Acute General Treatment

- Active cooling if hyperthermic (p. 421)
- General and/or specific treatment for intoxication, including discontinuation of drugs suspected to cause tremor.
- Correct metabolic and electrolyte abnormalities (e.g., hypocalcemia).
- Address active infection (p. 271).

Chronic Treatment

- Long-term glucocorticoid therapy is often necessary for inflammatory tremor syndromes and idiopathic glucocorticoid-responsive tremor syndrome (p. 530).
- Orthostatic tremor usually improves with phenobarbital or gabapentin administration.
- Supportive care is aimed at keeping animals safe and ensuring adequate caloric and water intake.

Possible Complications

Prolonged tremors may result in hyperthermia, hypoglycemia, dehydration, and anorexia.

Recommended Monitoring

Follow-up exam and serial diagnostic studies as directed by the animal's clinical condition

PROGNOSIS & OUTCOME

- Idiopathic generalized tremor syndrome usually responds within days to glucocorticoid therapy, but relapses may occur.
- Toxin and drug-induced tremors resolve if the animal survives the initial event.
- Recovery from metabolic or infectious disease varies.
- Hypomyelination of springer spaniels: males typically do not recover, but females between 2 and 12 months of age may recover completely (sex-linked disorder).
- Idiopathic head tremors may improve and become less frequent over time and rarely cause clinical dysfunction.
- Senile tremors generally do not interfere with normal function.
- Central axonopathy in Scottish terriers is progressive and associated with a poor prognosis.
- Lysosomal storage diseases are usually fatal.

PEARLS & CONSIDERATIONS

Comments

- Involuntary muscle contractions must be distinguished from seizure. Involuntary muscle contractions are not associated with autonomic dysfunction (urination, defecation, salivation). They are associated with normal mentation, and they can be consistent with a described clinical syndrome of muscle contractions.
- In some cases, such as those with seizures, a patient with a clinical syndrome of involuntary muscle contractions may respond to an anticonvulsant trial.

Technician Tips

- Generalized tremors can cause life-threatening hyperthermia. Body temperature must be monitored, and active cooling may be necessary.
- Minimizing stress and excitement in hospital is helpful in minimizing tremors.

Client Education

- Owners should be warned that excitement and exercise often precipitate or worsen tremors.

- Many tremor syndromes have a known or suspected inherited basis, and these animals should not be bred.

SUGGESTED READING

de Lahunta A, et al: Classifying involuntary muscle contractions. Compend Contin Educ Pract Vet 28:516-529, 2006.

AUTHOR: Greg Kilburn, DVM, DACVIM
EDITOR: Leah A. Cohn, DVM, PhD, DACVIM

Tricuspid Valve Dysplasia

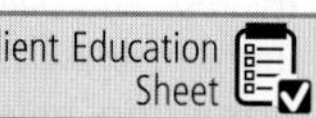

BASIC INFORMATION

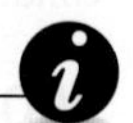

Definition

Congenital cardiac abnormality involving the right atrioventricular (AV) valve (tricuspid valve) and characterized by any or all of the following: thickened leaflets, foreshortened chordae tendineae, fused or underdeveloped right ventricular (RV) papillary muscles, leaflets (especially septal) tethered to underlying ventricular muscle, and redundancy of the parietal leaflet

Synonyms

TVD, congenital tricuspid valve malformation, Ebstein's anomaly (specific congenital tricuspid valve malformation characterized by atrialization of the right ventricle)

Epidemiology

SPECIES, AGE, SEX

- Dogs and cats of either sex
- Present at birth, but affected individuals are identified at any age based on first detection of a heart murmur or onset of clinical signs

GENETICS, BREED PREDISPOSITION

- Identified in several breeds, notably Labrador retrievers
- An autosomal dominant mode of inheritance with incomplete penetrance has been found only in the Labrador breed.
    - Affected Labrador retrievers (from different families) have had the same susceptibility locus, suggesting a founder effect.
- An autosomal recessive mode of inheritance has been suggested in the dogue de Bordeaux breed.

ASSOCIATED DISORDERS

Typically an isolated congenital heart defect; atrial septal defect, patent foramen ovale, mitral valve dysplasia, ventricular septal defect, pulmonic stenosis, and patent ductus arteriosus have coexisted.

Clinical Presentation

HISTORY, CHIEF COMPLAINT

- Often no clinical signs are detectable by the owner (incidental discovery of heart murmur on routine physical exam).
- Severe forms of the disease cause exercise intolerance/syncope, abdominal distention, dyspnea (due to pleural effusion), poor appetite, and weight loss.

PHYSICAL EXAM FINDINGS

- Typically, a right-sided systolic heart murmur of tricuspid regurgitation (TR) that is significantly softer or even inaudible over the left precordium, but severe TVD and RV dilation can shift the point of maximal intensity into the left precordium.
- Rarely, a soft diastolic murmur of tricuspid valve stenosis
- Tachycardia possible
- Jugular venous distention and pulsation if severe disease
- Abdominal palpation: hepatomegaly and a peritoneal fluid wave if right-sided congestive heart failure (R-CHF) is present
- Femoral pulse: usually normal; weak with severe disease associated with poor cardiac output
- Lung auscultation: usually normal; muffled lung sounds if pleural effusion
- Mucous membrane color: usually normal; pale with poor cardiac output; cyanotic if concurrent patent foramen ovale or septal defect

Etiology and Pathophysiology

During embryonic development, tricuspid valve leaflets are almost exclusively derived from ventricular myocardium by a process of undermining the RV inner wall.

- The inner layer of RV myocardium is undermined from the remainder to form a skirt in which perforations appear in the apical portion.
- These perforations enlarge until only the papillary muscles remain, and the initially muscular chordae tendineae become fibrous.
- Abnormalities during this process lead to TVD.

DIAGNOSIS

Diagnostic Overview

Physical exam findings are suggestive, and TR murmur in a pup or kitten should prompt referral. Echocardiography is required for confirmation, delineation of the defect's extent, and to identify other cardiac defects that may coexist.

Differential Diagnosis

- Myxomatous (degenerative) tricuspid valve disease: usually older dogs; concurrent (more severe) myxomatous mitral valve disease is often present
- Ventricular septal defect: produces a right precordial systolic murmur most commonly (p. 1036)
- Tricuspid valve endocarditis: rare in dogs and cats, typically associated with systemic illness and fever (can be waxing and waning)

Initial Database

Echocardiogram (p. 1094): diagnostic test of choice

- Two-dimensional imaging defines degree of leaflet thickening, adherence of the septal leaflet to the interventricular septum, redundancy of the parietal leaflet, presence of hyperechoic fibrous tissue at the annulus resulting in stenosis, and right atrial and RV dilation
- Doppler echocardiography documents the presence and degree of TR, presence/severity of concurrent pulmonary hypertension, and presence/severity of tricuspid stenosis.
- Concurrent defects can be identified.

Thoracic radiographs:

- Normal in mild disease
- Evidence of right atrial and RV enlargement in moderate to severe disease
- Enlargement of the caudal vena cava and possible pulmonary hypoperfusion in severe disease
- Hepatomegaly, peritoneal effusion, and pleural effusion can occur in severe cases (R-CHF).

Electrocardiogram (p. 1096):

- Normal in mild disease
- May exhibit fragmentation or splintering of the QRS complex, with a normal mean electrical axis
- Less commonly, classic right axis deviation of the QRS complex as seen with RV enlargement
- P waves may be tall and wide.
- May exhibit ventricular preexcitation or tachycardia associated with accessory pathway conduction
- Atrial reentrant tachyarrhythmias or atrial fibrillation possible with marked RA dilation

Blood pressure (p. 1065):

- Often normal
- May be decreased in R-CHF

Central venous pressure (CVP):

- Normal in mild and often in moderate disease
- Increased in severe disease as R-CHF ensues

Advanced or Confirmatory Testing

Holter monitoring to document intermittent tachyarrhythmias (p. 1120)

TREATMENT

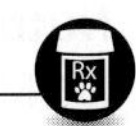

Treatment Overview

Goals of treatment are to control R-CHF if present and control associated tachyarrhythmias.

Acute General Treatment

- Abdominocentesis or abdominal drainage (p. 1056) for severe peritoneal effusion that can inhibit diaphragmatic movement
- Cage rest for severe R-CHF
- Antiarrhythmic treatment for acute control of tachyarrhythmias

Chronic Treatment

- Careful diuretic administration for CHF: furosemide 1-3 mg/kg PO q 8-12h or torsemide 0.2-0.4 mg/kg PO q 12h; spironolactone 1-2 mg/kg PO q 12h
- Angiotensin-converting enzyme (ACE) inhibition may be helpful (e.g., enalapril or benazepril 0.2-0.5 mg/kg PO q 12-24h)
- Pimobendan 0.2-0.3 mg/kg PO q 8-12h in the face of R-CHF or RV myocardial failure
- Various antiarrhythmic agents (tailored to a given case), depending on the diagnosed arrhythmia; consultation with a cardiologist is recommended
- Exercise restriction
- Surgical tricuspid valve repair/replacement has not generally been successful.

Nutrition/Diet

As appropriate for chronic R-CHF (p. 409) and cardiac cachexia, if present

Behavior/Exercise

Strict exercise restriction in the face of R-CHF or syncope

Drug Interactions

- Lowest effective dosage of diuretics to avoid compromising renal perfusion
- As indicated for chronic management of R-CHF (p. 409)

Possible Complications

- Excessive diuresis causing decreased forward output and weakness
- Electrolyte abnormalities and azotemia caused by renal hypoperfusion secondary to poor forward output and/or diuresis; hypokalemia can exacerbate certain arrhythmias
- Hypoalbuminemia secondary to cardiac cachexia and chronic peritoneal effusion

Recommended Monitoring

- As indicated for R-CHF (p. 409)
- Monitor for tachyarrhythmias (electrocardiogram, Holter monitoring if necessary).

PROGNOSIS & OUTCOME

- Better than is typically cited in the literature
- Dogs with mild disease and many with moderate disease can have a normal life span.
- Dogs with severe disease have shortened life spans, but some can live several years (5 or more years is possible).

PEARLS & CONSIDERATIONS

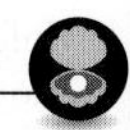

Comments

- TVD appears to be inherited as an autosomal dominant trait with reduced penetrance in Labradors, meaning it may be transmitted by the sire or the dam, and the extent to which offspring are affected varies individually.
- Carefully auscult young animals over the right precordium to detect this disease.
- Major complications in severe disease include CHF and tachyarrhythmias.

Technician Tips

Central venous pressure and systemic blood pressure monitoring are important in TVD dogs that are hospitalized for issues directly related to their heart or for other issues (e.g., gastrointestinal disease).

Client Education

At-risk breeds should be carefully screened, particularly before breeding, with echocardiography.

SUGGESTED READING

Adin D: Tricuspid valve dysplasia in the dog. In Bonagura JD, editor: Kirk's Current veterinary therapy XIV, St. Louis, 2012, Saunders, pp 762-765.

AUTHOR: Kathy Wright, DVM, DACVIM
EDITOR: Meg M. Sleeper, VMD, DACVIM

Tritrichomonas Infection

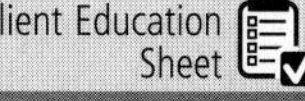

BASIC INFORMATION

Definition

Relatively common infection of the distal ileum and colon with the protozoan parasite *Tritrichomonas foetus* causing chronic or intermittent diarrhea in cats

Synonyms

Trichomoniasis, trichomonosis

Epidemiology

SPECIES, AGE, SEX

Cats of any age, breed, or sex can be infected. Clinical signs are more common in young cats (median age, 1 year), and older cats are more commonly subclinically infected. There is a single report of a dog infected with *T. foetus.*

GENETICS, BREED PREDISPOSITION

Purebred cats may be at increased risk for infection, likely due to dense housing conditions in catteries rather than genetics.

RISK FACTORS

- Dense population environments (e.g., shelters, catteries)
- Subclinically infected cats may be an important source of infection for other cats.

CONTAGION AND ZOONOSIS

Transmission from cats to humans has not been described.

GEOGRAPHY AND SEASONALITY

Worldwide

Clinical Presentation

HISTORY, CHIEF COMPLAINT

- Chronic or intermittent diarrhea is the most common complaint. Diarrhea is typically large-bowel, but some cats develop small-bowel diarrhea later in the disease course. The duration of diarrhea ranges between 1 day and 8 years.
- Diarrhea is typically refractory to standard antibiotic or antidiarrheal therapy, or might improve initially but recur shortly after treatment ends
- Most infected cats remain in good health and have a normal appetite, activity level, and body condition unless there are concurrent diseases.
- Involuntary dripping of feces may occur in cats with severe diarrhea.

PHYSICAL EXAM FINDINGS

- Usually normal unless other diseases are present
- Painful anal inflammation is possible in cats with chronic/recurrent diarrhea and tenesmus.

Etiology and Pathophysiology

- *T. foetus* is a single-cell, highly motile, flagellated protozoan parasite that exists only as a trophozoite (no cyst stage).
- Feline *T. foetus* isolates are similar to but genetically different from isolates that cause infertility and abortions in cattle.

- Infection occurs by direct fecal-oral transmission through ingestion of trophozoites.
- The pathophysiologic sequence is not fully understood, but organism, host, and environmental factors are likely involved.

DIAGNOSIS

Diagnostic Overview

- Suspected in any cat with diarrhea (especially large-bowel form)
- Confirmation requires direct fecal smear exam, specific culture, and/or fecal polymerase chain reaction (PCR) assay.

Differential Diagnosis

- Giardiasis or enteritis due to other protozoan parasites
- Intestinal parasitism
- Infectious causes of colitis
- Infiltrative intestinal disease (e.g., inflammatory bowel disease [IBD], intestinal lymphoma)
- Dietary intolerance or sensitivity
- Antibiotic-responsive diarrhea

Initial Database

- CBC, serum biochemistry profile, urinalysis: typically normal
- Direct fecal smear exam: multiple fresh smears from diarrheic feces or collected directly from the colon by flushing sterile saline should be examined
  - Insensitive (sensitivity ≈15%) but fairly specific for *T. foetus*. Negative results do not exclude infection.
  - A speck of fresh feces is mixed with a drop of saline on a microscope slide, covered with a coverslip, and microscopically examined using the 20× or 40× objective.
  - *T. foetus* is similar in size to and must be distinguished from *Giardia* (p. 386). It may be difficult to differentiate *T. foetus* from apathogenic *Pentatrichomonas hominis*.
  - Trophozoites of *T. foetus* have an undulating membrane and demonstrate directed forward movement; motility of *Giardia* resembles a falling leaf.
- Fecal flotation with or without *Giardia* ELISA to rule out other parasites and *Giardia*.
- *T. foetus* infection cannot be diagnosed with fecal flotation because it does not form cysts.
- Imaging (radiographs and ultrasound): generally unremarkable

Advanced or Confirmatory Testing

- Fecal PCR for *T. foetus* DNA: most sensitive and specific test. False-negative results may occur. To increase sensitivity, use fresh diarrheic feces or feces collected directly from the colon by flushing sterile saline.
- Fecal protozoal culture using the *T. foetus* InPouch TF ideally performed in house
  - More sensitive (sensitivity ≈55%) and specific than direct fecal smear exam but less sensitive than fecal PCR. To increase sensitivity, use fresh diarrheic feces or feces collected directly from the colon by flushing with sterile saline.
  - Negative results do not exclude infection, and test does not differentiate *T. foetus* from *P. hominis*.
  - Only *T. foetus* organisms can grow in the culture media. Positive results (confirmed by microscopic exam) are highly suggestive of infection.

TREATMENT

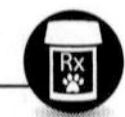

Treatment Overview

Treatment aims to resolve diarrhea and eradicate infection.

Acute and Chronic Treatment

- Standard antiprotozoal, antibacterial, and antidiarrheal therapies are ineffective, although transient clinical improvement may occur.
- Ronidazole 30 mg/kg PO q 24h × 2 weeks: treatment of choice.
  - Powdered drug (must be compounded), not FDA approved for use in cats in the United States; obtain informed consent from owner.
  - Most cats (72%-100%) show clinical improvement or resolution of diarrhea during appropriate treatment. However, a second 2-week treatment may be needed in some.
  - It is unclear how often eradication of infection occurs after treatment. Some cats show clinical improvement or resolution of the diarrhea but remain PCR positive.
  - Neurotoxicity (anorexia, lethargy, ataxia, seizures) is a serious adverse effect of ronidazole that is reported for 5% of cats treated with the recommended dosage. Onset of any neurologic deficit requires immediate termination of treatment.
- Treatment of clinically normal cats positive for *T. foetus* is not recommended because elimination of the carrier state may not be achieved.
- Post-treatment testing, ideally using fecal PCR, should be performed in cases where diarrhea persists or recurs soon after completing treatment. Post-treatment testing if diarrhea resolves is problematic because such cats can be PCR positive as subclinical carriers.
- Reasons for treatment failure after appropriate treatment include reinfection (e.g., from a subclinically infected cat) and resistance to ronidazole. The prevalence of ronidazole-resistant *T. foetus* is suspected to be high.

Nutrition/Diet

Highly digestible, high-protein/low-carbohydrate, or sometimes hypoallergenic diets suitable for IBD or other causes of enteritis are indicated.

Possible Complications

Chronic trichomoniasis is speculated, but not proved, to trigger development of idiopathic IBD.

PROGNOSIS & OUTCOME

- Untreated, chronic diarrhea can resolve spontaneously but may persist up to 2 years or longer. The majority of these cats can remain subclinical carriers or experience recurrent bouts of diarrhea after stress or immunosuppression. They remain infectious for other cats.
- If appropriately treated, chronic diarrhea typically resolves. Infection may be eradicated from some treated cats, but others remain subclinical carriers.

PEARLS & CONSIDERATIONS

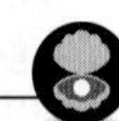

Comments

- Young cats with diarrhea, cats from population-dense environments, and cats unresponsive to treatments with antimicrobial or antiprotozoal drugs are highly suspected to have *T. foetus* infection.
- *T. foetus* and *Giardia* infections often coexist in cats.
- Close monitoring of cats receiving ronidazole for signs of neurotoxicosis is mandatory.
- If diarrhea persists more than 2 weeks after the end of treatment, consider retesting for *T. foetus* using PCR.
- PCR tests for *T. foetus* are often part of a multi-pathogen diarrhea panel used for cats.

Prevention

Appropriate hand/litter box hygiene and separation of carrier cats from young cats and kittens in multiple-cat households or catteries

Technician Tips

Trophozoites exhibiting forward motion on a fresh fecal smear is indicative of *T. foetus* infection rather than *Giardia* infection.

SUGGESTED READING

Gookin JL, et al: The conundrum of feline Trichomonosis. J Feline Med Surg 19:261, 2017.

AUTHOR: Panagiotis G. Xenoulis, DVM, Dr.med.vet., PhD
EDITOR: Rance K. Sellon, DVM, PhD, DACVIM

Tularemia

Client Education Sheet

BASIC INFORMATION

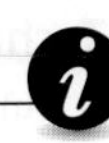

Definition

Acute zoonotic bacterial infection is caused by fastidious gram-negative aerobic intracellular coccobacilli, *Francisella tularensis* subsp *tularensis* (type A [more virulent]) or subsp *holarctica* (type B); uncommon in occurrence

Synonyms

Rabbit fever, deerfly fever, lemming fever

Epidemiology

SPECIES, AGE, SEX

- Extremely broad host range: affects > 300 species of wild and domestic mammals, amphibians, arthropods, birds, and humans
- Seroprevalence indicates that subclinical infection is common in dogs and cats in endemic areas.
- Clinical disease occurs occasionally in cats and rarely in dogs.
- Affected cats often are severely ill; dogs are more resistant and have milder signs; puppies and kittens are more susceptible than adults.

RISK FACTORS

- Outdoor pets with exposure to arthropod vectors or reservoirs of infection, especially wild rabbits or rodents
- Humans at greater risk include veterinarians, farmers, hunters, landscapers, meat handlers, cooks, and laboratory personnel.

CONTAGION AND ZOONOSIS

- Highly infectious zoonotic disease; the infectious dose for humans is < 100 organisms by cutaneous or conjunctival exposure and < 10 organisms via inhalation
- Transmission occurs through direct contact with infected animals, their tissues or excrement, and contaminated fomites; cat bites or scratches; insect bites (ticks, biting flies); ingestion of contaminated food (especially meat) or water; and inhalation of aerosolized organisms (bacterial cultures, contaminated plant material).

GEOGRAPHY AND SEASONALITY

- Different subtypes have a worldwide distribution. Type A occurs in North America only; type B occurs throughout the Northern Hemisphere.
- Occurs in distinct endemic areas, with a few cases in bordering areas; sporadic disease with 100-200 human cases per year in the United States
- Most human cases recognized in the central and Rocky Mountain states (i.e., AR, CO, KS, MO, OK, WY)
- Seasonality parallels level of outdoor activities/exposure; reduced in winter

Clinical Presentation

HISTORY, CHIEF COMPLAINT

- Subclinical to mild to fatal disease occurs 2-7 days after exposure.
- Cats presented for veterinary care often have severe acute disease with nonspecific signs (lethargy, anorexia).
- Dogs may present with anorexia, lethargy, weakness, and mucopurulent oculonasal discharge.
- Recent contact with rabbits or rabbit carcasses is common.

PHYSICAL EXAM FINDINGS

- Cats: fever, lymphadenopathy, oral or lingual ulcerations, splenomegaly, hepatomegaly, icterus. Occasionally, milder nonfatal form of disease may present as chronic draining cutaneous lesions.
- Dogs: fever, lymphadenomegaly, and oculonasal discharge

Etiology and Pathophysiology

- *F. tularensis* is a highly infectious, gram-negative intracellular bacterium found in water and mud.
- Two disease cycles are noted: a terrestrial cycle associated with transmission of type A (subsp *tularensis*) from infected rabbits, ticks (eastern and central United States), and biting flies (western United States), and an aquatic cycle associated with transmission of type B (subsp *holarctica*) from infected aquatic mammals (muskrat, beaver, voles) through contamination of water by carcasses or excrement or mechanical transmission by biting insects
- Transmission occurs through inoculation (cat or insect bite), ingestion, inhalation, or contact with skin or conjunctiva (able to penetrate intact skin).
- Ticks are a reservoir host and a true vector (transtadial transmission); other biting insects are mechanical vectors.
- At the site of inoculation, the organism multiplies locally and spreads to local lymph nodes, resulting in regional lymphadenopathy.
- Bacteremia with seeding of the organism to multiple organs throughout the body may follow, particularly in cats and humans.
- *Francisella* is an obligate intracellular organism: it invades and replicates in macrophages, facilitating persistence and systemic dissemination.

DIAGNOSIS

Diagnostic Overview

Tularemia should be considered in acutely febrile patients with regional or generalized lymphadenopathy, especially in endemic areas and/or if oral ulcerations or cutaneous abscesses are present and/or history of exposure to rabbits (common) or ticks.

Differential Diagnosis

- Cytauxzoonosis
- Plague *(Yersinia pestis)*
- Pseudotuberculosis *(Yersinia pseudotuberculosis)*
- Nocardiosis
- Mycobacterial infection
- Pasteurellosis
- Causes of icterus (p. 528)

Initial Database

- CBC: panleukopenia or leukocytosis with toxic neutrophils, thrombocytopenia
- Serum biochemistry profile: increased liver enzymes activities (alanine aminotransferase [ALT]), hyperbilirubinemia, hyperglycemia
- Cytologic exam of affected tissues: suppurative to pyogranulomatous inflammation

Advanced or Confirmatory Testing

- Serologic test: fourfold increase in titer or single markedly high titer (≥1 : 160 in humans); false-positives may occur because of cross-reactivity with *Brucella* and *Yersinia*. False-positive *Bartonella quintana* serology has been reported for a human with tularemia.
- Definitive diagnosis: demonstration of organism by polymerase chain reaction (PCR) assay, direct fluorescent antibody, or culture (culture is not usually recommended; warn laboratory of clinical suspicion). Use caution during diagnostic sampling and specimen handling because organism is highly infectious.
- Problems with culture identification include fastidious nature of organism and danger to lab personnel.

TREATMENT

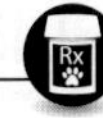

Treatment Overview

- Cats must be treated early and intensively; treat presumptively while awaiting test results.
- Antimicrobial treatment for eradication of *Francisella* organisms and supportive care for accompanying conditions (dehydration, septic shock [p. 907])
- Wear barrier attire (personal protective equipment [PPE]) and stringently avoid cutaneous contact with infected animals or splatter/aerosolization of patient blood, tissue, and excrement to prevent transmission of disease to humans and other animals.
- Canine cases are often mild.

Acute and Chronic Treatment

- Supportive therapy, including IV fluid administration

- Specific antimicrobial therapy is required, but comparative efficacy studies for cats are lacking. In humans, gentamicin, ciprofloxacin, or doxycycline is most commonly used, with relapse more commonly reported after treatment with bacteriostatic antimicrobials (tetracycline, chloramphenicol).
  - For cats, gentamicin (only once the patient is well hydrated), fluoroquinolones, tetracyclines, erythromycin, and chloramphenicol have been used.
  - Beta-lactam antibiotics and azithromycin are not effective.
  - Pradofloxacin 7.5 mg/kg PO q 24h for 10 days, *or*
  - Enrofloxacin 5 mg/kg IM, IV q 24h for 10 days (if IV, dilute with saline and administer slowly), *or*
  - Gentamicin 5-8 mg/kg IV, SQ, or IM q 24h for 7-14 days. Ensure hydration and normal renal function before treatment to reduce risk of nephrotoxicity; in animals with chronic kidney disease, decrease dose of aminoglycoside or choose another antibiotic.

Drug Interactions

- Aminoglycosides: avoid concurrent use of other renally excreted or potentially ototoxic drugs (e.g., furosemide, cephalosporins).
- Fluoroquinolones may alter metabolism of other drugs, leading to toxicosis (e.g., theophylline); avoid > 5 mg/kg/day of enrofloxacin in cats due to retinal toxicity.

Possible Complications

- Sepsis (p. 907)
- Disseminated intravascular coagulation (p. 269)
- Acute kidney injury/anuria (p. 23)

Recommended Monitoring

- Monitor temperature, heart rate, respiratory rate and effort, body weight and hydration status, and blood pressure; monitor for complications of sepsis.
- For patients receiving aminoglycosides, monitor urine sediment and serum blood urea nitrogen (BUN) and creatinine.

PROGNOSIS & OUTCOME

- Can be rapidly fatal in untreated cats with overt clinical signs
- Self-limited infection in most dogs
- Rapid resolution of fever follows administration of appropriate antibiotic.

PEARLS & CONSIDERATIONS

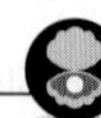

Comments

- May be underreported in dogs because of the mild, self-limited nature of disease.
- Highly infectious and zoonotic: multiple reports of tularemia in humans acquired by cat bite
- Centers for Disease Control and Prevention (CDC) class A pathogen; potential bioterrorism agent
- Tularemia awareness is important for veterinarians to (1) recognize, treat, and prevent disease in animal patients; (2) prevent disease exposure to themselves and other people in contact with infected animals; and (3) recognize potential bioterrorism in an unexplained increase in cases.
- Tularemia is a reportable disease in most U.S. states; many states require immediate reporting (within 3 hours). Reporting regulations vary by country, state, and within-state region and may change.

Prevention

- Control of arthropod vectors
- Limit exposure to rabbits, rodents, and other wild mammals.

Technician Tips

- Tularemia is extremely infectious and readily transmitted from infected animals to humans.
- Strict protective measures should be used in handling animals, their bedding, and all laboratory samples.
- Use of hoses to clean cages of infected animals, or blow dryers or fans in the proximity of the patient, is contraindicated. Resulting aerosols may cause exposure by inhalation and subsequent pneumonic tularemia, the most highly fatal form of the disease in people.

Client Education

- Multiple reports of transmission to humans from infected cats (cat bite, cat scratch, cutaneous contact) and from pet prairie dogs
- No recorded transmission from infected dogs to humans, but the possibility is not excluded

SUGGESTED READING

Larson MA, et al: *Francisella tularensis* bacteria associated with feline tularemia in the United States. Emerg Infect Dis 20:2068, 2014.

AUTHOR: Marcella D. Ridgway, VMD, MS, DACVIM
EDITOR: Joseph Taboada, DVM, DACVIM

Ulcerative and Erosive Skin Disorders

BASIC INFORMATION

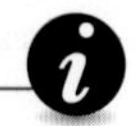

Definition

A *cutaneous erosion* is a shallow epidermal defect that does not penetrate the basement membrane. Erosions are usually associated with self-trauma or mild epidermal conditions. A *cutaneous ulcer* is produced by a break in the continuity of the epidermis, with exposure of the underlying dermis. Ulcers are usually a consequence of a deep and serious pathologic process. Healing ulcers typically result in scarring.

Epidemiology

SPECIES, AGE, SEX

Vary according to the underlying pathologic process

GENETICS, BREED PREDISPOSITION

Some diseases have a genetic basis or are related to anatomic defects (e.g., intertrigo in English bulldogs and Chinese Shar-peis).

Clinical Presentation

HISTORY, CHIEF COMPLAINT

A thorough history is important, considering the extensive list of differential diagnoses. Some clues may help pinpoint the condition:

- Travel history (e.g., leishmaniasis in dogs traveling to Europe), grooming and boarding (contagion risk such as herpesvirus infection in cats), and similar environmental factors may affect a patient's risk of developing a certain condition.
- Presence of signs of systemic illness (e.g., lethargy, anorexia, lameness) may narrow the differential diagnosis (e.g., systemic lupus erythematosus [SLE], leishmaniasis, systemic mycoses), and diagnostic methods are oriented differently.
- Prior treatments: response to prior treatment or therapy administered before onset of clinical signs allows the inclusion or exclusion of some dermatoses (e.g., cutaneous adverse drug reaction).

PHYSICAL EXAM FINDINGS

- Dermatologic exam for identifying erosive and ulcerative lesions and general physical exam to detect signs of underlying systemic diseases

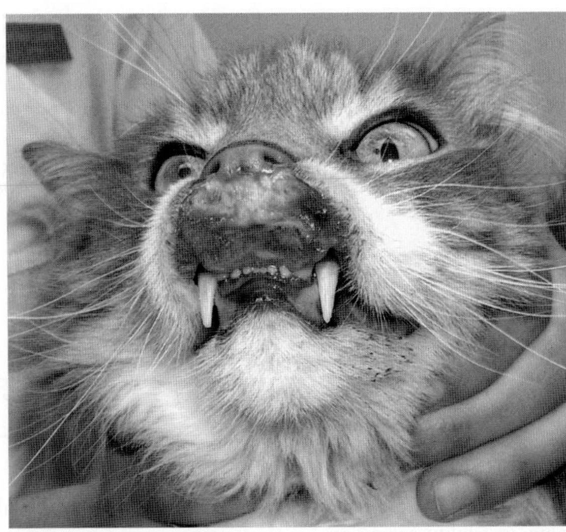

ULCERATIVE AND EROSIVE SKIN DISORDERS Severe indolent ulcer in a cat. (Copyright Dr. Manon Paradis.)

- The clinician should look for primary lesions such as vesicles, bullae and pustules, and the distribution of the lesions and involvement of the mucosa. This information can suggest a specific group of diseases.
- Secondary lesions such as crusts are common.
- Exact description of the lesions varies according to the underlying disease.

Etiology and Pathophysiology

Variable, depending on underlying cause

- Congenital, hereditary, and conformational defects: for example, erosions can result from skin friction (e.g., intertrigo), and ulcerations can be secondary to abnormal fragility of the dermoepidermal junction (e.g., epidermolysis bullosa [EB]).
- Infectious diseases (bacterial, viral, parasitic, fungal, rickettsial): some organisms infect and lyse keratinocytes (e.g., herpesvirus) or can cause epidermal necrosis secondary to vasculitis (e.g., canine Rocky Mountain spotted fever) or a substantial inflammatory reaction, leading to ulcerative dermatitis.
- Immune-mediated disorders: ulcers may follow the rupture of vesicles and bullae caused by the action of autoantibodies.
- Drug-induced conditions
- Self-induced lesions
- Environmental injuries (e.g., coagulation necrosis of the epidermis/dermis associated with thermal or chemical burns)
- Secondary to systemic diseases (e.g., uremia resulting from renal failure may cause oral ulceration)
- Ischemic disorders: any dermatopathy that interferes with vascular supply of the skin can potentially cause ulcers secondary to skin necrosis.
- Neoplasia: ulcerations noticed in skin tumors such as cutaneous epitheliotropic lymphoma or squamous cell carcinoma (SCC) are usually secondary to the infiltration of the skin by neoplastic cells.
- Idiopathic conditions

DIAGNOSIS

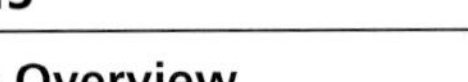

Diagnostic Overview

A definitive diagnosis is required in order to institute the appropriate treatment regimen (p. 1452).

Differential Diagnosis

- The list of differentials is extensive. Among the common conditions, consider feline eosinophilic granuloma complex (indolent ulcer, eosinophilic plaque, eosinophilic granuloma), bacterial skin infection (*Staphylococcus* sp), parasitic disorders (demodicosis), trauma (self-induced or not), immune-mediated disorders (pemphigus complex and lupus erythematosus), and cutaneous neoplasia.
- Congenital and hereditary: idiopathic facial dermatitis of Persian and Himalayan cats, aplasia cutis, EB, dermatomyositis
- Infectious/parasitic diseases: demodicosis, flea bite hypersensitivity, feline mosquito bite hypersensitivity, fly bite dermatitis; systemic mycoses, sporotrichosis, phaeohyphomycosis, zygomycosis, candidiasis, dermatophyte granuloma, pseudomycetoma, protothecosis, pythiosis, aspergillosis; deep pyoderma, mucocutaneous pyoderma, pyotraumatic dermatitis; feline leukemia virus (FeLV), feline cowpox, feline calicivirus (FCV), feline herpesvirus (FHV); canine Rocky Mountain spotted fever, leishmaniasis, and mycobacterial infection
- Immune-mediated disorders: pemphigus complex, bullous pemphigoid, erythema multiforme, toxic epidermal necrolysis, vasculitis, lupus erythematosus, EB acquisita, cold-agglutinin disease, and uveodermatologic syndrome
- Cutaneous adverse drug reactions
- Self-induced lesions: pruritic dermatoses, psychogenic dermatoses, neuropathies
- Environmental injuries: burns, frostbites
- Systemic diseases: superficial necrolytic dermatitis, calcinosis cutis, uremia
- Neoplasia: SCC, cutaneous epitheliotropic lymphoma, mast cell tumor, paraneoplastic alopecia
- Conformational dermatoses: intertrigo, pressure sores
- Iatrogenic: radiation therapy, thermal or tissue injury
- Miscellaneous: feline plasma cell pododermatitis, feline ulcerative dermatitis with linear subepidermal fibrosis, snake bite

Initial Database

- Patient history and physical exam are important in the diagnostic process.
- Cytologic exam of any exudate contents (see p. 1091): bacteria, inflammatory cells, acantholytic keratinocytes (pemphigus), fungal organisms, neoplastic cells
- CBC, serum biochemistry panel, and urinalysis if systemic signs are observed

Advanced or Confirmatory Testing

- Skin biopsies (p. 1091) for histopathologic exam are indicated in most cases of ulcerative dermatoses.
- Endocrine tests and serologic exam depend on suspected disease.
- Coombs' test: cold-agglutinin disease
- Antinuclear antibody (ANA) test: often positive for animals with SLE
- Imaging, if relevant, to confirm systemic disease or stage tumors
- Infectious disease testing, as appropriate

TREATMENT

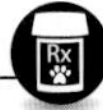

Treatment Overview

Varies considerably according to the disease. It must address the primary cause of the erosions or ulcers.

Acute and Chronic Treatment

- Immunosuppressive treatments are required in immune-mediated diseases, whereas infectious diseases require proper antimicrobial treatment.
- Antiparasitic treatments as required
- Neoplastic diseases should be addressed according to the type of tumor.
- Some patients with conformational dermatoses may need surgery to correct the skin defect.
- Supportive care may be required, especially in animals with severe lesions or systemic illness.

PROGNOSIS & OUTCOME

Ranges widely from good to poor, depending on the primary cause

PEARLS & CONSIDERATIONS

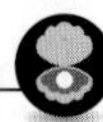

Comments

- Considering the wide range of treatments, making a definitive diagnosis to correctly address the disease is a wise approach, and

it prevents adverse effects of an improper treatment trial.
- Primary lesions (e.g., vesicles, bullae, pustules) or skin surrounding erosion/ulcer should be selected for skin biopsies.
- Some of these diseases are life-threatening.
- Be aware of the zoonotic potential of some of these diseases (e.g., sporotrichosis).

Technician Tips

- Prevent further aggravation of the lesions by body protection (e.g., body suit) or keeping the animal in a safe environment, especially when the epidermal detachment is severe.
- Keep the skin lesions clean.
- Isolation may be required if a contagious disease is suspected.

SUGGESTED READING

Mason IS: Erosions and ulcerations. In Ettinger SJ, Feldman EC, editors: Textbook of veterinary internal medicine, ed 7, St. Louis, 2010, Saunders, pp 79-83.

AUTHOR: Frédéric Sauvé, DMV, MSc, DACVD
EDITOR: Manon Paradis, DMV, MVSc, DACVD

Ulcers, Oral Mucosal

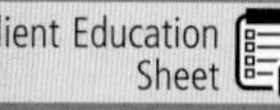

BASIC INFORMATION

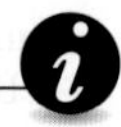

Definition

Mucosal ulcers are deep tissue defects that result in loss of surface tissue and extend through the basement membrane into the underlying submucosa. Mucosal ulcerations develop secondary to a wide range of causes.

Synonym

Oral ulcers

Epidemiology

SPECIES, AGE, SEX

Affected animals can include dogs and cats of any breed, age, or sex.

GENETICS, BREED PREDISPOSITION

- Maltese and cocker spaniels have a higher prevalence of chronic ulcerative paradental stomatitis (CUPS).
- Cats of any breed may be affected with feline gingivostomatitis (i.e., lymphocytic-plasmacytic gingivostomatitis [LPGS]).

RISK FACTORS

- Infectious diseases such as feline leukemia virus (FeLV), feline immunodeficiency virus (FIV), feline calicivirus (FCV), and feline herpesvirus (FHV)
- Dental disease (feline resorptive lesions, periodontal disease), immunosuppressive diseases, chronic immunosuppressive therapy, or gastroesophageal reflux disorders

CONTAGION AND ZOONOSIS

FeLV, FIV, FCV, and FHV are transmissible to other cats. *Bartonella henselae* can infect humans (cat scratch disease).

Clinical Presentation

DISEASE FORMS/SUBTYPES

Pattern of oral ulceration may be helpful in determining the underlying cause (p. 1261).

HISTORY, CHIEF COMPLAINT

- Reluctance to eat
- Hypersalivation
- Halitosis
- Weight loss
- Behavior changes such as pawing at the mouth, decreased grooming, irritability, aggression
- Dysphagia

PHYSICAL EXAM FINDINGS

A thorough oral exam may require sedation
- Oral pain
- Halatosis
- Ptyalism
- Thin body condition
- Dental plaque
- Gingivitis
- Periodontitis
- Stomatitis
- Faucitis (pharyngitis/tonsillitis)
- Focal to multifocal areas of oral ulceration ranging from the tongue, buccal mucosal surfaces, hard palate, and glossopalatine folds
- Rarely, systemic signs including dehydration, fever, lymphadenomegaly, lethargy

Etiology and Pathophysiology

- Ulcers represent denuded epithelium that penetrates the epithelial-connective tissue border and extends deeper into the submucosa. Ulcerated mucosa results in breakdown of the normal mucosal barrier and sets the stage for secondary infection and oral discomfort. A multitude of disease processes can result in or contribute to formation of oral ulcers.
- Infectious (fungal, viral, bacterial, rickettsial)
  - Viral: FeLV, FIV, FCV, FHV, feline syncytium-forming virus, and feline infectious peritonitis (FIP); feline panleukoepnia and canine distemper virus may cause stomatitis
  - Rickettsial: Rocky mountain spotted fever (RMSF)
  - Fungal: candidal stomatitis
  - Bacterial: aerobic/anaerobic, leptospirosis
- Immune-mediated disease: pemphigus vulgaris, bullous pemphigoid, systemic lupus erythematosus, erythema multiforme, vasculitis, and toxic epidermal necrosis
- Metabolic: kidney disease (uremic ulcers), endocrine disease (uncommon; hyperadrenocorticism, diabetes mellitus, hypothyroidism, hypoparathyroidism)
- Inflammatory: periodontal disease, dental tartar
- Trauma: foreign body, electrical cord chewing, gum chewers disease (chronic chewing of the cheeks)
- Neoplasia: epitheliotropic lymphoma, squamous cell carcinoma, melanoma, other oral tumors
- Toxins: acid or alkali ingestion, cationic detergents present in some disinfectants, potpourri ingestion, bleaches, plants (e.g., dieffenbachia, peace lily, calla lily)
- Nutritional: malnutrition, riboflavin deficiency
- Idiopathic
  - Eosinophilic granuloma complex (cats, Siberian Huskies, Alaskan Malamutes, Cavalier King Charles spaniel)
  - CUPS: hallmark lesions are contact ulcers or kissing ulcers
  - LPGS
  - Stomatitis (p. 943)

DIAGNOSIS

Diagnostic Overview

A thorough medical history and physical and oral exams help guide the clinician to selection of appropriate diagnostics.

Differential Diagnosis

If the animal presents with dysphagia, rule out other causes, including foreign bodies, neurologic disease (including rabies), dental malocclusion, and severe dental disease or dental abscess.

Initial Database

- Visual and tactile oral exam (may require sedation or anesthesia)
- CBC: mild nonregenerative anemia, neutropenia, or inflammatory leukogram may be present with inflammatory/infectious causes
- Serum biochemistry profile: evidence for metabolic disease (e.g., azotemia)
- Urinalysis: isosthenuric urine may support renal failure. Proteinuria may be evident with infectious, inflammatory, immune-mediated, or neoplastic causes.
- FeLV/FIV serology

Advanced or Confirmatory Testing

- Case-specific advanced diagnostics
  - If dental disease suspected: dental radiographs, teeth extraction
  - If neoplastic disease suspected: thoracic radiographs for metastasis
  - If infectious disease suspected: serology, polymerase chain reaction (PCR) assay
  - If immune-mediated disease suspected: antinuclear antibody titer
  - If metabolic disease suspected, consult individual disease chapters.
- Tissue biopsy and histopathology
- Cultures are rarely helpful.

TREATMENT

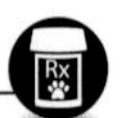

Treatment Overview

Focus should be on addressing underlying disease process. It is important to be mindful of nutritional support throughout the therapeutic period.

Acute General Treatment

- Address and treat underlying disease.
- Broad-spectrum antibiotic if secondary infection present: amoxicillin, clindamycin, or doxycycline is a good first choice.
- Pain control: buprenorphine 0.01-0.02 mg/kg PO q 8-12h
- Mouthwash for local pain relief: mix equal parts viscous lidocaine 2% and sucraflate suspension 1 g/10 mL; apply 2-5 mL to affected areas up to q 6h. There are many alternative “magic mouthwash” formulations, but caution should be used with ingredients and dose. The toxic dose of lidocaine is ≈6 mg/kg.
- Fluid therapy (IV or SQ) and hospitalization if patient is anorexic, dehydrated, ill
- Nutritional support (see below)

Chronic Treatment

- For CUPS and LPGS: dental extractions and meticulous dental hygiene are necessary.
- For immune-mediated disease: immunosuppressive therapy
- For identified infectious disease: appropriate antimicrobial, antiviral, or antifungal therapy
- For uremic ulcers: address chronic kidney disease (p. 169).
- Oral bovine lactoferrin was reported to have an antiinflammatory effect on chronic stomatitis in FIV-infected cats.

Nutrition/Diet

- Entice with highly palatable, aromatic foods. Baby food or blended food may be helpful.
- Severe cases with prolonged anorexia may require placement of a nasogastric or esophagostomy tube.

Drug Interactions

Immunosuppressive drugs should be avoided in FeLV/FIV-infected cats.

Possible Complications

Persistent inappetence to anorexia in cats may lead to hepatic lipidosis

PROGNOSIS & OUTCOME

- Depends on underlying cause
- Many of the idiopathic causes tend to be recurrent and respond poorly to therapy.

PEARLS & CONSIDERATIONS

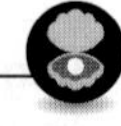

Comments

Identifying a definitive underlying condition is crucial for appropriate management.

Technician Tips

Imparting the importance of dental hygiene and demonstrating at-home dental cleaning are important in many of these cases.

SUGGESTED READING

Arzi B, et al: Oral manifestations of systemic disorders in dogs and cats. J Vet Clin Sci 1:112-124. 2008.

AUTHOR: Megan van Eeden, DVM
EDITOR: Leah A. Cohn, DVM, PhD, DACVIM

Umbilical Hernia

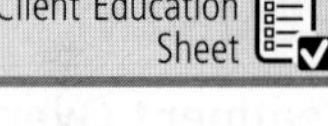

BASIC INFORMATION

Definition

Congenital midline defect of closure of the body wall at the umbilicus with various amounts of herniated contents

Epidemiology

SPECIES, AGE, SEX

- Most common abdominal hernia in small animals
- Dogs and cats of either sex; from birth but sometimes not identified until adulthood

GENETICS, BREED PREDISPOSITION

- Breed predisposition in dogs: Airedale terriers, basenjis, Pekingese, pointers, and Weimaraners
- Breed predisposition in cats: Cornish rex
- Umbilical hernias thought to be heritable, likely through polygenic inheritance

RISK FACTORS

- Excessive traction on umbilicus at birth
- Larger hernias more likely to result in organ entrapment, incarceration, or strangulation

ASSOCIATED DISORDERS

- Cryptorchidism
- Fucosidosis, an inherited, autosomal recessive neurovisceral lysosomal storage disease
- Ectodermal dysplasia
- Pentalogy of Cantrell
  - Sternal cleft
  - Cardiac defects
  - Peritoneopericardial diaphragmatic hernia
  - Ectopic cordis syndrome

Clinical Presentation

DISEASE FORMS/SUBTYPES

- Uncomplicated
  - Single umbilical hernia without organ incarceration or other anatomic abnormalities
- Complicated
  - Concurrent anatomic abnormalities
  - Strangulated or incarcerated abdominal viscera
- Omphalocele
  - Large midline umbilical and skin defect that allows abdominal viscera to protrude from the body
  - Most affected animals are euthanized or die before attempted surgical correction
- Gastroschisis
  - Grossly similar to omphalocele, although paramedian in location; almost always results in neonatal death

HISTORY, CHIEF COMPLAINT

- Typically an incidental finding on physical exam during routine puppy/kitten evaluation. The owner may report a soft swelling on midline that may change in size. It is usually nonpainful and may or may not be reducible.
- Systemic signs of illness may be present if abdominal viscera are strangulated.

PHYSICAL EXAM FINDINGS

- Soft, nonpainful swelling along midline at the site of the umbilicus
  - May or may not be reducible
  - Other clinical signs may be present, depending on what contents are within the hernia.
- Acute abdominal visceral herniation
  - Firm, painful mass, and possible abdominal pain
- Make sure to check for two descended testicles in the male dog/cat.

Etiology and Pathophysiology

- Umbilical hernia results when the lateral folds, principally the rectus abdominis muscle and fascia, fail to fuse or have delayed fusion after the midgut relocates in the sixth week of gestation.
- Herniation is usually limited to falciform ligament or omentum. Rarely are organ contents herniated.
- Umbilical hernia may diminish in size as the animal ages. Minimal size is usually achieved at approximately 6 months of age.

DIAGNOSIS

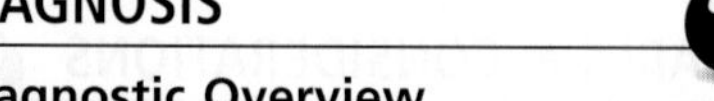

Diagnostic Overview

Diagnosis is typically made on physical exam alone. Radiographs can be performed in cases of large hernia or if concerned about hernia contents.

Differential Diagnosis

- Abscess
- Neoplasia (unlikely)
- Supraumbilical hernia
- Patent urachal remnant

Initial Database

CBC and chemistry panel are usually unremarkable, except if bowel is incarcerated.

Advanced or Confirmatory Testing

- For complicated hernias, radiographs can be taken to determine the hernia contents.
- Ultrasound can also be used if concern exists for abscess, although rarely used.

TREATMENT

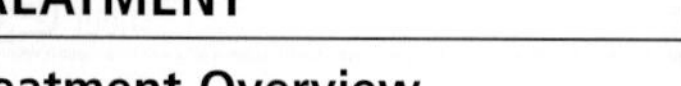

Treatment Overview

Treatment is aimed at replacement of herniated contents and closure of the defect with a tension-free closure. This is most commonly performed during at the time of routine sterilization procedure.

Acute General Treatment

- Conservative management
  - Small hernias that are easily reducible or have no hernial contents do not require repair.
  - An umbilical hernia identified early in life should be monitored.
  - Spontaneous closure may occur as late as 6 months of age.
- Simple umbilical hernias can be repaired primarily.
  - Incision is made over the hernia, and contents are replaced into the abdomen.
  - The edges do not need to be freshened before closure.
  - Primary closure is usually achieved as part of the closure of the abdominal cavity.
- Complicated hernia
  - Immediate surgical correction with evaluation of herniated viscera
  - If hernia is chronic or extremely large, muscle flaps or mesh may be needed to close abdominal cavity.

Possible Complications

- Incisional dehiscence
  - Rare
  - Large defect
  - Excessive tension on repair
- Gastroschisis and omphalocele
  - Early neonatal death due to contamination of abdominal cavity

Recommended Monitoring

When noted early in life, should be monitored frequently to determine if closure is necessary. Enlargement or acute swelling may indicate incarceration of abdominal viscera, which warrants immediate veterinary evaluation.

PROGNOSIS & OUTCOME

- Excellent with simple, uncomplicated hernias
- Guarded prognosis if large, complicated, or open
- Damage to herniated contents may change the prognosis.

PEARLS & CONSIDERATIONS

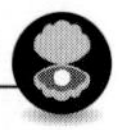

Comments

- Umbilical hernias are typically an incidental finding and usually can be repaired in an elective manner.
- Entrapment of abdominal viscera should be higher concern for larger defects.
- Always examine patients with umbilical hernias for other congenital defects.

Prevention

- Do not breed affected dogs or cats because this is likely an inherited defect.
- Minimal traction should be applied to umbilicus during parturition.

Technician Tips

- Umbilical hernias can usually wait until elective sterilization procedure to be repaired.
- Changes in size of the hernia can be an indication of changes in hernia contents and may warrant more rapid intervention.

Client Education

- Treatment may be conservative or herniorrhaphy to prevent complications.
- Veterinarians should train breeders in proper neonatal care.

SUGGESTED READING

Smeak DD: Abdominal wall reconstruction and hernias. In Johnston SA, et al, editors: Veterinary surgery: small animal, ed 2, St. Louis, 2017, Elsevier, pp 1564-1591.

AUTHOR: Jacob A. Rubin DVM, DACVS
EDITOR: Elizabeth A. Swanson DVM, MS, DACVS

Upper Airway Obstruction

Client Education Sheet

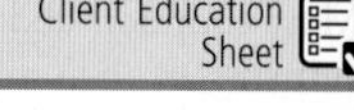

BASIC INFORMATION

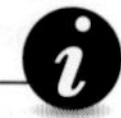

Definition

Inability to move air effectively through nose/mouth, pharynx, larynx, and/or trachea

Epidemiology

SPECIES, AGE, SEX

- Airway foreign body (FB) more likely in young dogs
- Nasopharyngeal polyps more likely in young cats and (rarely) dogs
- Laryngeal paralysis more likely in older dogs and (rarely) cats
- Neoplastic obstruction more likely in older adult dogs or cats

GENETICS, BREED PREDISPOSITION

- Brachycephalic animals are predisposed to airway obstruction.
- Breed predispositions exist for laryngeal paralysis (p. 574).

RISK FACTORS

Environmental factors: excitement, heat, and exercise, especially in animals with predisposition to obstruction (e.g., brachycephalic airway syndrome, laryngeal paralysis)

ASSOCIATED DISORDERS

Brachycephalic airway syndrome, laryngeal paralysis, neoplasia, nasopharyngeal polyp, pulmonary edema

Clinical Presentation

DISEASE FORMS/SUBTYPES

- Supraglottic structures: brachycephalic airway syndrome (p. 128), laryngeal paralysis (unilateral/bilateral), foreign bodies (pharyngeal/laryngeal), nasopharyngeal polyp (p. 681), laryngeal collapse, laryngeal edema or hemorrhage, laryngeal neoplasia (p. 573), epiglottic entrapment

- Subglottic structures: tracheal collapse (p. 194), FB, tracheal neoplasia, tracheal hypoplasia, trauma. Mass lesions external to the airway (e.g., thyroid carcinoma, cervical abscess) can cause narrowing or collapse of the airway.

HISTORY, CHIEF COMPLAINT

- Loud breathing (new stertor or stridor) is most consistent finding. Respiratory effort may be mild or severe. Acute distress after playing with an object (e.g., ball) suggests FB obstruction. Neoplasia may manifest as progressive dyspnea. Laryngeal paralysis often is accompanied by a change in the sound of the bark (dysphonia). Clinical signs often are exacerbated by exercise, excitement, or on a warm day.
- Foreign object (e.g., ball, marble, acorn) aspiration may be witnessed, although the mistaken belief that an FB has been aspirated is a common error that some clients believe passionately ("something stuck in the throat") even when the problem is clearly different (e.g., pulmonary edema, pleural effusion).

PHYSICAL EXAM FINDINGS

- Noisy, stridorous (laryngeal or subglottic) or stertorous (nasal or nasopharyngeal) breathing
  - Typically exaggerated inspiratory effort
  - Noise may be heard only on inspiratory (dynamic obstruction) or during both phases (fixed obstruction).
- Sometimes, orthopneic posture, cyanosis, paradoxic breathing (chest and abdomen move in opposition), bulging at thoracic inlet (lung lobe herniation), Horner's syndrome (nasopharyngeal polyp)
- Hyperthermia possible (excessive muscle activity, ineffective cooling)
- Specific conformations (e.g., short nose) raise the suspicion of associated malformations.
- Loud sounds may be referred to the lower airways; auscult over the trachea to help determine origin.
- Obesity may magnify clinical signs.

Etiology and Pathophysiology

- Most resistance to airflow occurs in the upper airways. Any fixed or dynamic obstruction in the upper airways increases resistance to breathing and, subsequently, the work of breathing.
- Inspiration against a partially or completely closed upper airway may cause noncardiogenic pulmonary edema as the alveoli become flooded with plasma due to negative pressure generated in the airways.

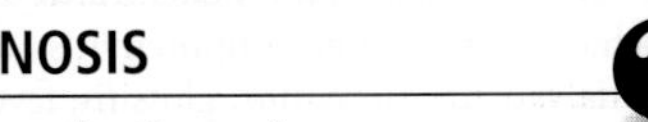

DIAGNOSIS

Diagnostic Overview

Upper airway obstruction is recognized on physical exam. Inspiratory dyspnea (restrictive breathing pattern characterized by a slow and deliberate inspiration and rapid exhalation), often with the point of stridor audible in the upper airway, helps localize the anatomic lesion. Stertor, in nonbrachycephic breeds, may be indicative of altered upper airway airflow. Signalment, history, and exam findings usually allow a refined differential diagnosis. Oral and laryngeal exam, diagnostic imaging, and endoscopy confirm the site (and sometimes nature) of the obstruction.

Differential Diagnosis

Occasionally, pleural effusion in cats mimics upper respiratory obstruction.

Initial Database

- Oral/laryngeal exam under sedation is the most important diagnostic test (p. 1125).
  - Be prepared for an emergent intubation or tracheostomy (and possibly positive-pressure ventilation if noncardiogenic pulmonary edema is present (pp. 1166 and 1185).
  - Doxapram 2.2 mg/kg IV can stimulate ventilation during exam but may result in glottic constriction requiring intubation.
- Ancillary testing includes radiographs (cervical and thoracic), CBC, serum biochemistry profile, and evaluation of oxygenation (pulse oximetry or arterial blood gas [ABG] analysis).

Advanced or Confirmatory Testing

Bronchoscopy (p. 1074), fluoroscopy, or CT may be useful for evaluating focal lesions and dynamic changes or for obtaining biopsies or cytologic specimens.

TREATMENT

Treatment Overview

Minimize stress while making diagnosis; sometimes the diagnosis and treatment occur simultaneously (e.g., FB is identified and removed). A general approach to treatment is provided on p. 1453.

Acute General Treatment

- Sedatives or analgesics, glucocorticoids at antiinflammatory doses, and oxygen supplementation (p. 1146) can be lifesaving.
- Secure airway patency if necessary (p. 1166).
- Hyperthermia (i.e., muscle activity or ineffective cooling, not true fever) can respond to physical cooling but not to antiinflammatory drugs (p. 421).
- Remove foreign object, if present.

Chronic Treatment

- Surgical correction: laryngeal tie-back procedure, remove nasopharyngeal polyp, repair stenotic nares, and so forth
- Medical management
  - Environmental control (e.g., avoid neck leads, avoid excessive heat)
  - Anxiolytic drugs (e.g., trazodone 2-7 mg/kg PO q 12h)

Nutrition/Diet

Weight loss diet may be indicated for long-term treatment of obesity.

Behavior/Exercise

Avoid heat stress.

Possible Complications

Recurrence of clinical signs, aspiration pneumonia, noncardiogenic pulmonary edema, and/or respiratory arrest

Recommended Monitoring

Monitor respiratory rate/effort, oxygenation, and ventilatory status.

PROGNOSIS & OUTCOME

- Depends on the underlying problem and severity of clinical signs
- Prognosis worse for cases with noncardiogenic pulmonary edema or pneumonia

PEARLS & CONSIDERATIONS

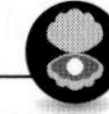

Comments

- Up to one-half the diameter of the airway can be compromised without obvious clinical signs.
- Major errors include underestimating the patient's distress, overzealous exam without a set action plan (e.g., having tools for intubation immediately available), and performance of tests or procedures that are detrimental to the condition of the patient at that time.
- A common radiographic misdiagnosis is the interpretation of a prominent or mineralized (but normal) larynx as an FB, especially if the neck is radiographed obliquely.
- Thoracic radiography and positive-pressure ventilation should be planned in case dyspnea and/or hypoxemia persist after relief of upper airway obstruction, as can occur when noncardiogenic pulmonary edema is also present.
- Dogs may be presented with pulmonary edema after a choking episode has resolved (e.g., "hanging" on chain).

Prevention

Avoid overexertion, prevent heat stress, and know the medical options that are available to help break the cycle of distress and dyspnea. Stenotic nares should be repaired early in life.

Technician Tips

Minimize stress by using minimal restraint and pursuing treatments in a stepwise manner. Procedures (e.g., catheter placement, blood sampling, individual radiographs) may need to be staged, depending on the stability of the animal. Injectable medications may be preferred to oral.

Client Education

Explain that brachycephalic animals are predisposed to upper airway problems. Dogs with untreated laryngeal paralysis must be maintained in cool environments, with activity minimized.

SUGGESTED READING

Costello MF: Upper airway disease. In Silverstein DC, et al, editors: Small animal critical care medicine, ed 1, St. Louis, 2009, Saunders, p 67.

AUTHOR: Megan Whelan, DVM, DACVECC, CVA
EDITOR: Benjamin M. Brainard, VMD, DACVAA, DACVECC

Upper Respiratory Infection (Cat)

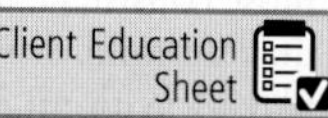

BASIC INFORMATION

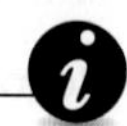

Definition

Upper respiratory infection is a common cause of upper respiratory tract signs and ocular abnormalities, including sneezing, nasal congestion, ocular and nasal discharge, conjunctivitis/keratitis, and oral ulcerations in cats. It is often the result of transmissible multiagent or single-agent infections, including feline herpesvirus 1 (FHV-1), feline calicivirus (FCV), *Bordetella bronchiseptica*, *Chlamydia felis*, and *Mycoplasma* species.

Synonyms

- Feline upper respiratory tract disease, feline infectious respiratory disease, feline respiratory disease complex, feline upper respiratory infection (URI)
- FHV-1: feline rhinotracheitis virus

Epidemiology

SPECIES, AGE, SEX

Young or elderly (debilitated) cats are typically the most severely affected.

GENETICS, BREED PREDISPOSITION

Brachycephalic purebred cats (Himalayans, Persians) appear to be at increased risk for developing chronic disease.

RISK FACTORS

- Multi-cat environments (boarding and breeding facilities, shelters, multi-cat households)
- Introduction of new cats to the home or facility
- Poor husbandry and overcrowding
- Lack of or inappropriate vaccination

CONTAGION AND ZOONOSIS

- Direct contact is the most common mode of transmission. FHV-1, FCV, and *B. bronchiseptica* are transmitted by ocular, nasal, and oral secretions, whereas ocular secretions are probably the most important medium for transmission of *C. felis*.
- Indirect (fomite) transmission may occur through cages, bowls, cleaning instruments, or personnel contaminated with secretions from infected cats. Fomites are a very important means of transmission of FCV.
- Aerosolization is an unlikely mode of transmission, but macrodroplets expelled during sneezing or coughing may allow transmission over distances of 1-2 meters.
- FHV-1 survives a maximum of 18 hours at room temperature and is readily inactivated by drying and most disinfectants. FCV is resistant to routine disinfection with quaternary ammonium compounds and survives in the environment for up to 1 month. *B. bronchiseptica* can persist longer than 10 days in the environment. The environment is less important than direct contact as a source of infection.
- *B. bronchiseptica* causes respiratory infections in cats, dogs, rabbits, and people. Transmission between dogs and cats may occur. There is zoonotic (minimal) potential in immunocompromised people.

GEOGRAPHY AND SEASONALITY

Worldwide distribution with no true seasonality

ASSOCIATED DISORDERS

- FHV-1 infection can cause osteolytic changes and permanent damage to the nasal turbinates predisposing to chronic upper respiratory tract disease and the development of keratoconjunctivitis sicca (KCS).
- Persistent FCV infection has been linked to chronic ulceroproliferative and lymphoplasmacytic stomatitis.

Clinical Presentation

DISEASE FORMS/SUBTYPES

- Herpesvirus: usually acute, severe upper respiratory signs in young animals; in chronic adult cases, it can manifest as a chronic conjunctivitis/keratitis with mild, recurrent upper respiratory signs or without respiratory signs. Feline herpesviral keratitis is discussed further on p. 464.
- Calicivirus: oral lesions (ulcers, stomatitis) predominate; ocular and respiratory signs are typically mild; isolated highly virulent strains that cause severe systemic disease and death

HISTORY, CHIEF COMPLAINT

- General signs of upper respiratory tract disease include sneezing, congestion, ocular and nasal discharge, epiphora, blepharospasm, hyporexia, and lethargy.
- Specific to calicivirus (p. 141), herpesvirus (p. 464), and *C. felis* (p. 157)

PHYSICAL EXAM FINDINGS

Respiratory disease complex:

- Serous to mucopurulent nasal and ocular discharge, nasal congestion
- Epiphora, blepharospasm, chemosis, conjunctival hyperemia
- Fever
- Sometimes dyspnea, increased airway sounds, wheezes, cough

Other:

- Specific to calicivirus (e.g., oral ulcers, lameness [p. 141]), herpesvirus (e.g., corneal lesions [p. 464]), and *C. felis* (e.g., conjunctivitis [p. 157])
- Virulent systemic calicivirus (rare): dermal necrosis and crusting, peripheral edema, evidence of shock
- *B. bronchiseptica*: lymphadenopathy, cyanosis if severe bronchopneumonia

Etiology and Pathophysiology

Feline herpesvirus:

- An alpha-herpesvirus specific to Felidae that attacks mucosal epithelial cells of the soft palate, tonsils, nasal turbinates, cornea, and conjunctiva, leading to multifocal epithelial necrosis and secondary clinical signs. Pulmonary involvement is rare.
- Incubation period is 2-6 days; disease usually runs its course in 10-20 days.
- Viral shedding has been detected as early as 24 hours after infection and persists for 1-3 weeks.
- Essentially all cats infected with FHV-1 become chronic carriers; the virus remains latent in the trigeminal ganglia. These cats act as an FHV-1 reservoir.
- Reactivation of shedding occurs in fewer than one-half of latently infected cats 4-12 days after stress. The mean duration of shedding is 7 days (up to 2 weeks). Shedding in carriers may occur with or without clinical signs.

Other infections:

- Feline calicivirus (p. 141)
- *B. bronchiseptica* (p. 125)
- *C. felis* (p. 157)

DIAGNOSIS

Diagnostic Overview

Usually the diagnosis is based on clinical presentation: sneezing, ocular and/or nasal discharge, coughing, conjunctivitis, anterior uveitis, faucitis, stomatitis, glossitis, fever, and/or lymphadenomegaly. History of exposure to other cats provides support for the diagnosis of viral respiratory disease, but because of recrudescence, exposure is not necessary to implicate viruses as the cause of clinical signs.

Identification of a causative agent is often not necessary because the disease is self-limited in most cats, but it is recommended in chronic and recurrent cases. Ruling out nonviral causes is important for treatment considerations.

Differential Diagnosis

- Nasal signs (p. 1255)
- Cough (p. 1209)
- Respiratory distress (p. 1219)
- Ocular signs: corneal and/or conjunctival trauma, corneal foreign body, neoplasia, KCS, uveitis, glaucoma

Initial Database

- CBC: often normal, but stress or inflammatory leukogram can occur
- Serum biochemistry profile and urinalysis: typically unremarkable; may reflect dehydration
- Thoracic radiographs: if lower respiratory signs are present

Advanced or Confirmatory Testing

- Serologic testing for herpesvirus and calicivirus is unrewarding because of widespread vaccination and exposure.
    - Serologic testing may be helpful in unvaccinated cats because affected animals typically have high titers.
- Virus isolation from nasal, conjunctival, or oropharyngeal swabs is the best diagnostic assay for FHV-1 and FCV; however, FCV is commonly isolated from the oral/respiratory mucosa of healthy cats, and positive viral culture should be supported by appropriate clinical presentation. Requires special swabs or media for transport.
    - Feline upper respiratory disease panel (www.idexx.com or www.antechdiagnostics.com); requires swab samples, depending on location of predominant clinical signs
- Conjunctival scrapes may demonstrate basophilic intracytoplasmic inclusions indicating *C. felis* infection.
- Polymerase chain reaction (PCR) assay of conjunctival swabs can also be used for ruling out *C. felis*. Special transport medium is required for culture.
- Transtracheal wash or bronchoalveolar lavage (p. 1073) with cytologic exam and culture and sensitivity are helpful in isolating *B. bronchiseptica* or other bacteria as causative agents of lower respiratory tract disease.
- Cryptococcal antigen titer to rule out cryptococcosis (p. 223) when chronic nasal signs present
- Nasal CT with rhinoscopy and nasal biopsy/culture can help to rule out neoplasia, fungal infection, dental disease, nasopharyngeal polyps, and deformities as causes of chronic respiratory signs (p. 678).

TREATMENT

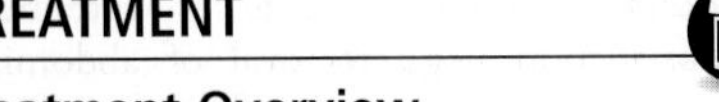

Treatment Overview

Treatment is typically supportive, with the goal of controlling secondary bacterial infections and maintaining comfort and appetite.

Acute General Treatment

Supportive care is the recommended treatment for cats presented with moderate to severe upper respiratory tract disease. Most cats with URIs can and should be managed at home by the owner to decrease pathogen dissemination in the hospital. Animals that are febrile, dehydrated, depressed, or compromised should be treated in isolation within the hospital until they are stable and can be sent home. Acute treatment includes

- IV or subcutaneous crystalloid fluid therapy
- Antibiotic therapy if a secondary bacterial infection is suspected (one of the following)
    - Amoxicillin-clavulanate 12.5 mg/kg PO q 12h
    - Azithromycin 5-10 mg/kg PO q 24-48h
    - Pradofloxacin 7.5 mg/kg PO q 24h
    - Marbofloxacin 2.75-5 mg/kg PO q 24h
    - Doxycycline 10 mg/kg PO q 24h (effective against *B. bronchiseptica, Mycoplasma* spp)
- Topical ophthalmic preparations
    - Artificial tears q 6h
    - I-Drop Vet (lubricant with 0.3% sodium hyaluronate): apply 1 drop q 8h
    - Antibiotic therapy: apply q 6-8h
        - Tetracycline ophthalmic preparations are the treatment of choice for *C. felis* and *Mycoplasma* spp conjunctivitis and in FHV-1–positive cats to prevent secondary bacterial infections. Topical tetracyclines can be irritating. Chloramphenicol, erythromycin, or ciprofloxacin topicals are alternative options.
        - Topical or systemic glucocorticoids should not be used in suspected FHV-1 keratitis.
        - Most triple-antibiotic ophthalmic preparations (neomycin, polymyxin, and bacitracin/gramicidin) are typically ineffective against *C. felis, Mycoplasma* spp, and FHV-1.
- Topical and systemic antiviral drugs for FHV-1 (p. 464)
- Treatment duration with antibiotics and antivirals should be determined on an individual case basis, but 2-4 weeks is often required while the viral disease runs its course.

Chronic Treatment

- Room humidification or inhalation of steam (putting the cat on a dry surface in a steamy bathroom) may aid in the removal of thick and viscous secretions and help ease nasal or airway congestion.
- FHV-1 carriers that have bouts of recrudescence can be treated on as-needed basis with oral antiviral therapy and/or L-lysine (250-500 mg PO/CAT q 24h) to decrease severity of outbreaks.

Nutrition/Diet

- Feed fresh, warm, highly palatable, and aromatic foods to overcome a decreased sense of smell from nasal congestion and reluctance to eat due to oral discomfort (p. 1199).
- Appetite stimulants may be necessary.
    - Mirtazapine 3.75 mg/CAT PO q 24-72h, *or*
    - Capromorelin 1-3 mg/kg PO q 24h for up to 21 days
- Placement of a feeding tube may be necessary in chronic cases with prolonged hyporexia or severe oral ulceration (p. 1106).

PROGNOSIS & OUTCOME

Except for very young or severely compromised cats or in cases of virulent calicivirus, prognosis is usually good for recovery from acute URI. Some animals develop chronic rhinitis, stomatitis, and/or KCS or have frequent recurrence of disease that requires lifelong management.

PEARLS & CONSIDERATIONS

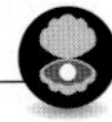

Comments

Indirect transmission may occur through cages, bowls, instruments, or personnel contaminated with secretions from infected cats. It is important to limit personnel exposure and the movement of cats suspected to have a URI.

Prevention

- Improve husbandry, decrease overcrowding and exposure to free-roaming or feral cats, and ensure appropriate cleaning and disinfection.
- Accelerated hydrogen peroxide disinfectants or dilute bleach (1 part bleach to 30 parts water) can be used to prevent FHV-1 and FCV spread in the hospital environment. FCV has shown resistance to common disinfectants such as quaternary ammonium compounds and chlorhexidine.
- Several modified live or inactivated virus vaccines are available and induce reasonable protection against clinical disease associated with FHV-1 and FCV infection. The vaccines are relatively successful in controlling disease and decreasing virus shedding, but they do not completely protect against infection or development of the carrier state.
    - Modified live vaccines (MLVs) may induce a mild form of respiratory disease.
- An intranasal MLV is available for *B. bronchiseptica* but is indicated only for cats at high risk for infection. Mild respiratory signs can occur after vaccination.
- MLV and killed vaccines are available for *C. felis*, but use is reserved for cats in multi-cat environments in which confirmed infections have been associated with clinical disease.

Technician Tips

Personnel should wear gloves, wash hands, and thoroughly clean and disinfect the room and any instruments, bowls, and/or cages that have been in contact with the cat.

Client Education

Owners should be instructed to minimize accumulation of mucus and saliva by cleaning the cat's face, mouth, and nares regularly.

SUGGESTED READING

Sykes JE: Feline respiratory viral infections. In Sykes JE, editor: Canine and feline infectious diseases, St. Louis, 2014, Elsevier, pp 239-251.

AUTHOR: Jon M. Fletcher, DVM, DACVIM
EDITOR: Joseph Taboada, DVM, DACVIM

Ureteral Obstruction

Client Education Sheet 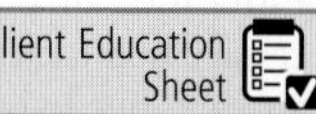

BASIC INFORMATION 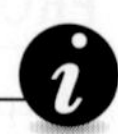

Definition

Obstruction of urine flow through one or both ureters; ureteral obstruction is recognized with increasing frequency, especially in cats

Epidemiology

SPECIES, AGE, SEX

Dogs or cats of any age or sex

GENETICS, BREED PREDISPOSITION

Certain breeds are overrepresented for some uroliths (important cause of ureteral obstruction) (pp. 1014, 1016, and 1019).

RISK FACTORS

- Intraluminal obstruction (e.g., urolith, trauma, inflammation, fibrosis/stricture, congenital stenosis, blood clots)
- Intramural obstruction (e.g., fibrosis/stenosis, ureterocele, fibroepithelial polyps, proliferative ureteritis, neoplasia)
- Extramural obstruction (e.g., retroperitoneal or pelvic masses, prostatic/bladder neoplasia, inadvertent ligation or fibrotic entrapment of ureter)

ASSOCIATED DISORDERS

- Renal failure ± uremia
- Hydronephrosis/hydroureter
- Pyelonephritis
- Uroabdomen (if ruptured ureter)

Clinical Presentation

DISEASE FORMS/SUBTYPES

- Partial or complete
- Unilateral or bilateral

HISTORY, CHIEF COMPLAINT

Clinical signs are often absent, especially with unilateral obstruction. When present, signs may be related to acute renal failure or to overt chronic kidney disease. Any of these may be seen:

- Lethargy/depression (due to uremia or renal pain)
- Anorexia/vomiting (due to uremia or renal pain)
- Polyuria and polydipsia (with chronic kidney disease)
- Dysuria, stranguria, pollakiuria, or hematuria
- Oliguria or anuria (bilateral obstruction [rare])

PHYSICAL EXAM FINDINGS

Physical exam is often normal; abnormalities can include

- Dehydration
- Poor body condition
- Enlarged kidney(s) due to hydronephrosis
- Abdominal discomfort or back pain (severity related to rate of onset of obstruction rather than degree of obstruction)
- Halitosis and/or oral ulceration due to uremia
- Abdominal fluid wave (if rupture and uroabdomen [rare])

Etiology and Pathophysiology

Urolithiasis is the most common cause of ureteral obstruction. However, there are many other potential causes (see above).

DIAGNOSIS

Diagnostic Overview

Ureteral obstruction may be discovered incidentally during imaging studies or (less often) may be identified as the cause of acute renal failure due to bilateral obstruction. Animals with subclinical or overt chronic kidney disease may be identified as having ureteral obstruction during imaging exams.

Differential Diagnosis

Other causes of renomegaly; other causes of acute kidney injury (p. 23)

Initial Database

- CBC generally unremarkable
  - Normocytic, normochromic, nonregenerative anemia (if chronic kidney disease or chronic inflammation)
  - Leukocytosis with left shift possible if concurrent pyelonephritis
- Serum biochemical profile abnormalities depend on degree of obstruction and/or nephron loss.
  - Azotemia
  - Hyperphosphatemia
  - Hyperkalemia
  - Metabolic acidosis
  - Increased symmetric dimethylarginine (SDMA)
- Urinalysis may be normal or may reveal isosthenuria, hematuria, pyuria, and/or crystalluria.
- Urine culture and susceptibility indicated even if sediment is inactive (occult infection)
- Blood pressure measurement to rule out systemic hypertension (p. 1065)
- Abdominal radiographs; renomegaly common; may also identify
  - Urolithiasis (calcium phosphate, calcium oxalate, and struvite uroliths)
  - Loss of retroperitoneal/abdominal contrast
  - Distended ureter
  - Mass (abdomen, bladder, ureter)

Advanced or Confirmatory Testing

- Abdominal ultrasound (sensitive and specific): pyelectasia (dilation of renal pelvis), hydronephrosis, hydroureter common
  - Often allows identification of a cause of ureteral obstruction (e.g., urolithiasis, mass)
- Excretory urography (EU), intravenous pyelography (p. 1101), percutaneous nephropyelography
  - Pyelectasia
  - Ureteral dilation or lack of filling (EU only)
- Renal scintigraphy or CT
  - Affected kidney contributes little to overall glomerular filtration rate (GFR).
- Quantitative analysis and culture of uroliths

TREATMENT 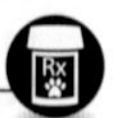

Treatment Overview

When unilateral obstruction is thought to be long-standing (e.g., absence of abdominal pain, absence of uroabdomen), therapy should still be considered to save existing renal function. Acute bilateral ureteral obstruction requires intervention to relieve obstruction and address consequences such as uremia, electrolyte, and acid-base disorders. If possible, attempts should be made to prevent further obstruction (e.g., prophylaxis of urolithiasis, correction of anatomic defects, removal of obstructive masses).

Acute General Treatment

- Bilateral obstruction is rare, but if present, requires interventional (radiological, surgical, endoscopic) treatment.
- Correct hydration, acid-base, and electrolyte disorders with crystalloid fluid therapy for azotemia, dehydration (p. 243).
  - Post-obstructive diuresis may require the ins-and-outs method of fluid rate adjustment (rate based on measured urine output) (p. 23).
  - Diuresis may flush out ureterolith.
  - Consider hemodialysis or peritoneal dialysis for stabilization.
- Percutaneous nephrostomy tubes may be used for preventing further renal damage while assessing renal function before surgical intervention.
  - Possible only if renal pelvis dilated
  - Placed with ultrasound guidance or via laparotomy
- Analgesia for abdominal pain (e.g., buprenorphine 0.01 mg/kg IM, IV, or SQ q 6-8h)
- Address uremic signs (pp. 23 and 169).
- Address urinary tract infection if present (pp. 232 and 849).

Chronic Treatment

- If obstruction is partial and there is adequate renal function and no infection, intervention is not routinely required but can be beneficial to save existing renal function.
- Address treatable causes of extramural obstruction (e.g., removal of abdominal tumors obstructing urine flow).
- Therapeutic or prophylactic measures for urolithiasis (pp. 1014, 1016, and 1019)

- Subcutaneous ureteral bypass (SUB) device (p. 1174)
    - Indicated for ureteral stenosis or ureterolithiasis, primarily in cats and small dogs
    - A newer treatment modality that may replace other treatment options but is not without complications
- Ureteral stent placed via interventional endoscopy or surgery
    - Limited availability; surgery is more widely available, which is important if the patient is unstable.
    - Primarily indicated for middle-sized to large dogs
- Ureteral surgery
    - Major complication is postoperative ureteral stricture formation.
    - Ureterotomy for intraluminal or intramural obstruction in the proximal third of the ureter
    - Ureteroneocystostomy for resection of distal ureter
    - Ureteroureterostomy to repair ureter after resection or transection (anastomosis of proximal ureter to distal portion of ureter on ipsilateral side), usually when proximal third cannot be implanted directly into bladder neck; highest incidence of postoperative obstruction
- Nephrectomy is reserved for animals with unilateral obstruction, adequate function in contralateral kidney, and loss of virtually all function in the affected kidney.

Nutrition/Diet

Diet appropriate for preventing specific urolith type

Possible Complications

- Renal failure (acute or chronic)
- Postoperative ureteral stenosis
- Urinary rupture and uroabdomen

Recommended Monitoring

- Repeat ultrasound at 2 weeks after initial evaluation and treatment, then monthly until resolved or stable. Remaining renal parenchymal changes are likely permanent.
- Animals with permanent hydroureter/hydronephrosis are monitored as for chronic kidney disease (pp. 23 and 169). Azotemic animals are monitored more intensively than nonazotemic animals.

PROGNOSIS & OUTCOME

- Depends on underlying cause, duration of obstruction, extent of renal parenchymal damage, presence of concurrent infection, and ability to resolve underlying cause
- Structural renal changes persisting 14-45 days or more after relief of ureteral obstruction are generally permanent.
- Complete bilateral obstruction of more than 3 days is fatal without appropriate treatment.

PEARLS & CONSIDERATIONS

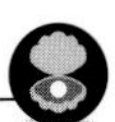

Comments

- Ureteral obstruction should be considered in the differential diagnosis for renal failure, especially in patients with evidence of nephrolithiasis or pyelonephritis.
- Bilateral ureteral obstruction is rare compared to unilateral obstruction but is life-threatening.
- Ureteral obstruction can recur, especially in the presence of existing nephroliths.

Prevention

Strategies that limit the formation of urolithiasis (pp. 1014, 1016, and 1019)

Technician Tips

Animals in acute renal failure should have urine output carefully quantified. One possible correctible cause of oliguria/anuria is bilateral ureteral obstruction.

Client Education

Strict adherence to dietary recommendations can minimize the risk of ureteral or urethral obstruction due to urolithiasis.

SUGGESTED READING

Berent A, et al: Subcutaneous ureteral bypass device placement for benign ureteral obstruction in cats: 137 cats (174 ureters). J Vet Intern Med 30:1539-1540, 2016.

AUTHOR: Adam Mordecai, DVM, MS, DACVIM
EDITOR: Leah A. Cohn, DVM, PhD, DACVIM

Urethral Obstruction

Client Education Sheet 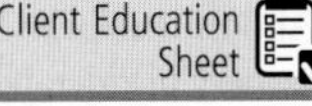

BASIC INFORMATION

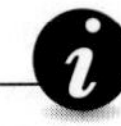

Definition

The common condition involves obstruction of the lower urinary tract and is usually due to urolith or matrix formation. Other causes (e.g., neoplasia, stricture, infections) are less common.

Epidemiology

SPECIES, AGE, SEX

- Cats and less commonly dogs of any age
- Males are anatomically predisposed to obstruction.

GENETICS, BREED PREDISPOSITION

- Certain breeds predisposed to specific urolith formation (e.g., Dalmatians: urate uroliths)
- Other breeds predisposed to urethral neoplasia (e.g., Scottish terrier)

RISK FACTORS

- Feline lower urinary tract signs/disease (FLUTS/D) (p. 332)
- Neoplasia
- Urinary tract infection
- Risk factors associated with urolithiasis (pp. 1014, 1016, and 1019)

ASSOCIATED DISORDERS

- Hydronephrosis
- Azotemia/uremia
- Hyperkalemic cardiac dysrhythmia
- Urinary bladder rupture
- Bladder atonia/hypotonia
- Urinary tract infection
- Postobstructive diuresis

Clinical Presentation

HISTORY, CHIEF COMPLAINT

- Urinary tract signs: pollakiuria, dysuria, stranguria, anuria/oliguria, hematuria, dribbling urine, licking prepuce/vulva (urethral discharge)
- Systemic signs: lethargy, anorexia, vocalization, restlessness, weakness, discomfort
- History of urinary infection or urolithiasis

PHYSICAL EXAM FINDINGS

- Enlarged, turgid urinary bladder (characteristic)
- Abdominal discomfort (common)
- Dribbling urine (occasionally)
- Bloody preputial/vulvar discharge (occasionally)
- Palpable urethral urolith or tumor (digital rectal exam in dogs) (occasionally)
- Bradycardia if severe hyperkalemia (in very advanced cases)

Etiology and Pathophysiology

- Urine supersaturation, urinary tract infection, certain disease states, and breed predisposition contribute to urolithiasis.
- In cats especially, urethral plugs may be composed of matrix (cellular debris, virus-like particles, ± bacteria, urinary crystals).
- Uroliths or plugs can obstruct the urethra; urethral anatomy favors obstruction in males.
- Neoplasia, especially transitional cell carcinoma (p. 991), may progress to cause obstruction.
- Urethritis may lead to urethral stricture.

DIAGNOSIS

Diagnostic Overview

The diagnosis of urethral obstruction is suspected in any patient that is straining to urinate and has an enlarged, firm urinary bladder present on abdominal palpation.

Differential Diagnosis

- Detrusor atony
- FLUTS/D
- Fungal granuloma
- Prostatic disease (male dogs)
- Reflex dyssynergia
- Trauma (pelvic fracture) with urethral damage, bladder entrapment hernia, penile fracture
- Urethral neoplasia
- Urethral stricture
- Urethral tissue valve/flap
- Urethritis
- Urolithiasis

Initial Database

- CBC: often unremarkable
- Serum biochemical profile: possible azotemia, hyperkalemia, ionized hypocalcemia, and findings consistent with predisposing conditions
- Urethral catheterization (pp. 1175 and 1176): distinguish functional from structural urethral obstruction, and localize structural obstruction; may relieve obstruction and provide urine for analysis
- Urinalysis: possible hematuria, crystalluria, pyuria, epithelial cells, dilute urine, bacteruria. Rarely, fungal hyphae or neoplastic cells
- Urine culture: if sample is obtained by catheterization, quantitative culture to distinguish contamination (<10^3 colony-forming units/mL) from infection
- Abdominal/pelvic radiographs: distended urinary bladder, possible radiopaque uroliths, renomegaly, ascites possible
- Abdominal ultrasound: possible uroliths, urinary bladder debris, pyelectasia, ascites
- Electrocardiogram: hyperkalemia signs (absent P waves, wide QRS complexes, bradycardia)

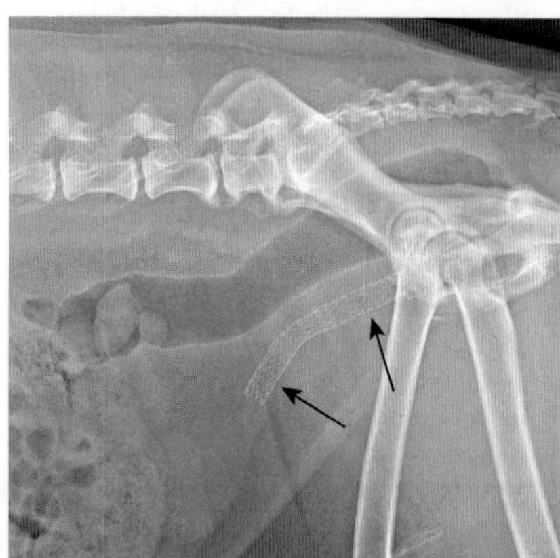

URETHRAL OBSTRUCTION A urethral stent *(arrows)* was placed in a male dog with urethral obstruction due to neoplastic infiltration.

Advanced or Confirmatory Testing

- Voiding cystourethrogram (p. 1181): determine location of urethral obstruction
- Retrieved uroliths: quantitative analysis, culture
- Other testing for conditions predisposing to urolith formation (e.g., bile acids as screen for portosystemic shunt)
- Cystoscopy to evaluate for masses, granuloma, etc.

TREATMENT

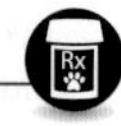

Treatment Overview

Treatment consists of relieving the urinary tract obstruction, which is generally done by passing a urinary catheter into the urinary bladder and draining the urine.

Acute General Treatment

- IV catheter for crystalloid fluid therapy, correcting electrolyte disorders, and administering sedation/anesthesia
    - Crystalloid fluids 5-10 mL/kg/h during sedation/anesthesia
    - Thereafter, rate should provide maintenance (40-60 mL/kg/day q 24h), correct dehydration, and match postobstructive diuresis losses.
        - Closed urine collection system to identify profound postobstructive diuresis, maintain sterility, and allow ins-and-outs fluid treatment plan
    - If serum potassium > 7 mEq/L, consider calcium gluconate, sodium bicarbonate, or insulin/dextrose therapy (p. 495).
- Small plug/urolith at the tip of the penis: remove by gentle massage (cats).
- Urethral catheterization can be attempted without sedation in male dogs; for cats, bitches, or dogs resistant to catheterization, sedation/anesthesia is usually required.
- Insert a sterile red rubber catheter, Slippery Sam tomcat catheter, or open-ended polypropylene catheter into the urethra to the point of obstruction. Once encountered, retropulse the urolith/debris into the urinary bladder using sterile saline or a 75% sterile saline and 25% sterile water-based lubricant mixture.
    - In male cats, a sterile, 22-gauge, 1-inch IV catheter (without stylet) may be used to dislodge urethral plug.
    - The urinary bladder is emptied; if debris is identified, lavage with sterile saline.
- An indwelling urinary catheter attached to a sterile, closed urine collection system is often indicated (e.g., pending correction of anatomic or functional obstruction, in cats with FLUTS/D, to prevent urolith movement back into urethra after retropulsion and pending cystotomy).
    - For indwelling purposes, polypropylene catheters should be replaced with red rubber or Foley catheters.
    - Ideally, radiographs are obtained to identify remaining radiopaque urethral/bladder uroliths and to evaluate appropriate catheter placement. The catheter should just enter the trigone.
- If a urinary catheter cannot be passed, decompressive cystocentesis can be performed to temporarily empty the urinary bladder pending definitive treatment.

Chronic Treatment

- Maintain indwelling urinary catheter appropriately (sterile, closed collection system): typically for 24-72 hours in cats with crystalluria or FLUTS/D (p. 1182)
- Phenoxybenzamine (dog 0.25 mg/kg PO q 12h; cat 2.5 mg/CAT PO q 12-24h) or prazosin (dog 1 mg/15 kg PO q 8-24h; cat 0.25-1 mg/CAT PO q 12-24h) may decrease urethral spasm (controversial).
- Antibiotic therapy based on urine culture/sensitivity; obtain culture when removing catheter.
- Address urolithiasis.
    - Diet/medical dissolution possible for some types but risk of repeated obstruction
    - Consider cystotomy, urohydropulsion (voiding, retrograde), cystoscopic-assisted retrieval, and laser lithotripsy.
- Perineal urethrostomy considered for male cats (or dogs) with recurrent obstruction
- Tube cystostomy or stents for urethral neoplasia (p. 1179)
- Stents can relieve obstruction due to stricture (p. 1179).

Nutrition/Diet

If uroliths are involved, specific dietary therapy may be warranted (pp. 1014, 1016, and 1019).

Possible Complications

- Complications of hyperkalemia
- Urethral tear
- Urinary bladder rupture
- Urethritis
- Urethral stricture
- Iatrogenic urinary tract infection
- Recurrent urinary tract infections with perineal urethrostomy and tube cystostomy
- Incontinence with stent placement

Recommended Monitoring

- Monitor urination once catheter is removed
- Daily bladder palpation during hospitalization after removing urinary catheter
- Repeat urinalysis and culture when catheter is removed and again 1 week later.
- Monitor as appropriate for underlying cause of obstruction.

PROGNOSIS & OUTCOME

- Urethral obstruction is rapidly life-threatening.
- If obstruction is alleviated and electrolyte disorders are addressed, prognosis is good (exception: neoplasia).
- Risk for recurrence is present regardless of cause and treatment.

PEARLS & CONSIDERATIONS

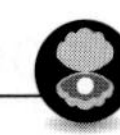

Comments

- In cats, FLUTS/D and urethral obstruction overlap substantially (cats can present with both simultaneously) but not completely. Increasingly, FLUTS/D is recognized as an environmental stress–associated disorder that causes urinary tract lesions. Long-term effective management may need to be centered on behavior and environmental enrichment, not on the urinary tract.
- Decompressive cystocentesis may facilitate urinary catheterization by reduction of back pressure.

Prevention

Dietary/medical therapy is indicated when uroliths are identified. Predisposing factors for urolith formation should be addressed directly whenever possible.

Technician Tips

- Overly aggressive attempts at manual expression of the bladder must be avoided because bladder rupture can result.
- Straining to urinate without producing a urine stream is highly suggestive of urethral obstruction.

Client Education

- Urinary tract obstruction is life-threatening. Stranguria or dysuria should prompt immediate veterinary attention.
- Adherence to dietary therapy for urolith dissolution must be strict.

SUGGESTED READING

Cooper ES: Controversies in the management of feline urethral obstruction. J Vet Emerg Crit Care 25:130-137, 2015.

AUTHOR: Anne M. Dalby, DVM, DACVIM
EDITOR: Leah A. Cohn, DVM, PhD, DACVIM

Urethral Sphincter Mechanism Incompetence

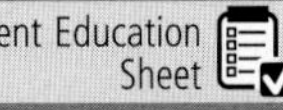

BASIC INFORMATION

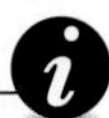

Definition

Urethral sphincter mechanism incompetence (USMI) is a very common cause of involuntary voiding of urine (urinary incontinence). It is most frequently identified in ovariohysterectomized bitches.

Synonyms

Estrogen-responsive or hormone-responsive incontinence, hormone-responsive urethral incompetence, spay incontinence

Epidemiology

SPECIES, AGE, SEX

Middle-aged spayed female dogs affected predominantly, although USMI occurs rarely in neutered adult males or intact bitches. Onset of incontinence may be months to years (median, 3.7 years) after ovariohysterectomy (OHE).

GENETICS, BREED PREDISPOSITION

Usually medium- to large-breed dogs. A positive association between tail docking and USMI has been demonstrated. Overrepresented breeds include boxer, Doberman pinscher, German shepherd, Old English sheepdog, rottweiler, springer spaniel, and Weimaraner.

RISK FACTORS

Intrapelvic bladder, short urethra, and obesity. Often occurs in association with ectopic ureter. Any cause of polyuria may initiate or exacerbate clinical signs. Early OHE in bitches expected to weigh > 25 kg as adults may increase risk.

ASSOCIATED DISORDERS

- Urinary tract infection
- USMI may accompany ectopic ureters in intact or neutered dogs and is a common reason for persistent incontinence after ectopic ureter surgical correction.

Clinical Presentation

HISTORY, CHIEF COMPLAINT

- Urinary incontinence: often most evident during rest (i.e., patients leave puddles after sleeping)
- Excessive licking of perineum
- Dogs can produce normal voluntary urine stream.

PHYSICAL EXAM FINDINGS

- Usually unremarkable. Neurologic exam should be conducted, including evaluation of tail and anal tone.
- Observed episode of urination is normal; bladder empties nearly completely after voluntary voiding.
- Perineal urine staining or perivulvar dermatitis sometimes observed

Etiology and Pathophysiology

- The vast majority of neutered bitches remain continent; it is unclear why a very small minority develops USMI.
- Sex hormones apparently sensitize the internal urethral sphincter to the effects of alpha-adrenergic stimulation.
- The bladder may be positioned in a relatively caudal position in neutered bitches, lessening the intraabdominal pressures on the urethra that help maintain urethral closure.
- USMI is commonly found in dogs with ectopic ureter and may account for continued incontinence after surgical correction of ectopia.

DIAGNOSIS

Diagnostic Overview

The diagnosis is suspected when an otherwise healthy, neutered bitch develops urinary leakage, especially during sleep. Ruling out other causes of incontinence and response to therapy are used to confirm the diagnosis.

Differential Diagnosis

- For inappropriate urination, distinguish between urinary incontinence and pollakiuria, polyuria, or behavioral disorders.
- Differentials for urinary incontinence: lower motor neuron disease/peripheral neuropathy, upper motor neuron disease, dysautonomia, urge incontinence, partial urethral obstruction, and congenital and acquired urinary tract structural defects (ectopic ureter[s], vaginal stricture/stenosis, urethrovaginal fistula)

Initial Database

- Complete neurologic exam (p. 1136): normal
- Rectal exam: normal
- CBC and serum biochemistry profile: unremarkable
- Complete urinalysis: occasionally, evidence of secondary cystitis
- Urine culture to rule out cystitis
- Abdominal radiographs or ultrasound of urinary structures: unremarkable, or bladder may display intrapelvic positioning.

Advanced or Confirmatory Testing

- Contrast studies and/or cystoscopy (p. 1085): not routinely required but can rule out structural causes of urinary incontinence. Unfortunately, USMI is difficult to recognize in dogs with ectopic ureter before surgical correction of ectopia.
- Urethral pressure profile (UPP) and/or leak point pressure (requires specialized equipment/expertise): not routinely used but can objectively identify urethral sphincter incompetence. May have prognostic utility in animals with ectopic ureter to predict resolution of incontinence after surgical correction
- Positive response to therapy is often used for supporting the diagnosis, but interpretation of result should be cautious because optimal

response may require dosage adjustment over weeks.

- Polyuria does not cause USMI; if present, identify underlying cause (p. 1271 and 1442).

TREATMENT

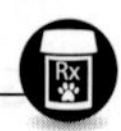

Treatment Overview

Medical treatment with phenylpropanolamine or hormone therapy usually results in control of incontinence. Endoscopic and surgical therapies are also options.

Acute General Treatment

- Medical therapy with phenylpropanolamine or estrogen compounds
- Treatment of secondary cystitis (p. 232)

Chronic Treatment

- Phenylpropanolamine is an alpha-agonist sympathomimetic used for increasing internal urethral sphincter tone. It is available as chewable tablets or oral solution 1-1.5 mg/kg PO q 8-12h or as time-released 75-mg capsules (<40 lb: one-half capsule q 24h; dogs 40-100 lb: 1 capsule q 24h; > 100 lb: 1.5 capsules q 24h). Discontinue if anxiety, hyperactivity, or tachycardia
- Estriol (Incurin) is a short-acting 17-beta-estradiol and estrone compound marketed for the treatment of sphincter mechanism incompetence. Regardless of size, dogs receive 2 mg PO q 24h × 14 days, followed by downward titration to lowest effective dose.
- Diethylstilbestrol (DES) is a synthetic estrogen that increases sensitivity of internal urethral sphincter to catecholamines. Dosage is empirical, with reduction in frequency and dose to least possible that controls clinical signs. Starting dose 0.1 mg (small dog), 0.3 mg (medium dog), or 0.7 mg (large dog) total daily dose PO q 24h for 3-5 days, then the same dose is given q 5-8 days as needed to control incontinence.
- Conjugated estrogens (e.g., Premarin 20 mcg/kg PO q 4 days) have been used in place of DES.
- Testosterone cypionate 2.2 mg/kg IM q 30 days can be used in castrated males (but phenylpropanolamine is preferred).
- Gonadotropin-releasing hormone (GnRH) analog can be used in place of DES but is less effective than phenylpropanolamine.
- Hormones may be administered concurrently with phenylpropanolamine when incontinence persists despite therapy (synergistic actions).
- Surgical therapies are usually reserved for refractory patients.
  - Percutaneously adjustable hydraulic urethral occluder placed at surgery
  - Cystoscopically administered periurethral injections of collagen or Teflon; likely needs to be repeated
  - Colposuspension, cystourethropexy, urethroplasty, transobturator vaginal tape, or urethral intussusception

Drug Interactions

- Hormone therapy may cause adverse reactions: estrogen compounds (e.g., bone marrow suppression), testosterone (e.g., prostatomegaly, behavioral changes)
- AVOID estradiol cypionate because of increased risk of marrow suppression.
- Phenylpropanolamine may cause adverse reactions (e.g., decreased appetite, gastrointestinal upset, hyperactivity, hypertension). Use with caution or avoid if there is systemic hypertension, heart disease, cardiac arrhythmias, or central nervous system disease or if monoamine oxidase inhibitors or other sympathomimetic agents are used.

Possible Complications

Secondary cystitis, perivulvar dermatitis

Recommended Monitoring

- Periodic urinalysis with Gram stain of sediment and/or bacterial culture and sensitivity if incontinence persists
- Periodic monitoring of blood pressure in dogs treated with phenylpropanolamine
- Periodic monitoring of CBC in dogs treated with estrogen drugs

PROGNOSIS & OUTCOME

Most dogs respond to medical therapy with improvement or resolution of clinical signs. Some dogs require more than a single type of medication, and ancillary surgical procedures may be required uncommonly.

PEARLS & CONSIDERATIONS

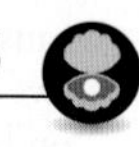

Comments

- USMI is the most common cause of acquired urinary incontinence in neutered bitches.
- Diagnosis is usually based on clinical presentation, ruling out other common causes of incontinence, and response to therapy.
- Minimal evaluation includes neurologic exam, observation of urination and palpation of bladder afterward, and urinalysis. Bladder imaging (radiographs or ultrasound) is ideal.

Prevention

- Early neutering does not increase the likelihood of incontinence in bitches predicted to weigh < 25 kg, but it may slightly increase risk in those that will weigh > 25 kg.
- Urethral occluders may be placed prophylactically at the time of corrective surgery for ectopic ureter.

Technician Tips

Questioning owners may help distinguish between urinary incontinence and a lack of house training. Often, incontinent bitches leave puddles where they sleep.

SUGGESTED READING

Byron JK, et al: Urethral sphincter mechanism incompetence in 163 neutered female dogs: diagnosis, treatment, and relationship of weight and age at neuter to development of disease. J Vet Intern Med 31:442-448, 2017.

AUTHOR & EDITOR: Leah A. Cohn, DVM, PhD, DACVIM

Uroabdomen

Client Education Sheet

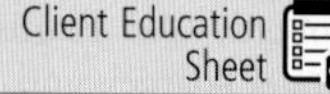

BASIC INFORMATION

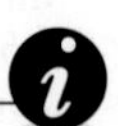

Definition

The condition is characterized by accumulation of urine within the peritoneal and/or retroperitoneal spaces and caused by leakage of urine from the kidneys, ureters, bladder, or proximal urethra.

Synonyms

Urinary tract rupture, uroperitoneum

Epidemiology

SPECIES, AGE, SEX

Any species or age and both sexes; males may be predisposed due to anatomic characteristics.

GENETICS, BREED PREDISPOSITION

Dogs with a tendency to develop urinary calculi are more likely to develop urinary obstruction. This includes dogs with portosystemic shunts (urate), Dalmatians (urate), shih tzu, miniature schnauzer, Bichon frisé, Lhasa apso, Yorkshire terrier (calcium oxalate), Newfoundland (cystine) (pp. 1014, 1016, and 1019).

RISK FACTORS

Pre-existing compromise of the urinary tract due to urinary obstruction (e.g., uroliths, neoplasia), iatrogenic causes (urethral catheterization, aggressive bladder palpation, surgical complication [laceration or ligation of urinary tract]), or abdominal or pelvic trauma (hit by car, pelvic fractures of any cause, penetrating abdominal wounds)

ASSOCIATED DISORDERS

- Hyperkalemia
- Metabolic acidosis
- Septic peritonitis (if concurrent urinary tract infection)
- Postrenal azotemia

Clinical Presentation

HISTORY, CHIEF COMPLAINT

- Nonspecific lethargy, anorexia, abdominal discomfort, vomiting
- Cause of urinary rupture may be known (e.g., witnessed being hit by a car) or suspected (stranguria)
- Ability to pass urine does not rule out urinary tract rupture or uroabdomen; patient may or may not have hematuria.

PHYSICAL EXAM FINDINGS

- Depression, dehydration common
- Abdominal pain
  - Lack of abdominal pain does not rule out uroabdomen, but because of chemical peritonitis, most are very painful.
  - Ascites may be detectable on abdominal palpation.
- Lack of a palpable bladder
  - Palpable bladder does not rule out urinary tract rupture/uroabdomen (small rupture, urethral rupture still potentially life-threatening).
- Bruising (perineum, ventral abdomen, and inguinal region)
- Bradycardia (from hyperkalemia)
  - Unlike dogs, cats may have severe hyperkalemia and maintain a normal or elevated heart rate.

Etiology and Pathophysiology

Accumulation of urine in the abdominal cavity results in the following consequences:

- Translocation of solutes that are normally higher in urine concentration (urea, creatinine, potassium, hydrogen) across the peritoneal lining into the extracellular fluid spaces and systemic circulation
- Postrenal azotemia
- Metabolic acidosis
- Hyperkalemia
- Chemical peritonitis

DIAGNOSIS

Diagnostic Overview

Definitive diagnosis is based on demonstration of urine in the abdomen. Plasma-to-abdominal fluid gradients of creatinine and potassium are helpful to differentiate uroabdomen from other causes of azotemia and ascites. A global approach to diagnosis and management is outlined elsewhere (p. 1454).

Differential Diagnosis

- Acute abdomen (p. 21)
- Ascites of other causes (e.g., hypoalbuminemia, cardiogenic, hemorrhage) (p. 79)
- Acute (oliguric/anuric) kidney injury (p. 23)

Initial Database

- CBC: generally unremarkable, sometimes hemoconcentration or leukocytosis
- Serum biochemistry profile: moderate or marked blood urea nitrogen (BUN), creatinine, and potassium elevations as well as low HCO_3^- are common. Hyponatremia may accompany ascites.
- Urinalysis: usually by catheterized sample, hematuria is the most common finding.
- Abdominal radiographs: loss of serosal detail
- Abdominal ultrasound: free abdominal fluid (anechoic); ultrasound contrast cystography may confirm bladder rupture (e.g., bladder bubble study). Visualization of bladder wall does not rule out rupture.
- Abdominocentesis (p. 1056): fluid:serum ratios for dogs
  - Creatinine concentration ratio ≥ 2:1 highly predictive of uroabdomen
  - Potassium concentration ratio ≥ 1.4:1 highly predictive of uroabdomen

Advanced or Confirmatory Testing

Positive-contrast cystourethrography (p. 1181) or IV excretory urography (p. 1101): most sensitive methods to confirm urine leakage and localize the site of leakage

TREATMENT

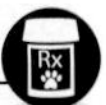

Treatment Overview

Immediately normalize perfusion and correct hyperkalemia, if present. Urinary diversion by urinary catheter ± peritoneal catheter is important in initial stabilization. After the animal is stable, surgical exploration is usually required for definitive repair. Urethral and ureteral surgery is technically demanding, and transfer of the patient to a center with advanced surgical facilities should be considered.

Acute General Treatment

- Intensive fluid therapy to treat shock if present and correct severe dehydration
  - Isotonic crystalloids are required for volume replacement and replacement of ongoing losses. Fluids with low concentrations of potassium (e.g., lactated Ringer's solution) should be used initially.
  - High fluid rates are often necessary for correction of dehydration and for management of postobstructive diuresis.
  - Fluid type and rate are continually reassessed based on physical monitoring and serial measurements of electrolyte concentrations.
- If the patient's serum potassium concentration > 7-8 mEq/L or there are clinical (e.g., bradycardia) or electrocardiographic (ECG) (e.g., no P waves in all ECG leads) changes due to hyperkalemia, immediate medical therapy and stabilization are required (p. 495).
- For animals with lower urinary tract injury and urine accumulation in the peritoneal space
  - Placement of peritoneal drainage catheter is simple and life-saving.
  - Placement of urethral catheter (bladder decompression and prevention of further urine leakage)
  - Placement of prepubic tube cystostomy in animals with severe urethral trauma
  - Analgesia and sedation as indicated; nonsteroidal antiinflammatory drugs should be avoided until azotemia has resolved and renal function has completely normalized.
  - If urinary tract infection is suspected, broad-spectrum antimicrobial drugs are indicated. Effort should be made to collect urine for culture, and ongoing antimicrobial use should be guided by culture and sensitivity (p. 232).

Chronic Treatment

- Fluid therapy to replace ongoing losses, including the presence of postobstructive diuresis
- Surgical correction of the leakage
- Some animals, especially cats with small leaks, can respond to medical management without surgery. In these cases, leave the catheter indwelling for 5-7 days, and then repeat positive-contrast cystogram to check for leaks.

Nutrition/Diet

All animals with uroabdomen, but especially cats, can have a long recovery from surgery. Consideration should be given to the placement of a feeding tube (nasoesophageal or esophageal [pp. 1106 and 1107]) at the time of surgery.

Drug Interactions

Do not add potassium chloride (KCl) to IV fluids until serum potassium level is normal or low.

Possible Complications

- Atrial standstill due to hyperkalemia
- Obstruction of the peritoneal drainage catheter with omentum
- Injury to other intraabdominal structures during placement of peritoneal drainage catheter
- Urethral stricture formation and urinary incontinence
- Persistent renal insufficiency

Recommended Monitoring

- Frequent monitoring of vital signs, including blood pressure (p. 1065)
- ECG monitoring if hyperkalemia (p. 1096)
- Fluid input and urine output from peritoneal drainage and urethral catheters q 2-4h; account for postobstructive diuresis in fluid therapy.
- Serum chemistry, venous blood gas, packed cell volume q 8-12h during initial stabilization
- Patient's weight q 12h

PROGNOSIS & OUTCOME

- Prognosis is good with early diagnosis, aggressive management, and definitive repair.

- The mortality rate is increased for animals with concurrent injuries or underlying neoplasia.

PEARLS & CONSIDERATIONS

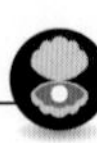

Comments

- Consider uroabdomen in animals with a history of abdominal or pelvic trauma, urinary obstruction, or urethral catheterization.
- A palpable bladder and the ability to void urine do not rule out uroabdomen.
- The abdominal fluid obtained is serosanguineous and may not look like urine; creatinine and potassium concentrations of the fluid (compared with serum or plasma) are diagnostic.
- Asepsis (urethral and peritoneal drainage catheters, sterile collection system) is essential for preventing secondary infection.
- In dogs and cats, lower urinary tract injuries are more common than renal/ureteral injuries. Contrast cystography and retrograde urethrography take precedence over IV excretory urography.
- Surgical repair should not be attempted until the animal has been stabilized with fluid therapy and abdominal drainage.

Technician Tips

Fluid therapy is a challenge in these patients, and accurate recording of fluid administration and fluid output is crucial. Patients with uroabdomen often have concurrent disease or injuries and may have a long recovery period; adequate attention to analgesia and nutrition benefits their recovery.

SUGGESTED READING

Stafford JR, et al: A clinical review of pathophysiology, diagnosis, and treatment of uroabdomen in the dog and cat. J Vet Emerg Crit Care 23:216-229, 2013.

AUTHOR: Gareth J. Buckley, VetMB, MA, DACVECC, DECVECC

EDITOR: Benjamin M. Brainard VMD, DACVAA, DACVECC

Urolithiasis, Oxalate

Client Education Sheet 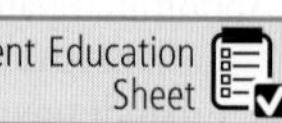

BASIC INFORMATION

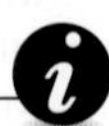

Definition

Urinary tract stones (uroliths) composed of calcium oxalate occur commonly in dogs and cats.

Synonyms

- Calcium oxalate dihydrate: weddellite
- Calcium oxalate monohydrate: whewellite

Epidemiology

SPECIES, AGE, SEX

Dogs:

- Increased frequency over the past 30 years; now the second most common canine urolith
- Incidence is greatest in middle-aged to older, castrated male dogs; tends to occur at a younger age in Bichon frisé dogs.

Cats:

- Second most common feline urolith
- Incidence greatest at 7-10 years of age; tends to occur at younger age in Siamese and Ragdolls; no sex predisposition
- More than 85% of nephroureteroliths are composed of calcium oxalate.

GENETICS, BREED PREDISPOSITION

- Increased risk (dogs): miniature schnauzer, Lhasa apso, Yorkshire terrier, Bichon frisé, Pomeranian, shih tzu, and miniature poodle
- Increased risk (cats): Ragdoll, British shorthair, foreign shorthair, Himalayan, Havana brown, Scottish fold, Persian, exotic shorthair

RISK FACTORS

- Hypercalcemia
- Acidic urine
- Highly concentrated urine
- Infrequent urination
- Primary hyperparathyroidism
- Hyperadrenocorticism
- Chronic metabolic acidosis
- Obesity
- Diets designed to minimize struvite formation in cats

ASSOCIATED DISORDERS

Feline lower urinary tract signs/disease (FLUTS/D), urethral obstruction, chronic kidney disease (CKD), urinary tract infection (UTI), nephroureterolithiasis

Clinical Presentation

HISTORY, CHIEF COMPLAINT

Clinical signs may be absent or include

- Hematuria
- Pollakiuria
- Dysuria
- Stranguria
- Inappropriate elimination (periuria)
- Rarely, systemic illness due to urinary obstruction
- Polyuria/polydipsia if concurrent hypercalcemia, CKD, or hyperadrenocorticism

PHYSICAL EXAM FINDINGS

Physical exam is usually unremarkable; abnormalities may include

- Hematuria (stains on prepuce, vulva, or hocks)
- Painful urinary bladder
- Palpable cystic calculi
- Palpable urethral calculi (by digital rectal exam in dogs)
- Enlarged, turgid bladder if urethral obstruction
- Renomegaly if secondary hydronephrosis or small irregular kidneys if CKD
- Findings associated with predisposing factors (e.g., hyperadrenocorticism: pot belly, alopecia, hepatomegaly [p. 485])

Etiology and Pathophysiology

- Hypercalciuria and/or hyperoxaluria promote formation of calcium oxalate uroliths.
- Hypercalciuria may result from increased intestinal absorption of calcium, increased

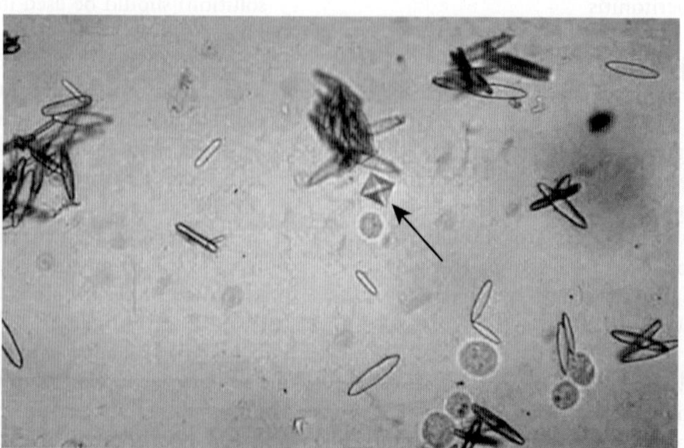

UROLITHIASIS, OXALATE Dozens of calcium oxalate monohydrate crystals are scattered throughout the microscope field in clumps and individually (picket fence board shape), and a single calcium oxalate dihydrate crystal is seen just to the upper right of the center of the image (*arrow;* Maltese cross/envelope shape).

renal excretion of calcium, or increased resorption of calcium from bone with or without hypercalcemia.

- Hypercalcemia is identified in 20%-35% of cats and ≈4% of dogs with calcium oxalate urolithiasis. Hypercalcemia in cats with calcium oxalate uroliths is usually idiopathic in nature; hypercalcemia in dogs with calcium oxalate uroliths is usually associated with primary hyperparathyroidism.
- Hyperadrenocorticism associated with calcium oxalate uroliths in dogs may or may not be associated with hypercalcemia.
- Hyperoxaluria in cats may be related to diet, inadequate vitamin B_6, and hepatic enzyme deficiencies.
- Urolith formation is potentiated by diminished concentrations of urinary crystallization inhibitors (e.g., nephrocalcin, citrate, pyrophosphate, glycosaminoglycans, Tamm-Horsfall mucoprotein).
- Diets with moderate fat and carbohydrate levels: increased risk of calcium oxalate stone formation (vs. diminished risk for diets high in moisture with a moderate magnesium, phosphorus, and calcium content)

DIAGNOSIS

Diagnostic Overview

Diagnosis is suspected in animals with radiopaque bladder stones and acidic urine or in animals with radiopaque nephroliths. Quantitative stone analysis is necessary for confirmation and an optimal treatment/prevention plan. More than 50% of patients with active calcium oxalate uroliths do not have concurrent crystalluria. A global approach to diagnosis and management is outlined on p. 1455.

Differential Diagnosis

- UTI, bacterial or fungal (p. 232)
- Other types of uroliths
- Urinary tract neoplasia (p. 991)

Initial Database

- CBC: unremarkable
- Serum biochemistry profile (including electrolytes) typically unremarkable
  - Hypercalcemia or evidence of endocrinopathy: uncommon
  - Azotemia, hyperkalemia, metabolic acidosis if urinary tract obstruction
- Urinalysis: acidic to neutral pH unless UTI; crystalluria (< 50%); hematuria and/or pyuria (occasional)
  - Storage of urine may lead to precipitation of oxalate crystals (artifact); urine sediment should be examined within 1 hour of collection.
  - Urine bacterial culture and susceptibility to rule out secondary infection
- Abdominal radiographs: radiopaque calculi most commonly located in bladder, sometimes urethra, ureter, or renal pelvis
  - Relative radiopacity of uroliths: struvite ≥ oxalate = $CaPO_4$ ≥ silica > cystine > urate
  - Shape varies from spiculated (dihydrate) to smooth (monohydrate). The perineum must be included in the radiographic field to identify uroliths in the urethra.

Advanced or Confirmatory Testing

- Abdominal ultrasound: little benefit beyond abdominal radiography but can confirm location, assess kidneys for evidence of pyelonephritis or hydronephrosis
- Urolith analysis: retrieved stones should be submitted for quantitative analysis (crystallography, x-ray diffraction, infrared spectroscopy) to determine urolith type.
- Urolith culture: if urine culture by cystocentesis is negative
- Cystoscopy with or without laser lithotripsy may facilitate stone removal for analysis and therapy (p. 1085).
- Specific diagnostic tests may be indicated to identify predisposing conditions (e.g., ionized calcium concentration, parathyroid hormone assay, adrenal function testing).

TREATMENT

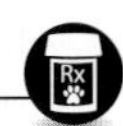

Treatment Overview

Urethral obstruction requires immediate relief. Oxalate stones cannot be dissolved with medical therapy, and uroliths in the bladder or urethra should be removed mechanically if they are causing clinical signs. Recurrence is common (up to 50% in 3 years in dogs).

Acute General Treatment

- Relieve urethral obstruction (pp. 1175 and 1176).
- Antibiotics (choice based on culture and susceptibility) if secondary UTI
- If uroliths are found incidentally in the absence of clinical signs, it is reasonable to omit removal and begin prevention to minimize growth of uroliths, including regular follow-up for urinalysis, urine culture, and radiography.
- Mechanical removal of bladder/urethral calculi producing clinical signs; radiographs should be repeated afterward to ensure complete removal.
  - Urohydropropulsion (voiding, retrograde [pp. 1175 and 1176]); avoid performing voiding urohydropropulsion in male cats.
  - Catheter-assisted retrieval
  - Cystoscopic-assisted retrieval (p. 1085)
  - Cystotomy/urethrotomy/urethrostomy/pyelotomy/nephrotomy/ureterectomy with neoureterocystostomy, ureteral stent, or subcutaneous ureteral bypass device implantation
  - Lithotripsy, intracorporeal or extracorporeal shock wave lithotripsy
- Calcium oxalate is the most common type of nephrolith/ureterolith. Because surgical removal of nephroliths can reduce renal function (p. 689), it is not uniformly indicated.

Chronic Treatment

- Identify underlying disorder (e.g., hyperadrenocorticism, hyperparathyroidism) if present, and treat appropriately.
- For cats with idiopathic hypercalcemia, high-fiber diet may be beneficial. To simultaneously alkalinize the urine, add potassium citrate 75 mg/kg PO q 12h, adjusted so urine pH = 6.5-7.0. Bisphosphonates (alendronate) may help control hypercalcemia: initially 2 mg/kg PO once weekly. Most cats respond to 10 mg/CAT. Follow with at least 6 mL of water PO after administration, and butter the lips to increase salivation and increase transit. Effects, if seen, occur in 3-4 weeks. Monitor serum ionized calcium (p. 491).
- Initiate measures to prevent recurrence (see Prevention below).

Nutrition/Diet

- Avoid calcium supplements, acidifying diets, and foods high in oxalate such as green leafy vegetables.

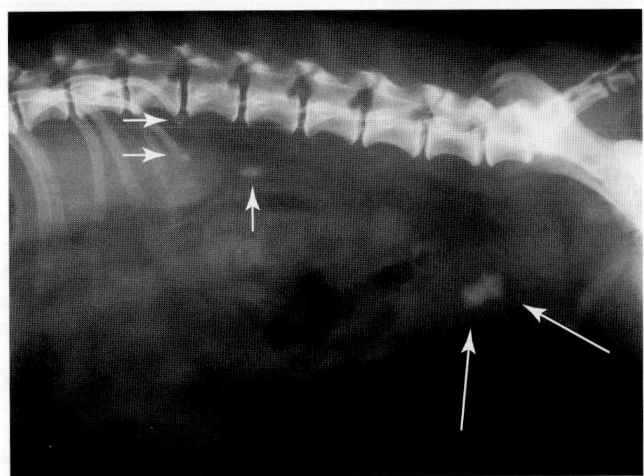

UROLITHIASIS, OXALATE Lateral abdominal radiograph of a dog with two large, irregular, mineral-opacity structures *(large arrows)* in the urinary bladder that are consistent with oxalate uroliths. A mineral opacity in the region of a ureter *(small single arrow)* and mineral opacities in both kidneys *(small arrows)* are also consistent with oxalate urolithiasis, but a dorsoventral or ventrodorsal view is necessary to differentiate ureterolithiasis from mineral in the gastrointestinal tract.

- Feed reduced-protein diets, which promote diuresis and formation of alkaline urine: Hill's u/d, w/d, or c/d, Royal Canin Urinary SO, Purina UR st/ox, Blue Buffalo WU (dogs) or Hill's Feline c/d Multicare, Royal Canin Urinary SO, Purina UR St/Ox, or Blue Buffalo WU (cats).
- Feed canned food, or add water to dry food when possible.

Possible Complications

- Urinary tract obstruction
- Hydronephrosis
- Hydroureter
- CKD (nephrolithiasis)
- UTI
- Some oxalate prevention diets are higher in fat than maintenance diets (obesity risk).

Recommended Monitoring

- Repeat urinalysis q 2 weeks, starting 2 weeks after removal of stones and initiation of dietary changes until urine pH = 7.0-8.0, specific gravity is less than 1.025, and no calcium oxalate crystals are found. If goals are not met, consider adding supplementary therapies (see Prevention below).
- Repeat abdominal radiographs and urinalysis q 3-6 months for first year, then q 6-12 months thereafter to evaluate for recurrence of uroliths.
- Monitor and treat any concurrent conditions (e.g., hypercalcemia, hyperadrenocorticism).

PROGNOSIS & OUTCOME

- Recurrence is common, and long-term monitoring and care are required.
- Nephrolithiasis may be associated with CKD.

PEARLS & CONSIDERATIONS

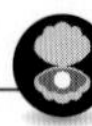

Comments

- Calcium oxalate uroliths frequently recur; long-term management and monitoring are recommended.
- Calcium oxalate crystalluria can be found in normal urine and does not necessarily correlate with the presence of calcium oxalate uroliths.
- In urine sediment, calcium oxalate dihydrate crystals (square envelope or Maltese cross shape: ⊠) are more commonly associated with nutritional or artifactual causes, whereas calcium oxalate monohydrate crystals (picket fence board or flattened hexagon shape: ⬭) are sometimes associated with ethylene glycol intoxication.
- Large quantities of calcium oxalate dihydrate crystals or large crystal aggregates warrant evaluation for hyperoxaluric or hypercalciuric conditions.
- The appearance of calcium oxalate monohydrate crystals in a dog presenting with acute kidney injury/acute uremia strongly suggests advanced ethylene glycol intoxication (p. 314). Because it is an acute intoxication, ethylene glycol ingestion does not lead to oxalate urolithiasis.

Prevention

- Treat any identified cause of hypercalcemia/ hypercalciuria.
- Initiate measures to prevent recurrence in a stepwise manner, adding the next measure when the first one is insufficient to produce urine with a pH between 7.0 and 8.0, a urine specific gravity less than 1.025, or prevent calcium oxalate crystal formation:
    - Promote water consumption (e.g., canned diet, wetted food, water fountains for cats).
    - Provide diet with restricted oxalate, sodium, and protein and which does not acidify the urine (see Nutrition/Diet above). Potassium citrate can be added if the urinary pH remains acidic (see Chronic Treatment above).
    - If calcium oxalate crystalluria persists, hydrochlorothiazide 2-4 mg/kg PO q 12h, chlorothiazide 20-40 mg/kg PO q 12h, or cyclothiazide 0.5-1 mg/kg PO q 24h or vitamin B_6 2-4 mg/kg PO q 12h can be added.
    - Avoid supplementation of vitamins C and D.
- For male cats with recurrent urethral obstruction, consider perineal urethrostomy.

Technician Tips

- When collecting voided urine sample for analysis, look closely for small voided stones; if recovered, these can be submitted for analysis.
- Oxalate uroliths cannot be dissolved by medical therapy.

Client Education

- Adherence to dietary therapy must be strict.
- Urethral obstruction is life-threatening. Stranguria should prompt immediate veterinary attention.

SUGGESTED READING

Lulich JP, et al: ACVIM Small Animal Consensus Recommendations on the Treatment and Prevention of Uroliths in Dogs and Cats. J Vet Intern Med 30:1564-1574, 2016.

AUTHOR: Joseph W. Bartges, DVM, PhD, DACVIM, DACVN
EDITOR: Leah A. Cohn, DVM, PhD, DACVIM

Urolithiasis, Struvite

Bonus Material Online 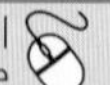 Client Education Sheet 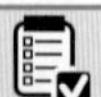

BASIC INFORMATION

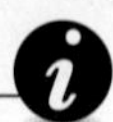

Definition

Urinary tract stones (uroliths) composed of magnesium ammonium phosphate. Struvite uroliths occur commonly in dogs and cats.

Synonyms

Magnesium ammonium phosphate stones, triple phosphate calculi/stones, urease calculi/stones, infection stones

Epidemiology

SPECIES, AGE, SEX

Dogs:

- The most common urolith of dogs, canine struvite uroliths are usually associated with urinary tract infections (UTIs) involving urease-producing bacteria, primarily *Staphylococcus.*
- Sterile struvite urolithiasis is rare in dogs.
- Any age; about twice as frequent in females as males because females are more likely to have UTIs

Cats:

- The most common urolith of cats; typically occur in sterile, alkaline urine
- Male cats may be at increased risk.
- Compared with calcium oxalate uroliths (second most common in cats), struvite uroliths occur in cats that are younger (4-7 years old) and are more likely to be neutered.

GENETICS, BREED PREDISPOSITION

- Dogs: any breed can be affected. Miniature schnauzer, shih tzu, Bichon frisé, miniature poodle, cocker spaniel, and Lhasa apso are overrepresented. English cocker spaniels may form sterile struvite uroliths.
- Cats: domestic shorthair, foreign shorthair, Ragdoll, Chartreux, Oriental shorthair, and Himalayan commonly affected

RISK FACTORS

Dogs:

- UTI with a urease-producing bacterial organism such as *Staphylococcus*, *Enterococcus*, or *Proteus*
- Highly concentrated urine
- Infrequent urination

Cats:

- Highly concentrated urine
- Alkaline urine
- Diet high in magnesium and phosphorous

ASSOCIATED DISORDERS

- Dogs: UTI (pp. 232 and 849)
- Cats: feline lower urinary tract signs/disease (FLUTS/D [p. 332]), urethral obstruction (p. 1009)

Clinical Presentation

HISTORY, CHIEF COMPLAINT

Clinical signs may be absent. When signs are apparent, they may include

- Hematuria
- Pollakiuria
- Dysuria
- Stranguria
- Inappropriate elimination (periuria)
- Rarely, systemic illness due to urinary tract obstruction, ascending infection causing pyelonephritis, or systemic illness that predisposes to UTI (e.g., diabetes mellitus)

PHYSICAL EXAM FINDINGS

Physical exam is usually unremarkable. Abnormalities may include

- Hematuria (stains on prepuce, vulva, or hocks)
- Painful urinary bladder
- Palpable cystic calculi
- Palpable urethral calculi (by digital rectal exam in dogs)
- Enlarged turgid bladder if urethral obstruction
- Renomegaly if secondary hydronephrosis

Etiology and Pathophysiology

Infection-associated struvite urolithiasis (mainly dogs):

- Bacterial urease converts urea to ammonia and carbonate.
  - The most common urease-producing pathogens are *Staphylococcus* and *Proteus* spp.
  - Other urease-producing pathogens include *Enterococcus, Pseudomonas, Klebsiella,* and *Ureaplasma* (urease-producing *Mycoplasma*) spp.
- Ammonia buffers H^+, converting to ammonium (NH_4^+) and increasing urine pH.
- Ammonium combines with phosphorus and magnesium, forming struvite crystals.
- Alkalinity decreases solubility of magnesium ammonium phosphate crystals.
- Calcium phosphate carbonate (i.e., calcium apatite) may be incorporated with infection-associated struvite, and urease degradation of urea results in CO_2 production; buffering yields a carbonate ion.
- Ammonium urate also may be incorporated with infection-associated struvite. Urease degradation of urea results in ammonia, and buffering yields ammonium, some of which binds uric acid to form ammonium urate.
- Crystals aggregate with organic material (including viable bacteria) and combine to form uroliths.
- Decreased presence of glycosaminoglycans may occur in some cases of FLUTS/D.

Sterile struvite urolithiasis (mainly cats): complex relationship of diet, water intake, individual predisposition, and subsequent urine pH and relative supersaturation

- Diets high in magnesium, phosphorus, calcium, chloride, and fiber with moderate protein content may predispose to struvite crystal formation.

DIAGNOSIS

Diagnostic Overview

Diagnosis is suspected in dogs with radiopaque bladder stones, alkaline urine, and/or UTI. The diagnosis is suspected in cats with radiopaque bladder stones, alkaline urine, and/or struvite crystalluria. Quantitative stone analysis is necessary to confirm the diagnosis and provide an optimal treatment/prevention plan, but emperic therapy may be appropriate. A global approach to diagnosis and management is outlined on p. 1456.

Differential Diagnosis

- UTI
- Other types of uroliths
- Urinary tract neoplasia

Initial Database

- CBC: unremarkable
- Serum biochemistry profile (including electrolytes): unremarkable unless urinary tract obstruction (p. 1009)
- Complete urinalysis: neutral or alkaline (common) pH, bacteria (especially likely in dogs), pyuria (especially likely in dogs), hematuria (inconsistent), and crystalluria (inconsistent) are possible.
  - Because storage of urine may lead to precipitation of struvite crystals, urine sediment should be examined within 1 hour of collection.
- Urine culture (identify uropathogen) and susceptibility (influence antimicrobial therapy)
- Abdominal radiographs
  - Generally radiopaque (radiopacity: struvite ≥ oxalate = $CaPO_4$ = silica > cystine > urate)
  - Often smooth or round in shape
  - Most commonly located in bladder; sometimes in urethra, ureter, or kidney

Advanced or Confirmatory Testing

- Abdominal ultrasound: little benefit beyond abdominal radiography; can confirm location, assess kidneys for evidence of pyelonephritis or hydronephrosis
- Urolith analysis: retrieved stones should be submitted for quantitative analysis (crystallography, x-ray diffraction, infrared spectroscopy) to determine urolith type.
- Urolith culture: retrieved stones can be cultured if urine culture obtained by cystocentesis is negative.
- If urine culture negative, bladder wall culture should be performed if stones are removed surgically or by cystoscopy.

TREATMENT

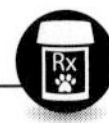

Treatment Overview

Although uncommon, urinary tract obstruction requires immediate relief. In the absence of urinary obstruction, treatment consists of a stone-dissolution diet or manual removal of stones and treatment of UTI.

Acute General Treatment

- Relieve urinary tract obstruction if present (pp. 1175 and 1176).
- Antibiotics for UTI are based on culture and susceptibility results (dogs > cats [p. 232]). Generally, antimicrobial therapy is continued until struvite urolith has dissolved or been removed.
- Choose between medical dissolution and mechanical calculi removal.
  - Urethral obstruction should be relieved mechanically.
  - Mechanical removal allows urolith analysis and culture.
  - Even large struvite uroliths can be amenable to medical dissolution.
  - Provided urethral obstruction is absent, trial of medical dissolution before mechanical removal is reasonable; potential drawbacks include risk of obstruction

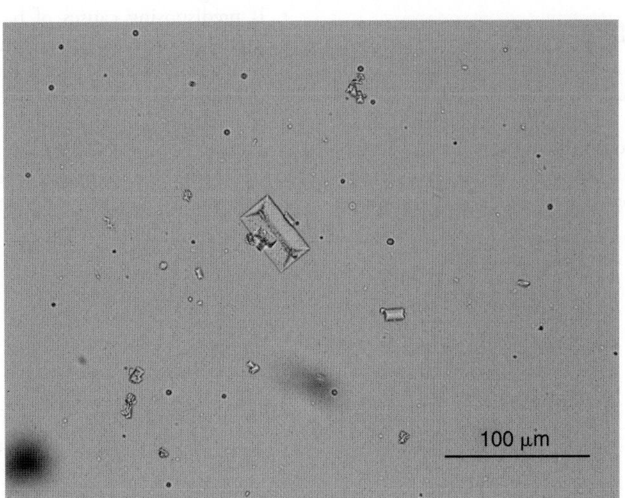

UROLITHIASIS, STRUVITE One large *(center)* and several smaller struvite crystals are seen. Note their characteristic rectangular coffin-lid shape.

before complete dissolution and ineffective dissolution.

- For medical dissolution, calculolytic diets (see Nutrition/Diet below) and appropriate antimicrobials are required.
  - Mean time to dissolution is 2-3 months (2-4 weeks for sterile uroliths, longer time for nephroliths than for cystoliths).
  - Urinalysis and urine culture should be repeated 5-7 days after initiating medical therapy. Goals are urine pH < 7.0, urine specific gravity of 1.010-1.020, and negative culture.
  - Medical therapy is continued 1 month beyond radiographic disappearance of uroliths.
  - Small uroliths may lodge in urethra (especially males) during urolith dissolution.
- Mechanical removal of uroliths
  - Urohydropropulsion (voiding, retrograde [pp. 1175 and 1176])
    - Avoid in male cats.
  - Catheter-assisted retrieval
  - Cystoscopy-assisted retrieval (p. 1085)
  - Cystotomy/urethrotomy/urethrostomy/pyelotomy/nephrotomy
  - Lithotripsy (intracorporeal laser lithotripsy or extracorporeal shock wave lithotripsy)

Chronic Treatment

- Predisposing causes of UTI should be addressed (e.g., control glucosuria in diabetic animals, treat hyperadrenocorticism).
- For animals with recurrent UTI, chronic prophylactic therapy may be considered after appropriate therapy of recognized infection (p. 232).
- Promote water consumption to avoid concentrated urine (e.g., canned food, wetting dry food, use of cat water fountains [p. 332]).
- Dietary therapy is crucial for sterile struvite urinary stones (see Nutrition/Diet below).
- Urinary acidifiers are seldom required if the pet is eating an appropriate diet and urinary tract infection is eliminated.

Nutrition/Diet

- Many commercial diets (e.g., Hill's Prescription Diet s/d, Royal Canin SO, Purina UR st/ox, Blue Buffalo WU) are designed to aid struvite urolith dissolution.
- Monitor urolith size periodically by radiographs (see Recommended Monitoring below).
- Some dissolution diets provide inadequate nutrition for long-term feeding. Calculolytic diet is continued 1 month past radiographic disappearance of uroliths.
- Other diets (e.g., Prescription Diet Multicare c/d and w/d, Royal Canin SO, Purina UR st/ox, Blue Buffalo WU) aid in the prevention of recurrent struvite urolithiasis and can be fed long term.

Possible Complications

- Risk of urethral obstruction from small stones or during medical dissolution as the stones become small enough to pass into the urethra (males)
  - Urinary tract obstruction
  - Hydronephrosis
  - Hydroureter
- UTI
- Urinary tract polyp formation
- Uroliths inadvertently may be left behind during surgery (up to 20% of stones are not removed).
- Some diets appropriate for treatment/prevention of struvite urolithiasis may predispose to calcium oxalate urolithiasis.
- Malnutrition due to long-term feeding of certain dissolution diets

Recommended Monitoring

- Repeat radiographs q 2-4 weeks during medical dissolution to evaluate urolith size and number.
- If no improvement is seen on radiographs after 4-8 weeks, mechanical removal is indicated.
- Repeat urinalysis 5-7 days after initiating medical dissolution therapy to ensure pH between 6.5 and 7, specific gravity between 1.010 and 1.020 (dogs) or 1.030-1.040 (cats) absent struvite crystals, and absent bacteruria.
- Ideally, urine culture is repeated 5-7 days after initiating medical dissolution therapy to ensure sterile urine.
- Repeat urine culture 5-7 days after stopping antibiotics to assess recurrence of infection, then again 3-4 weeks later.
- If predisposing causes of bacterial cystitis cannot be corrected or in animals with sterile struvite urolithiasis, repeat urinalysis q 4-6 months.
- If predisposing causes of bacterial cystitis cannot be corrected or in animals with sterile struvite urolithiasis, repeat abdominal radiographs initially q 3-6 months for 1 year, then q 6 months thereafter.

PROGNOSIS & OUTCOME

- Prognosis for dissolution of uroliths is good.
- Recurrence of struvite urolithiasis is common.

PEARLS & CONSIDERATIONS

Comments

- Struvite urolithiasis in dogs is routinely associated with UTI. Elimination of infection is crucial for dissolution of stones with a calculolytic diet.
- Struvite urolithiasis in cats is rarely associated with UTI; long-term diet modification is often necessary to prevent recurrence.
- If uroliths fail to resolve with medical therapy, consider
  - Inadequate infection control
  - Failure to comply with diet restrictions
  - Mixed or alternative urolith composition
- Struvite crystalluria can be found in normal urine and does not reliably predict struvite urolithiasis.

Prevention

- Dogs: if urinary infection can be eliminated, long-term diet change is not necessary.
- Cats: long-term use of canned struvite-management diets (e.g., Royal Canin SO, Purina UR st/ox, Prescription Diet c/d Multicare, Blue Buffalo WU) is best if recurrence noted.
- The merit of supplementing with glycosaminoglycans is unknown.

Technician Tips

Any voided urinary stone should be saved for analysis.

Client Education

- Adherence to dietary therapy must be strict in cases of sterile struvite urolithiasis.
- Prevention of UTI is the most important preventative measure for most dogs.
- Urethral obstruction is life-threatening. Stranguria should prompt immediate veterinary attention.

SUGGESTED READING

Lulich JP, et al: ACVIM Small Animal Consensus Recommendations on the Treatment and Prevention of Uroliths in Dogs and Cats. J Vet Intern Med 30:1564-1574, 2016.

AUTHOR: Joseph W. Bartges, DVM, PhD, DACVIM, DACVN
EDITOR: Leah A. Cohn, DVM, PhD, DACVIM

Urolithiasis, Urate

Bonus Material Online 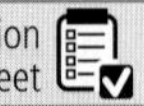 Client Education Sheet

BASIC INFORMATION

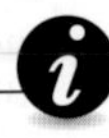

Definition

Urinary tract stones (uroliths) composed of uric acid and its salts (usually ammonium urate) comprise approximately 5%-10% of uroliths in dogs (except Dalmatians and English bulldogs) and cats.

Synonyms

Purine urolithiasis, ammonium urate urolithiasis, uric acid urolithiasis, urate calculi/stones

Epidemiology

SPECIES, AGE, SEX

- Most often seen in young to middle-aged adult dogs and young adult cats
- Urate uroliths are the most common urolith of Dalmatian dogs (≈35% of Dalmatians form urate uroliths) and occur predominantly in 3- to 4-year-old males.
- English bulldogs: ≈50% of uroliths in this breed composed of urate, ≈50% cystine
- Second most common mineral in uroliths from neonatal dogs and cats (after infection-induced struvite)
- Neonatal/young adult dogs and cats with portosystemic shunts (PSSs) or hepatic microvascular dysplasia (MVD).

GENETICS, BREED PREDISPOSITION

- High uric acid (HUA) Dalmatians (non–back-crossed) are unique in their excretion of uric acid instead of allantoin as an end product of purine metabolism, but only a subset develops urate urolithiasis. The tendency to form uroliths is heritable, although the genetics are incompletely understood. Back-crossed Dalmatians may be homozygous or heterozygous low uric acid (LUA) excreters; only homozygous HUA dogs are HUA excreters.
- Predisposed non-Dalmatian breeds include English bulldogs and Black Russian terriers.
- Due to congenital PSS, miniature schnauzers, shih tzus, and Yorkshire terriers are also overrepresented for having urate stones.

RISK FACTORS

- PSS (p. 814)
- Hepatic MVD (p. 655)
- Hepatic cirrhosis (p. 174)
- Acidic urine and/or urinary infection with urease-producing bacteria
- Breed and *SLC2A9* mutation

ASSOCIATED DISORDERS

- Urinary tract infection
- Ureteral or urethral obstruction
- Liver disease (see Risk Factors)

Clinical Presentation

HISTORY, CHIEF COMPLAINT

Clinical signs often absent. When apparent, may include

- Pollakiuria
- Hematuria
- Inappropriate elimination (periuria)
- Stranguria, dysuria
- If PSS and/or MVD is present, growth retardation
- If hepatic dysfunction is present, encephalopathy and/or hypoglycemia (e.g., altered mentation, seizures)
- Systemic illness due to urinary obstruction

PHYSICAL EXAM FINDINGS

Physical exam is usually unremarkable. Abnormalities may include

- Hematuria (stains on prepuce, vulva, hocks)
- Palpable cystic calculi
- Palpable urethral calculi (by digital rectal exam in dogs)
- Enlarged, turgid bladder if urethral obstruction present
- ± Signs of PSS, MVD, hepatic encephalopathy (p. 440)

Etiology and Pathophysiology

- Dalmatians
  - During protein catabolism in non-Dalmatian dogs, purine metabolism leads to uric acid oxidation by hepatic uricase, producing allantoin (excreted in urine).
  - Despite normal uricase activity, Dalmatians convert uric acid to allantoin inadequately, resulting in increased urinary excretion of poorly soluble uric acid.
  - This occurs due to a mutation in the *SCL2A9* gene that encodes for a hepatic transporter of uric acid. HUA Dalmatians and urate urolith–forming English bulldogs and Black Russian terriers are homozygous recessive for this mutation.
- Dogs with hepatic dysfunction: reduced uricase function and increased renal excretion of uric acid and ammonia resulting from reduced hepatic conversion/urea synthesis
- Non-Dalmatian, non–English bulldog, non–Black Russian terriers, and cats without hepatic dysfunction: unknown

DIAGNOSIS

Diagnostic Overview

Diagnosis is suspected in dogs with radiolucent uroliths and a breed predisposition or hepatic dysfunction. Diagnosis in cats and healthy dogs of other breeds is usually based on quantitative stone analysis.

Differential Diagnosis

- Urinary tract infection
- Other types of uroliths
- Urinary tract neoplasia

Initial Database

- CBC: often unremarkable, but PSS is associated with microcytosis.
- Serum biochemical profile: often unremarkable but may suggest hepatic dysfunction (pp. 174 and 814). Urinary tract obstruction

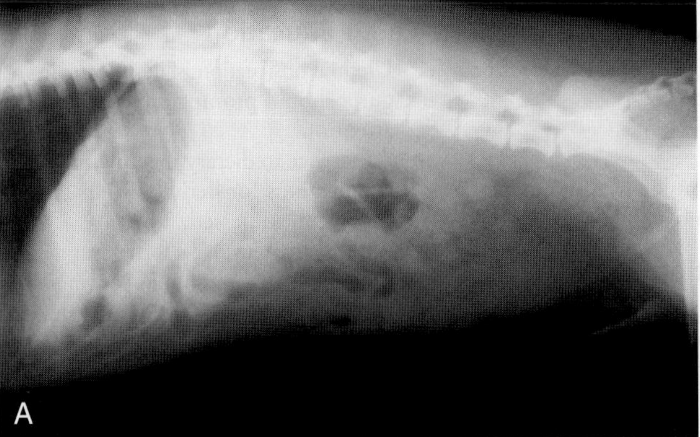

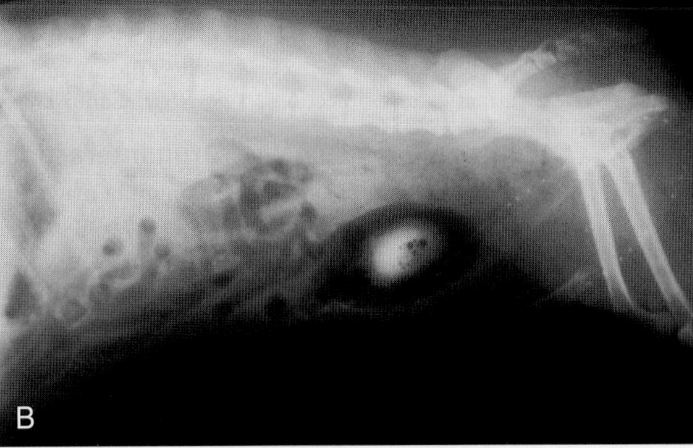

UROLITHIASIS, URATE Plain lateral abdominal radiograph (**A**) and double-contrast cystogram (**B**) show urate cystic calculi. Note the cranial displacement of the axis of the stomach, indicating microhepatica. This dog had an extrahepatic portosystemic shunt. The urethral catheter (containing air and positive contrast) in this male dog is seen as an incidental observation.

can lead to azotemia, hyperkalemia, and metabolic acidosis.
- Urinalysis: frequently aciduria; urate crystals sometimes identified; physical irritation and/or secondary infection sometimes leads to hematuria, pyuria, or bacteriuria
- Urine culture and sensitivity to rule out secondary infection
- Abdominal radiographs: urate uroliths are often radiolucent (radiopacity: struvite ≥ oxalate = $CaPO_4$ = silica > cystine > urate).
  - If visible, often few smooth, round uroliths identified
- Microhepatica is suggestive of PSS, MVD, or cirrhosis.
- Abdominal ultrasound: confirm urolithiasis, which may be missed on abdominal radiographs. Confirms location of uroliths within the urinary tract; may identify PSS or hepatic abnormalities

Advanced or Confirmatory Testing
- In non-Dalmatians or when appropriate: serum bile acids or other tests to rule out hepatic disease
- Contrast (or double-contrast) cystography, urethrography: alternative to ultrasound for confirmation/localization of radiolucent stones (p. 1181)
- Urolith analysis: retrieved stones submitted for quantitative analysis (crystallography, x-ray diffraction, infrared spectroscopy) to determine urolith type
- Cystoscopy may facilitate urolith removal for analysis and therapy (p. 1085).

TREATMENT

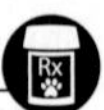

Treatment Overview
Urinary tract obstruction requires immediate relief. In the absence of urinary obstruction, treatment consists of medical stone dissolution or manual removal of stones, as well as treatment of underlying disorders (e.g., PSS) or preventive therapy. Medical dissolution often is ineffective in dogs and cats with PSS.

Acute General Treatment
- Relieve urinary tract obstruction (pp. 1175 and 1176) if present.
- If present, treat hepatic encephalopathy (p. 440).
- If present, treat urinary tract infection (pp. 232 and 849).
- Choose between medical dissolution (see Chronic Treatment below) and mechanical removal:
  - Urinary tract obstruction should be relieved mechanically.
  - Mechanical removal allows for urolith analysis, culture.
  - Cats are poorly amenable to medical dissolution of urate uroliths.
- Mechanical removal of calculi (pp. 1175 and 1176)
  - Urohydropropulsion (voiding, retrograde): avoid in male cats
  - Catheter-assisted retrieval
  - Cystoscopic-assisted retrieval (p. 1085)
  - Cystotomy/urethrotomy/urethrostomy/pyelotomy/nephrotomy
  - Lithotripsy

Chronic Treatment
- Animals with hepatic disease
  - Surgical correction of PSS prevents recurrence; cystotomy may be used to remove uroliths during surgical correction of hepatic shunt.
  - If hepatic disease cannot be corrected, institute medical management (including restricted-protein diet), and monitor for recurrence.
  - Allopurinol, which inhibits the conversion of xanthine to uric acid, is ineffective with PSS or MVD.
- Promote water consumption to avoid concentrated urine (e.g., canned food, wetting dry food, use of cat water fountains).
- Feed low-purine calculolytic diet (see Nutrition/Diet below).
- If urine remains acidic after diet change, consider adding sodium bicarbonate 25-50 mg/kg PO q 12h or potassium citrate 75 mg/kg PO q 12-24h, with dosage adjustment to maintain urine pH of 7.0-7.5.
- Allopurinol 15 mg/kg PO q 12h, with dosage reduction for azotemic dogs, for dissolution
- Medical dissolution is not effective in all dogs. For one-third, urate uroliths resolve in approximately 30 days. For another one-third of dogs, uroliths decrease in size and number, facilitating urolith retrieval by voiding urohydropropulsion or catheter-assisted retrieval. For the other one-third of dogs, uroliths increase in size and number due to xanthine formation.

Nutrition/Diet
Reduced-protein (therefore reduced-purine) diet:
- Dogs: for example, Hills u/d, Royal Canin Urinary UC Low Purine, Royal Canin Vegetarian Formula
- Cats: a diet formulated for chronic kidney disease, such as Prescription Diet k/d, Royal Canin Renal Support (A, D, E, F, S, or T) Purina NF, Blue Buffalo KM
- With PSS and MVD: a diet formulated for liver disease such as Prescription Diet l/d or Royal Canin Hepatic LS

Drug Interactions
Allopurinol may result in skin eruptions when used with ampicillin/amoxicillin.

Possible Complications
- Chronic use of low-purine diets may result in cardiomyopathy, perhaps related to carnitine or taurine deficiency (especially English bulldogs).
- Severely protein-restricted diets are inappropriate for growing, pregnant, or lactating animals.
- Xanthine urolith formation with allopurinol administration

Recommended Monitoring
- Serum biochemical profile and urinalysis 2 weeks after diet change. Goal is urine pH 7.0-8.0, specific gravity < 1.020, and absent crystals. Assuming adequate renal function and diet adherence, blood urea nitrogen (BUN) should be < 10 mg/dL. Monitor urinalysis q 2-4 weeks until uroliths resolved and q 3-6 months thereafter.
- Monitor dissolution of uroliths q 4 weeks with lower urinary tract contrast studies or ultrasound. Monitor for recurrence in like manner q 3-6 months for a year, then q 6-12 months.

PROGNOSIS & OUTCOME

- Prognosis for dissolution: fair (dogs)
- Recurrence is common unless cause resolved (e.g., PSS corrected).

PEARLS & CONSIDERATIONS

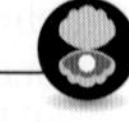

Comments
- Non-Dalmatian dogs with urate uroliths should be evaluated for hepatic disease, even when showing no overt signs of hepatopathy.
- Cats with urate urolithiasis have underlying hepatic disease less commonly than non-Dalmatian dogs.
- Apparently healthy dogs > 5 years of age with congenital PSS often develop clinical signs of urate urolithiasis rather than signs of hepatic encephalopathy.

Prevention
- Avoid high-protein diets in at-risk dogs (e.g., Dalmatian), but severely protein-restricted diets or allopurinol before a first episode of urate urolithiasis is not recommended.
- Heritability of tendency to form urate uroliths suggests breeding affected Dalmatian should be avoided.
- Long-term dietary ± allopurinol therapy 5-7 mg/kg PO q 12h is indicated for Dalmatian after first episode of urolithiasis.

Technician Tips
Dalmatian owners should be aware of this common issue in the breed.

Client Education
- Urethral obstruction is life-threatening. Stranguria should prompt immediate veterinary attention.
- Adherence to dietary therapy must be strict.
- Implications for heritability in Dalmatians should be addressed.
- After Dalmatians have formed urate uroliths, preventive therapy should continue lifelong.

SUGGESTED READING

Lulich JP, et al: ACVIM Small Animal Consensus Recommendations on the Treatment and Prevention of Uroliths in Dogs and Cats. J Vet Intern Med 30:1564-1574, 2016.

AUTHORS: Joseph W. Bartges, DVM, PhD, DACVIM, DACVN; Leah A. Cohn, DVM, PhD, DACVIM
EDITOR: Leah A. Cohn, DVM, PhD, DACVIM

Uterine Disorders, Non-neoplastic

Client Education Sheet

BASIC INFORMATION

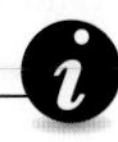

Definition

- Uterine torsion is an uncommon condition involving twisting of one or both uterine horns or the uterine body on its own axis.
- Uterine prolapse is a rare condition where the uterus everts through the cervix and vagina (one or both horns may be involved).

Epidemiology

SPECIES, AGE, SEX

Either condition may occur at any age or parity. Uterine torsion may occur unrelated to pregnancy. Prolapse is more common in queens.

RISK FACTORS

- Large litter size may predispose to torsion.
- Any condition causing excessive straining (e.g., dystocia, necrotic vaginitis, severe cystitis, diarrhea, constipation) may predispose to prolapse.

ASSOCIATED DISORDERS

Both may be associated with shock, sepsis, disseminated intravascular coagulation, multiple organ dysfunction syndrome, and systemic inflammatory response syndrome.

Clinical Presentation

DISEASE FORMS/SUBTYPES

- Torsion may involve one or both horns and/or the uterine body and may be from 90° to >2160° (six complete turns described in one report).
- Prolapse occurs in the puerperal period and may involve one or both horns, be partial or complete, and occurs rarely before delivery of all fetuses.

HISTORY, CHIEF COMPLAINT

Torsion:

- History of no progression from stage 1 to stage 2 of labor or cessation of ongoing stage 2 labor
- Acute abdominal pain
- Shock

Prolapse:

- History of prolonged straining (labor, other)
- Tissue protrudes from the vulvar lips.
- Queens may present up to 48 hours after delivery of last kitten.

PHYSICAL EXAM FINDINGS

- Acute abdominal pain and splinting
- Vocalization
- Hemorrhagic vulvar discharge
- Excessively vulvar licking
- Abdominal distention
- Tachycardia and tachypnea
- Pale mucous membranes with increased capillary refill time
- ± Collapse
- ± Devitalized prolapsed tissue

Etiology and Pathophysiology

- Torsion: unknown cause; may be due to fetal or bitch activity or abnormal uterine motility (inertia) with continued fetal activity; pyometra, mucometra, hydrometra, or hematometra; neoplasia
- Prolapse: eversion of the tip of a uterine horn followed by excessive straining (due to any cause) during uterine involution or eversion of the tip of a horn due to uterine inertia followed by normal uterine contraction patterns

DIAGNOSIS

Diagnostic Overview

- Torsion: based on cessation of labor or acute abdominal pain. Ultrasound may be supportive, but diagnosis is conclusively based on exploratory laparotomy.
- Prolapse: based on physical exam findings of prolapsed tissue from the vulvar lips after parturition. Inability to locate the uterus on ultrasound of the abdomen is confirmatory.

Differential Diagnosis

Uterine torsion:

- Pyometra
- Uterine rupture
- Uterine inertia (primary or secondary)
- Acute gastrointestinal disorders (bloat, gastric or mesenteric torsion), other causes of the acute abdomen

Uterine prolapse:

- Bladder or vaginal prolapse
- Vaginal rupture and evisceration
- Vaginal, cervical, or uterine neoplasia

Initial Database

- CBC: ± leukocytosis, ± toxic neutrophils, evidence of dehydration
- Serum biochemistry profile: normal to increased renal and hepatic values and electrolyte disturbance, depending on duration
- Abdominal ultrasonography
  - Hemorrhage into uterine lumen and edema (hypoechogenicity) of the uterine wall adjacent to the torsion
  - Fetuses may be viable or dead.
  - Intraluminal gas may be present.

TREATMENT

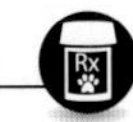

Treatment Overview

Treatment goals:

- Patient stabilization (IV fluid resuscitation, pain control)
- Exploratory laparotomy for correction of torsion (if tissue is not necrotic or severely ischemic), cesarean section to deliver remaining fetuses if still viable, or ovariohysterectomy (OHE) if tissue is devitalized
- Prolapsed tissue is cleaned and replaced with combination of manual manipulation externally and abdominal surgical approach. OHE may be necessary if tissue is devitalized.

Acute General Treatment

Torsion:

- Broad-spectrum antibiotics (ampicillin 10-22 mg/kg IV q 6-8h with enrofloxacin 10-15 mg/kg IM, SQ, or IV q 24h; maximum of 5 mg/kg q 24h IM in cats) as soon as diagnosis is confirmed and when devitalized tissue is present
- If the horn is severely ischemic or necrotic, do not detorse the affected horn(s) because this may result in reperfusion injury and allow systemic circulation of bacteria and toxin; perform OHE with torsion *in situ*.
- If only one horn is affected, partial OHE may be performed, oversewing the uterine body at the level of the bifurcation.

Prolapse:

- Initially, digital pressure and inversion of the horn into itself starting distally and working toward the tip. Applying 50% dextrose solution topically and waiting a few minutes for osmotic detumescence may decrease size of prolapsed tissue.
- Care should be taken to invert the entire horn to its tip (this should be confirmed visually).
- Oxytocin after complete inversion for uterine involution
- If manual reduction is impossible, uterine amputation is indicated.

Behavior/Exercise

If the dam is stable, she may be allowed to nurse any neonates.

Recommended Monitoring

CBC, serum biochemistry profile

PROGNOSIS & OUTCOME

- With early diagnosis, the prognosis is good for survival.
- With systemic illness, the prognosis for survival is guarded to poor.
- Recurrence is unlikely.

PEARLS & CONSIDERATIONS

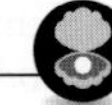

Comments

- Caution should be taken when handling either condition because the uterine wall may be friable.
- Do not administer calcium or oxytocin to patients suspected of torsion or prolapse.

Prevention

OHE

Technician Tips

Carefully monitor patients under anesthesia. Marked drop in blood pressure may occur from reperfusion injury. To avoid this, administer fluid bolus with crystalloid or colloid solutions and do not premedicate with hypotensive drugs (e.g., acepromazine, dexmedetomidine).

Client Education

- Failure of an animal to continue to progress through labor should instigate a veterinary exam.
- Bloody discharge or abdominal pain during or after delivery is abnormal.

SUGGESTED READING

Johnston SD, et al: Disorders of the canine uterus and uterine tubes, and disorders of the feline uterus and uterine tubes. In Johnston SD, editor: Canine and feline theriogenology, Philadelphia, 2001, Saunders, pp 206-463.

AUTHOR: Cheryl Lopate, MS, DVM, DACT
EDITOR: Michelle A. Kutzler, DVM, PhD, DACT

Uterine Neoplasia

Client Education Sheet 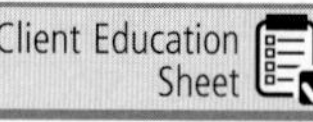

BASIC INFORMATION 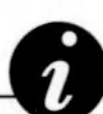

Definition

Benign or malignant cellular proliferations involving the uterus are uncommon in dogs and cats.

Synonyms

Uterine mass, nodule, or polyp

Epidemiology

SPECIES, AGE, SEX

- Most common in bitches > 10 years of age and queens between 5 and 10 years of age
- Accounts for 1%-19% of all reproductive tumors in dogs and 1%-2% of all reproductive tumors in cats

GENETICS, BREED PREDISPOSITION

Boxers may be overrepresented.

RISK FACTORS

Older age, intact reproductive tract

CONTAGION AND ZOONOSIS

Transmissible venereal tumor (TVT); uterine metastases can result in TVT dysgerminoma

ASSOCIATED DISORDERS

Uterine torsion and/or rupture

Clinical Presentation

DISEASE FORMS/SUBTYPES

May involve the endometrium (polyp); myometrium (leiomyoma, fibroma, fibroleiomyoma, fibroadenoma, adenoma, leiomyosarcoma, adenocarcinoma, adenoacanthoma, fibrocarcinoma); lipoma; or metastatic disease (lymphoma; TVT dysgerminoma)

HISTORY, CHIEF COMPLAINT

- Bloody, mucoid, mucopurulent, or mucohemorrhagic vulvar discharge
- Abdominal distention
- Ascites
- Depression or lethargy
- Vomiting
- Anorexia
- Dysuria
- Constipation
- Chronic low-grade fever: uncommon

PHYSICAL EXAM FINDINGS

- Bloody vulvar discharge
- Abdominal distention with palpable mid-caudal abdominal mass
- Weight loss
- Depression
- Lymph node enlargement (especially inguinal): uncommon

Etiology and Pathophysiology

- Uterine tumors may be of endometrial, myometrial, serosal origin; may be primary or metastatic
- Leiomyoma is the most common tumor and may be found incidentally or concurrent with pregnancy.

DIAGNOSIS 

Diagnostic Overview

Tumor is typically suspected with a history of bloody vulvar discharge with supportive cytologic findings and/or ultrasound evidence of a uterine mass. Histopathologic exam of a specimen from the mass is the confirmatory test of choice.

Differential Diagnosis

- Pyometra
- Segmental endometrial hyperplasia
- Uterine lithiasis
- Pregnancy
- Mummified fetus
- Subinvolution of placental sites (SIPS)
- Adenomyosis
- Granuloma
- Mural abscess
- Decidual reaction
- Remnant of the mesonephric duct
- Serosal inclusion cysts

Initial Database

- CBC, serum biochemistry profile, urinalysis (avoid unguided cystocentesis): results may be normal with benign tumors to abnormal with metastatic disease, depending on metastatic location.
- Cytologic exam of vulvar discharge may demonstrate neoplastic cells.
- Radiographs may reveal an enlarged caudal abdominal viscus.
- Abdominal ultrasound exam reveals a mass in the uterine, cervical, or vaginal lumen:
    - If mass appears solid (homogeneous, minimally vascularized), fine-needle aspiration for cytologic exam is appropriate.
- Thoracic radiographs for evidence of metastasis

Advanced or Confirmatory Testing

- Hysteroscopy may reveal a luminal or mural mass.
- Biopsy may be taken by transcervical endoscopic collection technique (TECT).
- MRI may better delineate the mass and provide further evidence of metastasis (rarely necessary).
- Laparoscopy may be useful for visualization and biopsy.

TREATMENT 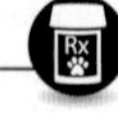

Treatment Overview

Ovariohysterectomy (OHE): partial or complete

Acute General Treatment

- Typically, complete OHE is recommended to ensure that any small masses not palpable or visible are removed at the time of initial surgery.
- Abdominal inguinal lymph nodes may be submitted for assessment of metastasis.
- For a long-standing tumor, necrosis of the uterine wall is possible, or adhesions to other abdominal tissues may require resection.

Chronic Treatment

Depending on tumor type and degree of metastasis, chemotherapy, immune modulators, or radiation therapy may be appropriate. Consultation with an oncologist is recommended.

Possible Complications

If malignancy is present, complications associated with tumor metastasis in other locations may occur.

Recommended Monitoring

If malignant, monitoring of other organ systems for metastasis may be required.

PROGNOSIS & OUTCOME

Good for benign tumors; guarded to poor for metastatic or malignant tumors

PEARLS & CONSIDERATIONS

Comments

Spayed females that have not undergone a complete hysterectomy (i.e., small portion of uterine tissue is remaining cranial to the cervix) are still susceptible to uterine neoplasia. As such, uterine neoplasia should be included as a differential diagnosis in all bitches presenting with these physical exam findings.

Prevention

Hysterectomy, ovariohysterectomy

Technician Tips

Abnormal cells noted on vaginal cytology should be brought to the attention of the veterinarian.

Client Education

Females, regardless of their age, should be spayed after the last litter to prevent tumors from developing.

SUGGESTED READING

Johnston SD, et al: Disorders of the canine uterus and uterine tubes. In Johnston SD, et al, editors: Canine and feline theriogenology, Philadelphia, 2001, Saunders, p 206.

AUTHOR: Cheryl Lopate, DVM, MS, DACT
EDITOR: Michelle A. Kutzler, DVM, PhD, DACT

Uveitis

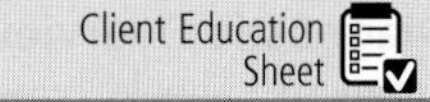

Client Education Sheet

BASIC INFORMATION

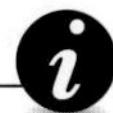

Definition

Uveitis is broadly defined as a breakdown in the uveal blood-ocular barrier, resulting in the abnormal presence of protein, white blood cells (WBCs), red blood cells (RBCs), and other compounds in the aqueous humor or vitreous with possible extension to other parts of the eye.

Synonyms

- Anterior uveitis: iridocyclitis, iritis, cyclitis
- Posterior uveitis: chorioretinitis, retinochoroiditis, choroiditis
- Panuveitis: concurrent anterior and posterior uveitis

Epidemiology

SPECIES, AGE, SEX

Dogs and cats; any age or sex, depending on the underlying cause

GENETICS, BREED PREDISPOSITION

- Most uveitic syndromes do not have a breed predisposition.
- Uveodermatologic (UVD) syndrome: Akitas, Samoyeds, Siberian Huskies
- Pigmentary and cystic glaucoma: golden retrievers

CONTAGION AND ZOONOSIS

- Underlying causes may have contagious and zoonotic potential.
- Contagious
  - Feline leukemia virus (FeLV)
  - Feline immunodeficiency virus (FIV)
  - Feline infectious peritonitis (FIP)
- Contagious and zoonotic
  - *Brucella canis*
  - Leptospirosis
  - *Toxoplasma gondii*

GEOGRAPHY AND SEASONALITY

Varies, depending on infectious agents (e.g., tick-borne diseases, systemic mycoses)

ASSOCIATED DISORDERS

- Systemic conditions: infectious or inflammatory disease, UVD syndrome, hypertension, systemic neoplasia (e.g., lymphoma)
- Ocular conditions: cataracts, trauma, intraocular neoplasia, retinal detachment

Clinical Presentation

DISEASE FORMS/SUBTYPES

- Any protein (seen as flare), whole blood (hyphema), WBCs (hypopyon), lipid, fibrin, or any combination of the above in the aqueous humor is consistent with uveitis (i.e., breakdown of the blood-aqueous barrier). Material also may be seen in the vitreous or the choroid/retina.
- Acute versus chronic

HISTORY, CHIEF COMPLAINT

- Various complaints, depending on duration, ocular signs, and systemic disease
- Ocular pain (photophobia, blepharospasm)
- Red eye
- Cloudy eye
- Diminished vision (especially if the condition is bilateral)

PHYSICAL EXAM FINDINGS

- Physical exam: varies depending on possible concurrent systemic illness
- Ophthalmic exam: findings vary tremendously, depending on severity, duration, and cause. Aqueous flare, including hypopyon, fibrin in the anterior chamber, hyphema and keratic precipitates are pathognomonic for anterior uveitis.
  - Aqueous flare
  - Hypopyon
  - Hyphema
  - Fibrin in anterior chamber
  - Keratic precipitates
  - Miosis
  - Synechia (anterior, posterior, dyscoria)
  - Varied intraocular pressure (IOP): decreased with acute uveitis, increased with secondary glaucoma
  - Corneal edema
  - Corneal vascularization
  - Iris change (e.g., reddening, darkening, depigmentation, thickening, iris bombé)
  - Conjunctival, episcleral injection
  - Cataract
  - Posterior segment changes: vitritis, chorioretinitis, retinal detachment, optic neuritis

Etiology and Pathophysiology

- Any opacification within the clear ocular media (e.g., blood, flare, WBCs) represents a disruption of the blood-ocular barrier, and empirical treatment with topical antiinflammatories (prednisolone acetate q 6-12h) can be started for the eye to try to reestablish the normal blood-ocular barrier if a corneal ulcer is not present.
- Material in the aqueous humor can lead to disruption of the normal flow by occluding the drainage angle of the eye, resulting in glaucoma. Regular monitoring (weekly initially while treating) should be performed, and glaucoma medications (dorzolamide/timolol q 8-12h) should be started when necessary.
- Ocular disease
  - Lens-induced uveitis
  - Corneal disease (e.g., infected ulcer, perforation)
  - Trauma
  - Primary intraocular neoplasia
  - Pigmentary and cystic glaucoma
  - Idiopathic/immune-mediated (60% of dogs and cats)
- Systemic disease
  - Secondary intraocular neoplasia (most common: lymphoma)
  - Infection (dog)
    - Tick-borne (*Ehrlichia*, Rocky Mountain spotted fever, Lyme disease)
    - Fungal (cryptococcosis, blastomycosis, histoplasmosis, coccidioidomycosis)
    - *Prototheca*
    - Leptospirosis
    - Brucellosis
    - Bacterial (septicemia, bacteremia)

- Infectious canine hepatitis
- Borreliosis
- Leishmaniasis
  - Infection (cat)
    - FeLV
    - FIV
    - FIP
    - Toxoplasmosis
    - Fungal (cryptococcosis, blastomycosis, histoplasmosis, coccidioidomycosis)
- UVD syndrome
- Hypertension
- Blood dyscrasias
- Aberrant metazoan parasites: *Dirofilaria immitis*, ascarids, fly larvae

DIAGNOSIS

Diagnostic Overview

Diagnostics should center on determining if there is an ocular cause for the uveitis by a complete ophthalmic exam and basic ophthalmic tests (Schirmer tear test [STT], fluorescein stain, tonometry). In the absence of a primary ocular cause, it is important to consider an underlying systemic illness. Client should be educated as to the possible risks of a missed diagnosis.

Differential Diagnosis

Other causes of a red eye:
- Primary glaucoma
- Conjunctivitis
- Episcleritis
- Keratitis
- Keratoconjunctivitis sicca

Initial Database

To rule in ocular causes of uveitis:
- Complete ophthalmic exam of both eyes, including a dilated fundic exam
- STT, fluorescein stain, tonometry

To rule in/out systemic causes of uveitis:
- Complete physical exam
- CBC
- Blood chemistry
- Urinalysis
- Blood pressure
- Infectious disease testing (retroviral testing for all cats; other testing based suspected disease)
- Thoracic radiographs
- Abdominal ultrasound

Advanced or Confirmatory Testing

- Lymph node aspirate
- Skin biopsy (UVD)
- Colonic scraping (protothecosis)
- Aqueocentesis, vitreocentesis (often referral test but rarely necessary)

TREATMENT

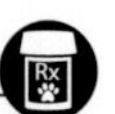

Treatment Overview

- Empirical treatment regardless of underlying cause is directed toward treating the eye and secondary complications.
- Frequency of antiinflammatories should be proportional to the degree of uveitis: less often (q 12-24h) for mild cases, more often (q 6-8h) for severe cases
- Ophthalmic steroids (prednisolone acetate or dexamethasone) should be used in moderate to severe cases unless corneal ulceration is present.
- Ophthalmic nonsteroidal antiinflammatories (NSAIDs) can be used in mild cases, if corneal disease precludes use of topical steroids, or in conjunction with steroids if uveitis is severe.
- Oral steroids or oral NSAIDs can be used concurrently with topical steroids or topical NSAIDs. For example, it is safe to treat with topical prednisolone acetate and oral carprofen.

Acute General Treatment

No corneal ulceration (no stain uptake):
- Topical prednisolone acetate 1% q 6-12h or topical dexamethasone q 6-12h (alone or in combination with antibiotics: neomycin, polymyxin B, or dexamethasone)

Corneal ulceration (stain uptake) (p. 209):
- Topical flurbiprofen or diclofenac (topical NSAID) q 6-8h
- Topical antibiotics given prophylactically or for active infection
- Systemic antiinflammatories if uveitis secondary to corneal disease is significant
- Topical atropine q 12-24h if IOP is low or low-normal
- Secondary glaucoma (IOP normal or > 25 mm Hg)
  - Topical dorzolamide-timolol q 8-12h

Refractory to topical therapy alone or considered free of systemic disease:
- Prednisone 0.5-1 mg/kg/day PO
- NSAIDS (e.g., carprofen, meloxicam)

Confirmed or suspected immune-mediated disease (e.g., UVD syndrome):
- Prednisone 1-2 mg/kg/day PO initially
- Azathioprine or other immunosuppressive medications as needed long term

Confirmed or suspected infectious disease:
- Appropriate antimicrobial therapy

Chronic Treatment

- Chronic treatment may be required if cause remains undetermined, cannot be corrected (e.g., lens-induced uveitis), or is related to chronic disease. The goal is to determine the minimum effective drug doses to keep the eye clear and comfortable.
- If the eye returns to normal on the course of antiinflammatories, the author will usually taper the topical antiinflammatories by a drop per day q 2 weeks (e.g., q 8h→q 12h × 2 weeks, q 12h→q24h × 2 weeks, q 24h→q 48h × 2 weeks). Regular monitoring should be performed during taper to check for flare-ups.

Recommended Monitoring

First recheck is typically in 1 week, to assess response and monitor for complications. If the eye is responding well, recheck times can be done q 2-4 weeks until the eye is normal or stable for at least 3-4 weeks. If the eye is responding poorly, consideration should be given to an alternative underlying cause. Enucleation is considered if prognosis for vision is poor and the eye remains painful.

PROGNOSIS & OUTCOME

- Prognosis for vision corresponds to severity, chronicity, and cause of uveitis. The prognosis is worse if the posterior segment is affected given possible involvement of the retina. Secondary glaucoma is a negative prognostic factor because it usually corresponds with severe uveitis or chronicity; glaucoma often permanently damages the optic nerve and retina.
- With prompt and aggressive treatment, most immune-mediated or idiopathic uveitis responds well.
- If there is no improvement in the face of treatment, a new search for systemic disease should be undertaken. If the prognosis for vision is poor, enucleation can relieve pain and provide diagnostic value with histopathologic exam and/or culture.

PEARLS & CONSIDERATIONS

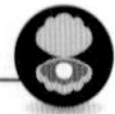

Comments

- An important diagnostic goal for uveitis is to determine whether there is a larger threat to

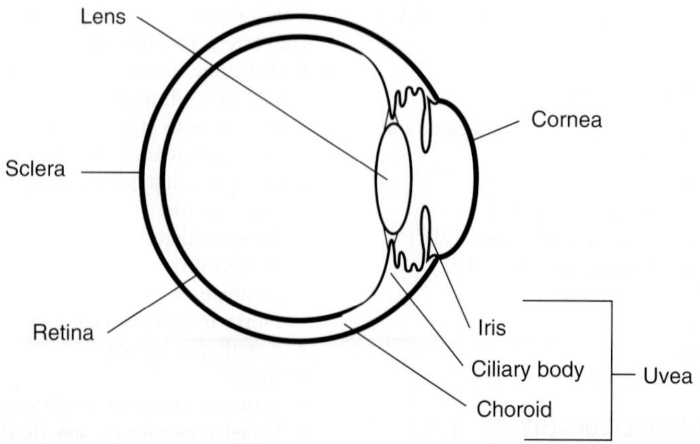

UVEITIS Sagittal section of the globe shows the anatomic relationships of the uvea with the other parts of the eye.

the patient's systemic health. This is especially important in areas of the country where fungal or tick-borne disease is prevalent.
- Idiopathic/immune-mediated uveitis is quite common, in which case systemic disease will not be identified.
- Inflammation may worsen as treatment frequency is tapered; close monitoring is indicated.

Prevention
- Preventive health care, including vaccinations and ectoparasite control.
- Refer animals with cataracts early so that surgical options can be discussed.
- Refer complicated ulcers/corneal perforations and lens luxations immediately if the eye is to be saved.

Technician Tips
Ensure that ancillary ocular diagnostics (fluorescein staining and IOP measurement) are performed for uveitis at all recheck visits.

Client Education
- Depending on the cause and response to therapy, uveitis may cause permanent blindness.
- Although a cause cannot always be determined, a search for the cause should be attempted because some causes are readily amenable to early treatment but can prove fatal if not addressed.
- Long-term treatment may be necessary.

SUGGESTED READING
Townsend WM: Canine and feline uveitis. Vet Clin North Am Small Anim Pract 38:323-346, 2008.

RELATED CLIENT EDUCATION SHEETS
Consent to Perform Abdominal Ultrasound
Consent to Perform Enucleation
How to Administer Eye Medications
How to Assemble and Use an Elizabethan Collar

AUTHOR: Thomas Chen, DVM, MS, DACVO
EDITOR: Diane V. H. Hendrix, DVM, DAVCO

Vacuolar Hepatopathy

Client Education Sheet 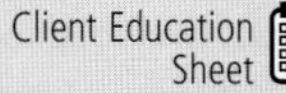 Bonus Material Online 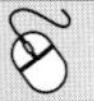

BASIC INFORMATION 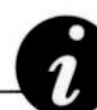

Definition
Vacuolar hepatopathy (VH) is a commonly detected canine liver syndrome characterized by the cytosolic accumulation of glycogen in hepatocytes, resulting in cell distention, fragility, and degeneration.

Synonyms
Steroid hepatopathy, glucocorticoid hepatopathy, hepatocellular steatosis, hepatocellular lipidosis

Epidemiology
SPECIES, AGE, SEX
- Dogs of any age, sex, or breed
  - Typically older dogs (median age, 9 years; range, 1-19 years)
  - Neutered females are overrepresented; neutered males are underrepresented.
- Rare in cats (p. 444)

GENETICS, BREED PREDISPOSITION
Vacuolar hepatopathy in Scottish terriers may be linked to adrenal steroidogenesis.

RISK FACTORS
- In one study, severe VH occurred three times more often in dogs exposed to glucocorticoids than other dogs, and 55% of dogs with VH had exogenous or excessive endogenous steroid hormone exposure.
- It is commonly diagnosed secondary to or concurrent with the following diseases:
  - Neoplastic diseases (28% of cases in one study)
  - Acquired hepatobiliary disease (13%)
  - Adrenal gland dysfunction (12%)
  - Neurologic diseases (11%)
  - Immune-mediated disease (10%)
  - Gastrointestinal diseases (9%)
  - Many less common conditions, including infections

ASSOCIATED DISORDERS
- Rarely, dogs develop hepatic insufficiency with biochemical evidence of cholestasis, parenchymal stromal collapse, and/or formation of regenerative nodules. Rarely, acquired portosystemic shunts, ascites, and even death have been reported, but these features might not have been due to VH.
- Dogs with VH have been reported to have biliary mucoceles (p. 374), but it is likely these conditions have a common underlying cause rather than VH causing biliary mucoceles.
- Scottish terriers with progressive VH seem to be predisposed to hepatocellular carcinoma (p. 446). Frequent serum biochemical analysis and ultrasonographic surveillance for early tumor detection is recommended for the breed.
- Progressive VH is seen with hepatocutaneous syndrome (p. 952).

Clinical Presentation
DISEASE FORMS/SUBTYPES
The severity of hepatocellular vacuolation is categorized as mild, moderate, or severe based on acinar zonal distribution of hepatocyte vacuolation on histopathology.

HISTORY, CHIEF COMPLAINT
- Clinical signs are often those associated with excess glucocorticoids (e.g., polyuria/polydipsia, polyphagia, panting, bilateral symmetric truncal alopecia [p. 485])
- In dogs with VH secondary to chronic illness, clinical signs are associated with the underlying disease process.

PHYSICAL EXAM FINDINGS
- Physical exam findings are typically associated with excess cortisol.
  - Overweight
  - Dermatologic abnormalities (e.g., truncal alopecia, pustules, striae)
  - Abdominal distention without fluid wave
  - Hepatomegaly with rounded liver border
- In dogs with VH secondary to chronic illness, findings can be markedly different and are associated with the underlying disease process.

Etiology and Pathophysiology
- Common liver disorder: in a review of hepatic biopsies from 500 dogs, VH was detected in 19%.
- VH is characterized by the cytosolic accumulation of glycogen in hepatocytes, resulting in cell distention, fragility, and degeneration.
- The majority (55% of dogs in one study) develop VH associated with iatrogenic, typical, or atypical hyperadrenocorticism.
  - The remaining dogs are theorized to develop VH secondary to stress-induced hypercortisolemia associated with illness, including cancer, infections, and inflammatory disease.
- Although previously considered a benign transformation, later observations raise the concern that VH may be associated with pathogenic scenarios, including hepatic insufficiency, hepatocellular carcinoma, or biliary mucoceles.

DIAGNOSIS

Diagnostic Overview

Usually, increased liver enzymes activities prompt hepatic ultrasound exam. Ultrasound findings are suggestive, although not pathognomonic, of VH. The diagnosis is confirmed by hepatic biopsy. For the majority of affected dogs, the medical history, exam, and minimum database are suggestive of endogenous or exogenous hyperadrenocorticism. If not, a diagnostic search for a primary disease process should be undertaken.

Differential Diagnosis

- Hepatotoxins (p. 1231)
- Adverse drug reactions
- Infectious agents (p. 1230)
- Inflammatory hepatopathies including hepatitis and cholangiohepatitis
- Copper storage hepatopathy (p. 458)
- Neoplasia (p. 1230)
- Cholestatic disease, including mucocele
- Ischemia/hypoxic injury, including surgical hypotension and hypoxia, liver lobe torsion or thromboembolic disease
- Severe systemic or metabolic disorders
  - Acute pancreatitis
  - Sepsis, septicemia, endotoxemia, heat stroke, trauma

Initial Database

Findings are typically associated with excess glucocorticoids. Review history for any exogenous steroid use, including topical preparations. In dogs with VH secondary to chronic stress or illness, the findings can be markedly different and are associated with the underlying disease process.

- CBC: often, components of a stress leukogram (lymphopenia, eosinopenia, neutrophilia, monocytosis) and thrombocytosis
- Serum biochemical profile
  - Very commonly, increased activities of alkaline phosphatase (ALP) and gamma-glutamyl transferase (GGT)
  - Lesser elevations of transaminases: aspartate aminotransferase (AST) and alanine aminotransferase (ALT)
  - Often, hypertriglyceridemia, hypercholesterolemia
  - Occasionally, decreased blood urea nitrogen (BUN) (noted with polyuria/polydipsia)
  - Mild hyperglycemia
  - Normal bilirubin, albumin
- Urinalysis: usually urine specific gravity < 1.020; moderate proteinuria (urine protein/creatinine ratio < 5)
- Abdominal radiography: evaluate hepatic size (subjective); hepatomegaly common
- Abdominal ultrasound: sensitive tool for evaluating hepatic parenchyma, the biliary system, and vascular structures
  - Permits guided sampling of liver
  - Hepatomegaly with a diffuse hyperechoic echogenicity typical of VH
  - Hypoechoic nodules are common.
  - Can reveal a coarse echotexture
  - Rarely, masses are secondary to VH (primary differential of a neoplasia)
  - Can identify abnormalities of adrenal size, symmetry
  - Can identify comorbid disease that might cause vacuolar hepatopathy (e.g., pancreatitis, extrahepatic abdominal tumors)
- Coagulation profile (p. 1325): rule out coagulopathy if biopsy anticipated
- Serum bile acids: normal to mild increase typical of VH
- If hyperadrenocorticism is suspected, screen by low-dose dexamethasone suppression or ACTH stimulation testing (pp. 485, 1300, and 1360).

Advanced or Confirmatory Testing

- Hepatic cytology (p. 1112)
  - Small sample size limits diagnostic accuracy.
  - Specificity is poor for VH, limiting the usefulness in confirming the diagnosis.
  - Most useful to rule out other hepatopathies, including diffuse neoplasia, bacterial abscesses, parasite infestations, and suppurative hepatitis
- Hepatic histopathology (p. 1128)
  - VH is characterized by hepatocytes distended with cytosolic glycogen, with or without discrete membrane-bound lipid inclusions. Severity is characterized as mild to severe and/or by the acinar zonal distribution of hepatocyte vacuolation. Acinar zonal distribution of vacuolation is variable, although a diffuse or predominantly zone 2 or 3 distribution is most common.
  - Because VH is confirmed only after biopsy interpretation, samples should be submitted for bacterial culture and copper quantification.
- Other diagnostic testing may be necessary to find an underlying cause for VH if endogenous or exogenous glucocorticoid excess is ruled out.

TREATMENT

Treatment Overview

For most dogs with VH, the focus of treatment is detecting, managing and if possible, reversing the underlying disease process. This can include stopping exogenous glucocorticoids (if possible), treating hyperadrenocorticism, and treating a condition resulting in stress-induced hypercortisolemia.

Acute General Treatment

Acute treatment is not typically required with VH, other than appropriate treatment of underlying or associated conditions (e.g., treatment of neoplasia, cholecystectomy to manage gallbladder mucoceles).

Chronic Treatment

- There is no specific therapy for VH.
- In most cases, reducing exogenous glucocorticoid administration or treating hyperadrenocorticism (pp. 485, 1426, and 1427) is appropriate.
- If another underlying disorder is recognized, it should be addressed.
- Although benefits are not proved, hepatoprotective therapies such as antioxidants have been used (p. 452).

Nutrition/Diet

Protein restriction, typical of liver-specific diets, is not required. Dietary therapy should be designed based on underlying conditions and to achieve and maintain an ideal body weight (p. 1077).

Drug Interactions

Any potentially hepatotoxic drug (e.g., nonsteroidal antiinflammatory drugs) should be avoided.

Possible Complications

Possible increased risk of thromboembolic disease and infections, considering the underlying or associated conditions

Recommended Monitoring

Protocols for monitoring patients with VH have not been established, other than as required by underlying disease. Exam and biochemical profile q 6 months seem reasonable for most affected dogs. In Scottish terriers, frequent ultrasonographic surveillance is recommended to screen for the possible development of hepatocellular carcinoma.

PROGNOSIS & OUTCOME

- Most dogs with vacuolar hepatopathy associated with excess glucocorticoids or steroidogenic hormones have a good prognosis.
- In dogs with vacuolar hepatopathy NOT associated with exogenous or excess endogenous glucocorticoids, the prognosis and outcome are based on the underlying condition.

PEARLS & CONSIDERATIONS

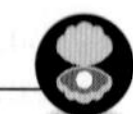

Comments

If elevated serum ALP and GGT activities persist after removing the source of excessive steroid hormones, other causes should be considered.

Prevention

- Use the lowest effective dose of glucocorticoids necessary.
- For disorders requiring chronic glucocorticoid use, consider steroid-sparing alternatives (e.g., cyclosporine for immune-mediated disease).

Technician Tips

Dogs with VH have a propensity for infections, delayed wound healing, and slow hair regrowth.

Client Education

Most dogs with VH secondary to hyperadrenocorticism do not require specific therapy for the hepatopathy.

SUGGESTED READING

Sepesy L, et al: Vacuolar hepatopathy in dogs: 336 cases (1993-2005). J Am Vet Med Assoc 229:246-252, 2006.

AUTHOR: Marnin A. Forman, DVM, DACVIM
EDITOR: Keith P. Richter, DVM, MSEL, DACVIM

Vaginal Congenital Abnormalities in the Bitch

BASIC INFORMATION

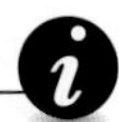

Definition

Malformations that reduce the diameter of the vestibulovaginal junction (bands) and may cause secondary infertility, vaginitis, or cystitis; include incomplete dissolution or fusion of the paramesonephric ducts (müllerian), hymenal remnants, and hypoplasia of the vestibulovaginal junction.

Epidemiology

SPECIES, AGE, SEX

Congenital vaginal abnormalities are present at birth but usually are undetected until the appearance of clinical signs. Young-adult female dogs are most commonly affected.

GENETICS, BREED PREDISPOSITION

Large-breed dogs may be overrepresented.

ASSOCIATED DISORDERS

Female dogs with ectopic ureters often have coincident congenital vaginal abnormalities.

Clinical Presentation

DISEASE FORMS/SUBTYPES

- Double vagina
- Hypoplasia of the vaginal vault
- Imperforate hymen
- Vaginal stenosis
- Vaginal stricture

HISTORY, CHIEF COMPLAINT

- Unsuccessful breeding attempts, obvious pain during breeding, avoidance of male during breeding attempts
- Purulent, often recurrent vaginal discharge
- Persistent or recurrent urinary tract infection (UTI), urine dribbling

PHYSICAL EXAM FINDINGS

- Vaginal discharge may be present.
- Narrowing of vestibulovaginal junction may be apparent during manual vaginal exam.

Etiology and Pathophysiology

- Incomplete fusion of the paramesonephric ducts can result in persistent dorsoventral bands.
- Vestibulovaginal hypoplasia causes concentric narrowing of the vestibulovaginal junction.
- Incomplete dissolution of the hymen can compromise the vestibulovaginal junction.
- Any type of vestibulovaginal stricture can interfere with breeding due to pain produced during penetration by a male dog.
- Anatomic abnormalities of the vestibulovaginal junction can inhibit drainage of vaginal secretions, which can lead to vaginitis or ascending UTI.

DIAGNOSIS

Diagnostic Overview

Clinicians should suspect vestibulovaginal abnormalities in bitches with a history of difficult or unsuccessful breeding. The diagnosis is usually made during vaginal exam.

Differential Diagnosis

- Behavioral abnormalities in breeding bitches in estrus who are reluctant to stand for a male
- Other causes of chronic UTI are more common.
- Vaginal discharge may be associated with juvenile-onset vaginitis or pyometra.

Initial Database

Digital vaginal exam

Advanced or Confirmatory Testing

- Vaginoscopy using a flexible or rigid endoscope (p. 1184), for which heavy sedation or general anesthesia is necessary
- Contrast radiography: retrograde vaginography

TREATMENT

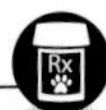

Treatment Overview

Remove obstruction/narrowing at vestibulovaginal junction.

Acute General Treatment

- Digital dilation of vestibulovaginal junction: effective for treatment of hymenal remnants or mild (membranous) vestibulovaginal stenosis
- Sharp resection of dorsoventral paramesonephric duct remnants or bands if present; can use scissor or laser excision
- For severe (fibrous) vestibulovaginal stenosis: resection and anastomosis of vestibulovaginal junction by an extended episiotomy

Chronic Treatment

After manual or surgical dilation, antibiotic therapy (based on culture and susceptibility [C&S] testing) may have to be extended up to 6 weeks for treatment of ascending UTI if present.

Behavior/Exercise

Bitches with previous painful breeding episodes may be reluctant to accept a male after treatment of vestibulovaginal abnormalities. Use of an experienced breeding male may be helpful.

Possible Complications

- Stricture secondary to resection and anastomosis

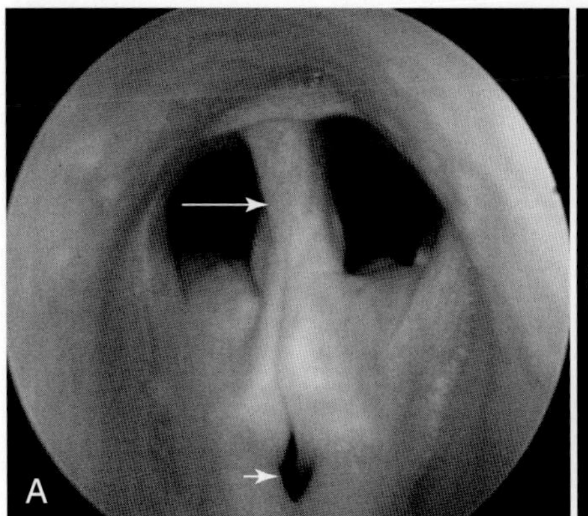

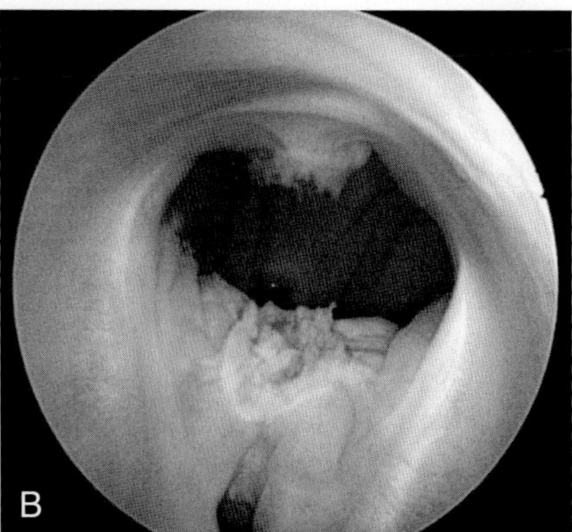

VAGINAL CONGENITAL ABNORMALITIES IN THE BITCH A, Vaginoscopic view of the vestibule of a female dog. Paramesonephric band *(long arrow)* spans the vaginal opening. Urethral orifice *(short arrow)* is unaffected by the paramesonephric band. **B,** Postoperative vaginoscopic view of the vestibule immediately after the paramesonephric band was excised using a holmium-YAG laser.

- Inadequate resection does not resolve clinical signs.

Recommended Monitoring

Observe the animal for recurrence of signs. Initial treatment may have to be repeated if stricture occurs secondary to resection or traumatic dilation.

PROGNOSIS & OUTCOME

- Prognosis is good if clinical signs are caused by hymenal remnants or mild vaginal stricture.
- Prognosis for resolution of clinical signs is fair to good for severe vaginal stricture treated by vestibulovaginal resection and anastomosis.

PEARLS & CONSIDERATIONS

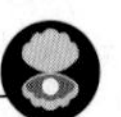

Comments

- Do not confuse normal narrowing at the vestibulovaginal junction with a pathologic condition.
    - The diameter of the vestibulovaginal junction must be less than 30% of the diameter of the maximal diameter of the vagina to be considered pathologic.
- Most congenital vaginal abnormalities do not cause clinical signs.
- Vestibulovaginal abnormalities (paramesonephric septal remnants, vaginal septa, double vagina) are very common in dogs with ectopic ureters.

Prevention

Because most vestibulovaginal abnormalities are congenital but not hereditary, there are no recommendations against breeding affected bitches after the abnormality is treated.

Technician Tips

Although digital vaginal exam is helpful in making a diagnosis of vestibulovaginal abnormality, direct visual inspection using vaginoscopy permits a much more accurate diagnosis.

Client Education

- Breeding bitches that are reluctant to stand for a male may have vestibulovaginal abnormalities that cause painful breeding.
- Congenital vaginal anomalies may be present without causing clinical signs.

SUGGESTED READING

Crawford JT, et al: Influence of vestibulovaginal stenosis, pelvic bladder, and recessed vulva on response to treatment for clinical signs of lower urinary tract disease in dogs: 38 cases (1990-1999). J Am Vet Med Assoc 221:995-999, 2002.

AUTHOR: James A. Flanders, DVM, DACVS
EDITOR: Michelle A. Kutzler, DVM, PhD, DACT

Vaginal Hyperplasia and Vaginal Prolapse

Client Education Sheet

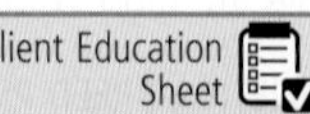

BASIC INFORMATION

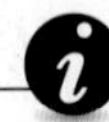

Definition

Edematous swelling of the vaginal mucosa cranial to the urethral orifice is an uncommon disorder that occurs during estrogen stimulation in the intact bitch. It may progress to vaginal protrusion through the vulvar lips.

Synonyms

Vaginal edema, hypertrophy, hyperplasia, eversion, or protrusion

Epidemiology

SPECIES, AGE, SEX

Intact bitch, 7 months to 16 years old

GENETICS, BREED PREDISPOSITION

- More common in large-breed dogs
- Predisposed breeds: bulldog, mastiff, boxer, Dalmatian, German shepherd, Saint Bernard, Labrador and Chesapeake Bay retrievers, Weimaraner, Walker hound, springer spaniel, Airedale terrier, and American pit bull terrier
- One case report of type III vaginal prolapse in a pregnant Maine coon cat

RISK FACTORS

- Young bitch under the influence of estrogen during proestrus or estrus; may occur or recur during diestrus, pregnancy, or parturition
- Can be observed as side effect of estrus induction with estrogen

ASSOCIATED DISORDERS

Markedly prolapsed vaginal tissue is subject to self-mutilation and may be dry, ulcerated, necrotic, and devascularized; possible dysuria or pollakiuria

Clinical Presentation

DISEASE FORMS/SUBTYPES

Vaginal hyperplasia:

- Type I: slight to moderate eversion of the vaginal floor cranial to the urethral orifice; confined to the vestibulum and appearing as a bulge at the perineum
- Type II: well-developed swelling of the vaginal floor, which may include the lateral vaginal walls, and protruding through the vulvar lips. The swelling appears dome shaped.
- Type III: well-developed protrusion of the entire circumference of the vaginal wall through the vulvar lips. The swelling appears doughnut-shaped and is a vaginal prolapse.

HISTORY, CHIEF COMPLAINT

- Previous occurrence of vaginal hyperplasia
- Onset of proestrus or estrus
- Licking or irritation of the vulva
- Mass protruding from vulva or bulge at the perineum
- Dysuria or pollakiuria
- Failure to allow intromission during breeding
- Tenesmus

PHYSICAL EXAM FINDINGS

Bulge at the perineum or protrusion of a pink, dome- or doughnut-shaped mass from vulva; surface of protrusion may be dry, necrotic, or ulcerated. Vaginal exam reveals:

- A urethral orifice located ventrally in all three types of vaginal hyperplasia
- Vaginal lumen is located dorsally in types I and II but centrally located in type III.
- In contrast, uterine prolapse is distinguished by the presence of tubular masses in the vagina or protruding from the vulva.

Etiology and Pathophysiology

- An exaggerated response of the vaginal mucosa to estrogen (hyperemia, edema, keratinization), the swelling begins as an eversion in the vaginal floor, cranial to the urethral orifice.
- Histopathologic exam of affected vaginal tissue is consistent with submucosal edema rather than hyperplasia or hypertrophy.

DIAGNOSIS

Diagnostic Overview

The diagnosis is suspected based on the presence of a vulvar swelling or protrusion in a young intact bitch. Typically, condition occurs during one of the first three estrous cycles.

Differential Diagnosis

- Benign or malignant vaginal neoplasia
- Vaginal polyp or cyst

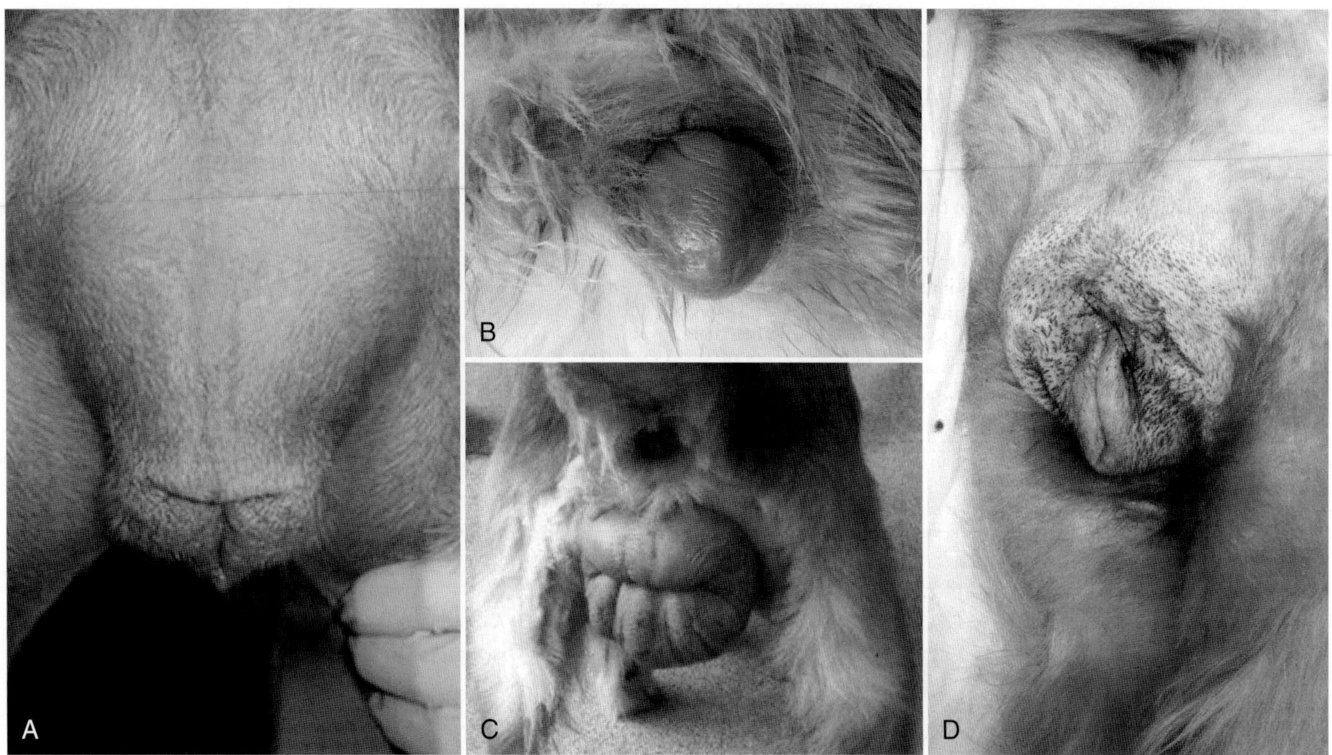

VAGINAL HYPERPLASIA AND VAGINAL PROLAPSE **A,** Type I vaginal hyperplasia: slight to moderate eversion of the vaginal floor cranial to the urethral orifice, appearing as a bulge at the perineum. **B,** Type II vaginal hyperplasia: well-developed swelling of vaginal floor, which may include lateral vaginal walls, protruding through vulvar lips. Swelling appears dome shaped. **C,** Type III vaginal hyperplasia: well-developed protrusion of entire circumference of vaginal wall through vulvar lips. Swelling appears doughnut shaped. **D,** Type III vaginal prolapse reduced to smaller size after 6 weeks. A stay suture was placed in vulvar lips to prevent recurrence protrusion of relaxed tissue for 2 additional weeks. At suture removal, there was no recurrence.

- True vaginal prolapse with concurrent entrapment of visceral organs (rare)
- Uterine prolapse
- Urethral neoplasia

Initial Database

- Stage of hormonal cycle based on vaginal cytologic exam
- Vaginal exam to locate the urethral orifice, vaginal lumen, origin of the protruding mass, and the size of its base
- Ensure that the animal is able to urinate.

Advanced or Confirmatory Testing

- Biopsy of vaginal mass confirms diagnosis in atypical bitches.
- In severe cases, survey radiographs can be used to evaluate visceral organ involvement; contrast radiography can confirm the location of the urethral orifice and vaginal lumen.

TREATMENT

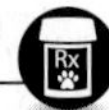

Treatment Overview

Treatment goals are to prevent drying, necrosis, and devitalization of exposed vaginal tissue; prevent future recurrence; and prevent urethral obstruction.

Acute General Treatment

- Insert a urethral catheter to relieve obstruction when present.
- Ensure that vaginal tissue is kept clean.
- Apply topical sterile, water-soluble lubrication or antibiotic ointment.
- Apply an Elizabethan collar or protective pants.
- Provide a clean environment to minimize tissue trauma.
- Schedule an ovariohysterectomy, which prevents recurrence and may hasten resolution; regression of tissue can occur within 21 days.
- Recognize that spontaneous regression at end of estrus is common.

Chronic Treatment

- Ovariohysterectomy prevents recurrence in nonbreeding bitches.
- Surgical excision of prolapsed vaginal tissue in bitches intended for breeding or in those with severely inflamed or devitalized vaginal tissue
    - May prevent recurrence during subsequent estrous cycles or at parturition
    - Various surgical techniques are described involving circumferential incision at the base of the prolapse.
    - Episiotomy may be needed.
- Manual reduction of prolapsed tissue and placement of stay sutures in the vagina do not prevent recurrence and may cause the bitch discomfort.
- Artificial insemination can be performed in breeding bitches.
- Regression of hyperplastic vaginal tissue should be expected within 1 week following ovulation. Induction of ovulation may hasten regression of vaginal tissue by decreasing estrogen stimulation. Gonadotropin-releasing hormone 2.2 mcg/kg IM repeated in 48 hours can be used for ovulation induction in nonbreeding cycles.

Drug Interactions

Avoidance of progestational drugs that contribute to pyometra.

Possible Complications

- Necrosis, infection, and devascularization of vaginal tissue
- Evisceration of abdominal organs
- Urination and defecation difficulties

Recommended Monitoring

- Monitor viability of prolapsed vaginal tissue.
- Evaluate ability to urinate.

PROGNOSIS & OUTCOME

- Good prognosis with ovariohysterectomy
- Recurrence rate is 66% in untreated bitches.

PEARLS & CONSIDERATIONS

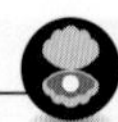

Comments

- Vaginal hyperplasia may progress to vaginal prolapse (type III). Forcible separation during breeding and excessive straining during parturition are other causes of vaginal prolapse.
- If excision of vaginal tissue is performed in late estrus or early diestrus, bleeding is minimized.
- If ovariohysterectomy is performed in anestrus (serum progesterone concentrations < 2 ng/mL), development of pseudopregnancy is minimized.
- Catheterize urethra during excision of vaginal tissue to help prevent inadvertent urethral trauma.

Prevention

- Ovariohysterectomy
- Surgical excision of redundant vaginal tissue may prevent recurrence during the next estrous cycle.

Technician Tips

Confirming ability to urinate and defecate is essential. Use of topical lubricant, an E-collar, and soft bedding minimize devitalization of exposed vaginal tissue.

Client Education

Discuss heritability and intended plans for the bitch. Ovariohysterectomy is the recommendation for nonbreeding bitches.

SUGGESTED READING

McNamara PS, et al: Chronic vaginocervical prolapse with visceral incarceration in a dog. J Am Anim Hosp Assoc 33:533-536, 1997.

AUTHOR: Kristine L. Gonzales, DVM, DACT
EDITOR: Michelle A. Kutzler, DVM, PhD, DACT

Vaginitis

Client Education Sheet 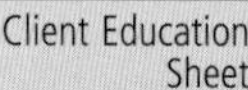 Bonus Material Online 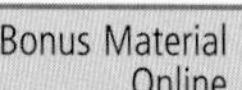

BASIC INFORMATION

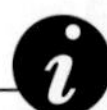

Definition

Inflammation/irritation of the vagina

Epidemiology

SPECIES, AGE, SEX

- Spayed or intact bitches or queens
- Prevalence: < 1% in bitches; rare in queens
- Juvenile onset: bitches 8 weeks to 1 year of age
- Adult onset: bitches > 1 year of age

RISK FACTORS

Anatomic abnormalities (vaginal strictures or septa), perivulvar dermatitis with atrophic juvenile vulva and excessive skin folds, perivulvar dermatitis in overweight dogs with urinary incontinence, systemic illness (e.g., diabetes mellitus, hyperadrenocorticism)

CONTAGION AND ZOONOSIS

Brucella canis, canine herpesvirus, transmissible venereal tumor

Clinical Presentation

DISEASE FORMS/SUBTYPES

- Juvenile onset versus adult onset
- Acute versus chronic (i.e., present for > 1 month)

HISTORY, CHIEF COMPLAINT

Juvenile onset:

- Most commonly scant whitish yellow vulvar discharge; occasionally large volume
- Excessive vulvar licking
- Females usually are not systemically ill.

Adult onset:

- Most commonly mucoid to purulent vaginal discharge
- More prevalent in spayed compared with intact females
- Pollakiuria, discomfort (e.g., excessive vulvar licking, pain when urinating)
- Clinical signs of concurrent disease (e.g., polyuria/polydipsia, urinary incontinence, pruritus)
- Vaginitis may be a contributing cause of infertility.

PHYSICAL EXAM FINDINGS

- Vulvar mucoid, purulent, or rarely blood-tinged discharge; occasionally no discharge
- Vulvar hyperemia
- Vaginal cytologic exam: white blood cells (WBCs) with or without bacteria
- Digital vaginal exam may reveal vaginal stenoses or septa.
- Atrophic or juvenile vulva with excessive skin folds with concurrent perivulvar dermatitis
- Overweight dogs with urinary incontinence with excessive perivulvar skin folds and persistent moisture and urine scalding

Etiology and Pathophysiology

- Many dogs have idiopathic vaginitis.
- Congenital anatomic abnormalities
  - Stenoses just cranial to the urethral papillae
  - Vaginal septa bands of tissues in the vaginal vault due to remnants of the medial walls of the müllerian (paramesonephric) ducts or abnormal merging with the caudal urogenital sinus
- Concurrent systemic diseases (e.g., diabetes mellitus, hyperadrenocorticism)
- *B. canis,* canine herpesvirus, transmissible venereal tumor
- Vaginal foreign body (e.g., grass awn, fetal bony fragment)

DIAGNOSIS

Diagnostic Overview

The diagnosis is generally suspected because of vulvar discharge (p. 1045). In the dog, vaginal palpation and vaginoscopy with sampling for cytologic exam are the cornerstones of establishing the diagnosis of vaginitis.

Differential Diagnosis

- Urinary tract infection (UTI; p. 232)
- Metritis
- Cystic endometrial hyperplasia/pyometra (p. 854)
- Uterine stump pyometra (p. 854)
- Vulvar, vaginal, or uterine tumor
- *B. canis*
- Canine herpesvirus (p. 466)
- Transmissible venereal tumor (p. 993)

Initial Database

- CBC, serum biochemistry profile: generally unremarkable
- Urinalysis: unless there are contraindications (e.g., coagulopathy, abdominal effusion, suspected urinary neoplasia, pyometra), obtain cystocentesis sample
  - Urine culture and susceptibility testing for UTI (common)
- Vaginoscopy (p. 1184) to assess discharge in the vagina; vesicular lesions (e.g., canine herpesvirus) or lymphoid follicles (nonspecific indicators of inflammation), urine pooling, masses, foreign bodies (e.g., fetal bone fragments, grass awns)
- Vaginal cytology (p. 1183)
  - In adult dogs, noncornified epithelial cells with WBCs (± bacteria) support a diagnosis of vaginitis.
  - A bloody discharge indicates a possible coagulopathy, blood-borne parasites (*Babesia* sp), foreign object, or tumor.
    - Rule out estrual sanguineous discharge in bitch if an ovarian remnant is possible.

Advanced or Confirmatory Testing

- Guarded bacterial culture from the cranial vagina: moderate to heavy growth of one or two bacterial types (more might suggest normal flora)
- Serologic titer for *B. canis* (p. 1319)
- Survey radiography assesses the pelvic canal for mineralized foreign bodies (e.g., fetal bone remnants)

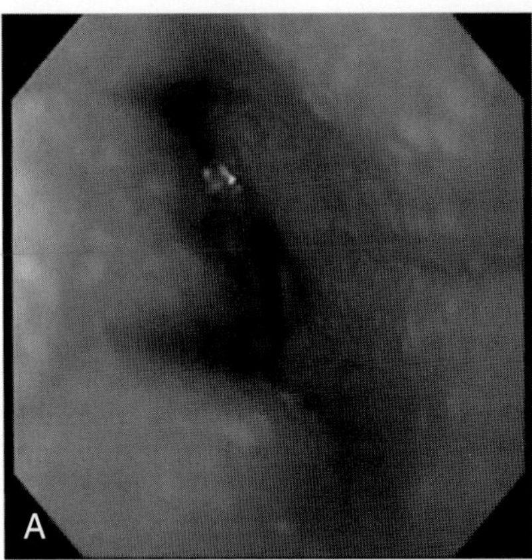

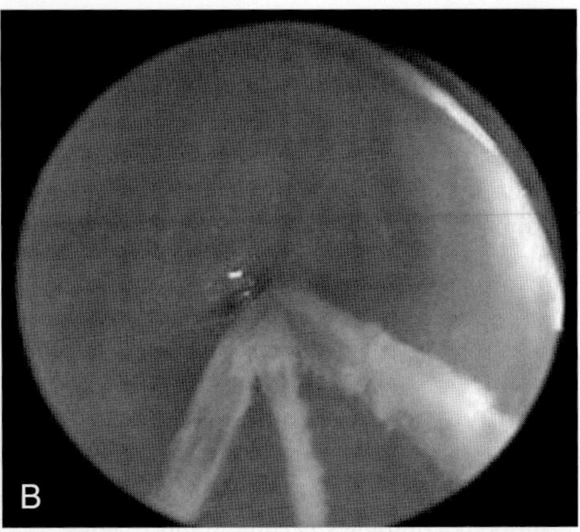

VAGINITIS A, Vaginoscopy of a bitch with chronic vaginitis shows prominent lymphoid follicles on the vaginal mucosa. **B,** Vaginoscopy of a bitch presenting with vaginitis shows a grass awn in the vaginal lumen. (Courtesy Dr. Autumn Davidson.)

- Contrast radiography
- Biopsy

TREATMENT

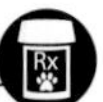

Treatment Overview

- Without an identifiable underlying primary cause, most cases of juvenile-onset and adult-onset vaginitis resolve spontaneously.
  - Treatment of the underlying cause, if identified, is usually curative.
- Most therapy for vaginitis is symptomatic because most cases are idiopathic.

Acute General Treatment

- In juvenile-onset and adult-onset vaginitis, antibiotic treatment, if used, should be based on results of culture and sensitivity (cranial vaginal guarded sample) and given for 4 weeks. Antibiotics are usually not warranted for mixed bacterial growth (a normal finding).
- Vaginal douches with antiseptics or antibiotics are unrewarding.
- If the primary problem is urinary incontinence
  - Urinary incontinence suspected due to urethral sphincter mechanism incompetence (up to 60% of adult cases): diethylstilbestrol (DES) 0.1-0.2 mg/kg, maximum dose of 1 mg PO q 24h for 5 days, tapering to 2 times per week, or phenylpropanolamine 1-1.5 mg/kg PO q 8-12h (p. 1011)
  - In overweight dogs with urinary incontinence with excessive perivulvar skin folds, persistent moisture, and urine scalding, vulvoplasty (episioplasty) is recommended.
  - Vaginal anatomic anomalies (up to 36% of cases): surgical repair may be indicated.
- If the primary problem is idiopathic
  - DES may be helpful to treat subclinical urinary incontinence and may enhance WBC migration to the vagina and increase vaginal elasticity. NOTE: do not use DES in dogs that have not reached full height because it may induce premature physeal closure of the long bones.
  - Glucocorticoids may be beneficial in some bitches. Do not use in cases of concurrent urinary incontinence.
- If history or clinical signs of concurrent atopic dermatitis (p. 91) and vaginitis coexist
  - May be beneficial to use hydroxyzine 1-2 mg/kg PO q 8-12h; decrease the dose if treatment is effective or if secondary effects such as sedation are pronounced

Chronic Treatment

- Owners should be instructed to keep the perivulvar skin folds clean.
- In mild to moderate cases of juvenile vaginitis, twice-daily cleaning with baby wipes may be beneficial.

Possible Complications

- Ascending UTI can result from chronic vaginitis.
- Self-mutilation can result from excessive licking of the perivulvar skin secondary to vaginitis.

Recommended Monitoring

Recheck animals showing any signs of systemic illness, and look for complications such as metritis.

PROGNOSIS & OUTCOME

- With spontaneous remission, future reproductive success is not compromised.
- In prepubertal dogs, vaginitis may or may not resolve after one or more estrous cycles, but ovariohysterectomy should be delayed until after the first cycle.

PEARLS & CONSIDERATIONS

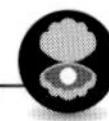

Comments

Limited understanding of the causes of vaginitis makes it difficult to predict when and if clinical signs will resolve.

Technician Tips

Excessive licking may be prevented using an Elizabethan collar; sedation (e.g., trazodone 2-3 mg/kg PO q 24h) may reduce scooting.

Client Education

Daily record of the frequency and severity of clinical signs (e.g., vulvar discharge, vulvar licking) can help the veterinarian to assess response to therapy.

SUGGESTED READING

Root Kustritz MV: Vaginitis in dogs: a simple approach to a complex condition. Vet Med 103:562-567, 2008.

AUTHOR: Carlos M. Gradil, DVM, MS, PhD, DACT
EDITOR: Michelle A. Kutzler, DVM, PhD, DACT

Vasculopathy, Cutaneous

Bonus Material Online 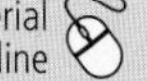 Client Education Sheet 

BASIC INFORMATION

Definition

The condition is characterized by blood vessel abnormalities that result in tissue necrosis. It can be divided into ischemic dermatopathies and cutaneous vasculitis (inflammatory process that targets the blood vessels).

Epidemiology

SPECIES, AGE, SEX

Dogs and cats of any age and either sex; dermatomyositis becomes manifest in young dogs (usually < 6 months)

GENETICS, BREED PREDISPOSITION

Any breed, but certain syndromes show breed predisposition:

- Familial cutaneous vasculopathy (autosomal recessive): Parson (Jack) Russell terrier, Scottish terrier, German shepherd
- Alabama rot: greyhounds
- Proliferative thrombovascular necrosis of the pinnae: dachshund, Weimaraner
- Rabies vaccine injection-site vasculitis (p. 550): miniature poodle, Bichon frisé, Yorkshire terrier

- Familial canine dermatomyositis: collie, Shetland sheepdog, corgi, and Beauceron shepherd
- Proliferative arteritis of the nasal philtrum: Saint-Bernard, giant schnauzers

RISK FACTORS

- Drug therapy
- Malignancy
- Infection (viral, bacterial, fungal, rickettsial)
- Immune-mediated diseases
- Insect bites
- Food allergy
- Vaccines
- Trauma, burns

ASSOCIATED DISORDERS

Systemic lupus erythematosus (SLE)

Clinical Presentation

DISEASE FORMS/SUBTYPES

- The lesions can be localized, regional, or multifocal to generalized.
- Vasculitis is categorized histologically as neutrophilic (leukocytoclastic, nonleukocytoclastic), eosinophilic, lymphocytic, granulomatous, or cell poor.

HISTORY, CHIEF COMPLAINT

Patients may present with crusted or ulcerative lesions that may be a cause for self-trauma. Patients with urticarial vasculitis may present with erythematous and often pruritic wheals.

PHYSICAL EXAM FINDINGS

- Description of the lesions varies according to the disease. Fever, anorexia, and lethargy may be present.
- Proliferative thrombovascular necrosis of the pinnae: notching of pinnal margins at tip and/or well-demarcated ulcers on the concave aspect of the pinna
- Idiopathic vasculitis: well-demarcated necrosis and ulceration, particularly at the extremities and pressure points; may include edema, alopecia, or crateriform ulcers on the central aspect of the footpads (some of these cases could be a rare manifestation of rabies vaccine–induced generalized ischemic dermatopathy)
- Urticarial vasculitis: generalized pruritus associated with papules, purpura, and wheals
- Familial canine dermatomyositis: erythema, ulceration, and mild crusting in the young dog. Affected areas include face, pinnae, pressure points, digits, and tail tip.
- Rabies vaccine–associated vasculitis

Etiology and Pathophysiology

- Type III hypersensitivity reaction is suspected as the primary pathomechanism. Antigen-antibody complexes become trapped along the basement membrane of vessel walls and activate the complement cascade. Type I and II hypersensitivity reactions may also be implicated.
- Other mechanisms include
    - Direct antibody binding to the vessel wall
    - Antineutrophil cytoplasmic antibodies (ANCA) binding to neutrophil granules and the subsequent release of toxic mediators, leading to a bystander reaction (granulomatosis with polyangiitis [Wegener's granulomatosis] in humans)

DIAGNOSIS

Diagnostic Overview

Cutaneous vasculopathy is first suspected based on the clinical presentation. The definitive diagnosis is based on a detailed history and skin biopsy.

Differential Diagnosis

- Cold-agglutinin disease
- Disseminated intravascular coagulation
- Frostbite
- Demodicosis (focal lesions)
- Dermatophytosis (focal lesions)

Initial Database

- Thorough history to assess risk of drug-induced vasculitis
- Routine CBC, serum biochemical profile, urinalysis: results are typically normal.
- Skin scrapings for focal (not ulcerated) lesions
- Diascopy for hemorrhagic lesions (e.g., vasculitis does not blanch when a glass slide is pressed over the top, in contrast to vascular dilation/congestion)
- Skin biopsy for histopathologic exam: it is often wise to submit tissue samples for fungal and bacterial culture at the same time.

Advanced or Confirmatory Testing

Selected according to signalment and clinical features of case:

- Bacterial serologic titers (dogs: *Rickettsia rickettsii, Ehrlichia canis, Borrelia burgdorferi*)
- Viral serologic titers (cats: feline leukemia virus [FeLV], feline immunodeficiency virus [FIV])
- Coagulation profile, Coombs' test, antinuclear antibody (ANA) test, and rheumatoid factor test may be indicated based on history, physical exam findings, and initial database supporting immune-mediated disease.
- Blood culture if sepsis is suspected
- Tissue culture of nodular or granulomatous lesions
- Hypoallergenic dietary trial (urticarial form of food hypersensitivity)

TREATMENT

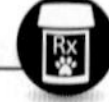

Treatment Overview

The goal is to improve circulation to the affected area, control self-trauma, and suppress the immune reaction while determining the inciting cause.

Acute General Treatment

- Discontinue current drug therapies.
- Bandage pressure points and keep wounds clean.
- Prevent self-trauma (Elizabethan collar).

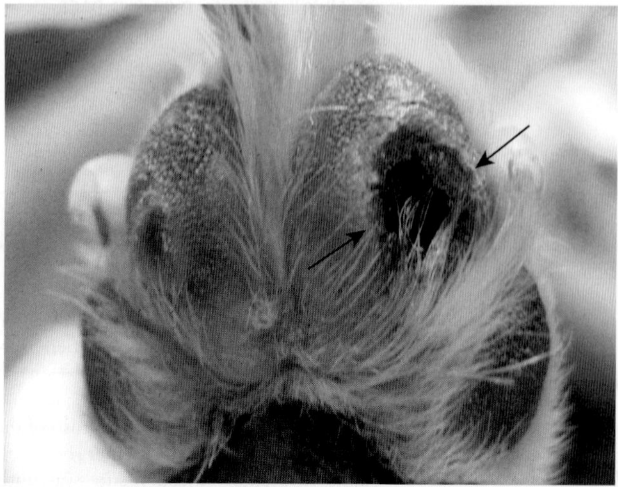

VASCULOPATHY, CUTANEOUS Typical punched-out paw pad lesion *(arrows)*.

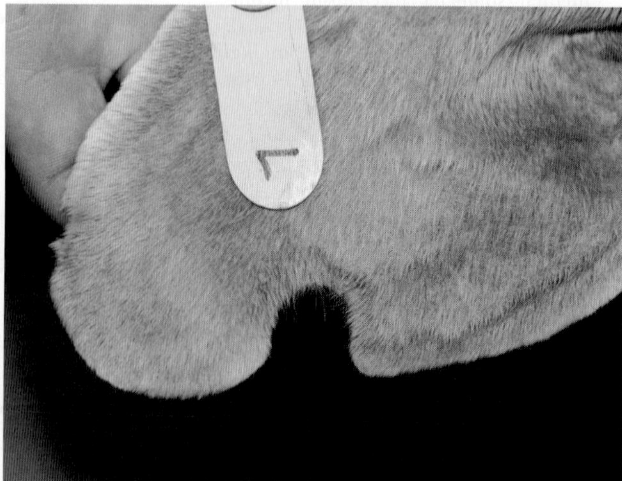

VASCULOPATHY, CUTANEOUS Weimaraner after a vasculitis episode. The dog responded to therapy but was left with a typical pinnal deformity.

Chronic Treatment

One or more may be indicated:

- Consider doxycycline while awaiting infectious disease titers.
- Pentoxifylline (increases erythrocyte plasticity) 15-25 mg/kg PO q 12h or 10-15 mg/kg q 8h; give after a meal
- Tetracycline and niacinamide >10 kg, 500 mg of each drug PO q 8h (<10 kg, 250 mg of each drug) for a minimum of 3 months; tapering is based on a favorable response.
- Prednisone or prednisolone 2-4 mg/kg PO q 24h starting dose, tapering is based on a favorable response.
- Azathioprine (dogs) 2.2 mg/kg PO q 24h for the first 1-3 weeks, then q 48h (with prednisone or prednisolone)
- Chlorambucil (cats) 0.1-0.2 mg/kg PO q 24-48h (with prednisolone)
- Dapsone (dogs) 1 mg/kg PO q 8h
- Sulfasalazine (dogs) 22-44 mg/kg PO q 8h
- Cyclosporine 5 mg/kg PO q 24h
- Tacrolimus 0.1% topically q 12h, can be considered in cases with focal disease, especially as a substitute for topical corticosteroids. Wear gloves to apply.

Possible Complications

Tissue necrosis and secondary infection; septicemia. Underlying cause of vasculitis might have nondermatologic manifestations (e.g., dermatomyositis can cause myositis; SLE can cause protein-losing nephropathy).

Recommended Monitoring

Depends on disease and treatment; monitor for adverse reactions to drug therapies as appropriate.

PROGNOSIS & OUTCOME

- Some cases resolve, whereas others are chronic or recurrent. Damage to other organs (renal, neurologic) also affects prognosis.
- Proliferative thrombovascular necrosis of the pinnae: varied response may require surgery.
- Idiopathic: may require long-term/indefinite treatment
- Urticarial: depends on identification of underlying cause; rule out food allergy (p. 345).

PEARLS & CONSIDERATIONS

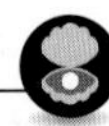

Comments

- Multiple skin biopsies are the key to diagnosis.
- Do not use drugs of similar classes to those used before development of the disease.
- Monitor closely for adverse reactions to therapy.

Prevention

Vaccinate dogs with caution if there is a history of rabies vaccine–induced vasculitis; repeat occurrences and risk of a generalized vasculitis or anaphylactic reaction have been suggested.

Technician Tips

To reduce the risk of a nondiagnostic sample, be careful not to biopsy the center of an ulcer; the margin of a lesion or an elliptical incision is recommended.

Client Education

Long-term treatment (4-6 months, sometimes indefinitely) is often needed.

SUGGESTED READING

Innera M: Cutaneous vasculitis in small animals. Vet Clin North Am Small Anim Pract 43:113-134, 2013.

AUTHOR: Stephen Waisglass, DVM, CertSAD, DACVD
EDITOR: Manon Paradis, DMV, MVSc, DACVD

Ventricular Arrhythmias

Bonus Material Online 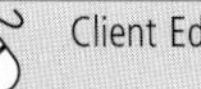 Client Education Sheet 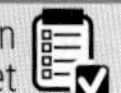

BASIC INFORMATION

Definition

- Ventricular arrhythmias are electrical discharges occurring spontaneously in the ventricles.
- The term *ventricular premature complex(es)* (VPCs) applies to one, two, or three consecutive premature ventricular impulses, whereas four or more in a row are defined as ventricular tachycardia (VT).
- VT involves a ventricular rate of 180 beats/min or more in dogs and 240 beats/min or more in cats.
- Strictly speaking, this chapter focuses on ventricular tachyarrhythmias (not ventricular escape rhythms); for simplicity, the term *ventricular arrhythmia* is used for designating VPCs and VT.

Synonyms

- Ventricular ectopy, extrasystoles, or tachyarrhythmias
- VPCs are synonymous with premature ventricular complexes (PVCs), premature ventricular depolarizations (PVDs), and similar variations.

Epidemiology

SPECIES, AGE, SEX

Any animal can be affected.

GENETICS, BREED PREDISPOSITION

- Boxers: arrhythmogenic cardiomyopathy (p. 76)
- Doberman pinschers and other dog breeds: dilated cardiomyopathy (p. 263)
- German shepherds: inherited VT of young adults
- Large-breed dogs: splenic masses, gastric dilation/volvulus (GDV)
- Cats (males > females): hypertrophic cardiomyopathy (p. 505)

RISK FACTORS

- Outdoor, roaming dogs: traumatic myocarditis (hit by car)
- Primary heart disease or systemic disturbance, if sufficiently severe, can cause ventricular arrhythmias.

GEOGRAPHY AND SEASONALITY

Chagas' disease: myocarditis (southern parts of the United States and Latin America)

ASSOCIATED DISORDERS

Syncope (rapid VT)

Clinical Presentation

DISEASE FORMS/SUBTYPES

- Incidental finding
- Clinically overt (e.g., causing syncope)
- Accelerated idioventricular rhythm (AIVR)

HISTORY, CHIEF COMPLAINT

Incidental finding (more common):

- Animal is presented for evaluation of a disorder other than syncope.
- Arrhythmia is noted during physical exam or subsequent monitoring.

Clinically overt:

- Syncope/episodic collapse
- Episodic stumbling, disorientation, confusion
- Animal may be well (and even playful and active) before and after episodes or may be lethargic, weak, or anorexic.

PHYSICAL EXAM FINDINGS

Incidental finding:

- Physical exam findings reflect the underlying disorder, but an arrhythmia is noted on physical exam.
- With VT, the arrhythmia is rapid and may be irregular (usually polymorphic on electrocardiogram [ECG]) or regular (usually monomorphic on ECG).
- Pulse deficit
  - Premature heartbeat ausculted, without a corresponding palpable pulse for that beat
  - Common with ventricular arrhythmias
  - Depends on the degree of prematurity of VPCs (how underfilled are the ventricles when the VPC causes contraction?)

Clinically overt:

- Wide range of presentations, from clinically normal and alert if arrhythmia is intermittent to profoundly weak and hemodynamically collapsed with very rapid, sustained VT
- Regularity or irregularity and pulse deficit as for incidental finding (see above)

Common Causes of Ventricular Arrhythmias

Hypokalemia[a,b]
Hypoxemia (e.g., due to cardiogenic pulmonary edema, pleural effusion, primary lung disease)[a]
Cardiomyopathy
Gastric dilation/volvulus[a]
Traumatic myocarditis/hit by car
Abdominal mass, especially splenic or hepatic[a]
Advanced valvular heart disease
Hypomagnesemia[a,b]
Acidosis[a]
Intoxication[a] (digitalis; oleander, foxglove, lily of the valley, azalea, and yew plants; many over-the-counter, prescription, or illicit drugs)

[a]Potentially correctable/curable.
[b]Presence may make ventricular antiarrhythmic drugs such as lidocaine, procainamide, and mexiletine ineffective.

Etiology and Pathophysiology

- Enhanced or abnormal automaticity, microreentry, and triggered activity (early or delayed after depolarizations) are mechanisms that underlie ventricular arrhythmias.
- These mechanisms can be activated or potentiated by systemic disturbances such as those previously listed (see Associated Disorders above).
- The result is one or more spontaneous electrical depolarizations originating prematurely in the ventricles. The prematurity is manifested on the ECG as a shorter R-R interval. The ventricular origin results in a QRS complex that is of a different shape from a sinus QRS complex.
- A greater degree of prematurity of VPCs (or more rapid VT) results in reduced diastolic filling time before contraction and ultimately a higher probability of clinical signs or hemodynamic deterioration (e.g., poor pulse, cerebral hypoperfusion) compared with slower ventricular arrhythmias.
- Accelerated idioventricular rhythms are seen commonly in hospitalized patients in association with noncardiac diseases (e.g., GDV surgery, splenic disease, immune-mediated hemolytic anemia, pancreatitis, post trauma, neurologic disease). They are typically benign, the rate is not rapid, and they usually do not require therapy.

DIAGNOSIS

Diagnostic Overview

Ventricular arrhythmias can be suspected on history (syncope), physical exam (premature beats, pulse deficits), and ECG (classically, wide and bizarre QRS complexes occurring prematurely). Careful inspection of the ECG allows differentiation from other similar-appearing but clinically different ECG deflections.

Differential Diagnosis

- VPCs can occur in many situations and do not automatically equate to a cardiac disorder. They can be seen in normal animals in low numbers (<50/24 hours). They are very commonly associated with noncardiac disease, possibly secondary to myocardial ischemia, electrolyte abnormalities, or other factors surrounding the underlying disease.
- Physical exam (irregular cardiac rhythm)
  - Supraventricular premature beats, marked respiratory sinus arrhythmia
- ECG (wide and bizarre QRS-T complexes)
  - Right or left bundle branch block
  - Ventricular escape rhythm
  - Right ventricular enlargement (if QRS predominantly negative in lead II)
  - Motion artifact
  - Accelerated idioventricular rhythm (ventricular rhythm at a rate of 120-170 beats/min). This is a fancy term for slow VT, but it is an appropriate name because a ventricular myocyte is firing as a pacemaker cell at an accelerated rate.

Initial Database

ECG (p. 1096) remains the gold standard for diagnosis of cardiac arrhythmias. Criteria for ventricular arrhythmias:

- VPC is substantially different from normal sinus QRS complexes.
  - Wide and bizarre QRS shape occurs because the impulse originates below the bundle of His and therefore cannot take advantage of the specialized conduction system. It must travel through the ventricular myocardium from muscle cell to muscle cell. This is slow and produces a wide, bizarre complex. QRS complexes can be positive in lead II or negative, depending on the site of origin in the ventricle.
  - VPC occurs prematurely. The R-R interval from the preceding normal sinus beat to the VPC is shorter than the interval between two normal sinus beats.
  - Large, bizarre T wave occurs because depolarization is abnormal; repolarization is also abnormal.
  - P waves continue to occur regularly during ventricular arrhythmias, but they are not related to VPCs and often are lost within the VPCs.

Advanced or Confirmatory Testing

- A 10- or 12-lead ECG: improved visualization of certain features of ventricular arrhythmias (e.g., better ability to see P waves not associated with the wide, bizarre QRS complexes of VPCs)
- CBC, serum biochemistry profile, urinalysis: especially to assess systemic proarrhythmic abnormalities such as hypokalemia
- Thoracic radiographs: particularly if suspicion of primary cardiac disease, hypoxemia, or thoracic trauma
- Echocardiogram (p. 1094): if a primary cardiac problem is suspected or no other cause is identified
- Abdominal imaging: if there is suspicion of an abdominal problem or a primary cause for the arrhythmia is not found
- Arterial blood gas (ABG) analysis: if acid-base or oxygenation abnormalities are suspected

TREATMENT

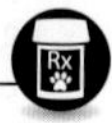

Treatment Overview

- Control arrhythmia to such a degree that adequate organ perfusion is present and there is a resolution or control of any arrhythmia-related clinical signs (e.g., syncope).
- Treatment decisions should be made based on whether the patient is experiencing or will experience hemodynamic compromise due to the arrhythmia. The goal is to treat the patient, not the ECG.
- The goal is not to abolish every VPC because overzealous treatment of arrhythmias may be detrimental.

Acute General Treatment

A treatment algorithm is provided on p. 1457.

- First, determine if the arrhythmia is a ventricular arrhythmia (VPC, VT) by ruling out common impostors (see Differential Diagnosis above).
- Second, identify and address any relevant underlying causes.
- Third, determine if there are overt clinical signs associated with the ventricular arrhythmia (e.g., syncope). If so, antiarrhythmic treatment is warranted.
- Fourth, if the ventricular arrhythmia is sustained at a rapid rate (>180 beats/min in large-breed dogs, > 220 beats/min in small-breed dogs, > 260 beats/min in cats), antiarrhythmic treatment is indicated.
- Medications
  - Lidocaine 1-2 mg/kg (dog) or 0.25-1 mg/kg (cat) IV bolus (can repeat up to three times in 10-15 minutes); can be followed with IV constant-rate infusion (CRI) at 40-80 mcg/kg/min (dog) or 10-20 mcg/kg/min (cat)
    - To make CRI of lidocaine: withdraw 25 mL from a 500-mL bag of crystalloid fluid (e.g., lactated Ringer's solution) and replace with 25 mL of 2% lidocaine. Concentration in bag is 1000 mcg/mL. Administer IV at usual fluid maintenance rate (66 mL/kg/day) assuming congestive heart failure (CHF) is not present. Infusion at this rate will be 50 mcg/kg/min.
  - Procainamide 6-15 mg/kg (dog) or 1-2 mg/kg (cat) slow IV bolus; may follow with IV CRI at 25-50 (dog) or 10-20 (cat) mcg/kg/min. Usually administered if lidocaine was ineffective despite normal electrolyte status, but both may be given together
- In patients who do not convert with IV lidocaine or procainamide, it is important to assess for any electrolyte abnormalities, particularly potassium, because antiarrhythmic agents are less effective when there is

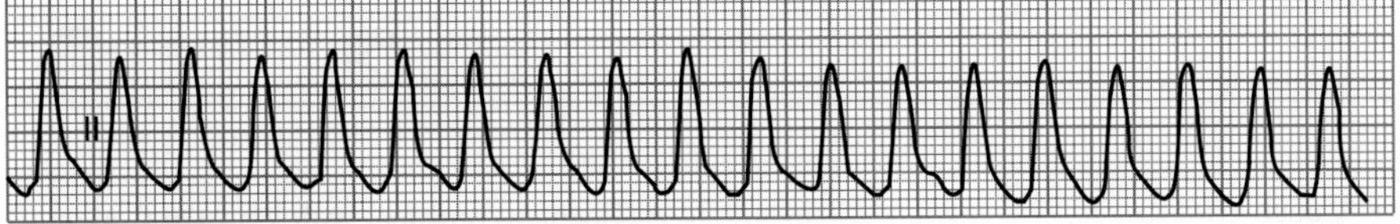

VENTRICULAR ARRHYTHMIAS Lead II ECG for a dog with ventricular tachycardia: 50 mm/s, 10 mm/mV. The ventricular tachycardia is monomorphic (ventricular premature complexes all of the same shape) and extremely rapid (375 beats/min) in this critically septic dog.

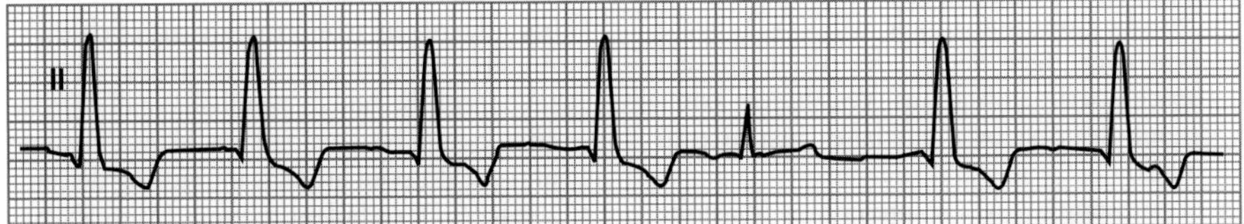

VENTRICULAR ARRHYTHMIAS Single-lead ECG for a dog with immune-mediated hemolytic anemia and an ausculted arrhythmia: 50 mm/s, 5 mm/mV. The fifth beat is a normal sinus beat; the remaining beats are of ventricular origin. Despite the ventricular arrhythmia, the rate is not rapid (115 beats/min) and likely only slightly faster than the underlying sinus rate. This is an accelerated idioventricular rhythm, a benign rhythm that does not require therapy beyond proactive treatment of its inciting cause (here, anemia).

hypokalemia. Hypomagnesemia can also promote dysrhythmias. For patients who do not convert, the authors will use the following:
- Sotalol 0.5-2 mg/kg PO q 12h (dogs); 10-20 mg/CAT PO q 12h for patients who are clinically stable
- Amiodarone (Nexterone) 3 mg/kg bolus over 15-20 minutes (dogs only); can be followed with IV CRI at 0.5 mg/kg/min (dogs only)

Chronic Treatment

- Ongoing management of the underlying cause
- Oral antiarrhythmic drugs may be used for treating rapid and/or clinically overt (syncopal) ventricular arrhythmia. Options include one of the following:
  - Sotalol 0.5-2 mg/kg PO q 12h (dogs); 10-20 mg/CAT PO q 12h; for small patients, can be compounded as a liquid formulation (e.g., 10 mg/mL). Clinical efficacy appears similar to tablet formulation and stable for up to 2 months.
  - Mexiletine 4-8 mg/kg PO q 8h and sotalol (see dose above) or atenolol 0.2-0.75 mg/kg PO q 12h (dogs)
  - Amiodarone 10 mg/kg PO q 12h for 1 week (loading), then 5-8 mg/kg PO q 24h (dogs)
  - Atenolol (cats) 6.25-12.5 mg/CAT PO q 12-24h

Nutrition/Diet

Administration of long-chain omega-3 fatty acids from fish oils (EPA, DHA) may reduce the number of VPCs. Effect on mortality unknown.

Behavior/Exercise

Exercise and the associated sympathetic drive may precipitate arrhythmias, but quality of life must also be strongly considered.

Drug Interactions

Digoxin can cause ventricular arrhythmias.

Possible Complications

Uncontrolled ventricular arrhythmias may progress to ventricular flutter and ventricular fibrillation (cardiac arrest), but normalization of the ECG to sinus rhythm using antiarrhythmic drugs alone has never been shown to improve the prognosis for survival. Complications can be minimized by treating/correcting inciting factors and reserving ventricular antiarrhythmic drugs for cases in which overt signs such as syncope are present or in which a very high rate (e.g., > 220 beats/min in dogs, > 260 beats/min in cats) is present despite management or correction of the underlying cause.

Recommended Monitoring

- ECG as dictated by clinical evaluation; monitoring ranges from continuous ECG with VT in an unstable, hospitalized animal to periodic ECG or Holter monitoring during recheck visits in stable animals
- Follow-up tests as listed for initial diagnosis to monitor underlying condition

PROGNOSIS & OUTCOME

- Ventricular arrhythmias that occur at a faster rate are more likely to produce clinical signs and carry a more guarded prognosis than slower ventricular arrhythmias.
- Ventricular arrhythmias that fail to respond to correction of the underlying problem (or for which the underlying problem cannot be corrected) usually indicate cardiac manifestations of a serious problem that carries a guarded short-term prognosis. Long-term prognosis depends on the exact nature of the underlying problem.

PEARLS & CONSIDERATIONS

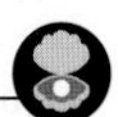

Comments

- Virtually any disease or disorder, if sufficiently severe to have systemic effects, can cause ventricular arrhythmias.
- Ventricular escape beats and VPCs often look identical. Ventricular escape beats occur at slow heart rates (20-40 beats/min for dogs, 40-100 beats/min for cats) or after a pause and are typically associated with second- or third-degree atrioventricular block or sinus pause/arrest. They are saving the heart from arrest and should never be treated with ventricular antiarrhythmics. In contrast, VPCs occur *prematurely* and are therefore in addition to the heart's usual rhythm.
- The most common correctable underlying causes of ventricular arrhythmias are hypokalemia, hypoxia, GDV, abdominal masses, anemia, metabolic acidosis, and pain.
- The most common treatable but noncorrectable causes of ventricular arrhythmias are cardiomyopathy and degenerative valvular heart disease.
- Ventricular arrhythmias most commonly are manifestations of an underlying disorder. Attempting to eliminate ventricular arrhythmias with antiarrhythmic drugs in a stable animal is analogous to shooting the messenger. Rather, the underlying cause needs to be addressed. Perhaps no antiarrhythmic drug is as beneficial to a patient with ventricular arrhythmias as correction of the underlying cause.

Prevention

Ventricular arrhythmias are clues to a primary cardiac or systemic disturbance. Preventing them relies on identifying and managing the underlying disease whenever possible.

Technician Tips

Impostors of ventricular arrhythmias are common on in-hospital telemetry monitors, but ventricular arrhythmias are an important signal requiring attention. Unusual-appearing heartbeats on an ECG monitor should be printed and reviewed with the attending veterinarian.

Client Education

Ventricular arrhythmias are serious disturbances of the cardiac rhythm. Their impact can range from minimal to life-threatening, and sudden cardiac death is always possible when an animal has a disorder that causes ventricular arrhythmias.

SUGGESTED READING

Côté E: Electrocardiography and cardiac arrhythmias. In Ettinger SJ, et al, editors: Textbook of veterinary internal medicine, ed 8, St. Louis, 2017, Elsevier, pp 1171-1187.

AUTHORS: Amara H. Estrada, DVM, DACVIM; Ashley E. Jones, DVM, DACVIM
EDITOR: Meg M. Sleeper, VMD, DACVIM

Ventricular Septal Defect

Video Available Client Education Sheet 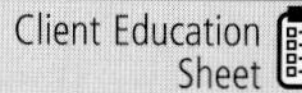

BASIC INFORMATION

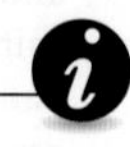

Definition

Anomalous communication between the right ventricle (RV) and left ventricle (LV), resulting in interventricular shunting of blood

Synonyms

Interventricular septal defect, VSD

Epidemiology

SPECIES, AGE, SEX

- Most common congenital heart defect in cats; fourth most common in dogs
- Typically diagnosed at a young age (median, 9-12 months)
- No sex predisposition

GENETICS, BREED PREDISPOSITION

- Predisposed dog breeds: Akita, basset hound, bloodhound, English and French bull dog, English springer spaniel, German shepherd, keeshond (hereditary), terrier breeds (border, fox, Jack Russell, Lakeland, West Highland white, Yorkshire)
- In cats, domestic shorthairs and Maine coons most frequently reported

ASSOCIATED DISORDERS

- Concurrent congenital cardiac defects present in up to 50% of cases, with pulmonic stenosis (PS) and as part of tetralogy of Fallot most common
- Aortic valvular insufficiency (AI) is common due to decreased support of aortic valve.

Clinical Presentation

DISEASE FORMS/SUBTYPES

- In dogs and cats, VSD most commonly involve the high membranous septum below the aortic valve on left side and cranial to the septal tricuspid valve leaflet on the right side (membranous or perimembranous VSD). Less common locations include below the pulmonic valve (juxtaarterial VSD) and in the muscular septum (muscular VSD).
- Left-to-right (L→R) shunting across the VSD is most common.
- Right-to-left (R→L, reverse shunting) may occur in cases accompanied by other defects that increase RV pressure (e.g., PS) or rarely with very large VSDs that result in pulmonary overcirculation and pulmonary hypertension (Eisenmenger's physiology).

HISTORY, CHIEF COMPLAINT

Frequently it is an incidental finding based on detection of a heart murmur. In the case of a large L→R VSD or in R→L VSD, the following may be observed:

- Exercise intolerance
- Dyspnea, tachypnea
- Cough (L→R)
- Cyanosis (R→L)
- Syncope

PHYSICAL EXAM FINDINGS

- Systolic murmur (grade III-V/VI) heard best over right ventral fourth intercostal space (perimembranous VSD); less commonly loudest over left base (juxtaarterial VSD)
- If substantial AI is present, a diastolic murmur may be heard over the left base.
- If congestive heart failure (CHF) is present: tachycardia, dyspnea, tachypnea, pulmonary crackles
- R→L shunt: cyanosis, generally no murmur unless another malformation is present

Etiology and Pathophysiology

- Magnitude and direction of shunting and the clinical consequences depend on size of defect, relative pulmonary and systemic vascular resistances, and presence of other cardiopulmonary defects.
- Small, isolated VSDs are most common and may result in minimal overcirculation and volume overload, whereas significant L→R shunting causes volume overload of pulmonary circulation and left side of the heart, potentially causing left-sided CHF and/or pulmonary hypertension (PH).
- R→L shunting VSD causes systemic arterial hypoxemia, leading to erythrocytosis and hyperviscosity syndrome.

DIAGNOSIS

Diagnostic Overview

Although strong clinical suspicion of VSD may be based on physical exam alone, definitive diagnosis requires echocardiography.

Differential Diagnosis

Tricuspid dysplasia (TVD), subaortic stenosis (SAS), PS, tetralogy of Fallot (of which VSD is one component), hypertrophic cardiomyopathy (HCM) in cats

Initial Database

CBC/serum biochemistry panel:

- Typically normal
- Erythrocytosis if R→L shunting

Thoracic radiographs:

- Normal with small VSD
- Larger L→R VSD: left-sided cardiomegaly, pulmonary overcirculation, ± pulmonary edema, ± right ventricular enlargement
- R→L VSD: right-sided cardiomegaly, variable pulmonary artery pattern (e.g., normal to enlarged if PH present; normal or small if PS present)

Electrocardiogram (ECG): often normal (p. 1096)

- Changes consistent with left atrial (LA) and/or LV enlargement if large L→R shunt or RV enlargement if R→L shunt
- ± Wide and/or notched Q wave, representing abnormal septal activation

Echocardiography (confirmatory test of choice):

- A visible defect in the interventricular septum (IVS) may be noted, although small defects often cannot be visualized (see *Videos*). Beware of tissue dropout artifacts mimicking defects.
- L→R VSD: turbulent jet from LV to RV on color Doppler echocardiography (see *Videos*), ± LA and LV enlargement
- Peak velocity (in m/s) of VSD jet measured with continuous-wave Doppler reflects the pressure gradient (ΔP [mm Hg]) between LV and RV according to modified Bernoulli equation ($\Delta P = 4V^2$), which generally speaks to size of defect (small VSD: $V > 4.5$ m/s; moderate-size VSD: $3 < V < 4.5$ m/s; large VSD: $V < 3$ m/s). Beware of underestimation of velocity due to malalignment with the VSD jet.
- R→L VSD: RV hypertrophy, flattening of the IVS, main pulmonary artery dilation
- ± AI on color and spectral Doppler echocardiography

Advanced or Confirmatory Testing

- Contrast echocardiography (saline bubble study) to confirm R→L shunt
- Cardiac catheterization for angiography, shunt quantification, and measurement of intracardiac pressures (only used pre-/intraoperative)

TREATMENT

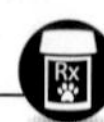

Treatment Overview

- Often no treatment is required because most VSDs are small and do not result in volume overload or other significant clinical consequences.
- Treatment of large L→R VSDs is directed at decreasing the shunt volume and preventing or eliminating the signs of CHF.
- Treatment of R→L VSDs is directed at reducing RV pressure and palliating the effects of erythrocytosis.

Acute and Chronic Treatment

L→R VSD with significant left-sided volume overload and risk or presence of CHF:

- Surgical repair by thoracotomy uncommon (requires cardiopulmonary bypass, available at very few referral institutions)
- Percutaneous transcatheter repair or hybrid techniques using a variety of devices have been described in dogs and may be available at some referral institutions.
- Pulmonary artery banding is a palliative surgical technique to decrease L→R shunt.

- If CHF present, use angiotensin-converting enzyme (ACE) inhibitors, furosemide, ± pimobendan (p. 408)

R→L VSD:

- Surgical repair contraindicated
- Phlebotomy is used to palliate signs and maintain packed cell volume (PCV) of 55%-65%. Hydroxyurea may be added if phlebotomy alone is insufficient.
- Sildenafil 1-2 mg/kg PO q 8-12h indicated if PH present

Possible Complications

- Left-sided CHF
- PH
- Shunt reversal (R→L) over time (Eisenmenger's physiology); rare
- Mural or valvular endocarditis: rare

Recommended Monitoring

- After diagnosis in puppies/kittens with no clinical signs, exam at 6 months, 1 year, and then yearly thereafter
- Frequent monitoring for animals with clinical signs and requiring treatment

PROGNOSIS & OUTCOME

- Excellent prognosis for small, isolated VSD
- Guarded prognosis for large VSD; risk of CHF and/or PH
- Concurrent substantial AI carries guarded prognosis
- Guarded to poor prognosis for R→L shunts; severe exercise limitations

PEARLS & CONSIDERATIONS

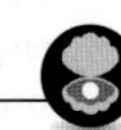

Comments

- In L→R VSD, the RV and pulmonary arterial circulation act as conduits for VSD flow. The LA and LV, however, receive increased venous return, resulting in increased diastolic pressures. Effective forward flow into the systemic circulation is reduced as a result of shunt flow. The latter two points account for the increased LV workload and predominant occurrence of left heart failure, not right heart failure, in L→R VSD.
- VSD and TVD are the two main differential diagnoses for a systolic murmur heard best on the right hemithorax in dogs or cats. Murmurs due to SAS may radiate prominently to the right side in some cases; HCM is another common differential in cats.
- Most VSDs are relatively small, with a loud murmur (grade IV/VI murmur or greater), well tolerated, and do not require therapy.

Prevention

Genetic basis is possible but unproven in most breeds. Consider discouraging breeding of affected animals.

Technician Tips

With isolated L→R VSD, the intensity of the murmur varies inversely with the size of the defect (the smaller the defect, the louder the murmur).

SUGGESTED READING

Beijerink BA, et al: Congenital heart disease. In Ettinger SJ, et al, editors: Textbook of veterinary internal medicine, ed 8, St. Louis, 2017, Elsevier, pp 1207-1248.

AUTHOR: M. Lynne O'Sullivan, DVM, DVSc, DACVIM
EDITOR: Meg M. Sleeper, VMD, DACVIM

Vestibular Disease

Client Education Sheet

BASIC INFORMATION

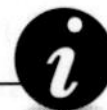

Definition

Category of disorders that affects the central or peripheral vestibular system of dogs and cats. They usually cause clinical signs of head tilt, nystagmus, and/or loss of balance.

Epidemiology

SPECIES, AGE, SEX

- Occurs in dogs and cats
- Idiopathic peripheral vestibular disease occurs in older dogs (usually > 8 years old) but in cats of any age.

ASSOCIATED DISORDERS

Nausea, vomiting

Clinical Presentation

DISEASE FORMS/SUBTYPES

- Peripheral vestibular disease (PVD): vestibulocochlear nerve lesion or inner ear disease
- Central vestibular disease (CVD): brainstem lesion (medulla oblongata)

HISTORY, CHIEF COMPLAINT

- Regardless of the underlying cause, most animals present with a peracute to subacute onset of clinical signs.
- The most common chief complaints are head tilt, nystagmus, and vestibular ataxia.
- Acute-onset vestibular disorders can produce such profound disequilibrium and ataxia that some owners believe their animal "had a stroke."

PHYSICAL EXAM FINDINGS

- Head tilt, nystagmus, and vestibular ataxia (can cause recumbency and whole-body rolling) are hallmarks of PVD and CVD.
- The most important aspect in localization of a lesion to the central vestibular system is identification of neurologic signs that cannot be attributed to PVD.
- Mental status
  - Central: often altered (depression, stupor, or coma)
  - Peripheral: animal should be alert and responsive but can often appear disoriented.
- Gait: vestibular ataxia (falling, veering, leaning, rolling, circling), usually toward the side of the lesion; seen with CVD and PVD. Hypermetria, intention tremors, and truncal sway can be observed if the cerebellum is affected (CVD).
- Head tilt: usually toward the side of the lesion; seen with CVD and PVD
- Spontaneous nystagmus: occurs with CVD and PVD. Vertical nystagmus occurs only in animals with CVD, and horizontal or rotary nystagmus can be seen with PVD or CVD. The fast phase of the nystagmus is usually away from the side of the lesion. Change in direction of the fast phase with altered head positions suggests CVD.
- Cranial nerve deficits: cranial nerve VII (facial nerve) paresis is sometimes seen in animals with PVD due to its proximity to peripheral vestibular structures. Cranial nerves V, VI, IX, and XII ipsilateral to lesion may be affected in animals with CVD but not PVD.
- Horner's syndrome: possible with PVD but rare with CVD; ipsilateral to lesion
- Postural reaction deficits are commonly seen with CVD, but should not be observed with PVD.
- Paradoxical CVD: lesion location as suggested by clinical signs related to the head (e.g., head tilt, nystagmus) does not match the lesion location suggested by the postural reaction deficits; the latter indicate the true side of the lesion (same side as hopping/proprioceptive deficit).
- Bilateral PVD: head tilt and nystagmus may not be present; animals can have wide side-to-side head excursions and walk with a crouched gait.
- Clinical signs related to disease in other central nervous system (CNS) locations, such as seizures, behavioral changes, or intention tremors, suggest multifocal central neurologic disease.

Etiology and Pathophysiology

- Basic neuroanatomy of the vestibular system
  - Peripheral: vestibular receptors (semicircular canals, saccule, utricle) located within the petrous temporal bone and cranial nerve VIII (vestibulocochlear nerve)
  - Central: vestibular nuclei in the dorsal portion of the medulla oblongata, vestibular pathways of the brainstem and spinal cord (medial longitudinal fasciculus, vestibulospinal tracts), vestibular components in the cerebellum, and vestibular pathways through the caudal cerebellar peduncle
- Cause of idiopathic peripheral vestibular disease in dogs and cats is unknown; an immune-mediated mechanism is suspected, but immunosuppressive drugs such as glucocorticoids have not been shown to help.

DIAGNOSIS

Diagnostic Overview

Clinical signs of vestibular disease are usually distinctive (see above). The diagnostic challenge consists of identifying peripheral versus central disease, which can be done on physical exam in most cases. The underlying cause is found using specific diagnostic tests ranging from hormonal assays (hypothyroidism) to advanced imaging (structural brain lesion).

Differential Diagnosis

Peripheral vestibular diseases:

- Otitis media/interna
- Idiopathic peripheral vestibular disease
- Nasopharyngeal polyps: cats > dogs
- Hypothyroidism: dogs
- Neoplasia: squamous cell carcinoma, ceruminous gland adenocarcinoma
- Ototoxicosis: topical chlorhexidine or iodine; systemic aminoglycosides, and other drugs; furosemide (rare)

Central vestibular diseases:

- Canine distemper virus (CDV) encephalomyelitis
- Feline infectious peritonitis (FIP)
- Rickettsial encephalitis: Rocky Mountain spotted fever (RMSF), ehrlichiosis
- Fungal encephalitis: *Cryptococcus neoformans* most common; blastomycosis or coccidioidomycosis in certain regions of North America
- Meningoencephalitis of unknown origin (MUO)
- Protozoal encephalitis: *Toxoplasma gondii*, *Neospora caninum*
- Neoplasia: meningioma, choroid plexus tumor, lymphoma, metastatic neoplasia
- Metronidazole toxicosis
- Cerebrovascular accident (infarct)

Initial Database

- CBC, serum biochemical analysis, urinalysis: results often normal
- Thyroid hormone analysis: low total thyroxine (T_4) and free T_4 and elevated thyroid-stimulating hormone (TSH) in dogs with hypothyroidism
- Otoscopic exam: evaluate tympanic membranes for integrity.

Advanced or Confirmatory Testing

- Bulla radiographs: dorsoventral, oblique lateral, and rostroventral-caudodorsal open-mouthed views. Abnormalities include soft-tissue or fluid opacity within the bulla and sclerosis of the tympanic bulla.
- Oropharyngeal and otoscopic exam under general anesthesia to identify nasopharyngeal polyps and otitis media. Abnormalities include soft-tissue or fluid opacity within the affected tympanic bulla (p. 681).
- Brainstem auditory evoked response (BAER) test may be useful for differentiating PVD from CVD.
- CT scan: useful for exam of the middle ear in patients with PVD. CT scans can also be used for CVD; however, beam-hardening artifacts in the caudal brain may preclude evaluation of the brainstem, and small lesions may not be visualized (MRI preferable for this location).
- MRI (p. 1132): useful for exam of peripheral and central vestibular structures; superior resolution of brain parenchyma
- Cerebrospinal fluid (CSF) analysis (pp. 1080 and 1323): used as an adjunct to advanced imaging, primarily to rule out encephalitis
- Infectious disease testing may be required in certain cases to rule out infectious encephalitis. CSF is the preferred sample for CDV, FIP, and cryptococcosis. Serum titers can be performed for *Toxoplasma* and *Neospora* spp.
- CSF culture and susceptibility (C&S) testing may be required for ruling out bacterial encephalitis (rare).
- Histopathologic exam is required for definitive diagnosis in many diseases causing structural lesions (e.g., masses). Tissue samples can be obtained via surgical excision or stereotactic brain biopsy.

TREATMENT

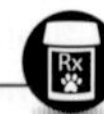

Treatment Overview

Definitive treatment for vestibular disease is based on diagnosis of the underlying cause.

Acute General Treatment

- Meclizine 25 mg/dose PO q 24h in dogs (12.5 mg/dose PO q 24h in cats) or maropitant 1 mg/kg SQ q 24h can help alleviate signs of nausea and vomiting. Meclizine causes less sedation than diphenhydramine and other antihistamines and can be purchased as an over-the-counter drug.
- Idiopathic PVD: clinical signs improve spontaneously over 1-2 weeks; no treatment has been shown to accelerate natural resolution of the disorder.
- Otitis media/interna: systemic antibiotics ± antifungals for 6-8 weeks, ideally based on C&S results. Surgical treatment (bulla osteotomy and total ear canal ablation) may be required to remove infected tissues.
- Nasopharyngeal polyps: bulla osteotomy (p. 681)
- Hypothyroidism: thyroid supplementation (p. 525)
- Neoplasia: surgical excision may be possible for meningioma and choroid plexus tumors, depending on lesion location. Surgical excision of tumors in the middle and inner ear may be possible but is difficult. Radiation therapy may provide some relief of clinical signs, and consultation with an oncologist is recommended in these cases (p. 557).
- CDV and FIP encephalomyelitis: no specific therapy is available but nonspecific supportive therapy with antibiotics and glucocorticoids may alleviate signs temporarily (pp. 271 and 327).
- Rickettsial encephalitis: doxycycline 5 mg/kg PO q 12h (pp. 285 and 891)
- Fungal encephalitis: fluconazole 5 mg/kg PO q 12h penetrates the CNS to a greater degree than other antifungal medications. Itraconazole and amphotericin B can be used for blastomycosis (pp. 121 and 184).
- MUO: immunosuppressive dose of prednisone, initially at 2 mg/kg PO q 12h for 1-2 days, then 1 mg/kg PO q 12h for at least 2 weeks. Then slowly taper the drug over 4-8 months to reach the minimal effective dose (p. 647).
- Protozoal encephalitis: clindamycin 10 mg/kg PO q 8-12h for 4 weeks or combination of trimethoprim-sulfadiazine 15 mg/kg PO q 12h and pyrimethamine 1 mg/kg PO q 24h (p. 984)
- Metronidazole toxicosis: discontinue metronidazole; diazepam 0.5 mg/kg IV once, then 0.5 mg/kg PO q 8h until resolution of signs; accelerates recovery; use extreme caution with oral dosing in cats due to idiosyncratic hepatic necrosis

Possible Complications

A permanent, mild head tilt may persist after resolution of other clinical signs.

Recommended Monitoring

- Serial neurologic exam every 4 weeks
- Serial infectious disease testing if indicated

PROGNOSIS & OUTCOME

- Prognosis for most PVDs is good with specific treatment, with the exception of neoplasia, which carries a guarded to poor prognosis.
- CDV and FIP encephalomyelitis: generally poor even with treatment
- Rickettsial and protozoal encephalitis: good with early and specific treatment
- Fungal encephalitis: fair to guarded; long-term treatment may be required to control clinical signs
- MUO: fair to guarded. Many dogs respond initially to treatment, but relapse is common.

In some dogs, glucocorticoids eventually can be discontinued.
- Neoplasia: generally poor long-term prognosis
- Metronidazole toxicosis: excellent

PEARLS & CONSIDERATIONS

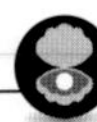

Comments

- Compensation for vestibular diseases will occur in many animals regardless of lesion location, and clinical signs may improve slightly even if the lesion is slow growing.
- The long-term prognosis for animals with CVD is variable depending upon the specific cause; however, treatment should be attempted to alleviate clinical signs.
- Additional information can be found in chapters on head tilt (p. 403), nystagmus (p. 698), and ataxia (p. 86).

Prevention

- Thyroid supplementation in dogs with hypothyroidism
- Avoid high doses and/or prolonged courses of metronidazole treatment. The recommendation is to limit the maximum daily dose to 15 mg/kg PO q 12h or less if hepatic function is compromised.

Technician Tips

The patient should be provided with thick bedding in a well-padded cage. Consider strapping the patient to a backboard for severe flailing or rolling. Use sling support until balance improves.

Client Education

Head tilt may persist.

SUGGESTED READING

Sanders SG: Disorders of hearing and balance: the vestibulocochlear nerve (CN VIII) and associated structures. In Dewey CW, et al, editors: A practical guide to canine and feline neurology, ed 3, Ames, IA, 2015, Wiley-Blackwell, pp 277-298.

AUTHOR: Mark T. Troxel, DVM, DACVIM
EDITOR: Karen R. Muñana, DVM, MS, DACVIM

Voice Change

BASIC INFORMATION

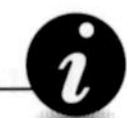

Definition

Condition is characterized by reduced vocalization and/or change in pitch of vocalization.

Epidemiology

SPECIES, AGE, SEX

- Canine and feline
- Apparent male predisposition (3:1) for idiopathic laryngeal paralysis

GENETICS, BREED PREDISPOSITION

- Hereditary laryngeal paralysis (Bouvier des Flandres, Siberian Husky, pit bull terrier)
- Generalized polyneuropathy (Dalmatian)
- Acquired laryngeal paralysis (giant and large breeds are overrepresented)
- Laryngeal edema/eversion of laryngeal saccules (brachycephalic breeds)

CONTAGION AND ZOONOSIS

If secondary to infectious diseases (e.g., infectious tracheobronchitis [kennel cough]), potential but rare zoonosis (e.g., immunocompromised persons) with *Bordetella bronchiseptica*

ASSOCIATED DISORDERS

Dogs:
- Infectious tracheobronchitis (kennel cough)
- Laryngeal paralysis
- Brachycephalic airway syndrome

Cats:
- Lymphoma
- Squamous cell carcinoma (SCC)
- Secondary to thyroidectomy
- Laryngeal paralysis

Clinical Presentation

HISTORY, CHIEF COMPLAINT

Voice change may be described as a change in pitch of bark or meow (dog/cat, respectively) or a persistent hoarseness.

- Variable voice changes, depending on condition
  - Peracute if traumatic
  - Acute if infectious
  - Subclinical and subtle if associated with neoplasia or with laryngeal paralysis
- May be associated with
  - Exercise intolerance if mild upper airway obstruction (structural or functional)
  - Inspiratory stridor and respiratory distress (dyspnea, cyanosis, syncope) if substantial upper airway obstruction (structural or functional)

PHYSICAL EXAM FINDINGS

Variable: depends on primary cause

Etiology and Pathophysiology

- Anatomic cause: structure of the larynx affected
- Functional cause: innervation of the larynx affected

DIAGNOSIS

Diagnostic Overview

Although most causes of voice change originate from a laryngeal/pharyngeal lesion (warranting a sedated laryngeal exam), systemic disturbances such as myasthenia gravis should be ruled out first, particularly if the history and physical exam are consistent with such disorders.

Differential Diagnosis

Anatomic causes:
- Laryngeal distortion
  - Blunt trauma (e.g., choke chain, hit by car, kicked by horse)
  - Penetrating trauma (e.g., stick, gunshot, dog/snake bite)
  - Osseous metaplasia
- Laryngeal edema (elongated soft palate, insect bite, chronic barking)
- Eversion of the laryngeal saccules
- Laryngeal/pharyngeal foreign body
- Laryngeal inflammation; laryngitis (traumatic, infectious [viral, bacterial], granulomatous, immune mediated, oral irritant exposure, polyp)
- Laryngeal neoplasia (mast cell tumor, SCC, leiomyoma/sarcoma, rhabdomyoma/sarcoma, fibroma/fibrosarcoma, lymphoma)

Functional causes:
- Dysfunction of the recurrent laryngeal nerve
  - Congenital/idiopathic laryngeal paralysis
  - Trauma to the nerve (direct or indirect):
    - Can occur after thyroidectomy or patent ductus arteriosus correction in cats.
  - Nerve compression (hematoma, abscess, tumor [thyroid carcinoma, lymphosarcoma])
  - Neuropathy, polyneuritis
- Myopathy (including cricoarytenoid dorsalis muscle)
- Neuromuscular disease (myasthenia gravis)

Initial Database

- CBC, serum biochemistry panel, and urinalysis: often unremarkable
- Cervical/thoracic imaging
  - Radiographs: the normal larynx, especially if mineralized, should not be mistaken for a foreign body. Laryngeal osseous metaplasia has been reported (rare).
  - Ultrasound (mass lesions, laryngeal paralysis)
- Oral/laryngeal/pharyngeal exam (visual ± endoscopy) (p. 1125); requires sedation depending on whether severe inspiratory dyspnea is present. With severe dyspnea, the laryngeal exam may be performed while the patient is awake because the patient is breathing with mouth and oropharynx is maximally opened. Direct per os laryngoscopy combined with the knowledge of the clinical history and physical exam is preferred to alternative techniques.

Advanced or Confirmatory Testing

Depending on prior results, any of these tests may be helpful:

- Ultrasound, CT, or MRI of larynx
- Serum acetylcholine receptor antibodies titer (myasthenia gravis [p. 668])
- Electromyography (myopathies)
- Exploratory surgery ± biopsy and histopathologic exam

TREATMENT

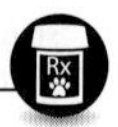

Treatment Overview

- Stabilize the patient if upper airway obstruction/dyspnea.
- Determine cause of voice change.
- Address primary cause of the condition.

Acute and Chronic Treatment

- Stabilization of the patient
  - If associated with mild inspiratory stridor
    - Sedation of the patient, oxygen supplementation if necessary (p. 1146)
  - If associated with severe inspiratory stridor and dyspnea
    - Sedation of the patient, oxygen supplementation, intubation/ventilation if necessary, emergency tracheostomy (p. 1166) if indicated
- Addressing the primary cause.
  - If secondary to anatomic cause
    - Tracheobronchitis (infectious) (p. 987)
    - Local trauma/inflammation: foreign body removal, antiinflammatory drugs (e.g., carprofen 2 mg/kg PO q 12h or meloxicam 0.1 mg/kg PO q 24h), antibiotics if indicated (penetrating wound; consider amoxicillin-clavulanate 12.5 mg/kg PO q 12h, then base the decision on aerobic and anaerobic culture and sensitivity [C&S]), soft palate resection if indicated
    - Eversion of laryngeal saccules: resection
    - Laryngeal mass: resection (ventriculocordectomy/partial laryngectomy), radiation therapy, or chemotherapy
    - If mass resection impossible: total laryngectomy with permanent tracheostomy
  - If secondary to functional cause
    - Laryngeal paralysis: unilateral cricoarytenoid lateralization
    - Surgical decompression of recurrent laryngeal nerve (hematoma, abscess drainage, mass excision)
    - Acquired neuropathy/neuromuscular disease: treat according to primary cause.

Possible Complications

Varies; depends on primary cause:

- Laryngeal paralysis: aspiration pneumonia
- Tumor: recurrence, progression of disease (local, regional, systemic)
- Inflammation, infection, or foreign body: airway obstruction, recurrence possible
- Trauma: potential irreversible nerve damage

Recommended Monitoring

Depends on primary cause

PROGNOSIS & OUTCOME

Varies, depending on condition:

- Infectious tracheobronchitis: excellent
- Trauma, inflammation, or foreign body: good to guarded
- Laryngeal paralysis: for life, good to guarded with surgery; voice change will not resolve
- Resectable laryngeal mass: good if benign and clean resection; poor if malignant, nonresectable, and/or not responsive to chemotherapy or radiation therapy

PEARLS & CONSIDERATIONS

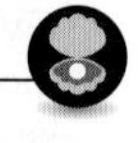

Comments

- A very common underlying cause in dogs is laryngeal paralysis.
- Ingestion of irritants (e.g., liquid potpourri) can cause oral ulceration along with laryngitis.

Technician Tips

Voice change is often the first sign of laryngeal paralysis. Ask owners of predisposed dogs (i.e., older retrievers) about any change in bark.

Client Education

If the cause is infectious tracheobronchitis, the affected dog should avoid contact with other dogs.

SUGGESTED READING

Monnet E: Surgical treatment of laryngeal paralysis. Vet Clin Small Anim 46:709-717, 2016.

AUTHOR: Bertrand Lussier, DMV, MSc, DACVS
EDITOR: Leah A. Cohn, DVM, PhD, DACVIM

Vomiting, Acute

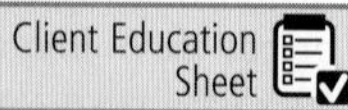

BASIC INFORMATION

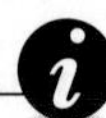

Definition

Active expulsion of stomach and sometimes duodenal contents is preceded by nausea and retching; duration is less than 7 days.

Synonym

Acute emesis

Epidemiology

SPECIES, AGE, SEX

- Any animal can be affected; patient demographics depend on the underlying cause.
- Young animals are more likely to ingest foreign bodies or acquire infectious diseases (viral and parasitic).

RISK FACTORS

Use of drugs such as nonsteroidal antiinflammatory drugs (NSAIDs) and chemotherapy; inadequate vaccination; dietary indiscretion

GEOGRAPHY AND SEASONALITY

Infectious causes often are more prevalent in specific geographic regions.

ASSOCIATED DISORDERS

The most common cause of acute vomiting is dietary indiscretion, but numerous gastrointestinal (GI) or systemic diseases can also cause vomiting.

Clinical Presentation

DISEASE FORMS/SUBTYPES

- Patients can be presented looking healthy with no concurrent signs of systemic disease. These are classified as nonserious cases.
- Patients can be presented while showing systemic clinical signs (e.g., lethargy, dehydration, abdominal distention, icterus, fever). These are classified as serious cases.

HISTORY, CHIEF COMPLAINT

It is important to differentiate vomiting (active abdominal movement, nausea) from dysphagia (difficulty swallowing) and regurgitation (passive movement of ingesta). Important components of the history:

- Vaccination status (parvoviral enteritis and canine distemper are more likely in unvaccinated dogs)
- Administration or ingestion of potentially ulcerogenic drugs such as NSAIDs or glucocorticoids
- Possibility of ingestion of a foreign body (e.g., exposure to objects that could be ingested; individual propensity to such ingestions)
- Dietary history (e.g., recent changes; content and volume of recent and typical meals)
- Description of the vomitus (e.g., hematemesis) and productiveness (e.g., nonproductive with gastric dilation/volvulus [GDV])
- Time relation of vomiting to food intake: if vomiting of undigested or partially digested food occurs 7-10 hours after ingestion, gastric outflow obstruction or gastric hypomotility is likely.

PHYSICAL EXAM FINDINGS

A thorough physical exam is mandatory. Specific points requiring extra attention:

- Hydration status
- Mouth inspection (e.g., linear foreign body in cats, ulcerations suggesting intoxication or uremia)
- Abdominal palpation (e.g., abdominal pain, abdominal distention, foreign body, mass, organomegaly, intussusception)
- Rectal exam (e.g., presence of melena, foreign material)

Etiology and Pathophysiology

- Stimulation of humoral (blood-borne substances) or neural (especially by receptors located throughout the GI tract) pathways can lead to activation of the vomiting center.
- Certain drugs (e.g., apomorphine [dogs], xylazine [cats]), uremic toxins, electrolyte, osmolar, or acid-base disorders can activate the chemoreceptor trigger zone, which triggers the vomiting center, causing vomiting.

DIAGNOSIS

Diagnostic Overview

A large proportion of patients presented for acute vomiting have benign, self-resolving illness. The extent of diagnostic testing is determined by presence or absence of signs of systemic illness; known inciting causes (e.g., overeating might prompt minimal investigation, whereas intoxication can warrant tests to evaluate body systems likely to be affected).

Differential Diagnosis

GI causes:

- Adverse food reactions (dietary indiscretion, intolerance)
- Obstruction (e.g., foreign body, intussusception)
- Gastritis: viral (parvovirus, coronavirus, distemper), bacterial
- Foreign body
- Parasites (*Physaloptera* spp, *Ollulanus tricuspis*)
- Motility disorders
- GDV (nonproductive)

Extra-GI causes:

- Extraabdominal disorders
  - Azotemia/uremia
  - Hypoadrenocorticism
  - Diabetic ketoacidosis
  - Intoxications
  - Drugs (e.g., NSAIDs, chemotherapy, glucocorticoids)
  - Neurologic disorders (especially vestibular)
- Intraabdominal disorders
  - Hepatic failure
  - Pancreatitis
  - Peritonitis
  - Pyometra

A detailed differential diagnosis is provided on p. 1293.

Initial Database

- If the animal is classified as a nonserious case: history and thorough physical exam are most important; further workup is determined by status and response to treatment.
- If the animal is classified as a serious case and/or vomiting was nonproductive, further diagnostic workup is always warranted:
  - CBC, serum chemistry profile (including sodium and potassium)
  - Urinalysis
  - Fecal exam
  - Medical imaging
    - Abdominal radiographs: radiopaque foreign bodies, signs of intestinal obstruction, ileus, GDV, or loss of abdominal detail suggesting pancreatitis or peritonitis
    - Abdominal ultrasound: changes associated with organomegaly, identification of origin and extent of masses, and other such findings
- With hematemesis: review medication/drug exposure history, search for cutaneous nodules (mastocytoma), and if relevant, consider coagulation profile, adrenocorticotropic hormone (ACTH) stimulation, and/or gastroduodenoscopy

Advanced or Confirmatory Testing

- If appropriate, infectious disease testing (e.g., parvoviral serology)
- If clinically relevant: liver function tests; ACTH stimulation test to rule out hypoadrenocorticism; toxicologic testing; neurologic exam; canine or feline pancreatic lipase immunoreactivity or 1,2-*O*-dilauryl-rac-glycero-3-glutaric acid-(6′-methylresorufin) ester (DGGR) study to rule out pancreatitis
- In some cases, especially to evaluate motility disorders or gastric outflow obstruction, GI contrast studies can be performed.
- If vomiting persists for more than 3-4 days or worsens, approach the animal as for chronic vomiting (p. 1042); endoscopy is often warranted if previous tests fail to identify the cause.

TREATMENT

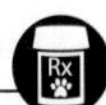

Treatment Overview

- Rehydrate the animal if needed.
- Implement treatment for systemic or life-threatening disorders (e.g., GDV, intoxications, uremia).
- Otherwise, allow the GI tract a short rest by giving nothing per os (NPO).

Acute General Treatment

Nonserious cases (animals generally treated as outpatients):

- NPO for 12-24 hours. If vomiting resolves, offer a small amount of water or a few ice cubes. Thereafter, initiate feeding with small quantities of a highly digestible, low-fat diet for several days. Gradually transition to the regular food.

Serious cases: hospitalize the animal and perform further diagnostic steps (see Initial Database and Advanced or Confirmatory Testing above).

- NPO, water, and food identical to nonserious cases
- IV fluid therapy (crystalloids): maintenance + replace dehydration + ongoing loss
- Antiemetics
  - Should be used only if the possibility of GI obstruction has been ruled out
  - Most useful when vomiting is severe and animal is at risk for dehydration or developing electrolyte/acid-base imbalances or reflux esophagitis
  - Maropitant 1 mg/kg q 24h SQ or IV or 2 mg/kg PO q 24h (selective neurokinin-1 receptor antagonist), *or*
  - Metoclopramide 0.2-0.5 mg/kg IM or SQ q 8h or as an IV CRI at 1-2 mg/kg/day (dopamine antagonist; central and peripheral antiemetic agent), *or*
  - Ondansetron 0.5-1 mg/kg PO or IV q 12 h (useful in refractory cases)
- Some causes of acute vomiting require surgical intervention (e.g., GDV, linear foreign body) or endoscopy (e.g., gastric foreign body)

Possible Complications

- Dehydration
- Reflux esophagitis
- Aspiration pneumonia
- Electrolyte and acid-base imbalances (especially hypokalemia and sometimes metabolic acidosis)

Recommended Monitoring

Signs of dehydration, body weight, abdominal pain, frequency of vomiting

PROGNOSIS & OUTCOME

Excellent with dietary indiscretion; otherwise, depends on underlying cause

PEARLS & CONSIDERATIONS

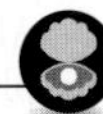

Comments

- Most cases of acute vomiting are self-limited and do not require further diagnostics, but it is important to not miss the more seriously ill animals and to recommend further workup and treatment if the vomiting does not subside within a few days.
- Use antiemetics carefully because they can mask progressive disease and response to primary therapy.

Technician Tips

Animals should be fed small amounts of bland food as soon as it is tolerated.

Client Education

Avoid feeding human food scraps and limit access to things that may be inappropriate for pets to eat (e.g., dietary indiscretion; garbage, animal carcasses).

SUGGESTED READING

Tello L, et al: Fluid and electrolyte therapy during vomiting and diarrhea. Vet Clin North Am Small Anim Pract 47:505-519, 2017.

AUTHORS: Sylvie Daminet, DVM, PhD, DACVIM, DECVIM

EDITOR: Leah A. Cohn, DVM, PhD, DACVIM

Vomiting, Chronic

Client Education Sheet

BASIC INFORMATION

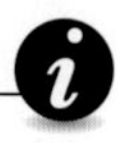

Definition

- Active expulsion of stomach and sometimes duodenal contents preceded by nausea and retching
- Intermittent or persistent vomiting for more than 7 days
- Chronic vomiting is a very common clinical sign and can be associated with a wide variety of gastrointestinal (GI) and non-GI disorders.

Synonym

Chronic emesis

Epidemiology

SPECIES, AGE, SEX

- Any animal can be affected; epidemiology depends on the underlying cause.
- Young animals are more likely to ingest foreign bodies; older animals are more likely to have neoplastic disease, hyperthyroidism, kidney failure.

GENETICS, BREED PREDISPOSITION

- Brachycephalic breeds: pyloric stenosis
- Airedale terrier: pancreatic carcinoma
- Shar-pei, rottweiler, German shepherd: inflammatory bowel disease (IBD)

RISK FACTORS

Depends on cause of vomiting (e.g., use of NSAIDs is risk factor for gastric ulcer; absent prophylaxis risk factor for parasites)

CONTAGION AND ZOONOSIS

Zoonotic potential of *Helicobacter heilmannii* and *Helicobacter felis* is unclear.

ASSOCIATED DISORDERS

Hypochloremic metabolic alkalosis, dehydration and hypovolemia, metabolic acidosis, weight loss

Clinical Presentation

DISEASE FORMS/SUBTYPES

Vomiting animals may appear healthy or may have signs of systemic disease (e.g., icterus, dehydration, depression).

HISTORY, CHIEF COMPLAINT

- It is important to differentiate vomiting from dysphagia and regurgitation.
  - Vomiting involves forceful retching and abdominal contraction and may produce bile-stained contents.
- Important questions
  - Description of vomiting (active retch), time in relation to food intake, character of the vomitus (e.g., possible hematemesis)
  - Diet history, including effect of various diets on clinical signs
  - Administration of potentially ulcerogenic drugs (e.g., NSAIDs, glucocorticoids)
  - Possibility of foreign body ingestion
  - Use of dewormers or prophylactic parasiticides
- If vomiting of undigested or partially digested food occurs 7-10 hours after ingestion, gastric outflow obstruction or gastric hypomotility is likely.

PHYSICAL EXAM FINDINGS

A thorough physical exam is mandatory but may be unremarkable. Extra attention is warranted regarding

- Hydration status
- Mouth inspection (sublingual linear foreign body in cats, ulcerations)
- Abdominal palpation (abdominal mass, thickened bowel loops)
- Rectal exam (presence of melena or hematochezia)
- Palpation of the neck for thyroid nodule (essential for cats > 6 years old)

Other findings may relate to cause of vomiting:

- Small kidneys in animal with uremic vomiting
- Enlarged salivary glands in dog with phenobarbital responsive sialadenitis
- Cutaneous nodules with mast cell–induced GI ulcers

Etiology and Pathophysiology

- Stimulation of humoral (blood-borne substances) or neural (especially by receptors located throughout the GI tract) pathways can lead to activation of the vomiting center.
- Certain drugs, uremic toxins, and electrolyte, osmolar, or acid-base disorders can activate the chemoreceptor trigger zone and cause vomiting.

DIAGNOSIS

Diagnostic Overview

Differentiation of systemic causes from GI causes begins with history and physical exam. Routine blood and urine tests and abdominal imaging (radiographs and/or ultrasonography) are warranted. If a cause is not found, specific tests (e.g., ACTH stimulation/resting cortisol in dogs, serum T_4 in adult cats) should be considered. Prophylactic broad-spectrum deworming and diet trial are usually indicated. Ultimately, failing a conclusive diagnosis from these measures, the proximal GI tract is assessed endoscopically and histologically.

Differential Diagnosis

A detailed differential diagnosis is provided on p. 1294.

- Extraabdominal disorders (e.g., uremia, hypoadrenocorticism, hyperthyroidism, heartworm infection [cats])
- Intraabdominal disorders (e.g., inflammatory bowel disease, hepatic disease, pancreatitis, food intolerance/allergy, foreign body, GI parasites, neoplasia)

Initial Database

CBC, serum biochemistry profile (including sodium and potassium), urinalysis, and fecal exam are indicated for essentially all pets with chronic vomiting.

- Serum T_4 (adult cats)
- Abdominal imaging: radiographs and/or ultrasound
- With hematemesis: check drug history, coagulation (p. 380)

Advanced or Confirmatory Testing

Additional diagnostics depend on results of screening tests. Commonly indicated tests:

- ACTH stimulation test: hypoadrenocorticism
- Canine or feline pancreatic lipase immunoreactivity or 1,2-*O*-dilauryl-rac-glycero-3-glutaric acid-(6′-methylresorufin) ester (DGGR) study: pancreatic disease
- Serum folate and cobalamin: small intestinal disease
- Heartworm antigen testing (cats)
- In rare cases, GI contrast studies may be indicated to evaluate motility disorders or gastric outflow obstruction.
- If tests fail to identify another cause for chronic vomiting, gastroduodenoscopy or exploratory celiotomy with GI and hepatic biopsies is indicated.

TREATMENT

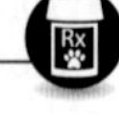

Treatment Overview

Goals are supportive treatment (if needed) and correction of the underlying cause.

Chronic Treatment

- Address any identified underlying disease or disorder, as appropriate.
- If the patient seems otherwise healthy and initial database fails to identify abnormalities, dietary therapy alone can be attempted. If the response is insufficient, further diagnostics are necessary, followed by specific treatment based on results.
  - Dietary manipulations (often low-fat, hypoallergenic diets containing a single and novel source of protein)
- Antiemetics (e.g., maropitant 1 mg/kg SQ or 2 mg/kg PO q 24h, maximum duration of 5 days, or metoclopramide 0.2-0.4 mg/kg SQ q 8h) can be used empirically after the presence of a foreign body is ruled out, but it does not substitute for addressing the cause of vomiting. Metoclopramide can cause lethargy and restlessness, especially in cats.

Drug Interactions

Ranitidine can interfere with hepatic metabolism of other drugs.

Possible Complications

- Weight loss due to malnutrition
- Dehydration
- Hypokalemia
- Sometimes, metabolic alkalosis with hypochloremia if a pyloric (sub) obstruction is present

PROGNOSIS & OUTCOME

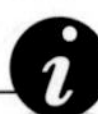

Depends on the cause

PEARLS & CONSIDERATIONS

Comments

- Concentrating only on the GI tract too early can lead to misdiagnosis and erroneous treatment.
- Vomiting can be caused by IBD even if there is no history of diarrhea or any abnormalities in the stomach. The small intestine should always be biopsied during endoscopy.
- The area under the tongue must be examined for a linear foreign body in every vomiting cat; this area is most easily visualized by pressing dorsally on the skin of the underside (ventral surface) of the mandible between the bodies of the mandible while the mouth is open.

Technician Tips

Emphasize to the owners the need to strictly follow nutrition guidelines.

SUGGESTED READING

Gallagher A: Vomiting and regurgitation. In Ettinger SJ, et al, editors: Textbook of veterinary internal medicine, ed 8, St. Louis, 2017, Elsevier, pp 158-164.

AUTHOR: Sylvie Daminet, DVM, PhD, DACVIM, DECVIM
EDITOR: Leah A. Cohn, DVM, PhD, DACVIM

von Willebrand Disease

BASIC INFORMATION

Definition

Hereditary primary hemostatic defect is caused by a quantitative or functional deficiency of von Willebrand factor (VWF). VWF is an adhesive protein required for normal platelet-collagen binding at sites of small vessel injury. Clinical expression varies in severity from a mild bleeding tendency after injury to more severe forms characterized by recurrent mucosal hemorrhage and prolonged bleeding from normal processes, such as deciduous tooth loss.

Synonyms

Factor VIII–related antigen (old terminology; protein is now referred to as von Willebrand factor [VWF]), VWD

Epidemiology

SPECIES, AGE, SEX

- von Willebrand disease (VWD) is the most common hereditary bleeding disorder of dogs. It is rare in cats.
- Severe forms typically manifest by 1 year of age, but milder forms may be inapparent unless the patient undergoes surgery or trauma.

GENETICS, BREED PREDISPOSITION

- Autosomal trait with three type classifications:
  - Type 1 VWD: mild to moderate; recessive or incomplete dominant inheritance
  - Types 2 and 3 VWD: severe; recessive inheritance
- Males and females express and transmit VWD with equal frequency.
- In recessive forms, affected pups inherit a VWF mutation from both dam and sire.
- Affected breeds
  - Type 1 VWD: Airedale, Akita, Bernese mountain dog, dachshund, Doberman pinscher, German shepherd, golden retriever, greyhound, Irish wolfhound, Kerry blue terrier, Manchester terrier, miniature pinscher, papillon, Pembroke Welsh corgi, poodle, schnauzer, and sporadic cases in any breed
  - Type 2 VWD: German short-haired pointer, German wirehaired pointer
  - Type 3 VWD: Chesapeake Bay retriever, Dutch kooiker, Scottish terrier, Shetland sheepdog, and sporadic cases (recent cases in Australian shepherd, border collie, cocker spaniel, Labrador retriever, Maltese)

Clinical Presentation

DISEASE FORMS/SUBTYPES

- Type 1 VWD: quantitative protein deficiency. Low plasma concentration of VWF (von Willebrand factor antigen [VWF:Ag]) with proportionate reduction in VWF function; the VWF protein has a full distribution of multimeric forms.
- Type 2 VWD: quantitative and functional protein deficiency; low plasma VWF:Ag level has a disproportionate decrease in VWF function measured by collagen binding or support of platelet agglutination. VWF protein lacks the high-molecular-weight multimers.
- Type 3 VWD: severe VWF deficiency, undetectable plasma VWF (VWF:Ag $< 0.1\%$)

HISTORY, CHIEF COMPLAINT

- Severe forms: recurrent mucosal bleeding, prolonged bleeding from loss of deciduous teeth or minor wounds, blood-loss anemia after surgery or trauma
- Mild forms: few spontaneous or severe bleeds; abnormal bleeding typically observed after surgical or traumatic injury

PHYSICAL EXAM FINDINGS

- Exam may be normal.
- Abnormal hemorrhage
  - Mucosal bleeding
  - Abnormal bleeding from traumatic/surgical wounds
- Pallor from blood loss anemia

Etiology and Pathophysiology

- Distinct VWF mutations causative for type 3 VWD have been described in Scottish terriers and Dutch kooiker dogs.
- Homozygosity for a mutation located at a splice site of the VWF gene has been associated with low VWF protein in type 1 VWD.
- Types 2 and 3 VWD cause a moderate to severe bleeding tendency.
- The clinical severity of type 1 VWD generally correlates with decrease in VWF concentration.
- VWF is an adhesive protein required for normal platelet-collagen binding and platelet aggregate formation at sites of small vessel injury under high shear.
- A lack of VWF impairs platelet plug formation and causes bleeding despite normal *in vitro* platelet numbers, normal platelet aggregation, and normal coagulation cascade parameters (normal coagulation profile).

DIAGNOSIS

Diagnostic Overview

VWD typically causes signs of mucosal hemorrhage and prolonged postoperative/traumatic hemorrhage. Platelet count and coagulation screening tests are normal.

Differential Diagnosis

- Primary hemostatic defects
  - Thrombocytopenia
  - Acquired or hereditary platelet dysfunction, thrombocytopathias (e.g., patient taking aspirin)
- Coagulation factor deficiency
- Vasculopathy or erosive/infiltrative vessel defect causing mucosal hemorrhage

Initial Database

- Thorough physical exam to define single versus multiple sites of hemorrhage
- Baseline hematocrit and plasma protein: normal, or decreased if bleeding is severe and chronic
- Platelet count or platelet estimate from blood smear: usually normal
- Point-of-care coagulation screening tests: usually normal
  - Activated clotting time (ACT)
  - Activated partial thromboplastin time (aPTT)
  - Prothrombin time (PT)
- Bleeding time (buccal mucosal bleeding time): increased (p. 1076)

Advanced or Confirmatory Testing

Diagnosis is based on specific measurement of plasma VWF concentration:

- VWF concentration (VWF:Ag)
  - VWF:Ag < 50% is evidence of VWF deficiency, but clinical bleeding tendency is usually seen in animals having more severe deficiency (<25%).
  - Types 1 and 2 VWD in dogs are characterized by the presence of low protein concentration, whereas type 3 VWD is characterized by a complete absence of VWF (VWF:Ag < 0.1%).
- Differentiation of types 1 and 2 VWD is based on the finding of dysfunctional and structurally abnormal protein in the type 2 form. Abnormal protein is identified based on the following tests:
  - VWF:CB = VWF collagen binding activity (functional assay)
  - VWF multimer analyses = Western blot to visualize VWF subunit structure
- Hereditary type 2 VWD has been identified in only two breeds: German wirehaired and short-haired pointers.
- An acquired type 2 VWD occurs in human beings with aortic stenosis. A study of mitral valve disease in Cavalier King Charles spaniels revealed abnormal VWF multimer distribution, compatible with type 2 VWD.

TREATMENT

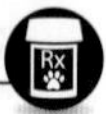

Treatment Overview

- Control active bleeding with transfusion therapy and local wound care.
- Avoid unnecessary surgery, trauma, and any drug therapy that inhibits platelet function or coagulation factor activity.
- Correct any underlying medical conditions that may impair hemostasis.

Acute General Treatment

A patient that had a normal preoperative platelet count but bleeds persistently during a surgical procedure, shows no physical evidence of severe systemic illness (vasculitis), and is not known to have been exposed to anticoagulant (e.g., rodenticide) or antiplatelet (e.g., aspirin) substances should be suspected of having VWD and may be treated as follows pending the results of confirmatory tests (see Advanced or Confirmatory Testing above):

- Transfusion (p. 1169) can supply hemostatic levels of VWF to control active hemorrhage refractory to local wound care. Patients with severe VWD (typically types 2 and 3 VWD) may require additional transfusions within the first 24 hours to sustain hemostasis after an initial response.
- Transfusion of plasma components reduces risk of volume overload or red cell sensitization while maximizing VWF replacement.
- Fresh-frozen plasma 10-15 mL/kg IV
  - Transfuse at the high end of dosage range for the initial transfusion.
  - Severely deficient patients may require repeated transfusions at q 8-12h intervals.
- Cryoprecipitate (unit dosage varies by supplier)
  - Prepared from fresh-frozen plasma and contains a 5- to 10-fold concentration of VWF in approximately one-tenth the volume of the starting plasma.
  - Cryoprecipitate's low volume eliminates the risk of volume overload if repeated transfusion is needed for high-dose VWF replacement.
- Fresh whole blood (12-20 mL/kg) can be used as a source of VWF replacement if plasma components are unavailable or replacement of red blood cells (RBCs) and VWF is desired to treat ongoing blood-loss anemia:
  - Risk of volume overload generally limits whole blood transfusion to q 24h intervals (p. 989).
- Packed RBC transfusion 6-12 mL/kg is indicated to treat severe blood-loss anemia.
- Use local wound care (suture, pressure wrap, tissue glue) to help control bleeding from superficial sites.

Chronic Treatment

- Intermittent transfusion may be needed to control hemorrhagic events in patients with severe (types 2 and 3) VWD.
- Preoperative transfusion to patients with type 2 or 3 VWD or severe expression of type 1 VWD to replace VWF before surgical procedures
  - Fresh-frozen plasma and cryoprecipitate are the best products for preoperative prophylaxis: same dose as described previously
  - Transfusion is administered just before the surgical procedure. Peak VWF is obtained immediately after transfusion, and values fall to baseline by 24 hours.
  - Close monitoring is required during the first 24 hours after the operation. Repeat transfusion (q 8-12h) may be required during this period for severe VWD.
- Desmopressin acetate (deamino-8-D-arginine vasopressin [DDAVP]) is a synthetic vasopressin analog that can be used preoperatively to enhance surgical hemostasis in patients with mild to moderate VWD (type 1 VWD); dosage is 1 mcg/kg SQ given 30 minutes preoperatively.
  - The response to DDAVP varies, and transfusion should be available if hemorrhage develops despite DDAVP therapy.
- Development of endocrinopathy (e.g., hypothyroidism, hypoadrenocorticism) or thrombocytopenia may exacerbate the bleeding tendency of VWF-deficient patients. Identification and correction of these disorders can reduce risk of clinical signs.

Behavior/Exercise

von Willebrand disease, unlike hemophilia and other hereditary coagulopathies, does not cause hemarthrosis. Exercise restrictions are unwarranted, but sharp sticks or chew toys should be avoided to prevent oral mucosal injuries.

Drug Interactions

Avoid drugs with anticoagulant or antiplatelet effects in animals with VWD:

- Nonsteroidal antiinflammatory drugs (NSAIDs)
- Sulfonamide antibiotics
- Heparin, warfarin (Coumadin)
- Plasma expanders
- Estrogens
- Cytotoxic drugs

Possible Complications

RBC sensitization causing transfusion reactions:

- Transfuse plasma components when possible.
- Dogs with severe VWD should be blood typed because repeated transfusion may be required. Choose type-matched donors for RBC or whole blood transfusions.
- Canine transfusion: after a first RBC transfusion, perform a cross-match before subsequent transfusions.

Recommended Monitoring

Demonstration of adequate VWF replacement:

- Cessation of active bleeding
- Stabilization of hematocrit/plasma protein

PROGNOSIS & OUTCOME

- Most dogs clinically affected with VWD have a good quality of life and require transfusions intermittently or rarely:
  - Animals with severe VWD (types 2 and 3 VWD) are most likely to develop spontaneous bleeding or require repeated transfusion. All dogs affected with types 2 and 3 VWD should receive a preoperative transfusion before surgical procedures.
  - Many dogs with type 1 VWD have mild disease expression. Clinical signs of abnormal bleeding are most likely to develop in dogs with VWF:Ag < 25%.
- Acute bleeding crises may require intensive transfusion support to rapidly provide hemostatic levels of VWF protein. Initial high-dose component therapy (fresh-frozen plasma or cryoprecipitate) is recommended to control severe bleeding.

Diseases and Disorders

PEARLS & CONSIDERATIONS 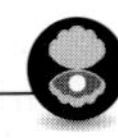

Comments

- Specific diagnosis of VWD requires measurement of plasma VWF concentration (VWF:Ag).
    - The findings of normal coagulation panel and platelet count do not rule out VWD.
- Signs of mucosal hemorrhage (rather than petechiae) are typical manifestations of VWD.

Prevention

- Screen animals preoperatively to determine baseline VWF:Ag for breeds or lines with a high prevalence of VWD. The risk of abnormal bleeding is greatest for dogs with VWF:Ag < 25%.
- Clinically affected dogs should not be used for breeding. Carriers of the VWD trait can be identified based on low level of VWF:Ag (<50%). The VWF protein assay is relatively fast and inexpensive and does not require knowledge of mutation type; however, values for carrier and clear dogs may overlap at the low end of the normal range (50%-70% VWF:Ag).
- A direct mutation detection strategy is offered for several breed variants of VWD by several commercial companies using DNA isolated from cheek swabs or blood samples. Using this method, dogs are classified as VWD affected if they are homozygous for a mutation or VWD carrier if they are heterozygous. DNA analyses provide unambiguous information on the presence, absence, and copy number of a specific mutation type.
- Selective breeding practices can reduce the prevalence or eliminate VWD from an affected pedigree. Breeding two clear parents is ideal and is expected to produce entire litters of clear pups. Breeding one carrier parent to a clear mate may be acceptable, and the clear pups produced from these matings can be used for subsequent generations. Carrier-to-carrier matings may produce affected pups and therefore should be avoided.

Technician Tips

Sample quality is important for obtaining valid VWF:Ag assay results. To avoid activation and depletion of VWF, blood samples should be drawn directly into tubes or syringes containing anticoagulant and centrifuged to separate plasma as soon as possible after collection.

Client Education

Owners and breeders should be aware of VWD and be advised to screen their pets to prevent propagation of the trait. Consider screening for VWD at puppy or wellness exams for breeds with high prevalence or severe forms of VWD (e.g., Doberman pinscher, Shetland sheepdog).

SUGGESTED READING

Brooks MB, et al: Von Willebrand disease. In Weiss DJ, et al, editors: Schalm's Veterinary hematology, Ames, IA, 2010, Wiley-Blackwell, pp 612-618.

AUTHOR: Marjory B. Brooks, DVM, DACVIM
EDITOR: Jonathan E. Fogle, DVM, PhD, DACVIM

Vulvar Discharge

Bonus Material Online 

BASIC INFORMATION 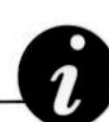

Definition

Discharge from the vulva usually originates from the reproductive tract (vagina or uterus) but may be seen with urinary tract disease. It may be abnormal or physiologically appropriate.

Epidemiology

SPECIES, AGE, SEX

More common in the bitch than queen (spayed or intact)

RISK FACTORS

- Sexually intact bitch
- Breeding bitch or queen (pregnancy loss, parturition)
- Vaginal stricture or septum, vaginal foreign body, vaginal neoplasia
- Ovarian remnant syndrome
- Urethral neoplasia, ectopic ureters, redundant lateral/dorsal vulvar fold
- Mibolerone treatment
- Exposure to transdermal hormone replacement therapy

CONTAGION AND ZOONOSIS

- *Brucella canis*
- *Campylobacter jejuni*
- Transmissible venereal tumor

ASSOCIATED DISORDERS

- Frequently associated with pyometra
- Often associated with abortion/premature labor, metritis, or endometritis
- May be occur with subinvolution of placental sites (SIPS) in the bitch
- Others: perivulvar pyoderma, urinary tract infection (UTI), urinary incontinence, urethritis, pseudohermaphroditism, hermaphroditism

Clinical Presentation

DISEASE FORMS/SUBTYPES

Canine brucellosis is caused by *B. canis*. However, dogs are susceptible to *Brucella abortus* and *Brucella suis* and may act as a reservoir.

HISTORY, CHIEF COMPLAINT

- Visible vulvar discharge
- Increased genital grooming
- Staining of carpet/bedding
- Scooting (rubbing perineum on floor)
- Pollakiuria
- Attracting males
- Hair staining in perineal area
- Lethargy, inappetence in cases of sepsis (e.g., pyometra)
- Polyuria and polydipsia (pyometra)

PHYSICAL EXAM FINDINGS

- Abnormalities are generally restricted to genital tract; exception is pyometra with secondary sepsis
- Inflamed, moist, red perivulvar skin ± moist or ulcerative pyoderma
- Red ± ulcerated vulvar mucosa; clitoral enlargement
- Classification of discharge type assists diagnostic approach
    - Color (colorless, brown, green, red, purulent)
    - Smell (malodorous or not)
    - Volume (mild, moderate)
- Discharge associated with bacterial infections is typically purulent/mucosanguineous and malodorous with moderate volume.
- Discharge due to inflammation is typically mucoid, white or clear, mild to moderate volume, and not malodorous.
- Rectal palpation may reveal foreign body or mass in the posterior vaginal vault and/or pelvic urethra.
- Digital vaginal exam may reveal discharge; small mucosal nodules (reactive lymphoid tissue) may be palpable with any inflammation and are not pathognomonic for any one cause.
- Most vaginal strictures are palpable at the level of the urethral papilla because this is where the müllerian ducts and urogenital sinus fuse during embryonic development.
- Fever, signs of septic shock, distended uterine horns, and/or abdominal discomfort may be noted with pyometra.
- Petechiae or bleeding may be present with thrombocytopenia or coagulopathy secondary to sepsis/disseminated intravascular coagulation related to pyometra.

Etiology and Pathophysiology

- Intact adult: purulent discharge is normal in estrous, abnormal in diestrous; may be secondary to pyometra (p. 854) or early

pregnancy loss. Mild hemorrhagic discharge is normal during proestrus in the bitch.
- Spayed adult: clear or purulent discharge often associated with secondary bacterial vaginitis due to anatomic abnormalities (lateral/dorsal vulvar fold dermatitis, vaginal stricture, septum), foreign body, or urinary tract infection with urethritis/vestibulitis. Neoplasia is more frequently associated with a hemorrhagic vaginal discharge (leiomyoma, leiomyosarcoma).
- Prepubertal dogs: lymphoplasmacytic vaginitis and juvenile-onset (puppy) vaginitis: unknown cause

DIAGNOSIS

Diagnostic Overview

- Purulent vaginal discharge in an intact patient should prompt an evaluation for pyometra during diestrous or metritis/endometritis in the periparturient period.
- Hemorrhagic vaginal discharge (with the exception of scant discharge during proestrus) warrants evaluation for systemic bleeding disorders (p. 433), SIPS in the postpartum bitch, and neoplasia.
- Chronic discharges should be evaluated with a thorough physical exam, including digital rectal and vaginal palpation, cytologic exam of the discharge, video vaginoscopy, and a routine database for detection of urinary tract infection, vulvar abnormalities, vaginal strictures, foreign body, and neoplastic change.

Differential Diagnosis

- Normal vaginal discharge; none should be malodorous
  - Estrus: hemorrhagic, low volume
  - Parturition: moderate to large volume, hemorrhagic, green or brown
  - Postpartum: low to moderate volume for up to 4-6 weeks, green initially then brown
- Endometritis/metritis: purulent, mucosanguineous, malodorous, moderate volume in association with a febrile postpartum bitch
- Subinvolution of placental sites (p. 950): hemorrhagic, moderate volume in association with periparturient period
- Juvenile-onset vaginitis: white, mucoid, and moderate volume
- Secondary bacterial vaginitis due to stricture, foreign body: mucoid, blood-tinged discharge; may be malodorous and scant to moderate volume
- Herpesvirus, *B. canis* infection (abortion), *C. jejuni*: abortion-associated discharge is typically brown, moderate volume.
- Urogenital neoplasia: varies; may be hemorrhagic, serous, or mucoid; scant to moderate volume
- Bleeding disorder: hemorrhagic; volume depends on degree of coagulation impairment
- Lymphoplasmacytic vaginitis: typically low volume, scant, and serous initially; may become mucoid with secondary bacterial infection; occasionally serosanguineous (p. 1030)
- Primary bacterial vaginitis (uncommon)
- Urinary tract infection/urethritis (p. 232)
- Perivulvar pyoderma: malodor is typically noted from the vulvar area; discharge may be mild to moderate in volume; mucoid and occasionally blood tinged
- Transmissible venereal tumor: vulvar mass typically noted; associated discharge is typically serosanguineous (p. 993).

Initial Database

- Physical exam, including evaluation of vulvar lip conformation, mucosa, and digital rectal and vaginal exams
- Vaginal cytologic exam (p. 1183)
- CBC: leukocytosis with left shift, toxic changes common with pyometra; leukopenia possible with endometritis; anemia may be noted postpartum or associated with SIPS
- Serum biochemical analysis: generally unremarkable unless systemic illness
- Urinalysis, sediment exam, and culture: assess for concurrent cystitis. Avoid cystocentesis if there is a possibility of pyometra or coagulopathy.
- Ultrasonographic evaluation of genitourinary tract: diagnostic test of choice for pyometra
- *Brucella* screening (p. 1319)

Advanced or Confirmatory Testing

- Guarded cranial vaginal aerobic/mycoplasma bacterial culture to evaluate bacterial population
- Retrograde double-contrast vaginocystourethrogram
- Cystoscopy (p. 1085) and video vaginoscopy (p. 1184), including exam of cervix: foreign body, congenital malformation, mass
- Vaginal biopsy ± mass biopsy
- Coagulation profile (if hemorrhagic discharge)
- Urethral pressure profile

TREATMENT

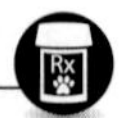

Treatment Overview

- Treatment goals are to restore patient's comfort, correct underlying cause, and prevent recurrence.

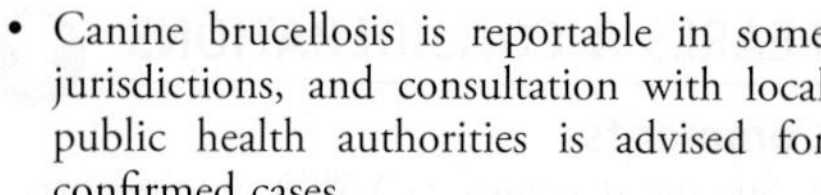

- Canine brucellosis is reportable in some jurisdictions, and consultation with local public health authorities is advised for confirmed cases.

Acute and Chronic Treatment

The nature and extent of treatment is determined by the underlying cause; vaginal discharge is simply a clue to underlying disease.

Behavior/Exercise

If discharge is associated with an infectious disease (e.g., *B. canis*, transmissible venereal tumor), bitch should be quarantined from other dogs to prevent transmission.

Possible Complications

Chronic estrogen exposure may cause myelotoxicosis.

Recommended Monitoring

- When diethylstilbestrol (DES) is used in high doses or for chronic therapy, regular evaluation of patient's CBC is advised (myelotoxicity).
- Clinical response for uncomplicated bacterial vaginitis
- Repeat exam and evaluation if complete resolution is not achieved after 14 days of therapy

PROGNOSIS & OUTCOME

- Good prognosis for secondary bacterial vaginitis if underlying cause is identified and corrected
- Idiopathic lymphoplasmacytic vaginitis is often recurrent but responsive to steroid therapy.

PEARLS & CONSIDERATIONS

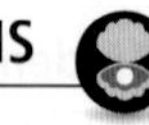

Comments

- Always rule out pyometra in an intact animal with vaginal discharge.
- Always perform digital vaginal and rectal palpation when initially evaluating a patient with vaginal discharge.

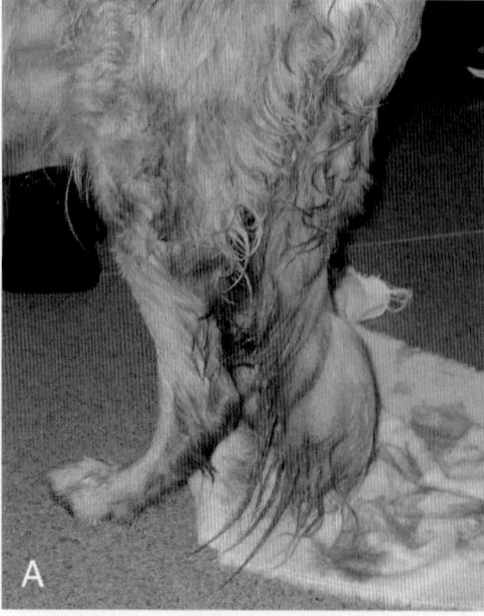

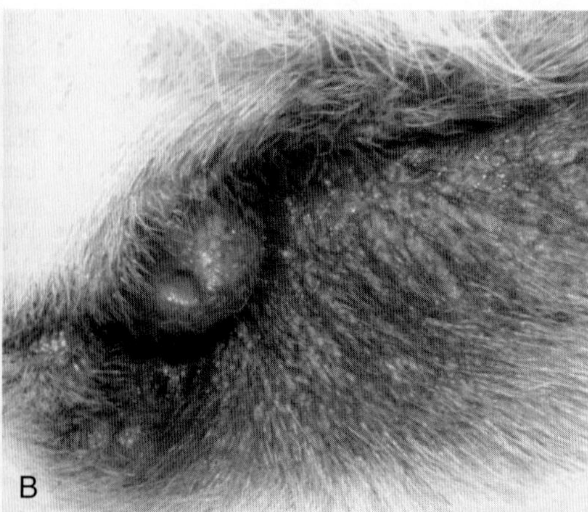

VULVAR DISCHARGE Normal postpartum vaginal discharge from a bitch 1 day (**A,** green discharge) and 1 week (**B,** brown discharge) after whelping.

- Normal vaginal flora is mixed (*Escherichia coli*, *Pasteurella multocida*, beta-hemolytic *Streptococcus* group G most common). Abnormal flora is typically a single isolate and/or heavy growth.
- Vaginal cytologic exam always helps to detect discharge due to estrus and the presence of estrogen influence in the bitch.
- Video vaginoscopy facilitates the evaluation of the entire canine vagina, which can be up to 35 cm long in some breeds.
- Surgical correction of strictures is not advised; clitorectomy is advised in cases of clitoral hypertrophy.

Prevention

Pyometra may be avoided by ovariectomy/ovariohysterectomy.

Technician Tips

- When providing services for the breeding bitch, always recommend regular *Brucella* screening.
- An empty 3-mL syringe case or an otoscope cone can be inserted between the vulvar lips and used as a sterile guard when collecting vaginal cultures.

Client Education

- Positive bacterial culture does not necessarily indicate infection.
- Prebreeding antibiotics do not prevent vaginitis or pyometra.
- Puppy vaginitis is usually self-limited and does not require antimicrobial treatment; antimicrobial treatment of puppy vaginitis may prolong resolution of the problem. These pups should be allowed to go through an estrous cycle before ovariohysterectomy.
- When using transdermal hormone replacement–containing estrogens, consult with your physician about a topical location for application that will not be in contact with pets.

SUGGESTED READING

Johnston SD, et al: Disorders of the canine vagina, vestibule, and vulva. In Johnston SD, et al, editors: Canine and feline theriogenology, Philadelphia, Saunders, 2001, pp 225-242.

AUTHOR: Sophie A. Grundy, BVSc (Hons), MANZCVS, DACVIM
EDITOR: Michelle A. Kutzler, DVM, PhD, DACT

Weight Loss

BASIC INFORMATION

Definition

Weight loss can be intentional or unintentional, but this chapter focuses on decreased body weight (BW) and/or muscle mass as the unintended consequence of disease.

Synonyms

Cachexia, emaciation, muscle wasting, catabolism

Epidemiology

SPECIES, AGE, SEX

Any species, any age, either sex

Clinical Presentation

DISEASE FORMS/SUBTYPES

- Accompanied or unaccompanied by localizing gastrointestinal (GI) signs
- Results from one or more mechanisms: decreased caloric intake, increased physiologic calorie utilization, catabolism associated with pathology, or nutrient loss.

HISTORY, CHIEF COMPLAINT

- Often, thin appearance, lethargy, decreased appetite, muscle atrophy
- It is important to determine
  - Quantity, quality, and appropriateness of the diet
  - Appetite (increased or decreased)
  - Daily activity/caloric expenditure
  - Presence of physiologic conditions that may increase energy requirements (e.g., extreme exercise, growth, pregnancy, lactation)
  - Presence of localizing GI signs (e.g., dysphagia, regurgitation, vomiting, diarrhea)

PHYSICAL EXAM FINDINGS

Poor body condition (or decrease compared with historic BW) ± poor haircoat, muscle atrophy, findings related to cause of weight loss (e.g., palpable mass might be present if cancer cachexia is cause for weight loss)

Etiology and Pathophysiology

- BW is affected by caloric intake, absorptive capacity, metabolic demand, and nutrient losses.
- Weight loss may result from
  - Inadequate quantity or quality of diet
  - Inability to prehend or swallow food
  - Regurgitation or vomiting of ingesta
  - Inappetence
  - Inability to digest or absorb ingested nutrients (e.g., exocrine pancreatic insufficiency [EPI], enteropathies)
  - Inability to use absorbed nutrients (e.g., diabetes mellitus, liver failure)
  - Increased metabolic rate (hyperthyroidism)
  - Increased catabolism (e.g., sepsis, neoplasia, heart failure, renal failure)
  - Loss of nutrients (e.g., protein-losing nephropathy or enteropathy)

DIAGNOSIS

Diagnostic Overview

Weight loss is a nonspecific clinical sign. When it is not deliberate, a broad systemic evaluation beginning with routine blood, urine, and fecal tests is indicated.

Differential Diagnosis

The differential diagnosis is provided on p. 1295.

Initial Database

- CBC, biochemistry panel, urinalysis, fecal parasite testing
- Cats: feline leukemia virus/feline immunodeficiency virus (FeLV/FIV) testing, thyroxine (T_4) level (>5 years old)

Advanced or Confirmatory Testing

Choice of testing is guided by preliminary data but often includes the following:

- Abdominal imaging (radiographs/ultrasound) to identify organomegaly, mass, effusion, GI tract thickening or intestinal layer loss, pancreatitis
- Urine protein-to-creatinine ratio to rule out protein-losing nephropathy
- Bile acids to rule out liver failure and portosystemic shunt (can exist even with normal biochemistry panel)
- Thoracic radiographs: rule out metastatic or other pulmonary disease
- Comprehensive thyroid testing (p. 503)
- ACTH stimulation test to rule out hypoadrenocorticism
- Trypsin-like immunoreactivity (TLI) to rule out EPI (especially if small bowel diarrhea)
- Fecal alpha$_1$-protease inhibitor activity if protein-losing enteropathy is suspected in the absence of diarrhea
- Upper GI endoscopy to rule out esophageal or gastric foreign body, ulcerations, luminal neoplasms, and lymphangiectasia
- GI biopsies by endoscopy, laparotomy, or laparoscopy
- Infectious disease testing when indicated

TREATMENT

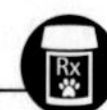

Treatment Overview

Treat underlying disease and provide nutritional support.

Acute General Treatment

Increase caloric intake:

- Dietary management
  - Increase palatability.
  - Increase caloric density.
  - Administer nutrition by feeding tube.
  - Rarely, partial or total parenteral nutrition (PPN or TPN)
- Pharmacologic management
  - Antinausea medications: maropitant, metoclopramide, ondansetron, phenothiazines. These medications may be contraindicated in some diseases.
  - Appetite stimulants: mirtazapine (dogs and cats), cyproheptadine (cats), capromorelin (dogs and cats), cannabis derivatives (data lacking currently)
  - Gastric acid reducers: proton pump inhibitors (omeprazole, pantoprazole, esomeprazole) are more effective than H2-receptor antagonists (famotidine, ranitidine) at increasing gastric pH.

Nutrition/Diet

- Enteral nutrition is preferred in animals that have a functioning GI tract.
- Feeding through a nasoesophageal, esophagostomy, gastrostomy, or jejunostomy tube may be required (pp. 1106, 1107, and 1109).
- Parenteral nutrition may be necessary in animals that cannot tolerate enteral feeding or if enteral feeding alone cannot meet caloric requirements (p. 1148).
- Caloric requirements (p. 1077) are estimated by calculating resting energy requirements (RER) and illness energy requirements (IER):
  - RER (in kcal) can be calculated as:
    - $70 \times (\text{BW [in kg]})^{0.75}$
  - IER is calculated by multiplying RER by an illness factor (1.2-1.4 for dogs; 1.1-1.2 for cats).

Drug Interactions

- Metoclopramide is contraindicated in patients with a physical obstruction of the GI tract or GI bleeding.
- Serotonin syndrome can result when any of the following are used in combination: mirtazapine, tramadol, trazodone, ondansetron/dolasetron, monoamine oxidase inhibitors (MAOIs) (e.g., selegiline), selective serotonin reuptake inhibitors (SSRIs) (e.g., fluoxetine) (p. 1281).
- Mirtazapine and tramadol may be less effective if used in combination with cyproheptadine.

Possible Complications

- Refeeding syndrome if anorexia is chronic and/or severe
- Aspiration pneumonia in patients that are regurgitating, vomiting, or being force-fed
- Hepatic encephalopathy if there is hepatocellular dysfunction

PROGNOSIS & OUTCOME

Depends on underlying disease process

PEARLS & CONSIDERATIONS

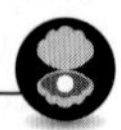

Comments

- Other clinical signs (e.g., vomiting, fever, cough) can provide more specific clues to the diagnosis than weight loss alone.
- Rarely, protein-losing enteropathies cause weight loss without diarrhea. Large-intestinal disease does not cause weight loss by itself; look for comorbidities or diffuse intestinal disease in a patient with weight loss and large-intestinal diarrhea.
- Record body condition score (BCS of 1-9; 5 is ideal) and muscle condition score (1-3; 3 is ideal) with every exam.
- Appetite stimulants are often ineffective in the presence of nausea or severe illness.

Technician Tips

- With hospitalized patients, use the same scale daily to keep an accurate trend of BW.
- When feeding by esophagostomy tube, if the patient begins to swallow, you are feeding too quickly.

Client Education

Weight loss is caused by a wide array of diseases; many are treatable, but obtaining a diagnosis might require extensive testing.

SUGGESTED READING

Baldwin K, et al: Special Report: 2010 AAHA Nutritional Assessment Guidelines for Dogs and Cats. J Am Anim Hosp Assoc 46:285-296, 2010. https://www.aaha.org/public_documents/professional/guidelines/nutritionalassessmentguidelines.pdf

AUTHOR: Bradley A. Green, DVM, DACVIM
EDITOR: Leah A. Cohn, DVM, PhD, DACVIM

Whipworm Infection

Client Education Sheet 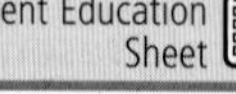

BASIC INFORMATION

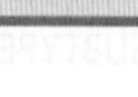

Definition

Infection of the cecum and possibly ileum and colon with *Trichuris vulpis* (dogs) or *Trichuris campanula* or *Trichuris serrata* (cats)

Synonym

Trichuriasis

Epidemiology

SPECIES, AGE, SEX

Primarily adult dogs; rare in cats

RISK FACTORS

- Roaming
- Exposure to feces or contaminated environment
- Poor health maintenance program, especially those lacking proper heartworm or intestinal parasite prevention

CONTAGION AND ZOONOSIS

Humans are rare aberrant hosts.

GEOGRAPHY AND SEASONALITY

- Common in the eastern and southern United States
- Ova are extremely resistant in the environment, surviving 4-5 years and demonstrating no seasonality.

Clinical Presentation

DISEASE FORMS/SUBTYPES

- Subclinical (common)
- Persistent or intermittent large-bowel diarrhea (mucoid stool, hematochezia, tenesmus) with various degrees of severity
- Hypoadrenocorticism-like syndrome: hyponatremia, hyperkalemia, azotemia, metabolic acidosis

HISTORY, CHIEF COMPLAINT

- None (incidental finding on fecal flotation)
- Clinical signs of large-bowel diarrhea: tenesmus; frequent, urgent defecation of loose or watery feces, possibly containing mucus or fresh blood (hematochezia); flatulence possible
- Occasionally associated with weight loss and protein-losing enteropathy
- In dogs with hypoadrenocorticism-like illness, lethargy, vomiting, or severe diarrhea may be present.

PHYSICAL EXAM FINDINGS

- Usually, animals with mild whipworm infections have a normal physical exam.
- Vague signs of mid-abdominal pain/tenderness, often characterized by flank licking, have been associated with granulomatous typhlitis.
- Rarely, physical signs of systemic disease (weight loss/cachexia) are present with

hypoadrenocorticism-like illness related to whipworm infection.

Etiology and Pathophysiology

- Direct life cycle begins with ingestion of embryonated eggs.
- Ova hatch in small intestine, and larvae burrow into mucosa for a 1-week period.
- Young adults emerge, relocate to the cecum/colon, and deeply embed the threadlike head (the whip) into the mucosa to feed on blood and tissue fluids.
- A 3-month prepatent period (range, 70-107 days) precedes appearance of ova in feces.
- Host response varies from mild localized inflammation to mucosal hyperplasia to granulomatous inflammation, resulting in variable degrees of gastrointestinal (GI) clinical signs.
- Affected animals can develop large-bowel diarrhea that ranges in severity from intermittent soft stool to severe, copious mucoid or hemorrhagic diarrhea with tenesmus.
- Whipworm-related enteritis may produce biochemical changes falsely suggesting hypoadrenocorticism.
  - Hyponatremia: due to concurrent diarrhea-associated sodium loss, water consumption, and anorexia
  - Hyperkalemia: due to metabolic acidosis, decreased kaliuresis from reduced flow in the distal renal tubules, and/or laboratory artifact (normal platelet K^+ release when clotting)
  - Primary enteritis-associated hyponatremia and hyperkalemia are not caused by aldosterone deficiency (hypoadrenocorticism), as confirmed by normal ACTH stimulation test results.
- Whipworm infection has been suggested as a cause of cecocolic intussusception.

DIAGNOSIS

Diagnostic Overview

Whipworm infection should be suspected in any dog with clinical signs of chronic colitis. Multiple fecal analyses should be pursued but may yield negative results despite infection (intermittent shedding). Monitoring the initial response to two courses of anthelminthic treatment (2 weeks apart), even with negative fecal analysis results, is an important step before pursuing costly diagnostics for any patient with solitary signs of intermittent large-bowel diarrhea.

Differential Diagnosis

- *Capillaria* spp infection (ova appear similar, but *Capillaria* spp do not cause enteritis)
- Dietary-responsive large-bowel diarrhea
- *Clostridium perfringens* enterotoxicosis
- Inflammatory bowel disease (large intestine)
- Chronic colitis (e.g., histiocytic ulcerative colitis)
- Eosinophilic colitis
- Histoplasmosis (large bowel)
- Neoplasia (carcinoma, lymphoma)
- Hypoadrenocorticism
- Protein-losing enteropathy
- Intussusception

Initial Database

- Serial fecal flotations to identify characteristic eggs (shed intermittently, often in low numbers). Dense flotation solution (specific gravity > 1.200, such as for sugar or zinc sulfate) is required.
- CBC: occasional eosinophilia and mild to moderate anemia
- Serum biochemistry profile: hyponatremia, hyperkalemia, azotemia, hypoalbuminemia, metabolic acidosis are occasionally seen.
- Rectal cytologic exam (p. 1157): insensitive for ova but may demonstrate clostridial spores, inflammatory cells, neoplastic cells, or fungal (*Histoplasma*) organisms
- Measuring basal cortisol concentration and following with ACTH response testing if basal cortisol is < 2 mcg/dL is recommended to rule out hypoadrenocorticism in dogs with hyponatremia and hyperkalemia (pp. 572 and 1300).

Advanced or Confirmatory Testing

An ELISA is available for coproantigen detection and offers a more cost-effective alternative than finding on colonoscopy.

TREATMENT

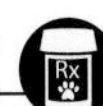

Treatment Overview

Therapeutic goal is elimination of parasites from the GI tract. Three treatments are needed to completely eliminate parasites due to prepatency period.

Acute General Treatment

- Anthelmintic therapy
  - Fenbendazole 50 mg/kg PO q 24h × 3 days is preferred.
  - Febantel 10 mg/kg PO q 24h × 3 days is an acceptable alternative.
  - Drontal Plus (contains febantel) is also appropriate.
- Current recommendations are to repeat treatment at 3 weeks and 3 months due to the long prepatent period and possibility of larval resistance.
- Supportive care (e.g., intravenous fluids) for electrolyte abnormalities and azotemia in severe cases
- Typhlectomy for granulomatous typhlitis or cecocolic intussusception (rare)

Chronic Treatment

Milbemycin oxime is an effective preventive for chronic, recurrent trichuriasis.

Drug Interactions

Dogs should be evaluated for heartworm infection before instituting milbemycin oxime.

Possible Complications

Possible adverse reaction with milbemycin oxime in heartworm-positive dogs

Recommended Monitoring

Frequent fecal exams for recurrent infections

PROGNOSIS & OUTCOME

- Excellent with appropriate therapy
- Reinfection likely as a result of environmental contamination with resistant ova.

PEARLS & CONSIDERATIONS

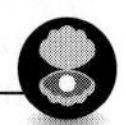

Comments

- *T. vulpis* is a common cause of large-bowel diarrhea in dogs in the eastern and southern United States.
- Empirical treatment is recommended in uncomplicated cases before pursuing a lengthy, expensive diagnostic workup.
- The potential for hypoadrenocorticism-like findings with trichuriasis must be recognized.
- Seizures have been reported in dogs with trichuriasis, most likely associated with profound hyponatremia.

Prevention

- Monthly administration of antiparasite products incorporating milbemycin oxime as a component is ideal in endemic areas and for chronic infections due to contaminated environments. These combination antiparasite medications often have the advantage of also preventing infection with *Dirofilaria immitis* and other endoparasites and ectoparasites.
- Moxidectin-containing antiparasite combinations can prevent *T. vulpis*, *Dirofilaria immitis*, and endoparasite and ectoparasite infections.
- In field trials, the cyclooctadepsipeptide emodepside has been effective against adult and immature forms of *T. vulpis* and other intestinal nematodes and cestodes.

Technician Tips

Characteristic microscopic appearance is large, ovoid, golden brown eggs with an operculum on each end. Eggs are heavy but can be found on fecal float using dense flotation solution (>1.020).

Client Education

Environmental contamination is the source for reinfection and is difficult to eliminate. Monthly prophylaxis is recommended after treatment.

SUGGESTED READING

Hall EJ: Diseases of the large intestine. In Ettinger SJ, et al, editors: Textbook of veterinary internal medicine, ed 8, St. Louis, 2017, Saunders, pp 1565-1592.

AUTHOR: Saralyn Smith-Carr, DVM, PhD, DACVIM
EDITOR: Rance K. Sellon, DVM, PhD, DACVIM

Xylitol Toxicosis

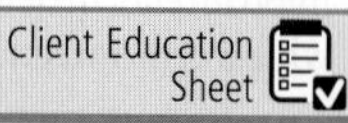

BASIC INFORMATION

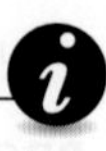

Definition

Xylitol is a 5-carbon sugar alcohol used as a sweetener in gums, candies, confectionery/baked goods, some peanut butters, and in some medications. Toxicosis is characterized by hypoglycemia leading to weakness, ataxia, lethargy, disorientation and seizures within minutes to hours after ingestion. Hepatotoxicosis can occur in 12-48 hours in some dogs and may be idiosyncratic (individual susceptibility). Toxicosis has been fatal in some dogs.

Synonyms

- Xylite, eutrit, newtol, xyliton
- Chemical names: 1,2,3,4,5-pentapentanol and 1,2,3,4,5-pentahydroxypentane
- Many sugar-free products contain xylitol as a sweetener.

Epidemiology

SPECIES, AGE, SEX

- Toxicosis has been documented in dogs only
- No known age, sex, or breed predisposition

RISK FACTORS

- Animals with pre-existing liver disease may be at increased risk for hepatotoxicosis.
- Young animals may be more prone to developing hypoglycemia.

Clinical Presentation

DISEASE FORMS/SUBTYPES

Xylitol toxicosis is an acute syndrome.

HISTORY, CHIEF COMPLAINT

- Evidence of chewed-up package; gum, or wrappers in vomitus/stool
- Vomiting, lethargy, weakness, disorientation, ataxia, seizures, typically 30 minutes to 12 hours after ingestion
- Some dogs develop hypoglycemia and acute liver failure. Other dogs do not show evidence of hypoglycemia but develop acute hepatic injury (p. 442) in 12-48 hours.

PHYSICAL EXAM FINDINGS

- Nonspecific lethargy, vomiting, weakness
- With marked hypoglycemia: ataxia, disorientation, seizures
- Evidence of bleeding disorder: petechiae, ecchymoses, gastrointestinal (GI) hemorrhage, oozing from venipuncture sites
- Vital signs (body temperature, respiratory rate and character, heart rate) are usually within normal range.

Etiology and Pathophysiology

- Toxicosis occurs acutely when dogs eat large amounts of xylitol-containing products.
- In humans, xylitol does not cause significant increase in insulin levels, but in dogs, xylitol causes a rapid and dose-dependent increase in blood insulin and concomitant hypoglycemia.
- Mechanism of hepatotoxicosis in dogs is unknown. Potential mechanisms include necrosis of hepatocytes due to adenosine triphosphate (ATP) depletion, resulting in cell necrosis; or production of reactive oxygen species, resulting in damage to cell membranes and macromolecules.

DIAGNOSIS

Diagnostic Overview

Diagnosis rests on history (observed or suspected ingestion), physical exam, and results of routine laboratory testing (hypoglycemia ± signs of acute liver injury +/− coagulopathy). No specific confirmatory test exists.

Differential Diagnosis

- Rule out other causes of hypoglycemia (p. 1240).
  - Toxicologic: insulin overdose, antidiabetic medications overdose (sulfonylureas)
  - Nontoxicologic: insulinoma, juvenile hypoglycemia, sepsis, others
- Rule out other causes of acute hepatic injury (p. 442).
  - Toxicologic: acetaminophen, blue-green algae, sago palm, hepatotoxic mushrooms, zinc phosphide, mycotoxin (aflatoxins), nonsteroidal antiinflammatory drug (NSAID) toxicosis
  - Nontoxicologic: bacterial hepatitis, idiopathic chronic hepatopathy, viral hepatitis, leptospirosis, others

Initial Database

- CBC: ± thrombocytopenia
- Serum biochemistry profile
  - Hypoglycemia (mild to severe; lowest reported is 26 mg/dL [1.5 mmol/L])
  - Increased liver enzymes (e.g., alanine aminotransferase [ALT]: 1000 to > 10,000 IU/L; normal < 120 IU/L)
  - Hyperbilirubinemia common (mean, 4.1 mg/dL; normal, < 0.6 mg/dL)
- Coagulation panel (if elevated liver enzymes)
  - Prothrombin time (PT) often elevated (36 to > 100 seconds)
  - Activated partial thromboplastin time (aPTT) markedly elevated (>100 seconds)

Advanced or Confirmatory Testing

Necropsy findings include icterus, hepatic necrosis, peritoneal and GI petechiae, and ecchymoses. Xylitol is metabolized quickly, and no residue is expected.

TREATMENT

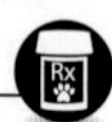

Treatment Overview

Mainstays of therapy are correction of hypoglycemia and addressing hepatotoxicity and coagulopathy. In asymptomatic animals exposed to a toxic dose, emesis can be induced if the exposure occurred within a few hours. The clinical presentation and evolution of the case determine treatment needs.

Acute General Treatment

- Decontamination of asymptomatic patient (p. 1087)
  - Induce vomiting (e.g., apomorphine [p. 1188]).
  - Do not give activated charcoal, which is not expected to be effective.
- Gastric lavage (p. 1117) is not typically recommended.
- Management of hypoglycemia and associated signs
  - 1-2 mL/kg of 50% dextrose (dilute in saline) bolus followed by 2 mL/kg/h IV; adjust according to blood glucose level. After blood glucose level is stable, continue to check q 2-4h.
  - Use oral source of dextrose (e.g., Karo syrup) to lick if dog is able to swallow; give small, frequent meals.
  - Seizures initially managed by normalizing blood glucose and/or addressing hepatic encephalopathy. Anticonvulsant drugs added if required (p. 903)
- Treat acute hepatic injury (p. 442). Consider *S*-adenosylmethionine (SAMe) or Denamarin q 8-12h for 24-48 hours. Use of *N*-acetylcysteine for 7 treatments may provide some benefits in preventing liver damage (same dose as used for acetaminophen toxicosis [p. 10]).
- Treat bleeding disorders.
  - Significant elevations in PT and/or aPTT (more than double, with or without overt bleeding): consider frozen or fresh-frozen plasma transfusion (p. 1169).
  - Hemorrhage addressed as appropriate (p. 433)

Chronic Treatment

SAMe 18 mg/kg PO q 24h for 1-3 months if evidence of hepatotoxicosis

Nutrition/Diet

- Karo syrup, honey, or corn syrup together with frequent feeding of small meals may be helpful initially for hypoglycemia.
- Optimal protein diet for liver damage

Drug Interactions

Metabolism and pharmacokinetic parameters of many medications can change due to liver damage. Dose adjustments should be made accordingly.

Possible Complications

- Coagulopathy secondary to acute liver failure and/or disseminated intravascular coagulation
- Hepatic encephalopathy (p. 440)
- Hyperthermia secondary to seizures

Recommended Monitoring

- Monitor blood glucose every 2-4 hours for 12-24 hours in all patients (whether showing overt signs of hypoglycemia or not).
- Recheck serum biochemistry profile (liver enzyme levels) at 24 hours. If elevated, monitor until they return to normal.
- Recheck coagulation profile at 24 hours if liver enzymes elevated. Monitor until return to normal.
- Neurologic signs of hypoglycemia

PROGNOSIS & OUTCOME

For dogs with hypoglycemia but no hepatic necrosis, prognosis is excellent. Guarded if hepatic necrosis and coagulopathy develops.

PEARLS & CONSIDERATIONS

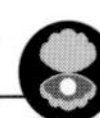

Comments

- Hypoglycemia can occur at xylitol dosages of > 100 mg/kg.
- Hepatotoxicity typically occurs at dosages > 500 mg/kg.
- Amount of xylitol in gums and candies varies widely; sugar-free gums can contain as little as 1 mg of xylitol per piece, and some brands may contain up to 2 g per piece.
- Some medications (liquids and chewables), rinses, toothpastes, foods (peanut butter, barbeque sauce), and throat lozenges may also contain xylitol (variable amounts).
- Sorbitol, mannitol, erythritol, or maltitol syrup present in some sugar-free products is not expected to induce hypoglycemia or liver damage in dogs.
- Splenda (sucralose), Sweet'n Low (saccharin, dextrose, and cream of tartar), and Equal (aspartame, dextrose, and maltodextrin) do not contain xylitol.

Prevention

Keep xylitol-containing products out of reach of dogs.

Technician Tips

Label may provide information on the amount of xylitol or other sugar-free alcohols in the product. In some cases, the label may be necessary because the same brand and similarly named products may be made with or without xylitol.

Client Education

Keep xylitol-containing gum, baked goods, oral hygiene products, and other sources away from dogs.

SUGGESTED READING

DuHadway MR, et al: Retrospective evaluation of xylitol ingestion in dogs: 192 cases (2007-2012). J Vet Emerg Crit Care 25:646-654, 2015.

AUTHOR: Irina D. Meadows, DVM, DABT
EDITOR: Tina Wismer, DVM, MS, DABT, DABVT

Zinc Phosphide Intoxication

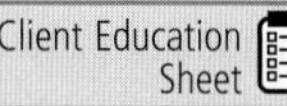

BASIC INFORMATION

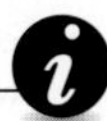

Definition

Zinc phosphide is a metallophosphide rodenticide available as 0.5%-10% bait. Acute toxicosis occurs from ingestion of bait and is characterized by vomiting (± blood), lethargy, respiratory distress, muscle tremors, seizures, and death.

Synonyms

Gopher or mole killer; Zn_3P_2, trizinc diphosphide

Epidemiology

SPECIES, AGE, SEX

All species are susceptible; dogs are more frequently involved.

GENETICS, BREED PREDISPOSITION

Animals that do not vomit are at greater risk for toxic effects.

CONTAGION AND ZOONOSIS

Public health significance to veterinary personnel and owners: human inhalation of phosphine gas can occur during decontamination or spontaneous emesis (risk of pulmonary and other effects in humans). The typical garlic or dead fish odor of phosphine may not be detectable at low but hazardous concentrations for humans. If handling a phosphine-intoxicated animal, ensure good ventilation, and contact human poison control (1-800-222-1222) if a human exposure has occurred (see Acute General Treatment below).

GEOGRAPHY AND SEASONALITY

Increased incidence during greater rodent activity and mobility after harvest

Clinical Presentation

HISTORY, CHIEF COMPLAINT

- History of exposure
- Vomiting with or without blood
- Agitation, abdominal discomfort
- Vocalization, teeth grinding
- Dyspnea
- Muscle tremors, seizure

PHYSICAL EXAM FINDINGS

As above, with potential of harsh lung sounds and crackles (due to pulmonary edema), cranial abdominal pain, cardiac arrhythmias, shock, slight garlic or rotten fish odor

Etiology and Pathophysiology

Source:

- Baits are available as commercial grain-based pellets, tracking powders, or paste (Sweeney's Poison Peanuts Mole and Gopher Bait, Dexol Gopher Killer Pellets, ZP Rodent Bait).

Mechanism of toxicosis:

- Onset of clinical signs in most cases is 15 minutes to 4 hours after ingestion; occasionally delayed up to 18 hours.
- Corrosive effects of zinc phosphide can cause signs of cranial abdominal (gastric) pain and bloody vomiting.
- Gastric acid hydrolysis of zinc phosphide liberates highly toxic phosphine gas, which is rapidly absorbed by passive diffusion.
- Phosphine disrupts cellular respiration by interfering with electron transport (cytochrome *c*) in the mitochondria, leading to cellular hypoxia, generation of reactive oxygen species, and lipid peroxidation, especially in tissues with high oxygen demand.
- Death is from cardiac arrest most commonly resulting from hypotensive shock, seizures, and pulmonary compromise.

DIAGNOSIS

Diagnostic Overview

Tentative diagnosis is based on history of exposure and clinical signs because timely testing is not available. Characteristic rotten fish or garlic smell supports diagnosis but poses risk of pulmonary toxicosis to humans. Diagnosis is confirmed by presence of zinc phosphide in the stomach contents, liver, or kidney (collect samples in airtight jar) by a diagnostic laboratory.

Differential Diagnosis

- Toxic: strychnine, metaldehyde, organophosphate or carbamate insecticides, arsenic
- Other: primary central nervous system (CNS) disease (e.g., neoplasia, encephalitis), hepatic encephalopathy

Initial Database

- Chest radiographs: pulmonary edema
- Acid-base status: respiratory and metabolic acidosis
- Electrocardiogram (ECG [p. 1096]): arrhythmias, nonspecific evidence of myocardial ischemia (e.g., ST-segment elevation or depression)
- Baseline CBC and serum chemistries generally unremarkable but decreased Mg^{2+}, Ca^{2+} possible
- Coagulation profile

Advanced or Confirmatory Testing

Freeze gastric contents, vomitus, liver, and kidney in airtight containers for zinc phosphide analysis at a diagnostic laboratory.

TREATMENT

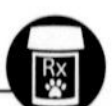

Treatment Overview

Because of human health risk of phosphine gas, owners or veterinary staff should decontaminate asymptomatic patients only in a well-ventilated area (outside if possible). Additional treatment is implemented based on the occurrence of signs: seizure control, treatment of noncardiogenic pulmonary edema, and supportive care to minimize or prevent renal/hepatic failure, while protecting the veterinarians and staff.

Acute General Treatment

- Reduce liberation of phosphine gas.
  - Magnesium hydroxide 10-60 mL/ANIMAL PO before presentation and vomiting induction can increase gastric pH. A commonly available preparation of magnesium hydroxide is Milk of Magnesia.
- Decontamination of patient (p. 1087)
  - Emesis (p. 1188) is indicated in patients not showing clinical signs. Apomorphine is preferred 0.04 mg/kg IM or IV or part of a crushed tablet dissolved in water instilled into conjunctival sac. NOTE: Use of 3% hydrogen peroxide 1-2 mL/kg PO (maximum of 45 mL/DOG) is not contraindicated for dogs, but it is possible that its use may enhance liberation of phosphine gas; weigh pros and cons before using in well-ventilated area, if at all.
  - Gastric lavage (p. 1117) can be risky due to public health hazard. Place a cuffed endotracheal tube. Consider only in patients in which emesis cannot be induced (comatose/obtunded animal). Use magnesium hydroxide as lavage fluid (use of water can increase phosphine liberation).
- Control seizures with one of the following:
  - Diazepam 0.5-2 mg/kg IV; repeat as needed
  - Pentobarbital 10-30 mg/kg IV to effect and repeat as needed or phenobarbital 3-30 mg/kg IV to effect
  - Propofol up to 3-6 mg/kg slow IV to effect, then constant-rate IV infusion 0.1-0.6 mg/kg/min titrated to effect
- Stabilize respiratory, cardiovascular, and neuromuscular systems.
  - Supplemental oxygen (p. 1146)
    - Place endotracheal tube if needed, with proper gas evacuation
    - If needed, positive-pressure ventilation (p. 1185)
  - Treat hypovolemic shock with crystalloid or colloid fluids; give one-fourth of crystalloid shock dose initially, and repeat as needed based on hemodynamic parameters up to the maximum shock dose (80-90 mL/kg/h for dogs, 40-60 mL/kg/h for cats). Synthetic colloid dose is approximately 20 mL/kg/d for dogs and 10-20 mL/kg/d for cats (adjust based on case parameters).
  - Monitor acid-base status, and correct metabolic or respiratory acidosis as needed.
  - Monitor electrolytes; correct any deficiency (Ca^{2+}, Mg^{2+}, and K^{+}).
- Gastrointestinal supportive care
  - Antiemetics: maropitant 0.5-1 mg/kg SQ q 24h
  - Gastroprotectants: omeprazole 0.5-1 mg/kg PO q 12-24h; sucralfate 0.25-1 g PO q 8-12h
  - Monitor serum biochemistry profiles for 72 hours for delayed hepatic and renal injury.
- Exogenous scavengers
  - *N*-acetylcysteine reduced liver injury in humans; loading dose 140-280 mg/kg PO or slow IV, then 70 mg/kg PO q 6h for six treatments.

Possible Complications

Renal, pulmonary, cardiac, and/or hepatic compromise; death

Recommended Monitoring

Closely monitor vital signs and basic chemistry parameters for 72 hours after exposure.

PROGNOSIS & OUTCOME

- Good for animals not showing clinical signs 8-16 hours after exposure
- Guarded to poor if cardiac arrhythmias, shock, or pulmonary edema develop; death usually within 6 hours
- Fair to good for cases surviving 24 hours

PEARLS & CONSIDERATIONS

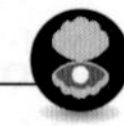

Comments

- Early vomiting (self-decontamination) may reduce risk of serious toxicosis in dogs.
- Human inhalation of phosphine off-gas during decontamination procedures is hazardous. Typical garlic/dead fish odor of phosphine may not be detectable at low but hazardous concentrations for humans.
- Baits may retain potency for 3 years in a dry environment.
- Toxic dose in dogs and cats is 20-40 mg/kg.
  - One tablespoon of 2% pellet bait contains approximately 180 mg of zinc phosphide, a significant risk for a 10-kg dog.
- Delayed hepatic or renal injury is possible 48-72 hours after exposure.
- Fumigants aluminum phosphide and magnesium phosphide are similar to zinc phosphide in toxicity.

Technician Tips

- As with any toxicosis, having the owner bring the container can confirm active ingredients (label and/or brand name search). Technicians who speak to owners on the telephone should encourage them to bring containers. Technicians should also recommend the owner take immediate measures to reduce phosphine gas if such exposure possible (see Acute General Treatment above).
- Do not wash vomitus down drain because water will liberate phosphine gas. Double-bag and dispose of vomitus in the trash.

Client Education

- Keep all baits away from dogs.
- Dogs can dig into mole/gopher holes and retrieve the bait in the yard/garden.

SUGGESTED READING

Knight MW: Zinc phosphide. In Peterson ME, et al, editors: Small animal toxicology, ed 3, St. Louis, 2013, Saunders, pp 853-864.

AUTHOR & EDITOR: Tina Wismer, DVM, MS, DABVT, DABT

Zinc Toxicosis

Client Education Sheet

BASIC INFORMATION

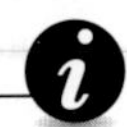

Definition

Syndrome occurs after ingestion of zinc-containing objects such as U.S. pennies minted after 1982, scrap metal pieces, galvanized wire, and hardware (e.g., washers, nuts). Clinical signs consist of acute gastrointestinal (GI) irritation, hemolysis, and/or possible renal, pancreatic and hepatic injury.

Epidemiology

SPECIES, AGE, SEX

Toxicosis is reported mostly for dogs (all breeds, any age, either sex) from ingesting zinc-containing objects. Birds are frequently exposed by chewing on galvanized wire cages, chains, and other sources.

Clinical Presentation

HISTORY, CHIEF COMPLAINT

- Inappetence, lethargy, protracted vomiting, diarrhea
- Dark-colored urine
- An animal may vomit or pass metallic objects in the feces.

PHYSICAL EXAM FINDINGS

- Abdominal discomfort/pain on palpation
- Pale mucous membranes
- Tachycardia, tachypnea, soft systolic murmur
- Icterus
- Discolored urine (hemoglobinuria)

Etiology and Pathophysiology

Source:

- Metallic zinc is used in galvanizing, welding, and soldering. Zinc salts are used as astringents, antiseptics, deodorants, wood preservatives, pigments, and insecticides. Zinc gluconate is ≈14% elemental zinc and often found in cough drops. Zinc oxide (10%-40%) is found in ointments, diaper rash creams, and sunblocks or sunscreens.
- U.S. pennies minted after 1982 weigh 2.5 g and are 97.6% zinc and 2.4% copper; 1982 pennies have various zinc contents, and pennies minted earlier have negligible zinc content. Canadian pennies made between 1997 and 2001 are 96% zinc and 4% copper.

Mechanism of toxicosis:

- Toxicosis occurs when zinc-containing objects are retained in the GI tract. Zinc leaches from metallic objects in an acidic pH of the stomach. Zinc is absorbed into the bloodstream, leading to oxidative damage to the erythrocytes and hemolysis.
- Zinc also causes direct GI mucosal irritation.

DIAGNOSIS

Diagnostic Overview

Suspicion of zinc toxicosis arises in one of three contexts: observed ingestion or vomiting/defecation of metallic objects; incidental finding of metallic object on abdominal palpation or radiography; or investigation of hemolytic anemia. Zinc levels can confirm toxicosis.

Differential Diagnosis

- Other substances causing oxidative injury: onions/garlic, acetaminophen, mothballs (naphthalene), local anesthetics
- Immune-mediated hemolytic anemia
- Tick-borne diseases
- Microangiopathic hemolysis (p. 59)
- Other causes of hemolysis (e.g., hypophosphatemia, hemolytic-uremic syndrome)

Initial Database

- CBC: regenerative anemia, Heinz bodies, hemoglobinemia, reticulocytosis, spherocytosis; neutrophilic leukocytosis
  - Regenerative response requires days to begin but is usually present by the time zinc-related anemia is detected.
- Serum biochemistry profile: elevation in serum bilirubin, liver enzymes, amylase, lipase, azotemia (if pigment nephropathy occurs)
- Urinalysis: hemoglobinuria, bilirubinuria, proteinuria
- Radiography to look for metallic object

Advanced or Confirmatory Testing

Definitive diagnosis depends on blood or tissue zinc levels:

- For blood collection, use special tubes (royal blue–top tube) and syringes without rubber grommets. Do not use traditional syringes, rubber grommets, and Vacutainer tubes, because the rubberized surfaces contain zinc.
- Toxic levels in dogs
  - Serum: 10-54 ppm (adequate levels 0.7-2 ppm)
  - Whole blood: 45 ppm has been fatal
  - Liver: 130-436 ppm (adequate levels 30-70 ppm)
  - Kidney: 175-295 ppm (adequate levels 16-30 ppm)
  - Urine: 10-25 ppm (adequate levels 2-5 ppm)

TREATMENT

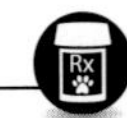

Treatment Overview

Life-threatening abnormalities must be identified and managed first. Severe anemia may require transfusion, pigment nephropathy (potentially resulting in acute kidney injury) should be addressed with intravenous fluids, and GI tract irritation may require treatment with antiemetics and GI protectants. After the patient is stabilized, the source of zinc should be removed from the GI tract. General supportive care is indicated during recovery. Chelation with calcium EDTA, dimercaprol, or D-penicillamine is rarely needed after the source of zinc has been removed.

Acute General Treatment

Management of life-threatening abnormalities if present:

- Anemia: if severe (e.g., hematocrit < 20% and/or clinical signs present), consider blood transfusion (p. 1169).
- Azotemia if concurrent with severe hemolysis: IV fluid therapy (e.g., 90-130 mL/kg/h, barring pre-existing heart disease [p. 23])
- Removal of zinc source from GI tract: endoscopy or gastrotomy
- Emesis (p. 1188): only if metallic object recognized in stomach in the absence of clinical signs related to intoxication (e.g., witnessed consumption)
- Because an acidic environment is needed for zinc absorption, antacids, H2-blockers, and/or proton pump inhibitors given soon after ingestion can decrease the stomach pH and therefore decrease the amount of zinc available for absorption. Activated charcoal is not indicated because like most metals, zinc is not adsorbed well.
- Early and sustained use of antacids until source is removed (calcium carbonate 70-185 mg/kg/day PO) and/or H2-blockers (famotidine 0.5-1 mg/kg PO q 12-24h) to decrease leaching and absorption of zinc

Chelation therapy: most cases of zinc poisoning do not require chelation therapy. Animals with zinc toxicosis usually respond well to fluid therapy and other supportive measures after the source of zinc has been removed. Serum zinc concentrations, clinical condition, hydration status, organ function, and whether the source of zinc is removed should be considered before deciding to chelate. In the rare case that requires chelation, options for chelation therapy include

- Calcium EDTA (6.6% solution = 66 mg/mL) in dogs: dilute to 10 mg CaEDTA/mL in 5% dextrose and give 25 mg/kg SQ at different sites q 6h for 2-5 days. Do not exceed 2 g/day, maximum of 5 consecutive days. In cats: give 27.5 mg/kg in 15 mL of 5% dextrose SQ q 6h for 5 days. Use with caution and monitoring because of risk of nephrotoxicosis, *or*
- Dimercaprol: 2-4 mg/kg SQ or IM q 8-12h for 2 days, *or*
- D-penicillamine: 110 mg/kg/day PO, divided q 6-8h for 1-2 weeks

Supportive care:

- IV fluids
- Control vomiting with maropitant 1 mg/kg SQ q 24h or 2 mg/kg PO q 24h for 5 days, or metoclopramide 0.2-0.5 mg/kg SQ q 8h if needed, provided GI obstruction is ruled out.

Possible Complications

Liver, pancreatic, and renal compromise

Recommended Monitoring

- CBC, serum biochemistry profile: packed cell volume (PCV), bilirubin, renal, pancreatic and liver values for 1-3 days or until resolution of signs
- Urinalysis (daily for resolution of pigmenturia)

PROGNOSIS & OUTCOME

- Good with supportive care after removing the source
- Poor if there is evidence of multiple organ system damage or failure (liver, kidney, and/or pancreas)

PEARLS & CONSIDERATIONS

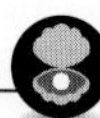

Comments

- Toxicosis is unlikely if zinc-containing objects move out of the GI tract quickly.
- The hematologic and clinical findings in animals with zinc toxicosis are similar to those found for immune-mediated hemolytic anemia (IMHA).
- U.S. dimes, nickels, and quarters do not contain significant amounts of zinc, so systemic zinc toxicosis is not expected from ingestion of these coins.
- The greatest amounts of zinc accumulate in blood, liver, kidney, skin, lung, brain, heart, and pancreas. Excretion of zinc occurs through bile and pancreatic secretions.
- Zinc toxicosis can cause a positive direct antiglobulin test (Coombs' test) result. Coombs' testing is not a reliable method of differentiating IMHA from zinc toxicosis.

Technician Tips

- Some radiopaque objects such as bismuth subsalicylate tablets (Pepto-Bismol) can resemble coins. Verify with client that medications have not been administered to the pet.
- Zinc gluconate cough/cold drops such as Cold Eeze rarely cause more than mild, self-limited GI upset.

SUGGESTED READING

Talcott PA: Zinc. In Peterson ME, et al, editors: Small animal toxicology, ed 3, St. Louis, 2013, Saunders, pp 847-885.

AUTHOR: Charlotte Means, DVM, MLIS, DABVT, DABT
EDITOR: Tina Wismer, DVM, MS, DABVT, DABT

SECTION II

Procedures and Techniques

EDITORS

Mark S. Thompson
DVM, DABVP

Leah A. Cohn
DVM, PhD, DACVIM (SAIM)

This section, Procedures and Techniques, presents approximately 150 different diagnostic and therapeutic interventions. The difficulty level is denoted as one diamond ◆ to three diamonds ◆◆◆. Techniques designated as ◆ are described in enough detail that a veterinarian should be able to open the book and complete the task immediately. At the other extreme, procedures designated as ◆◆◆ provide the practitioner with the type of "need to know" information that will facilitate client conversations before referral for more specialized care. Techniques designated as ◆◆ are very doable but might take a bit of practice with a more experienced colleague. Variants and alternatives exist for virtually all of them, and not every patient can undergo the exact same approach. The clinician should remember that written, informed consent should be provided by the animal's owner for virtually all of these, and many applicable consent forms can be found in associated online materials.

NOTE: The unit of measure of micron, sometimes denoted by the Greek letter μ, is abbreviated in this text by mc. For example, 1 mcL = 1 microliter; 1 mcg = 1 microgram.

Synonyms

Other names by which the procedure is known

Overview and Goal

An extremely brief summary of how the procedure is carried out (overview) and the intended result (goal)

Indications

The diseases and disorders for which a procedure should be considered

Contraindications

Diseases and disorders that the procedure could make worse. In the presence of such a disease or disorder, the procedure cannot safely be performed and must be withheld (absolute contraindication) or should only be considered if no other suitable alternatives exist (relative contraindication).

Equipment, Anesthesia

The equipment and materials required to perform the procedure, and whether the patient needs to be anesthetized, sedated, or neither (awake)

Anticipated Time

The expected duration of the procedure, including basic set-up, when performed by an experienced clinician skilled in carrying it out

Preparation: Important Checkpoints

Milestones encountered during preparation that can be overlooked, undervalued, or otherwise missed

Possible Complications and Common Errors to Avoid

In the author's experience, certain steps in a procedure have recurrently led to mistakes or oversights. This information is highlighted here as a precautionary step.

Procedure

The step-by-step description of how to perform the procedure

Postprocedure

Important steps to take after the procedure has been completed, typically to reduce complications and improve patient safety

Alternatives and Their Relative Merits

Other procedures that have similar goals and may be better suited in certain cases than the one being described

Pearls

Observations, pitfalls, and other items of critical information that the author has found to be most important regarding the procedure

Abdominocentesis

Difficulty level: ◆

Synonyms

Paracentesis, abdominal tap

Overview and Goal

Obtain abdominal fluid samples for diagnostic purposes.

Indications

- Abdominal distention with fluid wave
- Ultrasound (US)–identified free abdominal fluid
- Can be combined with abdominal drainage for relief of physical pressure due to ascites (p. 79)

Contraindications

- Coagulopathies (p. 1325); relative contraindication and benefit may outweigh small risk
- Abdominal distention due to mass or organomegaly rather than fluid

Equipment, Anesthesia

- +/− US unit (helpful for small volume or isolated fluid pockets)
- Sterile gloves
- Chlorhexidine scrub and solution
- If only diagnostic sampling planned: 22-gauge × 1-inch needle and 6- to 10-mL syringe
- If diagnostic procedure combined with therapeutic abdominal drainage:
  - Intravenous (IV) catheter or butterfly catheter set (depends on size of patient and amount of fluid)
  - Extension set
  - 3-way stopcock
  - Syringe (size depends on patient and amount of fluid)
  - Bowl for waste fluids
- Sample tubes (red top, purple top)
- +/− sedation, depends on patient's disposition

Anticipated Time

5-15 minutes

Preparation: Important Checkpoints

- Assess patient's risk of coagulopathy.
- If in doubt based on exam, confirm presence of abdominal fluid with US.
- Have supplies at the ready.

Possible Complications and Common Errors to Avoid

- Failure to obtain sample: use US guidance
- Potential laceration of visceral organs
  - Restrict needle movement to in-and-out motion, with minimal side-to-side motion
  - Use US guidance if small fluid volume
- Subcutaneous fluid accumulation: minor complication, typically resolves spontaneously

Procedure

- Positioning depends on patient comfort, temperament, and fluid volume. For large volume of fluid, lateral recumbency commonly used if animal is comfortable. Otherwise, standing allows fluid to pool ventrally but requires extra attention to restraint.
- Clip hair and aseptically prep site, typically selecting ventral aspect of the abdominal midline close to the umbilicus. Other sites may be chosen if US guidance is used to find isolated fluid pocket.
- If planning to remove a large volume: select appropriate catheter size for the patient and the amount of fluid to be obtained. With sterile gloves and technique, attach the extension set to the catheter on one end and the 3-way stopcock on the other for the syringe to attach to. An assistant may be necessary to aspirate.
  - If using an IV catheter, the stylet should be removed after insertion through the abdominal wall to prevent any lacerations of other organs. However, this may make it difficult to pull copious amounts of fluid, especially if using a small catheter. A butterfly catheter may be used for a shorter needle size.
- For diagnostic samples: connect syringe to needle
- Advance needle through the skin and body wall at an oblique angle with the needle pointing craniad (i.e., needle is not inserted straight in perpendicular to abdomen). Aspirate fluid and collect into a red and purple top for diagnostic tests.
- Remove the needle following the same direction as it was inserted; the oblique angle allows the tissue to close over the track.
- Always document the amount of fluid that has been removed, including a detailed description of the fluid.

Postprocedure

- Submit fluid for analysis (p. 1343). In addition to cytology, cell count, and total protein, other assays can include hematocrit, creatinine, potassium, triglyceride, culture, or polymerase chain reaction (PCR), depending on clinical suspicion.
- Monitor patient for subcutaneous fluid accumulation around collection site. An abdominal wrap may be placed if this occurs, being aware of patient's respiratory effort.

Alternatives and Their Relative Merits

- Abdominal drainage: to remove large volume of abdominal fluid that compromises patient comfort or respiration. Aliquots can be submitted for fluid analysis.
- Diagnostic peritoneal lavage: to retrieve diagnostic samples of small amounts of abdominal fluid. Often requires sedation and not always a guaranteed sample collection.

AUTHOR: Savanah Smith, RVT

EDITORS: Leah A. Cohn, DVM, PhD, DACVIM; Mark S. Thompson, DVM, DABVP

Acupuncture

Bonus Material Online

Difficulty level: 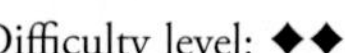

Overview and Goal

- Acupuncture may be used in concert with other methods of integrative pain management for the control of acute or chronic pain.
- Many clinicians report that acupuncture resolves the clinical problem or serves well as a maintenance therapy for a lifelong condition in ≈80% of cases.
- There are indications for the use of acupuncture as an adjunct treatment for specific visceral organ diseases.
- The many different techniques (e.g., heat, needles, laser, implant) used for stimulating an acupuncture point may be a source of confusion. Each method has its purpose and particular virtues in a given clinical setting.
- Several neurophysiologic mechanisms describe acupuncture effects. Spinal gates, central nervous system (CNS) endorphin release, and viscerocutaneous reflex arcs are a few of them.
- There are four different schools of acupuncture thought: *traditional Chinese medicine*

(TCM), *the eight principles, medical-empirical,* and *bioelectric acupuncture*. All systems use the same needles and insert them into the same acupuncture points. Differences in clinical outcome among these methodologies are difficult to measure and appear to be slight.

- The standards for education and certification in animal acupuncture are well established. Referral for this treatment should be to a veterinarian with appropriate credentials from the International Veterinary Acupuncture Society or the Chi Institute.

Indications

- Chronic orthopedic pain, especially
  - Hip dysplasia (p. 469)
  - Cranial cruciate ligament injury (p. 218)
  - Elbow dysplasia (p. 288)
  - Other degenerative joint disease
- Postoperative (acute) pain
- Back pain (including nonsurgical intervertebral disc disease [IVDD]) (p. 555)
- Lumbosacral syndrome (p. 592)
- Canine epilepsy (p. 301)
- Asthma syndromes
- Demodectic mange (p. 244)
- Acral (lick) granuloma (p. 16)
- Malaise of chemotherapy
- Inflammatory bowel disease (p. 543)

NOTE: In the abstract, acupuncture is capable of influencing virtually any disease process or organ system. Although we may accept the theoretical basis for this point of view, there are numerous medical and practical reasons to avoid considering acupuncture as an isolated treatment modality. Acupuncture may be helpful as a treatment for hypothyroidism, for example, but thyroid supplementation is known to be successful, low cost, and safe.

Contraindications

- Pregnancy and tumors are often cited as relative contraindications. Use of acupuncture therapy in patients with these conditions should be reserved for clinicians with advanced knowledge of safe protocols.
- There are specific cautions for the use of electroacupuncture, which should be understood by practitioners who use this modality.

Equipment, Anesthesia

- Needles: 28-38 gauge, sterile, disposable, solid, acupuncture needles
- Microamperage electrostimulator
- Moxa (herbal product)
- Milliwatt diode laser equipment is useful for younger animals, birds, ferrets, and pocket pets.
- Anesthesia is not indicated; sedation is rarely needed.

Anticipated Time

- Varies from 15 to 60 minutes for each treatment session
- Particular problems may be resolved after a single treatment, but most will need 3-8 treatments.
- Maintenance treatments for chronic conditions (e.g., hip dysplasia, epilepsy) may be performed at intervals of 1-6 months.

Preparation: Important Checkpoints

- Acupuncture may be performed on the sedated or anesthetized patient, but this is seldom necessary and may cause more problems than it prevents.
- Physical restraint for needle placement is seldom required and can make future treatments more difficult.
- Quiet surroundings and the presence of the owner can provide reassurance, especially for cats.
- There is no requirement for preparation of the skin at the site of needle insertion, even in immunosuppressed patients.

Possible Complications and Common Errors to Avoid

- Clinically relevant complications of acupuncture in animals are rare, and patients do not require hospitalization.
- It is common for patients to experience somnolence for 12-24 hours after treatment.
- A stuck or "frozen" needle (resists removal) often occurs: this is easily resolved by further manipulation of the needle for a few minutes.
- Immediately after the first treatment, patients may show a transient increase in disease signs of the condition being treated.
- Concurrent use of pharmaceuticals is not a contraindication for acupuncture.
- Local infection or seizures occur in < 0.1% of patients.

Procedure

- Acupuncture is normally performed on an outpatient basis.
- Although some practitioners find simple (minimal) methods of restraint to be needed for some cases, most patients will be treated without forceful or unpleasant restraint.
- Most patients do not feel most needles; when they do, the clinician may elect to remove the needle.
- Needles remain in place for an average of 10-20 minutes before removal.
- Treatments are repeated at intervals of 24 hours to several weeks.
- After the appearance of a useful response to treatment in the patient, supportive or maintenance treatments may be needed in some cases, especially for chronic pain conditions in older animals.
- For a number of visceral organ, immune system, or dermatologic conditions and cases of back pain, maintenance treatments may not be required.

Postprocedure

- Other than occasional somnolence, there are few postprocedure considerations after routine acupuncture.
- In cases where acupuncture is intended to eventually replace medication, the clinician should anticipate this by gradual dose reduction of systemic analgesic or antiinflammatory drugs.

Alternatives and Their Relative Merits

- The relative merit of pharmaceutical alternatives varies widely with the disease being treated.
- For treatment of pain, nonsteroidal antiinflammatory drugs (NSAIDs) can be effective but carry the risk of adverse drug reactions in a significant percentage of patients.
- Treatment of chronic orthopedic pain is best accomplished with multimodal therapies, and the combination of a low-dose NSAID and acupuncture is often very effective and reduces the likelihood of renal or gastrointestinal injury from the use of NSAIDs alone.
- For conditions likely to persist for the rest of the patient's life (e.g., osteoarthritis), it may be appropriate to place a permanent implant in the acupuncture points that have been successful in treatment of the problem. For example, small rods or spheres of sterile metallic 0.999 gold are often used in this way for long-term treatment of degenerative joint disease.
- When acupuncture fails to provide adequate clinical results or cannot be continued for other reasons, it may be necessary to consider pharmaceutical or surgical options.

SUGGESTED READING

Han JS: Acupuncture and endorphins. Neurosci Lett 36:258-261, 2004.

AUTHOR: Arthur I. Ortenburger, DVM, MS
EDITORS: Leah A. Cohn, DVM, PhD, DACVIM; Mark S. Thompson, DVM, DABVP

Procedures and Techniques

Arterial Blood Sampling and Arterial Catheterization

Difficulty level: ♦♦

Synonym

Arterial phlebotomy

Overview and Goal

To access a peripheral artery with a needle or catheter for blood sampling or direct arterial blood pressure monitoring

Indications

- Collection of arterial blood sample for analysis (most frequently arterial blood gas analysis [ABG])
- Placement of an arterial catheter for direct blood pressure measurement (typically in critically ill or anesthetized animals)

Contraindications

Coagulopathy: recommend coagulation evaluation before procedure, assess patient for overt signs of bleeding, question client regarding prior history of bleeding

Equipment, Anesthesia

Arterial catheter: chemical restraint not typically required, although placement is most frequently done after induction in anesthetized patients.

- One to two assistants for restraint
- Hair clippers
- Sterile scrub material
- 6-10 3 × 3 gauze squares
- Arterial catheter (standard over-the-needle IV-type catheter)
  - Cats, dogs < 10 kg: 24 or 25 gauge
  - Dogs 10-25 kg: 22 gauge
  - Dogs > 25 kg: 20 gauge
- 22-gauge needle to nick skin
- White tape, 2-cm (1-inch) width
- Heparinized sterile saline flush
- T-port/male adapter
- 3-way stopcock
- Pressure transducer and monitor (if continuously monitoring direct arterial pressure)

For arterial blood sample:

- Hair clippers
- Sterile scrub material
- 1-mL heparinized syringe (commercial or prepared by coating syringe with heparin and expelling remaining liquid)
- 20-25–gauge needles (guidelines for size same as for arterial catheters, above)
- Rubber stopper
- +/− Ice bath

Anticipated Time

- 3-5 minutes (arterial blood sample)
- 10-15 minutes (arterial catheter)

Preparation: Important Checkpoints

- Make sure patient is adequately restrained and all materials are nearby.
- For animals with increased respiratory effort, have supplemental O_2 available.

Possible Complications and Common Errors to Avoid

- Discomfort during placement: consider lidocaine bleb in the skin where catheter will be introduced
- Hemorrhage/hematoma formation during attempted placement or if inadequate pressure is applied to the puncture site after procedure
- Thrombosis of the vessel (unlikely to cause clinically significant ischemia)
- Spasm of the vessel preventing future phlebotomy attempts
- Infection of the catheter/site
- Pre-existing hypotension may make vessel identification more challenging.
- Excessive pressure during vessel palpation may lessen pulse pressure and limit vessel identification.
- Obtaining a mixture of venous and arterial blood from adjacent vessels confounds blood gas analysis.

Procedure

Arterial blood sampling:

- Restrain patient in lateral recumbency with vessel to be used exposed, typically dorsal metatarsal or femoral artery.
- Clip hair in the region of the intended puncture site, and sterile scrub site.
- Palpate pulse with nondominant hand; use middle and index fingers to assess the anatomic course of the artery.
- Use heparinized syringe with needle size appropriate to patient (see above).
- At a 45-degree angle to the skin, advance the needle through the skin and into the artery (some prefer to keep the bevel of the needle pointing down for arterial puncture).
- When the artery has been punctured, a flashback of blood will be seen, and the syringe self-fills due to arterial pressure. Fill syringe to approximately 0.5 mL for ABG analysis.
- Apply direct pressure to the phlebotomy site until all hemorrhage has stopped (usually 5 minutes).
- Remove any air bubbles from syringe, and place open needle into rubber stopper.
- Immediately perform ABG, or place syringe in an ice bath.

Arterial catheter placement:

- The dorsal metatarsal artery is the most commonly used and is described in detail below. Femoral, auricular, metacarpal, lingual, and coccygeal arteries may also be used.
- Restrain, clip, and scrub as above. Clip the dorsal surface of distal hindlimb from hock to beginning of phalanges.
- Have assistant hold limb in extended position. Do not occlude flow to the vessel (hold off).
- Palpate pulse with index and middle fingers of nondominant hand to convincingly determine the anatomic course of the artery. The artery lies between the third and fourth metatarsal bones.
- Nick the skin only above the intended insertion site using the bevel of a hypodermic needle.
- Over-the-needle IV catheter (IVC) sized appropriate to patient (see above) is held in the dominant hand.

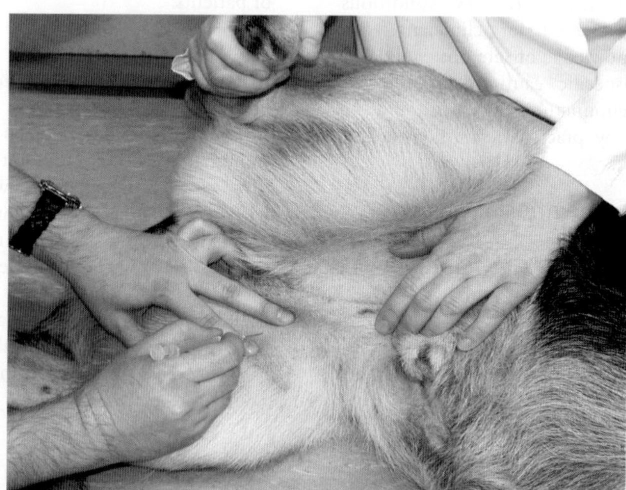

ARTERIAL BLOOD SAMPLING AND ARTERIAL CATHETERIZATION Blood sampling from femoral artery of a dog in left lateral recumbency. Cranial is to lower right. Assistant holds right hindlimb elevated and the prepuce retracted. Phlebotomist identifies course of left femoral artery between middle and index fingers by palpation of femoral pulse with both fingers and prepares to enter the artery, with the needle bevel down.

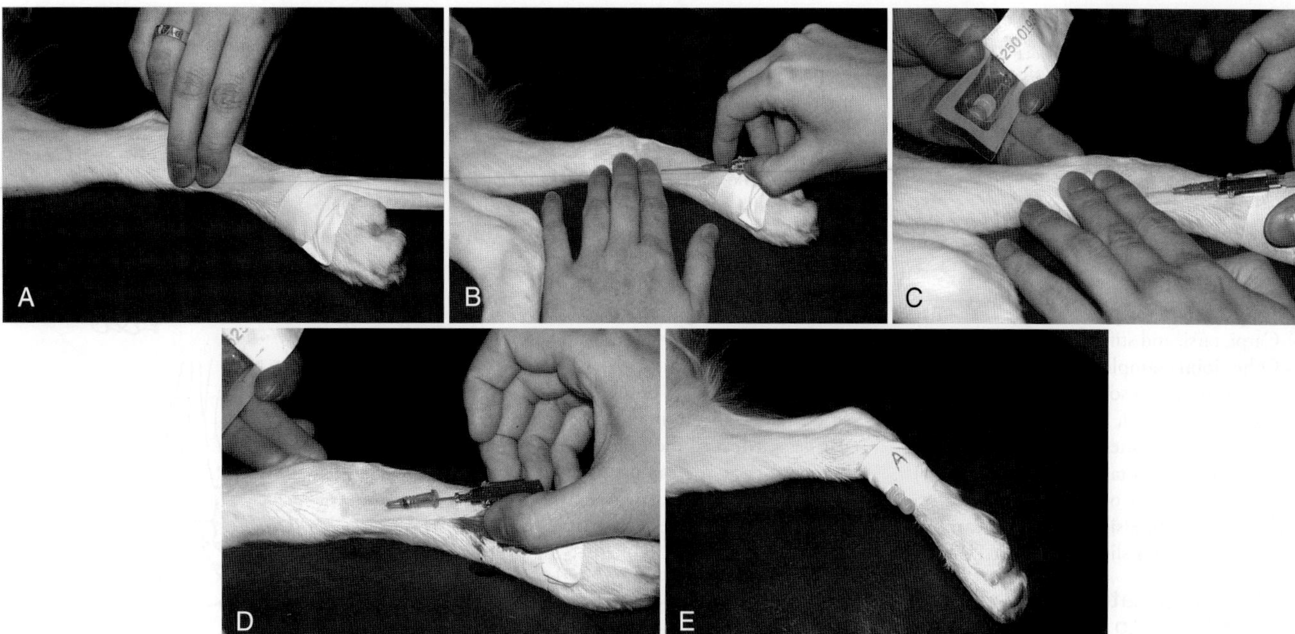

ARTERIAL BLOOD SAMPLING AND ARTERIAL CATHETERIZATION Placement of arterial catheter in a dog's right metatarsal artery. **A**, Palpation of arterial pulse. **B**, Introduction of catheter using right hand while simultaneously palpating arterial pulse for orientation using left hand (i.e., right-handed clinician). **C**, Flashback of blood confirms proper placement. **D**, Removal of stylet in preparation for placement of catheter cap. **E**, Capped catheter is flushed with heparinized saline, wrapped, and clearly marked as arterial.

- Insert IVC through the skin incision and into the artery at a 15-30–degree angle running parallel to the anatomic course (some prefer to keep the bevel of the needle pointing down for arterial puncture).
- When flashback or pulsatile flow (with open catheter) is seen, advance the catheter off the needle.
- Attach T-port and 3-way stopcock with male adapter.
- Flush with heparinized saline.
- Anchor to patient's leg using white tape. Clearly mark catheter and line as *arterial*.

Postprocedure

- Monitor for bleeding, inflammation, infection
- Ensure the catheter is not dislodged, or significant bleeding may ensue.
- Flush catheter after all blood draws; thrombosis/occlusion can occur.
- Label catheter clearly as arterial to prevent inadvertent injection of medications into the catheter, which could have dangerous complications.

Alternatives and Their Relative Merits

- Venous blood gas analysis
  - Technically easier to perform
  - PvO_2 less relevant
- Pulse oximetry
  - Noninvasive
  - Not always reliable
- Surgical cut-down procedure for arterial catheter placement
  - More invasive

SUGGESTED READING

Trim CM, et al: A survey of the use of arterial catheters in anesthetized dogs and cats: 267 cases. J Vet Emerg Crit Care 27:89-95, 2017.

AUTHOR: Lillian Good, DVM, DACVECC
EDITORS: Leah A. Cohn, DVM, PhD, DACVIM; Mark S. Thompson, DVM, DABVP

Arthrocentesis

Difficulty level: ♦♦

Synonyms

Joint aspirate, joint tap, synovial tap

Overview and Goal

A procedure to obtain a small amount of synovial (joint) fluid for diagnostic purposes, usually including cytologic evaluation ± bacterial culture

Indications

- Swollen joints (effusion)
- Painful joints unexplained by recognized orthopedic disease
- Stiff, stilted gait suggestive of polyarthritis (p. 803)
- Fever of unknown origin (p. 334)

Contraindications

Wound or pyoderma over the aspiration site; severe thrombocytopenia or coagulopathy

Equipment, Anesthesia

- Sedation usually required
- Clippers
- Gauze, alcohol and surgical scrub
- Microscope slides and #2 pencil for labeling
- 22-25 gauge needles (preferably plastic hub), at least one per joint
- 1-6 mL syringes, several
- Sterile gloves

- ± Red top tube, Culturette, or culture medium–containing vial
- ± Purple top tube for extra joint fluid

Anticipated Time

15-30 minutes

Preparation: Important Checkpoints

- Have patient fasted for sedation
- Choose joints to sample
  - For polyarthritis, typically sample 2-4 joints.
  - Carpi, tarsi, and stifles are most accessible.
  - Other joints sampled if there is a specific indication to do so (e.g., if a single joint is effusive/painful, it should be sampled)
  - Joint swelling often feels "puffy"; these spots are best to tap.
- Label slide and place on tray for quick access; include joint name/side (e.g., right carpus) and patient ID on slide label.

Possible Complications and Common Errors to Avoid

- Inability to retrieve fluid: effusive joints are best. May not be able to get sample from every joint
- Blood contamination of sample: release negative pressure before needle withdrawal. If gross blood contamination seen, sample another joint
- Hemarthrosis (rare with precautions): coagulopathy or < 40,000 platelets are contraindications.
- Introduction of bacteria (rare): aseptic technique is crucial
- Torn joint capsule (rare): sedation to prevent movement

Procedure

- While waiting for sedation to take effect, shave target joints, and perform preliminary skin cleaning.
- Don sterile gloves while an assistant performs aseptic skin prep on the joint. Keep glove wrapper clean to use as a sterile field.
- Carpus
  - Assistant should flex the carpus fully.
  - Palpate the cranial surface of the joint for a natural depression on the craniomedial aspect of the carpometacarpal or radiocarpal space, with the tendons of the extensor carpi radialis and common digital extensor on either side. Depending on the degree of joint effusion, this very small space (1-4 mm, depending on patient size) may be pushed out rather than a divot in.
- Tarsus (hock)
  - Assistant steadies the joint in a somewhat flexed position.
  - Medial and lateral access to the tarsal joint is available from the caudal aspect of the joint.
  - The lateral and medial malleoli of the distal tibia are palpated for a depression that occurs medial and caudal to each one. The depression is more or less sunken, depending on degree of effusion.
- Stifle
  - Assistant steadies the joint in a neutral position.
  - The joint is entered from the front to either medial or lateral side of the patellar tendon, directing the needle caudally toward the center of the tibial plateau.
- Place needle on syringe while maintaining sterility; the glove wrapper can be used to set open syringes on. Aspirate and expel a bit of air to break the seal on the syringe before performing the tap.
- Again palpate the landmarks on the aseptically prepared joint.
- Determine the angle of the joint space, and insert the needle, trying to avoid hitting the cartilage. Most of the time when you enter the joint space, you can tell there is a rubbery feel, and you do not hit a hard surface (bone). The needle goes in deeper when in the space than if over bone.
- If you do hit hard bone, gently pull the needle back a tiny bit, and move slightly, tapping along the way to reach the joint space when the bone ends (this is only millimeters).
- When the needle seems to have gone deep to enter the joint space, gently aspirate on the syringe without moving the needle (movement causes bleeding).
- If you do not get fluid right away, be patient, and wait at least 15-30 seconds before letting off the negative pressure. Joint fluid can be viscous, and especially when using a 25-gauge needle, it can take a moment to produce fluid.
- For cytology, only a very tiny volume is required, and you can stop after you see fluid in the needle hub. Culture takes only a bit more volume. Stop when you have the amount of fluid needed to reduce the risk of blood contamination.
- Release negative pressure, and pull the needle straight out as quickly as possible. If you aspirate while removing the needle, blood contamination is likely.
- If the only fluid is in the needle hub, remove the needle from the syringe, and fill the syringe with air. Reattach to the needle with sample in hub.
- Expel the contents of the needle, bevel side facing down, onto the microscope slides (a very tiny drop per slide is adequate). Use a clean slide to make a gentle smear.
- If culture is required, a drop of fluid can be placed on a Culturette, or fluid can be added to culture media. Large volumes (>0.1 mL) are occasionally obtained from large, effusive joints. Extra volume can be placed in a red top tube for culture submission or other analysis.
- The same procedure is repeated on another 1-3 joints, depending on clinical indication.

Postprocedure

- Assess gross appearance of joint fluid (clear or turbid, color, blood contamination)
- Assess viscosity while fluid is expelled from the needle or by placing a drop on one slide, covering with another, and separating the two. Normal synovial fluid is thick and sticky.

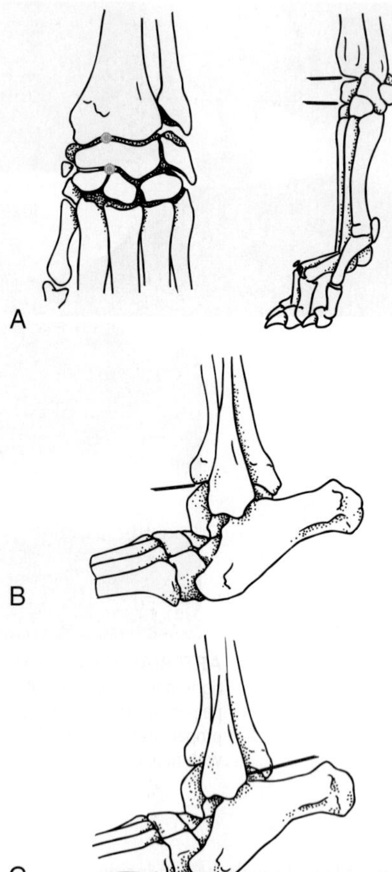

ARTHROCENTESIS Schematic representation of recommended sites for arthrocentesis in the dog and cat. **A**, Carpus: partially flex joint. Palpate and enter craniomedial aspect of carpometacarpal or radiocarpal space. **B**, Hock: cranial approach. Palpate space between tibia and tibiotarsal bone on craniolateral surface of hock; insert needle in shallow, palpable space. **C**, Hock: lateral approach. Partially flex joint, and insert needle under (distal to) lateral malleolus of fibula. (Reprinted with permission from Nelson RW, et al: Small animal internal medicine, ed 4, St. Louis, 2009, Mosby, pp 1122-1124.)

- Submit samples for cytologic assay and any other planned testing.

Alternatives and Their Relative Merits

- Joint radiographs: demonstrates bone erosion if present
- Bone scan: can identify which joints are inflamed/diseased
- Synovial biopsy: invasive technique useful if joint capsule thickened or deformed
- Arthroscopy: invasive technique to explore diseased joint, usually reserved for biopsy or planned therapeutic procedure

Pearls

Be patient during aspiration because joint fluid is viscous and can be slow in coming.

AUTHOR: Matthew Haight, CVT
EDITORS: Leah A. Cohn, DVM, PhD, DACVIM; Mark S. Thompson, DVM, DABVP

Artificial Insemination

Difficulty level: ◆

Overview and Goal

To effectively deliver fresh, chilled, or frozen-thawed semen into the cranial vagina

Indications

Convenience (geographic separation of dam and sire), maximizing use of valuable semen, ineffective natural mating (e.g., inexperienced/uncooperative male)

Contraindications

Poor timing/incorrect detection of estrus, systemic illness or other medical disorder likely to compromise successful fertilization, poor technique and/or materials and equipment, and semen quality that is not optimal and inadequate total number of viable sperm (arbitrarily, < 50 million motile sperm for small or toy breeds or < 100 million motile sperm for medium, large breeds) are relative contraindications, but acceptable results may be obtained, especially if switching to transcervical insemination (p. 1168) or surgical intrauterine insemination.

Equipment, Anesthesia

The procedure is generally performed awake. Required materials and equipment include

- Latex, nitrile or vinyl examination gloves
- Sterile, water-soluble, nonspermicidal lubricant
- Semen in sterile plastic pipette or tomcat catheter (toy breeds)
- Rubber-free (Air-Tite) sterile syringe for expelling the semen in the pipette

Anticipated Time

10 minutes

Preparation: Important Checkpoints

- Above all, the insemination process should be timed optimally, based on serial determinations of concentrations of blood progesterone. Luteinizing hormone assays can corroborate findings of blood progesterone levels. This means inseminating 1-4 days after ovulation.
- For optimal results, two inseminations should be planned 24-72 hours apart in this window of time.
- Methods for estrus detection and estimation of anticipated time of ovulation require hormonal assays, vaginoscopy (p. 1184), vaginal cytologic examinations (p. 1183), or a combination thereof.
- Semen that has been properly handled and is of good quality must be available.
- The help of one or two assistants for basic restraint and handling of the bitch.

Possible Complications and Common Errors to Avoid

- Urethral catheterization with the pipette: avoided by advancing the pipette along the lateral (left or right) aspect of the vagina, not the ventral aspect
- Vaginal injury or perforation: avoided by concurrent gentle palpation of the vagina and cervix abdominally and avoidance of pressure if resistance is met while advancing the pipette
- The semen should be deposited specifically in the cranial-most part of the vagina as close to the cervix as possible to increase the likelihood of success.

Procedure

- The bitch is placed standing in a location that is comfortable for the inseminator, typically an examination table for small dogs and the ground for medium- to large-breed dogs.
- An assistant restrains the bitch and draws her tail to one side (or this can be done by a second assistant).
- The inseminator dons gloves and holds the semen-filled pipette in the right hand if the inseminator is right-handed.
- The inseminator parts the labia and elevates the vulva dorsally using the hand not holding the pipette.
- The pipette tip is placed in the vestibule and elevated dorsal to the brim of the pelvis and lateral (left or right) to avoid the urethral papilla.
- The pipette is gently advanced dorsocranially. The inseminator releases the labia and uses the non-pipette hand to palpate the abdomen and locate the cervix.
- The pipette continues to be advanced until its tip is felt with the fingertips, transabdominally to be immediately caudal to the cervix.
- At this time, the bitch's hindquarters are elevated at a 30- to 45-degree angle; the inseminator then delivers the semen by depressing the plunger on the syringe connected to the pipette.

Postprocedure

- With insemination into the cranial vagina, maintain the bitch's hindquarters elevated for 1-10 minutes to improve delivery of semen to the uterus. In the dog, sperm first reach the uterus 30-120 seconds after insemination into the cranial vagina when the bitch is positioned with elevated hindquarters, but this process is hindered when the bitch is left in a horizontal (normal) posture after vaginal artificial insemination.
- Some practitioners advocate feathering of the vulva and perineum to induce uterine contractions and further favor movement of sperm into the uterus. However, this procedure is not scientifically justified or needed.

Alternatives and Their Relative Merits

Fertile dogs experience normal pregnancy rates and litter sizes after intravaginal inseminations; however, intracervical or surgical uterine inseminations may be advised for frozen-thawed semen or low-sperm doses. Surgical artificial insemination with fresh semen is relatively common in North America, but its ethical validity remains controversial.

SUGGESTED READING

Eilts BE, et al: Artificial insemination in the dog. In Root-Kustritz MV, editor: Small animal theriogenology, St. Louis, 2003, Butterworth/Heinemann, pp 61-95.

AUTHOR: Carlos R. F. Pinto, MedVet, PhD, DACT
EDITORS: Leah A. Cohn, DVM, PhD, DACVIM; Mark S. Thompson, DVM, DABVP

Procedures and Techniques

Barium Esophagram, Dynamic

Difficulty level: ♦♦♦

Synonyms

Barium swallow, fluoroscopic esophagram

Overview and Goal

To administer a contrast agent per os and observe the oral and pharyngeal phases of swallowing and esophageal transit using fluoroscopy. The goal of the study is to define abnormalities of swallowing and/or esophageal transit.

Indications

Functional abnormalities of swallowing (dysphagia [p. 277], abnormal esophageal motility). Can be used for evaluating mechanical abnormalities (mass, foreign body, extrinsic compression), but a static esophagram is usually sufficient for this purpose.

Contraindications

- Evidence or risk of esophageal perforation. Risk of esophageal perforation may be present in patients with a sharp/irregular esophageal foreign body or a foreign body that is present for longer than 24 hours.
- Megaesophagus: not an absolute contraindication, but the study is not needed for diagnosis, and there may be a risk for aspiration of the contrast agent. NOTE: Exception may be for diagnosis of lower esophageal achalasia as a cause of megaesophagus.

Equipment, Anesthesia

- Contrast agent
  - Liquid barium (30% weight/volume and higher density)
  - Iodinated contrast agent:
    - Non-ionic (iohexol, iopamidol, ioxaglate compounds)
    - Diluted 1 : 1 with water
- Highly palatable canned food
- Syringes for barium administration
- Bowl and utensil for mixing barium and food
- X-ray unit
  - Fluoroscopic capability
  - Spot film capability
  - Videorecording capability
- Protective clothing (lead aprons, gloves, thyroid shields) for personnel
- Paper towels or similar for cleanup of barium on animal and x-ray table

Anticipated Time

15-20 minutes

Preparation: Important Checkpoints

- Survey films of thorax and cervical region
  - If contraindications are present (as previously mentioned), study should not be performed.
  - If plain films are diagnostic (i.e., megaesophagus [p. 642]), the study may be unnecessary.
- Prepare contrast agents
  - Barium
    - Liquid barium in appropriately sized syringe
    - Liquid barium mixed with canned food. Only a small amount of barium (<5 mL) is needed, which keeps the solid consistency of the food.
  - Non-ionic iodinated contrast agent
    - Iohexol, iopamidol, ioxaglate compounds
    - Liquid diluted 1 : 1
    - Diluted liquid is mixed with canned food.
- Personnel needed for procedure (restraint and administration of contrast). This may require two to three people, depending on animal's size and temperament.
- All personnel should have appropriate lead protective apparel (aprons, thyroid shield, gloves).
- Paper towels or other barrier drapes to limit excess contrast agent on table and animal

Possible Complications and Common Errors to Avoid

- Aspiration of contrast agent: study is always begun with a liquid contrast agent and no food. Animals with disorders requiring these evaluations may be prone to dysphagia and aspiration of contrast. If a small amount of liquid contrast agent is aspirated, it can be coughed up. If the animal aspirates liquid contrast agent, the study should be aborted.
- Ionic iodinated contrast agents: use of these agents is CONTRAINDICATED because clinically significant, *potentially fatal* pulmonary edema can occur if they are aspirated. Ionic agents include diatrizoate, iothalamate, and iodamide compounds.
- *Non-ionic* iodinated contrast agents can be used if there is a suspicion of but not definite evidence of esophageal perforation.
- Leakage of contrast agent: evidence or risk of esophageal perforation is considered a contraindication for this study. If contrast agent leakage is suspected at any time, the study should be aborted.
- Assuming the procedure is not stopped because of aspiration of contrast agent or evidence of leakage of contrast agent, it is important to perform the study with liquid contrast agent and liquid contrast agent mixed with food to give as full an assessment of esophageal function as possible.
- Fluoroscopic procedures involve a substantial radiation dose to the animal and to personnel. Radiation safety (e.g., proper protective clothing, collimation so that personnel are not included in the primary beam) is paramount.

Procedure

Dynamic esophagram, barium:

- Survey films of thorax and cervical region (already described in preparation).
- Position animal in right lateral recumbency (if a C-arm fluoroscopy unit is used, it may be possible to place the animal in sternal recumbency or standing and use a horizontal beam) with appropriate restraint; special holding units for such studies available in some referral settings).
- Activate fluoroscopy unit briefly to determine correct positioning and collimation.
- Activate the videorecorder.
- Administer liquid barium PO 2-3 mL for a cat and 5-10 mL depending on the size of the dog), and activate fluoroscopic unit. Image the oral and pharyngeal phases of swallowing (progression of barium from mouth to esophagus) and esophageal transit (progression from upper esophageal sphincter to stomach). Repeat 2-3 times even if no abnormality is defined.
- Spot film any areas of abnormality; lateral views are generally sufficient.
- Administer barium and canned food mixture PO. Appropriately sized food balls (1-3 cm in diameter) may be fed to the animal or placed in the mouth. Activate fluoroscopic unit, and image the oral and pharyngeal phases of swallowing (progression of barium and food from mouth to esophagus) and esophageal transit (progression from upper esophageal sphincter to stomach). Repeat 2-3 times even if no abnormality is defined.
- Spot film any areas of abnormality; lateral views are generally sufficient.

Dynamic esophagram, *non-ionic* iodinated contrast agent:

- This study may be performed if esophageal rupture is suspected or if endoscopy is to be performed immediately after the esophagram. If an esophageal perforation is suspected, a static esophagram is usually performed instead, using a *non-ionic* iodinated compound.
- The dynamic esophagram using a *non-ionic* iodinated contrast agent follows the same procedure as the barium esophagram.

Postprocedure

Rarely, GI signs may occur but are typically mild and self-limited.

Alternatives and Their Relative Merits

Static esophagram: a static esophagram (administration of barium and obtaining routine films) can be used in place of a dynamic study for certain indications. A static study does not require the use of a fluoroscopy unit and is sufficient for most suspected mechanical abnormalities of the esophagus (e.g., esophageal foreign body, esophageal mass, esophageal stricture). However, abnormalities of swallowing and esophageal transit are rarely identified in this study, and it provides no information on the pharyngeal phase of swallowing.

SUGGESTED READING

O'Brien T: Esophagus. In O'Brien T, editor: Radiographic diagnosis of abdominal disorders in the dog and cat: radiographic interpretation, clinical signs, pathophysiology, Davis, CA, 1981, Covell Park Vet Company, p 141.

AUTHOR: Patricia L. Rose, DVM, MS, DACVR
EDITORS: Leah A. Cohn, DVM, PhD, DACVIM; Mark S. Thompson, DVM, DABVP

Behavioral Assessment

Bonus Material Online

Difficulty level: 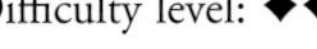

Overview and Goal

The goals are to re-establish the owner-animal bond and to protect the owner and the public from injury and loss of property.

Indications

Veterinarians should ask clients at every visit how satisfied they are with the pet. This allows early behavioral assessment and intervention. It is often too late to intervene after owners are contemplating getting rid of the pet.

Contraindications

If the dog or cat is very aggressive, re-homing is not an option. If the owner is unable or unwilling to work with a behaviorist on the issue, euthanasia may be indicated.

Equipment, Anesthesia

- Assess-A-Hand, a child-sized doll, a life-sized stuffed dog
- Closed circuit television (camera and time-lapse videorecorder)
- Food treats, water bowl, and toys

Anticipated Time

An hour for cats or 2 hours for dogs; appropriate assessment can be time-consuming.

Preparation: Important Checkpoints

- Have a history form, preferably one for each species. Pictures or videos of dogs and cats in various moods are very helpful.
- Have the most commonly used tools, such as basket muzzles, Gentle Leaders, ThunderShirts, Calming Caps, and Kong toys available, along with catalogs or websites of less commonly recommended products.

Possible Complications and Common Errors to Avoid

Dealing with aggressive animals is hazardous so liability is great, but do not neglect owner's problems, or a patient may be lost to euthanasia.

Procedure

The overall goals are to determine the exact nature of the problem and to allow appropriate intervention and prognosis when possible. With facsimile machines and electronic mail, sending and receiving histories before the consultation is a convenient and time-saving strategy. A sample set of history forms can be found at https://bform.habilis.net/canine-history/.

- Rule out medical disorders (e.g., urinary tract infection, interstitial cystitis, ectopic ureters [p. 282]) for periuria (house soiling [pp. 533 and 535]); metabolic, central neural, or thyroid disorders; and pain-producing conditions for aggression, and treat these appropriately if they are present.
- Clarify the nature of the environment surrounding the behavioral problem. Important environmental factors include the number of people and animals in the household and the amount of space the animal has at its disposal when the owners are home and when they are gone. In cats, the location, type, and contents of litter boxes are important. Has there been a change in the people or pets in the household or their schedules? If the presenting problem is destructive behavior, house soiling, or barking, an important step is to determine whether these events occur when the owners are at home or only when they are gone (p. 905).
- Clarify the reaction of the owners and others to the animal's misbehavior. Do they punish the animal (generally worsens/compounds the problem) or soothe it? Soothing efforts may reinforce phobias (p. 787).
- Help the owner to avoid misdirected interventions such as punishing after the fact, rewarding the dog for aggressive behavior, or rewarding jumping up.
- The owner should be given a reasonable treatment plan that does not involve a risk to the owner or the public.
- Behavior history forms for cats can be shorter than those for dogs because cats rarely are trained and do not require the attention that dogs do. Because cats are much less likely to demonstrate their misbehavior during an interview, a videorecording of the cat is very helpful. If the problem is periuria, time-lapse videorecording can elucidate which cat in a multi-cat household is soiling and what that cat's pre-elimination and post-elimination behavior is. Many cats visit the litter box but leave to eliminate elsewhere, indicating an aversion to the litter or to the box (p. 533).
- A detailed history should be obtained. Let us use a destructive dog as an example. It is important to determine just when and where the animal is destructive. The owners usually will have attempted to deal with the problem themselves, and the methods they have used should be recorded. It is always important to maintain a neutral attitude when taking a history because any criticism of the owners' methods may inhibit them from volunteering any additional information as the interview continues.
- For issues of aggression, it should be made clear to whom the aggression is directed: the owners, visitors, a specific type of person (e.g., male, female, wheelchair user), other dogs (or specific dogs), or other animals (in the home or outside the home).
- The animal's early history often gives a clue about the cause of misbehavior. For example, if a dog was obtained from a kennel at 6 months of age, it may never have been properly socialized to people during the socialization period of 7 to 14 weeks of age. If the dog was obtained as a 3-week-old puppy or was hand raised, it may be too dependent on people and not properly socialized to dogs. If the dog was obtained from an animal shelter, it may have been placed there because of destructive or aggressive behavior in the original home.
- Hand-raised kittens frequently are presented for aggression (p. 38) as adults and feral or free-ranging cats may be reluctant to remain indoors and may vocalize, claw, or spray when confined.
- Canine aggression (p. 40) is much more complicated. The victim, time, place, and circumstances of the aggressive episode must be known. The owner should be asked to describe the dog's posture (position of its ears and tail) as well as its vocalization and mouth position. Pupillary dilation and raised hackles indicate that the dog was experiencing sympathetic stimulation. A temperament test should be performed. A toddler-sized doll can be walked toward the dog. Although some dogs are frightened, aggressive ones bark or even bite the doll. An artificial hand (Assess-A-Hand) can be used for determining how responsive the dog is to touching of its head, abdomen, paws, and tail. The artificial

hand can also be used for pulling food or bones from the dog safely.

Postprocedure

Re-check in 3 and 6 weeks to determine the success of the treatment and compliance of the owner.

Alternatives and Their Relative Merits

Behavior problems can be referred to trainers, but there is no quality assurance. Herbal remedies also lack quality control or controlled studies of their efficacy. The more serious the behavioral issue, the more benefit there is to be gained from referral to a veterinary behavioral specialist.

AUTHOR: Katherine A. Houpt, VMD, PhD, DACVB
EDITORS: Leah A. Cohn, DVM, PhD, DACVIM; Mark S. Thompson, DVM, DABVP

Biopsy, Ultrasound-Guided Percutaneous

Difficulty level: ◆◆

Synonyms

Tissue core biopsy, Tru-Cut biopsy

Overview and Goal

Procedure to obtain tissue core sample using ultrasound guidance and real-time monitoring of needle instrument placement

Indications

- Ultrasonographic detection of focal mass lesion
- Physical, ultrasonographic, or biochemical detection of diffuse or focal parenchymal organ abnormalities

Contraindications

- Cavitated mass or bleeding disorder: risk of hemorrhage
- If abscess possible: risk of leakage, sepsis
- Intrathoracic masses not in contact with the chest wall: poor visualization
- Diffuse lung disease: risk of pneumothorax (p. 797)

Equipment, Anesthesia

- Biopsy instrument: typically 14- to 18-gauge needle
  - Automatic (biopsy gun using disposable needle)
    - Manually advanced to a point 1.5-2 cm superficial to lesion
    - When triggered, cutting needle and external shaft automatically advance a specific distance.
  - Semiautomatic (disposable, safest, most commonly used)
    - Inner cutting needle manually advanced to desired depth
    - When triggered, external shaft automatically advances over cutting needle.
  - Manual
    - Operator controls depth of needle and length of tissue sampled.
    - Requires two hands to operate device
- Formalin container and cassette
- A #11 scalpel blade to incise skin
- A set of 25-gauge standard injection needles or a 3-mL syringe filled with saline
- Hair clippers
- Surgical scrub, rubbing alcohol
- Sector or linear-array ultrasound transducer
  - Sector transducers allow sampling of deep structures.
  - Linear-array transducers provide better resolution of superficial structures.
- ± Biopsy guide: easiest method but angle of needle insertion fixed
- Anesthesia: intravenous (IV) or gas anesthesia usually required. Depending on the size and location of the lesion, light sedation and local anesthesia may be adequate.

Anticipated Time

The procedure time is 10-15 minutes plus anesthesia preparation/recovery time.

Preparation: Important Checkpoints

- Perform coagulation profile and platelet count.
- Place IV catheter.
- Ensure proper function of biopsy instrument.

Possible Complications and Common Errors to Avoid

- Avoid overly rapid advancement and activation of the instrument.
  - A common, serious error of inexperienced veterinarians is to advance and activate the instrument in one motion, which is contraindicated (poor placement/control of instrument tip).
  - The full extent of the instrument must be observed and monitored carefully and advanced with caution to the area to be sampled.
- Identify and avoid large vessels in the organ being sampled or in those adjacent to the structure to minimize hemorrhage.
- Avoid penetrating bowel lumen, especially with larger-gauge instruments, because of risk of peritonitis.
- Ensure that the ultrasound beam captures the full length and orientation of the instrument in the animal (p. 1112).
- Sample the left aspect of the liver when possible to avoid the gallbladder and hilar vessels on the right. If the liver is small or cranially located, consider a caudal intercostal approach.
- In cases of bilateral renal abnormalities, the left kidney should be sampled because of its more caudal location.
- Sample the caudal cortex of a kidney to avoid the medulla and arcuate and hilar vessels.
- Do not pass through an organ other than the one being sampled.
- Avoid using preanesthetic drugs that cause splenomegaly or panting (acepromazine/phenothiazines or hydromorphone/opiates, respectively) whenever possible.

Procedure

- Restrain the animal in dorsal or lateral recumbency. A padded U- or V-shaped trough can be used.
- Clip hair from the ventral abdomen.
- Thoroughly evaluate area of interest sonographically, characterize lesion, identify adjacent or internal vessels to be avoided, and determine least traumatic location and direction of needle placement.
- Prepare skin with surgical scrub.
- Obtain ultrasound image of area to be sampled with area of interest in focal zone of image.
- Ensure that probe marker location on screen corresponds with desired needle course.
- Prepare biopsy instrument.
- Make a small skin incision with a scalpel blade at the site needle will be introduced.
- Introduce needle parallel to plane of ultrasound beam, visualizing it as it is advanced.
- Slowly fan transducer side to side to identify needle as necessary.
- Automatic instrument
  - Note the *throw length* of the biopsy device before triggering it. This is the additional distance the instrument advances when triggered.
  - Manually advance the needle, stopping at this distance superficial to desired biopsy site. CAUTION: When triggered, needle will advance the full predetermined throw length to obtain biopsy.
  - Trigger needle: cutting needle and external shaft will advance the predetermined throw length to obtain sample.
- Semiautomatic instrument
  - Manually advance the inner cutting needle to desired biopsy depth.
  - Trigger needle: external shaft will automatically advance over cutting needle to obtain sample.

- Manual instrument
  - Manually advance the inner cutting needle to desired biopsy depth.
  - Manually advance the external shaft over the cutting needle to obtain sample.
  - Requires two hands to operate, and two people are required for biopsy procedure.
- Withdraw instrument from animal.
- Use a 25-gauge needle to gently lift sample from biopsy needle or gently flush the sample from the needle using a syringe filled with saline.
- Place sample in cassette and place in formalin container.
- Two to three samples of each organ or lesion are obtained.

Postprocedure

- Scan to evaluate for hemorrhage. A very small amount of hemorrhage is not uncommon.
- If small amount of hemorrhage is noted, re-evaluate after several additional minutes, ensuring that the patient is monitored (mucous membrane color, blood pressure) and is kept recumbent with the biopsied side down (e.g., sternal recumbency if a liver biopsy was near or on the ventral midline).
- Hematuria is common after renal biopsy.

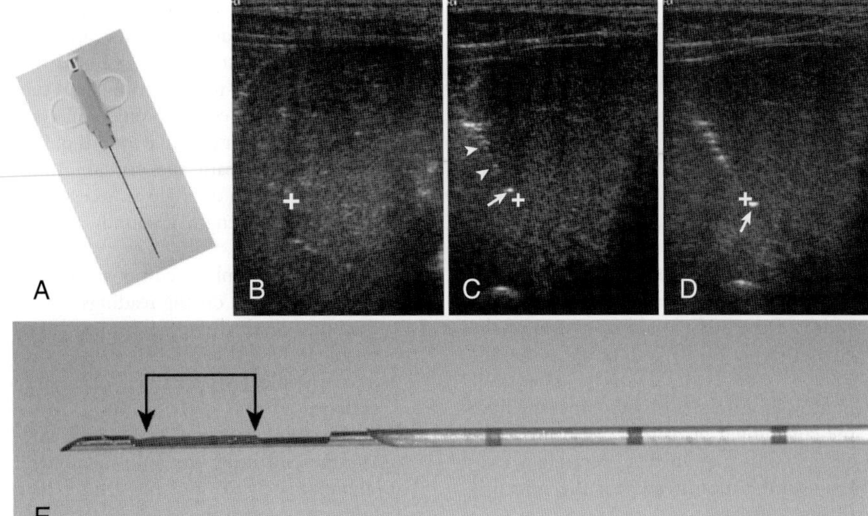

BIOPSY, ULTRASOUND-GUIDED PERCUTANEOUS A, Semiautomatic-type instrument used for ultrasound-guided core biopsy. **B,** Ultrasound of a dog's liver in preparation for core biopsy. Targeted area chosen for biopsy is marked (+). **C,** Ultrasound of same dog's liver, with the biopsy under way. Semiautomatic instrument shown in panel **A** has been advanced *(arrowheads)* until its tip *(arrow)* is immediately above the target. **D,** Internal stylet advancing. With instrument held immobile, internal stylet is slowly advanced, crossing through the targeted area or lesion. After the stylet is in the fully advanced/deployed position shown, the instrument can be triggered, which obtains the sample. **E,** Core of liver tissue *(between arrows)* is shown within chamber of stylet.

Alternatives and Their Relative Merits

Laparoscopic (p. 1128) and surgical biopsies are more invasive but have higher diagnostic quality in some cases.

Pearls

- Confirm that the patient has been properly fasted, with an empty stomach, before performing a liver biopsy. Distention of the gastric fundus can interfere with visualization of the left aspect of the liver.
- Performing a percutaneous biopsy can be difficult if the patient has moderate or marked peritoneal effusion. Laparoscopic or surgical biopsy may be preferred in those cases.
- If the liver is small and has highly irregular margins suggesting cirrhosis, laparoscopic biopsy or surgical biopsy may be preferred.

SUGGESTED READING

Mattoon JS, et al: Ultrasound-guided aspiration and biopsy procedures. In Mattoon JS, et al, editors: Small animal diagnostic ultrasound, ed 3, St. Louis, 2015, Saunders, pp 50-77.

AUTHOR: Wendy D. Fife, DVM, MS, DACVR
EDITORS: Leah A. Cohn, DVM, PhD, DACVIM; Mark S. Thompson, DVM, DABVP

Blood Pressure Measurement

Difficulty level: ♦

Overview and Goal

- The goal of noninvasive blood pressure (BP) assessment in animals in a veterinary setting is to accurately measure arterial BP and detect abnormal BP, particularly systemic hypertension.
- Doppler sphygmomanometric methods or automated oscillometric methods may be used.
- Doppler methods deliver systolic BP values.
- Oscillometric methods deliver systolic, diastolic, and mean BP values.
- Systolic BP is the value of interest in most clinical cases of systemic hypertension (p. 501).

Indications

- Presence of clinical signs of systemic hypertension (p. 501)
- Presence of systemic disease known to be associated with systemic hypertension (e.g., renal disease, hyperthyroidism [p. 503]), hyperadrenocorticism (p. 485), diabetes mellitus (p. 251), pheochromocytoma (p. 785)

Contraindications

Random BP screening in young, healthy animals is not recommended.

Equipment, Anesthesia

Doppler method (used in dogs and cats; the preferred method for cats):

- Commercial Doppler amplifier with attached piezoelectric crystal for detection of blood flow
- Sphygmomanometer previously calibrated for accuracy
- A variety of cuff sizes based on animal limb circumference
- Pliable measuring tape to measure animal limb circumference
- Ultrasound coupling gel
- Hair clippers and isopropyl alcohol, if desired, for preparation of site of piezoelectric crystal application

Oscillometric method (automated system used in dogs, less reliable in cats):

- Commercial automated oscillometric BP monitor with print or data storage capability
- A variety of cuff sizes based on animal limb circumference
- Pliable measuring tape to measure animal limb circumference

Anticipated Time

- Doppler method: approximately 10 minutes
- Oscillometric method: approximately 20 minutes

Preparation: Important Checkpoints

- Be sure the animal has acclimated to the clinic's environment and is calm and comfortable in lateral or sternal recumbency or sitting. BP values may be obtained in standing animals only if a tail cuff is used. Owner presence and assurance may help calm the animal.
- Be sure the cuff size used is appropriate and noted in the record for future reference. The width of the cuff should be ≈40% of the circumference of the limb or tail at the cuff site.
- During measurements with either method, the cuff should be at the level of the right atrium. This may involve elevating a forelimb during measurement if the animal is sitting.
- BP should be measured by well-trained individuals in the practice to maximize consistency. This is especially important when Doppler methods are used.

Possible Complications and Common Errors to Avoid

- Erratic oscillometric readings may be obtained if an arrhythmia or very high heart rate is present.
- Turn volume knob to low or zero before turning Doppler amplifier on; then gradually increase volume to search for the pulse after contact is established between the crystal and the patient's skin. Failing to do this can produce extremely loud static noise that is startling to the patient (if using speakers) or deafening to the operator (if using headphones).
- For maximal accuracy in Doppler readings, be sure the audible signal is strong before beginning cuff occlusions.

Procedure

Doppler method:

- Restrain the animal in a comfortable position, and allow time and reassurance for acclimation. The position of the animal depends on the animal's temperament and mobility and on the planned position of the cuff.
  - Cuff on forelimb at level of radius: sternal or lateral recumbency or sitting position
  - Cuff on hindlimb proximal to hock (tibial level) or distal hindlimb (metatarsal level): lateral recumbency preferred; sternal recumbency may be used if limb is in gentle extension during measurement.
- Measure the circumference of the limb or tail at the intended cuff site, and select an appropriately sized cuff (see above).
- Wrap the cuff snugly around the limb, and attach to sphygmomanometer.
- Clip or dampen hair as needed at site of Doppler crystal application distal to the cuff (palmar or plantar arterial arch, proximal to the metacarpal/metatarsal pad and slightly medial); apply coupling gel, and hold or tape crystal in position.
- The crystal is placed against the patient's skin concave side down; the flat aspect of the crystal faces outward.
- Turn volume knob to low setting, and turn amplifier on. Verify correct position of crystal by listening for clear pulsatile sounds of flow in the artery beneath the crystal. Adjust the crystal position or angle as necessary to improve signal strength if sounds are soft, distant, or muffled.
- Gently position limb so cuff is at the level of the right atrium during readings.
  - Sternum level if animal is in lateral position
  - Thoracic inlet level if animal is sternal or sitting
- While listening to sound of pulsatile flow, inflate the cuff using the bulb manometer to approximately 20 mm Hg greater than the pressure needed to cut off flow sounds.
- Slowly deflate the cuff (1-3 mm Hg per second), and note pressure at which pulsatile sounds of flow recur. This pressure is recorded as the systolic pressure.
- Completely deflate the cuff, and count the heart rate in the approximately 30 seconds between pressure readings. A contemporary heart rate can be recorded with each BP reading.
- Record at least 6 measurements in succession, allowing approximately 30 seconds to 1 minute between measurements to allow for limb reperfusion.
- Discard the first reading, and average the results of the remaining readings to obtain a representative number for systolic pressure and heart rate. High heart rate may indicate that increased levels of stress have affected readings. If the BP is trending down with successive measurements, extra measurements may be recorded, and the last 5 values averaged for a representative value.

Oscillometric method:

- Restrain the animal in a comfortable position, and allow time and reassurance for acclimatization. The position of the animal depends on animal's temperament and mobility and on the planned position of the cuff.
  - Cuff on forelimb at level of radius: sternal or lateral recumbency or sitting position
  - Cuff on distal hindlimb at level of metatarsus (median artery): lateral recumbency preferred; sternal recumbency may be used if limb is in gentle extension during measurement.
  - Cuff on proximal tail head: sternal or lateral recumbency or standing if animal is relatively immobile during readings (tail head is preferred cuff site for oscillometric measurement technique in cats).
  - Limb cuffs should not be used in standing animals.
- Measure the circumference of the limb or tail at the intended cuff site, and choose an appropriately sized cuff.
- Wrap the cuff snugly around the limb, with the center of the inflatable bladder of the cuff positioned over the artery, and attach to the BP monitor.
- Gently position limb so cuff is at the level of the right atrium during readings (no repositioning required if tail cuff is used).
  - Sternum level if animal is in lateral position
  - Thoracic inlet level if animal is sternal or sitting
- Record at least 6 measurements in succession, allowing approximately 30 seconds to 1 minute between measurements to allow for limb reperfusion.
- Discard the first reading and any readings with clearly spurious results, and average the results of the remaining readings to obtain a

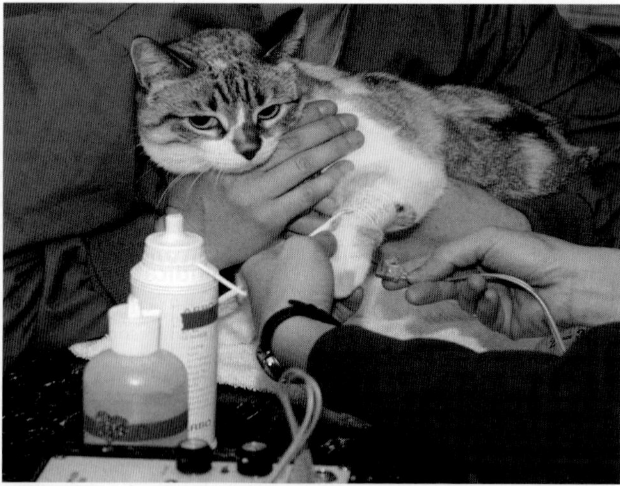

BLOOD PRESSURE MEASUREMENT Doppler method is used for estimating blood pressure (BP) in a cat. The patient is restrained in a calm, comfortable position. Cuff is applied to a distal forelimb, and limb is elevated such that cuff is at level of right atrium during readings. Coupling gel is applied to Doppler crystal (shown). After Doppler crystal is positioned over palmar arterial arch and a strong audible signal is obtained, bulb sphygmomanometer is used for inflating cuff and occluding arterial flow and then slowly deflated. Pressure at which arterial flow is again audible is recorded as the systolic BP.

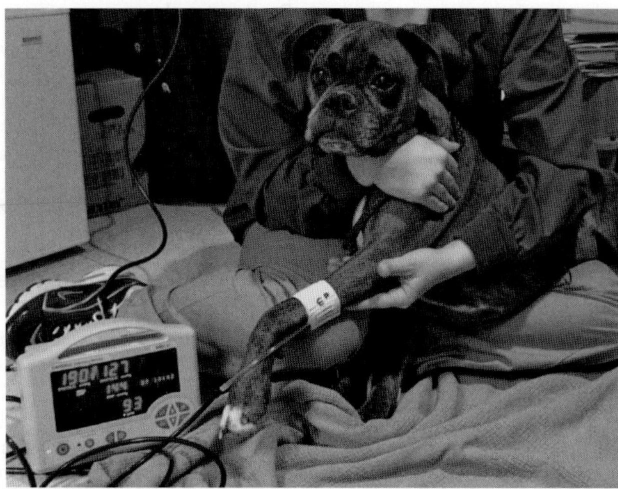

BLOOD PRESSURE MEASUREMENT Automated oscillometric method used with a forelimb cuff to obtain systolic, diastolic, and mean blood pressure in a dog. Dog is restrained in a comfortable position, with intended cuff-site limb gently extended. Cuff is positioned at mid-radius level, and limb is positioned such that cuff is at level of right atrium during readings.

representative number for systolic, diastolic, and mean pressures, respectively.
- If heart rate associated with a reading is clearly incorrect, BP values may be spurious. High heart rate during recording may indicate high animal stress levels and possible elevated BP due to stress of procedure. If heart rate is decreasing during serial measurements, take several more readings and average the final 5 values. If an arrhythmia is present, the heart rate may not be recorded and the results of that iteration should be discarded.

Postprocedure

- Record the average values in animal's record, with notation of method, cuff size, and cuff site used.
- Evaluate BP values in light of clinical findings and level of anxiety or excitement during BP measurement.

Alternatives and Their Relative Merits

Invasive BP measurement involves acute arterial puncture (typically femoral artery) with a small-gauge needle attached to a pressure transducer or catheter placement in a distal artery (typically dorsal pedal) and attachment to pressure tubing and a pressure transducer. A BP tracing is printed, and systolic and diastolic pressure can be determined from the pressure tracing.

- Highly accurate information because direct measurement is used
- Local anesthesia is used to minimize discomfort.
- Arterial puncture or arterial catheter placement requires more technical skill than noninvasive methods (p. 1058).
- Bleeding may occur at site of arterial puncture; apply pressure to puncture site for at least 5 minutes after the needle is withdrawn.
- Invasive methods are rarely used in conscious clinical patients, but indwelling arterial catheters are frequently used for continuous BP assessment in anesthetized or critically ill patients.

Pearls

Cuff location, cuff size, and animal position can affect measured BP values. Each of these should be noted for each patient and remain the same for future BP assessments.

SUGGESTED READING

Brown S, et al: Guidelines for the identification, evaluation, and management of systemic hypertension in dogs and cats. J Vet Intern Med 21:542-558, 2007.

AUTHOR: Rebecca L. Stepien, DVM, MS, DACVIM
EDITORS: Leah A. Cohn, DVM, PhD, DACVIM; Mark S. Thompson, DVM, DABVP

Bone Aspiration and Biopsy

Bonus Material Online 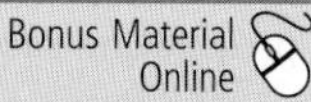

Difficulty level: ◆

Synonym

Bone fine-needle aspiration (FNA)

Overview and Goal

Minimally invasive sampling of bony mass or lesion identified radiographically

Indications

Used to obtain diagnosis of bony mass or radiographic aggressive bone lesion (pp. 165, 725, and 726). Simple aspiration often used first, moving on to a biopsy if diagnosis is not forthcoming.

Contraindications

- Contraindication to sedation or anesthesia (biopsy)
- Severe bleeding disorder
- Skin infection over bone sampling site

Equipment, Anesthesia

- Heavy sedation, neuroleptanalgesia, or general anesthesia with local analgesic for biopsy
  - Typical sedation protocol: dexmedetomidine 5 mcg/kg IM or IV with morphine 0.5 mg/kg IM or IV
  - Typical general anesthesia protocol: premedicate with above sedation drugs, induce with propofol 6 mg/kg IV to effect, maintenance with propofol as needed or isoflurane gas
  - Local analgesia: 9 : 1 mixture of 2% lidocaine HCl to sodium bicarbonate 1-2 mL infiltrated subcutaneous to periosteum
- Clippers
- Antiseptic scrub solution, isopropyl alcohol, gauze squares for skin preparation
- For aspiration: sterile or nonsterile gloves, hypodermic needles (18 or 20 gauge), 10-mL syringe, cytology slides (#10-#20)
- For biopsy: sterile gloves, #11 scalpel blade, Jamshidi needle or bone trocar, tissue jar, and 10% formalin

Anticipated Time

15-20 minutes

Preparation: Important Checkpoints

- Radiographs: confirm lesion and best sampling location
- Thoracic radiographs: to check for metastatic disease from primary bone tumors
- Discussion with owner of potential complications, including iatrogenic pathologic fracture

Possible Complications and Common Errors to Avoid

- Iatrogenic pathologic fracture: altering angle or location of multiple samples may reduce risk.

- Although bone aspirations have less risk of pathologic fracture, there is a lower likelihood of definitive diagnosis and does not allow for special stains or immunohistochemistry (IHC) on biopsy samples.
- Avoid using too small of a needle or biopsy instrument. Although bigger instruments will remove/damage larger pieces of bone, they also result in more tissue for diagnosis.
- If soft tissue prevents easy contact with bone, cut-down and dissection of vital soft tissues before aspiration or biopsy may be warranted. For aspiration, use radiographs to find an ideal location of cortical lysis/diseased bone to biopsy. Avoid major muscles.
- Minor complications include pain, bleeding, infection.

Procedure

- Place sedated/anesthetized animal in recumbency with easiest access to diseased bone, as identified by radiographs. An approximate measurement of the thickness of the lesion should be made from radiographs to anticipate desired depth of needle penetration.
- The skin over the lesion is clipped and aseptically scrubbed. Local analgesia is infused subcutaneously and deep to the periosteum.
- Brief aseptic scrub is repeated after local analgesia injection; clinician then dons gloves.

For aspiration:

- An 18- or 20-gauge needle is inserted into the diseased bone and a woodpecker technique is repeated until a sufficient sample has been obtained or blood begins to fill the hub of the needle.
- Remove needle, attach air-filled syringe, and immediately disperse sample onto microscope slides. If blood is visible in needle hub, place only a single drop of sample per slide.
- An additional blank slide is used to make smears; use care not to place too much pressure and smash the sample.

For biopsy:

- While wearing sterile gloves, remove stylet from the biopsy needle to ensure that needle is in working order and seal has been broken; replace stylet.
- Tent the skin, and make a stab incision with blade. CAUTION: ensure nerves and vessels do not course in the chosen area.
- Take biopsy needle in dominant hand, and work through subcutaneous tissues until contact is made with underlying bone. Seating (similar to a bone marrow biopsy) is likely not possible due to cortical loss in diseased bone. After the needle is advanced into diseased bone/tissue, remove stylet, and continue advancing biopsy needle. A clockwise-counterclockwise motion with firm, downward pressure may be necessary.
  - CAUTION: due to weakness of diseased bone, using index finger and thumb as a buffer will help prevent penetration through the bone or damage to surrounding soft-tissue structures. The biopsy needle should be palmed (butt of the needle in palm, needle shaft held firmly between index finger and thumb) so that the tips of the thumb and index finger pinching the needle shaft act as a buttress.
- After sufficient advancement (deep penetration into the diseased bone), slightly rock the needle in the same circular direction to break bone free from attachments.
- Continue to rotate (slight rock) needle as it is removed from the bone. A plug of tissue should be seen in biopsy needle.
- Tissue plug is removed using stylet inserted in normograde direction (bone trocar) or retrograde (Jamshidi-type needle, which is tapered at the tip) to push the tissue out into the formalin jar.
- Two or three samples are taken from one location to increase diagnostic yield. Skin sutures may be necessary for larger skin incisions.

Postprocedure

- Apply direct pressure and ice for 10-15 minutes to reduce hematoma development/bleeding.
- Ensure appropriate analgesics are available because patient will likely have pain after procedure.
- If there is concern about pathologic fracture, radiograph sample site.

Alternatives and Their Relative Merits

- Open biopsy: more invasive with higher risk of infection, but specimens will likely be larger.
- Amputation (if lesion on a limb): considered part of standard of care for primary bone malignancies; also necessary for pathologic fractures. Because amputation will limit treatment options (radiation, bisphosphonates, limb spare), thoroughly discuss differential diagnoses and prognosis with owner.

Pearls

- Larger-bore needles are helpful to penetrate through cortical bone for aspiration.
- Steadying/buffering biopsy needle with index finger and thumb prevents clinician from overpenetration and potential tissue damage during biopsy.
- Adequate pain medications will allow patients to remain comfortable while waiting for cytology or biopsy results.
- Use radiographs to find best location to aspirate or biopsy. Necrotic areas (complete absence of bone) may not be diagnostic, whereas sclerotic or proliferative areas may be too dense to biopsy.

AUTHORS: Brian K. Flesner, DVM, MS, DACVIM; Deborah J. Tate, RVT, VTS
EDITORS: Leah A. Cohn, DVM, PhD, DACVIM; Mark S. Thompson, DVM, DABVP

Bone Marrow Aspiration and Core Biopsy

Bonus Material Online 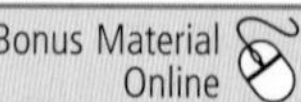

Difficulty level: ♦♦

Synonym

Bone marrow aspiration (BMA)

Overview and Goal

To obtain a sample of bone marrow cells for cytologic (aspiration) and/or histologic (core biopsy) analysis

Indications

- Cytopenias without identifiable underlying cause
- Abnormal blood cell number or morphology on blood smear
- Staging of neoplasia: lymphoma (pp. 607 and 609) or mast cell tumor (pp. 632 and 634) most common
- Diagnosis of feline leukemia virus (FeLV) infection (p. 329) with suspicious clinical presentation and negative peripheral test
- Unexplained gammopathy
- Infectious screening for fever of unknown origin (p. 334)

Contraindications

- Contraindications to sedation or anesthesia
- Skin infection over bone marrow sampling site
- Thrombocytopenia is *not* a contraindication

Equipment, Anesthesia

- Sedation, neuroleptanalgesia, or general anesthesia with local analgesia
  - Typical sedation: dexmedetomidine 5 mcg/kg IM or IV with morphine 0.5 mg/kg IM or IV
  - Typical general anesthesia: premedicate with above sedation drugs, and induce with propofol 6 mg/kg IV to effect; maintenance with propofol as needed or isoflurane gas
  - Local analgesia: 9:1 mixture of 2% lidocaine HCl to sodium bicarbonate; 1-2 mL infiltrated subcutaneous to periosteum

- Clippers
- Antiseptic scrub solution, isopropyl alcohol, gauze squares for skin preparation
- Sterile gloves
- #11 scalpel blade
- Bone marrow aspiration and/or biopsy needle (e.g., Jamshidi), typically 15-18 gauge
- 6-10 mL syringe
- Cytology slides (#20-#30): tilt most slides lengthwise to ≈45% angle, frosted end up, before starting procedure
- Tissue jar and 10% formalin for biopsy

Anticipated Time

15-20 minutes

Preparation: Important Checkpoints

CBC should be obtained the same day as the BMA/biopsy.

Possible Complications and Common Errors to Avoid

Aspirate:

- Inadvertent clotting of sample; preventable by reducing the time between aspiration and smearing to few seconds

Core biopsy:

- Not always required; BMA is less invasive and often adequate
- Loss of the sample on withdrawal of biopsy needle. This can be minimized by adequate rocking of the biopsy needle when it is fully embedded in the marrow to break off the deep attachments to the core.
- Although unlikely, bone fracture is possible.

BMA or core:

- Inadequate or nondiagnostic sample; be sure there are visible spicules for BMA or visible red marrow for the biopsy core
- Hematoma formation or bleeding is rare, even in thrombocytopenic animals.
- Sliding off the bone, causing soft-tissue trauma: prevented with use of anatomic landmarks and making good needle-to-bone contact before advancing needle into bone

Procedure

Humeral approach to BMA:

- For a right-handed clinician, patient is placed in left lateral recumbency. The skin over the point of the shoulder is clipped and aseptically scrubbed.
- Externally rotate the humerus, find the scapulohumeral joint, move finger distally from the joint, and locate flat surface of the proximal humerus (distal to the greater tubercle. Local analgesia is infused subcutaneously deep to the periosteum.
- Brief aseptic scrub is repeated after local analgesia injection; clinician then puts on sterile gloves.
- Before making stab incision, remove stylet from the biopsy needle to ensure that needle is in working order and seal has been broken; replace stylet.
- Using nondominant hand, externally rotate the humerus (can be done by assistant). With dominant hand, palpate the joint, move slightly distally, and find the flat surface of the humerus.
- Tent the skin, and make a stab incision.
- Take biopsy needle in dominant hand, and work through subcutaneous tissues until contact is made with underlying bone. This prevents slippage off of the bone.
- After the needle has made contact with the bone, the needle should be perpendicular to the surface of the humerus. Rotate the needle clockwise-counterclockwise with firm, downward pressure, avoiding any extraneous side-to-side motion.
- After good purchase into the bone has been made, the needle should be able to move the entire leg without the needle wiggling.
- After needle is seated into bone, remove cap and stylet (place them on sterile surface for potential further use), attach syringe, and aspirate with short, quick pulses of pressure.
- After blood/marrow is visualized in hub of syringe (typically only 1-3 short aspirates are required), stop aspiration, remove syringe from needle, and immediately disperse onto microscope slides.
- Individual droplets of blood/marrow are placed near frosted upper end of tilted slides. Excess blood contamination will drain down slide. You should be able to see spicules of marrow as small white/cream dots/clumps on the slide.
  - Any remaining sample collected into the syringe (accidental oversampling) can be placed on additional slides or in a purple top Vacutainer tube. Spicules can be removed later if slides are inadequate.
- An additional, blank slide is used to smear the samples, being careful not to place too much pressure on the sample during the squash preparation.
- Blood/marrow clots extremely fast, and the entire aspiration-to-slide preparation should be done very quickly to avoid clotted sample.
- If the clinician is satisfied with acquired sample, the needle can be removed from the bone. If not, another aspiration can be attempted.

Ilial approach to BMA:

- Ilial BMA is more suitable for medium and large dogs than for cats or small dogs and often requires minimal sedation or only local analgesia.
- Other than positioning and site of sample collection, the procedure is exactly as for humeral BMA.
- The animal is positioned in sternal recumbency.
- Palpate for the small, flat portion on the dorsum of the ilial wing; this is the target for aspiration, with no regard to using the right or left side.

Core biopsy, humerus or ilium:

- The same procedure as for bone marrow aspiration is followed up to the point of advancing the needle. Stop after the needle is partially seated because it will be further advanced through the marrow after the stylet has been removed.
- Remove cap and stylet from needle.
- Advance needle clockwise-counterclockwise with firm, downward pressure to fill several millimeters of the needle with bone marrow. The cap can be replaced, or thumb may be placed over end of the biopsy needle (where syringe is attached for aspiration).
- When full purchase has been made and the needle is deeply seated, rotate (slightly rock) the needle very slightly in the same, circular direction to break core of marrow and bone free from underlying attachments.
- Continue to rotate (slightly rock) needle as it is removed from the bone. A plug of marrow should be seen in biopsy needle.
- Insert the stylet retrograde through the needle to dislodge the tissue plug directly into 10% formalin. The core sample should have visible red marrow. If only white is seen, repeat the biopsy procedure to avoid a nondiagnostic sample.

Postprocedure

- Provide analgesia (e.g., tramadol or nonsteroidal antiinflammatory drugs) for 1-3 days, as appropriate.
- For animals with severe thrombocytopenia, apply pressure to site until bleeding stops.

Alternatives and Their Relative Merits

- Sternal BMA using 18-gauge hypodermic needle: can be performed on medium or large dogs with minimal sedation. Not amenable to biopsy from this site
- Repeated CBC to assess trends in cytopenias
- Buffy coat examination

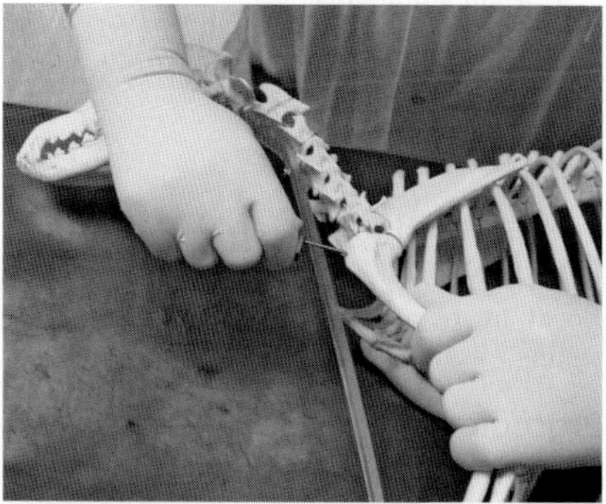

BONE MARROW ASPIRATION/CORE BIOPSY Position for bone marrow aspiration from the proximal humerus, using a skeleton for demonstration. This right-handed clinician is standing dorsal to the recumbent animal and is holding the humerus firmly. The needle tip is on the distal, lateral surface of the greater tubercle, ready to be advanced.

Pearls

- Aspirate is often adequate for cancer staging, assessment of megakaryocyte numbers, or recognition of infectious pathogens, but biopsy is needed for architectural detail of marrow.
- Tenting the skin and moving through layers of subcutaneous tissue *before* making contact with bone will alleviate slippage off of bone and soft-tissue trauma.
- As an alternative to placing aspirate on standing slides that allow blood to drain away, the entire sample can be placed on a watch glass in EDTA and a pipette used to pick out the spicules that are then transferred to microscope slides.
- Aspiration itself is the most painful part of the procedure but is over quickly. For nonsedated or lightly sedated animals, be prepared for a reaction during the actual aspiration.

AUTHORS: Brian K. Flesner, DVM, MS, DACVIM; Deborah J. Tate, RVT, VTS
EDITORS: Leah A. Cohn, DVM, PhD, DACVIM; Mark S. Thompson, DVM, DABVP

Breeding Soundness Exam: Female Dog

Difficulty level: ♦♦

Overview and Goal

Evaluate the physical and physiologic parameters of the breeding female to determine her likelihood for normal fertility.

Indications

- Before breeding, to ensure general health and likelihood of a healthy litter
- Prepurchase evaluation of a female intended for breeding
- A breeding female with a history of abnormal estrous cycles or failure to conceive when bred to a fertile male with appropriate breeding management

Equipment, Anesthesia

- Canine vaginal speculum
- Pediatric proctoscope and a penlight
- Cotton-tip swab, slides, and Romanowsky stain (Diff-Quik) for vaginal cytologic evaluation
- Double-guarded swabs for culture of the cranial vagina
- Blood collection supplies
- Ultrasound
- If vaginoscopy is required
    - Rigid endoscope
    - Sedation/anesthesia

Anticipated Time

30-90 minutes

Preparation: Important Checkpoints

Be aware of available breed-specific genetic testing.

Procedure

- Obtain a complete reproductive history; this information is used for determining the diagnostic approach required and should include
    - Fertility of dam, sire, and littermates
    - Date and age at first estrus
    - Duration of estrus
    - Duration of interestrus intervals
    - Progesterone/vaginal cytologic evaluation results and dates from previous estrous cycles
    - Insemination dates and semen evaluation (if performed)
    - Date(s) and method(s) of pregnancy diagnosis (p. 816)
    - Whelping dates and litter sizes
    - Dates and results of *Brucella canis* tests
    - Vaccination and general health history: take into account factors and diseases that could alter fertility, including thyroid disorders (p. 525), prolonged treatment with glucocorticoids (e.g., for skin problems), and potential exposure to reproductive pathogens such as canine herpesvirus.
- The following diagnostic samples should be collected.
    - Serum progesterone: result should coincide with the expected stage of the estrous cycle.
    - Vaginal cytologic sample: result should coincide with the stage of the estrous cycle (p. 1061) and could potentially reveal inflammation.
    - *Brucella canis* serologic testing should be performed every 12 months.
    - CBC and serum biochemistry profile, thyroid function tests
- A complete physical exam, including careful palpation of the mammary glands and a digital vaginal exam. Physical factors that may reduce fertility include abnormal vulvar conformation, vaginal strictures, and a persistent median septum. Potential hereditary disorders such as orthopedic disorders (hip dysplasia [p. 469], elbow dysplasia [p. 288], cranial cruciate ligament rupture [p. 218]), ophthalmic disorders, and heart conditions should be brought to the attention of the breeder.
- Vaginal speculum exam performed using a canine vaginal speculum and/or the pediatric proctoscope (p. 1184) allows visualization of the caudal vagina only. The degree of vaginal crenulation as well as the presence or absence of vaginitis can be observed.
- Vaginoscopy (p. 1184) requires a rigid or flexible endoscope at least 30 cm long (depending on the size of the bitch). This will allow visualization of the entire vagina and external cervical os. Strictures, persistent median septa, and other abnormalities may be observed.
- Vaginal culture should be obtained after a sterile prep of the vulva and careful retraction of the vulvar lips or insertion of a sterile vaginal speculum.
    - Contamination can be prevented by using a double-guarded swab.
    - Careful interpretation of the vaginal culture is required; if high numbers of potentially pathogenic bacteria are cultured, the result may be considered significant.
    - Culture should be interpreted together with the history and vaginal cytologic findings. If there is no evidence of infertility or inflammation, a positive culture—even with a potential pathogen—is most likely insignificant.
    - If *Mycoplasma canis* is a concern, the diagnostic lab should be contacted regarding the culture procedures and shipping requirements before obtaining a sample.
- Ultrasonography of the uterus and ovaries is part of a complete breeding soundness exam. In larger bitches, it can be difficult to image the ovaries consistently. The uterus is located dorsal to the bladder and should be followed to the horn tips.
    - The features of the uterus will vary with the stage of the estrous cycle. During proestrus and estrus, the uterus will be edematous and have a heterogeneous echotexture. There may be a small amount of fluid present in the lumen at this time. During diestrus, the uterus will have a more homogeneous echotexture and may have a convoluted course. The uterus will have a greater diameter during diestrus compared to proestrus or estrus. Cystic

structures within the endometrium are abnormal at any stage of the estrous cycle and may indicate cystic endometrial hyperplasia. The presence of luminal fluid in diestrus is also abnormal and indicates mucometra or pyometra. Ovarian structures should coincide with the stage of the estrous cycle. Follicles larger than 8 mm are most likely anovulatory follicles. They may be significant if signs of prolonged proestrus (p. 822) exist (estrogen exposure) and may be estrogen-producing cysts. During diestrus, the ovaries contain corpora lutea and some small follicles. During anestrus, the ovaries have only small follicles and may be difficult to locate.

Postprocedure

Additional tests:

- An abnormal or unexpected progesterone or vaginal cytologic analysis should be followed by serial tests every 2 days.
- A positive *Brucella* rapid slide agglutination test (RAST) or tube agglutination test (TAT) should be followed by a more specific test, such as agar gel immunodiffusion or culture.
- Suspected vaginal abnormalities can be further evaluated by a vaginography or vaginoscopy.
- Karyotyping should be performed on females with abnormal external or internal genitalia, irregular estrous cycles, or failure to cycle.
- Abnormal appearance of the uterus on ultrasound can be followed with exploratory laparotomy, which allows for a thorough evaluation of the uterus, ovaries, and uterine tubes. A uterine biopsy and culture can also be performed at this time. Uterine cytology may also contribute to diagnosis of uterine pathology.
- Doppler assessment of the hemodynamics of the uterine artery correlates with uterine health and fertility. Specifically, resistivity index and pulsatility index negatively correlate with fertility. Spectral morphology may also correlate with fertility, as in other species.

SUGGESTED READING

Johnston S, et al: Clinical approach to infertility in the bitch. In SD Johnston, et al. Canine and feline theriogenology, New York, 2001, Saunders, pp 257-273.

AUTHOR: Bronwyn Crane, DVM, MS, DACT
EDITORS: Leah A. Cohn, DVM, PhD, DACVIM; Mark S. Thompson, DVM, DABVP

Breeding Soundness Exam: Male Dog

Difficulty level: ♦♦

Overview and Goal

Evaluate the physical and physiologic parameters of the breeding male.

Indications

- Before breeding, especially with a virgin male; a male with a history of systemic disease; or when the male has not been used for breeding for several months
- Less than 50% whelping rate
- Prepurchase evaluation of a male intended for breeding

Equipment, Anesthesia

- Scrotal calipers
- A semen collection vessel such as
  - 15-mL centrifuge tube and plastic cone
  - Sterile urine cup
  - Whirl-Pak bag
- Microscope
- Morphology stain (eosin-nigrosin) and Romanowsky (Diff-Quik) stain for cytologic analysis
- Hemocytometer and Unopette system for white blood cell (WBC) count
- Ultrasound

Anticipated Time

30-90 minutes

Preparation: Important Checkpoints

- One-week sexual rest recommended before a breeding soundness exam (BSE)
- It is recommended to fill out an evaluation form when performing a BSE because it helps ensure all important points are covered and provides a valuable record. An evaluation form is available from the Society for Theriogenology.

Possible Complications and Common Errors to Avoid

- It is important to prevent thermal, mechanical, or chemical injury to the semen after collection.
- A poor-quality semen sample, especially one with low sperm numbers, should be interpreted with caution, because it may be an incomplete ejaculate. Seminal alkaline phosphatase (ALP) of epididymal origin can be used for distinguishing between an incomplete ejaculate and true azoospermia. Normal ALP concentration of a complete ejaculate is 5000-40,000 IU/L, whereas an incomplete ejaculate is typically < 1000 IU/L.

Procedure

- History
  - Obtain a general health history, including nutrition, vaccinations, systemic diseases, and previous illnesses with attention to anything that may have resulted in thermal injury (fever) or trauma to the penis or scrotum. Include all previous medications, especially glucocorticoids, anabolic steroids, chemotherapeutics, anthelmintics, and antifungal agents.
  - Obtain a thorough reproductive history, including libido, presence of a tie at each breeding, and the details for all bitches bred. This would include their age and parity, type of breeding management used, dates bred, method of pregnancy diagnosis, whelping dates, and litter sizes. The results from any previous semen evaluations, cytologic evaluation, and cultures should also be included.
- Perform a general physical exam, noting any musculoskeletal pain that may affect mating ability and potential hereditary or congenital defects. Chronic conditions such as obesity, skin disease, and endocrine disorders can also negatively impact fertility.
- Scrotal width should be measured with calipers. This correlates with testicular volume and sperm production.
- The testes and epididymides should be palpated for symmetry and consistency. The testes lie horizontally in the scrotum, with the tail of the epididymis at the caudal pole; the body and head of the epididymis lie along the cranial-dorsal aspect. It is abnormal for the testes to be soft or hard,

which may indicate degeneration, hypoplasia, neoplasia (p. 962), fibrosis, or abnormal development.

- Prostate evaluation involves rectal and abdominal palpation. For rectal palpation, it may be necessary to simultaneously exert dorsal pressure on the abdomen to lift the bladder and prostate higher into the pelvic inlet. On rectal exam, the prostate should be smooth and bilobed and lie 2-3 cm caudal to the brim of the pelvis. Size, texture, and pain should be evaluated.
  - An ultrasound exam is warranted if any abnormalities are noted. If the prostate cannot be reached by rectal exam, it may be evaluated by transabdominal ultrasound or radiography.
- Examine the prepuce for discharge or paraphimosis. Preputial discharge may be the result of posthitis or balanoposthitis. The penis is best examined during semen collection. If semen collection is not to be performed, the prepuce should be reflected and the penis evaluated.
- Semen collection
  - Before starting, the collection vessels should be within reach of the collector.
  - If possible, the male and teaser bitch should be allowed to interact. When the male becomes sexually excited, the collector should step in and begin to stimulate the penis through the prepuce.
  - The bulbus glandis is stimulated inside the prepuce until an erection is established; then the prepuce is retracted caudal to the bulbus glandis to expose the penis.
  - The collector encircles both hands around the base of the bulbus glandis. To simulate the tie, the dog may want to step over the collector's arm. The dorsal aspect of the penis remains dorsal as the collector turns the penis 180° until it is directed caudally.
  - The ejaculate should be fractionated, with each fraction collected in a separate vessel. The first fraction is the pre-sperm fraction consisting of 1-2 mL of clear prostatic fluid. The second fraction is the sperm-rich fraction and consists of 1-3 mL of an opaque to creamy white fluid. The third fraction is clear prostatic fluid and continues to be produced as long as the erection is maintained.
  - After the collection is complete, placing a small amount of water-soluble lubricant around the bulbus glandis will aid retraction into the prepuce.
- Semen evaluation
  - Color
    - The first and third fractions should be colorless, and the second should be slightly white to cream colored. In cases of prostatic disease, such as benign prostatic hyperplasia (BPH), the third fraction may be pink, red, or brown colored. A yellow color indicates urine contamination; an Azostix can be used for confirming the presence of urea.
  - Semen analysis
    - Motility is evaluated by placing a drop of semen on a warm slide and adding a cover slip. Gross motility is evaluated at low power (10-20×), and individual motility is evaluated at 40× magnification. Normal motility is > 70% with good forward progression.
    - A morphology slide is prepared by placing a drop of semen on a warm slide along with a drop of an eosin-nigrosin morphology stain. The two drops are mixed together, spread evenly across the slide, and allowed to air dry. Alternatively, the slide can be prepared by smearing the semen drop across the slide and stained using Diff-Quik. If this method is used, the slide should remain in the purple and red stain for 10 minutes each to ensure stain penetration of the sperm cells. The slide must be evaluated under oil immersion (100×). Normal morphology should be > 70%. Primary defects should not be greater than 10%, and secondary defects should not be greater than 20%.
    - A concentration is obtained by creating a 1:100 dilution, using a WBC Unopette or by manually pipetting 20 mcL of semen into 2 mL of distilled water and counting the central square on a hemocytometer. This is the concentration in million cells per milliliter.
    - Volume should be 1-30 mL total, with the sperm-rich fraction comprising 1-12 mL.
    - Total sperm/ejaculate should be 200 million to 2 billion. This depends on the body weight of the dog but should be > 22 million/kg body weight.
  - Cytologic analysis
    - Normal semen should contain < 2000 WBC/mcL; there should be < 6 leukocytes per high-power field in all portions of the ejaculate.
    - Abnormalities include red blood cells, tumor cells, and spermatocytes.
  - Culture
    - $>10^4$ gram-negative organisms/mL and an inflammatory cytologic profile indicate bacterial infection (typically prostatitis).
  - pH: between 6.3 and 6.7. Dogs with BPH have an elevated pH (≈7.5).
- Blood should be collected for a baseline database, including *Brucella canis* testing, CBC, serum biochemistry profile, and thyroid function tests.

Postprocedure

- If there is a high number of morphologically abnormal sperm, the semen analysis should be repeated in ≈60 days.
- Additional tests not part of a routine BSE but that can be performed to further investigate an infertility problem include
  - Staining for intact acrosomes
  - Computer-assisted semen analysis allows objective evaluation of motility.
  - Fluorescent stains, including evaluation for apoptosis (Annexin V assay) and DNA fragmentation (tunnel assay)
  - Flow cytometry for oxidative status of sperm and sperm chromatin structure assay
  - Sperm membrane integrity using the hypoosmotic swelling test (HOST)
  - Endocrine assays: testosterone concentrations may be lower in infertile dogs. Blood should be collected multiple times and pooled to avoid the natural highs and lows.
  - Karyotype
  - Testicular ultrasound supports diagnoses such as testicular neoplasia, hydrocele, and degeneration and allows precise calculation of testicular volume. Doppler evaluation of testicular artery blood flow can be correlated with fertility parameters.
  - Testicular biopsy

SUGGESTED READING

Johnston J, et al: Clinical approach to infertility in the male dog. In SD Johnston, et al. Canine and feline theriogenology, New York, 2001, Saunders, pp 370-387.

AUTHOR: Bronwyn Crane, DVM, MS, DACT
EDITORS: Leah A. Cohn, DVM, PhD, DACVIM; Mark S. Thompson, DVM, DABVP

Bronchoalveolar Lavage, Blind

Client Education Sheet  Video Available 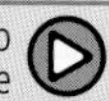

Difficulty level: ◆◆

Synonym

Blind bronchoalveolar lavage (BAL)

Overview and Goal

Simple technique, requiring no special equipment, to obtain bronchoalveolar lavage fluid (BALF) for cytology and culture in animals with respiratory disease

Indications

- Cats and small dogs suspected of having infectious or inflammatory respiratory diseases based on clinical signs and radiographic findings
- Most useful for diffuse lower airway or alveolar disease or when disease causes a productive cough

Contraindications

- Contraindication: coagulopathy. Respiratory distress is a relative contraindication.
- Not recommended for larger dogs (≥12 kg; difficult to obtain sample)
- For animals with disease localized to a specific lung lobe, collection of BALF by bronchoscopy is preferred (p. 1074).

Equipment, Anesthesia

- Laryngoscope
- Lidocaine or other topical anesthetic for laryngeal application (cats)
- Sterile endotracheal tube (ET)
- 8-12 Fr red rubber catheter
- Warm 0.9% sterile saline
- 20-mL syringes
- Two sterile collection tubes without additives
- Anesthesia: short-acting anesthesia (e.g., propofol) is sufficient.
- Oxygen source
- Ideally, pulse oximeter monitor
- Bronchodilator (e.g., terbutaline for injection, albuterol metered-dose inhaler); cats especially
- Emergency supplies in case resuscitation, ventilation, or thoracocentesis are required.

Anticipated Time

Depending on experience, 10 minutes or less

Preparation: Important Checkpoints

- Ensure that all supplies are available, including emergency needs.
- While maintaining sterility, cut the distal tip of the catheter using sharp sterile scissors or a blade to create an open end.
- Trim the other end of the red rubber catheter to ensure a tight fit with a 20-mL syringe.
- Pretreat cats with bronchodilator to minimize bronchospasm (e.g., terbutaline 0.02-0.04 mg/kg SQ 15-20 minutes before procedure).

Possible Complications and Common Errors to Avoid

- Hypoxia is expected but typically resolves quickly.
- More serious complications can include bronchospasm or pneumothorax (p. 797). Risk is minimized by pre-treating cats with terbutaline and by using a soft (i.e., red rubber) catheter.
- The distal end of the catheter must be wedged into a small airway to retrieve instilled saline. Inadequate wedging at the time of catheter placement or due to movement of the catheter after saline infusion may result in poor fluid return.
- Excessive suction applied to the syringe may collapse the small airway and impede fluid return.

Procedure

- Apply topical lidocaine on the arytenoids to minimize laryngospasm; cats especially
- Intubate the patient while taking care to avoid contact with the oral cavity to prevent contamination.
- Provide supplemental oxygen for several minutes before saline installation.
- Place the animal in lateral recumbency (either side) with the neck outstretched.
- Attach a syringe prefilled with warm saline to the red rubber, always keeping the distal end sterile.
  - 10-25 mL aliquots are typical, depending on size (most cats require 15-20 mL).
  - Hold the red rubber catheter with the open distal end up, and flush a small amount (≈0.5 mL) of saline through the red rubber to wet the end.
- Insert the red rubber into the ET while avoiding contact with the outer portion of the ET (see *Video*).
- Advance the red rubber until resistance is encountered, indicating that it is wedged in place.
  - When resistance is first encountered, give the catheter a small twist followed by gentle pressure; sometimes it catches on an airway bifurcation without wedging, and this helps avoid that error.
- Once wedged, quickly infuse the entire volume of saline.
- Without changing the syringe or moving the catheter, draw back on the syringe plunger in a gentle pulsatile fashion.
  - If the catheter is wedged, there may be negative pressure. Continue to draw back in a pulsatile fashion while very slowly withdrawing the red rubber.
  - After saline is flowing into the syringe, hold the catheter in the same spot, and continue aspirating until the flow is reduced or stops.
  - Slowly withdraw the catheter further while continuing to pull back the syringe plunger until no more fluid is retrieved. Time of insertion to completion should take no more than 30-60 seconds.
  - The volume of saline retrieved ranges from 30%-80% of the volume instilled; a good sample is > 50% recovered.
- Remove the catheter from the ET, and access sample quality grossly.
  - A good sample should contain surfactant, which appears as foam that rises to the top of the fluid.
  - If a good-quality sample is not achieved, the procedure can be repeated once, assuming the animal is oxygenating well (pulse oximetry is useful) and appears stable.
  - Flip the patient to the opposite side, and administer oxygen for several minutes before repeating procedure.
- When an adequate sample has been collected, the patient's hindquarters can be elevated so that an assistant can perform coupage to aid in drainage of fluid remaining the airways.
- Oxygen supplementation can be administered by ET until extubation

Postprocedure

- Oxygen supplementation (p. 1146) must be provided after the procedure during anesthetic recovery.
- Patients should be monitored closely for evidence of respiratory distress or cyanosis for 10 minutes after the procedure. Measurement of SpO_2 can be useful.
  - Cyanosis or distress associated with reduced lung sounds suggests pneumothorax (consider thoracocentesis [p. 1164]).
  - Cyanosis or distress with wheeze suggests bronchospasm (consider albuterol inhaler or terbutaline injection).
- Auscultation of pulmonary crackles after the procedure is expected.
- The BALF aliquots are submitted for cytologic evaluation and culture/susceptibility tests; other special tests (e.g., fungal antigen tests, viral polymerase chain reaction [PCR]) may be warranted in some cases.
- BALF samples should be analyzed promptly to avoid cell distortion. If the samples are sent to an outside laboratory, prepare an unstained slide by cytocentrifugation to submit along with the fluid sample.

Alternatives and Their Relative Merits

- Transtracheal wash: less invasive, does not require anesthesia
- Bronchoscopic-assisted BAL: allows visualization of the airways and direct sampling of specific lung lobes; preferred to blind BAL for medium to large dogs (p. 1074)

Pearls

Ideally suited for diffuse small airway disease (e.g., feline asthma) and productive alveolar disease (e.g., bacterial pneumonia) in stable cats or small dogs. Interstitial lung disease is less amenable to diagnosis by BALF but occasionally can be diagnostic (e.g., blastomycosis, pulmonary lymphoma).

RELATED CLIENT EDUCATION SHEET

Consent to Perform Bronchoalveolar Lavage (BAL)

AUTHOR: Aida I. Vientós-Plotts, DVM
EDITORS: Leah A. Cohn, DVM, PhD, DACVIM; Mark S. Thompson, DVM, DABVP

Bronchoscopy

Client Education Sheet

Difficulty level: ◆◆◆

Overview and Goal

To view and assess the anatomy (mucosal, structural) and function (dynamic collapse) of the airways from larynx to distal bronchi and to obtain samples from the distal airways for analysis

Indications

- Diagnostic: evaluation of lower airway and parenchymal disease (culture/cytologic examination, biopsy) and documentation of airway caliber disorders (malacia, collapse, compression, bronchiectasis, bronchial stenosis, torsion)
- Therapeutic: foreign body/secretion removal

Contraindications

- Major: severe hypoxemia, unstable cardiac arrhythmias, heart failure
- Minor: significant resting expiratory effort, bronchomalacia, inexperience

Equipment, Anesthesia

Equipment:

- Flexible endoscope: 3-5 mm in diameter, 55-85 cm long
- Mouth gag, sterile gauze, suction capabilities
- Sterile saline
  - Preloaded in 3 or 4 10-20 mL syringes for bronchoalveolar lavage (BAL)
  - For rinsing and cleaning
- Sterile, water-soluble lubricant
- Forceps: if foreign body removal or mucosal biopsy is required

Anesthesia:

- Pre-treatment with a bronchodilator is recommended, especially in small dogs and all cats; use injectable terbutaline 0.01 mg/kg SQ at least 15 minutes before the procedure.
- Intravenous (IV) catheter for administration of a short-acting, injectable anesthetic protocol: atropine 0.02-0.04 mg/kg IM or glycopyrrolate 0.01-0.02 mg/kg IM; in addition, butorphanol 0.05-0.1 mg/kg IM and diazepam 0.1 mg/kg IV, followed by propofol 3-6 mg/kg, slow IV titrated to effect, with repeated miniboluses of propofol (1 mg/kg) as needed over the duration of the procedure to maintain anesthetized state.
- Intubation is rarely used for the procedure; an anesthesia T-piece is required if the scope will be passed through the tube; jet ventilation can be used if available.
- Provide oxygen before, during, and after the procedure; insufflate oxygen through the endoscope channel or a 3-8 Fr sterile urinary catheter passed alongside the scope during the procedure; use a sterile endotracheal tube or a face mask for oxygen administration before and after.
- Topical 2% lidocaine if needed to decrease pharyngeal/laryngeal/tracheal sensation, excessive coughing, and movement
- Doxapram HCl 2.2 mg/kg IV once to assist with the evaluation of intrinsic laryngeal function prior to bronchoscopy, if functional laryngeal exam is indicated
- Electrocardiogram (ECG), oximetry, blood pressure (BP) cuff, and other monitoring equipment

Anticipated Time

A complete bronchoscopy and BAL procedure can be completed within 10-20 minutes by an experienced endoscopist; initial setup as well as animal recovery time is additional.

Preparation: Important Checkpoints

- The bronchoscopist must have a good understanding of normal bronchial mucosa and lung anatomy to diagnose subtle airway abnormalities.
- The bronchoscope should be cleaned and ready for use.
- Ensure all supplies and equipment are available before starting the procedure; anesthetic monitoring and image capture equipment should be turned on and ready to use.
- Antibiotics should be discontinued at least 5 days before the procedure for optimal culture results.
- Thoracic radiographs are useful to help identify specific lung regions for examination and for BAL.

Possible Complications and Common Errors to Avoid

- Contamination of the BAL sample is possible if care is not taken to avoid touching the upper airways during insertion of the scope. Guarded catheters may be used for decreasing the potential for BAL contamination, although catheter cost limits their use.
- Pulmonary barotrauma (tracheobronchial or lung rupture) is possible if the oxygen insufflation rate exceeds the ability of the gas to exit the lungs; this is of concern in smaller animals when the bronchoscope diameter is close to the tracheal size and pressure builds up in the lungs as active insufflation continues.
- Airway collapse during recovery can result in severe hypoxemia; anticipate when active expiratory effort is noted before anesthesia; slow recovery from anesthesia and topical lidocaine sprayed on the tracheobronchial mucosa help minimize this concern.

Procedure

- Sternal recumbency is recommended in cats and dogs.
- Topical 1%-2% lidocaine may be applied to the pharyngeal/laryngeal mucosa to minimize laryngospasm or excessive coughing.
- Provide oxygen as already outlined.
- Evaluate the oropharyngeal/laryngeal region; doxapram HCl (2.2 mg/kg IV once) to stimulate and confirm normal intrinsic laryngeal motion if indicated.
- Insert the bronchoscope into the airways, noting changes in shape (stenosis, stricture), dynamic caliber (malacia, collapse), and mucosa (secretions, erythema, edema, masses).
- In the normal animal, the dorsal tracheal membrane is taut so that there is little if any redundancy (no visible protrusion or collapse into the airway).
- The healthy tracheobronchial mucosa is a smooth, light pink surface with a rich supply of submucosal capillaries; if these capillaries are not visible, mucosal edema or cellular infiltration may be present.
- Healthy mucosa has a slightly glistening appearance; mucosal edema is readily apparent because it imparts a gelatinous appearance to the mucosal surface.
- The clinician should examine the carina for abnormalities (widening, compression, mucosal infiltration) before evaluating

each lobar and as many segmental and/or subsegmental bronchi as possible (as the animal and endoscope size can allow).

- Airway bifurcations beyond the carina are referred to simply as *spurs*. Like the carina, they should also form a sharp V, but they become widened and appear U-shaped with chronic airway inflammation and/or mucosal edema.
- Small polypoid mucosal nodules are commonly encountered in the bronchi of dogs with chronic bronchitis.
- Small amounts of white or slightly opaque mucus may be noted in a healthy animal, but larger accumulations or secretions of unusual color are abnormal.
- The normal monopodial branching system results in a gentle, smooth tapering of the airways. Changes may be focal or generalized and include those of shape and size of the airway lumen, such as an intraluminal stricture/tumor, external compression (tumor or lymphadenopathy), bronchiectasis, or dynamic collapse (malacia).
- Whether or not abnormalities are noted, samples should be obtained for culture and cytologic examination. After the initial airway evaluation, the endoscope is removed from the animal and cleaned by alternatively suctioning the channel with sterile saline and air immediately before reinsertion.
- The BAL site (lobe and bronchus) is chosen based on radiographic and gross bronchoscopic findings. If no site is clearly abnormal, BALs from both middle lung lobes should be collected.
- To perform a BAL, the bronchoscope is first gently wedged into a segmental or smaller bronchus. Aliquots of 10-20 mL of sterile saline (depending on the size of the animal) are instilled into the airway (by the suction channel or a washing pipette) and then immediately aspirated using slow, gentle hand suction.
- Ideally, at least two different sites (lung lobes) should be lavaged.
- A 40%-90% return of the volume instilled is expected. Difficulty in fluid recovery results when a proportionately large endoscope is used (prevents wedging into a small bronchus) or if malacic airways collapse when suction is applied.
- Collected fluid is often turbid and should have foam indicating surfactant in the sample.
- If there is enough time and anesthetic depth is appropriate, the nasopharynx also should be examined.

Postprocedure

- Provide supplemental oxygen (p. 1146) until fully recovered.
- Crackles are commonly noted on auscultation for a short time after a BAL procedure.
- Process samples immediately.
  - Quantitated aerobic cultures should be made if possible.
  - *Mycoplasma* and anaerobic cultures are processed using Amies transport media, or submit fluid in a sterile tube.
  - Cytologic analysis: total white blood cell (WBC) and differential cell counts should be done. The predominant cell in all species should be the alveolar macrophage (>70%), with usually < 3%-8% of all other cell types (except cats, which may have ≥ 15% eosinophils and still be normal).
- Handling the scope
  - Immediately rinse/wipe the scope down when finished to prevent secretions from drying.
  - Clean and sterilize the scope as outlined in the manufacturer's manual.
  - Store the scope hanging up (to fully dry it) in a protected space/closet.

Alternatives and Their Relative Merits

- Tracheal wash procedures are less expensive and easier to perform, but they lack the ability to direct sampling into specific sites; provide no information regarding anatomic, structural, or functional airway abnormalities; and offer no therapeutic capability.
- A technique of passing a 5-8 Fr sterile red rubber feeding tube into the lower trachea and wedging in a distal bronchus is called a *blind BAL*. The site sampled is unknown, and no visual assessment of the airways is made. The distal tip (side holes) of the catheter should be cut off, and the catheter is then passed until gently wedged in a distal airway. The BAL is performed as described above.
- Fine-needle lung aspiration biopsy has been used successfully to sample consolidated lung lobes and larger masses that are in contact with the chest wall.

Pearls

- In patients with pronounced expiratory effort, it is difficult to obtain a good return from a BAL. These patients are more likely to experience hypoxemia during recovery. Use very slow, gentle hand suction technique

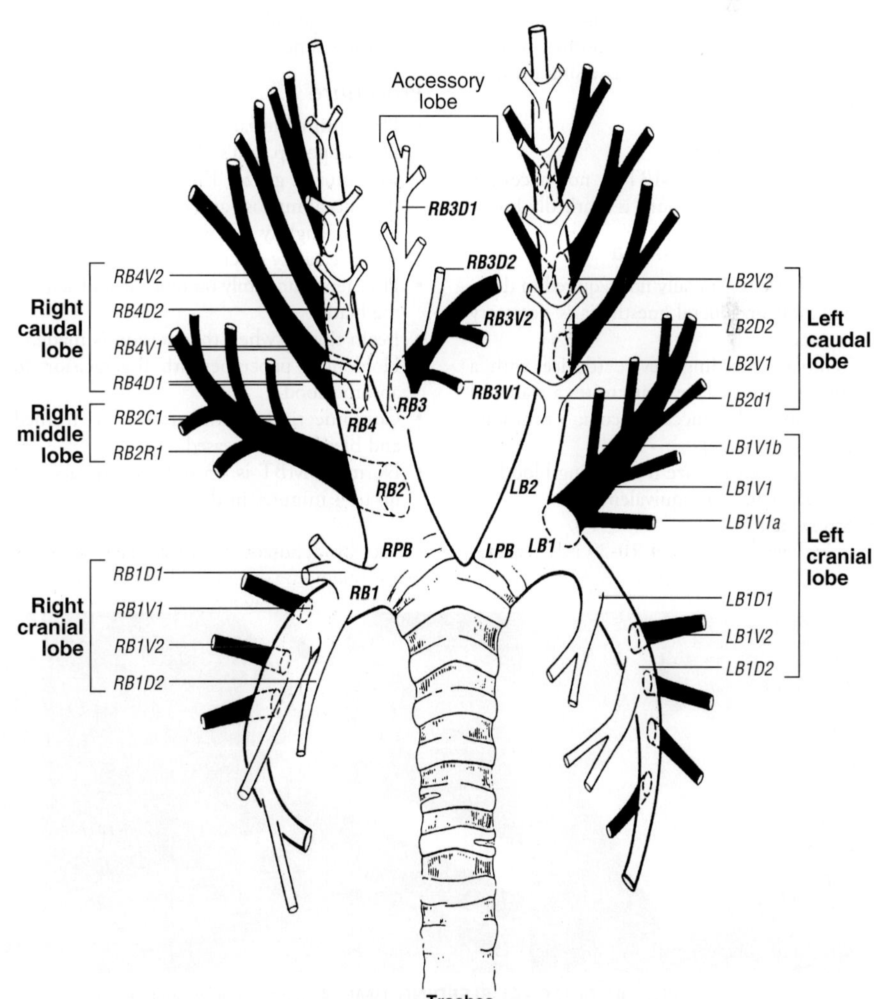

BRONCHOSCOPY Diagrammatic representation of the normal canine tracheobronchial tree. (Reprinted with permission from Amis T, et al: Systematic identification of endobronchial anatomy during bronchoscopy in the dog. Am J Vet Res 47:2649-2657, 1986.)

to obtain BAL fluid, allow slow anesthesia recovery, and oxygenate well until recovered.
- When one lung lobe is more affected than others, begin evaluation with the less affected lobes.

SUGGESTED READING

McKiernan B: Bronchoscopy. In McCarthy TC, editor: Veterinary endoscopy for the small animal veterinary practitioner, St. Louis, 2005, Saunders, pp 201-227.

Reproduced from the third edition in modified form.

AUTHOR: Brendan C. McKiernan, DVM, DACVIM
EDITORS: Leah A. Cohn, DVM, PhD, DACVIM; Mark S. Thompson, DVM, DABVP

Buccal Mucosal Bleeding Time

Difficulty level: ♦♦

Synonyms

Bleeding time, buccal mucosal bleeding time (BMBT)

Overview and Goal

To quickly and easily assess primary hemostasis (i.e., evaluate formation of a platelet plug)

Indications

Presence of mucosal hemorrhage (petechiae/ecchymoses, gingival bleeding, epistaxis, melena, hematuria) in animals with a normal platelet count and may be used for assessing primary hemostasis preoperatively

Contraindications

Thrombocytopenia (BMBT is not necessary or helpful if platelet count is markedly low)

Equipment, Anesthesia

- Anesthesia is generally not required in dogs.
- Sedation or general anesthesia is necessary in cats.
- Template bleeding device (device with a spring-loaded blade that creates a standard incision in the buccal mucosa; 5 mm long and 1 mm wide)
- Filter paper or gauze for blotting blood
- Muzzle gauze (or equivalent)
- Stopwatch

Anticipated Time

A total of 5-10 minutes

Preparation: Important Checkpoints

Evaluate platelet count before evaluating BMBT.

Possible Complications and Common Errors to Avoid

- Animal may become agitated; use sedation as needed to keep animal still for entire test.
- Do not manually disrupt clot while assessing clotting time.

Procedure

- Place animal in lateral recumbency.
- Evert upper lip, and secure in everted position with muzzle gauze. This allows exposure of the buccal mucosa and causes the vessels to become slightly engorged.
- Remove safety catch from template.
- Place template firmly on mucosa, and activate the blade.
- Begin timing when the incision is made.
- Hold filter paper beneath the incision to absorb blood.
- Continue timing until a clot has formed and bleeding has ceased.
- Normal BMBT is ≈3 minutes in cats and up to 4 minutes in dogs.

Postprocedure

After the clot has formed and the test is completed, it may be necessary to apply direct pressure as needed if the clot becomes disrupted and bleeding resumes.

Alternatives and Their Relative Merits

Cuticle ("toenail") bleeding time; less reliable as a measure of primary hemostasis and more painful to the animal

Pearls

- Avoid the temptation to place blotting material directly on the incision.
- High interoperator variability limits the accuracy of this test.

SUGGESTED READING

Couto G: Hemostasis. In Nelson R, et al, editors: Small animal internal medicine, ed 4, St. Louis, 2009, Mosby, pp 1245-1246.

Reproduced from the third edition in unabridged form.

AUTHOR: Erika de Papp, DVM, DACVIM
EDITORS: Leah A. Cohn, DVM, PhD, DACVIM; Mark S. Thompson, DVM, DABVP

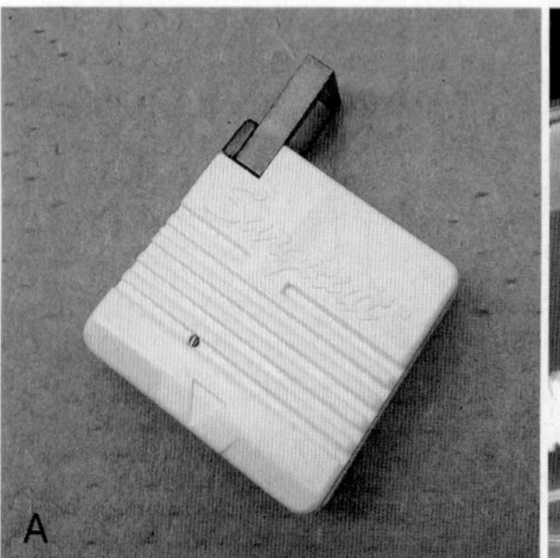

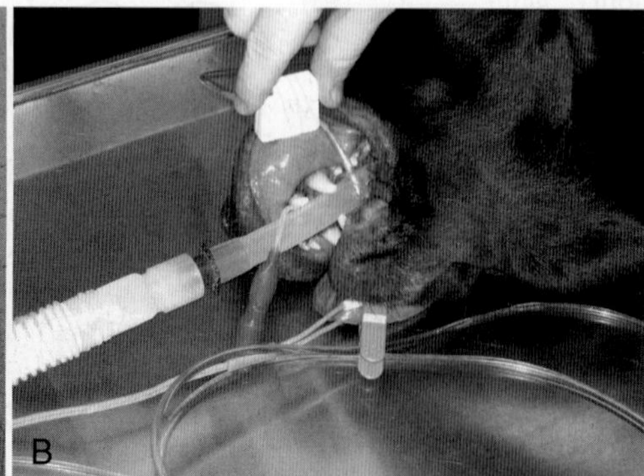

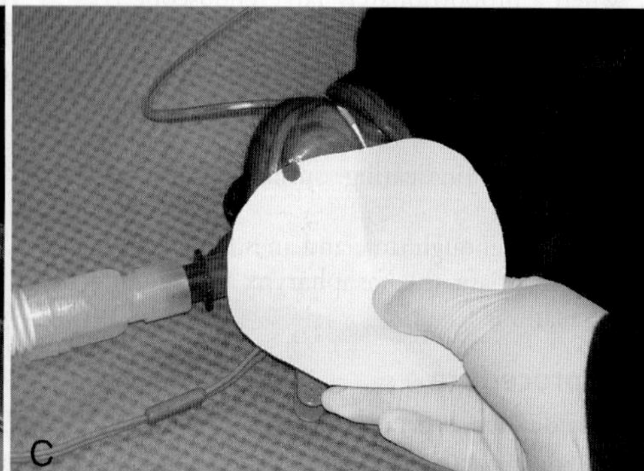

BUCCAL MUCOSAL BLEEDING TIME A, Template device before activation. **B,** Template bleeding device placed against buccal mucosa. **C,** Blotting blood below the incision.

Calorie Needs Calculation

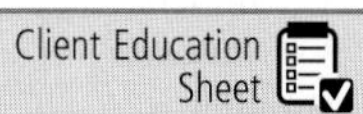

Difficulty level: ◆

Synonyms

Energy requirements, caloric requirements

Overview and Goal

The goal of calculation of estimated calorie needs is to provide client guidance on amounts to feed and to compare current or historical to expected intakes to more accurately evaluate unwanted weight loss or gain.

Indications

When providing new feeding recommendations for new pets, for pets switching diets, or for pets who have unintentionally lost or gained weight

Contraindications

If current intake can be accurately determined and correlated with serial body weight measurements, this is the best indicator of an individual's needs and is superior to equations.

Equipment, Anesthesia

Calculator or computer

Anticipated Time

Less than 1 minute to calculate estimated energy needs; variable time needed to collect and assess current calorie intake data from an individual diet history

Preparation: Important Checkpoints

- Body weight in kg
- If possible, complete a thorough diet history with exact diets, treats, supplements, and daily amounts fed

Possible Complications and Common Errors to Avoid

Equations provide only an estimate but are applied to patients with individual needs. Use only as a starting point, then use serial body weights at consistent intake to make appropriate adjustments in amount fed.

Procedure

- Measure body weight (BW) in kg.
- Calculate resting energy requirement (RER):
  - $RER = BW^{0.75} \times 70$
  - Hint: to raise BW to 0.75 power for 20-kg dog, use a smart phone or calculator, or enter this into an Internet browser: 20^0.75, then multiply answer by 70 to get RER
- Apply life stage/activity factor to estimate maintenance energy requirement (MER):
  - MER = RER × life stage/activity factor
  - Life stage/activity factors
    - Growing dog: 3 (<4 months) to 2 (>4 months)
    - Overweight-prone or sedentary dog: 1.0-1.2
    - Overweight-prone or sedentary cat: 0.8-1.0
    - Neutered dog: 1.4-1.6
    - Neutered cat: 1.0-1.2
    - Intact dog: 1.8
    - Intact cat: 1.4
- To achieve weight loss, see p. 700.

Postprocedure

- Measure serial body weights over time at consistent intake (repeat diet history at each visit).
- Apply body and muscle condition scoring at each visit.
- Adjust the amount fed as needed to achieve or maintain ideal body condition.

Alternatives and Their Relative Merits

A complete diet history and determination of total current calorie intake, ideally in consideration of body weight trends, is the best way to determine the needs of an individual.

Pearls

- Calorie content is often available on product websites, and is required to be provided on labels of packaged pet foods and treats per Association of American Feed Control Officials guidelines, which are law in many U.S. states.
- It is not unusual for true energy needs of individual patients to vary up to +/− 50% compared to estimates determined by equations.

SUGGESTED READING

Freeman L, et al: WSAVA nutritional assessment guidelines. Compend Contin Educ Vet 33(8):E1-E9, 2012.

RELATED CLIENT EDUCATION SHEETS

How to Change a Pet's Diet
How to Effectively Induce Weight Loss in a Dog or Cat

AUTHOR: Jennifer A. Larsen, DVM, PhD, DACVN
EDITORS: Leah A. Cohn, DVM, PhD, DACVIM; Mark S. Thompson, DVM, DABVP

Cardiopulmonary Resuscitation

Difficulty level: ◆◆

Synonyms

Cardiopulmonary resuscitation (CPR), cardiopulmonary cerebral resuscitation

Overview and Goal

CPR is used in apneic animals without signs of effective circulation (i.e., cardiopulmonary arrest [CPA]). It consists of basic life support (BLS) and advanced life support (ALS). BLS includes positive-pressure ventilation and external chest compressions. ALS includes monitoring, vascular access, drug administration, and defibrillation.

The immediate goals of CPR are 1) preserving organ function, foremost the heart and brain, and 2) restarting the heart. Its purpose is to provide the animal a chance for meaningful survival. The overall survival to hospital discharge rate is less than 10% for dogs or cats undergoing CPR, but it is markedly higher for anesthetized animals.

Indications

CPR is the only available treatment for CPA. Quick recognition of CPA and immediate administration of CPR is important for a favorable outcome.

Contraindications

- Do not resuscitate (DNR) order, provided by pet owner
- The CPA is precipitated by severe, irreversible disease.
- Clear signs of death (e.g., rigor mortis; dependent lividity)

Equipment, Anesthesia

A resuscitation environment should include an audited crash cart and cognitive aids.

- Equipment
  - Pressure bag for rapid fluid infusion
  - Manual resuscitator bag
  - Airway suction unit and supplies
  - Laryngoscope
  - Endotracheal tubes of various sizes, with ties
  - Electrocardiogram (ECG) monitor
  - Defibrillator
  - External and internal defibrillation paddles
  - Capnograph

Procedures and Techniques

- Clippers
- Footstool
- Supplies
  - Syringes and hypodermic needles
  - Intravenous catheters
  - Suture material
  - Tape and gauze
  - Conductive gel for defibrillator
- Drugs
  - Epinephrine
  - Vasopressin
  - Atropine
  - Amiodarone or lidocaine
  - Naloxone
  - Flumazenil
  - Atipamezole
  - Calcium gluconate
  - 50% dextrose
  - Sodium bicarbonate
- Cognitive aids
  - CPR algorithm
  - Dosing chart

Anticipated Time

- On recognition of CPA, CPR should be initiated with minimum delay and continued until return of spontaneous circulation (ROSC) is achieved, or extending the resuscitation effort further is considered futile or is abandoned due to owner choice.
- There is no definitive duration of CPR beyond which the resuscitation effort is futile. The decision to discontinue CPR should rather be based on comorbidities, the reversibility of the cause of CPA, and patient response to CPR (e.g., end-tidal CO_2 concentration [$ETCO_2$]).
- In animals with minimal pre-arrest morbidity (e.g., anesthetic overdose), it is reasonable to conduct CPR for at least 20 minutes.

Preparation: Important Checkpoints

- Staff should undergo theoretical and psychomotor skills training in CPR with refreshers every 6 months.
- Dosing chart and CPR algorithm displayed
- Audited crash cart
- Case record sheet to document the code
- Resuscitation code from pet owners for animals at risk of CPA or undergoing general anesthesia

Possible Complications and Common Errors to Avoid

- Delayed onset of CPR
- Poor quality of chest compressions
- Excessive ventilation
- Routine administration of resuscitative fluid volumes
- Delay to initiate open-chest CPR when indicated

Procedure

Recognize CPA:

- Nonanesthetized animal: unconscious and not breathing. You may assess the airway and feel for a pulse or heartbeat, but complete in 10-15 seconds.
- Anesthetized patient: use physiologic monitoring (e.g., ECG, capnography, esophageal stethoscope) to identify absence of effective circulation.
- Call for help.
- Initiate BLS immediately.

Start BLS with chest compressions:

- Animal in left or right lateral recumbency
- Position yourself on the dorsal side of the animal.
- Position shoulders vertically above the compression point.
- Elbows locked, with compression force originating from core muscles
- Stack your hands to generate one focal compression point.
- Compression point varies with chest conformation or size of animal:
  - Highest point of chest in round-chested dogs (e.g., Labrador)
  - Over the heart in keel-chested dogs (e.g., greyhound)
  - Over the heart in small dogs (<7 kg) or cats
  - Circumferential in small dogs or cats; one hand reaches around sternum to compress the heart, and the other reaches around the back
  - Over the mid-sternum in flat-chested dogs (e.g., English bulldog), with the animal in dorsal recumbency
- Compression rate: 100-120 compressions/min
- Compression depth: one-third to one-half of the chest width
- Allow the chest to fully expand between two chest compressions.
- Avoid or minimize interruption in chest compressions for intubation or vascular access.
- Deliver chest compressions in uninterrupted cycles of 2 minutes.

Intubate and ventilate as early as possible:

- Conduct orotracheal intubation, inflate the cuff, and secure the tube.
- Initiate ventilation as follows:
  - Self-inflatable resuscitator bag or the rebreathing bag of an anesthesia machine
  - Supplemental oxygen
  - 10 breaths/min
  - Inspiratory time: 1 second
  - Tidal volume: 10 mL/kg
  - No coordination with chest compressions required
- Only one rescuer present or intubation not possible:
  - Mouth-to-snout or bag-mask ventilation
  - Extend the animal's neck to align with back.
  - Firmly close the animal's mouth.
  - Form a seal with your mouth around the animal's nares or with the mask around the animal's muzzle.
  - Give 2 short breaths (inspiratory time: 1 second).
  - Immediately resume chest compressions.

ALS includes monitoring, vascular access, drug administration, and defibrillation and should minimally disrupt high-quality BLS.

- Monitoring includes ECG and capnography and should be initiated during the first CPR cycle.
  - A 3-lead ECG to determine the arrest rhythm
  - The rhythm guides drug administration and defibrillation.
  - Nonshockable rhythms: asystole and pulseless electrical activity (PEA)
  - Shockable rhythms: pulseless ventricular tachycardia (pVT) and ventricular fibrillation (VF)
  - Chest compressions need to be interrupted for ECG interpretation.
  - This 5-second pause for rhythm check should occur every 2 minutes.
  - $ETCO_2$ of < 10 mm Hg: poor efficacy
  - $ETCO_2$ of < 10 mm Hg: review CPR technique, and improve chest compression quality
  - A sudden increase in $ETCO_2$ indicates ROSC.
  - Pulse oximetry and noninvasive blood pressure measurement are not useful during CPR.
  - Collect a blood sample early, and analyze for electrolyte, acid-base, glucose, and severe anemia.
- Drug administration can occur by intravenous (IV), intraosseous (IO), or endotracheal (ET) route:
  - Place IV or IO access with minimal interruption of chest compressions.
  - Consider cut-down technique for venous cannulation.
  - IO access in very small or neonatal patients
  - Administer IO drugs and doses as for IV.
  - Chase IV/IO drugs with a flush of isotonic crystalloids (5 mL in cats and small dogs; 20 mL in a larger dog).
  - Double drug doses for ET.
  - Use long catheter to administer ET drugs, with the tip at the carina of the trachea, flush with isotonic saline.
  - Intracardiac injection is not recommended.
- Drug dosages should be displayed in the resuscitation area.
- Drugs include vasopressors, atropine, antagonists, bicarbonate, and antiarrhythmics.
  - Epinephrine and vasopressin can be used as vasopressor to improve coronary and cerebral perfusion. Both drugs can be used interchangeably. Give vasopressors in nonshockable rhythms and repeat every 3-5 minutes (i.e., every second CPR cycle).
  - Start with a low dose of epinephrine (0.01 mg/kg IV/IO).
  - Use only a high dose of epinephrine (0.1 mg/kg IV/IO) in prolonged CPR (e.g., > 10 minutes).
  - Consider atropine administration in animals with nonshockable rhythm, especially if a vagal cause of CPA is suspected.
  - Use reversal agents for opioids, benzodiazepines or alpha-2 adrenoceptor agonists, if appropriate.
  - Amiodarone is indicated when VF persists despite 2 or more defibrillation

attempts. Lidocaine is an alternative when amiodarone is not available.
  - Give sodium bicarbonate (1 mEq/kg IV/IO) when CPR is prolonged (e.g., > 10 minutes).
- Defibrillation is the treatment of choice for shockable rhythms (i.e., pVT or VF).
  - After a shockable rhythm is identified, defibrillate as early as possible while minimally interrupting chest compressions.
  - Apply ample amounts of defibrillator gel to the defibrillator electrodes (e.g., paddles).
  - Charge the defibrillator to the Joules appropriate for the animal's size.
  - Interrupt chest compressions, and position the paddles on either side of the chest over the heart.
  - Apply ample pressure on the paddles to reduce impedance to current.
  - Ensure that nobody is in contact with the animal (CLEAR!), and apply a single shock.
  - Resume chest compressions for a full 2-minute cycle of CPR until next rhythm analysis.
  - If VF/pVT persists, consider increasing defibrillator dose by 50%.
  - See electrical defibrillation (p. 1088).
- Identify and treat reversible causes of CPA.
  - Severe electrolyte abnormalities: hypokalemia; hyperkalemia; hypocalcemia
  - Severe metabolic acidosis: sodium bicarbonate (1 mEq/kg IV/IO)
  - Severe hypoglycemia: dextrose 50% (0.5 g/kg IV/IO)
  - Pneumothorax: open-chest CPR
  - Severe hemorrhage: resuscitative fluid therapy and blood transfusions

Discontinuation of CPR: high-quality CPR should be continued until one of the two occurs:

- CPR is abandoned for futility or on owner's decision
- ROSC is achieved, recognized by
  - Palpable femoral pulse
  - Marked increase in $ETCO_2$

Postprocedure

Postcardiac arrest (PCA) care is crucial for a positive outcome. It encompasses two phases:

- Prevention of re-arrest
  - Continue mechanical/manual ventilation to achieve normoventilation (i.e., $PaCO_2$ = 35-40 mm Hg; $ETCO_2$ = 30-35 mm Hg) and oxygen supplementation for an SpO_2 = 94%-98%.
  - Start an epinephrine CRI at 0.1 mcg/kg/min and titrate to maintain a mean arterial blood pressure of 80 mm Hg without inducing significant cardiac arrhythmias.
- Supportive care to minimize organ injury
  - Hemodynamic optimization: continue vasopressors, inotropes, fluid therapy; consider possible transfusion of red blood cells to maintain a normal blood pressure and to allow quick lactate clearance.
  - Respiratory optimization: support ventilation and oxygenation (normal $ETCO_2$ and SpO_2) until the animal regains normal respiratory function.
  - Targeted temperature management: maintain hypothermia (33°C-37°C) if comatose, and do not permit faster rewarming than 0.5°C/h.
  - Consider administration of phenobarbital to prevent seizures.
  - Correct significant acid-base/electrolyte abnormalities.
  - Provide analgesia and sedation as needed.
  - Refer to a facility that can provide 24-hour intensive care for further PCA care.

Alternatives and Their Relative Merits

CPR should be reserved for animals with comorbidity levels that render return to an acceptable quality of life possible. An advanced directive (e.g., resuscitation code) should be obtained from pet's owner for all animals at risk of CPA.

Pearls

- Do not delay initiation of CPR by using additional monitoring or testing. If in doubt, start CPR.
- Quality of chest compressions is most important for effective CPR. Training is essential!

Dosing Chart for Drugs Recommended for Cardiopulmonary Resuscitation

Treatment	Drug or Defibrillation Dosing	Dose	TOTAL DOSE (ML) BASED ON WEIGHT (KG [LB]) 2.5 (5)	5 (10)	10 (20)	15 (30)	20 (40)	25 (50)	30 (60)	35 (70)	40 (80)	45 (90)	50 (100)
Arrest	Epi low (1 mg/mL) every 3-5 min	0.01 mg/kg	0.03	0.05	0.1	0.15	0.2	0.25	0.3	0.35	0.4	0.45	0.5
	Epi high (1 mg/mL) for prolonged CPR	0.1 mg/kg	0.25	0.5	1	1.5	2	2.5	3	3.5	4	4.5	5
	Vasopressin (20 U/mL)	0.8 U/kg	0.1	0.2	0.4	0.6	0.8	1	1.2	1.4	1.6	1.8	2
	Atropine (0.54 mg/mL)	0.04 mg/kg	0.2	0.4	0.8	1.1	1.5	1.9	2.2	2.6	3	3.3	3.7
Antiarrhythmic	Amiodarone (50 mg/mL)	5 mg/kg	0.25	0.5	1	1.5	2	2.5	3	3.5	4	4.5	5
	Lidocaine (20 mg/mL)	2 mg/kg	0.25	0.5	1	1.5	2	2.5	3	3.5	4	4.5	5
Reversal	Naloxone (0.4 mg/mL)	0.04 mg/kg	0.25	0.5	1	1.5	2	2.5	3	3.5	4	4.5	5
	Flumazenil (0.1 mg/mL)	0.01 mg/kg	0.25	0.5	1	1.5	2	2.5	3	3.5	4	4.5	5
	Atipamezole (5 mg/mL)	100 mcg/kg	0.05	0.1	0.2	0.3	0.4	0.5	0.6	0.7	0.8	0.9	1
Defib Biphasic	External defib (J)	2-4 J/kg	5	10	20	30	40	50	60	70	80	90	100
	Internal defib (J)	0.2-0.4 J/kg	1	2	2	3	4	5	6	7	8	9	10

Defib, defibrillation; *Epi*, epinephrine.
(Modified from Fletcher DJ, et al: RECOVER evidence and knowledge gap analysis on veterinary CPR. Part 7: Clinical guidelines. J Vet Emerg Crit Care 22(suppl 1):S102-S131, 2012.)

- CPR requires an excellent team performance; conduct mock codes and debriefings.
- Do not expect animals to return to normal within hours after ROSC. Neurologic prognostication is difficult and not well defined for small animals. Neurologic progress should be assessed over several days before arriving at a definitive grave neurologic prognosis.

SUGGESTED READING

Fletcher DJ, et al: RECOVER evidence and knowledge gap analysis on veterinary CPR. Part 7: Clinical guidelines. J Vet Emerg Crit Care 22(suppl 1):S102-S131, 2012.

AUTHORS: Manuel Boller, Dr. med. vet., MTR, DACVECC; Daniel J. Fletcher, PhD, DVM, DACVECC
EDITORS: Leah A. Cohn, DVM, PhD, DACVIM; Mark S. Thompson, DVM, DABVP

Cerebrospinal Fluid Collection

Client Education Sheet 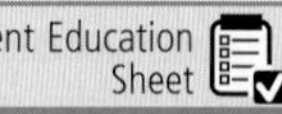

Difficulty level: ♦♦

Synonyms

Spinal tap, CSF tap

Overview and Goal

- To safely collect an uncontaminated sample of cerebrospinal fluid (CSF) from an animal with suspected central nervous system (CNS) disease
- CSF analysis is the single most valuable diagnostic test for evaluating inflammatory CNS disorders, and it aids in the diagnosis of other encephalopathies and myelopathies.

Indications

- Clinical signs consistent with CNS or nerve root dysfunction
- Monitoring treatment efficacy of confirmed inflammatory CNS disease
- Intrathecal administration of contrast material (myelography) or medications

Contraindications

Absolute:
- Increased intracranial pressure (depressed mental status, bradycardia, hypertension, miosis, anisocoria)
- Any condition in which general anesthesia is contraindicated

Relative:
- Advanced imaging results that identify a noninflammatory disease process consistent with the animal's clinical signs
- Coagulopathy

Equipment, Anesthesia

- General anesthesia and endotracheal intubation
- A few 20- or 22-gauge, 1½-inch spinal needles (2½-inch or 3½-inch needles may be needed for large dogs or for lumbar approach)
- Hair clippers
- Surgical scrub solution, isopropyl alcohol, and gauze
- Sterile surgical gloves
- Sterile collection tubes (do not use tubes containing EDTA [lavender-top tubes])
- An assistant to position the animal and stabilize the animal's head and neck
- Level stationary or locked table

Anticipated Time

About 30 minutes of anesthesia

Preparation: Important Checkpoints

- Performed preferably after advanced imaging has ruled out noninflammatory processes (neoplasia, malformation, vascular disorders) and obvious increased intracranial pressure (coning and caudal displacement of the cerebellum, flattening of gyri, loss of sulci)
- Make arrangements for laboratory transport within 30 minutes of collection, or have in-house analysis equipment prepared and calibrated.
- If immediate analysis of the CSF is not possible, special preservation techniques may be required (prior laboratory consultation is recommended).
- Warn owners of hair clipping and low risk of complications. Complications associated with the procedure, although rare, can be fatal.

Possible Complications and Common Errors to Avoid

- Blood contamination of the sample
- Iatrogenic neuronal injury
- Brain herniation
- Inadequate sample volume

Procedure

CEREBELLOMEDULLARY APPROACH

- General anesthesia and intubation
- Preparation and positioning for centesis from the cerebellomedullary cistern (preferred for ease and lower risk of blood contamination)
  - Shave and aseptically prepare the skin from the occipital protuberance to the spine of C3 and to the base of each pinna.
- Don sterile gloves.
- Patient in right lateral recumbency (right-handed clinician) or left lateral (left-handed clinician)
- An assistant holds the head with the neck flexed at a 90° angle and the head and neck parallel to the table. Care must be taken to not overflex the neck, which could result in obstruction of the endotracheal tube or compress the jugular veins and increase intracranial pressure. For the head to be parallel to the table, the assistant must hold the nose slightly elevated from the table.
- The assistant positions the dorsal aspect of the neck at the edge or slightly over the edge of the table.
- The clinician should sit on a stool or kneel to be at eye level with the animal's head.

Landmarking and puncture:
- The right-handed clinician places the left thumb on the right wing of the animal's atlas and the left middle/ring finger on the left wing of the atlas.
- The left index finger is used for identifying the midline by palpating the occipital protuberance and the dorsal spine of C2, drawing an invisible line between these points.
  - Many cats and toy-breed dogs do not have a well-defined occipital protuberance; instead, the spine of C2 should be used as the sole landmark for identifying the midline.
- The orientation of the needle's path should be parallel to the table's surface and toward the angle of the animal's mandible.
- For dogs, using the right hand, the needle with stylet in place is inserted through the skin along the midline just cranial to the wings of the atlas.
- In cats, the skin is often tough, and the distance between the skin and subarachnoid space is very small. Although the same point of insertion is identified, the skin should be tented before inserting the needle through the skin into the subcutaneous tissues.
- The needle is directed through subcutaneous fat and muscle toward the subarachnoid space, taking care to avoid lateral, caudal, or cranial deviation of the spinal needle.
- Occasionally, a loss of resistance to the needle insertion is felt as the needle passes through the fascial planes of the muscle and, eventually, the dorsal atlantooccipital membrane; this so-called pop is not reliable and should not be used as an indicator of appropriate depth of the needle.

- While maintaining a grip on the hub of the needle with the right hand, the clinician uses the left hand to grasp the needle near its insertion into the skin.
- The stylet is withdrawn with the right hand, and the needle hub is examined for CSF flow.
- If no CSF is present, the needle is first withdrawn a few millimeters while watching for the appearance of CSF to ensure the needle has not been inserted too deeply (into nervous tissue), and then the needle is advanced. The stylet need not be replaced at this point. (Although advancing the needle without the stylet creates a slight risk of creating a tissue plug in the needle, it decreases the risk of advancing the needle too deeply because CSF appears as soon as the subarachnoid space is entered.)
- As the needle is advanced, one of three things happens:
  - CSF appears in the hub of the needle and begins to drip out. The needle should then be advanced 1 mm farther to place the entire bevel in the cerebellomedullary cistern, and the needle is grasped firmly against the skin. The slight advancement and firm hold on the needle reduce the risk of blood contamination from meningeal vessels.
  - The needle hits bone. This is usually the occipital bone, and the needle should be redirected caudally to enter the cerebellomedullary cistern; if it strikes the atlas, the needle must be redirected cranially. The needle may be walked along the bone to find the cistern, bearing in mind that it will be only millimeters deeper, but this may result in blood contamination from trauma to the periosteum.
  - Frank blood appears in the hub. This most likely indicates that the needle is off midline and has punctured a venous sinus. In this case, the needle is removed and discarded, gloves are changed, the surgical prep is repeated, and the procedure is started again. NOTE: If blood is encountered, it is typically from a location outside the subarachnoid space and does not limit the ability to obtain an uncontaminated sample when the procedure is repeated.
- After CSF begins to drip from the hub, it is collected into two plain, sterile, red-top tubes. Ideally, an assistant collects the sample, and the examiner does not release the needle during collection.
- In general, 1 mL of CSF is required for assessment of the white blood cell (WBC) count, protein concentration, and cytologic examination (1 mL/5 kg of body weight can be obtained safely).
- If the animal weighs > 5 kg, additional CSF can and should be collected for possible culture or ancillary diagnostics, such as infectious titers, flow cytometry, or immunoglobulin indices.
- After the appropriate amount of CSF has been collected, the needle is removed.
- NOTE: If during the procedure the heart rate acutely decreases or fluid streams rather than drips from the hub when the subarachnoid space is entered, the needle should be removed and the procedure aborted.

LUMBAR APPROACH

- General anesthesia and intubation
- Preparation and positioning (for centesis from the lumbar subarachnoid space) is technically more difficult, yields less fluid, and is more likely to involve blood contamination but is more sensitive for focal thoracolumbar lesions.
- The skin is shaved and aseptically prepared over the dorsal midline from L3 cranially to the midsacrum caudally and the wings of the ilium laterally.
- Sterile gloves are worn, but the field is not usually draped.
- The animal is positioned in lateral recumbency with the hindlimbs and lumbar spine flexed (tucked posture).

Landmarking and puncture:

- The needle enters the L5-L6, or L6-L7 interspace in dogs or the L7-S1 interspace in cats.
- Except in very small or thin animals, the L6 dorsal spine is typically the most caudal and can be palpated just cranial to the wings of the ilium.
- If the L7 dorsal spine is palpable, it is usually much smaller than that of L6 and lies between the wings of the ilium.
- Radiographs can demonstrate individual differences in anatomy.
- The needle is inserted into the skin just caudolaterally to the caudal dorsal spine of the space to be entered (i.e., caudolaterally to L6 for puncture between L5 and L6).
- The needle is directed craniomedially to puncture the interarcuate space between the vertebrae.
- If bone is encountered, the needle is redirected (usually cranially) until the space is identified.
- If the needle is inserted to the hub and no bone is encountered, the needle is too short or directed too far laterally.
- Fluid can be collected from the dorsal subarachnoid space, but more often the needle is passed through the nervous tissue to the floor of the vertebral canal.
- The stylet is removed, and if CSF is not recovered, the needle is withdrawn slightly to enter the ventral subarachnoid space while the examiner watches for the appearance of fluid in the hub of the needle.
- CSF typically flows much more slowly from this site compared with the cerebellomedullary cistern.

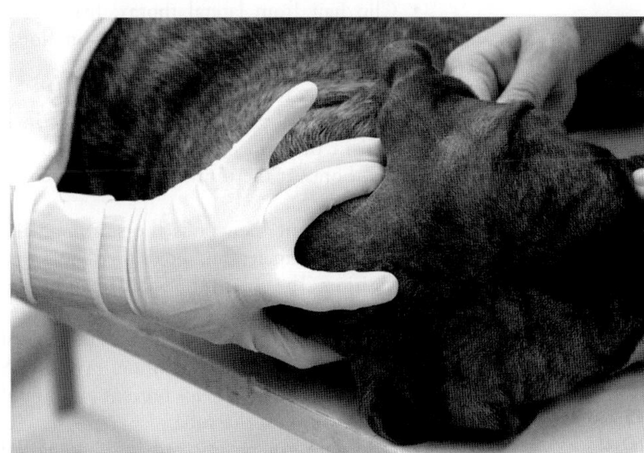

CEREBROSPINAL FLUID COLLECTION Landmarks for cerebellomedullary approach. Dog is in right lateral recumbency, head pointing to right. Right-handed clinician is using left hand to identify the occipital protuberance (index finger) and wings of the atlas (right wing of atlas: thumb; left wing of atlas: middle and ring fingers). Patient's neck is appropriately flexed (90°), and nose is elevated by an assistant so muzzle is parallel to table surface.

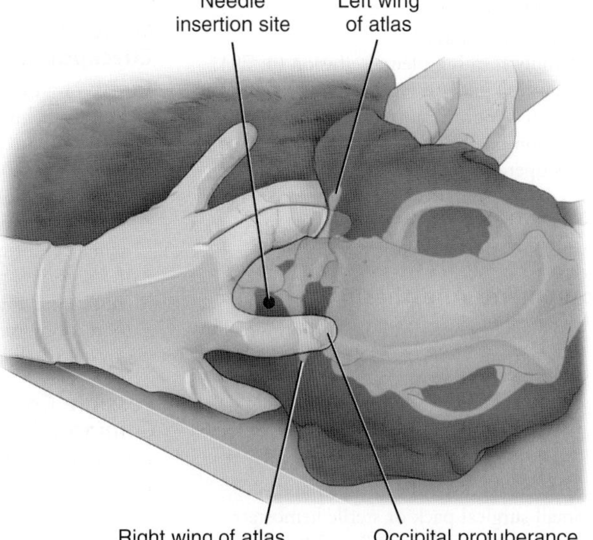

CEREBROSPINAL FLUID COLLECTION Diagram of same dog, showing bony landmarks and site of needle insertion.

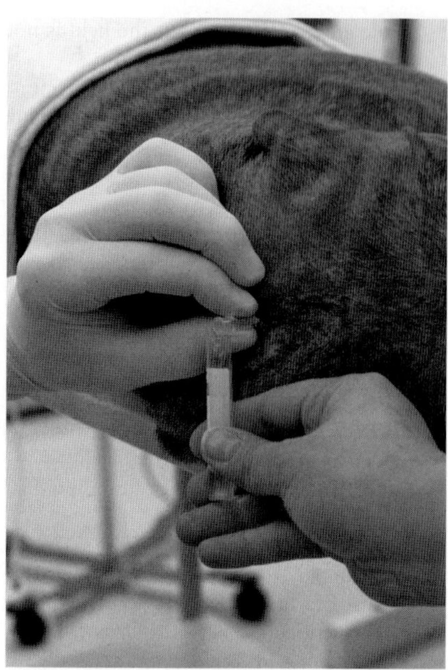

CEREBROSPINAL FLUID COLLECTION Same animal. While clinician holds the needle, an assistant collects the cerebrospinal fluid.

Postprocedure

- Routine postanesthetic monitoring
- Monitor for neurologic deficits due to iatrogenic trauma (respiratory difficulty or vestibular ataxia with puncture from the cerebellomedullary cistern; paresis and proprioceptive ataxia with lumbar puncture).

Alternatives and Their Relative Merits

MRI (p. 1132) or CT scan:

- Advanced imaging superior for the diagnosis of structural lesions
- May be strongly suggestive of inflammatory disease
- Typically used in addition to CSF analysis to fully evaluate disorders of the CNS

Serum infectious titers:

- Systemic disease not necessarily reflective of CNS disease
- For most inflammatory nervous system diseases, no infectious agent is identified.

Pearls

- In cats, tent the skin, and insert the needle through the skin first.
- Avoid overflexing the neck (may kink/obstruct the endotracheal tube).
- Ensure adequate spontaneous ventilation during recovery; procedural complications can result in hypoventilation.

RELATED CLIENT EDUCATION SHEETS

Consent to Perform Cerebrospinal Fluid Tap
Consent to Perform General Anesthesia

AUTHOR: Greg Kilburn, DVM, DACVIM
EDITORS: Leah A. Cohn, DVM, PhD, DACVIM; Mark S. Thompson, DVM, DABVP

Chest Tube Placement

Client Education Sheet 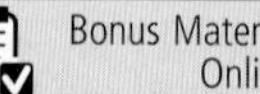 Bonus Material Online 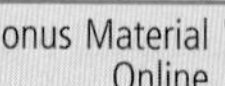

Difficulty level: ◆◆ 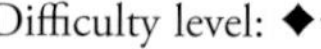

Synonym

Thoracostomy tube placement

Overview and Goal

To provide means for frequent or continuous drainage of fluid or air from the pleural cavity

Indications

- Pyothorax (p. 857)
- Rapidly forming pleural effusion (p. 791)
- Recurring pneumothorax (p. 797) requiring repeated thoracocentesis
- Tension pneumothorax
- Postoperative thoracotomy management

Contraindications

Severe bleeding disorder (p. 433)

Equipment, Anesthesia

- General anesthesia with intubation (ideally) or sedation
- Clippers
- Surgical scrub
- #11 scalpel blade
- Local anesthetic (e.g., 2% lidocaine, 0.1-0.25 mL/kg, SQ, maximum 7 mL)
- Small surgical pack or sterile hemostats
- Suture material (e.g., 2-0 to 3-0 nylon)
- An assistant (if possible)
- Thoracostomy tube
- Catheter adapter
- 3-way stopcock
- Injection caps
- ± Continuous drainage device
- 20-gauge orthopedic wire or plastic zip ties
- Wire twister and cutter if using orthopedic wire

Anticipated Time

About 15-45 minutes

Preparation: Important Checkpoints

- Make 3-5 extra drainage holes in chest tube with scalpel blade if thick or purulent fluid is present in pleural space (<50% of the diameter of tube). Be sure not to compromise the integrity of the tube with extra holes.
- Monitor animal's oxygenation with pulse oximetry during anesthesia and placement.
- If tension pneumothorax is present, continuous evacuation of pleural space by thoracocentesis until chest wall is opened can help stabilize animal.

Possible Complications and Common Errors to Avoid

- Improper (SQ) placement of tube
- Impaling the heart or lungs with the tube's stylet/trocar
- Pulmonary contusions
- Placement of the tube into the abdominal cavity, with abdominal organ trauma
    - Aforementioned complications are more common with the trocar method.
- Tube migration or premature removal of tube by animal
- Development of life-threatening pneumothorax if tube becomes open to atmosphere

Procedure

- General anesthesia (preferable) or sedation; lateral recumbency
- Clip hair from lateral thorax: from axilla cranially to last rib caudally and from dorsal spine to ventral midline.
- Aseptically prep and drape area.
- Using scalpel blade, make a small stab incision in the skin over the highest point of the thorax at the ninth or tenth intercostal space (ICS).
- The assistant then pulls the skin cranially several centimeters and holds the skin in that position. The chest tube will be placed into the thorax through the seventh or eighth ICS. When the skin is released after placement of the tube, there is a SQ tunnel of 2-3 ICS over the tube. This helps prevent air or fluid leakage around the tube.
- Lidocaine can be injected into intercostal muscle at the tube insertion site, or an intercostal nerve block can be performed, injecting lidocaine just ventral and caudal to the transverse processes of the thoracic vertebrae/head of ribs one space cranial and caudal and at the site of insertion. Before

injecting, aspirate back to determine that needle is not in the intercostal artery or vein.

- If the patient is anesthetized, stop manual ventilation while inserting tube into thorax to deflate lungs and decrease risk of lung trauma.
- With the skin still drawn cranially, hemostats are used for bluntly dissecting vertically into the pleural space, spreading the jaws wide enough for the tube to snugly fit through the opening. The tube is inserted through the jaws of the hemostat and advanced cranially and ventrally along the chest wall, making sure that all side holes in the tube are well within the thorax. The distance the tube is advanced can be measured with the stylet. The tip of the tube should be at the second or third ICS.
- Connect tube to a 3-way stopcock and injection caps or a pleural drainage system.
- Secure to skin with a purse-string suture around the tube at the entry site and a Chinese finger trap suture pattern (with or without tissue glue to affix the suture to the tube) to reduce sliding of the tube.
- Place sterile dressing and light bandage.
- Tube connection sites can be secured with orthopedic wire in figure-eight patterns or plastic zip ties.

Alternate method, trocar technique:

- Sedation/anesthesia, initial prep as previously described
- Tube and trocar/stylet within it are tunneled SQ by 2-3 rib spaces and then positioned perpendicular to the chest wall and grasped tightly 1-2 inches from distal tip.
- Top of the tube will be hit bluntly with the palm of the other hand, popping the tube through the thoracic wall and into pleural space; the other hand, grasping tube and trocar 1-2 inches from the distal tip, acts as a guard to prevent the tube from entering the thorax excessively.
- Tube is slid off the trocar/stylet cranially and ventrally along chest wall, then connected and secured as described previously.
- This very rapid placement technique is recommended in dogs only in emergency situations because of increased risk of iatrogenic trauma and is never recommended in cats because of their very compliant chest walls.

Alternate method: insertion of guide wire–based chest tube

- Local anesthesia (± sedation if needed)
- Seldinger technique: as for multilumen jugular catheters (p. 1123)
- An assistant pulls the skin cranially several centimeters and holds it in place while the tube is inserted. This creates a SQ tunnel once released. An 18- or 14-gauge catheter introducer is placed into the pleural space through the seventh or eighth ICS.
- A 60-cm guide wire is inserted through the catheter, leaving ≈20 cm or more outside the thorax.
- The catheter introducer is removed, leaving the guide wire in place.
- The 14-gauge catheter is inserted into the pleural space over the guide wire, the guide wire is removed, and the catheter is sutured in place.
- Small-diameter and flexible material make it well tolerated, especially in cats, small dogs, and animals with pneumothorax.
- Can become obstructed if effusion is thick or kink if placed in animals with a thick chest wall (large or obese dogs)

Postprocedure

- Thoracic radiographs (lateral and ventrodorsal or dorsoventral) to check tube(s) placement
- Bandage to secure tube(s)
- Pain management: injectable opioids versus intrathoracic bupivacaine (both modalities can be used for optimal pain control)
  - Bupivacaine can be given (1.5 mg/kg) diluted 1:1 with 0.9% NaCl through tube q 6-8h.
- Continuous monitoring as long as the chest tube is in place because of the risks of disconnection and development of pneumothorax

Alternatives and Their Relative Merits

Repeat thoracocentesis: may become difficult to manage animal if pleural evacuation is needed frequently

Pearls

The risk of impaling lung or heart can be minimized with the trocar technique if the operator holds the distal portion of the tube and trocar in a clenched fist, with 1-2 inches of tube and trocar protruding, to prevent excessive penetration into the thorax.

SUGGESTED READING

Lombardi R, et al: Pleural space drainage. In Burkitt Creedon JM, et al, editors: Advanced monitoring and procedures for small animal emergency and critical care, West Sussex, UK, 2012, Wiley-Blackwell, pp 378-392.

RELATED CLIENT EDUCATION SHEETS

Consent to Perform General Anesthesia
Consent to Perform Thoracocentesis

AUTHOR: Lori S. Waddell, DVM, DACVECC
EDITORS: Leah A. Cohn, DVM, PhD, DACVIM; Mark S. Thompson, DVM, DABVP

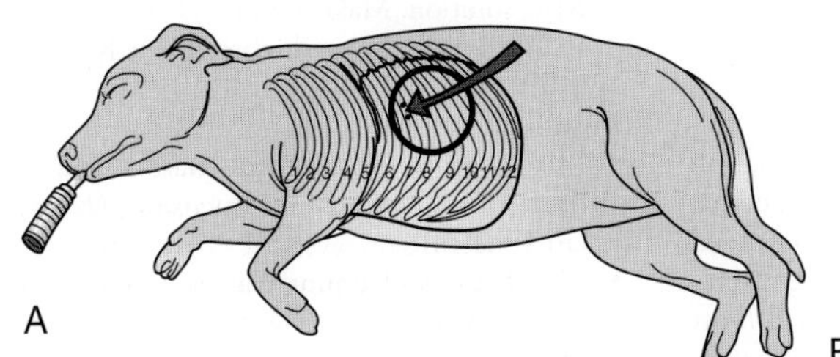

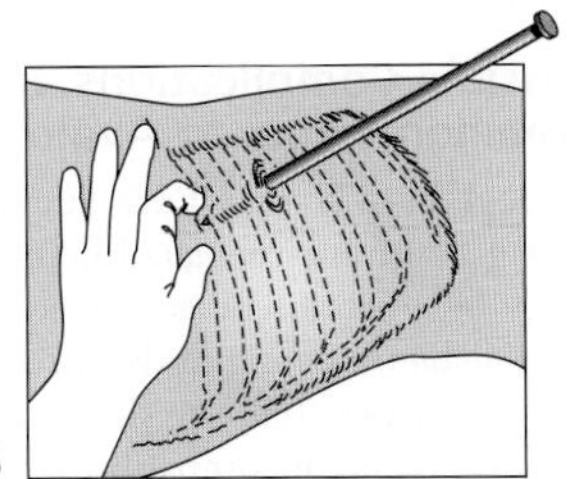

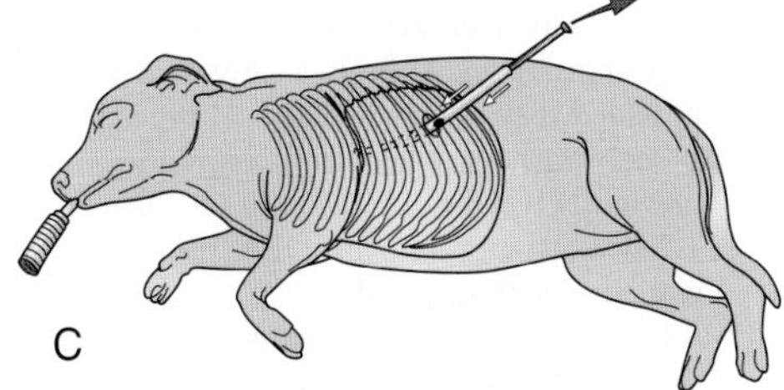

CHEST TUBE PLACEMENT A, For placement of a chest tube, animal is in lateral recumbency, and an incision is made in the skin at least two intercostal spaces (ICSs) caudal to planned site of entry into thorax. **B,** Chest tube and trocar within it are tunneled together SQ to the appropriate ICS, and chest is entered with the tube. **C,** Tube is then advanced off the trocar *(small arrows)* such that all side holes of the chest tube are within the pleural space and trocar has not advanced farther into chest. Trocar is then withdrawn *(large arrow),* and chest tube is capped and secured.

Cross-Match and Blood Typing

Difficulty level: ♦♦

Synonyms

- *Blood typing* determines presence or absence of antigens on the red blood cell (RBC) membrane. Clinically, blood group DEA 1 in dogs and the AB system in cats are most important.
- *Major cross-match* evaluates for antibodies in the recipient's plasma against the donor's RBCs and has greatest clinical significance.
- *Minor cross-match* evaluates for antibodies in the donor's plasma against the recipient's RBCs.

Overview and Goal

Cross-matching and/or blood typing eliminates most immunologic transfusion reactions (p. 989).

Indications

- Blood typing: perform before administering a blood transfusion (p. 1169) on all donors and recipients; minimizes sensitization and avoids hemolytic transfusion reactions
- Cross-match: performed before whole blood or packed RBC transfusions on all cats and on dogs that received a transfusion > 4 days previously (even if blood typed) or have an unknown transfusion history
  - First-time canine transfusions are considered safe without prior cross-matching; dogs do not possess clinically significant naturally occurring antibodies. Although mild immunologic incompatibilities have been documented in first-time transfusion recipients, their clinical importance needs further investigation.
  - Pregnancy does not sensitize dogs to RBC antigens. Dogs that have whelped can be used as blood donors and can receive a first transfusion without a cross-match provided they are properly blood typed.
  - Based on flow cytometry techniques, previously typed DEA 1.2-positive (DEA 1.2+) dogs appear to be DEA 1+ with weak antigenic expression.
  - A high percentage of Dobermans, Dalmatians, and possibly shih tzus are negative for the Dal blood type (Dal–), and most of the canine population is Dal positive (Dal+), including blood donors. Consider testing above breeds for Dal or performing cross-match because previously sensitized Dal– dogs may develop acute or delayed hemolytic reactions, and compatible blood may be difficult to find.
  - New canine blood types (Kai 1 and Kai 2) have been identified, but their clinical relevance is unknown.
  - Blood typing and cross-matching are recommended for all cats, even with first transfusion, because cats have naturally occurring antibodies to AB and Mik RBC antigens; an AB mismatch can be lethal to a type B recipient.
  - AB blood typing cannot detect Mik-related incompatibilities.

Equipment, Anesthesia

Blood typing:

- In-house canine DEA 1 and feline AB system blood-typing kits (Alvedia Quick Test, others)
  - Blood donor animals can be typed with a mail-out test along with other donor screening tests.
- Approximately ≥ 0.4 mL EDTA-anticoagulated (lavender-top tube) whole blood

Cross-match:

- 1-2 mL EDTA-anticoagulated blood from recipient and donor (or cross-match segments from units of blood)
- Tabletop centrifuge
- 3-mL test tubes (or red-top tubes)
- 0.9% saline
- Disposable pipettes or 1-mL syringes
- Test tube rack

Anticipated Time

- Blood typing: 2-5 minutes
- Major and minor cross-match: 30-40 minutes

Preparation: Important Checkpoints

- Ensure proper storage and check expiration dates.
- Blood type or cross-match EDTA blood samples within 2-3 days of collection; the physical integrity of RBCs is essential for correct results.
- Breed and geographic prevalence of blood types for dogs and cats vary.

Possible Complications and Common Errors to Avoid

- Dogs or cats that have autoagglutination (e.g., immune-mediated hemolytic anemia [p. 60]) cannot be accurately blood typed using blood-typing cards based on agglutination reaction (false-positive) and will most likely appear incompatible on cross-match.
- A patient cannot be accurately blood typed after recent blood transfusion using in-house blood-typing kits.
- Severely anemic cats or dogs (<10% hematocrit) may not show agglutination with blood-typing cards (prozone effect). Centrifuge sample, and remove plasma to concentrate RBCs before adding a drop to the test card.
- Any weakly to moderately positive DEA 1+ dog should be considered a DEA 1+ blood donor. For transfusion purposes, transfuse weakly positive DEA 1+ recipients with DEA 1– blood because it remains unknown if such patients could mount an immune response against strongly positive DEA 1+ blood.
- Feline blood-typing kits may not detect type AB cats.
- Cats with feline leukemia virus–related anemia (p. 329) may present discordant blood typing results depending on the technique used.

Procedure

- Blood typing: commercially available blood-typing kits (see package inserts)
- Cross-match: gel-based major and minor cross-match test kits are commercialized for in-practice use (see figure), and may decrease the subjectivity of interpreting results (see package inserts).

STANDARD CROSS-MATCH (MAJOR AND MINOR)

Step 1:

- Collect 1-2 mL of donor blood in an EDTA tube, or use an equivalent 1-2 mL of cross-match segments from desired unit of blood.
- Collect 1-2 mL of recipient blood in an EDTA tube.
- Centrifuge donor and recipient blood in separate labeled tubes for 5 minutes (1000 *g*).
- Remove plasma using a pipette, and save in separate labeled tubes for later use (use different pipettes for donor and recipient).
- Wash remaining packed RBCs three times by filling tubes with 0.9% saline, gently resuspending, centrifuging (1000 *g*) for 5 minutes, and decanting off the saline (discard the saline).
- After a third wash, add 0.2 mL of washed packed RBCs from the donor red-top tube to 4.8 mL of 0.9% saline (in a separate tube), and gently mix to obtain a 3%-5% RBC solution. Make a similar 3%-5% RBC solution with the washed recipient RBCs.

Step 2:

In separate test tubes:

- Mix 2 drops of recipient plasma and 1 drop of donor RBC suspension (major cross-match).
- Mix 2 drops of donor plasma and 1 drop of recipient RBC suspension (minor cross-match).
- Mix 2 drops of recipient plasma and 1 drop of recipient RBC suspension (autocontrol).
- Incubate at 37°C (ideally, but room temperature is acceptable) for 15-20 minutes.
- Centrifuge for 30 seconds.
- Observe the plasma for hemolysis. Gently resuspend the RBC button by tapping the tube, and examine for agglutination.
- Hemolysis or agglutination indicates incompatibility.

Postprocedure

- Administer type-specific blood to the patient. DEA 1+ dogs can receive DEA 1+ or DEA

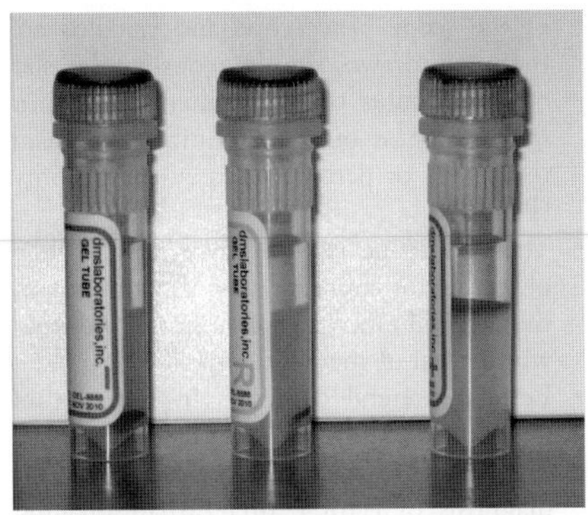

CROSS-MATCH AND BLOOD TYPING Gel-based major cross-match test kit (DMS Laboratories, Flemington, NJ).

1– blood, but DEA 1– dogs should only receive DEA 1– blood.

- When the recipient autocontrol shows hemolysis or agglutination, the cross-match cannot be interpreted. In such cases, use DEA 1– blood or *universal blood* (determined by extensive prior blood typing as a mail-out).
- If all available units are incompatible, the least reactive unit may need to be administered.
- Cats with a positive result in both wells of blood-typing cards should be retested; if result persists, they should be retested in a reference laboratory for the rare AB blood type.

Alternatives and Their Relative Merits

- Canine and feline EDTA-collected blood samples can be sent to commercial laboratories for extensive blood typing: advised for blood donors and prior transfusion incompatibilities. Different labs test for different dog erythrocyte antigens.
- A feline genetic mutation associated with the B blood group exists, and a DNA test has been developed. Cats can be tested at an early age from a buccal swab, which may be useful for cat breeders to avoid neonatal isoerythrolysis. The DNA test does not distinguish between types A and AB, however.

SUGGESTED READING

Tocci LJ: Canine recipient screening. In Yagi K, et al, editors. Manual of veterinary transfusion medicine and blood banking. Ames, IA, 2016, Wiley-Blackwell, pp 117-129.

AUTHORS: Søren R. Boysen, DVM, DACVECC; Marie-Claude Blais, DMV, DACVIM
EDITORS: Leah A. Cohn, DVM, PhD, DACVIM; Mark S. Thompson, DVM, DABVP

Procedures and Techniques

Cystoscopy

Client Education Sheet 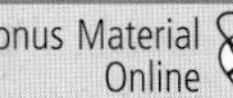 Bonus Material Online 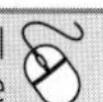

Difficulty level: ♦♦♦

Overview and Goal

Transurethral cystoscopy (urethrocystoscopy) involves the use of rigid or flexible endoscopes for examination of the lower urinary tract. Most anatomic structures can be visualized: vulvar vestibule, vagina, urethral orifice, urethra, urinary bladder, and ureteral orifices. Success is favored by proper training and experience. Several sizes and lengths of endoscopes need to be available to be prepared for the breadth of patient sizes and each sex. This procedure is done commonly in specialty practice.

Indications

Suspicion of any of the following disorders or presence of the listed clinical signs can be indications for transurethral cystoscopy:

- Anatomic abnormalities: vaginal strictures, persistent vaginal membranes (p. 1027), ectopic ureters (p. 282), urachal diverticula
- Cystitis: chronic infectious (p. 232), idiopathic, interstitial
- Posttraumatic or postoperative assessment: pelvic fractures, abdominal trauma, prior surgery
- Hematuria: examination to identify origin of bleeding and observation of ureteral orifices (unilateral vs. bilateral hematuria of renal origin)
- Urethritis: infectious, inflammatory, granulomatous/proliferative
- Stranguria, dysuria, pollakiuria, urinary incontinence: identification of possible causes; therapeutic periurethral submucosal injections of collagen for urethral sphincter mechanism incompetence (p. 538)
- Calculi: urethral or cystic calculi retrieval and identification (pp. 1014, 1016, and 1019)
- Cancer: urethra, bladder, prostate, vagina
- Urethral stricture: diagnosis, interventional dilation, and/or stent placement (p. 1179)
- Uncommon: removal of small polyps and tumors via endoscopic loops and electrocautery
- Ureteroscopy: for advanced endoscopists; requires concurrent fluoroscopy
- Holmium-doped yttrium, aluminum, garnet (Ho:YAG) laser: used for laser lithotripsy. CO_2 lasers are used for ablative treatment of intraluminal tumors and ectopic ureter.

Contraindications

- Animal size and sex are the most common limiting factors; the exact limitations depend on the endoscope's external diameter relative to the patient (see below).
- Known severe bacterial urinary tract infection (UTI) is a relative risk factor.
- Pre-existing perforation or rupture of bladder or urethra

Equipment, Anesthesia

To be prepared for most sizes and sex of patient may require a mix of six or seven rigid and flexible endoscopes.

- General anesthesia with tracheal intubation is required.
- Preparation of the preputial or perineal area by clipping interfering hair and gentle cleansing
- Between 1 and 2 L of body-temperature, sterile saline for flush and infusion during procedure using an intravenous (IV) infusion set. A second IV infusion set is used for drainage by collection from the opposite port.
- Water-soluble sterile lubricant with or without lidocaine jelly
- Bacterial culture tubes
- Biopsy jars with 10% buffered formalin
- Flexible-tipped ureteral guide wires can be helpful for bypassing obstructions, strictures, and tears (serving a stylet-type function), then allowing catheters to be passed over them. Human ureteral dilation catheters can be used with the guide wires if urethral stricture is present.
- Accessory implements include sterile brushes, guide wires, biopsy forceps, balloon catheters, sterile catheters, stone retrieval baskets, and polypectomy snares (with or without electrocautery).
- Appropriate light source and light cable
- Documentation equipment (digital video capture is most common, VCR)
- Flexible endoscopes
  - Size of scope selected varies by length and diameter of the segment to be assessed (e.g., measure from the cranial tip of filled bladder to perineum, and consider the diameter of the urethra).
  - Ancillary catheters, brushes, stone retrieval baskets, and biopsy forceps to fit selected scopes
  - Flexible endoscopes require more positioning and manipulation of the animal because they tend to be deflected easily by external pressures.
- Rigid endoscopes
  - A wide array of rigid endoscopes from human medicine can be used for transurethral cystoscopy, including purpose-designed cystoscopes, small laparoscopes, and adapted arthroscopes.

- Rigid endoscope sizes most commonly used range from 2.7-5 mm in diameter, with respective cannula (sheath) diameters ranging from 3.8-6 mm; length of the scopes ranges from 7-30 cm. The cannula usually includes the associated biopsy, infusion, and outflow ports. Smaller scopes may have the outer cannula and ports combined into one single unit.
- A 0° viewing angle may be better for viewing the urethra, and a 30° viewing angle may be preferred for viewing the bladder.
- A bridge is used for connecting some scopes with their cannulas and to provide additional access ports (generally one or two) for flushing or infusion of saline and passage of other instruments.
- The Albarrán lever is a deflecting bridge that forces flexible biopsy instruments to exit the bridge at an angle; this facilitates biopsy and grasping of structures that are almost parallel to the scope.
- The Ellik evacuator allows rapid saline lavage to provide for collection of small calculi when attached to a rigid cystoscope cannula.
- Rigid scopes tend to provide superior images.

Anticipated Time

About 30-75 minutes, depending on ease of passage, extent of lesions, and whether the procedure is diagnostic or also therapeutic (e.g., stone retrieval)

Preparation: Important Checkpoints

- Have clear goals for the procedure based on case assessment, and perform sonographic and radiographic imaging first.
- Know the appearance of normal structures in the lower urinary tract.
- Plan ahead for staff involvement with setup, procedural assistance, and cleaning the equipment.
- Discuss with owner the risks and that repeated procedures may be required (e.g., incomplete stone retrieval, failure to dilate stricture).
- Have alternative plans for surgery if warranted and goals are not achieved.
- Pre-procedure enemas can reduce interference by colorectal feces (can lessen mechanical depression of adjacent urinary structures but may increase risk of fecal contamination of perivulvar region) (p. 1099).

Possible Complications and Common Errors to Avoid

- Iatrogenic UTI
- Mistaking the fossa clitoridis in female dogs for the urethral orifice
- Prior digital- or catheter-induced trauma and edema to the urethral tubercle (papilla) or urethra can hinder entry of the endoscope into the urethra.
- Urinary tract rupture can result from inappropriate technique (e.g., overfilling, pushing without visual path) and/or weakness from pre-existing disease. Care should be taken during biopsy of abnormal tissue (e.g., the site of remnant urachal diverticula, intramural neoplasm).
- Urethral mucosal edema due to ongoing inherent trauma from endoscopy can be a limiting factor in uroendoscopy.
- Have available catheter or lubricated guide wire to use as stylet through tumor-narrowed passages.
- Do not rely on visual impressions, but obtain samples for histopathologic or cytologic assay.
- Might not achieve goals (diagnostic, therapeutic)

Procedure

- If the urine is turbid and dark or there is gross hematuria, it may be best to empty the bladder before the procedure.
- Ventral or dorsal recumbency; the author prefers dorsal recumbency, but it can be advantageous to reverse the initially selected position.
- The perineum and prepuce/vulva are cleansed.
- For female dogs and cats, the fiber endoscope or assembled rigid scope is placed in the vulva, and the vulvar skin is gently pinched externally by an assistant to create a seal; then a saline infusion is started until the vault is distended.
- Examine the vulvar and vaginal areas to the level of the cervical os, and identify the urethral orifice; then cannulate the urethra with the scope. The urethra is distended with inflow of saline as the scope is advanced to the bladder. The bladder is emptied as needed through the biopsy channel of the fiberscope or outflow port of the cannula.
- For male patients, the technique is similar, except that the prepuce is held to form a seal around a flexible fiberendoscope. The limiting diameter is the passage through the os penis. In some instances, male dogs may also have the pelvic and proximal urethral segments examined using a rigid urethrocystoscope through a temporary prepubic perineal urethrostomy.
- The bladder is examined in a methodical pattern to include the apex to the trigonal region. Adequate distention is created and maintained with saline flow through the inflow port. It is important to visualize the appearance of mucosa when the bladder is less distended and when filled.
- The ureteral orifices are identified, and in many cases, pulsatile flow of urine can be observed. Biopsies are taken for histopathologic evaluation and culture. Calculi may be examined and samples taken for analysis. Calculi may be larger than the lumen of the cannula channel. If smaller than the urethral limitation, these larger calculi may be drawn up to and held against the end of the scope. The scope and calculus are then withdrawn simultaneously. The size of the calculus or its fragments can limit the usefulness of this technique and lead to surgery or percutaneous cystolithotomy (PCCL).
- The endoscope is withdrawn slowly while observing for abnormalities. Visualization of the urethral mucosa is often superior during withdrawal of the endoscope.
- Ectopic ureteral openings in the urethra (sometimes multiple sites) can be identified. Cystoscopy can be more accurate for diagnosis of ectopic ureter than imaging studies.
- In the male dog, the colliculus seminalis is located dorsally and can be seen more prominently in intact dogs, along with the associated prostatic and deferent duct openings into the proximal urethra.
- The vaginal area is again reviewed, and if appropriate, this is the best time to obtain biopsies or brush cytologic samples or to perform procedures such as balloon bougienage.

Postprocedure

- Postprocedural urethral obstruction due to mucosal edema or inflammation occurs infrequently and is usually correlated to the severity of the pathology present. Monitor micturition until normal voiding is seen.
- Use appropriate pain management.

Alternatives and Their Relative Merits

Laparoscopic-assisted PCCL is more invasive and carries greater equipment requirements. It may be used when larger tumors obstruct the trigone or urethra, for removal of more calculi, or for placing a retrograde catheter or guide wire to facilitate antegrade catheterization of an obstructed urethra.

Pearls

- Be vigilant about the degree of filling of the bladder to avoid bladder overdistention or rupture.
- Try to avoid cystocentesis for 24 hours before cystoscopy because it can leave points of iatrogenic hemorrhage in the mucosa.
- Plan ahead if a retention urethral catheter should be placed after cystoscopy.
- Examine the contents of the outflow urine collection bag for small calculi that might have gone unseen initially.

SUGGESTED READING

Morgan M, et al: Cystoscopy in dogs and cats. Vet Clin North Am Small Anim Pract 45:665-701, 2015.

AUTHOR: Mark E. Hitt, DVM, MS, DACVIM
EDITORS: Leah A. Cohn, DVM, PhD, DACVIM; Mark S. Thompson, DVM, DABVP

Decontamination of Patients After Oral Exposure to Toxicants

Client Education Sheet

Difficulty level: ◆

Overview and Goal

These procedures are used to prevent or lessen the severity of clinical signs that may develop after ingestion of a toxicant.

Indications

- Emetics and gastric lavage are used for removing a toxicant from the gastrointestinal (GI) tract.
- Dilution is indicated when an irritating (e.g., some detergents, bleaches) or corrosive (e.g., alkali, acids) material has been ingested.
- Activated charcoal is used for binding (adsorbing) a toxicant in the GI tract to prevent systemic absorption and facilitate removal in the feces.

Contraindications

- Animals that are able to vomit safely include dogs, cats, ferrets, and potbelly pigs. Emetics should not be used in birds, rodents, rabbits, horses, or ruminants.
- If the patient has ingested a central nervous system stimulant and is already agitated, the additional stimulation of vomiting could trigger seizures.
- Induction of vomiting and gastric lavage are contraindicated with
  - Ingestion of corrosive agents, including alkalis and acids, due to esophageal and oral damage
  - Ingestion of petroleum distillates (volatile hydrocarbons) due to the risk of aspiration
- Dilution is not appropriate in patients who are at an increased risk for aspiration, including those who are actively seizing or obtunded.
- Activated charcoal does not bind all toxicants. Some chemicals that are not bound effectively by charcoal include ethanol, methanol, fertilizer, fluoride, petroleum distillates, most heavy metals, iodides, nitrates, nitrites, sodium chloride, and chlorate.
- Activated charcoal should not be given to animals that are actively vomiting or those that have ingested caustic or corrosive materials.

Equipment, Anesthesia

Unless the patient is already obtunded, gastric lavage usually requires sedation or general anesthesia.

Anticipated Time

The time varies depending on the procedure (see Procedure below).

Preparation: Important Checkpoints

- When deciding whether to induce emesis, the clinician must take into account any pre-existing conditions of the patient that can cause vomiting to be hazardous, including severe cardiac disease (vomiting is a strong vagal influence, and pre-existing bradycardia, such as the sick sinus syndrome, may be exacerbated), seizure disorder, or recent abdominal surgery.
- Emesis may not be needed if the animal has already vomited and is not appropriate if the animal is already exhibiting clinical signs such as ataxia, disorientation, coma, seizures, or recumbency, which make emesis hazardous.
- Obtain a baseline serum sodium concentration before administering activated charcoal due to risk of developing hypernatremia (an uncommon but serious idiosyncratic reaction seen in some dogs).

Possible Complications and Common Errors to Avoid

- Dilution: using an excessive volume can lead to vomiting and re-exposure of the esophagus to the damaging material.
- Emesis: if too much 3% hydrogen peroxide is used or more concentrated hydrogen peroxide (>3%) is used, protracted or hemorrhagic gastritis can result.
- Gastric lavage: risks associated with gastric lavage include esophageal or gastric damage or perforation, hypothermia and accidental placement of the tube in the trachea and instillation of fluid into the lungs. The tube should be well lubricated, advanced gently without encountering resistance, and checked repeatedly to ensure it is in the esophagus and stomach before administering any liquid or solution into the tube.
- Activated charcoal
  - Risk of aspiration if regurgitation or vomiting occurs after giving charcoal. If a patient does aspirate charcoal, the prognosis is poor. Pretreatment with an antiemetic can reduce the risk of aspiration.
  - If the activated charcoal is retained in the GI tract for an extensive period (e.g., due to ileus), it may release the compound it had adsorbed, leading to clinical signs. For this reason, activated charcoal products frequently also contain a cathartic.
  - Hypernatremia may occur due to an osmotic shift of water from the intracellular and extracellular spaces into the GI tract as a result of the activated charcoal solution.

Procedure

- Dilution: give a small amount (2-6 mL/kg in dogs, cats) of water, milk, or canned food orally.
- Emetics
  - Dogs: 3% hydrogen peroxide solution (over the counter): feed a small meal first and then give 2.2 mL/kg (1 mL/lb body weight) PO, maximum 45 mL (3 tablespoons) by cheek pouch using spoon, medicine cup, turkey baster, or oral syringe. Once given, encourage gentle exercise, such as on-leash walking. The patient normally vomits within 15-20 minutes (>90% of cases). If not, can repeat once, *or*
  - Dogs: apomorphine 0.03 mg/kg IV or 0.04 mg/kg IM (least preferred) or crush ¼ - ½ tablet, place in a syringe (without a needle), dissolve with a few drops of saline, and administer into the conjunctival sac. After sufficient vomiting occurs, rinse conjunctival sac. Sedation can be reversed with naloxone 0.04 mg/kg IV if needed.
  - Cats: xylazine 0.44 mg/kg IM (reverse with yohimbine 0.1-0.25 mg/kg slow IV after vomiting is complete) or dexmedetomidine 40 mcg/kg IM (reverse with equal volume of atipamezole)
- Gastric lavage (p. 1117): The patient is anesthetized unless already comatose; a cuffed endotracheal tube must be in place to prevent aspiration
  - A large-bore orogastric tube with a fenestrated end is inserted to a length equal to the distance from the nose to the xiphoid cartilage. Placement of the orogastric tube must be accurate to avoid infusion of water into the respiratory tract (fatal).
  - Body temperature (38°C; always < 40°C and > 35°C) tap water (5-10 mL/kg) is instilled. The head of the patient should be kept lower than the chest throughout the procedure.
  - Gravity is used to instill the water (by holding the tube higher than the patient) and then to drain the water and gastric contents by moving the tube to be lower than the patient.
  - The flushing process should be repeated multiple times until the lavage fluid runs clear. With each flush, approximately the same amount of fluid instilled should be removed. The free end of the tube should be occluded before tube removal to reduce the risk of aspiration.
- Activated charcoal 1-2 g/kg PO (use labeled dosage when using commercial products)
  - If asymptomatic: can be given with a large (35-60 mL) oral dosing syringe or can be mixed with a small amount of canned food or chicken broth and offered to the patient.
  - In symptomatic patients, it is administered by orogastric tube (general anesthesia if not comatose; a cuffed endotracheal tube is essential before passing orogastric tube).

Procedures and Techniques

When the administration is complete, the orogastric tube must be occluded when removing it to reduce the risk of aspiration.

Postprocedure

- After emesis, withhold food and water for several hours (or longer if clinically indicated), and monitor for signs of aspiration. Fluid therapy as indicated for dehydration and serum electrolyte disturbances
- After gastric lavage, monitor body temperature and for signs of aspiration. Fluid therapy as indicated for dehydration and serum electrolyte disturbances
- After activated charcoal administration, monitor serum sodium (for hypernatremia) and for signs of aspiration.

Alternatives and Their Relative Merits

Because decontamination procedures are not without risks, the clinician must decide in each case if the possible clinical outcome of an exposure to a toxicant warrants performing the procedure.

Pearls

- Emetics are usually most effective within 2-3 hours after the exposure, but in some cases, emesis may be effective even after that time frame. Substances that coalesce to form bezoars (e.g., chocolate or chewable medications) or time-released medications may be appropriately addressed with emesis induced > 3 hours after ingestion.
- Xylazine is an effective emetic in 42% of cats. Dexmedetomidine may be more effective at the labeled dosage (40 mcg/kg IM), with vomiting expected within 2-3 minutes of IM administration. The drug can be reversed with atipamezole immediately after vomiting so sedation does not persist.
- Some dogs will drink 3% hydrogen peroxide voluntarily when it is mixed with a small amount (5 mL, 1 teaspoon) of ice cream, peanut butter, chicken broth, or milk/yogurt. This may be especially helpful for recent ingestions by patients that are still asymptomatic and at home.
- Expired hydrogen peroxide may not effectively induce emesis.
- Concentrated (>3%) hydrogen peroxide can potentially cause severe bloody gastroenteritis and air embolism.
- On average, dogs vomit 3-4 times from hydrogen peroxide and apomorphine, and 48%-52% of the ingested toxicant is recovered in the vomitus.
  - Duration of emesis in dogs is 42 and 29 minutes after onset with hydrogen peroxide and apomorphine, respectively.
  - Persistent mild nausea, hypersalivation, and lethargy occur in 3% and 14% of dogs given hydrogen peroxide or apomorphine, respectively. Administration of gastroprotectants should be considered.
- Apomorphine is poorly effective as an emetic in cats.

SUGGESTED READING

DeClementi C: Prevention and treatment of poisoning. In Gupta RC, editor: Veterinary toxicology: basic and clinical principles, ed 2, London, 2012, Academic Press, pp 1361-1368.

AUTHOR: Camille DeClementi, VMD, DABT, DABVT
EDITORS: Leah A. Cohn, DVM, PhD, DACVIM; Tina Wismer, DVM, MS, DABVT, DABT

Defibrillation, Electrical

Bonus Material Online 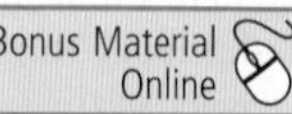

Difficulty level: ♦♦

Overview and Goal

Administration of a controlled electrical shock to a fibrillating heart depolarizes the heart muscle, places the myocytes into a transient refractory period, and stops the uncoordinated muscle activity. Restoration of a normal sinus rhythm or asystole is the desired outcome.

Indications

- Ventricular fibrillation
- Pulseless ventricular tachycardia

Contraindications

- Any rhythm other than ventricular fibrillation or pulseless ventricular tachycardia
  - Coarse or fine fibrillation may be present.
  - Patients with a fibrillation rhythm who are unconscious and do not have palpable pulses
  - The electrocardiographic (ECG) rhythm should be checked in more than one lead because fine fibrillation may be difficult to see in some leads.
- An inability to electrically isolate the patient from its surroundings

Equipment, Anesthesia

- ECG monitor
- Equipment necessary for cardiopulmonary resuscitation (CPR) (e.g., endotracheal [ET] tube, drugs, monitoring devices [p. 1077])
- Defibrillator, monophasic or biphasic
- Defibrillation gel
- Electrical outlet

Anticipated Time

1-10 minutes

Preparation: Important Checkpoints

- CPR has begun
- ECG demonstrates ventricular fibrillation
  - Patternless electrical activity with rapid undulations that may be coarse or fine
  - No synchronized activity/QRS complexes seen

Possible Complications and Common Errors to Avoid

- Inadvertent shock delivered to bystanders in direct or indirect contact with the patient. This can have dangerous consequences and lead to cardiac arrest.
- Burn to patient's body wall or damage to cardiac myocytes
- Fire
  - Oxygen should be disconnected from the patient before shock delivery.
  - Alcohol should not be used on ECG leads or elsewhere on patient.
- Delayed defibrillation
  - The likelihood of a successful defibrillation decreases rapidly with persistent fibrillation. In people, every minute of ventricular fibrillation results in a 10% decreased rate of hospital discharge.
- Poor body contact with paddles/gel
- Use of the wrong gel; ultrasound gel is not an appropriate option because it does not have effective conduction.

Procedure

- CPR is underway according to RECOVER guidelines (p. 1077).
- Ventricular fibrillation is noted on ECG.
  - If fibrillation has been present for < 4 minutes, immediately defibrillate.
  - If ventricular fibrillation is suspected to have been ongoing for > 4 minutes, perform a 2-minute cycle of CPR before the defibrillation attempt.
- Defibrillation gel is applied to both paddles.
- Energy requirement is determined/chosen. For external defibrillation, use
  - Biphasic defibrillator (preferred) 2-4 J/kg
  - Monophasic defibrillator 4-6 J/kg
- Patient is rotated into dorsal recumbency (foam or Plexiglas cradle ideal), and the paddles are firmly placed directly over the heart on opposite sides of the chest.
- The person discharging the shock must determine that no one is in contact with the patient, table, or any fluids/gels contacting the patient or table.
  - *After* confirming this, a statement of ALL CLEAR should be made.

- After each defibrillation attempt, the ECG pattern should be checked and CPR immediately resumed for a 2-minute cycle if defibrillation attempt did not successfully terminate the fibrillation rhythm.
- Consider increasing the shock delivered by 50% in subsequent defibrillation attempts if the first shock was unsuccessful.

Postprocedure

- Repeat 2-minute CPR cycle as needed.
- Repeat defibrillation attempts if ventricular fibrillation persists. Consider increasing the shock delivered by 50% in subsequent defibrillation attempts.
- Post-CPR care per RECOVER guidelines

Alternatives and Their Relative Merits

- Precordial thump: striking the patient's chest with the heel of the hand directly over the heart may result in mechanical defibrillation.
  - Minimal effect
  - Consider if electrical defibrillation is unavailable.
- Antiarrhythmic agents: amiodarone, lidocaine, magnesium sulfate
  - Consider as adjunctive therapy in refractory cases not responding to electrical defibrillation.
  - Of the pharmacologic options available, amiodarone may have the most consistent benefit.
  - Lidocaine may be considered when amiodarone is unavailable.
  - Magnesium sulfate may be considered for treatment of torsades de pointes.

SUGGESTED READING

Fletcher DJ, et al: RECOVER evidence and knowledge gap analysis on veterinary CPR. Part 7: clinical guidelines. J Vet Emerg Crit Care 22(suppl 1):S102-S131, 2012.

AUTHOR: Lillian I. Good, DVM, DACVECC
EDITORS: Leah A. Cohn, DVM, PhD, DACVIM; Mark S. Thompson, DVM, DABVP

Dental Extraction

Difficulty level: ♦

Synonym

Exodontics

Overview and Goal

- Removal of a tooth in a way that ensures complete removal of the roots and rapid healing of the dental alveolus and oral soft tissue
- Closed extraction is indicated for simple, rooted teeth, except canine teeth or any tooth that has already lost most of its attachment. Canines and multirooted teeth usually require open extraction.

Indications

- Nonvital (dead) teeth; teeth with exposure or contamination of the endodontic system
- Moderate to severe periodontal disease (p. 776)
- Stomatitis in cats (p. 943)
- Nonrestorable dental lesions: dental resorptions (p. 982), dental fractures (p. 980), dental caries
- Persistent primary teeth (p. 238) (if permanent teeth are present), retained roots or impacted teeth, some teeth involved in jaw fracture
- Dental traumatic malocclusions
- Oral surgery: removal of oral tumors (pp. 711 and 714), oral cysts

Contraindications

- When general anesthesia is contraindicated because of severe uncontrolled metabolic disease
- Animals with a bleeding disorder
- Animals undergoing chemotherapy or radiotherapy, or receiving bisphosphonate therapy

Equipment, Anesthesia

- General anesthesia and perioperative pain control; regional or local anesthesia as needed
- Closed extraction
  - Dental radiograph
  - A #11 or #15 scalpel blade
  - Dental elevators or dental luxators
  - Dental forceps
- Open extraction: as above plus
  - Periosteal elevator
  - Dental unit with high-speed handpiece and FG dental burs (no. 699-701 in regular, long shank and surgical lengths)
  - Bone rongeurs or bone rasp
  - Bone curette
  - Sterile saline with syringe and atraumatic needle
  - Soft-tissue scissors (LaGrange)
  - Tissue forceps
  - Needle holder, 4-0 resorbable suture material with swaged-on needle

Anticipated Time

About 5 minutes for most closed extractions and 20 minutes for most open extractions

Preparation: Important Checkpoints

Dental radiographs: check for the number of roots, their shape, and their structural integrity (root resorption); the condition of the surrounding bone; and the presence or absence of a periodontal ligament with possible root ankylosis.

Possible Complications and Common Errors to Avoid

- Oronasal fistula (p. 720): if occurs, should be closed with a mucoperiosteal flap at the time the extraction is done or as a delayed surgery if the gingival tissue is so inflamed that its capacity to hold sutures is questionable.
- Root fracture
  - Most easily prevented by examination of the preoperative radiographs and proper treatment planning. If the root is in advanced stage of resorption, is ankylosed, and has no evidence of periodontal or endodontic infection, it could be left in place for continued resorption.
  - Although the clinician should try to remove the entire root, the risk of damaging surrounding tissue should be weighed against the benefit of finding the very last piece of root material.
  - When a root fragment is left *in situ,* the owner should be informed of the outcome of the surgery, and follow-up radiographs should be planned. The risk of causing an abscess is higher when the root was infected or the fragment has been mobilized and its blood supply severed during its attempted extraction.
- Jaw fracture: usually the result of a blind attempt at extracting a tooth without preoperative dental radiographs and appropriate treatment planning. Small-breed dogs with severe periodontal disease of the first lower molars and cats during extraction of the mandibular canines are the most at risk for jaw fracture during dental extraction.
- Root fragments displaced into soft tissue, the nasal cavity, or the mandibular canal should be retrieved.

Procedure

Closed extraction:

- Circumferential incision of the gingival attachment around the tooth with a scalpel blade
- Mobilization of the tooth with dental elevators using first-class lever, wheel-and-axle, or wedge types of forces:
  - The tip of the elevator is used circumferentially as a wedge between the root and the bone to stretch the periodontal ligament or as a wheel-and-axle force with the side of the blade engaged under the enamel bulge mesial or distal to the tooth to elevate the tooth out of the alveolus.

- ◦ Use light forces over a longer period of time (at least 10 seconds each time) to break the attachment without fracturing the root.
  - ◦ Extend the index finger (of the hand holding the elevator) along the shaft of the elevator to protect deeper structures in case of slippage.
- Extraction with dental forceps after the tooth is mobile. Light rotation force around the long axis of the root may help.
- Check that extraction is complete; perform a postoperative radiograph if needed.
- Brief digital pressure to help hemostasis, reduce expansion of the alveolar wall caused by the extraction, and approximate the gingival margins
- Suture if needed.

Open extraction:

- Circumferential incision of the gingival attachment around the tooth with a #15 scalpel blade
- Preparation of a mucoperiosteal flap (long horizontal incision with one or two vertical incisions if needed); elevation with a periosteal elevator
- With a dental bur, buccal cortical bone and alveolar bone is removed to expose the root surface up to half of its length.
- On a multirooted tooth, the crown is sectioned between the roots.
- Each individual root with its attached piece of crown is luxated and elevated.
- Check that the extraction is complete (radiographs).
- Smooth the edge of the alveolar bone with a bone rongeur, rasp, or diamond bur; curette and flush debris out of the alveolus.
- Trim the border of the soft tissue if needed (LaGrange scissors).
- Suture with a simple interrupted suture pattern.
  - ◦ After a surgical extraction, the mucoperiosteal flap is sutured back in place, even in the case of an abscess.
  - ◦ It is important to cover the bone exposed during elevation of the soft tissue.

Postprocedure

- Surgical extractions: pain medication for 3-7 days, soft food for 10 days
- Antibiotics are not necessary in most cases, except when animal shows systemic clinical signs (e.g., fever, loss of appetite) or the condition has progressed to osteomyelitis.
- Recheck in 10-14 days.

Alternatives and Their Relative Merits

Endodontics, periodontics, and orthodontics are other alternative treatments. They have the advantage of preserving the teeth and are often a better option when the owner is interested in doing the necessary aftercare and home dental care.

AUTHOR: Yvan Dumais, DVM, DAVDC, FAVD
EDITORS: Leah A. Cohn, DVM, PhD, DACVIM; Mark S. Thompson, DVM, DABVP

Dental Prophylactic Treatment

Client Education Sheet

Difficulty level: ♦

Synonyms

Dental cleaning and polishing, dental prophylaxis

Overview and Goal

- Complete oral examination
- Removal of calculus and plaque buildup on teeth to create a healthier dentogingival environment
- Polishing teeth surfaces to make them less prone to calculus accumulation

Indications

- Plaque (soft) and calculus (hard) buildup on dental surfaces
- Treatment of gingivitis
- Prevention of periodontal disease
- Annual dental examination
- Part of the maintenance phase in the treatment of periodontitis

Contraindications

- Established periodontitis: animal should receive more involved diagnostic and treatment procedures rather than prophylactic treatment (p. 776).
- When general anesthesia is contraindicated because of systemic illness
- Old age is not a contraindication.
- NOTE: Dogs with mitral valve endocardiosis have not been shown to have a greater risk of dental procedure–associated bacterial endocarditis than dogs with normal heart valves.

Equipment, Anesthesia

- General anesthesia and endotracheal intubation
- Hand instruments
  - ◦ Scalers (H 6-7)
  - ◦ Curettes (Gracey ¾, Gracey 13⁄14, Mini-five ½)
  - ◦ Dental explorer and periodontal probe (XP-17/0W)
  - ◦ Dental mirror
  - ◦ Instrument tray
  - ◦ Ceramic sharpening stone
- Power instruments
  - ◦ Ultrasonic (magnetostrictive with metal stack, magnetostrictive with ferrite rods or piezoelectric) or sonic scaler
  - ◦ One tip for removal of supragingival calculus
  - ◦ One perio (or universal) tip for removal of subgingival calculus and debris. The energized water spray at the end of the tip also kills bacteria present in the gingival sulcus with what are referred to as *acoustic streaming* and the *cavitation effects of ultrasonic waves.*
  - ◦ A dental polisher of a dental unit (air or electric powered) with low-speed handpiece and contra-angle attachment. Because the speed of the prophy cup should be about 4000 rpm, a contra-angle attachment with a 4:1 gear ratio is usually necessary with air-driven units.
  - ◦ Prophy head, multi-use or single-use head
  - ◦ Rubber prophy cups; prophy paste (jars or unidose cups) or flour pumice (fine or medium grit)
- Chlorhexidine solution 0.12%
- Good lighting conditions, magnifying glasses
- Dental chart (p. 1140)

Anticipated Time

About 20 minutes for a cat and 45 minutes for a dog

Preparation: Important Checkpoints

Operator protection:

- Surgical mask, gloves, eye protection, scrub top or gown
- Instill 0.12% chlorhexidine solution in the animal's mouth before starting the procedure to reduce bacterial counts in the aerosols generated during power scaling.

Animal protection:

- Keep the animal warm because of the cooling effect of the water spray during power scaling. Protect the eyes (lubrication, towel), and sterilize the instruments. Appropriately inflate the cuff of the endotracheal tube, and use lubricating gel.
- Administer antibiotics only if animal is immunosuppressed or has a severe infection: ampicillin 20 mg/kg IV 1 hour before the procedure, or use clindamycin 5 mg/kg or

clavulanic acid–amoxicillin 13.5 mg/kg, PO 12 hours before the procedure.
- Place cotton gauze in the oropharynx to catch pieces of calculus that could otherwise enter the trachea after extubation.

Possible Complications and Common Errors to Avoid

- Forgetting to remove the cotton gauze in the oropharynx before extubation
- Causing thermal damage to the dental pulp by staying too long over a tooth during power scaling or polishing or inadequate water spray during power scaling
- Damaging the tooth surface by being heavy handed during scaling and polishing or by using burs (Rotosonics) to remove calculus
- Dental cusp (tip) fracture caused when using extraction forceps to chip away the calculus (not recommended)
- Power instrumentation: use the lowest effective intensity (power) setting; use a light touch; work with the last 3 mm at the end of the tip; keep the tip moving, with adequate water spray. Use the side of the tip. Use a gauge to check tip wear, and replace when 2 mm has been lost (50% loss of efficacy).

Procedure

- The anesthetized, intubated animal is placed in lateral recumbency. All stages of the procedure described here are performed on the labial side of the teeth on the nonrecumbent side and the lingual/palatal side of the teeth on the recumbent side. Then the animal is turned over, and the procedure can be repeated (avoids turning the animal multiple times).
- Remove very heavy calculus deposits with a dental scaler, hoe, or calculus forceps.
- Remove gross and moderate supragingival calculus using hand instrumentation (dental curette, scaler) or power instrumentation (sonic or ultrasonic with a heavier tip at moderate- to high-intensity setting).
- The working surface of the power scaler should be held parallel, not perpendicular, to the tooth surface.
- Remove light supragingival and subgingival calculus with hand instrumentation (dental curette) or power instrumentation (sonic or ultrasonic with slim perio or universal tip at low- to moderate-intensity setting).
- Check for residual dental calculus using a disclosing solution, air spray from an air/water syringe, or a dental curette.
- The teeth are polished with prophy paste or flour pumice.
- Dental examination with dental explorer; periodontal examination with periodontal probe. Chart all findings.
- Flush the gingival sulcus with an atraumatic needle and saline to remove the prophy paste or flour pumice, calculus debris, and bacteria.
- Perform final rinse with 0.12% chlorhexidine.

Postprocedure

- Discuss home oral care with owners, and find appropriate regimen.
- Provide the owner with information about the postoperative treatment plan, including the date of the next dental appointment.

Alternatives and Their Relative Merits

- The wrong alternative to preventing periodontal disease with dental prophylactic treatment and home dental care is to wait until periodontal disease has progressed and periodontal treatment is necessary to help control disease progression. This is obviously not an option that benefits the animal or owner.
- Brushing the teeth will not remove existing calculus.
- Dental prophylactic treatment performed without general anesthesia provides some cosmetic improvement but no long-term benefit.

RELATED CLIENT EDUCATION SHEETS

Consent to Perform Dental Cleaning
Consent to Perform General Anesthesia

AUTHOR: Yvan Dumais, DVM, DAVDC, FAVD
EDITORS: Leah A. Cohn, DVM, PhD, DACVIM; Mark S. Thompson, DVM, DABVP

Procedures and Techniques

Dermatologic Diagnostic Procedures

Difficulty level: ♦

Overview and Goal

- Tests that are performed to confirm a diagnosis and/or to rule out differential diagnoses for skin lesions
- The most common diagnostic procedures in dermatology are examination of the haircoat and skin with good lighting and magnification, flea combing, acetate tape preparation, skin scrapings, trichoscopy, skin cytologic examination, Wood's lamp examination, fungal culture for dermatophytes, and skin biopsies.

Indications

- Skin scrapings: used primarily to find mites and occasionally nematode infestation
- Skin cytologic examination: extremely useful diagnostic procedure indicated in almost every dermatology case. It can rapidly and inexpensively detect the presence of inflammation, infection (bacteria, fungi), autoimmune disease (acantholytic keratinocytes in pemphigus), or neoplasia.
- Wood's lamp examination: useful screening tool for dermatophytosis caused by *Microsporum canis*
- Dermatophyte culture: indicated when dermatophytosis is suspected and in virtually any cat with undiagnosed skin disease
- Trichoscopy (trichography, trichogram) is the microscopic examination of forcefully plucked hairs. Most useful for finding ectoparasites (particularly louse or *Cheyletiella* ova and *Demodex*), identifying hair shaft fracture (e.g., pruritic cats), and finding large melanin clumps suggesting color dilution alopecia and black hair follicular dysplasia. It is generally not useful for hair cycle arrest in dogs (except poodles, where most hairs are normally in anagen) because normal anagen/telogen ratios have not been established for most breeds.
- Skin biopsies: to confirm a diagnosis or provide direction (without always receiving a definitive diagnosis). Recommended for any neoplastic or suspected neoplastic lesion, any persistent or unusual lesion, any vesicular dermatosis, and any undiagnosed alopecia.

Equipment, Anesthesia

Simple equipment is required to perform veterinary dermatologic tests. Standard equipment and materials:

- One or two dull #10 or #21 scalpel blades
- Glass microscope slides and coverslips (22 × 40 or 22 × 50 mm)
- Mineral oil
- Cotton-tipped applicators
- Acetate tape (clear adhesive tape)
- Microscope
- Hemostat
- Handheld magnifying lens
- Flea combs
- Otoscope and several otoscopic cones
- Cytologic examination stain (e.g., Diff-Quick)
- Microbiological specimen collection and transport systems (e.g., culture swabs)
- Wood's lamp
- Dermatophyte test media
- Sterile toothbrushes
- Syringes
- A few 22-, 23-, and 25-gauge needles
- Biopsy kit, including 4- and 6-mm biopsy punches
- Local anesthetic (e.g., lidocaine 2%)
- Biopsy jars containing 10% neutral buffered formalin

Anticipated Time

The procedures take a few minutes.

Possible Complications and Common Errors to Avoid

- Skin scrapings: to avoid false-negative results, it is important to clip hair before performing skin scrapings. However, it is preferable to use scissors when surface mites such as *Cheyletiella* are suspected because they can be lost if electric clippers are used. NOTE: A positive scraping allows the clinician to find and identify a parasitic infestation, but its sensitivity in ruling out a diagnosis depends on the parasitic disease and the aggressiveness of sampling.
- Skin biopsies: do not scrub—or wipe or rub with alcohol or antiseptic—the surface of a biopsy site before performing punch biopsies. Pathologic changes on the skin surface, which often are critical in making a diagnosis, may be altered or removed. For the same reason, do not shave the area of interest; gently clip the hair with scissors if necessary. This does not apply for excisional biopsies.

Procedure

Skin scraping:

- Apply a few drops of mineral oil to the area of skin selected for scraping, or coat the dull scalpel blade that is used for performing the scraping with mineral oil. Broad superficial scrapings that collect scales and crusts should be performed when looking for mites living on the surface *(Cheyletiella, Demodex gatoi)* or in the superficial layers of the epidermis *(Sarcoptes, Notoedres)*. Deeper skin scrapings must be performed for deep-dwelling mites *(Demodex)*. In the latter case, the skin must be squeezed to help extrude the mites from the hair follicles first, and the scrapings should be deep enough to create capillary oozing.
- The skin scraping material that is collected on the scalpel blade is smeared on a glass slide; mineral oil is added and a coverslip mounted. Examination is done with 4× *(Cheyletiella, Sarcoptes, Notoedres)* or 10× *(Demodex)* objective. *Demodex* mites are part of the skin's normal flora, but it is rare to find them on skin scrapings in healthy dogs. If one or two mites are found, more deep skin scrapings should be taken to confirm the diagnosis of demodicosis. Conversely, numerous negative skin scrapings from appropriate areas should reliably exclude demodicosis and notoedric mange. In areas that are difficult to scrape (e.g., eyelids, paws), hair can be plucked and the proximal ends examined under a microscope for the presence of *Demodex* mites.
- Negative skin scrapings (even if several are performed) do not rule out sarcoptic mange or cheyletiellosis.

Skin cytologic examination:

- Allows microscopic examination of fluid or material collected from nodules, tumors, cysts, plaques, draining tracts, ulcers, pustules, vesicles, papules, and surface of the skin or ears. Several techniques may be used for obtaining samples:
  - Impression smears made from the surface of intact lesions or from cut surfaces of surgically excised nodules or tumors
  - Impression smears made after lancing pustules or papules or after lifting or gently scraping away a superficial crust or collerette
  - Fine-needle aspiration (FNA) of cells or material from lesions
  - Smears made by rolling the cotton-tipped applicator across a glass slide (particularly useful for ear specimens). Humidify the tip of applicator when lesions are dry.
  - Scrapings of surface epithelial cells and debris with a dry, dull scalpel blade. This material is then smeared onto a glass slide.
- After the specimen has dried, the slide is stained with a modified Wright's stain (e.g., Diff-Quik) and examined microscopically. When a drop of mineral oil is put on the stained dried specimen and then covered with a large coverslip (e.g., 22 × 40 mm), visualization of cells and most microorganisms with 40× objective is enhanced, and examination under oil immersion (100× objective) in not needed in most cases.

Wood's lamp examination:

- This ultraviolet light is a very useful tool for the diagnosis of dermatophytosis (p. 247). The animal should be examined in a dark room. In untreated animals, the majority of *M. canis* lesions fluoresced. This inherent property of *M. canis* causes infected hairs (not scales or crusts) to fluoresce an apple green color. It is a fast and inexpensive screening tool for dermatophytosis. False-positives are unfortunately frequent. Glowing hair should be plucked and the proximal end examined further with the Wood's lamp or used for culture or direct examination for fungal elements under microscope. A negative examination does not rule out dermatophytosis.

Dermatophyte culture (p. 247):

- Generally performed in clinics on commercial dermatophyte test medium (DTM), available in glass jars or flat plates. The culture medium consists of a Sabouraud-dextrose agar, antibacterial and antifungal agents to inhibit growth of contaminants, and phenol red (pH indicator).
- Pluck hairs from the edge of newly developing lesions. Broken or frayed hairs and those that fluoresce with Wood's lamp are the best specimens. The plucked hairs should be firmly pressed onto the surface of the medium. Alternatively, vigorous brushing of the haircoat with a sterile toothbrush or a small piece of sterile carpet can effectively collect hairs and scales (more useful to identify carriers not showing obvious lesions). Collected material is removed from the toothbrush with a sterile hemostat and placed into the culture medium. Alternately, if plates are used, the DTM is inoculated by gently embedding or repeatedly dabbing the toothbrush into the medium.
- Ideally, the culture medium should be incubated at 22°C-30°C (72°F-86°F) for 2 weeks and should be checked daily for fungal growth. Desiccation hinders growth. The culture medium should be kept for up to ≈3 weeks in animals with antifungal pretreatment or suboptimal culture environment fungal growth. Look for a whitish, fluffy to powdery colony with a red color change in the medium *around the same time* that the colony is first visible. Contaminants (environmental molds) eventually turn the media red; however, colony growth is usually well established before any color change appears in the medium. Most saprophyte colonies are pigmented (black, gray, green, or multicolored). Nonetheless, identification of the fungi is essential if a suspected dermatophyte is grown on culture. Macroconidia must be

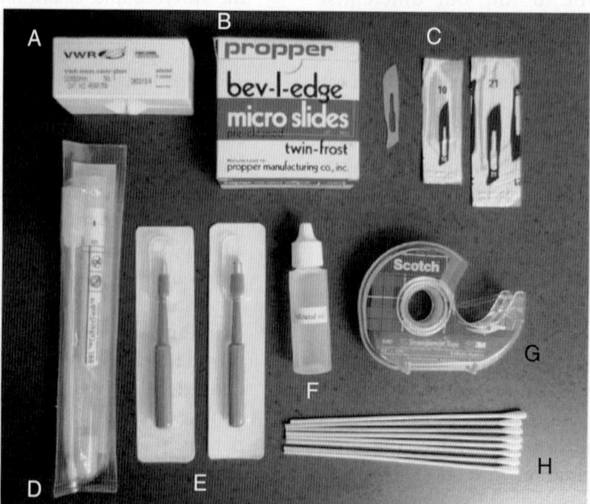

DERMATOLOGIC DIAGNOSTIC PROCEDURES Material used for performing dermatologic diagnostic tests. **A,** Cover glass. **B,** Glass microscope slides. **C,** #10 or #21 scalpel blades. **D,** Culture swab (collection and transport system). **E,** Biopsy punches. **F,** Mineral oil. **G,** Acetate tape (clear adhesive tape). **H,** Cotton-tipped applicators.

collected from the mycelial surface by gently applying the sticky side of clear acetate tape to the aerial surface. The tape with sample is then pressed onto a glass slide over a drop of methylene blue or lactophenol cotton blue stain and examined under microscope for characteristic macroconidia.

Bacterial culture and sensitivity (C&S) (p. 1333)

- Due to a recent increase of methicillin-resistant *Staphylococcus pseudintermedius*, C&S are performed much more commonly in canine pyoderma.
- The Culturette swabs are used for collecting moist exudates from pustules under crusts or epidermal collarettes.
- Otic cultures are generally performed when rods and neutrophils are seen on cytologic examination.

Skin biopsy:

- The biopsy technique selected (punch biopsy, wedge biopsy, excisional biopsy) varies according to the type of lesions.
- Site selection is crucial. Choose several representative lesions that may represent various stages of the same pathologic process or multiple problems, with emphasis on primary lesions if possible (e.g., pustules, vesicles).
- Punch biopsy specimens (usually 6 mm) can be obtained under local anesthesia (1 mL of 2% lidocaine per site injected SQ beneath the specimen; do not exceed 1 mL/5 kg of body weight). If a pustule or other small lesion is selected, it should be centered in the biopsy specimen. The biopsy punch should be rotated in only one direction to minimize shearing artifact. Handle the specimen carefully. The forceps should grasp the hairs of the biopsy sample or its deepest surface (e.g., subcutis), never the core of the biopsy sample. The specimen must be put rapidly (<2 minutes) in 10% neutral buffered formalin. Skin biopsy punch sites can be sutured with 1-2 interrupted sutures.
- Skin biopsies, along with a detailed history, animal description, biopsy sites, +/− photos, should be submitted to a veterinary dermatopathologist.

Allergy testing:

- Food allergy is most reliably diagnosed based on an elimination food trial followed by a provocation food trial (p. 345).
- Atopic dermatitis is most reliably diagnosed by intradermal skin testing (or serology testing) (p. 91).

Alternatives and Their Relative Merits

Therapeutic trials (e.g., antiparasitic, antimicrobial) can be valuable in establishing a diagnosis and are frequently performed in veterinary dermatology. For example, therapeutic trials with an acaricidal agent are indicated when sarcoptic mange is suspected but skin scrapings are negative.

SUGGESTED READING

Miller WH Jr, et al: Muller & Kirk's Small animal dermatology, ed 7, St. Louis, 2013, Saunders, pp 78–95.

AUTHOR: Manon Paradis, DMV, MVSc, DACVD
EDITORS: Leah A. Cohn, DVM, PhD, DACVIM; Mark S. Thompson, DVM, DABVP

Ear Cytology

Difficulty level: ♦

Synonym

Otic cytology

Overview and Goal

Ear cytology is a screening test to assess for microorganisms and the cellular character of the ear canal. It is an essential part of the examination of the ear canal in patients with suspected otitis externa (p. 728) and otitis media.

Indications

- Ear cytology should be performed on all patients with visible ear canal inflammation or exudate.
- Mineral oil preps of dark exudates may identify *Otodectes* or *Demodex* mites.
- Follow-up ear cytology is useful to assess response to therapy.

Contraindications

Patients that do not allow sampling of the ear canal with a swab due to pain-induced aggression

Equipment, Anesthesia

- Cotton swabs on wooden applicator sticks long and stiff enough to allow sampling from deep in vertical ear canal
- Glass microscope slides
- ± Lighter for heat fixing
- Modified Wright stain (Diff-Quik)
- Microscope for evaluation of slide
- Seldom requires sedation

Anticipated Time

15 minutes, including staining and viewing

Preparation: Important Checkpoints

- Assistant to restrain the patient
- Premark a slide so as to identify which side is up.

Possible Complications and Common Errors to Avoid

- Inadequate sample from not sampling deep into the vertical ear canal
- Difficulty in sampling a painful or aggressive patient. An experienced assistant should provide restraint rather than the pet owner.
- Ear canal too swollen or occluded to allow sampling

Procedure

Collection of the sample:

- Debris is collected from the vertical canal of each ear on a cotton swab.
- The swab from the right ear is rolled on the right side of the slide, and the swab of the left ear is rolled on the left side.
- Although heat fixing is a common practice, studies have shown it to be unnecessary. If the collected material is waxy, the slide may be heated briefly with the lighter to melt the wax and allow penetration of the sample by the stain.
- The slide is stained using the modified Wright stain (Diff-Quik).
- Dry, crumbly, black exudates are typical of ear mite infestation; another swab should be rolled into mineral oil and then covered with a coverslip to examine for mites.

Examination of the slides:

- Mineral oil preps are examined under low power (4× objective to orient the viewer and 10× to identify mites)
- Stained slides are examined under low power to orient the viewer and find areas of high cellularity/organisms. The slide is then examined under higher power (40× objective) to identify organisms such as *Malassezia pachydermatis*, bacterial rods or cocci, fungi such as *Candida* or *Aspergillus*, and neutrophils. Squamous cells and keratin are normally found in ear cytologies but may be seen in increased numbers with inflammation and in dog breeds predisposed to ceruminous otitis externa.

Postprocedure

Therapy depends on clinical presentation and interpretation of ear cytology.

Alternatives and Their Relative Merits

- *Otodectes* mites may be detected as small, white specks moving within the ear canal

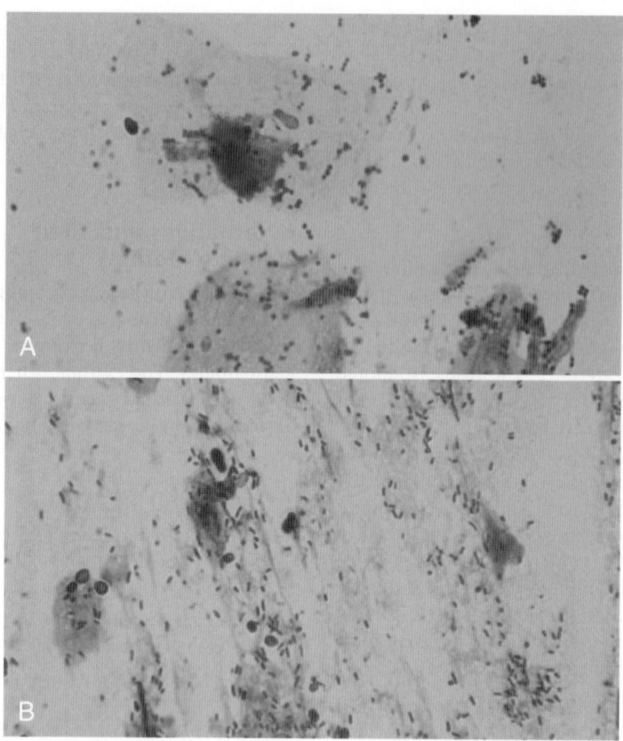

EAR CYTOLOGY Prepared cytology slides (40× magnification, Wright stain) showing mixed infection of a few *Malassezia* yeast and cocci bacteria (**A**) and *Malassezia* yeast with rod bacteria (**B**).

on otoscopy, but failure to visualize mites does not rule out infestation.
- Culture of the ear canal may be necessary with persistent infections. Ear cytology is typically performed first to confirm bacterial infection.

Pearls

- Ear cytologies can contain high numbers of bacteria or yeast without a neutrophilic response. The presence of neutrophils, especially if degenerative, indicates that rupture of the tympanic membrane and concurrent otitis media is likely and that the ear should be flushed with the patient under anesthesia.
- *Pseudomonas* otitis externa tends to be ulcerative. Rod bacteria on cytology surrounded by a blue- to purple-staining biofilm with the presence of neutrophils from an ulcerated ear canal is suspicious for *Pseudomonas*.

AUTHOR: Mark S. Thompson, DVM, DABVP
EDITOR: Leah A. Cohn, DVM, PhD, DACVIM

Echocardiography

Client Education Sheet 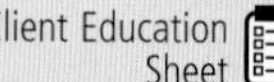 Bonus Material Online 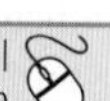

Difficulty level: ♦♦♦

Synonyms

Cardiac ultrasound, echo

Overview and Goal

A complete echocardiographic study should
- Reveal the pertinent congenital or adult-onset heart lesions
- Evaluate valvular function
- Quantify ventricular systolic and diastolic function
- Estimate the hemodynamic burden through quantification of chamber size (dilation, hypertrophy)

Indications

- Congenital or adult-onset cardiac disease (e.g., valvular, myocardial, pericardial), cardiac neoplasia, pulmonary hypertension, systemic hypertension, and pleural effusion or respiratory distress of uncertain cause
- Limited echo studies can be useful in selected emergency situations (e.g., pericardial effusion, estimation of atrial size, or ventricular ejection fraction during initial stabilization if other initial diagnostic modalities are hazardous or nondiagnostic [p. 1102]).

Contraindications

- Patient should be stable enough to handle restraint.
- Animals with life-threatening problems (e.g., respiratory distress due to pleural effusion or pulmonary edema) need to be stabilized first; limited echo study may be warranted to screen for effusions, extensive structural heart disease.

Equipment, Anesthesia

- Scanning table with holes cut out because examination from beneath the animal improves image quality
- Ultrasonic transmission gel
- Isopropyl alcohol
- Hair clippers might be needed.
- Ultrasound equipment; sector-scanning transducers preferred
  - For cats and small dogs: usually 7- or 8-MHz transducer; medium-sized dogs: 5-MHz transducer; large dogs: 2.5-3.5-MHz transducer
  - It may be necessary to use two different probes during one examination.
- The echocardiography machine should have M-mode, two-dimensional (2D), Doppler (pulsed wave, continuous wave, and color coded), and electrocardiogram (ECG) capabilities.
- Sedation/anesthesia is neither required nor desired except in very uncooperative animals.

Anticipated Time

Varies due to experience and case complexity (5-40 minutes)

Preparation: Important Checkpoints

- Dogs and cats usually require little preparation for echocardiographic examination.
- Fasting is not needed.
- Hair might be clipped over the right third to sixth intercostal spaces (ICSs) and left fourth to seventh ICS (precordial transducer locations); however, in most dogs and cats, satisfactory images can be obtained by parting the haircoat and applying isopropyl alcohol and transmission gel.

Possible Complications and Common Errors to Avoid

- Although the technique has no known physical hazard, there are risks associated with the improper interpretation or use of the results of the ultrasound.

- Use high-frequency transducers to obtain quality images of near-field structures.
- Use low-frequency transducers for quality Doppler (color, pulse wave, continuous wave) signals.
- Adjust depth of the real-time image to fill the field of view (reduce amount of lung field).
- Adjust gain to avoid producing a white, distorted image due to a high setting; too low a setting will produce a weak signal.
- Remember the concept of blue/away and red/toward (BART) for color-flow Doppler studies.

Procedure

- Image quality is improved in lateral recumbency; however, dogs and cats may be examined in a standing, sitting, or sternal position.
- The ultrasound machine's ECG clips are attached to the legs as recommended by the manufacturer for measurements and timing within the cardiac cycle.
- Starting in right lateral recumbency (animal's limbs toward the examiner), the right parasternal location (window) is between the right third and sixth ICS, between the sternum and costochondral junctions (landmark: palpate right precordial heartbeat and place transducer at this location to start). Attention is paid to having the assistant restrain the animal with the forelimbs drawn far enough cranially to open the axilla/acoustic window.
- Long-axis views: beam plane is oriented slightly clockwise from perpendicular to long axis of the body, parallel to the long axis of the heart, and with the transducer index mark pointing toward the heart base (craniodorsally, approximately toward the animal's shoulder). The following two views are obtained: first, a four-chamber view with the ventricles displayed to the left and the atria to the right; second, a view obtained by slight clockwise rotation of the transducer from the four-chamber view into a slightly more craniodorsal orientation, revealing the left ventricular outflow tract, aortic valve, and aortic root.
- Short-axis views: rotate the transducer ≈90° toward the sternum from the four-chamber view (keep probe in same position except for the rotation) such that the beam plane is oriented perpendicular to the long axis of the heart, with the transducer index mark pointing cranioventrally toward the animal's elbow (proper orientation identified by circular symmetry of the left ventricle [LV] or aortic root). Five standard transverse images (LV with papillary muscles, LV at mitral chordae tendineae level, LV at mitral valve level, heart base–aorta/left atrium level, and heart base–pulmonary artery) are obtained from this position by pivoting the transducer from the apex to the base of the heart (caudal/ventral to cranial/dorsal).
- Turn the animal over into left lateral recumbency, with the animal's limbs still toward the sonographer.
- Left caudal (apical) parasternal location: the location is between the left fifth and seventh ICS, as close to the sternum as possible (landmark: palpable left apical heartbeat).
    - Left apical two-chamber views: the transducer index mark points toward the heart base (dorsal), and the beam plane is parallel to the long axis of the heart to visualize the left side of the heart (left atrium, LV, and mitral valve). Slight rotation of the transducer into a craniodorsal to caudoventral orientation reveals LV, LV outflow tract, aortic valve, and aortic root in a long-axis view.
    - Left apical four-chamber views: this is the only view in which the transducer index mark points to the left and caudally, opposite of all other views. NOTE: The transducer should be as far caudally toward the apex of the heart as possible, often around the seventh ICS and tilted to point cranially. The beam plane is in a left caudal to right cranial orientation and then directed dorsally toward the heart base, revealing the ventricles in the near field closest to the transducer and the atria in the far field (heart is oriented vertically; LV, mitral valve, and left atrium should appear to the right). Modest cranial tilting of the beam from the above view will bring the left ventricular outflow region into view (five-chamber view).
- Left cranial parasternal location: the location is between the left third and fourth ICS, between the sternum and costochondral junctions.
    - Long-axis views: with the transducer index mark pointing cranially and the beam plane oriented parallel to the long axis of the body and heart, a view of the LV outflow tract, aortic valve, and ascending aorta is obtained (LV will be displayed to the left and aorta to the right). From this position, angling of the beam ventrally (toward the sternum) to the aorta brings out the right atrium/right auricle, tricuspid valve, and inflow region of the right ventricle (displayed to the right, with the LV noted to the left). Angling the transducer dorsally (transducer is almost horizontal and parallel with the table) in relation to the ascending aorta produces a view of the main pulmonary artery, pulmonary valve, and right ventricular outflow tract.
    - Short-axis views: remain in the same location as for the cranial long axis, and rotate the transducer until the transducer's index mark is toward the thoracic spine (dorsally, ≈90° from the location of long-axis view; aorta should appear circular in the center of the image). The right ventricular

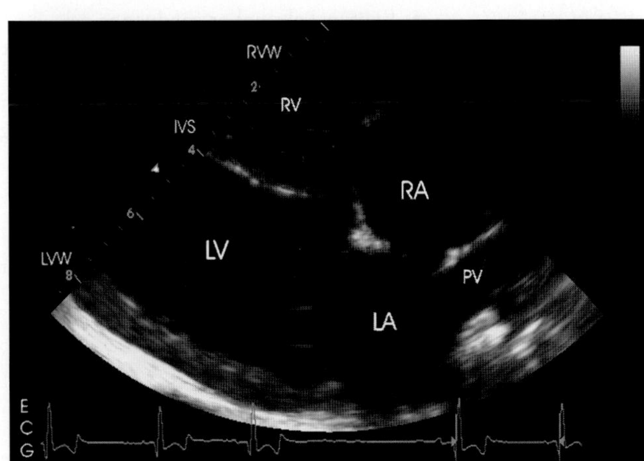

ECHOCARDIOGRAPHY Right parasternal, four-chamber, long-axis view in a normal dog (obtained without shaving). *IVS,* Interventricular septum; *LA,* left atrium; *LV,* left ventricle; *LVW,* left ventricular wall; *PV,* pulmonary vein; *RA,* right atrium; *RV,* right ventricle; *RVW,* right ventricular wall.

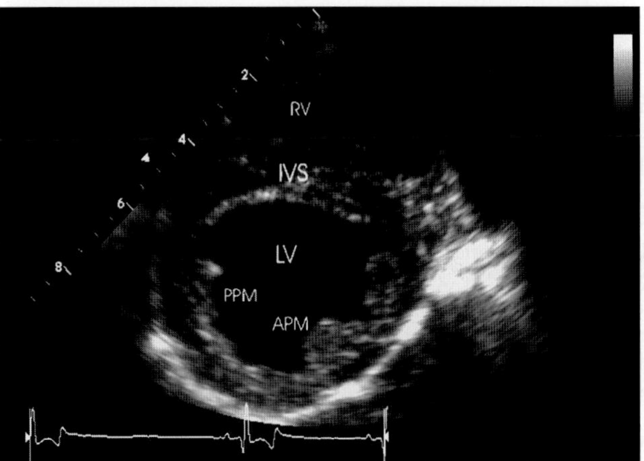

ECHOCARDIOGRAPHY Right parasternal, short-axis view at the left ventricular papillary muscle level in same dog. From this view, gentle pivoting motion (caudal/ventral to cranial/dorsal) of the transducer beam toward the base reveals the other four standard views obtained from this location. *APM,* Anterior papillary muscle; *IVS,* interventricular septum; *LV,* left ventricle; *PPM,* posterior papillary muscle; *RV,* right ventricle.

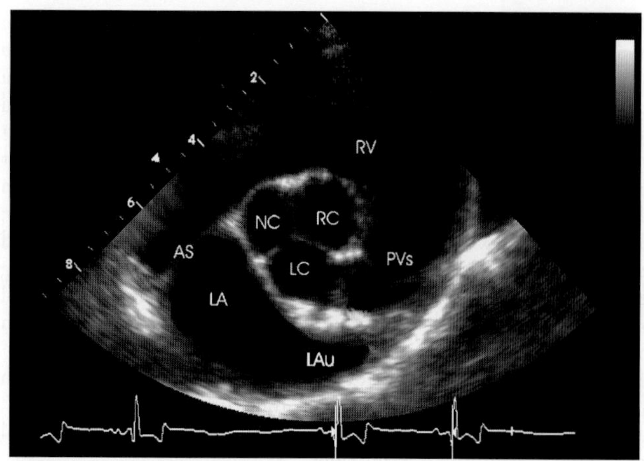

ECHOCARDIOGRAPHY Remaining in the same right parasternal window as the two previous views, gently pivoting toward the heart base, the right parasternal, short-axis view at the left atrium/aorta level was obtained in the same dog. *AS,* Atrial septum; *LA,* left atrium; *LAu,* left auricle; *LC,* left coronary cusp; *NC,* noncoronary cusp; *PVs,* pulmonic valve; *RC,* right coronary cusp; *RV,* right ventricle.

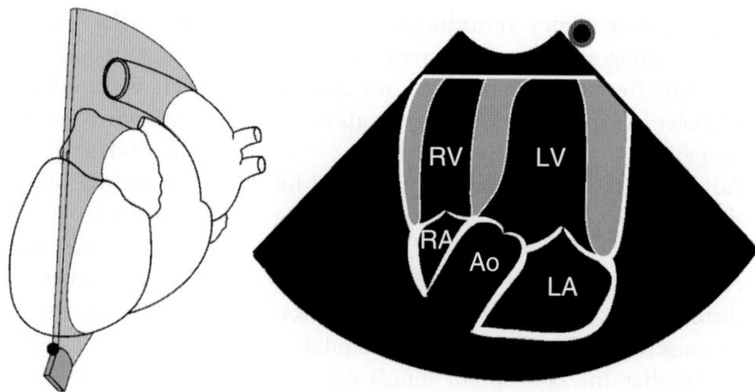

ECHOCARDIOGRAPHY Five-chamber view is obtained at left apical parasternal location. Left apical parasternal location is the only time during echocardiographic examination when the index mark on the head of transducer is directed caudally. *Ao,* Aorta; *LA,* left atrium; *LV,* left ventricle; *RA,* right atrium; *RV,* right ventricle.

inflow tract should be to the left and the outflow tract and pulmonary artery to the right.

Postprocedure

- Remove ECG clips.
- Wipe gel and alcohol from animal.

Alternatives and Their Relative Merits

Transesophageal echocardiography:

- Semi-invasive procedure
- Requires general anesthesia in animals
- Provides superb clarity and resolution

Pearls

- Patient positioning with the limbs toward the ultrasonographer in left or right lateral recumbency makes patient restraint easier if only one person is available to restrain the patient.
- The long axis of a cat's heart tends to become more parallel to the sternum as a cat ages; therefore, the angle of the ultrasound probe will be different for a 16-year-old cat versus a 2-year-old. Imaging the position of the heart in the thorax and how it changes with age allows better probe placement and reduces frustration greatly.
- Cardiac neoplasms may be best imaged when some pericardial fluid is present.
- To reduce the risk of false-positive (pseudotumor) and false-negative (missed lesion) results for neoplasms, it is critical to demonstrate a mass convincingly in more than one view.

SUGGESTED READING

Bélanger MC: Echocardiography. In Ettinger SJ, et al, editors: Textbook of veterinary internal medicine, ed 7, St. Louis, 2010, Saunders Elsevier, pp 415-431.

Reproduced from the third edition in unabridged form.

AUTHOR: Robert Prošek, DVM, MS, DACVIM, DECVIM
EDITORS: Leah A. Cohn, DVM, PhD, DACVIM; Mark S. Thompson, DVM, DABVP

Electrocardiography

Difficulty level: ♦♦

Synonyms

Electrocardiogram (ECG), EKG, electrocardiography

Overview and Goal

To assess the cardiac electrical activity and cardiac rhythm in a clinical setting and may provide some information about cardiac chamber enlargement, electrolyte abnormalities (hyperkalemia [p. 495]), or metabolic disturbances (hypoxia).

Indications

- Cardiac arrhythmia detected on physical examination (bradycardia, tachycardia, irregular rhythm)
- Part of routine monitoring or part of a preanesthetic evaluation for patients going under general anesthesia
- Syncope/weakness events
- Episodic clinical signs of uncertain type but that might represent syncope
- Screening of breeding or at-risk animals (boxers, Dobermans) for latent arrhythmias
- Evaluation of a patient with suspected hyperkalemia
- Monitoring during pericardiocentesis (p. 1150)

Contraindications

Tachypnea/dyspnea: relative contraindication for typical lateral restraint, but ECG can be done with patient standing or sternal rather than standard right lateral position if indicated

Equipment, Anesthesia

- ECG machine: machine, paper (if applicable), leads with atraumatic clips to connect to patient's skin
- Isopropyl alcohol or conducting gel
- ± Cutaneous cardiac electrode adhesive patches
- Nonconductive surface (i.e., mat on floor or top of table for patient to lay on, reducing electrical interference)

Anticipated Time

Five minutes, possibly longer if looking for infrequent arrhythmias, although a Holter monitor would be better for this (p. 1120)

Preparation: Important Checkpoints

- Input patient information into the machine, if applicable.
- Ensure sufficient paper loaded in the machine.
- Patient should be placed on mat in right lateral recumbency (standard normal values were derived from this position).

- If the reason for using cardiac monitoring is the occurrence of sporadic clinical signs, a complete medical evaluation is usually indicated in addition to the ECG:
  - CBC, serum biochemistry, urinalysis +/− urine culture: all cases; hypoglycemia, hypocalcemia (p. 515), urinary tract infection (p. 232), acid-base/metabolic disorders
  - Serum preprandial and postprandial bile acids (if consistent with case): hepatic encephalopathy (p. 440)
  - Thoracic radiographs, echocardiogram (p. 1094): all cases; assessment of cardiac structure, presence or absence of congestive heart failure
  - Troponin-I (p. 1389), tick panel, Chagas (if consistent with case): myocarditis (p. 675)

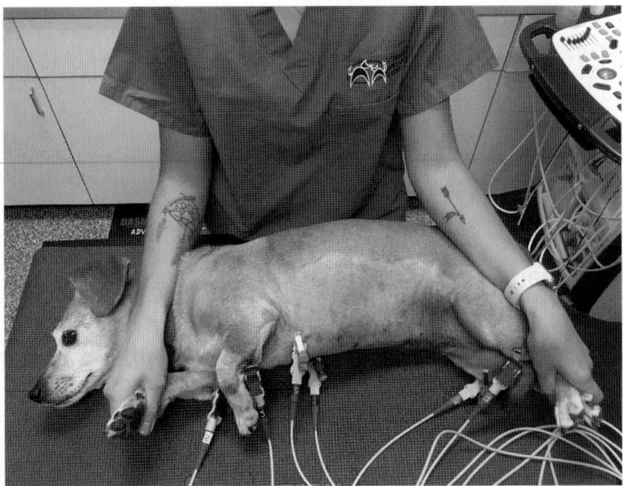

ELECTROCARDIOGRAPHY Patient is gently restrained in right lateral recumbency, with the legs perpendicular to the body. Patient is placed on a mat for insulation to reduce electrical interference. Standard limb leads are attached in addition to two precordial leads.

Possible Complications and Common Errors to Avoid

- Poor electrode/lead contact with skin: avoided by applying sufficient isopropyl alcohol to the skin at the location of lead contact, clipping fur if adhesive electrode patches applied
- Motion artifact (can mimic abnormal cardiac activity, leading to misdiagnosis): avoided by adequate patient restraint (+/− sedation if safe and necessary); apply leads to distal limbs to minimize respiratory motion artifact
- Electrical interference: avoided by placing patient on nonconductive surface, adjusting filter setting on ECG machine to eliminate 60-Hz cycle interference, avoid wire-to-wire and/or clip-to-clip contact
- Purring/shaking artifact: alcohol-soaked gauze in front of cat's nose, fear-free/calming techniques for shaking/nervous patients +/− sedation if safe and necessary
- Multiple leads should be evaluated rather than just one lead: lead II does not always provide clearest deflections/waves, and assessment of multiple leads provides various viewpoints around the heart to more thoroughly evaluate directionality of electrical activity, as well as artifact
- Cutaneous adhesive pads should be used for prolonged ECG monitoring (e.g., under general anesthesia, hospitalized patients) to avoid damage to the skin from prolonged attachment of lead clips.

Procedure

- Patient should be placed in right lateral recumbency. Other positions (sternal, sitting, standing) are also acceptable, but determination of mean electrical axis and criteria for chamber enlargement is applicable only if ECG performed with standard positioning.
- Typically at least two people are required to perform an ECG: an assistant to restrain the patient and a clinician to attach the leads and interpret the tracing.
- Leads are attached to skin of distal limbs according to color/label. Usually, white = right forelimb, black = left forelimb, green = right hindlimb, red = left hindlimb. Precordial leads may also be attached.
- Alcohol or conducting gel should be applied where leads are attached to patient (unless leads attached to adhesive electrode pads).
- A standard ECG includes tracings from all six limb leads (I, II, III, avR, aVL, aVF). Additional information may be gained from precordial lead tracings. Generally, the ECG is collected and monitored for 3 minutes for overt abnormalities/abnormal complexes. ECG settings should be noted and adjusted as needed (e.g., paper speed of 25 or 50 mm/sec); sensitivity of 10 mm/mV is standard, but half sensitivity (5 mm/mV) may be necessary when large QRS complexes present (e.g., tall R waves, deep S waves, or ventricular premature complexes). The tracing can be evaluated in more detail to perform specific interval and deflection measurements (e.g., PR interval, R-wave height, QRS duration) after completion of the procedure. Measurements ideally should be performed on 50-mm/sec paper speed for accuracy.

Postprocedure

Clips are carefully removed from the patient before release of restraint, or adhesive pads are removed after monitoring is complete.

Alternatives and Their Relative Merits

- Telemetry: for prolonged ECG monitoring (e.g., patients admitted to hospital or monitoring after anesthesia)
- Holter monitor: 24-hour ECG used for screening occurrence of infrequent arrhythmias, for antiarrhythmic therapy monitoring
- Event monitor: for long-term (days to months) monitoring
- Implantable event monitor (e.g., Reveal Plus [Medtronics]): allows an extended period of monitoring (up to 10 months). Devices are very small (size of a USB jump drive), and implantation is achieved with a subcutaneous pocket. Devices are available from Canpacers and relatively inexpensive. Access to a Medtronic programmer is necessary, however, to retrieve the stored information.
- Smart phone ECG application: smartphone case with electrodes can be purchased and used with the associated app (www.alivecor.com); allows owners to collect ECG tracing at home and transmit electronic PDF of ECG to veterinarian by email.

ECG Clip/Electrode Placement for Standard Limb Leads (I, II, III, aVR, aVL, aVF)

Electrode	Placement
RA, white	Right forelimb, clip to skin just proximal to the olecranon (caudal triceps region)
LA, black	Left forelimb, clip to skin just proximal to olecranon (caudal triceps region)
RL, green	Right hindlimb, clip to skin just proximal to the stifle (cranial thigh); ground wire
LL, red	Left hindlimb, clip to skin just proximal to the stifle (cranial thigh)

AUTHORS: Ashley E. Jones, DVM, DACVIM; Amara H. Estrada, DVM, DACVIM
EDITORS: Leah A. Cohn, DVM, PhD, DACVIM; Mark S. Thompson, DVM, DABVP

Endoscopy, Upper GI (Gastroduodenoscopy)

Client Education Sheet · Bonus Material Online

Difficulty level: ◆◆

Synonym

Upper gastrointestinal (GI) endoscopy

Overview and Goal

Minimally invasive endoscopic method of visualizing the mucosal surface of the stomach and proximal duodenum. This procedure offers the possibility of retrieving foreign bodies (p. 1115), performing mucosal biopsies, and placing a gastrostomy or jejunostomy tube (p. 1109).

Indications

- Chronic or acute vomiting
- Gastric/esophageal foreign body (p. 351)
- Suspicion of gastric or duodenal ulcer (p. 380)
- Suspicion of gastric or duodenal neoplasia (p. 379)
- Suspicion of inflammatory bowel disease (p. 543)
- Placement of percutaneous endoscopic gastrostomy (PEG) tube for enteral feeding

Contraindications

- Food or barium in stomach
- Large and/or sharp foreign body

Equipment, Anesthesia

- General anesthesia (with endotracheal intubation) required
- Mouth gag/speculum
- Flexible fiberoptic or video endoscope
  - Diameter of 9-10 mm and length of 1000-1250 mm are sufficient for gastroscopy and duodenoscopy of most medium- to large-sized dogs and for only gastroscopy of cats and small dogs.
  - A diameter of 5.5 mm or less is usually necessary to enter the duodenum of cats or small dogs. A length of 900-1000 mm is usually sufficient for cats and small dogs.
- Vacuum source for endoscopic suction
- Endoscopic biopsy forceps
- Endoscopic foreign-body retrieval forceps, snares, or baskets
- Biopsy jar with 10% buffered formalin; cassettes for placement of biopsies in formalin ideal

Anticipated Time

- Usually 60-90 minutes anesthesia time (30-60 minutes endoscopy time)
- Complex foreign-body retrieval may take > 60 minutes.

Preparation: Important Checkpoints

- Animal should have fasted for 12 hours before the procedure if possible.
- Simpler, less invasive diagnostic procedures are performed before diagnostic endoscopy (e.g., CBC, serum biochemistry profile, urinalysis, abdominal radiographs in all cases), abdominal ultrasound, fecal flotation, adrenocorticotropic hormone stimulation test (i.e., ACTH stimulation test), and others as indicated by the specific features of each case).

Possible Complications and Common Errors to Avoid

- Narcotic analgesics (e.g., morphine and butorphanol) increase motility of the pyloric antrum and may make passage of the endoscope into the duodenum difficult.
- If there is any possibility the stomach may contain food, perform an abdominal radiograph immediately before endoscopy to confirm the stomach is empty.
- Gastric or duodenal rupture
  - Usually only occurs when the wall is compromised by a deep ulcer or neoplasia. Avoid advancing the scope when the lumen cannot be seen.
- Overinsufflation, usually of the stomach, may cause potentially severe bradycardia due to abdominal compartment syndrome and creates the risk of gastric rupture.
- Prior administration of barium can make visualization difficult, and aspirating it through the endoscope may be damaging to the suction channel of the endoscope.
- Failure to recognize the major duodenal papilla as a normal structure (major and minor duodenal papillae in cats) could lead to inadvertent biopsy and potential fibrosis and obstruction of the pancreatic and common bile ducts.

Procedure

- Induce general anesthesia.
- Position the animal in left lateral recumbency.
- Place a mouth gag.
- Lubricate the endoscope with water-based lubricating jelly.
- Introduce the endoscope into the mouth, and feed it gently through the upper esophageal sphincter.
- Examine the esophageal mucosa as the scope is advanced down to the lower esophageal sphincter.
- Insufflate the esophagus with enough air to prevent the walls from collapsing on the scope and reducing visibility. An assistant may be required to gently occlude the upper esophagus by gently squeezing the cervical region externally, immediately cranial to the larynx, to prevent insufflated air from escaping out of the mouth. This will not be necessary after the tip of the endoscope is in the stomach.
- It is important to keep repositioning the scope as it is advanced so the scope is kept in the center of the lumen on the screen. This maximizes visibility and minimizes trauma to the gut wall.
- Thread the scope through the lower esophageal sphincter by keeping the opening to the stomach in the center of the screen/view piece while gently advancing the scope.
- After the distal end of the endoscope is in the stomach, insufflate the stomach with air to separate the walls and improve visibility. Insufflate until the rugal folds of the stomach are less prominent but still present. If the rugal folds are completely flattened by insufflation of air, there is risk of compromising respiration or rupturing the stomach.
- If duodenoscopy is to be performed, it is best to proceed directly to the pylorus. Prolonged insufflation or other activity in the stomach stimulates pyloric tone and motility, making threading the scope through the pylorus more difficult.
- Advancing the scope through the pylorus is usually the most difficult part of this procedure. The tone and degree of patency of the pylorus can be quite varied.
- If it is difficult to advance the scope to the opening of the pylorus (i.e., the scope is fed into the animal but advances no closer to the pylorus), suction some air out of the stomach—it may have been overinflated. This is common in large-breed dogs.
- If the pylorus is open, immediately advance the scope into the duodenum. If the pylorus is closed, maintain the opening to the pylorus in the middle of the screen while gently advancing the scope. If resistance is encountered, do not force the scope. Sometimes, insufflating some air at the opening of the pylorus will stimulate it to open (short puffs of air).
- If the pylorus is impossible to thread, try feeding a closed pair of endoscopic biopsy forceps through the pylorus. Use the threaded forceps as a guide wire to feed the scope into the duodenum.
- After the distal end of the endoscope is in the duodenum, advance the scope down to the limit of its length.
- Identify, if possible, the major duodenal papilla where the pancreatic duct and common bile duct empty into the duodenum. Do not biopsy this structure accidentally.
- Examine and identify any irregularities of the duodenal mucosa and any foreign bodies.
- Obtain multiple (6-12) mucosal biopsies using biopsy forceps. Store them in 10% formalin. Brushings or fluid samples for cytologic analysis or culture may be obtained now as well.
- Slowly withdraw the endoscope from the duodenum, and obtain mucosal biopsies periodically along its length.
- After the tip of the endoscope is back in the stomach, examine the entire stomach,

including obtaining a retroflexed view to visualize the gastric cardia. This maneuver requires maximal flexion of the endoscope tip such that the endoscope is seen emerging through the cardia. Identify any mucosal irregularities, masses, ulcers, or foreign bodies.
- Obtain multiple (6-12) biopsies of any irregular structures and normal mucosa. Be cautious about taking a biopsy of deep gastric ulcers, because this could cause perforation of the stomach wall.
- Deflate the stomach before withdrawing the endoscope into the esophagus.
- Deflate the esophagus while slowly continuing to withdraw the endoscope from the esophagus. Suction any fluid in the esophagus because it may be refluxed gastric acid that can ulcerate the esophagus if left behind.
- Take the scope out of the animal, remove the mouth gag, and recover the animal from anesthesia.

Postprocedure

- This procedure is minimally invasive, and analgesics are rarely required.
- Clean the endoscope (internal and external surfaces) immediately, before secretions and fluid have dried.

Alternatives and Their Relative Merits

Exploratory laparotomy:
- Large, full-thickness biopsies may be taken from anywhere in the GI tract.
- All the abdominal organs can be visualized and biopsied if needed.
- Virtually any foreign body may be retrieved anywhere in the stomach or intestine.
- Serosal surfaces and wall thickness can be evaluated.
- Gastrostomy tube or jejunostomy tube may be placed.
- Tumors or abnormal tissue may be surgically excised.

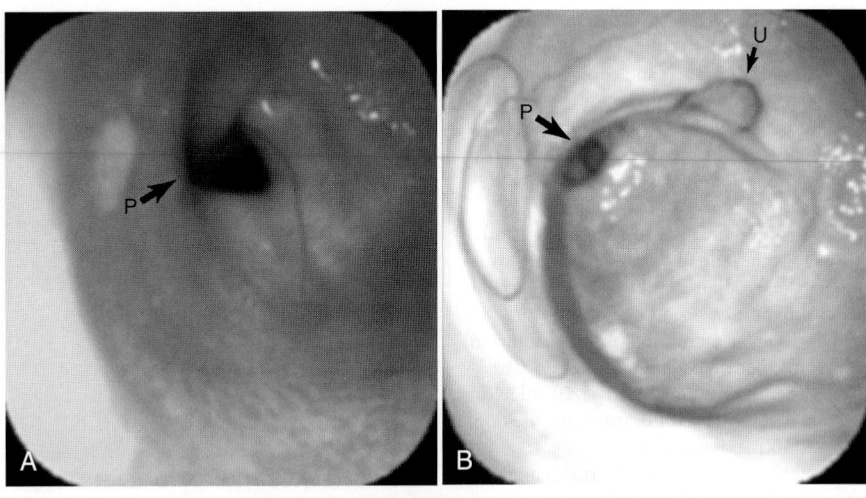

ENDOSCOPY, UPPER GI (GASTRODUODENOSCOPY) **A**, Endoscopic view of the normal pylorus (P). **B**, Endoscopic view of the pylorus (P) and a large crater-like gastric ulcer (U).

- More invasive, may be more costly, may be more time consuming
- More painful for the animal, longer recovery time
- Greater risk of peritonitis and incisional dehiscence
- Unable to visualize the esophagus
- Unable to visualize the mucosal surface of stomach or intestines unless a gastrotomy or an enterotomy is performed

Pearls

- Immediately before gastroscopy to retrieve a foreign body, always perform an abdominal radiograph to ensure the foreign body has not advanced beyond the endoscope's reach into the small or large intestine.
- If endoscopy is being planned for a dog with chronic vomiting, an ACTH stimulation test or baseline cortisol should be considered first, to rule out hypoadrenocorticism.
- It may be helpful for an assistant to feed the endoscope into or out of the patient while the veterinarian controls the rest of the endoscope with both hands. This is particularly the case with veterinarians new to the technology or during particularly delicate portions of the procedure.

SUGGESTED READING

Tolbert MK: Gastrointestinal endoscopy. In Ettinger SJ, et al, editors: Textbook of veterinary internal medicine, ed 8, St. Louis, 2017, Elsevier.

RELATED CLIENT EDUCATION SHEETS

Consent to Perform Endoscopy, Upper GI (Gastroduodenoscopy)
Inflammatory Bowel Disease
Lymphangiectasia
Lymphoma, Gastrointestinal

AUTHOR: Peter M. Foley, DVM, MSc, DACVIM
EDITORS: Leah A. Cohn, DVM, PhD, DACVIM; Mark S. Thompson, DVM, DABVP

Enema: Evacuation or Retention

Bonus Material Online 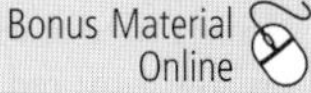

Difficulty level: ♦

Synonym

Introduction of fluid into the rectum and colon

Overview and Goal

To promote evacuation of feces or to administer medicinal substances

Indications

Evacuation enema:
- Constipation (p. 202) (especially in cats), obstipation, or colonic foreign body (rare)
- Patient preparation for colonoscopy
- Preparation for imaging procedures when the presence of fecal matter in the colon might interfere with image interpretation (e.g., contrast CT to identify ectopic ureter)

Retention enema:
- Fermentable substrate (e.g., lactulose), to adjust colonic pH for hepatic encephalopathy when animal is unable to swallow
- Administration of fecal microbiota transplant (p. 1105)
- Rarely, administration of medications (e.g., benzodiazepines for seizures, lactulose

Contraindications

- Rectal or anal pain
- Fractious animal
- Hypervolemic patient or risk for volume overload
- Cool water enemas are NOT recommended for treating heat stroke.
- Sodium phosphate enemas can cause hyperphosphatemia and hypocalcemia and are NOT recommended in cats and dogs.

Equipment, Anesthesia

- Materials
    - Rounded edge, nontraumatic tubing (e.g., red rubber catheter, Foley catheter)

- A 60-mL syringe for cats/small dogs or enema bucket with drain spout at the bottom (or funnel) and connection tubing for medium or large dogs
- Lubricant
- Access to outside or easily cleaned area
- Examination gloves
- Enema solutions
  - Warm water or isotonic saline 10-20 mL/kg; some add dioctyl sodium sulfosuccinate (emollient laxative) or water-soluble lubricant, *or*
  - 10%-20% lactulose (osmotic solution) 5 mL per cat and 10 mL per dog, *or*
  - Mineral oil (lubricant): 5-10 mL (cat, small dog), 10-20 mL (medium-size dog), 20-30 mL (large dog)
  - Other medication or solution, as indicated

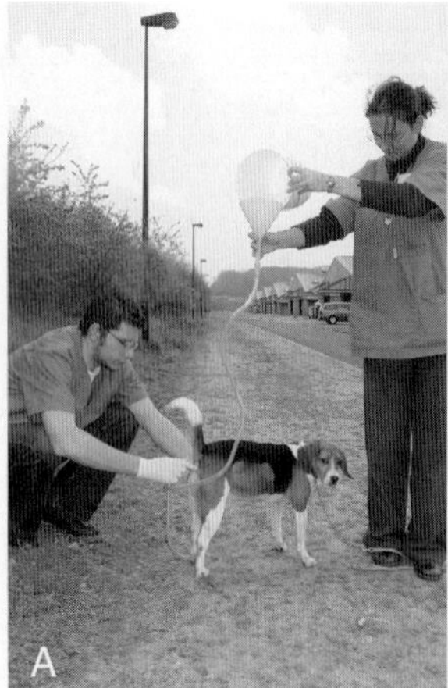
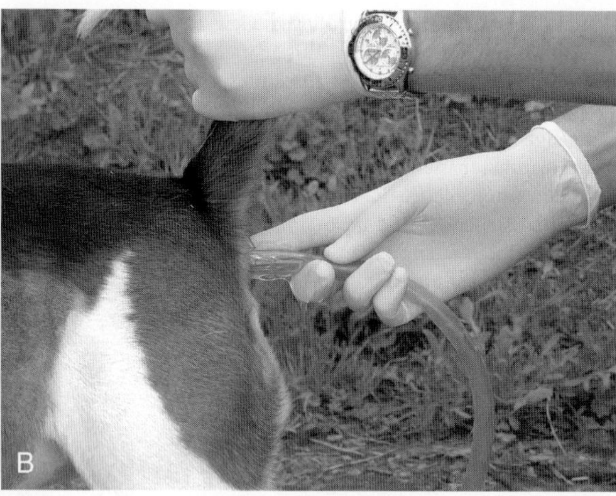

ENEMA (EVACUATION AND RETENTION) A, Large volumes of enema fluid are instilled using gravity, a funnel, and a tube. **B**, Enema tube that is well lubricated is passed into the anus and advanced without resistance to a point corresponding to the maximal distance from the anus to the last rib. (Courtesy Dr. Sylvie Daminet.)

Anticipated Time

Varies with size of the animal, typically 20-40 minutes, including preparation

Preparation: Important Checkpoints

- Ensure adequate hydration status.
- Choose an appropriate area for cleaning after procedure and for feces to be evacuated.
- Obtain assistance for appropriate animal restraint (manual, rarely chemical) and to hold enema solution container.
- Perform rectal exam first.
- For medication administration: appropriate size syringe and syringe with water to flush tubing after medication infused
- Anesthesia is not required in most patients.

Possible Complications and Common Errors to Avoid

- Do not stand immediately behind the animal.
- Excessive force may traumatize the colonic mucosa, and if the colon is diseased, a risk of perforation exists (rare).
- Excessive volume can be absorbed, causing fluid overload and pulmonary edema.
- Vomiting can occur with overly aggressive enema volumes or overfilling the colon.

Procedure

- Using a tube of appropriate size (range, 10-12 Fr [3-4 mm] red rubber catheter in an adult cat and small dog; 30 Fr [10 mm] tubing in a large dog for large volumes) and adequate lubricant to coat the tube.
- The well-lubricated catheter should be introduced gently into the rectum and advanced as far in as it can pass without resistance or resentment, likely to the level of the last rib.
- For evacuation enema, solution administered slowly over 2-5 minutes. Gently withdraw and advance the tubing a few centimeters as needed while the enema is administered to help loosen feces.
- Patients with severe constipation may, besides enemas, need manual extraction. After instillation of the enema under general anesthesia, the anus is kept closed for 5-15 minutes and the abdomen gently massaged.
- Repeat enemas no more than q 4-6h.
- For colonoscopy preparation: animals should be fasted for 24-36 hours and water restricted 2-4 hours before the procedure. An oral isosmotic gastrointestinal lavage solution should be given orally the day before the procedure (e.g., GoLytely/Colyte 2 doses of 30 mL/kg slowly by oroesophageal or nasoesophageal tube and given 2-4 hours apart the day before the procedure). The morning before colonoscopy, multiple warm water enemas are given until the colonic fluid is clear.
- Small-diameter tubes are used for administration of medications (e.g., benzodiazepines, lactulose). For medication administration, a syringe is attached to a red rubber catheter. The medication is infused, followed by an infusion of a few milliliters of water to ensure complete introduction of the medication into the colon. Large volumes should be avoided to reduce chance of immediate defecation.

Postprocedure

- Evacuation enema: allow the animal to recover in an area that is large enough to allow defecation and movement away from feces; diarrhea is expected.
- Retention enema: litter box should be removed for cats, and dogs should be caged to discourage defecation.

Alternatives and Their Relative Merits

- For obstipation or preparation for colonoscopy, constant rate infusion of Colyte (GoLytely) through a nasogastric tube has been successful.
- Oral administration of laxatives (e.g., lactulose) if animal is conscious and able to swallow; for mild cases of constipation, or prevention of constipation

Pearls

- Warm solutions to body temperature for comfort.
- Cats are higher risk for intravascular volume overload.
- When treating constipation, create a long-term medical plan.

SUGGESTED READING

Sherding RG: Diseases of the large intestine. In Tams TR editor: Small animal gastroenterology, ed 2, 2003, Saunders, pp 251-285.

AUTHOR: Sylvie Daminet, DVM, PhD, DACVIM, DECVIM

EDITORS: Leah A. Cohn, DVM, PhD, DACVIM; Mark S. Thompson, DVM, DABVP

Excretory Urogram

Difficulty level: ♦♦

Synonyms

Intravenous pyelogram (IVP), intravenous (IV) urogram

Overview and Goal

When the kidneys are difficult to assess by plain-film radiography or qualitative renal functional information is needed, an excretory urogram could be performed. On survey abdominal radiographs, the kidneys may not be visualized in animals that have decreased abdominal detail (young, thin, peritoneal fluid).

Indications

- Identify kidneys (if poor abdominal detail)
- Mass lesions of kidneys (or mass in region of kidney)
- Qualitative assessment of renal function (subjective)
- Patency, continuity of urinary tract
- Before nephrectomy
- Abnormal renal size, shape
- Persistent hematuria (p. 428)
- Suspected renal or ureteral calculi
- Suspected hydronephrosis (p. 483) or pyelonephritis (p. 849)
- Suspected ureteral ectopia (p. 282), ureterocele, ureteral rupture
- To evaluate the urinary bladder when it cannot be catheterized
- Postoperative assessment of urinary tract (patency, strictures, leakage)

Contraindications

- Dehydration
- Previous reaction to iodinated contrast medium (a nonionic medium should be used)
- Caution should be used in animals with the following conditions:
  - Diabetes mellitus (p. 251)
  - Multiple myeloma (p. 663)
  - Congestive heart failure (pp. 408 and 409)
  - Hypertension
  - Concurrent drug administration (cardiac glycosides)
  - Severe debilitation

Equipment, Anesthesia

- Many recommend the use of general anesthesia or heavy sedation; however, an excretory urogram can be performed in an unanesthetized animal.
- IV catheter
- Hair clippers
- Surgical scrub solution, rubbing alcohol, and gauze/sponges to prepare skin for catheter placement
- Tape/releasing elastic (Vetrap-type) bandage
- Iodinated contrast medium (sodium iothalamate, sodium diatrizoate)
- Nonionic contrast medium (iohexol, iopamidol) if clinically warranted
- Syringe
- Heparin/saline for flush
- Enema set
- Antianaphylactic agents (e.g., diphenhydramine, 2-4 mg/kg for IM injection)
- Oxygen and drug cart to address any possible procedural complication

Anticipated Time

Approximately 1 hour

Preparation: Important Checkpoints

- Advise owner that hair will be clipped from the site of IV catheter placement.
- Animal should be fasted for 24 hours before the procedure; water is given ad libitum.
- Enema (p. 1099) given at least 2 hours before study to remove a maximum of the fecal material from the colon, allowing visualization of kidneys and ureters
- Assess hydration: proceed only if normal.
- Standard aseptic placement of IV catheter in a cephalic vein; it is imperative that the catheter be properly placed.
- Secure the catheter in place with tape/releasing elastic (Vetrap-type) bandage.
- Draw 900 mg iodine per kg body weight of contrast material into syringe.
- Add an appropriate amount of heparin/saline flush into a syringe.

Possible Complications and Common Errors to Avoid

- Vomiting: this often occurs immediately after injection of the contrast medium. If the animal is muzzled, the muzzle should be removed immediately to avoid aspiration.
- Systemic hypotension, bradycardia
- Anaphylaxis (p. 54) (airway edema, vascular collapse, bronchospasm)
- Perivascular injection may result in sloughing of surrounding tissue.
- Contrast medium–induced kidney injury
- Administration of iodinated contrast media may affect urine specific gravity, urine sediment, and urine culture results for 24 hours after administration.
- Blood values (blood urea nitrogen [BUN], creatinine, prothrombin time [PT], activated partial thromboplastin time [aPTT], thromboplastin time [TT], and hematocrit) might also be affected for up to 24 hours after contrast administration.

Procedure

- Preliminary abdominal radiographs are made to determine adequate animal preparation and to set radiographic technique.
- The kilovoltage peak (kVp) should be set between 65 and 75 to maximize contrast.
- Flush the catheter to again ensure patency.
- Inject contrast material rapidly as a bolus.
- Flush catheter of residual contrast material using heparin/saline syringe.
- A ventrodorsal view is obtained at 20 seconds.
- Ventrodorsal and right lateral views are obtained at 5, 20, and 40 minutes.
- Oblique views are obtained at 5 minutes to visualize ureteral termination at the urinary bladder.

Postprocedure

- If general anesthesia is used: routine anesthetic recovery
- Maintain adequate hydration.
- The IV catheter should remain in place at least 15-20 minutes after the procedure. This allows venous access should an adverse reaction to the contrast medium occur.

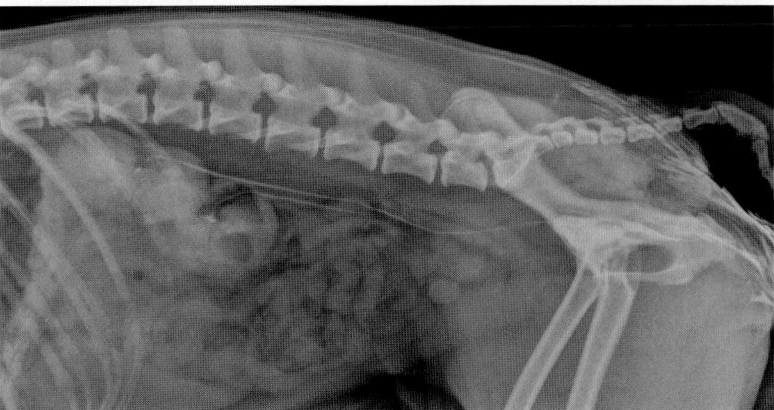

EXCRETORY UROGRAM Excretory urogram, lateral view. Both kidneys and ureters are clearly seen. The diagnosis was ectopic ureter, supported by the presence of contrast on the haircoat of the dog's hindquarters (the dog did not void voluntarily during the procedure).

Procedures and Techniques

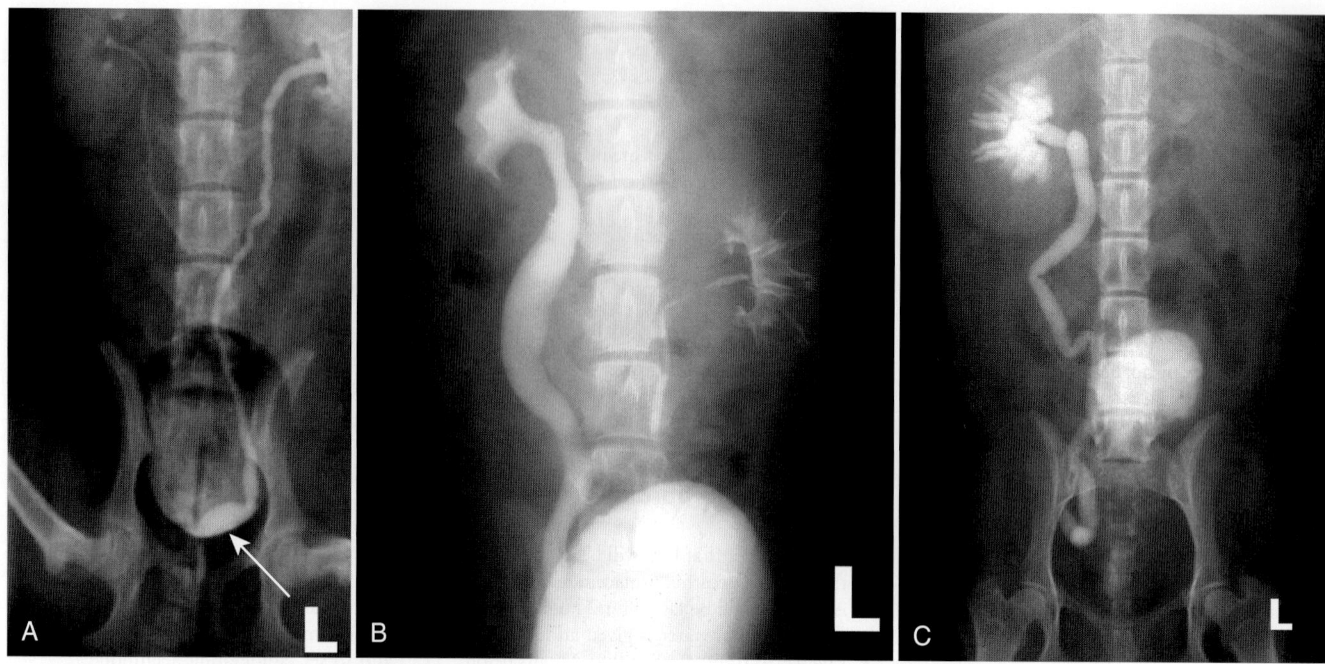

EXCRETORY UROGRAM Excretory urograms, ventrodorsal views. **A,** Ectopic ureter (left side), normal ureter (right side). Ectopic ureter is diffusely enlarged (hydroureter), especially distally where it inserts in an ectopic location *(arrow)*. **B,** Pyelonephritis (right side). Right-sided hydronephrosis and severe hydroureter are apparent. **C,** Additional example of hydronephrosis and hydroureter, affecting the right side. *L,* Left.

- Remove the IV catheter > 20 minutes after the procedure.

Alternatives and Their Relative Merits

- Plain abdominal radiographs: inexpensive means to survey the abdomen. Radiopaque renal or ureteral calculi can be visualized. Evaluate renal size and shape if abdominal detail is adequate and fecal material is not obscuring their visualization.
- Abdominal ultrasound: excellent potential for visualization of kidneys, especially in animals with poor radiographic abdominal detail. Renal size, shape, position, and echogenicity relative to the liver and spleen can be assessed. The size of the renal pelvis and internal architecture of the kidneys can be assessed. Ultrasound can determine if masses are solid or cystic. Resistive index can be calculated.
- Cystoscopy (p. 1085)/urethroscopy: excellent visualization of ectopic ureter(s); opportunity for therapeutic intervention (laser)
- Computed tomography (CT) provides excellent detail of size, shape, and margination of the kidneys. IV contrast media can be used for enhancing findings in the kidneys and/or ureters. CT is excellent for assessing ectopic ureters. CT is more costly to perform than other studies listed and may require general anesthesia.
- Nuclear scintigraphy (diethylenetriamine pentaacetate [DTPA]): to determine global and individual glomerular filtration rates, to evaluate the animal's response to treatment, to evaluate function of contralateral kidney before surgery and possible removal of diseased kidney, to identify and determine the severity of subclinical renal disease in an animal receiving nephrotoxic agents, and to examine renal perfusion by obtaining rapid serial images during first-pass circulation

Pearls

The likelihood of the animal vomiting can be decreased by injection of contrast as a slow bolus over 20-30 seconds.

SUGGESTED READING

Muhlbauer MC, et al: Radiography of the dog and cat: guide to making and interpreting radiographs, ed 1, Hoboken, NJ, 2013, Wiley-Blackwell.

AUTHOR: LeeAnn Pack, DVM, DACVR
EDITORS: Leah A. Cohn, DVM, PhD, DACVIM; Mark S. Thompson, DVM, DABVP

FAST Ultrasound Examinations

Video Available 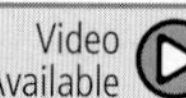

Difficulty level: ♦♦

Synonyms

Focused assessment with sonography for trauma, triage, and tracking (FAST), abdominal FAST (AFAST®), thoracic FAST (TFAST®)

Overview and Goals

- FAST scans aim to quickly identify pathology in emergency and critical care patients, determine its significance, and evaluate its progression.
- AFAST has a high sensitivity and specificity for detecting abdominal effusion.
- TFAST has a high sensitivity and specificity for the diagnosis of pneumothorax, pericardial, and pleural effusion. Can help distinguish between cardiac and noncardiac causes of respiratory distress.

- Lung ultrasound identifies interstitial/alveolar pathology.
- Aid in obtaining fluid samples for cytologic examination via ultrasound-guided aspiration

Indications

- Any trauma patient
- Critically ill or unstable patients
- Respiratory distress
- Change in patient status

Contraindications

None. Does not require sedation, shaving, or anesthesia; can be performed patient-side during stabilization without compromising patient stability because of special positioning, transport, or restraint.

Equipment, Anesthesia

- B-mode ultrasound with a 5- or 7.5-MHz curvilinear probe (former for larger dogs)
  - Linear array probes may help identify glide sign
- Alcohol and/or ultrasound gel

Anticipated Time

3-6 minutes for each of AFAST, TFAST, and lung ultrasound. Requires minimal training.

Preparation: Important Checkpoints

Do not need to clip hair

Possible Complications and Common Errors to Avoid

- A negative scan does not exclude pathology.
- Retroperitoneal and focal injury may be missed on AFAST scans.
- FAST scans do not identify the fluid type or its origin.
- False-positive results
  - Vascular structures, intestinal wall, and gallbladder can be confused for free fluid. Two views (long and short axes) decrease false-positive results.
  - Glide sign is difficult to identify in panting or severely tachypneic patients.
- False-negative results
  - Patients initially negative on emergency ultrasound scans may become positive over time. Re-evaluate in 2-4 hours (sooner if patient status changes).
  - Glide sign may be intermittent with low respiratory rates and absent during apnea.

Procedure

AFAST®

- Free fluid often appears as hypoechoic/anechoic (black) triangles.
- Left or right lateral recumbency preferred (but can be done standing)
- The ultrasound probe is placed on four regions of the abdomen in a consistent, systematic approach. At each site, the probe is fanned through an angle of 45° in long- and short-axis views and moved 1 inch (2.5 cm) in cranial, caudal, left, and right directions. Fanning increases likelihood that abdominal fluid is detected and that target organs are properly identified. The four locations are:
  - Diaphragmatic-hepatic (DH): at the subxiphoid, allows visualization of the diaphragm, liver lobes, and gallbladder
  - Splenorenal (SR): allows visualization of the spleen and left kidney
  - Cystocolic (CC): allows visualization of the bladder
  - Hepatorenal (HR): allows visualization of the liver and right kidney
- Fluid aspiration confirms fluid type (e.g., transudate, exudate, bile, blood, urine, chyle, septic, inflammatory) (pp. 79 and 1343).
- Abdominal fluid score (AFS) is specific to trauma patients.
  - AFS 1: positive fluid in one site; AFS 2: positive in any two sites; AFS 3: positive in any three sites; AFS 4: positive in all four sites
  - AFS aids in documenting fluid progression or resolution.
  - Short-term increase in AFS suggests ongoing intraabdominal hemorrhage; further patient evaluation is warranted.
  - Decrease in AFS indicates resolving hemorrhage.
  - AFS has been validated only in lateral positions.

TFAST®

- The probe is placed on five sites. Fanning the probe is not necessary for the chest tube site (CTS). The five locations are:
  - DH: with the probe directed cranially to observe the pericardium and pleural spaces (adjust depth to view heart)
  - CTS: left and right CTS at the level of the seventh to ninth intercostal spaces on the dorsolateral thoracic wall (closer to vertebrae)
  - PCS (pericardial site): left and right PCS over the heart at the level of the fifth and sixth intercostal spaces on the ventrolateral thoracic wall (closer to the sternum)
- Patients are placed in left or right lateral recumbency for the DH and nondependent thoracic site views (CTS and PCS views; see below) and then rolled into sternal recumbency for the contralateral thoracic site views. Patients in respiratory distress should be placed in sternal recumbency or scanned in standing position to obtain the four thoracic site views.
- The DH site can detect pericardial (p. 773) and pleural effusion (p. 791).
- The CTSs are used for detecting pneumothorax (p. 797), pleural effusion, and B-lines.
  - The probe is placed between two ribs. The characteristic image obtained is called the *bat sign*.
  - Bat sign: two adjacent ribs (hyperechoic arched structures with distal black shadowing) with the horizontal pleural line extending between and slightly distal to the two ribs. This line represents the interface between visceral pleura and parietal pleura.
  - The glide sign and/or B-lines can be identified between the two ribs at the level of the pleural line.

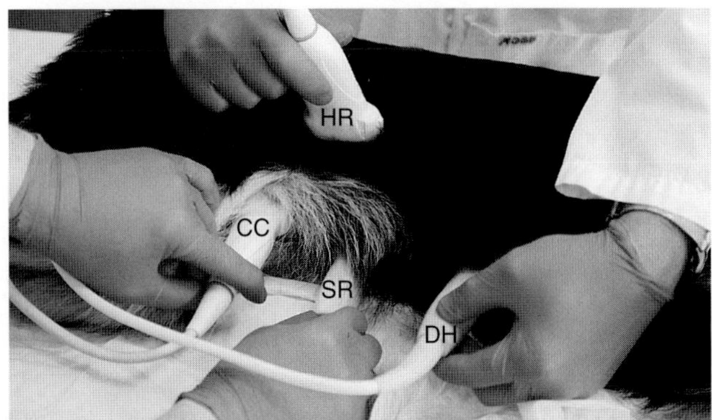

FAST ULTRASOUND EXAMINATIONS AFAST®: patient is in left lateral recumbency. The probe is placed on four regions of the abdomen: 1) diaphragmatic-hepatic (DH): at the subxiphoid; 2) splenorenal (SR) at left sublumbar region; 3) cystocolic (CC), on midline over the bladder; and 4) hepatorenal (HR) at right sublumbar region.

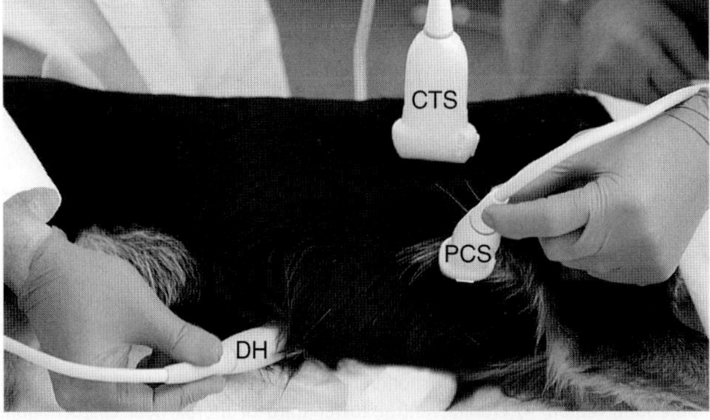

FAST ULTRASOUND EXAMINATIONS TFAST®: patient is in left lateral recumbency. The probe is placed on five sites: 1) diaphragmatic-hepatic (DH) at the subxiphoid, with the probe directed cranially to observe the pericardium and pleural spaces; 2) left and right chest tube site (CTS) at the level of the seventh to ninth intercostal spaces on the dorsolateral thoracic wall (closer to vertebrae); 3) left and right pericardial sites (PCS) over the heart at the level of the fifth to sixth intercostal spaces on the ventrolateral thoracic wall (closer to the sternum).

Procedures and Techniques

- Glide sign: normal to-and-fro motion of the pleural line as the parietal and visceral pleura slide past each other during respiration; identified as horizontal pendulous movement along the pleural line (see *Video*). The presence of a glide sign excludes pleural effusion and pneumothorax at the probe placement site. The absence of a glide sign suggests the presence of pneumothorax.

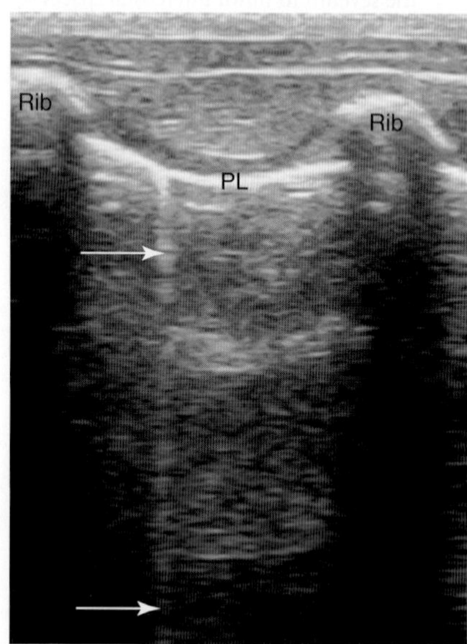

FAST ULTRASOUND EXAMINATIONS B-lines, glide sign, and bat sign. B-lines *(white horizontal arrows)* are reverberation artifacts originating from the pleural line (PL) extending to the edge of the far field image. NOTE: The PL of the image depicted in this figure can be seen in patients with or without a pneumothorax.

- B-lines: hyperechoic vertical streaks originating from the pleural line. They swing with the to-and-fro motion of the glide sign and do not fade distally, extending through the far field (see *Video*). They exclude pneumothorax at those focal probe placement sites. Multiple B-lines suggest alveolar-interstitial syndrome (AIS) such as pulmonary contusions, cardiogenic or noncardiogenic pulmonary edema (p. 836), pneumonia (pp. 793 and 795), or neoplasia.
- Lung point: location at which collapsed lung secondary to pneumothorax re-contacts the thoracic wall; increases the specificity of detecting pneumothorax (see *Video*). The probe should be walked cranially and ventrally to identify the lung point.

- The PCSs are used for detecting pleural and pericardial effusions.
  - The probe is placed to visualize the heart, pericardial sac, and pleural spaces.
- Ultrasound-guided, fine-needle aspiration can be safely performed for therapeutic and diagnostic purposes.

LUNG ULTRASOUND

- Two protocols have been described: a dorsal-ventral intercostal sliding protocol and Vet BLUE®.
- Intercostal sliding lung ultrasound:
  - Starting caudal dorsally at the 9th-10th intercostal space, the probe is placed perpendicular or parallel to the ribs and then passed in a dorsal to ventral direction within the intercostal spaces.
  - At the ventral margin of the lung/diaphragm interface, the probe is moved a rib cranially and passed in a ventral to dorsal direction within the intercostal space. The process is repeated, covering the entire thorax bilaterally.
- Vet BLUE involves four bilateral thoracic sites:
  - Caudal dorsal: upper third of thorax at 9th intercostal space or dorsal caudal lung region
  - Perihilar: 6th intercostal space at middle third of thorax or perihilar region
  - Caudal-cardiac: lower third of thorax near costochondral junction at 6th-8th intercostal space or middle lung region
  - Cranial-ventral: lower third of thorax near costochondral junction at 3rd-5th intercostal space or cranial lung region
- Vet BLUE: the probe is placed at each site and moved 1-2 rib spaces cranially/caudally to identify B lines:
  - In larger dogs, the probe can also be moved 1-2 cm dorsally/ventrally.
  - If B lines are visualized, the probe is held stationary, and the number of B-lines is recorded.
  - ≤3 B lines at a single site can be normal.
  - ≥3 B lines at a single site or that coalesce indicate AIS.
  - The more numerous the B-lines, the more severe AIS at that location

Postprocedure

Emergency ultrasound scans that are initially negative for fluid, air, or AIS may become positive over time. Serial scans are recommended 2-4 hours after the initial scan (sooner if unstable) and then as needed to decrease false-negatives.

Alternatives and Their Relative Merits

- Radiographs are complementary tests that should be considered in critically ill patients: use caution when restraining patients as patients may decompensate. Small amounts of air and/or effusion may be missed due to lack of sensitivity.
- Emergency ultrasound scans do not replace formal extensive ultrasound scans.
- Blind thoracocentesis (p. 1164) may be used in dyspneic patients with suspected pneumothorax and pleural effusion based

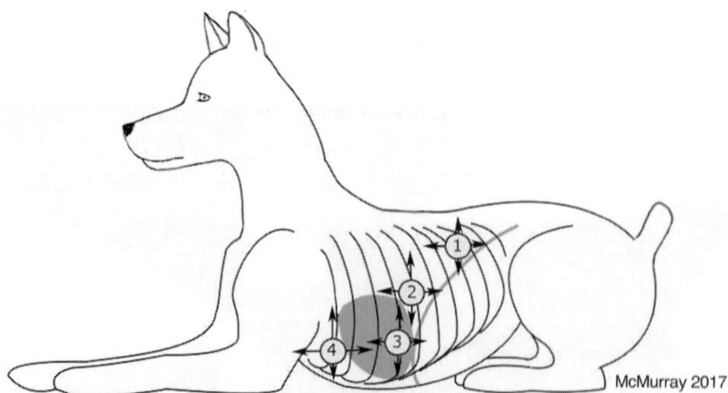

FAST ULTRASOUND EXAMINATIONS Vet BLUE®: 1) caudal dorsal: upper third of thorax at the 9th intercostal space or dorsal caudal lung region; 2) perihilar: 6th intercostal space at middle third of thorax or perihilar region; 3) caudal-cardiac: lower third of thorax near costochondral junction at 6th-8th intercostal space or middle lung region; 4) cranial-ventral: lower third of thorax near costochondral junction at 3rd-5th intercostal space or cranial lung region. At the middle lung site (3), if the heart obscures the field of view, the probe is moved caudally 1-2 rib spaces until the heart is no longer visible and the lung can be evaluated. At the cranial lung site (4), the probe is moved cranially one rib space at a time until the heart is no longer visible and lungs can be evaluated. The patient's forelimb can be pulled cranially to facilitate probe positioning. (Courtesy Dr. Jantina McMurray, Calgary, Alberta.)

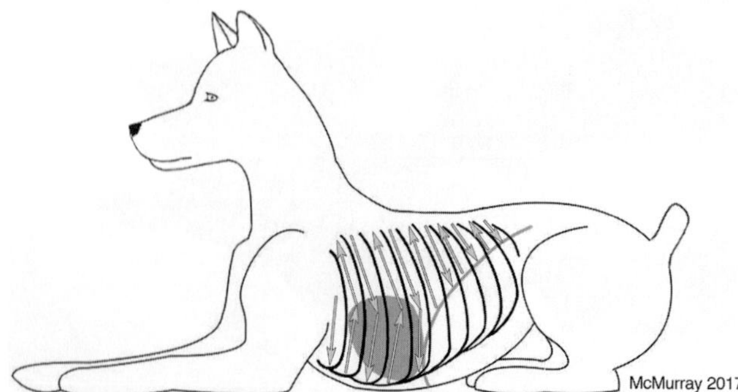

FAST ULTRASOUND EXAMINATIONS Intercostal sliding lung ultrasound. Starting caudal dorsally at the 9th-10th intercostal space, the probe is passed from a dorsal to ventral direction within the intercostal space. At the ventral margin of the lung/diaphragm interface the probe is moved a rib cranially and passed from a ventral to dorsal direction within the intercostal space. The process is repeated, covering the entire thorax bilaterally. (Courtesy Dr. Jantina McMurray, Calgary, Alberta.)

on history and physical exam; attendant risks must be considered (e.g., lung laceration).
- Computed tomography scan: gold standard for pneumothorax detection but involves anesthesia/heavy sedation and is not as widely available; cannot be performed cageside.

Pearls

- Not all patients produce pathology that is detectable on emergency ultrasound scans.
- FAST scans omit large areas of the abdomen and thorax and do not reliably exclude localized organ injury.
- Dorsal positioning of patients should be avoided because of a higher risk of worsening respiratory and/or cardiovascular compromise.
- Change the depth and focus at each location of the emergency ultrasound scan after the organs of interest are identified; helps identify smaller accumulations of fluid and improves image quality.
- TFAST is best evaluated when the patient takes a deep breath.
- Keep your hand, the patient, and the ultrasound probe still when assessing the glide sign to avoid a false-positive glide sign.
- Increase the depth to view the entire heart when differentiating pericardial from pleural effusion.
- The DH view helps differentiate pericardial and pleural effusion.
- The number of B-lines correlates to the severity of AIS.
- Practice improves skill.

SUGGESTED READING

Boysen SR, et al: The use of ultrasound for dogs and cats in the emergency room: AFAST and TFAST. Vet Clin Small Anim 43:773-797, 2013.

AUTHORS: Serge Chalhoub, DVM, DACVIM; Søren R. Boysen, DVM, DACVECC
EDITORS: Leah A. Cohn, DVM, PhD, DACVIM; Mark S. Thompson, DVM, DABVP

Fecal Transplant

Difficulty level: ◆

Synonyms

Fecal microbiota transplant (FMT), stool transplant

Overview and Goal

- The overall goal of fecal transplant is to alter the patient's gastrointestinal (GI) microbiome, thereby improving GI health.
- Stool from a healthy, screened donor is introduced into the GI tract of a patient with GI signs (usually chronic diarrhea) believed to be due to intestinal dysbiosis. The transplant can be given by retention enema (most common), delivered to the ileum by colonoscopy, delivered orally or by stomach tube, or through a combination of these routes.
- There is very sparse published data regarding optimal transplant procedures, safety, or efficacy of fecal transplant in dogs or cats, but the technique has gained in popularity due to anecdotal success stories.

Indications

Dogs or cats with chronic diarrhea that have failed to respond to the standard therapy, including food trials, probiotics, or antibiotics

Contraindications

- Recognized cause of GI signs for which there is a known, effective treatment
- Good response to food trials, probiotics, or antibiotics
- Known or suspected intestinal ulceration
- Immunocompromise is a relative contraindication.

Equipment, Anesthesia

Can be performed with or without sedation; sedation may encourage enema retention (goal ≥ 45 minutes).

Materials:

- Gloves
- Blender, or container and disposable spoon to mix feces
- Fresh stool from healthy, screened donor
- Measuring device or gram scale
- Milk (alternative: sterile saline or water)
- Sieve strainer device or gauze/cheese cloth
- Syringes with tip appropriate for tubing or with adaptor to connect syringe to enema tubing
  - Number and size depends on volume of transplant infusion
- Enema tubing: size depends on patient size but adequate in length to reach at least the transverse colon
  - For cats or small dogs, 8 to 12 Fr red rubber catheter appropriate
  - For larger dogs, larger-bore tubing appropriate
- Lubricant
- ± Canned, enticing food

Anticipated Time

60-90 minutes, including the transplant preparation and enema retention time

Preparation: Important Checkpoints

Donor selection criteria are not well established, but suggest

- Clinically healthy pet of same species
  - Ideally, pet from same household as is patient
  - Avoid using donors from institutional housing (e.g., clinic animals).
- Between 1 and 7 years of age
- Normal, well-formed stools absent of blood or excessive mucus
- No systemic antimicrobial exposure during the past 6 months
- Diet that does not include raw meat or animal-based treats
- Regular use of endoparasite prevention
- At a minimum, perform direct and flotation fecal parasite exam on donor stool within a week of use.
- Ideally, test donor stool for multiple GI pathogens (e.g., IDEXX Diarrhea RealPCR Panel, Antech Canine or Feline GI PCR Panel, fecal culture) within a week of use.

Patient preparation:

- Fast the patient overnight before the procedure.
- Allow patient to defecate before beginning the procedure.
- Ideally, avoid administering the transplant while the patient is receiving antimicrobials.

Possible Complications and Common Errors to Avoid

- Not having donor stool at the time of procedure: have the donor spend the day at the clinic, and do not allow them access/opportunity to defecate the morning of the procedure.
- Early evacuation of enema by recipient: consider sedation; avoid excessive volume or overly rapid infusion of enema; do not allow access to litter box (cat) or outdoors for at least 45 minutes after procedure.
- Iatrogenic transmission of pathogens: use only healthy donor with normal stool, and screen for parasites ± other pathogens within a week of transplant.
- Ineffective transplant: use fresh stool from donor that has not recently received antimicrobial drugs; avoid exposure of transplant liquid ("fecal shake") to bacteriostatic materials; avoid excessive exposure of fecal shake to air/oxygen because many of the normal microbes are anaerobic

Procedure

- Wear gloves while handling stool and during preparation and administration of the fecal shake.

- Allow donor animal to defecate naturally, and immediately recover stool, avoiding excessive contamination with litter, grass, or dirt.
- Blend fresh stool at a ratio of 1 part stool and 3-4 parts milk (or saline/water) using a blender or a spoon; the goal is to create an emulsion without large pieces of solid stool.
- Use a sieve (or gauze, cheese cloth) strain the emulsion to remove larger particulates that might clog the enema tubing.
- Draw up prepared fecal shake into syringes, with size and number appropriate to administer 10 mL/kg dose (e.g., for a 10-kg dog, you might use two 60-mL syringes, each containing 50 mL of fecal shake).
- Sedate the patient, if desired, and position (using restraint as needed) for enema administration. In sedated patient, lateral recumbency is used, but the procedure can be done in any position.
- Roughly measure the length of tubing required for the enema to reach the transverse colon or even the ileum.
- Lubricate the tubing, and gently insert per rectum. Advance slowly to the appropriate position (e.g., ileocolic junction to transverse colon).
- Administer the calculated volume of the fecal shake slowly, avoiding sudden pressure that might trigger patient defecation.
- For optimal results, the transplant should be retained in the colon for at least 45 minutes, but longer retention is ideal.
- Any remaining fecal shake solution may be offered to the patient for consumption, either as is or mixed with a tasty food. Many dogs willingly drink the fecal shake prepared with milk.

Postprocedure

Beyond keeping the patient quiet and trying to avoid allowing defecation for at least 45 minutes, there is no special care required.

Alternatives and Their Relative Merits

- Commercially available probiotics are always administered before turning to fecal transplant because there is no risk of iatrogenic disease transmission with probiotic administration.
- Alternative methods of fecal transplant include administration by colonoscopy directly into the ileum, administration by feeding fecal shake, or administration by stomach tube. Stomach acid may kill beneficial microbes, making administration by enema or colonoscopy preferred routes.

Pearls

- Owners should be warned that this is a largely untested procedure that is not without risk.
- For animals that respond well, improvement often occurs within several days.
- Transplant can be repeated if there is a partial response. Repetition once or twice for animals that fail to respond is reasonable, but if there is still no improvement, further transplants are unlikely to be effective.
- Send a fecal score chart home with the client and have them score and record in a log any changes in stool consistency.
- Because oxygen exposure is likely to kill beneficial anaerobic microbes, use of fresh stool (<4 hours after defecation) is best.

SUGGESTED READING

Schmitz S, et al. Understanding the canine intestinal microbiota and its modification by pro-, pre- and synbiotics—what is the evidence? Vet Med Sci 2(2):71-94, 2016.

AUTHOR: Matthew Haight, CVT
EDITORS: Leah A. Cohn, DVM, PhD, DACVIM; Mark S. Thompson, DVM, DABVP

Feeding Tube Placement: Esophagostomy

Client Education Sheet · Bonus Material Online

Difficulty level: ♦♦

Synonym

Esophageal feeding tube

Overview and Goal

To provide a route (days to weeks) for delivering enteral nutrition and oral medications to a patient unable or unwilling to eat on its own

Indications

- Nutritional support for anorexic patients
- Disorders of swallowing or mastication
- Route of evacuation of food material in cases of megaesophagus (p. 642)

Contraindications

- Frequent vomiting
- Coagulopathy
- Gastrointestinal (GI) obstruction

Equipment, Anesthesia

- General anesthesia or heavy sedation
- Clippers; materials for aseptic prep and scrub
- Mouth gag
- Sterile gloves
- Feeding tube (red rubber type), typically 10-Fr diameter for cats and small dogs, up to 18 Fr for larger dogs
- Christmas tree adapter and cap
- #11 scalpel blade
- Needle-holding forceps, suture scissors
- Long, curved hemostatic forceps (e.g., curved Kelly, Carmalt)
- Nonabsorbable 2-0 or 3-0 suture material (e.g., nylon)
- White surgical tape
- Bandage material: sterile gauze pad, roll gauze, Esmarch-type bandage (e.g., Vetrap)

Anticipated Time

20-30 minutes, including preparation

Preparation: Important Checkpoints

- Obtain owner consent: discuss cost, risks (anesthesia, bleeding, aspiration pneumonia [p. 793]), care of the tube and feeding at home.
- Identify landmarks. It is useful to have an assistant hold off the external jugular vein to ensure the incision will be far from its location.
- Trim the feeding tube to the correct length, if necessary. Ideally, the tube should extend from the incision to the 7th rib, plus 6-8 cm of tube that remains outside the patient. The tip of the tube should be the portion trimmed, not the syringe end of the tube.

Possible Complications and Common Errors to Avoid

- Make the incision small at first to keep the seal tight around the tube; you can always enlarge it if necessary.
- Landmarks: avoid jugular vein or close proximity to the larynx. They can be avoided by advancing the tip of the curved forceps to the midpoint between the point of the shoulder and the caudal edge of the mandible and elevating the esophagus with the tip of the curved forceps when they are in the esophagus.
- Avoid clogging of tube by injecting a few milliliters of tap water immediately after every feeding or medication administration.
- If the tube becomes clogged, several milliliters of a carbonated, unsweetened beverage (e.g., seltzer or club soda) can be instilled into the tube for several minutes to soften and dislodge the obstruction.

Procedure

- Induce general anesthesia, and intubate the patient.
- Place the animal in right lateral recumbency, and apply a mouth gag.
- Shave and disinfect the skin on the left side of the neck from the angle of the jaw to the

point of the shoulder and from the vertebral column to the ventral midline.
- Put on sterile gloves.
- Insert the curved Carmalt forceps into the mouth, with the tips closed and pointing up (away from the table), through the upper esophageal sphincter, and into the cervical esophagus.
- Advance the curved forceps until the tip is halfway between the caudal edge of the mandible and the point of the shoulder.
- Press the curved tip of the forceps into the lateral wall of the esophagus so that it forms a visible tenting of the skin on the left lateral surface of the neck midway between the caudal edge of the mandible and the point of the shoulder. Make sure the tenting of the skin is well dorsal to the jugular vein. Use the fingers of your right hand (if you are right handed) to palpate the tip of the curved forceps. The confluence of the linguofacial and maxillary veins into the external jugular vein lie close to the caudal edge of the mandible. These vessels must be avoided when making the stab incision into the esophagus.
- Using your extended left index finger, apply firm upward pressure to elevate the tip of the curved forceps. This movement pushes aside the external jugular vein as it tents the skin. An assistant may hold off the external jugular vein to make its location more apparent.
- Using a scalpel blade, make a small 2-4 mm wide stab incision over the tip of the forceps. Continue deepening the incision until the blade strikes the tips, allowing them to penetrate to the outside and be visible.
- Using your left hand, open the tips of the forceps, and use them to grasp the tip of the feeding tube.
- Being careful not to lose the grip on the tip of the feeding tube, slowly withdraw the forceps back out of the mouth, pulling the tip of the feeding tube through the skin, into the esophagus, and out of the patient's mouth. Keep pulling the tube through the skin until 6-8 cm of the flared, proximal end of the feeding tube remain protruding from the skin.
- Turn the tip of the feeding tube back toward the stomach, and insert the tip of the tube back down the patient's esophagus. Curved or straight hemostats or your finger can help guide the tube down the esophagus.
- Plug the proximal (external) end of the tube using a Christmas tree adapter and cap.
- Secure the tube to the skin by placing a white-tape butterfly and suturing it to the skin or using a Chinese finger trap pattern.
- Place a sterile dressing over the tube's insertion into the skin, and bandage the neck loosely with roll gauze and Esmarch-type bandage (e.g., Vetrap). Its purpose is to keep the site clean and prevent the tube from becoming dislodged.

Postprocedure

- Lateral cervical and thoracic radiographs should confirm the placement of the tube. The tube should not be kinked, and the tip should lie between the caudal edge of the heart and the diaphragm.
- Feeding can begin immediately using a liquid diet that flows easily down the tube. Each feeding or administration of medication down the tube should be followed by a bolus of 5-10 mL of water, and immediate capping of the tube to prevent reflux of food into the tube where it might dry and cause an obstruction.
- Most esophagostomy tubes are left in place for several days or weeks. If longer-term use is needed, a percutaneous endoscopic gastrostomy (PEG) (p. 1109) tube should be considered.
- There is no minimum time that the tube must be left in place, and if it is accidentally dislodged or needs to be removed immediately after placement, there is no danger.
- The tube may be removed without sedation in most animals. Simply remove the bandage material and sutures, kink the tube, and slowly pull the tube out. This causes minimal to no discomfort.
- The stoma left behind after removal of the tube will heal by second intention within 24-48 hours. It almost never needs to be sutured closed.

Alternatives and Their Relative Merits

- Syringe force feeding: less invasive but often more stressful and may lead to food aversion
- Nasoesophageal tube (p. 1107): requires less sedation or anesthesia but more irritating to the patient and more easily dislodged and clogged
- PEG tube: easier to maintain long term but more expensive equipment (endoscope) needed to place it and potentially more dangerous complications (septic peritonitis)
- Larger-bore tubes of different material (e.g., silicone tubing) can be used instead of red rubber catheters to facilitate feeding of blenderized diets in place of liquid diets.

Pearls

- Esophagostomy tubes are ideal for short-term provision of enteral nutrition.
- Tubes can be used by owners at home.
- Esophagostomy tube placement is rapid, has minimal risk of complications, and does not require complex equipment.
- The most challenging part of the tube placement is sliding the tip of the tube down to the caudal portion of the esophagus after it has been pulled out of the mouth. The external portion of the tube will flip from pointing caudally to pointing cranially when the tip of the tube is successfully slid into its final position in the caudal esophagus.
- Technician tip: warm the liquid diet to body temperature, and deliver with pet alert and in sternal position over 15-30 minutes.
- Technician tip: to free up time for other treatments, the meal can be delivered by syringe pump or frequent small doses.

SUGGESTED READING

Fink L, et al: Esophagostomy feeding tube placement in the dog and cat. J Vet Dent 31:133-138, 2014.

AUTHOR: Peter M. Foley, DVM, MSc, DACVIM
EDITORS: Leah A. Cohn, DVM, PhD, DACVIM; Mark S. Thompson, DVM, DABVP

Feeding Tube Placement: Nasoesophageal and Nasogastric

Difficulty level: ♦

Overview and Goal

Enteral nutrition prevents deleterious effects of malnourishment and can improve recovery from disease, postsurgical healing, immune function, and decrease duration of hospitalization. Placement of a feeding tube facilitates administration of daily caloric requirements and oral medications.

Indications

- Short-term, inexpensive enteral feeding during hospitalization (<7 days)
- Administration of oral liquid medication and fluids
- Suctioning of gastric fluid, gastric decompression, and prevention of gastric distention (nasogastric tube only)

Contraindications

- Severe facial injuries involving the nares and nasal turbinates
- Severe pharyngeal, laryngeal, or esophageal physical or functional abnormalities (e.g.,

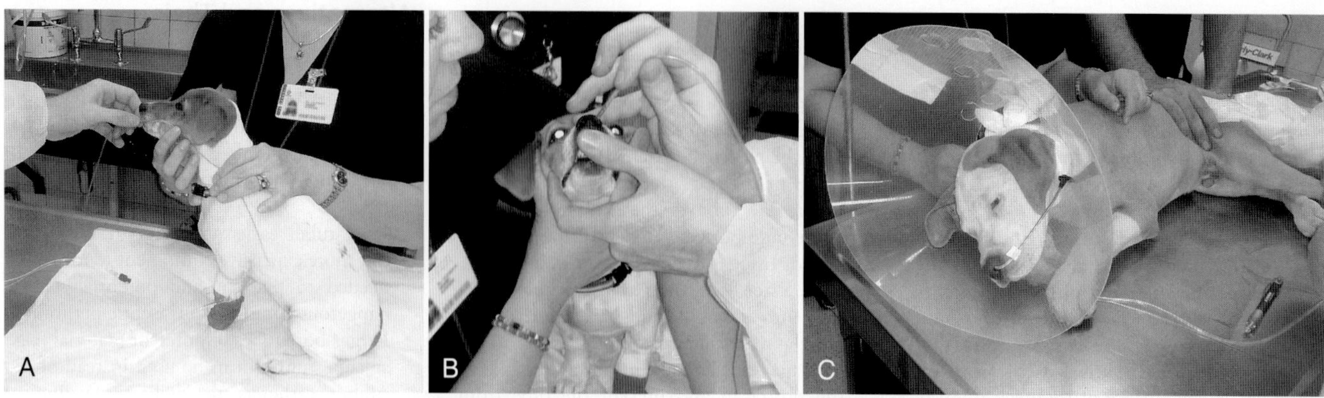

FEEDING TUBE PLACEMENT: NASOESOPHAGEAL AND NASOGASTRIC A, Measurement of feeding tube length. **B,** After instilling lidocaine into the nostrils, the clinician uses the left hand to push the nostril dorsally, and advances the tube in a medial, then caudal direction. **C,** Dog after placement of nasoesophageal tube and Elizabethan collar. The tube is glued in place and sutured (through the tape butterfly) to avoid dislodgement.

megaesophagus [p. 642], esophageal surgery or perforation [p. 309], absent gag reflex)
- Uncontrolled vomiting (pp. 1040 and 1042) or regurgitation (p. 873)
- Neurologic impairment
- Severe thrombocytopenia (p. 972) or coagulopathies
- Long-term feeding
- Aggressive patients

Equipment, Anesthesia

- Placed without sedation; for very fractious animals, sedation may be required
- Topical local anesthetic (2% [20 mg/mL] lidocaine)
- Syringe and needle
- Permanent marker or tape to mark tube length
- Water-based lubricating jelly
- Flexible feeding tube (polyvinyl, polyurethane, or silicone)
- Suture material or quick-drying glue
- Elizabethan collar
- Radiographic facilities

Anticipated Time

5-10 minutes

Preparation: Important Checkpoints

- Select largest tube that will pass through the nares. Guidelines: puppies and kittens, 3 Fr; cats and small dogs, 5 Fr; larger cats and dogs, 8 Fr or bigger; giant dog breeds, 12-18 Fr. If tube diameter is too small, feeding solutions cannot pass through.
- Premeasure and mark the length of the tube. For nasoesophageal intubation, measure from the nostril to the seventh intercostal space (ICS); for nasogastric intubation, measure up to the 10th ICS.

Possible Complications and Common Errors to Avoid

- Lidocaine intoxication in cats and possibly smaller dogs (approximate toxic dosage [topical]: 4 mg/kg)
- Tracheal, nasal or nasopharyngeal intubation
- Epistaxis
- Tube blockage with food particles, mucus, or esophageal or gastric mucosa
- Rhinitis or dacryocystitis within a few days of tube placement
- Esophageal reflux
- Vomiting or regurgitation with expulsion of the tube
- Aspiration pneumonia (p. 793)

Procedure

- Manual restraint of animal, with or without sedation
- Elevate the nose, and with the animal's mouth closed, instill 0.25-0.5 mL lidocaine in each nostril. Time the instillation to coincide with inhalation to minimize the amount of anesthetic blown or sneezed out of the nares. Both nostrils should be anesthetized at this time to avoid delay if it becomes necessary to use the other nostril. The head and restraint are released while allowing lidocaine to take effect (1-2 minutes).
- End of premeasured tube is coated with lubricating jelly.
- Tube is directed ventromedially into the nostril and passed by the ventral meatus. Tube is advanced up to the premeasured mark. Slight flexion of the neck enables the animal to swallow the distal end of the tube and facilitate proper placement.
- Check correct placement of tube in the esophagus or stomach.
  - Attempts to aspirate air from the tube with a syringe will create negative pressure if the tube lies in the esophagus. If air is easily withdrawn from the tube, it is likely in the airway.
  - Injecting air through the tube creates gurgling sounds on auscultation of the stomach if the tube was successfully placed into the stomach.
  - Capnography will detect a CO_2 curve with airway placement
  - The author prefers to obtain a lateral radiograph of the cervical and thoracic esophagus to visually confirm correct placement.
- The tube can be sutured or glued into place. The first point of attachment to the skin is as close to the nares as possible. Additional sutures or glue should be placed on the dorsum of the muzzle or on the cheek. Avoid the whiskers in cats to prevent irritation.
- Some animals do not tolerate the tubes, and an Elizabethan collar may be required.

Postprocedure

- Ensure that tube does not migrate out.
- Regularly flush tube with a volume of water equivalent to or greater than the volume of the tube itself to avoid blockage. This is indicated especially before and immediately after administering food or medications.
- Well-liquidized food should be warmed to body temperature and administered slowly or as a constant rate infusion to avoid rapid distention of the esophagus or stomach.
- Keep tube opening closed between feedings to avoid air buildup in the stomach.
- Use of a prokinetic (e.g., metoclopramide) could assist with functioning of the lower esophageal sphincter to minimize the risk of esophageal reflux.
- If obstruction of the tube with food or medication occurs, one or more instillations of a few milliliters of carbonated water (seltzer, mineral water, club soda) may dissolve the obstruction. If this is not successful, the tube must be replaced.
- Easily removed even within hours of placement

Alternatives and Their Relative Merits

Alternative feeding tubes can be placed with minor surgery and short general anesthesia (e.g., percutaneous endoscopic gastrostomy [PEG] tube [p. 1109], esophagostomy tube [p. 1106]) or in conjunction with major surgical procedures (e.g., gastrostomy and jejunostomy).

Pearls

- There is no difference in complication rates between the two tube locations (nasoesophageal or nasogastric).
- In dogs, the nasal planum can be pushed dorsally to ease initial insertion of the tube.
- Do not check tube placement by injecting water into the tube. Some animals are too weak to cough, and the majority of cats will not cough even when the tube is intratracheal.

SUGGESTED READING

Marks SL: Nasoesophageal, esophagostomy, gastrostomy, and jejunal tube placement techniques. In Côté E, et al, editors: Textbook of veterinary internal medicine, ed 8, St. Louis, 2017, Elsevier.

AUTHOR: Mirinda Nel van Schoor, BVSc, MMedVet
EDITORS: Leah A. Cohn, DVM, PhD, DACVIM; Mark S. Thompson, DVM, DABVP

Feeding Tube Placement: Percutaneous Endoscopic Gastrostomy (PEG)

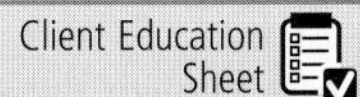

Client Education Sheet

Difficulty level: ♦♦

Overview and Goal

Placement of a percutaneous endoscopic gastrostomy (PEG) tube using minimally invasive techniques that provides a portal of entry into the stomach for administration of food and medications. These tubes typically can be left in place for weeks to many months.

Indications

To enable enteral nutrition and/or medication delivery in an animal that is unable or unwilling to eat on its own for an extended period (e.g., cat with hepatic lipidosis, animal with a jaw fracture) or if severe esophageal disease is present

Contraindications

- Intestinal obstruction
- Pancreatitis
- Abdominal effusion
- Patient cannot tolerate anesthesia

Equipment, Anesthesia

General anesthesia required

- Endoscope with a biopsy forceps
- Prepackaged PEG tube kit (Corflo, Cook Medical PEG-24 Pull or Vygon Vet, 16-20 Fr in diameter, according to animal size), which includes a tube with a distal pliable disk and a tapered proximal extremity prolonged by a wire with a loop at its end, a large-gauge needle, a thin cable with loop at the end, two flanges (one straight and one with a 90-degree angle allowing the tube to become parallel to the abdominal wall), and adapters to close the tube
- A sterile #11 scalpel blade
- Suture material for the skin (e.g., 2-0, 3-0 nylon)
- Suture scissors and needle holder

Anticipated Time

About 15-20 minutes of procedure and 30 minutes of anesthesia time

Preparation: Important Checkpoints

- Preparation of the animal: the left side of the abdomen is shaved and aseptically scrubbed.
- The animal is anesthetized and placed in right lateral recumbency.

Possible Complications and Common Errors to Avoid

- The pulling of the PEG tube through the gastric and abdominal wall can be facilitated by carefully opening the skin around the tube with a scalpel blade (opening should only be large enough to accommodate the tube).
- The disk of the PEG tube may be blocked at the level of the gastroesophageal sphincter. A firmer pull will allow the ampulla to pass this obstacle. NOTE: It is essential to brace this traction on the tube with counterpressure at the level of the body wall. If pulling the PEG tube into place with the right hand, the clinician's left thumb and forefinger are on the body wall, adjacent to the tube, and are exerting counterpressure to make sure the disk stops at the stomach wall and does not come out entirely.
- The PEG tube must be left in place for at least 2 weeks to allow fibrous tissue to surround the portion of the tube between the stomach and the abdominal wall, thereby sealing it off from the abdominal cavity. This is important for the safe removal of the PEG tube and minimizes the risk of peritonitis.
- Accidental dislodgment of the tube before 2 weeks requires emergent evaluation as peritonitis can result.
- Blockage of the PEG tube by dried food should be avoided by rinsing the tube after each use (i.e., follow food or medications with water). If blockage occurs, it can be addressed by repeatedly administering a few milliliters of carbonated water (seltzer, club soda, mineral water) into the tube until the obstruction dissolves.

Procedure

- The endoscope is introduced into the stomach, and the extremity of the endoscope should be pointing toward the left side of the antrum. The light at the endoscope tip should be visible through the skin.
- The stomach is then inflated with air until the skin becomes tense.

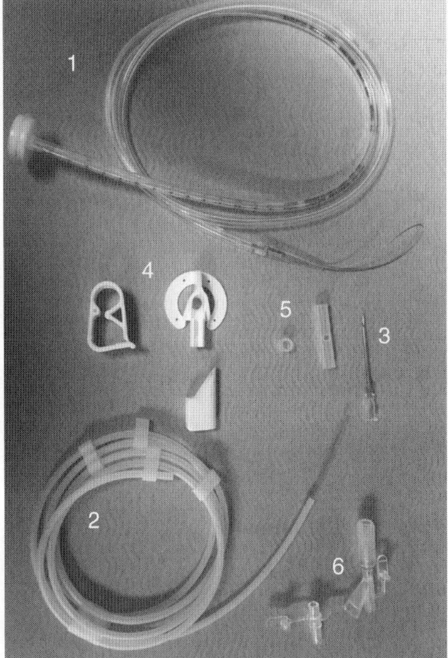

FEEDING TUBE PLACEMENT: PERCUTANEOUS ENDOSCOPIC GASTROSTOMY PEG kit (Corflo) includes a PEG tube with a tapered extremity prolonged with a wire with a loop at the end (1), a wire with a loop at the end (2), a needle (3), an L-shaped flange in two parts (4), a regular flange (5), and adapters to close the PEG tube (6). (Used with permission from Halyard Health.)

- The needle is introduced through the body wall into the gastric lumen, aiming for the light of the endoscope.
- After the needle tip is visible in the lumen of the stomach, the wire loop is introduced through the needle into the stomach.
- With the endoscope, the extremity of the loop of the wire inside the stomach is grabbed using the biopsy forceps of the endoscope; wire, biopsy forceps, and endoscope are pulled outside all together through the esophagus and the mouth. NOTE: Ensure that the proximal end of the wire is kept outside (e.g., clamp it with a mosquito hemostat) to avoid the whole length of the wire being pulled through.

- The loop at the tip of the PEG tube is then passed into the loop of the wire that is emerging from the animal's mouth.
- The PEG tube is then passed into its own loop and pulled to tighten the connection between the two loops.
- After this is done, the clinician can start to pull on the wire emerging on the abdominal side until the connected loops emerge from the abdominal wall.
- By continuing to pull on the wire, the tapered tip of the PEG tube soon appears through the skin. Here again, bracing with digital counterpressure at the abdominal wall is essential. To also allow the PEG tube to pass through the skin, the clinician often must widen the skin incision using a scalpel blade. Caution is warranted to avoid cutting the wire.
- The PEG tube must be pulled all the way until the disk lies against the gastric wall (this can be checked by endoscopy).
- After the PEG tube is fully pulled out with the disk and well in contact with the gastric wall, its extremity is cut and inserted through the two parts of the 90-degree flange. These two parts are then pushed all the way against the abdominal skin and assembled. The disk of the flange is then sutured to the skin. This flange reorients the PEG tube, which becomes parallel to the abdominal wall. Additional sutures can be used to keep the PEG tube in place against the flank.
- The adapter is then fitted to the extremity of the PEG tube.

Postprocedure

- An Elizabethan collar may be necessary to prevent removal of the tube by the animal.
- Water can be administered as soon as 18 hours after placement, and food 24 hours after placement of the tube.
- Removal of the PEG tube: no sooner than 2 weeks after the placement (as described) to avoid possible leakage of food from the stomach into the abdominal cavity.

Low-profile PEG tubes:

- For long-term use, the temporary PEG tube can be replaced by a low-profile PEG tube, also called gastrostomy button. To do that, wait at least 2 weeks (or preferably, 6 weeks) before removing the temporary PEG tube to allow the fibrous tunnel to become strong enough.
- After the temporary PEG tube is removed, the low-profile PEG tube is introduced directly through the fibrous tunnel. This tube is kept in place by inflating the distal balloon on the gastric side and by suturing the proximal side to the skin.

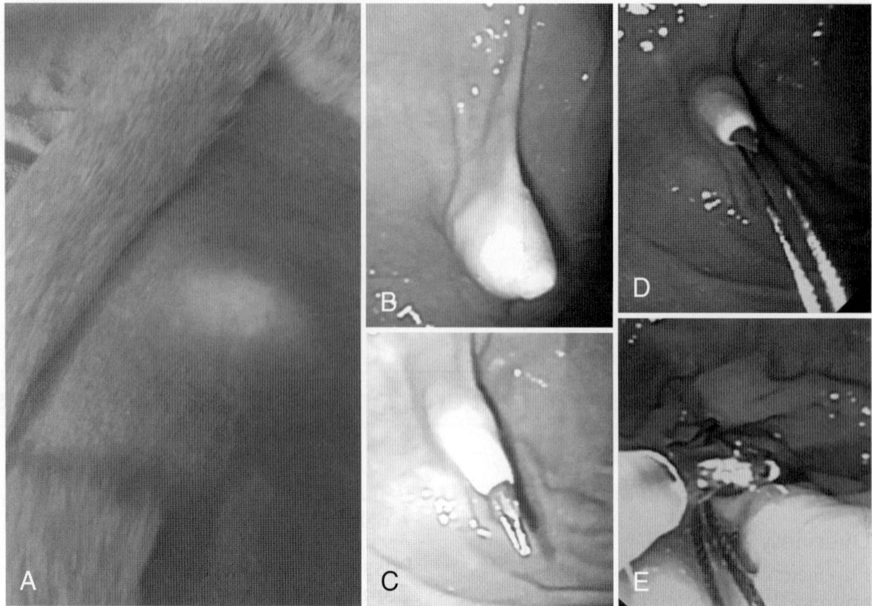

FEEDING TUBE PLACEMENT: PERCUTANEOUS ENDOSCOPIC GASTROSTOMY A, Anesthetized dog in right lateral recumbency, head to bottom. The light of the endoscope in the stomach is visible through the skin, indicating where the needle should be inserted and pointing toward. **B,** Endoscopic view of the tenting of the gastric wall created by the needle. **C,** The tip of the needle has entered the stomach. **D,** The loop of the wire is passed through the needle. **E,** This loop is grabbed using an endoscopic biopsy or grasping forceps.

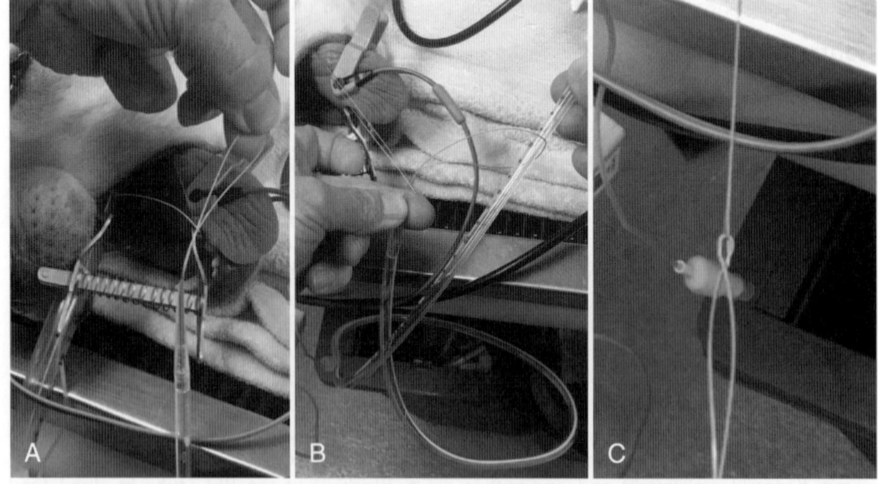

FEEDING TUBE PLACEMENT: PERCUTANEOUS ENDOSCOPIC GASTROSTOMY After the looped extremity of the wire is pulled from the mouth, the loop of the wire attached to the PEG is passed into it (**A**). The PEG is passed into its own loop (**B**), and the two wires are pulled to secure the connection (**C**).

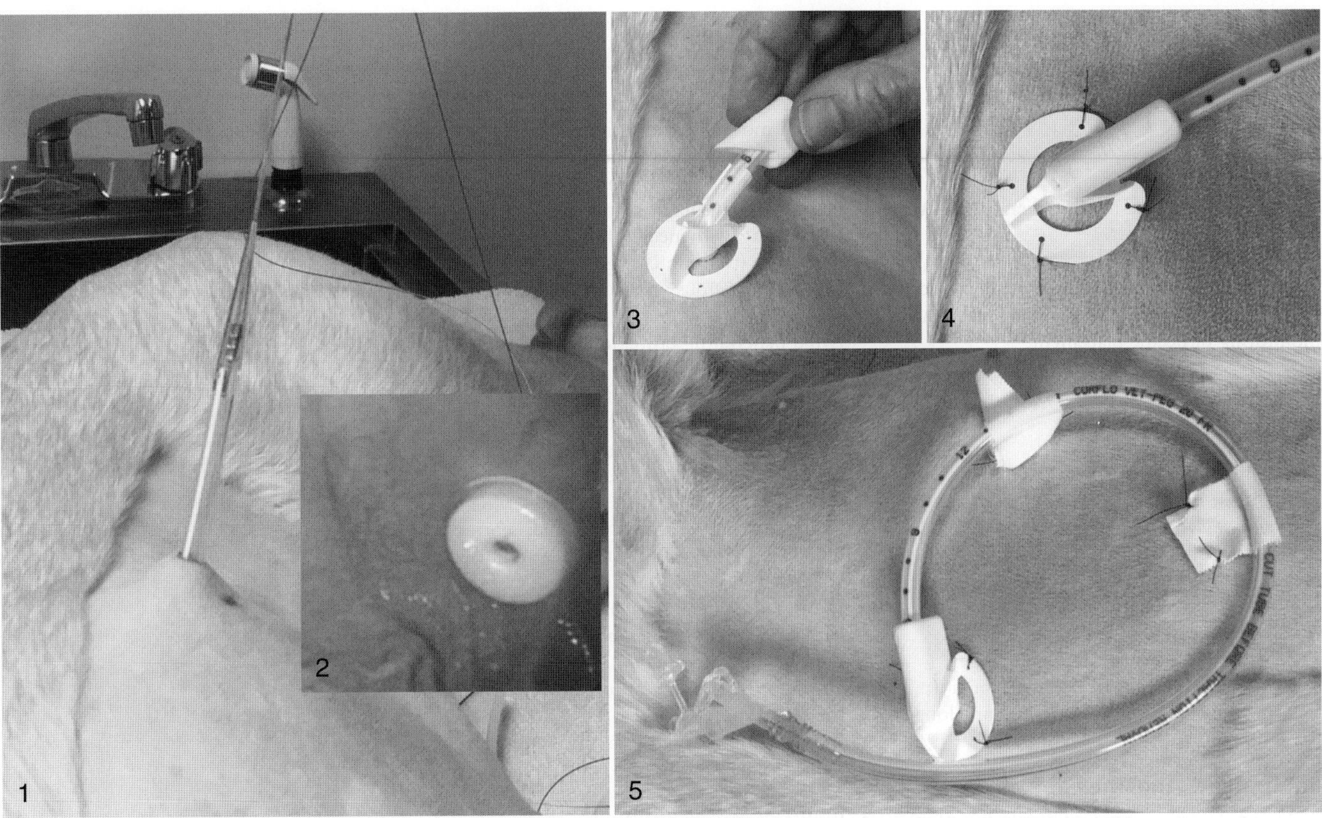

FEEDING TUBE PLACEMENT: PERCUTANEOUS ENDOSCOPIC GASTROSTOMY Anesthetized dog in right lateral recumbency, head to bottom *(panel 1)*. The percutaneous endoscopic gastrostomy (PEG) tube is being pulled until the disk is against the stomach wall *(panel 2)*. After cutting the extremity of the PEG tube, the two parts of the angled flange are fed over the tube until against the abdominal wall *(panel 3)*. After assembling the two parts, the disk of the flange is sutured to the skin *(panel 4)*. The PEG tube is then secured to the flank *(panel 5)*. The procedure is then complete.

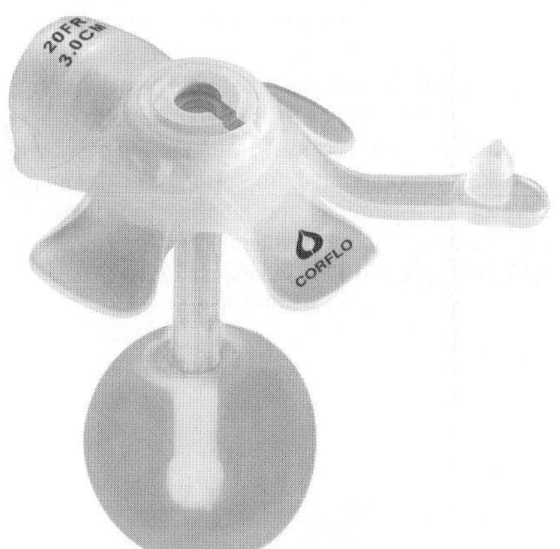

FEEDING TUBE PLACEMENT: PERCUTANEOUS ENDOSCOPIC GASTROSTOMY Low-profile PEG tube (Corflo gastrostomy button). One can see the balloon that can be deflated for insertion and reinflated after the button is in place. (Used with permission from Halyard Health.)

Alternatives and Their Relative Merits

- Pharyngostomy/esophageal tubes (p. 1106): do not require an endoscope for placement and are therefore less costly. They can be used or removed immediately and usually work for a few weeks. Their use requires normal esophageal function.
- Nasoesophageal tubes (p. 1107): provide a short-term solution (a few days). They are easy to place and easily removed by the animal. They are smaller in diameter, which can limit the rate of delivery of food.
- Jejunostomy tube: requires surgical or endoscopic placement. They are used for bypassing the stomach and providing enteric feedings in animals with pancreatitis, for example.
- Parenteral nutrition: not as complete as enteral nutrition; requires a central catheter

RELATED CLIENT EDUCATION SHEETS

Consent to Perform General Anesthesia

How to Use and Care for an Indwelling Feeding Tube

AUTHOR: Eric de Madron, DVM, DACVIM, DECVIM

EDITORS: Leah A. Cohn, DVM, PhD, DACVIM; Mark S. Thompson, DVM, DABVP

Fine-Needle Aspiration, Ultrasound-Guided

Difficulty level: ♦♦

Synonym

Needle aspiration, fine-needle aspiration (FNA)

Overview and Goal

Procedure to obtain small tissue or fluid samples using ultrasound guidance and real-time monitoring of needle placement

Indications

- Cytologic evaluation of
  - Mass or nodule
  - Diffuse parenchymal organ abnormalities
  - Diffuse infiltrative disease (e.g., mast cell disease, lymphoma) screening
- Drainage of cysts, abscesses, or fluid

Contraindications

- Cavitated mass: risk of hemorrhage
- Bleeding disorder: risk of hemorrhage
- Suspected transitional cell carcinoma (p. 991): possibility of seeding tumor along needle tract

Equipment, Anesthesia

- 22- or 25-gauge standard sterile injection needles, 1½ inches (4 cm) in length:
- 6-mL syringes
- Glass microscope slides
- Hair clippers
- Surgical scrub, rubbing alcohol
- Sector or linear-array ultrasound transducer
  - Sector transducers allow sampling of deep structures.
  - Linear-array transducers provide better resolution of superficial structures.
- Often done with manual restraint alone. Sedation or even anesthesia sometimes required (e.g., anxious animal, small structure in close proximity to large vessel)

Anticipated Time

5-10 minutes

Preparation: Important Checkpoints

- If at increased risk for bleeding, perform platelet count ± coagulation profile.
- Determine if sedation is required; place intravenous (IV) catheter if needed.
- Ensure proper animal restraint.

Possible Complications and Common Errors to Avoid

- To decrease hemodilution, avoid the suction method in sampling vascular organs (e.g., spleen).
- Identify and avoid large vessels.
- Hemorrhage is uncommon if 22- or 25-gauge needle is used and the movement of the needle through the entire procedure is one-dimensional (in and out only, with no side-to-side motion).
- Do not move the needle side to side within an organ because this can cause tissue trauma.
- If redirecting needle orientation, withdraw needle tip to subcutis and then reinsert. Redirecting with needle fully advanced is ineffective (position changes little or not at all) and dangerous (shearing of tissue with needle tip).
- Avoid penetrating bowel lumen due to risk of peritonitis.
- Sample the left aspect of the liver when possible to avoid the gallbladder and hilar vessels on the right. If the liver is small or cranially located, consider an intercostal approach.
- For renal aspirates, sample the caudal cortex of the kidney to avoid the medulla and hilar vessels.
- In cases of bilateral renal abnormalities, the left kidney should be sampled because of its more caudal location.
- Do not pass through an organ other than the one being aspirated.
- Avoid administering drugs that cause splenomegaly or panting (e.g., phenothiazines, some opiates).
- If aspirating an adrenal gland mass, be aware of possible blood pressure alterations and severe hemorrhage with pheochromocytoma (p. 785).
- Ensure contact between the lesion and chest wall when sampling a thoracic lesion to minimize risk of pneumothorax.

Procedure

- Restrain the animal in dorsal or lateral recumbency. A padded U- or V-shaped trough can be used to make the animal more comfortable.
- Clip hair at planned needle insertion site.
- Thoroughly evaluate area of interest, characterize lesion by ultrasound, identify vessels to be avoided, and determine shortest distance and safest direction of needle placement.
- Ensure that the area of interest is within the focal zone of the transducer.
- Prepare skin with surgical scrub.
- Obtain ultrasound image of area to be sampled.
- Ensure probe marker location on screen corresponds with desired needle course.

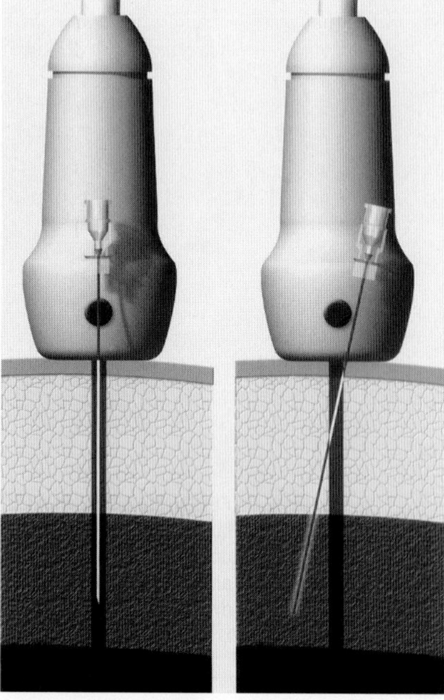

FINE-NEEDLE ASPIRATION, ULTRASOUND-GUIDED Importance of correct alignment between needle and ultrasound probe. *Left,* Correct alignment is present, and full extent of needle is seen. *Right,* Needle is not aligned with ultrasound beam, and only proximal portion of needle is seen. Trauma to deeper tissues is possible because location of the needle tip is unknown. (Reprinted from Fife WD: Abdominal ultrasound: aspirations and biopsies. In Ettinger SJ, et al, editors: Textbook of veterinary internal medicine, ed 7, St. Louis, 2010, Saunders, pp 376-379.)

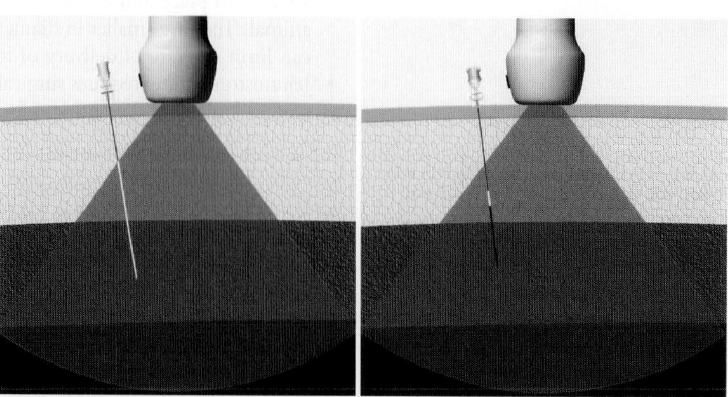

FINE-NEEDLE ASPIRATION, ULTRASOUND-GUIDED Views as seen on monitor of ultrasound machine, perpendicular to other figure. *Left,* Correct alignment produces complete visualization of needle. *Right,* Probe/needle malalignment underrepresents depth of needle.

- Freehand technique: hold transducer in nondominant hand, and insert needle with dominant hand.
- Without syringe suction (nonaspiration technique)
  - Attach a 6-mL syringe preloaded with 4-5 mL of room air to 22- or 25-gauge needle.
  - Introduce needle parallel to plane of ultrasound beam, visualizing needle as it is advanced.
  - Slowly fan transducer side to side to identify entire needle length to tip.
  - Rapidly advance and retract needle 3-4 times (poke tissue) to fill needle shaft with cells. Do not move needle in any direction except in and out.
  - Withdraw needle from animal and expel contents onto microscopic slide(s) immediately. Lightly smear using standard technique.
- With syringe suction (true aspiration technique)
  - Attach empty 6-mL syringe to needle.
  - Introduce needle parallel to plane of ultrasound beam, as described.
  - Apply suction to syringe three to four times while gently advancing and retracting needle.
  - Release suction before withdrawing needle from animal.
  - Disconnect syringe from needle.
  - Retract plunger to fill syringe with air, and reconnect syringe to needle.
  - Expel contents onto microscopic slide(s) immediately, and lightly smear using standard technique.
- Multiple samples of each organ or lesion should be obtained, using a new needle for each procedure.

Postprocedure

Scan to evaluate for hemorrhage (uncommon complication).

Alternatives and Their Relative Merits

Tissue-core and surgical biopsy are more invasive but produce larger tissue samples.

Pearls

- The nonsuction technique is often attempted first, and if a noncellular sample is obtained, the suction technique is then performed.
- The suction technique is useful for aspirates of less vascular structures (e.g., lymph node) but often results in hemodilution when aspirating vascular organs such as the spleen.
- Cells may dry and clot in the needle very quickly. When the needle is withdrawn, the expulsion of needle contents onto a microscope slide and the slide smearing technique should be completed within seconds.
- Obtaining an FNA of an organ may be challenging if large-volume effusion is present. In those cases, surgical or laparoscopic biopsy may be preferred.

SUGGESTED READING

Mattoon JS, et al: Ultrasound-guided aspiration and biopsy procedures. In Mattoon JS, et al, editors: Small animal diagnostic ultrasound, ed 3, St. Louis, 2015, Elsevier, pp 50-77.

AUTHOR: Wendy D. Fife, DVM, MS, DACVR
EDITORS: Leah A. Cohn, DVM, PhD, DACVIM; Mark S. Thompson, DVM, DABVP

Fine-Needle Sampling for Cytopathologic Analysis: Lung

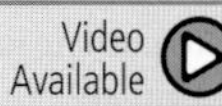

Difficulty level: ♦♦

Synonyms

Fine-needle aspiration (FNA) of the lung, lung aspirate, fine-needle lung sampling

Overview and Goal

Minimally invasive, safe, rapid technique to provide cells from lung lesions for cytopathologic diagnosis

Indications

Best suited for sample collection from nodules or consolidated lesions toward the periphery of the lung but can be used in animals with heavy, diffuse pulmonary infiltrates

Contraindications

- Coagulopathy
- Bullae
- Marked pulmonary hypertension (p. 838)
- Lesion too deep in the chest or adjacent to organs such as the heart or great vessels

Equipment, Anesthesia

Does not require anesthesia, but animal must be restrained and should not be in marked respiratory distress at time of sampling. Sedation or anesthesia can facilitate safe sampling when movement is an issue or if imaging studies (ultrasound [US], computed tomography [CT]) are used to guide collection of aspirates.

- Clippers and disinfectant for skin
- Sterile 22-gauge needle × 3; 1- to 1.5-inch length is typical to reach the lesion depth
- Sterile syringe, 6 to 12 mL, ideally with Luer-Lok
- Microscope glass slides (6-10) and a tray to hold them
- Pencil or marker (for slide identification)
- Appropriate Romanowsky-type stain (e.g., Diff-Quik) if immediate staining is desired
- Microscope, optimally with 4×, 10×, 20×, and a higher objective (50× or 100× oil objective)
- Optional: unstained slides may be submitted to an outside laboratory for review by a clinical pathologist
- Optional: fluid may be submitted for microbial culture or cytocentrifugation concentration for cytopathologic evaluation

Anticipated Time

Actual sample collection and processing time < 15 minutes; longer if anesthesia or direct imaging guidance is used

Preparation: Important Checkpoints

- Select appropriate needle size and length depending on predetermined (by imaging studies, such as thoracic radiographs) location of the lung mass.
- Have necessary collection (including US machine, if planning to use US guidance) and glass slide preparation equipment on hand.
- Have emergency supplies available for the rare complication of significant pneumothorax (p. 1164).

Possible Complications and Common Errors to Avoid

- Although generally safe, discuss possible complications with pet owner and obtain informed consent. Patients with diffuse pulmonary disease may be at increased risk for clinically decompensating after the procedure. Hemorrhage (hemothorax [p. 436]), hemoptysis, external hemorrhage, pneumothorax (p. 797), seeding of malignant cells, and rupture of pulmonary abscess (p. 5) are the most serious potential complications. Pet owners should also be warned that the technique may not provide a diagnosis.
- The needle should be inserted just in front of a rib to avoid intercostal vessels.
- Avoid placing needle into or through the diaphragm. It is not uncommon for clinical pathologists to receive slides with liver tissue from FNA of the lung.
- If blood is seen in the needle/syringe during aspiration, immediately withdraw the needle from the thorax.
- Excessive vacuum pressure during needle aspiration (cells may lyse)

- Excessive compression when spreading cells on slide (cells may lyse)
- Inadequate compression when spreading cells on slide (clumped cells cannot be evaluated)
- Sampling nondiagnostic areas, such as areas adjacent to the mass or areas of necrosis or fluid associated with a mass that contains solid tissue (may miss diagnostic cells)
- Having open container of formalin nearby (can alter staining of the cells, altering morphology and rendering smears useless)
- Contamination of the sample with materials such as ultrasound gel (or starch granules from powdered gloves, which are no longer available in the United States and limited use in Canada)
- Copious blood contamination can make cytologic interpretation difficult to impossible. A bloody sample may prompt repeat sampling, but the patient's status should be considered. If iatrogenic hemorrhage is sufficient to obscure microscopic interpretation, but the patient is stable with no evidence of inordinate hemorrhage/hemothorax, an additional collection can be attempted.
- Using heat fixing to help cells stick to the glass slide. More often than not, this can significantly alter cell morphology. Air-drying is recommended (see procedure, below).
- Failure to label the glass slides with appropriate patient identifier and location of the site sampled
- If sending to a reference laboratory, failure to place the glass slides in appropriate protective packaging

Procedure

- Locate nodule or consolidation on thoracic radiographs and assess
  - Side of thorax for lesion (right or left)
  - Rib space of lesion
  - Height of lesion (e.g., just above the costochondral junction)
  - Distance from skin to lesion (to choose needle length as well as guide placement)
  - Note surrounding structures (may abort procedure if vital structures very close to lesion)
- Sedation or anesthetic induction (if desired)
- For conscious animals, appropriate skilled restraint
- Oxygen supplementation provided for animals with diffuse lung disease or dyspnea
- Procedure may be performed with animal in sternal or lateral recumbency, depending on lesion location. Animals with respiratory disease are often more comfortable in a sternal position, which is generally preferred by the authors.
- Clip and disinfect the area of the skin overlying the lesion.
- Attach an empty syringe to the needle; break the seal on the syringe, but expel any air before proceeding.
- If using US or CT guidance, identify the lesion.

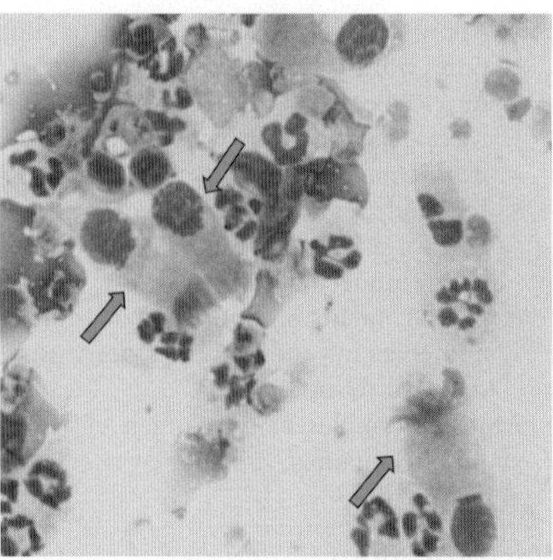

FINE-NEEDLE SAMPLING FOR CYTOPATHOLOGIC ANALYSIS: LUNG Lung FNA in a cat. Ciliated respiratory epithelial cells *(arrows)* can be present among inflammatory cells in lesions as shown. They can also be present in FNA of normal lung. Free cilia can exfoliate and resemble extracellular thin bacteria; caution is to be used when interpreting these aspirates.

- If using thoracic radiographs, use rib space and other landmarks to identify the area just overlying the lesion.
- If diffuse disease is present, aspirate on either side of the chest between the 7th and 9th ribs approximately one-third of the height of the chest down from the spine.
- Insert the needle through the skin only, just caudal to the area overlying the lesion.
- Advance the needle forward to just in front of the rib overlying the lesion.
- Gently plunge the needle through the intercostal muscles into the area of the lesion (estimated or as confirmed by imaging).
- Optional step: without redirecting to the side, gently move the needle in and out by a few millimeters.
- Apply repeated suction to the syringe several times in rapid succession (see *Video*).
- Pull the needle straight out of the animal.
- Remove the needle from the syringe.
- Fill the syringe with air and reattach to the needle.
- Expel the contents of the needle, and prepare the slides as for FNA of SQ mass.
- The procedure may be repeated if necessary. Because diagnostic yield is reduced with diffuse disease (as compared to a solid lesion), immediate repetition on the other side of the chest is useful.

Postprocedure

- Periodically monitor respiratory rate and effort and mucous membrane color for a few hours after the procedure.
- There is no need for routine repeat imaging studies, but these may be warranted by worsened respiratory distress.

Alternatives and Their Relative Merits

- Bronchoalveolar lavage (pp. 1073 and 1074) is more useful for diffuse airway or alveolar disease and less so for solid masses. For focal disease, it should be obtained with bronchoscopic guidance.
- Surgical biopsy (thoracotomy, thoracoscopy): much more invasive, expensive, with greater morbidity, but optimal diagnostic yield and potential for therapeutic benefit
- Relative merits of cytopathologic versus histopathologic evaluation

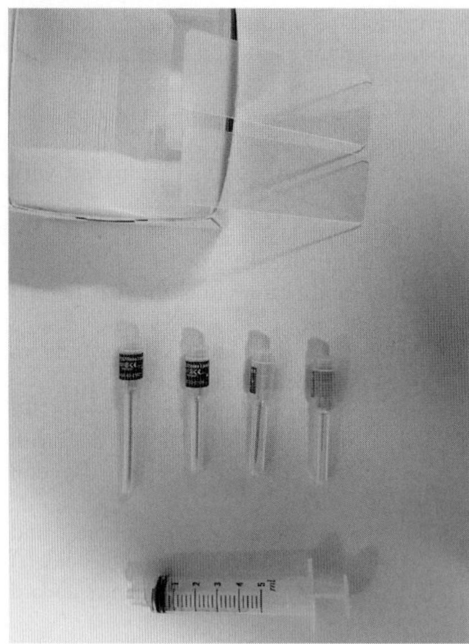

FINE-NEEDLE SAMPLING FOR CYTOPATHOLOGIC ANALYSIS: LUNG Lung FNA equipment. *Bottom,* 6-mL syringe with Luer-Lok. *Middle,* Four needles, top to bottom: 22 gauge, 1.5 inch; 22 gauge, 1 inch; 20 gauge, 1 inch; 25 gauge, 1 inch. *Top,* Microscope glass slides.

Pearls

- Diagnostic yield for solid lesion is up to 85% but is less for diffuse lung disease.
- Fine-needle aspirates of normal lung typically contain some degree of hemorrhage ± rare macrophages ± few respiratory epithelial cells.
- In addition to cells of interest, other materials (e.g., mucus, ruptured cellular debris) may be seen.
- Mixed inflammatory cells and hemosiderophages may coexist with neoplastic cells in tremendously variable proportions.
- Larger needles produce more cells for diagnosis but are also associated with greater morbidity.

SUGGESTED READING

DeBerry JD, et al: Correlation between fine-needle aspiration cytopathology and histopathology of the lung in dogs and cats. J Am Anim Hosp Assoc 38:327-336. 2002.

AUTHORS: Ryan M. Dickinson, DVM, DACVP; Leah A. Cohn, DVM, PhD, DACVIM
EDITORS: Leah A. Cohn, DVM, PhD, DACVIM; Mark S. Thompson, DVM, DABVP

Foreign Body Removal, Esophageal (Endoscopic)

Client Education Sheet

Difficulty level: ◆◆

Overview and Goal

- In dogs, objects causing esophageal obstruction are mostly found in one of three locations: at the thoracic inlet, at the level of the heart base, or caudal to the heart (most common) (p. 351).
- Most foreign bodies obstructing the esophagus can be removed without surgery. An attempt should be made to remove foreign bodies by esophageal endoscopy to avoid surgery and its complications (e.g., difficult access, limited healing ability, associated morbidity).
- If an object cannot be removed by the oral route, an attempt can be made to advance it into the stomach, provided complications such as esophageal perforation (from a sharp-edged foreign body, esophageal wall devitalization, or overly aggressive forward pressure) are avoided. Objects passed into the stomach may be removed by gastrotomy or left to be digested (in the case of digestible objects).

Indications

Foreign objects lodged in the esophagus (e.g., bones, fishhooks, needles, toys, hairballs)

Contraindications

Esophageal perforation (p. 309) is an absolute contraindication; thoracotomy is indicated in these cases.

Equipment, Anesthesia

- General anesthesia
- Cuffed endotracheal tube
- Mouth gag/speculum
- Rigid tube (overtube) with smooth edges for esophageal dilation (optional); typical external diameters are 2 cm (cat, small dog), 3 cm (medium-size dog), and 4 cm (large dog).
- Flexible fiberoptic endoscope (or rigid proctoscope)
- Endoscopic basket, grasping forceps (recommended), polypectomy snare or endoscopic biopsy forceps (second choice)
- Water-soluble lubricating jelly
- Polyethylene catheter or feeding tube (optional)
- Balloon catheter (optional)
- Suctioning apparatus

Anticipated Time

20-90 minutes, depending on size of object and ease with which it can be retrieved

Preparation: Important Checkpoints

- Confirm location of foreign body, presence of aspiration pneumonia (p. 793) and evidence of esophageal perforation by performing survey and contrast radiography using low-osmolality, nonionic contrast medium. Radiographs should be performed immediately before induction of general anesthesia to confirm that the foreign body has not spontaneously passed into the stomach.
- Endoscopic evaluation of location of foreign body and state of esophageal mucosa (p. 1098)
- Ensure adequate patient hydration and perfusion.
- Antibiotic therapy if indicated by aspiration pneumonia or esophageal perforation
- Advise the owner of possible complications.
    - Emergency thoracotomy may be required if perforation occurs or removal by the oral route is impossible; possible gastrotomy if the foreign body has to be pushed through into the stomach.

Possible Complications and Common Errors to Avoid

- Esophageal mucosal trauma (hemorrhage, erosion, ulceration) (p. 312)
- Esophageal perforation, pyothorax (p. 857), pleuritis, mediastinitis
- Aspiration pneumonia
- Tension pneumothorax (p. 797) (associated with esophageal insufflation)
- Bradycardia due to vagal stimulation
- Sepsis (p. 907) (due to aspiration or esophageal rupture)
- Esophageal stricture (p. 310) (clinically manifests > 2 weeks postprocedure)
- Bronchoesophageal fistulation (rare)

Procedure

- Classified as an emergency procedure
- General anesthesia
- Place endotracheal tube and inflate cuff to prevent aspiration of esophageal contents.
- Animal in sternal or left lateral recumbency
- Examine mouth and sublingual region for the presence of objects such as thread, needles, or fishhooks.
- Suction esophagus to remove any liquid contents and contrast medium.

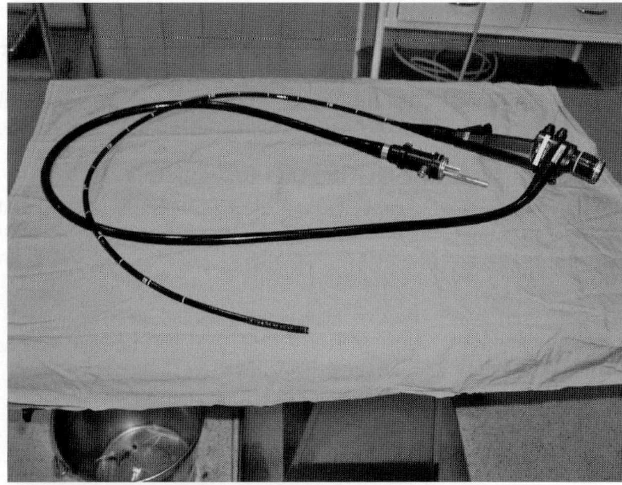

FOREIGN BODY REMOVAL, ESOPHAGEAL (ENDOSCOPIC) A 1-m flexible fiberoptic endoscope. This endoscope is adequate for esophageal procedures in dogs and cats of all body sizes.

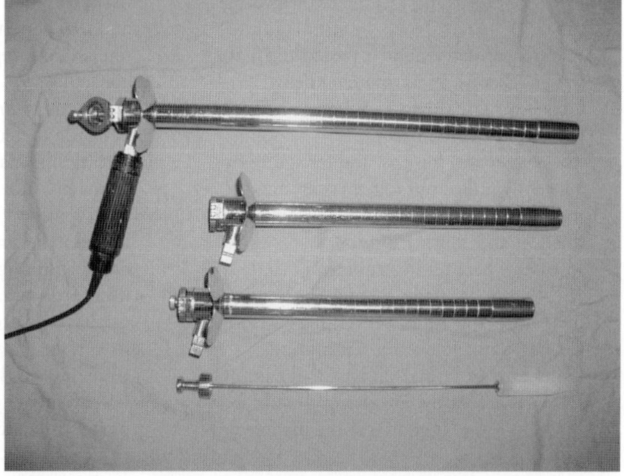

FOREIGN BODY REMOVAL, ESOPHAGEAL (ENDOSCOPIC) Large *(top)* and two small *(below)* rigid proctoscopes used for retrieving esophageal foreign bodies and small proctoscopic stylet *(bottom)*. Stylet is placed into proctoscope for advancing into esophagus. After the desired degree of insertion is achieved, stylet is withdrawn, and glass port (seen in the open position in the large proctoscope, *top*) may be closed for most effective visualization.

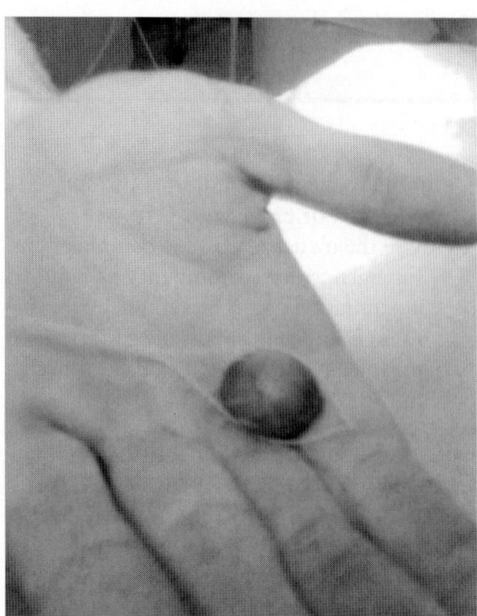

FOREIGN BODY REMOVAL, ESOPHAGEAL (ENDOSCOPIC) Polypectomy snare used to retrieve a palm seed.

- Insert mouth gag/speculum.
- Flexible fiberoptic endoscope technique:
  - For medium-size or larger dogs, a rigid lubricated stomach tube can be placed to assist in dilating the esophagus. The endoscope is passed through this tube.
  - Lubricate the endoscope.
  - Pass the endoscope to the level of the foreign body, visualizing the foreign body and assessing the integrity of the adjacent esophagus.
  - Insufflation of air will allow dilation of the esophagus around the foreign body. This may be useful in dislodging foreign bodies such as bones that are embedded in the esophageal wall.
  - Lubrication can be placed at the site of the foreign body, using a catheter or feeding tube.
  - A retrieval instrument is passed through the endoscope operating channel.
  - Grasp or snare the foreign body, and pull it close to the endoscope.
  - The endoscope, forceps, and foreign body are gently pulled out together through the mouth while ensuring adequate esophageal dilation and lubrication.
  - In cases where an overtube was inserted, an attempt is made to pull the foreign body into the tube, preventing it from causing damage during removal.
  - If the foreign body is lodged and cannot be retrieved easily, an attempt could be made to rotate it gently. If the maneuver results in dislodging the object, another attempt can be made to retrieve it.
  - With smooth, round foreign bodies, a cuffed catheter (e.g., Foley catheter) can be passed past the object, the cuff inflated on the aboral side, and the catheter used for pulling the object toward the mouth.
  - Fishhooks embedded in the mucosa can be removed if the tip can be grasped and the hook gently pulled through the mucosa. Fishhooks that penetrate the wall must be removed surgically. The surgeon cuts the protruding tip, and the endoscopist removes the endoesophageal section, thereby avoiding the need to cut into the esophagus.
  - If retrieval is not possible, an attempt could be made to push the foreign body into the stomach.
  - The esophageal mucosa is carefully examined endoscopically after removal of the foreign body.
- Rigid proctoscope technique
  - Lubricate proctoscope.
  - Pass the proctoscope into the esophagus to the level of the foreign body, visualizing the foreign body and assessing the integrity of the surrounding esophagus.
  - Lubricant can be placed at the site of the foreign body, using a polyethylene catheter.
  - Using grasping forceps, the foreign body is brought close to the end of the proctoscope.
  - If the foreign body is small enough, it can be pulled into the lumen of the proctoscope.
  - The foreign body, proctoscope, and grasping forceps are pulled out together by gentle manipulation and traction and with adequate lubrication.
  - Continuous visualization and gentleness of traction are essential to ensure that complications such as esophageal laceration or perforation are noticed immediately and that retrieval can be stopped and the foreign body repositioned or the procedure aborted.
  - If retrieval is not possible, an attempt could be made to gently push the foreign body into the stomach using a well-lubricated stomach tube, provided no evidence of esophageal devitalization (e.g., deep mucosal lacerations and discolorations, other signs of possibly imminent perforation) are seen and the foreign body does not have pointed or sharp protrusions on its surface.
  - Careful examination of the esophageal wall after foreign body removal; any suspicion of possible esophageal perforation warrants close radiographic and clinical monitoring.

Postprocedure

- If esophageal mucosa is damaged (suspected on endoscopic observation of darkened/discolored esophageal mucosa, deep mucosal lacerations, or after prolonged, difficult procedure; confirmation radiographically)
  - Lacerations that do not extend through the full thickness of the esophageal wall can be left to heal by epithelialization.
  - Full-thickness tears and necrosis require immediate surgical intervention.
- Withhold food and water for 24 hours.
- Maintain hydration and electrolyte balance.
- Pain management, antibiotics (as described), prokinetic agents, glucocorticoids, and/or gastric antacids may be indicated (p. 380).
- Gastrostomy feeding tube is placed distal to the site of the foreign body if prolonged withholding of food is indicated (p. 1109).
- After recovery, introduce liquids, followed by gruel if no adverse reactions are noted after liquids have been introduced.

Alternatives and Their Relative Merits

- Advancement of foreign body into stomach followed by gastrotomy
  - Sharp objects and objects such as toys should not be pushed into the stomach (risk of esophageal perforation). Follow-up radiography is advised to ensure that foreign bodies were digested or passed through the digestive tract.
- For cases in which esophageal perforation and its complications have already developed (p. 309), surgical removal of the foreign body by thoracotomy is the only alternative.
- Fluoroscopy-guided removal with balloon extraction or forceps manipulation
  - Disadvantages: not freely available in practice; lack of post-procedure visualization of esophageal mucosa

Pearls

- Preferred method makes use of flexible endoscopes.
- The use of biopsy forceps is discouraged because damage to the instrument is possible.

SUGGESTED READING

Tams TR, et al: Endoscopic removal of gastrointestinal foreign bodies. In Tams TR, et al, editors: Small animal endoscopy, ed 3, St. Louis, 2011, Mosby, 228-248.

AUTHOR: Mirinda Nel van Schoor, BVSc, MMedVet
EDITORS: Leah A. Cohn, DVM, PhD, DACVIM; Mark S. Thompson, DVM, DABVP

Gastric Intubation, Gavage, Lavage

Difficulty level: ♦♦

Synonyms

Gastric decompression, orogastric feeding, orogastric intubation

Overview and Goals

Passage of a hollow tube into the mouth and through the oropharynx into the stomach to facilitate decompression of gas, removal of stomach contents (lavage), or administration of large volumes of liquid, food, or medication (gavage)

Indications

- Gastric intubation
  - Preoperative stabilization of gastric dilation/volvulus (GDV); allows evacuation of gas and fluid, resulting in an improved hemodynamic state
  - Relief of discomfort associated with gaseous dilation (without torsion) of the stomach
- Gavage
  - Administration of large volumes of liquid medication, including
    - Activated charcoal after toxin ingestion (p. 1087)
    - Barium for gastrointestinal (GI) contrast radiography (p. 1172)
    - Hyperosmotic laxative agent before colonoscopy
  - Administration of formula to neonatal animals that are not nursing on their own
- Lavage
  - Removal of stomach contents with suspected intoxications
  - NOTE: Gastric lavage may not be indicated in all cases of toxin ingestion. Substance ingested, consistency, time since ingestion, and animal status influence whether gastric lavage is appropriate.
- Preoperative stabilization of GDV (p. 377). Removal of stomach contents may help decrease the speed of gas reaccumulation while the animal is being prepared for surgery, slowing or preventing cardiovascular deterioration.

Contraindications

- Esophageal disease may lead to tube-induced trauma or perforation. Conditions of concern include esophageal stricture (p. 310), neoplasia, ulceration, megaesophagus (p. 642), and recent esophageal surgery.
- Gastric disease may lead to tube-induced trauma or perforation. Conditions of concern include neoplasia (p. 379), ulceration (p. 380), and recent gastric surgery.
- Any swallowing disorder (e.g., megaesophagus, esophageal motility disorder), pharyngeal disorder, or laryngeal disorder (e.g., paralysis [p. 574], previous tie-back surgery) that could predispose a non-endotracheally intubated animal to aspiration
- If even one of these conditions is present, the risk of the procedure versus its benefits (which will vary from case to case) must be considered before deciding whether to perform the procedure.

Equipment, Anesthesia

Gastric intubation:

- Two assistants (minimum)
- Flexible plastic tubing of various lengths and diameters. The distal end must be smooth and atraumatic; smoothing may be achieved by brief heating of the end of the tube over a flame, cooling, and trimming edges with a scalpel blade. One to three side holes may facilitate evacuation of stomach contents by minimizing obstruction of a single distal hole with gastric mucosa or ingesta.
- A roll of clinic-type white cloth tape
- Water-soluble lubrication jelly
- Mouth gag/speculum

If gastric lavage, all of the above plus

- Funnel or stomach pump
- Container (e.g., bucket) to collect stomach contents and lavage fluid
- Lavage fluid: usually warm (body temperature) water

Anticipated Time

Depends on cooperation of animal; additional time may be needed for sedation or general anesthesia

- Gastric intubation: 2-5 minutes
- Gavage: 3-10 minutes
- Lavage: 10-60 minutes

Preparation: Important Checkpoints

- Ensure that adequate manual or chemical restraint for the procedure is planned. Personal preference and animal stability may dictate the degree of sedation or anesthesia chosen. NOTE: Some clinicians prefer to ensure a patent and protected airway to minimize the potential for aspiration pneumonia through the use of general anesthesia and a cuffed endotracheal (ET) tube when gastric lavage is performed.
- Maximize cardiovascular stability before the procedure.

Possible Complications and Common Errors to Avoid

- Inadvertent passage of the orogastric tube into the trachea can result in mild to severe complications.
  - Tracheal irritation leading to transient coughing or mucosal bleeding is possible.
  - Tracheal or bronchial placement of the gastric tube can result in airway obstruction until the tube is repositioned.
  - Tracheal or bronchial tearing can result in pneumomediastinum, pneumothorax, and death.
  - Tracheal or bronchial administration of gavage or lavage fluids can result in severe aspiration pneumonia and death.
  - The procedure (as explained below) describes avoidance of these complications.
- Oral, pharyngeal, laryngeal, esophageal, or gastric trauma can result if excessive force is used for passing the gastric tube. Full-thickness tearing is possible, especially with a pre-existing underlying disease.
- Inability to pass the tube into the stomach may reflect the choice of a tube with a diameter that is too large, esophageal obstruction (foreign body, stricture, neoplasia), torsion of the stomach, or excessive lower esophageal sphincter (LES) tone. Discontinuation of metoclopramide before elective gastric intubation is recommended to minimize LES tone.
- Inadequate sedation of an uncooperative animal will lead to longer procedure times and increased risk of injury to the animal and veterinary staff.
- Inability to effectively remove gastric contents through lavage may be related to excessive size or adhesive nature of gastric contents, gastric compartmentalization, or other factors.
- Regurgitation during lavage, gastric overfilling, or esophageal administration of large volumes of lavage fluid can result in aspiration if a cuffed ET tube is not in place.
- Excessive tube advancement can cause occlusion of the distal end of the tube against stomach mucosa. Palpation of the tube pressing against the stomach wall may indicate a need for partial retraction.

Procedure

- Manual restraint, sedation, or general anesthesia as indicated
- Position animal in sternal recumbency. If animal is uncomfortable, alternate positions (e.g., sitting, standing, lateral) may be better tolerated.
  - Placement of the animal on an elevated surface will allow gravity-assisted efflux of stomach contents and lavage fluid after the tube is in place.
- Choose appropriate tube diameter for esophageal size and procedure planned. For example, a tube with an outer diameter of 1.5 inches (3.5 cm) is appropriate for most medium-sized dogs (45 lb [20 kg]). A larger tube size may be necessary to facilitate effective lavage compared to gas decompression only.
- Measure the length of tube necessary to pass from the nose to the xiphoid. Mark this distance on the tube with a piece of tape or nontoxic marker.

Procedures and Techniques

- Place a mouth gag (speculum) to prevent the animal from chewing on the tube.
  - A roll of 2-inch (5-cm)–wide, clinic-type, white cloth tape works well in many animals. The tube will pass through the hole in the tape roll. Place tape roll on top of the tongue and behind all four canine teeth.
  - Have an assistant hold the mouth closed around the mouth gag.
  - Avoid using a gag that can damage the teeth.
- Generously lubricate the distal portion of the stomach tube.
- Pass the tube into the mouth through the mouth gag.
- Advance the tube through the oropharynx and into the esophagus. Steps to promote and confirm esophageal and subsequent gastric intubation include
  - Choice of a larger gastric tube size than appropriate ET tube size will lessen the possibility of tracheal intubation.
  - A neutral or very slightly ventroflexed position of the head (i.e., avoiding extension of the neck) will reduce the opportunity for the tube to pass into the trachea.
  - In the awake animal, allow the swallowing reflex to facilitate tube passage through the pharynx.
  - If substantial coughing occurs, reassess placement because the orogastric tube may be in the trachea.
  - Palpate the tube in the esophagus (separate from the tracheal rings).
  - Direct visualization of tube passage through the esophagus along the left side of the neck (in lean, short-haired patients).
  - Small amounts of air infused into the stomach tube result in a gurgling sound when the stomach is ausculted.
  - Mild suction applied to the tube should reveal negative pressure, stomach contents, or odorous gastric gas with proper gastric intubation, whereas airflow and absence of negative pressure suggest that the tube is in the airways.
- Pass the tube up to the marked point that indicates where the tube should have entered the stomach. Relief of gas pressure can be assessed through auditory, tactile, and olfactory observations.
  - Certain conditions such as GDV may inhibit tube passage into the stomach. Choice of a smaller tube, gentle rotational pressure on the tube, repositioning of the animal, or percutaneous needle gastric decompression may facilitate passage.

DECOMPRESSION

- Place the external portion of the stomach tube lower than the animal's head and body to allow gravity-assisted evacuation of stomach contents.
- Gentle massage of the stomach through the body wall may help to increase efflux.

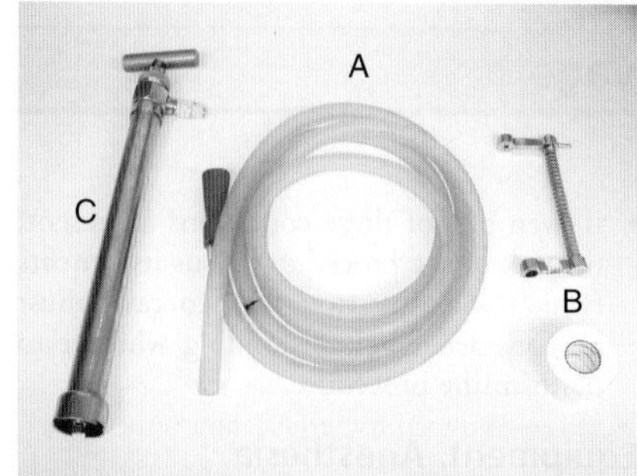

GASTRIC INTUBATION, GAVAGE, LAVAGE Materials and equipment used for gastric intubation and lavage. **A,** Orogastric tube. **B,** Metal speculum or roll of tape to be used as a mouth gag. **C,** Stomach pump for lavage.

GAVAGE

- Using a syringe, funnel, or stomach pump, instill the desired medication through the tube into the stomach.
- With administration of viscous materials, dilution with water may facilitate passage through the tube.
- Coughing, dyspnea, or cyanosis at any point suggests the tube may be in the respiratory tree. The procedure is terminated immediately, with kinking of the proximal tube to avoid leakage of tube contents during withdrawal, tube removal, and animal care (e.g., physical examination, thoracic radiography) as warranted.

LAVAGE

- Using a funnel or stomach pump, instill approximately 5-10 mL/kg of lukewarm (body temperature) water into the tube.
- Acute onset of coughing, dyspnea, or cyanosis warrants immediate termination, as previously described.
- Hold the tube higher than the animal's head to prevent efflux of the lavage fluid until desired.
- Gently massage the stomach to facilitate mixing of the stomach contents with the lavage fluid.
- Lower the stomach tube below the level of the head to allow the lavage fluid to efflux. Gentle manipulation of the tube forward or backward 1-3 cm may improve efflux.
- If the tube obstructs with stomach contents, flushing or manual breakdown may relieve the obstruction. If this is unsuccessful, the tube should be removed and the entire process repeated.
- Repeat lavage administration and efflux until the efflux is clear and the stomach contents have been removed.

REMOVAL

- Kink the tube during removal to prevent laryngeal/pharyngeal contamination with liquid remaining in the tube lumen.
- Remove the mouth gag.

Postprocedure

- Monitor recovery from sedation/anesthesia.
- Supportive care as indicated for the condition.

Alternatives and Their Relative Merits

- Nasoesophageal/nasogastric intubation
  - May be less stressful to the animal than orogastric intubation
  - Tube can be left in place for repeated aspirations/instillations.
  - Small tube diameter prevents administration of viscous substances and effective lavage. Withdrawal of large volumes of gastric contents is often not possible.
- Percutaneous needle decompression/ gastrocentesis
  - May be easier to perform in a fractious animal
  - Allows gastric gas decompression when degree of torsion or another esophageal obstruction prevents tube passage
  - Potential for splenic puncture/laceration, gastric vessel or wall laceration, or other abdominal trauma
  - Ineffective for removing ingesta or large volumes of gastric contents
- Manual oral administration of medications/ formula (pediatric animals)
  - Decreased chance of complications associated with orogastric intubation and gavage
  - Administration of large volumes to an uncooperative animal is labor intensive.
  - Risk of aspiration with force feeding
- Induced emesis to clear gastric contents (p. 1188)
  - Often more effective at removing stomach contents than lavage
  - Risk of aspiration, especially with decreased mentation or laryngeal/ pharyngeal dysfunction
  - Not indicated with caustic ingestions
  - Not effective in all animals

AUTHOR: Lillian I. Good, DVM, DACVECC
EDITORS: Leah A. Cohn, DVM, PhD, DACVIM; Mark S. Thompson, DVM, DABVP

Glucose Curve

Client Education Sheet 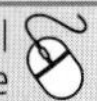 Bonus Material Online

Difficulty level: ◆

Synonyms

Blood glucose curve (BGC), serial blood glucose monitoring

Overview and Goal

A BGC is used in conjunction with clinical signs and changes in body weight to help monitor patients with diabetes mellitus (DM) and to guide changes to an insulin therapy protocol.

Indications

- Initial regulation of DM (p. 251)
- Poorly regulated DM
- Suspected hypoglycemia

Contraindications

- Bleeding disorder
- Concurrent illness (insulin requirement likely to decrease when the illness resolves)
- Fractious/stressed patient

Equipment, Anesthesia

- No sedation or anesthesia required
- Glucose monitor: as of this writing, AlphaTRAK 2 (Zoetis) is the only glucometer calibrated for dogs and cats and tested in peer-reviewed publications.
- Glucose test strips
- Adequate restraint
- Needle or lancet for obtaining capillary blood *or* needle and syringe to obtain venous blood
- Insulin (follow pet owners' normal regimen)

Anticipated Time

- If on twice-daily insulin, a 10-12 hour BGC typical
- A 24-hour BGC may be necessary for pet receiving once-daily insulin, if overnight hypoglycemia is suspected, or if the glucose nadir has not occurred within 12 hours.

Preparation: Important Checkpoints

- Obtain a history, and perform a physical examination; specifically note changes in urination, water intake, appetite, and weight.
- Determine if the pet will be fed/given insulin at home or in clinic. If at home, confirm that the patient has eaten and received morning insulin per the normal routine.
- Ensure that the glucometer is calibrated for the correct species (enter the relevant code on the vial into the glucometer before reading samples).
- Run a control solution on your glucometer once per month to ensure accurate readings.

Possible Complications and Common Errors to Avoid

- Unless hypoglycemia suspected, wait 5-7 days after each change in insulin dosage before performing a BGC.
- Stress-induced hyperglycemia (especially in cats) can lead to blood glucose (BG) concentrations that are higher than the patient's normal daily BG range. If a patient is easily stressed in a veterinary hospital, at-home monitoring and/or fructosamine measurement (p. 1345) should be considered.
  - Many cat owners can be taught to perform a BGC at home, with results provided to the veterinarian for interpretation.
- Ensure that a glucometer calibrated for canine/feline patients is used because glucometers designed for humans vary significantly in accuracy when used for dogs and cats.
- If insulin is administered in the hospital as part of the BGC, ensure the correct insulin syringe type is used (U-40 vs. U-100) to avoid overdosing/underdosing of insulin.

Procedure

- If the patient is unlikely to eat in the hospital, feeding and insulin administration at home is acceptable, following the normal schedule and presenting for the BGC immediately afterward.
  - This results in missing the pre-insulin BG measurement but is preferable to doing a BGC when the patient will not eat.
- If the animal is to be fed and given insulin in the clinic, obtain a pre-feeding and pre-insulin BG concentration, and record the value.
  - If BG < 150 mg/dL, do not give insulin. Recheck BG throughout the day to identify hypoglycemia.
  - Reduce the dose of insulin, and give the new insulin dose at the next 12-hour interval during which the BG > 200-250 mg/dL.
  - Consider remission in cats in which the BG does not increase within 12 hours.
- Feed the dog/cat its normal diet (same quantity) and give its normal insulin dose in the same order as usually done at home.
- If using a canine/feline glucometer, ensure that the code entered into the glucometer matches that of the correct species.
  - The calibration code for dogs and cats is often different and is typically listed on the test strip vial.
  - Obtain blood samples every 2 hours, and record the BG concentration.
  - Common sites for BG sampling include the inner pinna (cats and dogs), inside of the upper lip and the elbow pad (dogs), and the pisiform metacarpal pad (cats).
  - When the BG is less than 150 mg/dL, check the BG hourly.
  - If the BG measurement is unexpected, recheck using a different sample to confirm that it is an accurate reading.

Postprocedure

Interpretation of BG curve: BGC results MUST be interpreted in conjunction with the patient's clinical signs and weight changes. Insulin dose should not be increased based on results of the BGC alone.

- Ideal curve
  - All values between 100 and 250 mg/dL
  - No precipitous decline in BG after insulin administration
  - Duration of insulin action (time from administration through nadir and until BG > 250 mg/dL) ≈12 hours in patients receiving insulin q 12h.
- Short duration of insulin action
  - If duration of action is < 8-10 hours and the patient has clinical signs of unregulated DM, consider changing to a longer-acting insulin.
- Persistent hyperglycemia
  - If the BG level is persistently > 250 mg/dL (never below 100-150 mg/dL) *and* clinical signs are present, the insulin dose should be increased (usually ½ unit per dose in cats and 10%-25% per dose in dogs).
- Hypoglycemia
  - If the BG is < 70-80 mg/dL at any time (value confirmed), the insulin dose should be decreased.
  - Hypoglycemia often occurs between midnight and 3 AM. If a patient's clinical signs get worse despite increasing insulin doses, the patient may be experiencing insulin-induced hyperglycemia (formerly thought to be the Somogyi effect), in which the BGs are high during the day but drop below acceptable concentrations at night. If this is suspected, a 24-hour BGC or continuous BG monitoring is recommended.

Timing of the next BGC

- One to 2 weeks after each insulin dose adjustment until regulated
- If signs of hypoglycemia (lethargy, seizures, ataxia, coma) or hyperglycemia (polyuria and polydipsia [PU/PD], weight loss, polyphagia) are recognized
- If there are no clinical signs of DM and the patient is on an established insulin dose, consider fructosamine measurement or repeat BGC q 3-6 months.

Alternatives and Their Relative Merits

Clinical signs:

- BGCs and other monitoring tools must be interpreted in conjunction with clinical signs.

- Quantify daily water intake to help determine if patient regulated or change in regulation occurs.
- When initial insulin begun at low dose (0.25 U/kg for dogs and 1 U/CAT, q 12h) and clinical signs of hyperglycemia are unabated, can increase dose without prior BGC.
- Do not exceed dose of 0.5 U/kg in dogs and 2 U/CAT before performing a BGC.

At-home monitoring:

- At-home monitoring is frequently recommended so as to avoid the stress of a hospital visit.
- Home BG monitoring also is indicated to allow the owner to check a BG whenever hypoglycemia is suspected. Owners should be cautioned not to increase the insulin dose without consulting with their veterinarian.

Monitoring fructosamine concentrations:

- Fructosamine (FrAm) concentrations indicate average glycemic control over the previous 2 weeks. Because the FrAm concentrations in well-controlled diabetics vary from one patient to the next, it is most useful to monitor the trend in individual patients.
- FrAm concentrations are not reliable indicators of hypoglycemia.

Continuous blood glucose monitoring (CBGM):

- CBGM devices have been used in human medicine for around 20 years and are being used with increased frequency in veterinary patients, typically within the referral hospital setting.
- A sensor is placed in the subcutaneous tissue by means of a 22-guage needle, and BG is measured every few minutes. The sensor is connected to a transmitter that sends data to the monitor that displays real-time data.
- The CBGM devices can be left in place for days. This allows for more detailed data on insulin regulation and is particularly helpful in identifying brief hypoglycemic episodes that would be missed with a BGC.

Pearls

- Do not adjust insulin therapy purely based on increased BG concentrations but only in concert with clinical signs (e.g., PU/PD, polyphagia, weight loss or gain).
- Decrease the insulin dose in any patient with confirmed hypoglycemia.
- Minimize patient stress by performing blood sampling in a quiet, relaxing environment.

SUGGESTED READING

Reusch CE: Feline diabetes mellitus. In Feldman EC, et al, editors: Canine and feline endocrinology, ed 4, St. Louis, 2015, Saunders.

AUTHORS: Harry Cridge, MVB; Patty Lathan, VMD, MS
EDITORS: Leah A. Cohn, DVM, PhD, DACVIM; Mark S. Thompson, DVM, DABVP

Holter/Cardiac Event Monitoring

Difficulty level: ♦♦

Synonyms

Ambulatory electrocardiography, cardiac telemetry

Overview and Goal

Allows assessment of cardiac rhythm during an extended period. The monitor may record the cardiac rhythm continuously for 24-48 hours (Holter monitor) or only when triggered to record over a period of days to weeks (event monitor, loop recorder). With these devices, the pet is able to be at home, and the owner is able to observe pet behavior.

Indications

- Syncope (p. 953)
- Episodic clinical signs of uncertain type but that might represent syncope
- Screening of breeding or at-risk animals (boxers, Dobermans) for latent arrhythmia (arrhythmia not causing overt clinical signs)
- Monitoring of antiarrhythmic drug effects (Holter monitor only)

Contraindications

- Animals likely to damage a portable monitor
- Animal that will be bathed or will be swimming
- Animal too small to carry monitor (monitoring may still take place, but animal stays mainly in pet carrier or cage for recording period)

Equipment, Anesthesia

- Clippers for hair
- Isopropyl alcohol
- Gauze squares or cotton balls
- Cardiac electrode adhesive patches (cutaneous)
- Ultrasound gel
- Holter vest or one can be made with bandage material: Esmarch-type bandage material (e.g., Vetrap), 1- or 2-inch, white medical tape +/− cast padding, roll gauze, stretch adhesive cotton bandage (e.g., Elastoplast)
- Holter or event monitor, including wires to connect to animal, new batteries, and a blank digital card (Holter only)
- Interpretation system and printer or access to such a system

NOTE: Monitors are expensive systems not routinely owned by general practices. They are available for rental from many sources, including www.vetheart.com, www.idexx.com, and pet-cardiology.com. Some veterinary college cardiology services have mail-out Holter programs (subject to change). In North America, examples include

- Cornell University: www.vet.cornell.edu; 607-253-3060
- North Carolina State University: cardiologycarenetwork.com; 919-513-6975

Veterinary sources are preferred because knowledge of common veterinary diseases, normal veterinary findings (sinus arrhythmia, sinus tachycardia, sinus pauses during daytime rest), and common veterinary artifacts (purring, panting, shaking) are important parts of interpretation.

The monitor itself is typically sent by courier to the hospital for placement on the animal. Instructions for placement, and patient daily diaries are usually sent with the monitor. When the monitoring period is over, the monitor is mailed back or transmitted by transtelephonic signal (event monitor), and findings and interpretations are reported back. Some mail-out programs (mostly veterinary colleges) also provide consultation on the case as part of the service, along with the written Holter/event monitor report.

Anticipated Time

- Installation: 10 minutes (event monitor) or 20 minutes (Holter)
- Monitoring period: 24 or 48 hours (Holter); 7-30 days (event monitor, longer if battery is replaced; weeks to many months for surgically implanted event monitors/loop recorders)

Preparation: Important Checkpoints

If the reason for using cardiac monitoring is the occurrence of sporadic clinical signs, a complete medical evaluation is usually indicated first:

- CBC, serum biochemistry panel, urinalysis: to investigate for electrolyte/metabolic disorders (e.g., hypoglycemia, hypocalcemia [p. 515]) as alternative cause of signs
- Serum preprandial and postprandial bile acids (if consistent with case): hepatic encephalopathy (p. 440)
- Electrocardiogram (ECG; standard, in-hospital): all cases; the diagnosis may be apparent without the need for Holter or cardiac event monitoring
- Thoracic radiographs, echocardiogram: all cases; assessment of cardiac structure,

presence or absence of signs of congestive heart failure

Monitor use:

- The monitor itself is checked for proper function before preparing to install it on the animal. These instructions are usually sent with the monitor.
- Discussion of care of the monitor with the owner: the monitor must stay dry, clean, intact, and undamaged.
- It is customary to have the owner leave a deposit in the sum of the replacement cost of the monitor before leaving the hospital with the machine.

Possible Complications and Common Errors to Avoid

- Wet monitor: no swimming or bathing during the recording period. In the rain, a plastic bag should be placed over the monitor by the owner.
- Damaged/chewed monitor or wires: if the owner observes the animal damaging the monitor, an immediate recheck is warranted. The equipment can be examined, and subsequently, the monitor may simply be more heavily wrapped to prevent damage, or the monitoring period may be terminated and the monitor removed.
- Unstuck electrode patches or poor electrode patch contact with skin: prevented by cleaning and preparing the skin with isopropyl alcohol before patch placement or with use of tissue glue in extreme cases.
- Monitoring period is inexplicably shorter than expected: prevented by using new batteries every time. For audiotape Holter monitors, it is important to ensure that the audiotape is not put into the monitor backward.
- Poor triggering of event button (Holter) or record button (event monitor): prevented by carefully showing the owners how to trigger the event and record buttons on the monitor at the time of installation
- Letting batteries run out, causing the captured events to be deleted (event monitor): clients need to return 1 day before expected end of battery life to replace battery.

Procedure

Holter monitor (see *Video*):

- The animal's apex beat (heartbeat on the thorax) is palpated bilaterally. These will be the sites of electrode patch placement.
- The hair is clipped vertically over these areas, starting close to the sternum and working upward to ensure a generous clip; there must be room for the electrode patches and a few centimeters of space separating them.
- The hairless skin is wiped clean with isopropyl alcohol–soaked gauze or cotton and allowed to dry completely. Technician tip: the patient should be standing throughout application to ensure proper positioning of the leads and for taping purposes.
- The patches are attached to the animal's skin: three patches on the left (starting just left of the sternum) and two patches on the right, leaving a one-half inch to an inch between each electrode. For taping ease, make sure electrode snaps are all facing in the same direction. For very active patients, a tiny amount of tissue glue (<1 full drop) can be placed on opposite ends of the adhesive band of each electrode patch.
- Secure electrodes with 1-inch or 2-inch white tape. Wrap the tape all the way around the chest, covering the electrodes on both sides but leaving snaps exposed.
- The leads are attached to the patches according to the color scheme usually shown in the inside of the Holter recorder or within the instructions. Pressing the wire attachments directly onto the patches can be painful to the animal and is not recommended. Rather, after the patch is attached to the skin, the patch and underlying skin are elevated with the finger, and the electrode is pressed into the snap between thumb and forefinger, not between the thumb and the dog. If using a vest, put Holter monitor in vest pocket and pull leads through before attaching to patient.
- After the leads are connected, the wires are gathered on top of the spine, with the cable exiting to the right side (most Holter vests have the recorder pocket on the right side) and taped with 2-inch tape to the tape around the chest. The only wire left exposed is the cable that attaches to the recording system. If patient has long fur, cast padding can be applied under the tape.
- The monitor is attached to the animal as follows:
    - If a Holter vest is not available, the monitor is held in a dorsal midline location, and 2-inch tape is wrapped around the chest, incorporating the wires and monitor such that they emerge at the dorsal midline.
    - Cast padding or gauze is wrapped over the tape, around the thorax, as well as cranial to the shoulders in a figure-eight pattern, creating a vest of bandage material. The monitor is included in this layer.
    - Esmarch-type (e.g., Vetrap) bandage material is then wrapped over the gauze in a similar fashion.
    - Occasionally, elastic cotton adhesive (Elastikon-type) bandage material is used along the cranial and caudal borders of the Vetrap to secure to the animal.
    - Alternatively, a purpose-made Holter vest for dogs can be used.
    - The monitor's event button should still be visible and accessible to the owner, but connections onto the thorax, loops of wire, and the rest of the monitor itself should be protected.
- If a clock setting can be adjusted on the monitor, it is set to the current time. If not, the times at which the battery was installed and the recording began are noted as time zero in the medical record.
- Instruct the owner to keep a diary of the dog's activities, including the time of the observed activity. This includes normal activities and events thought to be of clinical relevance. The owner also may press the event button on the monitor if an episode of apparent significance (e.g., collapse)

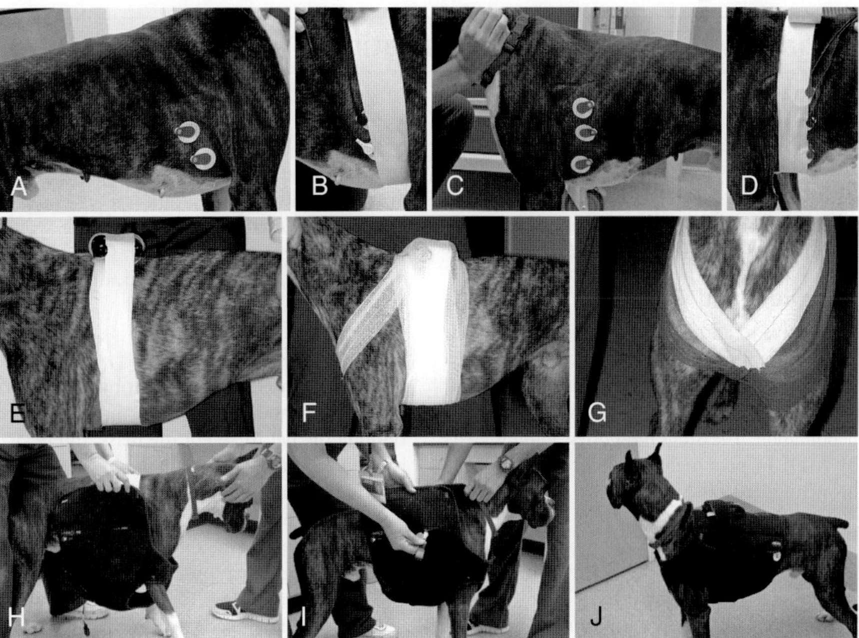

HOLTER/CARDIAC EVENT MONITORING A-J: *Top row,* Electrode patch placement for Holter monitor. Electrode connecting tips on the ends of Holter monitor wires should be arranged as follows: on dog's right *(top to bottom)*, black, white, and on the dog's left *(top to bottom),* red, green, brown. *Middle row,* Illustration of gauze, taping, and Vetrap for Holter monitor placement if Holter vest not available. *Bottom row,* Illustration of Holter monitor placement with a Holter vest.

occurs; it will be flagged on the Holter recording.

Event monitor:

- Animal preparation and patch preparation are the same as for Holter monitors (previously described).
- There are only two wires/electrodes and therefore only two electrode patches (white electrode typically attached to electrode patch on right hemithorax).
- The monitor is wrapped onto the animal as described above. It is essential to leave the record button visible and accessible.
- When the animal has an episode, the owner must press the record button. Doing so captures the ECG preceding and after the time the button was pressed. Typically, the monitors are set to store the preceding 45-second period of ECG and the subsequent 15 seconds, for a total of 1 minute of ECG spanning the clinical episode.
- Event monitors typically have a total memory of 5 minutes (i.e., five 1-minute episodes), although newer models can store 18 minutes or more.
- Newer models can be programmed to automatically store events if the owner is not present to witness the event. For example, the monitor can be programmed to record any heart rate lower than 40 or higher than 200 beats/min.
- Typically, batteries must be changed every 5-7 days.

Postprocedure

After the recording period (24-48 hours for Holter; 6 days to 8 weeks for Event monitors), the bandage material, monitor, wires, and electrode patches are removed without the use of scissors. The entire system is unwrapped to avoid cutting or damage to the leads and wires. Removal of the skin patches can be facilitated with isopropyl alcohol. The cassette or digital card (or in some cases, the entire monitor) is returned to the supplier or sent away for analysis. Some event monitor systems can transmit the stored information transtelephonically to the receiving station. If this is not done very soon after a recorded event, however, the batteries continue to be drained and the information eventually will be lost. Be sure to collect the Holter diary from the owner as well so that the recorded information can be interpreted in relation to the patient's activity level.

Alternatives and Their Relative Merits

- In-hospital ECG: less motion artifact but shorter duration and under artificial conditions
- Holter monitor instead of event monitor: screening for occurrence of latent arrhythmia; antiarrhythmic drug monitoring
- Event monitor instead of Holter monitor: long-term (days) monitoring; smaller animals; transtelephonic transmission of recorded information
- Implantable event monitor (Reveal Plus, Medtronic): allows an extended period of monitoring (up to 10 months). Devices are very small (size of a USB jump drive), and implantation is achieved with a subcutaneous pocket and local anesthesia in many cases. Devices are donated to a veterinary cardiology group (CanPacers) and are inexpensive. Access to a Medtronic programmer is necessary, however, to retrieve the stored information.
- Smartphone-based monitor for direct ECG recording (www.alivecorvet.com): portable, on-demand ECG recording, good-quality single-lead tracing, online storage of data; no reachback effect, rhythm may have returned to normal by the time owner applies the recorder
- Wireless, adhesive, waterproof, 14-day continuous recorder patch (Zio Patch): investigational

SUGGESTED READING

Petrie JP: Practical application of Holter monitoring in dogs and cats. Clin Tech Small Anim Pract 20:173-181, 2005.

AUTHORS: Amara H. Estrada, DVM, DACVIM; Ashley E. Jones, DVM, DACVIM
EDITORS: Leah A. Cohn, DVM, PhD, DACVIM; Mark S. Thompson, DVM, DABVP

Inhalant Medication Administration

Bonus Material Online 

Difficulty level: ◆

Synonyms

Metered-dose inhaler (MDI), aerosol medication, hydrofluoroalkane (HFA) inhaler

Overview and Goal

The goal is to administer drugs directly to the airways to minimize systemic effects. Although most such medications are administered by MDI, other drugs can be administered through nebulization. The drugs most often administered by MDI in pets include glucocorticoids and bronchodilators.

Indications

Delivery of aerosolized medication directly to the upper and lower airways:

- Rhinitis (allergic and immune mediated) (p. 890)
- Chronic bronchitis (p. 136)
- Collapsing trachea (p. 194)
- Feline asthma (p. 84)
- Other types of bronchopulmonary disease

Contraindications

- Known hypersensitivity to the medication to be administered
- Facial trauma/disfigurement that would prevent placement of mask
- Frightened, agitated, stressed, or untrained animal

Equipment, Anesthesia

MDI can be used in hospital or by pet owners at home. Although sedation is not necessary, training the pet to accept the mask and device is often required.

- MDI containing drug of choice
  - Albuterol available as 90 mcg/actuation
  - Fluticasone available as 44, 110, and 220 mcg/actuation
- Spacer/chamber device: although spacer devices made for humans can be adapted, veterinary-specific products are preferred.
  - Commercially available for dogs and cats (https://www.trudellmed.com/animal-health)
- Face mask: specific to size and shape of animal's muzzle; veterinary spacer devices typically sold with a face mask

Anticipated Time

Well-trained animal: 30-60 seconds per treatment

Preparation: Important Checkpoints

- The majority of dogs and cats can tolerate placement of the mask and spacer. Those that resist initially can usually (≈80% of cats, 95% of dogs) be trained to accept treatments.
- For a novice animal, expose it to the face mask and spacer/chamber before starting treatment with an MDI. Gradually introduce the mask with treats/peanut butter or butter on the inside of the mask. Practice several times a day.
- After the face mask is accepted, add on the spacer, holding the combination in place initially for 5 seconds and building up to

30 seconds/10 breaths at a time. This may take a few weeks.

Possible Complications and Common Errors to Avoid

- Some animals initially hold their breath; wait for 7-10 breaths for treatment
- Infection associated with inhaled glucocorticoid use
  - Oral candidiasis, reported in humans, has not been reported in pets.
  - Facial dermatophytosis in the area of the mask can occur.
- Some animals cough after receiving treatment; this is often self-resolving.
- Rarely, a mild contact dermatitis can form where the face mask contacts the face. It is minimized by wiping the face mask edge after each use.
- Untrained, struggling animals can injure their eyes on the edge of the face mask.
- Pet owners can be injured if treating untrained pets.
- Cats with severe bronchoconstriction can benefit from aerosolized bronchodilators even if administration requires very brief restraint/stress.
- Many topical treatments for human airway disease are not in the format of a self-propelled MDI. These medications (e.g., dry-powder inhalers) cannot be adapted to use in a pet animal. Be sure the drug formulation prescribed is in the form of an MDI that can fit the spacer device.

Procedure

- Vigorously shake MDI 3-5 times (approx. 5 seconds).
- Remove the lid, and attach MDI to the spacer/chamber with an appropriately sized face mask attached to the other end.
- Position the animal for gentle restraint to prevent side-to-side movement.
- Gently apply the mask to the animal's face, ensuring a snug fit covering the nose and corners of the mouth but not covering the eyes.
- Depress inhaler (actuate the MDI).
- Hold mask in place for 5-10 breaths (20-30 seconds), watching chest wall movements, one-way valve in spacer, or counting condensations of breath in the spacer.
- If a second dose is needed, wait 30-60 seconds in between, and repeat the procedure.

Postprocedure

- Wipe patient's face/muzzle with a paper towel or washcloth.
- Maintain cleanliness of MDI and spacer following manufacturer's recommendations; clean before first use and weekly.
- If the MDI does not have a built-in dose countdown feature, record number of doses used per canister to know when to refill medication. Number of doses per canister is on the packaging. A myth that a float test to determine medication remaining in a canister is inaccurate and may damage the canister.

Alternatives and Their Relative Merits

- Medication administered by another route, especially when acute antiinflammatory properties are needed. Inhaled glucocorticoids can take 7-10 days to reach full effect. Parenteral bronchodilators are indicated in a fractious animal or in an animal resistant to restraint.
- Nebulization does not offer superior drug administration compared with a face mask and spacer MDI combination but allows drugs unavailable as an MDI to be administered as an inhalant. Examples include antibiotics, lidocaine, and saline.

Pearls

- Use oral glucocorticoids for first 1-2 weeks concurrently with inhaled glucocorticoids in acute inflammatory conditions, and then taper oral medications.
- If an animal is intolerant to the sound of the actuated MDI, actuate the MDI, and then place the mask on the face. This will reduce the administered dose by approximately one-half.
- The manufacturers of veterinary aerosol delivery devices offer excellent client tutorial information, including video clips, on their websites (e.g., https://www.trudellmed.com/trudell-animal-health).
- Chronic, frequent use of racemic albuterol bronchodilators in asthma can be dangerous and should be avoided (p. 84).

SUGGESTED READING

Feline Asthma: Inhaled medications (website). http://www.fritzthebrave.com/meds/inhaled.html/.

AUTHOR: Christine Savidge, DVM, DACVIM
EDITORS: Leah A. Cohn, DVM, PhD, DACVIM; Mark S. Thompson, DVM, DABVP

Jugular Catheter Placement and Management

Bonus Material Online 

Difficulty level: ♦♦

Synonym

Central line

Overview and Goal

Jugular catheterization provides venous access for a critically ill patient that allows for needleless sampling and longer use of a single catheter for prolonged hospitalization.

Indications

- Needleless, simple blood sampling; especially useful when frequent sampling required (e.g., patients with diabetes ketoacidosis) or when sampling is difficult
- Measurement of central venous pressure (CVP) in hypovolemic patients or fluid-intolerant patients
- Infusion of multiple fluids concurrently, facilitated by catheters with multiple lumens
- Infusion of fluids that have a high osmolality (e.g., > 7.5% dextrose solutions, parenteral nutrition)
- Longer use of a single catheter for prolonged hospitalization. A jugular catheter typically eliminates the need to replace multiple peripheral catheters.

Contraindications

- Coagulopathy or severe thrombocytopenia
- Increased intracranial pressures (e.g., traumatic brain injury)
- Pyoderma or inflammation of the skin over the neck and jugular vein
- Caution in hypercoagulable states (e.g., hyperadrenocorticism, protein-losing nephropathy, immune-mediated hemolytic anemia) as thrombosis may occur

Equipment, Anesthesia

- Sedation is often not required in critically ill animals.
- In animals that would not lie still for the procedure, consider the following sedatives, depending on the animal's clinical condition and temperament: butorphanol 0.2-0.4 mg/kg IV/IM, midazolam or diazepam 0.2-0.5 mg/kg IV. Both of these drugs may be given individually or combined for better effect. Avoid benzodiazepines in animals that are agitated or fractious. Dexmedetomidine 1-5 mcg/kg IV may be used in stable clinical patients. Dexmedetomidine may make visualization of the vessel difficult due to vasoconstriction.
- Clippers, surgical scrub with gauze for aseptic preparation of insertion site
- Injectable lidocaine
- A #11 or #15 scalpel
- Sterile surgical gloves
- Sterile drape
- Suture material
- 0.9% NaCl flush (may contain heparin)
- Bandaging material

- Electrocardiogram (ECG) machine for monitoring
- Central line kit (MILA International; Cook and Arrow) using the Seldinger technique. The kit usually includes an introducer catheter (or needle), guide wire, dilator, and the central catheter. Some kits may also include scrub solution, scalpel, suture, and injectable lidocaine.
  - A through-the-needle central line kit may be used instead of the Seldinger technique kit. This chapter presents only the Seldinger technique.

Anticipated Time

30-60 minutes

Preparation: Important Checkpoints

- Assess platelet count, and if concern exists, coagulation profile before catheterization
- Ensure all equipment needed is available, and have one or (ideally) two assistants available.
- Assess the patient's requirement for sedation and have sedatives on hand if needed.

Possible Complications and Common Errors to Avoid

- Correct hypovolemia before placing catheter.
- Ventricular arrhythmias may develop during placement but are usually self-limiting.
- Although rare, hemorrhage or pneumomediastinum may develop, especially if catheter perforates through jugular vein.
- Infection and thrombosis are possible delayed complications.

Procedure

- Administer sedation if needed; often not required in critically ill animals.
- Place animal in lateral recumbency (or dorsal recumbency in heavily sedated animals).
- Shave wide area centered on jugular furrow, extending up to the ventral midline of the neck ventrally and dorsally. Shave cranially to the mandible and caudally to just before the thoracic inlet.
- Wearing exam gloves, perform surgical scrub and preparation of shaved area, focusing around the jugular vein.
- Perform hand hygiene, and don sterile gloves
- Have assistant stand behind the animal, with the spine facing the assistant. Have assistant hold the head of the animal, keeping it straight with one hand, while the other hand occludes the jugular vein outside the sterile field.
- Drape the area around the insertion site, which is usually around the proximal one-third of the jugular vein.
- OPTIONAL: infuse lidocaine aseptically into subcutaneous region around insertion site (0.1-0.5 mL should be sufficient for most dogs). Do not exceed 4 mg/kg in dogs. It is best to avoid lidocaine in cats due to risk of toxicity.
- Using sterile technique and a tape measure, have assistant measure from the insertion site to the 2nd-3rd intercostal space.
- Aseptically flush all lumens of the jugular catheter, and clamp off tubing after flushing.
- While assistant is holding off jugular vein around the thoracic inlet, place large-bore over-the-needle catheter (or needle, depending on what comes in the kit) into jugular vein with tip pointing toward the heart. Feed catheter over the stylet into the vein. In thick-skinned animals, you may need to insert catheter in skin first before inserting it into the vein. Note that introducer catheter may also be inserted after a mini or surgical cut-down procedure.
- Insert the J end of the guide wire into the catheter. To accomplish this, the guide wire is retracted into the plastic end of the sheath. The plastic end is then inserted into the end of the catheter, and the guide wire advanced through the catheter into the vein for about 4-15 cm, depending on the size of the dog. Watch ECG for ventricular arrhythmias during guide wire placement, and gently retract guide wire a few centimeters if arrhythmias are seen.
- Remove the over-the-needle catheter, and ensure that the guide wire does not back out or touch a nonsterile field. Ensure that the guide wire is always held on to during placement so that it does not inadvertently migrate completely into the jugular vein.
- Insert plastic dilator into the vessel by placing the guide wire through it and guiding it into the vessel. Passage of the dilator may be facilitated by tenting the skin and gently rotating the dilator into the vessel. A cut into the skin with a #11 scalpel blade next to the wire may ease insertion.
- Insert approximately one-half of the length of the dilator into the vessel, hold for a few seconds, and remove dilator from the guide wire. Expect bleeding from the insertion site, and use sterile gauze to apply pressure if needed.
- Insert the jugular catheter over the guide wire and guide it into the vessel to predetermined length (see above). Ensure the end of the wire is projecting out of the distal end of the catheter before advancement of the catheter into the vein. The wire should be held as the catheter is advanced into the vessel.
- Remove guide wire after catheter is at desired length in the jugular vein. Pull back on attached syringe to ensure blood flows though catheter easily, flush catheter, and secure jugular catheter using sutures.
- Cover insertion site with an adhesive or nonadhesive dressing, and then apply loose bandage.
- Obtain thoracic radiographs to evaluate for correct positioning of catheter. The tip of the jugular catheter should be in the cranial vena cava, just before the right atrium. If the catheter is in the heart, it should be backed out to the ideal position.

Postprocedure

- Monitor catheter insertion site daily for phlebitis, infection, or catheter backing out.
- Avoid neck leashes while jugular catheter is in place to prevent inadvertent removal.
- Flush unused lumens with 0.9% NaCl or heparinized 0.9% NaCl every 4-6 hours.
- Use three-syringe technique for blood draws.
  - Use a first syringe to evacuate a small volume of blood; this is discarded.
  - Attach a second syringe to collect blood for sampling.
  - Use a third syringe filled with 0.9% saline or heparinized saline solution to flush all blood from the catheter lumen.
- Remove jugular catheter as soon as it is no longer needed.
- Monitor patient for development of thrombosis associated with the jugular catheter (e.g., edema of the head).
- Ideally, patient should be monitored 24 hours/day to avoid bleeding if catheter is accidentally removed.

Alternatives and Their Relative Merits

- A central line can be placed in the lateral or medial saphenous vein extending to the caudal vena cava.
- A peripherally inserted central line (PICC) may be easier to place in animals that do not tolerate placement of a jugular catheter and may be safer if thrombocytopenia is present.

SUGGESTED READING

Campbell M, et al: Catheterization off the venous compartment. In Creedon JM, et al, editors: Advanced monitoring and procedures for small animal emergency and critical care, ed 1, West Sussex, UK, 2012, Wiley.

AUTHOR: Adesola Odunayo, DVM, MS, DACVECC
EDITORS: Leah A. Cohn, DVM, PhD, DACVIM; Mark S. Thompson, DVM, DABVP

Laryngeal, Pharyngeal, and Oral Examination

Difficulty level: ♦

Overview and Goal

The goal of nondental oral examination is to thoroughly evaluate the structure of the oral cavity, nasopharynx, and larynx and to assess laryngeal function. Facial symmetry, cranial nerve function, respiration, jaw movement, and swallowing reflexes are evaluated in the nonsedated animal. Thorough examination of the oral cavity usually requires general anesthesia or heavy sedation.

Indications

Diagnosis of neoplasia (pp. 711 and 714), inflammatory masses (p. 573), laryngeal collapse, laryngeal paralysis (p. 574), foreign bodies, fractures, elongated soft palate, oronasal fistulas (including cleft palates [p. 180]), trauma (p. 576), ranula, pharyngeal mucocele (p. 894), nasopharyngeal stenosis, epiglottic retroversion, and other oral conditions

Contraindications

Should not be attempted with respiratory distress until patient can be restrained safely for anesthetic induction and intubation

Equipment, Anesthesia

- Essentials
  - Anesthetic (e.g., propofol or inhalant), selection of endotracheal tubes
    - For laryngeal exam, propofol 6 mg/kg IV to effect and doxapram 1 mg/kg IV
    - Heavy sedation (e.g., dexmedetomidine combined with an opiate) acceptable if laryngeal function will not be evaluated
  - SpO_2 monitor and pulse Doppler for patient monitoring
  - IV access
  - Laryngoscope or flexible endoscope: high-quality, waterproof inspection cameras (e.g., Depstech, www.depstech.com); inexpensive and provide excellent visualization and lighting of the oropharynx
  - Gauze tie and sponge for jaw and tongue retraction, respectively
  - Gloves
  - Dental speculum or assistant
  - Cotton-tipped applicators or tongue depressor for soft-tissue retraction
- May also need
  - Stylet (e.g., polypropylene urinary catheter) for endotracheal tube if intubation will be difficult
  - Dental mirror if flexible endoscope not available
  - Focused light source (e.g., headlamp)
  - Needles and syringes, slides, cotton-tipped swabs, Tru-Cut biopsy needles, and formalin jars for cytology and histopathology samples
  - Surgical instruments if palate or mass resection or biopsy anticipated
  - Spay hook for palate retraction
  - Magnification glasses
  - Suction
  - Gauze sponges and Allis tissue forceps (sponge on a stick) for local tamponade
  - Otoscope

Anticipated Time

Approximately 15 minutes

Preparation: Important Checkpoints

- Expect general anesthesia for painful examinations and intubation for surgery or if airway compromise is a concern.
- Multiple sizes of cuffed endotracheal tubes in case airway is narrowed from obstruction or collapse. May need a stylet (see below)
- Preoxygenate before induction, and provide oxygen (intubation or flow-by) during the exam.
- Extra propofol for intubation after laryngeal function exam is complete
- IV doxapram is given if no motion (normal or paradoxical) is noted during laryngeal function exam.
- Be prepared for placement of temporary tracheostomy tube (p. 1166).
- Provide oxygen during recovery; nasal catheters may be needed (p. 1146).

Possible Complications and Common Errors to Avoid

- Laryngeal function exam: laryngeal paralysis can be falsely diagnosed in animals under too deep an anesthetic plane or that have not been given doxapram to stimulate deep inspiratory breaths. A diagnosis of laryngeal paralysis can be missed if laryngeal movement is not correlated with normal respiratory cycle (e.g., abduction on inhalation, adduction on exhalation) if paradoxical motion is present.
  - Laryngeal function is decreased in normal dogs when performed under acepromazine/propofol or ketamine/diazepam.
- Dyspnea can occur during recovery because of swelling, hemorrhage, or positional compression by normal soft tissues, particularly in heavily sedated animals. Anxiety on recovering can cause panting, which increases negative pressure on the airway, increasing the risk of swelling and obstruction.

Procedure

- Before anesthesia, evaluate facial symmetry, skull anatomy, skin, lymph nodes, salivary glands, globe retropulsion, respiration, nasal airflow, capillary refill time, mucous membrane color, cranial nerve function, jaw movement, and swallowing reflexes, and determine whether patient can extend and retract tongue and open mouth fully.
  - Full oral examination occurs only after airway patency is verified, laryngeal function is assessed, and intubation performed. With practice, the veterinarian can observe multiple parts of the airway while these three steps are occurring, as described below.
- Place an intravenous catheter, preferably without opioid or acepromazine sedation. Infuse propofol to effect (usually up to 6 mg/kg IV). Have an assistant pass gauze tie caudal to maxillary canines to hold head upwards.
- Under light anesthesia, open mouth with downward pressure on mandible. Note incisor/canine occlusion, ease of jaw retraction, noise with temporomandibular joint (TMJ) movement, and presence of odor or discharge.
  - When the mouth is closed, dogs and cats have a scissor bite: the crown of the maxillary canine is lateral and caudal to that of the mandibular canine; the tip of the mandibular canine rests in a recess rostrodorsal and lateral to the neck of the maxillary canine.
  - Acquired malocclusions can occur with TMJ luxation, jaw/joint fractures, tooth trauma, or neoplasia.
    - With unilateral rostrodorsal TMJ luxation (most common), mandible is shifted and tilted ventrally to unaffected side.
  - Resistance to opening mouth may occur with pain, swelling, neoplasia, foreign bodies, fractures, TMJ luxations, retrobulbar or ocular disease, ear disease, tetanus, masticatory myositis, craniomandibular osteopathy, TMJ ankyloses.
  - Inability to close mouth can occur with TMJ malformation or luxation, foreign body, soft-tissue swelling, neoplasia, tooth-to-tooth contact, trigeminal neuropathy.
- Grasp tongue with gauze sponge and pull outward, or flatten base of tongue with laryngoscope to visualize caudal oral cavity. Concurrently evaluate tongue.
  - If tongue is difficult to pull from mouth, look for ankyloglossia (short lingual frenulum), lingual or sublingual neoplasia, lingual trauma, lingual abscess, foreign body.
  - Dorsal surface of tongue is covered with papillae.
  - Lingual lesions: neoplasia, ulcers, trauma, foreign bodies, eosinophilic granuloma complex, calcinosis circumscripta, contact burns from caustic ingestion, calicivirus stomatitis, uremic glossitis, electrical cord burns, swelling from circumferential string or hair foreign body

- Evaluate palate length, shape, and position
  - Normal length: palate usually slightly overlaps the apex of the epiglottis; when the epiglottis is retracted ventrally by pressure with the laryngoscope blade near its base, the epiglottic tip easily disengages from the soft palate.
  - Elongated palate: palate extends caudal to epiglottis apex, contacting body of epiglottis when ventral to apex or extending beyond its lateral margins, contacting arytenoid cartilage when dorsal to apex.
  - Palate with oblong extension off caudal midline indicates elongated palate being suctioned into laryngeal ostium during inspiration.
  - Short palate: extends rostral to midpoint of tonsillar crypts.
  - Cleft soft palate: split along midline, down one side or both sides
  - Nasopharyngeal mass: palate may bulge ventrally
- Press downward at base of epiglottis with laryngoscope blade to disengage the epiglottic apex from its resting position on the soft palate. Evaluate shape, and position.
  - Normal epiglottis: spade-shaped from dorsal view. When disengaged from caudal border of soft palate, epiglottic lateral margins are oriented horizontally so that the laryngeal cartilages/ostium can be seen without needing to compress the epiglottis with the laryngoscope blade.
  - Abnormal epiglottic shape: neoplasia, calcification, swelling/edema
  - Epiglottic retroversion: because of hyoepiglotticus muscle weakness, the epiglottis is rotated dorsocaudally (vertically oriented), is diamond shaped from a front view, and covers the laryngeal ostium during inspiration.
- Examine larynx
  - Normal laryngeal ostium is diamond shaped with the corniculate processes ("horns") of the arytenoids framing the top, the cuneiform processes ("knees") framing the wider midpoints, and the vocal folds (extending ventrally from the caudal surface of the arytenoids) framing the ventral half of the diamond. Abaxial (lateral) to each vocal fold is a recess (laryngeal ventricle) lined by mucosa known as the *laryngeal saccule*.
  - Abnormal shape caused by neoplasia, inflammation, congenital cyst, trauma
  - Animals with inspiratory dyspnea may have swollen mucosa and everted laryngeal saccules.
  - Animals with laryngeal paralysis have a visible laryngeal ostium between breaths but is narrowed on inspiration.
  - In animals with laryngeal collapse, the saccules are usually everted, and the corniculate processes may be touching or overlapping on midline.
  - Dogs may have laryngeal webbing from debarking.
  - Look for puddle sign: pooling purulent exudate at ventral part of larynx or rostral trachea; present in 83% of dogs with tracheobronchial grass awns and absent in 80% of dogs with bacterial airway disease.
- Evaluate laryngeal function under light anesthesia to rule out laryngeal paralysis.
  - While assistant holds maxilla up with gauze tie, grasp tongue with gauze sponge in nondominant hand, and pull base of tongue and epiglottis downward with a laryngoscope blade (occasionally blade must be used on epiglottis itself, which may affect laryngeal function). Alternatively, insert an endoscope up and over epiglottis to view larynx without distorting local anatomy.
  - If normal movement (abduction synchronized with inhalation), paralysis ruled out
  - If paradoxical movement (arytenoids adduct on inspiration and blow open on exhalation), laryngeal paralysis diagnosed; can be unilateral
  - If no movement or unsure, give doxapram 1 mg/kg IV, and watch for deep inspiratory breath about 8 seconds after injection. On inhalation, cartilages should abduct; if they move inward (paradoxical), laryngeal paralysis present. If no movement seen, watch for active motion as anesthetic wears off. Some dogs with early laryngeal paralysis will have no motion, but vocal folds will quiver.

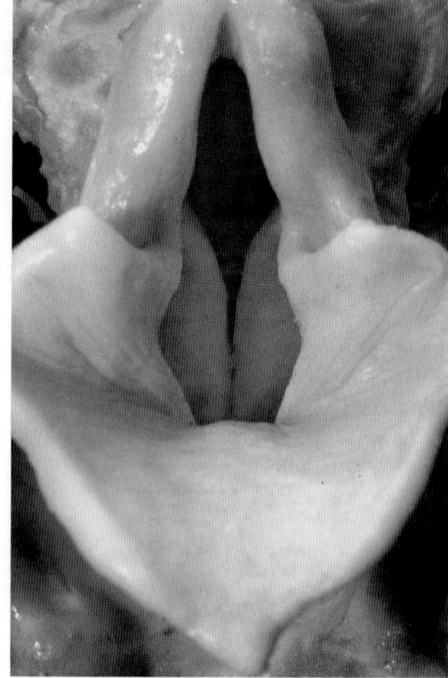

LARYNGEAL, PHARYNGEAL, AND ORAL EXAMINATION The normal laryngeal ostium is diamond shaped with the corniculate processes of the arytenoids framing the top, the cuneiform processes framing the wider midpoints, and the vocal folds (extending ventrally from the caudal surface of the arytenoids) framing the ventral half of the diamond. Abaxial (lateral) to each vocal fold is a recess (laryngeal ventricle) lined by mucosa known as the laryngeal saccule.

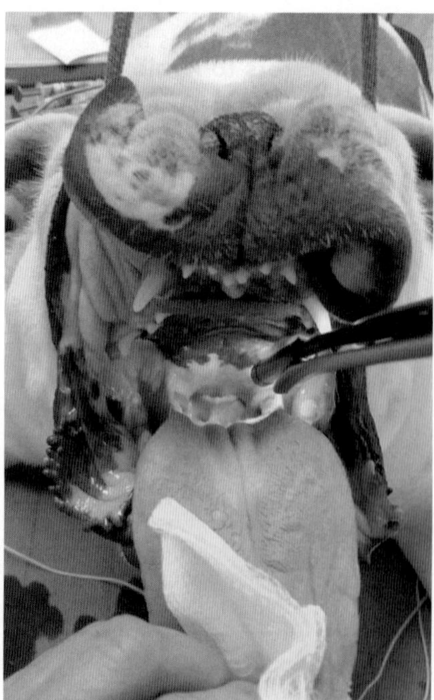

LARYNGEAL, PHARYNGEAL, AND ORAL EXAMINATION A palate of normal length usually slightly overlaps the apex of the epiglottis; when the epiglottis is retracted ventrally by pressure with the laryngoscope blade near its base, the epiglottic tip easily disengages from the soft palate.

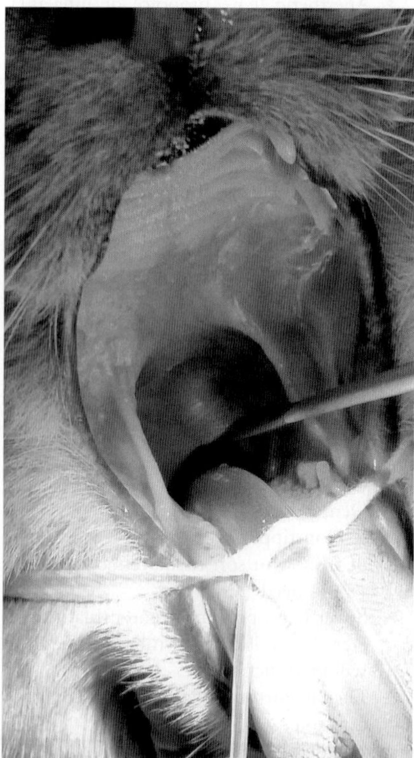

LARYNGEAL, PHARYNGEAL, AND ORAL EXAMINATION Examination of the nasopharynx is performed by retracting the soft palate rostrally with a spay hook (shown), stay suture, or Babcock forceps.

- Intubate the animal.
  - Arytenoid cartilages should be flexible enough to accommodate an appropriately sized tube. Cartilages may not be easily pushed aside if they are calcified, their connections fibrosed, or a mass is present.
  - If a nasopharyngeal mass blocks the laryngeal ostium, elevate the mass with an instrument or cotton-tipped swab, and insert about 4 inches of a long (e.g., 18-24 inch) polypropylene urinary catheter between the laryngeal cartilages into the trachea. While holding catheter tip end steady near the larynx, slide the endotracheal tube over the catheter. Remove the catheter after the tube is in.
- Retract the soft palate rostrally with a spay hook, stay suture, or Babcock forceps to examine the nasopharynx.
  - In a heavily sedated, nonanesthetized dog, retraction may not be possible due to gag reflex. In that case, palpate soft palate for bulges or masses, and press it dorsally. During dorsal depression, the soft palate should sink (indent) toward the skull into the three-sided trough created by the caudal nasal spine of palatine bone rostrally and bony ridges of palatine and pterygoid bones laterally. If this space is not palpable, there may be a mass or tissue thickening.
- With the palate retracted, examine tissues along dorsal and caudolateral aspects of nasopharynx and oropharynx for swelling, discharge, and discoloration.
  - Foreign bodies (e.g., sticks, needles) may penetrate these areas and embed or migrate caudally.
  - Pharyngeal mucoceles cause swelling dorsal to larynx that may obstruct the airway. Temporary treatment with a stab incision and suctioning of entrapped saliva or permanent treatment with sialadenectomy may be necessary for anesthetic recovery.
  - Nasal blastomycosis can cause nasopharyngitis.
  - Nasopharyngeal masses in cats include inflammatory polyps, tumors (e.g., oncocytoma).
  - Nasopharyngeal masses in dogs include melanoma, lymphoma, mast cell tumor, polyp, transmissible venereal tumor.
- Examine the space dorsal to soft palate and palatine bone with retroflexed endoscope or dental mirror.
  - The oval-shaped choanae are the openings of the two nasopharyngeal meatuses, and caudal to them is the intrapharyngeal ostium. There should be no visible turbinates in these spaces.
    - Nasopharyngeal turbinates have been reported as a contributing factor to inspiratory dyspnea in brachycephalic breeds.
  - Choanal atresia and nasopharyngeal stenosis: the choanae and intrapharyngeal ostium are not visible because of partial or complete membranous or osseous obstruction.
  - Nasopharyngeal dysgenesis (reported in dachshunds) results in a slitlike intrapharyngeal ostium.
- Return palate to its normal position, and evaluate tonsils. Palatine tonsils are usually partially to completely hidden from view because of their positions in tonsillar fossae. Tonsillar enlargement may be caused by inflammation, neoplasia, or negative pressure from inspiratory dyspnea.
- Examine hard palate for oronasal fistulae, ulcerations, trauma, and masses.
  - The incisive papilla is a normal mass of tissue on midline caudal to the maxillary incisors. On either side are openings of the incisive ducts, which lead to the vomer nasal organ.
  - Hard palate mucosa normally has transverse ridges.
- Examine the ventral surface of the tongue.
  - Sublingual and mandibular salivary ducts open at sublingual caruncle (a mucosal fold).
  - Cats have lingual molar salivary glands in a fold of tissue medial to the mandibular first molar.
  - Ranula are saliva-filled outpouchings from leakage of sublingual/mandibular salivary ducts. If ruptured, excess mucosal folds and blood may be seen.
  - Sublingual masses include neoplasia, traumatic proliferation, ectopic thyroid cysts.
- Examine the mandible, maxilla, buccal pouches, mucous membranes, lips for trauma; neoplasia; petechiae; erosions; vesiculobullous (autoimmune), ulcerative, or proliferative lesions.
  - Parotid and zygomatic ducts open at level of maxillary fourth premolars.
- Proceed to dental examination (p. 1140).

Postprocedure

- Monitor for dyspnea postoperatively.
- Cats with mouths held open fully by spring-loaded gags can develop cortical blindness and neurologic deficits.

Alternatives and Their Relative Merits

Other diagnostic modalities include laryngeal ultrasound for diagnosis of laryngeal paralysis (cats especially) and MRI or contrast CT for determining extent of lesions.

SUGGESTED READING

Kressin D: Oral examination of cats and dogs. Compend Contin Educ 31:72-85, 2009.

AUTHOR: Karen M. Tobias, DVM, MS, DACVS
EDITORS: Leah A. Cohn, DVM, PhD, DACVIM; Mark S. Thompson, DVM, DABVP

Lipid Emulsion for Intoxication

Difficulty level: ♦

Synonyms

Intralipid therapy, intravenous lipid emulsion (ILE) therapy

Overview and Goal

The goal of ILE is to use lipids supplied by fat emulsions (often used as part of parenteral nutrition) to reduce the severity of toxicoses and/or the length of treatment required for intoxication. The exact mechanism of action is unknown, but the lipid shuttle theory is the most accepted. With the infusion of ILE, a lipid phase is created in the aqueous portion of the blood. The lipid phase transiently sequesters the toxin, decreasing free (active) drug and then accelerates its movement from drug-susceptible organs to organs that can store (muscle, fat), detoxify (liver), or excrete (kidney, bladder) the toxin.

Indications

- Intoxications that do not have a good outcome using traditional therapies
- Severe or potentially severe clinical signs
- Lipophilic toxins (toxins that have a high log *P* value) more likely to benefit from this therapy. Other toxin properties can also affect efficacy, including charge at physiologic pH, protein binding, and volume of distribution.
- Toxins with positive outcomes (reported and anecdotal): marijuana, baclofen, calcium channel blockers, avermectins, local anesthetics, serotonergic medications

Contraindications

- Allergies to egg, soy, fish, safflower, or coconut: anaphylaxis
- Limited fat metabolism/elimination
- Coagulopathy
- Hypokalemia (p. 516)
- Hypophosphatemia

Equipment, Anesthesia

- 20% lipid emulsion
- Peripheral catheter
- Fluid pump

Anticipated Time

About 60-90 minutes for initial setup and bolus plus constant-rate infusion (CRI)

Preparation: Important Checkpoints

- Once opened, bag is good for only 24 hours.
- Use aseptic technique because there are no preservatives in the lipid emulsion.
- If volume overload is a concern, stop other fluids during administration of lipids.

Possible Complications and Common Errors to Avoid

- ILE has not been shown to be consistently effective in all cases of lipophilic drug toxicosis.
- Can antagonize/remove antidotal agents or other supportive therapies
- Volume overload
- Lipemia
- Pancreatitis (pp. 740 and 742)
- Hemolysis (oxidative damage)
- Corneal lipidosis (rare, reversible)
- Fat overload syndrome (hyperlipidemia, fat embolism, hepatomegaly, splenomegaly, thrombocytopenia, jaundice, coagulopathy, hemolysis) seen with excessive volumes or high administration rates

Procedure

- Place intravenous (IV) catheter
- 1.5 mL/kg bolus over 30 minutes (as fast as possible if asystole)
- 0.25 mg/kg/min CRI for 30-60 minutes
- Monitor for pyrogenic and allergic responses (especially first 20 minutes), and stop infusion immediately if this occurs.
- Check for lipemia in 4-6 hours. If no lipemia and animal is still symptomatic, repeat the CRI; if still lipemic, wait and recheck in a couple of hours.

Postprocedure

- Lipemia: do not redose unless serum is clear.
- Recurrence of toxicosis: lipids may be more quickly eliminated than the toxin; toxins with a large volume of distribution can redistribute and cause clinical signs.
- Hemolysis: rare

Alternatives and Their Relative Merits

Symptomatic and supportive care relevant to the specific toxicant

Pearls

- Lipids are relatively inexpensive and have about a 2-year shelf life.
- Hyperlipemia can interfere with laboratory testing.

SUGGESTED READING

Robben JH, et al: Lipid therapy for intoxications. Vet Clin North Am Small Anim Pract 47(2):435-450, 2017.

AUTHOR: Tina Wismer, DVM, MS, DABVT, DABT
EDITORS: Leah A. Cohn, DVM, PhD, DACVIM; Mark S. Thompson, DVM, DABVP

Liver Biopsy, Laparoscopic

Client Education Sheet

Difficulty level: ♦♦♦

Overview and Goal

- Visual inspection of all liver lobes to obtain biopsy samples and safe access to the gallbladder for aspiration
- Samples are superior in size to ultrasound-guided Tru-Cut samples
- Procedure time, with experience, should be less than that of an open laparotomy.

Indications

- Abnormal liver function
- Persistently elevated serum liver enzyme levels
- Ascites of unknown origin (p. 79)
- Abnormal sonographic findings of the liver
- Monitoring results of specific therapy (e.g., copper chelation)
- Suspected infectious or inflammatory biliary tract disease (cholecystocentesis)

Contraindications

- Conditions necessitating full abdominal exploration
- Abnormal clotting times
- Poor patient condition
- Patient size: very small

Equipment, Anesthesia

- Xenon light source and cable
- Carbon dioxide insufflator and tubing
- Video camera and monitor
- 5-mm 0° or 30° telescope
- Trocar cannulas (3) or single-site port
- Veress needle (optional)
- 5-mm oval cup biopsy forceps
- 14-16 gauge needle biopsy instrument
- 18-20 gauge spinal needle
- Blunt palpation probe
- Hemostatic agent
- General anesthesia is recommended, although sedation and local anesthesia may be used in compromised patients.

Anticipated Time

Uncomplicated procedure can be accomplished in less than 30 minutes with experience.

Preparation: Important Checkpoints

- Recent CBC with platelet count, coagulation profile, and serum biochemical profile
- ± Thromboelastography and buccal mucosal bleeding time
- Blood pressure
- List of samples to be obtained (e.g., liver tissue for histology, copper levels, and bacterial culture; bile for culture)

Possible Complications and Common Errors to Avoid

- Proper room setup and portal placement is paramount to a successful and seamless procedure.
- Splenic laceration on abdominal entry with the Veress needle
  - Use modified Hasson technique instead.
  - Hemorrhage is usually self-limiting.
- Aggressive sampling with the biopsy forceps can create excessive hemorrhage.
  - Use hemostatic material or apply compression with the blunt palpation probe.
- Patients showing respiratory compromise may require ventilatory support.
- Bile leakage after gallbladder aspiration is an uncommon complication.

Procedure

Liver biopsy:

- Establish pneumoperitoneum using a Veress needle or modified Hasson technique.
- Insufflate the abdomen with CO_2 with a maximum pressure of 15 mm Hg.
- Telescope placement may be on ventral midline caudal to the umbilicus or a right-sided midabdominal approach.
  - If the pancreas must be explored, the right-sided approach is preferred to avoid the falciform ligament.
  - For routine liver biopsies, a midline approach offers the most flexibility as the Hasson technique may be used, and the left lateral lobe is better visualized.
- A single-site port may be used for access for the telescope and for instruments.
- If a single-site port is not used, the instrument portal is established using the scope to visualize placement in the right cranial abdomen.

- Use the blunt probe placed into the instrument portal to evaluate all lobes.
- Remove the blunt probe, and insert the biopsy forceps into the instrument portal to sample multiple liver lobes.
- Position the cup forceps on the margin of a lobe, slowly twist the forceps and withdraw to sever the liver sample, and remove through the cannula.
- To sample the liver surface, open the forceps, direct at a 90° angle to the surface, push into the liver 5-1 0 mm, and close.
- Check all biopsy sites for excessive hemorrhage; the blunt probe or gel foam may be used for hemostasis.

Gallbladder aspiration:

- Insert a 20-gauge, 2-3 inch spinal needle using telescope guidance into the right ventrolateral abdomen, caudal to the last rib.
- Direct the needle through the apex in an avascular region of the gallbladder surface, and use a 3-5 mL syringe to aspirate as much fluid as possible to prevent leakage.
- Fluid should be submitted for aerobic and anaerobic bacterial culture.

Closure:

- Open all cannulas, and expel CO_2 from abdomen with gentle pressure on the abdomen before removal of the cannulas.
- Close port sites routinely in two- to three-layer closure.

Postprocedure

- The patient should be monitored for bleeding by packed cell volume/total solids and blood pressure.
- The patient may be monitored overnight or discharged from the hospital the same day.
- An e-collar should be placed and the patient activity level limited for 7-10 days.

Alternatives and Their Relative Merits

- Laparotomy: larger samples may be obtained, a full exploration may be performed, and therapeutic intervention such as liver lobectomy may be performed when appropriate. Longer procedure times and more invasive than laparotomy
- Ultrasound-guided liver biopsy: less invasive, may be performed using sedation, smaller samples obtained

Pearls

- Poorly placed portals prevent adequate visualization and access to the liver
- A 30° scope improves visualization over a 0° scope.
- Biopsy abnormal- and normal-appearing liver, and sample from at least two lobes.

SUGGESTED READING

McDevitt HL, et al: Short-term clinical outcome of laparoscopic liver biopsy in dogs: 106 cases (2003-2013). J Am Vet Med Assoc 248:1, 2016.

RELATED CLIENT EDUCATION SHEETS

Consent to Perform General Anesthesia
Consent to Perform Hepatic (Liver) Biopsy

AUTHOR: Jill K. Luther, DVM, MS, DACVS
EDITORS: Leah A. Cohn, DVM, PhD, DACVIM; Mark S. Thompson, DVM, DABVP

Local and Regional Anesthesia

Difficulty level: ◆

Synonym

Local blocks

Overview and Goals

- *Local anesthesia* and *regional anesthesia* refer to a broad range of techniques that use local anesthetic agents delivered to a discrete anatomic area (as opposed to systemic delivery).
- With these techniques, the local anesthetic agent inhibits pain by blocking transmission of noxious input (and other types of sensory input) before it ever reaches the brain. The animal's level of consciousness is not affected.
- This contrasts with general anesthesia, during which nociceptive processing continues to occur, but the animal is not able to perceive pain because of the unconscious state.

Indications

Infiltrative anesthesia:

- Incisional block: supplemental analgesia for a variety of surgical procedures (e.g., abdominal wall incisions, total ear canal ablation incisions)

Peripheral nerve blocks:

- Dental nerve block: supplemental analgesia for tooth extractions, maxillary/mandibular surgeries
- Brachial plexus block: supplemental analgesia for surgical procedures involving the forelimb distal to shoulder
- Distal radial, ulnar, and median nerve blocks: supplemental analgesia for feline onychectomy or any surgical procedure involving the distal forepaw
- Intercostal nerve blocks: supplemental analgesia after lateral thoracotomy or desensitizing area around isolated rib fractures

Other regional techniques:

- Intraarticular anesthesia/analgesia: supplemental analgesia for procedures involving the joint space (stifle most common)
- Interpleural anesthesia: supplemental analgesia for thoracic and cranial abdominal pain (especially pancreatitis)
- Intravenous (IV) regional anesthesia: desensitization of a distal limb to facilitate surgery

Contraindications

Infiltrative anesthesia, peripheral nerve blocks, others: injection into infected tissue

Equipment, Anesthesia

Local anesthetic agents:

- Lidocaine: duration ≈1-3 h; total dose ≤ 5 mg/kg (dog); ≤ 3 mg/kg (cat)
- Bupivicaine: duration ≈3-4 h; total dose ≤ 2 mg/kg (dog); ≤ 2 mg/kg (cat)
- Liposome encapsulated bupivacaine: gradual-release formulation with duration ≈72 h; approved for use at incision site for cruciate surgery (5.3 mg/kg [0.4 mL/kg] dogs) and for onychectomy (5.3 mg/kg per limb or 10.6 mg/kg [0.8 mL/kg] cats). May be diluted 1.1 with 0.9% sterile saline to increase injection volume for incisional infiltration

Infiltrative anesthesia:

- Incisional block
  - Hypodermic needle (22, 25 gauge), syringe, sterile gloves, local anesthetic
  - Animal is usually under general anesthesia, and block is done before incision is made or at the end of the surgery before complete closure.

Peripheral nerve blocks:

- Dental nerve block
  - Hypodermic needle (22, 25 gauge), syringe, local anesthetic
  - Animal is usually under general anesthesia.
- Brachial plexus block
  - Hypodermic needle (22 gauge) or spinal needle (22 gauge, 2-3 inches [5-8 cm]), syringe, local anesthetic
  - Specialized insulated needle (22 gauge, 3 inches) required if a nerve locator is to be used
  - Animal is usually sedated or under general anesthesia.
- Distal radial, ulnar, median nerve blocks
  - Hypodermic needle (22, 25 gauge), syringe, local anesthetic
  - Animal is usually under general anesthesia, and block is done before surgical procedure.
- Intercostal nerve block
  - Hypodermic needle (22, 25 gauge), syringe, local anesthetic

- Animal is usually sedated or under general anesthesia.
- Epidural anesthesia/analgesia

Other regional techniques:

- Intraarticular anesthesia/analgesia
  - Hypodermic needle (22 gauge), syringe, sterile gloves, local anesthetic (lidocaine, bupivacaine) ± opioid (morphine)
  - Animal is usually sedated or under general anesthesia.
- Interpleural anesthesia
  - Butterfly catheter (22 gauge) or through-the-needle catheter (20 gauge, 2 inches); preplaced chest tube or commercial interpleural anesthesia tray, syringe, sterile gloves, local anesthetic
  - Dosages: lidocaine ≤ 5 mg/kg (dog) q 2-4h; ≤ 3 mg/kg (cat) q 4h; bupivacaine ≤ 2 mg/kg (dog) initially, then ≤ 1 mg/kg q 6h; ≤ 1 mg/kg (cat) initially, then ≤ 0.5 mg/kg q 6h.
  - Animals are usually sedated or under general anesthesia.
- IV regional anesthesia
  - Cling-and-release bandage material (e.g., Vetrap), IV catheter (22 gauge), tourniquet, hypodermic needle (22 gauge), syringe, local anesthetic (lidocaine)
  - Dose: lidocaine 2.5-5 mg/kg (dog only)
  - Animal is usually sedated.

Anticipated Time

This time does not include clipping of hair and preparation of the site where indicated.

- Infiltrative anesthesia
  - Incisional block: < 1-2 minutes
- Peripheral nerve blocks
  - Dental nerve blocks: < 1-2 minutes
  - Brachial plexus block: < 5-10 minutes
  - Distal radial, ulnar, median nerve blocks: < 1-2 minutes
  - Intercostal nerve blocks: < 1-2 minutes
- Other regional techniques
  - Intraarticular anesthesia/analgesia: < 1-2 minutes
  - Interpleural anesthesia: < 5-10 minutes
  - IV regional anesthesia: < 5-10 minutes

Preparation: Important Checkpoints

- Ensure that injection site is clipped (if applicable) and aseptically prepared.
- Adhere to strict aseptic technique during all procedures; doing this is mandatory.
- Ensure that drug solutions are free from contamination (especially for epidural and intraarticular techniques).

Possible Complications and Common Errors to Avoid

- Systemic local anesthetic toxicosis is possible with any technique and is usually associated with inadvertent IV injection/excessive drug doses. Calculate total dose per animal.
- Infiltrative anesthesia
  - Incisional block: inadvertent IV or intraarterial injection, penetration of body cavities/organs
- Peripheral nerve blocks
  - Dental nerve block: self-mutilation after sensory loss to tongue and lips (rare)
  - Brachial plexus block: inadvertent IV or intraarterial injection or injection into the thoracic cavity with possible pneumothorax/pulmonary laceration
  - Distal radial, ulnar, median nerve blocks: self-mutilation after sensory loss to distal paws (rare)
  - Intercostal nerve block: inadvertent intrathoracic injection with possible pneumothorax/pulmonary laceration
- Other regional techniques
  - Intraarticular anesthesia/analgesia: articular cartilage damage
  - Interpleural anesthesia: pneumothorax, pulmonary laceration
  - IV regional anesthesia: ischemic limb damage; systemic local anesthetic toxicosis due to tourniquet failure

Procedure

For selected techniques only

- Peripheral nerve blocks
  - Dental nerve blocks
    - Infraorbital: palpate infraorbital foramen rostral and ventral to medial canthus of eye; insert needle into foramen and aspirate. If there is negative pressure (no blood), inject local anesthetic.
    - Mandibular: palpate mandibular foramen intraorally on the medial surface of the mandible, and insert needle percutaneously from the ventromedial aspect of the mandible toward the foramen and aspirate. If there is negative pressure (no blood), inject local anesthetic.
  - Brachial plexus block
    - From a cranial approach, insert the needle medial to the scapula just ventral to the body of the sixth cervical vertebra; advance until the tip of the needle is just beyond the first rib and aspirate. If there is negative pressure (no blood), inject one-fourth dose of a local anesthetic; withdraw needle partially, and aspirate. If there is negative pressure (no blood), inject another one-fourth dose of anesthetic; repeat until needle is completely withdrawn and all drug has been injected.
  - Distal radial, ulnar, median nerve blocks: three injections required per paw
    - On dorsal aspect, insert needle just proximal to the first phalanx and aspirate; if negative pressure (no blood), inject local anesthetic.
    - On palmar aspect, insert needle just medial to accessory carpal pad and aspirate; if negative pressure (no blood), inject local anesthetic.
    - Remove needle and insert just lateral and proximal to accessory carpal pad and aspirate; if negative pressure (no blood), inject local anesthetic.
- Other regional techniques
  - Interpleural anesthesia

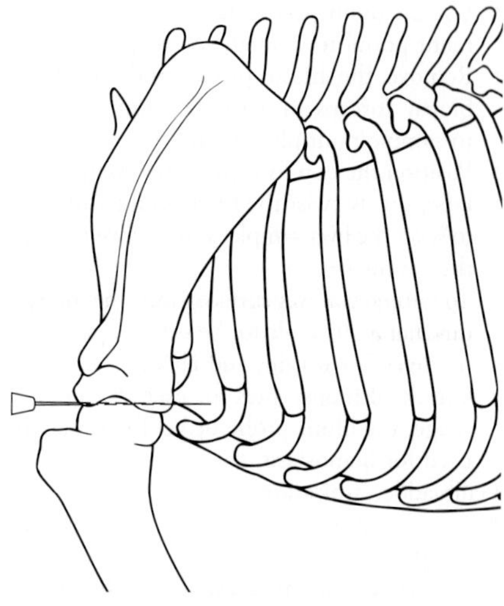

LOCAL AND REGIONAL ANESTHESIA Brachial plexus nerve block. Place needle medial to scapulohumeral joint, lateral to thoracic wall, toward costochondral junction, parallel to vertebral column. (From Fossum TW, et al: Small animal surgery, ed 2, St. Louis, 2002, Mosby.)

    - Insert catheter in the ninth intercostal space on the midlateral aspect of thorax.
    - Aspirate to remove air/blood.
    - Inject local anesthetic (lidocaine should be injected first in conscious animals to minimize discomfort and can be followed by bupivacaine if a long-duration block is desired).

Postprocedure

- If local/regional anesthesia is being used for supplementing analgesia in conjunction with general anesthesia, injectable and inhalation anesthetic requirements may be markedly reduced.
- Animals must be monitored for adequacy of analgesia and treated accordingly.

Alternatives and Their Relative Merits

- Pain associated with surgery, trauma, and a variety of medical conditions can usually be managed using systemic analgesics (e.g., opioids, nonsteroidal antiinflammatory drugs [NSAIDs]); however, these agents are not able to block peripheral nociceptive input.
- The inclusion of a local or regional technique constitutes a multimodal approach to anesthesia and pain management and is simply good medical practice.

SUGGESTED READING

Campoy L, et al: Canine and feline local anesthetic and analgesic techniques. In Grimm KA et al, editors: Veterinary anesthesia and analgesia, ed 5, Ames, IA, 2015, Wiley Blackwell, pp 827-856.

AUTHOR: Leigh A. Lamont, DVM, MS, DACVAA
EDITORS: Leah A. Cohn, DVM, PhD, DACVIM; Mark S. Thompson, DVM, DABVP

Local and Regional Anesthesia: Dentistry and Oral Surgery

Client Education Sheet

Difficulty level: ♦

Overview and Goals

- Saving medical expenses by reducing the concentration needed of an inhalation anesthetic
- Minimizing complications from hypotension, bradycardia, and hypoventilation
- Enabling faster recovery with fewer complications
- Providing analgesia in postoperative period

Indications

Procedures in dentistry, oral and maxillofacial surgery

Contraindications

- History of allergy to a local anesthetic agent
- Bleeding disorder (risk of hematoma formation and ischemic nerve damage)
- Pre-existing peripheral neuropathy (risk of permanent nerve damage)
- Infection at needle insertion site/pathway
- Inflammation at injection site (altering effect of anesthetic agent)

Equipment, Anesthesia

- Usually performed under general anesthesia
- Needles: 1¼ to 1½ inches long (3-3.5 cm) (depending on depth of penetration), 22- to 27-gauge (depending on whether going through skin or mucosa) on 1- to 3-mL syringes (depending on volume injected)
- Bupivacaine 0.5% (effective for up to 6-8 hours); lidocaine 2% (effective for up to 2 hours); onset time for analgesia longer with long-acting local anesthetics (few minutes for lidocaine, up to 15 minutes for bupivacaine)

Anticipated Time

1-2 minutes per block (including calculating dosage, preparing syringe/needle, and injecting local anesthetic)

Preparation: Important Checkpoints

Calculate total maximum dosages:

- Bupivacaine 2 mg/kg in cats and dogs
- Lidocaine 5 mg/kg in dogs, 1 mg/kg in cats
- 0.5% solution contains 5 mg/mL and 2% solution contains 20 mg/mL
- To benefit from both local anesthetics (i.e., short onset time and long acting), one can mix 0.2 mL lidocaine 2% with 0.8 mL bupivacaine 0.5% per 4.53 kg (10 lb) as maximum patient dosage.

Consider how many jaw quadrants (sites) need nerve blocks:

- Depending on oral examination findings
- Volumes per site of 0.2 (cats/small dogs) to 0.8 mL (large dogs) often sufficiently effective
- Repeating nerve blocks possible (considering total maximum dosage and length of procedure)

Possible Complications and Common Errors to Avoid

Iatrogenic failure:

- Overdose (calculate correct dosage)
- Injection into vessel lumen (aspirate before injecting, stop and withdraw if blood; otherwise, keep needle steady during injection)
- Vessel laceration (apply digital pressure with gauze if occurs; avoid bending of needle tip on bone)
- Hematoma (apply digital pressure with gauze if occurs)
- Infection (use sterile equipment for each injection site)
- Nerve damage (inject lowest effective volume; reinsert needle if abnormal resistance to injection is felt [possible intrafascicular placement of needle tip])
- Ocular trauma (avoid advancing needle too dorsal when blocking the maxillary nerve, and keep needle parallel to the hard palate when blocking the infraorbital nerve)

Self-mutilation:

- Pawing at mouth (consider placing e-collar)
- Biting on lip/cheek (after preoperative or postoperative presence of malocclusion)
- Biting on tongue (desensitization of tongue after inferior alveolar nerve block unlikely when proper technique employed)

Procedure

Local anesthesia:

- Topical gels: application of anesthetic gel onto mucosal surfaces; short-lived effects
- Splash block (wound irrigation): dropping of local anesthetic solution (0.05-0.1 mL/kg in cats and 0.1-0.2 mL/kg in dogs of a mixture of 0.25 mL phenylephrine 1% and 50 mL lidocaine 2%) onto a wound; for example, into nasal cavity after maxillectomy before or through nostrils after surgical closure
- Intraligamentous injection: into the periodontal ligament; cumbersome
- Injection near planned incision: around surgical site

Regional anesthesia: select one or more sites depending on location of lesion/intervention.

- Maxillary nerve block
    - Intraoral: insert needle through oral mucosa just caudal to last maxillary molar, and advance it in a dorsal direction (maxillary nerve enters infraorbital canal through maxillary foramen); slightly bending the needle 7-9 mm from its tip facilitates block placement and indicates how deep needle is placed.
    - Extraoral: insert needle through skin of the caudal cheek, and advance it in a medial and slightly dorsal direction (caudal to maxilla, ventral to zygomatic arch, and rostral to mandibular ramus).
    - Areas desensitized: incisive bone, maxilla and palatine bone, all maxillary teeth on

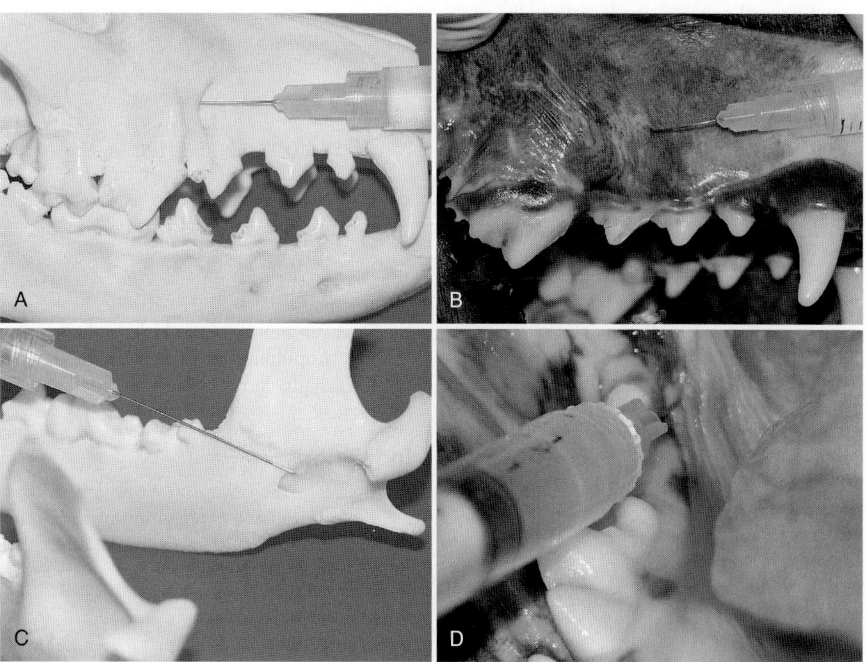

LOCAL AND REGIONAL ANESTHESIA: DENTISTRY AND ORAL SURGERY Skull (**A**) and cadaver (**B**) show infraorbital nerve block in a dog. Skull (**C**) and cadaver (**D**) show inferior alveolar nerve block in a dog. (Copyright Dr. Alexander M. Reiter.)

Procedures and Techniques

that side and adjacent soft tissues (including some nasal mucosa)
  - Do not inject into the eye!
- Infraorbital nerve block
  - Intraoral: insert needle through labial mucosa at the transverse level of the maxillary second/third premolar in a caudal direction toward the infraorbital foramen (keep needle parallel to the hard palate when advancing it into the infraorbital canal).
  - Extraoral: insert needle through lateral skin (similar to when going through mucosa but not recommended because larger needle is needed).
  - Areas desensitized: incisive bone and maxilla, maxillary incisors, canine, and premolars/molars and adjacent soft tissues (depending how far needle is advanced caudally into infraorbital canal; because infraorbital canal is short in cats, all maxillary tissues on that side can easily be desensitized)
  - Do not inject into the eye!
- Major palatine nerve block
  - Insert needle through palatal mucosa at the transverse level of the main cusp of the maxillary third premolar between the median plane and dental arch, and advance it caudally just rostral to the major palatine foramen (located palatal to the maxillary fourth premolar about halfway toward the median plane).
  - Areas desensitized: palatine shelf of the maxilla and adjacent soft tissues
  - Some resistance felt during injection is expected because palatal mucosa does not contain submucosa (slight bleb often visible after injection).
- Inferior alveolar nerve block
  - Intraoral: insert needle through oral mucosa immediately caudal to the last mandibular molar on the medial aspect of the mandible, and advance it along bone surface in a caudoventral direction toward the mandibular foramen.
  - Extraoral: insert needle through skin at an unnamed notch of the caudoventral mandible between its body and angular process, and advance it on the medial aspect along the bone surface toward the mandibular foramen.
  - Areas desensitized: mandibular body, all mandibular teeth and adjacent soft tissues
- Middle mental nerve block
  - Insert needle through labial mucosa rostral to a frenulum-like fold between the mandibular canine and first premolar (dog) or third premolar (cat), and advance it along the lateral bone surface in a caudoventral direction toward the middle mental foramen.
  - Extraoral: insert needle through lateral skin (similar to when going through mucosa but not recommended because larger needle is needed).
  - Areas desensitized: rostral mandibular body, teeth rostral to injection site (mandibular incisors +/− canine) and adjacent soft tissues
  - In larger patients, you may enter the mandibular canal through the middle mental foramen.

Postprocedure

- Apply digital pressure/perform brief massage of the injection site.
- Safely discard needle and syringe.
- Monitor the injection site for hematoma formation.

Pearls

- Technicians should master nerve block techniques for dental and oral surgical procedures.
- Use a fresh sterile needle for each individual injection.
  - Repeat use of same needle for more than one injection increases risk of infection.
  - Repeat bumping onto bone causes needle tip to bend, which may injure vessel/nerve upon needle retraction.
- Always aspirate before injection.
  - If no vacuum is felt when going through skin upon placing maxillary or inferior alveolar nerve blocks, needle tip may be located within oral cavity or oropharynx.
  - Aspirate for several seconds with thinner needles, as it may take longer for blood to appear within syringe if needle tip is indeed in vessel lumen.
- Keep needle steady during injection.
  - Ensure that needle is firmly attached to the syringe before injection.
  - Upon advancing the needle, one may enter a vessel and exit it again. For example, retracting needle during injection may position the needle tip back into a vessel lumen.

SUGGESTED READING

Beckman B: Anesthesia and pain management for small animals. Vet Clin North Am Small Anim Pract 43:669-688, 2013.

AUTHOR: Alexander M. Reiter, DVM, Dr. med. vet., DAVDC, DEVDC
EDITORS: Leah A. Cohn, DVM, PhD, DACVIM; Mark S. Thompson, DVM, DABVP

Magnetic Resonance Imaging Scan

Difficulty level: ♦♦♦

Synonyms

MRI, MR

Overview and Goal

- Magnetic resonance imaging (MRI) is a method of cross-sectional imaging that does not involve ionizing radiation. Compared to radiography, MRI allows improved evaluation of areas of complex anatomy by avoiding superimposition of multiple structures. The contrast resolution of MRI is vastly superior to that of radiography and computed tomography (CT).
- MRI can be used for assessing any area of the body. In veterinary medicine, common uses include assessment of the brain and spinal column. Musculoskeletal imaging (e.g., scapulohumeral joint, stifle) is also increasingly commonplace in small animal practice.

Indications

- Disease of the central nervous system; best method available for imaging of the brain
- Selected orthopedic, abdominal, and other soft-tissue disorders

Contraindications

- Inability to tolerate general anesthesia
- Presence of a pacemaker: in a minority of patients, the MRI magnetic field alters the pacemaker program or causes the pacemaker to oscillate in the patient. In human medicine, MRI suites bear warnings forbidding entry to any person with a pacemaker, and it is unlikely that an MRI technician would allow a veterinary patient with a pacemaker to be scanned.
- Presence of ferrous (iron-containing) metal, including implants and intestinal foreign bodies
  - Movement of the metal when in the magnetic field, causing soft-tissue trauma
- Presence of large metallic implants (nonferrous) in the area of interest:
  - Heating of the metallic implants → tissue damage.
  - Imaging artifact severely limits the value of the study.

GENERAL MRI SAFETY CONSIDERATIONS

- Injury to the patient and/or damage to the MRI magnet can occur if careful attention is not paid to basic safety regarding the presence of metallic objects within the MRI suite.
- The magnet is the core of the MRI unit, and the magnet is always on, 24 hours/day. It is never safe to have loose metallic objects in the vicinity of the magnet—that is, anywhere in the same room as the MRI unit (MRI suite).
- Because the chemical composition of metal objects (ferrous or nonferrous) may not be known, all metallic objects should be regarded as potential safety hazards and excluded from the MRI suite.
- All equipment used in the area of the MRI magnet must be constructed of plastic and/or nonferrous metal or must be kept a safe distance from the magnet and secured. Recorded instances of this guideline not being followed have produced injury and death in patients and hospital personnel through blunt trauma caused by large objects that transform into projectiles because of their strong attraction to the magnet.
- The safe distance from the magnet will depend on the field strength of the magnet, the shielding of the magnet, and the amount of ferrous metal in the object. A distance of 36 inches (≈1 meter) is generally sufficient for a magnet of 1.0 tesla or less field strength.
- Because of the safety hazards associated with MRI, it is best to limit the number of personnel in the MRI suite to the minimum necessary to perform the study and monitor the patient.

Equipment, Anesthesia

General anesthesia is required. MRI studies are prolonged and generally performed using gas anesthesia. Constant-rate infusion of intravenous (IV) anesthetic agents can be used, but gas anesthesia is preferred because of the duration of the procedure.

- Endotracheal tube, *not* wire reinforced
  - A laryngoscope can be used only if the patient is intubated in an area isolated from the MRI magnet.
- Anesthesia machine for gas anesthesia
  - Unit specified as being MRI safe (nonferrous metals and plastic used in construction)
  - Generic anesthesia unit with long breathing circuit; minimum distance to magnet ≈3 feet (1 meter)
- IV pump for constant-rate infusion
  - Unit specified as being MRI safe (nonferrous metals and plastic used in construction)
  - Generic infusion pump with extension tubing; minimum distance to magnet ≈3 feet (1 meter)

Monitoring equipment:

- Pulse oximeter
  - The patient attachment and cables must be specially constructed of nonferrous metal and/or plastic. Fiberoptic technology is employed; an example is the Nonin 7500 FO unit.
- Blood pressure/CO_2 measurements
  - The patient attachment and cables must be specially constructed of nonferrous metal and/or plastic (e.g., SurgiVet monitors)
- Electrocardiogram (ECG)
  - ECG electrodes for MRI use are available. Because of radiofrequency interference, usable ECG tracings cannot be acquired during image acquisition.
- Emergency kit
  - As with any procedure performed under general anesthesia, the equipment and drugs necessary for emergency cardiopulmonary cerebral resuscitation (CPCR) should be immediately available.
  - Great care should be exercised to ensure that metallic objects are not introduced near the magnet during CPCR. In case of emergency, the patient will need to be removed from the MRI suite and resuscitative efforts performed at a safe distance from the magnet.

Intravenous contrast agents:

- Paramagnetic agents
  - Gadolinium diethylenetriamine pentaacetic acid (Gd-DTPA): Magnevist
  - Gadodiamide: Omniscan
    - Nephrogenic systemic fibrosis has been reported as a sequela to the injection of intravenous paramagnetic contrast agents in human patients with renal insufficiency. This syndrome has not been reported in veterinary patients, but care should be taken when administering these agents to patients with renal dysfunction. Gadodiamide has a higher safety ratio than Gd-DTPA.
- Intravenous fluids
- Blankets/heated fluid pads or bags

Anticipated Time

The time required to perform the study depends on many factors:

- Field strength of the magnet: the higher the field strength of the magnet, the more quickly the study can be performed.
- Configuration/size of the radiofrequency coils
- Size of the area to be scanned
- Number and type of imaging sequences performed: with MRI, images are acquired in multiple planes and using multiple different imaging sequences; the more acquisitions performed, the longer the study

Approximate times (based on use of a 1.0-tesla magnet):

- Brain: 1-1.5 hours
- Spinal column
  - Cervical: 1-1.5 hours
  - T3-L3: 1.5-2 hours
  - Lumbar: 1-1.5 hours

Because of long scan times, it is important to determine neuroanatomic localization of spinal lesions so that only the affected area of the spinal column is scanned, particularly in large dogs.

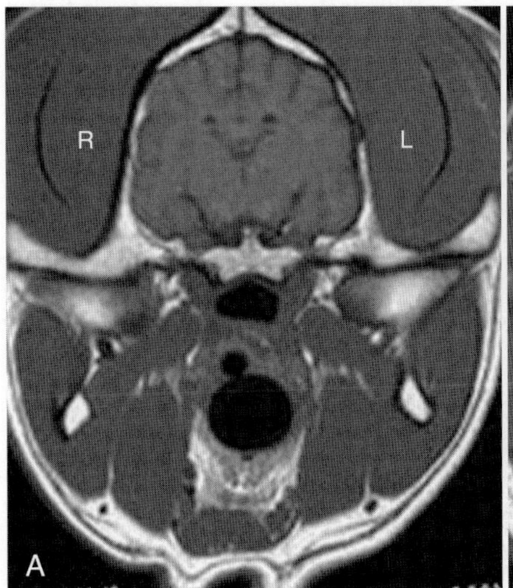

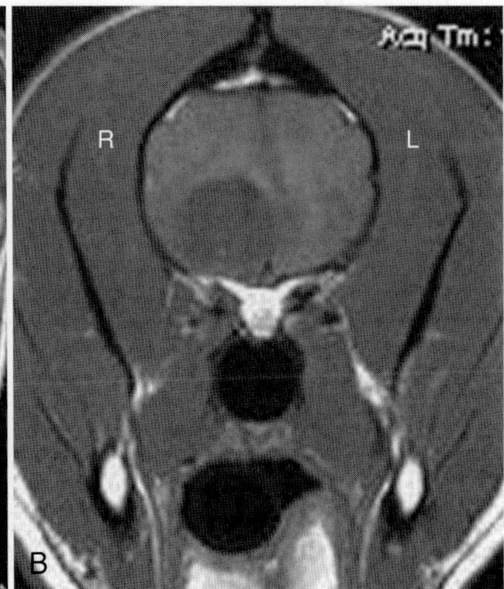

MAGNETIC RESONANCE IMAGING SCAN T1-weighted magnetic resonance images from a normal (**A**) and abnormal (**B**) canine brain. Images are from rostral to midcerebrum. In MRI, the imaging characteristics of tissues are determined by the imaging sequence used. To define the tissue characteristics of a lesion, multiple different imaging sequences are performed, and the appearance of the lesion in these images is compared. The term *intensity* is used for describing the appearance of tissues in scans. In the normal patient (**A**), there is a subtle difference in intensity between gray matter and white matter of the brain, and intensity of muscle is different from that of brain. This illustrates the level of soft-tissue contrast achieved with MRI. In the abnormal patient (**B**), note the large, round hypointense lesion with a slightly hyperintense rim in the right ventral cerebrum; the lesion causes left deviation of the falx cerebri. Differential diagnoses for mass lesions in the brain include neoplasia, granuloma formation, and abscess formation. In this case, the appearance of the lesion in multiple imaging sequences was consistent with a diagnosis of neoplasia with a central necrotic component.

Procedures and Techniques

Preparation: Important Checkpoints

- Obtain thorough patient history: pacemaker? nonferrous metallic implants/foreign bodies? ferrous metallic implants/foreign bodies?
- Routine laboratory evaluation: CBC, serum biochemistry panel
- +/− Thoracic radiographs
- +/− Abdominal radiographs or ultrasound
- Many patients undergoing MRI are older and may have multiple diseases. Routine laboratory evaluation and thoracic and abdominal screening may be indicated in these patients for two reasons: 1) to rule out the presence of concurrent disease that may affect the patient's ability to tolerate general anesthesia and 2) to identify the presence of any potentially life-shortening disease process unrelated to the primary complaint (e.g., incidental splenic mass).
- Make sure all needed equipment is available and functional. This is especially important if the study is to be performed at an outside (e.g., nonveterinary) facility.
- Preparation for general anesthesia
  - Routine preanesthetic fasting
  - Place IV catheter: when placing the catheter, the anticipated position of the patient in the MRI unit must be considered, and the catheter should be placed to allow easy access during the procedure. For example, in patients undergoing a scan of the head, it is convenient to have the IV catheter placed in the saphenous vein. This is, however, not an absolute requirement because the forelimb can be extended caudally for ease of access if the catheter is in a cephalic vein.
  - Clipping of hair in areas where monitoring devices are to be applied (depending on type of monitoring devices used)

Possible Complications and Common Errors to Avoid

- Complications associated with general anesthesia
- Burns induced by placement of cables
  - Objects within the magnet can become hot due to the effect of radiofrequency pulses. Monitoring cables within the magnet should not be coiled and should not be placed on the patient. Wrapping the cables in fabric (e.g., towels, blankets) will provide further protection.
- Injury to the patient and/or damage to the magnet can occur if careful attention is not paid to basic safety regarding the presence of metallic objects within range of the magnet (see above).

Procedure

- Anesthetize and intubate the patient.
- Move the patient to the MRI area and position within the gantry as dictated by the area of interest and the configuration of the radiofrequency coils.
- Connect IV fluids and monitoring devices; place blankets and water bottles.
- Scan.
- +/− Inject intravenous contrast agent.
  - Contrast is routinely used in brain imaging and sometimes used for imaging of the spinal column.
  - Gd-DTPA (Magnevist) 0.2 mL/kg IV bolus
  - Gadodiamide (Omniscan) 0.2 mL/kg IV bolus
- Rescan for postcontrast images.
- Briefly review images.
  - Evaluation of the images may suggest additional imaging sequences indicated in the particular case (e.g., obtaining T2*-weighted images in suspected hemorrhagic lesions).
  - Rarely, the images obtained will identify an additional area of concern that should be scanned before the patient is allowed to recover from general anesthesia.

Postprocedure

No additional considerations beyond routine monitoring of the patient during recovery from general anesthesia

Alternatives and Their Relative Merits

CT:

- Advantages
  - Shorter imaging time (and therefore shorter time under general anesthesia)
  - Better imaging of bone
- Disadvantages
  - Far inferior contrast resolution
  - Image acquisition is in only one plane.
  - Reformatted images have much lower spatial resolution than original images or MR images.
- If available, MRI is the preferred imaging method for evaluation of the central nervous system.

SUGGESTED READING

Gavin P, et al: Practical small animal MRI, Ames, IA, 2009, Wiley-Blackwell.

AUTHOR: Patricia L. Rose, DVM, MS, DACVR
EDITORS: Leah A. Cohn, DVM, PhD, DACVIM; Mark S. Thompson, DVM, DABVP

Nebulization, Coupage, and Respiratory Therapeutics

Difficulty Level: ♦♦

Synonyms

- Nebulization: aerosolization
- Coupage: thoracic wall percussion
- Pulmonary (chest) physical therapy
- Bronchial drainage/positioning

Overview and Goals

- Nebulizers are used for aerosolizing saline to humidify airway secretions or to aerosolize drugs to obtain high local concentrations while minimizing systemic absorption and toxicosis.
- Coupage aids in the removal of secretions from the tracheobronchial tree.
- Pulmonary (chest) physical therapy or bronchial drainage/positioning uses gravity-assisted positioning to assist mobilization of airway secretions.
- Early ambulation facilitates mobilization and clearance of airway secretions, changes the lung regions being ventilated, and maintains muscular tone and strength.
- Thoracic wall percussion/vibration moves loosened secretions from small airways to larger airways so they can be expectorated or suctioned.
- Airway suction is the active removal of airway secretions in patients with impaired mucociliary clearance. It reduces the risk of lower airway contamination from oropharyngeal contamination or atelectasis from mucus plugs.

Indications

Patients with inhalation injury (e.g., smoke inhalation [p. 919]) or retained secretions (recumbent patients, bacterial or fungal pneumonia [p. 795], asthma [p. 84], eosinophilic bronchopneumopathy, mechanically ventilated or intubated patients)

Contraindications

- Percussion/vibration usually is not suitable in patients with thoracic wall damage (i.e., fractured ribs or recent thoracotomy).
- Nebulized antibiotics are recommended in humans only for multidrug-resistant, gram-negative infections that are susceptible to aminoglycosides or polymyxin E (colistin); gram-positive bacterial infections are relative contraindications.

Equipment, Anesthesia

Three types of nebulizers:

- Jet nebulizers: employ oxygen under high pressure to generate the aerosol. Jet flow rate determines the rate of droplet generation and the droplet size distribution.
- Ultrasonic nebulizers: the aerosol is produced by the vibration of a piezoelectric crystal. Frequency and vibration amplitude determine drug output and droplet size.
- Vibrating mesh nebulizers: use a mesh or plate with multiple openings to generate the aerosol. Reported to have better lung parenchymal penetration

Drugs that are specifically formulated or reported to be aerosolized*:

- Antibiotics: aminoglycosides (amikacin, tobramycin/tobramycin solution for inhalation [TSI], and gentamicin), polymyxins (colistin or polymyxin E), and vancomycin
- Airway humidification: sterile 0.9% saline
- Antifungals: amphotericin B
- Bronchodilators: racemic epinephrine, beta-2 agonist (e.g., terbutaline, albuterol)
- Antiinflammatory: glucocorticoids, lidocaine
- Mucolytic drugs: *N*-acetylcysteine
- Oxygen free-radical scavengers: heparin/*N*-acetylcysteine combination

Anticipated Time

- Nebulization: 15-30 minutes to allow sufficient time for adequate drug delivery/effect. Longer times are generally not tolerated by the patient or the operator (poor compliance). Nebulization and coupage should be performed every 6-12 hours.
- Chest physical therapy, ambulation, percussion/vibration, and airway suctioning should be performed every 2-4 hours initially and gradually tapered as secretions improve.

Preparation: Important Checkpoints

- Keep equipment for nebulization and airway suction sterile. Gloves (sterile or clean) should be worn when manipulating equipment. Nebulization reservoirs should be replaced or cleaned daily and a new suction tip used for each suction.
- In-line suction units for mechanically ventilated patients can reduce the risk of iatrogenic infections.
- Clean and disinfect equipment between patients. Disposable parts (e.g., nebulization reservoirs) should be exchanged daily if contaminated and between patients.

*Information for most aerosolized drugs listed are extrapolated from experimental and human clinical studies, and use in dogs and cats is considered off-label.

Possible Complications and Common Errors to Avoid

Nebulization and coupage:

- Bronchoconstriction: most common and serious side effect. Using drug formulations not made for aerosolization increases the risk. Pretreatment or concurrent use of a bronchodilator may reduce the risk.
- Environmental waste: many nebulizers will continuously aerosolize drug even if the patient is not inhaling, allowing drug to be lost to the ambient air.
- Operator exposure: because of environmental contamination, operators may inhale some of the aerosolized drug or saline. A protective face mask can reduce the risk of exposure.
- Low deposition of certain drugs: to allow deep penetration to the lower airways, the majority of the droplets produced should be within the range of 1-5 micrometers. Nebulizer type, use of nonaerosolized drug formulations, and highly viscous solutions are causes of poor drug penetration.
- Iatrogenic infection: contamination of the nebulizer or drugs can effectively deliver potential pathogens into the deep airways of an already compromised patient.

Airway suctioning:

- Suctioning may cause tracheal irritation and bleeding, abrupt drop in partial pressure of oxygen, vagal stimulation, and bradycardia. Preoxygenating and limiting suction time have been shown to reduce the risk of hypoxemia.

Procedure

Nebulization and coupage:

- Follow manufacturer's instructions carefully to ensure proper use. In general, sterile 0.9% saline or the specific drug diluted with sterile 0.9% saline is instilled in the nebulizer reservoir. With the nebulizer on, place the reservoir approximately 2-3 inches (5-8 cm) from the patient's nose for 15-30 minutes. Face masks or tents can facilitate nebulization. Certain nebulizers can be attached to the inspiratory limb of a ventilation circuit, facilitating nebulization in mechanically ventilated patients.
- Perform coupage after nebulization by repeatedly percussing both sides of a patient's chest wall simultaneously, typically while standing above and behind the patient and using cupped hands and gentle force. Coupage for 15-30 seconds or less if coupage triggers repeated coughing

Pulmonary (chest) physical therapy:

- In the true sense, this involves 12 basic positions for postural drainage. The simplest and most practical form for clinical practice is to turn recumbent patients side to side every 2 hours to aid in mobilization of airway secretions.

Early ambulation:

- Assist and encourage patients to ambulate, even for short distances. In the author's experience, this is essential to the successful treatment of pneumonia in recumbent, large-breed dogs (e.g., wolfhounds).

Thoracic wall percussion/vibration:

- Manual or mechanical vibrations to vibrate the thoracic cage

Airway suctioning in comatose or anesthetized animals and/or animals with a tracheostomy:

- Preoxygenate with 100% oxygen for a minimum of 1 minute before suctioning.
- The patient should be positioned with the head raised at a 45° angle and the catheter inserted into the endotracheal/tracheostomy tube.
- Suction should begin while the catheter is gradually withdrawn from the airway. Do not suction for more than 15 seconds without reoxygenation. Oropharyngeal secretions should be suctioned after tracheal suctioning.

Postprocedure

- Monitor closely for desaturation and hypoxemia after the application/administration of any of the above therapies.
- Decompensation may occur as a result of bronchoconstriction, incomplete mobilization of mucus causing airway obstruction, tracheal irritation, or exhaustion.

Alternatives and Their Relative Merits

Metered-dose inhaler (MDI; p. 1122) is a more practical alternative for at-home delivery of specific medications. However, only certain medications are routinely available in MDI form.

SUGGESTED READING

Chow KE, et al: Scintigraphic assessment of deposition of radiolabeled fluticasone delivered from a nebulizer and metered dose inhaler in 10 healthy dogs. J Vet Intern Med 31(suppl 31), 2017, https://doi.org/10.1111/jvim.14832/.

AUTHOR: Michael Ethier, DVM, DVSc, DACVECC
EDITORS: Leah A. Cohn, DVM, PhD, DACVIM; Mark S. Thompson, DVM, DABVP

Neurologic Examination

Difficulty level: ♦

Overview and Goal

To evaluate a patient's neurologic function through clinical physical assessment of mentation, gait, posture, postural reactions, spinal nerve reflexes, and cranial nerve examination. The goal in a patient with a nervous system lesion is to establish the anatomic location of that lesion. The anatomic diagnosis will determine the differential diagnosis and the choice of ancillary studies to be recommended.

Indications

Reasons for an owner to present a patient for a neurologic examination:

- Seizures (p. 903), abnormal spontaneous uncontrolled movements, pacing, circling, head pressing, tremors (p. 994)
- Abnormal mentation: depressed to unresponsive, no recognition of owner, loss of trained habits, excreting indoors
- Abnormal gait: lame, paretic (pp. 756 and 757), ataxic (p. 86), paralyzed, collapsing
- Loss of balance, hearing, vision (p. 123)
- Head tilt (p. 403), unable to close eyelids, unable to prehend food or swallow, protruded third eyelid, pupil asymmetry, eye deviation
- Regurgitation (p. 873), dyspnea (p. 879)

Contraindications

- Aggressive patient
- Injured patient for whom manipulation may exacerbate the nervous system lesion and the examination is limited to the recumbent patient

Equipment, Anesthesia

- Quiet area
- Outdoor area or a room large enough to evaluate the gait
- Nonskid floor surface; indoor-outdoor carpet works well
- Pleximeter, source of bright light, small forceps

Anticipated Time

About 10-20 minutes

Preparation: Important Checkpoints

- Assess for contraindications (see above).
- NOTE: To avoid introducing bias, review existing diagnostic test results (e.g., lab tests, radiographs) *after* performing the neurologic examination.

Possible Complications and Common Errors to Avoid

- Do not be biased by a single abnormality.
- Do the same methodical, thorough evaluation on every patient, regardless of the complaint or the signs that are evident.

Procedure

There are five main components to the neurologic examination: sensorium, gait, postural reactions, spinal reflexes, and cranial nerves. The order in which the five components are evaluated depends on the patient's behavior and chief complaint.

- Sensorium: owners are best able to evaluate subtle changes in their animal's behavior or sensorium. In increasing severity, sensorium changes are depression, lethargy, obtundation, semicoma (stupor), and coma.
- Gait: diagnosis of gait disorders is based on pattern recognition for specific anatomic sites in the nervous system (and musculoskeletal system). They are best evaluated with the patient moving on grass or a rug where slipping is not a problem. As a rule, changes are best seen with the patient walking slowly and taking numerous slow turns. Two qualities of paresis and three qualities of ataxia are considered in gait analysis:
  - Paresis (neurogenic abnormality of muscle activity tone/strength)
    - Lower motor neuron (LMN) paresis causes a loss of ability to support weight, reflected in rapid, short strides with collapsing on the affected limb. The patient walks with a lame gait.
    - Upper motor neuron (UMN) paresis interferes with gait generation, delaying the protraction of the affected limb and lengthening the stride. This form of paresis cannot be separated from general proprioceptive (GP) ataxia because of the close association of the caudal projecting UMN tracts and cranial projecting GP tracts in any transverse section of the spinal cord and caudal brainstem.
  - Ataxia (incoordination)
    - GP ataxia creates the appearance of the patient not knowing where its limb(s) is/are located in space. This also results in a delay in protraction of the limb and a prolonged stride, and the patient may show an excessive medial (adduction) or lateral (abduction) excursion of the limb as it is protracted. Both UMN and GP deficits can cause the patient to occasionally stand on the dorsal aspect of its paw.
    - Vestibular ataxia is evident when the patient has a head tilt and drifts or stumbles to the side from loss of balance.
    - Cerebellar ataxia is characterized by a delay in protraction and an excessive response, a dysmetric abrupt gait generation that usually is associated with some balance loss. As a rule, sudden flexion movements predominate.
- Postural reactions: normal postural reactions require most components of the peripheral and central nervous systems to be intact. The most reliable of the postural reactions is the hopping response.
  - Hopping response: each limb is tested by holding the patient so that most of the weight is borne on the limb to be tested, and the patient is moved laterally on that limb:
    - First, straddle the patient so that you and the patient are facing in the same direction.
    - Palpate the thoracic limbs to determine if any denervation or disuse atrophy is present.
    - Flex and extend the limbs to determine range of motion and muscle tone.
    - Place the paw on its dorsal surface—the paw replacement test—and observe how quickly it is replaced. NOTE: This is not just a test of conscious proprioception (CP) because disorders of the UMN, LMN, and/or general somatic afferent cutaneous receptors can result in a delay in this response. A sole CP deficit cannot be determined, and that term should be discarded from the neurologic examination. Be aware that many normal patients may delay in replacing the paw to its supporting position.
    - Brace your own elbow on your ipsilateral knee and support the abdomen so that most of the patient's weight is on its thoracic limbs.
    - With your other arm, pick up the patient's thoracic limb on that side, and push the patient laterally away from that limb. This forces the patient to hop on the opposite thoracic limb.
    - After three or four hops, do not move, but just reverse both thoracic limbs so that you can pick up the opposite thoracic limb and hop the patient back on the contralateral thoracic limb.
    - Compare one thoracic limb with the other only when it is being hopped laterally.
    - Move back to the pelvic limbs, and repeat the muscle palpation, range of motion, and paw replacement.
    - At that time, check the tail and anus for tone and reflex response.
    - Stand beside the patient, and with one arm placed under the sternum, pick the patient up so it is standing on its pelvic limbs.
    - Pick up the closest pelvic limb, and push the patient away so that it hops laterally on the opposite pelvic limb.
    - Repeat this maneuver on the opposite side.

- Always compare the thoracic limbs with each other and then the pelvic limbs with each other because the response in the pelvic limbs normally tends to be slower than that of the thoracic limbs.
- For very large dogs, it is easier to make the same observations while the dog is hemiwalked.
- For hemiwalking, stand beside the patient, and pick up the ipsilateral thoracic and pelvic limbs so they are located at your side. Then push the patient gently away.
- These hopping responses are much more reliable than the paw replacement test.

- Spinal reflexes: for spinal reflex testing, the patient should be placed in lateral recumbency.
  - Manipulate the limbs to assess muscle tone.
  - With the patient relaxed and the stifle slightly flexed, elicit the patellar reflex by tapping on the patellar tendon. If it is not present in one or both limbs, always place the patient in the opposite recumbency, and repeat the patellar reflex before concluding that it is absent. Some old dogs with no neurologic complaints lack the patellar reflex. This is the only reliable tendon reflex because the other myotactic reflexes (e.g., triceps, biceps, extensor carpi radialis) may not be present in some normal animals.
  - The withdrawal-flexor reflex is routinely tested by gently compressing the base of the claw in each paw with forceps and observing the strength of the limb flexion and the patient's response (e.g., abrupt turning, vocalization) to the noxious stimulus. NOTE: The sensory modality that is tested is not pain. A noxious stimulus is used, and what is observed is the patient's reaction to this conscious perception (nociception). Pain is the patient's response to a noxious stimulus. It is often difficult to determine a patient's response to a minimal noxious stimulus, and there is no practical value to differentiating the patient's response to light and strong noxious stimuli (pp. 1257 and 1258).
- Cranial nerves: sitting down on the floor with your back against the wall and knees flexed is the best position from which to evaluate small dogs and cats. Place the patient between your thighs and hold its head while testing the function of the cranial nerves. You can perform this cranial nerve exam on larger dogs by straddling them so that you and the dog are both looking in the same direction. Proper evaluation requires a relaxed, almost motionless patient. Use a regional approach, starting with the eyes:
  - Menace response
    - The menace response assesses vision and facial nerve function as long as the stimulus of the hand thrust at the patient's face does not touch the face or whiskers or create excessive air movement.
    - If there is no response, be sure the eyelids are able to close (i.e., there is no facial paralysis).
    - If there is a normal palpebral reflex or spontaneous eyelid closure but still no menace response, tap the eyelids or face gently to get the patient's attention, and then repeat the menace gesture.
    - Failure to close the eyelids to a menace in a patient > 10 weeks old with normal facial nerve function or the lack of eyeball or head retraction in a patient with facial paralysis indicates a lesion in some part of the visual pathway from the eyeball to the occipital lobe.
    - Patients with significant cerebellar disorders that have no menace response are still visual.
    - Assessing the menace response before shining a light in the patient's eyes avoids falsely compromising the menace response with the glare of the light.
  - Pupil size and pupillary light reflex
    - With a strong light source, assess the size and symmetry of the pupils from a distance.
    - Bring the light to about 1-2 cm from the eye, and swing it from one eye to the other and back again.
    - Repeat this to be sure that with the light in one eye, the pupils of both eyes are constricting.
    - Deficits in this light reflex implicate a lesion in the eye/optic nerve (optic chiasm or tracts) and/or the general visceral efferent component of the oculomotor nerve.
  - Ocular position and movement
    - Observe the position of the eyeballs for strabismus, and test abduction (abducent, VI) and adduction (oculomotor, III) nerve function by moving the head side to side while observing the eyes.
    - Look for a resting nystagmus. If not present, look for a positional nystagmus with the head held flexed laterally to either side and then extended dorsally. Occasionally, it is worthwhile to look for this sign with the patient placed in dorsal recumbency.
  - Trigeminal nerve (V)
    - Palpate the muscles of mastication (motor, V) for denervation atrophy.
    - Recheck the palpebral reflex by stimulating the lateral and medial canthi with blunt forceps (sensory, V; motor, VII).
    - Place the blunt forceps against the nasal septum on each side to assess the ophthalmic (V) and the nociceptive pathway to the opposite somesthetic cortex.
    - Observe for ear movement and lip symmetry and tone (VII).
    - Open the mouth to assess muscle tone (motor, V) and range of motion.
  - Glossopharyngeal (IX), vagus (X), and hypoglossal (XII)
    - Observe the tongue for its size and movements (XII).
    - Place one finger in the oropharynx to determine the muscle tone and the patient's response to the presence of the finger—the gag reflex (IX and X).

Postprocedure

By establishing the anatomic diagnosis (location of the lesion in the nervous system), the results of the neurologic exam allow a differential diagnosis to be established and a diagnostic plan to be created.

SUGGESTED READING

de Lahunta A, et al: Veterinary neuroanatomy and clinical neurology, ed 3, St. Louis, 2009, Saunders.

AUTHOR: Alexander de Lahunta, DVM, PhD, DACVIM, DACVP

EDITORS: Leah A. Cohn, DVM, PhD, DACVIM; Mark S. Thompson, DVM, DABVP

Ophthalmic Examination

Difficulty level: ◆

Overview and Goal

Basic examination of the structure and function of the eyes and adnexa (surrounding structures) to establish an ophthalmic diagnosis, prognosis, and treatment plan and to evaluate the need for additional diagnostic testing or referral

Indications

- An abnormal appearance to the eye(s) or adnexa
- Ocular discomfort or trauma
- Vision impairment/loss
- Systemic disease that may have ocular manifestations

Contraindications

A very aggressive patient, particularly with a fragile eye, may not tolerate an awake ocular examination without injuring the patient or examiner.

Equipment, Anesthesia

- Exam table in a quiet room that can be darkened
- Bright focal light source (well-charged Finoff transilluminator or otoscope without a cone)
- Schirmer tear test (STT) strips
- Fluorescein dye–impregnated strips
- Rose Bengal dye–impregnated strips (optional)
- Sterile saline/eye irrigating solution
- Topical anesthetic (e.g., 0.5% proparacaine), often refrigerated
- Tonometer (e.g., Schiøtz, Tono-Pen, TonoVet)
- 1% tropicamide (optional)
- Magnifying or fundic lens (lens strength of 20-28 diopters [D] or a 2.2 lens good for general use) or direct ophthalmoscope
- Muzzle for aggressive patients
- Sedation and/or anesthesia are generally not necessary and may hinder a good examination.

Anticipated Time

About 10-20 minutes (longer if mydriatics are used)

Preparation: Important Checkpoints

- Adequate restraint greatly aids examination and is generally best performed by one or more assistants, not the owner. Muzzle dogs if necessary.
- Examine the animal at eye level (on exam table); large dogs may be examined on the floor, sitting up, and if necessary, backed into a corner.
- Cats especially can become enophthalmic during examination; frequent repositioning of the body or the use of other stimuli are often necessary to reduce enophthalmos.

Possible Complications and Common Errors to Avoid

- Fragile eyes (ruptured eyes, descemetoceles) should be handled extremely gently, if at all. NOTE: do not palpate, retropulse, or measure intraocular pressure in these eyes.
- Perform STT before any topicals are applied (these alter the wetness of the ocular surface); assess fluorescein staining before tonometry (tonometry may give false appearance of corneal lesions); assess pupillary motion before pharmacologic mydriasis. NOTE: do not give mydriatics if glaucoma (p. 387) is a possibility.
- Patient fear/anxiety and/or a weak light source are common causes for an apparently weak pupillary light response (PLR).

Procedure

- Grossly assess functional vision as the animal walks to/in the exam room: Does the animal navigate confidently, easily avoiding objects? Does it walk slowly and cautiously, using its whiskers and other senses to navigate? Is it easily startled by obstacles? Does vision appear to be worse on one side than the other?
- Test vision by dropping cotton balls or gauze into different areas of the visual field. Functional vision can also be tested using an obstacle course in an enclosed area. The best obstacles are relatively large, safe to bump into, and free of odor. Vary the course during the test. Do not provide excessive nonvisual guidance (sound, food). Repeat in dim light if indicated.
- Looking at the face head-on in room light, assess the overall appearance and symmetry of the head and orbits, resting pupil size, and globe size, position, and motility. Note any ocular discharge or tear staining.
  - Evaluate the eyelid shape and conformation before manipulating the head.
  - Palpate the muscles of mastication, and assess the degree of globe retropulsion through the closed lids. Palpate both eyes simultaneously to best assess symmetry.
  - Retropulsing each eye individually elevates the nictitans, which can then be evaluated for presence, shape, coloration, motility, and abnormalities.
- Assess the cranial nerves bilaterally (p. 1136)
  - Menace response (II afferent, VII efferent): covering one eye, perform a menacing gesture to the open eye to elicit a blink, without stimulating the vibrissae or face. Hold your hand flat and vertical with its lateral aspect toward the animal's eye or use just one finger to allow testing of smaller areas of the visual field while minimizing air motion.
    - Cerebellar disease may cause absence of the menace response without loss of vision.
    - Very young puppies and kittens normally do not menace.
  - Palpebral reflex (sensory V afferent, VII efferent): lightly touch the lateral and medial canthi to stimulate blinking. Observe for completeness of blinking.
    - In cases where the lids are unable to close but sensation is present (e.g., facial paralysis, exophthalmos), globe retraction and nictitans elevation (± III, IV, VI efferent) or head withdrawal may be seen instead.
  - Dazzle reflex (II afferent, VII efferent): rapidly apply a very bright focal light to one eye. This should cause the eye to blink (subcortical pathway). An intact dazzle does not alone signify vision so much as some degree of retinal and optic nerve function.
  - Pupillary light reflex (II afferent, III efferent): apply a bright light to one eye, and observe ipsilateral (direct PLR) and contralateral (indirect or consensual PLR) pupillary constriction. Note the degree and speed of pupillary constriction.
- If mucoid ocular discharge is present, measure tear production.
  - Gently wipe away very large clumps of discharge if they will obstruct placement of the tear test strip, without touching the lid margins or ocular surface.
  - Keeping the proximal end of the STT strip in the package, fold at the notch. Place the folded tip between the lower lid and globe. Close lids if necessary, keep strip in for 60 seconds, and immediately replace if blinked out.
  - Low is < 10 mm/min, borderline is 10-15 mm/min, normal is > 15 mm/min wetting in dogs and cats (sometimes even lower for many normal cats).
  - If a corneal herpetic lesion is suspected, apply Rose Bengal dye. Place a drop of sterile saline to a Rose Bengal–impregnated strip, and lightly touch (or allow a drop to fall on) to the dorsal bulbar conjunctiva. Allow the lids to blink. Examine the cornea with focal white light for dye retention, indicating the presence of nonvital epithelial cells, and for a characteristic dendritic dye uptake pattern.
- If corneal ulceration (p. 209) is suspected, apply fluorescein. Place a drop of sterile saline or proparacaine on a fluorescein strip, and lightly touch the strip (or allow a drop to fall on) to the dorsal bulbar conjunctiva. Allow the lids to blink. Flush excess fluorescein with saline to prevent false-positive results (ocular discharge, epithelialized but irregular corneal surfaces). Examine in a darkened room, ideally with cobalt light/Wood's lamp. Fluorescein uptake indicates an absence of corneal epithelium.
  - In 1-5 minutes, fluorescein may appear at the nostril(s) or mouth, indicating nasolacrimal patency (positive Jones test). NOTE: a negative Jones test result does not necessarily indicate nasolacrimal duct obstruction.
- Retroilluminate the eyes to identify opacities in the visual axis.
  - Hold the transilluminator above your ear, and shine it into the animal's eyes. Adjust your position (usually to below the level of the animal) until you see the tapetal reflection. Opacities in the clear ocular media will appear silhouetted.
- Carefully examine the surface and anterior segments of the eyes in dim light with a bright focal light or transilluminator. Note the lid margins, nasolacrimal puncta, bulbar and palpebral conjunctivae, cornea and anterior chamber, iris surface, pupil, and anterior lens.
  - Holding the light from the side (across the plane of the iris) will aid greatly in accentuating the three-dimensionality of anterior chamber structures.
- Examine the fundus, noting the optic nerve, retinal vessels, tapetum, and nontapetum.
  - A drop of tropicamide may be given for mydriasis (contraindicated if there is any suspicion of glaucoma). Wait 20-30 minutes after applying; effects will last for 2-4 hours.

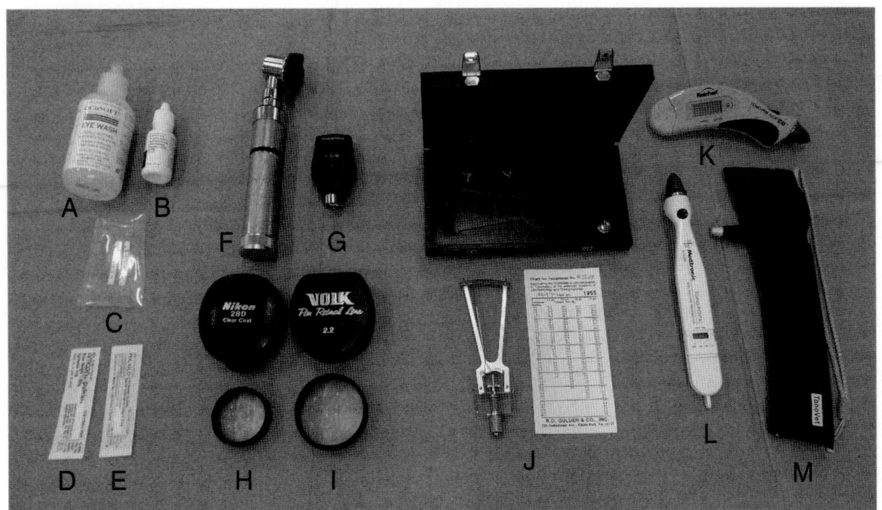

OPHTHALMIC EXAMINATION Selected equipment and materials that may be used during an ophthalmic examination. **A**, Sterile eye irrigating solution. **B**, A 0.5% proparacaine solution. **C**, Schirmer tear test (STT) strips in packaging. **D**, Rose Bengal strip in packaging. **E**, Fluorescein strip in packaging. **F**, Otoscope head on base of direct ophthalmoscope. **G**, Direct ophthalmoscope head. **H**, A 28 diopter (28D) fundic lens with case. **I**, A 2.2 fundic lens with case. **J.** Schiøtz tonometer with box, weights, test block, and conversion chart. **K**, Tono-Pen Avia tonometer. **J**, Tono-Pen tonometer. **M**, TonoVet tonometer (no probe tip loaded).

- Indirect ophthalmoscopy: the preferred method because it provides a wider view that is easier to interpret and is safer for the examiner:
  - Using a fundic lens and bright focal light or transilluminator, position yourself as for performing retroillumination (described above), an arm's length away from the animal. The assistant should hold the lids open. If using an aspheric fundic lens, hold the lens' flatter side (white rim) toward the animal. Place the lens 1-2 inches from the animal's eye, and then move it toward you slightly until the fundic view (inverted and backward) fills the lens. Examine the whole fundus, adjusting as if the fulcrum of the line of sight is at the animal's lens (e.g., move laterally for a more medial view).
- Direct ophthalmoscopy: provides a highly magnified view of very small areas of the fundus, with the examiner very close to the patient
  - To allow the widest area to be examined, use your right eye to examine the animal's right eye, and use your left eye to examine the animal's left eye.
  - With the largest white circle setting and the diopter dial set on 0, focus on the fundus by viewing the eye from 2-6 inches (5-15 cm) from the animal. View as many areas as possible. Adjust the focus if needed by changing diopter settings, which allow focusing at different depths when used at a fixed distance and any correction required by your eyes. The image is a direct image (not reversed).
  - If blepharospasm or resistance on the part of the animal is seen, dim the light, apply the polarizing filter, or use a smaller circle size.
  - The crosshairs in the fixation aperture may be used for measuring fundic structures. Size comparison may also be made to the size of the optic nerve head.
  - The red-free (green) filter allows for differentiation between fundic blood, which appears black, and melanin, which appears brown.
  - An optional cobalt filter may be used for detecting fluorescein-positive corneal lesions.
  - The slit-beam (thin, long rectangle) setting may help in detecting three-dimensionality of anterior segment lesions. View the beam on the eye directly and not through the ophthalmoscope window.

- If the eye is red or cloudy, the pupil is abnormal, or there is vision loss, perform tonometry. Palpation of the globes with the fingers alone is inadequate to measure intraocular pressure (IOP). Referral is necessary if you cannot perform tonometry when indicated. Apply a drop of topical anesthetic (may not be necessary with TonoVet tonometer). Avoid pressure on the ventral neck, lids, or globes.
  - Schiøtz: assemble the tonometer and clean the footplate. Test the tonometer by placing it on the included test block (gives a scale reading of 0). Position the animal with iris plane parallel to floor (dorsal recumbency or sitting up with nose pointed up). Holding the tonometer by the handles and keeping it vertical, gently rest the footplate on the central cornea (not the third eyelid or sclera) until a single reading is produced. Repeat two to three times, and use included chart to get actual IOP. If IOP is > 25 mm Hg, repeat with next additional smallest weight. Record IOP in mm Hg (not as scale readings). Clean after use.
  - Tono-Pen: Properly fit a clean tip cover, turn on, and calibrate if necessary. Gently touch the instrument tip to the cornea, making brief contact and keeping it perpendicular to the corneal surface; it does not need to be horizontal. Repeat several times until a long beep is heard. A bar over the 5% value at the bottom indicates a statistically acceptable reading in mm Hg.
  - TonoVet: Properly insert a new probe tip. Turn on and ensure that proper species calibration is on. Holding the instrument horizontal with the tip 4-8 mm from and perpendicular to the cornea, repeatedly press the button to take readings until a long beep is heard. A nonblinking *d* before the reading indicates a statistically significant, dog-/cat-calibrated reading.
  - Normal IOP in dogs and cats is 15-25 mm Hg.

Postprocedure

Flush corneas of excess fluorescein if necessary. Protect eyes from light if mydriatics were used.

AUTHOR: Jane Cho, DVM, DACVO
EDITORS: Leah A. Cohn, DVM, PhD, DACVIM; Mark S. Thompson, DVM, DABVP

Oral/Dental Examination and Charting

Bonus Material Online 

Difficulty Level: ◆

Overview and Goal

Inspection and palpation of extraoral and intraoral, hard and soft tissues should be performed in such a manner that an overall picture of oral health and disease can be drawn and further diagnostic measures and treatment options planned. A complete diagnosis and treatment plan can be formulated only after examination under sedation or general anesthesia.

Indications

An oral examination should be performed as part of each wellness visit and is necessary with any complaint relating to halitosis (p. 402), oral discomfort, pawing at the face, difficulty opening or closing the mouth, drooling (p. 833), oral bleeding, nasal or ocular signs, difficulty eating/drinking/swallowing, inappetence, weight loss, facial asymmetry, oral masses and swellings around the mouth, or a history of head trauma (p. 404).

Contraindications

- Vicious animals (examination under sedation/anesthesia if clinical signs warrant)
- Patients in severe pain (examination under sedation/anesthesia)

Equipment, Anesthesia

- Conscious oral examination
  - Inspection: good light source
  - Palpation: gloves, pen
- Oral examination under sedation/anesthesia
  - Inspection: good light source, magnifying loupes, headlamp
  - Palpation: gloves, dental explorer, periodontal probe, dental mirror
  - Dental radiography

Anticipated Time

- Patient history: 3-5 minutes
- Conscious oral examination: 3-5 minutes
- Oral examination under sedation/anesthesia: 2-4 minutes
  - With periodontal probing and dental exploration: additional 3-5 minutes
  - With dental radiography: additional 10-15 minutes for cats, additional 15-20 minutes for dogs

Preparation: Important Checkpoints

Obtain a full patient history:

- Diet and supplements
- Access to treats and toys
- Abnormal chewing patterns
- Home oral hygiene (e.g., tooth brushing, use of oral care products)
- Medications (and responsiveness to medications)
- Patient's environment (indoor/outdoor, other pets)
- Vaccination and neuter status
- Previous medical issues (including dental/oral care performed)
- Current medical issues
- Presenting complaint: as noted in Indications (above) and
  - Rapid lower jaw or tongue movements
  - Preferential chewing on one side of the mouth
  - Plaque and calculus accumulation on teeth (p. 776)
  - Mobile teeth, losing teeth, missing teeth
  - Dropping food from the mouth or nose
  - Sneezing, nasal discharge

Examining for systemic disease (to assess the anesthetic risk or to determine the possibility of dental/oral lesions being secondary to a systemic condition)

- Preanesthetic testing (p. 1196)
- Coagulation profile, buccal mucosal bleeding times (occasionally indicated) (pp. 1076 and 1325)
- Cardiac evaluation (pp. 1094 and 1096) or other complementary examinations performed as necessary
- Cats with acute or chronic oral inflammation (beyond gingivitis): tested for feline leukemia virus (FeLV [p. 329]), feline immunodeficiency virus (FIV [pp. 325]), and occasionally for feline bartonellosis (p. 111)

Know the deciduous and permanent dentitions in the cat and dog (using the modified Triadan system):

- Right maxillary quadrant = 100 (500 when referring to deciduous teeth)
- Left maxillary quadrant = 200 (600 when referring to deciduous teeth)
- Left mandibular quadrant = 300 (700 when referring to deciduous teeth)
- Right mandibular quadrant = 400 (800 when referring to deciduous teeth)
- Each tooth is assigned a number within each quadrant. Beginning with 01 for the first incisor (the one closest to the midline), teeth are consecutively numbered from mesial (the surface of the tooth that faces the midline of the dental arch) to distal (the surface of the tooth that faces away from the midline of the dental arch).
- Because the dog has a full set of permanent premolars, tooth numbering is consecutive from 01 to 10 on the upper jaw and 01 to 11 on the lower jaw. The canines (04), the fourth premolars (08) of the upper jaw, and the first molars (09) of the lower jaw represent reference teeth to allow counting forward or backward when numbering teeth.
- The permanent maxillary first premolar (05) and the permanent mandibular first (05) and second (06) premolars are absent in the cat. Because the maxillary fourth premolar (08) is the largest cheek tooth of the upper jaw, counting forward identifies the premolars between the canine and fourth premolar as the maxillary second and third premolars (06 and 07). Similarly, knowing that the mandibular first molar (09) is the largest cheek tooth of the lower jaw allows you to identify the mandibular premolars between the canine and first molar as the mandibular third and fourth premolars (07 and 08).
- Taking the quadrant and tooth number into consideration, three numbers are used for identifying a specific tooth. For example, the permanent right maxillary fourth premolar is tooth 108, and the permanent left maxillary second premolar is tooth 206. The deciduous right maxillary canine is tooth 504, and the deciduous right mandibular fourth premolar is tooth 808.

Possible Complications and Common Errors to Avoid

- Not being able to distinguish lesions from normal anatomic structures. For example, certain normal structures are often misidentified as tumors.
  - Unpaired incisive papilla in midline of most rostral hard palate
  - Lingual molar gland immediately caudolingual to mandibular first molar bilaterally
  - Unnamed frenulum-like structure attaching lower lip bilaterally to mandibles between canine and first premolar (dog) or third premolar (cat)
- Not being able to match a reported symptom with an identifiable sign if an oral examination is not completed
- Not charting (compiling data on computerized or paper clinical records) so that symptoms/signs, diagnostic tests performed/treatments instituted, and patient progression can be shared between professional veterinary health care providers
- Being injured by the patient during conscious or sedated/anesthetized oral examination
- Injuring the patient during conscious or sedated/anesthetized oral examination (do not use dental explorers and periodontal probes in conscious patients)

Procedure

Extraoral examination:

- Watch the animal eat and drink (if the owner reports abnormal eating and drinking).
- Inspect and palpate eyes, ears, nose, masticatory muscles, face, lips, and jaws.
- Evaluate the presence of airflow from each nostril (have one closed with a thumb while airflow from the other nostril is evaluated with a plucked tuft of the animal's hair or a chilled microscope slide).
- Observe discharge from oral, nasal, and ocular orifices, sinus tracts, and ears.

- Evaluate external skin lesions (traumatic, infectious, inflammatory, neoplastic).
- Note asymmetry (including muscle volume), facial swellings, exophthalmos or enophthalmos (check for ability to retropulse the eyes by gently pushing them through the closed eyelids into their orbits).
- Palpate the jaws, intermandibular tissues, zygomatic arches, and neck for pain, asymmetry, discontinuity, crepitus, and emphysema.
- Assess the range of mouth opening by measuring the distance between the incisive edges of the upper and lower incisors.

Intraoral examination (with mouth closed):

- Examine mucocutaneous areas, then retract the animal's upper and lower lips.
- Assess teeth for their presence, structural integrity (wear, fracture), root exposure (gingival recession vs. extrusion), deposits (plaque, calculus), color (external/internal stain), sensitivity (gently knock on teeth along the dental arch with a pen).
- Note moisture, integrity, color, pigmentation of the oral mucosa and the location, size, thickness, surface characteristics (e.g., texture, inflammation, bleeding), and symmetry of any abnormal lesions.

Intraoral examination (with mouth open):

- Mouth opening facilitated when the animal's head is rotated dorsally
  - Dog: hold muzzle with one hand, place thumb of that same hand just caudal to maxillary canine teeth against rostral hard palate, and rotate head dorsally.
  - Cat: hold entire head (in the area of the zygomatic arches) with one hand, and rotate it dorsally.
- Open mouth by pushing lower jaw ventrally with index finger of other hand.
- First, inspect structures that are not visible when the mouth is closed (i.e., palate, tongue, sublingual area, and lingual/palatal aspects of the teeth).
- Ventral surface of the tongue and sublingual tissues become more visible when carefully pushing the thumb of the second hand dorsally into the intermandibular area (which raises the tongue).
- Dorsal surface of the caudal tongue, soft palate, palatine tonsils, and oropharynx becomes more visible when tongue is pushed ventrally with index and middle fingers of that same hand.
- Nasopharynx is palpable when extending the middle finger of that same hand along the hard palate caudally and pushing it against the soft palate dorsally.

Intraoral examination (with mouth open in the sedated/anesthetized patient):

- Assess structural integrity of teeth with a dental explorer; the pointed tip can detect irregularities of the crown surface and determine whether pulp exposure has occurred in a fractured tooth (p. 980).
- Inspect gingiva and alveolar mucosa over the roots of teeth, and palpate for the presence of swellings and sinus tracts, which may indicate endodontic disease or neoplasia.
- Gently insert periodontal probe into the space between the tooth and gingiva (gingival sulcus), and obtain measurements around the entire circumference of each tooth.
  - Cat: not deeper than 0.5 mm
  - Dog: not deeper than 3 mm
  - Deeper measurements indicating presence of periodontal pockets or, in the case of gingival enlargement, pseudopockets
- Other periodontal parameters: plaque and calculus (tartar) accumulation, gingival index, gingival recession or enlargement, total attachment loss, tooth mobility, and missing teeth, tooth resorption (p. 982)
- Other abnormalities: persistent (retained) deciduous teeth, supernumerary teeth, dental or skeletal malocclusion, circumscribed ulcers, widespread oral inflammation, oral masses, lacerations, and other signs of trauma

Postprocedure

Dental and oral charts represent legal documents and are essential parts of every patient's medical record.

Pearls

- Become familiar with the Triadan tooth numbering system.
- Learn how to use a dental explorer and periodontal probe.
- Clinical signs may not be apparent to the owner until the disease is well advanced.
- Obvious lesions such as fractured teeth, moderate to severe periodontal disease,

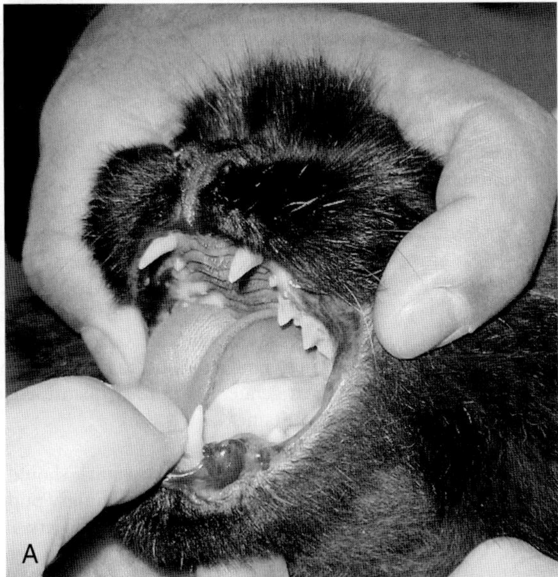

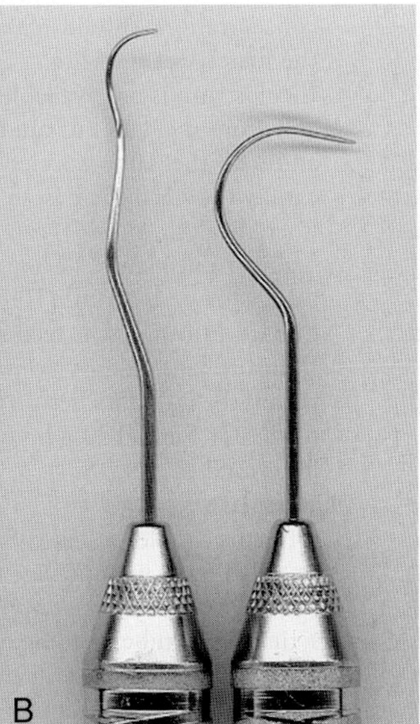

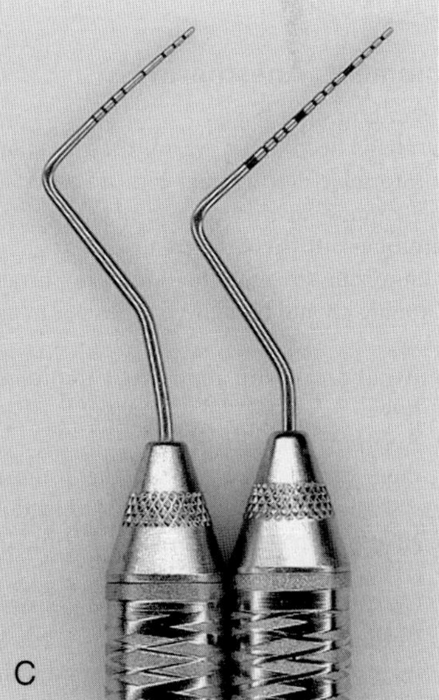

ORAL/DENTAL EXAMINATION AND CHARTING A, Mouth opening in a cat. The cat's head is held and rotated slightly dorsally with one hand, while the index finger of the other hand opens the mouth by pushing the lower jaw ventrally. Gently forcing the thumb of the same hand into the intermandibular area will raise the tongue, allowing inspection of its ventral surface and the sublingual tissues. **B**, Dental explorers (not to be used in conscious patients): the 11/12 ODU explorer on the left is preferred for use in cats and small dogs, and the shepherd's hook on the right is used in mid- to larger-sized dogs. **C**, Periodontal probes (not to be used in conscious patients): the Michigan O with Williams markings at 1, 2, 3, 5, 7, 8, 9, and 10 mm on the left is preferred in cats and small dogs, and the CP-15 UNC with markings at each millimeter and wide, black markings at 5, 10, and 15 mm on the right is preferred for mid- to larger-sized dogs. (Copyright Dr. Alexander M. Reiter.)

stomatitis, and oral masses can often be identified in the conscious patient.
- Sedation/anesthesia is usually required for a thorough intraoral examination and application of more sophisticated diagnostic tools.

SUGGESTED READING

Reiter AM, et al: Dentistry for the surgeon. In Tobias KM, et al, editors: Veterinary surgery: small animal, St. Louis, 2012, Elsevier, pp 1037-1053.

AUTHOR: Alexander M. Reiter, DVM, Dr. med. vet., DAVDC, DEVDC
EDITORS: Leah A. Cohn, DVM, PhD, DACVIM; Mark S. Thompson, DVM, DABVP

Orphaned Puppy and Kitten Care

Bonus Material Online

Difficulty level: ◆

Overview and Goal

A common assumption is that most neonate orphan fatalities are due to infectious disease. However, the majority of orphan puppy and kitten fatalities are from caregiver error secondary to inadequate husbandry.

Indications

- Death of the dam
- Dam with agalactia, mastitis (p. 618), or other debilitating disease
- Large litter and dam is incapable of feeding all offspring adequately
- Neonates that are much smaller or weaker than their siblings and have difficulty competing

Contraindications

- Hand rearing orphaned puppies and kittens is laborious and expensive.
- Hand-reared offspring tend to be poorly socialized with others of their species, as evidenced by behavioral problems in the future.

Equipment, Anesthesia

Whelping/nesting box:
- Orphans need a dry, warm, draft-free, and comfortable nesting box, with sides that are tall enough to prevent the neonates from climbing out (hypothermia risk).
- Minimizing stressful situations is important. Orphans should be allowed to sleep, eat, and grow.
    - Avoid areas with much foot traffic and noise.
    - Avoid overhandling.
    - High stress levels impair the immune system, increasing the risk of infection, and can have potentially detrimental effects on future socialization.
    - Consider minimizing neonatal stress through the use of pheromone diffusers in the nursery area (Feliway for kittens and Adaptil for puppies).

Bedding:
- Bedding material should be soft, absorbent, nonabrasive, and should comfortably insulate the neonate from heat loss. Bedding should provide good footing and be incapable of bunching up and trapping the neonate. Bedding material must be kept clean and changed frequently.

Temperature (e.g., lamps, heating pad):
- Due to lack of a shivering reflex (2 weeks of life) and limited brown fat for thermogenesis, newborn puppies and kittens must be kept in an ambient temperature of 29.5°C-35°C (85°F-95°F).

Hygiene (antiseptic soap, disinfectant cleaning solution):
- Proper hygiene is vital because orphaned puppies and kittens are more susceptible to infectious disease. Caregivers should be meticulous about cleanliness of bedding and feeding supplies.

Colostrum:
- Since only negligible amounts of maternal antibodies (<5%) are passed through the placenta to the developing fetus, an adequate ingestion of colostrum must occur within the first 24 hours to acquire passive immunity from the mother. If the colostrum intake is questionable, serum concentrations of alkaline phosphatase (ALP) and gamma-glutamyltransferase (GGT) can be checked. If colostrum has been ingested, these serum concentrations should remain high during the first 2 weeks of life.
- If colostrum is not available, serum (preferably from the dam but can be from another adult of the same species in the kennel/cattery provided there is no risk of neonatal isoerythrolysis [p. 686]) can be administered orally to a neonate < 12 hours old by feeding tube. Dosage is 15 mL/100 g body weight, divided into multiple feedings.
- If the orphans did not receive any colostrum within the 24 hours, serum can be administered SQ: 5 mL/100 g body weight q 6-8h for a total of 3 doses.

Milk replacer:
- Orphans should be fed 6-8 times each day (q 3-4h) until weaning age (4-4.5 weeks of age). This can be accomplished by bottle, syringe, or tube feeding an appropriate milk-replacement diet.
- Commercial replacement diets (e.g., Esbilac, Just Borne, KMR, Veta-Lac) are recommended because of their balanced nutritional content. Homemade diets can be made, but formulating a nutritionally balanced homemade milk replacer is difficult. Administering improper replacement diets (e.g., cow's milk) leads to poor nutrition with inadequate rates of growth and is usually accompanied by the onset of diarrhea and attendant fluid and electrolyte losses that quickly become critical.

Tube feeding: 5- or 8-Fr red rubber catheter, syringe (p. 687)
- If a neonate is not gaining weight from bottle feeding, it should be supplemented by tube feeding.

Anticipated Time

- Orphans need intensive management until weaning (4-4.5 weeks of age).
- Depending on the size of the litter and whether bottle or tube feeding is used, each elimination/weighing/feeding/elimination session could take up to or over 60 minutes.

Preparation: Important Checkpoints

Hygiene:
- Before handling orphans, caregivers should wash their hands with an antiseptic soap.

Elimination:
- Before and after each meal, orphans need to be stimulated to urinate and defecate by rubbing the perineal and preputial areas with a warm, damp cotton ball (until age 3 weeks and voluntary control of these functions has developed).

Milk replacer:
- Food must be warmed before feeding and should be at maternal body temperature (101.5°F [38.6°F]). Cold food can stimulate vomiting, induce hypothermia, and inhibit absorption by slowing peristalsis. Food that is too hot can burn the neonate's mouth, esophagus, and stomach. Caregivers should mix only enough formula to last 24-48 hours and refrigerate any unused quantities in a glass container.

Weight gain:
- Neonates (including orphans) should be vigorous, squirmy, and fat. Hungry puppies and kittens are restless and will cry until fed. Weight loss or failure to gain should immediately alert the caregiver of a possible health problem that warrants investigation.
- Orphans should be weighed morning and night. Puppies and kittens should gain 5% to 10% of body weight daily. This equates to 1-3 g per day per pound (2-7 g/day/kg) anticipated adult weight for puppies and 50-100 g weekly for kittens. They should double their weight by 10 days of age.

Possible Complications and Common Errors to Avoid

- Orphans may be immunocompromised by stress and/or inadequate colostral antibody consumption.
- Neonates being supplemented with milk replacers need to be monitored for constipation. Warm water enemas can be performed if needed.

Procedure

Tube feeding:

- First, measure the distance from the tip of the nose to the last rib. Then, with a permanent marker, mark 75% of that measurement on the catheter. This mark guides the length of the tube's insertion so that it correctly reaches the stomach and avoids kinking of the tube.
- While holding the neonate upright or with it in ventral recumbancy, insert the tip of the tube along the roof of the mouth, following the path of least resistance. No force is needed, and most neonates swallow the feeding tube easily. If the catheter is accidentally inserted into the trachea, the neonate may cough as a sign of the incorrect placement. Another indication of incorrect catheter placement is inability to fully insert the tube to the premeasured mark. After the tube has been inserted, a syringe containing the milk replacer is attached to the end of the catheter. Correct placement of the feeding tube is supported by the presence of negative pressure using the syringe on the end of the tube.
- Warm an appropriate amount of commercial milk replacer (based on the size and age of the neonate; see label) and slowly feed it to the neonate over 1-2 minutes. Monitor for gastric distention. Average stomach capacity in neonates is 0.7 fluid ounces (4 tsp) per pound of body weight (1 mL/20 g body weight).

Postprocedure

Tube feeding:

- After the feeding is complete, the catheter is manually kinked (to avoid milk dripping out of it during removal, causing aspiration) and removed.
- Stimulate urination and defecation again.

Alternatives and Their Relative Merits

In the right circumstances, cross-fostering of orphans can be successful. If orphans are accepted by their new dam and are of similar size to their new siblings, this alternative provides ideal nourishment and nurturing. However, cross-fostered orphans can be rejected or severely injured by the new dam, and caregivers must be cautious until a maternal bond is clearly established.

Pearls

- It is extremely important to make sure that the body temperature of the neonate is above 96°F before feeding. If the body temperature is too low, ileus develops, and the ingested material will start to ferment instead of being digested, resulting in a bloated and distressed neonate.
- Cleaning and disinfecting should not be considered as synonymous because few disinfectants work well in the face of organic debris; therefore, proper cleaning should occur before disinfecting the area. Proper selection of disinfectants is important, and care should be taken to keep them from becoming environmental toxins. Neonates have very thin skin, and transdermal absorption of toxins occurs more readily than in adults. Many disinfectants are significant respiratory irritants at higher concentrations. The caregiver should be particularly careful with cleaning agents that contain pine oils or phenols.

SUGGESTED READING

Peterson ME: Care of the orphaned puppy and kitten. In Peterson ME, et al, editors: Small animal pediatrics: the first 12 months of life, St. Louis, 2011, Saunders, pp 67-73.

AUTHOR: Michelle A. Kutzler, DVM, PhD, DACT
EDITORS: Leah A. Cohn, DVM, PhD, DACVIM; Mark S. Thompson, DVM, DABVP

Procedures and Techniques

Orthopedic Examination

Difficulty level: ♦

Overview and Goal

To identify and localize an orthopedic disorder by performing a thorough and reproducible exam of the axial and appendicular skeleton, joints, and musculature

Indications

Any animal with abnormal musculoskeletal function due to injury, joint, muscle, or bone-related disease

Contraindications

In trauma cases, life-threatening problems should be addressed and animal stabilization ensured before performing a detailed orthopedic evaluation.

Equipment, Anesthesia

- Specialized equipment is usually not required.
- Goniometer to measure joint angles is optional.
- Sedation/general anesthesia is rarely necessary.

Anticipated Time

About 20-30 minutes

Preparation: Important Checkpoints

Detailed history tailored to the individual case, including:

- Signalment (p. 1262)
  - Breed-specific orthopedic disorders
- Owner assessment of problem
- Duration of problem
- Speed of onset
- Relationship to trauma, exercise, or time of day
- Course of problem
- Influence of rest or medications
- Associated or independent systemic disease
- Previous orthopedic problems and associated treatments and outcomes
- Family history
- Diet and exercise regimen
- Observation in the exam room noting how the animal sits, stands, and moves around
- Observation of different gaits in an open area with nonslip flooring

Possible Complications and Common Errors to Avoid

- Do not overinterpret breed-specific disorders.
- Beware of misinterpretation of neurologic disorders for orthopedic problems and vice versa:
  - Postural reactions such as proprioceptive testing and tactile placement responses, together with spinal cord reflexes, can help differentiate orthopedic from neurologic disorders.
- Perform neurologic exam after orthopedic exam (p. 1136).

Procedure

- Strive to palpate entire musculoskeletal system.
- Palpate all joints for swelling, thickening, crepitus, pain, and instability.
- Palpate all muscles for swelling, atrophy, pain, and asymmetry.
- Palpate bones for irregularity, pain, and instability.
- Palpate entire spine (including flexion, extension, and lateral deviation of the head and neck; tail head flexion and flexion and extension of the lumbosacral joint) for pain and sensitivity.
- Place all joints through a full range of motion.

- Know normal range of motion for all joints.
- When appropriate, use opposite limb as normal for comparison, best achieved in a standing position.
- Specific orthopedic tests include an Ortolani maneuver for hip joint laxity and a cranial drawer/sign test or a tibial thrust test for stifle joint instability.
- Ortolani maneuver
  - The femur is forced dorsally and perpendicular to the spine in an attempt to subluxate the hip joint.
  - Slow abduction of the limb allows the femoral head to return to the acetabulum.
  - An audible or palpable clunk is a positive sign, suggesting hip laxity.
- Cranial drawer/sign test (p. 218)
  - The examiner places a finger and thumb of one hand on the patella and lateral fabella proximal to the joint; the finger and thumb of the other hand are placed on the fibular head and tibial crest distal to the joint.
  - Cranial translation of the tibia can be applied to the joint in stifle flexion and extension. A torn cranial cruciate ligament produces cranial subluxation (cranial movement) of the tibia relative to the femur.
- Tibial thrust test (p. 218)
  - Evaluates the same instability as a cranial drawer test (i.e., tests mainly for cranial cruciate ligament integrity)
  - Dorsiflexion of the hock while the stifle is in slight flexion
  - Positive result consists of a tibial thrust motion (cranial movement of the tibial plateau relative to the rest of the stifle), appreciated by placement of an index finger on the tibial crest.
  - Animal cooperation will determine whether the exam requires sedation or general anesthesia.
- Perform a rectal exam in cases of pelvic trauma.

Postprocedure

- Inform owner that some animals may be sore or painful after an orthopedic exam.
- Use nonsteroidal antiinflammatory drugs (NSAIDs) if the animal shows evidence of discomfort or pain (e.g., lameness) after manipulation.

Alternatives and Their Relative Merits

- Plain radiographs
  - May require sedation
  - Minimum of two views of the localized region
  - Normal opposite limb can be useful as a control for comparison.
  - In trauma patients, thoracic radiographs should precede orthopedic radiographs as part of a minimum database.
  - Initial radiographic assessment of spinal injuries should ideally be performed without sedation.
  - Radiographic information and clinical/physical exam are complementary; one cannot entirely replace the other because some animals with radiographically severe lesions are clinically mildly affected and vice versa.
  - Specific radiographic studies may be indicated (e.g., PennHIP, dorsal acetabular rim [DAR] view of pelvis, hyperflexed or hyperextended view of joint).
- Arthrocentesis (p. 1059)
  - Where joint swelling is palpated, arthrocentesis may be indicated for cytologic evaluation of synovial fluid.
- CT scan and MRI (p. 1132) techniques can be extremely useful in specific cases.
  - Rule in or rule out diagnosis that is unclear from exam and routine testing
  - CT scan is usually preferred for bone analysis, and MRI is usually preferred for soft-tissue analysis, including ligament and articular cartilage damage.
  - Requires general anesthesia
  - Cost or availability may be prohibitive.
- Bone scan and nuclear scintigraphy
  - Helpful to localize an occult orthopedic lameness
  - Highly sensitive but nonspecific
  - Requires sedation and hospitalization of "hot" animal, and cost or availability may be prohibitive.
- Diagnostic ultrasound
  - In skilled hands, can identify biceps, supraspinatus, infraspinatus, triceps, Achilles and iliopsoas tendon lesions
- Arthroscopy
  - Allows minimally invasive visualization and diagnosis ± surgical repair of a joint disorder
  - Requires general anesthesia, and cost or availability may be prohibitive.

AUTHOR: Nicholas J. Trout, VetMB, MA, DACVS, DECVS
EDITORS: Leah A. Cohn, DVM, PhD, DACVIM; Mark S. Thompson, DVM, DABVP

Otoscopy, Video

Bonus Material Online 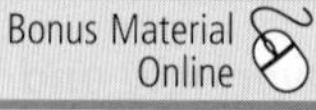

Difficulty level: ♦♦

Overview and Goal

Video otoscopy is a visually superior technique over traditional, handheld otoscopy for examining the ear canal. It facilitates

- Image capture for improving client compliance and therapeutic monitoring
- Constant visualization during deep canal flushing
- Examination of the middle ear
- Myringotomy and medical treatment of otitis media
- Intralesional injection of corticosteroids for severely stenotic canals
- Removal of polyps and foreign bodies
- Biopsy of masses

Indications

- Diagnostic workup of
  - Otitis (externa and media) (p. 728)
  - Head shaking
  - Deafness (p. 237)
  - Horner's syndrome
  - Vestibular disease (p. 1037)
- Management and monitoring of unresponsive or recurring otitis
- Myringotomy for treatment of otitis media

Contraindications

Very painful ears without analgesia and pharmacologic restraint

Equipment, Anesthesia

Otoscopy:

- Video-otoscope
- Anti-fog agent (the author uses a drop of liquid hand soap rubbed on lens)
- Skilled restrainer
- Sedation and analgesia if the patient's ears are painful
- Cotton-tipped swabs to collect samples for cytology

Deep ear flushing:

- Requires an assistant; this can be the same person who is monitoring anesthesia
- Requires intubation to protect the lower respiratory tract
- Video-otoscope
- Intraprocedural analgesia to prevent patient response to stimulus
- Ceruminolytic agent such as squalene before premedicating
- Warm soapy (chlorhexidine based) water
- Sterile physiologic saline solution (warmed to body temperature)
- Three large-volume syringes (>60 mL) to push solutions at variable pressures into the canal
- 5-Fr polypropylene urinary catheter or red rubber feeding tube with the tip cut, converting it into an open-ended catheter (heat the cut end briefly over a flame to dull it)
- Videoscopic curettes, biopsy forceps, and grasper

Myringotomy:
- 5½-inch, open-ended tomcat catheter
- Sterile culturettes for submission of samples for culture and sensitivity
- Sterile saline
- Injectible antibiotic for infusion into bulla
- Optional: suction unit, flushing and suction apparatus, three-way stopcock, a third large-volume syringe or intravenous (IV) fluid administration set

Anticipated Time

- Ear examination: <5 minutes per ear in a conscious, nonsedate animal
- Ear flushing: 10-20 minutes per ear
- Myringotomy/biopsy: 10-20 minutes additional to ear flushing

Preparation: Important Checkpoints

Ear examination:
- Avoid instilling topical medication or cleaning solutions in the ear 48 to 72 hours before.

Ear flushing:
- Consider antiinflammatory doses of systemic corticosteroids (e.g., prednisone 0.5-1 mg/kg PO q 24h) for 4-5 days before to prevent procedural-induced canal stenosis.
- Collect cytologic and culture samples of the external canal before cleaning.
- Pretreat canal with a ceruminolytic agent before administering preanesthetic medication.

Possible Complications and Common Errors to Avoid

- Otoscopy: causing pain
- Ear flushing: vestibular signs, deafness, Horner's syndrome, and inadvertent tympanic membrane rupture are uncommon but possible complications and usually are transient. These can be avoided through adequate analgesia/anesthesia, excellent visualization, and careful manipulation of instruments in proximity of the tympanum.
- Not using systemic corticosteroids before ear flushing can prevent adequate access to the tympanum and results in a higher risk of procedural-induced stenosis. In severe and chronic cases, repeated intralesional corticosteroid injections may be needed to render the canal accessible for video-otoscopic access. However, if the otitis is that severe, ablation surgery is probably indicated.

Procedure

- Use disinfected otoscope tips for each animal (follow manufacturer recommendation for video-otoscopes).
- Examine the good ear first, even if the patient presents with unilateral disease.
- For painful ears, injectable sedation and analgesia are essential (see back cover for protocols).
- Collect cytologic samples from both canals. Submit cultures from canals that are refractory to treatment or frequently relapse.
- Otoscopy in the awake patient is the same for handheld and video:
  - Use adequate restraint of the head to minimize movement.
  - Position the head so the muzzle is angled slightly toward the side opposite of you.
  - Pull the pinna away from the skull to straighten the canal.
  - Gently introduce the scope tip into the canal via the intertragic incisure (just caudal to the tragus), then visually guide the scope deeper into the canal, examining the walls as you move toward and then past the vertical-horizontal canal junction. Be aware of the Noxon fold at the dorsal aspect of this junction, and maneuver the scope gently past it.
- Ear flushing
  - Collect cytologic and culture samples first.
  - Pretreat canal(s) with a ceruminolytic agent.
  - Premedicate, induce general anesthesia, and intubate.
  - Patient is positioned in lateral recumbency, ideally on a tub table.
  - Position yourself dorsal to the patient's head.
  - Remember to examine the "good" ear first.
  - Introduce the modified 5-Fr urinary catheter through the working channel of the otoscope until the tip is visible.
  - Assistant fills and attaches the large-volume syringe containing soapy water to the other end and proceeds to flush using small pulses while you direct catheter tip as needed to dislodge debris. Use graspers for larger chunks of debris. Remove debris adhered to the tympanum using the blunt catheter tip and curette to reveal the tympanic membrane.
  - Suction the canal, flush with warm water, suction again, flush with warm saline solution, and then suction completely dry before making a final assessment of the tympanum. When viewing the tympanum through a fluid interface, even the normal eardrum appears white and opaque because light is refracted as it passes through the fluid-ear interface demarcated by the tympanum.
  - At this point, be prepared to perform other procedures such as biopsy, polyp removal, or myringotomy (when the tympanum is opaque or not intact).

Myringotomy if indicated:
  - Change flush catheter to 5½-inch, open-ended tomcat catheter.
  - Repeatedly flush, then suction sterile saline (1-mL volumes) to clear out infectious debris.
  - Save the first 1 mL for culture.

Procedures and Techniques

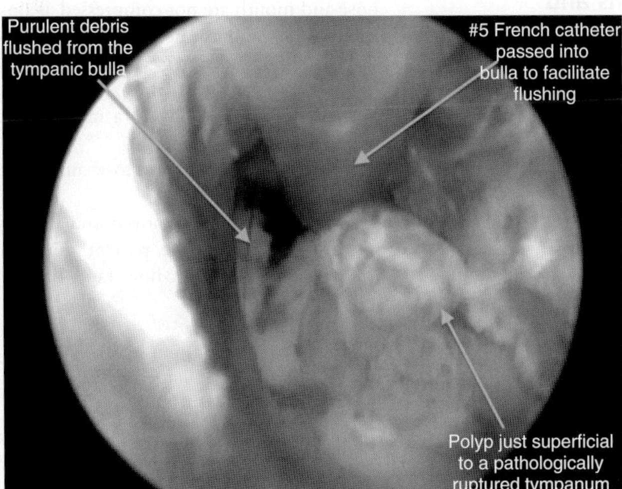

OTOSCOPY Intractable and chronic otitis treated by total ablation and lateral bullectomy. (Courtesy Dr. Jeffrey M. Person.)

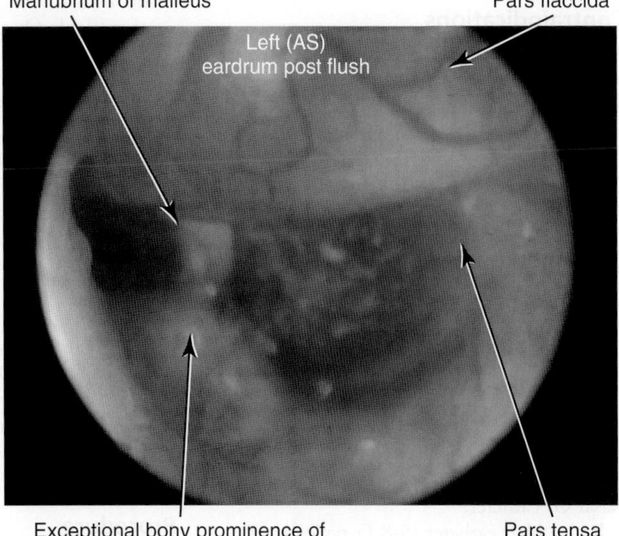

OTOSCOPY Otoscopic view of a normal proximal ear canal and tympanum. (Courtesy Dr. Jeffrey M. Person.)

- After bulla flushed clean and completely suctioned, infuse antibiotic medication.
- Suction residual fluid from the canal.
- Instill topical medication if appropriate.
- Recover the patient.

Postprocedure

- Topical +/− systemic corticosteroids to reduce the iatrogenic-induced inflammation.
- Instruct owners to start treating the ear the next day.
- Analgesics are paramount to manage post-procedural pain and to facilitate treatments at home by the owner.

Alternatives and Their Relative Merits

Handheld otoscopes are less expensive and very portable and are adequate for cursory examinations of the ear canal but are useless for ear-flushing procedures

Advantages of video-otoscope:

- Greatly improved visualization of the canal due to optics, light, and magnification
- Can increase client compliance when you share images with the client
- Allows image documentation for medical records
- Vastly superior for ear-flush procedures
- Allows for precise and thus safer placement of instruments for tympanic curettage, biopsy, myringotomy, foreign-body and polyp removal

Pearls

- Do not scope a painful ear.
- Recommend video-otoscopic flushing sooner rather than later for ears that are refractory to treatment or for ears that have relapsed within a shorter than expected period.
- Make your final assessment of the tympanum from a dry canal to eliminate the visual artifact caused by refraction of light from your light source.

SUGGESTED READING

Angus JC, et al: Uses and indications for video-otoscopy in small animal practice. Vet Clin North Am Small Anim Pract 31(4):809-828, 2001.

AUTHOR: Jeffrey M. Person, DVM
EDITORS: Leah A. Cohn, DVM, PhD, DACVIM; Mark S. Thompson, DVM, DABVP

Oxygen Supplementation

Bonus Material Online 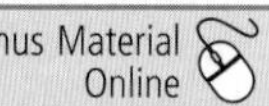

Difficulty level: ♦

Overview and Goal

Oxygen (O_2) supplementation aims to increase inspired O_2 content, thereby increasing O_2 diffusion to the blood to correct or improve hypoxemia.

Indications

- Respiratory distress: increased respiratory rate or effort, paradoxical breathing, orthopnea
- Hypoxemia: cyanosis, $PaO_2 \leq 80$ mm Hg, pulse oximetry (SpO_2) reading < 95%
- During triage and initial assessment of severe/critical injury or illness

Contraindications

The only true contraindication is open flame, but caution should be used.

- Nasal O_2 catheters in traumatic brain injury patients can increase intracranial pressure.
- Rapid correction of chronic hypoxemia can alter respiratory drive that has been based on hypoxemia rather than normal hypercapnia.

Equipment, Anesthesia

Equipment needed depends on method chosen for supplementation. All require an O_2 source.

- O_2 tanks, central O_2 source with outlets, or O_2 generator
- A source for humidification of O_2 needed if continued for more than an hour
- Tubing from O_2 source to delivery method (e.g., cage, mask, tent)

Nasal O_2 catheter:

- Red rubber catheter (5-8 Fr typical)
- Lubricant (lidocaine gel ideal)
- Proparacaine drops or lidocaine
- Suture material or tissue staples
- Adapter to fit between red rubber and O_2 tubing
- Elizabethan collar (e-collar)

Other methods may require face mask, oxygen tent, oxygen cage, incubator, or other supplies.

Anticipated Time

Varies with type and duration of required supplementation; flow-by or face mask O_2 delivery can begin almost instantly

Preparation: Important Checkpoints

- Ensure O_2 source is available (e.g., full tanks) at all times.
- Be familiar with the setup and maintenance of available O_2 cage or incubator.

Possible Complications and Common Errors to Avoid

- O_2 toxicity can occur if fraction of inspired O_2 (FIO_2) > 50% for prolonged period. Toxicity can occur in 12 hours with 100% O_2 or 18 hours with 80% O_2.
  - Actual FIO_2 may not be known, depending on method of supplementation (e.g., FIO_2 not quantified for flow-by, nasal catheter)
  - Room air is 21% FIO_2; many hypoxemic animals are comfortable with FIO_2 of 40%, but FIO_2 > 40% may be required for severely hypoxemic patients.
  - Use the lowest flow rate (nasal catheter) or FIO_2 (O_2 cage) to maintain adequate O_2 saturation (e.g., $SpO_2 \geq 94\%$).

Procedure

Flow-by O_2 supplementation:

- Easiest method of providing short-term O_2 supplementation (e.g., during triage or while preparing for a more sustainable method of supplementation)
- Mild to modest increase in O_2 concentration
- Well tolerated by most
- Leads to O_2 waste
- The O_2 source (hose or tubing) is placed close (1-5 cm) to the patient's nose/mouth.
- FIO_2 ≈25%-40%, depending on the O_2 flow rate (3-15 L/min) and how close the O_2 source is to the patient's nose/mouth.

Face mask:

- Quick and simple way to provide short-term O_2 supplementation
- A mask can increase the FIO_2 to 50%-60%, especially when using high flow rates of ≈8-12 L/min.
- Anesthetic face mask connected to O_2 source is held over the patient's face. Ensure that the nose and mouth are not compressed against the wall of the mask because this can have severe consequences on gas flow through the mask and patient ventilation.
- Some patients resist having a mask placed on their faces.
- Tight-fitting masks may lead to accumulation of carbon dioxide (CO_2).
- The mask should be removed and flow-by O_2 implemented if the patient does not tolerate it due to high flow rates or CO_2 accumulation.

Tents and hoods:

- Commercial O_2 tents can be used for recumbent animals, with the tent placed loosely over the animal's head.
- O_2 tubing is run into a precut hole in the tent, and flow rates are generally as high as 10-15 L/min.
- O_2 hoods can be assembled using an e-collar and plastic food wrap. The transparent wrap

covers about 80% of the e-collar, with room left open for elimination of CO_2 and to prevent hyperthermia.
- An O_2 tubing is run on the inside of the e-collar, and flow rates set at 3-10 L/min, depending on the size of the patient.
- Both methods are inexpensive and easy to set up but use a lot of O_2.

Cages and incubators:
- O_2 cages and incubators offer a low-stress means of O_2 supplementation for the short term and for longer durations.
- Immediate placement of a dyspneic animal into a clear O_2 cage can be calming to the animal, provide needed O_2, and can allow safe observation of respiratory effort and pattern.
- O_2 cages prevent ready access without opening the door or window, rapidly dropping the ambient O_2 concentration to that of room air.
- Many different models of O_2 cages and incubators are available, including commercial models and makeshift setups.
- Capable of delivering high concentrations of O_2 (≥40%-60%), many are sold with O_2 regulator that allows the clinician to set the desired FIO_2
- Some cages are able to effectively eliminate CO_2 and regulate humidity and temperature. Incubators are usually not regulated as easily as cages, but O_2 sensors, thermometers, and hygrometers can help monitor internal conditions.
- Ensure incubators are not so tightly sealed that they prevent CO_2 elimination.
- O_2 cages use large volumes of O_2.

Nasal prongs:
- Nasal prongs can be used in dogs to supply O_2 supplementation for hours to days.
- Various sizes of prongs fit into the nostrils and are secured behind the ears.
- The tubing can be taped or stapled in place but are more easily removed (and replaced) than nasal catheter.
- Compared to nasal catheters (see below), higher flow rates are typically used with nasal prongs.
- Not suitable for cats or small dogs

Nasal catheter:
- Relatively simple to place and generally well tolerated for O_2 supplementation lasting a few to many days
- Often performed without, but sedatives may facilitate placement in resistant animals (butorphanol 0.2-0.4 mg/kg IV/IM once). An assistant is usually required to help restrain the patient during placement.
- With the nose pointed up, place a few proparacaine drops or topical lidocaine drops inside the nostril.
- Red rubber catheters are generally used for nasal insufflation. Small-breed dogs and cats may use a 5-Fr catheter (cats may not tolerate nasal O_2 catheters well); medium-sized to large-breed dogs do well with an 8-Fr catheter.
- Use the catheter to measure from the external naris to the medial canthus of the eye; mark with a permanent marker or tape.
- Lubricate the catheter tip with KY gel or lidocaine gel.
- While the assistant is holding the patient's head with the nose pointed toward the ceiling, the catheter should be advanced in a ventromedial direction to the premeasured mark.
- The tube is then secured to the nostril with sutures or staples. The tube should also be secured (with either suture or staples) on the side of the face or up the bridge of the nose.
- The end of the tube is then connected to an O_2 source, usually requiring an adaptor or Christmas tree.
- The O_2 flow rate for nasal catheters is usually 50-150 mL/kg/min. For a 20-kg dog, flow rates will be between 1-3 L/min.
- Bilateral nasal O_2 tubes can be used in dogs with severe hypoxemia or dogs that do not respond adequately to one nasal O_2 catheter. The flow rate can be doubled when two catheters are present.
- An e-collar should be placed to prevent inadvertent removal.

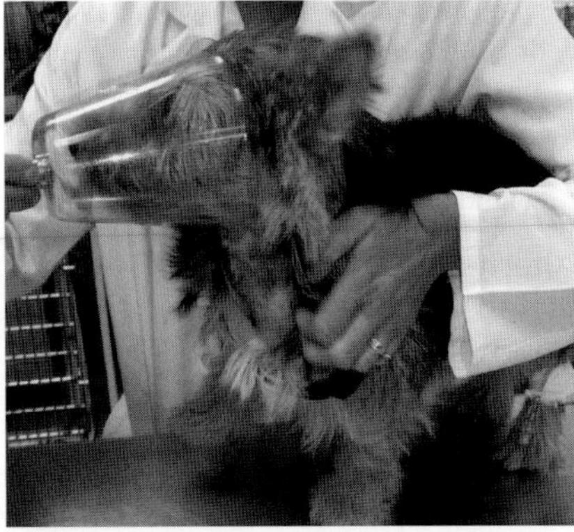

OXYGEN SUPPLEMENTATION Face masks also offer a simple, rapid, but short-term method of O_2 supplementation.

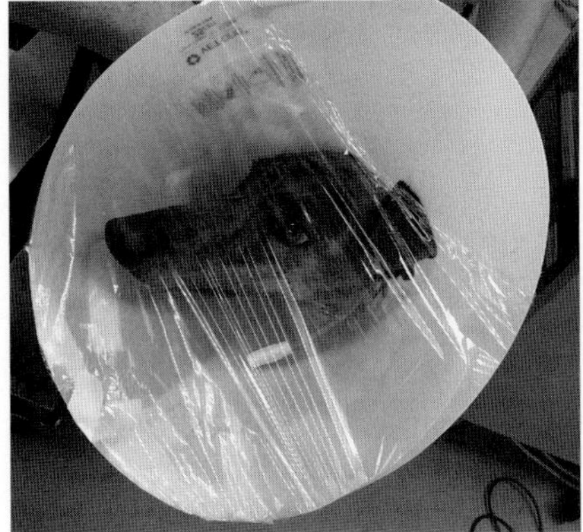

OXYGEN SUPPLEMENTATION O_2 supplementation can be achieved by covering ≈¾ of an Elizabethan collar with plastic wrap and inserting the oxygen tubing under the collar.

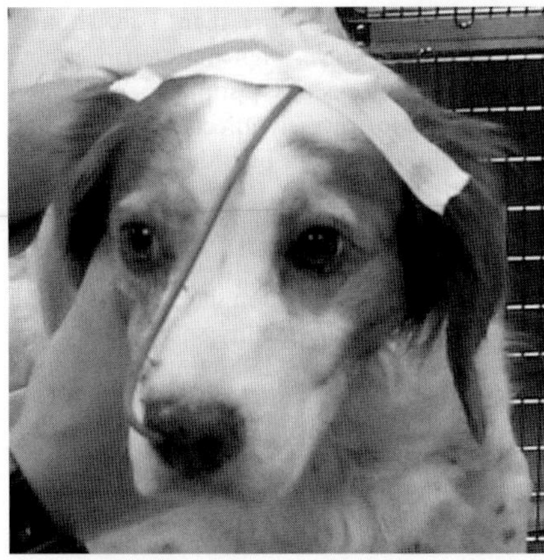

OXYGEN SUPPLEMENTATION Nasal catheters offer a simple but effective method of O_2 supplementation for a few to many days. Bilateral catheters can be placed if additional O_2 is required.

Tracheal catheter:
- Patients with upper airway obstruction can benefit from tracheal O_2 supplementation.
- It may also be helpful when there are contraindications to nasal catheter placement (animals with traumatic brain injury or nasal neoplasia).
- The ventral neck should be shaved and aseptically prepared.
- Wearing sterile gloves, a 14- to 20-gauge, 1-1.5 inch over-the-needle catheter is placed into the tracheal lumen through the tracheal cartilages. It is usually easier to lift up the skin and pass the catheter through the skin first before passing the catheter through the tracheal ring.
- An O_2 source is attached to the catheter after the stylet is removed.
- O_2 flow rates of 1-3 L/min can give an FIO_2 of 60%-80%.
- Tracheal catheters are simple to place and are typically well tolerated, but they can be challenging to secure and may fall out in mobile patients.

Endotracheal intubation:
- Requires induction of general anesthesia such as propofol 2-6 mg/kg IV or ketamine 2-10 mg/kg IV combined with diazepam/midazolam 0.1-0.5 mg/kg IV
- Anesthesia is maintained with inhalant or chemical drugs.
- Mechanical ventilation can be manual or by mechanical ventilator machine.
- Can provide 100% O_2 for patients unresponsive to other means of O_2 supplementation
- Facilitates mechanical ventilation (p. 1185); mechanical ventilation can be lifesaving for animals unable to sustain respiratory rate/effort despite less aggressive means of O_2 supplementation
- Patient should be intubated if arterial blood gas or pulse oximetry shows progressive hypoxemia with $SpO_2 < 90\%$ or $PaO_2 <$ 60 mm Hg despite O_2 supplementation.
- Prolonged high FIO_2 exposure is toxic.

- If performed for more than a few hours, this is an invasive, high maintenance, and expensive means of O_2 supplementation.
- Reserved for severely affected animals and in facilities that can provide intensive care.

Postprocedure

- Ideally, animals requiring more than short-term O_2 supplementation should be managed in a 24-hour care facility so that they can be closely monitored for improvement or deterioration.
- Assessment of oxygenation is important, whether by arterial blood gas analysis (p. 1058) or pulse oximetry.
- Animals requiring more than a day or two of O_2 supplementation usually require gradual weaning off O_2 over 12-72 hours by turning down the flow rate (or FIO_2 for O_2 cages) with repeat assessment of clinical condition.

Alternatives and Their Relative Merits

- There are no good alternatives to O_2 supplementation for treatment of hypoxemia.
- Animals with anemia can have tissue hypoxia without having hypoxemia and can benefit from transfusion therapy.

Pearls

Nasal O_2 supplementation is extremely useful but less so for cats, brachiocephalic dog breeds, and dogs that consistently breathe through the mouth.

SUGGESTED READING

Boyle J: Oxygen therapy. In Creedon JM, et al, editors: Advanced monitoring and procedures for small animal emergency and critical care, ed 1, West Sussex, UK, 2012, John Wiley & Sons.

AUTHOR: Adesola Odunayo, DVM, MS, DACVECC
EDITORS: Leah A. Cohn, DVM, PhD, DACVIM; Mark S. Thompson, DVM, DABVP

Parenteral Nutrition

Bonus Material Online 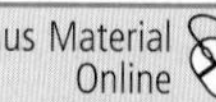

Difficulty level: ♦♦

Synonyms

Total parenteral nutrition (TPN), partial parenteral nutrition (PPN), peripheral parenteral nutrition (PPN)

Overview and Goals

- Parenteral nutrition (PN) is nutrition delivered by the intravenous (IV) route.
- Used when enteral feeding is not possible and the need for nourishment is a critical factor in clinical outcome.

Indications

Patients need nutritional support when
- Enteral nutrition is contraindicated (e.g., severe gastrointestinal [GI] dysfunction)
- Sufficient nutrition cannot be provided by the enteral route alone (e.g., severe malabsorptive disease).

Contraindications

- Patients that can be fed safely and effectively by an enteral route, even if feeding tubes are required
- Patients that are at risk with catheter placement
  - Central venous catheters in patients at high risk for thromboembolic disease (e.g., protein-losing nephropathy or enteropathy [p. 600], hyperadrenocorticism [p. 485], disseminated intravascular coagulopathy [p. 269])
  - Jugular catheters in patients with increased cerebral pressure (e.g., head trauma)
- Patients at risk of fluid overload (e.g., patients with heart failure, oliguria, or severe hypoproteinemia)

Equipment, Anesthesia

- Venous access
  - A dedicated catheter is required for nutrient solution delivery to avoid septic complications and drug-nutrient interactions.
  - Treat catheter placement as a surgical procedure (p. 1123).
  - A central venous catheter is preferred to deliver PN because the nutrient solution is hyperosmolar. Dilute solutions can be used for peripheral venous infusion, but the resulting large volume can be a limiting factor.
  - Catheters made of nonthrombogenic materials (polyurethane or silicone) are preferred, particularly for peripheral infusion.
  - Multilumen central or peripherally placed central catheters (PICC lines) can be used if one of the ports is dedicated for PN.
- Nutrient admixture
  - Amino acid solutions (3%-10%) are used for providing protein. These solutions come with and without added electrolytes.
  - Nonprotein calories can be provided by a combination of lipid emulsions (10% or 20%) and dextrose (10%-50%) or dextrose alone.
  - Electrolytes can be added to the nutrient solution as needed or provided separately in the patient's crystalloid fluid therapy. The latter allows greater flexibility. Alternatively, a combination amino acid and electrolyte solution can be used.
  - Special parenteral vitamin and mineral preparations are available. However, because most companion animals receive PN for relatively short periods (<2 weeks), only certain vitamins and minerals are commonly added to the nutrient admixture (B complex ± potassium phosphate and magnesium sulfate).
- Monitoring and nursing care
  - PN is best delivered continuously (although not absolutely necessary), and 24-hour nursing care is desirable for administration and for catheter vigilance/catheter care.
  - Many of the complications of PN can be life-threatening, and careful monitoring of the patient is mandated. This includes frequent checks of serum glucose and electrolyte concentrations; some in-house serum chemistry analyses necessary.

Anticipated Time

- Patient assessment and PN prescription formulation can take 30-60 minutes depending on the complexity of the case and the PN formulation.
- Nutrient admixture compounding can take 30-60 minutes depending on the facilities and equipment available.
- The overall duration of parenteral nutritional support will depend on the underlying disease and the patient's response.

Preparation: Important Checkpoints

Nutrient admixture:
- Prepare PN solutions under aseptic conditions. Solutions must be compounded in a specific sequence and carefully mixed.
- Use the services of a home infusion service or a human hospital pharmacy to compound PN solutions when the veterinary practice lacks the facilities and expertise.

Possible Complications and Common Errors to Avoid

- Common metabolic complications
  - When addressing electrolyte abnormalities, delivering supplements in the IV fluids rather than in the PN solution allows greater flexibility. Later, when the amount of supplementation for maintenance is established, it can be included in the PN formulation.
  - Hyperglycemia: if present, reduce the percentage of nonprotein calories from dextrose, or give regular insulin (p. 251).

- Hypokalemia: if present, supplement IV fluids with potassium chloride (p. 516). Monitor for hypomagnesemia.
- Hypophosphatemia: if present, supplement IV fluids with potassium phosphate, or add potassium phosphate to PN formulation.
- Hypomagnesemia: if present, supplement IV fluids with magnesium sulfate, or add magnesium sulfate to PN formulations.
- Hyperlipidemia: if present, reduce or omit the lipid emulsion.

- Catheter complications
  - Loss of venous access secondary to catheter malposition or thrombosis: if occurs, replace catheter.
  - Thrombophlebitis: if occurs, replace catheter. Select peripheral catheters that are long and made of nonthrombogenic materials, especially with peripheral infusions.
  - Infection: if occurs, remove catheter and culture the tip. Replace with a new catheter in a new location.

Procedure

PN prescription formulation:

- Choose between central or peripheral venous administration.
  - Central is preferred for smaller volumes of PN and lower risk of thrombophlebitis.
  - Peripheral is possible if central is not available, but the patient must be fluid tolerant because required lower tonicity means a larger volume of infusate.
- Calculating the caloric goal
  - Calculate the resting energy requirement (RER) using the patient's current body weight (or the animal's estimated ideal weight if overweight, such as body condition score > 6/9).
  - Formula: RER = 70 + 30 × (body weight in kilograms) for patients weighing 2-30 kg; use 70 × (body weight in kilograms)$^{0.75}$ for patients that weigh outside this range.
  - Start with a caloric goal of the RER, and adjust based on patient response.
- Decide which percentage of calories will be delivered as protein, depending on the patient's level of protein tolerance or deficiency.
  - Dogs: provide 15%-25% of goal calories as protein (4-6 g/100 kcal).
  - Cats: provide 25%-35% of goal calories as protein (6-8 g/100 kcal).
  - Amino acid solutions: provide 4 kcal/g.
  - To calculate the volume of amino acid solution required
    - Divide the protein calories by 4 kcal/g = grams of amino acids required
    - Divide the grams of amino acids required by the grams of amino acids per milliliter in the solution = volume of amino acid solution
  - NOTE: for peripheral infusion, use ≤ 6% amino acid solutions because of high osmolarity.
- Decide which percentage of nonprotein calories will be delivered as dextrose, with the remainder to be delivered as lipid.
  - 100% of the nonprotein calories can be delivered as dextrose, but hyperglycemia is a common sequela; 50% dextrose provides 1.7 kcal/mL.
  - Alternatively, lipid emulsions can be used for delivering 50%-70% of the nonprotein calories; 20% lipid emulsions provide 2 kcal/mL.
  - NOTE: for peripheral venous infusion, a high percentage of nonprotein calories from lipid is preferred because the lipid emulsions are iso-osmolar. They are also more calorically dense than dextrose solutions that can be safely infused peripherally (≤20% dextrose).
- Add 0.2 mL/100 mL total infusate of vitamin B complex.
- Decide whether electrolytes will be added.
  - Supplementation may not be necessary if amino acid solutions containing additional electrolytes are used.
  - CAUTION: supplementation is contraindicated in patients with kidney disease/renal failure.
  - Potassium phosphate: 8 mEq/1000 kcal
  - Magnesium sulfate: 0.8 mEq/100 kcal
- Calculate the hourly infusion rate by dividing the total volume by 24.

Sample Worksheet for a 17.5-kg (39-lb) Dog: Centrally Administered Parenteral Nutrition Calculation

CANINE HIGH-PROTEIN REGIMEN

Weight: 17.5 kg	Resting energy requirement (RER) = 600 kcal/day
Day 1 goal	50% RER = 0.5(600) = 300 kcal
Day 2 goal	100% RER = 600 kcal
% Protein calories	25%
Nonprotein calories	50% from lipid, 50% from dextrose

Solutions

8.5% Amino acids (without electrolytes)

50% Dextrose

20% Lipid emulsion

Potassium phosphate (3 mM/mL)

Injectable B complex

Day 1 Calculations

Amino Acids

0.25 × 300 kcal = 75 kcal from protein

There are 4 kcal/g protein; therefore, the patient needs 18.75 g of protein: 75 kcal ÷ 4 kcal/g = 18.75 g

8.5% amino acid solution = 0.085 g protein/mL; therefore, the animal needs 220 mL 8.5% amino acid solution: 18.75 g ÷ 0.085 g/mL = 220 mL

Nonprotein Calories

0.75 × 300 kcal = 225 kcal

50% dextrose to provide 50% nonprotein calories = 112.5 kcal. 50% dextrose solution = 1.7 kcal/mL; therefore, the patient needs 66 mL 50% dextrose solution: 112.5 kcal ÷ 1.7 kcal/mL = 66 mL

20% lipid emulsion to provide 50% nonprotein calories = 112.5 kcal. 20% lipid emulsion = 2 kcal/mL; therefore, the patient needs 56 mL 20% lipid emulsion: 112.5 kcal ÷ 2 kcal/mL = 56 mL

Potassium Phosphate

Dosed at 8 mM/1000 kcal delivered; therefore, the patient needs 2.4 mM potassium phosphate: (8 mM × 300 kcal) ÷ 1000 kcal = 2.4 mM

Potassium phosphate solution = 3 mM/mL; therefore, the patient needs 0.8 mL potassium phosphate: 2.4 mM ÷ 3 mM/mL = 0.8 mL

Vitamin B Complex

Dosed at approximately 2 mL/L infused

Total infusate for day 1 = 343 mL; therefore, 1 mL B complex should be sufficient.

Infusion Rate

343 mL ÷ 24 h = 14 mL/h

Day 2 Calculations

Same calculations as those for day 1, but substitute 600 kcal for 300 kcal.

Postprocedure

- Delivery
  - Deliver the solution at a constant rate using an infusion pump.
  - Administer 50% of the goal infusion, and monitor for metabolic complications the first day, advancing to the goal rate the next day if no problems occur that cannot be addressed.

Procedures and Techniques

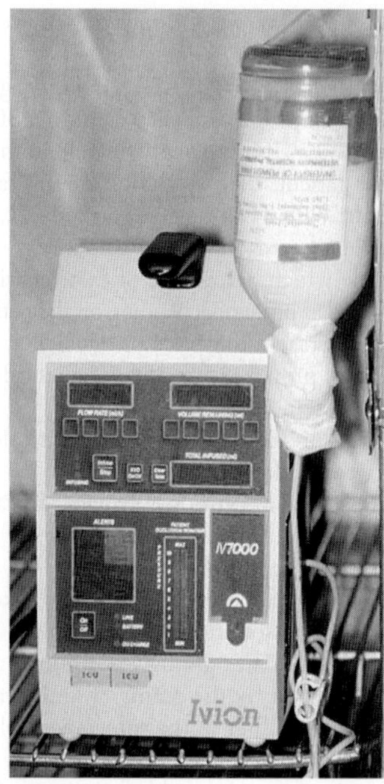

PARENTERAL NUTRITION Infusion pump and prepared parenteral nutrition solution ready for administration. (Courtesy Dr. Lesley King.)

- Do not discontinue PN abruptly, especially in patients that are not eating. If a patient cannot be weaned, monitor for hypoglycemia.
- Catheter care
  - Examine the catheter site at least daily for signs of phlebitis or infection, changing the dressing as needed.
  - Change the drip set every day.
  - Never use the catheter for any purpose other than the delivery of PN (e.g., no blood sampling, administering medications or fluids).
- Monitoring
  - In addition to the routine monitoring appropriate for any animal on IV fluid therapy, patients receiving PN should be monitored for metabolic complications.
  - Blood glucose monitored at least q 12h and serum electrolytes at least q 24h
  - When a packed cell volume (PCV) test is performed, the serum should be examined for evidence of lipemia.
  - CBC and serum biochemistry profile as indicated and at least once weekly

Alternatives and Their Relative Merits

Enteral nutrition:

- In general, nutrient delivery by the enteral route is safer and less costly than PN.
- Enteral nutrition has trophic effects on the GI tract and supports the structure and function of the mucosa and the barrier function of the gut.
- Preferred over PN whenever feasible

SUGGESTED READING

Michel KE, et al: Parenteral nutrition. In Silverstein DC, et al, editors: Small animal critical care medicine. ed 2, St. Louis, 2015, Elsevier, pp 687-690.

AUTHOR: Kathryn E. Michel, DVM, MS, MSED, DACVN
EDITORS: Leah A. Cohn, DVM, PhD, DACVIM; Mark S. Thompson, DVM, DABVP

Pericardiocentesis

Bonus Material Online 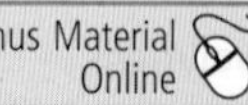

Difficulty level: ♦♦

Synonym

Pericardial tap

Overview and Goal

Removal of pericardial effusion (PE) for diagnostic investigation and for therapeutic relief of signs related to cardiac tamponade

Indications

- Cardiac tamponade: when PE elevates intrapericardial pressure above pressure in the right heart, resulting in lethargy, collapse or near collapse, abdominal distention, or dyspnea
- Diagnostic investigation of the cause of PE by fluid analysis and cytology

Contraindications

- Small-volume effusion where the risk of cardiac puncture is high (caution in cats because volume of effusion often is small)
- Caution in cases of suspected left atrial tears (which seldom result in tamponade and may, with pericardiocentesis, promote continued hemorrhage from the left atrium)

Equipment, Anesthesia

- Manual restraint is often sufficient, but light sedation (e.g.. butorphanol) may be warranted to reduce patient movement. Avoid agents that cause excessive panting.
- Clippers, surgical scrub, isopropyl alcohol, and gauze pads for clipping and preparing the skin
- Lidocaine 0.5-3 mL for local block +/− for ventricular arrhythmias
- 3-mL syringe for local block
- Ultrasound machine for location selection
- Electrocardiographic (ECG) monitoring
- 14-18 gauge, 2-5¼ inch over-the-needle catheter
  - 21-gauge, 1-inch butterfly catheter preferred in cats
- #11 scalpel blade
- Sterile gloves
- 6-mL syringe
- 20-35 mL syringe(s)
- Optional extension tubing and 3-way stopcock
- Bowl for collecting drained effusate
- Red- and lavender-top tubes

Anticipated Time

10-60 minutes

Preparation: Important Checkpoints

- Diagnostic evaluation of the cause of PE (by echocardiogram, fluid analysis and cytology, chest radiographs, CBC, chemistry profile, urinalysis, T_4 [cats], +/− abdominal ultrasound) is encouraged (p. 773).
- Clients should be educated about potential complications but should also be told that the benefit of pericardiocentesis in relieving cardiac tamponade outweighs the risks.
- For stable patients, cursory echocardiogram is performed before centesis because cardiac tumors are more easily visible with an outline of anechoic PE.
- A peripheral intravenous (IV) catheter is placed for sedation, antiarrhythmic doses of lidocaine, or emergency use.
- Continuous ECG monitoring should be employed whenever possible, both during and just after pericardiocentesis.
- Assistants are necessary to provide manual restraint and should be encouraged to stay vigilant because many dogs feel relief within only a few moments of removing PE and may attempt to move.

Possible Complications and Common Errors to Avoid

- Ventricular arrhythmias warranting vigilant ECG monitoring and ready availability of lidocaine.
- Re-effusion: risk depends on cause with variable time frame
- Rare risk of chamber or tumor puncture causing acute hemorrhage, cardiovascular collapse, or death

Procedure

- Restrain patient in left lateral recumbency because catheter entry from the right side of the thorax is less likely to lacerate lung

tissue or a coronary artery. A wide site covering approximately the 2nd to 8th intercostal spaces is clipped and aseptically prepared.
- The site of entry is chosen by ultrasound guidance or by approximating the location of the right-sided cardiac notch.
  - Notch is at the 4th or 5th intercostal space ventral to the costochondral junction (the point of contact between the flexed elbow and the thoracic wall).
- Local block: a 3-mL syringe and 22-gauge needle are used to infuse lidocaine (0.5-3 mL, based on patient size) through the intercostal musculature down to the pleura. The author prefers to advance the needle to the pleura first, aspirate to avoid pleural effusion, and then infuse lidocaine as the needle is withdrawn to the level of the skin, ensuring all layers of tissue are blocked. The needle is redirected, and the procedure is continued until a 2-cm perimeter around the site of entry is infused.
- The clinician is sterilely gloved before handling the blade or catheter.
- A #11 scalpel blade is used to make a 0.5-1 cm deep stab incision at the site of entry to ease catheter advancement.
- The same #11 blade can optionally be used to create a side hole in the large 14-18 gauge catheter to promote flow. The side hole should not exceed 30% of the catheter circumference, and it should be at least 0.5 cm away from the point of tapering in order to maintain catheter integrity.
- A 6-mL syringe is attached to the stylet inside the large catheter. The needle and catheter, held perpendicular to the body wall and just off the *cranial* edge of the rib, are advanced together through the stab incision while negative pressure is applied to the 6-mL syringe.
- Fluid (most commonly hemorrhagic in appearance) is visible in the syringe as soon as the metal stylet (but not the plastic catheter) has penetrated the pericardium. Slowly advance the stylet and catheter together another 2-4 mm before threading the catheter off the stylet and removing the stylet from the thorax.
- A 20-35 mL syringe is attached to the end of the catheter to aspirate PE. Once full, this syringe can be exchanged for another. Optionally, extension tubing and a 3-way stopcock can be used to expel fluid into a collecting bowl without the need for syringe exchange.
- An assistant must evaluate the removed fluid for clotting, which indicates chamber puncture or an acute/active hemorrhage.
- ECG is monitored for ventricular arrhythmias, which may arise from disease or if the catheter tip contacts the myocardium. This often simultaneously produces palpable friction, in which case the catheter should be slightly withdrawn/repositioned. When this friction becomes unavoidable and/or when effusion is no longer aspirated into the syringe, the catheter is withdrawn from the thorax.

Postprocedure

- Aliquots of fluid should be assayed for type and examined microscopically (p. 1343). If there is any suspicion that PE is infectious in origin, fluid should also be submitted for bacterial ± fungal culture and susceptibility testing.
- Although rarely necessary, skin glue, a staple, or nonabsorbable suture can be used to close the skin over the catheter entry site.
- Diagnostic echocardiogram and a re-evaluation are recommended in the 12-24 hours after pericardiocentesis because rapid re-effusion is possible. ECG monitoring is recommended throughout this period.
- Abdominal effusion associated with cardiac tamponade often resorbs within 48 hours after pericardiocentesis. Therapeutic abdominocentesis is performed only if necessary to rapidly improve patient comfort.
- IV fluid therapy is indicated for patients that are clinically dehydrated or have been hyporexic.

Alternatives and Their Relative Merits

- Surgical pericardectomy or less commonly percutaneous balloon pericardiotomy may be indicated, depending on the cause of the effusion. This reduces the risk that effusion will recur and/or that chronic or recurrent PE will cause constrictive pericarditis.
- Diuretics are indicated only in the rare instances where PE occurs as a manifestation of congestive heart failure (cats). Otherwise, diuretics are not effective in evacuating PE and can adversely reduce preload, exacerbating clinical signs of poor cardiac output.

Pearls

- Although most PEs appear red, blood can be distinguished from PE by the fact that blood will clot and PE will not clot, unless PE is due to a very recent bleeding event. Packed cell volume of the PE is usually less than that of peripheral blood.
- Samples saved in the red- and lavender-top tubes should be taken first from the fluid removed to preserve sterility.
- After the pericardium is penetrated with a catheter, the tautness of that tissue is reduced, which makes repeated puncture very difficult. If a catheter penetrated the pericardium, the fluid can escape through the catheter entry site into the thorax, making multiple attempts unnecessary.

SUGGESTED READING

Gidlewski J, et al: Therapeutic pericardiocentesis in the dog and cat. Clin Tech Small Anim Pract 20:151, 2005.

AUTHOR: Erin L. Anderson, VMD, MSc, DACVIM
EDITORS: Leah A. Cohn, DVM, PhD, DACVIM; Mark S. Thompson, DVM, DABVP

Procedures and Techniques

Postpartum Management of the Bitch/Queen

Client Education Sheet 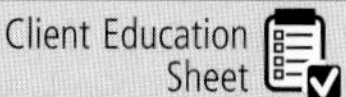

Difficulty Level: ◆

Synonyms

- Postparturient care
- Postwhelping/queening management
- Postnatal care

Overview and Goals

- Care of the dam and offspring after parturition
- To wean as many healthy pups/kittens as possible

Indications

- Owner requests information on postpartum management
- Natural birth
- Cesarean section at hospital

Equipment, Anesthesia

- Whelping box/nesting area
- Thermometer: to aid in regulating the temperature of the environment. Thermometer should be placed at the level of the puppies or kittens
- Dry towels: For vigorous rubbing of neonates and to keep the dam clean
- Suction: a suction bulb or an Argyle DeLee suction catheter for cleaning neonate airways
- Indirect mechanisms for temperature regulation (Bair Hugger, warm water bottles, and/or heating pad/lamp)
  - Ambient temperature in the pup/kitten area should be maintained at 29.5°C-35°C (85°F-95°F) with space away from the pups/kittens available for the bitch/queen.

  - Important: any heating implement used needs to be monitored closely with a way for the young to get away from the heat if it is excessive.
- Nonslip absorbent surfaces (blankets, towels, pee pads)
- Anesthesia
  - If a cesarean section was performed, careful monitoring of the bitch/queen after anesthesia should continue until the bitch/queen is completely conscious. The addition of postcesarean pain medication should strongly be considered (e.g., tramadol 1-4 mg/kg, carprofen 4.4 mg/kg, meloxicam 0.1 mg/kg).

Anticipated Time

- Owners should implement unobtrusive monitoring and not leave first-time mothers or nervous bitches/queens alone with offspring until they are sure the dam will not cannibalize the young.
  - Typically, it takes 2-3 days, especially after a cesarean section, before a bitch/queen can be left alone.
  - Dog Appeasing Pheromone (diffuser or collar) or Feliway (diffuser or wipes) may help to calm nervous or agitated bitches or queens, respectively.

Preparation: Important Checkpoints

- Prepare an area that is safe and quiet (e.g., whelping box/nesting area).
- Attention to hygiene (washing hands, changing clothes, keeping other dogs/cats away) reduces the risk of infection for the dam and offspring.
- It may be necessary to assist the pups/kittens to suckle initially.
  - If the bitch/queen continues to refuse to accept the pups/kittens, she should be evaluated for mammary discomfort resulting from mastitis (p. 618).
- Nutrition
  - It is important during lactation to provide enough energy and protein to the dam. She will need to produce enough milk for the offspring while maintaining her own body weight.
  - Small dog breeds have higher nutrient requirements per pound of body weight than large dog breeds.
  - The first week, feed 1½ times the regular maintenance diet; the second week, feed two times maintenance; and the third week, feed three times maintenance.
  - Good-quality, nutrient-dense, easily digestible food is recommended.
- Because the bitch/queen may express reluctance to leave the whelping box/nesting area and her pups/kittens, food and fresh water may need to be made available in the whelping box/nesting area.
- The bitch/queen should be encouraged to get some time away from the offspring while the whelping box/nesting area is being cleaned.
- Prepartum dental health should not be ignored.
  - Remember that the dam uses her mouth to clean the offspring and tear the umbilical cord. If the dam has poor oral hygiene, she is more likely to introduce bacteria to the umbilicus.

Possible Complications and Common Errors to Avoid

- Most problems can be clarified and some fully diagnosed with a thorough history (environmental, medical) and physical exam of the dam and offspring.
- Postpartum risks
  - Toy-breed dogs are at a greater risk for postparturient hypocalcemia.
  - Excessively large dog litters may predispose dams to eclampsia (p. 281).
    - More than 6 pups for small-breed dogs (<9 kg)
    - More than 9 pups for medium-breed dogs (9-20 kg)
    - More than 10 pups for large-breed dogs (20-40 kg)
    - More than 12 pups for giant-breed dogs (>40 kg)
  - Maiden bitches/queens do not always have good mothering instincts.
  - Maiden bitches are susceptible to subinvolution of placental sites (SIPS [p. 950]).
  - Older bitches/queens are more predisposed to postpartum disorders (e.g., mastitis [p. 618], acute metritis).
    - Acute metritis is an ascending bacterial infection (typically gram negative) of the uterus in the immediate postpartum period that can be life-threatening. Clinical signs include fever, dehydration, depression, anorexia, agalactia, disinterest in offspring, and a deep port wine to black malodorous vaginal discharge.
- Postpartum complications
  - Abnormal exam findings in the dam may include depression, inappetence, poor mothering, inadequate lactation (evidenced by anxious or distressed offspring), prolonged or abnormal vaginal discharge, and engorged or inflamed mammary glands.
  - Mammary glands should be evaluated daily for heat, pain, or changes in consistency (p. 618).
  - Postpartum rectal temperature normally may be elevated for 24-48 hours but should not exceed 39.4°C (103°F).
  - Postpartum lochia (vaginal discharge, normal endometrial drainage) can be obvious for 4-6 weeks and may last as long as 12 weeks.
    - Normal: green-black to brick red with no significant odor (should become

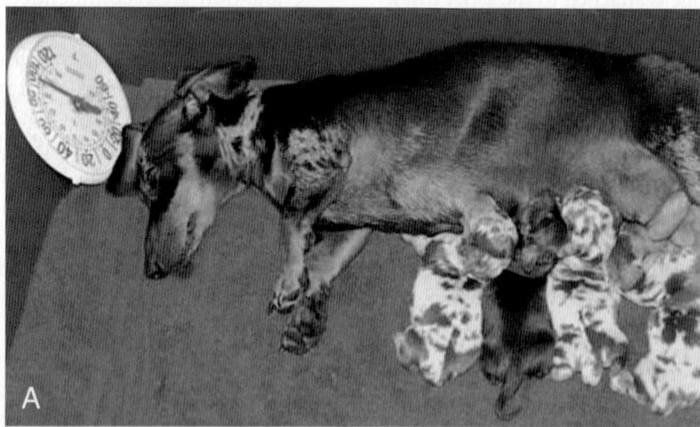

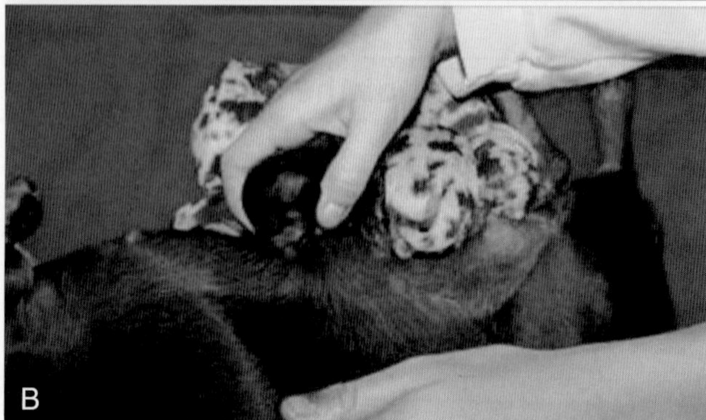

POSTPARTUM MANAGEMENT OF THE BITCH/QUEEN A, A thermometer should be placed in the whelping/nesting box at the level of the puppies or kittens. The temperature should be maintained at 29.5°C-35°C (85°F-95°F), with a temperature gradient so that puppies/kittens can move to a warmer or cooler area if desired. **B**, It may be necessary to assist the puppies or kittens to suckle initially. (Courtesy Michelle A. Kutzler.)

more red/brown and scant over time)
- Abnormal: cream colored or any of the above with a significant odor

Procedure

- Perform a postpartum physical exam of dam and offspring.
  - Exam allows early detection of periparturient disorders if they arise.
  - Lactating dam and offspring have an increased susceptibility to infectious disease.
- Based on physical exam findings, decide whether a postpartum problem exists.
  - Often, postpartum problems present as problems with offspring.
- Weight of dam, pups/kittens should be ascertained at birth and recorded daily for the first few weeks to document/address changes.
- Some differential diagnoses to consider based on exam findings:
  - Prolonged or abnormal-appearing vaginal discharge: SIPS, metritis, retained placenta
  - Swollen mammary glands: mastitis, galactostasis, agalactia, hypogalactia
- Diagnostic testing may be necessary to address a suspected problem.
  - CBC, serum biochemistry panel, fibrinogen: healthy postpartum dams may be slightly anemic, with an elevated fibrinogen and normal chemistry profile.
  - Vaginal cytologic exam: healthy dams typically have erythrocytes and hemosiderophages present in vaginal discharge for 4-6 weeks postpartum.
  - Vaginal culture: healthy postpartum dams have positive bacterial cultures for normal vaginal flora, similar to all healthy bitches; overgrowth of a single organism may be cause for concern.
  - Milk cytologic exam, pH, and culture
- Abdominal ultrasonography and/or radiographs
  - Check for retained placenta or retained fetus.
- Sometimes, additional treatments are necessary.
  - For postpartum dams, breeders may request a "clean-out shot," meaning an oxytocin injection. This is no longer considered necessary because suckling offspring have the same effect.
    - A dose of 2-10 units (up to a maximum of 20 units) oxytocin IM or intranasal aids in uterine involution if retained placentas are suspected or offspring are born dead.
    - Do not give until an obstructive dystocia is ruled out.

Postprocedure

- The dam and offspring should be rechecked at 3 and 6 weeks.
- After caesarean section, dam and offspring can continue to be monitored at home.
- Strict adherence to biosecurity procedures helps to keep dam and offspring healthy.
- Many drugs are excreted into the milk, which can then be ingested at high (even toxic) levels by the nursing offspring. Verification of the potential for milk excretion and the effects of the drug on the neonates is essential before prescribing a drug to a lactating dam.

Alternatives and Their Relative Merits

The dam can be allowed to give birth without any intervention.

Pearls

- Keeping the bitch/queen in a clean, comfortable, warm, and safe environment with plenty of fresh water is in her best interest.
- Cooked pumpkin is a useful food additive to help correct diarrhea after placental ingestion.
- Do not neglect the importance of proper nutrition while the bitch/queen is pregnant and while nursing her offspring.
- Feeding raw diets during pregnancy and in postpartum period is discouraged.
- Temperature plays a huge role in successful postpartum health of dam and puppies/kittens; pay close attention to the environmental temperature.
- Know the signs of postpartum conditions such as eclampsia.
  - Signs of eclampsia include tremors, weakness, and a form of paralysis called puerperal tetany, characterized by stiff limbs and an inability to stand or walk.
- Do not leave first-time mothers or nervous bitches/queens alone with offspring until you are sure the dam will not cannibalize the young.

SUGGESTED READING

Johnston SD, et al: Periparturient disorders in the bitch. In Johnston SD, et al, editors: Canine and feline theriogenology, Philadelphia, 2001, Saunders, pp 129-145.

AUTHOR: Clare M. Scully, DVM, MA, MS, DACT
EDITORS: Leah A. Cohn, DVM, PhD, DACVIM; Michelle A. Kutzler, DVM, PhD, DACT

Prostatic Diagnostic Sampling

Client Education Sheet 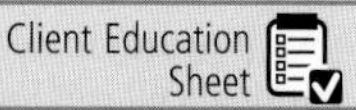

Difficulty level: ♦♦

Overview and Goal

Nonsurgical techniques for obtaining prostate tissue samples for culture, cytologic analysis, and/or histopathologic examination

Indications

- Pyuria
- Hematuria
- Penile/urethral discharge
- Prostate enlargement
- Prostatic mineralization
- Asymmetrical/irregular/nodular prostate

Contraindications

- Inadequate restraint
- Bleeding disorder
- Prostate abscess (for automated needle biopsy and large-needle aspirate)
- Acute prostatitis (relative contraindication)
- Suspicion or possibility of urethral transitional cell carcinoma (for fine-needle aspiration [FNA] and automated needle biopsy). Diagnostic (traumatic) catheterization would be a safer option in this case to reduce the risk of tumor seeding.

Equipment, Anesthesia

FNA:
- 18-gauge needle
- 12-mL syringe
- Usually does not require sedation
- Ultrasound machine

Automated needle biopsy:
- Automated biopsy needle (14-20 gauge)
- General anesthesia
- Ultrasound machine

Prostatic massage:
- Urinary catheter that is long enough to reach the urinary bladder
- Two 5-mL syringes
- Two 5-mL aliquots of sterile saline
- Two sterile sample containers capable of holding at least 5 mL of fluid
- Manual restraint to general anesthesia, depending on the demeanor of the patient
- Ultrasound guidance is helpful.

Diagnostic catheterization:
- Urinary catheter that is long enough to reach the prostatic urethra
- 60-mL syringe
- Sedation pending patient
- Ultrasound is helpful.

Anticipated Time

- Abdominal ultrasound takes 10-40 minutes, depending on operator expertise.
- FNA takes about 5 minutes.
- Automated needle biopsy with anesthesia, prostatic massage, or diagnostic catheterization takes 20-30 minutes.

Preparation: Important Checkpoints

- Lateral or dorsal recumbency
- These procedures usually require the attending veterinarian and one or two assistants.
- Needle aspiration can be performed on a fully awake animal, provided the animal is adequately restrained.
- Automated needle biopsies require heavy sedation with analgesia or general anesthesia.
- For prostatic massage and diagnostic catheterization, digital rectal palpation and urethral catheterization are necessary. If the patient resists these procedures, sedation is advised.
- A soft red rubber (Sovereign type) feeding tube is less traumatic than a polypropylene catheter.

Possible Complications and Common Errors to Avoid

- FNA and automated needle biopsy procedures require the placement of a needle or biopsy instrument directly into the prostate. Adjacent large vessels such as the distal abdominal aorta and caudal vena cava can be lacerated with patient movement or a biopsy miss.
- These procedures should not be performed on animals with inadequate coagulation systems.
- If acute bacterial prostatitis (p. 827) is present, prostatic massage can result in release of bacteria into the bloodstream and septicemia.
- Diagnostic catheterization and automated needle biopsy may lacerate the urethra.
- If an abscess or cyst is present, rupture is possible secondary to all of these procedures.
- With prostatic neoplasia (particularly transitional cell carcinoma [pp. 828 and 991]), there is a risk of tumor seeding along needle or biopsy tract.

Procedure

FNA, nonguided:

- If the prostate is sufficiently enlarged that it can be palpated externally (abdominally) and stabilized by caudal abdominal palpation, the procedure can be performed without the use of ultrasound (nonguided).
- The external surface of the skin overlying the region of the enlarged prostate is clipped of hair and aseptically prepared with surgical scrub.
- The needle is affixed to the syringe, the needle tip is placed through the prepared skin, and the tip is advanced into the prostate gland.
- Material is aspirated into the needle by drawing on the syringe plunger to create negative pressure in the syringe.
- Negative pressure is released before withdrawing the needle.
- The needle and syringe are then withdrawn quickly, the syringe is detached from the needle and filled with air, and the syringe is reattached to the needle. The contents are vigorously expelled onto a microscope slide to make fresh smears for cytologic evaluation.
- A portion of the material can be placed in appropriate media for culture and susceptibility (C&S) testing instead of being smeared, or the procedure can be repeated to obtain more material for this purpose.

FNA, guided:

- The animal should undergo a full abdominal ultrasound evaluation, and an appropriate area for aspiration should be identified.
- The skin is clipped of hair and aseptically prepared with surgical scrub.
- The needle with a syringe attached is then advanced through the skin into the prostate under ultrasound guidance.
- The prostate gland is aspirated, and the sample is handled for evaluation (as described).

Automated needle biopsy:

- Automated needle biopsies (guided or nonguided) are attained as described above for needle aspiration. Because this is a more invasive and painful procedure, general anesthesia is recommended.
- Care must be taken not to transect the urethra with this full-thickness biopsy procedure. With this in mind, the biopsy should be taken in an orientation angled away from the urethra, not perpendicular to the urethra.
- A portion of the biopsy is taken for culture. The biopsy is then rolled on a slide for cytologic analysis. The sample is then placed in formalin and processed for histopathologic examination.

Prostatic massage:

- The tip of the penis is extended from the prepuce and cleaned with a mild disinfectant.
- A urinary catheter is placed into the bladder, and the urine is completely removed.
- Sterile saline (5 mL) is instilled into the bladder. This fluid is then aspirated and placed in a sterile tube labeled *tube #1*.
- The veterinarian then places an index finger in the rectum and palpates the prostate and the catheter. The catheter is retracted until the tip can be felt caudal to the prostate. Ultrasound can also be used for confirming catheter placement at the level of the prostate gland. The prostate is then massaged for 1 minute.
- The palpating finger is retracted until it is caudal to the holes in the catheter. Pressure is applied to the catheter rectally so that fluid injected into the catheter does not leak out of the penis but moves forward into the bladder.
- Another 5 mL of sterile saline is injected into the catheter. The fluid flows across the prostatic urethra into the bladder.
- The catheter is then pushed into the bladder, and the fluid is aspirated into a syringe and placed into a sterile tube labeled *tube #2*. Both tubes are presented for fluid analysis and culture.
- Sample #1 will have only bladder material, whereas sample #2 will have both prostate and bladder material. Comparing the two samples allows the clinician to localize the disease process to the prostate and/or the urinary bladder.

Diagnostic catheterization:

- Prepare the penis, and empty the bladder as above.
- The urinary catheter is placed into the prostatic urethra. Correct catheter placement can be verified by digital rectal examination or by ultrasound.
- A 60-mL syringe is attached to the end of the catheter, and negative pressure is applied so that prostate tissue is aspirated into the holes of the catheter. Quickly pull the catheter back and forth within the urethra at the level of the prostate gland while suction on the 60-mL syringe is maintained. This tears tissue from the prostate gland that is aspirated into the catheter.
- While maintaining negative pressure on the syringe, remove the catheter from the urethra. This prostatic tissue can be evaluated by cytologic evaluation, and sometimes a large enough piece is obtained for histopathologic evaluation.

Postprocedure

- These are outpatient procedures, and the client may be sent home the same day provided that its clinical condition allows.
- The patient should be sent home on an antibiotic if bacteria are identified from urine or prostate pending culture and susceptibility; antibiotics with adequate prostatic penetration should be used (e.g., enrofloxacin).
- The client should be counseled that there may be hematuria transiently after the procedure.

Alternatives and Their Relative Merits

A technique for performing a needle aspiration biopsy of the prostate per rectum using a guarded needle has been described. This technique has the problem of injecting bacteria directly into the prostate because the colon cannot be sterilized. The advent of ultrasound-guided techniques has made this procedure obsolete.

Pearls

- Diagnostic catheterization is easier if the patient is sedated.
- These nonsurgical biopsy techniques have made surgical biopsy techniques almost obsolete.

SUGGESTED READING

Nyland TG, et al: Needle-tract implantation following ultrasound-guided fine-needle aspiration biopsy of transitional cell carcinoma of the bladder, urethra, and prostate. Vet Radiol Ultrasound 43:50-53, 2002.

Reproduced from the third edition in modified form.

RELATED CLIENT EDUCATION SHEETS

Consent to Perform Abdominal Ultrasound
Consent to Perform Castration, Canine
Consent to Perform Cystocentesis
Consent to Perform General Anesthesia
Consent to Perform Fine-Needle Aspiration of Masses

AUTHORS: Donald R. Krawiec, DVM, PhD, DACVIM; Lenore Mohammadian, DVM, MSpVM, DACVR
EDITORS: Leah A. Cohn, DVM, PhD, DACVIM; Mark S. Thompson, DVM, DABVP

Radiographic Interpretation, Thorax

Client Education Sheet Bonus Material Online 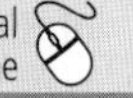

Difficulty level: ♦

Overview and Goal

Stepwise interpretation of thoracic radiographs to curate a list of differential diagnoses

Anticipated Time

Anticipated time to evaluate thoracic radiographs is 15 minutes.

Preparation: Important Checkpoints

- Ventrodorsal (VD) and dorsoventral (DV) views have different advantages and disadvantages that can be weighed before taking radiographs.
  - A DV view is useful in cardiovascular evaluation due to consistent positioning of the heart and clear visualization of the pulmonary vessels, especially in barrel-chested patients.
  - The DV view is preferred for patients in respiratory distress.
- Right and left lateral views vary slightly in appearance and can be used in a complementary fashion for optimal evaluation.

Possible Complications and Common Errors to Avoid

- Do not base a diagnosis on incomplete or poor-quality radiographic studies.
- Evaluate the entire image, not only the intrathoracic structures. Lesions such as bone lysis or discospondylitis can otherwise be missed.
- Distinguish cutaneous structures such as skin tags from pulmonary nodules by applying barium to the cutaneous structures and repeating radiographs.

Procedure

General:

- At least two orthogonal views (lateral and VD/DV) should be evaluated. Three views (right lateral, left lateral, and VD/DV) are necessary for assessment for aspiration pneumonia or metastases.
- Use a systematic approach. For example, an inside-out approach starts with evaluation of the cardiac silhouette and ends in the periphery of the radiograph with the body wall and musculoskeletal structures.
- Assess for proper patient positioning and radiographic technique. Rotation may cause inaccurate assessment of cardiac size.
- The appearance of the canine thorax varies significantly with breed.
- Assess patient's body condition; excess fat may obscure the lung fields.

Heart:

- The clock-face analogy is used to evaluate the cardiac silhouette. Enlargements in the cardiac chambers, aorta, pulmonary artery, as well as cardiac masses can result in a convex appearance in that specific region of the cardiac silhouette.

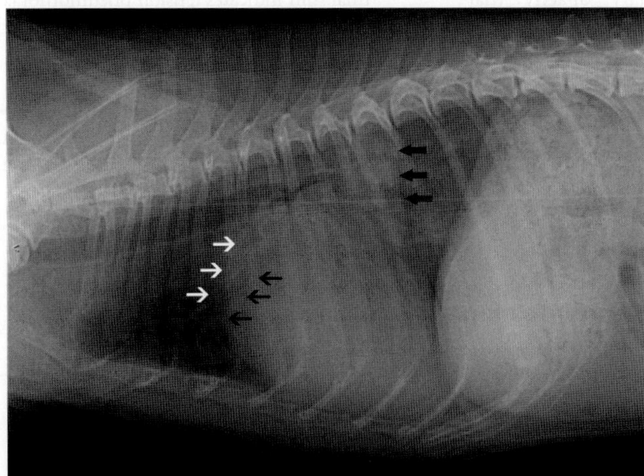

RADIOGRAPHIC INTERPRETATION, THORAX Left-sided congestive heart failure (CHF). Lateral thoracic radiograph of a 13-year-old Maltese terrier cross with left-sided CHF. Note the severe left atrial enlargement *(thick black arrows)* and left ventricular enlargement characterized by the dorsal displacement of the trachea. Pulmonary veins *(thin black arrows)* are enlarged compared with the corresponding arteries *(white arrows)*, and a caudodorsally distributed unstructured interstitial pulmonary pattern is seen.

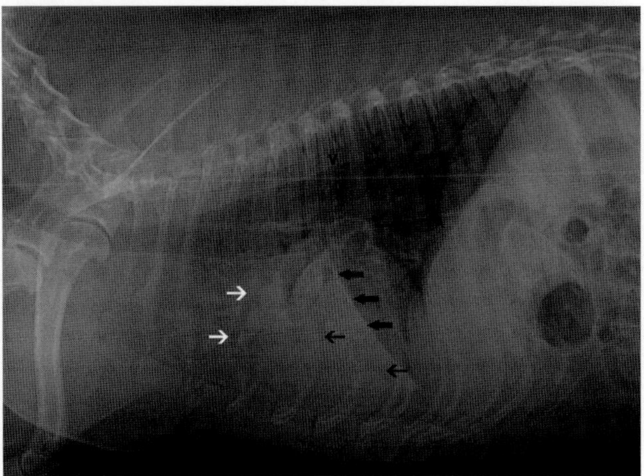

RADIOGRAPHIC INTERPRETATION, THORAX Megaesophagus with aspiration pneumonia. Left lateral thoracic radiograph of a 9-year-old beagle with regurgitation and hypersalivation. Note the generalized esophageal dilation *(Vs)*. A lobar sign *(thick black arrows)* is seen between the right middle and right caudal lung lobes. Prominent air bronchograms can be seen in the right cranial *(white arrows)* and right middle lung lobes *(thin black arrows)*. Polyradiculoneuritis was suspected.

- Vertebral heart score can be used to objectively assess cardiac size (p. 1187).
- Dog: lateral view, heart length: 2.5 (deep-chested) to 3.5 (round-chested) intercostal spaces.
- Dog: VD/DV view, heart width: ≤ ⅔ of the thoracic width.
- Dog: left atrial (LA) enlargement on the lateral view leads to a convexity at the caudodorsal aspect of the cardiac silhouette. LA enlargement on the VD/DV view may cause the mainstem bronchi to spread apart.
- Cat: heart length = distance from the cranial aspect of the fifth rib to the caudal aspect of the seventh rib
- Cat: LA enlargement confers a kidney bean shape to the heart on the lateral view. LA or biatrial enlargement may create a valentine-shaped heart on the VD/DV view.
- A globoid shape to the cardiac silhouette may indicate pericardial effusion, right- and left-sided cardiac disease, dilated cardiomyopathy, or a peritoneal pericardial diaphragmatic hernia.
- Evaluate the cardiac silhouette, the pulmonary vessels, and lungs concurrently for suspicious of left-sided heart failure. Evaluate the cardiac silhouette, caudal vena cava, and the abdomen concurrently for suspicion of right-sided heart failure.
- Hypovolemia (e.g., dehydration, hypoadrenocorticism) may cause microcardia.

Vessels:

- Caudal vena cava diameter varies with the cardiorespiratory phase but should be similar to aortic diameter.
- A pulmonary artery and its corresponding vein should be similar in diameter when measured at the same level. The cranial pulmonary vessels are best evaluated on the left lateral view.
- On the lateral view, the cranial pulmonary vessels should be smaller than the diameter of the proximal fourth rib.
- On the VD/DV view, the caudal pulmonary vessels normally may be up to 1.2 times the diameter of the ninth rib.

Lung:

- A lesion in dependent lung lobes may silhouette with the surrounding atelectatic lung and not be seen. In a nondependent position, the lesion will be surrounded by aerated lung, allowing its detection.
- Lung lesions create patterns categorized as alveolar, bronchial, and interstitial.
- Distinguish further among differential diagnoses based on lesion location.
- Recumbent atelectasis is common. Features: interstitial or alveolar pattern with ipsilateral mediastinal shift
- Benign pulmonary osseous metaplasia can be distinguished from pulmonary nodules based on their small size and mineral opacity.
- Alveolar pattern
  - Silhouetting (border effacement): increased pulmonary opacity prevents the clear demarcation between abnormal lung and an abutting soft-tissue–opacity structure (e.g., cardiac silhouette, body wall).
  - Lobar sign: increased opacity in an abnormal lung lobe creates a sharp demarcation against an abutting normal lung lobe.
  - Air bronchogram/"trees in the fog": increased lung opacity (fog) effaces the pulmonary vessels, and only the airways (trees) can be distinguished.
- Bronchial pattern
  - Faint airway markings are normal.
  - Thickened airways create the appearance of doughnuts and tram tracks when the airways are viewed end-on or from the side, respectively.
- Interstitial pattern
  - Structured interstitial pattern: soft-tissue–opacity nodules that can be various sizes, ranging from miliary (pinpoint) to nodules (<2 cm in diameter). Structures > 2 cm are masses.
  - Unstructured interstitial pattern: a mild increase in pulmonary opacity that causes difficulty in seeing clear margins to the pulmonary vessels. The opacity is not enough to cause effacement of the pulmonary vessels or silhouetting.
  - Many artifacts can cause an unstructured interstitial pulmonary pattern.
  - The unstructured interstitial pattern can be transient, seen early in a disease process or when a disease is resolving.
  - Severe bronchial disease may lead to a concurrent structured interstitial pattern if airway plugging occurs.

Mediastinum:

- Evaluate the position of the mediastinum. Evaluate for structures that are normally seen and that are not normally seen.
- Pneumomediastinum reveals mediastinal structures that are not normally seen (e.g., brachiocephalic trunk).
- Pneumomediastinum can cause pneumothorax (not vice versa).
- LA enlargement and tracheobronchial lymphadenopathy cause splaying of the mainstem bronchi; the former causes dorsal displacement of the trachea, and the latter causes ventral displacement.
- If megaesophagus is seen, distinguish segmental from generalized dilation to narrow the differential list.
- Evaluate for tracheal narrowing.

Pleural space:

- Pleural effusion
  - VD view (rather than DV) allows better assessment of the cardiac silhouette when effusion is present.
  - Pleural fissure lines and retraction of the lung lobes that results in a scalloped appearance along the lung periphery.
- Pneumothorax
  - Cardiac silhouette separated from the sternum on the lateral view. A space exists between the lung lobe and the body wall where normal bronchial markings are not seen.
  - Pneumothorax with a contralateral mediastinal shift indicates tension pneumothorax. Emergency thoracocentesis is warranted (p. 1164).

Body wall and abdomen:

- Assess the diaphragm and other musculoskeletal structures for evidence of trauma, congenital diseases, neuromuscular disease, or neoplasia.

Causes of an Alveolar Pulmonary Pattern

Cause	Distribution*	Prevalence
Pneumonia	Ventral	Common
Cardiogenic pulmonary edema	Variable	Common
Noncardiogenic pulmonary edema	Dorsocaudal	Less common
Hemorrhage		
Trauma	Variable	Common
Coagulopathy	Variable	Less common
Thromboembolism	Variable	Less common
Atelectasis	Variable	Common
Allergy (eosinophilic)	Variable	Rare
Primary lung tumor	Variable	Rare

*Disease distributions are generalizations, and the specific distribution of any disease leading to an alveolar pattern is variable.

From Thrall DE: The canine and feline lung. In Thrall DE, editor: Textbook of veterinary diagnostic radiology, ed 6, St. Louis, 2013, Saunders.

Causes of a Bronchial Pulmonary Pattern

Cause	Prevalence
Allergic airway disease	Common
Infection	
Bacterial	Less common
Parasitic	Rare
Chronic irritation	Less common
Cardiogenic pulmonary edema	Less common
Diffuse tumor	Rare

From Thrall DE: The canine and feline lung. In Thrall DE, editor: Textbook of veterinary diagnostic radiology, ed 6, St. Louis, 2013, Saunders.

Causes of Interstitial Nodules and Masses

Finding	Cause	Prevalence
Multiple solid nodules	Metastasis Mycosis Septic emboli	Common Varies with region Rare
Solitary solid mass	Primary tumor Abscess	Common Rare
Multiple cavitary nodules	Metastasis Parasite Bullae	Rare Rare Uncommon
Solitary cavitary mass	Primary tumor Abscess Bulla	Common Rare Uncommon

From Thrall DE: The canine and feline lung. In Thrall DE, editor: Textbook of veterinary diagnostic radiology, ed 6, St. Louis, 2013, Saunders.

Causes of an Unstructured Interstitial Pattern

Cause	Prevalence
Poor radiographic technique	Common
Poor ventilation	Common
Body habitus	Common
Cardiogenic edema	Common
Lymphoma	Uncommon
Solid tumor metastasis	Uncommon
Deep mycosis	Uncommon

Adapted from Thrall DE: The canine and feline lung. In Thrall DE, editor: Textbook of veterinary diagnostic radiology, ed 6, St. Louis, 2013, Saunders.

- Use the extrapleural sign to distinguish extrathoracic lesions from pulmonary lesions. A broad-based mass extending into the thorax is likely of body wall or extrapleural origin. A thoracic mass contacting the body wall at an acute angle is likely intrathoracic or pulmonary in origin.

Postprocedure

Additional imaging studies or other diagnostic tests may be required for a definitive disease diagnosis.

Alternatives and Their Relative Merits

- CT: precludes superimposition, can better characterize anatomic relationships, and is better able to detect pulmonary metastasis. Routine CT is not ideal for cardiac evaluation.
- Ultrasound: further characterizes lesions, guides fine-needle aspiration, and evaluates blood flow; reverberation artifact makes investigation of intrathoracic lesions difficult.
- Echocardiography: characterizes cardiac structure and function.

SUGGESTED READING

Thrall DE, editor: Textbook of veterinary diagnostic radiology, ed 7, St. Louis, 2018, Saunders.

AUTHOR: Aisha N. Young, DVM, MVSc, DACVR
EDITORS: Leah A. Cohn, DVM, PhD, DACVIM; Mark S. Thompson, DVM, DABVP

Rectal Scraping

Difficulty level: ◆

Synonyms

Rectal scrape, rectal cytologic analysis

Overview and Goal

The goal of rectal scraping is to obtain samples of mucosal tissue for cytologic examination.

Indications

- Animals with signs of disease of the rectum or distal colon, such as hematochezia and tenesmus, especially when rectal mucosa has a diffusely thickened or cobblestone feel on rectal palpation
- Most commonly indicated for the diagnosis of rectal histoplasmosis, protothecosis, pythiosis, or neoplasia

Contraindications

Suspicion of rectal perforation or deep ulceration

Equipment, Anesthesia

- Often performed without anesthesia or sedation. Sedation may be required for animals with pain on rectal palpation or for animals with an uncooperative temperament.
- Wooden tongue depressor (alternatively, cotton-tipped applicator or blunt-tipped metal spatula such as those for pharmacy use)
- Exam glove
- Lubricant
- Microscope slides

Anticipated Time

5-10 minutes

Preparation: Important Checkpoints

The rectum should be empty of formed fecal matter. Allowing the animal to defecate shortly before the procedure or manual evacuation of the rectum is sufficient (i.e., bowel cleansing or enemas are not required).

Possible Complications and Common Errors to Avoid

- Rectal perforation is possible with vigorous scraping or overzealous insertion of the instrument.
- Splintered or sharp edges of the tongue depressor should be smoothed or covered with a gloved finger.

Procedure

- Depending on the size of the patient, the tongue depressor may be left intact or broken lengthwise to a smaller width.

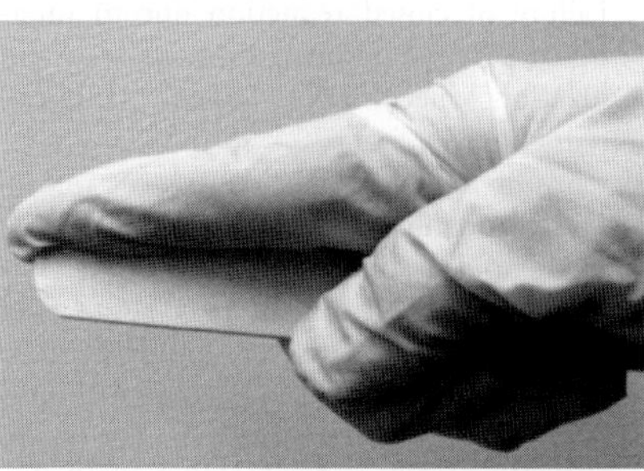

RECTAL SCRAPING One side of a tongue depressor is covered with a gloved finger before insertion of the lubricated finger and the depressor approximately 2 inches (5 cm) into the rectum. Once in the rectum, gentle pressure is used to move the depressor in an arcing motion to obtain tissue for cytologic examination.

- The depressor is held in a gloved hand to the length of an outstretched index finger. If the depressor has been broken, the finger should cover the roughened edge.
- Lubricant is applied to the finger but not to the tongue depressor.
- The finger and depressor are inserted approximately 2 inches (5 cm) into the rectum.
- The finger is used for applying gentle but firm pressure to the tongue depressor while making two to three sweeping motions covering 20%-50% of the circumference of the rectum.
- The gloved finger and tongue depressor are removed.
- The edge of the tongue depressor is scraped against a microscope slide.
- Gentle smears are made from the material gathered during the scraping. Try to minimize the amount of lubricant that contaminates the slide.
- Slides are processed for cytologic examination in a routine fashion.
- For animals with extremely friable rectal tissue or for very small animals, a cotton-tipped applicator can be used in place of the tongue depressor.

Postprocedure

Special care is not required afterward, but the animal should be monitored for worsened pain or systemic signs that may indicate rectal perforation.

Alternatives and Their Relative Merits

- Noninvasive fecal flotation or examination of direct fecal smear may detect intestinal parasites responsible for large-bowel signs.
- Tissue biopsy provides larger samples with intact architecture but requires general anesthesia and bowel cleansing.
- Serologic tests with varying sensitivity and specificity are available for histoplasmosis and pythiosis.

AUTHOR: Leah A. Cohn, DVM, PhD, DACVIM
EDITOR: Mark S. Thompson, DVM, DABVP

Reduction (Closed): Shoulder, Elbow, or Hip

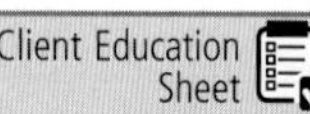

Difficulty level: ♦♦

Synonyms

Coxofemoral luxation (hip); dislocated shoulder, elbow, or hip; scapulohumeral luxation (shoulder)

Overview and Goals

- Severe joint trauma can cause ligament/joint capsule damage, resulting in displacement of the bones of a joint.
- Closed reduction aims to restore the normal alignment of the joint without surgical intervention and to maintain stability until these soft tissues heal.

Indications

- Traumatic luxation of normal shoulder, elbow, hip joints (pp. 291, 472, and 913)
- Acute luxation (<5 days)

Contraindications

- Luxation associated with severe ligament damage or avulsion fractures that impede normal joint function and/or leave the joint unstable after closed reduction
- Failure of closed reduction due to interposed soft tissue, hematoma, or recurrent luxation necessitates open (surgical) reduction.
- Chronic luxation (>5-7 days)
- Dysplastic joint
  - Glenoid dysplasia
  - Total hip replacement may be a better option in cases of severe hip dysplasia.
- Femoral head and neck ostectomy (FHO) may be an acceptable alternative to closed/open hip reduction in a small dog or cat.

Equipment, Anesthesia

- General anesthesia
- Rope or leash to provide counterpressure (hip luxation)
- Assistant
- Bandage material

Anticipated Time

About 10-30 minutes

Preparation: Important Checkpoints

- Advise owner of aftercare and possible drawbacks:
  - Recurrence
  - Degenerative joint disease
  - Decreased range of motion
  - Possible need for open reduction
  - Postreduction bandage care
  - Postreduction exercise restriction

After anesthetic induction:

- Minimum of two views of the joint to confirm luxation versus fracture
- Animal in lateral recumbency, affected limb up (affected limb on the nonrecumbent side)
- Hanging the affected limb can be useful (elbow luxation) for 5-10 minutes. Secure the carpus, and hoist the limb vertically with traction. Be sure to secure the limb proximal to the metacarpi and use a thick, soft rope (or roll gauze) in a double-loop technique, rather than a single loop, to distribute pressure evenly on the distal limb. These measures reduce the risk of iatrogenic damage.

Possible Complications and Common Errors to Avoid

- If there is excessive instability after closed reduction, open reduction should be performed.
- Failure to critically evaluate plain radiographs to assess joint anatomy or damage, avulsion fragments and intraarticular debris
- Trying to reduce a luxation with sedation alone
- Failure to appropriately bandage the luxation
- Removal of bandage too soon
- Inadequate patient exercise restriction
- When hanging the forelimb to help with elbow luxation reduction, be sure to secure the limb proximal to the metacarpi and use a thick, soft rope (or roll gauze) in a double-loop technique to distribute pressure evenly on the distal limb. These measures reduce the risk of iatrogenic damage.

Procedure

All luxation reductions are performed with the animal under general anesthesia and in lateral recumbency, with affected side up (nondependent).

- Shoulder
  - Forelimb held in extension (in a ventral direction perpendicular to the long axis of the body, as in the standing animal)
  - For lateral luxation of the humeral head, apply medial pressure to the head at the same time as lateral pressure on the scapula.
  - Check range of motion and stability.
  - Place leg in a spica splint.
  - For medial luxation of the humeral head, apply lateral pressure to the head at the same time as medial pressure on the scapula.
  - Check range of motion and stability.
  - Place the leg in a Velpeau sling.
  - Splint or sling can be removed after 2 weeks.
  - Passive range-of-motion exercises can begin after bandage removal, but restricted exercise is essential for another 2-4 weeks.
- Elbow
  - Radius and ulna are usually luxated laterally relative to the distal humerus.
  - With the elbow in flexion, inwardly rotate the antebrachium.
  - Combined with elbow flexion, this movement enables the anconeal process of the ulna (caudal-most extent of the trochlear notch in the ulna) to hook into the olecranon fossa of the humerus. This maneuver is followed by careful extension of the elbow.

- Hook the anconeal process of the ulna between the humeral condyles, and carefully extend the elbow. With this part of the maneuver, the joint should be reduced.
- Passive range-of-motion exercises can begin after bandage removal, but restricted exercise is essential for 4-6 weeks, followed by 2 weeks of leash exercise only.
- Hip
  - Assistant stands on opposite side of animal, holding the ends of a padded rope or leash placed in the animal's groin to provide counterpressure.
  - Craniodorsal hip luxation (more common):
    - The tarsus is grasped and externally rotated while the femur is pulled caudally.
    - The head of the femur rides up (moves laterally and then caudally) and over the dorsal acetabular rim.
    - Internal rotation while maintaining distal traction on the femur, together with direct pressure on the greater trochanter, seats the head in the acetabulum.
    - Place hip in an Ehmer or modified Ehmer sling for 2 weeks.
  - Caudoventral luxation
    - The femur should be abducted and externally rotated to seat the femoral head in the acetabulum.
    - Hobbles may be applied for 10-14 days.
  - Medially directed pressure can be applied to the reduced proximal femur as the hip is passively flexed and extended in an attempt to drive debris from the acetabulum.

Postprocedure

- Radiograph to evaluate the reduction.
- Toes should be accessible or visible to monitor for heat, cold, swelling, or pain.
- Bandage needs to be protected from moisture and kept clean and dry.

Alternatives and Their Relative Merits

- Open reduction
  - Requires surgical intervention
  - Greater cost
  - Carries a higher rate of success than closed reduction for the shoulder, elbow, and hip
- FHO may be worth considering for cats and small dogs because the possibility of hip reluxation is eliminated.
- Arthrodesis can provide pain relief for a chronically unstable joint. Aside from cost, complications include nonunion, stress fractures, implant failure, and infection.
- Excision glenoid arthroplasty for the shoulder joint. There are few reports of glenoid arthroplasty, but an abnormal gait is to be expected.
- Amputation

RELATED CLIENT EDUCATION SHEETS

Consent to Perform General Anesthesia
How to Assist a Pet That Is Unable to Rise and Walk
How to Perform Range-of-Motion Exercises
How to Provide Bandage Care and Upkeep at Home

AUTHOR: Nicholas J. Trout, VetMB, MA, DACVS, DECVS
EDITORS: Leah A. Cohn, DVM, PhD, DACVIM; Mark S. Thompson, DVM, DABVP

Rhinoscopy

Client Education Sheet 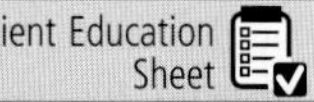

Difficulty level: ♦♦♦

Overview and Goal

Minimally invasive, endoscopic approach to the nasal cavity for visual examination and biopsy procedures

Indications

- Chronic nasal discharge
- Chronic sneezing
- Epistaxis, after ruling out coagulopathy, hypertension, or ehrlichiosis (p. 305)
- Nasal foreign body (identification and removal)
- Stertor
- Maxillary, nasal, or facial deformity
- Sample collection to confirm clinical suspicion (biopsy for histopathology or deep nasal culture)

Contraindications

Coagulopathy (primary/secondary); severe hypertension

Equipment, Anesthesia

- General anesthesia and endotracheal intubation with optimal endotracheal tube cuff seal
- Maxillary local block, 2% lidocaine
- Mouth gag or cut needle cap for cat/small dogs
- Sterile, water-soluble lubricant
- Sterile saline solution for flush
- Gauze for packing off oropharynx
- Flexible endoscope (small < 3 mm diameter maximum for patients < 10 kg) for retrograde pharyngoscopy to evaluate the nasopharynx
- Flexible or 1.9-2.7 mm, 30° oblique, rigid endoscope for anterograde cranial rhinoscopy
- Vacuum source for suction
- Culture container with growth media
- Biopsy forceps (intraendoscopic or separate clamshell or cup biopsy forceps)
- Biopsy jar with 10% buffered formalin
- Phenylephrine (e.g., Neo-Synephrine drops) for postoperative epistaxis

Anticipated Time

- 60-90 minutes anesthesia time, 30-60 minutes for endoscopy
- Up to 3-4 hours for complex foreign bodies and/or copious flushing

Preparation: Important Checkpoints

- Advise owners that epistaxis is expected for 1-3 days after the procedure.
- Assess coagulation (e.g., platelet count, coagulation profile [p. 1325])
- Measure blood pressure (p. 1065)
- Serology for canine ehrlichiosis or fungal exposure based on geography
- Advanced imaging (CT/MRI) where available

Possible Complications and Common Errors to Avoid

- Biopsy sample not representative of disease process; risk minimized by advanced imaging
- Inability to examine caudal conchae if endoscope is too big (especially cats and small dogs), or to see choanae during nasopharyngeal exam (especially in dolichocephalic dogs)
- Hemorrhage after biopsy; low risk of serious blood loss. Rarely, hemorrhage warrants a blood transfusion, or if bleeding persists, ipsilateral carotid ligation.
- Penetration of compromised cribriform plate, traumatizing the brain. Measure distance from tip of the nostril to medial canthus of the eye. This measured length on endoscope is the maximal length of insertion.
- Aspiration of fluid, prevented by a well-fitted endotracheal tube with adequately inflated cuff and packing the pharynx during the procedure plus oropharyngeal suctioning and lowering the nose for drainage after the procedure.
- Superficial bacterial culture or culture of nasal flush will likely differ from caudal nasal cavity cultures.

Procedure

- Sternal recumbency with animal facing endoscopist; head at edge of table,

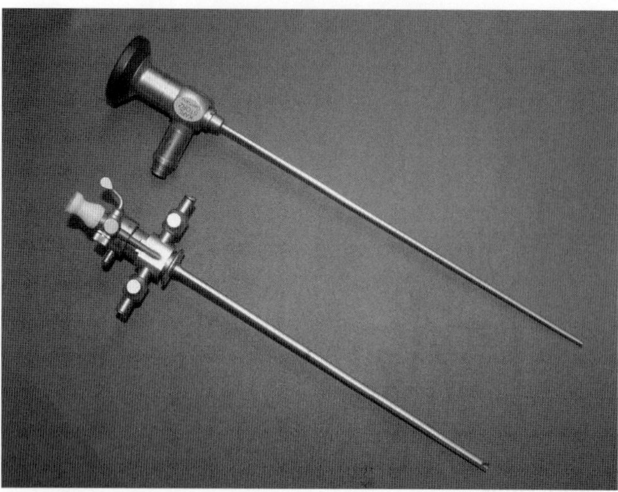

RHINOSCOPY Karl Storz 2.7-mm, 30° visual field, rigid endoscope: telescope, and outer sheath with cannulas for concurrent flushing and introduction of a biopsy instrument.

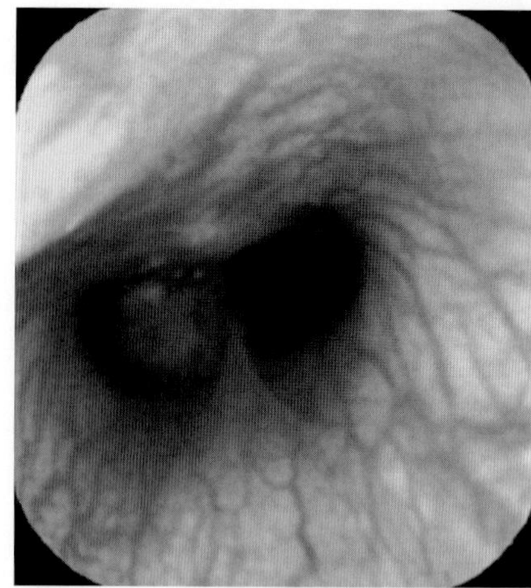

RHINOSCOPY Endoscopic view, retroflexed behind the soft palate to show the choanae. Dog's right is on left side of the image. A fleshy mass is seen in the right choana.

with waste bucket directly underneath, elevated on folded towels with nose pointed down
- Prop mouth open with mouth gag/needle cap, and ensure appropriate inflation of endotracheal cuff.
- Enter oral cavity with endoscope in a flexed J position, and rotate the tip of the endoscope at the caudal edge of the soft palate to visualize the nasopharynx. Pull endoscopic rostrally for closer view of choanae, assessing for mucosal fragility, discharge, hyperemia, masses, erosions, or ulcers. Biopsy suspect tissue before removing flexible scope.
- Pack oropharynx with gauze; count in and count out to ensure retrieval of all gauze after the procedure.
- Measure length from tip of nostril to medial canthus of eye; this is the maximal length of insertion of the endoscope or biopsy instruments to prevent penetration of a compromised cribriform plate and brain trauma. Can mark instrument with tape to avoid accidental overinsertion.
- Advance endoscope into one nostril, medial and ventral and then immediately dorsal, entering alongside the nasal septum. Usually begin on the least affected side.
- Begin saline infusion through endoscope for improved visualization and flushing.
- Examine ventral, middle, and dorsal meatus systematically, assessing mucosal changes, turbinate structure, discharge, and meatal size (open with destruction as with rhinitis or narrowed with obstruction with edema and proliferative neoplasms).
- Biopsy as indicated through endoscope biopsy port or blindly after procedure with cup biopsy forceps. Biopsy may be delayed until all areas have been visualized to minimize blood obscuring the view.
- Remove gauze sponges (count out), and suction oropharynx.
- Instill phenylephrine (few drops in each nostril) for voluminous epistaxis.

Postprocedure

Recover patient with nose tipped down, head elevated; extubate as late as safely possible with cuff inflated until last minute. Placing an ice pack on the muzzle may help reduce hemorrhage. If bleeding continues, phenylephrine can be repeated.

- Sedation/analgesia to minimize stress and sneezing (butorphanol or micro dose acepromazine/dexmedetomidine)
- Discharge same or next day, depending on bleeding
- If bleeding substantial, monitor packed cell volume/total solids to assess blood loss

Alternatives and Their Relative Merits

- CT/MRI: can localize lesion, may give indication of neoplasm, foreign body, or aspergillosis
- Blind nasal biopsy: quick, reasonable yield if biopsy guided by imaging but can miss region of interest
- Nasal flush: minimal tissue disruption, can dislodge foreign material, discharge, or with force, tumor cells
- Nasal swab/culture: poor cytologic yield in awake animal, superficial culture often shows normal flora
- Rhinotomy: most invasive but can yield definitive diagnosis if other methods fail

Pearls

- Pushing the nostril dorsally with a thumb and inserting the endoscope next to the nasal septum eases endoscope entrance.
- Rhinoscopy without imaging or biopsy is not a useful diagnostic tool except when removing foreign material. Most causes of rhinitis cannot be differentiated by gross examination but require biopsy and histopathology.

SUGGESTED READING

Saylor DK, et al: Rhinoscopy. In Tams TR, et al, editors: Small animal endoscopy, ed 3, St. Louis, 2011, Mosby.

AUTHOR: Christine Savidge, DVM, DACVIM
EDITORS: Leah A. Cohn, DVM, PhD, DACVIM; Mark S. Thompson, DVM, DABVP

Slings, Casts, and Other Forms of Immobilization

Client Education Sheet

Difficulty level: ◆

Synonym

External coaptation

Overview and Goal

To provide appropriate temporary support and allow healing of musculoskeletal injuries, alone or as augmentation of surgical repairs

Indications

- Robert Jones bandage: temporary immobilization of unstable fractures; control of edema and swelling; appropriate for open fractures after wound dressing
- Splints: temporary immobilization of fractures or peripheral joint luxations (p. 1158); also used after surgery for joint injuries, arthrodeses, or tendon injuries
- Casts: immobilization of distal limb fractures when mechanically stable; also appropriate after surgical repair (similar to splints)
- Slings: partial immobilization of all joints of the limb and prevention of weight bearing. Ehmer sling is used primarily after reduction of hip luxation to prevent recurrence.

Contraindications

Excessive duration of immobilization may lead to muscle and joint contracture and permanent loss of mobility. Use with caution, especially in pediatric animals.

Equipment, Anesthesia

Sedation may be required for appropriate placement of splints and bandages if animal is in pain or uncooperative. General anesthesia is required for reduction of fractures or joint luxations before immobilization. Amounts and widths of required materials depend on animal size:

- Appropriate wound dressing, if needed
- A 0.5- or 1-inch (1.25- or 2.5-cm) width roll of tape
- Rolls of cast padding, 2-6 inches (5-15 cm) width
- Rolls of conforming gauze, 2-6 inches (5-15 cm) width
- Rolls of self-adherent stretch tape

Additional materials:

- Roll of cotton, 12-inch (30-cm) width (for Robert Jones bandage)
- Fiberglass resin or plaster-impregnated casting tape, 2-4 inches (5-10 cm) wide for casts
- Stretch stockinette (for casts, optional)
- Rigid Mason metasplint, lateral plastic limb splint, fiberglass or thermoplastic splint (for splints)

Anticipated Time

About 10-30 minutes for application of most casts, splints, and slings

Preparation: Important Checkpoints

Wounds should be treated and an appropriate dressing applied before splinting or bandaging.

Possible Complications and Common Errors to Avoid

- The distal third and fourth digits should be left visible whenever possible to allow monitoring for coolness, swelling, cyanosis, or discharge, any of which warrants removal of the splint, cast, or bandage for closer evaluation of the soft tissues.
- All bandages, splints, slings, and casts should be checked frequently for limb swelling or discoloration, skin abrasions, loosening or slippage, moisture, or odor.
- Severe ischemia can result from poor application or management.

Procedure

Robert Jones bandage:

- Divide bulky roll cotton lengthwise and in thickness; reroll to create several smaller, narrower rolls.
- Apply adhesive tape stirrups directly to the skin of the medial and lateral or cranial and caudal surfaces of the distal limb, extending from the carpus or tarsus distally 4-6 inches (10-15 cm) beyond the toes.
- Apply cotton, winding it around the limb from distal to proximal as far as possible into the axillary or inguinal space.
- Each turn of the cotton should overlap the previous layer by 50%.
- Wrap the cotton as evenly as possible.
- Apply conforming gauze around the cotton as tightly as possible, working from distal to proximal.
- Cotton should be evenly compressed until the bandage is firm to the touch.
- Pull the tape stirrups proximally, and apply them onto the bandage. Their purpose is to prevent the bandage from slipping off the limb.
- Cover with a tertiary layer of conforming tape.
- Goal of this bandage is even compression and firm support over the entire limb.
- Properly applied, the finished bandage should make a thumping sound like a ripe melon when it is percussed.
- Tips of digits must be visible for monitoring. Due to high compression, this bandage can cause severe ischemic injury if applied poorly.

Splints:

- Apply tape stirrups as for the Robert Jones bandage.
- Apply cast padding, starting distally and winding around the limb as far proximally as needed.
- Apply a layer of conforming gauze from distal to proximal area.
- Place rigid splint material, usually on the caudal or lateral side of the limb.
- Repeat another one to two layers of conforming gauze.
- Cover with an outer layer of conforming tape.

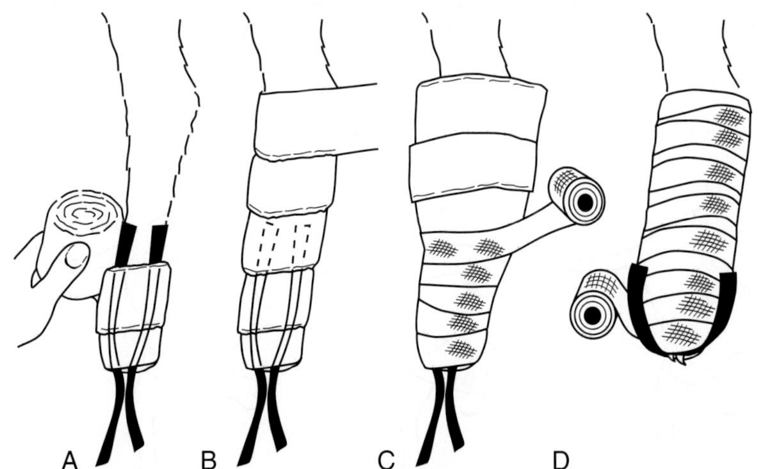

SLINGS, CASTS, AND OTHER FORMS OF IMMOBILIZATION Robert Jones bandage. **A**, Adhesive tape stirrups *(black)* are applied to skin on opposite sides of distal limb. Wound dressing is applied as needed. Roll cotton (or for small patients, cast padding) is wrapped evenly around paw. **B**, Cotton is continued proximally, well above site of injury, and with overlap of about 50% at each turn to create the full length of the bandage. **C**, Conforming gauze is applied in the same manner from distal to proximal but pulled tightly at each turn. Cotton should be evenly compressed. **D**, Tape stirrups are reflected proximally and stuck to bandage. An outer tertiary layer of conforming elastic tape is applied over the cotton. Finished bandage should be firm with even compression over entire surface. Digits must be visible for monitoring.

Casts:

- Apply adhesive tape stirrups.
- Roll stockinette over the limb, allowing extra length proximally and distally. Stockinette is optional but does give the cast a more finished appearance.
- Apply a light layer of cast padding over stockinette.
- Apply roll gauze with light and even compression.
- Apply casting tape over the gauze in distal-to-proximal direction, overlapping by 50% and avoiding digital pressure and wrinkles during application. Layer as needed for appropriate strength.
- Support the limb at multiple points while hardening to avoid dents or incorrect alignment.
- Roll stockinette ends over the cast ends.
- Apply the stirrups to the cast. Their purpose is to prevent the cast from slipping off the limb.
- Cover with an outer tertiary layer of elastic conforming tape.

Slings:

- Velpeau sling (forelimb)
  - Lightly pad the foot and carpus with cast padding to prevent excessive flexion.
  - Wrap conforming gauze around the foot from medial to lateral.
  - Hold the limb adducted against the body wall with the carpus, elbow, and shoulder in flexion.
  - Roll the conforming roll gauze around the limb and thorax, passing caudally to the opposite forelimb to prevent slipping.
  - Continue on the same pattern for two to three layers, incorporating the entire carpus and paw.
  - Apply a light tertiary layer of conforming tape over the gauze in the same pattern.
  - The easiest way to perform these steps is with the patient awake and standing.
  - To avoid joint contracture, the sling should not be used for more than 2 weeks.
- Ehmer sling (hindlimb)
  - Lightly pad the metatarsal region with cast padding.
  - Hold the stifle and tarsus in flexion.
  - Pass adhesive tape around the padded metatarsal region, coming up the lateral side of the metatarsus.
  - Twist tape 180° to keep the adhesive side against the skin, and pass it medially to the stifle.
  - Pass the tape over the lateral thigh as far proximally into the inguinal region as possible.
  - Again twist the tape to keep the adhesive against the skin, and pass it distally medial to the hock.
  - Continue tape back up to the starting point at the lateral side of the metatarsal region.
  - Repeat the pattern two or three times to layer the tape.
  - If maintaining hip reduction, following the last pattern, pass the tape over the lateral side of the flexed leg over the back and around the abdomen as a belly band; stick the tape to itself on the abdominal wall, taking care to exclude the prepuce in males. NOTE: Adhesive tape must be stuck directly to haired skin to avoid slippage.
  - To avoid joint contracture, the sling should not be used for more than 2 weeks.
  - The limb must be monitored frequently for swelling or skin abrasion.

Postprocedure

- Check digits and distal limb at least q 12h for any signs of ischemic injury.

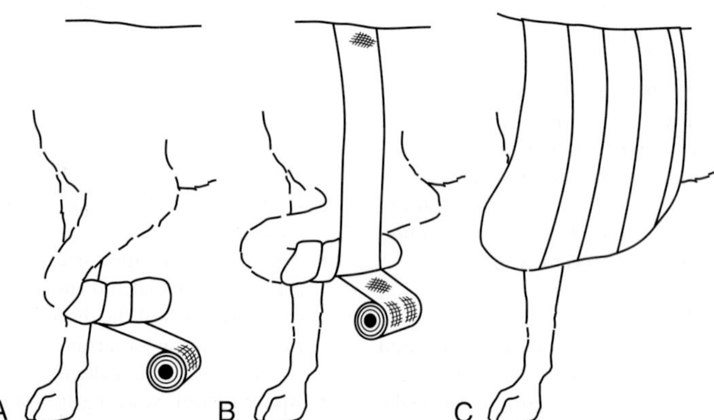

SLINGS, CASTS, AND OTHER FORMS OF IMMOBILIZATION Velpeau sling. **A**, Conforming gauze bandage material is wrapped loosely around the paw, with direction of wrapping causing the gauze to pass from medial to lateral on the dorsal surface of the paw. **B**, With carpus, elbow, and shoulder all flexed, gauze is brought from paw over the lateral aspect of limb and shoulder, over thorax and dorsum, and caudal to the opposite axilla. It then continues across the ventral thorax, back to the starting point. **C**, Several more layers of gauze are applied in a similar manner, and a few layers are brought around (cranial to) the flexed carpus to prevent extension of the elbow because extension could force the distal limb out of the bandage. Wide elastic tape is used for covering the gauze in a pattern similar to that used for the gauze application, which completes application of the splint.

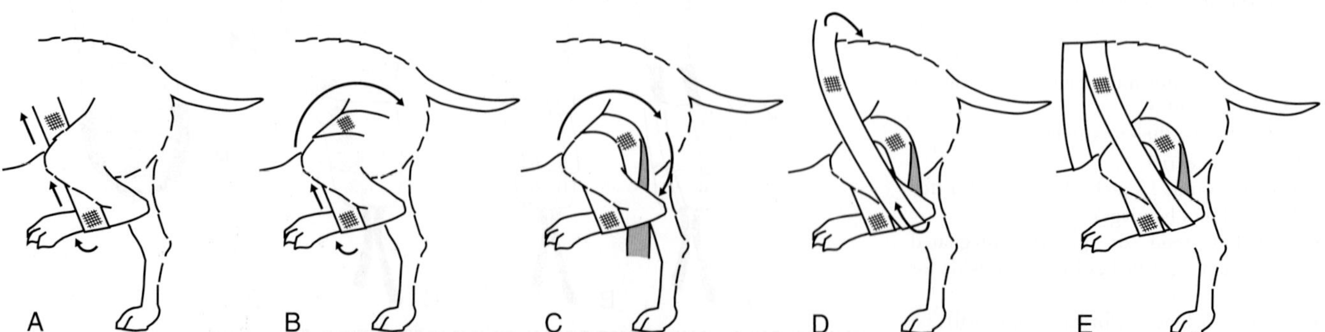

SLINGS, CASTS, AND OTHER FORMS OF IMMOBILIZATION Ehmer sling. **A**, Adhesive tape is passed around the lightly padded metatarsal region, coming up the lateral side of the metatarsus. **B**, Tape is twisted 180°, and stifle and tarsus are held in flexion. Adhesive side of tape is applied to medial side of stifle, continuing up and over thigh as proximal into inguinal space as possible. **C**, Tape is again twisted 180° to keep adhesive side against skin and is applied to medial side of hock and then around to starting point on lateral side of metatarsals. Tape is continued for another 1-2 layers over same pattern for greater support. **D**, To support hip reduction, tape may be continued over the back, with the hip in slight abduction. **E**, Tape is passed once around the body and stuck to itself as a belly band.

- Monitor contact points of bandage materials, especially around bony prominences and joints.

Pearls

- Well-adhered tape stirrups are essential for preventing slippage and loss of Robert Jones bandages and casts.
- Ease of application and risk of complications have improved with the use of commercially available alternatives (DogLeggs vest with Ehmer sling and DogLeggs Velpeau sling, DogLeggs Therapeutic Rehabilitative Products, Washington, DC).

SUGGESTED READING

Swaim SF, et al: Small animal bandaging, casting, and splinting techniques. Ames, IA, 2011, Wiley-Blackwell.

AUTHOR: Peter Moak, DVM
EDITORS: Leah A. Cohn, DVM, PhD, DACVIM; Mark S. Thompson, DVM, DABVP

Sterilization, Surgical: Gonad Sparing

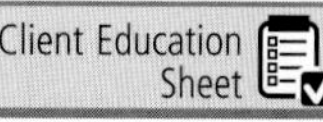

Difficulty level: ◆◆

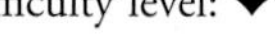

Synonyms

- Ovary-sparing spay
- Hysterectomy
- Vasectomy

Overview and Goals

- Prevention of pregnancy
- Sterilization
- Preservation of hormones

Indications

Method of surgically sterilizing dogs without removing gonads, for which the beneficial health impacts are only recently beginning to be understood

Contraindications

Dogs used for breeding programs

Equipment, Anesthesia

- General anesthesia
- Surgical pack
- Spay hook
- #10 scalpel blade
- Suture (surgeon's discretion)
- Sterile gown/gloves
- Surgical scrub
- Clippers

Anticipated Time

- Will depend on experience of the surgeon
- Ovary-sparing spay
  - Due to the importance of making sure that all uterine tissue has been removed and the additional suture time for a longer incision, the procedure may take slightly longer than a routine spay.
- Vasectomy
  - Relatively quick procedure; shorter than a routine castration

Preparation: Important Checkpoints

Preanesthetic bloodwork

Possible Complications and Common Errors to Avoid

- Ovary-sparing spay
  - As with any surgery, complications may arise from the use of general anesthesia.
  - If any part of the uterus remains after surgery, the dog will be at risk for developing a stump pyometra (p. 854), which can be life-threatening.
  - Leaving the ovaries may contribute to an increased risk of mammary tumors (p. 623) in the future.
- Vasectomy
  - Sperm granulomas
  - Short-term possible complications include infection, bruising, and bleeding into the scrotum, resulting in a hematoma.
  - In rare cases, the ductus deferens may recannulize.

Procedure

- Ovary-sparing spay
  - The anesthetized patient is positioned in dorsal recumbency, and the surgical site is sterilely prepared and draped.
  - Before beginning an incision, the incision site should be carefully planned.
    - The incision will typically be made directly over the midline, 1-3 finger widths caudal to the umbilicus, depending on the size of the patient. A larger, more caudal incision will be made than for a traditional spay, allowing the complete uterus and cervix to be fully exteriorized from the incision.
  - With a #10 scalpel blade, a midline incision is made through the skin, subcutaneous tissues, and linea alba, similar to a traditional spay.
  - After the abdomen is entered, the uterus must be located.
    - This can be done using a spay hook or the surgeon's finger.
    - To confirm that the uterus has been located, trace the structure cranially to the ovary or caudally to the bifurcation.
    - After the uterine horn is identified, it should be exteriorized while leaving the ovary in the abdomen. NOTE: do not break down the ovarian suspensory ligaments.
    - Gentle traction is placed on the horn upward while the ovary is palpated digitally. After the ovary is isolated, identify the ovarian bursa and uterine tube.
    - These landmarks help the surgeon decide where to create a window through the broad ligament so that the cranial vasculature to the uterine horn may be transfixed and ligated.
      - Place a transfixing ligature across the uterine tubes.
    - Take time to ensure that all uterine tissue is caudal to the ligatures and can be removed when transected.
    - Transect distal to the ligatures, and repeat this procedure on the contralateral side.
  - After both horns are free from the ovaries, follow the uterus caudally to identify the cervix.
    - The cervix is identified as a firm, white bulge demarcating the lower extent of the uterine body.
    - Ligatures can be placed on the cervix or distal to the cervix (cranial vagina).
      - A large, crushing clamp is temporarily placed across the cervix or vagina to demarcate the intended cut line.
      - A transfixing ligature is tied in the crushed tissue at the site of the previously placed clamp.
      - A clamp is then placed approximately one-half inch further down the cervix or vagina cranially to act as a guide for cutting as the entire uterine body is excised, again taking the time to ensure that all the uterine tissue is removed.
    - Before beginning the routine abdominal closure, the abdomen is evaluated to be certain that no bleeding is evident.
- Vasectomy
  - The anesthetized patient is positioned in dorsal recumbency, and the surgical site is sterilely prepared and draped.
  - With a #10 blade, make a 1-2 cm incision into the skin over the spermatic cord between the scrotum and inguinal ring.
    - This incision is midway between and parallel to both spermatic cords, permitting blunt dissection of these structures.
    - The spermatic cord is identified by direct observation and exteriorization

(prescrotal) or by laparoscopy (abdominal) during the procedure.
  - Locate the spermatic cord, incise the vaginal tunic, and isolate the ductus deferens by blunt dissection.
    - The ductus deferens is located lateral to the prepuce and penis between the inguinal rings.
    - The ductus deferens is a white, cordlike structure ≈3 mm in diameter.
  - Double ligate the ductus deferens and resect a 1.0-cm section of ductus between the ligatures.
  - Repeat the procedure on the opposite cord, and close the skin incision with simple interrupted suture pattern.

Postprocedure

- Patients should be assessed at the completion of the surgical procedure to determine whether any conditions need to be immediately addressed or communicated to recovery personnel.
- Postoperative analgesia requirements will vary among individual patients because of differences in surgical complexity, surgical technique, patient age, and individual responses to pain and analgesic agents but need to be considered in every case.
- Keep the dog quiet and indoors for approximately 2 weeks after she/he returns home from the hospital to allow time to heal. Prevent rough housing, and do not allow excessively activity.
- Monitor the incision daily for signs of redness, swelling, or discharge.
- Do not allow the dog to lick or chew at the incision.
- Skin sutures, if present, will be removed in 10-14 days.
- If the hysterectomy/vasectomy was performed for reasons other than preventing reproduction, further treatment and/or monitoring may be necessary.

Alternatives and Their Relative Merits

- Ovariohysterectomy: when performed properly, removes both ovaries and the entire uterus, eliminating risk of ovarian and/or uterine diseases in the future
- Ovariectomy: when performed properly, removes both ovaries, eliminating risk of ovarian diseases in the future
- Castration: removal of both testes eliminates the risk of testicular and some prostatic diseases in the future.
- Intratesticular injection (chemical castration): can be performed with or without sedation but does not require general anesthesia; retains some testosterone production

Pearls

- In general, finding the uterus with a spay hook is easier on the right side because this avoids the spleen. However, it can be found and picked up on either side.
- Place the resected piece of ductus deferens on a cover slip to identify sperm for confirmation that ductus deferens was the tissue removed.
- When prepping the patient for surgery, clip the hair, vacuum, and then use a lint roller to remove any remaining hair.
- Reminding the surgeon to implement proper preoperative and postoperative pain control may lead to better outcomes for patients.
- If it is impossible to stop the dog from licking, offer an Elizabethan collar or e-collar for the recovery time to prevent irritating the area.

SUGGESTED READING

Cooley DM, et al: Endogenous gonadal hormone exposure and bone sarcoma risk. Cancer Epidemiol Biomarkers Prev 11:1434-1440, 2002.

AUTHOR: Clare M. Scully, DVM, MA, MS, DACT
EDITORS: Leah A. Cohn, DVM, PhD, DACVIM; Michelle A. Kutzler, DVM, PhD, DACT

Thoracocentesis

Difficulty Level: ◆

Synonyms

Chest tap, pleural tap, thoracentesis (human medicine)

Overview and Goal

Rapid and technically easy procedure that is therapeutic (removing air or fluid from the pleural space) and diagnostic (confirming the presence of air or fluid; obtaining samples of fluid for analysis)

Indications

- Animals with respiratory distress (increased respiratory rate and effort) and suspected (e.g., dull lung sounds, paradoxic breathing, hyperresonance or hyporesonance on thoracic percussion) or confirmed (radiographs, ultrasound) pleural effusion or pneumothorax
- May also be used diagnostically to obtain samples of smaller-volume pleural effusions (p. 791) that are not causing significant clinical signs (technically more challenging)

Contraindications

Severe bleeding disorder; fractious behavior

Equipment, Anesthesia

- Clippers
- Antiseptic scrub (e.g., chlorhexidine)
- Sterile gloves
- Large syringe (10-60 mL, depending on size of animal)
- A 3-way stopcock
- Sterile extension tubing and a sterile needle, catheter, or butterfly catheter
  - Large dogs: 1½-inch (4-cm) needle or longer catheter, 18-22 gauge
  - Medium dogs, large cats: 1-inch (2.5-cm) needle or catheter, 20-22 gauge
  - Cats, small dogs: ¾- to ⅞-inch (2- to 3.5-cm) butterfly needle, 22-23 gauge; 25-gauge needle can be used for diagnostic centesis
- Bowl (for fluid)
- Red- and purple-top tubes for fluid sample submission
- Sedation may be needed, depending on animal's disposition and stability.

Anticipated Time

Procedure is relatively fast (<5 minutes), although it can be prolonged (45-60 minutes) if a large amount of fluid or air (i.e., several liters) must be removed or the effusion is viscous, contains fibrin clumps or blood clots, or is compartmentalized.

Preparation: Important Checkpoints

- If the patient is in severe respiratory distress and has dull lung sounds on auscultation, thoracocentesis should be performed before thoracic radiographs.
- In cases when respiratory signs are less severe, thoracic radiographs can be used for confirming the presence of fluid or air in the pleural space before thoracocentesis.
- Ultrasound is less stressful and can be used to confirm the presence and location of fluid and/or air and used to guide thoracocentesis (p. 1102).
- Discuss possible complications with owners.
- Rule out bleeding disorder as likely cause of respiratory signs first (from history, physical examination, ± coagulation screening).
- Prepare equipment and supplies.
- Patient must be kept relatively still, either with restraint or sedation, to minimize risk of iatrogenic pneumothorax or hemothorax.

Possible Complications and Common Errors to Avoid

- Iatrogenic pneumothorax
- Intrathoracic hemorrhage
- Re-expansion pulmonary edema in situations of chronic pleural space disease
- Acute death from stress of restraint in animals with severe respiratory compromise

Procedure

- Position animal, preferably in sternal recumbency or standing, but lateral recumbency is also acceptable for pneumothorax.
- Provide supplemental oxygen if needed (p. 1146).
- Have assistant available to restrain animal or give sedation as needed.
  - Consider brief, quiet rest in oxygen cage if patient is anxious and extremely dyspneic.
  - For mild or no dyspnea, butorphanol 0.1-0.2 mg/kg IV may be used for light sedation; protocols for heavy sedation or anesthesia (e.g., propofol) likely require intubation.
- Clip and aseptically prepare appropriate rib space.
  - If expecting fluid or if unsure (fluid vs. air), clip at the seventh or eighth intercostal space (ICS), about at the level of the costochondral junction.
  - If expecting air, clip at the eighth or ninth ICS, approximately one-third of the way down the chest.
- Wear sterile gloves for the insertion of the appropriate-size needle or butterfly catheter.
- Attach needle to syringe or extension set with 3-way stopcock and syringe.
- Insert needle slowly, bevel side up, just cranial to the rib to avoid intercostal blood vessels. When through skin (beveled edge of needle is no longer visible), begin aspirating with a few tenths of 1 mL of negative pressure for a cat or small dog or 1-2 mL of negative pressure for larger patients.
- If air is expected, the needle can be directed dorsally so that the needle is almost parallel to the chest wall. If fluid is expected, the needle can be directed ventrally.
- Observe hub of needle for fluid (flashback).
  - If a small amount of frank blood is aspirated or the lungs can be felt rubbing against needle, the needle should be moved to a different location.
  - If large amount of blood is obtained, place 1-2 mL in a red-top tube to see if it clots.
  - Blood from hemothorax should not clot; blood from the heart or a vessel should clot if the animal is not coagulopathic.
- For other types of fluid, aspiration should continue until no more can be removed.
- Directing the needle ventrally, rolling the animal slightly to the side on which thoracocentesis is being performed, and reaspirating from a more ventral location can facilitate removal of as much fluid as possible.
- Ultrasound guidance can identify small fluid pockets for diagnostic thoracocentesis.
- Fluid is submitted for fluid analysis and cytologic examination and is saved for bacterial culture and susceptibility (C&S) (aerobic, anaerobic) tests if cytologic examination suggests septic exudate or paired triglyceride levels (compared to serum) if it appears chylous.
- Aspiration of air will turn the tubing a slightly foggy white color as the warm air from the thoracic cavity encounters the room-temperature tubing:
  - Aspirate until negative pressure is reached.
  - If negative pressure is never obtained, a tension pneumothorax may be present, and chest tubes with continuous suction are needed (p. 1082).

Postprocedure

Monitor for returning signs of respiratory distress, which could represent return of underlying pleural disease or iatrogenic pneumothorax or hemothorax. Thoracic ultrasound or radiographs can identify residual volume of fluid/air and assess for lung pathology.

Alternatives and Their Relative Merits

- Chest tube placement (p. 1082): continuous removal of fluid and air. More invasive, greater risk of iatrogenic complications

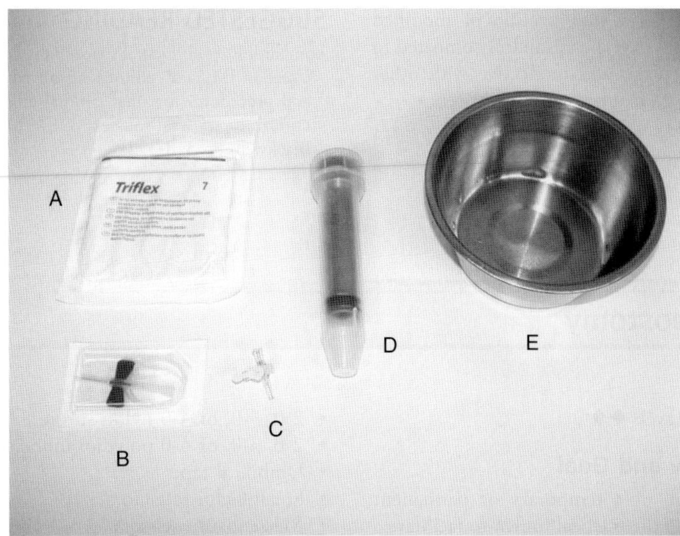

THORACOCENTESIS Materials used for thoracocentesis for a cat or small dog. **A,** Sterile gloves. **B,** Butterfly-type catheter. **C,** A 3-way stopcock. **D,** Large syringe. **E,** Bowl.

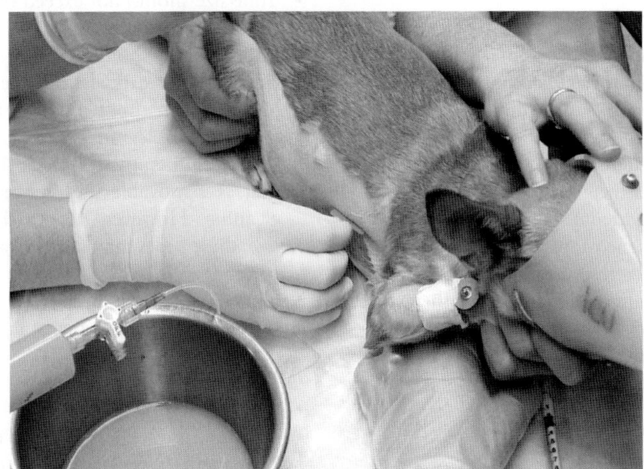

THORACOCENTESIS Thoracocentesis for removal of turbid (septic) pleural effusion from a Chihuahua. The dog's head is to the right, and an open muzzle is placed loosely for protection of staff without compromising the animal's respirations. A butterfly catheter with 3-way stopcock and a 60-mL syringe are in use. The entry site is at the right seventh or eighth intercostal space, approximately at the level of the costochondral junction.

Procedures and Techniques

- Diuretics: slow mobilization of modified transudates (e.g., heart failure) compared to thoracocentesis and ineffective with other causes (e.g., exudates, hemorrhage)

SUGGESTED READING

Lombardi R, et al: Pleural space drainage. In Burkitt Creedon JM, et al, editors: Advanced monitoring and procedures for small animal emergency and critical care, West Sussex, UK, 2012, Wiley-Blackwell, pp 378-392.

AUTHOR: Lori S. Waddell, DVM, DACVECC
EDITORS: Leah A. Cohn, DVM, PhD, DACVIM; Mark S. Thompson, DVM, DABVP

Tracheostomy

Client Education Sheet

Bonus Material Online 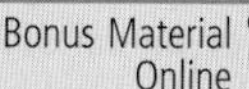

Difficulty Level: ♦♦

Overview and Goal

The creation of a temporary or permanent opening into the tracheal lumen to facilitate a patent airway and provide a conduit for airflow when blockage or collapse of the nasal cavity, oral cavity, nasopharynx, and/or larynx has compromised respiration

Indications

Temporary tube tracheostomy:
- Upper respiratory collapse
- Upper respiratory obstruction
- Surgery of the head and neck
- Laryngeal edema
- Anaphylaxis (p. 54)
- Ventilator patients

Permanent tracheostomy:
- Severe upper respiratory compromise that cannot be effectively treated with medical management
- Most commonly placed in patients with neoplasia, severe trauma, or laryngeal collapse

Contraindications

Lower airway disease

Equipment, Anesthesia

Anesthesia:
- If performing on elective basis, general anesthesia is recommended.
- Local anesthesia (+/− analgesia/sedative) if patient is too unstable for general anesthesia
- In patients that are unconscious due to upper airway obstruction, a tracheostomy may be performed in the absence of local or general anesthesia. However, after the tracheostomy procedure is complete, anesthesia and analgesia are instituted before the return of consciousness.

Surgical preparation (elective):
- Nonsterile exam gloves
- Hair clippers
- Surgical scrub solution, saline, gauze sponges

Instruments and supplies:
- Sterile gloves
- Sterile gauze
- Sterile drape
- Towel clamps
- #10 and #15 scalpel blades
- Scalpel handle
- Brown-Adson tissue forceps
- 2-0, 3-0, or 4-0 nylon suture
- 2-0, 3-0, or 4-0 polydioxanone suture
- Umbilical tape
- Small Gelpi retractors
- Metzenbaum scissors
- Mosquito or Kelly hemostatic forceps
- Suture scissors
- Needle drivers

Tracheostomy tubes:
- Tube size should not exceed one-half of the tracheal diameter.
- Tube length should extend six to seven tracheal rings caudal from the stoma.
- Single-lumen tubes must be removed and replaced for cleaning.
- Double-lumen tubes have an inner cannula that is removable and more efficient for cleaning. However, due to the large bore size, these tubes may not be feasible in small patients.
- Cuffed tubes are used when mechanical ventilator support is necessary.

Anticipated Time

- Surgical prep: 5 minutes
- Temporary tracheostomy: 10 minutes
- Permanent tracheostomy: 30 minutes

Preparation: Important Checkpoints

- Educate clients on potential risks and complications and the long-term prognosis of the underlying disease process.
- Organize all instruments before the beginning of the procedure if time allows (preferably all supplies needed to perform a tracheostomy should be kept in a designated surgery suite to allow quick and efficient access).
- Place the patient in dorsal recumbency with towels folded and placed under the cervical region to elevate and stabilize the neck
- Perform a routine sterile preparation (if time permits) of the ventral cervical region from the ventral ramus of the mandible to the manubrium.

Potential Complications and Common Errors to Avoid

- Infection
- Hemorrhage
- Dehiscence
- Subcutaneous emphysema, pneumomediastinum, pneumothorax
- Tracheal malacia
- Excessive mucus production
- Temporary (tube) tracheostomy
  - Gagging, retching, coughing, and vomiting
  - Tube obstruction
  - Spontaneous extubation
  - Aberrant tube placement
  - Tracheal irritation leading to tracheocutaneous and/or tracheoesophageal fistula
  - Vascular erosion
  - Stricture, stenosis, and mucosal erosions from pressure necrosis
- Permanent tracheostomy
  - Mucocutaneous dehiscence
  - Stenosis and/or stricture
  - Acute stomal obstruction from mucus plug or excessive skin folds
  - Excessive mucus production and accumulation
  - Tracheal irritation leading to coughing, gagging, and mucosal erosions

Procedure

Temporary tracheostomy:
- Make a ventral, cervical midline skin incision extending 3-5 cm in length from the most caudal aspect of the larynx. Continue the incision by blunt dissection through the subcutaneous tissues to expose the underlying paired sternohyoid muscles.
- The ventral aspect of the trachea can be exposed by bluntly separating the sternohyoid muscles along their midline aponeurosis and retracting the muscle bellies and skin laterally. Retraction can be aided by the placement of Gelpi retractors.
- After the ventral aspect of the trachea is exposed, proper positioning of the tracheostomy should be determined by locating the annular ligament between the 3rd and 4th tracheal rings.
- A horizontal tracheostomy can be made into the annular ligament between the 3rd and 4th tracheal rings. The width of the incision should not exceed one-half of the tracheal circumference due to potential damage of the laryngeal nerves.
- A vertical tracheostomy can be made by a midline incision through the 3rd through 5th tracheal cartilages.
- A tracheal flap tracheostomy can be performed by making a U-shaped incision starting at the 3rd tracheal cartilage and

extending to the 5th tracheal cartilage. This tracheostomy technique should be used only when conversion to a permanent tracheostomy is not warranted due to the potential damage to the tracheal mucosa.

- After the tracheostomy is complete, two stay sutures should be placed at each edge of the incision and appropriately labeled (cranial/caudal or medial/lateral). The stay sutures will be used to stabilize the trachea during tube insertion and during tube exchanges.
- Secure the tracheostomy tube using umbilical tape tied around the patient's neck.
- The cranial and caudal skin edges may be sutured together if necessary.
- The stoma around the tube is gently covered with antibiotic ointment.

Permanent tracheostomy:

- Make a ventral, cervical midline skin incision extending 6-8 cm in length from the most caudal aspect of the larynx. Continue the incision by blunt dissection through the subcutaneous tissues to expose the underlying paired sternohyoid muscles.
- The ventral aspect of the trachea can be exposed by bluntly separating the sternohyoid muscles along their midline aponeurosis and retracting the muscle bellies and skin laterally. Retraction can be aided by the placement of Gelpi retractors.
- After the ventral aspect of the trachea is exposed, proper positioning of the tracheostomy should be determined by locating the 3rd through 6th tracheal rings.
- Create a small tunnel dorsal to the trachea by blunt dissection.
- The paired sternohyoid muscles can be apposed dorsally to the trachea by placing mattress sutures using polydioxanone through the tunnel. The dorsal apposition of the sternohyoid muscles induces a ventral deviation of the trachea and aids in tension relief when apposing the tracheal mucosa to the skin.
- The ventral aspects of the 3rd through 6th tracheal rings are removed by incising the tracheal cartilages to the level of the mucosa and gently dissecting the free edges of the cartilage rings using the back of a scalpel blade and thumb forceps.
- The width of the cartilage removed should be no wider than one-half of the tracheal circumference. Care should be taken during the removal of the tracheal rings to try to preserve the integrity of the tracheal mucosa.
- Perimucosal tissue may be apposed to the dermis surrounding the tracheostomy site using 2-0, 3-0, or 4-0 polydioxanone sutures. The apposition of these tissues before the mucocutaneous apposition of the tracheostomy is critical in order to provide a tension-free closure.
- Make an I- or H-shaped incision into the tracheal mucosa.
- Appose the skin edges cranial and caudal to the tracheostomy site.
- Fold the mucosa over the free cartilage edges, and suture the mucosa to the skin edge using simple interrupted sutures at each corner of the tracheostomy.
- The remainder of the mucocutaneous apposition may be performed by using simple interrupted sutures or in a simple continuous pattern using 4-0 polydioxanone.
- Peritracheostomy skin folds may warrant resection if the risk of tracheostomy occlusion is foreseen. Caution should be exercised when removing skin folds not to remove too much tissue and create tension across the tracheostomy site.

Postprocedure

Temporary tracheostomy tube care:

- Proper tracheostomy site care is critical to ensure proper healing, prevent airway infection, and reduce the risk of acute obstruction.
- Aseptic technique should be practiced by all personnel who are involved with tracheostomy care (unless emergency).
- Tracheostomy tubes should be removed and cleaned or replaced every 12-24 hours (or as needed). Tubes should be soaked in 2% chlorhexidine solution and thoroughly rinsed before replacement.
- Before any non-emergent tube care procedure, patients should be preoxygenated for 2-5 minutes to help reduce hypoxemia.
- A sterile suction catheter no greater than one-half the diameter of the tracheostomy tube with a blunt end and side suction holes should be used for tube maintenance. The catheter should be inserted to the level of the obstruction before the initiation of suction. Intermittent suction should be used while rotating the catheter as is it is removed to eliminate any debris causing obstruction. Try to limit the time the catheter is in the trachea to 10-15 seconds per cleaning.
- The frequency of catheter suctioning is determined by the degree of mucus production. Initial maintenance may be necessary q 15 minutes but is usually q 4-6h.
- Nebulization and coupage q 4h can aid in removal of mucus and debris.

Temporary tracheostomy tube removal:

- Tracheostomy tube removal should be prioritized as soon as adequate upper airway flow has been re-established.
- To ensure that adequate airflow through the upper airway has returned, the patient should be challenged for 10-15 minutes with the tracheal tube removed. During this trial period, the patient should be carefully observed for signs associated with respiratory distress and/or obstruction. If the respiratory rate and effort are satisfactory during this trial, the tube is removed.
- No closure of the tracheostomy site is recommended, and the stoma should be allowed to heal by second intention.
- For flap tracheostomy, any excess granulation tissue should be debrided, and the flap should be sutured back into its anatomic location using 4-0 polydioxanone.

Permanent tracheostomy care:

- Frequent cleaning of the stoma is necessary to keep the area free of mucus, debris, and foreign material.
- Long-term maintenance includes routine clipping of the hair surrounding the stoma.
- Patients should not be allowed to swim or be kept in environments with high particulate debris.

Cuffed tubes:

- Inflation of cuffs is necessary to seal the airway during positive-pressure ventilation. Auscultation of the airway during positive-pressure ventilation should be performed to ensure no leaks are present.
- Cuff deflation is not recommended unless positive-pressure ventilation cannot be achieved.

Alternatives and Their Relative Merits

- Oxygen supplementation (p. 1146): should be initiated in all patients with respiratory distress, even though it may not be adequate as sole therapy. Oxygen supplementation before the initiation of more invasive measures can help reduce the oxygen deficit and provide some level of initial stabilization.
- Oral/endotracheal intubation: due to the ease and noninvasive nature, this method of management should be attempted first in patients with upper airway obstruction.

Pearls

- Overweight patients or those with redundant skin folds along the ventral neck are at increased risk for tube complications and physical obstruction of the tracheostomy stoma. Extra attention should be paid when tube placement or exchange is performed.
- Always have a replacement tube and a full set of replacement supplies readily available for any patient with a tracheostomy due to the fact that obstruction may be very acute, and rapid response times are critical.
- Dogs tend to do better than cats with permanent tracheostomy.

SUGGESTED READING

Mazzafero EM: Temporary tracheostomy. Top Companion Anim Med 28(3):74-78, 2013.

AUTHOR: K. David Hutcheson, DVM
EDITORS: Leah A. Cohn, DVM, PhD, DACVIM; Mark S. Thompson, DVM, DABVP

Transcervical Insemination

Difficulty Level: ◆◆

Overview and Goals

- Transcervical insemination (TCI) involves the endoscopic visualization of the cervix and its catheterization. Semen is then injected through the catheter and into the uterine lumen.
- The two primary methods of intrauterine insemination are catheterization of the cervix by TCI or injection of semen into the uterine lumen by laparotomy.
- TCI requires specific equipment and careful breeding management.

Indications

- Intrauterine insemination is required when using frozen-thawed semen.
- Female subfertility
- Cases in which the semen is reduced in viability or dosage (<150 million progressively motile, morphologically normal sperm)
- TCI can be used for ruling out vaginal or cervical abnormalities through visualization of these areas and catheterization of the cervix.

Contraindications

If the bitch is not in late estrus, the vaginal wall is more sensitive, and the procedure is uncomfortable and more likely to require sedation.

Equipment, Anesthesia

- Endoscope
  - Extended-length, rigid cystourethroscope with a working length of 29 cm and 22 Fr diameter; ideal for dogs 25-75 lb (12-35 kg). It should have a 30° viewing angle with a sheath and a bridge. Use with urinary catheters 6-8 Fr in diameter.
  - Cold light source and cable
- Camera and video tower system
- Adjustable-height exam table with nonslip surface
- Anesthesia or sedation is not usually required; a bitch in estrus tolerates the procedure very well. Smaller breeds are more likely to require sedation.

Anticipated Time

10-40 minutes

Preparation: Important Checkpoints

Breeding management and insemination timing:

- The ideal timing for TCI is days 5-7 after the luteinizing hormone (LH) surge (LH surge = day 0). This is based on oocyte viability and the degree of cervical relaxation required for catheterization. Secondary oocytes are present only after day 4-5, and by day 8, the oocytes become senescent. Before day 4, the cervix will be difficult to catheterize.
- The LH surge can be timed directly by testing LH or indirectly by monitoring serum progesterone and looking for the rise above 1.5-3 ng/mL.
- When timing insemination, it is important to consider the longevity of the semen based on its handling and state (fresh vs. cooled shipped vs. frozen).
- Typical breeding management with any type of semen includes two inseminations between days 4 and 7:
  - The frequency of insemination using TCI is limited only by the ability to catheterize the cervix. Once-daily inseminations, although not usually necessary, are possible during days 4-7 or as long as the cervix can be catheterized.

Semen preparation and evaluation:

- The minimal intrauterine dose of semen is 75 million morphologically normal, progressively motile sperm. Optimal pregnancy rates are obtained with doses > 100 million morphologically normal, progressively normal sperm.
- The volume of semen injected into the uterine lumen should be between 1 mL and 3 mL. The size of the bitch and the capacity of the uterus will determine the ideal insemination volume.
- If using freshly collected semen, every effort should be made to fractionate the collection to separate the sperm-rich portion. The volume of the sperm-rich fraction is usually less than 3-5 mL. If TCI is scheduled to occur within a short time, the unextended sperm-rich fraction can be used. If additional volume is needed, the prostatic fluid can be used to follow the semen into the uterus and flush the catheter.
- If using cooled shipped semen or semen extended to a volume greater than 5 mL, the semen should be centrifuged at 900 *g* for ½ min/mL. The supernatant should be drawn off until the ideal volume is achieved, and the remaining pellet is resuspended.
- Frozen semen should not be thawed until the cervix is successfully catheterized. Thaw instructions and procedures should be followed. It is recommended to prepare for thawing in advance to ensure that insemination occurs within a few minutes of catheterization of the cervix.

Possible Complications and Common Errors to Avoid

- Occasionally, it is not possible to catheterize the cervix. This is affected by factors such as the stage of the estrous cycle, size of the female, and parity. It may also be necessary to use a catheter with a narrower diameter.
- The anatomy is challenging because the natural angle of the cervical canal is craniodorsal. Adjusting the angle of the endoscope can straighten the vagina and cervix.
- Inadequate insufflation can result in poor visualization of the external cervical os.
- Excessive serosanguineous discharge, especially in early estrus, can hinder visualization. If needed, this discharge may be aspirated through the scope or by urinary catheter.

Procedure

- Equipment and semen should be prepared in advance to limit the time the dog is restrained.
- The dog is restrained in a standing position on a table. Restraint should include a person or device to limit forward movement and

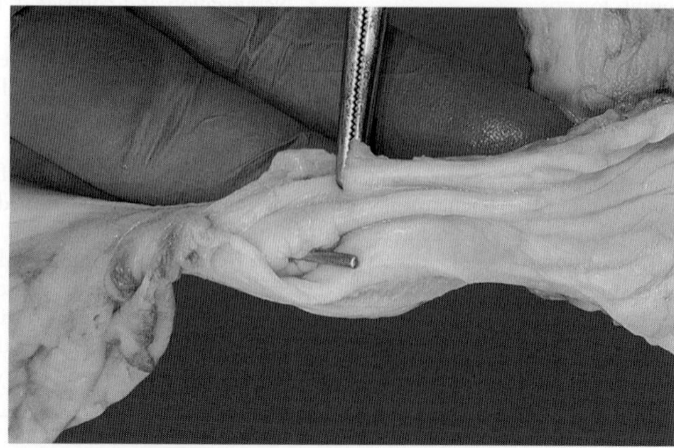

TRANSCERVICAL INSEMINATION Morphologic/anatomic specimen shows the external cervical opening in a bitch, located at the cranial ventral portion of the dorsal vaginal fold. A metal probe has been passed through the cervical canal, illustrating the special challenge faced during transcervical insemination. (Copyright Dr. Robert Lofstedt.)

side-to-side movement, and to prevent sitting or lying. The table is adjusted to a comfortable height for the inseminator.

- The rigid endoscope is placed at the vulvar lips and advanced, noting important anatomic landmarks.
  - The caudal vagina of the bitch has a steep incline as it extends caudally over the pubic bone.
  - The scope should be advanced with mild pressure against the dorsal surface of the caudal vagina to avoid the sensitive clitoris and urethra.
  - In the cranial vagina, the vaginal folds become longitudinal, and the prominent dorsal vaginal fold or pseudocervix can be visualized.
  - The cervix is located on the dorsal vaginal wall at the cranial extent of the dorsal vaginal fold. It typically angles in caudoventral direction. The tissue of the cervix will appear more fibrous and sharply creased than the surrounding vaginal tissue. The cervix is often described as having a rosette appearance.
  - The vaginal fornix extends cranial to the cervix and is a blind pocket.
  - Location within the vagina can also be determined by transabdominal palpation.
- It is often necessary to insufflate the vagina to improve visualization as the scope is advanced. The vulvar lips may need to be held shut to prevent air from escaping.
- After the cervix is visualized, the catheter is advanced, and the external os of the cervix is probed. A gentle twisting motion can help the catheter penetrate the cervix.
- The catheter should be visualized as it is advanced through the cervix. It should be placed as far as it can be advanced into the uterine lumen, as long as no resistance is felt. A distance of 2-5 cm is recommended to ensure semen is deposited at least in the cranial uterine body.
- After the catheter is in place, the semen is injected gradually. If backflow is observed through the cervix, the catheter should be repositioned and the injection of semen continued. The catheter should be flushed with an appropriate amount of air, extender, or prostatic fluid to ensure all of the semen has entered the uterine lumen.
- The catheter is withdrawn, and the rigid endoscope then is retracted.

Postprocedure

It has been recommended to elevate the hindquarters for 10 minutes to facilitate movement of the semen from the uterus into the uterine tubes. Alternatively, the table on which the dog is standing may be adjusted so the hindquarters are elevated by 30°.

Alternatives and Their Relative Merits

- Surgical insemination involves the direct injection of semen through the uterine wall into the lumen. This method is precise but invasive and should be performed only once per estrous cycle.
- Laparoscopic insemination also involves the direct injection of semen through the uterine wall. The technique has been compared to natural insemination, with no significant differences when using freshly collected semen. This technique requires specialized equipment as used for laparoscopic procedures.
- Norwegian intrauterine insemination catheters are rigid catheters that are 20-50 cm long, with a tip diameter of 0.5-1 mm. The catheters are advanced into the cervix blindly, with the operator relying only on transabdominal palpation for correct placement. This procedure requires an extensive level of operator experience and risks traumatizing the vagina and cervix, but it does eliminate the need for expensive equipment.

SUGGESTED READING

Wilson MS: Transcervical insemination techniques in the bitch. Vet Clin North Am Small Anim Pract 31(2):291-303, 2001.

AUTHOR: Bronwyn Crane, DVM, MS, DACT
EDITORS: Leah A. Cohn, DVM, PhD, DACVIM; Mark S. Thompson, DVM, DABVP

Transfusion Therapy and Collection Techniques for Blood Banking

Bonus Material Online

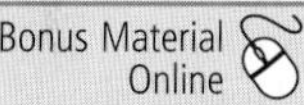

Difficulty Level: ◆◆

Synonyms

Blood transfusion, blood component therapy

Overview and Goal

Safely collect and administer blood products

Indications

Fresh whole blood:

- Improve oxygen delivery
  - Hemolysis
  - Blood loss
  - Nonregenerative anemia
  - Autologous blood patch pleurodesis (p. 797)
- Provide clotting factors
  - Anticoagulant rodenticide toxicity (p. 69)
  - Liver failure
  - von Willebrand disease (VWD) (p. 1043)
  - Disseminated intravascular coagulation (DIC) (p. 269)
  - Hemophilia A (p. 431)
  - Other factor deficiencies
- Support oncotic pressure
  - Protein-losing disease (enteropathy, nephropathy, massive skin wounds or burns, serosal inflammation)
- Fresh whole blood is not recommended for treatment of thrombocytopenia unless marked active hemorrhage and anemia exist.

Stored whole blood:

- Same as for fresh whole blood except do not use for VWD, liver disease, hemophilia A, and DIC; after 6 hours of storage, platelets, factors V and VIII, and von Willebrand factor decrease.
- Fresh blood is preferred over stored for animals with hepatic encephalopathy.

Packed red blood cells (PRBCs):

- Improve oxygen delivery
  - When oncotic support and clotting factors are not required
  - When volume overload is a concern (cardiac disease, renal failure, chronic anemia)

Fresh-frozen plasma (FFP):

- Provide clotting factors (same as fresh whole blood)
- Support oncotic pressure (same as fresh whole blood)
- Pancreatitis (controversial) or colostrum replacement
- Must be separated and frozen within 6 hours of collection

Frozen plasma (plasma frozen > 6 hours after collection or FFP stored > 1 year):

- Anticoagulant rodenticide toxicity and hemophilia B (factors II, VII, IX, and X preserved)
- Support oncotic pressure
- Pancreatitis (controversial) or colostrum replacement

Others:

- Platelet-rich plasma and platelet concentrate are rarely used in private practice (labor intensive, 2- to 3-day storage times, special storage conditions).
- Frozen platelet concentrate or freeze dried platelets are occasionally used for massive or life-threatening hemorrhage associated with extreme thrombocytopenia.

Contraindications

- Animals with normal to increased packed cell volume (PCV)
- Administer cautiously in patients with volume overload, heart disease, or kidney disease/oliguria/anuria.
- Incompatible recipients
    - Cross-match dogs that have received a transfusion more than 4 days earlier, even if using the same previously cross-matched compatible donor.
    - Cats: all require blood typing and/or cross-matching before transfusion (p. 1084) due to presence of preformed antibodies.
- First-time transfusions in dogs are usually safe without prior blood typing and/or cross-matching, although compatibility testing is still recommended to decrease future incompatibilities.

Equipment, Anesthesia

BLOOD COLLECTION

- Hair clippers and material for sterile prep

Dogs:

- Donors should be healthy adults, weigh > 30 kg, have a normal physical exam, and (at a minimum) negative heartworm and rickettsial serologic test results. Ideally, dogs used regularly for donation should be blood typed as negative for DEA 1.1, 1.2, 3, 5, and 7 but positive for DEA 4 (p. 1204).
- Butorphanol 0.1-0.2 mg/kg for IV use
- Sterile 450-mL collection bag with tubing, needle, and anticoagulant (commercially available)
- Digital gram scale
- Hemostat forceps
- Scissors
- Hemoclips and stripper sealer (optional)

Cats:

- Donors should be healthy adults, weigh > 4 kg, have a normal physical exam and blood smear, and (at a minimum) be negative for feline leukemia virus (FeLV) and feline immunodeficiency virus (FIV) serologies. Blood type of donor cats should be known, as should type of recipient (p. 1203).
- Ketamine HCl 1-2 mg/kg for IV use
- Two 35-mL syringes (60-mL syringe may collapse the vein)
- Anticoagulant (citrate-phosphate-dextrose-adenine 1 [CPDA-1] or adenine-citrate-dextrose [ACD])
- A 19-gauge butterfly needle
- NOTE: heparin (300 units/50 mL blood collected) can be used in an emergency.
    - Dilute heparin in 3 mL of saline to facilitate mixing.
    - Heparin contains no preservatives: administer blood within 24 hours.
    - Heparin activates platelets; avoid in thrombocytopenic animals.

BLOOD ADMINISTRATION

- IV or intraosseous (IO) catheter
- Transfusion set with filter (dogs)
- A 170-micron syringe filter and an IV extension set (cats)

Anticipated Time

- Whole blood collection: 20-40 minutes
- Administration: maximum of 4 hours, depending on animal's condition

Preparation: Important Checkpoints

- Check PCV of recipient and donor before transfusion.
- Save hematocrit tube containing recipient plasma for future comparison if hemolytic reactions occur.
- Aseptic technique is essential.

Possible Complications and Common Errors to Avoid

Transfusion reactions (p. 989):

- Monitor temperature, heart rate, and respiratory rate every 10 minutes for 30 minutes, then every 60 minutes until transfusion is completed.
- If cross-matched, adverse reactions are uncommon (3%) and rarely fatal (<1%)
- Stop transfusion if adverse reaction observed. Evaluate signs; if mild without evidence of hemolysis or bacterial contamination, restart transfusion at a slower rate, and monitor closely.
- Risk of reactions is reduced by
    - Using donor dogs negative for DEA 1.1 and DEA 7
    - Cross-matching all donors with recipients
    - Using proper collection, administration, and storage techniques
    - Not adding anything other than 0.9% saline to blood products

Hemolytic transfusion reaction:

- May be acute (restlessness, fever, tachycardia, vomiting within 20 minutes of starting transfusion) or delayed (3-14 days after transfusion; shortened duration of benefit of transfusion but no other overt signs) (p. 989).

Anaphylactic reactions:

- Usually mild: fever, urticaria, erythema, pruritus
- Stop transfusion; administer antihistamines (e.g., diphenhydramine 1-2 mg/kg IM) and glucocorticoids (e.g., dexamethasone SP 0.1-0.2 mg/kg IV).
- Can usually restart transfusion at a slower rate

Volume overload:

- Cough, dyspnea, jugular distention
- Stop transfusion.
- Administer furosemide (e.g., 2 mg/kg IV) ± oxygen supplementation.

Bacterial contamination:

- Examine blood for discoloration, and submit blood for culture and Gram stain if fever persists after transfusion.

Other concerns:

- Dogs that receive a first-time cross-matched, compatible transfusion can develop antibodies against the donor blood in 1-2 weeks; any subsequent transfusion (even if using the same donor) should be cross-matched.

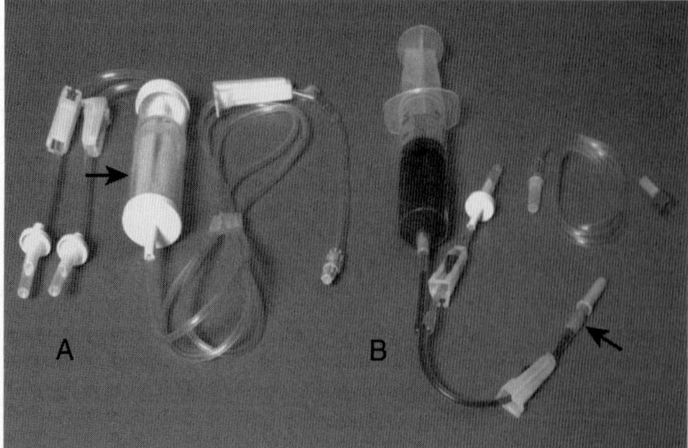

TRANSFUSION THERAPY Two blood transfusion systems, with filters indicated by *arrows*. **A,** A transfusion set with filter chamber typically used for larger volumes (medium- and large-breed dogs). **B,** A 170-mm syringe filter and intravenous extension set typically used for cats and toy-breed dogs.

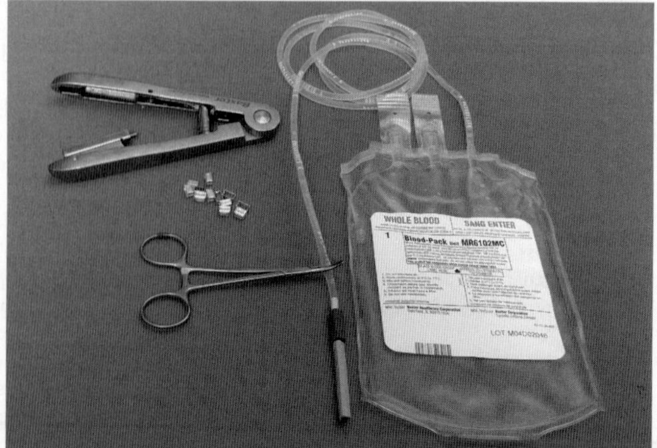

TRANSFUSION THERAPY Materials for blood collection. A blood collection bag, tubing, and needle *(right)* are shown with a hemostatic clamp placed on the tubing to prevent leakage of the anticoagulant. Hemoclips and a stripper-sealer *(left)* are shown.

- Microembolism
- Hypothermia
- Acidosis
- Citrate toxicosis
- Hyperammonemia (stored blood in patient with hepatic failure)

Procedure

Blood collection for banking: blood donor dogs:
- Administer butorphanol 0.2 mg/kg IV.
- Place in lateral recumbency on an elevated surface.
- Clip ventral neck (center over jugular furrow).
- Perform sterile scrub.
- Place collection bag on the scale at a level below the animal (blood collects by gravity).
- Zero the scale (collection bag ± anticoagulant ≈85 g).
- NOTE: If less than 450 mL of blood is to be collected, anticoagulant must be expressed from the collection bag to maintain the 1:7 anticoagulant-to-blood ratio (e.g., to collect 225 mL blood, discard one-half of the anticoagulant [32 g]).
- Clamp tubing with hemostat (near needle).
- Hold off jugular vein for visualization.
- Remove needle cap and insert needle (16-17 gauge) into jugular vein.
- Remove hemostat; collection begins.
- During collection, gently rock the bag intermittently to mix blood with anticoagulant.
- Rotate/adjust needle delicately if flow stops.
- Continue collection until scale reads 450 g (± 45 g).
- Release jugular vein pressure.
- Reclamp tubing near needle.
- Remove needle from jugular vein.
- Carefully recap needle.
- Strip blood from tubing into bag to mix with anticoagulant.
- Allow tubing to refill to prepare short segments of tube with blood for later cross-match.
- Tie/hemoclip tubing at 6- to 10-cm intervals for storage and cross-match. This allows access to small blood sample without penetrating stored blood bag.
- Remove hemostat.
- If collection technique is questionable, blood should be used within 24 hours.

Blood collection for banking: blood donor cats:
- Sedate (1-2 mg/kg ketamine IV; may add diazepam 0.1 mg/kg IV if necessary).
- Clip ventral neck (center over jugular furrow).
- Perform sterile scrub.
- Use a separate needle to put 4 mL ACD or CPDA-1 into each sterile 35-mL syringe.
- Connect one 35-mL syringe to a butterfly needle.
- Hold off jugular vein to visualize.
- Remove needle guard.
- Insert butterfly needle into jugular vein.
- Gently aspirate 27 mL of blood while slowly rocking the syringe to mix anticoagulant and blood.
- Disconnect syringe from butterfly catheter.
- Cap syringe with a sterile needle.
- Attach second anticoagulant-filled syringe, and gently aspirate 27 mL of blood as already described.
- Release jugular pressure.
- Remove needle from jugular vein.
- NOTE: A similar technique can be used in dogs (60-mL syringe with 7 mL ACD or CPDA-1) if collection bags are unavailable; refrigerate and use within 24 hours.

Transfusion of blood products:
- For all blood products
  - Always use a filter.
  - Start slowly (0.5 mL/kg/h) for 15-20 minutes.
  - Monitor for reactions.
  - Increase rate if no reactions occur.
  - Complete transfusion by 4 hours (decreases bacterial contamination).
  - Typical rate is 5-10 mL/kg/h.
  - Can increase to 20 mL/kg/h in unstable hypovolemic animals
  - Can administer as rapidly as possible in a crisis
  - For heart disease, renal failure, or potential volume overload, administer at 1-4 mL/kg/h, and monitor for volume overload (see above).
  - Can divide dosage into smaller aliquots and refrigerate up to 24 hours (allows slower administration with minimal risk of bacterial contamination)
- From a syringe
  - Attach syringe filter to syringe.
  - Attach IV extension set to filter.
  - Prime system with blood product.
  - Connect extension set to IV catheter.
  - Use syringe pump or intermittent slow bolus administration (i.e., healthy cats: 5 mL over 5 minutes, then wait 6-12 minutes and repeat).
- From a collection bag
  - Use blood administration set with filter (see manufacturer's instructions).
  - Prime administration set with blood product.
  - Attach to IV catheter.
  - Set drip rate.
  - Some infusion pumps can be used; check manufacturer specifications.
- Dosages
  - Whole blood: 10-20 mL/kg
    - Generally, 2 mL/kg increases PCV ≈1%.
  - PRBCs: 5-10 mL/kg
    - Generally, 1 mL/kg increases PCV ≈1%.
    - Can dilute with 50-125 mL 0.9% saline to decrease viscosity
  - Alternatively, PRBCs or whole blood (milliliters) dose = BW (kilograms) × 90 × (PCV desired − PCV recipient)/PCV of donor blood; substitute 90 with 60 for cats.
  - Oncotic support
    - 45 mL/kg FFP generally increases serum albumin by 1 g/dL (10 g/L).
- Warming whole blood or PRBCs is not essential; indications to warm
  - Multiple transfusions
  - Hypothermic animals
  - Neonates
  - Warm by room air or water bath (*never* microwave); place blood in waterproof bag for water bath immersion.
  - Do not exceed 37°C (hemolysis).
- FFP/frozen plasma, 10-20 mL/kg:
  - Plastic is fragile when frozen; handle frozen units delicately.
  - Thaw in 37°C water bath in a waterproof plastic bag.
  - Give within 4 hours for clotting factors.
  - Can store 24 hours in refrigerator after thawing if clotting factors not required
  - Repeat dosage if coagulopathy persists.

Postprocedure

- Blood donors: place neck wrap (for several hours) to minimize hematoma formation. Offer food and water. Administer fluids if hypovolemic (tachycardia, pale mucous membranes, prolonged capillary refill time) or the fluid equivalent if more than 2% of the body weight in kilograms is collected.
- Patients/recipients: check PCV 2 hours after the transfusion is complete. Check coagulation profile after administering plasma for coagulopathies.

Alternatives and Their Relative Merits

- Polymerized hemoglobin (e.g., Oxyglobin):
  - Improves oxygen delivery
  - Provides colloidal support but no other plasma benefits
  - Dogs: 10-30 mL/kg at a maximum of 10 mL/kg/h
  - Cats: 5-10 mL/kg at a maximum of 5 mL/kg/h
  - Monitor closely for signs of volume overload, especially in cats.
  - Product has been on and then off the commercial market; may not be available
- Colloids
  - Hypoalbuminemia requires large volumes of whole blood or plasma to correct.
  - Synthetic colloids (dextrans, gelatins, and hydroxyethyl starches): controversial due to risk of acute kidney injury in people. Still frequently used to support colloidal pressure in cats and dogs (bolus 5-20 mL/kg, then 10-20 mL/kg/day; use lower doses for cats).
  - Human albumin: role is controversial; use with caution because fatal reactions reported. Suggested guidelines if used: dogs, 2-7 mL/kg of 25% or 10-35 mL/kg of 5% over 4-6 hours. Canine-specific albumin may be safer, but studies are lacking, and availability is limited. Dosage is the same as for human albumin.
- Lyophilized canine products
  - Lyophilized canine albumin has been used in hypoproteinemic dogs (Animal Blood Resources International, Dixon, CA). Reconstitute 800 mg/kg with 0.9%

saline to yield 5%, 10%, or 16% solution, and administer IV over 6 hours (per manufacturer's directions). Further studies are required to assess efficacy and safety.
  - Lyophilized canine platelets administered per manufacturer's directions have been transfused in dogs with minimal complications (Animal Blood Resources International, Stockbridge, MI). Further studies are needed to determine efficacy.
  - Xenotransfusion of DEA 1–negative canine blood to cats with blood compatibility issues to feline donors and in life or death situations has been reported. Recommended only in extreme situations, when no other options exist; RBC life span of transfused canine blood to cats is very short, and transfusion reactions, including hemolysis, should be expected. Repeat xenotransfusions in cats often results in acute fatal reactions. Major and minor cross-matching is recommended with xenotransfusions.

SUGGESTED READING

Yagi K, et al, editors: Manual of veterinary transfusion medicine and blood banking, Ames, IA, 2016, Wiley-Blackwell.

AUTHOR: Søren R. Boysen, DVM, DACVECC
EDITORS: Leah A. Cohn, DVM, PhD, DACVIM; Mark S. Thompson, DVM, DABVP

Upper Gastrointestinal Radiographic Contrast Series

Difficulty level: ♦

Synonyms

Barium series, UGI

Overview and Goals

- To identify morphologic and/or functional abnormalities of the stomach and/or small-intestinal tract
- The upper gastrointestinal (UGI) radiographic contrast series is most commonly performed using barium, which gives the best mucosal detail and therefore the best evaluation of morphology. The study may be performed with an iodinated contrast agent; these do not give good mucosal detail and are most useful for evaluating gastrointestinal (GI) patency.

Indications

- Severe or protracted vomiting
- Hematemesis or melena
- Abdominal pain
- Abnormalities of survey radiographs requiring further investigation
- Determine location of GI structures (i.e., herniation)
- Assessment of GI motility

Contraindications

- Survey radiographic evidence of perforation
  - If perforation is suspected, a barium study should not be performed. Iodinated contrast agents can be used, but because of their relatively poor opacity, these agents may fail to demonstrate GI leakage. In the case of suspected GI perforation, exploratory laparotomy is recommended.
- Survey radiographic evidence of obstruction
  - Not an absolute contraindication, but the study is not needed for diagnosis
- Projectile vomiting or frequent regurgitation
  - The risk of aspiration of contrast outweighs the potential benefits.
- Prior use of motility-altering drugs
  - Accurate assessment of GI function is not possible, and this may lead to a false diagnosis of obstruction.

Equipment, Anesthesia

- Contrast agent
  - Liquid barium (30% weight/volume: dose 10 mL/kg PO once); in very obese patients, dose for optimal rather than actual weight.
  - Nonionic iodinated contrast agent (preferred to an ionic iodinated agent)
    - Iohexol (Omnipaque) 10 mL/kg PO of diluted iohexol (240-875 mg I/mL, diluted 1 : 1 to 1 : 3 with tap water)
    - The greater the iodine concentration of the iohexol, the better the mucosal detail.
    - Administration of undiluted iohexol causes vomiting.
  - Ionic iodinated contrast agent, such as Renografin (used for IV injection but can be given orally): Renografin 2-7 mL/kg PO, total dose not to exceed 50 mL
- Syringes for contrast administration
- Orogastric tube of the appropriate size
- X-ray unit
- Protective clothing (lead aprons, gloves, thyroid shields) for personnel
- Paper towels or similar material for cleanup of barium on animal and x-ray table
- Drugs for restraint (used only if absolutely necessary). The following agents have been shown to have the least effect on motility and should be used if a motility disorder is suspected. Because the effect on GI motility of other, newer sedative drugs has not been proved, they cannot be recommended:
  - Dogs: acepromazine 0.05-0.1 mg/kg IV; avoid if animal is elderly or systemically ill
  - Cats: given IM 20 minutes before procedure, ketamine 13.2 mg/kg with midazolam 0.44 mg/kg *or* acepromazine 0.22 mg/kg

Anticipated Time

- Barium: ≈6 hours to complete the study; actual time performing the study is ≈1.5 hours
- Iodinated contrast agents: 2-3 hours to complete the study; actual time performing the study is ≈1 hour.
- ± Additional film at 24 hours after contrast administration

Preparation: Important Checkpoints

Empty GI tract (see Common Errors below):
- Fasting to empty the stomach
- Remove any excess fluid from stomach by tube
- Enema, only if colon is very full

Possible Complications and Common Errors to Avoid

Complications:
- Aspiration of barium: if the animal has projectile vomiting and/or radiographic evidence of severe gastric fluid retention, the risks outweigh the potential benefits.
- Aspiration of iodinated contrast agents: ionic iodinated contrast agents can cause severe (i.e., fatal) pulmonary edema if aspirated. *Ionic iodinated contrast agents should be administered only by orogastric intubation.*
- Leakage of contrast into the abdominal cavity. If leakage of barium occurs, immediate exploratory laparotomy is indicated to remove as much barium from the abdominal cavity as possible and address the cause of the leakage.

Common errors:
- Administration of too small a volume of barium
  - This is the *most common technical error* (occurs more often than administration of proper volume of barium).
  - Accurate evaluation of gastric emptying time is not possible, and full distention

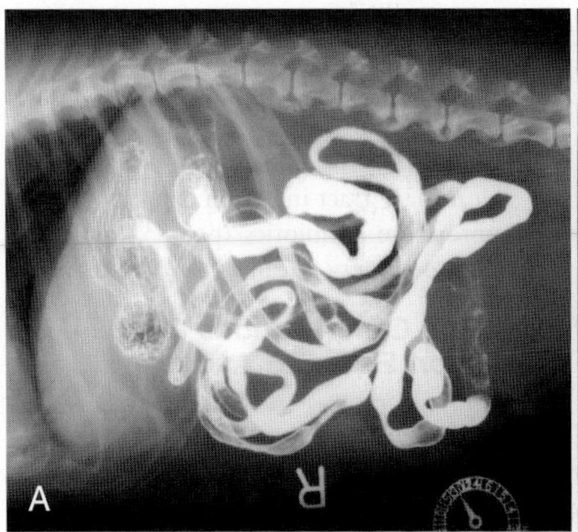

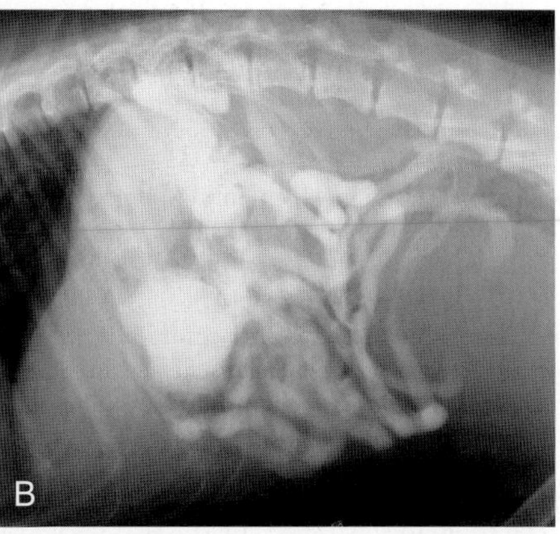

UPPER GASTROINTESTINAL RADIOGRAPHIC CONTRAST SERIES A, Right lateral radiograph obtained 30 minutes after administration of liquid barium. Note high opacity of contrast agent and good mucosal detail. **B**, Right lateral radiograph obtained 30 minutes after administration of iohexol. Contrast agent is much less opaque, and mucosal surface is poorly defined.

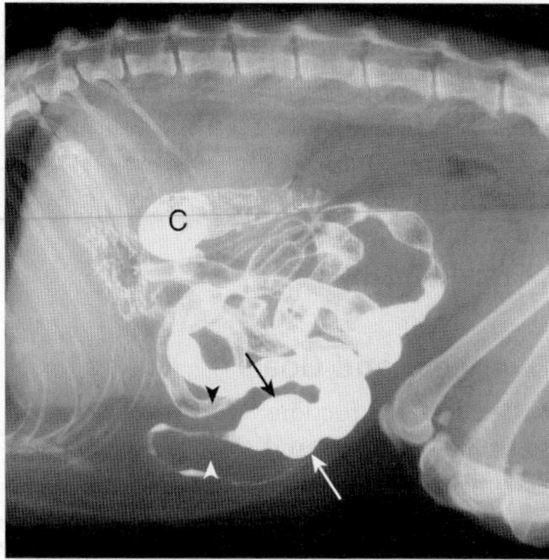

UPPER GASTROINTESTINAL RADIOGRAPHIC CONTRAST SERIES Right lateral radiograph obtained 2 hours after administration of liquid barium. Distended segment of small intestine *(arrows)* suddenly narrows at an area of intramural thickening *(arrowheads)* caused by a circumferential soft-tissue mass in this cat. Barium is seen in cecum *(C)*, indicating bowel is patent.

of the intestinal segments is not achieved if the volume of barium is too low. This can lead to serious misinterpretation of the study.

- Failure to empty the stomach of food before administration of barium is also a common technical error. The presence of food in the stomach makes accurate assessment of gastric emptying time impossible.
- Failure to obtain appropriately timed images
- Administration of barium before abdominal ultrasound or endoscopy may interfere with these procedures.

Procedure

- Obtain survey (plain) right lateral and ventrodorsal (VD) radiographs of the abdomen.
- Administer contrast.
  - Barium: 10 mL/kg PO administration by orogastric tube is preferred, but barium may be administered per os; *or*
  - Iodinated contrast agent: iohexol 10 mL/kg PO of diluted iohexol (240-875 mg I/mL diluted 1 : 1 to 1 : 3) *or* Renografin 2-7 mL/kg PO, with total dose not to exceed 50 mL. Administration by orogastric tube is necessary with the use of ionic iodinated agents to avoid aspiration and preferred with the use of nonionic iodinated contrast agents.
- Barium: obtain film sequence following a routine timetable. The timing of films can be altered as the study progresses, based on the findings of the study.
  - Immediate: right and left lateral, VD, and dorsoventral (DV)
    - The DV view provides evaluation of the body and pyloric region of the stomach, and it is important to obtain this view in the immediate film series. However, it can be difficult to position the patient for a DV view, and VD views are preferred for the remainder of the film series.
  - 30 minutes: right lateral and VD
  - 60 minutes: right lateral and VD
  - 90 minutes: right lateral and VD
  - 3 hours: right lateral and VD
  - 5 hours: right lateral and VD
  - ± 24 hours: right lateral and VD
- Iodinated contrast agents: obtain film sequence using a routine timetable. The timing of films can be altered as the study progresses, based on what is found in the study:
  - Immediate: right and left lateral, VD, and DV:
    - The DV view provides evaluation of the body and pyloric region of the stomach, and it is important to obtain this view in the immediate film series. However, it can be difficult to position the patient for a DV view, and VD views are preferred for the remainder of the film series.
  - 15 minutes: right lateral and VD
  - 30 minutes: right lateral and VD
  - 60 minutes: right lateral and VD
  - 2 hours: right lateral and VD
- By definition, the UGI radiographic contrast series is considered to be complete when contrast has almost completely emptied from the stomach and has entered the large intestine.
- In a patient with retention of barium in the stomach and contrast in the large intestine, the UGI radiographic contrast series should be continued until the stomach empties or an abnormality to account for the barium retention is noted.
- If an abnormality (i.e., obstruction) is identified, the study is considered to be complete even if barium is still in the stomach and/or has not entered the large intestine.

Postprocedure

- Inform the client that stools may have a paler color for several defecations after the procedure.
- The findings of the UGI radiographic contrast series may lead to additional diagnostic tests such as exploratory laparotomy or endoscopy.

Alternatives and Their Relative Merits

- Endoscopy
  - Endoscopy allows visualization of the mucosal surface of the stomach and duodenum and allows tissue biopsy.
  - Endoscopy does not evaluate the entire small-intestinal tract and requires the use of general anesthesia.
- Abdominal ultrasonography
  - Ultrasonography is rapid and noninvasive and does not involve ionizing radiation.
  - However, ultrasonographic evaluation of the GI tract can be severely limited by gas in the tract. Interpretation of ultrasound images of the GI tract requires an experienced sonographer, and GI disease may not cause significant changes in the ultrasonographic appearance of the intestine.
- Exploratory laparotomy
  - Allows assessment of the entire length of the GI tract, full-thickness gastric and intestinal biopsies, and treatment of obstruction. However, general anesthesia, invasiveness, and recovery/incision healing time make laparotomy a second-order diagnostic modality after less invasive evaluations such as plain radiography, UGI radiographic contrast series, ultrasonography, and/or endoscopy.

SUGGESTED READING

O'Brien T: Esophagus. In O'Brien T, editor: Radiographic diagnosis of abdominal disorders in the dog and cat: radiographic interpretation, clinical signs, pathophysiology, Davis, CA, 1981, Covell Park Vet Company, p 141.

AUTHOR: Patricia L. Rose, DVM, MS, DACVR
EDITORS: Leah A. Cohn, DVM, PhD, DACVIM; Mark S. Thompson, DVM, DABVP

Ureteral Occlusion, Subcutaneous Ureteral Bypass

Client Education Sheet 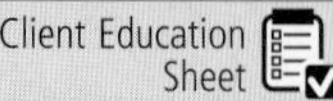

Difficulty level: ♦♦♦

Synonym

SUB

Overview and Goals

- Ureteral obstructions are a major clinical problem in cats and dogs, and are most commonly associated with ureteroliths, ureteral strictures, or trigonal neoplasia of the ureterovesicular junction. Traditional surgical treatment options are more invasive and are reported to have greater morbidity than the newer interventional options such as ureteral stent placement or subcutaneous ureteral bypass (SUB) device.
- In the author's experience, use of the SUB device is preferred for cats over placement of ureteral stents, and it can be used in specific cases in dogs. In the past 9 years, the author has placed > 500 SUB devices with good to excellent results (especially in cats) in the short and long term.

Indications

- Cats with any cause of a ureteral obstruction (e.g., ureteroliths [p. 1008], strictures, tumors, extraluminal ureteral compression). A SUB device can be predictably placed in cats regardless of the cat's size or severity of obstruction.
- In dogs, SUB can be considered instead of ureteral stent placement if there is a ureteral stent reaction, ureteral surgery is too complicated, or a radical surgery is being considered for removal of transitional cell carcinoma.
- Interventional procedures are especially helpful for cats that could benefit from reduced anesthesia time or cases that could be challenging using traditional ureteral surgery, such as proximal ureteral obstructions (stones/stricture), numerous ureterolithiasis requiring multiple ureterotomies, extensive ureteral injury, or trauma associated with ureteral calculi in which only a short segment of proximal ureter remains.

Contraindications

- Although not an absolute contraindication, mineralization of an SUB device in dogs is more common than mineralization of ureteral stents resulting in re-occlusion. Therefore, stent placement usually is preferred in dogs.
- A small-diameter renal pelvis (<8 mm) does require the nephrostomy tube to be modified as a ureterostomy tube, but this does not preclude placement of the SUB device. The author has successfully placed SUB devices in cats with a renal pelvis under 3 mm in diameter.

Equipment, Anesthesia

- General anesthesia is required.
- SUB device: a polyurethane catheter (6.5 Fr) that is composed of a locking-loop nephrostomy and cystostomy catheter and a metallic shunting port that connects the catheters subcutaneously, allowing for drainage and system flushing/sampling
- A traditional fluoroscopic C-arm is sufficient for visualization during ureteral interventions.
- Various guide wires and catheters are needed for each procedure.

Anticipated Time

In experienced hands, an SUB device can be placed, on average, in 45 minutes unilaterally, and 60 minutes bilaterally. Typically, an esophagostomy tube is placed after surgery is complete, which can add an additional 10 minutes to the procedure time.

Preparation: Important Checkpoints

- Appropriate hydration prior to anesthesia should be a goal. Many patients are overhydrated and minimal additional fluids are needed during surgery.
- If a urinary tract infection is present, begin appropriate antibiotics (pp. 232 and 849) prior to surgery, ideally 48-72 hours prior.

Possible Complications and Common Errors to Avoid

- Technical error is avoided by proper training.
- Mineralization of the device (24% of cats) is minimized by use of a tetra-sodium EDTA flush q 3 months. Despite mineralization of the device, only 12% of cats needed an SUB exchange due to development of ureteral patency and failure or ureteral re-obstruction. Mineralization is more likely in dogs than cats after SUB placement.
- Chronic urinary tract infections (8% of cats) are minimized by use of a tetra-sodium EDTA flush q 3 months and amenable to use of antimicrobial drugs chosen on the basis of urine culture and susceptibility testing. It is usually unnecessary to treat asymptomatic bacteriuria associated with *Enterococcus* spp (most common potential pathogen isolated from these cats).
- Dysuria is rare (<5%) after SUB device placement.

Procedure

The procedure should be done by trained interventionalists using fluoroscopic guidance and surgical assistance.

Postprocedure

- Esophagostomy tube (p. 1106) is usually placed to ensure appropriate nutrition, medications, and hydration, ultimately shortening hospitalization time (median, 4 days).
- Flush each SUB device regularly, typically at 1 week, 1 month, and then every 3 months thereafter using the tetra-sodium EDTA solution to help avoid mineralization and chronic urinary tract infections.
- Urinary tract ultrasounds should be done every few months for all patients with a history of a ureteral obstruction due to the high risk of the contralateral kidney being obstructed.

Alternatives and Their Relative Merits

The decision about the best procedure for each patient should be based on the operator's experience and the cause of obstruction.

- Traditional ureteral surgery: more invasive, longer anesthesia times, reported to have higher perioperative morbidity and mortality rates, and not readily applicable for all causes of ureteral obstruction (e.g., stricture, numerous stones, stone location, tumors). Surgical or interventional options are operator dependent. Decisions about

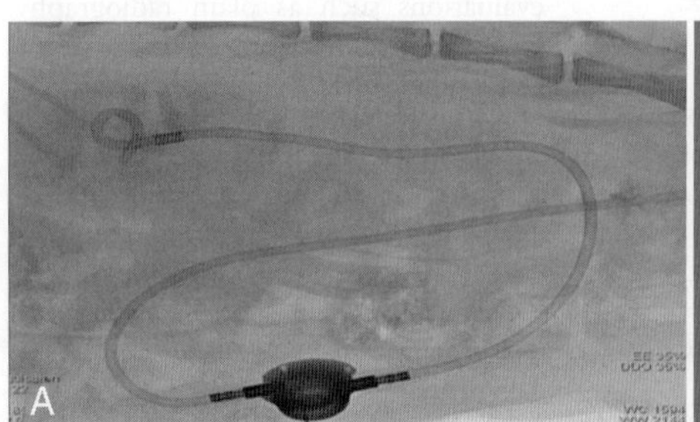

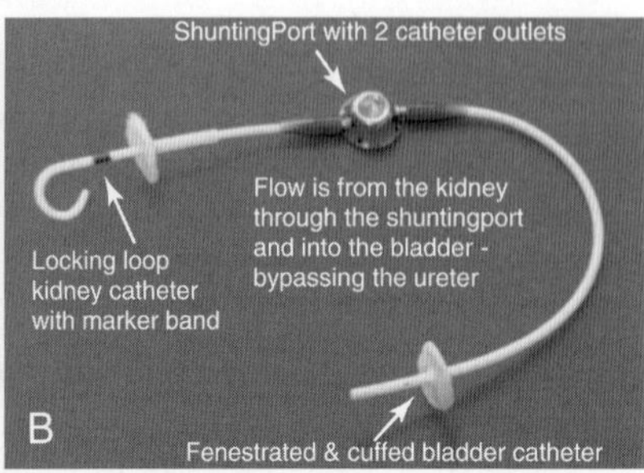

URETERAL OCCLUSION, SUBCUTANEOUS URETERAL BYPASS A, A lateral fluoroscopy image of a SUB device after implantation. Notice the locking-loop nephrostomy tube in the renal pelvis and the cystostomy tube in the urinary bladder. Both are hooked to a subcutaneous shunting port. **B**, The SUB device.

approach must consider skill level and availability.
- Ureteral stent placement: preferred for most dogs but associated with more long-term complications in cats.

Pearls

- No preoperative imaging or biochemical data can predict the overall outcome or renal function, but prognosis for long-term survival of cats with a benign cause of ureteral obstruction treated with stent placement is excellent.
- SUB placement in cats is associated with minimal morbidity and mortality rates.

SUGGESTED READING

Berent A, et al: The use of a subcutaneous ureteral bypass (SUB) device for the treatment of benign ureteral obstructions in cats: 137 cats, 174 ureters (2009-2015). J Am Vet Med Assoc 253(10):1309-1327, 2018.

AUTHOR: Allyson Berent, DVM, DACVIM
EDITORS: Leah A. Cohn, DVM, PhD, DACVIM; Mark S. Thompson, DVM, DABVP

Procedures and Techniques

Urethral Obstruction (Canine): Medical Management

Client Education Sheet

Difficulty level: ♦♦

Overview and Goal

Complete urethral obstruction is a potentially life-threatening event, culminating in death from uremia within 2-5 days if untreated. Although most causes of urethral obstruction are intraluminal (e.g., urethroliths, foreign material, urethral plugs [p. 1009]), mural (e.g., urethral and prostatic tumors [p. 828], urethral strictures) and extramural causes (e.g., pelvic fractures, perineal hernia [p. 774], compressive masses, iatrogenic urethral ligation) and functional disorders (e.g., detrusor-sphincter dyssynergia [p. 871]) result in similar clinical consequences.

Indications

- Urethroliths (common)
- Urethral/prostatic neoplasia
- Blood clots
- Intraurethral foreign bodies
- Matrix-crystalline urethral plugs (uncommon)

Contraindications

Retrograde hydropropulsion in patients with lower urinary tract rupture may inadvertently result in fluid accumulation in abdominal, retroperitoneal, perineal, or scrotal spaces.

Equipment, Anesthesia

- The type and degree of sedation/anesthesia varies, depending on patient status and veterinarian's preference.
- Cardiovascular stabilization
  - Warming pad
  - Intravenous (IV) catheter
  - Warm IV replacement fluids
  - Sodium bicarbonate
- Decompressive cystocentesis
  - A sterile 1½-inch, 22-gauge needle
  - IV extension tubing
  - 3-way stopcock
  - Large syringe (20-60 mL)
- Retrograde urethral flushing
  - Sterile isotonic nonirritating solutions (e.g., normal saline, lactated Ringer's solution)
  - Long, flexible, large-bore sterile catheter (e.g., 8 Fr, 22-inch red rubber feeding tube)
  - Large, sterile syringe (12-60 mL)
  - Moistened gauze sponges
- Indwelling catheter placement
  - Nonabsorbable suture and needle holders
  - Soft, flexible, inert, sterile urinary catheter

Anticipated Time

About 20 minutes to 1 hour

Preparation: Important Checkpoints

- Inform owners of the possibility of urinary bladder rupture and guarded short-term prognosis with or without therapy.
- Inform owners that in many cases, surgery or lithotripsy will be needed to correct intraluminal causes of obstruction. Urethral stenting (p. 1179) may be needed to manage mural urethral occlusion and extramural urethral compression.

Possible Complications and Common Errors to Avoid

- Appropriate medical imaging (e.g., survey radiography, contrast urethrography [p. 1181]) or urethroscopy (p. 1085) is essential to verify, localize, and search for the underlying cause of obstruction. Diagnostic evaluations should be obtained early in the diagnostic process before initiation of therapy.
- Unsuccessful transurethral insertion and passage of urinary catheters is an unreliable and sometimes unsafe (i.e., urethral tear, rupture, and subsequent stricture) method of confirming and localizing urethral obstruction.

Procedure

- Sedate or anesthetize animal.
- Decompressive cystocentesis
  - Attach a 1.5-inch, 22-gauge needle, IV extension tubing, and 3-way stopcock; then use a large-volume syringe (20-60 mL) to remove urine from bladder, entering at the center of the bladder with the needle directed obliquely (caudodorsally).
  - By using the IV extension tubing and 3-way stopcock between the needle and syringe, the urinary bladder will not have to be repunctured to empty a syringe full of urine.
  - Excessive digital pressure should not be applied to the bladder wall while the needle is in the lumen to prevent urine from being forced around the needle into the peritoneal cavity.
  - Attempting complete evacuation of the bladder lumen is undesirable because the sharp point of the needle may damage the bladder wall. We recommend that 10-15 mL of urine remain in the bladder.
  - Cystocentesis should not contribute to bladder rupture. Excessive manipulation or compression of a devitalized, overdistended bladder or excessive abdominal compression by a painful, inadequately anesthetized patient is usually the cause of bladder rupture.
  - Advantages
    - Obtaining a pre-treatment urine sample for analysis and culture
    - Temporarily halting the adverse metabolic consequences of obstruction
    - Reducing intraluminal bladder pressure to facilitate retropulsion
    - Reducing pain associated with bladder overdistention
  - Disadvantages
    - Potential extravasation of urine into peritoneal cavity
    - Bladder wall trauma
- Retrograde urethral flushing
  - Lubricate around the urethroliths
    - Fill one 12-mL syringe with 5 mL of saline and another 12-mL syringe with 5 mL of sterile water-soluble lubricant.
    - Attach these two syringes with a 3-way stopcock.
    - Mix the contents of both syringes by emptying one syringe into the other, back and forth several times.
    - After inserting a urethral catheter, inject 3-8 mL of mixture to lubricate around uroliths. This step is not always necessary.

- Insert a lubricated, large-bore flexible catheter into the distal urethra. The tip of the catheter should remain distal to urethroliths.
- Occlude pelvic urethra proximal to urethroliths: insert a gloved index finger into the rectum, and occlude the urethral lumen by compressing the urethra against the floor of the bony pelvis.
- Occlude distal urethra: with a moistened gauze sponge, occlude the distal urethra by compressing the distal tip of penis around the catheter.
- Forcefully flush fluid through catheter.
  - Fill a large syringe (20-60 mL) with sterile isotonic solution (e.g., saline, lactated Ringer's solution). The normal bladder holds approximately 7-11 mL/kg of the patient's weight.
  - With the syringe attached to the flexible catheter, turn it upside down, and place the top of the plunger against the tabletop.
  - Hold the syringe by the barrel, and forcefully push it down over the plunger with the goal of rapidly and forcefully emptying the syringe and subsequently dilating the urethral lumen with saline.
- Relieve occlusion of pelvic urethra: after the urethra becomes dilated, digital pressure applied to the pelvic urethra (but not the penile urethra) should be rapidly released.
- Continue flushing
  - Continue flushing fluid through the catheter and urethral lumen to propel urethroliths into the urinary bladder. Use caution not to overdistend the bladder lumen with saline.
  - If the technique is repeated, accumulation of saline in the bladder lumen necessitates repeating decompressive cystocentesis.
- To perform this technique in female dogs, insert the index finger into the vagina, and apply digital pressure; occlude the distal urethra over the catheter at the urethral papilla. Inserting the index finger in the rectum and applying digital pressure over the catheter in the pelvic urethra can also achieve distal urethral occlusion.

Postprocedure

- Medical imaging
  - Radiography provides an appropriate method of assessing whether all radiopaque uroliths have been flushed into the bladder lumen.
  - Transurethral catheterization is not a reliable method of verifying that all uroliths have been flushed out of the urethra.
- Pain medication (e.g., butorphanol, hydromorphone) is indicated for a short duration (1-2 days). Nonsteroidal antiinflammatory drugs (NSAIDs) are contraindicated in animals with compromised renal function or dehydration.
- Prevent negative fluid balance associated with postobstructive diuresis by administering parenteral fluids.

Alternatives and Their Relative Merits

To minimize surgical disfigurement of the urethra (e.g., urethrotomy, urethrostomy), consider lithotripsy to shatter obstructing urethroliths if retrograde urohydropropulsion is not successful.

Pearls

- This procedure should be performed only in dogs that are adequately anesthetized; urethral manipulation is very painful.
- Instilling lidocaine in the flushing solution is unlikely to be helpful because topical anesthetics require prolonged contact (>5 minutes) with the urothelium to be effective.

SUGGESTED READING

Osborne CA, et al: Canine retrograde urohydropropulsion. Lessons from 25 years of experience. Vet Clin North Am Small Anim Pract 29:267-281, 1999.

RELATED CLIENT EDUCATION SHEETS

Consent to Perform Cystocentesis
Consent to Perform General Anesthesia
Urolithiasis

AUTHORS: Jody P. Lulich, DVM, PhD, DACVIM; Carl A. Osborne, DVM, PhD, DACVIM
EDITORS: Leah A. Cohn, DVM, PhD, DACVIM; Mark S. Thompson, DVM, DABVP

Urethral Obstruction (Feline): Medical Management

Difficulty level: ♦

Overview and Goal

Complete urethral obstruction (p. 1009) is a potentially life-threatening event, culminating in death from uremia within 2-5 days if untreated. Although most causes of urethral obstruction are intraluminal (e.g., urethral plugs, urethroliths, foreign material), mural (e.g., tumors, urethral strictures), and extramural (e.g., pelvic fractures, iatrogenic urethral ligation), they result in identical clinical consequences.

Indications

- Matrix-crystalline urethral plugs (common)
- Urethroliths (common)
- Blood clots
- Intraurethral foreign bodies (i.e., buckshot)

Contraindications

Retrograde hydropropulsion in patients with lower urinary tract rupture may inadvertently result in fluid accumulation in abdominal, retroperitoneal, or perineal region.

Equipment, Anesthesia

- The type and degree of sedation/anesthesia vary, depending on patient status and veterinarian's preference.
- Cardiovascular stabilization
  - Warming pad
  - Intravenous (IV) catheter
  - Lukewarm IV replacement fluids
  - Sodium bicarbonate
  - Insulin and glucose to manage hyperkalemia
  - Calcium gluconate to manage hyperkalemia (p. 495)
- Decompressive cystocentesis
  - Sterile 1½-inch, 22-gauge needle
  - IV extension tubing
  - 3-way stopcock
  - Several syringes (3-20 mL)
- Retrograde urethral flushing
  - Sterile, nonirritating isotonic solutions (e.g., normal saline, lactated Ringer's solution)
  - Sterile, open-ended catheter (e.g., Minnesota olive-tip catheter)
  - IV extension tubing
  - Large syringe (12-35 mL)
  - Moistened gauze sponges
- Indwelling urinary catheter placement
  - Nonabsorbable suture and needle holders
  - Soft, flexible, inert sterile urinary catheter
  - Elizabethan collar

Anticipated Time

About 20 minutes to 1 hour

Preparation: Important Checkpoints

- Ensure cardiovascular stabilization before general anesthesia or urethral flushing.
- Prevalence of potentially life-threatening abnormalities in cats with urethral obstruction
  - Hypothermia (<100°F [37.8°C]) = 39%
  - Acidemia (pH < 7.2) = 16%
  - Bradycardia (<149 beats/min) = 12%
  - Hyperkalemia (>8 mEq/L) = 12%
  - Hypocalcemia (<0.8 mmol/L) = 6%-12%

- Inform owners of the possibility of urinary bladder rupture and guarded short-term prognosis with or without therapy.

Possible Complications and Common Errors to Avoid

- Cats with urethral obstruction and cardiovascular collapse rarely show overt signs referable to the urinary system at the time of presentation. Assessment of urinary bladder size (i.e., palpation or medical imaging) is essential to avoid overlooking urethral obstruction as the primary cause for cardiovascular or respiratory distress.
- Survey radiography is essential to verify, localize, and search for the underlying cause of obstruction; radiographs should be performed early in the diagnostic process before initiation of therapy. Non-obstructed dysuric cats usually have small urinary bladders.
- Unsuccessful bladder expression is an unreliable and sometimes unsafe (i.e., bladder rupture) method of confirming urethral obstruction.
- Unsuccessful transurethral insertion of urinary catheters is an unreliable and sometimes unsafe (i.e., urethral tear, rupture, and subsequent stricture) method of confirming and localizing urethral obstruction.
- Caustic, strongly acidic flushing solutions are contraindicated.

Procedure

- Sedate or anesthetize the patient. Consider epidural anesthesia to locally control pain and thereby minimize the quantity and risk of general anesthetics.
- To fragment urethral plugs, gently massage the distal urethra and cautiously compress the urinary bladder with the goal of promoting expulsion of plugs. This is easy to perform but not commonly effective.
- Decompressive cystocentesis
  - Attach a 1½-inch, 22-gauge needle, IV extension tubing, and a 3-way stopcock. Then use a large-volume syringe (20-35 mL) to remove urine from bladder, inserting the needle at the center of the bladder with the needle directed obliquely (caudodorsally).
  - By using the IV extension tubing and 3-way stopcock between the needle and syringe, the urinary bladder will not have to be repunctured to empty a syringe full of urine.
  - Excessive digital pressure should not be applied to the bladder wall while the needle is in the lumen to prevent urine from being forced around the needle into the peritoneal cavity.
  - Attempting complete evacuation of the bladder lumen is undesirable because the sharp point of the needle may damage the bladder wall. The authors recommend that 5-15 mL of urine remain in the bladder.
  - Properly performed cystocentesis should not contribute to bladder rupture. Excessive manipulation or compression of a devitalized, overdistended bladder wall or excessive abdominal compression by a painful, inadequately anesthetized patient may promote rupture.
  - Advantages of decompressive cystocentesis
    - Obtaining urine sample for analysis and culture
    - Temporarily halting the adverse metabolic effects of obstruction
    - Reducing intraluminal bladder pressure to facilitate retropulsion
    - Reducing pain associated with bladder overdistention
  - Disadvantages of decompressive cystocentesis
    - Potential extravasation of urine into peritoneal cavity
    - Bladder wall trauma
- Flushing plug contents out the external urethral orifice
  - Attach open-ended catheter, IV extension tubing, and large (35-mL) fluid-filled syringe in that order. Displace air in the tubing by filling tubing and catheter with fluid from the syringe before insertion in the urethra.
  - Insert tip of catheter into distal urethral opening.
  - Flush a large quantity of sterile isotonic solution into the urethral lumen, allowing it to reflux out the external urethral orifice. The goal is to break up a urethral plug, similar to massaging the urethra.
  - Subsequent application of steady but gentle digital pressure to the bladder wall may result in expulsion of a urethral plug.
  - This method is unlikely to flush uroliths back into the urinary bladder.
- Retrograde urethral flushing (to propel intraluminal contents into urinary bladder)
  - Attach open-ended catheter, IV extension tubing, and fluid-filled syringe (3-12 mL) in that order. Displace air in the tubing by filling tubing and catheter with fluid from the syringe before insertion in the urethra.
  - Insert tip of catheter into distal urethral opening.
  - With a moistened gauze sponge, occlude the distal urethra around the catheter.
  - Pull the penile urethra caudally to extend it parallel to the vertebral column.
  - Flush fluid vigorously by emptying syringe.
  - Repeat urethral flushing if needed while also remembering to repeat decompressive cystocentesis if bladder lumen becomes distended with flushing solution.
  - The greatest pressure to retrograde hydropropulse is achieved with the smallest syringe.
- In some cases, radiographs are indicated to verify return of uroliths into urinary bladder or assess catheter placement.

Postprocedure

Indwelling transurethral catheters:

- Not always indicated
- When indicated, 3- or 5-Fr, flexible feeding tubes composed of material that minimizes foreign body inflammatory response are preferred.
- To minimize urethral trauma, avoid open-end catheters with sharp stylets.
- Indications
  - Inadequate/poor urine stream after urethral flushing
    - Urethral spasm/swelling (≈1-3 days)
    - Excessive urinary precipitates (≈1-2 days)
  - Assist correction of postrenal azotemia (≈1-2 days).
  - Promote recovery of detrusor contractility (≈1-5 days).
  - Promote repair of urothelial urethral tear (≈3-10 days).
- Care and management
  - Place as atraumatically and cleanly as possible.
  - Maintain a closed collection system.
  - Remove indwelling catheters as soon as possible.
  - If urine is initially sterile, avoid antimicrobial therapy until catheter is removed.
  - If urine is initially infected, treat the infection (p. 232).
  - Treat potentially life-threatening infections.
  - Do not give the cat corticosteroids.
- Nutritional therapy to dissolve struvite crystals, urethral plugs, or small struvite uroliths (p. 1016)
- Analgesia (1-2 days). Nonsteroidal antiinflammatory drugs (NSAIDs) are contraindicated in cats with compromised renal function or dehydration.
- Prevent negative fluid balance associated with postobstructive diuresis by giving parenteral fluids.
- The following drugs are commonly administered to cats without proven efficacy, safety, or physiologic justification: urethral smooth-muscle relaxants (e.g., phenoxybenzamine, prazosin), urethral antispasmodics (e.g., propantheline, oxybutynin), parasympathomimetics (e.g., bethanechol), and skeletal muscle relaxants (e.g., diazepam, dantrolene). If used at all, should be closely monitored.

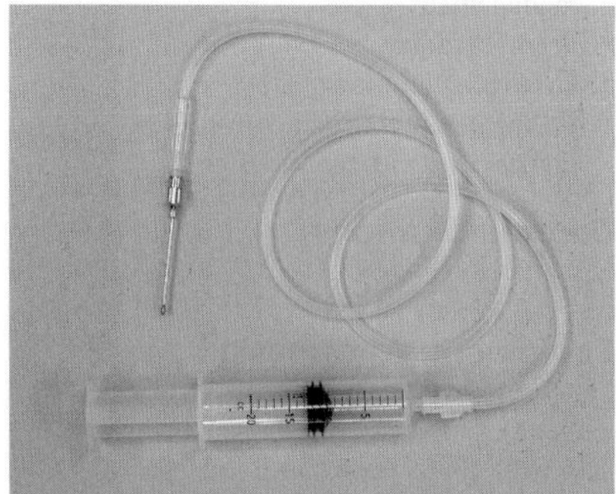

URETHRAL OBSTRUCTION (FELINE): MEDICAL MANAGEMENT Assembled catheter, IV extension tubing, and syringe to facilitate removing obstruction in the urethra of cats.

Procedures and Techniques

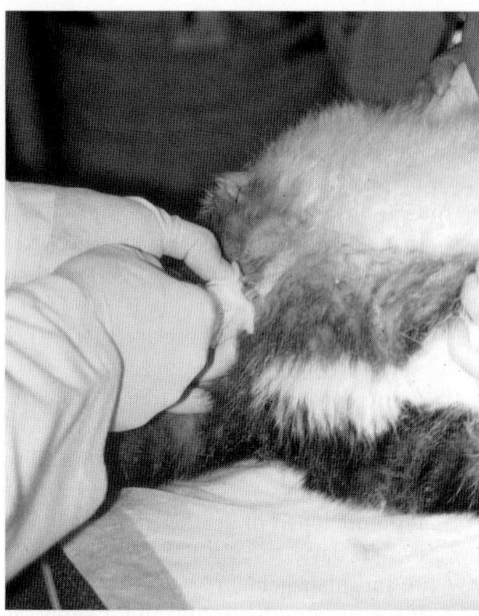

URETHRAL OBSTRUCTION (FELINE): MEDICAL MANAGEMENT Perineum of an anesthetized cat undergoing medical management of urethral obstruction. Cat is in dorsal recumbency; cranial is to right of the photograph. Occluding the distal urethra around the catheter and pulling the urethra caudally and dorsally to displace urethral kinking facilitates retrograde flushing of plugs and stones into the urinary bladder.

Alternatives and Their Relative Merits

- A pharmacologic approach using acepromazine, buprenorphine, and medetomidine with repeat decompressive cystocentesis has been reported for alleviating idiopathic urethral obstruction (p. 332).
- Urethrostomy may be indicated if obstruction cannot be corrected. Contrast urethrography (p. 1181) is indicated to localize the site(s) of obstruction and to select the location of surgery.

Pearls

- Medical imaging of the urethra before treatment (e.g., catheterization) is essential to understand the cause and best approach for patient care.
- Most cats are insufficiently anesthetized to safely unobstruct the urethra. This is understandable because a deep plane of anesthesia may cause further cardiac and metabolic decompensation of the patient. Consider epidural anesthesia to sufficiently anesthetize the perineal region to safely and more successfully clear the urethra.

SUGGESTED READING

O'Hearn AK, et al: Coccygeal epidural with local anesthetic for catheterization and pain management in the treatment of feline urethral obstruction. J Vet Emerg Crit Care 21:50-52, 2011.

AUTHORS: Jody P. Lulich, DVM, PhD, DACVIM; Carl A. Osborne, DVM, PhD, DACVIM
EDITORS: Leah A. Cohn, DVM, PhD, DACVIM; Mark S. Thompson, DVM, DABVP

Urethral Occluder Placement

Client Education Sheet 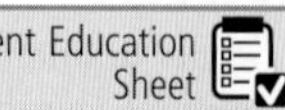

Difficulty level: ♦♦♦

Synonym

Artificial urethral sphincter

Overview and Goal

The artificial urethral sphincter (AUS) is indicated for the treatment of refractory urinary incontinence secondary to urethral sphincter mechanism incompetence in dogs.

Indications

- Urethral sphincter mechanism incompetence (p. 1011) refractory to medical management
- Pelvic bladder
- Urethral hypoplasia
- Refractory incontinence following surgical management of ectopic ureters

Contraindications

Patient unstable for surgery

Equipment, Anesthesia

- General anesthesia is required
- Artificial urethral sphincter port system (Norfolk Vet Products)
  - AUS
  - Huber point needles
  - Vascular access port (Companion port, three sizes available)
- Stainless steel reusable backfill catheter (Norfolk Vet Products) or syringe
- Routine equipment needed for celiotomy

Anticipated Time

Expected procedure time is 60-90 minutes

Preparation: Important Checkpoints

- CBC, serum chemistry panel, urinalysis, and urine bacterial culture within 2 weeks of the procedure
- Abdominal radiographs
- Ensure appropriately sized AUS and vascular access port are available and sterile.

Possible Complications and Common Errors to Avoid

- Avoid excessive dissection around the urethra to minimize trauma to the blood supply.
- Postoperative urethral obstruction, dysuria, and urinary tract infection have been reported.

Procedure

- The patient's skin is aseptically prepared from xiphoid to pubis.
- A caudal approach to the abdomen is performed by ventral midline celiotomy from the umbilicus to the pubic symphysis for maximal exposure of the urethra.
- A stay suture is placed in the apex of the bladder and retracted cranially.
- A 2-cm section of urethra is isolated using right-angle forceps at least 2 cm caudal to the bladder neck in the female dog and 1 cm caudal to the prostate in the male dog.
- Use a strand of suture or a Penrose drain to measure the urethral circumference.
- The AUS should be roughly 50% of the circumference (urethra = 20 mm and AUS = 10 mm).
- The AUS is primed with sterile saline to flush out the air using a syringe or a backfill catheter. The fluid is then removed and the tubing clamped.
- The vascular access port is flushed with sterile saline using a Huber point needle.
- The AUS is secured to the vascular access port and inflated to check for leaks.
- The AUS is fully deflated and passed around the urethra.
- The cuff must be oriented such that the actuating tubing is directed cranially.
- The port is disconnected from the AUS temporarily to tunnel the tubing through the abdominal wall lateral to the rectus abdominis muscle, where the port will be secured to the external rectus fascia.
- The tubing is reconnected to the port, the blue boot is advanced, and the port is sutured to the fascia using polypropylene suture.

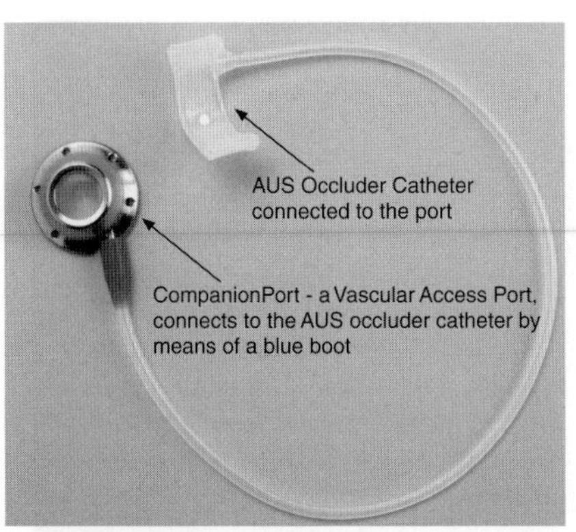

URETHRAL OCCLUDER PLACEMENT Artificial urethral sphincter (i.e., urethral occluder) device for implantation. The metallic port is used to attach a Huber point needle for addition or removal of fluid in the occluder portion, which is surgically placed around the urethra. (Copyright 2011, Norfolk Vet Products, Skokie, IL.)

- The 2-0 polypropylene suture is threaded through the eyelets of the AUS and tied to close the cuff.
- Calibration of the occluder
  - The port is flushed with sterile saline to remove all air trapped in the diaphragm, and then all saline is removed.
  - Saline is then gradually introduced 0.1 mL at a time to determine the degree of occlusion achieved with each 0.1-mL infusion.
  - Maximum fluid volume is noted in the medical record.
- The AUS should remain completely deflated for 6 weeks after surgery to allow for resolution of inflammation and revascularization of periurethral tissue.

Postprocedure

- The patient remains in the hospital until urination without straining is observed.
- Recheck examination at 6 weeks postoperatively to begin inflating the cuff in 0.05-0.2 mL increments.

Alternatives and Their Relative Merits

- Submucosal urethral injections of bulking agents: less invasive, temporary effects
- Culposuspension: no implants needed, up to 55% reported success rate
- Urethropexy, cystourethropexy: may have a 70% success rate combined with culposuspension, 21% complication rate
- Transobturator vaginal tape: invasive, 33% postoperative dysuria rate, delayed fistula formation
- Transpelvic urethral sling: invasive, less than 50% long-term continence rate, fistula formation

Pearls

- Err on the side of oversizing rather than undersizing the AUS to avoid urethral obstruction.
- Huber point needles must be used through the vascular access port.

SUGGESTED READING

Currao RL, et al: Use of a percutaneously controlled urethral hydraulic occluder for treatment of refractory urinary incontinence in 18 female dogs. Vet Surg 42:4, 2012.

AUTHOR: Jill K. Luther, DVM, MS, DACVS
EDITORS: Leah A. Cohn, DVM, PhD, DACVIM; Mark S. Thompson, DVM, DABVP

Procedures and Techniques

Urethral Stent Placement

Client Education Sheet 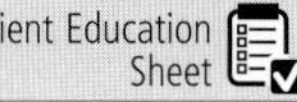

Difficulty level: ♦♦♦

Overview and Goal

Placement of a permanent, expandable stent to relieve urethral obstruction and re-establish urine stream in a patient with partial or complete obstruction

Indications

Urethral obstruction (p. 1009) refractory to standard of care:

- Urethral/bladder trigonal neoplasia (p. 991)
- Benign urethral stricture
- Prostatic neoplasia (p. 828) causing urethral obstruction
- Sustained urethral spasm refractory to medical therapy

Contraindications

- Self-expanding nitinol urethral stents are permanent; they are not amenable to removal.
- If the obstruction can be relieved through another means without requiring a permanent implant, it should be done. A removable urethral stent can be considered in this situation.

Equipment, Anesthesia

- General anesthesia is required.
- Fluoroscopy or digital radiology. Fluoroscopy is preferred because it provides real-time imaging, allowing faster and more precise stent placement.
- Software package for making measurements from fluoroscopic images or calculator for manual measurements
- Appropriately sized, self-expanding, metallic urethral stent (Vet-Stent-Urethra by Infiniti Medical, Menlo Park, CA). An inventory of various lengths and diameters of stents allows diagnosis and placement to occur under the same anesthesia.
- A removable, silicone-covered nitinol stent (Allium Medical Caesarea Industrial Park South, Caesarea, Israel) has been used in a few veterinary patients with promising results.
- Iodinated contrast medium, introducer sheath (generally 8 Fr), marker catheter, 0.035-inch hydrophilic guide wire (HGW), Berenstein catheter

Anticipated Time

60-90 minutes

Preparation: Important Checkpoints

- Ensure multiple-sized urethral stents are available.
- Ensure the owner understands urinary incontinence can occur (25% in females/males after placement of a urethral stent for obstructive neoplasia).

Possible Complications and Common Errors to Avoid

Patients should be referred to a formally trained and experienced specialist.

- An inappropriately small stent increases the risk of stent migration.
- Misplaced stent or one not spanning the entire obstruction can result in persistent urethral obstruction.
- After stent placement, care must be taken when performing a rectal palpation or taking a rectal temperature because the stent could become damaged or compressed.

Procedure

- Under general anesthesia, place animal in lateral recumbency.
- The prepuce or vulvar region is aseptically prepared.
- A marker catheter is advanced into the terminal portion of the colon over a 0.035-inch-diameter HGW. This marker catheter allows correction of magnification and is essential in selection of stent size. The marker catheter can be placed in a 14-Fr red rubber catheter to protect it from kinking.
- Proper catheter and patient positioning is verified by fluoroscopy.
- A 0.035-inch HGW is inserted into the urethra and advanced into the bladder under fluoroscopic guidance.

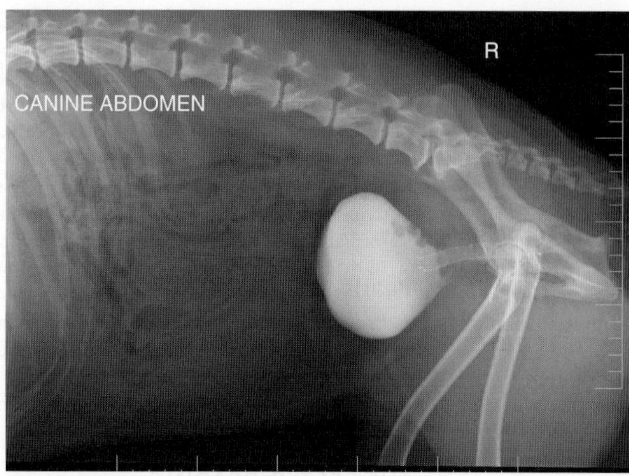

URETHRAL STENT PLACEMENT Urethral stent placed in a female dog with urethral and substantial trigonal transitional cell carcinoma. The stent is visible as a fine mesh tube over and cranial to the pubis; several filling defects in the trigone region are caused by the neoplastic mass.

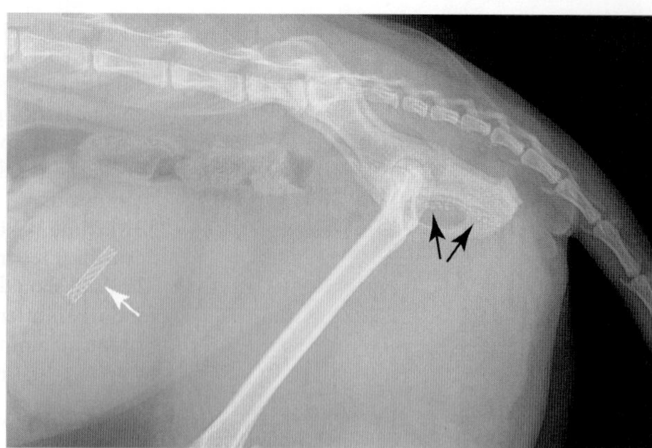

URETHRAL STENT PLACEMENT Two urethral stents were placed in a male cat with sustained urethral spasm. One year later, the cat received several enemas due to constipation. After the procedure, it was found that his urine stream had decreased. A radiograph revealed complications involving both stents. The cranial-most stent had migrated into the bladder *(white arrow)*, and the stent remaining in the urethra was damaged (fractured and flattened, *black arrows*). This case illustrates the importance of a careful, gentle approach when performing certain manipulations (enemas, rectal palpation, rectal temperature) in animals that have urethral stents.

- An appropriately sized introducer sheath (usually 8 Fr) is slid along the guide wire into the distal urethra.

Contrast cystourethrogram:
- In females, this can be done through the introducer sheath with the HGW in place.
- In male dogs, a Berenstein catheter is advanced over the HGW and through the introducer sheath that has been sutured to the prepuce. The HGW is removed, and contrast (50:50 mixture of iodinated contrast and 0.9% sterile saline) is injected through the Berenstein catheter.
- Contrast is injected into the urinary bladder to ensure full bladder distention, allowing clear distinction between the urethra, trigone, and bladder.
- The catheter is then withdrawn into the proximal urethra, and contrast is continuously injected while withdrawing the catheter under fluoroscopic guidance. The catheter is withdrawn to the distal portion of the urethra (in males) or the vestibule (in females while maintaining HGW access).
- The site and length of the obstruction can be determined along with measurement of the maximal urethral diameter.
- A voiding cystourethrogram (manually compressing the bladder under fluoroscopic guidance) can further assist in visualizing the obstruction, but radiation safety principles must be respected (i.e., keep compressing hand away from x-ray beam).

Stent selection:
- A diameter stent 10%-15% greater than the maximal diameter of the urethra near the obstruction is selected.
- The length of the obstruction is calculated, and the stent length is chosen to extend 0.5-1 cm both cranial and caudal to the obstruction.
- The stent is passed over the guide wire and into position under fluoroscopic guidance and then deployed.
- The stent is not reconstrainable, and after deployment has been initiated, it cannot be stopped or replaced.
- Patency is verified by performing another contrast cystourethrogram.
- The stent delivery system, the sheath, HGW, and marker catheter are withdrawn.
- If the urethra cannot be catheterized (e.g., obstructive urethral transitional cell carcinoma), an antegrade approach through the bladder can be used to pass the HGW and gain access to the bladder and urethra. In male cats, this antegrade approach can be used to pass the stent as the small diameter of the penile urethra prevents retrograde passage of the stent.

Postprocedure

- Patients can be discharged the same day.
- Long-standing urethral obstruction can be associated with bladder atony. Bethanechol 5-15 mg/DOG total dose PO q 8h for 7-10 days after the procedure can assist in reestablishing detrusor function.
- Analgesia: nonsteroidal antiinflammatory drugs (NSAIDs), buprenorphine, or tramadol can be administered for 4-5 days after the procedure.
  - NSAIDs can be part of a chemotherapy protocol for transitional cell and prostatic carcinoma.
- Ongoing chemotherapy is indicated in the presence of bladder/urethral/prostatic neoplasia (stent only palliative).

Alternatives and Their Relative Merits

- Urethral catheterization: short-term option to relieve urethral obstruction
- Cystostomy tube: the tube can be placed by a percutaneous approach or surgically and emptied by the owner 2-3 times/day; no incontinence, high rate of urinary tract infections
- Manual bladder evacuation at home: requires dedicated and skilled owner, risk of bladder trauma/rupture; some patients with complete urethral obstruction cannot be manually emptied

Pearls

- Good bladder filling during the voiding urethrocystogram is essential because it allows identification of the urethra and trigone. Placing a stent in the trigone is inappropriate and may result in stent migration into the bladder.
- A longer stent is easier to place and more likely to span the obstructed area.
- There is no association between the length of the stent placed and the incontinence rate.
- No predictors of incontinence have been identified.

RELATED CLIENT EDUCATION SHEETS

Consent to Perform General Anesthesia
Prostatic Diseases

AUTHOR: Marilyn Dunn, DMV, MVSc, DACVIM
EDITORS: Leah A. Cohn, DVM, PhD, DACVIM; Mark S. Thompson, DVM, DABVP

Urethrogram

Difficulty level: ◆◆

Overview and Goals

- The urethra cannot be seen on survey radiographs, and a positive-contrast examination is necessary for radiographic evaluation.
- Ultrasound can be used for visualizing small portions of the urethra in the male; however, adequate diagnostic imaging of the entire urethra requires radiographic assessment with the injection of iodinated contrast material.
- A simple urethrogram is quick and easy to perform.
- A vaginocystourethrogram is usually performed in the female because of the difficulty of catheterizing the female urethra.

Indications

- Clinical signs
  - Dysuria, stranguria
  - Difficulty catheterizing, urethral obstruction
  - Trauma to pelvis or os penis
  - Hematuria in a voided or catheterized urine sample but normal urine on cystocentesis
  - Hemorrhagic preputial discharge with a normal penile/preputial physical exam
- Differential diagnosis
  - Urethral calculi (especially important with radiolucent calculi)
  - Urethral tear/rupture, stricture, neoplasia, or fistula (p. 1009)
  - Iatrogenic urethral trauma
  - Other urethral mucosal abnormalities
  - Penile or extrapelvic urethral disease
  - Congenital anomalies
  - Postoperative evaluation of urethra to assess patency and completeness of healing
  - Evaluation of perineal or caudal abdominal masses

Contraindications

Relative contraindications include active lower urinary infection, emphysematous cystitis, or allergy to radiopaque contrast.

Equipment, Anesthesia

- Heavy sedation is often adequate to perform the study in male dogs; general anesthesia can be used if necessary. The male cat should be under general anesthesia.
- Mild surgical scrub solution and gauze/sponges for disinfecting the penis before catheterization
- Urinary catheter (preferably with inflatable balloon), such as a Foley catheter
- Iodinated contrast medium (sodium iothalamate, sodium diatrizoate) or low-osmolar, nonionic, water-soluble iodines such as iohexol or iopamidol (180-300 mg iodine/mL most common) can be used.
- Sterile lubricating jelly
- Sterile syringe for contrast (e.g., 12 mL)
- Sterile syringe for inflating the catheter balloon
- Sterile catheter adapter (Christmas-tree type)
- Sterile 3-way stopcock
- Sterile saline
- Sterile gloves
- Enema bag/set
- Open-ended tomcat catheter (e.g., 3.5 Fr) used for male cats

Anticipated Time

Approximately 20-30 minutes

Preparation: Important Checkpoints

- An enema (p. 1099) is indicated approximately 2 hours before the study to ensure the removal of fecal material from the colon (could compromise visualization of the urethra).
- Dilute iodinated contrast media to 50% solution with sterile saline.
- Sterile gloves should be worn from this point forward in the preparation.
- Draw 12 mL of diluted contrast material into 12-mL syringe.
- Remove Foley catheter from packaging in a sterile manner, and remove guide wire.
- Attach catheter adapter (Christmas tree) to the open port (lumen) of the Foley catheter.
- Attach 3-way stopcock to catheter adapter.
- Load syringe with air for inflating balloon later by drawing appropriate amount of air into the syringe (based on recommendation of Foley balloon size).
- Test integrity of the balloon.
  - Attach syringe containing air to side port (going to balloon, not the catheter lumen).
  - Infuse air into the balloon, filling it to the recommended level to ensure balloon is intact, and hold for a few seconds (to test inflation).
  - After it is clear the balloon will hold air, withdraw the air from the balloon back into the syringe.
- Attach syringe with contrast material onto 3-way stopcock, and fill the Foley catheter with contrast material. If this step is bypassed, air bubbles will be injected, resulting in a suboptimal study.
- Close the stopcock to the contrast material.
- In male cats, diluted contrast material is drawn into the syringe, and the syringe is attached directly to the tomcat catheter.

Possible Complications and Common Errors to Avoid

- Trauma due to overdistention of the balloon
- Rupture of the urethra: forceful injection when the urethra is obstructed can lead to urethral rupture. Resistance to injection should prompt adjustment of the catheter or termination of the procedure.
- Mild, transient submucosal hemorrhage secondary to balloon: avoid leaving urethral catheter in place longer than 15 minutes (urethral trauma caused by local ischemia and mechanical trauma)
- Urinary bladder–associated complications (hemorrhagic cystitis, catheter kinking or knotting in the bladder lumen, pulmonary air embolism, bladder rupture secondary to overdistention of the bladder) are rare because the catheter remains in distal urethra.
- Bacterial contamination
- False results: catheter in too far (past lesion site), too little contrast, air bubbles
- Contrast media reactions (absorbed systemically though mucosa)
- Anaphylactic reactions (rare)

Procedure

- Preliminary caudal abdominal radiographs (lateral and oblique ventrodorsal) are made to set radiographic technique and ensure adequate preparation of the animal.
- The kilovoltage peak (kVp) should be set between 65 and 75 to maximize contrast.
- The dog should be placed in left lateral recumbency (to reduce the risk of pulmonary air embolism).
- An assistant should then extrude the penis from the prepuce.
- The penis should be prepped with a mild surgical scrub solution.
- Sterile lubricating jelly is placed onto the tip of the Foley catheter.
- Insert Foley catheter into the distal urethra until the balloon can no longer be seen, but no further. The procedure is conducted with the catheter inserted into the urethra a very short distance to avoid passing beyond the site of the lesion.
- Inject air into balloon to inflate and then close the stopcock to maintain inflation. A suitable volume of air should meet little resistance and yet should provide enough of a seal to prevent backflow of contrast out the urethra during injection.
- Tug very lightly on the catheter to ensure the balloon seal is tight, and adjust inflation (increase or decrease) accordingly.
- With the dog's hindlimbs pulled forward to allow an unobstructed radiographic projection of the urethra, inject 12 mL of contrast material rapidly into the urethral catheter. NOTE: The contrast material should flow smoothly and with no resistance; if resistance is met, stop the injection, and make the radiographic exposure.
- Make radiographic exposure just before the end of injection.

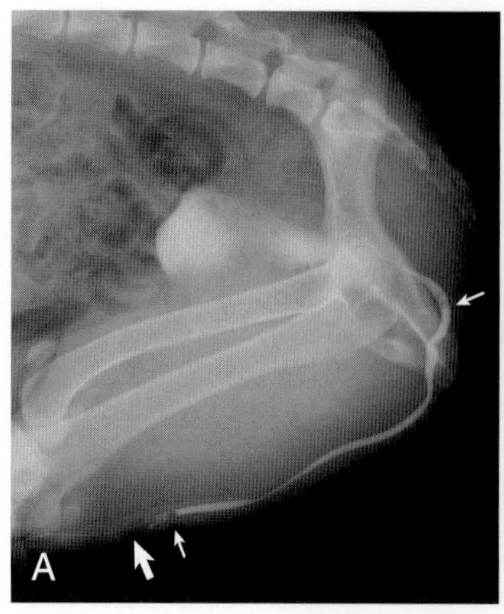

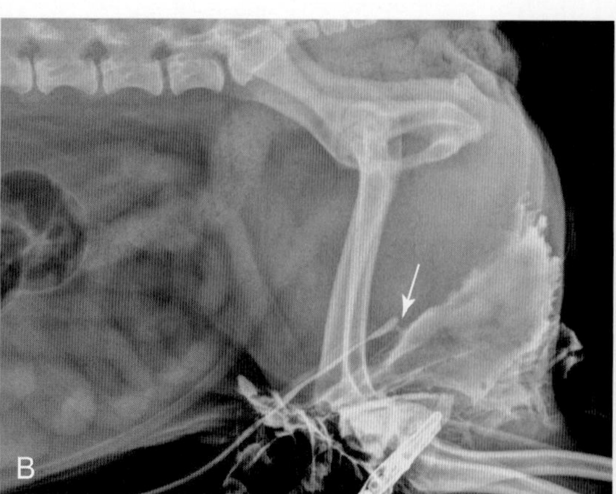

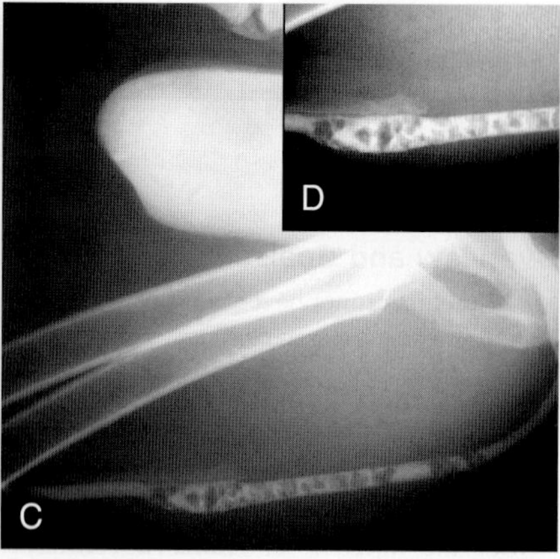

URETHROGRAM A, Normal canine male urethrogram (lateral view, cranial to left). Small air bubbles are seen in the membranous urethra and penile urethra *(small arrows)*, and the inflated balloon of the Foley catheter can be seen *(large arrow)*. **B**, Male dog with urethral rupture (lateral view, cranial to left). Contrast material is seen leaking from the urethra *(arrow)* into the soft tissues as a result of the ruptured urethra (bottom right of image). **C**, Male dog with urethroliths (lateral view, cranial to upper left). **D**, Zoomed view, showing multiple urethroliths.

- Close the stopcock to the syringe that contained the contrast material, and remove syringe.
- Refill syringe with diluted contrast material in preparation for second injection, and reattach syringe to stopcock; open stopcock to allow contrast flow.
- Place dog in an oblique ventrodorsal position, and inject 12 mL of contrast material rapidly.
- Make radiographic exposure just before the end of injection.
- For male cats, animal preparation and survey radiographs are the same as the dog. The penis is extruded and prepped, a lubricated tomcat catheter is placed just inside the distal urethra, and contrast material is injected as described (but typically 3 mL volume instead of 12 mL).

Postprocedure

- After the study is complete, the air should be removed from the Foley balloon before the catheter is withdrawn from the penis.
- If general anesthesia was used: routine anesthetic recovery

Alternatives and Their Relative Merits

- Plain abdominal radiographs: inexpensive means to survey the urethra for radiopaque urethral calculi. Otherwise, contrast medium is needed to visualize the urethra and most of its associated lesions.
- Abdominal ultrasound: can be used for assessing a portion of the urethra.

Pearls

- Start a stopwatch when the Foley balloon is inflated inside the penis to be certain 15 minutes are not exceeded.
- Air bubbles are perfectly round, and urethral calculi generally are not.

SUGGESTED READING

Holt P: Urological disorders of the dog and cat, London, 2012, Manson Publishing.

AUTHOR: LeeAnn Pack, DVM, DACVR
EDITORS: Leah A. Cohn, DVM, PhD, DACVIM; Mark S. Thompson, DVM, DABVP

Urinary Catheter Care, Indwelling

Bonus Material Online 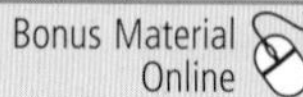

Difficulty level: ♦

Overview and Goal

Indwelling urinary catheters are used in hospitalized patients to maintain patient cleanliness (recumbent patients), to allow urinary drainage from patients with urethral obstructive diseases (p. 1009), and to monitor urinary output of critically ill patients. Appropriate care is required to prevent infection, ensure patient comfort, and maximize catheter longevity.

Indications

All patients with an indwelling urinary catheter

Equipment, Anesthesia

Surgical scrub, water, gauze pads, sterile saline, exam gloves, and 0.05% chlorhexidine solution

Anticipated Time

10-15 minutes

Preparation: Important Checkpoints

Ensure all supplies are available, and have an available assistant.

Possible Complications and Common Errors to Avoid

Overzealous handling of the urinary catheter may lead to inadvertent removal.

Procedure

- Indwelling urinary catheter maintenance should be performed every 8 hours for hospitalized patients. Gross contamination with blood, feces, urine, or dirt should be addressed as soon as it occurs.
- All indwelling urinary catheters should be attached to a closed collection system. This can be easily and cheaply accomplished by using an empty fluid bag (e.g., emptied 1-L bag of lactated Ringer's solution), along with a new fluid line and an adaptor to attach the line to the urinary catheter. A closed collection system reduces the risk for ascending bacterial infection, keeps the patient clean, and allows easy assessment of urine production.
- The collection bag should be kept lower than the patient to prevent retrograde flow of urine back to the patient, which may predispose to urinary tract infections.

- The collection bag should be emptied based on a predetermined schedule (e.g., q 1-8h) or when it is almost full.
- Wash hands before and after handling the urinary catheter or collection system.
- Put on exam gloves. Evaluate the urinary catheter and collection system, and ensure that the catheter is still in place and there are no leaks in the system.
- Use surgical scrub to clean skin around the vulva/prepuce, as well as exposed area of the catheter and collection system. Follow by rinsing with gauze and water.
- Wipe the skin around the vulva/prepuce, as well as exposed area of the catheter and collection system with gauze and 0.05% chlorhexidine solution. Flush the vulva/prepuce with 0.05% chlorhexidine solution.
- Empty closed collection system (if needed).
- The urine collection line and bag should be replaced when there is gross contamination that cannot be easily cleaned.

Postprocedure

Ensure that all disconnected bags or lines are properly connected after collection bag is emptied.

Pearls

- Clamps attached to fluid lines are usually removed to prevent them from being accidentally closed, preventing urine flow. However, temporarily clamping the line during animal transport can prevent retrograde flow of urine back into the animal.
- When moving a patient with an indwelling urinary catheter, ensure that the collection bag is always below the patient to prevent retrograde flow of urine back to the animal.

SUGGESTED READING

Aldrich J: Urethral catheterization. In Creedon JM, et al, editors: Advanced monitoring and procedures for small animal emergency and critical care, ed 1, West Sussex, UK, 2012, John Wiley & Sons.

AUTHOR: Adesola Odunayo, DVM, MS, DACVECC
EDITORS: Leah A. Cohn, DVM, PhD, DACVIM; Mark S. Thompson, DVM, DABVP

Vaginal Cytology

Bonus Material Online 

Difficulty level: ◆

Synonym

Colpocytology

Overview and Goal

Examination of cells exfoliated from the vaginal epithelium can assist in determining reproductive status and local inflammatory conditions (vaginitis). In clinical practice, it is important to determine whether the bitch has a keratinizing (proestrus) or keratinized vaginal epithelium (estrus).

Indications

- Staging the bitch's reproductive status for breeding management
- Assisting in determining whether a previously spayed bitch is experiencing estrual symptoms resulting from ovarian remnant syndrome (p. 732) or exposure to exogenous hormone. Vaginal keratinization (cornification) is a bioassay for estrogen.
- Evaluating the nature of any vulvar discharge

Contraindications

None; care and strict aseptic technique must be used when sampling the pregnant bitch.

Equipment, Anesthesia

- Cotton- or rayon-tipped swab, preferably with a (semiflexible) plastic shaft (polystyrene) that is 6 inches long. Sudden movements by uncooperative bitches may cause the wooden-shaft, cotton-tipped swabs to break during the specimen collection procedure.
- A 3-mL syringe with saline solution to wet the cotton tip
- A glass slide (preferably a premium precleaned glass slide with frosted end for patient identification)
- A fast Romanowsky-type stain kit (e.g., Diff-Quik)
- A booklet of bibulous paper
- A brightfield microscope

Anticipated Time

Total procedure: < 10 minutes

- Sample collection: 10-60 seconds
- Making of slide smear and staining: ≤ 4 minutes
- Reading of slide and interpretation: ≤ 2 minutes

Preparation: Important Checkpoints

- Have a kit with main supplies for collecting the vaginal specimen: a box of glass slides, a 3-mL syringe that has been prefilled with saline solution, a permanent marker or pencil to write the patient's ID in the glass slide
- Ensure a stain kit and a microscope are available for use.

Possible Complications and Common Errors to Avoid

- Avoid inadvertently introducing the swab into the bitch's urethra. When that happens, a diagnosis of nonkeratinized (cornified) vaginal smear is made. To avoid it, ensure the swab is introduced into the bitch's vagina just ventral to the dorsal vulvar commissure.
- For vaginal smears without enough cells for interpretation, repeat the procedure to ensure enough cells are collected.
- Vaginal smears with too many spindle-shaped cells likely indicate that vestibular or clitoral fossa cells, not vaginal epithelial cells, were collected. For proper reading and interpretation, cells must be collected from the middle to cranial vaginal regions.

Procedure

- Wet the cotton-tipped swab with a couple of drops of saline solution.
- Introduce the swab just ventral to the dorsal vulvar commissure into the vaginal vault.
- Advance the swab 0.5-3 cm (depending on dog breed and size) horizontally into the vestibular area, and then immediately tip it at ≥ 45° angle (almost toward to the anus) and advance it craniodorsally until in the vagina proper.
- The swab is then repositioned horizontally, and adequate exfoliation of vaginal epithelium cells can be accomplished by moving the swab tip back and forth and by twirling the swab shaft a couple of times.
- The swab is then quickly withdrawn from the bitch's vagina and rolled onto the glass smear in two or three streaks; do not roll the swab tip back and forth on the same area.
- Air-dry and proceed to staining (according to the manufacturer's instructions).
- Blot the wet, stained slide onto a sheet of bibulous paper, and proceed to brightfield microscopy.
- Initial screening of the slide is done at 100× magnification for an overall assessment of types of cells (i.e., determination of the percentage of cornified vs. noncornified vaginal epithelial cells).
- Intermediate stages of epithelial cells or microorganisms (fungal, bacterial) can be further examined at 400× or 1000× (under immersion oil) if needed.
- Noncornified cells (parabasal and small, intermediate-stage cells) are small, round cells with a large, stippled nucleus. Noncornified cells have large nucleus-to-cytoplasm ratios. Cornified cells (large, intermediate-stage and superficial cells) have a more angular shape, and the nucleus is pyknotic or not apparent

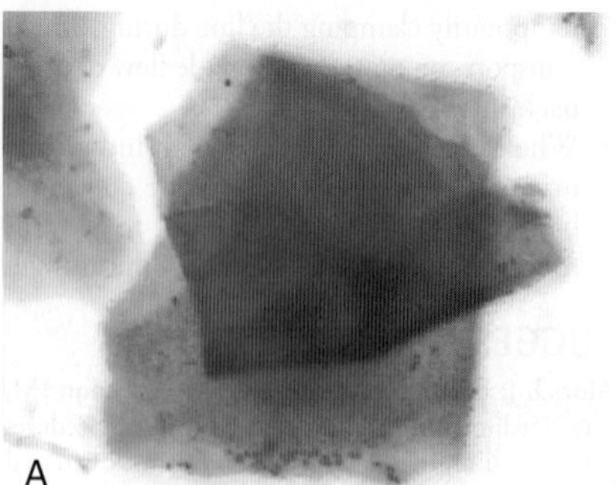

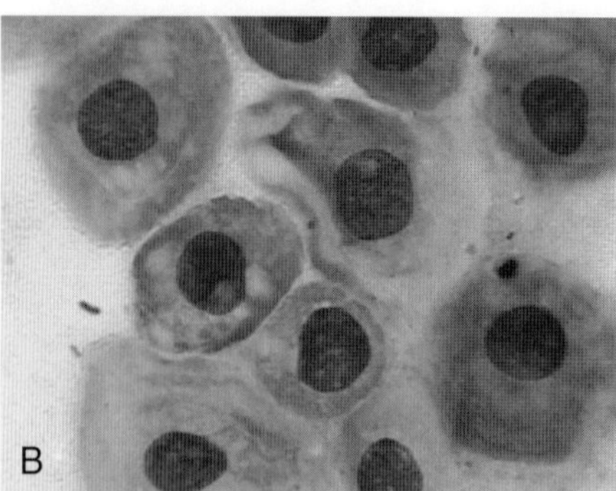

VAGINAL CYTOLOGY Vaginal smears stained with Romanowsky stain and observed with brightfield microscopy. **A**, Estrus: superficial epithelial cells observed at 1000× magnification. **B**, Diestrus: parabasal epithelial cells observed at 400× magnification.

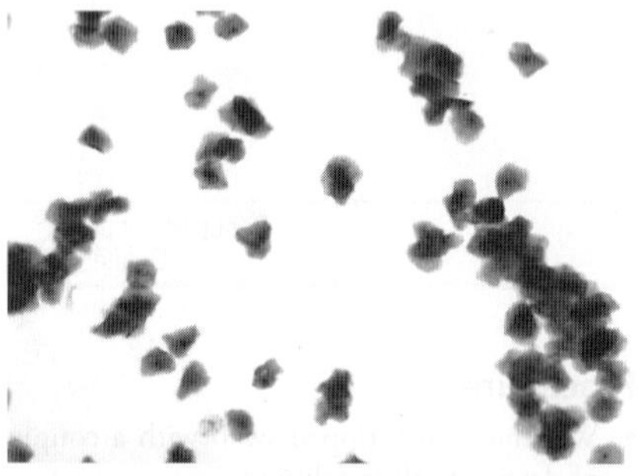

VAGINAL CYTOLOGY Vaginal smear depicts 100% cornification (superficial and large, intermediate-stage squames) that is consistent with estrus. Smear stained with Romanowsky stain and observed with brightfield microscopy at 100× magnification.

due to being poorly stained. The percentage of cornified cells increases approximately 10% per day during proestrus, reaching 90%-100% (full cornification) by the onset of estrus. At the end of estrus, the first day of cytologic diestrus is characterized by an abrupt (overnight) decline in the percentage of cornified cells and the appearance of a significant number of noncornified cells and influx of leukocytes. The vaginal epithelium is virtually 100% noncornified during diestrus or anestrus and in spayed bitches.

Postprocedure

None

Pearls

- A small vaginal speculum may be used to aid placing the swab into the vagina proper, thereby bypassing the vestibular area and preventing inadvertent entry into the urethra. However, the use of proper technique virtually prevents improper catheterization of the urethra or excessive collection of vestibular cells, making speculum use unnecessary.
- Use of a cytobrush is an efficient approach to exfoliate and collect vaginal epithelial cells. However, when using a cytobrush, it is essential to also use a vaginal speculum because most bitches will resent the cytobrush being placed in the vagina without the aid of a speculum.
- The proper use of cotton-tipped swabs ensures the collection of plenty of vaginal epithelial cells, making the use of cytobrushes not essential.
- Ovarian remnants or exposure to estrogen creams could cause a spayed dog to present with vaginal cornification.

SUGGESTED READING

Canine vaginal cytology (website). http://therio.vetmed.lsu.edu/k-9__vaginal_cytology.htm

AUTHOR: Carlos R. F. Pinto, MedVet, PhD, DACT
EDITORS: Leah A. Cohn, DVM, PhD, DACVIM; Mark S. Thompson, DVM, DABVP

Vaginoscopy

Difficulty level: ♦

Overview and Goal

Visual inspection of the surface of the vaginal mucosa can be accomplished through a plastic or metal speculum or is most rewarding with a fiberoptic endoscope.

Indications

- Examining the physical changes associated with hormonal events of the canine reproductive cycle
- Evaluating abnormal conditions of the caudal reproductive tract (vestibule, vagina, and caudal cervix). Common disorders of the caudal reproductive tract include vaginal septa, vaginovestibular stenosis (strictures) (p. 1027), paramesonephric septal remnants, tumors, foreign bodies, lymphoid inflammation or hyperplasia, and ectopic ureters (p. 282).
- To facilitate catheterization of the cervix for intrauterine artificial insemination (p. 1061)

Equipment, Anesthesia

Bitches in estrus tolerate vaginal procedures well; bitches in early proestrus or anestrus may need sedation or even general anesthesia, depending on the medical reasons to perform the vaginoscopy.

Equipment:

- Endoscope or speculum: size of rigid endoscope should be compatible with the size of the bitch
- Canine vaginal shunt system (best for bitches in estrus; TCI Shunt System)
- Sterile water-soluble lubricant
- Light source if not integral part of endoscope/speculum
- Swabs
- Microscope slides

Anticipated Time

5-20 minutes

Preparation: Important Checkpoints

- Apply lubricant copiously to the endoscope or speculum before introducing it.
- Position: if in estrus, most bitches remain standing during vaginoscopy, especially if transcervical insemination is the goal. In anestrous or spayed dogs, care should be taken to not traumatize the vaginal walls, especially if a rigid endoscope is being used.
- Anesthetized dogs may be positioned in lateral, ventral, or dorsal recumbency; the latter prevents inadvertent fecal contamination of the perineovulvar area.

Procedure

- After the perineum is cleansed and excessive hair clipped, the vulvar labia are separated, and the lubricated instrument is introduced at a craniodorsal angle to avoid the clitoral fossa until the vestibule and vagina are observed.
- Estrual bitches will tolerate the use of a vaginal shunt to facilitate air insufflation and distention of mid-cranial vagina.
- Areas to be inspected: urethral opening, vaginovestibular junction (cingulum), vagina, vaginal dorsal median fold that leads to the narrow cranial vagina, vaginal fornix, paracervical area, and cervical caudal os (ostium uteri externum)
- Physical changes due to circulating hormones cause dramatic changes in the appearance of the vaginal mucosa, especially during proestrus and estrus.

- Under the influence of estrogens produced by ovarian follicles, the vaginal epithelium undergoes hyperplasia and metaplasia during proestrus. The vaginal mucosa becomes edematous, swollen, and appears smooth, round, and plump.
- As the bitch advances into late proestrus and estrus, declining concentrations of serum estrogens result in a wrinkling and shrinking of the vaginal mucosal folds, progressing to a markedly angulated and crenulated outline during mid to late estrus.

Postprocedure

- Submission of samples
- Microscopic review of smears

Alternatives and Their Relative Merits

- Digital vaginal palpation: conveys the changes in texture of the vaginal mucosa and reveals vaginal strictures but is not as informative as vaginoscopy.
- Serum progesterone assay (p. 1375): often used in conjunction with vaginoscopy; the appearance of the mucosa and cornification of cells (p. 1183) indicate when to begin measuring serum progesterone. Conversely, visual inspection of the vaginal mucosa can serve to corroborate hormonal findings (luteinizing hormone and/or progesterone levels). During the fertile period in the bitch, the vaginal wall is characteristically crenulated as a result of low and high blood levels of estrogen and progesterone, respectively.

Pearls

- Vaginal procedures are best performed during proestrus and estrus.
- When not in estrus, most bitches resent vaginal exams.
- Sedation may be required for uncooperative bitches, whether in estrus or not.
- A minute amount of petroleum jelly may facilitate the introduction of the vaginoscope (and vaginal shunt whenever applicable) in a patient resenting the procedure.

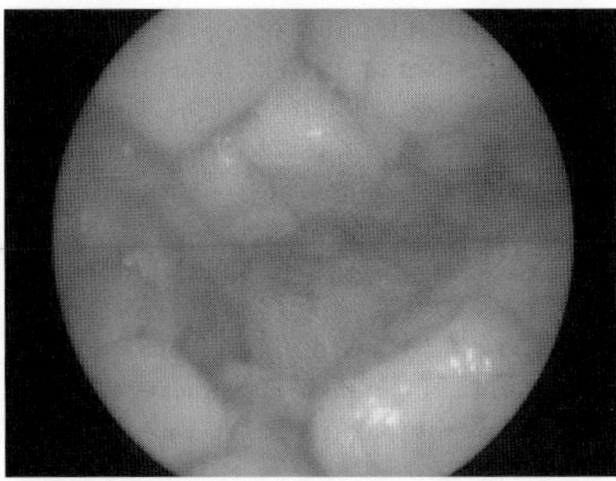

VAGINOSCOPY Endoscopic view of the canine vagina in midestrus.

SUGGESTED READING

Lévy X. Videovaginoscopy of the canine vagina. Reprod Domest Anim 51(Suppl 1):31-36, 2016.

AUTHOR: Carlos R.F. Pinto, MedVet, PhD, DACT
EDITORS: Leah A. Cohn, DVM, PhD, DACVIM; Mark S. Thompson, DVM, DABVP

Ventilation, Positive Pressure

Difficulty level: ♦♦♦

Synonyms

Artificial ventilation, assisted ventilation, mechanical ventilation, positive-pressure ventilation (PPV)

Overview and Goals

- Maintain normal arterial oxygen (PaO_2) and carbon dioxide ($PaCO_2$) pressure until an underlying disease can be identified and treated.
- Therapeutic targets (using the least aggressive ventilator settings)
  - PaO_2 > 60 mm Hg (minimum, > 80 mm Hg preferred)
  - $PaCO_2$ 35-50 mm Hg
  - End-tidal CO_2 35-50 mm Hg
  - Arterial oxygen saturation (SaO_2) > 90% (minimum, > 94% preferred)
  - Measure PaO_2 and $PaCO_2$ with arterial blood gases (ABGs); measure end-tidal CO_2 with capnometry (inserted between endotracheal tube and breathing device) and SaO_2 with pulse oximetry (attached to the tongue). The PaO_2/FIO_2 ratio is helpful in predicting prognosis and severity of the underlying disease.
- Prognosis varies with underlying disease.
  - A reasonable goal is to discharge 25%-40% of mechanically ventilated cases. Survival rates of dogs with PaO_2/FIO_2 less than 200 mm Hg at 4 and 12 hours after initiation of positive-pressure ventilation (PPV) are 15% and 6%, respectively.
  - Animals with ventilatory failure and normal lung function (e.g., opioid or barbiturate overdose, certain toxins, tick paralysis, botulism) have the best prognosis. Survival rates with respiratory failure are 20%-30%, and patients with ventilatory failure have a 50%-70% survival rate.

Indications

Early intervention carries a better prognosis.

- Ventilatory failure: $PaCO_2$ > 55 mm Hg and pH < 7.3
  - Some can be managed with short-term PPV (e.g., reversible opioid overdose).
- Respiratory failure: PaO_2 < 60 mm Hg or SaO_2 < 90% despite supplemental oxygen
  - Often requires > 12 hours of PPV
- Animals with sustained, extreme respiratory distress: increased work of breathing
  - Often requires > 12 hours of PPV

Contraindications

- Irreversible underlying disease
- Lack of trained personnel
- If > 6-12 hours of PPV is anticipated, initiating manual PPV is questionable if mechanical PPV is not available.
- Not having a 24-hour, on-site trained technician (with the animal) and veterinarian

Equipment, Anesthesia

- PPV requires intensive 24-hour monitoring and nursing care but can be lifesaving.
  - Owner communication and highly trained staff are essential.
  - Manual PPV requires a person to continually deliver manual breaths to the animal.
  - Mechanical PPV involves a machine to deliver breaths.
  - Manual PPV is practical only for short-term use (up to several hours), whereas mechanical PPV is required for long-term care (>6-12 hours).
- Intubation
  - Animals can be ventilated via inflated endotracheal or tracheostomy (p. 1166) tubes.
  - Low-pressure, high-volume cuffs are preferred.
  - Endotracheal intubation is more common (familiarity, ease of procedure, minimal risk of tissue damage).
  - If PPV exceeds 24 hours or when heavy sedation is not desired, tracheostomy may be preferred (allows some dogs to eat and drink).
- Sedation (IV, as needed; more common with concurrent endotracheal intubation); options include
  - Pentobarbital 2 mg/kg boluses to effect (up to 12 mg/kg) q 4-6h or as needed to maintain sedation
  - Fentanyl 5 mcg/kg boluses to effect up to 50 mcg/kg, then 5-7 mcg/kg/h constant-rate infusion (CRI) (can add diazepam)
  - Propofol 2-8 mg/kg bolus to effect, then 0.1-0.3 mg/kg/min CRI

- Alfaxalone 0.5 mg/kg boluses IV titrated to effect up to 3 mg/kg total dose in dogs and cats, followed by CRI (6-10 mg/kg/h) to effect. In cats, it is not recommended as a single agent IV due to the potential for rough recoveries, which may exacerbate dyspnea. Can be combined with other drugs for balanced total IV anesthesia
- Close cardiovascular monitoring is required in animals under heavy sedation.
- Minimum recommended monitoring
  - Vital signs
  - Level of consciousness
  - ABGs or pulse oximetry and end-tidal CO_2
  - Arterial blood pressure (BP) (p. 1065)
  - Continuous ECG (p. 1096)
  - Volume of fluids in and out (urinary catheter)
  - Hematocrit, total protein, glucose, and urine specific gravity
  - Ventilator settings should be recorded every hour.

Manual:

- Ambu bag and attached oxygen
  - Inexpensive
  - Readily available
  - Pediatric-sized bag most common (typically 450-950 mL volume)
  - Can be used without supplemental oxygen (not ideal)
  - Excellent for short-term use (i.e., during cardiopulmonary resuscitation [CPR])
  - Can add positive end-expiratory valves, which create positive end-expiratory pressure (PEEP) to recruit collapsed alveoli and improve oxygen exchange (typically in 0-10 cm or 0-20 cm H_2O sizes)
  - Some Ambu bags have a removable safety valve that opens when a specific airway pressure is exceeded (typically 40 cm H_2O).
  - Difficult to determine tidal volume and airway pressures delivered (vary with size and degree of manual pressure applied to the bag)
- Anesthesia machine with manual ventilation
  - Readily available
  - Estimate tidal volume delivered with the size of the reservoir bag
  - Can monitor airway pressure with attached pressure gauge
  - Can apply adjustable PEEP valves (typical range, 0-40 cm H_2O)

Mechanical:

- Anesthesia ventilators
  - Limited choice of ventilator modes
  - Typically deliver only 100% inspired oxygen concentrations (FIO_2)
  - Increased risk of oxygen toxicosis if ventilating > 12 hours
- Mechanical ventilators
  - Allow greatest control over type of breath delivered (pressure, volume, flow rate, FIO_2, respiratory rate, sensitivity to trigger a breath, and PEEP)
  - Supply humidified oxygen
  - Can be used for long-term care (days to weeks)
  - Relatively expensive

Anticipated Time

- Can take several minutes to set up mechanical ventilators.
- Initiate manual PPV (takes seconds to initiate) while mechanical ventilators are being set up.
- Duration of ventilation time varies with the underlying disease and animal's response.

Preparation: Important Checkpoints

- Ensure oxygen source, monitoring equipment, and suction devices are available.
- Nutritional support should be available for long-term cases.
- Pleural space disease (pneumothorax, pleural effusion) should be identified and treated before ventilation.
  - Thoracocentesis (p. 1164) in suspected cases; untreated pleural space disease is associated with higher incidence of ventilatory complications (p. 1102).
- Check that Ambu bag valves are functioning properly (not sticking) between uses.
- Check anesthetic machine and anesthesia ventilator, and check that mechanical ventilator tubing is correctly connected, valves are functioning, humidifiers are full, and there are no leaks in the system.

Possible Complications and Common Errors to Avoid

- Barotrauma: avoid airway pressure > 30 cm H_2O.
- Cardiovascular effects: PPV increases intrathoracic pressures, which may impede venous return and subsequently decrease cardiac output; at a minimum, monitor heart rate and BP closely.
- Oxygen toxicosis: substantial risk after 12 hours if FIO_2 remains > 60%
- Ventilator-associated pneumonia: monitor for deterioration of respiratory function or unexplained fever.
  - Confirm diagnosis with radiographs, lung ultrasound, and endotracheal wash (p. 1073).
- Pneumothorax: more common with high airway pressures (>30 cm H_2O)
  - Can cause acute deterioration in ventilatory parameters
  - Auscultation usually reveals dull breath sounds in upper parts of thorax (e.g., dorsally when animal is in sternal recumbency).
  - The absence of a glide sign with thoracic focused assessment of sonography for trauma (TFAST) strongly suggests pneumothorax (p. 1102).
  - Perform thoracocentesis in suspected cases (p. 1164).
  - Tension pneumothorax causes a severe decrease in cardiac output and hypotension; check for tension pneumothorax in ventilated animals that suddenly develop shock.
- Oral and ocular ulcers: usually avoided with good nursing care
  - Use sterile eye lubricant, and cleanse mouth with 0.1% chlorhexidine solution–soaked gauze sponges every 4 hours.

Procedure

NOTE: Step-by-step guidelines to initiate PPV are beyond the scope of this text. Clinicians should consult more extensive reviews to become familiar with different ventilator modes and their indications. The following are suggested guidelines for starting PPV. Adjust settings based on patient response. Most cases do better in sternal recumbency.

- Ambu bag
  - Bag size (in milliliters) should be at least 15 × body weight (kilograms) to deliver adequate tidal volumes.
  - Set oxygen flow rates at 10-15 L/min (delivers 50%-90% oxygen levels).
  - Attach adjustable PEEP valve to exhaust limb if PEEP desired (requires compatible attachment site). Adjust PEEP by turning valve to the desired level (start with 5 cm H_2O).
  - Higher (90%-100%) inspired oxygen levels can be achieved with an oxygen reservoir bag.
  - Animals can breathe spontaneously while connected to Ambu bags, although airway resistance is higher.
- Anesthetic machine with manual ventilation
  - Insert adjustable PEEP valve in the expiratory limb of tubing (bidirectional valves eliminate the risk of occlusion associated with backward insertion of unidirectional valves) if PEEP is desired.

Suggested initial PPV setting guidelines

- Inspired oxygen concentration (FIO_2): start with 100% FIO_2.
  - For long-term (many hours) use, decrease to the lowest FIO_2 that maintains desired PaO_2/SaO_2 to reduce the risk of oxygen toxicosis.
- Respiratory rate (RR): 8-20 breaths/min
  - Increase the RR to decrease the $PaCO_2$ if > 50 mm Hg.
  - New RR = RR × $PaCO_2$/desired $PaCO_2$
  - RR often > 20 breaths/min if underlying pulmonary disease is present
- Oxygen flow rates: start with 0.5-1 L/kg/min.
  - Often need to increase if underlying pulmonary disease is present
- Tidal volume (amount of air delivered with each breath). Normal values: 10-15 mL/kg.
  - Values of 4-6 mL/kg are associated with fewer lung injuries in people.
  - Volumes in excess of 20 mL/kg are likely to cause lung injury (barotrauma and volutrauma).
  - May need to increase tidal volume if $PaCO_2$ does not respond to increased RR

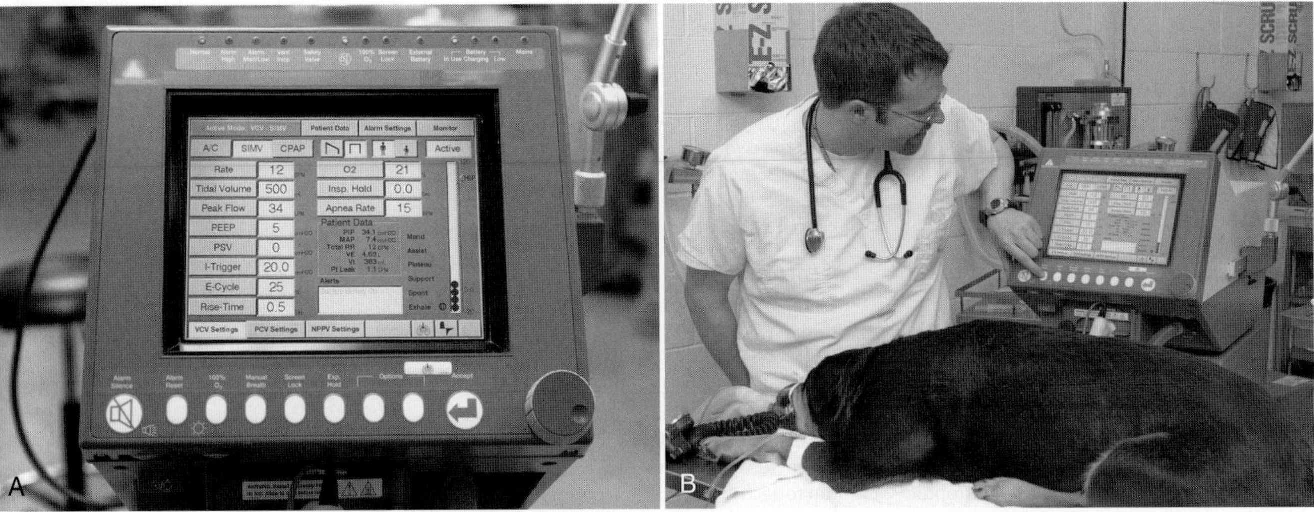

VENTILATION, POSITIVE PRESSURE A, Potential ventilator settings for a 40- to 60-kg animal. Volume-control ventilation (VCV) with synchronized intermittent mandatory ventilation (SIMV) is shown. The inspired oxygen content is 21% (room air). The peak inspiratory pressure (PIP) is high (34 cm H_2O), and efforts should be made to decrease this value by decreasing tidal volume, increasing peak flow rate, or decreasing positive end-expiratory pressure (PEEP). **B,** Ventilator in use.

 - General rule: use lowest volume possible to achieve oxygen and carbon dioxide goals.
- Airway pressure
  - Monitor if pressure gauge available
  - Normal airway pressures reach 15-20 cm H_2O.
  - Avoid values > 30 cm H_2O (likely to result in lung injury).
- Inspiratory time: normally 1.5-2.5 seconds
- Inspiratory-to-expiratory (I:E) ratio: start with values of 1 : 2-1 : 4.
  - A ratio >1 : 2 is preferred to prevent the next breath being delivered before exhalation is complete.
  - Increasing RR or tidal volume will decrease I:E ratio.
  - Increasing oxygen flow rates will increase I:E ratio.
  - Changing one parameter may require a change in another to maintain desired I:E ratio.
- PEEP
  - Healthy lungs do not require PEEP.
  - Adding PEEP to diseased lungs often improves oxygenation, prevents further alveolar collapse, and reduces ventilator-induced lung injury.
  - Often start at 3 cm H_2O.
  - If 3 cm H_2O does not achieve desired results (based on PaO_2/SaO_2), increase PEEP by 2-4 cm H_2O until desired values are achieved.
  - Exceeding 15 cm H_2O of PEEP increases the risk of lung injury and may decrease cardiac output.

Postprocedure

- Supplemental oxygen is often required after weaning from ventilation (p. 1146).
  - Oxygen supplementation should be set up before extubation (nasal oxygen is frequently used).

Alternatives and Their Relative Merits

Liquid ventilation using perfluorocarbons shows promise in managing some forms of respiratory failure in people but is cost-prohibitive.

SUGGESTED READING

Campbell VL, et al: Pulmonary function, ventilator management, and outcome of dogs with thoracic trauma and pulmonary contusions: 10 cases (1994-1998). J Am Vet Med Assoc 217(10):1505-1509, 2000.

AUTHOR: Søren R. Boysen, DVM, DACVECC
EDITORS: Leah A. Cohn, DVM, PhD, DACVIM; Mark S. Thompson, DVM, DABVP

Vertebral Heart Score Measurement

Difficulty level: ♦

Synonym

VHS

Overview and Goal

The purpose of performing a vertebral heart score (VHS) is to provide an objective measurement of the cardiac silhouette and provide a quantitative method to track the size of the cardiac silhouette over time. The goal of this procedure is to reduce errors associated with subjective assessment and interpatient variability. Although this procedure has been described using ventrodorsal and dorsoventral radiographs, lateral views are recommended because they exhibit lower measurement variability.

Indications

Any pet with possible heart disease

Contraindications

- Poor technique or positioning on thoracic radiographs
- Severe lung pathology or pleural effusion may obscure visualization of the cardiac silhouette.

Equipment, Anesthesia

- No anesthesia required. A VHS can be performed on a lateral view of any thoracic radiograph with good technique and positioning.
- The procedure requires a measurement device (i.e., ruler, calipers, piece of paper and pen, or measurement tools included with imaging software).

Anticipated Time

<1 minute

Preparation: Important Checkpoints

A lateral thoracic radiograph is required.

Possible Complications and Common Errors to Avoid

- Be careful not to include the sternopericardial ligament when measuring the long axis of the cardiac silhouette.
- Measurements should be performed on the same recumbent view for consistency, particularly when comparing measurements over time.
- A normal VHS does not rule out the presence of heart disease, particularly in cats due to the frequent occurrence of hypertrophic cardiomyopathy.
- Consider breed; there is some degree of breed-related variability in normal VHS.

Procedure

- Measure the long axis of the cardiac silhouette by drawing a line from the ventral aspect of the left mainstem bronchus to the cardiac apex.
- Measure the short axis of the cardiac silhouette by drawing a line perpendicular to the first line at the widest aspect of the heart. A common reference point for the caudal border of this line is halfway between the dorsal and ventral points of the caudal vena cava.
- Reposition the long- and short-axis measurements over the thoracic vertebrae, starting at the cranial endplate of T4.
- Measure the number of vertebrae covered by the long- and short-axis measurements, and sum the two values, rounded to the nearest 0.1 vertebra. One vertebral unit (V) is the distance from one cranial endplate to the cranial endplate of the following vertebra.

Postprocedure

- Compare the value to established reference values (8.5-10.6 V in dogs, 6.7-8.1 V in cats).
- Be cognizant of breed differences and breed-specific reference ranges. Breeds that may normally exceed 10.6 V include German shepherd dogs (up to 11.2 V), dachshunds (up to 11.6 V), Labrador retrievers and Cavalier King Charles spaniels (up to 11.7 V), and boxers (up to 12.6 V). Multiple breeds do not have an established reference range but are documented to have a higher mean VHS (greyhounds, beagles, Pomeranians, pugs, Boston terriers).

Alternatives and Their Relative Merits

- Evaluating the width of the cardiac silhouette using a guide of 2.5-3.5 rib spaces on a lateral thoracic radiograph is common and easy to perform, although it is widely influenced by breed and thoracic conformation.
- Measurement of the cardiothoracic ratio has been described using linear and area comparisons of cardiac and thoracic dimensions. Both methods vary significantly, depending on the phase of respiration, and linear measurements also vary significantly between breeds. Area measurements have been evaluated in only one breed (German shepherd dogs), and further studies are indicated.

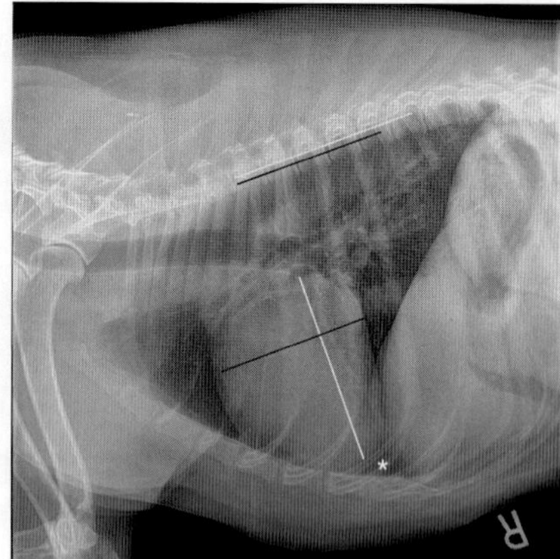

VERTEBRAL HEART SCORE A VHS is performed by measuring the long and short axis of the cardiac silhouette and transposing them over the spine, beginning at the cranial endplate of T4. This dog has a normal VHS of 10.4 V. The *asterisk* denotes the sternopericardial ligament, which should not be included in the measurement of the long axis.

AUTHOR: Lyndsay Kong, DVM
EDITORS: Leah A. Cohn, DVM, PhD, DACVIM; Mark S. Thompson, DVM, DABVP

Vomiting, Induction of

Difficulty level: ♦

Synonym

Emesis induction

Overview and Goal

Deliberate, safe induction of vomiting to reduce exposure to ingested toxicants

Indications

Suspected or confirmed ingestion of a toxin in an asymptomatic animal

Contraindications

- Do not induce vomiting in a symptomatic animal (e.g., sedated, depressed, reduced gag reflex, tremors, dyspnea, seizures) due to increased risk of aspiration. If the animal already has clinical signs of intoxication, the time frame since ingestion is too long for emesis to be beneficial.
- Do not induce vomiting after ingestion of a corrosive agent (acid, alkali, cationic detergent) due to increased risk of esophageal damage.
- Do not induce vomiting after ingestion of a hydrocarbon due to increased risk of aspiration.
- Do not induce vomiting after ingestion of sharp objects due to risk of esophageal perforation.

Equipment, Anesthesia

- Anesthesia and sedation are *contraindicated* (animal must be able to protect its airway)
- Dogs: 3% hydrogen peroxide or apomorphine
- Cats: dexmedetomidine (preferred) or xylazine

Anticipated Time

5-10 minutes

Preparation: Important Checkpoints

- If animal has not eaten recently, feed a small meal to increase emesis production.
- Monitor animal so that it does not re-ingest the vomitus.

Possible Complications and Common Errors to Avoid

- Risk of aspiration: monitor for dyspnea, coughing, lethargy, and fever after emesis. Pursue thoracic radiographs if symptomatic.
- Gastric irritation is common, but usually benign.
- Gastric ulceration/hemorrhage is rare but can be seen with excessive doses of hydrogen peroxide in the dog or after hydrogen peroxide use in the cat.
- Esophagitis: rare
- Esophageal stricture: rare, usually secondary to ingestion of a corrosive or sharp foreign body
- Use of outdated/inactive hydrogen peroxide does not cause emesis (should be bubbly).

Procedure

Calculate dose of emetic (choose one):

- 3% Hydrogen peroxide (dogs) 2.2 mL/kg PO once (maximum of 45 mL/dog), wait 10-15 minutes; if no emesis and still asymptomatic, can repeat once. Emesis occurs in 90% of dogs (median time, 14.5 minutes), *or*
- Apomorphine (dogs) 0.03 mg/kg IV, or $\frac{1}{4}$-1 tablet per dog, dissolved in sterile saline and instilled in conjunctival sac; rinse eye with saline solution after emesis. Emesis occurs in 94% of dogs (median time, 18.6 minutes), *or*
- Dexmedetomidine (cats) 0.007-0.04 mg/kg IM. Emesis occurs within 5 minutes for 92% of cats. Reverse sedative effects with atipamezole 0.4 mg/kg IM, *or*
- Xylazine (cats) 0.44 mg/kg IM. Reverse sedative effects with atipamezole 0.4 mg/kg IM or yohimbine 0.11 mg/kg IV. Less effective than dexmedetomidine
- If instructing owners to give 3% hydrogen peroxide at home, recommend that they give it into the side of the mouth (cheek pouch) to reduce the risk of aspiration. If no dosing syringes are available, a plastic or paper cup or turkey baster can be used. One teaspoon = 5 mL; 1 tablespoon = 15 mL.

Postprocedure

Check vomitus for evidence of the toxin.

- An antiemetic can be given if needed (especially if activated charcoal is to be given).
- Gastroprotectants can be started prophylactically (e.g., proton pump inhibitor such as omeprazole).

Alternatives and Their Relative Merits

- Activated charcoal (p. 1087): can be given after emesis or in place of emesis to reduce absorption of toxin. No effect on corrosives, heavy metals, or petroleum distillates
- Gastric lavage (p. 1117) can be performed in some cases when emesis is contraindicated. Use inflated endotracheal tube to protect airway.
    - No benefit over emesis in amount of ingesta returned
    - Risk of hypothermia and electrolyte abnormalities
    - Contraindicated with corrosives or petroleum distillates
- Table salt is not recommended due to risk of hypernatremia if emesis is not successful.
- Dish detergent is a poor emetic.

Pearls

Time frame during which emesis is useful will vary with the substance ingested. For example, pain or cold medications reach blood levels in 10-60 minutes, but rodenticides can stay in the stomach for up to 4 hours and chocolate for up to 12 hours.

SUGGESTED READING

Khan SA, et al: Effectiveness and adverse effects of the use of apomorphine and 3% hydrogen peroxide solution to induce emesis in dogs. J Am Vet Med Assoc 241(9):1179-1184, 2012.

AUTHOR: Tina Wismer, DVM, MS, DABVT, DABT
EDITORS: Leah A. Cohn, DVM, PhD, DACVIM; Mark S. Thompson, DVM, DABVP

Wound Care

Client Education Sheet 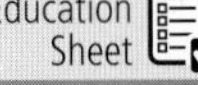

Difficulty level: ♦

Synonym

Wound management

Overview and Goal

The main tenets of wound care are to convert a contaminated wound into a clean wound that can be closed surgically or allowed to heal on its own. The desired outcome is to re-establish the epithelium at the wound site to maintain or restore function to the affected body part.

Indications

Any injury that results in a loss of continuity in the skin ± underlying tissues

Contraindications

Hemodynamically unstable patient

Equipment, Anesthesia

- Clippers
- Sterile lubricating jelly
- Surgical scrub
- Sterile surgical instruments (surgical pack or wound pack): scalpel, Metzenbaum and Mayo scissors, needle holders, hemostats, thumb forceps, drape material, towel clamps, gauze
- Sterile gloves
- Sterile flush (0.9% NaCl or lactated Ringer's solution)
- Bandage materials
- ± Suture material, laparotomy pads, splint materials
- General anesthesia recommended for most wound care
- Heavy sedation ± local anesthesia for minor wounds

Anticipated Time

20 minutes to 2 hours, depends on severity and number of wounds

Preparation: Important Checkpoints

- Discuss all aspects of wound care with owners; open wound management may take several weeks and incur large expense.
- Be prepared to handle wounds aseptically.
- Wear exam gloves to treat/handle wound patients.

Possible Complications and Common Errors to Avoid

- Infection
- Inadequate clipping and prepping of wounds
- Inappropriate closure
- Failure to cover/protect wounds/drains

Procedure

Initial wound care (stable patient) under general anesthesia (heavy sedation if minor wound):

- Apply a liberal amount of sterile lubricant into the wound. Alternatively, pack large wounds with moistened sterile gauze and temporarily close with staples or suture.
- Clip *widely* around all wounds (e.g., 5 cm around wounds on trunk, circumference of limb).
- Perform a sterile prep of skin surrounding wound(s) with chlorhexidine or Betadine scrub. Do not allow the scrub solution to contact the wound bed.
- Copiously lavage wound(s) with sterile lactated Ringer's solution or saline solution to remove gel, entrapped hair, and other debris (use caution if penetration of a body cavity or joint space is suspected).
    - Do NOT force lavage fluids into puncture wounds.
- Using sterile instruments and sterile technique, gently probe wound(s) with hemostats, looking for the extent of subcutaneous pockets and depth of wound penetration.
- Surgically debride debris and devitalized/severely damaged tissue. Leave any questionable tissues. Reassess daily and debride if nonviable.
- Obtain samples for aerobic and anaerobic culture and susceptibility (culture swab and tissue) after the wound is cleaned.

Wound closure:

- Assess for ability to close wound(s).
    - Primary closure: considered for fresh (<6 hours or minimal to no contamination)

wounds that can be adequately flushed and debrided. Wounds with questionable viability and simple puncture wounds should not be closed primarily.
  - Delayed primary closure: for wound with mild to moderate contamination or devitalization. Open wound management initially but converted to a clean wound and closed before granulation tissue has formed
  - Secondary closure: moderate to severe contamination or devitalization. Open wound management until healthy granulation bed has formed and then closed over the granulation bed
  - Wound closure options: apposition of adjacent tissues, skin flaps (rotation or pedicle), skin grafts
- Open wound management (p. 909):
  - Bandages are used to administer topical medication; keep the wound surface clean, protected, warm, and moist, and wick away excessive wound fluids/exudate.
  - Devitalized tissues should be removed as they become evident.
  - Frequency of bandage changes depends on type of bandage used.
  - Always handle open wounds in a sterile manner.
- Drain placement
  - Place a drain to close dead space, if present, and monitor effusion.
  - Closed suction drains (e.g., Jackson-Pratt for large pockets; TLS drain or homemade version using a butterfly catheter and Vacutainer for small pockets)
    - Remove when drainage < 1-2 mL/kg/day
  - Passive drains (e.g., Penrose drains) must be covered by a bandage at all times, greater risk of ascending infection
    - Remove after drainage has significantly decreased (typically 3-5 days).
  - Drains should exit at a site separate from the suture line.
  - Do not place drain directly underneath suture line because it causes increased risk of dehiscence.

Postprocedure

- Monitor for dehiscence, signs of infection, bandage slipping, bandage strikethrough (change if noted)
- Provide appropriate pain management
- Bandage changes as appropriate for type of bandage
- Antibiosis: broad spectrum initially, adjust based on culture and susceptibility if needed
- If appearance of wound changes for the worse, consider bacterial culture and susceptibility testing.

Alternatives and Their Relative Merits

- Many wound care systems are commercially available.
- Vacuum-assisted closure (VAC) (negative-pressure wound therapy) improves granulation tissue formation and provides wound drainage.

Pearls

- Clip widely around wounds.
- Handle all wounds aseptically.
- Do not close wound beds until they are healthy to maximize success.
- Scar tissue is prone to repeat injury/neoplasia. Consider flaps/grafts for more robust closure of large wounds.

SUGGESTED READING

Balsa IM, et al: Wound care. Vet Clin North Am Small Anim Pract 45:1049-1065, 2015.

AUTHOR: Elizabeth A. Swanson, DVM, MS, DACVS
EDITORS: Leah A. Cohn, DVM, PhD, DACVIM, and Mark S. Thompson, DVM, DABVP

SECTION III

Differentials, Lists, and Mnemonics

EDITORS

Leah A. Cohn
DVM, PhD, DACVIM (SAIM)

Etienne Côté
DVM, DACVIM (Cardiology, SAIM)

Abdominal Distention

Cause	Feature
Abdominal effusion	Ballotable fluid wave if voluminous; abdominal imaging; abdominocentesis
Organomegaly	Careful abdominal palpation; abdominal radiographs and/or ultrasound
Mass (neoplastic, hematoma, abscess, cyst, granuloma)	Careful abdominal palpation; abdominal radiographs and/or ultrasound
Intraabdominal lymphadenopathy	Careful abdominal palpation; palpation of superficial lymph nodes (variable association with abdominal lymphadenopathy); abdominal radiographs and/or ultrasound
Gastrointestinal tract overdistention	History (e.g., acute, persistent, nonproductive retching with gastric dilation/volvulus), abdominal radiographs
Obesity	Physical examination; other concurrent signs (panting, exercise intolerance, heat intolerance); exclusion of other Dx
Muscular weakness	Physical examination: loss of muscle mass also apparent in limbs, other signs of hyperadrenocorticism or muscle-wasting disease
Pneumoperitoneum	Abdominal radiographs
Urinary bladder distention	Abdominal palpation; radiographs or ultrasound
Pyometra/hydrometra/mucometra	Complete blood count (pyometra); abdominal ultrasound (pyometra, hydrometra, mucometra)
Pregnancy	Palpation of fetuses; radiographs or ultrasound

AUTHORS: Etienne Côté, DVM, DACVIM; Leah A. Cohn, DVM, PhD, DACVIM

Abdominal Distention: Mnemonic

The 5 F's

Fat—obesity
Fetus—pregnancy
Fluid—ascites or other effusion
Firm—organomegaly or mass effect
Flatulence—distended viscus organ (i.e., gastric dilatation, distended bladder)

Acidosis, Lactic

Type A: Hypoxic
- Increased oxygen demand
  - Intense physical exertion
  - Seizures
- Decreased oxygen availability
  - Reduced tissue perfusion
    - Cardiac arrest, cardiopulmonary cerebral resuscitation
    - Shock
    - Hypovolemia
    - Low cardiac output
    - Thromboembolic disease
  - Reduced arterial oxygen content
    - Critical hypoxemia ($PO_2 < 30$ mm Hg)
    - Extremely severe anemia (packed cell volume [PCV] < 10%)

Type B: Nonhypoxic
- Drugs and toxins
  - Phenformin
  - Salicylates
  - Ethylene glycol
  - Many others
- Diabetes mellitus
- Liver failure
- Neoplasia (e.g., lymphoma)
- Sepsis
- Uremia
- Hypoglycemia
- Hereditary defects
  - Mitochondrial myopathies
  - Defects in gluconeogenesis

Modified from DiBartola S: Fluid, electrolyte, and acid-base disorders in small animal practice, ed 4, St. Louis, 2012, Saunders.

Acidosis, Metabolic

Increased Anion Gap (Normochloremic)	Normal Anion Gap (Hyperchloremic)
Ethylene glycol intoxication	Diarrhea
Salicylate intoxication	Renal tubular acidosis
Other rare intoxications (e.g., paraldehyde, methanol)	Carbonic anhydrase inhibitors (e.g., acetazolamide)
Diabetic ketoacidosis*	Ammonium chloride
Uremic acidosis†	Cationic amino acids (e.g., lysine, arginine, histidine)
Lactic acidosis	Posthypocapnic metabolic acidosis
	Dilutional acidosis (e.g., rapid administration of 0.9% saline)
	Hypoadrenocorticism‡

*Patients with diabetic ketoacidosis may have some component of hyperchloremic metabolic acidosis in conjunction with increased anion gap acidosis.
†The metabolic acidosis early in kidney disease may be hyperchloremic and later convert to typical increased anion gap acidosis.
‡Patients with hypoadrenocorticism typically present with hypochloremia due to impaired water excretion, absence of aldosterone, impaired renal function, and lactic acidosis. These factors prevent manifestation of hyperchloremia.
From DiBartola S: Fluid, electrolyte, and acid-base disorders in small animal practice, ed 4, St. Louis, 2012, Saunders.

Acidosis, Respiratory

Airway Obstruction
- Aspiration (e.g., foreign body, vomitus)
- Mass (e.g., neoplasia, abscess)
- Collapsing trachea
- Bronchiectasis
- Asthma
- Obstructed endotracheal tube
- Brachycephalic airway syndrome
- Laryngeal paralysis/laryngospasm

Respiratory Center Depression
- Neurologic disease (e.g., brainstem, high cervical spinal cord lesion)
- Drugs (e.g., narcotics, sedatives, barbiturates, inhalation anesthetics)

Increased CO_2 Production With Impaired Alveolar Ventilation
- Cardiopulmonary arrest
- Heatstroke
- Malignant hyperthermia

Neuromuscular Defects
- Myasthenia gravis
- Tetanus
- Botulism
- Polyradiculoneuritis
- Polymyositis
- Tick paralysis
- Hypokalemic myopathy in cats
- Hypokalemic periodic paralysis in Burmese cats
- Drug-induced (neuromuscular blocking agents, aminoglycosides with anesthetics, organophosphates)

Restrictive Extrapulmonary Disorders
- Diaphragmatic hernia
- Pleural space disease
- Chest wall trauma/flail chest

Intrinsic Pulmonary and Small Airway Disease
- Acute respiratory distress syndrome
- Bronchiectasis
- Asthma
- Severe pulmonary edema
- Pulmonary thromboembolism
- Pneumonia
- Pulmonary fibrosis
- Diffuse metastatic disease
- Smoke inhalation

Inadequate Mechanical Ventilation

Marked Obesity (Pickwickian Syndrome)

From DiBartola S: Fluid, electrolyte, and acid-base disorders in small animal practice, ed 4, St. Louis, 2012, Saunders.

Acute Kidney Injury

PRERENAL/ HEMODYNAMIC
- Anesthesia
- Cardiovascular shock
- Dehydration*
- Hemorrhagic shock
- Hypoadrenocorticism*
- Hypoalbuminemia
- Hypotensive shock
- Hypovolemic shock
- Renal vascular occlusion/thrombi
- Septic shock
- Surgery
- Trauma
- Vasculitis

INTRINSIC RENAL

Infectious Disease
- Babesiosis
- Borreliosis
- Feline infectious peritonitis
- Leishmaniasis
- Leptospirosis
- Pyelonephritis
- Rickettsial infections

Nephrotoxins (Not Exhaustive)
- Allopurinol
- Aminoglycosides
- Amphotericin B
- Bisphosphonates
- Cisplatin/carboplatin
- Dextran 40
- Diuretics
- Ethylene glycol
- Grapes/raisins
- Heavy metals
- Hemoglobinuria
- Lilies (cats)
- Methotrexate
- Myoglobinuria
- Nonsteroidal antiinflammatory drugs (NSAIDs)
- Penicillamine
- Radiocontrast agents
- Venom (snake, bee)
- Vitamin D analogs

Other Conditions
- Disseminated intravascular coagulation
- Glomerulonephritis
- Heatstroke
- Hepatorenal syndrome
- Hypercalcemia
- Lymphoma
- Malignant hypertension
- Malignant hyperthermia
- Pancreatitis
- Pigmenturia (hemoglobin/myoglobin)
- Renal arterial thromboembolism
- Systemic inflammatory response syndrome
- Systemic lupus erythematosus
- Trauma
- Vasculitis

POSTRENAL
- Bilateral renal calculi
- Bilateral ureteral calculi
- Extraluminal obstruction
- Prostatic disease
- Rupture of outflow tracts
- Urethral calculi
- Urethral neoplasia

*Hypoadrenocorticism, diuretic treatment, and diabetes mellitus may cause azotemia with isosthenuria in the absence of kidney disease.
Modified from Bonagura J: Kirk's Current veterinary therapy XIII, St. Louis, 2000, Saunders.

Acute Respiratory Distress Syndrome (ARDS)

Causes, Predispositions, and Risk Factors*
- Drugs (often idiosyncratic)
- Electrocution
- Near drowning
- Neurologic insult (e.g., brain injury)
- Noxious gas inhalation (e.g., phosphine toxicosis)
- Oxygen toxicosis
- Pancreatitis
- Pneumonia (aspiration, other)
- Pulmonary contusions
- Pulmonary embolism
- Sepsis (e.g., secondary to parvoviral enteritis or other processes)
- Smoke inhalation
- Strangulation
- Stem cell transplantation
- Transfusion
- Trauma (massive)
- Upper airway obstruction (laryngeal paralysis, elongated soft palate, foreign body, mass)
- Uremia
- Vasculitis/systemic inflammatory response syndrome (SIRS) (e.g., secondary to necrotizing pancreatitis or other generalized inflammatory states)
- Venous air embolism

*Risk factors may apply to veterinary patients, human patients, or both.

Adrenal Mass/Nodule

Adrenal Cortex
- Nodular hyperplasia
- Adenoma
- Carcinoma

Adrenal Medulla
- Pheochromocytoma
- Ganglioneuroma

Extra-adrenal Masses
- Extra-adrenal pheochromocytoma (paraganglioma)

Other Adrenal Masses
- Myelolipoma
- Granulomatous disease (fungal, feline infectious peritonitis [FIP])
- Teratoma
- Adrenal cyst
- Hematoma

Metastasis
- Mammary gland tumors
- Lymphoma
- Leukemia
- Pulmonary adenocarcinoma
- Other carcinomas (prostate, bladder, gastric)

Pseudoadrenal Masses
- Arising from kidney, pancreas, lymph nodes, and blood vessels

Technical Artifacts

From Bonagura J: Kirk's Current veterinary therapy XIII, St. Louis, 2000, Saunders.

Alkalosis, Metabolic

Chloride Responsive
- Vomiting of stomach contents
- Diuretic therapy
- Post-hypercapnia

Chloride Resistant
- Primary hyperaldosteronism
- Hyperadrenocorticism

Alkali Administration
- Oral administration of sodium bicarbonate or other organic anions (e.g., lactate, citrate, gluconate, acetate)
- Oral administration of cation exchange resin with nonabsorbable alkali (e.g., phosphorus binder)

Miscellaneous
- Refeeding after fasting
- High-dose penicillin
- Severe potassium or magnesium deficiency

From DiBartola S: Fluid, electrolyte, and acid-base disorders in small animal practice, ed 4, St. Louis, 2012, Saunders.

Alkalosis, Respiratory

Hypoxemia (stimulation of peripheral chemoreceptors by decreased oxygen delivery)
- Right-to-left shunting
- Decreased PiO_2 (e.g., high altitude)
- Congestive heart failure
- Severe anemia
- Severe hypotension
- Decreased cardiac output
- Pulmonary diseases with ventilation-perfusion mismatch
  - Pneumonia
  - Pulmonary thromboembolism
  - Pulmonary fibrosis
  - Pulmonary edema
  - Acute pulmonary distress syndrome (ARDS)

Pulmonary Disease (stimulation of stretch/nociceptors independent of hypoxemia)
- Pneumonia
- Pulmonary thromboembolism
- Interstitial lung disease
- Pulmonary edema
- ARDS

Centrally Mediated Hyperventilation
- Liver disease
- Gram-negative sepsis
- Drugs: salicylate intoxication, progesterone (pregnancy), xanthines (e.g., aminophylline)
- Recovery from metabolic acidosis
- Central neurologic disease
  - Trauma
  - Neoplasia
  - Infection
  - Inflammation
  - Cerebrovascular accident
- Exercise
- Heatstroke

Muscle Metaboreceptor Overactivity
- Congestive heart failure

Overzealous Mechanical Ventilation

Situations Causing Pain, Fear, or Anxiety

From DiBartola S: Fluid, electrolyte, and acid-base disorders in small animal practice, ed 4, St. Louis, 2012, Saunders.

Alopecia, Canine Symmetrical

Disorders Causing Symmetrical Alopecia in Dogs

Disorders	Signs Apart From Alopecia	Common Clinicopathologic Abnormalities	Diagnostic Tests
Alopecia X	Skin hyperpigmentation, hair regrowth at the biopsy site	None	Signalment, rule out other causes, skin biopsies (large number of flame follicles suggestive)
Anagen defluxion	Related to severe systemic disease or to cytotoxic therapy	Related to the underlying disorder	History, trichogram
Breed-specific follicular dysplasia	Secondary pyoderma	None	Signalment, trichogram, skin biopsy
Canine recurrent flank alopecia	None	None	Signalment, history, skin biopsy
Color dilution alopecia	Comedones, secondary pyoderma	None	Signalment, trichogram, skin biopsy
Congenital alopecia	Anomalies of dentition	None	Signalment, skin biopsy

Continued

(Continued from previous page)

Disorders Causing Symmetrical Alopecia in Dogs—cont'd

Disorders	Signs Apart From Alopecia	Common Clinicopathologic Abnormalities	Diagnostic Tests
Hyperadrenocorticism	Atrophic skin, calcinosis cutis, comedones, prominent cutaneous blood vessels, phlebectasia PU/PD, polyphagia, panting, pot belly, muscle atrophy, lethargy, testicular atrophy, abnormal estrus	Stress leukogram, increased serum alkaline phosphatase, hypercholesterolemia, hyposthenuria, urinary tract infection	History, physical findings, ACTH stimulation test, low-dose dexamethasone suppression test, high-dose dexamethasone suppression test, ultrasonography, urine cortisol/creatinine ratio
Hyperestrogenism	Skin hyperpigmentation, linear preputial dermatosis Enlarged vulva, gynecomastia Abnormal estrus, abnormal sexual behavior	Bone marrow suppression	Signalment (often older cryptorchid male or intact female), physical findings, ultrasonography/radiography, histopathology (gonads)
Hypothyroidism	Dull haircoat, scaling, myxedema, lethargy, obesity Rat tail appearance common	Hypercholesterolemia, mild nonregenerative anemia	Total T_4, free T_4, TSH, (+/– TgAA, TSH stimulation test with hrTSH)
Pattern alopecia	None	None	Signalment, skin biopsy
Pituitary dwarfism	Skin hyperpigmentation, secondary pyoderma Proportionate dwarfism, clinical signs of hypothyroidism (if concomitant TSH deficiency), hypogonadism (if concomitant LH and FSH deficiency)	None	Signalment, physical findings, basal and poststimulation GH measurement, total T_4 or free T_4
Sebaceous adenitis	Scaling, follicular casts	None	Skin biopsy, trichogram
Telogen effluvium	Only if systemic disease or physiologic stress is present	None	History, trichogram, skin biopsy

ACTH, Adrenocorticotropic hormone; *FSH,* follicle stimulating hormone; *GH,* growth hormone; *hrTSH,* human recombinant thyroid stimulating hormone; *LH,* luteinizing hormone; *PU/PD,* polyuria/polydipsia; *T_4,* thyroxine; *TgAA,* antithyroglobulin antibodies; *TSH,* thyroid stimulating hormone.
Reproduced from the third edition in unabridged form.

THIRD EDITION AUTHOR: Manon Paradis, DMV, MVSc, DACVD

American Society of Anesthesiologists Classification System

American Society of Anesthesiologists: Classification System for Physical Status and Recommended Tests for Each Class

Physical Status	Definition	Examples	RECOMMENDED LABORATORY TESTS: Minor*	Major†	Prognosis
I	Healthy with no organic disease	Elective procedures, not necessary for health (e.g., ovariohysterectomy)	PCV, TP, urine specific gravity	CBC, U/A, surgical panel‡	Excellent
II	Local disease with no systemic signs	Healthy nonelective surgery (e.g., skin laceration, simple fracture)	PCV, TP, urine specific gravity	CBC, U/A, surgical panel‡	Good
III	Disease causes moderate systemic signs that limit function	Heart murmur, anemia, pneumonia, mild chest trauma, moderate dehydration	CBC, U/A, surgical panel‡	CBC, U/A, biochemical panel§	Fair
IV	Disease causes severe systemic signs that threaten life	Gastric torsion, diaphragmatic hernia, severe chest trauma, severe anemia or dehydration	CBC, U/A, biochemical panel§	CBC, U/A, biochemical panel§	Guarded
V	Moribund, not expected to live for more than 24 hours with or without surgery	Endotoxic shock, severe trauma, multiorgan failure	CBC, U/A, biochemical panel§	CBC, U/A, biochemical panel§	Grave
E	Emergency	Qualifier of above classes	PCV, TP, urine specific gravity	Depends on facilities available	Variable

*Minor is duration less than 60 minutes.
†Major is duration longer than 60 minutes or concerns patients older than 7 years.
‡Surgical panel: urea, creatinine, alkaline phosphatase, alanine aminotransferase, glucose, sodium, potassium, chloride, total protein.
§Biochemical panel: full panel includes surgical panel tests plus bicarbonate, anion gap, calcium, phosphorus, cholesterol, total bilirubin, gamma-glutamyltransferase, and albumin.
CBC, Complete blood cell count; *PCV,* packed cell volume; *TP,* total protein; *U/A,* urinalysis.
From Tobias KM, Johnson SA: Veterinary surgery: small animal, St. Louis, 2012, Saunders; Slatter D: Textbook of small animal surgery, ed 3, Philadelphia, 2003, Saunders.

Amyloidosis

Diseases Reported in Association With Amyloidosis in Dogs

INFECTIOUS
- **Bacterial**
  - Pyelonephritis
  - Pyometra
  - Pyoderma
  - Other chronic bacterial infections
- **Protozoal**
  - Hepatozoonosis
  - Leishmaniasis
- **Parasitic**
  - Dirofilariasis
- **Fungal**
  - Blastomycosis
  - Coccidioidomycosis

INFLAMMATORY
- Dermatitis, chronic
- Dermatomyositis
- Inflammatory bowel disease
- Pancreatitis
- Periodontal disease
- Polyarthritis
- Systemic lupus erythematosus

NEOPLASTIC
- Lymphoma
- Myeloma
- Other neoplasms

MISCELLANEOUS
- Hyperlipidemia (?)
- Congenital C3 deficiency (MPGN)
- Chronic insulin infusion
- Cyclic hematopoiesis in gray collies

FAMILIAL
- Shar-pei dog
- Abyssinian cat
- Siamese cat

IDIOPATHIC

Modified from Ettinger S, Feldman E: Textbook of veterinary internal medicine, ed 7, St. Louis, 2010, Saunders.

Anemia, Immune-Mediated

Examples of Underlying Disorders and Triggers

Infectious
- Bacterial: bartonellosis, ehrlichiosis, anaplasmosis, salmonellosis, feline hemotropic mycoplasmosis, various acute and chronic infections (e.g., abscess, pyometra, discospondylitis)
- Parasitic: babesiosis, dirofilariasis, *Trichuris vulpis* infection, *Ancylostoma caninum*, bee stings

Drugs/Toxins
- Levamisole
- Cephalosporins
- Carprofen
- Vaccines
- Propylthiouracil (cats)
- Methimazole (cats)
- Griseofulvin
- Bee-sting envenomation

Neoplasia
- Hemolymphatic: leukemias, lymphoma, multiple myeloma
- Soft-tissue sarcoma, bronchoalveolar carcinoma, mast cell tumor, splenic hemangioma

Inflammatory Disorders
- SLE
- Prostatitis/cystitis
- Pancreatitis

Genetic Predisposition
- American cocker spaniel (one-third of all cases)
- English springer spaniel
- Old English sheepdog
- Irish setter
- Poodle
- Dachshund

SLE, Systemic lupus erythematosus.
Modified from Ettinger S, Feldman E: Textbook of veterinary internal medicine, ed 7, St. Louis, 2010, Saunders.

Anemia: Causes

Hemorrhage

Surgery/Trauma

Bleeding Disorder

- von Willebrand disease/thrombopathia
- Thrombocytopenia
- Factor deficiency (hemophilia, liver failure)
  - DIC

Ectoparasitosis (Fleas, Ticks, Lice)

Gastrointestinal Bleeding

- Hookworms
- Peptic ulcer
- GI neoplasia
- Heatstroke

Renal Bleeding

- Primary renal hematuria
- Renal telangiectasia
- Sterile hemorrhagic cystitis

Epistaxis

Neoplasia (Hemangiosarcoma)

Hemolysis

Antibody-Mediated

- Primary immune-mediated hemolytic anemia
- Secondary immune-mediated hemolytic anemia
- Neonatal isoerythrolysis
- Transfusion reaction

Congenital

- Phosphofructokinase deficiency (English springer spaniels, American cocker spaniel)
- Familial nonspherocytic, hemolytic anemia (poodles)
- Elliptocytosis (one crossbred dog)
- NADH methemoglobin reductase deficiency (several breeds of dogs)
- Hemolytic anemia secondary to RBC membrane defect (beagles)
- Pyruvate kinase deficiency (beagles, basenjis, West Highland white terriers, giant schnauzers, Abyssinians)
- Vitamin B_{12} deficiency (giant schnauzers)
- Predisposition to oxidant injury, high erythrocyte potassium and low glutathione levels (Akitas, shiba inus)

Toxin/Drug-Induced

- Propylthiouracil
- Lead
- DL-methionine
- Cephalosporins
- Fenbendazole
- Dapsone
- Gold salts
- MLV vaccines
- Oxidants
- Onions
- Acetaminophen
- Methylene blue
- Phenacetin
- Propylene glycol
- Phenol compounds (mothballs)
- Benzocaine
- Hydroxyurea
- Vitamin K_3

RBC Parasites

- Hematoprotozoal *Mycoplasma* spp
- Cytauxzoonosis
- Babesiosis

Microangiopathic

- Splenic torsion
- Cava syndrome
- Hemangiosarcoma
- Vasculitis
- DIC

Decreased Production

Bone Marrow Disorder

- Hematopoietic malignancy
- Myelofibrosis
- Idiopathic aplastic anemia
- Irradiation
- Aplastic anemia
- Pure red cell aplasia
- Immune-mediated RBC precursor destruction
- Myelodysplasia

Infectious Disease

- *Ehrlichia canis*
- Feline leukemia virus
- Histoplasmosis
- Parvovirus/panleukopenia

Systemic Disease

- Anemia of chronic disease/inflammation
- Chronic kidney disease
- Liver disease
- Endocrine disease (hypothyroidism, hypoadrenocorticism)
- Neoplasia

Toxin/Drug

- Estrogen
- Chemotherapy
- Azathioprine
- Phenylbutazone
- Fenbendazole
- TMS
- Phenobarbital
- Griseofulvin
- Quinidine
- Thiacetarsamide
- NSAIDs
- Skunk musk
- Others

Nutritional

- Mineral deficiency (iron)
- Vitamin deficiency (B complex)
- Inadequate protein intake

DIC, Disseminated intravascular coagulation; *GI,* gastrointestinal; *IHA,* immune-mediated hemolytic anemia; *MLV,* modified live virus; *NSAIDs,* nonsteroidal antiinflammatory drugs; *RBC,* red blood cell; *TMS,* trimethoprim/sulfadiazine.

Modified from Bonagura J: Kirk's Current veterinary therapy XII: small animal practice, ed 12, St. Louis, 1995, Saunders, p 448.

Anorexia

Cause	Salient Characteristic
Primary Anorexia	Disinterested in eating; rare; primary disease of the appetite and/or satiety centers
Secondary Anorexia caused by various systemic diseases (virtually any), including metabolic, endocrine, infectious, inflammatory, and neoplastic	Disinterested in eating; common; many causes will be identified with a thorough history, complete physical exam, and minimum laboratory database (complete blood count, biochemistry panel, urinalysis)
Secondary Anorexia Associated With Nausea	Vomiting, lip licking, drooling often seen; food avoidance common (may push food away in cage)
Gastrointestinal (GI) inflammatory disease	Other GI signs usually present, including vomiting, diarrhea
Ileus	Radiographs may be suggestive; abdominal ultrasound to verify lack of motility; may be localized or diffuse, adynamic/paralytic, or obstructive
Delayed gastric emptying	Vomiting of food hours after ingestion; radiographs confirm the retention of food/fluid in the stomach > 8 hours; contrast studies, ultrasonography, and/or endoscopy to identify cause
Vestibular disease	Head tilt, nystagmus, circling, vestibular ataxia
Medication adverse effect	Many drugs; review medication history, especially regarding antibiotics, NSAIDs, and chemotherapeutics
Food aversion	Important in cats; typically associated with episode of pain, vomiting, or nausea
Pseudoanorexia (reluctance to eat)	Interested in eating but difficult/painful to prehend/masticate/swallow; initial interest when food provided; complete oral exam may require sedation/anesthesia
Retrobulbar (apical tooth root) abscess	Acute unilateral facial swelling; pain on opening mouth; dental exam and radiographs
Intraoral masses/foreign bodies	Halitosis; oral/facial swelling possible; sedation/anesthesia may be necessary for complete oral exam
Mandibular fractures/temporomandibular joint disease	History of trauma; careful palpation (pain, crepitus); radiographic or CT examination
Masticatory myositis	Difficulty/inability to open mouth; acute (painful muscle swelling) or chronic (muscle atrophy); high 2M fiber serum antibody titer; temporal/masseter muscle biopsy
Periodontal disease, gingivostomatitis	Oral examination; symmetrical inflammation of the caudal oropharynx differentiates caudal stomatitis from periodontal disease
Salivary gland disorders (e.g., mucocele, neoplasia)	Paracentesis of lesion reveals a stringy, sometimes blood-tinged fluid with low cell numbers consistent with a mucocele (often young dogs); neoplasia is uncommon
Oropharyngeal dysphagia	Oral dysphagia: difficulty prehending food, food may be dropped. Pharyngeal dysphagia: normal prehension with repeated attempts at swallowing, flexion/extension of the neck; thorough oral exam, neck radiographs, fluoroscopy, +/– contrast study
Esophageal disease (masses, foreign bodies)	Ptyalism; regurgitation; odynophagia (repeated, painful attempts at swallowing); radiographs +/– esophagoscopy
Nasal disease	Sense of smell impacts willingness to eat (cats especially); nasal congestion/obstruction/discharge on physical exam
Behavioral	Thorough history; anxiety disorders; social conflict (e.g., dominance aggression); emotional stress (e.g., loss of companion); rule out medical conditions first

CT, Computed tomography; *NSAIDs,* nonsteroidal antiinflammatory drugs.
Reproduced from the third edition in modified form.

THIRD EDITION AUTHOR: **Julio Lopez, DVM, DACVIM**

Anorexia: Tips for Coax Feeding

- Minimize stress at mealtimes.
- Approximate the patient's routine feeding management as much as possible.
- Control nausea, including the use of antemetic drugs.
- Recognize the signs of food aversion and modify/temporarily suspend active feeding accordingly.
- Choose complete and balanced, energy-dense foods that are appropriate for the patient's medical condition.
- When medically appropriate, choose foods the patient is familiar with.
- Warm the food slightly.
- Offer modest portions of fresh foods frequently.
- Offer one food item at a time.
- Attempt both hand feeding and leaving food with pet for short periods.
- Do not leave food with the patient for extended periods of time.
- Try novel foods if the patient seems averse to his/her typical diet.
- Offer various textures/consistencies of food.
- If pet foods are not accepted, may try enticing human foods (e.g., meat-based baby foods, canned tuna).
- Give clear feeding instructions that include the specific diet to be fed, portion size, and meal frequency.
- Appetite stimulant drugs (e.g., capromorelin, mirtazapine) may be useful.

Modified from the third edition.

THIRD EDITION AUTHOR: **Kathryn E. Michel, DVM, MS, DACVN**

Antidotes and Reversal Agents

Antidotes can be divided into four broad categories: chemical (C), receptor (R), dispositional (D), and functional (F). The category may change, depending on the usage. Chemical antidotes act directly on the toxicant to make it less toxic and/or to increase excretion. Receptor antidotes prevent the toxin from binding to the receptor site (can bind directly or change the conformation of the receptor, preventing binding). Dispositional antidotes reduce the amount of toxin available to tissues by altering absorption, metabolism, distribution, or excretion of the toxicant. Functional antidotes act on the symptoms caused by the toxicant.

Reversal Agent/Antidote	Toxicant/Main Indication	Dose	Comment(s)
2-PAM (Pralidoxime)	OP toxicosis (nicotinic signs)	20 mg/kg IM or slow IV, q 8h	C; most beneficial within 24 hours of exposure, may still be useful beyond this time; discontinue after 3 doses if no benefit
Activated charcoal	Most organic compounds	1-2 g/kg PO	D; does not bind alcohols, heavy metals, nitrates, chlorates
Antivenins	Pit vipers, coral snakes, etc.	See product insert for directions	C; multiple products available
Atipamezole (Antisedan)	Amitraz, brimonidine, clonidine, detomidine, dexmedetomidine, imidazoline decongestants, medetomidine, tizanidine, xylazine	50-200 mcg/kg IM or IV	R; preferred over yohimbine due to longer duration of effect
Atropine sulfate	OPs and carbamate toxicosis (muscarinic signs); muscarinic mushrooms	0.02-0.04 mg/kg IV or IM (mushrooms); 0.1-0.05 mg/kg, ¼ dose IV with remainder IM or SQ (cholinergic toxicosis)	R; avoid atropinization (hyperthermia, tachycardia, mydriasis)
BAL (British anti-Lewisite; dimercaprol)	Lead, arsenic, inorganic mercury, gold, copper	3-6 mg/kg IM q 6-8h	C; nephrotoxic; injection can be irritating and painful; helps remove lead from CNS
Calcium disodium EDTA (Calcium disodium versenate)	Lead, zinc, cadmium, iron, copper, nickel, chromium, manganese	Dog: 100 mg/kg SQ q 24h for 2-5 days (divide dose into 4 portions and dilute to 10 mg CaEDTA/mL with 5% dextrose) Cat: 27.5 mg/kg SQ q 6h for 5 days (dilute in 15 mL 5% dextrose)	C; nephrotoxic; painful injections; do not use if metal still present in GI tract
Cholestyramine	Cholecalciferol, naproxen	300 mg/kg PO q 8h for 2-4 days	D; binds to bile acids needed for enterohepatic recirculation of some toxins
Cyproheptadine (Periactin)	Serotonin syndrome	Dogs: 1.1 mg/kg PO or rectally q 6h for a max of 2 doses Cats: 2-4 mg (total) PO or rectally q 6h for a max of 2 doses	R; appetite stimulant in cats
Dantrolene	Hops (dogs)	1-15 mg/kg PO q 8-12h; 1 mg/kg IV	F; reverses the malignant hyperthermia-like reaction
Deferoxamine (Desferal)	Iron	40 mg/kg IM q 4-8h	C; most effective in first 24 hours; urine may turn wine color (vin rose) during chelation
Digoxin immune Fab (Digibind)	Digitalis, cardiac glycoside plants, toad toxins	Start with 1-2 vials IV over 30 minutes and increase as needed	C; expensive but rapid acting and efficacious
D-penicillamine (Cuprimine)	Lead, copper, iron, mercury, zinc, cobalt, manganese	Dog: 110 mg/kg/d PO divided q 6-8h for 1-2 weeks Cat: 125 mg (total) q 12h PO for 5 days	C; do not use when metal is still present in the GI tract; vomiting is common; nephrotoxic
Ethanol	Ethylene glycol	CRI dosing: 7% ethanol; loading dose of 8.6 mL/kg, then 1.43 mL/kg/h Bolus dosing: 20% ethanol; Dog: 5.5 mL/kg IV q 4h for 5 treatments, then q 6h for 4 treatments Cats: 5 mL/kg IV q 6h for 5 treatments, then q 8h for 4 treatments	D; proof is double the percentage of alcohol
Flumazenil (Romazicon)	Benzodiazepines	0.01 mg/kg IV	R; reverses severe CNS depression; short half-life; repeat in 1-3 hours if needed
Folinic acid (Leucovorin)	Methotrexate, trimethoprim, pyrimethamine, *Gyromitra* mushrooms (false morels)	If known quantity of methotrexate, give on a mg-to-mg basis (1 : 1); if unknown, 25-250 mg/m^2 q 6h IV, IM for up to 72 hours	F; folinic acid is active form of folic acid
Fomepizole (4-methylpyrazole; 4-MP)	Ethylene glycol	Dogs: 20 mg/kg slow IV over 15-30 minutes, 15 mg/kg at 12 hours and 24 hours, 5 mg/kg at 36 hours Cats: 125 mg/kg slow IV, 31.25 mg/kg at 12, 24, 36 hours	D; must be compounded; no longer commercially produced

(Continued from previous page)

Reversal Agent/Antidote	Toxicant/Main Indication	Dose	Comment(s)
Lipid emulsion 20%	Fat soluble toxicants	1.5 mL/kg bolus, then 0.25 mL/kg/min for 30-60 minutes	D; check for lipemia in 4 hours; if none, can repeat (p. 1127)
Methocarbamol (Robaxin)	Permethrin, bifenthrin, metaldehyde, tremorgenic mycotoxin, serotonergic medications (tremors)	50-150 mg/kg PO or IV	F; not an anticonvulsant; can be given rectally if needed
N-acetylcysteine (Mucomyst)	Acetaminophen/paracetamol, *Amanita* mushrooms, xylitol, sago palm	140 mg/kg IV or PO, then 70 mg/kg q 6h for 7+ treatments	C, D; comes as 10% and 20% solutions; dilute to 5% before administration
Naloxone (Narcan)	Opioids/opiates	0.04-0.1 mg/kg IV	R; reverse respiratory/CNS depression; short half-life; repeat in 1-3 hours if needed
Pamidronate (Aredia)	Cholecalciferol, calcipotriene; calcitriol	1.2-2 mg/kg diluted in 250 mL 0.95 NaCl, administer over 2 hours	F; inhibits osteoclastic bone resorption; treats hypercalcemia
Physostigmine	Atropine and other anticholinergics; ivermectin, antihistamines	1 mg (total) IV q 12h	F; short duration of action (30-60 minutes), repeated dosing can cause seizures
Protamine	Heparin	1-1.5 mg for each mg (100 U) of heparin, slow IV; reduce dose by $\frac{1}{2}$ for each 30 minutes that has passed	C; rapid neutralization of heparin; too rapid administration causes hypotension, anaphylactoid-like reaction
Pyridoxine (vitamin B_6)	Isoniazid toxicosis in dogs; *Gyromitra* mushrooms (false morels)	If known quantity of isoniazid, give on a mg-to-mg basis (1 : 1); if unknown, start at 71 mg/kg at a 5%-10% IV infusion over 30-60 minutes	F, D; potential adjunct therapy for ethylene glycol toxicosis
S-adenosylmethionine (SAMe; Denosyl)	Hepatotoxic agents (acetaminophen, *Amanita* mushrooms, xylitol, sago palm)	18 mg/kg q 24h	F; protects against oxidative stress
Succimer (2-3-dimercaptosuccinic acid; Chemet)	Lead, arsenic, mercury	10 mg/kg PO q 8h for 5 days (cats) or 10 days (dogs)	C; less nephrotoxic than other lead chelators; can be used when ingested lead is still present in the GI tract
Vitamin K_1 (phytonadione)	Anticoagulants (warfarin, brodifacoum, bromadiolone), sulfaquinoxaline	2.5-5 mg/kg PO, IM, SQ divided	F; IV use can cause allergic reaction; better absorption with fatty food
Yohimbine (Yobine)	Amitraz, brimonidine, clonidine, detomidine, dexmedetomidine, imidazoline decongestants, medetomidine, tizanidine, xylazine	0.11 mg/kg IV	R; shorter half-life and less specific than atipamezole

Note: The unit of measure of micron, sometimes denoted by the Greek letter μ, is abbreviated in this text by mc. For example, 1 mcL = 1 microliter; 1 mcg = 1 microgram.
CNS, Central nervous system; *GI*, gastrointestinal; *OP*, organophosphate.

AUTHOR: **Tina Wismer, DVM, DABVT, DABT, MS**

Ataxia

Differential Diagnosis Item	Key Feature(s)
Intervertebral disc extrusion	Commonly acute and focally painful at the site (patients commonly show abdominal tensing with spinal palpation)
Fibrocartilaginous embolism	Peracute onset; usually occurs during exercise; asymmetrical; not progressive or painful after 24 hours; micturition problems common; Horner's syndrome ipsilaterally with cervical lesions
Degenerative myelopathy	Insidious onset, slow progression; mildly asymmetrical; nonpainful; may cause patellar reflex deficit
Cervical spondylomyelopathy/"wobbler syndrome"	Acute or chronic; short, stiff thoracic limb strides and long ataxic pelvic limb strides; variable hyperesthesia
Myelitis	Focal or multifocal signs; typically acute and rapidly progressive over days
Syringomyelia	Cervical scoliosis common; often asymmetrical; focal or multifocal; phantom scratching and cervical hyperesthesia common
Neoplasia	Often insidious and progressive; variable hyperesthesia
Vestibular	Usually accompanied by heat tilt and nystagmus; maybe central or peripheral vestibular disorder
Cerebellar	Hypermetric gait; intention tremors common

Reproduced from the third edition in modified form.

THIRD EDITION AUTHOR: **Greg Kilburn, DVM, DACVIM**

Back Pain

Differential Diagnoses	Key Feature(s)
Intervertebral disc disease (IVDD)	Variable degree of pain on palpation, often accompanied by proprioceptive deficits, ataxia, paresis, or paralysis
Acute noncompressive nucleus pulposus extrusion (ANNPE, Type III IVDD)	Acute or peracute onset; variable degrees of pain on palpation, proprioceptive deficits, ataxia, paresis, or paralysis
Vertebral fracture/luxation	History or suspicion of trauma warrants early screening, spinal radiographs, but treat life-threatening injuries first; neurologic status important for prognosis
Meningitis/meningomyelitis	Often multifocal neurologic localization; may include signs of encephalitis
Discospondylitis/vertebral osteomyelitis	Usually progressive over days to weeks; fever may accompany pain without radiographic changes early in the course of disease
Neoplasia	Most often chronic but may be acute presentation; primary or metastatic; spinal pain more common with vertebral origin than meningeal or nerve parenchymal tumors
Ischemic myelopathy	Acute but transient pain, resolving within hours; neurologic deficits may be asymmetrical; lower motor neuron deficits associated with poorer prognosis
Orthopedic spinal pain	Spondylosis deformans, articular facet degenerative joint disease, psoas muscle injury (lumbar)
Pain not localized to spinal column	Aortic thromboembolism (cats), abdominal pain may mimic spinal pain, kidney pain, polyarthritis (multiple joint effusion and pain), polymyopathy (diffuse muscle pain)

AUTHOR: Peter Moak, DVM

Bleeding Disorders: Expected Findings

Disorder	Clinical Picture		Plt#	BMBT	PT	aPTT	D-dimer, FDP
Primary	Petechiae, ecchymosis, hyphema, epistaxis, GI bleeding	Thrombocytopenia	↓	↑	N	N	N
		Thrombocytopathy	N to ↓	↑	N	N	N
Secondary	Spontaneous bleeding, hematoma, intracavitary bleeding, ecchymosis, hemarthrosis	Vitamin K antagonism, deficiency*	N to ↓	N	↑	↑	N to ↑
		Failure of hepatic synthesis	N	N	↑	↑	N to mild ↑
		Hemophilia A and B (factor VIII, IX deficiency)	N	N	N	↑	N
		Factor XII deficiency†	N	N	N	↑	N
Other	Any type of bleeding	DIC	↓	↑	↑	↑	↑
	Bleeding following trauma‡	von Willebrand disease	N	↑	N	N to mild ↑	N
	Bruising, oozing at wound site (often delayed 24-48 h)	Early fibrinolysis	N	N	N	N	↑

BMBT, Buccal mucosal bleeding time; *DIC,* disseminated intravascular coagulation; *FDP,* fibrin/fibrinogen degradation products; *N,* normal; *plt#,* platelet count.
*PT prolonged before aPTT.
†Does not cause bleeding, but can cause confusion when detected incidentally (e.g., investigation of cholestatic disease).
‡Types 2 and 3, or severe type 1, can cause spontaneous hemorrhage.

Bleeding Disorders: Primary versus Secondary

Primary Hemostatic Defect	Secondary Hemostatic Defect
Petechiae common	Petechiae rare
Hematomas rare	Hematomas common
Bleeding at mucosal membranes, bleeding from multiple sites	Bleeding into muscles, joints, and body cavities
Bleeding immediately after venipuncture	Delayed bleeding after venipuncture
Mechanism: failure of platelet plug formation	Mechanism: platelet plug forms, but there is failure of platelet plug stabilization by coagulation factors
Examples: immune-mediated thrombocytopenia, aspirin therapy, von Willebrand disease	Examples: anticoagulant rodenticide intoxication, coagulopathy of hepatic insufficiency, hemophilias

From Bonagura J: Kirk's Current veterinary therapy XII: small animal practice, St. Louis, 1995, Saunders, p 459.

Blood Type Frequencies, Cats

Breed	% Type A*	% Type B*
Abyssinian	84-100	0-16
Birman	82-100	0-18
British shorthair	64	36
Burmese	93-100	0-3
Chartreux	77	18
Cornish rex	66-100	0-33
Devon rex	59	41
Exotic shorthair	73	27
Himalayan	94	6
Japanese bobtail	84	16
Maine coon	97	3
Norwegian forest cat	93	7
Oriental shorthair	100	0
Persian	86	14
Ragdoll	77-80	5-20
Russian blue	80	20
Scottish fold	81	19
Siamese	100	0
Somali	71-82	18-24
Sphinx	83	17
Tonkinese	100	0
Turkish Angora	54	46
Turkish Van	40-42	57-60

Geographic Location†	% Type A*	% Type B*
Australia	62-74	26-36
Austria	88-97	3-12
Argentina	97	3
Brazil	95	3
Finland	100	0
France	85	15
Italy	89-91	7-11
Germany	94-99	1-6
Greece	78	20
Hungary	100	0
Portugal	80-90	4-7
Netherlands	96	4
Scotland	97	3
Switzerland	99	0.4
Turkey	73	25
United Kingdom/England	54-97	3-40
USA—Northeast	99	<1
USA—North central	99	<1
USA—Southeast	99	1.5
USA—Southwest	98	2.5
USA—West Coast	95	5

*Percentages given as range based on one to several studies; % type AB not included.

†Geographical proportions affected by breeds included at location (e.g., British shorthair have high proportion of B type blood, impacting geographic distribution in some studies from the United Kingdom).

Differentials, Lists, and Mnemonics

Blood Type Groups, Dogs

Dog Erythrocyte Antigen (DEA) Systems and Blood Types

Antigen	Estimated Population Prevalence	Comment
DEA 1.1	62%	DEA 1.x antigens are most associated with ITR
DEA 1.2	2%	
DEA 1.3	0.1%	
DEA 3	5%	Most likely in greyhounds and Japanese-bred dogs
DEA 4	98%	ITR to antigen extremely rare due to high prevalence
DEA 5	15%	Most likely in greyhounds and Japanese-bred dogs
DEA 6	96%	No commercial typing system for recognition
DEA 7	40%-55%	Can be found unassociated with RBC
DEA 8	20%-40%	No commercial typing system for recognition
Dal	98%	Lack of Dal in Dalmatians (11.7%), shih tzus (57.1%), and Doberman pinschers (42.4%) increases risk of transfusion reaction in these breeds

ITR, Immunologic transfusion reaction; *RBC*, red blood cell.

Bone Diseases, Congenital

Congenital Skeletal Disorders of Small Animals

Generalized Bone Malformations

- Osteopetrosis—dense bones
- Osteogenesis imperfecta—osteopenia and bone fragility
- Mucopolysaccharidosis—lysosomal enzyme defects
- Dwarfism—osteochondrodysplasias (Scottish fold) and pituitary
- Congenital hypothyroidism
- Retained cartilage cores
- Craniomandibular osteopathy
- Multiple cartilaginous exostoses
- Avascular necrosis of the femoral head

Malformations of Individual Bones

- Hemimelia—radial or tibial agenesis
- Congenital amputation—absence of distal limb portion
- Phocomelia—missing segment of limb
- Amelia—absence of complete limb

Malformations of Bone Combinations

- Syndactyly—fused digits
- Polydactyly—extra digits
- Ectrodactyly—split or lobster claw deformity

Adapted from Ettinger S, Feldman E: Textbook of veterinary internal medicine, ed 6, St. Louis, 2005, Saunders, p 1970.

Bradycardia

Causes of Bradycardia in Dogs and Cats

A. **Arrhythmias**
  1. Second-degree AV block
  2. Third-degree AV block
  3. Sick sinus syndrome/sinus node dysfunction
  4. Atrial standstill (hyperkalemia, atrial myopathy)

B. **Hypothermia**

C. **Hypothyroidism**

D. **Organophosphate toxicosis**

E. **Pharmacologic** (e.g., due to beta-blockers, calcium channel blockers, digitalis, opiates, alpha-2 agonist drugs)

F. **Vagal tone high: normal**
  1. Brachycephalic breed
  2. Athletic animal at rest
  3. Sleep

G. **Vagal tone high: abnormal**
  1. GI disturbances
  2. Upper respiratory obstruction (e.g., foreign body, laryngeal paralysis, elongated soft palate, laryngeal collapse, airway edema, mass, anesthetic circuit problem)
  3. Neurologic lesions (central and severe: usually comatose patient)

AV, Atrioventricular; *bpm*, beats per minute; *GI*, gastrointestinal.

Notes: First-degree AV block does not affect the heart rate.

In critically ill or anesthetized animals, an acute transition from tachycardia to bradycardia may indicate an immediate transition to cardiac arrest.

Definition of bradycardia in the clinical setting: heart rate < 60 bpm (large-breed dogs), < 70 bpm (medium-breed dogs), < 90 bpm (small-breed dogs), < 130 bpm (cats).

Calcium Content of Calcium Salts

Calcium Salt	CALCIUM CONTENT PER GRAM mg	mmol	mEq
Calcium acetate (anhydrous)	253	6.3	12.6
Calcium carbonate	400	10.0	20.0
Calcium chloride (dihydrate)	273	6.8	13.6
Calcium chloride (hexahydrate)	183	4.6	9.1
Calcium citrate (tetrahydrate)	211	5.3	10.5
Calcium glubionate (monohydrate)	66	1.6	3.3
Calcium gluceptate (anhydrous)	82	2.0	4.1
Calcium gluconate (monohydrate)	89	2.2	4.5
Calcium glycerophosphate (anhydrous)	191	4.8	9.5
Calcium hydrogen phosphate (dihydrate)	233	5.8	11.6
Calcium lactate (anhydrous)	184	4.6	9.2
Calcium lactate (trihydrate)	147	3.7	7.3
Calcium lactate (pentahydrate)	130	3.2	6.5
Calcium lactate gluconate (dihydrate)	129	3.2	6.4
Calcium lactobionate (dihydrate)	51	1.3	2.5
Calcium levulinate (dihydrate)	131	3.3	6.5
Calcium phosphate [$10CaO.3P_2O_5.H_2O$]	399	10.0	19.9
Calcium pidolate (anhydrous)	135	3.4	6.7
Calcium silicate [$CaSiO_3$]	345	8.6	17.2
Calcium sodium lactate (tetrahydrate)	78	1.9	3.9

Reproduced with permission from Sweetman SC: Martindale: The complete drug reference, ed 38, London, 2014, Pharmaceutical Press, p 1785.

Chronic Kidney Disease: IRIS Staging

SERUM CREATININE mg/dL (mcmol/L)		
Dog	**Cat**	**Stage**
<1.4 (<125)	<1.6 (<140)	1
1.4-2.0 (125-180)	1.6-2.8 (140-250)	2
2.1-5.0 (181-440)	2.9-5.0 (251-440)	3
>5.0 (>440)	>5.0 (>440)	4
SUBSTAGE (PROTEINURIA) URINE PROTEIN/CREATININE RATIO		
Dog	**Cat**	**Substage**
<0.2	<0.2	Nonproteinuric
0.2 to 0.5	0.2 to 0.4	Borderline
>0.5	>0.4	Proteinuric
SUBSTAGE (HYPERTENSION) SYSTOLIC BLOOD PRESSURE mm Hg		
Both Dogs and Cats		**Substage**
<150		Nonhypertensive
150 to 159		Borderline
160 to 179		Hypertensive
≥180		Severely hypertensive

NOTE: Staging applies to animals with suspected chronic kidney disease. For animals with normal creatinine, this might include imaging abnormalities of the kidneys, symmetric dimethylarginine (SDMA) concentrations > 14 mcg/dL, or persistently isosthenuric urine with no alternative explanation.
NOTE: The unit of measure of micron, sometimes denoted by the Greek letter μ, is abbreviated in this text by mc. For example, 1 mcL = 1 microliter; 1 mcg = 1 microgram.
IRIS, International Renal Interest Society.

Chronic Kidney Disease: Complications and Comorbidities

Complications of Chronic Kidney Disease
- Anemia
- Anorexia
- Dehydration
- Hypermagnesemia
- Hyperparathyroidism
- Hyperphosphatemia
- Hypocalcemia or hypercalcemia
- Hypokalemia
- Malnutrition
- Metabolic acidosis
- Proteinuria
- Systemic hypertension
- Uremic encephalopathy
- Uremic gastritis, gastric ulcers
- Uremic pneumonitis
- Uremic stomatitis
- Weight loss

Comorbid Conditions: Common
- Cardiac disease
- Degenerative joint disease
- Dental and oral diseases
- Hyperthyroidism (cats)
- Nephroliths and ureteroliths
- Urinary tract infections

Adapted from Ettinger S, Feldman E: Textbook of veterinary internal medicine, ed 7, St. Louis, 2010, Saunders.

Collapse

Differential Diagnosis Item	Typical Key Feature(s)
Ruptured splenic mass	Common cause of collapse in large-breed dogs. Hypotension, pallor, tachycardia—hemorrhagic shock; hemoabdomen, cavitated splenic mass on ultrasound. Some: concurrent right atrial mass, cardiac tamponade.
Syncope	Inadequate cerebral blood flow. Severe bradycardia or tachycardia, pulmonary hypertension, or heart failure. Mucous membranes pale during collapse but normal when recovered. Collapse is brief (<60 sec). Normal once recovered. Murmur, arrhythmia, or normal between episodes.
Metabolic causes of collapse	Weakness due to anemia, sepsis, hypoglycemia, hypocalcemia, hypokalemia, cortisol deficiency. Weakness typically persistent but may be exercise-induced initially. Treat cause once discovered; rapid response expected.
Respiratory distress	Severe dyspnea, often with cyanosis during collapse. Increased effort during obstructive phase breathing. Inspiratory dyspnea: pharyngeal/laryngeal disorder (with stridor); pleural space disorder (quiet). Inspiratory/expiratory dyspnea: pulmonary, collapsing trachea, upper and lower airway. Expiratory dyspnea: small airway disease, asthma.
Pericardial effusion/cardiac tamponade	Typically causes weak pulse, muffled heart sounds, tachycardia; abdominal distention also common (from cardiac tamponade or concurrent abdominal mass rupture).
Partial seizures	Can resemble episodes of collapse. Consciousness maintained, ataxia possible, falling/crawling possible. Occasionally stereotypical movements. Postictal phase possible, including blindness/altered mentation. Paroxysmal, recurrent. Normal between seizures if due to epilepsy.
Other nervous system disease	Structural spinal cord or brain lesion causes localizing neurologic signs. Polyradiculoneuritis, botulism, and tick paralysis cause profound generalized weakness and loss of reflexes. Myasthenia gravis and muscle diseases cause weakness with normal proprioception and reflexes. Palpebral reflex may be fatigable in myasthenia gravis.
Bone/joint disease	Bone or joint pain or fractures cause reluctance or inability to stand/walk. Pain in multiple joints is common with polyarthritis.
Exercise-induced collapse	Inherited in Labrador retrievers, others. Collapse during strenuous exercise, especially in hot environment; primarily affects hindlimbs, lasts 10-30 minutes; normal between episodes. Genetic test is available; only homozygous dogs collapse.

Reproduced from the third edition in unabridged form.

THIRD EDITION AUTHOR: **Susan M. Taylor, DVM, DACVIM**

Coma

Cause	Salient Characteristic
Intracranial—Acute/Rapidly Progressive	
Trauma*	History and presence of other traumatic injuries is confirmatory. Most common cause of coma in dogs and cats.
Granuloma	Often a diagnosis of exclusion. Rule out other causes. Often multifocal with a history of seizures, although focal forms exist. MRI, +/– CT scan may be helpful.
Hemorrhage	Suspected in patients with hypertension (check blood pressure), hypocoagulable states, and intracranial tumors (particularly hemangiosarcoma). Coagulation testing (TEG, PT/PTT, BMBT) and MRI often required.
Status epilepticus	History and physical examination are confirmatory.
Embolism/ischemic encephalopathy	Suspected in patients with predisposing hypercoagulable states (IMHA, hyperadrenocorticism, glomerular disease, heart disease, etc.). Hypercoagulable TEG tracings in patients with predisposing disease. MRI, +/– CT scan often required for confirmation.
Intracranial—Chronic/Slowly Progressive	
Tumor*	Often older dogs with a history of seizures, circling, and behavioral changes. MRI, +/– CT scan confirms the diagnosis.
Abscess	Possible history of bite wounds, prior infections (parvovirus), or trauma. Rule out other causes. MRI, +/– CT scan required.
Developmental disorders (hydrocephalus, storage diseases)	Suspected in young patients with progressive onset and domed skull conformation. Ultrasound (through fontanelle) or MRI required.
Systemic Infectious	
Rabies	Vaccination status, geographic exposure risk, history and clinical signs
Feline infectious peritonitis	Definitive diagnosis on histopathologic evaluation
Canine distemper	History, gastrointestinal signs, often progressive and multifocal. Immunofluorescent antibody testing or anti-CDV antibody titers in CSF. More common in developing countries.
Fungal	CSF culture and cytology, MRI
Parasitic	Fecal, CSF cytology, MRI

(Continued from previous page)

Cause	Salient Characteristic
Systemic Noninfectious	
Toxins[†]	
Lead	History, radiographic metallic foreign bodies, red blood cell abnormalities, concurrent GI signs, whole blood lead concentration
Barbiturates	History of exposure, blood concentrations
Antidepressants	History of exposure
Tranquilizers	History of exposure
Alcohol	History of exposure, blood levels, severe metabolic acidosis
Ethylene glycol	History, ethylene glycol testing, severe metabolic acidosis, calcium oxalate crystalluria
Metabolic	
Hypoglycemia*	Serum glucose concentration
Hypernatremia	Serum sodium concentration
Hyponatremia	Serum sodium concentration
Diabetic ketoacidosis	Serum and/or urine ketones
Hyperosmolar diabetes mellitus	Calculate osmolality (sodium and glucose), predisposing cause of decreased GFR (kidney disease, hypovolemia, heart failure, shock)
Hepatic encephalopathy*	History, serum ammonium, pre- and post-serum bile acids, urine bile acids. Often in cats with hepatic lipidosis and young dogs with portosystemic shunts.
Uremic encephalopathy*	BUN, creatinine, USG, potential history of previous chronic kidney disease
Hypoadrenocorticism	ACTH stimulation test, basal cortisol
Myxedema coma	Serum T_4 and TSH
Miscellaneous	
Severe hypovolemia/shock*	Assessment of physical perfusion parameters, lactate, base excess
Post-cardiac arrest	History of cardiorespiratory arrest
Heat stroke	History, environmental temperature, rectal temperature
Erythrocytosis	PCV
Hyperglobulinemia	Globulin levels on chemistry panel

*Common causes of coma in small animals.
[†]Can evaluate with over-the-counter drug testing kit or human hospital toxicology screen.
ACTH, Adrenocorticotropic hormone; *BMBT,* buccal mucosal bleeding time; *BUN,* blood urea nitrogen; *CDV,* canine distemper virus; *CSF,* cerebrospinal fluid; *CT,* computed tomography; *GFR,* glomerular filtration rate; *GI,* gastrointestinal; *IMHA,* immune-mediated hemolytic anemia; *MRI,* magnetic resonance imaging; *PCV,* packed cell volume; *PT,* prothrombin time; *PTT,* partial thromboplastin time; T_4, thyroxine; *TEG,* thromboelastography; *TSH,* thyroid-stimulating hormone; *USG,* urine specific gravity.
Reproduced from the third edition in unabridged form.

THIRD EDITION AUTHOR: Søren R. Boysen, DVM, DACVECC

Congenital Heart Disease: Breed Predilections

Breed	Condition
Basset hound	Pulmonic stenosis (PS)
Beagle	PS
Bichon frisé	Patent ductus arteriosus (PDA)
Boxer	Subaortic stenosis (SAS), PS, atrial septal defect (ASD)
Boykin spaniel	PS
Bull terrier	Mitral dysplasia (MVD), SAS
Chihuahua	PS, PDA
Chow chow	PS, cor triatriatum dexter (CTD)
Cocker spaniel	PDA, PS
Collie	PDA
Doberman pinscher	ASD
English bulldog	PS, ventricular septal defect (VSD), tetralogy of Fallot (ToF)
English springer spaniel	PDA, VSD
German shepherd	SAS, PDA, tricuspid valve dysplasia (TVD), mitral valve dysplasia (MVD)
German shorthaired pointer	SAS
Golden retriever	SAS, TVD, MVD
Great Dane	SAS, MVD, TVD
Keeshond	PDA, ToF
Labrador retriever	TVD, PDA, PS
Maltese	PDA
Mastiff	PS, MVD
Miniature schnauzer	PS
Newfoundland	SAS, MVD, PS
Pomeranian	PDA
Poodle	PDA
Rottweiler	SAS
Samoyed	PS, SAS, ASD
Shetland sheepdog	PDA
Terrier breeds	PS
Weimaraner	TVD, peritoneopericardial diaphragmatic hernia
Welsh corgi	PDA
West Highland white terrier	PS, VSD
Yorkshire terrier	PDA

Reproduced from Beijerink NJ, Oyama MA, Bonagura JD. Congenital heart disease. In Ettinger SJ, Feldman EC, Côte E, eds. Textbook of veterinary internal medicine, 8th ed, St. Louis, Saunders, 2017, p. 1207.

Constipation

Differential Diagnosis of Constipation in the Cat

Neuromuscular Dysfunction

- Colonic smooth muscle: idiopathic megacolon, aging
- Spinal cord disease: lumbosacral disease, cauda equina syndrome, sacral spinal cord deformity (Manx cat)
- Hypogastric or pelvic nerve disorders: traumatic injury, malignant disease, dysautonomia
- Submucosal or myenteric plexus neuropathy: dysautonomia, aging

Mechanical Obstruction

- Intraluminal: foreign material (bones, plant material, fur), neoplasia, rectal diverticulum, perineal hernia, anorectal stricture
- Intramural: neoplasia
- Extraluminal: pelvic fracture, neoplasia

Inflammation

- Perianal fistula, proctitis, anal sac abscess, anorectal foreign body, perianal bite wound

Metabolic and Endocrine

- Metabolic: dehydration, hypokalemia, hypercalcemia
- Endocrine: hypothyroidism, obesity, nutritional secondary hyperparathyroidism

Pharmacologic

- Opioid agonists, cholinergic antagonists, diuretics, beta-agonists, phenothiazines

Environmental and Behavioral

- Soiled litter box, inactivity, hospitalization, change in environment

Adapted from Washabau RJ, Day MJ: Canine and feline gastroenterology, St. Louis, 2013, Elsevier Saunders.

Corneal Ulcer

Underlying Causes of Corneal Ulceration in Dogs and Cats

- Cranial nerve V and/or VII deficits
- Distichiasis
- Ectopic cilia
- Entropion
- Exophthalmos
- Foreign body
- Herpes virus, feline
- Keratoconjunctivitis sicca (KCS)
- Lagophthalmos
- Ocular trauma
- Other lid defects
- Qualitative tear film deficiencies (mucin and/or lipid)
- Severe debilitation

Modified from Maggs DJ, Miller PE, Ofri R: Slatter's Fundamentals of veterinary ophthalmology, ed 5, St. Louis, 2013.

Cough

Cause	Onset	Salient Feature
Aspiration pneumonia	Acute	History suggestive (e.g., anesthesia, regurgitation); harsh/loud sounds ± crackles; right middle or caudal portion of left cranial lobes often involved but radiographic changes lag up to 24 hours
Cardiogenic pulmonary edema (dogs only)	Acute	Heart murmur ± arrhythmia; harsh/loud sounds ± crackles; venous distention, perihilar infiltrate on thoracic radiographs; heart disease confirmed on echocardiography; rare to have cough + comfortable respirations due to cardiogenic pulmonary edema (especially uncommon in small breeds), usually dyspnea +/- cough
Noncardiogenic pulmonary edema/acute respiratory distress syndrome	Acute	History of inciting trigger (smoke inhalation, electrocution, sepsis, etc.); respiratory distress and hypoxemia; harsh/loud sounds ± crackles; alveolar pattern on thoracic radiographs with normal heart/blood vessels
Pulmonary hemorrhage	Acute	History (notably anticoagulant exposure); evidence of systemic bleeding diathesis; harsh/loud sounds ± crackles; thoracic radiographs alveolar pattern
Pulmonary thromboembolism (PTE)	Acute	Suspected or confirmed hypercoagulable state (cancer, heartworm disease, protein-losing nephropathy or enteropathy, immune-mediated hemolytic anemia); respiratory distress and hypoxemia common; normal thoracic radiographs simultaneously = strongly suggestive of PTE; other radiographic findings possible (e.g., hypoperfused lung lobe, alveolar pattern)
Tracheal/bronchial foreign body	Acute	Lateral cervical radiograph and/or tracheoscopy
Tracheobronchitis	Acute	Patient usually feels well; recent history of interaction with new/different dogs (contagion)
Pneumonia (bacterial, fungal, protozoal)	Acute or insidious	Often systemic illness; harsh/loud sounds ± crackles; thoracic radiographs suggestive; transtracheal wash or bronchoalveolar lavage to isolate organisms
Eosinophilic bronchopneumopathy	Acute or insidious	Marked eosinophilic infiltrate on bronchoalveolar lavage; uncommon; radiographic lung infiltrates can be dramatic
Heartworm disease	Acute or insidious	Thoracic radiographs ± arterial distention and right-sided enlargement; heartworm antigen test (dog); heartworm antibody and antigen test (heat treated) and/or echocardiography (cat)
Interstitial lung disease (e.g., pulmonary fibrosis, BOOP)	Acute or insidious	Variable radiographic findings; rule out other conditions; biopsy required for confirmation of most types
Mediastinal mass	Acute or insidious	Noncompliant cranial thorax (cats); thoracic radiographs or thoracic ultrasound; FeLV antigen test in cats; evidence of lymphoma elsewhere
Tracheobronchial lymphadenopathy	Acute or insidious	Often systemic illness; thoracic radiographs confirm lymphadenopathy ± other abnormalities (e.g., miliary pattern from fungal pneumonia)
Collapsing trachea (dogs)	Insidious	Disproportionately loud; often small-breed (+/– obese) dogs; worse with excitement; apparent on radiographs, fluoroscopy, and/or bronchoscopy
Asthma/allergic airway disease (cats)	Insidious	Wax/wane cough (often mistaken for hairballs); ± respiratory distress, wheeze; airway eosinophilia is supportive (rule out lungworms and heartworms)
Bronchiectasis	Insidious	Radiographic diagnosis, often coexisting with chronic sterile bronchitis or other airway/lung disease
Chronic sterile bronchitis	Insidious	Disproportionately loud; often small-breed (+/– obese) dogs; no dyspnea at rest; bronchoscopy identifies mucosal edema, no infection but neutrophilic inflammation
Gastroesophageal reflux disease	Insidious	Diagnosis based on exclusion of other disorders and response to aggressive gastric acid control
Left atrial enlargement	Insidious	Mitral heart murmur; confirm enlargement on thoracic radiographs/echocardiogram; contested as cause of cough since dogs with or without left atrial enlargement show no difference in cough or degree of airway inflammation cytologically
Lungworms	Insidious	Systemically well; endemic region; Baermann fecal (but shedding can be intermittent) + fecal flotation; response to anthelmintic treatment trial
Pulmonary neoplasia (metastatic or primary)	Insidious	If metastatic, weight loss common ± primary site found on examination; thoracic radiographs and/or computed tomography (more sensitive); fine-needle aspirate, airway lavage, or biopsy to confirm
Tracheal mass/stenosis	Insidious	Lateral cervical radiograph and/or tracheoscopy

BOOP, bronchiolitis obliterans with organizing pneumonia, also known as cryptogenic organizing pneumonia; *FeLV*, feline leukemia virus.

AUTHORS: Etienne Côté, DVM, DACVIM and Leah A. Cohn, DVM, PhD, DACVIM

Cranial Nerve Deficits

Nerve	Clinical Signs	Clinical Tests	Normal Response	Abnormal Response
I. Olfactory	Hyposmia or anosmia	Smell of food or nonirritating, volatile substance	Interest in food; sniff, recoil, or nose lick with volatile substance	No response
II. Optic	Visual impairment and hesitancy in moving	1. Obstacle test 2. Visual placing reaction 3. Menace reaction 4. Following movement test	1. Avoidance of obstacle 2. Visual placement of limbs 3. Eye blink 4. Eyes following objects	1. Bumping objects 2-4. No response
III. Oculomotor	Ventrolateral strabismus	1. Ocular movement in horizontal and vertical planes	1. Normal ocular excursion	1. Impaired movements of affected eye
	Paralysis of upper eyelid (ptosis), mydriasis	2. Point source of light in each eye	2. Direct and consensual pupillary light reflexes	2. On affected side, direct pupillary reflex absent, consensual reflex present; on normal side, direct pupillary reflex present, consensual reflex absent
Sympathetic control of pupillary function	Constricted pupil (miosis), enophthalmos, prolapse of third eyelid, ptosis of upper lid			
IV. Trochlear	Usually not noted			
V. Trigeminal (motor and sensory)	Atrophy of masticatory muscles Inability to close mouth	1. Jaw tone 2. Palpate and observe masticatory muscles 3. Palpebral reflex 4. Corneal reflex 5. Probe nasal mucosa 6. Touch face	1. Resistance to opening jaws 2. Normal muscle contour and resilience 3. Eye blink 4. Eye blink and globe retraction 5. Recoil 6. No reaction	1. Lack of resistance 2. Atrophy, hypotonia 3-5. No response 6. Intense discomfort
VI. Abducent	Medial strabismus	Ocular movements in horizontal plane	Normal ocular excursion	Impaired lateral movement of affected eye
VII. Facial	Asymmetry of facial expression Inability to close eyelids Lip commissure paralysis Ear paralysis	1. Palpebral reflex 2. Corneal reflex 3. Menace reaction 4. Tickle ear	1-3. Eye blink 4. Ear flick	1-4. No response
VIII. Vestibulocochlear Vestibular	Nystagmus, head tilt, circling Falling and rolling	1. Ocular movements in horizontal and vertical planes 2. Caloric and rotatory test 3. Righting reactions	1-2. Normal physiologic nystagmus 3. Normal righting	1-3. No response, ventrolateral strabismus on dorsal extension of head
Cochlear	Deafness	Hand clap	Startle reaction, blink, ear contraction	No response
IX. Glossopharyngeal	Dysphagia	Gag reflex	Swallowing response	No response
X. Vagus	Dysphagia Abnormal vocalizing Inspiratory dyspnea Megaesophagus	1. Gag reflex 2. Laryngeal reflex 3. Oculocardiac reflex	1. Swallow 2. Cough 3. Bradycardia	1-3. No response
XI. Spinal accessory	Usually not noted			
XII. Hypoglossal	Deviation of tongue	1. Tongue stretch 2. Nose rub	1. Retraction 2. Lick response	1-2. No response

Cutaneous Masses

Epithelial Neoplastic and Non-Neoplastic Skin Masses

Epidermal Origin
- Viral papilloma
- Squamous cell carcinoma
- Basal cell carcinoma
- Dermoid cyst (Rhodesian ridgeback)

Follicular Origin
- Follicular cyst (infundibular cyst)
- Follicular hamartoma
- Trichoblastoma
- Trichoepithelioma
- Trichofolliculoma
- Infundibular keratinizing acanthoma (intracutaneous cornifying epithelioma, keratoacanthoma)
- Pilomatricoma

Melanocytic Origin
- Melanocytoma
- Melanoma

Sebaceous Origin
- Sebaceous hamartoma/nevus
- Sebaceous gland hyperplasia/adenoma
- Sebaceous epithelioma
- Sebaceous carcinoma
- Perianal (hepatoid) gland hyperplasia and adenoma
- Perianal gland epithelioma
- Perianal gland carcinoma

Sweat Gland Origin
- Apocrine cyst
- Apocrine adenoma
- Apocrine adenocarcinoma
- Eccrine carcinoma

Mesenchymal Neoplastic and Non-Neoplastic Skin Masses

Fibrous Origin
- Collagenous hamartoma/nevus
- Canine nodular dermatofibrosis (German shepherd)
- Acrochordon (skin tag)
- Fibroma
- Fibrosarcoma

Vascular and Perivascular Origin
- Hemangioma
- Hemangiosarcoma
- Lymphangiosarcoma
- Hemangiopericytoma

Lipocytic Origin
- Lipoma
- Liposarcoma

Muscular Origin
- Leiomyoma
- Leiomyosarcoma

Neural and Perineural Origin
- Merkel cell tumor

Lymphohistiocytic Skin Masses

Histiocytic Origin
- Canine cutaneous histiocytoma
- Canine reactive histiocytosis (cutaneous, systemic)
- Histiocytic sarcoma

Lymphocytic Origin
- Plasmacytoma
- Epitheliotropic lymphoma
- Nonepitheliotropic lymphoma
- Cutaneous lymphomatosis

Miscellaneous Origins
- Mast cell tumor
- Transmissible venereal tumor
- Cutaneous metastases

For noninflammatory and infectious processes, see algorithm of Nodular Dermatitis.
Reproduced from the third edition in unabridged form.

THIRD EDITION AUTHOR: Manon Paradis, DMV, MVSc, DACVD

Cyanosis: Causation

Cause	Examples	Considerations
Decreased inspired oxygen (FiO_2)	Smoke inhalation, asphyxiating gas, anesthetic mishap	History suggestive; responds to O_2 supplementation
Decreased peripheral perfusion	Shock, aortic thromboembolism (saddle thrombus), hypothermia	Only area of reduced blood flow affected (e.g., hind paw pads with saddle thrombus)
Disordered control of breathing	Coma, brain trauma	History and examination, including neurologic examination
Erythrocytosis	Polycythemia vera, Eisenmenger's complex, right-to-left patent ductus arteriosus, renal carcinoma	Absolute concentration of deoxygenated hemoglobin >4 to 5 g/dL; normal respiratory effort; normal thoracic imaging
Heart disease (right-to-left shunting)	Tetralogy of Fallot, Eisenmenger's complex, right-to-left patent ductus arteriosus	Differential cyanosis (pink oral and conjunctival mucous membranes; cyanotic vulvar/preputial mucosa) is characteristic of right-to-left shunting patent ductus arteriosus; other causes generalized.
Hypoventilation	Botulism, polyradiculoneuritis, severe obesity, chest wall deformity, excessively deep anesthetic plane	History and examination crucial; $PaCO_2$ increased
Intrinsic lung disease	Interstitial lung disease, pneumonia, pulmonary edema, pulmonary neoplasia	Adventitial sounds common; thoracic imaging usually supportive of pulmonary dysfunction
Lower airway obstruction	Asthma, severe tracheal collapse, bronchial carcinoma	Cough and wheeze are characteristic; bronchointerstitial infiltrates common but not consistent
Methemoglobinemia	Congenital, acquired oxidative RBC injury (e.g., drugs, skunk musk, *Allium* species foods)	SpO_2 reading often 75% to 85% and normal PaO_2; respiratory effort often normal; thoracic imaging normal; chocolate-brown blood when methemoglobin >10%
Pleural space disease	Pleural effusion, pneumothorax, flail chest	Muffled lung/heart sounds, TFAST scan or radiographs diagnostic
Pulmonary hypertension	Stage C or > myxomatous mitral valve disease, heartworms, pulmonary fibrosis, bronchomalacia, severe tracheal collapse, pulmonary neoplasia, right-to-left patent ductus arteriosus	Right heart enlargement sometimes seen on radiographs; tricuspid murmur possible; tricuspid valve regurgitation velocity ≥2.7 m/s, high-velocity pulmonic insufficiency ± "notching" on Doppler echocardiography

Continued

(Continued from previous page)

Cause	Examples	Considerations
Pulmonary vascular disease	Pulmonary thromboembolism, pulmonary veno-occlusive disease (PVOD), pulmonary capillary hemangiomatosis (PCH)	Acute-onset cough and respiratory effort; history of predisposing disease (e.g., immune-mediated hemolysis, protein-losing nephropathy); concurrent pulmonary hypertension with PVOD and PCH that is refractory to or progresses to congestive heart failure with PDE5 inhibition
Upper airway obstruction	Laryngeal paralysis, brachycephalic airway syndrome, foreign body, polyp	Stridor is characteristic; laryngoscopy and/or cervical imaging useful

Diabetes Insipidus, Nephrogenic

CONGENITAL (Primary)
ACQUIRED (Secondary)
- **Functional**
  - Drugs
    - Glucocorticoids
    - Lithium
    - Demeclocycline
    - Methoxyflurane
    - Diuretics
  - Infections
    - *Escherichia coli* endotoxin (e.g., pyelonephritis, pyometra)
    - Leptospirosis
  - Electrolyte/mineral disturbances
    - Hypokalemia
    - Hypercalcemia
  - Altered medullary hypertonicity
    - Hypoadrenocorticism
    - Portosystemic shunt
  - Multifactorial or unknown mechanism
    - Hepatic insufficiency
    - Hyperthyroidism
    - Hyperadrenocorticism
  - Postobstructive diuresis
  - Acromegaly
  - Pheochromocytoma
  - Primary hyperaldosteronism
  - Leiomyosarcoma
- **Structural**
  - Medullary interstitial amyloidosis (e.g., in cats, Shar-pei dogs)
  - Polycystic kidney disease
  - Chronic pyelonephritis
  - Chronic interstitial nephritis

Modified from DiBartola S: Fluid, electrolyte, and acid-base disorders in small animal practice, ed 4, St. Louis, 2012, Saunders Elsevier.

Diabetes Mellitus: Complications

Complications in Dogs and Cats

Common
- Iatrogenic hypoglycemia
- Persistent polyuria and polydipsia (PU/PD)
- Weight loss
- Cataracts (dogs)
- Bacterial infections, especially of the urinary tract
- Pancreatitis
- Ketoacidosis
- Hepatic lipidosis
- Peripheral neuropathy (cat)

Uncommon
- Peripheral neuropathy (dog)
- Glomerulonephropathy, glomerulosclerosis
- Retinopathy
- Systemic hypertension
- Exocrine pancreatic insufficiency
- Gastric paresis
- Diabetic diarrhea
- Diabetic dermatopathy (dog) (i.e., superficial necrolytic dermatitis/ hepatocutaneous syndrome)

Modified from Feldman E, Nelson R: Canine and feline endocrinology and reproduction, ed 3, St. Louis, 2004, Saunders.

Diabetic Ketoacidosis: Triggers

Triggers and Predisposing Conditions

Acromegaly
Chronic kidney disease
Congestive heart failure
Epinephrine release
Glucagonoma
Glucocorticoid treatment
Hepatitis/cholangiohepatitis
Hyperadrenocorticism
Infection
- Abscess (subcutaneous, other)
- Periodontal/oral
- Pneumonia
- Pyoderma
- Pyometra
- Urinary tract infection

Insulin absence/resistance/misadministration
Pancreatitis
Progesterone (diestrus; progestogen treatment)

Diarrhea

Differential Diagnosis	Characteristic Features
Dietary	
Food intolerance/allergy	Recent diet change, +/– new protein source
Abrupt diet change/dietary indiscretion	History; no treatment vs. empirical therapy for comfort
Overeating	History
Poor quality food	History; abdominal distention, borborygmi, flatulence
Infectious	
Parasitic: • Hookworms—*Ancylostoma/Uncinaria* spp • Whipworms—*Trichuris vulpis* • Roundworms—*Toxocara* spp, *Strongyloides* spp • *Trichinella* spp • Protozoa (*Isospora* spp—coccidiosis; *Giardia* spp; *Cryptosporidium parvum; Pentatrichomonas/Tritrichomonas foetus; Balantidium coli; Entamoeba histolytica)*	Fecal flotation(s): 1 may suffice if positive, but at least 3 (up to 5) recommended if negative. Emperic deworming often used before proceeding to advanced diagnostic testing.
Bacterial: • *Campylobacter jejuni* • *Clostridium* spp *(perfringens, difficile, upsaliensis)* • *Escherichia coli* • *Salmonella* spp • *Yersinia enterocolitica* • *Shigella* spp • *Bacillus piliformis* • Dysbiosis (antibiotic-responsive diarrhea)/Enterobacteriaceae	Consider possibility of primary underlying disorder with secondary bacterial enteritis. Fecal cytology: presence of *Campylobacter* or *Clostridium* spp does not equate with cause of diarrhea as many are nonpathogenic.
Viral: • Coronaviruses • Canine distemper • Canine parvovirus • Feline leukemia virus (FeLV) • Feline immunodeficiency virus (FIV) • Feline infectious peritonitis (FIP) • Feline panleukopenia	Species-specific viral infections: ELISA test readily available (FeLV, FIV, feline panleukopenia, canine parvovirus)

Continued

(Continued from previous page)

Differential Diagnosis	Characteristic Features
Fungal: • Histoplasmosis • Mycotoxins (spoiled foods) • Cryptococcosis • Pythiosis/lagenidiosis • Protothecosis	Patient usually very ill; geographic location (histoplasmosis, pythiosis/lagenidiosis, protothecosis, +/− cryptococcosis), identification of organism in lesion is confirmatory
Rickettsial: *Neorickettsia helminthoeca* (salmon poisoning)	Patient usually febrile, ill; geographic distribution (e.g., Pacific northwestern United States)
Inflammatory	
Inflammatory bowel disease (diet responsive, antibiotic responsive, steroid responsive, and nonresponsive)	Weight loss, GI signs, palpably thickened intestine: highly variable; rule out concurrent/primary disorders first (food intolerance/allergy, parasitic disease, dysbiosis) before U/S and biopsy for histologic confirmation
Hemorrhagic gastroenteritis	Acute episode; elevated PCV without concomitant elevation in total solids
Lymphangiectasia	Yorkshire terriers predisposed; panhypoproteinemia common; GI signs variable; effusion or neurologic/respiratory signs possible (embolism)
Chronic/histiocytic ulcerative colitis	Boxers predisposed; highly responsive to enrofloxacin
Breed-specific (Shar-pei, basenji, soft-coated Wheaten terrier)	Often associated with PLE. Soft-coated Wheaten terriers may have concomitant protein-losing nephropathy.
Hypereosinophilic syndrome	Cats; peripheral eosinophilia, other organs often infiltrated
Other	
Villous atrophy	Associated with gastrinoma, gluten-sensitive enteropathy, or idiopathic
Neoplasia: • Lymphoma • Adenocarcinoma • Mast cell tumor • Leiomyoma/leiomyosarcoma	Systemic signs (e.g., weight loss, inappetence) possible; abdominal U/S may be strongly supportive; confirmation is histopathologic.
Intestinal foreign body	Abdominal XR, U/S: obstructive pattern, foreign body may be visible.
Intussusception	Concurrent enteropathy is common. Bull's-eye appearance on U/S is pathognomonic.
Mesenteric volvulus	Acute pain, hypotension. XR: generalized ileus. Surgical confirmation.
Irritable bowel syndrome	Diagnosis by exclusion. Stress common (e.g., working dogs).
Extraintestinal Causes	
Toxins/drugs: • NSAIDs • Organophosphates • Antibiotics • Lactulose • Antineoplastic chemotherapy • Heavy metals	History of exposure/ingestion; gastric perforation possible (NSAIDs); hypersalivation, muscle tremors likely with organophosphates; therapeutic intent and intolerance are typical with antibiotics, lactulose, chemotherapy
Acute pancreatitis	Cranial abdominal pain variable; serum spec PLI, abdominal U/S
Hepatobiliary disease	Serum transaminase activity, serum bile acids, abdominal U/S
Kidney disease	Serum creatinine, urinalysis
Exocrine pancreatic insufficiency	Two common scenarios are weight loss with steatorrhea, or insulin-resistant diabetes mellitus. Serum TLI is confirmatory.
Hypoadrenocorticism	Wax-wane clinical course in adult dog is typical; hyponatremia, hyperkalemia supportive; ACTH stimulation to confirm
Diabetic ketosis	Glucosuria and ketonuria to confirm
Hyperthyroidism (cats)	Weight loss with good appetite is typical; T_4 +/− fT_4 to confirm

ACTH, Adrenocorticotropic hormone; *fT_4,* free thyroxine by equilibrium dialysis; *NSAIDs,* nonsteroidal antiinflammatory drugs; *PCV,* packed cell volume; *PLE,* protein-losing enteropathy; *PLI,* species-specific pancreatic lipase immunoreactivity; *T_4,* thyroxine; *TLI,* trypsin-like immunoreactivity; *U/S,* ultrasound; *XR,* radiograph.
Reproduced from the third edition in unabridged form.

THIRD EDITION AUTHOR: Lisa Carioto, DVM, DVSc, DACVIM

Diarrhea, Neonatal

Causes of Neonatal Diarrhea in Puppies and Kittens

Dietary
- Abrupt change in diet
- Overfeeding
- Indiscretion: garbage ingestion
- Ingestion of abrasive or indigestible material
- Food intolerance
- Intolerance of lactose ingested as milk

Endoparasitic
- Helminths: ascarids, hookworms, whipworms, *Strongyloides*
- Others: cestodes, trematodes, *Trichinella*
- Protozoa: coccidia (*Cystoisospora*), *Cryptosporidium, Giardia intestinalis*
- Others: *Pentatrichomonas, Entamoeba, Balantidium*, rickettsial organisms
- Salmon poisoning disease

Obstructive
- Intestinal foreign body
- Intussusception
- Mesenteric volvulus

Drug- and Toxin-Induced
- Antiinflammatory drugs
- Antimicrobials
- Anthelmintics
- Heavy metals: lead, arsenic, thallium
- Insecticides: organophosphates
- Plants

Infectious
- Viral: parvoviruses, coronaviruses, rotaviruses, canine distemper, FeLV, FIV, FIP
- Bacterial: *Salmonella* spp, *Campylobacter* spp, *Yersinia enterocolitica, Bacillus piliformis, Escherichia coli, Clostridium* spp

Extraintestinal
- Uremia
- Hepatic disease
- Hypoadrenocorticism
- Acute pancreatitis
- Diabetes mellitus

Idiopathic Chronic Diarrhea in Young Cats

FeLV, Feline leukemia virus; *FIP*, feline infectious peritonitis; *FIV*, feline immunodeficiency virus.
Modified from Bonagura J: Kirk's Current veterinary therapy XIII, St. Louis, 2000, Saunders.

Diarrhea: Small Intestinal versus Large Intestinal

Characteristic	Small Intestine	Large Intestine
Defecation		
Frequency	Normal to mildly increased (2-4 times/d)	Greatly increased (4-10 times/d)
Dyschezia (inability to defecate without straining or signs of pain)	Absent	Dogs: frequent. Cats: less common
Tenesmus (straining)	Absent	Dogs: common. Cats: less common (rule out stranguria/urethral obstruction)
Urgency	Uncommon (unless severe acute enteritis)	Frequent
Feces		
Mucus	Uncommon	Common
Hematochezia (fresh blood in/on feces)	Absent	Common
Melena (digested blood in feces)	Occasional	Absent
Volume	Often increased	Normal to decreased (due to increased frequency)
Quality	Loose to watery; ± undigested food/fat	Loose to semisolid
Steatorrhea (undigested fat in feces)	Possible (with maldigestion or malabsorption)	Absent
Associated Signs		
Weight loss	Common	Uncommon (more likely with diffuse neoplasia, histoplasmosis, pythiosis)
Vomiting	Possible	Uncommon (with acute colitis even before onset of abnormal stools)
Appetite	May be normal, ↑ or ↓ depending on cause	Normal or ↓ depending on cause
Halitosis	Possible (maldigestion/malabsorption)	Absent
Borborygmus	Possible	Absent
Flatulence	Possible	Possible
Fecal incontinence	Rare	Possible
"Scooting" or chewing of perianal area	Absent	Possible (with proctitis)

Reproduced from the third edition in modified form.

THIRD EDITION AUTHOR: Lisa Carioto, DVM, DVSc, DACVIM

Diet Assessment

Relevant Considerations	
Inquire about specific varieties and amounts of what the patient is typically fed and what it is currently being fed, including: Commercial pet foods Home-prepared diets Table foods or scraps Treats Dietary supplements Foods used to deliver medications or supplements	Establish who lives in the household and whether there have been any recent changes, including: People and other pets Inquire about how the patient is fed and whether there have been any recent changes, including: Who feeds the pet Timing of meals Free choice versus meal feeding Ask about the patient's feeding behavior

Reproduced from the third edition in unabridged form.

THIRD EDITION AUTHOR: Kathryn E. Michel, DVM, MS, DACVN

Discolored Urine

Urine Color	Cause	Differentials (Examples)	Useful Findings
Colorless	Dilute urine	Chronic kidney disease, diabetes mellitus, diabetes insipidus, glucocorticoid (endogenous or exogenous)	Hyposthenuric, isosthenuric, or minimally concentrated
Yellow/orange	Normal concentrated urine	NA	Diagnosis of exclusion; concentrated specific gravity, UA otherwise unremarkable
	Bilirubinuria (prehepatic)	Hemolytic anemia of any cause	Anemia, RBC shape changes common; hyperbilirubinemia (plasma yellow)
	Bilirubinuria (hepatic)	Hepatic disease (e.g., chronic hepatitis, cirrhosis, hepatotoxicity, hepatic neoplasia, hepatic lipidosis)	Elevated liver enzymes, hyperbilirubinemia (plasma yellow) with normal hematocrit
	Bilirubinuria (posthepatic)	Cholestatic disease (cholangiohepatitis, gallbladder mucocele), biliary rupture	Elevated liver enzymes, hyperbilirubinemia (plasma yellow) with normal hematocrit, ultrasound imaging of biliary tree
	Drugs or dyes	Phenazopyridine, fluorescein, nitrofurantoin, others	History
Cloudy, variable opaque	Pyuria	UTI, sterile cystitis, pyometra	WBC on sediment
	Lipiduria	Hepatic lipidosis (cats), hyperlipidemia of any cause, healthy pets	Lipid droplets on urinalysis, ± hyperlipidemia
	Crystalluria	Related to UTI, idiopathic, artifact	Crystals on sediment
Pink/red	Renal, ureteral disease	Primary renal hematuria, glomerulonephritis, renal telangiectasia, renal neoplasia	RBC on sediment, imaging findings, cystoscopy
	Bladder, urethral disease	UTI, sterile hemorrhagic cystitis, urolithiasis, urethritis, feline idiopathic cystitis, transitional cell carcinoma	RBC on sediment, imaging findings
	Reproductive disease/condition	Prostatitis, prostatic neoplasia, estrus	RBC on sediment, imaging findings, free catch vs. cystocentesis or catheter sample (not discolored)
	Coagulopathy	Thrombocytopenia, DIC, vitamin K antagonism	RBC on sediment, evidence of bleeding elsewhere, thrombocytopenia, increased BMBT, or prolonged PT/aPTT
	Hemoglobin	Intravascular hemolysis of any cause, synthetic hemoglobin administration	RBC absent on UA, hemoglobinemia (pink plasma)
	Drugs or dyes	Phenazopyridine, phenolsulfonphthalein, beets, rhubarb	History
	Trauma	Abdominal trauma	History and examination, imaging studies

(Continued from previous page)

Urine Color	Cause	Differentials (Examples)	Useful Findings
Brown, black	Myoglobin	Crush injury, prolonged seizure, severe myopathy, heatstroke	RBC absent on UA, plasma clear, history, ammonium sulfate test
	Methemoglobin	Congenital, oxidative injury to RBC	Chocolate-colored blood, fixed SpO_2 (75%-85%)
	Bilirubinuria	See yellow/orange	See yellow/orange
	Hemoglobin	See pink/red	See pink/red
	Trauma	See pink/red	See pink/red
	Drugs or dyes	Phenolic compounds, nitrites, sulfasalazine, aniline dyes, others	History
	Melanin	Melanoma	Examination, imaging studies
Other colors (blue, green, any)	Water-soluble pigments	Consumption of food dyes, water-soluble markers, foods (e.g., beets), or drugs (e.g., rifampin, methylene blue, propofol)	UA otherwise unremarkable; colors may be unnatural (e.g., fluorescent); history helpful
	Biliverdin	Severe hepatic disease	Elevated liver enzymes, imaging studies
	Pseudomonas infections		Bacteriuria, pyuria
	Porphyrias	Inherited or acquired disorders within the heme biosynthetic pathway	Various other issues, depending on specific disorder

BMBT, Buccal mucosal bleeding time; *RBC,* red blood cell; *UA,* urinalysis; *WBC,* white blood cell.

Disinfectants, Antimicrobial Spectrum

Agent*	Alcohols	Aldehydes	Alkalis: Ammonia	Biguanides: Chlorhexidine	Halogens: Hypochlorite (Bleach)	Oxidizing Agents	Phenolics	Quaternary Ammonium Compounds
Mycoplasmas	++	++	++	++	++	++	++	+
Gram-positive bacteria	++	++	+	++	++	++	++	++
Gram-negative bacteria	++	++	+	+	++	++	++	+
Pseudomonads	++	++	+	±	++	++	++	±
Enveloped viruses	+	++	+	++	++	++	++	+
Non-enveloped viruses	–	+	±	–	++	+	±†	–
Fungal spores	±	+	+	±	+	±	+	±
Mycobacteria	+	++	+	–	+	±	++	–
Bacterial spores	–	+	±	–	++	+	–	–

*Examples of microorganisms from each category: **Mycoplasmas**: *Mycoplasma cynos, Mycoplasma felis*; **gram-positive bacteria**: *Staphylococcus* spp, *Streptococcus* spp; **gram-negative bacteria**: *Bordetella bronchiseptica, Salmonella* spp; **pseudomonads**: *Pseudomonas aeruginosa*; **enveloped viruses**: influenza virus, herpesvirus; **non-enveloped viruses**: feline panleukopenia virus, canine parvovirus, feline calicivirus; **fungal spores**: *Aspergillus* spp; **acid-fast bacteria**: *Mycobacterium fortuitum*; **bacterial spores**: *Clostridium difficile, Clostridium perfringens.*

†In general, phenols are not active against non-enveloped viruses but they do have some activity against rotaviruses. Activity against parvoviruses has not been documented.

++, Highly effective; +, effective; ±, limited activity; –, no activity.

Modified from the Canadian Committee on Antibiotic Resistance. Infection Prevention and Control Best Practices for Small Animal Veterinary Clinics, 2008; https://www.wormsandgermsblog.com/files/2008/12/CCAR-Guidelines-Final1.pdf. Last accessed April 24, 2018.

Disseminated Intravascular Coagulation (DIC)

Associated Conditions

Inflammatory/Toxic
- Acute hepatic injury
- Sepsis
- Acute kidney injury
- Fever of unknown origin
- Meningitis
- Pancreatitis
- Pneumonia
- Pyometra
- Snakebite
- Heatstroke

Immune-Mediated
- Immune-mediated thrombocytopenia
- Immune-mediated hemolytic anemia

Neoplastic
- Lymphoma
- Mammary adenocarcinoma/mammary tumor
- Hemangiosarcoma
- Splenic mass (type unknown)
- Heart base tumor
- Intra-abdominal sarcoma
- Malignant histiocytosis
- Mast cell tumor
- Oral carcinoma
- Perianal adenocarcinoma
- Pulmonary carcinoma
- Nasal squamous cell carcinoma
- Squamous papilloma (vulvar)
- Bladder tumor

Parasitic
- *Angiostrongylus vasorum* infection

Other
- Hemorrhagic gastroenteritis
- Cold agglutinin disease
- Multitrauma
- Gastric dilation/volvulus
- Diabetes mellitus

Dysphagia

Anatomic Location	Key Feature(s)
Oropharyngeal Dysphagia	Oral examination and observation of attempts to eat/drink Oral lesion: • Difficulty with prehension • Pain on prehension • Food dropping from mouth Pharyngeal/cricopharyngeal lesion: • Normal prehension • Repeated attempts to swallow • Choking/gagging common
Oral stage	Ddx: oral masses, retrobulbar abscess, FB, trauma (e.g., mandibular/maxillary fracture), TMJ disorders (luxation, fracture, craniomandibular osteopathy), dental pain, glossitis, stomatitis, cleft palate, lingual frenulum lesion, masticatory myositis, myopathy, cranial nerve V, VII, and XII dysfunction (any cause, including rabies) Consider: sedated/anesthetized oral exam, dental radiographs, survey skull/neck radiographs (special attention to mandibles, temporomandibular joint and teeth), advanced imaging (CT or MRI)
Pharyngeal stage	Ddx: pharyngeal inflammation (trauma, abscess, eosinophilic granuloma, pharyngeal sialocele), cranial nerve V, VII, IX, and X dysfunction, FB, lymphadenopathy, neoplasia Consider: palpate pharynx and neck for masses, asymmetry, or pain; sedated/anesthetized pharyngeal examination; pharyngeal region radiographs to rule out mass lesions, FB; barium contrast and video fluoroscopy (pharyngeal dysfunction)
Cricopharyngeal stage	Ddx: cricopharyngeal achalasia, cricopharyngeal asynchrony Consider: breed (cocker and springer spaniels, toy breeds, golden retrievers), differentiation via fluoroscopic contrast study
Esophageal Dysphagia	Characterized by regurgitation Ddx: primary (idiopathic) megaesophagus, secondary megaesophagus, esophageal stricture, extraesophageal compression (e.g., vascular ring anomaly), esophageal diverticulum Consider: cervical and thoracic radiograph (megaesophagus and to rule out aspiration pneumonia), esophagoscopy for esophagitis, FB (which can be retrieved) and strictures (which can be balloon-dilated), specific tests for cause of megaesophagus (if present)
Gastroesophageal Dysphagia	Ddx: reflux esophagitis, hiatal hernia, periesophageal hernia, gastroesophageal intussusception Consider: thoracic and abdominal radiographs, abdominal ultrasound, flouroscopy, endoscopy

Ddx, Differential diagnosis; *FB*, foreign body; *TMJ*, temporomandibular joint.
Reproduced from the third edition in modified form.

THIRD EDITION AUTHOR: Oriana D. Raab, DVM, DACVIM

Dyspnea

Upper Airway Disorders
- Nasal cavity*
  - Stenotic nares
  - Obstruction (infection, inflammation, neoplasia, trauma, bleeding disorder, foreign body)
- Pharynx, larynx
  - Elongated or edematous soft palate
  - Epiglottic retroversion
  - Pharyngeal polyp (cat > dog)
  - Laryngeal edema, collapse, foreign body, inflammation, trauma, paralysis, spasm, neoplasia, vocal-fold webbing
  - Pharyngeal collapse
  - Everted laryngeal saccules
- Cervical trachea
  - Collapse, stenosis
  - Trauma, foreign body
  - Neoplasia, osteochondral dysplasia
  - Parasites (*Oslerus osleri*)

Lower Airway Disorders
- Thoracic trachea (see Cervical trachea, above)
  - Extraluminal compression (lymphadenopathy, heart-based tumors, +/– enlarged left atrium)
- Bronchial disease (allergic, infectious, parasitic, chronic obstructive pulmonary disease)

Pulmonary Parenchymal Disorders
- Edema (cardiogenic, noncardiogenic)
- Pneumonia (infectious, parasitic, aspiration)
- Neoplasia
- Allergy (allergic pneumonitis, including heartworm)
- Eosinophilic (eosinophilic granuloma, eosinophilic bronchopneumopathy)
- Embolism (lymphoma or other neoplasia, dirofilariasis, hyperadrenocorticism, disseminated intravascular coagulation, immune-mediated hemolytic anemia, protein-losing nephropathy or enteropathy)
- Trauma, bleeding disorders

Pleural/Body Wall Disorders
- Pneumothorax
- Pleural effusion
- Congenital body wall disorders (pectus excavatum)
- Thoracic wall trauma
- Thoracic wall neoplasia
- Thoracic wall paralysis
- Diaphragmatic hernia (congenital, acquired)

Mediastinal Disorders
- Hemorrhage
- Infection
- Trauma, including pneumomediastinum
- Neoplasia (lymphoma, thymoma, other)

Peritoneal Cavity Disorders
- Organomegaly, obesity
- Effusion (marked)
- Gastric torsion, dilation/volvulus

Hemoglobin Disorders
- Anemia
- Methemoglobinemia
- Cyanosis

Miscellaneous
- Central nervous system (brain, spinal cord)
- Peripheral nerve, neuromuscular, muscular
- Metabolic (acidemia; severe hypokalemia in cats)
- Anxiety/fear
- Pain

*Only likely to cause dyspnea if the animal is a semiobligate nasal breather (e.g., cats).
Modified from Ettinger S, Feldman E: Textbook of veterinary internal medicine, ed 5, St. Louis, 2000, Saunders.

Dystocia: Causes

Causes in Bitches and Queens

Cause	Bitch (%)	Queen (%)
Maternal	75.3	67.1
Primary complete inertia	48.9	36.8
Primary partial inertia	23.1	22.6
Birth canal too narrow	1.1	5.2
Uterine torsion	1.1	—
Uterine prolapse	—	0.6
Uterine strangulation	—	0.6
Hydrallantois	0.5	—
Vaginal septum formation	0.5	—
Fetal	24.7	29.7
Malpresentations	15.4	15.5
Malformations	1.6	7.7
Fetal oversize	6.6	1.9
Fetal death	1.1	1.1

From Feldman EC, Nelson RW: Canine and feline endocrinology and reproduction, ed 3, St. Louis, 2004, Saunders.

Edema

Cause	Contributing Factor	Specific Clinical Syndromes
Increased hydrostatic pressure	Impaired venous return	Congestive heart failure (CHF) Pericardial disease (pericardial effusion, constrictive pericarditis, pericardial cyst or neoplasm) Portal hypertension Venous obstruction or compression (thrombosis, external pressure, extremity inactivity)
	Small-caliber arteriolar dilation	Heat Neurohumoral dysregulation
Reduced plasma oncotic pressure	Hypoproteinemia	Protein-losing nephropathy (amyloidosis, glomerulonephritis) Synthetic failure (chronic liver disease) Malnutrition Protein-losing gastroenteropathy
Lymphatic obstruction	Decreased lymphatic drainage of interstitium	Various inflammatory conditions Congenital (lymphedema) Neoplastic Postsurgical Postirradiation
Sodium retention	Excess dietary intake with renal insufficiency	
	Increased tubular sodium resorption	Renal hypoperfusion Increased renin-angiotensin-aldosterone secretion
Inflammation	Acute inflammation Chronic inflammation Angiogenesis Vasculitis	

Modified from Kumar V, et al, editors: Robbins and Cotran's Pathologic basis of disease, ed 8, Philadelphia, 2009, Saunders.

Differentials, Lists, and Mnemonics

Effusions

Parameter	Transudate	Modified Transudate	Exudate	Hemorrhage
Specific gravity	<1.018	1.018-1.025	>1.025	>1.025
Protein (g/dL)	<2.5	2.5-6.0	>2.5	>2.5
Appearance	Clear and watery	Clear to serosanguineous	Turbid, serosanguineous, serofibrinous	Serosanguineous, sanguineous
Cellularity (cells/mm^3)	<1000	>2500	>5000	>5000
Cytologic examination	Macrophages, mesothelial cells, and occasional neutrophils	Macrophages, mesothelial cells, and occasional neutrophils and erythrocytes	Variable	Primarily erythrocytes
Examples	Hypoalbuminemia (renal loss, GI loss, hepatic synthetic failure, massive skin wound/burn loss), prehepatic congestion/obstruction (e.g., portal vein thrombosis)	Heart failure, posthepatic vascular obstruction (e.g., caudal vena caval thrombosis), neoplasia, chyle	Septic (bacterial infection [aerobic, anaerobic]), nonseptic (e.g., FIP)	Anticoagulant rodenticide toxicosis, ruptured neoplasm, trauma

FIP, Feline infectious peritonitis; *GI*, gastrointestinal.
Modified with permission from Kittleson MD, Kienle RD, editors: Pericardial disease and cardiac neoplasia. In Small animal cardiovascular medicine, St. Louis, 1998, Mosby, p 420.

Effusions, Bicavitary

Conditions Associated With Bicavitary Effusions

Cardiovascular Conditions
- Cardiac tamponade: pericardial effusion of any cause (e.g., neoplastic, idiopathic, toxic [anticoagulant])
- Constrictive pericardial disease
- Right-sided congestive failure: dilated cardiomyopathy, tricuspid regurgitation of any cause (tricuspid dysplasia, myxomatous tricuspid valve disease/endocardiosis, other), severe pulmonic stenosis, cor pulmonale of any cause (heartworm disease/caval syndrome, idiopathic pulmonary hypertension, other), tricuspid valve stenosis
- Caudal vena cava thromboembolism or tumor

Congenital Obstruction
- Caudal vena cava, cor triatriatum dexter, Budd-Chiari syndrome

Hypoalbuminemia (Severe)
- Protein-losing nephropathy, protein-losing enteropathy, advanced hepatic disease, pancreatitis, extensive burns

Bleeding disorders (Secondary Hemostasis)
- DIC, hemophilia, rodenticide intoxication, hepatic failure

Bile Peritonitis (more often abdominal only)

Chylous effusion (more often pleural only)

Vasculitis
- FIP
- Rickettsial disease
- Immune-mediated vasculitis
- Uremic vasculitis

Neoplastic Conditions
- Right atrial fibroma
- Metastatic adenocarcinoma
- Lymphoma
- Hemangiosarcoma
- Mesothelioma
- Cholangiocellular carcinoma
- Chemodectoma
- Prostatic adenocarcinoma
- Diffuse carcinomatosis

DIC, Disseminated intravascular coagulation; *FIP*, feline infectious peritonitis.
Modified from Willard M, Tvedten H: Small animal clinical diagnosis by laboratory methods, ed 5, St. Louis, 2012, Saunders.

Endocarditis

Frequency of Isolation of Bacteria From Positive Blood Culture

Bacteria	Canine Endocarditis (% of Cases)
Gram Positive	
Staphylococcus pseudintermedius	6-33
Streptococcus spp	12-26
Corynebacterium spp	19
Gram Negative	
Escherichia coli	6-30
Bartonella spp	28
Anaerobic	
Propionibacterium acnes	6
Fusobacterium spp	6

Modified from Greene C: Infectious diseases of the dog and cat, ed 4, St. Louis, 2012, Saunders.

Eosinophilia: Potential Causes

Asthma (cats)
Atopic and related hypersensitivity disorders
Drug reaction (e.g., tetracycline)
Eosinophilic bronchopneumopathy (various syndromes)
Eosinophilic enterocolitis (allergic colitis)
Eosinophilic granuloma complex
Eosinophilic rhinitis/conjunctivitis
Hypereosinophilic syndrome, idiopathic
Hypoadrenocorticism (Addison's disease)
Infections (e.g., *Aspergillus* spp, *Pneumocystis carinii, Hepatozoon americanum*)
Leukemia, eosinophilic
Mast cell tumor/mastocytosis
Myositis, eosinophilic
Nonparasitic dermatologic disease
Panosteitis
Paraneoplastic (lymphoma, others)
Parasitism* (e.g., heartworm disease, gastrointestinal parasites, ectoparasites)
Pyometra
Uterine disease
Vasculitis, eosinophilic

*Most common cause.
Modified from Feldman E, Nelson R: Canine and feline endocrinology and reproduction, ed 3, St. Louis, 2004, Saunders.

Epistaxis

Cause	Salient Characteristics
Nasal Disease	
Neoplasia	Very common cause of acute and recurrent epistaxis. Carcinoma most common but mesenchymal, transmissible venereal tumors, and lymphoma also reported (lymphoma common in cats). Often starts unilateral but may become bilateral with time.
Trauma	Acute onset of epistaxis, often with suggestive history; physical examination may reveal other evidence of trauma
Foreign body	Such as grass awn; more likely in acute setting than recurrent; usually unilateral
Fungal infection	*Aspergillus* causes acute or recurrent epistaxis in dogs; bleeding due to fungal rhinitis less common in cats (*Cryptococcus, Rhinosporidium, Aspergillus).* Often starts unilateral but may become bilateral with time.
Other infection	Viral rhinitis or secondary bacterial infections are uncommon cause of epistaxis
Inflammation	Lymphoplasmacytic, eosinophilic, or neutrophilic rhinitis can cause unilateral or bilateral bleeding, usually recurrent.
Dental disease	Tooth root (periapical) abscess, oronasal fistulas; usually unilateral, recurrent
Vascular malformations	Arteriovenous fistulas; usually unilateral, recurrent
Systemic Disease	
Primary hemostatic disorder: thrombocytopenia	Other evidence of bleeding (petechiae, ecchymosis) commonly identified; confirmed by blood smear review
Primary hemostatic disorder thrombocytopathy	Petechiae and ecchymosis less consistently identified than with thrombocytopenia; may be detected by prolonged mucosal bleeding times, specific platelet function testing
Secondary hemostatic disorder	May be other evidence of bleeding, such as melena or hematuria. Prothrombin time (PT) and/or aPTT prolonged
Hyperviscosity	Marked erythrocytosis or hyperglobulinemia; may be evidence of underlying cause (e.g., multiple myeloma, ehrlichiosis, leishmaniasis)
Rickettsial disease	Expect additional evidence of illness. Serologic titers and/or PCR, as appropriate based on geographic area and clinical signs. Monocytic ehrlichiosis particularly important cause.
Leishmaniasis	Common cause of epistaxis in endemic areas; can cause hyperviscosity, thrombocytopenia
Systemic hypertension	Link with epistaxis not well documented in dogs or cats; ruled out by blood pressure measurement

Erythrocytosis

Relative
- Acute hemorrhagic diarrhea syndrome
- Dehydration
- Splenic contraction

Absolute
- Hypoxemia (respiratory disease, obesity, high altitude)
- Renal neoplasm
- Pyelonephritis
- Renal cyst
- Hydronephrosis
- Hepatoma
- Right-to-left shunting cardiovascular malformation (Eisenmenger's physiology)
  - Tetralogy of Fallot
  - Right-to-left patent ductus arteriosus
  - Septal defect with concurrent severe pulmonic stenosis or pulmonary hypertension
  - Double outlet right ventricle
  - Transposition of the great arteries
- Polycythemia vera

NOTE: Strictly speaking, the correct term is *erythrocytosis* (an increase in number of red blood cells). However, the term *polycythemia* (increase in numbers of all blood cell lines) still is used interchangeably.

Facial Muscle Wasting

Developmental	
• Muscular dystrophy	• X-linked, weakness and altered gait within first few weeks of age, glucocorticoids have no effect, clinical deterioration slows after 6 months
• Centronuclear myopathy	• Present between 2-6 months of age; DNA test is commercially available
• Dermatomyositis	• Myositis often develops after dermal lesions
Neuropathy	
• Idiopathic trigeminal neuropathy	• Lack of facial sensation on ipsilateral side of nerve lesion
• Brainstem lesion at level of trigeminal nerve (e.g., trigeminal nerve tumor)	• Other cranial nerves, particularly abducens and facial, may be affected; MRI required to support diagnosis
Infectious	Associated with generalized muscle atrophy and concurrent signs of primary disease
• Toxoplasmosis	• Rare
• Neosporosis	• Rare
• Hepatozoonosis	• More common in puppies, tick-borne
• Trypanosomiasis	• Endemic areas; diagnosis based on organism identification
• Leptospirosis	• Hepatic and renal dysfunction, possible coagulation defects
• Ehrlichiosis	• Concurrent thrombocytopenia, anemia, lymphadenopathy, leukopenia
• Leishmaniasis	• Endemic areas; lymphadenopathy
Immune-Mediated	
• Systemic lupus erythematosus	• Myositis occurs in only 6% of canine cases
• Paraneoplastic polymyositis	• Associated with boxers
• Idiopathic polymyositis	• Although cause is unknown, it may be associated with thymomas, cimetidine, trimethoprim-sulfas, or penicillamine
• Masticatory myositis	• Initial masticatory muscle swelling; early treatment allows better prognosis for functional recovery
Iatrogenic	
• Glucocorticoid administration	• Drug history important; associated with generalized muscle atrophy and other signs of hyperadrenocorticism, more commonly seen with chronic use (always use glucocorticoid at lowest effective dose)
Metabolic	Associated with findings specific for the differential
• Hyperadrenocorticism	• Polyuria/polydipsia, truncal alopecia, potbellied appearance common
• Cardiac cachexia	• Diffuse muscle atrophy, exercise intolerance, tachycardia, weak femoral pulses, ascites, coughing
Neoplastic	Cachexia and protein energy malnutrition resulting in diffuse muscle atrophy are features of many neoplastic and chronic inflammatory conditions
Disuse Atrophy	
• TMJ dysplasia	• TMJ radiographs or computed tomography required for diagnosis
• Traumatic luxation of the TMJ (cats)	• Associated with previous trauma
• TMJ ankylosis (cats)	• Associated with chronic inflammatory process of the TMJ

Reproduced from the third edition in modified form.

THIRD EDITION AUTHOR: Paolo Pazzi, BVSc, MMedVet, DECVIM-CA

Feline Leukemia Virus and Feline Immunodeficiency Virus: Associated Disorders

- Abortion/fetal resorption/thymic atrophy (FeLV ≫ FIV)
- Anemia; hemolytic/aplastic (FeLV ≫ FIV)
- Anisocoria
- Anterior uveitis/pars planitis/glaucoma (FIV ≫ FeLV)
- Behavioral changes/dementia
- Chronic fever
- Chronic progressive polyarthritis
- Diarrhea/panleukopenia-like syndrome
- Gingivitis/stomatitis (FIV > FeLV)
- Glomerulonephritis
- Hypergammaglobulinemia (FIV > FeLV)
- Immune-mediated disease
- Immunosuppression with opportunistic infections
- Lymphoma/lymphoid leukemias (FeLV ≫ FIV)
- Lymphopenia/neutropenia
- Myeloproliferative disease/erythroleukemia (FeLV ≫ FIV)
- Peripheral neuropathies
- Thrombocytopenia (FeLV ≫ FIV)
- Urinary incontinence
- Weight loss/cachexia

FeLV, Feline leukemia virus; *FIV,* feline immunodeficiency virus.
Modified from Ettinger S, Feldman E: Textbook of veterinary internal medicine, ed 5, St. Louis, 2000, Saunders.

Fever of Unknown Origin

Differential Diagnosis	Key Feature(s)
Localized Infections/Inflammation	
Abscess/cellulitis (bite wound, retrobulbar, apical tooth root, hepatic) (dog, cat)	Carefully palpate the entire patient for any swellings or painful sites. An original puncture/bite wound may no longer be apparent.
Cholangiohepatitis (cat), hepatitis (dog)	Patients present with weight loss, vomiting, anorexia, lethargy, and variable degrees of icterus. Ultrasonographic sludge in gallbladder highly suggestive (cats).
Discospondylitis (dog)	A collapsed intervertebral disc space with vertebral endplate erosion (radiographic) and spinal hyperpathia are suggestive.
Endocarditis (dog)	New-onset murmur, especially diastolic, is suggestive.
Osteomyelitis (dog, cat)	Perform radiographs when evaluating chronic draining tracts to evaluate for underlying osteolysis and proliferative bony changes.
Peritonitis (dog, cat)	Blood glucose levels >20 mg/dL (>1.1 mmol/L) compared to peritoneal fluid, and peritoneal fluid lactate levels >2.5 mmol/L compared to blood levels, are highly suggestive.
Pneumonia (dog, cat)	Patients with radiographic aspiration pattern suggesting pneumonia that do not have a history of vomiting should be evaluated for esophageal dysmotility.
Prostatitis (dog)	Extremely unlikely to occur in a castrated patient
Pyelonephritis (dog, cat)	May be present despite an unremarkable CBC, biochemical profile, and urine sediment
Pyometra (dog, cat)	All febrile female dogs should have imaging of the uterus or uterine stump.
Pyothorax (dog, cat)	"Sulfur granules" in the pleural fluid: highly suggestive of infection with either *Actinomyces* or *Nocardia*
Sepsis (dog, cat)	Persistent neutropenia or congenital/acquired immunodeficiency may predispose patients to sepsis without an apparent nidus for the infection.
Bacterial Infections	
Bartonellosis (dog, cat)	A new-onset heart murmur or generalized lymphadenopathy is suggestive.
Borreliosis (dog)	Shifting leg lameness and lymphadenopathy, proteinuria, or both are suggestive.
Brucellosis (dog)	Any intact male or female dog with a history of breeding should be screened.
Leptospirosis (dog)	Fever in combination with renal and/or hepatic insufficiency is suggestive.
Mycobacteriosis, L-form bacteria (cat)	Chronic, nonhealing skin lesions and draining tracts that do not respond to typical antibiotic therapy are suggestive.
Mycoplasmosis (dog, cat)	May cause respiratory signs or hemolytic anemia
Salmonellosis (dog, cat)	Severe, acute gastroenteritis in patients fed a raw food diet is suggestive.
Tularemia (cat > dog)	Patients may have a history of contact with rabbits or rabbit carcasses.
Yersiniosis (cat > dog)	Cats may have a history of hunting, ingesting wild rodents, or being exposed to fleas.
Viral Infections	
Canine distemper (dog)	Respiratory signs followed by gastrointestinal signs and central nervous system signs in an unvaccinated dog are suggestive.
Canine influenza (dog)	Respiratory signs and a history of exposure to high-density dog populations (e.g., dog show) are suggestive.

Continued

(Continued from previous page)

Differential Diagnosis	Key Feature(s)
Feline calicivirus, feline herpesvirus-1 (cat)	Fever may precede the development of classic upper respiratory signs.
Feline infectious peritonitis (cat)	A polyclonal gammopathy is suggestive. However, antemortem diagnosis can be elusive.
FeLV, FIV (cat)	All ill cats of unknown retrovirus status or cats with potential for exposure since last test (e.g., outdoor access) should be ELISA tested.
Rickettsial Infections	
Salmon poisoning (dog)	Hemorrhagic gastroenteritis and lymphadenopathy occurring in dogs in the Pacific northwestern United States are suggestive.
Tick-borne disease (anaplasmosis, ehrlichiosis, Rocky Mountain spotted fever) (dog)	Generalized lymphadenopathy, petechiae/ecchymoses, and cytopenias in endemic areas are suggestive.
Fungal Infections	
Systemic aspergillosis (dog)	A German shepherd dog with chronic weight loss, neurologic deficits, radiographic evidence of bony lesions or discospondylitis is suggestive.
Systemic mycoses (blastomycosis, coccidioidomycosis, cryptococcosis, histoplasmosis) (dog, cat)	Respiratory, gastrointestinal, or neurologic signs with pyogranulomatous infection in endemic areas are suggestive.
Protozoal	
Babesiosis (dog)	Hemolytic anemia in a dog with a history of tick exposure, recent blood transfusion, dogfighting, or splenectomy is suggestive.
Cytauxzoonosis (cat)	Fever, jaundice, and pallor in an outdoor cat in endemic areas are suggestive.
Hepatozoonosis (dog)	Extreme leukocytosis with cachexia, myalgia, and periosteal reaction in endemic areas is suggestive.
Leishmaniasis (dog)	Chronic weight loss, lymphadenopathy, ulcerative skin lesions, uveitis, and epistaxis are suggestive.
Neosporosis (dog)	Acute, ascending paralysis in puppies is typical.
Toxoplasmosis (dog, cat)	Respiratory, CNS, or ocular signs with a positive IgM titer are suggestive.
Trypanosomiasis (dog)	Fever can occur in the acute stage of infection, before the onset of dilated cardiomyopathy.
Immune-Mediated	
Immune-mediated hemolytic anemia (dog, cat)	Spherocytosis, anemia, and positive agglutination test are suggestive.
Immune-mediated neutropenia (dog)	Primary immune-mediated neutropenia is a diagnosis of exclusion of other causes of neutropenia.
Immune-mediated polyarthritis (dog, cat)	May not cause clinically apparent joint swelling and is a very common cause of FUO; therefore, arthrocentesis should be considered in the diagnostic workup of all FUO cases.
Immune-mediated thrombocytopenia (dog, cat)	Most likely cause of severe thrombocytopenia (<25,000/mcL) in an otherwise healthy-appearing animal
Steroid-responsive meningitis-arteritis (dog)	"Walking on eggshells" gait in a young adult dog is suggestive.
Meningoencephalitis (granulomatous, necrotizing) (dog)	Forebrain neurologic signs in a small-breed dog are suggestive.
Pemphigus (dog, cat)	Progressive dermatitis that does not respond to antibiotic treatment and edema of the limbs in a middle-aged patient is suggestive.
Systemic lupus erythematosus (dog, cat)	Manifestations can vary from patient to patient, but polyarthritis is the most common clinical sign.
Rheumatoid arthritis (dog, cat)	Polyarthritis with erosion of articular cartilage is suggestive.
Vasculitis (dog, cat)	Erythema and edema of the skin, particularly in gravity-dependent areas
Inflammatory	
Hypertrophic osteodystrophy (dog)	"Double physeal" line on long-bone radiographs is pathognomonic.
Juvenile cellulitis (dog)	Facial swelling and pustules with granulomatous lymphadenitis in a puppy are suggestive.
Pancreatitis (dog, cat)	Measurement of species-specific serum pancreatic lipase immunoreactivity is the most sensitive and specific laboratory test currently available, but the final diagnosis requires integration of all clinical data available.
Panniculitis (dog)	Painful subcutaneous swellings or nodules that may have developed draining tracts are suggestive.
Panosteitis (dog)	Patchy areas of increased intramedullary opacity of the long bones in young large-breed dogs are suggestive.
Pansteatitis (dog, cat)	A diet containing large amounts of raw fish is suggestive.
Neoplastic	
Solid tumors (dog, cat)	Tumors that are necrotic, elicit an inflammatory response, or have widespread metastases are more likely to cause a fever.
Hematopoietic tumors (histiocytic sarcoma, lymphoma, leukemia, myeloma) (dog, cat)	Fever may be intermittent or continuous.

(Continued from previous page)

Differential Diagnosis	Key Feature(s)
Miscellaneous	
Drug reaction/toxin (e.g., penicillins, sulfas, tetracyclines) (dog, cat)	A detailed drug and supplement history should be obtained from all patients with FUO.
Hyperthyroidism (cat ≫ dog)	Weight loss, gastrointestinal signs, tachycardia, behavioral change, and increased shedding are suggestive.
Hypothalamic disease (dog, cat)	Patients with a hypothalamic lesion may also exhibit changes in appetite and endocrine disturbances.
Portosystemic shunt (dog, cat)	Elevated postprandial bile acids are suggestive.
Shar-pei fever (dog)	Self-limiting fever and hock swelling in a Shar-pei are suggestive.

NOTE: The unit of measure of micron, sometimes denoted by the Greek letter μ, is abbreviated in this text by mc. For example, 1 mcL = 1 microliter; 1 mcg = 1 microgram.
CBC, Complete blood count; *CNS,* central nervous system; *ELISA,* enzyme-linked immunosorbent assay; *FeLV,* feline leukemia virus; *FIV,* feline immunodeficiency virus; *FUO,* fever of unknown origin.

AUTHOR: Karen M. Tefft, DVM, MVSc, DACVIM

Flatulence

Differential Diagnosis Item	Key Feature(s)
Anatomic	Excessive aerophagia (risk factor for flatulence) is common in brachycephalic breeds. Surgical correction of stenotic nares and elongated soft palate may help reduce aerophagia.
Dietary	Substrates for bacterial gas production include dietary fiber (decreased dry matter digestibility), poorly digestible protein, and carbohydrates (notably non-absorbable oligosaccharides [e.g., raffinose]). Fresh or dried foods containing fructose, resistant starches, and fermentable fiber can also increase intestinal gas production (e.g., apples, prunes, and bananas), as can dietary sources high in sulfur and/or protein (e.g., nuts, spices, cruciferous vegetables). Aerophagia may be reduced by feeding several small meals daily rather than a single large meal; feeding in quiet, isolated areas; and feeding a mixture of moist and dry foods.
Activity/Exercise	Dogs should be allowed out to relieve themselves within 30 minutes of meals to encourage defecation and elimination of gas. Active outdoor dogs have been shown to exhibit less flatulence while with owners; however, vigorous exercise, as observed in working and sporting canine breeds, may lead to excessive gastrointestinal gas.

Reproduced from the third edition in unabridged form.

THIRD EDITION AUTHOR: Oriana D. Raab, DVM, DACVIM

Gastrointestinal Ulceration

Conditions Associated with GI Ulceration in Small Animals

Drugs
- NSAIDs*
- Corticosteroids

Stress
- Shock
- Sepsis
- Trauma
- Major surgery

Neurologic Disease
- Head trauma
- Intervertebral disc disease†

Metabolic Disorders
- Liver disease
- Uremia
- Hypoadrenocorticism
- DIC

Inflammatory Bowel Disease

GI Neoplasia
- Solid tumors (leiomyoma, adenocarcinoma)
- Lymphoma
- Mast cell tumor (anywhere; degranulation causes ulceration)
- Gastrinoma and other APUDomas

Gastric Motility Disorders

Miscellaneous Disorders
- Endurance exercise (sled dogs)
- GI foreign body
- *Helicobacter* infection (role undetermined)
- Caustic substance ingestion

*NSAIDs that have been associated with GI ulcers in small animals include aspirin, indomethacin, phenylbutazone, flunixin, ibuprofen, deracoxib, meloxicam, naproxen, piroxicam, firocoxib, ketorolac, and meclofenamic acid.
†Treated with corticosteroids.
APUDoma, Amine precursor uptake and decarboxylase neoplasm; *DIC,* disseminated intravascular coagulation; *GI,* gastrointestinal; *NSAIDs,* nonsteroidal antiinflammatory drugs.
Modified from Ettinger S, Feldman E: Textbook of veterinary internal medicine, ed 7, St. Louis, 2010, Saunders.

Genetic and Hereditary Disease Testing

For current information on available genetic disease testing in pets, see the PennGen website: https://www.vet.upenn.edu/research/academic-departments/clinical-sciences-advanced-medicine/research-labs-centers/penngen/tests-worldwide

Glomerular Diseases, Cats

Associated Diseases Reported in Cats

Infectious
- Bacterial
  - Chronic bacterial infections
  - Mycoplasmal polyarthritis
- Viral
  - FIV
  - FIP (MN)
  - FeLV (MN)

Inflammatory
- Pancreatitis
- Cholangiohepatitis
- Chronic progressive polyarthritis
- SLE (MN)
- Other immune-mediated diseases

Neoplastic
- Leukemia (MN)
- Lymphoma (MN)
- Mastocytosis
- Other neoplasms

Miscellaneous
- Acromegaly (?)
- Mercury toxicosis (MN)

Familial (MN)

Idiopathic (MN)

FeLV, Feline leukemia virus; *FIP,* feline infectious peritonitis; *FIV,* feline immunodeficiency virus; *MN,* membranous nephropathy; *SLE,* systemic lupus erythematosus; *?,* uncertain association.
From Ettinger S, Feldman E: Textbook of veterinary internal medicine, ed 7, St. Louis, 2010, Saunders.

Glomerulonephritis, Dogs

Associated Diseases Reported in Dogs

Infectious
- Bacterial
  - Bartonellosis
  - Borreliosis (MPGN)
  - Brucellosis
  - Endocarditis
  - Pyometra
  - Pyoderma
  - Other chronic bacterial infections
- Rickettsial
  - Ehrlichiosis
  - Anaplasmosis
- Protozoal
  - Babesiosis (MPGN)
  - Hepatozoonosis
  - Leishmaniasis (MPGN, MN, P-E, and P-M)
  - Trypanosomiasis
- Viral
  - Canine adenovirus type 1 (P-M)
- Parasitic
  - Dirofilariasis (MPGN, MN)
- Fungal
  - Blastomycosis
  - Coccidioidomycosis

Inflammatory
- Chronic dermatitis
- Inflammatory bowel disease
- Pancreatitis
- Periodontal disease
- Polyarthritis
- SLE (MPGN, MN, P-E, and P-M)
- Other immune-mediated diseases

Neoplastic
- Leukemia
- Lymphoma
- Mastocytosis
- Primary erythrocytosis (MCD?)
- Systemic histiocytosis
- Other neoplasms

Miscellaneous
- Corticosteroid excess
- Trimethoprim-sulfa therapy
- Hyperlipidemia (?)
- Congenital C3 deficiency
- Cyclic hematopoiesis
- Mercury toxicity

Familial
- Beagle
- Bernese mountain dog
- Bull terrier
- Bullmastiff
- Cocker spaniel
- Dalmatian
- Doberman pinscher
- English foxhound
- French mastiff
- Greyhound
- Newfoundland
- Pembroke Welsh corgi
- Rottweiler
- Samoyed
- Shar-pei
- Soft-coated wheaten terrier

Idiopathic (MN, MCD, P-E, or M)

MCD, Minimal change disease; *MN,* membranous nephropathy; *MPGN,* membranoproliferative (mesangiocapillary) glomerulonephritis; *P,* proliferative (*E,* endocapillary; *M,* mesangial); *SLE,* systemic lupus erythematosus; *?,* association uncertain.
Modified from Ettinger S, Feldman E: Textbook of veterinary internal medicine, ed 7, St. Louis, 2012, Saunders.

Glucosuria

Causes in Dogs and Cats

Blood glucose concentration exceeding renal threshold (common)	Diabetes mellitus Stress (especially in cats) Infusion of dextrose-containing fluids Hyperadrenocorticism (rarely causes glucose >180 mg/dL [>10 mmol/L]) Pheochromocytoma (rare)
Abnormal proximal renal tubular function	Aminoglycoside toxicosis Acute kidney injury Fanconi syndrome Primary renal glucosuria
Contamination	Urinary hemorrhage in an animal with mild hyperglycemia
Artifact	Pseudoglucosuria in cats with urethral obstruction

From Willard M, Tvedten H: Small animal clinical diagnosis by laboratory methods, ed 5, St. Louis, 2012, Saunders.

Halitosis

Oral Diseases
- Periodontal disease (gingivitis, periodontitis, abscessation)
- Neoplasia (melanoma, fibrosarcoma, SCC)
- Foreign body or trauma (fractures, electrical cord injury)
- Pharyngitis
- Stomatitis, lymphocytic-plasmacytic feline stomatitis

Respiratory Diseases
- Rhinitis and/or sinusitis
- Neoplasia
- Pneumonia or pulmonary abscess

Dermatologic Diseases
- Lip fold pyoderma
- Ulcerative mucocutaneous pyoderma
- Feline or canine eosinophilic granulomas
- Pemphigus complex, bullous pemphigoid, systemic lupus erythematosus
- Drug eruptions
- Cutaneous lymphoma
- Exposure to DMSO

Metabolic Diseases
- Uremia
- Diabetic ketoacidosis

Gastrointestinal Diseases
- Megaesophagus
- Inflammatory bowel disease
- Exocrine pancreatic insufficiency
- Neoplasia
- Constipation

Dietary
- Aromatic foods (onions, garlic)
- Fetid foodstuffs (e.g., ingestion of carrion)
- Coprophagy

Grooming Behavior
- Anal sacculitis
- Vaginitis/balanoposthitis
- Lower UTI

DMSO, Dimethyl sulfoxide; *SCC,* squamous cell carcinoma; *UTI,* urinary tract infection.
Adapted from Veterinary clinical guide to odor and disease: the oral cavity and dermatology, Yardley, PA, 1997, Veterinary Learning Systems.

Heart Murmur, Nonpathologic: Mnemonic

The 6 S's

Soft—usually grade 1 or 2/6
Systolic—invariably systolic in nature
Short—early to midsystole; does not cover the first or second heart sound
Single—no additional audible abnormalities (e.g., no click, gallop, arrhythmia)
Sensitive—intensity less at rest than with exercise; may change with positioning or phase of respiration
Small—limited to one location, typically the left heart base; does not radiate

Modified from Bronzetti G, Corzani A. The seven "S" murmurs: an alliteration about innocent murmurs in cardiac auscultation. Clin Pediatr (Phila). 49:713, 2010, © 2010 by SAGE Publications. Reprinted by permission of SAGE Publications, and Côté E, Edwards NJ, Ettinger SJ, et al. Management of incidentally detected heart murmurs in dogs and cats. J Am Vet Med Assoc 246:1076-1088, 2015.

Heart Murmurs: Nonpathologic Versus Pathologic

Characteristics Associated With Nonpathologic Heart Murmurs Versus Murmurs Associated With Congenital Heart Disease

Nonpathologic ("Innocent," "Juvenile," "Benign") Murmur
- Grade usually < III/VI
- Systolic
- PMI: usually left base
- Murmur characteristics may change with animal position
- Murmur intensity may increase or decrease with increasing heart rate
- Decreased intensity (or full resolution) with age
- Generally inaudible after ≈16 weeks of age
- Animal clinically normal

Congenital Heart Disease
- Any grade
- Any timing possible
- PMI: any possible
- Similar murmur characteristics in all body positions
- Murmur intensity increases with increase in heart rate
- Same or increasing intensity up to and beyond 16 weeks of age
- Persists after ≈16 weeks of age
- Stunting, unthriftiness, cyanosis, or signs of heart failure may be present

PMI, Point of maximal murmur intensity.
Modified from Côté E, Edwards NJ, Ettinger SJ, et al. Management of incidentally detected heart murmurs in dogs and cats. J Am Vet Med Assoc 246:1076-1088, 2015.

Differentials, Lists, and Mnemonics

Heartworm Disease: Complications

Untreated
- Eosinophilic granulomatosis
- Eosinophilic pneumonitis
- Right-sided congestive heart failure*
- Hemoglobinuria, "pigment nephropathy"*
- Hemolytic anemia*
- Pulmonary thromboembolism

During or Shortly After Treatment Period

Acute (Surgical Removal)
- Anaphylaxis
- Hypotension
- Cardiac arrest

Subacute (Medical Treatment)
- Eosinophilic pneumonitis
- Pain at injection site (melarsomine)
- Pulmonary thromboembolism (possibly massive, especially if inadequate exercise restriction)
- Sudden death (especially if inadequate exercise restriction)

*Together, comprise the "caval syndrome" of heartworm disease.

Hematemesis

Coagulopathy (1o, 2o, or Mixed)
- Disseminated intravascular coagulation
- Thrombocytopenia/thrombocytopathy
- Congenital coagulation factor deficiencies
- Acquired coagulation factor disorders (e.g., anticoagulant exposure)

Upper Airway Bleeding
- Nasal neoplasia
- Aspergillosis
- Inflammatory rhinitis

Esophageal Disorders
- Esophagitis
- Esophageal neoplasia
- Esophageal foreign bodies

Gastric or Duodenal Ulcerations
- Drugs (e.g., NSAIDs, glucocorticoids)
- Uremia
- Hepatic failure
- Hypoadrenocorticism
- Gastrinoma
- Mastocytosis/mast cell tumor
- Exercise induced (sled dogs)
- Spinal surgery/severe stress
- Sepsis, shock

Gastric/Duodenal Foreign Bodies

Hemorrhagic Gastroenteritis

Heavy Metal Intoxication

Infectious Disorders
- GI parasitism
- Viral gastroenteritis
- Bacterial gastroenteritis

Perioperative Hemorrhage

Infiltrative Disease
- Neoplasia
- Inflammatory bowel disease
- Phycomycosis

Metabolic Disorders
- Renal disease
- Liver disease
- Hypoadrenocorticism

Neoplastic GI Disease
- Gastric neoplasia
- Esophageal neoplasia

GI, Gastrointestinal; *NSAIDs*, nonsteroidal antiinflammatory drugs.

Hematochezia

Causes of Hematochezia

Unclassified
- Acute hemorrhagic diarrhea syndrome (formerly hemorrhagic gastroenteritis)

Inflammatory
- Inflammatory bowel disease
- Histiocytic ulcerative colitis
- Idiopathic colitis
- Perianal fistula
- Mucocutaneous lupus erythematosus

Infectious
- Bacterial: *Campylobacter, Clostridium, Mycobacterium, Salmonella*
- Fungal/algal: *Cryptococcus, Histoplasma, Pythium, Prototheca*
- Parasitic: *Ancylostoma, Uncinaria, Trichuris,* coccidia, *Tritrichomonas, Leishmania, Heterobilharzia americana, Entamoeba histolytica*
- Viral: parvovirus

Ischemic/Traumatic
- Hypovolemic shock
- Thrombosis/infarction
- Intussusception
- Cecal inversion
- Volvulus
- Foreign body
- Pelvic fracture
- Rectoanal stricture
- Racing sled dogs

Drug-Induced
- Glucocorticoids
- Nonsteroidal antiinflammatory drugs
- Cytotoxic chemotherapy drugs

Neoplastic
- Adenocarcinoma
- Gastrointestinal stromal tumor
- Leiomyoma/leiomyosarcoma
- Lymphoma
- Plasmacytoma
- Colorectal polyp

Vascular
- Vascular ectasia/angiodysplasia
- Arteriovenous fistula

Metabolic
- Hypoadrenocorticism
- Uremic kidney disease
- Liver disease, particularly with portal hypertension or portosystemic shunt(s)
- Pancreatitis

Bleeding Disorder
- Thrombocytopenia
- Thrombocytopathia
- Disseminated intravascular coagulation
- Rodenticide intoxication
- Specific factor deficiencies

Modified from Tefft KM: Melena and hematochezia. In Ettinger SJ, Feldman EC, Côté E, editors: Textbook of veterinary internal medicine: diseases of the dog and cat, ed 8, St. Louis, 2017, Elsevier.

Hematuria

Urinary Tract Origin (Kidneys, Ureters, Bladder, Urethra)

- Trauma
  - Traumatic collection (e.g., catheter, cystocentesis)
  - Renal biopsy
  - Blunt trauma (e.g., hit by car)
- Urolithiasis
- Neoplasia (any area of genitourinary tract)
- Inflammatory disease
- Urinary tract infection
- Feline lower urinary tract signs/disease/interstitial cystitis
- Chemically induced inflammation (e.g., cyclophosphamide-induced cystitis)
- Glomerulonephritis*
- Parasites
  - *Dioctophyma renale*
  - *Capillaria plica*
- Bleeding disorder
  - Anticoagulant intoxication
  - Disseminated intravascular coagulation
  - Hemophilia
  - Hepatic failure
  - Thrombocytopenia
- Renal infarction
- Renal granuloma
- Renal pelvic hematoma
- Polycystic kidneys*
- Renal dysplasia*
- Vascular malformation
  - Renal telangiectasia (Welsh corgi)
  - Idiopathic renal hematuria

Genital Tract Contamination

- Estrus
- Uterine subinvolution
- Inflammatory, neoplastic, and traumatic lesions of the prostate, prepuce, or vagina

*Often only microscopic hematuria.
Modified from Ettinger S, Feldman E: Textbook of veterinary internal medicine, ed 6, St. Louis, 2005, Saunders.

Hemoptysis

Differential Diagnosis Item	Key Feature(s)
Airway foreign body	Often acute onset; history may be suggestive (e.g., hunting in tall grass), tracheobronchoscopy useful
Bacterial pneumonia	Systemic signs common, underlying/predisposing cause (e.g., regurgitation, bronchiectasis) common
Bronchiectasis	Uncommonly causes hemoptysis; history of chronic cough or respiratory disease
Chronic bronchitis	Uncommonly causes hemoptysis unless coughing is extreme
Coagulation factor deficiency	May be other sites of bleeding; confirm by coagulation profile (PT, aPTT)
Congestive heart failure	Severe respiratory distress and expectoration of bloody fluid or foam from left-sided failure, heart murmur and harsh/loud lung sounds, crackles on auscultation
Eosinophilic bronchopneumopathy	Uncommonly causes hemoptysis; peripheral eosinophilia possible
Fungal pneumonia	Likelihood of diagnosis depends on geography, travel history, lifestyle, history of recent soil excavation, etc. Thoracic radiographs: multiple pulmonary patterns can occur, but multifocal nodular pattern can be confused with metastatic neoplasia.
Heartworm infection	Uncommonly causes hemoptysis; consider geography, travel, and deworming history
Iatrogenic	Consistent patient history (e.g., intubation, lung aspirate, or biopsy)
Lung lobe torsion	Emergent condition, often with pleural effusion; Afghan hound and pug overrepresented
Neoplasia (primary)	Pulmonary or tracheal; nodule or mass identified on thoracic radiographs
Neoplasia (metastatic)	Weight loss common, other tumor may be identified on exam (e.g., splenic hemangiosarcoma), thoracic radiographs highly suggestive
Parasitic infection	Consider geography, travel, and deworming history
Pulmonary hypertension	Uncommonly causes hemoptysis; echocardiographic identification of high-velocity tricuspid regurgitation
Pulmonary thromboembolism	Uncommonly causes hemoptysis; diagnosis can be challenging; predisposing causes (e.g., heartworm disease, systemic hypercoagulable states) are important clues
Thrombocytopenia/thrombocytopathy	Uncommonly causes hemoptysis; petechiae/ecchymosis often seen
Trauma	Patient history and lifestyle (e.g., off leash, roaming behavior), physical evidence of trauma

Reproduced from the third edition in modified form.

THIRD EDITION AUTHOR: **Kelly Mitchell, DVM, DVSc, DACVIM**

Hemothorax

Trauma	Pulmonary abscessation	Costal exostosis*
Malignancy	Recent surgery	Endometriosis*
Bleeding disorder	Aortic aneurysm	Foreign body
Diaphragmatic hernia	Swan-Ganz catheter placement*	Heartworm disease
Lung lobe torsion	Tube thoracostomy*	Central venous catheter placement
Pulmonary infarction	Hemopneumothorax*	

*Reported only in human literature.
Modified with permission from King L: Textbook of respiratory disease in dogs and cats, St. Louis, 2004, Saunders, p 611.

Hepatic Infections and Abscesses

Aerobic Cultures (n = 659) (Positive Cultures: n = 171)*

n ≥ 30 each
- *Escherichia coli*
- *Enterococcus* spp

n ≥ 10
- *Staphylococcus pseudintermedius*
- *Streptococcus* group D enterococci

n ≥ 5 each
- *Klebsiella pneumoniae*
- *Staphylococcus aureus*
- Beta-hemolytic streptococci
- *Serratia marcescens*
- *Staphylococcus epidermidis*
- *Enterobacter aerogenes*
- *Pseudomonas aeruginosa*
- *Citrobacter freundii*

n = 2 each*
- *Acinetobacter* spp
- *Candida* spp
- *Enterobacter agglomerans*
- *Pasteurella multocida*
- *Pseudomonas fluorescens*
- *Nocardia*
- *Bacillus* spp

n = 1 each
- *Bordetella bronchiseptica*
- *Campylobacter jejuni*
- *Escherichia hermanii*
- *Klebsiella oxytoca*
- *Lactobacillus*
- *Moraxella phenylpyruvica*
- *Morganella morganii*
- *Prevotella* (previously a *Bacteroides*)
- *Proteus*
- *Pseudomonas fluorescens*
- Beta-hemolytic *Streptococcus*
- *Staphylococcus* spp
- *Salmonella*

Anaerobic Cultures (n = 569) (Positive Cultures: n = 71)*

n ≥ 10 each
- *Clostridium perfringens*
- *Clostridium* spp
- *Propionibacterium acnes*

n ≥ 4 each*
- *Actinomyces*
- *Corynebacterium* spp
- *Bacteroides* spp
- *Peptostreptococcus*

n = 1 each
- *Fusobacterium*
- Anaerobic streptococci
- *Bacillus*

Additional Microbes Reported Elsewhere (Case Reports)
- *Bacillus piliformis*
- *Francisella tularensis*
- *Listeria monocytogenes*
- *Neisseria* spp (Eugenic fermenter-4 bacilli)

Other Proven Noncultured Infectious Agents Based on Antibody Titers, Histopathology, and/or Molecular Testing and Response to Treatment
- *Leptospira* serovars
- *Borrelia burgdorferi*
- *Ehrlichia* spp
- *Rickettsia rickettsii*
- *Toxoplasma gondii*
- *Babesia* spp
- Trematodes

*In order from most to least common.
Data acquired from case records from 1985 to 2010, Companion Animal Hospital, College of Veterinary Medicine, Cornell University, Ithaca, NY.
From Greene C: Infectious diseases of the dog and cat, ed 4, St. Louis, 2012, Saunders.

Hepatic Neoplasia

Dogs*

Primary Hepatic Tumors (26%)
- Hepatocellular carcinoma
- Hepatocellular adenoma
- Hepatic hemangiosarcoma
- Biliary carcinoma

Other
- Leiomyosarcoma
- Liposarcoma
- Myxosarcoma
- Fibrosarcoma
- Biliary adenoma
- Hepatic carcinoid

Hemolymphatic Neoplasia (28%)
- Lymphoma
- MCT
- Plasma cell tumor

Metastatic Neoplasia (46%)

Cats

***Primary Hepatic Tumors (20%)**
- Biliary carcinoma
- Hepatocellular carcinoma
- Hepatic hemangiosarcoma

Other
- Biliary cystadenoma
- Myelolipoma
- Hepatic carcinoid

Hemolymphatic Neoplasia (60%)
- Lymphoma
- MCT
- Plasma cell tumor

Metastatic Neoplasia (20%)

*Primary tumors: in order of prevalence, from most prevalent to least.
MCT, Mast cell tumor.
From Ettinger S, Feldman E: Textbook of veterinary internal medicine, ed 6, St. Louis, 2005, Saunders.

Hepatomegaly

Category	Differential Diagnosis (examples)
Benign causes	Nodular hyperplasia, extramedullary hematopoiesis, individual variation
Breed related	Bedlington terrier, Labrador retriever, Doberman pinscher, cocker spaniels
Congestion	Right heart failure, cardiac tamponade, Budd-Chiari syndrome, liver lobe torsion, veno-occlusive disease
Drugs or toxins	Glucocorticoids, phenobarbital, numerous other drugs and hepatotoxins
Endocrine	Hyperadrenocorticism, diabetes mellitus
Immune mediated	Immune-mediated hemolytic anemia, immune-mediated thrombocytopenia
Inflammatory	Cholangitis/cholangiohepatitis complex (cat), chronic hepatitis (dog)
Infectious	Bacterial: bartonellosis, leptospirosis, abscess, many others
	Viral: feline infectious peritonitis, canine adenovirus-1
	Protozoal: toxoplasmosis, cytauxzoonosis, babesiosis
	Fungal: histoplasmosis, coccidioidomycosis
	Parasitic: hepatic fluke, visceral larval migrans, *Heterobilharzia americana*
Neoplastic	Hepatic: hepatocellular carcinoma, malignant histiocytosis, bile duct carcinoma
	Metastatic: lymphoma, mast cell tumor
Metabolic	Hepatic lipidosis, amyloidosis, lysosomal storage disorder
Miscellaneous	"Hepatotracheal syndrome" (airway-associated liver disease), cystic disorders
Mistaken identity	Splenomegaly, pancreatic mass, non-hepatic granuloma, thoracic structures pushing liver caudad (e.g., deep inspiration, emphysema, pleural effusion), brachycephalic/chondrodystrophic confirmation

Hepatotoxins

Drugs

(For additional details see *Hepatotoxic Drugs in Dogs and Cats,* section 3, web content.)

- Acetaminophen
- Amiodarone
- Aspirin
- Azathioprine
- Azole antifungal drugs
- Benzodiazepines
- Carprofen
- Diazepam (cats)
- Griseofulvin (cats)
- Halothane
- Intranasal *Bordetella* injections given IM/SQ
- Iron
- Itraconazole
- Ketoconazole
- Lomustine
- Methimazole
- Phenobarbital
- Phenytoin
- Primidone
- Tetracyclines
- Trimethoprim sulfa (dogs)

Plants

- *Amanita* mushrooms and other genera
- Blue-green algae (*Microcystis* cyanobacteria)
- Cycad palms (Sago palms)
- Castor bean seeds (used in jewelry)
- Many others not commonly ingested by pets

Other

- Aflatoxins
- Carbon tetrachloride
- Dimethylnitrosamine
- Envenomation
- Fungicides (some types)
- Heavy metals (Cu, Fe, Pb)
- Herbicides (some types)
- Insecticides (some types)
- Metaldehyde
- Organic solvents (e.g., CCl_4)
- Phenol (clay pigeons, roofing material, Lysol products)
- Rodenticides (some types)
- Xylitol
- Zinc phosphide
- β-methylamino L-alanine

Horner's Syndrome

Location	Example of Lesion	Associated Neurologic Deficit
Cervical spinal cord	Focal myelopathy External injury Fibrocartilaginous embolism Intervertebral disc disease	Spastic tetraplegia, dyspnea Spastic hemiplegia
T1–T3 spinal cord	Focal myelopathy External injury Fibrocartilaginous embolism Neoplasia Diffuse myelomalacia	Tetraparesis and ataxia, or tetraplegia, with LMN deficit in thoracic limbs and UMN and GP deficits in pelvic limb
T1–T3 ventral roots, proximal spinal nerves	Avulsion of roots of brachial plexus Lymphoma	LMN paresis or paralysis of the ipsilateral thoracic limb with variable loss of nociception
Cranial thoracic sympathetic trunk, cervicothoracic ganglion, middle cervical ganglion	Lymphoma Nerve sheath neoplasm Abscess	None if confined to the trunk or ganglia
Cervical sympathetic trunk	Injury by surgery, jugular venipuncture, dog bites	None if unilateral; bilateral lesions interfere with laryngeal and esophageal functions because of vagal nerve involvement
Middle ear cavity	Otitis media Neoplasia	Clinical signs of peripheral vestibular dysfunction; ipsilateral ataxia, head tilt, abnormal nystagmus, facial paresis or paralysis, facial tetanus
Retrobulbar	Injury, abscess Neoplasm	Varies with degree of involvement of optic and oculomotor nerves, which influence pupillary size and vision

LMN, Lower motor neuron; *GP*, general proprioceptive; *UMN*, upper motor neuron.
Modified from de Lahunta A, Glass E: Veterinary neuroanatomy and clinical neurology, ed 3, St. Louis, 2009, Saunders.

Hypercalcemia

Condition	Characteristic Feature
Lymphoma	Usually mediastinal
Chronic kidney disease (CKD)	Less than 5% of all CKD cases
Primary hyperparathyroidism	Rarely clinically ill; PU/PD is primary complaint
Hypoadrenocorticism	Increase in Ca parallels increase in K
Vitamin D toxicosis	Increases in both Ca and PO_4
Apocrine gland carcinoma of the anal sacs	Careful rectal palpation of all hypercalcemic dogs
Multiple myeloma	Often dramatic increase in serum globulins
Variety of other carcinomas	Dogs are usually ill
Idiopathic (feline)	Diagnosis of exclusion

PU/PD, Polyuria/polydipsia.
Reproduced from the third edition in unabridged form.

THIRD EDITION AUTHOR: **Edward C. Feldman, DVM, DACVIM**

Hypercalcemia: Laboratory Findings

	PTH	PTHrP	Ionized Calcium	Phosphorus	Vitamin D	BUN
Parathyroid adenoma	N to +++	–	+++	–	N/++	N/+
Hypercalcemia of malignancy	–	++	++	–	N	N/+
Hypoadrenocorticism	N	N	+	N/+	N	N/+
Vitamin D toxicosis	–	–	+++	++	+++	N/+
Renal secondary hyperparathyroidism	++	N/++	+	++	N	+++
Granulomatous disease	–/N	?	+	N	N/+	N
Parathyroid hyperplasia	N to +++	–	+++	–	N/++	N/+

BUN, Blood urea nitrogen; *N,* normal blood concentration; *PTH,* parathyroid hormone; *PTHrP,* PTH-related protein; (–), below normal blood concentration; (+), greater than normal blood concentration.
Modified from Slatter D: Textbook of small animal surgery, ed 3, Philadelphia, 2003, Saunders.

Hypercalcemia: Mnemonics

Hypercalcemia: HARD IONS

- **H**—hyperparathyroidism
- **A**—Addison's disease
- **R**—renal failure
- **D**—D vitamin and granuloma
- **I**—idiopathic
- **O**—osteolytic lesions
- **N**—neoplasia
- **S**—spurious

Hypercalcemia: HOGS IN YARD

- **H**—hyperparathyroidism
- **O**—osteolytic lesions
- **G**—granulomatous disease
- **S**—spurious
- **I**—idiopathic
- **N**—neoplastic disease
- **Y**—young, growing dogs
- **A**—Addison's disease
- **R**—renal failure
- **D**—vitamin D

Hypercapnia

Hypoventilation
- Neuromuscular disorder
- Medullary dysfunction (e.g., excessive depth of anesthesia, intracranial disease)
- Cervical disease or neuromuscular disease

Airway Obstruction
- Large-airway obstruction (e.g., laryngeal paralysis, tracheal collapse)
- Small-airway obstruction (e.g., chronic airway disease, bronchoconstriction)

Thoracic Wall Problems
- Open pneumothorax
- Flail chest
- Anterior displacement of the diaphragm by abdominal space filling disorders
- Pleural space filling disorder (e.g., air, fluid, diaphragmatic hernia)

Pleural Fibrosis

Pulmonary Parenchymal Disease (Late)

Inappropriate Ventilator Settings

Dead-Space Rebreathing

Recent Bicarbonate Therapy (in Ventilatory Compromised Animals)

Compensation for Metabolic Acidosis

Increased Carbon Dioxide Production
- Fever/hyperthermia
- Thyrotoxicossi
- Increased catabolism (e.g., sepsis, steroids)

Definition of hypercapnia (synonym: hypercarbia): abnormally increased arterial carbon dioxide tension (e.g., in dogs: PCO_2 >50 mm Hg [venous], >44 mm Hg [arterial]; in cats: PCO_2 >45 mm Hg [venous], >32 mm Hg [arterial]).
Modified from King L: Textbook of respiratory disease in dogs and cats, St. Louis, 2004, Saunders, p. 184.

Differentials, Lists, and Mnemonics

Hyperchloremia

Pseudohyperchloremia
- Lipemic samples (colorimetric methods)
- Potassium bromide therapy

Excessive Loss of Sodium Relative to Chloride
- Diarrhea (very common cause)

Excessive Gain of Chloride Relative to Sodium
- Therapy with chloride salts (NH_4Cl, KCl)
- Total parenteral nutrition
- Fluid therapy (e.g., 0.9% NaCl, hypertonic saline, KCl-supplemented fluids)
- Salt poisoning

Renal Chloride Retention
- Renal failure
- Renal tubular acidosis
- Hypoadrenocorticism*
- Diabetes mellitus*
- Chronic respiratory alkalosis
- Drug-induced: acetazolamide, spironolactone

Other Causes
- Exercise

*May be associated with corrected hypochloremia in cats.
Cl^- (corrected) = Cl^- (measured) × (Na^+ [normal]/Na^+ [measured]).
Modified from de Morais HSA: Chloride ion in small animal practice: the forgotten ion. J Vet Emerg Crit Care 2:11-24, 1992.

Hypercholesterolemia: Mnemonic

Having pepperoni pizza @ night can cause instant death.
H—hypothyroidism
P—postprandial
P—pancreatitis
N—nephrotic syndrome
C—Cushing's
C—cholestasis
I—idiopathic breed related
D—diabetes mellitus

Hyperemia

Differential Diagnosis Item	Key Feature(s)
Generalized Hyperemia	
Hyperthermia-induced	Potentially incidental finding unless supported by the presence of other infectious, inflammatory, immune-mediated, neurogenic, environmental, or toxic etiologies
Carbon monoxide intoxication	History; otherwise, confirmation requires co-oximetry (very limited availability). Can occur with extreme hemolysis, resulting in hyperemia despite anemia.
Anaphylaxis/drug reaction	History of exposure and presence of supporting clinical signs
Mast cell tumor, pheochromocytoma	Episodic hyperemic episodes
Contact dermatitis	History of exposure to potential allergen
Cardiac, hepatic, venous occlusion	Decreased venous return states also associated with additional clinical signs
Hyperdynamic phase of shock	Evidence of severe illness such as sepsis or heatstroke
Drugs and toxins	Alpha-adrenergic receptor blocker, alcohol ingestion, cyanide, acepromazine
Erythrocytosis	Primary or secondary causes of erythrocytosis; confirmed with CBC or packed cell volume
Hemoglobinemia	Hemolysis or administration of synthetic hemoglobin
Regional Hyperemia	
External constriction	Examine for presence of a rubber band, collar, identification band, tight bandaging.
Allergen exposure	Insect bites may result in localized swelling, usually the face in dogs and paws in cats. Check for history and presence of exposure, such as urticaria, vomiting, poor peripheral perfusion.
Internal obstruction	Comparative pulse oximetry and blood pressure readings are suggestive, supported by ultrasound evaluation.

Reproduced from the third edition in edited form.

THIRD EDITION AUTHOR: Lisa M. Abbott, DVM, MRCVS

Hyperglobulinemia

Polyclonal
- **Infections**
  - Bacterial*†
    - Brucellosis
    - Pyoderma
    - Bacterial endocarditis
    - Actinomycosis /nocardiosis
  - Viral
    - FIP‡
    - FIV
    - FeLV
  - Fungal*†
    - Systemic fungal infections (e.g., blastomycosis, histoplasmosis, coccidioidomycosis)
  - Rickettsial†‡
    - Ehrlichiosis
    - Salmon poisoning disease
  - Protozoal
    - *Hepatozoon canis, H. americanum*
  - Parasitic
    - Dirofilariasis*†
    - Demodicosis
    - Scabies
    - Echinococcosis
- **Immune-Mediated Disease**
  - Infections (immune complex)
    - Dirofilariasis*†
    - Feline cholangitis/cholangiohepatitis
    - Pyometra
  - SLE, including glomerulonephritis, IMHA, IMT, and polyarthritis*
  - IMHA, IMT (unrelated to SLE)*
  - Pemphigus complex, bullous pemphigoid*
  - Rheumatoid arthritis*
- **Neoplasia**†‡

Monoclonal
- **Infections**
  - Ehrlichiosis (can be polyclonal)†‡
  - Leishmaniasis (can be polyclonal)†‡
  - FIP (rarely monoclonal)
- **Idiopathic**†‡
  - Benign monoclonal gammopathy
- **Neoplasia**†‡
  - Multiple myeloma‡
  - Macroglobulinemia
  - Lymphoma
  - Extramedullary plasmacytoma (rare)
- **Miscellaneous**
  - Cutaneous amyloidosis
  - Plasmacytic gastroenterocolitis*

*Mild (4–5 g/dL [40-50 mg/mL]).
†Moderate (5–6 g/dL [50-60 mg/mL]).
‡Severe (>6 g/dL [>60 mg/mL]).
Effect of age should be considered when assessing globulin value.
FeLV, Feline leukemia virus; *FIP,* feline infectious peritonitis; *FIV,* feline immunodeficiency virus; *IMHA,* immune-mediated hemolytic anemia; *IMT,* immune-mediated thrombocytopenia; *SLE,* systemic lupus erythematosus.
Modified from Willard M, Tvedten H: Small animal clinical diagnosis by laboratory methods, ed 5, St. Louis, 2012, Saunders.

Hyperglycemia

- Diabetes mellitus*
- "Stress"/aggression/fear (cat)*
- Postprandial (propylene glycol, corn syrup)
- Hyperadrenocorticism*
- Acromegaly (cat)
- Diestrus (bitch)
- Pheochromocytoma (dog)
- Pancreatitis
- Exocrine pancreatic neoplasia
- Acute kidney injury
- Drug therapy*
  - Glucocorticoids
  - Progestogens
  - Megestrol acetate
  - Thiazide diuretics
  - Others
- Parenteral nutrition
  - Dextrose-containing fluids*

*Common.
Modified from Willard M, Tvedten H: Small animal clinical diagnosis by laboratory methods, ed 5, St. Louis, 2012, Saunders.

Hyperkalemia

Increased Potassium Intake

Iatrogenic

Caused by oversupplementation in intravenous (IV) maintenance fluid bag, failing to disperse newly added potassium in IV fluids, and/or failing to close the fluid line to the patient while adding potassium to the IV fluid bag.

Potassium Translocation from the Intracellular Fluid (ICF) to the Extracellular Fluid (ECF) Spaces

Mineral Acid–Associated Metabolic Acidosis

Inorganic anions (ammonium chloride, hydrochloric acid, azotemia) associated with protons being unable to enter cells as organic (ketones) anions can. As a result, potassium shifts extracellularly to maintain electroneutrality across the cell membrane. Blood gas analysis shows low pH, a large base deficit, and an elevated TCO_2.

Insulin Deficiency

Diabetes mellitus. Insulin allows intracellular transport of potassium across the cell membrane, whereas its absence allows potassium to leave the cell. Insulin also has its own independent means of moving potassium into the intracellular space whereby it stimulates the Na^+-H^+ antiporter and secondarily the Na^+-K^+-ATPase pump at the cell membranes of insulin-dependent cells.

Hypertonicity/Hyperosmolality

Hyperosmolar nonketotic and ketoacidotic diabetes mellitus, or administration of hyperosmolar drugs or substances. Hyperosmolality causes intracellular water to exit the ICF and enter the ECF; solvent drag carries potassium into the ECF.

Massive Tissue Destruction ("Crush Syndrome"), Rhabdomyolysis

Results from crushing or rapid necrosis of tissue that allows cellular potassium to migrate into the ECF. This in association with acute kidney injury can cause

Continued

(Continued from previous page)

hyperkalemia. High serum CK, AST, and LDH concentrations, and myoglobinuria, are expected if the disorder is sufficiently severe as to cause hyperkalemia.

Acute Tumor Lysis Syndrome

This syndrome can occur when cancer chemotherapy causes massive tumor cell death and a massive release of cellular contents, including potassium. Treatment history, hyperphosphatemia, azotemia are consistent.

Hyperkalemic Periodic Paralysis

A very rare familial muscular disease characterized by cellular membrane leakage of potassium that occurs intermittently. The clinical sign is severe muscle weakness. The undulating course of clinical signs with coexisting hyperkalemia is highly suggestive of this disorder.

Pseudohyperkalemia

Thrombocytosis, Leukocytosis, Hemolysis

Hyperkalemia caused by escape of potassium from white blood cells, red blood cells (relevant to hyperkalemia when they contain very high intracellular potassium concentrations, as with Japanese dog breeds: shiba inu, Akita, Tosa inu), and/or platelets into the serum. Complete blood count indicating high cell numbers is suggestive; repeating the potassium measurement on a plasma sample or a nonhemolyzed sample will show the correct blood potassium level.

Decreased Excretion

Hypoaldosteronism

Hallmark of typical (not solely glucocorticoid-deficient) hypoadrenocorticism/Addison's disease, which causes aldosterone deficiency. In the absence of adequate aldosterone, potassium excretion and sodium resorption at the distal renal tubule are compromised. Coexisting hyponatremia and azotemia are supportive; the definitive diagnosis is obtained with an ACTH stimulation test.

Acute Kidney Injury (AKI)

Caused by any of several renal insults affecting renal blood flow, glomerulotubular balance, or renal vascular integrity. Azotemia, serum electrolyte abnormalities, and impaired urine concentration ability are expected if the disorder is sufficiently severe to cause hyperkalemia.

Urinary Bladder Rupture and/or Urinary Tract Outflow Obstruction

A history of trauma or stranguria is usually present. Abdominal radiographs, ultrasonography, and/or contrast urography are indicated. High concentrations of potassium, creatinine, or both in ascites (>1.4 times higher than serum) are consistent with uroabdomen.

Type 4 Renal Tubular Acidosis

Rare condition where hyperkalemia is associated with normal ACTH stimulation test results. Azotemia and urine specific gravity vary, depending on stage of disease. Urine fractional excretion studies along with urine anion gap measurements lead to the diagnosis.

Certain Drugs

History may reveal usage, or ingestion of toxic amounts of, certain potassium-sparing diuretics and/or ACE inhibitors (impairing renal potassium excretion) or beta-adrenergic blocking drugs (impairing catecholamine activity and therefore potassium transfer from ECF to ICF).

Other Conditions

Case reports/short case series describe "pseudoaddison's disease" associated with parasitic enterocolitis (whipworms), chylothorax and other pleural effusions, ascites, and term pregnancy in dogs. Mechanism remains unexplained for most of these conditions, but the results of ACTH stimulation are normal. Hyperkalemia occurring with these disorders, along with normal ACTH stimulation test results, suggests the diagnosis of pseudoaddison's disease.

Laboratory and blood collection errors (e.g., collection into a lavender-top tube, which contains the anticoagulant tripotassium EDTA) should always be considered as etiologies for hyperkalemia when there is no explanation for hyperkalemia. Perhaps this should be the first query before needless diagnostic tests are done.

ACE, Angiotensin-converting enzyme; *ACTH*, adrenocorticotropic hormone; *AST*, aspartate aminotransferase; *CK*, creatine kinase; *LDH*, lactate dehydrogenase; *TCO_2*, total carbon dioxide.

THIRD EDITION AUTHOR: Michael Schaer, DVM, DACVIM, DACVECC

Hyperlipidemia

Diseases and Conditions That Cause Hypertriglyceridemia or Hypercholesterolemia

Causes of Hypertriglyceridemia

Increased Triglyceride Production

- By hepatocytes
- By enterocytes:
  - Postprandial hyperlipidemia

Decreased Lipolysis or Intravascular Processing of Lipoproteins

- Hypothyroidism
- Nephrotic syndrome
- Lipoprotein lipase deficiency (rare in cats, very rare in dogs)

Other, Unknown, or Multiple Mechanisms

- Acute pancreatitis
- Diabetes mellitus
- High-lipid diet
- Hyperadrenocorticism or excess glucocorticoids
- Hyperlipidemia in a Brittany spaniel
- Idiopathic hyperlipidemia of miniature schnauzers

Causes of Hypercholesterolemia

Increased Cholesterol Production

- By hepatocytes:
  - Nephrotic syndrome or protein-losing nephropathy
- By enterocytes:
  - Postprandial hyperlipidemia

Decreased Lipolysis or Intravascular Processing of Lipoproteins

- Hypothyroidism
- Nephrotic syndrome or protein-losing nephropathy
- Lipoprotein lipase deficiency (very rare in dogs)

Other, Unknown, or Multiple Mechanisms

- Acute pancreatitis
- Cholestasis (obstructive)
- Diabetes mellitus
- Hyperadrenocorticism
- Hypercholesterolemia in briards
- Idiopathic hyperlipidemia of miniature schnauzers

Data from Stockham FL, Scott MA: Lipids. In Fundamentals of veterinary clinical pathology, Ames, Iowa, 2002, Iowa State Press, pp 521–537.

Hypernatremia

Pure Water Deficit
- Primary hypodipsia (e.g., in miniature schnauzers)
- Diabetes insipidus:
  - Central
  - Nephrogenic
- High environmental temperature
- Fever
- Inadequate access to water

Impermeable Solute Gain
- Salt poisoning
- Hypertonic fluids
  - Hypertonic saline
  - Sodium bicarbonate
  - Parenteral nutrition
  - Sodium phosphate enema
- Hyperaldosteronism
- Hyperadrenocorticism

Hypotonic Fluid Loss
- Extrarenal
  - Gastrointestinal
    - Vomiting
    - Diarrhea
    - Small-intestinal obstruction
  - Third-space loss
    - Peritonitis
    - Pancreatitis
  - Cutaneous
    - Burns
- Renal
  - Osmotic diuresis
    - Diabetes mellitus
    - Mannitol infusion
  - Chemical diuretics
  - Chronic kidney disease
  - Nonoliguric acute kidney injury
  - Postobstructive diuresis

From DiBartola S: Fluid, electrolyte, and acid-base disorders in small animal practice, ed 4, St. Louis, 2012, Saunders.

Hyperphosphatemia

Maldistribution (Translocation)
- Tumor cell lysis
- Tissue trauma or rhabdomyolysis
- Hemolysis
- Metabolic acidosis

Increased Intake
- Gastrointestinal
  - Phosphate enemas
  - Vitamin D intoxication
- Parenteral
  - IV phosphate

Decreased Loss
- Acute or chronic kidney disease
- Uroabdomen or urethral obstruction
- Hypoparathyroidism
- Acromegaly*
- Hyperthyroidism

Physiologic: young growing animal

Laboratory Error (e.g., lipemia or hyperproteinemia, depending on methodology)

*Importance in veterinary medicine uncertain.
From DiBartola S: Fluid, electrolyte, and acid-base disorders in small animal practice, ed 4, St. Louis, 2012, Saunders.

Hyperproteinemia (Increased Serum Total Protein)

Inflammation
- Infectious
  - Bacterial (e.g., deep pyoderma, brucellosis)
  - Viral (e.g., feline infectious peritonitis, feline immunodeficiency virus)
  - Protozoal (e.g., leishmaniasis, hepatozoonosis)
  - Rickettsial (e.g., ehrlichiosis)
  - Fungal (e.g., blastomycosis, histoplasmosis)
- Noninfectious
  - Neoplasia (especially if necrotic areas are present)
  - Foreign-body granuloma
  - Antigenic response (e.g., inflammatory bowel disease, systemic lupus erythamatosus)

Paraneoplastic Protein Synthesis
- Multiple myeloma
- Lymphoma

Dehydration
- Hemoconcentration can elevate both albumin and globulin fractions.
- Dehydration/hemoconcentration is the only differential diagnosis to explain hyperalbuminemia.

Modified from Cowell R: Veterinary clinical pathology secrets, St. Louis, 2004, Mosby, p 56.

Hypersensitivity

Types and Examples

Features: Type and Mechanism	Examples	Pathophysiology	Signs
Type I Immediate (anaphylactic)	Food allergy Atopy dermatitis Insect bite hypersensitivity Adverse vaccine reaction Adverse drug reaction	Acute, systemic inflammation is triggered by IgE-mediated degranulation of mast cells and basophils; degranulation releases histamine, leukotrienes, interleukins, and other vasodilatory and inflammatory substances.	Urticaria (plaques of skin swelling) Angioedema (regional or diffuse cutaneous or visceral swelling) Pruritus If severe: hypotension and shock (dogs) or dyspnea (cats)
Type II Cytotoxic	Immune-mediated hemolytic anemia Immune-mediated thrombocytopenia Hypothyroidism (lymphocytic thyroiditis) Hemolytic reaction (incompatible transfusion donor-recipient match; neonatal isoerythrolysis) Pemphigus Adverse drug reaction	Antibody (IgM or IgG) binds to surface molecules (rightly or wrongly perceived as antigenic) on cells of body tissues. The antibody-tagged cells are destroyed by the mononuclear-phagocytic (reticuloendothelial) system.	Signs depend on body tissue cells involved. Examples include hemolysis and cutaneous lesions.
Type III Immune complex–mediated	Systemic lupus erythematosus Rheumatoid arthritis Feline infectious peritonitis Glomerulonephritis	Complexing of antibody with soluble antigen (slight excess of antigen causes the most intense reactions). Deposition of antigen-antibody complexes in tissues elicits neutrophil release of enzymes and free radicals, causing tissue damage. Common sites of tissue damage include glomeruli, synovium, and vascular endothelium.	Signs of protein-losing nephropathy, polyarthritis, polyarteritis
Type IV Delayed (cell-mediated)	Contact hypersensitivity Transplanted organ rejection	T lymphocyte–mediated (rather than primarily antibody-mediated) interaction with antigen. "Delayed" refers to late onset of reaction (>12 hours after beginning of exposure) due to mobilization and infiltration of T lymphocytes, usually "memory T cells" from prior or ongoing exposure to antigen. These T lymphocytes secrete inflammatory substances and attract macrophages and more lymphocytes, leading to tissue destruction.	Signs depend on body tissue involved. Examples include cutaneous lesions (contact hypersensitivity) and organ dysfunction (transplant rejection).

Hypertension, Systemic: Mnemonic

Can Having High Pressure Kill A Pet?

- **C**—Cushing's syndrome
- **H**—Hyperthyroidism
- **P**—pheochromocytoma
- **K**—kidney disease
- **A**—aortic coarctation
- **P**—primary hypertension

Hyperthermia, Nonfebrile

- Airway obstruction
- Drugs (e.g., ketamine, phenothiazines, anticholinergics, amphetamines)
- Excitement/stress
- Exercise, mild—some Labrador retrievers
- Exercise, strenuous
- High ambient temperature
- Hyperthyroidism
- Hypothalamic tumor
- Malignant hyperthermia
- Pheochromocytoma
- Seizures
- Serotonin syndrome
- Tetanus
- Tremors

Hypoalbuminemia

Mechanism	Examples	Key Feature
Decreased production	Hepatic insufficiency	Common cause of severe ↓; liver enzymes usually ↑; ± icterus; abnormal hepatic imaging common
	Starvation	Mild to moderate ↓; weight loss; ± GI signs; may be associated with maldigestion/malabsorption
	Acute phase inflammation (negative acute phase protein)	Mild to moderate ↓; inflammatory leukogram; hyperglobulinemia; infectious and/or inflammatory disease often recognized
	Hypoadrenocorticism	Mild to moderate ↓; absence of stress leukogram; Na^+↓K^+↑ (if typical); waxing and waning GI signs sometimes recognized
Dilution	Iatrogenic fluid use	Mild to moderate ↓; in-hospital weight gain; history supportive
	Fluid-retaining states	Mild to moderate ↓; evidence of underlying disease (e.g., congestive heart failure, cirrhosis, kidney failure)
	SIADH	Mild to moderate ↓; Na^+↓ with hypo-osmolality; inappropriate urine Na^+ retention; evidence of underlying disease or drug (e.g., nervous system disorders, neoplasia, lung disease, and drug induced)
Loss	Protein-losing nephropathy	Very common cause of severe ↓; proteinuria with inactive urine sediment and UPC >0.4 (cat) or 0.5 (dog)
	Protein-losing enteropathy	Very common cause of severe ↓; globulin ↓; GI signs common
	Protein-losing dermatopathy	Can cause severe ↓; readily apparent on physical examination (e.g., burns, major skin sloughing)
	Blood loss	Chronic blood loss more relevant than acute; GI bleeding or *Ancylostoma* spp infestation important causes
Sequestration	Effusion into body cavities	Mild to marked ↓; abdominal and/or pleural effusion, especially high protein or chylous effusions
	Vasculitis	Mild to moderate ↓; thrombocytopenia common

GI, Gastrointestinal; *SIADH,* syndrome of inappropriate antidiuretic hormone; *UPC,* urine protein creatinine ratio.

Hypocalcemia

Differential Diagnosis	Key Feature(s)
Primary hypoparathyroidism (immune-mediated, idiopathic)*	Clinical signs of hypocalcemia usually are present. Normal to increased phosphorus. Normal to decreased parathyroid hormone (PTH). Normal renal function.
Primary hypoparathyroidism (post-op parathyroidectomy or bilateral thyroidectomy)*	Clinical signs of hypocalcemia may be present. May occur 1-3 days post-op parathyroidectomy to treat hyperparathyroidism or bilateral thyroidectomy to treat hyperthyroidism.
Eclampsia*	Clinical signs of hypocalcemia usually are present. Normal to decreased phosphorus. Usually occurs in small-breed dogs in the first few weeks of lactation.
Acute kidney injury/chronic kidney disease	Ionized calcium is normal, except in advanced disease. Usually asymptomatic for hypocalcemia. Increased phosphorus. Azotemia.
Ethylene glycol toxicity*	Clinical signs of hypocalcemia may be present. Azotemia. Monohydrate calcium oxalate crystals may be seen on urinalysis.
Acute pancreatitis*	Usually asymptomatic for hypocalcemia. Occurs with severe, acute pancreatitis.
Intestinal malabsorption*	Clinical signs of hypocalcemia may be present. May have concurrent hypomagnesemia and/or hypovitaminosis D.
Hypoalbuminemia	Ionized calcium is normal. Does not cause clinical signs.
Hypomagnesemia*	Clinical signs of hypocalcemia may be present. Occurs secondary to decreased absorption or increased gastrointestinal or renal loss.
Rhabdomyolysis*	Usually asymptomatic for hypocalcemia. Myoglobinuria and increased AST and CK may be observed.
Tumor lysis syndrome*	Clinical signs of hypocalcemia may be present. Occurs during the period of maximum cytolysis (usually 5-7 days after initiation of chemotherapy) in dogs with large tumor burden. Hyperkalemia and hyperphosphatemia may also be present.
Nutritional secondary hyperparathyroidism*	Usually asymptomatic for hypocalcemia but exhibit pain and skeletal abnormalities. Hypophosphatemia. Increased PTH. History of a homemade diet.
Hypovitaminosis D*	Clinical signs of hypocalcemia may be present. Occurs from intestinal malabsorption or a homemade diet.
Phosphate-containing enemas*	Clinical signs of hypocalcemia may be present. History is confirmatory.
Massive blood transfusion*	Clinical signs of hypocalcemia may be present. Can occur after multiple transfusions with citrated blood.
Laboratory error	Ionized calcium is normal. Does not cause clinical signs. Repeat measurement of total calcium is normal.

*Ionized serum calcium concentration is also low.
Clinical signs of hypocalcemia include muscle fasciculations, ear twitching, facial rubbing, anxiety, and seizures.

AUTHOR: Karen M. Tefft, DVM, MVSc, DACVIM

Hypoglycemia: Causes

- Artifact
  - Glucometers (especially those designed for humans)
  - Delayed serum/plasma separation*
  - Laboratory error
- Beta-cell tumor (insulinoma)*
- Chronic kidney disease (rarely)
- Erythrocytosis (severe)
- Extrapancreatic neoplasia
  - Hepatocellular carcinoma, hepatoma
  - Renal adenocarcinoma
  - Leiomyosarcoma, leiomyoma
  - Hemangiosarcoma (rarely)
  - Others
- Exocrine pancreatic neoplasia
- Hepatic insufficiency
  - Portocaval shunts*
  - Chronic fibrosis, cirrhosis
  - Acute hepatic failure
- Hepatic enzyme deficiencies
  - von Gierke's disease (type 1 glycogen storage disease)
  - Cori's disease (type 3 glycogen storage disease)
- Hypoadrenocorticism
- Hypopituitarism
- Iatrogenic
  - Insulin therapy*
  - Sulfonylurea therapy/accidental exposure
  - Ethanol
  - Ethylene glycol
- Idiopathic hypoglycemia
  - Neonatal hypoglycemia
  - Juvenile hypoglycemia (esp. toy breeds)*
  - Hunting dog hypoglycemia (exercise)
- Infection
  - Sepsis*
  - *Babesia canis*
  - Bartonellosis
  - *Trypanoxoma congolense*
- Leukocytosis (severe)
- Starvation (prolonged)
- Toxins
  - Xylitol*
  - Oleander
  - Ethanol/ethylene-glycol
  - Alpha-lipoic acid

*Particularly important causes of hypoglycemia.

Hypokalemia*: Causes

Decreased Intake or Absorption
- Decreased intake (unlikely as sole factor)
- Administration of potassium-free (e.g., 0.9% NaCl, 5% dextrose in water) or deficient fluids (e.g., lactated Ringer's solution over several days)
- Bentonite clay ingestion (e.g., cat litter)

Translocation (ECF → ICF)
- Alkalemia
- Insulin/glucose-containing fluids
- Catecholamines
- Thyrotoxicosis
- Hypothermia
- Hypokalemic periodic paralysis (Burmese cats)
- Total parenteral nutrition
- Refeeding syndrome

Increased Loss
- Vomiting of stomach contents
- Diarrhea
- Osmotic diuresis (e.g., uncontrolled diabetes mellitus)
- Chronic renal failure in cats
- Diet-induced hypokalemic nephropathy in cats
- Distal (type I) renal tubular acidosis (RTA)
- Proximal (type II) RTA after $NaHCO_3$ treatment
- Fanconi syndrome
- Postobstructive diuresis
- Dialysis
- Plasmapheresis
- Hyperadrenocorticism (mineralocorticoid excess)
- Primary hyperaldosteronism (adenoma, adenocarcinoma, hyperplasia)
- Hereditary disorders as yet undescribed in dogs or cats (e.g., Bartter syndrome, Gitelman syndrome, Liddle syndrome)

Drugs and Toxins
- Loop diuretics (e.g., furosemide, ethacrynic acid)
- Thiazide diuretics (e.g., chlorothiazide, hydrochlorothiazide)
- Insulin
- Beta-2 agonists (e.g., albuterol, terbutaline, dobutamine)
- Theophylline intoxication
- Amphotericin B
- Penicillins
- Rattlesnake envenomation
- Pseudoephedrine, ephedrine
- Granulocyte colony stimulating factor (pharmacologic dosage)
- Licorice ingestion (natural licorice, not common candies)
- Sodium phosphate enemas

*Hypomagnesemia is a common concurrent electrolyte disturbance that can be caused by the same initiating factor as hypokalemia and that can itself increase urinary potassium loss.
Modified from DiBartola SP, De Morais HA: Disorders of potassium, hypokalemia and hyperkalemia. In DiBartola SP: Fluid, electrolyte, and acid-base disorders in small animal practice, ed 4, St. Louis, 2012, Saunders.

Hypomagnesemia

Gastrointestinal
- Reduced intake/starvation/malnutrition
- Chronic diarrhea
- Gastric suction
- Malabsorption syndromes
- Short bowel syndrome
- Gastric bypass surgery
- Colonic neoplasia
- Familial or inherited

Renal
- Diabetes mellitus/diabetic ketoacidosis
- Diuretics (except potassium-sparing agents)
- Osmotic agents (including hyperglycemia)
- Intrinsic renal causes of diuresis
  - Postobstructive
  - Polyuric acute kidney injury/uremia
  - Hyperaldosteronism
  - Hyperthyroidism
- Renal tubular acidosis
- Concurrent electrolyte disorders
  - Hypokalemia
  - Hypercalcemia/hyperparathyroidism
  - Hypophosphatemia
- Drugs
  - Gentamicin
  - Carbenicillin
  - Ticarcillin
  - Cyclosporin
  - Cisplatin
- Postrenal transplantation
- Familial or inherited

Miscellaneous
- Excessive loss from
  - Sweat
  - Lactation
- Redistribution
  - Acute myocardial infarction
  - Acute pancreatitis
  - Insulin
  - Catecholamine excess
- Idiopathic

From DiBartola S: Fluid, electrolyte, and acid-base disorders in small animal practice, ed 4, St. Louis, 2012, Saunders.

Hyponatremia

Differential Diagnosis Item	Key Feature(s)
Hyperglycemia	Seen most often in conjunction with DKA: hyperglycemia increases plasma hyperosmolality, drawing water into the vascular space by osmosis, which dilutes Na^+. Corrected Na^+ = (Measured Na^+) + 1.6[(Serum glucose − 100)/100].
Mannitol infusion	Treatment history is definitive; exogenous hyperosmolar infusion draws water into the vascular space, causing dilutional hyponatremia.
Hepatic cirrhosis/severe liver disease	Patients are hypervolemic and may present icteric with elevated liver enzymes or with encephalopathy, evidence of reduced hepatic synthetic function (low albumin, glucose, cholesterol, BUN concentrations).
Congestive heart failure	Radiographic evidence of pulmonary edema and cardiomegaly (and/or ascites if right-sided failure): common
Kidney disease	Patients are hypervolemic, azotemic with isosthenuric urine. Excess excretion of Na^+ can occur with tubular diseases or pyelonephritis.
Nephrotic syndrome	Patients are hypervolemic with proteinuria, hyperlipidemia, hypoalbuminemia, and interstitial edema/body cavity effusion.
Psychogenic polydipsia	Patients are normovolemic with low plasma osmolality and polyuria; no other signs of systemic illness.
Syndrome of inappropriate ADH secretion	Patients are normovolemic with low plasma osmolality, high urine osmolality, and natriuresis with normal renal, adrenal, and thyroid function and no edema or ascites. Can occur with neurologic, pulmonary, or neoplastic disorders.
Diuretic administration	Patients are hypovolemic, as diuretics promote renal sodium; a rare cause of hyponatremia since sodium and free water loss equilibrate.
Hypoadrenocorticism	Distal tubular Na^+ and Cl^- loss due to aldosterone deficiency. Hypovolemia, hypotension, hypochloremia, and hyperkalemia common; ACTH stimulation test is diagnostic.
Cutaneous loss	Extensive burns cause hypovolemia via large fluid losses through wounds.
Myxedema coma	In addition to the normal signs of hypothyroidism, patients have dull to obtunded mentation, hypothermia, bradycardia, and hypotension.
Hypotonic fluid administration	Hospitalized patients treated with hypotonic fluids can develop normovolemic hyponatremia; anxiety, stress, pain, anesthetic drugs can increase vasopressin levels, causing decreased renal water excretion, potentiating the hyponatremia.
Gastrointestinal loss	Vomiting, diarrhea, sequestration, excess salivation causes a loss of isotonic ECF, which, when replaced by renal water retention and water drinking, dilutes the remaining plasma Na^+.
Third-space loss	Seen in pancreatitis, peritonitis, uroabdomen, pleural effusion, peritoneal effusion due to acute loss of isotonic fluid from the vascular space.
Pseudohyponatremia	Artifactual change due to lipemia and/or hyperproteinemia

ACTH, Adrenocorticotropic hormone; *ADH,* antidiuretic hormone; *BUN,* blood urea nitrogen; *DKA,* diabetic ketoacidosis; *ECF,* extracellular fluid.
Reproduced from the third edition in unabridged form.

THIRD EDITION AUTHOR: Yonáira Cortés, DVM, DACVECC

Hypophosphatemia

Maldistribution (Translocation)
- Treatment of diabetic ketoacidosis
- Carbohydrate load or insulin administration
- Respiratory alkalosis or hyperventilation
- Parenteral nutrition or nutritional recovery
- Hypothermia

Increased Loss (Reduced Renal Resorption)
- Primary hyperparathyroidism
- Renal transplantation
- Major hepatic resection (?)
- Renal tubular disorders (e.g., Fanconi syndrome)
- Proximally acting diuretics (e.g., carbonic anhydrase inhibitors) (?)
- Eclampsia
- Hyperadrenocorticism (?)

Decreased Intake (Reduced Intestinal Absorption)
- Dietary deficiency (?)
- Vomiting (?)
- Malabsorption (?)
- Phosphate binders
- Vitamin D deficiency

Laboratory Error

Renal Replacement Therapy

(?), Importance in veterinary medicine uncertain.
Modified from DiBartola S: Fluid, electrolyte, and acid-base disorders in small animal practice, ed 4, St. Louis, 2012, Saunders.

Differentials, Lists, and Mnemonics

Hypotension, Systemic

Decreased Preload
- Hypovolemia
  - Hemorrhage
  - Trauma
  - Gastrointestinal losses
  - Polyuria
  - Hypoadrenocorticism
  - Effusions or other third spacing of fluid
  - Burns
  - Heatstroke
  - Pulmonary arterial hypertension (severe)
- Decreased Venous Return
  - Pericardial effusion/cardiac tamponade
  - Constrictive pericarditis
  - Severe pneumothorax
  - Positive-pressure ventilation
  - Gastric dilation/volvulus
  - Heartworm disease (caval syndrome)

Decreased Cardiac Function
- Cardiomyopathy
- Valvular disease
- Obstruction/stenosis
- Bradyarrhythmias
- Tachyarrhythmias
- Electrolyte abnormalities
- Acid-base disturbances
- Severe hypoxemia

Decreased Vascular Tone
- SIRS
- Anaphylaxis
- Neurogenic
- Drug-induced (anesthetic agents, vasodilators, beta-blockers, calcium channel blockers)
- Electrolyte abnormalities
- Acid-base disturbances
- Severe hypoxemia

SIRS, Sepsis/systemic inflammatory response syndrome.
Modified from Ettinger S, Feldman E: Textbook of veterinary internal medicine, ed 7, St. Louis, 2010, Saunders.

Hypothermia

Iatrogenic
- Surgery
- Anesthesia
- Overzealous treatment of hyperthermia

Systemic Disease
- Cardiac disease
- Hypothyroidism
- Sepsis (cats > dogs)
- Shock
- Chronic kidney disease
- Hypoadrenocorticism
- Malnutrition
- Hypoglycemia
- Neurologic disease:
  - Head trauma
  - Neoplasia
  - Cerebrovascular accident

Environmental
- Exposure
- Trauma

Modified with permission from Bonagura J: Kirk's Current veterinary therapy XII: small animal practice, St. Louis, 1995, Saunders, p 159.

Hypothyroidism, Neurologic Associations

- Neuromuscular weakness (slowly progressive)
- Muscle atrophy (scapular, masticatory)
- Facial nerve paralysis
- Vestibular signs (peripheral)
- Laryngeal paralysis
- Megaesophagus
- Cognitive dysfunction (congenital; cretinism)

Hypoxemia

Mechanism	Examples	Key Features
Decreased FiO_2	Anesthetic mishap, suffocation, altitude	History suggestive; completely responsive to O_2
Hypoventilation	Airway obstruction (e.g., laryngeal paralysis); pleural space disease (e.g., pneumothorax, pleural effusion); chest wall disease (e.g., flail chest); neurologic disease (e.g., botulism, CNS lesion); drugs/toxins (e.g., anesthetic agents, sedatives, opioids)	Cause often apparent on physical exam; $PaCO_2$ always ↑; responsive to O_2, but cause must be addressed (e.g., bypass airway obstruction)
Diffusion barrier impairment	Disorders that cause diffuse thickening of the alveolar barrier (e.g., pulmonary fibrosis, pulmonary neoplasia)	Adventitial lung sounds common; pulmonary imaging typically abnormal; $PaCO_2$ normal or slightly ↓
Ventilation-perfusion mismatch	Abnormal distribution of perfusion (e.g., pulmonary thromboembolism) and/or ventilation impairment (e.g., atelectasis, pleural space disease, pneumonia, pulmonary edema, pulmonary hemorrhage)	A-a oxygen gradient ↑; pulmonary imaging abnormalities often present; perfusion impairment often difficult to prove without advanced testing
Right-to-left shunt (intrapulmonary or extrapulmonary)	Causes of intrapulmonary shunt similar to ventilation-perfusion mismatching (e.g., atelectasis, pneumonia, pulmonary edema); extrapulmonary shunts due to congenital heart disease (e.g., reverse PDA)	Poorly responsive to O_2 administration; cardiac or pulmonary imaging abnormalities often present

A-a gradient, alveolar-arterial gradient; *FiO_2,* fractional inspired oxygen; *PDA,* patent ductus arteriosus.
Simplified oxygen A-a gradient equation when patient is breathing room air = $(150 - PaCO_2/0.8) - PaO_2$; should be <15.
The most common mechanisms of hypoxemia are hypoventilation and ventilation-perfusion mismatch, and more than one mechanism may be present in the same patient.

Icterus

Icterus	Prehepatic	Hepatic	Posthepatic	
Mechanism	Hemolysis	Hepatocellular dysfunction	Biliary obstruction (intra- or extrahepatic)	Biliary rupture
Examples	IMHA—Primary or secondary (e.g., RBC parasites, neonatal isoerythrolysis, neoplasia) Hemolytic toxins (e.g., Zn, acetaminophen) Fragmentation (e.g., caudal caval syndrome, splenic torsion) Hereditary disorders (e.g., PK or PFK deficiency, osmotic fragility)	Inflammatory liver disease (e.g., chronic hepatitis) Infection (e.g., leptospirosis, histoplasmosis, ICH, FIP) Toxins/drugs (e.g., sago palm, blue-green algae, phenobarbital) Neoplasia Hereditary and breed-related disorders (e.g., copper hepatopathy) Cirrhosis Sepsis*	Mucocele Cholelith Cholangitis Hepatic lipidosis* Pancreatitis Biliary neoplasia Duodenal infiltrative disease	Trauma Complication of biliary obstruction (e.g., mucocele)
Key laboratory findings	Marked anemia; ± hemoglobinemia, hemoglobinuria; RBC morphology aberrations common	ALT↑> ALP↑; ± cholesterol ↓; ± albumin, BUN, glucose ↓; leukon variable; ± ammonia ↑	ALP↑>ALT↑; cholesterol ↑; GGT↑ (exception: hepatic lipidosis); leukon variable	Abdominal effusion supportive of bile peritonitis; ALP↑>ALT↑; GGT↑; inflammatory leukogram
Bile acids	Normal	Not useful	Not useful	Not useful
Key imaging findings	Spleen may be enlarged	Liver size may be small, normal, or enlarged/mass; ± altered echogenicity on US	US evidence of GB disease or bile duct obstruction	Abdominal fluid (US may be required to identify small volume effusion); gallbladder rupture may or may not be identified on US

*Multiple mechanisms for icterus may be involved.

ALP, Alkaline phosphatase; *ALT,* alanine aminotransferase; *BUN,* blood urea nitrogen; *FIP,* feline infectious peritonitis; *ICH,* infectious canine hepatitis; *IMHA,* immune-mediated hemolytic anemia; *PK,* pyruvate kinase; *PFK,* phosphofructokinase; *RBC,* red blood cell; *US,* ultrasound; *Zn,* zinc.

Ileus

Functional
- Abdominal surgery
- Ischemia
- Irritable bowel syndrome (diarrhea is more likely)
- Pancreatitis

Inflammatory
- Fulminant bacterial enteritis
- Parvovirus
- Peritonitis

Metabolic
- Diabetes mellitus
- Endotoxemia
- Hypokalemia
- Uremia

Neuromuscular
- Anticholinergic drugs
- Opioid drugs
- Dysautonomia
- Spinal cord injury
- Visceral myopathy
- Visceral neuropathy

Physical
- Intestinal obstruction
  - Foreign body
  - Intussusception
  - Masses—neoplasia, granuloma
  - Mechanical—torsion, volvulus, incarceration in hernia, adhesions
- Overdistention by aerophagia

From Ettinger S, Feldman E: Textbook of veterinary internal medicine, ed 7, St. Louis, 2010, Saunders.

Immunodeficiency Syndromes: Acquired

Drugs
- Antineoplastics
- Glucocorticoids
- Other immunosuppressive agents (e.g., azathioprine, cyclosporine)

Malnutrition
- Intestinal parasitism
- Inflammatory bowel disease
- Protein-calorie deficiency
- Vitamin D deficiency
- Obesity

Infections
- Viral infection (FeLV, FIV, FIP, CDV, parvovirus)
- Rickettsial infections
- Leishmaniasis

Endocrine Disease
- Hyperadrenocorticism
- Diabetes mellitus

Neoplasia

Miscellaneous
- Neonatal colostrum deprivation

CDV, Canine distemper virus; *FeLV,* feline leukemia virus; *FIP,* feline infectious peritonitis; *FIV,* feline immunodeficiency virus.

Modified from Bonagura J: Kirk's Current veterinary therapy XIII, St. Louis, 2000, Saunders.

Differentials, Lists, and Mnemonics

Immunodeficiency Syndromes: Congenital*

Disease (Synonyms)	Inheritance†	Breeds	Defect	Characterization
Barrier Defects				
Ciliary dyskinesia (immotile cilia syndrome)	AR	Many breeds†	Functional and morphologic cilia abnormalities CDC39	Rhinosinusitis, bronchopneumonia with bronchiectasis, situs inversus
Neutrophil Defects				
Bactericidal neutrophil defect	U	Doberman pinscher	Unknown	Upper respiratory infections, reduced bactericidal activity, ciliary dyskinesia not excluded
Trapped neutrophil syndrome	AR	Border collie	Unknown	Fever, neutropenia (despite myeloid hyperplasia), failure to thrive, and sometimes lameness; genetic test available
Cyclic hematopoiesis (cyclic neutropenia)	AR	Collie (gray), basset hound	Hematopoietic growth factors defect	Severe neutropenia every 12-14 days, reactive amyloidosis, DNA-mutation test
Chronic idiopathic neutropenia	U	Rottweiler	G-CSF deficiency	Recurrent fever, sepsis, polyarthritis, pyoderma
Leukocyte adhesion deficiency	AR	Irish setter, red and white setter, domestic medium hair cat	CD11/18 deficiency, beta-chain (CD18) deficiency	Severe leukocytosis, infection with limited pus formation, lack of neutrophil adhesion, DNA-mutation test
Pelger-Huët anomaly	AD	Australian shepherd, foxhound, Persian cats, others	Unknown	No immunodeficiency, hyposegmented granulocytes
Leukocyte granulation	U	Birman cats	Unknown	No immunodeficiency, acidophilic granules
Complement component 3 deficiency (C3 deficiency)	AR	Brittany spaniel	C3 deficiency	Pyogenic infections, lack of C-mediated phagocytosis in colony of dogs with neuromuscular disease
Chédiak-Higashi syndrome	AR	Persian cats	Unknown	No immunodeficiency, large granules in phagocytes, bleeding tendency
Reactive (AA) amyloidosis	U	Abyssinian cats	Unknown	Reactive (AA) amyloidosis, renal failure
Increased susceptibility to *Pneumocystis* pneumonia	AR	Dachshund, Cavalier King Charles spaniel	Unknown	*Pneumocystis* pneumonia
Susceptibility to fungal and rickettsial infections; pyoderma	U	German shepherd	Possible macrophage or T-cell defect	Severe ehrlichiosis, Rocky Mountain spotted fever, disseminated aspergillosis, deep pyoderma
Immune vasculitis, amyloidosis	U	Shar-pei, Abyssinian cats, Oriental shorthair cats	Elevated IL-6	Arthritis, amyloidosis, kidney injury/ chronic kidney disease, hepatic rupture, hypoproteinemia
Lethal acrodermatitis	AR	Bull terrier	Zinc metabolism defect	Zinc deficiency, hyperkeratosis
Increased susceptibility to parvoviral infection	U	Rottweiler, Doberman pinscher	Unknown	Parvovirus infection
Vaccine-exacerbated immune disturbance	U	Akita, Weimaraner	Unknown	Variable meningitis, polyarthritis, amyloidosis
Humoral Immune Defects				
X-linked severe combined immunodeficiency (X-SCID)	XR	Basset hound, Cardigan Welsh corgi	Common gamma-chain of IL-2 and other cytokines	Severe bacterial and viral infections, no IgG and IgA, deficient lymphocyte blastogenesis, DNA-mutation test
SCID	AR	Jack Russell terrier	DNA-protein kinase catalytic subunit	Severe serum immunoglobulin deficiency, hypoplasia of lymphoid tissues, DNA-mutation test
SCID	AR	Frisian water dog	RAG1 gene defect alters antigen-recognition	Severe IgM, IgG, and IgA deficiency and lymphopenia, DNA mutation test
Combined immunodeficiency	U	Shar-pei	T-cell and B-cell defects, low IL-6 and IL-2	Skin, respiratory, and gastrointestinal infections
Thymic abnormalities and dwarfism	U	Weimaraner	Unknown	Reduced growth, thymosine responsive

*In addition to the listed syndromes, bone marrow dyscrasias have been described in miniature and toy poodles and transient hypogammaglobulinemia in Samoyeds, but less is known of these disorders.
†For example, springer spaniel, Old English sheepdog, English setter, West Highland white terrier, pointer.
AD, Autosomal dominant; *AR,* autosomal recessive; *G-CSF,* granulocyte colony-stimulating factor; *IL,* interleukin; *U,* unknown; *XR,* X-linked recessive.
Modified from Greene CE: Infectious diseases of the dog and cat, ed 4, St. Louis, 2012, Saunders.

Inappropriate Urination

Urine Collected From Pet by Owner at Home	Characteristic Features
Specific Gravity >1.025 (not PU)	
Lower urinary tract disease Infection Urolithiasis Neoplasia (e.g., transitional cell carcinoma of the urinary bladder) Anatomic defect (pelvic bladder, ectopic ureter, etc.) Neurologic disorder (e.g., intervertebral disc disease)	• Often combined with dysuria. Besides urine sediment examination and culture, rectal palpation, vaginal/preputial examination, abdominal imaging of value
Positive for glucose (is PU)	• Measure blood glucose. Increased: diabetes mellitus. Normal: renal glycosuria.
Behavioral	• Medical evaluation unremarkable; consult with behaviorist
Specific Gravity <1.020 (PU)	
Step 1: if specific gravity = 1.008-1.012, or as high as 1.020 with dehydration:	• Evaluate for chronic kidney disease (serum biochemical profile + urinalysis)
Step 2: if no evidence of chronic kidney disease:	
Pyometra	• Stage of estrous cycle
Hyperadrenocorticism	• Other classic signs
Hypercalcemia	• Serum Ca
Hepatic insufficiency	• Serum glucose, cholesterol, urea, albumin, bile acids
Hyperthyroidism	• Serum thyroxine
Hypoadrenocorticism	• Low serum Na, high serum K; ACTH stimulation test
Hypokalemia	• Serum K
Pyelonephritis	• Specific gravity usually 1.010-1.020; urine culture (± pyelocentesis)
Diabetes insipidus	• Increased serum osmolality
Psychogenic polydipsia	• Decreased serum osmolality
Postobstructive	

PU, Polyuric.
Reproduced from the third edition in modified form.

THIRD EDITION AUTHOR: Edward C. Feldman, DVM, DACVIM

Differentials, Lists, and Mnemonics

Incontinence, Fecal

Disorder	Salient Feature
Sphincter Incontinence: Differentiate non-neurogenic from neurogenic causes	
Non-Neurogenic Sphincter Incontinence:	Structural damage to anal sphincter (internal and external), levator ani, and coccygeus muscles; abnormal rectal exam with normal neurologic exam
Perianal trauma or surgery (e.g., anal sac, rectal resection, perineal urethrostomy)	Medical history; digital rectal exam +/– pelvic radiographs may reveal abnormalities suggestive of trauma
Neoplasia	Abnormal digital rectal exam; most commonly involves the anal sac
Perianal fistula	Painful; single or multiple ulcerated draining tracts; can involve considerable amount of adjacent tissue
Rectovaginal fistula	Usually congenital; passing of urine from the anus during voiding; recurrent UTI; English bulldogs predisposed
Perineal hernia	Digital rectal exam reveals defect in the pelvic diaphragm; reducible perianal swelling ventrolateral to anus; usually unilateral, R > L; tenesmus often part of recent history
Neurogenic Sphincter Incontinence:	Normal anal sphincter anatomy; neurologic deficits reflect lesion localization (i.e., UMN vs. LMN); concurrent urinary incontinence is suggestive
Degenerative lumbosacral vertebral canal stenosis/"cauda equina" syndrome	Common cause of fecal incontinence in adult, large-breed dogs; lumbosacral pain on manipulation is characteristic; LMN signs with normal/exaggerated patellar reflexes; abnormal sensation of the perineum/extremities possible
Infection (discospondylitis)	Extreme pain over affected vertebrae; adult male dogs most commonly; associated with UTI or bacteremia (with systemic signs, e.g., anorexia, fever)
Neoplasia	Vertebral or surrounding soft-tissue tumors; infiltrative spinal cord neoplasia (lymphoma in cats); hemangiopericytoma/malignant peripheral nerve sheath tumors in dogs
Intervertebral disc disease (type II), trauma	History; pain on manipulation of affected area; radiographs to evaluate for lumbosacral fracture/luxation

Continued

(Continued from previous page)

Disorder	Salient Feature
Fibrocartilaginous embolism	Large- to giant-breed dogs; acute-onset nonprogressive deficits; variable pain during examination (often none); bilateral, asymmetrical neurologic deficits
Congenital (spina bifida, sacrococcygeal hypoplasia)	Spina bifida: Manx cat and bulldog predispositions; neurologic signs only if concurrent spinal cord malformation Sacrococcygeal hypoplasia: common in Manx cats; increased risk of clinical signs if all coccygeal vertebrae absent
Intracranial or spinal cord disease involving UMN pathways cranial to L4	Less common cause; UMN signs; abnormal cranial nerve exam, behavior or mentation indicative of intracranial disease
Peripheral neuromuscular disease	Usually diffuse involvement reflecting generalized weakness and LMN dysfunction
Autonomic dysfunction: dysautonomia	Gastrointestinal (GI) signs common; pupillary light reflex may be absent despite normal vision; heart rate may not increase after atropine administration
Reservoir Incontinence: Awareness of urge to defecate but conscious control to defecate is overwhelmed; patient postures to defecate every time (showing awareness of passing feces); normal sphincter and neurologic exam	
Inflammatory (proctitis, colitis), infectious or neoplastic colorectal disease	Signs of GI disease (e.g., weight loss, anorexia, vomiting, tenesmus, and/or dyschezia); feces usually abnormal (e.g., diarrhea, hematochezia); digital rectal exam may reveal pain, mucosal irregularities, tumors
Diets or diseases causing diarrhea	Overwhelming fecal volume; responds to a bland, limited-ingredient, or low-residue diet trial
Subtotal colectomy	Medical history; decreased rectal capacity causing frequent, urgent defecation
Constipation (overflow incontinence)	Radiographs to confirm; diarrhea passes around formed feces
Conditions affecting locomotion	Observe gait, sitting/standing, and urination/defecation attempts; complete orthopedic examination
Behavioral Incontinence: Conscious defecation in inappropriate locations with normal posturing and frequency; physical exam usually unremarkable; rule out medical conditions first	
Inadequate/inappropriate housetraining	Usually young or newly adopted pets
Separation anxiety	Only occurs in the absence of the owner; usually associated with other destructive behaviors
Litter box aversions	Inadequate privacy; inter-cat aggression; litter box, substrate, or location preferences; poor litter box hygiene
Cognitive dysfunction	Geriatric animal; changes in interactive or social behavior, and sleep cycles; anxiety or excessive/repetitive locomotion

L, Left; *L4*, fourth lumbar vertebra; *LMN*, lower motor neuron; *R*, right; *UMN*, upper motor neuron; *UTI*, urinary tract infection.
Reproduced from the third edition in unabridged form.

THIRD EDITION AUTHOR: **Julio Lopez, DVM, DACVIM**

Incontinence, Urinary

Size of Bladder Immediately After Voiding	Salient Features
Big Bladder (i.e., Urine Retention)	
UMN disorders	Often neurologic dysfunction obvious (e.g., paresis); bladder difficult to express
LMN disorders	Often neurologic dysfunction obvious (e.g., paresis); pelvic trauma/disease may be recognized; bladder easily expressed
Dysautonomia	Additional signs typical (e.g., megaesophagus, fixed pupils, vomiting, dry eyes)
Bladder atony	Follows any cause of urine retention; may be temporary or permanent
Detrusor-sphincter dyssynergia	Typically adult large-breed dog; urine stream starts then quickly stops; repeated attempts at urination
Partial urethral obstruction	Overflow dribbling of urine; obstruction/difficulty passing urinary catheter; imaging often identifies cause (e.g., prostatic enlargement, urethral stone, mass effect)
Little Bladder (i.e., Complete Voiding)	
USMI	Very common in middle-aged to older spayed dogs; begins as puddle while sleeping; often responds to treatment trial
Ectopic ureters	Congenital; may be mistaken for housebreaking issues; confirmed by contrast imaging or cystoscopy
Patent urachus	Congenital; may be mistaken for housebreaking issues; wetness/dribbling from near umbilicus
Urge incontinence	Associated with stranguria, pollakiuria; active urinary sediment typical; infection common but not consistent
Pelvic bladder	Usually not a problem unless combined with other disorder (e.g., mild USMI, polyuria)
Vaginal diverticulum/stricture	Relatively mild incontinence; digital vaginal examination and vaginoscopy can confirm
Feline leukemia virus	Test all incontinent cats for retrovirus infection
Behavioral	Rule out medical conditions; behavioral assessment

LMN, Lower motor neuron; *UMN*, upper motor neuron; *USMI*, urethral sphincter mechanism incompetence.

Infertility, Male

Congenital
- **Chromosomal/developmental**
  - Cryptorchidism
  - Ductular hypoplasia/aplasia
    - Epididymis or vas
  - Penis, prepuce abnormality
  - Testicular hypoplasia/aplasia
- **Hormonal**
  - Hypopituitarism
  - Hypothyroidism
- **Primary ciliary dyskinesia (Kartagener's syndrome)**

Acquired
- **Abstinence, prolonged**
- **Ejaculatory failure**
  - Neurologic
  - Pain
  - Physical/anatomical
- **Fever**
- **Fluid accumulations**
  - Hematocele
  - Hydrocele
  - Varicocele
- **Fucosidosis**
- **Immune-mediated orchitis/epididymitis**
- **Hormonal**
  - Hypopituitarism or hypogonadism
  - Hyperadrenocorticism
- **Infectious**
  - Orchitis/epididymitis
    - Bacterial
      - Brucellosis
      - *E. coli, Klebsiella, Pseudomonas, Staphylococcus, Streptococcus, Mycoplasma, Ureaplasma, Proteus, Haemophilus,* plus many more
    - Fungal—*Blastomyces dermatitidis, Coccidioides immitis, Cryptococcus neoformans, Histoplasma capsulatum*
    - Viral—Herpesvirus
- **Medications**
  - Anabolic steroids
  - Chemotherapeutic agents
  - Cimetidine
  - Clomipramine
  - Estrogens
  - Glucocorticoids
  - GnRH antagonists
  - Gossypol
  - Ketoconazole
  - Progestogens
  - Spironolactone
  - Sulfasalazine
- **Metabolic**
  - Renal
  - Hepatic
  - Sepsis/endotoxemia
- **Neoplasia**
  - Testicular, epididymal, scrotal, ductular, prostatic
    - Endocrine (Sertoli cell tumor)
- **Nutritional**
- **Overuse**
- **Pain**
  - Musculoskeletal
  - Neurologic
  - Posthitis/balanoposthitis
- **Prostatic disease**
  - Benign prostatic hyperplasia
  - Prostatic cyst (intraprostatic or periprostatic)
  - Prostatitis or prostatic abscess
- **Psychological**
  - Apprehension
  - Fear
- **Retrograde ejaculation**
- **Scrotal trauma or dermatitis**
- **Sperm granuloma**
- **Toxin**
  - Chemical
  - Environmental
- **Trauma**
  - Testicular compression
  - Testicular hyperthermia
- **Urethral prolapse**
- **Vascular insult or infarct**

Inflammatory Bowel Diseases

Causes of Chronic Small Bowel Inflammation

Chronic Infection
- *Giardia* sp
- *Histoplasma* sp
- *Toxoplasma* sp
- *Mycobacterium* sp
- Protothecosis
- Pythiosis
- Pathogenic bacteria (*Campylobacter, Salmonella* spp, pathogenic *Escherichia coli*)

Food Allergy

Small Bowel Inflammation Associated With Other Primary Gastrointestinal Diseases
- Lymphoma
- Lymphangiectasia

Idiopathic Causes
- Lymphocytic-plasmacytic enteritis (LPE)
- Eosinophilic gastroenterocolitis (EGE)
- Granulomatous enteritis (same as regional enteritis?)
- Neutrophilic enteritis (possibly secondary to bacterial invasion)

From Hall EJ, Day MJ: Diseases of the small intestine. In Ettinger SJ, Feldman EC, Côté E: Textbook of veterinary internal medicine: diseases of the dog and cat, ed 8, St. Louis, 2017, Elsevier.

Differentials, Lists, and Mnemonics

Insulin Resistance

Causes of Insulin Ineffectiveness or Insulin Resistance in Diabetic Dogs and Cats

Caused by Insulin Therapy
- Inactive insulin
- Diluted insulin
- Improper administration technique
- Inadequate dose
- Somogyi effect
- Inadequate frequency of insulin administration
- Impaired insulin absorption, especially Ultralente insulin
- Antiinsulin antibody excess

Caused by Concurrent Disorder
- Acromegaly (cat)*
- Congestive heart failure
- Chronic inflammation, especially pancreatitis or bowel
- Chronic kidney disease
- Diabetogenic drugs, including glucocorticoids*
- Diestrus (bitch)*
- Glucagonoma (dog)
- Hepatobiliary disease
- Hyperadrenocorticism*
- Hyperlipidemia
- Hyperthyroidism (cat)
- Hypothyroidism (dog)
- Infection, especially of oral cavity and urinary tract
- Neoplasia
- Obesity
- Pancreatic exocrine insufficiency
- Pheochromocytoma
- Progesterone excess (endogenous or exogenous)*

*Marked insulin resistance
Modified from Feldman E, Nelson R: Canine and feline endocrinology and reproduction, ed 3, St. Louis, 2004, Saunders.

Iron Abnormalities

	Serum [Iron]	TIBC	Ferritin
Normal	N	N	N
Hemolytic anemia	↑	↑	↑
Anemia of chronic disease	N or ↓	N or ↓	N or ↑
Iron deficiency (= chronic blood loss)	↓	N or ↑	↓*
Inflammation	↓	↓	↑
Glucocorticoid treatment/ excess	↑	N	—
Iron overload/toxicosis	↑	↓	↑
Artifact (sample contamination)	↑ (serum Fe > TIBC)	↓ or N	—

*Concurrent inflammation or other disorders may raise ferritin level into normal range.
N, Normal; *TIBC*, total iron-binding capacity (equivalent to saturated transferrin concentration).

Keratoconjunctivitis Sicca (KCS)

- Immune-mediated adenitis: most common (dogs)
- Breed predisposition
- Congenital anomaly
- Drug-induced (transient KCS): general anesthesia, topical anesthesia, atropine
- Drug toxicosis (transient or permanent KCS): sulfa drugs, phenazopyridine, aminosalicylic acid, etodolac
- Iatrogenic:
  - Removal of the gland of the third eyelid
- Idiopathic
- Infectious agents:
  - Canine distemper virus
  - Feline herpesvirus
- Metabolic disease (hypothyroidism, hyperadrenocorticism, diabetes mellitus)
- Chronic blepharoconjunctivitis (chemosis/ascending infection from lacrimal gland, causing lacrimal ductal obstruction)
- Neurogenic
- Radiation therapy for nasal or intracranial neoplasms
- Trauma to orbit or eye

Modified with permission from Bonagura J: Kirk's Current veterinary therapy XII: small animal practice, Philadelphia, 1995 Saunders, p 1232.

Ketonuria

- Diabetes mellitus/diabetic ketoacidosis
- Starvation
- Lactation
- Pregnancy
- Fever
- Renal glucosuria
- Severely carbohydrate-restricted diet
- Glycogen storage disease
- Extreme exercise
- False-positive: hematuria, hemoglobinuria, aciduria, highly concentrated urine

Lameness

Cause	Features
Degenerative	
Degenerative joint disease (DJD)	Waxing and waning chronic lameness of any limb; exacerbated by exercise; characterized by joint thickening and decreased ROM; confirm radiographically as DJD with osteophytosis and sclerosis
Cranial cruciate ligament rupture	Hindlimb lameness; often waxing and waning but progressive; may be acute; stifle joint effusion; joint thickening, particularly medially (medial buttress); pain on hyperextension; cranial drawer in extension/flexion; partial tears of caudolateral band of cranial cruciate ligament produce all signs of cruciate ligament disease except cranial drawer
Hip dysplasia	Degenerative joint disease of the hips characterized by joint laxity and progressive DJD; bimodal presentation—young dogs with severe laxity and hip pain, and middle-age to older dogs with worsening chronic hindlimb lameness; short-strided gait hindlimbs; bunny hopping gait; difficulty with rising; may walk with limbs adducted (narrow base); decreased ROM on extension; pain on hip extension; confirmed radiographically as DJD or laxity on VD hip extended radiograph; PennHIP evaluation best for documenting laxity and screening for breeding
Anomalous (Heritable, Congenital)	
Osteochondritis dissecans (OCD)	Defect of endochondral ossification resulting in thickened articular cartilage, cartilage fissure, and development of osteochondral flap; age of presentation 4-8 months; radiographically appears as flattened area of articular surface; joint effusion; pain on joint flexion/extension; common sites caudal humeral head, medial trochlear ridge talus, humeral condyle, femoral condyle; diagnosis of OCD of hock aided with skyline radiographs of talus with joint flexed; for shoulder, supinated and pronated views of shoulder useful
Hip dysplasia	Described above
Elbow dysplasia	A group of diseases affecting the elbow: ununited anconeal process (UAP), OCD of the humeral condyle, fragmented medial coronoid process (FMCP), joint incongruity; age of presentation 4-12 months; radiographs may identify UAP >5 months of age, OCD of humeral condyle, joint incongruity >4-5 mm, FMCP may be difficult to identify on radiographs alone; FMCP characterized by medial compartment DJD, CT or arthroscopy may be needed for confirmation; occasionally may present in older patients as DJD in the elbows with signs of elbow pain and decreased ROM
Patellar luxation	Age of presentation 6 months and up; dogs and cats; intermittent lameness may progress to constant lameness with cartilage wear exposing subchondral bone; reluctance to jump or climb stairs; palpable medial or lateral patellar instability
Radial agenesis	Very early age with severe carpal/forelimb deformity; confirmed radiographically
Congenital elbow luxation	Very early age, thickening of elbow, abnormal ROM; confirmed radiographically
Metabolic	
Panosteitis	Age of presentation 5-14 months; large-breed, fast-growing dogs; waxing, waning, often shifting-leg lameness; diaphyseal long-bone pain on palpation; confirm radiographically with patchy increased medullary opacity in long bones, often centered on nutrient foramen; cause unknown, genetics, rapid growth, and diet suspected factors
Hypertrophic osteodystrophy (HOD)	Age of presentation 2-7 months; large- and giant-breed dogs; acute onset of lameness and in severe cases reluctance to walk; fever; metaphyseal bone pain; radiographs show "double physis" from cancellous bone necrosis adjacent to physis; severe cases can lead to mortality or later growth deformity from physeal bridging
Hypokalemia/hypomagnesemia	Generalized weakness; ventroflexion of neck possible (notably cats); confirmation via bloodwork
Diabetic neuropathy (cats)	History of diabetes mellitus, progressive hindlimb weakness, characterized by sciatic weakness, and plantigrade stance in hindlimbs
Neoplastic	
Osteosarcoma (appendicular)	Most common neoplastic cause of lameness; middle-age to older patients; pain on palpation of site in bone; aggressive bone lesion radiographically with lysis, sclerosis, and periosteal reaction; must be diagnosed by biopsy, especially in areas endemic for fungal disease; common sites include proximal humerus, distal radius, distal femur, tibia (proximal and distal); prognosis ≈12-18 months medial survival with intensive treatment in dogs; good in cats, amputation may be curative
Synovial cell sarcoma	Age of presentation middle age to older, severe joint thickening, pain; radiographs may show soft-tissue swelling of joint, and lysis of articular surfaces; diagnosis by cytology or biopsy; histiocytic joint neoplasia may present similarly; differentiated on biopsy
Soft-tissue sarcoma/carcinoma	Periarticular or neoplasia of soft tissues may cause lameness in dogs or cats; firm soft-tissue swelling identified; possible mass or mineralization on radiography; diagnosis by biopsy
Digit neoplasia	Relatively common cause of lameness; painful digital swelling, often note lysis of P3; most common are squamous cell carcinoma and melanoma
Metastatic	Mammary neoplasia in cats can be metastatic to digits; pulmonary osteopathy may be a paraneoplastic syndrome with primary pulmonary tumors
Inflammatory/Infectious/Immune	
Bacterial infection/cellulitis	Fever is common; progressive soft-tissue swelling; limb edema more common in dogs; abscess and bite wounds are common cause of lameness in outdoor cats
Septic arthritis	Septic arthritis very painful condition; young dogs and cats <1 yr of age; solitary or multiple joints affected; possible fever; joint effusion—suppurative inflammation with degenerative neutrophils; bacteria not always seen; positive joint fluid culture; occasionally seen in older patients with immunosuppression as polyarthropathy; or in solitary joint with severe pre-existing DJD
Tick-borne polyarthritis	Walking on eggshells; short-strided gait; severe cases present with fever and unwillingness to walk; multiple joint effusion and pain; (+) tick serologic titers; acute suppurative inflammation on joint tap—nonseptic; rapid improvement within 48 hours of starting doxycycline treatment

Continued

Differentials, Lists, and Mnemonics

(Continued from previous page)

Cause	Features
Immune-mediated polyarthritis	Similar to infectious polyarthritis; (–) tick serologic titers; +/– (+) ANA or RF; acute suppurative or lymphoplasmacytic inflammation on arthrocentesis—nonseptic, incomplete response to doxycycline, responds to high-dose steroids; clients should be informed lifelong management needed
Bacterial osteomyelitis	May occur hematogenously in young animals but is uncommon; acute or chronic traumatic osteomyelitis includes trauma and postsurgical infections, treatment with appropriate antibiotics based on culture and possibly surgery for debridement or stabilization; treatment may be needed for months; typically until at least 1 month post radiographic resolution
Fungal osteomyelitis	Must be considered in endemic areas; characterized by bony lysis, sclerosis, and periosteal changes; identification of fungal organisms on cytology or biopsy; endemic regions helpful
Trauma	
Fracture/ligament rupture	History of traumatic event, i.e., hit by car, fall, etc.; identification of abrasions, bruises, or lacerations; gross instability or crepitus associated with fracture/luxation/ligament rupture; radiographic evidence of fracture/luxation or joint instability
Wound	Although external wounds may be obvious, small wounds may be hidden under the fur or between the toes

ANA, Antinuclear antibody test; *CT,* computed tomography scan; *RF,* rheumatoid factor; *ROM,* range of motion; *VD,* ventrodorsal.
Reproduced from the third edition in unabridged form.

THIRD EDITION AUTHOR: David A. Puerto, DVM, DACVS

Lethargy

Differential Diagnosis Item	Key Feature(s)
Metabolic	Accumulation of metabolic by-products, cytokines, and electrolyte and acid-base disturbances. Among the most common: renal disease, hepatic disease, GI disease (note vomiting/diarrhea in history), pancreatic disease, peritonitis (systemic signs usually severe), hemoabdomen (centesis confirmatory), urinary tract obstruction (history of stranguria and/or abdominal trauma [bladder rupture]), and anemia (pallor) can result in lethargy via several pathways. Complete history and physical examination can help direct diagnostic testing. CBC, serum biochemistry, urinalysis, pre- and postprandial bile acids, urine protein/creatinine ratio, urine culture and susceptibility.
Neoplastic	Neoplasia in any organ system can be accompanied by inflammation, a negative energy balance, cytokine production, and electrolyte and acid-base disorders. Cytokines and cachexins (such as TNF-alpha) can result in fatigue, suppress hunger, and promote muscle wasting. Complete physical examination, CBC, serum biochemistry, urinalysis, imaging (e.g., ultrasound, CT scan), and histopathologic analysis of biopsy samples can provide diagnosis.
Nutritional	Specific vitamin and/or mineral deficiencies as a result of inadequate or inappropriate diet. Cachexia can result from chronic conditions and involve anorexia, weight loss, and muscle wasting. Obesity can also result in a less active pet. Carefully evaluate diet history, including all supplements, and calculate caloric requirements to ensure adequate daily intake. Record body condition score and muscle condition at each veterinary visit.
Infectious disease	Bacterial, viral, fungal, rickettsial, protozoal, or parasitic agents can affect any organ and have specific or nonspecific clinical signs. A thorough physical and neurologic examination is key. CBC, serum biochemistry, and urinalysis may help to identify affected body system. Imaging (e.g., radiographs or ultrasound) and specific disease testing (e.g., serologic titers, 4Dx Snap test), culture, and susceptibility often important.
Central nervous system	Careful neurologic examination and lesion localization are essential. CNS dysfunction can result from inflammatory (e.g., sterile meningoencephalitis), infectious (e.g., bacterial meningitis—very uncommon), immune-mediated, vascular (e.g., embolism), or space-occupying lesions (e.g., neoplasia). Advanced imaging (e.g., MRI), infectious disease testing (e.g., *Toxoplasma* serologic titer), and cerebrospinal fluid analysis, including culture and susceptibility, can help to identify underlying disease.
Cardiac	Lethargy can be the result of decreased cardiac output and diminished tissue oxygen delivery; typically preceded or concurrent with exercise intolerance. Can be seen in association with cardiac arrhythmias, bacterial endocarditis, heart failure (right or left), hypertension or hypotension, and pericardial effusion. Abnormalities on careful physical examination (e.g., arrhythmia on cardiac auscultation or decreased heart sounds with pericardial effusion). Consider ECG, blood pressure measurement, thoracic radiographs, echocardiogram.
Endocrine	Can be a clinical sign of most endocrine diseases, including diabetes mellitus, hypoadrenocorticism, or hypothyroidism. CBC, serum biochemistry profile, and urinalysis with history and physical examination can direct diagnostic testing for specific endocrine dysfunction (e.g., ACTH stimulation test, T_4/TSH).
Drugs	Many medications can result in lethargy (e.g., anticonvulsants, narcotics, and cardiovascular drugs [beta-blockers, digoxin, etc.]). Complete medication history is important.
Pain	Chronic pain is usually accompanied by anatomically specific signs (e.g., lameness with polyarthritis); physical exam is most important.
Behavior	Interindividual variations in normal behavior can be interpreted by clients as lethargy or laziness. History often includes very active other pet (past or present). Physical exam unremarkable. Animals tend to become more sedentary with age.

Reproduced from the third edition in modified form.

THIRD EDITION AUTHOR: Julie Walter, DVM

Lymphadenopathy

Differential Diagnosis	Key Features
Generalized Lymphadenopathy	
Reactive:	
• Infectious (incomplete list)	• The majority of these conditions have concurrent supportive findings:
• Rickettsial infection	• Thrombocytopenia, leukopenia, nonregenerative anemia, hyperglobulinemia
• Leishmaniasis	• Endemic areas, amastigotes may be detected in lymph node aspirates
• Feline leukemia virus, feline immunodeficiency virus	• Leukopenia, nonregenerative anemia; point-of-care testing positive
• Systemic mycoses (histoplasmosis, blastomycosis, cryptococcosis, sporotrichosis, coccidioidomycosis, aspergillosis)	• Endemic areas, immunosuppressed patients, localized fungal infection with sudden deterioration in condition
• External parasites	• Skin scrape for *Sarcoptes scabiei, Demodex* sp, etc.
• Generalized dermatopathy	• Apparent on examination
• Noninfectious/inflammatory	• May occur with recent trauma or autoimmune-related disorders
Neoplasia:	
• Lymphoma, systemic mastocytosis, leukemia, multiple myeloma	• Fine-needle aspirate of the popliteal or superficial cervical (prescapular) lymph nodes is recommended; certain neoplasms (lymphoma, myeloma notably) may be associated with hypercalcemia, hyperglobulinemia, thrombocytopenia
Nonspecific Hyperplasia	• Cause may be undetermined; associated with retrovirus infections in cats and leishmaniasis in dogs
Solitary or Regional Lymphadenopathy	
Superficial:	
• Inflammatory conditions of the drained region resulting in lymphadenitis (e.g., abscessation, wounds, tick bites, dermatitis, periodontal disease)	• If only one lymph node is affected, carefully examine the drainage area of the lymph node for the underlying cause (p. 598)
• Metastatic neoplasia	
Deep (Visceral):	
• Systemic mycoses	• Associated with (often marked) systemic illness
• Metastatic neoplasia	• Identify primary neoplasm via physical exam, ultrasound, radiography. Fine-needle aspirate or biopsy required for final diagnosis
• Inflammatory conditions of the drained region (e.g., enteritis, hepatitis)	• Clinical, biochemistry, and/or imaging signs often supportive of primary problem

Reproduced from the third edition in modified form.

THIRD EDITION AUTHOR: Paolo Pazzi, BVSc, MMedVet

Lymphatic Disorders

Lymphangitis, Lymphedema, Lymphadenitis, Lymphadenopathy
- Infection
- Neoplasia
- Reactive hyperplasia
- Granuloma

Lymphedema
- **Primary Developmental Abnormality of Lymphatics**
  - Hypoplasia
  - Aplasia
  - Lymphangiectasia
  - Hyperplasia
- **Secondary Acquired Abnormality of Lymphatics**
  - Surgical excision of lymphatics or lymph nodes
  - Posttraumatic lymphangiopathy
  - Neoplastic invasion
  - Extrinsic compression of lymph vessels or tissue
  - Acute obstructive lymphadenitis
  - Chronic sclerosing lymphadenitis/lymphangitis
  - Lymphatic atrophy with interstitial fibrosis
  - Radiation therapy

Lymphocyst
- Cystic hygroma, lymphoceles, pseudocyst

Lymphangiomas

Lymphangiosarcomas

From Ettinger S, Feldman E: Textbook of veterinary internal medicine, ed 7, St. Louis, 2010, Saunders.

Lymphoma Staging Classification

The World Health Organization (WHO) Clinical Staging System for Lymphoma

Stage	Description
Stage I	Single lymph node
Stage II	Multiple regional lymph nodes
Stage III	Generalized lymphadenopathy
Stage IV	Liver and/or splenic involvement with or without stages I-III
Stage V	Blood and/or bone marrow involvement and/or extranodal involvement; with or without stages I-IV

Substage A: no overt clinical signs of disease
Substage B: overt clinical signs of disease

From Withrow S, Vail D, Page R: Withrow & MacEwen's Small animal clinical oncology, ed 5, St. Louis, 2013, Saunders.

Differentials, Lists, and Mnemonics

Megaesophagus

Associated Diseases and Causes in Dogs

Central Nervous System
- Canine distemper
- Cervical spondylomyelopathy with leukomalacia
- Brainstem lesions
- Neoplasia
- Trauma

Peripheral Neuropathies
- Polyneuritis
- Polyradiculoneuritis
- Ganglioradiculitis
- Dysautonomia
- Giant cell axonal neuropathy
- Spinal muscular atrophy
- Intoxication:
  - Lead
  - Thallium
  - Acrylamide
- Bilateral vagal damage
- Tetanus
- Botulism

Neuromuscular Junction
- Myasthenia gravis
- Botulism
- Tetanus
- Anticholinesterase toxicity

Esophageal Obstruction
- Esophageal stricture
- Persistent aortic arch
- Esophageal tumor
- Esophageal granuloma
- Lower esophageal sphincter achalasia-like syndrome
- *Spirocerca lupi*
- Hiatal hernia
- Thymoma

Esophageal Musculature
- Esophagitis
- Systemic lupus erythematosus
- Glycogen storage disease
- Polymyositis
- Dermatomyositis
- Cachexia
- Trypanosomiasis
- Hypoadrenocorticism
- Hypothyroidism?

Genetic
- Miniature schnauzer, golden retriever, German shepherd, Great Dane, Newfoundland, Shar-pei
- Muscular dystrophy (golden retriever)

Miscellaneous
- Pyloric stenosis
- Gastric dilation/volvulus
- Pituitary dwarfism
- Thymoma
- Mediastinitis

Idiopathic

?, Cause-and-effect relationship not established.

Modified from Bonagura J: Kirk's Current veterinary therapy XIII, St. Louis, 2000, Saunders.

Melena

Causes of Melena

Ingestion of Blood
- Sinonasal lesions
- Pulmonary lesions
- Oral/pharyngeal lesions
- Diet

Inflammatory
- Esophagitis
- Gastroenteritis
- Eosinophilic gastritis
- Inflammatory bowel disease

Infectious
- Bacterial: *Campylobacter, Clostridium, Mycobacterium, Neorickettsia helminthoeca, Salmonella*
- Fungal/algal: *Cryptococcus, Histoplasma, Pythium, Prototheca*
- Parasitic: *Spirocerca, Physaloptera, Ancylostoma, Uncinaria*
- Viral: parvovirus

Ischemic/Traumatic
- Hypovolemic shock
- Thrombosis/infarction
- Intussusception
- Volvulus
- Foreign body
- Racing sled dogs

Postsurgical
- Enterotomy
- Gastric invagination postcorrection of gastric dilation/volvulus
- Percutaneous endoscopic gastrostomy tube placement

Drug-Induced
- Corticosteroids
- Nonsteroidal antiinflammatory drugs

Neoplastic
- Adenocarcinoma
- Gastrointestinal stromal tumor
- Leiomyoma/leiomyosarcoma
- Lymphoma
- Mast cell tumor
- Gastrinoma

Vascular
- Vascular ectasia/angiodysplasia
- Arteriovenous fistula
- Gastric or esophageal varices (rare)

Metabolic
- Hypoadrenocorticism
- Uremic kidney disease
- Liver disease, particularly with portal hypertension or portosystemic shunt(s)
- Pancreatitis
- Hypereosinophilic syndrome

Bleeding Disorder
- Thrombocytopenia
- Thrombocytopathia
- Disseminated intravascular coagulation
- Rodenticide intoxication
- Specific factor deficiencies

Modified from Tefft KM: Melena and hematochezia. In Ettinger SJ, Feldman EC, Côté E, editors: Textbook of veterinary internal medicine: diseases of the dog and cat, ed 8, St. Louis, 2017, Elsevier.

Monoclonal Gammopathy

Associated Conditions

Multiple myeloma
Waldenstrom's macroglobulinemia
B-cell lymphoma/leukemia
Plasma cell leukemia
Nonsecretory myeloma
Extramedullary plasmacytoma
Monoclonal gammopathy of undetermined significance
Chronic lymphocytic leukemia
Leishmaniasis
Lymphoma
Feline infectious peritonitis
Ehrlichiosis
Amyloidosis
Lymphocytic enteritis

Modified from Bonagura J: Kirk's Current veterinary therapy XII: small animal practice, St. Louis, 1995, Saunders, p 525.

Myocarditis

Viral
- Canine distemper virus (neonate)
- Canine herpesvirus
- Canine parvovirus (prenatal, neonate)
- West Nile virus

Rickettsial
- *Rickettsia rickettsii*

Bacterial
- Numerous genera
- *Borrelia burgdorferi*
- *Bartonella henselae*
- *Bartonella vinsonii* subsp *berkhoffii*

Algal
- *Prototheca* spp

Fungal
- *Blastomyces dermatitidis*
- *Cryptococcus neoformans*
- *Coccidioides immitis*
- *Aspergillus terreus*
- *Paecilomyces variotii*

Protozoal
- *Trypanosoma cruzi*
- *Toxoplasma gondii*
- *Hepatozoon americanum*
- *Neospora caninum*

Traumatic
- Hit by car
- Injury from falling
- Penetrating trauma
- Cardiac catheterization

Immune-Mediated Conditions
- Rarely reported in veterinary medicine

Unknown
- Transmissible myocarditis-diaphragmitis of cats

Modified with permission from Greene C: Infectious disease of the dog and cat, ed 4, St. Louis, 2012, Saunders.

Myopathies

Classification

Inflammatory
- Infectious
  - Bacterial: leptospirosis
  - Protozoal: toxoplasmosis, neosporosis
  - Parasitic: *Toxocara*, others
- Immune-Mediated
  - Masticatory myositis
  - Polymyositis
  - Dermatomyositis

Degenerative
- Acquired
  - Endocrine:
    - Hyperadrenocorticism
    - Hypothyroidism
    - Hypokalemic polymyopathy (cats)
  - Fibrotic/ossifying myopathies
  - Ischemic
  - Nutritional
  - Neoplastic
  - Toxic (e.g., monensin, glucocorticoid)
- Inherited
  - Muscular dystrophy:
    - Exercise-induced collapse in Labrador retrievers
    - X-linked muscular dystrophy (dystrophin deficient)
    - Other muscular dystrophies (dystrophin positive)
  - Myotonia
  - Metabolic:
    - Pyruvate dehydrogenase phosphatase 1 deficiency in Clumber and Sussex spaniels
    - Glycogen storage disease
      - Mitochondrial myopathy
      - Lipidic myopathy
      - Malignant hyperthermia
  - Centronuclear myopathy (Labrador retriever)
  - Hypertonicity in Cavalier King Charles spaniels
  - Inherited myopathy of Great Danes
  - Others (e.g., Irish terriers, German shepherds, miniature schnauzer)

From Ettinger S, Feldman E: Textbook of veterinary internal medicine, ed 6, St. Louis, 2005, Saunders; and Shelton D: What's new in muscle and peripheral nerve disease. Vet Comp Orthop Traumatol 20:249-255, 2007.

Myopathies, Feline Congenital

Characteristics

Disease	Affected Breeds and Geographical Provenance	Mode of Inheritance	Underlying Defect	Clinical Signs	Prognosis
Congenital myotonia	DSH (NZ, US)	Autosomal recessive	Probable defect in chloride channels	Stiff gait, hyperactivity of selected muscle groups when startled, percussion dimple	Fair to good (nonprogressive condition, cats enjoy a normal quality of life)
Devon rex and sphynx myopathy	Devon rex (AUS, GB), sphynx	Autosomal recessive	COLQ variant	Cervical ventroflexion; generalized muscle weakness; abnormal gait; megaesophagus	Poor (many cats die of asphyxiation)
Dystrophin-deficient myopathy	DSH (US, NL, CH)	X-linked recessive	Dystrophin deficiency	Skeletal muscle hypertrophy with possible complications, sensitivity to stress, stiff gait	Guarded to fair (cats can have an almost normal quality of life but may require more frequent veterinary visits)
Glycogen storage disease type IV	Norwegian forest cats (US, Europe)	Autosomal recessive	GBE deficiency	Stillbirth, muscle tremor, muscle atrophy; cardiomyopathy	Poor (all cats eventually die from the condition)
Hypokalemic myopathy	Burmese (AUS, NZ, GB, NL)	Probably autosomal recessive	Unknown	Transient, paroxysmal clinical signs with generalized muscle weakness, cervical ventroflexion	Good response to potassium supplementation
Malignant hyperthermia	DSH	Unknown	Unknown	Severe hyperthermia during anesthesia (halothane)	Poor (two reported cases in which cats died)
Merosin-deficient myopathy	DSH, Siamese (US)	Unknown	Merosin (laminin-2) deficiency	Hindlimb weakness from 6 months old, worsening to muscle atrophy and contractures at 1 year old	Poor (both cats in the two reported cases were euthanized before 2 years of age)
MG	DSH	Unknown	Lack of ACH receptors	Generalized muscle weakness	Fair, generally good response to therapy
Nemaline myopathy	DSH (US)	Possibly autosomal recessive	Unknown	Progressive weakness (6-18 months); rapid, choppy, hypermetric gait; tremor, exercise intolerance	Poor (five reported cats died or were euthanized)

ACH, Acetylcholine; *AUS*, Australia; *CH*, Switzerland; *DSH*, domestic shorthair; *GB*, Great Britain; *GBE*, glycogen branching enzyme; *MG*, myasthenia gravis; *NL*, Netherlands; *NZ*, New Zealand; *US*, United States.
Modified from Gaschen F, Jaggy A, Jones B: Congenital diseases of feline muscle and neuromuscular junction. J Feline Med Surg 6:355-366, 2004.

Myositis, Infectious

Microorganisms Associated With Musculoskeletal Infections

Hepatozoon americanum
Hepatozoon canis
Toxoplasma gondii
Neospora caninum
Borrelia burgdorferi
Rickettsia rickettsii
Ehrlichia canis
Babesia canis
Leishmania infantum
Cytauxzoon felis
Sarcocystis
Toxigenic *Streptococcus canis*
Leptospirosis
Feline immunodeficiency virus
Numerous other bacteria (e.g., *Staphylococci* [dogs], *Pasteurella multocida* [cats])

Nasal Discharge

	Unilateral	Bilateral
Serous		• Stress • Nasal mites • Allergy • Irritants (e.g., cleaning products, cigarette smoke) • Early viral infection (i.e., FCV, FHV-1) • Congestive heart failure
Mucoid or mucopurulent	• Oronasal/periodontal disease (e.g., tooth-root abscess, oronasal fistula) • Foreign body (e.g., grass awn, sticks) • Early nasal neoplasia (e.g., adenocarcinoma, undifferentiated carcinoma, lymphoma) • Early fungal rhinitis (e.g., *Cryptococcus* spp, *Aspergillus* spp, *Penicillium* spp) • Neurogenic rhinitis (e.g., usually concurrent to ipsilateral KCS) • Parasitic (e.g., *Cuterebra* spp) • Idiopathic lymphoplasmacytic rhinitis (can be unilateral)	• Systemic disease (e.g., vomiting, regurgitation, pneumonia, viral respiratory infections, dysautonomia) • Oronasal/periodontal disease (e.g., cleft palate, bilateral tooth-root abscesses) • Nasopharyngeal stenosis • Fungal rhinitis (e.g., *Cryptococcus* spp, *Aspergillus* spp, *Penicillium* spp, *Rhinosporidium* spp) • Nasal neoplasia (e.g., adenocarcinoma, chondrosarcoma, lymphoma) • Nasopharyngeal polyp (cats > dogs) • Idiopathic lymphoplasmacytic rhinitis • Secondary bacterial rhinitis

Epistaxis	• Fungal rhinitis
	• Nasal neoplasia
	• Hemostatic defect (often bilateral, but may begin as unilateral epistaxis)
	• Trauma
	• Foreign body (typically becomes mucoid or mucopurulent with time)
		• Hemostatic defect
		  • Primary (thrombocytopenia, thrombocytopathy)
		  • Secondary (e.g., vitamin K rodenticide, liver failure)
		• Severe systemic hypertension (rare)
		• Vasculitis (infectious, immune mediated, idiopathic)
		  • Infectious (e.g., ehrlichiosis)
		  • Immune mediated
		  • Idiopathic
		• Fungal rhinitis
		• Nasal neoplasia

AUTHOR: Jared Jaffey, DVM, MS, DACVIM

Nasal Discharge/Obstruction in Cats, Chronic

Viral rhinitis with or without secondary bacterial infection
- Herpesvirus (feline viral rhinotracheitis)
- Calicivirus

Neoplasia (nasal lymphoma, adenocarcinoma, other)
Lymphoplasmacytic rhinitis
Foreign body (often plant material, grass)
Cryptococcal rhinitis
Tooth root abscess
Oronasal fistulae
Nasopharyngeal stenosis
Esophageal motility dysfunction
Nasopharyngeal polyp
Cleft palate, congenital (uncommon)

Cause often remains undetermined even after diagnostic investigation.

Nasal Neoplasia

Malignant Tumors of the Canine and Feline Nasal Cavity and Paranasal Sinuses

Canine
- Adenocarcinoma
  - Differentiated
  - Undifferentiated
- Transitional cell carcinoma
- Squamous cell carcinoma
- Chondrosarcoma
- Fibrosarcoma
- Lymphoma

Feline
- Adenocarcinoma
- Lymphoma

Infrequently Reported
- Osteosarcoma
- Hemangiosarcoma
- Rhabdomyosarcoma
- Leiomyosarcoma
- Nerve sheath tumors
- Neuroblastoma

Modified from Bonagura J: Kirk's Current veterinary therapy XIII, St. Louis, 2000, Saunders.

Neck Pain: Common Causes

Intervertebral disc disease	Chondrodystrophic breeds >2-3 years of age; no history of trauma, no fever, acute onset of pain/paresis
Meningitis (inflammatory or infectious)	Cranial cervical pain; possible fever, negative findings on spinal imaging (CT or MRI), neutrophilic or mixed inflammation in CSF; breeds: Bernese mountain dog, boxer, beagle, Nova Scotia duck tolling retriever; infections: cryptococcosis, neosporosis, toxoplasmosis
Cervical spondylomyelopathy	Typically large- or giant-breed dogs; UMN deficits to limbs common
Foreign body/abscess	Focal pain, swelling or heat; possible fever, hypersalivation; progressive swelling with abscess/cellulitis; dogs with history of chewing objects and stick play; cats that are indoor/outdoor or multi-cat household
Trauma/fracture	Trauma history; acute onset of pain/paresis; survey radiographs showing fracture/subluxation in cervical spine
Neoplasia	Older dog or cat; should be high on the differential list for non-chondrodystrophic breeds without cervical spondylomyelopathy (large-/giant-breed dogs)
Atlantoaxial instability	Young small-breed dogs
Discospondylitis	May be febrile; often apparent on radiographs; brucellosis testing and blood culture recommended

Apparent neck pain can be due to disease other than the cervical spine (thorax, head, nerve sheath tumor).
CSF, Cerebrospinal fluid; *CT,* computed tomography; *MRI,* magnetic resonance imaging; *UMN,* upper motor neuron.
Reproduced from the third edition in modified form.

THIRD EDITION AUTHOR: **David A. Puerto, DVM, DACVS**

Nephrotoxic Agents

Class of Agent	Examples
Antibacterials	Aminoglycosides, cephalosporins (cephaloridine, cefazolin, cephalothin), penicillins, sulfonamides, fluoroquinolones, tetracyclines, vancomycin, carbapenems, aztreonam, rifampin, nafcillin, polymyxin
Antiprotozoals	Trimethoprim-sulfamethoxazole, sulfadiazine, thiacetarsamide, pentamidine, dapsone
Antifungals	Amphotericin B
Antivirals	Acyclovir, foscarnet
Chemotherapeutics	Cisplatin or carboplatin, doxorubicin, azathioprine, methotrexate
Immunosuppressives	Cyclosporine, interleukin-2
Nonsteroidal antiinflammatories	All
Angiotensin-converting enzyme inhibitors	All
Diuretics	All
Radiocontrast agents	All iodinated radiographic contrast agents
Miscellaneous therapeutics	Allopurinol, cimetidine, apomorphine, Dextran 40, penicillamine, EDTA, streptokinase, methoxyflurane, tricyclic antidepressants, lipid-lowering agents, calcium antagonists, vitamin D_3 analogs (psoriasis medications), lithium, phosphorus-containing urinary acidifiers
Heavy metals	Mercury, uranium, lead, bismuth salts, chromium, arsenic, gold, cadmium, thallium, copper, silver, nickel, antimony
Organic compounds	Ethylene glycol, chloroform, pesticides, herbicides, solvents, carbon tetrachloride and other chlorinated hydrocarbons
Miscellaneous toxins	Gallium nitrate, bisphosphonates, mushrooms, grapes, raisins, snake venom, bee venom, lilies, vitamin D_3–containing rodenticides, sodium fluoride, superphosphate fertilizer
Endogenous toxins	Hemoglobin, myoglobin

From Langston CE: Acute kidney injury. In Ettinger SJ, Feldman EC, Côté E, editors: Textbook of veterinary internal medicine: diseases of the dog and cat, ed 8, St. Louis, 2017, Elsevier.

Nerves of the Forelimb: Cutaneous Distribution

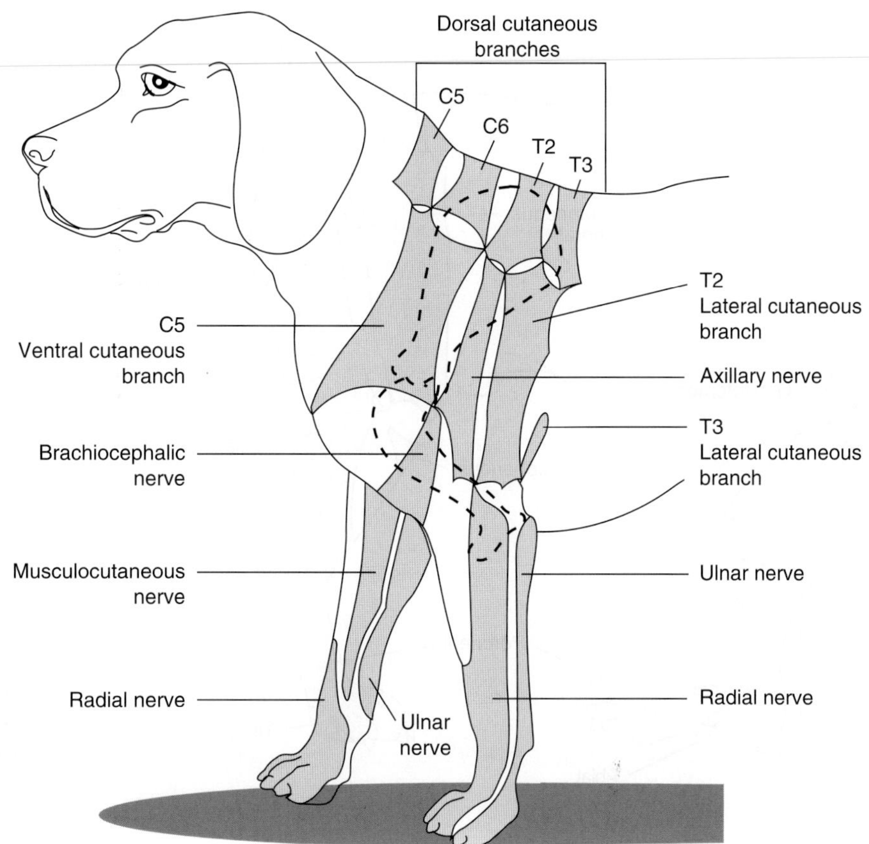

(Figure reproduced from De Lahunta A, Glass E: Veterinary neuroanatomy and clinical neurology, ed 3, St. Louis, 2009, Saunders, with permission.)

Nerves of the Forelimb: Localization of Contributing Spinal Cord Segments

Nerve	Spinal Cord Segments
Phrenic	C5, 6, 7
Cranial pectoral	C6, 7, 8
Suprascapular	C6, 7
Subscapular	C6, 7
Musculocutaneous	C6, 7, 8
Axillary	C7, 8
Thoracodorsal	C8
Lateral thoracic	C8, T1
Radial	C7, 8, T1, 2
Median and ulnar	C8, T1, 2
Caudal pectoral	C8, T1, 2
Sympathetics (Horner's)	T1, 2, 3

From Evans H, de Lahunta A: Guide to the dissection of the dog, ed 7, St. Louis, 2010, Saunders.

Nerves of the Hindlimb: Cutaneous Distribution

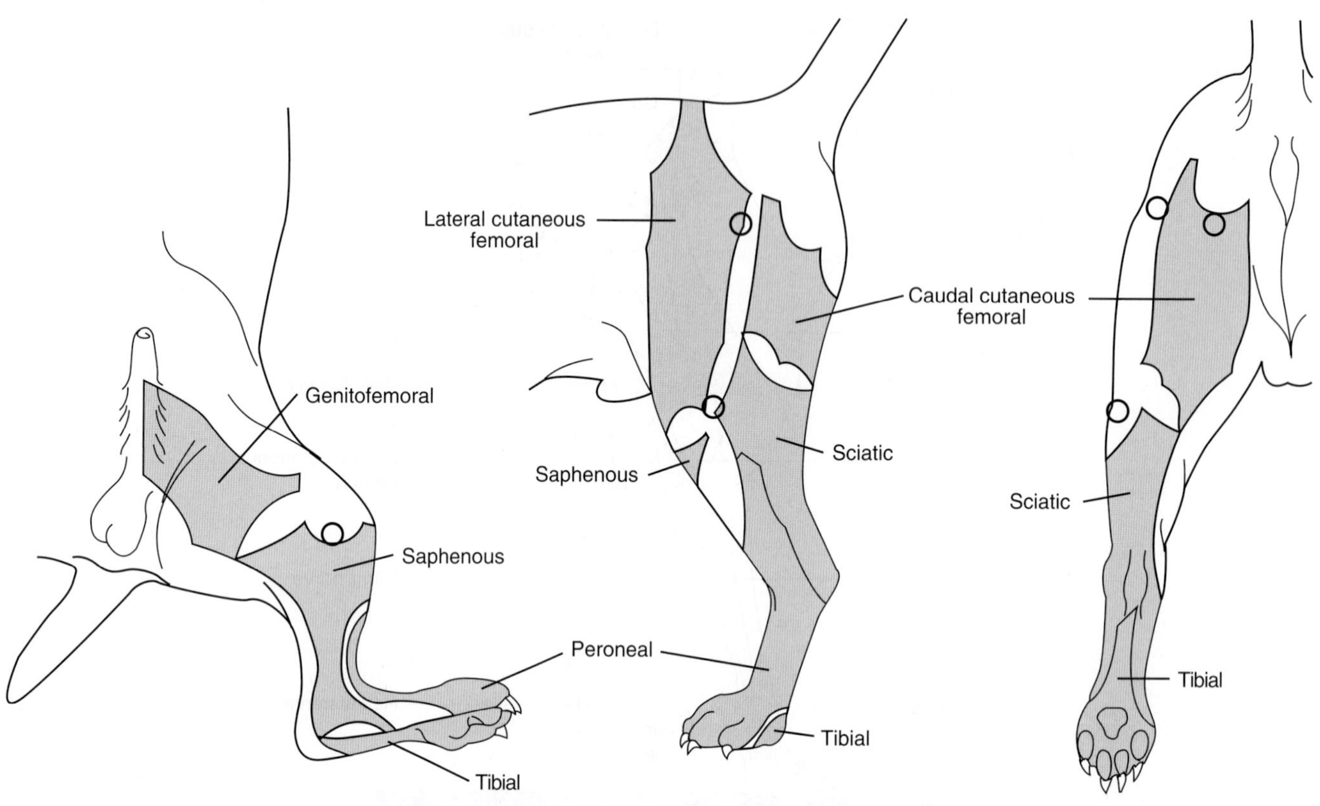

○ Palpable bony landmarks

(Figure reproduced from De Lahunta A, Glass E: Veterinary neuroanatomy and clinical neurology, ed 3, St. Louis, 2009, Saunders, with permission.)

Nerves of the Hindlimb: Localization of Contributing Spinal Cord Segments

Nerve	Spinal Cord Segments
Femoral	L4, 5, 6
Obturator	L(4), 5, 6
Cranial gluteal	L6, 7, S1
Caudal gluteal	L7, S1, 2
Sciatic	L6, 7, S1, 2
Pudendal	S1, 2, 3

From Evans H, de Lahunta A: Guide to the dissection of the dog, ed 7, St. Louis, 2010, Saunders.

Neurologic Signs: Brain

Relationship of Clinical Signs to Anatomic Site of Lesion

Clinical Signs	Functional System	Anatomic Location
Inability to prehend	Masticatory and tongue muscles	CN V, XII, pons-medulla
Dysphagia	Tongue, palatal, pharyngeal, and esophageal muscles	CN IX, X, XI, XII, medulla
Drooling	Facial paralysis, dysphagia	CN VII, middle ear, medulla
		CN IX, X, medulla
Head tilt, nystagmus, loss of balance, rolling	Vestibular system	CN VIII: inner ear, medulla, cerebellum
Strabismus	CN to extraocular muscles, vestibular system	CN III, IV, VI, midbrain-medulla
		Inner ear-medulla-cerebellum
Circling		
With loss of balance	Vestibular system	Inner ear, medulla, cerebellum
Without loss of balance	Limbic system (?)	Frontal lobe, rostral thalamus
Head and eye deviation—turning to one side	Limbic system (?)	Frontal lobe, rostral thalamus
Pacing, head pressing	Limbic system	Frontal lobe, rostral thalamus
Opisthotonos	Upper motor neuron	Rostral cerebellum, midbrain
Blindness	Visual system	
	Dilated unresponsive pupils	Eyeball, optic nerves
	Normal pupils	Visual cortex–cerebrum (midbrain)
Depression, semicoma, coma	Ascending reticular activating system	Pons to thalamus–cerebral cortex
Seizures	Cerebrum, thalamus-hypothalamus	
Hyperesthesia, hyperactivity to external stimuli	Ascending reticular activating system	Thalamus, cerebrum
Aggressive behavior, mania-hysteria, odontoprisis	Limbic system	Thalamus, cerebrum
Tremor		
Associated with movements, head, and neck	Cerebellar system	Cerebellum
Associated with movements, head, trunk, limbs	Multiple systems	Diffuse CNS
Episodic, not associated with movements, head, trunk, limbs		Thalamus, cerebrum
Bradycardia, hypothermia, hyperthermia	UMN for general visceral efferent system	Hypothalamus
Irregular-ataxic respirations	UMN for respiratory muscle LMN	Pons-medulla

CN, Cranial nerve; *CNS,* central nervous system; *LMN,* lower motor neuron; *UMN,* upper motor neuron; *?,* may occur with lesion in this location.
From de Lahunta A, Glass E: Veterinary neuroanatomy and clinical neurology, ed 3, St. Louis, 2009, Saunders.

Neuromuscular Diseases

Diseases of the Lower Motor Neuron

- Neuromuscular Junction—Junctionopathies
  - Myasthenia gravis
  - Drugs and toxins:
    - Botulinum toxin
    - Blue-green algae (anatoxins)
    - Aminoglycosides
    - Polymyxins
    - Ionophores (lasalocid)
    - Black widow spider venom
    - Organophosphates
    - Snake venoms
    - Tick bite paralysis
- Peripheral Nerves—Neuropathies
  - Degenerative/inherited:
    - Alaskan malamute/greyhound polyneuropathy
    - Dancing Doberman disease
    - Distal sensorimotor neuropathy
    - Birman cat polyneuropathy
    - Boxer dog axonopathy
    - Giant axonal neuropathy
    - Laryngeal paralysis/polyneuropathy complex
    - Inherited polyneuropathy of Leonberger dogs
    - Laryngeal paralysis
    - Distal denervating disease
    - Golden retriever hypomyelinating polyneuropathy
    - Miniature schnauzer demyelinating polyneuropathy
    - Hypertrophic neuropathy
    - Megaesophagus
    - Idiopathic facial paralysis
    - Sensory neuropathy
    - Idiopathic self-mutilation
    - Spinal muscular atrophy
    - Dysautonomia
    - Lysosomal storage disease
  - Anomalous/developmental:
    - Optic nerve hypoplasia
  - Metabolic:
    - Diabetic neuropathy
    - Hyperadrenocorticoid neuropathy
    - Hyperchylomicronemia (cats)
    - Hyperoxaluria (cats)
    - Hypothyroid neuropathy
  - Neoplastic:
    - Paraneoplastic neuropathy
    - Malignant nerve sheath tumors
    - Mononuclear cell neoplasia
  - Inflammatory/infectious, autoimmune:
    - Brachial plexus neuritis/neuropathy
    - Optic neuritis
    - Polyradiculoneuritis
    - Chronic inflammatory demyelinating polyneuropathy/chronic relapsing polyneuropathy
    - Protozoal polyradiculoneuritis
    - Sensory ganglioradiculoneuritis
    - Trigeminal neuritis
    - Hemifacial spasm
    - Ischemic neuromyopathy
  - Traumatic:
    - Isolated nerve injury
    - Compartment syndrome
    - Brachial plexus injury
  - Toxic:
    - Thallium poisoning
    - Pyridoxine poisoning
    - Vincristine neuropathy
    - Delayed organophosphate toxicity (cats)
    - Walker hound mononeuropathy
    - Salinomycin toxicity (cats)

Muscle Disease-Myopathies

- Degenerative/Developmental:
  - Muscular dystrophy
  - Centronuclear myopathy
  - Exercise-induced intolerance and collapse of Labrador retrievers
  - Distal myopathy of rottweilers
  - Myotonia congenital
  - Fibrotic myopathy
  - Nemaline myopathy
  - Myositis ossificans (fibrodysplasia ossificans progressive)
  - Pharyngeal/esophageal dysfunction of Bouviers
  - Polysystemic disorder of English springer spaniels
  - Cricopharyngeal achalasia
  - Episodic muscle hypertonicity ("cramp")
  - Myokymia and neuromyotonia
- Metabolic:
  - Hypokalemic myopathy
  - Hyperkalemic periodic paralysis
  - Hyperadrenocorticoid (Cushing's) myopathy
  - Hypothyroid myopathy
  - Malignant hyperthermia
  - Exertional myopathy
  - Lipid storage/mitochondrial myopathies
  - Glycogen storage disorders (glycogenoses)
- Inflammatory/Infectious:
  - Masticatory myositis
  - Extraocular myositis
  - Laryngeal/pharyngeal myositis
  - Autoimmune polymyositis
  - Dermatomyositis
  - Feline hyperesthesia syndrome
  - Infectious myositis
  - Tetanus
- Ischemic:
  - Ischemic neuromyopathy
- Traumatic:
  - Infraspinatus contracture
  - Iliopsoas muscle injury
  - Quadriceps contracture
  - Coccygeal muscle injury

Neutrophil Dysfunction

Causes of Congenital and Acquired Neutrophil Dysfunction

Dysfunction	Species
Chemotactic Factor Generation	
Congenital	
C3 deficiency (Brittany spaniel)	Dog
Adherence	
Congenital	
CD11–CD18 adhesion protein deficiency (Irish setter)	Dog
Acquired	
Diabetes mellitus (poorly regulated)	Dog
Chemotaxis	
Congenital	
C3 deficiency (Brittany spaniel)	Dog
CD11–CD18 adhesion protein deficiency (Irish setter)	Dog
Chédiak-Higashi syndrome (Persian)	Cat
Pelger-Huët anomaly?	Dog*
Primary ciliary dyskinesia	Dog
Recurrent infections (Weimaraner)	Dog
Acquired	
Bacterial pyoderma	Dog
Demodicosis (serum inhibitor?)	Dog
FeLV infection	Cat
FIP	Cat
Hyperalimentation-induced hypophosphatemia	Dog
Protothecosis (serum inhibitor?)	Dog
Phagocytosis	
Congenital	
C3 deficiency (Brittany spaniel)	Dog
CD11–CD18 adhesion protein deficiency (Irish setter)	Dog
Recurrent and persistent infections (Weimaraner)	Dog
Acquired	
Continuous-flow centrifugation and filtration-leukapheresis	
Collected neutrophils (few hours after pheresis)	Dog
Hyperalimentation-induced hypophosphatemia	Dog
Aging	Dog
Bacterial Killing	
Congenital	
CD11–CD18 adhesion protein deficiency (Irish setter)	Dog
Cyclic neutropenia (gray collies)	Dog
Recurrent and persistent infections (Weimaraner)	Dog
Rhinitis-pneumonia syndrome (Doberman pinscher)	Dog
Acquired	
FeLV infection	Cat
Hyperalimentation-induced hypophosphatemia	Dog
Lead toxicosis	Dog
Turpentine-induced inflammation	Dog
Chemotherapy	Dog
Kidney failure	Dog

*Neutrophil chemotaxis was tested in only one of four English-American (Walker) foxhounds with Pelger-Huët anomaly; defective chemotaxis has not been found in other dogs, including foxhounds, with the anomaly.

FeLV, Feline leukemia virus; *FIP*, feline infectious peritonitis.

Modified from Bonagura J: Kirk's Current veterinary therapy XIII, St. Louis, 2000, Saunders.

Obesity: Causes and Contributors

Excess caloric intake (most common)	Hyperadrenocorticism
Insufficient physical activity	Hypothalamic disorders
Neutering	Chronic steroid or antiepileptic drug use
Hypothyroidism	Orthopedic disease

Reproduced from the third edition in modified form.

THIRD EDITION AUTHOR: **Kathryn E. Michel, DVM, MS, DACVN**

Oral Ulcers

Comparison of Ulcerative Lesions in Oral Cavities of Dogs and Cats

Cause	Species	Lesion Location
Excessive licking (eosinophilic ulcer)	C	Upper incisor or carnassial area of lip, near philtrum, roof of mouth (hard palate)
Autoimmune diseases (e.g., bullous pemphigoid, pemphigus vulgaris, systemic lupus erythematosus, erythema multiforme)	D	Roof of mouth, lips, cheeks, often symmetrical; other mucocutaneous regions, footpads
Irritants, uremia	B	Tip of tongue
Viral (parvoviral), rickettsial (RMSF)	D	Multifocal lingual
Contact mucositis (AKA contact mucosal ulceration, chronic ulcerative paradental stomatitis [CUPS], ulcerative stomatitis, idiopathic stomatitis, lymphocytic plasmacytic stomatitis, and plaque-reactive stomatitis). Breed predisposition Maltese dog, greyhound, Cavalier King Charles spaniel, and Scottish terrier.	D > C	Mucosa apical to the maxillary canines and 4th premolars most likely involved. Marked inflammation with or without ulceration and necrosis of the vestibular mucosa in areas that contact tooth surfaces are also affected.
Dental tartar, periodontal disease	B	Periodontal regions (gingival margins)
Traumatic (e.g., malocclusion, foreign body, injury from bone/stick)	B	Any area affected
Chemical (e.g., liquid potpourri, acids, caustic substances, quaternary ammonium disinfectants, pancreatic enzyme supplements)	B	In shelter settings, oral ulcers and drooling associated with overzealous use of disinfectants can be mistaken for calicivirus in cats.
Herpesvirus	C	Tongue, palate, multifocal
Calicivirus	C	Acute: dorsal tongue surface Chronic: caudal mucositis (inflammation of the caudal oral cavity lateral to the palatoglossal folds), extending rostrally into gingiva, alveolar mucosa and labial, buccal and sublingual mucosa
Spirochete-induced aphthous ulcers	D	Bright red ulcers
Immunosuppression: hyperadrenocorticism, leukopenia, FeLV, FIV	B	Periodontal region, may spread to gums and cheeks
Electrocution	C	Lips, labial mucosa, alveolar mucosa and gingiva, tongue (often in linear pattern), hard palate mucosa
Metabolic disease (e.g., uremia)	B	Tongue tip
Nutritional disorders (e.g., protein calorie malnutrition, riboflavin deficiency)	B	Variable

B, Both cat and dog; *C,* cats; *D,* dogs; *FeLV,* feline leukemia virus; *FIV,* feline immunodeficiency virus; *RMSF,* Rocky Mountain spotted fever.
Modified from Greene C: Infectious diseases of the dog and cat, ed 4, St. Louis, 2012, Saunders.

Orthopedic Disorders: Common Signalment Profiles

Young (≤1 Year Old) Little Dogs

Forelimb
- Congenital medial shoulder luxation
- Lateral humeral condylar fractures
- Elbow incongruities
- Congenital elbow luxations
- Septic arthritis
- Distal radius/ulna fractures

Hindlimb
- Aseptic necrosis of the femoral head (Legg-Calvé-Perthes disease)
- Femoral capital physeal fractures
- Patellar luxation
- Septic arthritis
- Pes varus (dachshunds)

Adult Little Dogs

Forelimb
- Congenital medial shoulder luxation
- Osteoarthritis from elbow incongruities
- Distal radius/ulna fractures
- Carpal hyperextension
- Polyarthritis

Hindlimb
- Patellar luxation
- Cranial cruciate ligament rupture (often with static drawer)
- Tarsal hyperflexion from rupture of the plantar tarsal ligament

Young (≤1.5 Years Old) Big Dogs

Forelimb
- OCD of the humeral head
- Panosteitis
- Lateral humeral condylar fractures
- Congenital elbow luxations
- Septic arthritis
- Ununited anconeal process
- Fragmented medial coronoid process
- Elbow incongruities
- OCD of the medial aspect of the humeral condyle
- Hypertrophic osteodystrophy
- Puppy carpal laxity and flexural deformity syndromes

Hindlimb
- Hip dysplasia
- Septic arthritis
- Capital femoral physeal fractures
- Panosteitis
- Patellar luxation
- Cranial cruciate ligament rupture (uncommon this young)
- OCD of the lateral femoral condyle
- OCD of the medial ridge of the talus (also the lateral ridge in rottweilers)

Adult Big Dogs

Forelimb
- Infraspinatus contracture/tendinopathy
- Supraspinatus tendinopathy
- Medial glenohumeral ligament tears
- Biceps tendinopathies
- Subscapularis tendon ruptures
- Osteosarcoma: proximal humerus, distal radius
- Lateral humeral condylar fractures (especially spaniels)
- Osteoarthritis due to elbow incongruity, elbow dysplasias
- Carpal hyperextension
- Abductor pollicis longus stenosing tenosynovitis
- Polyarthritis

Hindlimb
- Lumbosacral compressive disease causing lameness
- Iliopsoas strain
- Osteoarthritis due to hip dysplasia
- Osteosarcoma: proximal and distal femur, proximal and distal tibia
- Fibrotic myopathy of the caudal thigh muscles
- Patellar luxation
- Cranial cruciate ligament rupture
- Osteoarthritis from talar OCD
- Gastrocnemius apparatus ruptures
- Tarsal hyperflexion from rupture of the plantar tarsal ligament
- Superficial digital flexor tendon luxation
- Digital tendon ruptures

Young Cats (≤2 Years of Age)

Forelimb
- Septic arthritis
- Radius/ulna fractures
- Radial hemimelia

Hindlimb
- Femoral capital physeal fractures (especially castrated males 1-2 years old)
- Patellar luxation
- Clubfoot condition

Adult Cats

Forelimb
- Osteosarcoma
- Osteochondromatosis: shoulder, elbow
- Cat bite abscesses
- Septic arthritis, osteomyelitis
- Carpal hyperextension
- Contracture of carpal/digital flexor muscles
- Lameness subsequent to declawing surgery

Hindlimb
- Patellar luxation
- Cranial cruciate ligament rupture
- Gastrocnemius apparatus ruptures
- Osteochondromatosis of the stifle

OCD, Osteochondritis dissecans.
Reproduced from the third edition in unabridged form.

THIRD EDITION AUTHOR: Kathleen Linn, DVM, MS, DACVS

Osteomyelitis

Causes in Dogs

Bacterial

Aerobes
- *Escherichia coli*
- *Klebsiella* spp
- *Pasteurella* spp
- *Proteus* spp
- *Pseudomonas* spp
- *Staphylococcus* spp (most common of the bacteria that cause osteomyelitis)
  - *S. pseudintermedius*
- *Streptococcus* spp

Anaerobes
- *Actinomyces* spp
- *Bacteroides* spp
- *Clostridium* spp
- *Fusobacterium* spp
- *Nocardia* spp
- *Peptostreptococcus* spp

Viral
- Canine distemper virus

Fungal
- *Aspergillus* spp
- *Blastomyces dermatitidis*
- *Candida* spp
- *Coccidioides immitis*
- *Cryptococcus neoformans*
- *Histoplasma capsulatum*

Ototoxic Agents

Potential to Cause Cochlear or Vestibular Damage

Ototoxic Agents	Comments
Aminoglycoside antibiotics (streptomycin, neomycin, kanamycin, amikacin, gentamicin, tobramycin)	Affects cochlear or vestibular apparatus; can be unilateral or bilateral; ototoxicity occurs mostly with repeated use; affects higher-frequency range first, followed by lower-frequency range
Other antibiotics (erythromycin; chloramphenicol; polymyxin B; minocycline; vancomycin, hygromycin B)	IV or large oral doses of erythromycin reversible; minocycline reversible; topical administration of polymyxin or some aminoglycosides in patients with perforated tympanic membrane; hygromycin B fed to three collies for 10 months
Tea tree oil	Possible if concentrated oil administered in the ear for treating otitis externa; high risk in patients with perforated tympanic membrane
Chemotherapeutic agents (cisplatin, carboplatin, nitrogen mustard)	Likely with repeated doses or high acute administration
Salicylate analgesics	Possible with large acute ingestion; reversible
Diuretics (furosemide, ethacrynic acid)	Can affect stria vascularis in cochlea; possible with rapid IV use, especially in human kidney disease patients; toxicosis not reported in small animals
Antiseptics (quaternary ammonium compounds such as benzethonium chloride, benzalkonium chloride, and cetrimide; ethanol, iodine or iodophors in 70% alcohol; chlorhexidine)	Possible with topical use; higher risk in patients with perforated tympanic membrane
Heavy metals (lead, mercury, arsenic)	Directly toxic to neural tissues; may affect hearing; ototoxicity not well documented in small animals
Quinine (antimalarial)	Likely not an issue in small animals
Propylene glycol	Possible with 100% solution used topically
Arsenic	Damage to stria vascularis
Lead	Directly toxic to neural tissues
Mercury	Atrophy of cerebral and cerebellar cortices

Panting

Elevated ambient temperature
Overweight/obesity
Fever, hyperthermia
Anxiety, nervousness
Excitement
Pain
Anemia
Hemoglobinopathy (e.g., methemoglobinemia)
Hyperadrenocorticism
Glucocorticoid therapy
Pheochromocytoma
Hepatic encephalopathy
Hyperthyroidism
Hypocalcemia
Narcotic administration
Cardiac disease/tachyarrhythmias
Brain disease

Modified with permission from King L: Textbook of respiratory disease in dogs and cats, St. Louis, 2004, Saunders, p 47.

Paraneoplastic Syndromes

Gastrointestinal Manifestations of Cancer

Cancer Cachexia
- Multiple tumor types

Gastroduodenal Ulceration
- Mast cell tumor
- Gastrinoma

Endocrinologic Manifestations of Cancer

Hypercalcemia of Malignancy
- Lymphoma
- Anal sac apocrine gland adenocarcinoma
- Multiple myeloma
- Parathyroid tumors
- Mammary tumors
- Thymoma
- Others

Hypoglycemia
- Insulinoma
- Hepatic tumors
- Salivary tumors
- Leiomyoma/leiomyosarcoma
- Plasma cell tumors
- Lymphoma
- Mammary tumors
- Others

Ectopic ACTH
- Primary lung tumors

Hematologic Manifestations of Cancer

Hypergammaglobulinemia
- Multiple myeloma
- Lymphoma

Anemia
- Multiple tumors

Continued

(Continued from previous page)

Erythrocytosis
- Renal tumors (increased erythropoietin)
- Lymphoma
- Nasal fibrosarcoma
- TVT
- Hepatic tumors

Neutrophilic Leukocytosis
- Lymphoma
- Multiple tumors

Thrombocytopenia/Coagulopathies/DIC
- Lymphoma
- Mast cell tumor
- Hemangiosarcoma
- Thyroid tumors
- Mammary tumors
- Nasal tumors
- Inflammatory carcinomas
- Others

Cutaneous Manifestations of Cancer

Alopecia
- Pancreatic carcinoma (feline)
- Others

Flushing
- Mast cell tumor
- Pheochromocytoma
- Others

Nodular Dermatofibrosis
- Renal cystadenoma/cystadenocarcinoma

Necrolytic Migratory Erythema/Superficial Necrolytic Dermatitis
- Glucagonoma

Cutaneous Necrosis of the Hind Paws
- Lymphoma (cat)

Pemphigus Vulgaris
- Lymphoma (dog and horse)

Renal Manifestations of Cancer

Glomerulonephritis/Nephrotic Syndrome
- Multiple myeloma
- Polycythemia vera
- Lymphocytic leukemia
- Others

Neurologic Manifestations of Cancer

Myasthenia Gravis
- Thymoma
- Osteosarcoma
- Biliary carcinoma
- Others

Peripheral Neuropathy
- Insulinoma
- Others

Miscellaneous Manifestations of Cancer

Hypertrophic Osteopathy
- Primary lung tumor
- Urinary bladder rhabdomyosarcoma
- Esophageal tumors
- Metastatic tumors
- Others

Fever
- Multiple tumors

ACTH, Adrenocorticotropic hormone; *DIC,* disseminated intravascular coagulation; *TVT,* transmissible venereal tumor.
From Withrow S, et al: Withrow & MacEwen's Small animal clinical oncology, ed 5, St. Louis, 2013, Saunders.

Paresis, Forelimb

Differential Diagnosis Item	Key Feature(s)
Intervertebral disc disease	Variable pain on spinal palpation, paresis, ataxia, proprioceptive deficits; clinical signs often asymmetrical; forelimb lameness/monoparesis may indicate nerve root entrapment (nerve root signature); MRI, CT, myelogram or CT/myelogram for confirmation
Cervical spondylomyelopathy	Chronic progressive cervical pain and proprioceptive ataxia; short-strided, spastic thoracic limb gait and pelvic limb ataxia are characteristic; forelimb lameness or paresis may indicate nerve root entrapment (nerve root signature). MRI reveals signal changes in the spinal cord parenchyma.
Vertebral anomaly (hemivertebra, block vertebra, butterfly vertebra)	Screw-tailed dog breeds most commonly affected; kyphosis, lordosis, scoliosis, and/or spinal cord and nerve root compression possible; Dx with survey spinal radiography, MRI to determine degree of spinal cord compression
Vertebral, spinal cord, or meningeal neoplasia (lymphoma, meningioma, osteosarcoma, nephroblastoma, metastatic neoplasia)	Chronic, progressive paresis and/or ataxia, less commonly acute (hemorrhage, ischemia); focal pain on spinal palpation; often asymmetrical and variable clinical signs relating to neuroanatomic location of lesion. Canine: middle-aged to older large breeds. Feline: young; lymphoma common. MRI is imaging modality of choice. Histopathologic evaluation for definitive diagnosis; FNA or biopsy obtained by fluoroscopic or CT guidance vs. open surgical approach.
Nerve root or peripheral nerve neoplasia (primary peripheral nerve sheath tumor or secondary tumor)	Chronic progressive unilateral lameness (nerve root signature), localized muscle atrophy, and variable neurologic deficits. Mass may only be palpable in advanced stage; MRI is imaging modality of choice. Uncommon in cats.
Bacterial infection (discospondylitis, meningitis)	Discospondylitis: acute to subacute, rapidly progressive, symmetrical or asymmetrical signs; focal spinal pain is common. Variable fever, anorexia, lethargy, and reluctance to exercise. CT is superior to radiographs for evaluation of vertebral lysis; blood, urine, +/− disc aspirate C&S indicated +/− *Brucella* titer. Meningitis: cervical pain, low head carriage, fever, vomiting, lethargy, anorexia are common. Urine/blood culture, CSF analysis/culture, +/− eubacteria PCR recommended.
Viral meningomyelitis (canine distemper virus, feline infectious peritonitis, rabies)	Distemper: flexor spasms of the limbs and neck strongly suggestive. Immunohistochemical staining of skin biopsy, viral inclusion bodies seen on postmortem CNS histopathology for definitive diagnosis. FIP: spinal cord deficits possible; Dx supported by CSF analysis/PCR; periventricular/meningeal contrast enhancement on MRI. Definitive diagnosis obtained histologically +/− immunohistochemical staining.
Fungal meningomyelitis (*Cryptococcus, Coccidioides, Blastomyces, Histoplasma*)	*Cryptococcus:* dog/cat, regional, uncommon cause of paresis. *Coccidioides/Blastomyces/Histoplasma:* dog, regional, rare causes of paresis.
Protozoal meningomyelitis (*Neospora caninum, Toxoplasma gondii*)	Young (<1 year) or immunocompromised dogs. Multifocal neurologic signs; predominantly pelvic limb LMN deficits and muscle wasting due to myositis-polyradiculoneuritis; serial increases in IgG titers > 1 : 64 support active infection; Dx with a combination of serum/CSF serology and CSF PCR.

(Continued from previous page)

Differential Diagnosis Item	Key Feature(s)
Meningomyelitis (steroid-responsive meningitis-arteritis [SRMA], granulomatous meningoencephalomyelitis [GME])	SRMA: dogs typically 6-18 months old; acute signs (severe cervical pain/stiffness, fever, depression, stiff gait) or chronic signs (ataxia, paresis). CSF pleocytosis, elevated protein (acute) or mononuclear/mixed cell population (chronic). GME: acute, progressive, focal/multifocal disease; mean age in dogs = 55 months. Disseminated form is rapidly progressive; focal form is slowly progressive. CSF mild to severe mononuclear pleocytosis with elevated protein; multifocal lesions of parenchyma and meninges on MRI with predilection for white matter (disseminated form) or single space-occupying mass lesion (focal form).
Vertebral trauma (fracture, luxation)	History of major trauma (hit by car ≈50%); thoracolumbar spine most often affected. Multiple spinal fractures/luxations in up to 20% of cases, warranting survey spinal radiographs as initial test (CAUTION: Radiographs may underestimate degree of spinal displacement at time of injury). Presence of nociception is most important prognostic factor.
Brachial plexus abnormalities (avulsion, neuritis)	Avulsion: history of trauma; peracute, nonprogressive; most involve the radial nerve. Ipsilateral Horner's syndrome and loss of cutaneous trunci reflex are common. Caudal avulsion (C8-T2 nerve roots): non–weight-bearing, carpus and elbow flexed. Complete avulsion (C6-T2 nerve roots) = non–weight-bearing, knuckled paw, drags limb. Serial electromyography, nerve conduction velocity useful for diagnosis and prognosis.
Peripheral nerve injury (e.g., radial nerve)	Radial nerve injury: loss of extension of elbow, carpus, and digit; non–weight-bearing; knuckling of paw, loss of sensation to dorsal surface of paw
Ischemic myelopathy (fibrocartilaginous embolism [FCE], thromboembolism [e.g., brachial artery embolus])	FCE: most common in young large-breed dogs. May be proceeded by mild trauma or vigorous activity. Commonly peracute to acute onset, nonpainful, nonprogressive after 24 hours and asymmetrical paresis. MRI is imaging modality of choice to evaluate intramedullary hyperintensity (T2-weighted), which can be prognostic and presumptively diagnostic. Definitive diagnosis made only by histopathologic exam. Brachial artery embolus: variable paresis and pain; knuckled paw; absent brachial pulse; foot pad cyanotic and cool.

C&S, Bacterial culture and susceptibility; *CNS,* central nervous system; *CSF,* cerebrospinal fluid; *CT,* computed tomography; *FIP,* feline infectious peritonitis; *FNA,* fine-needle aspiration; *IgG,* immunoglobulin G; *LMN,* lower motor neuron; *MRI,* magnetic resonance imaging; *PCR,* polymerase chain reaction.
Reproduced from the third edition in unabridged form.

THIRD EDITION AUTHOR: **Dan Polidoro, DVM, DACVS**

Paresis, Hindlimb

Differential Diagnosis Item	Key Feature(s)
Intervertebral disc disease	Variable pain on spinal palpation, paresis, ataxia, proprioceptive deficits; clinical signs often asymmetrical; hindlimb lameness/monoparesis may indicate nerve root entrapment (nerve root signature); MRI, CT, myelogram or CT/myelogram for confirmation
Degenerative myelopathy	Chronic, progressive, nonpainful, UMN paraparesis and proprioceptive ataxia in dogs usually 8 years or older. Dx of exclusion of other neurologic disorders causing progressive myelopathy. Genetic testing for superoxide dismutase 1 (SOD1) gene mutation.
Lumbosacral disease	Male, medium- to large-breed and working dogs overrepresented. Pain on dorsal or ventral (via rectal exam) palpation of lumbosacral disc space (L7–S1). Exercise intolerance or reluctance to exercise is common. MRI is imaging modality of choice to confirm Dx, but poor correlation between degree of cauda equina compression on imaging and clinical severity of disease.
Vertebral anomaly (hemivertebra, block vertebra, butterfly vertebra)	Screw-tailed dog breeds most commonly affected; kyphosis, lordosis, scoliosis, and/or spinal cord and nerve root compression possible; Dx with survey spinal radiography, MRI to determine degree of spinal cord compression
Endocrine neuropathy (diabetes mellitus)	Poorly controlled diabetes mellitus in cats may result in sciatic neuropathy; plantigrade stance in hindlimbs.
Vertebral, spinal cord, or meningeal neoplasia (lymphoma, meningioma, osteosarcoma, nephroblastoma, metastatic neoplasia)	Chronic, progressive paresis and/or ataxia, less commonly acute (hemorrhage, ischemia); focal pain on spinal palpation; often asymmetrical and variable clinical signs relating to neuroanatomic location of lesion. Canine: middle-aged to older large breeds. Feline: young; lymphoma common. MRI is imaging modality of choice. Histopathologic exam for definitive diagnosis; FNA or biopsy obtained by fluoroscopic or CT guidance versus open surgical approach.
Nerve root or peripheral nerve neoplasia	More common in thoracic limb and nerve root
Bacterial meningomyelitis (discospondylitis, meningitis, epidural empyema)	Discospondylitis: acute to subacute, rapidly progressive, symmetrical or asymmetrical signs; focal spinal pain is common. Variable fever, anorexia, lethargy, and reluctance to exercise. CT is superior to radiographs for evaluation of vertebral lysis; blood, urine, +/– disc aspirate C&S indicated +/– *Brucella* titer. Meningitis: cervical pain, low head carriage, fever, vomiting, lethargy, anorexia are common. Urine/blood culture, CSF analysis/culture, +/– eubacteria PCR recommended.

Continued

(Continued from previous page)

Differential Diagnosis Item	Key Feature(s)
Viral meningomyelitis (canine distemper virus, feline infectious peritonitis, rabies)	Distemper: flexor spasms of the limbs and neck strongly suggestive. Immunohistochemical staining of skin biopsy, viral inclusion bodies seen on postmortem CNS histopathology for definitive diagnosis. FIP: spinal cord deficits possible; Dx supported by CSF analysis/PCR; periventricular/meningeal contrast enhancement on MRI. Definitive diagnosis obtained histologically +/– immunohistochemical staining.
Fungal meningomyelitis *(Cryptococcus, Coccidioides, Blastomyces, Histoplasma)*	*Cryptococcus* = dog/cat, regional, uncommon cause of paresis. *Coccidioides/Blastomyces/Histoplasma* = dog, regional, rare causes of paresis.
Protozoal meningomyelitis *(Neospora caninum, Toxoplasma gondii)*	Young (<1 year) or immunocompromised dogs. Multifocal neurologic signs; predominantly pelvic limb LMN deficits and muscle wasting due to myositis-polyradiculoneuritis; serial increases in IgG titers > 1:64 support active infection; Dx with a combination of serum/CSF serologic titer and CSF PCR.
Meningomyelitis (steroid-responsive meningitis-arteritis [SRMA], granulomatous meningoencephalomyelitis [GME])	SRMA: dogs typically 6-18 months old; acute signs (severe cervical pain/stiffness, fever, depression, stiff gait) or chronic signs (ataxia, paresis). CSF pleocytosis, elevated protein (acute) or mononuclear/mixed cell population (chronic). GME: acute, progressive, focal/multifocal disease; mean age in dogs = 55 months. Disseminated form is rapidly progressive; focal form is slowly progressive. CSF mild to severe mononuclear pleocytosis with elevated protein; multifocal lesions of parenchyma and meninges on MRI with predilection for white matter (disseminated form) or single space-occupying mass lesion (focal form).
Vertebral trauma (fracture, luxation)	History of major trauma (hit by car ≈50%); thoracolumbar spine most often affected. Multiple spinal fractures/luxations in up to 20% of cases, warranting survey spinal radiographs as initial test (CAUTION: Radiographs may underestimate degree of spinal displacement at time of injury). Presence of nociception is most important prognostic factor.
Peripheral nerve injury (sciatic, peroneal, tibial, femoral)	Sciatic nerve injury: severe monoparesis but weight bearing preserved, knuckled paw; hock and digits do not flex or extend, absent withdrawal reflex, loss of sensation to paw except medially. Femoral nerve injury: cannot extend stifle so non–weight-bearing, absent sensation medial paw. Tibial nerve injury: dropped hock. Peroneal nerve injury: hyperextended hock; knuckled paw.
Ischemic myelopathy (fibrocartilaginous embolism [FCE], aortic thromboembolism)	FCE: most common in young large-breed dogs. May be preceded by mild trauma or vigorous activity. Commonly peracute to acute onset, nonpainful, nonprogressive after 24 hours, and asymmetrical paresis. MRI is imaging modality of choice to evaluate intramedullary hyperintensity (T2-weighted), which can be prognostic and presumptively diagnostic. Definitive diagnosis made only by histopathologic exam. Aortic thromboembolism: variable paresis; painful; absent or decreased femoral pulse; firm and painful pelvic limb muscles; cool, cyanotic nail beds and foot pads.

C&S, Bacterial culture and susceptibility; *CNS,* central nervous system; *CSF,* cerebrospinal fluid; *CT,* computed tomography; *FNA,* fine-needle aspiration; *FIP,* feline infectious peritonitis; *IgG,* immunoglobulin G; *LMN,* lower motor neuron; *MRI,* magnetic resonance imaging; *PCR,* polymerase chain reaction; *UMN,* upper motor neuron.
Reproduced from the third edition in unabridged form.

THIRD EDITION AUTHOR: Dan Polidoro, DVM, DACVS

Pericardial Diseases

Congenital Disorders
- Pericardial Defects
  - Peritoneopericardial diaphragmatic hernia
  - Pericardial cyst

Acquired Disorders
- Pericardial Effusion
  - Hydropericardium (transudate)*
    - Congestive heart failure
    - Hypoalbuminemia
    - Peritoneopericardial diaphragmatic hernia
  - Pericarditis
    - Infectious (bacterial, fungal)
    - Sterile (idiopathic, metabolic, viral; exudate rare)
  - Hemopericardium (hemorrhage)
    - Neoplastic
    - Traumatic
    - Cardiac rupture (especially left atrial)
    - Idiopathic

Pericardial Mass Lesions (± Effusion)
- Neoplastic
- Granulomatous (actinomycosis, coccidioidomycosis)
- Pericardial abscess

Constrictive Pericardial Disease
- Idiopathic
- Infectious
- Pericardial foreign body
- Neoplastic

*Conditions that rarely compromise cardiac function.
From Kittleson M, Kienle R: Small animal cardiovascular medicine, St. Louis, 1998, Mosby, p 417.

Peritonitis

Aseptic Peritonitis
- Chemical peritonitis:
  - Bile peritonitis
  - Uroperitoneum
- Peritoneal foreign body
- Starch granulomatous peritonitis
- Sclerosing encapsulating peritonitis
- Mechanical peritonitis

Septic Peritonitis
- Leakage of gastrointestinal contents:
  - Perforating intestinal foreign body
  - Gastric rupture in gastric dilation/volvulus
  - Perforating gastric or intestinal ulcers
  - Colonic perforation (steroidal or nonsteroidal antiinflammatory drug–induced)
  - Dehiscence of intestinal surgical wound
- Iatrogenic perforation:
  - Intraperitoneal alimentation
- Penetrating abdominal wounds
- Blunt abdominal trauma
- Ischemic intestinal injury
- Pancreatitis
- Ruptured pyometra
- Ruptured non-viable pregnancy
- Uterine torsion
- Ruptured prostatic abscess
- Liver abscess or hepatitis
- Splenic abscess or splenitis
- Splenic torsion
- Mesenteric lymph node abscess
- Ruptured gallbladder or bile duct with bacterobilia
- Ruptured bladder with cystitis
- Umbilical abscess
- Surgical peritoneal contamination
- Peritoneal dialysis

Modified from Slatter D: Textbook of small animal surgery, ed 3, Philadelphia, 2003, Saunders.

Plant Toxicoses

Toxic Plants: Common Garden and Household Plants Toxic to Dogs and Cats

Botanical Name	Common Name	Toxic Principle	Clinical Signs
CNS Stimulation			
Brunfelsia spp	Yesterday-today-and-tomorrow	Hopeanine, brunfelsamide	(*Brunfelsia* Toxicosis)
Ipomoea spp	Morning glory	Lysergic acid	Seeds; vomiting, agitation, tachycardia, hallucinations (rare)
Psilocybe spp	Magic mushrooms	Psilocybin	(Mushroom Toxicosis; see p. 667)
CNS Depression			
Cannabis sativa	Marijuana, pot	Delta-9-THC	(Marijuana Toxicosis; see p. 625)
Macadamia integrifolia	Macadamia nuts	Unknown	(Macadamia Nut Toxicosis; see p. 613)
Mixed CNS Effects			
Amanita muscaria		Muscimol, ibotenic acid	(Mushroom Toxicosis; see p. 667)
Nicotiana spp	Tobacco	Nicotine	(Nicotine Toxicosis)
Hepatotoxic			
Amanita phalloides	Death cap mushroom	Amatoxins	(Mushroom Toxicosis; see p. 667)
Cycas spp *Zamia* spp	Cycad palm Sago palm	Cycasin	(Palm [Cycad/Sago] Toxicosis; see p. 737)
Cardiovascular and Respiratory Effects			
Adenium obesum *Asclepias* spp *Convallaria majalis* *Digitalis purpurea* *Hellebore* spp *Kalanchoe* spp *Nerium oleander* *Thevetia* spp	Desert rose Milkweed Lily-of-the-valley Foxglove Hellebore Kalanchoe Oleander Yellow oleander	Cardiac glycosides	(Cardiotoxic Plants; see p. 143)
Kalmia spp *Leucothoe* spp *Pieris* spp *Rhododendron* spp	Laurel Black laurel Pieris Azalea, rhododendron	Grayanotoxins	(Cardiotoxic Plants; see p. 143)
Malus spp *Nandina domestica* *Prunus* spp *Pyrus* spp *Hydrangea* spp	Apple, crabapple Heavenly bamboo Cherry, almond, apricot Pear Hydrangea	Cyanogenic glycosides	Seeds/pits, plant material; generally only cause mild GI signs; cyanide poisoning unlikely in nonruminants; seed coat must be broken to cause clinical signs
Phoradendron spp	Mistletoe	Toxalbumin, phoratoxin	Vomiting, diarrhea, dyspnea, bradycardia (rare)
Taxus spp	Yew	Taxine	(Yew Toxicosis)

Continued

Differentials, Lists, and Mnemonics

(Continued from previous page)

Toxic Plants: Common Garden and Household Plants Toxic to Dogs and Cats—cont'd

Botanical Name	Common Name	Toxic Principle	Clinical Signs
Nephrotoxic			
Hemerocallis spp *Lilium* spp	Day lily Lily, Easter lily, Asiatic lily, tiger lily	Unknown	Cats only (Lily Toxicosis; see p. 590)
Oxalis spp *Rheum* spp	Shamrock, dock, sorrel Rhubarb	Soluble calcium oxalates	Drooling, vomiting; acute renal damage rare in nonruminants
Vitis spp	Grapes, raisins	Unknown	(Grapes and Raisins Toxicosis; see p. 396)
Hemolysis			
Allium spp	Onions, garlic, chives	N-propyl disulfide	(Onion or Garlic Toxicosis; see p. 707)
Severe GI Signs With Potential Systemic Involvement			
Amaryllis spp *Narcissus* spp	Amaryllis Daffodil, jonquil, narcissus, paperwhite	Lycorine and other alkaloids	Bulbs most toxic; vomiting, diarrhea, hypotension
Clitocybe spp *Inocybe* spp		Muscarine	(Mushroom Toxicosis; see p. 667)
Colchicum autumnale	Autumn crocus	Colchicine	Hemorrhagic enteritis, bone marrow suppression, tremors, seizures, death
Cyclamen spp	Cyclamen	Triterpenoid saponins	Rhizomes most toxic; vomiting, diarrhea, seizures (rare)
Humulus lupulus	Hops		
Hyacinthus spp	Hyacinth	Alkaloids, calcium oxalates	Bulbs most toxic; vomiting, diarrhea, hypotension
Ilex spp	Holly	Saponins, alkaloids, triterpenes	Vomiting, diarrhea, abdominal pain
Ricinus communis	Castor bean	Ricin	(Castor Bean Toxicosis)
Mild to Moderate GI Signs			
Alocasia spp *Aglaonema modestum* *Anthurium* spp *Caladium* spp *Dieffenbachia* spp *Epipremnum* spp *Monstera* spp *Philodendron* spp *Schefflera* spp *Spathiphyllum* spp *Zantedeschia* spp	Elephant's ear Chinese evergreen Flamingo flower Caladium, angel wings Dieffenbachia, dumb cane Pothos, devil's ivy Swiss cheese plant, cutleaf philodendron Philodendron Schefflera, umbrella plant Peace lily Calla lily	Insoluble calcium oxalates	Oral irritation, vomiting, drooling, oral pain, rarely pharyngeal swelling
Persea americana	Avocado	Persin	Vomiting, diarrhea, pit foreign body (cardiotoxic in birds)
Ficus spp	Ficus, weeping fig	Furocoumarins, triterpenes	Sap; vomiting, dermatitis
Iris spp	Iris, flag	Pentacyclic terpenoids	Rhizomes most toxic; vomiting, diarrhea, drooling
Sansevieria spp	Mother-in-law's tongue, snake plant	Saponins, organic acids	Vomiting, diarrhea
Tulipa spp	Tulip	Tulipalin A and B	Vomiting, drooling, diarrhea; highest concentration in bulb
Aloe vera *Dracaena* spp *Hedera* spp *Hosta* spp	Aloe Dracaena, corn plant English ivy Hosta	Saponins	Vomiting, diarrhea
Crassula spp	Jade	Unknown	Vomiting, ataxia (cats)
Chrysanthemum spp	Chrysanthemum, mum	Pyrethrins	Vomiting, drooling
Euphorbia pulcherrima	Poinsettia	Irritant latex sap	Vomiting, diarrhea

AUTHOR: Tina Wismer, DVM, DABVT, DABT, MS

Pleural Effusion

Cause	Appearance	Total Protein*	Cytologic Examination	Other Tests
Pyothorax *(septic exudate)*	Cloudy, tomato soup appearance, malodor	>4 g/dL	Degenerative neutrophils, intracellular and extracellular bacteria, macrophages, RBCs	Aerobic and anaerobic C&S
Idiopathic chylothorax *(modified transudate)*	Milky white[†]	3 g/dL	Mature lymphocytes, few RBCs, few macrophages, few neutrophils	Effusion and serum triglyceride levels
Right-sided (± left-sided in cats) heart failure *(modified transudate)*	Clear	2 g/dL	Very few cells: RBCs, lymphocytes	Echocardiogram
Lymphoma *(modified transudate or nonseptic exudate)*	Clear, milky, serosanguineous	2-4 g/dL	Immature lymphoblasts, few mature lymphocytes, few RBCs	Thoracic radiographs, thoracic ultrasound, aspirate/cytologic examination of mass
Thymoma *(modified transudate or nonseptic exudate)*	Clear, milky, serosanguineous	2-4 g/dL	Mesothelial cells, mature lymphocytes, few RBCs, few macrophages	Thoracic radiographs, thoracic ultrasound, aspirate/cytologic examination of mass
Other neoplasia (e.g., carcinoma) *(modified transudate or nonseptic exudate)*	Clear, cloudy, serosanguineous, bloody	2-4 g/dL	Clumps of neoplastic cells	Thoracic radiographs, thoracic ultrasound
Hypoalbuminemia *(pure transudate)*	Clear, watery	<2.5 g/dL	Mononuclear cells (mesothelial cells, lymphocytes, macrophages)	Serum albumin, urine protein/creatinine ratio, bile acids
FIP (cats) *(nonseptic exudate)*	Straw-colored, cloudy	>4 g/dL	Macrophages, lymphocytes, RBCs, fibrin	FIP PCR on fluid

*To convert from g/dL to mg/mL, multiply g/dL by 10.
[†]Occasionally translucent; definitive diagnosis via triglyceride concentration, which is higher in chylous effusions than in blood.
C&S, Culture and susceptibility; *FIP,* feline infectious peritonitis; *PCR,* polymerase chain reaction; *RBCs,* red blood cells.
Modified with permission from King L: Textbook of respiratory disease in dogs and cats, St. Louis, 2004, Saunders, p 16.

Pneumonia, Aspiration

Conditions Predisposing an Animal to Aspiration of Stomach Contents

Impairment of Protective Airway Reflexes
- Coma
- Head trauma
- Metabolic derangements
- Central depressant medications (sedation, general anesthesia)
- Muscle relaxants
- Seizures
- Airway trauma
- Laryngeal dysfunction (including laryngeal paralysis before and after surgical treatment)
- Pharyngeal dysfunction
- General anesthesia

Large Volumes of Intragastric Food/Fluid
- Delayed gastric emptying:
  - Ileus
  - Bowel obstruction
  - Pain
  - Anxiety
  - Opioid medication
  - Peristaltic abnormalities
  - Pregnancy
  - Obesity
- Overfeeding by enteral tube
- Recent meal (before emergency anesthesia/surgery)

Impaired Function of Gastroesophageal Sphincter
- Presence of a nasogastric feeding tube
- Achalasia
- Esophageal obstruction
- Abnormalities of esophageal function:
  - Megaesophagus
  - Reflux esophagitis
  - Myasthenia gravis
  - Esophageal dysmotility

Modified from King L: Textbook of respiratory disease in dogs and cats, St. Louis, 2004, Saunders, p 423.

Pollakiuria and Stranguria

Differential Diagnosis	Key Feature(s)
Bladder neoplasia (e.g., transitional cell carcinoma)	Scottish terrier predisposed; +/– RBC, WBC, atypical epithelial cells on UA (avoid cystocentesis); mass effect (most often trigone area) on ultrasound or contrast cystogram; traumatic/diagnostic catheterization for cytology (unless atypia identified on UA); *BRAF* gene mutation (urine assay)
Cystic calculi	RBC, WBC, +/– crystals on UA; culture may be positive (particularly with struvite stones); radiographs (i.e., struvite, calcium based); ultrasound or contrast cystogram for radiolucent stones (e.g., urate)
Cystitis, bacterial or fungal	WBC, RBC, and bacteria/fungi on UA; culture positive; imaging normal, bladder wall thickening, or emphysematous cystitis
Cystitis, nonbacterial	± History of causative insult (e.g., cyclophosphamide); RBC +/– WBC, no bacteria on UA; bacterial culture negative; imaging variable (e.g., normal, thickened, polypoid, emphysematous)
Feline lower urinary tract signs/idiopathic cystitis	Often indoor cat; RBC but no WBC or bacteria on UA; culture negative; imaging normal or bladder wall thickening
Prostatic disease	Male castrated (prostatic carcinoma) or intact (prostatitis, benign prostatic hyperplasia, cyst, abscess, carcinoma); variable urine sediment exam; abnormal rectal ± abdominal palpation; prostatomegaly on radiographs; size/parenchymal abnormalities on US; prostatic wash or ejaculate for cytology and culture
Urethral disease	+/– RBC or WBC on UA; culture negative; urethra prominent on rectal exam; contrast urethrogram shows obstruction (stone, mass) or irregular tissue (inflammation, neoplasia). Causes include neoplasia (transitional cell carcinoma, squamous cell carcinoma), urethrolithiasis, trauma, urethrorectal fistula, urethral prolapse, urethritis

RBC, Red blood cells; *UA,* urinalysis; *WBC,* white blood cells.

Polyarthritis, Inflammatory

Infectious
- *Ehrlichia ewingii*
- *Anaplasma phagocytophilum*
- *Rickettsia rickettsii*
- *Borrelia burgdorferi*
- *Mycoplasma* spp (erosive or nonerosive)
- West Nile virus
- Septic arthritis (more often a monoarthropathy)
- Leishmaniasis
- Feline syncytium-forming virus/feline leukemia virus
- Calicivirus-associated (cats)

Immune Mediated
- Rheumatoid arthritis (erosive)
- Periosteal proliferative polyarthritis (erosive, cats)
- Polyarthritis of greyhounds (erosive)
- Systemic lupus erythematosus
- Polyarthritis/polymyositis
- Steroid-responsive meningitis-arteritis
- Akita dogs juvenile arthritis
- Shar-pei fever (swollen hock syndrome)
- Polyarteritis nodosa
- Idiopathic immune-mediated polyarthritis (IMPA)
  - Type I (idiopathic)
  - Type II (infection associated)
  - Type III (enteropathic)
  - Type IV (malignancy associated)

Miscellaneous
- Vaccination "reactions"
- Plasmacytic/lymphocytic synovitis
- Drug induced:
  - Sulfonamides (Doberman pinschers)
  - Erythropoietin
  - Penicillins
  - Phenobarbital
  - Lincomycin

Polyphagia

Differential Diagnosis Item	Key Feature(s)
Common	
Drug induced/iatrogenic	Any age; phenobarbital, glucocorticoids, progestins, benzodiazepines, antihistamines and appetite stimulants (cyproheptadine, mirtazapine), exogenous insulin. Determined by history.
Intestinal parasitism	Fecal flotation/fresh saline smear, fecal ELISA
Hyperadrenocorticism (HAC)	46%-57% of dogs with HAC are polyphagic, without concurrent weight loss; confirmed with ACTH stimulation test or low-dose dexamethasone suppression test.
Diabetes mellitus	Concurrent weight loss, polyuria/polydipsia very common; diagnosis with persistent hyperglycemia, glucosuria, +/– elevated fructosamine (for confirmation in cats)
Exocrine pancreatic insufficiency	Weight loss, steatorrhea, or diarrhea present; German shepherd most common breed but others affected; diagnosis confirmed with low 12-hour-fasted serum TLI.

(Continued from previous page)

Differential Diagnosis Item	Key Feature(s)
Behavioral or physiologic	Risk factors include overfeeding, gluttony/high satiety threshold, highly palatable food, response to a stressful event, low-calorie food, high activity level, and pregnancy/lactation.
Hyperthyroidism	Common in adult cats, rare in dogs; weight loss, thyroid nodule palpable in ≈90% of hyperthyroid cats; measure serum T_4 and if inconclusive, serum free T_4 by equilibrium dialysis.
Gastrointestinal infiltration	Increased suspicion if intestinal wall thickening on palpation and/or ultrasound; biopsy is confirmatory.
Sudden acquired retinal degeneration	Concurrent acute visual deficits/blindness +/− HAC; mechanism unknown
Uncommon/Rare	
Lesion of hypothalamic satiety center	Other neurologic deficits expected
Cold ambient temperature	Environmental history
Acromegaly	Concurrent diabetes mellitus almost always present

HAC, Hyperadrenocorticism; *T_4,* thyroxine; *TLI,* trypsin-like immunoreactivity.
Modified from the third edition in unabridged form.

THIRD EDITION AUTHOR: Christine Savidge, DVM

Polyuria and Polydipsia: Differential Diagnosis

Disorder	Diagnostic Aids
Diabetes mellitus	Fasting blood glucose, urinalysis
Renal glycosuria	Fasting blood glucose, urinalysis
Chronic kidney disease	BUN, creatinine, Ca:P, urinalysis
Postobstructive diuresis	History, monitoring urine output
Pyometra	History, CBC, abdominal radiography, abdominal ultrasonography
Escherichia coli septicemia	Blood, urine, or other bacterial cultures
Hypercalcemia	Serum calcium
Hepatic insufficiency	Biochemistry panel, bile acids, ammonia tolerance test, abdominal radiography and ultrasonography
Hyperadrenocorticism	History, ACTH stimulation test, dexamethasone suppression test, urine cortisol/creatinine ratio
Primary hyperaldosteronism	Serum sodium and potassium, BP, abdominal ultrasonography, ACTH stimulation test (aldosterone)
Bacterial pyelonephritis	Urine culture, abdominal ultrasonography, excretory urography
Hypokalemia	Serum potassium
Hyponatremia	Serum sodium
Hypoadrenocorticism	Na:K, ACTH stimulation test
Hyperthyroidism	Serum thyroxine
Diabetes insipidus	Trial treatment; modified water deprivation test
Psychogenic PD	Modified water deprivation test
Polycythemia/erythrocytosis	CBC
Acromegaly	Serum GH and IGF-1, CT scan
Paraneoplastic disorders:	
Intestinal leiomyosarcoma	Abdominal ultrasonography, biopsy
Iatrogenic disorders	History
Very low-protein diet	History

ACTH, Adrenocorticotropic hormone; *BP,* blood pressure; *BUN,* blood urea nitrogen; *CBC,* complete blood count; *GH,* growth hormone; *IGF-1,* insulin-like growth factor 1; *PD,* polydipsia.
From Feldman E, Nelson R: Canine and feline endocrinology and reproduction, ed 3, St. Louis, 2004, Saunders.

Portosystemic Shunts

Breeds
- More commonly single, intrahepatic in large-breed dogs
- More commonly single, extrahepatic in small-breed dogs and cats

Multiple Shunts
- Multiple shunts are extrahepatic and are most commonly acquired rather than congenital. They occur secondary to portal hypertension induced by chronic hepatopathies or surgical intervention in an animal with hepatic microvascular dysplasia.

Location on Portogram
- If shunt is cranial to T13, more likely intrahepatic
- If any part of the shunt is caudal to T13, more likely extrahepatic

Preputial Discharge

Urine
- PU/PD
- Ectopic ureters
- Urethral sphincter mechanism incompetence
- UTI
- Urolithiasis

Hemorrhagic
- Bleeding disorder (thrombocytopenia, coagulopathy, vessel wall disruption)
- Neoplasia (bladder, urethra, prostate, testicle)
- Inflammation/infection (bladder, urethra, prostate, testicle, penis/prepuce [balanoposthitis])
- Foreign body (bladder, urethra, prepuce)
- Trauma
- Urolithiasis

Mucopurulent
- Penile and preputial inflammation/infection (balanoposthitis)
- Neoplasia
- Foreign body (preputial, urethral)
- Phimosis

PU/PD, Polyuria/polydipsia; *UTI,* urinary tract infection.

Differentials, Lists, and Mnemonics

Prostatomegaly

Disorder	Signalment	CHARACTERISTICS OF PROSTATIC PALPATION				
		Size*	Symmetry	Texture	Mobility	Pain
BPH	Older MI	≤ +++	Symmetric	Normal	Normal	Absent
Acute prostatitis	Any age MI	+ to ++	Symmetric	Normal	Normal	Moderate to marked
Chronic prostatitis	Any age MI	+ to ++	Symmetric	Normal	Normal	Absent to mild
Cyst	Any age MI	≤ ++++	Asymmetric	± Fluctuant	Normal	Absent to mild
Abscess	Any age MI	≤ ++	± Asymmetric	± Fluctuant	Normal	Mild to marked
Neoplasia	Older MC or MI	≤ ++	± Asymmetric	Firm	Fixed	Absent to mild

*BPH is common in older, intact males, so concomitant BPH with any other cause of prostatic disease could result in a larger than expected prostate.
BPH, Benign prostatic hyperplasia; *MC,* male castrate; *MI,* male intact.

Proteinuria

Mechanism	Examples
PRERENAL	
Physiologic	Strenuous exercise, fever, hyperthermia, venous congestion, seizures
Excessive load	Paraproteinemia, myoglobinemia, hemoglobinemia, severe hyperproteinemia
RENAL	
Glomerular	
Glomerulonephritis	
Infectious	Lyme, brucellosis, dirofilariasis, ehrlichiosis, anaplasmosis, chronic bacterial infections (e.g., endocarditis, pyoderma, gingivitis), leishmaniasis
Immune mediated	SLE, membranoproliferative glomerulonephritis
Familial	Many breeds (e.g., soft-coated wheaten terrier, bullmastiff, bull terrier, Dalmatian)
Neoplastic	Leukemia, lymphoma, mastocytosis, histiocytosis
Inflammatory	Chronic dermatitis, pancreatitis, polyarthritis, periodontitis, inflammatory bowel disease
Idiopathic	Minimal change disease, membranous nephropathy
Glomerulosclerosis	Systemic hypertension, hyperadrenocorticism, diabetes mellitus
Amyloidosis	Familial, inflammatory (e.g., SLE, hepatozoonosis), idiopathic
Tubular	Fanconi syndrome, tubular necrosis
POSTRENAL	
Lower urinary	Infectious or sterile cystitis, transitional cell carcinoma, urolithiasis, hemorrhagic cystitis
Genital	Prostatitis, pyometra, vaginitis, perivulvar dermatitis

SLE, Systemic lupus erythematosus.

Pruritic Canine Dermatoses

Disease	Site	Lesions
Flea allergy dermatitis C, R, S	Bilaterally symmetrical, dorsal lumbosacral, caudal thighs, groin, axilla, caudal half of body	Papules, macules, alopecia, erythema, lichenification, hyperpigmentation, excoriations, fibropruritic nodules
Canine scabies C	Ventrum, pinnae margins, face, elbows, partially bilaterally symmetrical	Macules, papules, erythema, alopecia, crusts, excoriations
Demodicosis C	Periorbital, commissures of mouth, forelegs, generalized	Alopecia, erythema, crusts, follicular plugging, hyperpigmentation, secondary pyoderma
Pyoderma C	Groin, axilla, ventrum, interdigital webs, generalized, pressure points	Pustules, crusted papules, erythema, alopecia, target lesions, coalescing collarettes, hyperpigmentation
Atopic dermatitis C, S	Face, periorbital, ears, caudal carpi and tarsi, feet (dorsum), otitis externa, axillae, generalized	Erythema, alopecia, excoriations, lack of primary lesions, lichenification, hyperpigmentation
Malassezia dermatitis C, R, S	Ventral neck, groin, skin folds, face, feet, ventrum	Erythema, exudative or dry, alopecia, hyperpigmentation, lichenification
Otodectic acariosis (ear mites) C	Ear canal, pinnae	Erythema, brown otic discharge, excoriation, alopecia
Food allergy L	Face, feet, ears, generalized	Erythema, alopecia, excoriations, lack of primary lesions
Cheyletiellosis L, R	Dorsum of thorax, generalized	Large scales, crusts, alopecia, erythema
Cornification defects L	Generalized, ears, preen body	Scales, crusts, alopecia, erythematous plaques
Acral lick dermatitis L	Anterior carpal, metacarpal, radial, metatarsal, tibial regions	Firm alopecic plaque, central irregular ulcer, hyperpigmented halo
Contact dermatitis U	Hairless areas, feet (ventrum), genitals, groin, axilla, generalized	Erythema, exudation, lichenification, hyperpigmentation, papules
Drug eruptions U	Anywhere, localized or generalized, face, ears, scrotum	Pleomorphic, erythema, papules, coalescing target lesions
Pediculosis U, R, S	Dorsum, generalized	Scales, crusts, alopecia, papules
Harvest mites (chiggers, trombiculiasis) U, R, S	Ventrum, legs, anywhere	Erythema, scales, crusts, papules, alopecia
Endoparasitic migration in puppies U	Face, feet, generalized	Erythema, alopecia, excoriations, lack of primary lesions
Pelodera dermatitis U, R, S	Ventrum, legs, groin	Erythema, papules, alopecia, crusts
Superficial necrolytic dermatitis (hepatocutaneous syndrome) U	Footpads, face, mucocutaneous junctions, genitals, groin	Adherent crusts, ulcers, erythema, excoriations, fissured pads
Epitheliotropic lymphoma U	Mucocutaneous, generalized	Erythema, alopecia, scaling, ulcers, nodules
Calcinosis cutis U	Dorsal neck, anywhere	Papules, plaques, erythema, crusting
Tail-dock neuroma U	Previously docked tail	Erythema, excoriations, alopecia

C, Common; *L,* less common; *R,* regional (geographically variable); *S,* seasonal; *U,* uncommon.
Modified from Ettinger S, Feldman E: Textbook of veterinary internal medicine, ed 6, St. Louis, 2005, Saunders.

Pruritic Feline Dermatoses

Disease	Site	Lesions
Flea allergy dermatitis C, R, S	Neck, dorsum, lumbosacral, caudal and medial thighs, groin, ears	"Miliary dermatitis," erythema, alopecia, eosinophilic plaques
Eosinophilic plaque C, R, S	Ventral abdomen, medial thighs, anywhere	Raised, ulcerated, erythematous alopecic plaques secondary to allergy (primarily flea allergy dermatitis)
Otodectic acariosis (ear mites) C	Ears, head, neck, rarely generalized	Otitis externa, excoriations, "miliary dermatitis"
Food allergy C	Head, neck, ears, generalized	Erythema, excoriations, alopecia, lack of primary lesions, "miliary dermatitis," eosinophilic plaque
Self-induced pruritic hair loss (atopic dermatitis, food allergy, flea allergy) L	Bilaterally symmetrical, caudal and lateral thighs, ventral abdomen, perineum	Alopecia, hair stubble, erythema, papules, underlying skin may be normal
Atopic dermatitis L, S	Head, neck, ears, generalized	"Miliary dermatitis," erythema, excoriations, alopecia, eosinophilic plaque

Continued

Differentials, Lists, and Mnemonics

(Continued from previous page)

Disease	Site	Lesions
Self-induced psychogenic hair loss L	Bilaterally symmetrical, stripe(s) on dorsal thorax, caudal and lateral thighs, ventral abdomen, perineum, forelegs	Alopecia, hair stubble, normal underlying skin
Cheyletiellosis L, R	Dorsum of thorax, generalized	Large scales, crusts, seborrhea, "miliary dermatitis"
Demodicosis L, R	Trunk, ventral, generalized	Alopecia, scaling
Mosquito-bite hypersensitivity U, R, S	Bilaterally symmetrical, dorsal muzzle, planum nasale	Papules, crusts, alopecia, erosion, exudation, periorbital, pinnae, paw pad margins fistulation
Pediculosis U, R, S	Dorsum, generalized	Scales, crusts, alopecia
Notoedric acariosis (feline scabies) U, R	Head, ears, neck, generalized	Erythema, papules, crusts, excoriations, partially bilaterally symmetrical alopecia
Harvest mites (chiggers, trombiculiasis) U, R, S	Ventrum, legs, anywhere	Erythema, scales, crusts, papules, alopecia
Pruritic dermatophytosis U	Head, neck, ears, generalized	Erythema, alopecia, hair stubble, "miliary dermatitis," hyperpigmentation
Drug eruptions U	Anywhere, localized or generalized, pinnae, face	Pleomorphic, erythema, papules, coalescing target lesions
Pemphigus foliaceus U	Bilaterally symmetrical, face, planum nasale, ears, interdigital webs, nipples, generalized	Pustules, epidermal collarettes, crusts, alopecia

C, Common; *L,* less common; *R,* regional; *S,* seasonal; *U,* uncommon.
Modified from Ettinger S, Feldman E: Textbook of veterinary internal medicine, ed 6, St. Louis, 2005, Saunders.

Ptyalism

Cause	Salient Characteristics
Conformational drooling	Chronic. Normal amount of saliva produced but retained by lip conformation. Often large, slack-lipped breeds.
Oral lesions	Possible signs of mouth pain, pawing at face, halitosis. Look for abscess, masses, foreign body, dental disease, gingivitis, burns, ulcers. Check FIV status if stomatitis present in cats.
Neurologic disease	Perform cranial nerve exam. Decreased gag reflex possible. Difficulty in prehending, chewing, or swallowing. History of trauma, seizures, abnormal behavior.
Neuromuscular	Regurgitation (myasthenia), bilateral or unilateral temporal or masseter muscle atrophy. Sardonic grin (tetanus). Inability to open or close mouth (temporomandibular joint disease, masticatory muscle myositis, trigeminal neuropathy).
Metabolic	Hepatic disease/portosystemic shunt (cats may have copper-colored iris), renal (uremic ulcers, halitosis), nausea-associated.
Toxins or drugs	Acute onset. Caustic or noxious exposure. Acute vitamin A toxicosis, pesticides (organophosphates), poisonous toads, mushrooms, cannabis/marijuana, prescription or over-the-counter medications (e.g., pilocarpine, ketamine), others.
Immune	Ulcerative stomatitis, mucocutaneous lesions.
Pain, anxiety, fear	Acute. Physical appearance/behavior supportive. Historical association with inciting events.
Salivary gland disorders	Phenobarbital responsive sialadenosis (firm, large salivary glands, often with vomiting or gagging), sialadenitis (painful), salivary neoplasia (unilateral).
Esophageal disease	Esophagitis or megaesophagus (regurgitation).
Infectious disease	Rabies (zoonosis), feline calicivirus, feline herpes virus, any infection causing nausea or oral ulcers.

FIV, Feline immunodeficiency virus.
Reproduced from the third edition in modified form.

THIRD EDITION AUTHOR: **Diana M. Schropp, DVM, DACVECC**

Pulmonary Hypertension: Causes and Associated Disorders

Airway or pulmonary parenchymal disease (chronic)
Branch pulmonary artery stenosis (congenital)
Congestive heart failure (chronic left-sided)
Heartworm disease
Hypoxemia (chronic): high altitude, chronic airway obstruction
Idiopathic/"primary"
Left-to-right shunting congenital malformations
Persistently underdeveloped/"fetal" pulmonary circulation
Pulmonary thromboembolism

Pulmonary Markings

Bronchial Pattern
- Allergic airway disease
- Chronic bronchitis (irritant, bacterial, parasitic)
- Calcification
- Peribronchial cuffing (edema, bronchopneumonia, eosinophilic bronchopneumopathy)

Interstitial Pattern

Nodular
- Neoplasia
- Granuloma (eosinophilic, fungal, parasitic- or heartworm-associated, foreign body)
- Bulla with fluid
- Hematoma, abscess, cyst
- Mucus-filled bronchus
- Bronchiectasis

Hazy and Unstructured, Diffuse
- Artifact (underexposure, obesity, end-expiratory film)
- Poor ventilation
- Degenerative changes
- Neoplasia (lymphoma, metastasis)
- Pneumonitis (toxic, inhalant, metabolic, viral, parasitic)
- ARDS
- Cardiogenic edema
- Transitional stages of disease, such as edema, hemorrhage, bronchopneumonia

Hazy and Unstructured, Localized
- Hemorrhage
- PTE
- Foreign body
- Partial atelectasis
- Transitional stages of disease, such as edema, bronchopneumonia, hemorrhage, or parasites

Alveolar Pattern

Diffuse
- Edema (cardiogenic or noncardiogenic)
- Bronchopneumonia
- Hemorrhage
- Smoke inhalation
- Near-drowning incident
- ARDS

Localized
- Edema
- Bronchopneumonia
- Hemorrhage
- Thromboembolism
- Primary lung tumor or metastasis
- Lobar collapse or atelectasis
- Heartworm disease
- Infarct

ARDS, Acute respiratory distress syndrome; *PTE,* pulmonary thromboembolism.
Modified from Ettinger S, Feldman E: Textbook of veterinary internal medicine, ed 7, St. Louis, 2010, Saunders.

Pulse Abnormalities

Differential Diagnosis Item	Causes
Hyperkinetic pulse	Increased sympathetic tone Anemia Aortic insufficiency Patent ductus arteriosus Bradyarrhythmias Hyperthyroidism Pregnancy Aorticopulmonary window Arteriovenous fistulae/anastomoses
Hypokinetic pulse	Hypovolemia Reduced systolic function Aortic/subaortic stenosis Dynamic left ventricular outflow tract obstruction
Decrease in pulse volume with inspiration	Pericardial effusion with cardiac tamponade Exaggerated variation in intrapleural pressure (airway obstruction)
Pulse deficits	Atrial fibrillation Atrial/supraventricular premature complexes Ventricular premature complexes Pulsus alternans (alternating normal pulse and pulse deficits with myocardial failure)
Irregular pulse rhythm	Atrial fibrillation (rapid) Atrial/supraventricular premature complexes (rapid) Ventricular premature complexes (rapid) Sinus arrhythmia (slow) Second-degree atrioventricular block (slow)
Regional pulse variation	Arterial thromboembolism

Reproduced from the third edition in unabridged form.

THIRD EDITION AUTHOR: Virginia Luis Fuentes, MA, VetMB, PhD, DVC, DACVIM, DECVIM

Pyoderma

Surface Pyoderma

Pyotraumatic dermatitis (acute moist dermatitis, hot spots):

Pyotraumatic folliculitis and furunculosis, demodicosis, dermatophytosis, neoplasia, cutaneous metastasis, fixed drug eruption, early necrotizing form of idiopathic nodular panniculitis, early localized vasculitis

Intertrigo (skinfold pyoderma):

Localized demodicosis, mucocutaneous pyoderma, dermatophytosis, *Malassezia* dermatitis, candidiasis, superficial necrolytic dermatitis, zinc-responsive dermatosis

Bacterial overgrowth:

Malassezia dermatitis, atopic dermatitis, food allergy

Superficial Pyoderma

Impetigo (puppy pyoderma):

Superficial bacterial folliculitis, demodicosis, dermatophytosis, early scabies

Superficial bacterial folliculitis:

Impetigo, exfoliative superficial pyoderma, dermatophytosis, demodicosis, sarcoptic acariasis, flea allergy dermatitis, pemphigus foliaceus, urticaria, drug eruption, erythema multiforme, sterile eosinophilic pustulosis, leishmaniasis

Exfoliative superficial pyoderma:

Superficial bacterial folliculitis, dermatophytosis, demodicosis, pemphigus foliaceus

Mucocutaneous pyoderma:

Intertrigo, *Malassezia* dermatitis, localized demodicosis, early discoid lupus erythematosus, zinc-responsive dermatosis, autoimmune skin diseases (DLE, SLE, PV, BP), epitheliotropic lymphoma (mycosis fungoides)

Deep Pyoderma

Pyotraumatic folliculitis and furunculosis:

Pyotraumatic dermatitis/acute moist dermatitis (hot spot), demodicosis, neoplasia, cutaneous metastasis, fixed drug eruption, idiopathic nodular panniculitis, localized vasculitis

Muzzle folliculitis and furunculosis (canine acne):

Localized demodicosis, dermatophytosis, early juvenile cellulitis, eosinophilic furunculosis, contact dermatitis

Pedal folliculitis and furunculosis:

Pelodera dermatitis, dermatophytosis, subcutaneous and systemic mycoses, opportunistic fungal diseases, mycobacterial diseases, interdigital pyogranulomas, neoplasia

Callus/pressure-point pyoderma: acral lick dermatitis, focal actinic comedones, sarcoptic acariasis

German shepherd dog pyoderma:

Demodicosis with secondary deep pyoderma, subcutaneous and deep mycoses, opportunistic fungal infection, idiopathic nodular panniculitis, vasculitis

BP, Bullous pemphigoid; *DLE,* discoid lupus erythematosus; *PV,* pemphigus vulgaris; *SLE,* systemic lupus erythematosus.
Reproduced from the third edition in unabridged form.

THIRD EDITION AUTHOR: Manon Paradis, DMV, MVSc, DACVD

Red Eye: Differential Diagnosis

Parameter	Anterior Uveitis	Conjunctivitis	Superficial Keratitis	Glaucoma
Conjunctiva	Not thickened, vessels easily seen	Thick, folded, and hyperemic, vessels concealed	Not thickened	Not thickened
Conjunctival vessels	Circumcorneal and straight, not movable with conjunctiva	Superficial, diffuse, and tortuous	Diffuse, vessels form fine network in vicinity of cornea	Diffuse, superficial, and prominent
Secretion or discharge	None	Moderate to copious	Serous to purulent	None
Pain	Moderate	Severe	Moderate to severe	Severe to acute
Photophobia	Moderate	None	Severe	Slight
Cornea	Clear to steamy	Clear	Clouded to opaque	Steamy
Pupil size	Small, sluggish, irregular, or fixed	Normal	Normal	Dilated, moderate to complete, and fixed
Pupillary light reflex	Poor	Normal	Normal	Absent
Intraocular pressure	Variable; typically low/diminished acutely	Normal	Normal	Elevated

NOTE: These disorders often do not exist in isolation, and features of two or more disorders may be present simultaneously, may negate each other, or may be additive.
With permission from Lavignette AM: Differential diagnosis and treatment of anterior uveitis. Vet Clin North Am 3:504, 1973. Modified from Slatter D: Fundamentals of veterinary ophthalmology, St. Louis, 2001, Saunders.

Regurgitation

Differential Diagnosis	Key Feature(s)
Regurgitation as the Primary Presenting Complaint	
Megaesophagus (idiopathic)	Regurgitation can be immediately postprandial or delayed. Esophageal dilation on imaging. Diagnosis of exclusion.
Esophagitis	History of risk factors (recent general anesthesia; vomiting; oral antibiotics). Increased swallowing movements and salivation. Inappetence due to pain. Radiographs may be normal. Diagnosis on endoscopy.
Esophageal foreign body	History of foreign body ingestion. Acute onset increased swallowing movements, salivation, pain. Radiographs may show foreign body. Endoscopy for confirmation.
Esophageal neoplasia	Chronic regurgitation. Increased swallowing movements. Pain on swallowing. Endoscopy for diagnosis.
Infectious (*Spirocerca lupi; Pythium insidiosum*)	Enlarged salivary glands. Chronic regurgitation. Increased swallowing movements. Confirmed with endoscopy.
Esophageal diverticulum	Partial dilation seen on contrast radiographs or endoscopy.
Esophageal stricture/stenosis	History of risk factors (recent general anesthesia; vomiting; oral antibiotics; foreign body removed). Increased swallowing movements and salivation. Inappetence due to pain. Regurgitation immediate after eating. Liquids kept down. Contrast radiographs or endoscopy is diagnostic.
Vascular ring anomaly	Young animals after weaning. History of regurgitation starting shortly after introduction of solids. Usually ravenous appetite but poor growth. Diagnoses made on plain dorsoventral thoracic radiograph.
Pharyngeal obstruction	Increased swallowing movements. Pawing at throat. Inappetence. Endoscopy may help but fluoroscopy best.
Pyloric outflow obstruction	Congenital: 4-12 months old. Boston terriers and English bulldogs. Acquired: 4- to 7-year-old small-breed dogs. Chronic vomiting/regurgitation. Ultrasound; contrast radiographs or endoscopy for diagnosis.
Hiatal hernia	Shar-pei and brachycephalic dogs overrepresented. Chronic clinical signs. Fluoroscopy or endoscopy for diagnosis.
Regurgitation as Part of Systemic Illness	
Gastroesophageal intussusception	Rare. German shepherds overrepresented. Severe pain. Vomiting and regurgitation. Thoracic radiographs may help. Endoscopy for confirmation.
Thoracic neoplasia (e.g., thymoma)	Usually over 8 years of age. Dyspnea. Hypercalcemia often present. Thoracic radiographs show cranial mediastinal mass.
Myasthenia gravis	Congenital <8 weeks of age in Jack Russell and smooth fox terriers. Acquired—German shepherds, golden retrievers, German short-haired pointers, others. In cats, +/– history of methimazole treatment. Generalized limb weakness (worse with exercise) often present. Can cause regurgitation alone. Acetylcholine receptor antibody test for confirmation.
Botulism	Possible history of ingestion of contaminated food or carrion. Acute and rapid generalized weakness. Tail wag is maintained.
Tetanus	History of wound or teething. Sensitive to touch and noise. Muscle spasm of the face and jaw. Rigid paresis. Mild hyperthermia.
Organophosphate intoxication	Acute. Vomiting/regurgitation and diarrhea. Generalized weakness. Muscle tremors. Miosis. Acetylcholinesterase levels for confirmation.
Dysautonomia	Mostly young adults. Vomiting/regurgitation; diarrhea, dysuria, mydriasis, coughing and nasal discharge may be present. Ocular pilocarpine test rules out anticholinergic intoxication. Confirmation: histopathologic exam of autonomic ganglia.
Polyradiculoneuritis	Lower motor neuron paralysis beginning in hindlimbs and progressing to full paralysis within 10 days. Nociception maintained +/– enhanced.
Tick paralysis	Finding a tick or tick crater. Hindlimb weakness with progression to generalized weakness—usually acute. Tail wag preserved. Voice change and nystagmus may be present. Dysphagia. Rapid (hours) improvement in signs with tick removal.
Lead	History of potential or confirmed exposure. Neurologic signs, vomiting, diarrhea, abdominal pain. Hypochromic anemia. Signs can be acute or chronic. Blood lead level for confirmation.
Thallium	Rare. Vomiting; diarrhea; regurgitation. Alopecia. Neurologic deficits include tremors and ataxia. Thallium concentrations in hair and blood can confirm.
Systemic lupus erythematosus	Young to middle age. Skin and oral mucosal lesions. Numerous other immune-mediated conditions: polyarthritis; hemolytic anemia; thrombocytopenia. A positive ANA titer.
Polymyositis	Middle-aged large-breed dogs. Acute or chronic signs. Weakness worsens with exercise. Stiff gait. EMG and muscle biopsies can help confirm.
Dermatomyositis	Young <1-year-old dogs. Collies and Shetland sheepdogs. Skin lesions on extremities. Muscle atrophy. Weakness and lameness. Painful and inappetent. Skin and muscle biopsies diagnostic.
Hypoadrenocorticism	Young to middle-aged dogs. Weakness and lethargy with anorexia and vomiting often wax and wane. Suspect if hyperkalemia and hyponatremia. Lack of stress leukogram (eosinophilia). ACTH stimulation test for confirmation.
Hypothyroidism	Other presenting signs include mental dullness, weakness and exercise intolerance. Seborrhea and bilateral symmetrical hair loss with a "rat tail." Measure T_4 in conjunction with TSH.

ACTH, Adrenocorticotropic hormone; *ANA,* antinuclear antibody; *EMG,* electromyogram; *T_4,* thyroxine; *TSH,* thyroid-stimulating hormone.
Reproduced from the third edition in modified form.

THIRD EDITION AUTHOR: Ninette Keller, BVSc, MMedVet

Differentials, Lists, and Mnemonics

Renomegaly

	Normal Shape	Abnormal Shape
Unilateral enlargement	Compensatory hypertrophy Diffuse infiltrative neoplasia (e.g., lymphoma) Edema/inflammation Perinephric pseudocysts Intracapsular hemorrhage Hydronephrosis	Non-diffuse neoplasia Abscess Cyst Hematoma Polycystic kidney disease
Bilateral enlargement	Amyloidosis Diffuse infiltrative neoplasia Edema/inflammation Perinephric pseudocysts Hydronephrosis	Non-diffuse neoplasia Polycystic kidney disease

Reproduced from the third edition in modified form.

THIRD EDITION AUTHOR: Darcy H. Shaw, DVM, MVSc, MBA, DACVIM

Respiratory Parasites

Parasite (Host)	Comment
Aelurostrongylus abstrusus (cats)	Coughing, sneezing, lethargy possible but usually no signs
Eucoleus aerophilus (formerly *Capillaria aerophila*) (dogs, cats)	Chronic cough or no clinical signs
Crenosoma vulpis (wild canids; rarely dogs)	Chronic cough clinically mimicking chronic sterile bronchitis
Eucoleus boehmi (dogs, cats)	Chronic sneezing, nasal discharge, facial rubbing
Filaroides hirthi (dogs only)	Breeding kennels; zinc sulfate flotation is best (not Baermann)
Oslerus osleri (wild canids; rarely dogs)	Nodules in large airway mucosa; treatment difficult
Paragonimus kellicotti (dogs, cats)	Chronic cough ± pneumothorax; rust-colored pharyngeal phlegm
Pneumonyssoides caninum (dogs)	Nasal mite; sensitive to parenteral (and presumably oral) ivermectin
Troglostrongylus brevior (cats)	Bronchi and bronchiolar infection; larvae in feces difficult to distinguish from other metastrongyloids

Retinopathies

Common Systemic Disorders Affecting the Retina
Dog
Blastomycosis
Coccidioidomycosis
Cryptococcosis
Distemper
Ehrlichiosis
Rocky Mountain spotted fever
Histoplasmosis
Systemic hypertension
Larva migrans (*Toxocara* spp)
Leishmaniasis
Lymphoma
Multiple myeloma
Toxoplasmosis
Uveodermatologic syndrome
Cat
Blastomycosis
Cryptococcosis
FIP
Histoplasmosis
Multiple myeloma
Systemic hypertension
Lymphoma (both FeLV-positive and -negative)
Toxoplasmosis
Tuberculosis

FeLV, Feline leukemia virus; *FIP,* feline infectious peritonitis.
Modified from Slatter D: Fundamentals of veterinary ophthalmology, St. Louis, 2001, Saunders.

Root Signature (Nerve)

Differential Diagnosis Item	Key Feature(s)
Nerve sheath neoplasia	Insidious onset and progressive lameness (usually forelimb) and atrophy followed by neck pain; ipsilateral Horner's syndrome and cutaneous trunci deficit possible
Lymphoma	More common in cats; lymphoma often evident elsewhere (kidney, gastrointestinal tract)
Lateral and foraminal disc extrusion (intervertebral disc disease)	Acute onset; chondrodystrophic breed; paravertebral pain present from the onset
Neuritis	Acute onset; rare
Degenerative lumbosacral stenosis	Hindlimb lameness often worsens with exercise; sciatic deficit; tail dysfunction and incontinence common

Reproduced from the third edition in unabridged form.

THIRD EDITION AUTHOR: Greg Kilburn, DVM, DACVIM

Salter-Harris Fracture Classification

Salter-Harris Classification of Separations or Fracture-Separations Involving a Growth Plate and the Adjacent Metaphysis and Epiphysis

Type of Fracture	Radiographic Findings	Principal Anatomic Region Involved
Type 1	Physeal separation, displacement of the epiphysis from the metaphysis at the growth plate	Proximal humerus and femur, distal femur
Type 2	Small corner of the metaphyseal bone fractured, with displacement of the epiphysis from the metaphysis at the growth plate	Distal femur and humerus, proximal humerus, proximal tibia
Type 3	Fracture through the epiphysis and part of the growth plate, with the metaphysis unaffected	Distal humerus
Type 4	Fracture through the epiphysis, growth plate, and metaphysis; several fracture lines possible	Distal femur, distal humerus
Type 5	Compression of the growth plate. Soft-tissue swelling but no bony abnormalities seen following the injury.	Distal ulna, distal radius, distal femur

Modified from Piermattei D, et al: Brinker, Piermattei, and Flo's Handbook of small animal orthopedics and fracture repair, ed 4, St. Louis, 2006, Saunders.

Seizures: Causes

EXTRACRANIAL
- **Hypoglycemia**
  - Glycogen storage diseases
  - Beta-cell neoplasm of pancreas/insulinoma
  - Youth and malnutrition (especially small or toy breeds)
  - Youth and GI disease (especially small or toy breeds)
  - Insulin excess (iatrogenic)
  - Intestinal leiomyosarcoma
  - Hunting dog hypoglycemia
  - Xylitol intoxication
- **Hyperglycemia/hyperosmolar nonketotic diabetes mellitus**
- **Hypoxemia**
- **Hepatoencephalopathy**
- **Renal disease**
  - Uremia
  - Nephrotic syndrome (embolism)
- **Electrolyte disorders**
  - Hypocalcemia
  - Hyperkalemia
  - Hyponatremia
  - Hypomagnesemia
  - Rapid change in serum osmolality
- **Hyperlipoproteinemia**
- **GI disease**
  - Parasitism
  - "Garbage intoxication"
- **Erythrocytosis**
  - Right-to-left shunt (e.g., reversed patent ductus arteriosus, tetralogy of Fallot, atrial or ventricular septal defect with concurrent pulmonic stenosis or pulmonary hypertension)
  - Renal neoplasm (erythropoietin-producing)
  - Chronic lung disease
  - Polycythemia vera
- **Intoxications**
  - Arsenic, amphetamines, blue-green algae, chlorinated hydrocarbons, chocolate, ethanol/methanol/fermented materials (e.g., bread dough), ethylene glycol, hexachlorophene, lead, marijuana, metaldehyde, mercury, organophosphates, radiopaque media for myelography, tremorgenic mycotoxins (penitrem A, roquefortine), prescription human medications

INTRACRANIAL
- **Inflammatory, Infectious**
  - Protozoal: toxoplasmosis, neosporosis, cytauxzoonosis
  - Viral encephalitides: canine distemper encephalitis, rabies, FIP meningoencephalitis
  - Fungal: cryptococcosis, coccidioidomycosis
  - Bacterial: uncommon
- **Inflammatory, Noninfectious**
  - Meningoencephalomyelitis of unknown origin (MUO)
    - Granulomatous meningoencephalomyelitis (GME)
    - Necrotizing meningoencephalitis (NME)
    - Necrotizing leukoencephalitis (NLE)
  - Eosinophilic encephalitis
  - Steroid-responsive meningitis-arteritis
- **Neoplasia**
  - Primary or metastatic
- **Malformation**
  - Hydrocephalus
  - Lissencephaly-pachygyria
- **Injury/trauma**
- **Intracranial hemorrhage**
- **Degeneration**
  - Thiamine deficiency in cats
  - Cerebral infarction in cats

IDIOPATHIC EPILEPSY

FIP, Feline infectious peritonitis; *GI*, gastrointestinal.
Modified from de Lahunta A, Glass E: Veterinary neuroanatomy and clinical neurology, ed 3, St. Louis, 2009, Saunders.

Differentials, Lists, and Mnemonics

Seizures: Characteristics and Differentiation

Seizures, Differentiation From Other Events

	Seizure (Grand Mal)	Seizure (Partial)	Syncope	Episodic Weakness	Narcolepsy/ Cataplexy
Precipitating event	Usually none; can occur during rest	Usually none	Exertion, pain, micturition, defecation, cough, stressful event	Exertion or none	Excitement, feeding
Prodrome	Minutes to days; atypical behavior (e.g., anxious, more withdrawn, attention-seeking) ± vomiting		Seconds; acute weakness, staggering, vocalization, autonomic stimulation	None (disorder is neuromuscular)	None
Aura	None	Marks onset of partial seizure	None	None	None
Event features	Chomping, hypersalivation, tonic-clonic limb motion; duration often 1-2 minutes but duration >5 minutes is consistent with seizure and highly inconsistent with syncope	Localized signs	Motionlessness; flaccid or rigid extension of limbs; opisthotonos possible; no tonic-clonic activity; duration generally transient (<1 minute)	Gradual or sudden loss of muscle tone, causing recumbency; mentation and consciousness remain normal; no tonic-clonic activity	Instantaneous loss of muscle tone; animal is immobile (sleeping) but appears to be aware of its surroundings.
Recovery	Slowness returning to consciousness; disorientation (commonly 10 minutes or longer); blindness, circling, and other signs of central nervous system dysfunction common	Varies	Rapid recovery of normal mentation; often able to walk (and considered back to normal by owner) within minutes	Highly variable; generally reflective of course of onset (gradual onset associated with slow recovery); in some cases, rapid-onset disorders may have a protracted course	Fairly rapid (several seconds to 1 minute), with appearance of waking from sleep

Convulsive syncope (anoxic or anoxic-epileptic seizures) are syncopal events generally caused by cardiac arrhythmias that produce profound syncope, temporary cerebral hypoxia, and seizures. Therefore, clarification of the type of event observed by the owner (syncope versus seizure) may be difficult and generally rests on the observation of an episode, the presence of heart disease, and the documentation of a severe bradycardia or tachycardia during the event. Videotaping of an episode by the owner and cardiac event monitoring (pager-size portable electrocardiographic [ECG] unit that is triggered by the owner when an event occurs) can be invaluable in clarifying whether an animal is experiencing seizures versus syncope.
Modified from Ettinger SJ, Feldman EC: Textbook of veterinary internal medicine, ed 6, St. Louis, 2005, Saunders, p 27.

Seizures, Refractory or Poorly Controlled

Factors Responsible for Inadequate Control of Seizures

Medication and Dosage
- Improper choice of drug
- Insufficient drug dosage
- Delayed increase in dosage
- Inadequate increase in dosage
- Too rapid change of medication
- Too rapid reduction of dosage
- Excessive fluctuations in serum concentrations
- Inappropriately combined drugs
- Failure to monitor serum levels
- Noncompliance
- Drug-drug interactions

Other Precipitating Factors
- Additional medications
- Additional diseases
- Physical or psychological stress

Diagnostic Failures
- Extracerebral causes of seizures
- Progressive brain lesions
- Misidentification of episodes
  - Syncope
  - Myasthenia gravis
  - Narcolepsy/cataplexy

Modified with permission from Kirk RW, Bonagura JD, editors: Kirk's Current veterinary therapy XI: small animal practice, St. Louis, 1993, Saunders, p 986.

Serotonin Syndrome–Inducing Agents

Agent	General Comments
Foods or supplements: L-5-HTP, L-tryptophan, *Griffonia* seed extract Aged cheese, chicken liver	• L-5-HTP is an OTC supplement used in humans for depression, insomnia; serotonin syndrome (SS) reported as a result of accidental ingestion in dogs. • Tyramine present in certain foods can interfere with MAO inhibitors' action and enhance their toxicity.
Medications that increase presynaptic release of serotonin: Amphetamine Methylphenidate Ecstasy (MDMA; 3,4-methylenedioxymethamphetamine) Bromocriptine L-dopa *Presynaptic reuptake inhibitors, selective serotonin reuptake inhibitors (SSRIs), and tricyclic antidepressants:* Fluoxetine Bupropion Duloxetine Fentanyl Pethidine Paroxetine Sertraline Citalopram Fluvoxamine Amitriptyline Clomipramine Tramadol Chlorpheniramine Venlafaxine Dextromethorphan Meperidine *Serotonin metabolism inhibitors:* Selegiline (MAO-B inhibitor; Anipryl) Amitraz *Serotonin agonists at postsynaptic membrane:* Buspirone Lithium LSD (lysergic acid diethylamide)	• In addition to CNS excitation from amphetamine, signs of confusion, disorientation, hallucination, and rigidity may be due to SS. • SS is a clinical entity characterized by presence of some GI signs, CNS signs (hyperreflexia, tremors, rigidity, confusion, agitation, excitation, seizures), and mydriasis, tachycardia, hyperthermia. • SS can be seen with acute large overdose or with repeated therapeutic treatment. • Cyproheptadine, 1.1 mg/kg for dogs and 2-4 mg/CAT PO or per rectum q 6-8h, can be used for treating signs of SS; discontinue after 2-3 treatments if no relief. • Chlorpromazine and other phenothiazines possess some antiserotonin effects. • Selegiline recommended for use in dogs for cognitive dysfunction. Interaction likely when selegiline used concurrently with tricyclic antidepressants, amitraz, meperidine, or SSRIs.

CNS, Central nervous system; *GI,* gastrointestinal; *MAO,* monoamine oxidase; *OTC,* over-the-counter.

From Crowell-Davis SL, Poggiagliolmi S: Understanding behavior: serotonin syndrome. Compend Contin Educ Vet 30:490-493, 2008; Mohammad-Zadeh LF, Moses L, Gwaltney-Brant SM: Serotonin: a review. J Vet Pharmacol Ther 31:187-199, 2008.

SIADH Causes: Mnemonic

S—surgery
I—intracranial disease
A—alveolar (lung disease)
D—drugs (e.g., opiates, cytotoxic drugs, anticonvulsants)
H—hormonal (hypothyroid, hypoadrenocorticism)

SIADH, Syndrome of inappropriate antidiuretic hormone.

Splenic Diseases: Infectious

Infectious Causes of Splenomegaly/Splenitis*		
Viral Diseases FIP (C) FeLV (C) FIV (C) Systemic calicivirosis (C) Infectious canine hepatitis (D) **Rickettsial and Mycoplasmal Diseases** Ehrlichiosis and anaplasmosis (canine and feline) RMSF (*Rickettsia rickettsii*) (D) Q fever (*Coxiella burnetii*) Hemotropic mycoplasmosis (*Mycoplasma haemofelis;* others) **Bacterial Infections** Canine brucellosis (D) Florida borreliosis	Plague Tularemia Streptococcosis Staphylococcosis Salmonellosis Endotoxemia Mycobacterial infections Bartonellosis Lyme borreliosis (D) Melioidosis Nocardiosis Bacteremias (various/virtually any) **Fungal Diseases** Cryptococcosis Histoplasmosis	Blastomycosis Sporotrichosis Paecilomycosis Systemic candidiasis *Monocillium indicum* (D) **Protozoal Diseases** Toxoplasmosis Cytauxzoonosis (C) Babesiosis (D) Leishmaniasis (D) Hepatozoonosis (D) Trypanosomiasis (D)

*Infectious disease may affect the spleen directly or indirectly cause splenomegaly by causing chronic anemia, chronic antigen stimulation, or disturbances in blood flow (e.g., endotoxemia).
C, Cats; *D,* dogs; *FeLV,* feline leukemia virus; *FIP,* feline infectious peritonitis; *FIV,* feline immunodeficiency virus; *RMSF,* Rocky Mountain spotted fever.
Modified from Ettinger S, Feldman E: Textbook of veterinary internal medicine, ed 7, St. Louis, 2010, Saunders.

Splenomegaly

Infiltration	
Neoplastic: acute and chronic leukemia, systemic mastocytosis (more common in cats), lymphoma, multiple myeloma	Splenic fine-needle aspirate for cytologic analysis, together with clinical findings, most frequently result in a diagnosis or guide further diagnostic steps in suspected neoplastic and non-neoplastic diseases.
Non-neoplastic: amyloidosis	
Congestion	
Iatrogenic/anesthetic: barbiturates, halothane	Anesthetics comprising acepromazine and opiate premedication with propofol induction cause significantly less engorgement than protocols using dexmedetomidine, diazepam, ketamine, or thiopentone.
Splenic torsion (alone or in association with GDV)	"Feathery" or "Swiss cheese" appearance of spleen on ultrasound, not to be confused with diffuse neoplasia (check splenic blood flow with Doppler)
Right-sided heart failure	Presence of positive jugular pulse, ascites, hepatomegaly, and, invariably, enlarged hepatic veins on abdominal ultrasound
Portal hypertension (liver-related)	Acute or chronic liver failure as evidenced by increased postprandial serum bile acids and either hepatomegaly (acute) or ascites and a small, irregular liver (chronic) on ultrasound
Inflammation/Infection	
Suppurative: hematogenous dissemination of bacterial infection	Fever, neutrophilia (with or without left shift)
Necrotizing: gas-forming anaerobes associated with splenic torsion	Neutrophilia (with or without left shift)
Eosinophilic: hypereosinophilic syndrome (cats)	Eosinophilia possible but not always present
Lymphoplasmacytic: ehrlichiosis, babesiosis, infectious canine hepatitis	Thrombocytopenia, anemia, hyperglobulinemia; endemic region
Granulomatous: systemic mycoses	Endemic region; demonstration of organism cytologically (caution regarding needlestick/public health risks)
Pyogranulomatous: FIP	Hyperglobulinemia, ascites, icterus
Lymphoreticular Hyperplasia	
Chronic bacteremic conditions: discospondylitis, brucellosis	Spinal pain, neutrophilia, concurrent granulomatous lesions
Immune-mediated disorders: IMHA, ITP	Associated with regenerative anemia, positive in-saline agglutination test, and/or severe thrombocytopenia
Systemic lupus erythematosus	Common concomitant clinical findings: nonerosive polyarthritis, fever, dermatologic signs
Extramedullary Hematopoiesis	Associated with concomitant anemia, leukopenia, or thrombocytopenia

FIP, Feline infectious peritonitis; *GDV,* gastric dilation/volvulus; *IMHA,* immune-mediated hemolytic anemia; *ITP,* immune-mediated thrombocytopenia.
Reproduced from the third edition in unabridged form.

THIRD EDITION AUTHOR: Paolo Pazzi, BVSc, MMedVet

Stomatitis

Causes of Stomatitis

Conditions associated with immune system depression or dysfunction	Necrotizing ulcerative gingivostomatitis Mycotic infections (commonly candidiasis) Neutrophil dysfunction, gray collie syndrome, drug therapy, viral infection (e.g., FeLV)
Autoimmune disorders	Vesiculobullous skin diseases (e.g., pemphigus and pemphigoid) Systemic or discoid lupus erythematosus Sjögren-like syndrome
Hypersensitivity	Drug eruptions Insect stings
Viral infections	FeLV FIV Calicivirus
Miscellaneous conditions	Eosinophilic granuloma complex Feline chronic gingivostomatitis Familial ulcerative stomatitis (Maltese)

FeLV, Feline leukemia virus; *FIV,* feline immunodeficiency virus.
Modified from Slatter D: Textbook of small animal surgery, ed 3, Philadelphia, 2003, Saunders.

Stress Leukogram: Mnemonic

Smiled
*S*egments and *m*onocytes *i*ncrease; *l*ymphocytes and *e*osinophils *d*ecrease.

Stridor

Differential Diagnosis	Key Features
Airway stenosis/webbing (pharyngeal, laryngeal, or tracheal)	Uncommon cause of stridor; usually follows insult or injury to the airway; recognized on laryngoscopy/tracheoscopy
Brachycephalic syndrome	More often characterized by stertor than stridor; breed-related congenital and acquired anatomic defects (not all defects present in affected dog—stenotic nares, elongated soft palate, everted laryngeal saccules, and hypoplastic trachea); chronic signs
Coagulopathy	Acute onset of stridor due to hematoma formation; more likely related to secondary (e.g., anticoagulant rodenticide intoxication) than primary hemostatic defect; unless other evidence of bleeding identified, may not be recognized before sedated airway exam
Epiglottic retroversion	Epiglottis episodically retroflexed into the rima glottidis; easily missed on pharyngeal/laryngeal exam due to episodic nature and self-correction when tongue is extended forward; seemingly uncommon
Extraluminal laryngeal compression	Compression from mass, lymphadenomegaly, abscess, or granuloma; can have either acute or insidious onset of clinical signs, depending on cause
Extraluminal tracheal compression	Compression from mass, lymphadenomegaly, abscess, or granuloma; can develop acute or insidious onset of clinical signs; careful palpation of the neck may reveal mass
Foreign body	Material lodged in pharynx, larynx, or upper portion of trachea; depending on density, may be identified on cervical radiographs; laryngoscopy/tracheoscopy diagnostic and therapeutic
Laryngeal collapse	Breed related in Norwich terriers; can occur as complication of brachycephalic airway syndrome; confirmed via imaging studies ± laryngoscopy
Laryngeal edema	Acute onset typical; can follow envenomation/bite or exposure to caustic chemical (e.g., liquid potpourri); confirmed via laryngoscopy; depending on cause, glucocorticoids may be helpful but temporary tracheostomy occasionally required

Continued

(Continued from previous page)

Differential Diagnosis	Key Features
Laryngeal paralysis (most common cause of stridor in dogs)	Very common cause of stridor in older dogs (Labrador retrievers overrepresented) but also occurs in young dogs and cats; change in bark may precede stridor; distress episodes precipitated by heat or excitement; confirmed by laryngoscopy under light sedation; can be idiopathic (common) or caused by any form of neuropathy/junctionopathy/myopathy (e.g., tick paralysis, myasthenia gravis)
Nasopharyngeal polyp	More often seen in cats than dogs; more common in young cats, but any age can be affected; often follows chronic upper airway inflammation; otic exam may be abnormal unilaterally; Horner's syndrome sometimes identified; laryngoscopy under anesthesia with retraction of the soft palate to examine nasopharynx to confirm; CT or sometimes skull radiographs also useful but not always necessary
Neoplasia	Intra- or extraluminal neoplasia/tumor; in cats, squamous cell carcinoma common; tissue biopsy required for diagnosis

Syncope

Causes	Key Features
Bradyarrhythmias	Syncope results after >6-8 second pause in electrical activity (i.e., failure of subsidiary pacemaker in third-degree AV block, or sinus arrest with subsidiary pacemaker failure in sick sinus syndrome). Auscultation, resting and ambulatory ECG helpful in diagnosis.
Tachyarrhythmias	Rates >300 bpm for >6 seconds (i.e., supraventricular or ventricular tachycardia). Heart rate and time necessary for syncope depend on underlying cardiac structure. Auscultation, resting and ambulatory ECG helpful in diagnosis.
Outflow obstructions	Commonly seen with severe pulmonic and aortic stenosis and pulmonary hypertension. Typically, syncope occurs with excitement or exertion. Echocardiogram is necessary to confirm diagnosis.
Cyanotic heart disease	Syncope is due to hypoxemia, hyperviscosity, or arrhythmia. Echocardiogram +/– contrast study is necessary to confirm diagnosis. PCV/TS is indicated to determine therapy.
Masses obstructing inflow/outflow of blood	Mass may be associated with the interior or exterior of the heart, potentially compromising cardiac output. Echocardiogram is necessary to determine tumor location/likely etiology and hemodynamic significance.
Congestive heart failure	Syncope may be first sign that animal is in heart failure before overt infiltrates are noted radiographically. Mechanism not well understood. Small-breed, white dogs appear overrepresented.
Neurologic	Caused by increased intracranial pressure with decreased cerebral perfusion. Uncommon cause of syncope, more likely seizures.
Metabolic	Abrupt decrease in oxygen or nutrient delivery. Serum biochemistry profile is indicated. Seizures more common than syncope.
Tussive	Small-breed dogs with upper and lower respiratory tract problems. Consider cough suppressant +/– bronchodilator trial.
Autonomic dysfunction	Excessive baroreflex causing bradycardia and hypotension.
Peripheral vasomotor dysfunction	Also known as postural hypotension. More common in people.

AV, Atrioventricular; *ECG,* electrocardiogram; *PCV,* packed cell volume; *TS,* total solids.
Reproduced from the third edition in modified form.

THIRD EDITION AUTHOR: Sarah J. Miller, DVM, DACVIM

Tachycardia

Sinus tachycardia
- Excitement
- Pain
- Toxicosis (e.g., chocolate; aminophylline/theophylline; pseudoephedrine, phenylpropanolamine, and related compounds; Bufo toad)
- Sepsis
- Hypotension
- Congestive heart failure
- Systemic illness (e.g., hyperthyroidism, fever, anemia)

Atrial flutter
Atrial fibrillation
Atrial/junctional tachycardias
Atrioventricular reentrant tachycardias (Wolff-Parkinson-White syndrome, others)
Ventricular tachycardia
Ventricular flutter
Torsade de pointes

Tenesmus

Differential Diagnosis	Characteristic Feature
Anal sac impaction/sacculitis/abscess	Distention of perianal area laterally and ventrally if severely impacted; rectal palpation strongly supportive
Perianal gland tumors	Location and appearance are suggestive; histopathologic confirmation (or regression after castration for adenoma)
Perineal hernia	Intact males predisposed. Visible perianal swelling less common in cats. Surgical repair and castration to decrease serum testosterone concentration.
Perianal fistula	German shepherds predisposed. May be present externally and/or internally.
Colonic or rectal polyp	Mucosal mass. Excision, histopathologic confirmation.
Rectal stricture	Small, flattened, ribbonlike stools, ± diarrhea
Anal sac adenocarcinoma	Always repalpate after draining anal sacs to rule out a mass/nodule. Fibrotic tissue may mimic a mass; palpate dorsally for sublumbar lymphadenopathy. Ultrasound of perineal region/anal sacs (experienced radiologist). Hypercalcemia in 25%-50% of cases in dogs.
Pseudocoprostasis	Anal obstruction due to severe matting of fur with feces. Evaluate haircoat, animal's environment (high stress, number of pets in household), etc., for deterrent to normal defecation.
Large bowel diarrhea	Mucoid feces, hematochezia, increased urgency
Genitourinary tract • Prostatic disorders • Idiopathic cystitis (cats) • UTI • Urethritis • Vaginitis • Urethral or urinary calculi • Neoplasia (TCC adenocarcinoma, leiomyo[sarco]ma, TVT)	In general, genitourinary abnormalities other than those causing prostatomegaly produce disorders of urination rather than tenesmus. Careful history and examination for accurate diagnosis.
Caudal abdominal cavity disorders	Abdominal palpation, rectal palpation, abdominal radiographs and/or ultrasound
Mass (organ compression)	Abdominal palpation, rectal palpation, abdominal radiographs and/or ultrasound
Pelvic fractures (misaligned healing of old pelvic fractures)	Orthopedic examination, rectal palpation, pelvic radiographs
Pelvic neoplasia	Rectal palpation, pelvic radiographs, biopsy with histopathologic diagnosis, rarely nuclear scintigraphy
Lumbosacral disease	Painful posturing to urinate and/or defecate, pollakiuria, inconsistent urine stream, incomplete voiding of bladder. Rectal palpation, neurologic exam, rule out UTI.

TCC, Transitional cell carcinoma; *TVT*, transmissible venereal tumor; *UTI*, urinary tract infection.
Modified from the third edition.

THIRD EDITION AUTHOR: Lisa Carioto, DVM, DVSc, DACVIM

Testicular Size Abnormalities

Large Testes	Small Testes
Neoplasia	Hypoplasia
Acute infection	Chronic inflammation
Testicular torsion	Cryptorchidism
Inguinoscrotal hernia	Degeneration
Sperm granuloma	Intersex

From Bonagura J: Kirk's Current veterinary therapy XIII, St. Louis, 2000, Saunders.

Differentials, Lists, and Mnemonics

Third Eyelid (Nictitating Membrane) Abnormalities

Prominent Third Eyelid With Focal Abnormality

- Curled or scrolled leading edge: excise abnormal cartilage.
- Pink, fleshy mass protruding between globe and third eyelid in a young dog ("cherry eye"): surgically reposition the gland.
- Pink, fleshy mass protruding between globe and third eyelid in an old dog: possible neoplasia; biopsy or complete excision of third eyelid.
- Mass within or on anterior surface of third eyelid: biopsy or local excision with or without adjunctive therapy; larger masses may require complete excision of third eyelid.

Generalized Enlargement of Third Eyelid

- Thickened and depigmented; may have corneal involvement (chronic superficial keratoconjunctivitis; "pannus"): conjunctival scraping or biopsy; treat with topical corticosteroids, cyclosporine.
- Thickened and inflamed with firm, fibrous nodules; cornea, episclera, and bulbar conjunctiva are also often involved: biopsy; treat on basis of breed and biopsy results (collie: nodular granulomatous episclerokeratitis; other breeds: ocular nodular fasciitis).
- Diffuse, generalized enlargement of third eyelid or gland of the third eyelid: aspiration or biopsy; lymphoma or other systemic neoplasia.

Prominent Third Eyelid Only

- Nonpigmented leading edge: appears prominent but needs no therapy
- Secondary to pain: check for corneal ulcer, foreign body, or other source of ocular or intraocular pain.
- Horner's syndrome: look for other signs of miosis, ptosis, and enophthalmos; attempt to localize lesion and treat if needed.
- Secondary to orbital disease: enophthalmos may lead to passive protrusion or orbital mass; cellulitis or myositis may displace third eyelid, causing protrusion.
- Systemic disease, such as tetanus
- Nonpigmented leading edge/margin (seen congenitally as a normal variant): appears prominent but needs no therapy

From Slatter D: Textbook of small animal surgery, ed 3, Philadelphia, 2003, Saunders.

Thromboembolism

Causes of and Predisposing Factors for Thrombosis and Thromboembolism

Vascular Endothelial Damage

- Arteriosclerosis
- Atherosclerosis
- Vasculitis
- Heartworm disease
- Catheterization (arterial or venous)
- Injection of irritating substances
- Neoplasia
- Vascular incarceration/compression
- Hyperhomocysteinemia
- Feline ischemic encephalopathy
- Fibrocartilaginous embolism

Hypercoagulability

- Infection/sepsis/abscess
- Neoplasia
- Hyperadrenocorticism
- Protein-losing nephropathy
- Protein-losing enteropathy
- Disseminated intravascular coagulation
- Thrombocytosis
- Platelet hyperreactivity
- Immune-mediated hemolytic anemia
- Parvovirus infection

Abnormal Blood Flow

- Neoplasia
- Cardiomyopathy
- Congestive heart failure
- Endocarditis
- Hypovolemia
- Shock
- Anemia
- Polycythemia
- Dehydration
- Hyperviscosity

Modified from Ettinger S, Feldman E: Textbook of veterinary internal medicine, ed 6, St. Louis, 2005, Saunders.

Thyroid Hormone Alterations

Variables That May Affect Baseline Serum Thyroid Hormone Function Test Results in Dogs

Variable	Effect
Age	Inversely proportional effect
Neonate (<3 months)	Increased T_4
Aged (>6 years)	Decreased T_4, increased TSH
Body size	Inversely proportional effect
Small (<10 kg)	Increased T_4
Large (>30 kg)	Decreased T_4
Breed:	
Sight hounds (e.g., greyhound), Nordic breeds (e.g., Siberian husky), basenjis, other breeds	T_4 and free T_4 lower than normal range established for dogs; no difference for TSH
Sex	T_4 higher in females during diestrus
Time of day	No effect
Weight gain/obesity	Increased
Weight loss/fasting	Decreased T_4, no effect on free T_4
Strenuous exercise	Increased T_4, decreased TSH, no effect on free T_4

(Continued from previous page)

Variables That May Affect Baseline Serum Thyroid Hormone Function Test Results in Dogs—cont'd

Estrus (estrogen)	No effect on T_4
Pregnancy (progesterone)	Increased T_4
Surgery/anesthesia	Decreased T_4
Concurrent illness*	Decreased T_4 and free T_4; depending on illness, TSH may increase, decrease, or not change
Moderate/severe osteoarthritis	No effect on T_4, free T_4, or TSH
Drugs:	
Aspirin	Decreased T_4, free T_4; no effect on TSH
Carprofen	Decreased T_4, free T_4, and TSH
Cephalexin	No effect on T_4, free T_4, or TSH
Clomipramine	Decreased T_4, free T_4; no effect on TSH
Deracoxib	No effect on T_4, free T_4, or TSH
Etodolac	No effect on T_4, free T_4, or TSH
Glucocorticoids	Decreased T_4 and free T_4; decreased or no effect on TSH
Furosemide	Decreased T_4
Ipodate	Increased T_4, decreased T_3
Methimazole	Decreased T_4 and free T_4; increased TSH
Phenobarbital	Decreased T_4 and free T_4; delayed increase in TSH
Phenylbutazone	Decreased T_4
Potassium bromide	No effect on T_4, free T_4, or TSH
Progestogens	Decreased T_4
Propylthiouracil	Decreased T_4 and free T_4; increased TSH
Sulfonamides	Decreased T_4 and free T_4; increased TSH
Dietary iodine intake	If excessive, decreased T_4, and free T_4; increased TSH
Dietary consumption of thyroid tissues	Increased T_4, free T_4, decreased TSH
Thyroid hormone autoantibodies	Increased or decreased T_4; no effect on free T_4 or TSH

*There is a direct correlation between the severity and systemic nature of illness and suppression of serum T_4 and free T_4 concentrations.
T_3, Triiodothyronine; *T_4*, thyroxine; *TSH*, thyroid-stimulating hormone.
Modified from Nelson RW, Couto GC: Small animal internal medicine, ed 4, St. Louis, 2009, Mosby.

Tonsillar Disorders

Differential Diagnosis Item	Key Feature(s)
Primary viral tonsillitis	Bilaterally symmetrical enlargement; clinical signs of underlying disease present (e.g., ocular and nasal discharge and sneezing); fever common; virus isolation or PCR possible for confirmation but rarely necessary
Primary bacterial tonsillitis	Bilaterally symmetrical enlargement; coughing present if *Bordetella bronchiseptica*; bacterial culture and sensitivity necessary to confirm
Secondary tonsillitis	Bilaterally symmetrical enlargement; chronic vomiting, regurgitation, or coughing due to other concurrent disease; palate disorder (elongated or cleft); oropharyngeal contamination from periodontal disease, or licking at inflamed anal sacs or pyoderma
Foreign body	Unilateral enlargement; grass awn, splinter, or porcupine quill visible on examination of tonsillar crypt
Tonsillar cyst	Unilateral enlargement; fluctuant, fluid-filled mass; rare
Squamous cell carcinoma	Unilateral irregular mass; biopsy required for confirmation
Lymphoma	Bilateral enlargement; often other lymphoid organs are affected (e.g., lymph nodes, spleen); fine-needle aspiration of tonsils for cytologic evaluation is possible under general anesthesia, but aspiration of other organs (e.g., lymph node) is often easier

PCR, Polymerase chain reaction.
Reproduced from the third edition in unabridged form.

THIRD EDITION AUTHOR: **Peter M. Foley, MSc, DVM, DACVIM**

Toxicants, Radiopaque

Name of Substance/Toxicant	Comments
Zinc	U.S. pennies minted after 1982; zinc-coated wires, nuts, bolts, screws
Lead	Fishing sinkers, some curtain weights, slug shots, pet toys (some)
Cadmium	Batteries (metal poisoning unlikely)
Mercury	Uncommon occurrence; difficult to see, since mercury from a broken thermometer can evaporate
Iron	Multivitamin pills containing iron; helpful for determining if exposure has occurred or not
Bismuth subsalicylates and other bismuth salts	Pills containing bismuth salts; pills may resemble pennies on radiograph.
Copper	Pennies (outer coating); copper-containing metallic objects (systemic copper poisoning from copper objects not likely; could see gastrointestinal [GI] signs)
Enteric-coated pills (e.g., aspirin)	May help confirm exposure on plain radiograph
Paradichlorobenzene-type mothballs	Naphthalene-type mothballs are not radiopaque.
Barium sulfate or other barium salts	Used for contrast radiography
Iodine crystals	Sometimes used for contrast studies
Some sustained-release or extended-release medications (e.g., tricyclic antidepressants, phenothiazines)	Ingestion of large amounts can be seen on the plain radiograph early on; this can help determine exposure.
Chloral hydrate	Crystals; no longer commonly used or available
Expandable polyurethane glue	Glues containing cyanates or isocyanates as active ingredients; glue can expand and cover entire stomach; glue not radiopaque but will be visible as a foreign-body object
Aluminum	Could see GI signs; systemic aluminum toxicosis from aluminum-containing products not likely
Nickel	U.S. coins (nickel, dime, quarter); could see GI signs; systemic nickel poisoning not expected
Calcium, magnesium, or aluminum-containing salts (antacids)	Antacid pills containing calcium carbonate, aluminum hydroxide, or magnesium hydroxide may be visible on radiograph early on.

Tracheal Neoplasia

Malignant Tumors of the Canine and Feline Trachea	
Lymphoma	Adenocarcinoma
Squamous cell carcinoma	Osteosarcoma
Mast cell tumor	Anaplastic carcinoma
Chondrosarcoma	Leiomyoma

Modified from Bonagura JD: Kirk's Current veterinary therapy XIII, ed 13, St. Louis, 1999, Saunders, p 503.

Tremors

Physiologic Tremor
- Fear
- Pain
- Weakness

Pathologic Tremor
- **Metabolic tremor**
  - Hypocalcemia
  - Hypoglycemia
  - Hepatic encephalopathy
  - Uremic encephalopathy
- **Toxins and drugs (partial list)**
  - Metaldehyde
  - Organophosphate
  - Pyrethrins
  - Mycotoxins
  - Hexachlorophene
  - Heavy metals
  - 5-Fluorouracil
  - Fentanyl/droperidol
  - Epinephrine
  - Blue-green algae
  - Metoclopramide
  - Diphenhydramine
  - Isoproterenol
  - Trazodone
  - Fluoxetine
  - Numerous illicit drugs
- **Intention tremor**
  - Cerebellar disease of any cause
- **Senile tremor (older dogs)**
- **Breed-related tremor syndromes**
  - Shetland sheepdog
  - Scottish terriers (central axonopathy)
  - Doberman pinscher (head tremor)
  - English bulldog (head tremor)
- **Idiopathic glucocorticoid responsive tremor syndrome**
  - Often smaller breeds; sometimes called "white shaker syndrome," though affected dogs need not be white.
- **Idiopathic head tremor syndrome (young adult dogs of several breeds)**
- **Orthostatic tremor (young adult giant-breed dogs)**
- **Myelination disorder (congenital disorder in several breeds)**
  - Hypomyelination
  - Dysmyelination

Ulcerative/Erosive Skin Lesions

Differential Diagnosis of Ulcers and Erosions Affecting Skin and Mucous Membranes

Canine Diseases

Infectious
- Bacterial pyoderma:
  - Surface:
    - Acute moist dermatitis (pyotraumatic dermatitis)
    - Intertrigo
  - Deep:
    - Folliculitis/furunculosis (including pyotraumatic folliculitis)
    - Oral bacterial infections (aerobic/anaerobic)
- Fungal:
  - Yeast infections (*Malassezia pachydermatis, Candida* spp)
  - Systemic/subcutaneous
- Parasitic:
  - Demodicosis

Metabolic
- Calcinosis cutis (hyperadrenocorticism)
- Uremia/renal failure
- Necrolytic migratory erythema/metabolic epidermal necrosis/hepatocutaneous syndrome

Neoplastic
- Epitheliotropic lymphoma
- Squamous cell carcinoma

Physical, Chemical
- Drug reactions
- Solar injury
- Thermal injury (freeze or burn)
- Urine scald

Immune Mediated/Autoimmune
- Discoid lupus erythematosus
- Vesicular cutaneous lupus erythematosus
- Pemphigus group
- Uveodermatologic syndrome
- Perianal fistulae
- Miscellaneous autoimmune subepidermal vesiculobullous diseases:
  - Bullous pemphigoid
  - Epidermolysis bullosa acquisita
  - Linear immunoglobulin A (IgA) bullous disease
  - Mucocutaneous pemphigoid
  - Bullous systemic lupus type 1

Miscellaneous
- Arthropod bites
- Urine scald
- Dermatomyositis
- Dystrophic epidermolysis bullosa
- Junctional epidermolysis bullosa
- Toxic epidermal necrolysis/erythema multiforme
- Acral mutilation syndrome (French spaniel, German and English pointers)
- Cutaneous asthenia (Ehlers-Danlos syndrome)

Feline Diseases

Infectious
- Viral:
  - Calicivirus and herpesvirus
- Bacterial:
  - Atypical mycobacteriosis
- Fungal:
  - Subcutaneous mycoses (e.g., sporotrichosis)
  - Systemic mycoses (e.g., cryptococcosis)

Metabolic
- Uremia/renal disease

Neoplastic
- Fibrosarcoma
- Lymphoma
- Squamous cell carcinoma

Physical/Chemical
- Drug reactions
- Thermal injury (burn or frostbite)

Immune Mediated/Autoimmune
- Bullous pemphigoid
- Pemphigus foliaceus
- Toxic epidermal necrolysis/erythema multiforme

Miscellaneous/Idiopathic
- Arthropod bites
- Dystrophic epidermolysis bullosa
- Eosinophilic plaque
- Idiopathic ulceration of dorsal neck
- Indolent ulcer
- Junctional epidermolysis bullosa
- Skin fragility syndrome
- Cutaneous asthenia (Ehlers-Danlos syndrome)

Modified from Ettinger S, Feldman E: Textbook of veterinary internal medicine, ed 7, St. Louis, 2010, Saunders.

Ulcers and Erosions (Cutaneous), Distribution

Distribution of Ulcers and Erosions as a Diagnostic Clue

Axillary/Inguinal
- Fungal (*Malassezia pachydermatis, Candida* spp) (D)
- Vesicular cutaneous lupus erythematosus (D)
- Intertrigo (D)
- Urine scald (D)

Focal/Multifocal
- Calcinosis cutis (D)
- Demodicosis (D)
- Eosinophilic plaque (C)
- Indolent ulcer (C)
- Intertrigo (D)
- Neoplasia (D, C)
- Pyoderma (principally pyotraumatic dermatitis or folliculitis) (D)
- Systemic/subcutaneous mycosis (D, C)

Facial
- Arthropod bites (D, C)
- Bullous pemphigoid (D, C)
- Deep pyoderma (D)
- Demodicosis (D)
- Dermatomyositis (D)
- Discoid lupus erythematosus (D)
- Linear immunoglobulin A (IgA) bullous disease (D)
- Pemphigus foliaceus/erythematosus (D, C)
- Solar injury (D, C)
- Squamous cell carcinoma (C)
- Systemic/subcutaneous mycosis (D, C)
- Uveodermatologic syndrome (D)

Mucocutaneous
- Bacteria (aerobic/anaerobic) (D, C)
- Bullous pemphigoid (D, C)
- Bullous systemic lupus type 1
- Epidermolysis bullosa acquisita (D)
- Epitheliotropic lymphoma (D)
- Fungal (*M. pachydermatis, Candida* spp) (D)
- Mucocutaneous pyoderma (D)
- Mucocutaneous pemphigoid (D)
- Pemphigus vulgaris (D)
- Toxic epidermal necrosis/erythema multiforme (D, C)
- Uremia (D, C)
- Viral infection (calicivirus/herpesvirus) (C)

Generalized/Extensive
- Bullous pemphigoid (D)
- Deep pyoderma (D)
- Demodicosis (D)
- Drug reaction (D, C)
- Epitheliotropic lymphoma (D)
- *Malassezia* dermatitis (D)
- Pemphigus group (D, C)
- Thermal injury (D, C)
- Toxic epidermal necrolysis/erythema multiforme (D, C)

C, Cat; *D*, dog.
Modified from Ettinger S, Feldman E: Textbook of veterinary internal medicine, ed 7, St. Louis, 2010, Saunders.

Upper Respiratory Infection, Feline

Feature	FVR	FCV*	FCh	Bb
Lethargy	+++	+	+	+
Sneezing	+++	+	+	++
Conjunctivitis	++	++	+++[†]	–
Hypersalivation	++	–[‡]	–	–
Ocular discharge	+++	++	+++	(+)
Nasal discharge	+++	++	+	++
Oral ulceration	+	+++	–	–
Keratitis	+	–	–	–
Coughing	(+)	–	–	++
Pneumonia	(+)	+	±	+
Lameness	–	++	–	–

*Strain variation.
[†]Often persistent.
[‡]Slight wetness may be seen around the mouth if ulcers present.
Bb, Bordetella bronchiseptica infection; *FCh, Chlamydia felis* (formerly *Chlamydophila felis* and *Chlamydia psittaci*) infection; *FCV*, feline calicivirus infection; *FVR*, feline viral rhinotracheitis (feline herpesvirus infection); (+), uncommon but may occur; ±, lesions may be present but are not usually seen clinically.
Adapted from Gaskell RM, Bennett M: Feline and canine infectious diseases, Oxford, 1996, Blackwell Science, p 8.

Urinary Crystals

Name	Description	Significance
Struvite (magnesium ammonium phosphate)	Colorless prisms with three to six sides (coffin lid)	Common in mildly acidic to alkaline urine in normal dogs and cats; may be associated with struvite calculi and infection with urease-producing bacteria
Calcium oxalate (monohydrate)	Dumbbells or small spindles	May be normal (especially if delay in analysis after urine collection) or due to ethylene glycol intoxication; may be associated with oxalate calculi
Calcium oxalate (dihydrate)	Colorless envelopes or small stars	May be normal (especially if delay in analysis after urine collection) or due to ethylene glycol intoxication; may be associated with oxalate calculi
Calcium phosphate	Prisms (long) or amorphous	May be normal or associated with calculi
Ammonium urate	Yellow-brown "thorn apples"	Normal in Dalmatians and English bulldogs; associated with hepatic insufficiency and portosystemic shunts; may be associated with urate calculi
Uric acid	Yellow to yellow-brown prisms, diamonds, or rosettes	Same as ammonium urate
Bilirubin	Golden yellow to brown needles or granules	May be present in normal dogs with concentrated urine or may be due to bilirubinuria
Cystine	Colorless flat hexagonal plates	Due to cystinuria; may be associated with calculi
Cholesterol	Colorless flat, notched plates	May be found in normal dogs and cats
Hippuric acid	Prisms (four to six sides with rounded corners)	Uncertain; have been confused with calcium oxalate monohydrate crystals
Sulfonamide	Clear to brown eccentrically bound needles in sheaves	Associated with sulfonamide administration
Xanthine	Amorphous, spheroid, or ovoid; yellow-brown	Difficult to differentiate from amorphous urates; can form during allopurinol therapy
Crystals associated with melamine toxicosis	Yellow-brown spherical crystals with radial striations	Present in urine from animals fed melamine/cyanuric acid–contaminated diets

NOTE: See p. 1131 for composite diagram of crystals found in urinary sediment.
Modified from Willard M, Tvedten H: Small animal clinical diagnosis by laboratory methods, ed 5, St. Louis, 2012, Saunders.

Urinary Tract Infections, Recurrent and Persistent

Cause	Means of Diagnosis
Lack of owner compliance in drug administration	History (count remaining doses of medication)
Upper UTI	Abdominal ultrasound showing dilated renal pelvis, culture urine from renal pelvis, urinalysis demonstrating WBC casts, isosthenuria common, azotemia
Calculi	Survey and/or contrast radiographs, ultrasonography, cystoscopy
Prostatitis	Rectal palpation, ejaculate cytologic examination and culture, prostatic aspirate, prostatic biopsy, ultrasonography
Neoplasm	Rectal palpation, vaginal palpation, cytologic examination of urine sediment, contrast radiographs, biopsy, ultrasonography, urethrocystoscopy
Diverticulum	Positive-contrast radiographs
Granuloma	Contrast radiographs, urethrocystoscopy, biopsy
Urinary incontinence or urine retention due to any cause	History, physical examination, determination of residual urine volume
Decreased resistance to infection	History, physical exam, medical evaluation to detect hyperadrenocorticism, diabetes mellitus, retroviral infection in cats, or other causes of immune compromise
Incorrect antibiotic selection	Urine C&S
Urinary catheterization	History, physical examination
Antibiotic resistance	Urine C&S
Foreign body	Ultrasound, cystoscopy
PU/PD (severe): antibiotic fails to attain adequate concentration in urine	Measure water intake; urinalysis
Vulvar or preputial conformational abnormalities (common, and commonly overlooked)	Physical exam, including vaginal palpation. Careful attention to recessed or hooded vulvar confirmation

C&S, Culture and susceptibility; *PU/PD*, polyuria and polydipsia; *UTI*, urinary tract infection; *WBC*, white blood cell.
Modified from Willard M, Tvedten H: Small animal clinical diagnosis by laboratory methods, ed 5, St. Louis, 2012, Saunders.

Urolith Radiopacity: Mnemonic

"I Can't "See" You" (from more to less radiopaque):
I—Infection stones (struvite uroliths)
C—Calcium oxalate uroliths
C—Cysteine uroliths
U—Urate uroliths

Uroliths: Radiographic and Physical Appearance

Radiographic Characteristics of Common Uroliths

Mineral Type	Degree of Radiopacity	Shape
Cystine	+ to ++	Smooth, usually small, round to oval
Calcium oxalate dihydrate	++++	Often rough, round to oval (occasionally jackstone)
Calcium oxalate monohydrate	+++	Often smooth, round (occasionally jackstone)
Struvite	+ to ++++	Smooth, round or faceted; sometimes assumes shape of renal pelvis, ureter, bladder, or urethra; sometimes laminated
Calcium phosphate	++++	Smooth, round or faceted
Ammonium urate and uric acid	0 to ++	Smooth but occasionally irregular; round or oval
Silica*	++ to ++++	Typically jackstone
Mixed and compound	+ to ++++	Varies with composition; may have detectable nucleus and shell
Matrix	0 to +	Usually round but may be influenced by location

*Not observed as a primary mineral in cats.
From Slatter D: Textbook of small animal surgery, ed 3, Philadelphia, 2003, Saunders.

Differentials, Lists, and Mnemonics

Uveitis

Causes of Anterior Uveitis in Cats and Dogs

Systemic Infection
- Bacterial
  - Bacteremia or septicemia (e.g., pyometra, abscess) (D, C)
  - Brucellosis (D)
  - Bartonellosis (D, C)
  - Leptospirosis (D)
  - Borreliosis (Lyme disease) (D)
- Rickettsial
  - Ehrlichiosis (D, C)
  - Rocky Mountain spotted fever (D)
- Viral
  - Canine adenovirus 1 (D)
  - Feline leukemia virus (C)
  - Feline immunodeficiency virus (C)
  - Feline infectious peritonitis (C)
- Mycotic
  - Blastomycosis (D, C)
  - Histoplasmosis (D, C)
  - Coccidioidomycosis (D, C)
  - Cryptomycosis (D, C)
  - Aspergillosis (D)
- Algal
  - Protothecosis (D)
- Parasitic
  - Aberrant nematode larval migration
  - *Toxocara* (ocular larval migrans) (D, C)
  - *Dirofilaria* larvae (D)
  - Others
- Protozoan
  - Toxoplasmosis (D, C)—primarily cats
  - Leishmaniasis (D, C)

Immune Mediated
- Lens-induced uveitis (D, C)
- Canine adenovirus vaccine (CAV-1 or CAV-2) reaction (D)
- Uveodermatologic syndrome (D)—primarily Akita and Arctic breeds of dogs
- Pigmentary uveitis (D) primarily golden retrievers
- Idiopathic anterior uveitis (D, C)

Neoplasia
- Primary (D, C)
- Metastatic—lymphoma most common (D, C)

Metabolic
- Diabetes mellitus—primarily through cataract and lens-induced uveitis (D)
- Hyperlipidemia (D)

Trauma
- Blunt or sharp trauma to the globe

Miscellaneous Causes of Blood-Eye Barrier Disruption
- Hyperviscosity syndrome (D, C)
- Hypertension (D, C)
- Scleritis (D)
- Ulcerative keratitis (D, C)

C, Cat; *D*, dog.
From Bonagura JD, Twedt DC, editors: Kirk's Current veterinary therapy XIV, St. Louis, 2009, Saunders.

Vaccine Failure

Host Factors
- Immunodeficiencies
- Maternal antibody interference
- Age: very young or very old
- Pregnancy
- Concurrent illness
- Fever, hypothermia
- Incubating disease at time of vaccination
- Drugs: cytotoxic, glucocorticoids
- Anesthesia?

Vaccine Factors
- Rendered ineffective during handling
- Improper storage
- Vaccines do not protect 100% of population (biological variation)
- Disinfectant used on needles and syringes
- Wrong strain
- Excessive attenuation
- Overwhelming exposure

Human Error
- Improper mixing of products
- Exposed at time of vaccination
- Concurrent use of antimicrobials or immunosuppressive drugs
- Simultaneous use of antisera
- Too frequent administration (<2-week interval)
- Wrong route of administration
- Delay between vaccines in initial series
- Omission of booster vaccination

Modified from Greene C: Infectious diseases of the dog and cat, ed 4, St. Louis, 2012, Saunders.

Vascular Disorders

Diseases of Arteries and Arterioles
- Occlusive Diseases
  - Arterial embolism
  - Arterial thrombosis
  - Angiitis, vasculitis
  - Vasospasm (traumatic, toxic)
  - Diabetic arteriopathy
- Nonocclusive Diseases
  - Arteriovenous (AV) fistula
  - Arterial aneurysm
  - Arterial calcification
  - Arteriosclerosis, hyalinosis, amyloidosis
  - Atherosclerosis
  - Vasculitis

Diseases of Veins
- Phlebectasia
- Varicosis
- Phlebitis and thrombophlebitis
- Venous thrombosis
- Venous malformations

Diseases of Lymphatics
- Lymphangitis
- Lymphedema
- Lymphangiectasia
- Lymphatic hypoplasia, aplasia, hyperplasia
- Lymphangioma, lymphocysts
- Lymphangiosarcoma

Tumors of Peripheral Blood Vessels
- Angioma, hemangioma, hemangiosarcoma

From Ettinger S, Feldman E: Textbook of veterinary internal medicine, eds 6 and 7, St. Louis, 2005 and 2010, Saunders.

Vestibular Disease: Central Versus Peripheral

	Central	Peripheral
Loss of balance	Yes	Yes
Head tilt	Yes	Yes
Falling/rolling	Yes (greater tendency to roll)	Yes
Nystagmus	Yes	Yes
Horizontal	Yes	Yes
Rotatory	Yes	Yes
Vertical	Yes	No
Positional	Yes	No
Strabismus (ventrolateral)	Yes	Yes
Cranial nerve deficits	Possible I-XII, especially V, VI, VII	Possible VII
Horner's syndrome	No	Possible
Cerebellar signs	Possible	No
Mental depression	Possible	No
Hemiparesis with ipsilateral postural reaction deficits	Possible	No

Modified with permission from Braund KG: Clinical syndromes in veterinary neurology, St. Louis, 1994, Mosby, p. 65.

Voice Change

Differential Diagnosis Item	Key Feature(s)
Anatomic Causes	
Laryngeal distortion	Laryngeal collapse as visualized via laryngoscopy
Laryngeal edema	Edema of corniculate/cuneiform processes as visualized via laryngoscopy
Eversion of the laryngeal saccules	Uni- or bilateral saccules visualized ventrally
Laryngeal/pharyngeal foreign body	As visualized via laryngoscopy
Laryngeal inflammation	Common with infectious tracheitis
Laryngeal neoplasia	Mass visualized via laryngoscopy
Functional Causes	
Dysfunction of the recurrent laryngeal nerve or congenital/idiopathic laryngeal paralysis	Laryngeal paralysis/paresis common in older large-breed dogs
Trauma to the nerve	Evidence of cervical trauma (wound, blunt trauma, or previous surgery)
Nerve compression	Hematoma, abscess, tumor on cervical/thoracic radiographs/ultrasound/CT or MRI
Neuropathy, polyneuritis	Signs of general weakness are usually present, megaesophagus
Myopathy	Evidence of muscular disease on EMG and on histopathologic evaluation of muscle biopsies
Neuromuscular disease (myasthenia gravis)	As per neuropathy/polyneuritis and serum acetylcholine receptor antibodies titer elevated

CT, Computed tomography; *EMG*, electromyogram; *MRI*, magnetic resonance imaging.
Reproduced from the third edition in unabridged form.

THIRD EDITION AUTHOR: **Bertrand Lussier, DMV, MSc, DACVS**

Vomiting, Causes of

Gastrointestinal Causes

- Obstruction
  - Physical
    - Intraluminal (e.g., foreign body, pyloric outflow obstruction)
    - Extraluminal (e.g., abdominal tumor)
  - Functional (e.g., dysautonomia, ileus)
- Infiltration
  - Neoplastic (e.g., GI lymphoma)
  - Inflammatory (e.g., inflammatory bowel disease)
  - Edema (e.g., right heart failure)
- Infection
  - Viral (e.g., parvovirus)
  - Bacterial (e.g., salmonellosis)
  - Fungal (e.g., histoplasmosis)
  - Parasitic (e.g., *Physaloptera*)
  - Oomycete (e.g., pythiosis)
- Peptic ulcer (e.g., NSAID use, gastrinoma)
- Gastrointestinal pain/distention
- Dietary intolerance
- Dietary indiscretion

Nongastrointestinal Causes

- Activation of CRTZ
  - Endogenous (e.g., uremia, hepatic failure)
  - Exogenous (e.g., chemotherapy drugs, antibiotics, narcotics)
- Abdominal inflammatory disorders (e.g., pancreatitis, peritonitis)
- Vestibular disorders (central or peripheral)
- Endocrinopathy (hypoadrenocorticism, hyperthyroidism, diabetic ketosis)
- Intracranial disease (e.g., increased intracranial pressure, brain tumor)
- Abdominal inflammatory disease (e.g., pancreatitis, peritonitis)
- Miscellaneous
  - Sepsis
  - Pain
  - Fear

Vomiting, Chronic

Category	Disorder	Salient Feature
Systemic: extra-abdominal	Uremia	Serum biochemistry profile + urinalysis: azotemia + isosthenuria
	Hypoadrenocorticism	Wax-wane clinical course is common; absence of stress leukogram in ill dog; ACTH stimulation test confirms
	Diabetic ketoacidosis	Hyperglycemia, glucosuria, ketonuria, and acidosis
	Hypercalcemia	Serum calcium concentration
	Hyperthyroidism (cats)	Serum thyroxine concentration
	Heartworm disease (cats; variable)	*D. immitis* antibody and antigen test, echocardiography, or all
Systemic: intraabdominal	Hepatobiliary disease	Icterus; serum liver enzyme concentrations, serum bile acids concentrations
	Pancreatitis	Pancreatic lipase immunoreactivity, abdominal ultrasound
	Peritonitis	Inflammation/infection on abdominocentesis cytology
Gastrointestinal causes	Chronic gastritis	Endoscopic (with biopsy, histopathology) diagnosis
	Food intolerance/allergy	Evidence of polysystemic allergies common (otitis/atopic dermatitis, allergic rhinitis/ bronchitis, etc.), dietary elimination trial confirmatory
	Foreign body	Behavior ("Does this dog like to mouth objects?"), history, radiographic obstructive pattern
	Intussusception	Abdominal ultrasound (target/bull's-eye appearance of intussusceptum within intussuscipiens)
	Parasites (*Physaloptera* spp, *Ollulanus tricuspis*)	Serial fecal flotations and/or empirical anthelmintic treatment; usually acts otherwise well
	Neoplasia	Abdominal imaging +/− needle aspirate; endoscopic or laparotomy (with biopsy, histopathology) diagnosis
	Inflammatory bowel disease	Endoscopic or laparotomy (with biopsy, histopathology) diagnosis
	Bilious vomiting syndrome	History of recurrent early-morning/preprandial vomiting suggestive; response to frequent, smaller feedings
	Motility disorders	Radiographic evidence of persistent functional ileus without identifiable cause; diagnosis of exclusion
	Colitis (up to 30% of dogs with colitis vomit)	Colitis signs prominent (tenesmus, mucoid stools, dyschezia, hematochezia)
	Gastrinoma	Evidence of gastric ulceration (usually endoscopic), laparotomy for excision of pancreatic neoplasm and/or hypergastrinemia confirmatory
	Hiatal hernia	Serial radiographs (assuming dynamic/"sliding" hiatal hernia)
	Pyloric stenosis	Delayed gastric emptying on plain or barium-contrast radiographs or flouroscopy; endoscopic/laparotomy diagnosis
	Gastric antral mucosal hyperplasia	Endoscopy

AUTHORS: Sylvie Daminet, DVM, PhD, DACVIM, DECVIM; Etienne Côté, DVM, DACVIM

Vulvar Discharge, Hemorrhagic

Hemorrhagic Vulvar Discharge in the Bitch and Queen	
With Mainly Superficial (Mature) Epithelial Cells (Estrogen Influence)	**Without Superficial (Mature) Epithelial Cells (No Estrogen Influence)**
Normal estrus, late proestrus, or early diestrus (most common)	Normal lochia, early postpartum (most common)
Ovarian remnant (common)	Subinvoluted placental sites, late postpartum (young, primiparous bitches)
Ovarian pathologic condition (i.e., cystic follicles, functional ovarian tumor)	Vaginal laceration
Exogenous estrogen	Neoplasia of vagina or uterus (most common cause in elderly bitches)
	Uterine torsion
	Bleeding disorder (especially primary hemostatic defects)

Modified from Willard MD, Tvedten H: Small animal clinical diagnosis by laboratory methods, ed 5, St. Louis, 2012, Elsevier.

Weakness

Major Causes		
Anemia	Hemorrhage	Neuromuscular/polyneuropathies
Cardiovascular disorders	Infectious disease states	Nutritional disorders
Chronic wasting diseases	Fever	Orthopedic disorders
Drug or toxin	Metabolic dysfunction states	Overactivity
Electrolyte disorders	Myopathic disorders	Pain
Endocrine disorders	Neoplasia	Pulmonary diseases
	Neurologic disorders	

Modified from Ettinger S, Feldman E: Textbook of veterinary internal medicine, ed 5, St. Louis, 2000, Saunders.

Weight Loss

Category	Disorder	Key Feature
Adequate calorie intake absent GI signs		
	Inadequate calorie provision	Dietary history, including amount fed
	Physiologic increases in energy demand (e.g., exercise, pregnancy, lactation, growth)	History and physical exam
	Pathologic increases in energy demand (e.g., hyperthyroidism)	History and physical exam; serum T_4
Compromised Ability to Eat or Retain Food		
	Unwilling or unable to prehend or masticate food	Shows interest in food; observe animal eating; thorough oral exam (sedation may be required)
	Dysphagia	Observe eating and ability to swallow; neurologic exam; dynamic barium esophagram under fluoroscopy
	Regurgitation	History of frequent regurgitation (differentiate from vomiting-passive); thoracic radiographs to r/o megaesophagus
	Vomiting, chronic	History of frequent vomiting (differentiate from regurgitation-active); pursue diagnostic evaluation
	Small bowel diarrhea, chronic	History of small bowel diarrhea; pursue diagnostic evaluation
Anorexia/Decreased Appetite		
	Nausea related to GI disease (e.g., ulcers, IBD, partial obstruction, GI neoplasia)	Can have weight loss even with infrequent or absent vomiting; lip licking or drooling; physical exam; abdominal imaging
	Nausea due to stimulation of CRTZ (e.g., uremia, hepatic failure, drugs)	Can have weight loss even with infrequent or absent vomiting; lip licking or drooling; history and exam often helpful; biochemical testing and imaging studies
	Nausea of any other cause (e.g., chronic pancreatitis, CNS disease, vestibular disease, pain, hypoadrenocorticism)	Can have weight loss even with infrequent or absent vomiting; lip licking or drooling; history and exam often helpful; biochemical testing and imaging studies
Maldigestive/Malabsorptive Conditions		
	Exocrine pancreatic insufficiency	Though a good appetite is common, poor appetite does not rule out EPI; trypsinlike immunoreactivity is diagnostic
	Infiltrative small intestinal disease (e.g., IBD, lymphoma, pythiosis)	Physical exam; abdominal imaging; endoscopy and biopsy
Inability to Utilize Nutrients		
	Diabetes mellitus	Blood glucose concentration; urinalysis for glucose, ketones
Cachexic Conditions		
	Neoplasia (cancer cachexia)	Physical exam may be suggestive; imaging studies as indicated; aspirate or biopsy
	Heart failure (cardiac cachexia)	History and physical exam suggestive; thoracic radiographs; echocardiography
	Kidney failure (renal cachexia)	History and physical exam suggestive; biochemical profile; urinalysis
	Chronic infections (septic cachexia)	Physical exam findings indicative; CBC generally indicates toxic WBC changes, left shift, or both
	Brain tumor	Neurologic deficits that indicate intracranial disease are almost always present when a brain tumor is responsible for weight loss

Continued

Differentials, Lists, and Mnemonics

(Continued from previous page)

Category	Disorder	Key Feature
Nutrient Loss		
	Protein-losing nephropathy	Urinalysis and serum biochemistry profile; urine protein-to-creatinine ratio
	Protein-losing enteropathy	Panhypoproteinemia; abdominal ultrasound; fecal alpha-1 protease inhibitor; biopsy for diagnosis
	Protein-losing dermatopathy (e.g., burn, TEN)	Obvious on physical examination
	Chronic blood loss (e.g., GI bleeding, heavy burden of blood-sucking parasites)	Physical exam including rectal exam; CBC with anemia and hypoproteinemia; fecal examination

CBC, Complete blood count; *GI,* gastrointestinal; *TLI,* trypsinlike immunoreactivity; T_4, thyroxine; *WBC,* white blood cell count; *r/o,* rule out.

AUTHORS: Bradley A. Green, DVM, DACVIM; Helio Autran de Morais, DVM, PhD, DACVIM; Etienne Côté, DVM, DACVIM

Zoonotic Diseases (Select)

Directly Transmitted Zoonoses Most Commonly Affecting Immunocompromised People*

Disease and Pet	Diagnosis	Treatment	Precautions
Toxoplasmosis: C	NR: fecal exam—oocysts rarely found; serology—cannot predict oocyst shedding; seropositive generally protected because of previous exposure	NR: clindamycin—reduces oocyst shedding; bathing—feces not often on fur	R: litter box hygiene—daily cleaning by immunocompetent assistant; preventing cat from hunting or eating raw meat
Giardiasis: C, D	R: test pups, kittens, diarrheic pets; zinc sulfate method, ELISA point-of-care, PCR	R: metronidazole, albendazole, fenbendazole	R: litter box hygiene; handling feces with gloves
Cryptosporidiosis: C, D	R: acid-fast or direct FA staining of feces, PCR	R: paromomycin; untreated may shed for 2 weeks	R: litter box hygiene; handling feces with gloves
Campylobacteriosis, helicobacteriosis: C, D	R: fecal culture NR: culture stomach contents or biopsy, histopathology with silver stains	R: I—erythromycin, chloramphenicol	R: preventing ingestion of raw meat
		R: G—metronidazole, ampicillin, bismuth subsalicylate	R: preventing ingestion of raw meat
Salmonellosis: C, D	R: fecal culture, selective media, PCR	NR: quinolones	R: preventing hunting and carrion or raw meat ingestion; if positive, temporarily removing animal from household
Bartonellosis: C, D	R: blood culture (C) or PCR	R: quinolones, doxycycline, rifampin	R: strict flea control, screening or avoiding kittens, avoiding bites or scratches and washing immediately if they occur
	NR: antibody testing		
Bordetellosis: C, D	NR: endotracheal wash and culture	R: tetracyclines	R: avoiding exposure to boarding kennels, dog shows, and congregated dogs; vaccinating if exposure likely

*For additional recommendations see Scheftel JM, et al: Compendium of veterinary standard precautions for zoonotic disease prevention in veterinary personnel. J Am Vet Med Assoc 237:1403–1422, 2010.
C, Cat; *D,* dog; *FA,* fluorescent antibody; *G,* gastric *Helicobacter* organisms; *I,* intestinal *Campylobacter* organisms; *NR,* not recommended; *PCR,* polymerase chain reaction; *R,* recommended.
Modified from Glaser CA, et al: Zoonotic infections of medical importance in immunocompromised humans. In Greene CE, editor: Infectious diseases of dogs and cats, ed 4, St. Louis, 2012, Elsevier.

SECTION IV

Laboratory Tests

EDITOR

Lois Roth-Johnson
DVM, PhD, DACVP

This section, Laboratory Tests, groups over 150 diagnostic tests that are used widely in small-animal practice. Information is drawn from both basic science and applied clinical medicine to provide a brief summary of each test. The facts and interpretations necessary to understand these tests under most circumstances are included. **NOTE:** The unit of measure of micron, sometimes denoted by the Greek letter μ, is abbreviated in this text by mc. For example, 1 mcL = 1 microliter; 1 mcg = 1 microgram.

Each topic is organized in a consistent manner. Sections for each entry include:

Definition

A concise explanation of the nature of the test

Synonym

When applicable, other names by which the test is known

Physiology

A brief description of the natural processes underlying the analyte being measured and specific application of the test

Reference Interval

A broad reference interval for normal results. Exact ranges are laboratory specific and may even be population or test kit specific. The ranges published here should be considered only a guide.

Causes of Abnormally High/Low Levels

The common differential diagnoses for values falling outside the normal range

Next Diagnostic Steps to Consider if Levels are High/Low

Recommended tests or procedures that typically are indicated if the current test is not the definitive test of choice

Important Interspecies Differences

Relevant physiologic or test-associated variation

Drug Effects

Alterations in test results that may be expected when a patient is receiving certain medications

Lab Artifacts

Extraneous factors that may produce a false reading and should be considered by the clinician when interpreting test results

Specimen Collection and Handling

The sample required to perform the test

Relative Cost

A price scale is included to provide a relative indication of test costs. Necessarily, the exact cost will vary from one laboratory or institution to another and one geographic region to another, and changes over time will alter these values within any laboratory. Nevertheless, by comparing tests to each other according to their costs, the price scale can provide a relative sense of the expense associated with each test. The scale used is based on costs of tests submitted to a full-service reference laboratory in North America in 2018, as follows:

$: <$50
$$: $50-100
$$$: $100-200
$$$$: >$200

Pearls

Tips, important reminders, or explanations generally acquired through experience. These are clinically important but otherwise often escape publication.

Acanthocyte

Definition

Erythrocyte morphologic abnormality characterized by irregularly spaced, usually blunt projections from the normally smooth round cell membrane with loss of normal erythrocyte central pallor (from the Greek *akantha,* meaning "thorn").

Synonyms

Burr cell, spur cell, echinoacanthocyte

Physiology

Altered red blood cell shape may be an artifact of blood film preparation. True acanthocyte morphology is associated with altered lipid metabolism, sometimes due to liver disease, resulting in abnormalities in the lipid structure of the red blood cell membrane. Vascular disease (vasculitis, DIC) may also disrupt normal red blood cell shape.

Reference Interval

Not reported unless seen on blood film. Healthy dogs and cats should not have appreciable numbers of circulating acanthocytes on properly prepared, fresh blood films.

Causes of Abnormally High Levels

Hemangiosarcoma; liver, splenic, or renal disease; artifact of blood film preparation

Next Diagnostic Steps to Consider if Levels Are High

Repeat CBC to confirm; if consistent finding, evaluate for liver, splenic, or renal disease and metabolic abnormalities as suggested by clinical signs. Evaluation of a saline preparation can help differentiate artifactual erythrocyte shape change from *in vivo* changes in erythrocyte shape.

Lab Artifacts

Specimen age artifact (delay in preparing blood film, sample not refrigerated); artifact of blood film preparation

Specimen Collection and Handling

Whole blood in EDTA (lavender top tube) or heparin (green top tube); include a blood film prepared when specimen was collected to help rule out specimen age artifact

Relative Cost: $/$$ (depending on reflex testing included in CBC panel)

Pearls

- Considered nonspecific and a common artifact; should be evaluated in a second, fresh specimen before drawing diagnostic conclusions.
- Acanthocytes can be difficult to differentiate from crenation. Crenated erythrocytes have regularly placed "tent-shaped" projections and retain an area of central pallor.

AUTHOR: Sharon M. Dial, DVM, PhD, DACVP
EDITOR: Lois Roth-Johnson, DVM, PhD, DACVP

Acetylcholine Receptor Antibody Test

Definition

Detection of serum autoantibodies aimed at skeletal muscle acetylcholine receptors (AChR). Used to confirm the presence of acquired myasthenia gravis (MG).

Synonym(s)

MG test, AchRAb titer

Physiology

Acetylcholine is used to transduce signals from nerves to skeletal muscle. Functional AChR on skeletal muscle (the post-synaptic membrane in the neuromuscular junction) are necessary for normal signal transduction. In acquired (immune mediated) MG, autoantibodies deplete AChR. An immunoprecipitation radioimmunoassay is used to detect these autoantibodies.

Reference Interval

0-0.6 nmol/L in dogs, 0-0.3 nmol/L in cats

Causes of Abnormally High Levels

High levels of AChR autoantibodies indicate the patient has acquired MG.

Next Diagnostic Steps to Consider if Levels Are High

An increased value is considered confirmatory for myasthenia gravis. Thoracic imaging is recommended to assess for the presence of a cranial mediastinal mass (thymoma associated MG) and to evaluate the patient for potential megaesophagus, a common problem in MG patients. General health screening and evaluation for other forms of neoplasia coinciding with acquired MG may also be prudent (p. 668).

Next Diagnostic Steps to Consider if Levels Are Low

AChR antibody testing is the gold standard for diagnosing MG. If the result is negative but MG is still suspected clinically, consider retesting in a few weeks. It is rare for acquired MG patients to be seronegative. Repeating neuromuscular examination, use of electrophysiologic testing, and muscle biopsy can be considered if other neuromuscular disorders have not been satisfactorily ruled out.

Important Interspecies Differences

Acquired MG is more common in dogs than cats.

Drug Effects

Recent immunosuppressive therapy can decrease the titer, potentially causing a false-negative result.

Lab Artifacts

Lipemia and hemolysis may cause false-positive results.

Specimen Collection and Handling

Serum, 2 mL (red top tube, separated from cells as soon as possible) should be submitted with a cold pack overnight. Fasting patient prior to blood draw is recommended to minimize risk of lipemia. Serum is stable for testing up to a week at 2°C to 8°C, longer if frozen.

Relative Cost: $$$

AUTHOR: Angela Royal, DVM, MS, DACVP
EDITOR: Lois Roth-Johnson, DVM, PhD, DACVP

Acetylcholinesterase Level

Definition

Enzyme that hydrolyzes choline ester neurotransmitters. Measured to confirm organophosphate or carbamate toxicity when clinical signs and response to therapy suggest this diagnosis.

Synonym(s)

Cholinesterase, AChE level

Physiology

The neurotransmitter acetylcholine (ACh) is released from presynaptic cell membranes. AChE at postsynaptic membranes degrades excess ACh to limit its activity. Organophosphate and carbamate pesticides inhibit AChE activity, leading to continued cholinergic signaling (depolarization of the cell membrane). Continuous depolarization may initially be stimulatory, but eventually becomes inhibitory/paralyzing as repolarization of the membrane is ineffective.

Reference Interval

Will vary by laboratory. Example: 1895-5240 U/L (dogs); 736-3016 U/L (cats)

Next Diagnostic Steps to Consider if Levels Are High

If organophosphate or carbamate exposure was suspected but AChE level is within reference range, assessment of stomach contents, vomitus, or suspected baits for these toxins may be helpful. The reversible nature of carbamate binding to AChE can result in higher-than-expected AChE levels, particularly if the sample was handled improperly.

Causes of Abnormally Low Levels

Organophosphate or carbamate toxicity; other toxin exposures are possible, including zinc phosphide and anatoxin-a(s).

Next Diagnostic Steps to Consider if Levels Are Low

Levels <50% of normal are suspicious for organophosphate or carbamate exposure, and levels <25% of normal are essentially diagnostic.

Lab Artifacts

Check with lab for possible artifacts. Anemic patients may have lower AChE activity in whole blood, owing to lesser amounts of erythrocyte AChE.

Specimen Collection and Handling

Heparinized whole blood, 1 mL (green top tube) or EDTA anticoagulated whole blood (lavender top tube). Check with lab to see which is preferred. Keep sample refrigerated and ship on ice overnight. Refrigerated serum or frozen brain (caudate nucleus, 5 grams) can be submitted from deceased patients.

Relative Cost: Whole blood $; blood and brain $$; brain $$

AUTHOR: Angela Royal, DVM, MS, DACVP
EDITOR: Lois Roth-Johnson, DVM, PhD, DACVP

ACTH (Adrenocorticotrophic Hormone), Endogenous

Definition

ACTH is a pituitary-derived peptide hormone occasionally measured to differentiate pituitary-dependent hyperadrenocorticism (PDH) from functional adrenal cortical neoplasia.

Synonym

Corticotropin

Physiology

Corticotropin-releasing hormone from the hypothalamus triggers release of ACTH from the corticotrophs of the anterior pituitary. ACTH stimulates production of cortisol from the adrenal cortex. Normally, cortisol then provides negative feedback to decrease ACTH production. Neoplastic corticotrophs are not constrained by this regulation. Accordingly, in PDH excessive ACTH is produced despite the concurrent increased concentration of cortisol in blood. See pp. 485 and 487.

Reference Interval

Varies by laboratory.

Causes of Abnormally High Levels

Pituitary micro- or macroadenomas can produce excessive ACTH, causing PDH. Alternatively, persistent hypocortisolemia in primary hypoadrenocorticism will result in increased ACTH production as an appropriate attempt to increase cortisol production.

Next Diagnostic Steps to Consider if Levels Are High

ACTH concentration would be measured only after confirming a patient has hyperadrenocorticism. In these patients, ACTH concentrations within or above the reference interval would confirm PDH.

Causes of Abnormally Low Levels

Hypercortisolemia suppresses the hypothalamic-pituitary-adrenal axis, decreasing ACTH concentration. This may occur in cases of functional adrenal cortical neoplasia causing hyperadrenocorticism or with exogenous administration of corticosteroids. Rarely, pituitary trauma, inflammation, or neoplasia can cause inability of corticotrophs to produce adequate ACTH (secondary hypoadrenocorticism).

Next Diagnostic Steps to Consider if Levels Are Low

In a patient with hyperadrenocorticism, low ACTH concentration suggests functional adrenal cortical neoplasia. Confirm with abdominal imaging.

Important Interspecies Differences

Most commonly measured in dogs.

Drug Effects

Administration of corticosteroids can suppress the hypothalamic-pituitary-adrenal axis, decreasing plasma ACTH concentration.

Lab Artifacts

ACTH is not stable in whole blood, glass tubes, or at room temperature or above. Failure to separate plasma from blood cells promptly or failure to keep the sample frozen or at least chilled during shipment will result in falsely decreased ACTH measurement.

Specimen Collection and Handling

Collect blood into a plastic or siliconized glass EDTA tube (lavender top), and immediately centrifuge tube to allow for prompt removal of plasma from blood cells. Transfer plasma to a plastic tube and freeze. Ship sample overnight, and package to ensure that plasma stays frozen or at minimum very chilled during transit.

Relative Cost: $$

Pearls

Rarely used in clinical practice

AUTHOR: Angela Royal, DVM, MS, DACVP
EDITOR: Lois Roth-Johnson, DVM, PhD, DACVP

ACTH (Adrenocorticotropic Hormone) Stimulation Test

Definition

The ACTH stimulation test involves measurement of blood cortisol concentration before and after administration of exogenous ACTH. The test is commonly used (1) for diagnosis of hyperadrenocorticism (HAC), (2) to monitor response to treatment of HAC, and (3) for diagnosis of hypoadrenocorticism.

Synonym

ACTH stim test

Physiology

In the hypothalamic-pituitary-adrenal axis, ACTH is secreted from the anterior pituitary gland in response to hypothalamic release of corticotrophin-releasing hormone. In turn, ACTH causes the adrenal cortex to release glucocorticoids and, to a lesser extent, other hormones. Administration of exogenous ACTH to a healthy dog or cat results in increased serum/plasma cortisol concentrations that remain within an established reference range. In uncontrolled HAC, the cortisol concentration should exceed the norm after ACTH administration, while in hypoadrenocorticism, cortisol concentration both before and after ACTH administration will be below the reference interval.

Reference Interval

- Reference intervals depend on the laboratory; to convert units to nmol/L multiply by 27.6.
- In dogs, they are approximately:
  - Baseline: 1-6 mcg/dL
  - Post-stimulation: 8-18 mcg/dL (gray zone 18-22 mcg/dL)
- In cats, they are approximately:
  - Baseline: 0.5-4 mcg/dL
  - Post-stimulation: 8-12 mcg/dL

Causes of Abnormally High Levels

- A baseline result in or above the reference interval rules out hypoadrenocorticism.
- A baseline result above the reference interval cannot be used to diagnose hyperadrenocorticism; elevated baseline levels are often due to stress.
- A post-stimulation result above the reference interval, and especially above the "gray zone," is compatible with hyperadrenocorticism.

Next Diagnostic Steps to Consider if Levels Are High

- If clinical signs are compatible with hyperadrenocorticism, a differentiating test should be performed to determine if the disease is adrenal- or pituitary-dependent (p. 485).

Causes of Abnormally Low Levels

- Both baseline and post-stimulation values below the reference interval suggest either hypoadrenocorticism or iatrogenic suppression of adrenal function.

Next Diagnostic Steps to Consider if Levels Are Low

- Careful medication history (including topical glucocorticoids) to rule out iatrogenic hyperadrenocorticism
- Evaluation of serum electrolytes and, if atypical hypoadrenocorticism present, measurement of endogenous ACTH (p. 512)

Important Interspecies Differences

- The dose of cosyntropin and reference ranges vary between dogs and cats.

Drug Effects

- Many glucocorticoids (exceptions: dexamethasone, triamcinolone) cross-react on the assay used to measure cortisol and can produce an artificially elevated cortisol concentration. They should not be given for 24 hours prior to performing an ACTH stimulation test.
- Exogenous glucocorticoids, even those applied topically, can cause adrenocortical atrophy. Despite signs of cortisol excess, affected animals have suppressed ACTH stimulation results (i.e., iatrogenic Cushing's syndrome).

Specimen Collection and Handling

- Use of Cortrosyn is preferred.
- Obtain a baseline sample (serum or plasma).
- For dogs to diagnose hyperadrenocorticism or hypoadrenocorticism:
  - Administer 5 mcg/kg Cortrosyn IV or IM (IV preferred), *or* 2.2 IU/kg (max 40 IU) ACTH gel IM. If monitoring mitotane or trilostane therapy, administer 1 mcg/kg Cortrosyn IV.
  - Obtain a second sample 1 h after Cortrosyn or 1 and 2 h after ACTH gel administration.
- For cats:
  - Administer 125 mcg/CAT Cortrosyn IV or IM (IV preferred), *or* 2.2 IU/kg ACTH gel IM.
  - Obtain a second sample 1 h after Cortrosyn or 1 and 2 h after ACTH gel administration.

Relative Cost: $$$

Pearls

- Compounded corticotropin formulations may not be as efficacious in stimulating a response as is cosyntropin and the time of peak cortisol concentration is not as consistent.
- In dogs, when clinical signs suggest hypercortisolism but prior testing does not support the diagnosis, consider ACTH administration followed by assessment of a full adrenal profile (i.e., cortisol, androstenedione, estradiol, progesterone, 17-OH progesterone, testosterone) rather than simple measurement of cortisol (https://vetmed.tennessee.edu/vmc/dls/Pages/Search-Lab-Test.aspx) (p. 490).
- If hypoadrenocorticism must be ruled out but is considered to be not likely, measurement of baseline cortisol may save the expense of ACTH stimulation testing. If hypoadrenocorticism seems likely, proceed with ACTH stimulation immediately.
- Cosyntropin is costly; leftover reconstituted cosyntropin can be stored at -20°C for up to 6 months. It should be stored as 50-mcg aliquots in plastic (e.g., syringe) rather than glass. Any thawed, unused cosyntropin should be discarded. Alternatively, the vial can be initially divided into 0.2-mL aliquots and stored frozen to reduce waste by removing only as much as is needed at one time.

AUTHOR: Leah A. Cohn, DVM, PhD, DACVIM
EDITOR: Ellen N. Behrend, VMD, PhD, DACVIM

Activated Coagulation Time (ACT)

Definition

The time interval from *in vitro* contact of blood with diatomaceous earth pellets to visible clot formation. ACT evaluates the intrinsic and common coagulation pathways but is less sensitive than activated partial thromboplastin time (aPTT).

Physiology

Contact activation occurs when whole blood is drawn into a warmed (37°C) tube containing diatomaceous earth pellets.

Reference Interval

Dogs: < 120 seconds; cats: < 165 seconds

Causes of Abnormally High Levels

Decreased concentration (less than 5% of normal) of any coagulation factor of the intrinsic or common coagulation pathways (all factors except VII); severe thrombocytopenia (<10,000 platelets/mcL); uremia. Critically ill dogs may have prolonged ACT due to inflammatory disease without bleeding tendency.

Next Diagnostic Steps to Consider if Levels Are High

Confirm with more sensitive tests (e.g., aPTT, platelet count).

Drug Effects

Prolonged by anticoagulant therapy (e.g., heparin), some antibiotics (newer lipoglycopeptide antibiotics, rarely used in veterinary medicine, may interfere with factor Xa).

Lab Artifacts

An in-office test. Any variation in protocol may alter results. Endpoint (visual clot detection) is subject to observer variability. Difficult venipuncture causing exposure to tissue factor and platelet activation may falsely shorten ACT.

Specimen Collection and Handling

Whole blood into siliceous (gray top) tube, prewarmed to 37°C. Mix by inversion, incubate at 37°C (purpose made heating block, water bath, or human axilla) and check for clot formation every 5-10 seconds. Do not incubate in a closed palm, as it does not provide a consistent 37°C environment.

Relative Cost: $

Pearls

- Insensitive test that may be useful cage side for suspected warfarin-intoxicated dogs if aPTT unavailable.
- Carriers of hemophilia (coagulation factors are 40%-60% of normal) and beagles with hereditary factor VII deficiency will not be detected.

AUTHOR & EDITOR: Lois Roth-Johnson, DVM, PhD, DACVP

Activated Partial Thromboplastin Time (aPTT)

Definition

Screening test for disorders of intrinsic and common coagulation pathways. Named for additives (e.g., partial thromboplastins, surface activators) used to activate coagulation *in vitro*. During testing calcium is added to overcome the effect of citrate, and aPTT is the time from addition of calcium chloride to clot detection.

Synonym(s)

aPTT, APTT, PTT

Physiology

There is extensive cross talk between the intrinsic and extrinsic coagulation cascades *in vivo*. Separation of the two in laboratory testing (e.g., PT, aPTT) is artifactual but useful to narrow differentials for coagulopathy. aPTT screens for deficiencies in intrinsic/contact (PK, XII, XI, IX, VIII) and common (X, V, II, fibrinogen) pathway factors and is prolonged when activity of a single factor is decreased by 70% or with multiple factor deficiencies.

Reference Interval

Laboratory, instrument, and species specific reference intervals must be used. Approximate intervals, dogs: 9-17 seconds; cats: 15-19 seconds

Causes of Abnormally High Levels

- Single factor deficiency: any intrinsic/contact or common pathway factor (e.g., hemophilia A [VIII], hemophilia B [IX] in dogs, and XII deficiency in cats)
- Multiple factor deficiencies: disseminated intravascular coagulation (DIC), liver disease (cholestatic, failure), vitamin K deficiency/antagonism, factor dilution (massive transfusion/fluid replacement)
- Severe von Willebrand disease: von Willebrand factor stabilizes factor VIII, so severe deficiency (<30%) can lead to increased aPTT.
- Anticoagulant therapy (e.g., heparin, warfarin)

Next Diagnostic Steps to Consider if Levels Are High

Interpret with signalment, history (e.g., drug/toxin exposure) and examination findings, other laboratory findings, and other markers of hemostasis (e.g., platelets, PT, fibrinogen) (p. 433).

Next Diagnostic Steps to Consider if Levels Are Low

Shortened aPTT cannot be used to confirm hypercoagulability.

Important Interspecies Differences

Cats: factor XII deficiency causes prolongation in aPTT with normal PT and normal hemostasis. Prolonged aPTT from unknown causes in cats with effective hemostasis has also been described.

Drug Effects

Increased: anticoagulant therapy (e.g., heparin, warfarin)

Lab Artifacts

- Shortened or normalized
  - Inappropriate ratio of plasma to citrate: overfilling citrate tube, severe anemia
  - Sample collection: difficult/traumatic venipuncture
- Prolonged:
  - Inappropriate ratio of plasma to citrate: underfilling of citrate tube, polycythemia
  - Sample collection: Difficult/traumatic venipuncture, improper storage
  - Anti-phospholipid antibodies: rarely documented in animals, but may interfere with phospholipids in testing phase even though animals don't have signs of hypocoagulation

Specimen Collection and Handling

Citrated whole blood (blue top tube) collected via atraumatic phlebotomy. Fill to the appropriate level (markings may vary by manufacturer). Centrifuge and separate plasma within 1 hour, store/ship refrigerated in plastic tube (additive free). If testing > 4 hours from collection, freeze for storage/shipment. Contact laboratory before collection as sample handling policy may vary.

Relative Cost: $-$$

Pearls

- Low aPTT values do not indicate a procoagulant state.
- Unfractionated heparin will prolong aPTT but not PT.
- Prolonged aPTT may be seen with a normal PT in the early stages of DIC.

AUTHOR: Mary Leissinger, DVM, MS, DACVP
EDITOR: Lois Roth-Johnson, DVM, PhD, DACVP

Alanine Aminotransferase (ALT)

Definition

Enzyme in hepatocyte cytoplasm

Synonym(s)

Glutamic pyruvate transaminase (GPT)—obsolete

Physiology

ALT is released from the cytoplasm following hepatocyte cell membrane injury. Low concentrations in erythrocytes or skeletal muscle may cause minor (usually clinically insignificant) increases in hemolytic diseases or with muscle injury, respectively.

Reference Interval

Reference interval is variable among laboratories and dependent upon analyzers/methodologies.

Causes of Abnormally High Levels

Hepatocellular injury from any cause. May be primary (e.g., hepatitis, lipidosis, neoplasia, blunt trauma, hepatotoxins) or secondary to gastrointestinal disease (e.g., pancreatitis, inflammatory bowel disease), hypoxia (e.g., congestive heart failure, hypotension, severe anemia), endocrinopathy (e.g., hyperthyroidism, diabetes mellitus), or systemic infections. Increases from muscle injury are uncommon, but may occur with muscular dystrophy.

Next Diagnostic Steps to Consider if Levels Are High

If values > 3 times the upper limit of reference interval or persistently increased, assess history for exposure to hepatotoxins (including medications) or support for secondary causes (e.g., gastrointestinal disease, endocrinopathy). If none, assess hepatic structure (e.g., abdominal radiographs, ultrasound) and function (e.g., pre- and postprandial serum bile acids). Consider biopsy if values remain increased or if hepatic abnormalities are identified with the aforementioned testing.

Causes of Abnormally Low Levels

Low values are of no clinical significance.

Drug Effects

Many drugs can induce hepatocellular injury, including azathioprine, glucocorticoids, carprofen, phenobarbital, methimazole, megestrol acetate, itra-/ketoconazole, lomustine (CCNU) and tetracycline.

Lab Artifacts

Increase: hemolysis (*in vivo* or artifactual).

Specimen Collection and Handling

Serum (red top tube). Heparinized or EDTA anticoagulated plasma may be substituted.

Relative Cost: $

Pearls

- Increased ALT indicates hepatocyte damage but is not a test of hepatic function, nor does it predict reversibility of hepatocyte injury.
- Minimally increased ALT may indicate serious disease processes or relatively benign conditions; correlating values with other clinical and laboratory findings and monitoring trends are essential for properly interpreting high ALT values.

AUTHOR: Mary Leissinger, DVM, MS, DACVP
EDITOR: Lois Roth-Johnson, DVM, PhD, DACVP

Albumin

Definition

Albumin is the predominant protein in peripheral blood.

Physiology

Albumin is synthesized by the liver. It is the major contributor to plasma oncotic pressure and also functions as a transport protein for ions, bilirubin, thyroxine, numerous drugs, and other compounds.

Reference Interval

Dogs and cats: 2.8-4.2 g/dL (28 to 42 g/L)

Causes of Abnormally High Levels

Dehydration or volume contraction secondary to fluid loss is most common. In dogs, hyperalbuminemia has rarely been reported with hepatocellular carcinoma. Glucocorticoid administration may cause a mild increase in albumin concentration.

Next Diagnostic Steps to Consider if Levels Are High

Assess hydration status. If normal, recheck results. Review the history/medical record for glucocorticoid usage.

Causes of Abnormally Low Levels

- Decreased production. Marked decrease in liver function (>80%), portosystemic shunt, acute phase response (inflammation), severe malnutrition/starvation, cachectic state, hypoadrenocorticism.
- Increased loss. May be loss of only albumin (selective) or all proteins (nonselective).
    - Selective. Protein-losing glomerulopathy. Albumin lost while globulins maintained.
    - Nonselective. Protein-losing enteropathy, hemorrhage, severe exudative dermatopathy/burns. Both albumin and globulins lost, but if concurrent inflammation present, globulins may not fall below reference range.
- Sequestration. Third space loss into body cavities with effusion or vasculitis.
- Dilution. Iatrogenic fluid overload, pathologic fluid retention (e.g., congestive heart failure, cirrhosis, syndrome of inappropriate antidiuretic hormone secretion)

Next Diagnostic Steps to Consider if Levels Are Low

Review history and physical exam with respect to intestinal, renal, and liver function. Assess in conjunction with hematocrit, total protein, globulins, liver values, and markers of renal function. If evidence of significant inflammation, consider acute-phase response. If a cause is not determined, consider additional diagnostics to assess GI/urinary protein loss and liver function (e.g., fecal flotation, urinalysis, urine protein/creatinine ratio, bile acids, serum folate/cobalamin).

See p. 1239.

Drug Effects

Increases in albumin are reported in dogs administered glucocorticoids in experimental studies. Effect may be mediated by increased glucocorticoid production and/or free water loss from corticosteroid-induced polyuria.

Lab Artifacts

- Hemolysis and/or lipemia may cause hyperalbuminemia, but impact is analyzer/method dependent.
- Use of reagents for human testing. Bromocresol purple used in human medicine does not reliably bind to albumin molecules in other species, resulting in artifactually low albumin measurements.

- Use of plasma samples. If heparinized/EDTA anticoagulated plasma is substituted, values may be higher from nonspecific binding of the reagent bromocresol green to globulins.

Specimen Collection and Handling

Serum (red top tube). Heparinized or EDTA anticoagulated plasma may be substituted.

Relative Cost: $

Pearls

- Concentrations may be slightly lower in very young and in geriatric patients.
- Interpret together with serum globulins to formulate differential diagnoses and clinical workup for abnormal values.
- Other than dehydration, high albumin is not associated with specific disease states.
- If hypoalbuminemia is detected by human lab, repeat test in veterinary lab.

AUTHOR: Mary Leissinger, DVM, MS, DACVP
EDITOR: Lois Roth-Johnson, DVM, PhD, DACVP

Albuminuria and Proteinuria

Definition

The detection and estimation of protein and albumin present in the urine.

Synonym(s)

Urine protein quantification, microalbuminuria testing, bumintest

Physiology

- Small proteins (<68,000 kDa) may pass through the glomerular filtration barrier or may be normal mucoproteins secreted by the renal tubules (Tamm-Horsfall proteins).
- Albumin, produced by the liver, is the main oncotic force within the vasculature. Because of its molecular weight (approximately 66-70 kDa) and charge, albumin is minimally filtered through the glomeruli and is thus preserved within the vasculature during health. The small amount of albumin filtered at the glomerulus is reabsorbed in the proximal tubules via pinocytosis.
- Proteinuria and albuminuria can be measured in several ways.

Reference Interval

- Wet chemistry instrument methods: 4-95 mg/dL protein
- Urine dipstick: negative, trace, 1+ (30 mg/dL), 2+ (100 mg/dL), 3+ (>300 mg/dL)
- SSA turbidity test: this method detects albuminuria and Bence Jones proteins better than globulins. Results are assessed on a turbidity scale; 1 to 4+
- Microalbuminuria: ELISA and nephelometric assays; detects albumin at concentrations < 30 mg/dL

Causes of Abnormally High Levels

Proteinuria can be divided into four major categories grouped based on origin: (1) prerenal, (2) glomerular, (3) tubular, and (4) hemorrhagic or inflammatory (postrenal) (p. 1444).

Next Diagnostic Steps to Consider if Levels Are High

- Examine urine sediment for evidence of hemorrhage and/or inflammation.
- Rule out muscle damage (elevated CK >20,000) or hemolysis (serum).
- Measure serum proteins (hyperproteinemia, hyperglobulinemia, or hypoalbuminemia).
- If Bence Jones proteinuria is suspected, consider urine or serum protein electrophoresis.
- Urine protein/creatinine ratio (p. 1391)

Drug Effects

- Dipstick method: falsely increased from quaternary ammonium salts or chlorhexidine
- SSA testing: increased from X-contrast media, tolbutamide, penicillin (large dose), sulfisoxazole, tolmetin sodium, and co-precipitation of crystals.

Lab Artifacts

- Dipstick method falsely increased
  - Highly buffered alkaline urine (>8.0) or in highly concentrated and moderately alkaline urine
  - Pigmenturia or abnormal urine color may interfere with reagent color interpretation.
- SSA testing
  - Decreased from highly buffered alkaline urine

Specimen Collection and Handling

Clean urine collection container; midstream catch, catheterized sample, or cystocentesis can be used. Microalbuminuria measured via point-of-care kit or as mail-out test.

Relative Cost: $

Pearls

- Urine protein should always be interpreted in light of the urine specific gravity, pH values, and sedimentation findings (inactive sediment: absence of pyuria and hematuria).
- Trace results on dipstick in concentrated urine (>1.025) are common.
- Cloudy urine should be ultracentrifuged before performing SSA testing.
- Microalbuminuria is more sensitive and specific for albuminuria than is dipstick assay.
  - Microalbuminuria is not unique to glomerular disease and should be interpreted in the context of the clinical presentation.
  - It may be useful as a screening/monitoring tool in breeds predisposed to protein-losing nephropathy (PLN) or in the presence of disease that predisposes to PLN before overt proteinuria is recognized.

AUTHOR: Erin N. Burton, DVM, MS, DACVP
EDITOR: Lois Roth-Johnson, DVM, PhD, DACVP

Aldosterone, Endogenous

Definition

Aldosterone is a mineralocorticoid hormone produced by the adrenal gland that is an integral part of the renin-angiotensin system that regulates water homeostasis and blood pressure. Endogenous aldosterone concentrations determine the amount of circulating aldosterone.

Physiology

Aldosterone is released by the zona glomerulosa in response to angiotensin II promoting the reabsorption of sodium, accompanied by water in exchange for potassium, at the level of the kidney (mainly distal tubules).

Reference Interval

- Dogs: 14-957 pmol/L (resting); 197-210 pmol/L3 (post–ACTH stimulation)
- Cats: 194-388 pmol/L (resting); 277-721 pmol/L (post–ACTH stimulation)

Causes of Abnormally High Levels

Adrenal neoplasia, low sodium intake, non-adrenal diseases that result in hypovolemia or hyponatremia

Next Diagnostic Steps to Consider if Levels Are High

Abdominal ultrasound to rule out adrenal neoplasia.

Causes of Abnormally Low Levels

Hypoadrenocorticism (Addison's disease), adrenal atrophy (idiopathic, secondary to medication, pituitary disease), high sodium intake

Next Diagnostic Steps to Consider if Levels Are Low

Rule out medication administration. Adrenocorticotropic hormone stimulation test (ACTH stim) to evaluate the hypothalamic-pituitary-adrenal axis.

Drug Effects

- Decrease: ACE inhibitors and nonsteroidal antiinflammatory drugs
- Increase: spironolactone

Specimen Collection and Handling

Plasma collected from EDTA tube (lavender top tube) or heparin (green top tube). Plasma should be separated from the erythrocyte mass as soon as possible and frozen until shipment. Ship on ice.

Relative Cost: $$

Pearls

- This test is rarely indicated as other simpler methods are available for discovery of hyperaldosteronism (e.g., ultrasonographic imaging of adrenal mass).
- Plasma aldosterone to renin ratios may aid in interpretation of inappropriate versus appropriate circulating values. However, may have limited clinical value due to availability of renin assay and collection requirements.

AUTHOR: Erin N. Burton, DVM, MS
EDITOR: Lois Roth-Johnson, DVM, PhD, DACVP

Alkaline Phosphatase (ALP)

Definition

Membrane-associated enzyme found in liver, bone, colostrum, and many other tissues. Physiologic role is not established.

Synonyms

AKP, sALP, SAP, ALKP

Physiology

Total ALP activity in most domestic mammals results from two isoforms of a single isoenzyme produced by the tissue-nonspecific ALP gene: liver (and biliary) associated (L-ALP) and bone associated (B-ALP). The tissue-specific (intestinal associated) isoenzyme produced by the I-ALP gene does not result in increases in total serum ALP activity. A third isoform, corticosteroid-induced ALP (C-ALP), is unique to the dog. Its activity is stimulated by endogenous and exogenous corticosteroids. Most ALP assays include total enzyme activity, but specific tests for liver and corticosteroid isoenzymes of ALP are available.

Reference Interval

Dogs: 0 to 150 U/L; cats: 4 to 80 U/L

Causes of Abnormally High Levels

Cholestasis, endocrinopathy (e.g., hyperadrenocorticism, hyperthyroidism in cats), drug (glucocorticoids, phenobarbital), osteoblast activity (bone growth, fracture repair, osteosarcoma)

Next Diagnostic Steps to Consider if Levels Are High

Review medication history; evaluate hepatobiliary structure and function; pursue possible causes based on relevant history, exam, and other clinicopathologic findings. Young, healthy dogs may have slightly to moderately elevated ALP attributed to bone growth.

Important Interspecies Differences

- Dogs: corticosteroid induction unique to dogs
- Cats: up to 75% of hyperthyroid cats have increased ALP activity caused by L- and B-ALP. Short serum half-life (6 hours in cats vs. 3 days in dogs), so slightly increased serum ALP activity in cats may be more clinically significant than a slight increase in dogs.

Drug Effects

Increase: corticosteroids, phenobarbital, primidone, prednisone, thyroxine

Specimen Collection and Handling

Serum (red top tube); allow to clot, centrifuge, collect serum, refrigerate, ship chilled. Can also be assessed from plasma (green top tube).

Relative Cost: $ (total serum); $$ (C-ALP specific)

Pearls

- Most dogs with increased ALP activity do not have hyperadrenocorticism. Increased ALP warrants a detailed review of history and physical examination before determining whether testing for hyperadrenocorticism is justified.
- C-ALP is used as a screening test but is not specific for hyperadrenocorticism, as stress or an iatrogenically administered corticosteroid may increase C-ALP.
- Increased ALP activity, especially without increased bilirubin, warrants investigation for hyperthyroidism in older cats.
- Benign familial increase in ALP (B-ALP) has been reported in related Siberian Husky puppies.
- Scottish terriers are more likely to have increased ALP with and without associated disease compared to other dog breeds.

AUTHOR: Carrie L. Flint, DVM, DACVP
EDITOR: Lois Roth-Johnson, DVM, PhD, DACVP

Ammonia

Definition

Nitrogenous product of protein catabolism

Synonyms

Though commonly referred to as ammonia (NH_3), the dominant form in blood is ammonium (NH_4^+).

Physiology

Ammonia is produced in the gastrointestinal tract by bacterial metabolism of dietary amino acids and carried via the portal circulation to the liver, where most is converted to urea in the urea cycle.

Reference Interval

Variable among laboratories but generally less than 90-100 mcg/dL (53-59 mcmol/L) in dogs and cats.

Causes of Abnormally High Levels

- Artifact: inappropriate sample handling and sample condition (common)
- Physiologic: high protein meal or extreme exercise
- Pathophysiologic: abnormalities in hepatic portal blood flow (acquired or congenital shunts), decreased liver function, urea cycle abnormalities (rare), cobalamin deficiency

Next Diagnostic Steps to Consider if Levels Are High

Review history, examination, complete blood count, serum biochemistry panel, and abdominal imaging results for signs of hepatobiliary disease and portal circulation abnormalities. Exclude physiologic or artifactual causes.

Drug Effects

Decrease: antibiotics that affect gastrointestinal flora, lactulose, *Lactobacillus acidophilus* culture, enema.

Lab Artifacts

- Increase: delay in harvesting plasma (>30 minutes), inappropriate submission to laboratory (see specimen collection and handling), or sample hemolysis. Interference from icterus/lipemia is method/analyzer dependent.
- Decrease: inappropriately filled or stoppered tube (loss of ammonia gas)

Specimen Collection and Handling

Twelve-hour fasting specimen preferred. Collect heparinized whole blood (green top tube), separate plasma from cells immediately, store on ice. Some laboratories may accept EDTA (purple top tube) plasma or serum. Must test or freeze (−20°C) within 3 hours. If frozen, ship on dry ice so sample does not thaw in shipment. Arterial samples preferred but not essential. Concurrent submission of a sample from a healthy control animal for comparison is generally recommended or required to exclude artifact as a cause of abnormal values.

Relative Cost: $$

Pearls

- Given the many preanalytic factors that may impact ammonia measurement, always contact the laboratory or be aware of laboratory sample handling policy before submission to ensure best results.
- Ammonia is superior to bile acids for assessing hepatic function if cholestasis is present.

AUTHOR: Mary Leissinger, DVM, MS, DACVP
EDITOR: Lois Roth-Johnson, DVM, PhD, DACVP

Laboratory Tests

Amylase

Definition

Enzyme that hydrolyzes complex carbohydrates. Measured in serum or plasma as a marker for acute pancreatitis, though it lacks specificity and sensitivity for this condition.

Physiology

Amylase is a cytosolic enzyme produced by multiple tissue types, most notably pancreatic acinar epithelium, intestine, and liver. Accordingly, damage to pancreatic acinar epithelium can result in leakage of amylase to the blood. Renal excretion/inactivation and hepatic clearance are both involved in clearing amylase from the blood.

Reference Interval

Varies by laboratory, often < 1600 U/L

Causes of Abnormally High Levels

Acute pancreatitis (and the resultant pancreatic acinar epithelial damage) is the most common cause of moderate to markedly increased values. Decreases in glomerular filtration rate (GFR; acute or chronic kidney disease, hypovolemia) often cause mild hyperamylasemia. Pancreatic neoplasia is an uncommon cause.

Next Diagnostic Steps to Consider if Levels Are High

If history, clinical signs, and other initial diagnostics are compatible with pancreatitis, abdominal imaging, pancreas-specific lipase immunoreactivity, or DGGR lipase measurement may be considered.

Important Interspecies Differences

Amylase is of little value in assessing cats for pancreatitis. Salivary amylase (present in some species) is not found in dogs or cats.

Drug Effects

Administration of dexamethasone or prednisone may decrease amylase activity level.

Lab Artifacts

Marked lipemia, hemolysis, or icterus may cause erroneous results. Use of EDTA, citrate, or fluoride oxalate tubes for sample collection results in decreased amylase results (amylase activity is calcium dependent).

Specimen Collection and Handling

Serum (red top tube) or heparinized plasma (green top tube) may be used. Fasting patient to minimize risk of lipemia is recommended. Separate serum or plasma from cells if shipping to a laboratory. Stable at 2°C - 8°C for 1 month.

Relative Cost: $

Pearls

- Mild hyperamylasemia has very poor specificity for diagnosis of pancreatitis. The greater the magnitude of hyperamylasemia, the more likely acute pancreatitis or pancreatic neoplasia becomes.
- Pancreatitis can be present even if amylase is within reference interval.

AUTHOR: Angela Royal, DVM, MS, DACVP
EDITOR: Lois Roth-Johnson, DVM, PhD, DACVP

Anaplasma Serologic Testing

Definition

- *Anaplasma* serologic testing detects circulating antibodies for *Anaplasma* spp. in serum or plasma.
- *Anaplasma phagocytophilum* is a tick-borne intracellular, gram-negative bacterium transmitted through *Ixodes* sp. ticks (p. 393).
- *Anaplasma platys* is a tick-borne intracellular, gram-negative bacterium transmitted by *Rhipicephalus sanguineus* (brown dog tick) ticks.

Synonyms

- *A. phagocytophilum*: anaplasmosis, canine granulocytic anaplasmosis
- *A. platys:* canine cyclic thrombocytopenia

Physiology

After tick inoculation, the bacteria enter the bloodstream and invades neutrophils (*A. phagocytophilum*) or platelets (*A. platys*). Morulae visualization in either platelets or neutrophils generally precedes antibody response. Antibodies can be detected approximately 1-2 weeks following initial infection.

Reference Interval

Qualitative SNAP ELISA testing to antibodies for *Anaplasma* spp. (detects both *A. phagocytophilum* and *A. platys*): positive or negative

Immunofluorescent antibody (IFA) technique for detection of *Anaplasma* spp. (detects both *A. phagocytophilum* and *A. platys*): acute and convalescent titers with a fourfold increase

Causes of Abnormally High Levels

A single positive test indicates exposure but not necessarily active infection. Seroconversion or a fourfold increase in antibody titers on acute and convalescent titers, in combination with clinical signs, can confirm infection.

Next Diagnostic Steps to Consider if Levels Are High

- Evaluate for clinical disease (fever, lethargy, polyarthropathy).
- CBC with blood smear evaluation for morulae (phagocytes or platelets) or thrombocytopenia
- Consider treatment or additional evaluation (p. 393).
- Re-evaluate ectoparasites control.

Causes of Abnormally Low Levels

- Uninfected
- Inadequate time for seroconversion

Next Diagnostic Steps to Consider if Levels Are Low

- If anaplasmosis is suspected based on clinical signs but titer is negative:
  - Repeat serology testing in 1-2 weeks.
  - PCR testing for *Anaplasma* spp.
  - Examine blood smear for morulae.
  - Consider empirical antimicrobial therapy.
  - Consider vector-borne disease with similar signs (e.g., Lyme disease, granulocytic ehrlichiosis).

Important Interspecies Differences

Cats can be infected with *Anaplasma* but rarely show clinical disease.

Drug Effects

- Animals can remain positive for months to years following antimicrobial administration for clinical illness.
- Initiation of empirical drug therapy will decrease sensitivity of molecular confirmation testing (e.g., PCR).

Specimen Collection and Handling

- In-clinic SNAP ELISA: serum (red top tube), plasma or whole blood (lavender or green top tube), fresh or refrigerated, test with 7 days of collection. Separate from cells and freeze for longer storage. Sample must be at room temperature for testing. Follow manufacturer instructions.
- IFA: serum (red top tube). Separate serum from clot, refrigerate, and ship chilled.

Relative Cost: \$ (In-clinic SNAP ELISA) and \$\$-\$\$\$ (IFA)

Pearls

- *A. phagocytophilum*: morulae are seen 4 days and IgG is detected 8 days after exposure. *A. phagocytophilum* morulae are indistinguishable from *Ehrlichia ewingii* morulae on cytology.
- *A. platys* morulae are uncommonly identified on blood smear evaluation and can easily be confused for platelet dense granules.
- Dogs are commonly co-infected with other tick-borne illnesses, especially *Borrelia burgdorferi* (the cause of Lyme disease).

AUTHOR: Erin N. Burton, DVM, MS, DACVP
EDITOR: Lois Roth-Johnson, DVM, PhD, DACVP

Anemia, Nonregenerative

Definition

Anemia characterized by inadequate reticulocytosis

Physiology

Decreased erythrocyte production is the primary cause. If decreased production is the sole cause of anemia, it may take weeks to months for anemia to be clinically evident. In anemia of chronic disease, inflammatory cytokines may decrease erythrocyte life span and release of erythropoietin (EPO) from the kidney, resulting in decreased erythrocyte production. Hepcidin, an acute-phase protein that regulates iron homeostasis, is suspected to be the key mediator of anemia of chronic disease. Nonregenerative anemia can also be caused by bone marrow disorders (infectious, neoplastic, or other types of injury); lack of EPO, iron, or cobalamin; or other factors.

Reference Interval

- Packed cell volume (PCV) 40%-54% (dogs) or 30%-40% (cats)
- Absolute reticulocyte counts < 80,000/mcL (dogs) or < 60,000/mcL (cats) associated with nonregenerative anemia. Reticulocyte percentage estimates are corrected for degree of anemia; < 1% corrected indicates nonregenerative anemia. (Corrected reticulocyte % = [patient's PCV/normal animal's PCV] × uncorrected reticulocyte %; dog normal PCV ≈45% dogs)

Causes of Abnormally Low Levels

Acute-onset anemia requires at least 3 days before regeneration becomes evident. Causes of nonregenerative anemia include chronic disease (many: kidney disease, endocrinopathies, neoplasia, infection, inflammation), primary bone marrow disease, pure red cell aplasia, immune-mediated destruction of RBC precursors, therapeutic agents (e.g., hydroxyurea, phenylbutazone, estrogen), nutritional deficiency (iron, folate, or vitamin B_{12})

Next Diagnostic Steps to Consider if Levels Are Low

Identification of underlying cause: serum biochemistry profile, urinalysis, feline retroviral testing, diagnostic imaging to find chronic disease. Advanced diagnostic testing may include bone marrow evaluation, serologic tests or PCR for infectious disease (e.g., ehrlichiosis), thyroid function tests, serum ferritin or folate.

Specimen Collection and Handling

EDTA anticoagulated blood (lavender top tube) for CBC and absolute reticulocyte count; freshly made direct blood smear for morphologic evaluation

Relative Cost: $ (reticulocyte count); $$ (CBC; reticulocyte count included in some CBC panels)

Pearls

- Anemia due to early or acute hemolysis and blood loss initially appears nonregenerative before the bone marrow has had time to respond. It takes ≈2-3 days after acute hemolysis or blood loss for reticulocytosis to be evident, and 7 days for an optimum response. Therefore, in nonregenerative anemia of recent onset, serial CBC, blood smear evaluation, and reticulocyte counts are recommended.
- Slow blood loss via the gastrointestinal tract (e.g., hookworms, gastric or intestinal ulceration) may also be associated with a nonregenerative anemia due to iron deficiency.

AUTHOR: Fidelia R. Fernandez, DVM, MS, DACVP
EDITOR: Lois Roth-Johnson, DVM, PhD, DACVP

Anemia, Regenerative

Definition

Anemia characterized by reticulocytosis; may be accompanied by basophilic stippling, Howell-Jolly bodies, and nucleated red blood cells (normoblastemia)

Synonym

Responsive anemia

Physiology

Hypoxemia induced by decreased red cell mass stimulates erythropoietin production in the kidney and, subsequently, erythropoiesis.

Reference Interval

Packed cell volume (PCV) (dogs: 40%-55%; cats: 30%-40%); absolute reticulocyte counts (percent reticulocyte × red blood cell count/mcL) of > 50,000/mcL (cats) and > 60,000/mcL (dogs) indicate regeneration. Reticulocyte percentage estimates are corrected for degree of anemia; > 1% corrected indicates regenerative anemia. (Corrected reticulocyte % = [patient's PCV/normal animal's PCV] × uncorrected reticulocyte %; dog normal PCV ≈45% dogs)

Causes of Abnormally High Levels

Blood loss and/or hemolysis

Next Diagnostic Steps to Consider if Levels Are High

Physical examination for evidence of blood loss (e.g., melena, ectoparasites); blood smear evaluation of red cell morphology for evidence of size, color, and shape changes, spherocytosis, agglutination, and parasitic inclusions. Serologic or PCR tests for infectious disease (e.g., hemotropic mycoplasmas, babesiosis). Coombs' test.

See pp. 57, 59, and 60.

Lab Artifacts

Presence of *Mycoplasma haemofelis* inclusions may falsely increase flow cytometric reticulocyte counts.

Specimen Collection and Handling

EDTA anticoagulated blood (lavender top tube) for CBC and reticulocyte count; fresh direct blood smear for morphologic evaluation of red cells

Relative Cost: $ (reticulocyte count); $$ (CBC; reticulocyte count included in some CBC panels)

Pearls

- An absolute reticulocyte count is the most reliable means of assessing red cell regeneration. In the absence of a reticulocyte count, a blood smear should be evaluated for polychromasia, but polychromasia does not necessarily reflect the adequacy of regenerative response.
- Reticulocytosis in the absence of anemia has been reported in association with the use of NSAIDs and immunosuppressive drugs.
- Polychromasia and a high red cell distribution width (RDW) more accurately identify regenerative anemias in dogs than do red cell indices such as MCV.

AUTHOR: Fidelia R. Fernandez, DVM, MS, DACVP
EDITOR: Lois Roth-Johnson, DVM, PhD, DACVP

Anion Gap

Definition

Calculated value using the formula $[(Na^+ + K^+) - (Cl^- + HCO_3^-)]$. Represents the negatively charged atoms and molecules in the bloodstream other than those in the formula.

Physiology

The total of positive and negative charges in blood must be equal. Routine serum biochemistry profile measures only some cations and anions. "Unmeasured anions" (e.g., lactate, charged proteins) and "unmeasured cations" (e.g., magnesium, calcium) exist. *Unmeasured* refers to anything other than the four ions included in the anion-gap formula. Measured cations (Na^+, K^+) normally exceed measured anions (Cl^-, HCO_3^-) by about 5-15 mEq/L (equivalent to the value of a "normal" anion gap). In health, the unmeasured anions are mostly charges on proteins. Organic acid (e.g., lactic acid) accumulation increases the anion gap in disease states.

Reference Interval

Dogs and cats: approximately 5-15 mEq/L (1 mEq/L = 1 mmol/L)

Causes of Abnormally High Levels

Conditions usually causing metabolic acidosis, most commonly lactic acidosis, uremia, ketoacidosis, ethylene glycol toxicosis

Next Diagnostic Steps to Consider if Levels Are High

Review history for ethylene glycol exposure. Evaluate serum biochemistry profile for azotemia, hyperglycemia. Collect urine for specific gravity, ketone measurement, examination for calcium oxalate monohydrate crystals. Perform blood gas analysis. Consider measuring lactate.

Drug Effects

Potassium bromide may falsely increase serum chloride measurement, decreasing the anion gap and often producing a negative number.

Lab Artifacts

Anything interfering with the measurement of the ions included in the anion-gap calculation will alter the anion-gap value (e.g., lipemia, hemolysis).

Specimen Collection and Handling

Serum (red top tube) for routine chemistry/electrolyte profile

Relative Cost: $$

Pearls

- The anion gap is commonly used for differentiating between bicarbonate loss (normal anion gap) and organic acid accumulation (high anion gap) in patients with metabolic acidosis.
- In mixed acid-base disorders, an animal may have metabolic acidosis with a normal or high pH because of competing factors. In this situation, a high anion gap helps identify "occult" acidosis.

AUTHOR: Sharon M. Dial, DVM, PhD, DACVP
EDITOR: Lois Roth-Johnson, DVM, PhD, DACVP

Antimullerian Hormone

Definition

Test for the presence of antimullerian hormone (AMH) in serum

Physiology

Antimullerian hormone is produced exclusively by the ovaries and the sustentacular cells (Sertoli cells) of the testicle. It is present in sexually mature females regardless of the stage of the estrus cycle. Detectable concentrations in serum indicate the presence of ovarian tissue or ovarian tumors. Preliminary evaluation indicates AMH is useful for evaluation of cryptorchidism and Sertoli cell tumors of the testicle in dogs.

Reference Interval

Reported as positive or negative

Causes of Abnormally High Levels

Intact female; ovarian remnants in spayed female; Sertoli cell tumor (male)

Next Diagnostic Steps to Consider if Levels Are High

Surgical removal of ovarian remnants or Sertoli tumor/retained testicle

Causes of Abnormally Low Levels

Intact female: not yet sexually mature

Next Diagnostic Steps to Consider if Levels Are Low

Retest if sexual maturity is questionable.

Drug Effects

Estrogen treatment or ingestion of estrogen-containing plants/supplements causes false-positives.

Specimen Collection and Handling

Serum (red top tube) 0.5 mL minimum. Submit frozen on ice. Sample must be received frozen or minimally thawed.

Relative Cost: $$

Pearls

Considered a reliable test for evaluating for ovarian remnants in both dogs and cats.

Assessment for cryptorchism and Sertoli cell tumors currently is preliminary.

AUTHOR & EDITOR: Lois Roth-Johnson, DVM, PhD, DACVP

Antinuclear Antibody (ANA)

Definition

Indirect immunofluorescent antibody (IFA) test to detect antibodies specific for DNA, RNA, and nucleoprotein

Physiology

Antinuclear antibodies are associated with autoimmune disorders, most notably systemic lupus erythematosus (p. 955).

Reference Interval

Reported as negative or positive; positive results reflect titer values and staining pattern (homogeneous nuclear, speckled nuclear, nuclear rim, or nucleolar).

Causes of Abnormally High Levels

SLE, some infections (e.g., ehrlichiosis, leishmaniasis, heartworms)

Next Diagnostic Steps to Consider if Levels Are High

Assess for skin lesions or systemic signs (e.g., glomerulonephritis, liver abnormalities, polyarthritis) consistent with SLE; rule out potential infections.

Important Interspecies Differences

Requires use of species-specific fluorescent antibody

Drug Effects

- False-negative: cytotoxic drugs, high doses of corticosteroids
- False-positive: sulfonamides, tetracycline, hydralazine, procainamide, griseofulvin, propylthiouracil, methimazole. Some infectious diseases.

Specimen Collection and Handling

Serum (red top tube). Store at 2°C-8°C (refrigeration).

Relative Cost: $$

Pearls

- Significance of pattern of fluorescence in domestic animals is unclear.
- Positive ANA titers support a clinical diagnosis of SLE in dogs but are not specific.
- Low positive titers can be seen with various diseases and in older animals.
- ANA titer is much more sensitive (better screening test) for SLE than the LE prep.

AUTHOR & EDITOR: Lois Roth-Johnson, DVM, PhD, DACVP

Antithrombin (AT)

Definition

Endogenous anticoagulant. Major plasma inhibitor of serine protease factors of the coagulation cascade (factors IX, X, XI, XII; thrombin and plasmin).

Synonyms

Antithrombin III (outdated), heparin cofactor

Physiology

Synthesized in liver; AT binds to thrombin, preventing conversion of fibrinogen to fibrin; heparin and heparin-like compounds accelerate the reaction between AT and thrombin. AT inactivates several additional coagulation factors as well. Decreased AT (due to loss or consumption) can result in a hypercoagulable state and increased risk of thrombosis.

Reference Interval

Measured as a percentage of species-specific pooled samples. Dogs: 75%-120%; cats: 75%-110%.

Causes of Abnormally High Levels

Exogenous glucocorticoid administration (dogs), inflammation (as part of positive acute-phase response in cats)

Next Diagnostic Steps to Consider if Levels Are High

Increased plasma AT concentration is not clinically significant.

Causes of Abnormally Low Levels

Increased loss (e.g., protein-losing nephropathy, protein-losing enteropathy), increased hepatic clearance of AT enzyme complexes (e.g., disseminated intravascular coagulation [DIC], sepsis), decreased production (e.g., liver failure)

Next Diagnostic Steps to Consider if Levels Are Low

Assess other aspects of the coagulation cascade (activated partial thromboplastin time and prothrombin time), platelet count, fibrinogen level, D-dimers, fibrin degradation products and, if available, thromboelastography. A procoagulant state may exist because of low AT levels alone or in conjunction with other disorders (e.g., DIC).

Drug Effects

Plasma AT is decreased in dogs with hyperadrenocorticism (hyperadrenocorticism can be associated with thromboembolic disease). L-asparaginase can decrease AT production.

Lab Artifacts

- Age: Lower levels of AT have been reported in young animals.
- Assay differences: AT may be overestimated in certain thrombin chromogenic assays (heparin cofactor II activity in addition to AT is detected).

Specimen Collection and Handling

Citrate (blue top tube), separate plasma (within 1 hour of sample collection) and transfer to plastic tube; freeze (store at 0°C-4°C). The citrate tube must be filled completely, as the ratio of blood to citrate is important for accurate testing.

Relative Cost: $$

Pearls

Patients with DIC, thrombosis, or nephrotic syndrome commonly have decreased levels. If the AT activity is <70% of the control, the animal may require anticoagulation using drugs other than heparin.

AUTHOR: Deborah G. Davis, DVM, DACVP
EDITOR: Lois Roth-Johnson, DVM, PhD, DACVP

Aspergillus spp. Serology

Definition

Specific tests may detect either antibodies to *Aspergillus* spp. (by ELISA, agarose gel immunodiffusion [AGID], or counter immunoelectrophoresis) or the presence of *Aspergillus* galactomannan antigen (GMA) (ELISA) in the serum or urine.

Physiology

- *Aspergillus* spp. are common environmental fungi (saprophytes) and opportunistic pathogens (dogs >> cats). Sinonasal aspergillosis (*A. fumigatus*) is far more common than disseminated aspergillosis (*A. terreus, A. flavus,* others) (p. 81).
- Nasal imaging showing turbinate destruction and areas of radiolucency in coordination with rhinoscopy for direct visualization of fungal plaques and to obtain specimens for analysis (cytologic, histopathologic, or microbiological) are the most informative tests for sinonasal infection, but AGID is sometimes useful.
- GMA ELISA is more useful for systemic aspergillosis (≈85%-90% sensitive and specific) than for sinonasal infection (≈24% sensitive).

Causes of Abnormally High Levels

- Antibody tests: presence of antibodies indicates exposure, but not necessarily active infection.
- Antigen: presence of serum or urine antigen indicates systemic infection, colonization, or may be a false-positive.

Important Interspecies Differences

Serologic tests often use species-specific antibodies; confirm that test used is valid for the species in question.

Lab Artifacts

False-positive results for the GMA ELISA are seen in dogs given Plasmalyte crystalloid fluids or some *Penicillium*-derived antibiotics.

Specimen Collection and Handling

Serum, 1 mL (red top tube); stable at 2°-8°C for five days; freeze at 20°C for longer storage.

Relative Cost: $$$

Pearls

- False-positive and false-negative results can occur with all tests for aspergillosis (including culture, cytologic analysis, and histopathologic analysis).
- *Penicillium* spp. is another genus of fungus that can cause nasal disease in dogs. The organisms appear similar and can only be differentiated via culture or serologic testing, not cytologic appearance. Serologic tests that detect antibody to either antigen are preferred.
- Both *Penicillium* spp. and *Aspergillus* spp. are ubiquitous in the environment.
- *Aspergillus* GMA ELISA in serum or urine is more sensitive in detecting systemic disease than localized nasal or pulmonary disease, and false-positive results are seen in dogs with other systemic fungal diseases.

AUTHOR: Sharon M. Dial, DVM, PhD, DACVP
EDITOR: Lois Roth-Johnson, DVM, PhD, DACVP

Baermann Fecal Examination

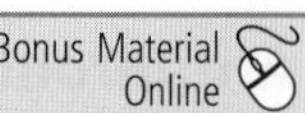

Definition

The Baermann fecal examination is used to detect living larvae, most commonly lungworm, in feces.

Physiology

The Baermann apparatus is a funnel clamped to a metal stand with clamped rubber tubing attached. Fresh feces are suspended in the funnel using a wire mesh sieve or in a double layer of cheesecloth while being submerged in lukewarm water for 8-12 hours. After incubation, the clamp on the tubing is released to allow the water to flow into a centrifuge tube. The centrifuge tube is spun, supernatant discarded, and the sediment is used for microscopic detection of larvae. This test relies on the tendency for larvae to migrate from feces to warm water.

Reference Interval

Reported as no nematode larvae seen or positive with genus or species identification.

Causes of Abnormally High Levels

Lungworm larvae, such as *Filaroides hirthi*, *Filaroides osleri*, *Crenosoma vulpis*, *Angiostrongylus vasorum*, and *Aelurostrongylus abstrusus* can be detected using this method.

Next Diagnostic Steps to Consider if Levels Are High

Positive larval identification is considered definitive.

Causes of Abnormally Low Levels

Diarrheic samples may not have a sufficient solid component.

Next Diagnostic Steps to Consider if Levels Are Low

This test is not sensitive, and a negative result does not rule out infection. Repetition of the test on several occasions will improve detection of parasites.

Drug Effects

Anthelmintic drugs may decrease larval shedding.

Lab Artifacts

Delayed processing of the sample may make interpretation difficult as free living nematode larvae or larvae from nematode eggs that hatch quickly in the environment (e.g., hookworms, strongylid, *Strongyloides* sp.) can be easily confused for lungworm larvae.

Specimen Collection

5 grams of fresh (<24 hours) feces that have had < 30 minutes of ground contact collected into a dry container devoid of preservatives

Relative Cost: $$

Pearls

- Bronchoscopy may be a more sensitive method for detection of *Filaroides osleri* in dogs; however, this method can be costly, time consuming, and requires general anesthesia.
- *Filaroides hirthi, Filaroides osleri, Strongyloides* sp. and *Dictyocaulus* sp. larvae and *Eucoleus* sp. ova are better recovered using flotation techniques.
- Baermann technique is preferred over fecal flotation for the detection of nematode larvae.

AUTHOR: Erin N. Burton, DVM, MS
EDITOR: Lois Roth-Johnson, DVM, PhD, DACVP

Bartonella Testing

Definition

Bartonella spp. are a group of vector-transmitted, intraerythrocytic bacterial organisms that can induce persistent infections in dogs, cats, and humans.

Physiology

Following vector transmission, chronic intravascular infections may produce no clinical signs or may cause acute, life-threatening disease or chronic debilitating illness (p. 111).

Reference Interval

- Immunofluorescence antibody (IFA) test for *Bartonella* spp. Negative titer is < 1:64.
- PCR: Reported as positive or negative

Causes of Abnormally High Levels

Seropositivity indicates exposure to *Bartonella* spp., but not necessarily current infection. Cross-reactivity with *Coxiella, Chlamydophila,* and nonpathogenic *Bartonella* spp. may confound IFA results. Positive standard PCR or PCR/culture in enrichment media (ePCR™) is consistent with current infection.

Next Diagnostic Steps to Consider if Levels Are High

- Submission of whole blood or fresh/frozen tissue for pre-enrichment culture (with BAPGM) followed by PCR and subculture onto agar plates (available at GALAXY Diagnostics, www.galaxydx.com).
- Submission of tissue biopsy for histopathologic analysis and PCR.

Causes of Abnormally Low Levels

Infected animals may be seronegative; therefore, ePCR™ should be considered if there is clinical suspicion of bartonellosis. Cyclic bacteremia or low numbers of organisms can result in false-negatives for ePCR™. A combination of both serology and ePCR™ is ideal.

Next Diagnostic Steps to Consider if Levels Are Low

Testing of three blood samples by ePCR™ is recommended, or empirical treatment if indicated.

Important Interspecies Differences

Cats: chronic infection is common in healthy cats with flea exposure, so IFA is of limited value. ePCR™ is considered the gold standard, but may require multiple attempts since bacteremia is intermittent; multiple samples are more important for the detection of infection in dogs than in cats.

Drug Effects

Effective antibiotic treatment may decrease serologic titers. Use of antibiotics before sample collection may result in a false-negative standard PCR or ePCR™, even if the antibiotic is not sufficient for the treatment of infection.

Lab Artifacts

PCR: false-positive results via contamination of samples or mispriming; false-negative results due to degradation of nucleic acids by improper sample handling and storage or low numbers of circulating organisms

Specimen Collection and Handling

Contact laboratory for specific instructions. IFA: submit 1 mL serum (red top tube). Standard PCR: submit 2 mL whole blood collected via aseptic technique in EDTA (lavender top tube) frozen at -20°C or refrigerated at 2-8°C. .ePCR™: submit 2-4 mL whole blood collected via aseptic technique in EDTA (lavender top tube); 3 draws over 1 week (triple blood draw) collected in EDTA frozen at -20°C or refrigerated at 2-8°C; 0.5-1.0 gram fresh or frozen tissue.

Relative Cost: $$ (IFA, standard PCR); $$$ (ePCR™)

Pearls

ePCR™ is the gold standard for diagnosis because some infected dogs and cats are seronegative, and culturing *Bartonella* spp. in dogs using routine microbiologic techniques is often unsuccessful. In most cases, diagnosis must be pursued concurrently with response to treatment because test results may take weeks.

AUTHOR: Patty J. Ewing, DVM, MS, DACVP
EDITOR: Lois Roth-Johnson, DVM, PhD, DACVP

Basophils

Definition

Granulocytic leukocytes that have an elongate, segmented nucleus and light purple to lavender granules in cytoplasm of dogs and cats. Basophils are the largest granulocytic leukocyte. Basophils are rarely encountered in the blood of healthy animals.

Physiology

Basophilic precursors undergo differentiation in the bone marrow, enter peripheral blood circulation for a few hours, and then enter tissue. Basophils produce leukotrienes and release histamine, heparin, and other mediators from their granules. Basophils participate in immunoglobulin E–mediated hypersensitivity reactions. They are similar in morphology to mast cells, but mast cells have a nonsegmented nucleus and primarily reside in tissue.

Reference Interval

Dogs and cats: 0-0.1 × 10^3 basophils/mcL

Causes of Abnormally High Levels

Allergic reactions (e.g., food, insect sting); parasitism (e.g., dirofilariasis, flea infestation); neoplasms (e.g., mast cell neoplasms, chronic basophilic leukemia); chronic myeloproliferative diseases (e.g., essential thrombocythemia, polycythemia vera)

Next Diagnostic Steps to Consider if Levels Are High

Additional tests directed by history, physical exam findings, and results of ancillary diagnostic tests

Important Interspecies Differences

Granules in feline basophils stain lighter violet than canine granules. Because canine basophils have fewer purple granules, gray basophilic cytoplasm, and are large in size, they could be misidentified as monocytes on blood smear.

Lab Artifacts

Hematology analyzers, even those that offer five-part differential leukocyte counts, do not reliably detect canine or feline basophils; blood smear examination is required to accurately detect basophilia.

Specimen Collection and Handling

EDTA whole blood (lavender top tube) and freshly prepared blood smear

Relative Cost: $$ (reported as part of CBC)

Pearls

Basophilia often accompanies eosinophilia, a further indication of allergic or parasitic disease. Careful examination is necessary to identify basophils; rapid aqueous-based Romanowsky stains (e.g., Diff-Quik) are poorly effective for staining the cytoplasmic granules of canine basophils.

AUTHOR: Stephen D. Gaunt, DVM, PhD, DACVP
EDITOR: Lois Roth-Johnson, DVM, PhD, DACVP

Bence Jones Proteinuria

Definition

The presence of excessive immunoglobulin light chains in urine.

Synonyms

Paraproteinuria, M-proteinuria, light chain proteinuria

Physiology

B-lymphocytes and plasma cells produce immunoglobulins that consist of two heavy chains and two light chains linked through disulfide bonds. During hyperplastic or neoplastic states, monoclonal lymphocytes or plasma cells can secrete excessive amounts of entire immunoglobulins or a portion of the immunoglobulin (i.e., solely the heavy chain or light chain), known as the M-protein (monoclonal protein) or paraprotein. The accumulation of these paraproteins by a monoclonal population typically results in hyperglobulinemia and a monoclonal gammopathy. The light chain proteins are of low molecular weight and can pass freely through the glomerulus. Bence Jones proteins are not readily detected on urine dipstick reagents, but rather with immunoprecipitation or urine protein electrophoresis.

Reference Interval

A positive result is abnormal in both cats and dogs.

Causes of Abnormally High Levels

Lymphoproliferative diseases (e.g., multiple myeloma, myeloma-related disease, lymphoma) and some chronic infectious diseases (e.g., leishmaniasis, ehrlichiosis, babesiosis)

Next Diagnostic Steps to Consider if Levels Are High

Evaluate for multiple myeloma/myeloma-related disease via serum and urine protein electrophoresis, radiographic evidence of osteolysis, and bone marrow evaluation for plasma cell neoplasm. See p. 663.

Important Interspecies Differences

Approximately 25%-40% of dogs and 40% of cats with multiple myeloma will have Bence Jones proteinuria.

Specimen Collection and Handling

Refrigerate for storage.

Relative Cost: $$

AUTHOR: Shannon D. Dehghanpir, DVM, MS, DACVP
EDITOR: Lois Roth-Johnson, DVM, PhD, DACVP

Bicarbonate

Definition

An anion that is the major extracellular buffer in blood. It is a calculated value, provided as part of a blood gas analysis.

Synonyms

HCO_3, bicarb

Physiology

Bicarbonate is formed from the conversion of carbon dioxide and water to carbonic acid by carbonic anhydrase. Carbonic acid dissociates into bicarbonate and hydrogen ion. During metabolic acidosis, bicarbonate minimizes pH changes by binding to excess H^+. Binding excess H^+ decreases measurable HCO_3^-.

Reference Interval

Dogs: 18-26 mEq/L (18-26 mmol/L)
Cats: 14-22 mEq/L (14-22 mmol/L)

Causes of Abnormally High Levels

- Metabolic alkalosis
  - Primary: gastric vomiting
  - Compensatory: secondary to respiratory acidosis (causes: pulmonary restrictive disease [pleural effusion, pneumothorax, diaphragmatic hernia], hypoventilation/central nervous system depression [anesthesia, narcotics, central neurologic disease], lower motor neuron disease, cervical spinal cord injury, myopathy/muscle fatigue, airway obstruction)
  - Iatrogenic: bicarbonate-containing solutions, loop diuretics (e.g., furosemide)

See p. 1195.

Next Diagnostic Steps to Consider if Levels Are High

Evaluate arterial blood gas profile (particularly pH and PCO_2) to differentiate between primary metabolic alkalosis (high pH, high HCO_3^-, high PCO_2) and metabolic compensation for respiratory acidosis (low pH, high PCO_2, high HCO_3^-). Evaluate for underlying causes listed above.

Causes of Abnormally Low Levels

- Primary metabolic acidosis
  - Bicarbonate loss: with gastrointestinal disease (e.g., vomiting, diarrhea, fluid sequestration) or renal loss or decreased hydrogen excretion (e.g., proximal and distal renal tubular acidosis, hypoadrenocorticism)
  - Titration of bicarbonate: ketoacidosis, lactic acidosis, retained renal acids (various causes of azotemia), and certain toxicities (ethylene glycol, salicylates, paraldehyde, methanol)
- Compensatory metabolic acidosis: occurs secondary to respiratory alkalosis (causes: pulmonary disease [pneumonia, pulmonary edema], significant hypoxemia, direct stimulation of central nervous system [pain, anxiety, central nervous system disease], sepsis)

See pp. 1192 and 1193.

Next Diagnostic Steps to Consider if Levels Are Low

Evaluate arterial blood gas profile to differentiate between primary metabolic acidosis (low pH, low HCO_3^-, low PCO_2) and metabolic compensation for respiratory alkalosis (high pH, low PCO_2, low HCO_3^-). Evaluate with serum biochemistry, and consider causes listed above. Increased anion gap indicates titration of bicarbonate.

Lab Artifacts

Decrease: processing delay or exposure to air

Specimen Collection and Handling

Whole blood in a heparinized syringe, avoiding exposure to room air, as described for blood gas analysis. Specimens analyzed within 15 minutes of collections are preferred. Storage in a capped syringe on ice at 4°C for up to 2 hours is acceptable.

Relative Cost: $$ (part of blood gas analysis)

Pearls

- Total carbon dioxide (TCO_2) estimates plasma bicarbonate and is part of most serum biochemistry profiles. TCO_2 is usually slightly higher (1-2 mEq/L) than bicarbonate on a blood gas profile, but is considered a clinically accurate assessment of bicarbonate.
- May not be practical to submit to a reference laboratory, owing to sensitivity of specimen to environmental influences and time constraints for accurate test results. Handheld instruments for cage-side use are available.
- Evaluate together with PCO_2, pH, serum chloride, and anion gap for optimal interpretation.

AUTHOR: Mary Leissinger, DVM, MS, DACVP
EDITOR: Lois Roth-Johnson, DVM, PhD, DACVP

Bile Acids (Blood, Urine)

Definition

Detergent-like compounds (predominantly cholic acid and chenodeoxycholic acid) synthesized in the liver from cholesterol and secreted in bile to aid in digestion and absorption of dietary fat.

Physiology

Bile acids (BAs) are the primary organic component of bile. In this form, they are stored in the gallbladder and released following feeding. An efficient enterohepatic circulation recycles BAs released into the portal circulation, with only a small amount appearing in the systemic circulation in health. Serum BAs are typically evaluated in paired samples (fasting and 2 hours postprandial). The urine BA/creatinine ratio (UBA:crt), which could reflect nonsulfated (NSBA) or sulfated bile acids (SBA) or both, is measured in a single random sample and reflects average serum BA concentration.

Reference Interval

Serum BAs

- Fasting BAs normally < 5 mcmol/L
  - Fasting BAs > 15 mcmol/L and/or postprandial BAs > 30 mcmol/L are abnormal.

Urine BAs

- Dogs: NSBA:crt > 1 and total UBA:crt > 7 are abnormal.
- Cats: NSBA:crt > 2 and total UBA:crt > 4 are abnormal.

Causes of Abnormally High Levels

- Decreased BA clearance from portal blood (decreased functional liver mass or compromised portal circulation [congenital or acquired portosystemic shunt])
- Cholestasis (hepatic or posthepatic) due to obstruction, cirrhosis, inflammation
- Biliary rupture

Next Diagnostic Steps to Consider if Levels Are High

Assess for cholestasis (bilirubin, alkaline phosphatase), portosystemic shunt (imaging), other liver diseases (alanine aminotransferase, imaging, liver biopsy)

Important Interspecies Differences

Increased serum BA concentrations have been reported in healthy Maltese dogs.

Drug Effects

Ursodiol, a synthetic BA, will increase serum BA measurements. Heparin may cause a false decrease.

Lab Artifacts

Hemolysis: false decrease

Lipemia: variable effect

Specimen Collection and Handling

Serum (red top tube): 12-hour fasting sample and 2-hour postprandial sample recommended; separate serum from erythrocytes as soon as possible. Store at 2°C-8°C (refrigeration).

Urine: fresh urine, avoid blood contamination

Relative Cost: Serum (single), $$; serum (paired), $$; urine BA:crt, $$

Pearls

- Only a small amount of food (10 mL for small and 30 mL for large dogs) is required for gallbladder contraction.
- Serum BA should not be assayed if cholestasis is present (icterus in the absence of hemolysis; hyperbilirubinemia) as results will not provide any additional information.
- Increased BA concentrations are a good indicator of hepatobiliary dysfunction, but are not specific for either severity or the type of underlying disease.
- Mildly increased serum BA concentrations can occur with extrahepatic disorders (e.g., gastrointestinal disease, hyperadrenocorticism).
- Lack of increased BA concentrations does not rule out liver disease.
- Spontaneous gallbladder contraction can result in fasting BA concentrations that exceed postprandial concentrations; interpretation of the higher value compared with reference intervals for postprandial samples is recommended.
- Urine test has low diagnostic sensitivity (false-negatives common) but good specificity (few false-positives).

AUTHOR: Carrie L. Flint, DVM, DACVP
EDITOR: Lois Roth-Johnson, DVM, PhD, DACVP

Bilirubin

Definition

Pigment produced by degradation of the heme portion of hemoglobin (and, to a lesser extent, other porphyrin-containing compounds)

Physiology

During red blood cell breakdown (either senescent or pathologic hemolysis), heme is oxidized to biliverdin and iron is released. Biliverdin is then reduced to unconjugated bilirubin, predominantly in macrophages of the spleen, bone marrow, and liver. Unconjugated bilirubin is released into the circulation, where it is bound to albumin and transported to the liver for uptake, conjugation, and secretion into bile. Conjugation renders bilirubin water-soluble. Laboratory assays include total serum bilirubin, direct (conjugated) bilirubin, and indirect (unconjugated) bilirubin.

Reference Interval

Dogs and cats: 0-0.3 mg/dL (0-5.13 mcmol/L)

Causes of Abnormally High Levels

- Hemolysis: may occur with intravascular or extravascular causes
- Liver disease: decreased hepatic uptake, decreased functional liver mass
- Cholestasis: may be from an intrahepatic (e.g., lipidosis) or extrahepatic (e.g., cholelithiasis, pancreatic mass/inflammation) obstruction. Can also result from a functional defect in bile salt or bilirubin transporters in the absence of physical obstruction, as seen with endotoxemia/sepsis. Biliary rupture will also lead to hyperbilirubinemia.
- Anorexia: increase is minimal, most often at or just greater than upper limit of the reference interval

Next Diagnostic Steps to Consider if Levels Are High

Rule out hemolytic disease first (e.g., CBC). Interpret with markers of hepatic injury, function, and cholestasis (e.g., ALT, AST, ammonia, ALP, GGT). Consider abdominal imaging +/- liver biopsy. Consider endotoxemia/sepsis if physical examination/laboratory data are suggestive.

Lab Artifacts

- Hemolysis: method dependent, may increase or decrease
- Lipemia: method dependent, may increase
- Light degrades bilirubin (up to 50% in 1 hour in direct sunlight or fluorescent light).

Specimen Collection and Handling

Serum (red top tube). Plasma (heparin or EDTA) may be substituted. Avoid hemolysis and separate serum from red blood cells as soon as possible. Store at 2°C-8°C (refrigeration). Protect from light.

Relative Cost: $ (single test); $$ (included in full chemistry or liver panel)

Pearls

- Hyperbilirubinemia is not present in all animals with hemolytic disease, but is more typical with rapid severe hemolysis.
- Delta bilirubin is protein-bound conjugated bilirubin that increases with cholestasis when hepatic secretion of conjugated bilirubin is impaired. It is not reported, but thought to be the cause of persistent hyperbilirubinemia in patients without hyperbilirubinuria.
- Although bile acids are a sensitive test of liver function, they typically add little useful information in animals with hyperbilirubinemia.

AUTHOR: Mary Leissinger, DVM, MS, DACVP
EDITOR: Lois Roth-Johnson, DVM, PhD, DACVP

Bilirubinuria

Definition

The presence of bilirubin, usually conjugated, in urine

Physiology

The mononuclear phagocyte system degrades hemoglobin from senescent erythrocytes into iron, amino acids, and unconjugated bilirubin. Hydrophobic in nature, unconjugated bilirubin must be albumin-bound for transport to the liver for conjugation. Conjugated bilirubin is water-soluble, transported to bile for fat emulsification, and degraded to urobilinogen by the intestinal tract. Conjugated bilirubin and urobilinogen can be absorbed into the portal circulation and become recycled for biliary excretion or remain in the plasma to be filtered by the glomerulus. Unconjugated bilirubin is not freely filtered by the glomerulus, as it is albumin-bound.

Reference Interval

- Trace to 1+ bilirubin can be observed in concentrated urine of healthy dogs
- Any degree of bilirubinuria is significant in cats

Causes of Abnormally High Levels

- Cholestatic disease (impaired bile flow) or biliary rupture allows conjugated bilirubin to leak into systemic circulation, with subsequent renal excretion.
- Excessive hemolysis (extravascular or intravascular) leads to increased hemoglobin breakdown and bilirubin formation.

Next Diagnostic Steps to Consider if Levels Are High

In dogs, assess degree of bilirubinuria and urine concentration as limited bilirubinuria can be normal in the species. Rule out a hemolytic anemia (e.g., decreased hematocrit, morphologic changes such as spherocytes, reticulocytosis). Evaluate a biochemistry panel for cholestasis (elevated alkaline phosphatase, gamma-glutamyl transferase, total bilirubin, and/or cholesterol). See p. 528.

Important Interspecies Differences

Dogs have a low renal threshold for bilirubin; additionally, canine renal tubular epithelium has the ability to conjugate bilirubin. Thus, low levels of bilirubin can be observed in healthy dogs, and bilirubinuria can precede hyperbilirubinemia.

Lab Artifacts

False-negative reactions can occur with high concentrations of ascorbic acid or nitrite (urinary tract infection), delayed sampling (due to hydrolysis of bilirubin to the undetectable unconjugated form), and exposure to UV light (which converts bilirubin to undetectable biliverdin).

Specimen Collection and Handling

Process or refrigerate within 30 minutes.

Relative Cost: $ (as part of urinalysis)

Pearls

Bilirubinuria is never normal in cats

AUTHOR NAME: Shannon D. Dehghanpir, DVM, MS, DACVP
EDITOR NAME: Lois Roth-Johnson, DVM, PhD, DACVP

Blastomyces Testing

Bonus Material Available 

Definition

Blastomycosis is a systemic fungal infection caused by the dimorphic fungus *Blastomyces dermatitidis*.

Physiology

Inhalation of *Blastomyces* spores results in a primary lung infection. Subsequent dissemination occurs via blood and lymphatics to multiple tissues, most notably skin, eye, bone, and lymph nodes.

Reference Interval

- Consult the laboratory conducting the test for information regarding reference range for agar gel immunodiffusion (AGID).
- Reference range for enzyme immunoassay (EIA) antigen test is < 0.2 ng/mL; 0.2-0.9 ng/mL is a low positive (many false-positives; positive predictive value [PPV] 36%); > 1 ng/mL is moderate-high positive (infection highly likely; PPV 91%). Sensitivity and specificity reported as 93.5% and 98%, respectively. (EIA available at MiraVista Diagnostics, www.miravistalabs.com)

Causes of Abnormally High Levels

A positive AGID test indicates exposure to *Blastomyces*. A positive EIA antigen indicates *Blastomyces* infection or infection with a cross-reactive fungus (e.g., histoplasmosis).

Next Diagnostic Steps to Consider if Levels Are High

Correlate results with clinical signs and radiographic findings. Demonstration of the organism in cytologic or tissue biopsy samples is preferred for definitive diagnosis (cytology should be prepared from any enlarged lymph nodes or draining skin tracts). Culture is slow to grow, requires special handling, and is rarely performed.

Causes of Abnormally Low Levels

Negative test result indicates lack of exposure, early infection, inadequate immune response to exposure or false-negative EIA antigen (10% of cases, mostly localized infections).

Next Diagnostic Steps to Consider if Levels Are Low

If high clinical suspicion of *Blastomyces* spp. exists but AGID and antigen tests are negative, consider cytology/histopathology of lesions, repeat urine and serum EIA antigen test in 1-2 weeks, or IgG antibody EIA test.

Drug Effects

Effective antifungal treatment will decrease antigen levels in EIA test.

Lab Artifacts

Interfering substances for the EIA test include Sputolysin, sodium hydroxide, EDTA, rheumatoid factor, and heterophile antibodies.

Specimen Collection and Handling

Submit 1 mL of serum (red top tube) for AGID and ≥0.25 mL for EIA antibody test. Submit ≥0.5 mL urine (preferred sample), ≥1.2 mL serum (red top tube), ≥0.5 mL bronchoalveolar lavage fluid, cerebrospinal fluid, or sterile body fluid for EIA test. Sample for EIA is stable for 2 weeks at room temperature or 2°C-8°C, and indefinitely if frozen.

Relative Cost: $$ (AGID); $$$ (EIA)

Pearls

- EIA antigen test has higher sensitivity than AGID for diagnosing canine blastomycosis.

- EIA antigen test possible cross-reactions with histoplasmosis (high cross-reactivity), coccidioidomycosis, aspergillosis and sporotrichosis
- EIA testing of urine is slightly more sensitive than serum/plasma; other samples, such as bronchoalveolar lavage fluid, may be more sensitive depending on disease presentation.
- EIA antigen test may be used for monitoring response to therapy and for early detection of relapse.

AUTHOR: Patty J. Ewing, DVM, MS, DACVP
EDITOR: Lois Roth-Johnson, DVM, PhD, DACVP

Blood Gas Analysis

Definition

Evaluation of blood pH, PCO_2, PO_2, and bicarbonate (HCO_3^-)

Synonym

Acid-base analysis

Physiology

Arterial PO_2 is used to assess hypoxemia and pulmonary function.

Physiologic buffers maintain blood pH within a narrow range. PCO_2 and HCO_3^- are used to detect respiratory and metabolic derangements, respectively. Initial interpretation is for significant changes of pH. PCO_2 and HCO_3^- are subsequently assessed to see if alterations are due to respiratory or metabolic abnormalities. In simple acid-base disorders, changes in the unaffected buffer system occur to compensate (e.g., if HCO_3- [metabolic base] decreases, causing metabolic acidosis, PCO_2 [respiratory acid] will decrease as compensation).

Reference Interval

- Arterial pH: dog, 7.35-7.45; cat, 7.30-7.42
- PCO_2 (mm Hg): dog, 32-42; cat, 25-37
- PO_2 (arterial, breathing room air; mm Hg): dog, 90-100; cat, 90-100
- HCO_3^- (mmol/L): dog, 19-26; cat, 14-21

Causes of Abnormally High Levels

Increased pH (alkalemia) with decreased PCO_2 indicates respiratory alkalosis.

Increased pH (alkalemia) with increased HCO_3^- indicates metabolic alkalosis.

Next Diagnostic Steps to Consider if Levels Are High

See p. 1397.

Causes of Abnormally Low Levels

Decreased pH (acidemia) with increased PCO_2 indicates respiratory acidosis.

Decreased pH (acidemia) with decreased HCO_3^- indicates metabolic acidosis.

Next Diagnostic Steps to Consider if Levels Are Low

See p. 1397.

Drug Effects

Drugs affecting respiratory function:
- Depression: (anesthetics, narcotics, sedatives) → respiratory acidosis
- Stimulation (salicylates, aminophylline) = respiratory alkalosis

Drugs that can cause a metabolic alkalosis:
- Administration of sodium bicarbonate
- Diuretics such as furosemide

Lab Artifacts

Exposure to room air will result in falsely decreased PCO_2, increased pH; possibly increased PO_2

Failure to analyze samples promptly can result in decreases in pH and PO_2.

Specimen Collection and Handling

Whole blood collected in heparinized syringe. Avoid bubbles, and cap end of syringe to limit exposure to room air.

Specimens analyzed within 15 minutes of collection are preferred. Storage in a capped syringe on ice at 4°C for up to 1 hour is acceptable.

Relative Cost: $$

Pearls

- Point-of-care analyzers are available for use in clinics.
- Venous blood samples are sufficient for routine evaluation of acid-base status (pH, PCO_2, and HCO_3^-).
- Arterial samples are more difficult to obtain but necessary to assess oxygenation.
- Use of reference point (midpoint of RI) can simplify interpretation.
- Mixed acid-base disorders can complicate interpretation.

AUTHOR & EDITOR: Lois Roth-Johnson, DVM, PhD, DACVP

Blood pH

Definition

Measurement of hydrogen ion (H^+) concentration (acidity) of blood

Physiology

There is an inverse relationship between blood pH and H^+ concentration. Increased H^+ = decreased blood pH.

Reference Interval

- Dog (venous): RI: 7.35-7.42; RP: 7.4
- Cat (venous): RI: 7.31-7.37; RP: 7.35

Reference point (midreference interval) is helpful.

Causes of Abnormally High Levels

Increased pH indicates alkalosis, either respiratory (decreased PCO_2) or metabolic (increased bicarbonate).

Metabolic causes include vomiting, diuretics, refeeding syndrome, overadministration of bicarbonate.

Respiratory causes include hyperventilation due to pulmonary disease, panting (pain, anxiety, thermoregulation, neurologic disorder), septicemia, mechanical overventilation.

Next Diagnostic Steps to Consider if Levels Are High

Thorough history and examination, serum chemistry, CBC, possible thoracic imaging

Causes of Abnormally Low Levels

Decreased pH indicates acidosis, either metabolic (low bicarbonate) or respiratory (increased PCO_2).

Metabolic causes include bicarbonate loss and/or production of endogenous acids due to lactic acidosis, ketoacidosis, renal disorders, ingestion of exogenous toxins (ethylene glycol), diarrhea.

Respiratory causes include pulmonary parenchymal disease, pulmonary restrictive disease (pleural effusion, pneumothorax, diaphragmatic hernia), central nervous system depression (anesthesia, narcotics, brainstem disease), hypoventilation, airway obstruction.

Next Diagnostic Steps to Consider if Levels Are Low

Thorough history and examination, serum chemistry, blood lactate, CBC, possible thoracic imaging

Metabolic acidosis:

Calculate anion gap to determine if due to loss of bicarbonate (anion gap normal; e.g., diarrhea, renal tubular acidosis) or accumulation of organic acid (high anion gap; e.g., diabetic ketoacidosis, lactic acidosis, uremic acidosis).

Drug Effects

- Decrease: sedative, narcotic, general anesthetics causing respiratory depression
- Increase: bicarbonate or diuretic administration

Lab Artifacts

- Decrease: delayed analysis (longer than 15 minutes for room temperature samples or greater than 1 hour for samples kept on ice [4°C]), excessive heparin in collection syringe
- Increase: Exposure to air (uncapped samples or samples with air bubbles) results in loss of CO_2.

Specimen Collection and Handling

Whole blood collected in an appropriately heparinized syringe. Cap syringe immediately to avoid air contamination. Samples analyzed within 15 minutes of collection are ideal, but samples kept at 4°C and analyzed within an hour are acceptable.

Relative Cost: Reported as part of blood gas analysis

Pearls

Because disturbances of blood pH can be life threatening, periodic monitoring during prolonged anesthesia and in patients with significant metabolic disease (e.g., severe vomiting or diarrhea) is suggested.

Mixed acid-base disturbances may occur, wherein any combination of respiratory or metabolic acidosis and respiratory or metabolic alkalosis occur simultaneously.

AUTHOR & EDITOR: Lois Roth-Johnson, DVM, PhD, DACVP

Blood Typing

Definition

Identification of specific inherited characteristic cell surface antigens on erythrocyte membranes. See also p. 1084.

Physiology

- Canine: Multiple blood groups systems exist. Dog erythrocyte antigen (DEA) 1.1 and 1.2 can induce acute hemolytic reactions in sensitized dogs. Delayed hemolytic reactions occur with other blood types. Blood type is identified by monoclonal or polyclonal antibodies on card agglutination assays, immunochromatographic cartridges, or gel-based methods.
- Feline: AB blood group system, composed of types A, AB, and B; defined by pre-existing, naturally occurring isoantibodies against the antigen they lack; type AB lacks isoantibodies; card agglutination, immunochromatographic cartridges, gel-based assays, and DNA testing (for b allele) exist.

Reference Interval

- Canine: dog erythrocyte antigen (DEA) 1.1 (the "A" system); reported as positive or negative, but may be a continuum from negative to positive. Any level of positive reaction should be considered DEA 1 positive.
- Feline: type A (most common), type B (less common), type AB (rare); prevalence varies with breed and geographic region.

Causes of Abnormally High Levels

Result is individual animal's blood type

Important Interspecies Differences

- Dogs do not have naturally occurring, pre-formed antierythrocyte surface antigen antibodies; a first transfusion will not usually cause a hemolytic reaction regardless of blood type. See p. 1169.
- All type B cats > 3 months of age have high titers of naturally occurring type A antibodies that act as strong hemagglutinins and hemolysins. Every cat should be blood typed before even a first blood transfusion. Type A or AB kittens born to type B queens are at risk of developing neonatal isoerythrolysis. Before breeding, cats from breeds with a large prevalence of type B should be screened for blood type. See p. 686.

Lab Artifacts

- False-positive: autoagglutination (card-based methods)
- False-negative: marked anemia

Specimen Collection and Handling

- EDTA whole blood (lavender top tube). Blood typing tests include both cage-side (cards, gel column agglutination) and mail-out options (immunochromatographic, genetic testing).
- Typing cards are species-specific. Dog blood typing cards can be used for determining DEA 1.1 antigen status, and cards for cats can be used for determining type A, B, or AB.

Relative Cost: $$$

Pearls

- Dogs: DEA 1.1 is the most antigenic; DEA 1.1 negative dogs are recommended as donors.
- Cats: Because of naturally occurring erythrocyte antigens, blood from blood donor and recipient cat should be typed.
- The Mik erythrocyte antigen recently has been identified in cats, resulting in an incompatibility cross-match even if A, B, or AB blood types are matched. Routine screening not currently available. Ideally, cats should be cross-matched before transfusion.
- The Dal erythrocyte antigen has been identified in dogs but is not detected by routine blood typing.

AUTHOR: Deborah G. Davis, DVM, DACVP
EDITOR: Lois Roth-Johnson, DVM, PhD, DACVP

Blood Urea Nitrogen (BUN)

Definition

Concentration of urea in serum, plasma, or whole blood (usually measured in serum)

Synonyms

BUN, urea, serum urea nitrogen (SUN)

Physiology

Most of serum urea is synthesized via the hepatic urea cycle, which converts ammonium derived from bacterial metabolism of dietary protein to urea. Minimal ammonium is derived from deamination of amino acids. The kidneys excrete urea. Urea is freely filtered by glomeruli; some is resorbed by tubular epithelial cells to establish (with sodium) the medullary concentration gradient.

Reference Interval

- Dogs: 10-30 mg/dL (3.6-11 mmol/L)
- Cats: 15-35 mg/dL (5.4-12.5 mmol/L)

Causes of Abnormally High Levels

- Decreased glomerular filtration rate (GFR): azotemia from prerenal causes (e.g., dehydration, decreased cardiac output, shock), renal disease, or postrenal causes (e.g., urinary outflow obstruction, rupture)
- Increased protein catabolism: fever, starvation, exercise
- Increased protein digestion: hemorrhage into the GI tract, high protein diet

Next Diagnostic Steps to Consider if Levels Are High

Evaluate with creatinine as these values often parallel. If creatinine is not increased, consider early azotemia, increased protein catabolism, gastrointestinal hemorrhage, or dietary cause. Also consider with urine specific gravity. Well-concentrated urine suggests prerenal causes. Isosthenuric or minimally concentrated urine supports renal and postrenal etiologies, as well as conditions that may impair urine-concentrating ability (e.g., hypoadrenocorticism, diuretic use, hypercalcemia, diabetes insipidus).

Causes of Abnormally Low Levels

Hepatic dysfunction (e.g., liver disease, portosystemic shunt), increased urea excretion (polyuria of any cause), decreased dietary protein (including low-protein therapeutic diets), physiologic (e.g., young animals), congenital deficiency of urea cycle enzymes (rare)

Next Diagnotic Steps to Consider if Levels Are Low

Check history for polyuria/polydipsia and information on diet. Check the chemistry panel for evidence of hepatocellular injury and/or decreased liver function. Assess urine specific gravity, urine output, water intake, serum concentrations of electrolytes.

Specimen Collection and Handling

Serum (red top tube) preferred. Heparinized plasma (green top tube) acceptable. Some methods can use EDTA plasma (lavender top tube).

Relative Cost: $$ (part of chemistry or renal panel); $ (single test)

Pearls

- High doses of gastroduodenal ulcerogenic drugs (corticosteroids, nonsteroidal anti-inflammatory drugs) may cause intestinal hemorrhage, increasing BUN with little effect on creatinine.
- Increased BUN with concurrent isosthenuria raises concern for compromised renal function, but other causes of impaired urine concentration ability/ADH responsiveness (e.g., hypoadrenocorticism, hypercalcemia, diuretic use, diabetes insipidus) must also be considered.

AUTHOR: Mary Leissinger, DVM, MS, DACVP
EDITOR: Lois Roth-Johnson, DVM, PhD, DACVP

Bone Marrow Cytology

Definition

Microscopic evaluation allowing assessment of blood precursor cell production and morphology. See p. 1068 for bone marrow aspiration protocol.

Physiology

Bone marrow contains trabecular bone with marrow spaces containing capillaries, hematopoietic cells, and adipocytes. Hematopoietic activity occurs in response to peripheral demand. Bone marrow aspiration is indicated when there are unexplained cytopenias (nonregenerative anemia, neutropenia, and/or thrombocytopenia), hyperglobulinemia, suspicion of certain types of neoplasia, or as part of staging of confirmed lymphoma and systemic mastocytosis.

Reference Interval

Marrow particles should contain 25%-75% hematopoietic cells, with all cell lines exhibiting orderly, complete maturation and normal shape, size, and features (morphology). The normal myeloid/erythroid ratio (M:E) is ≈1:1, and can range from 0.6:1 to 4:1.

Causes of Abnormally High Levels

Hyperplasia of one or more cell lines may occur secondary to increased peripheral demand for cells due to cell destruction, increased utilization, or loss. Neoplasia such as acute or chronic leukemia (with or without maturation and morphologic abnormalities) results in high marrow cellularity and effacement of normal marrow tissue. Lymphocytes and plasma cells may be increased in marrow because of antigenic stimulation or neoplasia. Iron stores may be increased with anemia of chronic disease and hemolytic anemia. Inflammation, infiltrating neoplasia, or hemophagocytic disease also results in increased cellularity of the marrow.

Next Diagnostic Steps to Consider if Levels Are High

Dependent on differential diagnosis based on history, physical exam findings, and results of CBC, serum biochemistry profile, and other diagnostic tests

Causes of Abnormally Low Levels

- Marrow hypoplasia indicates decreased cell production. Causes include anemia of chronic disease, chronic kidney disease, ehrlichiosis (dogs), drug-induced or immune-mediated destruction of precursor cells in the marrow, toxic insult (e.g., sulfa antibiotics, albendazole, phenylbutazone), viral infection (i.e., feline leukemia virus, parvovirus, canine distemper), myelofibrosis.
- Maturation arrest and dysplastic changes of erythrocytes occur with viral infection, iron deficiency, myelodysplastic syndrome, or toxic insult.
- Iron stores are decreased with blood loss and iron deficiency.

Next Diagnostic Steps to Consider if Levels Are Low

Dependent on differential diagnosis based on history, physical exam findings, and results of

CBC, serum biochemistry profile, and other diagnostic tests. Bone marrow aspiration often is the final diagnostic step for confirming hematopoietic disorders; core biopsy with histopathologic evaluation may be required for accurate determination of cellularity in disorders resulting in marrow hypoplasia/aplasia or myelofibrosis.

Important Interspecies Differences

Iron stores are not usually visible in cat bone marrow and cannot be evaluated cytologically.

Specimen Collection and Handling

Aspirated marrow should immediately be made into fresh smears and some placed in an EDTA (lavender top) tube. Proper collection and preparation of slides are essential for accurate interpretation. Hematopoietic cells degenerate rapidly after collection. Slides must be prepared immediately (before a clot forms) or within 30 minutes after collection if anticoagulant is used. A good bone marrow aspirate has several marrow particles for evaluation, with spreading of the cells in a monolayer for evaluation of morphology.

Relative Cost: $$$

Pearls

- Bone marrow aspirates must be interpreted concurrently with CBC (ideally, obtained same day) results.
- An accompanying bone marrow core biopsy may help in the interpretation of overall cellularity of the bone marrow, which complements the evaluation of morphology and maturation sequence from the marrow aspirate.
- A fresh smear of the marrow aspirate should be stained and examined for the presence of marrow spicules/cells while the animal is still sedated; if spicules are not adequate, the procedure may be repeated immediately.
- Sometimes, pathogens (e.g., *Histoplasma*) or overtly neoplastic cells are identified by microscopic marrow exam.

AUTHOR: Ruanna E. Gossett, DVM, PhD, DACVP
EDITOR: Lois Roth-Johnson, DVM, PhD, DACVP

Borrelia (Lyme Disease) Serology

Definition

Lyme borreliosis is a tick-borne disease of dogs and humans that is caused by the spirochete *Borrelia burgdorferi.*

Physiology

Borrelia spp. organisms are inoculated via an *Ixodes* tick bite. After local proliferation, organisms spread in connective tissues, including joints. Persistent infections are common; they may produce no clinical signs or may result in chronic debilitating disease such as arthritis or meningitis. Immune response to infection occasionally results in potentially fatal protein-losing nephropathy (p. 596).

Reference Interval

- In-clinic SNAP qualitative ELISA for antibody to the C_6 peptide of *B. burgdorferi* antigen (SNAP® 4Dx® Plus): positive or negative result
- Quantitative C_6 antibody ELISA (Lyme Quant C6®) test (reference laboratory): < 30 units/mL
- Multiplex assay (fluorescent bead technology): negative, vaccine, or infection
- IFA/ELISA (whole spirochetes): negative or positive for spirochete antibodies

Causes of Abnormally High Levels

- C_6 peptide: SNAP® 4Dx® Plus positive test indicates natural exposure to *B. burgdorferi*, while magnitude of increase in quantitative C_6 can be used to help determine relevance of antibody response and to monitor therapeutic response.
- Multiplex assay differentiates vaccinated, early infection and chronic infection in some but not all patients.
- Positive IFA/ELISA indicates exposure but does not differentiate self-limiting or subclinical infection, active infection, Lyme vaccination, or cross-reacting bacteria (*Leptospira* sp.). Western blot: presence of 3-6 Lyme-specific bands suggests exposure or infection. Antibodies against several specific proteins are more typical of natural infection than vaccination; however, reliable differentiation is questionable. Interpretation of banding patterns is not always clear-cut.

Next Diagnostic Steps to Consider if Levels Are High

All positive tests should prompt urinalysis to detect proteinuria, and ideally CBC and chemistry profile as well. If SNAP® 4Dx® Plus is positive, consider the Lyme Quant C_6® to help decide if treatment is warranted in healthy dogs, or to establish a baseline for monitoring response to treatment. Increasing levels of C_6 antibodies reflect active infection, while antibodies should decline with treatment. If IFA/ELISA is positive, consider qualitative or quantitative C_6. Neither PCR nor blood culture is recommended due to low sensitivity.

Causes of Abnormally Low Levels

Early infection or uninfected

Next Diagnostic Steps to Consider if Levels Are Low

Consider repeating C_6 antibody test or multiplex in 3-5 weeks if clinically appropriate (recent tick exposure).

Important Interspecies Differences

Despite evidence of seropositivity for *Borrelia* in cats (including C_6 ELISA assay), natural disease has not been described. Polyarthritis and meningitis have been observed in some experimentally infected cats.

Drug Effects

Lyme Quant C_6® level should decrease > 50% within 3-6 months following treatment.

Specimen Collection and Handling

The IDEXX SNAP® 4Dx® Plus test requires 0.3 mL of serum or plasma (red top or lavender top tube), using manufacturer's directions for in-clinic test. Lyme Quant C_6® requires 1 mL of serum (red top tube). Multiplex assay: 2 mL serum. IFA and Western blot: 1 mL of serum (red top tube). Samples are stable for up to 5-7 days at refrigerator temperature or several weeks when frozen.

Relative Cost: $ (IDEXX SNAP® 4Dx® Plus), $$ (Lyme Quant C_6®), $$$ (Western blot)

Pearls

- Most dogs exposed to *Borrelia* (and therefore, having a positive test result) do not develop clinical signs of Lyme disease; the decision to treat should be based on clinical signs, clinically significant Lyme Quant C_6® level (>30 units/mL, or increasing level), and/or presence of proteinuria.

AUTHOR: Patty J. Ewing, DVM, MS, DACVP
EDITOR: Lois Roth-Johnson, DVM, PhD, DACVP

Bromide

Definition
Active ingredient in potassium (KBr) or sodium bromide (NaBr), drugs used for treating seizure disorders

Physiology
The precise mechanism of action in seizure control has not been elucidated. It is believed that preferential transport of bromide rather than chloride across cell membranes results in neuronal hyperpolarization and depressed neuron excitability, and therefore an increased seizure threshold.

Reference Interval
Target serum concentration range (interpret in conjunction with clinical signs):
- As sole anticonvulsant: 100-300 mg/dL
- In combination with phenobarbital: 80-200 mg/dL

Causes of Abnormally High Levels
Excessive dosage leads to bromide toxicosis

Next Diagnostic Steps to Consider if Levels Are High
Lower dosage

Important Interspecies Differences
Used primarily in dogs; should be used sparingly in cats as they are more prone to exhibiting toxic side effects, particularly pneumonitis.

Drug Effects
Additive sedation if other central nervous system (CNS) sedatives are used. Diuretics may enhance excretion, increasing bromide dose required for seizure control. Keep dietary chloride constant during treatment; excessive chloride can result decrease seizure control, whereas markedly decreased chloride (in some low-salt diets) can result in toxicosis.

Lab Artifacts
Increase: ion-selective electrode method of measurement (chloride interference)

Specimen Collection and Handling
Serum (red top tube), refrigerate. Submit first sample within 1 week of loading dose, second at 1 month; monitor every 3-6 months. If no loading performed, measure after 1 month and again at 2-3 months for steady-state concentration.

Relative Cost: $$

Pearls
- Older animals, those with other diseases, and those with renal dysfunction may be more prone to adverse reactions.
- Bromides are not approved by the U.S. Food and Drug Administration for use in animals.
- Bromide has a small therapeutic window, and serum concentrations should not be used as sole indicator of toxicity.

AUTHOR: Carrie L. Flint, DVM, DACVP
EDITOR: Lois Roth-Johnson, DVM, PhD, DACVP

Brucella Slide Agglutination

Definition
ELISA test for detection of *Brucella canis* antibody in serum

Synonym
Rapid slide agglutination test (RSAT)

Physiology
Highly sensitive screening test used to detect *B. canis* infection. Patient serum is mixed with heat killed *B. ovis* on slide and evaluated for agglutination.

Reference Interval
Agglutination indicates positive test (patient serum contains antibodies to *B. canis*); serum from noninfected dogs fails to agglutinate.

Causes of Abnormally High Levels
B. canis infection; false-positive test may occur in patients with antibodies to *Bordetella bronchiseptica, Pseudomonas* spp., *Moraxella* spp., or other gram-negative bacteria. Only ≈40% of positive tests are associated with true *B. canis* infection.

Next Diagnostic Steps to Consider if Levels Are High
Confirm positive test results with 2-mercaptoethanol tube agglutination, agar gel immunodiffusion (AGID), tube agglutination (TAT), indirect fluorescent antibody test (IFAT), or culture. Appropriate culture samples (vaginal exudate, aborted pups, semen) depend on clinical signs and associated available tissues or specimens.

Causes of Abnormally Low Levels
For the first 3-4 weeks after infection, serologic test results may be negative even with bacteremia.

Next Diagnostic Steps to Consider if Levels Are Low
If exposure or disease is suspected, retesting after 30 days is suggested before admission to breeding kennels. Low or intermediate titers may indicate previous disease or recent exposure. Follow-up blood culture may be helpful in these animals.

Lab Artifacts
Gross hemolysis interferes with interpretation.

Specimen Collection and Handling
Serum (red top tube), 1 mL; separate serum from clot; stable at 2-8 °C for four days.

Relative Cost: $$

Pearls
- Humans are susceptible (zoonosis), but human *B. canis* infections are rare.
- After bacteremia, organisms may concentrate in prostate and epididymis. Agglutination titers decline.
- Chronically infected female dogs typically have recurrent bacteremia and highest titers during proestrus, estrus, pregnancy, or abortion. Testing is suggested at these times.
- The test has a high sensitivity and thus is a reasonable screening test. All breeding dogs should be tested regularly.
- Test result required by some countries (New Zealand, Australia) for entry of dogs. Import requirements change and vary, so check for most recent regulations.
- Infection with other species of *Brucella* besides *B. canis* may not be detected.

AUTHOR: Sharon M. Dial, DVM, PhD, DACVP
EDITOR: Lois Roth-Johnson, DVM, PhD, DACVP

Buffy Coat

Definition

The thin white layer of packed leukocytes and platelets found atop the packed erythrocytes following high-speed centrifugation of anticoagulated blood

Physiology

Leukocytes and platelets are less dense than erythrocytes, so they deposit above the packed erythrocytes following centrifugation.

Reference Interval

Typically not measured. The height of this layer in a spun blood specimen can be a crude index of the total leukocyte count.

Causes of Abnormally High Levels

Any condition causing leukocytosis or thrombocytosis can increase the thickness of the buffy coat layer.

Next Diagnostic Steps to Consider if Levels Are High

CBC with blood smear examination, smear with evaluation of buffy coat itself

Specimen Collection and Handling

EDTA whole blood (lavender top tube), or immediately filled and spun hematocrit tube

Relative Cost: $$

Pearls

- Smears of buffy coat cells can be used for concentrating abnormal leukocytes that occur in very low numbers. Examples: detection of mastocytemia as a staging tool in dogs with mast cell neoplasm, detection of infectious agents in neutrophils or monocytes (e.g., *Histoplasma* in dogs and cats, *Hepatozoon americanum* or Ehrlichia morulae in dogs)
- In dogs with babesiosis, infected erythrocytes are less dense than normal erythrocytes and can occur in higher numbers on buffy coat smears.
- Low numbers of circulating mast cells detected on buffy coat smears occur as an incidental finding in dogs (and rarely in cats) with various inflammatory diseases. Therefore, buffy coat detection of mast cells is seldom used to screen for mast cell neoplasms.

AUTHOR: Stephen D. Gaunt, DVM, PhD, DACVP
EDITOR: Lois Roth-Johnson, DVM, PhD, DACVP

Calcium, Serum

Definition

Essential mineral with important regulatory functions (cell signaling). Serum total calcium (tCa^{2+}) includes protein-bound (35%-40%), anion-complexed (10%), and ionized (iCa^{2+}) (50%-55%) fractions.

Synonyms

Ca, Ca^{2+}

Physiology

Serum levels are regulated by parathyroid hormone (PTH) and calcitriol (vitamin D metabolite), affecting intestine, kidney, and bone. Dietary absorption depends on calcitriol. Glomeruli filter non–protein-bound Ca^{2+}; 98% is reabsorbed by tubules. Low [iCa^{2+}] stimulates PTH production, mobilizing Ca^{2+} from bone, increasing renal tubular resorption, stimulating calcitriol synthesis. In hypercalcemia of malignancy, PTH-related peptide (PTHrP) mimics actions of PTH. iCa^{2+} is the biologically active form.

Reference Interval

- Total Ca^{2+}: 8.5-11 mg/dL; 4.2-5.5 mEq/L (2.1-2.75 mmol/L)
- Ionized Ca^{2+}: 4.5-6 mg/dL; 2.2-3 mEq/L (1.1-1.5 mmol/L)

Causes of Abnormally High Levels

Hypercalcemia of malignancy, primary hyperparathyroidism, osteolysis, granulomatous diseases, hypervitaminosis D, kidney disease/kidney injury (including grape/raisin intoxication), idiopathic (cats), hypoadrenocorticism, hyperproteinemia, excess supplementation, physiologic (young dogs). See p. 1232.

Next Diagnostic Steps to Consider if Levels are High

Interpret with serum [phosphorus], physical exam (including rectal palpation for anal sac neoplasm and careful lymph node palpation), and other laboratory data. Measure serum [iCa^{2+}]. If ionized hypercalcemia, consider measuring PTH, PTHrP.

Causes of Abnormally Low Levels

Hypoalbuminemia (iCa^{2+} normal despite low tCa^{2+}), puerperal tetany, hypoparathyroidism, 2° hyperparathyroidism, hyperadrenocorticism, ethylene glycol intoxication, pancreatitis, malabsorption syndromes, hypomagnesemia, hypovitaminosis D (including renal disease), acute tumor lysis syndrome, severe tissue trauma, sepsis. See p. 1239.

Next Diagnostic Steps to Consider if Levels are Low

Measure serum [iCa^{2+}], albumin. Interpret with physical exam, relevant history, and other laboratory data. Measurement of PTH, Mg^{2+} may be of use in select cases.

Important Interspecies Differences

Cats may have idiopathic increase in iCa^{2+}

Drug Effects

- Increase: thiazide diuretics, supplements or rodenticides containing vitamin D, excess oral phosphate binders, antipsoriasis creams
- Decrease: furosemide, glucocorticoids, phosphate enemas, calcitonin, mithramycin, Ca^{2+}-binding anticoagulants (in blood transfusion products), bicarbonate administration

Lab Artifacts

- Decreased: inappropriate anticoagulant (EDTA, citrate, oxalate bind Ca^{2+} *in vitro*)
- Decreased [iCa^{2+}]; aerobic sample handling, over heparinization
- Increased [iCa^{2+}]; prolonged exposure to erythrocytes, use of serum separator tubes (SST). The gel plugs of SST are reported to leak calcium into the serum sample.
- Effects of bilirubin, lipemia, and hemolysis are instrument/assay dependent

Specimen Collection and Handling

- Serum (red top tube) preferred; heparinized plasma (green top tube) may be used.
- iCa^{2+}: anaerobic handling necessary. Harvest serum or plasma within 1 hour. Serum is preferred. Do not use serum separator tubes. Do not freeze. Heparin concentration should not exceed 4% of blood volume in tube. Heparinized whole blood used by some portable point-of-care analyzers

Relative Cost: $ (single test); $$ (as part of panel)

Pearls

- Use of correction formula in hypoalbuminemic dogs does not predict [iCa^{2+}] and is not recommended.
- Hypocalcemia is common in critically ill patients. It is not always predicted by [tCa^{2+}], and is best assessed by measurement of [iCa^{2+}].
- Treatment decisions for calcium disorders should be based upon derangements in [iCa^{2+}] rather than [tCa^{2+}].

AUTHOR: Mary Leissinger, DVM, MS, DACVP
EDITOR: Lois Roth-Johnson, DVM, PhD, DACVP

Canine Distemper Testing

Definition

Canine distemper is a multisystemic disease caused by canine distemper virus (CDV), a *Morbillivirus*.

Physiology

Following inhalation, the virus attaches to upper respiratory tract epithelium and replicates in macrophages. It spreads to regional lymph nodes, then to bone marrow, thymus, spleen, mesenteric lymph nodes, and gastrointestinal tract. One to two weeks later, the virus spreads to epithelium and the central nervous system. See p. 271.

Reference Interval

Refer to laboratory conducting the tests. Available tests include serum or cytologic immunofluorescent antibody test (IFA) titer, ELISA, direct IFA, viral neutralization assay, and PCR or quantitative RT-PCR.

Causes of Abnormally High Levels

- Positive IFA immunoglobulin (Ig) M titer indicates recent exposure to vaccine or acute natural infection. IgM is detectable from 1-4 weeks postexposure. Positive IFA IgG titer indicates exposure to vaccine, presence of maternal antibody, or chronic natural infection. Serum viral neutralization assay is preferred for determining protective antibody response to vaccination.
- Positive direct IFA on cytologic or histopathologic sample is diagnostic of infection.
- Positive PCR or RT-PCR indicates recent vaccination (up to 10 days) or natural infection.
- Positive RT-PCR result may be quantified to differentiate wildtype infection from vaccine strain. If indeterminate result, retest in a few days.

Next Diagnostic Steps to Consider if Levels are High

- Direct immunofluorescence or in-clinic ELISA is used for detecting antigen (acute distemper) in cytologic smears of conjunctival, tonsillar, genital, or urinary bladder epithelium; in cerebrospinal fluid (CSF); or in white blood cells (buffy coat or bone marrow).
- Increased anti-CDV antibody in CSF compared to serum may be helpful in diagnosing chronic distemper.
- PCR/RT-PCR: Buffy coat or conjunctival swab positive usually indicates acute infection, while urine, blood, or CSF positive usually indicates chronic infection.
- Routine cytologic evaluation of conjunctival or blood smears for inclusions (routine staining, with or without IFA) is often unrewarding.

Causes of Abnormally Low Levels

Lack of protective vaccine antibody titer or early infection. Improper sample handling or insufficient primers may result in a false-negative by PCR.

Next Diagnostic Steps to Consider if Levels are Low

- If clinically indicated, evaluate IgM titer or repeat IgG titer in 2-3 weeks (expect increase if original low/absent level was due to early infection). A negative result does not exclude a diagnosis.
- Histopathology and immunohistochemistry may be diagnostic (generally reserved for postmortem evaluation).

Specimen Collection and Handling

- Serologic tests: 1 mL of serum (red top tube). Stable for 5 days at 2°C-8°C or up to months frozen.
- IFA: conjunctival, urinary sediment, buffy coat smears (or whole blood in EDTA [lavender top tube] stored < 48 hours refrigerated), air-dried and preferably fixed in acetone × 5 minutes.
- PCR/RT-PCR: minimum 0.3 mL of CSF, tracheal wash fluid, or whole blood in EDTA (lavender top tube), minimum 3 mL urine (store at 2°C-8°C), tissue collected aseptically into sterile saline; freeze immediately to prevent RNA degradation.
- Quantitative RT-PCR: deep pharyngeal and conjunctival swabs in red top or sterile plastic tube; stable for 10 days at 2°-8°C.

Relative Cost: $$ (IFA, PCR)

Pearls

- Serum neutralization test remains the gold standard for measuring protective antibody. Titers correlate well with level of protection.
- Quantitative RT-PCR may assist in differentiating exposure to vaccine strain from CDV wildtype infection.

AUTHOR: Patty J. Ewing, DVM, MS, DACVP
EDITOR: Lois Roth-Johnson, DVM, PhD, DACVP

Laboratory Tests

Canine Parvovirus Testing

Definition

Canine parvoviral enteritis is a highly infectious, often fatal disease of Canidae caused by a small, nonenveloped DNA virus, CPV-2, which requires rapidly dividing cells for replication.

Physiology

See p. 760. Viremia develops 1-5 days following oronasal exposure to contaminated feces. Spread to lymphoid tissue and bone marrow causes necrosis, leukopenia, and immunosuppression.

Reference Interval

Commonly available tests: fecal antigen ELISA (negative or positive; in-clinic point-of-care test); serum immunoglobulin (Ig)M and IgG IFA, serum antibody by hemagglutination inhibition (HI) or ELISA (serologic titers); PCR (negative/positive +/- strain identification as 2a, b or c) RT-PCR (negative or positive result)

Causes of Abnormally High Levels

- Positive fecal ELISA test indicates viral antigen shedding due to natural infection (usually strong positive) or recent (4-8 days) vaccination with modified live vaccine (usually weak positive); one study showed no vaccine cross-reactivity with the SNAP® Parvo ELISA.
- Positive fecal PCR indicates natural infection or recent vaccination (for at least 2 weeks postvaccination). Quantitative RT-PCR test assists in differentiating vaccine and wildtype virus by incorporating a technical cut-off to prevent reporting of positives at the low levels seen in vaccinated dogs. Positive serum IgM by IFA indicates recent exposure (natural or vaccination); usually positive by the time clinical signs are present.
- Positive IgG titer by IFA indicates exposure (natural or vaccination); can demonstrate rising titer in acute and 10- to 14-day convalescent serum samples.
- Serum antibody titer by HI of ≥ 1:64 indicates previous exposure (natural or vaccination) and protective antibody.

Next Diagnostic Steps to Consider if Levels are High

Positive fecal ELISA or PCR with appropriate clinical signs is generally diagnostic.

Causes of Abnormally Low Levels

- Negative fecal ELISA indicates uninfected, very early postexposure, or end of viral shedding (shedding decreases by 8-12 days post-natural infection and/or 5-7 days after onset of clinical signs).
- False-negative fecal ELISA may occur if sample not freshly collected or if viral antigen is bound to antibody.
- False-negative PCR possible from degradation of nucleic acids via improper sample handling and storage.
- Negative serologic result indicates lack of exposure to virus, early infection before seroconversion, or inadequate vaccine protection.

Next Diagnostic Steps to Consider if Levels are Low

If clinical signs and laboratory findings are consistent, but initial test negative, repeat test, alternative test or electron microscopic evaluation of feces (expensive, not always readily available). Histopathologic evaluation and tissue culture can provide definitive diagnosis, but require biopsy.

Drug Effects

Recent vaccination may cause weak positive ELISA or positive PCR result.

Lab Artifacts

Severe hemolysis and lipemia interfere with IFA.

Specimen Collection and Handling

ELISA: rectal swab for in-clinic test per kit instructions; 3-5 g fresh feces in plastic container stored for ≤24 hours (2°-8°C) or longer if frozen. HI, IFA: 1 mL serum (red top tube), can be stored at 2°C-8°C up to 4 days. PCR/RT-PCR: fecal swab (minimum 1 g) or 5 g of feces in sterile container; stable for 10 days at 2°-8°C.

Relative Cost: $ (fecal antigen ELISA), $$ (serology, PCR/RT-PCR)

Pearls

- In-clinic ELISA and PCR tests are most often used to confirm clinical diagnosis.
- Some ELISA tests for canine parvovirus also detect feline parvovirus (panleukopenia) from cats that are shedding virus.
- Laboratory-based HI is necessary for assessment of likely protective antibody (sometimes used in lieu of revaccination).

AUTHOR: Patty J. Ewing, DVM, MS, DACVP
EDITOR: Lois Roth-Johnson, DVM, PhD, DACVP

Casts, Urine Sediment

Definition

Cylindrical aggregates of mucoprotein with or without cells that form in the lumen of the renal tubules.

Synonyms

Cylindruria

Physiology

The formation of casts is initiated by excess precipitated mucoprotein (Tamm-Horsfall mucoprotein), which is normally secreted in small quantities by the renal tubular epithelial cells. Highly concentrated and acidic urine, decreased urine flow, and excessive serum protein promote the precipitation of mucoprotein. Hyaline casts are pure precipitates of mucoprotein. When sloughed renal tubular epithelial cells become entrapped within the mucoprotein matrix, cellular casts result. These cellular (or fatty) casts undergo degrees of degeneration within the renal tubular lumen, resulting in coarsely granular, finely granular, to waxy casts. As waxy casts require urinary stasis for formation, their presence often signifies oliguric renal failure. White blood cell and red blood cell casts indicate inflammation and hemorrhage, respectively.

Reference Interval

- 1-2 hyaline and 0-1 granular casts per low-power field can be observed in concentrated urine of clinically normal dogs and cats.
- Cellular and waxy casts are pathologic.

Causes of Abnormally High Levels

- Hyaline casts: prerenal or renal proteinuria
- Cellular and granular casts: acute renal tubular injury (necrosis, nephrotoxicity, or ischemia)
- Waxy casts: persistent tubular injury, typically in patients with decreased urine output

Next Diagnostic Steps to Consider if Levels are High

Rule out nephrotoxicity; review history for exposure to nephrotoxin; serum chemistry profile; renal imaging +/- renal biopsy if indicated clinically

Lab Artifacts

Dissolution and false-negative results can occur with delayed processing or dilute or alkaline urine.

Specimen Collection and Handling

Process or refrigerate urine within 30 minutes.

Relative Cost: $ (as part of urinalysis)

AUTHOR: Shannon D. Dehghanpir, DVM, MS, DACVP
EDITOR: Lois Roth-Johnson, DVM, PhD, DACVP

Cerebrospinal Fluid Analysis (CSF)

Definition
Cerebrospinal fluid (CSF) is the aqueous fluid that surrounds the brain and spinal cord. *Pleocytosis* refers to an increased cellularity of the CSF sample. *Xanthochromia* refers to yellow discoloration of the sample, typically from blood that has been present in the CSF for days or longer. *Albuminocytologic dissociation* refers to a disproportionate elevation of CSF protein compared to minimally elevated or normal CSF cell count.

Physiology
CSF provides support and protection for neural structures, serves as a transport medium for metabolic products to and from the brain, and provides a barrier to control the microenvironment of the nervous system. It is normally colorless, clear, and almost acellular. Cytocentrifugation is required for cytologic evaluation of cells to assess for inflammation, hemorrhage, and infectious agents. Protein (primarily albumin) concentration is normally very low and requires microprotein assays for accurate assessment. When CSF is submitted for analysis, aliquots are often also submitted for infectious disease testing.

Reference Interval
- Dogs: red blood cell (RBC), < 30/mL; white blood cell (WBC), 0-4/mL; protein, < 35 mg/dL
- Cats: RBC, < 30/mL; WBC, 0-4/mL; protein, < 36 mg/dL

Causes of Abnormally High Levels
- Increased protein: hemorrhage, increased permeability of the blood-CSF barrier, or localized production of immunoglobulins
- Increased protein with normal cellularity: trauma, degenerative disease, intervertebral disc disease, fibrocartilaginous embolism, cervical spondylomyelopathy, neoplasia, and viral infections
- Increased protein and cell counts: inflammation, infection (viral, fungal, protozoal, bacterial, rickettsial, parasitic), granulomatous meningoencephalitis, steroid-responsive meningitis, neoplasia, immune-mediated disease, vasculitis, and necrotizing meningoencephalitis. Neoplastic cells are rare in CSF; lymphoma is the most commonly identified neoplasm.

Next Diagnostic Steps to Consider if Levels are High
Correlate CSF findings with history, general physical, neurologic, and imaging findings. Consider infectious disease titers (e.g., canine distemper virus, Neospora) on blood and/or CSF.

Drug Effects
Glucocorticoids may reduce inflammatory cell counts, but may be required for patient stabilization if a high degree of suspicion exists for steroid-responsive disease. Provided CSF tap occurs < 24 hours after initiation of glucocorticoids, accurate CSF cell counts are expected.

Specimen Collection and Handling
CSF in EDTA (lavender top tube) or red top tube; refrigerate. Analysis should be performed as soon as possible; cells deteriorate and lyse rapidly because of the low protein concentration. Addition of autologous serum to CSF (1:1) helps preserve cells for cytologic evaluation. However, a separate aliquot of CSF must be submitted for protein determination and cell counts. Any specimens with additives should be labeled with additive type and quantity.

Relative Cost: $$$; CSF protein only: $$

Pearls
- Many patients with neurologic disease may have no cytologic abnormalities in CSF samples. Examples include idiopathic epilepsy, hydrocephalus, intoxication or metabolic disease, vertebral disease, trauma, myelomalacia, and neoplasia.
- Blood contamination from sample collection can cause increase in protein and cells in CSF; as a general rule, hemorrhage may account for 1 WBC for every 500 RBC in CSF.

AUTHOR: Ruanna E. Gossett, DVM, PhD, DACVP
EDITOR: Lois Roth-Johnson, DVM, PhD, DACVP

Chloride

Definition
Major extracellular fluid (ECF) anion. Serum [Cl^-] essentially equals ECF [Cl^-]. Cl^- concentrations influenced by Na^+, HCO_3^-

Synonyms
Cl, Cl^-

Physiology
Major component of gastric secretions; intestinal resorption is coupled to Na^+ resorption, HCO_3^- secretion. Kidneys play major regulatory role: filtered by glomeruli, reabsorbed in renal tubules following Na^+ and water. Acid-base status affects serum levels: there is an inverse relationship between serum [Cl^-] and [HCO_3^-]. Serum [Na^+] and [Cl^-] usually change proportionally, but a selective increase in [Cl^-] causes hyperchloremic acidosis; a selective decrease causes hypochloremic alkalosis.

Reference Interval
Dogs: 105-115 mEq/L. Cats: 114-123 mEq/L
Unit conversion: 1 mEq/L = 1 mmol/L

Causes of Abnormally High Levels
- With proportional [Na^+] increase: same as hypernatremia (see pp. 1234 and 1382).
- Without proportional increase in [Na^+]: hyperchloremic metabolic acidosis
  - Primary: caused by loss of HCO_3^- via gastrointestinal (e.g., diarrhea) or kidneys (e.g., renal failure, renal tubular acidosis)
  - Compensatory: renal retention secondary to primary respiratory alkalosis (chronic)

Next Diagnostic Steps to Consider if Levels are High
- Evaluate in relation to serum [Na^+], acid-base balance.
- Calculate serum $[Cl^-]_{corrected}$ to determine if proportional change relative to [Na^+]:

$$\text{Corrected } Cl^- = (\text{mean normal } Na^+/\text{measured } Na^+) \times \text{Measured } Cl^-$$

Reference interval for $[Cl^-]_{corrected}$ is the same as for [Cl^-].

Causes of Abnormally Low Levels
- With proportional decrease in serum [Na^+]: same as hyponatremia (see p. 1382).
- Without proportional decrease in [Na^+]:
  - Primary hypochloremic metabolic alkalosis: gastrointestinal loss/sequestration (gastric vomiting, upper GI obstruction)
  - Compensatory hypochloremic metabolic alkalosis: renal loss secondary to chronic respiratory acidosis
  - Other: hyperadrenocorticism

Next Diagnostic Steps to Consider if Levels are Low

- Evaluate in relation to [Na^+], acid-base balance.
- Calculate corrected serum [Cl^-] to determine if proportional change.

Drug Effects

- Decreased: thiazide or loop diuretics, $NaHCO_3^-$, glucocorticoids
- Increased: NH_4Cl, KCl, hypertonic saline, acetazolamide, spironolactone. Halides cause artifactual increase.

Lab Artifacts

- Marked hyperlipidemia or hyperglobulinemia may decrease measured [Cl^-] by electrolyte exclusion effect (if using indirect potentiometry). Serum osmolality is normal.
- False increase: halides (bromide, iodide) are measured as Cl^- if using potentiometry.
- Sample handling: Cl^- increases if free water loss from improperly stoppered tube.

Specimen Collection and Handling

Serum (red top tube) preferred; heparinized plasma (green top tube) may be used.

Relative Cost: Individual test, electrolyte panel or other partial panels: \$; included in full chemistry panel: \$\$

Pearls

- If corrected chloride is within reference interval, changes in chloride are due to changes in free water and differentials for hyponatremia or hypernatremia are investigated. Corrected chloride outside reference interval suggests an acid-base disturbance and should be interpreted with HCO_3^- and anion gap.
- Most reference laboratory methods are subject to electrolyte exclusion effect artifacts. Portable point-of-care analyzer methods usually not affected.

AUTHOR: Mary Leissinger, DVM, MS, DACVP
EDITOR: Lois Roth-Johnson, DVM, PhD, DACVP

Cholesterol

Definition

- Lipid found only in animal tissues. Test measures circulating blood (serum) concentration.
- *Hyperlipidemia* signifies hypercholesterolemia and/or hypertriglyceridemia.

Physiology

Synthesized by the liver or absorbed from diet in the intestines, cholesterol is essential to life as a major component of cell membranes and precursor for synthesis of steroid hormones and bile acids. The liver is the major site of cholesterol synthesis, excretion, and catabolism. Cholesterol and other lipids are insoluble in water. They are transported in blood attached to apoproteins. Lipid–apoprotein complexes are called *lipoproteins*. They contain variable proportions of triglycerides, cholesterol, cholesterol esters, and phospholipid. In laboratory analysis, lipoproteins can be separated by ultracentrifugation into chylomicra, high-density lipoproteins (HDL), intermediate-density lipoproteins, low-density lipoproteins (LDL), and very-low-density lipoproteins (VLDL), but the clinical importance of lipoprotein profiling in small animal medicine is minimal compared to human medicine.

Reference Interval

Dogs: 112-328 mg/dL. Cats: 82-218 mg/dL. Unit conversion: 38.7 mg/dL = 1 mmol/L.

Causes of Abnormally High Levels

- Primary hyperlipidemia: idiopathic in schnauzer dogs; hypercholesterolemia of Briard dogs, Doberman pinschers, and rottweilers; familial hyperchylomicronemia of cats
- Secondary hyperlipidemia: postprandial (most common), hypothyroidism, diabetes mellitus, liver disease, cholestasis, hyperadrenocorticism, pancreatitis, nephrotic syndrome
- See pp. 496 and 1236.

Next Diagnostic Steps to Consider if Levels are High

- Ensure that blood sample was drawn after ≥ 12-hour fast.
- Assess for causes of secondary hyperlipidemia (endocrine or metabolic disease). If no cause is identified, consider primary hyperlipidemia.

Causes of Abnormally Low Levels

Chronic liver disease, hypoadrenocorticism, intestinal lymphangiectasia, starvation

Next Diagnostic Steps to Consider if Levels are Low

Clinical evaluation for disorders listed above.

Important Interspecies Differences

Dogs and cats are resistant to atherosclerosis, partly owing to the low concentration of very-low-density lipoproteins in these species. High-density lipoproteins are the major lipoproteins in dogs and cats.

Drug Effects

- Increase: exogenous corticosteroids, phenytoin, methimazole
- Decrease: lipid-lowering diets, bile acid sequestrants, hepatic hydroxymethylglutaryl coenzyme A reductase inhibitors (statins), and dirlotapide lower serum cholesterol levels

Lab Artifacts

Increase: hemolysis

Specimen Collection and Handling

- 10- to 12-hour fast is required, but postprandial hypercholesterolemia is mild (usually < 2 times the reference interval).
- Serum (red top tube), heparinized plasma (green top tube), or EDTA plasma (lavender top tube). Stable for 1 week at 2°C-8°C and 4 weeks at −20°C

Relative Cost: Single test \$; included in a variety of panels \$-\$\$

Pearls

- The most common cause for hypercholesterolemia and no other CBC/serum biochemistry abnormalities in an adult, fasted dog is hypothyroidism.
- In icteric dogs, increased cholesterol supports cholestasis while decreased cholesterol supports liver failure.

AUTHOR: Ruanna E. Gossett, DVM, PhD, DACVP
EDITOR: Lois Roth-Johnson, DVM, PhD, DACVP

Coagulation Profile

Definition
Series of tests designed to assess the coagulation pathway and localize specific disorders of coagulation factors that result in hemostatic defects. Consists of prothrombin time (PT), activated partial thromboplastin time (aPTT), and sometimes activated clotting time (ACT).

Synonym
Clotting profile

Physiology
PT, aPTT, and ACT are tests that help evaluate key coagulation factors that make up the coagulation cascade. Coagulation factors are a cascade of enzymes requiring sequential activation. They eventually convert fibrinogen to fibrin, stabilizing the platelet plug. The coagulation cascade is divided into overlapping intrinsic, extrinsic, and common pathways. Activation of the extrinsic pathway is through tissue thromboplastin (released from cell surface membranes of injured tissues), and the intrinsic pathway is initiated by contact activation of injured vessel basement membrane by negatively charged surfaces of collagen or platelets.

Reference Interval
- ACT: specific for tube/activator used
- aPTT: typically 8.6-12.9 seconds (dogs) and 13.7-30.2 seconds (cats)
- PT: typically 5.1-7.9 seconds (dogs) and 8.4-10.8 seconds (cats)

Causes of Abnormally High Levels
- Prolonged PT: extrinsic (factor VII) or common coagulation (X, V, II, thrombin, and fibrinogen) pathway defect; most sensitive test of anticoagulant rodenticide intoxication; vitamin K deficiency/antagonism, decrease/absence of extrinsic or common pathway factors, disseminated intravascular coagulation (DIC), antiphospholipid antibodies, antibodies to coagulation factors, biliary obstruction, liver failure
- Prolonged aPTT: defects in intrinsic pathway (factors XII, XI, IX, VIII); hemophilia, severe von Willebrand disease (von Willebrand factor is carrier protein for factor VIII), DIC, vitamin K antagonism or absence, bile insufficiency, infiltrative bowel disease, exocrine pancreatic insufficiency, or liver failure
- Prolonged ACT: any disorder that sufficiently increases PT, aPTT, or both (common pathway), marked thrombocytopenia

Next Diagnostic Steps to Consider if Levels are High
Platelet count, fibrin degradation products, specific factor analysis

See pp. 431, 433, and 1202.

Important Interspecies Differences
Factor XII deficiency will cause markedly prolonged aPTT without hemorrhage in cats.

Drug Effects
Increased: warfarin toxicity, anticoagulant drugs (e.g., heparin, factor Xa inhibitors)

Lab Artifacts
Increase: inadequately filled tubes (causes specimen dilution by anticoagulant); traumatic venipuncture

Specimen Collection and Handling
Citrated plasma (blue top tube) for PT and aPTT. Fill tubes completely, refrigerate, send to lab on ice. Commercial ACT tube (various available) test performed in clinic.

Relative Cost: $$

Pearls
- A coagulation profile is indicated if the patient is bleeding into muscles or joints, has unexplained bleeding into body cavities, or develops hematomas after blood draw.
- A coagulation profile is indicated before liver biopsy.
- ACT is a poorly sensitive point-of-care test that should be followed up with PT and aPTT.
- Low PT, aPTT, ACT values are not reliable to detect a procoagulant or thrombogenic state.

AUTHOR: Deborah G. Davis, DVM, DACVP
EDITOR: Lois Roth-Johnson, DVM, PhD, DACVP

Cobalamin

Definition
Water-soluble vitamin with a porphyrin ring

Synonyms
Cyanocobalamin, vitamin B_{12}

Physiology
Source is dietary. Released from food during gastric digestion and bound to R-proteins. Transferred to intrinsic factor (IF) in alkaline intestinal pH. IF is produced by gastric parietal cells in dogs and by the exocrine pancreas in dogs and cats; it enhances ileal cobalamin absorption. Cobalamin has hepatic storage. It is a required cofactor in pathways involving folate and formation of succinyl coenzyme A. If the latter is impaired by cobalamin deficiency or decreased intracellular availability, methylmalonic acid accumulates, and defective formation of neuronal lipids causes neurologic disease.

Reference Interval
- Dogs: 250-910 ng/L; cats: 290-1500 ng/L
- Unit conversion: 1 pg/mL = 0.1 ng/dL; 1 pg/mL × 0.7378 = pmol/L

Causes of Abnormally High Levels
Uncommon; dietary supplementation and possibly hepatocellular necrosis

Next Diagnostic Steps to Consider if Levels are High
Review oral or parenteral supplements; assess for hepatic disease.

Causes of Abnormally Low Levels
Decreased absorption due to ileal diseases such as inflammation, villous atrophy, neoplasia; decreased IF production due to gastric disease in dogs and exocrine pancreatic insufficiency in dogs and cats; congenital hypocobalaminemia due to malabsorption or insufficiency of IF in giant schnauzers, border collies, other canine breeds, and rarely cats; small intestinal bacterial overgrowth (intestinal dysbiosis) as enteric bacteria bind cobalamin.

Next Diagnostic Steps to Consider if Levels are Low
Rule out artifact due to sample light exposure. Assess for intestinal diseases and for exocrine pancreatic insufficiency (serum trypsin-like immunoreactivity).

Drug Effects
Oral or parenteral supplements increase concentration.

Lab Artifacts
- Falsely decreased by excessive light exposure
- Assays for human samples are unreliable in dogs and cats.

Specimen Collection and Handling

Serum (red top tube), 1 mL, collected after overnight fast; separate serum from clot. Store refrigerated. Freeze if greater than 24 hours before testing.

Relative Cost: $$ (cobalamin only); $$$ (cobalamin and folate); $$$ (cobalamin, folate, and trypsin-like immunoreactivity)

Pearls

- Evaluate in conjunction with folate and trypsin-like immunoreactivity.
- Dietary deficiency is uncommon as cobalamin is abundant in commercial pet foods.
- Although low values may be seen, assessment of cobalamin levels is no longer considered reliable for the diagnosis of intestinal bacterial overgrowth/dysbiosis.
- Cobalamin concentration within the reference interval does not rule out intestinal disease.
- Gastrointestinal diseases often respond to treatment poorly until cobalamin supplementation is begun.

AUTHOR: Shelley Burton, DVM, MSc, DACVP
EDITOR: Lois Roth-Johnson, DVM, PhD, DACVP

Coccidiodes Serology

Definition

Coccidioides immitis is a dimorphic soil fungus that is found in the lower Sonoran life zone (Arizona, Southern California, and New Mexico in the southwestern United States and in parts of Mexico); it can cause serious illness in infected dogs. Serologic testing is used to help confirm suspected infection and is especially useful when cytologic samples from diseased tissue are not readily available or when organism is not visualized.

Synonyms

Coccidioidomycosis, Valley fever

Physiology

Infection is acquired via inhalation of anthroconidia/anthrospores from soil, followed by development of pulmonary disease with potential dissemination to skeletal system, lymph nodes, eyes, heart, lungs, central nervous system, and other visceral organs.

Reference Interval

Reference intervals vary among laboratories and test methodologies. Both IgG (chronic) and IgM (acute) testing can be performed, as can antigen assays (less sensitive than antibody assays).

Causes of Abnormally High Levels

Interpretation of reported values is highly dependent on test methodology. Check with specific laboratory.

- Agar gel immunodiffusion (AGID): can detect IgM and/or IgG antibodies. False-positive results (especially at low titer) are common.
- Latex agglutination: detects immunoglobulin M (IgM) that occurs early in infection. False-positive results common.
- Enzyme-linked immunosorbent assay (ELISA): cross-reactive with antibody to other fungi
  - IgM: ≈15% false-positive; occurs early in infection
  - IgG: indicates chronic infection

Less commonly used tests:

- Complement fixation antibody: detects IgM. Positive in early infection
- Tube precipitation antibody: detects IgG. Positive with active infections and postexposure. Titers ≥64 are seen more commonly with severe pulmonary or disseminated disease.
- *Coccidioides* galactomannan antigen assay: poor sensitivity

Next Diagnostic Steps to Consider if Levels are High

Consider confirmation with cytology or histology if feasible. Culture is not recommended, especially in a private clinical setting, as the organism is highly infectious to humans. See p. 184.

Causes of Abnormally Low Levels

- Uninfected animal
- False-negative results: insufficient time for seroconversion, severely immunocompromised, other

Important Interspecies Differences

Antibodies may persist in cats for years even with therapy (dependent on assay type).

Lab Artifacts

- Cross-reactivity with *Blastomyces* sp. is possible in ELISA tests.
- False-negative complement fixation antibody test in dogs may be due to interference from anticomplement factors in 15%-25% of normal dog sera.

Specimen Collection and Handling

Serum (red top tube), single sample or paired samples obtained 4-6 weeks apart. Refrigerate. Titers can be run on cerebrospinal fluid.

Relative Cost: $$

Pearls

- Rising titers over time may suggest poor drug therapeutic response.

AUTHOR: Erin N. Burton, DVM, MS, DACVP
EDITOR: Lois Roth-Johnson, DVM, PhD, DACVP

Colloid Osmotic Pressure (COP)

Definition

The pressure exerted by large non-permeant proteins that promotes intravascular fluid retention and maintains blood volume.

Synonym

Oncotic pressure

Physiology

The movement of fluid across capillary membranes is mediated through Starling's forces, which include hydrostatic and colloid osmotic pressures generated both intravascularly and interstitially. Albumin is responsible for ≈80% of the colloid osmotic pressure (COP), with minor contributions from globulins and fibrinogen. With normal vascular integrity, these proteins are unable to traverse the vascular membrane, preventing fluid movement to the interstitial space. COP also stimulates intravascular fluid shifting through an osmotic effect, the Gibbs-Donnan effect. As plasma colloidal proteins are anions, permeant cations (e.g., sodium) will readily diffuse into the intravascular space, maintaining electroneutrality and increasing plasma osmolality.

Reference Interval

- Dog: 14-27 mm Hg
- Cat: 21-34 mm Hg

Causes of Abnormally High Levels

Not clinically significant. Hemoglobinemia (hemolysis), recent treatment with colloid solutions (e.g., plasma, Hetastarch), and hyperglobulinemia (e.g., feline infectious peritonitis, multiple myeloma)

Next Diagnostic Steps to Consider if Levels are High

Rule out recent treatment with colloid solutions. Assess for hemolytic anemia and hyperglobulinemia.

Causes of Abnormally Low Levels

Hypoalbuminemia (hemorrhage, exudative lesions, hepatic failure, intestinal or renal loss [p. 1239]); acidemia (decreases the Gibbs-Donnan effect)

Next Diagnostic Steps to Consider if Levels are Low

Evaluate for blood/albumin loss, hepatic failure, sepsis/systemic inflammatory response syndrome, acidemia.

Drug Effects

Colloid solutions will increase the COP. The oncotic effects of plasma last longer than synthetic colloids (e.g., Hetastarch) as albumin has a longer circulating half-life than synthetic colloids.

Lab Artifacts

In vitro hemolysis may cause a falsely increased COP.

Specimen Collection and Handling

Serum (red top tube) or plasma (lavender top tube); separate from cells as soon as possible. COP is measured with a commercial colloid osmometer.

Relative Cost: $$

Pearls

- Patients with acute decreases in COP (e.g., secondary to acute hemorrhage) are more likely to develop hypovolemia, hypoxia, and edema compared to patients with chronic hypoalbuminemia (e.g., secondary to protein-losing enteropathy or nephropathy).
- Not offered by most reference laboratories; may be available through teaching hospitals or specialty/emergency hospitals or clinics.

AUTHOR: Shannon D. Dehghanpir, DVM, MS, DACVP
EDITOR: Lois Roth-Johnson, DVM, PhD, DACVP

Complete Blood Count (CBC)

Definition

A group of routine hematologic tests for measuring several parameters of erythrocytes, leukocytes, and platelets. Tests include indicators of circulating erythrocyte mass (e.g., hematocrit, hemoglobin, erythrocyte concentration), measurement of erythrocyte size and hemoglobin concentration (e.g., MCV, MCHC), reticulocytes, total and differential leukocyte concentrations, platelet concentration and size, and evaluation of morphology of blood cells on a stained blood smear. A refractometric total plasma protein concentration is often included.

Synonyms

CBC, hemogram

Physiology

Leukocytes, erythrocytes, and platelets are produced in the bone marrow and then enter peripheral circulation for various lengths of time. Increased or decreased numbers of cells in an aliquot of blood can be relative or absolute. Abnormalities in cell numbers often suggest specific disorders, including systemic disease or, less often, bone marrow disorders. In addition to changes in cell number, microscopic examination of cell size and shape, or the presence of cellular inclusions, can provide crucial clues as to disease presence.

Reference Interval

See specific cell types.

Specimen Collection and Handling

EDTA (lavender top tube) blood sample and freshly prepared blood smear for lab to stain. If in-clinic hematology analyzer is available, follow manufacturer recommendations and examine a stained blood smear.

Relative Cost: $$

Abnormal Erythrocyte	Appearance	Clinical Relevance
Acanthocyte (spur cell)		Associated with vascular, liver, or renal disease
Codocyte (target cell)		Regenerative anemia; liver or renal disease; abnormal lipid metabolism
Eccentrocyte		Oxidative injury
Keratocyte		Vascular disease, including hemangiosarcoma and disseminated intravascular coagulation
Heinz body		Oxidative injury
Leptocyte		Iron deficiency
Schistocyte		Vascular disease including hemangiosarcoma, disseminated intravascular coagulation
Spherocyte		Immune-mediated hemolysis or partial phagocytosis; unlike small red blood cells (microcytosis), spherocytes have no central pallor

COMPLETE BLOOD COUNT Erythrocyte abnormalities. See discussion of various red blood cell morphologic abnormalities (i.e., poikilocytosis).

Pearls

Know how the laboratory you use determines differential leukocyte concentrations and whether blood smears are examined routinely. Although automated hematology analyzers provide three- or five-part differential leukocyte counts as part of a CBC, the differential counts obtained from microscopic examination of stained blood smears remain the most accurate method for differentiating leukocytes, detecting left shifts and toxic changes in neutrophils, and for recognition of shape changes.

See discussion of various red blood cell morphologic abnormalities (p. 1374).

AUTHOR: Stephen D. Gaunt, DVM, PhD, DACVP
EDITOR: Lois Roth-Johnson, DVM, PhD, DACVP

Coombs' Test

Definition

Detects immunoglobulin or complement bound to the surface of erythrocytes to aid in the diagnosis of primary or secondary immune-mediated hemolytic anemia

Synonym

Direct antiglobulin test (DAT)

Physiology

Patient erythrocytes are washed with saline to remove nonspecific bound surface proteins. Species-specific Coombs' reagent is added that includes polyvalent antisera that will bind to IgM, IgG, and complement (C3) bound to the surface of the patient's erythrocytes, resulting in agglutination.

Reference Interval

Reported as "no agglutination" or "agglutination observed" at a specific titer. Typically incubated to body temperature, but some laboratories report room temperature results as well (i.e., cold agglutinins)

Causes of Abnormally High Levels

Primary or secondary immune-mediated hemolytic anemia (IMHA), prior blood transfusion

Next Diagnostic Steps to Consider if Levels are High

See p. 60.

Causes of Abnormally Low Levels

Look for non–immune-mediated causes of hemolysis (see p. 59), but false-negative tests occur, so negative test cannot rule out IMHA.

Important Interspecies Differences

Species-specific reagents are required to perform this test.

Drug Effects

Treatment with glucocorticoids or other immunosuppressive drugs may result in a false-negative test. Prior transfusions can cause positive result.

Lab Artifacts

- Prozone reaction is common when the ratio of antibody to antigen is inappropriate, resulting in false-positives.
- Hemolysis suggests that there was formation of immune complexes between antisera and surface-bound immunoglobulins
- False-negative may occur with low surface-bound immunoglobulins and/or C3, weakly bound immune complexes that were eluted during washing, or detachment of immunoglobulin or C3 from sample aging.

Specimen Collection and Handling

Whole blood collected in EDTA (lavender top tube). Store at 8°C. Test as soon as possible.

Relative Cost: $$

Pearls

- Coombs' testing is not standardized and is often unnecessary given other clinical pathology data.
- Negative Coombs' testing does not rule out IMHA.
- Positive test results do not confirm primary IMHA, and secondary causes, such as infectious disease or neoplasia, should be ruled out.
- Coombs' test provides no information regarding immune-mediated disease other than IMHA.

AUTHOR: Erin N. Burton, DVM, MS, DACVP
EDITOR: Lois Roth-Johnson, DVM, PhD, DACVP

Cortisol

Definition

Cortisol is a glucocorticoid that has far-reaching effects on gluconeogenesis, lipolysis, immune responses, and water balance, among other things. Cortisol measurement is useful in diagnosing patients with hypoadrenocorticism and hyperadrenocorticism. Baseline value alone is insufficient for diagnosis and instead is compared with another value (example, cortisol to ACTH ratio or urine cortisol to creatinine ratio) or measured at multiple time points during the ACTH stimulation test, low-dose dexamethasone suppression test, or high-dose dexamethasone suppression test.

Physiology

ACTH release from the pituitary promotes adrenocortical secretion of cortisol. Increasing cortisol concentration in the blood will normally inhibit further ACTH production, facilitating homeostasis. Cortisol concentration fluctuates throughout the day and can be affected by disease states, other stressors, and drug administration. Pathologic hypercortisolemia is the main feature of hyperadrenocorticism, attributable to either overproduction of ACTH or direct overproduction of cortisol from a functional adrenal cortical neoplasm. Atrophy or destruction of the adrenal cortices results in hypoadrenocorticism, including hypocortisolemia.

Reference Interval

Varies by laboratory, and commonly expressed as either mcg/dL or nmol/L. Interpret in light of established reference interval for species by given laboratory and testing methodology.

Causes of Abnormally High Levels

Hyperadrenocorticism, general illness, or other stressors

Next Diagnostic Steps to Consider if Levels are High

In a patient with suspected hyperadrenocorticism, baseline cortisol concentration is of limited value. Instead, ACTH stimulation testing or low-dose dexamethasone suppression testing should be performed (p. 485).

Causes of Abnormally Low Levels

Hypoadrenocorticism, administration of steroids, or treatment with ketoconazole, trilostane, mitotane

Next Diagnostic Steps to Consider if Levels are Low

If hypoadrenocorticism is suspected, ACTH stimulation testing should be performed for confirmation (p. 512).

Drug Effects

Cortisol assays may cross-react with pharmacologic steroids administered within 24 hours, including prednisolone, 11-deoxycortisol, prednisone, and others. Ketoconazole inhibits steroid synthesis. Trilostane and mitotane are used therapeutically to decrease cortisol production.

Lab Artifacts

- Do not use serum separator tubes for blood collection; gel from serum separator tubes can interfere with cortisol measurement.
- EDTA contamination and icterus invalidate results. Multiple assay types available; use a reputable laboratory with validated results for dogs and cats.

Specimen Collection and Handling

Collect blood into plain red top tubes, allow to clot, centrifuge, and transfer serum to a separate tube clearly labeled with the sample ID/time. Ship samples frozen or refrigerated, on ice.

Relative Cost: Cortisol $$; urine cortisol: creatinine ratio $$

Pearls

- Baseline cortisol concentration can fluctuate and so is of limited value.
- Baseline cortisol > 2 mcg/dL effectively rules out hypoadrenocorticism, but cortisol below this cut-off warrants confirmatory testing (generally ACTH stimulation test).
- Urine cortisol to creatinine ratio can be used as a screening test for hyperadrenocorticism; however, diagnosis requires ACTH stimulation testing or low-dose dexamethasone suppression testing.

AUTHOR: Angela Royal, MS, DVM, DACVP
EDITOR: Lois Roth-Johnson, DVM, PhD, DACVP

Creatine Kinase (CK)

Definition

Cytosolic enzyme with highest activity in skeletal muscle, cardiac muscle, smooth muscle, brain, and nerves. Skeletal muscle injury is responsible for clinically significant increases in serum concentrations in dogs and cats.

Synonym

Creatine phosphokinase (CPK)

Physiology

- CK is critical for energy production causing muscle contraction.
- CK catalyzes the formation of adenosine triphosphate (ATP) by transfer of high-energy phosphate from creatine phosphate to adenosine diphosphate (ADP). Catalyzes the reverse reaction when muscles are at rest
- Serum CK activity is primarily of muscle origin, and is a sensitive indicator of skeletal muscle damage.
- CK is released into the interstitium when muscle membranes become damaged. Plasma concentration increases 4-6 hours after injury and peaks at approximately 12 hours. Values return to normal within 24-48 hours.
- The half-life in blood is approximately 2-4 hours. Persistently increased serum CK concentrations indicate ongoing muscle damage.
- CK isoenzymes may be measured to more specifically localize muscle damage to cardiac or skeletal muscle. CK isoenzyme measurements are not routinely used in veterinary medicine. In human cardiology, other biomarkers have superseded CK (pp. 1369 and 1389).

Reference Interval

Dogs: 10-200 U/L; cats: 64-440 U/L

Causes of Abnormally High Levels

Trauma, exertion, seizures, malignant hyperthermia, intramuscular injections, degenerative muscle disease, infectious and noninfectious (metabolic, toxic, immune-mediated, nutritional) myopathies, muscle ischemia/necrosis (e.g., arterial thromboembolism), anorexia in cats resulting in muscle catabolism

Next Diagnostic Steps to Consider if Levels are High

Evaluate for muscle disease or injury, or muscle catabolism. In dogs, as in people, serum cardiac troponin-I levels are probably more sensitive and specific for myocardial damage than CK myocardial isoenzyme.

Important Interspecies Differences

Increased serum CK is common in anorexic cats.

Lab Artifacts

- Increase: hemolysis, lipemia, hyperbilirubinemia, contamination of blood with muscle fluid during difficult venipuncture; dilution of samples (attributed to dilution of CK inhibitors in serum)
- Decrease: collection in citrate (blue top tube) or sodium fluoride (gray top tube)

Specimen Collection and Handling

Serum (red top tube), heparinized plasma (green top tube), or EDTA plasma (lavender top tube). Refrigerated samples are stable for 8-12 hours; samples stored at −20°C are stable for 2-3 days.

Relative Cost: $

Pearls

Persistent exceedingly high CK levels (e.g., > 200,000 U/L) are strongly suggestive of muscular dystrophy.

AUTHOR: Ruanna E. Gossett, DVM, PhD, DACVP
EDITOR: Lois Roth-Johnson, DVM, PhD, DACVP

Creatinine

Definition

Creatinine is a waste product from degradation of muscle creatine.

Physiology

Creatinine is continuously produced from degradation of muscle phosphocreatine and creatine, and is excreted in urine. It is freely filtered by glomeruli and is not resorbed by renal tubular cells.

Reference Interval

Dogs 0.6-1.5 mg/dL (53-133 μmol/L); cats: 0.6-2.0 mg/dL (53-177 mcmol/L)

Causes of Abnormally High Levels

- Decreased glomerular filtration rate (prerenal, renal, or postrenal)
- Animals with greater muscle mass (e.g., greyhounds) or recent high-protein meal (e.g., cooked meat) may have mild increase.
- Artifact (e.g., vitamin C)

Next Diagnostic Steps to Consider if Levels are High

Check serum urea (BUN) concentration and urine specific gravity concurrently. Urea and creatinine concentrations increase in parallel in most renal/urinary disorders; isosthenuria and parallel increase in BUN support renal azotemia. Check medication history and possible sources of artifact if creatinine increased but BUN normal.

Causes of Abnormally Low Levels

- Thin body condition/muscle
- Increased glomerular filtration rate
- Artifact (e.g., severe icterus)

Next Diagnostic Steps to Consider if Levels are Low

Evaluate for muscle loss/pathologic weight loss. Exclude normal variation (e.g., young animals) or artifact.

Drug Effects

Cephalosporins, vitamin C may cause spurious increase.

Lab Artifacts

Severe icterus may artifactually lower values. High levels of certain chromogens (e.g., glucose, ketones, vitamin C) may artifactually increase values.

Specimen Collection and Handling

Serum (red top tube) or heparinized plasma (green top tube)

Relative Cost: $$ (part of full panel); $ (single test)

Pearls

The creatinine reference interval is wide, though values for an individual healthy patient are maintained tightly. Therefore, trend of increase in a single patient's creatinine is clinically important even when total remains within reference interval.

AUTHOR: Mary Leissinger, DVM, MS, DACVP
EDITOR: Lois Roth-Johnson, DVM, PhD, DACVP

Cross-Matching

Definition

Laboratory procedure to detect antibodies between a patient and a potential blood donor. The *major cross-match* involves patient's serum and donor blood cells; the *minor cross-match* uses donor serum and the patient's blood cells.

Physiology

Major cross-match determines if there are agglutinating and/or hemolytic antibodies in a potential blood recipient that would react with antigens on donor blood cells. Antibodies may be naturally occurring (all cats) or induced by a previous mismatched transfusion (any species). Incompatible transfusion can lead to adverse outcome, though incompatible minor cross-match is seldom associated with severe transfusion reactions.

Reference Interval

Lack of agglutination or hemolysis indicates recipient-donor compatibility.

Causes of Abnormally High Levels

Agglutination (either macroscopic or microscopic) or significant hemolysis in the cross-match tubes but not in control indicates an incompatible donor.

Important Interspecies Differences

Cats have naturally occurring antibodies, and cross-matching should always be performed before transfusion, regardless of previous transfusion history. Transfusion of type A blood into type B cats causes hemolysis (in minutes to 2 days) and severe anaphylaxis.

Drug Effects

Glucocorticoids and other immunosuppressants may mask incompatibility.

Lab Artifacts

Agglutination in the control tubes (patient serum added to patient red blood cells [RBCs] or donor serum added to donor RBCs) indicates reagent contamination or autoagglutination.

Specimen Collection and Handling

Two tubes are preferred, one EDTA (lavender top tube) and one tube without anticoagulant (red top tube or serum separator tube).

Relative Cost: $$

Pearls

- A compatible cross-match does not indicate that the animal and the donor have the same blood type; it merely means that erythrocyte antibodies were not detected. Therefore blood typing remains essential in all donors and recipients.
- Cross-match should be performed before all repeat transfusions performed more than a few days apart, regardless of blood type or results of prior cross-match.
- This test does not identify antibodies against WBCs, platelets, or plasma proteins.
- Cross-match can be performed in clinic (p. 1084)

AUTHOR: Deborah G. Davis, DVM, DACVP
EDITOR: Lois Roth-Johnson, DVM, PhD, DACVP

Cryptococcus Antigen Test

Definition

Cryptococcus is an environmental saprophytic, dimorphic fungus with worldwide distribution. The *Cryptococcus* antigen test detects cryptococcal polysaccharide capsular antigen, in the yeast form, within serum or cerebrospinal fluid (CSF).

Physiology

Inhalation of organisms is the presumed method of transmission. Clinical presentation depends on the size of the inoculum, virulence of the strain, and host defenses. Nasal or pulmonary infections are most common, but dissemination to the central nervous system (CNS), eyes, skin, bones, and lymph nodes also occurs. The organism's variably thick, polysaccharide capsule inhibits phagocytosis; thus degree of inflammation observed on cytology or histopathology can vary.

Reference Interval

Initial screening done on undiluted samples; positive serum or CSF usually titered to endpoint values. Positive titer values vary by reference laboratory.

Causes of Abnormally High Levels

Latex agglutination test (LAT) for cryptococcal polysaccharide capsular antigen is widely available in most reference laboratories. Sensitivity and specificity of these assays is approximately 90%; however, false-positives can occur.

Next Diagnostic Steps to Consider if Levels are High

Histopathologic evaluation, cytologic diagnosis, or culture may be helpful to confirm and is recommended with low titers (typically <200). See p. 223.

Lab Artifacts

Serum separator tube (SST) gel, lipemia, hemolysis, specimen turbidity, and anticoagulants interfere with testing.

Specimen Collection and Handling

- Collect blood in a plain red top tube; do not use SST. Spin and collect serum. Fasted samples are preferred. Serum is stable for up to 48 hours if stored at 2°C-8°C. Freeze (non–frost-free freezer to avoid defrost cycles) for longer sample storage. CSF, 1 mL, collected in a sterile tube with no additives; process immediately or freeze.
- CSF is preferred if CNS signs are present; may be more sensitive.

Relative Cost: $$

Pearls

- LAT can be used to monitor therapy as titers should decrease to zero with disease resolution.
- Titers from different laboratories using different methodologies can vary considerably; using the same methodology is necessary for serial titer interpretation.

AUTHOR: Erin N. Burton, DVM, MS
EDITOR: Lois Roth-Johnson, DVM, PhD, DACVP

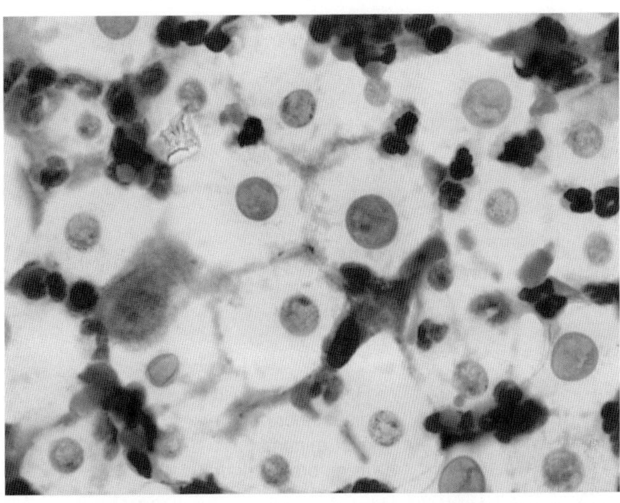

***CRYPTOCOCCUS* ANTIGEN TESTING.** Modified Wright Giemsa at 100x objective. Cytologic specimens from a nasal mass in a cat with *Cryptococcus* sp. suspected *Cryptococcus neoformans.*

Crystals, Urine Sediment

Definition

Precipitation of urinary solutes

Synonyms

Crystalluria

Physiology

Urinary crystal formation depends on several factors, including the concentration of urinary solutes, urine pH, urinary flow rate, temperature, and storage. Supersaturation of urinary solutes is influenced by hydration status, diet, and medications. Urine pH and solubility factors are helpful tools in identifying crystals. Inorganic salts (e.g., phosphate, ammonium, magnesium) are less soluble in neutral or alkaline pH, while organic solutes (e.g., bilirubin, uric acid, cystine) more commonly crystallize in acidic urine. Decreased urine flow and temperatures (refrigeration) can promote crystal formation.

Reference Interval

- Reported as the number of specific crystals per 40x microscopic field objective
- Some crystals can be observed in the urine of healthy dogs and cats (see below).

Causes of Abnormally High Levels

- Struvite, calcium oxalate dihydrate, and brushite: healthy dog or cat, urolithiasis
- Ammonium biurate and uric acid: portosystemic shunt, hepatic dysfunction
- Bilirubin: healthy dog, bilirubinuria
- Calcium oxalate monohydrate and dihydrate: ethylene glycol toxicosis, hyperoxaluria/calciuria
- Cystine: inherited defect of urinary cystine transport (cystinuria)

Next Diagnostic Steps to Consider if Levels are High

Review signalment, diet, and medication history. Evaluate for hepatic failure or acute kidney injury. Perform urine culture and sensitivity if indicated (e.g., struvite crystalluria).

Important Interspecies Differences

Ammonium biurate crystals may be found in healthy Dalmatians and English bulldogs.

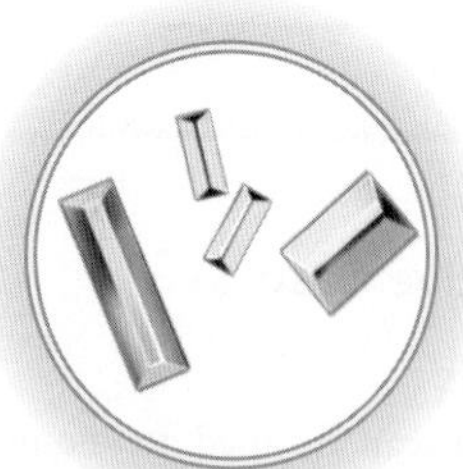

Common in dogs (infection) and cats (nutrition), especially with alkaline urine or as artifact

Ammonium magnesium phosphate (triple phosphate, struvite)

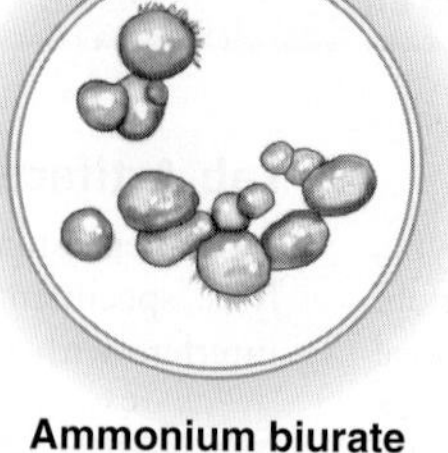

Infrequent in healthy patients except Dalmatians and English bulldogs; if numerous, suggests liver dysfunction or shunt in dogs and cats

Ammonium biurate

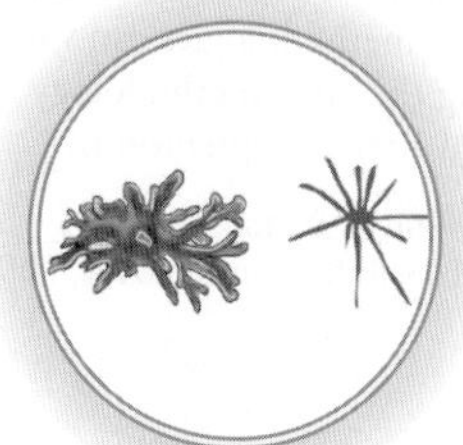

Associated with bilirubinuria

Bilirubin

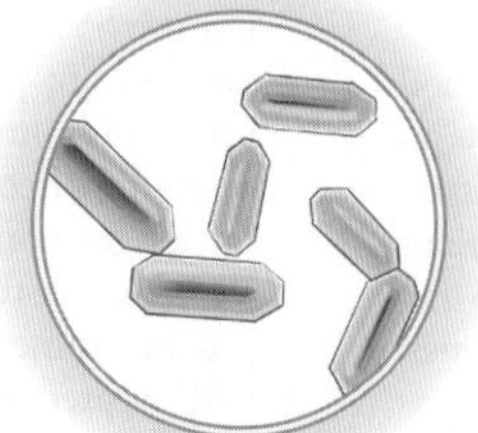

Suggests ethylene glycol intoxication

Calcium oxalate monohydrate

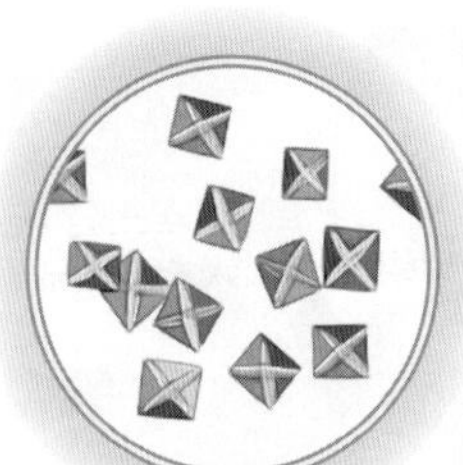

Seen in healthy patients; suggests ethylene glycol intoxication

Calcium oxalate dihydrate

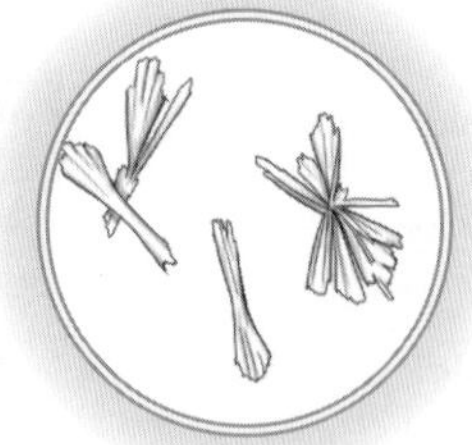

Seen in healthy dogs

Calcium phosphate

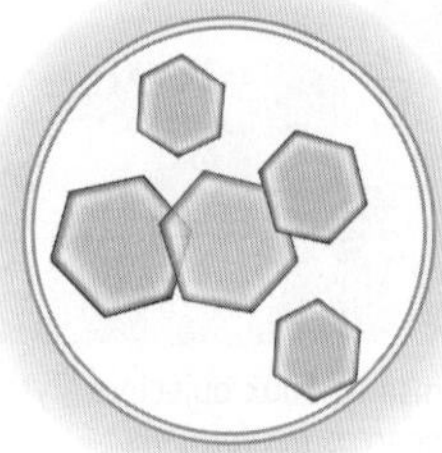

Rare; suggests liver disease or primary cyst(e)inuria (e.g., breed-related)

Cyst(e)ine

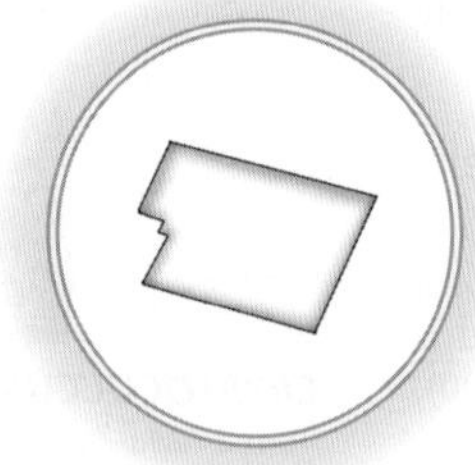

Uncommon in healthy dogs; may occur with hypercholesterolemia or renal disease

Cholesterol

Sulfa, contrast media; renal elimination of material

Drug crystals

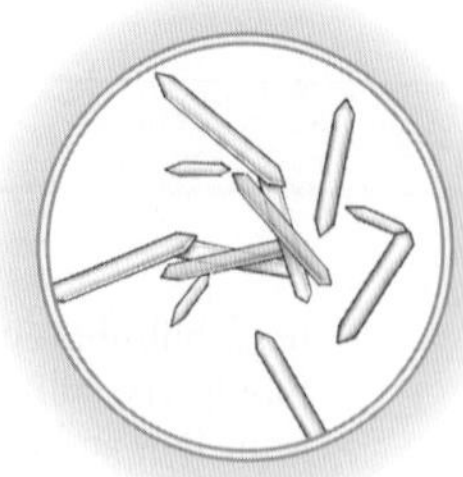

Rare; should be distinguished from calcium oxalate monohydrate (history, physical exam)

Hippuric acid

CRYSTALS IN URINE SEDIMENT

Drug Effects

Crystals may form with urinary excretion of certain antibiotics (e.g., sulfonamides) and radiographic contrast agents.

Lab Artifacts

Evaluation of fresh urine yields most accurate results, as delayed sampling and refrigeration (storage) can dissolve or promote crystal formation, respectively.

Specimen Collection and Handling

Process immediately for best results. If refrigerated, allow urine to reach room temperature before analyzing.

Relative Cost: $ (as part of urinalysis)

Pearls

There are several variations of calcium oxalate monohydrate crystals. Care must be taken to avoid misidentifying calcium oxalate monohydrate crystals as calcium carbonate crystals, which do not occur in the urine of cats and dogs.

AUTHOR: Shannon D. Dehghanpir, DVM, MS, DACVP
EDITOR: Lois Roth-Johnson, DVM, PhD, DACVP

Culture and Sensitivity, Bacterial

Definition

Bacterial culture techniques grow *(in vitro),* isolate, and characterize potential bacterial pathogens from biological specimens. Bacterial sensitivity (i.e., susceptibility) techniques aid in determination of potential antimicrobial effectiveness against isolated bacterial species.

Synonyms

Culture and susceptibility, C/S

Physiology

For routine bacterial culture, the biological specimen is streaked onto a blood and MacConkey agar culture media and incubated for 24-48 hours. Resultant bacterial colonies are isolated and identified. For antimicrobial susceptibility testing, each bacterial type is exposed to various antimicrobials at a variety of concentrations to assess the ability of each to inhibit bacterial growth.

Reference Interval

- Bacterial isolates are identified by genus and/or species.
- There are multiple ways to determine and report antibacterial susceptibility. These include:
  - Broth dilution method: the isolate is cultured in serial dilutions of antimicrobial compounds. The lowest concentration of antimicrobial that inhibits bacterial growth is the Minimum Inhibitory Concentration (MIC). A predetermined range of acceptable MIC for each pathogen can be used to classify the organism as susceptible, intermediate, or resistant to a given antimicrobial compound. The lower the MIC concentration, the more likely the pathogen is to be responsive to a given antimicrobial compound.
  - Kirby Bauer disk diffusion: a plate of growth media is evenly streaked with the bacterial isolate. Commercially prepared disks impregnated with standard concentrations of antimicrobial compounds are spaced around the plate, which is then incubated. The size of the ring of growth inhibition around the disk correlates with the ability of the compound to inhibit growth, but true MIC cannot be determined.
  - E-test: Commercially available plastic test strips impregnated with gradually decreasing concentration of antimicrobial compounds can be placed on a plate of growth media streaked with bacterial isolate. The strip allows semi-quantitative determination of the ability of the antimicrobial to inhibit bacterial growth.
  - Automated susceptibility testing systems: Various commercial systems used in large laboratories provide automated susceptibility data, usually with an MIC provided.
  - Genotypic methods: though not standard, genotypic methods such as PCR can be used to detect DNA sequences characteristic of antimicrobial resistance.

Causes of Abnormally High Levels

Infection or contamination by bacteria produces growth.

Next Diagnostic Steps to Consider if Levels are High

Multiple factors beyond sensitivity results must be considered when selecting antimicrobials. These include likely *in vivo* response in a given environment (e.g., purulent material inactivates some antimicrobial compounds), bioavailability of the drug in target tissue (e.g., beta-lactams achieve high concentrations in the urinary bladder), specific host factors (e.g., nephrotoxic drugs should be avoided in animals with renal compromise), potential drug interactions or toxicities, route of administration, available formulations, costs, potential drug toxicities, and others.

Causes of Abnormally Low Levels

Inhibition of growth by antimicrobial drugs or other molecules, overgrowth of other bacteria (pathogenic or contaminants), poorly representative specimen or mishandling of specimen, absence of infection

Drug Effects

Previous or ongoing antimicrobial administration may result in false-negative results.

Lab Artifacts

- Contamination (during collection by use of nonsterile containers, prolonged storage at room temperature, or delays in shipment) may result in overgrowth.
- Delays in culture may result in absent growth.
- Contaminant organisms may inhibit growth of more fastidious organisms.

Specimen Collection and Handling

Fresh tissue or fluid in sterile container; culture swab is acceptable for both aerobic and anaerobic culture. Blood specimens should be collected in blood specimen vials containing growth media. Tubes containing microbial preservative are available for urine cultures where a delay in plating is anticipated. Consult laboratory for any specific questions on ideal collection and transport conditions.

Relative Cost: $$

Pearls

- Not all bacteria are easily detected using routine bacteria culture techniques. Fastidious organisms may need special growth media, incubation and atmospheric conditions.
- Microbial susceptibility is seldom provided for anaerobic isolates.
- Special media may be appropriate for sample submission. For example, special blood culture media contain beads that bind and inhibit antimicrobial drugs, improving the chance of bacterial growth in animals that have received antibiotic treatment.
- MIC *in vitro* may not predict resolution of an infection *in vivo*.
- In some instances, use of a drug with a "high MIC" may be appropriate.
- For infections resistant to many antimicrobial compounds, consultation with a specialist is recommended.

AUTHOR: Erin N. Burton, DVM, MS
EDITOR: Lois Roth-Johnson, DVM, PhD, DACVP

Cyclosporine Blood Levels

Definition

Cyclosporine is a potent immunosuppressant drug that impairs T-lymphocyte activation and the downstream immune responses of several inflammatory cells; blood levels are measured as a marker for reaching a therapeutic target.

Physiology

Cyclosporine is used to treat a variety of autoimmune disorders (dermatologic, hematologic), as well as perianal fistulas. Variable pharmacokinetics requires routine monitoring of blood levels, often including both trough and peak samples. Cyclosporine is metabolized in the liver, so patients with liver disease may require dose adjustments. At least 50% of cyclosporine in blood is within erythrocytes.

Reference Interval

Canine range: peak (1.5-2 hours postdose) 800-1400 ng/mL; trough (immediately before next 12-hour dose): 400-600 ng/mL (immunosuppression), 100-300 ng/mL (perianal fistula), 250 ng/mL (inflammatory bowel disease)

Causes of Abnormally High Levels

Overdosage, hepatic dysfunction, interaction with drugs (see below)

Causes of Abnormally Low Levels

Interaction with drugs (see below), insufficient dosage, poor gastrointestinal absorption

Drug Effects

- Coadministration of phenobarbital, phenytoin, trimethoprim-sulfamethoxazole, rifampin, famotidine, octreotide, terbinafine, cyclophosphamide, clindamycin, and azathioprine lower blood cyclosporine levels.
- Coadministration of azole antifungals, amphotericin B, azithromycin, acetazolamide, cisapride, ciprofloxacin/enrofloxacin, corticosteroids, and metronidazole increase blood cyclosporine levels.

Specimen Collection and Handling

EDTA whole blood (lavender top tube). Ship overnight on ice. Check within 3-5 days of initiating therapy, then at 2- to 4-week intervals until steady therapeutic response. Though peak and trough levels are ideal initially, single 2-hour peak sample may be sufficient for long-term monitoring.

Heparinized tubes (green top) are used for pharmacodynamic monitoring.

Relative Cost: $$$$ (peak and trough); $$$ (single sample)

Pearls

- Metabolites may be active, so monitor response to therapy in addition to blood levels of parent compound to reduce risk of toxicosis.
- High Performance Liquid Chromatography (HPLC) was previously considered the gold standard assay for cyclosporine determination but has largely been replaced by Fluorescence Polarization Immunoassay (FPIA).
- Pharmacodynamic monitoring may be used as an alternative: http://www.cvm.msstate.edu/animal-health-center/pharmacodynamic-laboratory

AUTHOR: Carrie L. Flint, DVM, DACVP
EDITOR: Lois Roth-Johnson, DVM, PhD, DACVP

D-Dimer

Definition

Protein fragments that form from the degradation of cross-linked fibrin; increased D-dimer concentrations indicate active coagulation and fibrinolysis.

Physiology

D-dimers form when plasmin digests cross-linked fibrin; the test is more specific than fibrinogen degradation products (FDPs) and indicates both thrombin and plasmin generation.

Reference Interval

Normal < 250 ng/mL

Causes of Abnormally High Levels

Increased fibrinolysis or decreased clearance of fibrin degradation products by the liver or mononuclear phagocytic system; specific causes include local and disseminated intravascular coagulation, internal hemorrhage, liver disease, chronic kidney disease, and thromboembolic disease.

Next Diagnostic Steps to Consider if Levels are High

Evaluation of the coagulation system: platelet count, activated partial thromboplastin time (aPTT), prothrombin time (PT); consider also thromboelastography (TEG), antithrombin, or thrombin time (TT), fibrinogen. Further evaluation for thromboembolism if clinical suspicion exists (pp. 842 and 1286)

Lab Artifacts

- Decrease: inadequately filled tube causes specimen dilution by anticoagulant
- Increase: *in vitro* clot formation

Specimen Collection and Handling

Citrated plasma (blue top tube); it is important that venipuncture be atraumatic to prevent activation of platelets and the coagulation systems; blood and anticoagulant should be mixed thoroughly immediately after collection. Tubes should be filled completely.

Relative Cost: $$

Pearls

D-dimers can be increased in patients without hypercoagulability. Only recommended when disseminated intravascular coagulation (DIC), hypercoagulability, or thrombosis is suspected

AUTHOR: Deborah G. Davis, DVM, DACVP
EDITOR: Lois Roth-Johnson, DVM, PhD, DACVP

Digoxin, Serum Level

Definition

Cardiac glycoside used in the management of supraventricular tachycardias, atrial fibrillation, and to a lesser degree heart failure

Synonym

Digitalis

Physiology

Serum monitoring is recommended due to widely variable interpatient pharmacokinetics and narrow therapeutic window. There is variable gastrointestinal (GI) absorption following oral dosing (presence of food may delay absorption). Digoxin undergoes slight metabolism but is mostly excreted by the kidneys. Signs of toxicity include other arrhythmias, worsening heart failure, GI signs, and weight loss.

Reference Interval

Therapeutic range (dog and cat): 1.0-2.0 ng/mL. Correlates with clinical effectiveness.

Toxicity signs typically seen with values > 2.5 ng/mL, but some dogs can exhibit signs at lower concentrations.

Causes of Abnormally High Levels

Overdose

Causes of Abnormally Low Levels

Correlate with clinical effectiveness, as minimum effective level not established. Hypokalemia potentiates digoxin-induced arrhythmias. If toxicosis is evident but the serum concentration is not excessive, serum potassium should be evaluated.

Next Diagnostic Steps to Consider if Levels are Low

If therapeutic intent is achieved, low levels are not of concern.

Important Interspecies Differences

Contraindicated in cats with hypertrophic cardiomyopathy

Drug Effects

Oral antacids, metoclopramide, phenobarbital, and sucralfate, among others, may decrease serum digoxin levels. Several drugs and herbs may increase digoxin concentrations, including furosemide, quinidine, tetracycline, and verapamil. Consult with pharmacist for complete list.

Specimen Collection and Handling

Serum (red top tube); do not use serum separator tubes; store at 2°C-8°C.

Relative Cost: $$

Pearls

- Use a lower dose for animals with large body size, obesity (digoxin not distributed in fat), and renal disease (due to elimination route) to avoid toxicosis.
- Dosing based on body surface area is recommended.
- The half-life of cardiac glycosides is highly variable among patients and is often long (12-20 hours in dogs, 48 hours in cats).

AUTHOR: Carrie L. Flint, DVM, DACVP
EDITOR: Lois Roth-Johnson, DVM, PhD, DACVP

Eccentrocyte

Definition

Erythrocyte damaged by oxidants. Characterized by focal area of fused membranes with eccentric displacement of hemoglobinized cytosol and loss of any central pallor. The collapsed area with fused membranes appears as a clear area at periphery of erythrocyte, which is outlined by a barely visible cell membrane.

Synonyms

Bite cell, hemighost

Physiology

During oxidative damage, hemichromes (oxidized forms of hemoglobin) bind to the band 3 protein of the membrane cytoskeleton. This creates cross-linking and fusion of the erythrocyte cytoskeleton and alters the membrane, with externalization of antigenic proteins and attachment of autoantibodies. Hemichromes can also precipitate to form Heinz bodies.

Reference Interval

Absent in health

Causes of Abnormally High Levels

- Oxidative erythrocyte injury: acetaminophen, onions, and benzocaine in dogs and cats, zinc and garlic in dogs. Heinz bodies may be seen concurrently.
- Also reported in dogs with vitamin K antagonist intoxication, T-cell lymphoma, and diabetic ketoacidosis. Certain illnesses apparently induce increased formation of endogenous oxidants, leading to eccentrocytes in absence of toxins typically associated with oxidative damage.
- Decreased antioxidant activity of erythrocytes (rare): congenital deficiency of glucose-6-phosphate dehydrogenase, with decreased production of reduced nicotinamide adenine dinucleotide phosphate (NADPH) in erythrocytes

Next Diagnostic Steps to Consider if Levels Are High

Evaluate history for source of oxidative damage to erythrocytes.

Drug Effects

Associated with previously used formulations of propofol that contained compound(s) that induced oxidative damage in dogs and cats

Specimen Collection and Handling

EDTA whole blood (lavender top tube) and freshly prepared blood smear for lab to stain

Relative Cost: $$ (reported as part of CBC)

AUTHOR: Stephen D. Gaunt, DVM, PhD, DACVP
EDITOR: Lois Roth-Johnson, DVM, PhD, DACVP

Ehrlichia Serologic Testing

Definition

Detection of serum antibodies directed against *Ehrlichia* spp.

Physiology

Ehrlichia spp. are rickettsial agents that infect dogs and, rarely, cats. Monocytic (*E. canis*) infection can cause acute illness, typically followed by a long period of subclinical infection. In some dogs, chronic disease manifestations follow. Granulocytic ehrlichiosis (*E. ewingii*) is most often associated with either unapparent infection or acute, febrile polyarthropathy. Other species of *Ehrlichia* may cause infection in dogs or cats with minimal clinical consequence.

Reference Interval

Reporting differs among reference laboratories; consult with laboratory for proper interpretation of serologic titer.

Causes of Abnormally High Levels

- The presence of antibodies indicates exposure to *E. canis* or related organisms. Some tests also detect antibodies to *E. ewingii* and *E. chaffeensis* (human monocytic ehrlichiosis).
- A positive titer is not proof that current clinical signs are due to active infection.
- A positive titer may persist indefinitely, despite treatment with appropriate antimicrobials.

Next Diagnostic Steps to Consider if Levels Are High

See p. 285.

Causes of Abnormally Low Levels

Acute infection (before antibody formation); infection with *Ehrlichia* spp. not reactive on test; uninfected animal

Next Diagnostic Steps to Consider if Levels Are Low

If a clinical suspicion for ehrlichiosis persists, consider either alternative forms of testing (e.g., PCR, different serologic test), repeat testing in 2 weeks, or empirical treatment.

Important Interspecies Differences

Check with lab for use of canine tests on feline patients. The point-of-care SNAP® (IDEXX Laboratories, Westbrook, ME) test for dogs can be used on cats.

Specimen Collection and Handling

Serum (red top tube, 1 mL); stable at 2°C-8°C for up to five days, or follow manufacturer's directions for point-of-care tests.

Relative Cost: $$

Pearls

- Some dogs maintain persistent titers for years despite appropriate therapy and apparent resolution of disease.
- Point-of-care serologic testing appears to have high specificity when compared with immunofluorescent assay, but may not detect low titers.
- *Ehrlichia* serologic testing is much more sensitive (i.e., better screening test) than evaluating a blood smear for the presence of ehrlichial inclusions (i.e., morulae) in leukocytes.

AUTHOR: Sharon M. Dial, DVM, PhD, DACVP
EDITOR: Lois Roth-Johnson, DVM, PhD, DACVP

Eosinophils

Definition

Granulocytic leukocyte with prominent eosinophilic granules in cytoplasm and a segmented nucleus

Physiology

Eosinophilic precursors develop in the marrow under influence of interleukin 5 (IL-5). Mature eosinophils are released into blood to circulate for a few hours and then enter tissue. Eosinophils contain major basic protein, which is important in attacking helminthic parasites. Eosinophils can both promote and inhibit hypersensitivity reactions. Eosinophilic inflammation occurs most often in cutaneous, respiratory, and intestinal tissues.

Reference Interval

Dogs: 0.1-1.3 × 10^3 eosinophils/mcL; cats: 0-1.5 × 10^3 eosinophils/mcL

Causes of Abnormally High Levels

Parasitism (e.g., dirofilariasis, larval migration in tissues); allergic reactions (e.g., flea bite hypersensitivity); idiopathic eosinophilic inflammation (e.g., hypereosinophilic syndrome, eosinophilic bronchitis); hypoadrenocorticism ("relaxed" leukogram, which is the unexpected absence of stress leukogram with eosinopenia in an ill patient); paraneoplastic (e.g., mast cell neoplasm, B or T cell lymphoma); chronic eosinophilic leukemia (rare)

Next Diagnostic Steps to Consider if Levels Are High

Use history and physical exam findings to assess for causes listed.

Causes of Abnormally Low Levels

Stress leukogram from endogenous or exogenous glucocorticoids; acute inflammation

Next Diagnostic Steps to Consider if Levels Are Low

Low values are rarely clinically significant.

Important Interspecies Differences

- In canine eosinophils, the granules are round and can vary considerably in size and number. In some dogs (greyhounds, but also other sighthounds and a few golden retrievers), eosinophils have clear vacuoles with a more apparent basophilic cytoplasm (instead of many eosinophilic granules), which are described as "gray eosinophils."
- Feline eosinophils have distinctive rod-shaped eosinophilic granules. Cats with gray eosinophils are reported rarely.

Drug Effects

Glucocorticoids cause increased sequestration of eosinophils in tissues, with resultant eosinopenia.

Specimen Collection and Handling

EDTA whole blood (lavender top tube) and freshly prepared blood smear for lab to stain

Relative Cost: $$ (reported as part of CBC)

AUTHOR: Stephen D. Gaunt, DVM, PhD, DACVP
EDITOR: Lois Roth-Johnson, DVM, PhD, DACVP

Erythrocytosis

Definition

Increased circulating erythrocyte mass, with increased hematocrit (or packed cell volume [PCV]), hemoglobin concentration, and/or blood erythrocyte count. Occurs from increase in the circulating erythrocytes only (relative erythrocytosis) or an increase in both circulating erythrocytes and erythropoietic cells (absolute erythrocytosis)

Physiology

- Relative erythrocytosis occurs most commonly when there is decreased plasma volume (e.g., dehydration) or with release of sequestered erythrocytes following epinephrine-induced splenic contraction.
- Absolute erythrocytosis indicates an increase in circulating and erythropoietic cells as a result of increased erythropoietin concentration or heightened response to erythropoietin.

- *Appropriate* increase in erythropoietin occurs secondary to hypoxemia.
- *Inappropriate* production of erythropoietin occurs uncommonly from hypoxia restricted to kidneys (e.g., right-to-left shunting patent ductus arteriosus [PDA]) or, rarely, paraneoplastic expression of erythropoietin).
- Polycythemia vera (p. 806) is a chronic myeloproliferative disease resulting from clonal proliferation of well-differentiated erythrocytes without an increase in basal levels of erythropoietin.
- Marked erythrocytosis, especially with absolute erythrocytosis, can cause hyperviscosity and resultant tissue hypoxia and thrombosis.

Causes of Abnormally High Levels

- Relative: dehydration; splenic contraction
- Absolute: high altitude; most right-to-left cardiac shunts; chronic pulmonary diseases; renal hypoxia due to right-to-left shunting PDA or renal tumor; paraneoplastic production of erythropoietin reported rarely with renal lymphoma, renal and hepatocellular carcinoma, and nasal fibrosarcoma; polycythemia vera. See p. 1222.

Next Diagnostic Steps to Consider if Levels Are High

Verify instrument hematocrit with manual test (packed cell volume). After ruling out the more common causes of relative erythrocytosis (e.g., physical exam and evaluation of serum albumin concentration for dehydration), consider arterial PO_2 measurement or SpO_2, urinalysis and abdominal ultrasound (evaluate kidneys), chest radiographs, echocardiography, +/− erythropoietin assay.

Important Interspecies Differences

- Erythrocytosis caused by epinephrine-induced splenic contraction is more likely in cats.
- Certain breeds of dogs, especially sighthounds (e.g., greyhounds) and some others (e.g., dachshunds), have a higher upper limit of the reference interval for hematocrit. See p. 1351.

Specimen Collection and Handling

EDTA whole blood (lavender top tube)

Pearls

- "Polycythemia" has commonly, but incorrectly, been used for describing the condition of increased red blood cell mass; "erythrocytosis" is the correct term, whereas "polycythemia" describes the state in which all blood cell lines are increased.
- Hypovolemia/dehydration is the most common cause of erythrocytosis in dogs and cats.

AUTHOR: Stephen D. Gaunt, DVM, PhD, DACVP
EDITOR: Lois Roth-Johnson, DVM, PhD, DACVP

Erythropoietin

Definition

Renal hormone that stimulates erythropoiesis in the bone marrow in response to tissue hypoxia

Synonym

EPO

Physiology

EPO is produced primarily by the kidney (sole source in dogs), with small amounts produced by the liver in some species. Tissue hypoxia stimulates EPO production. EPO induces differentiation of erythroid progenitor cells to rubriblasts, stimulates mitosis of erythroid cells, reduces maturation time, and accelerates bone marrow release of reticulocytes.

Reference Interval

Radioimmunoassay method: dogs, 8.4-28 mU/mL; cats, 10-30 mU/mL

Causes of Abnormally High Levels

Hypoxemia-inducing cardiovascular or pulmonary disease; hypoxemia due to high altitude; inappropriate EPO production due to EPO-producing neoplasm (leiomyoma, leiomyosarcoma, renal carcinoma, others), renal cyst, pyelonephritis, or hydronephrosis; hyperthyroidism; EPO therapy. Regardless of cause, secondary erythrocytosis is the result.

Next Diagnostic Steps to Consider if Levels Are High

- Confirm erythrocytosis. If absent, EPO result may be spurious or represent early disease. Serial monitoring of hematocrit is warranted in these cases.
- Identify cause of any hypoxemia-inducing condition: arterial blood gas measurement, thoracic imaging, possibly echocardiography
- Evaluate for neoplasia, kidney lesions, and endocrinopathy.

Causes of Abnormally Low Levels

Decreased EPO in the presence of erythrocytosis and normal PaO_2 suggests polycythemia vera; although measurement of EPO is not clinically indicated in anemia, low EPO would be expected with chronic kidney disease–associated anemia.

Next Diagnostic Steps to Consider if Levels Are Low

Assess renal structure (diagnostic imaging) and function.

Lab Artifacts

Increased: hemolyzed or lipemic specimens

Specimen Collection and Handling

Serum (red top tube) or heparinized plasma (green top tube); separate serum or plasma from erythrocytes, freeze, and transport frozen. Do not use serum separator tubes.

Relative Cost: $$$

Pearls

- Measurement of serum EPO levels is an appropriate test in patients with repeatable absolute erythrocytosis without hypoxemia.
- "Polycythemia" refers to increase in all circulating cell lines but is often used for referring to erythrocytosis, an increase in circulating red blood cells.

AUTHOR: Fidelia R. Fernandez, DVM, MS, DACVP
EDITOR: Lois Roth-Johnson, DVM, PhD, DACVP

Estradiol/Estrogen, Serum Levels

Definition

Hormone synthesized and secreted by developing ovarian follicles

Physiology

Dogs: Proestrus is under the influence of progressively increasing circulating concentrations of estradiol, which is produced by the developing ovarian follicles. A rising estradiol level correlates with development of marked changes in the vaginal mucosa, vulva, and uterus. Serum estradiol concentrations start to increase just before proestrus becomes clinically detectable. Estradiol concentrations above 25 pg/mL are typical of early proestrus, and concentrations greater than 60-70 pg/dL are typical of late proestrus. Peak estradiol serum concentrations are reached 24-48 hours before the end of proestrus before standing heat (estrus). Male dogs with Sertoli cell tumors and male feminization syndrome have increased production of estrogens by testicular tumor cells, or increased androgenous hormone conversion to estrogens by metabolic tissues (e.g., liver, neural tissue) or testicular cells, or normal estrogen levels are concurrent with decreased androgen levels. In male dogs with Sertoli cell tumors, estrogens are typically not measured. Typically, the feminizing syndrome is recognized through overt clinical signs, and the underlying tumor is surgically removed without serologic testing.

Cats: Anestrus and interestrus periods typically are associated with estradiol serum concentrations < 12-15 pg/mL. Estradiol concentrations > 20 pg/mL typically accompany follicular activity (follicular phase of the feline cycle averages 7.0-7.7 days, depending on whether coitus is experienced and whether ovulation is induced). Day 1 of the follicular phase of estrus typically is associated with an estradiol concentration ≈25 pg/mL; at day 3 it is ≈45 pg/mL, at day 5 it is ≈50 pg/mL or above, at day 7 it is ≈20-25 pg/mL, and by day 8 it has returned to ≈10 pg/mL.

Reference Interval

Dog: baseline during anestrus is 5-15 pg/mL. Unit conversion formula: 1 pg/mL × 3.67 = 1 pmol/L

Causes of Abnormally High Levels

- Dog/intact: mid to late proestrus
- Cat/intact: midfollicular phase of estrus cycle
- Spayed/suspected spayed dog or cat: ovarian remnant

Causes of Abnormally Low Levels

- Ovariectomy
- Measurement during anestrus or diestrus phase of cycle

Next Diagnostic Steps to Consider if Levels Are High

In suspected ovariectomized cats administer hCG to cause luteolysis of follicles; check for increasing progesterone. If progesterone increases above 2.5 ng/mL 5-7 days later, exploratory surgery is recommended (persistent ovarian tissue). This test is not used in dogs.

Important Interspecies Differences

- Cats are induced ovulators and are seasonally polyestrous.
- Dogs are spontaneous ovulators and have a typical interestrus interval of 7-12 months.

Lab Artifacts

Increased values in hemolyzed or lipemic samples; gel from serum separator tubes causes variable interference

Specimen Collection and Handling

Serum (2 mL minimum) collected in a red top tube (do not use serum separator tubes).

Analyte is stable in serum sample maintained at 2°C-4°C for up to 48 hours. Specimens should be frozen if analysis interval is longer.

Relative Cost: $$

Pearls

- Antimullarian hormone is the preferred test for assessing for ovarian remnants or spay status.
- Luteinizing hormone may also be used to determine spay status in a patient not currently showing signs of heat.

AUTHOR & EDITOR: Lois Roth-Johnson, DVM, PhD, DACVP

Ethylene Glycol Testing

Definition

Point-of-care/cage-side test kits for the diagnosis of ethylene glycol (antifreeze) toxicity

Physiology

Ethylene glycol (antifreeze) is not toxic in its pure state, but the breakdown products from oxidation within the kidney and the liver result in glycolic acid and oxalate accumulation and subsequent nephrotoxicosis and metabolic acidosis. The available test kits only detect plasma ethylene glycol concentration, not the nephrotoxic metabolites.

Reference Interval

- Kacey Ethylene Glycol Test Strips (Kacey, Inc.): reported as negative, 20, 50, or 75 mg/dL. Positive result is ≥ 20 mg/dL (cat) and ≥ 50 mg/dL (dog).
- VetSpec Ethylene Glycol Qualitative Reagent Test Kit (Catachem, Inc.): reported as negative or positive (quantified at ≈5 mg/dL, ≈150 mg/dL, or ≥ 300 mg/dL)

Causes of Abnormally High Levels

Consumption of ethylene glycol (usually within 12 hours)

Next Diagnostic Steps to Consider if Levels Are High

Ethylene glycol toxicity results in marked acid-base, electrolyte, and osmolality derangements along with acute kidney injury. Blood gas and electrolyte panels to identify a marked metabolic acidosis, electrolyte derangements (hypochloremia/hyperkalemia), and possible hypocalcemia. Renal panels and urinalysis for evidence of acute kidney injury (azotemia). Urine calcium oxalate monohydrate crystals may be present in the first few hours of toxicities. See p. 314.

Causes of Abnormally Low Levels

Ethylene glycol is rapidly metabolized and cleared from the bloodstream; test is negative if exposure has been > 12-18 hours.

Next Diagnostic Steps to Consider if Levels Are Low

If clinical history suggests intoxication, evaluate renal parameters, electrolytes, and acid-base status. Determine serum levels of metabolites (glycolic acid).

Important Interspecies Differences

Both tests are approved for dogs and cats.

Drug Effects

Propylene glycol, glycerol, and ethanol can interfere with these tests, resulting in a false-positive (Kacey).

Specimen Collection and Handling

- Kacey: 20 mcL (1 drop) of plasma. Separate 0.5-1 mL of whole blood in an EDTA (lavender top tube) or lithium heparin (green top tube) for 3-5 minutes for plasma.
- Catachem: 0.1 mL of plasma. Separate 0.5-1 mL of whole blood in an EDTA (lavender top tube) or lithium heparin (green top tube) for 3-5 minutes for plasma.

Relative Cost: $$$

Pearls

- Cats are more susceptible to ethylene glycol toxicity (minimum lethal dose = 1.4-6.6 mL/kg) than dogs (minimum lethal dose = 4.4 mL/kg).
- Gas chromatography is considered the gold standard, but is not always practical for clinical settings.
- Local hospitals may be able to perform this assay. The chemical detected is the same in both humans and animals.

AUTHOR: Erin N. Burton, DVM, MS, DACVP
EDITOR: Lois Roth-Johnson, DVM, PhD, DACVP

Factor Xa Inhibition

Definition

Inhibition of Factor Xa is the mechanism for certain direct-acting oral anticoagulants (e.g., rivaroxaban, apixaban). The action of these drugs can't be assessed by classical coagulation tests. Plasma concentration is the current method for evaluation for appropriate therapeutic levels or overdose.

Physiology

Factor Xa inhibitors, used to control thromboembolic conditions, act directly without needing cofactors for activation. Most of these drugs are up to 60% bioavailable in dogs. Therapeutic activity generally correlates with plasma concentration. Classical coagulation tests (PT, aPTT) do not correlate with blood levels. Therefore, monitoring is done by measuring plasma anti-Xa activity rather than traditional coagulation assays. Specific assays are required for different drug (e.g., heparin, rivaroxaban) monitoring.

Reference Interval

Send out test for veterinary reference lab; may have to use human lab or local human hospital

Causes of Abnormally High Levels

Overadministration

Causes of Abnormally Low Levels

Underdosing

Specimen Collection and Handling

Plasma (green top tube), 1 mL minimum. Spin, collect plasma immediately and freeze.

Relative Cost: Check with reference lab or local human hospital labs.

Pearls

- PT may suffice for qualitative measurement of patient clotting ability (i.e., clot intensity), but a drug-specific assay is needed for monitoring and assessing blood levels.
- Thromboelastography may serve as an alternate means of assessing anticoagulation if Factor Xa inhibition assay is unavailable.
- These assays can also be used to assess the efficacy of heparin anticoagulation.

AUTHOR & EDITOR: Lois Roth-Johnson, DVM, PhD, DACVP

Fecal Culture

Definition

Microbiologic evaluation of feces for growth of enteric bacterial pathogens

Synonym

Stool culture

Physiology

Enteric dysbiosis and diarrhea in small animal may be caused by bacterial pathogens or pathobionts. Routine aerobic and anaerobic cultures are often of limited utility in complex bacterial communities such as feces. Alternative culture techniques are often necessary for the identification of enteric pathogens in fecal samples.

Reference Interval

Reported as negative or degree (light, moderate, heavy) of growth of specific pathogens. Microbial susceptibility may also be provided.

Causes of Abnormally High Levels

Common small animal enteric pathogens include *Salmonella* spp, *Shigella* spp, *Campylobacter* spp, *E. coli* O157:H7, *Clostridium difficle*, *Yersinia* spp. Culture results that include normal enteric flora are not diagnostically useful.

Next Diagnostic Steps to Consider if Levels are High

See pp. 182, 260, and 898.

Causes of Abnormally Low Levels

Growth may be absent despite infection, especially after antimicrobial therapy. Alternatively, the cause for signs may not be due to bacterial infection.

Next Diagnostic Steps to Consider if Levels are Low

Intermittent shedding of pathogen may cause false-negative results. If clinical signs continue to suggest enteric bacterial disease, consider PCR assay or repeat culture.

Drug Effects

Antimicrobial therapies, even low levels, may inhibit or alter culture growth.

Lab Artifacts

False-negative:

- Pre-analytical error from delay in shipping or setting up culture, omission of suspected fastidious organisms on submission form to guide laboratory personnel on appropriate media selection, inappropriate shipping media, and exposure of anaerobes to oxygen

- Contamination or overgrowth of normal flora

Specimen Collection and Handling

Fresh feces in a sterile container strongly preferred over rectal swabs. Many of the listed bacterial isolates require special transport medium. Contact reference laboratory to obtain appropriate media and transport instructions.

Relative Cost: $$

Pearls

- Many of these pathogens are slow growing and may take several days before a result can be provided.
- Several laboratories now offer "diarrhea panels" with PCR tests for multiple enteric pathogens; these have increasingly replaced the use of traditional fecal culture.
- As whole genome and/or metagenomic 16S rRNA PCR sequencing techniques become more readily available in reference laboratories, these may provide more complete characterization of the fecal microbiota profile than routine fecal culture techniques.

AUTHOR: Erin N. Burton, DVM, MS, DACVP
EDITOR: Lois Roth-Johnson, DVM, PhD, DACVP

Fecal Flotation

Definition

Screening test for the identification of parasitic ova or cysts in feces

Synonyms

Qualitative fecal exam, simple or passive fecal flotation, centrifugal fecal flotation

Physiology

The specific gravity of a solution coupled with gravity (simple or passive) or centripetal (centrifugal) motion result in the flotation of parasitic eggs to the surface. Depending on the method, the parasitic ova will adhere to the coverslip placed over the vial or are extracted from the meniscus with a microbiological loop. The coverslip or extracted fluid is examined at low (10× obj.) and high (40× obj.) power for parasitic ova or cysts.

Reference Interval

Reported as "no ova seen" or positive with genus or family identification

Causes of Abnormally High Levels

Gastrointestinal (or uncommonly respiratory) parasitic infections. Ova from various nematodes (e.g., ascarids, hookworms, whipworms), cestodes, trematodes, or protozoan oocysts (coccidians) or cysts (*Giardia* sp.) can be identified.

Next Diagnostic Steps to Consider if Levels are High

Positive test result correlates with infection.

Causes of Abnormally Low Levels

- Intermittent shedding of ova or pre-patent period for pathogen
- For parasites with "heavy" ova, or low numbers of ova, fecal flotation may not be sensitive. In general, the higher the specific gravity, the greater the variety of parasitic ova that can be detected

Next Diagnostic Steps to Consider if Levels are Low

Serial fecal flotation, other gastrointestinal or respiratory diagnostic testing

Drug Effects

Administration of anthelmintic may decrease ova or cyst shedding.

Lab Artifacts

- Flotation solutions with high specific gravities may distort ova or cyst morphology.
- Plant debris and pollen are common pseudoparasites.

Specimen Collection and Handling

Gross examination of the feces is an important first step of the fecal examination for the identification of cestode proglottids or adult helminths. A minimum of 3-5 g of fresh feces (within hours) or refrigerated (<24 hours) is preferred. All specimens submitted to a reference laboratory should be transported with cold packs. Helminth eggs can be preserved in feces with an equal volume of 5%-10% buffered formalin. Samples that have been fixed should be denoted on submission form.

Relative Cost: $

Pearls

- Ova burden does not always correlate well to worm burden as some species are more prolific egg layers than others; thus serial testing is often necessary.
- Preservation in buffer formalin offers the potential benefit of inactivating many other infectious agents.

AUTHOR: Erin N. Burton, DVM, MS
EDITOR: Lois Roth-Johnson, DVM, PhD, DACVP

Feline Coronavirus Testing

Definition

Feline coronavirus (FCoV) infection refers to two distinct entities: feline infectious peritonitis (FIP) and feline enteric coronaviral (FECV) enteritis. FIP is a systemic viral disease of high mortality characterized by insidious onset, fever, disseminated pyogranulomatous inflammation, and in some cases, proteinaceous effusions in body cavities ("wet form"). FECV causes mild transient diarrhea and/or vomiting and, less commonly, chronic or severe diarrhea.

Synonym

FIP titers

Physiology

In FIP, FCoV is ingested and then replicates in intestinal epithelial cells and probably tonsils and oropharynx. In some cats, a mutated virus infects macrophages, with subsequent extension to multiple tissues. Antiviral antibodies are produced such that immune complexes form and are deposited in blood vessels of serosal surfaces, uvea, kidney, liver, and other tissues. A pyogranulomatous response ensues. Proteinaceous abdominal or thoracic effusion results from increased vascular permeability. FIP-type is thought to represent a spontaneous mutation of FCoV that occurs *in vivo* in some cats.

Reference Interval

- Serologic titer by IFA or ELISA: refer to testing laboratory

- Quantitative mRNA RT-PCR results reported as negative, high positive (>50 copies/specimen), or low positive (<50 copies/specimen)
- RT-PCR results negative or positive with biotyping

Causes of Abnormally High Levels

Positive FCoV titer (IFA or ELISA) indicates nonspecific exposure to any of the following: FIPV, FECV, other coronaviruses, or FIP vaccine. Very high titers (>1 : 16,000) may increase suspicion of FIP when compatible clinical signs are present, but the result is not confirmatory.

Next Diagnostic Steps to Consider if Levels are High

Correlate with history, physical exam findings, and other laboratory data. Cytologic evaluation, PCR, or IFA on effusion fluid may be supportive but not definitive. RT-PCR biotyping or simultaneous testing of blood, feces, and effusion or tissue aspirates may assist in differentiating FIP from FECV. Histopathologic and immunohistochemical analysis of biopsy or necropsy tissue remains the gold standard for FIP diagnosis. See p. 327.

Causes of Abnormally Low Levels

False-negative serologic test results may arise from peracute infection, low level or lack of antibody production (especially in immunosuppressed cats), or antibody bound within immune complexes. False-negative RT-PCR results due to low nuclei acid load or unknown strain variation.

Next Diagnostic Steps to Consider if Levels are Low

If FIPV is still suspected, consider same diagnostic steps as described above or submitting alternative specimen type for RT-PCR.

Lab Artifacts

RT-PCR: false-positive results due to specimen contamination; false-negative results due to degradation of nucleic acids via improper sample handling or storage

Specimen Collection and Handling

0.5-1 mL serum (red top tube) or CSF for IFA or ELISA. Samples stable for days to weeks at 4°C or for months at −20°C. For mRNA RT-PCR, submit ≥ 0.5 mL of EDTA blood (lavender top tube) and/or body cavity fluid, fecal swab (for exclusion of FECV), tissue aspirates/biopsies in special sample buffer (obtained from Auburn University, www.vetmed.auburn.edu/wp-content/uploads/2015/03/FIP-virus.pdf). Keep samples for RT-PCR at room temperature (do not freeze). For FIPV RealPCR™, refer to https://idexxcom-live-b02da1e51e754c9cb292133b-9c56c33.aldryn-media.com/filer_public/dd/81/dd8192c9-ae9b-4d1b-841a-06748adc75ac/feline-infectious-peritonitis-virus.pdf.

Relative Cost: $$ (IFA serum antibody, PCR), $$$ (IFA tissue, RT-PCR)

Pearls

- A negative titer does not rule out FIP, nor does a positive titer confirm FIP. Multiple site sampling and evaluation via the RT-PCR increases sensitivity and specificity.
- FCoV testing is not useful to predict future illness in healthy cats.

AUTHOR: Patty J. Ewing, DVM, MS, DACVP
EDITOR: Lois Roth-Johnson, DVM, PhD, DACVP

Feline Immunodeficiency Virus (FIV) Testing

Definition

Feline immunodeficiency virus (FIV) is a lentivirus that attacks the immune system of cats, resulting in progressive immunosuppression.

Physiology

FIV is inoculated via saliva or blood from bite wounds. There are three phases of infection. *Acute:* FIV initially infects T lymphocytes and salivary glands, then other mononuclear cells; cats may have fever, leukopenia, and lymphadenopathy. *Subclinical:* cats may be without clinical signs for years. *Chronic:* progressive immunosuppression with various clinical disorders (see p. 325)

Reference Interval

ELISA, IFA, Western blot or RT-PCR: positive or negative

Causes of Abnormally High Levels

ELISA and immunochromatogenic assays are screening tests for antibody. Positive result indicates exposure to FIV or FIV vaccine. Due to maternally transferred antibody, FIV testing of kittens ≤ 6 months old born to FIV-positive queens is unreliable (false-positives).

Next Diagnostic Steps to Consider if Levels are High

- Confirmatory tests: Western blot or IFA may or may not differentiate between maternal antibody, vaccination, or infection.
- RT-PCR test may be a useful test for differentiating some vaccine exposures or maternal antibody from true infection.

Causes of Abnormally Low Levels

Negative ELISA, IFA, or Western blot indicates lack of exposure, acute or subacute infection, or undetectable levels of antibody due to immunosuppression. Negative RT-PCR indicates lack of infection, nucleic acid below limit of detection of assay, or uncommon strain not detected by assay.

Next Diagnostic Steps to Consider if Levels are Low

If clinical signs suggest FIV infection, test via a second method or retest in 4-12 weeks.

Lab Artifacts

RT-PCR: false-positive results due to contamination of samples; false-negative results due to degradation of nucleic acids via improper sample handling and storage

Specimen Collection and Handling

- ELISA, Western blot, IFA: 1.0 mL serum (red top tube); stable at 2°C-8°C for 7 days or weeks to months if frozen. Most ELISA tests are run as point-of-care kits per manufacturer's directions.
- RT-PCR: 2 mL whole blood (lavender top tube), 0.5 mL CSF; stable for 10 days at 2°C-8°C or weeks to months frozen

Relative Cost: $$ (IFA, ELISA); $$$ (Western blot)

Pearls

- Seroconversion may take up to 3 months, so when screening healthy cats via ELISA, retesting is recommended > 2 months after potential exposure.
- FIV-vaccinated cats test positive as early as 28 days postvaccination and remain positive for at least 1 year. RT-PCR may help identify FIV-infected cats that have been vaccinated or have unknown vaccination history and test positive on ELISA, IFA, or Western blot.

AUTHOR: Patty J. Ewing, DVM, MS, DACVP
EDITOR: Lois Roth-Johnson, DVM, PhD, DACVP

Feline Leukemia Virus (FeLV) Testing

Definition

Feline leukemia virus (FeLV) is a gammaretrovirus of cats that causes hematopoietic neoplasia, immunosuppression, and/or anemia.

Physiology

Following oronasal exposure to FeLV, the virus replicates in oropharyngeal lymphoid tissue. The virus may be cleared with an effective immune response (abortive infection). An ineffective immune response results in viremia and replication in bone marrow and lymphoid cells. Infected cats may be transiently viremic with latent virus residing in the marrow (regressive infection), or may become persistently viremic (progressive infection). ELISAs and other immunochromatographic assays become positive during the primary viremic phase, before bone marrow infection. See p. 329.

Reference Interval

ELISA, IFA, and PCR/RT-PCR: reported as positive or negative

Causes of Abnormally High Levels

- ELISA (screening test) detects the free soluble FeLV core antigen p27 as early as 30 days after infection; a positive ELISA indicates viremia, but viremia may be transient. False-positives occur infrequently (usually due to technical error; sensitivity = 90%-98%; specificity = 98%-99%). IFA (confirmatory test) detects the cell-associated FeLV core antigen p27 as early as 6 weeks after infection; a positive IFA indicates persistent bone marrow infection.
- Discordant results are possible. Positive ELISA with negative IFA is suggestive of early infection that may persist or become latent. Negative ELISA with positive IFA suggests false result, and both tests should be repeated, or perform RT-PCR. Positive ELISA with negative RT-PCR suggests viral nucleic acid below limit of detection, an uncommon strain not detected by PCR, or falsely positive ELISA.

Next Diagnostic Steps to Consider if Levels are High

If ELISA screening test is positive, repeat ELISA in 6-8 weeks or confirm with IFA test or PCR/RT-PCR.

Causes of Abnormally Low Levels

A negative ELISA or IFA may be present with either early infection or regressive infection, or in uninfected cats.

Next Diagnostic Steps to Consider if Levels are Low

If the cat was recently exposed to an FeLV-positive cat but the ELISA is negative, retesting in 30-90 days is recommended. PCR for proviral DNA may be indicated if latent FeLV infection is suspected or for potential blood donors. If positive ELISA and negative IFA, repeat both tests in 6-8 weeks. PCR/RT-PCR can also be performed.

Lab Artifacts

Hemolysis or lipemia may cause a false-positive or false-negative ELISA result. Marked thrombocytopenia or neutropenia may cause a false-negative IFA. Use of excessively thick buffy coat or bone marrow smears may cause a false-positive IFA test. False-positive RT-PCR results may be due to specimen contamination, and false-negative results may be due to degradation of nucleic acids via improper sample handling and storage or aged sample.

Specimen Collection and Handling

ELISA: 1 mL serum (red top tube) or EDTA plasma (lavender top tube). Stable for 7 days at 2°C-8°C or months if frozen. Performed as in-clinic test kit, or mail out. IFA: 1 mL EDTA plasma (lavender top tube), buffy coat smear, or unstained, unfixed bone marrow smear. Stable for 48 hours at 2°C-8°C (whole blood); store slides at room temperature. PCR: 2 mL EDTA whole blood (lavender top tube); stable for 10 days at 2°-8°C; fresh tissue 24 hours at 2°C-8°C or frozen for longer.

Relative Cost: $ (ELISA), $$ (IFA, PCR/RT-PCR)

Pearls

- Vaccination for FeLV involves a different component of the virus than the one detected by ELISA, IFA, or PCR. Therefore, prior vaccination does not affect test results.
- ELISA test is more sensitive (more likely to catch all FeLV-positive cases) compared to IFA, but less specific (may erroneously identify a few FeLV negative cats as positive, especially in populations with low prevalence of FeLV).
- Only highly reliable laboratories should be entrusted with FeLV PCR testing; they should provide information on reliability of testing.

AUTHOR: Patty J. Ewing, DVM, MS, DACVP
EDITOR: Lois Roth-Johnson, DVM, PhD, DACVP

Fibrin or Fibrinogen Degradation Products (FDP)

Definition

Fibrin or fibrinogen degradation products (FDPs) are protein fragments of fibrin or fibrinogen that have been cleaved by plasmin as part of fibrinolysis. Assays to detect FDPs are used for identifying increased fibrin or fibrinogen breakdown that is seen with excessive coagulation (disseminated intravascular coagulation [DIC]). Plasmin can act on both fibrinogen and fibrin. Assays for FDPs do not differentiate between fibrinolysis and fibrinogenolysis.

Physiology

- Plasmin breaks down fibrin and fibrinogen into Fragments D and E (FDPs). FDPs inhibit coagulation by competing with fibrinogen for active sites on thrombin and interfering with the conversion of fibrinogen to fibrin.
- FDPs interfere with platelet aggregation by binding to the fibrinogen binding site on platelets.
- FDPs are eliminated by the liver and kidney. Patients with hepatic or renal disease can have increased FDPs in the absence of significant fibrin(ogen)olysis.

Reference Interval

Semiquantitative normal values: dogs, 0-10 mcg/mL; cats, 0-8 mcg/mL. Abnormal values are reported as moderately increased or markedly increased.

Causes of Abnormally High Levels

- Increased fibrinolysis: internal hemorrhage, thromboembolism, DIC, sepsis, hyperadrenocorticism, protein-losing nephropathy or enteropathy, pancreatitis, parvoviral infection (dogs)
- Increased fibrinogenolysis: rattlesnake envenomation
- Decreased FDP clearance: hepatic disease, kidney disease

Next Diagnostic Steps to Consider if Levels are High

- CBC with platelet count, serum biochemistry profile, urinalysis
- Coagulation profile: activated partial thromboplastin time, prothrombin time,

thrombin time, antithrombin, and D-dimer levels

Important Interspecies Differences

Plasma FDP testing is currently only validated in the dog

Drug Effects

Fibrinolytic drugs (e.g., streptokinase) can increase FDP concentrations.

Lab Artifacts

False increases can occur when FDP generation occurs during collection (traumatic venipuncture).

Specimen Collection and Handling

- Serum assay: special tubes filled with thrombin, or reptilase (snake venom) with soybean trypsin inhibitor or aprotinin (light blue top tubes with yellow label)
- Plasma assays: citrated (light blue top tube). Tubes must be completely filled. Most reference laboratories will supply collection tubes.

Relative Cost: $$

Pearls

- Serum (plain red top tube) specimens cannot be used because clot formation consumes FDPs, lowering measurement. A clot in the citrate tube will interfere with accuracy of the plasma assay.
- Traditional FDP assays do not differentiate between fibrinolysis and fibrinogenolysis; D-dimer assays are specific for fibrinolysis.
- Most often used to help support diagnosis of DIC

AUTHOR: Deborah G. Davis, DVM, DACVP
EDITOR: Lois Roth-Johnson, DVM, PhD, DACVP

Fibrinogen

Definition

Glycoprotein important in hemostasis; a positive acute-phase protein that increases due to inflammation or tissue injury; important in tissue repair

Physiology

Made in the liver; production is upregulated with inflammation or tissue damage (due to cytokines interleukin [IL]-1, IL-6, and tumor necrosis factor [TNF]). It is a nonenzymatic coagulation factor (factor I), cleaved (activated) by thrombin to form fibrin and promote stable clot formation.

Reference Interval

Dogs: 150-300 mg/dL; cats: 150-300 mg/dL

Causes of Abnormally High Levels

Major causes: dehydration (hemoconcentration) and increased hepatic production due to inflammation or tissue damage. Can also increase with hyperadrenocorticism, pregnancy, and nephrotic syndrome

Next Diagnostic Steps to Consider if Levels are High

Look for source of inflammation/tissue injury: review history and physical exam; CBC (determine if inflammatory leukogram is present), serum biochemistry profile; if hyperglobulinemia, serum protein electrophoresis is warranted (polyclonal gammopathy suggests inflammatory process; p. 1375).

Causes of Abnormally Low Levels

Increased consumption in disseminated intravascular coagulation (DIC) or increased fibrinogenolysis, decreased hepatic fibrinogen synthesis, inherited/congenital disorders (documented in Bichon frisé, Bernese mountain dog, Lhasa apso, Vizsla, and collie).

Next Diagnostic Steps to Consider if Levels are Low

Full coagulation profile (activated partial thromboplastin time, prothrombin time, thrombin time, platelet count, and fibrinogen degradation products [FDPs]) to assess for DIC. Serum biochemistry profile and serum bile acids to evaluate hepatic function

Drug Effects

Heparin can decrease fibrinogen concentration.

Lab Artifacts

False decreases can occur with hemolysis, lipemia, and high levels of FDPs.

Specimen Collection and Handling

Quantitative measurement requires citrated plasma. Centrifuge and remove plasma within 1 hour of collection and transfer to plain red top tube. Label as plasma. Test as soon as possible. Stable at 2°C-8°C for 24 hours; freeze if there is a longer time interval before testing.

Relative Cost: $$

Pearls

Fibrinogen can be measured by heat precipitation (not recommended in dogs and cats; unreliable for low fibrinogen), coagulation methods (quantitative), and immunologic assays (to detect rare dysfibrinogenemic disorders).

AUTHOR: Deborah G. Davis, DVM, DACVP
EDITOR: Lois Roth-Johnson, DVM, PhD, DACVP

Fluid Analysis

Definition

The evaluation of fluid that accumulates in a body cavity secondary to altered hemodynamics, decreased oncotic pressure, inflammation, neoplasia, hemorrhage, or lymphatic disease

Physiology

The pleural, pericardial, and peritoneal cavities lie between two thin mesothelium-lined serous membranes that cover the viscera and body wall. Normally, a scant amount of fluid between these membranes serves as a lubricant. An effusion or accumulation of fluid into a body cavity will form with increased submesothelial capillary permeability or hydrostatic pressure, decreased submesothelial capillary oncotic pressure, or impaired lymphatic drainage. Mechanistic classification of effusions based on either transudation, exudation, or vessel/viscus leakage helps limit the list of differential diagnoses and is based on the total protein (TP) quantification, total nucleated cell counts (TNCC) and red blood cell (RBC) counts, and physical and chemical evaluation.

Reference Interval

- Normal: TNCC < 3000 cells/mcL and TP < 2.5 g/dL. Scant in amount
- Transudate: TNCC < 3000 cells/mcL and TP < 2.5 g/dL
- Protein-enriched ("modified") transudate: TNCC < 3000 cells/mcL and TP ≥ 2.5 g/dL
- Exudate: TNCC > 3000 cells/mcL and TP typically > 2.5 g/dL (unless hypoalbuminemia is present). The character of exudate varies more than transudate or modified transudate, depending on cause.

Causes of Abnormally High Levels

- Transudate: hypoalbuminemia, pre-sinusoidal hypertension. Typically clear and colorless
- Protein-enriched ("modified") transudate: heart failure, post-sinusoidal hypertension. Typically clear and amber
- Exudate: inflammation (e.g., pancreatitis), infection (e.g., bacterial peritonitis), neoplasia (e.g., mesothelioma), hemorrhage (e.g., splenic rupture), lymphatic disease. Typically turbid and white to brown
- Specific effusions with variable TNCC and TP:
  - Feline infectious peritonitis: low TNCC (<3000 cells/mcL) with markedly high TP (>4.5 g/dL). Typically clear and yellow
  - Hemorrhage: high RBC; TNCC is comparable to blood. Typically red and does not clot
  - Chylous effusion/lymphorrhage: Small lymphocytes predominate +/- increased neutrophils and lipid-laden macrophages if chronic. Typically white
  - Neoplasia (e.g., carcinoma, mesothelioma, lymphoma); variable appearance
  - Uroperitoneum; may have concurrent hemorrhage
  - Bile peritonitis; typically yellow to green

Next Diagnostic Steps to Consider if Levels are High

- Ancillary biochemical analysis:
  - Chylous effusion/lymphorrhage: measure fluid triglycerides to determine if chylous (> 100 mg/dL)
  - Neoplasia: immunocytochemistry can help categorize carcinoma, mesothelioma, lymphoma, etc.
  - Uroperitoneum: measure fluid creatinine (> 2× plasma creatinine).
  - Bile peritonitis: measure fluid bilirubin (> 2× plasma bilirubin).

Specimen Collection and Handling

Submit fluid in EDTA (preferable) and red top tube. Submit direct smears prepared at time of sample collection.

Relative Cost: $$

Pearls

- Malodorous fluid or fluid containing degenerate neutrophils +/- bacteria should be submitted for culture.
- Though often white, chylous effusion may be clear in anorexic animals.
- Though often yellow/brown, effusion from a biliary tract rupture can be clear (i.e., white bile).
- Very small amounts of bleeding can cause a pink or red effusion due to a nonhemorrhagic cause.

AUTHOR: Shannon D. Dehghanpir, DVM, MS, DACVP
EDITOR: Lois Roth-Johnson, DVM, PhD, DACVP

Folate

Definition

Anionic form of folic acid

Synonyms

Folic acid, vitamin B_9

Physiology

Primary source is diet; also produced by enteric bacteria. Ingested folate is released from food and hydrolyzed in proximal small intestine. Dietary and bacterial origin folate is taken up by proximal intestinal epithelium, metabolized, and absorbed into blood.

Reference Interval

Dogs: 7.7-24.4 mcg/L; cats: 9.7-21.6 mcg/L. Unit conversion: mcg/L × 2.226 = nmol/L.

Causes of Abnormally High Levels

Small intestinal bacterial overgrowth (intestinal dysbiosis) with/without exocrine pancreatic insufficiency (EPI), impaired gastric acid secretion, low intestinal pH due to EPI or excessive gastric acid production, oversupplementation, cobalamin deficiency

Next Diagnostic Steps to Consider if Levels are High

Rule out sample hemolysis. Test for EPI with trypsin-like immunoreactivity (TLI) measurement. Check history for dietary supplementation.

Causes of Abnormally Low Levels

Small intestinal mucosal disease, antibiotics depleting intestinal flora, rarely dietary deficiency, possibly extensive neoplasia (as folate is used in DNA synthesis)

Next Diagnostic Steps to Consider if Levels are Low

Rule out artifact due to sample light exposure. Evaluate diet, medication history. Assess for inflammatory or other bowel diseases. Assess for EPI with TLI measurement.

Important Interspecies Differences

Increased folate (due to bacterial overgrowth) associated with low IgA in German shepherd dogs.

Drug Effects

Antibiotics depleting intestinal flora could decrease levels. Phenytoin and sulfasalazine can decrease levels in humans; unconfirmed in animals.

Lab Artifacts

- False increase: hemolyzed specimens (released from erythrocytes)
- Falsely decreased: excessive light exposure

Specimen Collection and Handling

Serum (red top tube). Fast animal and separate serum from clot as soon as possible to avoid hemolysis. Store frozen (preferred) or refrigerate up to 48 hours only.

Relative Cost: $ (folate); $$$ (folate, cobalamin, trypsin-like immunoreactivity)

Pearls

- Evaluate folate in conjunction with cobalamin and TLI. Reference laboratories typically offer panels that include all three tests.
- Cobalamin deficiency may cause normal or increased folate concentrations (it may accumulate when cobalamin is unavailable to act with it as a cofactor).
- Dietary deficiency is uncommon as folate is abundant in commercial pet foods.
- Although high levels may be seen, assessment of folate levels is no longer considered reliable for the diagnosis of bacterial overgrowth/dysbiosis.
- Human maternal folate deficiency is associated with congenital malformations, but there is no evidence of this in dogs and cats.

AUTHOR: Shelley Burton, DVM, MSc, DACVP
EDITOR: Lois Roth-Johnson, DVM, PhD, DACVP

Fructosamine

Definition

Fructosamine is a composite measurement of glycated serum proteins (mainly albumin). It is measured to strengthen the suspicion of diabetes mellitus (especially in cats) or to monitor glycemic control in known diabetics.

Physiology

The degree of increase in fructosamine concentration is dependent on the magnitude and duration of hyperglycemia over the span of the previous 2-3 weeks. Transient hyperglycemia (i.e., stress or epinephrine-mediated hyperglycemia) will not increase fructosamine concentration over the reference interval. Altering the amount or half-life of albumin and other serum proteins will accordingly change the fructosamine concentration.

Reference Interval

Varies by laboratory. Example: 142-450 mcmol/L

Causes of Abnormally High Levels

Persistent hyperglycemia (diabetes mellitus). Hypothyroidism can also cause a mild increase.

Next Diagnostic Steps to Consider if Levels are High

- When hyperglycemia is measured a single time, increased fructosamine concentration is supportive of a diagnosis of diabetes mellitus as opposed to stress-related hyperglycemia (cats).
- Magnitude of increased fructosamine concentration in a known diabetic can help determine if insulin therapy and other glycemic management protocols may need to be optimized. Serial glucose measurements (glucose curve) may be necessary to better tailor therapy.

Causes of Abnormally Low Levels

Persistent hypoglycemia (for example, a patient with insulinoma), hypoproteinemia, and/or decreased half-life of serum proteins (as seen in hyperthyroidism). Not normally run in animals with hypoglycemia

Next Diagnostic Steps to Consider if Levels are Low

A low fructosamine concentration in a diabetic patient receiving insulin suggests therapy has been causing periods of hypoglycemia. Treatment protocol should be re-evaluated, and serial glucose measurements (glucose curve) warranted.

Drug Effects

Levodopa can falsely increase fructosamine measurement.

Lab Artifacts

Check with laboratory to see if hemolysis or lipemia may interfere with the specific methodology used.

Specimen Collection and Handling

If mailing sample to outside laboratory, collect blood into red top tube, allow to clot, centrifuge, transfer serum to separate tube, and refrigerate until shipment. Ship overnight with cold packs. Some laboratories will accept either serum or heparinized plasma.

Relative Cost: $$

AUTHOR: Angela Royal, MS, DVM, DACVP
EDITOR: Lois Roth-Johnson, DVM, PhD, DACVP

Fungal Culture

Definition

Microbiologic analysis of tissue or exudate for growth of fungal organisms

Physiology

Laboratory conditions enhance growth of pathogens and allow isolation of fungal colonies and their subsequent identification by morphologic features and chemical tests. Specimens from animals suspected of cryptococcosis, blastomycosis, histoplasmosis, or coccidioidomycosis should not undergo fungal culture in the veterinary clinical setting due to health risk to veterinary personnel. Fungal culture is commonly employed for dermatophytosis (p. 247) or saprophytic infections.

Reference Interval

Reported as negative or degree (light, moderate, heavy) of growth of specific pathogens

Causes of Abnormally High Levels

Fungal infection or contamination

Next Diagnostic Steps to Consider if Levels are High

Culture is definitive. Used as a confirmatory test for dermatophytes. *Aspergillus* spp. may be cultured for specific identification if organisms are seen in cytologic or histologic specimens.

Important Interspecies Differences

Dermatophytes may cause pseudomycetoma (deep granulomatous or pyogranulomatous lesions) in cats, especially Persian cats, and nodular dermatophytosis (kerion) in dogs. Culture of superficial scrapings or hair typically is negative in these cases.

Drug Effects

Corticosteroids and other immunosuppressive therapies may enhance organism growth.

Lab Artifacts

False-negative: improper media or growth conditions

Specimen Collection and Handling

- Dermatophytes: hair plucked from affected areas should be submitted in dermatophyte test media or sterile dry containers.
- Tissue or exudate: sterile, dry container

Relative Cost: $$

AUTHOR: Sharon M. Dial, DVM, PhD, DACVP
EDITOR: Lois Roth-Johnson, DVM, PhD, DACVP

Gamma-Glutamyl Transferase (GGT)

Definition

Serum enzyme, marker for liver disease associated with cholestasis or biliary hyperplasia

Synonyms

GGT, gamma-glutamyltransferase

Physiology

Membrane-associated enzyme present in most cell types. Greatest activity found in biliary and renal tubular epithelial cells. Increased serum concentration is primarily associated with biliary and hepatic disease. Increased urine GGT/creatinine ratio can provide evidence for renal tubular damage.

Reference Interval

Dogs: 0-13 U/L; cats: 0-6 U/L

Causes of Abnormally High Levels

Cholestasis, biliary hyperplasia, ingestion of colostrum in neonates (some species); may be induced by corticosteroid administration in dogs.

Next Diagnostic Steps to Consider if Levels Are High

- Evaluate recent drug administration.
- Interpret in light of serum chemistry profile, including alkaline phosphatase (ALP), alanine transaminase (ALT), and bilirubin; bile acids (if hyperbilirubinemia absent); abdominal ultrasound +/− liver biopsy.

Important Interspecies Differences

- Serum GGT is significantly increased within 24 hours of suckling in pups (not kittens); levels fall to within reference intervals by 10 days of age.
- Elevated GGT activity generally considered to have better diagnostic sensitivity than ALP for cholestasis in horses and cattle.

Drug Effects

Corticosteroids cause elevated GGT activity in dogs. May see mild elevation with phenobarbital use.

Lab Artifacts

Variable effects of hemolysis depending on assay type (can falsely increase or falsely decrease results)

Specimen Collection and Handling

Serum (red-top tube); separate as soon as possible, store at 8°C

Relative Cost: $ (as individual test); often included in chemistry profiles

Pearls

- GGT is more sensitive but less specific for liver disease than ALP in the cat and more specific but less sensitive in the dog. However, the combination of minimal or no increase in GGT and significant increase in ALP is associated with hepatic lipidosis in the cat.
- Uncommon cause of increased GGT is neoplasia (hepatic, pancreatic, renal).
- Increased urine GGT/creatinine ratio has been associated with renal disease in dogs and ponies, but could also be caused by decreased GFR.

AUTHOR: Carrie L. Flint, DVM, DACVP
EDITOR: Lois Roth-Johnson, DVM, PhD, DACVP

Gastrin

Definition

Group of peptide hormones secreted by G cells of gastric antrum and duodenum in response to protein meal. Gastrin stimulates parietal cell secretion of gastric acid and histamine release by enterochromaffin cells. Also stimulates pancreatic acinar cells when bound to cholecystokinin.

Synonyms

G-34 (big gastrin), G-17 (little gastrin), G-14 (mini gastrin)

Physiology

Ingestion of protein meal stimulates release. Binds to receptors in parietal, enterochromaffin cells, regulating gastric acid release for protein digestion. Enhances digestion by stimulating gastric blood flow, antral motility, and pancreatic secretion. Stimulates DNA, RNA production, and proliferation of parietal cells and gastric mucosa.

Reference Interval

Overnight fasting sample: less than 27.8 ng/L

Normal dogs may have undetectable concentrations.

Causes of Abnormally High Levels

Excess secretion associated with gastric mucosa hypertrophy, gastric and duodenal ulceration. The underlying cause is typically a neoplasm of pancreatic islet delta cells (gastrinoma); when these cells undergo neoplastic transformation, they regain the ability to produce gastrin (normally only occurs in delta cells of the fetus). Renal failure leads to gastrin accumulation that can cause gastrointestinal ulcer and upset. Other gastrointestinal disorders may cause excess gastrin (e.g., upper gastrointestinal obstruction, previous small intestine resection, gastric dilatation/volvulus, *Helicobacter pylori*).

Next Diagnostic Steps to Consider if Levels Are High

Evaluate gastric mucosa (endoscopy) for hypertrophy, ulceration; assess for pancreatic islet (delta cell) tumor (abdominal ultrasound or CT and, with a pancreatic mass or liver lesions suggestive of metastases, laparotomy).

Drug Effects

Increased: H_2 blockers, antacids, and proton pump inhibitors

Specimen Collection and Handling

Gastrin is not stable at room temperature. Separate serum from clot as soon as possible and transfer from a red top tube to a plastic tube. Freeze immediately and ship on dry ice. 1 mL of serum, minimum.

Relative Cost: $$

Pearls

- Send out test to specialized gastrointestinal laboratories.
- The recommended cutoff value for diagnosis of gastrinoma is 10 times the upper limit of the reference interval.

AUTHOR & EDITOR: Lois Roth-Johnson, DVM, PhD, DACVP

Giardia Testing

Definition

Giardiasis is a diarrheal disease caused by the protozoan *Giardia* in animals and humans. *Giardia duodenalis* is the most common species that affects dogs; however, there are numerous assemblages with various infectivity for animals and humans. Fecal-oral exposures via food, water, or fomite transmission are common routes of infection.

Synonym

Beaver fever

Physiology

Giardia cysts are ingested by the animal. Bile acids degrade the cyst wall in the small intestine, resulting in the release of trophozoites that attach to the apices of small intestinal villi. Attachment leads to villus blunting and ultimately malabsorption and diarrhea. As trophozoites move toward the colon, they become encysted and pass in feces.

- Direct fecal smears use a drop of saline with a minuscule amount of diarrheic stool to identify motile trophozoites using microscopy visualization. Lugol's iodine can be added to enhance visualization.
- Zinc sulfate ($ZnSO_4$) fecal flotation relies on accurate identification of cysts that have floated to the surface when feces have been mixed with $ZnSO_4$ via simple or centrifugal methods.
- *Giardia* fecal ELISA detects the *Giardia* antigen in feces.
- Fecal direct immunofluorescence assay uses *Giardia*-specific fluorescently labeled antibodies to detect *Giardia* cysts in feces.
- Real-time polymerase chain reaction (RT-PCR) detects *Giardia*-specific amplified DNA sequences on feces.

Reference Interval

- Direct fecal smear: positive or no trophozoites or cysts seen
- Fecal flotation with centrifugation: positive or no cysts seen
- *Giardia* fecal ELISA: positive or negative
- Direct IFA: positive or no cysts seen
- RT-PCR: positive or below detectable limit

Causes of Abnormally High Levels

Evidence of intestinal infection

Next Diagnostic Steps to Consider if Levels Are High

In symptomatic animals, initiation of antiprotozoal therapy is recommended. See p. 386.

Causes of Abnormally Low Levels

Intermittent shedding of the organism; concurrent or previous antiprotozoal administration; not infected

Next Diagnostic Steps to Consider if Levels Are Low

Repeat testing in symptomatic animals, possibly using an alternative testing method.

Important Interspecies Differences

Dog strains are not known to infect cats. Cat strains are not known to infect dogs. Human infection as the result of exposure to canine giardiasis is considered a rare occurrence.

Drug Effects

Administration of antiprotozoal drugs may decrease *Giardia* shedding.

Lab Artifacts

On fecal flotation and direct fecal smear, yeast can appear similar in morphology and size to *Giardia* cysts, but yeast lacks internal structures (i.e., median bodies and two to four nuclei) and is often seen budding.

Specimen Collection and Handling

Fresh unrefrigerated feces collected within 30 minutes for direct smear. Fresh feces (within 24 hours) and stored between 2°C-8°C for all other *Giardia* testing.

Relative Cost: $ to $$

Pearls

- *Giardia* testing should be performed only on symptomatic animals.
- Zinc sulfate is the preferred solution for fecal flotation. Sugar solutions tend to distort and collapse *Giardia* cysts.
- *Tritrichomonas* sp. trophozoites in cats can appear morphologically similar to *Giardia* sp. trophozoites. *Giardia* sp. trophozoites have a "falling leaf" motion versus the erratic movements of *Tritrichomonas*. Trophozoites die within 30 minutes of defecation or collection.
- *Giardia* sp. cysts are similar in size to a canine RBC and easiest to visualize at 40x objective.

AUTHOR: Erin N. Burton, DVM, MS, DACVP
EDITOR: Lois Roth-Johnson, DVM, PhD, DACVP

Globulins

Definition

Globulins are all of the non-albumin proteins found in blood. They can be further classified as alpha, beta, or gamma via protein electrophoresis.

Physiology

Globulins are a heterogeneous group of serum proteins that include immunoglobulins, coagulation factors, complement, many acute-phase proteins, and lipoproteins, with a wide variety of physiologic functions.

Reference Interval

Dogs: 2-4 g/dL (20-40 g/L). Cats: 2.5-5 g/dL (25-50 g/L)

Causes of Abnormally High Levels

- Polyclonal gammopathy: any cause of chronic inflammation, hepatic disease, feline infectious peritonitis, occult heartworm disease, immune-mediated disease
- Monoclonal gammopathy: usually lymphoid malignancy such as multiple myeloma, lymphoma, or lymphoid leukemia. Rarely reported with non-neoplastic conditions including canine ehrlichiosis, leishmaniasis, lymphoplasmacytic enteritis and dermatitis
- If concurrent hyperalbuminemia: dehydration

Next Diagnostic Steps to Consider if Levels Are High

- If hyperalbuminemia and supportive physical exam findings, consider dehydration. If hydration status adequate, interpret with other lab work (e.g., CBC, chemistry panel) and physical exam to prioritize differentials.
- Protein electrophoresis and/or immunoelectrophoresis to differentiate monoclonal from polyclonal gammopathy

Causes of Abnormally Low Levels

- Primary/inherited and acquired immunodeficiencies, including failure of passive transfer
- If concurrent hypoalbuminemia (panhypoproteinemia): consider hemorrhage, protein-losing enteropathy, exudative dermatopathy/burns, and severe malnutrition/starvation. Albumin and globulin values are variable with liver disease.

Next Diagnostic Steps to Consider if Levels Are Low

Consider with signalment, presenting complaint, and biochemistry values, particularly albumin, to prioritize differentials. If hypoalbuminemia is present, interpret along with physical exam findings and CBC results to determine likely cause of panhypoproteinemia.

Lab Artifacts

Globulins are calculated by subtracting the measured albumin concentration from measured serum total protein concentration. If there is concern for inaccuracy in either of these reported values, the globulin value should be questioned. Sample hemolysis and/or lipemia may impact results, but sources of interference vary with analyzer and method.

Specimen Collection and Handling

Serum (red-top tube). If heparinized plasma is substituted, total protein and calculated globulins will be higher due to the presence of fibrinogen.

Relative Cost: $$ (must order total protein and albumin, or a panel)

Pearls

Electrophoretic evaluation is necessary to determine increases in specific globulin fractions.

AUTHOR: Mary Leissinger, DVM, MS, DACVP
EDITOR: Lois Roth-Johnson, DVM, PhD, DACVP

Glucose, Blood

Definition

Blood concentration of the sugar utilized for energy production

Physiology

Carbohydrates in the diet are catabolized to glucose for absorption and transport to tissues. The liver produces glucose via gluconeogenesis and glycogenolysis, and stores glucose as glycogen or converts glucose to amino acids and lipids. Blood glucose is primarily regulated by dietary intake and the hormones insulin and glucagon, which regulate its hepatic storage, release, and tissue utilization.

Reference Interval

- Dogs: 60-125 mg/dL (3.3-6.9 mmol/L); cats: 70-150 mg/dL (3.9-8.3 mmol/L)
- To convert from mg/dL to mmol/L, multiply by 0.0555.

Causes of Abnormally High Levels

Diabetes mellitus, glucose-containing fluids, hyperadrenocorticism, hyperthyroidism, acromegaly/hyperpituitarism, acute pancreatitis, excitement-induced epinephrine release (primarily cats), postprandial (minor elevation). See p. 1235.

Next Diagnostic Steps to Consider if Levels Are High

Assess for persistent hyperglycemia, glucosuria, ketonuria, +/- serum fructosamine.

Causes of Abnormally Low Levels

Paraneoplastic (insulinoma, leiomyosarcoma, others), insulin overdose, neonatal or juvenile hypoglycemia, advanced liver disease, congenital portosystemic shunt, extreme exertion, sepsis, hypoadrenocorticism, hypopituitarism, long-term starvation (rare cause of hypoglycemia in adults) or malabsorption, glycogen storage diseases, intoxication (e.g., xylitol, oleander), artifact (delay in separating red blood cells from serum/plasma, erythrocytosis or extreme leukocytosis). See p. 1240.

Next Diagnostic Steps to Consider if Levels Are Low

Resample to verify persistent hypoglycemia. Correlate with other clinical and laboratory findings. Evaluate for insulinoma (p. 552).

Important Interspecies Differences

Hyperglycemia due to excitement-induced epinephrine release is common in cats.

Drug Effects

- Increase: glucocorticoids, adrenocorticotropic hormone, intravenous fluids containing dextrose, growth hormone, glucagon, megestrol acetate, thiazide diuretics, xylazine, ketamine (cats), morphine, and phenothiazine tranquilizers
- Decrease: excess insulin (exogenous or insulinoma), ethanol toxicity, treatment with salicylates, sulfonylurea, xylitol, o,p'-DDD

Lab Artifacts

- Decrease: delayed separation of serum or plasma from red blood cells results in artificial depression due to utilization of glucose by blood cells.
- Increase: lipemia
- Point-of-care glucometers often underestimate blood glucose (especially those designed for use in humans).

Specimen Collection and Handling

Serum (red top tube) or heparinized plasma (green top tube). Separate from cells within 30 minutes after sample collection. Use fluoride oxalate anticoagulant (gray top tube) if plasma separation is not possible: stable at 2°C-8°C for 4 days.

Relative Cost: Single test $; included in many chemistry panels $-$$$

AUTHOR: Ruanna E. Gossett, DVM, PhD, DACVP
EDITOR: Lois Roth-Johnson, DVM, PhD, DACVP

Glucosuria

Definition

The presence of glucose in urine secondary to overwhelmed or defective renal tubular reabsorption

Synonym

Glycosuria

Physiology

Glucose is freely filtered by the glomerulus and is subsequently reabsorbed by the proximal renal tubular epithelial cells. Glucose reabsorption is dependent upon the glomerular filtration rate, tubular reabsorption rate, and urine flow. During hyperglycemic states, the increased concentration of glucose in the ultrafiltrate exceeds the maximum reabsorptive capacity of the renal tubules. The point at which the reabsorptive capacity of the renal tubules is exceeded is termed the renal threshold and differs among species.

Reference Interval

Negative in healthy patients; stressed cats may have transient glucosuria. Positive results are reported in semi-quantitative values.

Causes of Abnormally High Levels

- With concurrent hyperglycemia: diabetes mellitus, hyperadrenocorticism, stress (cats), pancreatitis, pheochromocytoma
- With concurrent euglycemia: renal tubular damage (e.g., nephrotoxicity), Fanconi syndrome, primary renal glucosuria

Next Diagnostic Steps to Consider if Levels Are High

Measure plasma glucose and/or fructosamine to exclude diabetes mellitus.

Important Interspecies Differences

The renal tubular threshold for glucose is ≈180 mg/dL in dogs and ≈280 mg/dL in cats.

Drug Effects

False-negative results can occur with high concentrations of ascorbic acid.

Lab Artifacts

Contamination with oxidizing agents (e.g., bleach) can result in false-positive results.

Specimen Collection and Handling

Avoid collection of urine off exam table or floor to prevent potential contamination with oxidizing agents. If refrigerated for storage, allow the sample to reach room temperature before processing.

Relative Cost: $ (reported as part of urinalysis)

Pearls

- Owners of diabetic dogs should be discouraged from altering insulin dose based on home monitoring of glucosuria.
- Owners of diabetic cats who notice glucosuria consistently absent via home monitoring should contact their veterinarian as disease may be in remission.

AUTHOR: Shannon D. Dehghanpir, DVM, MS, DACVP
EDITOR: Lois Roth-Johnson, DVM, PhD, DACVP

Glycated Hemoglobin

Definition

Hemoglobin (Hgb) with nonenzymatically added glucose is referred to as glycated or glycosylated Hgb. Can be used to monitor therapy in diabetic patients; however, use of fructosamine for this purpose is far more common. Results usually reported as the % glycated Hgb out of total Hgb but may instead be reported as the total concentration of glycated Hgb.

Synonyms

Glycosylated Hgb. Hgb A_{1c} is a specific form.

Physiology

The degree of increase in glycated Hgb concentration in a patient is dependent on the magnitude and duration of hyperglycemia over the span of approximately 2 months. Altering the total Hgb concentration (anemia, erythrocytosis) will accordingly change the total glycated Hgb concentration.

Reference Interval

Varies by laboratory. Example: 1.7%-4.9% (dogs)

Causes of Abnormally High Levels

Persistent hyperglycemia (diabetes mellitus)

Next Diagnostic Steps to Consider if Levels Are High

Increased glycated Hgb indicates insulin therapy and other glycemic management protocols may need to be optimized. Serial glucose measurements (glucose curve) may be necessary to better tailor therapy.

Causes of Abnormally Low Levels

Persistent hypoglycemia, recent hemorrhage or hemolysis resulting in a skewed proportion of young erythrocytes (and thus less glycated Hgb), anemia of any type will decrease total glycated Hgb concentration.

Next Diagnostic Steps to Consider if Levels Are Low

Decreased glycated Hgb in a diabetic patient receiving insulin suggests that therapy has been causing periods of hypoglycemia. Treatment protocol should be re-evaluated, and serial glucose measurements (glucose curve) may be warranted.

Important Interspecies Differences

Not all human Hgb A_{1c} assays are validated for use in veterinary species.

Lab Artifacts

Varies with methodology used; contact your laboratory for more information.

Specimen Collection and Handling

- Collect blood into an EDTA (purple top) tube. Refrigerate and ship sample with cold packs. Refrigerated blood is considered stable for a week before analysis. Storage at room temperature may decrease results.
- Recently, an A1c test kit has been marketed for dogs and cats (A1Care, Baycom Diagnostics). A drop of whole blood is applied to a test card that is mailed out for analysis.

Relative Cost: $$

AUTHOR: Angela Royal, MS, DVM, DACVP
EDITOR: Lois Roth-Johnson, DVM, PhD, DACVP

Heartworm Microfilarial Filter Testing

Definition

Diagnostic testing for the qualification of microfilariae such as *Dirofilaria immitis*

Synonyms

Knott's test, heartworm filter test

Physiology

This test enhances the sensitivity of identification of microfilariae in the blood via concentration and lyses of erythrocytes via trapping the microfilariae (L1) on a polycarbonate filter.

Reference Interval

Reported as "No microfilariae observed" or "Microfilariae observed"

Causes of Abnormally High Levels

Microfilarial loads from *Dirofilaria* spp. or *Acanthocheilonema reconditum* infection

Next Diagnostic Steps to Consider if Levels Are High

Differentiation of *D. immitis* from *A. reconditum* and *D. repens*. *A. reconditum* larva's body is generally smaller in diameter than a canine erythrocyte (≈8 mcm), while *D. immitis* is approximately the same diameter or slightly larger. *D. repens* is an uncommon infection in the United States. Confirmation with a heartworm antigen test and/or advanced imaging (echocardiogram, thoracic radiograph) is recommended. Consider staging the patient for heartworm disease using the American Heartworm Society guidelines (https://www.heartwormsociety.org/).

Causes of Abnormally Low Levels

Occult infections (the presence of adult heartworm without a microfilaremia) result from single-sex infections, prepatent infection, destruction of microfilariae by monthly heartworm preventatives, or host immune destruction of microfilariae.

Next Diagnostic Steps to Consider if Levels Are Low

Consider a heartworm antigen test to rule out an occult infection.

Important Interspecies Differences

Cats usually have occult heartworm infections; thus other heartworm testing (e.g., antibody and/or antigen test or advanced imaging) is recommended.

Drug Effects

Concurrent heartworm preventative medications decrease the sensitivity of this test secondary to destruction of microfilariae.

Specimen Collection and Handling

Approximately 1 to 2 mL of anticoagulated whole blood (EDTA, heparin, citrate) is necessary to perform this test.

Relative Cost: $

Pearls

- Knowledge of microfilarial morphology is necessary for interpretation of this test, as in some areas of the United States and world, *D. immitis* is not the only microfilarial that can be identified in circulation. Other commonly identified microfilariae include *Dirofilaria repens* and *Acanthocheilonema reconditum*.
- The availability of this test has become variable in reference laboratories with the advent of more sensitive and specific point-of-care *Dirofilaria immitis* testing.

AUTHOR: Erin N. Burton, DVM, MS, DACVP
EDITOR: Lois Roth-Johnson, DVM, PhD, DACVP

Heartworm Serology Testing

Definition

Antigen and antibody testing for *Dirofilaria immitis*

Synonym

Occult heartworm testing

Physiology

- Antigen tests detect the adult female nematodes of *Dirofilaria immitis*.
- Antibody testing detects the species-specific antibodies resulting from immature, adult male, adult female, and single-sex nematode *D. immitis* infections.

Reference Interval

- Antigen tests are reported as positive or no antigen detected.
- Antibody test are reported as positive or no antibodies detected.

Causes of Abnormally High Levels

- Antigen: infection with adult nematodes; false-positive results may occur with marked hemolysis
- Antibody: indicates exposure to larvae or adult nematodes. Seroconversion in cats can be detected as early as 60 days postinfection.

Next Diagnostic Steps to Consider if Levels Are High

Consider staging the patient for heartworm disease using the American Heartworm Society guidelines (https://www.heartwormsociety.org/veterinary-resources/american-heartworm-society-guidelines).

Causes of Abnormally Low Levels

- Antigen: false-negatives result from low worm burden (<3 female worms), male-only infections, or if only immature stages are present. Natural antibody-antigen complexes have been documented to interfere with test.
- Antibody: false-negatives result from insufficient antibody production or conversion time (<60 days postinfection). Each antibody test varies at level of sensitivity for different stages of nematode maturation.

Next Diagnostic Steps to Consider if Levels Are Low

If clinical signs are present, consider other diagnostics such advanced imaging (thoracic radiographs, echocardiogram), CBC/biochemistry panel with a complete urinalysis, or request heat treatment of serum sample before antigen testing.

Important Interspecies Differences

The sensitivity of the heartworm antigen and antibody testing in cats is markedly lower than dogs, thus negative results should be interpreted with caution. Using both antibody and antigen testing in cats may improve the accuracy of diagnosis in this species.

Drug Effects

The antigen test can remain positive for up to 6 months post-adulticide treatment.

Lab Artifacts

- Improper storage of the antigen test kits may interfere with test results.
- Improper handling or storage of the sample may result in degradation of the antigen.

Specimen Collection and Handling

- Antigen: whole blood, serum, or plasma depending on kit; specimens may be refrigerated for up to five days or frozen for longer storage.
- Antibody: serum, 1 mL. Specimens may be refrigerated for up to five days or frozen for longer storage.

Relative Cost: Antigen or antibody $; combined antibody and antigen panel $$

Pearls

- The color intensity of antigen tests does not correlate well with the degree of worm burden.
- Positive antibody test conveys only exposure. Not all animals that have had exposure have clinical disease.
- False-negative antigen tests after "slow kill" therapy are possible. If suspected, send samples to laboratory for heat treatment before testing.
- Kits for in-clinic testing may decrease cost per test if a high number of tests are done.
- Current information and guidelines can be found online from the American Heartworm Society; https://heartwormsociety.org.

AUTHOR: Erin N. Burton, DVM, MS, DACVP
EDITOR: Lois Roth-Johnson, DVM, PhD, DACVP

Heinz Bodies

Definition

Single or multiple precipitated denatured hemoglobin particles on the erythrocyte membrane, often associated with oxidative damage. See p. 1327.

Synonyms

Erythrocyte refractile body or ER body, HB, Schmauch body

Physiology

Oxidants may cause irreversible denaturation of hemoglobin molecule, causing Heinz body (HB) formation. HBs have affinity for, and form a complex with, membrane protein band 3 on both the internal and external erythrocyte membrane. HBs also make erythrocytes rigid and less deformable (via cross-linking of spectrin and hemoglobin), making affected erythrocytes prone to intravascular and/or extravascular hemolysis (erythophagocytosis by splenic macrophages).

Reference Interval

Low proportion seen in erythrocytes of normal cats; uncommon in normal dogs

Causes of Abnormally High Levels

Drugs (see Drug Effects) and chemicals in food (onions, garlic, chives) or other substances (zinc, propylene glycol, skunk musk); deficiency of enzymes that protect against oxidants

Next Diagnostic Steps to Consider if Levels Are High

- Review patient history (diet, drug or toxin exposure, ingestion of metallic [zinc] foreign objects, exposure to skunk musk).
- CBC, urinalysis, biochemistry profile: anemia, hemolysis.

Important Interspecies Differences

- Normal in feline erythrocytes because of innately unstable hemoglobin structure, predisposition to form methemoglobin (low methemoglobin reductase activity), and inefficient removal by spleen. Normally occurring HBs are not associated with regenerative anemia or hemolysis. Increased HB formation may occur without substantial anemia in diabetes mellitus, hyperthyroidism, and lymphoma.
- In other species, increased numbers of HBs may be seen post-splenectomy.

Drug Effects

Acetaminophen, benzocaine-containing products, DL-methionine, methylene blue, phenacetin, phenazopyridine, phenothiazine, and vitamin K_3 cause HB formation and hemolytic anemia.

Specimen Collection and Handling

EDTA whole blood (lavender top tube) for CBC, Wright- and new methylene blue–stained blood smears

Relative Cost: $$ (reported as part of CBC)

Pearls

- Free HBs may falsely increase instrument platelet counts and hemoglobin measurement.
- HBs may occur concurrently with eccentrocytes (also a result of oxidative injury) and spherocytes (due to splenic removal of HBs from red cell membranes).

AUTHOR: Fidelia R. Fernandez, DVM, MS, DACVP
EDITOR: Lois Roth-Johnson, DVM, PhD, DACVP

Hematocrit

Definition

The percentage of blood composed of erythrocytes. Electronic cell counters calculate hematocrit using this formula: (MCV × RBC)/10 = HCT, where HCT is hematocrit, MCV is mean corpuscular volume (in femtoliters [fL]), and RBC is erythrocyte count ($\times 10^6$/fL). Provided Hb (hemoglobin) reading is accurate (i.e., no interference from hemolysis, lipemia, Heinz bodies, etc.), HCT = Hb × 3.

Physiology

HCT values are slightly less than packed cell volume (PCV, from centrifugation) because there is no trapped plasma in an HCT calculation, as can occur with spun PCVs. Sources of variation:

- Due to the variable MCV of domestic animals, values for HCT may be erroneous if the instrument is not calibrated for specific species.
- Abnormal plasma osmolality and electrolyte balance may also result in a difference between HCT and PCV that is generally not clinically significant.
- Although PCV measures changes in erythrocyte volume as they occur *in vivo*, dilution of erythrocytes with normal saline and standing in hematology instruments may cause erythrocytes to return to their normal volume.

Reference Interval

Dogs: 36%-60%; cats: 29%-48%

Causes of Abnormally High Levels

Erythrocytosis due to breed (sighthounds), dehydration, splenic contraction ("relative polycythemia"), hypoxemia, independent erythropoietin production (e.g., renal neoplasia), or polycythemia vera (myeloproliferative disease of erythrocytes or primary absolute erythrocytosis)

Next Diagnostic Steps to Consider if Levels Are High

Assess hydration status, review clinical history, assess oxygenation, and evaluate for causes of erythrocytosis/polycythemia.

Causes of Abnormally Low Levels

Anemia, overhydration

Next Diagnostic Steps to Consider if Levels Are Low

Blood smear evaluation for type of anemia and evidence of regeneration (e.g., polychromasia), absolute reticulocyte count, then further testing as indicated

Important Interspecies Differences

Greyhounds, whippets, salukis, Afghan hounds, and dachshunds have slightly higher normal values (up to 65% is considered normal, with some individuals exceeding even this level).

Drug Effects

Erythropoietin injections increase HCT; drugs toxic to bone marrow (hydroxyurea, methimazole, many others) and drugs that cause hemolysis (e.g., zinc, methylene blue, benzocaine) can decrease HCT.

Lab Artifacts

- Hemolysis, lipemia, and specimen clotting prevent accurate reading.
- Insufficient filling of EDTA (lavender top) tube dilutes specimen, decreasing HCT; tubes should be filled to capacity for accurate results.

Specimen Collection and Handling

EDTA anticoagulated blood (lavender top tube); two capillary tubes for PCV; Vacutainer tubes must be completely filled. Transport at room temperature or refrigerate.

Relative Cost: $

Pearls

- The differences between HCT and PCV values are not clinically significant except at very high values (PCV/HCT > 65%), where plasma trapping becomes substantial.
- "Polycythemia" refers to an increase in all circulating cell lines, but this term is often used interchangeably with "erythrocytosis," the correct term to indicate an increase in HCT.

AUTHOR: Fidelia R. Fernandez, DVM, MS, DACVP
EDITOR: Lois Roth-Johnson, DVM, PhD, DACVP

Hemoglobinuria and Hematuria

Definition

Hemoglobinuria is the presence of hemoglobin in urine and is associated with red to brown urine that persists in the specimen even after centrifugation. *Hematuria* is the presence of erythrocytes in urine and is associated with red, cloudy urine that clears with centrifugation. Either one may cause a positive reaction on the blood reagent square of a urine dipstick.

Physiology

- Free hemoglobin in the plasma binds haptoglobin; the complex is cleared in the liver. When haptoglobin becomes saturated, free hemoglobin splits into dimers that are excreted by the kidneys. Hemoglobin in glomerular filtrate is absorbed by proximal tubules and metabolized to bilirubin, iron, and globin. Unabsorbed hemoglobin appears in urine (hemoglobinuria).
- Erythrocytes may appear in the urine from upper urinary (renal, rarely ureteral), lower urinary (bladder, urethra), urogenital (prostate, testes, prepuce, uterus, vagina, vulva), or artifactual (traumatic sampling) sources.

Reference Interval

- Hemoglobin is not found in normal urine.
- Finding < 5 erythrocytes/HPF is considered normal in urine sediment.

Causes of Abnormally High Levels

- Hemoglobinuria: severe intravascular hemolysis. Free hemoglobin also may appear in urine in cases of hematuria if erythrocytes lyse in very dilute (specific gravity ≤ 1.008) or alkaline urine.
- Hematuria may be associated with urinary tract hemorrhage, trauma, infection, inflammation, or bleeding neoplasia (p. 1229).

Next Diagnostic Steps to Consider if Levels Are High

- Hemoglobinuria: identify cause of hemolysis by blood smear evaluation for hemic parasites, Heinz bodies, eccentrocytes and spherocytes. Evaluate CBC, serum biochemistry profile, RBC enzyme deficiency, and abdominal and thoracic imaging for triggers of hemolytic anemia. Evaluate history for spider bite, viper/coral snake envenomation, bee sting or exposure to toxins.
- Hematuria: rule out coagulopathy. Determine when hematuria occurs during micturition (beginning of urination suggests lower urinary/genital origin; end of urination, bladder origin; throughout urination suggests renal disease, diffuse bladder disease, prostatic disease). Renal/bladder ultrasonographic evaluations often helpful. See pp. 428 and 1229.

Drug Effects

Drugs causing intravascular hemolysis can also result in hemoglobinuria.

Specimen Collection and Handling

Urine (5 mL) in a clean specimen container. Indicate collection method.

Relative Cost: $ (reported as part of standard urinalysis)

Pearls

- Avoid cystocentesis if gross hematuria appreciated until coagulopathy and bladder neoplasia have been ruled out.
- Cystocentesis and catheterization are frequently associated with iatrogenic, microscopic hematuria. These collection methods are not recommended for monitoring remission or progression of hematuria.
- Free-catch urine from bitches in heat (proestrus) may also be contaminated with blood.
- A urine reagent strip that is positive for blood in the absence of red cells on urine sediment warrants evaluation for hemoglobinuria or myoglobinuria (p. 1367).

AUTHOR: Fidelia R. Fernandez, DVM, MS, DACVP
EDITOR: Lois Roth-Johnson, DVM, PhD, DACVP

Hemolysis

Definition

Hemolysis is rupture of erythrocytes, releasing hemoglobin. It results in red discoloration of serum or plasma.

Physiology

Hemolysis is most commonly an *in vitro* artifact from traumatic venipuncture or improper sample handling. It may also occur *in vivo* with pathologic erythrocyte injury (especially intravascular injury). Hemolysis may interfere with laboratory assays by sample discoloration, altering spectrophotometric assay results, dilution of normal substances in serum, or leakage of analytes from erythrocytes. The degree of hemolysis may affect some analytes more than others (see individual test entries in this section of the textbook). The analytes affected and degree of interference depend on the method and type of analyzer.

Lab Artifacts

- Hemolysis causes an artifactual increase in hemoglobin, mean corpuscular hemoglobin concentration, calcium, potassium, alanine aminotransferase, aspartate aminotransferase, creatine kinase, lactate dehydrogenase, triglycerides, and total protein.
- Hemolysis causes an artifactual decrease in RBC count, hematocrit, glucose, creatinine, total bilirubin, bile acids, alkaline phosphatase, gamma-glutamyltransferase, amylase, and lipase.

Pearls

Ways to prevent *in vitro* hemolysis include:

- Avoid traumatic venipuncture.
- Avoid using a needle with an inappropriately small diameter. Use a 21-gauge or larger

bore needle to transfer or introduce blood specimens into Vacutainer tubes to avoid excess turbulence/foaming and resultant hemolysis.
- Avoid excess negative pressure when drawing blood into syringe and excessive agitation of the sample in the tube.
- Ensure prompt separation of serum from the clot and proper storage of sample (refrigeration; avoid freezing).
- Avoid delay in sample analysis or delayed transport of samples to the laboratory for analysis.
- Avoid exposing sample to temperature extremes.

AUTHOR: Ruanna E. Gossett, DVM, PhD, DACVP
EDITOR: Lois Roth-Johnson, DVM, PhD, DACVP

High-Dose Dexamethasone Suppression Test

Definition

The high-dose dexamethasone suppression test (HDDST) is a dynamic test of the hypothalamic-pituitary-adrenal axis used to differentiate between pituitary-dependent hyperadrenocorticism (PDH) and the presence of a functional adrenal cortical neoplasm in a patient known to have hyperadrenocorticism. Baseline and post-dexamethasone blood samples are collected for cortisol measurement.

Synonym

HDDST

Physiology

Administration of dexamethasone should suppress pituitary ACTH production and thus adrenocortical cortisol production. Functional adrenal neoplasms and some (≈35%) pituitary neoplasms will continue to autonomously secrete cortisol and ACTH, respectively.

Reference Interval

Varies by laboratory. Examples of guidelines for "adequate" suppression of cortisol levels post-dexamethasone administration are < 1.4 mcg/dL or suppression by more than half of baseline cortisol concentration. Cortisol measured as either mcg/dL (common unit) or nmol/L (SI unit).

Causes of Abnormally High Levels

Failure of HDDST to suppress cortisol often indicates the presence of functional adrenal cortical neoplasia. Failure to suppress cortisol can also be seen with some (≈35%) PDH and very rarely in patients with ectopic ACTH production from a nonpituitary neoplasm.

Next Diagnostic Steps to Consider if Levels Are High

Abdominal imaging to elucidate whether one adrenal gland is enlarged (supportive of functional adrenal cortical neoplasm), or if there is bilateral adrenomegaly (supportive of PDH). Consider measurement of endogenous ACTH concentration if confusion still exists. See pp. 34, 485, and 487.

Causes of Abnormally Low Levels

Adequate suppression during HDDST indicates pituitary micro- or macroadenoma causing PDH.

Next Diagnostic Steps to Consider if Levels Are Low

Suppression of cortisol production with the HDDST in a patient known to have hyperadrenocorticism confirms PDH.

Important Interspecies Differences

Dose of dexamethasone differs between species.

Drug Effects

Cortisol assays may cross-react with pharmacologic steroids administered within 24 hours, including prednisolone, 11-deoxycortisol, prednisone, and others.

Lab Artifacts

- Do not use serum separator tubes for blood collection; gel from serum separator tubes can interfere with cortisol measurement.
- EDTA and icterus also interfere with assay.

Specimen Collection and Handling

Three blood samples for cortisol measurement are collected. For each, collect blood into plain red top tubes, allow to clot, centrifuge, and transfer serum to a separate tube clearly labeled with the sample ID/time. Ship samples frozen or refrigerated, on ice.
- Baseline cortisol sample drawn in morning
- Administer 0.1 mg/kg dexamethasone IV (dogs) or 1 mg/kg dexamethasone IV (cats).
- Collect additional blood sample at 4 hours and again at 8 hours post-dexamethasone administration.

Relative Cost: $$

Pearls

- Due to ready accessibility of advanced imaging, HDDST is now seldom used to discriminate between adrenal and pituitary-dependent hyperadrenocorticism.
- HDDST is not used for the diagnosis of hyperadrenocorticism and should be performed only after confirming that hyperadrenocorticism is present.
- Though suppression of cortisol concentration confirms PDH, failure to suppress does not discriminate between functional adrenal cortical neoplasia and PDH.

AUTHOR: Angela Royal, MS, DVM, DACVP
EDITOR: Lois Roth-Johnson, DVM, PhD, DACVP

Howell-Jolly Bodies

Definition

Retained erythrocyte nuclear fragments. Basophilic intraerythrocytic inclusions that are generally single, spherical, and ≈0.5 to 1 mcm in diameter

Physiology

During development in the bone marrow, mammalian erythroid progenitor cells contain nuclei. Howell-Jolly bodies represent nuclear fragments that have separated from the nucleus of the developing erythrocyte. They are removed by the spleen.

Reference Interval

Howell-Jolly bodies are occasionally found in the erythrocytes of healthy animals, more often in cats than dogs. Only reported on blood smear review if excessive

Causes of Abnormally High Levels

Regenerative anemia, decreased splenic function/splenectomy, hereditary macrocytosis of poodles, myelodysplastic syndrome, or drugs (e.g., glucocorticoids, chemotherapeutics)

Next Diagnostic Steps to Consider if Levels Are High

If a strongly regenerative anemia is present, no further investigation is necessary. Review history for prior splenectomy and current medications. Consider macrocytosis of poodles (MCV may range from 90-100 fL). Myelodysplastic syndromes are uncommon in veterinary medicine, and in these conditions Howell-Jolly bodies would be accompanied by dysplastic features and cytopenias in one or more hematologic cell lines. If myelodysplastic syndrome is suspected, the sample should be submitted for review by a clinical pathologist.

Important Interspecies Differences

Howell-Jolly bodies are generally absent in the peripheral blood of healthy dogs owing to the presence of a sinusoidal spleen in this species, which effectively removes the inclusions from erythrocytes. The non-sinusoidal spleen of cats is not as efficient at removal, so low numbers of inclusions may be found in the peripheral blood of healthy cats.

Drug Effects

Glucocorticoid therapy or chemotherapeutic agents can increase numbers.

Specimen Collection and Handling

Anticoagulated blood sample, as for routine CBC with blood smear

Relative Cost: $$ (reported as part of CBC, and only if excessive)

Pearls

Occasionally inclusions may appear atypical and difficult to distinguish from inclusions of pathologic significance (e.g., parasites). If numerous or atypical, consider review by a clinical pathologist.

AUTHOR: Mary Leissinger, DVM, MS, DACVP
EDITOR: Lois Roth-Johnson, DVM, PhD, DACVP

Insulin, Serum Level

Definition

Insulin is a polypeptide hormone that promotes uptake of glucose by a variety of cell types.

Physiology

Insulin is produced by pancreatic islet beta-cells. Normally a rise in blood glucose concentration (but also growth hormone, amino acid concentration, and others) will cause release of insulin to the blood. Major effects of insulin include promotion of myocyte and adipocyte glucose uptake, increased production of glycogen in hepatocytes and myocytes, and decreased lipolysis and proteolysis. Depletion of pancreatic beta-cells results in inadequate insulin production (type I diabetes mellitus). Persistent insulin antagonism (for instance, in hyperadrenocorticism) will initially cause concurrent hyperglycemia and hyperinsulinemia. Measurement of insulin in diabetic patients is not common. Instead, serum insulin is usually measured concurrently with glucose concentration to investigate hypoglycemia in a patient with suspected insulinoma (functional beta-cell neoplasm).

Reference Interval

Varies by laboratory

Causes of Abnormally High Levels

In a hyperglycemic patient

- Expected response to hyperglycemia. If persistent, indicates insulin resistance/insensitivity.
  - Concurrently increased insulin and progesterone concentration in a newly diagnosed diabetic intact female dog suggests diestrus may be causing the insulin insensitivity. This form of diabetes mellitus may not require medical management post-ovariohysterectomy.

In a hypoglycemic patient

- Overproduction of insulin
  - Insulinoma
  - Xylitol toxicosis

Next Diagnostic Steps to Consider if Levels Are High

In a patient suspected to have insulinoma, abdominal imaging to identify a potential neoplasm is warranted. See p. 552.

Causes of Abnormally Low Levels

Low levels are expected in a hypoglycemic patient or in patients with type I diabetes mellitus.

Next Diagnostic Steps to Consider if Levels Are Low

If insulin level or insulin to glucose ratio is low in a hypoglycemic patient, evaluation for other causes of hypoglycemia is warranted. Assuming CBC and chemistry panel do not support the possibility of hypoadrenocorticism, hepatic insufficiency, portosystemic shunt, sepsis, or other known causes of hypoglycemia, imaging/assessment of the patient for neoplasia is still recommended. Paraneoplastic hypoglycemia is sometimes related to factors other than insulin itself. For example, overproduction of insulin-like growth factor 2 (IGF-2) has been reported in some canine tumors.

Drug Effects

Administration of exogenous insulin or insulin antagonists may increase results.

Lab Artifacts

Presence of patient anti-insulin antibodies may falsely increase or decrease results depending on test methodology.

Specimen Collection and Handling

Collect blood into a red top tube at a point when the patient is hypoglycemic, ideally < 65 mg/dL (if assessing for insulinoma). Spin and collect serum, refrigerate or freeze, and submit on ice overnight. Plasma from heparin tubes (green top) or EDTA tubes (lavender top) may be acceptable; check with your lab for specific guidelines. Hemolysis will interfere with some assays; clear serum or plasma is preferred.

Relative Cost: $-$$

AUTHOR: Angela Royal, MS, DVM, DACVP
EDITOR: Lois Roth-Johnson, DVM, PhD, DACVP

Iron Profile

Definition

Iron profiles can help characterize whether an animal has an iron-deficient or iron-overload state.

- Serum iron (Fe): circulating Fe bound to transferrin
- Total iron-binding capacity (TIBC): measurement of plasma's capacity to carry Fe in serum by estimating the concentration of Fe carrying serum and plasma proteins in blood
- Unbound iron-binding capacity (UIBC): calculated value; TIBC minus serum Fe
- Stainable iron in macrophages of the bone marrow, spleen, or liver: subjective visual assessment of bone marrow aspirates and/or bone marrow core sections for free or stainable iron
- Serum ferritin: an intracellular iron-binding protein that changes in proportion to body stores
- Serum transferrin: a circulating transport protein for iron. Transferrin concentration (mg/dL) can be converted to TIBC (mcg/dL) by multiplying by 1.389.
- % Transferrin saturation: estimates the percentage of Fe-binding sites occupied by Fe on apotransferrin (unsaturated transferrin molecule) by calculating serum Fe × 100 divided by TIBC.

Synonyms

Iron profile, iron panel, iron testing, Fe profile

Physiology

Iron is an essential mineral that is taken up by small intestinal enterocytes and transferred to the bone marrow and other tissues by the acute-phase plasma protein transferrin. Iron (Fe^{3+}) is stored in the cytoplasm of numerous cells (muscle, macrophages, enterocytes) by an intracytoplasmic protein (ferritin). Most (75%) plasma iron is transferred to the bone marrow for erythropoiesis; the remainder is stored in various organs (mainly liver). The majority of total body iron (≈65%) is found in hemoglobin, with much of the remainder stored as ferritin and hemosiderin within macrophages. Far smaller quantities are stored in muscles (myoglobin), plasma proteins and enzymes, and only 0.1% bound to transferrin in the plasma.

Reference Interval

Dog: serum iron 125-225 mcg/dL; TIBC 225-325 mcg/dL; ferritin 525-1100 mcg/dL

Causes of Abnormally High Levels

- Serum Fe: Fe overload from excess intake (diet or iatrogenic), increased glucocorticoid (endogenous or exogenous)
- TIBC: Fe deficiency, Fe overload from excess intake (diet or iatrogenic),
- Stainable iron: inflammation, pathologic hemolysis, Fe overload from excess intake (diet or iatrogenic)
- Serum ferritin: inflammation, Fe overload from excess intake (diet or iatrogenic), pathologic hemolysis, hepatic insufficiency, hepatocyte necrosis
- % transferrin saturation: increased serum Fe, decreased TIBC

Next Diagnostic Steps to Consider if Levels Are High

Rule out supplementation/intoxication, liver disease; consider referral.

Causes of Abnormally Low Levels

- Serum Fe: Fe deficiency, inflammation, young animal (kittens)
- TIBC: hepatic insufficiency, inflammation, protein-losing nephropathy, protein-losing enteropathy
- Stainable iron: Fe deficiency, young animals
- Serum ferritin: Fe deficiency, young animals, hepatic insufficiency
- % transferrin saturation: decreased serum Fe, increased TIBC

Next Diagnostic Steps to Consider if Levels Are Low

- Investigate for underlying cause, depending on signalment and clinical signs (e.g., anemia, chronic inflammatory conditions, liver or renal disease)

Important Interspecies Differences

- Cats do not typically have visual stainable iron in the bone marrow on aspiration or core tissue biopsy.

Drug Effects

Glucocorticoids increase serum iron levels in dogs (unknown mechanism).

Lab Artifacts

Hemolysis falsely increases serum iron concentrations.

Specimen Collection and Handling

Fast patient overnight. Collect in serum (red top) tube; spin and separate cells from serum within 2 hours; transfer serum to plastic tube. Freeze and ship to lab on ice. Specimen must be free of hemolysis.

Relative Cost: $$

Pearls

- Serum iron profiles are seldom used in small animal veterinary medicine.
- Iron deficiency may cause anemia characterized by microcytosis and hypochromasia.
- Serum Fe concentrations are often an unreliable measurement of total body iron status.
- Assessment of an animal's Fe status is enhanced when laboratory tests are grouped as a profile.
- In young animals, intestinal parasitism is a common cause of Fe-deficiency anemia.
- In older animals, chronic gastrointestinal bleeding is a common cause of Fe-deficiency anemia.
- Animals with anemia of inflammatory disease typically have normal to low serum iron, TIBC, and normal to high serum ferritin.

AUTHOR: Erin N. Burton, DVM, MS, DACVP
EDITOR: Lois Roth-Johnson, DVM, PhD, DACVP

Ketonuria

Definition

The presence of ketones (beta-hydroxybutyrate, acetoacetate, acetone) in the urine

Physiology

Ketogenesis is initiated during states of limited carbohydrate availability. Ketonuria develops when the blood ketone concentration exceeds the renal threshold allowing ketones to enter the urine through glomerular filtration and tubular secretion. Urine ketones can be measured via urine dipstick or the Acetest®; however, beta-hydroxybutyrate is not detected by either of these methods.

Reference Interval

Negative in healthy patients; positive results are reported in semi-quantitative values.

Causes of Abnormally High Levels

Diabetes mellitus, starvation/negative energy balance, persistent hypoglycemia. See p. 1248.

Next Diagnostic Steps to Consider if Levels Are High

Evaluate for diabetes mellitus/diabetic ketoacidosis (p. 251). Perform confirmatory Acetest®.

Lab Artifacts

Hematuria, hemoglobinuria, and highly concentrated, acidic urine may cause false-positive results.

Specimen Collection and Handling

Perform with fresh urine.

Relative Cost: $ (reported as part of urinalysis)

Pearls

Serum or plasma can also be used to detect ketonemia. Blood ketones typically resolve before ketonuria during treatment of ketotic diabetes mellitus. See p. 254.

AUTHOR: Shannon D. Dehghanpir, DVM, MS, DACVP
EDITOR: Lois Roth-Johnson, DVM, PhD, DACVP

Lactate

Definition

Metabolic end product of anaerobic glycolysis

Synonym

Lactic acid

Physiology

Lactate production increases with hypoxia (especially from skeletal muscle and GI tract) or abnormal carbohydrate metabolism associated with some diseases. Liver, kidney, and heart consume lactate. Hyperlactemia (usually L-lactate) occurs when production exceeds utilization, potentially causing lactic acidosis. D-lactate is produced by bacteria; D-lactic acidosis is less common.

Reference Interval

< 2 mEq/L, < 2 mmol/L (experimental studies). Unit conversion: mg/dL × 0.112 = mEq/L; 1 mmol/L = 1 mEq/L.

Causes of Abnormally High Levels

- Hypoxemic (type A): strenuous exercise, seizures, any cause of decreased oxygen availability (shock, hypovolemia, cardiac disease, pulmonary edema)
- Nonhypoxemic (type B): gastric dilatation/volvulus, diabetes mellitus, liver failure, neoplasia, sepsis, renal failure, hypoglycemia, babesiosis, rare hereditary defects (mitochondrial myopathy, pyruvate dehydrogenase deficiency)
- Lactic acidosis should be suspected when there is an unexplained increase in the anion gap.

Next Diagnostic Steps to Consider if Levels Are High

Evaluate for underlying cause, depending on clinical signs and history.

Drug Effects

- Increase: ethylene glycol intoxication
- Decrease: bromide/potassium bromide

Lab Artifacts

- Increase: delayed plasma harvest, venous stasis (e.g., prolonged venous occlusion during venipuncture), struggling during venipuncture
- Decrease: free hemoglobin; metamizole (dipyrone) therapy

Specimen Collection and Handling

Plasma collected in lithium heparin (green top tube) or sodium fluoride (gray top tube); must be centrifuged immediately and plasma removed from erythrocytes. Refrigerate immediately or freeze. Some blood gas and point-of-care analyzers use whole blood.

Relative Cost: $

Pearls

- Not measured as part of routine biochemical profile, but cage-side testing is increasingly common in emergency/critical care settings.
- Markedly elevated lactate concentrations have been associated with a poor prognosis in critical care settings. For example, in dogs with gastric dilatation/volvulus, an initial plasma lactate > 7.4 mmol/L predicts a poor outcome with 88% accuracy.
- Most methods measure L-lactate but not D-lactate.

AUTHOR & EDITOR: Lois Roth-Johnson, DVM, PhD, DACVP

Lactate Dehydrogenase (LDH)

Definition

Cytosolic enzyme found in most cells in the body

Physiology

LDH catalyzes the oxidation of L-lactate to pyruvate and the reverse reaction. LDH is present in many tissues, notably heart, skeletal muscle, liver, kidney, and erythrocytes. Leakage into the blood and extracellular space occurs with tissue injury. It also increases with even slight sample hemolysis. There are five site-specific LDH isoenzymes that can be separated electrophoretically: heart (LDH1); reticuloendothelial system (LDH2); lung (LDH3); kidney, placental, pancreas (LDH4); and skeletal muscle and liver (LDH5). In veterinary medicine, LDH isoenzyme measurement is usually restricted to research applications because other markers of muscle and hepatic injury exist that are more sensitive and specific.

Reference Interval

Dogs: 50-380 U/L; cats: 46-350 U/L

Causes of Abnormally High Levels

Cardiac disease, skeletal muscle disease, renal injury, liver disease, and hemolysis

Next Diagnostic Steps to Consider if Levels Are High

Evaluate for muscle injury, hepatic disease, or hemolytic anemia.

Lab Artifacts

Hemolysis results in a false increase because erythrocytes contain LDH.

Specimen Collection and Handling

Serum (red top tube), 1 mL. Store at 4°C.

Relative Cost: Single test $; included in many biochemistry profiles $$ - $$$

Pearls

Total serum LDH does not identify site-specific isoenzymes, which requires electrophoresis. Inspection for hemolysis and evaluation in conjunction with clinical signs and other serum chemistry values are often sufficient for identifying the source of increased serum LDH.

AUTHOR: Ruanna E. Gossett, DVM, PhD, DACVP
EDITOR: Lois Roth-Johnson, DVM, PhD, DACVP

Lead, Blood Level

Definition

Whole blood lead levels are the diagnostic test of choice to confirm or eliminate the diagnosis of lead intoxication.

Physiology

Lead is generally poorly absorbed from the GI tract but once absorbed, it is retained in soft tissues and bone for months to years. Lead has deleterious effects on several physiologic processes, including enzymes, erythrocyte and mitochondrial metabolism, and antioxidants. Blood lead is found primarily within erythrocytes; levels decline over time, but half-life is variable. Elimination in dogs is primarily via bile and feces. Erythrocyte abnormalities expected with toxicity include basophilic stippling and rubricytosis in the absence of anemia. See p. 578.

Reference Interval

Typical toxic range in whole blood

- 0.6 ppm or greater is diagnostic of toxicity.
- 0.35 ppm or greater with signs and confirmatory tests (D-aminolevulinic acid [ALA] or fecal lead) is also diagnostic.
- > 20 mcg/mL (point-of-care analyzer, LeadCare II)

Causes of Abnormally High Levels

Exposure to lead

Next Diagnostic Steps to Consider if Levels Are High

Consider radiographs to assess for metallic foreign bodies (20% of affected dogs) in the gastrointestinal tract.

Specimen Collection and Handling

Whole blood (heparinized [green top tube] or EDTA [lavender top tube]). Refrigerated samples or those older than 24 hours can result in falsely decreased blood lead level (LeadCare II analyzer).

Relative Cost: $$$ (blood or tissue)

Pearls

- Kidney, liver, GI tissue or feed may be submitted. Kidney considered preferable (≥ 10 ppm is diagnostic). Formalin-fixed samples are acceptable.
- In animals, chronic exposure is more common than acute exposure.
- Blood levels and clinical signs do not always correlate.

AUTHOR: Carrie L. Flint, DVM, DAVCP
EDITOR: Lois Roth-Johnson, DVM, PhD, DACVP

Left Shift

Definition

The presence of band neutrophils (or earlier neutrophilic precursors such as metamyelocytes or myelocytes) in peripheral blood, which indicates active inflammation. It is clinically useful to define the type of left shift present in leukograms. When segmented neutrophils are also increased, the left shift can be described as "regenerative," suggesting an appropriate marrow response. When the segmented neutrophil count is within or below reference range, the left shift is described as "degenerative," suggesting the granulopoietic response of marrow is outweighed by tissue demand.

Physiology

Band neutrophils, metamyelocytes, and myelocytes are late neutrophilic precursors that normally remain in the marrow storage pool to differentiate into segmented neutrophils there. When intense tissue demand for neutrophils during inflammation depletes segmented neutrophils from the marrow storage pool and/or induces granulocytic hyperplasia of the marrow, increased numbers of band neutrophils (and earlier precursors) are released into blood. The cause of active inflammation inducing a left shift can vary from infectious (e.g., bacterial, fungal) to noninfectious (e.g., pancreatitis, IMHA) causes.

Reference Interval

Dogs: 0-0.3 × 10^3 band neutrophils/mcL; cats: 0-0.2 × 10^3 band neutrophils/mcL

Causes of Abnormally High Levels

Acute or active inflammation, granulocytic leukemia

Next Diagnostic Steps to Consider if Levels Are High

Identify source of inflammation; if none is found despite comprehensive evaluation and repeated assessments, a bone marrow aspirate and core biopsy could be indicated to assess for myelodysplastic syndrome or granulocytic leukemia (very rare).

Specimen Collection and Handling

EDTA whole blood (lavender top tube) and freshly prepared blood smear for laboratory to stain

Pearls

- Always examine a stained blood smear for band neutrophils, because the neutrophil counts generated by automated hematology analyzers do not distinguish between segmented and band neutrophils. Toxic change in neutrophils, another indicator of intense inflammation that can accompany a left shift, is also detected only on blood smear examination.
- Although it mimics a left shift, the hyposegmentation of neutrophils in Pelger-Huët anomaly (see p. 1371) is not considered a left shift.

AUTHOR: Stephen D. Gaunt, DVM, PhD, DACVP
EDITOR: Lois Roth-Johnson, DVM, PhD, DACVP

Leptospira Diagnostic Tests

Definition

Leptospirosis is a zoonotic disease caused by pathogenic serovars of *Leptospira interrogans,* a motile, spiral-shaped bacterium (spirochete). Multiple serovars cause clinical disease.

Physiology

- Organisms penetrate abraded skin and/or mucous membranes, replicate in the bloodstream, and rapidly disseminate to multiple organs, most importantly liver and kidney (allows shedding in urine). Organisms replicate in the renal tubular epithelium, causing chronic tubulointerstitial nephritis and a persistent carrier state if untreated. See p. 583.
- Serovars included in vaccines: *canicola, icterohaemorrhagiae, grippotyphosa,* and *pomona.*

Reference Interval

- Microscopic agglutination test (MAT): reported as titer values; panel of serovars varies among laboratories.
- Rapid IgM immunochromatographic lateral flow assay (IgM LFA), ELISA for antibody and PCR/RT-PCR: positive or negative result

Causes of Abnormally High Levels

- MAT: active disease suggested by a fourfold rise (paired serum samples 2-4 weeks apart). A single titer of ≥ 1:800 in a nonvaccinated dog, or dog vaccinated > 6 months prior, is also suggestive of infection. Vaccine-induced titers may be as high as 1:3200, but are usually much lower by 3-6 months postvaccine (≤1:400).
- Positive ELISA or IgM LFA: exposure to *Leptospira* spp. or vaccination (<6 months interference postvaccination for IgM LFA and > 1 year for ELISA).
- Positive PCR: supportive of infection

Next Diagnostic Steps to Consider if Levels Are High

- Treat if signs suggest active disease. Consider PCR/RT-PCR (urine, blood, cerebrospinal fluid, aqueous humor, or tissue); direct fluorescent antibody testing on tissue (kidney, liver) collected before antibiotic administration.
- Darkfield microscopy or culture (blood, urine) is technically difficult and not widely available.

Causes of Abnormally Low Levels

Serologic tests: early infection, antibiotic treatment, infecting serovar not included in test. Negative PCR/RT-PCR due to insufficient nucleic acid, chronic carrier state, antibiotic treatment, or occurrence of new strains/serovars

Next Diagnostic Steps to Consider if Levels Are Low

Repeat IgM LFA in 3-7 days or MAT titer or ELISA in 1-2 weeks. PCR can detect infection earlier than MAT or ELISA.

Important Interspecies Differences

Cats are less susceptible than dogs to clinical disease, but may have positive titers.

Drug Effects

Antibiotic therapy may cause a blunt rise in serologic titer and cause negative PCR and culture results.

Specimen Collection and Handling

MAT: 2 mL of serum (red top tube). Stable 5 days at 2°C-8°C or longer if frozen. ELISA or IgM LFA: 1 mL of serum (red top tube). Stable 7 days at 2°C-8°C. PCR/RT-PCR: 2 mL EDTA whole blood (lavender top tube) and 2 mL urine in sterile container. Stable 10 days at 2°C-8°C or longer if frozen. For in-clinic tests, follow manufacturer's directions.

Relative Cost: $ (ELISA and IgM LFA); $$ (MAT)

Pearls

- The diagnosis can be missed if relevant serovars are excluded from serologic testing, because there is no consistent serologic cross-reactivity from one serovar to another. Serovars currently recommended for testing: *canicola, pomona, grippotyphosa, bratislava, icterohaemorrhagiae, hardjo,* and *autumnalis.*
- It may be useful to evaluate urine PCR and serologic tests concurrently. Vaccination interferes with IgM LFA test for shorter period of time (most are negative by 12-16 weeks postvaccination) than ELISA or MAT (several months to ≥1 year).

AUTHOR: Patty J. Ewing, DVM, MS, DACVP
EDITOR: Lois Roth-Johnson, DVM, PhD, DACVP

Leukocyte Function Tests

Definition

Tests of the *in vitro* ability of neutrophils, monocytes, and lymphocytes to perform specific functions unique to that cell type. These tests are not routinely available. For several tests, the specific leukocyte must be freshly isolated from blood and tested within hours.

Physiology

- Neutrophil function tests include measuring response to chemotactic stimuli, oxidative burst and release of oxidative metabolites, phagocytosis and killing of bacteria, and expression of adhesion and activation cell markers (e.g., CD18). See p. 1260.
- Monocytes are tested for ability to phagocytose particles and for cellular markers.
- Lymphocyte tests include proliferative response to specific mitogens (i.e., lymphocyte blastogenesis), expression of B- and T-cell receptors and other markers, and quantitation of serum antibodies.

Causes of Abnormally Low Levels

Though both congenital and acquired causes of leukocyte dysfunction exist, these tests are most often performed in young dogs or cats with suspected congenital immunodeficiency (e.g., canine leukocyte adhesion defect, severe combined immunodeficiency), or in a research setting.

Specimen Collection and Handling

The laboratory performing tests should be contacted for specific sample collection and shipment handling; many function tests must be performed on freshly isolated cells.

Relative Cost: $$-$$$

Pearls

Animals with suspected congenital immunodeficiency states (e.g., pups or kittens with recurrent infections) are best evaluated in a referral setting.

AUTHOR: Stephen D. Gaunt, DVM, PhD, DACVP
EDITOR: Lois Roth-Johnson, DVM, PhD, DACVP

Leukocytes (Leukocytosis/Leukopenia)

Definition

Leukocyte refers to a blood cell that can be categorized as either granulocytic (neutrophils, eosinophils, and basophils) or mononuclear (lymphocytes and monocytes). *Leukocytosis* indicates an increase above the reference interval; *leukopenia* indicates a decrease below the reference interval.

Synonym

White blood cells (WBCs)

Physiology

Encompasses several different types of cells with different functions and kinetics. More specific analysis of neutrophils, lymphocytes, monocytes, eosinophils, and basophils is indicated (see respective topics). Changes in the number and morphology of each different leukocyte should be investigated.

Reference Interval

Dogs: 6-17 × 10^3 leukocytes/mcL; cats: 6-19 × 10^3 leukocytes/mcL

Causes of Abnormally High Levels

Leukocytosis is usually due to increased neutrophils (neutrophilia) or lymphocytes (lymphocytosis). Leukocytosis does not automatically equal inflammation; a stress leukogram (due to cortisol release) is common in dogs, while physiologic leukocytosis (due to epinephrine release) is common in cats. Leukocytosis caused by inflammation can also be accompanied by band neutrophils (left shift), toxic neutrophilic changes, or both. Leukocytosis should be interpreted with physical exam findings, magnitude of increase, and other laboratory test results.

Next Diagnostic Steps to Consider if Levels Are High

Evaluate the absolute concentrations of each leukocyte type to determine the specific cause of leukocytosis.

Causes of Abnormally Low Levels

Leukopenia is most often attributed to neutropenia or lymphopenia.

Next Diagnostic Steps to Consider if Levels Are Low

- Evaluate the absolute concentration of each leukocyte type to determine the specific cause of leukopenia.
- In dogs with persistent neutropenia without an identifiable cause, consider bone marrow aspiration for cytologic evaluation; in cats, retroviral testing (feline leukemia virus, feline immunodeficiency virus) should be performed first.

Lab Artifacts

Nucleated erythrocytes (nRBCs) cannot be accurately differentiated from leukocytes by automated leukocyte counting methods, so nRBCs falsely add to the total leukocyte concentration. A correction formula is used for calculating the concentration of total leukocytes when nRBCs are present: correct WBC/mcL = counted WBC/mcL × 100/(100 + number of nRBCs per 100 WBCs). Not all laboratories necessarily make this correction on the final CBC report, and "leukocytosis" in the presence of nRBC should prompt investigation of this possible artifact.

Specimen Collection and Handling

EDTA whole blood (lavender top tube) and freshly prepared blood smear for laboratory to stain

Relative Cost: $$ (reported as part of CBC)

Pearls

- Rather than total leukocyte count, the absolute concentrations of individual leukocytes should be evaluated: neutrophil, lymphocyte, monocyte, eosinophil, and basophil.
- Severe leukocytosis (>50,000/mcL), regardless of cause, is generally associated with a guarded prognosis.

AUTHOR: Stephen D. Gaunt, DVM, PhD, DACVP
EDITOR: Lois Roth-Johnson, DVM, PhD, DACVP

Laboratory Tests

Lipase

Definition

Enzyme that hydrolyzes triglycerides to fatty acids and glycerol

Synonyms

For pancreas-specific lipase immunoreactivity (spec cPLI and spec fPLI), see p. 1370.

Physiology

Lipase is present in pancreas, adipose tissue, gastric mucosa, and duodenal mucosa. Pancreatic lipase catabolizes triglycerides into fatty acids and glycerol, monoglycerides, and diglycerides in the proximal small intestine. Bile salts and colipase enhance the efficiency of lipase activity. The pancreas is considered the primary source of serum lipase concentration, although other tissues may contribute.

Reference Interval

Serum lipase activity based on enzymatic activity:

- Dogs: 100-750 IU/L
- Cats: 10-195 IU/L

Causes of Abnormally High Levels

Pancreatitis, kidney disease, azotemia, hepatic disease, gastrointestinal disease (gastroenteritis, duodenal obstruction, peritonitis, inflammatory bowel disease [IBD]), neoplasia

Next Diagnostic Steps to Consider if Levels Are High

If clinical signs suggest pancreatitis (dogs and cats), with or without increase in serum amylase (dogs only), assess pancreatic lipase immunoreactivity (spec cPLI, fPLI) and/or abdominal ultrasound. Evaluate for concurrent disease (IBD, gastroenteritis, proximal intestinal foreign body, hepatic disease, neoplasia, and especially in cats, cholangiohepatitis and hepatic lipidosis).

Causes of Abnormally Low Levels

Exocrine pancreatic insufficiency

Next Diagnostic Steps to Consider if Levels Are Low

Serum trypsin-like immunoreactivity, cobalamin, folate

Important Interspecies Differences

Total serum lipase levels are not a reliable indicator of pancreatitis in cats; spec PLI is much more sensitive and specific in both dogs and cats.

Drug Effects

Dexamethasone and prednisone therapy increase lipase activity, without concurrent increase in amylase.

Lab Artifacts

Decrease: lipemia, hemolysis, icterus

Specimen Collection and Handling

Serum (red top tube) or serum separator tube (red top SST). Fasted sample preferred.

Stable at 2°C-8°C for 3 weeks. Avoid freeze/thaw.

Relative Cost: $ (serum lipase)

Pearls

- Degree of increase of lipase in serum does not correlate with severity of pancreatitis. Rather than using individual values, continued increases, decreases, or plateaus of levels are more meaningful.
- Spec PLI may be measured serially in a confirmed pancreatitis patient (dog or cat) to assess disease progression.

AUTHOR: Ruanna E. Gossett, DVM, PhD, DACVP
EDITOR: Lois Roth-Johnson, DVM, PhD, DACVP

Lipemia

Definition

Lipemia is the increased concentration of triglyceride-rich lipoproteins (chylomicra and very-low-density lipoproteins) in blood, resulting in the cloudy/turbid appearance of serum or plasma.

Physiology

Lipemia may interfere with certain laboratory assays by causing dilution of substances in serum, or turbidity of the sample, which affects the results of spectrophotometric assays. Lipemia causes hemolysis, which further contributes to interference with laboratory assays. Lipemia may be normal (i.e., postprandial) or pathologic.

Reference Interval

Normally absent from a fasting blood sample

Causes of Abnormally High Levels

Postprandial specimens, primary or secondary hyperlipidemias. See pp. 496 and 1236.

Next Diagnostic Steps to Consider if Levels Are High

- Confirm animal was fasted (12-24 hours) before sample collection. If lipemia in dogs persists with fasting, it may be cleared (to eliminate lipemia-related artifacts) by injection of 100 U/kg of sodium heparin intravenously and collection of the blood sample 15 minutes later. Triglycerides should be measured in an aliquot of fasting lipemic serum before clearing. Ultracentrifugation may clear lipemic serum to avoid laboratory interference with other assays.
- Evaluation for causes of secondary hyperlipidemia (p. 1236) is indicated if lipemia is present in a fasted blood sample. If no evidence of these conditions is found, consider primary hyperlipidemia.

Pearls

- Many laboratories report the presence and degree of lipemia, as well as the expected severity of interference and analytes affected.
- Analytes that can be artifactually *increased* by lipemia include hemoglobin, MCHC, triglycerides, plasma protein measured by refractometer, and spectrophotometric assays for glucose, calcium, phosphorus, alanine aminotransferase (ALT), creatine kinase (CK), and total bilirubin.
- Analytes that can be artifactually *decreased* by lipemia include lipase, amylase, and albumin.
- Hypercholesterolemia does not cause lipemia.

AUTHOR: Ruanna E. Gossett, DVM, PhD, DACVP
EDITOR: Lois Roth-Johnson, DVM, PhD, DACVP

Low-Dose Dexamethasone Suppression Test

Definition

The low-dose dexamethasone suppression test (LDDST) is a screening test for hyperadrenocorticism. It sometimes also discriminates between pituitary-dependent hyperadrenocorticism (PDH) and adrenal tumor (AT) hyperadrenocorticism (4-hour sample result) in dogs.

Physiology

Patients with hyperadrenocorticism are resistant to negative feedback of cortisol on the hypothalamic-pituitary-adrenal axis, resulting in inadequate suppression of cortisol concentrations following administration of dexamethasone (dogs: 0.01 mg/kg IV; cats: 0.1 mg/kg IV). Blood is sampled just before, and 4 and 8 hours postinjection. In healthy dogs, release of hypothalamic corticotropin-releasing hormone (CRH), pituitary adrenocorticotropic hormone (ACTH), and subsequent adrenal cortisol are suppressed for up to 48 hours. See p. 485.

Reference Interval

Baseline cortisol: 0.4-6 mcg/dL (dogs); 0.4-4 mcg/dL (cats). Unit conversion: 1 mcg/dL × 27.6 = 1 nmol/L. Depending on laboratory, suppression is often regarded as < 1.0 to 1.4 mcg/dL.

Causes of Abnormally High Levels

Serum cortisol levels:

- 4-hour and 8-hour cortisol: failure to suppress to < 50% of baseline or < 1.4 mcg/dL: may be PDH or AT, or technical error with injection
- 4-hour cortisol < 1.4 mcg/dL but 8-hour cortisol > 1.4 mcg/dL: consistent with PDH
- 4-hour or both 4-hour and 8-hour cortisol(s) < 50% of baseline (indicating suppression) but both > 1 mcg/dL and 8-hour > 4-hour: likely PDH
- 4-hour and 8-hour cortisol both < 1.4 mcg/dL: normal
- False increase: icterus, recent administration of glucocorticoid detected by assay

Next Diagnostic Steps to Consider if Levels Are High

- If needed, consider tests to discriminate between PDH and AT
  - Imaging studies
  - High-dose dexamethasone suppression test (HDDST) or endogenous ACTH measurement

Causes of Abnormally Low Levels

If 8-hour suppressed by > 50% below baseline (or < 1.4 mcg/dL), hyperadrenocorticism may be absent or atypical, but false-negative result also possible. See p. 487.

Next Diagnostic Steps to Consider if Levels Are Low

If hyperadrenocorticism remains on the differential diagnosis, can perform ACTH stimulation test or LDDST may be repeated 1-3 months later. Abdominal imaging can also help by defining adrenal size. See pp. 485 and 487.

Important Interspecies Differences

Hyperadrenocorticism is rare in cats. Cats require administration of 0.1 mg/kg dexamethasone IV because 15%-20% of healthy cats fail to suppress with the 0.01 mg/kg dosage used in dogs.

Drug Effects

- Long-term use of glucocorticoids leads to suppression of cortisol secretion.
- Immunoassays for cortisol measurement have significant cross-reactivity with other glucocorticoids and drugs. Prednisolone is highly cross-reactive (69%), while dexamethasone is minimally so (<0.1%).
- Ketoconazole inhibits steroid biosynthesis, causing low cortisol concentrations.
- Mitotane and trilostane reduce cortisol production; LDDS is not used as a tool to monitor therapy with these drugs.

Specimen Collection and Handling

Serum, 1 mL (red top tube); EDTA plasma (lavender top tube) can be used in some but not all test methodologies (e.g., avoid EDTA for commonly used Immulite assay). Cortisol in EDTA plasma is more stable than in serum. Cool specimens are more stable than warm samples.

Relative Cost: $$ to $$$ (depending on test methodology)

Pearls

- Chronic stress and nonadrenal illness can cause false-positive test results; LDDST is best done once nonadrenal illness is resolved (if possible) or controlled.
- ACTH stimulation testing is generally preferred over LDDST for ruling out hyperadrenocorticism in diabetic patients.
- ACTH stimulation testing is the only method to diagnose iatrogenic hyperadrenocorticism.
- Very small volumes of dexamethasone are used (e.g., 0.01 mg/kg using dexamethasone 4 mg/mL equals 0.01 mL for a 4-kg [9-lb] dog). Therefore, dead space in a regular syringe and needle hub should be considered. Either dilution (add dexamethasone to diluent, not the other way around) or use of an insulin syringe (no dead space in hub) should be considered.
- Dexamethasone-SP must be dosed on the basis of the dexamethasone component only (4 mg/mL Dex-SP equivalent to 3 mg/mL dexamethasone).

AUTHOR: Carrie Flint, DVM, DACVP
EDITOR: Lois Roth-Johnson, DVM, PhD, DACVP

Lupus Erythematosus Preparation (LE Prep)

Definition

Preparation of incubated clotted blood crushed through a wire sieve. Blood is collected and centrifuged; buffy coat is mixed with equal amounts of serum, smeared, and stained with Wright stain or new methylene blue. Preparations positive for lupus erythematosus (LE) show rosetting of neutrophils around nuclear material and LE cells (neutrophils with phagocytized homogeneous, magenta-staining nuclear material on a Wright-stained smear).

Physiology

LE cell formation occurs in the presence of sufficient immunoglobulin G antibody reactive to deoxyribonucleoprotein along with complement. This antinuclear antibody binds the nuclei of traumatized or nonviable leukocytes. Viable neutrophils then phagocytize the opsonized nuclear material, forming the LE cell.

Reference Interval

Reported as negative or positive

Causes of Abnormally High Levels

Positive test indicates active disease (systemic lupus erythematosus [SLE]).

Next Diagnostic Steps to Consider if Levels Are High

Diagnostic evaluation for SLE (p. 955)

Lab Artifacts

Mere phagocytosis of nuclear material with intact chromatin pattern (tart cell) does not constitute an LE cell.

Specimen Collection and Handling

5-10 mL of blood in a glass test tube. Heparinized blood (green top tube) may also be used.

Relative Cost: $$

Pearls

- LE cells may occur in skin lesions and joint fluid of patients with active SLE.
- Absence of LE cells does not rule out SLE. The test is specific for SLE (positive is true positive) but is a very poor screening test (low sensitivity; most patients with SLE are negative by this test).
- ANA testing and correlation with clinical signs are needed for diagnosis of SLE.

AUTHOR: Fidelia R. Fernandez, DVM, MS, DACVP
EDITOR: Lois Roth-Johnson, DVM, PhD, DACVP

Luteinizing Hormone (LH)

Definition

Glycoprotein gonadotrophin produced by the anterior pituitary

Physiology

In females, LH synergizes with follicle-stimulating hormone (FSH) to initiate ovulation and secretion of progesterone. LH is essential for corpus luteum formation. In males, LH is important for normal growth and function of testicular interstitial (Leydig) cells, which secrete testosterone. Spayed dogs and cats maintain baseline concentrations since there is no inhibition from ovarian estradiol secretion. Values in intact bitches are low until just before ovulation. Low concentration is maintained in intact cats until ovulation is induced.

Reference Interval

2-29 ng/mL; considerable variability during anestrus

Causes of Abnormally High Levels

Preovulation, ovarian cysts

Next Diagnostic Steps to Consider if Levels Are High

A marked increase in serum LH concentration occurs approximately 48 hours before ovulation. Progesterone concentration should remain high if pregnancy has occurred. Evaluation for cystic ovaries with abdominal ultrasound if inappropriate/persistent elevation

Causes of Abnormally Low Levels

Low values are associated with anestrus.

Next Diagnostic Steps to Consider if Levels Are Low

Evaluate for anestrus.

Lab Artifacts

ELISA method: hemolyzed or lipemic samples should not be used; however, hemolysis does not interfere with radioimmunoassay.

Specimen Collection and Handling

Serum, 1 mL. Collect blood in red top tube, spin, and collect serum. Sample should be free of hemolysis and lipemia. Store at 2°C-4°C for 24 hours; freeze for longer storage. Ship frozen or on ice. Cage-side test kits are also available.

Relative Cost: $$

Pearls

To facilitate ovulation timing, once visible signs of estrus have begun and vaginal cytology reveals > 70% cornified cells, serum LH levels should be measured daily to ensure detection of the preovulatory LH surge and optimal timing of breeding/insemination.

Antimullarian hormone evaluation is better for assessment of spay status or for ovarian remnants.

AUTHOR & EDITOR: Lois Roth-Johnson, DVM, PhD, DACVP

Lymphocytes (Lymphocytosis, Lymphopenia)

Definition

The mononuclear leukocytes that mediate immune responses. Most lymphocytes are small with condensed chromatin and scant basophilic cytoplasm, although very low numbers have more cytoplasm with fine red to magenta granules clustered near nucleus (granular lymphocytes). On a blood smear, the nucleus of a small lymphocyte in dog or cat is typically similar or slightly larger in size compared to erythrocytes or smaller than neutrophils.

Physiology

Lymphocytes migrate from blood into lymphoid tissues, circulate in the lymphatic system, and reenter the venous circulation via the thoracic duct. Using surface receptors as markers, lymphocytes can be classified as T lymphocytes (e.g., CD3-positive) that mediate cell-mediated responses, B lymphocytes (e.g., CD79a-positive) that mediate humoral responses, or natural killer lymphocytes (null cells) that mediate cytotoxicity. Most of the circulating lymphocytes in blood are T lymphocytes. Granular lymphocytes include cytotoxic T cells and natural killer cells.

Reference Interval

Dogs: 1.0-5.0 × 10^3 lymphocytes/mcL; cats: 1.5-7.0 × 10^3 lymphocytes/mcL

Causes of Abnormally High Levels

- Excitement/physiologic leukocytosis from epinephrine release (especially young cats)
- Lymphoid neoplasms (e.g., lymphoid leukemias, stage V lymphoma)
- Inflammatory diseases with antigenic stimulation (especially infections such as *Ehrlichia canis* or *Spirocerca lupi*)
- Hypoadrenocorticism ("relaxed" leukogram: lymphocytosis without neutrophilia in an obviously stressed animal, i.e., conspicuous absence of a stress leukogram)

Next Diagnostic Steps to Consider if Levels Are High

- Evaluate for causes listed, depending on clinical signs.
- The PCR for antigen receptor rearrangement (PARR) test evaluates clonality of T and B lymphocyte antigen receptor genes and is a sensitive method to detect neoplastic lymphocytes.

Causes of Abnormally Low Levels

- Endogenous or exogenous glucocorticoids (stress leukogram)
- Acute inflammation (especially viral infections)
- Disruption of lymphatic flow (e.g., chylothorax, lymphangiectasia)
- Immunodeficiency (e.g., severe combined immunodeficiency)

Next Diagnostic Steps to Consider if Levels Are Low

Evaluate for causes listed, depending on clinical signs.

Drug Effects

Glucocorticoids cause lymphopenia by causing sequestration of lymphocytes in lymphoid tissue and lympholysis (minor).

Specimen Collection and Handling

EDTA whole blood (lavender-top tube) and freshly prepared blood smear for laboratory to stain

Relative Cost: $$ (reported as part of CBC)

Pearls

- In evaluating lymphocytosis, cell morphology is important. Markedly increased numbers of large or atypical lymphocytes indicate acute lymphoid leukemia/stage V lymphoma, whereas a marked increase in small, well-differentiated lymphocytes occurs with chronic lymphoid leukemia/stage V lymphoma or non-neoplastic causes of lymphocytosis.
- Neoplastic granular lymphocytes occur in blood with lymphomas that usually originate in the small intestine of cats or liver/spleen of dogs.

AUTHOR: Stephen D. Gaunt, DVM, PhD, DACVP
EDITOR: Lois Roth-Johnson, DVM, PhD, DACVP

Lymphoma Flow Cytometry

Definition

Flow cytometry allows identification and quantification of specific cell populations in complex fluids such as blood or aspirates of lymph node or bone marrow. Cells in suspension are tagged with antibodies and then passed single-file through an electronic detection apparatus; these cells interrupt (scatter) a signal, allowing cell size and complexity to be measured. This method can be used to assist in the diagnosis and subtyping of lymphoma, among other uses.

Physiology

Lymphoma is a neoplastic proliferation of lymphocytes that can be categorized based on lymphocyte type (T cell vs. B cell) and cell size (large cell vs. small cell). Membrane surface molecules, marked by fluorescence-labeled antibodies, can be used to further identify lymphocyte populations using flow cytometry. Examples of commonly used cell surface markers are:

- B cell (dog) CD1, CD21, CD45RA, CD90, and MHC class II
- T cell (dog) CD3, CD4, CD8, and αβ-TCR or γδ-TCR

Causes of Abnormally High Levels

Lymphoma and lymphoid leukemia are associated with expansion of homogeneous populations of a single phenotype and size (e.g., homogeneous population of large CD21+ B cells).

Next Diagnostic Steps to Consider if Levels Are High

See pp. 607 and 609.

Important Interspecies Differences

The antibodies used in flow cytometry are a combination of species-specific antibodies and antibodies that cross-react among several species.

Lab Artifacts

Cytoplasmic fragments from fragile neoplastic lymphocytes can interfere with accurate quantitation of cells.

Specimen Collection and Handling

Blood, bone marrow aspirates in EDTA (lavender top tube), and lymph node aspirates in transport media or serum spiked saline. Overnight shipping on ice is necessary. Most laboratories request a concurrent blood film and CBC for blood and bone marrow aspirates. Do not ship on Friday, and do not freeze the sample. Contact the laboratory for specific sample and shipping needs.

Relative Cost: $$$$

Pearls

- Flow cytometry should be used in addition to histologic and/or cytologic diagnostic techniques in the diagnosis of lymphoma, not as a primary diagnostic test. It is not useful in the diagnosis and characterization of lymphoid neoplasia that has mixed populations such as T-cell rich B-cell lymphoma.
- Persistent lymphocytosis can occur in canine ehrlichiosis, with expansion of CD8+ T cells. On the blood film, the lymphocytes show morphology consistent with large granular lymphocytes.

AUTHOR: Sharon M. Dial, DVM, PhD, DACVP
EDITOR: Lois Roth-Johnson, DVM, PhD, DACVP

Lymphoma Polymerase Chain Reaction (PARR)

Definition

This test amplifies a targeted portion of the lymphocyte DNA, the T cell and B cell receptors, to determine if a population of lymphocytes is monoclonal (likely neoplastic) or polyclonal (likely reactive/nonneoplastic).

Synonym

Polymerase chain reaction for antigen receptor rearrangements (PARR)

Physiology

- Normal lymphocyte maturation confers a wide range of heterogeneity to T- and B-cell receptor genes.
- Extraction and amplification of DNA of these receptor genes via polymerase chain reaction (PCR) produces a myriad of different length amplification segments (amplicons) in healthy individuals.
- In contrast, PCR analysis of lymphocytes that have expanded monoclonally from a single precursor cell, as in lymphoma, produces amplicons that are all of the same length.
- Occasionally, a neoplastic expansion of lymphocytes can produce a few subpopulations of neoplastic cells with slightly different sequences and an oligoclonal expansion.

Causes of Abnormally High Levels

Single or small number of broad amplicon bands: neoplasia

Next Diagnostic Steps to Consider if Levels Are High

Positive clonal expansion of a lymphocyte population is diagnostic for lymphoma, warranting lymphoma staging and treatment (pp. 607 and 609).

Important Interspecies Differences

The test is dependent on DNA sequences that are species-specific, requiring species-specific PCR primers.

Lab Artifacts

- Samples with a background of inflammatory cells can mask a clonal expansion, depending on the specific primers used in the test.
- Amplification of a sample with a small number of lymphocytes can result in a pseudoclonal PCR profile.

Specimen Collection and Handling

Fresh blood, bone marrow, body cavity fluids, lymph node aspirates, tissue, and, in some cases, formalin fixed tissues and air-dried or prestained cytologic slide preparations can be submitted. Contact the laboratory for specific sample requirements.

Relative Cost: $$$$

Pearls

- Tests offered by different laboratories can vary substantially in the number of gene sequences that are recognized by their PCR primers. A negative clonality test does not rule out neoplasia; some assays produce up to 25% false-negative results.
- This is an ancillary test for the identification and characterization of lymphoma. The results of the test must be interpreted in light of histopathologic/cytologic, immunohistochemical, and clinical findings.
- The test is most commonly used for differentiating reactive small lymphocytes from neoplastic small lymphocytes when microscopic morphology alone cannot provide a definitive diagnosis of neoplasia.

AUTHOR: Sharon M. Dial, DVM, PhD, DACVP
EDITOR: Lois Roth-Johnson, DVM, PhD, DACVP

Magnesium

Definition

Essential nutrient and major divalent cation. Serum total magnesium includes protein bound (30%), anion-complexed (15%), and ionized (55%) fractions.

Synonyms

Mg, Mg^{2+}

Physiology

Absorbed in small intestine from dietary sources and excreted in urine, feces, and milk. Most (99%) Mg^{2+} is intracellular; serum level may not reflect total body Mg. Ionized Mg (iMg^{2+}) is the biologically active form. Kidneys control Mg^{2+} balance; filtered by glomerulus and reabsorbed in tubules. Mg^{2+} is essential for many cellular processes, including membrane ion pumps that control intracellular [K^+] and [Ca^+].

Reference Interval

Dogs and cats: 1.4-2.3 mg/dL; 1.2-1.9 mEq/L (0.58-0.95 mmol/L)

Causes of Abnormally High Levels

- Decreased urinary excretion: decline in GFR of any cause (e.g., prerenal, renal, postrenal)
- Drug-induced: excess supplementation (e.g., diet, antacids, intravenous), ACE inhibitors, spironolactone
- Extracellular shifting: may rarely occur with severe tissue damage (e.g., rhabdomyolysis, severe hemolysis) and release of intracellular stores

Next Diagnostic Steps to Consider if Levels are High

Evaluate for dehydration, renal function, urinary disease; review oral and parenteral supplements; exclude artifact.

Causes of Abnormally Low Levels

- Hypoalbuminemia: decreases protein-bound Mg^{2+}; no effect on [iMg^{2+}]
- Excess excretion: generally from renal system, as with diuresis (e.g., renal disease, fluids, diuretics, osmotic diuresis) and diseases that affect renal handling (e.g., diabetes mellitus, hyperparathyroidism, hyperthyroidism). May occur with lactation
- Inadequate gastrointestinal (GI) absorption: chronic diarrhea, malabsorption syndromes, deficient diet, prolonged anorexia
- Intracellular shifting: administration of insulin or glucose
- Iatrogenic: magnesium-poor fluids or total parenteral nutrition

Next Diagnostic Steps to Consider if Levels are Low

Measure serum albumin. Evaluate for renal causes, GI disease.

Drug Effects

- Decrease: loop and osmotic diuretics, drugs that induce renal tubular injury
- Increase: administration of Mg^{2+}-containing laxatives, antacids, ACE inhibitors, spironolactone

Lab Artifacts

- Falsely increased by hemolysis or delayed serum separation
- Falsely decreased if anticoagulants that bind Mg^{2+} are used (EDTA, citrate, oxalate)

Specimen Collection and Handling

Serum preferred (red top tube); heparinized plasma (green top tube) may be used. Remove serum/plasma from erythrocytes promptly.

Relative Cost: $

Pearls

- Low serum [Mg^{2+}] is common in critical care settings.
- Concurrent hypocalcemia, hypokalemia may be refractory to therapy until hypomagnesemia is corrected.
- Consider EDTA contamination if result is unexpected and concurrent hypocalcemia and hyperkalemia are present.

AUTHOR: Mary Leissinger, DVM, MS, DACVP
EDITOR: Lois Roth-Johnson, DVM, PhD, DACVP

Mast Cell Tumor Prognostic Panel

Definition

Panel of histochemical stains that identify proliferation markers, genetic mutations, and staining patterns in mast cell tumors (MCTs) in a way that increases the precision and accuracy of the prognosis

Physiology

- Histologically, most MCTs in dogs and cats are of intermediate grade (grade II), with highly variable treatment response within this grade. Test panels can help clarify prognosis.
- Proliferating cell nuclear antigen (PCNA) is a subunit of a DNA polymerase that is expressed at high levels in the S-phase of the cell cycle; Ki-67 is a nuclear protein not expressed in noncycling cells; and AgNORs are argyrophilic nucleolar organizational regions associated with transcription of ribosomal RNA, which increase in number during cell proliferation.
- Mutations in c-KIT (the proto-oncogene that encodes KIT, the tyrosine kinase receptor) and abnormal cytoplasmic localization of KIT are associated with more aggressive tumor behavior.
- In addition to providing prognostic information, c-KIT mutations indicate favorable response to tyrosine kinase inhibitors.

Causes of Abnormally High Levels

Increased expression of PCNA, Ki-67, and AgNORs and the presence of c-KIT mutation and/or increased cytoplasmic expression of KIT are indicative of increased potential for aggressive tumor behavior. This is a general result, and specific median survival times associated with varying combinations and levels of these results remain to be proven.

Next Diagnostic Steps to Consider if Levels are High

Stains are prognostic and do not require additional diagnostic testing.

Lab Artifacts

Prolonged exposure to formalin (>7-8 weeks) may alter both immunohistochemical staining and DNA integrity, resulting in false-negative results. In practice, this is rarely a concern because tissue specimens are paraffin embedded promptly after fixation, not kept in formalin long-term.

Specimen Collection and Handling

Formalin fixed tissue (biopsy specimen) or paraffin blocks

Relative Cost: $$$$

Pearls

- The prognostic value of a panel of stains exceeds the prognostic value of any individual stain.
- Several laboratories offer various mast cell tumor panels, the results of which cannot be compared directly. Selection of a single laboratory is recommended, and a comprehensive interpretation from a board-certified pathologist should be provided.
- Other than c-KIT PCR to identify potential response to tyrosine kinase inhibitors in high-grade tumors, the mast cell tumor panels have limited utility in MCTs that are clearly low grade or high grade.

AUTHOR: Sharon M. Dial, DVM, PhD, DACVP
EDITOR: Lois Roth-Johnson, DVM, PhD, DACVP

Methemoglobinemia, Methemoglobinuria

Definition

Methemoglobin (MetHb) has an iron moiety that has been oxidized to the ferric (Fe^{3+}) state from the normal ferrous (Fe^{2+}) state in hemoglobin.

Methemoglobinemia: accumulation of MetHb in blood

Methemoglobinuria: presence of MetHb in urine

Synonym

MetHb

Physiology

Increased production of MetHb results from exposure to oxidant chemicals, drugs, plants, or decreased reduction of MetHb due to a hereditary enzyme deficiency. MetHb cannot bind and carry oxygen to tissue.

Reference Interval

MetHb spot test: drop of venous blood on a white paper towel normally is bright red; if methemoglobin concentration is > 10%, spot remains dark with a brown tinge. Actual value measured with co-oximetry; normally represents < 2% of total hemoglobin in blood/urine

Causes of Abnormally High Levels

Hereditary deficiency of methemoglobin reductase or exposure to oxidant chemicals (nitrite, copper), drugs (e.g., acetaminophen, benzocaine, phenazopyridine, zinc), or plants

Next Diagnostic Steps to Consider if Levels are High

- If spot test is positive, consider co-oximetry to measure concentrations of MetHb as a percentage of the total hemoglobin concentration in the blood sample. Arterial blood gas to measure oxygen tension; pulse oximetry not reliable but will be low in methemoglobinemia
- CBC with smear review to determine if hemolytic anemia is present, because it is a common sequela to oxidant injury of erythrocytes
- Evaluation of red blood cell morphology for Heinz bodies and eccentrocytes (hallmarks of oxidant injury)
- MetHb reductase determination or genetic testing if hereditary deficiency is suspected

Specimen Collection and Handling

Anticoagulated whole blood for spot test; 0.5 mL minimum

Co-oximetry on fresh whole blood on ice may be run at nearby human lab/hospital within 2 hours

MetHb reductase determination: prior arrangements must be made with a laboratory. Whole blood (1 mL in EDTA [lavender top tube]) should be refrigerated and sent chilled (not frozen) with assay done the same day specimen collected. One or more samples collected from normal animals submitted as control. Not offered by most veterinary reference labs; may be run in human lab if erythrocyte lysing agent does not cause MetHb formation

Relative Cost:

Check with local human reference lab/hospital ($-$$).

Pearls

- Severe methemoglobinemia produces chocolate-brown discoloration of the blood.
- Spot testing is rapid, inexpensive, and may be done in-house.
- Most chemicals producing methemoglobinemia also produce Heinz body hemolytic anemia.
- "Saturation gap" occurs when there is a difference between SpO_2 and PaO_2 in animals with methemoglobinemia.
- Methemoglobinemia may cause cyanosis in animals without respiratory distress.

AUTHOR & EDITOR: Lois Roth-Johnson, DVM, PhD, DACVP

MiraVista Fungal Testing

Definition

MiraVista is a reference laboratory headquartered in Indianapolis, IN, that specializes in tests that identify fungal antigen in body fluids. Some of these tests offer significant advantages to other serodiagnostic methods of mycotic infection.

Synonym

Fungal antigen tests

Physiology

During invasive systemic/disseminated fungal disease, fungal agents can shed specific structural antigens (e.g., cell wall galactomannan) into body cavity fluids, specifically serum, urine, CSF, and bronchoalveolar lavage (BAL) fluid. Current tests offered include *Aspergillus* spp, *Blastomycosis dermatitidis, Coccidioides* spp, *Cryptococcus neoformans, Histoplasmosis capsulatum*. Of these, galactomannan antigen assays offer an advantage over other serodiagnostics for systemic aspergillosis, blastomycosis, and histoplasmosis. There is considerable cross-reactivity between the dimorphic fungi.

Reference Interval

Depends on specific test; may be reported as positive or negative, or with numerical value and laboratory-supplied suggested interpretation

Causes of Abnormally High Levels

Fungal infection, usually systemic or invasive

Next Diagnostic Steps to Consider if Levels are High

See pp. 81, 121, 184, 223, and 476.

Drug Effects

Aspergillus antigen test: piperacillin-tazobactam, amoxicillin/clavulanic acid, and fluids containing sodium gluconate (e.g., Plasma-Lyte) causing false-positive results.

Specimen Collection and Handling

For *B. dermatitidis* and *H. capsulatum*, urine antigen determination is more sensitive than is serum/plasma. Fluids other than blood should be collected in a sterile screw-top tube. CSF specimen requirement is 0.8 mL; other fluids (BAL, urine specimen) requirement is 0.5 mL. Treatment of the sample with mucolytic and keratolytic agents can degrade most fungal antigens. BAL samples that are too viscous to pipette are rejected. For blood samples, collect serum (1.2 mL) in a red top tube, allow to clot for 30 minutes, centrifuge, transfer serum to a plastic screw-cap tube. Plasma samples (1.2 mL) should be collected in EDTA and spun for 15 minutes. Transfer plasma to plastic screw-top tube. Samples are stable at 2°C-8°C for 2 weeks, or 5 months if frozen.

Relative Cost: $$$

Pearls

- Cytologic or histopathologic identification of fungal elements is preferred, but serology is valuable for support of diagnosis when organism cannot be identified.
- Urine antigen tests can be serially monitored to assure clinical response to antifungal therapy.
- A negative result for any fungal antigen test does not rule out fungal disease.
- At present, alternative serodiagnostic tests are preferred over galactomannan assay for sino-nasal aspergillosis, *C. immitis* and *C. neoformans*.
- Utilize the diagnostic laboratory website for test-specific information relating to appropriate sample, collection technique, sample stability, and submission (http://miravistalabs.com/veterinary-fungal-infections/).

AUTHOR: Sharon M. Dial, DVM, PhD, DACVP
EDITOR: Lois Roth-Johnson, DVM, PhD, DACVP

Monocytes (Monocytosis, Monocytopenia)

Definition

Largest leukocyte on blood smear. They have lobulated to occasionally indented, oval nuclei and gray basophilic cytoplasm with fine azurophilic granules and occasionally clear vacuoles. Monocytes become macrophages upon entering tissues and fluids.

Physiology

Monocytes are produced in the marrow, with a short transit time from monoblast to monocyte, which quickly enters blood. Monocytes and macrophages are involved in killing bacteria and fungi, presenting antigens to lymphocytes, removal of necrotic and apoptotic cell debris, and destruction of senescent or abnormal erythrocytes. Dendritic cells (antigen-presenting cells in tissue) also derive from monocytic precursors in marrow.

Reference Interval

Dogs: 0.1-1.5 $\times$ 10^3 monocytes/mcL; cats: 0-1 $\times$ 10^3 monocytes/mcL

Causes of Abnormally High Levels

- Inflammation, acute or chronic
- Stress leukogram, from endogenous or exogenous glucocorticoids
- Monocytic leukemia, myelomonocytic leukemia, hemophagic histiocytic sarcoma

Next Diagnostic Steps to Consider if Levels are High

Evaluate for given causes, depending on signalment, history and physical exam.

Causes of Abnormally Low Levels

Monocytopenia is not considered a clinically significant abnormality, because monocytes often occur in very low numbers naturally.

Specimen Collection and Handling

EDTA whole blood (lavender top tube) and freshly prepared blood smear for laboratory to stain

Relative Cost: $$ (reported as part of CBC)

Pearls

After acute onset of neutropenia caused by transient suppression of hematopoiesis (e.g., anticancer chemotherapy), monocytes return to high levels in blood sooner than neutrophils since monocytopoiesis is more rapid than granulopoiesis. Therefore, in neutropenic patients, even mild monocytosis can signal hematopoietic recovery and impending resolution of neutropenia.

AUTHOR: Stephen D. Gaunt, DVM, PhD, DACVP
EDITOR: Lois Roth-Johnson, DVM, PhD, DACVP

Mycobacterial Culture

Definition

Laboratory growth, isolation, and identification of *Mycobacterium* spp.

Physiology

Mycobacterium spp. cause uncommon but important opportunistic infections in dogs and cats. Organisms may be shed intermittently in respiratory specimens (tracheal exudate) or present constantly in solid tissue specimens (skin, lymph node) during infection. The organism must be grown in specific media, and growth and identification of these fastidious organisms may take 2-4 months.

Reference Interval

Reported as growth or no growth, with identification of organisms

Causes of Abnormally High Levels

Infection with *Mycobacterium* spp. Common sites of infection include skin (leproid) and respiratory tract. Infections may become systemic, involving lymphatics and bone marrow.

Next Diagnostic Steps to Consider if Levels are High

See p. 670.

Important Interspecies Differences

- Feline leprosy *(M. lepraemurium)* and atypical mycobacteriosis (*M. avium, M. fortuitum, M. thermoresistibile, M. xenopi, M. phlei,* and *M. smegmatis*) are considered unique to the cat.
- Dogs, especially basset hounds, are susceptible to systemic disease caused by *M. avium*.
- Dogs are not a reservoir for *Mycobacteria sp.* Rare infection with *M. bovis* and very rare infection with *M. tuberculosis* is attributed to contact with infected people.

Drug Effects

Concurrent or recent antibiotic therapy may inhibit growth.

Lab Artifacts

Contamination or overgrowth by commensal organisms may mask growth.

Specimen Collection and Handling

Tissue or exudate from lesion in a sterile container. If zoonotic *Mycobacterium* spp. are suspected, the container should have a screw top and a double outer container should be used; label as biohazard. Submit to laboratory as soon as possible and warn lab of suspected diagnosis.

Relative Cost: $$

Pearls

- Cutaneous or localized infections are more likely to become systemic in immunocompromised hosts. Immunocompromised owners may be more susceptible to zoonotic infection.
- Fine-needle aspirates of solid tissue lesions are characterized by macrophages containing rod-shaped organisms that appear as negative images with Wright-Giemsa or Diff-Quik stains.
- Organisms will stain with acid-fast stains.
- PCR testing for detection of DNA is available for some of the zoonotic strains of *Mycobacterium* spp., but culture and susceptibility testing remain the gold standard.

AUTHOR: Sharon M. Dial, DVM, PhD, DACVP
EDITOR: Lois Roth-Johnson, DVM, PhD, DACVP

Mycoplasma spp Culture

Definition

Laboratory growth of infectious *Mycoplasma* spp agents for isolation and identification

Physiology

Mycoplasma spp are the smallest, simplest self-replicating bacteria. These organisms are fastidious and grow slowly in culture, so confirmation of infection is often made via more rapid PCR testing instead of bacterial culture. A subset of potential pathogens known as hemotropic *Mycoplasma* spp (previously called *Haemobartonella* spp) may be associated with hemolytic anemia, but bacterial culture is rarely used for disease confirmation.

Reference Interval

Reported as no growth or growth with identification of pathogens; *Mycoplasma* growth may or may not be speciated, depending on the laboratory used.

Causes of Abnormally High Levels

Infection is associated with upper/lower respiratory disease, conjunctivitis, arthritis, and hemolytic disease (hemotropic *Mycoplasma* spp).

Next Diagnostic Steps to Consider if Levels are High

See pp. 199, 438, and 987.

Causes of Abnormally Low Levels

Overgrowth of other organisms; improper handling or culture conditions; prior use of antimicrobial drugs; uninfected animal

Drug Effects

Glucocorticoid or other immunosuppressive therapies may enhance culture recovery of organism. Antimicrobial drugs that act by means other than cell wall inhibition impede culture.

Lab Artifacts

Contamination with commensals may mask growth. Organism grows slowly in culture, and cultures may be discarded inadvertently if laboratory personnel are not informed that *Mycoplasma* spp infection is suspected.

Specimen Collection and Handling

Swabs, exudate, or tissue should be submitted in specific transport media to enhance growth. Laboratory should be contacted to obtain media for sample submission.

Relative Cost: $$

Pearls

- Mycoplasmal conjunctivitis and respiratory disease are more likely to occur in cats; arthritis is more likely to occur in dogs. Co-infection with other pathogens is common in *Mycoplasma* infection.
- Growth in culture may take up to 2 weeks; serologic tests or PCR is more commonly used for disease diagnosis.
- Culture is rarely used for documentation of hemotropic *Mycoplasma;* microscopic visualization of organisms and/or PCR is used instead.

AUTHOR: Sharon M. Dial, DVM, PhD, DACVP
EDITOR: Lois Roth-Johnson, DVM, PhD, DACVP

Myoglobinemia, Myoglobinuria

Definition

Myoglobin is a low-molecular-weight heme protein found in muscle tissue.

Physiology

Myoglobin stores and transports oxygen in muscle fibers. It is released from muscle when there is severe disruption of the muscle membrane or necrosis. Myoglobin is detected in the serum 2-4 hours after injury. It does not significantly bind serum proteins. It passes quickly through the glomerulus and is excreted in urine. Red to brown urine discoloration due to myoglobinuria occurs before plasma discoloration. Myoglobinuria causes a positive occult blood test result on a urine dipstick.

Reference Interval

Serum myoglobin in dogs: < 10-13.6 ng/mL. Cats: < 10-13.8 ng/mL. Not present in urine of healthy animals

Causes of Abnormally High Levels

Trauma, ischemia, toxic injury, or necrosis of muscle tissue

Next Diagnostic Steps to Consider if Levels are High

Evaluate for muscle injury or necrosis (e.g., serum creatine kinase level) versus laboratory evidence of hemolysis.

Lab Artifacts

Must distinguish myoglobinuria from other causes of positive reaction for blood on urine dipstick such as hematuria, hemoglobinuria, and substances that cause a false-positive reaction (high bilirubin concentration, contamination of urine with oxidizing agents in disinfectants, leukocytes, bacteria, peroxidase, or iodine)

Specimen Collection and Handling

- Myoglobinemia: serum (red top tube), heparinized plasma (green top tube), or EDTA plasma (lavender top tube). Refrigerate at 2°C-8°C.
- Myoglobinuria: 1 mL urine (clean container without additives)

Relative Cost: $$$

Pearls

- Myoglobinuria may be distinguished from hemoglobinuria and hematuria by checking the urine sediment for the presence (hematuria) or absence of red blood cells and evaluating the color of the plasma or serum for a pink discoloration (hemoglobinemia). Hemoglobin in plasma binds haptoglobin and is largely retained in the circulation (not readily cleared by glomerular filtration). Pink discoloration of the serum indicates hemolysis and suggests hemoglobinuria as cause for positive urine dipstick blood result. Myoglobin is readily excreted in the urine, so the serum is usually clear to yellow. If there are no red blood cells in urine sediment and no evidence of hemoglobinemia, a positive blood result on urine dipstick suggests myoglobinuria by process of elimination.
- Myoglobinuria may be confirmed with an ammonium sulfate precipitation test on urine, and checking for additional evidence of muscle damage (e.g., elevation of serum creatine kinase). Addition of ammonium sulfate to urine to 80% concentration will cause hemoglobin to precipitate. Myoglobin does not precipitate and will continue to give a positive occult blood result on urine dipstick.

AUTHOR: Ruanna E. Gossett, DVM, PhD, DACVP
EDITOR: Lois Roth-Johnson, DVM, PhD, DACVP

Neospora Serology

Definition

Detection of serum antibody to *Neospora caninum* by IFA or ELISA

Physiology

N. caninum is a coccidian parasite whose morphology is identical to *Toxoplasma gondii* under light microscopy. Clinical manifestations of *N. caninum* in dogs are primarily neurologic and musculoskeletal. Transplacental and environmental transmission occurs.

Causes of Abnormally High Levels

- Infection with or prior exposure to *N. caninum*. Rising titer (>4-fold) confirms active infection. Positive cerebrospinal fluid titers are suggestive of disease.
- IFA tests have little cross-reactivity with other parasites, including *T. gondii*. However, cross-reactivity depends on the antigen source used for the assay (among other laboratory-based factors) and may vary.
- Most dogs with confirmed neosporosis have titers ≥ 1:200. High titers have been found in clinically normal dogs, suggesting subclinical disease.

Next Diagnostic Steps to Consider if Levels Are High

Treatment for neosporosis if clinical signs are compatible with this disease. See p. 984.

Important Interspecies Differences

Serologic tests use species-specific reagents and must be adapted for the species of interest. Cats have been experimentally infected, but clinically, neosporosis in cats is unknown; natural disease in small animals is mainly seen in dogs. *N. caninum* is an important cause of abortion in ruminants.

Specimen Collection and Handling

Serum, 1 mL (red top tube), refrigerated

Relative Cost: $$$

Pearls

- Diagnosis is sometimes made via observation of tachyzoites of *N. caninum* in biopsy/necropsy tissue or in cytologic preparations. Although the morphology of the tachyzoites of *N. caninum* and *T. gondii* is identical, differentiation can be made via direct fluorescent antibody, immunohistochemical staining of tissue samples, or PCR.
- Almost all commercially available laboratory tests for antibody are for immunoglobulin G (IgG).

AUTHOR: Sharon M. Dial, DVM, PhD, DACVP
EDITOR: Lois Roth-Johnson, DVM, PhD, DACVP

Neutrophils (Neutrophilia, Neutropenia)

Definition

Granulocytic leukocytes with segmented nuclei and inconspicuous cytoplasmic granules. Their primary functions during inflammation are bacterial phagocytosis and killing.

Synonyms

Polymorphonuclear neutrophil (PMN), segmented neutrophil

Physiology

Precursors in bone marrow respond to colony-stimulating factors, and production is increased during inflammatory and immune responses. Mature neutrophils can be found in the marrow (storage pool), in peripheral blood (circulation pool), or associated with vascular endothelial cells (marginal pool). Neutrophils circulate for only a few hours before leaving the vascular space for tissues. In blood samples collected for CBC, only neutrophils in the circulating pool are counted.

Reference Interval

Dogs: 3-11.5 × 10^3 neutrophils/mcL; cats: 2.5-12.5 × 10^3 neutrophils/mcL

Causes of Abnormally High Levels

- Inflammation, whether acute or chronic, infectious or noninfectious. If acute inflammation, left shift and/or toxic changes may be present.
- Stress leukogram (glucocorticoids shift neutrophils from marrow storage pool and from marginal pool into circulating pool)
- Excitement leukocytosis (increased blood flow shifts neutrophils from marginal to circulating pool).
- Paraneoplastic production of colony-stimulating factor
- Chronic granulocytic leukemia
- Canine leukocyte adhesion deficiency (rare)

Next Diagnostic Steps to Consider if Levels Are High

Assess for cause depending on clinical signs.

Causes of Abnormally Low Levels

- Intense inflammation, especially if bacterial cause (increased tissue demand)
- Decreased granulopoiesis (e.g., feline leukemia virus [FeLV] or feline immunodeficiency virus [FIV] infection, drugs [see below], myelophthisis)
- Acute parvoviral infection (decreased marrow production and endotoxemia)
- Endotoxemia and severe hypothermia can transiently shift neutrophils from circulating to marginal pool.
- Destruction of mature neutrophils (e.g., immune-mediated neutropenia)

Next Diagnostic Steps to Consider if Levels Are Low

In absence of identifiable infection/inflammation, consider bone marrow aspirate or core biopsy

Important Interspecies Differences

- Neutrophilia from excitement is more likely in young cats, whereas neutrophilia from glucocorticoids (stress leukogram) is more likely in dogs.
- Dogs typically have greater degree of neutrophilia than cats.
- Cats may have benign idiopathic neutropenia (diagnosis of exclusion).

Drug Effects

- Increase: glucocorticoids
- Decrease: albendazole, methimazole, trimethoprim-sulfa, phenobarbital, many chemotherapeutic anticancer agents

Specimen Collection and Handling

EDTA whole blood (lavender top tube) and freshly prepared blood smear for laboratory to stain

Relative Cost: $$ (reported as part of CBC)

Pearls

- Inflammation is not the only cause of neutrophilia; other common causes are stress leukogram and excitement leukocytosis.
- Extreme neutrophilia (>50,000 neutrophils/mcL) is more often reported in dogs with localized inflammation at sites/lesions that start with a "p" (especially pyometra, but also pancreatitis, prostatitis, pleuritis, peritonitis). Other inflammatory diseases associated with extreme neutrophilia include hepatozoonosis and immune-mediated hemolytic anemias.
- Mature neutrophilia can be a useful descriptive term, as it indicates that no bands or left shift is present.

AUTHOR: Stephen D. Gaunt, DVM, PhD, DACVP
EDITOR: Lois Roth-Johnson, DVM, PhD, DACVP

N-Terminal Pro-B-Type Natriuretic Peptide (NT-proBNP)

Definition

Circulating biomarker for cardiac disease in dogs and cats

Synonym

BNP

Physiology

Natriuretic peptides of both A- and B-type (ANP, BNP) are produced by myocardial tissue and released into circulation in response to increased pressure and wall stress. BNP occurs in circulation in two forms: biologically active but unstable C-terminal BNP and biologically inactive NT-proBNP. The NT-proBNP form has a longer half-life, and increased serum concentration has been correlated with cardiac disease in dogs and cats. Daily variation is reported.

Reference Interval

Dog:

- < 900 pmol/L within reference interval
- 900-1800 pmol/L slight increase; cardiac workup suggested if clinical signs present
- > 1800 pmol/L consistent with heart disease

Cat:

- < 100 pmol/L within reference interval
- 100-270 pmol/L slight increase; cardiac workup suggested if clinical signs present
- > 270 pmol/L consistent with heart disease

Causes of Abnormally High Levels

Increased intracardiac hydrostatic pressure. Lung disease, presumably by causing cor pulmonale (minimal increases). Azotemia (renal, prerenal) and dehydration may cause slight increases.

Important Interspecies Differences

The assay is a species-specific ELISA test; the canine assay cannot be used on feline blood or vice versa, nor can the human assay be used on blood from either species.

Drug Effects

Drugs used for treating cardiac disease (diuretics, angiotensin-converting enzyme inhibitors, beta-adrenergic receptor blockers, vasodilators, antiarrhythmics) may decrease values slightly.

Lab Artifacts

Prolonged contact with glass, delayed separation of cells from plasma, and improper or prolonged storage will decrease values.

Specimen Collection and Handling

Plasma (preferred in dogs) or serum. Contact laboratory for specific specimen requirements. Special protease-inhibitor (pink top) tubes required previously, now generally unnecessary. For in-clinic tests, follow manufacturer's instructions.

Relative Cost: $$

Pearls

- Patients with pulmonary hypertension or renal disease may have elevated NT-proBNP concentrations.
- Serum NT-proBNP levels help differentiate between dyspneic patients with cardiogenic pulmonary edema (high NT-proBNP) and dyspneic patients with noncardiac disease (normal NT-proBNP) in both dogs and cats.

- Daily variation may occur secondary to physical exertion, fluid intake, and (likely) circadian rhythm.
- NT-proBNP shows promise for distinguishing cats with physiologic heart murmurs (result within reference interval) from cats with heart murmurs due to cardiomyopathy (increased NT-proBNP): 71% sensitivity, 100% specificity in one study.
- Dobermans with NT-proBNP > 735 pmol/L may be at increased risk of occult dilated cardiomyopathy. Echocardiography and EKG or Holter monitor recommended.

AUTHOR: Carrie L. Flint, DVM, DACVP
EDITOR: Lois Roth-Johnson, DVM, PhD, DACVP

Pancreatic Lipase

Definition

Lipase produced only by the pancreas. Species-specific assays for canine pancreatic lipase (cPL) or feline pancreatic lipase (fPL) include rapid semiquantitative point-of-care tests (SNAP cPL, SNAP fPL, IDEXX Laboratories) or a quantitative test (Spec cPL, Spec fPL, IDEXX Laboratories or Gastrointestinal Laboratory, Texas A&M University). These two tests correlate well in dogs; the manufacturer reports high agreement for the feline assay, but independent evaluation is pending.

Synonyms

Pancreatic lipase immunoreactivity (PLI), pancreatic-specific lipase (PSL), canine pancreatic lipase (cPL), feline pancreatic lipase (fPL)

Physiology

Leakage from pancreatic exocrine cells occurs with pancreatitis and likely neoplasia, hypoperfusion and trauma. In individual healthy dogs there is considerable biologic variation, so only increases of ≈5-fold or greater are considered clinically significant. cPL is cleared rapidly (<24 hours), so values reflect current exocrine pancreatic cell leakage.

Reference Interval

- Canine Spec cPL: 0-200 mcg/L; feline Spec fPL: 0-3.5 mcg/L
- Gray zone values (201-399 mcg/L in dogs, 3.6-5.3 mcg/L in cats) suggest pancreatitis; retesting is recommended.
- Higher values (>400 mcg/L in dogs, >5.4 mcg/L in cats) are consistent with pancreatitis.

Causes of Abnormally High Levels

Pancreatitis, especially if acute. Potentially also pancreatic neoplasia, hypoperfusion, or trauma. Animals with the following conditions may have high values with or without concurrent pancreatitis: miniature schnauzers with hypertriglyceridemia; overweight/obese dogs; dogs with heart failure, acute abdominal disease, hyperadrenocorticism or parvoviral enteritis; cats with diabetes mellitus or inflammatory bowel disease. Intraindividual variability exists in healthy dogs, accounting for gray zone or up to 6% false-positive results.

Next Diagnostic Steps to Consider if Levels are High

Assess clinical signs, routine laboratory tests and abdominal ultrasonography. Consider quantitative Spec test or DGGR lipase activity measurement.

Causes of Abnormally Low Levels

Exocrine pancreatic insufficiency in dogs (trypsin-like immunoreactivity is a superior test; p. 1390). Chronic pancreatitis (decreased exocrine tissue).

Drug Effects

Dogs treated with phenobarbital, potassium bromide, or prednisolone may have increased cPL; unknown if drug effect or due to pancreatitis.

Specimen Collection and Handling

Serum, 1 mL minimum (red top tube). Unless fasting is clinically contraindicated, fast for 12 hours, collect blood and remove serum from clot. Store refrigerated up to 8 days or frozen. SNAP test is performed on serum.

Relative Cost: $$

Pearls

- Currently the most sensitive and specific blood test for pancreatitis in both dogs and cats.
- Sensitivity is higher than specificity. Negative SNAP cPL or normal Spec cPL results typically rule out pancreatitis. When results are positive, clinical signs, routine laboratory tests, and ultrasonography should help differentiate pancreatitis from other conditions.
- Lipemia, bilirubin, or hemolysis does not interfere with the assay.

AUTHOR: Shelley Burton, DVM, MSc, DACVP
EDITOR: Lois Roth-Johnson, DVM, PhD, DACVP

Parathyroid Hormone

Definition

Hormone produced by parathyroid glands in response to low blood calcium levels; important in the rapid and precise regulation of calcium

Synonyms

Parathormone, PTH

Physiology

Parathyroid hormone (PTH) acts directly on bone and kidney and indirectly on the gastrointestinal (GI) tract to increase serum calcium levels. In the kidney, renal excretion of phosphate increases, tubular resorption of calcium increases, and vitamin D precursors are converted to active vitamin D (which, along with PTH, increases calcium absorption from the GI tract). PTH mobilizes calcium and phosphate from bone. Ultimately, these actions increase blood calcium and reduce phosphate.

Reference Interval

Dogs and cats: 2-13 pmol/L (approximate; exact range is laboratory specific)

Causes of Abnormally High Levels

Hyperparathyroidism: primary hyperparathyroidism (parathyroid adenoma/hyperplasia); multiple endocrine neoplasia, chronic kidney disease (renal secondary hyperparathyroidism); pseudohyperparathyroidism (decreased PTH-receptor receptiveness). Rare: nutritional secondary hyperparathyroidism.

Next Diagnostic Steps to Consider if Levels are High

See p. 499.

Causes of Abnormally Low Levels

Parathyroid inflammation and degeneration (lymphocytic parathyroiditis); inadvertent surgical removal of parathyroid (thyroidectomy in cats); decreased PTH production due to inhibition (hypervitaminosis D, hypercalcemic disorders other than primary hyperparathyroidism); congenital hypoparathyroidism (rare)

Next Diagnostic Steps to Consider if Levels are Low

See p. 519.

Lab Artifacts

Prolonged storage (>2 months) or thawing of sample may alter results, either increased or decreased. Lipemia and hemolysis falsely decrease measurement. EDTA plasma samples have higher values.

Specimen Collection and Handling

Contact laboratory; serum (red top tube without additive; do not use serum separator tube) is frequently used for the assay. Samples should be centrifuged immediately after clotting, frozen, and shipped frozen as soon as possible.

Relative Cost: $$$

Pearls

- It is important to know serum iCa to correctly interpret PTH results. Normal PTH with high iCa is physiologically inappropriate (hypercalcemia feedback inhibition should suppress PTH) and suggests hyperparathyroidism.
- Kidney disease and secondary hyperparathyroidism is typically associated with normal to low iCa and increased PTH.

AUTHOR: Deborah G. Davis, DVM, DACVP
EDITOR: Lois Roth-Johnson, DVM, PhD, DACVP

Parathyroid Hormone–Related Protein (PTHrP)

Definition

Humoral factor with a molecular structure similar to parathyroid hormone (PTH); can bind to PTH receptors. It plays an important role in humoral hypercalcemia of malignancy.

Synonym

PTHrP

Physiology

Has important endocrine and paracrine actions in the fetus but produced in insignificant amounts in adult tissues. In humoral hypercalcemia of malignancy, neoplastic cells secrete excess amounts of PTHrP and other cytokines. PTHrP binds to PTH receptors in bone and kidney and mimics the effects of PTH: osteoclastic bone resorption, increased renal resorption of calcium, and decreased renal resorption of phosphate. Malignancies associated with increased PTHrP include T-cell lymphoma, thymoma, apocrine gland adenocarcinoma of the anal sac, squamous cell carcinoma (cat), and sporadic cases of other carcinomas.

Reference Interval

Not normally found circulating in the blood. Dogs: < 2 pmol/L

Causes of Abnormally High Levels

Humoral hypercalcemia of malignancy. See p. 754.

Next Diagnostic Steps to Consider if Levels are High

Generally measured along with serum ionized calcium (iCa), phosphorus, serum PTH. Review physical exam, including rectal palpation in dogs (perianal mass, sublumbar lymphadenopathy). CBC, serum biochemistry profile, urinalysis, and diagnostic imaging, including thoracic radiographs to identify neoplastic disease and its complications

Lab Artifacts

Repeated thawing causes degradation of the protein and interferes with validity of results (either falsely increasing or decreasing). Proteases in serum can degrade PTHrP and cause false-negative results. False-positives can occur with hemolysis.

Specimen Collection and Handling

Contact laboratory for specifics. If serum is sent, immediately spin the sample after it clots, separate serum, transfer to plastic tube, and freeze. Ship frozen. If plasma is required, collect blood in EDTA (lavender top tube), separate plasma from erythrocytes, transfer to a plastic tube, and ship frozen.

Relative Cost: $$$

Pearls

Three mechanisms can cause cancer-associated hypercalcemia: humoral hypercalcemia of malignancy, local bone resorption induced by hematologic neoplasms in bone marrow (e.g., multiple myeloma), and bone resorption induced by metastatic bone lesions. Humoral hypercalcemia of malignancy usually causes an elevated serum ionized calcium level, a low PTH level, and a low phosphorus level.

AUTHOR: Deborah G. Davis, DVM, DACVP
EDITOR: Lois Roth-Johnson, DVM, PhD, DACVP

Pelger Huët

Definition

A congenital defect in nuclear lobulation of leukocytes that is rare in dogs and cats. The characteristic appearance of a hyposegmented nucleus is most evident in neutrophils but also occurs in eosinophils, basophils, monocytes, and megakaryocytes. The nuclear shape of blood neutrophils in affected animals are bilobed ("pince-nez" cell), band, or round (similar to early neutrophilic precursors), but the nuclear chromatin of affected neutrophils is coarsely condensed, similar to mature neutrophils.

Synonyms

Pelger Huët syndrome

Physiology

Segmented neutrophils in dogs and cats typically have 3-5 nuclear lobes. Heterozygotes for the congenital Pelger Huët anomaly exhibit hyposegmented neutrophils, many of which resemble band neutrophils. The heterozygous condition is benign, and affected animals have no ill effects with minimal alteration of neutrophil function. The low incidence of homozygotes is attributed to embryonic death. The genetic defect in people is linked to mutations of the laminin B receptor, as B-type laminin mediates nuclear shape by binding the nuclear membrane to chromatin. Rarely, genetically normal animals develop hyposegmentation of neutrophils in response to inflammation, B vitamin deficiency, neoplastic disease, or other illness ("pseudo" Pelger Huët). In such cases, hyposegmentation may be transient.

Reference Interval

Reported if present on slide review

Specimen Collection and Handling

EDTA whole blood (lavender top tube) and freshly prepared blood smear for laboratory to stain

Pearls

- When an otherwise unremarkable CBC report has a substantial number of "bands" or "metamyelocytes" in an apparently healthy dog or cat, consider the likelihood of Pelger Huët.
- Pelger Huët is essentially an incidental finding, with no adverse clinical effect.
- Since the hyposegmented neutrophils in cats and dogs with Pelger Huët do not reflect neutrophilic precursors released from the marrow, the term "left shift" is not applicable.

AUTHOR: Stephen D. Gaunt, DVM, PhD, DACVP
EDITOR: Lois Roth-Johnson, DVM, PhD, DACVP

Phenobarbital Serum Level

Definition

Serum levels of anticonvulsant barbiturate used to monitor treated patients

Physiology

Phenobarbital is slowly absorbed from GI system, with good bioavailability (peak 4-8 hours after administration). It undergoes hepatic metabolism with a widely variable elimination half-life (dogs 12-125 hours, average 48 hours; half-life cats 35-56 hours). Diet, body weight and composition, and concurrent drug use can alter pharmacokinetics. Can result in hepatotoxicity

Reference Interval

Therapeutic target: 15 to 40 mcg/mL dogs; 23 to 28 mcg/mL cats

Causes of Abnormally High Levels

> 40 mcg/mL may indicate toxicosis, but there is considerable variability, and some dogs may develop toxicosis at lower concentrations.

Next Diagnostic Steps to Consider if Levels are High

Consider dose reduction if seizures well-controlled. If seizures continue, consider addition/substitution of alternative anticonvulsant drug. See p. 903. Consider effects of comorbidities and concurrently administered drugs. Evaluate liver enzymes/function (i.e., bile acids).

Causes of Abnormally Low Levels

Serum levels < 10 mcg/mL typically are subtherapeutic, with considerable variability in responses among dogs.

Next Diagnostic Steps to Consider if Levels are Low

Correlate drug levels with seizure control to decide whether to increase dose, replace/supplement with another anticonvulsant, or discontinue.

Drug Effects

Concurrent administration of many other drugs, such as certain antibiotics (e.g., doxycycline, chloramphenicol, metronidazole), anticoagulants (warfarin), cardiopulmonary drugs (e.g., aminophylline/theophylline, certain beta-blockers, quinidine), glucocorticoids (prednisone, others), and many others, alters levels of phenobarbital. Consult a pharmacology textbook or pharmacist for information regarding specific drug interactions.

Lab Artifacts

Avoid serum separator tube, which can cause falsely decreased phenobarbital concentrations.

Specimen Collection and Handling

Serum (red top tube); avoid serum separator tube. Sample can be collected any time relative to dosing.

Relative Cost: $$

Pearls

- Phenobarbital is involved in many drug interactions; consult pharmacology textbook or pharmacist if multiple medications.
- Considerable variability in clinical response occurs; blood level does not always correlate with clinical response or hepatic toxicosis.
- Blood levels are not as useful when combining with bromide or levetiracetam since a therapeutic effect likely can be achieved with lower levels of phenobarbital.

AUTHOR: Carrie L. Flint, DVM, DACVP
EDITOR: Lois Roth-Johnson, DVM, PhD, DACVP

Phosphorus

Definition

Inorganic form of phosphate; the major intracellular anion; primarily located in bone (as hydroxyapatite), with the remainder in soft tissues and in circulation

Synonyms

Phosphate, PO_4^{2-}

Physiology

Clinical assays measure only the total inorganic phosphorus, although both organic and inorganic phosphorus are present (depending on pH). Blood levels are affected by intestinal absorption, shifting between intracellular and extracellular compartments, renal clearance, and animal's age. Parathyroid hormone (PTH) triggers phosphaturia.

Reference Interval

Dogs: 3.2-8.1 mg/dL. Cats: 3.2-6.5 mg/dL. Unit conversion: 1 mg/dL = 0.323 mmol/L

Causes of Abnormally High Levels

Misdistribution (e.g., tumor lysis syndrome, myopathies, metabolic alkalosis); increased intake (e.g., phosphate enema, increased vitamin D); decreased loss (e.g., decreased renal excretion, ruptured bladder, hypoparathyroidism); bone metabolism (e.g., growing animal, osteolytic bone lesions). See p. 1237.

Next Diagnostic Steps to Consider if Levels are High

- Rule out artifact (repeat test).
- CBC/chemistry profile/urinalysis (rule out urinary, other metabolic disease); consider endocrine testing (PTH levels, thyroid hormone [cats]); ionized calcium; survey skeletal radiographs

Causes of Abnormally Low Levels

Misdistribution (e.g., during treatment for diabetic ketoacidosis); increased loss (e.g., Fanconi syndrome in dogs, primary hyperparathyroidism); decreased intake (e.g., hypovitaminosis D, prolonged anorexia). See p. 1241.

Next Diagnostic Steps to Consider if Levels are Low

Repeat to rule out artifact. CBC/chemistry profile/urinalysis; ionized calcium

Drug Effects

- Decrease: phosphate binding antacids, anesthetics, diuretics, insulin, anticonvulsants, bicarbonate, mithramycin, salicylates, glucocorticoids
- Increase: phosphate enemas, intravenous supplementation, furosemide, vitamin D or vitamin D–containing toxins (p. 164), hydrochlorothiazide, minocycline

Lab Artifacts

- Increase: hemolysis *(in vivo* or *in vitro),* delayed separation of serum from clot, hyperlipidemia, monoclonal gammopathy, thrombocytosis
- Decrease: postprandial carbohydrates (mild), hyperbilirubinemia (with certain assays)

Specimen Collection and Handling

Serum (red top tube) preferred; can also be measured in heparinized plasma (green top tube) and urine

Relative Cost: $

Pearls

- Healthy animals < 1 year of age may normally have serum phosphorus levels that exceed the reference interval for adults.
- Acute hypophosphatemia (e.g., during initial management of diabetic ketoacidosis) can cause severe hemolytic anemia.

AUTHOR: Deborah G. Davis, DVM, DACVP
EDITOR: Lois Roth-Johnson, DVM, PhD, DACVP

Platelets

Definition

- Thrombocytopenia: decreased platelet count
- Thrombocytosis: increased platelet count
- Thrombopathia: abnormal platelet function

Physiology

Platelets are discoid, anucleate cytoplasmic fragments, 5-7 mcm in diameter, important in primary hemostasis. Produced from megakaryocytes in bone marrow, spleen, and lung. They adhere to subendothelium by the binding of von Willebrand factor (vWF) to platelet glycoprotein Ib (GPIb). Aggregation occurs through binding of platelet membrane $a_{IIb}b_3$ with fibrinogen or vWF. Activated platelets release granule contents (fibrinogen, factor V, ADP, ATP, plasminogen), thromboxane A2, and arachidonic acid. Mediator release and reactions with leukocytes are important in inflammation and wound healing.

Reference Interval

- Dogs: 150,000-500,000/mcL
- Cats: 150,000-400,000/mcL
- 9-15 platelets per 100× field (blood film) associated with adequate platelet numbers

Causes of Abnormally High Levels

Redistribution (exercise, epinephrine release), neoplasia (essential thrombocythemia, acute megakaryocytic leukemia), increased production (inflammation, iron deficiency, rebound from thrombocytopenia), hyperadrenocorticism, immune-mediated hemolytic anemia

Next Diagnostic Steps to Consider if Levels are High

Examine blood film to confirm increase; CBC/serum biochemistry profile for evidence of inflammation (neutrophilia with left shift, elevated globulins); +/− serum iron profile; +/− bone marrow aspirate

Causes of Abnormally Low Levels

- Decreased production: FeLV, myelotoxic drugs, infiltrative bone marrow disease (neoplastic, infectious), myelofibrosis
- Destruction: immune-mediated thrombocytopenia, infectious disease (e.g., *Anaplasma platys*, babesiosis)
- Consumption: vasculitis (e.g., immune-mediated, Rocky Mountain spotted fever), disseminated intravascular coagulation, massive bleeding or thrombosis
- Sequestration (often mild to moderate in severity): hypersplenism, heartworm disease
- Breed related

Next Diagnostic Steps to Consider if Levels are Low

Blood film evaluation to rule out clumping and look for hemotropic infectious agents or macroplatelets; assess history and physical exam to identify underlying disorder/trigger; coagulation profile to rule out coagulopathy, DIC; serologic titers or PCR for infectious agents; bone marrow aspirate

Important Interspecies Differences

- Greyhounds have lower platelet counts.
- β-1 tubulin defect in Cavalier King Charles spaniels, cairn and Norfolk terriers
- Cats: strong propensity for platelet clumping

Drug Effects

- Thrombocytosis: vincristine, vinblastine, exogenous corticosteroids
- Thrombocytopenia: chemotherapeutic agents, estrogens, phenylbutazone, certain diuretics, certain antibiotics/antimicrobials

Lab Artifacts

- Clumping: traumatic venipuncture, clots/microclots in tube, heparinized sample
- Macroplatelets (decrease due to undercounting by automated analyzers)
- Severe anemia may cause platelets to appear increased in blood smears.

Specimen Collection and Handling

EDTA whole blood (lavender top tube) preferred; citrated whole blood (blue-top tube) can be used.

Relative Cost: $ (manual platelet count); automated platelet counts and estimates are reported with CBC ($$)

Pearls

- Breed-related thrombocytopenia does not result in bleeding, but breed-related thrombocytopathia often does result in abnormal bleeding.
- Thrombopathia should be considered in a bleeding patient with prolonged buccal mucosal bleeding time when platelet count, hematocrit, coagulation parameters (prothrombin time, activated partial thromboplastin time), and vWF are normal. Document with specific platelet function tests.

AUTHOR: Deborah G. Davis, DVM, DACVP
EDITOR: Lois Roth-Johnson, DVM, PhD, DACVP

Poikilocytes

Definition

General term for abnormally shaped mature erythrocytes in blood. This shape change can be artifactual (e.g., crenation) or pathologic (e.g., spherocytes, schistocytes). See p. 1327.

Physiology

Normal shape of mature erythrocyte is discocyte (biconcave disk). With damage to cell membrane (e.g., antibodies, toxins, lipid accumulation), damage to hemoglobin (e.g., oxidation), or interaction with sinusoidal macrophages of spleen or liver, the plasma membrane and/or protein cytoskeleton of the erythrocyte is/are altered, and an abnormal erythrocyte shape results.

Reference Interval

- Only artifactually induced poikilocytes (e.g., crenation) should be observed in the blood of healthy animals.
- The presence of even low numbers of the other types of poikilocytes should prompt consideration of their associated conditions or diseases.

Causes of Abnormally High Levels

Immune-mediated hemolytic anemias (spherocytes), erythrocyte fragmentation (schistocytes, acanthocytes, prekeratocytes, keratocytes), oxidative damage (Heinz bodies, eccentrocytes, pyknocytes), hepatic diseases (acanthocytes), venomous snake bite (echinocytes, spherocytes), bee sting (spherocytes), congenital defect in erythrocyte membrane proteins (elliptocytes, spherocytes).

Next Diagnostic Steps to Consider if Levels are High

Based on specific poikilocyte(s) identified, investigate associated diseases or conditions associated with that poikilocyte.

Important Interspecies Differences

Crenation (artifact) occurs more commonly in feline erythrocytes. Spherocytosis is more easily detected in the erythrocytes of dogs, because normal canine erythrocytes have a prominent central pallor that is lacking in spherocytes.

Lab Artifacts

- Poorly prepared blood smears will distort canine erythrocytes so that central pallor is lost and cells may resemble spherocytes.
- Erythrocytes on blood smears allowed to slowly air-dry during preparation could have refractile markings and distortion; best to rapidly dry smears by waving or use heat block.
- Lipemia causes lysis and distortion of erythrocyte morphology.
- Crenation often occurs from effects of smear preparation on erythrocytes.
- Reticulocytes have excess cell membrane, which can produce an abnormal shape; clinically relevant shape changes should only be evaluated in mature erythrocytes.

Specimen Collection and Handling

EDTA whole blood (lavender top tube) and freshly prepared blood smear for laboratory to stain

Pearls

See p. 1327 for a differential diagnosis diagram of various poikilocytes.

AUTHOR: Stephen D. Gaunt, DVM, PhD, DACVP
EDITOR: Lois Roth-Johnson, DVM, PhD, DACVP

Potassium

Definition

Major intracellular cation continually pumped into cell by energy-dependent sodium/potassium-ATPase pump at cell membrane; important in cardiac and neuromuscular membrane potentials/excitability

Synonym

K^+

Physiology

Influenced by acid-base status. Metabolic acidosis (e.g., with chronic kidney disease) causes extracellular shift and hyperkalemia. Under normal conditions, excess plasma K^+ is excreted in the urine. Hyperkalemia is uncommon if renal function is normal (exceptions: postrenal lesions, hypoadrenocorticism, iatrogenic). Potassium is released during normal platelet coagulation, potentially causing pseudohyperkalemia.

Reference Interval

Typically 3.5-5.5 mEq/L (mmol/L)

Causes of Abnormally High Levels

Decreased renal excretion (oliguric/anuric renal failure, urinary tract obstruction or rupture), hypoadrenocorticism, artifact gastrointestinal disease (salmonellosis, trichuriasis), pleural effusion with repeated drainage, tumor lysis syndrome, diabetic ketoacidosis, metabolic acidosis (due to inorganic acids), rhabdomyolysis

Next Diagnostic Steps to Consider if Levels are High

Repeat measurement using green top tube (heparin) if sample was collected in a red top tube; CBC, serum biochemistry profile, and urinalysis; evaluate for drugs that can cause hyperkalemia; abdominal ultrasound/radiographs (check integrity of urinary tract); ACTH stimulation test to rule out hypoadrenocorticism if clinically compatible; blood gas determination to assess acid-base status. See p. 495.

Causes of Abnormally Low Levels

Increased loss (vomiting, diarrhea), chronic kidney disease (cats), postobstructive diuresis, inappropriate fluid therapy (dilutional hypokalemia), polyuria associated with diabetes mellitus, ketoacidosis, hyperadrenocorticism, hyperaldosteronism, alkalemia, and hypokalemic periodic paralysis of Burmese cats

Next Diagnostic Steps to Consider if Levels are Low

See p. 516.

Drug Effects

- Hyperkalemia: angiotensin-converting enzyme inhibitors, potassium-sparing diuretics (e.g., spironolactone), K^+ penicillin, oversupplementation of fluids with K^+, o,p′-DDD (iatrogenic hypoadrenocorticism), trimethoprim
- Hypokalemia: loop diuretics (furosemide), thiazide diuretics, amphotericin B, penicillin, administration of K^+-free fluids (dilutional)

Lab Artifacts

Serum K^+ is higher than plasma K^+, especially if thrombocytosis is present; marked hemolysis in dog breeds (Akitas, English springer spaniels) with high K^+ red blood cell concentration;

marked leukocytosis or reticulocytosis; incomplete separation of plasma. Drawing blood through an intravenous catheter may dilute sample, resulting in false decrease. Use of lavender top tubes (K_3EDTA anticoagulant) causes false increase. Severe lipemia can cause mild hypokalemia on standard chemistry panels.

Specimen Collection and Handling

Serum (red top tube); K^+ remains stable for extended periods of time, but platelet activation-induced K^+ release makes sampling into heparin (green top tube) and separation of plasma from red cells preferable.

Relative Cost: $

Pearls

- Assess the acid-base status of hypokalemic/hyperkalemic animals.
- Normal K^+ levels in the presence of metabolic acidemia suggest low K^+ stores. Normal K^+ in an alkalotic animal suggests increased total body K^+.
- Hemolysis alone rarely causes artifactual hyperkalemia, and when it does, the patient is generally of a breed that has unusually high intra-RBC K^+ stores (e.g., Asian dog breeds).

AUTHOR: Deborah G. Davis, DVM, DACVP
EDITOR: Lois Roth-Johnson, DVM, PhD, DACVP

Progesterone

Definition

Steroid hormone secreted by corpora lutea of the ovaries and by the placenta

Physiology

Progesterone is secreted by the cells of developing corpus luteum, the presence of which indicates pregnancy, diestrus, or an ovarian lesion (e.g., cyst or neoplasm). Concentrations greater than those of anestrus (i.e., >2 ng/mL) are used for predicting time of ovulation in bitches. Progesterone, secreted by the placenta, is needed to maintain pregnancy. Decreasing progesterone concentrations (<2 ng/mL) usually indicate impending parturition (within 24 hours).

Reference Interval

- Anestrus/proestrus: < 1.0 ng/mL
- Pre-LH surge: 1.0-1.9 ng/mL
- LH surge (24-48 hours preovulation): 2.0-3.0 ng/mL
- Post-LH surge, preovulation: 3.1-4.9 ng/mL
- Ovulation: 5.0-12.0 ng/mL
- Diestrus: > 12 ng/mL

Causes of Abnormally High Levels

Developing corpora lutea followed by pregnancy; residual ovarian tissue in a patient thought to have been spayed; luteal cysts; granulosa cell tumor

Next Diagnostic Steps to Consider if Levels are High

Confirm the presence of ovarian abnormalities (e.g., abdominal ultrasound) if not evaluating a breeding bitch.

Causes of Abnormally Low Levels

Depends on stage of cycle; may indicate normal anestrus or failure to ovulate, failure to become pregnant or maintain pregnancy, or impending parturition

Next Diagnostic Steps to Consider if Levels are Low

Evaluate for causes of infertility or abortion if repeated failure to maintain pregnancy.

Important Interspecies Differences

Test used primarily in dogs; not used in cats because they are induced ovulators

Drug Effects

Minimal interference by deoxycortisol, deoxycortisone, and dihydroprogesterone

Lab Artifacts

Falsely decreased with storage at room temperature or delay in separation of serum or plasma from red blood cells (separation should be performed immediately); lipemia interference if measured by chemiluminescence; use of serum separator tubes falsely decreases values

Specimen Collection and Handling

Depends on the laboratory; serum (red top tube) or heparinized (green top tube) or EDTA plasma (lavender top tube) may be used. Do not use serum separator tubes. Separate serum or plasma from red blood cells immediately. May store at 2°C-8°C for up to 7 days; frozen for 3 months.

Relative Cost: $$

AUTHOR & EDITOR: Lois Roth-Johnson, DVM, PhD, DACVP

Protein Electrophoresis

Definition

Qualitative and quantitative determination of proteins, typically measured in serum but may also be performed on cerebrospinal fluid or urine. Proteins separate into groups (fractions) based on their rate of migration in an electric field. Protein charge and size determine migration rate.

Physiology

The five major fractions of soluble body proteins are albumin and the four globulin fractions: alpha 1, alpha 2, beta, and gamma; beta and gamma globulins each have two fractions. Albumin is the largest fraction in healthy animals. The alpha 1 globulin fraction primarily contains acute-phase proteins. The alpha 2 globulin and beta globulin fractions contain acute-phase proteins, lipoproteins, and some immunoglobulins. The gamma globulin fraction contains immunoglobulin (Ig) A, IgG, and IgM. Increased gamma globulins appear on the electrophoresis tracing as a broad-based peak (polyclonal) or a single narrow peak (monoclonal).

Reference Interval

	Dogs	Cats
alpha1	0.2-0.5 g/dL	0.2-1.1 g/dL
alpha2	0.3-1.1 g/dL	0.4-0.9 g/dL
beta1	0.6-1.2 g/dL	0.3-0.9 g/dL
beta2	0.6-1.4 g/dL	0.6-1.0 g/dL
gamma1	0.5-1.3 g/dL	0.6-1.0 g/dL
gamma2	0.4-0.9 g/dL	1.4-1.9 g/dL

Unit conversion: g/dL × 10 = mg/mL

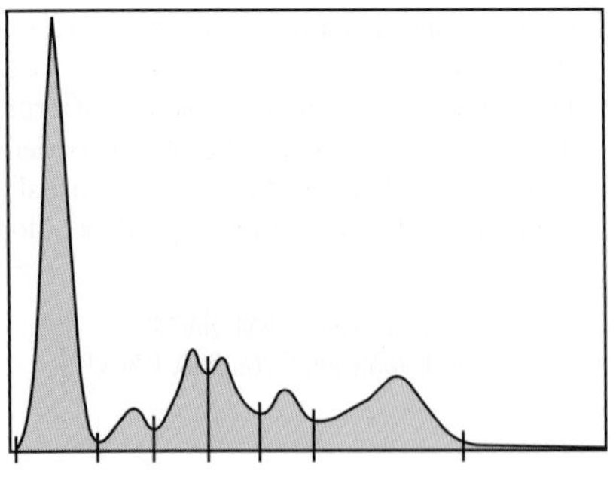

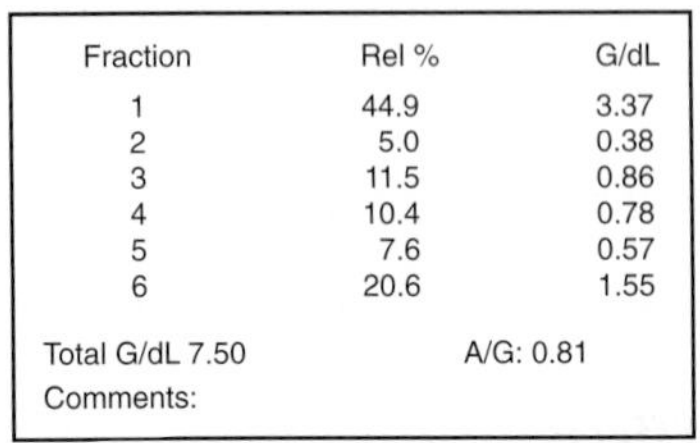

Fraction	Rel %	G/dL
1	44.9	3.37
2	5.0	0.38
3	11.5	0.86
4	10.4	0.78
5	7.6	0.57
6	20.6	1.55

Total G/dL 7.50 A/G: 0.81
Comments:

PROTEIN ELECTROPHORESIS, NORMAL Serum protein electrophoresis tracing demonstrating a normal distribution of serum proteins.

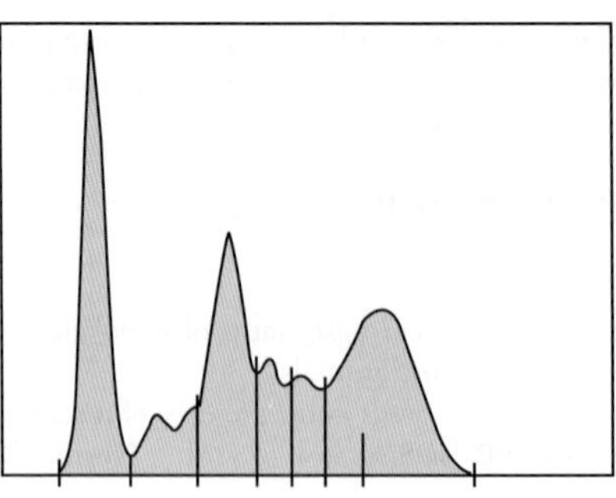

Fraction	Rel %	G/dL
1	28.8	2.97
2	7.1	0.73
3	20.1	2.07
4	7.5	0.77
5	6.4	0.66
6	30.1	3.10

Total G/dL 10.30 A/G: 0.40
Comments:

PROTEIN ELECTROPHORESIS, POLYCLONAL Serum protein electrophoresis tracing demonstrating hyperglobulinemia that is polyclonal in distribution, as is typical of inflammation.

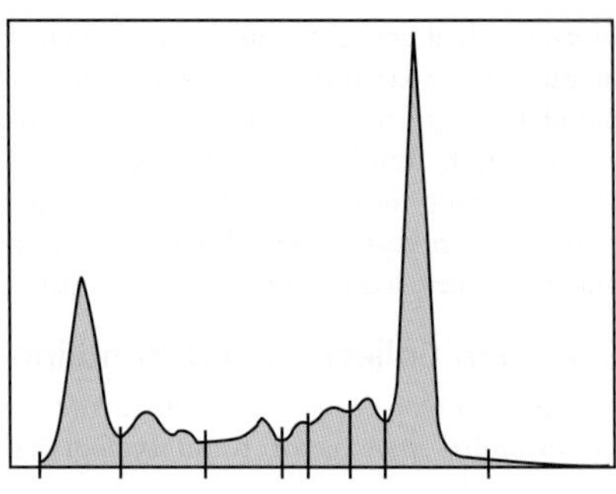

Fraction	Rel %	G/dL
1	23.4	2.41
2	10.4	1.07
3	7.7	0.79
4	3.2	0.33
5	7.0	0.72
6	6.7	0.69
7	41.7	4.30

Total G/dL 10.30 A/G: 0.31
Comments:

PROTEIN ELECTROPHORESIS, MONOCLONAL Serum protein electrophoresis tracing demonstrating hyperglobulinemia that is monoclonal in distribution (single peak). This patient had multiple myeloma.

Causes of Abnormally High Levels

- Increased alpha globulin: acute inflammation, nephrotic syndrome, corticosteroid administration
- Increased beta globulin: acute inflammation, nephrotic syndrome, liver disease, immune responses, neoplasia
- Increased gamma globulins: immune stimulation, neoplasia

Next Diagnostic Steps to Consider if Levels are High

- Polyclonal gammopathy: assess for inflammation, infection, immune-mediated disease, liver disease, neoplasia (neoplasia less commonly polyclonal)
- Monoclonal gammopathy: assess for multiple myeloma, B-cell lymphoma, lymphocytic leukemia; inflammatory or infectious disease (infection less commonly monoclonal; ehrlichiosis, feline infectious peritonitis, leishmaniasis, feline stomatitis, lymphoplasmacytic enterocolitis)

Causes of Abnormally Low Levels

- Albumin: acute-phase response, glomerular disease, liver disease, starvation, cachexia
- Albumin and globulins: gastrointestinal disease (protein-losing enteropathy), blood loss, sequestration in body cavity effusion, severe exudative skin disease, excess fluid therapy or water intake
- Globulins: failure of passive transfer (FPT), inherited or acquired immunodeficiency

Next Diagnostic Steps to Consider if Levels are Low

Based on which fraction(s) is/are low, investigate for albumin loss or decreased albumin synthesis, globulin loss, FPT, acquired or inherited immunodeficiency

Lab Artifacts

Hemolysis artificially elevates beta globulins, because hemoglobin migrates in this region on electrophoresis; lipemia promotes hemolysis.

Specimen Collection and Handling

Serum (red top tube), refrigerate. Heparinized plasma (green top tube) is acceptable.

Relative Cost: $$

Pearls

The numeric values obtained from protein electrophoresis must be assessed in conjunction with the tracing. The values alone do not differentiate between monoclonal and polyclonal gammopathies.

AUTHOR: Ruanna E. Gossett, DVM, PhD, DACVP
EDITOR: Lois Roth-Johnson, DVM, PhD, DACVP

Proteins Induced by Vitamin K Absence or Antagonism (PIVKA)

Definition

Proteins induced by vitamin K absence or antagonism (PIVKAs) are inactive precursor coagulation proteins that accumulate in the peripheral blood when vitamin K is absent or inhibited.

Synonym

Thrombotest

Physiology

Factors II, VII, IX, X, and proteins C, S, and Z are all vitamin K–dependent proteins involved in coagulation homeostasis. Synthesized as inactive precursors in the liver, they require vitamin K for activation. Vitamin K epoxide reductase is critical for this reaction. In the absence of vitamin K or if vitamin K epoxide reductase is inhibited (e.g., by anticoagulant rodenticides), the inactive coagulation precursors (PIVKAs) accumulate in the blood. The thrombotest, which is actually a modification of the prothrombin test, is sensitive to PIVKAs but does not directly measure them.

Reference Interval

Dogs: 12-20 seconds; cats: 20-30 seconds

Causes of Abnormally High Levels

Decreased vitamin K (e.g., neonate born to malnourished mother, prolonged anorexia), malabsorption of vitamin K (e.g., cholestasis, infiltrative bowel disease), or vitamin K antagonism (e.g., anticoagulant rodenticides, therapeutic Coumadin)

Next Diagnostic Steps to Consider if Levels are High

CBC/profile, urinalysis (avoid cystocentesis), coagulation profile, determine if recent exposure to drugs or anticoagulant rodenticides. Draw blood from a compressible vein (e.g., limb) in patients with suspected/confirmed bleeding tendencies.

Important Interspecies Differences

Cats with hepatic, biliary, or inflammatory bowel diseases can have prolonged results without bleeding tendencies.

Drug Effects

Prolonged results: vitamin K antagonists (e.g., warfarin, heparin) and antimicrobials (gut sterilization causing vitamin K deficiency)

Lab Artifacts

Citrate (blue top) tube must be filled to capacity or the results will be falsely prolonged.

Specimen Collection and Handling

Plasma from minimally traumatic venipuncture collected in citrate (blue top tube). Spin and separate plasma. Refrigerate specimens that will be analyzed within 3 hours; freeze if > 3 hours.

Relative Cost: $$

Pearls

PIVKA test may be slightly more sensitive than prothrombin time, but it is not specific for vitamin K–dependent disorders. For example, it can be prolonged with DIC or inherited factor VII deficiency.

AUTHOR: Deborah G. Davis, DVM, DACVP
EDITOR: Lois Roth-Johnson, DVM, PhD, DACVP

Prothrombin Time (PT)

Definition

Screening coagulation test of the extrinsic and common coagulation pathways

Synonyms

One-stage prothrombin time (OSPT), PT

Physiology

Plasma is warmed and mixed with a Ca^{2+}-thromboplastin reagent, allowing tissue factor in the reagent to activate factor VII in the plasma. This initiates the extrinsic and common coagulation pathways. The resulting fibrin clot is detected by an instrument. The prothrombin time (PT) is the time from the plasma and reagent mixing to the formation of the clot.

Reference Interval

Values are approximate (reference intervals are laboratory and instrument specific). Dogs: 7-11 seconds; cats: 5-8 seconds.

Causes of Abnormally High Levels

Hepatic disease, vitamin K deficiency or antagonism, disseminated intravascular coagulation (DIC), anticoagulant intoxication, hereditary defects in extrinsic or common pathway (factors VII, X, V, II, and I), heparin, presence of fibrin degradation products (FDPs), antibodies to phospholipids or coagulation factors

Next Diagnostic Steps to Consider if Levels are High

Rule out causes (p. 433); specific coagulation factor assays are rarely done.

Causes of Abnormally Low Levels

- PT may be shortened (due to high fibrinogen) with inflammation. Decreased PT does not indicate hypercoagulability; rather, it is usually a result of suboptimal phlebotomy (sample collection artifact).

Drug Effects

Therapeutic Coumadin/warfarin should prolong PT by 1.5- to 2.5-fold, and vitamin K_1 should return it to normal.

Lab Artifacts

Improper blood/citrate ratios impact results (too little blood can prolong, and too much blood can shorten PT).

Specimen Collection and Handling

Citrated plasma (blue top tube). Avoid traumatic venipuncture (can artifactually prolong PT). Fill tube to capacity without overfilling. Immediately mix the blood and anticoagulant by repeated gentle inversion.

Relative Cost: $$

Pearls

- Antagonism or absence of vitamin K–dependent coagulation factors, as occurs in anticoagulant rodenticide intoxication, warfarin treatment, or hepatic disease, tends to increase PT before activated partial thromboplastin time (aPTT). This is due to the short half-life of factor VII.
- Prolonged PT and normal aPTT can be seen in cats with DIC. Dogs with DIC can have normal PT.

AUTHOR: Deborah G. Davis, DVM, DACVP
EDITOR: Lois Roth-Johnson, DVM, PhD, DACVP

Pyuria

Definition

Increased numbers of leukocytes, specifically in the urine secondary to urogenital tract inflammation

Synonym

Leukocyturia

Physiology

Leukocytes migrate from the blood to the urinary tract secondary to inflammation from infectious or noninfectious etiologies. Identification of leukocytes in urine is performed through microscopic evaluation of the urine sediment. Results are recorded as number of leukocytes per 40× objective (hpf). Individual leukocytes cannot be identified on wet mount cytology preparations alone; staining of urine either through Sedi-Stain™ or Romanowsky stains is necessary.

Reference Interval

Healthy patients have < 5 leukocytes/hpf.

Causes of Abnormally High Levels

- Neutrophils: cystitis/pyelonephritis, urinary tract neoplasia, urolithiasis, contamination from the genital tract
- Lymphocytes: polypoid cystitis, lymphoma
- Eosinophils: drug-induced acute tubulointerstitial nephritis; polypoid or eosinophilic cystitis

Next Diagnostic Steps to Consider if Levels are High

Ensure sterile collection of urine. Exclude urinary tract infection by submitting sterile urine for microbial culture and sensitivity. Consider abdominal ultrasound to evaluate for calculi or neoplasm.

Specimen Collection and Handling

Unless there is a suspected hemostatic defect or epithelial neoplasm, sterile collection via cystocentesis is recommended to exclude genital tract contamination. Process immediately as leukocytes deteriorate within a few hours.

Relative Cost: $ (reported as part of urinalysis)

Pearls

- Some dogs with diabetes mellitus or hyperadrenocorticism may have positive bacterial cultures without pyuria, suggestive of defective chemotaxis.
- Urine dipstick assessment of pyuria is notoriously unreliable in dogs and cats and should not be used.

AUTHOR: Shannon D. Dehghanpir, DVM, MS, DACVP
EDITOR: Lois Roth-Johnson, DVM, PhD, DACVP

Rabies Diagnostic Testing

Definition

Evaluation of presence or absence of rabies virus infection

Physiology

Rabies is an acute encephalitis caused by an RNA virus of the rhabdovirus family. Virus localizes to the central nervous system. Direct IFA testing of brain tissue is used for definitive diagnosis. Submission of appropriate specimens requires necropsy examination. The test detects viral antigen in the neural tissue of infected animals.

Reference Interval

Results are reported as positive or negative.

Causes of Abnormally High Levels

Viral infection

Next Diagnostic Steps to Consider if Levels Are High

Exposed personnel should consult their physicians and/or their State Public Health Department immediately. Exposed animals should be quarantined and observed for development of clinical signs (p. 861).

Specimen Collection and Handling

Fresh brain tissue. NOTE: Aerosolization of rabies virus is possible during craniotomy portion of necropsy or during removal of head (exposure of spinal cord). Therefore, removal of head or brain should, ideally, be reserved for qualified personnel (e.g., pathologist or state veterinarian). Body of rabies suspect should be chilled (refrigerated), not frozen. If practitioner must cut the brain, cut in sagittal (longitudinal) section. Submit half in clean, dry double bag for IFA test. Clearly label as rabies suspect. Contact the laboratory performing the testing for appropriate packaging instructions.

Relative Cost: $$—$$$$ (charges vary widely among state labs)

Pearls

- All personnel who participate in sample collection should have been vaccinated and have a known, adequate vaccination titer.
- Personal protective equipment during tissue collection should include heavy rubber gloves, laboratory gown, and waterproof apron, boots, surgical masks, protective sleeves, and a face shield.
- Most testing is done at state diagnostic laboratories.
- Half the brain should be submitted in formalin to assess for other diseases if rabies testing is negative.
- Brain tissue is the only suitable specimen; other tissues such as whiskers or peripheral nerve are not.
- There are no reliable antemortem tests for rabies virus in animals.
- Dogs and cats that have an implanted microchip, are currently vaccinated for rabies, and have a suitable titer certified by the FVNA Laboratory at Kansas State University or the Veterinary Command Food and Diagnostic Laboratory, Fort Sam Houston, Texas, may avoid quarantine when traveling from the continental United States to Hawaii or the United Kingdom if they meet other criteria. For more details regarding pet travel, refer to https://www.aphis.usda.gov/aphis/pet-travel/.

AUTHOR: Sharon M. Dial, DVM, PhD, DACVP
EDITOR: Lois Roth-Johnson, DVM, PhD, DACVP

Relaxin

Definition

Peptide hormone produced by the reproductive tract of many species during pregnancy

Physiology

Relaxin may be produced by the corpus luteum (CL), placenta, or uterus, depending on species and stage of reproductive cycle. In pregnant dogs, relaxin is initially produced by the CL, followed by the placenta. It is produced by the placenta in cats. The primary effects of relaxin occur during implantation and later during parturition. Relaxin promotes uterine, cervical, and vaginal growth during pregnancy. It may also play an important role in mammary development in some species. Additionally, relaxin is involved in nonreproductive processes such as fibrosis, wound healing, and protection against myocardial ischemia.

Reference Interval

- Reported as positive or negative
- Dogs (pregnant): may be positive as early as 14 days postmating; consistently positive 25 days postmating
- Cats (pregnant): may be positive as early as 25 days postmating; consistently positive 31 days postmating

Causes of Abnormally High Levels

- Pregnancy
- High concentration may persist following abortion.
- Ovarian cysts in nonpregnant animals

Next Diagnostic Steps to Consider if Levels Are High

Evaluate for pregnancy (e.g., ultrasound).

Lab Artifacts

Hemolysis, lipemia may cause false-negative results.

Specimen Collection and Handling

Plasma or serum, 1 mL. Collect blood in EDTA (lavender top tube), citrate (blue top tube), or heparin (green top tube) or serum (red top tube). Spin down, collect plasma or serum, and transfer to a clean tube without additives and label plasma or serum. Store at 2°C-8°C up to 48 hours; freeze for longer storage. Do not use whole blood, hemolyzed or lipemic samples.

Relative Cost: $$$

Pearls

Relaxin is the only protein found to be associated specifically with pregnancy in dogs and cats. It is also useful for ruling out pseudocyesis/pseudopregnancy (nondetectable in pseudopregnant patients).

AUTHOR & EDITOR: Lois Roth-Johnson, DVM, PhD, DACVP

Reticulocytes

Definition

Erythroid precursors that have expelled their nuclei and have larger volume, more ribosomes and RNA, and less hemoglobin than mature erythrocytes (that is, immature erythrocytes). Name derived from reticulum that forms after RNA is precipitated by supravital dyes (e.g., new methylene blue). See p. 1327.

Synonym

Polychromatophilic erythrocyte

Physiology

With increased erythropoietin and proliferation of erythroid precursors, increased numbers of reticulocytes are released into blood. In cats, two forms of maturating reticulocytes are identified with supravital stains (e.g., new methylene blue). *Aggregate* reticulocytes have increased RNA that forms a prominent reticulum; these correspond to polychromatophilic erythrocytes on Romanowsky-stained smears and reticulocytes detected by hematology analyzers. *Punctate* reticulocytes have less RNA that forms pinpoint inclusions and are not apparent on Romanowsky-stained smears or included in automated reticulocyte counts. This distinction has limited clinical significance since manual reticulocyte counts are performed infrequently in cats.

Reference Interval

- Dogs: (nonanemic): < 80-95 × 10^3 reticulocytes/mcL (or × 10^9/L)
- Cats: (nonanemic): < 60 × 10^3 reticulocytes/mcL (or × 10^9/L)

Causes of Abnormally High Levels

Regenerative anemias from blood loss or hemolysis (p. 1307) are the most common cause of reticulocytosis. Increased reticulocytes in the absence of anemia could suggest compensatory response for low-grade hypoxia or hemolysis. However, reticulocytosis without anemia is increasingly linked to drug therapy (e.g., glucocorticoids, NSAIDs) or dietary supplements (e.g., glucosamine, omega-3 fatty acids) that stimulate erythropoiesis.

Next Diagnostic Steps to Consider if Levels Are High

Determine specific cause of blood loss or hemolysis if the patient is anemic. Reticulocytosis without anemia may reflect an incidental finding (see above).

Causes of Abnormally Low Levels

Nonregenerative anemias (p. 1306) or recent onset of anemia (≈3-7 days is required for regenerative response)

Next Diagnostic Steps to Consider if Levels Are Low

See p. 63. Bone marrow aspirate or core biopsy often useful for nonregenerative anemia.

Important Interspecies Differences

Dogs mount a higher reticulocyte response than cats during regenerative anemias. Cats demonstrate different types of reticulocytes (see Physiology).

Lab Artifacts

Autoagglutination may decrease the number of detectable reticulocytes. Presence of intraerythrocytic inclusions (e.g., basophilic stippling, siderotic or Pappenheimer bodies, Heinz bodies, leukemic cell fragments, *Babesia* spp inclusions) or large or clumped platelets could falsely increase the reticulocyte concentration.

Specimen Collection and Handling

EDTA whole blood (lavender top tube) for flow cytometric counting by analyzers (preferred) or manual counting of supravital stained smears

Relative Cost: $ (reflex reticulocyte counts in anemic animals part of some CBC profiles)

Pearls

- An increase in absolute concentration (rather than percentage) of reticulocytes is the gold standard for determining whether anemia is regenerative or nonregenerative.
- Because the absolute number of reticulocytes is preferred over reticulocyte percentage, correction equations for anemic animals are no longer in widespread use. Reticulocyte count may not be included in routine CBC; request count when CBC performed on anemic patients.
- Following acute blood loss or hemolysis, increased numbers of reticulocytes are not expected to occur in peripheral blood until at least 3 days afterward.

AUTHOR: Stephen D. Gaunt, DVM, PhD, DACVP
EDITOR: Lois Roth-Johnson, DVM, PhD, DACVP

Rheumatoid Factor (RF)

Definition

Autoantibodies to the Fc portion of autologous immunoglobulin (Ig)G

Physiology

Immunoglobulins (predominantly IgM) form complexes with RF in peripheral circulation, synovial fluid, and synovial tissues. Ongoing inflammation results in destruction of articular cartilage.

Reference Interval

Reported as negative or positive; positive results are associated with titers, and interpretation is specific for each reference laboratory.

Causes of Abnormally High Levels

- Rheumatoid arthritis. False-positive results are common and occur in animals with (non-autoimmune) polyarthritis, heartworm disease, pyometra, leishmaniasis, and systemic lupus erythematosus (SLE).

- Other disorders causing antigenic stimulation cause false-positive: osteoarthritis, fibrositis, polyarteritis nodosa.

Next Diagnostic Steps to Consider if Levels Are High

Synovial fluid analysis +/- synovial biopsy; serologic testing for infectious diseases (rickettsial, borreliosis, fungal, parasitic [heartworm] disease); radiograph affected joint(s)

Important Interspecies Differences

Rarely evaluated in cats. Low positive titers associated with retrovirus infection and SLE

Lab Artifacts

- Freezing specimen destroys RF activity
- Avoid hemolysis and lipemia

Specimen Collection and Handling

Serum (red top tube); do not freeze

Relative Cost: $$

Pearls

Unreliable. Neither sensitive nor specific for diagnostic use. Dogs with rheumatoid-like arthritis tend to have naturally low RF levels and detectable serum RF is present in only about 25% of affected dogs.

AUTHOR: Carrie L. Flint, DVM, DACVP
EDITOR: Lois Roth-Johnson, DVM, PhD, DACVP

Rocky Mountain Spotted Fever Serologic Tests

Definition

Rocky Mountain spotted fever (RMSF) is a tick-borne acute systemic disease caused by *Rickettsia rickettsii*. It is characterized by fever, anorexia, thrombocytopenia, joint effusion, uveitis, neurological signs, and vasculitis in dogs (p. 891).

Physiology

R. rickettsii is inoculated via a tick bite, enters the circulatory system, and replicates within vascular endothelial cells, where it induces vasculitis. This leads to vascular permeability, microvascular hemorrhage, thrombocytopenia, edema, and ultimately multiple organ damage.

Reference Interval

IFA: refer to testing laboratory. PCR/RT-PCR: negative or positive result

Causes of Abnormally High Levels

A positive titer indicates exposure to either *R. rickettsii* or avirulent rickettsiae that cross-react. In the presence of characteristic acute clinical signs, a very high single immunoglobulin (Ig) G titer (≥ 1 : 1024), a fourfold increase in paired IgG titers (2-4 weeks apart), or a positive IgM titer supports active infection. A positive titer without signs of acute vasculitis is likely due to exposure to cross-reactive rickettsiae.

Next Diagnostic Steps to Consider if Levels Are High

PCR/RT-PCR (whole blood, tissue, or CSF), direct FA staining of infected tissues, and tissue culture are available but are not necessary if clinical signs are compatible with RMSF and the titer(s) is/are positive.

Causes of Abnormally Low Levels

A negative titer indicates either early/acute infection or lack of exposure. Negative PCR/RT-PCR due to lack of infection, nucleic acid below limit of detection, antibiotic treatment, or new strain variations; because rickettsiae do not infect blood cells, false-negative PCR can occur on blood samples.

Next Diagnostic Steps to Consider if Levels Are Low

If clinical signs of RMSF are present and initial titer is negative, submit a convalescent titer in 2-4 weeks. Treatment should not be delayed while awaiting confirmation.

Drug Effects

Effective antibiotic treatment may blunt serologic titers but seldom hinder serologic diagnosis. Even a single dose of effective antibiotic before sample collection can cause false-negative PCR/RT-PCR result.

Specimen Collection and Handling

IFA: 2 mL serum; stable for 5 days at 2°C-8°C or 0°C for several weeks; paired/sequential serum samples may be submitted to the same laboratory for testing at the same time. PCR/RT-PCR: 2 mL whole blood or 0.5 mL CSF (lavender top tube); stable 10 days at 2°C-8°C; fresh tissue 24 hours at 2°C-8°C or frozen.

Relative Cost: $$ (IFA, PCR/RT-PCR)

Pearls

- Because of the rapid progression of clinical RMSF, treatment is initiated based on clinical suspicion. The turnaround time of RMSF serology and the frequent need for convalescent titers mean that confirmatory diagnosis is often retrospective.
- Serology is generally preferred over PCR.
- Positive serology in a dog with chronic disease is likely not meaningful.

AUTHOR: Patty J. Ewing, DVM, MS, DACVP
EDITOR: Lois Roth-Johnson, DVM, PhD, DACVP

Schistocytes

Definition

Erythrocyte fragments that are considered to be the hallmark of microangiopathic hemolysis

Synonym

Schizocytes

Physiology

Schistocytes result from shredding of erythrocytes as they pass through microvasculature containing fibrin thrombi or altered endothelium. Any traumatic or physical injury to erythrocytes can cause schistocyte formation. See p. 1327.

Causes of Abnormally High Levels

Disseminated intravascular coagulation (DIC), vasculitis, hemangiosarcoma, dirofilariasis, intravenous catheters, burns, endocarditis, myelofibrosis, glomerulonephritis, and severe iron-deficiency anemia (increased erythrocyte fragility causes fragmentation)

Next Diagnostic Steps to Consider if Levels are High

Evaluate clinical history and physical exam as well as coagulation profile; consider imaging studies and infectious disease testing (e.g., heartworm, tick-borne disease).

Important Interspecies Differences

Schistocytes uncommon in cats with DIC, possibly because their smaller erythrocytes are less likely to be damaged by fibrin in vascular spaces.

Specimen Collection and Handling

EDTA whole blood (lavender top tube) for CBC and fresh blood smear for morphologic evaluation

Relative Cost: $$ (reported as part of CBC)

Pearls

- Even small numbers of schistocytes are clinically significant, indicating underlying microangiopathy; unlikely to be induced artifactually by smear preparation technique.
- Absence of schistocytes does not rule out DIC (correlate with coagulation profile).
- A CBC report of *poikilocytosis* (a broad term that refers to the presence of any circulating, abnormally shaped RBCs) warrants pathologist review of blood smear to define the shape change and identify any schistocytes.
- Submission of blood smear prepared at time of sample collection will minimize artifacts of morphology due to specimen age.

AUTHOR: Fidelia R. Fernandez, DVM, MS, DACVP
EDITOR: Lois Roth-Johnson, DVM, PhD, DACVP

SDMA

Definition

A biomarker that aids in the early detection of renal disease in dogs and cats

Synonym

Symmetric dimethylarginine

Physiology

SDMA is a variant of the amino acid arginine that is produced at a constant rate by all nucleated cells and is excreted primarily by the kidneys. The molecule is a specific marker for renal function as it is freely filtered by the glomerulus, is not reabsorbed by the renal tubules, and correlates well with the glomerular filtration rate. SDMA is more sensitive than creatinine in early detection of chronic kidney disease. An increase in SDMA occurs with ≈40% loss of renal function (versus ≈75% for creatinine). Additionally, unlike creatinine, SDMA is not influenced by muscle mass. This latter attribute provides a major advantage compared to creatinine, which is dependent on muscle mass and is often within reference interval in poorly muscled/cachectic patients with chronic kidney disease. SDMA is currently offered only by IDEXX Laboratories, as an individual test and as part of routine biochemistry panels, and has been added to the International Renal Interest Society (IRIS) staging guidelines for chronic renal disease.

Reference Interval

Healthy dogs and cats: ≤ 14 mcg/dL

Causes of Abnormally High Levels

Renal disease (values > 20 mcg/dL are essentially diagnostic for renal disease)

Next Diagnostic Steps to Consider if Levels are High

Assess for renal disease and underlying cause via urinalysis, serum biochemistry panel, urine protein/creatinine ratio, and/or abdominal imaging. See pp. 167 and 169.

Important Interspecies Differences

Healthy puppies, kittens, and greyhounds may have slightly increased values.

Specimen Collection and Handling

Serum (preferred) or heparinized plasma. Stable at room temperature for 4 days, longer (14 days) if refrigerated

Relative Cost: $$ (test performed by IDEXX Laboratories)

AUTHOR: Shannon D. Dehghanpir, DVM, MS, DACVP
EDITOR: Lois Roth-Johnson, DVM, PhD, DACVP

Semen Analysis

Definition

Assessment of male ejaculate for volume, sperm quantity and morphology, percent of live sperm, presence of other cells, bacteria, and, occasionally, alkaline phosphatase. Used primarily as part of assessment of male fertility. Also used to assess prostatic disease in intact male dogs.

Physiology

Ejaculate is divided into three fractions. First and third fractions are mostly prostatic secretion; the second sperm-rich fraction should be used for evaluation.

Reference Interval

Normal total sperm count is roughly 10 million per 1 pound of body weight, where total number = concentration × volume collected. Motility, which is often considered an indicator of viability, should be ≥ 80%; motility patterns are random. Sperm should have single heads of uniform shape and size; free heads should be rare; tails are normally straight to slightly curved. Abnormal sperm have hooked, kinked, or multiple tails and should be less than 20% of the population. It is common to see a few urethral, prostatic, or squamous epithelial cells; low numbers of bacteria are also common. Alkaline phosphatase > 10,000 U/L.

Causes of Abnormally Low Levels

Decreased numbers of normal viable sperm suggest testicular injury, neoplasia, or atrophy. Decreased concentration of seminal alkaline phosphatase indicates obstruction of genital tubular structures.

Next Diagnostic Steps to Consider if Levels are Low

Examination of testicle and epididymis on physical examination and using ultrasound; measurement of resting plasma testosterone

Lab Artifacts

Aged sample or exposure to temperature extremes invalidates physical and biochemical analysis.

Specimen Collection and Handling

Motility must be evaluated immediately and cannot be assessed in specimens transported to a reference laboratory. Physical analysis (color, morphology, sperm count): 1 mL semen from sperm-rich fraction in sterile container. Include volume of sperm-rich fraction collected. Alkaline phosphatase: 1 mL semen in sterile container. Store at room temperature. Specimens < 2 hours old are considered best. Maximum collection to examination interval is 72 hours.

Relative Cost: $$ (physical analysis); $ (alkaline phosphatase)

Pearls

- History is an important aspect of fertility assessment; relying on a single test invites error.
- Semen alkaline phosphatase concentration is significantly greater than serum concentration and may exceed the sensitivity of many in-clinic instruments.

AUTHOR & EDITOR: Lois Roth-Johnson, DVM, PhD, DACVP

SNAP Tests

Definition

Point-of-care testing based on ELISA technology designed for a wide variety of common small animal infections and biomarkers.

Physiology

Proprietary (IDEXX Laboratories, Inc., Westbrook, Maine) test kits contain conjugate solution, tube for sample-conjugate incubation, and a SNAP® device. Depending on the test type, feces, serum, plasma, and whole blood are incubated with the conjugate solution and then poured into the test well of the SNAP device. The conjugate-sample solution diffuses across the test window until it reaches an "activation circle" and is then depressed or "snapped" to release the wash solution and substrate in reverse flow across the same testing window. A color change spot, generally blue, within the testing window will appear and is compared to the product insert for interpretation.

Reference Interval

Varies depending on the specific test. Results may be positive or negative. For some tests, the degree or darkness of the color change observed may correlate to a semiquantitative value.

Next Diagnostic Steps to Consider if Levels are High

SNAP® tests are often used as screening tools for various diseases. Depending on the clinical presentation, confirmatory testing, such as PCR, culture and sensitivity, and advanced imaging, may be necessary for confirmation of diagnosis.

Lab Artifacts

These test kits are susceptible to improper storage and shipping. Mishandling of reagents and/ or kits may result in false-positives or false-negatives, depending on the test. Improper mixing of conjugate with patient sample may result in false-positive or false-negative test results.

Specimen Collection and Handling

Anticoagulated whole blood (lavender or green top tube), serum (red top tube; separated), plasma (lavender or green top tube), or feces, depending on tests. Follow manufacturer's instructions.

Relative Cost: Packs that include multiple test kits: $$$-$$$$; kits for individual tests when purchased in bulk: $

Pearls

- SNAP® tests are in-clinic screening tests. Tests may also be run at reference laboratories, but the advantage of obtaining a rapid response is lost.
- Common SNAP tests include metabolic/ biomarker (fPL, cPL, feline and canine proBNP, canine and feline total T_4, canine cortisol, and canine and feline bile acids), vector borne (*Anaplasma* spp, *Ehrlichia* spp, heartworm [canine and feline], Lyme) infections, diarrheal (giardiasis, canine parvovirus), leptospirosis, and retroviral diseases (feline leukemia and feline immunodeficiency virus).
- The term *SNAP* is specific to the tests and testing devices made by IDEXX Laboratories, Inc., but the term is sometimes used colloquially for any point-of-care diagnostic test.

AUTHOR: Erin N. Burton, DVM, MS, DACVP
EDITOR: Lois Roth-Johnson, DVM, PhD, DACVP

Sodium

Definition

Major extracellular fluid (ECF) cation. Serum [Na^+] essentially equals ECF [Na^+]. Serum [Na^+] is relative to hydration status and ECF volume but does not indicate total body Na^+ content.

Synonyms

Na, Na^+

Physiology

Serum [Na^+] is net balance of oral intake, excretion, and water shifts between ECF and ICF (intracellular fluid). Na^+ and water are lost via kidneys, intestine, skin, and respiratory tract. Serum [Na^+] depends on circulating blood volume and plasma osmolality. With hypovolemia, aldosterone promotes renal Na^+ resorption and antidiuretic hormone (ADH, vasopressin) promotes renal water resorption. Hypo-osmolality causes decreased water intake, increased renal water excretion. Hypervolemia reduces Na^+ resorption. Hyperosmolality promotes water intake, ADH-mediated renal water resorption. Osmotic water shifting from ICF to ECF dilutes serum [Na^+].

Reference Interval

Dogs: 144-152 mEq/L. Cats: 150-160 mEq/L. Unit conversion: 1 mEq/L = 1 mmol/L.

Causes of Abnormally High Levels

- Water deficit (most common)
  - Loss of hypotonic fluid: via respiratory (fever, panting), gastrointestinal (vomiting, diarrhea), or renal system (any cause of polyuria, including osmotic diuresis, renal disease, central/nephrogenic diabetes insipidus) or uncommonly with cutaneous (severe burns), third space loss (pancreatitis, peritonitis), or toxicosis (paintball ingestion, phosphate enema)
  - Decreased intake: neurologic disease causing decreased thirst response (primary adipsia/hypodipsia), lack of access to water

- Sodium gain: excess ingestion (e.g., seawater, beef jerky, salt-flour dough mixtures), hypertonic fluid or sodium bicarbonate administration, hyperaldosteronism
- See p. 1237.

Next Diagnostic Steps to Consider if Levels are High

Evaluate hydration status; evaluate for listed diseases.

Causes of Abnormally Low Levels

- With high measured osmolality: hyperglycemia, mannitol administration
- With normal measured osmolality: artifactual (hyperlipidemia, hyperglobulinemia)
- With low measured osmolality:
  - Hypovolemia: vomiting, diarrhea, peritonitis, pleural effusion, uroabdomen, hypoadrenocorticism, prolonged diuretic administration, ketonuria, Na^+-wasting nephropathy
  - Hypervolemia: heart failure, severe hepatopathy, nephrotic syndrome, advanced kidney disease (oliguric/anuric)
  - Normovolemia: hypotonic fluid therapy, psychogenic polydipsia, syndrome of inappropriate antidiuretic hormone secretion (SIADH; rare)
- Intracellular shifting: Na^+ may shift intracellularly when severe tissue damage (e.g., rhabdomyolysis) or hypokalemia is present
- See p. 1241.

Next Diagnostic Steps to Consider if Levels are Low

Evaluate hydration status; evaluate for listed diseases; measure plasma osmolality.

Drug Effects

- Increase: osmotic diuretics, furosemide, phosphate enema, corticosteroids
- Decrease: chronic diuretic use

Lab Artifacts

- Marked hyperlipidemia or hyperglobulinemia may decrease measured Na^+ by electrolyte exclusion effect (if using indirect potentiometry).
- Marked hemolysis: may interfere; effect is method dependent
- Sample handling: Na^+ increases if free water loss from improperly stoppered tube

Specimen Collection and Handling

Serum (red top tube) preferred. Heparinized plasma may be used (lithium or ammonium heparin, green top tube).

Relative Cost: Individual test, electrolyte panel, or other partial panels: $; included in full chemistry panel: $$

Pearls

- Sampling from an improperly cleared intravenous catheter commonly causes inaccurate values.
- Most reference laboratory methods are subject to electrolyte exclusion effect artifacts. Portable point-of-care analyzer methods usually not affected.
- Hypovolemia causing both hypo- and hypernatremia may seem paradoxical. Loss of hypotonic fluid may initially result in volume depletion and a relative hypernatremia. Subsequent water intake and renal water conservation may effectively dilute serum [Na^+].
- Chronic hypo- or hypernatremia must be corrected slowly to prevent brain injury.

AUTHOR: Mary Leissinger, DVM, MS, DACVP
EDITOR: Lois Roth-Johnson, DVM, PhD, DACVP

Spherocytes

Definition

Small, dense-staining erythrocytes with no central pallor, considered the hallmark of immune-mediated hemolytic anemia (IMHA) or a normal finding after blood transfusion (p. 1327)

Physiology

Partial phagocytosis of antibody-coated erythrocytes by macrophages causes loss of surface membrane without loss of volume, resulting in spherocyte formation. Pitting (excision) of Heinz bodies in the spleen also leads to spherocyte formation. May also be seen in cases of canine babesiosis and hemotropic mycoplasmosis in cats and dogs.

Causes of Abnormally High Levels

Immune-mediated hemolysis, viper and bee sting envenomation, hemoparasitism, zinc toxicosis, neoplasia, or idiopathic; normal phenomenon beginning 2-3 days after transfusion of erythrocytes (even if properly cross-matched)

Next Diagnostic Steps to Consider if Levels are High

Evaluate history for causes of anemia; slide autoagglutination test +/- Coombs' test if IMHA suspected

Important Interspecies Differences

Spherocytes are easily detected in dogs because of normally prominent central pallor; difficult to identify in cats, which normally have no central pallor in their erythrocytes. Some breeds of dogs (shiba inu and Akita) normally have microcytic erythrocytes that should not be confused with spherocytes.

Specimen Collection and Handling

EDTA whole blood (lavender top tube) for evaluation of gross agglutination and CBC, fresh blood smear for morphologic evaluation

Relative Cost: $$ (reported as part of CBC)

Pearls

- Microcytic erythrocytes of severe iron-deficiency anemia differ from spherocytes in that they are hypochromic and truly microcytic (mean corpuscular volume is decreased); spherocytes have normal red cell volume and appear hyperchromic.
- In anemic patients, a CBC and/or fresh blood smears to screen for spherocytosis (suggesting IMHA) should always be obtained before transfusion. Spherocytosis after transfusion does not discriminate between IMHA and normal post-transfusion phenomenon.
- Spherocytic anemia or IMHA may not always be accompanied by a positive Coombs' test (false-negative result in some cases).
- Lack of spherocytes does not rule out IMHA.
- Submission of fresh direct blood smear at time of blood collection is recommended to minimize artifacts of morphology due to sample aging.

AUTHOR: Fidelia R. Fernandez, DVM, MS, DACVP
EDITOR: Lois Roth-Johnson, DVM, PhD, DACVP

Synovial Fluid Analysis

Definition

Gross, physicochemical, and microscopic assessment of a sample of joint fluid

Physiology

Analysis includes assessment of viscosity, mucin clot test, cell counts, protein concentration, and cytologic evaluation. Microscopic examination assesses cell population distribution and may detect infectious agents.

Reference Interval

Normal synovial fluid is colorless to pale yellow, viscous, has high mucin (hyaluronic acid) content, and does not clot. Erythrocytes are absent. Nucleated cell counts vary among species and the joint sampled but are usually 500/mcL (up to 3000 cells/mcL occasionally reported in normal joints). Synoviocytes and macrophages predominate. Protein concentration ranges from 1.8-4.8 g/dL (18-48 mg/mL) by refractometer.

Causes of Abnormally High Levels

- Increased erythrocyte count indicates iatrogenic blood contamination or hemarthrosis.
- Increased nucleated cell count occurs with degenerative and inflammatory arthropathies, and may occur with neoplasia.
    - Mononuclear cells predominate in degenerative arthropathy or joint instability. Causes include trauma, osteoarthrosis, osteochondritis dissecans, and aseptic necrosis of the femoral head.
    - Neutrophils predominate in inflammatory arthropathies (infectious, noninfectious such as crystal induced, immune mediated). Bacterial infection is usually monoarticular due to penetrating trauma. Polyarticular infection may be due to systemic bacterial infection, tick-borne disease, fungal infection, viral infection, and (rarely) mycoplasmal infection. Noninfectious inflammatory arthropathies typically are polyarticular (immune-mediated diseases; chronic progressive polyarthritis in cats).

Next Diagnostic Steps to Consider if Levels are High

- Hemorrhage: distinguish iatrogenic versus pathologic. Erythrophagocytosis suggests hemarthrosis. If hemarthrosis, evaluate for trauma versus bleeding disorder.
- Degenerative arthropathy: joint radiographs, assess for joint instability/ligament tear.
- Inflammatory arthropathy: serologic tests and/or PCR (e.g., *Borrelia* spp, *Ehrlichia* spp, *Anaplasma* spp); culture synovial fluid (especially if monoarticular); if other disease signs present, assess for systemic disease (e.g., serum antinuclear antibody test if proteinuria, other signs of systemic lupus erythematosus; p. 955); joint radiographs to assess for erosive lesions

Next Diagnostic Steps to Consider if Levels are Low

Occasionally patients with degenerative joint disease or joint instability do not have abnormalities detected in cytologic preparations. For polyarthropathy, multiple joints should be sampled simultaneously to improve test sensitivity.

Specimen Collection and Handling

Fluid in EDTA (lavender top tube) for cell counts, cytologic evaluation; red top tube (culture); refrigerate

Relative Cost: $$ (Most laboratories apply lower prices for specimens from multiple joints submitted at the same time.)

Pearls

Some samples are very viscous, and the addition of a drop of crystalline hyaluronidase allows for a more accurate assessment of cell counts. Addition of hyaluronidase should be done at the reference laboratory after viscosity and protein concentration are measured and after the mucin clot test is done and slides for cytologic evaluation are prepared.

AUTHOR: Ruanna E. Gossett, DVM, PhD, DACVP
EDITOR: Lois Roth-Johnson, DVM, PhD, DACVP

Taurine Blood Levels

Definition

Amino acid having an important role in myocardial and retinal metabolism

Physiology

Low blood levels of taurine have been associated with dilated cardiomyopathy in cats and some dog breeds (cocker spaniels, retrievers, and some giant dog breeds such as Newfoundlands). Determination of plasma and/or whole blood levels of taurine may be useful in patients with dilated cardiomyopathy that might benefit from supplementation. Taurine-deficient cats (but not dogs) may develop degenerative retinal lesions.

Reference Interval

- Plasma, cats and dogs: 60-120 nmol/mL (critical level is <40)
- Whole blood, cat: 300-600 nmol/mL (critical level is <200)
- Whole blood, dog: 200-350 nmol/mL (critical level is <150)

Causes of Abnormally Low Levels

Dietary deficiency, poor bioavailability, excessive loss of metabolic precursors (cysteine), malabsorptive intestinal disease and/or familial predisposition

Next Diagnostic Steps to Consider if Levels are Low

Provide taurine supplementation, evaluate diet, consider potential causes of deficiency, monitor, address heart disease if needed.

Drug Effects

Fasting may decrease plasma but not whole blood levels of taurine; therefore, whole blood is preferred.

Lab Artifacts

Decreased

Specimen Collection and Handling

- Whole blood: 1 mL heparinized whole blood (green top tube). Do not spin or separate; refrigerate sample.
- Plasma: 1 mL frozen heparinized plasma. Spin, separate plasma immediately without disturbing buffy coat and transfer plasma to plastic tube. Freeze immediately.

Relative Cost: $$$$

Pearls

Dogs can develop taurine-deficient dilated cardiomyopathy even on taurine replete diet; poor bioavailability (e.g., binding by rice husks, intestinal malabsorption) and excess urinary excretion of taurine precursors (e.g., cysteine) proposed as mechanisms.

Low taurine levels are not used as a screening test for cardiomyopathy.

Breed differences may exist for taurine levels. Example: Cocker spaniels with dilated cardiomyopathy may not have blood taurine levels below the reference interval, yet still may benefit from taurine supplementation.

AUTHOR & EDITOR: Lois Roth-Johnson, DVM, PhD, DACVP

Testosterone

Definition

Testosterone is an anabolic steroid hormone derived from cholesterol. Most often measured to differentiate castrated males from cryptorchid males, but is also included on adrenal sex hormone panels

Physiology

- Testosterone is an androgen and accordingly has key roles in male gonadal development and fertility. Testicular Leydig/interstitial cells in intact males produce the majority of testosterone, so castrated males and females are expected to have very low testosterone concentrations.
- Aberrations in steroidal hormone enzymes can occur in adrenal cortical neoplasms, potentially leading to increased adrenal testosterone production.

Reference Interval

Varies by laboratory. One example states that intact male dogs and cats should have testosterone concentrations of > 0.1 ng/mL, whereas castrated males and females should have concentrations < 0.01 ng/mL. Basal testosterone concentration can fluctuate in normal intact males, and accordingly, sometimes a baseline sample is collected and compared with a second sample following administration of human chorionic gonadotropin (hCG) or gonadotropin releasing hormone (GnRH); either should increase testosterone concentration.

Causes of Abnormally High Levels

In a male patient who is thought to be castrated, increased testosterone concentration suggests the presence of remaining Leydig/interstitial cells (cryptorchid or remnant testicular tissue). Slightly increased concentration may require additional testing for clarification (hCG stimulation testing, measurement of antimullerian hormone).

Next Diagnostic Steps to Consider if Levels are High

Abdominal imaging to locate cryptorchid testicle(s).

Causes of Abnormally Low Levels

Low concentration is expected in castrated males and females. In an intact male, decreased testosterone concentration may indicate a primary infertility disorder or could be seen with the presence of a Sertoli cell tumor.

Next Diagnostic Steps to Consider if Levels are Low

In intact male, consider assessment of other sex hormones and evaluation of the patient for the presence of a Sertoli cell tumor.

Drug Effects

Administration of testosterone compounds will increase results.

Lab Artifacts

Serum separator tubes may interfere with results; use plain red top tubes for blood collection.

Specimen Collection and Handling

Collect blood in a red top tube, and harvest serum. Submit serum on ice, ideally overnight.

Relative Cost: $$

AUTHOR: Angela Royal, MS, DVM, DACVP
EDITOR: Lois Roth-Johnson, DVM, PhD, DACVP

Thyroglobulin Antibody (TgAA)

Definition

Autoantibodies directed at thyroglobulin, associated with canine autoimmune thyroiditis. TgAA is generally included as part of a thyroid testing panel rather than measured as a stand-alone test.

Physiology

Lymphocytes involved in autoimmune thyroiditis can produce antibodies directed at a variety of epitopes along thyroglobulin molecules. Collectively these antibodies are termed TgAA. The presence of circulating TgAA indicates autoimmune thyroiditis is present, but does not alone predict whether the patient has hypothyroidism. In some cases, detectable TgAA may be found with normal thyroid hormone and TSH concentrations. A subset of these patients will proceed to clinical hypothyroidism. OFA Thyroid Registry certification requires normal TgAA results (along with fT_4 and TSH results) as autoimmune thyroiditis is a heritable condition.

Reference Interval

Will be provided by your laboratory. Example: 0%-35%, with results interpreted as negative, positive, or inconclusive.

Causes of Abnormally High Levels

Increased TgAA results indicate the presence of autoimmune thyroiditis, or rarely may be associated with thyroid neoplasia.

Next Diagnostic Steps to Consider if Levels are High

TgAA is generally included as part of a thyroid testing panel. Increased TgAA should be interpreted in light of the other tests on the panel to determine whether the patient is truly hypothyroid. Patients with high TgAA but normal thyroid hormone status should be rechecked in the future for the potential emergence of hypothyroidism.

Next Diagnostic Steps to Consider if Levels are Low

TgAA will remain within normal limits in some hypothyroid dogs. The remainder of the panel results should be used to decide whether hypothyroidism is still likely for the patient. Low TgAA also does not entirely rule out the possibility of autoimmune thyroiditis.

Important Interspecies Differences

Measured in dogs only

Lab Artifacts

Nonspecific binding of immunoglobulins can falsely increase TgAA results; however, nonspecific binding can be quantified and TgAA results adjusted accordingly to negate this interference.

Specimen Collection and Handling

Collect blood into a plain red top tube or serum separator tube, allow to clot, centrifuge, and remove serum. Freeze serum (or keep refrigerated if shipping the day of collection) and submit serum alone, on ice, overnight. In general, gross hemolysis or lipemia should be avoided.

Relative Cost: $$

Pearls

- Increased TgAA is a common finding in hypothyroid dogs and indicates autoimmune thyroiditis is present.
- Not all dogs with hypothyroidism will have increased TgAA.
- Increased TgAA can be seen in patients without hypothyroidism.

- Increased TgAA increases suspicion of hypothyroidism, but is not confirmatory for diagnosis.
- Patients with increased TgAA but normal thyroid hormone status may proceed to clinical hypothyroidism in the future, but some do not.

AUTHOR: Angela Royal, MS, DVM, DACVP
EDITOR: Lois Roth-Johnson, DVM, PhD, DACVP

Thyroid-Stimulating Hormone (TSH)

Definition

Pituitary-derived hormone that acts on the thyroid gland, causing production and secretion of thyroid hormones

Synonyms

Thyrotropin, TSH

Physiology

Thyroid-stimulating hormone (TSH) is released from the pituitary after stimulation by thyrotropin-releasing hormone (TRH). TSH acts on the thyroid to stimulate synthesis and secretion of thyroxine (T_4) and triiodothyronine (T_3). In turn, T_3 and T_4 provide negative feedback to reduce TSH and TRH secretion.

Reference Interval

Dogs: 0-0.5 ng/mL

Causes of Abnormally High Levels

Hypothyroidism (primary); mild increases with some nonthyroidal illnesses or drugs

Next Diagnostic Steps to Consider if Levels are High

Generally measured with total T_4; consider free T_4 (by equilibrium dialysis). See p. 525.

Causes of Abnormally Low Levels

Test sensitivity is insufficient to differentiate normal from low concentrations.

Important Interspecies Differences

Species-specific immunoassay. No specific feline TSH assay is available, but the canine assay detects increased levels (due to cross-reactivity) in cats.

Drug Effects

Mild increases may be seen with corticosteroids, phenobarbital, and potentially other drugs.

Specimen Collection and Handling

Serum (red top tube), 1 mL. To avoid interference by fibrin, allow full clot formation before centrifugation and removal of serum. Store refrigerated up to 7 days.

Relative Cost: $$

Pearls

- 75% of hypothyroid dogs have increased TSH. High TSH and concurrently low T_4 or free T_4 are diagnostic for hypothyroidism. However, hypothyroidism is not ruled out if TSH is within the reference interval.
- Although not well standardized, an expected decrease in TSH levels can be used along with T_4 levels to monitor thyroid replacement therapy in canine hypothyroidism.
- Using the canine TSH assay for cats can be helpful to detect high concentrations in iatrogenic hypothyroid states.

AUTHOR: Shelley Burton, DVM, MSc, DACVP
EDITOR: Lois Roth-Johnson, DVM, PhD, DACVP

Thyroxine (Total T_4), Free Thyroxine by Equilibrium Dialysis

Definition

Total thyroxine (T_4, TT_4) is the major storage form of thyroid hormone. Free T_4 (fT_4) is the biologically available non–protein-bound form.

Synonym

T_4, tetraiodothyronine

Physiology

Thyroxine is highly protein bound in circulation and not biologically active. In cells, thyroxine is deiodinated to the active form of the hormone (T_3), which increases metabolic rate.

Reference Interval

- Approximate; check specific laboratory reference interval. Common unit (mcg/dL) × 12.87 = SI unit (nmol/L)
  - Dogs: T_4: 1.2-3.9 mcg/dL (15-50 nmol/L); fT_4: 0.8-3.2 mcg/dL (10-41 pmol/L)
  - Cats: T_4: 0.8-3.5 mcg/dL (10-45 nmol/L); fT_4: 0.6-2.2 mcg/dL (8-28 pmol/L)

Causes of Abnormally High Levels

Hyperthyroidism; presence of autoantibodies to T_4; exogenous T_4, TSH, or TRH; rarely, administration of iodine-containing compounds or raw food diet

Next Diagnostic Steps to Consider if Levels are High

- If hyperthyroidism suspected: see p. 503.
- If autoantibodies suspected: measure T_4 autoantibody levels.
- Evaluate diet, supplements for iodine content.

Causes of Abnormally Low Levels

Spontaneous or iatrogenic hypothyroidism; nonthyroidal illness; drugs

Next Diagnostic Steps to Consider if Levels are Low

Measure serum TSH levels (p. 525); evaluate for nonthyroidal diseases or drug administration.

Important Interspecies Differences

- Spontaneous hypothyroidism is extremely rare in cats, so a low T_4 or fT_4 is typically due to nonthyroidal illness, drug administration, or iatrogenic hypothyroidism.
- Hyperthyroidism is uncommon in dogs. Consider thyroid neoplasia, thyroid-rich diet (such as some raw diets), or T_4 autoantibodies.

Drug Effects

Many drugs, including but not limited to glucocorticoids and phenobarbital, may decrease total T_4 concentration, with less (or no) effect on fT_4.

Lab Artifacts

- Artifactual increase of free and total T_4 if stored in glass tubes at 37°C
- Severe hyperbilirubinemia can artifactually increase T_4 in some assays.

Specimen Collection and Handling

Serum (red top tube), 1 mL. To avoid interference by fibrin, allow full clot formation before centrifugation. Remove serum and transfer to plastic tube. Store refrigerated up to 7 days. Frozen samples are stable for up to 1 month.

Relative Cost: Total T_4: $; fT_4: $$

Pearls

- T_4 and fT_4 can be markedly lower in sighthounds and older dogs; puppies up to 6 months and small breeds tend to have higher levels.
- Approximately 5% of dogs with clinical hypothyroidism have T_4 values within but at the low end of the reference interval.
- Approximately 10% of cats with clinical hyperthyroidism have T_4 values within the upper end of the reference interval due to T_4 fluctuations. Recheck T_4 if hyperthyroidsim suspected.
- Total T_4 within the reference interval supports euthyroidism in dogs, but a low T_4 is not specific for hypothyroidism, as drugs and nonthyroidal illness also decrease it.
- Free T_4 is not as likely as T_4 to be affected by nonthyroidal illness or drugs, so a very low level supports hypothyroidism.
- High T_4 is diagnostic for hyperthyroidism in cats; fT_4 is more sensitive but less specific for the diagnosis, and should be interpreted along with TT4.
- Unpredictable diurnal fluctuations in dogs can slightly decrease T_4 values.
- Ensure use of a standard or modified equilibrium dialysis fT_4 method.
- Given assay variability, use one laboratory for ongoing patient testing.

AUTHOR: Shelley Burton, DVM, MSc, DACVP
EDITOR: Lois Roth-Johnson, DVM, PhD, DACVP

Total Protein (Serum)

Definition

Serum proteins consist of albumin, antibodies, complement, enzymes, coagulation factors, and transport proteins. Albumin and globulin make up the majority of serum total proteins. Fibrinogen, factor V, and factor VIII are proteins present in plasma but not in serum, because they are utilized in clot formation.

Synonym

Total solids, TP, TS

Physiology

The proteins in serum are important for maintaining colloid osmotic pressure (primarily albumin), buffering to maintain blood pH, hemostasis, transport of molecules (hormones, drugs, calcium, bilirubin, hemoglobin, other proteins, lipids, and metal ions), acute-phase response to inflammation, and immune response. Most are synthesized in the liver or immune system.

Reference Interval

Dogs: 5.1-7.8 g/dL. Cats: 5.9-8.5 g/dL. Unit conversion: g/dL × 10 = mg/mL.

Causes of Abnormally High Levels

Increased globulin: acute and chronic inflammation or infection (rickettsial, bacterial, viral, fungal, protozoal, parasitic), immune-mediated disease, chronic hepatic disease, nephrotic syndrome, and neoplasia (myeloma, lymphoma, lymphocytic leukemia, and rarely solitary plasma cell tumors). Increased albumin occurs with dehydration and is "relative."

Next Diagnostic Steps to Consider if Levels are High

Characterize hyperproteinemia by measuring serum albumin and globulin levels; assess hydration status; perform serum protein electrophoresis if hyperglobulinemia is absolute (normal albumin level) and repeatable.

Causes of Abnormally Low Levels

Low albumin without a decrease in globulins occurs with protein-losing nephropathy and chronic hepatopathies. Both hypoalbuminemia and hypoglobulinemia occur with protein-losing enteropathy, whole blood loss (gastrointestinal, lacerations/trauma, other hemorrhage), exudative skin disease, massive burns, and effusive disease. Hypoglobulinemia with normal albumin occurs with decreased immunoglobulin concentration due to failure of passive transfer or inherited or acquired immune deficiency.

Next Diagnostic Steps to Consider if Levels are Low

Characterize hypoproteinemia by measuring serum albumin and globulin levels. As indicated clinically, evaluate for gastrointestinal, hepatic, renal (glomerular) disease.

Drug Effects

- Increased: testosterone, estrogens, growth hormone
- Decreased: thyroxine, cortisol

Lab Artifacts

Increase (globulin fraction): lipemia, hemolysis, and hyperbilirubinemia

Specimen Collection and Handling

Serum (red top tube) preferred. Heparinized plasma (green top tube) or EDTA plasma (lavender top tube). Stable for 1 month at 2°C-8°C

Relative Cost: Single test: $; included in many chemistry panels: $-$$

Pearl

Reference intervals based on serum values. If measured in plasma (heparin or EDTA) samples, values may be slightly higher.

AUTHOR: Ruanna E. Gossett, DVM, PhD, DACVP
EDITOR: Lois Roth-Johnson, DVM, PhD, DACVP

Laboratory Tests

Toxoplasma Serologic Testing

Definition

Toxoplasmosis is a protozoal disease caused by *Toxoplasma gondii*, an intracellular parasite that infects many tissues of birds and mammals, including humans (p. 984).

Physiology

Transmission to cats and dogs occurs via ingestion of tissue cysts within intermediate hosts. Most infections are latent with no clinical signs, but infection persists for life as tissue-encysted bradyzoites. Enteroepithelial phase of primary infection in the definitive host (cat) results in fecal shedding of oocytes. Immunosuppression in the dog or cat may lead to cyst rupture, multiplication of tachyzoites, and fulminant systemic clinical disease.

Reference Interval

Reported as titer values with interpretation

Causes of Abnormally High Levels

ELISA or IFA: positive IgG with negative IgM titer most consistent with chronic exposure to *T. gondii (≥ 2 weeks post-infection)*. Recent exposure or active infection typically results in positive IgM with negative IgG titer (1-2 weeks post-infection) or both positive IgM and IgG titer. Up to 20% of cats may not develop positive IgM titer during active infection. Conversely, some cats, especially those concurrently infected with feline immunodeficiency virus, may have IgM titers that persist for months to years after infection. Since infected animals harbor tissue cysts for life, a long-term measurable IgG titer is expected. Positive titer does not indicate oocyst shedding.

Next Diagnostic Steps to Consider if Levels are High

If IgG titer is positive, evaluate IgM titer or paired IgG titers (2-3 weeks apart). Greater than fourfold increase in paired IgG titers indicates recent exposure. Some infectious disease specialists recommend response to treatment (e.g., with clindamycin) as a diagnostic test in patients with compatible clinical signs and a positive IgM or rising IgG titer.

PCR test on cerebrospinal fluid (CSF), aqueous humor, whole blood, respiratory lavage fluid, or fresh tissue to demonstrate presence of *Toxoplasma* DNA. Definitive diagnosis requires demonstration of tachyzoites or cysts cytologically or histopathologically (with immunohistochemistry) and/or PCR, or rarely via animal or cell culture inoculation.

Causes of Abnormally Low Levels

Negative IgG and IgM titers indicate absence of exposure, peracute infection, or insufficient immune response to infection.

Next Diagnostic Steps to Consider if Levels are Low

If clinical signs are suggestive of acute toxoplasmosis, re-evaluate IgM and IgG titers in 3-6 weeks or consider alternative testing (p. 984).

Drug Effects

Clindamycin may decrease IgM titer, but will not affect IgG titer. High doses of corticosteroids administered to cats with latent infection may decrease IgG titers and increase IgM titers.

Lab Artifacts

False-positive ELISA: lipemia and hemolysis

Specimen Collection and Handling

Serum (red top tube), 1 mL. CSF or aqueous humor (lavender top tube), 0.5 mL. Stable for 5 days at 2°C-8°C or longer frozen. Paired serum samples should be submitted to the same laboratory for testing at the same time.

Relative Cost: $$ (ELISA, PCR, IFA)

Pearls

- Value of a single IgG measurement is very limited because approximately 30% of healthy cats and dogs have a positive titer.
- No single serologic assay can definitively confirm a diagnosis. IFA has more false-positives than ELISA; at low dilutions the specificity of ELISA may be lower than IFA.
- IgG-seropositive, IgM-seronegative cats are unlikely to be shedding oocytes. IgM-seropositive cats might or might not be shedding oocysts (period of shedding occurs briefly soon after infection).

AUTHOR: Patty J. Ewing, DVM, MS, DACVP
EDITOR: Lois Roth-Johnson, DVM, PhD, DACVP

Triglycerides

Definition

Main storage form of long-chain fatty acids

Synonym

Triacylglycerol

Physiology

Three fatty acid molecules are bound (esterified) to a glycerol backbone to form a triglyceride molecule, the main lipid in adipose tissue/body fat. Primary sites of triglyceride synthesis are liver, small intestine, adipose tissue, and mammary gland, but synthesis occurs in most cells. Triglycerides are transported in the blood bound to apoproteins, forming complexes called *lipoproteins*. Circulating triglyceride levels reflect a balance of absorption and synthesis by the small intestine, synthesis and secretion by hepatocytes, and uptake by adipose tissue. These processes are affected by dietary fat intake and hormones (insulin, glucagon).

Reference Interval

Serum levels, dogs: 20-150 mg/dL; cats: 20-90 mg/dL. Unit conversion: 1 mg/dL = 0.0113 mmol/L.

Causes of Abnormally High Levels

- Primary hyperlipidemia: idiopathic hyperlipidemia (schnauzer, beagles, and rarely in Brittany spaniels, mixed-breed dogs and cats); familial hyperchylomicronemia in cats
- Secondary hyperlipidemia: postprandial, hypothyroidism (dogs), diabetes mellitus, pancreatitis, hepatic disease, nephrotic syndrome, hyperadrenocorticism, high-fat diet, acromegaly (cats)

Next Diagnostic Steps to Consider if Levels are High

- Measure fasting levels (minimum 12-hour fast) to rule out postprandial hyperlipidemia. If persistent, assess for causes of secondary hyperlipidemia. If secondary hyperlipidemia is ruled out, primary hyperlipidemia is diagnosis of exclusion. See pp. 496 and 1236.

Causes of Abnormally Low Levels

Malabsorption/maldigestion; hepatic synthetic failure (chronic hepatopathies)

Next Diagnostic Steps to Consider if Levels are Low

Serum trypsin-like immunoreactivity (TLI), cobalamin (vitamin B_{12}) and folate levels; assess for panhypoproteinemia; serum bile acids (pre- and postprandial)

Important Interspecies Differences

Hyperlipidemia may occur in cholestatic liver disease. Cats with hepatic lipidosis do not have hyperlipidemia.

Drug Effects

- Increased: doxorubicin, exogenous corticosteroids, megestrol acetate
- Decreased: lipid-lowering diets, supplementation with fish oils, nicotinic acid and fibric acid derivatives such as gemfibrozil

Lab Artifacts

Hemolysis, lipemia, increased fluid viscosity, and glycerol artificially elevate triglyceride levels.

Specimen Collection and Handling

Ensure sample collected after 12-hour fast. Serum (red top tube), heparinized plasma (green top tube), or EDTA plasma (lavender top tube). Stable at 2°C-8°C for 1 week, 3 months frozen at −20°C

Relative Cost: $$

Pearls

- Triglyceride levels may be measured in suspected chylous effusions. Triglyceride levels in the effusion that are greater than serum triglyceride levels indicate chylous effusion, even if the effusion is not opaque white.

- Marked hypertriglyceridemia can predispose to pancreatitis in dogs, so dietary intervention is warranted.

AUTHOR: Ruanna E. Gossett, DVM, PhD, DACVP
EDITOR: Lois Roth-Johnson, DVM, PhD, DACVP

Triiodothyronine (T_3)

Definition

Active form of iodine-containing thyroid hormone; primary function is to increase rate of cell metabolism. Rarely measured as diagnostic test

Synonym

3,5,3′-triiodothyronine

Physiology

Approximately 20% of T_3 is produced in the thyroid gland; the rest is from conversion of T_4 to T_3 in cells. Thyroxine (T_4) is 99% protein-bound in circulation. T_4 dissociates to the more biologically active free T_3 to enter cells. Binding to intracellular receptor proteins causes an increased metabolic rate.

Reference Interval

Dogs and cats: 0.5-1.8 ng/mL. Unit conversion: 1 ng/mL × 1.536 = 1 nmol/L (SI unit).

Causes of Abnormally High Levels

Hyperthyroidism; presence of autoantibodies to T_3; exogenous T_3, TSH, or TRH; rarely, administration of iodine-containing compounds

Next Diagnostic Steps to Consider if Levels are High

- If hyperthyroidism suspected: clinical evaluation (p. 503)
- If autoantibodies suspected: measure T_3 autoantibody levels.
- Evaluate diet and supplements for iodine content, raw foods.

Causes of Abnormally Low Levels

Spontaneous or iatrogenic hypothyroidism; non-thyroidal illness; drugs

Next Diagnostic Steps to Consider if Levels are Low

Measure TSH and T_4 or free T_4 by equilibrium dialysis; evaluate for non-thyroidal diseases and drug administration.

Drug Effects

Many drugs, including glucocorticoids and phenobarbital, decrease T_3 concentration. Not as thoroughly studied as for T_4, but consider that many drugs may have this effect.

Specimen Collection and Handling

Serum (red top tube), 1 mL. To avoid interference by fibrin, allow full clot formation before centrifugation and removal of serum. Store refrigerated up to 7 days. Frozen samples are stable for up to 2 months.

Relative Cost: $

Pearls

- T_3 is of little value in diagnosis of hypothyroidism due to broad overlap in T_3 serum levels between euthyroid, hypothyroid, and euthyroid sick dogs (insensitive and nonspecific).
- Serum T_3 decreases later in the course of hypothyroidism than T_4.

AUTHOR: Shelley Burton, DVM, MSc, DACVP
EDITOR: Lois Roth-Johnson, DVM, PhD, DACVP

Troponins, Cardiac

Definition

Troponins are intracellular myofibrillar proteins expressed in cardiac and skeletal muscle. Cardiac troponin I (cTnI) is the most diagnostically relevant.

Physiology

- Troponins regulate the contractility of striated muscle. They mediate the interaction between the sarcomeric proteins actin and myosin. The troponin complex is composed of three proteins: *troponin I* is the inhibitory component that prevents interaction between actin and myosin until intracellular calcium is bound by *troponin C; troponin T* is the tropomyosin-binding element that binds troponin I to the actin filament.
- The cardiac isoforms of troponins I and T are specific markers for myocardial injury because they are antigenically distinct from skeletal muscle troponins. Cardiac troponins are released into the circulation during cardiac ischemia and necrosis. They increase in proportion to the degree of myocardial injury, regardless of cause. Troponins increase in circulation within 4-6 hours after myocyte injury and may persist up to 1 or 2 weeks; renal function affects clearance. They are sensitive and specific markers of myocardial injury.

Reference Interval

Different diagnostic instruments assess different parts of the cTnI molecule such that normal reference ranges are instrument-specific. Contact laboratory for reference range information. Sample normal ranges:

- Dogs: < 0.2 ng/mL (cTnI), 0.01-0.15 ng/mL (cTnT), 0.05-0.21 ng/mL (cTnC)
- Cats: 0.03-0.16 ng/mL (cTnI), 0.05-0.22 ng/mL (cTnT)

Causes of Abnormally High Levels

- Dogs: pericardial effusion caused by hemangiosarcoma or idiopathic pericarditis (serum levels greater with hemangiosarcoma, though substantial overlap), arrhythmogenic right ventricular cardiomyopathy of boxers, gastric dilation/volvulus, doxorubicin cardiotoxicosis, babesiosis, acute pulmonary thromboembolism
- Dogs and cats: myocardial contusion, myocarditis, arrhythmias, structural heart disease associated with congestive heart failure
- Cats: hyperthyroidism, hypertrophic cardiomyopathy

Specimen Collection and Handling

Serum (red top tube), heparinized plasma (green top tube), or EDTA plasma (lavender top tube); refrigerate or freeze at −20°C.

Relative Cost: $$

Pearls

Elevated cardiac troponin indicates myocardial injury, but not etiologically specific. Further evaluation is required to determine the underlying cause.

AUTHOR: Ruanna E. Gossett, DVM, PhD, DACVP
EDITOR: Lois Roth-Johnson, DVM, PhD, DACVP

Trypsin-Like Immunoreactivity (TLI)

Definition

Species-specific immunologic assay used to diagnose exocrine pancreatic insufficiency (EPI)

Synonyms

TLI, fTLI (feline specific), cTLI (canine specific)

Physiology

The assay detects trypsinogen, trypsin, and trypsin bound to a proteinase inhibitor. Trypsinogen, the inactive form of trypsin, is produced by pancreatic acinar epithelial cells and is present in low concentrations in the blood of normal patients. EPI leads to reduced amounts of trypsinogen released into circulation.

Reference Interval

Dogs: 5-45 mcg/L; cats: 12-82 mcg/L

Causes of Abnormally High Levels

Pancreatitis, decreased glomerular filtration rate (GFR), malnourished patients (usually dogs)

Next Diagnostic Steps to Consider if Levels are High

- TLI > 50 mcg/L (dogs) or > 100 mcg/L (cats) is consistent with pancreatitis, although TLI is not recommended for diagnosis of pancreatitis; species-specific pancreatic lipase (PLI) assay is the preferred test.
- Evaluate for pancreatitis (e.g., PLI; see pp. 740, 742, and 1370).
- Evaluate for decreased GFR.

Causes of Abnormally Low Levels

Exocrine pancreatic insufficiency (EPI)

Next Diagnostic Steps to Consider if Levels are Low

Results < 2.5 mcg/L (dogs) and < 8 mcg/L (cats) are diagnostic for EPI.

- Evaluate serum cobalamin (B_{12}) and folate (associated abnormalities common).
- See p. 317.

Values of 2.5-5 mcg/L (dogs) or 8-12 mcg/L (cats) are equivocal:

- If GFR decreased, low concentration from EPI may increase into equivocal range.
- Ensure fasting (12-18 hours) sample.
- Repeat TLI assay in 4 weeks.

Important Interspecies Differences

An association between increased TLI and cobalamin deficiency can exist in the cat, and cobalamin supplementation variably improves TLI results.

Lab Artifacts

High temperatures will cause artifactual decrease in TLI.

Specimen Collection and Handling

Serum (red top tube), nonhemolyzed, fasting (12-18 hours) sample

Relative Cost: $$

Pearls

- Ensure that species-specific assays are performed.
- Oral supplementation with pancreatic extracts does not interfere with TLI assays.

AUTHOR: Carrie L. Flint, DVM, DACVP
EDITOR: Lois Roth-Johnson, DVM, PhD, DACVP

Urinalysis

Definition

The physical, chemical, and microscopic evaluation of urine

Synonym

UA

Physiology

Urine can be collected via the following techniques: free-catch (voided), table collection (i.e., aspirated from clean table or floor after voiding), catheterization, and cystocentesis. Submission of urine collected by cystocentesis is ideal, as contamination from the environment or distal urogenital tract is less likely. Physical properties of urine include the evaluation of color, clarity, and solute concentration (specific gravity). Chemical analysis is commonly performed with a urine dipstick (test strip) and includes measurements of urine pH, protein, glucose, ketones, blood, and bilirubin. Lastly, the urine sediment is examined microscopically for the presence of casts, crystals, red blood cells, white blood cells, epithelial cells, bacteria, yeast, parasites, lipid, and/or sperm. A urinalysis provides insight to the patient's hydration status and renal function as well as the presence of disease (e.g., protein-losing nephropathy, urinary tract infection).

Reference Interval

The following values are observed in healthy dogs and cats:

- Color: yellow to amber
- Clarity: clear
- Specific gravity: 1.015-1.045 (dog) and 1.035-1.060 (cat)
- pH: 6.0-7.5
- Protein, glucose, ketones, blood: negative
- Bilirubin: Can be low positive in healthy dogs. Any positive result is significant in cats.
- Casts: 1-2 hyaline and 0-1 granular
- Crystals: struvite, calcium oxalate dihydrate, and brushite crystals can be observed in healthy dogs or cats.

- RBCs and WBCs: < 5/hpf
- Epithelial cells: variable, depending on sample collection
- Bacteria, yeast, parasites: negative, unless contamination present
- Lipid: positive or negative
- Sperm: can be observed in intact males

Causes of Abnormally High Levels

Refer to the following chapters in Section 4 of this textbook: Urine Specific Gravity, Urine pH Abnormalities, Bilirubinuria, Glucosuria, Ketonuria, Casts in the Urine Sediment, Crystals in Urine, and Pyuria.

Causes of Abnormally Low Levels

Refer to the following chapters in Section 4 of this textbook: Urine Specific Gravity, Urine pH Abnormalities

Specimen Collection and Handling

- Process immediately (ideal) or refrigerate for storage. If refrigerated, allow urine to reach room temperature before analyzing.
- Samples should be regimented via centrifugation before microscopic cell analysis.

Relative Cost: $

Pearls

- Multiple brands of urine dipsticks are available for veterinary medicine. Read the package insert to ensure correct interpretation.
- The following urine dipstick reagents are unreliable in veterinary medicine: urobilinogen, nitrite, leukocyte esterase, and specific gravity.
- Tabletop collection of samples should be a last choice, since contamination from the environment may be significant.
- Gross debris should be wiped from external genitalia before collecting free-catch samples. Aim for "midstream" catch to minimize initial contamination of urine from genitalia.
- Cystocentesis should be avoided if hemostatic disorder or bladder cancer is suspected.

AUTHOR: Shannon D. Dehghanpir, DVM, MS, DACVP
EDITOR: Lois Roth-Johnson, DVM, PhD, DACVP

Urine Cortisol/Creatinine Ratio

Definition

Screening test for hyperadrenocorticism that measures the ratio of urine cortisol to urine creatinine

Synonym

Urine cortisol/urine creatinine ratio (UC/UC)

Physiology

Because urinary excretion of creatinine is fairly constant, its ratio to urine cortisol reflects serum cortisol levels over the time of urine formation.

Reference Interval

- Dogs and cats: < 13 × 10–6 (ratio reference intervals have no units). Values for cats are not well established but may be higher than for dogs (further study needed).
- Ratios within the reference interval help rule out hyperadrenocorticism.

Causes of Abnormally High Levels

Physiologic stress, many nonadrenal diseases, and hyperadrenocorticism

Next Diagnostic Steps to Consider if Levels are High

Review history, routine laboratory test results, and physical examination findings for signs of hyperadrenocorticism. Adrenocorticotropic hormone (ACTH) stimulation test and/or low-dose dexamethasone suppression test (LDDST) if indicated. See p. 485.

Important Interspecies Differences

Test experience is limited in cats.

Drug Effects

- Increased ratio: corticosteroid administration (especially prednisolone and prednisone) variably cross-reacts with the cortisol assay.

Lab Artifacts

Depends on assay method; bilirubin can falsely increase

Specimen Collection and Handling

Fresh urine, 3 mL minimum in a clean plastic container. Ideally, urine from first morning voiding is obtained by clients at home to minimize stress-associated increases. Unclear if food intake increases ratio; fasting may be optimal.

Relative Cost: $$

Pearls

- Increased ratio is a sensitive but very nonspecific test for hyperadrenocorticism.
- A ratio within the reference interval means that hyperadrenocorticism is unlikely, but a high ratio cannot be used for diagnosis. Best used when there is a low index of suspicion for hyperadrenocorticism.
    - Recent studies suggest that UC/UC may not be as sensitive as once believed (perhaps only 70% sensitive).
- Ratio cannot be used for monitoring therapy.

AUTHOR: Shelley Burton, DVM, MSc, DACVP
EDITOR: Lois Roth-Johnson, DVM, PhD, DACVP

Laboratory Tests

Urine pH Abnormalities

Definition

Urine acidity (pH < 7.0) or alkalinity (pH > 7.0)

Synonyms

Aciduria or alkalinuria

Physiology

The kidneys regulate acid-base balance by selectively excreting acids or bases. In conjunction with a blood gas analysis and biochemistry panel, evaluation of urine pH helps gauge acid-base balance. Urine pH can help determine calculus type in urolithiasis, and modification of urine pH via diet can inhibit urolith formation in patients prone to urinary calculi. The stability of formed elements (e.g., crystals, casts, cells) is dependent upon urine pH.

Reference Interval

Dogs and cats: 6.0 to 7.5; however, urine pH can change with food or medications. Aciduria and alkalinuria are not always associated with disease.

Causes of Abnormally High Levels

Alkalinuria: alkaloses, urea degradation (i.e., effect of storage, urease-containing bacteria), distal renal tubular acidosis

Next Diagnostic Steps to Consider if Levels are High

Ensure use of fresh urine. Evaluate for urinary tract infection via urine sediment and bacterial culture.

Causes of Abnormally Low Levels

Aciduria: acidoses, paradoxic aciduria (secondary to hypochloremic metabolic alkalosis), proximal renal tubular acidosis, hypokalemia

Next Diagnostic Steps to Consider if Levels are Low

Consider history (including drugs) and clinical signs. Evaluate for an acid-base disturbance with a blood gas analysis and biochemistry panel.

Drug Effects

Loop and thiazide diuretics promote aciduria secondary to potassium-wasting (i.e., H^+ is excreted in exchange for K^+ retention).

Lab Artifacts

Pigmenturia can interfere with interpretation. Prolonged storage of urine may raise pH.

Specimen Collection and Handling

Perform with fresh urine as urine alkalinizes over time.

Relative Cost: $ (reported as part of urinalysis)

Pearls

- Alkalinuria may cause false proteinuria via dipstick reagent pad.
- Reagent test strips measure pH in increments of 0.5 between the range of 5.0 and 8.5.

AUTHOR: Shannon D. Dehghanpir, DVM, MS, DACVP
EDITOR: Lois Roth-Johnson, DVM, PhD, DACVP

Urine Protein/Creatinine Ratio

Definition

A quantitative measurement of protein in the urine that is unaffected by urine concentration

Synonyms

UPC, UP:UC

Physiology

Most serum proteins cannot pass through the glomerular filtration barrier due to their large size. Small proteins that pass through the glomerulus are typically reabsorbed by the renal tubules. Thus, sources of proteinuria include increased delivery of small proteins to the glomerulus, glomerular disease, tubular disease, or post-glomerular sources of protein (i.e., hemorrhage or inflammation of the urogenital tract). The UPC is calculated by dividing the urine total protein (mg/dL) by the urine creatinine (mg/dL). As the renal excretion of creatinine is relatively constant, any increase in the UPC reflects increased protein excretion. UPCs are generally performed after documentation of proteinuria via urine dipstick in absence of a pre-renal or post-renal cause.

Reference Interval

- Healthy dogs and cats: < 0.2
- Borderline proteinuria: 0.2-0.5 (dogs) and 0.2-0.4 (cats)
- Proteinuria: > 0.5 (dogs) and > 0.4 (cats)

Causes of Abnormally High Levels

- Pre-renal (overflow) proteinuria: hemoglobinuria, myoglobinuria, Bence Jones proteinuria
- Renal proteinuria: glomerular disease (e.g., glomerulonephritis, amyloidosis, glomerulosclerosis), tubular disease (e.g., Fanconi syndrome, acute kidney injury), transient proteinuria (secondary to fever, stress, exercise)
- Post-renal proteinuria: inflammation or hemorrhage of the urogenital tract

Next Diagnostic Steps to Consider if Levels are High

- Exclude pre-renal (e.g., hemoglobinuria, myoglobinuria) or post-renal (e.g., hematuria, pyuria, bacteriuria) protein sources.
- If first abnormal UPC, repeat testing to exclude transient cause.
- See pp. 51 and 390.

Specimen Collection and Handling

Perform on fresh urine with inactive sediment. Urine can be collected via free-catch or cystocentesis. Pooled samples are preferable to single ("spot") samples. Urine samples can be collected by the pet owner and stored frozen before submission; the veterinarian can combine equal volumes from each urine sample for analysis. Hospital collection (versus home collection) may increase results, likely due to transient stress proteinuria.

Relative Cost: $$

Pearls

- A UPC > 2 is typically associated with glomerular disease (assuming pre- and post-renal causes excluded).
- Proteinuria secondary to tubular disease is often mild (UPC < 2).
- Do not perform UPC in the face of recognized lower urinary tract inflammation or when gross hematuria is present.
- UPC has replaced 24-hour urine quantification for assessment of proteinuria.

AUTHOR: Shannon D. Dehghanpir, DVM, MS, DACVP
EDITOR: Lois Roth-Johnson, DVM, PhD, DACVP

Urine Specific Gravity (USG)

Definition

The measurement of urine solute concentration based on the density of urine compared to water

Synonym

Urine density

Physiology

Glomerular filtrate is modified by the renal tubules through reabsorption or secretion of water or solutes (e.g., urea, creatinine, K^+). Reabsorption of water requires functional antidiuretic hormone and medullary hypertonicity. Urine solute concentration is measured by urine specific gravity (USG) or osmolality (the gold standard) and is used to assess the concentrating ability of the kidneys. USG is typically measured indirectly via refractometry. Always interpret the USG in conjunction with the patient's hydration status, presence or absence of azotemia (i.e., elevated BUN, creatinine), and urinary and therapeutic history.

Reference Interval

- Healthy, euhydrated patient: 1.015-1.045 (dog) and 1.035-1.060 (cat)
- Dehydrated patient with adequate concentrating ability: > 1.030 (dog) and > 1.035 (cat)
- Dehydrated patient with inadequate concentrating ability: 1.013-1.029 (dog) and 1.013-1.034 (cat)
- Isosthenuria: 1.008-1.012
- Dilute urine/hyposthenuria: < 1.008

Causes of Abnormally High Levels

> 1.030 (dog) and > 1.035 (cat) with azotemia: dehydration

Next Diagnostic Steps to Consider if Levels are High

Evaluate hydration status.

Causes of Abnormally Low Levels

- < 1.030 (dog) and < 1.035 (cat) in a dehydrated patient: diuretic/fluid therapy, osmotic/postobstructive diuresis, hyperadrenocorticism, hypercalcemia, pyometra, pyelonephritis, medullary washout (e.g., liver dysfunction, hypoadrenocorticism), hypokalemia, and potentially, renal disease
- Isosthenuria with azotemia is suggestive of renal disease.
- Dilute urine/hyposthenuria does not typically indicate renal disease, but can be observed with overhydration, central diabetes insipidus, and primary polydipsia in addition to some of the aforementioned causes.

Next Diagnostic Steps to Consider if Levels are Low

Exclude drug effects (e.g., diuretic or fluid therapy). Assess for glucosuria. Perform complete blood count and biochemistry panel to evaluate for azotemia and other abnormalities. Evaluate water intake and urinary history. Perform abdominal imaging. Consider urine culture, leptospira titers, urine cortisol/creatinine ratio.

Important Interspecies Differences

Cats produce more concentrated urine than dogs.

Drug Effects

Fluid, glucocorticoid, or diuretic therapy will decrease the USG.

Lab Artifacts

- USG measurements via dipstick reagent are inaccurate.
- Use of a refractometer with a feline-specific calibration scale may result in falsely lowered USGs in cats. The canine or human scale should be used for feline urine.

Specimen Collection and Handling

Process or refrigerate immediately. Temperature-compensated refractometers should be used to measure USG.

Relative Cost: $ (reported as part of urinalysis)

Pearls

- Dilute urine/hyposthenuria may cause lysis of urinary formed elements (e.g., cells, casts).
- Glucosuria and proteinuria will increase the USG; 1 g/dL of either substance can increase the USG by ≈0.003 units.

AUTHOR: Shannon D. Dehghanpir, DVM, MS, DACVP
EDITOR: Lois Roth-Johnson, DVM, PhD, DACVP

von Willebrand Factor Assay

Definition

Diagnostic test for measuring von Willebrand factor (vWF). Decreased functional vWF causes prolonged bleeding time and abnormal primary hemostasis, known as von Willebrand disease (vWD).

Physiology

- vWF is produced by endothelial cells and megakaryocytes. It circulates with factor VIII (prolongs factor VIII stability). Stored in endothelial cells and platelet alpha-granules, vWF bridges the exposed subendothelial collagen and platelets, and among platelets. Platelet binding of vWF triggers a cascade of hemostatic and thrombotic events. Low levels of vWF result in lack of platelet activation (p. 1043).
- Type 1 vWD: quantitative vWF deficiency. Type 2 vWD: quantitative vWF deficiency and concurrent functional deficiencies of remaining vWF. Type 3 vWD: no detectable vWF.
- Measured by quantitative ELISA with species-specific antibodies to vWF +/− qualitative multimeric analysis (separates the different vWF multimers) to identify type 2 vWD. Functional assays (platelet aggregation or collagen binding assays) are available but rarely used in clinical settings.

Reference Interval

Dogs (quantitative ELISA): 60%-172% of normal pooled plasma

Causes of Abnormally High Levels

Azotemia, liver disease

Causes of Abnormally Low Levels

vWD is the most common heritable bleeding disorder in dogs. Typically, vWF levels < 35% are indicative of type 1 vWD. Patients with type 2 vWD can have low to normal vWF concentrations and variable vWF function. Concentrations between 30% and 70% suggest a carrier.

Next Diagnostic Steps to Consider if Levels are Low

For several dog breeds, genetic tests can detect mutations and identify heterozygotes (i.e., carriers).

Important Interspecies Differences

Feline platelets contain vWF; canine platelets do not contain significant levels. Thrombocytopenia does not affect vWF values in dogs.

Drug Effects

Epinephrine, endotoxin, and 1-deamino-8-D-arginine vasopressin (DDAVP) can increase vWF.

Lab Artifacts

Decrease: hemolysis, clotting

Specimen Collection and Handling

Collect blood in sodium citrate (blue top tube) or EDTA (lavender top tube). After centrifugation, plasma should be promptly collected, frozen, and shipped overnight.

Relative Cost: $$$

Pearls

- If the platelet count and coagulation time are normal and there is no evidence of vasculitis or platelet dysfunction (e.g., aspirin), prolonged buccal mucosal bleeding time is screening test for vWD.
- DNA testing is breed-specific and used to identify potential carriers but does not predict the degree to which a dog will be clinically affected. The value obtained from factor assay better predicts the likelihood of clinical signs. DNA test does not help to diagnose type 3 vWD.
- Breeding should be discouraged for any dog with factor levels < 70%.

AUTHOR: Deborah G. Davis, DVM, DACVP
EDITOR: Lois Roth-Johnson, DVM, PhD, DACVP

Warfarin

Definition

Warfarin and related second-generation compounds have been a commonly used rodenticides but are being phased out of use; similar compounds are also used to treat people with hypercoagulable states. Warfarin testing is typically for retrospective confirmation (e.g., identification and prevention of future reintoxication or for legal purposes). Animals suspected of active hemorrhage due to ingestion of warfarin or other anticoagulant intoxicants should be evaluated with prothrombin time (PT) or assessment of proteins inhibited by vitamin K absence/antagonism (PIVKA) because turnaround time for warfarin assay is long.

Synonyms

First-generation compounds: warfarin (i.e., Coumadin), indanedione-containing rodenticides

Second-generation compounds: coumarin-based generics (brodifacoum, difenacoum, bromadiolone) and the indanedione, diphacinone

Physiology

Well but slowly absorbed following oral administration; plasma levels peak in 6-12 hours. Most is protein bound, but high concentrations in liver, spleen, kidney. Elimination rate via hepatic metabolism depends on compound, amount ingested; may accumulate if small amounts ingested over several days. Warfarin half-life in dog plasma is 14.5 hours; the half-life of diphacinone is suspected to be days. Brodifacoum is assumed to be similar or longer than that of diphacinone. The differences in residual half-lives have important therapeutic implications. Compounds interfere with coagulation by decreasing active coagulation factors II, VII, IX, and X (competitive inhibition of vitamin K epoxide-reductase).

Reference Interval

Consult laboratory for reference interval and for inclusion of both first- and second-generation compounds in test panel.

Causes of Abnormally High Levels

Ingestion of compounds or animals that have consumed compounds. Relay toxicosis (incurred from consumption of prey [e.g., rodents] that have eaten warfarin) rarely occurs with second-generation anticoagulants other than diphacinone.

Next Diagnostic Steps to Consider if Levels Are High

Inquire about potential exposure to rodenticide or human drugs; remove source; administer vitamin K; whole blood transfusion (p. 69)

Drug Effects

Oxyphenbutazone, phenylbutazone, diphenylhydantoin, sulfonamides, and corticosteroids increase susceptibility to toxicity.

Specimen Collection and Handling

Chemical detection of specific anticoagulants in vomitus or baits. Liver tissue (frozen) for postmortem diagnosis. Unclotted blood, stomach contents, intestinal content, feces, spleen, and kidney may also be submitted.

Relative Cost: $$ (Send out test for most veterinary reference laboratories; additional fees may apply.)

Pearls

Conditions enhancing susceptibility are high dietary fat (fatty acids displace the plasma protein-bound anticoagulant), prolonged oral antibiotic therapy, biliary obstruction, liver disease, hypoalbuminemia (warfarin is highly plasma protein bound), renal disease.

Most veterinary reference laboratories do not do rodenticide testing. When testing is offered, results are usually not available for several days or weeks. Testing is typically confirmatory rather than proactively diagnostic.

AUTHOR & EDITOR: Lois Roth-Johnson, DVM, PhD, DACVP

Zinc, Serum Level

Definition

Zinc is an essential trace mineral required for proper function of many enzyme systems. Deficiency and toxicosis are imbalances that can be seen clinically.

Physiology

Dietary zinc is absorbed in the intestine, metabolized in the liver, and exported to peripheral tissues for use and storage. Zinc-responsive dermatosis is a deficiency of zinc presenting as a dermatologic disorder in dogs. Zinc toxicity typically occurs following ingestion of zinc-containing products.

Reference Interval

Normal serum zinc concentration is < 2 mcg/mL; liver wet weight is < 30-70 ppm. Check with laboratory for values consistent with intoxication.

Causes of Abnormally High Levels

Ingestion of metal pieces, zinc-containing topical ointments (e.g., diaper creams), zinc phosphide rodenticides, or U.S. pennies minted after 1982.

Next Diagnostic Steps to Consider if Levels are High

History, specifically regarding exposure to zinc-containing creams and rodenticides; abdominal radiography (for ingested metal). Hemolysis and multiorgan failure can be sequelae of zinc poisoning. See pp. 1051 and 1053.

Causes of Abnormally Low Levels

Malnutrition, malabsorption, animals receiving total parenteral nutrition

Next Diagnostic Steps to Consider if Levels are Low

See Zinc-Responsive Dermatosis (web edition).

Important Interspecies Differences

- Zinc-responsive dermatosis occurs as a familial form (plush-coated northern dog breeds) and in puppies fed zinc-deficient diets (or those containing excessive calcium).
- Lethal acrodermatitis is a rare inherited disorder of zinc metabolism in bull terriers that does not respond to zinc supplementation and is invariably fatal.

Drug Effects

Chelation therapy may decrease serum zinc concentrations

Specimen Collection and Handling

- Serum: avoid tubes with rubber tops (contain zinc stearate).
- Tissue: liver, kidney, GI contents can be used to rule out intoxication; skin biopsy for suspected zinc-deficient dermatosis

Relative Cost: $$$

Pearls

- CAUTION: In zinc phosphide intoxication, there may be a characteristic acetylene odor to the gastric contents (which may be bloody), and this gas is harmful to humans. Zinc phosphide causes emesis in dogs and cats, so fatal intoxication is not frequent.

AUTHOR: Carrie L. Flint, DVM, DACVP
EDITOR: Lois Roth-Johnson, DVM, PhD, DACVP

SECTION V

Clinical Algorithms

EDITORS

Leah A. Cohn
DVM, PhD, DACVIM (SAIM)

Etienne Côté
DVM, DACVIM (Cardiology, SAIM)

Abortion: Diagnostic Approach

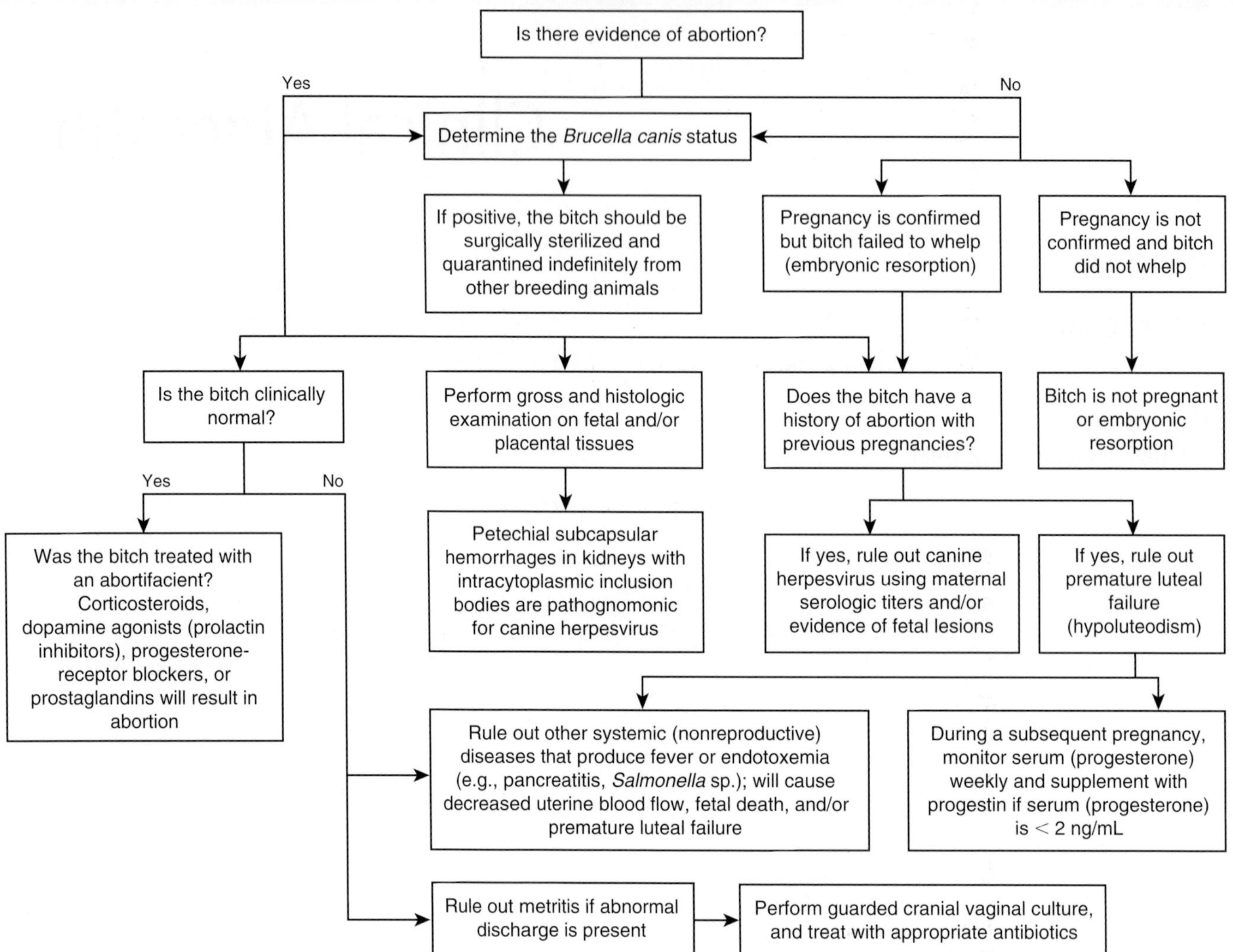

Acid-Base Disorders

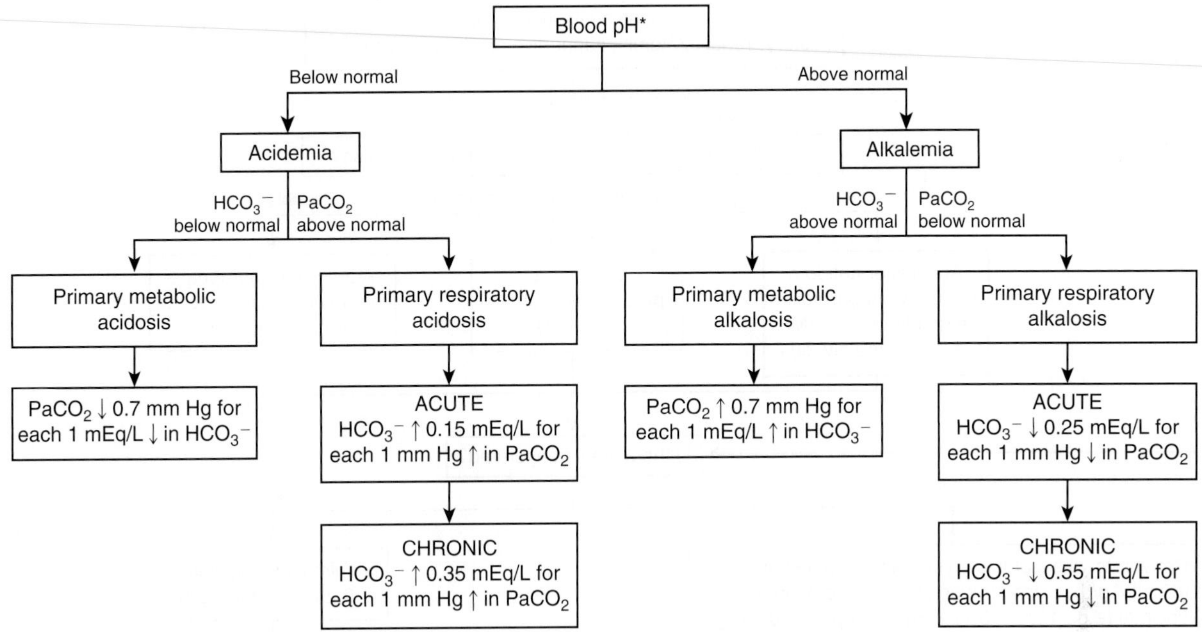

*pH may be in reference range due to compensation or mixed acid-base disorders.
(From Slatter DH: Textbook of small animal surgery, ed 3, St. Louis, 2003, Saunders.)

Clinical Algorithms

Acute Kidney Injury

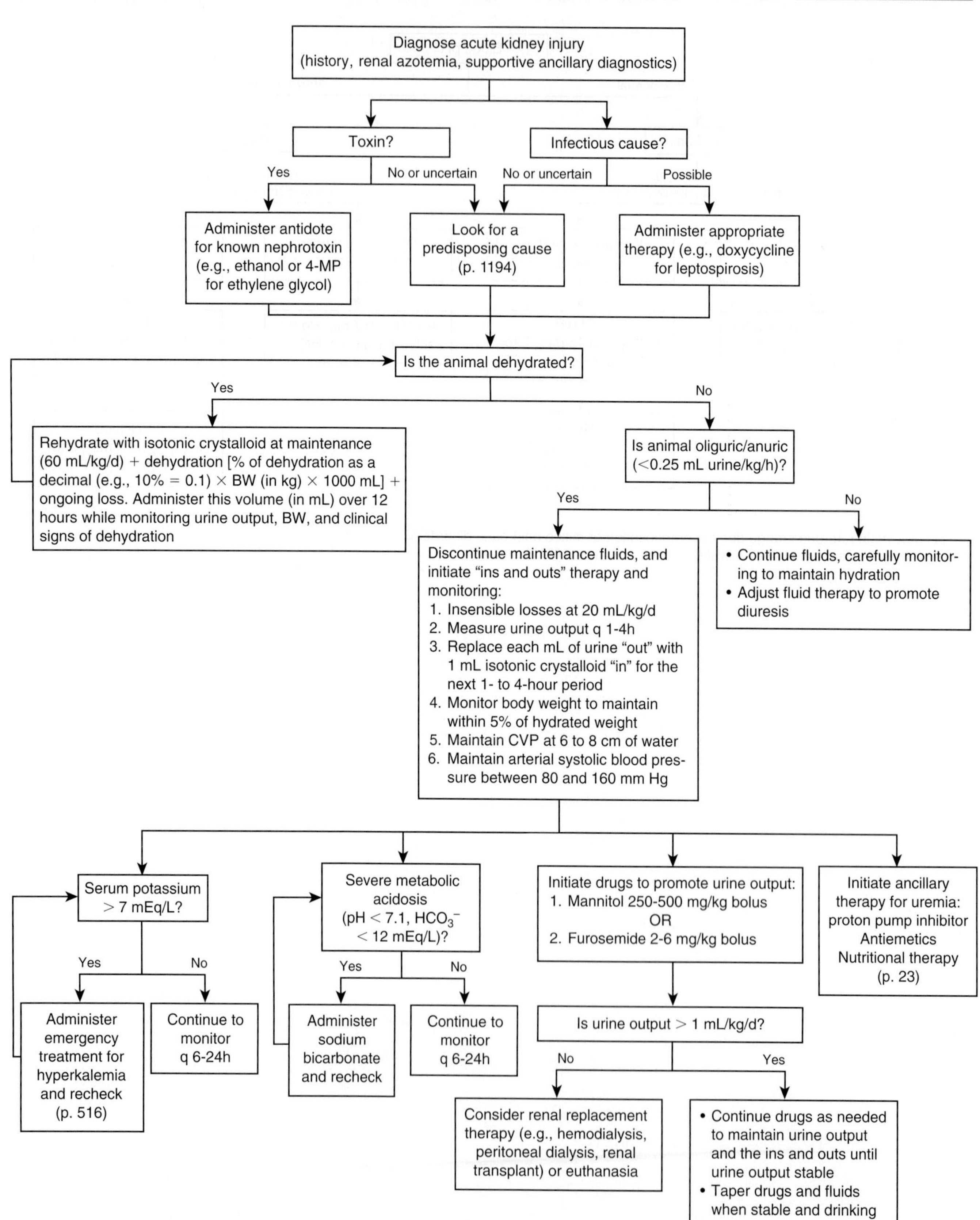

4-MP, 4-methylpyrazole; *BW*, body weight; *CVP*, central venous pressure.

UPDATED AND EDITED BY: Leah A. Cohn, DVM, PhD, DACVIM
ORIGINALLY WRITTEN BY: Marie E. Kerl, DVM, MPH, DACVECC, DACVIM

Adenocarcinoma of the Anal Sacs

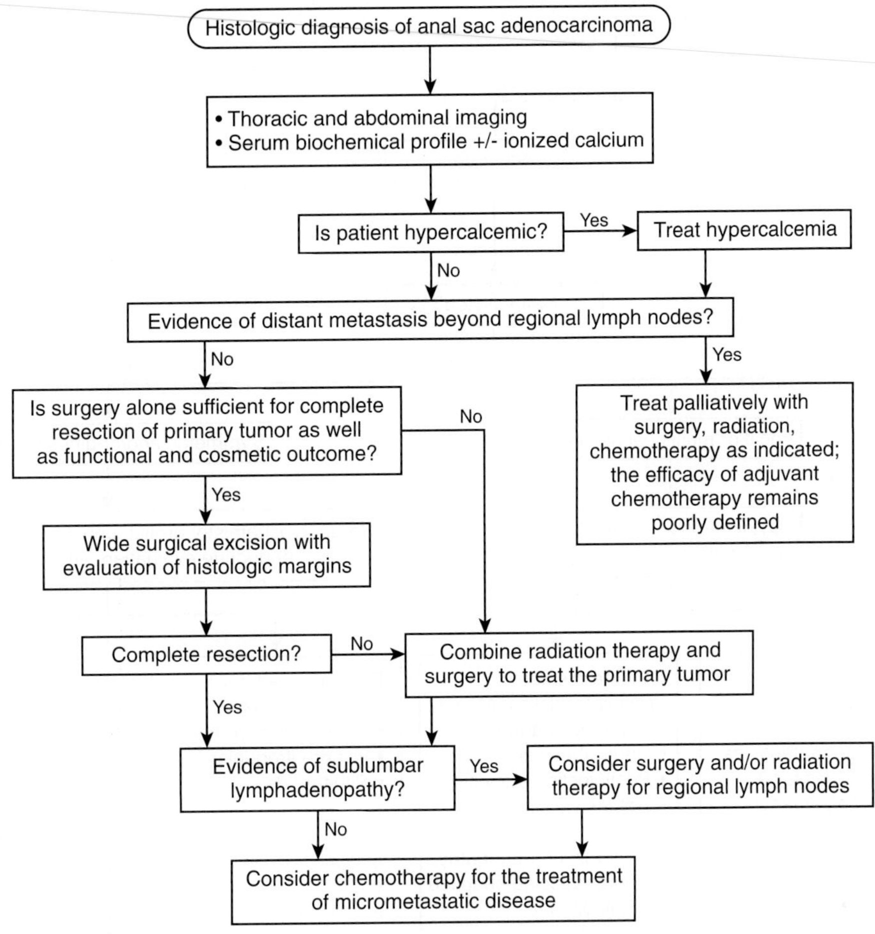

UPDATED AND EDITED BY: Leah A. Cohn, DVM, PhD, DACVIM
ORIGINALLY WRITTEN BY: Elizabeth A. McNiel, DVM, PhD, DACVIM, DACVR

Clinical Algorithms

Alopecia, Canine

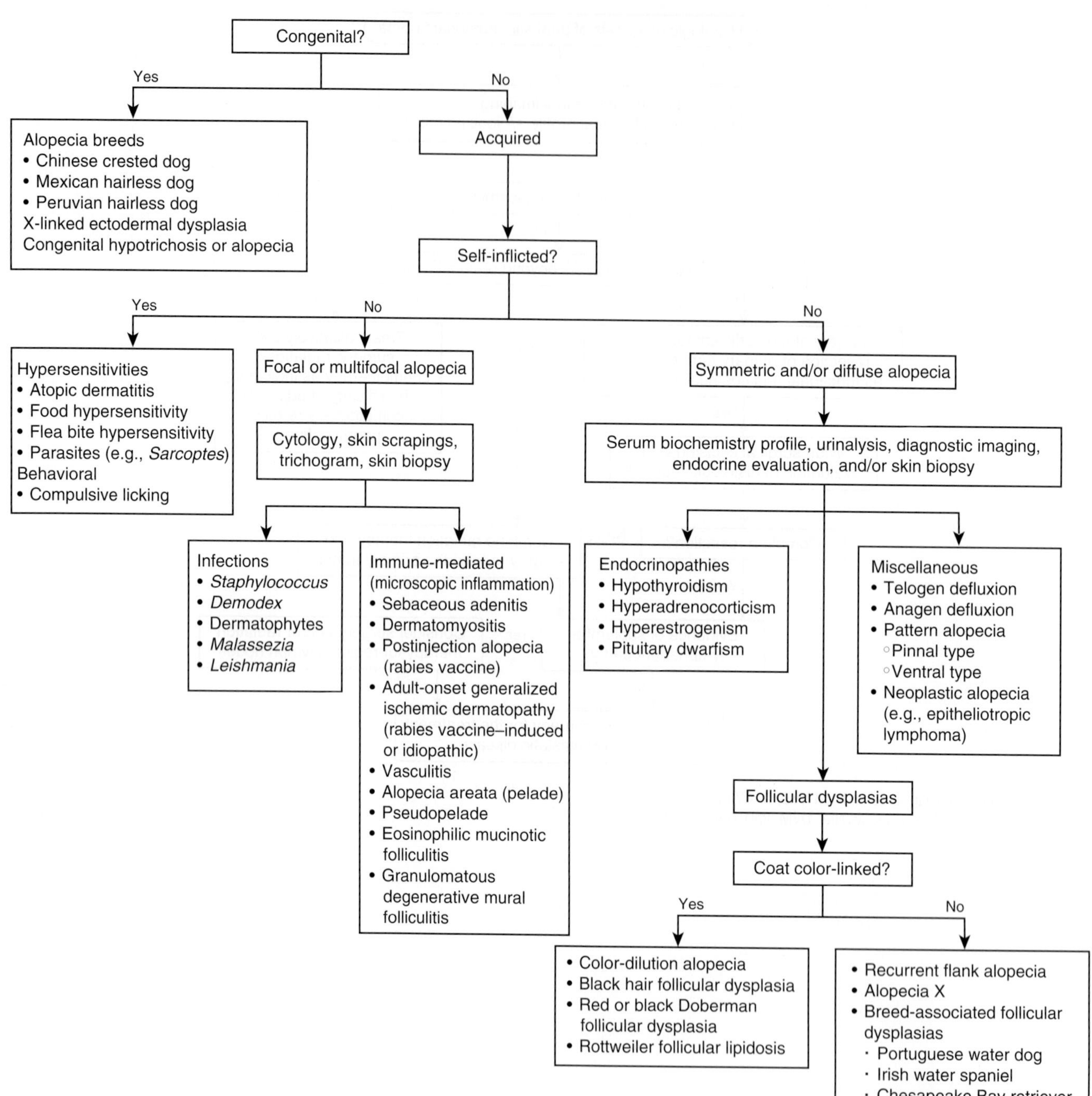

UPDATED AND EDITED BY: Leah A. Cohn, DVM, PhD, DACVIM
ORIGINALLY WRITTEN BY: Manon Paradis, DVM, MVSc, DACVD

Alopecia, Feline

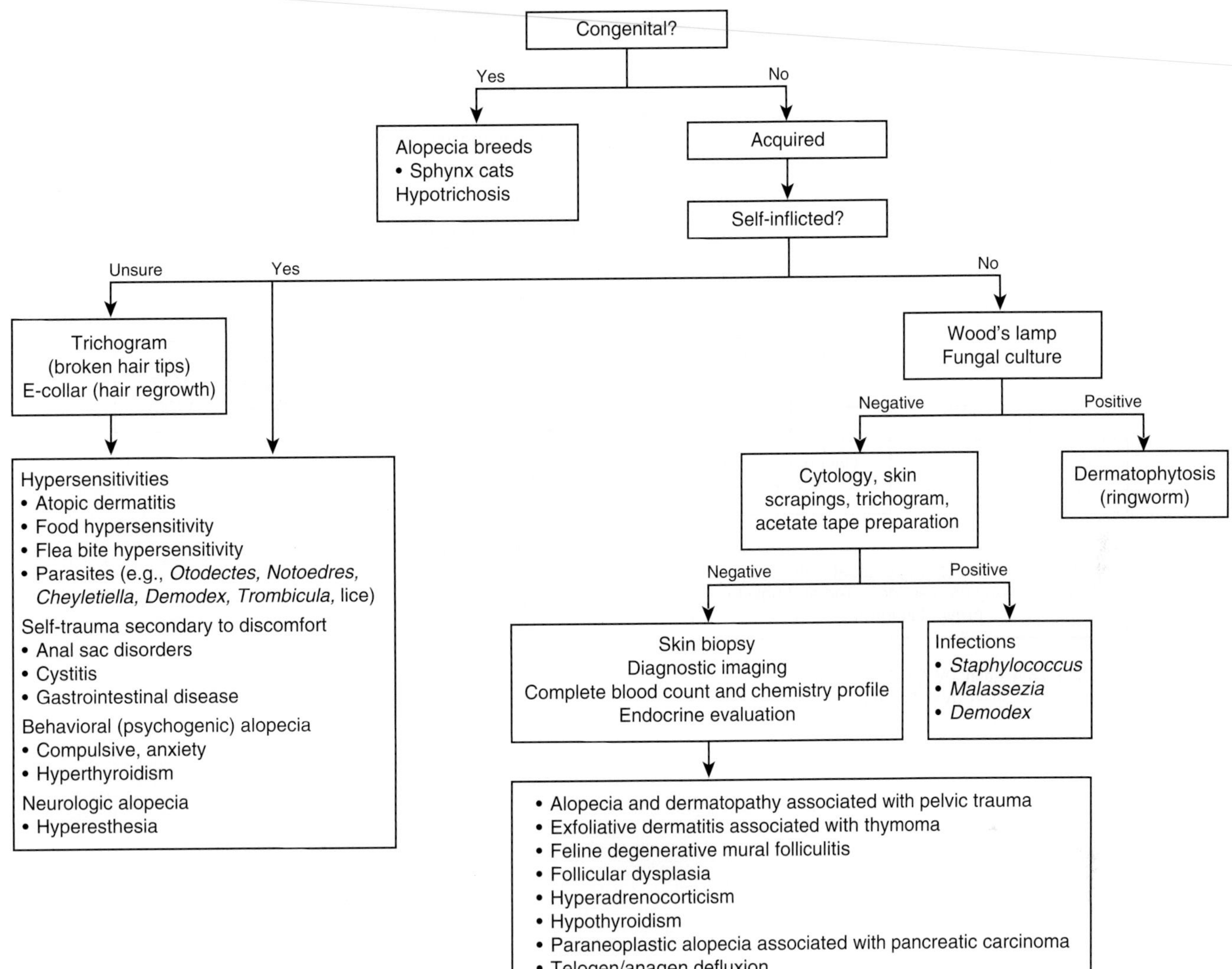

EDITED BY: Leah A. Cohn, DVM, PhD, DACVIM
ORIGINALLY WRITTEN BY: Manon Paradis, DVM, MVSc, DACVD

Anesthetic Complications

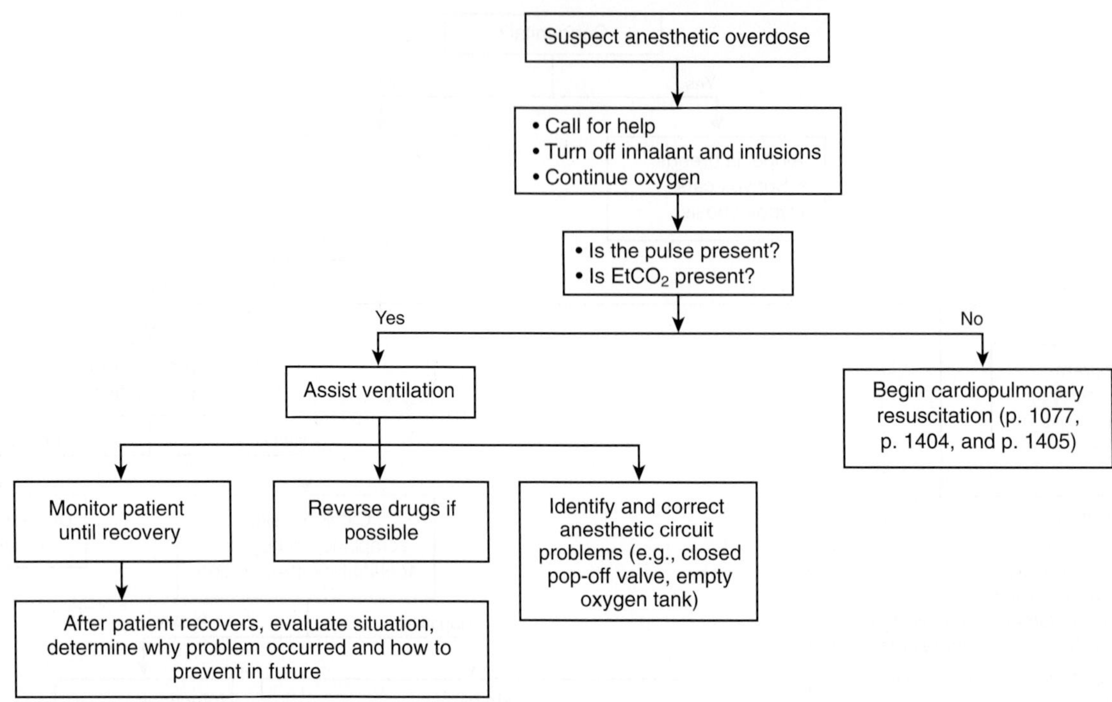

UPDATED AND EDITED BY: Leah A. Cohn, DVM, PhD, DACVIM
ORIGINALLY WRITTEN BY: Scott P. Shaw, DVM, DACVECC

Asthma

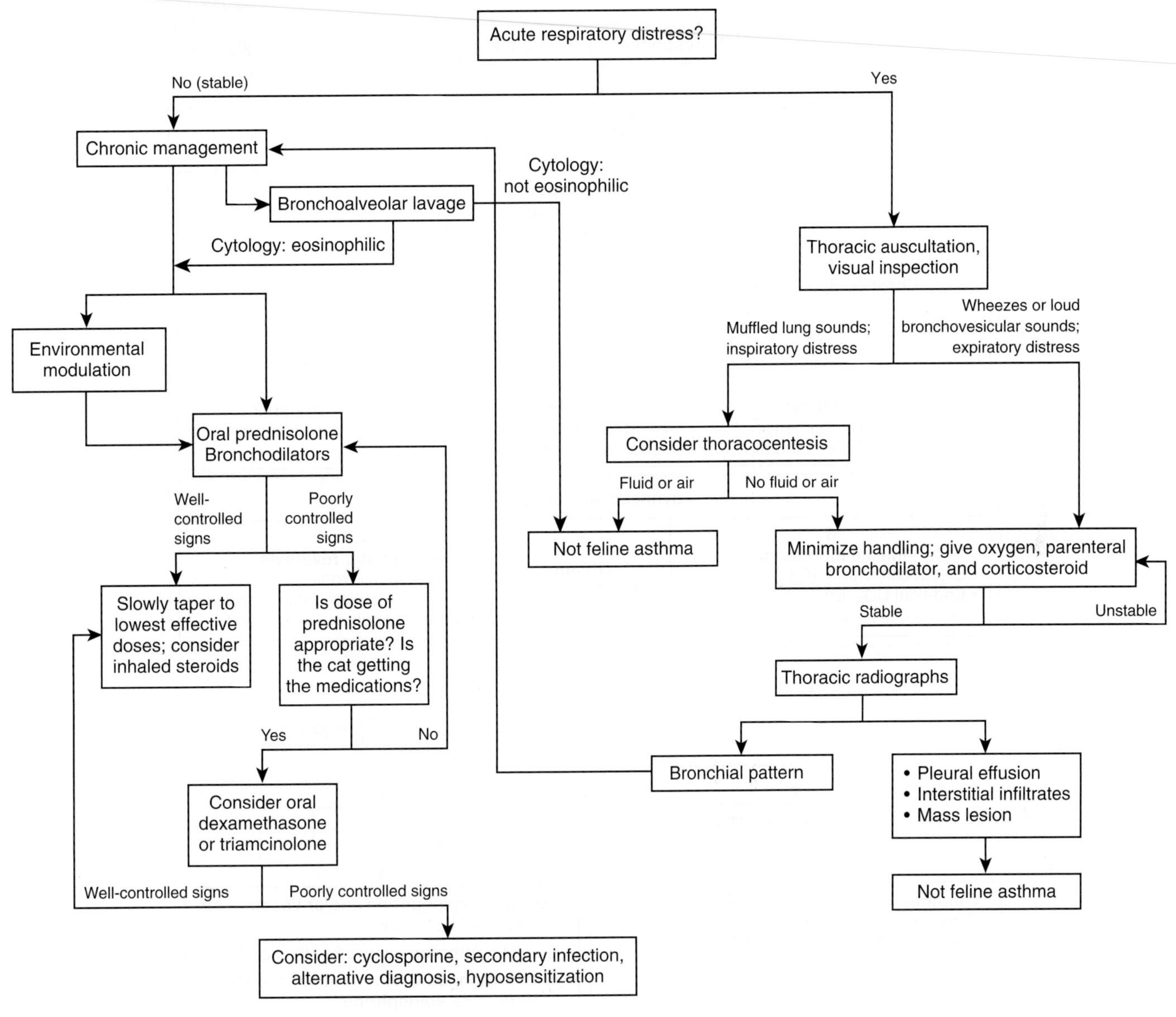

UPDATED AND EDITED BY: Leah A. Cohn, DVM, PhD, DACVIM
ORIGINALLY WRITTEN BY: Carol Reinero, DVM, PhD, DACVIM

Clinical Algorithms

Cardiopulmonary Cerebral Resuscitation

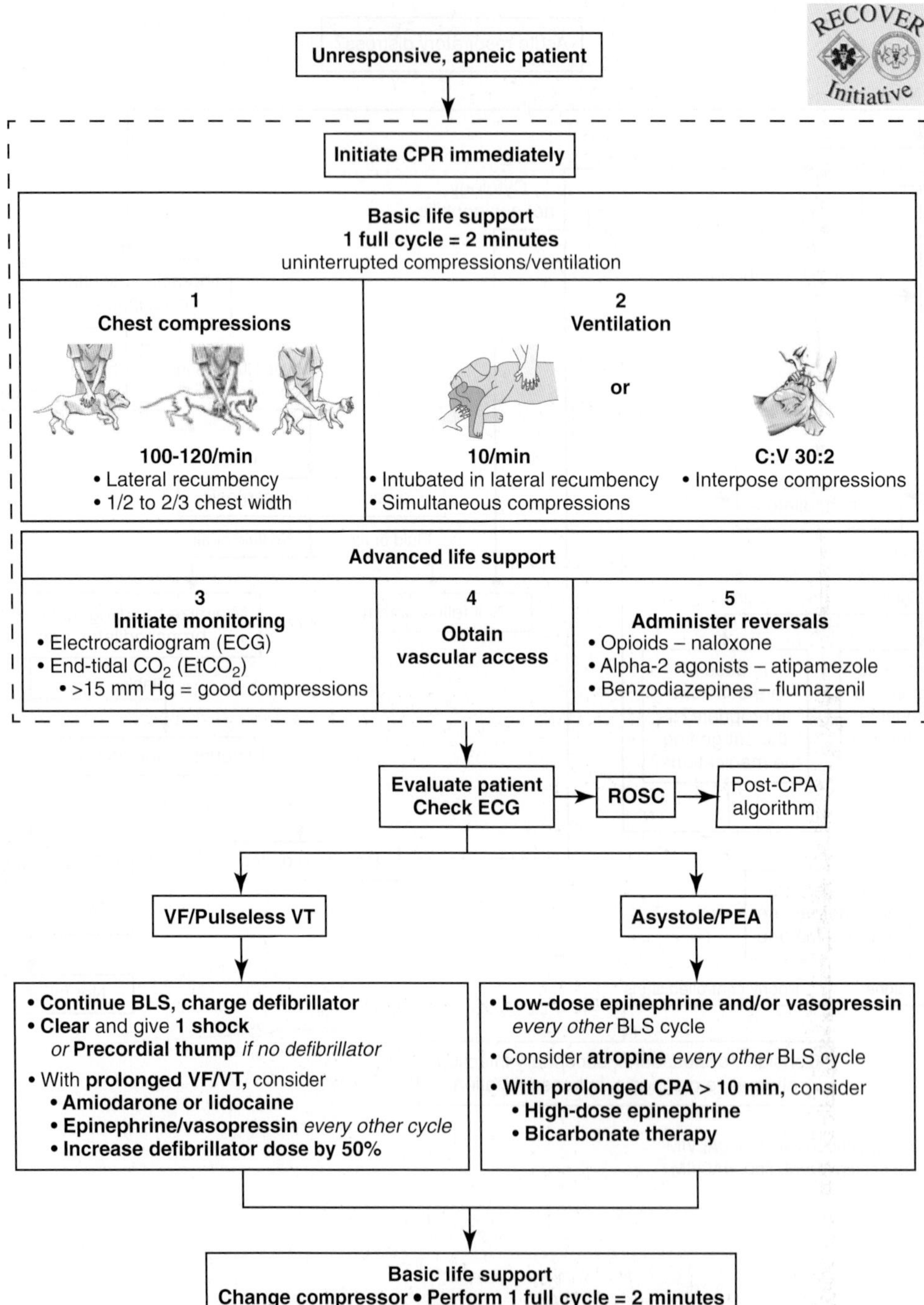

CPR algorithm chart. This chart summarizes the clinical guidelines most relevant to the patient presenting acutely in CPA. The box surrounded by the gray dashed line contains, in order, the initial BLS and ALS actions to be taken when a patient is diagnosed with CPA: (1) administration of chest compressions, (2) ventilation support, (3) initiation of ECG and $EtCO_2$ monitoring, (4) obtaining vascular access for drug administration, and (5) administration of reversal agents if any anesthetic/sedative agents have been administered. The algorithm then enters a loop of 2-minute cycles of CPR with brief pauses between to rotate compressors, to evaluate the patient for signs of ROSC, and to evaluate the ECG for a rhythm diagnosis. Patients in PEA or asystole should be treated with vasopressors and, potentially, anticholinergic drugs. These drugs should be administered no more often than every other cycle of CPR. Patients in VF or pulseless VT should be electrically defibrillated if a defibrillator is available, or mechanically defibrillated with a precordial thump if an electrical defibrillator is not available. Immediately after defibrillation, another 2-minute cycle of BLS should be started. The defibrillator dose can be increased by 50% after the first shock if a second shock is necessary. *ALS*, Advanced life support; *BLS*, basic life support; *CPA*, cardiopulmonary arrest; *CPR*, cardiopulmomary resuscitation; *C:V*, compression-to-ventilation ratio; *$EtCO_2$*, end-tidal CO_2; *PEA*, pulseless electrical activity; *ROSC*, return of spontaneous circulation; *VF*, ventricular fibrillation; *VT*, ventricular tachycardia.

(Modified from Fletcher DJ, et al: RECOVER evidence and knowledge gap analysis on veterinary CPR. Part 7: Clinical guidelines. *J Vet Emerg Crit Care.* 22(S1):S102–S131, 2012.)

Cardiopulmonary Cerebral Resuscitation Post-Arrest Care

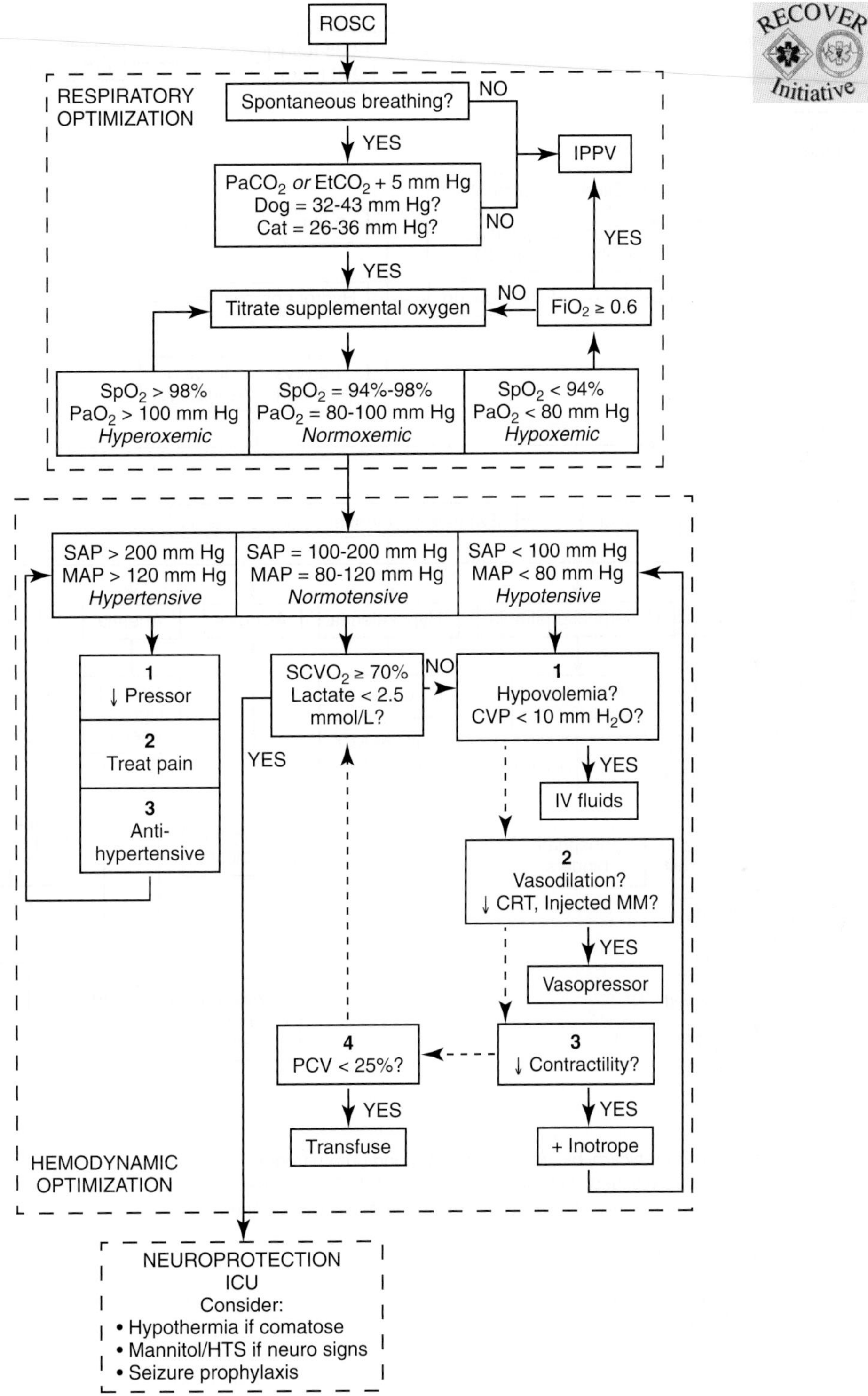

Post-cardiac arrest (PCA) care algorithm. This chart summarizes a comprehensive treatment protocol for PCA care that includes components of controlled ventilation and oxygenation, goal-directed hemodynamic optimization, and neuroprotective strategies. The sequence shown reflects the order in which each component should be assessed and treatment initiated. Assessment and initiation of treatment for the subsequent component will likely commence before the endpoints of the previous component have been completely met. Thus respiratory, hemodynamic, and neuroprotective treatment strategies will be initiated in parallel in most cases.

CRT, Capillary refill time; *CVP*, central venous pressure; *$EtCO_2$*, end-tidal carbon dioxide; *HTS*, hypertonic saline; *ICU, intensive care unit; IPPV*, intermittent positive pressure ventilation; *MAP*, mean arterial pressure; *MM*, mucous membrane color; *PaO_2*, partial pressure of oxygen, arterial; *PCV*, packed cell volume; *ROSC*, return of spontaneous circulation; *SAP*, systolic arterial pressure; *$SCVO_2$*, central venous oxygen saturation; *SpO_2*, peripheral capillary oxygen saturation.

(From Fletcher DJ, et al: RECOVER evidence and knowledge gap analysis on veterinary CPR. Part 7: Clinical guidelines. *J Vet Emerg Crit Care.* 22(S1):S102–S131, 2012.)

Clinical Algorithms

Chronic Kidney Disease: Management

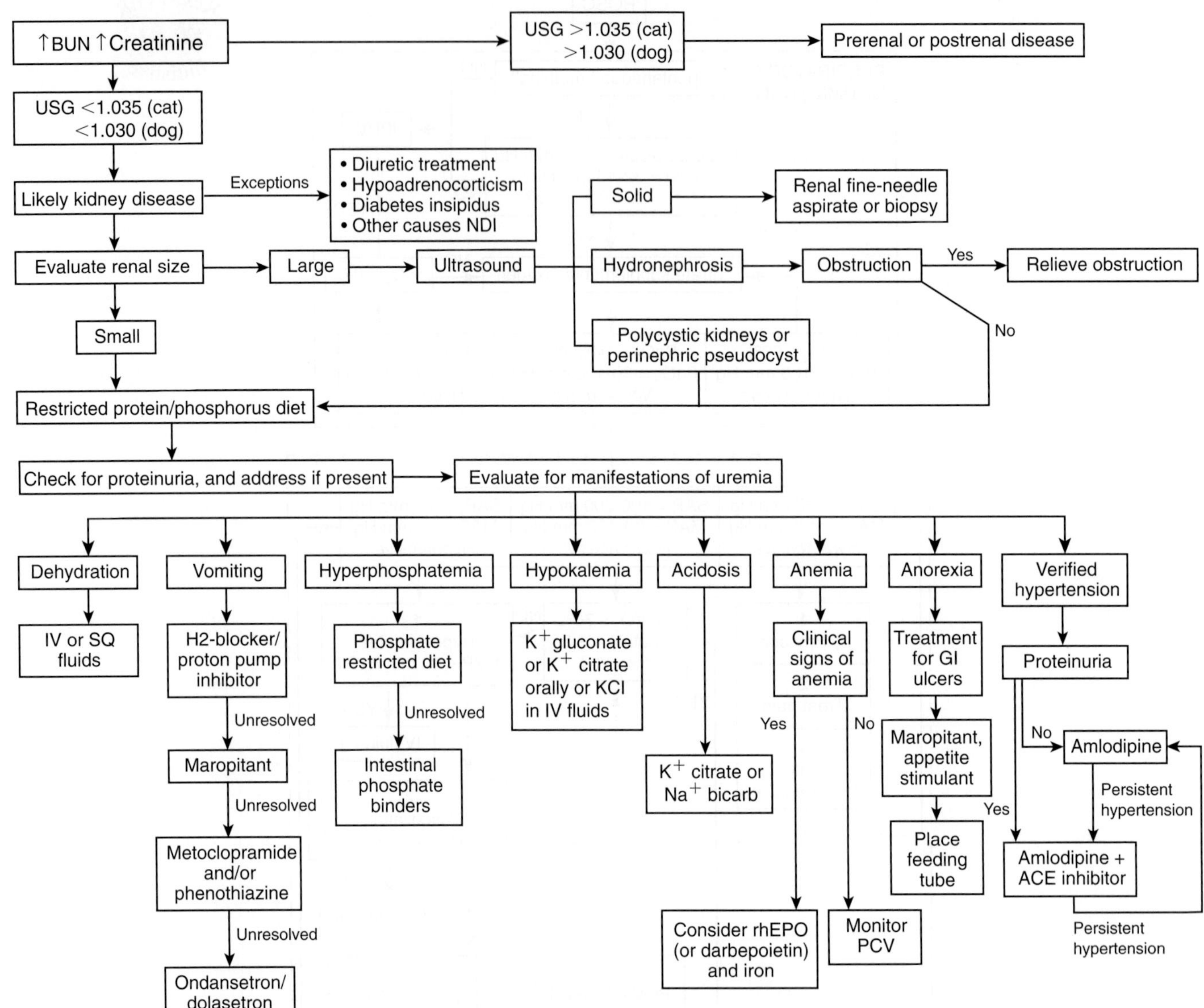

ACE, Angiotensin-converting enzyme; *bicarb*, bicarbonate; *BUN*, blood urea nitrogen; *GI*, gastrointestinal; *IV*, intravenous; *NDI*, nephrogenic diabetes insipidus; *PCV*, packed cell volume; *rhEPO*, recombinant human erythropoietin; *SQ*, subcutaneous, *USG*, urine specific gravity.

Reproduced from the third edition in modified form

THIRD EDITION AUTHOR: Cathy E. Langston, DVM, DACVIM
EDITOR: Leah A. Cohn, DVM, PhD, DACVIM

Constipation, Obstipation, and Megacolon

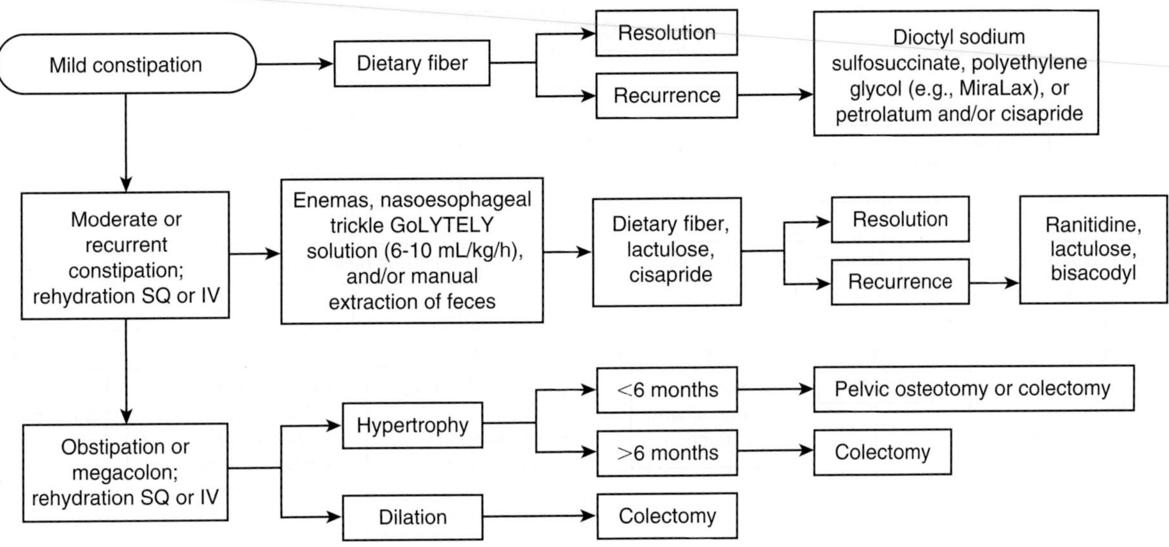

Modified from Slatter DH: Textbook of small animal surgery, ed 3, St. Louis, 2003, Saunders.

Cyanosis

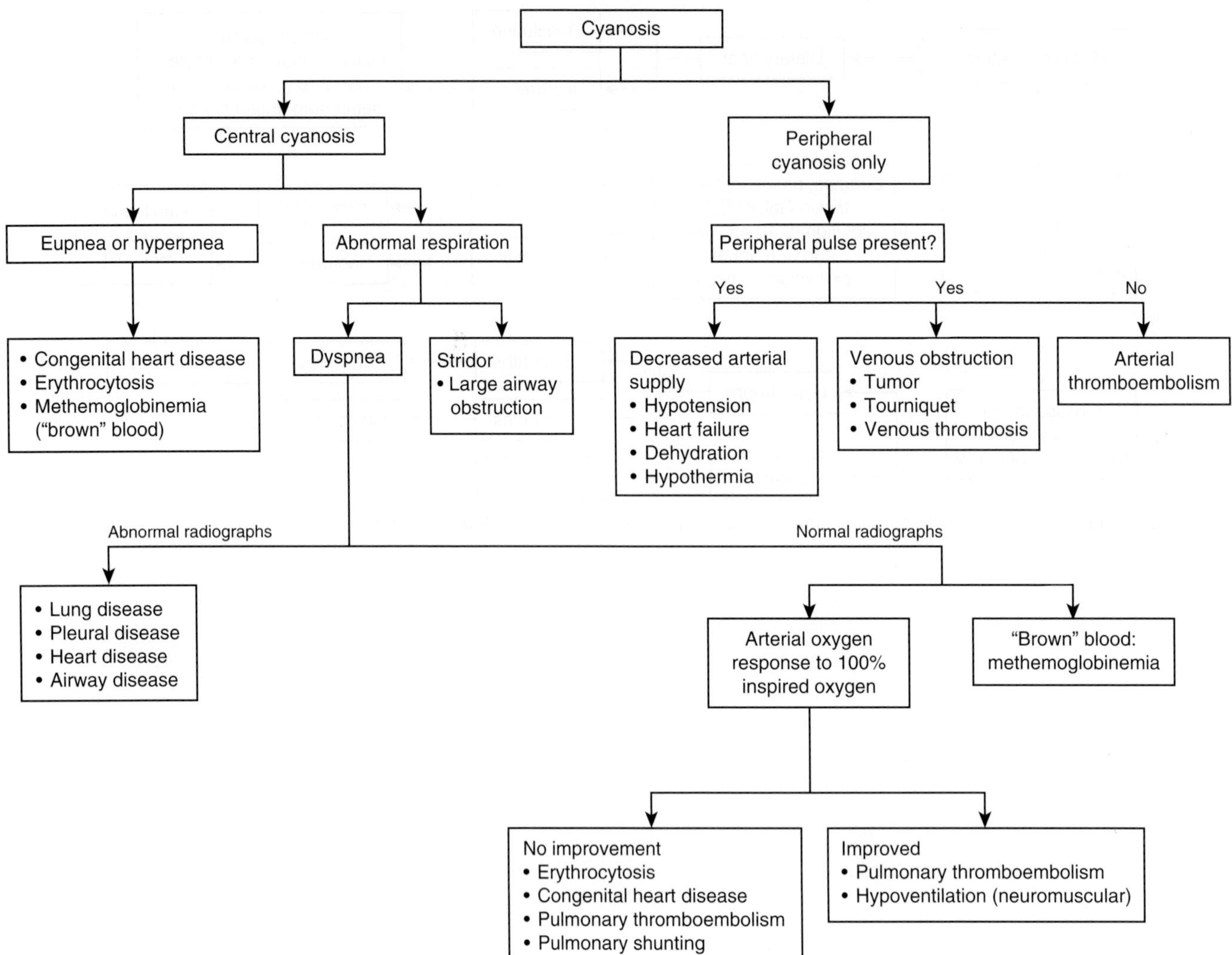
Cyanosis
Central cyanosis
Peripheral cyanosis only
Eupnea or hyperpnea
Abnormal respiration
Peripheral pulse present?
Yes
Yes
No
• Congenital heart disease
• Erythrocytosis
• Methemoglobinemia ("brown" blood)
Dyspnea
Stridor
• Large airway obstruction
Decreased arterial supply
• Hypotension
• Heart failure
• Dehydration
• Hypothermia
Venous obstruction
• Tumor
• Tourniquet
• Venous thrombosis
Arterial thromboembolism
Abnormal radiographs
Normal radiographs
• Lung disease
• Pleural disease
• Heart disease
• Airway disease
Arterial oxygen response to 100% inspired oxygen
"Brown" blood: methemoglobinemia
No improvement
• Erythrocytosis
• Congenital heart disease
• Pulmonary thromboembolism
• Pulmonary shunting
Improved
• Pulmonary thromboembolism
• Hypoventilation (neuromuscular)

Diabetes Insipidus

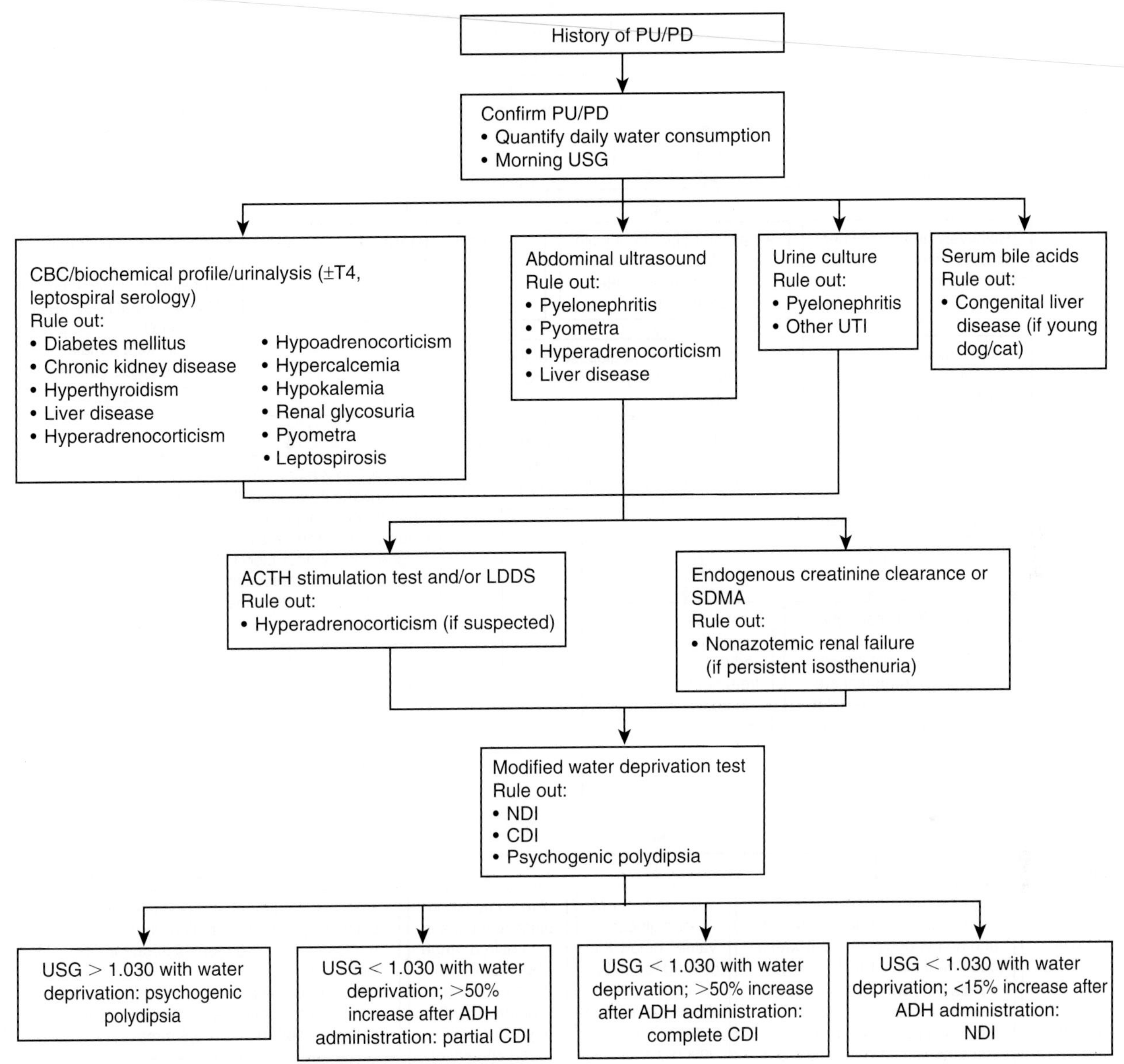

ACTH, Adrenocorticotropic hormone; *ADH,* antidiuretic hormone; *CBC,* complete blood count; *CDI,* central diabetes insipidus; *LDDS,* low-dose dexamethasone suppression test; *NDI,* nephrogenic diabetes insipidus; *PU/PD,* polyuria/polydipsia; *SDMA,* symmetric dimethylarginine; *USG,* urine specific gravity; *UTI,* urinary tract infection.

UPDATED AND EDITED BY: Leah A. Cohn, DVM, PhD, DACVIM
ORIGINALLY WRITTEN BY: Sarah L. Naidoo, DVM, MSc, DACVIM

Clinical Algorithms

Diabetes Mellitus: Treatment

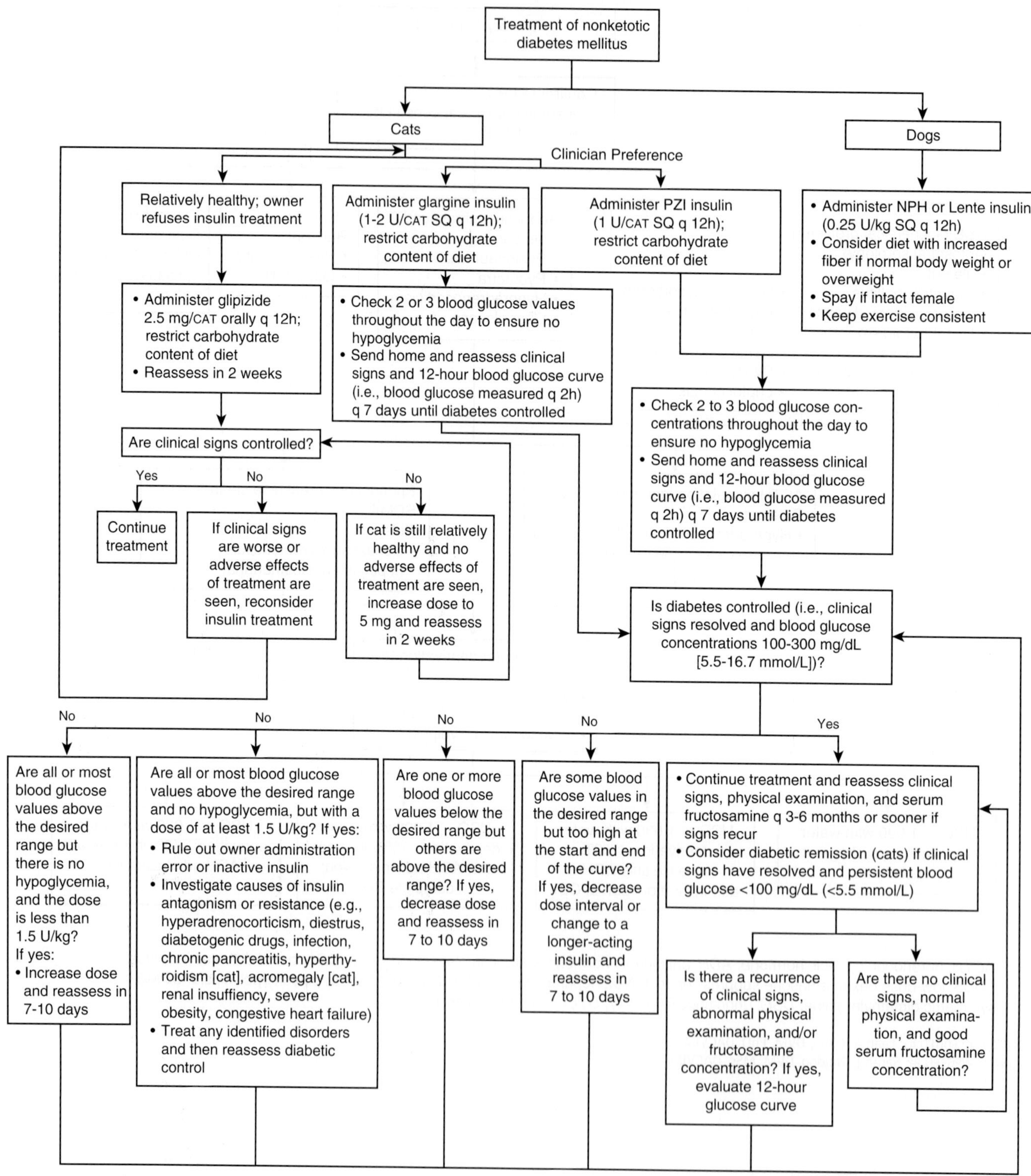

NPH, Neutral protamine Hagedorn; *PZI*, protamine zinc insulin; *SQ*, subcutaneous.

UPDATED AND EDITED BY: Leah A. Cohn, DVM, PhD, DACVIM
ORIGINALLY WRITTEN BY: Sherri Ihle

Diarrhea, Large Bowel

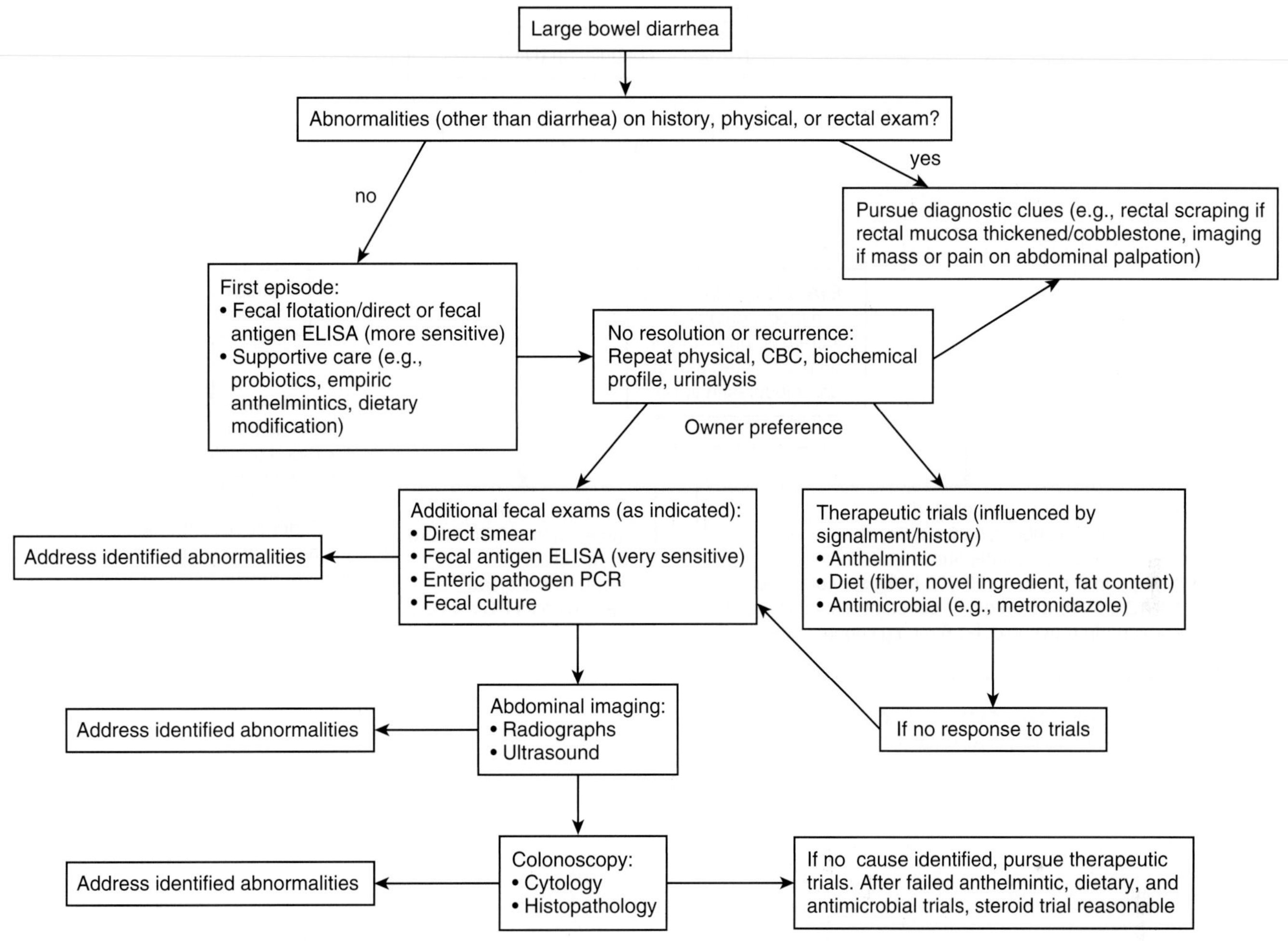

Clinical Algorithms

Disseminated Intravascular Coagulation

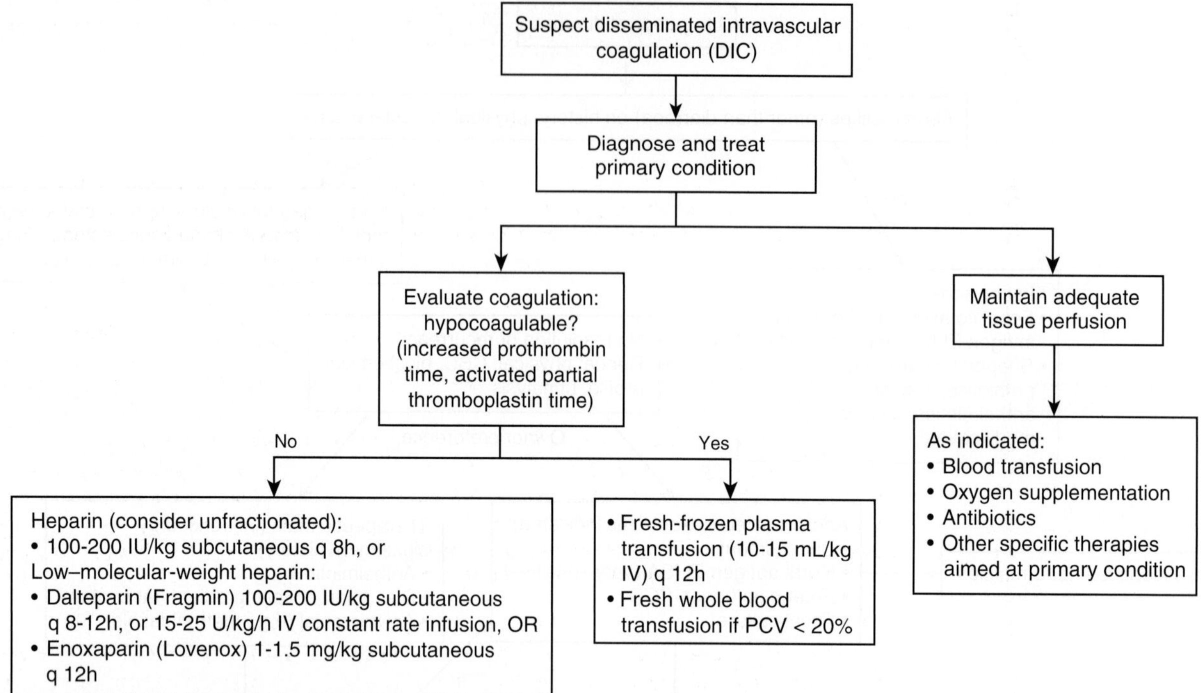

UPDATED AND EDITED BY: Leah A. Cohn, DVM, PhD, DACVIM
ORIGINALLY WRITTEN BY: Scott P. Shaw, DVM, DACVECC

Draining Tracts, Cutaneous

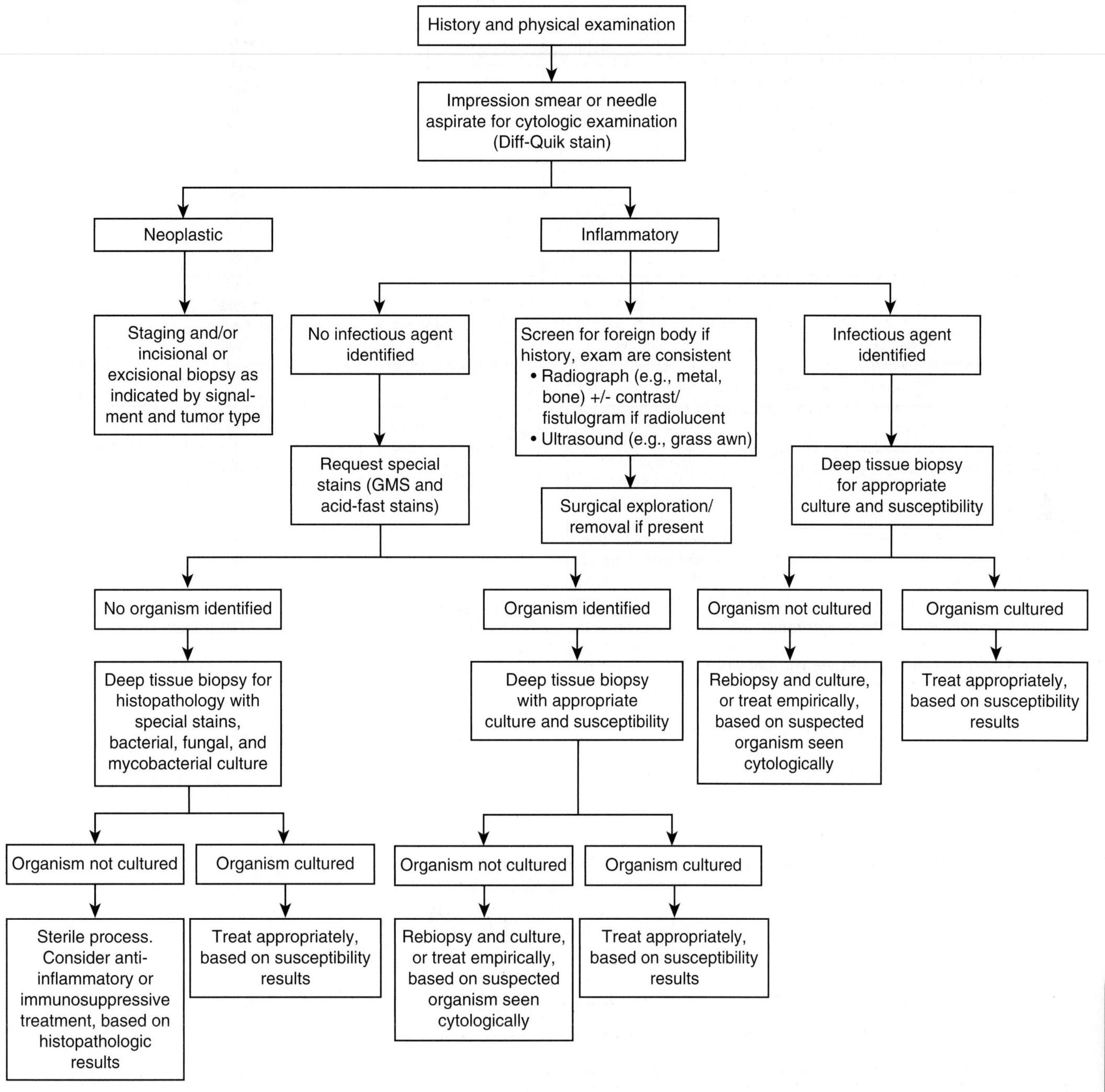

GMS, Gömöri methenamine silver.
(Reproduced from the third edition in unabridged form)

THIRD EDITION AUTHOR: Andrew Lowe, DVM, MSc, DACVD
THIRD EDITION EDITOR: Manon Paradis, DVM, MVSc, DACVD

Clinical Algorithms

Dyspnea and Respiratory Distress: Hospital-Acquired

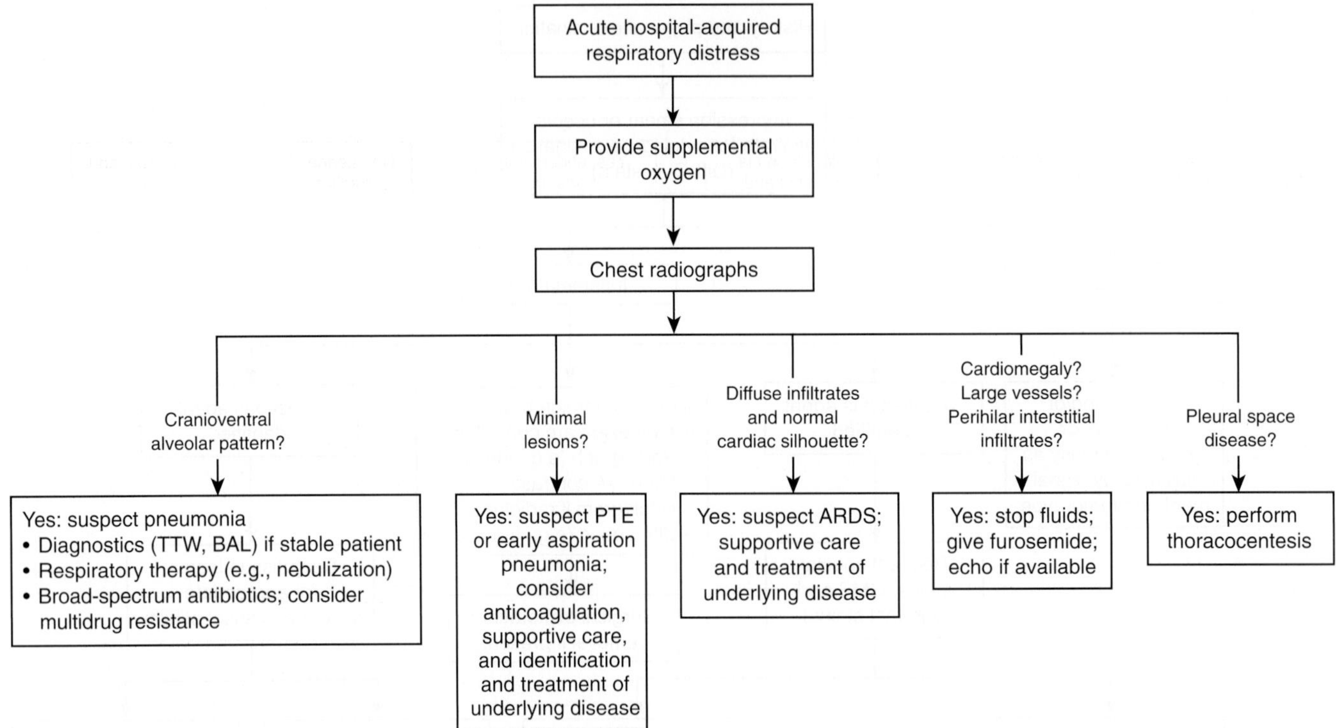

ARDS, Acute respiratory distress syndrome; *BAL,* bronchoalveolar lavage; *PTE,* pulmonary thromboembolism; *TTW,* transtracheal wash.

UPDATED AND EDITED BY: Leah A. Cohn, DVM, PhD, DACVIM
ORIGINALLY WRITTEN BY: Scott P. Shaw, DVM, DACVECC

Dystocia

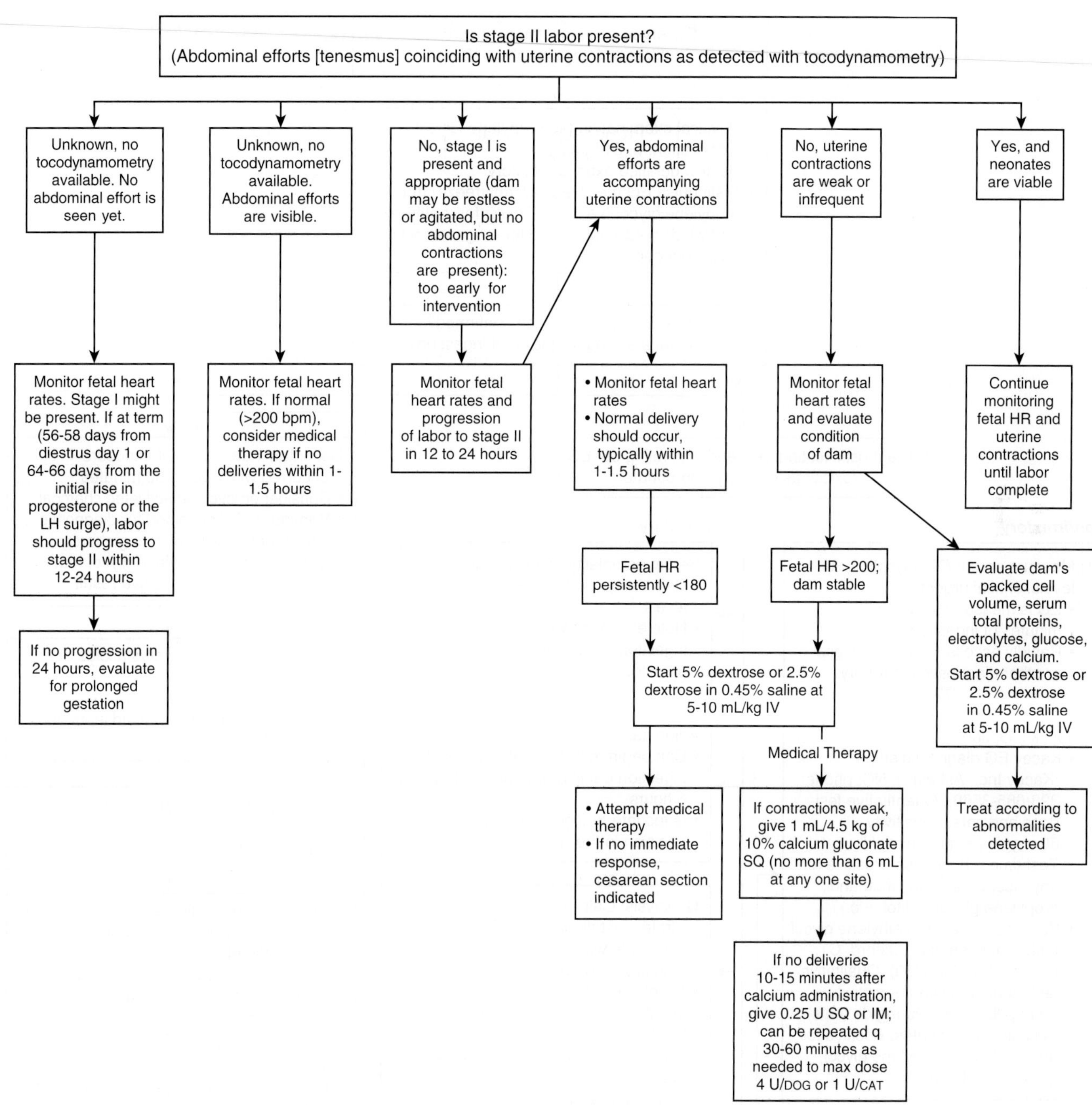

AUTHOR: Autumn P. Davidson, DVM, MS, DACVIM
EDITOR: Michelle A. Kutzler, DVM, PhD, DACT

Clinical Algorithms

Ethylene Glycol Intoxication

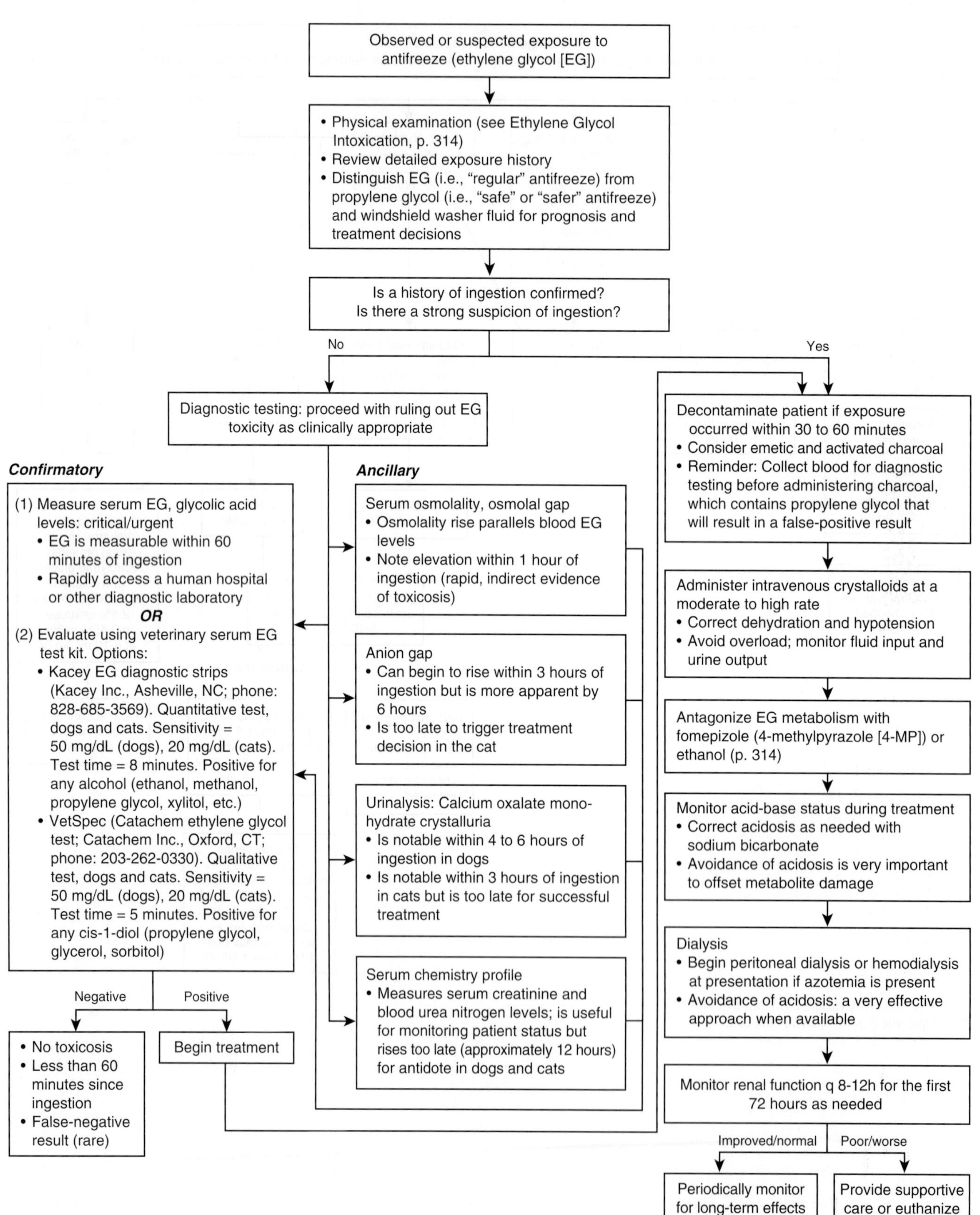

UPDATED AND EDITED BY: Leah A. Cohn, DVM, PhD, DACVIM
ORIGINALLY WRITTEN BY: Michael W. Knight, DVM, DABVT, DABT

Feline Lower Urinary Tract Signs

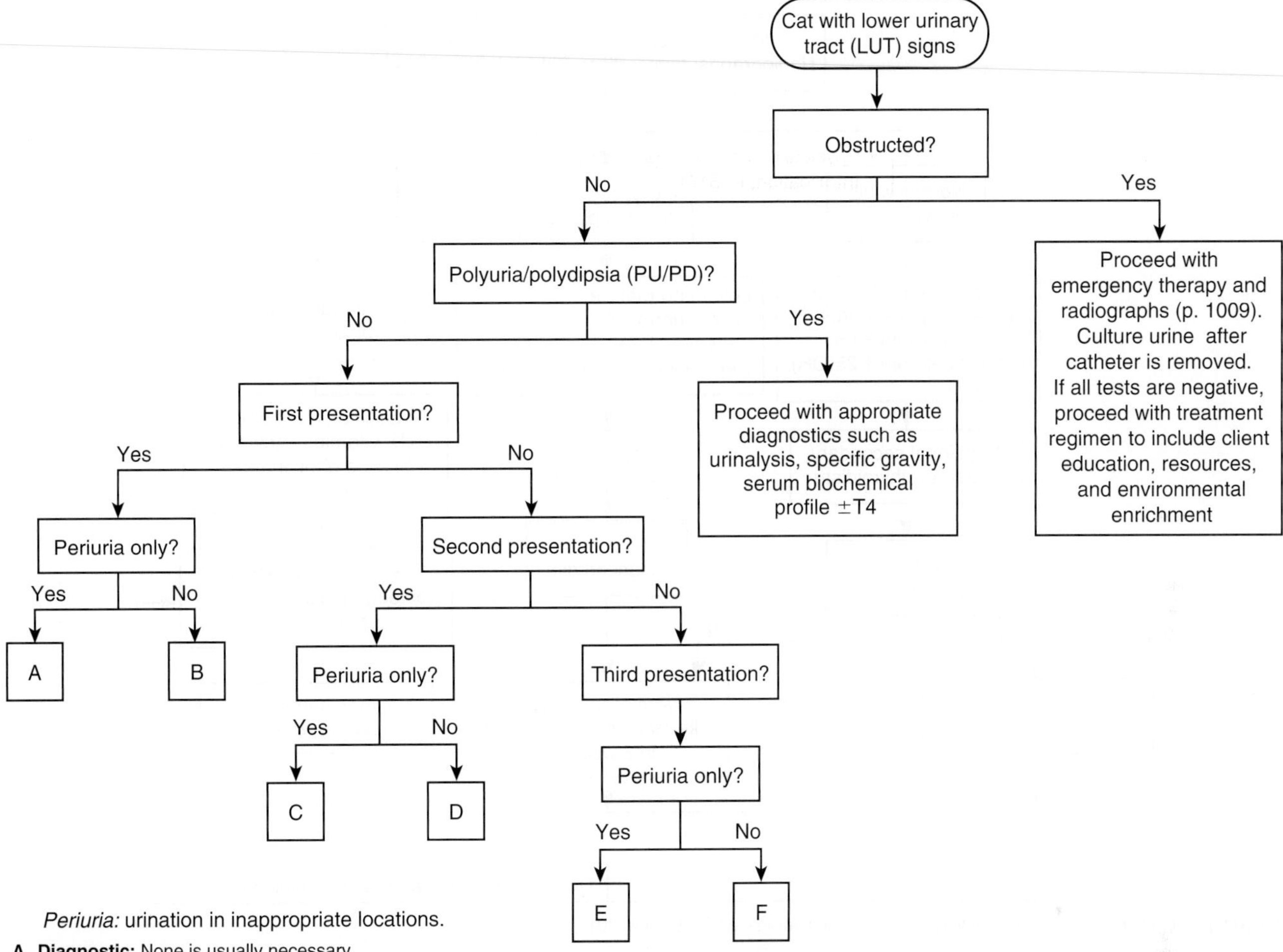

Periuria: urination in inappropriate locations.

A Diagnostic: None is usually necessary.
Treatment: Address litter box management and cleaning of soiled areas. (see Inappropriate Elimination, Cat p. 533)
Medications: No medications are recommended.

B Diagnostic: A radiograph should be considered, especially if hematuria is present.
Treatment: If the radiograph is negative, therapy should include analgesia for 2 to 3 days during the acute episode. Litter box management and cleaning of soiled areas should be addressed.
Medications: No medications are recommended.

C Diagnostic: A urinalysis is recommended. If submaximal urine specific gravity is present, then appropriate diagnostics are needed.
Treatment: If diagnostic tests are negative, then the resource checklist* should be reviewed and additional areas that were not previously addressed should be incorporated.
Medications: Pheromone therapy is recommended.

D Diagnostic: A radiograph, urinalysis, and urine culture are recommended.
Treatment: If all tests are negative, analgesia should be provided for 2 to 3 days during acute episode. Canned food is encouraged for the cat in addition to litter box management and cleaning of soiled areas. The cat's urine specity gravity is monitored for 3 to 4 weeks to assess the cat's water intake.
Medications: Pheromone therapy is recommended.

E Diagnostic: A urinalysis should be performed if it has not already been done. Radiographs, urine culture, and biochemical profile are also recommended.
Treatment: If all tests are negative, then the resource checklist* is formally reviewed and those areas that have not already been addressed should be incorporated. Further information for cleaning soiled areas should be provided. Additional resources (websites, books) on how to provide an enhanced indoor environment for cats should be provided to clients. Intercat conflict issues should also be addressed.
Medications: Pheromone therapy should be used in conjunction with behavior-altering medications such as tricyclic antidepressants (TCAs) or buspirone. The medication should be taken for 4 weeks; if no improvement is seen, a referral for further diagnostics and consultation should be considered.

F Diagnostic: A radiograph, a urinalysis, and a urine culture should be performed. A complete blood count (CBC) and biochemical profile should also be submitted. If all tests are negative, a contrast study or abdominal ultrasound of the bladder and urethra should be considered to rule out radiolucent calculi and other mass lesions.
Treatment: If all diagnostics are negative, analgesia should be provided for 2 to 3 days during acute episode. In addition to canned food, ensure that water consumption is sufficient. Water should be viewed as a "drug," and the cat's urine specific gravity should be monitored (goal: submaximal concentration, e.g., urine specific gravity < 1.040) to evaluate water intake. The resource checklist* should be formally reviewed, and those areas that have not already been addressed should be incorporated. Additional resources (websites, books) on how to provide an enhanced indoor environment for cats and information on litterbox hygiene should be provided (see client handout How to Reduce Inappropriate Elimination by Litterbox Hygiene) to clients. Intercat conflict issues should also be addressed. Follow-up and support for clients are essential.
Medications: Pheromone therapy should be used in conjunction with behavior-altering medications such as TCAs or anxiolytics. Medication should be taken for 4 weeks; if no improvement is seen, a referral for further diagnostics such as a cystoscopy should be considered.

*Additional materials available at http://indoorpet.osu.edu/index.cfm.
(Modified from Ettinger SJ, Feldman EC: Textbook of veterinary internal medicine, ed 6, St. Louis, 2005, Saunders.)

Clinical Algorithms

Fractures, Multiple Pathologic

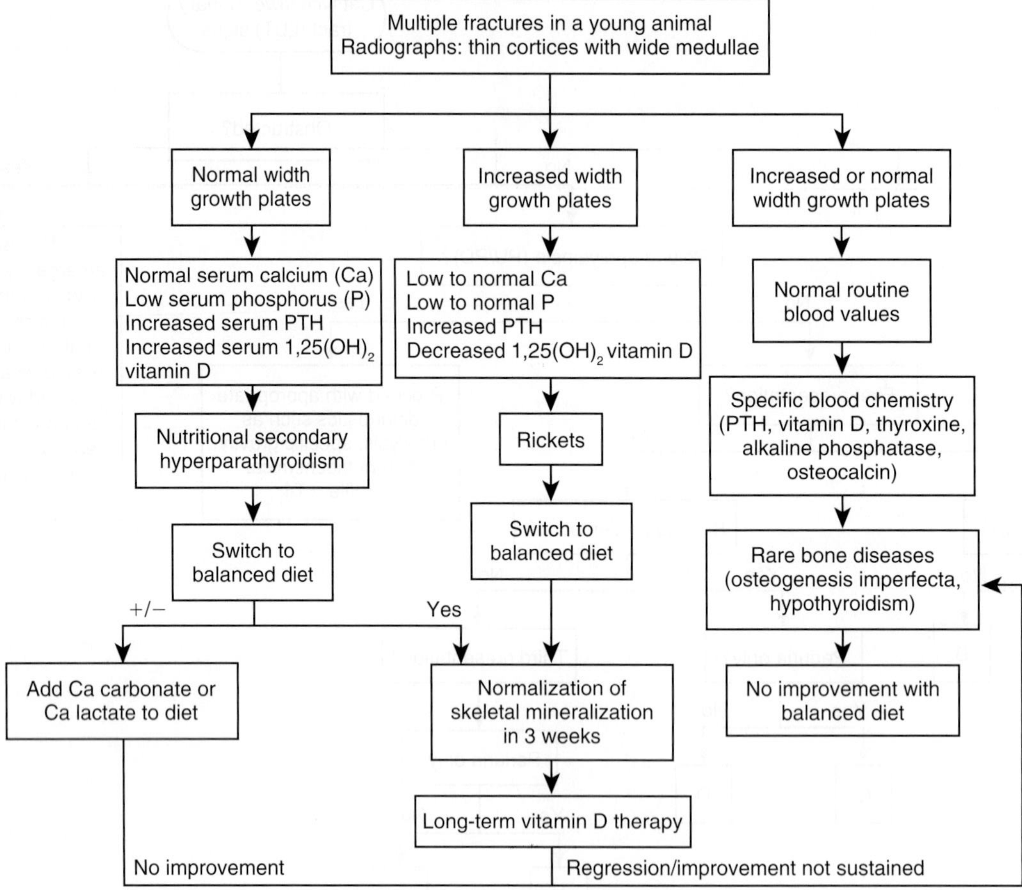

(From Ettinger SJ, Feldman EC: Textbook of veterinary internal medicine, ed 7, St. Louis, 2010, Elsevier.)

Glaucoma

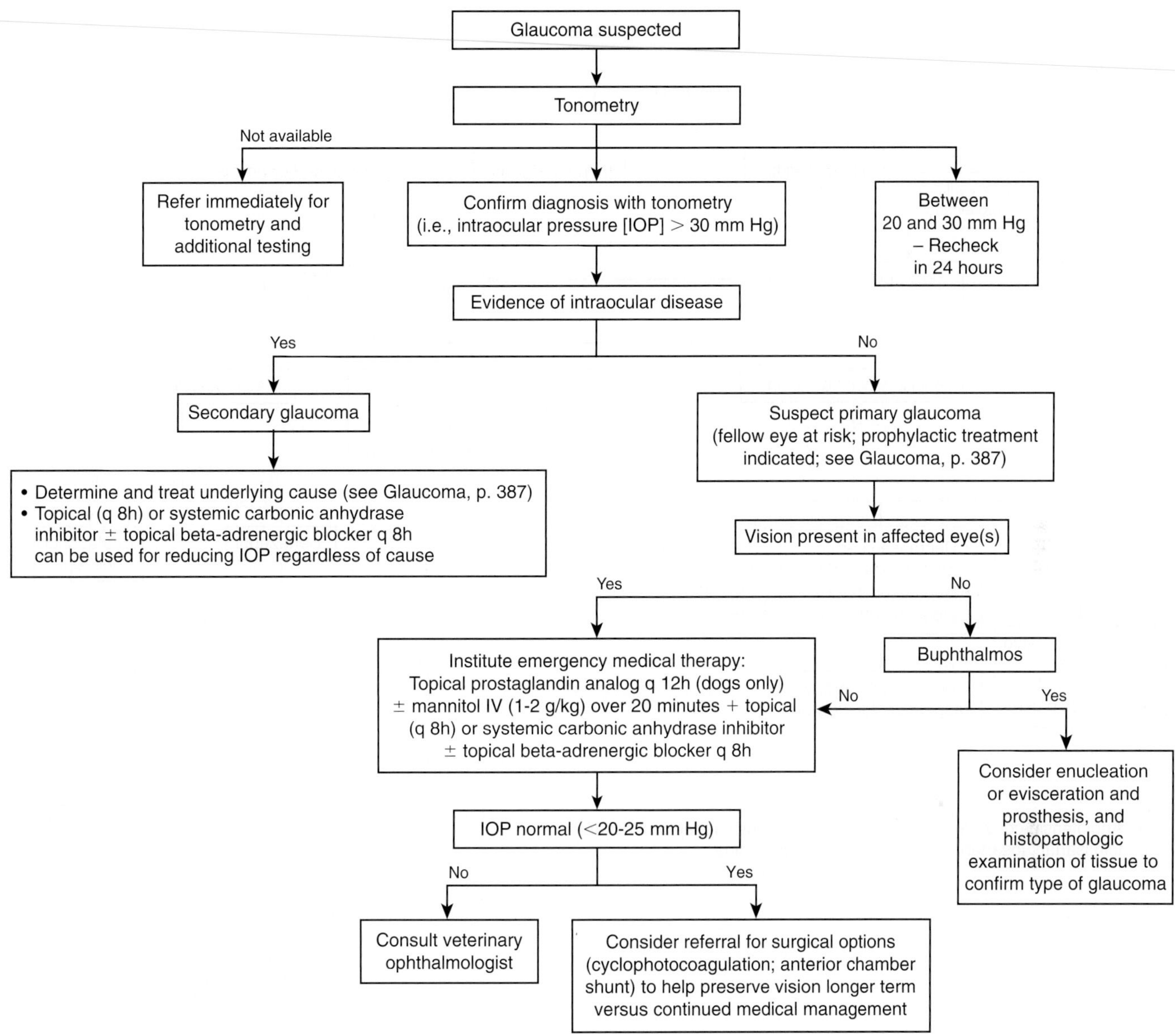

UPDATED AND EDITED BY: Leah A. Cohn, DVM, PhD, DACVIM
ORIGINALLY WRITTEN BY: Cheryl L. Cullen, DVM, MVetSc, DACVO

Glomerulonephritis: Management

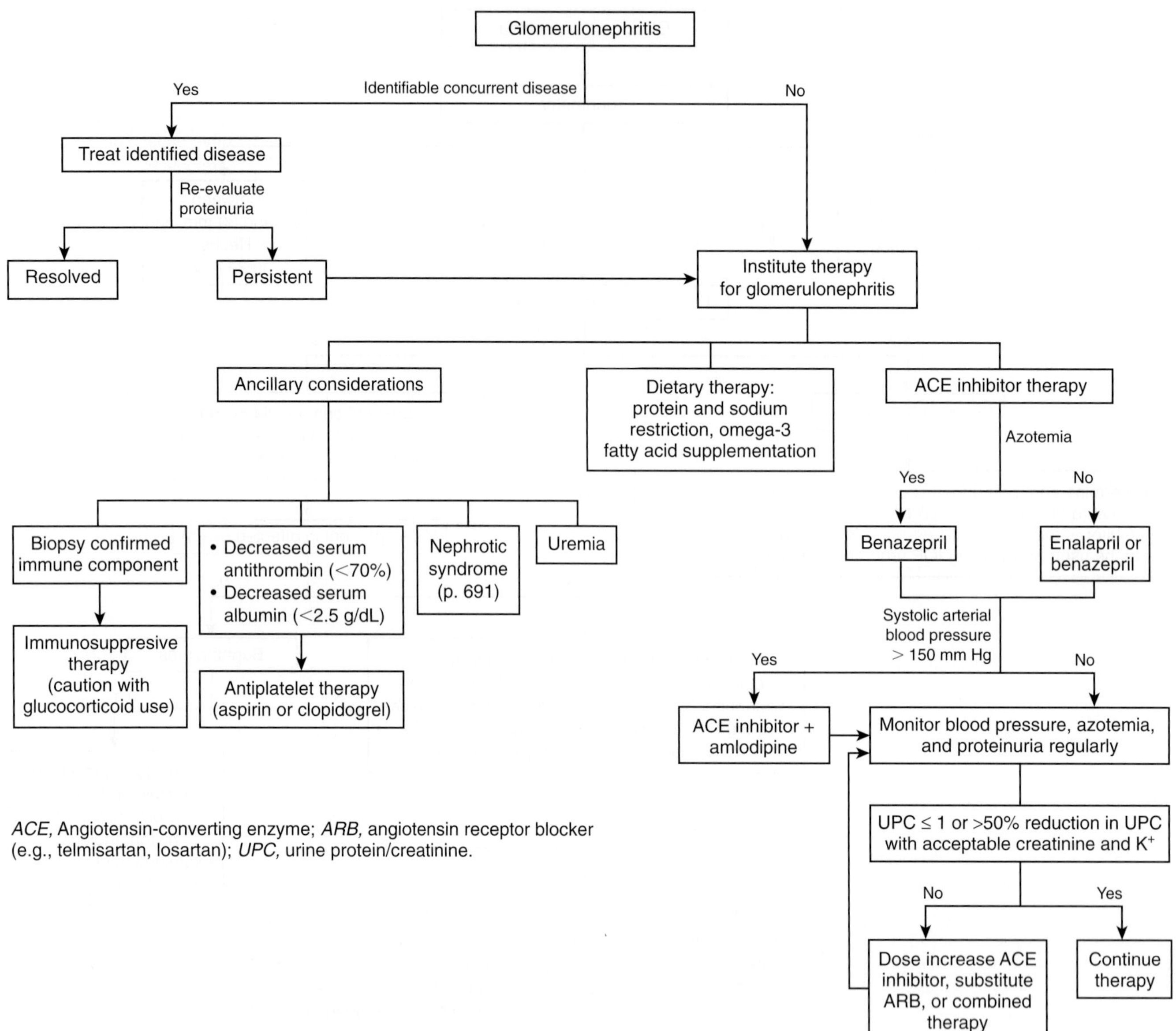

ACE, Angiotensin-converting enzyme; *ARB,* angiotensin receptor blocker (e.g., telmisartan, losartan); *UPC,* urine protein/creatinine.

UPDATED AND EDITED BY: Leah A. Cohn, DVM, PhD, DACVIM
ORIGINALLY WRITTEN BY: Anne M. Dalby, DVM, DACVIM

Head Trauma

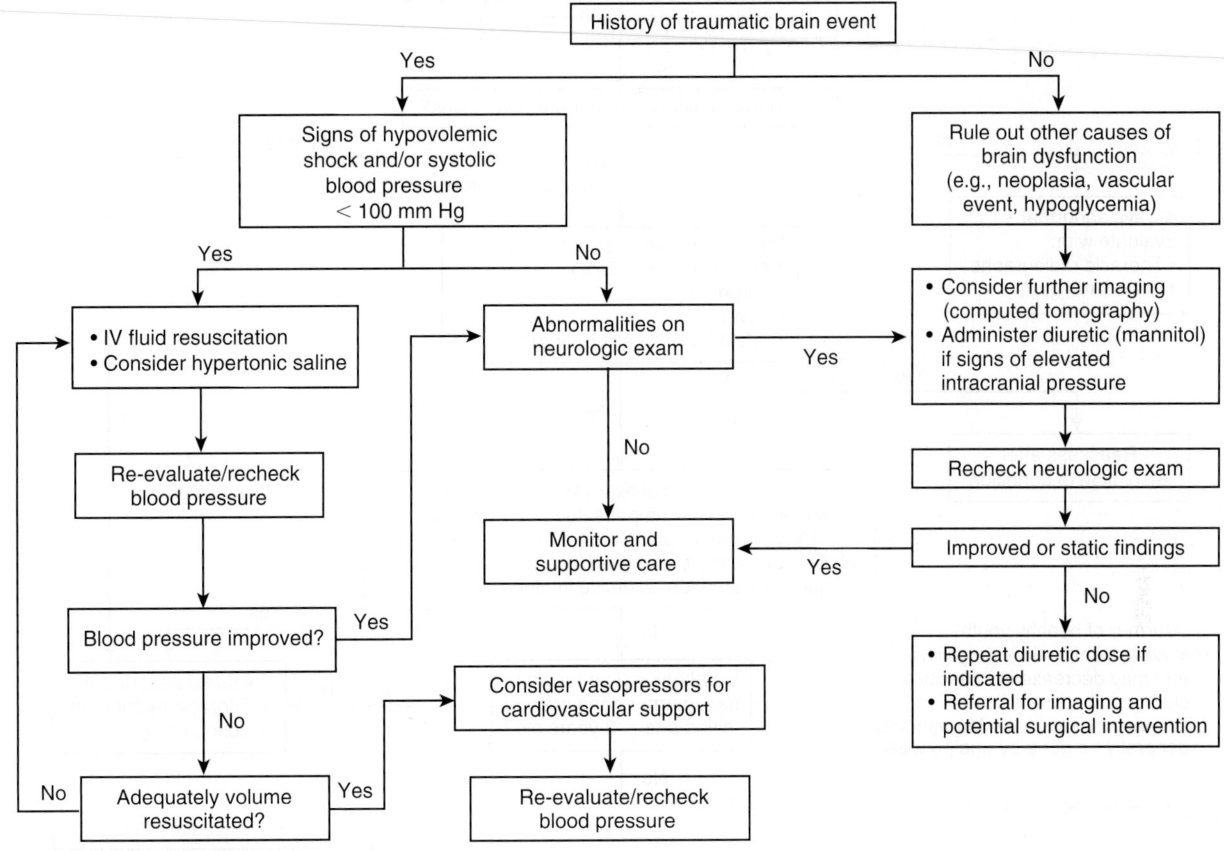

EDITED BY: Leah A. Cohn, DVM, PhD, DACVIM
ORIGINALLY WRITTEN BY: Scott P. Shaw, DVM, DACVECC

Clinical Algorithms

Heart Murmur: Incidental Finding ("Asymptomatic")

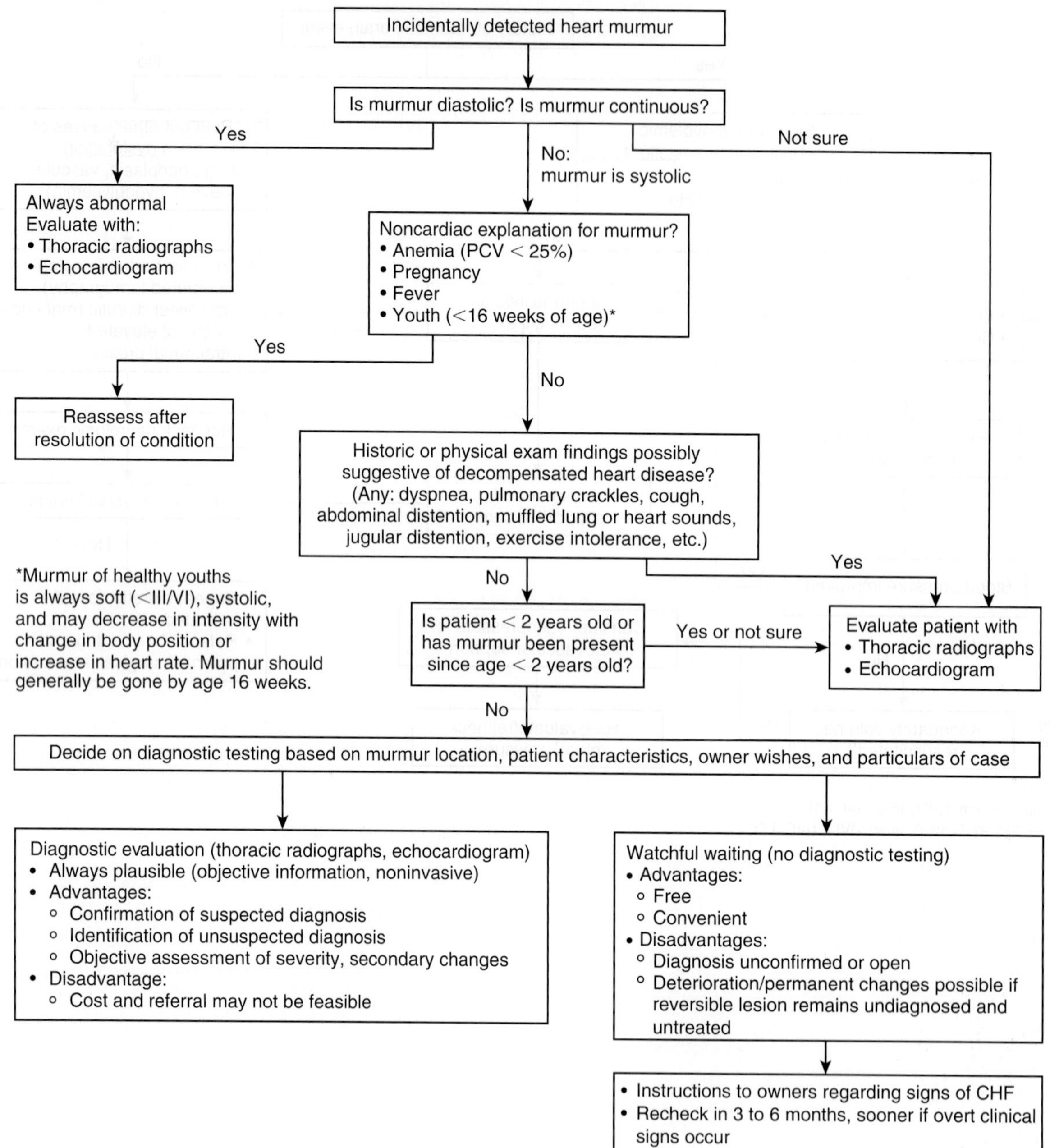

CHF, Congestive heart failure; *PCV*, packed cell volume.

AUTHOR & EDITOR: Etienne Côté, DVM, DACVIM

Heartworm Disease: Management

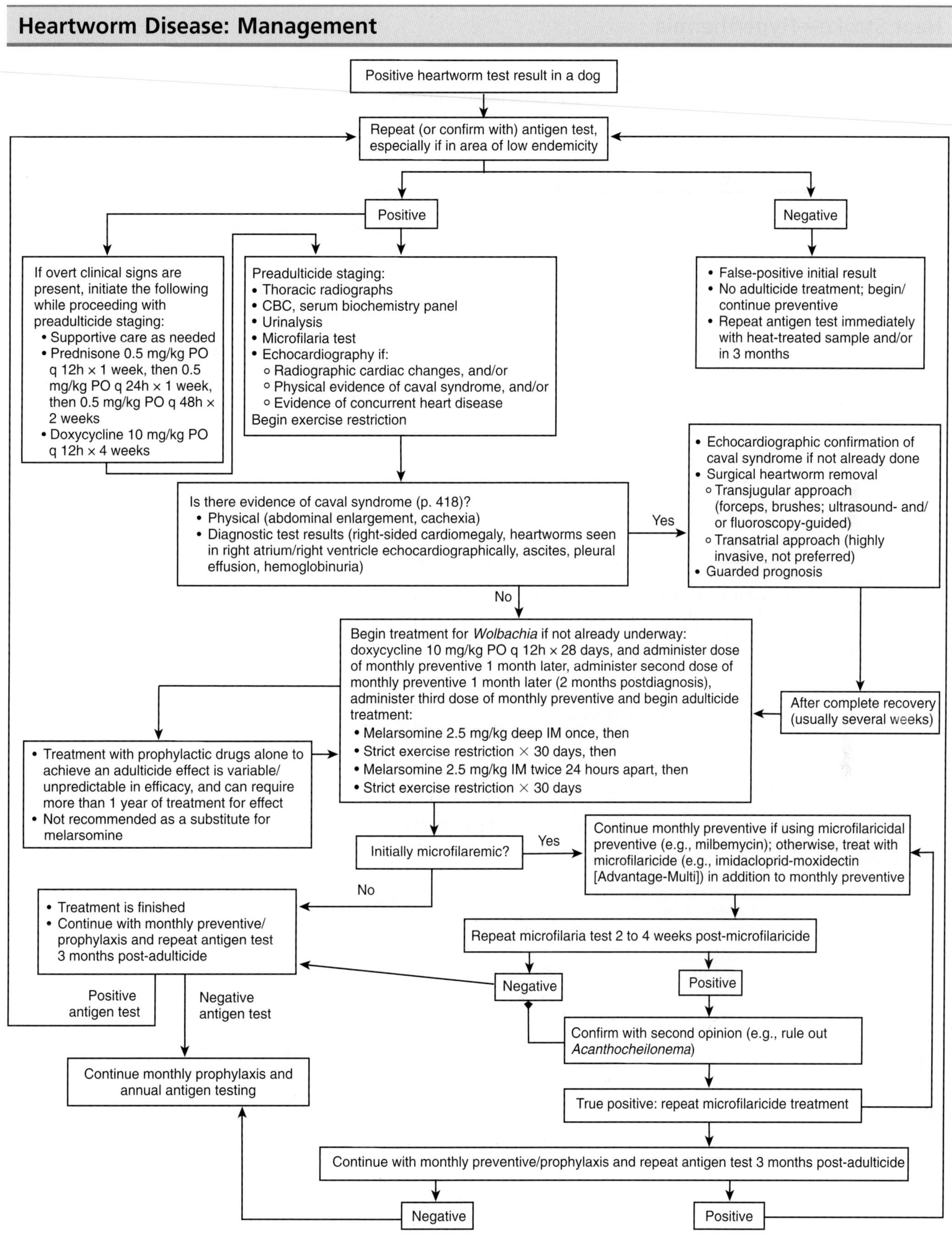

CBC, Complete blood count; *IM,* intramuscular.
Additional information available on the American Heartworm Society website: www.heartwormsociety.org.

AUTHOR & EDITOR: Etienne Côté, DVM, DACVIM

Heat Stroke—Hyperthermia

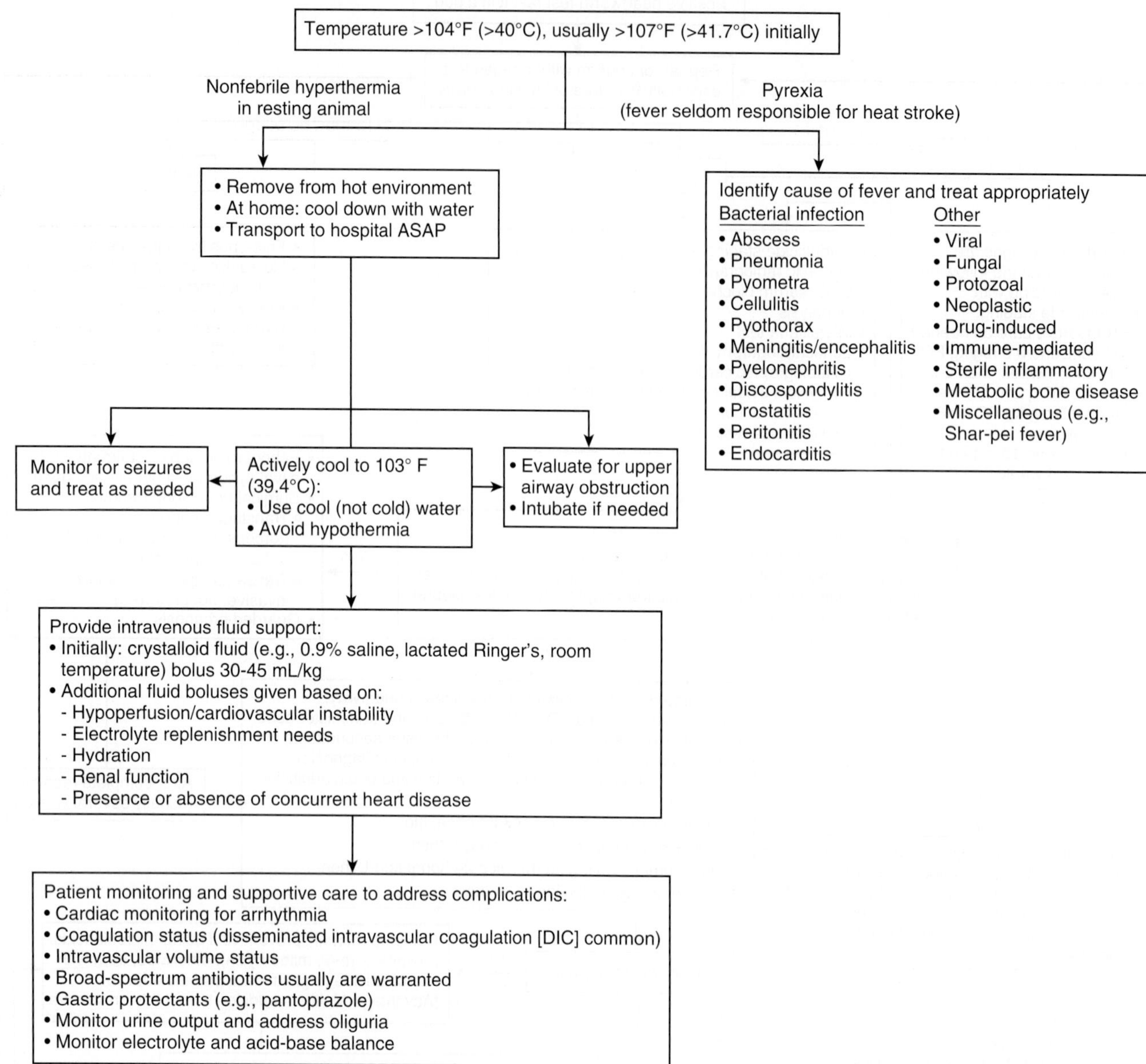

UPDATED AND EDITED BY: Leah A. Cohn, DVM, PhD, DACVIM
ORIGINALLY WRITTEN BY: Scott P. Shaw, DVM, DACVECC

Hip Dysplasia

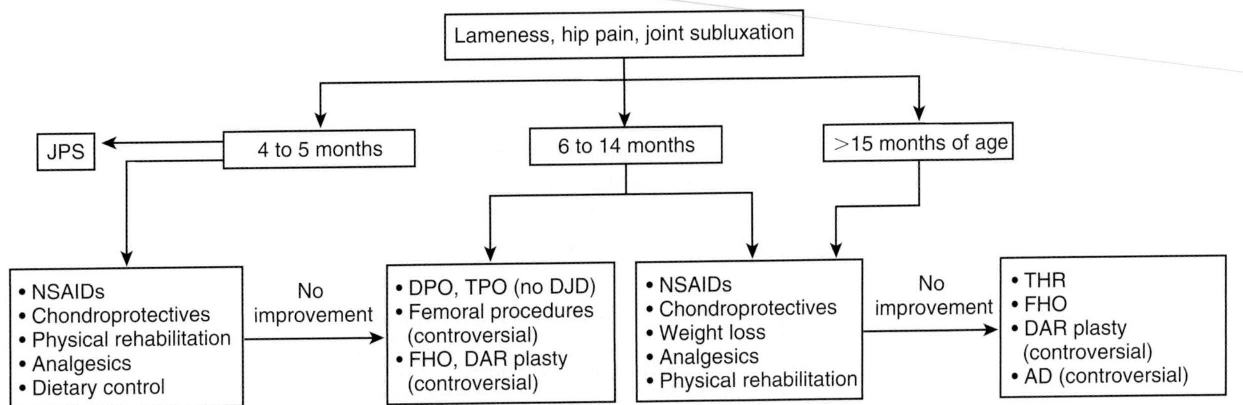

AD, Acetabulum denervation; *DAR* plasty, dorsal acetabular rim arthroplasty; *DJD,* degenerative joint disease; *DPO,* double pelvic osteotomy; *FHO,* femoral head/neck ostectomy; *JPS,* juvenile pubic symphysiodesis; *NSAIDs,* nonsteroidal antiinflammatory drugs; *THR,* total hip replacement; *TPO,* triple pelvic osteotomy.

EDITED BY: Leah A. Cohn, DVM, PhD, DACVIM
ORIGINALLY WRITTEN BY: Joseph Harari, DVM, MS, DACVS

Hit by Car

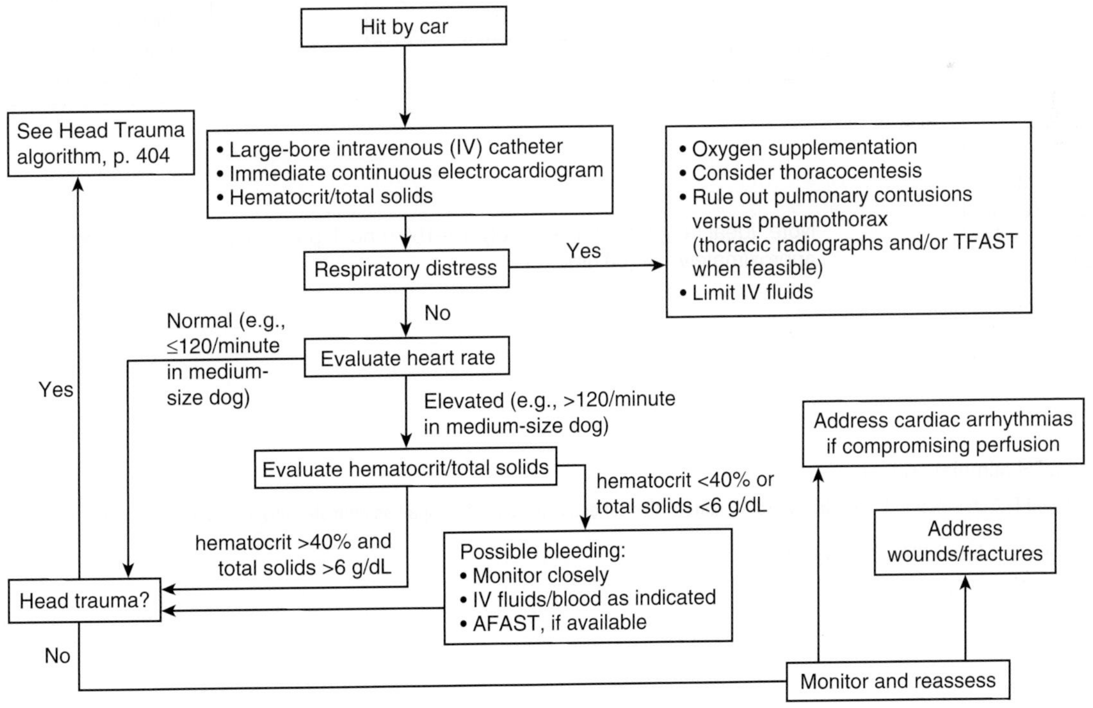

AFAST, Abdominal focused ultrasound for triage/trauma; *TFAST,* thoracic focused ultrasound for triage/trauma.

UPDATED AND EDITED BY: Leah A. Cohn, DVM, PhD, DACVIM
ORIGINALLY WRITTEN BY: Scott P. Shaw, DVM, DACVECC

Clinical Algorithms

Hyperadrenocorticism: Mitotane Induction for Pituitary Disease

See also the *Mitotane Maintenance for Pituitary Disease* algorithm.

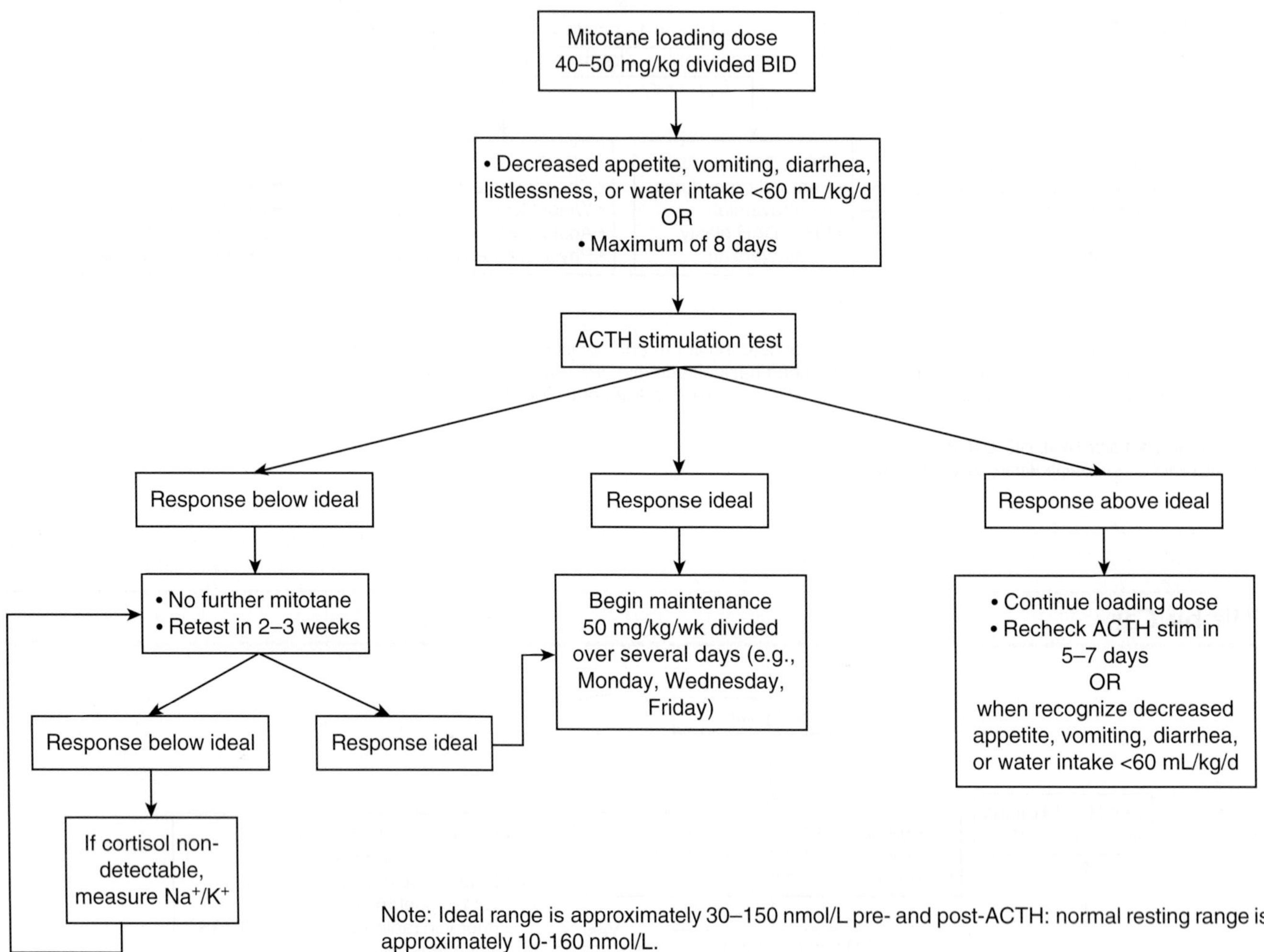

ACTH stim, ACTH stimulation test.

(From Rand J, Behrend E, Gunn-Moore D, Campbell-Ward M, editors: Clinical endocrinology of companion animals. New York: Wiley-Blackwell, 2013.)

AUTHOR & EDITOR: Ellen N. Behrend, VMD, PhD, DACVIM

Hyperadrenocorticism: Trilostane Therapy

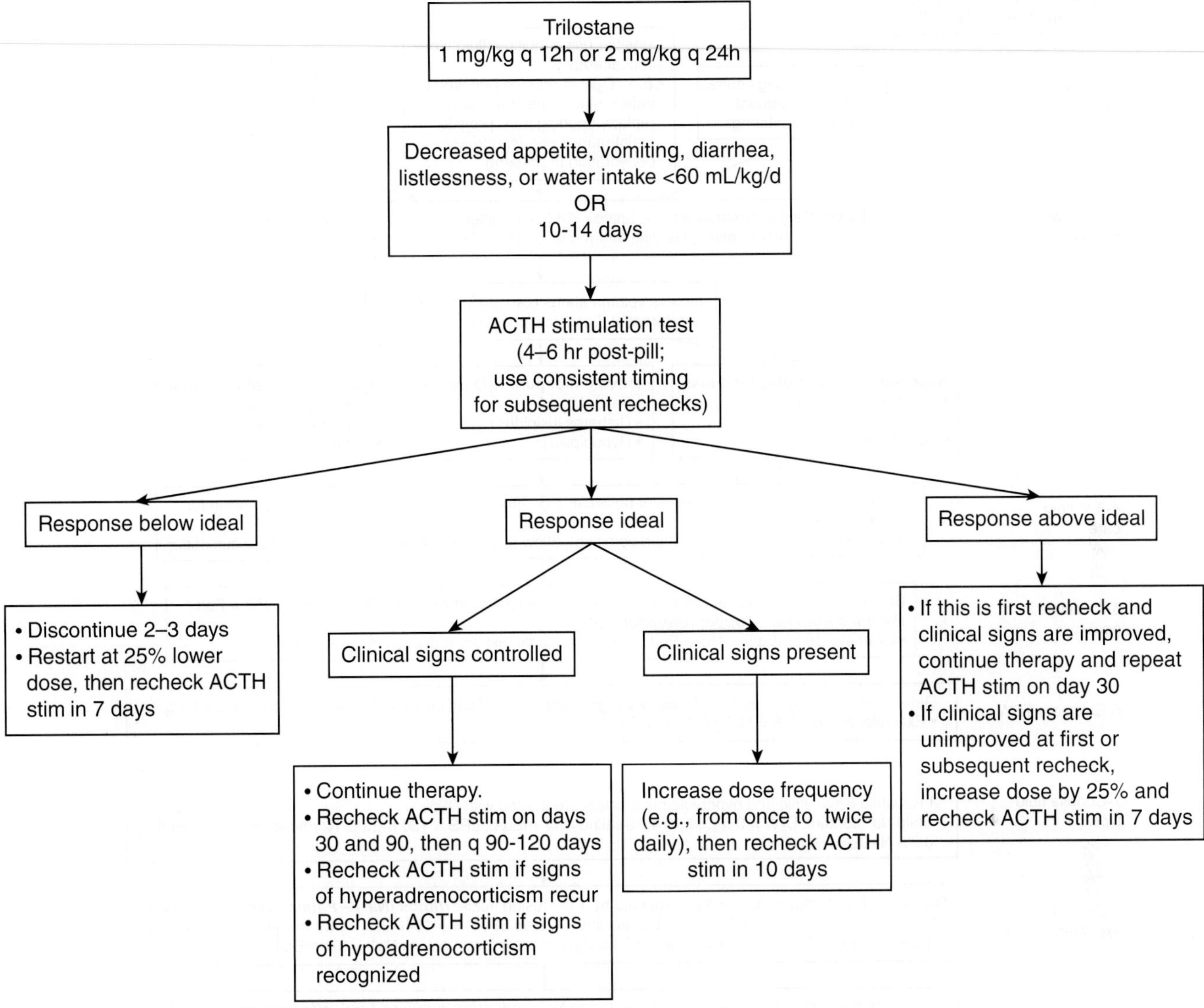

Note: Ideal range is 30–150 nmol/L pre- and post-ACTH; normal resting range is 10–160 nmol/L.
ACTH stim, ACTH stimulation test.

(From Rand J, Behrend E, Gunn-Moore D, Campbell-Ward M, editors: Clinical endocrinology of companion animals. New York: Wiley-Blackwell, 2013.)

AUTHOR & EDITOR: Ellen N. Behrend, VMD, PhD, DACVIM

Hypernatremia, Correction of

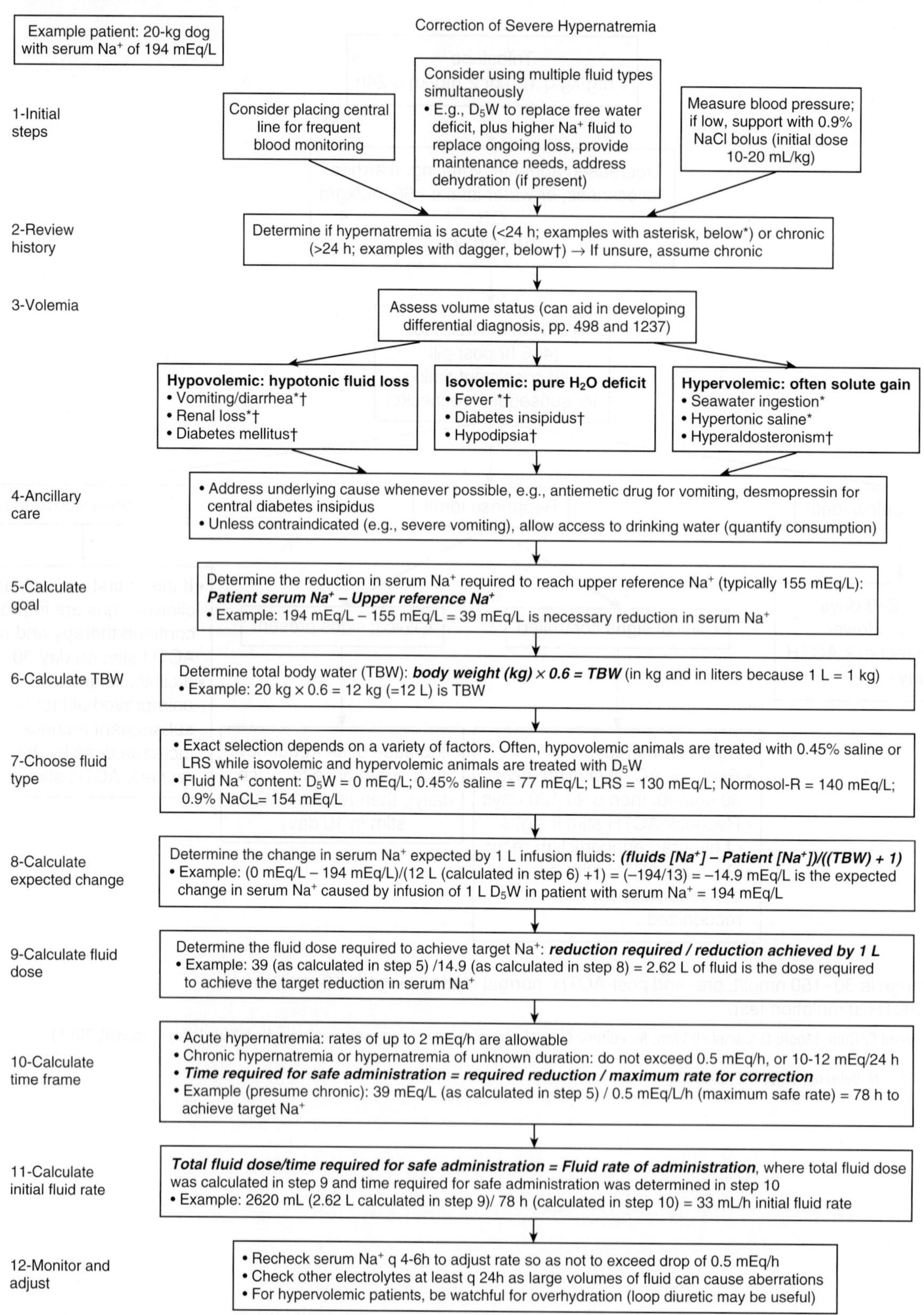

Alternative methods: 1) Same as above, but initially only perform calculations for the first 24 h of care. That is, in step 5 instead of targeting the eventual goal 155 mEq/L Na^+, target a serum Na^+ that is 10 to 12 mEq/L lower than the starting Na^+. In our example case, the 24 h target would be 194 – 12 = 182 mEq/L. At the end of 24 h, recheck serum Na^+ and perform calculations again for the next 24 h. 2) Calculation of water deficit for freewater replacement (may underestimate deficit); water deficit = 0.6 × body weight (kg) × ([patient Na^+/normal Na^+] – 1). 3) Rule of thumb: 3.7 mL/kg/h of D_5W will reduce serum Na^+ by 1 mEq/L/h

AUTHOR & EDITOR: Leah A. Cohn, DVM, PhD, DACVIM

Hypoadrenocorticism

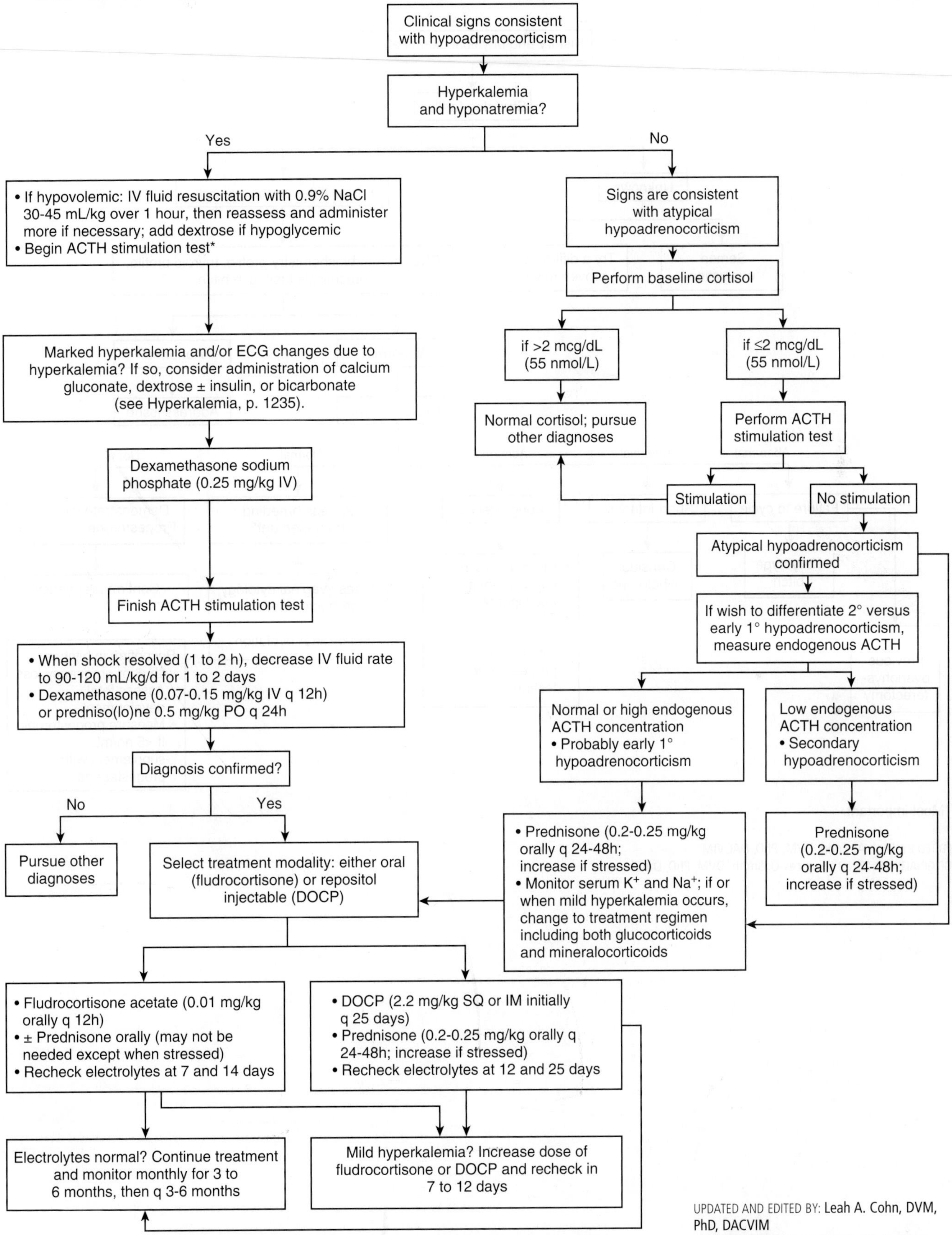

Clinical signs consistent with hypoadrenocorticism

Hyperkalemia and hyponatremia?

Yes

- If hypovolemic: IV fluid resuscitation with 0.9% NaCl 30-45 mL/kg over 1 hour, then reassess and administer more if necessary; add dextrose if hypoglycemic
- Begin ACTH stimulation test*

Marked hyperkalemia and/or ECG changes due to hyperkalemia? If so, consider administration of calcium gluconate, dextrose ± insulin, or bicarbonate (see Hyperkalemia, p. 1235).

Dexamethasone sodium phosphate (0.25 mg/kg IV)

Finish ACTH stimulation test

- When shock resolved (1 to 2 h), decrease IV fluid rate to 90-120 mL/kg/d for 1 to 2 days
- Dexamethasone (0.07-0.15 mg/kg IV q 12h) or predniso(lo)ne 0.5 mg/kg PO q 24h

Diagnosis confirmed?

No: Pursue other diagnoses

Yes: Select treatment modality: either oral (fludrocortisone) or repositol injectable (DOCP)

- Fludrocortisone acetate (0.01 mg/kg orally q 12h)
- ± Prednisone orally (may not be needed except when stressed)
- Recheck electrolytes at 7 and 14 days

- DOCP (2.2 mg/kg SQ or IM initially q 25 days)
- Prednisone (0.2-0.25 mg/kg orally q 24-48h; increase if stressed)
- Recheck electrolytes at 12 and 25 days

Electrolytes normal? Continue treatment and monitor monthly for 3 to 6 months, then q 3-6 months

Mild hyperkalemia? Increase dose of fludrocortisone or DOCP and recheck in 7 to 12 days

No

Signs are consistent with atypical hypoadrenocorticism

Perform baseline cortisol

if >2 mcg/dL (55 nmol/L)

Normal cortisol; pursue other diagnoses

if ≤2 mcg/dL (55 nmol/L)

Perform ACTH stimulation test

Stimulation

No stimulation

Atypical hypoadrenocorticism confirmed

If wish to differentiate 2° versus early 1° hypoadrenocorticism, measure endogenous ACTH

Normal or high endogenous ACTH concentration
- Probably early 1° hypoadrenocorticism

Low endogenous ACTH concentration
- Secondary hypoadrenocorticism

- Prednisone (0.2-0.25 mg/kg orally q 24-48h; increase if stressed)
- Monitor serum K^+ and Na^+; if or when mild hyperkalemia occurs, change to treatment regimen including both glucocorticoids and mineralocorticoids

Prednisone (0.2-0.25 mg/kg orally q 24-48h; increase if stressed)

ACTH, Adrenocorticotropic hormone; *DOCP*, desoxycorticosterone pivalate.

UPDATED AND EDITED BY: Leah A. Cohn, DVM, PhD, DACVIM
ORIGINALLY WRITTEN BY: Cary L. M. Bassett, DVM, DACVIM

Infertility in the Female Dog

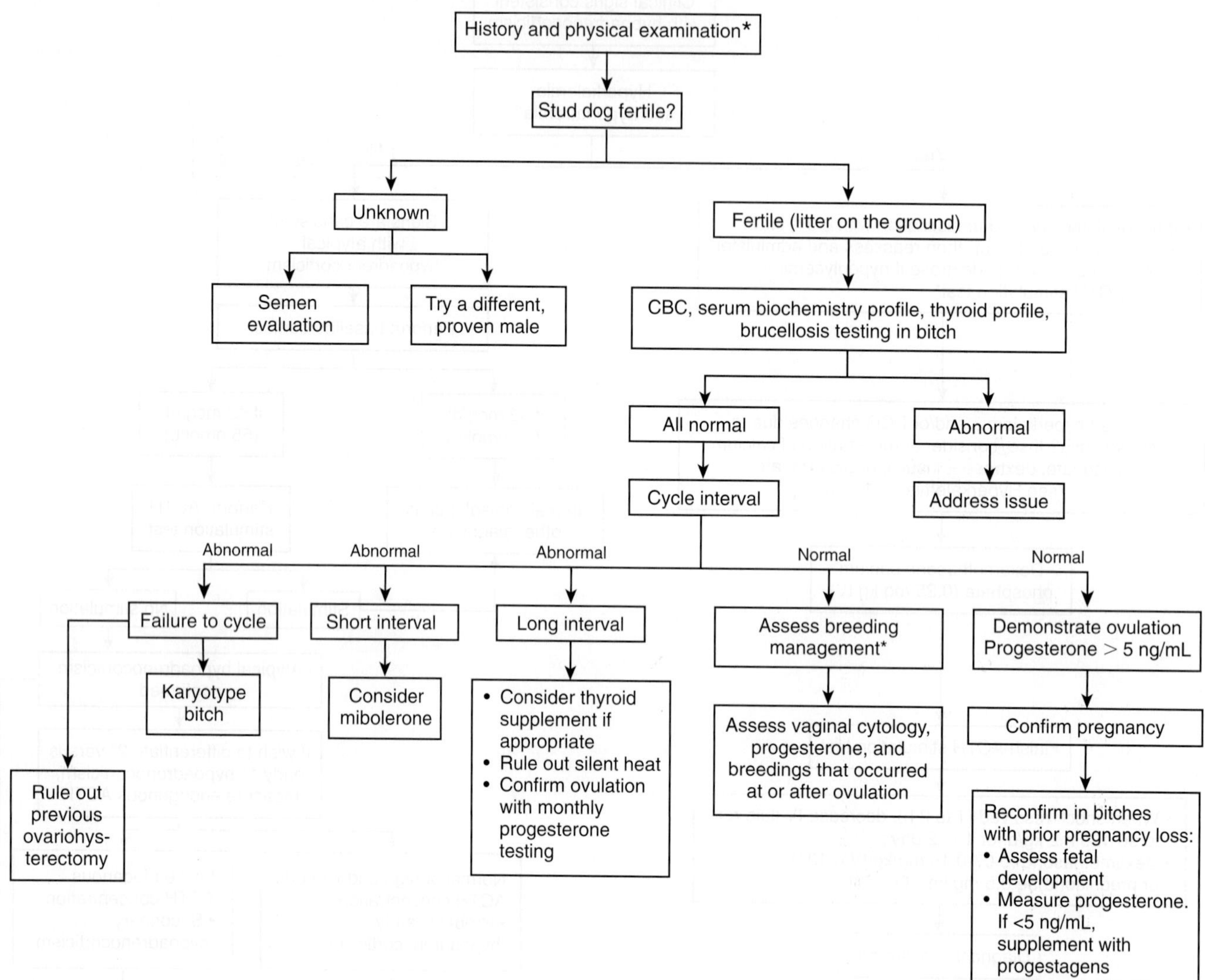

*Most important.

EDITED BY: Leah A. Cohn, DVM, PhD, DACVIM
ORIGINALLY WRITTEN BY: Frances O. Smith, DVM, PhD, DACT

Intervertebral Disc Disease

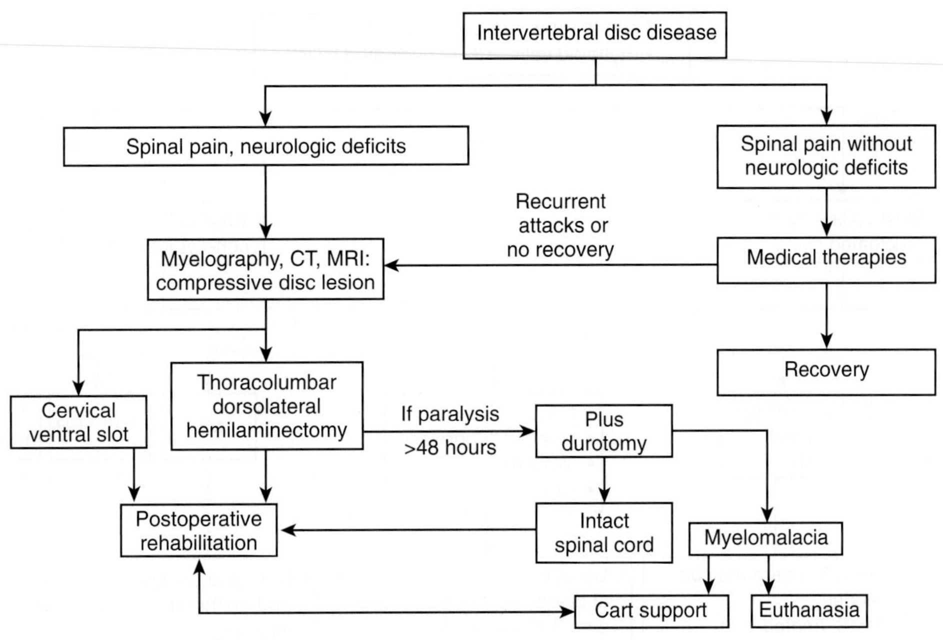

CT, Computed tomography; *K9*, canine; *MRI*, magnetic resonance imaging.

EDITED BY: Leah A. Cohn, DVM, PhD, DACVIM
ORIGINALLY WRITTEN BY: Joseph Harari, DVM, MS, DACVS

Clinical Algorithms

Leukemias: Classification and Treatment

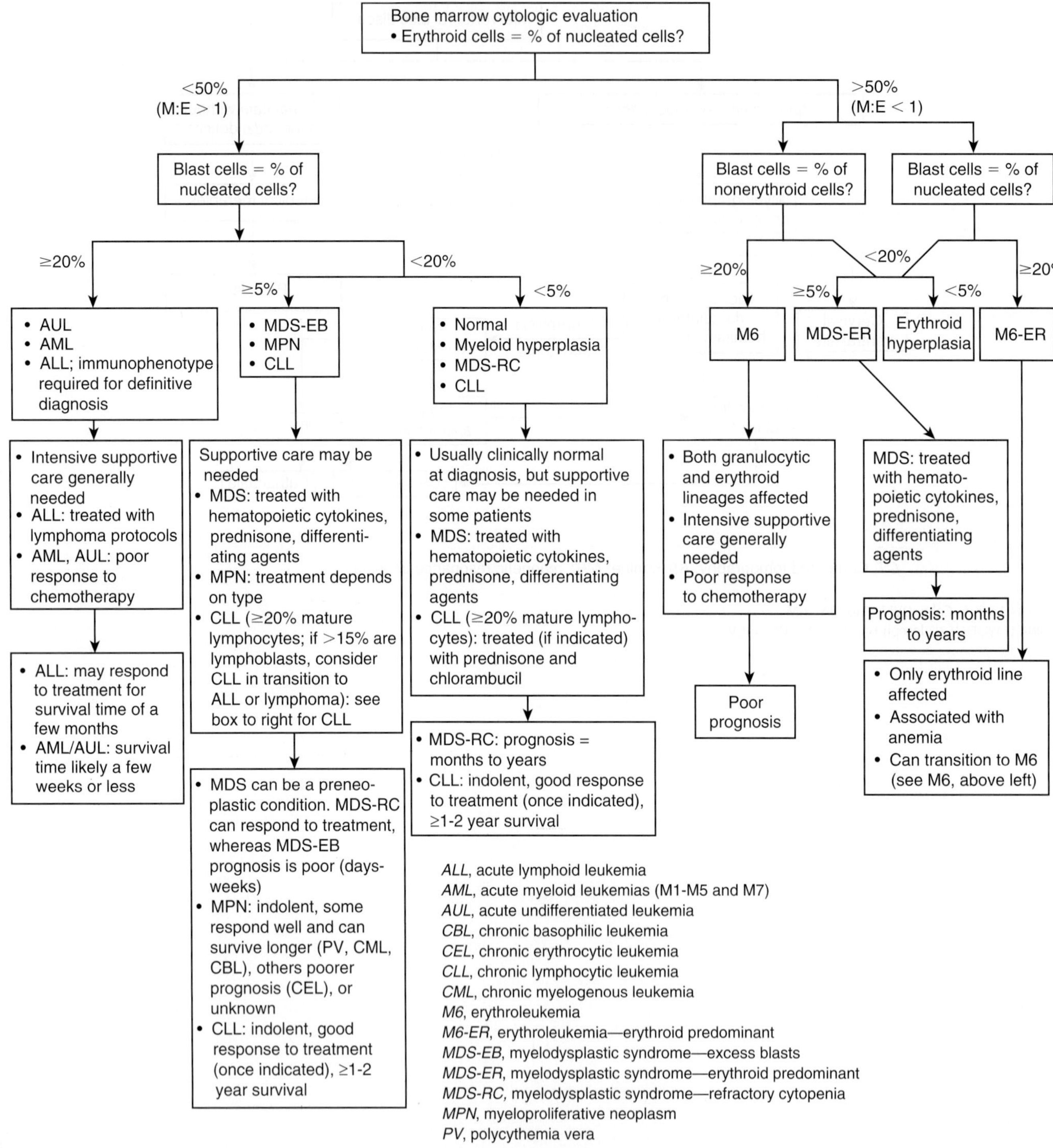

Based on the Animal Leukemia Study Group criteria for classification of acute myeloid leukemias in dogs and cats, and modified from Jacobs RM, et al: Tumors of the hemolymphatic system. In Meuten DJ, editor: Tumors in domestic animals, ed 4, Ames, IA, 2002, Iowa State Press, pp 119–198.

EDITED BY: Leah A. Cohn, DVM, PhD, DACVIM
ORIGINALLY WRITTEN BY: Nicole C. Northrup, DVM, DACVIM

Mammary Gland Tumors, Cat

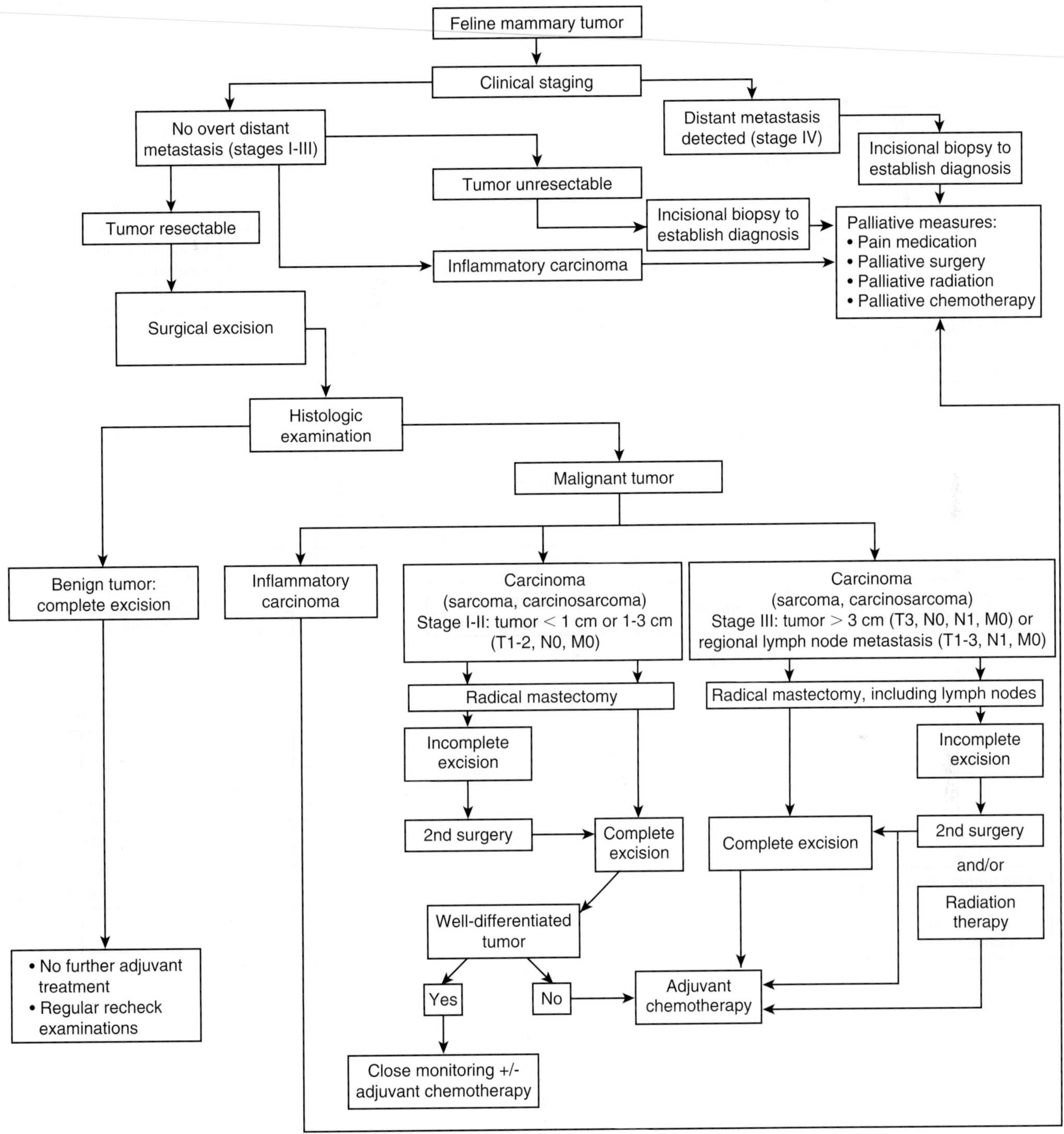

EDITED BY: Leah A. Cohn, DVM, PhD, DACVIM

Mammary Gland Tumors, Dog

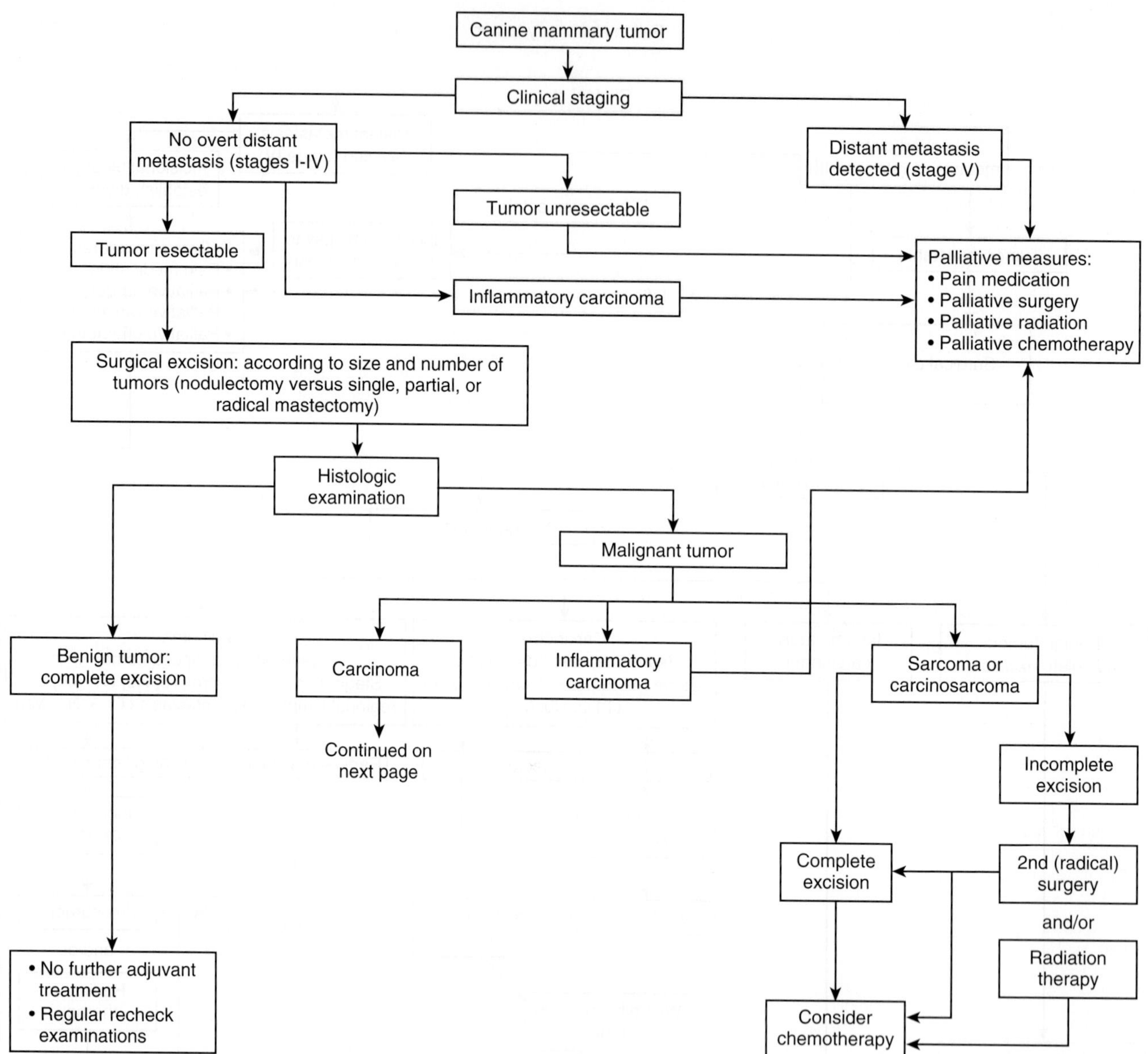

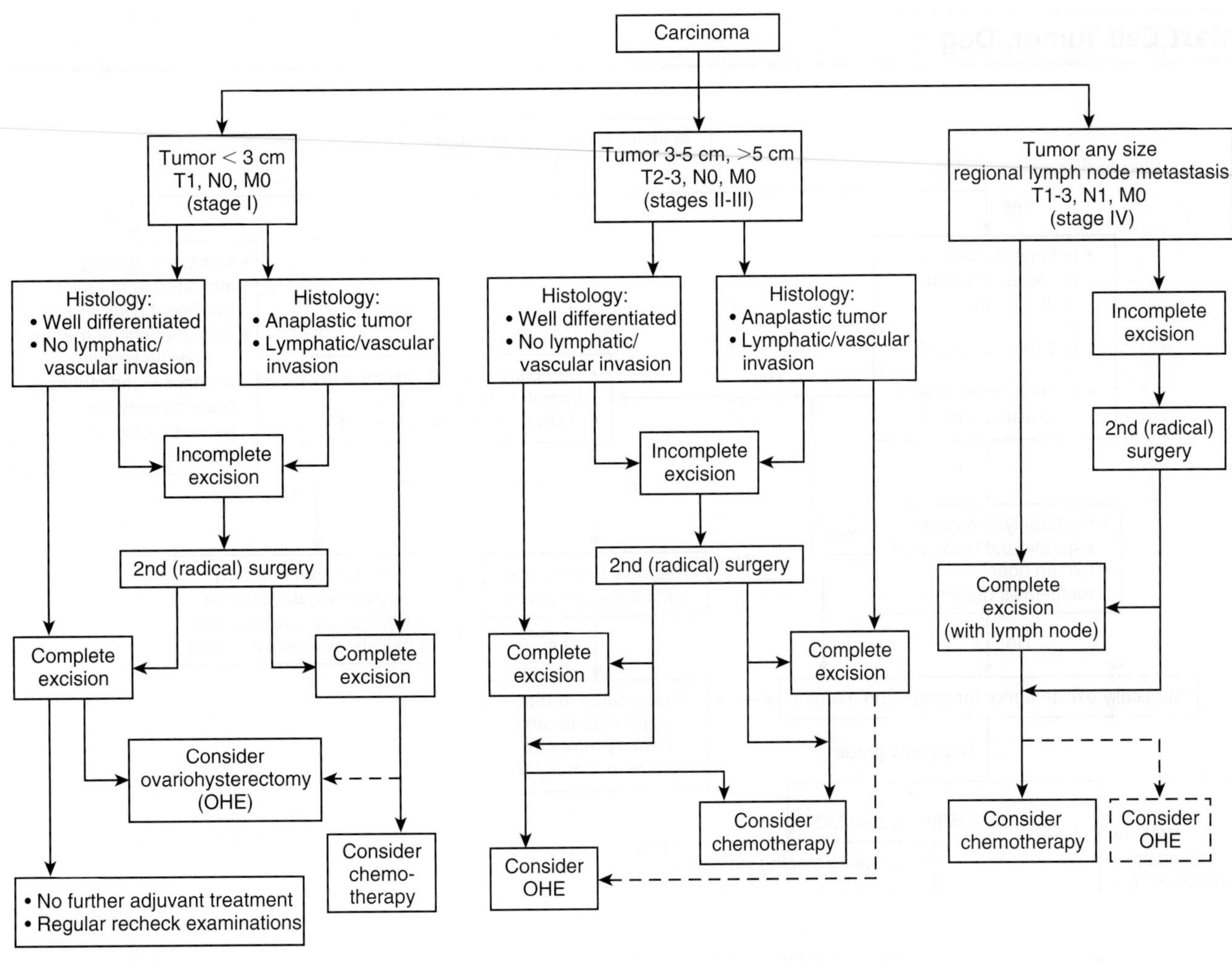

Dashed lines represent possible but nonessential courses of action.

EDITED BY: Leah A. Cohn, DVM, PhD, DACVIM

Mast Cell Tumor, Dog

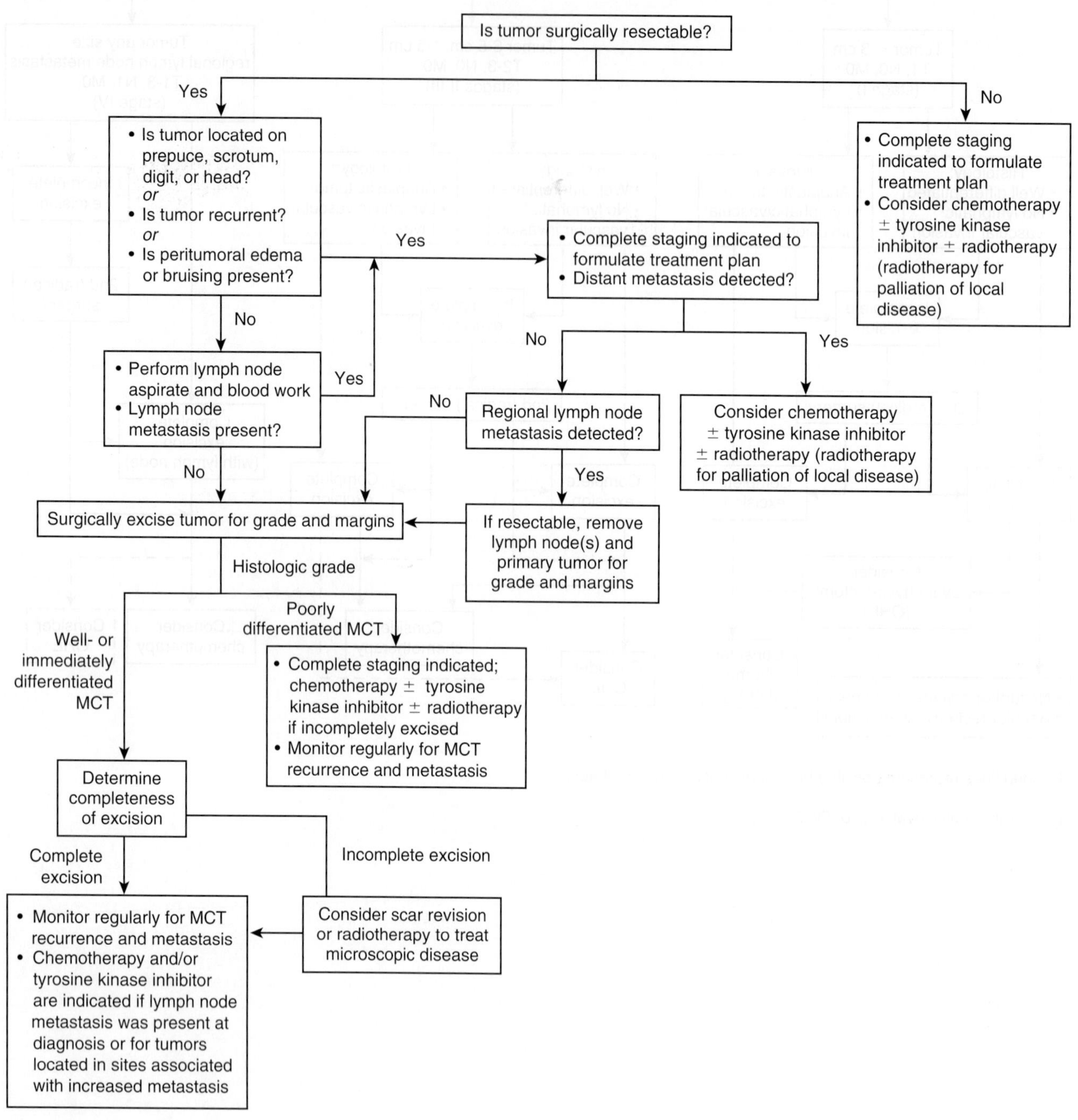

MCT, Mast cell tumor.

EDITED BY: Leah A. Cohn, DVM, PhD, DACVIM
ORIGINALLY WRITTEN BY: Tracy Gieger, DVM, DACVIM, DACVR

Melanoma

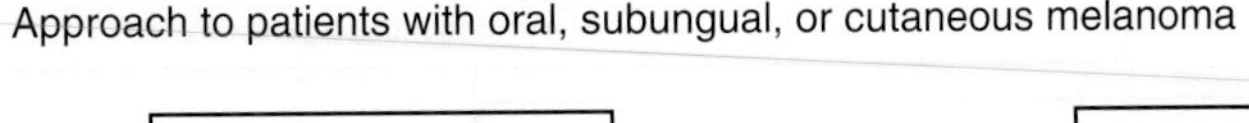

Oral melanoma
→ Staging including blood work, lymph node aspiration, thoracic radiographs, ± CT scan

Subungual (nailbed) melanoma
→ Staging including blood work, lymph node aspiration, thoracic radiographs, ± abdominal ultrasound

Cutaneous melanoma
→ What is mitotic index?
- ≥3 per high-power field → Staging including blood work, lymph node aspiration, thoracic radiographs, ± abdominal ultrasound
- <3 per high-power field →
  - Surgical excision
  - Monitor for local recurrence
  - No further therapy

All three staging boxes → **Is distant metastasis identified?**

- **Yes** → Treatment options:
  - Palliative radiotherapy to tumor (if significant clinical signs from tumor) *and/or*
  - Melanoma vaccine and platinum chemotherapy (survival benefit of chemotherapy controversial) *or*
  - No treatment; palliation of signs only
- **No** → **Is regional lymph node metastasis identified?**
  - **Yes** → Treatment options:
    - Marginal excision of primary tumor and lymph node followed by radiotherapy
    - Limb amputation if subungual or cutaneous tumor on limb *and*
    - Platinum chemotherapy
    - Melanoma vaccine
  - **No** → **Is excision of macroscopic tumor possible?**
    - **No** → Treatment options:
      - Radiotherapy of macroscopic tumor, melanoma vaccine, and platinum chemotherapy
    - **Yes** → **Is radical excision (>2 cm) of tumor possible?**
      - **Yes** → Treatment options:
        - Radical excision of primary tumor and adjuvant chemotherapy *or*
        - Marginal excision of primary tumor followed by radiotherapy, melanoma vaccine, and platinum chemotherapy
      - **No** → Treatment options:
        - Marginal excision of primary tumor followed by radiotherapy, melanoma vaccine, and platinum chemotherapy

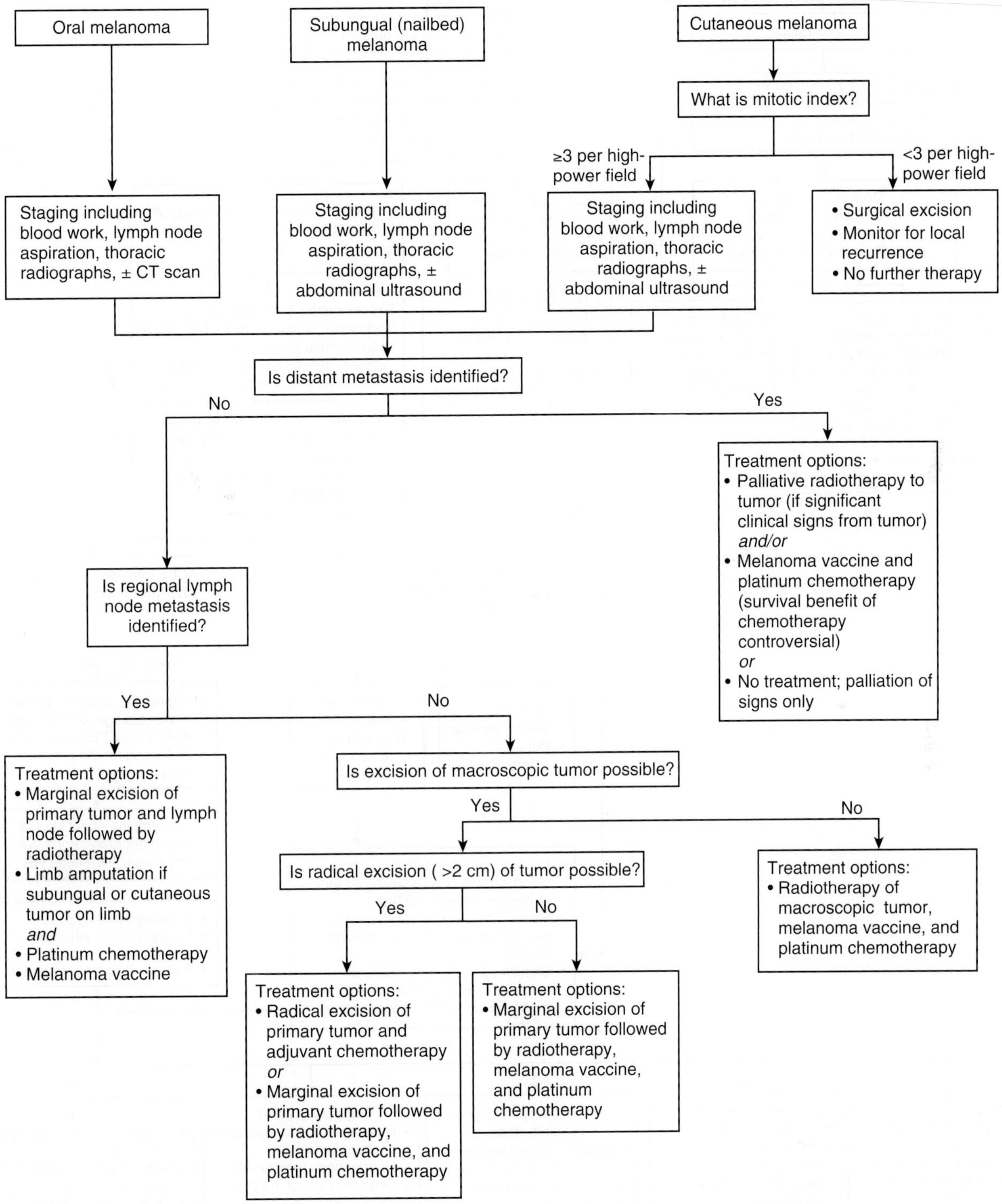

CT, Computed tomography.

UPDATED AND EDITED BY: Leah A. Cohn, DVM, PhD, DACVIM
ORIGINALLY WRITTEN BY: David R. Proulx, DVM, DACVIM

Organophosphate and Carbamate Intoxication

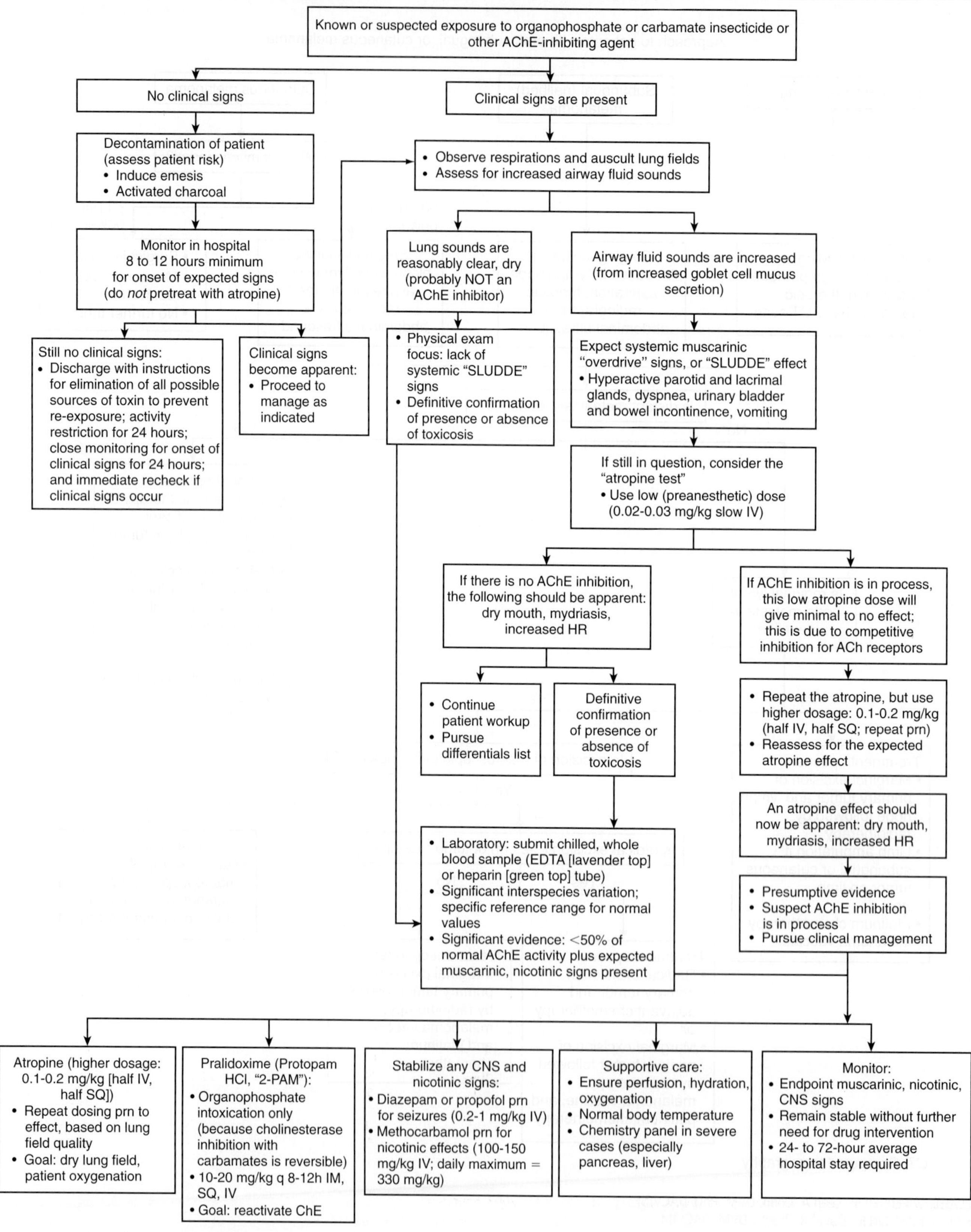

ACh, Acetylcholine; *AChE*, acetylcholinesterase; *CNS*, central nervous system; *HR*, heart rate; *IM;* intramuscular; *IV*, intravenous; *prn*, as needed; *SLUDDE*, salivation, lacrimation, urination, diarrhea, dyspnea, emesis; *SQ*, subcutaneous.

EDITED BY: Leah A. Cohn, DVM, PhD, DACVIM
ORIGINALLY WRITTEN BY: Michael W. Knight, DVM, DABVT, DABT

Peritonitis, Septic

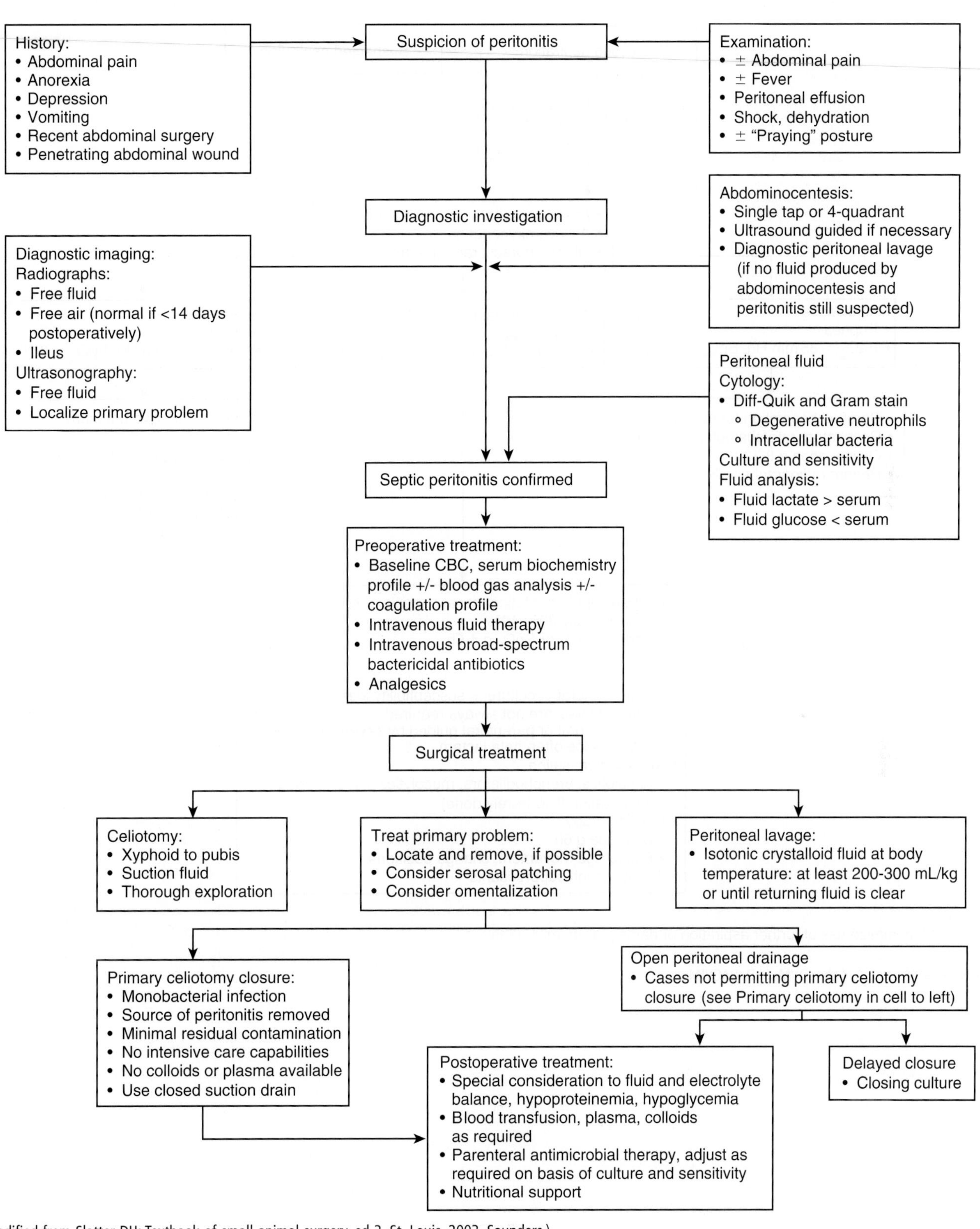

(Modified from Slatter DH: Textbook of small animal surgery, ed 3, St. Louis, 2003, Saunders.)

Pneumonia, Aspiration

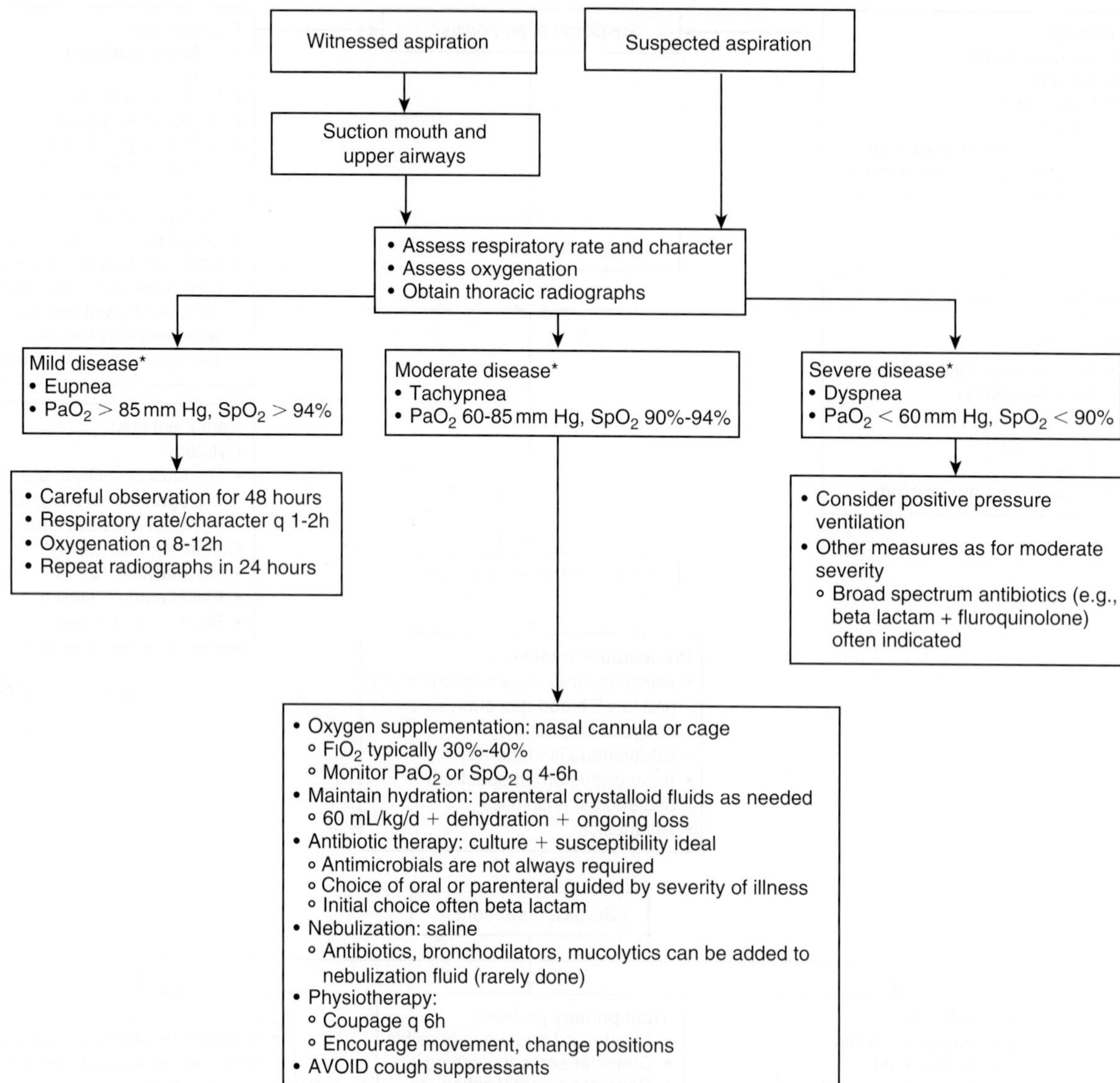

*For all, minimize risk of further aspiration or damage from aspiration.

AUTHOR & EDITOR: Leah A. Cohn, DVM, PhD, DACVIM

Polyarthritis

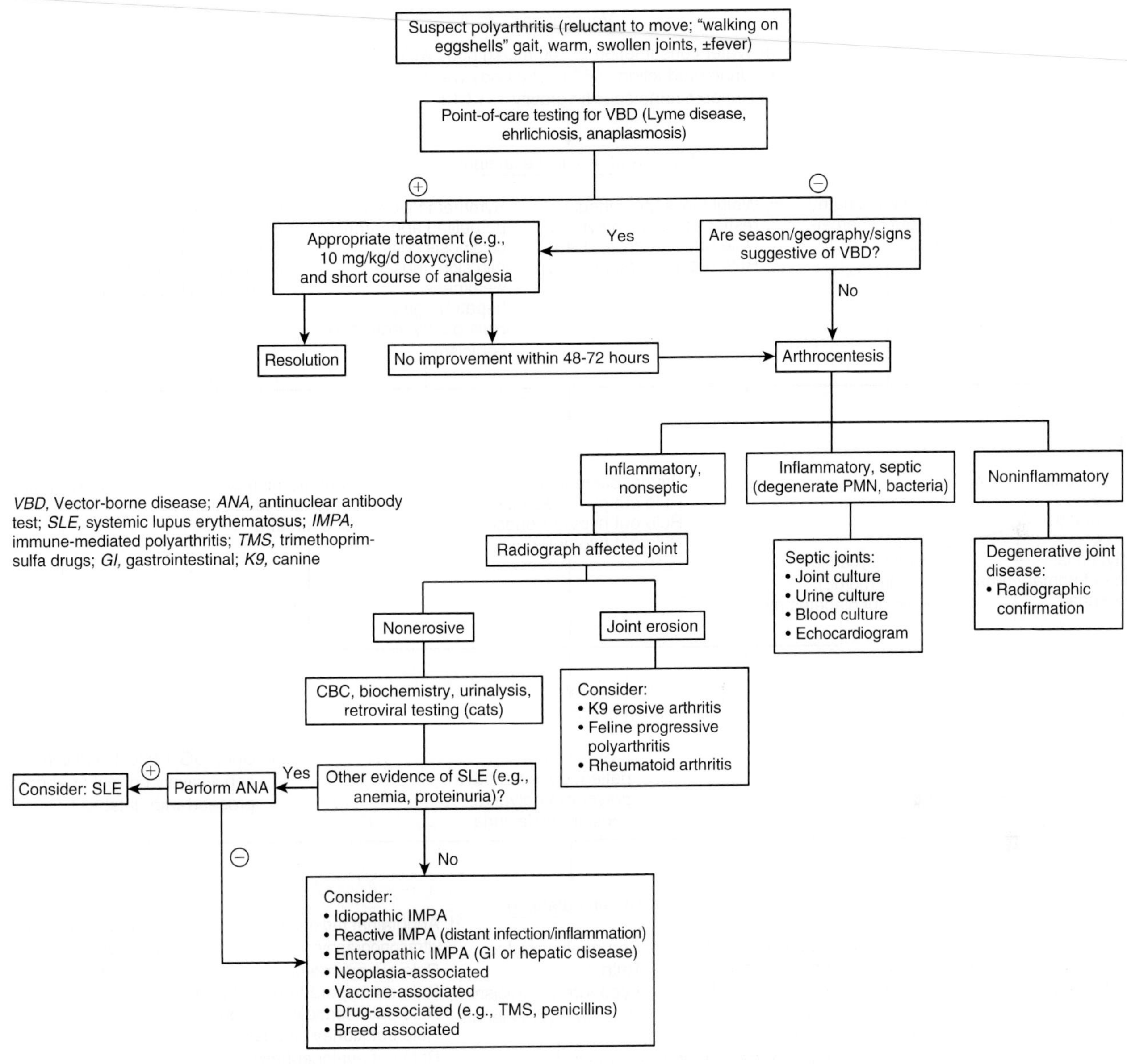

VBD, Vector-borne disease; *ANA*, antinuclear antibody test; *SLE*, systemic lupus erythematosus; *IMPA*, immune-mediated polyarthritis; *TMS*, trimethoprim-sulfa drugs; *GI*, gastrointestinal; *K9*, canine

AUTHOR & EDITOR: Leah A. Cohn, DVM, PhD, DACVIM

Polyuria and Polydipsia

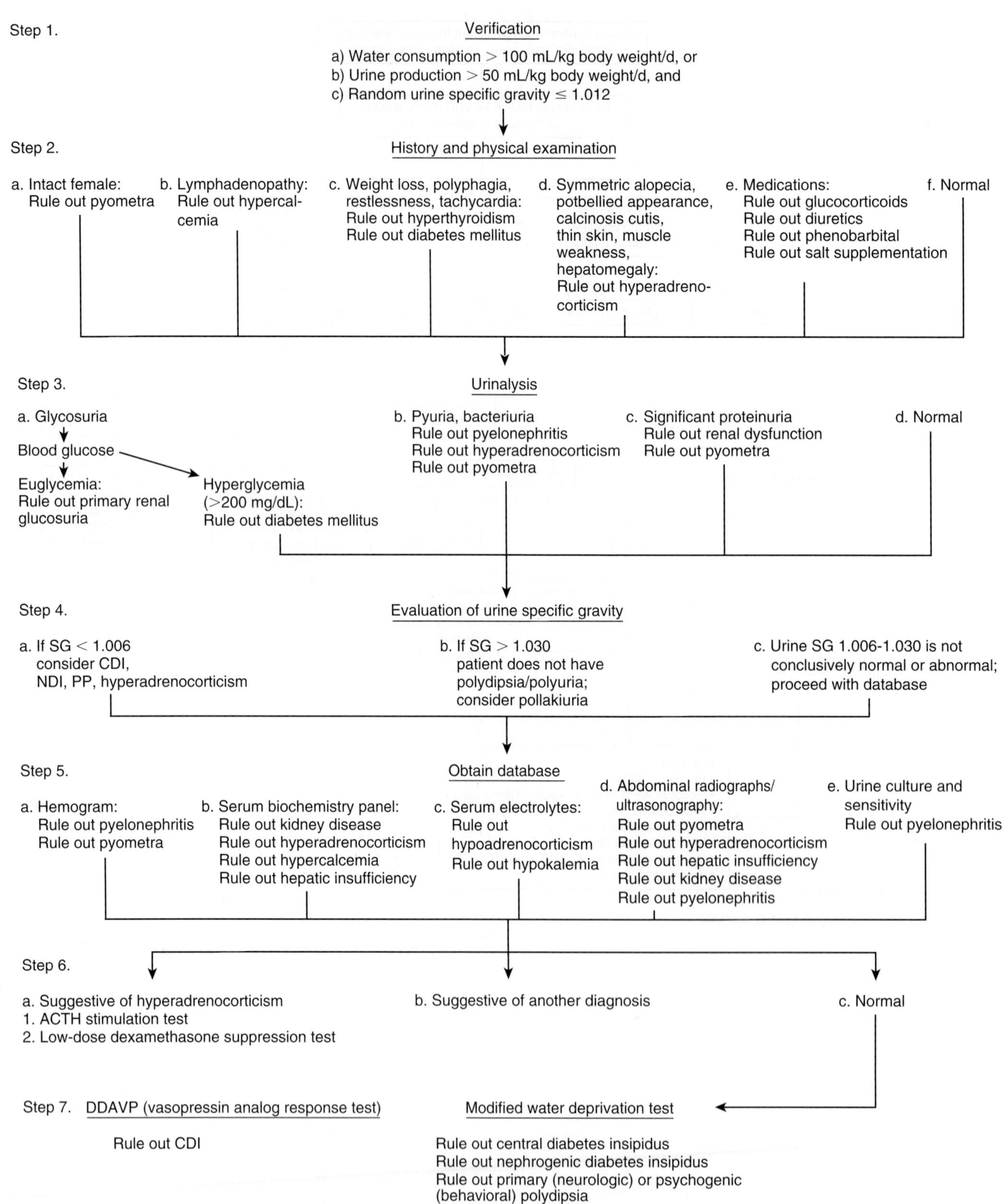

CDI, Central diabetes insipidus; *NDI,* nephrogenic diabetes insipidus; *PP,* primary or psychogenic polydipsia; *SG,* specific gravity.
(Modified from Feldman EC, Nelson RW: Canine and feline endocrinology and reproduction, ed 3, St. Louis, 2004, Saunders.)

Prostatitis

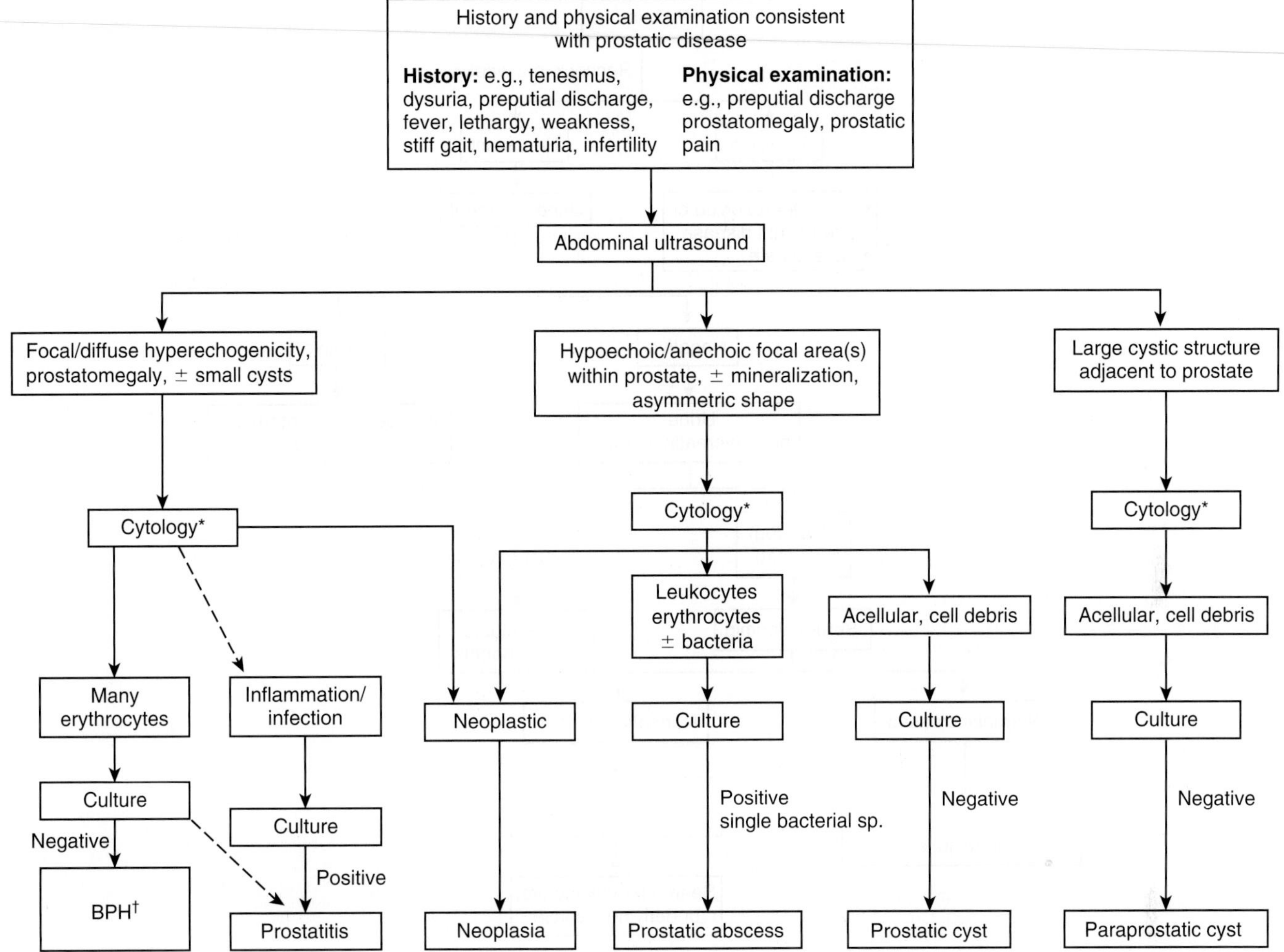

*Cytology can be obtained from a fine-needle aspirate, a prostatic massage, or an ejaculate depending on circumstances.
†Highly unlikely in castrated male.
BPH, Benign prostatic hyperplasia.

EDITED BY: Leah A. Cohn, DVM, PhD, DACVIM
ORIGINALLY WRITTEN BY: Lisa A. Brownlee, DVM, MS, DACVIM

Protein-Losing Nephropathy

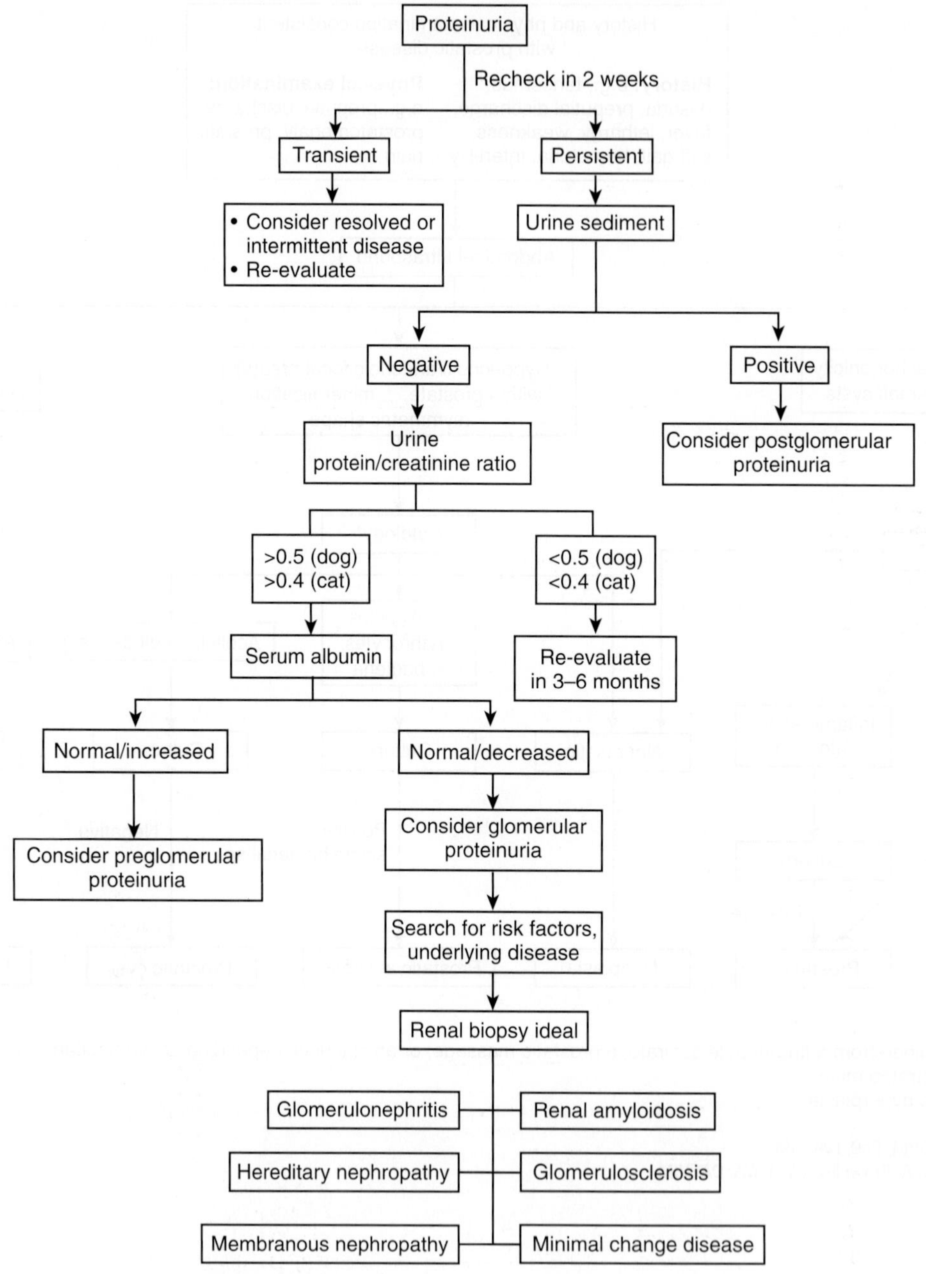

UPDATED AND EDITED BY: Leah A. Cohn, DVM, PhD, DACVIM
ORIGINALLY WRITTEN BY: Anne M. Dalby, DVM, DACVIM

Pruritus

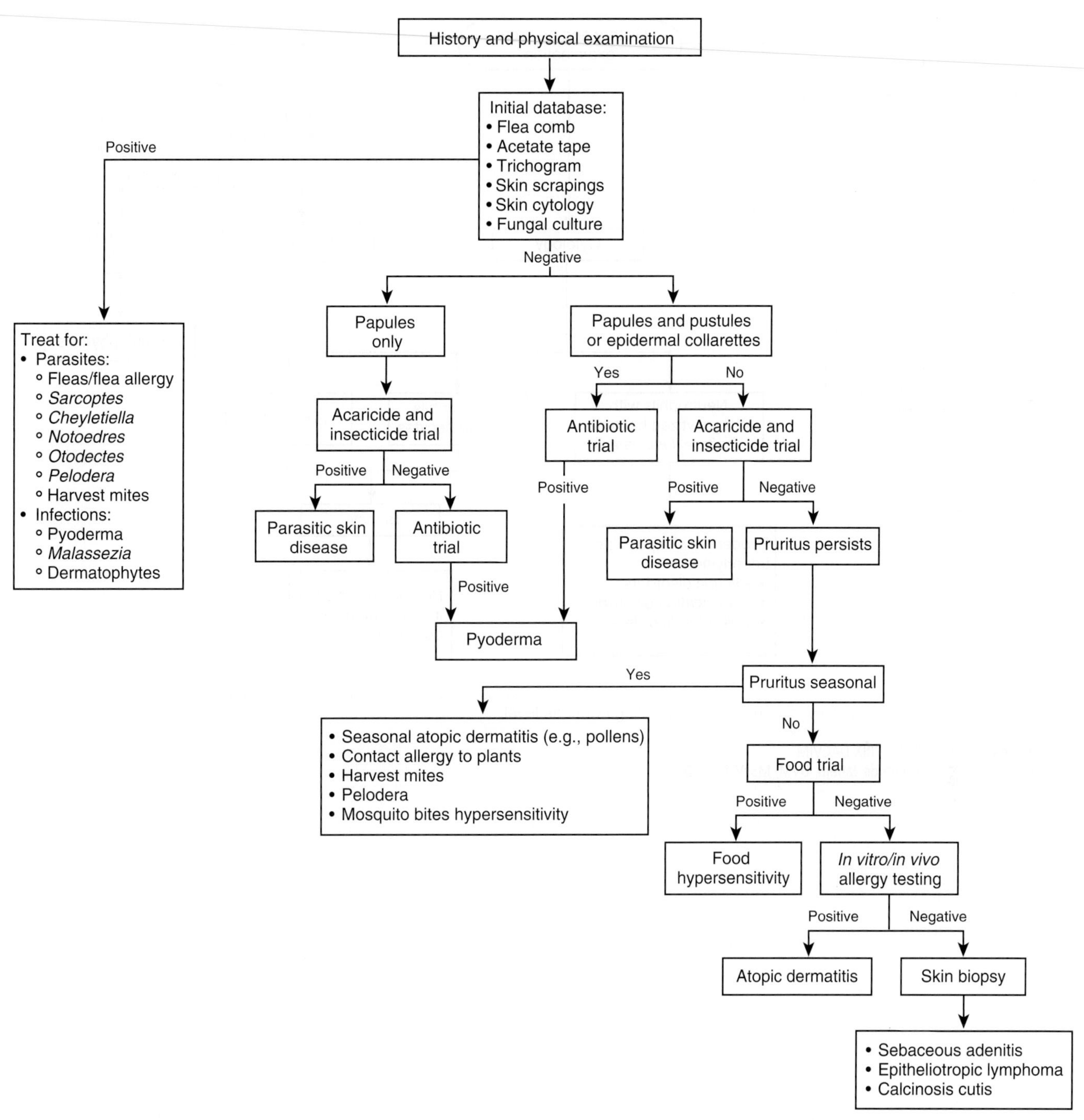

EDITED BY: Leah A. Cohn, DVM, PhD, DACVIM
ORIGINALLY WRITTEN BY: Manon Paradis, DVM, MVSc, DACVD

Pustular and Crusting Skin Disorders

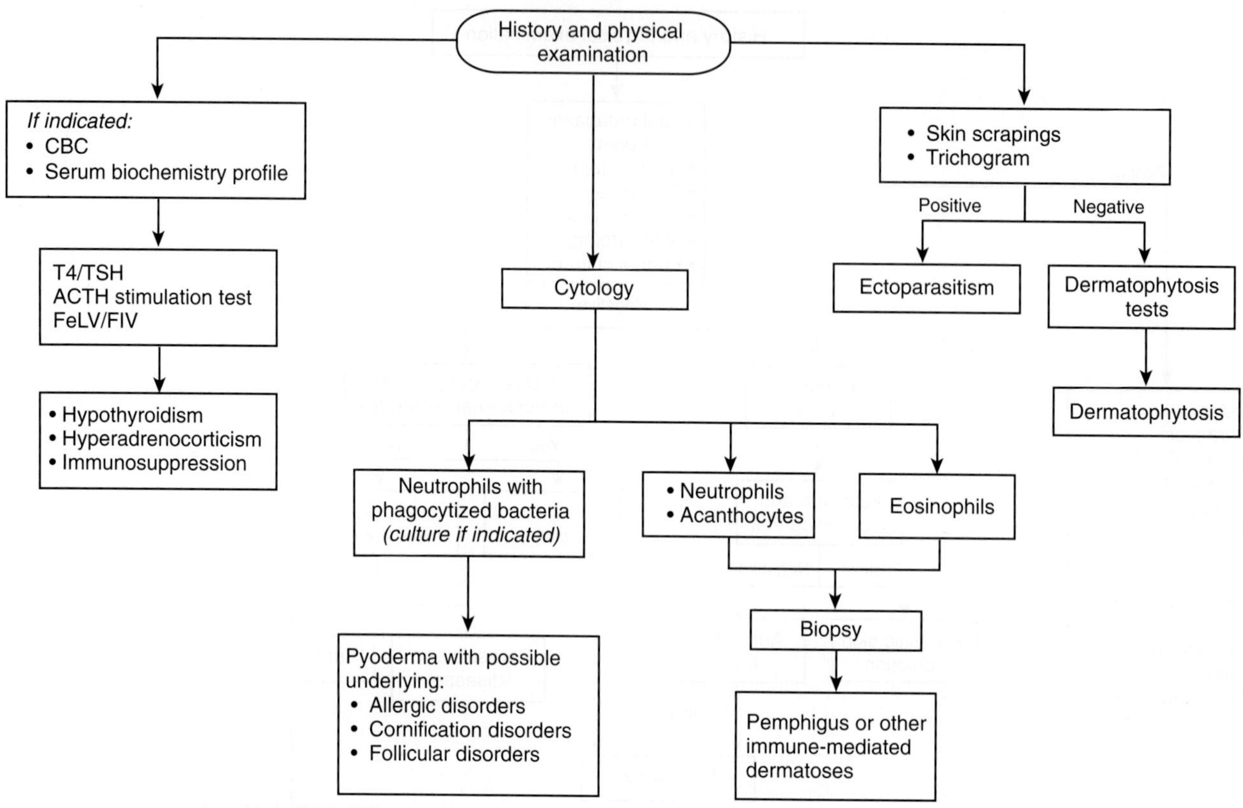

ACTH, Adrenocorticotropic hormone; *CBC,* complete blood count; *FeLV,* feline leukemia virus; *FIV,* feline immunodeficiency virus; *T4,* serum thyroxine level; *TSH,* serum thyroid-stimulating hormone level.

EDITED BY: Leah A. Cohn, DVM, PhD, DACVIM
ORIGINALLY WRITTEN BY: Caroline de Jaham, DVM, MScV, DACVD

Red Eye, Acute

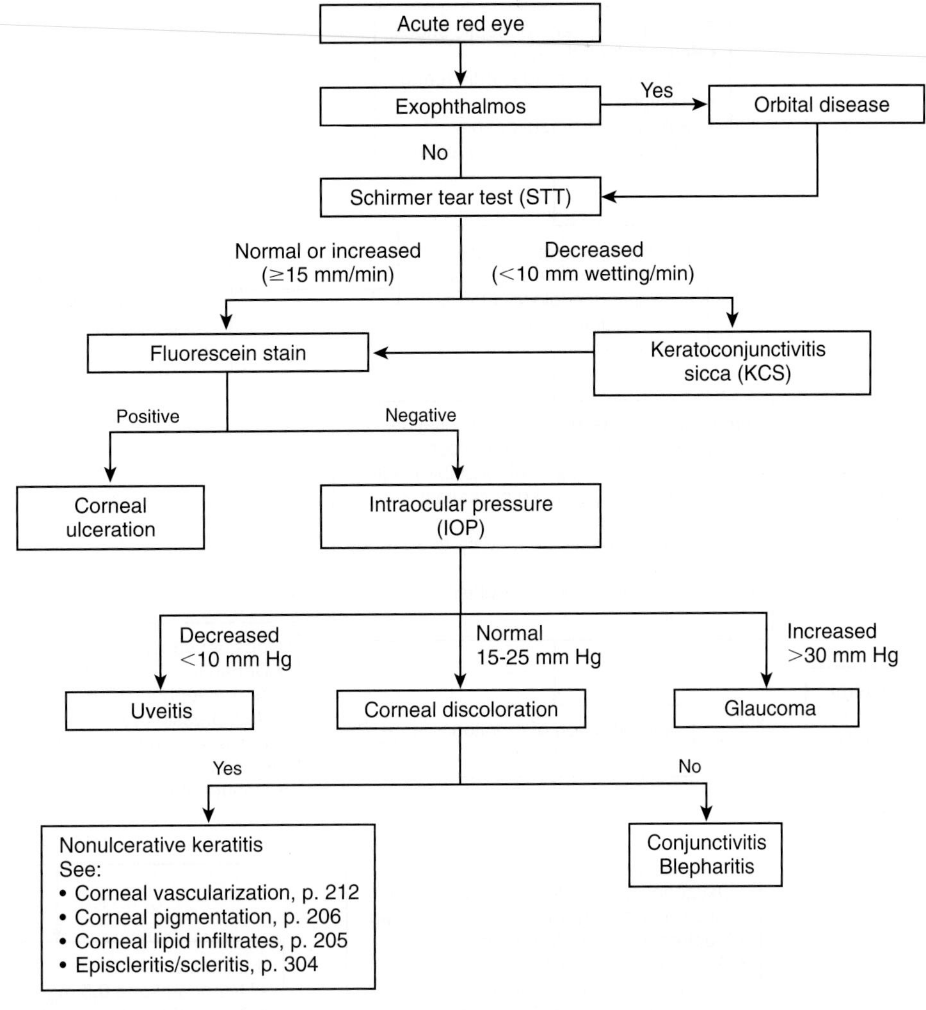

Note: STT values ≥ 10 but < 15 mm wetting/minute may be normal or indicative of early KCS; IOPs between 10-15 and 25-30 mm Hg may be normal for some animals (interpret STT values and IOPs in light of other ophthalmic findings).

EDITED BY: Leah A. Cohn, DVM, PhD, DACVIM
ORIGINALLY WRITTEN BY: Cheryl L. Cullen, DVM, MVetSc, DACVO

Clinical Algorithms

Sepsis and Septic Shock

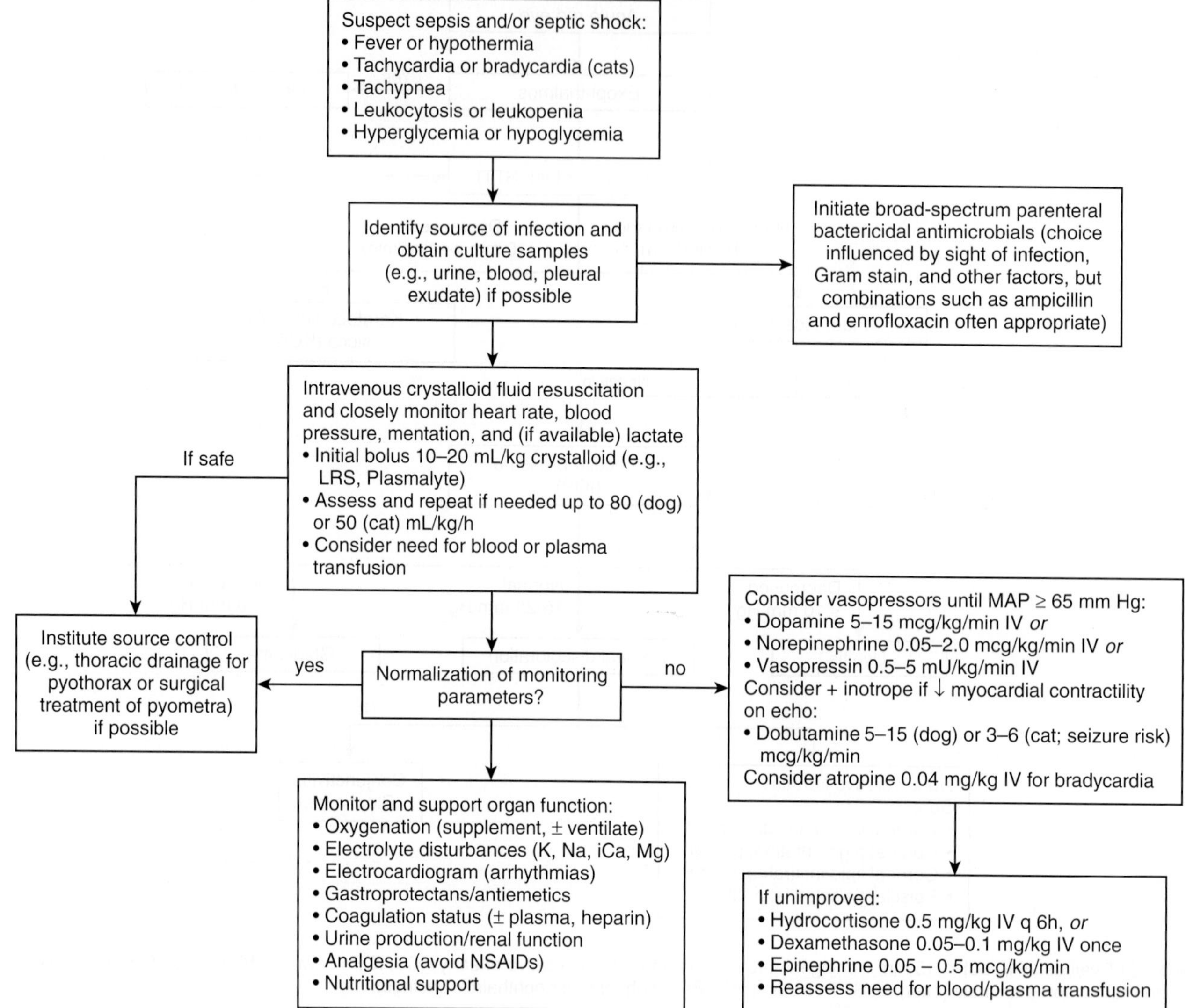

Shock, Hypovolemic

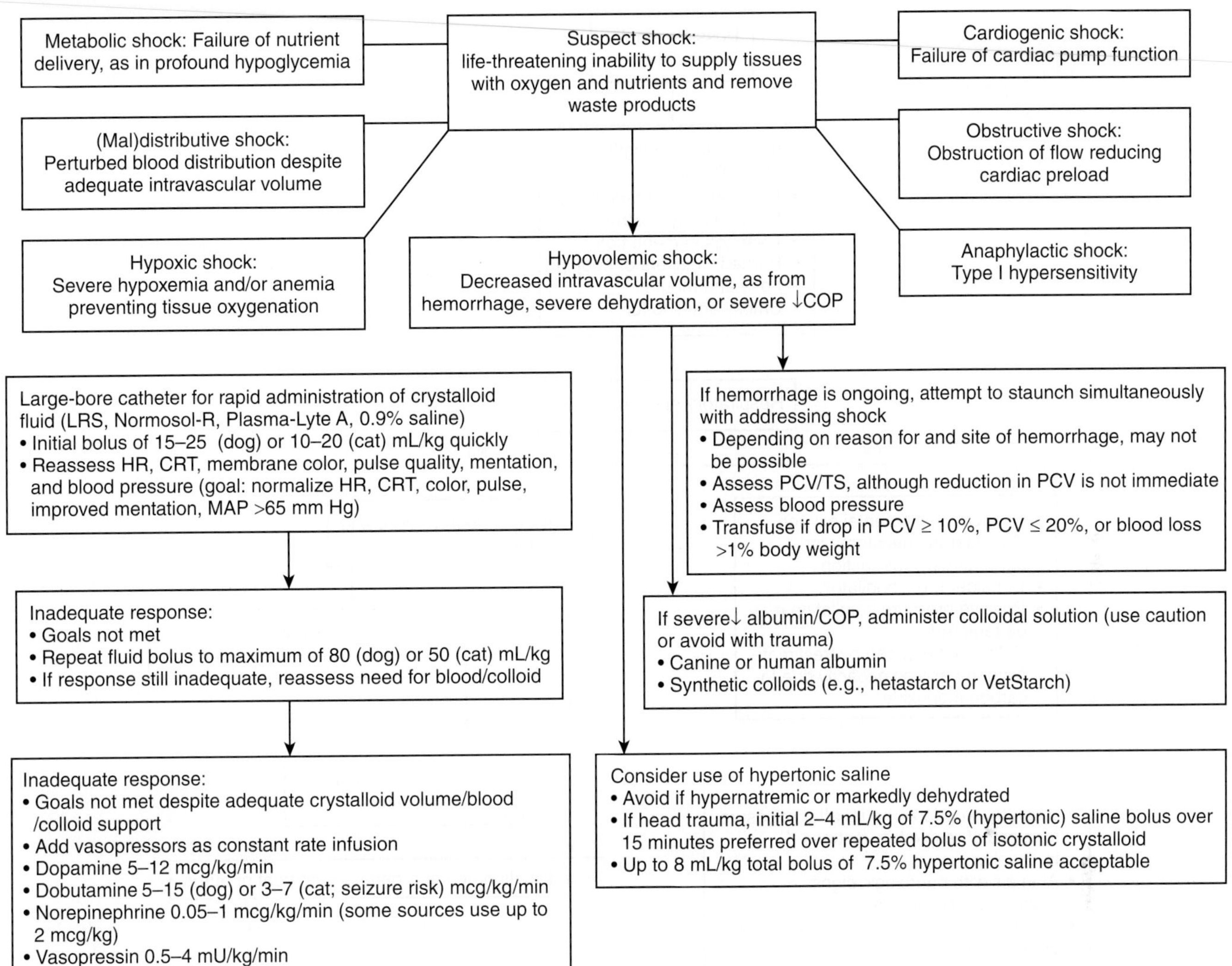

COP, Colloid oncotic pressure; *CRT*, capillary refill time; *HR*, heart rate; *LRS*, lactated Ringer's solution; *MAP*, mean arterial pressure; *PCV*, packed cell volume; *TS*, total solids.

Smoke Inhalation

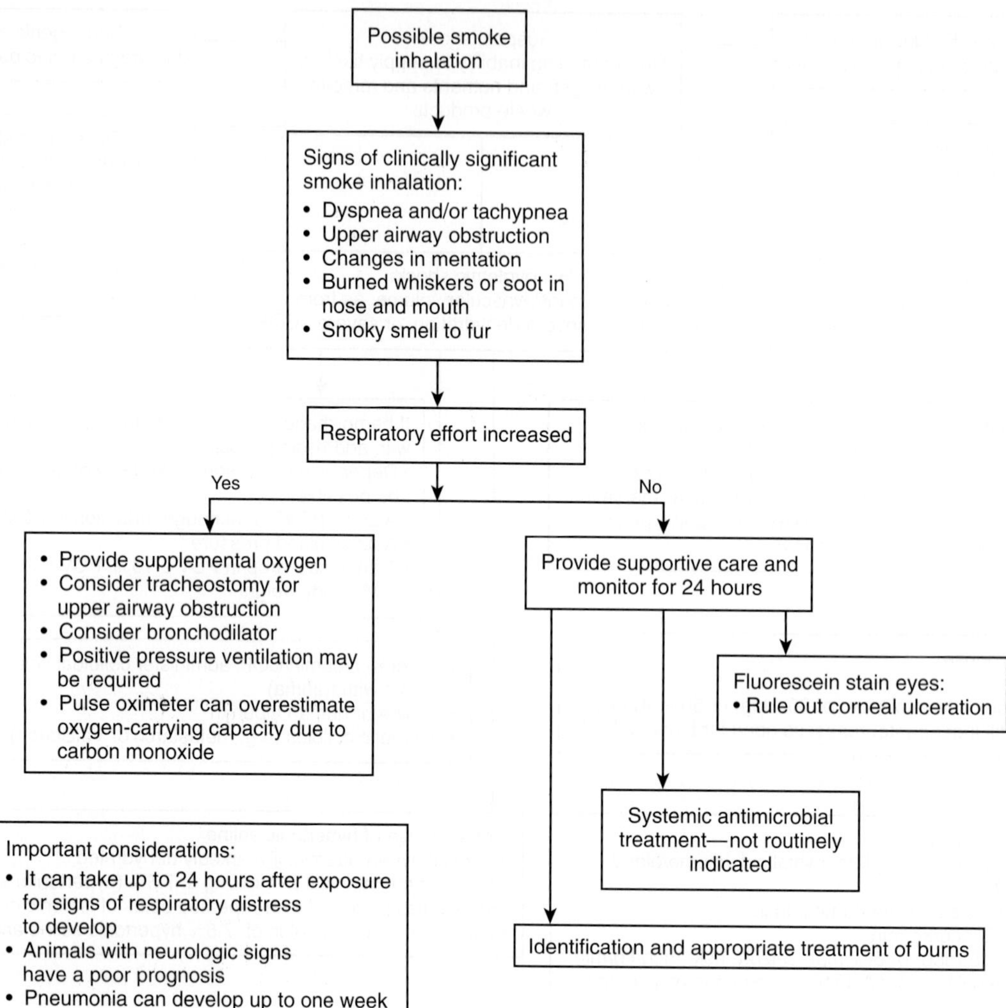

UPDATED AND EDITED BY: Leah A. Cohn, DVM, PhD, DACVIM
ORIGINALLY WRITTEN BY: Scott P. Shaw, DVM, DACVECC

Soft-Tissue Sarcoma: Diagnostic and Therapeutic Approach

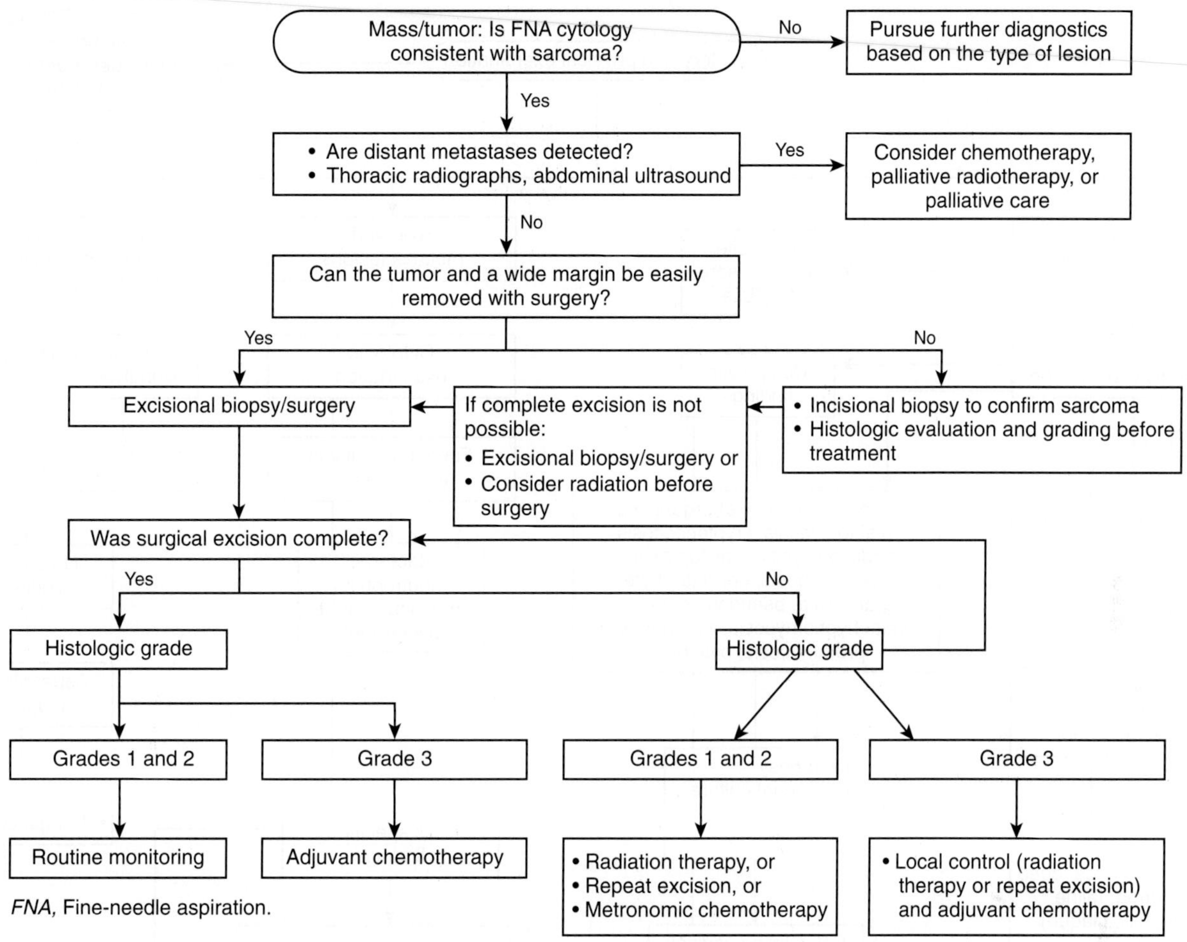

FNA, Fine-needle aspiration.

EDITED BY: Leah A. Cohn, DVM, PhD, DACVIM
ORIGINALLY WRITTEN BY: John Farrelly, DVM, MS, DACVIM, DACVR

Clinical Algorithms

Ulcerative and Erosive Dermatoses

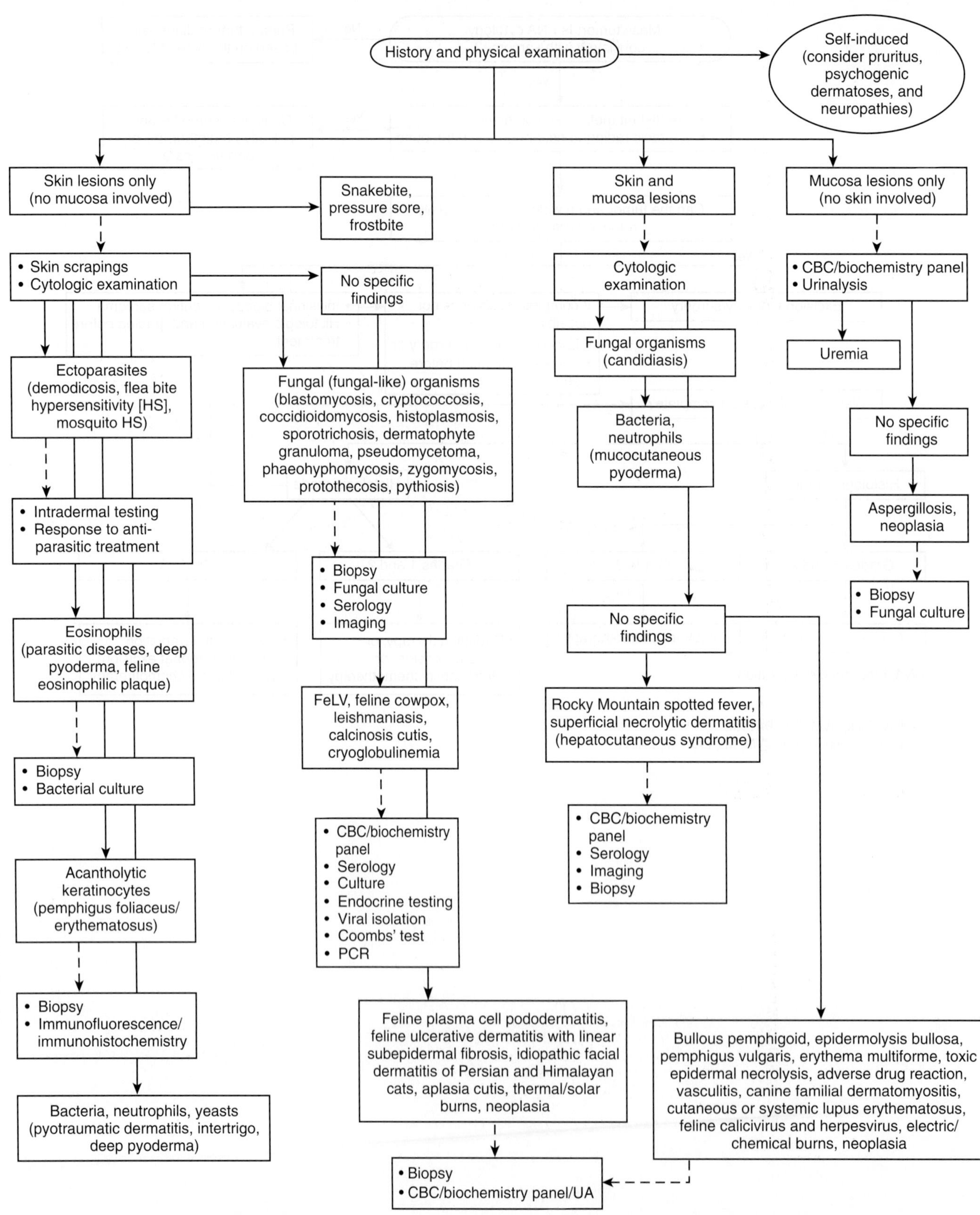

CBC, Complete blood count; *FeLV,* feline leukemia virus; *PCR,* polymerase chain reaction; *UA,* urinalysis. Dashed lines indicate diagnostic procedures.

EDITED BY: Leah A. Cohn, DVM, PhD, DACVIM
ORIGINALLY WRITTEN BY: Frédéric Sauvé, DMV, MSc, DACVD

Upper Airway Obstruction/Choking

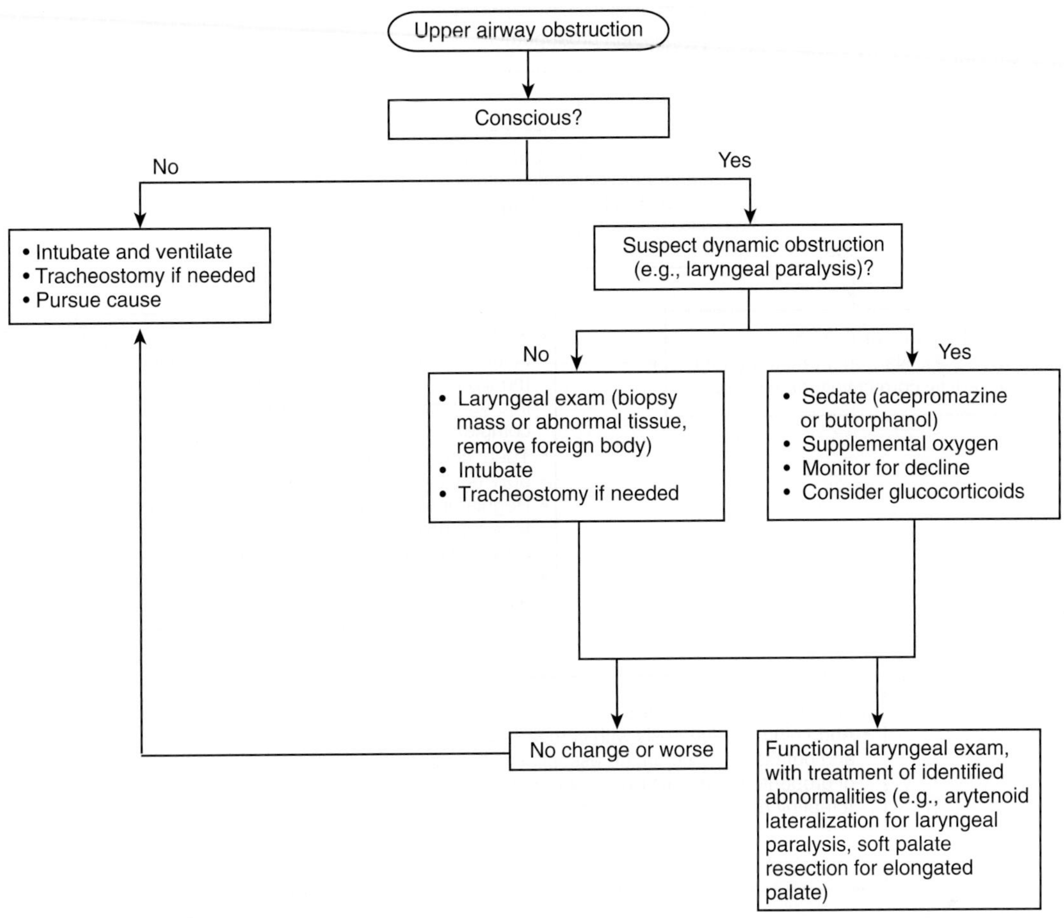

UPDATED AND EDITED BY: Leah A. Cohn, DVM, PhD, DACVIM
ORIGINALLY WRITTEN BY: Scott P. Shaw, DVM, DACVECC

Uroabdomen

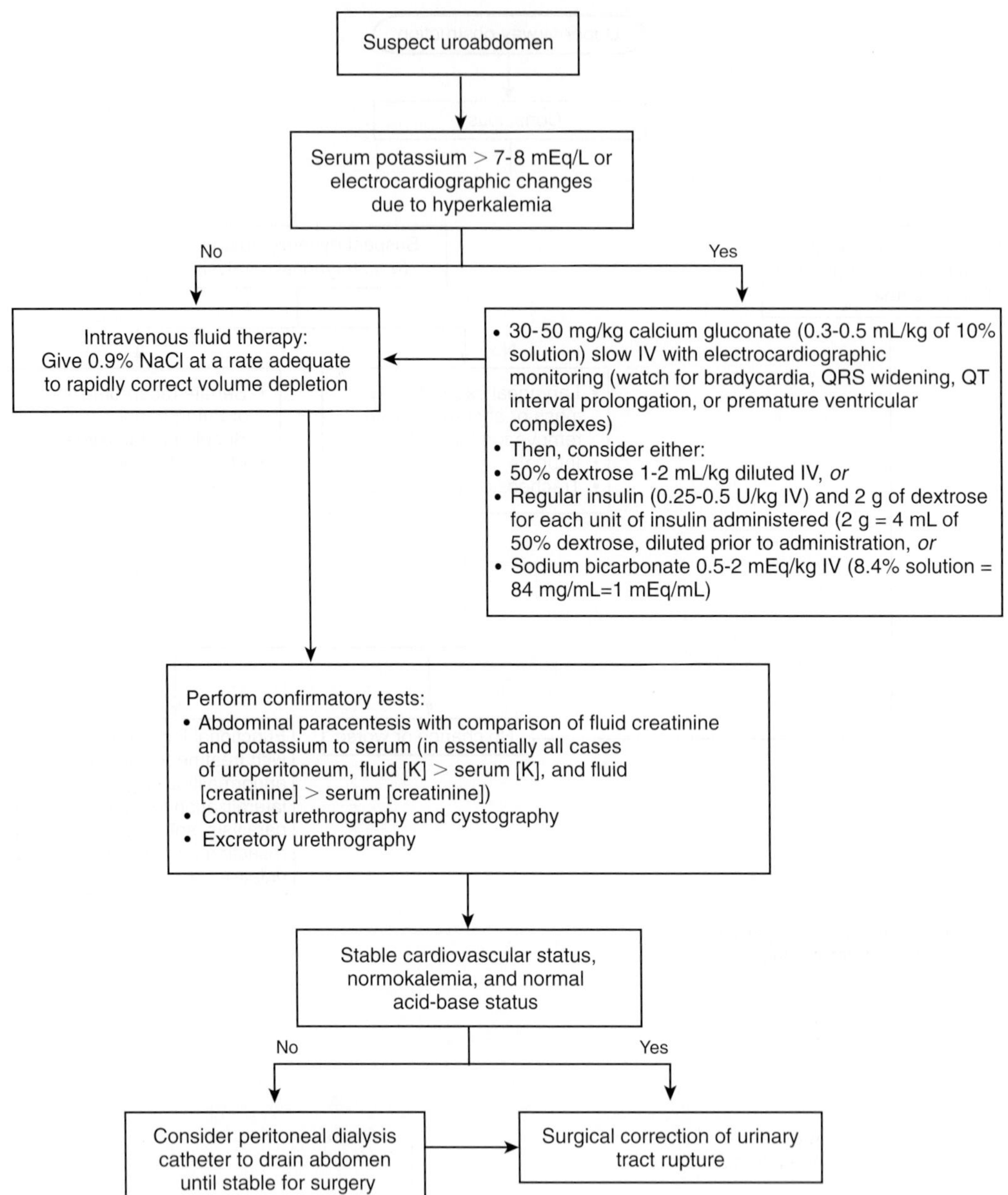

EDITED BY: Leah A. Cohn, DVM, PhD, DACVIM
ORIGINALLY WRITTEN BY: Scott P. Shaw, DVM, DACVECC

Uroliths, Oxalate

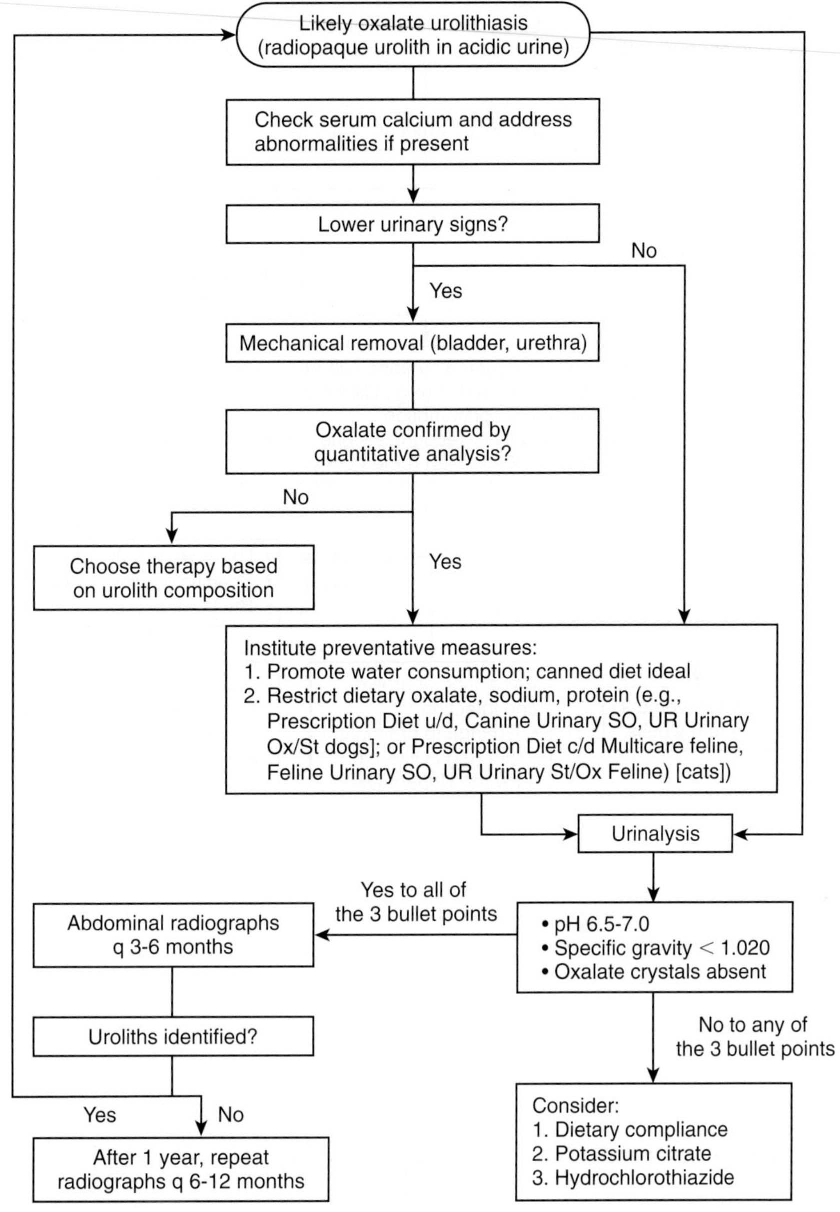

AUTHOR & EDITOR: Leah A. Cohn, DVM, PhD, DACVIM

Clinical Algorithms

Uroliths, Struvite

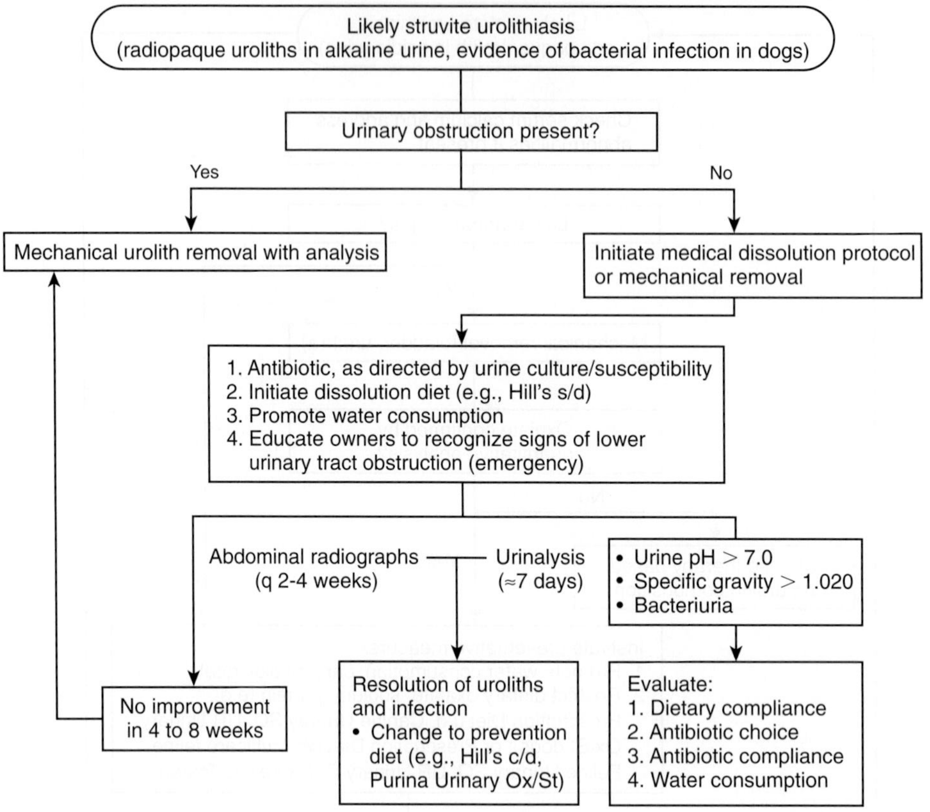

AUTHOR & EDITOR: Leah A. Cohn, DVM, PhD, DACVIM

Ventricular Tachycardia: Management

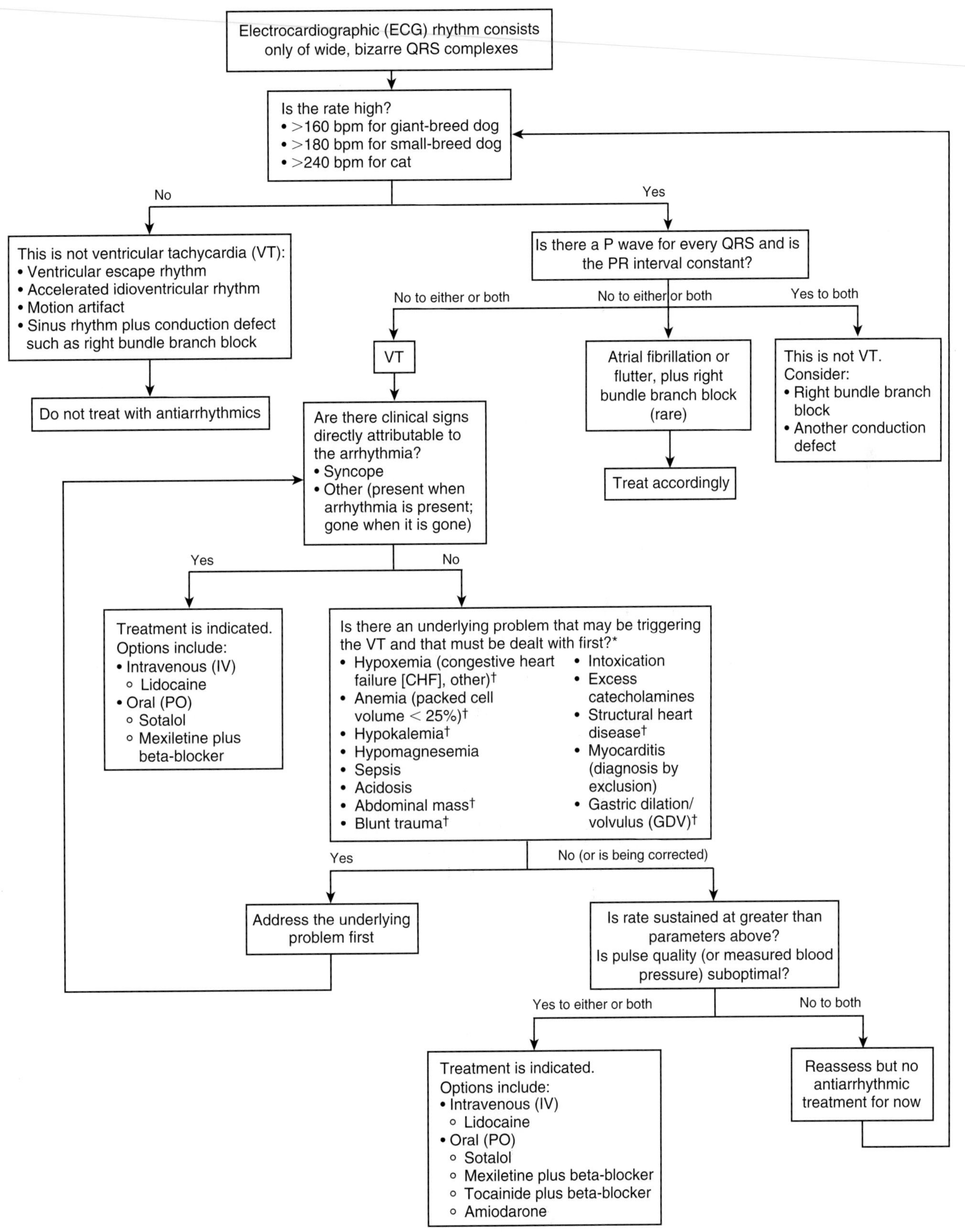

*Virtually any medical problem, if severe enough, can cause ventricular arrhythmias.

†Most common.

(Modified from Ettinger SJ, Feldman EC: Textbook of veterinary internal medicine, ed 8, St. Louis, 2017, Elsevier.)

SECTION VI

Drug Compendium

EDITORS

Gigi Davidson
BSPharm, DICVP

Leah A. Cohn
DVM, PhD, DACVIM (SAIM)

Drug Formulary

The drugs listed in this formulary represent a compilation of many of the therapeutic agents used in small animal practice, without implying endorsement (or lack thereof) of specific medications. Not all drugs used in veterinary practice are included, and some of those listed may be used infrequently. Drugs are organized in alphabetical order by generic names, with trade names or often used synonyms in parentheses. The web version of the text also includes a cross-reference with many of the trade names/synonyms listed alphabetically. We hope that this can help you to find the drug of interest on those occasions in which the brand name (e.g., Prozac) is commonly used and the generic name (e.g., fluoxetine) just does not come readily to mind. Abbreviations used in the formulary are first defined on this page for the reader's reference.

Canine and feline dosages are listed separately in the second and third columns, respectively. (The unit of measure of micron, sometimes denoted by the Greek letter μ, is abbreviated in this text by mc. For example, 1 mcL = 1 microliter; 1 mcg = 1 microgram.) The fourth column, titled Adverse Effects/Warnings, describes important side effects or contraindications for each drug. A fifth column, titled Administration/Availability, includes formulations and important notes about administration. This column also denotes the Controlled Substance Schedules (CSS) as listed by the U.S. Drug Enforcement Administration.

While every effort has been made to include clinically useful, important, and accurate information, a comprehensive review of the details of individual drugs is too voluminous to be listed in this format. Therefore, it remains the clinician's responsibility to ensure that the particulars of any drug are appropriate for the intended application. The clinician should recheck drug dosages for accuracy as well as for specific indications, contraindications, and warnings. Again, the clinician needs to identify the specific and recommended indications for each drug by reviewing relevant information (e.g., product insert, primary sources) before prescribing, recommending, or using a drug.

Although limitations of space do not allow inclusion in print, we encourage readers to avail themselves of additional drug-related information found in the web version of this text. This includes information regarding important interactions between veterinary drugs, drugs of concern when administered to dogs with *MDR1/ABCB1-Δ*, charts comparing composition of fluid types, relative potency of various preparations of glucocorticoids, and more.

Materials presented are taken from several sources: 1) drug-related information from the other sections of this textbook; 2) the clinical experience of the editors and previous redactors of this formulary; 3) Plumb DC: Veterinary Drug Handbook, ed 9, Ames, IA, 2018, Wiley; 4) Papich MG: Saunders Handbook of Veterinary Drugs: Small and Large Animal, ed 3, St. Louis, 2011; 5) Ramsey I: BSAVA Formulary, Part A: Canine and Feline, ed 9, 2017, Wiley; 6) VIN Veterinary Drug Handbook, www.vin.com. The editors thank Drs. Steve Ettinger and Wayne Schwark for their important contributions to the original version of this Formulary in the first edition of this textbook.

ABBREVIATIONS

AAFP: American Association of Feline Practitioners
BSA: body surface area
BW: body weight
CHF: congestive heart failure
CNS: central nervous system
CRI: constant rate infusion
CSS: controlled substance schedule
D_5W: sterile 5% dextrose in water
DCM: dilated cardiomyopathy
DKA: diabetic ketoacidosis
DM: diabetes mellitus
FDA: Food and Drug Administration
GI: gastrointestinal
h: hour(s)
HDDST: high-dose dexamethasone suppression test
IBD: inflammatory bowel disease
IM: intramuscular
IV: intravenous
IVDD: intervertebral disc disease
KCS: keratoconjunctivitis sicca
LDDST: low-dose dexamethasone suppression test
MAO: monamine oxidase
mcg: microgram
mcL: microliter
MDR1/ABCB1-Δ: genetic mutation of P-glycoprotein
MUE: meningitis encephalitis of unknown etiology
NIOSH: National Institute for Occupational Safety and Health
NSAIDs: nonsteroidal antiinflammatory drugs
OA: affected eye
OTC: over-the-counter
PCV: packed cell volume
PO: per os (oral)
prn: as needed
PU/PD: polyuria/polydipsia
q: every
SQ: subcutaneous
SVT: supraventricular tachycardia
U: unit(s)

A

Generic Name (Brand Name, Synonyms)	Canine Dosages	Feline Dosages	Adverse Effects/Warnings	Administration/ Availability
Acarbose (Precose)	Hypoglycemic agent: 12.5-25 mg/DOG orally q 12h with each meal. Can increase dose to 50 mg/DOG q 12h.	Hypoglycemic agent: 12.5 mg/CAT orally with each meal q 12h. Can increase dose to 25 mg/CAT q 12h.	Flatulence, diarrhea common. May contribute to episodes of hypoglycemia.	Tablets. Give with food.
Acetylcysteine (Mucomyst, N-acetylcysteine, NAC, ACC)	Hepatoprotection/antidote: Dilute 10% sterile NAC with sterile saline 1:4; administer 140 mg/kg IV over 20 minutes, then 70 mg/kg IV q 6h Degenerative myelopathy: 25 mg/kg PO q 8h for 2 weeks, then q 8h q other day given concurrently with aminocaproic acid Corneal ulceration: 2%-6% solution topically q 2h for 24 hours, then q 6-8h for 1 week	Hepatoprotection: Dilute 10% sterile NAC with sterile saline 1:4; administer 140 mg/kg IV over 20 minutes, then 70 mg/kg IV q 12h	Sulfurlike odor, bronchospasm if inhaled, GI distress for oral routes.	Tablets, solutions for inhalation. Solutions must be sterilized with a 0.22-micron filter before injection or use in the eye. Dilute 10% solutions 1:4 with saline before IV administration.

Generic Name (Brand Name, Synonyms)	Canine Dosages	Feline Dosages	Adverse Effects/Warnings	Administration/ Availability
Acepromazine (Aceproject, ACE)	Premedication or as sedative: 0.025-0.05 mg/kg IV, 0.05-0.15 mg/kg SQ or IM; oral tablets 0.5-1 mg/kg PO	Premedication or as sedative: 0.025-0.05 mg/kg IV, 0.01-0.1 mg/kg SQ or IM; oral tablets 0.5-1 mg/kg PO	Can cause hypotension and cardiovascular collapse. Do not use to treat noise phobias (e.g., thunderstorms, fireworks).	Tablets, solutions (differing concentrations)
Acetaminophen (Tylenol)	Analgesia: 10-15 mg/kg PO q 8-12h (other analgesics preferred)	Do not use in cats.	Oxidant damage to cells, hepatotoxicity, allergic reactions, cytopenias, facial edema, and KCS may occur in dogs. Cats are deficient in enzyme needed to conjugate and excrete drug (do not use in cats).	Tablets, capsules, liquid formulations OTC
Acetaminophen with codeine (Tylenol #3)	Analgesia: 1-2 mg/kg as based on codeine component (as long as acetaminophen ≤15 mg/kg) PO q 12h	Do not use in cats.	Oxidant damage to cells, hepatotoxicity, allergic reactions, cytopenias, facial edema, and KCS may occur in dogs. Cats are deficient in enzyme needed to conjugate and excrete drug (do not use in cats).	Tablets, oral solution with variable concentrations of each drug. CSS-III.
Acitretin (Soriatane)	Keratinization disorders: 0.5-1.32 mg/kg PO q 24h	Keratinization disorders: 3 mg/kg or one 10-mg capsule/CAT q 24h	Teratogen. Do not use in pregnant animals, and avoid use in households with pregnant women.	Oral capsules
ACTH: see Cortrosyn				
Albendazole (Albenza, Valbazen)	Giardia when other treatments have failed: 25 mg/kg PO q 12h for 3-5 days	Giardia when other treatments have failed: 15-25 mg/kg PO q 12h for 3-5 days	Not recommended in dogs or cats due to high risk of myelosuppression.	Tablets, oral suspension. Give with food.
Albuterol (Proventil, Ventolin)	Bronchodilation: 0.02-0.05 mg/kg (20-50 mcg/kg) PO q 8-12h as needed. Inhalation via metered-dose inhaler (1-2 puffs of 90 mcg q 8-12h) or nebulization for short-term or occasional use.	Acute asthma: 1 puff (90 mcg) with an appropriate spacer and mask. May repeat q 30 minutes for up to 4-6 hours in acute episodes.	Use with caution in patients with cardiac dysrhythmias or dysfunction, seizure disorders, hypertension, or hyperthyroidism. Intoxication can cause severe hypokalemia. Chronic, frequent inhalational use should be avoided due to proinflammatory effects.	Tablets, extended-release tablets, oral syrup, and metered-dose inhalers. Inhalers must be used in combination with an appropriate spacer and face mask.
Alendronate (Fosamax)	Refractory hypercalcemia or to reduce pain associated with bone tumors (extra-label): 0.5-1 mg/kg PO q 24h on an empty stomach	Idiopathic hypercalcemia: 5-10 mg/CAT PO once weekly and adjusted to effect	May cause esophageal erosions, GI upset, jaw and auditory canal osteonecrosis, and musculoskeletal pain. Perform necessary dental work before starting therapy.	Tablets, solution. Give on empty stomach (12-hour fast) to maximize bioavailability. Avoid splitting tablets to reduce risk of esophageal damage. Follow tablet administration with 6 mL water.
Allopurinol (Zyloprim)	Dissolution of urate uroliths: 10 mg/kg PO q 8h or 15 mg/kg PO q 12h for up to 4 weeks; 10 mg/kg PO q 24h to prevent recurrence Leishmaniasis: 5-20 mg/kg PO q 12h alone or in combination with meglumine antimoniate or miltefosine	Leishmaniasis: 10-20 mg/kg PO q 12-24h	Use with caution in patients with renal or hepatic dysfunction. Less common adverse effects include bone marrow suppression, severe dermatologic reactions, hepatitis, and vasculitis.	Tablets, injection
Alprazolam (Xanax)	Behavioral disorders: 0.02-0.1 mg/kg (usually 0.02-0.05 mg/kg initially) PO q 6-12h as needed	Behavioral disorders: 0.125–0.25 mg/CAT q 8-24h Sedation for transportation: 0.5–1 mg/CAT 1 hour before leaving for veterinary visit	Sedation is common. Use with caution in hepatic or renal disease.	Tablets, extended-release tablets, orally disintegrating tablets, oral solution. CSS-IV.
Aluminum hydroxide (Amphojel)	Hyperphosphatemia: Initial dose of 30-40 mg/kg per day in divided doses and mixed with food; titrate up to 100 mg/kg as necessary	Hyperphosphatemia: Initial dose of 30-40 mg/kg per day in divided doses and mixed with food; titrate up to 100 mg/kg as necessary	Avoid giving concurrently with other medications to avoid drug interactions.	Oral suspension. Compounding pharmacies may compound capsules or provide metered scoops of dry powder for addition to food. Give with meals 1 hour before or 2 hours after other drugs.

Generic Name (Brand Name, Synonyms)	Canine Dosages	Feline Dosages	Adverse Effects/Warnings	Administration/ Availability
Amantadine (Symmetrel)	Adjunct analgesia: 2-5 mg/kg PO q 24h	Adjunct analgesia: 2–5 mg/kg PO once q 24h	GI upset occurs commonly in dogs at onset of treatment. Use with caution in patients with hepatic disease, renal disease (dosage adjustment may be required), CHF, active psychoses, eczematoid dermatitis, or seizure disorders.	Tablets, capsules, syrup
Amikacin sulfate (Amikin, Amiglyde-V)	Susceptible infections: 15-30 mg/kg IV, IM, or SQ q 24h	Susceptible infections: 10-15 mg/kg IV, IM, or SQ q 24h	Adverse effects include nephrotoxicity, ototoxicity, neuromuscular blockade; these adverse effects may be worse in cats. Use carefully (if at all) in animals that have renal insufficiency or are dehydrated. Dose reduction has been suggested for sighthounds.	Injection. For intravenous administration, should be further diluted with normal saline or D_5W and administered over 30-60 minutes.
Amino acids 3% and glycerin injection with electrolytes (ProcalAmine)	Partial parenteral nutrition: Maintenance rate Hepatocutaneous syndrome: 25 mL/kg IV over 8 hours	Partial parenteral nutrition: Maintenance rate	Thrombophlebitis, fever, and GI signs are potential complications.	No longer commercially available. Pure amino acid injections (8.5%, 10%) are still available.
Aminocaproic acid (Amicar)	Antifibrinolytic: 50-100 mg/kg PO, IV q 6-8h. May also be used as prophylaxis prior to surgery in sighthound breeds. Degenerative myelopathy: 500 mg PO q 8h given concurrently with acetylcysteine	Use is not described in cats	May cause GI upset in dogs initially. Contraindicated in dogs with active clotting disorders, including disseminated intravascular coagulation.	Tablets (expensive), injection. The injectable formulation may be mixed with vitamin solutions and given orally. Injectable formulations can also be diluted in 0.9% saline for infusion over 30 minutes.
Aminophylline	Bronchodilator: 5-10 mg/kg PO q 8-24h; can be given IM or diluted for slow IV administration for emergent bronchodilation	Bronchodilator: 4-5 mg/kg PO q 8-24h	CNS stimulation and GI upset	Tablets are no longer commercially available, though compounding pharmacists may prepare oral capsules from the powder. The injectable formulation may be given orally followed by at least 6 mL of water or food.
Amiodarone (Cordarone, Pacerone)	Arrhythmias: Initial loading dosage of 8-10 mg/kg PO q 12h for 1 week and then reduced to 5-10 mg/kg PO q 24h thereafter	Use in cats is not described.	GI upset is common. Corneal deposits, neutropenia, thrombocytopenia, bradycardia, hepatotoxicity, and positive Coombs' tests have also been reported.	Tablets, injection. Some brands of intravenous products may cause serious histamine reaction in dogs.
Amitraz (Mitaban)	Demodicosis: Dilute 10.6 mL per 2 gallons of water, and apply topically q 14 days for 3-6 treatments until mites are gone. Wet coat thoroughly and allow to air-dry.	Do not use on cats.	Transient sedation, skin irritation are possible. Ingestion can cause salivation, vomiting, hyperglycemia, bradycardia, and respiratory depression. HIGHLY TOXIC to cats. MAO inhibitor activity. Do not use with interacting drugs (e.g., TCAs, SSRIs, selegiline).	Solution for dipping. Also found in some tick collars for dogs.
Amitriptyline HCl (Elavil)	Adjunctive therapy for behavioral disorders: 1-2 mg/kg PO q 12h Adjunctive analgesic therapy: 3-4 mg/kg PO q 12h	Anxiolytic for lower urinary tract syndrome: 5-10 mg/CAT (0.5-1 mg/kg) PO q 24h (can be divided twice daily)	Anticholinergic side effects are common. Do not use with MAO inhibitors (e.g., amitraz). Use with caution in patients with thyroid disorders, urinary retention, hepatic disorders, KCS, glaucoma, cardiac rhythm disorders, DM, or adrenal tumors due to anticholinergic adverse effects.	Tablets

Generic Name (Brand Name, Synonyms)	Canine Dosages	Feline Dosages	Adverse Effects/Warnings	Administration/ Availability
Amlodipine (Norvasc, Istin)	Hypertension: 0.1-0.5 mg/kg PO q 12-24h; titrate up to effect with maximum dose 1 mg/kg/day	Hypertension: 0.625 mg/CAT PO q 12-24h, or 0.125-0.25 mg/kg PO q 24h up to 0.5 mg/kg as needed	Titrate dose upward as needed to reduce risk of anorexia and syncope (cats). Gingival hyperplasia has been reported in dogs. Hypotension and bradycardia are possible in dogs and cats.	Tablets. May be compounded into a stable oral suspension.
Ammonium chloride (Uroeze)	Urinary acidification: 20 mg/kg PO q 8-12h Intoxication benefiting from acidification: 50 mg/kg PO q 6h Ammonia tolerance test: 100 mg/kg PO or by enema once (check fasting ammonia first; if increased, test should not be performed)	Urinary acidification: 20 mg/kg PO q 12h	Most common adverse effect is GI upset. May result in metabolic acidosis. Contraindicated in patients with uremia or hepatic encephalopathy (tolerance test dangerous and not necessary if fasting ammonia is elevated).	Tablets. Compounding pharmacies may supply metered scoops of bulk powder for addition to food.
Amoxicillin (Amoxil, Amoxi-Tabs, Amoxi-Drop)	Susceptible infections: 11-20 mg/kg PO q 8-12h Borreliosis infections: 20 mg/kg PO q 8h for 30 days	Susceptible infections: 11-15 mg/kg PO q 8-12h	Most common adverse effect is GI upset. Hypersensitivity reactions have been reported.	Tablets, capsules, powder for oral suspension
Amoxicillin/clavulanic acid (Clavamox, Augmentin)	Susceptible infections: 12.5-25 mg/kg PO q 8-12h Staphylococcal endocarditis: 22 mg/kg PO q 8h for 6-8 weeks	Susceptible infections: 12.5-25 mg/kg PO q 8-12h Upper respiratory infection: 12.5 mg/kg PO q 12h	Most common adverse effect is GI upset. Hypersensitivity reactions have been reported. Neurotoxicity in dogs has been reported after use of high doses.	Tablets, oral suspensions. If using fractions of tablets, wrap remainder tightly in foil before next use.
Amphotericin B deoxycholate (Fungizone)	Susceptible mycotic or algal infections: 0.25-0.5 mg/kg diluted in 5% dextrose (final concentration ≤0.1 mg/mL) and give IV over 4 to 6 hours q 48h to total cumulative dose of 8-12 mg/kg or first signs of nephrotoxicosis. Alternative route of administration is to dilute dose in 500 mL of 0.45% saline/2.5% dextrose (<20 mg/liter concentration) for SQ administration q 48h	Susceptible mycotic or algal infections: 0.25-0.5 mg/kg diluted in 5% dextrose to final concentration of 0.1 mg/mL and give IV over 4-6 hours q 48h to total cumulative dose of 6-10 mg/kg or first signs of nephrotoxicosis	Some degree of dose-related nephrotoxicity is inevitable; lipid-complexed and liposome-encapsulated amphotericin B is less nephrotoxic.	Injection for reconstitution. Do not mix with 0.9 % saline. Some clinicians diurese with saline before treatment.
Amphotericin B liposomal encapsulated (AmBisome, Abelcet)	Susceptible mycotic or algal infections: 1-3.3 mg/kg diluted (≤1 mg/mL) in D_5W given IV over 2 hours administered q 48h to total cumulative dose of 12-20 mg/kg or first signs of nephrotoxicosis	Susceptible mycotic or algal infections: 1 mg/kg diluted (≤1 mg/mL) in D_5W given IV over 2 hours administered q 48h to total cumulative dose of 8-12 mg/kg or first signs of nephrotoxicosis	Lipid-complexed and liposome-encapsulated amphotericin B is less nephrotoxic than conventional formulation and therefore may be used in a higher cumulative dose. However, infusion reactions such as phlebitis are more common.	Injection for reconstitution. Dilute calculated dose in D_5W to ≤1 mg/mL.
Ampicillin (Princillin, Omnipen, Polyflex)	Susceptible infections: 20-40 mg/kg IV q 6-8h. Higher dosages required for many enterococcal infections.	Susceptible infections: 20-40 mg/kg IV q 6-8h. Higher dosages required for many enterococcal infections.	Adverse events are usually GI; hypersensitivity has been reported. Many dosing references to IV ampicillin are appropriate only for ampicillin sodium solutions for injection. Ampicillin trihydrate suspension for injection (Polyflex) should not be given IV.	Injection, capsules. Amoxicillin is preferred over ampicillin for oral administration.
Ampicillin + sulbactam (Unasyn)	Susceptible infections: 20-30 mg/kg IV q 6-8h	Susceptible infections: 20-30 mg/kg IV q 6-8h	Injections can cause pain (IM and SQ) or thrombophlebitis (IV). Hepatotoxicity has been reported in humans and anecdotally observed in dogs. Hypersensitivity reactions occasionally reported.	Injection
Amprolium (Corid)	Coccidiosis: Adults 300-400 mg/DOG PO q 24h for 7-12 days; puppies 60 to 200 mg/PUP PO q 24h	Coccidiosis: 60-100 mg/CAT PO q 24h for 7 days	Ensure that patient swallows entire dose as it is extremely bitter. Prolonged high doses or overdoses may cause thiamine deficiency.	Oral solution, soluble oral powder

Generic Name (Brand Name, Synonyms)	Canine Dosages	Feline Dosages	Adverse Effects/Warnings	Administration/ Availability
Apomorphine (Apometic, Apokyn)	Emesis induction: 0.03 mg/kg IV, 0.04 mg/kg IM (least preferred), or ¼ to 1 tablet/DOG crushed and dissolved in small volume sterile saline instilled in conjunctival sac (rinse eye after emesis)	Do not use in cats.	Overdoses in dogs may result in cardiorespiratory depression, CNS stimulation/depression and protracted vomiting. Naloxone reverses CNS and respiratory symptoms, but does not affect vomiting. Contraindicated in cats.	Usually compounded. Tablets or injectable product for humans is not readily available for veterinary use.
Ascorbic acid (vitamin C)	Antioxidant: 20-30 mg/kg PO, IM, or slow IV q 6-8h for 2-3 days	Antioxidant: 20-30 mg/kg PO, IM, or slow IV q 6-8h for 2-3 days	Use to reverse methemoglobinemia is controversial.	Tablets, injection
Asparaginase (Elspar)	Chemotherapy for lymphoma: 400 units/kg, or 10,000 units/m^2 (NOT units/kg) IM or SQ	Chemotherapy for lymphoma: 400 units/kg IM, SQ, or IP	Antihistamine or glucocorticoid pre-treatment indicated to mitigate risk of severe hypersensitivity reaction. Asparaginase is intermittently commercially available as an FDA-approved product but may be purchased from FDA-registered 503B outsourcing facilities. Because asparaginase is used in cancer chemotherapy, it was once considered a hazardous drug; however, it was removed from the NIOSH list of hazardous drugs in 2016.	Available from sterile compounding outsourcing facilities as 10,000-U vial. No longer classified as a hazardous drug by NIOSH.
Aspirin	Antithrombotic: 0.5-2 mg/kg PO q 12-24h Analgesia: 10 mg/kg PO q 12h (alternative analgesics preferred)	Analgesic/antipyretic/antiinflammatory: 10 mg/kg PO q 48-72h Antithrombotic: 5 mg/CAT PO q 72h	Enteric-coated tablets for humans may be released erratically or not at all in dogs and cats. Highly protein bound; use lower doses in hypoalbuminemic patients. Dogs are more sensitive to GI ulceration than cats. Aspirin has an extended half-life (30 hours) in cats.	Plain or enteric-coated tablets or effervescent tablets for dissolution in water
Atenolol (Tenormin)	Cardiovascular indications: 0.25-1.5 mg/kg PO q 12h	Cardiovascular indications, including hypertension: 6.25 mg/CAT (¼ of a 25-mg tablet) PO q 12h. Dosage may be titrated upward to maximum of 25 mg q 12h.	Adverse effects include bradycardia, inappetence, lethargy and depression, impaired AV conduction, CHF, hypotension, and hypoglycemia.	Tablets. Compounding pharmacies may prepare stable oral suspensions. Reduce dose with renal dysfunction.
Atipamezole (Antisedan)	Alpha-adrenergic reversal: 3750 mcg/m^2 IM once; practically, mL for mL volume equivalent to dexmedetomidine or medetomidine used Amitraz toxicity: 50 mcg/kg IM up to q 4h prn	Alpha-adrenergic reversal agent: mL for mL volume equivalent to medetomidine	Occasionally GI signs, hypersalivation, or tremors are seen. Reversal is rapid, so exercise caution as animal may be briefly hyperexcitable or hyper-reactive.	Injection
Atovaquone (Mepron, Malarone)	Susceptible infection: 15 mg/kg PO q 8h with a fatty meal; often combined with azithromycin	Cytauxzoonosis: 15 mg/kg PO q 8h, with azithromycin	Oral suspension is very viscous and opaque; suspension drawn up into oral dosing syringes should be allowed to settle, undisturbed, protected from light to ensure that all air bubbles have dissipated so that an accurate dose can be achieved.	Oral suspension (preferred) or oral tablets in combination with proguanil. Best absorbed with food.
Atropine sulfate	Bradycardia: 0.04 mg/kg IV (during cardiopulmonary resuscitation; can be given intratracheal or intraosseous if no vascular access), or divided IV and IM Organophosphate intoxication: 0.1-0.5 mg/kg; give ¼ dose IV and the remainder SQ or IM Preanesthetic: 0.01- 0.02 mg/kg IM or IV	Bradycardia or toxicoses: 0.04 mg/kg IV (during cardiopulmonary resuscitation; can be given intratracheal or intraosseous if no vascular access), or divided IV and IM Preanesthetic: 0.01- 0.02 mg/kg IM or IV	Adverse effects are dose related and include dry mouth, increased viscosity of secretions, dysphagia, constipation, vomiting, thirst, urinary retention, CNS effects, arrhythmias, and others.	Injection
Atropine sulfate ophthalmic	Mydriasis: 1 drop solution or ⅛ inch ointment per affected eye q 8-12h, then q 24-48h prn	Mydriasis: 1 drop solution or ⅛ inch ointment per affected eye q 8-12h, then q 24-48h prn	Hypersalivation, irritation, and sensitivity to bright light are potential adverse effects.	1% ointment or solution

Generic Name (Brand Name, Synonyms)	Canine Dosages	Feline Dosages	Adverse Effects/Warnings	Administration/ Availability
Auranofin (Ridaura)	Immune-mediated skin diseases: 0.05-0.2 mg/kg PO q 12h (up to 9 mg/day total dose)	Immune-mediated skin diseases: 0.2-0.3 mg/kg PO q 12h	Can cause a variety of dose-related immune-mediated or GI side effects, and on rare occasions renal and hepatic toxicity and dermal eruptions.	Capsules
Azathioprine (Imuran)	Immunosuppression: 2 mg/kg PO q 24h for 1-3 weeks followed by dose reduction, often to 1 mg/kg q 24h, followed by gradual further reduction with switch to q other day dosing Perianal fistulas: 1-2 mg/kg PO q 24h until lesions improve, then q 48h	Do not use in cats.	Adverse effects include GI effects, bone marrow suppression, pancreatitis, and hepatotoxicity (monitor CBC and liver enzymes). Avoid use with ACE inhibitors, sulfa-containing antibiotics, and allopurinol. Azathioprine poses a high risk of myelotoxicity in cats and in some dogs.	Tablets
Azithromycin (Zithromax)	Susceptible infections: 5-10 mg/kg PO q 24h for 3-7 days; 7-15 mg/kg PO q 12h for 5-7 days (cryptosporidiosis); combined with atovaquone for hematoprotozoal infection (e.g., *Babesia gibsoni*, 10 mg/kg q 24h for 10 days)	Susceptible infections: 5-10 mg/kg PO q 12h first day then q 24h for 3 days; ongoing treatment q 72h has been suggested for chronic upper respiratory infection; combined with atovaquone for hematoprotozoal infection (e.g., *Cytauxzoon felis*, 10 mg/kg q 24h for 10 days)	Can cause GI upset. Hypersensitivity reactions possible, especially with IV administration.	Tablets, powder for oral suspension, oral powder packets, injection. Some brands of injection may cause severe histamine reactions in dogs.

B

Generic Name (Brand Name, Synonyms)	Canine Dosages	Feline Dosages	Adverse Effects/Warnings	Administration/ Availability
Benazepril (Fortekor, Lotensin)	ACE inhibition: 0.25- 0.5 mg/kg PO q 24h, titrated prn to 1 mg/kg q 12h	ACE inhibition: 0.25-1 mg/kg PO q 12-24h	Adverse effects include GI upset, azotemia, hyperkalemia, and hypotension. Rashes, cough, neutropenia, and agranulocytosis have been reported in humans.	Tablets
Bethanechol (Urecholine)	Parasympathetic agonist (GI or urinary muscle stimulation): 5-25 mg/DOG PO q 8h	Parasympathetic agonist: 1.25-7.5 mg/CAT PO q 8h	Adverse effects include ptyalism, GI upset, and bronchoconstriction; contraindicated in the presence of GI or urinary obstruction.	Tablets
Bisacodyl (Dulcolax)	Laxative: 5-20 mg/DOG PO q 24h	Laxative: 5 mg/CAT PO q 24h	Can cause cramping; short-term use only.	Tablets OTC
Bismuth subsalicylate (Pepto-Bismol)	Antidiarrheal: 1 mL per 4 kg BW PO q 6-8h	Caution due to salicylate	Causes dark-colored stool (resembles melena).	Tablets, liquids OTC
Bleomycin (Blenoxane)	Antineoplastic: 10 units/m^2 IV or SQ q 24h × 3 days, then 10 units/m^2 q 7 days; maximum total = 200 units/m^2	Use is not described for cats.	Pulmonary damage is the most serious adverse effect. Allergic reactions, fever, anorexia, and vomiting; delayed toxic effects include dermatologic effects, stomatitis, pneumonitis, pulmonary fibrosis. NIOSH hazardous drug and should be prepared, administered, and disposed of in accordance with federal and local requirements.	Lyophilized powder for injection. Reconstitute 15-unit or 30-unit vial with 5 mL or 10 mL, respectively, of sodium chloride injection, 0.9%, USP, and administered slowly over 10 minutes. Cytotoxic, NIOSH-listed hazardous drug and should be prepared, administered, and disposed of in accordance with federal and local requirements.
Bromide: see potassium bromide				
Budesonide (Entocort EC)	IBD: 3 mg/m^2 PO q 24h (not to exceed 3 mg), or 0.5-3 mg/DOG q 24h	IBD: 1 mg/CAT PO q 24h Asthma: 400 mcg inhaled q 12h	Although budesonide causes less suppression of the HPA axis in humans, this may not be the case in dogs. Adverse effects associated with other glucocorticoid types can be seen.	Extended-release enteric capsules and also through compounding, or as compound for nebulization.

Generic Name (Brand Name, Synonyms)	Canine Dosages	Feline Dosages	Adverse Effects/Warnings	Administration/ Availability
Buprenorphine HCl (Buprenex, Simbadol)	Analgesia: 5-40 mcg/kg (0.005-0.04 mg/kg) IV, IM, or SQ q 6-12h	Postoperative analgesia with Simbadol: 0.24 mg/kg SQ q 24h up to 3 days Analgesia: 10-30 mcg/kg (0.01-0.03 mg/kg) IM, IV, or oral transmucosal q 6-8h	Respiratory depression is the most likely adverse effect, and vomiting and behavioral changes can occur in dogs or cats. In dogs, salivation, bradycardia, hypothermia, miosis, tachycardia, and high blood pressure have been reported. In cats, mydriasis and hyperthermia have been reported.	Injection and extended-release injection on FDA's Index of Legally Marketed Unapproved New Animal Drugs for Minor Species. CSS-III.
Buspirone (BuSpar)	Behavioral disorders: 0.5-2 mg/kg PO q 8-12h	Behavioral disorders: 0.5-1 mg/kg (or 2.5 mg/CAT) PO q 8-12h	Generally, well tolerated but bradycardia, GI disturbances, and stereotypic behaviors have been reported. Undesirable behavioral changes may result from disinhibition.	Tablets
Busulfan (Myleran, Busulfex)	Antineoplastic: 3-4 mg/m^2 PO q 24h	Antineoplastic: 2-4 mg/m^2 PO q 24h	Myelosuppression is common and potentially severe. Pulmonary fibrosis, hepatotoxicity, and hyperpigmentation of skin may occur. Uric acid levels should be monitored.	Tablets. Cytotoxic, NIOSH-listed hazardous drug and should be prepared, administered, and disposed of in accordance with federal and local requirements.
Butorphanol tartrate (Stadol, Torbutrol, Torbugesic)	Analgesia, sedation: 0.2-1 mg/kg PO, IM, SQ q 6-12h; 0.1-0.2 mg/kg IV. At dose of 0.1-0.5 mg/kg IV, IM can be combined with acepromazine 0.025-0.05 mg/kg mixed in same syringe Antitussive: 0.5-1 mg/kg PO q 6-12h	Analgesia: 0.1-0.5 mg/kg q 6-12h IV, IM, SQ	Reduce dose in dogs with *MDR1/ABCB1-Δ* mutation. Potential adverse effects include sedation, ataxia, anorexia, vomiting, or diarrhea (rarely).	Tablets, injection. CSS-IV.

C

Generic Name (Brand Name, Synonyms)	Canine Dosages	Feline Dosages	Adverse Effects/Warnings	Administration/ Availability
Cabergoline (Dostinex, Galastop)	Prolactin inhibition: 5 mcg/kg (0.005 mg/kg) PO q 8h	Prolactin inhibition: 25-50 mcg/CAT or 5-10 mcg/kg PO q 24h	Vomiting is the most common adverse effect. Has caused changes in coat color.	Available only through compounding in the United States; oral solution available in Europe.
Calcitonin (Miacalcin, Calcimar)	Hypercalcemia of malignancy: 4-8 units/kg IV, IM, or SQ q 12h	Hypercalcemia of malignancy: 4-8 units/kg IV, IM, or SQ q 12h	Anorexia and vomiting are the most common adverse effects. Pain at injection site is also reported.	Injection, metered-dose inhaler. Expensive.
Calcitriol (Rocaltrol, Calcijex)	Hypoparathyroidism: 0.03-0.06 mcg/kg PO q 24h, then 0.005-0.015 mcg/kg PO q 24h, with oral calcium and adjusted prn CKD: 2-2.5 ng/kg PO q 24h on empty stomach, adjusted upward prn not to exceed 7 ng/kg/d, or pulse dose of 20 ng/kg twice weekly at bedtime on empty stomach	CKD: Initial dosage 1.65-3.63 ng/kg (= 0.00165-0.00363 mcg/kg) PO q 24h on empty stomach, adjusted upward prn	May cause hypercalcemia or hyperphosphatemia (monitor levels closely).	Capsules, oral solution, and injection. A dilute solution may be prepared from the concentrated oral solution to better achieve small doses. Oil can be removed from capsule and diluted in corn oil and stored for up to 2 weeks.
Calcium carbonate (Tums, Epakitin)	Calcium supplementation/ phosphate binder: 90-150 mg/kg/d PO divided and given with food or just before each meal Epakitin phosphorous binder: 1 g/5 kg BW PO q 12h with food	Calcium supplementation/ phosphate binder: 90-150 mg/kg/d PO divided and given with food or just before each meal Epakitin phosphorous binder: 1 g/5 kg BW PO q 12h with food	Hypercalcemia is possible with overdosing or prolonged dosing. Interacts with many drugs and must be given 1 hour before or 2 hours after other drugs.	Tablets OTC, powder (Epakitin). Administer 1 hour before or 2 hours after other medications.
Calcium Disodium EDTA (Calcium Disodium Versenate)	Heavy metal poisoning: 25 mg/kg SQ q 6h diluted in 5% dextrose for 2-5 days	Heavy metal poisoning: 27.5 mg/kg SQ in 15 mL 5% dextrose q 6h for 5 days; rest for 5 days, repeat if needed	Painful on IM injection. Do not confuse with Sodium EDTA.	Available only through compounding. Dilute to 10 mg/mL in D_5W before administration.

Generic Name (Brand Name, Synonyms)	Canine Dosages	Feline Dosages	Adverse Effects/Warnings	Administration/ Availability
Capromorelin (Entyce)	Appetite stimulant: 3 mg/kg PO q 24h	Appetite stimulant: 1-3 mg/kg PO q 24h for up to 21 days	Well tolerated, but can cause GI upset, polydipsia, hypersalivation, abdominal discomfort, head shaking, lethargy, elevated BUN and phosphorus.	Oral solution
Carboplatin (Paraplatin)	Antineoplastic: 300 mg/m^2 IV in D_5W over 15 minutes q 3 weeks for 4 treatments	Unlike cisplatin, carboplatin may be used in cats. Antineoplastic: 200 mg/m^2 IV in D_5W over 15 minutes q 4 weeks. Carboplatin degrades to cisplatin in saline solutions.	Adverse events commonly include GI toxicity and myelosuppression. In dogs two nadirs occur around day 7-10 and 16-21 post carboplatin therapy.	Injection; rapidly degrades to cisplatin in saline solutions. Cytotoxic, NIOSH-listed hazardous drug and should be prepared, administered, and disposed of in accordance with federal and local requirements.
Carnitine: see L-carnitine				
Carprofen (Rimadyl, Novox, Quellin, Vetprofen)	Antiinflammatory/analgesic NSAID: 4.4 mg/kg PO q 24h OR divided and given as 2.2 mg/kg PO q 12h	Not recommended for use in cats due to nephrotoxicity. Not approved for use in cats in USA, but UK label: 4.4 mg/kg IV or SQ once	Adverse effects commonly include GI upset. Hepatocellular necrosis occurs in 0.05% of dogs treated. Other reported adverse effects include neurotoxicity and hematologic and behavioral changes.	Oral caplets, chewable tablets, and injection. Oral liquids may be prepared from tablets.
Carvedilol (Coreg)	Valvular heart disease: initial dose 0.15-0.2 mg/kg PO q 12h for 1 week. After evaluating blood pressure and heart rate, the dose can be increased to 0.3 mg/kg PO q 12h.	Dosing in cats is not described.	Use with caution if at all in dogs with CHF as carvedilol is a negative inotrope. Other side effects include lethargy, inappetence, and hypotension.	Tablets, extended-release oral capsules
Cefadroxil (Cefa-Tabs, Cefa-Drops, Duricef)	Susceptible infections: 22 mg/kg PO q 12h Superficial pyoderma: 22-35 mg/kg PO q 12h for 28-42 days	Susceptible infections: 22 mg/kg PO q 12-24h	Well tolerated, but most common adverse effect is GI upset. Hypersensitivity reactions have been reported.	Tablets, capsules, and powder for oral suspension
Cefazolin sodium (Ancef, Kefzol)	Susceptible infections or surgical prophylaxis: 22-35 mg/kg IM, IV, SQ q 6-8h. CRI 1.3 mg/kg loading dose, followed by 1.2 mg/kg/h	Susceptible infections or surgical prophylaxis: 22-35 mg/kg IM, IV q 8-12h	Well tolerated, but adverse effects include GI upset and pain on IM injection. Hypersensitivity occurs rarely. Consider dose reduction in advanced renal failure.	Injection, injection for reconstitution
Cefotaxime (Claforan)	Susceptible infections: 20-80 mg/kg (often 40 mg/kg) IV, SQ, or IM q 6-12h CRI with an initial IV load of 3.2 mg/kg IV followed by a CRI of 5 mg/kg/h GI surgical prophylaxis: 30 mg/kg IV 30-60 minutes before incision	Susceptible infections: 20-80 mg/kg (often 40 mg/kg) IV, SQ, or IM q 6-12h CRI with an initial IV load of 3.2 mg/kg IV followed by a CRI of 5 mg/kg/h	Generally well tolerated. IM and SQ injections may be painful. Rare adverse effects include neurotoxicity, cytopenias, hepatitis, and renal damage.	Injection
Cefotetan (Cefotan)	Susceptible infections: 30 mg/kg IV or SQ q 8-12h GI surgical prophylaxis: 30 mg/kg IV 30-60 minutes before incision	Susceptible infections: 30 mg/kg IV or SQ q 8-12h GI surgical prophylaxis: 30 mg/kg IV 30-60 minutes before incision	Generally well tolerated. IM and SQ injections may be painful. Rare adverse effects include neurotoxicity, cytopenias, hepatitis, and renal damage.	Injection
Cefovecin (Convenia)	Susceptible infections: 8 mg/kg SQ once; can be repeated once in 1 to 2 weeks if partial resolution of infection	Susceptible infections: 8 mg/kg SQ once	Well tolerated but adverse effects include anorexia, depression, and vomiting. Hypersensitivity reactions have occurred. Cefovecin is highly protein bound and should be used cautiously with other drugs that are highly bound to plasma proteins.	Injection for reconstitution in sterile water; keep refrigerated and protect from light. Reconstituted product darkens on storage but can be kept for 2 months.
Cefoxitin	Susceptible infections: 30 mg/kg q 6-8h IM or IV Presurgical prophylaxis: 20-30 mg/kg IV, IM 30 minutes before surgery; may repeat in 3-6 h	Susceptible infections: 30 mg/kg q 6-8h IM or IV Presurgical prophylaxis: 20-30 mg/kg IV, IM 30 minutes before surgery; may repeat in 3-6 h	Rare hypersensitivity reactions	Injection (powder for reconstitution or solution). Once reconstituted, stable for 24 h at room temperature or up to 1 week if refrigerated. Solution can be frozen immediately once for longer storage up to 45 days.

Generic Name (Brand Name, Synonyms)	Canine Dosages	Feline Dosages	Adverse Effects/Warnings	Administration/ Availability
Cefpodoxime (Simplicef, Vantin)	Susceptible skin and soft tissue infections: 5-10 mg/kg PO q 24h	Susceptible skin and soft tissue infections: 5-10 mg/kg PO q 24h	Well tolerated but adverse effects include inappetence, GI upset, and lethargy. Hypersensitivity and pemphigus-like drug reactions are rare, but possible.	Tablets
Ceftazidime (Ceptaz, Fortaz, Tazicef)	Susceptible infections (usually *Pseudomonas*): 30 mg/kg IV, IM, SQ q 6-8h or as a continuous IV infusion (CRI) with a loading dose of 4.4 mg/kg and a CRI infusion rate of 4.1 mg/kg/h Infections other than *Pseudomonas*: 30-50 mg/kg IV or IM q 6-12h	Susceptible infections (usually *Pseudomonas*): 30 mg/kg IV, IM, SQ q 8h or as a continuous IV infusion (CRI) with a loading dose of 4.4 mg/kg and a CRI infusion rate of 4.1 mg/kg/h	Painful on IM injection. May cause GI upset or dysbiosis. Hypersensitivity has been reported.	Injection
Cephalexin (Keflex, Cepexin, cefalexin)	Susceptible infections: 22-40 mg/kg PO q 8-12h	Susceptible infections: 15-30 mg/kg PO q 8-12h	Well tolerated, but adverse effects include GI upset. Hypersensitivity or blood dyscrasias occur rarely. Consider dose reduction in advanced renal failure.	Capsules, tablets, powder for oral suspension
Cetirizine (Zyrtec)	Antipruritic antihistamine: 5-10 mg/DOG (up to maximum 2 mg/kg) PO q 12h	Antipruritic antihistamine: 5 mg/CAT PO q 24h	Generally well tolerated. Sedation, hypersalivation and ataxia may occur in animals despite being a "nonsedating" antihistamine.	Tablet, oral solution OTC
Charcoal, activated	GI adsorbent for acute poisoning: 1-2 g/kg PO or by stomach tube (preferred); use labeled dose when using commercial product. Can be mixed with small amount of canned food or broth and offered for voluntary consumption, or mixed with water (1 g/5 mL) for syringe or tube administration	GI adsorbent for acute poisoning: 1-2 g/kg PO or by stomach tube (preferred); use labeled dose when using commercial product. Can be mixed with small amount of canned food or broth and offered for voluntary consumption, or mixed with water (1 g/5 mL) for syringe or tube administration	Do not administer to animals that are vomiting (aspiration risk) or that have ingested caustic or corrosive materials. Charcoal combined with cathartic can cause hypernatremia (especially in smaller animals). Rapid administration may cause vomiting/aspiration. Not effective for all toxicants (e.g., mineral acids or alkalis, ethanol, fertilizer). Stains clothing.	Granules and oral suspensions combined with sorbitol cathartic to encourage evacuation of charcoal-bound toxicant
Chitosan-based phosphate binder (Epakitin)	Phosphate binder: 1 g/5 kg BW PO q 12h	Phosphate binder: 1 g/5 kg BW PO q 12h	Contains lactose, calcium carbonate, chitosan, and hydrolyzed soy protein.	Scoopable powder to add to food
Chlorambucil (Leukeran)	Antineoplastic: 2 mg/m^2 PO q 24h for 3 weeks beyond remission; then 1.5 mg/m^2 PO q 24h for 15 days and then q third day; or 0.1-0.2 mg/kg PO q 24-72h, or 15-20 mg/m^2 PO q 2 weeks	Antineoplastic: 15 mg/m^2 PO q 24h for 4 days, repeated q 3 weeks, or 2 mg/CAT PO q 48h, or 20 mg/m^2 PO q 2 weeks. Often administered with prednisolone.	Adverse events commonly include GI toxicity and myelosuppression.	Tablets. Cytotoxic, NIOSH-listed hazardous drug and should be prepared, administered, and disposed of in accordance with federal and local requirements. Although can be compounded, advisability of using compounded liquids is questionable due to possible human exposure.
Chloramphenicol (Viceton)	Susceptible infections: 40-60 mg/kg PO, IM, IV q 6-8h	Susceptible infections: 15-50 mg/kg PO, IM, IV q 12h	Can cause bone marrow suppression, as well as GI upset. Use with extreme caution in patients with pre-existing hematologic disorders, pregnancy, hepatic failure, and in neonates. Lower doses used in cats as they are at higher risk for adverse events, especially if used >14 days. Multiple drug interactions. Risk of aplasia in humans who are susceptible.	Tablets, capsules, oral suspension, injection, and ophthalmic ointment. Owner should be cautioned to wear gloves and wash hands after administration.
Chorionic gonadotropin, human (Chorulon, HCG)	Cryptorchidism: 100-1000 units/DOG IM q 3-4 days × 4 treatments Testosterone stimulation for gonadal status testing: Measure testosterone before and 24 hours after 750 units IV (regardless of body weight) Male infertility (controversial): 500-1000 units/DOG IM q 2 weeks	Induction of ovulation: 500 units IM on day 1 or days 1 and 2 of estrus. Alternatively, 250 units IM on days 2 and 3 of estrus, coupled with mating 3 times per day at 3-hour intervals for the first 3 days of estrus.	Contraindicated in androgen-responsive neoplasias or hypersensitivity to the drug.	Injection

Generic Name (Brand Name, Synonyms)	Canine Dosages	Feline Dosages	Adverse Effects/Warnings	Administration/ Availability
Cimetidine (Tagamet)	H_2 blocking antacid: 5-10 mg/kg PO or IV q 6-8h	H_2 blocking antacid: 2.5-5 mg/kg PO q 6-12h	Multiple drug interactions and limited efficacy mean that this drug is now rarely used in dogs or cats.	Tablets, oral solution (both OTC), and injection
Ciprofloxacin (Cipro)	Susceptible infections: 25-30 mg/kg PO q 24h, or 20-25 mg/kg IV q 24h	Susceptible infections: 20-25 mg/kg PO q 24h, or 20-25 mg/kg IV q 24h	Well tolerated but can cause GI distress, CNS stimulation, crystalluria, urolithiasis, and hypersensitivity. Intact tablets have variable bioavailability in dogs, but using higher dosage and crushing tablets often permits therapeutically effective blood levels. Like other fluoroquinolones, it is relatively contraindicated for young, growing animals due to cartilage abnormalities. Use with caution in hepatic or renal insufficiency, dehydration.	Tablets (crush before administration), injection, and ophthalmic preparations
Cisapride	Prokinetic: 0.5 mg/kg PO q 8-12h; can gradually increase to 1 mg/kg PO q 8h	Prokinetic: 2.5 mg/CAT PO q 12h initially, gradually increasing up to 7.5 mg/CAT q 8h if needed. Often combined with lactulose for treatment of constipation.	Generally well tolerated in animals but GI upset can occur. Contraindicated in GI obstruction. Discontinued for human use due to QT interval prolongation.	Available only through compounding
Cisplatin (Platinol-AQ)	Antineoplastic: 50-70 mg/m^2 slow IV infusion q 3-5 weeks accompanied with saline diuresis Intrapleural instillation: 50 mg/m^2 diluted in saline to volume of 250 mL/m^2, warmed to body temperature, and infused into pleural space q 3-4 weeks prn to control malignant effusion	Do not use in cats.	Never use in cats due to risk of fatal pulmonary edema. Adverse effects in dogs include GI upset, nephrotoxicity, ototoxicity, and myelosuppression.	Injection for infusion; must be given as slow IV infusion to dogs with fluid diuresis before and after infusion. Cytotoxic, NIOSH-listed hazardous drug and should be prepared, administered, and disposed of in accordance with federal and local requirements.
Clarithromycin (Biaxin)	Susceptible infections: 5-12.5 mg/kg PO q 12h	Susceptible infections: 7.5 mg/kg or 62.5 mg/CAT PO q 12h	Generally well tolerated other than GI upset. Many drug interactions.	Tablets, oral suspension
Clindamycin (Antirobe, Cleocin)	Susceptible infections: 11-33 mg/kg PO q 12h; 10-15 mg/kg IV q 12h	Susceptible infections including toxoplasmosis: 11-33 mg/kg PO q 24h	Adverse effects include GI upset or esophageal injuries (esophagitis, strictures) when solid dosage forms were given without food or a water bolus. Cats may show hypersalivation or lip smacking after administration of the oral liquid due to the unpleasant taste.	Tablets, capsules, oral solution, powder, topical solutions, and injection
Clofazimine (Lamprene)	*M. avium*-intracellulare complex infections, or opportunistic mycobacteriosis: 4-8 mg/kg PO q 24h for 4 weeks, usually as part of a multidrug protocol	*M. avium*-intracellulare complex infections, feline leprosy, or opportunistic mycobacteriosis: 4-10 mg/kg, or 25-50 mg/CAT PO q 24-48h for 4 weeks, usually as part of a multidrug protocol	Adverse effects are usually GI upset (may be dose-limiting). Clofazimine stains skin, eyes, bodily fluids, and excreta. Treatment duration often for weeks to months.	Tablets. May be difficult for veterinarians to obtain due to restricted distribution systems.
Clomipramine (Clomicalm, Anafranil)	Behavior modification: 1-2 mg/kg PO q 12h initially and eventually up to 3 mg/kg PO q 12-24h	Behavior modification: 0.25-1 mg/kg PO q 24h; begin at lower dose and titrate up prn	Avoid use in animals exposed to MAO inhibitors (e.g., amitraz and l-deprenyl). Adverse effects include GI upset, sedation, anticholinergic effects; cats may be more sensitive than dogs. Use with caution in liver disease, cardiac rate and rhythm disorders, urinary retention, or reduced GI motility. Avoid use in breeding males.	Tablets

Generic Name (Brand Name, Synonyms)	Canine Dosages	Feline Dosages	Adverse Effects/Warnings	Administration/ Availability
Clonazepam (Klonopin)	Anxiolytic: 0.5-1 mg/kg PO q 8-12h Antiepileptic: up to 2 mg/kg PO q 12h	Anxiolytic and antiepileptic: 0.02-0.5 mg/kg PO q 8-12h	Adverse effects include hypersalivation, hypersecretion in upper respiratory passages, GI effects, transient elevations of liver enzymes, and hematologic effects. Tolerance to the antiseizure effects has been reported in dogs. Cats may develop hepatocellular necrosis, but this is not as likely as with oral diazepam.	Tablets and rapidly disintegrating tablets. CSS-IV.
Clonidine (Duraclon, Catapres)	Behavior modification and anxiolytic: 0.01-0.05 mg/kg PO approximately 1.5 to 2 hours before the triggering event; start with lower dose and titrate up if necessary	Adjunctive antidiarrheal: 5-10 mcg/kg 2-3 times a day, SQ or PO	Adverse effects may include transient hyperglycemia, dry mouth, constipation, sedation, paradoxical arousal, hypotension, collapse, and bradycardia.	Tablets, injection, transdermal patch
Clopidogrel (Plavix)	Thromboprophylaxis: 1-2 mg/kg PO q 24h, or 10 mg/kg PO on day 1, then 2-3 mg/kg PO q 24h thereafter	Thromboprophylaxis: 18.75 mg/CAT PO q 24h; higher doses have been used	Generally well tolerated. Adverse effects may include vomiting or bleeding.	Tablets
Clorazepate (Tranxene-SD, Gen-Xene)	Anxiolytic and adjunct antiepileptic: 0.5-2 mg/kg PO q 8-12h. Tolerance can occur with continued use.	Anxiolytic: 0.02-0.4 mg/kg PO q 12-24h Antiepileptic: 3.75-7.5 mg/CAT PO q 12-24h	Adverse effects include sedation and ataxia. May exacerbate myasthenia gravis. Use with caution in liver disease. May worsen aggression through disinhibition.	Tablets
Cosyntropin (ACTH, Cortrosyn)	ACTH stimulation test: 5 mcg/kg solution IV once. Can use entire vial of Cortrosyn per dog regardless of size.	ACTH stimulation test: 125 mcg/CAT	Rare hypersensitivity reactions.	Dry powder for reconstitution. Compounded solutions may not be as efficacious and time of peak response may be less consistent. Gel no longer available.
Cyanocobalamin (vitamin B_{12})	Hypocobalaminemia: 25 mcg/kg SQ q 1 week for 6 weeks, then once more in 4 weeks. Recheck cobalamin status. Alternatively, for dogs <9 kg give 250 mcg, for dogs 9-18 kg give 500 mcg, or dogs >18 kg give 1000 mcg PO q 24h for 12 weeks, then check cobalamin status.	Hypocobalaminemia: 250 mcg/CAT SQ once a week for 6 weeks, then q 1-2 months based on cobalamin levels, or 250 mcg PO q 24h for 12 weeks then recheck status	Very well tolerated	Tablets, injection
Cyclophosphamide (Cytoxan, Neosar)	Antineoplastic: 10-15 mg/m^2 (as a daily metronomic dose), or 50 mg/m^2 PO q 24h for 3 to 4 days of each week, or 250-300 mg/m^2 once q 3 weeks	Antineoplastic: 10-15 mg/m^2 (as a daily metronomic dose) to 50 mg/m^2 PO q 24h for 3 to 4 days each week to larger dosages of 250-300 mg/m^2 once q 3 weeks	Adverse effects are myelosuppression, GI effects, alopecia in cyclical hair-growing breeds, and sterile hemorrhagic cystitis. Pulmonary fibrosis and secondary cancers may occur. Adjunctive treatment with furosemide is used as prophylaxis for hemorrhagic cystitis.	Tablets, injection. Cytotoxic, NIOSH-listed hazardous drug and should be prepared, administered, and disposed of in accordance with federal and local requirements.
Cyclosporine-systemic (Atopica, Neoral, Sandimmune)	Atopic dermatitis: 5 mg/kg PO q 24h (or if given concurrently with ketoconazole 2.5-3 mg/kg PO q 24h) Immunosuppression: 5 mg/kg PO q 12-24h, adjusted based on functional or pharmacologic monitoring KCS: 0.5 cm of ophthalmic ointment on affected eye q 12h	Eosinophilic granuloma, asthma, or allergic dermatitis: 4-7 mg/kg or 25 mg/CAT PO q 24h	GI upset is commonly reported initially. Giving the drug with a small amount of food or placing doses in the freezer for 30-60 minutes before administration anecdotally alleviates vomiting, or may use antiemetic such as maropitant first several days of treatment. Gingival hypertrophy, papillomatosis, protein-losing nephropathy, and secondary infection (e.g., toxoplasmosis) or malignancy have been reported.	Capsules, oral solution, injection, and ophthalmic ointments. Injections may cause a severe histamine reaction in dogs. Administer with food in dogs and on an empty stomach in cats. Do not interchange Sandimmune with Atopica/Neoral/Gengraf products as Sandimmune is not bioequivalent.

Generic Name (Brand Name, Synonyms)	Canine Dosages	Feline Dosages	Adverse Effects/Warnings	Administration/ Availability
Cyproheptadine (Periactin)	Dysphoria of serotonin syndrome or toxicoses: 1.1 mg/kg PO; doses may be repeated q 4-6h as needed until signs have resolved Appetite stimulation: 0.2 mg/kg PO q 12h	Appetite stimulant: 1-4 mg/CAT PO q 8-25h (largely obsolete use) Dysphoria of serotonin syndrome or toxicoses: 2-4 mg/CAT PO; doses may be repeated q 4-6h as needed until signs have resolved	Agents such as capromorelin (for dogs) and mirtazapine (for dogs and cats) have made use of cyproheptadine as an appetite stimulant obsolete. Use of cyproheptadine in small animals as an antihistamine is becoming rare. Adverse effects include sedation and anticholinergic effects. Cats may exhibit paradoxical hyperstimulation; some reports of hemolytic anemia in cats.	Tablets, oral solution
Cytarabine (Cytosar-U)	Antineoplastic: 300 mg/m² SQ divided into 3 or 4 doses q 24h over 3-4 days, or IV as a continuous infusion (lasting 4-8 hours) once weekly Inflammatory brain disease (MUE): 50 mg/m² SQ q 12h for 2 consecutive days, or 25 mg/m² per hour for an 8-hour CRI; may be repeated q 3-4 weeks	Antineoplastic: 100 mg/m² SQ q 12h for 2 to 4 days. Use in cats is not well-described.	Adverse effects are primarily GI and myelosuppression.	Injection. Cytotoxic, NIOSH-listed hazardous drug and should be prepared, administered, and disposed of in accordance with federal and local requirements.

D

Generic Name (Brand Name, Synonyms)	Canine Dosages	Feline Dosages	Adverse Effects/Warnings	Administration/ Availability
Dacarbazine (DTIC)	Antineoplastic: 800-1000 mg/m² IV over 4-8 hours q 2-3 weeks OR lower dosage 200-250 mg/m² q 24h IV for 5 days with the treatment cycle repeated q 3-4 weeks	Do not use in cats.	Adverse effects include GI toxicity and myelosuppression. Usually reserved for cases not responsive to more conventional therapies.	Injection. Cytotoxic, NIOSH-listed hazardous drug and should be prepared, administered, and disposed of in accordance with federal and local requirements.
Dactinomycin (Cosmegen, actinomycin-D)	Antineoplastic: 0.5-1 mg/m² IV over 20 minutes; repeated at 1- to 3-week intervals	Dosing is not described for cats.	Adverse effects are primarily GI toxicity and myelosuppression.	Injection. Cytotoxic, NIOSH-listed hazardous drug and should be prepared, administered, and disposed of in accordance with federal and local requirements.
Dalteparin (Fragmin, LMWH)	Thromboprophylaxis: 100-150 units/kg SQ q 8-12h	Thromboprophylaxis: No consensus dosing described, but 100-175 units/kg SQ q 6-12h described	Can cause or worsen bleeding; contraindicated with severe thrombocytopenia. Available in broad range of concentrations; ensure correct dosing.	Injection (expensive). U-100 insulin syringes useful for providing accurate dosing.
Dapsone (Avlosulfon)	Mycobacteriosis: 1.1. mg/kg PO q 6h until remission, then 0.3 mg/kg q 8-12h Spider envenomation: 1 mg/kg PO q 24h for 10 days (inhibits neutrophil migration)	Do not use in cats.	Due to its adverse effect profile (hepatotoxicity, dose-dependent methemoglobinemia, hemolytic anemia, thrombocytopenia, neutropenia, GI effects, cutaneous drug eruptions, and neuropathies), dapsone is rarely used in veterinary medicine. Dapsone is a potential carcinogen.	Tablets
Darbepoetin (Aranesp)	Erythropoiesis: 0.45-1.5 mcg/kg SQ once weekly until the target PCV is attained, then extending interdose interval as tolerated (q 2-3 weeks typical). Administer iron supplement.	Erythropoiesis: 0.7-1.8 mcg/kg SQ once weekly until the target PCV is attained, then extending interdose interval as tolerated (q 2-3 weeks typical). Administer iron supplement.	Anti-erythropoietin antibody formation with resultant pure red blood cell aplasia (PRCA) may occur as well as injection-site reactions, polycythemia, hypertension, seizures, or iron deficiency.	Injection

Generic Name (Brand Name, Synonyms)	Canine Dosages	Feline Dosages	Adverse Effects/Warnings	Administration/ Availability
Decoquinate (Deccox)	Hepatozoonosis: 10-20 mg/kg PO q 12h mixed in food	Dosing is not described for cats.	Generally well tolerated. Must be given for >2 years to treat hepatozoonosis.	Powdered feed additive OTC
Deferoxamine (Desferal)	Iron chelator: 15 mg/kg/h IV; or 40 mg/kg IM q 4-8h for 48-72 hours until serum iron is <300 mcg/dL. Most effective within 24 hours of intoxication.	Iron chelator: 15 mg/kg/h IV; or 40 mg/kg IM q 4-8h for 48-72 hours until serum iron is <300 mcg/dL. Most effective within 24 hours of intoxication.	Adverse effects include hypersensitivity reactions, auditory neurotoxicity, pain or swelling at injection sites, and GI distress. Contraindicated in severe chronic kidney disease and anuria unless used with dialysis. Will turn urine a pink color during iron chelation.	Injection; difficult to obtain
Denamarin: see silymarin				
Deracoxib (Deramaxx)	Analgesic/antiinflammatory NSAID: 1-2 mg/kg PO q 24h (long-term use); 3-4 mg/kg PO q 24h (maximum 7 days)	Do not use in cats.	Adverse effects are primarily GI and renal, though hepatic and dermatologic events have been reported. Do not use with other NSAIDs or corticosteroids.	Tablets
Desmopressin acetate (DDAVP)	Diabetes insipidus: 1 drop of 0.01% solution in the conjunctival sac q 12-24h. Up to 4 drops per dose may be required in some patients; 1-2 mcg/kg SQ q 12-24h; 0.1 mg/DOG PO q 8h (tablets)	Diabetes insipidus: 1 drop of the 0.01% solution in the conjunctival sac q 12-24h; 0.25-0.5 mg/CAT PO q 8-12h (tablets)	Well tolerated. Occasionally, hypersensitivity reactions have been reported.	Tablets and solution for nasal inhalation. Expensive.
Desoxycorticosterone pivalate (DOCP, Percorten-V, Zycortal)	Hypoadrenocorticism: 2.2 mg/kg IM or SQ initially and then as needed for disease control (typically once a month)	Hypoadrenocorticism: 10-12.5 mg/CAT IM per month or as needed to control signs	Supplemental glucocorticoid therapy usually required. The injection should be shaken vigorously for 3-4 minutes before use to ensure uniformity of dose. Well tolerated, though lethargy, GI upset, and other events can occur.	Injectable suspension
Dexamethasone sodium phosphate (Azium, Dexate, Decadron)	Glucocorticoid; effects (and uses) vary with dose Anaphylaxis: 0.5 mg/kg IV once Antiinflammatory: 0.1-0.2 mg/kg PO, SQ, or IV q 24h Immunosuppressive: 0.2-0.5 mg/kg PO, SQ, or IV q 24h Hypoadrenocortical crisis: 0.1-0.5 mg/kg IV; maintenance: <0.1 mg/kg PO prn up to q 24h LDDST: 0.01 mg/kg IV once HDDST: 0.1 mg/kg IV once	Glucocorticoid; effects (and uses) vary with dose Anaphylaxis: 0.5 mg/kg IV once Antiinflammatory: 0.1-0.2 mg/kg PO, SQ, or IV q 24h Immunosuppressive: 0.2-0.5 mg/kg PO, SQ, or IV q 24h LDDST: 0.1 mg/kg IV once	Glucocorticoid 7-10× more potent than prednisone. Adverse effects are those typical of glucocorticoids (e.g., PU/PD, polyphagia, GI ulceration, HPA axis suppression, hyperglycemia). Often used for short duration, substituting an intermediate-acting glucocorticoid (e.g., prednisone or prednisolone) if chronic therapy required. Do not combine with NSAIDs.	Tablets, oral solution, ophthalmic, and injection
Dexmedetomidine (Dexdomitor, Sileo)	Sedation/analgesia: 5-10 mcg/kg IM or IV Preanesthetic: 125-375 mcg/m^2 IM Treatment of noise aversion using the oromucosal gel (Sileo): 125 mcg/m^2 BSA administered onto the oral mucosa between the dog's cheek and gum. The first dose should be administered approximately 30-60 minutes before onset of fear stimulus.	Sedation: 10-20 mcg/kg IM Emesis induction: 7 mcg/kg IM or 3.5 mcg/kg IV, and reverse after emesis (which occurs before sedation)	Adverse effects include bradycardia (does not usually require treatment), AV block, decreased respiration, hypothermia, urination, vomiting, hyperglycemia, and pain on IM injection. Prolonged sedation, paradoxical excitation, hypersensitivity, apnea, and death from circulatory failure may occur, although rarely. Often combined with butorphanol or hydromorphone for profound sedation. Adverse effects of oromucosal gel are typically limited to mild sedation.	Injection, oromucosal gel
Dexrazoxane (Zinecard, Cardioxane)	Prevention of doxorubicin cardiotoxicity: 10× the administered milligram dose of doxorubicin IV 5-10 minutes before doxorubicin Doxorubicin extravasation: 1000 mg/m^2 IV within 6 hours and again on day 2. Infuse 500 mg/m^2 IV on day 3.	Dosing is not described for cats.	May reduce efficacy of doxorubicin and increase myelosuppression.	Injection. Wear gloves when handling. Generics available but very expensive.

Generic Name (Brand Name, Synonyms)	Canine Dosages	Feline Dosages	Adverse Effects/Warnings	Administration/ Availability
Diazepam (Valium, Diastat)	Cluster seizures or status epilepticus: 0.5-1 mg/kg rectally; 0.5 mg/kg intranasally; 0.5-1 mg/kg IV, 0.1-2 mg/kg/h IV as a CRI Adjunctive treatment of metronidazole toxicity (CNS): 0.43 mg/kg IV and then PO q 8h for 3 days Premedication in combination with other sedatives: 0.1-0.3 mg/kg IV	Due to fatal idiosyncratic hepatic failure in some cats, many clinicians avoid use of oral diazepam in cats. For anesthesia in combination with other drugs: 0.1-0.3 mg/kg IV	Adverse effects include sedation, ataxia, CNS excitement (dogs), increased appetite, hepatic failure (cats). Tolerance to the antiepileptic effects over time limits usefulness. Use with caution in hepatic or renal disease; in aggressive, debilitated, or geriatric patients; or in patients with significant respiratory depression. Diazepam injection is physically incompatible with many other injectable drugs.	Tablets, injection, or rectal gel. CSS-IV.
Diazoxide (Proglycem)	Insulinoma: Initially 5 mg/kg PO q 12h. May gradually increase to 50 mg/kg PO q 12h.	Malignancy-associated hypoglycemia: Initially 5 mg/kg PO q 12h. May gradually increase to 40 mg/kg PO q 12h.	Adverse effects are more likely in dogs with hepatic dysfunction and include GI upset, tachycardia, hematologic abnormalities, DM, cataracts, and sodium and water retention. Contraindicated in hypoglycemia secondary to insulin overdosage. Use with extreme caution in CHF or renal disease.	Oral suspension
Diethylstilbestrol (DES)	Sphincter mechanism incompetence: 0.1-1 mg/DOG (0.02 mg/kg, to a maximum of 1 mg) PO q 24h for 3-5 days as an induction dose and then decreased to lowest dose that will maintain urinary continence, often once or twice a week	Use is not described in cats.	Adverse effects include blood dyscrasias, GI effects, and pyometra (nonspayed females). DES was removed from the human market due to carcinogenicity in the offspring of exposed pregnant women. Other drugs usually preferred to DES for urinary incontinence (e.g., phenylpropanolamine, estriol).	Available only through compounding
Digoxin (Lanoxin)	Atrial fibrillation: Initially, 0.0025-0.005 mg/kg PO q 12h (alternatively in dogs weighing > 20 kg, dose digoxin using BSA at 0.22 mg/m^2). Do not exceed 0.25 mg/DOG (regardless of size) in a 12-hour period. Base dose on lean BW.	CHF associated with DCM: cats <3 kg, ¼ of a 0.125-mg tablet PO q 48h; cats 3-6 kg, ¼ of a 0.125-mg tablet PO q 24h; cats >6 kg, ¼ of a 0.125-mg tablet PO q 12-24h	GI upset is commonly associated with high blood concentration, and arrhythmias may occur. Use with extreme caution in animals with renal disease, complex ventricular arrhythmia, or subaortic stenosis. Digoxin is relatively contraindicated in cats with hypertrophic cardiomyopathy. Monitor blood concentrations. Toxicity more likely with hypokalemia.	Tablets and oral elixir
Dihydrotachysterol	Hypoparathyroidism: Initially, give 0.03 mg/kg PO q 24h until effect is demonstrated, then 0.02 mg/kg PO q 24h for 2 days, then 0.01 mg/kg/d PO thereafter	Hypoparathyroidism: Initially, give 0.03 mg/kg PO q 24h until effect is demonstrated, then 0.02 mg/kg PO q 24h for 2 days, then 0.01 mg/kg/d PO thereafter	Hypercalcemia, nephrocalcinosis, and hyperphosphatemia can occur. May only be obtained through compounding. Use with extreme caution in hyperphosphatemia, renal dysfunction (when receiving the drug for nonrenal indications).	Available only through compounding
Diltiazem hydrochloride (Cardizem, Dilacor XR)	Acute SVT: 0.05 mg/kg IV over 1-2 minutes; repeat prn to total dose of 0.75 mg/kg IV Chronic supraventricular tachycardia: Initially, 1 mg/kg PO q 8h and titrated upward to a maximum of 4 mg/kg PO q 8h Tachycardia of atrial fibrillation: 0.5-1.5 mg/kg PO q 8h of immediate-release tablets; or 3-5 mg/kg PO q 12h for sustained-release products	Arrhythmias of HCM: 0.8-2.5 mg/kg PO q 12h to q 8h; 10 mg/kg PO q 24h, in sustained-release form	Oral diltiazem is available in a wide variety of dosage forms with different release profiles. Clinicians should ensure that the correct dosage form is dispensed. XR capsules contain inner tablets that may be fractionated for dosing cats and small dogs. Contraindicated in severe hypotension, sick sinus syndrome, or second- and third-degree AV block, acute myocardial infarction (MI), radiographically documented pulmonary congestion. Use with caution in geriatric patients or in those with heart failure (particularly if also receiving beta-blockers) or with hepatic or renal impairment.	Available in immediate-release and sustained-release tablets, and injection

Generic Name (Brand Name, Synonyms)	Canine Dosages	Feline Dosages	Adverse Effects/Warnings	Administration/ Availability
Dimenhydrinate (Dramamine, Gravol)	Motion sickness: 4-8 mg/kg PO, IM, or IV q 8h	Motion sickness: 12.5 mg/CAT PO, IM, IV q 8h	Can cause CNS depression, anticholinergic effects, and GI upset. Use with caution in GI or urinary obstruction, hyperthyroidism, seizure disorders, cardiovascular disease or hypertension. Less effective than maropitant.	Tablets, injections. Injections should be diluted before administration.
Dimethyl sulfoxide (DMSO)	Amyloidosis: 80 mg/kg SQ q 48h or 300 mg/kg PO q 24h	Use in cats is not described.	Can cause contact irritation, sulfurous odor. Teratogenic. Efficacy poorly established.	No approved dosage forms; FDA import alert. Often illegally marketed and difficult to obtain quality product. Nonsterile solution, gel, topical. Sterilize solution with 0.22-micron sterilizing filter; dilute 1 : 4 with sterile water for SQ injection. Wear gloves.
Dimercaprol (BAL in Oil, British anti-lewisite)	Chelating agent (e.g., arsenicals): 2.5-5 mg/kg IM q 4h for the first 2 days of treatment, then q 12h until recovery	Chelating agent (e.g., arsenicals): 2.5-5 mg/kg IM q 4h for the first 2 days of treatment, then q 12h until recovery	Adverse effects may include vomiting, seizures with higher dosages, increased blood pressure, and tachycardia. Contraindicated with impaired hepatic function (unless secondary to acute arsenic toxicity) and iron, cadmium, or selenium poisoning. Use with caution with impaired renal function. Alkalinize urine to prevent reabsorption. Administer deep IM (painful).	Injection
Diminazene (Berenil)	Babesiosis, trypanosomiasis: 4.2 mg/kg IM q 21 days	Cytauxzoonosis: 2 mg/kg IM repeated in 7 days	Adverse effects include tremors, itching, sweating, convulsions, dyspnea, recumbency, hypotension, and diarrhea.	Not available in the United States. Available in other countries as injection and powder for oral solution, but imports into the United States may be seized by the FDA and U.S. Customs.
Dinoprost tromethamine (Lutalyse)	Pyometra (use is very controversial): Day 1, give 0.1 mg/kg SQ once; Day 2, give 0.2 mg/kg SQ once; Days 3-7, give 0.25 mg/kg SQ q 24h Abortifacient up to 30 days after breeding: 0.1 mg/kg SQ q 8h for 3 days and then 0.2 mg/kg SQ q 8h to effect, usually in combination with misoprostol	Pyometra: 0.1 mg/kg SQ on the first day, then 0.25 mg/kg SQ q 24h for 5 days	Absolutely contraindicated in any desired pregnancy. Adverse effects include abdominal pain, emesis, defecation, urination, and pupillary dilation followed by constriction, tachycardias, restlessness and anxiety, fever, hypersalivation, dyspnea, and panting. Cats may also exhibit increased vocalization and intense grooming behavior.	Injection
Dioctyl sodium sulfosuccinate (DSS, Colace, Docusate)	Stool softener: 25-100 mg/DOG (depending on size) PO q 12-24h or 60-90 mL (10 mg/docusate/mL) per rectum	Stool softener: 50 mg /CAT PO q 24h, or 60 mL (8 mg/mL solution) per rectum	Well tolerated but can cause cramping, diarrhea, and GI mucosal damage.	Capsules, liquids (for use PO or per rectum) OTC.
Diphenhydramine HCl (Benadryl)	Antihistamine: 2-4 mg/kg PO q 8-12h or 0.5-2 mg/kg IM, SQ, or IV Vestibular disease: 4-8 mg/kg PO q 24h	Antihistamine: 2-4 mg/kg PO q 8-12h	Sedation and GI upset may be seen. Cats may experience paradoxical CNS stimulation. Contraindicated in GI or urinary obstruction, hyperthyroidism, seizure disorders, cardiovascular disease, or hypertension.	Tablets, capsules, and oral liquids OTC, and injections
Diphenoxylate HCl with atropine (Lomotil)	Antidiarrheal: Dosage is based on the diphenoxylate component: 0.05-0.2 mg/kg PO q 8-12h Antitussive: 0.25 mg/kg PO q 8-12h	Not usually recommended for cats due to opioid stimulation	Adverse opioid effects include constipation, bloat, and sedation. Do not use in patients receiving MAO inhibitors (e.g., amitraz, l-deprenyl) or in patients with *MDR1/ABCB1-Δ* mutants. Use with caution in respiratory disease, hepatic encephalopathy, hypothyroidism, severe renal insufficiency, adrenocortical insufficiency, head injuries, increased intracranial pressure, acute abdominal conditions, and in geriatric or severely debilitated patients.	Tablets, oral liquid. CSS-V.

Generic Name (Brand Name, Synonyms)	Canine Dosages	Feline Dosages	Adverse Effects/Warnings	Administration/ Availability
DL-methionine	Urinary acidification: 100 mg/kg PO q 12h	Urinary acidification: 1000-1500 mg/CAT PO q 24h	Adverse effects include GI distress (food may alleviate), Heinz-body hemolytic anemia (cats). Contraindicated in renal failure, pancreatic disease, hepatic insufficiency, pre-existing acidosis, oxalate or urate calculi.	Tablets, powder, gel; give with food
Dobutamine HCl (Dobutrex)	Hypotension (after volume resuscitation): CRI IV of 2.5-20 mcg/kg/min titrated upward to effect in sterile LRS, 0.9% NaCl or D_5W	Hypotension (after volume resuscitation): CRI IV of 2.5-20 mcg/kg/min titrated upward to effect in sterile LRS, 0.9% NaCl or D_5W	Use for no longer than 48 hours; may increase heart rate—monitor for arrhythmias; cats are very sensitive to dobutamine and may have seizures; doses >10 mcg/kg/min in dogs are more likely to be arrhythmogenic.	Injection
Dopamine HCl (Intropin)	Hypotension (after volume resuscitation): CRI IV of 2-2.5 mcg/kg/min titrated upward to effect, often in 7-15 mcg/kg/min range	Hypotension (after volume resuscitation): CRI IV of 2-2.5 mcg/kg/min titrated upward to effect, often in 7-15 mcg/kg/min range	GI upset, arrhythmia, hypotension or hypertension, dyspnea, and vasoconstriction can occur. Contraindicated in pheochromocytoma, ventricular fibrillation, and uncorrected tachyarrhythmia. Extravasation can cause severe tissue damage.	Injection
Doramectin (Dectomax)	Demodectic and sarcoptic mange: 0.6 mg/kg PO or SQ q 7 days; continue treatment until remission of clinical signs and no evidence of mites on 2 successive skin scrapings 14 days apart; 0.3 mg/kg SQ q 3-4 days may be better tolerated than 0.6 mg/kg q 7 days	Demodicosis: 400-600 mcg/kg (0.4-0.6 mg/kg) SQ q 7 days for 4 weeks past 2 consecutive negative skin scrapings 4-6 weeks apart	Contraindicated in dogs with the *MDR1/ABCB1-Δ* genetic mutation. Adverse effects are rare in nonmutant dogs, but include pupil dilation, lethargy, blindness, or coma.	Injection
Dorzolamide (Trusopt)	Glaucoma: 1 drop OA q 8-12h	Glaucoma: 1 drop OA q 8-12h	Adverse effects include burning and stinging upon application (due to low pH), superficial punctate keratitis, local hypersensitivity reactions, and corneal edema.	Ophthalmic solution, sometimes combined with timolol
Doxapram (Dopram-V)	Laryngeal function exam: 2.2 mg/kg IV Stimulate respiration during anesthesia: 1.1 mg/kg (with gas anesthesia) or 5.5-11 mg/kg (with barbiturate anesthesia) IV Stimulate respiration in neonates: 0.1 mL (2 mg) IV in umbilical vein (IM or sublingual also possible)	Laryngeal function exam: 2.2 mg/kg IV Stimulate respiration during anesthesia: 1.1 mg/kg (with gas anesthesia) or 5.5-11 mg/kg (with barbiturate anesthesia) IV Stimulate respiration in neonates: 0.1 mL (2 mg) IV in umbilical vein (IM or sublingual also possible)	Adverse effects include hypertension, arrhythmias, seizures, hypersensitivity, and respiratory alkalosis. Contraindicated in mechanical ventilation, seizure disorders, head trauma, respiratory failure secondary to neuromuscular disorders, airway obstruction, pulmonary embolism, pneumothorax, acute asthma, dyspnea, or whenever hypoxia is not associated with hypercapnia.	Injection
Doxepin (Sinequan)	Psychogenic dermatoses: 3-5 mg/kg (not more than 50 mg/DOG) PO q 12h tapered to lowest effective dose	Psychogenic dermatoses: 0.5-1 mg/kg PO q 12-24h tapered to lowest effective dose	Contraindicated in animals currently or recently (within 2 weeks) exposed to MAO inhibitors or fluoxetine. Adverse effects include hyperexcitability, GI distress, or lethargy, and a dose-related ventricular tachycardia.	Tablets, capsules, oral solution
Doxorubicin (Adriamycin, Doxil)	Antineoplastic: 30 mg/m^2 IV q 2-3 weeks. Maximum cumulative dose = 180-240 mg/m^2 depending on breed and risk factors.	Antineoplastic: 20-25 mg/m^2 or 1 mg/kg IV q 3-5 weeks. Maximum cumulative dose suggested 180 mg/m^2.	Adverse effects include myelosuppression, cardiac toxicity (dogs), nephrotoxicity (cats), alopecia, gastroenteritis (vomiting, diarrhea), and stomatitis. Some brands cause hypersensitivity in dogs. Use with caution in patients with impaired hepatic function (dosage adjustments necessary), and in dogs with *MDR1/ABCB1-Δ* mutations. Extravasation can cause severe tissue damage (dexrazoxane treatment indicated).	Injection administered by IV catheter with 0.9% saline or 5% dextrose infusion over ≥15 minutes. Cytotoxic, NIOSH-listed hazardous drug and should be prepared, administered, and disposed of in accordance with federal and local requirements. Extravasations should be treated with dexrazoxane.

Generic Name (Brand Name, Synonyms)	Canine Dosages	Feline Dosages	Adverse Effects/Warnings	Administration/ Availability
Doxycycline (Doxirobe, Vibramycin)	Susceptible infections: 5-10 mg/kg PO or 5 mg/kg IV q 12-24h Immune-mediated dermatosis: 5 mg/kg PO q 12-24h with niacinamide	Susceptible infections: 5-10 mg/kg PO q 24h	GI upset, hepatopathy, and hypersensitivity can occur, as can enamel staining in puppies/kittens. May cause anorexia and hyperthermia in cats. Solid dosage forms may cause esophageal erosion/stricture (especially cats). Administer with food or follow with at least 6 mL of liquid. GI protectants can reduce absorption. Compounded liquid stability limited.	Tablets, capsules, gel, oral suspension, or injection. Injection must be diluted to not more than 1 mg/mL for IV administration; do not administer IM or SQ.
D-penicillamine	Copper hepatopathy: 10-15 mg/kg PO q 12h on an empty stomach (at least 20-30 minutes before feeding) Lead intoxication: 30-110 mg/kg divided into 6 doses for 7 days	Lead poisoning: Limited dosing information; 10-15 mg/kg or 125 mg/CAT PO q 12h for 5 days	May cause vomiting, skin eruptions, vascular lesions, or cytopenias; monitor CBC and supplement pyridoxine (vitamin B_6) 25 mg PO q 24h.	Available only through compounding. Administer on empty stomach if tolerated, or give with a small amount of food if GI upset.

E

Generic Name (Brand Name, Synonyms)	Canine Dosages	Feline Dosages	Adverse Effects/Warnings	Administration/ Availability
Edrophonium (Tensilon, Enlon)	Test for myasthenia gravis: 0.1-0.2 mg/kg IV Reversal of nondepolarizing neuromuscular blockade: 0.25-0.5 mg/kg IV using low dose first; repeat once if necessary	Test for myasthenia gravis: 0.25-0.5 mg/CAT IV	Can cause cholinergic signs; pretreat (0.02-0.04 mg/kg IV) or have atropine available during use. Relatively contraindicated in asthma or mechanical urinary or intestinal tract obstruction. Use with caution in bradycardias or atrioventricular block.	Injection
Enalapril maleate (Enacard, Vasotec)	ACE inhibition for CHF: 0.5 mg/kg PO q 24h, can increase to q 12h if needed Proteinuria: 0.25-0.5 mg/kg PO q 12-24h initially, increasing prn up to 2 mg/kg daily	ACE inhibition for CHF: 0.25-0.5 mg/kg PO q 24h Proteinuria: 0.25-1 mg/kg PO q 12-24h	Adverse effects include GI upset, azotemia, hyperkalemia; cough is reported in humans. Use with caution in renal insufficiency (dosages may need to be reduced) and in patients with hyponatremia, hypotension, pre-existing hematologic abnormalities, or a collagen vascular disease.	Tablets, oral solution, and injection (as enalaprilat)
Enoxaparin (Lovenox)	Thromboprophylaxis: 0.8-1 mg/kg SQ q 6-8h	Thromboprophylaxis: 0.75-1.5 mg/kg SQ q 6-8h	Can cause or worsen bleeding. Must be given SQ. Available in broad range of concentrations; ensure correct dosing. Monitor via Xa activity.	Injection. U-100 insulin syringes are useful for providing accurate doses. Expensive.
Enrofloxacin (Baytril, Enroflox)	Susceptible infections: 10-20 mg/kg q 24h PO, IM. Can be given off label as diluted product by SQ or IV route	Due to the risk of irreversible retinal blindness, other fluoroquinolones are preferred for use in cats. If used, doses must not exceed 5 mg/kg/d and should not be used by parenteral route	Well tolerated in dogs at approved route/dose. Can cause GI upset, CNS stimulation, pain on injection. Can cause blindness in cats after parenteral injection or at doses >5 mg/kg/d (less toxic fluoroquinolone agents are available for use in cats). Risk of cartilage damage in young, growing animals (consider risk/benefit ratio). IV administration of undiluted enrofloxacin may cause dogs to vomit. Use with caution in hepatic or renal insufficiency. Many potential drug interactions. Use of large animal enrofloxacin injection in small animals may cause severe phlebitis and sloughing at injection site due to extremely alkaline pH, and will cause mucosal ulceration if given orally.	Tablets, injections approved for small animals. Do not use large animal injections by any route in small animals. Compounding pharmacies can prepare stable oral suspensions. Oral dosing best on an empty stomach to avoid chelation (especially dairy). Must be diluted to 10× the volume (e.g., 2.27 mg/mL final concentration) in saline before SQ or IV administration.

Generic Name (Brand Name, Synonyms)	Canine Dosages	Feline Dosages	Adverse Effects/Warnings	Administration/ Availability
Ephedrine	Anesthesia-related hypotension: 0.15-0.25 mg/kg diluted into 5 mL of a balanced electrolyte solution or saline, and give small-increment IV boluses to effect	Anesthesia-related hypotension: 0.15-0.25 mg/kg diluted into 5 mL of a balanced electrolyte solution or saline, and give small-increment IV boluses to effect	Can cause CNS stimulation, tachycardia, hypertension, or anorexia. Use with extreme caution if at all in nursing animals. Contraindicated in severe cardiovascular disease and arrhythmias. Use with caution in glaucoma, prostatic hypertrophy, hyperthyroidism, DM, cardiovascular disorders, or hypertension.	Injection (tablets no longer available). Dilute dose into 5 mL of saline or other electrolyte solution, and give in small IV boluses.
Epinephrine (Adrenalin)	Anaphylaxis: 1-5 mL (1:10,000 solution = 0.1 mg/mL) SQ, or 0.01 mg/kg IM CPR: 0.01 mg/kg IV q 3-5 minutes early in CPR; 0.1 mg/kg IV may be considered after prolonged CPR. Intratracheal alternative 0.03-0.1 mg/kg	Anaphylaxis: 20 mcg/kg IV CPR: 0.01 mg/kg IV q 3-5 minutes early in CPR; up to 0.1 mg/kg IV may be considered after prolonged CPR	Can cause anxiety, tremor, excitability, vomiting, hypertension, arrhythmias. Contraindicated in shock due to nonanaphylactoid causes, during general anesthesia with halogenated hydrocarbons, DCM or coronary insufficiency; cases in which vasopressor drugs are contraindicated (e.g., thyrotoxicosis, hypertension). Use extreme caution in patients with a prefibrillatory cardiac rhythm.	Injection; confirm concentration before use. New labeling standards in some locations now avoid ratio expressions used formerly; what was called 1:1000 epinephrine is now labeled as 1 mg/mL, while 1:10,000 epinephrine is 0.1 mg/mL.
Ergocalciferol (Calciferol, Drisdol)	Hypocalcemic tetany: 4000-6000 units/kg PO q 24h initially and then 1000-2000 units/kg PO q 24h to once weekly	Hypocalcemic tetany: 4000-6000 units/kg PO q 24h initially and then 1000-2000 units/kg PO q 24h to once weekly	Can cause hypercalcemia. Calcitriol is safer and generally preferred over ergocalciferol; however, ergocalciferol may be less expensive.	Tablets, capsules
Erythromycin	Promotility agent: 0.5-1 mg/kg PO q 8h Susceptible infections: 10-20 mg/kg PO q 8-12h	Promotility agent: 0.5-1 mg/kg PO q 8h Susceptible infections: 10-20 mg/kg PO q 8-12h	GI upset or pain is the most common adverse effect. Allergic reactions are rare. Painful on IM injection. Multiple drug interactions.	Injection, tablets, topical. Currently injection and tablets are difficult to obtain for veterinary use. Although formerly cost effective, it has become expensive.
Erythropoietin (EPO, rHuEPO, Epogen, Procrit)	Erythropoiesis: 100 units/kg SQ 3×/wk until the low end of the target hematocrit range is achieved, then once weekly.	Erythropoiesis: 100 units/kg SQ 3×/wk until the low end of the target hematocrit range is achieved, then once weekly.	Adverse effects include autoantibody development, causing worsened anemia, vomiting, hypertension, seizures, uveitis, iron depletion, local reactions at injection sites, fever, arthralgia, and mucocutaneous ulcers. Contraindicated in uncontrolled hypertension.	Injection. Iron supplementation suggested.
Esmolol (Brevibloc)	Short-term control of SVT: 0.05-0.1 mg/kg/min IV CRI, titrated to effect. Can administer intermittent IV bolus of 0.05-0.1 mg/kg q 5 minutes up to a maximum of 0.5 mg/kg	Short-term control of SVT: 0.05-0.1 mg/kg/min IV CRI, titrated to effect	Can cause hypotension or bradycardia. Contraindicated in overt cardiac failure, 2nd- or 3rd-degree AV block, bradycardia, or in cardiogenic shock. Use with caution in CHF, bronchoconstrictive lung disease, or DM.	Injection vials or premixed ready-to-administer bags. Injection diluted in saline or D_5W before administration.
Esomeprazole (Nexium)	Proton pump inhibitor antacid: 1 mg/kg PO q 24h	Use is not described for cats.	Seldom used in dogs. Use caution in patients with hepatopathy. Multiple drug interactions.	Tablets OTC
Estriol (Incurin)	Hormone-responsive urinary incontinence: 2 mg PO q 24h for 14 days then taper to lowest effective dose	Dosing in cats is not described.	Adverse effects are GI- and estrogen-related; bone marrow depression risk appears to be low with this estrogen.	Tablets

Generic Name (Brand Name, Synonyms)	Canine Dosages	Feline Dosages	Adverse Effects/Warnings	Administration/ Availability
Ethanol	Ethylene glycol poisoning—CRI or intermittent-dose strategy: CRI: loading dose of 8.6 mL/kg slow IV of 7% alcohol solution, followed by 1.43-2.86 mL/kg/h CRI for 48 hours Intermittent-dose strategy: 5.5 mL/kg of a 20% solution IV over 1 hour q 4h for 5 treatments, then q 6h for four additional treatments, each dose being given over 1 hour	Ethylene glycol poisoning—CRI or intermittent-dose strategy: CRI: loading dose of 8.6 mL/kg slow IV of 7% alcohol solution, followed by 1.43-2.86 mL/kg/h CRI for 48 hours Intermittent-dose strategy: 5.5 mL/kg of a 20% solution IV over 1 hour q 4h for 5 treatments, then q 6h for four additional treatments, each dose being given over 1 hour	Fomepizole is preferred for both species (higher dose for cats), but availability and expense may prevent use. Adverse effects of ethanol include CNS and respiratory depression, hypoglycemia, diuresis, as well as pain and infection at the injection site. Avoid extravasation. Monitor fluid, electrolyte, and respiratory status; monitor blood alcohol levels.	Use either Everclear (190 proof, equals 95% ethanol) or plain vodka (80 proof, equals 40% ethanol). To make ethanol solution, divide desired final % solution by ethanol % in product and multiply by mL of fluid in bag (e.g., 5% dextrose) to give the volume of fluid to be replaced by ethanol. For example, to make 7% ethanol using Everclear, (7%/95%) × 1000 mL D_5W - 74 mL, meaning remove 74 mL of fluid from liter bag and add 74 mL of Everclear. To make 20% solution using 80 proof (40% ethanol) vodka in a 1-liter bag of D_5W, (20%/40%) × 1000 mL = 500 mL, remove 500 mL of fluid from bag and replace with 500 mL of vodka.
Etidronate (Didronel)	Hypercalcemia of malignancy: 5-30 mg/kg PO q 24h or divided q 12h	Hypercalcemia of malignancy: 5-20 mg/kg PO q 24h or divided q 12h	Adverse effects include esophagitis, GI upset, renal damage, and bone pain. Contraindicated in renal impairment, delayed esophageal emptying, upper GI inflammation or ulcers, and bone fractures.	Tablets; give on empty stomach.

F

Generic Name (Brand Name, Synonyms)	Canine Dosages	Feline Dosages	Adverse Effects/Warnings	Administration/ Availability
Famciclovir (Famvir)	Dosing in dogs is not described.	Feline herpesvirus type 1 (FHV-1): 90 mg/kg PO q 12h, or 125 mg/CAT PO q 8h	Generally well tolerated, but anorexia and polydipsia have been noted in some cats.	Tablets
Famotidine (Pepcid)	H_2 antagonist antacid: 0.5-1.1 mg/kg PO, IM, SQ, or IV q 12-24h	H_2 antagonist antacid: 0.5-1.1 mg/kg PO, IM, SQ, or IV q 12-24h	Well tolerated, but use with caution in severe cardiac, hepatic, or renal dysfunction (consider dose reduction). Rapid IV administration might cause bradycardia or hemolysis (cats).	Tablets, chewable tablets, disintegrating tablets, coated tablets, oral suspension, and injection. Oral forms OTC.
Felbamate (Felbatol)	Adjunctive antiepileptic: 15-20 mg/kg PO q 8h, up to 70-80 mg/kg PO q 8h	Dosing in cats is not described.	Generally well tolerated. Use is typically after multiple other agents have failed.	Tablets, oral suspension
Fenbendazole (Panacur, Safe-Guard)	Susceptible helminth infections: 50 mg/kg PO q 24h; duration usually longer for respiratory (7 days) than GI (3 days) parasites Prophylaxis in pregnant bitch: 25 mg/kg PO q 24h from 40 days of pregnancy until 2 days after whelping	Susceptible helminth infections: 50 mg/kg PO q 24h (not FDA approved in cats)	Adverse effects include GI upset; bone marrow suppression rarely reported.	Oral granules, oral suspension. OTC formulations.

Generic Name (Brand Name, Synonyms)	Canine Dosages	Feline Dosages	Adverse Effects/Warnings	Administration/ Availability
Fentanyl (Sublimaze, Duragesic)	Analgesia: Injection—0.01-0.04 mg/kg SQ, IM, IV; CRI—0.003-0.006 mg/kg/h (3-6 mcg/kg/h) IV; Patches—5-10 kg = 25 mcg/h; 10-20 kg = 50 mcg/h; 20-30 kg = 75 mcg/h; >30 kg = 100 mcg/h	Analgesia: Injection—0.01-0.04 mg/kg SQ, IM, IV; CRI—0.003-0.006 mg/kg/h (3-6 mcg/kg/h) IV; Patches—2.5-mg patch (= 25 mcg/h)	Use with caution in geriatric, ill, or debilitated patients and in those with a pre-existing respiratory problem or CNS depression. Adverse effects include dose-related respiratory, CNS, and circulatory depression (bradycardia); also urine retention, constipation, dysphoria, or agitation. Naloxone can reverse mu but not kappa-receptor effects. Dogs may become dysphoric when used as a postoperative CRI. Avoid human exposure when handling. Potential for human abuse.	Injection, transdermal patches. CSS-II.
Ferrous sulfate (Fer-In-Sol, Feosol)	Iron-deficiency anemia: 100-300 mg/DOG PO q 24h	Iron-deficiency anemia: 50-100 mg/CAT PO once q 24h	GI upset is common but can be lessened by administration with food. Overdosage can be fatal.	Tablets, oral solution; give with food. OTC.
Filgrastim (Neupogen)	Neutropenia: 5 mcg/kg SQ q 24h	Neutropenia: 5 mcg/kg SQ q 24h	Occasionally, irritation at the injection site may occur. Bone or musculoskeletal pain, splenomegaly (including splenic rupture), glomerulonephritis, capillary leak syndrome, and hypotension have been reported in humans. Antibody formation may occur.	Injection (concentrations variable)
Finasteride (Proscar, Propecia)	Benign prostatic hypertrophy: 0.1-1 mg/kg PO q 24h	Dosing in cats is not described.	Adverse effects include GI upset and minor sexual side effects. Use with caution in hepatic impairment.	Tablets
Firocoxib (Previcox, Equioxx)	Antiinflammatory/analgesic NSAID: 5 mg/kg PO q 24h	Not recommended for use in cats.	Can cause GI upset, but serious gastric ulcer/perforation is possible. Do not combine with other NSAIDs or corticosteroids.	Tablets (give with food), chewable tablets, injection
Fluconazole (Diflucan)	Susceptible mycotic infection, including fungal cystitis: 5-10 mg/kg PO, IV q 12-24h	Susceptible mycotic infection, including fungal cystitis: 5-10 mg/kg PO, IV q 12-24h CNS cryptococcosis: 50-100 mg/CAT PO, IV q 12h	GI upset, CNS, and skin effects can occur. Multiple drug interactions. Not effective for all fungal infection (e.g., not effective for aspergillosis).	Tablet, powder for oral suspension, injection
Flucytosine (Ancobon)	Generally not recommended for use in dogs due to severe toxicity For life-threatening cryptococcosis: 50-75 mg/kg PO q 8h (much lower doses, 25 mg/kg, sometimes recommended). Must be administered with a polyene or azole antifungal agent.	Life-threatening cryptococcosis: 25-50 mg/kg PO q 6h or 50-65 mg/kg PO q 8h. Must be administered with a polyene or azole antifungal agent	Adverse effects include GI upset, bone marrow suppression, cutaneous eruption and rash, oral ulceration, increased hepatic enzymes, and CNS effects in cats. Use with extreme caution if at all for renal impairment, pre-existing bone marrow depression, or hematologic diseases or in patients receiving other bone marrow suppressant drugs.	Capsules
Fludrocortisone (Florinef)	Hypoadrenocorticism: 0.1 mg/5 kg or 0.01 mg/kg PO q 24h, adjusted according to response	Hypoadrenocorticism: 0.05-0.1 mg/CAT PO q 24h adjusted according to response	Adverse effects are dose related and include PU/PD, hypertension, edema, and hypokalemia. GI discomfort may occur and can be lessened with food.	Tablets; give with food.
Flumazenil (Romazicon)	Reversal of benzodiazepines: 0.01 mg/kg IV and repeat q h if needed	Reversal of benzodiazepines: 0.01 mg/kg IV and repeat q h if needed	Adverse effects include injection site reactions, vomiting, cutaneous vasodilation, vertigo, ataxia, and blurred vision; seizures and cardiac arrhythmias have been reported in humans. Use extreme caution in mixed overdoses as rapid withdrawal of benzodiazepines may precipitate seizures if used to control epilepsy.	Injection

Generic Name (Brand Name, Synonyms)	Canine Dosages	Feline Dosages	Adverse Effects/Warnings	Administration/ Availability
Fluorouracil (Adrucil, 5-FU)	Antineoplastic: 150 mg/m^2 IV weekly, or 5-10 mg/kg IV weekly	Do not use in cats.	Contraindicated in poor nutritional states, with bone marrow suppression, or with serious infections. Adverse effects include dose-dependent myelosuppression, GI toxicity, and neurotoxicity.	Injection, topical cream. Cytotoxic, NIOSH-listed hazardous drug and should be prepared, administered, and disposed of in accordance with federal and local requirements.
Fluoxetine (Prozac, Reconcile)	Behavioral disorders: 1-2 mg/kg PO q 24h	Behavioral disorders: 0.5-1 mg/kg or 2 mg/CAT PO q 24h	Do not use in patients receiving MAO inhibitors (e.g., amitraz, l-deprenyl). Use with caution in DM or seizure disorders; dosages may need to be reduced in patients with severe hepatic impairment. Adverse effects include anorexia, lethargy, GI effects, anxiety, irritability, insomnia, hyperactivity, panting, or hyperreactivity.	Tablets, oral solution
Flurbiprofen (Ocufen)	Ocular NSAID: 1 drop in affected eye q 6-24h	Ocular NSAID: 1 drop in affected eye q 6-24h	Minor ocular irritation or discomfort, miosis, or mydriasis can be seen. Contraindicated in hypersensitivity.	Ophthalmic solution
Fluticasone (Flovent, Flixotide)	Glucocorticoid for inflammatory airway disease: 1 puff (110 or 220 mcg/puff strength) q 12-24h using an appropriate spacer and mask	Glucocorticoid for inflammatory airway disease: 1 puff (usually 110 mcg/puff strength, but some prefer 220 mcg/puff) q 12-24h using an appropriate spacer and mask	Well tolerated, although HPA axis suppression is possible. Demodicosis has been reported in contact areas on muzzle.	Metered-dose inhaler in three strengths. Use with appropriate face mask and spacer device, allowing 10 breaths after actuation. Also available as intranasal spray, ointments, and topical creams, or in combination with other drugs (e.g., salmeterol) for inhalational administration.
Folic acid (folate, vitamin B_9)	Folate deficiency: 1-5 mg PO, SQ weekly Poorly regenerative anemia: 1-5 mg PO q 24h (anecdotal)	Folate deficiency: 1-5 mg PO, SQ weekly Supplement during prolonged trimethoprim/sulfa treatment: 2 mg/CAT q 24h	Very well tolerated	Tablets OTC, injection
Fomepizole (Antizol-Vet, 4-MP)	Ethylene glycol poisoning: 20 mg/kg IV, then 15 mg/kg IV 12 and 24 hours later, then final dose of 5 mg/kg 36 hours after initial dose; may give additional 5 mg/kg doses as necessary	Ethylene glycol poisoning: 125 mg/kg slow IV, then 31.25 mg/kg IV at 12, 24, and 36 hours. Cats must be treated within 3 hours of ingestion.	Adverse effects after rapid IV infusion include phlebitis and phlebosclerosis; anaphylaxis is possible. Monitor and treat acid/base, fluid, and electrolyte imbalances. May inhibit elimination of ethanol (and vice versa).	Injection. Veterinary product discontinued and human product very expensive. Dilute with saline or D_5W and administer by slow IV infusion.
Fondaparinux (Arixtra)	Use not described for dogs.	Anticoagulant; thromboprophylaxis: 0.06 mg/kg SQ q 12h	Selectively binds antithrombin, inactivating factor Xa. No effect on platelet function. No clinical trials to establish safety or efficacy in cats at this time, but bleeding is a potential complication of use.	Injection
Furosemide	Loop diuretic: Initial 2 mg/kg q 8-12h IV, IM, SQ, or PO. Can increase dose or frequency if needed in treatment of CHF up to 6 mg/kg. Alternatively, initial bolus followed by 0.1-1 mg/kg/h CRI. Titrate to lowest effective dose/frequency for chronic use.	Loop diuretic: Initially 1 mg/kg IV, IM, SQ, or PO q 8-24h; may increase if needed up to 4 mg/kg. Titrate to lowest effective dose/frequency for chronic use.	Electrolyte depletion; dehydration; may increase toxicity of other drugs (e.g., amphotericin B, aminoglycosides, ACE inhibitors, glucocorticoids)	Injection, tablets, syrup. Tablets can be split. Check pH of various products before administering SQ. Human-labeled products have a pH of 8-9.3 and are painful on SQ injection.

G

Generic Name (Brand Name, Synonyms)	Canine Dosages	Feline Dosages	Adverse Effects/Warnings	Administration/ Availability
Gabapentin (Neurontin)	Adjunctive analgesia: 10-20 mg/kg PO q 8-12h Adjunctive therapy for refractory epilepsy: 10-30 mg/kg PO q 6-8h	Adjunctive analgesia: 5-10 mg/kg PO q 8-12h Adjunctive anticonvulsant: 5-20 mg/kg PO q 6-12h Reduce fear responses and anxiety associated with veterinary examinations: 50-100 mg/CAT PO once before visit	Human liquid dosage forms may contain xylitol; do not use these in dogs. Sedation and ataxia are the most common adverse effects.	Tablets, capsules, and oral solution. Compounding pharmacies may prepare xylitol-free oral liquids.
Gemcitabine (Gemzar)	Antineoplastic: 45 mg/m^2-900 mg/m^2, usually given IV over 30-60 minutes q 7-14 days (consult veterinary oncologist before use)	Antineoplastic: 25 mg/m^2 diluted and given IV slowly twice weekly (consult veterinary oncologist before use)	Adverse effects are primarily GI toxicity and myelosuppression.	Injection; cytotoxic, NIOSH-listed hazardous drug and should be prepared, administered, and disposed of in accordance with federal and local requirements.
Gemfibrozil (Lopid)	Hyperlipidemia: 150-300 mg/DOG or 10 mg/kg PO q 12h	Hyperlipidemia: 7.5-10 mg/kg PO q 12h (anecdotal)	Generally well tolerated but abdominal pain, GI upset, and abnormal liver function tests have been reported.	Tablets; give 30 minutes before a meal.
Gentamicin (Gentocin, Garamycin)	Susceptible infections: 9-14 mg/kg IV, IM, or SQ q 24h Sighthounds: 6 mg/kg IV q 24h or 9 mg/kg SQ, IM q 24h Otitis: apply q 8h Susceptible ocular infections: apply q 8h Chemical enucleation: 25 mg injected into vitreous	Susceptible infections: 5-8 mg/kg IV, IM, or SQ q 24h Otitis: Apply q 8h Susceptible ocular infections: Apply q 8h Chemical enucleation: 25 mg injected into vitreous	Nephrotoxicity, ototoxicity, and neuromuscular blockade. Cats may be more sensitive to toxic effects, especially vestibular effects. Risk of nephrotoxicity increased in animals with dehydration, pre-existing renal disease, extremes of age, hypokalemia, and with treatment duration. Some ophthalmic preparations contain steroids and should not be used in fungal keratitis.	Injection, ophthalmic and otic preparations, and topical creams
Glipizide (Glucotrol)	Do not use in dogs.	Diabetes mellitus: 2.5-5 mg/CAT PO q 12h with food	Adverse effects include GI upset, hypoglycemia, and liver toxicity. May take 4-8 weeks to achieve full effect, and loss of efficacy is common. Contraindicated in ketoacidosis or with severe illness. Use with caution in cats with concurrent endocrinopathy.	Tablets; give with meals.
Glucosamine-chondroitin sulfate (Cosequin)	Adjunctive therapy of osteoarthritis: 15-30 mg/kg (of the chondroitin component) PO q 24h then taper to lowest effective dose	Adjunctive therapy of osteoarthritis and lower urinary disease: 15-30 mg/kg (of the chondroitin component) PO q 24h then taper to lowest effective dose	Effects may take 4-6 weeks. Dietary supplements are not regulated by the FDA and are of varying quality. Do not switch brands. Ingredients are from natural sources (e.g., blue crab, exoskeletons, cartilage), and hypersensitivity is possible. Some products contain high levels of potassium. GI upset is mild and self-limiting.	Tablets, capsules, and powders; give with food.
Glycopyrrolate (Robinul)	Treatment of muscarinic signs of organophosphate poisoning: 0.01-0.02 mg/kg SQ, IM, IV prn q 8-12h	Treatment of muscarinic signs of organophosphate poisoning: 0.01-0.02 mg/kg SQ, IM, IV prn q 8-12h	Rarely used in small animals; may be useful as an adjunct in treating muscarinic signs of organophosphate or carbamate toxicity. Adverse effects include tachycardia, arrhythmias, intestinal ileus, mydriasis, and photophobia.	Injection, tablets
Glycosaminoglycan-polysulfated (Adequan, Chondroprotec)	Degenerative joint disease: 4.4 mg/kg IM twice weekly for up to 4 weeks	Chondroprotective: 2 mg/kg IM q 3-5 days for 4-6 treatments	Occasional pain at injection site. May disrupt hemostasis in dogs.	Injection
GoLYTELY (polyethylene glycol-electrolyte solution)	Large bowel cathartic: 22-33 mL/kg PO or via stomach tube twice, 2 hours apart, 12 hours before GI endoscopy. Some dogs will drink willingly if mixed with broth.	Large bowel cathartic: 20-30 mL/kg via stomach tube twice, 2 hours apart, 12 hours before GI endoscopy	Withhold food; pretreatment with antiemetic should be considered. Aspiration can be fatal.	Powder for solution

Generic Name (Brand Name, Synonyms)	Canine Dosages	Feline Dosages	Adverse Effects/Warnings	Administration/ Availability
Gonadotropin-releasing hormone (GnRH, gonadorelin, Cystorelin)	Male infertility or test for cryptorchidism: 2.2-3.3 mcg/kg IM	Male infertility or test for cryptorchidism: 25 mcg/CAT IM	Response may be clinical (overt physical signs) or endocrine (2- to 4-fold increase in serum testosterone levels).	Injection
Granisetron (Kytril)	Antiemetic: 0.1-0.5 mg/kg PO or IV q 12-24h	Antiemetic: 0.1-0.5 mg/kg PO or IV q 12-24h	Use in veterinary medicine is uncommon due to availability of other antiemetics such as maropitant.	Tablets, injection, and transdermal patch
Grapiprant (Galliprant)	Analgesia/antiinflammatory: 2 mg/kg PO q 24h (dose in ½ tablet increments according to label directions)	Grapiprant is not labeled for cats; however, 3-15 mg/kg PO q 24h for 28 days appeared safe	Well tolerated but GI adverse effects are possible from this prostaglandin receptor antagonist. Avoid combination with glucocorticoids or COX-inhibiting NSAIDs.	Tablets
Griseofulvin (Fulvicin, Gris-Peg)	Dermatophytosis (rarely used): microsize forms—50 mg/kg PO q 24h or divided and given q 12h; ultramicrosize forms—5-10 mg/kg PO q 24h	Do not use in cats.	Azole antifungals and terbinafine have replaced griseofulvin for use in treating dermatophytosis. Ultramicrosize is 1.5 times more potent than microsize. Contraindicated in pregnancy, known hypersensitivity, or hepatocellular failure. Known teratogen in cats. Adverse effects include anorexia, vomiting, diarrhea, anemia, neutropenia, leukopenia, thrombocytopenia, depression, ataxia, hepatotoxicity, or dermatitis/photosensitivity.	Microsize and ultramicrosize oral suspension; give with a fatty meal.
Growth hormone, human (somatotropin)	Hypopituitary dwarfism: 0.1 units/kg (0.05 mg/kg) SQ 3 times per week for 4-6 weeks Alopecia X: 0.15 units/kg of porcine growth hormone SQ 2 times weekly for 6 weeks	Use is not described for cats.	May cause DM; blood and urine glucose should be monitored. Hypersensitivity reactions are possible, but less so if using porcine origin product. Long-term use of high doses may cause acromegaly.	Injection

H

Generic Name (Brand Name, Synonyms)	Canine Dosages	Feline Dosages	Adverse Effects/Warnings	Administration/ Availability
Heparin, unfractionated	Anticoagulant dose adjusted based on response, with usual goal of 1.5 to 2× increase in aPTT: Initial dose 150-300 units/kg SQ q 6-8h, or loading dose of 100 units/kg IV followed by 20-50 units/kg/h IV CRI	Thromboprophylaxis: 50-100 units/kg (low-dose) or 200-300 units/kg (high-dose) SQ q 6-8h	Can cause or worsen bleeding; contraindicated in severe thrombocytopenia. Protamine sulfate may be used as antidote. Not effective if antithrombin depleted.	Injection (variable concentrations—check labels carefully)
Heparin, low-molecular-weight: see dalteparin and enoxaparin				
Hetastarch 6% (Hespan)	Colloid: 5-10 mL/kg IV bolus, followed by 1 mL/kg/h IV CRI	Colloid: 10-15 mL/kg/d IV CRI	Adverse effects include volume overload, disturbed coagulation, allergic reaction, and possible nephrotoxicity. Rapid administration to cats can cause vomiting.	Solution for infusion

Generic Name (Brand Name, Synonyms)	Canine Dosages	Feline Dosages	Adverse Effects/Warnings	Administration/ Availability
Hydralazine (Apresoline)	CHF due to valvular disease: 0.5-3 mg/kg PO q 12h, titrating from lowest dose prn	Vasodilation in CHF: 2.5 mg/CAT PO q 12h, titrated prn to a maximum of 10 mg/CAT q 12h	Adverse effects include hypotension, reflex tachycardia, sodium/water retention (if not given concurrently with a diuretic), or GI upset (common). Use with caution in dogs receiving ACE inhibitors, with severe renal disease, intracerebral bleeding, or pre-existing autoimmune diseases. Contraindicated with hypovolemia or pre-existing hypotension.	Tablets, injection
Hydrochlorothiazide (HydroDIURIL, Microzide, HCTZ)	Systemic hypertension: 1 mg/kg PO q 12-24h (may combine with spironolactone 1-2 mg/kg PO q 12h to reduce potassium loss) Malignancy-associated hypoglycemia: 2-4 mg/kg PO q 24h in conjunction with diazoxide 5-20 mg/kg q 12h Prevention of calcium oxalate uroliths: 2-3 mg/kg PO q 12h Diabetes insipidus: 2 mg/kg PO q 12h	CHF refractory to furosemide alone: 1-2 mg/kg PO q 12h Prevention of oxalate uroliths: 1 mg/kg PO q 12h Diabetes insipidus: 12.5-25 mg/CAT PO q 12-24h	GI upset, hypokalemia, hypochloremic alkalosis, and other electrolyte imbalances can occur. Ensure that tablets do not contain spironolactone when treating cats. Contraindicated in pregnancy. Avoid with severe renal disease, pre-existing electrolyte and water balance abnormalities, impaired hepatic function, hyperuricemia, systemic lupus, or diabetes mellitus. Multiple drug interactions.	Tablets and capsules, and in combination with spironolactone.
Hydrocodone bitartrate (Tussigon, Hycodan)	Antitussive: 0.2-0.5 mg/kg PO q 6-12h	Rarely used in cats. Many products also contain acetaminophen.	Adverse effects include sedation, constipation (with chronic therapy), vomiting, or other GI disturbances. Contraindicated in patients receiving MAO inhibitors (e.g., amitraz and l-deprenyl), and in patients with diarrhea caused by a toxic ingestion. Any combination product containing acetaminophen must NOT be used in cats. Use with caution in hypothyroidism, severe renal insufficiency, hypoadrenocorticism, increased intracranial pressure, acute abdominal conditions, and geriatric or severely debilitated patients.	Tablets and oral solutions; often combined with acetaminophen. CSS-II.
Hydrocortisone acetate (Cortef, Solu-Cortef)	Glucocorticoid. Hypoadrenocorticism: 0.4-0.8 mg/kg PO q 12-24h Post-CPR recovery: 1 mg/kg IV followed by either 1 mg/kg q 6h IV or 0.15 mg/kg/h IV CRI, then tapered as the patient's condition allows	Glucocorticoid. Hypoadrenocorticism: 0.4-0.8 mg/kg PO q 12-24h Post-CPR recovery: 1 mg/kg IV followed by either 1 mg/kg q 6h IV or 0.15 mg/kg/h IV CRI, then tapered as the patient's condition allows	Adverse effects are those associated with glucocorticoid use (e.g., PU/PD). Oral forms may cause GI upset and gastric ulceration.	Tablets, injection, and topical creams (some OTC). Often compounded.
Hydrogen peroxide 3% (H_2O_2)	Emetic: 2.2 mL/kg PO, to a maximum of 45 mL/DOG; may repeat once in 15 minutes Topically: Used for wound cleaning	Do not use as an emetic in cats.	Emesis induction is not appropriate for all toxin ingestions and is often not helpful after onset of signs due to intoxication. Can cause esophageal or gastric irritation, and aspiration is possible. Do not use in dogs with severe lethargy, megaesophagus, debilitation (e.g., respiratory distress, decreased swallowing reflex, bradycardia), seizures, or in dogs that have had recent abdominal surgery.	Solution OTC
Hydromorphone (Dilaudid)	Analgesia: 0.05-0.2 mg/kg IV, IM, or SQ q 2-4h or given as a CRI with an initial dose of 0.05-0.1 mg/kg IV and then as CRI at 0.01-0.05 mg/kg/h IV	Analgesic: 0.05-0.1 mg/kg IV, IM, or SQ q 2-6h or given as a CRI at 0.01-0.05 mg/kg/h IV	Dogs: Nausea, vomiting, defecation, panting, vocalization, and sedation are common; CNS and respiratory depression, bradycardia, decreased GI motility possible. Cats: Nausea, ataxia, hyperesthesia, hyperthermia (monitor temperature), and behavioral changes.	Injection. CSS-II.

Generic Name (Brand Name, Synonyms)	Canine Dosages	Feline Dosages	Adverse Effects/Warnings	Administration/ Availability
Hydroxyurea (Hydrea, Droxia, Mylocel)	Polycythemia: initially 30-60 mg/kg PO q 24h (or divided twice daily) for 1-2 weeks until PCV is normalized, then tapered to lowest effective dose q other day Malignancies: variable (consult veterinary oncologist)	Polycythemia: 10-15 mg/kg PO q 12h for 1-2 weeks until PCV normalized, then tapered to lowest effective dose q other day	Use with caution in anemia, bone marrow suppression, history of urate stones, infection, impaired renal function, or in patients receiving other chemotherapy or radiotherapy. Adverse effects include GI upset, stomatitis, sloughing of nails, alopecia, and dysuria; most serious are bone marrow suppression and pulmonary fibrosis.	Capsules
Hydroxyzine (Atarax, Vistaril)	Antihistamine: 2 mg/kg PO q 12h Antipruritic: 0.5 to 2 mg/kg PO q 6-12h	Antihistamine: 5-10 mg/CAT PO q 12h or 2 mg/kg PO q 12h	The most common adverse effect is sedation. Pamoate salts are more lipophilic and are more likely to cross the blood-brain barrier, causing CNS effects. Use with caution in patients with prostatic hypertrophy, bladder neck obstruction, severe cardiac failure, angle-closure glaucoma, or pyeloduodenal obstruction. Largely replaced by alternative treatments.	Tablets, capsules

I–K

Generic Name (Brand Name, Synonyms)	Canine Dosages	Feline Dosages	Adverse Effects/Warnings	Administration/ Availability
Ifosfamide (Ifex)	Antineoplastic: For dogs <10 kg give 350 mg/m^2 and for dogs >10 kg give 375 mg/m^2 as infusion during aggressive saline diuresis. Begin diuresis at least 30 minutes before drug administration, and continue at least 5 hours after drug administration. Mesna at a dose of 20% of the ifosfamide dose is given as an IV bolus at the start of the IV infusion and again 2 and 5 hours after the ifosfamide infusion. Can repeat q 3 weeks.	Antineoplastic: 900 mg/m^2 as infusion during aggressive saline diuresis. Begin diuresis at least 30 minutes before drug administration, and continue at least 5 hours after drug administration. Mesna urothelial protectant dosed at 20% of the patient's calculated mg dose of ifosfamide and administered at time zero (immediately before ifosfamide administration), and then repeated 2 and 5 hours after ifosfamide. Can repeat q 3 weeks.	Must be given with saline diuresis and bladder-protective agent (i.e., mesna). Adverse effects include myelosuppression, renal and bladder toxicity, neurotoxicity, and GI upset. Nadirs in dogs and cats are typically seen in 5-7 days but may be delayed for as much as 14-21 days.	Injection; must be diluted to ≤20 mg/mL for use. Cytotoxic, NIOSH-listed hazardous drug and should be prepared, administered, and disposed of in accordance with federal and local requirements. Mesna is purchased separately as an injection.
Imidocarb (Imizol)	Babesia: 6.6 mg/kg IM or SQ; repeat dose in 2 weeks. Pretreat with atropine at 0.05 mg/kg SQ to mitigate the muscarinic effects.	Cytauxzoon: 5 mg/kg IM once and repeated in 14 days. Pretreat with atropine at 0.05 mg/kg SQ to mitigate the muscarinic effects. Less optimal than atovaquone and azithromycin.	Never administer IV. Cholinergic signs are common and can be mitigated with atropine or glycopyrrolate pre-treatment. Do not use imidocarb in patients exposed to cholinesterase-inhibiting drugs, pesticides, or chemicals. Use extreme caution in dogs with impaired lung, hepatic, or renal function. Less commonly reported effects include panting, diarrhea, restlessness, and injection site inflammation (more common after the second dose, and rarely may ulcerate). Hypoglycemia has been reported. Rarely, severe renal tubular or hepatic necrosis, and severe cholinergic signs have occurred.	Injection

Generic Name (Brand Name, Synonyms)	Canine Dosages	Feline Dosages	Adverse Effects/Warnings	Administration/ Availability
Imipenem-cilastatin (Primaxin)	Susceptible infections: 5-10 mg/kg IV q 6-8h	Susceptible infections: 5-10 mg/kg IV q 6-8h	Use with caution in renal impairment (dosage adjustment may be required) and in CNS disorders (e.g., seizures, head trauma). Adverse effects include GI upset, CNS toxicity (seizures, tremors), hypersensitivity, and infusion reactions (thrombophlebitis). Too rapid IV infusions may cause GI or CNS toxicity, or other untoward effects. Rarely, increases in serum creatinine, BUN, hepatic enzymes, hypotension, and tachycardia have been reported.	Powder for injection; reconstituted imipenem solution should be further diluted in a compatible IV solution and infused over 20-60 minutes.
Imipramine (Tofranil)	Narcolepsy/cataplexy: 0.5-1 mg/kg PO q 8-12h Behavioral disorders: 2.2-4.4 mg/kg PO q 24h Urethral incompetence: 5-15 mg/DOG PO q 12h	Behavioral modification: 0.5-1 mg/kg PO q 12-24h Urethral incompetence: 2.5-5 mg/CAT PO q 12h	Anticholinergic side effects are common. Do not use with MAO inhibitors (e.g., amitraz). May lower seizure threshold. Use with caution in patients with thyroid disorders, urinary retention, hepatic disorders, KCS, glaucoma, cardiac rhythm disorders, DM, or adrenal tumors due to anticholinergic adverse effects.	Tablets, capsules
Immunoglobulin (IGIV, IVIG, hIVIG)	Immune-mediated blood disorder: 0.5-1.5 g/kg IV over 6-12 hours	Dosing in cats is not described.	Adverse effects are often associated with too rapid IV administration (administer over 6-12 hours). Can cause anaphylaxis, perhaps associated with trace amounts of human albumin. Can cause increased blood pressure or local reactions at or near the injection site. Volume overload is possible. IVIG may promote hypercoagulability and an inflammatory state.	Injection; infused over a 6- to 12-hour period. Very expensive.
Insulin, regular (Humulin-R, Novolin-R)	DKA or hyperosmolar syndrome: 0.2 units/kg/h IV CRI, or prepare in saline as described (see administration) and begin infusion at 10 mL/h IV CRI, adjusting prn based on frequent glucose assessment (see Diabetic Ketoacidosis). Dextrose supplementation begun when glucose is <250. Alternative intermittent IM dosing: 0.1-0.2 units/kg IM into muscles of the rear legs; repeat IM doses of 0.1 units/kg q 1h until glucose <250 mg/dL, then IM q 4-6h or SQ q 6-8h until ready to switch to longer-acting insulin upon return of appetite	DKA: Prepare in saline as described (see administration), and begin infusion at 10 mL/h IV CRI, adjusting prn based on frequent glucose assessment (see Diabetic Ketoacidosis). Dextrose supplementation begun when glucose is <250; or intermittent IM dosing as for dog starting with 0.1 units/kg Hyperkalemia: ¼ units/kg IV bolus, or 1 units/CAT with dextrose supplementation (2 g dextrose per unit of insulin, ½ by bolus and ½ in IV fluids)	Hypoglycemia is most important adverse effect. Other adverse effects include insulin-induced hyperglycemia (Somogyi effect), insulin antagonism/resistance, rapid insulin metabolism, and local hypersensitivity reactions.	Injection. To prepare CRI, add 1.1 units/kg (cat) or 2.2 units/kg (dog) to bag of 0.9% saline then run diluted insulin solution through IV tubing and discard the first 50 mL of fluid (due to adsorption onto plastic tubing) before attaching to the patient.
Insulin, detemir (Levemir)	DM: 0.1 units/kg SQ q 12h, adjusted prn. Rarely used in dogs.	DM: 0.25 units/kg SQ q 12h, adjusted prn. Rarely used in cats.	Hypoglycemia is most important adverse effect. More potent in dogs than other commonly used insulin types. Other adverse effects include insulin-induced hyperglycemia (Somogyi effect), insulin antagonism/resistance, rapid insulin metabolism, and local hypersensitivity reactions.	Injection; use U100 syringes for injection. Vial should be rolled to mix and not shaken. Also available as insulin pen.

Generic Name (Brand Name, Synonyms)	Canine Dosages	Feline Dosages	Adverse Effects/Warnings	Administration/ Availability
Insulin, glargine (Lantus)	DM: 0.3 units/kg q 12h, adjusted prn. Not generally recommended for dogs.	DM: 0.25 units/kg or 1 unit/CAT q 12h, adjusted prn. A preferred insulin for cats.	Hypoglycemia is most important adverse effect. Other adverse effects include insulin-induced hyperglycemia (Somogyi effect), insulin antagonism/resistance, rapid insulin metabolism, and local hypersensitivity reactions.	Injection; use U100 syringes for injection. Vial should be rolled to mix and not shaken. Also available as insulin pen (stored at controlled room temperature after opening). NOTE: Basaglar may not be a therapeutic equivalent to Lantus in cats.
Insulin, NPH (Humulin-N, Novolin-N)	DM: 0.25-0.5 units/kg SQ q 12h, adjusted prn. A preferred insulin for dogs.	Rarely used for cats.	Hypoglycemia is most important adverse effect. Other adverse effects include insulin-induced hyperglycemia (Somogyi effect), insulin antagonism/resistance, rapid insulin metabolism, and local hypersensitivity reactions.	Injection; use U100 syringes for injection. Vial should be rolled to mix and not shaken.
Insulin, lente (Vetsulin)	DM: 0.25-0.5 units/kg SQ q 12h, adjusted prn. A preferred insulin for dogs.	DM: 0.25-0.5 units/kg, or 1 unit/CAT SQ q 12h	Hypoglycemia is most important adverse effect. Other adverse effects include insulin-induced hyperglycemia (Somogyi effect), insulin antagonism/resistance, rapid insulin metabolism, and local hypersensitivity reactions.	Injection; use U40 insulin syringes for injection. Unlike other insulins, vial should be well shaken to mix. Also available with insulin pen.
Insulin, PZI (Prozinc)	DM: 0.25-0.5 units/kg SQ q 12h, adjusted prn. Not generally recommended for dogs.	DM: 1 unit/CAT SQ q 12h, adjusted prn. A preferred insulin for cats.	Hypoglycemia is most important adverse effect. Other adverse effects include insulin-induced hyperglycemia (Somogyi effect), insulin antagonism/resistance, rapid insulin metabolism, and local hypersensitivity reactions.	Injection; use U40 insulin syringes for injection. Vial should be rolled to mix and not shaken.
Interferon-alfa (hulFN-alfa Intron-A)	Cutaneous or oral papillomas: 1.5-2 million units/m^2 SQ 3 times weekly	Antiviral cytokine: 10 units/kg PO q 24h, or 30-50 units/CAT, or 10,000 units/kg SQ q 24h; may be continued 1 week on treatment, one week off treatment.	Oral dosing seems to be very well tolerated. Injectable high doses in cats may cause malaise, fever, allergic reactions, myelotoxicity, myalgia, and injection site reactions. Use with caution in pre-existing autoimmune disease, severe cardiac disease, pulmonary disease, uncontrolled DM, herpes infections, hypersensitivity to the drug, or CNS disorders.	Injection; may be further diluted in saline for SQ or oral use.
Interferon-omega (Virbagen Omega, Recombinant Omega Interferon of Feline Origin, rFelFN-ω, Virbagen)	Antiviral cytokine (parvovirus): 2.5 million units/kg IV q 24h for 3 days	Antiviral cytokine (retrovirus): 1 million units/kg SQ q 24h for 5 days, repeated again 2 weeks and 2 months later	Well tolerated but GI upset and post-treatment hyperthermia have been reported. Intravenous administration to cats may cause increased incidence and severity of adverse effects. Do not vaccinate animals currently undergoing treatment. Dogs may develop antibodies to this recombinant feline product. Expensive.	Injection. No approved product in the United States, but available in European Union, Asia. Expensive.
Irbesartan (Avapro)	Hypertension: 5 mg/kg PO q 12h	Hypertension: 5 mg/kg PO q 12h	Little known about use in veterinary patients. Adverse effects include diarrhea, dyspepsia, fatigue, orthostatic dizziness, and hypotension.	Tablets; tablets with HCTZ
Iron-dextran injection	Iron supplementation: 10-20 mg/kg (maximum 300 mg/DOG) IM once monthly or converted to oral ferrous sulfate	Iron supplementation: 10 mg/kg IM once monthly or converted to oral ferrous sulfate	Causes pain on IM injection. Chronic overdosage can cause cirrhosis. Do not use in patients with acute pyelonephritis, and should not be used in conjunction with oral iron supplements.	Injection

Generic Name (Brand Name, Synonyms)	Canine Dosages	Feline Dosages	Adverse Effects/Warnings	Administration/ Availability
Isoproterenol (Isoprenaline, Isuprel)	Sinus bradycardia, complete AV block: 0.02-0.5 mcg/kg/min IV, or 0.04-0.08 mcg/kg/min IV CRI	Sinus bradycardia, complete AV block: 0.02-0.5 mcg/kg/min IV, or 0.04-0.08 mcg/kg/min IV CRI	Can cause tachycardia, anxiety, tremors, and GI upset. More arrhythmogenic than alternative drugs and therefore rarely used in veterinary medicine. Contraindicated in tachycardia or AV block caused by cardiac glycoside intoxication.	Injection. Dilute 1 mg into 500 mL of D_5W to make a 2 mcg/mL solution.
Isosorbide dinitrate (Isordil, Ismo, Imdur)	Adjunctive therapy for CHF: As the dinitrate salt 8-10 mg/kg PO q 12h; as the mononitrate 0.5-2 mg/DOG PO q 12h	Adjunctive therapy for CHF: As the dinitrate salt 8-10 mg/kg PO q 12h; as the mononitrate 0.5-2 mg/CAT PO q 12h	Adverse effects include tachycardia, restlessness, or GI effects. Use with extreme caution in patients with low blood pressure or hypovolemia. Do not use as a monotherapy.	Tablets, extended-release tablets
Isotretinoin (Accutane)	Sebaceous skin disorders: 1 mg/kg PO q 12-24h	Feline acne: 5-10 mg/CAT PO q 24h	Do not use in homes with a pregnant woman. Use with extreme caution in hypertriglyceridemia, severe renal or hepatic disease. Hairless skin may sunburn more easily. Adverse effects include KCS in dogs, GI distress, behavioral changes from CNS effects, and pruritus. Cats have more severe reactions, including blepharospasm, periocular crusting, erythema, diarrhea, and weight loss due to anorexia.	Capsules; give with food.
Itraconazole (Itrafungol, Sporanox)	Susceptible systemic mycoses: 5-10 mg/kg PO q 24h, or 5 mg/kg PO q 12h	Susceptible systemic mycoses: 50-100 mg/CAT or 5-10 mg/kg PO q 24h, or 5 mg/kg PO q 12h	Adverse effects include anorexia, GI upset, hepatotoxicity. Oral solutions contain 15% propylene glycol and may cause Heinz body formation in cats. In dogs, erythema multiforme or toxic epidermal necrolysis occurs rarely, and ulcerative skin lesions, vasculitis, and limb edema may occur at higher dosages. Use with caution in hepatic impairment and in animals with reduced cardiac function.	Capsules and oral solutions; give with fatty meal. Compounded forms prepared from the bulk powder are not bioavailable in dogs and cats and do not achieve appropriate therapeutic blood levels.
Ivermectin (Ivomec, Heartgard)	Heartworm prevention: 0.006 mg/kg PO q month Sarcoptic mange: 0.2-0.4 mg/kg PO or SQ q 7 days for 4 treatments Ear mites: Otic preparation topically once or twice	Heartworm prevention: 0.024 mg/kg PO q month Sarcoptic mange: 0.2-0.4 mg/kg PO or SQ q 7 days for 4 treatments Ear mites: Otic preparation topically once or twice	Adverse effects are dose related, with low dosages found in heartworm prevention well tolerated. Higher dosages can cause neurologic adverse effects and should be avoided in dogs with *MDR1/ABCB1*-Δ mutation. Multiple drug interactions possible. Off-label use of large animal products in dogs or cats can cause severe adverse reactions, including death.	Tablets, chewable tablets, oral paste, oral solutions, pour-on, injectable solutions, otic preparations (multiple formulations for different purposes in different species). Ivermectin for small animals found at low dose in heartworm preventatives, sometimes combined with other anthelmintics.
Kaolin-pectin (Kaopectolin)	Diarrhea: 1-2 mL/kg PO q 4-6h prn	Diarrhea: 1-2 mL/kg PO q 4-6h prn	Generally well tolerated. Transient constipation may occur with high doses. Impacts absorption of other medications. Do not use for severe diarrhea.	Oral suspension OTC

Generic Name (Brand Name, Synonyms)	Canine Dosages	Feline Dosages	Adverse Effects/Warnings	Administration/ Availability
Ketamine HCl (Ketaset, Ketaflo, Vetalar)	Restraint: 3 mg/kg IV with diazepam or midazolam 0.1 mg/kg IV (can be combined in same syringe)	Restraint: 5-10 mg/kg IM; can be supplemented with 2 mg/kg IV if needed. Often combined with other agents for sedation/anesthesia for minor procedures: ketamine 3 mg/kg IV plus diazepam or midazolam 0.1 mg/kg IV (can be combined in same syringe), or ketamine plus butorphanol 0.1-0.5 mg/kg IM, IV, or buprenorphine 0.005-0.02 mg/kg IM, IV	Adverse effects include pain on IM injection; increased heart rate, blood pressure, and myocardial oxygen consumption. Eyes should be protected from injury with an ocular lubricant. Does not provide muscle relaxation and should not be used alone for major surgery. Contraindicated where increased intraocular pressure or open globe injuries are present. Use with caution in animals with pre-existing seizure disorders, cardiovascular and renal compromise.	Injection. CSS-III.
Ketoconazole (Nizoral)	Susceptible mycotic infection (not recommended for most systemic mycosis): 5-10 mg/kg PO q 12-24h Long-term pulse dosing for onychomycosis: 5-10 mg/kg PO 3 days on and 4 days off Cyclosporin dose reduction adjunct: 2.5-5 mg/kg PO q 24h	Generally not recommended for cats.	Adverse effects include GI upset, dose-related hepatotoxicity, and adrenal suppression. Use with caution in hepatic disease or thrombocytopenia. Long-term use has been associated with cataracts.	Tablets; give with a fatty meal.
Ketoprofen (Ketofen, Anafen)	Antiinflammatory/analgesic NSAID: 2 mg/kg IM, IV, or SQ once (postoperative pain control), followed by 1 mg/kg PO q 24h prn or lowest effective dose	Antiinflammatory/analgesic NSAID: 1-2 mg/kg IM, IV, or SQ once (postoperative pain control), followed by 1 mg/kg PO q 24h prn or lowest effective dose. Alternative analgesics usually preferred in cats.	Adverse effects include GI upset and ulcers, renal necrosis, hepatitis, and platelet inhibition. Do not administer with glucocorticoids or other NSAIDs. Rarely used in small animals.	Tablets, capsules and injection. Oral forms given with food.

L

Generic Name (Brand Name, Synonyms)	Canine Dosages	Feline Dosages	Adverse Effects/Warnings	Administration/Availability
Lactulose (Cephulac, Kristalose)	Hepatic encephalopathy: 0.25-0.5 mL/kg PO q 6-8h until stools are loose Enema: 3 parts lactulose and 7 parts warm water and give 1-10 mL/kg as a retention enema for 20-30 minutes	Hepatic encephalopathy: 0.25-0.5 mL/kg PO q 6-8h until stools are loose Constipation: ½ - ¾ teaspoon q 12h mixed with food, adjusted to obtain desired stool consistency	Adverse effects include flatulence, gastric distention, and cramping. Contraindicated in intestinal obstruction. Use with caution in diabetic patients. Cats may be easier to medicate with the oral crystals (1 g crystals = 1.5 mL liquid).	Oral liquid or crystals
Lansoprazole (Prevacid)	Proton pump inhibitor antacid: 1-2 mg/kg to maximum of 20 mg/day IV or PO q 24h	Proton pump inhibitor antacid: 1 mg/kg IV or PO q 24h	Adverse effects not well documented in dogs or cats; dizziness, irregular heart rate, weakness, "jitters," and seizures described in humans.	Delayed-release orally disintegrating tablets, capsules, both OTC, and injection. Give on empty stomach each morning.
Lanthanum (Fosrenol, Lantharenol)	Phosphate binder: 5-20 mg/kg PO q 12h; titrate to effect	Phosphate binder: 15-45 mg/kg/d PO divided with meals, or 200 mg/CAT q 12h	Contraindicated in intestinal obstruction, ileus, or fecal impaction. Use with caution in presence of colitis or ulcers. Adverse effects include vomiting and food avoidance. May impact absorption of some drugs (e.g., famotidine).	Tablets; give with meals.
Laxative paste (Laxatone)	Constipation: per label instructions	Constipation or hairballs: per label instructions, or 2.5-5 mL PO initially, then 1-2.5 mL PO 2-3 times per week	Aspiration	Oral gel OTC

Generic Name (Brand Name, Synonyms)	Canine Dosages	Feline Dosages	Adverse Effects/Warnings	Administration/Availability
L-carnitine (Carnitor, levocarnitine)	Deficiency causing cardiomyopathy: 50-200 mg/kg PO q 8h	Hepatic lipidosis: 250-500 mg/CAT PO q 24h	Dose-related GI upset.	Tablets, oral powder, or oral solution OTC, and injection. Give oral forms with food.
Leflunomide (Arava)	Immunosuppression: 3-4 mg/kg PO q 24h	Immunosuppression: 2-3 mg/kg PO q 24h	Adverse effects include GI upset, lethargy, bone marrow suppression, and hypercholesterolemia. Contraindicated in pregnancy and hepatic impairment.	Tablets; give with food.
Levamisole (Levasole, Tramisol)	Adjunct for systemic lupus (SLE): 2-5 mg/kg PO q 48h not to exceed 150 mg/DOG. Rarely used as anthelmintic	Rarely used in cats	Adverse effects include GI upset, neurotoxicity, hematologic toxicity, mydriasis, lethargy, and hypersalivation. Avoid in animals with significant renal or hepatic impairment.	Soluble powders OTC; give with food.
Levetiracetam (Keppra)	Anticonvulsant: 15-20 mg/kg PO q 8h for immediate-release tablets; 30 mg/kg PO q 12-24h for extended-release tablets Status epilepticus: 30-60 mg/kg IV slow bolus	Anticonvulsant: 20-30 mg/kg PO q 8h Status epilepticus: 20 mg/kg IV once by slow bolus	Adverse effects include mild sedation and GI upset. Human extended-release generic products may not be bioequivalent. Use with caution in renal impairment.	Immediate- and extended-release tablets, oral solution, and injection. Oral forms may be given with or without food. Extended-release products should not be broken or crushed. Administer IV bolus over 5-15 minutes.
Levothyroxine sodium (Thyro-Tabs Canine, Synthroid)	Hypothyroidism: 0.02 mg/kg PO q 12h (adjust as needed based on T_4) Myxedema crisis: 5 mcg/kg IV q 12h until oral treatment possible	Hypothyroidism: 0.02-0.04 mg/kg PO q 12-24h (adjust based on T_4)	Use with caution with cardiac disease, DM, or in elderly patients. Dogs with hypoadrenocorticism should receive replacement of mineralocorticoid and glucocorticoid therapy before receiving levothyroxine as an increased basal metabolic rate may exacerbate electrolyte disturbances.	Available in tablets and chewables, powder, and injection. Administer consistently either with or without food. Do not add injection to other fluids.
Lidocaine (Xylocaine, Lignocaine)	Arrhythmias: 2-4 mg/kg IV over 1-2 minutes, then 0.5-2 mg/kg q 20-60 minutes, or 0.04-0.08 mg/kg/min (40-80 mcg/kg/min) CRI IV Regional anesthesia: up to 4 mg/kg local injection Epidural: 1 mL of 2% lidocaine per 4.5 kg BW	Cats are very sensitive and develop cardiodepression. Arrhythmias: 0.25-0.75 mg/kg slowly over 5 minutes; give 1-4 mg bolus maximum over 5 minutes; use diluted solution as CRI 0.01-0.04 mg/kg/min Regional anesthesia: 2-4 mg/kg local injection Urethral catheterization: sterile gel applied to catheter	Ensure product for IV use does not contain epinephrine. Use IV with caution in patients with liver disease (reduce dose 50%), CHF, shock, hypovolemia, severe respiratory depression, marked hypoxia, bradycardia or incomplete heart block.	Injection, transdermal patch, gel, and ready-to-administer premixed bags in D_5W. Administer IV slowly. Do not administer epinephrine-containing products IV.
Liothyronine, T_3 (Cytomel, Triostat)	Hypothyroidism nonresponsive to levothyroxine: 4-6 mcg/kg PO q 8h	T_3 suppression test: 25 mcg/CAT PO q 8h for 7 doses. Measure T_4 2-6 hours after last dose.	Use with caution in patients with liver disease (reduce dose 50%), CHF, shock, hypovolemia, severe respiratory depression, marked hypoxia, bradycardia or incomplete heart block having VPCs. For IV use ensure that products do not contain epinephrine.	Tablets or injection; administer consistently either with or without food. Do not add injection to other fluids.
Lisinopril (Prinivil, Zestril)	ACE inhibitor used for CHF: 0.5 mg/kg PO q 12h	Adjunctive treatment of CHF: 0.25-0.5 mg/kg PO q 24h	GI distress, cough, weakness, hypotension, renal dysfunction, and hyperkalemia possible. Rashes, neutropenia, and agranulocytosis have been reported in humans. Use with caution in coronary or cerebrovascular insufficiency, pre-existing hematologic abnormalities, electrolyte disorders, or collagen vascular disease.	Tablets; give with food.
Lomustine (CCNU, Gleostine, CeeNU)	Antineoplastic: 50-90 mg/m^2 q 2-6 weeks. Consult with veterinary oncologist.	Antineoplastic: 40-60 mg/m^2 q 3-6 weeks or as a single 10-mg dose q 3 weeks. DO NOT administer with alpha-lipoic acid as has been suggested for dogs. Consult with veterinary oncologist.	Adverse effects are serious and include bone marrow depression, hepatotoxicity, and lung injury.	Capsules. NIOSH classifies lomustine as antineoplastic agent that represents an occupational hazard to health care workers and that should always be handled with use of recommended engineering controls and personal protective equipment (PPE), regardless of formulation.

Generic Name (Brand Name, Synonyms)	Canine Dosages	Feline Dosages	Adverse Effects/Warnings	Administration/Availability
Loperamide (Imodium)	Antidiarrheal: 0.1-0.2 mg/kg PO q 8-12h	Antidiarrheal: 0.05-0.16 mg/kg PO q 8-12h	Do not administer to dogs with *MDR1/ABCB1-Δ* mutation (naloxone may be used to reverse effects). Cats may experience a paradoxical CNS excitation. Use with caution if at all in animals with increased cranial pressure or acute abdomen. Use with extreme caution in hepatic impairment. Constipation, bloat, and sedation are the most likely effects in dogs. Multiple reported drug interactions.	Tablets, capsules, and oral liquid OTC
Losartan (Cozaar)	Angiotensin receptor blocker: non-azotemic dogs 0.5 mg/kg PO q 24h, titrating up to 1 mg/kg/d prn; azotemic dogs, 0.125 mg/kg PO q 24h, titrating up to 0.5 mg/kg/d	Use not described for cats.	Adverse effects not well described in dogs or cats. Hypotension, cough, hyperkalemia, and azotemia can occur in humans.	Tablets; also available combined with hydrochlorothiazide.
Lorazepam (Ativan)	Behavioral modification: 0.02-0.5 mg/kg PO q 8-24h Status epilepticus: 0.2 mg/kg IV or intranasally	Behavioral modification: 0.025-0.25 mg/kg or 0.125-0.25 mg/CAT PO q 8-24h	Polyphagia, aggression, sedation, and ataxia can occur. Sudden discontinuation may result in return of unwanted behaviors. Use injection with care in cats as the injection contains propylene glycol and benzyl alcohol.	Tablets, oral solution, and injection. CSS-IV.
Lovastatin (Mevacor)	Hypercholesterolemia: 10-20 mg/DOG PO q 24h	Use not described for cats.	Lethargy, GI upset, muscle pain, and hepatotoxicity are possible.	Tablet; give with food.
Lysine (l-lysine, Enisyl-F, Felisyl)	No well-described use in dogs.	Herpes (FHV-1) viral infection: 250-500 mg/CAT q 12-24h	Renal dysfunction reported in humans. Efficacy questionable for FHV-1.	Chewable treats, oral paste or gel, powder OTC

M

Generic Name (Brand Name, Synonyms)	Canine Dosages	Feline Dosages	Adverse Effects/Warnings	Administration/Availability
Magnesium hydroxide (Milk of Magnesia)	Hypomagnesemia/hypocalcemia: 5-15 mL/DOG PO q 12-24h	Hypomagnesemia/hypocalcemia: 5 mL/CAT PO q 12-24h	Can cause diarrhea, electrolyte disturbances, and interferes with many orally administered drugs. Contraindicated in renal insufficiency.	Oral suspension OTC
Magnesium sulfate	Hypomagnesemia: 0.75 mEq/kg/d (or 0.375 mmol/kg/d) IV	Hypomagnesemia: 0.75 mEq/kg/d (or 0.375 mmol/kg/d) IV. Used in addition to potassium supplementation.	Use with caution in patients with renal failure; dosage reduction of 50%-75% recommended. Adverse effects are from hypermagnesemia and include drowsiness, muscular weakness, bradycardia, hypotension, hypocalcemia, respiratory depression, and increased Q-T intervals.	Injection. Give IV slowly (over 10-20 minutes) and then as a CRI to desired effect.
Mannitol (Osmitrol)	Cerebral edema, oliguric renal failure, or adjunctive treatment of glaucoma: 0.25-0.5 g/kg as a slow IV bolus over 10-20 minutes	Cerebral edema, oliguric renal failure, or adjunctive treatment of glaucoma: 0.25-0.5 g/kg as a slow IV bolus over 10-20 minutes	Volume depletion, volume overload in oliguric patients, hypernatremia, hypokalemia, and metabolic acidosis are the most severe adverse effects. Use with caution in oliguric renal failure. Other adverse effects may include GI upset, CHF, tachycardia, acute kidney injury (if osmolality >320 mOsm/L), and CNS effects.	Injection. Inspect for crystals before administration (warming will dissolve crystals). Do not give mannitol with whole blood products unless at least 20 mEq/L of sodium chloride is added to the mannitol solution or pseudoagglutination may result.

Generic Name (Brand Name, Synonyms)	Canine Dosages	Feline Dosages	Adverse Effects/Warnings	Administration/ Availability
Marbofloxacin (Zeniquin)	Susceptible infections: 2.75-5.5 mg/kg PO or SQ q 24h Leishmaniasis: 2 mg/kg PO q 24h for 28 days	Susceptible infections: 2.75-5.5 mg/kg PO q 24h	Well tolerated, but adverse effects include GI distress, CNS stimulation, or hypersensitivity. Consider benefit/risk in young, growing animals because of damage to cartilage. May increase seizure risk. Does not cause retinopathy in cats at recommended dose. Use with caution in hepatic or renal insufficiency and dehydration.	Tablets, injection. Compounding pharmacies may prepare stable oral suspensions. Give on an empty stomach, but can give with nondairy foods to minimize GI upset if necessary.
Maropitant (Cerenia)	Antiemetic: 1 mg/kg SQ or IV (slow injection) or 2 mg/kg PO q 24h Prevention of motion sickness: 8 mg/kg PO 2 hours before travel then q 24h up to 2 days Adjunct antitussive (controversial use): 2 mg/kg PO q 48h	Antiemetic: 1 mg/kg PO, SQ, or IV (over 1-2 minutes) Prevention of vomiting with CKD: 4 mg/CAT PO q 24-48h	Generally well tolerated. SQ injection can cause pain (refrigerate to minimize). May cause myelosuppression in puppies <11 weeks of age. Use with caution in hepatic failure or with cardiovascular disease. Do not use in GI obstruction or acute intoxications. Human caregivers should wear gloves as maropitant causes contact dermatitis in many humans.	Tablets (give on empty stomach), injection. Keep refrigerated to minimize pain on injection. If given IV, solutions should be administered over 1-2 minutes.
Mastinib (Masivet, Kinavet)	Antineoplastic (especially mast cell tumor): 12.5 mg/kg PO q 24h	Not recommended for use in cats.	Not FDA approved. Proteinuria and neutropenia are relevant adverse events.	Not available in the United States.
Meclizine (Bonine, Dramamine II, Antivert)	Prophylaxis of vestibular syndromes, motion sickness: 4 mg/kg or 25 mg/DOG PO q 24h	Prophylaxis of vestibular syndromes: 6.25-12.5 mg/CAT PO q 24h	Adverse effects include dry mouth, dry eyes, tachycardia. Paradoxical CNS stimulation has also occurred. Due to its anticholinergic side effects, meclizine should be used cautiously in prostatic hypertrophy, bladder neck obstruction, severe cardiac failure, glaucoma, or pyeloduodenal obstruction.	Tablets OTC
Medetomidine (Domitor)	Sedation/restraint: 0.005-0.02 mg/kg (5-20 mcg/kg) IM as a single agent	Sedation/restraint: 0.02 mg/kg (20 mcg/kg) IM	Adverse effects are dose related and include bradycardia, depressed respiration, hypothermia, urination, vomiting, hyperglycemia, and pain on IM injection. May increase ocular pressure in dogs but not cats.	Injection
Medroxyprogesterone acetate (Provera)	Alopecia X: 5-7 mg/kg SQ q 4 weeks for 4 treatments Long-term reproductive control: 2.5-3 mg/kg IM q 5 months	Adjunctive therapy to refractory urine marking in neutered male cats: 5-20 mg/kg SQ or IM 3-4× yearly Long-term reproductive control: 2 mg/kg IM q 5 months	Drug rarely used due to adverse event profile, including PU/PD, lethargy, endocrinopathy, and pyometra. It may predispose animals to DM and should not be used in diabetics. May suppress adrenal function; treated animals may require supplemental corticosteroids in stressful situations.	Tablets, injection. Injections administered SQ should be given in visually inconspicuous area as it may cause permanent alopecia at the injection site.
Meglumine antimonite (Glucantime, N-methyl-glucamine antimoniate)	Leishmaniasis: 100 mg/kg SQ q 24h for 4 weeks +/- allopurinol	Use in cats is not described.	Use in renal, hepatic, or cardiac failure carries a higher risk of adverse effects, including the risk of worsening renal function through damage to renal tubules. Other adverse effects include injection site reactions, lethargy, GI effects, and elevated liver enzymes.	Not available in the United States. May be obtained through Centers for Disease Control and Prevention or imported from Europe.

Generic Name (Brand Name, Synonyms)	Canine Dosages	Feline Dosages	Adverse Effects/Warnings	Administration/ Availability
Melarsomine (Immiticide, Diroban)	Heartworm infection (class 1): 2.5 mg/kg deep IM in the lumbar epaxial muscles twice, 24 hours apart, or as for class 2-3 Heartworm disease (class 2, 3): 2.5 mg/kg deep IM in the lumbar epaxial muscles; enforce strict rest for 1 month, then repeat 2 more doses 24 hours apart (total of 3 injections)	Do not use in cats.	Pain at injection site and reluctance to move following treatment is common. Other adverse effects include coughing, gagging, depression, inappetence, fever, lung congestion, and vomiting. Do not administer to dogs with caval syndrome. Post-treatment thrombotic events are strongly correlated with activity. Strict cage rest should be imposed for at least 2-4 weeks after treatment.	Injection. Administer deep IM strictly following the manufacturer's package insert. Wear appropriate personal protective equipment (e.g., gloves, gowns, face mask) to protect from exposure.
Melatonin (Regulin, PrimeX, Dermatonin)	Alopecia X: 3-12 mg/DOG PO q 8-24h, or using the implants 8 mg (dogs <9 kg), 12 mg (dogs 9-18 kg), and 18 mg (dogs >18 kg) implanted SQ 1-2× yearly as needed Adjunct for immune-mediated blood disorder: 3 mg/DOG for dogs <20 kg, and 6 mg/DOG for dogs >20 kg PO q 12h	Nocturnal hyperactivity: 1.5-6 mg/CAT PO before bedtime	Generally very well tolerated. May cause sedation. Implants are occasionally associated with injection site reactions.	Tablets OTC, implants
Meloxicam (Metacam, Mobic, OroCam)	Antiinflammatory/analgesic NSAID: 0.2 mg/kg PO, IV, or SQ initially, followed by 0.1 mg/kg PO q 24h	Product bears a black box warning about use in cats. ISFM and AAFP support low dosing for chronic pain. Chronic antiinflammatory/ analgesic NSAID: 0.1 mg/ kg PO initially, followed by 0.05 mg/kg PO q 24h tapered to lowest effective dose	Adverse events are similar to other NSAIDs and include GI upset, ulceration, perforation, and renal toxicity. Do not combine with other NSAIDs or glucocorticoids. Manufacturers state that there is no known safe dosing of this drug in cats; however, it is often used as an analgesic for chronic conditions such as osteoarthritis in cats.	Tablets, oral suspension, injection, transmucosal oral solution. Oral forms given with food.
Melphalan (Alkeran)	Antineoplastic: 2 mg/m^2 PO q 24h for 2 weeks, then 2-4 mg/m^2 PO q 48h; or 0.1 mg/kg PO q 24h for 10 days, then 0.05 mg/kg PO q 24h; or 1.5 mg/m^2 PO q 24h for 7-10 days; or 7 mg/m^2 q 24h for 5 days q 3 weeks	Antineoplastic: 2 mg/m^2 PO q other day; or 0.1 mg/kg PO q 24h for 2 weeks, then q 48h	Use with caution in patients with leukopenia, thrombocytopenia, previous radiotherapy, impaired hepatic or renal function. Adverse effects include GI upset, pulmonary infiltrates or fibrosis, and myelosuppression.	Tablets. Cytotoxic, NIOSH-listed hazardous drug and should be prepared, administered, and disposed of in accordance with federal and local requirements.
Memantine (Namenda)	Behavioral disorders: 0.3-0.5 mg/kg PO q 12h	Use is not described in cats.	Poor evidence for clinical efficacy or safety in veterinary patients, though no specific adverse effects described.	Tablets
Meropenem (Merrem)	Multidrug-resistant infections: 8.5-12 mg/kg SQ q 12h or 24 mg/kg IV q 12h; increase to q 8h if neutropenia and pathogen minimum inhibitory concentration >1	Multidrug-resistant infections: 10 mg/kg q 12h SQ, IV	Generally well tolerated. Alopecia or hair color change may occur at SQ injection sites. GI upset and seizures have been reported. Do not use in animals that have known allergies to beta-lactam antimicrobials.	Injection. Stable at 50 mg/mL in refrigerator for up to 25 days.
Mesalamine (5-ASA, Asacol, Pentasa)	IBD: 10-20 mg/kg PO q 8h	Use is not described in cats.	Not commonly used in veterinary medicine.	Controlled-release capsules
Mesna (Mesnex)	Adjunctive therapy to ifosfamide for antineoplastic therapy: Give mesna at 20% of the ifosfamide dose as an IV bolus initially with ifosfamide infusion; repeat at 2 and 5 hours after the ifosfamide infusion. Treatment is repeated q 3 weeks.	Adjunctive therapy to ifosfamide for antineoplastic therapy: Give mesna at 20% of the ifosfamide dose as an IV bolus initially with ifosfamide infusion; repeat at 2 and 5 hours after the ifosfamide infusion. Because the dose of ifosfamide is significantly greater for cats, the dose of mesna will also be comparatively larger. Treatment is repeated q 3 weeks.	Used as an adjunctive therapy with ifosfamide administration and saline diuresis to prevent hemorrhagic cystitis.	Injection. Dilute 20 mg/mL before administration at 20% of ifosfamide dose.

Generic Name (Brand Name, Synonyms)	Canine Dosages	Feline Dosages	Adverse Effects/Warnings	Administration/ Availability
Methadone (Dolophine)	Analgesia: Loading dose of 0.1-0.2 mg/kg IV, followed by 0.12 mg/kg/h IV CRI Perioperative and postoperative analgesia: 0.1-1 mg/kg IV, SQ, or IM q 4-8h	Analgesia: Loading dose of 0.1-0.2 mg/kg IV, followed by 0.12 mg/kg/h IV CRI Perioperative and postoperative analgesia: 0.05-0.5 mg/kg IV, SQ, or IM q 4-6h	Adverse effects are typical for opioids and include panting, whining, sedation, defecation, constipation, bradycardia, CNS excitation, histamine response, and respiratory depression. Use with extreme caution in hypothyroidism, severe renal insufficiency, hypoadrenocorticism, in geriatric or severely debilitated patients, head injuries, increased intracerebral pressure, acute abdominal conditions, respiratory disease or acute respiratory dysfunction.	Injection. Dilute in saline for CRI infusions. CSS-II.
Methazolamide (Neptazane)	Glaucoma: 2-5 mg/kg PO 2-3×/d	Glaucoma: 1-4 mg/kg PO 2-3×/d	May cause mild metabolic acidosis (bicarbonaturia); GI, CNS adverse effects possible.	Tablets. Very expensive. Use may be obsolete due to cost and compared to more efficacious topical therapies with fewer side effects.
Methimazole (Tapazole, Felimazole)	Functional thyroid neoplasia: 2.5-5 mg/DOG PO q 12h (other treatments indicated)	Hyperthyroidism: 2.5 mg/CAT PO or by transdermal gel q 12h initial dose, adjusted based on response to therapy. Response to transdermal may take several weeks.	Adverse effects include GI upset, blood dyscrasias, facial excoriations (requires discontinuation of therapy), and rarely hepatotoxicity and myasthenia gravis. Avoid use in autoimmune disease, primary liver disease, hematologic disorders or coagulopathies, or pregnant/lactating queens. May unmask underlying renal failure.	Tablets. Compounding pharmacists may provide oral suspensions and transdermal gels. Give oral preparations with food. Use gloves when applying topically to inner pinnae.
Methionine, DL: see DL-methionine				
Methocarbamol (Robaxin)	Muscle relaxation: 20-45 mg/kg PO q 8-12h; Muscle tremors of toxicoses: 44-220 mg/kg slow IV; use high end of dose range if strychnine, metaldehyde, tetanus; maximum 330 mg/kg/day	Muscle relaxation: 20-45 mg/kg PO q 8-12h	Adverse effects include sedation, salivation, emesis, lethargy, weakness, and ataxia.	Tablets, injection. Avoid IM or SQ injection due to pain, and administer slowly by IV infusion, being careful to avoid extravasation.
Methotrexate	Antineoplastic: 0.06 mg/kg PO q 24-48h; or 2.5 mg/m^2 PO q 24-48h	Antineoplastic: 2.5 mg/m^2 PO q 2-3 days	Adverse effects include leukopenia, GI bleeding, hepatotoxicity. Contraindicated in bone marrow depression, severe hepatic or renal insufficiency.	Tablets, injection. Cytotoxic, NIOSH-listed hazardous drug and should be prepared, administered, and disposed of in accordance with federal and local requirements.
Methylene blue (new methylene blue)	Methemoglobinemia: 1 mg/kg IV for short-term use, or 1.5 mg/kg PO q 24-48h for chronic use	Use in cats is not described.	Oxidant compound that can result in magnified oxidative damage and hemolysis. Use with caution, and consider consultation with veterinary toxicologist or internist.	Available through compounding
Methylphenidate (Ritalin)	Narcolepsy: 0.1-0.25 mg/kg PO q 8-24h	Use in cats is not described.	Adverse effects include CNS stimulation, hyperthermia, tremors, tachycardia, tachypnea, and anorexia. Use with caution in seizure disorders, cardiac disease, hypertension, or in aggressive animals.	Tablets, oral solution, oral suspension. A drug of high abuse by humans; prescriptions limited to 30 days. CSS-II.

Generic Name (Brand Name, Synonyms)	Canine Dosages	Feline Dosages	Adverse Effects/Warnings	Administration/ Availability
Methylprednisolone acetate (Medrol, Depo-Medrol)	Antiinflammatory long-acting glucocorticoid: 1-2 mg/kg IM, SQ repeated as needed up to q several weeks. Intermediate-duration glucocorticoids (e.g., predniso[lo]ne) preferred in most situations. Can be used as intralesional injection.	Antiinflammatory long-acting glucocorticoid: 10-20 mg/CAT IM, SQ repeated as needed up to q several weeks. Intermediate-duration glucocorticoids (e.g., prednisolone) preferred in most situations. Can be used as intralesional injection.	Adverse effects are those typical of glucocorticoids (e.g., PU/PD, polyphagia, hypothalamic-pituitary axis suppression). Can precipitate DM. Contraindicated in active infections, GI ulceration, and hyperadrenocorticism. Do not use concurrently with NSAIDs or other glucocorticoids. Use with caution in hypertension, CHF, renal insufficiency.	Injectable suspension. Shake well before using.
Methylprednisolone sodium succinate (Solu-Medrol)	Rapid-acting parenteral glucocorticoid: 30 mg/kg slow IV once, then 15 mg/kg IV q 6h prn up to 48 hours (use in shock and IVDD controversial)	Rapid-acting parenteral glucocorticoid: 30 mg/kg slow IV once, then 15 mg/kg IV q 6h prn up to 48 hours (use in shock controversial)	Adverse effects include GI ulceration. Typically used only in acute care, so longer-term adverse effects of glucocorticoids may not have been recognized. Active infection, GI ulceration, and hyperadrenocorticism are contraindications. Do not use concurrently with NSAIDs. Use with caution in hypertension, CHF, renal insufficiency.	Injection
Methyltestosterone (Android, Methitest)	Testosterone-responsive alopecia: 1 mg/kg (up to 30 mg/DOG) PO q 24-48h until hair regrowth, then lowest effective dose 1-2×/wk Hormone-responsive incontinence in male dogs: 0.5 mg/kg PO q 24h (other treatments preferred)	Do not use in cats.	May cause premature closure of epiphyseal plates in growing animals. Contraindicated in hepatic failure and pregnancy. Use with caution in heart failure.	Tablets, capsules
Metoclopramide (Reglan)	Antiemetic and gastric prokinetic: 0.2-0.5 mg/kg PO, SQ, or IM q 6-8h, or 0.01-0.09 mg/kg/h IV CRI	Not preferred for cats. Antiemetic and gastric prokinetic: 0.2-0.5 mg/kg q 6-8h PO, SQ, or IM; or 0.01-0.09 mg/kg/h IV CRI	Adverse effects include frenzied behavior, disorientation, constipation; these are more likely in cats than dogs. Contraindicated in patients with GI hemorrhage, obstruction, or perforation. May trigger hypertensive crisis in pheochromocytoma. Use with extreme caution if at all in presence of seizures or head trauma. Do not use concurrently with phenothiazines. Use with caution and reduce dose in CHF or renal failure.	Tablets, oral solution, injection. Dilute IV doses in saline and administer slowly to minimize CNS adverse effects.
Metoprolol (Lopressor)	Noncongestive heart failure: 0.2 mg/kg PO q 12h slowly titrated upward (as tolerated) q 2-3 weeks	Beta-blocker: 2-15 mg/CAT PO q 8h	Contraindicated in 2nd- or 3rd-degree heart block and sinus bradycardia. Adverse effects may include bradycardia, lethargy, weakness, depression, impaired AV conduction, worsening of heart failure, hypotension, hypoglycemia, syncope, and diarrhea.	Tablets
Metronidazole (Flagyl)	Susceptible anaerobic infections or IBD: 10-15 mg/kg PO q 12h (do not exceed 60 mg/kg/day) Anaerobic sepsis: 15 mg/kg IV over 30-60 minutes q 12h Giardiasis: 15-25 mg/kg PO q 12-24h for 5 -7 days	Susceptible anaerobic infections or IBD: 10-15 mg/kg PO q 12h Anaerobic sepsis: 15 mg/kg IV over 30-60 minutes q 12h Giardiasis: 15-25 mg/kg PO q 12-24h for 5-7 days	Adverse effects include neurotoxicity (rare in cats), blood dyscrasias, GI upset, and hepatopathy. Use with caution and reduce dose by 50% in hepatic failure and decrease frequency to q 24h. Dogs may experience neurotoxicity in doses >60 mg/kg/day.	Tablets, oral solution, injection. Compounding pharmacists may prepare palatable preparations of metronidazole benzoate, which requires multiplying the dose of metronidazole by 1.6. Tablets are extremely bitter. Injections should not be refrigerated. Dilute IV doses in saline and administer over 30-60 minutes.

Generic Name (Brand Name, Synonyms)	Canine Dosages	Feline Dosages	Adverse Effects/Warnings	Administration/ Availability
Mexiletine (Mexitil)	Ventricular arrhythmias: 5-10 mg/kg PO q 8-12h. Avoid use or reduce dose in *MDR1/ABCB1-Δ* mutants.	Ventricular arrhythmias: 4-10 mg/kg PO q 8-12h. Cats are more likely to experience adverse effects than dogs.	GI upset is the most common adverse effect and may be minimized by giving with food. Use with extreme caution if at all in patients with 2nd- or 3rd-degree AV block or cardiogenic shock. Avoid use or reduce dose in *MDR1/ABCB1-Δ* mutants.	Capsules; give with food.
Miconazole (Conofite)	Susceptible mycotic lesions: Apply q 12h for 2 weeks beyond resolution	Susceptible mycotic lesions: Apply q 12h for 2 weeks beyond resolution	Well tolerated. Some owners experience contact sensitivity.	Solution and cream OTC
Midazolam (Versed)	Sedation/restraint: 0.1 mg/kg IV combined with ketamine 3 mg/kg, or combined with butorphanol 0.1-0.5 mg/kg, or combined with hydromorphone 0.05-0.2 mg/kg Premedication for anesthesia: 0.1-0.3 mg/kg SQ, IM, IV Status epilepticus: 0.1-0.3 mg/kg IM or IV, or 0.2-1.0 mg/kg intranasally, or 0.05-0.5 mg/kg as a CRI	Premedication for anesthesia: 0.1-0.3 mg/kg SQ, IM, IV Status epilepticus: 0.1-0.3 mg/kg IM or IV, or 0.2-0.5 mg/kg intranasally	The most common adverse effect is respiratory depression. Can cause anxiety or excitement in dogs. Use with caution in hepatic and renal insufficiency or glaucoma.	Injection. Can combine with ketamine in same syringe. Dilute in saline for CRI infusions. CSS-IV.
Miltefosine (Milteforan, Impavido)	Leishmaniasis: 2 mg/kg PO q 24h concurrently with allopurinol × 28 days.	Use in cats is not described.	Vomiting and diarrhea are very common. Contraindicated in pregnancy. Use with caution in hepatic insufficiency.	Available as an orphan drug (capsules) in the United States; may be difficult for veterinarians to obtain.
Minocycline (Minocin)	Susceptible infections: 7-12.5 mg/kg PO q 12h	Susceptible infections: 8-12.5 mg/kg PO q 12h, or 50 mg/CAT PO q 24h followed by at least 6 mL of liquid	Adverse events are usually GI, but minocycline also may cause elevation in hepatic enzymes or hyperthermia (cats), and is a photosensitizing agent. Relative contraindication in pregnancy and animals <6 months old. Used as a replacement for doxycycline for economic reasons. Urinary concentrations are low; not recommended for treating UTI.	Capsules, oral suspension. Give on an empty stomach if possible, but can give with nondairy food to minimize GI upset if necessary. Follow capsule with at least 6 mL of liquid to ensure passage to through the esophagus.
Mirtazapine (Remeron)	Appetite stimulant: 1.1-1.3 mg/kg PO q 24h, not to exceed 30 mg/DOG per day.	Appetite stimulant: 1.88 mg/CAT PO q 24-48h initially; can increase dose to 3.75 mg/CAT PO q 24h prn, or 7.5 mg/CAT transdermally q 24h. Reduce dose by 30%-50% for renal impairment.	Adverse events include sedation and increase in liver enzymes. Do not administer to patients that have received an MAO inhibitor in the previous 14 days. Combination with serotonergic medications (e.g., tramadol, fluoxetine) can cause serotonin syndrome. Dosage reduction may be required in hepatic and renal failure.	Tablets and orally disintegrating tablets (disintegrating tablets are difficult to fraction). Compounding pharmacists may prepare transdermal gels.
Misoprostol (Cytotec)	GI protectant with NSAID therapy: 2-7.5 mcg/kg PO q 8-12h	GI protectant with NSAID therapy: 2-5 mcg/kg PO q 8-12h	The most common adverse effect is GI upset. Contraindicated in pregnancy. Do not use in households with pregnant women.	Tablets; may give with food to minimize GI upset.
Mitotane (Lysodren, o,p'-DDD)	Hyperadrenocorticism: Induction phase—30-50 mg/kg/d PO with a meal q 24h or divided q 12h until induction is achieved (≈5-10 days, based on ACTH stimulation testing). Maintenance dose—35-50 mg/kg/wk in 2-3 divided doses	Do not use in cats.	The most common adverse effects are lethargy, ataxia, weakness, and GI upset; should be stopped immediately if these signs occur and ACTH stimulation test performed. Use with extreme caution in patients with DM or hepatic failure. Do not use in households with pregnant women. Dosage form greatly affects bioavailability. Suspensions in oil are ≈40× more bioavailable than solid tablets.	Tablets. Give with a fatty meal. Cytotoxic, NIOSH-listed hazardous drug and should be prepared, administered, and disposed of in accordance with federal and local requirements. Owner should wear gloves when handling.

Generic Name (Brand Name, Synonyms)	Canine Dosages	Feline Dosages	Adverse Effects/Warnings	Administration/ Availability
Mitoxantrone (Novantrone)	Antineoplastic: 5-6 mg/m^2 IV once q 3 weeks	Antineoplastic: 5-6.25 mg/m^2 IV once q 3 weeks	Adverse effects are dose dependent GI upset, hepatotoxicity, and myelosuppression. Neutropenia nadir usually occurs at about 10 days. Seizures have occurred in cats. Avoid extravasation. Use with caution in patients with myelosuppression, concurrent infection, hyperuricemia or hyperuricuria, and impaired hepatic function.	Injection. Cytotoxic, NIOSH-listed hazardous drug and should be prepared, administered, and disposed of in accordance with federal and local requirements.
Morphine sulfate	Analgesia: 0.5-1 mg/kg IM, SQ, or IV; or 0.1-0.2 mg/kg/h IV CRI Epidural use: 0.1 mg/kg in 0.3 mL/kg saline (max of 6 mL) Palliative analgesia: immediate-release morphine 1 mg/kg PO q 4-6h; sustained-release morphine 2-5 mg/kg PO q 12h	Not commonly used in cats due to vomiting and hyperexcitability Analgesia: 0.05-0.2 mg/kg IM, SQ q 2-6h	Adverse events commonly include vomiting and decreased intestinal peristalsis. Dogs are likely to experience CNS and respiratory depression; cats are likely to experience CNS hyperstimulation. Cats may experience hyperthermia. Morphine should not be used in patients that have received an MAO inhibitor in the previous 14 days. Contraindicated in GI obstruction. May cause histamine release; do not use in envenomation toxicities or animals with mast cell tumors.	Tablets, extended-release tablets (do not split or crush), oral solutions, injection, extended-release injection. Administer IV doses slowly to minimize histamine release. Controlled substance. CSS-II.
Mycophenolate mofetil (Cellcept, MMF)	Immunosuppression: 6-15 mg/kg IV or PO q 12h	Do not use in cats (limited metabolism).	Adverse effects usually include GI upset and hemorrhagic diarrhea. Myelosuppression is also possible. Reduce dosage in severe renal impairment. Avoid combination with azathioprine due to similar mechanism of action.	Capsules, compounded oral suspension, injection. Injection diluted with D_5W for slow IV infusion over 2 hours (never bolus). Infusion incompatible with other drugs.

N

Generic Name (Brand Name, Synonyms)	Canine Dosages	Feline Dosages	Adverse Effects/Warnings	Administration/ Availability
Naloxone (Narcan)	Opioid reversal: 0.01-0.04 mg/kg IV, IM, SQ; duration of action is 45-90 minutes; repeat as needed for opioids with long half-lives	Opioid reversal: 0.01-0.04 mg/kg IV, IM, SQ; duration of action is 45-90 minutes; repeat prn Postanesthetic hyperthermia: 0.01 mg/kg IM or SQ	Generally well tolerated; however, hyperalgesia may occur when opioids are reversed. Rapid opioid reversal may result in tachycardia, blood pressure changes, ventricular arrhythmias, pulmonary edema, and seizures. Does not work orally due to large first-pass effect.	Injection
Naltrexone (Trexan, ReVia)	Opioid antagonism: 0.0025-0.003 mg/kg IV Behavioral disorders: 2-5 mg/kg PO q 24h	Behavioral disorders: 25-50 mg/CAT PO q 24h	Generally well tolerated; however, hyperalgesia may occur when opioids are reversed. Contraindicated in hepatic insufficiency. Negates antitussive effect of opioids.	Tablets, injection
Neomycin (Biosol, Neomix)	Hepatic encephalopathy: 10-20 mg/kg PO q 8-12h	Hepatic encephalopathy: 10-20 mg/kg PO q 8-12h	Ototoxicity (especially cats) and nephrotoxicity are not high risk after oral administration; however, these may occur if intestinal disease is present and neomycin is systemically absorbed. Avoid in azotemic patients.	Oral solution; give with food.

Generic Name (Brand Name, Synonyms)	Canine Dosages	Feline Dosages	Adverse Effects/Warnings	Administration/ Availability
Neostigmine (Prostigmin)	Myasthenia gravis: 0.01-0.05 mg/kg IM, SQ q 6h or prn	Myasthenia gravis: 0.01-0.05 mg/kg IM, SQ q 6h or prn	Contraindicated in peritonitis, intestinal or urinary tract obstructions. Use with caution in patients with epilepsy, peptic ulcer disease, bronchial asthma, cardiac arrhythmias, hyperthyroidism, vagotonia, or megacolon. Adverse muscarinic effects can be reversed with atropine.	Injection
Niacinamide (nicotinamide, vitamin B_3)	Immune-mediated dermatopathies (in combination with doxycycline): Empirically dosed, <5 kg—100 mg/DOG PO q 8h; 5-10 kg—250 mg/DOG PO q 8h; >10 kg—500 mg/DOG PO q 8h	Use in cats is not described.	Contraindicated in liver disease and gastric ulcers. Generally well tolerated, but adverse effects may include anorexia, vomiting, diarrhea, and lethargy. Hepatic enzyme elevation may occur. Do not confuse with niacin.	Tablets and capsules
Nitrofurantoin (Macrodantin, Macrobid)	Susceptible urinary infection: 4 mg/kg PO q 8h	Susceptible urinary infection: 4 mg/kg PO q 8h	Adverse effects include GI upset, peripheral neuropathy, pulmonary hypersensitivity reactions, hepatopathy, and neurotoxicity (rare). Contraindicated in renal impairment.	Capsules; give with food.
Nitroglycerin (NTG, Nitro-bid, Minitran)	Adjunct therapy for acute heart failure: Empirically dosed for small dogs—¼ - ½ inch; medium dogs—½ -1 inch; large dogs—1-2 inches q 6-12h on hairless skin	Adjunct therapy for acute heart failure: Empirically dosed for cats—⅛ - ¼ inch q 6-12h on hairless skin	Can cause rash at application site or hypotension. Use with extreme caution in cerebral hemorrhage, head trauma, diuretic-induced hypovolemia, or other hypotensive conditions. Tolerance to effects occurs with 2-3 days of use. Avoid contact with human skin.	Ointment. While wearing gloves, apply to a hairless region, such as the inside of the ear flap or groin.
Nitroprusside (Nitropress)	Hypertensive crisis: 1-7 mcg/kg/min IV CRI	Hypertensive crisis: 1-2 mcg/kg/min IV CRI	Adverse effects include hypotension, GI upset, restlessness, muscle twitching, and dizziness. Use with caution in patients with hepatic insufficiency, severe renal impairment, hyponatremia, or hypothyroidism.	Injection. After reconstitution dilute in D_5W, and give IV slowly as a CRI. Do not flush IV line as this may cause overdose. Avoid extravasation.
Norepinephrine (Levophed)	Profound hypotension: 0.05-0.2 mcg/kg/min IV CRI, titrated to effect (maximum 1-2 mcg/kg/min)	Profound hypotension: 0.05-0.1 mcg/kg/min IV CRI then titrate to effect using not more than 1-2 mcg/kg/min	Do not use as a substitute for blood or fluid replacement. Without appropriate blood or fluid replacement, peripheral and visceral vasoconstriction, decreased renal perfusion and urine output, and poor systemic blood flow can result. Arrhythmias and hypertension can also occur. Cats are more likely than dogs to suffer these adverse events.	Injection. Dilute with D_5W (not saline) for IV injection. Typically a 4-mg vial is added to a 250-mL bag of D_5W to make a 16-mcg/mL solution. Discard injections with a pinkish or yellowish tint.
Nystatin (Nilstat)	Candidiasis: 50,000-150,000 units/DOG PO q 6-8h	Candidiasis: 50,000 units/CAT PO q 6-8h	Generally well tolerated with occasional GI upset.	Oral suspension. Shake well before using.
Nitenpyram (Capstar)	Fleas (immediate kill): Dogs up to 11 kg, one 11.4-mg tablet PO once; dogs >11 kg, one 57-mg tablet once (can repeat q 24h)	Fleas (immediate kill): 11.4-mg tablet/CAT PO once (can repeat q 24h)	Rare reports of lethargy/hyperactivity, GI upset, hypersalivation, vocalization.	Tablets

O

Generic Name (Brand Name, Synonyms)	Canine Dosages	Feline Dosages	Adverse Effects/Warnings	Administration/ Availability
Oclacitinib (Apoquel)	Atopic dermatitis: 0.4-0.6 mg/kg PO q 12h for up to 14 days and then q 24h	Hypersensitivity dermatitis: 0.4-0.6 mg/kg PO q 12h for up to 14 days and then q 24h	Do not use in animals <12 months old or pregnant. Adverse effects include GI upset, PU/PD, and lethargy. Benign cutaneous and subcutaneous masses have also been reported. May increase susceptibility to infection or neoplasia. Monitor CBC, biochemical profile, and urinalysis periodically.	Tablets; give with food. Wash hands after handling. Pregnant women should avoid contact with this drug.
Octreotide (Sandostatin)	Insulinoma: 10-40 mcg/DOG SQ q 8-12h; sustained-release injection: 0.5 mcg/kg IM q 28 days	Chylothorax: 10-20 mcg/kg SQ q 8-12h	Use with extreme caution in biliary tract dysfunction; may inhibit gallbladder contraction. Generally well tolerated. May cause anorexia.	Injection (sustained and immediate release)
Ofloxacin (Ocuflox)	Ocular infection: 1 drop topically in affected eye q 12h	Ocular infection: 1 drop topically in affected eye q 12h	Can cause irritation.	Ophthalmic solution
Olsalazine (Dipentum)	IBD: 5-20 mg/kg PO q 8h	Use is not described for cats.	Adverse effects include GI upset and keratoconjunctivitis sicca. Use with caution in animals with renal disease.	Capsules; give with food.
Omeprazole (GastroGard, UlcerGard, Prilosec)	Proton pump inhibitor antacid: 0.7-1.5 mg/kg PO q 12h; doses up to 2 mg/kg q 12h can be used	Proton pump inhibitor antacid: 0.5-1.5 mg/kg PO q 12-24h	Well tolerated but may cause GI upset, CNS disturbance, hematologic abnormalities, or proteinuria. Dosage may need to be reduced in patients with severe hepatic or renal disease.	Tablets and capsules OTC, or compounded into oral suspensions. Give 30 minutes before a meal.
Ondansetron (Zofran)	Antiemetic: 0.5-1 mg/kg PO or IV (slowly over 2-15 minutes) q 8-12h; avoid use in dogs with *MDR1/ABCB1-Δ* mutation	Antiemetic: 0.1-1 mg/kg IV (slowly), SQ, IM, or PO q 6-12h	Generally well tolerated but sedation, constipation, tremors, and arrhythmias reported. May prolong QT interval; use cautiously in animals with heart disease and with other arrhythmogenic drugs. Dosage reduction may be required in severe hepatic dysfunction. Avoid use in dogs with *MDR1/ABCB1-Δ* mutation.	Tablets, disintegrating tablets, injection, or compounded into transdermal gel. Dilute in saline and give over 2-15 minutes when giving IV injection.
o,p'-DDD: see mitotane				
Orbifloxacin (Orbax)	Susceptible infections: 2.5 mg/kg-7.5 mg/kg, PO q 24h	Susceptible infections: 2.5 mg/kg-7.5 mg/kg, PO q 24h	Can cause GI upset or retinal lesions in cats (less likely than enrofloxacin). May lower seizure threshold. Use with caution in hepatic dysfunction. Avoid in rapidly growing animals.	Tablets; give with food (no iron, dairy, or antacids).
Ormetoprim-sulfadimethoxine (Primor)	Susceptible infections: 55 mg/kg PO once, then 27.5 mg/kg PO q 24h	Coccidiosis: 60 mg/kg PO q 24h	Adverse effects include GI upset, hypersensitivity, KCS, and crystalluria. Use with caution in Doberman pinschers due to idiosyncratic polyarthritis.	Tablets
Oseltamivir (Tamiflu)	Canine influenza: 2 mg/kg PO q 12h for 5 days	Use is not described for cats.	Not effective if used >40 hours after onset of signs. Use in dogs is controversial. Adverse effects include GI upset and ataxia.	Capsules and oral suspension
Oxymorphone (Numorphan)	Preanesthesia: 0.1-0.2 mg/kg IM, SQ; 0.05-0.22 mg/kg IV Analgesia: 0.05-0.2 mg/kg IV, IM, SQ q 2-4h prn	Analgesia: 0.01-0.05 mg/kg IV, IM, SQ q 2-4h prn	Can cause respiratory and CNS depression, hypotension, sedation, bradycardia, hyperexcitability (cats), panting (dogs); reverse with naloxone.	Injections (tablets and suppository not used in animals). Injections may be difficult to obtain as many manufacturers have stopped producing. CSS-II.
Oxytocin (Pitocin)	Induction of labor: mini doses: 0.25-0.5 units/DOG q 15-30 minutes Induction of lactation: 2-10 units/DOG IM or intranasally	Induction of labor: mini doses: 0.25-0.5 units/CAT q 15-30 minutes, or 2-5 units/CAT IV, IM, or SQ once Induction of lactation: 2-10 units/CAT IM, SQ, or intranasally once	Generally well tolerated but contraindicated with uterine or vaginal obstruction or abnormal fetus presentation. Correct hypoglycemia or hypocalcemia before use.	Injection

P

Generic Name (Brand Name, Synonyms)	Canine Dosages	Feline Dosages	Adverse Effects/Warnings	Administration/ Availability
Pamidronate (Aredia)	Refractory hypercalcemia: 1.3-2.3 mg/kg (diluted in 150-250 mL of 0.9% sodium chloride and administered IV over 2-4 hours). Can repeat as soon as 1 week prn (typically q 3-6 weeks).	Refractory hypercalcemia: 1.3-2.3 mg/kg (diluted in 150-250 mL of 0.9% sodium chloride and administered IV over 2-4 hours)	Adverse effects include electrolyte imbalance and nephrotoxicity, especially if administered too rapidly. Use with caution in patients with impaired renal function. Use with caution in young or growing animals and in those animals healing from bone fracture.	Injection. Must be diluted in 150-250 mL saline and administered over 2-4 hours for IV dosing.
Pancreatic enzymes (Viokase, Pancrezyme)	Pancreatic insufficiency: 2-3 crushed tablets or ¾ -2 teaspoonfuls of powder with each meal immediately before feeding; incubation is not necessary	Pancreatic insufficiency: ½ -1 crushed tablet or ¼ - ¾ teaspoonful of powder with each meal immediately before feeding; incubation is not necessary.	Do not administer PO without mixing in food as oromucosal damage can result. Clients should avoid inhaling powder or getting in eyes. GI upset is the major adverse effect.	Powder (preferred), tablets. Crush tablets before mixing with food. Mix either powder or crushed tablets with food to minimize oral or esophageal erosion.
Pantoprazole (Protonix)	Proton pump inhibitor antacid: 0.7-1 mg/kg IV slowly (over 15 minutes) q 24h	Proton pump inhibitor antacid: 0.7-1 mg/kg IV slowly (over 15 minutes) q 24h	Generally well tolerated. Diarrhea may occur. Hyperglycemia has also been reported.	Injection for IV use only; administer IV slowly over 15 minutes.
Paroxetine (Paxil)	Behavioral disorders: 0.5-3 mg/kg PO q 24h	Behavioral disorders: 0.25-1.25 mg/kg PO q 24h	Do not administer to patients who have received MAO inhibitors within the previous 14 days. Use with caution in patients with seizure disorders or severe cardiac, hepatic, or renal disease. If used in these conditions, dosages must be reduced. Adverse effects include lethargy, salivation, GI upset, anxiety, irritability, insomnia, hyperactivity, or panting. In cats, behavioral changes, anorexia, constipation, and changes in elimination patterns may occur.	Tablets, oral suspension
Penicillamine: see D-penicillamine				
Penicillin G potassium or sodium (PfizerPen)	Susceptible infections: 20,000-40,000 units/kg IV or IM q 4-8h	Susceptible infections: 20,000-40,000 units/kg IV or IM q 4-8h	Penicillin is generally well tolerated. Allergic reactions can occur. Large IV doses of penicillin potassium and sodium can cause electrolyte imbalances. Physically incompatible with many other drugs in solution.	Injection for IV use only. Administer slowly to avoid electrolyte imbalances.
Penicillin G procaine (Wycillin)	Susceptible infections: 20,000-40,000 units/kg IM, SQ q 12-24h	Susceptible infections: 20,000-40,000 units/kg IM, SQ q 12-24h	Generally well tolerated. Allergic reactions may occur. Do not give IV. May cause injection site reactions.	Injectable suspension. Shake vigorously before use, and never administer IV.
Pentobarbital (Nembutal)	Anesthesia: 10-30 mg/kg IV slowly to effect Seizures: 3-15 mg/kg IV slowly to effect	Anesthesia: 10-30 mg/kg IV slowly to effect Seizures: 3-15 mg/kg IV slowly to effect	Adverse effects include respiratory depression, hypothermia, and postanesthetic hyperexcitation. Contraindicated in severe liver disease, nephritis, or respiratory depression. Use with caution in hypovolemia, anemia, hypoadrenocorticism, or cardiac disease.	Injection for IV use only. Avoid extravasation. When giving IV for induction of anesthesia, administer ⅓ to ½ of dose as bolus followed by slow infusion of the remainder to effect. Expensive. CSS-II.
Pentosan polysulfate (PPS, Cartrophen-Vet, Elmiron)	Chondroprotective: 3 mg/kg SQ or IM once weekly for 4 weeks	Chondroprotective: 3 mg/kg SQ or IM once weekly for 4 weeks	Generally well tolerated, but GI upset is reported. Mild anticoagulant effects. Contraindicated in advanced liver or kidney impairment, evidence of infection, blood or coagulation disorders, or malignancy. Avoid several days before planned surgery.	Injection. Not approved in the United States but can be imported.
Pentoxifylline (PTX, Trental)	Inflammatory dermatoses or vasculitis: 15-25 mg/kg PO q 8-12h or 30 mg/kg PO q 12h	Inflammatory dermatoses or vasculitis: 100 mg/CAT PO q 12h	Well tolerated, but GI upset and CNS stimulation can occur. Use with caution in severe hepatic or renal impairment and in patients at risk for hemorrhage.	Tablets

Generic Name (Brand Name, Synonyms)	Canine Dosages	Feline Dosages	Adverse Effects/Warnings	Administration/ Availability
Phenobarbital	Antiepileptic: 2.5-3 mg/kg PO q 12h and adjusted with target range of trough serum levels 15-45 mcg/mL. Loading dose: 12-24 mg/kg IV once and then 3-4 mg/kg IV q 20 minutes until target blood level is achieved. Sialadenosis: 2.6-6 mg/kg PO q 12h, tapered with response	Antiepileptic: 1-3 mg/kg PO q 12h and adjusted with target range of trough serum levels 15-45 mcg/mL. Loading dose: 12-24 mg/kg IV once and then 3-4 mg/kg IV q 20 minutes until target blood level is achieved.	Adverse effects include sedation, PU/PD, polyphagia, blood dyscrasias, and hepatopathy. Cats may experience facial excoriations and coagulopathies. Use cautiously in animals with hepatic or renal insufficiency and in animals with respiratory compromise. Multiple drug interactions.	Tablets, injection. Compounding pharmacists may prepare a stable oral suspension. Avoid rapid IV administration (>50 mg/min); parenteral solutions are highly alkaline; avoid extravasation. CSS-IV.
Phenoxybenzamine HCl (Dibenzyline)	Functional urethral outflow obstruction: 0.25 mg/kg PO q 12h Pheochromocytoma: 0.25-0.5 mg/kg PO q 12h then increased to effect up to a maximum of 2.5 mg/kg PO q 12h	Functional urethral outflow obstruction: 2.5-7.5 mg/CAT PO q 12-24h	Adverse effects include hypotension, weakness/dizziness, GI upset, miosis, increased intraocular pressure, tachycardia, sodium retention and nasal congestion. Use with caution in patients with hypotension or CHF.	Capsules. Commercial product very expensive. USP-grade powder for compounding is less costly.
Phenylephrine (Neo-Synephrine)	Rhinitis: 1-2 drops IN q 8-24 h Hypotension: 1-3 mcg/kg/min as IV CRI, adjusted to effect	Hypotension: 1-2 mcg/kg/min IV CRI	Adverse effects include CNS stimulation, arrhythmias, and hypertension (blood pressure should be monitored when administering IV). Contraindicated in severe hypertension and ventricular tachycardia. Use with caution in patients with hyperthyroidism and heart disease.	Topical nose drops (OTC), injection. Oral tablets are available for human use, but use is not described for animals. Topical use with pediatric ($\frac{1}{8}$th% = 0.125%) or diluted products. IV solutions are typically diluted to 0.1-0.4 mg/mL in normal saline.
Phenylpropanolamine (Proin)	Urethral sphincter mechanism incompetence: 1-2 mg/kg PO q 8h	Urethral sphincter mechanism incompetence: 1-2 mg/kg PO q 8-12h	Generally well tolerated, but adverse effects include GI upset, anxiety, urine retention, tachycardia, and hypertension. Use with extreme caution in glaucoma, hyperthyroidism, DM, cardiovascular disorders, kidney insufficiency, or hypertension.	Flavored tablets. Oral liquids are available in Canada, but must be compounded in the United States.
Phenytoin (Dilantin)	Ventricular arrhythmias: 10 mg/kg slowly IV; 30-50 mg/kg PO q 8h (rarely indicated) Anticonvulsant: No longer recommended	Do not use in cats.	Adverse effects include GI upset, ataxia, sedation, hepatopathy, and gingival hyperplasia. Not effective as an anticonvulsant. IV use contraindicated in 2nd- or 3rd-degree heart block, sinoatrial block, or sinus bradycardia. Multiple drug interactions.	Tablets, capsules, oral suspension, injection. Doses administered IV are undiluted at a rate of not more than 50 mg/min.
Phytonadione: see vitamin K				
Pimobendan (Vetmedin)	CHF: 0.25 mg/kg PO q 12h, adjusted upward as indicated by clinical response	CHF: 0.25 mg/kg PO q 12h, adjusted upward as indicated by clinical response	Well tolerated, but adverse effects include GI upset and worsening of arrhythmias. Contraindicated in conditions for which increased cardiac output poses risk.	Tablets. Give on empty stomach.
Piperacillin + tazobactam (Zosyn)	Susceptible bacterial sepsis: 40-100 mg/kg IV over 30 minutes q 6-8h	Susceptible bacterial sepsis: 40-100 mg/kg IV over 30 minutes q 6-8h	Reduce dosage (both dose and frequency) in renal impairment. Use with caution in patients with hypernatremia (high sodium content). Adverse effects include injection site reactions and hypersensitivity.	Injection. Solutions for IV administration are typically diluted in a volume of 50 mL normal saline.
Piroxicam (Feldene)	Antiinflammatory/analgesic NSAID with antiangiogenic/antineoplastic properties: 0.3 mg/kg PO q 24h	Antiinflammatory/analgesic NSAID with antiangiogenic/antineoplastic properties: 0.3 mg/kg PO q 24-72h	Adverse effects include GI ulceration, bleeding, and nephrotoxicity (especially cats). Use with caution in patients that have a history of GI bleeding, kidney or liver dysfunction. Do not use with other NSAIDs or glucocorticoids.	Capsules; usually must be compounded to achieve desired doses. Give with food.
Plerixafor (Mozobil)	Use is not described for dogs.	FIV: 0.5 mg/kg SQ q 12h	Adverse effects include diarrhea, nausea, fatigue, injection site reactions, headache, arthralgia, dizziness, and vomiting.	Injection. Expensive.

Generic Name (Brand Name, Synonyms)	Canine Dosages	Feline Dosages	Adverse Effects/Warnings	Administration/ Availability
Ponazuril (Toltrazuril sulfone, Marquis)	Neospora or toxoplasmosis: 7.5-15 mg/kg PO q 24h × 28 days, or 50 mg/kg q 24h once, repeated in 7 days Coccidiosis: 20 mg/kg PO q 24h × 3 days	Neospora or toxoplasmosis: 7.5-15 mg/kg PO q 24h × 28 days, or 50 mg/kg q 24h once, repeated in 7 days Coccidiosis: 20 mg/kg PO q 24h × 3 days	Adverse effects are usually GI in nature but may include neurotoxicity from folate depletion. KCS has been reported.	Oral paste
Potassium bromide	Idiopathic epilepsy: Loading dose 400-600 mg/kg PO divided over 5 days with food. Maintenance: 25-35 mg/kg PO q 24h to achieve therapeutic serum levels of 1-3 mg/mL	Do not use in cats.	Contraindicated in cats due to adverse respiratory effects. Adverse effects include transient sedation and GI upset. Overdoses cause ataxia, tremors, mydriasis, or other CNS manifestations of bromism. Avoid fluctuations in chloride intake once therapeutic blood levels are reached.	A commercially available tablet preparation is available but is not FDA approved. Compounding pharmacists may also prepare stable capsules and solutions. Give with food to minimize GI upset. Elevate food bowls until tolerance to sedation has occurred.
Potassium citrate (Urocit-K)	Urinary alkalinizer/potassium supplement: 50-75 mg/kg PO q 12h	Urinary alkalinizer/potassium supplement: 50-75 mg/kg PO q 12h	Adverse effects include GI upset and ulceration, hyperkalemia. Use with caution in patients prone to GI ulceration or esophageal strictures. Follow doses with at least 6 mL of liquid or food. Contraindicated in hyperkalemia and UTIs with struvite stones.	Tablets. Follow with 6 mL of liquid or food to prevent esophageal ulceration.
Potassium gluconate (Tumil-K)	Potassium supplement: 0.5-1 mEq/kg PO q 12h	Potassium supplement: 0.5-1 mEq/kg PO q 12h	Contraindicated in hyperkalemia and UTIs with struvite stones. Use with caution in patients prone to GI ulceration or esophageal strictures. Follow doses with at least 6 mL of liquid or food. Adverse effects include GI upset, GI ulceration, and hyperkalemia.	Tablets, powders, oral gels. Follow tablets with 6 mL of liquid or food to prevent esophageal ulceration.
Potassium phosphate	Hypophosphatemia: 0.01-0.03 mmol/kg/h IV CRI	Hypophosphatemia: 0.01-0.03 mmol/kg/h IV CRI	Adverse effects include hyperphosphatemia (and related hypocalcemia), hypotension, renal failure, or soft tissue mineralization. Contraindicated in hyperphosphatemia, hypocalcemia, and oliguric renal failure.	Concentrated injection for dilution in normal saline (do not dilute with calcium- or magnesium-containing fluids).
Pradofloxacin (Veraflox)	Susceptible bacterial infection: 3 mg/kg PO q 24h. Although available for dogs elsewhere, NOT approved for use in dogs in the United States.	Susceptible infections: 7.5 mg/kg PO q 24h	Generally well tolerated, with GI upset sometimes seen. Blood dyscrasias are possible in dogs and in cats that receive therapy longer than 6 weeks or with high dosages. Rapid growth is a relative contraindication due to possible adverse cartilage effects. Use with caution with renal or hepatic insufficiency. May cause photosensitivity.	Only oral suspension in the United States; tablets and suspension elsewhere. Give on an empty stomach if tolerated, or with nondairy foods if necessary due to GI upset.
Pralidoxime chloride (2-PAM, Protopam)	Organophosphate poisoning: 20-50 mg/kg IM or SQ; repeated q 8-12h prn	Organophosphate poisoning: 20-50 mg/kg IM or SQ; repeated q 8-12h prn	Adverse effects include GI upset, tachycardia, and muscle weakness. Use with extreme caution in patients with myasthenia gravis. Monitor patients for effect and repeat as needed.	Injections for SQ or IM administration. Ideally initiated within 24 hours of organophosphate exposure.
Praziquantel (Droncit, Drontal)	Tapeworms: 5-12.6 mg/kg PO or SQ once Salmon poisoning flukes: 10-30 mg/kg PO or SQ once Paragonimus: 23 mg/kg PO q 8h × 3 days	Tapeworms: 5.7 mg/kg PO or SQ once	Oral forms are generally well tolerated but may cause GI upset. Injectable forms can cause pain on injection, vomiting, and ataxia. Use with caution in patients with history of seizures.	Tablets, injection. Some forms OTC.
Prazosin (Minipress)	Urethral relaxation: 0.07 mg/kg, or 0.5-4 mg/DOG PO q 8-12h Afterload reduction in CHF: dogs <15 kg, 1 mg, or dogs >15 kg, 2 mg PO q 8h titrated to effect	Urethral relaxation: 0.25-1 mg/CAT PO q 8-12h	Adverse effects include CNS depression, GI upset, tachycardia, and nictitans elevation. Contraindicated in hypotension. Some dogs with the *MDR1/ABCB1-Δ* mutation may be sensitive; use with caution in known mutants.	Capsules, or compounded (usually necessary for feline dosing). Give with food.

Generic Name (Brand Name, Synonyms)	Canine Dosages	Feline Dosages	Adverse Effects/Warnings	Administration/ Availability
Prednisolone sodium succinate	Glucocorticoid. Shock of multiple causes: 5-11 mg/kg IV slow bolus; repeat up to q 6h	Glucocorticoid. Shock of multiple causes: 5-11 mg/kg IV slow bolus; repeat up to q 6h	Contraindicated in the presence of viral or systemic fungal infections, GI ulceration, and hyperadrenocorticism. Do not use concurrently with NSAIDs. Use with caution in hypertension, CHF, renal insufficiency. Can cause GI ulceration.	Injection. IV doses are typically further diluted in normal saline before administration.
Prednisolone, prednisone (Cortef)	Glucocorticoid effects (and uses) vary with dose. Physiologic replacement: 0.2-0.3 mg/kg PO q 24h Antiinflammatory: 0.5-1 mg/kg PO q 24h Immunosuppression: 2-4 mg/kg PO q 24h Adjunct therapy for neoplasia: 40 mg/m^2 PO q 24h for 7 days; then 20 mg/m^2 PO q 48h	Glucocorticoid effects (and uses) vary with dose. Physiologic replacement: 0.2-0.3 mg/kg PO q 24h Antiinflammatory: 0.5-1 mg/kg PO q 24h Immunosuppression: 2-4 mg/kg PO q 24h Adjunct therapy for neoplasia: 40 mg/m^2 PO q 24h for 7 days; then 20 mg/m^2 PO q 48h	Dose-dependent adverse effects include PU/PD, polyphagia, and suppression of the hypothalamic pituitary axis. Contraindicated in the presence of active infections, GI ulceration, and hyperadrenocorticism. Do not use concurrently with NSAIDs or other glucocorticoids. Use with caution in hypertension, CHF, DM, and renal insufficiency.	Tablets, oral solution. Give with food, usually in morning. Topical, ophthalmic, and otic preparations of prednisolone available. For cats, prednisolone preferred over prednisone by any route.
Pregabalin (Lyrica)	Neuropathic pain: 2-4 mg/kg PO q 8-12h	Use is not described for cats.	The most common adverse effects are sedation and ataxia. Use with caution in patients with renal insufficiency or heart failure.	Capsules, oral solution. CSS-V.
Procarbazine (Matulane)	Antineoplastic: 25-50 mg/m^2 PO q 24h	Antineoplastic: 50 mg/m^2 PO q 24-48h	GI upset, hepatotoxicity, and myelosuppression are the most common adverse effects. May also cause CNS depression. Platelet nadir usually occurs at 3-4 weeks.	Capsules. Cytotoxic, NIOSH-listed hazardous drug and should be prepared, administered, and disposed of in accordance with federal and local requirements.
Propantheline (Pro-Banthine)	Antimuscarinic for sinus bradycardia: 0.25-5 mg/kg PO q 8-12h Detrusor hypercontractility: 0.25-0.5 mg/kg PO q 8-12h	Detrusor hypercontractility: 0.25-0.5 mg/kg or 7.5 mg/CAT PO q 8-12h	Adverse effects are dose-related and are similar to those of atropine (e.g., dry mouth and eyes, tachycardia, constipation). GI upset and hypersalivation are reported in cats. High dose can cause ileus. Use with caution in hepatic disease, renal disease, hyperthyroidism, hypertension, CHF, tachyarrhythmias, prostatic hypertrophy, esophageal reflux, or hot environmental conditions (heat prostration).	Tablets
Propofol (PropoFlo, Diprivan, PropoFlo-28)	Ultrashort anesthetic: 3-6 mg/kg IV; 0.2-0.5 mg/kg/min IV CRI, titrated to effect	Ultrashort anesthetic: 3-6 mg/kg IV; 0.2-0.5 mg/kg/min IV CRI, titrated to effect	Adverse effects include respiratory depression, hypothermia, and seizurelike activity. Cats, greyhounds, and very thin animals may have more profound effects. Prolonged CRIs may cause Heinz body formation in cats. Some formulations contain excipients that may cause histamine release in dogs. Some formulations contain high levels of benzyl alcohol, which may be problematic in cats. Use with caution in animals with cardiovascular or respiratory depression.	Injection. Administer IV slowly over 60-90 seconds to avoid apnea, titrating to effect.
Propranolol (Inderal)	Susceptible tachyarrhythmias: IV: 0.02 mg/kg IV slowly over 2-3 minutes; titrate dose up to effect (to a maximum of 0.1 mg/kg), repeated in 8 hours prn; or 0.1-0.2 mg/kg PO q 8h, titrated to effect up to a maximum of 1.5 mg/kg PO q 8h	Susceptible tachyarrhythmias: IV: 0.02 mg/kg IV slowly over 2-3 minutes; titrate dose up to effect (to a maximum of 0.1 mg/kg); 2.5 mg/CAT PO q 8-12h, maximum 10 mg/CAT/dose	Adverse effects include GI upset, syncope, bradycardia, depression, impaired AV conduction, CHF, hypotension, hypoglycemia, and bronchoconstriction. Contraindicated in CHF, bradyarrhythmias, and bronchospasm. Reduce dosing in hepatic insufficiency. Use cautiously in diabetics.	Tablets, capsules, oral solution, injection. Dilute IV doses in D_5W and administer slowly at not more than 1 mg/min.

Generic Name (Brand Name, Synonyms)	Canine Dosages	Feline Dosages	Adverse Effects/Warnings	Administration/ Availability
Protamine sulfate	Heparin overdose: 1 mg protamine/100 U of heparin overdose. Ideally given immediately by slow IV infusion. Can repeat prn, reducing protamine dose 50% for q 30-60 minutes post heparin overdose.	Heparin overdose: 1 mg protamine/100 U of heparin overdose. Ideally given immediately by slow IV infusion. Can repeat prn, reducing protamine dose 50% for q 30-60 minutes post heparin overdose.	Generally well tolerated. Acute hypotension, bradycardia, pulmonary hypertension, and dyspnea may occur if injected IV rapidly.	Injection. Can dilute in normal saline or D_5W for slow IV injection at a rate of not more than 50 mg/10 min.
Psyllium mucilloid (Metamucil)	Bulk laxative: 0.5-5 g, or 1-3 teaspoons, PO q 12-24h in moistened food	Bulk laxative: 2-4 teaspoons PO q 12-24h, in moistened food	Adverse effects may include flatulence. Bowel obstruction may occur if animal is not well hydrated. Contraindicated in intestinal obstruction.	Powder OTC. Give with food and ensure hydration.
Pyrantel pamoate (Strongid T, Nemex)	Roundworms/hookworms: 5-10 mg/kg PO with food; repeat in 7-10 days	Susceptible intestinal parasites: 10-20 mg/kg PO; repeat as needed	Generally well tolerated. Do not administer to severely debilitated animals. Adverse effects are mostly due to GI upset.	Tablets, oral suspension. Give with food. OTC forms available.
Pyridostigmine bromide (Mestinon, Regonol)	Myasthenia gravis: 0.2-2 mg/kg PO q 8-12h with food; 0.01-0.03 mg/kg/h IV CRI for fulminant disease	Myasthenia gravis: 0.25-2.0 mg/kg PO q 24h with food	Adverse effects are dose-related and include increased GI motility, salivation, urination, abdominal pain, diarrhea, bradycardia, and increased lacrimation. Use with caution in patients with bronchospastic disease, epilepsy, hyperthyroidism, bradycardia or other arrhythmias, vagotonia, or GI ulcer diseases. Reduce dosage in renal impairment.	Tablets, extended-release tablets, oral syrup, injection. Give oral forms with food. IV doses should be administered slowly as a CRI.
Pyrimethamine (Daraprim)	Susceptible protozoal infection: 0.5-1 mg/kg PO q 24h for 48 hours, then 0.25-0.5 mg/kg PO q 24h for 14 days	Use with caution in cats due to adverse effect profile. Susceptible protozoal infection: 0.5-1 mg/kg PO q 24h for 48 hours, then 0.25 mg/kg PO q 24h for 14 days	Adverse effects include anorexia, malaise, vomiting, depression, and bone marrow depression, which may be more severe in cats. Oral administration of folinic acid at 1 mg/kg PO or folic acid 5 mg/day may alleviate the adverse hematologic and neurologic effects. Use cautiously in animals with pre-existing folate deficiencies.	Tablets. Pregnant women should avoid handling.

Q-R

Generic Name (Brand Name, Synonyms)	Canine Dosages	Feline Dosages	Adverse Effects/Warnings	Administration/ Availability
Quinidine (Quinaglute, Quinidex)	Ventricular arrhythmias: 6-16 mg/kg PO or IM q 6-8h	Do not use in cats.	Dose-related adverse effects include weakness, GI upset, hypotension, and arrhythmia. Contraindicated in myasthenia gravis, complete AV block with pacemaker, QRS widening disorders, digitalis intoxication, aberrant ectopic impulses, or abnormal rhythms secondary to escape mechanisms. Do not use with digoxin.	Tablets, injection (do not give IV)
Rabeprazole (AcipHex)	Acid suppression: 0.7-1 mg/kg PO q 24h	Use is not described for cats.	Well tolerated but may cause GI upset, CNS disturbance, hematologic abnormalities, or proteinuria. Dosage may need to be reduced in patients with severe hepatic or renal disease.	Tablets

Generic Name (Brand Name, Synonyms)	Canine Dosages	Feline Dosages	Adverse Effects/Warnings	Administration/ Availability
Ramipril (Altace, Vasotop)	Heart failure: 0.125-0.25 mg/kg PO q 12h	Arterial hypertension: 0.5 mg/kg PO q 24h	Well tolerated but GI upset can occur. Weakness, hypotension, or hyperkalemia are also possible.	Capsules
Ranitidine HCl (Zantac)	H_2 antagonist antacid and prokinetic: 1-4 mg/kg PO, SQ, IM, or slow IV q 8-12h	H_2 antagonist antacid and prokinetic: 2.5 mg/kg slow IV q 12h, or 3.5 mg/kg PO q 12h	Generally well tolerated but rapid IV doses may cause arrhythmias, vomiting, and hypotension in cats. May cause elevated liver enzymes with chronic use. Use lower doses in renal insufficiency. Antacid efficacy limited.	Tablets (OTC), injection (give slowly IV)
Rifampin (Rifadin)	Adjunctive therapy for susceptible infections: 5-15 mg/kg PO or IV q 12-24h	Susceptible infection: 10-15 mg/kg PO or IV q 24h	Adverse effects include GI upset and hepatopathies. Use with caution in hepatic insufficiency; rifampin hepatotoxicity can be fatal. Will stain tears, urine, saliva, and feces a red-orange color. Usually used in combination with other antimicrobial drugs.	Capsules, injection. Compounding pharmacists may prepare stable oral suspensions. Give with food. IV doses should be diluted with normal saline or D_5W and infused slowly.
Rivaroxaban (Xarelto)	Oral anticoagulant: 0.5-1 mg/kg PO q 12-24h (anecdotal dose)	Oral anticoagulant: 2.5 mg/CAT q 24h (anecdotal dose)	Clinical experience in pets is limited. Hemorrhage is predominant adverse effect and is more likely when combined with platelet inhibition.	Tablets
Robenacoxib (Onsior)	Antiinflammatory/analgesic NSAID: 1-2 mg/kg PO q 24h Perioperative analgesia: 2 mg/kg SQ once or PO q 24h for 3 days	Antiinflammatory/analgesic NSAID: 1-2.4 mg/kg PO q 24h Perioperative analgesia: 2 mg/kg SQ q 24h × 3 doses or 1-2.4 mg/kg PO q 24h up to 6 days	Adverse events are usually GI in nature but may also include nephrotoxicity and hepatotoxicity. Use with caution in animals with dehydration, hypotension, or with impaired cardiac, renal, or hepatic function. Do not use concurrently with glucocorticoids or other NSAIDs. Cats must be monitored closely for renal toxicity.	Tablets (give with food), injection
Ronidazole	Giardiasis (not first-line treatment): 30-50 mg PO q 12h for 7 days	Tritrichomonas foetus: 30 mg/kg PO q 24h for 14 days	Neurotoxicity has been reported in cats and manifests as tremors, lethargy, anorexia, ataxia, nystagmus, seizures, hyperthermia, or behavioral change. GI upset may also occur.	Available only through compounding. Give with food. Wear gloves when administering, and wash hands afterward.
Rutin (Bioflavonoids)	Lymphedema: 50 mg/kg PO q 8h	Chylothorax: 50 mg/kg or 250 mg/CAT PO q 8h initially, reducing to q 12h if effective	Generally well tolerated	Tablets, capsules OTC

S

Generic Name (Brand Name, Synonyms)	Canine Dosages	Feline Dosages	Adverse Effects/Warnings	Administration/ Availability
S-adenosyl methionine (SAMe, Denosyl)	Hepatoprotectant: 20 mg/kg PO q 24h	Hepatoprotectant: 20 mg/kg PO q 24h	Generally well tolerated. GI upset may occur.	Capsules; give on empty stomach
Selegiline (deprenyl, Anipryl, Eldepryl)	Cognitive dysfunction: 0.5 mg/kg PO q 24h Narcolepsy: 2 mg/kg PO q 24h	Do not use in cats.	Do not use with other MAO inhibitors, opioids, SSRIs, or tricyclic antidepressants. Adverse effects include GI upset, CNS effects, and aggression. Efficacy is questionable.	Tablets
Sertraline (Zoloft)	Behavior modification: 0.5-4 mg/kg PO q 12-24h	Behavior modification: 0.25-1.5 mg/kg PO q 12-24h	Do not use with other MAO inhibitors. Adverse effects include GI upset, CNS effects, and heightened reactivity. Avoid abrupt withdrawal.	Tablets, oral solution

Generic Name (Brand Name, Synonyms)	Canine Dosages	Feline Dosages	Adverse Effects/Warnings	Administration/ Availability
Sildenafil (Viagra, Revatio)	Pulmonary hypertension: 1-3 mg/kg PO q 8-12h	Pulmonary hypertension: 0.25 to 1.6 mg/kg PO q 12h	Most common adverse effect is GI upset. Do not use concurrently with nitrates. Use with extreme caution in patients with resting hypotension, fluid depletion, severe left ventricular outflow obstruction, or autonomic dysfunction.	Tablets. Compounding pharmacists may prepare stable oral suspensions.
Silymarin (milk thistle, Marin Plus)	Hepatoprotectant: 20-50 mg/kg PO q 24h	Hepatoprotectant: 10-50 mg/ kg PO q 24h	Generally well tolerated. GI upset may occur.	Tablets, capsules, powder; give on empty stomach. Some forms OTC.
Silver sulfadiazine (SSD, Silvadene)	Dermal injury including burns: apply topically q 12-24h	Dermal injury including burns: apply topically q 12-24h	Hypersensitivity can occur. If used on large wounds, toxicities associated with sulfa-based antibiotics (e.g., KCS, blood dyscrasia) are possible.	Topical cream. Use dressings or Elizabethan collars to prevent licking.
Sodium bicarbonate	Metabolic acidosis: mEq bicarbonate required = 0.5 × BW (kg) × (desired CO_2 mEq/L - TCO_2 mEq/L); give ¼ calculated dose slowly IV, and repeat dosing if required 4 hours later Urine alkalinization: 25-50 mg/ kg PO q 12h Renal tubular acidosis: 1-10 mEq/kg/day in divided doses PO, titrated to effect and with potassium supplementation	Metabolic acidosis: mEq bicarbonate required = 0.5 × BW (kg) × (desired CO_2 mEq/L - TCO_2 mEq/L); give ¼ calculated dose slowly IV, and repeat dosing if required 4 hours later	Use with caution as can cause metabolic alkalosis, electrolyte disorders, CHF, paradoxical CNS acidosis. Contraindicated in alkalosis or with excessive GI chloride loss. Use with extreme caution in DKA, hypocalcemia, CHF, nephrotic syndrome, hypertension, oliguria, volume overload. Multiple drug interactions.	Tablets (OTC), injection. Oral solution can be prepared from baking soda.
Sodium iodide	Sporotrichosis: 40 mg/kg PO q 8-12h	Sporotrichosis: 2.5 mg/kg PO q 24h; increase dose in 2.5 mg/kg increments to effect q 5 days. Other treatments preferred.	May cause iodism, which manifests as GI upset, depression/lethargy, twitching, hypothermia, and cardiovascular failure; more likely in cats. Do not use in animals with renal failure or severe dehydration.	Powder, oral tincture, injection. Give with food.
Sodium stibogluconate (Pentostam)	Cutaneous leishmaniasis: 30-50 mg/kg IV or SQ q 24h for 3-4 weeks	Use is not described in cats.	Adverse effects include pain on injection, thrombophlebitis, musculoskeletal pain, hemolytic anemia, leukopenia, GI upset, pancreatitis, myocardial injury and arrhythmias, renal toxicity, shock, and sudden death. Contraindicated in renal failure and cardiac arrhythmias.	Not available in the United States but can be imported from other countries or supplied by the Centers for Disease Control and Prevention if public health threat recognized.
Sodium thiosulfate	Cyanide toxicity: 40-50 mg/ kg IV, or 150-500 mg/kg IV bolus, or 150-500 mg/kg CRI +/-sodium nitrite	Cyanide toxicity: 150-500 mg/ kg IV bolus or CRI +/-sodium nitrite IV; contact animal poison control center for guidance	Generally well tolerated, but hypernatremia, hypotension, GI upset, and metabolic acidosis may occur.	Injection
Sotalol (Betapace)	Tachyarrhythmia: 1-3 mg/kg PO q 12h titrated upward to effect	Tachyarrhythmia: 1-3 mg/kg PO q 12h titrated upward to effect	Adverse effects include dyspnea, bronchospasm, fatigue/dizziness, nausea, vomiting, and worsening of arrhythmias. Contraindicated in bradyarrhythmia, asthma, long Q-T syndromes, cardiogenic shock or uncontrolled CHF. Use with caution in patients with DM, hyperthyroidism, and renal insufficiency.	Tablets; give on empty stomach.
Spironolactone (Aldactone)	Adjunctive therapy of CHF: 1-2 mg/kg PO q 12-24h; not first-line diuretic	Hyperaldosteronism: 2 mg/kg PO q 12h titrated prn Adjunctive for cardiomyopathy: 1-3 mg/kg PO q 12-24h	Adverse effects include GI upset and electrolyte imbalance. Severe facial excoriations may limit use in cats. Contraindicated in hypoadrenocorticism, hyperkalemia, or hyponatremia. Do not administer spironolactone in conjunction with NSAIDs to dogs with renal insufficiency.	Tablets

Generic Name (Brand Name, Synonyms)	Canine Dosages	Feline Dosages	Adverse Effects/Warnings	Administration/ Availability
Stanozolol (Winstrol-V)	Anabolic steroid: 1-4 mg/DOG PO q 12h	Do not use in cats.	Contraindicated in pregnancy and breeding animals. Cats may suffer severe hepatotoxicity. Adverse effects include electrolyte imbalance, behavioral change, GI upset, and hepatotoxicity.	No longer available in the United States. Compounding pharmacists may prepare oral dosage forms. CSS-III.
Streptozotocin (Streptozotocin, Zanosar)	Insulinoma: 500 mg/m^2 infusion preceded and followed by extensive IV fluid diuresis	Do not use in cats.	Use with extreme caution in patients with decreased renal, bone marrow, or hepatic function. May cause permanent DM. Adverse effects are typically GI upset and hepatotoxicity. Myelosuppression may also occur.	Injection. Cytotoxic, NIOSH-listed hazardous drug and should be prepared, administered, and disposed of in accordance with federal and local requirements.
Sucralfate (Carafate)	Esophageal/gastric protectant: 0.25-1 g/DOG PO q 4-12h; use suspension for esophageal disease	Esophageal/gastric protectant: 0.25-0.5 g/CAT PO q 4-12h	Generally well tolerated. Constipation or vomiting (cats) can occur. May impair absorption of several oral medications (separate dosing by 2 hours when possible).	Tablets (can be dissolved in water just before administration), oral suspension; give on empty stomach 30 minutes before meals.
Sulfadimethoxine/ormetoprim (Primor)	Susceptible infections: 55 mg/kg PO initially, then 27.5 mg/kg PO q 24h	Do not use in cats.	Adverse effects include KCS, GI upset, blood dyscrasia, and hypersensitivity reactions. Doberman pinschers are more susceptible to polyarthritis caused by sulfonamides; use with caution in this breed.	Tablets
Sulfamethoxazole/ trimethoprim (TMS, co-trimoxazole, Tribrissen)	Susceptible infections: 15-30 mg/kg PO q 12h; higher dose for nocardiosis	Susceptible infections: 15-30 mg/kg PO q 12-24h	Adverse effects include KCS, GI upset, blood dyscrasia, and hypersensitivity reactions. Doberman pinschers are more susceptible to polyarthritis caused by sulfonamides; use with caution in this breed.	Tablets, oral suspension
Sulfasalazine (Azulfidine)	IBD: 20-50 mg/kg PO q 8-12h Adjunct therapy for vasculitis: 20-40 mg/kg PO q 8h	IBD: 10-20 mg/kg PO q 12-24h	Adverse effects include KCS, GI upset, blood dyscrasia, and hypersensitivity reactions. Doberman pinschers are more susceptible to polyarthritis caused by sulfonamides; use with caution in this breed.	Tablets; give with food.

T

Generic Name (Brand Name, Synonyms)	Canine Dosages	Feline Dosages	Adverse Effects/Warnings	Administration/ Availability
Tacrolimus	Perianal fistulae or other immunologically mediated skin disorder: Applied to site of affected skin (use gloves) q 12h initially, reducing frequency once disease improves	Use in cats is not described.	Avoid human contact. Well tolerated for topical skin application.	Topical ointment. Owner must wear gloves and avoid contact (increased risk for cancers in humans).
Tadalafil (Cialis)	Pulmonary hypertension: 2-3 mg/kg PO q 24h; can be titrated up	Use in cats is not described.	Adverse effects are typically GI upset. Do not use concurrently with nitrates. Use with extreme caution in patients with resting hypotension, fluid depletion, severe left ventricular outflow obstruction, or autonomic dysfunction.	Tablets
Tamsulosin (Flomax)	Urethral relaxant: 0.01-0.2 mg/kg PO q 24h	Urethral relaxant: 0.004-0.006 mg/kg PO q 12-24h	Sustained-release dosage forms make extrapolation to small animals difficult. Adverse effects may include hypotension.	Sustained-release capsules
Taurine	DCM: 0.5-1 g/DOG PO q 8-12h for dogs weighing <25 kg and 1-2 g/DOG PO q 8-12h for dogs weighing >25 kg	DCM: 250-500 mg/CAT PO q 12h	Well tolerated.	Tablets OTC

Generic Name (Brand Name, Synonyms)	Canine Dosages	Feline Dosages	Adverse Effects/Warnings	Administration/ Availability
Telmisartan (Semintra, Micardis)	Proteinuria: 0.5-1 mg/kg PO q 12-24h; titrate up prn to maximum 5 mg/kg/d	Proteinuria: 1 mg/kg PO q 24h	Adverse effects include hypotension, GI upset, and anemias. Contraindicated in pregnancy. Do not use in uncorrected hypovolemia or electrolyte imbalance.	Tablets, compounded oral solution. Expensive.
Terbinafine (Lamisil)	Susceptible systemic mycoses: 30-35 mg/kg PO q 8-12h, often combined with other antifungal Malassezia: 30 mg/kg PO q 24h	Susceptible dermatologic mycosis: 20-30 mg/kg PO q 24h for 7 days, skip 21 days and repeat pulse dosing	Generally well tolerated, but GI upset, facial dermatitis, or swelling can occur. Use with caution and adjust dosing in patients with renal and hepatic insufficiency.	Tablets, granules; give with food.
Terbutaline (Brethine)	Bronchodilator, beta agonist: 1.25-5 mg/DOG PO q 8-12h; commonly used scheme 0.625-1.25 mg for small dogs; 1.25-2.5 mg for medium dogs; 2.5-5 mg for large dogs; PO q 12h Tocolytic for premature labor: 0.03 mg/kg PO q 8h	Bronchodilator, beta agonist acute use: 0.01 mg/kg SQ or IM once; chronic use: 0.625-1.25 mg/CAT PO q 12h	Adverse effects include increased heart rate, tremors, CNS excitement, and dizziness. Use with caution if at all in DM, hyperthyroidism, hypertension, seizure disorders, or cardiac disease. Do not administer injections IV.	Tablets, injection (do not administer injections IV)
Testosterone	Hormone-responsive urinary incontinence in males: 2.2 mg/kg IM q 30 days	Use in cats is not described.	Contraindicated in pregnancy. Use with caution in patients with renal, cardiac, or hepatic dysfunction. Not for use in female animals. Adverse effects include perianal adenomas, perineal hernias, prostatic disorders, and behavioral changes (aggression).	Injection (tablets available but dosing not described in animals). CSS-III.
Theophylline	Bronchodilator: 10 mg/kg PO q 12h	Bronchodilator: 15-25 mg/kg PO q 24h	Adverse effects include CNS stimulation and GI upset. Other adverse effects include insomnia, increased gastric acid secretion, diarrhea, PU/PD. Use with extreme caution in severe cardiac disease, seizure disorders, gastric ulcers, hyperthyroidism, renal or hepatic disease (50% dosage reduction), severe hypoxia, or severe hypertension.	Give with food to minimize GI upset. Sustained-release tablets are no longer available. Immediate-release capsules may be prepared by compounding pharmacists.
Thiamine (vitamin B_1)	Thiamine deficiency: 10-100 mg/DOG IM, IV, PO q 12h	Thiamine deficiency: 50-100 mg/CAT IM, IV, PO q 12h	Generally well tolerated. Pain on injection has been reported. Hypersensitivity to excipients may cause anaphylactoid reactions.	Tablets OTC, injection
Ticarcillin-clavulanate (Timentin)	Susceptible infection: 20-50 mg/kg IV q 6-8h	Susceptible infection: 20-50 mg/kg IV q 6-8h	Generally well tolerated but can cause anaphylaxis or allergic reactions.	Not commercially available at present
Tiletamine zolazepam (Telazol)	Sedation for minor procedures: 9.9-13.2 mg/kg IM (lower dose may be adequate for restraint)	Sedation for minor procedures: 9.9-13.2 mg/kg IM	Respiratory depression, pain on injection, and tachycardia often occur. Contraindicated in animals with severe cardiac, pulmonary, or pancreatic disease. May cause prolonged recoveries in animals with renal disease.	Injection. CSS-III.
Timolol (Timoptic)	Glaucoma: 1 drop in the affected eye(s) q 12h	Glaucoma: 1 drop in the affected eye(s) q 12h	May cause transient burning, stinging, and irritation upon application. May cause slight miosis. Timolol maleate may trigger attacks in cats with asthma and should not be used in cats with heart disease due to bradycardia.	Ophthalmic solution
Toceranib (Palladia)	Antineoplastic: 2.4-2.75 mg/kg PO q 48h is better tolerated with less toxicities than the labeled dose	Antineoplastic: 2.75 mg/kg PO q 48h or on a Monday-Wednesday-Friday type schedule	Adverse GI effects are likely, and the manufacturer recommends concurrent treatment with prokinetics and gastroprotectants. Other adverse effects include muscle cramping/pain, neutropenia, hypoalbuminemia, thromboembolic disease, vasculitis, pancreatitis, nasal depigmentation, change in coat or skin color, epistaxis, seizures, pruritus, and increased systolic blood pressure. May cause thromboemboli and edema. Mast cell degranulation during treatment may require discontinuation of therapy. Do not use in pregnant animals.	Tablets; give with food.

Generic Name (Brand Name, Synonyms)	Canine Dosages	Feline Dosages	Adverse Effects/Warnings	Administration/ Availability
Topiramate (Topamax)	Adjunctive antiepileptic: 5-10 mg/kg PO q 8-12h	Refractory epilepsy: 12.5-25 mg/CAT PO q 12h	Adverse effects include GI distress, sedation, ataxia, inappetence, and irritability. In cats, sedation and inappetence have been noted. Use with caution in hepatic insufficiency.	Tablets, capsules, and extended-release sprinkle capsules
Torsemide (Demadex)	Diuretic for CHF: 0.1-0.4 mg/kg PO q 12-24h	Diuretic for CHF: 0.2-0.3 mg/kg PO q 12-24h	Can cause dehydration and potentially severe electrolyte disturbances. Use cautiously in significant hepatic dysfunction, hyperuricemia, or DM. Torsemide is 10× more potent than furosemide. Ensure adequate hydration.	Tablets. Compounding pharmacists may prepare stable oral suspensions. Ensure that plenty of fresh drinking water is available at all times.
Tramadol (Ultram)	Analgesia: 4-10 mg/kg PO q 8h; begin at lower end of dose range and titrate upward if needed; analgesic effect may be delayed by days to weeks	Analgesia: 1-2 mg/kg PO q 12h, questionable efficacy	Well tolerated but adverse effects include sedation, respiratory depression, and hypersalivation from the extremely bitter taste. Use with caution in presence of respiratory depression. Use with caution in animals with a history of seizures.	Tablets. Compounding pharmacists may prepare stable oral suspensions. Salty flavors may mask bitter taste for cats. CSS-IV.
Trazodone (Desyrel)	Anxiolytic: 5-7 mg/kg PO q 12h starting dose, adjusted prn. If given with tramadol, daily dose should be reduced to 3.5 mg/kg PO q 12h until tramadol is discontinued.	Pre-stressor anxiolytic: 50 mg/CAT PO 60-90 minutes before event (e.g., travel to veterinary clinic). Doses up to 100 mg/CAT can be used if needed.	Do not use with MAO inhibitors (e.g., amitraz or selegiline) to avoid hypertension from serotonin syndrome. Well tolerated but adverse effects can include sedation (most common), ataxia, priapism, cardiac conduction disturbances, increased anxiety, and hyperreactivity.	Tablets. Compounding pharmacists may prepare stable oral suspensions.
Triamcinolone (Vetalog)	Antiinflammatory glucocorticoid: 0.4-0.8 mg/kg IM, SQ, PO q 24h, tapered Immunosuppressive: 1.5-2.0 mg/kg PO, IM, SQ q 24h, tapered Intralesional injection of long-acting acetonide: 0.6 mg at one site, maximum 1.8 mg total dose, q 3-4 weeks at most	Antiinflammatory glucocorticoid: 0.4-1 mg/kg IM, SQ, PO q 24h, tapered Immunosuppressive: 1.5-3.0 mg/kg PO, IM, SQ q 24h, tapered Intralesional injection of long-acting acetonide: 0.6 mg at one site, maximum 1.8 mg total dose, q 3-4 weeks at most	Adverse effects are usually GI upset after oral use and those typical of glucocorticoid use (e.g., PU/PD, polyphagia, hypothalamic-pituitary suppression). Contraindicated during active infection or GI ulceration. Use with caution in DM, hypertension, CHF, renal insufficiency. No mineralocorticoid activity, so oral forms sometimes better tolerated than oral predniso(lo)ne. Do not use concurrently with NSAIDs.	Tablets, powder, inhalants, ointments and creams, injection. Give oral products with food. Less potent than dexamethasone but more potent than prednisolone; available in intermediate- and long-acting (acetonide) forms.
Trientine (Syprine)	Copper chelation: 10-15 mg/kg PO q 12h	Use in cats is not described.	Generally well tolerated. Acute kidney injury has occurred in dogs. Chronic dosing has resulted in dystonias, muscle spasms, and iron-deficiency anemia.	Capsules; give 1-2 hours before meals. Very expensive.
Trilostane (Vetoryl)	Hyperadrenocorticism: 2.2-7.0 mg/kg/d, may divide q 12h; adjust based on ACTH stimulation test and clinical response	Hyperadrenocorticism: 3.0-5.0 mg/kg PO q 12-24h; adjust based on ACTH stimulation test and clinical response	Generally well tolerated. Adverse effects include GI upset and mild hyponatremia/hyperkalemia. Adrenal necrosis and death have occurred.	Capsules. Can be compounded into stable solution. Give with food.
Trimethoprim/sulfamethoxazole: see sulfamethoxazole/trimethoprim				
Trimeprazine with prednisolone (Temaril-P)	Antihistamine with glucocorticoid: 1 tab/5 kg BW PO q 12h for 4-7 days, then 1 tab/5 kg BW PO q 24h for 4-7 days, then 1 tab/5 kg BW PO q 48h	Antihistamine with glucocorticoid: 1 tab/CAT PO q 12h (5 mg trimeprazine/2 mg prednisolone)	Adverse effects are sedation, GI upset, and adverse effects of glucocorticoids (e.g., PU/PD, polyphagia). Contraindicated in presence of viral or systemic fungal infections, GI ulceration, and hyperadrenocorticism. Use with caution in hypertension, CHF, renal insufficiency. Do not use concurrently with NSAIDs.	Tablets; give with food.
Tropicamide (Mydriacyl)	Mydriasis: 1 drop in the affected eye(s) q 8-12h	Mydriasis: 1 drop in the affected eye(s) q 8-12h	Adverse effects include sensitivity to bright light, burning and irritation upon application, and superficial punctate keratitis. Hypersalivation may also occur.	Ophthalmic solution
Tylosin (Tylan)	Antibiotic-responsive diarrhea: 11-25 mg/kg PO q 24h; 11 mg/kg PO q 12h for 28 days (cryptosporidiosis)	Use in cats is not described.	Generally well tolerated. May cause mild GI upset.	Powder; give with food.

U-Z

Generic Name (Brand Name, Synonyms)	Canine Dosages	Feline Dosages	Adverse Effects/Warnings	Administration/ Availability
Ursodiol (Actigall, ursodeoxycholic acid)	Adjunct therapy for chronic hepatitis: 10-15 mg/kg PO q 12-24h	Adjunct therapy for chronic hepatitis: 10-15 mg/kg PO q 12-24h	Contraindicated in bile duct obstruction. Generally well tolerated. Diarrhea and abdominal pain have been reported.	Tablets, capsules; give with food. Compounding pharmacists may prepare stable oral suspensions.
Vancomycin (Vancocin)	Susceptible gram-positive, life-threatening infections: 15-20 mg/kg IV over 30-60 minutes q 6-8h, or 3.5 mg/kg IV bolus followed by 1.5 mg/kg/h IV CRI. Consult veterinary microbiologist or internist before use.	Susceptible gram-positive, life-threatening infections: 15-20 mg/kg IV over 30-60 minutes q 6-8h, or 3.5 mg/kg IV bolus followed by 1.5 mg/kg/h IV CRI. Consult veterinary microbiologist or internist before use.	Adverse effects include nephrotoxicity and ototoxicity. Thrombophlebitis, severe hypotension, and cardiac arrest following IV administration have been reported. Reserve for life-threatening gram-positive infections that are resistant to other agents. Reduce doses in renal failure.	Injection (tablets have no utility in veterinary medicine). Do not give IM, SQ, or IP as severe tissue damage and pain may occur. IV doses are diluted in normal saline or D_5W to concentrations of <5 mg/mL and administered slowly.
Vasopressin (Pitressin, arginine vasopressin, antidiuretic hormone, ADH)	CPR: 0.6-0.8 units/kg IV, or 1.2 units/kg intratracheal, or 0.8 units/kg IV q 3-5 minutes prn Refractory shock states: 0.5-4 mU/kg/min IV to effect Diagnostic for diabetes insipidus: 0.5 units/kg IM to maximum 5 units after 5% weight loss from water deprivation	CPR: 0.6-0.8 units/kg IV, or 1.2 units/kg intratracheal, or 0.8 units/kg IV q 3-5 minutes prn Refractory shock states: 0.5-4 mU/kg/min IV to effect Diagnostic for diabetes insipidus: 0.5 units/kg IM to maximum 5 units after 5% weight loss from water deprivation	Use with caution in patients with vascular disease, seizure disorders, heart failure, or asthma. Serious adverse effects are possible, including anaphylaxis, cardiac arrhythmia or arrest, GI upset, tremors, and smooth muscle contractions.	Aqueous injection
Verapamil (Calan, Isoptin, Verelan)	Calcium channel blocker used for SVT: 0.05 mg/kg IV q 5-10 minutes up to total dose of 0.15 mg/kg, or 2-10 mcg/kg/min CRI, or 0.5-3 mg/kg PO q 8h	SVT: 0.025 mg/kg slow IV q 5-10 minutes up to total dose of 0.15 mg/kg, or 2-10 mcg/kg/min CRI, or 0.5-1 mg/kg PO q 8h	Contraindicated in patients with cardiogenic shock or severe CHF (unless secondary to a SVT amenable to verapamil therapy), hypotension, sick sinus syndrome, second- or third-degree AV block, digoxin intoxication, and *MDR1/ABCB1-Δ* mutation. Use with caution in patients with heart failure, hypertrophic cardiomyopathy (common in cats), and hepatic or renal impairment. Toxicity may be potentiated in patients with hepatic dysfunction. It should be used cautiously in patients with atrial fibrillation. Multiple drug interactions.	Injection (tablets, capsules seldom used in veterinary medicine). For IV dosing, give only as a slow infusion over at least 2 minutes with continuous EKG and blood pressure monitoring.
Vinblastine (Velban)	Antineoplastic: 1.5-3 mg/m² IV q 1-2 weeks	Antineoplastic: 1.5-3 mg/m² IV q 1-2 weeks	Adverse events are GI toxicity and myelosuppression. Cats can develop neurotoxicity that can be associated with constipation or paralytic ileus, thereby aggravating anorexia. Irritating if extravasated. Contraindicated in neutropenia. Dosage reduction required in hepatic failure (50%) and in dogs with *MDR1/ABCB1-Δ* mutation (25%-30%).	Injection. Cytotoxic, NIOSH-listed hazardous drug that should be prepared, administered, and disposed of in accordance with federal and local requirements.
Vincristine (Oncovin, Vincasar PFS)	Antineoplastic: 0.5-0.75 mg/m² IV q 1-2 weeks Transmissible venereal tumor: 0.025 mg/kg IV weekly, maximum 1 mg/dose Immune-mediated thrombocytopenia: 0.02 mg/kg or 0.5 mg/m² IV once	Antineoplastic: 0.5-0.75 mg/m² IV q 1-2 weeks	Adverse events are GI toxicity and myelosuppression. Cats can develop neurotoxicity that can be associated with constipation or paralytic ileus, thereby aggravating anorexia. Irritating if extravasated. Contraindicated in neutropenia. Dosage reduction required in hepatic failure (50%) and in dogs with *MDR1/ABCB1-Δ* mutation (25%-30%).	Injection. Cytotoxic, NIOSH-listed hazardous drug and should be prepared, administered, and disposed of in accordance with federal and local requirements.

Vitamin B_1: see thiamine

Vitamin B_3: see niacinamide

Generic Name (Brand Name, Synonyms)	Canine Dosages	Feline Dosages	Adverse Effects/Warnings	Administration/ Availability
Vitamin B_9: see folic acid				
Vitamin B_{12}: see cyanocobalamin				
Vitamin C: see ascorbic acid				
Vitamin K_1 (phytonadione, Mephyton)	Anticoagulant rodenticide intoxication: Prophylaxis—1.5-2.5 mg/kg PO q 12h; treatment of bleeding—one injection of 1.5-2.5 mg/kg IM or SQ with small needle, followed by 2.5 mg/kg PO dosing. Duration of treatment depends on type of rodenticide ingested.	Anticoagulant rodenticide intoxication: as for dogs Hepatic disease with prolonged coagulation: 1 mg/kg SQ q 12h before biopsy (recheck coagulation times)	Excipients in injectable products may cause anaphylactoid reactions after IV administration. Adverse events include anaphylactoid reactions from some injectable products and bleeding at the injection site. Limit volume of injection at each site. Transfusion often required initially for actively bleeding animals.	Tablets, capsules, and injection. Use small-gauge needles when injecting and avoid IV injection.
Voriconazole (Vfend)	Susceptible mycotic infections: 4-5 mg/kg PO q 12-24h	Do not use in cats.	Cats experience severe adverse reactions. Adverse reactions include hepatotoxicity and extreme changes in blood pressure. Use with caution in patients with hepatic dysfunction or proarrhythmic conditions. Multiple drug interactions.	Tablets, powder for suspension or solution (IV use not described for clinical use in dogs)
Warfarin (Coumadin)	Thromboprophylaxis: 0.05-0.2 mg/kg PO q 24h with PT target of 1.5-2 times baseline or INR target of 2-3	Do not use in cats.	Can cause dose-related hemorrhage. Contraindicated with active bleeding, hypertension, hepatic insufficiency, pericardial effusion, or pregnancy. Multiple drug interactions. Treatment must be carefully monitored by PT or international normalized ratio.	Tablets. Multiple drug/food interactions.
Xylazine (Rompun)	No longer used in dogs.	Emetic agent: 0.44-1.1 mg/kg IM or IV once	Do not use concurrently with epinephrine. Use with caution in pre-existing cardiac dysfunction, hypotension or shock, respiratory dysfunction, severe hepatic or renal insufficiency, pre-existing seizure disorders, or if severely debilitated. Yohimbine is antagonist.	Injection
Yohimbine (Yobine, Antagonil)	Amitraz toxicity: 0.11 mg/kg IV or 0.25 mg/kg IM with atipamezole 50 mcg/kg IM	After xylazine-induced emesis: 0.1-0.2 mg/kg IV once	Use cautiously in seizure disorders. Use carefully in patients with renal disease.	Injection
Zafirlukast (Accolate)	Leukotriene inhibitor: dogs <11.4 kg 5 mg, dogs 11.4-22.3 kg 10 mg, dogs 22.7-34.1 kg 20 mg PO q 12h	Leukotriene inhibitor: 5 mg/CAT PO q 12-24h; questionable efficacy.	Adverse effects not well established in cats or dogs. Efficacy has not been established for feline asthma.	Tablets; give on empty stomach.
Zinc sulfate, acetate, gluconate, or methionine	Zn responsive dermatosis: 2 mg/kg PO q 24h (or divided bid if stomach upset) elemental Zn Adjunctive treatment for copper toxicosis: 5-10 mg/kg elemental Zn q 12h for 3 months, then 50 mg PO q 12h	Severe hepatic lipidosis: 7-10 mg/kg elemental Zn PO q 24h	GI upset, or hemolysis with large dose. Drug absorption interactions occur.	Tablets, capsules, or compounded. Usually combined with other nutraceuticals. OTC preparations available.
Zonisamide (Zonegran)	Adjunctive anticonvulsant: 2-10 mg/kg PO q 12h	Adjunctive anticonvulsant: 5-10 mg/kg PO q 24h	Adverse effects include sedation (usually transient), ataxia, and inappetence. Dogs may develop idiopathic hepatic necrosis, urinary calculi, hepatopathy, acute tubular acidosis, and erythema multiforme.	Capsules. Compounding pharmacists may prepare a stable oral suspension.

Index

Boldface page numbers indicate chapter titles. Page numbers followed by *a* indicate algorithms; *b*, boxes; *e*, electronic content; *f*, figures; and *t*, tables.

U

V

W

Sedation and Chemical Restraint in Small Animal Practice

Keith Branson, DVM, MS

Disclaimer: *The following drugs and applications are recommended based on published reports and clinical experience. Specific use must be guided by appropriate and reasonable precautions, preparation, and information on the part of the veterinarian using or advocating the use of these products. Descriptions of drug effects and parameters of usage are likely to vary from one patient to the next, and the description of the drug characteristics listed here applies to patients that are otherwise healthy.*

Acepromazine

Expected observable effect: tranquilization, ± hypotension. With encouragement, the animal should still be able to rise and walk but with obvious mental depression.
Dosage and route (dog or cat): 0.025-0.05 mg/kg IV or 0.05-0.15 mg/kg IM or SQ (oral tablet dosage is 5-10 times higher)
Pain control: none
Time to desired effect of sedation: 2-3 minutes (IV), 5-15 minutes (IM or SQ), 10-20 minutes (oral)
Indications: tranquilization of otherwise healthy, young- to middle-aged dogs and cats
Contraindications (relative): old age; hypotension; most heart, liver, or kidney diseases and other disorders in which arterial hypoperfusion could be deleterious
Advantages: substantial, effective sedation/mental depression; effect is often prolonged
Drawbacks: no analgesia, no antianxiety effects; highly variable/unpredictable duration and intensity of effect, especially in older or systemically ill patients. Rare manic/hyperaggressive reactions
Expected duration of effect/recovery: 30 minutes to several hours
Alternative: for milder sedation: butorphanol + either diazepam or midazolam (e.g., healthy but older dog or cat)—see below
Notes and comments: seizure threshold-lowering effects are unproven

Butorphanol + Acepromazine

Expected observable effect: mild to moderate sedation. Does not cause immobilization, but prolongs the duration and degree of tolerance to restraint
Dosage and route (dog or cat): butorphanol 0.1-0.5 mg/kg IV or IM + acepromazine 0.025-0.05 mg/kg IV or IM. Butorphanol and acepromazine can be mixed in the same syringe for immediate use.
Pain control: mild
Time to desired effect of sedation: < 1 minute (IV) or 10-15 minutes (IM)
Indications: sedation and immobilization for minimally painful procedures. Useful for very active or agitated young animals
Contraindications: older animals (relative contraindication to acepromazine); hypovolemia, dehydration, hypotension, most heart diseases, marked acid-base imbalance, or other instances of systemic illness
Advantages: prolonged sustained sedation; flexibility of IM or IV route
Drawbacks: prolonged recovery period and interindividual variability of effect, especially when combined with acepromazine
Expected duration of effect/recovery: 20-30 minutes (IV use), variable up to hours (IM route when combined with acepromazine)
Alternatives: for slightly greater sedation butorphanol + diazepam/midazolam (e.g., healthy but older dog or cat)—see below. For greater sedation: add acepromazine 0.025-0.05 mg/kg IV or 0.05-0.15 mg/kg IM (e.g., healthy young dog or cat).
Notes and comments: butorphanol + acepromazine 0.05 mg/kg + glycopyrrolate 0.01 mg/kg are commonly added together to create a preanesthetic combination ("B-A-G") for healthy dogs and cats. Reduce dose for dogs with *MDR1/ABCB1-Δ*.

Buprenorphine

Expected observable effect: prolonged mild to moderate sedation; the animal may be roused with stimulation, but quickly reverts to being quiet and less responsive
Dosage and route (dog or cat): 0.005-0.02 mg/kg IV or IM. Alternatively, 0.01 mg/kg sublingually (transmucosal absorption) is possible in cats.
Pain control: mild to moderate
Time to desired effect of sedation: 15-30 minutes (longer to achieve peak analgesic effects). Clinical sedation may be apparent sooner when buprenorphine is combined with other sedatives/tranquilizers.
Indications: sedation and immobilization for minimally painful procedures. Useful for very active or agitated young animals
Contraindications: older animals (relative contraindication); hypovolemia, dehydration, hypotension, most severe heart diseases, marked acid-base imbalance, or other instances of systemic illness
Expected duration of effect/recovery: up to 6-8 hours with higher dosage of buprenorphine combined with acepromazine, IM
Alternatives: for greater sedation (e.g., diagnostic imaging in a very agitated but stable puppy), add acepromazine 0.02-0.05 mg/kg (IM or IV)
Combinations: can be combined with dexmedetomidine (0.005-0.01 mg/kg) as a premedication or heavy sedation protocol
Notes and comments: this is a long-acting opioid and its effects are not easily reversed with naloxone. Buprenorphine is used frequently for postoperative analgesia due to the prolonged dosing interval that is required. A once-a-day formulation is available (Simbadol). The time to onset for Simbadol is comparable to the conventional product.

Butorphanol + Diazepam (or Butorphanol + Midazolam)

Expected observable effect: the animal becomes quieter but remains responsive to sound and is less likely to react to mild noxious stimuli or to struggle during manual restraint.
Dosage and route (dog or cat): butorphanol 0.1-0.5 mg/kg IV or IM + either diazepam 0.1-0.2 mg/kg IV or midazolam 0.1-0.2 mg/mg IV or IM. Avoid combining other drugs in the same syringe with diazepam due to propylene glycol in diazepam's formulation.
Pain control: mild.
Time to desired effect of sedation: <1 minute (IV) or 5-15 minutes (IM)
Indications: mild sedation and analgesia (e.g., ultrasound exam or radiographs of very restless young animal or of mildly fractious cat)
Contraindications: liver disease (diazepam, midazolam); hypovolemia, dehydration, marked acid-base imbalance, or other instances of severe systemic illness
Advantages: provides light sedation
Drawbacks: IV administration (diazepam); short duration of action
Expected duration of effect/recovery: animals that are otherwise healthy generally remain able to ambulate with this protocol or regain the ability to do so within 15-20 minutes of administration (IV use).
Alternatives: for greater sedation, omit diazepam/midazolam and replace with dexmedetomidine 0.005 mg/kg IM or IV, or omit butorphanol and replace with hydromorphone 0.1-0.2 mg/kg IM or IV, or add acepromazine 0.025-0.05 mg/kg IM or IV.
Notes and comments: midazolam historically was expensive but is now available as generic (cost is similar to diazepam). Midazolam is better tolerated for IM injection and the absorption is less variable.

Hydromorphone

Expected observable effect: mild to moderate sedation. Generally, the animal still will be able to walk. Hyperresponsiveness to sound is common (avoid loud noises).
Dosage and route (dog or cat): 0.05-0.2 mg/kg IV or IM
Pain control: moderate
Time to desired effect of sedation: 1-2 minutes (IV) or 5-15 minutes (IM)
Indications: analgesia and sedation (mild or moderate)
Contraindications: vomiting/nauseated patient; noisy environment; hypovolemia, dehydration, marked acid-base imbalance, or other instances of severe systemic illness
Advantages: minimal cardiovascular depression; analgesic properties
Drawbacks: nausea, panting, increases vagal tone (causing bradycardia). When used in cats, it may cause hyperthermia and excitement if used alone.
Expected duration of effect/recovery: sedative effects typically are longer than butorphanol. Animals regain the ability to walk within 30 minutes of administration. Repeated dosing for analgesia is q 4-6h.
Alternatives: for greater sedation, add diazepam/midazolam (see below) or acepromazine (see above).
Notes and comments: emetic effects appear less pronounced in painful animals when administered IV.
Reversal: can be revsersed with naloxone